Third Edition

TEXTBOOK OF PRIMARY CARE MEDICINE

Editor-in-Chief
John Noble, M.D.
Director, Center for Primary Care
Professor of Medicine
Boston University School of Medicine
Boston, Massachusetts

Senior Editors
Harry L. Greene, II, M.D.
Executive Vice President
Massachusetts Medical Society
Waltham, Massachusetts

Wendy Levinson, M.D.
Chief, Section of General Internal Medicine
Professor of Medicine
University of Chicago
Chicago, Illinois

Geoffrey A. Modest, M.D.
Clinical Professor of Medicine
Boston University School of Medicine
Medical Director
Upham's Corner Health Center
Dorchester, Massachusetts

Cynthia D. Mulrow, M.D., M.Sc.
Senior Research Associate, Veterans Administration
Professor of Medicine, University of Texas Health Sciences Center at San Antonio
Veterans Administration
Audie L. Murphy Memorial Veterans Hospital
San Antonio, Texas

Joseph E. Scherger, M.D., M.P.H.
Chair, Department of Family Medicine
Associate Dean for Clinical Affairs
Department of Family Medicine
College of Medicine
University of California at Irvine
Orange, California

Mark J. Young, M.D.
Chairman, Community Health and Health Studies
Lehigh Valley Hospital
Allentown, Pennsylvania

with more than 700 illustrations and 98 color plates

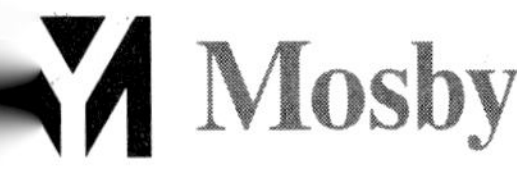

A Harcourt Health Sciences Company
St. Louis London Philadelphia Sydney Toronto

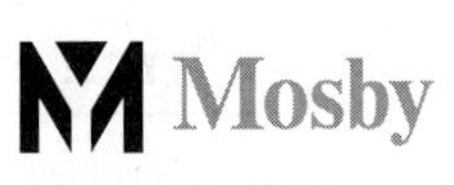

A Harcourt Health Sciences Company

Editor: Elizabeth Fathman
Senior Managing Editor: Kathy Falk
Project Manager: Carol Sullivan Weis
Production Editor: David Stein
Designer: Mark A. Oberkrom

Third Edition

NOTICE

Medicine is an ever-changing field. Standard safety precautions must be followed, but as new research and clinical experience broaden our knowledge, changes in treatment and drug therapy may become necessary or appropriate. Readers are advised to check the most current product information provided by the manufacturer of each drug to be administered to verify the recommended dose, the method and duration of administration, and contraindications. It is the responsibility of the licensed prescriber, relying on experience and knowledge of the patient, to determine dosages and the best treatment for each individual patient. Neither the publisher nor the editor assumes any liability for any injury and/or damage to persons or property arising from this publication.

Mosby, Inc.
A Harcourt Health Sciences Company
11830 Westline Industrial Drive
St. Louis, Missouri 63146

Printed in the United States of America

International Standard Book Number 0-323-00828-3

00 01 02 03 04 GW/KPT 9 8 7 6 5 4 3 2 1

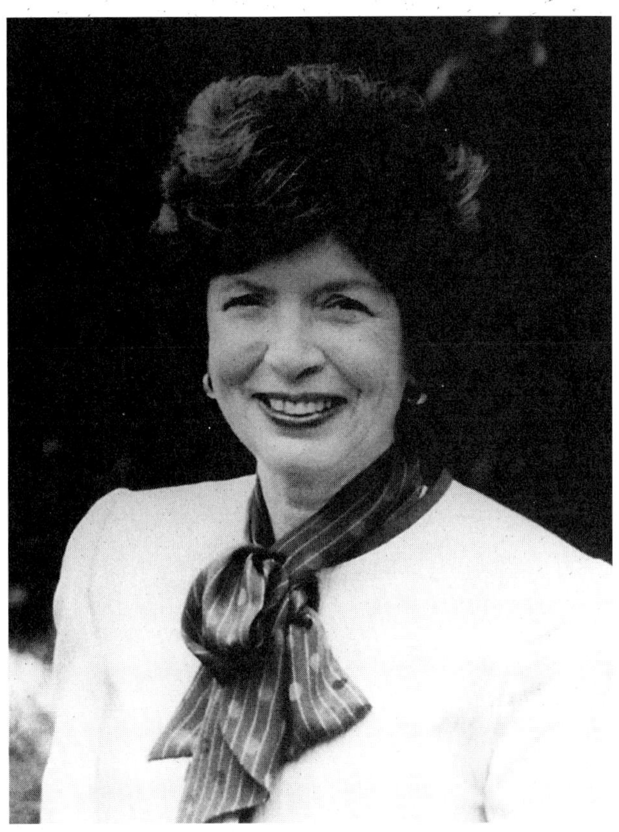

Ann Sullivan Baker
1938-1996

A superb clinician, gifted teacher, and internationally recognized expert in infectious diseases of the eye and head and neck, Ann was an outstanding generalist and specialist. Her lectures were exceptional and her handouts were treasured. It was from one of her lectures and the accompanying handout that she developed her chapter on Bites, Stings, and Irritations *published in the first and second editions of this text.*

Ann Baker was a pioneer for women in medicine; she gracefully combined a distinguished career in medicine with a full life as mother, spouse, and marvelous friend.

Contributors

Sapana P. Adhikari, B.S.
Department of Obstetrics and Gynecology, Boston University School of Medicine, Boston, Massachusetts

Nezam H. Afdhal, M.D.
Chief of Hepatology, Director of the Liver Center, Beth Israel Deaconess Medical Center, Associate Professor, Harvard Medical School, Boston, Massachusetts

Elizabeth A. Alexander, M.D., M.S.
Professor, Department of Family Practice, Michigan State University, East Lansing, Michigan; Physician Staff, Department of Family Practice, Sparrow Health System, Lansing, Michigan

Jack E. Ansell, M.D.
Professor of Medicine, Boston University School of Medicine, Vice Chairman of Clinical Affairs, Department of Medicine, Boston Medical Center, Boston, Massachusetts

Louis J. Aronne, M.D.
Clinical Associate Professor, Department of Medicine, Cornell University Medical College; Assistant Attending Physician, Department of Medicine, New York Presbyterian, New York, New York

Subhas Banerjee, M.B.B.S., M.R.C.P.
Clinical Fellow in Medicine, Division of Gastroenterology, Department of Medicine, Harvard Medical School; Fellow in Gastroenterology, Division of Gastroenterology, Beth Israel Deaconess Medical Center, Boston, Massachusetts

Patricia P. Barry, M.D., M.P.H.
Executive Director, Merck Institute of Aging and Health, Merck and Company, Inc., Washington, D.C.

Bahar Bastani, M.D.
Associate Professor of Medicine and Nephrology, Department of Internal Medicine-Nephrology, St. Louis University School of Medicine, St. Louis University Health Sciences Center, St. Louis, Missouri

Kenneth L. Baughman, M.D.
Director, Division of Cardiology; Professor of Medicine, The Johns Hopkins University School of Medicine, The Johns Hopkins Hospital, Baltimore, Maryland

Umar Beejay, M.D.
Section of Gastroenterology, Boston University School of Medicine, Boston Medical Center, Boston, Massachusetts

David M. Benedek, M.D.
Assistant Professor, Department of Psychiatry, Uniformed Services University of the Health Sciences, F. Edward Hebert School of Medicine, Bethesda, Maryland; Assistant Chief, Inpatient Psychiatry Service, Department of Psychiatry, Walter Reed Army Medical Center, Washington, DC

Michael S. Benninger, M.D.
Chairman, Department of Otolaryngology-Head and Neck Surgery, Henry Ford Hospital, Detroit, Michigan

Timothy J. Benstead, M.D., FRCP
Associate Professor, Division of Neurology, Dalhousie University, Halifax, Nova Scotia, Canada

Jennifer R. Berman, M.D.
Instructor of Urology, Department of Urology, Director of Women's Sexual Health Clinic, Boston University, Boston, Massachusetts

John H. Bland, M.D.
Professor of Medicine-Rheumatology, Emeritus, Department of Medicine, University of Vermont Medical Center; Hospital of Vermont, Department of Medicine, Burlington, Vermont

James Boyd, M.D.
Resident, Department of Neurology, University of Vermont-College of Medicine, Resident, Department of Neurology, Fletcher Allen Health Care, MCVH, Burlington, Vermont

Sharon B. Brodie, M.D.
Instructor in Medicine, Harvard Medical School, Instructor in Medicine, Division of Infectious Disease, Beth Israel Deaconess Medical Center, Boston, Massachusetts

Robert V. Brody, M.D.
Department of Public Health
San Francisco General Hospital
San Francisco, California

Frank W. Brown, M.D., M.B.A.
Associate Professor of Psychiatry and Behavioral Sciences, Department of Psychiatry and Behavioral Sciences, Emory University School of Medicine; Medical Director, Wesley Woods Geriatric Hospital, Atlanta, Georgia

Melanie J. Brunt, M.D., M.P.H.
Clinical Instructor in Medicine, Harvard Medical School, Boston, Massachusetts; Chief of Endocrinology, Department of Medicine, The Cambridge and Somerville Hospitals, Cambridge, Massachusetts

Robert Burakoff, M.D.
Professor of Medicine, Department of Medicine, State University of New York at Stony Brook, Health Sciences Center, Stony Brook, New York; Chief, Academic Gastroenterology, Division of Gastroenterology, Hepatology, & Nutrition, Department of Medicine, Winthrop-University Hospital, Mineola, New York

Michael Burnett, M.D.
Resident, Section of Otolaryngology-Head and Neck Surgery, Penn State University, Milton S. Hershey Medical Center, Hershey, Pennsylvania

Jaime Burkle, M.D.
Clinical Fellow in Cardiovascular Diseases, Division of Cardiology, Mount Sinai Medical Center, Miami Beach, Florida

John W. Burress, M.D., M.P.H., FACOEM
Preceptor; Member Resident's Advisory Committee, Department of Occupational and Environmental Medicine, Harvard School of Public Health, Boston, Massachusetts; Staff, Department of Family Practice, Newton-Wellesley Hospital, Newton, Massachusetts

Thomas J. Byrd, M.D.
Assistant Clinical Professor, Kresge Eye Institute, Wayne State University Medical School, Detroit, Michigan; Staff Surgeon (Ophthalmologist), Department of Surgery, Henry Ford Wyandotte Hospital, Wyandotte, Michigan

Lisa Rowland Callahan, M.D.
Assistant Professor, Department of Medicine, Cornell University Medical College; Medical Director, Women's Sports Medicine Center, Hospital for Special Surgery, New York, New York

Thomas L. Campbell, M.D.
Professor, Department of Family Medicine and Psychiatry, University of Rochester School of Medicine, Rochester, New York

Juan J. Canoso, M.D.
Director, Clinical Rheumatology, New England Medical Center, Boston, Massachusetts

J. Chris Carey, M.D.
Vice Chair OB-GYN, University of Pennsylvania, Hershey Medical Center, Hershey, Pennsylvania

Joseph T. Chambers, Ph.D., M.D.
Associate Professor, Department of Obstetrics and Gynecology, Division of Gynecologic Oncology, Yale University School of Medicine, New Haven, Connecticut

Setsuko K. Chambers, M.D.
Associate Professor, Department of Obstetrics and Gynecology, Division of Gynecologic Oncology, Yale University School of Medicine, New Haven, Connecticut

Ru-fong Cheng, M.D.
Assistant Professor, Department of Obstetrics and Gynecology, University of Pennsylvania, Philadelphia, Pennsylvania

David C. Christiani, M.D.
Professor of Occupational Medicine and Epidemiology, Department of Environmental Health, Harvard School of Public Health, Physician, Pulmonary and Critical Care Unit, Massachusetts General Hospital, Boston, Massachusetts

Murray D. Christianson, M.D., FRCS, FACS
Division Head, Ophthalmic Plastic and Reconstructive Surgery, Eye Care Services Department, Henry Ford Hospital, Detroit, Michigan

William D. Clark, M.D.
Lecturer, Department of Medicine, Harvard Medical School, Boston, Massachusetts; Medical Director, Addiction Resource Center, Mid Coast Hospital, Bath, Maine

Jay D. Coffman, M.D.
Professor of Medicine, Department of Medicine, Boston University School of Medicine; Chief, Vascular Medicine Section, Department of Medicine, Boston Medical Center, Boston, Massachusetts

Steven A. Cole, M.D.
Professor, Department of Psychiatry, Albert Einstein College of Medicine (Long Island Jewish Division), Glen Oaks, New York; Vice President and Medical Director, Care Management Group of Greater New York, Inc., Lake Success, New York

Wilson S. Colucci, M.D.
Professor, Department of Medicine and Physiology, Boston University School of Medicine; Chief, Department of Cardiovascular Medicine, Boston Medical Center, Boston, Massachusetts

Joshua A. Copel, M.D.
Professor, Department of Obstetrics and Gynecology, Section Head, Maternal-Fetal Medicine, Yale University School of Medicine; Director of Obstetrics, Department of Obstetrics and Gynecology, Yale-New Haven Hospital, New Haven, Connecticut

James M. Coumas, M.D.
Musculoskeletal Radiologist, Charlotte Radiology, Department of Radiology, Carolina Medical Center, Carolina Health Care System, Charlotte, North Carolina

Burke A. Cunha, M.D.
Chief, Infectious Disease Division, Winthrop-University Hospital, Mineola, New York

Deborah A. Darnley-Fisch, M.D.
Senior Staff Ophthalmologist-Glaucoma Division, Department of Eye Care Services, Henry Ford Health System, Detroit, Michigan

James A. Delmez, M.D.
Professor of Medicine, Department of Internal Medicine, Renal Division, Washington University School of Medicine; Physician, Department of Internal Medicine, Barnes-Jewish Hospital, St. Louis, Missouri

Fernando Coste Delvecchio, M.D.
Endourology Fellow, Department of Urology, Duke University Medical Center, Durham, North Carolina

Susan Tobey Denman, M.D.
Clinical Instructor, Department of Dermatology, Oregon Health Sciences University; Active Staff, Department of Dermatology, St. Vincent's Hospital, Portland, Oregon

Richard A. DeRemee, M.D.
Professor (Emeritus), Department of Pulmonary and Critical Care, Mayo Clinic, Rochester, Minnesota

Uday R. Desai, M.D.
Director of Vitreoretinal Service, Department of Ophthalmology, Henry Ford Health System, Detroit, Michigan

Dennis D. Diaz, M.D., FACS
Assistant Professor of Surgery, Section of Otolaryngology Head and Neck Surgery, Pennsylvania State Geisinger Health System, Milton S. Hershey Medical Center, Hershey, Pennsylvania

Michael F. Dillingham, M.D.
Executive Director, Sports Medicine Program, Stanford University; Clinical Professor, Department of Functional Restoration, Stanford Health Services, Stanford, California

Stephen Dolan, M.D., FCCP
Assistant Professor of Medicine, Department of Pulmonary and Critical Care Medicine, Medical College of Wisconsin; Director, Respiratory Therapy, Pulmonary and Critical Care Medicine, VAMC – Milwaukee, Milwaukee, Wisconsin

Keith Doram, M.D., M.B.A., FACP
Associate Professor of Clinical Medicine, Department of Medicine, Penn State College of Medicine, Hershey, Pennsylvania; Chief, Division of General Internal Medicine, Department of Medicine, Lehigh Valley Hospital, Allentown, Pennsylvania

Michael J. Droller, M.D.
Professor and Chairman, Department of Urology, The Mount Sinai Medical Center, The Mount Sinai School of Medicine; Director of Urology; Attending Physician, Department of Urology, The Mount Sinai Hospital, New York, New York

Susana A. Ebner, M.D.
Assistant Professor of Medicine, Boston University School of Medicine; Attending Physician, Department of Medicine, Section of Endocrinology, Boston Medical Center, Boston, Massachusetts

Kathryn L. Edmiston, M.D.
Associate Professor of Medicine, Department of Internal Medicine, University of Massachusetts Medical Center, Worcester, Massachusetts

Richard M. Effros, M.D.
Chief of Pulmonary Medicine, Medical College of Wisconsin, Froedtert Hospital, Milwaukee, Wisconsin

Charles C. Engel, Jr., M.D., M.P.H.
Assistant Professor of Psychiatry, Department of Psychiatry, Uniformed Services University, Bethesda, Maryland; Chief, Gulf War Health Center, Walter Reed Army Medical Center, Washington, DC

Arthur H. Eskew, M.D.
Assistant Professor of Medicine, Department of Medicine, Boston University School of Medicine, Boston Medical Center, Boston, Massachusetts

John J. W. Fangman, M.D.
Instructor in Internal Medicine and Pediatrics, Harvard Medical School, Massachusetts General Hospital, Boston, Massachusetts

Alan P. Farwell, M.D., FACP
Associate Professor of Medicine, Department of Medicine, University of Massachusetts Medical School; Staff Physician, Department of Medicine, UMass Memorial Health Care, Worcester, Massachusetts

Fred G. Fedok, M.D.
Division Chief and Associate Professor of Otolaryngology, Pennsylvania State Geisinger Health System, Milton S. Hershey Medical Center, Hershey, Pennsylvania

Leonor Fernandez, M.D.
Instructor of Medicine, Harvard Medical School; Staff Physician, Department of Medicine, Beth Israel Deaconess Medical Center, Boston, Massachusetts

Robert G. Frykberg, D.P.M., M.P.H.
Dean for Clinical Affairs, College of Podiatric Medicine and Surgery, Des Moines University Osteopathic Medical Center, Des Moines, Iowa

Akira Funahashi, M.D.
Professor of Medicine Emeritus, Medical College of Wisconsin, Division of Pulmonary Medicine, Milwaukee, Wisconsin

Nelson M. Gantz, M.D.
Clinical Professor of Medicine, Department of Medicine, Allegheny University of the Health Sciences, Philadelphia, Pennsylvania; Chairman, Department of Medicine and Chief, Division of Infectious Diseases, Department of Medicine, Pinnacle Health Hospitals, Harrisburg, Pennsylvania

Ann Gateley, M.D.
Associate Professor of Medicine, Department of Internal Medicine, University of New Mexico, Albuquerque, New Mexico

David F. Giansiracusa, M.D.
Professor, Department of Medicine, University of Massachusetts Medical School; Attending Physician, Department of Medicine and Rheumatology, University of Massachusetts Memorial Medical Center, Inc., Worcester, Massachusetts

Michael M. Givertz, M.D.
Assistant Professor of Medicine, Department of Medicine; Boston University School of Medicine; Clinical Director, Cardiomyopathy Program, Department of Medicine, Boston Medical Center, Boston, Massachusetts

Irwin Goldstein, M.D.
Professor of Urology, Department of Urology, Boston University School of Medicine, Boston, Massachusetts

Michael G. Goldstein, M.D.
Adjunct Professor, Department of Psychiatry and Human Behavior, Brown University School of Medicine, Providence, Rhode Island; Associate Director, Bayer Institute for Health Care Communication, West Haven, Connecticut

Norton J. Greenberger, M.D.
Professor and Chairman, Department of Internal Medicine, Kansas University School of Medicine, Kansas University Medical Center, Kansas City, Kansas

Jerry M. Greene, M.D.
Instructor in Medicine, Department of Medicine, Harvard Medical School, Boston, Massachusetts; Chief, Rheumatology Section, Department of Medical Service, Brockton/West Roxbury, Department of Veterans Affairs Medical Center, West Roxbury, Massachusetts

Carrie J. Guise, Ph.D.
Clinical Assistant Professor, Department of Psychiatry, New York University School of Medicine; Medical Education Coordinator (Behavioral Medicine), Department of Medicine, Lenox Hill Hospital, New York, New York

Elizabeth Haase, M.D.
Assistant Clinical Professor of Psychiatry, Attending Physician, Department of Psychiatry, Columbia Presbyterian Medical Center, Columbia University, New York, New York

Carolyn I. Hale, M.D.
Associate, Department of Dermatology, Oregon Health Sciences University, Department of Internal Medicine, Salem Hospital, Salem, Oregon

David A. Halle, M.D.
Instructor of Medicine, Section of General Internal Medicine, Boston University School of Medicine, Boston, Massachusetts

Leslie R. Harrold, M.D., M.P.H.
Assistant Professor of Medicine, Department of Medicine, University of Massachusetts Medical School; Assistant Professor of Medicine, Department of Medicine, UMass Memorial Health Care, Worcester, Massachusetts

James J. Heffernan, M.D.
Medical Director, Health Care Associates, Beth Israel Hospital, Boston, Massachusetts

Janet B. Henrich, M.D.
Associate Professor of Medicine, Associate Professor of Obstetrics and Gynecology, Yale University School of Medicine, Department of Internal Medicine, Attending Physician, Department of Medicine, Yale-New Haven Hospital, New Haven, Connecticut

Irl B. Hirsch, M.D.
Associate Professor of Medicine, University of Washington, Medical Director, Diabetes Care Center, University of Washington Medical Center, Seattle, Washington

Richard M. Hoffman, M.D., M.P.H.
Assistant Professor, Department of Medicine, University of New Mexico; Staff Physician, Department of General Internal Medicine, Albuquerque VAMC, Albuquerque, New Mexico

Michael F. Holick, M.D., Ph.D.
Professor of Medicine, Dermatology and Physiology, Department of Medicine, Boston University Medical Center, Boston, Massachusetts

Brian A. Howard, M.B., ChB(HONS)
Osteoradiologist, Department of Radiology, Carolinas Medical Center, Charlotte, North Carolina

Edward H. Illions, M.D.
Director of Reproductive Endocrinology, Fertility Institute of Ft. Lauderdale, Sheridan Healthcorp, Hollywood, Florida

Robin R. Ingalls, M.D.
Assistant Professor of Medicine, Boston University School of Medicine, Department of Medicine, Section of Infectious Diseases, Boston Medical Center, Boston, Massachusetts

Richard S. Irwin, M.D.
Professor of Medicine, Department of Medicine, University of Massachusetts Medical School; Director, Division of Pulmonary Allergy, and Critical Care Medicine, Department of Medicine, UMass Memorial Health Care, Worcester, Massachusetts

Eric W. Jacobson, M.D.
Associate Professor of Medicine, Department of Medicine, University of Massachusetts Medical School; Associate Professor of Medicine, Department of Medicine, Division of Rheumatology, University of Massachusetts Memorial Health Care, Worcester, Massachusetts

Manoj Jain, M.D., M.P.H.
Clinical Assistant Professor of Medicine, Department of Internal Medicine, University of Tennessee, Consultant Physician, Department of Internal Medicine, Baptist Memorial Hospital, Memphis, Tennessee

Diane H. Johnson, M.D.
Assistant Professor, Department of Medicine, State University of New York School of Medicine at Stony Brook, Stony Brook, New York, Assistant Director, Infectious Disease Division, Winthrop University Hospital, Mineola, New York

Nirmal Joshi, M.D.
Assistant Professor of Medicine, Department of Medicine, Physician, Section of General Internal Medicine, Milton S. Hershey Medical Center, Hershey, Pennsylvania

Leslie E. Kahl, M.D.
Associate Professor of Medicine, Associate Dean for Student Affairs, Department of Medicine, Washington University School of Medicine, Barnes Jewish Hospital, St. Louis, Missouri

Wishwa N. Kapoor, M.D., M.P.H.
Falk Professor of Medicine; Chief, Division of General Internal Medicine, Department of Medicine, University of Pittsburgh Medical Center, Pittsburgh, Pennsylvania

Curtis Kapsner, M.D.
Vice-Chairman, Department of Internal Medicine, University of New Mexico; Staff Physician, Department of Medical Service, Albuquerque VAMC, Albuquerque, New Mexico

Edward K. Kasper, M.D., FACC
Associate Professor of Medicine, Department of Cardiology Division, Johns Hopkins School of Medicine; Director, Johns Hopkins Cardiomyopathy & Heart Transplant Service, Cardiology Division, Johns Hopkins Hospital, Baltimore, Maryland

Wayne J. Katon, M.D.
Professor and Vice Chair, Department of Psychiatry, University of Washington Medical School; Professor, Vice Chair, Chief of Division of Health Services and Psychiatric Epidemiology, Department of Psychiatry, University of Washington, Seattle, Washington

Michael Katzman, M.D.
Assistant Professor, Departments of Medicine (Section of Infectious Diseases) and Department of Microbiology and Immunology, Pennsylvania State University College of Medicine, Milton S. Hershey Medical Center, Hershey, Pennsylvania

Jack Kaufman, M.D.
Professor, Department of Medicine, Medical College of Wisconsin, Froedtert Memorial Lutheran Hospital, Milwaukee, Wisconsin

Julie Kaufmann, M.D., Ph.D.
Assistant Clinical Professor of Medicine, Section of General Internal Medicine, Boston University School of Medicine, Boston, Massachusetts

Andrew M. Kaunitz, M.D.
Professor and Assistant Chair, Department of Obstetrics and Gynecology, University of Florida Health Science Center, Jacksonville, Jacksonville, Florida

David L. Keefe, M.D.
Associate Professor, Department of Obstetrics and Gynecology, Women and Infants Hospital and Brown University Medical School; Director Division of Reproductive Medicine and Infertility, Department of Obstetrics and Gynecology, Women and Infants Hospital, Providence, Rhode Island

Ciarán P. Kelly, M.D.
Assistant Professor of Medicine, Department of Gastroenterology, Harvard Medical School; Director, Fellowship Training, Department of Gastroenterology, Beth Israel Deaconess Medical Center, Boston, Massachusetts

Mumtaz J. Khan, M.D.
Department of Otolaryngology Head and Neck Surgery, Henry Ford Hospital, Detroit, Michigan

Kenneth A. Kingsly
Chief Resident, Department of Urology, Tufts University School of Medicine, Department of Urology, New England Medical Center, Boston, Massachusetts

Saulo Klahr, M.D.
Simon Professor of Medicine, Washington University School of Medicine, Barnes-Jewish Hospital, St. Louis, Missouri

Natalie C. Klein, M.D.
Assistant Professor, Department of Medicine, State University of New York School of Medicine at Stony Brook, Stony Brook, New York; Associate Director, Infectious Disease Division, Winthrop-University Hospital, Mineola, New York

Sharon K. Knight, M.D.
Instructor, Division of Gynecology, Department of Obstetrics & Gynecology, University of Tennessee, Memphis, Tennessee

Jarol B. Knowles, M.D., M.P.H.
Assistant Professor of Medicine, Division of Digestive Diseases and Nutrition, University of North Carolina, Chapel Hill, North Carolina

Kathleen C. Kobashi, M.D.
Fellow, Female Urology, Urodynamics and Reconstructive Urology, Department of Urology, Tower Urology Institute for Continence, Cedars-Sinai Medical Center, Los Angeles, California

Raymond S. Koff, M.D.
Professor of Medicine, Department of Medicine, University of Massachusetts Medical School, Worcester, Massachusetts; Chairman, Department of Medicine, MetroWest Medical Center, Framingham, Massachusetts

Robert J. Krane, M.D.
Professor of Surgery, Harvard Medical School, Director of Neurology, Massachusetts General Hospital, Boston, Massachusetts

Dennis H. Kraus, M.D.
Associate Professor, Department of Otorhinolaryngology, Cornell University Medical Center, Associate Attending, Head and Neck Service, Director, Speech and Hearing Center, Department of Surgery, Memorial Sloan-Kettering Cancer Center, New York, New York

Talya H. Kupin, M.D.
Senior Staff Ophthalmologist, Department of Ophthalmology, Henry Ford Hospital, Detroit, Michigan

Edward V. Lally, M.D.
Associate Professor of Medicine, Department of Medicine, Boston University School of Medicine, Boston, Massachusetts; Director, Division of Rheumatology, Department of Medicine, Roger Williams Medical Center, Providence, Rhode Island

Eric S. Lambright, M.D.
Assistant Instructor of Surgery, Department of Surgery, Hospital of the University of Pennsylvania, Philadelphia, Pennsylvania

J. Thomas Lamont, M.D.
Charlette F. And Irving W. Rabb Professor of Medicine, Department of Medicine, Harvard Medical School; Chief of Gastroenterology, Department of Medicine, Beth Israel Deaconess Medical Center, Boston, Massachusetts

Michael D. LaSalle, M.D.
Clinical Assistant Professor of Urology, Section of Urology, Department of Surgery, The University of Medicine and Dentistry of New Jersey, Newark, New Jersey; Former Fellow—Erectile Dysfunction and Male Reproductive Medicine and Surgery, Department of Urology, Boston University School of Medicine, Boston, Massachusetts

Alex C. Lau, M.D.
S.O.A.R. Clinic, Fellow, Department of Functional Restoration, Stanford Medical Center, Menlo Park, California

Gary E. Leach, M.D.
Clinical Professor of Urology, Department of Urology, University of Southern California; Director, Tower Urology Institute for Continence, Cedars-Sinai Medical Center, Los Angeles, Californi

Joseph M. Lenehan, M.D.
Staff Surgeon, Department of Plastic Surgery, South Shore Hospital, South Weymouth, Massachusetts

Herbert Lepor, M.D.
Professor and Martin Spatz Chairman, Department of Urology, NYU Medical Center, Chief, Urology, Department of Urology, Tisch Hospital, New York, New York

Loren Leshan, M.D.
Associate Professor, Program Director, St. Mary's Family Practic Residency Program, Department of Family & Community Medicine, Medical College of Wisconsin; Department of Family Medicine, St. Mary's Hospital, Milwaukee, Wisconsin

G. Robert Lesser, M.D.
Director, Glaucoma Service, Department of Ophthalmology, Henry Ford Health Sciences Center, Detroit, Michigan

Claire A. Levesque, M.D.
Assistant Professor of Neurology, Department of Neurology, Boston University; Clinical Director, NeuroBehavior Program, Jewish Memorial Hospital, Boston, Massachusetts

Sharon A. Levine, M.D.
Associate Professor of Medicine, Attending Physician, Geriatric Section, Department of Medicine, Boston University School of Medicine, Boston Medical Center, Boston, Massachusetts

Matthew E. Levison, M.D.
Professor, Department of Medicine and Public Health, School of Medicine, MCP Hahnemann University; Chief, Division of Infectious Diseases, Department of Medicine, Medical College of Pennsylvania Hospital, Philadelphia, Pennsylvania

Howard Libman, M.D.
Associate Professor of Medicine, Harvard Medical School; Associate in Medicine, Beth Israel Deaconess Medical Center, Boston, Massachusetts

David Lichtenstein, M.D.
Assistant Professor of Medicine, Boston University School of Medicine; Director of Endoscopy, Department of Medicine, Boston Medical Center, Boston, Massachusetts

Eric H. Lieberman, M.D.
Pending, Department of Medicine, University of Miami, Miami, Florida; Director, Clinical Cardiology Practice, Division of Cardiology, Mount Sinai Medical Center, Miami Beach, Florida

Leonard S. Lilly, M.D.
Associate Professor of Medicine, Harvard Medical School; Cardiologist, Brigham & Women's Hospital, Boston, Massachusetts

Frank W. Ling, M.D.
Faculty Professor and Chairman, University of Tennessee Medical Group; Professor and Chair, Department of Obstetrics & Gynecology, University of Tennessee, Memphis, Tennessee

Randolph J. Lipchik, M.D.
Associate Professor of Medicine, Division of Pulmonary and Critical Care Medicine, Medical College of Wisconsin, Milwaukee, Wisconsin

Scott David Lippe, M.D.
Senior Gastroenterology Fellow, Department of Medicine, Division of Gastroenterology, Nepatology, & Nutrition, Winthrop-University Hospital, Mineola, New York

Gary H. Lipscomb, M.D.
Professor and Director, Division of Gynecology, Department of Obstetrics & Gynecology, University of Tennessee, Memphis, Tennessee

Nancy Y.N. Liu, M.D.
Assistant Professor of Medicine, Department of Medicine, Division of Rheumatology, University of Massachusetts Medical School, Worcester, Massachusetts

Ana Maria Lopez, M.D., M.P.H.
Assistant Professor of Clinical Medicine and Pathology, Arizona Cancer Center, University of Arizona, Medical Director, Women's Health Initiative, Arizona Telemedicine Program, Departments of Clinical Medicine and Pathology, University Medical Center, Tucson, Arizona

Joseph Loscalzo, M.D., Ph.D.
Wade Professor and Chairman, Department of Medicine, Boston University School of Medicine; Physician-in-Chief, Department of Medicine, Boston Medical Center, Boston, Massachusetts

Robert C. Lowe, M.D.
Instructor in Medicine, Harvard Medical School, Associate Physician, Department of Medicine, Brigham and Women's Hospital, Boston, Massachusetts

Philip A. Lowry, M.D.
Associate Physician, Oncology and Hematology, Centre Medical Associates State College, Pennsylvania

Debra M. Lundquist, M.S.N., R.N., CS, OCN
Nurse Practitioner, Department of Hematology/Oncology, University of Massachusetts Medical Center, Worcester, Massachusetts

J. Mark Madison, M.D.
Associate Professor of Medicine and Physiology, Department of Medicine, University of Massachusetts Medical School; Director, Pulmonary Diagnostic Laboratory, Department of Medicine, UMass Memorial Health Care, Worcester, Massachusetts

Urania Magriples, M.D.
Assistant Professor, Department of Obstetrics and Gynecology, Maternal Fetal Medicine, Yale University School of Medicine; Attending Physician and Director of Out-patient Clinics, Department of Obstetrics and Gynecology, Yale-New Haven Hospital, New Haven, Connecticut

James Malone, M.D.
Resident Physician, Department of Otolaryngology, Head and Neck Surgery, Pennsylvania State University; Resident Physician, Department of Otolaryngology, Head and Neck Surgery, Pennsylvania State Geisinger Health System, Milton S. Hershey Medical Center, Hershey, Pennsylvania

David T. Martin, M.D.
Lahey Clinic Medical Center, Burlington, Massachusetts

Kevin J. Martin, M.B., B.Ch.
Professor of Internal Medicine, Director, Division of Nephrology, St. Louis University, Department of Internal Medicine, St. Louis University Hospital, St. Louis, Missouri

David McAneny, M.D., FACS
Associate Professor of Surgery, Department of Surgery, Boston University; Staff Surgeon, Department of Surgery, Section of Surgical Oncology, Boston Medical Center, Boston, Massachusetts

Susan H. McDaniel, Ph.D.
Professor of Family Medicine and Psychiatry, University of Rochester School of Medicine and Dentistry, Rochester, New York

James L. McGuire, M.D.
Former Chairman, Department of Medicine, Mt. Auburn Hospital, Cambridge, Massachusetts
Deceased

Patrick McKinney, M.D., FACMT
Assistant Professor, Medical Director, New Mexico Poison Center, Department of Emergency Medicine, College of Pharmacy, University of New Mexico, Albuquerque, New Mexico

James C. Melby, M.D.
Professor of Medicine and Physiology, Boston University School of Medicine, Boston, Massachusetts

Pierre F. Michetti, M.D.
Assistant Professor, Harvard Medical School; Assistant Physician, Department of Medicine, Gastroenterology, Beth Israel Deaconess Medical Center, Boston, Massachusetts

Samuel A. Mickelson, M.D., FACS
Atlanta Ear, Nose and Throat Associates, Atlanta, Georgia

Yehia Mishriki, M.D.
Professor of Clinical Medicine, Department of Medicine, Penn State University College of Medicine, Hershey, Pennsylvania; General Internist, Department of Medicine, Lehigh Valley Hospital, Allentown, Pennsylvania

Elinor A. Mody, M.D.
Staff Physician, Department of Rheumatology, Brigham and Women's Hospital, Boston, Massachusetts

Lynne H. Morrison, M.D.
Assistant Professor of Dermatology, Department of Dermatology, Oregon Health Sciences University, Active Staff; Assistant Professor of Dermatology, Department of Dermatology, Oregon Health Sciences University and Portland Veteran's Administration Hospital, Portland, Oregon

Ronald A. Morton, M.D.
Assistant Professor of Urology, Director of Laboratories, The Baylor Prostate Center, Baylor College of Medicine, Houston, Texas

T. Jock Murray, O.C., M.D., FRCPC, MACP
Professor of Medical Humanities, Director, MS Research Unit, Dalhousie Medical School, Halifax, Nova Scotia, Canada

Philip R. Muskin, M.D.
Associate Professor of Clinical Psychiatry, Department of Psychiatry, Columbia University, College of Physicians & Surgeons; Associate Chief, Department of Consultation-Liaison Psychiatry, Columbia-Presbyterian Medical Center, New York, New York

Wadie Najm, M.D.
Assistant Clinical Professor, Department of Family Medicine, University of California, Irvine, Orange, California

Julian J. Nussbaum, M.D.
Chairman, Eye Care Services Department, Henry Ford Medical Group, Detroit, Michigan

Robert D. Oates, M.D.
Associate Professor of Urology, Department of Urology, Boston University School of Medicine, Boston, Massachusetts

Thomas A. O'Bryan, M.D.
Assistant Professor of Medicine, Department of Medicine, Physician, Section of General Internal Medicine, Milton S. Hershey Medical Center, Hershey, Pennsylvania

Glennon O'Grady, M.D.
Vice Chair for Clinical Affairs, Department of Family Medicine, Boston University School of Medicine, Boston Medical Center, Boston, Massachusetts

Ann L. Parke, M.B.B.S.
Professor of Medicine, Department of Medicine, Division of Rheumatology, University of Connecticut Health Center; Professor of Medicine, Department of Medicine, Division of Rheumatology, John Dempsey Hospital, Farmington, Connecticut

Frank Parker, M.D.
Professor of Dermatology, Department of Dermatology, Oregon Health Sciences University, Portland, Oregon

David G. Pfister, M.D.
Associate Professor of Medicine, Weill-Cornell University Medical College; Associate Attending Physician, Memorial Sloan Kettering Cancer Center, New York, New York

Glenn M. Preminger, M.D.
Professor of Urologic Surgery, Department of Urology, Duke University Medical Center; Director, Duke Comprehensive Kidney Stone Center, Department of Urology, Duke University Medical Center, Durham, North Carolina

Kenneth W. Presberg, M.D.
Associate Professor of Medicine, Division of Pulmonary and Critical Care Medicine, Department of Medicine, Medical College of Wisconsin; Co-Director, Medical Intensive Care Unit, Department of Medicine, Froedtert Memorial Lutheran Hospital, Milwaukee, Wisconsin

William Pryse-Phillips, M.D., FRCP, FRCPC
Professor of Medicine, Department of Neurology, Faculty of Medicine, Memorial University of Newfoundland; Neurologist, Department of Neurology, Health Sciences Center, St. John's, New Foundland, Canada

Timothy E. Quill, M.D.
Professor of Medicine and Psychiatry, Department of Medicine, University of Rochester; Associate Chief of Medicine, Department of Medicine, The Genesee Hospital, Rochester, New York

Sanford T. Reikes, M.D.
Assistant Professor of Internal Medicine; Assistant Director of Dialysis, Department of Nephrology, St. Louis University School of Medicine, St. Louis University Health Sciences Center, St. Louis, Missouri

Lynn F. Reinke, M.S.N., R.N.-CS
Adult Nurse Practitioner, Department of Pulmonary and Critical Care Medicine, VA Medical Center, Milwaukee, Wisconsin

Michael Reiss, M.D.
Director, Breast Cancer Research Program, Yale Cancer Center, Department of Medicine (Section of Medical Oncology), Yale University School of Medicine, New Haven, Connecticut

Peter A. Rice, M.D.
Professor of Medicine and Microbiology, Boston University School of Medicine; Chief, Section of Infectious Diseases, Department of Medicine, Boston Medical Center, Boston, Massachusetts

Phoebe Rich, M.D.
Associate Professor of Dermatology, Department of Dermatology, Oregon Health Science University, Portland, Oregon

W. Scott Richardson, M.D.
Associate Professor of Medicine, Department of Medicine, University of Texas Health Science Center at San Antonio; Member, Division of General Medicine, Department of Ambulatory Care, Audie L. Murphy Memorial Veterans Hospital, San Antonio, Texas

Kim Riordan, M.D.
Chicago Abused Women Coalition, Hospital Crisis Intervention Project, Chicago, Illinois

David H. Roberts, M.D.
Clinical and Research Fellow, Pulmonary and Critical Care Department, Harvard Medical School; Clinical and Research Fellow, Pulmonary and Critical Care Department, Massachusetts General Hospital, Boston, Massachusetts

Janet Roberts, M.D.
Clinical Professor of Dermatology, Department of Dermatology, Oregon Health Sciences University, Portland, Oregon

David Rosenzweig, M.D., FACP
Associate Professor Emeritus, Department of Medicine, Medical College of Wisconsin; Senior Attending Physician, Froedtert Memorial Lutheran Hospital, Department of Medicine, Milwaukee, Wisconsin

Richard I. Rothstein, M.D.
Associate Professor of Medicine, Dartmouth Medical School, Hanover, New Hampshire, Chief, Gastroenterology, Dartmouth-Hitchcock Medical Center, Lebanon, New Hampshire

Thomas D. Sabin, M.D.
Professor of Neurology, Tufts University School of Medicine, Director, Neurology Residency Program, New England Medical Center, Boston, Massachusetts

R. Mark Sadler, M.D.
Associate Professor of Medicine (Neurology), Department of Medicine, Dalhousie University, Halifax, Nova Scotia, Canada; Active Staff, Department of Medicine, Queen Elizabeth II Heal Sciences Centre, Halifax, Nova Scotia, Canada

Grannum R. Sant, M.D.
Charles M. Whitney Professor and Chair, Department of Urolog Tufts University School of Medicine; Urologist-in-Chief, New England Medical Center, Boston, Massachusetts

Diane Savarese, M.D.
Assistant Professor of Medicine, Hematology Oncology Division, Department of Medicine, University of Massachusetts Medical School; Assistant Professor of Medicine, Division of Hematology-Oncology, UMass Memorial Health Care, Worcester, Massachusetts

Ralph M. Schapira, M.D.
Associate Professor of Medicine, Department of Internal Medicine, Medical College of Wisconsin; Staff Physician and Chief, Section of Pulmonary/Critical Care Section, Froedtert Memorial Lutheran Hospital, Milwaukee, Wisconsin

Edgar C. Schick, Jr., M.D.
Director, Echocardiography Laboratory, Lahey Clinic Medical Center, Burlington, Massachusetts

Harold B. Schiff, M.D.
Associate Clinical Professor of Neurology, Tuft's Medical School, Department of Neurology, Newton-Wellesley Hospital, Newton Lower Falls, Massachusetts

Rhett M. Schiffman, M.D., M.S.
Associate Director of Research, Department of Ophthalmology, Henry Ford Hospital, Detroit, Michigan

Janet Schlechte, M.D.
Professor of Medicine, Department of Internal Medicine, University of Iowa Hospitals and Clinics, Iowa City, Iowa

Donald P. Schlueter, M.D.
Emeritus Professor of Medicine, Department of Medicine, Medical College of Wisconsin; Senior Attending Staff, Department of Medicine, Froedtert Memorial Lutheran Hospital, Milwaukee, Wisconsin

Paul G. Schmitz, M.D.
Associate Professor of Internal Medicine, Department of Internal Medicine, Division of Nephrology, St. Louis University School of Medicine, St. Louis University Health Sciences Center, St. Louis, Missouri

Paul C. Schroy, III, M.D., M.P.H.
Associate Professor of Medicine, Department of Medicine, Boston University School of Medicine; Clinical Director, Associate Visiting Physician, Department of Medicine, Section of Gastroenterology, Boston Medical Center, Boston, Massachusetts

David B. Seaburn, M.S.
Assistant Professor, Psychiatry and Family Medicine, University of Rochester School of Medicine, Strong Memorial Hospital, Rochester, New York

Michael D. Seidman, M.D.
Clinical Associate Professor, Department of Otolaryngology, Wayne State University; Director, Division of Otology/Neurotology Surgery, Department of Otolaryngology-Head and Neck Surgery, Henry Ford Health System, Detroit, Michigan

Andrew Shapiro, M.D.
Clinical Assistant Professor, Department of Surgery, Penn State University, Section of Otolaryngology, Milton S. Hershey Medical Center, Hershey, Pennsylvania

James C. Shaw, M.D.
Associate Professor of Clinical Medicine; Chief, Section of Dermatology, University of Chicago, Chicago, Illinois

Tammi L. Shlotzhauer, M.D.
Clinical Instructor, Department of Medicine, University of Rochester; Chairman, Department of Rheumatology, Unity Health System, Rochester, New York

George T. Simpson, II, M.D., M.P.H.
Professor of Otolaryngology, State University of New York at Buffalo; Chief of Otolaryngology/Head and Neck Surgery, Department of Surgery, Buffalo, New York

Barry Skarf, M.D., Ph.D.
Director, Neuro-Ophthalmology Service, Department of Eye Care Services, Henry Ford Health System, Detroit, Michigan; Adjunct Associate Professor, Department of Ophthalmology, University of Toronto, Toronto, Ontario, Canada

Jay S. Skyler, M.D.
Professor of Medicine, University of Miami School of Medicine, Miami, Florida

Gerald W. Smetana, M.D.
Health Care Associates, Beth Israel Hospital, Boston, Massachusetts

Steven Sondheimer, M.D.
Professor of Obstetrics and Gynecology, Department of Obstetrics and Gynecology, University of Pennsylvania School of Medicine, Philadelphia, Pennsylvania

Virginia D. Steen, M.D.
Professor of Medicine, Department of Internal Medicine, Georgetown University, Georgetown University Hospital, Washington, DC

Linda M. Sutton, M.D.
Assistant Professor of Medicine, Director, Oncology Network, Department of Medicine, Duke University Medical Center, Durham, North Carolina

Robert M. Swift, M.D., Ph.D.
Psychiatrist-in-Chief, Roger Williams Medical Center; Associate Professor of Psychiatry & Human Behavior, Brown University Medical School, Providence, Rhode Island

Irma O. Szymanski, M.D.
Professor of Pathology, University of Massachusetts Medical School, Director, Transfusion Services, Hospital Laboratories, UMass Memorial Medical Center, Worcester, Massachusetts

Bert G. Tavelli, M.D.
Clinical Associate Professor, Department of Dermatology, Oregon Health Sciences University, Portland, Oregon

Basil Varkey, M.D., FRCP(C), FCCP
Professor of Medicine, Department of Medicine, Pulmonary and Critical Care Division, Medical College of Wisconsin; Associate Program Director, Internal Medicine Residency, Department of Medicine, Medical College of Wisconsin, VA Medical Center, Milwaukee, Wisconsin

Nagagopal Venna, M.D., M.R.C.P.(I), M.R.C.P.(UK)
Associate Professor of Neurology, Department of Neurology, Boston University School of Medicine; Director, Ambulatory Neurology Clinic, Department of Neurology, Massachusetts General Hospital, Boston, Massachusetts

Barbara A. Ward, M.D.
Associate Professor of Surgery, Yale University School of Medicine; Attending Surgeon, Yale-New Haven Hospital, New Haven, Connecticut

Carole Warshaw, M.D.
Associate Professor, Department of Psychiatry, University of Illinois; Director of Behavioral Science, Primary Care Internal Medicine, Department of Internal Medicine, Cook County Hospital, Chicago, Illinois

Bruce R. Weinstein, M.D.
Associate Professor of Medicine, Department of Medicine, University of Massachusetts Medical School, UMass Memorial Health Care, Worcester, Massachusetts

Jocelyn C. White, M.D., FACP
Assistant Professor, Department of Medicine, Oregon Health Sciences University; Faculty, Department of Medicine, Legacy Portland Hospitals, Portland, Oregon

Cynthia J. Whitener, M.D.
Assistant Professor of Medicine, Division of Infectious Diseases and Epidemiology, Pennsylvania State University College of Medicine, Milton S. Hershey Medical Center, Hershey, Pennsylvania

Charles Telfer Williams, M.D.
Clinical Instructor, Department of Family Medicine, Boston University School of Medicine; Associate Medical Director, Department of Family Medicine, Boston Medical Center, Boston, Massachusetts

Noel N. Williams, M.D. M.Ch., FRCSI, FRCS (Gen)
Assistant Professor in Surgery, Department of Surgery, Hospital of the University of Pennsylvania, Philadelphia, Pennsylvania

David W. Windus, M.D.
Associate Professor of Medicine, Department of Internal Medicine, Renal Division, Washington University; Associate Professor of Medicine, Department of Medicine, Barnes-Jewish Hospital, St. Louis, Missouri

Thomas N. Wise, M.D.
Professor of Psychiatry, Johns Hopkins School of Medicine, Baltimore, Maryland; Medical Director, Behavioral Services, Inova Health Systems, Boston, Massachusetts

Robert A. Witzburg, M.D.
Professor and Vice Chair, Department of Medicine, Boston University School of Medicine, Chief, Section of Community Medicine, Department of Medicine, Boston Medical Center, Boston, Massachusetts

M. Michael Wolfe, M.D.
Professor and Chief, Section of Gastroenterology, Boston Medical Center, Boston, Massachusetts

Steven R. Ytterberg, M.D.
Associate Professor, Mayo Medical School, Department of Internal Medicine, Division of Rheumatology, Mayo Medical School, Staff Consultant, Department of Internal Medicine, Division of Rheumatology, Mayo Clinic, Rochester, Minnesota

Bernard Zimmermann, III, M.D.
Associate Professor of Medicine, Department of Medicine, Boston University School of Medicine, Boston, Massachusetts; Rheumatologist, Roger Williams Medical Center; Chief, Rheumatology Section, Providence VA Medical Center, Providence, Rhode Island

John J. Zurlo, M.D.
Associate Professor, Division of Infectious Diseases and Epidemiology, Pennsylvania State University College of Medicine, Milton S. Hershey Medical Center, Hershey, Pennsylvania

Preface

The clinical presentation and management of the illnesses and problems of primary care as it is actually practiced are the major focus for the third edition of *Textbook of Primary Care Medicine*. The principles to be followed and the pitfalls to be avoided in diagnosis and treatment are stressed. This edition has been completely reorganized and rewritten to provide up-to-date information on the broad field of primary care medicine. The distinguished list of editors and contributors to this edition are recognized as leaders in their fields. New contributors to this edition bring a fresh perspective to many chapters. Although many are specialists, they write from a generalist's perspective.

This edition consists of 183 chapters organized into two main parts: (1) General issues and approach to disease in primary care medicine and (2) Disease state management by organ system. Over 30 chapters are new to this edition including 12 chapters in the new *signs and symptoms* section. The text and algorithms in this section guide the reader in evaluating physical findings and specific laboratory tests to determine what intervention(s) is called for. A new section on neurology focuses on the neurologic problems that present to generalist physicians. Other new chapters cover primary care of adolescents, alternative medicine, mental disorders in general practice, personality disorders, sexual disorders, and dermatologic diagnosis. A new chapter is included on *Evidence-Based Medicine,* and many chapters include best-evidence medicine sections. Chapters in *Part 2, Disease State Management by Organ System,* follow a standard format to make it easy to locate information quickly. The liberal use of tables, boxes, and bulleted text also provides quick access to information. Managed care guides are included throughout the text. As such, the text represents one component of a total medical information system.

The other element of this state-of-the-art medical information system on primary care is the optional CD-ROM. It not only includes the complete third edition of this text, but also includes *Mosby's GenRx* (a pharmacopoeia hyperlinked to the text), videos of clinical procedures that can be performed by the primary care physician in the office setting, patient teaching guides, and questions and answers for review. Using the CD, the practitioner can access the primary care website for web-linked updates and Medline references.

Textbook of Primary Care Medicine is intended to serve as a valuable reference in the office, clinic, and emergency room. The information contained in this edition reflects the commonality of medical experience shared by the generalist and specialist physicians, physician assistants, and nurse practitioners. My colleagues and I have sought to create an extensive source of knowledge and experience to aid all who practice general medicine, family practice, and primary care.

John Noble

Acknowledgments

Textbook of Primary Care Medicine, in its third edition, is the product of careful planning and the scholarship of many individuals: chapter authors, section editors, senior editors, and the publishers. In addition to many new contributors, this edition includes several new editors. New Senior Editors include Joseph E. Scherger and Cynthia D. Mulrow. Our new Section Editors include Joseph Loscalzo, *Cardiology;* Steven A. Cole, *Psychiatry;* Jay S. Skyler, *Endocrinology;* Nezam H. Afdhal, *Gastroenterology;* and T. Jock Murray, *Neurology.* Evidence-based principles have been introduced throughout most chapters with the guidance of Cynthia D. Mulrow and W. Scott Richardson.

Our team at Mosby has been a delight to work with. Led by Liz Fathman, Acquisitions Editor, and Kathy Falk, Senior Managing Editor, it has been possible not only to create a thoroughly updated and revised text but also to develop an electronic and CD base for the text that greatly expands the breadth and depth of its content. Carol Sullivan Weis, Project Manager, and David Stein, Senior Production Editor, have taken the manuscript through production to its final book form, on time, on target regarding length, and with top quality. Bob Boehringer, Senior Marketing Manager, and Lana VanLaningham, Multimedia Producer, have designed our marketing program and the new dimensions of multimedia for *Textbook of Primary Care Medicine.* On behalf of our Senior Editors and myself, congratulations and many thanks to all.

JOHN NOBLE

Contents

PART ONE

General Issues and Approach to Disease in Primary Care Medicine

I Core Issues and Special Groups in Primary Care

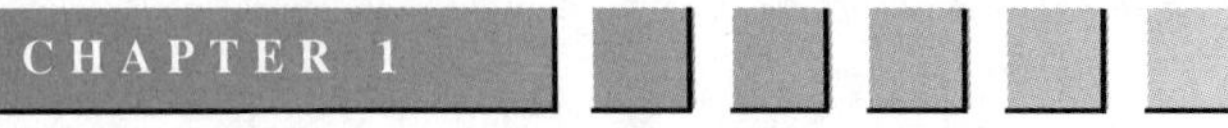

Lifelong Learning and Evidence-Based Medicine for Primary Care

W. Scott Richardson
Cynthia D. Mulrow

Excellent primary care physicians are handmade. They fashion themselves, with the help of teachers, colleagues and patients, by building skills, attitudes, and knowledge of many kinds. They sharpen and resharpen their abilities throughout their careers, carrying out their own programs of lifelong learning.[1,4] Indeed, the commitment to lifelong study is a central value for a career in the health professions.[14] This textbook aims to help primary care physicians keep that commitment to their profession, their patients, and themselves.

Throughout their careers, excellent primary care physicians learn and use many kinds of knowledge, some of which are depicted in Fig. 1-1. For instance, in caring for a patient with advancing heart failure, a physician might draw on: clinical experience to quickly recognize the progression of symptoms despite treatment; human pathophysiology to identify possible causes of the worsening; research evidence to estimate the patient's prognosis; clinical ethics and the patient's perspective to plan advance directives; and the context of care, to know what palliative services are available in the community. Each form of knowledge may have strengths and limitations, and no single form can supply all that physicians need for every decision. Thus wise physicians become comfortable learning several forms of knowledge and use clinical judgment to select, weigh, and integrate these forms for the care of individual persons.[2]

These forms of knowledge all change over time, but three in particular change rapidly: the context of care, human biology, and clinical care research. The yearly volume of new knowledge in any one of these areas is overwhelming, and together they outstrip human mental capacity. No one person can read it all and know it all. Thus we need methods to select the relatively small proportion of new knowledge in each field that warrants our attention. This chapter concerns such methods for selecting knowledge from clinical care research.

In addition to confronting the sheer volume of research publications, primary care physicians attempting to understand and use evidence from clinical care research face other challenges. When this research is examined critically, only about 2% of it represents evidence that is sufficiently valid and clinically applicable to warrant a change in practice.[11] Without some help, physicians are more likely to encounter information that *should not* change their practice than information that should. Even in the face of this "plenty," many clinical questions arise during patient care that go unanswered,[23] and with time the cumulative effect of not learning is obsolescence.[7,18] Unfortunately, traditional continuing education based on passive learning methods, such as didactic lectures, does little to stop the inexorable decline in our clinical knowledge or actual performance.[5]

Evidence-based medicine (EBM) is a relatively new approach to lifelong learning and clinical practice that holds much promise for primary care. EBM is "the conscientious and judicious use of current best evidence from clinical care research in the management of individual patients," and practicing it means integrating current best evidence along with clinical expertise, patients' perspectives, and other knowledge.[12] EBM provides clinicians with tools for finding, understanding, and using evidence from research that is scientifically valid and clinically useful. Thus evidence-based practicing and learning can help primary care physicians carry out their programs of lifelong learning.

After finishing formal postgraduate training, primary care physicians find themselves in two situations in which evidence from clinical care research can be learned and integrated: when trying to keep current and when solving patient problems. Although there is much overlap, these two situations have some differences in emphasis and require that we plan our learning differently. This chapter summarizes the skills and resources of EBM for lifelong learning in primary care and intersperses tips on how to use them for keeping current and for solving problems.

EBM EVIDENCE-BASED MEDICINE STEPS AND SKILLS (Box 1-1)

Recognizing Information Needs

The first step in using research evidence is to recognize when it is needed. Several kinds of knowledge for primary care are needed, and much of the time, we already possess and can readily use this knowledge. The sense of satisfaction that goes with knowing what we need to know has been called *cognitive resonance*.[16] At times, caring for patients brings unfamiliar clinical circumstances or challenging information

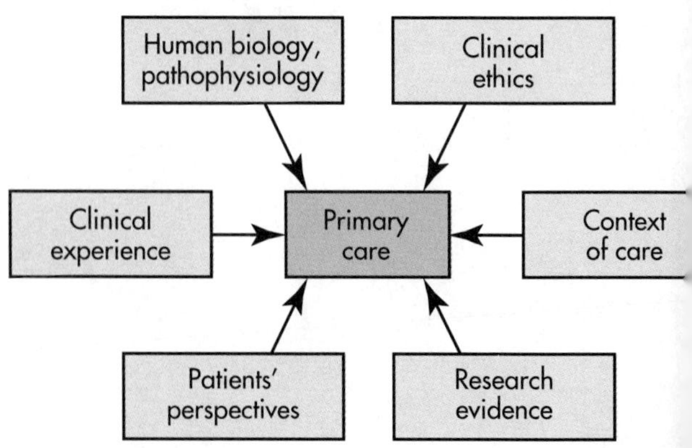

Fig. 1-1. Selected forms of knowledge used in primary care.

and at some level we become aware that our knowledge stores do not have the necessary information. The disturbing feelings such situations provoke have been called *cognitive dissonance,* and these sensations can motivate us to learn.[16] Being alert to our own cognitive dissonance can help us recognize when we need new knowledge.

Since knowledge of several kinds is used for primary care, not every information need will be a gap of evidence from the medical literature. Sometimes cognitive dissonance is a signal that we lack information about our patient's preferences or that we lack sufficient experience with a disorder. Often, however, cognitive dissonance is a signal that new knowledge from clinical care research is needed in order to make sensible clinical decisions. These moments are opportunities for evidence-based learning, and with practice we can recognize them in our everyday work.

Box 1-1. EBM Evidence-Based Medicine Steps and Skills

Recognizing information needs
Asking answerable clinical questions
Finding answers to questions
Appraising research evidence
Understanding research evidence
Applying research evidence to individual patients
Putting evidence into practice in lifelong learning

Asking Answerable Clinical Questions

Having found a gap in knowledge, we convert the information need into a clinical question, the answer to which should fill the gap. Clinical questions about knowledge come in infinite variety, but most can be loosely classified as either background or foreground questions (Fig. 1-2). Background questions ask about the disorder itself, such as "What is essential hypertension?" or "When do the complications of hypertension occur?" Note that background questions usually have two components: a question root (who, what, where, when, how, and why) with a verb, and the disorder (or an aspect of it) under study. Questions about background knowledge are especially useful when we have little familiarity with the disorder under study.

In contrast, foreground questions ask about caring for patients with the disorder, such as "In elderly patients with isolated systolic hypertension, does antihypertensive drug therapy reduce stroke, cardiovascular disease, and total mortality enough to be worth its adverse effects?" Note that foreground questions usually have three or four components: the patient and/or problem (in this example, elderly patients with isolated systolic hypertension); the intervention, test, or exposure (antihypertensive drug therapy); comparison inter-

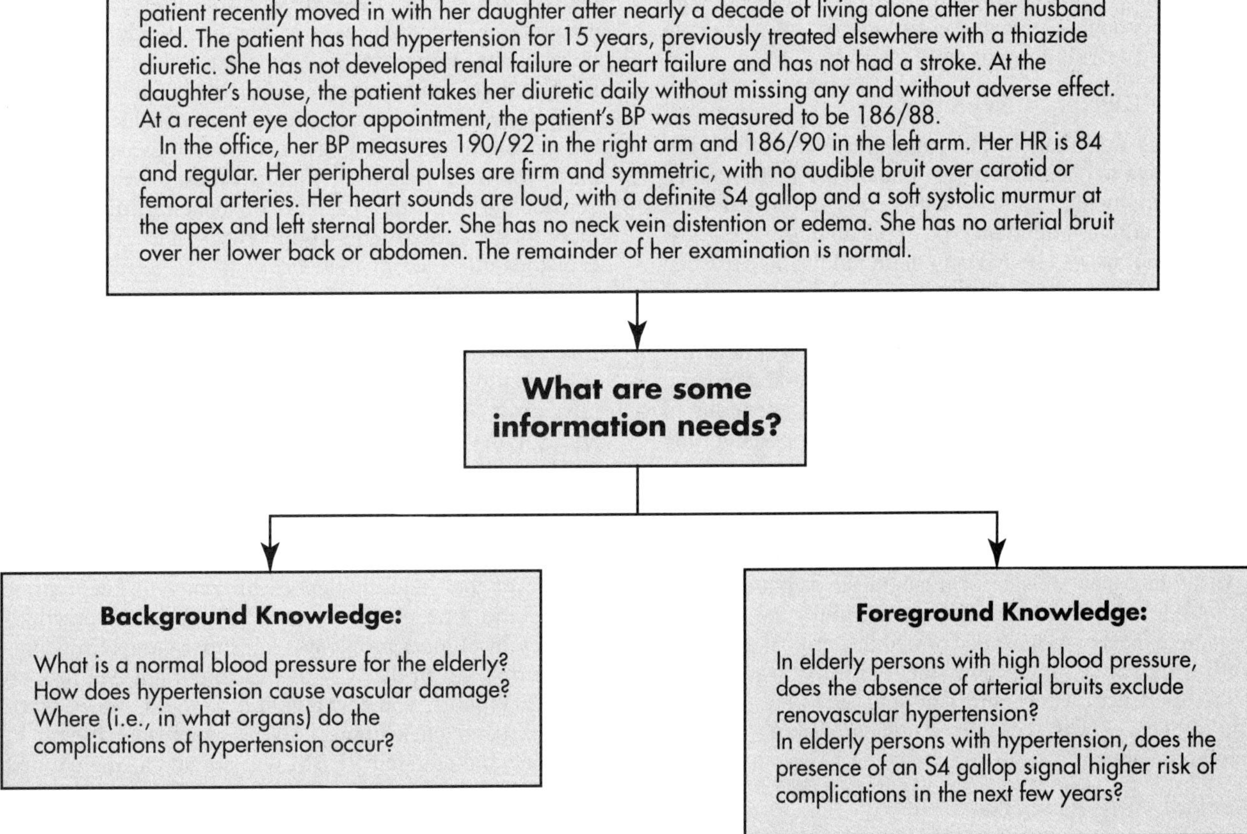

Fig. 1-2. Illustrative case.

ventions, when relevant (implied comparison to no drug); and the clinical outcomes of interest (stroke, cardiovascular disease, mortality, adverse effects). Questions about foreground knowledge are useful when we are already familiar with the background knowledge about the disorder.

Asking questions in this manner takes practice, but with time it can become second nature. Good questions can pay off by helping us focus our scarce reading time for learning that is directly relevant to our patients' illnesses and our learning needs; suggesting the forms that good answers will take; leading directly to efficient search strategies; and improving communication with other clinicians in consultation and when learning.[17,19,20] Expert physicians recognize innumerable questions that could be asked about patients and their problems. Rather than trying to answer every one, we should focus on those questions that seem most urgent for a particular patient's care, most appropriate to personal knowledge needs, or most feasible to answer in the available time.

Finding Answers to Questions

Having chosen a question and phrased it clearly, we can begin finding answers. Because time is short, it makes sense to start the search with resources that have the highest chance of yielding the needed answers. Since questions will vary, so should resource use. For background questions, the best sources are up-to-date summaries about the disease in question, as might be found in a recent text chapter or narrative review. For foreground questions, the most useful sources are up-to-date summaries of the best evidence informing the management of patients with the disease, as would be found in recent systematic review or evidence-based practice guideline. Good searching skills, although beyond the scope of this chapter, can be developed with practice and coaching and are essential for sustaining an evidence-based learning program.

Appraising Research Evidence

Having found information that may yield the necessary answer, we have to decide whether or not to use it. To do this, we make judgments about whether this information is sufficiently credible, important, and applicable to the clinical situation to warrant its use. Making these judgments has been termed *critical appraisal,* and involves applying some rules of evidence along with common sense, within a framework that balances open-mindedness with healthy skepticism.[21] Box 1-2 lists critical appraisal issues for several common forms of evidence in the form of checklists of questions to ask.[22] We can use these checklists when appraising the evidence ourselves or when reviewing the appraisal portions of evidence summarized by others.

When applying the evidence-based clinical routines and practice policies that others develop, we cannot and should not expect to repeat this critical appraisal step ourselves; those who summarized the evidence and built the practice policies are expected to have performed this critical appraisal carefully, making explicit how the evidence was found, how the evidence was appraised, and how the strength of the evidence was considered when making clinical recommendations.

Understanding Research Evidence

We can apply evidence-based clinical routines and practice policies without an intimate knowledge of the raw results of the underlying research. Often, though, when estimating the expected benefits and possible harms of applying the recommended test or treatment, we need to understand what the research results are and what they mean. Such results may be reported in quantitative terms, including some that may not be familiar. Some definitions, explanations, and tips for understanding these numerical results of evidence about diagnosis and therapy are presented in Boxes 1-3[10] and 1-4.[15] More complete discussions of these topics are available; some of them are listed at the end of the chapter.

Applying Research Evidence to Individual Patients

Having decided that the evidence warrants use, we now apply the intervention to our patients. Each patient is an individual person, with a unique blend of biologic, psychologic, and sociologic factors that may influence the outcomes of illness and the responsiveness to our interventions. We can never foretell with absolute certainty whether our patient will respond in the same way as the patients in whom the intervention was studied. Even so, we can extrapolate evidence from studies to our patients, if we do it carefully and sensibly. To help decide whether extrapolation is wise, we might ask the following questions[9]:

Is my patient so different from those in the study tha results cannot be applied?
Is the treatment feasible in my setting?
What are the likely benefits and harms from the treatment
How will my patient's values influence the decision?

Most of the time variations in human risk and responsive ness are matters of degree, in that we differ quantitatively i amount of risk or chances of responding. Seldom do we diffe in absolute terms in risk or responsiveness, such th interventions produce opposite effects. Thus we can usuall apply the evidence to our patients, after considering how the unique biology, psychology, and sociology adjust our est mates of their risk and responsiveness. We can then ad consideration of the balance of benefits and harms ar incorporate our patients' preferences into patient-centere decisions informed by evidence.

Putting Evidence into Practice in Lifelong Learning

When building a plan for lifelong learning in primary ca physicians face two main learning situations: keeping curre and solving patient problems. Research evidence can understood and used for both learning situations, and t strategies and tactics of EBM can help you do this. We ha gathered our own and others' tips for keeping current a solving patient problems into Fig. 1-3.[3,6,8,13,22]

One of the great challenges in trying to keep current finding the time to devote to it. The pace of practice, urgency of clinical problems, and other competing demar all seem to get in the way of this important, yet less urg activity. Whether you get an hour per month, per week, or day to spend on keeping current, your time is still fin Learning and practicing EBM will not add a single minute your hour, but it can help you use your limited learning ti wisely and efficiently. Thus we emphasize managing ti well, learning some evidence-based learning skills, managing the evidence literature well.

Box 1-2. Critical Appraisal of Selected Types of Evidence

Individual Trials of Therapy

Validity

1. Was the assignment of patients to treatment randomized? Was the randomization list concealed?
2. Were all patients who entered the trial accounted for at its conclusion? Were they analyzed in the groups to which they were randomized?
3. Were patients, physicians, and study personnel kept "blind" to which treatment was being received?
4. Aside from the experimental treatment, were the groups treated equally?
5. Were the groups similar at the start of the trial?

Importance

1. What is the magnitude of the treatment effect?
2. How precise is the estimate of treatment effect?

Applicability

1. Do these results apply to my patient?
   Is my patient so different from those in the trial that its results cannot help me?
   How great would the potential benefit of therapy actually be for my patient?
2. Are my patient's values and preferences satisfied by the regimen and its consequences?
   Do we have a clear assessment of these values and preferences?
   Are they met by this regimen and its consequences?

Systematic Review of Therapy Trials

Validity

1. Is this a review of randomized trials of the treatment of interest?
2. Does it include a *methods* section that describes:
   a. Finding and including all relevant trials?
   b. Assessing their individual validity?
3. Were the results consistent from study to study?

Importance

1. What is the magnitude of the treatment effect?
2. How precise is the estimate of treatment effect?

Applicability

1. Do these results apply to my patient?
   Is my patient so different from those in the trial that its results cannot help me?
   How great would the potential benefit of therapy actually be for my patient?
2. Are my patient's values and preferences satisfied by the regimen and its consequences?
   Do we have a clear assessment of these values and preferences?
   Are they met by this regimen and its consequences?

Practice Guidelines

Validity

1. Were all important decision options and outcomes clearly specified?
2. Was the evidence relevant to each decision option identified, validated, and combined in a sensible and explicit way?
3. Are the relative preferences that key stakeholders attach to the outcomes of decisions (including benefits, harms, and costs) identified and explicitly considered?
4. Are the guideline's recommendations unaffected by clinically sensible variations in patients' outcomes and values?

Importance

1. Does this guideline offer an opportunity for significant improvement in the quality of health care practice?
   Is there a large variation in current practice?
   Does the guideline contain new evidence (or old evidence not yet acted on) that could have an important effect on management?
   Would the guideline affect the management of so many people, or concern individuals at such high risk, or involve such high costs that even small changes in practice could have major impacts on health outcomes of resources (including opportunity costs)?

Applicability

1. What barriers exist to implementing this guideline? Can they be overcome?
2. Can I enlist the collaboration of key colleagues?
3. Can I meet the following educational, administrative, and economic conditions that are likely to determine the success or failure of implementing the strategy:
   a. Credible synthesis of evidence by a respected body
   b. Respected, influential local exemplars already implementing the strategy
   c. Consistent information from all relevant sources
   d. Opportunity for individual discussions about the strategy with an authority
   e. User-friendly format for guidelines
   f. Implementable within target group of physicians (without need for extensive outside collaboration)
   g. Freedom from conflict with economic incentives, administrative incentives, patient expectations, and community expectations.

Diagnostic Tests

Validity

1. Was there an independent, blind comparison with a reference gold standard of diagnosis?
2. Was the diagnostic test evaluated in an appropriate spectrum of patients (patients similar to those in whom it would be used in practice)?
3. Was the reference standard applied regardless of the diagnostic test result?

Importance

1. How powerful is this diagnostic test (in likelihood ratios or sensitivity and specificity)?

Applicability

1. Is the diagnostic test available, affordable, accurate, and precise in my setting?
2. Can I generate a clinically sensible estimate of my patient's pretest probability (from personal experience, practice data, this report, or other literature)?
3. Will the resulting posttest probabilities affect my management and help my patient?
   Could it move me across a threshold for testing or treatment?

Continued

Box 1-2. Critical Appraisal of Selected Types of Evidence—cont'd

Would my patient be a willing partner in carrying it out?
4. Would the consequences of the test help my patient?

Harm/Etiology
Validity

1. Were there clearly defined groups of patients, similar in all important ways other than exposure to the treatment or other suspected cause?
2. Were the exposures and clinical outcomes measured the same ways in both groups? Was the assessment of outcomes either objective or blinded to exposure?
3. Was patient follow-up sufficiently long and complete?
4. Do the results satisfy some "tests of causation"?
   Did exposure clearly precede the onset of the outcome?
   Is there a dose-response gradient?
   Is there positive evidence from a "dechallenge/rechallenge" study?
   Is the association consistent from study to study?
   Does the association make biologic sense?

Importance

1. How strong is the association between exposure and outcome?
2. How precise is the estimate of strength of association?

Applicability

1. Can the study results be extrapolated to my patient?
2. What are my patient's risks of the adverse outcome?
3. What, if any, benefits might my patient forego if we stop the exposure?
4. (For harm from therapy) What alternative treatments are available?

Prognosis
Validity

1. Was a well-defined, representative sample of patients assembled at a common (usually early) point in the course of disease?
2. Was patient follow-up sufficiently long and complete?
3. Were objective outcome criteria applied in a "blind" fashion?
4. If subgroups with different prognoses are identified:
   Was there adjustment for important prognostic factors?
   Was there validation in an independent group ("test set") of patients?

Importance

1. How likely are the outcomes over time?
2. How precise are the prognostic estimates?

Applicability

1. Were the study patients similar to mine?
2. Will this evidence have a clinically important impact on what to offer or tell my patient?

Box 1-3. Understanding Evidence About Diagnostic Tests*

		Target Disorder (Iron Deficiency)		
		Present	Absent	Totals
Diagnostic test result	Positive (<65 mmol/L)	731 a	270 b	1001 a + b
(Serum ferritin)	Negative (>65 mmol/L)	78 c	1500 d	1578 c + d
	Totals	809 a + c	1770 b + d	2579 a + b + c + d

Sensitivity = a/(a + c) = 731/809 = 90%
Specificity = d/(b + d) = 1500/1770 = 85%
Positive predictive value = a/(a + b) = 731/1001 = 73%
Negative predictive value = d/(c + d) = 1500/1578 = 95%

Pretest probability (here, = prevalence) = (a + c)/(a + b + c + d) = 809/2579 = 32%
Posttest probability after positive result = a/(a + b) = 731/1001 = 73%
Posttest probability after negative result = c/(c + d) = 78/1578 = 5%

Likelihood ratio for positive test result:
LR + = sensitivity(1 − specificity) = 90%/15% = 6
Likelihood ratio for negative test result:
LR − = (1 − sensitivity)/specificity = 10%/85% = 0.12

Pretest odds = prevalence/(1 − prevalence) = 32%/68% = 0.47
Posttest odds = pretest odds × likelihood ratio

Posttest probability = posttest odds/(posttest odds + 1)

How much can likelihood ratios change disease likelihood?
LR's of >10 or <0.1 cause large changes, often ruling in or ruling out disease
LR's of 5-10 or 0.1-0.2 cause moderate changes
LR's of 2-5 or 0.2-0.5 cause small changes
LR's of <2 or >0.5 cause tiny changes
LR's of 1.0 cause no change at all

Estimates of pretest probability can come from:
Remembered clinical experience with similar patients
Data from practice setting
Prevalence of target disorder in article about diagnostic test (e.g., above, where prevalence of iron deficiency was 32%)
Published studies of disease probability
Population vital statistics

*Sample data from Guyatt GH, Oxman AD, Ali M, et al: Laboratory diagnosis of iron-deficiency anemia: an overview, *J Gen Intern Med* 7:145-153, 1992.

Box 1-4. Understanding Evidence About Therapy*

NASCET 2-Year Outcomes

		Outcome + **(Any major stroke or death)**	**Outcome −** **(No stroke or death)**	**Totals**
Treatment allocation	Experimental (surgical)	19 a	309 b	328 a + b
	Control (medical)	38 c	293 d	331 c + d
	Totals	57 a + c	602 b + d	659 a + b + c + d

The rates of outcome events in experimental and control groups are:
Experimental event rate (EER) = a/(a + b) = 19/328 = 0.080
Control event rate (CER) = c/(c + d) = 38/331 = 0.181

Some ways you will find these two event rates compared:

1. **As a simple difference:** Subtracting the experimental event rate from the control event rate expresses the absolute size of the difference between the two rates. This is known as risk difference or absolute risk reduction (ARR).
   ARR = CER − EER = 0.181 − 0.080 = 0.101
   Using the ARR preserves the information about the absolute size of the treatment effect and about the baseline risk without treatment (CER).

2. **As the difference with a twist:** To make the ARR more friendly, transform it by dividing it into 1, yielding the number needed to treat (NNT).
   NNT = 1/ARR = 1/0.101 = 10
   This NNT of 10 means that 10 patients need to be treated with endarterectomy to prevent one additional major stroke or death over 2 years.

3. **As the difference compared with control:** To estimate the relative benefit of treatment compared with control, the difference in event rates can be divided by the control event rate, yielding the relative risk reduction (RRR).
   RRR = ARR/CER = (CER − EER)/CER = 0.101/0.181 = 56%
   Using the RRR gives a sense of relative benefit and can be used to compare across interventions for a disorder, but it obscures the baseline risk without active treatment (CER is literally divided out) and the absolute size of the difference in event rates.

4. **As a ratio of rates:** Another estimate in relative terms can be made by creating a ratio of the event rates, known as the risk ratio or relative risk (RR).
   RR = EER/CER = 0.80/0.181 = 0.44

5. **As a ratio of odds:** If desired, outcomes could be described in terms of odds, rather than event rates. Thus the odds of the outcome in experimental group are a/b, and the odds of the outcome in the control group are c/d. Making a ratio of the two yields the odds ratio (OR).
   OR = (a/b)/(c/d) = ad/bc = (19 × 293)/(309 × 38) = 0.47
   Odds ratios are sometimes used in summaries of systematic reviews, as well as in studies of risk of harm from various exposures.

*Sample data from NASCET study, NASCET Collaborators: Beneficial effect of carotid endarterectomy in symptomatic patients with high-grade stenosis, *N Engl J Med* 325:445-453, 1991.

Time is even more critical when solving patient problems. ot only is there little time to carry out learning, but :casionally the clinical situations impose short deadlines by hich decisions must be made. Often, however, the pace of ıtpatient illness is such that learning to solve patient oblems can be accomplished between visits, rather than all once. Our advice emphasizes preparing by developing ills and resources, carrying out evidence-based learning hen (not if) the situations arise, and using the evidence in tient care. The accumulated learning from many such teractions is great, and being patient-based, it may be easier r us to remember. According to an old proverb, "long ırneys begin with a single step," to which we would add nd they continue in the same manner, one step at a time."

Together, keeping up-to-date and solving patient problems mpose most of our individual work for lifelong learning. If choose them carefully, formal continuing medical educan (CME) activities can be useful supplements for our erall learning program. As we mentioned earlier, CME grams based on passive methods such as lectures simply not work. Continuing education can be effective, however, if it relies on methods shown in trials to be effective, including individualized audit and feedback on actual practice; individualized advice on practice from a respected, evidence-based teacher; academic detailing using evidence-based recommendations; and mini-sabbaticals to clinical sites that practice up-to-date, evidence-based care.[5] Moreover, we suggest selecting CME that allows us to target our specific learning needs; allows us to integrate new knowledge with prior experience; allows us to plan and practice our behavior changes; provides coaching and constructive feedback; and encourages us to plan follow-up on our learning at a later time.[1,16]

EBM LEARNING MORE ABOUT EVIDENCE-BASED MEDICINE

As with most clinical skills, evidence-based learning takes practice. This chapter provides only an introduction, and we suggest you learn more about the concepts and skills of EBM by using the resources listed in Box 1-5 and in the References and Additional Readings. As with any other clinical field,

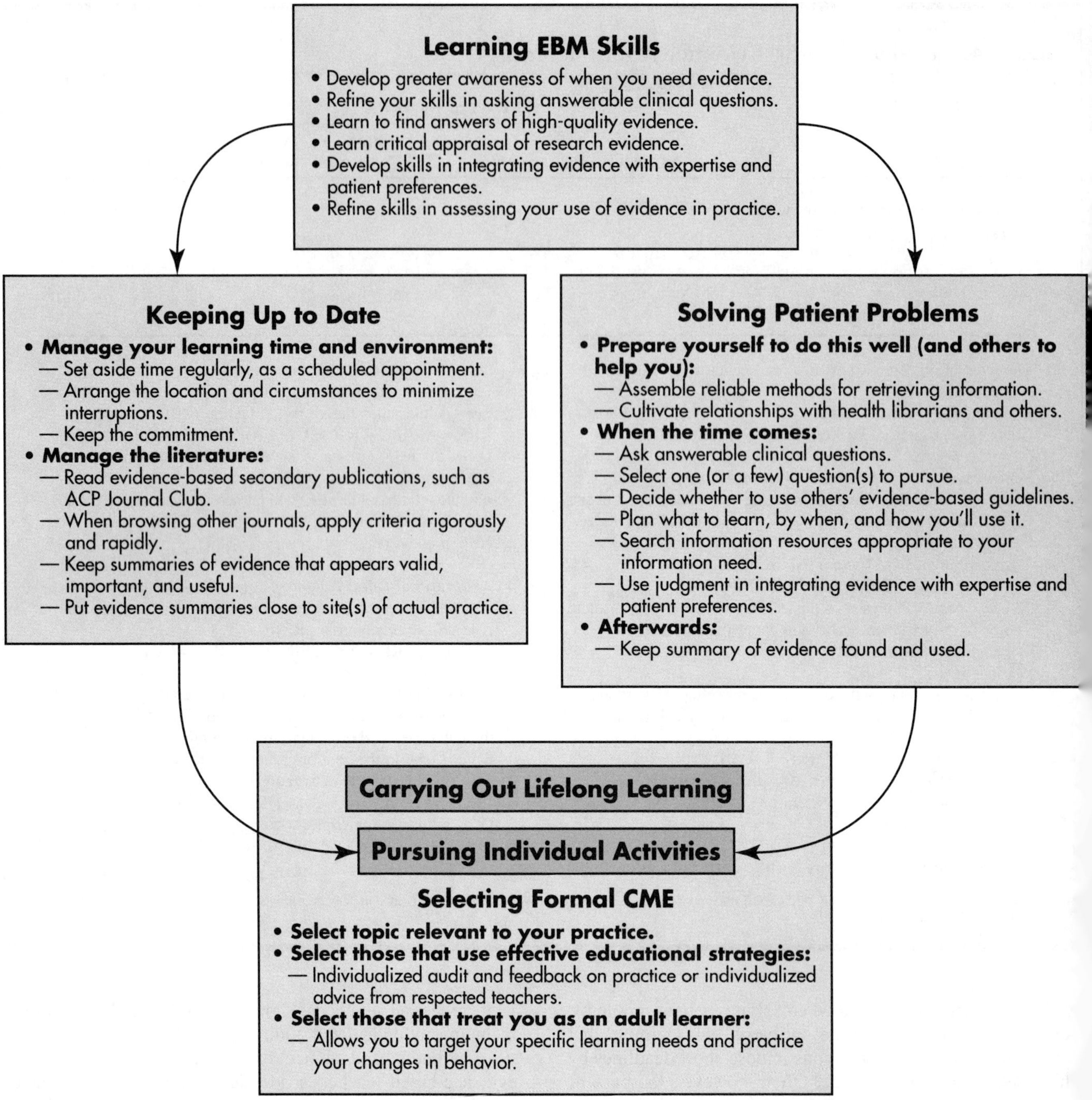

Learning EBM Skills

- Develop greater awareness of when you need evidence.
- Refine your skills in asking answerable clinical questions.
- Learn to find answers of high-quality evidence.
- Learn critical appraisal of research evidence.
- Develop skills in integrating evidence with expertise and patient preferences.
- Refine skills in assessing your use of evidence in practice.

Keeping Up to Date

- **Manage your learning time and environment:**
  - — Set aside time regularly, as a scheduled appointment.
  - — Arrange the location and circumstances to minimize interruptions.
  - — Keep the commitment.
- **Manage the literature:**
  - — Read evidence-based secondary publications, such as ACP Journal Club.
  - — When browsing other journals, apply criteria rigorously and rapidly.
  - — Keep summaries of evidence that appears valid, important, and useful.
  - — Put evidence summaries close to site(s) of actual practice.

Solving Patient Problems

- **Prepare yourself to do this well (and others to help you):**
  - — Assemble reliable methods for retrieving information.
  - — Cultivate relationships with health librarians and others.
- **When the time comes:**
  - — Ask answerable clinical questions.
  - — Select one (or a few) question(s) to pursue.
  - — Decide whether to use others' evidence-based guidelines.
  - — Plan what to learn, by when, and how you'll use it.
  - — Search information resources appropriate to your information need.
  - — Use judgment in integrating evidence with expertise and patient preferences.
- **Afterwards:**
  - — Keep summary of evidence found and used.

Carrying Out Lifelong Learning

Pursuing Individual Activities

Selecting Formal CME

- **Select topic relevant to your practice.**
- **Select those that use effective educational strategies:**
  - — Individualized audit and feedback on practice or individualized advice from respected teachers.
- **Select those that treat you as an adult learner:**
  - — Allows you to target your specific learning needs and practice your changes in behavior.

Fig. 1-3. Using EBM for lifelong learning in primary care.

Box 1-5. EBM Surfing the Net

Evidence-Based Care	http://hiru.hirunet.mcmaster.ca/ebm/
Centre for EBM (UK)	http://cebm.jr2.ox.ac.uk/
ScHARR	http://www.shef.ac.uk/uni/academic/R-Z/scharr/ir/netting
Cochrane	http://hiru.mcmaster.ca/cochrane/default.html
Bandolier	http://www.jr2.ox.ac.uk/bandolier/index/html

keep watch for new developments in EBM that make it easi and faster to stay excellent as primary care physicians.

SUMMARY

EBM represents a way of practicing in which we c integrate valid and important new research findings with c other knowledge to solve patient problems and ke up-to-date. Practicing EBM builds on, rather than replac our clinical expertise and enhances our abilities to dec with our patients which management plans best fit th preferences. Using EBM skills for lifelong learning can h us provide primary care that is clinically expert, eviden based, and person-centered.

REFERENCES

1. Candy PC: *Self-direction for lifelong learning: a comprehensive guide to theory and practice,* San Francisco, 1991, Jossey-Bass.
2. Cassell EJ: *Doctoring: the nature of primary care medicine,* New York, 1997, Oxford University.
3. Cook DJ, Meade MO, Fink MP, for the Evidence-Based Medicine in Critical Care Group: How to keep up with the critical care literature and avoid being buried alive, *Crit Care Med* 24:1757-1768, 1996.
4. Davis DA, Fox RD, editors: *The physician as learner: linking research to practice,* Chicago, 1994, AMA.
5. Davis DA, Thompson MA, Oxman AD, et al: Changing physician performance: a systematic review of the effect of continuing medical education strategies, *JAMA* 274:700-705, 1995.
6. Davidoff FM: Continuing medical education resources, *J Gen Intern Med* 12[Suppl. 2]:S15-S19, 1997.
7. Evans CE, Haynes RB, Birkett NJ, et al: Does a mailed continuing education program improve clinician performance? Results of a randomized trial in antihypertensive care, *JAMA* 255:501-504, 1986.
8. Fletcher RH, Fletcher SW: Evidence-based approach to the medical literature, *J Gen Intern Med* 12[Suppl. 2]:S5-S14, 1997.
9. Glasziou P, Guyatt GH, Dans AL, et al: Applying the results of trials and systematic reviews to individual patients [Editorial], *ACP J Club* 129(3):A15-A16, 1998.
10. Guyatt GH, Oxman AD, Ali M, et al: Laboratory diagnosis of iron-deficiency anemia: an overview, *J Gen Intern Med* 7:145-153, 1992.

1. Haynes RB: Where's the meat in clinical journals? [Editorial], *ACP J Club* 119:A22-A23, 1993.

2. Haynes RB, Sackett DL, Gray JAM, et al: Transferring evidence from research into practice: 1. The role of clinical care research evidence in clinical decisions [Editorial], *ACP J Club* 125:A14-A16, 1996.

3. Larson EB: How can clinicians incorporate research advances into practice? *J Gen Intern Med* 12[Suppl. 2]:S20-S24, 1997.

4. Napodano RJ: *Values in medical practice,* New York, 1986, Human Sciences.

5. NASCET Collaborators: Beneficial effect of carotid endarterectomy in symptomatic patients with high-grade stenosis, *N Engl J Med* 325:445-453, 1991.

6. Neighbour R: *The inner apprentice,* Newbury, UK, 1996, Petroc.

7. Oxman AD, Sackett DL, Guyatt GH, for the Evidence-Based Medicine Working Group: Users' guides to the medical literature: I. How to get started, *JAMA* 270:2093-2095, 1993.

. Ramsey PG, Carline JD, Inui TS, et al: Changes over time in the knowledge base of practicing internists, *JAMA* 266:1103-1107, 1991.

. Richardson WS: Ask, and ye shall retrieve [EBM Note], *Evidence-Based Medicine* 3:100-101, 1998.

. Richardson WS, Wilson MC, Nishikawa J, et al: The well-built clinical question: a key to evidence-based decisions [Editorial], *ACP J Club* 123:A12-A13, 1995.

Sackett DL, Haynes RB, Guyatt GH, et al, editors: *Clinical epidemiology: a basic science for clinical medicine,* ed 2, Boston, 1991, Little, Brown.

Sackett DL, Richardson WS, Rosenberg WMC, et al: editors: *Evidence-based medicine: how to practice and teach EBM,* New York, 1997, Churchill-Livingstone.

Smith R: What clinical information do doctors need? *Br Med J* 313:1062-1068, 1996.

DITIONAL READINGS

dland D, Go AS, Davoren JB, et al: *Evidence-based medicine: a framework for clinical practice,* Stamford, Conn, 1998, Appleton Lange.

enhalgh T: *How to read a paper,* London, 1997, BMJ Books.

gy C, Haines A, editors: *Evidence-based practice in primary care,* London, 1998, BMJ Books.

us SE, Badenoch D, Richardson WS, et al: *Practising evidence-based medicine: learner's manual,* ed 3, Oxford, UK, 1998, Radcliffe Medical.

CHAPTER 2

Generalist's Approach to the Medical Interview

Wendy Levinson

The relationship between physician and patient forms the basis for high-quality medical care in any setting. Without a trusting relationship, physicians cannot accurately diagnose patients' problems and develop approaches to treatment of illness and health prevention. Trusting relationships are truly the bedrock for the practice of general medicine. The era of managed care has presented challenges to the physician-patient relationship, with many patients unsure whether the physician is working exclusively in their best interest. Patients wonder whether physicians have pressures to control cost that unduly influence the physicians' judgment. Simultaneously, physicians are under increasing pressure to see more patients in a limited period of time. More than ever, physicians need to communicate both efficiently and effectively with patients to maximize outcomes.

The medical interview is the primary care physician's tool for developing a trusting relationship, diagnosing illness, developing a treatment plan, educating patients about illness and health, and motivating behavior change. Effective interviewing skills lead to improved outcomes including greater patient satisfaction, greater patient adherence to treatment, enhanced biologic outcomes, and decreased risk of malpractice suits. In general, research demonstrates that patients prefer *patient-centered* interviewing. This style of interviewing encourages patients to become active partners in their medical care by being informed and helping select treatment options they believe best suited for their needs. A physician interview style that includes actively listening to patients' concerns, asking their opinions, presenting options, and letting patients choose is preferable for the majority of patients. *Activated patients* may actually have better biologic outcomes than patients who take a more passive role in care.

This chapter discusses the critical elements of the medical interview that make it both efficient and effective. It includes a discussion of the three major functions of the interview: data gathering, building a positive relationship and addressing patients' emotions, and educating and motivating patients. It suggests specific skills demonstrated to be effective in the interview and addresses particular communication strategies useful in challenging situations in managed care.

WHAT MAKES AN INTERVIEW EFFICIENT?

Several factors make the interview and patient care process efficient. Most important among these are getting the problem straight to begin with, listening and observing actively at several levels simultaneously (e.g., the story, how it is told, affect, and mental status), detecting and correcting barriers to communication (e.g., patient deafness, delirium), creating an efficient structure, completing the three functions of the interview, and using correct technique. The interview's structural elements and three functions are shown in Box 2-1. Table 2-1 describes some common errors leading to inefficiency, as well as possible solutions.

STRUCTURE

Preparing Self and Environment

Effective preparation of the office environment, the medical data, and oneself can make the interview more efficient and effective. Usually patients first come in contact with the office by phone and then by interacting with office staff in the reception area or waiting room. The quality of all these initial interactions can have a significant effect on patients before they even meet the physician. Patients who have waited for a long time without explanation or who have had negative interactions with the office staff may be irritated, making a barrier to effective communication (Fig. 2-1). The environment of the consultation or examination room may also be important to the interview. Ensuring privacy, avoiding unnecessary distractions, and creating a comfortable seating environment for patients indicate concern and readiness on the part of the physician to address patient needs.

Preparation of the medical data can significantly increase the efficiency of the interview. Use of structured questionnaires that patients complete before meeting with the physician may provide clues about issues patients want to discuss. These forms can be particularly useful with new patients for efficient collection of data related to family history, allergies, and pertinent social history, but they generate many false-positives and false-negatives. For return patients, reviewing recent laboratory data, x-ray reports, and other results before the interview can help the physician maximize use of the interview time. Review of pertinent medical data before the visit also indicates that the physician has been thoughtful about the patient's problem since the last visit. This communicates the physician's concern for the patient and may enhance the sense of trust.

In addition to preparing the environment and the data, the physician is well advised to take a moment for self preparation. There are many distractions in a busy day, and taking a moment on the threshold of the consultation room to look at the chart, take a deep breath, and prepare psychologically to work with the next patient increases effectiveness by focusing attention on the present task.

Box 2-1. Structure and Functions of the Interview

Structural Elements

Preparing
- Self
- Office environment

Opening
Setting the agenda for the visit
Allowing patients to tell the story in their own words; establishing narrative thread
Using open to closed cones of questions
Understanding the patient as a person
Understanding the setting of the illness
Eliciting patients' beliefs about the problem
Summarizing finding and opinion
Planning treatment
Closure

Functions

Gathering information
Developing and maintaining a relationship
Educating and motivating behavior change

Table 2-1. Common Practices Leading to Inefficiency

	Problem	Potential solution
Early part of interview	Being distracted by other patient concerns	Take a moment to get prepared, hand off beeper, take no calls
	Keeping patient waiting	Inform patients about delays and apologize to them
	Lacking medical data (e.g., lab)	Review relevant data beforehand
	Not knowing patient's name	Check beforehand
	Overlooking patient discomfort or distress	Observe and address directly
	Premature interruptions	Allow time for patient to complete opening statement
	Not eliciting all reasons for visit early on	Ask "What else?"
	Imposing own agenda	Negotiate
Middle of interview	Long lists of close-ended questions	Open-ended questions; use open to closed cone
	Delaying social history until after history of present problem	Interweave social history naturally
	Interrupting patient story and directing conversation	Allow patient to tell story; build narrative thread
End of interview	Assuming patient can remember everything	Write instructions Give pamphlets on diseases
	Failing to check patient beliefs about diagnosis	Ask what patient thinks
	Not checking for patient questions	Ask if patient has questions
	Assuming patient agrees with treatment	Elicit patient opinion
	Assuming patient can implement	Ask what parts will be difficult
	Giving too much treatment advice at once	Simplify; write it down; give patient pamphlets about problem

The Opening

The opening moments of the interview are critical in the relationship between the physician and patient and the effectiveness of the visit. From the moment the examination room door opens, the physician starts learning about the patient by actively observing mood, grooming, style of dress, and other nonverbal factors. These clues help in understanding the patient. The physician can use these initial nonverbal clues to make the patient more comfortable (e.g., "You look like you are in some discomfort. Can I help to make you more comfortable before we begin?").

The physician starts the visit by greeting the patient and introducing himself or herself to new patients. These greetings set the tone, helping the patient to feel welcome. Asking patients what they prefer to be called (e.g., Ms., Mr., Dr., first name), communicates respect for patient preferences.

After introductions, we usually begin by eliciting the reason for the visit with open-ended questions like, "What is the problem that brings you here today?" or "What concerns have led to your visit today?" Studies support the importance of letting patients complete the opening statement about their concerns uninterrupted. Interrupting the patient before completion of the initial statement may be interpreted as a lack of interest or a lack of time. Furthermore, interrupting early in the interview may lead the patient to delay expressing real concerns until late in the visit or not at all. Although physicians often worry that the patient will take too long, most patients complete their opening statement within 90 seconds and provide important historic details.

After the patient has explained the initial concern, it is effective to ask the patient, "What else concerns you?" This is important, since on average patients have three problems at a first visit, and often the concern mentioned initially is not the most important. Allowing the patient to express all concerns at the beginning of the interview enhances efficiency because (1) the physician learns all of the problems that the patient is hoping to cover in the visit, instead of discovering them at the end of the visit (last-minute problems ["Oh, by the way..."] can be particularly frustrating to the physician); (2) the patient may remind himself or herself about concerns that have been forgotten initially; (3) this strategy enables the physician to prepare to negotiate with the patient about what concerns can be covered in this visit and what will be dealt with at a later time. After eliciting all of the patient's concerns, the physician can summarize before proceeding to in-depth questioning about any one of the problems. This communicates to the patient that the physician has listened attentively and allows the physician a moment to organize the problem list mentally.

Setting the Agenda for the Visit

Once the physician knows all of the patient's concerns, it may be necessary to work with the patient to negotiate the priorities for the visit. Particular concerns may be a high priority for the patient and must be addressed during that visit for the patient to feel the time was well spent. The physician may have other concerns, particularly about urgent medical problems. A typical sequence of dialogue follows:

Physician: So I understand that there are four concerns you would like to address today: your headache, shoulder pain, heart palpitations, and constipation. In the time we have available today, we may not be able to cover all of these. Which is most important to address today?

Patient: I would like to make sure we talk about my headaches.

Physician: That's fine. I'd be happy to address that. In addition, I want to discuss your heart palpitations just to be sure that everything is okay there. Why don't we start with those two and plan to address the shoulder pain and constipation at a follow-up visit if we don't have time today? Would that be all right?

Patient: That sounds fine as long as you can help me get an appointment about the other problems within a few weeks.

Physician: I think we can arrange that before you leave.

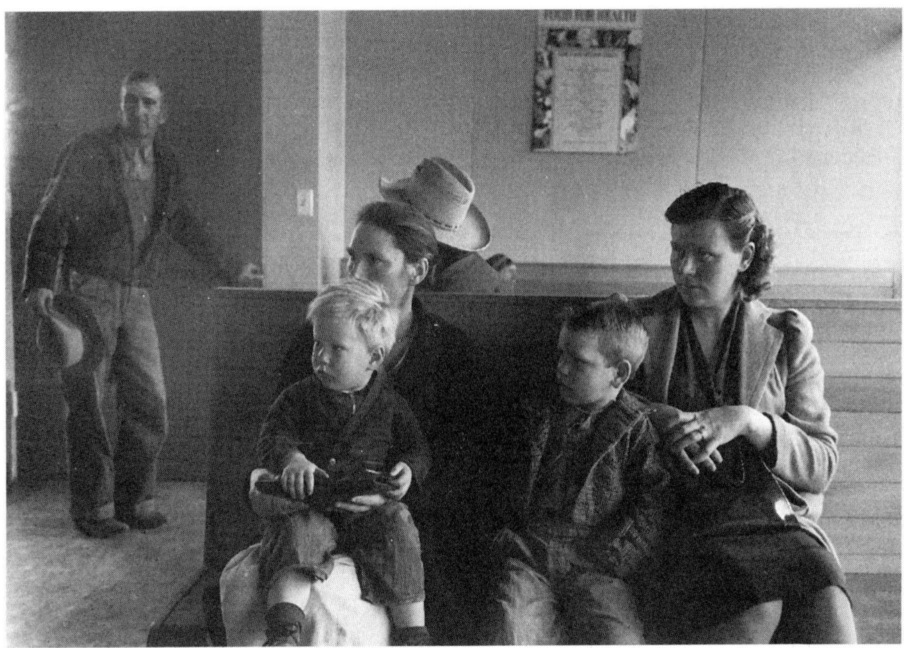

Fig. 2-1. Patients in waiting room. (From the Collections of the Library of Congress.)

Negotiation allows the physician and patient to plan together how to use the time available. In this manner the patient is assured that the important problems will be addressed and the physician is assured that there is adequate time for investigation of medical concerns.

Allowing the Patient to Tell a Story

Allowing the patient to tell the story of the illness in his or her own words is the most efficient and comfortable way to begin to assess a problem. The patient frames what he or she perceives as relevant, revealing personal views of cause and effect. The patient mentions details and facts a physician would not think to ask about. While the patient is talking, the physician can be thinking about what is said and developing hypotheses about the nature of the problem and approaches to ruling in and ruling out these hypotheses. Inviting the patient to tell the story of the illness also reveals the context of the illness—the nature of the patient's work, the home in its complexity, and important relationships. This understanding is needed in planning approaches to care. Telling a story also improves patient recall because it places the patient's attention in a remembered context, where the fine details are accessible to recall.

This storytelling is initiated by asking the patient, "So, tell me what happened," or "Let's go back to the beginning and tell me the story of your problem." This creates a *narrative thread* that organizes the interview. Once the patient is telling the story, the physician can quietly ask for elaboration on points about the person, the context, and relationships; learn as much as needed ("Tell me more about your husband"), and then return to the narrative thread by asking, "And then what happened?"

Progressing from Open- to Closed-Ended Questions

Note that the above questions begin with "Tell me" and little else. This is because it is more efficient and more thorough to begin each line of inquiry with an open-ended question, which invites a free-form response to a query rather than a short, specific answer (e.g., "Tell me about your chest pain" rather than "Where does it hurt?"). Studies have documented that open-ended questions produce more information, more efficiently, with greater satisfaction for both physician and patient. In addition, the patient includes unanticipated information and connections. Initially the advantages of open-ended questions seemed counterintuitive to us, but our experience has borne them out. Once the patient has responded, the physician can then begin to focus on smaller aspects of the situation. Once the open-ended approach has been exhausted (often quickly), one then can ask close-ended questions about facts not covered. Use of specific routine questions to screen risk behaviors is helpful. Effective screening questions are presented in Table 2-2.

Understanding the Patient as a Person

Although the importance of understanding the patient as a person in the process of assessing the problem cannot be overstated, the process of acquiring that understanding can be highly efficient and minimalistic. The opening observation often reveals ethnicity, style, socioeconomic status, and sometimes work and marital status. The content and presentation of speech provides information about the patient's reasoning and beliefs. The affect (e.g., a frown or sadness) shows feelings about the subject, as does gesturing (e.g., covering the face, looking down and away, suddenly brightening).

Understanding the Setting of the Illness

One cannot be sure in advance what aspects of the patient's life will be crucial or contributory. Several dimensions are usually relevant in most patients. First is social setting—who is at home (if there is a home), who is close or painfully distant, what are the supports. Environmental features may be critical, such as type of work and location of home or work (e.g., isolated in the country, a fifth-floor walk-up, a violent neighborhood with strong pressures to drink or use drugs). Ethnic and cultural background may determine health care–seeking behavior, adherence to agreed plans, or use of dangerous remedies.

Eliciting the Patient's Beliefs About the Problem

The patient's beliefs about the problem, health care in general, and how to relate to physicians can be crucial to the outcomes of care. If the patient believes the problem is due to an excess of hot or cold humors, as some Puerto Rican believe, then prescribing the wrong remedy (e.g., a hot remedy for a hot disease, such as orange juice with potassium supplementation for hypertensive patients on diuretics) leads to total noncompliance. Therefore it is necessary to check, probably several times, to what the patient attributes the problem. Similarly, if the patient believes that physicians are

Table 2-2. Screening Questions

Condition	Specific questions	Indicator
Alcohol	CAGE: Have you even tried to *C*ut down on your drinking? Are you ever *A*nnoyed when people comment on your drinking? Have you ever felt *G*uilty about something you've done after drinking? Do you ever have an *E*ye opener?	Screen all new patients
Sexual preference	Are you sexually active? Is this with men, women, *or both?*	Screen all new patients
Domestic violence	During the last year has anyone hit, kicked, or punched you?	Screen all female patients (particularly important emergency room setting)
Guns	Do you have a gun in your home?	Screen all new patients

judgmental, are not to be trusted, or are out to do things only for money, he or she will reveal less and cooperate less. If the patient's culture dictates that seeking care is shameful, he or she will not come for care soon enough, even for emergencies. If the patient believes that the physician should not be upset, the difficult facts will be hidden (e.g., by many persons of orthodox or authoritarian background and by some traditional Chinese).

This method deviates from the idea that one should collect the social history separately. This is because when social and personal information are collected simultaneously with biomedical information, more is revealed, patient recall is improved, and the process proves more efficient. One can always complete information not elicited later.

Summary of Thoughts and Findings

The end of the consultation is pivotal in most interviews. The patient feels increasingly vulnerable, since the physician now has information he or she does not—information the patient fears may be bad news. At this point plans must be created and negotiated with the patient. Therefore it is always important at this stage to summarize thoughts, findings, and preliminary ideas about the next steps in discussion and planning.

After the physician presents ideas and thoughts about the patient's diagnosis, it is important to check the patient's feelings and reactions. The patient may have beliefs about the nature of the illness that either fit or are in disagreement with the physician's opinion. To explore the patient's reactions and beliefs, the physician might ask a sequence of questions:

> *Physician:* I've explained to you that I think your symptoms may be due to a peptic ulcer. How does that fit with your ideas about your stomach pain?
>
> *Patient:* I'm a bit uncertain; I thought that ulcers only occurred when people were stressed and I feel like everything is going well in my life. How could I have an ulcer?
>
> *Physician:* That's a good question, since lots of people believe that stress and ulcers are related. In fact, a number of factors contribute to the formation of ulcers, such as fatigue, a genetic disposition, and a stomach infection. So people commonly develop ulcers even without stress.

A simple explanation helps the patient accept the hysician's diagnosis and be more prepared to work with the hysician to plan the treatment course. In other cases it is cessary to integrate the patient's beliefs into the diagnostic xplanation, even if the patient's ideas come from a different ame of reference than the physician's. For example, patients ay have beliefs about illnesses due to certain food bstances that do not fit with the physician's scientific proach to the nature of the illness. Whenever the physician n accept the patient's beliefs as possible and can integrate ese beliefs with a scientific explanation, the patient may be ore likely to collaborate in the treatment plan.

anning Treatment

with the presentation of the diagnosis, the physician often esents the options for treatment. It is essential to involve the ient in the planning process. If a patient does not believe t the treatment plan is likely to succeed or does not derstand the details of the treatment, follow-through is ikely. It is important for the physician to check the ient's beliefs and feelings about the treatment options just as he or she checked beliefs about the diagnosis. Then the physician can engage in a dialogue with the patient about which treatment the patient believes is most appropriate.

> *Physician:* I've suggested that you use these pills to treat your peptic ulcer disease. What do you think of that?
>
> *Patient:* It seems reasonable to me, although I've always heard that diet is important for ulcer treatment. Couldn't I treat this by avoiding certain foods and not use the pills?

By probing the patient's beliefs, the physician can identify barriers that might lead the patient to leave the physician's office without intending to fill the prescription or follow the treatment plan. If the patient and physician are in agreement about the treatment, it is useful to help the patient anticipate the problems in implementing the treatment.

> *Physician:* It's difficult to remember pills three times a day. What do you think the hard part of this will be for you? How might you provide reminders to yourself?

This gives the patient permission to express the possibility of forgetting the pills and allows an opportunity for the doctor and patient to discuss ways to help the patient remember.

Other simple strategies can help the patient in the planning phase, including writing down instructions, referring patients to educational programs available in the health care facility or in public, giving the patient educational pamphlets pertinent to the illness, and sending a visiting nurse to follow up (e.g., with a new diabetic patient).

It is essential to ask the patient whether there are questions and to have the patient review the main points before moving to the closing phase of the interview. By having the patient reiterate and the physician clarify before ending the interview, the physician can increase the likelihood that the patient will understand and comply with the treatment planned. Ultimately this makes the physician's work much more efficient by avoiding unnecessary treatment failures.

Closure

After the educational phase of the interview, the final few moments are spent in closure. During closure the physician reviews the immediate next steps: "Now I'd like you to go to the reception desk with this laboratory slip. They will direct you to the laboratory." The physician also can reiterate the plan for the timing of the next visit, checking with the patient about whether that seems appropriate: "Perhaps we can see each other in approximately 4 weeks. Does that seem about the right length of time from your perspective?" The physician can outline the plan for contact in the interim between visits if this is appropriate. Understanding how to reach the physician in an emergency or how to get the results of pertinent laboratory tests can save time-consuming phone calls to the office. Finally, in saying goodbye to the patient, the physician often sets the tone for the next visit and can do some planning: "I look forward to seeing you in a month and will be eager to see your headache diary so we can explore this problem further."

Other Issues

Should the interview continue during the physical? Does this common practice enhance time efficiency or does it breed error? No one really knows, although both are likely to some extent. The argument against talking during the physical examination is that it distracts the examiner, thereby decreasing sensitivity and causing him or her to miss physical findings, especially on auscultation and palpation.

The reality, however, is that most physicians do talk before and during the examination. It is very helpful to the patient to have the examination introduced and to explain what is being done, especially if painful, unusual, or in difficult areas (rectal and genital examinations). Clearly the physician's perceptions should be directed toward the examination. Social talk, chatting, or pursuing a review of systems will distract unduly.

Should a physical examination always be done? Obviously, there are some follow-up visits that do not require a physical reexamination. But there are several reasons to err on the side of examining. First, things change, sometimes unexpectedly. Second, it has become very clear that the act of physical touch has a reassuring, calming, and perhaps healing effect; if done gently and caringly, it also improves the physician-patient relationship and rapport. Third, patients expect to be examined. Failure to do so when the patient expects it leads to loss of trust in the physician's caring or competence, unless explained effectively. This then affects healing, comfort, and satisfaction. Many patients find the absence of physical examination unacceptable regardless of explanation.

FUNCTIONS

The broad functions of the interview fall into three categories: gathering data, developing a relationship and dealing with patient feelings, and educating the patient about diagnosis and treatment and encouraging behavior change. The process of data collection has been described in the previous section.

Developing and Maintaining a Relationship

Patients seeking care from their primary care physician often are worried about their health problems or have emotional distress about issues in their personal lives. They may come to the appointment feeling sadness, anger, frustration, or anxiety. To build trust and make the interview most effective, the physician must recognize and address patient feelings. This may be the most challenging task for the physician. It is often neglected.

The expression of empathy and understanding for patient feelings is a powerful communication skill that deepens the therapeutic relationship. Empathic listening indicates that the physician cares and understands the challenges in a patient's life. Demonstration of compassion and respect is key to providing a trusting environment that is therapeutic for patients. This communication skill, the expression of empathy, is one of the most important skills of doctoring and is at the heart of clinical medicine.[2]

When patients are experiencing strong emotions, the physician may fear that discussing these emotions directly will slow the interview down by "opening a can of worms." What to do if the patient expresses deep feelings of loneliness and the physician cannot fix the situation or make the patient feel better? What if the patient is angry and directs this at the physician? Often a physician's personal feelings or worries serve as barriers to discussing these emotional issues. In fact, studies show that talking to patients about their feelings and understanding their emotional experience is therapeutic and builds the relationship between patients and physicians.

It is best to address feelings when they first appear in the interview. This can be accomplished by first commenting directly on the feelings and then making a statement that indicates understanding the patient's experience.

Physician: You seem pretty sad about these recent events.

Patient: Yes, I feel so terrible. I had hoped this would never happen.

Physician: I can understand feeling like that. It must feel so disappointing to you to have it turn out this way.

Such brief comments by the physician indicate recognition of the patient's pain and an understanding about the life experience of the patient. Furthermore, if appropriate, the physician can make a further statement of empathy, such as "I would feel the same way in your position" or "Many people would feel as you do in this situation." These statements are appropriate only if genuine. Even if the physician disagrees with the patient's point of view, certain statements indicate understanding, for example, "I can understand your feeling frustrated or angry if you have felt that I have not been taking your complaints seriously" or "I can understand feeling angry with the delay in getting an appointment when you were worried there was something seriously wrong with your health." In these examples the physician accepts how the patient feels even though he or she would not have had the same reaction as the patient in a similar situation or believes the patient's response is unreasonable.

In addition to direct discussion of patient feelings, a physician can indicate acceptance of a patient by echoing the patient's words or reiterating what the patient has said. Brief phrases can indicate attention and caring. For example, the physician listening to a patient's worries about an episode of shortness of breath can say "Sounds like it was frightening for you."

Nonverbal indicators of concern can also be powerful in building the relationship with the patient. This can include maintaining a relaxed and nondefensive posture when patient is expressing anger directly at the physician. Body posture may indicate acceptance. Also, touching the patient as an expression of caring (e.g., a patient who is crying) is often a strong statement of a physical and psychologic connection.

EDUCATING AND MOTIVATING PATIENTS

One of the most important roles of the medical interview is to inform the patient about the diagnosis and treatment options. In fact, studies of patient satisfaction frequently reveal that patients believe that they do not receive an adequate amount of information from their physician. Particularly as the pressures to see an increasing number of patients intensifies, physicians may tend to allocate the majority of their time gathering information and performing the physical examination, hence cutting short the time available for educating patients. It is essential to budget time to allow an adequate period for discussion and to permit patients an opportunity to ask questions. In addition, physicians should consider the language used to describe medical problems and avoid medical jargon. Selection of simple nonmedical words helps ensure that patients understand the meaning of a physician's explanation.

As discussed previously, it is particularly important to check how the explanations of the disease or the treatment fit with the patient's own beliefs. A recent study demonstrated that, overall, patients visit alternative medicine providers twice as frequently as they do traditional primary care physicians. Patients are also unlikely to disclose information about the treatment prescribed by alternative medicine healers. Careful nonjudgmental inquiry may allow patients to share discussions about herbal remedies, acupuncture, or dietary programs that they are either using or would prefer. Obtaining this information enables physicians to tailor their instructions appropriately.

During the last few years a useful approach to motivating patients to change risk behaviors has been developed based on a model by Prochaska and Demeclenti. Although most of the research pertaining to *motivational interviewing* has been tested in alcohol use, there is an increasing amount of information about the utility of this model in a variety of risk behaviors including smoking, weight reduction, and dietary changes.

The model proposes that certain patients are in different stages of "readiness to change" at any particular time. Patients may be in a stage of precontemplation, contemplation, preparation, action, maintenance, or relapse. A patient in the *precontemplation* stage may appear defensive and totally uninterested in changing smoking habits. A patient in the *contemplation* stage may have thought about the pros and cons of stopping smoking but has not done anything about it. A patient in the *preparation* stage has not only thought about stopping but has started to make some plans concerning how to do it; however, those plans have not been implemented yet. A patient in the *action* stage has implemented the plans and is making a genuine effort to stop. A patient in the *maintenance* stage has had a period of maintaining the appropriate behavior and is consciously trying to avoid falling back into the old pattern. A patient in the *relapse* stage has successfully stopped for a period of time but is now smoking again. Using this model the role of the physician is to help identify the stage of change for a particular patient at a point in time and encourage the patient to move to the next stage. Hence it is unrealistic to expect every patient to be willing to move to an action stage after several brief discussions with the physician, since many patients may be in the precontemplation stage and are not prepared to move to the action stage. In fact, studies demonstrate that it often takes patients several weeks, months, or years to move into the action and maintenance stages, and most likely patients will relapse and reenter the cycle several more times in order to ultimately become successful. Details of this model are provided in Chapter 51.

MANAGED CARE AND THE PHYSICIAN-PATIENT RELATIONSHIP

Managed care presents specific challenges in the routine practice of medicine (Table 2-3). Both patients and physicians are confronted with situations that may be unique to the managed care setting or more challenging than in the previous fee-for-service environment. For example, patients frequently have to change their primary care physician, leaving a longstanding trusting relationship for a new physician found on a provider list. In another instance patients may suspect that a managed care physician has a financial incentive that limits the use of diagnostic procedures. Patients may wonder if the reason the physician is not ordering a test is to avoid cost. Similarly the patient may believe that the primary care physician is limiting referrals to a particular specialist for cost reasons rather than quality-of-care reasons.

Table 2-3. Communication Dilemmas Common in Managed Care

Problem	Example
Time constraints	Oh by the way doctor, I still have other things bothering me. I'm hoping we can spend at least 30 minutes together to discuss all of these problems.
Misguided requests	I would prefer that newer antibiotic even though it is not on the formula rate. My friends have told me that it works a lot better than the old standard antibiotics.
Specialists' referral	I know how my insurance works. I need to get an authorization from you, but my gynecologist has always managed these problems and I want to go back to her.
Bending the rules	Doc, I haven't seen a dentist in years and I can't afford to go now. My plan will pay for it if you say I need it because of my diabetes.
Financial incentives	I've been reading in the newspaper about HMO's paying doctors to do fewer tests. I certainly don't want that to happen to me. Are you in one of those HMO's?

These types of situations place the physician in an awkward position and raise challenging questions for the physician. How can a physician maintain the trust of a patient while disclosing the internal utilization review process the health organization uses for consideration of referral requests? Should physicians discuss possible financial conflicts of interest with their patients? Although there are no straightforward answers to these questions, communication skills of negotiation are critically important to resolving potential conflicts. It is essential that physicians understand the patients' perspective, validate their concerns, and find a common goal for both patient and physician. This is an example of a patient with diabetes seeing a new primary care physician.

Patient: I have always been careful with my diabetes and seen my ophthalmologist and cardiologist every 6 months. In addition, I see the diabetes specialist who helps me adjust my insulin dose. I hope you will complete referral forms for these providers for me.

Physician: It sounds like you take good care of your diabetes and that's excellent. It also sounds like you have a lot of trust in the specialists who have helped you take care of your diabetes. I would like to help you continue to receive the highest quality care for your diabetes and to work with your specialist. I would also like to help coordinate your care as a primary care provider. Perhaps we can work together to determine what role I will play in coordinating your diabetic care and the role your specialist will have. After we do that, we can decide which of the referrals to the specialists seems important. How does that sound to you?

Patient: That's fine as long as there is an opportunity for me to see the specialists that I have relationships with.

Physician: I'm sure that we can arrange things so that you will continue to work with those doctors in an appropriate and ongoing fashion. Let's start by working together so that we get to know each other and I understand your health and your diabetes.

Through the process of negotiation the doctor and patient may be able to establish a common goal and avoid the conflicts that result from differences in doctors' and patients' expectations. This kind of negotiation requires physicians to have excellent communication skills.

COMMUNICATION AND MALPRACTICE

Not only is the quality of the physician-patient relationship important to patient satisfaction, adherence, and biologic outcomes, it is particularly important to medical malpractice prevention. Patients initiate medical malpractice suits not only when there has been a breach in the quality of medical care, but also when they believe that the physician was not as attentive or caring as he or she should have been. The best evidence supporting the relationship of communication to medical malpractice in different specialties is derived from two recent studies. A study by Entman et al[1] compared obstetricians/gynecologists who had never been sued with those with prior suits. It demonstrated that patients of sued physicians had twice as many complaints about their care, including feeling rushed, ignored, and inadequately informed about their medical condition.

Along with several colleagues, I conducted a major study examining the differences between the communication style of physicians who have and those who have not been sued. The study included examination of 1265 audio tapes of routine visits between primary care physicians and patients and between surgeons (orthopedic and general surgery) and their patients. The data revealed that the communication styles of primary care physicians who had never been sued differed significantly from the styles of the physicians who had been sued. Never-sued primary care physicians used more facilitative language (encouraging the patients to talk, asking their opinions), laughed more, oriented the patient to medical care (explaining what was going on in the course of care), and elicited more information about therapy for their patients than sued physicians. Although there were no statistically significant differences between sued and never-sued surgeons, similar trends were evident. Table 2-4 summarizes the characteristics of never-sued primary care visits.

Table 2-4. Characteristics of Never-sued Primary Care Physician Visits

Characteristic/communication behavior	Description/example
Physician facilitates conversation	Asks patient's opinion and checks understanding
Physician orients patient	Directs and instructs patient regarding the medical visit process
Physician laughs or exhibits humor	Physician displays comfort with humor
Patient provides more therapeutic information	Patient shares important clinical information about treatment
Visits last longer	18.3 minutes vs. 15 minutes for sued physicians

In conclusion, it is evident that communication breakdowns between physicians and patients may contribute to the initiation of medical malpractice litigation. Whether individual physicians can prevent malpractice risks by communication skills training has not been proven, but such training could help physicians modify many of the high-risk communication behaviors.

REFERENCES

1. Entman SS, Glass CA, Hickson GB, et al: The relationship between malpractice claims history and subsequent obstetric care, *JAMA* 272:1588-1591, 1994.
2. Squier RW: A model of empathic understanding and adherence to treatment regimen in practitioner-patient relationships, Soc Sci Med 30:325-339, 1990.

ADDITIONAL READINGS

Kaplan SH, Greenfield S, Ware JE: Assessing the effects of physician-patient interactions on the outcomes of chronic disease, *Med Care* 27:S110-S127, 1989.

Levinson W, Roter D, Mullooly J, et al: Physician-patient communication: the relationship with malpractice claims among primary care physicians and surgeons, *JAMA* 227:553-559, 1997.

Lipkin M, Putnam SM, Lazare A, editors: The medical interview: clinical care, education, and research, New York, 1995, Springer.

O'Connell D: Behavior change. In *Behavioral medicine in primary care—a practical guide,* Stamford, Conn, 1997, Appleton & Lange pp 125-135.

CHAPTER 3

Medical Adherence: The Physician-Patient Relationship

Geoffrey A. Modest

Medical adherence, or *compliance,* is the extent to whic patients follow the suggestions of their health care provider Lack of compliance is a remarkably common problem. recent study[1] using electronic medication monitors h confirmed many prior studies, finding that 50% to 60% patients are adherent and take their medications more th 80% of the time, 5% to 10% are nonadherent and ta medications less than 20% of the time, and 30% to 40% a partially adherent. Adherence decreases with time: more th 50% of newly diagnosed hypertensive patients drop out treatment within 1 year and 74% by 5 years. In spite of t heightened public awareness of cardiac risk factors, t recent Sixth Report of the Joint National Committee Hypertension[11] found a downward trend in hypertensi control, with only 27% of hypertensive patients in go control. Twenty percent of patients receiving prescriptions not even fill them. Dietary interventions seem to be even l effective: only one third of patients are still on the diet a 1 year. Therapy for acute, symptomatic conditions is much better. The initial medication adherence in patie given a 10-day course of antibiotics for an acute infection, for example, approaches 75%, yet fewer than 25% of patients complete the full course of therapy. In general, therapy for existing medical conditions (secondary prevention) is associated with higher rates of adherence than for potential diseases (primary prevention).

Physicians are no better than 50/50 in estimating the adherence of their patients. The statistics are not much better for patients well known by their physician and selected specifically as likely to be adherent. In general, the patient's age, gender, race, marital status, income level, intelligence, and educational level are not helpful in predicting adherence.

Medical nonadherence has many adverse consequences. It may be directly harmful to patients: not only will the underlying medical problem remain untreated, but patients risk potentially life-threatening overmedication as they are given more and more medications to treat their problem. In addition, nonadherent patients may be seen more often in the office and may receive a more extensive laboratory evaluation (e.g., as the physician searches for reasons for a patient's "nonresponsive" condition). Estimates of the overall cost of noncompliance exceed $100 billion annually, largely through lost productivity and preventable hospital admissions. One study[6] found that one third of hospital admissions for congestive heart failure resulted from medication and/or dietary nonadherence.

ASSESSING COMPLIANCE

The first task for the physician is to suspect that a patient is nonadherent. There are many situations in which adherence is unlikely. For example:

- A patient who misses office appointments or drops out of care
- A patient who is unable to state correctly how to take the medications (e.g., the patient who needs to look at the label on the medication bottle to see how many times a day he or she is supposed to take that medication)
- A medication bottle with more than the expected number of pills on a return visit
- The lack of anticipated clinical response to a therapeutic intervention
- A medication level (e.g., serum, urine) below expectation for a given dose of medication
- Lack of an expected concurrent medication effect for a given dose of medication (e.g., a patient with a rapid pulse on a high dose of a β-blocker)
- A patient who has alcoholism, other substance abuse, or an underlying psychiatric disorder

It is important to note that adherence may be erratic. For example, patients typically take medications at a higher frequency just before and just after a visit with a medical provider. Therefore a patient may have a seizure between office visits because of inadequate serum medication levels, yet may have therapeutic levels at the time of the next office visit.

What is the best way to determine whether or not the patient is adherent? It is clear that in order to obtain accurate information as well as to reinforce the physician-patient relationship, the question of adherence must be phrased in a nonaccusatory, open-ended manner. When done in this way, approximately 50% of nonadherent patients will admit it. This subgroup, not surprisingly, is the most responsive to attempts to improve adherence.

Nonthreatening ways to ask the question of medication adherence can be almost as accurate as measuring medication levels.[9] One approach is to establish the context of medication-taking as a general problem by saying, for example, "Many people have trouble remembering to take medicines. How often do you miss or forget to take your blood pressure pill?" If the patient does not have an expected therapeutic response to a medication, one might comment, "You aren't doing quite as well as I had hoped, and I'm wondering if there are any problems with the medication that I didn't explain?" This would deflect the blame from the patient. Pill counts are reasonably accurate when done infrequently and unannounced, but also run the risk of undercutting physician-patient rapport.

Once nonadherence has been identified, it is important to ask the patient what he or she believes are the obstacles to taking the medication. Patients, however, may not reveal the true causes, for example, if they are embarrassed to admit that the medication costs more than they can afford.

There is a great deal of literature on issues of medical adherence, with a recent systematic review of the randomized clinical intervention trials.[4] It is notable that the approaches are so diverse that a true meta-analysis is not possible, with many of the interventions being short term as well as so complex and time-consuming as to be impractical. Given these limitations, the rest of this chapter will present an arbitrary division of many of the reasons that patients may be nonadherent and several of the accepted approaches and interventions to address them.

MECHANICAL/BEHAVIORAL ISSUES

Concrete Obstacles

Nonadherence may result if the medications cost too much, the medical appointments are not at convenient times (e.g., the patient has to miss work), the waiting times at the office are too long, transportation to the office is costly or difficult, or the medication vials are too difficult to open (especially true when arthritic patients are given childproof medication bottles). Certain medication formulations might be problematic: adherence rates for inhalers are typically lower than for pills. Obstacles to care, such as unfriendly or unhelpful staff or excessively long waiting times to get an appointment, may translate into nonadherence both for appointments and medication-taking. Solutions to these problems include:

- Arranging office appointments at convenient times
- Educating office staff to a pro-consumer orientation
- Utilizing less expensive medications or arranging for free medications from pharmaceutical companies when possible
- Requesting easy-to-open vials for arthritic patients
- Implementing reminder phone calls or appointment cards
- Contacting the patient when appointments are missed, since adherence is very poor in patients who drop out of care
- Making sure that the physician is seen as accessible to his or her patients

Complex Medication Regimens

Simplified medication regimens are easier for patients, less intrusive, and lead to improved adherence. One study,[1] which confirmed prior studies, documented improved medication adherence as the medication frequency decreased from three times per day (59% adherence) to one time per day (84% adherence). In addition, a study of diabetic patients found the frequency of medication errors increased from 15% when patients were given one medication to 25% with two to three medications to more than 35% with more than five medications.[5] It is helpful that the recent Joint National Committee on Hypertension[11] promoted the use of combination medications. In some cases, medications can be given parenterally or in a supervised way for guaranteed adherence (e.g., intramuscular benzathine penicillin for syphilis, depot injection of fluphenazine for schizophrenia, or directly-observed therapy for tuberculosis). Therefore medication adherence has been shown to improve with:

- Less frequent dosing schedules
- Fewer numbers of medications
- Directly observed therapy

Forgetting to Take Medications

Forgetting to take one's medications is especially common in the elderly, although it is a problem at all ages. Successful interventions include:

- Cueing medication taking (*tailoring* the medication regimen) to some personal established habit of the specific patient
- Using daily medication dispensers
- Using computer-generated medication reminders, especially if medication taking is likely to diminish between office visits
- Reinforcing the need to take the medications and reviewing how to do so

EDUCATION ISSUES

A necessary component of medical adherence is that the patient understand exactly what is expected of him or her. In this context, it is important to realize that less than 5 minutes after seeing a physician, the patient forgets 50% of the physician's statements. Patient recall deteriorates as the number of physician instructions increases and if those instructions are embedded in the middle of the interview. Recall is optimized by reiterating the most important physician suggestions at the end of the interview and providing written instructions.

It is well documented that adherence improves when patients receive a *clear presentation of medical instructions* from a physician whom they respect. Directions on how to take medications should be unambiguous and medical terminology should be avoided. Instructions should be given as specific, concrete advice and not as general recommendations. When giving dietary counseling for hypercholesterolemia, for example, it is better to find out exactly which foods the patient is eating and give specific suggestions than to generalize that the patient should avoid such foods as eggs or cheese. Information should be given in a relaxed setting, with good eye contact, and responding to the patient's verbal issues and nonverbal cues. In order to impart a consistent message, it makes sense that all recommendations be filtered through one physician, usually the primary care provider. It is counterproductive, for example, to have a specialist make one recommendation and the primary care physician make another. When giving medications, it is best to give specific times of the day that the medication should be taken. In one study, only 36% of patients understood what "every 6 hours" meant. These specific instructions should incorporate the unique needs of the individual patient (e.g., patients may not want to take diuretics in the morning if they must go on public transportation soon thereafter). It is often helpful to give the patient written instructions or pill charts indicating which times to take which medication.

Medication side effects represent a fairly common reason that patients do not take medications. For example, the British Medical Research Council Working Party, in its study of hypertension therapy, found that 20% of its subjects withdrew from the study because of side effects from either the diuretic or β-blocker therapy. Physicians should inquire about common side effects (e.g., constipation with verapamil), as well as possibly embarrassing ones (e.g., sexual dysfunction with diuretics), in case the patient is reluctant to volunteer this information. It is important to phrase the issue of side effects, when possible, in the context that there are other choices of medications available that do not have the same side effects. Since most clinical trials have been done with male subjects, female patients may experience side effects that are not well documented in the medical literature.

Patient education is clearly a desirable goal. Patients who do not understand their physician's instructions take medications less reliably than those who do (15% vs. 60%). It should be pointed out, however, that some studies have shown that successful educational interventions alone do not necessarily translate into improved adherence.

PSYCHOSOCIAL ISSUES

There is an array of psychosocial issues that undercut the patient's ability to understand and adhere to medical suggestions. Patients who are psychotic, depressed, manic, or paranoid are less likely to take medications and may need the assistance of a case manager. Patient denial may also be a major obstacle. In general, nonadherent patients do not perceive themselves as susceptible to disease or else consider the disease less severe than its reality. Hence it is important to inquire about the patient's understanding of the disease. It is also useful to ask the patient if he or she is/was emotionally close to others with the same disease, since denial may occur when the patient has unresolved issues with that family member or friend. In addition, there are studies documenting that patients who are having difficulty dealing with their life stressors may not take their medications or change their lifestyle as suggested by the physician.

CULTURAL ISSUES

Everyone comes from his or her own culture with his or her own *health belief system.* It is important to emphasize that this health belief system, or the patient's *explanatory model* of what is going on, is often fragmentary, incomplete, and self-contradictory, and changes over time. There are four factors related to the health belief model that help predict whether a person is likely to be adherent: (1) the degree to which the patient is concerned about health issues; (2) the perceived susceptibility to an illness or adverse outcome; (3) the seriousness of the consequences of an adverse outcome through nonadherence; and (4) the benefits and costs of the recommended actions, including emotional costs, inconvenience to the patient, or possibility of adverse effects.

Recommended changes in behavior must be congruent with the patient's health belief system. New health habits (e.g., dietary changes) must be acceptable within the broad framework of that belief system. If a person feels that tuberculosis results from sorcery,[10] for example, he or she might not take the prescribed medications. It is especially important in patients from non-Western cultures to acknowledge and incorporate, whenever possible, the role of non-Western remedies (see Chapter 12). Many people have already tried home remedies or seen traditional healers before coming to see their physician. Simply acknowledging that it is alright to take garlic pills for hypertension may create a more substantial alliance with the patient and lead to more medication taking as well. When it seems inappropriate to incorporate traditional remedies into the care plan, or when the patient seems particularly refractory to necessary Western medications, it is useful to identify the "health expert" of the family. When possible, this person should be encouraged to return with the patient for a group discussion in which the specifics of the health care plan, including traditional and Western approaches, can be negotiated.

GENERAL APPROACH

The cornerstone to educating a patient with regard to a disease and its management is to assess the patient's understanding. A wealth of important information is provided by simply asking patients to explain, in their own words, their understanding of the disease and its therapy. This provides a quick check that the instructions were given in a clear manner, in language the patient can understand, and in a culturally congruent way, and that there were no evident obstacles to that understanding (e.g., depression or denial). Patients should be encouraged to ask questions and express confusion. Physician monologues are much less useful than interactive communication with patient participation. This communication is optimized with good eye contact and with the use of personal language. Instructions should be phrased specifically to the patient and not as generalities (e.g., "It would be helpful if you could..." instead of "People with hypertension should...").

Many nonadherent patients make conscious, considered, "intelligent" decisions to be nonadherent. It is important for the physician to understand the patient's perspective. Eighty percent of patients in one study stated they understood that patients with hypertension are unable to tell when their blood pressure is elevated, yet 92% of these same patients believed that they themselves could tell when their blood pressure was elevated. In a study of partially adherent patients, 18% feared that taking medications regularly would lead to a worsening of health status and 22.5% feared side effects of medications. Furthermore, patients may believe (and correctly so) that the medication prescribed is incorrect or that their particular case is different from the "average case" on which data on therapy are based.

Case management strategies—often organized around nursing personnel and associated with intensified patient education, frequent telephone calls to educate and "check in" with the high-risk patients, and home visits—have been shown to dramatically improve health status and patient quality of life and decrease expensive resource utilization, especially in patients with coronary artery disease, congestive heart failure, hypertension, and asthma. One study,[2] which used an asthma outreach nurse as the case manager only 8 hours a week, achieved a 79% decrease in emergency room visits and 86% decrease in admissions for 53 children followed 2 years. Newer studies in individuals with the human immunodeficiency virus (HIV), where medication adherence is so crucial, have found benefit from individualized case management consisting of close home-based and telephone contact performed routinely and soon after any medication adjustment.

PHYSICIAN-PATIENT RELATIONSHIP

The key issue with medical adherence revolves around the nature of the physician's relationship with the patient. In this regard, the use of the term *compliance* is problematic since it connotes an authoritative and paternalistic relationship with the patient.[12] Less value-laden terms such as *medication taking* or *adherence* are more neutral and reflect better a concept of shared goals.

It is clear from several studies that the content of the physician-patient relationship has a direct bearing on medication taking. For example, a study showed that mothers give more prescribed medication to their children when they believe that their physician is understanding and friendly and interacts in a manner that is satisfying to them. Patients take medications at increased frequency when they are given by their primary care physician instead of by a covering or emergency room physician, presumably reflecting the strength of the physician-patient bond in therapy.

The patient should believe that there is an atmosphere of openness of communication, a *mutual respect* in which the physician has listened to his or her concerns and addressed them. Patients follow physician advice more often when they think the encounter was long enough and allowed for them to deal with their agenda as well as that of the physician.

The physician should also *involve patients in their own care*. There have been several important studies that suggest that empowering patients in monitoring their disease leads to improved medication taking. Even in selected "noncompliant" patients, self-monitoring of blood pressure was associated with a 20% to 30% improvement in documented medication taking. Similarly, studies have shown improved medication taking with the use of physician-patient agreements, wherein the physician and patient collectively target medical problems and negotiate a mechanism to resolve them. The patient is encouraged to choose specifically which of the behavioral changes he or she thinks is personally most appropriate. For example, the patient might decide such things as the best time to take a medication or the relative role of diet vs. medication. The physician might then negotiate an appropriate goal blood pressure and the frequency of office visits, teach the patient empowering activities (e.g., doing home glucose monitoring), and, whenever possible, establish guidelines for the patient to modify his or her own therapy. The recent asthma guidelines[3] emphasize that adequate asthma therapy requires a partnership between the physician and patient. Of note, adults enrolled in an asthma self-management strategy to deal with asthma exacerbations had a threefold decrease of asthma readmissions over a 32-month period.[2] This view of adherence is an interactional one, based on mutual understanding, rapport, and trust, and allows the patient to assume some responsibility for his or her own health.

FAMILY AND COMMUNITY APPROACH

Sickness of one family member has a ripple effect throughout the family (see Chapter 6), as well as in the broader community of the patient (e.g., work, friends). There are obvious benefits to involving the family in the care of the individual attempting behavior modification. It is extremely difficult to change a person's diet, for example, if the cook of the family is not involved, or to get someone to quit smoking when others at home smoke. Furthermore, a study with multiple educational interventions[7] found the most dramatic effect on appointment keeping, diet, weight control, and blood pressure occurred in the subgroup assigned to family involvement, much more so than in the patients assigned to either small group discussions or in-depth exit interviews. Family members in that subgroup were given a booklet describing how they could provide support for the patient in controlling hypertension. The chosen family members understood that the patient needed to take the medications even when he or she was feeling well, made a commitment to help the patient remember to take the medications and keep appointments, and identified at least three concrete ways that they could assist the patient in taking medications. Therefore sometimes the most significant approach to nonadherence is simply to ask the patient to invite key family members to discuss the patient's problem and involve them in the solutions. It is often important to involve the patient's broader community in the care as well. Many community-based organizations are available. Group discussions with other people afflicted with the same problem (e.g., self-help groups dealing with smoking cessation) have been shown to improve behavior modification. In addition, recruiting the help of the local pharmacist or visiting nurse can significantly improve compliance. These professionals often have a detailed understanding of whether a patient is refilling his or her medications at appropriate intervals or if there are problems with any of the medications (e.g., a visiting nurse may know that the patient will not take diuretics because the patient has arthritis and the bedroom is physically distant from the bathroom). Sometimes physicians can be involved in discussing changes in the patient's work structure with the employer (e.g., changing the lunchtime of a diabetic patient so that he or she eats at an appropriate time each day). Sometimes physicians can help promote larger community-oriented approaches (e.g., encouraging the creation of smoke-free institutions).

PRIMARY PREVENTION STRATEGY

It is better to prevent problems with medication taking than to attempt to detect and change them. In principle, when initiating a therapeutic regimen, the following points will minimize problems:

- Simplified medication regimen
- Brief, explicit, personal instructions repeated at the end of the encounter
- Medication regimen tailored to the individual's needs and habits
- Printed instructions and education material
- Development of physician-patient rapport (e.g., when possible, changing medications should be avoided on a first encounter with a patient)
- Asking the patient to verbalize his or her understanding of the disease process and the therapeutic regimen, in order to correct misunderstandings
- Use of medication containers with compartments to organize multiple medications and minimize the risk of medication errors
- Asking the patient to bring in his or her medications ("brown bag review"), asking what he or she is taking and how, reviewing misunderstandings, and getting rid of old medications
- Enlisting family members/community support (including pharmacists, case managers)

SUMMARY

There are several recent review articles on the subject of medical adherence[4,6,8,9] and the cultural issues involved.[10] The key to adherence is an individualized approach. Most patients do take medicines appropriately. However, a substantial minority do not. When a problem is identified, the physician can screen for the simple, mechanical obstacles, such as complexity of therapeutic regimen, cost of medications, or side effects. If the problem lies beyond those issues, simply asking the patient what his or her understanding of the disease and its therapy is will indicate if there is a significant educational deficit. The problem often lies in some aspect of the relationship between the physician and the patient. For whatever reason, the patient may not be able to "hear" what the physician is saying, and/or the physician is unable to "hear" the real issues of the patient. An important step here is conceptualizing the encounter as an interactional one, with open communication and open negotiations leading to empowering the patient in the broader context of his or her family and community.

REFERENCES

1. Eisen SA, Miller DK, Woodward RS, et al: The effect of prescribed daily dose frequency on patient medication compliance, *Arch Intern Med* 150:1881-1884, 1990.
2. Greineder DK, Loane KC, Parks P: Reduction in resource utilization by an asthma outreach program, *Arch Pediatr Adolesc Med* 149:415-420, 1995.
3. Guidelines for the diagnosis and management of asthma, highlights of the expert panel report II, *National Heart, Lung, and Blood Institute*, February 1997.
4. Haynes RB, McKibbon KA, Kanani R: Systematic review of randomised trials of interventions to assist patients to follow prescriptions for medications, *Lancet* 348:383-386, 1996.
5. Hulka BS, Kupper LL, Cassel JC, et al: Medication use and misuse: physician-patient discrepancies, *J Chronic Dis* 28:7-21, 1975.
6. Miller NH: Compliance with treatment regimens in chronic asymptomatic diseases, *Am J Med* 102(2A):43-49, 1997.
7. Morisky DE, DeMuth NM, Field-Fass M, et al: Evaluation of family health education to build social support for long-term control of high blood pressure, *Health Educ Quar* 12:35-50, 1985.
8. Rudd P: Clinicians and patients with hypertension: unsettled issues about compliance, *Am Heart J* 130:572-579, 1995.
9. Sackett DL, Haynes RB, Guyatt GH, et al: Helping patients follow the treatments you prescribe. In *Clinical epidemiology: a basic science for clinical medicine*, ed 2, Boston, 1991, Little, Brown, pp 249-281.
10. Sumartojo E: When tuberculosis treatment fails: a social behavioral account of patient adherence, *Am Rev Respir Dis* 147:1311-1320, 1993.
11. The Sixth Report of the Joint National Committee on Prevention, Detection, Evaluation, and Treatment of High Blood Pressure, *Arch Intern Med* 157:2413-2446, 1997.
12. Trostle JA: Medical compliance as an ideology, *Soc Sci Med* 27:1299-1308, 1988.

CHAPTER 4

Periodic Health Examination

Arthur H. Eskew

Even though the concept of prevention is inherent throughout medical care, it has traditionally focused on tertiary prevention in individuals with symptomatic illness. The periodic health examination emphasizes primary and secondary prevention. It involves the performance of tasks that include history and physical examination, laboratory and other tests, and procedures designed to determine an individual's risk for certain preventable conditions and provide guidance to reduce or avoid additional risk or to diagnose those conditions in an early, presymptomatic state in the hope of reducing morbidity and mortality.

The recent compilation of available evidence regarding a broad spectrum of preventive health procedures, largely attributable to the work of the Canadian Task Force on the Periodic Health Examination and the U.S. Preventive Services Task Force (USPSTF), makes it possible for providers and patients to make more informed decisions regarding the risks and benefits of many procedures. Although the benefit of many other commonly recommended screening and preventive procedures remains unproven, the physician has a wealth of expert consensus on which to draw in designing a screening strategy[10] (Fig. 4-1).

This chapter on periodic health examination outlines an approach to evaluating various preventive procedures by discussing barriers and suggesting strategies to ensure that the physician achieves a high rate of compliance with these procedures. Important issues and areas in which physicians can provide support and anticipatory guidance are discussed.

THE PERIODIC HEALTH EXAMINATION VS. THE ANNUAL PHYSICAL EXAMINATION

The periodic health examination is distinct from the routine or annual physical examination in that it involves the delivery of specific services and procedures based on an individual's age, sex, and estimated risk for disease. It is a process of collecting data, estimating risks and determining specific diseases and conditions for which a patient is at risk, and focusing clinical, cognitive, and diagnostic resources in a fashion that would provide most benefit. It can seldom be accomplished in a single visit or contact with the patient. The concept of an "annual physical" is not obsolete, but rather needs to be modified to incorporate the process and goals of periodic health examination. The history and physical examination provide both the foundation of data on which the preventive care strategy is based and the opportunity to carry out some of that care. When the annual physical reveals an opportunity for intervention, appropriate follow-up visits should be scheduled to emphasize the importance of prevention and reinforce adherence.

Notably, most patient visits are symptom-or disease-related. Therefore any successful preventive health strategy in practice must rely on integrating the periodic health examination into symptom-and disease-related care. This represents a challenge in terms of organizing oneself to carry out the preventive care agenda efficiently.

PREVENTIVE CARE

Prevention in the primary care setting refers to care that is directed at preserving the health of an individual patient and the community in which the provider practices. The importance and potential effect of preventive care is evident, given the estimate that as much as 50% of the mortality from the 10 leading causes of death in the United States is attributable to potentially modifiable lifestyle factors. The proficient performance of preventive health care requires the physician to possess a firm understanding of clinical epidemiology, the performance characteristics of a broad array of tests and procedures, and clinical decision making. Also necessary is a detailed understanding of an individual's risks, social situation, values, and preferences, as well as knowledge of the incidence and prevalence of conditions and diseases that are important causes of morbidity and mortality in the surrounding community.

Types of Prevention

Prevention can be divided into several categories. *Primary prevention* refers to services directed at the prevention of disease before its onset. Examples include immunizations to prevent infectious diseases or counseling to prevent unwanted pregnancy in teenagers. *Secondary prevention* would involve maneuvers designed to detect diseases at an earlier, presymptomatic stage, so as to decrease morbidity and mortality. The use of mammography to detect early breast cancer before it is palpable or metastasizes is an example. *Tertiary prevention* is the care directly associated with preventing complications or undue morbidity in persons with established symptomatic chronic disease, for example, using angiotensin-converting enzyme inhibitors to reduce symptoms and prolong survival in chronic congestive heart failure patients. The goal is to provide primary prevention whenever practical or possible, and to fall back on secondary preventive care when it is not. Tertiary prevention is employed when both primary and secondary preventive care for a given condition are either not available, have not been done, or have failed.

Deciding Which Preventive Services to Provide

In approaching the provision of comprehensive preventive care, the physician is faced with selecting from a large number of screening and early detection strategies and anticipatory interventions for a large number of important conditions and diseases. For those conditions that are potentially amenable to screening, early detection, or anticipatory guidance, the following criteria need to be met:

1. The condition should be an important cause of morbidity and mortality in the screened population.
2. The condition should have a high enough prevalence so as to be suitable for screening. This criterion is important because prevalence will determine the number of false-positives and false-negatives (and hence the positive and negative predictive values) for any given screening test for that procedure. Rare conditions will yield higher false-positive rates on screening tests, regardless of the characteristics of those tests.
3. An effective screening test or procedure must exist for the condition. This test should be sensitive enough to detect

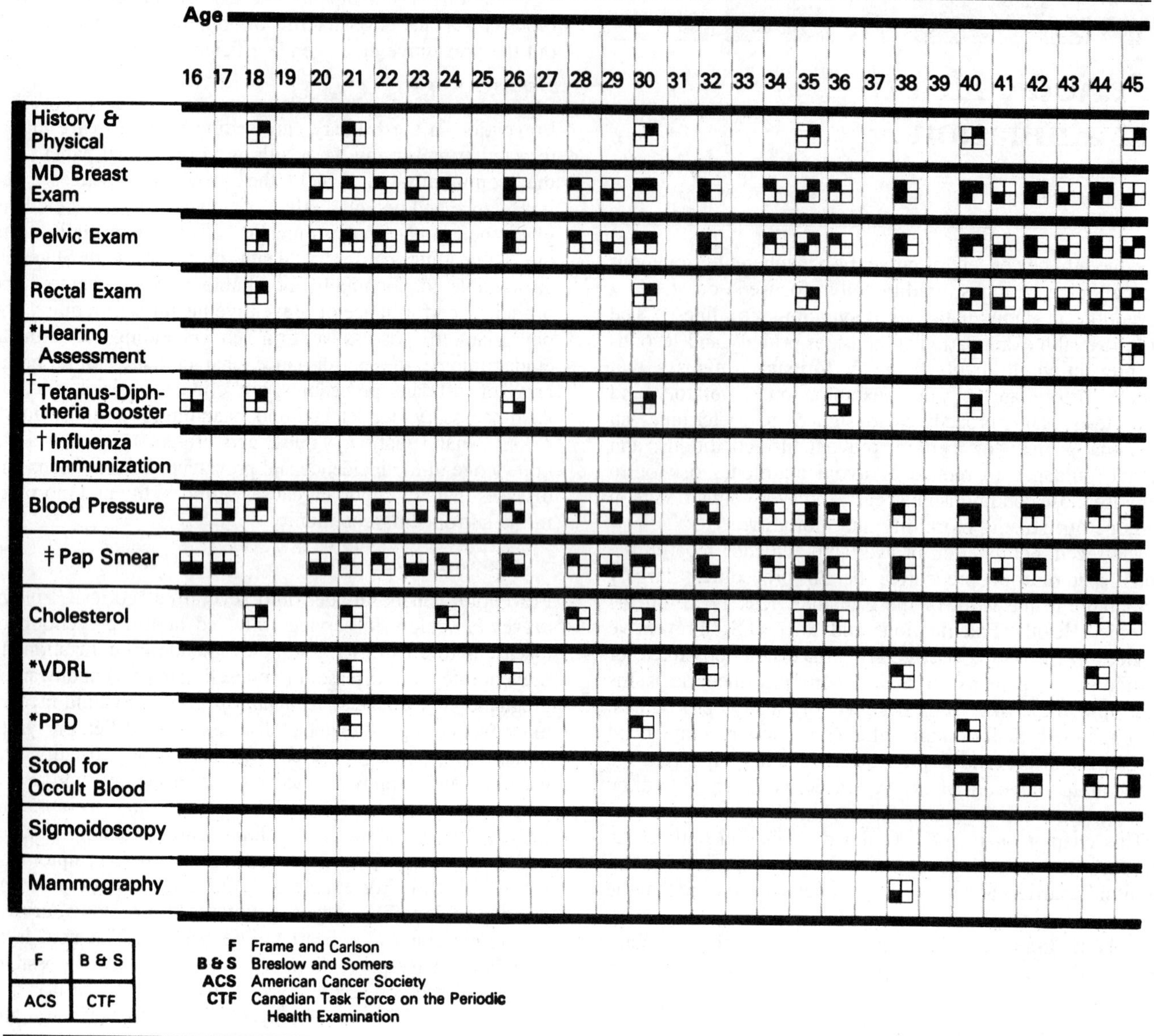

Fig. 4-1. Summary of recommendations of the four major studies. *Canadian Task Force recommends that this be done on the basis of clinical judgment. †Centers for Disease Control and Prevention recommends that at first visit physician check immunization history for rubella, mumps, poliomyelitis, diphtheria/tetanus toxoids, and pertussis. ‡If sexually active. A blackened square indicates that a study has considered the maneuver and recommended it. Empty squares indicate that the maneuver was either not considered or considered but not recommended. (From Hayward RA, et al: *Ann Intern Med* 114:758, 1991.)

most cases and specific enough to keep the number of individuals misdiagnosed with the condition to a minimum. Ideally, the test should be demonstrated to be effective in controlled clinical trials and in practice situations.

4. The screening test should be low risk and acceptable to individuals undergoing the procedure. The risks attendant to screening can include the direct physical risk of the screening procedure or of subsequent procedures that are performed as a result of a positive screening test (e.g., the risk of bowel perforation with colonoscopy performed to evaluate a positive test for fecal occult blood) or less tangible risks (e.g., the unnecessary anxiety caused if an individual is incorrectly diagnosed with a condition, such as a malignancy). Although usually difficult to quantify, the risk of false reassurance (e.g., a patient ignores symptoms because of a recent negative screening test) also needs to be considered.
5. There should be a benefit to early intervention for the condition. The most definitive evidence of efficacy for a screening procedure comes from controlled clinical trials demonstrating a reduction in cause-specific mortality resulting from the screening procedure in question. Unfortunately, such evidence exists for few screening tests (e.g., mammography and breast examination for women between the ages of 50 and 74, fecal occult blood testing for individuals past the age of 50). In most instances the physician must rely on indirect evidence, such as case-control or observational studies and expert opinion. Authorities such as the Canadian Task Force on Preventive

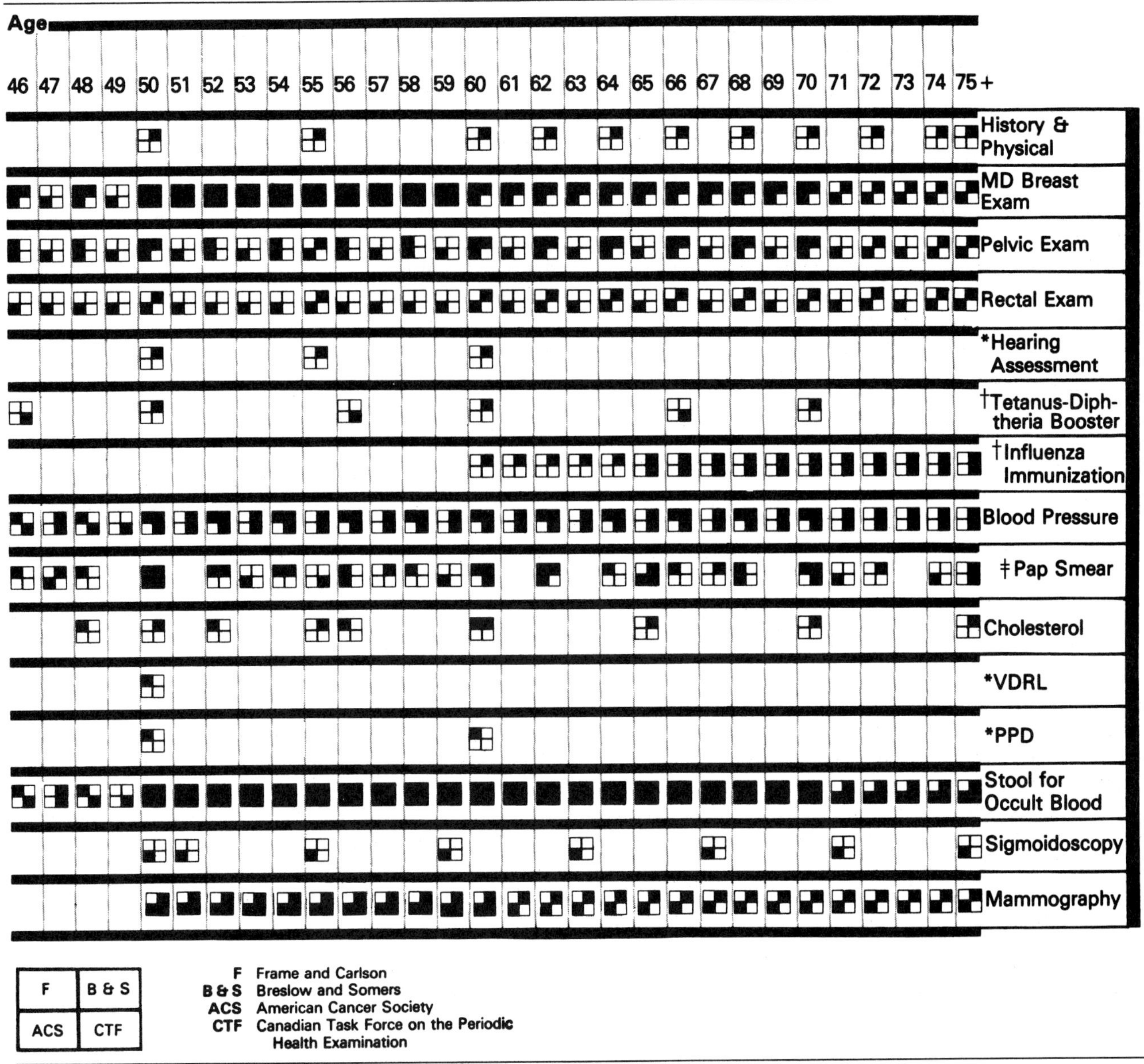

Fig. 4-1, cont'd. For legend see opposite page.

Services, the USPSTF, and the American College of Physicians have published recommendations and practice guidelines based on rigorous and methodic review of published evidence on a broad variety of screening procedures and preventive services. Other organizations such as the American Cancer Society have relied more heavily on consensus and expert opinion. Such published guidelines form the foundation for the provision of preventive services in general practice. In considering the quality of indirect evidence from observational studies and consensus, the physician must be aware of the common biases in studies involving screening and early detection, such as *lead time bias, length time bias,* and *over-detection bias. Lead time bias* refers to the phenomenon by which screening-detected diseases such as cancer will appear to be associated with improved survival in comparison with cases of the same disease that are diagnosed because of clinical symptoms. This is because the disease is detected at an earlier point in its natural history. Actual survival, however, may or may not be affected. *Length time bias* is introduced because diseases with a longer latency period (and which therefore presumably progress more slowly) are more likely to be detected by screening than diseases with a shorter latency and more rapidly progressive course (and therefore shorter survival). *Over-detection* bias occurs when screening detects preclinical disease that, if undetected, would not have contributed to the mortality of the affected individuals.

6. The screening test or procedure should be affordable and/or cost-effective. Such information is rarely available

directly but has been estimated for many procedures and has been incorporated into guidelines such as those published by the Canadian Task Force (CTF) and USPSTF.

ELEMENTS OF THE PERIODIC HEALTH EXAMINATION

Risk Assessment

Building the Database. One of the most important aspects of providing effective preventive care during the periodic health examination is a complete and comprehensive clinical database, one used to assess risk of disease and direct anticipatory guidance and screening procedures. Collecting data can be a time-consuming task, part of which the physician may want to delegate to the patient or to office staff through the use of self-completed history forms or questionnaires. They can be completed before the appointment or while the patient is in the waiting room. The form should then be reviewed and clarified with the patient during the examination. The self-completed history form also may alert the physician to a patient's limited English proficiency or illiteracy.

Medical History. Perhaps the most central part of any medical database involves the collection of information regarding previous medical diagnoses, their treatment and response to treatment, current and previous medications and allergies, history of immunizations and childhood illnesses, and prior surgical history including response to anesthesia. This is generally accomplished through patient interview, through review of immediately available medical records, and by formally requesting medical records from previous providers or hospitals at which the patient was treated. The information obtained should be recorded on a problem list, which is generally organized into active and inactive problems, and prominently located in the patient's office chart.

Family History. A detailed family history is essential for gauging the patient's susceptibility to a variety of important and potentially preventable conditions, and thus determines the primary and secondary preventive efforts (Box 4-1). It may also help the physician to understand the patient's experience and concerns with serious illness in his or her family.

Box 4-1. Common Conditions in Which Family History Contributes to Risk

- Cancer, especially breast, colon, prostate, and ovarian
- Hypertension
- Diabetes
- Hyperlipidemia, atherosclerosis, coronary artery disease
- Alcoholism
- Mental illness
- Autoimmune disease
- Multiple endocrinopathies
- Tuberculosis, hepatitis B, or other prevalent infectious diseases that pose increased risk to family members

Social History. Providing individualized and attentive health care depends on thorough knowledge of the patients and their circumstances. It is also increasingly recognized that there is a correlation between socioeconomic conditions and the risk of cardiovascular disease, cancer, substance abuse, and violence. In addition to occupation, the physician should inquire about education, military service, marital status, relationships, household members, leisure activities, and travel. Any use of alcohol, tobacco, and other psychoactive substances also should be noted.

Occupational and Environmental History (See Chapter 11). It has been estimated recently that 390,000 cases of occupation-related illnesses and 100,000 occupational illness–related deaths occur in the United States annually. However, only a small percentage of the illnesses responsible for those deaths are recognized as being related to workplace exposures, since the clinical presentation is rarely diagnostic of occupational disease. Primary care physicians should take an occupational history of each patient as part of a periodic health examination, concentrating on both present and any previous long-term jobs. Efforts should be made to determine the exact nature of the patient's job and to specifically ask about exposure to dust, fumes, solvents or chemicals, noise, vibration, or repetitive motion. The physician should consider the possibility of an occupational cause of illness in patients with dermatologic problems, respiratory illnesses, cardiovascular diseases, emotional disturbances, musculoskeletal pains, malignancies, neurologic problems, hearing losses, traumatic injuries, and certain infectious diseases, such as hepatitis or human immunodeficiency virus (HIV).[1]

The Sexual History. The sexual history of a patient is an essential part of the periodic health examination. A large number of medical, social, and psychiatric conditions can manifest themselves as sexual problems or dysfunction through the life cycle, and yet patients often will not volunteer such information. The physician who cares for adolescents realizes that sexuality is a central focus for them (see Chapter 7). The opportunity to offer preventive guidance against sexually transmitted diseases, unwanted pregnancy, and sexual abuse depends on the physician establishing an atmosphere in which sexual problems, concerns, and questions can be openly discussed (see Chapter 56). Sexual dysfunction is a problem in the middle aged and elderly, and an often overlooked yet treatable cause of a decreased quality of life.

With the advent of the acquired immunodeficiency syndrome (AIDS) epidemic, as well as high rates of a variety of sexually transmitted infections, it is crucial that the physician ask not only about sexual function but also about sexual orientation and behavior. An effective approach might be to begin a general discussion about high-risk behaviors with a patient and then afford the opportunity for the patient to ask questions. The physician may appropriately choose to collect sensitive information and counsel the patient at follow-up visits rather than at the first encounter, unless a specific complaint dictates otherwise. Although it is common for patients to be reticent regarding their reproductive health concerns, most open up later if the provider establishes that such concerns are welcomed for discussion. See Chapter 34 for more information on effective techniques for taking the sexual history.

Maintaining and Tracking Data

Many studies have established the utility of using a system of reminders to prompt the physician when certain indicated periodic preventive procedures are due. An example would be a paper spreadsheet in which patient-specific preventive health procedures and proposed frequency are listed in the left-hand margin and dates are listed across the top (Fig. 4-2). As a procedure is performed it is recorded, thus providing a prompt to perform that procedure again after a specified amount of time has elapsed. An effective strategy is to send letters or postcards to patients reminding them that preventive care is due and to call for an appointment. Such applications are perfect for small computers, which can track dates and provide automatic reminders to both patients and physicians. There is some evidence that the use of computerized reminders can enhance performance.[8] With the increasing practicality and use of electronic patient records in the office setting, it is likely that the automation of these tasks will become standard.

Regardless of whether a paper or an electronic system is used to keep track of preventive health care, certain characteristics are essential for success. The reminder should be readily available at the time of the patient encounter, and the physician should have the ability to instantaneously update the patient's prevention database. The prevention profile should be customized for each patient, with the physician having the option to suppress reminders when they are no longer warranted. The physician should be able to derive summary statistics so as to gauge overall performance. Peer review mechanisms can be devised within a practice to ensure maximum compliance with previously established guidelines.

Most routine prevention can be organized or carried out by office staff or midlevel practitioners and thus incorporated into waiting time or an exit interview with a nurse. Literature and pamphlets emphasizing the importance of preventive care are often effective in increasing patient awareness and interest and can be prominently displayed in the waiting area and examining rooms.

Anticipatory Guidance

Diet and Exercise. During periodic health examinations, the physician should take the opportunity to provide advice regarding proper nutrition, weight maintenance, and aerobic exercise. Proper diet is being increasingly recognized as central to any preventive strategy. Dietary fat and cholesterol play a major causal role in atherogenesis, and saturated fat intake has been implicated in increasing the risk of colon and breast cancer. Severe obesity (30% above ideal body weight [IBW]) is a risk factor for increased mortality, largely through an increase in cardiovascular and cerebrovascular disease.

The physician should include a baseline dietary assessment in each patient's database. Dietary guidelines appropriate for the general population should be promulgated (e.g., the American Heart Association Step I diet) (see Chapter 71). Most patients can be advised to cut down on fatty meats by substituting chicken, fish, and lean meats; to select more fruits and vegetables; and to substitute low or nonfat dairy products for whole fat ones. The maintenance of body weight in the basal state requires approximately 1500 to 1800 calories per day. Patients should reach and maintain their approximate ideal body weight by adjusting intake according to their activity level.

Aerobic exercise is beneficial in reducing cardiovascular risk and helps to reduce stress and promote a sense of well being. In postmenopausal women, weight-bearing aerobic exercise can aid in preventing osteoporosis. Spending as little as 15 minutes a day 3 days a week on modest aerobic exercise such as brisk walking may be beneficial and can be recommended to most patients.

Alcohol, Tobacco, and Other Substance Use and Abuse. When one considers the prevalence of alcohol, nicotine, and other chemical dependence, and their propensity to predispose to serious health problems (e.g., trauma, liver disease, cancer, heart disease), it is not so difficult to accept that substance abuse is a major contributor to death and morbidity in the United States.

Alcohol Use and Abuse. The primary care physician must be aware of not only the high prevalence of alcohol abuse but also of the highly variable and frequently subtle clinical presentation. Alcohol is toxic to virtually every organ system in the body and can result in a multitude of health effects. The provider should be alert to the potential role of serious alcohol abuse in patients presenting with:

- Excitability or anxiety
- Gastrointestinal tract complaints, such as dyspepsia, heartburn, or recurrent diarrhea
- Hypertension (especially with poor response to treatment)
- Dysrhythmias (especially atrial fibrillation), palpitations, or cardiomyopathy
- Depression
- Sleep disturbances
- Sexual dysfunction
- Recurrent major or minor trauma
- Multiple somatic complaints
- Work absenteeism, interpersonal problems, or marital difficulties

Since an individual's alcohol abuse frequently affects the family, the primary care physician may receive the first hints of a problem from the presenting complaints, often subtle, of those nearest the patient.

There are varying definitions of alcohol abuse and dependency. All of them emphasize the consequences of the individual's alcohol intake rather than the frequency or amount of intake and loss of control over drinking despite these adverse consequences. *Dependency* is distinguished from abuse in that it implies physiologic tolerance and the onset of withdrawal symptoms with abstinence. *Harmful drinking* is continued heavy consumption of alcohol-containing beverages despite adverse physical or social consequences, but does not necessarily involve physiologic dependence on alcohol. *Hazardous drinking* is the frequent consumption of 40 to 60 grams of alcohol (about three to four drinks) in men and 28 to 40 grams of alcohol (about two to three drinks) in women. This correlates roughly with drinking to the point of intoxication. Hazardous drinkers are at high risk of progressing to harmful drinking or dependence, and should therefore receive advice to cut down or abstain.

ROUTINE HEALTH MAINTENANCE CHECKLIST

Indicate Dates Done/Results

	Date	
	Comprehensive Hx. & P.E.	
HABITS	Smoking/Tobacco Use	
	Alcohol Consumption	
	Other Substance Use	
	Diet	
	Regular Exercise	
	Breast Self-Exam / Testicle Self-Exam } Teach/Review	
EXAMINATION	Height (Stocking Feet)	
	Weight (No Shoes)	
	Blood Pressure, sitting	
	Breast Examination	
	Pelvic Examination/Pap Smear	
	Rectal Examination	
TESTING	Mammography	
	Hemoccult x 3	
	Sigmoidoscopy/Colonoscopy	
	Tonometry/Ophthalmology Exam	
	Tuberculin Test (PPD)	
	Syphilis Serology (RPR)	
	Total Cholesterol/HDL-C	
	Hgb/Hct	
	Creatinine	
	Urinalysis	
IMMUNIZATIONS	Td	
	MMR	
	Serology	
	Hepatitis B	
	Serology	
	Pneumovax	
	Influenza	

Fig. 4-2. Example of a prevention flow sheet. (From Boston Medical Center.)

Denial is prevalent, and patients who are harmful drinkers usually will not attribute their problems to a continued use of alcohol, despite overwhelming evidence to the contrary. Adult and adolescent patients should be asked about their use of alcoholic beverages. Those who respond positively should have a more in-depth history taken, one that focuses on the association between alcohol consumption and other events, such as injuries, traffic violations or accidents, arguments, interpersonal conflicts or marital problems, and school or job problems (e.g., absenteeism). In addition, a number of instruments such as the CAGE questionnaire (Box 4-2) or the longer Michigan Alcohol Screening Test (MAST) are available to physicians to screen for dysfunctional alcohol use. The CAGE questionnaire is popular because of its brevity, the ease with which it can be memorized, and the reasonably good sensitivity and specificity when two positive responses are elicited. One positive response also may indicate a significant alcohol abuse problem and is worthy of further investigation. Those patients with a family history of alcoholism, particularly in one or both parents, are at higher risk of becoming alcoholic and should be periodically rescreened (Chapter 51). Physicians should consider advising abstinence in patients with such history.

For many patients with problem drinking, there is evidence that office-based intervention by primary care physicians can significantly reduce hazardous and untoward alcohol consumption. A recent randomized controlled study has indicated that a brief intervention on the part of primary care physicians can significantly impact on drinking on the part of nondependent problem drinkers.[7] Outcomes that are improved include number of drinks per week and frequency of binge drinking, as well as number of days of hospitalization. Long-term improvement and improvement in other alcohol-related outcomes (e.g., injuries and accidents) were not measured, since the follow-up period was relatively brief. Despite the modest effect on frequency and intensity of drinking, routine physician intervention in hazardous and harmful drinkers is supported by the fact that most alcohol-related medical and social problems occur in nondependent problem drinkers, as well as by the low risk posed by advice-giving and counseling.

Useful office-based interventions characteristically involve advising abstinence, or in instances where patients do not have abstinence as a goal, advice on limiting consumption to amounts not generally considered harmful (one to two drinks per day in men and zero to one drink per day in women). Possible untoward effects and contributions of alcohol on current health problems or symptoms should be emphasized.

Box 4-2. The CAGE Questionnaire

C: "Have you ever felt the need to *C*ut down on your drinking?"
A: "Have people *A*nnoyed you by criticizing your drinking?"
G: "Have you ever felt bad or *G*uilty about your drinking?"
E: "Have you ever had a drink first thing in the morning to steady your nerves or get rid of a hangover? (*E*ye-opener)"

Tobacco (Nicotine) Dependency. Despite increasing public knowledge about the adverse consequences of tobacco use, smoking continues to contribute to an enormous burden of suffering in the United States (see Chapter 57). It is important that the primary care physician ask all patients regularly about tobacco use. Those who do smoke should be educated about both its adverse effects and the health and economic benefits of quitting (e.g., a one-pack-per-day smoker now spends about $1000 a year on cigarettes), and should be advised to quit. A small but significant number of patients quit simply because their physician advised them to do so. See Chapter 57 for smoking cessation techniques.

Other Substances. The clinical presentation of the abuse of substances other than alcohol varies with the chemical in question, but abuse syndromes share a common ground of social and relationship dysfunction, financial problems, and trauma (see Chapter 52). Cocaine use can cause catastrophic cardiovascular and neurologic events, as well as depression and panic disorder. Marijuana smoking can lead to chronic lung disease. Injection drug use is a leading cause of HIV infection, hepatitis, endocarditis, and local infectious complications.

As with alcohol, the primary care physician should ask about other substance use and take a more in-depth history of those patients responding affirmatively. Treatment referral should be offered to patients who continue their abuse. Patients who use a substance despite evidence of significant medical or social consequences or whose history suggests a loss of control over the substance should be strongly urged to seek treatment.

Domestic Violence. Domestic violence traditionally has been an underreported and underrecognized problem in primary care populations. Although as many as 2 to 4 million women are battered by their husbands or significant others, only about one in 20 is diagnosed with the battering syndrome by a physician, since few women disclose abuse, despite the fact that many consider their physician as a source of help. Homes in which domestic violence is perpetrated by men against women (the vast majority of domestic violence) are far more likely to include abused and neglected children, and those children are apt to grow up to abuse their spouses and children. Domestic violence is a major cause of suicide among women and homicide committed by women against their husbands or significant others. There is a strong association between domestic violence and alcohol and substance abuse, both on the part of the perpetrator and the victim (see Chapter 59).

Victims of battering occasionally present with recurring physical evidence of trauma but more commonly present with nonspecific constellations of symptoms, such as depression, fatigue, unexplained abdominal or pelvic pain, or multiple somatic complaints that are frequently atypical. The prevalence of physical, emotional, or sexual abuse in these patients may be as high as 45%.

The most effective strategy for detecting domestic violence is to ask, since patients rarely volunteer the information. Statements such as "Marriages (or relationships) are frequently very difficult" and "Does your husband (or partner) ever strike you or make you feel bad about yourself?" convey a message of concern, letting the patient know that the physician is willing to discuss such subjects. Surveys on the issue indicate that most patients not only do not mind being asked, but actually expect the inquiry. It is important to assure patients about the confidentiality of the conversation, since they may fear reprisal. Younger women who are beginning the coupling process should be asked in a neutral fashion if they have been coerced into performing sexual acts through intimidation or physical violence. Children and adolescents should be asked about arguments at home and their consequences, as well as about their parents' usual methods of punishment.[22]

Although it is tempting to do so, the primary care physician should avoid the urge to rescue the victim. The provider's main role is that of counselor and supporter. The victim should receive the message that violence is wrong and illegal and that there are laws offering protection. Careful documentation of the history and physical findings (including photographs, if possible), as well as x-rays done to evaluate injuries, may assist the patient in pursuing legal protection later. The physician should at least provide the telephone number of a local violence hotline or battered person's shelter. If the situation is more urgent, the patient should be encouraged to notify the local authorities. In some instances the actions taken by the physician are governed by local mandated reporting laws, such as in cases of suspected abuse of a minor or an older adult. The treatment of victims with severe physical and psychologic sequelae should be referred to providers experienced in the management of domestic violence. See Chapter 59 for further discussion.

Adolescent Health Issues. Adolescence is a time of rapid emotional and physical change, when many lifestyle factors that are likely to influence long-term health are established. Health issues of particular salience to adolescents include teenage pregnancy; sexually transmitted diseases (STDs); violence and injuries; substance abuse, including alcohol and tobacco; physical and sexual abuse; depression and suicide; eating disorders and proper nutrition; and exercise. Despite the apparent opportunity for meaningful primary prevention, adolescents remain medically underserved. Young men, in particular, are unlikely to see physicians except for sporadic, symptom-related care, while young women may be seen more frequently for routine gynecologic and family planning visits. These occasions should be viewed as an opportunity to ask about concerns, to screen for possible problems, and to provide appropriate anticipatory guidance and referral as necessary. The primary care physician should be familiar with and comfortable asking about these issues. Participation in school-based programs and clinics such as those providing presports participation physicals may afford the opportunity to intervene with a broader sample of the adolescent population in a community.

Teenage Pregnancy and Sexually Transmitted Disease (STD) Prevention. Unwanted teenage pregnancy is occurring in epidemic proportions. Forty percent of young women in the United States become pregnant by the time they are 19 years old, 20% become mothers, and 15% have therapeutic abortions. The teenage abortion rate in the United States exceeds the teenage pregnancy rate in other Western countries (e.g., in Sweden, a young woman is half as likely to become pregnant despite a sexual activity rate 50% higher than that of adolescent women in the United States). This statistic has been attributed to the greater availability and acceptance of contraceptives in the European teenage population. The potential for increasing contraceptive use is apparent when one considers that 51% of American teenagers do not use contraception on first intercourse, and 20% of the young women who become pregnant do so within 1 month of first intercourse.

The primary care physician may wish to become active on a communitywide basis by advocating school-based educational programs and by breaking down barriers that inhibit the availability of contraceptives for teens. In the absence of such programs, the physicians themselves are the major source of contraceptive information for teens. Unfortunately teens are unlikely to initiate a discussion about sexual concerns, leaving it to the physician to inquire in a neutral, nonthreatening fashion at unrelated visits (e.g., a routine gynecologic appointment). Phrasing questions such as "Many women (or men) your age have questions about sex and avoiding pregnancy. I would be happy to answer any questions you have today or in the future if you would like" creates an atmosphere in which teenagers can feel that the subject of sexuality is fair territory for discussion and that their provider is an ally. Toward this end, the physician should stress the confidentiality of the discussion and avoid adopting a judgmental or moralizing attitude. Physicians should familiarize themselves with state laws regarding the treatment of minors, but in general it is unlikely that a physician will be subject to legal recourse for prescribing birth control to a teen who requests it. Federally funded facilities are required to provide birth control to a minor who requests it, and although individual physicians have the right to refuse, they are required to provide referral to a facility or physician who will.[23]

Primary and secondary prevention of both teenage pregnancy and STDs should include a discussion about the physiology of reproduction and about transmission of STDs, and information about behaviors and contraceptives. Oral contraceptives (OCPs), although effective at preventing conception, may not be an ideal method for teens, in that they require advanced planning and strict compliance, and provide no protection against STDs. Barrier methods, particularly condoms, are better in the latter regard, but less effective in the former. Therefore condoms plus another method, such as OCPs, should be recommended for adolescents who choose to remain sexually active. The physician should stress that no contraceptive method other than abstinence is 100% effective in preventing HIV transmission. It is important to discuss the intense social, emotional, and physical impact of becoming sexually aware and to educate teens on the potential advantage of postponing sexual intimacy until later in adulthood.

Violence, Risk-Taking Behavior, and Injury Prevention. Homicide is the third leading cause of death among 15-to 24-year-old men in the United States and is now recognized as a major health problem. Physicians should routinely ask about fighting and injuries, and the circumstances under which they occur. The possibility of substance abuse and its relationship to fighting or injuries should be explored, and the connection emphasized to the patient. The association of substance abuse with domestic violence must be kept in mind, and patients should be routinely questioned regarding their homelife and their parents' attitudes toward punishment. The teen with a history of violence should be warned about the risk of death and/or serious injury, and given gener advice regarding nonviolent techniques for resolving conflicts. Those with a history of alcohol or drug use should be offered referral for treatment.[24]

Injuries are the leading cause of death in persons 1 to 44 years old, and automobile-related accidents are the most important source of injury.[21] Physicians should routinely point out the effectiveness of seatbelts, especially those with shoulder restraints, and encourage their use even for brief trips. The use of child restraint seats should be encouraged, since an unrestrained child is 11 times more likely to die in an accident than a restrained one. Fortunately, the physician is assisted in these endeavors as more and more states invoke mandatory seatbelt and child restraint laws. Alcohol use is at the root of approximately 50% of all traffic fatalities, and adolescents should be advised against drinking and driving.

Physicians also should promote the use of other appropriate protective equipment (e.g., head, wrist, elbow, and knee protection during in-line skating, and bicycle and motorcycle helmets).[17]

Depression and Suicide. Suicide is the second leading cause of death among persons 15 to 24 years old. Young women attempt suicide more frequently than young men; however, men are more likely to succeed, and therefore account for the vast majority of suicide-related deaths in this group. Physicians should be aware of the association between an adolescent's suicidal behavior and major life stressors, such as school difficulties, domestic discord and abuse, parental divorce, and relationship problems. Additional factors include substance abuse, antisocial behavior, homosexuality, and major depression. The history of prior suicide attempts is the strongest risk factor. None of the other factors alone or in combination have been found to have value in defining a high-risk individual. The periodic health examination of the adolescent should include routine questioning about social functioning, home life, and mood, as well as screening questions for the vegetative signs of depression. Those who report serious suicidal ideation should be further assessed for the "lethality" of their plan (e.g., having a specific method in mind, having already obtained the planned means). Those who are determined to act must be hospitalized; those less intent can be managed as outpatients. The complexity of the average teenager's social and maturational hurdles, as well as the frequent need to include parents and other family members in the treatment plan, makes referral to a provider skilled in this area almost always a necessity.

Eating Disorders. As a result of definitional and reporting problems, the exact incidence of eating disorders is unknown; however, it is believed to have increased dramatically in the past 2 decades. The reasons for this are unclear but are believed to be associated with the current trend equating thinness with beauty. Women outnumber men with these disorders by as much as 25 to 1. Anorexia nervosa and bulimia nervosa may present quite overtly in their severe forms or subtly with minor degrees of severity. The routine care of the adolescent should include a dietary history, not only to provide anticipatory guidance regarding nutritional habits, but also to screen for unusual attitudes and obsessions about food, eating, distorted body image, or inappropriate self-perception that the adolescent is overweight. Adolescents with eating disorders frequently present with depressed mood and/or anxiety and hyperactivity. They often experience problems at home, in school, and at work, and may be socially isolated. Any of these signs should raise suspicion. Additionally, the physician should be aware of the possibility of an eating disorder in an adolescent who presents with unexplained electrolyte abnormalities, especially hypokalemia, who is remarkably underweight (more than 15% below IBW); shows a delay or plateau in the development of secondary sex characteristics; has primary or secondary amenorrhea; displays severe periodontal disease (a result of habitual purging of stomach contents); or has difficulty adjusting socially. Patients with bulimia nervosa may show wide swings in body weight over months or years, but most often present at or near their IBW. Bulimics suffer the most severe metabolic derangements, which may be life-threatening. Hospitalization for fluid and electrolyte replacement is indicated in extreme cases, even without the patient's consent if his or her refusal constitutes an immediate threat to survival. Management of less severe cases can be done on an outpatient basis, although referral to a clinician experienced in these disorders (usually a psychiatrist, psychiatric nurse, or psychologist) is wise. See Chapter 55 for more information on the diagnosis and treatment of eating disorders.

Office-Based Screening

A comprehensive discussion of all screening procedures that the primary care physician may wish to consider is beyond the scope of this chapter; however, several of the major targets of screening in primary care practice are discussed here.

Colorectal Cancer Screening. Colon cancer is the second most common lethal cancer in the United States, affecting both men and women equally. Lifetime incidence for persons of average risk is approximately 6%, but is two to three times higher for persons with an affected first-degree relative. Patients with a familial polyposis syndrome have a risk 20 to 30 times higher, virtually a 100% lifetime risk. Persons with ulcerative or Crohn's colitis also have a greatly increased risk, as much as fivefold to sixfold lifetime risk.

There is mounting evidence that colorectal cancer may be linked to certain dietary factors and therefore may be somewhat preventable. Treatment of advanced disease remains unsatisfactory, placing an emphasis on screening to detect early, potentially curable disease.

The physician has a relatively wide array of useful screening procedures that vary dramatically in terms of availability, acceptability, efficacy, and cost. For most of these procedures, controlled, prospective data demonstrating a reduction in mortality from colorectal cancer are lacking. Therefore a screening strategy must be chosen based on a patient's estimated risk and preferences.[5]

Digital Rectal Examination. The digital rectal examination (DRE), in which the examiner inserts a gloved finger into the rectum to detect palpable neoplasia, is probably of minimal efficacy, since only about 10% of lesions arise within 7 cm of the anal verge. The main utilities are that the DRE allows direct palpation of the prostate gland in men and can be combined with office stool guaiac testing (although some recommend against office-based screening because of the potential of inducing bleeding by insertion of the examiner's finger). There is no convincing evidence either for or against the routine performance of DRE.[27]

Stool Guaiac Testing (Fecal Occult Blood Testing [FOBT]). Stool guaiac testing is based on the detection of peroxidase-like activity in the stool, a result of the presence of occult blood. Procedurally, the patient is instructed to test three consecutive stools by sampling two different areas of each stool using a wooden spatula or similar implement and applying it to the two slide windows of a guaiac testing card. One card is needed for each of the three bowel movements. The cards are subsequently developed by placing a few drops of a hydrogen peroxide solution onto them. A test is positive when any of the six slide windows turn blue, denoting the presence of heme. One week before testing it is recommended that the patient be placed on a meat-free diet that also omits foods high in peroxidase (e.g., horseradish, melons, and cauliflower). To minimize the false-negative rate, the cards should be developed within 1 week of sampling. Controversy has surrounded rehydrating the slides by placing a drop of deionized water on the slide before adding the developer solution. This increases the sensitivity of the test but also raises the false-positive rate and lowers the positive predictive value. Stool guaiac testing has an approximate sensitivity of 50% to 60% for malignancy (lower for polyps), and a positive test has a 5% to 10% positive predictive value for malignancy and 15% to 45% for polyps. Any patient with a positive result should be further investigated with colonoscopy or air contrast barium enema with a flexible sigmoidoscopy (see Chapter 105).

There is evidence from a randomized controlled study by Mandel and colleagues (the Minnesota Study) showing a 33% reduction in cause-specific mortality through annual stool guaiac testing with rehydration before developing the cards.[18] Two more recent European studies of biennial screening without rehydration have shown a smaller treatment effect of 16% and 18% reduction respectively in cause-specific mortality.[9,15] Similarly a recent meta-analysis of screening trials found a 16% reduction.[25]

Sigmoidoscopy. The use of sigmoidoscopy to screen for colorectal cancer is being reevaluated. The American Cancer Society recommends flexible sigmoidoscopy every 3 to 5 years following two negative examinations 1 year apart for persons of usual risk over the age of 50, based on data from uncontrolled, observational studies. The USPSTF and National Cancer Institute have not recommended routine sigmoidoscopy, citing a lack of evidence of efficacy. The theoretic advantage and intuitive appeal of sigmoidoscopy stem from the well-accepted natural history of colorectal cancer, in which most invasive cancers arise from premalignant, adenomatous polyps, a process that is believed to take an average of 7 to 10 years. Using a sigmoidoscope, the examiner can identify, biopsy, and/or remove suspicious lesions within reach of the instrument. Sigmoidoscopy can be considered therefore to be virtually 100% sensitive and specific within its reach, and 60% of all potential cancers arise within reach of a 65-cm flexible sigmoidoscope. Although there are no prospective controlled studies demonstrating that screening with sigmoidoscopy reduces mortality from colorectal cancer, studies do demonstrate that malignant lesions discovered during sigmoidoscopic screening are less advanced (Duke's stages A and B) than lesions that present with symptoms, a trend also demonstrated with stool guaiac screening. If one accepts this shift toward less advanced lesions as a surrogate end point, then the evidence strongly supports the use of sigmoidoscopy for screening.

Weighed against the use of sigmoidoscopy are its relatively low availability (although this procedure is well within the purview of the generalist), its significant cost, greater discomfort, and the risk of bleeding or perforation from the procedure. If performed, the sigmoidoscopy should be combined with annual stool guaiac testing.

Colonoscopy. The use of colonoscopy to screen for colorectal cancer offers the advantage of direct visualization of the entire colon from rectum to cecum, with the removal or biopsy of all suspicious lesions. This is achieved through greater discomfort, a more difficult bowel preparation, much greater cost, and higher risk of perforation. Furthermore, it is estimated that the increase in efficacy over a program of stool guaiacs, DRE, and sigmoidoscopy is marginal. For all of these reasons colonoscopy is rarely used purely for screening in persons of usual risk, but is quite reasonable and frequently recommended for persons at much greater risk (e.g., first-degree relative with colon cancer, familial polyposis syndromes, or inflammatory bowel disease [IBD]).

In summary, primary care physicians should place emphasis on colorectal screening as an important avenue to reduced morbidity and mortality in their practice population. Many organizations recommend that annual FOBT and flexible sigmoidoscopy every 3 to 5 years should be offered to persons of usual risk beginning at age 50. The USPSTF concludes that there is strong evidence in favor of screening, but it is unclear if the optimal strategy is FOBT or sigmoidoscopy or both. Colonoscopy every 10 years may be a reasonable alternative, but the lack of trial data, increased risk, and cost need to be considered. Persons with a family history of colon cancer, particularly in first-degree relatives with onset before age 60, should begin screening at age 40 with either FOBT annually and sigmoidoscopy every 3 to 5 years or colonoscopy every 10 years. If there is suspicion or history of familial polyposis or hereditary nonpolyposis colorectal cancer, referral should be made for surveillance colonoscopy as well as genetic counseling and testing.

Cervical Cancer Screening. A woman of average risk in the United States has an approximately 0.7% cumulative lifetime risk of developing invasive carcinoma of the uterine cervix, and a 2% lifetime risk of carcinoma in situ. Although these risks are relatively low in comparison with other important malignancies, they are heavily affected by screening, and, according to estimates, would be two to three times higher in an unscreened population. The risk is increased in African-Americans and Latinas, as well as with early age of first intercourse, multiple sexual partners, cigarette smoking, and oral contraceptive use.

Based on a wealth of empiric evidence, the efficacy of cervical cancer screening using the Pap smear is widely accepted. Numerous population-based reports looking at the effects of widespread screening studies have demonstrated a dramatic impact on the incidence of invasive cervical carcinoma and carcinoma in situ.[4]

Some controversy remains regarding the age to begin screening, the age to end screening, and the optimal frequency at which to screen. It appears that to maintain most of its efficacy, screening should begin in a patient's early 20s at the latest and continue until the age of 65. Beginning at age 17 or continuing until age 75 results in only marginal gains at a substantial cost, if considered on a population-wide basis. Notably, the efficacy of screening from age 65 to 75 or later is much higher if the woman has not had a prior Pap smear. Likewise, screening annually rather than every 3 years results in marginal benefit. At intervals greater than every 3 years th benefit falls off significantly, but screening still retains approximately 65% efficacy at an interval of every 10 years. Ultimately, decisions regarding the age to begin screening and the interval at which to screen should be based on the patient's preferences, as well as on an assessment of her baseline risk. Current recommendations are for screenings to begin at age 18 or at the beginning of sexual activity, with annual examinations through the age of 65. This protocol is estimated to reduce invasive cervical cancer by more than 90%.

Breast Cancer Screening. Breast cancer is currently the second most common cause of cancer death among women. At present, a woman of average risk has a one in nine cumulative lifetime risk of developing breast cancer, with the risk increasing two to three times in those who have a first-degree relative afflicted. Of those who develop breast cancer, approximately one half will die from the disease. In the absence of knowledge regarding effective primary prevention, the primary care physician must emphasize early detection and cure. Fortunately, effective screening strategies exist that utilize one-and two-view mammography, singularly and in combination with physician-performed breast examination. However, many unanswered questions and controversies remain.[19]

The evidence for the efficacy of mammography with and without physician-performed breast palpation in lowering breast cancer–related mortality for women between the ages of 50 and 74 has been demonstrated by a number of large randomized trials and is accepted by most authorities. The magnitude of this reduction ranges from approximately 15% to 30% and may be higher for women in the 50- to 60-year-old age group.[11] Standard recommendations for women of average risk include annual two-view mammography in combination with at least annual physician-performed breast palpation beginning at age 50.

Controversies in Breast Cancer Screening

Screening in younger women. No study has definitively demonstrated a benefit of mammography with or without breast palpation in the 40- to 49-year-old age bracket, although several studies have strongly suggested an emerging trend. A recent meta-analysis of the available randomized controlled trials also found no evidence of a benefit in women between 40 and 49 in terms of cause-specific mortality.[12] Factors contributing to a lesser efficacy of screening in this cohort include a lower incidence of breast cancer in younger women, radiographically denser breasts that may conceal important mammographic abnormalities, and the detection of tumors that may be less amenable to therapy. Factors that further weigh against mammographic screening in this age group include potentially higher risk of radiation-induced breast cancer, both through higher sensitivity of the breast tissue and through a longer period of time over which a woman will be exposed.

The USPSTF currently finds that there is insufficient evidence to recommend for or against mammographic screening of women of usual risk in this age group.[26] The American Cancer Society, American College of Obstetrics and Gynecology, National Cancer Institute, and American Medical Association are in favor of screening. The American College of Physicians and the Canadian Task Force on the Periodic Health Examination recommend *against* screening in women less than 50 years old.[28]

Screening in older women. Most available studies address the use of breast palpation and mammography in women 40 to 75 years old. Evidence suggests that women between the ages of 50 and 69 derive the majority of mammography's benefit. A possible reason for a lack of efficacy for mammography in older women is the tendency for postmenopausal breast cancer to behave in a less aggressive manner and to respond readily to hormonal therapy. The use of mammography in women over the age of 75 should therefore be individualized. Most authorities recommend the continued use of physician-performed breast palpation with or without breast self-examination in women older than 75, while recommendations regarding mammography vary.[28]

Breast self-examination. Although widely recommended and taught, breast self-examination (BSE) has not been subjected to enough scientific study to allow specific recommendations regarding its use. It is likely that efficacy is linked to technique, method of instruction, and reinforcement. The most favorable estimates place sensitivity at approximately 25%. Since the false-positive rate, and hence specificity, is unknown, its value as a screening procedure, either alone or in combination with other modalities, cannot be determined. However, BSE may have higher sensitivity in younger women for whom mammography may be less desirable. If employed, it is best used either as a sole screening strategy when other modalities are unavailable or impractical or in combination with mammography and physician-performed breast examination, where it has the potential to detect interval tumors (cancers that become manifest between screening visits).[20]

Frequency of screening. The optimal frequency of screening is unknown, but data from several studies suggest that the mortality reduction increases as the interval between screenings decreases. Annual mammography is most widely recommended, BSE is generally recommended at monthly intervals, and a physician-performed breast palpation should be done at least annually.

Prostate Cancer. Prostate cancer is currently the most common malignancy, and the second most common cause of cancer-related death, in men in the United States (see Chapter 152). The incidence of prostate cancer increases steadily with advancing age, and may approach 100% in men past 90, if one includes small microscopic foci of disease. Since effective primary prevention is unclear, early diagnosis in the hopes of curative therapy has been emphasized as an effective strategy to combat this disease, which accounts for more than 35,000 deaths in the United States annually. The lifetime cumulative risk of developing prostate cancer is approximately 10% in men of average risk. Risk doubles for men who have a first-degree relative affected by prostate cancer, and the risk redoubles for each additional first-degree relative affected. For reasons that are not understood, African-Americans have a 50% increased risk of developing prostate cancer.

Despite the significant burden of disease from prostate cancer, poor knowledge regarding natural history and prognostic factors, as well as a lack of prospectively determined proof of the efficacy of screening in terms of disease-specific mortality reduction, poses significant decision-making difficulties for the physician regarding the potential benefit of screening.[14] Therefore the standard screening modalities are discussed in terms of their characteristics and potential efficacy in detecting disease, and remaining controversies and limitations are emphasized.

Digital Rectal Examination. An annual DRE is recommended for men over the age of 40 by the American Cancer Society, both to detect prostate cancer and to act as part of a screening strategy for colorectal cancer. Early studies suggested benefit for populations screened for prostate cancer by this method based on survival comparisons with historic controls. Furthermore, there seems to be a shift toward the detection of disease confined to the gland in serially screened patients. Although the sensitivity, specificity, and positive predictive values of DRE have been estimated, they are likely to be overestimates. Tumors arising in the medial lobe and transitional zones (approximately 30% of significant tumors) are not readily detectable. The DRE's ability to detect disease confined to the gland is apparently limited, since approximately 50% of tumors detected by DRE that have clinically limited-stage disease (stages A and B) are found to have more advanced disease after surgical staging. In addition, there is large interobserver variability. Despite this, 30% of significant prostate cancers are potentially detectable at a curable stage by DRE.

Prostate-Specific Antigen. The prostate-specific antigen (PSA) is a serine protease produced only in the prostate gland and detectable in the serum. Because both normal and malignant prostatic cells produce PSA, it can be elevated in a variety of prostate disorders, most commonly benign prostatic hyperplasia (BPH). Although the degree of elevation is generally higher with prostate cancer, there is enough overlap between benign and malignant disease, particularly early malignant disease, to necessitate further investigation. Values between 0 and 4 ng/ml are considered normal, although they are not inconsistent with early cancer. Values greater than 10 are highly specific for prostate cancer, although many patients with values in this range already have incurable disease. In the range from 4 to 10 ng/ml, the PSA levels generated by most curable prostate cancers, there is maximal overlap between benign and malignant disease, making interpretation difficult. Thus PSA has neither a sufficient sensitivity nor specificity to be useful as a sole screening method, and its routine use remains controversial for men of usual risk. If used, it should be combined with the DRE, since the combination of tests has improved sensitivity over either test alone.

Percent Free PSA. Percent free PSA compares the amount of free PSA to bound (complexed with protease inhibitors) in the serum. Free PSA is expressed as a percentage of total serum PSA. For those men whose PSA is between 4 and 10 ng/ml, and whose DRE is not suspicious for malignancy, measuring the percent free PSA can improve specificity to the point where approximately 20% of unnecessary biopsies can be avoided.[2]

Transrectal Ultrasound. Like DRE and PSA, transrectal ultrasound (TRUS) lacks the adequate sensitivity and specificity to be used as a sole screening method, especially considering its cost and lesser acceptability. Although it has the ability to detect many tumors missed by DRE, TRUS adds little when both the DRE and PSA are normal. At present, the main role of TRUS is in guiding biopsies.

Current Recommendations. The USPSTF and Canadian Task Force do not recommend screening for prostate cancer. The American Cancer Society and American Urological Association are in favor of screening men between the ages of 50 and 60. Most other authorities recommend counseling on risks and unknown benefits of screening prior to proceeding.[29]

Screening for Coronary Heart Disease Risk with Serum Cholesterol. Coronary heart disease (CHD) is the most common cause of death in the United States and in many Western countries and causes a large amount of morbidity. The established risk factors for CHD include male sex, family history of premature CHD, hypertension, cigarette smoking, sedentary lifestyle, obesity, diabetes, and elevated serum cholesterol. There is accumulating evidence elevated homocysteine levels are another important risk factor, which may be modifiable through vitamin supplementation, especially folate, pyridoxine, and vitamin B_{12}. Screening for elevated serum cholesterol has become a central focus of the periodic health examination. This is a result of the importance of CHD in the population; the establishment of a causal link between elevated serum cholesterol (specifically the low-density lipoprotein [LDL] fraction) and CHD; the synergy with and interplay between elevated serum cholesterol and other modifiable cardiovascular risk factors; the availability of management strategies that can significantly lower total and LDL cholesterol; and the growing amount of experimental evidence that interventions lowering serum total and LDL cholesterol result in a reduced risk of CHD and CHD-related mortality, and even overall mortality.

The National Cholesterol Education Program of the National Heart, Blood, and Lung Institute has issued guidelines for routine screening, detection, and follow-up and treatment of persons with elevated serum (LDL) cholesterol.[6] Although the optimal interval is not firmly established, screenings are recommended at least every 5 years for all adults over the age of 20, regardless of other cardiovascular risk factors. Screening is accomplished through the measurement of a random total serum cholesterol and a random high-density lipoprotein (HDL) cholesterol. Individuals with a total serum cholesterol under 200 mg/dl are considered to have a desirable cholesterol. Total serum cholesterols between 200 and 239 mg/dl are considered borderline, and a total serum cholesterol of 240 mg/dl or more is considered to be elevated. An HDL less than 35 mg/dl adds an additional risk factor to be used in following the guideline, while an HDL greater than 60 mg/dl subtracts a risk factor. A reanalysis of the subjects in the placebo arms of the Lipid Research Clinics Coronary Primary Prevention Trial[16] and participants in the Framingham study found that using the total cholesterol to HDL cholesterol ratio was superior to the LDL level in predicting risk of CHD events. A cutoff of 5.6 for women and 6.4 for men was suggested as identifying individuals at increased risk (roughly the 90th percentile).[13] Individuals with a ratio less than 4 are at lower than average risk, and this may be an appropriate time for primary prevention.

For individuals with either borderline or elevated total serum cholesterol, further investigation with a fasting lipoprotein electrophoresis and triglyceride is recommended in order to determine the LDL cholesterol and HDL cholesterol. LDL values less than 130 are desirable and do not warrant further specific intervention. Individuals with either borderline (130 to 159 mg%) or elevated (greater than 160 mg%) are candidates for varying degrees of dietary intervention and possibly drug therapy, depending on response to diet and the presence or absence of established atherosclerosis or other cardiovascular risk factors. The reader is referred to Chapter 71 for more information on the detection and management of lipid disorders.

Laboratory Testing. There is no evidence to support widespread screening with blood work or urinalysis in adults without specific clinical conditions or risk factors (except serum cholesterol, above). Many physicians, for example, believe that obtaining routine complete blood counts (CBCs) is indicated in premenopausal women, since as many as 30% may be iron deficient. Similarly, although the prevalence of both subclinical and overt hypothyroidism varies markedly among studies, up to 10% of women greater than 40 years old may be subclinically hypothyroid and 1% to 2% may be overtly hypothyroid. Some physicians therefore routinely assess thyroid-stimulating hormone (TSH) levels on women over 40 years of age. Although there is no experimental evidence of efficacy, this procedure may be cost-effective for older women.[3] Routine urinalysis, although not rigorously evaluated and not recommended by the USPSTF, is performed by some physicians in hopes of detecting early renal and bladder malignancies. Most physicians obtain a rapid plasma reagin test (RPR) or venereal disease research laboratories test (VDRL) at least once on adults, and periodically if the patients engage in high-risk sexual practices, have a history of STD, or reside in urban areas.

Immunizations and Chemoprophylaxis

Providing immunizations is one of the most important functions of the primary care physician. This important topic is addressed fully in Chapter 5 (Immunization), as are travel-related immunization procedures and chemoprophylaxis.

In light of the recent increase in incidence of tuberculosis, purified protein derivative (PPD) testing is an important preventive procedure both for certain individuals and for the community at large. Persons with known exposures, who are employed in health care–related fields or who have immigrated from endemic areas, should be screened and considered for appropriate chemoprophylaxis if positive. Nursing home residents should be screened with a two-step procedure on admission and annually. For a full discussion see Chapter 74.

SPECIAL ISSUES IN THE ELDERLY

Prevention

Prevention in the elderly should generally be focused on attempts to deter frailty and functional decline. The causal factors behind loss of vitality in the elderly include the realms of lifestyle, social factors, and the accumulation of chronic illness, in addition to the loss of physiologic reserve that is part of normative aging. Early research suggests that attention to modifiable factors such as proper diet, exercise, and avoidance of tobacco and alcohol, as well as attention to such common geriatric problems as sensory loss, social isolation, and depression, may go far in improving the aging process. Many of the topics touched on in this chapter are discussed more fully in the section on geriatric medicine in Chapter 8.

Whether or not an "elderly" person should be subjected to routine preventive services recommended for all adults deserves special consideration. There is a paucity of evidence regarding the risks and benefits of common preventive services in the elderly (here defined as individuals over the age of 75). The decisions should probably not be made based on some arbitrary age cutoff, but rather based on the patients' functional status and general health, some consideration of actuarial survival, the natural history and epidemiology of the target disorder, and the known magnitude of the potential benefits and risks in patients in whom the intervention has been studied.

Hearing Impairment

More than one third of all individuals over the age of 65 have audiometrically detectable hearing loss, and a substantial proportion report a significant decrease in the quality of their lives as a result. There is evidence linking hearing loss to social isolation, and possibly to depression and cognitive decline.

Given this significant burden of suffering, efforts at screening and detection seem advisable. However, such common bedside examination techniques as the whisper test, the finger rub test, and the tuning fork test are unlikely to be either sensitive or specific enough to serve as reliable screening tests. There is good evidence that a handheld audioscope performs very well in this regard, provided it is combined with visual inspection of the auditory canals and removal of any obstructing earwax. In addition, standardized questionnaires have been developed that focus on social or communication impairment as a result of hearing loss.

Once a potential hearing problem is uncovered through the use of a screening tool, formal audiologic evaluation should be arranged. Despite the real concerns about hearing aid compliance and the cost of these devices in the absence of Medicare reimbursement, many patients benefit greatly.

Visual Impairment

The suffering from visual impairment in older individuals is probably similar to that from hearing impairment. However, because glasses are less socially stigmatizing than hearing aids, and decreasing visual acuity interferes more with important activities like reading and driving, many persons seek eye examinations and corrective prescriptions from ophthalmologists and optometrists directly.

The major causes of visual decline in the elderly, other than refractive error, include glaucoma, senile macular degeneration, cataracts, and diabetic retinopathy. There is probably benefit to early detection of glaucoma, although the primary care physician is relatively limited in screening options. Schiøtz's tonometry is not widely recommended for screening, a result of its relative difficulty, operator dependency, and questionable reliability. Thus screening still lies in the hands of the specialist. As there is no effective treatment for senile macular degeneration, screening for this disease is probably unwarranted. Laser therapy for early proliferative diabetic retinopathy is effective in reducing the incidence of severe visual loss by as much as 50%; however, routine funduscopic examination is not sensitive enough to detect most instances of this disease in its early stages, before visual acuity is lost. Cataracts are readily detectable on routine ophthalmoscopic examination, but determining the amount of visual impairment attributable to them requires sophisticated methods, and there is probably no benefit to early treatment.

This is not to imply that primary care physicians should

not routinely ask about or examine their elderly patients' vision. Visual loss that has developed gradually may go unnoticed or unreported, or the patient may accept it as part of being old. Visual loss may be an important, yet reversible factor in patients presenting with depression, cognitive decline, falls and injuries, or other functional decline. Visual acuity is readily testable using a Snellen's wall chart or pocket visual screener. Patients with best corrected vision less than 20/40 or with decline since their last examination should be referred for further evaluation.

All patients older than 40 should probably have a routine eye examination by an ophthalmologist, with a follow-up examination at least every few years for patients with no problems uncovered. Patients with diabetes should have annual eye examinations by an ophthalmologist to screen for proliferative diabetic retinopathy and also in light of the higher incidence of glaucoma.

Screening for Cognitive Impairment

Recent studies have suggested that approximately 10% of all individuals over the age of 65 have dementia. That prevalence may increase to almost 50% in individuals over the age of 85. The vast majority of these individuals have Alzheimer's disease or other primary degenerative dementia; however, a substantial minority has a vascular cause. Despite the staggering prevalence, in most instances mild degrees of cognitive impairment go unrecognized by physicians. Most likely this is because the usual screening questions about orientation to person, place, and time, although meaningful when they are abnormal, lack sufficient sensitivity to detect most cases.

A number of brief, simple instruments are available to screen for dementia. One of the most widely used and best validated is the Folstein Mini-Mental Status Examination (MMSE) (see Box 8-2 in Chapter 8). It consists of 11 questions and tasks with a total possible score of 30. Scores greater than 24 are considered normal, whereas scores less than 24 are indicative of dementia and usually warrant further evaluation. The MMSE is relatively insensitive to the early loss of higher executive function, especially in individuals with a high educational background. A "normal" score cutoff should be adjusted downward for individuals with little formal education (see Chapters 8 and 158).

The value of early detection of dementia lies in the fact that a small number (perhaps one in 10 in some instances) are the result of reversible causes (e.g., vitamin B_{12} deficiency, thyroid disease) and may become irreversible if not recognized early. Vascular dementias may stabilize with aggressive control of cardiovascular risk factors, especially cigarette smoking and hypertension. The physician should always pay careful attention to potentially offending drugs, including alcohol. Even with an Alzheimer's-type dementia, in which no effective treatment of the underlying process exists, early diagnosis may lead to the prevention of unnecessary comorbidity and caregiver stress, through early referral to community-based services and home-care services. Symptomatic drug therapies are available that are most efficacious when employed in the earlier stages of disease.

Depression

Although no major authority recommends routine screening for depression in asymptomatic individuals, depression in the elderly may be quite subtle, making recognition and diagnosis difficult. It should be recognized that the elderly, particularly men, account for a disproportionate number of suicides, the majority of which are associated with depression and/or anxiety. Depression is commonly associated with early dementia, where it serves to increase the severity of symptoms, and, in general, is a common concomitant or cause of functional decline. Depression itself may present as cognitive decline, which may be erroneously attributed to a primary dementia. This pseudodementia, as it is commonly called, is an important cause of reversible dementia. Depression is extremely common following stroke in the elderly, in which case it may impede or prevent maximal recovery.

For all of these reasons, the physician should consider screening elderly patients for depressive symptoms. A simple, validated questionnaire (e.g., the geriatric depression scale) is useful in this regard. Once diagnosed, depression is readily treatable in the primary care setting, with referral or hospitalization reserved for patients who represent diagnostic or management dilemmas or who are actively suicidal. See Chapter 48 for a complete discussion of depression and its management.

Falls

Falls are a major cause of morbidity and mortality in community-dwelling elderly. One in three persons over the age of 75 falls each year, one fourth of those will suffer a serious injury, and one twentieth will suffer a fracture. The highest risk exists in patients with a history of falling. Other important risk factors include the use of sedative medication cognitive impairment, polypharmacy, abnormalities of balance and gait, and urinary incontinence. Environmenta hazards such as poor lighting, loose rugs, extension cords and low furniture also frequently play a role.

Although there may be some overlap, fall syndrome should be distinguished from syncope, which has its ow differential diagnosis and should prompt hospitalization i most instances. Physicians should ask older patients abou falls routinely, and follow up positive responses wit questions designed to accurately characterize the even keeping in mind that patients often give nonspecific answe (e.g., "I must have slipped").

The primary and secondary prevention of falls includes routine history and physical, with attention paid to excludin previously unrecognized acute illness, and evaluating ar simplifying the patient's medication regimen, eliminatir sedatives whenever possible. Orthostatic hypotension, whic can be caused by a variety of medications and medic conditions, should be sought out and offending agents conditions removed or treated. Vision, hearing, and cogniti status should be evaluated, and intervention or referral carri out when appropriate. Physical therapy or an exerci program may be of benefit in improving strength, gait, ar balance. Patients should be counseled about the value improving lighting, removing low furniture, and taping do loose rugs and lamp cords. The physician should consic the potential benefit of a home visit by the physician, o home evaluation from a certified home health agency (s Chapter 8).

Urinary Incontinence

The prevalence of urinary incontinence rises steadily w age, and women are more frequently affected than m Urinary incontinence is the single most common fac precipitating institutionalization in the elderly. Other important impairments and morbidity that can result from established urinary incontinence include social isolation, depression, and falls.

Urinary incontinence is a distressing and embarrassing problem that frequently is not volunteered by the patient. The physician should routinely ask in a neutral and direct fashion about difficulty with bladder control, paying attention to timing (diurnal vs. nocturnal), amount voided, dribbling, and any association between coughing or laughing and dribbling. A history of urgency or dysuria is also important to consider. Often, the office history and physical examination lead to a diagnosis and effective intervention without referral. For a more detailed discussion of the evaluation and treatment of urinary incontinence, see Chapters 8 and 151.

REFERENCES

1. Baker DB, Landrigan PJ: Occupationally related disorders, *Med Clin North Am* 74(2):441, 1990.
2. Catalona WJ, Partin AW, et al: Use of percentage of free prostate-specific antigen to enhance differentiation of prostate cancer from benign disease: a prospective multicenter clinical trial, *JAMA* 279:1542-1547, 1998.
3. Danese MD, Powe NR, et al: Screening for mild thyroid failure at the periodic health examination: a decision and cost-effectiveness analysis, *JAMA* 276:285-292, 1996.
4. Eddy DM: Screening for cervical cancer, *Ann Intern Med* 113:214, 1990.
5. Eddy DM: Screening for colorectal cancer, *Ann Intern Med* 113:373, 1990.
6. Expert Panel on Detection, Evaluation, and Treatment of High Blood Cholesterol in Adults: Summary of the Second Report of the National Cholesterol Education Program (NCEP) (Adult Treatment Panel II), *JAMA* 269:3015-3023, 1993.
7. Flemming MF, Manwell LB, et al: Brief physician advice for problem alcohol drinkers: a randomized controlled trial in community-based primary care practices, *JAMA* 277:1039-1045, 1997.
8. Frame PS: Can computerized reminder systems have an impact on preventive services in practice? *J Gen Intern Med* 5(Suppl):S112, 1990.
9. Hardcastle JD, Chamberlain JO, Robinson MHE, et al: Randomised controlled trial of faecal-occult-blood screening for colorectal cancer, *Lancet* 348:1472-1477, 1996.
10. Hayward RS, et al: Preventive care guidelines: 1991, *Ann Intern Med* 114:758, 1991.
11. Hurley SF, Kaldor JM: The benefits and risks of mammographic screening for breast cancer, *Epidemiol Rev* 14:101, 1992.
12. Kerlikowske K, Grady D, et al: Efficacy of screening mammography: a meta-analysis, *JAMA* 273:149-154, 1995.
13. Kinosian B, Glick H, Garland G: Cholesterol and coronary heart disease: predicting risks by levels and ratios, *Ann Intern Med* 121(9):641-647, 1994.
14. Kramer BS, et al: Prostate cancer screening: what we know and what we need to know, *Ann Intern Med* 119:914, 1993.
15. Kronborg O, Fenger C, Olsen J, et al: Randomised study of screening for colorectal cancer with faecal-occult-blood test, *Lancet* 348:1467-1471, 1996.
16. Lipid Research Clinics Program: The Lipid Research Clinics Coronary Primary Prevention Trial results: I. Reduction in incidence of coronary heart disease, *JAMA* 251:351-364, 1984.
17. Lowenstein SR, Hunt D: Injury prevention in primary care, *Ann Intern Med* 113(4):261, 1990.
18. Mandel JS, Bond JH, Church TR, et al: Reducing mortality from colorectal cancer by screening for fecal occult blood, *N Engl J Med* 328:1365-1371, 1993.
19. Morrison AS: Screening for cancer of the breast, *Epidemiol Rev* 15(1):244, 1993.
20. O'Malley MS, Fletcher SW: Screening for breast cancer with breast self-examination: a critical review, *JAMA* 257:2196, 1987.
21. Polen MR, Friedman GD: United States Preventive Services Task Force: automobile injury—selected risk factors and prevention in the health care setting, *JAMA* 259(1):76, 1988.
22. Sassetti MR: Domestic violence, *Prim Care* 20(2):289, 1993.
23. Slap GB: The periodic health examination and adolescent pregnancy, *Ann Intern Med* 109(9):692, 1988.
24. Stringham P, Weitzman M: Violence counseling in the routine health care of adolescents, *J Adolesc Health Care* 9:389, 1988.
25. Towler BP, Irwig L, Glasziou P, et al: Screening for colorectal cancer using the faecal occult blood test, Hemocult (Cochrane Review). In *The Cochrane Library*, 4, 1998; Oxford: Update Software.
26. US Preventive Services Task Force: *Guide to clinical preventive services*, ed 2, Alexandria, Va, 1996, International Medical, p 73.
27. US Preventive Services Task Force: *Guide to clinical preventive services*, ed 2, Alexandria, Va, 1996, International Medical, pp 89-90.
28. US Public Health Service: *Clinician's handbook of preventive services*, ed 2, Washington, DC, 1998, US Government Printing Office, pp 259-260.
29. US Public Health Service: *Clinician's handbook of preventive services*, ed 2, Washington, DC, 1998, US Government Printing Office, p 278.

CHAPTER 5

Immunizations and Travel

Julie Kaufmann

Immunizations are one of the most cost-effective medical interventions for an individual and the public health. Although the prevention of disease in an individual is readily achievable, the ultimate goal is the elimination of disease by maintaining a high level of immunity in the population. Unfortunately, immunizations are not a part of routine care in many adult medicine practices. As a result, a substantial proportion of the morbidity and mortality from vaccine-preventable diseases occurs in older adolescents and in adults.

GENERAL CONSIDERATIONS

The recommendations for vaccinations in the United States come from the Advisory Committee on Immunization Practices (ACIP). The American College of Physicians also publishes guidelines. Recommendations are based on an individual's risk of exposure to the disease, susceptibility to the disease, and the risk of transmitting the disease to others. The characteristics of the immunobiologic (vaccine or immune globulin), scientific knowledge about the principles of immunization, and the risk, benefit, and cost of the immunobiologic are also considered.

Most vaccine-preventable illnesses and disease exposures requiring postexposure prophylaxis must be reported to the local or state health department. Public health officials rely on the reporting of vaccine-preventable illnesses to evaluate and plan prevention strategies on a local level. In addition, the data are used to evaluate national policies, practices, and strategies for future vaccination programs.

Principles of Vaccination

Active immunization uses immunogens to simulate a natural infection, which results in an antitoxic, antiinvasive, or neutralizing activity in the recipient. Such immunogens include live attenuated virus, inactivated virus, and bacterial proteins or polysaccharides. Some agents induce lifelong protection, some provide partial protection, and some must be readministered for continued effectiveness. The efficacy of the vaccine is defined by the protection against natural disease. The antibody response is an indirect measure of protection because in some cases the immunologic reaction responsible for protection is poorly understood; in this instance the serum antibody concentrations are not always predictive of protection.

Passive immunization with immune globulin (IG) is used (1) to provide immediate antibody levels for individuals who have recently been exposed or who soon may be exposed to a disease; (2) to provide antibody for individuals who are immunocompromised and would be expected to have a poor immunogenic response to an illness exposure or to a previous active immunization; or (3) to help suppress the effects of a toxin when a disease is already present. Pooled IG is derived from a large pool of donors so is likely to contain antibodies to hepatitis A and measles. The disease-specific immune globulins HBIG, TIG, HRIG, and VZIG are derived from selected donor pools with high titers to the desired antibody (Box 5-1).

Records, Route, Site, and Dosage

Physicians should maintain a permanent vaccination record for each patient as required by law. This record should include type of immunization, site and route of vaccination, lot number and expiration date, and date given. Patients should be given information on the risks and benefits of immunization and a copy of their own vaccination record for future reference.

The route of immunization is important for each vaccine. Vaccines developed for intramuscular (IM) use should not be given subcutaneously because the immune response may be decreased, and risks include local irritation, inflammation, and necrosis from the adjuvant in the vaccine. The preferred site for adult IM injections is the deltoid muscle, where the risk of vascular and neural injury is low. It is preferable to avoid giving two IM injections in the same limb, especially if one is known to cause a local reaction. Except for the administration of large doses of IG, the buttock should not be used routinely as a site for IM injection because of proximity of the sciatic nerve and because the depth of fat may make performing a true IM injection difficult. If the buttock must be used to accommodate large-volume injections (e.g., IG) or multiple doses of vaccines, the upper outer quadrant is preferred. In general, no more than 5 ml should be given at one site.

If it is necessary to give more than one vaccine in a limb, the vaccine sites should be at least 1 to 2 inches (2.5 to 5 cm) apart. Whenever administering any vaccine with an IG, the sites chosen should be remote from each other (e.g., deltoid for vaccine, buttock for IG).

When pooled IG is indicated and IM injections are contraindicated, such as in patients with severe thrombocytopenia or severe coagulation disorder (e.g., hemophilia), an intravenous preparation can be used at a dosage of 110 mg/kg. Because intravenous IG preparations are derived from smaller donor pools, they may not be as effective for hepatitis A or measles prophylaxis, and their efficacy for these purposes is unknown.

In adults a 20- to 25-gauge, 1- to 1½-inch needle is used for IM injections (care should be taken to perform a true IM injection in obese patients); a 23- to 25-gauge, ⅝- to ¾-inch needle for subcutaneous injections; and a 25- to 27-gauge, ⅜- to ¾-inch needle for intradermal injections.

Vaccine Schedules and Missed Doses

The recommendations for the dosage of vaccines are derived from clinical experience, experimental trials, and theoretic considerations. Adherence to the recommended schedules provides the most predictable outcome in terms of side effects and clinical efficacy. If a dose is delayed during a vaccination series, the schedule should be continued and not restarted, since generally no decline occurs in final antibody levels. Giving doses at less than the recommended interval, however, should be avoided because it may weaken the immune response, and some vaccines are more likely to produce local or systemic symptoms if given too soon. If a vaccine is given earlier than the recommended time interval, it should not be considered part of a series.

Minor illness with or without fever is not a contraindication to receiving a vaccine, especially if poor compliance is a

Box 5-1. Agencies and Abbreviations

Agencies

Morbidity and Mortality Weekly Report (MMWR)
http://www2.cdc.gov/mmwr

US Department of Health and Human Services
Public Health Service
Centers for Disease Control and Prevention (CDC)
National Center for Prevention Services
Division of Quarantine
Atlanta, GA 30333
1-404-639-3311
http://www.cdc.gov/nip

Traveler's hotline: CDC
1-404-332-4559
http://www.cdc.gov (select traveler's health)

Vaccine Adverse Event Reporting System (VAERS)
PO Box 1100
Rockville, MD 20849-1100
1-800-822-7967
http://www.cdc.gov/nip/VAERS.htm

Abbreviations

ACIP Advisory Committee on Immunization Practices
WHO World Health Organization
Td tetanus and diphtheria vaccine
MMR measles, mumps, and rubella vaccine
IPV inactivated poliovirus vaccine
HBV hepatitis B vaccine
HAV hepatitis A vaccine
HbCV hemophilus influenza *(Haemophilus influenzae)* b conjugate vaccine

IG immune globulin
HBIG hepatitis B IG
VZIG varicella-zoster IG
TIG tetanus IG
HRIG human rabies IG

concern. Moderate or severe illness with or without fever is a contraindication. Vaccination should be delayed, if possible, so that symptoms of the illness are not mistaken for side effects of the vaccine, and to ensure an optimum immune response to the vaccine.

Multiple Vaccines and Immune Globulins

The administration of multiple vaccines is often desirable to minimize patient visits for vaccination and increase compliance, especially if patient follow-up is uncertain. It may also be necessary if several vaccinations are needed in a short time in preparation for travel abroad. Table 5-1 summarizes recommendations for the simultaneous and nonsimultaneous administration of immunobiologics. If the recommended time intervals cannot be followed, serologic testing should be performed or the second vaccination repeated subsequently.

IG preparations and other antibody-containing blood products do not interfere with the immune response to inactivated vaccines, but they do interfere with the antibody response to live vaccines, with the exception of oral typhoid and yellow fever vaccine. Since the immune response to a live vaccine occurs 1 to 2 weeks after vaccination, any IG-containing product should be given 2 weeks after an MMR or 3 weeks after varicella vaccine. The time interval between administering an IG-containing product and then a measles-containing vaccine appears to be dose dependent. The suggested intervals are based on the interference of the immune response to measles vaccine for 5 months after a dose of 80 mg/kg of IG (half-life about 30 days). In general the ranges and intervals are as follows: for up to 10 mg IG/kg, wait 3 months; for 20 mg IG/kg, 4 months; 25 to 50 mg IG/kg, 5 months; 60 to 100 mg IG/kg, 6 months; 160 mg IG/kg, 7 months; 400 mg IG/kg, 8 months; 1000 mg IG/kg, 10 months; and for 2000 mg IG/kg, wait 11 months. Packed red blood cells have an estimated 60 mg IG/kg, and platelet products have 160 mg IG/kg. For simplicity, the CDC recommends waiting 5 months after any IG-containing product and the administration of varicella vaccine. If a live vaccine must be administered within the recommended interval, serologic testing should be performed to ensure an adequate response, or the vaccination should be repeated after the appropriate interval.

Hypersensitivity and Local Reactions

Some vaccines contain small amounts of antibiotics, preservatives, and animal protein that may induce hypersensitivity reactions (see Contraindications in Table 5-2). Any person with a known anaphylactic response to these components should not receive the vaccine. Most often an allergy to neomycin is not an anaphylactic response but a contact dermatitis. This cell-mediated response is not a contraindication for vaccines containing neomycin. Some vaccines (e.g., tetanus/diptheria, varicella, parenteral typhoid, cholera, plague) typically cause fever, local redness, and soreness. These reactions appear to be toxic rather than hypersensitive. If an urticarial reaction to any vaccine is noted or if a person has a history of a hypersensitivity reaction to a vaccine component, the recipient should have skin testing before a decision is made to continue or discontinue the vaccine.

Intramuscular preparations of IG can be associated with minor reactions (e.g., headache, chills, flushing, nausea) and a pyogenic reaction with high fever. Rarely a hypersensitivity reaction can occur, most often in people with immunoglobulin A (IgA) deficiency. None of the IG preparations has been associated with the transmission of hepatitis B or human immunodeficiency virus (HIV). One product was associated with hepatitis C transmission, but the manufacturing process has been changed.

The Vaccine Adverse Event Reporting System (VAERS) monitors serious adverse reactions to immunobiologics (see Box 5-1). The reported information helps both to improve the general knowledge about adverse reactions, since these reactions are indeed rare, and to provide a database for reactions to newer vaccines. VAERS is also used to stimulate research to confirm a causal association and to identify risk factors for adverse events. Any unusual or severe reaction should be reported to VAERS.

GENERAL RECOMMENDATIONS

To reduce the morbidity and mortality of vaccine-preventable illnesses, vaccination surveillance should continue throughout adolescence and adulthood and should be part of every routine and episodic visit. The ACIP specifically recommends a systematic immunization review at age 50 to improve

Table 5-1. Administration of Multiple Vaccines

Vaccine combination	Recommended minimum interval between doses
[Tw]o or more killed vaccines	None. May be administered simultaneously or at any interval between doses. (If possible cholera, parenteral typhoid and plague vaccines should be given on separate occasions to avoid accentuating their side effects.)
[Ki]lled and live vaccines	None. May be administered simultaneously or at any interval between doses. (Cholera vaccine with yellow fever vaccine is the exception. These vaccines should be given separately at least 3 weeks apart, or antibody response to each may be suboptimal.*)
[Tw]o or more live vaccines*	May be administered simultaneously. If given separately, they must be separated by at least 4 weeks. Oral typhoid vaccine can be administered at any time before, with, or after parenteral live vaccines.
[Liv]e vaccine and purified protein derivative (PPD)*	May be administered simultaneously. If given separately, PPD should be given 4 to 6 weeks after live vaccine.

[*If g]uidelines for time intervals cannot be followed, vaccine should be repeated after appropriate interval, or vaccine antibody titers should be measured.
[Mod]ified from CDC: General recommendations on immunization: recommendations of the Advisory Committee on Immunization Practices (ACIP), *MMWR* 43(RR-1):15 and 16, 1994.

immunization rates in adults. To ensure patients' optimal protection against vaccine-preventable illnesses, physicians must learn to evaluate patients according to age criteria and individual risks for specific illnesses. These risks include concomitant medical illnesses, lifestyle, occupational and environmental exposures, ethnicity, and travel plans. Foreign-born persons need to be evaluated for vaccines that they may not have received in childhood (Table 5-2).

All adults should have received a primary tetanus and diphtheria toxoid series (Td) and should be given a booster every 10 years starting in adolescence. Some authorities recommend a single booster at age 50. If the primary series status is unknown, it should be given.

Adults born before 1957 can be considered immune to measles and mumps. In this age group, women of childbearing potential should be tested for rubella antibody and should be vaccinated if not immune. Persons born after 1956 should have been given one dose of measles, mumps, and rubella (MMR) vaccine in childhood at or after 12 months of age or should have laboratory evidence of immunity to all three components of the vaccine. For measles and mumps but not rubella, a physician-diagnosed case may also serve as evidence for immunity.

All adults should be immune to varicella. This can be documented by a reported illness or laboratory immunity. If neither is present, the vaccine should be given.

Adults who are 65 years or older should receive a single dose of pneumococcal vaccine and a yearly influenza vaccine. Their caregivers and household and close family members should be given influenza vaccine as well.

SPECIAL RECOMMENDATIONS

Certain vaccines may be recommended for persons with particular medical conditions, living situations, or lifestyles. Other vaccines are to be avoided.

Pregnancy and Breast-feeding

Since many young women receive care in obstetrics and gynecology or family-planning practices, health care providers in these settings should be well versed in vaccination principles and strategies. As part of ongoing preventive health, all women should be evaluated for their risk of vaccine-preventable illnesses and updated on their immunizations.

In addition to any other vaccines that are indicated, women of childbearing age in particular should be current for measles, rubella, and varicella vaccination recommendations because these infections can result in morbidity and mortality in the fetus and newborn. Pregnant women should be tested for hepatitis B infection, and if they are infected, the newborn and household and sexual contacts should be evaluated and treated appropriately. The influenza vaccine should be given to pregnant women who will be beyond their first trimester during the influenza season because of the higher risk for hospitalization. In addition, pregnant women who have medical conditions that increase their risk of complications of influenza should be vaccinated regardless of the stage of pregnancy.

Certain inactivated viral or bacterial vaccines and toxoids are thought to be safe during pregnancy, but some are better studied than others (see Table 5-2). It is prudent to wait until the second trimester to reduce the theoretic risk of teratogenicity. Vaccination should not be delayed, however, if developing the vaccine-preventable illnesses is a risk during the first trimester. Live vaccines should not be given to a pregnant woman or a woman planning to become pregnant within 3 months (1 month for varicella). Household contacts of pregnant women can receive live vaccines. The inadvertent MMR to a pregnant woman has not been associated as yet with congenital rubella syndrome, but the risk of spontaneous abortion is increased in the first trimester. (See sections on individual vaccines for administering the live vaccines yellow fever and oral typhoid during pregnancy.) There is no known risk to the fetus from passive immunization with any IG preparation; they are safe to give in pregnancy and should be used as indicated.

A pregnant woman who needs a varicella, measles, mumps, or rubella vaccination should receive these vaccines immediately after delivery, even if she has received anti-Rh_0 IG or any IG-containing products, so that the opportunity for vaccination is not lost. In this instance, serologic testing should be performed to ensure adequate immune response or the vaccination repeated at the appropriate time interval (see Multiple Vaccines and Immune Globulins).

Inactivated vaccines pose no special risk to breast-feeding mothers or their infants. Live vaccines multiply in the body, but most are not excreted in breast milk. Although rubella can be excreted in the breast milk, it causes only an asymptomatic infection. No data are available for the varicella vaccine, but it is believed to be safe. Giving yellow fever vaccine or oral typhoid vaccine is not contraindicated in breast-feeding women.

Immunocompromise and Other High-Risk Medical Conditions

Immunocompromise may be the result of infection with HIV, hematologic or generalized malignancies, chemotherapeutic or immunosuppressive agents, radiation, steroids, functional or anatomic asplenia, and complement or immunoglobulin deficiencies. Certain medical conditions ar associated with defects in host defense and therefore with higher incidence of illness or with increased morbidity an mortality from illness because of poor physiologic reserv The degree of immunocompromise can vary with stage c disease and treatment and should be determined on a individual basis.

Immunizations should be given early in the course of th disease to optimize the immune response. In general, patien can be divided into those with HIV, those with seve immunocompromise not resulting from HIV, and those who illness does not dictate the avoidance of any vaccine but do necessitate additional vaccines not given to healthy adul Table 5-3 lists the vaccines recommended for the individuals as well as contraindicated vaccines.

Human Immunodeficiency Virus Infection. Persc with HIV should be evaluated for their vaccination histc and their risk of vaccine-preventable illnesses, as outlined all adults. In addition, certain vaccines are especia recommended because of increased disease susceptibility severity.

Inactivated viral or bacterial vaccines and toxoids can given to HIV patients. In general, HIV-infected individu should not be given live virus vaccines because of the risk uncontrolled viral replication. If indicated, however, an M is recommended for those with asymptomatic HIV infec

Text continued on p

... United States 18 Years of Age and Older

Name	Primary schedule and booster(s)	Indications*	Side effects	Contraindications*	Pregnancy†
Tetanus and diphtheria adsorbed toxoid (Td)	Two 0.5-ml IM doses 1 month apart; third dose 6-12 months after second; booster every 10 years (see Table 5-4 for postexposure prophylaxis).	All adults; check for receipt of primary series in refugees, immigrants, and foreign-born patients.	Local erythema and pain; rarely, anaphylaxis, neuropathy encephalitis, Guillain-Barré syndrome.	Neurologic or anaphylactic reaction to previous dose (can be given TIG for postexposure prophylaxis).	Use if indicated; no confirmed risk to fetus.
Measles (as MMR) live virus	One 0.5 ml SC dose; second dose at least 1 month later (or immunity by antibody titer or physician-diagnosed measles).	Adults born after 1956 need one dose; additional dose on entering school, long-term correctional facility, or health care work; during outbreaks; and for foreign travel. Adults born before 1957 are considered immune, but giving one dose to health care workers at risk of exposure may be prudent.	Local erythema and pain, low-grade fever, rash, arthralgias 1 to 21 days after vaccination; rarely, high fever 5-12 days after vaccination; extremely rarely, anaphylaxis and thrombocytopenia within 2 months.	Anaphylaxis to chicken eggs, gelatin, neomycin, or previous dose.	Contraindicated, but no confirmed risk to fetus.
Mumps (as MMR) live virus	One 0.5-ml SC dose (or immunity by antibody titer or physician-diagnosed mumps).	All adults born after 1956. Adults born before 1957 are considered immune.	As for measles.	As for measles.	As for measles.
Rubella (as MMR) live virus	One 0.5-ml SC dose (or immunity by antibody titer).	Adults born after 1956; women of childbearing potential.	As for measles.	As for measles. Rubella vaccine from human diploid cells can be given to persons with anaphylaxis to chicken eggs.	As for measles.
Varicella live virus	Two 0.5-ml SC doses separated by 1 or 2 months (or immunity by reported illness or antibody titers).	All adults.	Typically, local pain and erythema; occasionally fever and varicella-like rash; rarely, zoster.	Anaphylaxis to gelatin, neomycin, or previous dose.	Contraindicated —unknown risk to fetus
Hepatitis B recombinant DNA–derived surface antigen particles	Two 1.0-ml IM doses 1 month apart; third dose 5 months after second; higher dose and more frequent schedule for persons with chronic renal failure or immunocompromise. Engerix also approved for dosing at 0, 1, 2, and 12 months to give three doses for upcoming exposure.	Persons with multiple sex partners or sexually transmitted diseases; male homosexuals; injection drug users, persons whose sex partner is in high-risk group; frequent recipients of blood products; hemodialysis patients; health care or public safety workers with frequent blood or body fluid exposures; institutionalized, developmentally disabled patients and their staff; household and sexual contacts of chronically infected carriers (for contacts of acutely infected persons, see Table 5-5); certain travelers to high-risk areas. Consider for persons from endemic area residing in U.S. community with similar culture.	Local erythema and pain; rarely, fever; extemely rarely, anaphylaxis.	Anaphylactic reaction to common baker's yeast, thimerosal, or previous dose.	Use if indicated; no reported risk to fetus.

Modified and updated from CDC: Update on adult immunization: recommendations of the Advisory Committee on Immunization Practices (ACIP), *MMWR* 40(RR-12):60-66 and 82-86, 1991.
IM, Intramuscular; *SC*, subcutaneous.
*See text and Table 5-3 for recommendations and contraindications regarding persons with HIV, severe immunocompromise, or special medical conditions. See Travel and Table 5-7 for more specific travel recommendations.
†If able, it is prudent to wait to vaccinate until after first trimester to minimize concern about teratogenicity. As a contraindication, "pregnancy" also includes the time 3 months (1 month for varicella vaccine) before conception. Breast-feeding is not a contraindication to any vaccine, but more information is available about some vaccines than others (see text).

Continued

Table 5-2. Immunizations for Adults in the United States 18 Years of Age and Older—cont'd

Name	Primary schedule and booster(s)	Indications*	Side effects	Contraindications*	Pregnancy†
Hepatitis A inactivated virus	Two 1.0-ml IM doses given 6 to 12 months apart.	Male homosexuals, bisexuals, injection drug users, persons with chronic liver disease or frequently receiving clotting factor concentrates, certain travelers to high-risk areas.	Local erythema and pain; headache, malaise.	Severe reaction to previous dose.	Use if indicated; unknown risk to fetus.
Pneumococcal bacterial polysaccharide	One 0.5-ml IM or SC dose; single revaccination after 5 years for persons with functional or anatomic asplenia, chronic renal failure, nephrotic syndrome, organ transplants, HIV, or severe immunocompromise and for those vaccinated 5 years ago when younger than 65 years and now older than 65 years.	Persons 65 years and older; patients with chronic pulmonary (except asthma) or cardiovascular disease, diabetes, alcoholism, cirrhosis, chronic renal failure, nephrotic syndrome, organ transplantation, asplenia, or immunocompromise from any cause; homeless persons, Native Alaskans; Apache Native Americans.	Local erythema and pain; low-grade fever.	More severe local reactions in persons revaccinated in less than 24 months; anaphylaxis to previous dose or any vaccine component.	Use if indicated; unknown risk to fetus.
Influenza inactivated virus	One 0.5-ml IM dose, seasonally.	As for pneumococcal vaccine (except Native Americans); asthmatic patients, caregivers and household contacts of vaccine candidates, health care workers, any adult desiring to reduce risk, travelers to tropics or southern hemisphere at risk of poor outcome.	Local pain and erythema; malaise; low-grade fever; headache.	Severe reaction to previous dose; anaphylaxis to chicken eggs.	Given to women in second or third trimester during influenza season, or if high risk give in first trimester; no confirmed risk to fetus.
Hemophilus influenza type b (HbCV) bacterial polysaccharide, conjugated	Dose for adults has not been determined; generally, one 0.5-ml IM dose is used.	Adults at highest theoretic risk; functional or anatomic asplenia; Hodgkin's disease; consider for HIV-infected persons.	Local erythema and pain; malaise; fever.	Hypersensitivity reaction to conjugated-protein carriers.	Use if indicated; no reported risk to fetus.
Meningococcal bacterial polysaccharide (serogroups A,C, W135, and Y)	One 0.5-ml SC dose; consider revaccination at 3 to 5 years.	Adults with functional or anatomic asplenia or with terminal complement component deficiency; prophylaxis during outbreaks if serogroup represented in vaccine; travelers to endemic areas; consider for college students living in dormatories.	Local erythema and pain.	Severe reaction to previous dose.	Use if indicated; no reported risk to fetus.
Lyme recombinant DNA–derived lipoprotein	Three 0.5-ml IM doses given at 0, 1, and 12 months.	Adults who live and work in wooded or grassy areas that harbor Lyme-bearing ticks.	Local pain and erythema; low-grade fever; arthralgias.	Anaphylaxis to yeast, kanamycin, or previous dose.	Register with manufacturer; unknown risk to fetus.
Rabies human diploid cell (HDCV), rabies vaccine adsorbed (RVA), chick embryo cell culture (PCEC); inactivated virus	Preexposure prophylaxis: 1.0-ml IM doses on days 0, 7, and 28; or 0.1-ml ID doses (HDCV only) on days 0, 7, and 21 or 28; booster dose or antibody titers every 2 years.	Veterinarians, animal handlers, certain laboratory workers, spelunkers, travelers for longer than 1 month to countries where rabies is endemic in domesticated and wild animals.	Local erythema and pain (in 75%), malaise; fever; headache; abdominal pain; myalgias; dizziness (5%-40%); anaphylaxis (0.1%); mild immune complex hypersensitivity reaction in persons given	Severe reaction to previous dose. Consult public health department if postexposure prophylaxis is needed.	Use if indicated; unknown risk to fetus.

	preexposure prophylaxis or previous postexposure prophylaxis, two 1.0-ml IM doses on days 0 and 3; or (2) all other persons, HRIG (20 IU/kg) up to half dose to infiltrate wound and remaining dose IM, with five 1.0-ml IM vaccine doses on days 0, 3, 7, 14, and 28.				
Polio inactivated virus (IPV)	IPV preferred for primary vaccination; two 0.5-ml SC doses 1-2 months apart; third dose 6-12 months after second; one booster dose for previously immunized travelers. For accelerated schedule see text.	Travelers to high-risk countries, health care workers exposed to virus.	Rarely, poliomyelitis (OPV); local pain and erythema; rarely, fever (IPV).	Anaphylactic reaction to previous dose, to neomycin or streptomycin (and for IPV, polymixin B). Household contacts and nursing personnel of immunocompromised persons should be given IPV, not OPV.	Use if high risk of infection, no confirmed risk to fetus.
Typhoid live bacteria (oral), inactivated whole bacteria (SC), bacterial polysaccharide (IM)	Four oral doses on days 0, 2, 4, and 6 with series repeated every 5 years; or two 0.5-ml SC doses 4 weeks apart or three SC doses weekly with booster every 3 years; or one 1.0-ml IM dose with a booster every 2 years.	Certain travelers to high-risk areas, certain laboratory workers, household contacts of chronic carrier	Live: nausea, abdominal discomfort, rash; inactivated: local pain and erythema; rarely, fever, malaise, headache.	Severe reaction to previous dose.	Use parenteral form if high risk of infection; no confirmed risk to fetus.
Yellow fever live virus	One 0.5-ml SC dose 10 days to 10 years before travel; booster dose every 10 years.	Certain travelers to areas where yellow fever is endemic.	Low-grade fever; headache; myalgias (2%-5%); extremely rarely, encephalitis.	Severe reaction to previous dose; anaphylaxis to chicken eggs.	Postponement of travel is preferable. Vaccinate if at high risk; attempt waiver if at low risk; unknown risk to fetus.
Japanese encephalitis inactivated virus	Three 0.5-ml SC doses on days 0, 7, and 30; need for booster doses unknown.	Certain travelers to areas where Japanese encephalitis is endemic.	Local erythema and pain; fever; malaise nausea; abdominal discomfort: anaphylaxis precautions.	Severe reaction to a previous dose. Persons with atopy are at risk of severe reactions.	Weigh risk vs benefit; unknown risk to fetus.
Cholera inactivated bacteria	Two 0.5-ml IM or SC doses; or two 0.2-ml ID doses given 1 to 4 weeks apart; booster dose every 6 months.	Travelers to areas that require vaccination or certain travelers at high risk.	Local erythema and pain; fever; malaise.	Severe reaction to previous dose.	Use if high risk of infection; unknown risk to fetus.

Modified and updated from CDC: Update on adult immunization: recommendations of the Advisory Committee on Immunization Practices (ACIP), *MMWR* 40(RR-12):60-66 and 82-86, 1991.
ID, intradermal; *TIG*, tetanus immune globulin; *HIV*, human immunodeficiency virus; *HRIG*, human rabies immune globulin.

Table 5-3. Recommendations for Persons with Medical Conditions Requiring Special Vaccination Considerations

Condition	Td	MMR	Varicella	HBV	HAV	Pneumovax§	Influenza‖	HbCV	Meningococcal	IPV	Other live vaccines#	Other killed vaccines**
HIV infection	Rou	Rou/Contr*	Contr†	Rou‡	Rou	Rec	Rec	Cons	Rou	Rou	Contr	Rou
Severe immunocompromise§§	Rou	Contr	Contr†	Rou‡	Rou	Rec	Rec	Rou‖‖	Rou	Rou	Contr	Rou
Renal failure	Rou	Rou	Rou	Rec‡	Rou	Rec	Rec	Rou	Rou	Rou	Rou	Rou
Diabetes	Rou	Rou	Rou	Rou	Rou	Rec	Rec	Rou	Rou	Rou	Rou	Rou
Chronic liver disease	Rou	Rou	Rou	Rou	Rec	Rec	Rec	Rou	Rou	Rou	Rou	Rou
Cardiac disease	Rou	Rou	Rou	Rou	Rou	Rec	Rec	Rou	Rou	Rou	Rou	Rou
Pulmonary disease	Rou	Rou	Rou	Rou	Rou	Rec	Rec	Rou	Rou	Rou	Rou	Rou
Alcoholism	Rou	Rou	Rou	Rou	Rou	Rec	Rec	Rou	Rou	Rou	Rou	Rou
Functional/anatomic asplenia	Rou	Rou	Rou	Rou	Rou	Rec##	Rec	Rec##	Rec##	Rou	Rou	Rou
Terminal complement deficiency	Rou	Rou	Rou	Rou	Rou	Rou	Rou	Rou	Rec	Rou	Rou	
Clotting factor disorders	Rou	Rou	Rou	Rec	Rec	Rou	Rou	Rou	Rou	Rou	Rou	Rou

Modified and updated from CDC: Recommendations of the Advisory Committee on Immunization Practices (ACIP): use of vaccines and immune globulins in persons with altered immunocompetence, *MMWR* 42(RR-4):16 and 17, 1993.

Rou, Routine as outlined for all adults; *Contr,* contraindicated; *Rec,* recommended; *Cons,* consider vaccination; see Box 5-1 for vaccine abbreviations.

*For asymtomatic, nonseverely immunocompromised persons with human immunodeficiency virus (HIV), MMR can be used; it is contraindicated in severely immunocompromised persons. MMR can be considered in symptomatic HIV patients without severe immunocompromise.

†Varicella can be given to household members and caregivers, but if varicella-like rash develops after vaccination, contact should be avoided.

‡Recommended for persons with severe chronic renal failure approaching or already receiving dialysis, and higher doses should be given. Antibody titers should be measured after vaccination in these patients and in those with HIV or severe immunocompromise (who may require higher doses) to ensure adequate response. Yearly titers should be measured in dialysis patients.

§Pneumovax should be repeated in 5 years for patients in whom vaccine is recommended. Asthma without chronic obstructive pulmonary disease is not an indication for the vaccine.

‖Influenza vaccine should also be given to caregivers and household members.

#Includes bacille Calmette-Guérin, vaccinia, oral typhoid, yellow fever (if exposure cannot be avoided, persons with HIV can be given yellow fever vaccine; see text).

**Includes rabies (check postvaccination titers in HIV or severely immunocompromised persons), Lyme, inactivated typhoid, cholera, plague, and anthrax.

§§Severe immunocompromise can result from congenital immunodeficiency, leukemia, lymphoma, malignancy, organ transplant, chemotherapy, radiation therapy, or high-dose corticosteroids.

‖‖Only for persons with Hodgkin's disease.

##Give at least 2 weeks in advance of elective splenectomy.

without evidence of severe immunosuppression because of a high risk of exposure to measles. Measles infection in these patients can be serious, and in limited studies the vaccine has been safe. For symptomatic patients without evidence of severe immunosuppression, the vaccine should be considered in high-risk situations. The vaccine is contraindicated for those with severe immunosuppression because of poor efficacy. Measles pneumonitis has occurred in a severely immunosuppressed HIV patient, and vaccine-induced morbidity has occurred in other immunocompromised patients.

Any needed immunization should be given early in the course of the disease rather than later, when the immune response may be suboptimal. The efficacy of vaccines in this group of patients has not been studied. In theory, people who do not respond adequately to initial vaccination may respond to higher doses of vaccine or to additional doses, but this also has not been evaluated.

Severe Immunocompromise Without HIV Infection. Individuals can be severely immunocompromised as a result of hematologic or general malignancy, chemotherapy, radiation therapy, high doses of corticosteroids (generally the equivalent of 20 mg/day prednisone for longer than 2 weeks), or other immunosuppressive therapies. The degree of immunocompromise should be evaluated on an individual basis. Steroids given for less than 2 weeks; alternate-day therapy with short-acting, low-dose preparations; physiologic replacement doses; topical preparations used for either skin, eye, or lung; or injections into joints are not considered immunosuppressive for the purpose of vaccination decisions. Vaccines should be given early in the course of a disease rather than later, when the immune response may be suboptimal.

Ideally any vaccination should precede chemotherapy or radiation therapy by more than 2 weeks and should be avoided during chemotherapy because of a potential suboptimal response. A vaccine should be given at least 3 months after chemotherapy; however, the ability to mount an immune response may be compromised for up to a year. For patients receiving high-dose corticosteroids for more than 2 weeks, vaccines should be given 3 months after discontinuation of the drug. If the duration of the high-dose corticosteroid use is less than 2 weeks, waiting 2 weeks may suffice. If the strength of a patient's immune response is in doubt, antibody titers may be helpful, or the vaccination can be repeated.

Individuals with severe immunocompromise should be evaluated for their vaccination history and their risk of vaccine-preventable illnesses, as outlined for all adults. In addition, certain vaccines are recommended especially for them.

Inactivated viral or bacterial vaccines and toxoids are safe for all severely immunocompromised patients. Live vaccines are contraindicated unless the immunocompromise is reversible (steroids, chemotherapy, radiation therapy, or other immunosuppressive therapy) and an appropriate interval has elapsed between discontinuation of therapy and administration of live vaccine.

Lifestyle and Environmental Risk

Homosexual and bisexual men and injection drug users are at increased risk for hepatitis A and B infection; 35% to 80% have serologic evidence of hepatitis B exposure. They should be screened for hepatitis A and B exposure; if not already immune or infected, they should be vaccinated. People should be evaluated early because continued exposure increases the chance of infection; 10% to 20% of homosexual men are infected with hepatitis B each year. Hepatitis B vaccine is also recommended for prostitutes, heterosexuals with multiple sex partners, and individuals with sexually transmitted diseases (STDs). Persons in these risk groups should be evaluated for hepatitis C, HIV, and other STDs because of concomitant risk. Injection drug users have an increased incidence of tetanus; physicians should be diligent in giving a Td to these patients.

Inmates of long-term correctional facilities have a high prevalence of hepatitis B, ranging from 10% to 80%, largely because of injection drug use and male homosexual activity. They should be screened for hepatitis B exposure and associated diseases. In addition, measles and rubella outbreaks have occurred in these facilities, and all inmates should be evaluated for immunity or vaccinated as appropriate if at increased risk.

The prevalence of hepatitis B in large institutions for developmentally disabled patients is 35% to 80%. Residents should be screened for hepatitis B exposure; if not already immune or infected, they should be vaccinated. Newly admitted persons should be vaccinated for hepatitis B. All residents should be given a yearly influenza vaccine because some residents may have medical illnesses that make influenza more serious. The staff should also be given hepatitis B and influenza vaccines.

Homeless persons are at risk for pneumococcal disease and influenza and should be vaccinated. Shelter staff should also be given influenza vaccine. There is a high prevalence of hepatitis B in the Native Alaskan population. These individuals should be screened for hepatitis B exposure; if not already immune or infected, they should be vaccinated. Also, Native Alaskan and some Native American populations are at increased risk for invasive pneumococcal disease and should be vaccinated.

Occupational Risk

Health care workers not only are at increased risk of exposure to illness but also can transmit the illness to susceptible patients.

Health care workers born after 1956 should either (1) have been vaccinated twice for measles and once for mumps and rubella after their first birthday, (2) have had physician-diagnosed measles and mumps, or (3) have laboratory immunity to all three diseases. In addition, health care facilities should consider requiring one dose of measles vaccine for employees born before 1957 unless they have serologic proof of measles immunity or have had physician-diagnosed measles. A significant number of cases of measles are reported in health care workers born before 1957.

Although all adults are recommended to have immunity to varicella, this is especially important in health care workers, and verified through reported illness, laboratory immunity, or vaccination. The employee who develops a varicella-like rash after immunization should avoid patient exposure until the lesions crust over. All health care workers and support staff who have patient contact should also be given a yearly influenza vaccine.

People with direct patient contact and laboratory personnel

working with blood or body fluids should be immunized against hepatitis B. Individuals with frequent exposure to blood in this setting have a 15% to 30% prevalence of hepatitis B infection, compared with less than 5% in the general population. An antibody titer should be measured after the vaccine series because it is useful in determining postexposure prophylaxis.

Bacille Calmette-Guérin (BCG) vaccine is recommended for health care workers exposed to multidrug-resistant tuberculosis when other efforts to decrease transmission have failed.

Hepatitis B vaccine is recommended for public safety personnel (e.g., police, firefighters, emergency medical technicians) who may be exposed to blood and secretions. It is also recommended for the staff of institutions for developmentally disabled persons because of the high prevalence of hepatitis B in the patients and the risk of exposure through bites or contact with blood, saliva, skin lesions, or other infectious secretions. These staff workers should also be given a yearly influenza vaccine.

Preexposure rabies vaccine should be given to laboratory workers who handle the virus, to veterinarians, and to animal handlers and field personnel who work with dogs, cats, raccoons, bats, and skunks. Those with avocations that bring them into contact with potentially rabid animals should also be considered for immunization. Preexposure vaccination eliminates the need for postexposure human rabies IG and reduces the number of rabies vaccines needed.

Laboratory personnel who may handle specimens containing poliovirus, smallpox or other orthopoxviruses, hepatitis A virus, *Yersinia pestis,* or *Bacillus anthracis* should be vaccinated for these illnesses. Anyone working with imported hides, furs, wools, and animal hair should receive anthrax vaccine. Field personnel dealing with rodents, rabbits, or their fleas should receive plague vaccine.

Students

Students in colleges, universities, or other postgraduate institutions should be evaluated on entry for any needed vaccination, as outlined for adults. Foreign students should provide documentation of prior vaccination or should be considered unvaccinated. Because of measles epidemics in universities, students born after 1956 should have been given two doses of measles vaccine after their first birthday, have had physician-diagnosed measles, or have serologic evidence of immunity. Meningococcal vaccine can be considered for college students living in dormitories. Students entering the health care profession also should be evaluated as for health care workers.

Immigrants and Refugees

In many countries, routine vaccines are not given. Foreigners entering the United States should provide documentation or receive vaccinations appropriate to their age and concomitant risk. For some vaccines, this may require a primary series. People from areas endemic for hepatitis B (see Table 5-7) should be screened for the virus; if they are carriers, susceptible household members and sexual partners should be evaluated. Individuals from countries with endemic hepatitis B who reside in a similar cultural community in the United States should be given hepatitis B vaccine if they are not already immune or infected.

VACCINE-PREVENTABLE ILLNESSES, VACCINES, AND POSTEXPOSURE PROPHYLAXIS

The following sections discuss vaccines individually. Table 5-2 summarizes vaccines, dose schedules, indications, contraindications, and side effects.

Tetanus and Diphtheria

Tetanus vaccine became available in the United States in the middle-to-late 1940s. Its use has contributed to a 90% reduction in the incidence of tetanus morbidity and mortality. The shift in population from rural to urban areas (resulting in a decreased exposure to spores), improved wound care, and postexposure prophylaxis have also contributed to this phenomenon. Vaccination of school-age children is required in 47 states, and since 1980 more than 95% of students have received a primary series.

Vaccination of adults is much more sporadic. Between 31% and 71% of older adults lack antibody to tetanus. Of the 50 to 100 cases of tetanus in the United States reported annually, 94% occur in adults over 20 years old and 70% in adults 50 years or older. Many of these individuals were born outside the United States and never had a primary immunization series. Of those with a known vaccination history, 93% have not received a primary series or booster dose. The case fatality rate is approximately 25% and increases with age; all recently reported deaths have occurred in adults older than 40 years.

Most individuals with reported tetanus have an identifiable acute injury: puncture, laceration, abrasion, bite, or scratch. Other sources of entry include chronic ulceration, abscess, or history of injection drug use. Only one third of those with tetanus sought medical care after an injury; of these, 75% were not appropriately managed according to current recommendations. The incubation period for clinical disease in most cases is 3 days to 3 weeks, with an average of 8 days.

Diphtheria is rare in the United States. Until recently, an average of only two cases per year have been reported, the majority in persons older than 20 years. Between 40% and 80% of adults older than 60 years lack protective antibody

Td, a combined preparation of adsorbed tetanus toxoi derived from the bacterium *Clostridium tetani* and diphtheri toxoid derived from *Corynebacterium diphtheriae,* is recom mended for adults. It contains tetanus toxoid and 25% les diphtheria toxoid than the childhood immunization to reduc side effects (the childhood vaccine is denoted DT). Th vaccine is almost 100% effective in preventing tetanus an 85% effective in preventing diphtheria. The vaccine does n contain any pertussis immunogens because the curre whole-cell preparation has an unacceptably high frequency side effects. An acellular preparation of *Bordetella pertuss* is being studied in adults in an effort to decrease the spread the disease by asymptomatic adult carriers.

People who develop urticaria or anaphylaxis to the vacci should be tested for allergy before further doses are restricte If an acute exposure occurs in these individuals, tetan immune globulin (TIG) should be given.

Table 5-4 summarizes the management of postexposu prophylaxis for tetanus. Immune prophylaxis should administered as soon as possible, ideally within 3 days, can be given later if delay is unavoidable. Local wound ca is important. The need for a Td and TIG depends on patient's vaccination status and the type of injury sustain

Table 5-4. Postexposure Immunoprophylaxis for Tetanus

Tetanus vaccine doses	Clean, minor wounds		All other wounds*	
	Td	**TIG**	**Td**	**TIG**
Uncertain or less than three†	Yes	No	Yes	Yes
Three or more‡	No§	No	No‖	No

Modified from CDC: Update on adult immunization: recommendations of the Advisory Committee on Immunization Practices (ACIP), *MMWR* 40(RR-12):70, 1991.
Td, Adsorbed tetanus and diphtheria toxoid for adult use (0.5 ml intramuscularly) as soon as possible and preferably within 3 days.
TIG, Tetanus immune globulin (250 U intramuscularly) as soon as possible and preferably within 3 days.
*Including but not limited to wounds contaminated with dirt, feces, soil, or saliva, as well as puncture wounds, avulsions, or wounds resulting from missiles, crushing, burns, or frostbite.
†Follow-up arrangements should be made to complete primary series.
‡If only three doses of a fluid toxoid have been received (used in some countries but less effective), a fourth dose of adsorbed tetanus toxoid should be given regardless of type of wound.
§Yes, if more than 10 years since last dose.
‖Yes, if more than 5 years since last dose.

The physician must determine exactly how many doses of vaccine the patient received in the past. In particular, immigrants, refugees, and foreign students should be evaluated to ensure that they received the primary series (often not routinely given during childhood in other countries). If receipt of a full primary series is uncertain, the patient should be managed as if unvaccinated. If a person has had a primary series, evaluating the date of the last dose given is important. If a Td is indicated after an exposure but is contraindicated because of a previous severe reaction, TIG should be given instead. If TIG (250 U intramuscularly) is to be given with a Td, separate sites should be used. Arrangements should be made to have patients complete a primary series if they have not done so previously. If TIG is given, ideally an MMR vaccine should not be given until 3 months later and varicella vaccine not until 5 months later.

Measles, Mumps, and Rubella

The U.S. Public Health Service has called for the elimination of measles, rubella, and congenital rubella by the year 2000 and has established initiatives for widespread vaccination to accomplish this goal.

Measles. Measles vaccine became available in the United States in 1963, and subsequently the cases of measles declined by 99%, to a low of 3600 in 1988. In 1989 and 1990, however, outbreaks of measles occurred, and the reported cases rose to 28,000. Two major types of outbreaks were noted: (1) among unvaccinated school-age children, including those younger than the recommended age for vaccination (less than 12 months), and (2) among vaccinated school-age children. Also, in 1989 a substantial number of cases occurred among students and personnel on college campuses. In response to these outbreaks, it was recommended in 1990 that children receive two doses of measles vaccine. Two doses were also recommended for adolescents, adults born after 1956, and high-risk groups. Subsequently the number of measles cases declined to 508 in 1996, of which 65 were imported. Only 100 cases were reported in 1998. A similar two-dose regimen used in Finland for more than 12 years has virtually eliminated the disease in that country.

Persons born before 1957 are generally considered immune, although serologic testing of hospital workers in 1989 and 1990 revealed that up to 9% born before 1957 were not immune. Of the health care workers who developed measles during 1985 to 1990, 29% were born before 1957. Encephalitis or death from measles occurs in one per 1000 cases.

Measles infection during pregnancy can result in spontaneous abortion, premature labor, and low birth weight. Although malformations have been reported in association with measles infection, no specific syndrome has been described.

Mumps. Live mumps vaccine was available in 1967, but because of cost, it was not routinely used until 1977. The number of reported cases of mumps declined from 185,000 in 1968 to 2000 in 1985 but rose in 1987 to 12,000 because of an unvaccinated cohort of young adults. The number of cases has been declining since then, and 666 cases were reported in 1998. Mumps is generally a self-limiting illness. Although orchitis can occur in postpubertal males, sterility is rare.

Rubella. The live rubella vaccine was licensed in the United States in 1969. The incidence of rubella infection declined from 56,000 cases in 1969 to 225 in 1988 but rose to 930 cases in 1990, with outbreaks in prisons and colleges. An estimated 6% to 11% of adolescents and young adults are susceptible to rubella. Of the cases reported in 1992 to 1997, averaging 200 to 300, more than 65% were in young adults.

The goal of vaccination is to prevent fetal infection and congenital rubella syndrome (CRS). Of infants infected during the first trimester, 25% will develop CRS that is recognizable at birth, and another 55% will have milder debilitating defects. Defects are rare when infections occur after 20 weeks' gestation. Pooled IG given as postexposure prophylaxis has no proven benefit in preventing fetal malformations.

Vaccine. When a measles, mumps, or rubella vaccine is indicated, the live trivalent vaccine (MMR), which contains all three immunogens, should be used because it provides additional protection against two other diseases. A single dose of an MMR provides long-lasting immunity in 90% to 95% of recipients, whereas two doses provides 99%. Of note, rubella vaccine grown in human diploid cell cultures rather than chicken embryos is available and safe for those with anaphylactic reactions to chicken eggs who need the rubella vaccine. Because it is a live virus vaccine, certain principles apply to giving an MMR and other live vaccines or IGs (see Multiple Vaccines and Immune Globulins on p. 37) to pregnant or immunocompromised persons (see Special Recommendations on p. 38).

Prophylaxis. Postexposure prophylaxis for measles should be given to any susceptible person and any patient with severe immunocompromise or symptomatic HIV regardless of vaccination status. Although no data exist on benefits to the fetus, special consideration should be given for administration of pooled IG to susceptible pregnant women exposed to measles.

The incubation period after exposure is generally 8 to 12 days. People are contagious for 1 to 2 days before the onset of symptoms (3 to 5 days before the rash) and up to 4 days after the appearance of the rash. Measles is transmitted by direct contact with infectious droplets and less often by airborne spread. Susceptible individuals exposed to measles should avoid contact with susceptible health care workers, pregnant women, and patients, as well as severely immunocompromised or symptomatic patients with HIV regardless of vaccination status, for 5 to 21 days after the exposure, even if postexposure prophylaxis is given. People who are ill with measles should avoid such contact for 7 days after they have developed the rash.

Measles illness may be modified in susceptible contacts by giving an MMR within 72 hours of exposure. Giving an MMR has the advantage of providing protection against subsequent measles exposure. If giving an MMR is contraindicated (e.g., pregnancy, symptomatic HIV, severe immunocompromise), or if the person is unlikely to mount an adequate immune response, pooled IG should be given within 6 days of exposure.

The dose of pooled IG for measles exposure in a healthy adult is 0.25 ml/kg (equivalent to 40 mg IG/kg) intramuscularly (IM), to a maximum of 15 ml. Severely immunocompromised patients and symptomatic patients with HIV should receive pooled IG regardless of their vaccination history at twice the dose given to healthy people, or 0.50 ml/kg (equivalent to 80 mg IG/kg) IM, to a maximum of 15 ml. If an immunocompromised patient is receiving a standard dose (100 to 400 mg/kg) of intravenous IG for other reasons at regular intervals, and if the last dose was given within 3 weeks of the measles exposure, this may be sufficient to prevent measles. When pooled IG is indicated and IM injection is contraindicated, as in patients with severe thrombocytopenia or a coagulation disorder (e.g., hemophilia), an intravenous preparation can be used at a dose of 110 mg/kg. Because these intravenous IG preparations are derived from smaller donor pools, they may not be as effective for measles prophylaxis. Their efficacy for these purposes is unknown, and therefore no specific recommendation exists.

If pooled IG is used for measles prophylaxis, an MMR should be given to healthy people after 5 months and to immunocompromised or symptomatic HIV patients after 6 months if it is not contraindicated at that time. If intravenous IG was used, an MMR vaccine should not be given until after 6 months for a 100-mg dose and up to 8 months later for a 400-mg dose. A second MMR may be indicated for those born after 1956 if they are at high risk of subsequent measles exposure.

Varicella

Varicella is a highly contagious childhood illness, with secondary attack rates in household members of up to 90%. Infection confers lifelong immunity, except in rare cases of reinfection in immunocompromised persons. In adults the disease is more serious than in children and can have associated pneumonitis, bacterial superinfections, encephalitis, hepatitis, and death. The severity is increased in older individuals and severely immunocompromised patients.

Varicella infection in a woman during the first half of pregnancy can result in embryopathy in up to 2% of cases. Varicella infection in women 5 days before and up to 2 days after delivery can result in disease in 30% of newborns, which is often severe.

Up to 15% of adults will develop varicella-zoster infection, which can become disseminated in immunocompromised patients.

In the United States, more than 90% of adults are immune, although the rates are lower for those in tropical or subtropical regions. Of those who report a history of varicella, 97% to 99% have serologic immunity, and of those who report a negative history, 71% to 93% will have antibody. Reported illness or laboratory evidence confers immunity in healthy and immunocompromised persons, except for bone marrow recipients, who are never considered immune, and for immunocompromised persons who received multiple transfusions and who have a negative history with a low varicella titer, because the antibody could have been acquired passively.

The live virus vaccine was licensed in 1995 and is recommended for all children and nonimmune adults, especially persons who live and work in environments where transmission of varicella is likely (i.e., households with children, colleges, prisons, day-care, medical facilities), nonpregnant women of childbearing age, and international travelers. One dose of the vaccine induces a seroconversion rate of 78% to 82%, and a second dose induces 99%. Salicylate ingestion should be avoided for up to 6 weeks after vaccination because of the Reye's syndrome associated with wild varicella. If a varicella-like rash develops after vaccination, contact with all susceptible persons should be avoided, and health care workers should probably be furloughed. In this setting, VZIG is not recommended for susceptible contacts because transmission is rare and disease is expected to be mild.

The vaccine is 70% effective in preventing any disease and 95% effective in preventing serious disease. Persons who develop varicella despite vaccination generally have fewer lesions, shorter illness, and less fever. The vaccine is effective in children for at least 20 years. The need for booster doses is unknown but is continually monitored, especially since the illness in adults is more severe than in children. It is no known whether the vaccine will decrease the incidence o zoster.

Because it is a live virus vaccine, certain principle apply to giving a varicella vaccine and other liv vaccines or IGs (see Multiple Vaccines and Immun Globulins on p. 37) to pregnant or immunocompromise persons (see Special Recommendations on p. 38).

A significant exposure to a person with chickenpo includes household contact, close indoor contact longer tha an hour, sharing a hospital room, or prolonged face-to-fac contact (e.g., physician and patient). The period of highe risk of contagion is 1 to 2 days before the onset of the ras and for 5 days after or until the last eruptions form a crus Immunocompromised patients may have an extended peric of new eruptions and therefore are contagious longer. significant exposure to a person with shingles results fro direct contact with uncovered lesions; airborne spread is rar An immunocompromised patient with shingles, howeve may shed a large viral load that can be aerosolized; in th setting, significant exposure may occur, as described for chickenpox.

Any person with wild or vaccine-associated varicella should avoid contact with susceptible persons for at least 5 days after the onset of the rash and for the duration of any new eruptions or until all the lesions have crusted over, whichever is longer. The incubation period is generally 14 to 16 days but can be anytime from 11 to 20 days. Exposed, susceptible people should avoid other susceptible persons for 10 to 21 days after the development of the rash in the index patient. *Those who receive varicella-zoster immune globulin (VZIG) for postexposure prophylaxis should avoid contact with susceptible individuals for 28 days because VZIG may prolong the incubation period of clinical disease.*

The decision regarding the administration of postexposure prophylaxis for varicella has been simplified because the vaccine is now approved for this purpose. VZIG can be used for those persons who cannot receive the vaccine: immunocompromised persons or pregnant women. The decision to administer VZIG for postexposure prophylaxis is based on the significance of the exposure as discussed above and the likelihood that an individual is susceptible to varicella. Even if IG aborts clinical disease in a pregnant woman, it is not known whether this protects the infant from infection and malformation.

Susceptibility to the illness needs to be evaluated on an individual basis. Even with negative histories, elder siblings in large families, parents whose children have had chickenpox, or those who have had other significant exposure to chickenpox are probably immune. It is preferable to measure a varicella antibody titer in people with an unknown susceptibility to determine their immune status, if this will not delay the administration of the vaccine beyond 72 hours or VZIG beyond 48 hours (except for specific immunocompromised persons and bone marrow recipients as noted above). In persons who were previously immunized (initial expected positive titer in 99%) who have a negative titer, no VZIG is needed because the disease is expected to be mild. There is currently no recommendation regarding giving the vaccine as these persons may or may not have an anamnestic response.

For postexposure prophylaxis to prevent or modify the disease, the varicella vaccine is 90% effective if given within days. It may still be effective up to 5 days. The second dose of the vaccine should be given in 1 or 2 months to complete the series. The dose of VZIG is 12.5 U/kg to a maximum of 25 U (the ideal dose has not been determined for immunocompromised individuals) given within 48 hours of exposure and preferably not beyond 96 hours. VZIG prophylaxis in this setting may last up to 3 weeks. If clinical disease does not develop and there is a new exposure after this time, another dose should be given. People who receive VZIG and who do not develop clinical disease may develop serologic immunity, but it is not known whether this is protective against future exposures. If VZIG is given, ideally varicella or MMR vaccine should not be given until 5 months later.

Hepatitis B

In certain areas of the world (see Table 5-7), hepatitis B is endemic, with the virus predominantly transmitted perinatally and during childhood. In the United States, most affected people acquire hepatitis B infection during late adolescence or young adulthood through body secretions or blood exposure; more than 89% of the cases occur in individuals older than 20 years. The lifetime risk of developing hepatitis B in the United States is less than 5% for the general population. In high-risk groups, such as injection drug users, it can approach 80%. Approximately 300,000 cases of acute hepatitis B infections occur each year in the United States, resulting in 10,000 hospitalizations and 250 deaths. The rate at which persons become chronic carriers is age dependent; infection in adults is associated with a 6% to 10% chronic carrier rate, infection in childhood with a rate as high as 60%, and perinatal infection with a rate as high as 90%.

Each year in the United States, 4000 people die of cirrhosis and 800 people die of liver cancer related to hepatitis B infection. Because Native Alaskans have a high incidence of hepatitis B, they were the subjects of a perinatal and adult vaccination program in 1982. The incidence of acute hepatitis B was reduced by 99%. In some countries with endemic hepatitis B, widespread vaccination has correlated with a reduction in chronic liver disease and hepatocellular carcinoma.

Previously, high-risk groups were targeted for vaccination in an effort to decrease the incidence of disease, but the incidence continued to rise. Since 1990 it has been recommended that all newborns in the United States be given hepatitis B vaccine. The vaccine also is recommended for all adolescents and certain adults in high-risk groups (see Table 5-2) and for certain travelers (see Table 5-7). Travelers to countries where hepatitis B is endemic can minimize exposure by avoiding intimate contact with the native population, especially contact involving blood, sex, and prolonged household contact.

Prevaccination screening for active disease should be done for high-risk groups, such as homosexual men, injection drug users, hemodialysis patients, recipients of multiple infusions of clotting factor concentrates or whole blood, and immigrants from high-risk countries, to identify people who are infected and who may benefit from treatment, as well as their household and sexual contacts who are at risk. Using any one serologic marker for screening is imperfect. Screening for *hepatitis B surface antigen* (HBsAg) alone would identify those who are currently infected, but not those who are immune and do not require vaccination. Screening for *hepatitis B surface antibody* (anti-HBs) alone would identify most of those who are immune, but not those who are infected, for whom treatment and evaluation of sexual or household contacts are important.

Screening for *hepatitis B core antibody* (anti-HBc) alone identifies anyone infected but does not differentiate between carriers and noncarriers. Anti-HBc could be tested if the goal of screening is to eliminate individuals who theoretically do not require vaccination. This is problematic, however, because people who have anti-HBc alone cannot necessarily be considered immune. In a study of United States blood donors with a relatively low incidence of hepatitis B, one quarter of patients who had isolated anti-HBc alone were shown to have a false-positive test. In several studies of populations with endemic hepatitis B, people with anti-HBc alone that was persistent and reproducible had a variable response to vaccination. Less than 20% had an anamnestic response, suggesting that more than 80% were not immune.

In addition, 10% to 40% had no response to a full series, suggesting a low-level carrier state. These studies suggest that people with anti-HBc alone and their at-risk contacts should be included in vaccination programs targeting high-risk groups. Therefore, to screen persons from high-risk groups, it is prudent to measure at least HBsAg and anti-HBs.

The vaccines used in the United States today contain purified HBsAg made with recombinant DNA technology. In adults the vaccine series is greater than 90% effective in preventing clinical disease. In some studies the antibody response to vaccination is reduced in older adults and in smokers or obese persons (perhaps a function of inadequate IM injection). If doses are missed in the usual series of 0, 1, and 6 months, the second and third doses should be given at least 2 months apart. A higher dose formulation is available for persons who may have a poor immune response to the standard vaccine (e.g., HIV, severe immunocompromise, approaching or on dialysis).

Postvaccination antibody testing is recommended for anyone at occupational risk to aid in deciding postexposure prophylaxis, as well as for immunocompromised persons and persons with renal failure who may have suboptimal response to the vaccine. Postvaccination titers should be evaluated at least 1 month after the series is completed. In one study of nonresponders to the vaccine series, 15% to 25% developed an adequate antibody titer to one additional dose. An additional 30% to 50% developed an adequate antibody response to another series. Revaccination with one or more doses should be considered for nonresponders after the presence of HBsAg has been excluded.

In healthy individuals, immunologic memory seems to persist for up to 15 years despite antibody titers below the threshold for immunity, as demonstrated by the absence of clinical disease and HBsAg in the serum during this time period. Currently, booster doses are not recommended for healthy individuals, although this may change in the future. Yearly antibody titers should be measured in hemodialysis patients because of the rapid decline in their antibody titers. A booster should be given if the antibody titer falls below 10 U/ml.

Tables 5-5 and 5-6 summarize recommendations for postexposure management of hepatitis B. Sexual and household contacts of a person with chronic hepatitis B should be evaluated for immunity and infection; if they have neither, they should receive hepatitis B vaccine (HBV). Sexual contacts of someone with acute hepatitis B should receive hepatitis B immune globulin (HBIG) as soon as possible and within 2 weeks of the last exposure; this is 75% effective in preventing disease. Contacts can be tested for an already-acquired infection if testing will not delay giving HBIG or HBV more than a few days. If sexual contact is not likely to continue and the exposed person is otherwise at low risk for exposure to hepatitis B in the future, one dose of HBIG is sufficient (adding one dose of HBV may increase effectiveness). HBIG should be given with HBV and the series of HBV completed if sexual contact is likely to continue. Alternatively, HBIG can be given (adding one dose of HBV may increase effectiveness) and the index person retested in 3 months. If the index person is not still infectious, nothing further is needed. If the index person is still infectious, a second HBIG should be given and the HBV series started in the partner. Household contacts of someone with acute hepatitis B who have a known exposure, such as blood contact through toothbrushes or razors, should be treated similarly to those with sexual exposure.

Table 5-5. Postexposure Immunoprophylaxis for Hepatitis B Virus in Susceptible Contacts After Sexual or Household Exposure

Index person	Exposure type	Immunoprophylaxis
Chronically infected	Household or sexual	Vaccination series
Acutely infected	Household with no blood exposure	None unless blood exposure
Acutely infected	Sexual or household with blood exposure	HBIG with or without vaccination series*

Modified from CDC: Hepatitis B virus: a comprehensive strategy for eliminating transmission in the United States through universal childhood vaccination: recommendations of the Immunization Practices Advisory Committee (ACIP), *MMWR* 40(RR-13):9, 1991.

HBIG, Hepatitis B immune globulin (0.06 ml/kg intramuscularly) as soon as possible and within 2 weeks of last sexual or household exposure.

Hepatitis B vaccine (1.0 ml intramuscularly) as soon as possible and within 2 weeks of last exposure to acutely infected person and as soon as possible after exposure to chronically infected person.

*See text.

Table 5-6 summarizes the management of percutaneous (needle-stick, laceration, or bite) or permucosal (ocular or mucous membrane) exposure to hepatitis B. If needed, HBIG and/or HBV should be given as soon as possible and at separate sites if both are given. In this setting the usefulness of giving them later than 1 week after exposure is not known. Two doses of HBIG are then 75% effective in preventing hepatitis B.

Individuals with hepatitis B and their contacts should also be evaluated for hepatitis C and HIV (if concomitant risk) and other STDs (with sexual exposure). The source person in a needle-stick injury should be evaluated for hepatitis C and abnormal liver function as well as HIV, especially if at high risk for these illnesses. The usefulness of giving pooled IG to prevent hepatitis C transmission is unknown. If HBIG is given, ideally an MMR vaccine should not be given until 3 months later and varicella vaccine not until 5 months later. For postexposure prophylaxis of HIV infection, see Chapter 32.

Hepatitis A

Hepatitis A is spread from person to person through fecal contamination and oral ingestion. It is endemic in developing countries, and sporadic outbreaks occur in the United States. The clinically identifiable sources of spread are 22% to 26% household or sexual contacts, 14% child care settings, 6% travel, 2% to 3% food or water sources, 4% homosexual or bisexual men, and 3% injection drug users. In the U.S. population, 33% of adults have natural immunity, which increases with age and decreases with higher income. Natural immunity is even higher in developing countries. Prevaccination titers are probably cost-effective in persons from high-risk groups, those over age 40, and persons from developing countries.

The highest degree of viral shedding occurs 1 to 2 weeks before clinical illness and is minimal 1 week after the onset of jaundice. Any person with active disease should be excluded

Table 5-6. Immunoprophylaxis for Hepatitis B Virus After Percutaneous or Permucosal Exposure to Blood

	Treatment, when source is:		
Exposed person	**HBsAg positive**	**HBsAg negative**	**Unknown**
Unvaccinated	HBIG and vaccine series*	Vaccine series*	Vaccine series*
Previously vaccinated			
Known responder	None	None	None
Known nonresponder	HBIG at 0 and 1 month, or HBIG and vaccine series*	None	If high-risk source, treat as HBsAg positive
Response unknown	Test exposed person for anti-HBs titer: 1. If adequate, none 2. If inadequate, HBIG and vaccine series*	Test exposed person for anti-HBs titer for future exposure management	Test exposed person for anti-HBs titer: 1. If adequate, none. 2. If inadequate, vaccine series*

Modified from CDC: Immunization of health care workers: recommendations of the Advisory Committee on Immunization Practices (ACIP) and the Hospital Infection Control Practices Advisory Committee (HICPAC), *MMWR* 46(RR-18):23, 1997.
HBsAg, Hepatitis B surface antigen; *anti-HBs,* Hepatatitis B surface antibody; adequate anti-HBs titer >10 mIU.
HBIG, Hepatitis B immune globulin (0.06 ml/kg intramuscularly) as soon as possible and within 24 hours of exposure. Unclear efficacy if given after 1 week of exposure.
Hepatitis B vaccine (1.0 ml intramuscularly) as soon as possible and within 1 week of exposure.
*Check for antibody titer at least 1 month after series to guide management of future exposures.

from attending day-care facilities, isolated if in a custodial institution, or furloughed from food-handling or health care employment until 1 week after the onset of symptoms or until the jaundice disappears, whichever is longer.

The hepatitis A vaccine is derived from purified viral antigens. The seroconversion rate after the first dose is 88% and after the second dose 100%. The vaccine is 95% to 100% effective in preventing clinical disease. The duration of immunity is at least 7 years. For travelers to high-risk countries, either vaccine or pooled IG is given. The vaccine is used when at least one dose can be given 4 weeks before departure. Otherwise, pooled IG is used: 0.02 ml/kg (3.3 mg IG/kg) IM for travel of 3 months or less; 0.06 ml/kg (10 mg IG/kg) IM for travel longer than 3 months, with revaccination every 5 months. Travelers should be educated to avoid exposure through careful food and water selection (see Travel). The vaccine is not recommended for persons who work with food or in child care because cases are sporadic in these settings.

Pooled IG (0.02 ml/kg IM) for postexposure prophylaxis of hepatitis A should be given as soon as possible and within 2 weeks of exposure. It is 85% effective in preventing disease and has its greatest effect early in the incubation period. When pooled IG is indicated and IM injection is contraindicated, as in patients with severe thrombocytopenia or a coagulation disorder (e.g., hemophilia), an intravenous preparation of 110 mg/kg can be used. Because these intravenous IG preparations are derived from smaller donor pools, they may not be as effective for hepatitis A. Therefore no specific recommendation exists.

Close household or sexual contacts of a person with acute hepatitis A should be given pooled IG. If a custodial institution has an outbreak of hepatitis A, selected staff in close contact with the index patient and clients should be given pooled IG. Co-workers of food handlers with hepatitis A should be given pooled IG. If a day-care center has an outbreak of hepatitis A, the staff and children as well as household contacts of diapered children should be given pooled IG. If pooled IG is given for hepatitis A prophylaxis, an MMR vaccine should not be given until 3 months later and varicella vaccine not until 5 months later.

The hepatitis A vaccine is not recommended for postexposure prophylaxis but has been useful in reducing cases during disease outbreaks in some populations.

Pneumococcus

Pneumococcal disease in the United States annually causes an estimated 150,000 to 570,000 cases of pneumonia, 2600 to 6200 cases of meningitis, and about 40,000 deaths. The mortality is highest in elderly people, patients with debilitating medical illnesses, and those who develop either meningitis or bacteremia. Pneumococcal disease in combination with influenza is the sixth leading cause of death in the United States. Up to two thirds of patients hospitalized with serious pneumococcal disease have been hospitalized in the previous 4 years and have not been vaccinated as recommended. With the emergence of drug-resistant strains of bacteria, prevention of disease has become even more important. Despite recommendations, vaccine rates are less than 30% in elderly persons.

The pneumococcal vaccine contains capsular antigens of the 23 types of *Streptococcus pneumoniae* that cause 88% of pneumococcal bacteremia. It is estimated to be at least 60% effective in preventing disease in immunocompetent adults older than 65 years. This degree of efficacy has been shown using cohort analysis for persons with diabetes, congestive heart failure, coronary vascular disease, and asplenia. Data for immunocompromised patients and those with alcoholism or cirrhosis suggest that the efficacy is less.

The vaccine's efficacy lasts for up to 9 years but is less in certain groups. Revaccination is recommended at 5 years for those who are most susceptible to a fatal disease or for those whose antibody levels decline at a rapid rate. It is also recommended at 5 years for persons vaccinated for any reason before age 65 and for those 65 years or older. Administration of more than two doses of the vaccine has not been studied and will be evaluated in the future.

Influenza

Influenza infection causes serious morbidity and mortality in the United States, especially in elderly persons and those with underlying medical illnesses. During influenza season, hospitalizations for comorbid conditions increase, and more cardiopulmonary deaths are associated with influenza and concomitant pneumonia. The average number of deaths attributable to influenza is estimated at 20,000 per year in the United States, with an estimated 110,000 hospitalizations. Up to 40,000 deaths occur during years with severe epidemics.

The efficacy of the influenza vaccine varies. In young healthy adults it is up to 90% effective in preventing disease, and it is cost-effective for employers to offer the vaccine to their workers. In elderly persons or those with chronic illnesses the antibody response can be much lower. In these individuals the vaccine is more effective in preventing lower tract disease and disease severity than the disease itself. The vaccine has been shown to be 50% effective in reducing influenza-related illnesses, 32% to 45% effective in preventing hospitalization, 31% to 65% effective in reducing hospital respiratory deaths, and 27% to 30% in reducing deaths from all causes. Despite this, 35% of adults over age 64 are not immunized each year.

Influenza A and B viruses are classified into subtypes according to two surface antigens: neuraminidase and hemagglutinin. Immunity to one subtype confers little or no protection against viruses of another subtype. Furthermore, antigenic variation within a subtype may occur, so vaccination with one strain may not protect against another distantly related strain of the same subtype. Because influenza season is April to September in the southern hemisphere and all year long in the tropics, worldwide surveillance and antigenic characterization of the circulating strains of influenza provide the basis for predicting which viral strains are most likely to cause illness in the United States in a given year. The inactivated vaccine, derived from two strains of influenza A and one strain of influenza B, contains either whole virus, viral antigen, or split virus (treated with lipid solvents), all initially grown in chicken embryos. The whole virus vaccine causes more febrile reactions in children and therefore is not recommended for them. Unlike the 1976 swine flu vaccine, no clear association exists between any subsequent influenza A and B vaccine and the Guillain-Barré syndrome.

Influenza season in the United States typically begins in December and peaks in January and February, so the vaccine is usually given from mid-October to early November. The vaccine can be used (1) as long as influenza is documented in a community and (2) as late as April. Antibodies to the influenza vaccine develop within 2 weeks. Although immunity typically lasts up to 10 months, it may last considerably less in medically ill or immunocompromised patients. Because immunity to the vaccine is short-lived and because strains of the virus in circulation may change, an annual vaccination is recommended. For treatment of susceptible individuals exposed to influenza A, see Chapter 33.

Hemophilus Influenza b

Invasive disease caused by hemophilus influenza type b occurs mostly in childhood, with 85% of cases occurring in children under age 5 years. The vaccine is given routinely in pediatric practice. Invasive hemophilus influenza disease is rare in adults and occurs predominantly in those with conditions that predispose them to infection with encapsulated organisms. Even so, less than half of the invasive disease in these individuals is caused by the type b bacteria used in the vaccine.

The vaccine is derived from a type b capsular polysaccharide of hemophilus influenza type b. It is conjugated to protein carriers to induce a greater immune response. The protein carriers include diphtheria toxoid or the outer membrane protein complex of *Neisseria meningitidis*. The clinical efficacy in adults is not known and the need for boosters not established, but in splenectomy patients vaccinated 2 weeks preoperatively, the vaccine is immunogenic in 87%. For postexposure prophylaxis of hemophilus influenza type b, see Chapter 27.

Meningococcus

In the United States, meningococcal disease occurs seasonally in late winter or early spring. It infects primarily children under age 5 years, with peak incidence between ages 6 and 12 months. One third of cases, however, occur in persons older than 20 years. The vaccine can be used to reduce the number of secondary cases during outbreaks if the responsible serogroups in the index case are represented by the vaccine. In the United States, serogroups B and C cause 30% and 50% of the cases respectively, and serotypes Y and W135 cause most of the rest.

The vaccine contains polysaccharides of *N. meningitidis* serotypes A, C, Y, and W135. The need for booster doses has not been studied, and the duration of protection varies for the individual serotypes; adults should be considered for revaccination in 3 to 5 years. For postexposure prophylaxis of *N. meningitidis,* see Chapter 27.

Lyme Disease

Lyme disease, the most common vector-borne disease in the United States, is principally caused by *Borrelia burgdorferi* and transmitted by *Ixodes* ticks that normally feed on deer. The illness was described in Europe in the early 1900s and first described in the United States in 1970, although serologic studies identify it as far back as 1962. Since 1982, more than 100,000 cases have been reported, and the number increases each year. Cases are mostly from northeastern, mid-Atlantic, north-central, and western Pacific states, although the prevalence within states varies greatly. The primary risk for developing the disease is residing in or traveling to woodland or grassy areas that harbor the tick. Late spring and early summer are the peak times for transmission, when the nymphs emerge to feed, but the risk continues throughout the year as the adults feed. The ticks are about the size of a pinhead, depending on their age (see Chapter 94).

The vaccine is a recombinant DNA–derived lipoprotein, OspA, which is the most immunogenic of the bacterium's outer surface proteins. The clinical efficacy in preventing Lyme disease after two doses is 50% and after three doses 78%. After two doses, 99% of patients develop vaccine antibody, which wanes to 83% by the third dose. The third dose results in 100% seroconversion, which lasts at least 7 months. The duration of clinical efficacy is at least 2 years and is being evaluated further. The immune response to the vaccine can cause a positive immunoglobulin G enzyme-linked immunosorbent assay (IgG ELISA) in the absence of true disease; therefore a confirmatory test for disease exposure is required. Previous infection may not confer protective immunity. Persons should be instructed how to avoid tick exposure (see Travel).

Rabies

Since rabies in domesticated animals was controlled in the 1940s and 1950s, only two or three cases of human rabies are reported each year. An epidemic of rabies infection in certain wild animals has spread to many parts of the United States in recent years. In the United States, more than 85% of rabies transmission is through carnivorous wild animals, such as skunks, raccoons, foxes, coyotes, and bats, and except for the woodchuck, rarely through rodents. In developing countries, rabies is transmitted primarily through domesticated animals, primarily the dog; wild animals harbor it as well. Rabies is usually transmitted through a bite, but saliva in contact with open wounds or mucous membranes may transmit the disease. In addition, airborne transmission probably has occurred in bat caves. The incubation period for rabies is generally 10 to 90 days but can be up to 1 year. The infection is almost uniformly fatal.

The three licensed inactivated rabies vaccines are grown in (1) human diploid cells (HDCV), (2) rhesus lung cell cultures (RVA), and (3) chick embryo cell cultures (PCEC). Anaphylaxis occurs in 0.1% of recipients and is a reason to discontinue the primary series. The serum sickness–like reaction seen with HDCV may not occur with the other types of rabies vaccine. Chloroquine and similar compounds (e.g., mefloquine) can interfere with the immune response to rabies vaccine when it is given intradermally. Travelers planning to take these antimalarials should receive at least three doses of the intradermal vaccine before taking the medication. If this cannot be accomplished, the IM route should be used, giving as much of the series as possible. Immunocompromised individuals who receive preexposure prophylaxis should have an antibody titer checked 1 month after the series. Giving a booster dose or checking the titer is recommended every 2 years for any person with frequent exposure. Although substituting different vaccine preparations during a series is not recommended, booster doses from one type seem to produce an anamnestic response in another.

The local or state health department should be contacted about any questionable exposure to rabies. Wild animals and ill domesticated animals are killed, whereas healthy domestic animals are observed for 10 days. If a quarantined animal develops signs of rabies, if an animal that likely has rabies cannot be located, or if a killed animal is shown to harbor rabies, postexposure prophylaxis is given.

The postexposure treatment of rabies begins with local wound care. Because the virus may localize at the entry site for a time, wound care is extremely important in preventing the virus from entering neural tissue. All wounds should be flushed and cleaned with soap and water and should not be sutured if possible. Antibiotic prophylaxis for the bacteria associated with the animal's bite should also be given. Table 5-2 summarizes immunoprophylaxis. HRIG should be given as soon as possible, but average delays of 5 days have not been associated with failures. In a low-risk situation when laboratory analysis of the suspected animal will be available within 48 hours, postexposure prophylaxis may wait pending these results. If indicated, HRIG should be given within 7 days of the first vaccine because after that time the immune response to the vaccine is expected to occur and HRIG is less useful. The dose of HRIG should not exceed the recommended dose because this can interfere with the immune response to the vaccine. Immunocompromised persons should have antibody titers measured 2 to 4 weeks after postexposure prophylaxis. If HRIG is given, ideally an MMR vaccine should not be given until 4 months later and a varicella vaccine not until 5 months later.

Poliomyelitis

In the United States the incidence of poliomyelitis is low because of the maintenance of very high vaccination rates (95% of children) since the vaccine became available in the mid-1950s and early 1960s. The last polio epidemic occurred in 1979 in a group who refused vaccination. Since that time the only cases of poliomyelitis in the United States (less than 10 per year) have been vaccine associated, of which 78% occur after the first dose. Likewise, in other parts of the western hemisphere, no wild poliovirus infections have been reported since 1991. Poliomyelitis is much more prevalent in most developing countries. In temperate areas, poliomyelitis occurs primarily during summer and fall, but in the tropics it can occur at any time.

The polio vaccine is available as an inactivated trivalent virus vaccine (IPV) containing virus types 1, 2, and 3. The oral, live trivalent virus vaccine is no longer manufactured in the United States. The primary series of IPV is three doses. If time does not allow for three doses as specified, the vaccine should be given as a series of three doses, each a month apart, giving as many of the doses as possible before travel. The primary series should then be completed subsequently. If travelers have already received a primary series, they should be given a booster dose. The vaccine series is 95% effective in preventing clinical disease.

Typhoid

Approximately 450 cases of typhoid fever occur annually in the United States, 70% of which are acquired through foreign travel. Typhoid vaccine is recommended for certain travelers (see Table 5-7). Travelers should be educated to avoid exposure through careful food and water selection (see Travel). The vaccine is also recommended for persons having continued household contact with a known carrier and for laboratory workers handling the bacterium.

Several preparations of the vaccine are derived from the bacterium *Salmonella typhi*. The vaccine series is 70% to 90% effective. No data exist on the safety of these vaccines during pregnancy. The oral live vaccine should not be given to immunocompromised patients, but the inactivated vaccine theoretically is considered safe.

Because the oral typhoid vaccine is a live vaccine, certain principles apply (see Multiple Vaccines and Immune Globulins). Parenteral typhoid, cholera, and plague vaccines typically cause local or systemic reactions; therefore the simultaneous administration of these vaccines should be avoided if possible. The antimalarial mefloquine may interfere with the immune response to oral typhoid; therefore the vaccine should be given 24 hours before or after mefloquine. Likewise, oral antibiotics should not be given within 7 days of oral typhoid.

Yellow Fever

Yellow fever has been reported in central Africa and central South America (see Table 5-7). The virus is transmitted by mosquito vector. The vaccine is available only at an approved yellow fever vaccination center, which can be located by contacting the local health department. Vaccinated persons should receive a validated International Certificate of Vaccination. Failure to document prior vaccination may result in revaccination, quarantine, or refusal of entry. Travelers should also be educated on how to avoid mosquitoes (see Travel).

The vaccine is an attenuated live virus vaccine grown in chicken embryos. Booster doses are recommended every 10 years, although recent evidence suggests that serologic immunity lasts for at least 30 years.

If a pregnant woman or a woman planning to become pregnant within 3 months intends to travel to endemic areas, yellow fever vaccine can be given if travel plans cannot be delayed and exposure is imminent. Even though it is a live vaccine, there is no known risk to the fetus, and disease in the mother has serious morbidity and mortality. Yellow fever vaccine should not be given to immunocompromised or symptomatic HIV-infected patients, although no data exist on adverse reactions. If the risk of yellow fever is high, asymptomatic HIV-infected individuals should be advised of the risk vs. benefit of vaccination and given the choice of vaccination.

Yellow fever vaccine is a live virus vaccine, so special principles apply to its administration (see Multiple Vaccines and Immune Globulins). Yellow fever and cholera vaccines should be given at least 3 weeks apart; simultaneous administration can diminish the antibody response to both vaccines.

Japanese Encephalitis

The mosquito-borne Japanese encephalitis virus is the leading cause of viral encephalitis in Asia. This encephalitis also occurs in the Indian subcontinent and in Oceania. The viral infection appears most often in native populations and leads to encephalitis in one of 20 to 1000 cases, with death occurring in 25% of those infected and neurologic sequelae in 30%. By adulthood, almost everyone in endemic countries has serologic evidence of exposure. The virus is transmitted seasonally in temperate regions, mainly during summer and early fall. In tropical areas, transmission can be year-round. The risk of acquiring infection is low for most travelers to these areas. However, the vaccine is recommended for travelers spending at least a month during the transmission season, especially if traveling in rural areas, and for those spending less time but most of it outdoors in rural areas (see Table 5-7). Travelers should also be educated about mosquito bites (see Travel).

The vaccine is composed of inactivated virus derived from virus-infected mouse brain. If there are time constraints and the recommended series cannot be completed, the vaccine can be given on days 0, 7, and 14. The vaccine is 80% to 90% effective in preventing encephalitis. A serious reaction to the vaccine consists of generalized urticaria and angioedema, which can occur up to 2 weeks postvaccination and at a rate of five in 1000 patients. Medications to treat anaphylaxis should be on hand at the vaccination, and the recipient should be observed for 30 minutes. Recipients should be warned of the symptoms of anaphylaxis and advised to seek medical attention if any occur in the ensuing weeks. Individuals with a history of hypersensitivity phenomena appear to be at increased risk. Vaccine-associated encephalitis is rare; only one or two cases per million vaccines have been documented. The need for booster doses is unknown, but immunity appears to last for at least 2 years.

Cholera

Cholera is a risk to travelers in more remote areas of Africa, Asia, and Latin America. The vaccine series is recommended for travelers to these countries who are at high risk. Although no country currently requires the vaccine, some local authorities may require it (see Table 5-7). The current vaccine series is only 50% effective in preventing clinical illness for 3 to 6 months. Travelers should be educated to avoid exposure through careful food and water selection (see Travel).

The vaccine is derived from the inactivated bacterium, *Vibrio cholerae*. A single dose satisfies requirements in most areas. A person at high risk, however, should receive the series. Yellow fever and cholera vaccines should be given at least 3 weeks apart; if given together, the antibody response to both vaccines can be diminished. In addition, cholera, parenteral typhoid, and plague vaccines often cause local or systemic reactions; therefore the simultaneous administration of these vaccines should be avoided if possible.

Plague, Anthrax, Vaccinia, and Bacille Calmette-Guérin

These vaccines are used only in highly selective circumstances. Plague (inactivated bacteria) and vaccinia (live virus) are recommended for laboratory workers who handle these organisms, anthrax (inactivated bacteria) for persons working with imported animal hides and furs, and BCG (live bacteria) for health care workers highly susceptible to multidrug-resistant *Mycobacterium tuberculosis* or high-risk travelers without access to purified protein derivative (PPD) screening. The manufacturer's guidelines should be consulted for doses, routes, and contraindications.

TRAVEL

International travelers should be evaluated at least 6 weeks before departure to obtain health information on the countries they plan to visit and any recommended vaccinations. Travelers should have a written summary of their medications, allergies, and health problems. They should bring a supply of medications and extra eyeglasses as needed. They should contact their health insurer regarding policies for urgent health care needs abroad.

Travel prophylaxis recommendations are based on WHO and CDC disease surveillance data. The data are based on information that generally underestimates the incidence of disease. Underreporting occurs in many countries because (1) the countries may have no mechanism for reporting and recording cases, (2) medical personnel may not always report cases, (3) infected individuals do not always seek medical attention, and (4) no medical personnel may be available in the area. In underdeveloped countries, poor living conditions and sanitation, lack of hygiene, and nonavailability of vaccines may result in a higher prevalence of some diseases. The risk of infection varies considerably within countries.

Many of the recommendations for vaccinating and educating travelers are not required by other countries but are advisable to prevent illness. Travelers must have the recommended immunizations for their age and any specia

Disease*	Areas affected[†]	Prophylaxis recommended[‡]	Ideal time between last vaccine dose and travel
Tetanus	All	All travelers; vaccine series/booster.	Probably 30 days for series Anamnestic response to booster
Measles	All	Born after 1956; ensure immunity by antibody titer, diagnosed measles, or two doses of vaccine.	As MMR, 7-14 days
Rubella	All	Born after 1956 and any female of childbearing age; rubella titer or one dose of vaccine.	As MMR, 7-14 days
Mumps	All	Born after 1956; ensure immunity by antibody titer, diagnosed mumps, or one dose of vaccine.	As MMR, 7-14 days
Varicella	All	All travelers; antibody titer, reported illness, or vaccine series.	7-14 days
Hepatitis B	5%-20% of population are carriers in Africa, Middle East except Israel, all Southeast Asia, Amazon basin, Haiti, and Dominican Republic; 1%-5% of population are carriers in south-central and southwest Asia, Israel, Japan, Americas, Russia, and eastern and southern Europe.	Travelers for more than 6 months in close contact with population or for less time but with high-risk activities (close household contact, seeking dental or medical care, sex); vaccine series.	Probably 30 days
Hepatitis A	Developing countries.	Travelers to rural areas; eating and drinking in settings of poor sanitation; vaccine or pooled immune globulin (IG).	Vaccine, 30 days Pooled IG, 2 days
Influenza	Tropics throughout the year; southern hemisphere from April to September.	Travelers for whom vaccine is otherwise indicated; give current vaccine and revaccinate in fall as usual.	7-14 days
Meningococcus*	Sub-Saharan Africa "belt" (Senegal to Ethiopia) from December to June; required for pilgrims to Saudi Arabia during Haj; epidemics reported in other African nations, India, Nepal, and Mongolia.	All travelers; vaccine.	7-10 days
Rabies	Endemic dog rabies exists in Mexico, El Salvador, Guatemala, Peru, Columbia, Ecuador, India, Nepal, Phillipines, Sri Lanka, Thailand, and Vietnam.	Travelers staying for more than 30 days or at high risk of exposure to domestic or wild animals; vaccine series/booster.	7-14 days
Poliomyelitis	Developing countries not in western hemisphere; at risk all year in tropics; in temperate zones, incidence increases in summer and fall.	All travelers; vaccine series/booster.	Parenteral vaccine series, 28 days (see text) Anamnestic response to booster
Typhoid fever	Many countries in Asia, Africa, Central America, and South America.	Travelers with prolonged stay in rural areas with poor sanitation; vaccine series/booster.	Oral vaccine, 7 days Parenteral vaccine, probably 14 days
Yellow fever*	North and central South America, forest-savannah zones of Africa; some countries in Africa, Asia, and Middle East require travelers from endemic areas to be vaccinated.	All travelers; vaccine/booster at approved yellow fever vaccination center.	10 days
Japanese encephalitis	Seasonally in most areas of Asia, Indian subcontinent, and western Pacific islands; in temperate zones, incidence increases in summer and early fall; in tropics, year-round incidence.	Travelers staying for more than 30 days in high-risk rural areas; staying outdoors during transmission season; vaccine series.	10 days
Cholera*	Certain undeveloped countries.	If required by local authorities, one dose usually suffices; primary series only for those living in high-risk areas under poor sanitary conditions or those with compromised gastric defense mechanisms (achlorhydria, antacid therapy, previous ulcer surgery); booster every 6 months.	Probably 30 days
Plague	Africa, Asia, and Americas in rural mountainous or upland areas.	Travelers whose research or field activities bring them in contact with rodents; vaccine series/booster; consider taking tetracycline (500 mg four times a day) for chemoprophylaxis (inferred from clinical experience in treating plague).	Probably 30 days

*Only yellow fever vaccine is required for entry by any country; cholera vaccine may be required by some local authorities; and meningococcus vaccine is required for pilgrims to Mecca, Saudia Arabia, during Haj. However, it is important to follow CDC recommendations for all vaccines to prevent disease. If a required vaccine is contraindicated or withheld for any reason, attempts should be made to obtain a waiver from the country's consulate or embassy.

[†]Because areas affected can change, and for more specific details, consult CDC's traveler's hotline (see Box 5-1).

[‡]For detailed information concerning administration of individual vaccines, see text under each vaccine and Table 5-2.

immunizations that may apply to them, since the prevalence of vaccine-preventable illness is higher in many other countries. The majority of travelers do not need additional vaccines. In some countries where the prevalence of measles, mumps, rubella, hepatitis A and B, influenza, meningococcus, rabies (carried by domesticated animals), polio, typhoid, yellow fever, Japanese encephalitis, cholera, or plague is high, special vaccines are recommended. Table 5-7 lists the vaccines and IGs recommended for travelers (see Table 5-2 for specific doses). Table 5-7 is general because recommendations change periodically according to disease surveillance. Health care providers should consult the CDC's traveler's hotline or web site for up-to-date information on vaccine-preventable illnesses in a specific area (see Box 5-1).

If a vaccine is contraindicated or withheld for any reason and the country requires a vaccination certificate or the local authorities require documentation of the vaccine, travelers should attempt to obtain a waiver from the country's embassy or consulate. Noncompliance with these requirements can result in quarantine on arrival.

Travelers often can minimize disease exposure. Many illnesses are transmitted through contaminated food and water. Any food should be cooked or boiled thoroughly or should be peeled. When drinking bottled water, the top should be wiped clean and dry. Ice cubes should be avoided. Iodine preparations can be brought to purify water in remote areas. Certain toxins, such as ciguatera, cannot be cooked away, so vectors should be avoided (e.g., barracuda, West Indian and Pacific Island fish). For recommendations regarding prophylaxis of traveler's diarrhea, see Chapter 111.

Insect vectors such as mosquitoes usually feed at dusk and dawn, and travelers should avoid going outdoors at these times. Clothes should cover most of the body and can be treated with the insect repellent permethrin. Diethylmethyltoluamide (DEET) in concentrations of 30% to 35% (which usually last 4 hours) should be applied sparingly to the skin, avoiding mucous membranes, eyes, and irritated skin. For the preexposure prophylaxis of malaria, see Chapter 30.

Avoiding sandals, tucking pants into shoes, using permethrin-treated clothing, and self-inspection after outdoor exposure can prevent tick-borne and flea-borne illnesses. If found, a tick should be removed with forceps or gloved hands, pulling straight out; twisting may lead to retained head parts. The skin should be cleansed thoroughly.

Contact with both wild and domesticated animals can promote rabies. Any bite should be promptly cleaned with soap and water and health care sought. The traveler should be reevaluated on return to the United States for the adequacy of the postexposure prophylaxis, since immunobiologics used in other countries may not be as effective.

Blood-borne illnesses such as hepatitis B and HIV are more common in many other countries. Condoms should be used for any sexual contact. If living in a household in a country with endemic hepatitis B, sharing razors or toothbrushes should be avoided. General safety measures to avoid accidents are extremely important, since the medical and blood supplies in other countries may be less safe. In many situations, blood transfusions should be avoided; instead, colloid or crystalloid plasma expanders are preferred. Urgent evacuation may be necessary.

ADDITIONAL READINGS

American Academy of Pediatrics. In Peter G, editor: *Red book: report of the Committee on Infectious Diseases,* ed 24, Elk Grove Village, Ill, 1998, The Academy.

American College of Physicians Task Force on Adult Immunization, Infectious Diseases Society of North America: *Guide for adult immunization,* ed 3, Philadelphia, 1994, The College.

Centers for Disease Control and Prevention (CDC): General recommendations on immunization: recommendations of the Advisory Committee on Immunization Practices (ACIP), *MMWR* 43(RR-1), 1994.

CDC: Immunization of health care workers: recommendations of the Advisory Committee on Immunization Practices (ACIP) and the Hospital Infection Control Practices Advisory Committee (HICPAC), *MMWR* 46(RR-18), 1997.

CDC: Measles, mumps, and rubella—vaccine use and strategies for elimination of measles, rubella, and congenital rubella syndrome and control of mumps: recommendations of the Advisory Committee on Immunization Practices (ACIP), *MMWR* 47(RR-8):1-57, 1998.

CDC: Prevention of hepatitis A through active or passive immunization: recommendations of the Advisory Committee on Immunization Practices (ACIP), *MMWR* 48(RR-12):1-37, 1999.

CDC: Prevention of varicella updated recommendations of the Advisory Committee on Immunization Practices (ACIP), *MMWR* 48(RR-06):1-5, 1999.

CDC: Recommendations of the Advisory Committee on Immunization Practices (ACIP): use of vaccines and immune globulins in persons with altered immunocompetence, *MMWR* 42(RR-4), 1993.

CDC: Update on adult immunization: recommendations of the Advisory Committee on Immunization Practices (ACIP), *MMWR* 40(RR-12), 1991.

CDC: Update on vaccine side effects: recommendations of the Advisory Committee on Immunization Practices (ACIP), *MMWR* 45(RR-12), 1996.

US Department of Health and Human Services, Centers for Disease Control and Prevention, National Center for Infectious Disease: *Health information for international travel 1996-97,* HHS pub no 95-8280, Atlanta, 1997, CDC.

CHAPTER 6

Family Health

Thomas L. Campbell
David B. Seaburn
Susan H. McDaniel

Despite rapid societal changes in the structure and function of families, the family remains the most important relational unit in society and provides individuals with their most basic needs for physical and emotional safety, health, and well-being. The family plays an essential role in all aspects of health, illness, and medical care. In health care, family members may act as informants, customers for treatment, consultants, or part of the problem.

We define *family* as "any group of people related either biologically, emotionally, or legally."[13] This includes all forms of traditional and nontraditional families, such as blended families, unmarried couples, and gay and lesbian couples. The relevant family context may include family members who live a distance from the patient or all the residents of a community home for developmentally delayed persons. In daily practice, primary care physicians are most involved with family members who live in the same household.

This chapter presents a primary care approach to family health. We discuss the role of the family as an important source of stress, social support, health beliefs, and health behaviors and as the primary caregivers in chronic illness. The impact of serious illness on the family and the family's influence on the course of an illness are emphasized. We outline the basic principles of working with families in primary care, including how to understand the family context of presenting symptoms, the use of genograms, the role of family meetings and conferences, and the importance of working collaboratively with mental health professionals. These principles are illustrated with a case example from primary care.

The task of the family-oriented primary care physician is to consider the patient within the family context, to gain a broader understanding of the presenting problem or illness, and to access more resources for treatment. A family orientation does not mean always seeing family members together in the office. This chapter addresses both how to treat the individual patient from a family perspective and how to involve other family members in the patient's care when needed.

FAMILY HEALTH AND ILLNESS CYCLE

One way to consider the multiple ways in which the family plays an important role in health is the family health and illness cycle (Fig. 6-1). This model organizes the literature on families and health and provides a temporal sequence for families' experiences with health and illness.[8] It also emphasizes the constant interaction between family members and health care professionals in all aspects of health and illness. Starting with health promotion and disease prevention, this section reviews the relevant research and clinical implications for each phase.

Health Promotion and Disease Prevention

The family is the social context in which health promotion and disease prevention occur. The World Health Organization has characterized the family as the "primary social agent in the promotion of health and well-being."[20] A healthy lifestyle is usually developed, maintained, or changed within the family setting. Behavioral risk factors tend to cluster within families because members share similar diets, physical activities, and tobacco and alcohol use.[8] In a 1985 Gallup survey of health-related behaviors, more than 1000 adults reported that their spouse or significant other was more likely to influence their health habits than anyone else, including their family physician.

Nutrition is an obvious family activity. Despite changes in traditional family roles, women still do most of the meal planning and preparation for the entire family. To counsel men with elevated cholesterol about dietary changes without involving their wives is unlikely to be successful. It is well documented that family members consume similar amounts of salt, calories, cholesterol, and saturated fats. Several randomized controlled trials have shown that involving the spouse in weight reduction programs significantly improves long-term weight loss.[1] A number of "family heart" studies have demonstrated the effectiveness of health promotion programs targeted at families rather than individuals.[4]

The initiation, maintenance, and cessation of *smoking* are strongly influenced by family relationships. Smokers are much more likely to marry other smokers, smoke the same number of cigarettes, and quit at the same time.[19] Smokers who are married to nonsmokers or ex-smokers are more likely to quit and remain abstinent than smokers married to smokers. Support from the spouse or partner is associated with successful smoking cessation.[6] In particular, supportive behaviors involving cooperative participation, such as talking a smoker out of smoking a cigarette, and reinforcement, such as expressing pleasure at the smoker's efforts to quit, predict

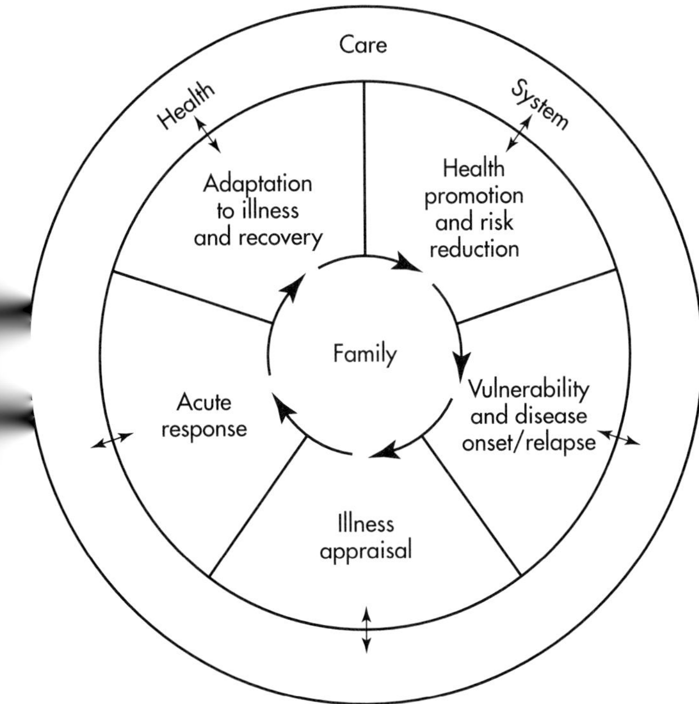

Fig. 6-1. Family health and illness cycle. (From Doherty WA, Campbell TL: *Families and health,* Beverly Hills, Calif, 1988, Sage.)

successful quitting. Negative behaviors, such as nagging the smoker and complaining about the smoking, predict relapse.[7]

In clinical practice it is more efficient and effective to conceptualize health promotion as a family activity and to counsel patients and their families together about healthy lifestyles. Other family members can be used as a valuable resource in facilitating changes in health behaviors. Exploring the family context, physicians can gain a better understanding and use more effective interventions to facilitate compliance with behavioral changes.

Vulnerability and Disease Onset/Relapse

As the most intimate social environment, the family is the major source of both stress and social support for most people. Most stressful life events, such as those ranked in the Holmes and Rahe Life Events Scale,[12] occur within the family. The adverse effects of the two most stressful life events, the death of a spouse and divorce, are well documented. Family members, particularly the spouse, are the most important social relationships and account for most of the association between social support and health. The quality of the marriage seems to have a particularly strong influence on overall health.

Symptoms and health problems seen by the primary care physician are often related to stress within the family setting. Patients, however, rarely identify family stress as a source of their symptoms. Using a biopsychosocial approach, the astute physician can accurately assess the role that family stress may play in a patient's symptoms and decide what interventions are most appropriate and effective.

Illness Appraisal

Most health problems are managed at home, in the family context, without any involvement of the health care system. The appraisal of physical symptoms is a complex personal and social activity that occurs outside the professional setting. As every physician knows, some patients consult their physicians frequently about minor self-limiting problems, whereas others do not contact the physician until they are "at death's door." Understanding how patients and families assess symptoms and decide whether to consult a physician can help the primary care physician better understand the patient's concerns and develop more effective treatment plans.

Most families have a "family health expert," usually the wife-mother or grandmother, who is assigned and assumes the role as the expert in health matters.[10] This individual is often consulted when a family member becomes ill, deciding what treatment should be given and whether a health professional should be consulted. Sometimes a patient may present to the physician solely at the request of another family member. For example, a middle-aged man may request a complete physical examination because his wife wants to make sure he does not have cardiovascular disease or other health problems. In such cases the physician should determine who is the "customer" and who is requesting the services.

Families usually have their own beliefs about health and illness, which may differ from medical knowledge or beliefs. These beliefs may affect whether a health professional is consulted and what treatments are used. If the physician's recommendations for treatment conflict with the family's belief system or the advice of the family health expert, the patient is unlikely to comply. Therefore the physician may inquire routinely about advice and recommendations the patient has received from others, particularly family members. When noncompliance is suspected, the patient and family's health beliefs should be assessed.

Acute Response

The diagnosis of a serious illness is one of the most feared and disruptive crises for families and challenges their coping skills. Few adults have escaped the dreaded phone call informing them of a health emergency, diagnosis of cancer, a heart attack, or death of a parent or other family member. The family's response to the crisis is influenced by their appraisal of the situation and their resources. Families may go through a period of disorganization, when their coping responses are inadequate to deal with the problems. Family members often assemble from around the country and put aside past problems and conflicts to help support and care for the ill family member.

What family members request and need most from health professionals during this acute period is medical information and emotional support. Lack of information about the condition, the treatment, or the prognosis of a loved one can be one of the most stressful aspects of the crisis. At this time, meeting with the entire family can be enormously beneficial, giving the essential medical information in a clear, concise manner and providing emotional support.[13] Even when care of the patient is being provided by other medical specialists, such as surgeons or oncologists, the primary care physician can play an important role explaining the medical situation to the family and providing support.

Adaptation to Illness and Recovery

Many families cope effectively with the crisis stage of a serious illness but may have more difficulty coping with chronic illness. Chronic illness has become a nearly universal part of family life and requires families to reorganize themselves around the illness. One half of all persons over age 65 are limited in their activities by some chronic condition, and family members are the primary caregivers for these persons. Not only does chronic illness have an enormous impact on the family, particularly the primary caregiver, but how the family copes with the illness can influence the course of the illness.

The challenge for families with a chronically ill family member is to reorganize to meet the needs of the chronic illness without sacrificing the needs of other family members. The chronic illness can be viewed as another family member who disrupts normal family routines and demands special time and attention.[11] Some families may try to ignore the illness, pretend that it does not exist, and avoid any changes in family life. Others may totally reorganize around the illness, always putting the needs of the illness and the patient first and neglecting the needs of other family members. At times, family members may become overprotective of the ill family member and overresponsible for care of the illness. In response, the patient may fail to assume the appropriate responsibility for the illness.

The primary care physician can help families adapt to the long-term demands of a chronic illness by meeting with them as a family or a couple and encouraging them to talk about the illness, especially their fears and emotional responses. Many families have never discussed the impact of a serious illness on their lives and can be profoundly affected by such meetings. Each family member can be encouraged to share feelings about the illness and its effects. The physician can help families decide whether they have achieved the desired balance between the patient's needs and the family's needs.

The following case example illustrates the interaction between family issues and development of cardiovascular disease.

Jim Goldner, 47 years old, had multiple cardiac risk factors and had not seen a physician in more than 10 years. Although both his father and his grandfather died of acute myocardial infarction (MI) in their 50s, Jim continued to smoke a pack of cigarettes a day and rarely exercised. His family always believed that the men died early from heart disease and that little could be done to prevent it. Jim's father had quit smoking after his first heart attack but suffered a second and fatal MI a year later. Jim was not worried about his health because he felt well and could still beat his 12-and 15-year-old sons in basketball.

On the other hand, Jim's wife, Betsy, was very worried about her husband's health. She was constantly hiding and throwing out his cigarettes and had placed the entire family on a low-cholesterol, low-fat diet despite complaints from her husband and sons. She continually tried to have Jim see their family's primary care physician and even made an appointment for him, which he canceled.

Ted, Jim and Betsy's 15-year-old son, was having difficulties in high school and at home. The previous year he had flunked several of his classes and was repeating his sophomore year. He was frequently out past his curfew on Saturday nights, and his parents had caught him smoking and drinking. He had frequent verbal arguments with his father, who was furious at him for his behavior and tried to punish him by imposing stricter limits.

One Saturday night Ted returned home drunk at 2 AM, 2 hours after his curfew. Jim was enraged and began shouting at his son and shoving him against the wall. Betsy tried to restrain and reason with her husband, who simply yelled back at her. In the midst of this family argument, Jim began experiencing dull chest pressure. At first Jim ignored his symptoms, but as the pain increased, he became short of breath and had to sit. Betsy immediately called an ambulance, despite her husband's protest. In the emergency room, his electrocardiogram showed that Jim was having an acute anterior wall MI.

PRINCIPLES OF FAMILY HEALTH

This section outlines the basic principles of family health and illustrates their use through the case of the Goldner family. These principles are relevant for all types of primary care and for a variety of problems, ranging from simple self-limiting health conditions to complex biopsychosocial issues.

Use Biopsychosocial Approach

Since a family-oriented approach is based on the biopsychosocial model, the primary care physician must avoid a split between biomedical and psychosocial issues or problems in patient care. Using a completely integrated, biopsychosocial approach is difficult in clinical practice. Western culture and medical training place great emphasis on diagnosing problems as either physical or emotional and often focus exclusively on one aspect of the problem. The challenge for the physician is to evaluate simultaneously the biomedical and psychosocial aspects of the problem and to decide at which level or levels of the biopsychosocial model to intervene. The family-oriented physician assumes that the family context will be relevant to most clinical problems, as illustrated in Jim Goldner's case.

Dr. C had known the Goldner family for almost 20 years. He saw Betsy regularly for her Pap smears and to monitor her hypothyroidism. He had seen Jim twice almost 10 years earlier. He had initially seen Jim for tendinitis in his hand and had convinced him to return for a complete physical examination. At that time, Dr. C talked to Jim about his coronary risk factors, stressing the importance of stopping smoking. Jim never returned for his fasting lipid profile or follow-up. Dr. C was aware of Betsy's concerns about her husband's health and her son's problems.

In his initial history, Dr. C learned about the family conflict that had precipitated Jim's symptoms. He realized that these family issues would have to be dealt with after Jim's condition had stabilized and he was out of the intensive care unit (ICU). Dr. C met with the Goldner family—Betsy, the children, and Jim's sister—at the hospital the following morning. He explained the event medically, Jim's current condition, and the treatment plans. He answered their questions and encouraged them to share their fears about Jim dying. Dr. C reassured them that Jim was stable, that thrombolysis had been started promptly enough to prevent serious damage, and that they would be contacted immediately about any change. Dr. C wanted to meet with them again to discuss Jim's ongoing care after he was out of the ICU.

Assess Family Context of Presenting Symptoms

Since most health problems are influenced by, and also influence, the family, the physician should have some understanding of the family context of every patient. This may be as simple as knowing who is in the household, what treatments other family members have recommended, or who is the patient's primary caregiver.

Patients may have physical symptoms that are related to family stress or family problems. These physical symptoms may represent a stress-related illness, an exacerbation of an underlying chronic illness, or some type of somatization for which no physiologic abnormalities can be found. Experienced primary care physicians are aware of "red flags" that indicate the need for more complete exploration of the problem. These red flags may include stress-related symptoms (e.g., chronic headaches), unexplained or inconsistent physical symptoms, the patient's mood, or who accompanies the patient to the visit. In these situations the physician might ask the patient, "Have you had to deal with any recent changes or stresses at home?"

A few other simple questions can be used to assess the family context quickly. "How has this problem affected you and your family?" allows the physician to assess the impact of the illness on the patient and family. Family health beliefs can be explored by asking, "What does your family think may have caused or could treat this problem?" "How could your family be helpful to you in dealing with this problem?" or "What suggestions have family members made to you about this problem?" can begin the discussion of how to use family members as a resource. By being alert to red flags and addressing routine family assessment issues, the physician can begin to assess the situation effectively and efficiently.

Use Genogram for Family Assessment

The genogram, or family tree, is the most basic and useful tool in family-oriented primary care. It is a simple method for obtaining and recording basic family information that provides a visual record of the family[16] (Fig. 6-2). Although similar to the family pedigree, used to obtain family histories of genetic diseases, the genogram also provides information about family structure, relationship patterns, developmental issues, life cycle stages, and stressful life events. Fig. 6-3

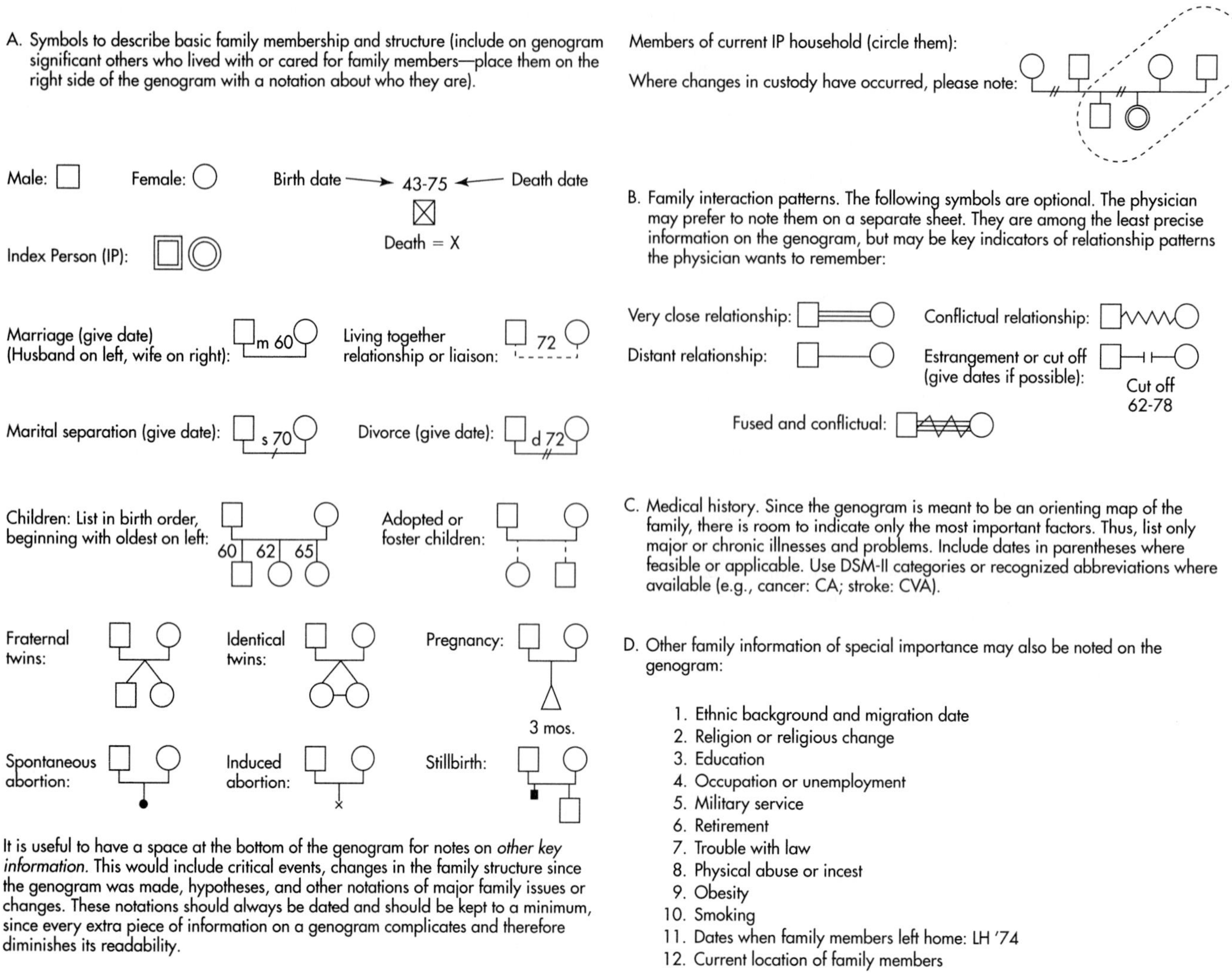

A. Symbols to describe basic family membership and structure (include on genogram significant others who lived with or cared for family members—place them on the right side of the genogram with a notation about who they are).

Male: Female: Birth date → 43-75 ← Death date

Death = X

Index Person (IP):

Marriage (give date) (Husband on left, wife on right): m 60

Living together relationship or liaison: 72

Marital separation (give date): s 70

Divorce (give date): d 72

Children: List in birth order, beginning with oldest on left: 60 62 65

Adopted or foster children:

Fraternal twins:

Identical twins:

Pregnancy: 3 mos.

Spontaneous abortion:

Induced abortion:

Stillbirth:

It is useful to have a space at the bottom of the genogram for notes on *other key information.* This would include critical events, changes in the family structure since the genogram was made, hypotheses, and other notations of major family issues or changes. These notations should always be dated and should be kept to a minimum, since every extra piece of information on a genogram complicates and therefore diminishes its readability.

Members of current IP household (circle them):

Where changes in custody have occurred, please note:

B. Family interaction patterns. The following symbols are optional. The physician may prefer to note them on a separate sheet. They are among the least precise information on the genogram, but may be key indicators of relationship patterns the physician wants to remember:

Very close relationship:

Conflictual relationship:

Distant relationship:

Estrangement or cut off (give dates if possible): Cut off 62-78

Fused and conflictual:

C. Medical history. Since the genogram is meant to be an orienting map of the family, there is room to indicate only the most important factors. Thus, list only major or chronic illnesses and problems. Include dates in parentheses where feasible or applicable. Use DSM-II categories or recognized abbreviations where available (e.g., cancer: CA; stroke: CVA).

D. Other family information of special importance may also be noted on the genogram:

1. Ethnic background and migration date
2. Religion or religious change
3. Education
4. Occupation or unemployment
5. Military service
6. Retirement
7. Trouble with law
8. Physical abuse or incest
9. Obesity
10. Smoking
11. Dates when family members left home: LH '74
12. Current location of family members

Fig. 6-2. Genogram format. (Redrawn from McGoldrick MSW, Gerson R: *Genograms in family assessment,* New York, 1986, Norton.)

shows the genogram of the Goldner family. Glancing at a patient's genogram gives the physician a "snapshot" of the patient's context and the family issues that may be relevant to that visit.

Many family-oriented physicians do a brief, skeletal genogram as part of the family and social history during the initial visit or physical examination. With practice, such a genogram can be obtained in less than 5 minutes and added to on subsequent visits. Patients are usually comfortable with providing family information and helpful in constructing the family tree. The genogram shows the patient that the physician is interested in all aspects of the patient's life. It also helps the physician to identify risk factors for inherited diseases and other problems. When the genogram is obtained as a part of routine practice, patients are more likely to reveal sensitive and important family issues, such as substance abuse or domestic violence.

The genogram is also helpful in caring for difficult and frustrating patients with complex medical problems. Little may be known about these patients' family and context. Using one appointment or 15 minutes to obtain a more detailed genogram can provide useful data about these patients and their problems. The genogram can help the patient and physician begin the gradual shift from a narrow focus on physical symptoms to a broader view of the patient's life circumstances.

> Jim's condition stabilized in the ICU, and he underwent cardiac catheterization, which showed distal narrowing in a branch of his left anterior descending coronary artery. During visits to the ICU, Dr. C began to talk with Jim about the events that precipitated his MI and about his cardiac risk factors. Dr. C obtained a more complete genogram related to heart disease in Jim's family. In the process, Jim talked about his conflict with his father and how Jim's father had dealt with his heart disease. Jim agreed to meet as a family with Dr. C to discuss his illness and how his family could help.

Explore Family's Developmental Challenges and Stresses

With the genogram and the ages of family members, the primary care physician can obtain a good sense of what developmental issues the family is likely to confront and whether these normative stresses are affecting the health of family members. The *family life cycle* is a useful conceptual framework for understanding family development.[5] Similar to the individual life cycle, the family life cycle assumes that families go through different stages for which specific developmental tasks must be accomplished. Families who d

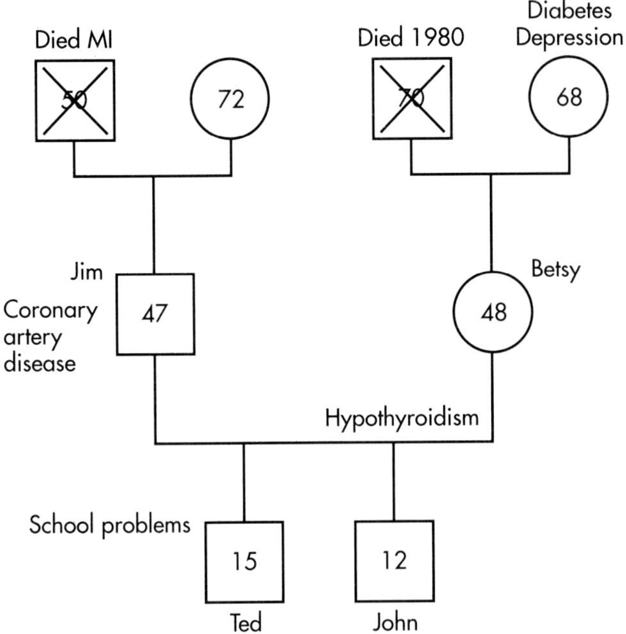

Fig. 6-3. Goldner family genogram.

not accomplish these developmental tasks at one stage may develop difficulties with subsequent family development. For example, some families have difficulties allowing young adult members to establish personal autonomy and independence. Young women sometimes become pregnant as a way to separate from their parents and start their own families. These women experience enormous stress as they try to live on their own, form an intimate relationship with a partner, and raise a child, all at the same time. They are at high risk for developing physical or emotional health problems.

Many normative family life transitions can be very stressful and can precipitate or exacerbate health problems. Many women and some men in their 40s are faced with the demands of caring for elderly and disabled parents while raising young children. The genogram allows the physician to identify quickly and explore these types of developmental stressors.

> Dr. C was aware of many developmental stresses faced by the Goldner family. The most immediate was their fear of Jim's premature death or disability. His wife was particularly concerned about whether he could return to his work as an automobile sales manager, which was very stressful. Ted's struggles to develop a sense of autonomy within his family and peer group was an obvious source of ongoing stress. Betsy's father had died 5 years previously, and her mother was declining physically and emotionally. Jim and Betsy had been contemplating whether to have her mother move in with them or find a supervised apartment for her. Betsy had recently gone through menopause and was concerned whether Jim still found her physically and sexually attractive.

Meet with Family Members

For many health problems, it may be helpful to meet and consult with a family member during a regularly scheduled office visit. Research has shown that family members often accompany the patient to the medical office, either remaining in the waiting room or joining the patient in the examination room. In the Direct Observation of Primary Care study, Medalie et al[17] evaluated the content of more than 4000 office visits to 138 family physicians. They found that another family member was present during 32% of visits, most often when the patient was a child under 13 (97%) or elderly (25%) but also 12% of the time with adult patients. Overall, another family member's health problem was discussed at 18% of these visits. Botelho et al[2] found that 39% of patients came to a family medicine center with a family member or friend and that two thirds of these accompanied the patient into the examination room. In a study of family practices in Ontario, one third of patients were accompanied by a family member or friend, who was usually described as an advocate for the patient.[3] This research documents that family members frequently accompany patients into the examination room or are present in the waiting room.

Meeting and consulting with family members during a routine visit can be helpful whenever the health problem is likely to have a significant impact on other family members or when family members can be a resource in the treatment plan. The most relevant family member for adult patients is usually the spouse. Inviting the partner or spouse to accompany the patient should be considered with (1) diagnosis of a serious condition during a chronic illness, (2) noncompliance with treatment recommendations, (3) somatization or unexplained medical symptoms, and (4) health problems that have a significant interpersonal component (e.g., marital problems, sexual dysfunction).

Involving family members in a routine medical visit rarely takes extra time. Visits may even be more efficient when a family member can provide important information about the health problem. The examination or consultation room must have an extra chair for the family member.

When a patient has a complaint related to an interpersonal problem, the physician tends to support and empathize with the patient, inadvertently taking sides in the conflict. The challenge for the primary care physician working with families is to maintain a positive relationship or alliance with each family member and avoid taking sides in any conflict or problem, except when the patient's safety is at risk. The physician must avoid blaming other family members or siding with the patient against another family member. To listen repeatedly to a patient complain about another family member is similar to only prescribing pain medication for a peptic ulcer; the patient feels better acutely while the underlying problem worsens. Meeting with the patient and other family members can help the physician avoid taking sides in a family conflict and maintain positive relationships with everyone involved.

Meet with Extended Family

Although the primary care physician can use a family-oriented approach while seeing an individual patient or meeting with family members during a routine office visit, at times it is helpful to convene the entire family for a more extended family conference. The decision to convene a family conference usually depends on the seriousness of the health problem and its impact on the family. During a hospitalization the physician should meet with the family at least twice, on admission and shortly before discharge. Family members can often provide valuable information about the events leading up to the admission, and they want information about the patient's medical condition. Before discharge the physician can review the course of the hospitalization and the plans for outpatient care and can elicit any family concerns about the patient returning home. This latter visit recognizes that the family usually must assume care of the patient after discharge.

It is particularly important to meet with the family when the diagnosis of a terminal illness is made or when a patient dies. Family members are often in a state of shock and need information and support. Because of the strong emotions surrounding death in a family, often a high degree of denial can interfere with effective communication and the sharing of feelings. Death is often viewed as a failure by the physician and is often accompanied by feelings of guilt. This guilt may result in the physician avoiding the family when it is most important for both parties to meet. Physicians should routinely see family members for follow-up during the first 6 months after a loss.

Dr. C met with the entire Goldner family before Jim left the hospital. He reviewed the events at the hospital and the treatment plans. At Dr. C's request, Betsy participated in the hospital cardiac rehabilitation program with her husband and agreed to continue as an outpatient. She went to the informational lectures and even used the treadmill to experience the exertion her husband could safely tolerate. The couple met with the hospital nutritionist to review Jim's diet, and they agreed to work together to help Jim stop smoking. Dr. C met with the couple alone to discuss how to resume their sexual activity. He made an appointment for outpatient follow-up for 1 month.

At the follow-up visit, Jim was doing well. He was actively participating in the cardiac rehabilitation program and had not smoked any cigarettes. Betsy was concerned, however, that Jim was doing too much physical activity too soon. He had returned to work full time and had put up the storm windows on their house the previous weekend. Jim complained that Betsy was always nagging him to "take it easy" and telling what he should and should not do. Dr. C helped the couple to negotiate a compromise. Jim agreed to cut back on some of his activities that were excessive and frightening his wife, and Betsy agreed not to monitor Jim's behavior. They agreed to return as a family in 1 month.

Assess Levels of Working with Families

When working with families in primary care, physicians should determine their level of involvement. As in other primary care areas, physicians must decide what level of skills and knowledge they have or want to have in a particular area. For example, when treating cardiac patients, physicians must decide whether they have the skills and interests to treat complicated post-MI patients in the ICU or whether they want to limit treatment to outpatient care of uncomplicated cardiac problems and refer other patients to a cardiologist.

Doherty and Baird[9] have outlined five levels of physicians' involvement with families and the knowledge, personal development, and skills needed for each (Box 6-1). This classification was developed to recognize that all physicians work with families at some level and that some problems require the expertise of a trained family therapist. Most primary care physicians usually work at level two, providing ongoing medical information and advice to families, and level three, eliciting feelings and providing support to families. Level four, performing systematic assessment and planned intervention, usually requires additional training in family systems theory and its application. At this level, physicians can provide brief and focused primary care family counseling for uncomplicated family problems. More complex and chronic family problems demand family therapy, a specialty service that requires 3 to 5 years of training and supervision and that is beyond the interest and training of most primary care physicians.

Deciding whether to treat a family or marital problem with primary care counseling depends on the physician's interests, expertise, and availability. The physician who does not have the interest, time, or additional training in family counseling should refer these problems to a skilled therapist. Many family physicians, however, find these problems interesting, challenging, and enriching to their practice and want to counsel families.[15] Box 6-2 shows the types of problems that typically can be managed in primary care counseling and those that usually require consultation and often referral to a mental health professional.

Dr. C met with the Goldner family again 3 months after Jim's heart attack. For the first few weeks after Jim's return from the hospital, Ted had been on his best behavior, not wanting to upset his father. As Jim resumed his usual activities and returned to work, however, Ted resumed his previous behaviors, and the arguments flared up again. Dr. C explored the problem with the Goldners, asking each about the issues. He recognized that the family problems were serious and longstanding. It was clear that Ted was abusing alcohol and perhaps drugs and would need further evaluation. Dr. C also suspected that Ted's behavior had kept his parents' focus on him and that they were not dealing with serious underlying marital problems.

Dr. C recommended that the Goldners see Dr. M, a psychologist and family therapist with whom Dr. C often collaborated. Dr. C explained that he thought their issues were serious, could affect Jim's health, and deserved treatment by an expert in family relations. Because Dr. C had established their trust during Jim's hospitalization, they agreed to see the family therapist. An appointment was made with Dr. M while they were in the office, and a follow-up appointment was made with Dr. C for several weeks after that.

Many family and marital problems are too chronic, complex, or time consuming for the family physician to counsel. These problems necessitate referral to a marriage and family therapist.[14,18] This specialty requires several years of supervised training after residency. Unlike the medical specialists whom family physicians meet and work with in the hospital, skilled therapists are not as easily found in the community. The most frequently used method for finding a good therapist is to ask respected colleagues whom they use and why. The American Association of Marriage and Family Therapy, the accrediting organization for family therapists, issues a directory of certified family therapists by city. Perhaps the most useful way to find a good and trusted therapist in the community is to arrange face-to-face meetings with several recommended therapists to learn about their interactive approaches, their theoretic orientations, and their interests and experience in interfacing with the medical system.

Counseling for referral is an important skill for primary care physicians to learn. It involves identifying key problems faced by the patient and family, including as many family members as reasonable in clarifying a desire for change, and contacting the appropriate family-oriented mental health professional. Patients are more likely to follow through on such referrals if the physician knows the professional by name. The physician should clarify the collaborative relationship with the therapist and that they will work as a team to provide care for the patient and family.

Box 6-1. Levels of Physician Involvement with Families

Level One: Minimal Emphasis on Family

The baseline level of involvement consists of dealing with families only as necessary for practical and medicolegal reasons, but not viewing communication with families as integral to the physician's role or as involving skills for the physician to develop. This level presumably characterizes most medical school training, in which biomedical issues are the sole conscious focus of patient care.

Level Two: Ongoing Medical Information and Advice

Knowledge base

Primarily medical, plus awareness of the triangular dimension of the physician-patient relationship

Personal development

Openness to engage patients and families in a collaborative way

Skills

1. Regularly and clearly communicating medical findings and treatment options to family members
2. Asking family members questions that elicit relevant diagnostic and treatment information
3. Attentively listening to family members' questions and concerns
4. Advising families about how to handle the patient's medical and rehabilitation needs
5. For large or demanding families, knowing how to channel communication through one or two key members
6. Identifying gross family dysfunction that interferes with medical treatment, and referring the family to a therapist

Level Three: Feelings and Support

Knowledge base

Normal family development and reactions to stress

Personal development

Awareness of one's own feelings in relationship to the patient and family

Skills

1. Asking questions that elicit family members' expressions of concerns and feelings related to the patient's condition and its effect on the family
2. Empathically listening to family members' concerns and feelings, and normalizing them where appropriate
3. Forming a preliminary assessment of the family's level of functioning as it relates to the patient's problem
4. Encouraging family members in their efforts to cope as a family with their situation
5. Tailoring medical advice to the family's unique needs, concerns, and feelings
6. Identifying family dysfunction, and fitting a referral recommendation to the family's unique situation

Level Four: Systematic Assessment and Planned Intervention

Knowledge base

Family systems

Personal development

Awareness of one's own participation in systems, including the therapeutic triangle, medical system, one's own family system, and larger community systems

Skills

1. Engaging family members, including reluctant ones, in a planned family conference or a series of conferences
2. Structuring a conference with even a poorly communicating family in such a way that all members have a chance to express themselves
3. Systematically assessing the family's level of functioning
4. Supporting individual members while avoiding coalitions
5. Reframing the family's definition of their problem in a way that makes problem solving more achievable
6. Helping the family members view their difficulty as one that requires new forms of collaborative efforts
7. Helping family members generate alternative, mutually acceptable ways to cope with their difficulty
8. Helping the family balance their coping efforts by calibrating their various roles in a way that allows support without sacrificing anyone's autonomy
9. Identifying family dysfunction that lies beyond primary care treatment, and orchestrating a referral by educating the family and the therapist about what to expect from one another

Level Five: Family Therapy

Knowledge base

Family systems and patterns whereby dysfunctional families interact with professionals and other health care systems

Personal development

Ability to handle intense emotions in families and self and to maintain neutrality in the face of strong pressure from family members or other professionals

Skills

The following is not an exhaustive list of family therapy skills but rather several key skills that distinguish level five involvement from primary care involvement with families.

1. Interviewing families or family members who are difficult to engage
2. Efficiently generating and testing hypotheses about the family's difficulties and interaction patterns
3. Escalating conflict in the family to break a family impasse
4. Temporarily siding with one family member against another
5. Constructively dealing with a family's strong resistance to change
6. Negotiating collaborative relationships with other professionals and other systems who are working with the family, even when these groups are at odds with one another

From Doherty WJ, Baird MA, editors: *Family-centered medical care: a clinical casebook,* New York, 1987, Guilford.

When referring a patient, couple, or family to a therapist, it is helpful to consult the therapist early in the process to share ideas and strategies and clarify the consultation or referral question. If the referral is the physician's idea rather than the patient's, it is often necessary to maximize the patient's motivation to see the therapist. Using the patient's language and understanding of the problem can help pitch the referral. Referring for an "evaluation" or "consultation" is

Box 6-2. Problems Addressed in Primary Care and Referred to Specialists

Problems Typically Seen in Primary Care Counseling

Adjustment to diagnosis of new illness
Other adjustment or situational disorders
Crises of limited severity or duration
Behavioral problems
Mild depressive reactions
Mild anxiety reactions
Uncomplicated grief reactions

Problems Usually Referred to Mental Health Specialist

Suicidal or homicidal ideation, intent, or behavior
Psychotic behavior
Sexual or physical abuse
Substance abuse
Somatic fixation
Moderate to severe marital and sexual problems
Multiproblem family situations
Problems resistant to change in primary care counseling

usually more acceptable than for "family therapy." Some patients hear a referral for family therapy as meaning that their family is bad or in some way responsible for the current problem. Having the patient make the appointment with the therapist while still in the physician's office can also help facilitate the referral. With reluctant, difficult, or somatizing patients, a joint session with the therapist may be extremely helpful in facilitating a referral.

The timing of a referral to a therapist is important. With some patients and families, it may take months or years to reach an agreement about a therapy referral. After the couple or family members have gone for consultation or ongoing therapy, the referring physician must communicate regularly with the therapist and inform the patient and family that the physician will continue to see the patient and collaborate with the therapist. Regular communication between the physician and psychotherapist helps avoid confusion or triangulation and facilitates clear treatment planning and division of labor.

SUMMARY

To use a family health approach to primary care, the physician must know the multiple factors that contribute to a patient's problems. The physician then can decide which problems can be addressed directly and which should be referred to a mental health professional. A family orientation does not mean that the primary care physician must treat all the family's problems.

Family health focuses on the family context of a patient's health problems and offers new opportunities for working with patients and their families. Families are viewed not only as potential sources of stress in patients' lives but also as important resources in patient care. Working collaboratively with families can be a rewarding aspect of primary care and is easily incorporated into the physician's practice.

REFERENCES

1. Black DR, Gleser LJ, Kooyers KJ: A meta-analytic evaluation of couples' weight-loss programs, *Health Psychol* 9:330-347, 1990.
2. Botelho RJ, Lue B, Fiscella K: Family involvement in routine health care: a survey of patients' behaviors and preferences, *J Fam Pract* 42:572-576, 1996.
3. Brown JB, Brett P, Stewart M, Marshall JN: Roles and influence of people who accompany patients on visits to the doctor, *Can Fam Physician* 44:1644-1650, 1998.
4. Campbell TL, Patterson JM: The effectiveness of family interventions in the treatment of physical illness, *J Marital Fam Ther* 21:545-584, 1995.
5. Carter E, McGoldrick M: *The expanding family life cycle: individual, family and social perspectives,* ed 3, New York, 1998, Prentice Hall.
6. Cohen S, Lichtenstein E: Partner behaviors that support quitting smoking, *J Consult Clin Psychol* 58:304-309, 1990.
7. Coppotelli HC, Orleans CT: Partner support and other determinants of smoking cessation maintenance among women, *J Consult Clin Psychol* 53:455-460, 1985.
8. Doherty WA, Campbell TL: *Families and health,* Beverly Hills, Calif, 1988, Sage.
9. Doherty WJ, Baird MA: Developmental levels in family-centered medical care, *Fam Med* 18:153-156, 1986.
10. Doherty WJ, Baird MA:*Family therapy and family medicine: toward the primary care of families,* New York, 1983, Guilford.
11. Gonzalez S, Steinglass P, Reiss D: Putting the illness in its place: discussion groups for families with chronic medical illnesses, *Fam Process* 28:69-87, 1989.
12. Holmes TH, Rahe RH: The social readjustment rating scale, *J Psychosom Res* 11:213-218, 1967.
13. McDaniel S, Campbell T, Seaburn D: *Family-oriented primary care: a manual for medical providers,* New York, 1992, Springer-Verlag.
14. McDaniel SH, Hepworth J, Doherty WJ: *Medical family therapy,* New York, 1992, Guilford.
15. McDaniel SH, Landau-Stanton J, Seaburn D, Campbell T: Family-oriented care for psychosocial problems of adolescents. In McAnarney E, Kreiger R, Orr D, Commerci G, editors: *Textbook of adolescent medicine,* New York, 1991, Saunders.
16. McGoldrick M, Gerson R, Shellenberger S: *Genograms: assessment and intervention,* ed 2, New York, 1999, Norton.
17. Medalie JH, Zyzanski SJ, Langa D, Stange KC: The family in family practice: is it a reality? *J Fam Pract* 46:390-396, 1998.
18. Seaburn DB, Gawinski BA, Gunn W, Lorenz A: *Models of collaboration: a guide for family therapists practicing with health care professionals,* New York, 1996, Basic Books.
19. Venters MH, Jacobs DR Jr, Luepker RV, et al: Spouse concordance of smoking patterns: the Minnesota Heart Survey, *Am J Epidemiol* 120:608-616, 1984.
20. World Health Organization: *Statistical indices of family health,* Geneva, 1976, WHO.

CHAPTER 7

Adolescents and Young Adults

Elizabeth A. Alexander

Unlike other age groups in the population, adolescents (age 13 to 21 years) are the only subgroup for whom mortality ha[s] not declined significantly in the past 30 years and for whom significant morbidity has increased. Also unlike other ag[e] groups, the major causes of morbidity and mortality ar[e] usually preventable (Fig. 7-1).[16] Rather than purely organi[c]

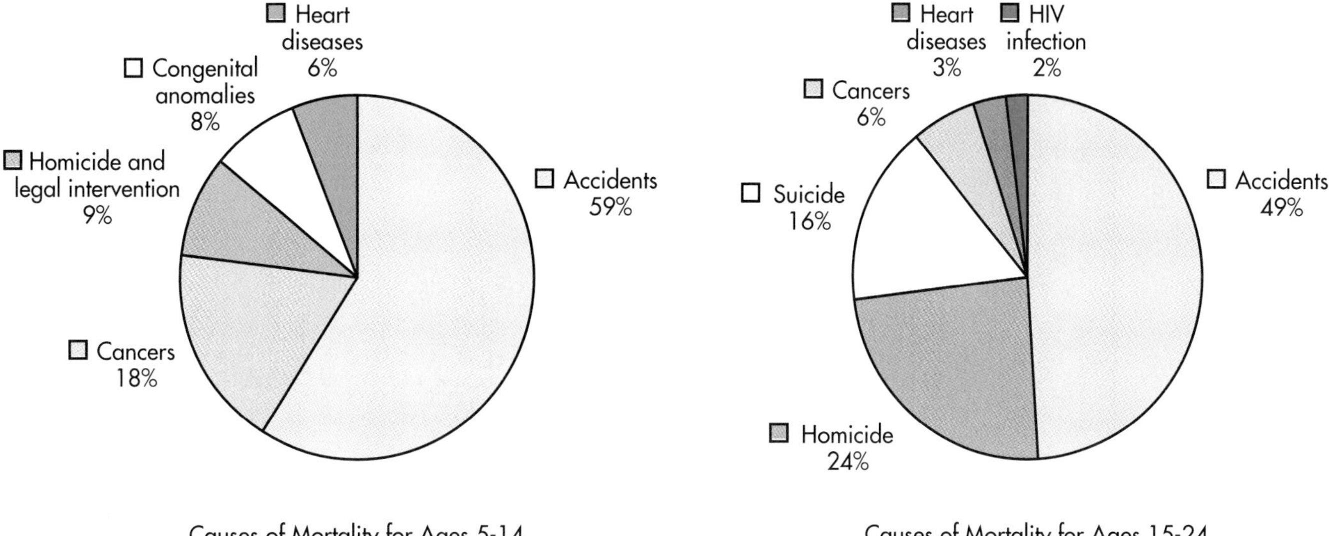

Fig. 7-1. Causes of child and adolescent mortality. *HIV*, Human immunodeficiency virus. (From Ventura SJ, Peters KD, Martin JA, et al: *Monthly Vital Statistics Report* 46 [suppl 2]:32-33, 1997.)

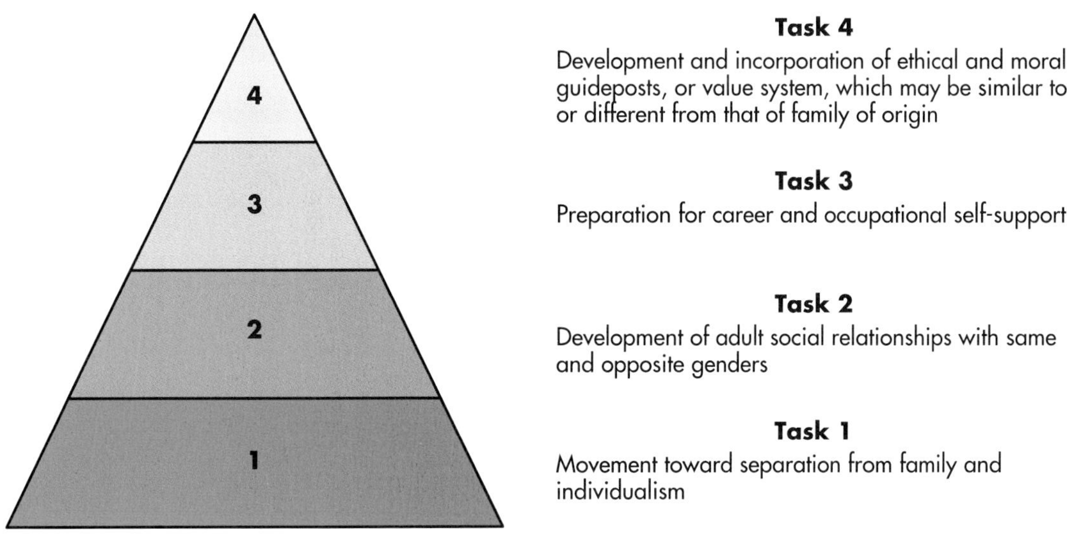

4
3
2
1
Task 4
Development and incorporation of ethical and moral guideposts, or value system, which may be similar to or different from that of family of origin
Task 3
Preparation for career and occupational self-support
Task 2
Development of adult social relationships with same and opposite genders
Task 1
Movement toward separation from family and individualism

Fig. 7-2. Erikson's model of developmental tasks for adolescents and young adults.

processes impairing health, as in other age groups, most preventable illnesses and deaths in adolescents are related to intersecting behavioral and developmental issues, or "pubertal hazards" that do not occur at other points in the life cycle. Health-related behavioral patterns established in adolescence also affect lifetime health patterns of many adults and thus have a secondary impact on morbidity and mortality as persons age.

Theoretically, 75% of the deaths in adolescents and young adults are preventable, and the cumulative impact of many adolescent behaviors on health into adulthood is modifiable. Many behavioral issues that cause mortality and morbidity in adolescence, however, are deeply rooted in complex social issues and cannot be resolved only in the health care setting. In addition to physicians' care, public policy change, community interventions, and protective factors that impact the health of adolescents and young adults are critical in addressing "behavioral epidemics" that impair health in these age groups and later in life.

DEVELOPMENTAL CONTEXT

Any approach to the care of adolescents and young adults requires an understanding of the developmental context in which this care occurs (Fig. 7-2). Struggling with and progressing toward mastery of these tasks often help explain risk-taking behavior in young people who previously have not engaged in unhealthy behaviors. For example, when a young adult rides in a car with an alcohol-impaired driver, the desire to be accepted by peers (task 2) may be more critical at that point in life than distantly perceived risks, such as death or impairment from an accident. Adolescents, in struggling with both developmental tasks 1 and 2, adopt a *relative-risk model*. This view is generally short term rather than long range, and the "data" in the risk assessment are

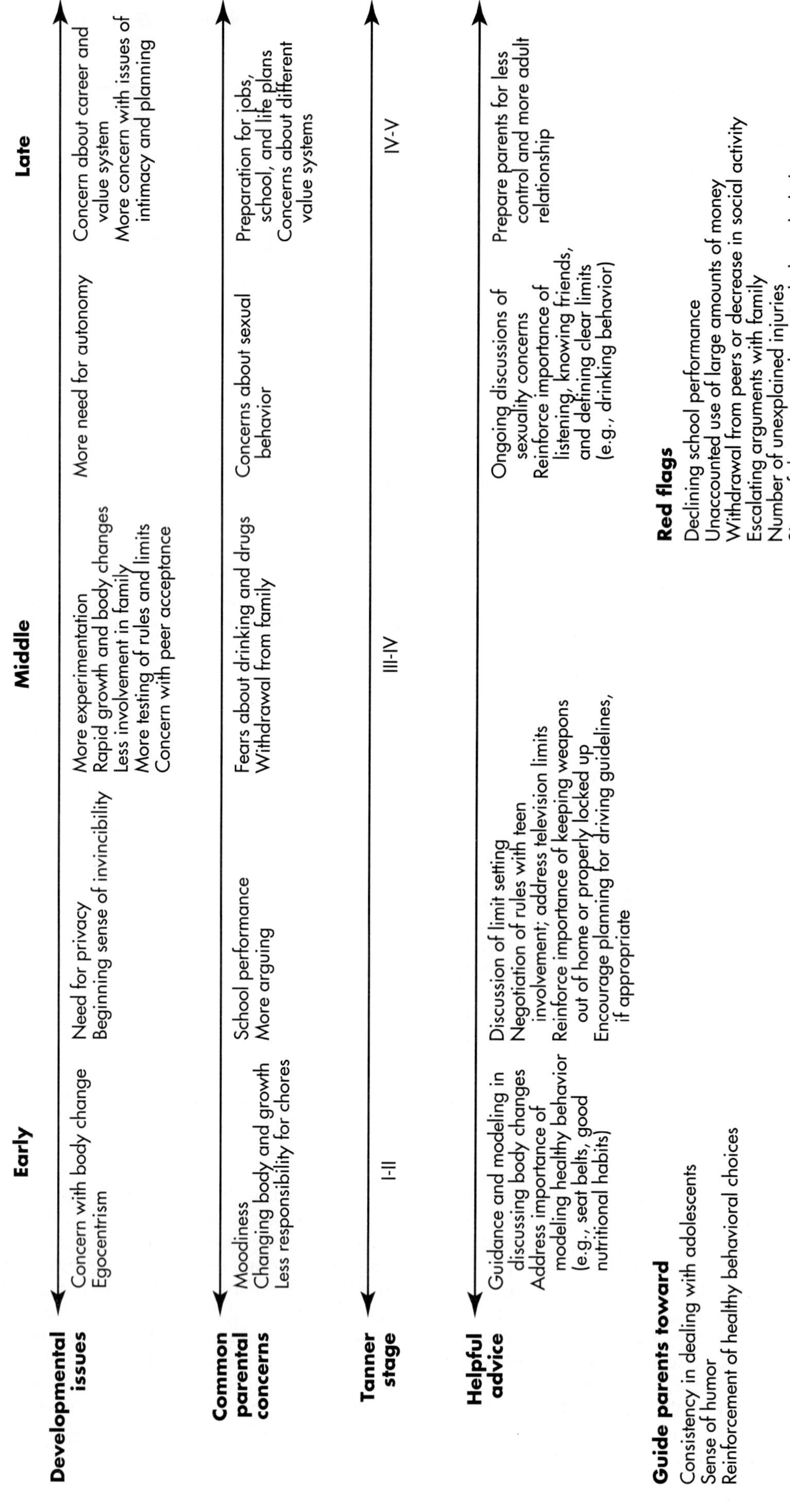

Early
Middle
Late
Developmental issues
Concern with body change
Egocentrism
Need for privacy
Beginning sense of invincibility
More experimentation
Rapid growth and body changes
Less involvement in family
More testing of rules and limits
Concern with peer acceptance
More need for autonomy
Concern about career and value system
More concern with issues of intimacy and planning
Common parental concerns
Moodiness
Changing body and growth
Less responsibility for chores
School performance
More arguing
Fears about drinking and drugs
Withdrawal from family
Concerns about sexual behavior
Preparation for jobs, school, and life plans
Concerns about different value systems
Tanner stage
I-II
III-IV
IV-V
Helpful advice
Guidance and modeling in discussing body changes
Address importance of modeling healthy behavior (e.g., seat belts, good nutritional habits)
Discussion of limit setting
Negotiation of rules with teen involvement; address television limits
Reinforce importance of keeping weapons out of home or properly locked up
Encourage planning for driving guidelines, if appropriate
Ongoing discussions of sexuality concerns
Reinforce importance of listening, knowing friends, and defining clear limits (e.g., drinking behavior)
Prepare parents for less control and more adult relationship
Guide parents toward
Consistency in dealing with adolescents
Sense of humor
Reinforcement of healthy behavioral choices
Red flags
Declining school performance
Unaccounted use of large amounts of money
Withdrawal from peers or decrease in social activity
Escalating arguments with family
Number of unexplained injuries
Signs of drug use or abuse, including alcohol

Fig. 7-3. Developmental issues in early, middle, and late adolescence into young adulthood, with parental concerns, corresponding Tanner stages, and counseling recommendations.

often either exaggerated or underestimated. Primary care physicians should therefore help young people assess whether they are making decisions based on good data, with consideration of the long-range view.

A second model describing the interface between developmental issues and risk-taking behaviors divides adolescence into three consecutive stages: early, middle, and late (Fig. 7-3).

HEALTH SCREENING AND PREVENTION

Settings

Adolescents may seek health care in a variety of settings, including primary care offices, school-based clinics, community clinics, and athletic "batch" screening programs. Unfortunately, some adolescents (12%) do not have access to any regular source of health care. Furthermore, although adolescents (ages 11 to 20) constitute about 17% of the population, they account for only 11% of health care visits.[6] Common barriers to care for this age group include discomfort with the setting (e.g., pediatrician's offices, offices that allow little privacy), inefficiency of clinical care, inconvenient hours, and problems with transportation. Many young people also do not know how to negotiate appointment systems in provider offices and simply forego care rather than persist with a scheduling system that puts their needs "on hold." To reach this group for preventive and long-term care, office-based providers might consider (1) special time blocks on Saturdays or after school reserved for adolescents, (2) special training of receptionists in dealing with adolescents who call directly, (3) artwork on walls that is inviting and relevant to this age group, and (4) alternate mechanisms for billing when confidentiality is requested.

Confidentiality

Several studies have shown that adolescents will not discuss ersonal health concerns without clear assurance of confiden-iality. Although the laws vary from state to state, most states rotect confidentiality for adolescents in the health care etting, unless there is a serious threat to life or long-term ealth. Minimally, providers must be clear about the issues nd agreements regarding confidentiality with both adoles-ents and their parents. The discussion about confidentiality referably should occur with both youth and parents together, efore the need for privacy arises. Part of this discussion also volves explicitly identifying issues that are exempt from nfidentiality, as well as care issues exempt from consent of ther parents or adolescents. Finally, discussion about issues payment when confidentiality is expected can prevent advertent disclosure of information through billings sent to rents. Box 7-1 provides an example form that may help to arify for parents and youth the boundaries of confidentiality th their physicians.[2]

isk Factors

e health care of adolescents should be guided primarily by tors that impair their health and development. The three idelines for justification of screening in the health care ting require that (1) the screening occur for conditions that ve significant burden in terms of morbidity or mortality; (2) effective means of screening is available; and (3) effective erventions are available to reduce risk when screening is sitive. When these screening guidelines are applied to the lth care of adolescents, the first and second requirements are straightforward, with the third more challenging. In the last decade, however, research has improved on the effectiveness of programs that protect the health of young people. This knowledge likely will increase over the next few years, making this third guideline more readily attainable.

The other dilemma in health screening for youth is that with so many preventable causes of disease and death, deciding *which* issues deserve attention within the constraints of limited contacts and time requires careful judgment. Because adolescents do not seek health care frequently, "premium" clinical time must focus on the most likely risks for a particular patient. For example, with inner-city youth, screening for alcohol-related driving behavior might yield fewer positive responses than screening for weapon availability or use. Finally, as in assessing risk factors, the physician also must assess protective factors that may balance the hazards of risk factors for many adolescents and young adults. Fig. 7-4 offers a paradigm for such assessment.

Box 7-1. Informed Consent for Parents of Adolescents

Dear Parent,

Many of your sons and daughters, in the next 5 to 10 years, may want the opportunity to discuss with me issues related to their development. Included in the concerns that adolescents often bring to their physician are questions (and potential decisions) about sexuality and sexual behavior, including sexually transmitted disease and contraceptive information, questions or concerns about substance abuse, issues related to the ability to handle peer pressure, and concerns about the family. Although, as their family physician, I cannot make decisions for them, I can make sure that they have access to accurate information about their health and have the opportunity to have another concerned adult listen to them and talk with them.

In order for young people to feel free to discuss personal issues with a physician, these conversations and treatment must remain confidential and private. If there is ever a concern that involves serious threat to life or will be likely to involve serious impairment of health to your son or daughter, you can be assured that we will involve you in these conversations. Otherwise, I will consider what your son or daughter tells me in this office as privileged information, just as I consider my conversations with you to be private and confidential.

It is my goal to be available as another trusted adult who is available to your son or daughter and to work in partnership with him or her toward a healthy adulthood. I also will continue to encourage your sons and daughters to discuss with you matters of importance in their lives. However, should they wish to come to me for care or guidance and request confidentiality in the professional relationship, I hope you will give your vote of confidence and permission for this kind of involvement in their care.

Sincerely yours,

I, ______________, give permission for ______________ to treat ______________, my son or daughter, and respect the privacy of the physician-patient relationship, so that what my child chooses to discuss with the physician will be kept confidential, except in instances that are life threatening.

From Alexander B: Sexual concerns of adolescents. In Taylor RE, editor: *Family medicine: principles and practice,* ed 5, New York, 1998, Springer.

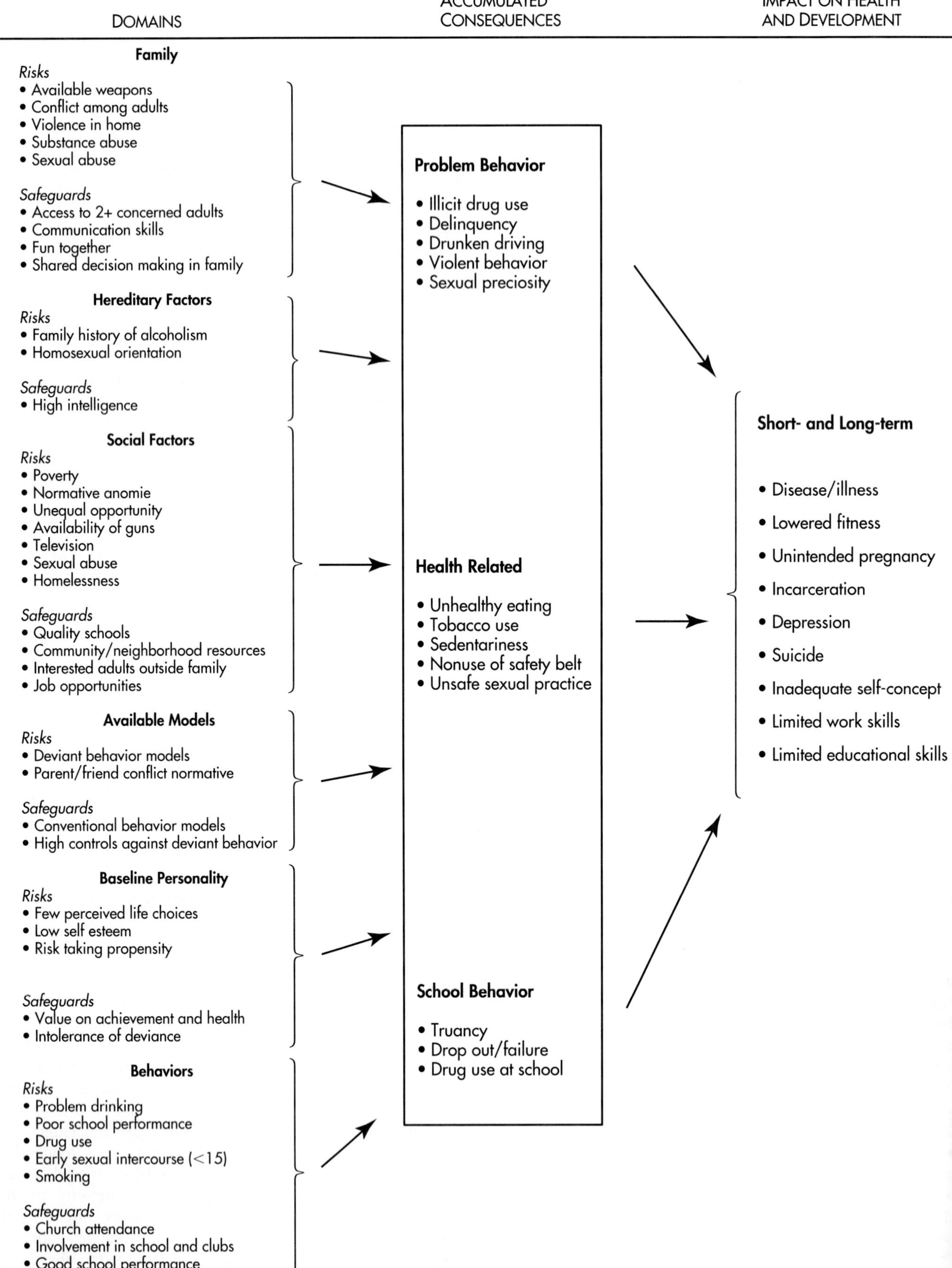
DOMAINS
ACCUMULATED CONSEQUENCES
IMPACT ON HEALTH AND DEVELOPMENT
Family
Risks
• Available weapons
• Conflict among adults
• Violence in home
• Substance abuse
• Sexual abuse
Safeguards
• Access to 2+ concerned adults
• Communication skills
• Fun together
• Shared decision making in family
Hereditary Factors
Risks
• Family history of alcoholism
• Homosexual orientation
Safeguards
• High intelligence
Social Factors
Risks
• Poverty
• Normative anomie
• Unequal opportunity
• Availability of guns
• Television
• Sexual abuse
• Homelessness
Safeguards
• Quality schools
• Community/neighborhood resources
• Interested adults outside family
• Job opportunities
Available Models
Risks
• Deviant behavior models
• Parent/friend conflict normative
Safeguards
• Conventional behavior models
• High controls against deviant behavior
Baseline Personality
Risks
• Few perceived life choices
• Low self esteem
• Risk taking propensity
Safeguards
• Value on achievement and health
• Intolerance of deviance
Behaviors
Risks
• Problem drinking
• Poor school performance
• Drug use
• Early sexual intercourse (<15)
• Smoking
Safeguards
• Church attendance
• Involvement in school and clubs
• Good school performance
• Plans for future
Problem Behavior
• Illicit drug use
• Delinquency
• Drunken driving
• Violent behavior
• Sexual preciosity
Health Related
• Unhealthy eating
• Tobacco use
• Sedentariness
• Nonuse of safety belt
• Unsafe sexual practice
School Behavior
• Truancy
• Drop out/failure
• Drug use at school
Short- and Long-term
• Disease/illness
• Lowered fitness
• Unintended pregnancy
• Incarceration
• Depression
• Suicide
• Inadequate self-concept
• Limited work skills
• Limited educational skills

Fig. 7-4. Assessment on health of multiple risks and safeguards in lives of adolescents. (Adapted from Jessor R: *J Adolesc Health* 12:602, 19

Table 7-1. Health Care Interventions for Adolescents and Young Adults with Degree of Supportive Evidence

Issue/intervention	No evidence to support	Some evidence to support	Clear evidence to support
Sexuality education	Withholding of information Fear-based tactics	Peer counseling Group education On-line interactional groups	Reduction in early onset of coitus and risky sexual behaviors with good information
Violence	Expulsion from school for students with weapons	Development of conflict-resolution skills	Presence of caring adults outside family Family counseling Involvement in extracurricular programs
Nutrition and eating disorders	Diet drugs Strict calorie control Fad diets	Adequate nutrition information Calcium intake assessment	Exercise programs Adult involvement with diet and exercise
Accident prevention	Preaching Scare tactics	Driver's education Peer normative and development programs	Laws on seat belts, helmet use, and older driving age Strict laws on penalties for drinking and driving
Depression and mood disorders	Screening routinely through testing Routine patient education	Attention to substance use; changes in school performance; parent education	Attention to cluster suicides Family history Programs that build skills for youth Adult mentoring programs
Alcohol and drug use	Abstinence programs Preaching, scolding	Media and advertising education Health education approach Family history	Clear and strict enforcement of drinking and driving penalties Peer normative and counseling programs Drug-free and alcohol-free alternatives for social activity

Outcomes

Although good research is limited on outcome markers for health care screening and preventive guidance for adolescents and young adults, some studies suggest that certain interventions make a positive difference on their health status (Table 7-1).

An equally important consideration in the use of health care resources involves what is *not* effective for youth. This information is also included, although even less research has been done in this area. Generally, preaching, scolding, threatening, withholding of information, and denial of care based on moral beliefs are not effective means of influencing the behavior of adolescents or young adults. Education, accurate information, and developmentally relevant information increase the chances of successfully partnering with youth in efforts to protect and preserve their health.

SPECIAL ISSUES

Sexuality and Reproductive Health

Data confirm that adolescents and young adults of the last decade continue to initiate intercourse earlier than did youth of previous generations. A synopsis of data* relevant to the sexual health of youth indicates the following[1,18]:

- The number of years of sexual intercourse (i.e., age at onset of coitus) correlates with increased numbers of sexual partners and with all sexual health risks, including human immunodeficiency virus (HIV) infection, sexually transmitted diseases (STDs), and unintended pregnancy. Therefore, knowing the age at first onset of coitus provides a proxy for estimation of risk.
- The median age of onset of coitus for youth is about 16, with a great increase in those who begin coitus between 14 and 16. About 7.2% of youth begin coitus before age 13.
- About 70% to 80% of youth have experienced intercourse by age 18.
- By grade 12, one fourth of all students have had intercourse with four or more partners.
- Sexually active youth have a 10% to 26% positive rate for some STDs (*Chlamydia,* gonorrhea, herpes, *Trichomonas*), depending on the study.
- HIV seroprevalence of homeless youth in areas of high HIV prevalence is 11%.
- About 16% to 20% of all diagnosed STDs infect adolescents.

Despite these data, clinicians often avoid screening youth for sexual risk-taking behaviors. Reasons for this avoidance include the pressure of time, poor reimbursement for preventive health, and a belief that the physician's patients are at lower risk than the general adolescent population. Millstein et al[9] reported that primary care physicians provide gynecologic and STD services to youth far below the recommended guidelines, with 31% providing STD/HIV education and only 40% regularly screening for sexual activity, 17% for numbers of sexual partners, 12% for sexual orientation, and 10% for casual sex. Because risk-taking behavior in sexuality and reproductive health has a wide range, the physician is faced with how best to assess risk efficiently, how often to screen, and the best screening methods. Fig. 7-5 presents a paradigm based on data and recommendations from several national groups, including the Adolescent Health Division of the American Medical Association (AMA) and the Centers for Disease Control and Prevention (CDC).[4]

For all adolescents, topics necessary for adequate screening and education for STDs include how they make

*Because research on youth uses heterosexual intercourse as the marker for sexual activity, these data reflect that research. Clinicians should be aware that some youth engage in sexual behaviors that would not be reflected in this definition.

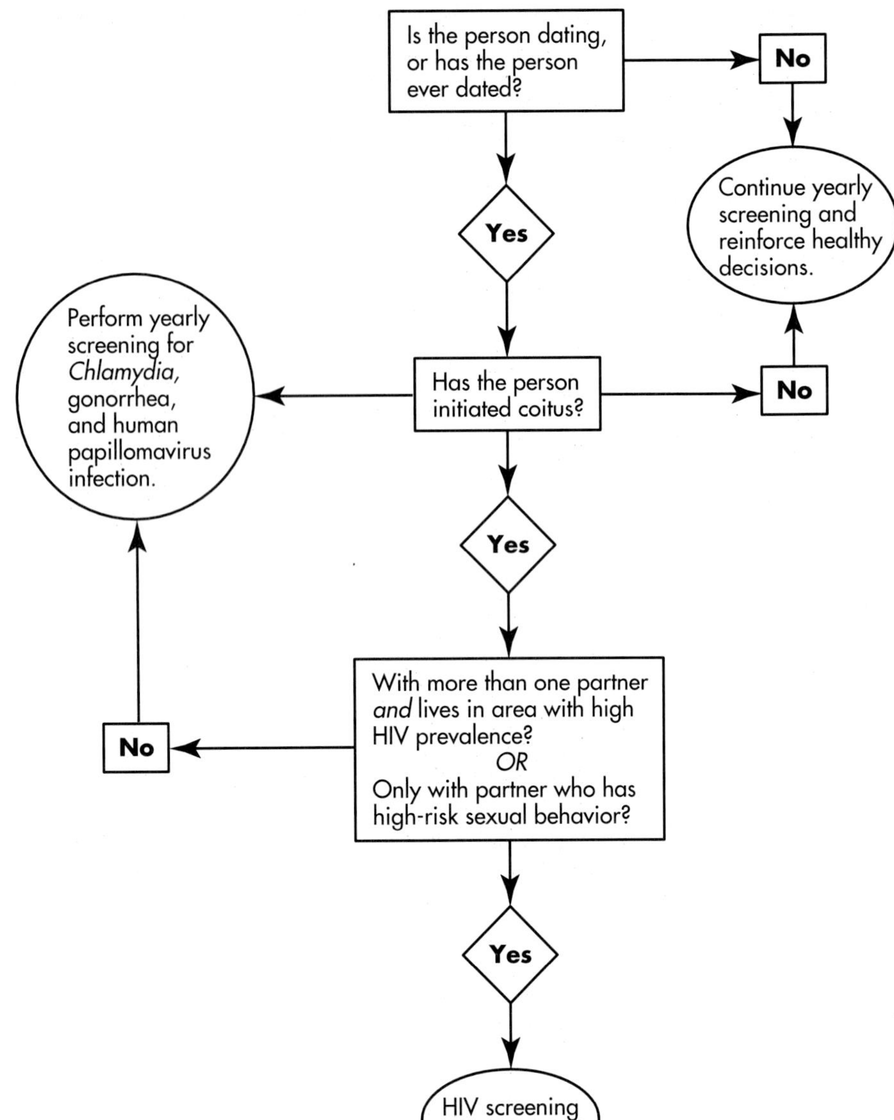

Fig. 7-5. Clinical decision-making approach to sexually transmitted disease (STD) screening for adolescents. *HIV,* Human immunodeficiency virus.

decisions about their sexual health, when they consider initiating intercourse, how they determine if a potential partner is safe, and how they insist on condom use if they choose to become sexually active. Predictors of STDs in teens include socioeconomic status, contraceptive method, frequency of intercourse, multiple partners, age at first intercourse, and sex with a partner who has symptoms of an STD. Of these, age of first coitus and lifetime number of partners have the highest positive predictability for STD and HIV risk.

New advances in STD testing for both men and women now permit screening and follow-up for gonorrhea, *Chlamydia,* and *Trichomonas* infection based on urine tests; a swab specimen from the cervix is not required in women. This laboratory option allows for easy follow-up of treated patients and more frequent testing than the annual gynecologic examination in youth with risk factors. Routine screening for *Chlamydia* infection and gonorrhea has been determined to be cost-effective when the prevalence of disease in the population is greater than 2%. Even in sexually active adolescents at lowest risk, the prevalence is 6%, so th cost-effectiveness of routine screening is well documented.[1]

Contraception. When a young person is sexually activ and requests a prescription method of contraception i addition to condoms, the physician's options include th diaphragm, oral contraceptives, depot progesterone prepara tions, and intrauterine device (IUD). Each has advantages an disadvantages, which must be individualized to the patien Regardless of the prescription contraceptive, the physicia still must reinforce the importance of condoms as a method minimizing the risk of STDs if a young person engages coitus. Table 7-2 lists the options for contraception, the effectiveness, side effects, benefits, and costs.

Gay, Lesbian, and Bisexual Youth. Little good r search is available on gay, lesbian, and bisexual youth. So adolescents and young adults struggle with the issue of sex orientation, with some ultimately self-identifying as g lesbian, or bisexual. Health risks that occur more frequen

Table 7-2. Options for Contraception

Method	Effectiveness	Benefits	Common side effects	Annual cost in addition to examination
Condoms and jelly	95%	Protective against STDs Widely available	Incorrect use Inconsistent use	$100
Diaphragm	95%	Inexpensive Some barrier protection	Urinary tract infection Vaginal irritation Cumbersome to use	$20
Intrauterine device (IUD)	98%	Convenient	Higher risk of infertility when STDs contracted	$60, if retained for 3-5 years
Oral contraceptives	99%+	Convenient	Smoking a relative contraindication	$200-$240
Depot progesterone	99%+	Convenient	Weight gain Depression	$220

STDs, Sexually transmitted diseases.

for this group than for heterosexual youth should guide their screening and care. These known risks, with available supporting data, include the following[5,15]:

- *Depression and suicide:* 33% of adolescents who self-identify as gay or lesbian attempt suicide during adolescence, and 30% of all adolescent suicides are committed by gay or lesbian youth.
- *Homelessness:* many homeless youth are gay, lesbian, or bisexual and have left or been forced to leave their homes because of conflict over this issue.
- *Sexual victimization:* a significant number of gay or lesbian youth, particularly the homeless population, are victimized sexually in exchange for food, money, or shelter. More gay and lesbian youth have a history of sexual abuse as children than do heterosexual youth.
- *Substance abuse:* 9% to 14% of gay, lesbian, and bisexual youth have histories of problematic substance use that involves risk to health; half of gay youth report alcohol misuse.
- *Violence:* 40% of gay youth report being victims of violence related to their sexual orientation; most (75%) of these incidents are not reported to adults because of fear.
- *School dropout:* 28% of gay youth withdraw from school because of harassment.

Although uncomfortable for some, it is important to consider and ask about the issue of sexual orientation of youth with a screening question such as, "Do you find yourself romantically attracted to boys, girls, or both?" If screening yields questions or concerns in this area, follow-up with attention to the more prevalent risk factors is critical. In caring for gay, lesbian, or bisexual youth, a safe physician confidant can be protective for young people who feel isolated without adult support.

Disordered Eating

The number of youth with disordered eating continues to rise in the United States. Asking youth how they feel about their weight or doing a 24-hour recall on dietary intake frequently yields positive results in screening. *Obesity,* defined as a body mass index greater than 95% for age and gender norms, affects 12% of all adolescents.[7] Data also indicate that less than 5% of obese teenagers manage to lose weight and maintain weight loss for 2 years. Many more youth *perceive* themselves as overweight, with 61.5% of adolescent girls and 21.5% of adolescent boys attempting weight loss at any one time. Caucasian girls are more likely to perceive themselves as overweight than other racial groups and subsequently engage more often in unhealthy eating patterns.[12] Accompanying the data on weight is a corresponding drop in physical activity, with the steepest decline between midchildhood and adolescence.

Cardiovascular Disease

A significant number (30%) of youth have at least one modifiable risk factor for coronary artery disease (elevated cholesterol, hypertension, smoking, or obesity), and 5% to 10% of youth have two or more risk factors. Long-term cardiovascular health should become a consideration before diet and exercise habits are firmly established or before disease has progressed. Thus screening for and discussing cardiovascular health are appropriate in adolescence. The National Cholesterol Education Project recommends that adolescents with a family history of hyperlipidemia or premature cardiovascular disease be screened earlier and that all adolescents have lipid screening by age 21. For low-density lipoprotein (LDL) cholesterol in adolescents, below 110 is normal, 110 to 129 is borderline, and above 130 is elevated. As with adults, the recommendation for initial treatment is diet and exercise.[11]

Skin Care

Acne is one of adolescents' most common health-related concerns. Skin care evaluation and treatment provide an opportunity for additional education related to smoking and sun exposure prevention and for access to youth on other health issues. When youth have acne, explaining the physiologic mechanisms, the principles of treatment, and regular follow-up is important (Table 7-3) (see Chapter 84).

Substance Use

Many physicians underestimate the age of onset of substance and their ability to detect problematic use through screening. They also are bereft of strategies for effective intervention

Table 7-3. Medications for Acne

Medications	Indications	Advantages	Common drugs
Topical astringents	Oily skin, papular acne	Cheap, convenient	Benzoyl peroxide
Topical antibiotics	Papular acne, minor cysts	Cheap, convenient	Erythromycin, clindamycin
Topical retinoids	Oily skin, papular acne, comedomes	Convenient	Retin A gel
Oral antibiotics	Papular acne	Convenient	Tetracycline, erythromycin
Oral retinoids	Cystic, scarring acne	Often curative	Isotretinoin (Accutane)*

*Patient must be using effective method of birth control, have written and oral informed consent, and be monitored for lipids while taking isotretinoin.

when they do uncover a problem. The following principles should guide the conversation about this topic with youth[10,13]:

- The *average age* of onset of alcohol use is 14 years, so beginning the conversation about substance use early (age 11 to 12) is appropriate.
- The problematic use of substances has covariance with other behavioral clusters, including accidents, school underperformance, delinquency, and sexual risk taking. These other clinical presentations should prompt questions about substance use.
- The best screening technique for substance use may be to ask a young person about friends' alcohol use (assuming use), then proceeding with more specific and personal questions regarding binge drinking and associated risk behaviors when using substances.
- The progression from casual or binge drinking to physiologic addiction occurs more rapidly with young people; thus the earlier the onset of drinking, the more likely drinking proceeds to addiction in youth.
- The biologic and laboratory markers for alcohol misuse are γ-glutamyltransferase (GGT), probably the most sensitive marker; serum iron; and mean corpuscular volume (MCV). The combined use of carbohydrate-deficient transferrin (CDT) with GGT to screen for excessive alcohol intake has a sensitivity of 75% and specificity of 85%.

The use of inhaled and smokeless tobacco often precedes alcohol misuse; thus tobacco is considered a "gateway drug," or early marker for subsequent problematic substance use (see Chapters 51 and 57).

Mood Disorders

Suicide is the third leading cause of death among adolescents and has tripled in the last 20 years. Firearm suicides have increased dramatically, and the availability of guns in the home is an independent risk factor for adolescent suicide. Across all ages, suicides increase in the spring, and with youth, most suicides (70%) occur in the home, where the primary means of attempt is kept. Sixty percent of all youth report having some suicidal ideation, and 8% to 9% report having made some attempt. Estimates of attempts among youth range from 50,000 to 500,000 a year, with the attempt-to-completion ratio about 100 to 1. Prior suicide attempts, male gender, history of substance abuse, family dysfunction, and access to weapons all are risk factors that increase the likelihood of suicide in youth.

The connection between suicide and psychologic diagnoses, including depressive disorders, is more complex. The diagnoses with the most positive predictive weight for suicide in adolescence are conduct disorder and substance abuse; mood disorders are correlated less strongly with suicide. Compared with depressed adults, adolescents with depression have less melancholia, less impairment of functioning, less likelihood of psychotic disorder, fewer suicide attempts connected to depression, and a lower lethality with attempts. Depressed adolescents describe more anxiety, phobias, somatic complaints, and behavioral problems than depressed adults. Other predictors and comorbid factors for depression include a family history of mood disorders and family conflict. Depression in adolescents typically resolves within 12 to 18 months of onset, with 70% of these youth having another episode within 5 years of the initial presentation. Selective serotonin reuptake inhibitors (SSRIs) are the most effective antidepressant choice for adolescents. Tricyclics have not been shown to be as efficacious in treating depression in adolescents as SSRIs and carry a higher risk for lethality if used in a suicide attempt.[3,17]

Health care providers fail to identify depression and suicide risk in youth often because of the belief that adolescents are normally in turmoil, they are normally healthy, and their worries are inconsequential. Time and training also constrain many providers. Effective screening for depression is direct, often with questions such as "Do you ever feel down?" "What usually causes that?" and "How do you handle your down feelings?" Predictive life events with a positive correlation for depression and suicide in youth include the recent death of a close friend or relative, parental divorce, sexual assault, and relocation.

REFERENCES

1. Alan Guttenmacher Institute: *Sex and America's teenagers,* New York 1994, The Institute.
2. Alexander B: Sexual concerns of adolescents. In Taylor RE, edito *Family medicine: principles and practice,* ed 5, New York, 199 Springer.
3. Birhauer B, Ryan ND, Williamson DE, et al: Childhood and adolesce depression: a review of the past 10 years. Part I, *J Am Acad Chi Adolesc Psychiatry* 35:1427-1439, 1996.
4. Committee on Prevention and Control of STDs: The hidden epidemi confronting sexually transmitted diseases, *SIECUS,* 25:4-17, 1997.
5. Eggleston V: Notes from the field: serving gay, lesbian, bisexu transgender and questioning youth, *SIECUS* 24:7-8, 1995.
6. Gilchrist V, Alexander E: Preventative health care for adolescents, *Pr Care* 21:759-779, 1994.
7. Hammer SL: Obesity: the search goes on, *J Adolesc Health* 20:4 1997.
8. Reference deleted in pages.
9. Millstein SG, Igra V, Gans J: Delivery of STD/HIV preventative servi to adolescents by primary care physicians, *J Adolesc Health* 19:249-2 1996.

10. Morrison SF, Rogers PD, Thomas MH: Alcohol and adolescents, *Pediatr Clin North Am* 42:371-387, 1995.
11. National Cholesterol Education Project: *Report of the Expert Panel on Blood Cholesterol Levels in Children and Adolescents,* NIH Pub No 91-2732, Washington, DC, 1991, US Department of Health and Human Services.
12. Neff LJ, Sargent RG, McKeown RE, et al: Black-white differences in body size perceptions and weight management practices among adolescent females, *J Adolesc Health* 20:459-465, 1997.
13. O'Malley PM, Johnston LD, Bachman JG: Adolescent substance use, *Pediatr Clin North Am* 42:241-259, 1995.
14. Orr DP: Urine-based diagnosis of sexually transmitted infections using amplified DNA techniques: a shift in paradigms? *J Adolesc Health* 20:3-5, 1997.
15. Saewyc EM, Bearinger LH, Heinz PA, et al: Gender differences in health and risk behaviors among bisexual and homosexual adolescents, *J Adolesc Health* 23:181-188, 1998.
16. Ventura SJ, Peters KD, Martin JA, et al: Births and deaths: United States, 1996, *Monthly Vital Statistics Report,* 46(suppl 2):32-33, 1997.
17. Walter G: Depression in adolescence, *Aust Fam Physician* 25:1575-1582, 1996.
18. Youth risk behavior surveillance—United States, 1997, *MMWR* 41:1-31, 1998.

CHAPTER 8

Geriatric Patients

Sharon A. Levine
Patricia P. Barry

DEMOGRAPHICS

Life expectancy has improved dramatically during the twentieth century in the United States, largely because of decreases in deaths from acute illness, infectious diseases, and accidents and better prevention of chronic disease. In 1900, 3.1 million Americans, or about 4% of the population, were 65 or older. At present the number is more than 34 million, or 12.5% of the population. By 2050 the group is projected to grow to 78.9 million. The oldest old are the fastest growing population segment. The survivors of the baby-boom generation will become a great-grandparent boom, resulting in a huge increase in the number of people aged 85 and older. That cohort is expected to number 18 million, or 5% of the population, by 2050. Centenarians, 100 years and older, are expected to increase dramatically in number, from 32,000 in 1982 to 597,000 in 2040. The ranks of the elderly are therefore increasing both in absolute terms and relative to the population (Fig. 8-1).

A person who turned 65 in 1900 had a life expectancy of 76.9 years; in general a 65 year old in 1995 had a life expectancy of 82.4 years. Whites outlive African-Americans: life expectancy in 1996 was 79.6 years for white women, 74.2 for African-American women, 73.8 for white men, and 66.1 for African-American men.

The gender gap in life expectancy means a preponderance of women in the elderly population. The gender ratio for elderly persons, or the number of men per 100 women, has been dropping over recent decades. It also decreases dramatically with age. As a result, elderly women are more likely than men to be living alone and to depend on nonspousal family or formal supports for care.

Despite decreased mortality and longer life, chronic illnesses continue to have a major impact on the elderly. Chronic conditions such as arthritis, hypertension, hearing impairments, and heart disease represent 60% of ailments plaguing community-dwelling elderly patients. In addition to addressing the three major causes of death in older Americans—cardiovascular disease, cancer, and stroke, which account for almost 80% of deaths among elderly persons—primary care physicians of the twenty-first century must confront issues of dependency and functional impairment in an older, sicker patient population with a multitude of coincident problems. Even without providing cures for chronic illnesses, a physician who improves sight, hearing,

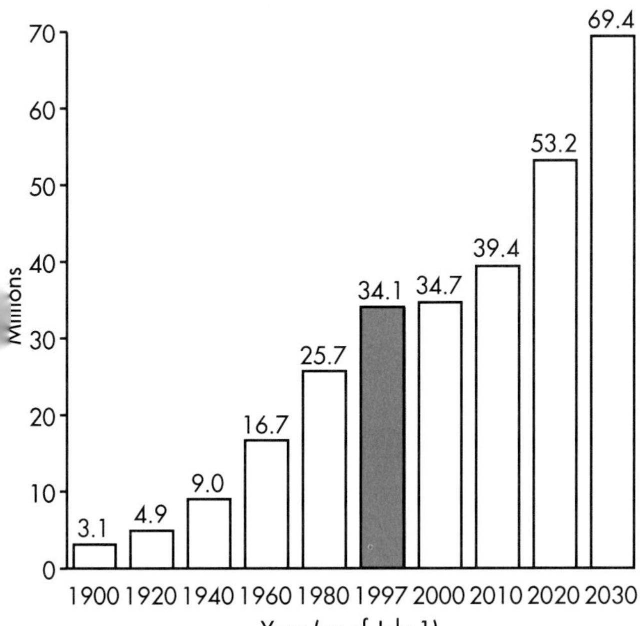

Fig. 8-1. Number (in millions) of persons 65 years of age and older from 1900 to 2030, based on data from the U.S. Bureau of the Census. Note that increments in years are uneven.

ambulation, or continence may enable a patient to remain in the community and avoid long-term institutionalization.

Many functionally impaired elderly currently reside in the community and are in need of primary care: only 5% of people over 65 are in nursing homes, and most of these are older than 85. Although the majority of noninstitutionalized elderly people function well physically, dependency needs do increase with age. Long-term care survey data indicate that 9.5 million people older than 50 living in the community have limitations in one or more of their activities of daily living (ADLs), which include bathing, toileting, feeding, and dressing, or instrumental activities of daily living (IADLs), which enable elders to live independently in the community and include managing finances, taking medications, preparing meals, housekeeping, and shopping.[10]

For those aged 65 to 74, only 6.7% depend on others for care. At 85 or older that number soars to 44%. In this age group, personal care assistance is required by 9.6% of those living alone, 18.8% of those who live with a spouse, and 25% of those living with others. Caregiver stress among family members on whom these elders depend has been well documented. Spouses often are elderly and disabled themselves, and children juggle work and childrearing with providing care for aging parents. The primary care physician must be sensitive to the burdens placed on family and friends. The physician should function as a resource for community services and exploration of possible long-term institutionalization.

APPROACH TO THE ELDERLY PATIENT

Environment

The environment where the history and physical examination take place should be adapted for the elderly patient. Rooms should be warm so that patients can comfortably disrobe. Lighting should be adequate, with minimal shadows and glare, to maximize sight for visually impaired patients. Rooms should be located away from noisy corridors and have adequate sound insulation so that hearing-impaired patients are not at a disadvantage. Doorways should be wide enough to accommodate adaptive devices such as wheelchairs. Chairs should have firm backs, high seats, and arms that make sitting and rising easy, especially for patients with arthritis or proximal lower extremity muscle weakness. Examination tables should be low enough for patients to mount and dismount safely. Pillows can be used to elevate the heads of patients with kyphoscoliosis.

Patients should be encouraged to wear eyeglasses and hearing aids. Amplification aids can be kept in the office for hearing-impaired patients. The use of adaptive aids such as walkers, canes, and wheelchairs should be encouraged and provided for those who need them.

History Taking

In eliciting the history from an older person, the physician should consider the maxim of geriatric medicine that atypical presentation of disease is typical. Many conditions, such as myocardial infarction, pneumonia, and sepsis, develop without their familiar symptoms or present as vague discomfort. Nonspecific complaints (e.g., malaise, fatigue, weakness) often are the only symptoms of potentially serious conditions. New confusion, falls, incontinence, or other subtle changes from the patient's baseline must alert the physician to possible underlying illness presenting atypically.

The examiner should speak slowly and clearly. Providers with high-pitched voices should be aware that high-frequency hearing loss is common among persons and should lower their voice accordingly. History taking can be time-consuming. The patient should first be interviewed alone to allow an opportunity for discussion of private matters. Well-meaning family members may try to answer questions posed to cognitively impaired or frail patients, but an attempt should be made to use the patient as a primary source when possible. It is also important, however, to gather data from medical records, family members, friends, and formal caregivers. Family observations are particularly significant, and when cognitive impairment is present, these may be much more sensitive than general screening tests for intellectual function.

When taking the history, the physician should adapt the usual format in order to focus on specific issues of the elderly. The social history should be expanded and functional status carefully assessed. The history should include a targeted review of systems and questions about nutrition, medications, immunizations, and advance directives (Table 8-1).

Affect Measurement

Affect measurement usually attempts to identify depression, which is common, treatable, and an important cause of dysfunction in elderly persons. The geriatric depression scale (GDS) has been validated in the clinical setting and was developed specifically for elderly patients (Fig. 8-2).

Physical Examination

The examiner should note the patient's personal hygiene and mood, which can provide clues to overall functional status (Box 8-1).

Height and weight should be recorded at the first visit and weight at subsequent visits to uncover problems with nutrition and to monitor fluid overload or overdiuresis in patients with congestive heart failure. Unintentional weight loss may indicate abuse, neglect, underlying malignancy, thyroid disease, or depression.

Postural blood pressure and pulse are noted. *Postural hypotension,* although present in 10% of healthy community-dwelling elderly, may indicate changes in volume status or medication side effects, both of which may predispose the patient to falls. *Orthostatic hypotension* is defined as a 20–mm Hg decrease in systolic pressure or a 10–mm Hg decrease in diastolic pressure 3 minutes after the patient has risen from supine to standing. *Systolic hypertension* is a systolic blood pressure of 160 mm Hg or greater; diastolic hypertension is 90 mm Hg or above. Stiff, atherosclerotic brachial arteries may give elevated blood pressure measurements even when intraarterial measurements are normal *(pseudohypertension). Osler's maneuver* should be employed *when pseudohypertension* is suspected. To perform the maneuver, the cuff should be inflated above the first Korotkoff sound. If the radial or brachial artery does not collapse and is still palpable, this may indicate rigid arteries mimicking hypertension. This maneuver is especially helpful in a patient who has no retinal findings or cardiac changes suggestive of longstanding hypertension.

Visual acuity should be assessed with a Snellen eye char[t]. The prevalence of cataracts, glaucoma, macular degeneratio[n], and refractive errors increases with age. Examination of gro[ss] visual fields by confrontation may reveal deficits caused b[y]

Table 8-1. Adaptation of Medical History for Geriatric Patients

Activity	Specific areas	Rationale
Expand social history.	Cover family, friends, caregivers, living arrangements, pets, religious community involvement, driving, caregiving responsibilities, financial status, substance abuse, and elder abuse.	Responses may shed light on such issues as whether patient has resources to remain safely in community, which supports would be needed to maximize patient's functional status at home, and whether placement in long-term care facility is warranted.
Assess functional status.	Measure activities of daily living (ADLs) and, for community-dwelling elderly patients, instrumental ADLs (IADLs), which require higher level of function. ADLs include critical elements of self-care: bathing, toileting, feeding, dressing, and transferring or ambulating. IADLs include managing finances, managing medication, preparing meals, housekeeping, shopping, using telephone, and arranging transportation.	Responses may indicate which services or types of adaptive equipment are needed for assistance. Measurements of IADLs may identify impairment at earlier stage.
Conduct targeted review of systems.	Inquire specifically about near and far vision, including ability to read, drive, and watch television, and hearing loss. Arthritis, incontinence, falls, gait problems, memory impairment, behavior changes, depression, and abuse, if suspected, should all be addressed. Sexual and substance abuse history should not be omitted simply because of age.	These problems are common and treatable in elderly patients but often are not volunteered during the history.
Assess nutritional status.	Inquire about appetite changes, and ask who buys and prepares meals.	Nutrition history can uncover poverty and functional disabilities and may provide clues to managing conditions such as deficiencies in vitamins B_{12} and D, congestive heart failure, diabetes, and hypertension.
Review medications.	Review of indications, dosage, schedule, and side effects of all over-the-counter and prescription drugs is mandatory, with a "brown bag" review (i.e., review of actual containers or dispensers) providing most accurate information. The home is best place to obtain medication review.	Responses may uncover errors of omission or duplication. Adverse drug reactions may be caused by prescribed or over-the-counter medications.
Review immunizations.	Inquire about immunizations for pneumococcal infections, influenza, and tetanus (see Chapter 5).	Immunizations are critical part of preventive care.
Review patient values.	Discuss advance directives and preferences for end-of-life care (see Chapter 9).	Timely discussion of these issues prevents confusion during catastrophic illnesses.

glaucoma, cerebrovascular events, or mass lesions. *Ectropion* (eversion of the eyelid) or *entropion* (inversion of the eyelid) may be present. *Arcus senilis* (depigmentation of the iris) occurs with normal aging. Dilated funduscopic examination may reveal increased cup-to-disc ratios associated with glaucoma or retinopathy from diabetes or hypertension.

Hearing can be assessed by the whisper test or a hand-held audioscope, which has excellent specificity and sensitivity. External auditory canals should be examined for cerumen impaction. Inspection and palpation of the oral cavity include evaluation of dentition and detection of gum disease, poorly fitting dentures, and abnormal lesions or masses.

Examination of the neck includes range of motion, which is important for driving skills and may give clues to vertebrobasilar insufficiency in patients with falls or near-syncope. The thyroid should be inspected and palpated for nodules or goiter. Auscultation of the carotids can reveal bruits or radiation of cardiac murmurs.

Because of the increasing incidence of breast cancer with age, yearly breast examinations for elderly women are important. Intertriginous areas also should be inspected for dermatitis or fungal infection.

Chest examination includes inspection for kyphosis and scoliosis and palpation of vertebral spines for tenderness. Otherwise the examination is the same as for younger adults.

The cardiac examination commonly *reveals* systolic murmurs, which occur *in 30% to 80% of patients 65* and older. The differential diagnosis includes aortic sclerosis, aortic stenosis, idiopathic hypertrophic subaortic stenosis, and mitral regurgitation. Aortic sclerosis usually has an early peaking systolic murmur that may radiate to the carotids. The murmur of aortic stenosis is late peaking, radiates to the carotids, and may be associated with delayed carotid upstroke and an S_4 heart sound. Delayed upstroke suggests significant aortic stenosis and should be documented promptly by echocardiography, since advanced age is not a contraindication to aortic valve replacement. *In elderly patients, however, the carotid upstroke may be brisker than expected because of stiff arteries, and significant aortic stenosis may be associated with an apparently normal carotid upstroke.* An S_4 sound is often found in healthy elderly persons and is caused by decreased ventricular compliance. For a patient who is unable to squat, the physician can simply raise the patient's lower extremities to increase venous return as a way of determining the characteristics of a murmur. *Diastolic murmurs are never considered normal in elderly patients.*

1. Are you basically satisfied with your life? N = 1
2. Have you dropped any of your activities or interests? Y = 1
3. Do you feel that your life is empty? Y = 1
4. Do you often get bored? Y = 1
5. Are you hopeful about the future? N = 1
6. Are you bothered by thoughts you can't get out of your head? Y = 1
7. Are you in good spirits most of the time? N = 1
8. Are you afraid that something bad is going to happen to you? Y = 1
9. Do you feel happy most of the time? N = 1
10. Do you often feel helpless? Y = 1
11. Do you often get restless and fidgety? Y = 1
12. Do you prefer to stay at home, rather than going out and doing new things? Y = 1
13. Do you frequently worry about the future? Y = 1
14. Do you feel you have more problems with memory than most? Y = 1
15. Do you think it is wonderful to be alive now? N = 1
16. Do you often feel downhearted and blue? Y = 1
17. Do you feel pretty worthless the way you are now? Y = 1
18. Do you worry a lot about the past? Y = 1
19. Do you find life very exciting? N = 1
20. Is it hard for you to get started on new projects? Y = 1
21. Do you feel full of energy? N = 1
22. Do you feel that your situation is hopeless? Y = 1
23. Do you think that most people are better off than you are? Y = 1
24. Do you frequently get upset over little things? Y = 1
25. Do you frequently feel like crying? Y = 1
26. Do you have trouble concentrating? Y = 1
27. Do you enjoy getting up in the morning? N = 1
28. Do you prefer to avoid social gatherings? Y = 1
29. Is it easy for you to make decisions? N = 1
30. Is your mind as clear as it used to be? N = 1

A score of 11 has been shown to be useful in the diagnosis of depression.

Fig. 8-2. Geriatric depression scale (GDS), with points for "No" *(N)* and "Yes" *(Y)* responses. (Modified from Yesavage JA et al: *J Psychiatr Res* 17:37, 1982.)

Box 8-1. Focused Physical Examination

- General: hygiene, mood
- Height and weight
- Vital signs: pulse and postural blood pressure, supine to standing
- Eyes: visual acuity, visual fields, ectropion, entropion, cataracts, increased cup-to-disc ratio, retinopathy
- Ears: audioscopy or whisper test, cerumen
- Oropharynx (with and without dentures): teeth, denture fit, exudates, lesions, gum disease
- Neck: range of motion, thyroid nodules or enlargement
- Chest: breasts, intertriginous areas, kyphoscoliosis, tenderness of vertebral spines
- Cardiac: murmurs
- Abdomen: scars, masses including aneurysms, bladder palpation, hernias
- Rectal: prostate examination, impaction, hemorrhoids, masses, fecal occult blood testing
- Pelvic: atrophic vaginitis, cystocele, urethrocele, rectocele, uterine prolapse, Pap smear, bimanual examination (ovaries should be nonpalpable)
- Extremities (with and without shoes): range of motion, deformities, venous stasis disease, peripheral pulses, edema, corns, calluses, bunions, hammer toes, warts, fungal infection, toenails, shoe fit
- Neurologic: mental status screening, sensorimotor examination, reflexes, gait
- Performance-oriented tests of gait and balance: "get up and go" test, Tinetti Performance-Oriented Assessment of Gait and Balance
- Skin: ulcers, stasis changes, cellulitis, actinic keratoses, basal cell carcinoma, malignant melanoma, pressure sores

The abdomen should be inspected for scars, which may indicate surgery that the patient has neglected to mention. An aortic aneurysm can be detected as a pulsatile mass greater than 3 cm, often with an associated bruit. The bladder can be palpated to assess for urinary retention when the history suggests this. Inguinal canals and femoral triangles should be examined for hernias. Yearly digital rectal examinations (DREs), which can be comfortably performed with the patient in the left lateral decubitus position, may detect prostate nodules and hyperplasia in men and fecal impaction, rectal masses, and occult blood in all elderly patients. Pathology in the prostate's median lobe, which is not accessible to the examining finger, may be missed on DRE. Prostate size on DRE does not correlate with outlet obstruction.

The gynecologic examination is still part of the routine evaluation of the elderly woman. For a patient with kyphosis a pillow under the head and neck makes the examination more comfortable. For patients with degenerative joint disease who cannot tolerate the dorsal lithotomy position even with leg-rest extenders, the left lateral decubitus position is helpful. The patient should be examined for the presence of atrophic vaginitis, cystocele, rectocele, urethrocele, and uterine prolapse. All women should have speculum examinations even if they have undergone hysterectomies, since in the past many hysterectomies were performed as supracervical procedures, leaving an intact cervix in which a carcinoma may develop. Frequency of Pap smears is discussed in Chapter 4. In a normal elderly woman the ovaries should be nonpalpable; if appreciated on bimanual examination, there may be ovarian malignancy.

Extremities should be inspected and joints put through active and passive range of motion. Common skin findings such as venous stasis changes, including hyperpigmentation and stasis ulcers, may be noted. Peripheral pulses should be assessed, and if absent, the distal extremity should be examined for signs of arterial insufficiency, such as pallor, dependent rubor, or coolness. *Pitting edema below the knee may indicate right-sided heart failure, venous stasis, or diseases associated with hypoalbuminemia.* The podiatric examination includes evaluation for corns, calluses, bunions, hammer toes, plantar warts, tinea pedis, and nails infected by fungus or simply overgrown. Determining the condition of the feet is essential in the evaluation of falls and gait disturbances. In addition, diabetic patients and others with peripheral neuropathies may be unaware of potentially dangerous foot ulcers or sores. *Patients should be examined with and without shoes to ensure that the shoes fit properly and are in good repair.*

Box 8-2. Folstein Mini-Mental State Examination

Orientation (maximum score 10)

"What is the _______ ?"Date (1)
Month (1)
Day (1)
Season (1)
Year (1)
"What is the name of this hospital?" (1)
"What floor are we on?" (1)
"What town (or city) are we in?" (1)
"What county are we in?" (1)
"What state are we in?" (1)

Registration (maximum score 3)

Say *ball, flag,* and *tree* clearly and slowly, about 1 second for each. After you have said all three words, ask the patient to repeat them. This determines the score (1-3). Keep repeating the words (up to six trials) until the patient can repeat all three. If all three are not learned, recall cannot be meaningfully tested.

Ball (1) Flag (1) Tree (1)

Attention and Calculation (maximum score 5)

Ask the patient to begin at 100 and count backward by 7, stopping after 5 subtractions. Score one point for each.

93 (1) 86 (1) 79 (1) 72 (1) 65 (1)

If the patient cannot or will not perform this task, ask him or her to spell *world* backward (D-L-R-O-W). The score is one point for each correctly placed letter.

D (1) L (1) R (1) O (1) W (1)

Recall (maximum score 3)

Ask the patient to recall the three words you previously asked him or her to remember.

Ball (1) Flag (1) Tree (1)

Language (maximum score 9)

Naming

Show the subject a wristwatch and a pencil, asking in turn, "What is this?" Score one point for each item.

Watch (1) Pencil (1)

Repetition

Ask the patient to repeat, "No ifs, ands, or buts." Score one point if correct.

Repetition (1)

Three-stage command

Give the subject a piece of blank paper and say, "Take the paper in your right hand, fold it in half, and put it on the floor." Score one point for each action performed correctly.

Takes in right hand (1) Folds in half (1) Puts on floor (1)

Reading

On a blank piece of paper, print the sentence "Close your eyes" in large letters. Ask the patient to read it and do what it says. Score if he or she actually closes the eyes.

Closes eyes (1)

Writing

Give the patient a blank piece of paper and ask him or her to write a sentence. It must contain a subject and a verb and make sense. Ignore grammar, spelling, and punctuation.

Writes sentence (1)

Copying

On a clean piece of paper, draw intersecting pentagons, each side about 1 inch, and ask patient to copy it exactly as it is. All 10 angles must be present, and two must intersect to score 1 point.

Draws pentagons (1)

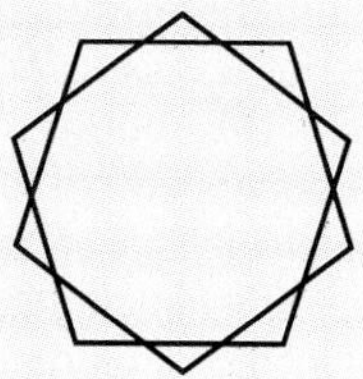

Total Score

Thirty points are possible. A score of 23 or less correlates well with moderate or worse cognitive function.

Modified from Folstein MF, Folstein ME, McHugh PR: *J Psychiatr Res* 12: 189, 1975.

The neurologic examination should include an office ssessment of mental status, such as the Folstein Mini-Mental tate Examination (Box 8-2), during which subtle well-ompensated dementia can be unmasked and severe memory npairment recognized and quantified. Such instruments nable the physician to establish a baseline and follow ɔgnitive function objectively over time. The cranial nerve, ensorimotor, and reflex examinations are performed as usual. ommon findings in healthy elderly persons include primi-ve reflexes such as the snout, glabellar, and palmomental flexes, which are nonpathologic in the absence of other ndings, and symmetrically diminished vibratory sense and kle jerks. Cranial nerve changes include diminished ac-mmodation, pupillary response to light, and upward gaze. Although motor strength is decreased in the elderly, this finding should not have clinical manifestations unless the patient has joint pain, decreased range of motion, or weakness. The neuromuscular examination may be normal in patients who have functional limitations. For example, hip and knee flexors may be normal in patients who have difficulty sitting down. Therefore it is imperative to use performance-based assessments to identify patients with functional disability, especially those who fall or have gait and balance problems. The Tinetti Performance-Oriented Assessment of Gait and Balance can easily be performed during an office evaluation with little time added to the visit (see Falls).

Skin should be inspected for xerosis, cellulitis, stasis dermatitis and ulcers, actinic keratoses, basal cell carcinomas, malignant melanoma, and pressure sores.

ASSESSMENT OF GERIATRIC CONDITIONS

Many older patients suffer from multiple disabilities and illnesses. Because of the complexity of their problems, a diagnosis-oriented approach may be inadequate for assessing and maintaining overall health and functional status. The physician needs information not only about individual ailments, but also about their interacting physical, mental, and social aspects. To answer that need, a coordinated multidisciplinary approach has evolved, known as *geriatric assessment,* which typically involves a physician, nurse, and social worker. Information is obtained and organized regarding five basic domains: (1) physical health, (2) performance of ADLs (basic and instrumental), (3) mental health, (4) socioeconomic resources, and (5) the patient's environment, with special emphasis on the relationships among the factors. Techniques for assessing the first four of these have been previously described (see Approach to the Elderly Patient).

The environmental assessment covers factors such as the convenience, safety, and availability of services and social supports. A home visit by the physician or other health care professional often provides essential information regarding the need for specific interventions, including physical equipment (ramps, grab bars), special services (homemakers, meals), and increased social activity (visitors, day care) (see Home Care).

In 1988 the National Institutes of Health sponsored the Consensus Development Conference on Geriatric Assessment Methods for Clinical Decision-Making. The consensus statement noted that the goals of assessment often are interdependent; diagnostic accuracy leads to appropriate interventions and better use of available services, resulting in improved function and optimal patient placement. Geriatric assessment should be performed in many different clinical settings, both institutional and community. The consensus statement pointed out that two aspects of geriatric assessment are particularly important: (1) targeting patients most likely to benefit, especially those who are frail but not terminally ill and those at critical transition points (e.g., change in living situation, loss of loved one or caregiver), and (2) linking assessment with care management and follow-up services to implement the recommendations resulting from assessment. Geriatric assessment is thus a *process* involving referral, collection of information, assessment, and development and implementation of a care plan, with periodic reassessment and modification of that plan.

In the past decade, geriatric assessment programs have been implemented and evaluated in inpatient units, outpatient and home care programs, and long-term care facilities. Well-designed studies have demonstrated the value of assessment in improving diagnostic and therapeutic outcomes in some settings, usually involving assessment by multidisciplinary teams and follow-up case management. Evaluation of geriatric assessment in outpatient settings has yielded inconsistent results. A 1993 meta-analysis of 28 controlled trials of five types of geriatric assessment concluded that some programs linking evaluation with strong long-term management are effective for improving survival and function in older persons.[14] However, comprehensive geriatric assessment is not widely available and is not adequately reimbursed.

The impact on outcome depends on the ability to target appropriate patients and to identify resources and services necessary for follow-up care. A better understanding of which components are likely to yield the most information is needed. Techniques that facilitate evaluation and management by primary care physicians should be developed before geriatric assessment is widely implemented in primary care.

FALLS

Falls are a common and morbid problem among both community-dwelling and institutionalized elderly. Falls can result in minor to severe acute injuries, prolonged physical and psychologic disability, institutionalization, and death. As with many geriatric conditions, causes of falls are often multifactorial and reversible with intervention. The tendency to fall represents a confluence of factors, including physical illness, disability, medications, and environmental hazards, often with a minor event tipping the balance. Most recent geriatrics literature uses the Kellogg International Work Group definition, in which the term *falls* excludes incidents resulting from intrinsic factors (e.g., syncope, stroke) or sequelae of violent acts (e.g., blows to head).[7]

Epidemiology

Worldwide, approximately one third of community-dwelling elderly over age 65 fall each year. That percentage rises with advancing age; the rate approaches 50% for those 80 and older. The number also rises with institutionalization: these patients have an average of 1.6 to 2.0 falls per year. Women fall more often than men until age 75, when the frequencies become the same, but men die more often from their falls. Half of those who fall do so more than once. Falls precipitate most injuries in people over 65, an age group for whom injuries are the seventh leading cause of death.

About 5% to 10% of falls lead to serious soft tissue injury, such as bruises, lacerations, hematomas, sprains, and joint dislocations. About 5% of falls result in fractures, usually of the hip, pelvis, wrist, or humerus. One in 100 falls results in a hip fracture, with this morbid and sometimes fatal complication occurring in one in 10 elderly over age 80 who fall. In one study, 12% of falls that did not cause serious injury resulted in the individual being on the floor at least 30 minutes, which creates a risk for rhabdomyolysis, pressure sores, pneumonia, and dehydration.[16]

Perhaps as devastating as the physical injuries and disabilities caused by falls are the psychologic and social sequelae. Fear of falling develops in almost 50% of those who have fallen, and 26% curtail their activities because of fear.[17] They withdraw from activities, losing functional ability, becoming further deconditioned, and increasing their risk of falling. This cycle can be a contributing factor in the ultimate institutionalization of a patient. One study of a cohort of older adults (mean age 80) found that those who had one fall without serious injury during the previous 3 months were 3.1 times more likely to be admitted to a skilled nursing facility than those who had not fallen during that period. Patients who had more than two such falls were 5.5 times more likely, and those who had falls with serious injuries during the 3-month period were 10.2 times more likely to be admitted to such a facility. The risks were adjusted for multiple confounders.[15]

Pathophysiology and Risk Factors

Falls are often caused by a complex interaction of intrinsic age-related or disease-related changes and extrinsic or environmental factors (Box 8-3). Gait, balance, and the

Box 8-3. Predisposing and Risk Factors for Falls

- Sensory deficits: vision, hearing, proprioception, vibration, vestibular function
- Orthostatic hypotension
- Gait and balance changes
- Musculoskeletal changes
- Cognitive impairment
- Medications
- Environmental hazards

Box 8-4. Medications Implicated in Falls

- Narcotics
- Hypnotics
- Benzodiazepines (especially long acting)
- Phenothiazines
- Tricyclic antidepressants
- Diuretics
- Vasodilators
- Alcohol

From Kellogg International Work Group: *Dan Med Bull* 34(suppl 4):1, 1987.

capacity to avoid a fall by regaining stability are affected by interrelated changes in the visual, neurosensory, and musculoskeletal systems. Gait changes include short steps, decreased velocity, decreased step height, and decreased arm swing. A senile gait is described as small stepped and wide based, with decreased arm swing and stooped posture, flexed hips and knees, uncertainty and stiffness in turning and sometimes difficulty initiating steps, and a tendency to fall without a clear reason.

Aging results in increased sway and decreased balance on one leg, but conditions such as Parkinson's disease, hemiplegia, neuropathies, myelopathies, and severe orthopedic deformities of feet, knees, and hips also affect gait (see Chapters 156, 163, and 169). There is a 20% to 40% decrease in isometric strength for ages 60 to 80.

Changes in vision caused by normal aging include decreased accommodation, acuity, contrast sensitivity, and adaptation to dark as well as glare intolerance. This situation is worsened by pathologic conditions commonly found in the elderly, such as presbyopia, cataracts, macular degeneration, retinopathy, and glaucoma. Vestibular function may decline from age-related changes such as disruption of vestibuloocular reflexes. Vestibulospinal function may be altered in patients with peripheral and central lesions from vestibulotoxins, including furosemide, aminoglycosides, aspirin, quinine, and ethanol. Proprioception may be affected by loss of proprioceptors in cervical or weight-bearing joints. Older persons' peripheral nervous systems have delayed motor and sensory nerve conduction velocities compared with those in young persons. The same is true of somatosensory-evoked potentials. Decreased vibration in toes and ankles has been documented. However, peripheral neuropathies from vitamin B_{12} deficiency, diabetes, alcoholism, and syphilis are common in the elderly and may contribute to problems with gait and balance.

Cognitive impairment can lead to loss of awareness of the environment and predispose people to falls. Falls occur three times more frequently in patients with senile dementia of the Alzheimer type (SDAT) than in healthy elderly.

Orthostatic hypotension occurs in 10% of community-dwelling elderly and is associated with 2% to 15% of falls. Causes of postural hypotension include autonomic dysfunction due to age, central nervous system damage, diabetes mellitus, hypovolemia, and decreased cardiac output. Metabolic and endocrine disorders, including Addison's disease, can cause orthostasis. Age-related physiologic changes, such as decreased renin-angiotensin response and decreased baroreceptor sensitivity, may contribute. Postprandial hypotension has been well documented. Drop attacks, reportedly associated with up to 10% of falls, result in sudden falls while walking or standing, without loss of consciousness. These may be caused by vertebral artery insufficiency secondary to atherosclerosis or compression by cervical spondylosis.

Several medications have been implicated in falls (Box 8-4). A recent systematic review and meta-analysis of 40 studies (not randomized controlled trials) of psychotropic drug use and falls in older people showed a small but consistent association between increased risk of falls and use of neuroleptics, antidepressants (mostly tricyclics), sedatives/hypnotics, and benzodiazepines. The use of more than one psychotropic drug increased the risk.[8] A similar review of 29 studies (also not randomized controlled trials) critically evaluating the evidence linking cardiac and analgesic drugs to falls showed that digoxin, diuretics, and type IA antiarrhythmics (antidysrhythmics) were associated with falls. The use of more than three or four drugs increased the risk of falls.[9] This meta-analysis indicated that no other class of cardiovascular drugs or analgesics was associated with increased risk of falls. In other studies, however, calcium channel blockers, β-blockers, centrally acting α-adrenergic agents, and narcotics have been implicated in falls.

From 40% to 50% of accidental falls are related to environmental hazards.[17] Furthermore, falls resulting in injury are more often related to environmental causes than falls that do not produce injury, particularly in younger and more active patients. Environmental factors include stairs (descent is especially hazardous where edges of steps are unclear); slippery, icy, uneven, or wet surfaces; poor lighting; unexpected obstacles such as children, toys, and pets; poorly fitting footwear and trousers; low beds, chairs, and toilets; loose rugs; wire; and clutter.

However, falls are usually caused by the combined effects of many factors. Sedatives, cognitive impairment, disability to the lower extremities, presence of a palmomental reflex, abnormalities of gait and balance, and foot problems pose the greatest risks. In addition, the risk of falling increases linearly with the number of these risk factors.

History

Questions about falls should be part of a routine history in patients 65 and older. A detailed history, including the what, when, where, and why of a fall, can reveal high-risk conditions or behaviors as well as patterns for recurrent problems. Open-ended questions such as, "Tell me about this fall and others you have had," may be very revealing. It is helpful to ask for a demonstration of the patient's positions before, during, and after a fall. The examiner also should ask about problems with gait, balance, or walking secondary to joint or foot conditions. Premonitory symptoms such as dizziness, lightheadedness, and vertigo can indicate hypotension, vestibular problems, hypoglycemia, or drug side effects. Incontinence causes falls by creating slippery surfaces. Chest pain associated with arrhythmias (dysrhythmias) or ischemia can cause hypotension. Questions about eyesight, hearing, sensation, memory problems, and depression also are relevant. If a patient is too cognitively impaired to give a meaningful history, information should be obtained from family, friends, and caregivers. Review of all over-the-counter and prescription drugs is essential. Questions about recreational drugs and alcohol are important. A medical history covering all medical and surgical conditions may identify patients who are at high risk.

Physical Examination

Supine-to-standing blood pressure after a 3-minute interval should be obtained to rule out symptomatic postural hypotension. Skin examination for turgor, pallor, and trauma is necessary. The head examination should include tests for visual acuity and fields, gaze preferences, nystagmus, and hearing loss. During the neck examination the physician should listen for carotid bruits and check for range of motion at the cervical spine. Pulmonary status can be assessed by listening for rales or egophony. The cardiac examination includes appreciation of murmurs, especially aortic stenosis, dysrhythmias, and gallops. Extremities should be evaluated for joint deformities, range of motion, corns, calluses, ulcers, bunions, long toenails, poorly fitting shoes, and signs of fractures. Range of motion and stability of the thoracic and lumbar spine also are important.

A neurologic evaluation for mental status, focal motor deficits, paresis, tremor, rigidity, decreased proprioception, and vibration should be carefully performed, although the standard neuromuscular examination may not reveal functional impairments. For example, knee and hip flexion may be normal most of the time, even when a patient remains functionally impaired and has difficulty sitting or standing. It is therefore important to perform functional assessments of gait and balance required for daily activities. In the "Get Up and Go" test the patient is instructed to arise from a chair without using the hands, walk 15 to 30 m, return, stand still, and then sit down. This test or the Tinetti Performance-Oriented Assessment of Gait and Balance can be performed easily in a few minutes during a home or office evaluation (Boxes 8-5 and 8-6).

Box 8-5. Performance-Oriented Assessment of Balance

- Sitting balance
- Arising from chair
- Immediate standing balance within 5 seconds
- Prolonged standing balance with eyes closed and feet close together
- Turning balance (360 degrees)
- Sternal nudge
- Neck turning side to side
- One leg standing balance
- Back extension
- Reaching up as if retrieving object from high shelf
- Bending down as if to pick up object from floor
- Sitting down

Modified from Tinetti ME, Ginter SF: *J Am Geriatr Soc* 34:119, 1986.

Box 8-6. Performance-Oriented Assessment of Gait

- Initiation of gait
- Step height
- Step length
- Step symmetry
- Step continuity
- Path deviation
- Trunk stability
- Walk stance
- Turning while walking

Modified from Tinetti ME, Ginter SF: *J Am Geriatr Soc* 34:119, 1986.

Environmental Assessment

Because the majority of falls in community-dwelling elderly persons occur at home during normal ADLs and because 40% to 50% of accidental falls are related to environmental hazards, a home evaluation by a physician, nurse, or physical therapist is essential in the workup of falls. Falls by healthier older adults often are associated with environmental factors. This group also has a higher frequency of falls that lead to injuries. Environmental checklists have been designed to evaluate the home for safety hazards (Box 8-7).

Laboratory Tests and Diagnostic Evaluation

The diagnostic workup should be guided by the history and physical examination (Box 8-8). Holter monitoring has not been shown to be useful in the routine evaluation of nonsyncopal episodes without cardiac symptoms; both fallers and nonfallers have a high incidence of ventricular and supraventricular dysrhythmias, and treatment of unclear value is fraught with side effects that can lead to falls.

Management and Interventions

Since up to 10% of falls unrelated to syncope are related to atypical presentation of acute illnesses in elderly patients such as pneumonia, stroke, anemia, or dehydration, it is important to rule out illness in a patient who suddenly starts falling. Patients at high risk for falls because of their physical or mental status or environmental factors should have their charts flagged for intervention. When prescribing medications, the physician should weigh the benefits of treatment with possible reactions affecting gait, balance, and mental status and should adjust dosages based on age-related changes in drug metabolism (see Drug Prescribing, p. 84). The physician should carefully review all over-the-counter, recreational, and prescribed drugs.

Patients who fall should also be treated for underlying dysrhythmias clearly associated with the fall, heart bloc

Box 8-7. Environmental Safety Checklist

Home

- Ensure adequate lighting, especially of stairs, walkways, door thresholds, and bathrooms.
- Remove clutter, toys, and low furniture.
- Secure carpet and tile edges.
- Remove throw rugs.
- Clearly mark or remove door thresholds.
- Remove cords and wires from floors.
- Avoid floor wax.
- Install grab bars in tub and shower and by toilet.
- Use rubber tub mats.
- Ensure that steps are even and edges are clearly marked.

Institution

- Adjust beds, chairs, and toilets to appropriate height.
- Provide adequate lighting of bathrooms and hallways.
- Ensure nonskid footwear that fits.

Outside

- Repair uneven, cracked, or broken sidewalks and steps.
- Cut back overgrown shrubbery blocking walkways.
- Provide handrails on steps.
- Ensure adequate illumination of walkways and steps.

Modified from Rubenstein LZ et al: *J Am Geriatr Soc* 36:266, 1988.

Box 8-8. Laboratory and Diagnostic Workup after Falls

- Complete blood count (CBC): infection, anemia
- Electrolytes, blood urea nitrogen (BUN), creatinine: volume status
- Glucose: diabetes, hypoglycemia
- Calcium: delirium
- Vitamin B_{12} and rapid plasma reagin (RPR): peripheral neuropathy, dementia
- Thyroid function tests: hypothyroidism, hyperthyroidism, muscle weakness
- Creatine kinase, calcium, potassium, phosphate, magnesium: muscle weakness
- Urinalysis: infection if indicated
- Electrocardiogram (ECG): arrhythmia (dysrhythmia), myocardial infarction
- Chest radiograph: congestive heart failure, pneumonia
- Computed tomography (CT) or magnetic resonance imaging (MRI) of head: subdural hematoma, hydrocephalus, tumor
- Toxicology screen and ethanol level
- Echocardiogram: valvular lesion, congestive heart failure

ɔlume loss, and Parkinson's disease. Patients with ortho-atic hypotension should receive education about raising the ɛad of the bed to decrease the incidence of hypotensive falls ɩ standing. These patients may find it helpful to wear graded ɛssure stockings to decrease venous pooling, to sit at the edge of the bed before standing, and to liberalize dietary salt. Mineralocorticoids may be helpful. Osteoporosis should be treated to help prevent fractures from falls. Drop attacks from vertebrobasilar insufficiency may be helped by a cervical collar. Glasses, hearing aids, new shoes, and assistive devices should be supplied when necessary.

Education regarding community services (e.g., adult day care, social senior centers) where patients can be more closely supervised, transportation, medical alert devices, and nutrition and alcohol counseling should be initiated. Physical or occupational therapy and specific strength and balance training may be beneficial. A meta-analysis of the effect of the multisite FICSIT (Fraility and Injuries: Cooperative Studies of Intervention Techniques) study showed that general exercise and balance training decreased the risk of falls by 10% and 17%, respectively.[12] In one of the FICSIT sites a multidisciplinary risk abatement program resulted in a reduction of falls by 31% at 1 year. The 301 subjects ages 70 and older were randomized to receive either home interventions to identify risk factors or social visits. Interventions included an environmental hazards assessment, medication review, treatment of postural hypotension, and physical therapy to improve strength, balance, and gait.[18] The study's success shows the need for a multidisciplinary approach to the primary and secondary prevention of falls. Finally, the patient should be instructed in how to arise from a fall and should be provided with a medical alert device.

URINARY INCONTINENCE

Epidemiology

Urinary incontinence represents a major cause of disability, social isolation, and institutionalization in elderly patients. It affects 5% to 15% of those over age 65 living in the community and 50% or more of those living in long-term care facilities. Neurologic impairment, immobility, and female gender are the major independent risk factors. Some 40% of hospitalized elderly are reported to be incontinent; much of this is transient and reversible if recognized and appropriately evaluated. Urinary incontinence is frequently cited by families as the major factor leading to the decision to place an elder in a nursing home. Institutionalized incontinent patients are much more difficult to care for than continent patients because of increased secondary problems (e.g., falls, skin breakdown) and expanded nursing care needs.

Pathophysiology

Continence requires structurally intact and functional detrusor and sphincter muscles as well as the reflexes that coordinate them. The onset of urinary incontinence is not part of normal aging, but age-related physiologic changes may predispose to incontinence (Box 8-9). Any of these in combination with another medical or physiologic problem may result in incontinence.

Proper function of the lower urinary tract depends greatly on normal function of the autonomic nervous system. The detrusor and sphincter are innervated by parasympathetic cholinergic fibers that emerge from the spinal cord at the S2-S4 level and travel via the pelvic splanchnic nerves, as well as sympathetic noradrenergic fibers via the paraaortic sympathetic chain. Parasympathetic stimulation results in detrusor contraction, sphincter relaxation, and voiding. Sympathetic stimulation inhibits detrusor contractions and increases the tone of the involuntary sphincter, thus promoting the storage of urine. The balance between the two sides of the autonomic nervous system and thus the control of the micturition reflex is mediated by several micturition centers located in the lower spinal cord, brainstem, and cerebral cortex. The cerebral cortex is the site of voluntary control and exerts an inhibitory influence on voiding. Injury, disease, or pharmacologic side effects at any point in the neurologic circuit can result in a disorder of either storage or voiding of urine and therefore can cause incontinence.

History and Physical Examination

The initial evaluation of the elderly incontinent patient includes a thorough history and physical examination, which often includes obtaining information from family members. The history should focus on the frequency, timing (diurnal versus nocturnal), volume, and symptoms associated with incontinence episodes. An incontinence chart or diary can be useful diagnostically and in the development of a treatment plan (Fig. 8-3).

Urinary incontinence can be triggered or perpetuated by a broad variety of medical and psychologic illnesses, most of which are not directly related to the function of the lower urinary tract. Because local structural and neurologic abnormalities frequently coexist with and contribute to incontinence, however, the physician should be particularly attentive to certain aspects of the neurologic and abdomino-pelvic examination. Sacral levels 2 through 4, which carry parasympathetic fibers to the detrusor and sphincter, can be examined by assessing rectal tone, perianal sensation, and the bulbocavernosus reflex. Abnormalities suggest significant spinal cord or cauda equina pathology. The abdomen should be carefully palpated and percussed for a suprapubic mass suggestive of a distended bladder. The rectal, and in women pelvic, examination is essential in excluding causes such as fecal impaction, rectal or pelvic masses, pelvic floor abnormalities (e.g., uterine prolapse), and cystocele or urethrocele. Vaginal infection should be excluded or treated and atrophic changes noted. Laboratory evaluation should include urinalysis and culture as appropriate. Chemistries to evaluate the patient's metabolic status, especially blood sugar and calcium, and renal function are important.

Careful review of medications and their indications is essential to any initial evaluation. Many prescription and over-the-counter drugs affect detrusor and sphincter function and may cause subtle degrees of delirium and cognitive dysfunction (Box 8-10).

Box 8-9. Physiologic Changes that Predispose to Incontinence

- Decreased bladder capacity
- Decreased ability to postpone voiding
- Decreased urethral and bladder compliance
- Decreased maximal urethral closing pressure
- Decreased urinary flow rate
- Increased postvoid residual (PVR)
- Increased uninhibited detrusor contractions
- Benign prostatic hypertrophy
- Atrophic vaginitis and urethritis

Classification and Etiology

Transient incontinence accounts for approximately 75% of new-onset incontinence and is most likely to have a reversible cause. The etiology usually is not readily referrable to the urinary tract, with the notable exception of urinary tract infection. Transient incontinence is common in elderly hospitalized patients. The DIAPPERS mnemonic helps in recalling the common causes of transient incontinence (Box 8-11).

Established incontinence refers to chronic incontinence caused by dysfunction of the detrusor, the outlet, or the neurologic pathways controlling them. Established incontinence is commonly divided into three general clinical syndromes to provide a framework for diagnosis and

Name ______________________ Week Starting ____ / ____ / ____
Month Day Year

Instructions:

Mark **D** for **"Dry"** each time urination occurs without leakage

Mark **W** for **"Wet"** each time leakage occurs
(If you cannot tell when the leakage occurred, mark **W** at the time closest to when you find the wetness.)

	7am	8am	9am	10am	11am	12n.	1pm	2pm	3pm	4pm	5pm	6pm	7pm	8pm	9pm	10pm	11pm	12am	1am	2am	3am	4am	5am	6a
Mon																								
Tues																								
Wed																								
Thur																								
Fri																								
Sat																								
Sun																								
	Morning					Afternoon						Evening					Night							

Fig. 8-3. Bladder record for outpatient settings.

management: (1) *urge* (from detrusor overactivity with uninhibited bladder contractions), (2) *stress* (from failure of the sphincter to remain closed during bladder filling), and (3) *overflow* (from impaired detrusor contractility, bladder obstruction, or both).

Incontinence that may be transient can become established if not promptly identified and managed or if assumed to be established from the outset. Established incontinence is less likely to be completely reversible, although management can ameliorate symptoms and reduce social impairment.

Urge Incontinence. Urge incontinence represents the most common clinical incontinence syndrome in the elderly. The history reveals a warning sensation occurring seconds to minutes before the involuntary voiding of moderate to large volumes of urine. Increased urinary frequency and nocturnal incontinence are common features. The postvoid residual (PVR) is typically low, and cystometry demonstrates contraction at low bladder volumes. The physician may find no objective neurologic signs, although this clinical pattern of incontinence is commonly associated with an underlying neurologic problem.

The cause of urge incontinence is usually *detrusor overactivity* (DO), either primary or secondary. Primary DO is an age-related change. The differential diagnosis of secondary DO includes stroke, Alzheimer's disease, parkinsonism, central nervous system tumors, and local bladder irritation (e.g., infection, stones, inflammation, tumors). DO may coexist with impaired detrusor contractility (detrusor hyperactivity with incomplete contractions, or DHIC). There is an increased PVR without outlet obstruction.

The evaluation of a patient with urge incontinence begins with a routine urinalysis and, if indicated, urine culture. The evaluation of women includes a pelvic examination with attention to contributory conditions, such as infectious or atrophic vaginitis. When infection or atrophy is diagnosed and treated, incontinence may resolve or greatly improve. For men a DRE with careful palpation of the prostate gland is essential. Although the size of the prostate gland correlates poorly with the presence or absence of outlet obstruction, the finding of a large gland is usually important. In addition, any finding of asymmetry, nodularity, or stony hardness warrants further investigation with prostate-specific antigen (PSA) testing and possible referral for transrectal ultrasound (TRU) and biopsy, if appropriate.

In most patients the initial evaluation of urge incontinence should also include a PVR volume determination. Volumes greater than 100 ml may indicate DHIC or obstruction and should prompt consideration of further investigation or referral. An empiric pharmacologic trial in such a setting carries a high risk of inducing urinary retention in male patients and is probably best avoided; for female patients there is much less risk. The finding of a normal PVR (less than 50 ml) is reassuring but does not exclude the possibility that urinary retention will occur, especially in men, in whom a normal PVR can be seen with significant prostate enlargement. Devices that measure urine flow during voiding can be used to screen for male patients with significant mechanical obstruction before a drug trial. When such measurements are not possible, men should be referred for

Box 8-10. Medications that Can Cause Incontinence

Antihypertensives
Antiadrenergics

Clonidine, α-methyldopa, β-blockers: decreased sphincter tone, cognitive dysfunction, depression

Calcium channel blockers

Verapamil, nifedipine, diltiazem, others: decreased detrusor contractility, constipation, fecal impaction

Angiotensin-converting enzyme (ACE) inhibitors

Captopril, others: drug-induced cough

Diuretics

Hydrochlorothiazide, furosemide, others: increased urine production, glucose intolerance

Sedative-Hypnotics

Benzodiazepines, chloral hydrate, antihistamines (e.g., diphenhydramine): cognitive dysfunction (delirium), anticholinergic effects

Antidepressants

Tricyclic agents (e.g., amitriptyline): anticholinergic side effects, cognitive dysfunction

Neuroleptics

Haloperidol, others: cognitive dysfunction, parkinsonism, anticholinergic effects, especially in low potency neuroleptics (e.g., thioridazine)

Narcotic Analgesics

Various: cognitive dysfunction

Ethanol

Cognitive, motor dysfunction, increased urine production

Decongestants

Ephedrine, pseudoephedrine, phenylpropanolamine: sphincter dysfunction, decreased detrusor contractility

Antihistamines

Diphenhydramine, chlorpheniramine, others: anticholinergic effects

Box 8-11. Common Causes of Transient Incontinence

D—Delirium
I—Infection
A—Atrophic vaginitis, urethritis
P—Pharmacy (drugs)
P—Psychologic (e.g., depression)
E—Excess excretion
R—Restricted mobility
S—Stool (fecal) impaction

From Resnick NM, Yalla SV: *N Engl J Med* 313:800, 1985.

cystoscopy and urodynamics before any pharmacologic intervention.

A bedside urodynamics test may detect DO and determine bladder capacity. A Foley catheter is inserted into the patient's bladder and attached to a syringe, which is used to fill the bladder with saline. A rise in the salination level in the syringe column is used to diagnose DO. Although bedside cystometry is moderately sensitive and specific for DO, its usefulness is unclear. When the diagnosis is uncertain, patients should be referred for formal testing.

The management of urge incontinence is aimed at treating underlying predisposing conditions when possible or appropriate; otherwise, treatment is aimed at managing symptoms. Assistive devices such as bedside commodes and urinals help to manage nocturnal symptoms. Toileting regimens based on completion of an incontinence chart are often effective for patients who can cooperate (see Fig. 8-3). Instructing patients to limit fluids, especially caffeinated beverages and alcohol, can restore control and confidence. Diuretic use should be avoided or minimized.

A logical clinical approach leads to the satisfactory management of most patients without referral, as well as the appropriate referral of a subset of patients who need further investigation. Table 8-2 provides evidence supporting the efficacy of various pharmacologic and behavioral treatments used for urge incontinence. Randomized controlled trials have shown that behavioral management for DO decreases incontinence episodes.[3] Patients who are cognitively intact can employ timed voiding while awake and can suppress precipitant urges through visualization and concentration. For patients with cognitive impairment, habit traini scheduled voiding, and prompted voiding are success techniques. Empiric pharmacologic intervention is eff tive in urge incontinence if implemented with appropri caution (Box 8-12).

Therapy is aimed at decreasing the contractility a suppressing spontaneous contractions of the detrusor. T can be accomplished with drugs such as oxybutynin a tolterodine, which have been shown to result in fev episodes of incontinence compared with placebo in rando ized controlled trials. Other drugs that have been shown decrease incontinence in case-control studies include antich linergics and tricyclic agents such as imipramine.[3] T selection of an agent depends on consideration of side effe and cost, as well as comorbid conditions. Dosing should initiated at the lower end of the stated range for each age until symptoms are ameliorated, side effects are encountere or the upper end of the dosage range is reached withc discernible effect.

Stress Incontinence. Stress incontinence is the mc common presenting pattern of urinary incontinence women. It is relatively uncommon in men, unless traumatic surgical damage has occurred to the urinary sphinct Patients complain of intermittent leakage of small amounts urine associated with laughing, coughing, or lifting hea objects. The cause is usually related to impaired urethr closure from a postmenopausal decrease in estrogen, wi subsequent atrophy and thinning of the urinary sphincter a pelvic floor muscles. The bladder neck and sphincter, whi

Table 8-2. Efficacy of Behavioral and Pharmacologic Treatments for Urge Incontinence

Treatment	Target population	Efficacy	Evidence*
Behavioral			
Bladder retraining	Cognitively intact	≥ 50% decrease in episodes in 75% of women	A
Prompted voiding	Dependent; cognitively impaired	Average reduction 0.8-1.8 episodes daily	A
Habit training	Voiding record available	≥ 25% decrease in episodes in one third of patients	B
Scheduling toileting	Unable to toilet independently	30%-80% decrease in episodes	C
Pelvic muscle exercises	Women only	Even in conjunction with bladder retraining, efficacy less than that for stress incontinence; limited data	B
Pharmacologic			
Oxybutynin	Unresponsive to behavioral treatment alone	15%-60% decrease in episodes over placebo; side effects common	A
Tolterodine	Unresponsive to behavioral therapy alone	12%-18% decrease in episodes over placebo; side effects approximately 20% less than with other muscarinic agents	A
Propantheline	Unresponsive to behavioral treatment alone	13%-17% decrease in episodes over placebo (nursing home data only); side effects common	B
Dicyclomine	Unresponsive to behavioral treatment alone	42% improvement over placebo	B
Tricyclic antidepressants	Other reasons to take these drugs	Decrease in nocturnal incontinence; side effects common	B
Hyoscyamine; calcium channel blockers	Unknown	Insufficient data	C
Nonsteroidal antiinflammatory drugs	Unknown	Limited data in women; 25% decrease in episodes over placebo	C
Flavoxate	—	Not efficacious	A
Vasopressin	Nocturnal enuresis	Insufficient data in adults	C

Modified from Cobbs EL, Duthie EH, Murphy JB: *Geriatrics review syllabus: a core curriculum in geriatric medicine,* ed 4, Dubuque, Iowa, 1999, Kendall/Hunt.
*A, Randomized controlled studies; *B,* case-control studies; *C,* case descriptions or expert opinion.

are normally located within the pelvis and are therefore intraabdominal, can descend out of the pelvis. In this situation, transient increases in intraabdominal pressure, rather than reinforcing the resting tone of the urinary sphincter, instead overwhelm it, resulting in the expulsion of urine.

Another variant of stress incontinence is stress-induced DO, in which coughing, laughing, lifting, or other maneuvers that produce a sudden rise in intraabdominal pressure result in an uninhibited contraction of the bladder. Several features distinguish this condition from simple stress incontinence: (1) the volume leaked is moderate to large; (2) nighttime incontinence is more common; (3) a brief but detectable delay may occur between the stress-inducing maneuver and the passage of urine; and (4) the patient may experience urgency.

The diagnosis of stress incontinence is based largely on history and physical examination. Pelvic and rectal examinations are indicated to detect evidence of estrogen deficiency and to exclude anatomic problems such as urethrocele or vesicocele, which might warrant surgical intervention. During the examination the patient should be asked to strain or cough, and the leakage of any urine should be noted. The patient then can be asked to repeat the maneuver after the examiner has inserted a finger in the vagina and elevated the bladder neck by exerting gentle pressure anteriorly. In a positive test the leakage of urine is corrected by bladder elevation.

The management of stress incontinence depends on the underlying cause, and the majority of patients respond to conservative therapy. Weight loss is indicated in obese patients and results in decreased pressure on the pelvic floor. The patient should be taught pelvic muscle exercises (PMEs), which involve isometric contraction of the pelvic sling muscles and can increase the strength and resting tone of the urinary sphincter. In randomized controlled trials, PMEs have resulted in 56% to 95% decreases in incontinence episodes. Biofeedback used in conjunction with PMEs has resulted in 50% to 87% reductions.[3]

Estrogen therapy, either topical or systemic, has been effective in case-control studies, especially for women with clinical evidence of estrogen deficiency, such as atrophic vaginitis and hot flashes. In patients who do not respond to these therapies a trial of α-adrenergic agonists, such as long-acting phenylpropanolamine, can be given (Box 8-13). However, the side effects of these agents in elderly patients can be considerable. Estrogen plus an α-adrenergic agonist is more effective than an α-agonist alone. Table 8-3 provides evidence supporting the efficacy of behavioral and pharmacologic treatments for stress and mixed stress and urge incontinence. In mixed stress and urge incontinence a sudden rise in intraabdominal pressure triggers detrusor contractions. The management is essentially the same as for urge incontinence, although the diagnosis is frequently difficult to make clinically. This is because the delay between the stress and the detrusor contraction may be extremely brief, although the volume voided usually is greater than with pure stress incontinence. Imipramine may be effective in the treatment of stress-induced DO because it combines sympathomimetic effects on the urinary sphincter with anticholinergic effects on the detrusor. The data on imipramine for mixed stress and urge incontinence, however, are insufficient at this time.

A variety of surgical procedures are available for selected patients who fail medical management. When surgery is not possible, a vaginal pessary or penile clamp may restore continence.

Overflow Incontinence. Overflow incontinence refers to incontinence that occurs in the setting of abnormally high bladder volumes and incomplete emptying. The most common underlying condition in men is mechanical outlet obstruction, usually benign prostatic hypertrophy, but other causes include urethral stricture and prostate cancer. An underactive detrusor may result from fibrotic tissue replacement of the detrusor or neurologic disease. Neurologic causes include peripheral neuropathy (from alcoholism, diabetes, pernicious anemia, or tabes dorsalis) or damage to spinal detrusor afferent nerves. By definition the PVR is high, and patients report constant or frequent dribbling, which may be exacerbated by stress, and decreased force of the urinary stream. Patients also may report the sensation of incomplete bladder emptying and the need to strain to void. Physical findings may include a palpable bladder or suprapubic dullness to percussion in addition to any underlying neurologic deficits. As determined by DRE, prostate size correlates poorly with the presence of outlet obstruction. If the PVR is greater than 200 ml, hydronephrosis should be excluded by ultrasound, and tests for renal function should be done to rule out renal failure.

The performance of urodynamics is particularly important in suspected overflow incontinence. Peak flow urine rates greater than 12 ml/second exclude obstruction. Cystoscopy is necessary to determine the presence and site of a mechanical obstruction. Management includes eliminating medications that decrease detrusor contractility or increase external sphinctor tone, if possible. Mechanical obstruction with acute urinary retention should be relieved by medical or surgical means, followed by a voiding trial. If the bladder does not regain contractility, continued catheterization (preferably intermittent) may be necessary. Management may also

Box 8-12. Drugs Used to Treat Urge Incontinence

Oxybutynin: 2.5-5 mg bid-tid
Oxybutinin XL: 5-30 mg qd
Tolterodine: 1-2 mg bid
Propantheline: 15-30 mg tid
Imipramine: 25-50 mg tid*
Dicyclomine: 10-20 mg tid

tid, Three times a day; *bid,* twice a day.
*Should be begun at lower doses (e.g., 10-25 mg daily) and gradually titrated upward; can cause serious cardiac conduction problems.

Box 8-13. α-Adrenergic Agents Used to Treat Stress Incontinence

Pseudoephedrine: 15-30 mg tid
Long-acting phenylpropanolamine: 25-75 mg bid

Table 8-3. Efficacy of Behavioral and Pharmacologic Treatments for Stress and for Mixed Urge and Stress Incontinence

Treatment	Target population	Efficacy	Evidence*
Behavioral			
PME	Women	56%-95% decrease in episodes; efficacy depends on program intensity	A
PME and biofeedback	Women	50%-87% improvement	A
	Men, after prostatectomy	Limited data	C
PME and vaginal cones	Women	68%-80% cured or greatly improved; no data on postmenopausal women	B
Electrical stimulation	Women, stress with or without urge UI	50%-94% cured or improved	B
Bladder retraining	Mixed UI, cognitively intact	≥50% decrease in episodes in 75% of patients	A
Prompted voiding	Mixed UI, dependent, cognitively impaired	Average reduction 0.8-1.8 episodes daily	A
Habit training	Mixed UI, voiding record available	≥25% decrease in episodes in one third of patients	B
Scheduled toileting	Mixed UI, unable to toilet independently	30%-80% decrease in episodes	C
Pharmacologic			
α-Adrenergic agonists	Women	0%-14% cure; 20%-60% patients with subjective improvement over placebo	A
α-Adrenergic agonists plus estrogen	Women	More efficacious than α-adrenergic agonists alone	A
Estrogens	Women	30% decrease in episodes over placebo; other systemic benefits may exist	B
Imipramine	Unknown	Very limited data	C
Propranolol	Unknown	Insufficient data	C

Modified from Cobbs EL, Duthie EH, Murphy JB: *Geriatrics review syllabus: a core curriculum in geriatric medicine,* ed 4, Dubuque, Iowa, 1999, Kendall/Hunt.
PME, Pelvic muscle exercises; *UI,* urinary incontinence.
**A,* Randomized controlled studies; *B,* case-control studies; *C,* case descriptions or expert opinion.

include cholinergic agents to increase bladder contractility (if the patient must continue taking antipsychotic or antidepressant medications with anticholinergic properties) and α-adrenergic blockers to decrease resting sphincter tone and decrease prostatic obstruction.

Functional Incontinence. Functional incontinence refers to incontinence that occurs because an individual has lost the capacity to move to an appropriate place to void in a timely manner. This definition incorporates both individuals with normally functioning urinary tracts and those with impaired function. An obvious example would be a patient who is hospitalized with a hip fracture and is placed in traction with an intravenous infusion. The patient is likely to become incontinent unless supplied with aids such as a bedside urinal or bedpan, prompt assistance from hospital staff, and aggressive restorative services such as physical and occupational therapy. Although usually less overt, global functional problems such as visual and auditory impairment, mobility problems, and deconditioning are frequently contributory factors in both transient and established incontinence. Identification and management of these functional difficulties are essential.

Use of Assistive Devices

The judicious use of adult incontinence briefs can provide substantial independence and prevent homeboundedness, functional decline, and institutionalization. Overuse can lead to skin maceration and breakdown, along with urinary and vaginal infections. The use of an indwelling or suprapubic Foley catheter should be reserved for patients in whom all other approaches have failed or are unacceptable. For those with hypocontractile bladders and retention as a cause of their incontinence, intermittent self-catheterization is a preferred method, with a lower infection rate.

Given the potential complications and loss of dignity, the use of Foley catheters and adult incontinence garments in acutely ill patients with transient incontinence is rarely appropriate, since the risk usually outweighs the benefit. Such management should not be invoked only for the convenience of the hospital or nursing home staff.

DRUG PRESCRIBING

The elderly use a disproportionately high volume of medications; the elderly constitute13% of the U.S. population but consume about 30% of all prescription drugs. Thus the primary care physician who has older patients is likely to encounter problems of adverse drug reactions (ADRs) and polypharmacy. The higher probability of ADRs in old age seems to relate more to clinical status than chronologic age, with an increased number of medications used in patients reflecting poorer clinical status.[4] Data on drug effects in elderly patients are limited because drug trials often exclude women and older persons.[5] Also, since the majority of studies have surveyed hospital admissions or inpatient populations, limited information is available on ADRs in outpatients. The most important factor in ADRs is the number of medications taken.

Idiosyncratic and allergic reactions appear to occur with the same frequency in elderly patients as in younger adult patients. Toxicity and side effects, however, are more common in older patients. Some elderly patients have diminished physiologic reserves because of disease, leading to decreased ability to tolerate stress and to respond appropriately to medications. Also, disease is more prevalent in the elderly, resulting in the need for more therapeutic interventions. Deficits in memory, sensation, and function increase the likelihood that patients will make medication errors. Certain illnesses appear to increase the risk of ADRs, including sensory loss, cognitive dysfunction, and diseases of the kidneys, liver, and heart.

Polypharmacy adds another dimension to the problem of ADRs. It increases the risk of individual ADRs and the likelihood of drug-drug interactions. If multiple drugs are prescribed and regimens are complex, prescribing errors (e.g., incorrect dosages) are also more likely to occur, and patients have more difficulty with adherence (see Chapter 3).

Drug responses are influenced by altered pharmacokinetics and pharmacodynamics. Pharmacokinetic changes with aging have been well described (Box 8-14). Since most drugs are absorbed by passive diffusion, absorption is generally unchanged if gastric mucosa is intact, but many poorly absorbed drugs have not been studied. Changes in body composition may affect drug distribution: lipid-soluble drugs may have a larger volume of distribution and thus a prolonged duration of action; water-soluble drugs may have a decreased volume of distribution, resulting in higher concentrations at standard dosages. The most important changes with age are those that affect drug clearance. Decreased phase I hepatic metabolism has variable effects and is influenced by other factors (e.g., smoking, alcohol consumption) but may result in prolonged clearance of active forms of many drugs. Phase II metabolism, such as conjugation, shows little or no change with aging. Renal elimination, correlated with creatinine clearance, may be decreased with age, resulting in higher concentrations of many drugs.

Pharmacodynamic effects depend on drug action at the receptor site and have not been well studied in the elderly. In general, most drug effects are similar to or greater than those in younger patients; effects may be magnified when disease states further alter drug elimination or response. For example, although cardiovascular β-adrenergic receptors appear to be less responsive, central nervous system receptors are often more sensitive, especially in patients with dementia.[6]

Sedation and confusion are common drug complications in elderly patients, especially from medications with anticholinergic effects and sedative-hypnotics that affect the central nervous system. Other disturbances that suggest ADRs include orthostasis, falls, depression, urinary retention or incontinence, constipation, anorexia, and metabolic abnormalities, such as hypoglycemia, hypokalemia or hyperkalemia, hyponatremia or hypernatremia, and azotemia. Box 8-15 lists useful guidelines in prescribing drugs for elderly patients.

Box 8-14. Pharmacokinetic Changes of Aging

Absorption: generally unchanged if gastric mucosa is intact.
Distribution: lipid-soluble drugs may have greater volume of distribution and prolonged duration of action; water-soluble drugs may have decreased volume of distribution and higher concentrations.
Metabolism: decreased phase I hepatic metabolism may result in prolonged clearance; phase II metabolism (e.g., conjugation) does not appear to change significantly.
Renal elimination: correlates with creatinine clearance and may be decreased with age, resulting in higher concentrations of renally excreted drugs.

Box 8-15. Guidelines in Prescribing Drugs for Elderly Patients

1. Take thorough medication history; have patient bring all medications.
2. Prescribe only when necessary; consider alternatives to medications whenever possible.
3. Choose medications carefully; "start low, go slow," considering the following:
   a. Toxicity
   b. Drug and disease interactions
   c. Compliance and cost
4. Give careful instructions, both verbal and written.
5. Initiate therapy one drug at a time.
6. Titrate dosage carefully.
7. Monitor effects and toxicity closely; monitor serum levels when appropriate.
8. Stop nonessential medications.
9. Review indications for all drugs.
10. Review for evidence of efficacy.
11. Always consider drugs as a cause of morbidity and toxicity.

HOME CARE

Until the 1940s, primary care was often delivered in the home. As medical technology grew more complex and patients became more mobile, care switched to hospitals, clinics, and offices; the prevalence of house calls gradually diminished. With prospective payment systems now encouraging early discharge and Medicare allowing home services without prior hospitalization, the provision of home care is rising meteorically. The home care industry has been the fastest growing U.S. service industry. From 1990 to 1997, Medicare home care expenditures increased from $3.9 billion to an estimated $17.2 billion. At the same time, because of a demographic increase in the number of elderly, more functionally impaired elders are residing in the community. About 9.5 million older people with limitations in their ADLs are currently noninstitutionalized. Survey data show that these elders and their families prefer the home as the primary site for care.[11]

Home care is the provision of a wide range of services and equipment to the patient in the home setting to restore and maintain the maximal level of comfort, function, and health.

Homebound patients are community-dwelling individuals who depend on the assistance of others to perform some ADLs because of acute or chronic medical conditions or disabilities. In the absence of this help, they would be at high risk of institutionalization. An impressive array of professional, ancillary, and diagnostic services can be provided in the home, as well as advanced technology (Box 8-16). Funding for these services comes from a variety of sources, including federal and state governments (e.g., Medicare [Box 8-17], Medicaid, Title XX of Social Security Act, Title III of Older Americans Act, Veterans Administration, research and demonstration grants), charities, Blue Cross and other commercial carriers, and private out-of-pocket payments.

Indications for a home care referral include advanced age and frailty, multiple comorbidities, recurrent and frequent admissions, homeboundedness, and impaired psychosocial or functional status. Often the first sign of decline in status is the inability to keep scheduled office or clinic appointments. A house call as part of comprehensive geriatric assessment helps to identify medical, psychosocial, and environmental factors that affect functional ability (Box 8-18). In a randomized controlled trial with 1-year follow-up, veterans 70 or older were screened by a physician assistant or registered nurse for medical, functional, and social problems. The results included the discovery of four new or suboptimally treated problems in each patient, on average, and an improvement in immunization rate and IADL scores.[2] The house call can be used for diagnostic purposes, for emergency evaluations that otherwise would require a trip to the emergency department, or for ongoing primary care of the homebound population, including home hospice care.

The home is the ideal nonthreatening location to identify the elder's strengths, abilities, and formal and informal supports. These factors are important in developing a care plan that can be put into operation realistically and complies with the patient's and family's wishes. A team approach and use of a home care coordinator for case management are essential in implementing complex plans, which may include referrals, services, and patient and family education. These approaches also allow continuous assessment of outcomes

Box 8-16. Services Available in the Home

Professional

- Physician
- Nurse
- Dentist
- Podiatrist
- Optometrist
- Rehabilitation therapists: occupational, physical, speech, respiratory
- Psychologist
- Dietitian
- Pharmacist
- Social worker

Ancillary/Supportive

- Home health aides
- Personal care assistants
- Homemakers
- Chore aides
- Volunteers
- Home-delivered meals

Diagnostic

- Phlebotomy
- Radiographs
- Electrocardiograms
- Holter monitoring
- Oximetry
- Blood cultures

Medical Equipment

- Intravenous infusion for chemotherapy, blood transfusion, antibiotics, total parenteral nutrition, pain management and other medications
- Ventilators
- Hemodialysis
- Medical alert devices
- Glucometers

Box 8-17. Services Covered by Medicare

Part A (100%)

- Home health aide
- Visiting nurse: RN observation/assessment, management, and evaluation of care plan
- Social service
- Physical therapy, occupational therapy, speech therapy if associated with skilled nursing need

Part B (20% Copayment)

- Physician visit
- Certain durable medical equipment
- Some diagnostic tests, electrocardiography, radiographs

Box 8-18. Problems Identified by House Calls

Medical

- Alcoholism
- Incontinence
- Sensory impairment
- Pain
- Compliance and medication errors
- Falls
- Depression

Other

- Safety/environmental
- Psychobehavioral
- Caregiver stress
- Elder abuse and neglect
- Nutrition
- Finances
- Limitations in ADLs/IADLs

er time so that the plan can be revised as the patient's needs d health status change. A prospective randomized trial ng a nurse-directed multidisciplinary intervention in pa- nts 70 or older hospitalized for congestive heart failure ulted in better survival in the intervention group, fewer admissions, better quality of life scores, and lower costs.[13]

LDER MISTREATMENT

pidemiology and Definition

istreatment of the elderly is found among all racial, ethnic, d socioeconomic groups and occurs in both community and stitutional settings. Incidence and prevalence rates in the mmunity vary, largely because of the lack of uniform finitions of elder abuse and neglect, particularly among tes and municipalities where reporting is mandatory. Lack awareness or denial of this problem by public and health re professionals can result in underreporting. Victims who quire heavy care may not report abuse or neglect for fear at they will hasten their placement in nursing homes, or ey may be embarrassed to admit to mistreatment. Studies dicate that 1 to 2 million elderly per year are victims of use (physical, psychologic, financial) or neglect. Inclusion those receiving inadequate care, which is a less restrictive finition, expands these numbers substantially.

Abuse or neglect can be *active,* as in the conscious thholding of food, clothing, shelter, or medicine, or *ssive,* perhaps because the caregiver is unable to bathe, ess, or feed the patient. A less judgmental approach is to gard the situation as a mismatch between the elderly rson's care needs and the services received. The problem of adequate care must be dealt with, however, regardless of the use.

tiology

everal theories explain abuse and neglect. The *dependency eory* states that the more physically and mentally impaired e patient, the greater the risk for abuse, although pendency alone is an insufficient cause. The *stressed-regiver theory* proposes that a threshold is exceeded by care eds, and this triggers abusive behavior. Superimposed ternal stresses, such as job loss or illness, exacerbate these regiving burdens to the point where abusive behavior is iggered. The *transgenerational family violence theory* holds at children who are abused learn violence as a behavior and use their own children and elderly parents. Social isolation n set the stage, since patients have little access to social pports or confidants. The *pathologic abuser theory* states at the psychopathology of the abuser is the etiology of mily violence, especially when alcohol, substance abuse, or sychiatric illness is involved.

No difference exists between the incidence in women and at in men, and age and level of cognition do not appear to e factors. The most significant risk factors are a history of revious family violence and evidence of substance abuse in e perpetrator. These risk factors, superimposed on an lderly person with heavy care needs, limited family esources, and stresses from juggling job and care duties, can ad to a multifactorial etiology for the abuse.

listory

everal clues from the patient history may be of help in the iagnosis of elder abuse and neglect. Inconsistent or nplausible explanations for disease or injury should alert the astute physician to possible elder mistreatment. Several hospital admissions or emergency room visits (often to different facilities) for illness or trauma, with explanations such as the elderly person being accident prone, should raise a red flag. The caregiver's insistence on providing the history or refusal to leave the room should also arouse suspicion. The patient's functional status in terms of ADLs and IADLs is important. Recent family stresses, such as loss of a loved one or job, the presence of family violence, and substance abuse, also indicate high-risk patients.

The patient should be interviewed in private so as not to be intimidated by possibly abusive caregivers. Specific questions should be asked about being hit, kicked, restrained, unfed, or left in soiled clothes. A sexual history, including questions about rape and incest, should also be elicited. A nonjudgmental, nonaccusatory interview with the suspected abuser should also occur in private. It is important to know if the alleged abuser is the patient's caregiver. The health care provider should determine the degree of the patient's dependence on the caregiver, as well as whether a fiduciary relationship exists (i.e., whether the provider is reimbursed for care or depends on the elderly person's income).

Physical Examination

Careful documentation of injuries and appearance should be recorded with narrative, drawings, or photographs. Dementia or delirium should be determined by mental status examination at the outset with an instrument such as the Folstein Mini-Mental State Examination (see Box 8-2). Box 8-19 lists signs of abuse.

Intervention and Treatment

The approach to elder abuse, neglect, and inadequate care usually involves a multidisciplinary team, including the skills of physicians, nurses, and social workers. Health professionals are mandated to report suspected cases of mistreatment in most states. State agencies often support elderly protective service programs that employ workers to make home

Box 8-19. Signs of Abuse, Neglect, and Inadequate Care

- Contusions
- Lacerations
- Abrasions
- Fractures
- Sprains
- Dislocations
- Burns
- Oversedation
- Anxiety
- Overmedication or undermedication
- Decubiti
- Untreated but previously diagnosed problems
- Dehydration
- Misuse of medications
- Malnutrition
- Hypothermia or hyperthermia
- Poor hygiene
- Depression

assessments. These visits can be made under the guise of assessing care needs that may be met by outside agencies. If needs are not being met and the competent patient wants to be relocated or separated from an abuser, arrangements can be made to find alternate living situations or to remove the perpetrator. If the patient is competent and resists intervention (which is often the case), the health care provider must clarify that the person need not remain in such an environment and that help can be provided. This assistance can be home care services (e.g., home health aides, visiting nurses, delivered meals) or can involve respite, counseling, and education for the caregiver. If the patient does not have the mental capacity for decision making, a court-appointed guardian or conservator may be necessary. Often, education, counseling, and support services for a stressed caregiver, even one who cares for a patient with severe dementia, can end the cycle of abuse. For an elder who lives with a pathologic abuser, interventions aimed at the abuser (e.g., counseling, job training, order to evacuate) may be necessary.

The American Medical Association has provided guidelines to the diagnosis and treatment of elder abuse.[1] Many complex ethical issues in the evaluation and treatment of elder abuse involve the patient's autonomy and right to refuse treatment as well as the confidentiality of the physician-patient relationship.

REFERENCES

1. American Medical Association: *Diagnostic and treatment guidelines on elder abuse and neglect,* Chicago, 1992, The American Medical Association.
2. Fabacher D, Josephson K, Pietruszka F, et al: An in-home preventive assessment program for independent older adults: a randomized controlled trial, *J Am Geriatr Soc* 42:630-638, 1994.
3. Fantl JA, Newman DK, Colling J, et al: *Urinary incontinence in adults: acute and chronic management,* Clinical practice guideline no. 2, AHCPR pub no. 96-0682, Rockville, Md, 1996, Agency for Health Care Policy and Research, Public Health Service, US Department of Health and Human Services.
4. Gurwitz JH, Avorn J: The ambiguous relation between aging and adverse drug reactions, *Ann Intern Med* 114:956-966, 1991.
5. Gurwitz JH, Col NF, Avorn J: The exclusion of the elderly and women from clinical trials in acute myocardial infarction, *JAMA* 268:1417-1422, 1992.
6. Hammerlein A, Derendorf H, Lowenthal DT: Pharmacokinetic and pharmacodynamic changes in the elderly: clinical implications, *Clin Pharmacokinet* 35:49-64, 1998.
7. Kellogg International Work Group on the Prevention of Falls by the Elderly: The prevention of falls in later life, *Dan Med Bull* 34(suppl 4):1, 1987.
8. Leipzig RM, Cumming RG, Tinetti ME: Drugs and falls in older people: a systematic review and meta-analysis. I. Psychotropic drugs, *J Am Geriatr Soc* 47:30-39, 1999.
9. Leipzig RM, Cumming RG, Tinetti ME: Drugs and falls in older people: a systematic review and meta-analysis. II. Cardiac and analgesic drugs, *J Am Geriatr Soc* 47:40-50, 1999.
10. The Lewin Group analysis of the 1994 National Health Interview Survey of Disability, Phase 1, 1994. In Kassner E, Bectel RW: *Midlife and older Americans with disabilities: who gets help?* Lakewood, Calif, 1998, American Association of Retired Persons.
11. Long Term Care Excel insert: Tabulation report, 1997. In Kassner E, Bectel RW: *Midlife and older Americans with disabilities: who gets help?* Lakewood, Calif, 1998, American Association of Retired Persons.
12. Province MA, Hadley EC, Hornbrook MC, et al: The effects of exercise on falls in elderly patients: a preplanned meta-analysis of FICSIT trials, *JAMA* 273:1341, 1994.
13. Rich MW, Beckham V, Wittenberg C, et al: A multidisciplinary intervention to prevent readmission of elderly patients with congestive heart failure, *N Engl J Med* 333:1190-1195, 1995.
14. Stuck AE, Siu AL, Wieland GD, et al: Comprehensive geri assessment: a meta-analysis of controlled trials, *Lancet* 342:1032-1 1993.
15. Tinetti ME, Williams CS: Falls: injuries due to falls and the ris admission to a nursing home, *N Engl J Med* 337:1279-1284, 1997.
16. Tinetti ME, Liu W, Claus EB: Predictors and prognosis of inability to up after falls among elderly persons, *JAMA* 269:65-70, 1993.
17. Tinetti ME, Speechley M, Ginter SF: Risk factors for fall among eld persons living in the community, *N Engl J Med* 319:1701-1707, 1
18. Tinetti ME, Baker DI, McAvay G, et al: A multifactorial interventio reduce the risk of falling among elderly people living in the commu *N Engl J Med* 331:821-827, 1994.

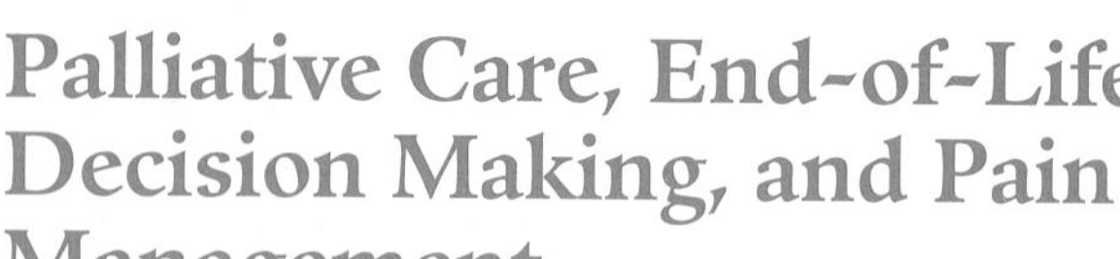

Palliative Care, End-of-Life Decision Making, and Pain Management

Timothy E. Quill
Robert V. Brody

Excellent patient care requires that physicians recognize a respond appropriately to the inevitability of death. Medi training concentrates on the pathophysiologic manifestatio of disease; physicians are much less prepared for t psychologic, social, spiritual, and symptomatic aspects incurable illness.

The goal of both palliative medicine and hospice is achieve the best possible quality of life for patients and th families.[1,7] Excellent management of pain and ot discomforting physical symptoms is followed by addressi the psychologic, social, spiritual, and existential dimensio of the patient's and family's suffering. In the United State hospice is further defined by legislation as an organizatior arrangement devoted to caring for terminally ill patients w (1) accept that they are dying, (2) are expected to li 6 months or less, and (3) are willing to forego invasiv disease-driven therapy. Hospice also emphasizes multidis plinary, coordinated care to support the patient and family home if possible, giving them the opportunity to find pea and acceptance before death.[6,22]

Hospice also implies a capitated Medicare benefit th reinforces supportive care at the end of life but militat against expensive, intrusive, complicated interventior including hospitalization. In contrast, palliative medicine h no particular organizational arrangement or reimburseme scheme. It incorporates highly technical and invasi approaches when appropriate and does not require th patients forego aggressive, disease-driven therapy. Palliati medicine is recognized as a subspecialty in the Unite Kingdom and Canada but not in the United States. The goa and values of palliative medicine and hospice are relevant the treatment of *all* severely ill patients, including those w want to continue complex treatment.[10] Expert pain ar symptom management and exploration of other dimensior of suffering are essential medical skills for all physicians w care for severely ill patients.

EPIDEMIOLOGY OF DYING

People in Western populations are living longer but are also experiencing increasing disability and dependence before death, including loss of decision-making capacity. The probability of facing ethically complex end-of-life decisions is therefore increasing, including whether to use highly technical, invasive treatments (e.g., cardiopulmonary resuscitation, dialysis) or even relatively noninvasive treatments (e.g., antibiotics, artificial feeding) with profound potential effects.

The hospice Medicare benefit is based on a prognostic model that requires death to be predicted with relative certainty within 6 months. This prognostic requirement may apply to some cancers (e.g., metastatic colon cancer) but is not well suited for other cancers with more uncertain prognoses (e.g., chronic hematologic malignancies) or for other common causes of death (e.g., congestive heart failure, chronic obstructive lung disease, dementia, stroke). Many of these patients would welcome a palliative approach that emphasizes enhancing quality of life, but they also want to continue some or all of their disease-driven treatments. Therefore new models of care are needed that allow for a hospicelike benefit for those who have a more uncertain prognosis (50% chance of dying within 6 months but 25% chance of being alive in 2 years, as with severe congestive heart failure), as well as for those who simultaneously want to keep open the options of aggressive treatment, including hospitalization with invasive procedures, if indicated.[10]

Undertreatment of pain by primary care physicians and specialists in a variety of settings is well documented, even when patients are severely ill and near death, despite clear agreement among experts about what constitutes adequate care.[1,8,9] Physician barriers include lack of proper training, unrealistic concern about opioid addiction, fear of review by regulatory agencies, and worries about hastening death. Similarly, many physicians avoid talking with their patients about the possibility of death and continue burdensome, unwanted medical technologies beyond any chance of success.[19] About 80% of deaths now occur in hospitals or chronic care facilities, often far removed from caring families and familiar surroundings. The same medical technology that can save and prolong meaningful life can, paradoxically, prolong the process of dying.[15] Physicians report that they frequently use too much medical technology at the end of life, but they often do not know how to stop. Hospice care tends to be offered late, if at all. In this context, primary care physicians are in a unique position to take an active role in informing, caring for, treating, and advocating for their severely ill and dying patients.

BASIC END-OF-LIFE ETHICAL PRECEPTS

Despite gaps between principle and practice, considerable ethical and legal progress has improved care options for severely ill and dying patients. There is widespread ethical and legal agreement about the domains discussed next.

1. Right to full disclosure.[1,4,12] Physicians have a clear obligation to help patients understand their clinical condition, including prognosis, and their options for disease-driven and palliative treatments. Although truth telling, even about terminal illnesses, is the standard of care in the United States, physicians should allow for special circumstances when a patient may choose *not* to have some information or for a family who may want to protect a vulnerable patient because of special cultural or personal circumstances. Physicians should critically explore these unusual circumstances, keeping the patient's values and interests in the center of these discussions.

2. Right to refuse treatment.[1,12] Patients have the right to make informed decisions about matters that affect their bodies, including the right to accept or reject potentially effective treatment according to their values and beliefs. The right to refuse effective, lifesaving treatment applies even when death is certain without treatment and when the patient's goal is to die. When a patient's decision is at odds with the physician's recommendations, the reasons for the discrepancies should be fully explored. Final decisions, however, rest with patients. This right has been extended to surrogate decision makers when the patient is mentally incapacitated and when the surrogates are acting according to the patient's expressed values or best interests.

3. Right to have treatment withdrawn once started.[3,12] Some clinicians are more reluctant about stopping life-sustaining treatments once started (e.g., ventilator, feeding tube, dialysis) than about not starting them. The experience of withdrawing treatment may be difficult for physicians partly because of the proximity of the physician's action to the patient's death. The patient may also need intensive treatment of subsequent symptoms, such as severe shortness of breath when a respirator is discontinued.[3] Nonetheless, this option allows patients to undergo limited trials of life-sustaining treatment without being obligated to continue them indefinitely. It also allows the patient's goals, circumstances, and choices to change over time. Competent patients or surrogate decision makers if patients are incapacitated should be supported in their rights to have unwanted ongoing treatment stopped, even if that treatment is life sustaining.

4. Substituted judgment for incompetent patients.[2] When a patient has lost the mental capacity to make decisions, caregivers should attempt to reconstruct the patient's values and philosophies to make decisions as the patient would if able to comprehend the medical situation and options available. Since only about 10% of Americans have formally expressed their end-of-life philosophy through an advance directive (health care proxy or living will), such determinations are often approximations at best. The proxy decision maker's role is not to express what they would want for the patient or for themselves but what the patient would want. Only when no clue exists to what the patient would have decided should a generic view of the patient's "best interests" be invoked.

5. Right to adequate pain management.[5,8,9] The vast majority of pain in severely ill patients can be managed using basic step care protocols (see later discussion). Good pain management not only improves the patient's quality of life but also may increase length of life and reduce unnecessary hospitalization. Potent opioid analgesics should be used to relieve the patient's pain, even if the high dosages required could inadvertently or indirectly contribute to the patient's death. The possible unintended contribution to the patient's death is justified under the principle of *double effect* (actions initiated with good intentions can have unintended bad consequences but can still be ethically and morally appropriate). Patients who fear physical pain should be reassured that the physician will diligently and aggressively work with them to find a regimen that effectively manages their pain.

6. Right to palliative care.[5] The 1997 U.S. Supreme Court decision denying a constitutionally protected right to physician-assisted suicide suggested that patients have a protected right to treatments directed at relieving pain and suffering. Palliative care is best delivered in hospice programs, which utilize the resources of a multidisciplinary team, including nurses, social workers, clergy, health aides, volunteers, and others, to help relieve uncomfortable symptoms and to help the patient prepare for death. Although clearly relevant when a patient is in the terminal stages of illness, palliative care approaches are also important for severely ill, suffering patients who want to continue some disease-driven therapies but have a significant but less certain likelihood of dying in the near future. Offering patients the hospice philosophy of care should not depend on their acceptance into a formal program, since it can be implemented in virtually any setting.

7. Duty not to abandon.[17] Since any dying patient's course is uncertain, a physician's most significant commitment is not to abandon. This implies an obligation to be available to the patient until death, to continue to problem solve, to support the caregivers (both family and professional), and to be helpful regardless of the circumstances. This commitment can take some of the fear out of this profound process. A continued clinical presence is at the core of providing humane care for dying patients.

COMMON END-OF-LIFE DECISIONS

1. Advance directive discussions.[2] The *living will* involves setting out a person's philosophy and specific directives toward health care should that person lose decision-making capacity in the future (Fig. 9-1). The *health care proxy* involves naming an individual to represent the patient for health care decisions should the patient lose decision-making capacity in the future (Fig. 9-2). Both have gained substantial ethical and legal standing throughout the United States. In some states the *durable power of attorney for health care* can be used for both functions.

Only 10% to 15% of the population have completed such documents. Barriers include the inherent difficulty defining an end-of-life philosophy and contemplating one's death, conflicts within families, the complexity of the forms and concepts, and the sustained effort needed to complete the document. Physicians should initiate discussion as part of routine care for all patients, as part of a physical examination, when considering health maintenance, or when the issue of severe illness arises. These discussions can be more difficult and frightening if considered for the first time when the patient is severely ill and at immediate risk for losing decision-making capacity. The discussion is crucial, however, if the patient's values are to remain central to health care decisions.

If the patient has trusted family or friends, many favor the health care proxy over the living will because of its increased flexibility to deal with unanticipated conditions. Proxies who are uninformed about patient wishes, however, may have a difficult time remaining true to the patient's values. The living will has the advantage of being a direct expression of the patient's philosophy; the disadvantage is that it may not explicitly cover the patient's actual condition. The safest approach may be for the patient to complete both documents or the durable power of attorney for health care.

Advance directives have no relevance to the care of competent patients, since these persons can directly participate in their own medical decision making. Advance directives are activated only when patients lose this capacity.

2. "Bad news," ineffective treatment, uncertainty about future.[4,12] Physicians regularly encounter patients who are working through these crises. There is no preset formula about how to proceed, except to say that telling the truth, even in the face of uncertainty or a poor prognosis, is usually critical to informed decision making. Whenever possible, the physician should follow the patient's lead about how rapidly and in what detail to convey the medical situation. Sometimes the process must be accelerated because of the immediacy of the patient's condition and the need for rapid decision making, but more often time can be allowed to enable the patient to integrate enough information to make a good decision. Attention should be paid to each patient's unique emotional responses, information needs, and support.

When the news is overwhelming (e.g., new, unexpected diagnosis of cancer or HIV), it is prudent initially to develop a "miniplan" to cover the first few hours or days (how to tell close family members, where to go from the office, how to handle fear) before making major treatment decisions or learning about the illness. When the patient has integrated the relevant medical information and is ready to make medical decisions, all reasonable treatment options should be explored, from the most aggressively curative to those that emphasize comfort and symptom relief. Physicians should share their own opinions, biases, and recommendations while reinforcing that the final decision rests with the patient. Early in the patient's course, primary care physicians must convey their commitment to work with the patient through the illness no matter what choices are made.

Sometimes family members and even physicians believe that telling the truth when the prognosis is poor may deprive the patient of hope. Most providers and ethicists in the United States believe that physicians should fully inform unless a compelling reason exists not to inform. Frequently, protective secrets tend to isolate family members from the patient and may deprive the patient of the opportunity to make informed medical decisions, to settle affairs, or to say goodbye. Since medical treatment is only one avenue for finding hope, the patient may also be deprived of the opportunity to seek it in other domains (e.g., spirituality or religion). The physician should respectfully explore the reasons for not telling a patient the truth but ultimately should follow the patient's lead in deciding whether and in what detail to inform.

3. Do not *attempt* resuscitation (DN*AR*).[20] Although this decision technically applies only to attempting cardiopulmonary resuscitation (CPR), it often represents a complex amalgam of decisions and meanings. DNAR discussions may be the first open acknowledgment to the patient and the family that treatment is not working and that death is likely in the near future. Since CPR is usually ineffective in patients with metastatic cancer and other noncardiac multisystem diseases, patients and families should not anguish over resuscitation decisions. Some institutions have changed the default resuscitation order, requiring physicians to write an order to resuscitate any patient hospitalized more than 24 hours. Others allow the patient and physician to decline specific parts of CPR, such as indicating "no chest compression" or "no intubation."

Unfortunately, DNAR emphasizes what will not be done and says nothing about what treatment will be tried

DIRECTIVE REGARDING FUTURE USE OF EXTRAORDINARY LIFE SUPPORT PROCEDURES
(Equivalent to Living Will)

To: My Family, my Physicians, my Lawyer, any Medical Facility in whose care I happen to be, any Individual who may become responsible for my Health Affairs, and All Others Whom It May Concern:

I, being of sound mind and over 18 years of age, hereby issue a directive, which I intend to be legally binding, *which shall become effective at some future time, only under the following circumstances:*

1. When I become unable to make my own decisions or express my wishes; *AND*

2. CHOOSE ALL THAT YOU WANT TO APPLY

☐ If I have a terminal illness; and/or
☐ I am permanently unconscious; and/or
☐ If extraordinary life support procedures or "heroic measures" would be medically futile; and/or
☐ Under the following circumstances (Please specify, for example, dementia, severe neurological illness or other permanent disabling condition to which you want this Directive to apply.):

____
____
____
____

Then I direct that my dying not be unreasonably prolonged; *AND*
CHOOSE *ONE*

☐ I wish to have COMFORT CARE ONLY, which is directed only toward relieving pain and suffering, regardless of the progress of my disease.
☐ I want CONSERVATIVE CARE, which is usual treatment (such as antibiotics) *but not* extraordinary treatment (such as cardiopulmonary resuscitation, mechanical ventilation, kidney dialysis, etc.)

OPTIONAL: I wish to make additional directives (about life support equipment or other matters):

____
____
____
____

PLEASE NOTE: If, at some future time, you cannot make decisions for yourself, New York State law prohibits withholding artificial nutrition and hydration from you, unless you have already made your wishes known.

If I cannot eat or drink enough because of my irreversible medical conditions: (☐ I DO / ☐ I DO NOT) want artificial nutrition (intravenous or tube feeding) and hydration (intravenous fluids).

In the absence of my ability to give directions regarding the aforementioned life sustaining procedures, it is my intention that this directive shall be honored as the final expression of my legal right to refuse medical treatment and to accept the consequences of such refusal.

I understand the full importance of this directive and I have signed it after thorough consideration of the nature and consequences of my refusal of such extraordinary life support procedures, including their benefits and disadvantages. This directive is in accordance with my strong convictions and beliefs and is made freely without any inducement or coercion from any person or institution.

____________________	____________________
Signature	Date

I hereby certify that I am over 18 years of age and that I have witnessed the above declarant's signature.

____________________	____________________
Witness	Witness
Printed Witness Name	Printed Witness Name
Date	Date

Fig. 9-1. Equivalent of a living will. (Modified from Genesee Hospital, Rochester, NY.)

Therefore the DNAR decision is often confused by patients, families, and medical personnel with abandonment ("do nothing"). To avoid this confusion, discussions about resuscitation must also include an explanation of what treatments will be provided. For some patients this might include all curative and pathophysiologically directed treatments except CPR (potentially including antibiotics, fluids, chemotherapy, blood products, radiation, and even intensive care or surgery), whereas for others a more exclusively palliative approach is appropriate. The treatment

HEALTH CARE PROXY

I, ____________________________ hereby appoint the following person as my HEALTH CARE AGENT, to make any and all health care decisions for me except for any restrictions I have noted below. This Proxy shall take effect when and if I become unable to make my own health care decisions.

____ _______________________

Health Care Agent Name/Address — Phone

____ _______________________

Alternate Health Care Agent Name/Address — Phone

Optional instructions or limitations on the Health Care Agent's authority, if any:

____

____

Unless I revoke it, this proxy shall remain in effect indefinitely. (Or until the date or condition stated below, if any.)

____

____

> PLEASE NOTE: If, at some future time, you cannot make decisions for yourself, New York State law prohibits your Health Care Agent from making decisions about withholding artificial nutrition and hydration from you, unless you have already made your wishes known.
>
> If I cannot eat or drink enough because of my irreversible medical conditions: (☐ I DO / ☐ I DO NOT) want artificial nutrition (intravenous or tube feeding) and hydration (intravenous fluids).

_______________________________ _______________________________

Signature — Date

____

Address

I hereby certify that I am over 18 years of age, and that the person who signed this Proxy appeared to do so willingly and free from duress and that he or she signed (or asked another to sign for him or her) this Proxy in my presence.

_______________________________ _______________________________

Witness — Witness

_______________________________ _______________________________

Printed Witness Name — Printed Witness Name

_______________________________ _______________________________

Date — Date

Fig. 9-2. Example of a health care proxy. (Modified from Genesee Hospital, Rochester, NY.)

plan should be individualized, tailored to the patient's values, goals, and medical condition.

4. Choosing hospice care.[1,13,22] Referral to a formal hospice program is frequently offered to patients only after all possible medical interventions have been exhausted and death is imminent. Physicians should discuss palliative care and potential hospice referral as possibilities much earlier in the course of a patient's illness, especially when the chances of effective treatment diminish or when treatment burdens outweigh expected benefits. The potential of palliative care and hospice should also be explored when patients raise fears about dying, reassuring them about the possibility of a more humane and less technologically dominated approach. Hospice care should not be equated with giving up. Instead, hospice care is an alternative medical approach emphasizing intensive caring for patients and an explicit focus on relieving suffering and symptoms rather than treating disease.

5. Opportunities for growth and healing at the end of life.[6,15] Although the end of life is frequently associated with loss and grief, opportunities for life closure can also make the process emotionally rich and personally meaningful for patient, family, and caregivers. For some patients, spiritual and religious issues predominate; others see it as an opportunity for families to come together and achieve closure. Physicians or other members of the health care team should explore these areas in an open-ended way with the patient and family and refer them to people with appropriate interest and expertise as appropriate. Sometimes the simple process of *life review,* where patients recount their life story from childhood to the present into a tape recorder as part of a family archive, can be meaningful. As always, the patient should decide whether and to what depth to implement this exploration.

6. Wanting to die.[14] Relatively few severely ill patients actually choose to intentionally end their lives, but many have transient or sustained wishes for death during intense suffering. The physician is in a unique position to lessen the isolation and despair that often accompany such feelings and to explore their underlying origins. Sometimes physicians are asked about their willingness to help patients die, now or in the future. Rather than responding with a "yes" or "no" based on assumptions about what the patient might actually be asking, the physician should explore the request in detail including a consideration of why it is occurring at that particular time. Special attention should be paid to underlying depression, anxiety, or pain and to the emergence of unaddressed psychologic, social, or spiritual issues.

Sometime in their careers, physicians may encounter patients whose suffering is intolerable, whose request is rational, and for whom palliative care alternatives are ineffective or unacceptable. Physicians' responsibilities in caring for such patients are currently under intense debate in the United States (see next section). An open discussion of the issue when raised by a patient and a wide-ranging search for palliative care alternatives are essential and uncontroversial. Thoroughly exploring a patient's request for a physician-assisted death does not imply an obligation for the physician to accede. Physicians must consider their own values, the status of the law, and their relationship with the patient before responding.

END-OF-LIFE CHALLENGES AND CONTROVERSIES

Two main public policy challenges remain to be solved in the care of dying patients. These issues are interrelated, but both are essential if physicians are to reassure patients that they will die with as much comfort, dignity, and meaning as possible.

1. Improving access to and delivery of palliative care for all dying patients.[1,5,6,10] Palliative care is the standard of care for dying patients, including pain and symptom management, patient and family support, and the opportunity for life closure. Multidisciplinary hospice programs are the models against which other systems of care should be measured, but they are underused among eligible patients and are only available to those who will likely die within 6 months. Although much is made about the potential cost savings of using hospice and avoiding deaths in the acute hospital setting, these savings are mainly in the last 2 months of life, and costs of palliative care increase relative to traditional care the longer the patient is in the program. New models of palliative care must be developed that can coexist with continued disease-driven care and must be used for patients whose prognosis is longer and more uncertain, such as those with congestive heart failure, chronic obstructive pulmonary disease, stroke, amyotrophic lateral sclerosis, and dementia.

Palliative care and hospice promote a multidisciplinary team to support the patient and family in the last phase of the patient's life. Unfortunately, physicians are often the weakest link in this team, in part because of inadequate education about available palliative measures to relieve pain and other forms of suffering, and in part because they are inadequately trained in the complex communication issues involved in end-of-life care. There is considerable momentum nationally to remedy this situation, but many challenges remain. Since comprehensive palliative care is the standard of care for dying persons, all physicians who care for severely ill patients must learn how to communicate with patients and families and then deliver what has been agreed on.

2. Expanding the range of options available when palliative care is failing and patients are ready to die.[13,15,18] What are the options if the patient's suffering is intolerable, palliative care alternatives have been exhausted, and the patient is requesting a hastened death? If the problem is severe pain or shortness of breath, legal and ethical experts generally agree that opioid pain relievers can be increased until the symptom is relieved or the patient is sedated. The purpose of this intervention is primarily to relieve the patient's symptoms, not to hasten death, even though that may be what the patient is requesting. If the patient is receiving life-supporting treatments, such as mechanical ventilators, dialysis, feeding tubes, or dexamethasone for brain swelling, these can be discontinued even if the patient's wish is to hasten death.

If these options are unavailable, the physician can consider providing terminal sedation to relieve other severe symptoms of suffering. The patient is sedated to unconsciousness with a benzodiazepine or barbiturate infusion to relieve the symptoms consistent with the double effect, then life-prolonging interventions such as artificial hydration and nutrition are withheld. The Supreme Court suggested that terminal sedation would be legally permitted. Its ethical status is currently being debated, but the practice is supported by hospice and geriatrics groups as a last-resort alternative to physician-assisted suicide. As an additional possibility, the patient can choose to stop eating and drinking, even though physically capable; the physician's role is passive, ensuring informed consent and that the patient is competent and all alternatives exhausted.

Physician-assisted suicide, in which the physician provides a potentially lethal prescription at the patient's request that the patient may then independently take, could also be an option. As of 2000, the practice is illegal in the United States except in Oregon. Although physician-assisted suicide is supported by a majority of people in public opinion polls, its ethical status as an intervention of last resort remains controversial. If considering this type of assistance, the physician should be aware of the law, carefully assess the patient, and speak with experienced and trusted colleagues to ensure that all alternatives have been explored. Safeguards for any of these interventions include a careful assessment of the patient's mental capacity, a full understanding of the patient's suffering including what makes it intolerable, and a careful search for standard palliative care alternatives.[18] If any question remains about the patient's mental capacity, second opinions by palliative care specialists, by those with experience in caring for dying patients, and by mental health professionals are essential.

PAIN MANAGEMENT

All physicians must become skilled at pain and symptom management to care for severely ill and dying patients. Although pain specialists are available at many major medical centers to help with unusual or intractable problems, pain can usually be managed using basic principles and techniques by the primary treating physician. These include caregiver continuity and commitment, careful assessments over time, and individually tailored treatment regimens that often combine pharmacologic and psychosocial/behavioral techniques (Box 9-1).

Pain Assessment

The patient's pain is always subjective, usually experienced by the person as an integrated biologic, psychologic, and social experience. Physicians should attempt to assess its multiple dimensions simultaneously. The patient's report of pain is the most reliable information available.

Pain has consequences. In addition to the unnecessary suffering, patients with unrelieved pain become catabolic, respond less well to other treatments, have greater complication rates, show more emotional disturbance, and sometimes die sooner. Cultural and psychologic factors influence the expression of and tolerance for pain. Factors that aggravate pain include insomnia, fatigue, nausea, anxiety, fear, misunderstanding, anger, shame, sadness, depression, memory of past pain, and expectation that pain will recur. Conversely, pain may be lessened with sleep, rest, sympathy, understanding, diversion, relief of other symptoms, and around-the-clock pain medication.

Acute pain has a well-defined temporal onset and may be associated with autonomic nervous system activity such as tachycardia, diaphoresis, elevated blood pressure, pallor, and pupil dilation. It may serve as a warning or protective purpose. Acute pain is best treated by recognizing and addressing the underlying cause directly and by using analgesics, which should be both administered around the clock to maintain steady analgesic blood levels and supplemented as needed for breakthrough pain. Acute, episodic pain that is associated with procedures (e.g., chest tube insertion or removal, dressing changes, bone marrow aspiration or biopsy, lumbar puncture) can be anticipated and treated prophylactically.

Chronic pain may not have a well-defined temporal onset, may last months to years, and frequently has no signs of autonomic nervous system hyperactivity. Instead, chronic pain is often associated with the signs and symptoms of depression, including hopelessness, helplessness, anhedonia, appetite and weight changes, sleep disturbances, and decreased social interaction. The underlying causes may not be treatable and in some circumstances not clearly identifiable. Chronic pain should be prevented whenever possible and treated aggressively once identified.

The assessment of pain and pain therapy requires regular, accurate measurement. Pain can be followed over time on a 10-point numeric scale, with 0 being no pain and 10 being the worst imaginable pain (Fig. 9-3). After any therapeutic intervention, one needs to learn how much relief was achieved (i.e., where did the pain rating move on the scale) and how long the relief lasted. Intervals between analgesic dosages are adjusted so that the analgesic effect is uninterrupted. The goal of pain management is not necessarily complete absence of pain, but rather a maximally functional patient. The patient is the ultimate arbitrator of whether pain relief goals have been achieved.[1,8,9]

Box 9-1. Goals of Pain Management

1. Identify and address the cause of pain.
2. Prevent chronic pain.
3. Erase the memory and expectation of pain.
4. Allow the patient to remain alert and to function.
5. Allow the patient to experience feelings other than pain.
6. Intervene as noninvasively as possible.

Treatment

Pain treatment almost always involves a combination of pharmacologic and psychosocial/behavioral techniques.

Psychosocial and Behavioral Approaches.[9,12,22] Meditation, self-hypnosis, distraction, humor, psychotherapy, spiritual exploration, hobbies, biofeedback, music, art, and many other approaches can be very effective and helpful in treating pain. The choice of technique depends on the patient's interests and condition and the presence of skilled practitioners or partners. For some patients, pain may be very tolerable when in the presence of others but intolerable when alone. Therefore, although pharmacologic approaches are vitally important and effective, other psychosocial factors might influence a patient's pain.

Pharmacologic Treatments.[7-9,22] Medications are generally effective provided they are used skillfully, with knowledge of the underlying pharmacokinetics and without

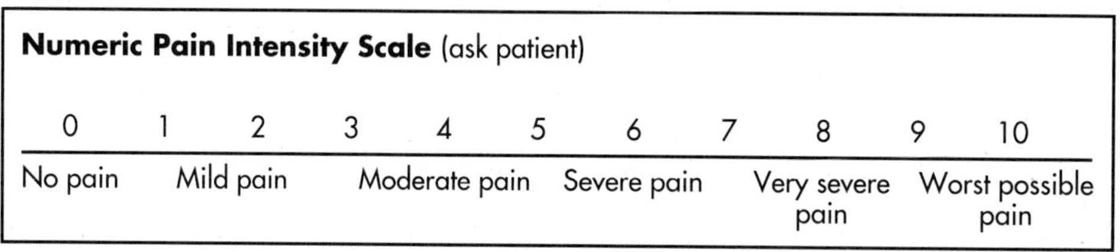

(Ruler front)

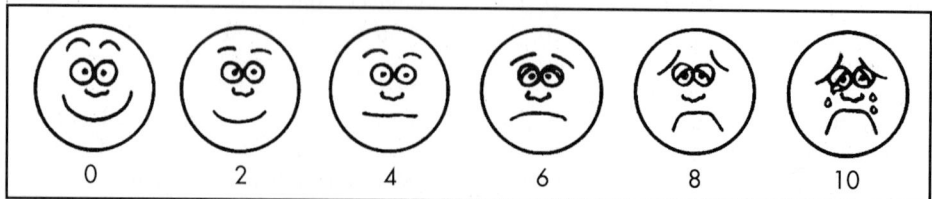

(Ruler back)

Fig. 9-3. Ruler for assessment of potential pain.

unnecessary fear or restraint. Table 9-1 shows an analgesic ladder of progressively stronger medications in the management of chronic pain; the higher the step, the greater the analgesic effect, while adverse reactions also become more likely. To treat any chronic pain, analgesics should be taken around the clock. Chronic pain should not be managed solely with as-needed dosing, although such dosages should be provided for breakthrough pain between regular dosing intervals. The initial drug dosage and interval are determined by the pharmacologic properties of the specific drug, but the final regimen of any drug should be individualized. Onset, peak effect, and duration of analgesia may vary from person to person because of differences in absorption, organ dysfunction, or tolerance.

The biologic half-life of the analgesic agent must be considered when adjusting the dosage and interval. The maximum effect of a given dose may not be seen until the drug has been administered over four or five half-lives. In addition, the duration of analgesia may be shorter than the half-life, which may be prolonged in renal or hepatic failure, when short-acting agents usually are administered at longer intervals.

Oral medications are preferred. Physicians should also be familiar with unique routes of administration (e.g., highly concentrated oral solutions, transdermal patches, subcutaneous infusions) that may be effective in special situations. Subcutaneous, intravenous, and intramuscular injections should be avoided if possible to enhance patient comfort and to minimize the risk to caregivers. *Patient-controlled analgesia* (within professionally established limits) has been shown to lessen postoperative pain, decrease complications, lead to earlier discharge, and lessen the overall opiate level consumed. This concept has been applied most frequently to parenteral pumps but also reinforces active patient participation in the selection, assessment, and control of analgesic regimens.

With step 2 and step 3 drugs (see Table 9-1), side effects must be anticipated. Constipation is predictable and should be treated prophylactically (Table 9-2). Box 9-2 outlines guidelines for analgesic use.

Special Patients

Loss of Ability to Swallow.[7,22] As patients near death or when they develop complications, they may lose the ability to ingest medications that were adequately controlling their pain. The physician should change to an equianalgesic amount of the same or a different medication. The options include, in general order of preference, oral concentrate (can be absorbed through oral mucosa), transdermal patch, subcutaneous infusion, and transrectal suppository. The physician must choose the best available route of delivery, then calculate the equivalent amount of medication needed (see Table 9-1). The total dose equivalent is generally reduced by 25% to 30% (to allow for individual differences) and given around the clock at intervals determined by usual drug half-lives. Ten to fifteen percent of the total daily dose is made available on an as-needed basis every few hours (see Box 9-2). Physicians who are unfamiliar with dose conversions should seek guidance from palliative care or pain specialists or consult with a knowledgeable pharmacist.

Invasive Options.[7] Intraspinal (epidural or intrathecal) opiates can provide analgesia at lower dosages and may reduce systemic side effects in special situations, but they tend to be invasive and expensive and require close monitoring. Nerve blocks, such as celiac block for the pain of pancreatic cancer, or other sympathetic or neurolytic blocks may also be useful when pain is well localized, especially when systemic analgesia fails because of unacceptable side effects. Anesthesiologists who specialize in pain management should be consulted if the patient might benefit from these approaches.

Neuropathic Pain.[8,9] Neuropathic pain is characterized by burning, tingling, numbness, and electrical and pins-and-needles qualities. It accompanies many medical and surgical conditions, is often underdiagnosed, and may also coexist with other forms of pain. Neuropathic pain does not respond well to conventional analgesics. Tricyclic agents are useful because they have a specific analgesic effect lacking in other classes of antidepressants. Compared with the antidepressant effect, pain relief occurs at lower dosages (10 to 25 mg for pain vs. 150 to 300 mg for depression) and sooner (1 to 3 days vs. 2 to 4 weeks for depression). These drugs are usually started at a low dosage and titrated up to relief of neuropathic pain or the development of side effects. Dosing at night may help with sleeplessness. These drugs may treat coexisting depression, which can aggravate pain.

Anticonvulsants such as carbamazepine, phenytoin, valproic acid, gabapentin, and clonazepam are used to treat neuropathic pain. The analgesic dosage is usually the same as the anticonvulsant dosage but may be less. The physician should start low and follow blood levels until adequate analgesia or a therapeutic range is reached. Mexiletine, an orally administered form of lidocaine, and capsaicin, a topical substance P inhibitor derived from chili peppers, have also been used to treat neuropathic pain. Conventional analgesics may be used if these more specific approaches are neither effective nor tolerated.

Anxiety and Depressive Disorders.[7] These conditions, often seen in the general population, are frequently associated with chronic pain or terminal diseases. Anxiety and depression contribute to considerable suffering, can aggravate chronic pain, and usually respond to treatment (see Chapter 48). It is important not to overnormalize (e.g., "Of course he's depressed, he's dying") because even depression secondary to terminal illness may respond to treatment. On the other hand, not all sadness or anxiety that accompanies grief, loss, or the dying process is part of a disorder. Each patient's unique circumstances should be thoroughly explored with the hope of finding a way to lessen suffering.

Substance Abuse.[7] Whether the substance is opiates, alcohol, or other chemicals, substance abusers present complex pain management dilemmas. The history should include the drug(s) of choice, route, dosage, and frequency of use, including time of last dose. Withdrawal must be recognized and treated. Because of physiologic tolerance, regular users of opiates require stronger analgesics and larger dosages to achieve the same analgesic effect. Effective pain management cannot occur until acute substance abuse issues, such as prevention and treatment of withdrawal, are addressed and brought under control. However, drug rehabilitation during an acute hospitalization for other major medical or surgical problems is seldom appropriate.

Table 9-1. Analgesic Ladder for Pain Management

Drug	Equianalgesic dose (mg)		Usual starting doses (mg)		Half-life (hours)	Duration (hours)	Comments
	IM/IV	PO	IM/IV	PO			
Step 1: Drug equivalents for mild pain†							
Acetaminophen (Tylenol, Datril, Panadol)	*	650	*	650 q4-6h	2	4	No antiinflammatory effect; does not inhibit platelet function; avoid in liver failure.
Aspirin, ASA	*	650	*	650 q4-6h	3-12	2-4	Avoid during pregnancy, in hemostatic disorders, in GI or GU bleeding, preoperatively, and in patients under age 18; may precipitate asthma.
Nonsteroidal antiinflammatory drug (NSAID) (various)	*	Varies	*	Varies	*	*	As with ASA; also useful with opiates for pain of bone metastases; upper GI toxicity common.
Ketorolac (Toradol)	30	10	30 q6h	10 q6h	4-7	6-8	IM preparation with all NSAID side effects; expensive; reduce dose with renal insufficiency.
Celecoxib (Celebrex)	*	200	*	200 qd	11	24	Cox 2 inhibitor-antiinflammatory effect similar to NSAID, but less GI toxicity; expensive.
Rofecoxib (Vioxx)	*	25	*	25 qd	17	24	Cox 2 inhibitor-antiinflammatory effect similar to NSAID, but less GI toxicity; expensive.
Step 2: Drug equivalents for moderate pain‡							
Codeine	120	200	30 q3-4h	30-60 q3-4h	3	4-6	Often used in combination with acetaminophen or ASA (325 mg); analgesic effect plateaus in adults receiving more than 120 mg q4h.
Hydrocodone (Hycodan)	*	30	*	5-10 q4-6h	3.3-4.5	4-6	Combined with acetaminophen (500 mg) (Vicodin).
Oxycodone (Roxicodone)	*	30	*	10 q4-6h	No data	4-6	Used in combination with ASA (Percodan, Roxiprin) or acetaminophen (Percocet, Tylox, Roxicet); upper limit of dosing not defined except for combination preparations.
Meperidine (Demerol)	75-100	300	75 q2-3h	NR	3-4	2-4	Short acting (about 2 hr); toxic metabolite causes irritability and seizures with repeated dosing; parenteral dose ⅓ oral dose; NR.
Propoxyphene	*	100	*	NR	6-12	4-6	Opiate with potentially toxic metabolite; used with acetaminophen (Darvocet-N); does not inhibit platelet function or cause GI upset or bleeding; may be habituating; NR.

		[illegible] naïve)	[illegible] q3-4h	[illegible] q3-4h	1.5-2	3-7	Standard against which all other analgesics are judged; available as several different preparations.§
Hydromorphone (Dilaudid)	1.5	7.5	1-2 q3-4h	4-8 q3-4h	2-3	4-5	As with morphine; duration of action 3-4 hr; 2-, 3-, 4-, 8-mg tablets, 3-mg rectal suppositories, and 1-, 2-, 4-, 10-mg/ml parenteral solutions available.
Methadone (Dolophine)	10	20	NR	5-10 q12h	15-30	4-6	Give q6-8h for pain, not qd; will accumulate with repeated dosing; equianalgesic dosage may cause unacceptable persistent sedation, so should be reduced on the third or fourth day of titration; inexpensive.
Fentanyl (Duragesic)	100 μg (single dose) 200 μg (continuous infusion)	100 μg/hr; transdermal patch equivalent to 180 mg morphine/24 hr	100 μg IV q1-2h	25-mg transdermal patch q72h	12 (transdermal)	48-72 (transdermal) 1-2 (IV)	25-, 50-, 75-, and 100-μg patches (Duragesic); 25-μg patch approximates 10 mg morphine PO q4h; with transdermal patch, steady state reached only after 24 hr, so other analgesics needed in interim; replace q72h at different site; fever may lead to increased levels; skin reservoir causes long half-life (50% 17 hr after removal), so careful monitoring required; most useful in stable chronic pain situations.

IM/IV, Intramuscular/intravenous; *PO,* oral; *q4-6h,* every 4 to 6 hours; *qd,* daily; *GI,* gastrointestinal; *GU,* genitourinary; *NR,* not recommended.
*Not available or not applicable.
†Equianalgesic dose: approximate comparisons with other step 1 drugs.
‡Equianalgesic dose: equivalent to 10 mg of parenteral morphine.
§Morphine preparations: Oral solution (MSIR), 2-4 mg/ml, when low doses needed.
Concentrated oral solution (Roxanol, OMS concentrate, MSIR concentrate), 20 mg/ml, absorbed sublingually when patient has no oral intake or difficulty swallowing; used when higher doses indicated.
Sustained-release (SR) tablet (MS Contin, Oramorph SR); 15, 30, 60, 100 mg; lasts 8-12 hr instead of 3-4 hr; titrate first with rapid-acting preparations for 24 hr, then divide into 2-3 doses for around-the-clock administration of SR tablet; continue short-acting preparation as needed for breakthrough pain; may be used rectally; do not crush tablet.
Immediate-release tablet (MSIR tablets), 15 and 30 mg, short acting.
Rectal suppositories (MS/S or RMS), short acting; 5, 10, 20, 30 mg per suppository.
Also indicated for intractable dyspnea; no upper limit to morphine dosing but relatively ineffective for neuropathic pain.

Table 9-2. Opioid Side Effects and Treatment

Side effect	Treatment	Comments
Constipation	Bisacodyl (Ducolax, 250 mg), senna (Senekot), or magnesium hydroxide (Milk of Magnesia, 30-60 ml) once or twice daily	Prophylaxis is better than as-needed dosing for steps 2 and 3 drugs (see Table 9-1); avoid bulk laxatives.
Sedation	Decrease dosage or increase interval of opiate; dextroamphetamine, 2.5-7.5 mg every 6 hours	Tolerance to sedation usually develops in 24-72 hr; sedation usually appears well before respiratory depression; avoid naloxone (Narcan) except in emergencies, as it will cause major withdrawal. If Narcan is needed, dilute 0.4 mg with 9 ml NS and give slowly to desired effect.
Nausea	Antihistamines, phenothiazines, butyrophenones, scopolamine, metoclopramide, steroids	Use trial-and-error approach: be sure nausea is not secondary to constipation; be aware of drug-specific side effects (e.g., dystonic reaction with phenothiazines or metoclopramide).

Box 9-2. Analgesic Guidelines

1. Pain is evaluated in all patients using 1 to 10 scale when other vital signs are measured.
   a. Mild pain: 1-4
   b. Moderate pain: 5-7
   c. Severe pain: 8-10
2. For chronic moderate or severe pain:
   a. Administer baseline medications around the clock.
   b. Give 10%-15% of total daily dose as needed every 1-2 hours for oral dose and every 30-60 minutes for subcutaneous and intravenous doses.
   c. Adjust baseline upward daily in amount equivalent to total dose.
   d. Negotiate target level of relief with patient (usually less than 5).
3. In general, oral route is preferable, then transcutaneous, subcutaneous, and lastly intravenous.
4. When converting from one opioid to another, some experts recommend reducing the equianalgesic dose by one third to one half, then titrating as in guideline 2.
5. Elderly patients and those with severe renal or liver disease should initially receive half the usual starting dose.

Including substance abuse caregivers in the plan of care is usually helpful.

The patient in recovery from abuse who develops a chronic pain problem requires an open discussion regarding the risks and benefits of opioid analgesics, including the potential of addiction relapse. If opioids are needed, active and recovering substance users may best be treated with a long-acting oral preparation given at scheduled times. Needles can be the environmental trigger for drug craving and generally are avoided. Prescribing rules and contracts are often helpful, including mutually agreed amounts and dosages renewed at fixed, relatively frequent intervals and statements that lost or stolen medications will not be replaced except at these intervals.

Patients without a history of abuse almost never become addicted when opiates are prescribed for acute or chronic pain. Health care providers must not allow concern or ignorance about addiction to prevent patients in their care from receiving adequate analgesia. Some patients exhibit drug-seeking behavior because no physician has adequately assessed or provided treatment for their pain.

OTHER PHYSICAL SYMPTOMS

Nausea, vomiting, diarrhea, constipation, open wounds, confusion, incontinence, and other symptoms may develop in severely ill or dying patients. Alone or in combination, each may aggravate pain or suffering and may undermine quality of life.[7,22] Experienced hospice and palliative care physicians and nurses should be consulted when a patient has developed an intractable physical symptom. Although not all such symptoms can be relieved with available interventions, many can be improved or at least made tolerable.

FINAL RECOMMENDATIONS

Caring for dying patients and their families can be a uniquely rewarding facet of clinical practice. Although dying is physiologically destructive, it may be psychologically, socially, and spiritually constructive. Facilitating this growth can be enormously gratifying. Dying patients need a knowledgeable guide, witness, and friend who will commit to facing the unknown with them through the entire process. Having known the patient when healthy and weathered disease processes together, the primary care physician is often in an ideal position to assume this role.

To prepare for this responsibility, physicians should undertake several activities. First, they should articulate their own personal end-of-life philosophy in some form of written advance directive. Physicians who have not personally been through this process are often unpersuasive in encouraging their patients to complete their own advance directives, and they may be less open about their own beliefs and recommendations as they help those who are facing death. Second, all physicians caring for severely ill patients must become skilled in palliative care, including basic measures to relieve severe pain and other symptoms. Third, if a patient has been cared for by multiple physicians in the course of the illness and is moving to the terminal phase, a specific physician should be identified to work through this phase of illness with the patient and family. That physician must commit to working with the health care team to care for the patient and family regardless of the illness course until the patient's death. The promise not to abandon may be the most fundamental aspect of primary care physicians' commitment to their dying patients.

REFERENCES

1. American Board of Internal Medicine: *Caring for the dying: identification and promotion of physician competency,* Philadelphia, 1996, American Board of Internal Medicine.
2. Annas G: The health care proxy and the living will, *N Engl J Med* 324:1210, 1991.
3. Brody H, Campbell ML, Faber-Langendoen K, et al: Withdrawing intensive life-sustaining treatment: recommendations for compassionate clinical management, *N Engl J Med* 336:652, 1997.
4. Buckman R: *How to break bad news: a guide for health care professionals,* Baltimore, 1992, Johns Hopkins University Press.
5. Burt RA: The Supreme Court speaks: not assisted suicide but a constitutional right to palliative care, *N Engl J Med* 337:1234, 1997.
6. Byock I: *Dying well: the prospect for growth at the end of life,* New York, 1997, Riverhead Books.
7. Doyle D, Hands GWC, MacDonald N, editors: *Oxford textbook of palliative medicine,* ed 2, New York, 1998, Oxford University Press.
8. Foley K: The treatment of cancer pain, *N Engl J Med* 313:84, 1985.
9. Jacox A, Carr DB, Payne R, et al: *Management of cancer pain,* Clinical practice guideline no 9, ACHPAR pub no 94-0592, Rockville, Md, 1994, Agency for Health Policy and Research, Public Health Service, US Department of Health and Human Services.
10. Lynn J: Caring at the end of our lives, *N Engl J Med* 335:201, 1996 (editorial).
11. Meisel A: Legal myths about terminating life support, *Arch Intern Med* 151:1497, 1991.
12. Quill TE: Bad news: delivery, dialogue and dilemmas, *Arch Intern Med* 151:463, 1990.
13. Quill TE: *Death and dignity: making choices and taking charge,* New York, 1993, WW Norton.
14. Quill TE: "Doctor, I want to die. Will you help me?" *JAMA* 270:841, 1993.
15. Quill TE: *A midwife through the dying process: stories of healing and hard choices at the end of life,* Baltimore, 1996, Johns Hopkins University Press.
16. Quill TE, Brody RV: "You promised me I wouldn't die like this": a bad death as a medical emergency, *Arch Intern Med* 155:1250, 1995.
17. Quill TE, Cassel CK: Nonabandonment: a central obligation for physicians, *Ann Intern Med* 122:368, 1995.
18. Quill TE, Lo B, Brock D: Palliative options of last resort: a comparison of voluntarily stopping eating and drinking, terminal sedation, physician-assisted suicide and voluntary active euthanasia, *JAMA* 278:2099, 1997.
19. Solomon MZ, O'Connell L, Jennings B, et al: Decisions near the end of life: professional views on life-sustaining treatment, *Am J Public Health* 83:14, 1993.
20. Tomlinson T, Brody H: Ethics and communication in do-not-resuscitate orders, *N Engl J Med* 318:43, 1988.
21. Waller A, Caroline NL: *Handbook of palliative care in cancer,* Boston, 1996, Butterworth-Heinemann.
22. Wallston KA, Burger C, Smith RA, et al: Comparing the quality of death for hospice and nonhospice cancer patients, *Med Care* 26:177, 1986.

CHAPTER 10

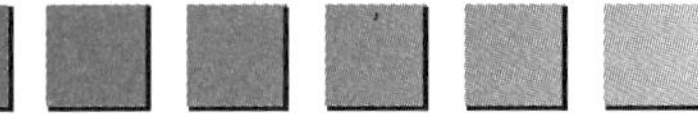

Community Health

Loren Leshan

Regardless of ever-changing health care delivery systems and beliefs, the main question guiding our medical practices continues to be "How do we provide the best care to *all* of our patients?"[9] The purpose of this chapter is to point to ways that "new" imperatives in medicine help us realize this oldest and best desire of our profession. Community medicine, which draws on the gold standard of population studies, offers an underutilized source of answers to that question.

Rather than being a buzzword or a fad, community medicine is intrinsically a part of what good doctors do, have always done, and will continue to do. It leads not only to better health for the patient and a stronger medical practice but also to improved satisfaction for the practitioner.[2] The philosophies and systems approach of community medicine offer ideas for potentially far-reaching public health ventures and also practical methods to improve health care in the community of one's clinical practice.[5,9] Community health practice, then, is a matter of enlightened patient, community, and self-interest.

This chapter gives the broadest overview of community health in the context of an "average" physician's practice in the United States. Instead of concentrating on providing a template for a formal system or a theoretic framework, it shows some of the ways physicians can use population data, community health principles, clinical guidelines, and evidence-based medicine to improve their everyday practice patterns, as well as to improve community health.

BACKGROUND

Community health practice is deeply embedded in the traditions of medicine.[6] One of the basic principles of community medicine is that for primary care physicians to provide effective health care over the long run, they need to view the whole panorama of their patients' lives, not just the isolated disease that brings the patients into medical care. This means integrating into health care an understanding of patients' families and the communities that constitute their physical environment and influence their beliefs, behaviors, and opportunities.

Medical history, lore, and personal experience are rich with stories of physicians making a difference in their communities. Both Aristotle and Maimonides stressed the importance of the environment and family. A more recent role model was William N. Pickles.[7a] Pickles studied the epidemiology of disease in his country practice in the Aysgarth Rural District of England. Like his colleague, Sir James MacKenzie, Pickles was able not only to care for the residents of his communities, but also to study the epidemiology of their illnesses. He understood that the context in which his patients lived, their community, was inseparable from their health concerns.

Changing Scene

Primary care in the United States has focused on *primary* patients, and most health care delivery models, although currently in the process of change, have been designed for individual health care, while public health departments have shouldered much of the responsibility for the health of populations. These departments have effectively, efficiently, and at low cost monitored the environment. They have spearheaded efforts to control environmental pollutants such as lead, disease vectors such as contaminated water, and outbreaks of infectious disease such as polio.

The separation of public and private health is artificial, however, and does not always lead to the best health care.[3] With changing social and financial structures, physicians are learning that by networking with community agencies, they can leverage their own effectiveness in preventing and solving problems for their patients.

REAL LIFE NEEDS LEAD TO COMMUNITY MEDICINE PRACTICES

Most physicians enter the world of community medicine when they identify a problem that is occurring commonly among patients in their community, and realize that individual treatment plans are not achieving the results they would like. The following composite vignette exemplifies how community health practices can evolve out of a recognized need.

Late one Saturday night, Dr. Gomez admitted a very sick asthmatic woman to the intensive care unit (ICU) for possible intubation. On his way home, after spending several harrowing hours with his patient, Dr. Gomez reflected on his many poorly controlled asthmatic patients and his fears for their lives. He wondered why it was so difficult to control their symptoms, prevent exacerbations, and manage their chronic asthma. The next morning at church, a group of parishioners overheard him expressing his concerns to their minister. They became interested and asked if there was anything they could do as a group of volunteers. The minister suggested that the doctor ask his patient what might be helpful. Later, when the patient was recovering, Dr. Gomez talked to her. She told him that the hardest task for her was creating the clean home environment described in the patient care booklet. Vacuuming and dusting in her apartment led to coughing fits and midnight emergency room visits. She was not sure the landlord would let her remove the carpeting.

One of the volunteers, the mother of an asthmatic child, was experienced in "environmental control." With a group of volunteers, she visited the patient with buckets and mops in hand. They talked to the landlord, who agreed to let them take up the carpeting and paint the floor. The volunteers not only cleaned and "decluttered" the apartment, but also helped find appropriate bedding. After the initial cleaning, a small group of volunteers spent 2 hours a month cleaning for the patient. She compensated them with babysitting, cooking, doing laundry, and other tasks that did not trigger her asthma.

The patient asked Dr. Gomez if she could help form a support group for asthmatic patients in his office. Dr. Gomez used his billing system to generate a list of his patients with asthma and sent them letters inviting them to the first meeting. With the help of clinic staff, the group created a patient diary to record peak airflows. Most patients had been told to measure their peak flows but few had been told what to do with the information.

Dr. Gomez then realized that he had given very few patients a "plan of care" to help them decide what to do when their peak flows were low. Although the National Institutes of Health (NIH) has disseminated asthma clinical guidelines suggesting the use of asthma "plans of care," Dr. Gomez had not implemented them. The support group and nursing staff helped Dr. Gomez develop a patient education sheet to give to patients with their individual "plan of care." The asthma support group was also successful in starting a cleaning cooperative. They helped each other maintain clean environments in exchange for services such as babysitting. Over the next 12 months, Dr. Gomez noticed that the patients in the support group experienced fewer asthma exacerbations and fewer symptoms.

This story illustrates several ways that physicians can work within their practices to build a healthier community of patients, as well as to improve patient care by following clinical guidelines. By focusing on common concerns and using common resources, the asthmatic patients and their physician were able to work together to manage a common condition that impacted all their lives. In time, the support group, physician, and nursing staff shared their asthma control program with others outside the practice through their religious organizations, health department, and schools.

DEFINITIONS

Populations are groups of people who can be described by epidemiologic or demographic factors such as infant mortality rate, literacy rate, economic level, age, and employment status.[10] Other important aspects that impact population in geographic communities are environmental factors such as air and water pollution; housing stock; and availability of opportunities for recreation, education, or employment.

A *community* is a group of individuals who are conscious of a shared unifying trait, such as common geographic boundaries, culture, history, language, age, race, religion, or special needs.

Community health is defined by population data: rates of infant mortality, fertility, and other vital statistics usually collected by the census bureau or health departments. Managed care organizations and other insurers can facilitate both the collection of data and the improvement of these rates. They can supply additional information about hospitalization, immunization rates, physicians' prescribing practices, and use of diagnostic tests.[10] These data can be used to improve clinical practice patterns and to monitor and improve patient outcomes. This chapter includes some ways this kind of population data can be used to improve physician practice patterns, as well as community health (Box 10-1).

A physician's practice is, in a sense, a special population,[1] unified by being served by the practice. The population of both patients who have presented for care and those who have not been seen is called the *denominator. Numerators* include any subsets of the denominator.

A *healthy community* would be one in which members interact and cooperate in helping each other grow, learn, and succeed. The physical environment would be nontoxic; health statistics and economic conditions would be favorable for all members of the community. Such a community would be considered a desirable place to live. Clearly, physicians can serve important leadership roles in improving the health and well being of the community and its members.

Box 10-1. Expanded Definitions of Community

People may be born into a geographic or circumstantial community (a small village in Mexico or people with Down syndrome).

Community can be created around people, or they may enter a community created by history, events, and circumstances (e.g., becoming a parent, contracting the human immunodeficiency virus [HIV], surviving the Holocaust). People also choose communities according to interest (e.g., doctors, fans of the Yankees).

Communities are sometimes described as having developmental cycles. For instance, when a group of immigrants settles into an area, they are often marginalized from the majority community. As they begin to adjust to their new homeland, they form neighborhood groups or associations. Over time, they usually adapt to fit into the mainstream. Eventually they may lose their "old ways," although they may maintain their identity through cultural and religious associations.

DEVELOPING COMMUNITY HEALTH CARE

Community-Oriented Primary Care

During the last 30 years, the World Health Organization (WHO) and the community health center movement have supported broad efforts to improve the health of populations through redesign of health care delivery systems. The method most often suggested for integrating traditional public health with primary care in order to provide more comprehensive and coordinated services on a community level is *community-oriented primary care* (COPC), also called responsive primary care (Box 10-2).

Although COPC can be used to apply epidemiologic and evidence-based medicine to a specific population in a specific practice, in reality most physicians lack the time, training, and incentive to fully implement the model as originally conceived by Kark.[4] Fortunately, it is not necessary to implement the entire model to realize benefits in most practices.[7] Pathman has found that most doctors do incorporate elements of community medicine into their practices. These commonly applied practices include (1) identifying and intervening in the health problems facing communities, (2) responding to the particular health issues of local cultural groups when caring for patients, (3) coordinating local community health resources in the care of patients, and (4) assimilating into the community and its organizations.

Although the first dimension may seem daunting in the press of daily practice, the second and third dimensions, responding to local cultural groups' health needs and coordinating resources for particular patient needs, are common practices. The fourth dimension, assimilating into the community and its organizations, often happens naturally as physicians pursue their personal and family lives.

Examples and Benefits

Identifying and Intervening in Health Problems Facing Communities. A common current practice involves routinely screening for lead in areas where the homes of most of the physician's patient population were built before 1978. Less common, but eliciting a response in places where the threat is high is recognizing a pattern of cancers common among workers at a local workplace and then identifying exposures to carcinogens. The physician would additionally help in efforts to eliminate the particular carcinogen from the workplace or lead from homes.

Responding to the Particular Health Issues of Local Cultural Groups When Caring for Patients. Examples of responsiveness include providing patient education materials that are culturally and linguistically appropriate to the background or educational levels of one's patients, or having evening or Saturday hours to accommodate the work schedules of the patient population. Such efforts build physicians' practices and patient adherence by increasing patient satisfaction.

Coordinating Local Community Health Resources in the Care of Patients. Examples of ways in which physicians coordinate resources in the care of patients include referring chemically dependent patients or survivors of domestic violence to appropriate resources.

Assimilating into the Community and its Organizations. Such common and rewarding activities as getting involved with the efforts of one's personal religious organization or the school system to address teen sexuality or substance abuse are assimilating activities. Physicians not only find their niche in their own communities through assimilation, they also provide leadership and expertise. The vignette earlier in this chapter also illustrates physician involvement in Pathman's dimensions. Dr. Gomez had joined one of the local community churches. He used that involvement to help coordinate local community health resources, in this case other church members. He responded to the health needs of a special group in his practice (people with asthma) by forming a support group in his community. Asthma was identified as a common health problem in the community. Subsequent intervention included educating children, teachers, and parents in the schools, and assisting in communitywide efforts to monitor and decrease the air pollution.

COMMUNITY MEDICINE AND QUALITY MANAGEMENT

A systematic methodology for optimizing patient care for common problems in primary care is described by Rivo.[9] He uses a four-step method (Box 10-3) and employs the principles of continuous quality improvement (CQI) or total quality management (TQM).

The vignette demonstrates the use of these steps. Dr. Gomez chose a common condition and identified patients within the practice with that condition (steps 1 and 2). He used NIH asthma care guidelines to guide the care of patients (step 3). The patient support group helped to define measurable outcomes by developing a patient record and plan of care. Over time patients were given peak flow meters and an individualized plan of care; they seemed to improve and had fewer symptoms and exacerbations. These were

Box 10-2. Steps in COPC Process

1. Defining and characterizing the community (or population)
2. Identifying and prioritizing community health problems
3. Involving the community in the design and implementation of interventions to improve community health
4. Monitoring and evaluating the impact of interventions

Modified from Nutting PA, et al: *Community oriented primary care: from principle to practice*, Albuquerque, 1990, University of New Mexico.

Box 10-3. Rivo's Steps for CQI/TQM

1. Choose common conditions that lend themselves to systems approach to care (see Box 10-4).
2. Identify patients in the practice with those conditions.
3. Choose measurable outcomes that reflect the best evidenced-based medical practice.
4. Regularly measure and try to improve these outcomes.

Modified from Rivo ML: It's time to start practicing population-based health care, *Fam Pract Man* June 1998.

Box 10-4. Common Conditions that Lend Themselves to a Population Approach

Prevention

Counseling and education
Screening
Immunizations and prophylaxis

Care of Chronic Conditions

Diseases such as diabetes, asthma, congestive heart failure, and hypertension
Chronic pain syndromes such as low back pain, headache, and chronic pelvic pain

Care of Common Acute Conditions or Problems

Urinary tract infection, sexually transmitted diseases (STDs), upper respiratory infections (URIs), low back pain, headache, otitis media, bronchitis, sprains, and strains

Management of Common Normal Conditions

Pregnancy and contraception

Modified from Rivo ML: It's time to start practicing population-based health care, *Fam Pract Man*, June, 1998.

measurable outcomes, which could have been used to monitor and improve care (steps 3 and 4).

Congestive heart failure and low back pain are examples of other conditions lending themselves to this approach. This clinical system can also be used to improve the delivery of prevention services such as immunizations or screenings (Box 10-4). By following a systems approach, physicians can lead the "community" of their practice to improve the clinical care of their patients.

ARENAS OF INVOLVEMENT: WHERE COMMUNITY MEDICINE TAKES PLACE

Reif and others have categorized physician involvement in their communities as levels or arenas of involvement[8] (Fig. 10-1). The first arena is the examination room. Here, in assessing and planning care, the physician must be aware of population characteristics, patterns of illness, risk, and injury. In getting to know the communities they serve, good physicians are aware of common cultural patterns, occupations, health-seeking behavior, and lifestyle. The good physician uses this awareness in developing diagnoses as well as care plans. Follow-up visits monitor the effectiveness of this approach.

The second arena is the clinic or health center. There, the focus is on the population of patients in the practice, whether they have been in the center for care or not. By following evidenced-based guidelines, physicians can ensure the best care for all the patients in the system. Using CQI and data from billing or insurers or demographic sources, physicians can monitor and improve primary care services within their practice system, much as Dr. Gomez did.

The third arena is the network of agencies and organizations within the neighborhood of the practice used to provide ancillary services such as counseling, home care, drug treatment, day care, domestic violence shelters, and hospice and other patient care needs. By knowing and working with this network, physicians are better able to meet the many needs of their patients. A good working relationship with the agencies within the network means that services are coordinated more efficiently and at lower cost, allowing physicians to leverage their own effectiveness.

An example of this might be managing the survivor of domestic violence identified at a patient visit. The physician usually does not have sufficient time in a busy day to do more than to identify a survivor of domestic violence. However, by knowing the network of agencies serving the needs of this population, the physician can refer the patient to further sources of help. Obviously, this does not mean the physician is handing the patient off, but rather that he or she is referring patients to other experts, while continuing the supportive, ongoing physician-patient relationship. This network works best if all providers work together to evaluate and improve their services.

On a community level, physicians can respond to the public health concerns by engaging in strategic planning and health campaigns with officials and community leadership. The impact of these efforts is measured by epidemiologic data. Decreasing teenage pregnancy or new human immunodeficiency virus (HIV) infections through community education campaigns is an example. The effectiveness of such efforts can be measured by monitoring the rates of teenage pregnancy and new HIV cases, which may be done by the local board of health. In broader arenas, physicians can help develop and support policies that improve the health of the state or nation, or even the world. In times of increasing health care costs, physicians can use community medicine principles to help ensure appropriate distribution of diminishing resources based on epidemiology and effectiveness.

COST-EFFECTIVENESS AND ETHICS

Maintaining Ethical Balances When Needs Compete

Increasing value and efficiency are not the only challenge arising from economic conditions. As health care has shifte from fee-for-service toward capitated delivery systems, physicians are increasingly being expected to maintain an ethica balance between the needs and resources of patients an families and those of communities. This mandate is sti informal, and the means to accomplish it are uncle Furthermore, most physicians have not been trained provide health care based on community needs and ou comes.[11] However, changes in the financial structure of t health care delivery system have once again underscored t importance of the community and family context, whi shapes our patients' lives and their illnesses.

Championing Cost-Effective Health Promotio

The shift to integrated health delivery systems and manag care has also shed light on the use of community hea principles to help guide the practice of medicine. A notal example is the use of technology. The rapid development medicine from technology to pharmaceuticals has gi physicians a wide and confusing array of choices diagnosis and treatment. It is often unclear which choice lead to the best outcomes for individual patients, let al

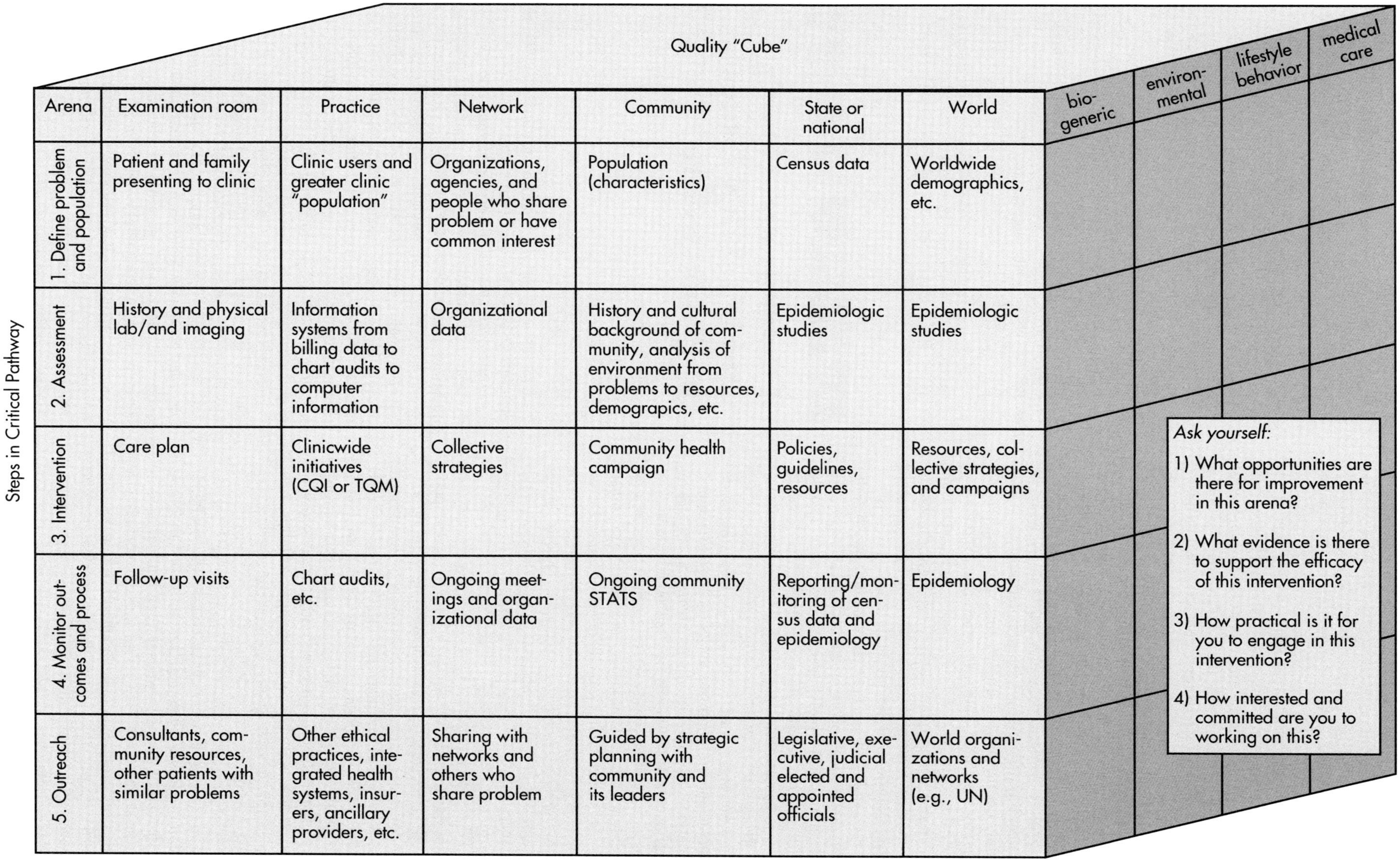

Quality "Cube"

Steps in Critical Pathway

Arena	Examination room	Practice	Network	Community	State or national	World
1. Define problem and population	Patient and family presenting to clinic	Clinic users and greater clinic "population"	Organizations, agencies, and people who share problem or have common interest	Population (characteristics)	Census data	Worldwide demographics, etc.
2. Assessment	History and physical lab/and imaging	Information systems from billing data to chart audits to computer information	Organizational data	History and cultural background of community, analysis of environment from problems to resources, demograpics, etc.	Epidemiologic studies	Epidemiologic studies
3. Intervention	Care plan	Clinicwide initiatives (CQI or TQM)	Collective strategies	Community health campaign	Policies, guidelines, resources	Resources, collective strategies, and campaigns
4. Monitor outcomes and process	Follow-up visits	Chart audits, etc.	Ongoing meetings and organizational data	Ongoing community STATS	Reporting/monitoring of census data and epidemiology	Epidemiology
5. Outreach	Consultants, community resources, other patients with similar problems	Other ethical practices, integrated health systems, insurers, ancillary providers, etc.	Sharing with networks and others who share problem	Guided by strategic planning with community and its leaders	Legislative, executive, judicial elected and appointed officials	World organizations and networks (e.g., UN)

bio-generic | environmental | lifestyle behavior | medical care

Ask yourself:

1) What opportunities are there for improvement in this arena?

2) What evidence is there to support the efficacy of this intervention?

3) How practical is it for you to engage in this intervention?

4) How interested and committed are you to working on this?

Fig. 10-1. Arenas of involvement in community medicine. (Courtesy Christopher Reif, MD, MPH.)

society. By basing the use of technology, pharmaceuticals, and treatments or interventions on their proven effectiveness in and across populations of people, physicians should be better able to control costs while maintaining or improving quality.[9]

In fact, randomized clinical control trials, the gold standard for evaluating technology and pharmacology, are population studies. Although the study population is usually adult men, physicians can apply their knowledge of their practice population's characteristics in deciding which tests or treatments are most useful in individual patients. For instance, the use of screening tests such as mammograms and cholesterol is based on the incidence of these cancers in the age and ethnic group of the particular patient. Another example is deciding when and whether to screen for diabetes. The increased prevalence of type 2 diabetes in African-Americans, Native Americans, and Mexican-Americans argues for screening patients in those populations.

By learning community characteristics, physicians can develop outcomes-oriented medical practices to enhance health and health care in both the short and long run. Although managed care organizations and insurers sometimes focus on short-term profits, ultimately it is cheaper to prevent disease and promote health, both of which are most successfully accomplished in a context of community health. However, viewing patients as members of a population has not always been the priority of physician or insurer. People currently shift in and out of different health maintenance organizations and physicians' practices, giving an apparent disincentive to consider prevention and population needs. Yet the changing groups continue to be drawn from the same geographic areas and community subsets in those areas, and overall population characteristics do not change as rapidly as the individual names do. By applying their understanding of the demographics and other characteristics of the populations they serve, physicians can improve the health of those communities. By documenting the outcomes of their efforts, they may also lead payers to realize the lower long-term costs and, perhaps, greater profits as patients benefit from prevention, care of chronic conditions, rehabilitation, and health maintenance.

Filling Gaps in the Safety Net

Finally, as the existing social support network for the poor and uninsured is revised, we look increasingly to public-private alliances to coordinate systems to provide health and social services more efficiently and effectively. Because prevention, diagnosis, and management of illness and health are enhanced by the functional interconnectedness of strong communities, physicians can work with others to coordinate services and resources and to build stronger and healthier communities for the benefit of all.

SUMMARY

This chapter gives a brief overview of community health. It does not intend to provide a template for action or a theoretic framework. Instead, it points to ways a "new" imperative in medicine helps realize and lead us to the oldest and best desires of our profession: giving each and all of our patients the best health care possible. Hopefully, these ideas will be useful to physicians in improving health delivery systems and the health of communities.

REFERENCES

1. Garr D, Rhyne R: Primary care and the community, *J Fam Pract* 46:291-292, 1998.
2. Greenlick MR: Educating physicians for population-based clinical practice, *JAMA* 267:1645-1648, 1992.
3. Institute of Medicine, Committee on the Future of Primary Care: *Primary care: America's health in a new era,* Washington, DC, 1996, National Academy.
4. Kark SL: *The practice of community oriented primary care,* Hemel Hempstead, England, 1984, Prentice Hall.
5. Nutting PA, Nagle J, Dudley T: Epidemiology and practice management: an example of community-oriented primary care, *Fam Med* 23:218-226, 1991.
6. Nutting PA, et al: *Community oriented primary care: from principle to practice,* Albuquerque, 1990, University of New Mexico.
7. Pathman D, et al: The four community dimensions of primary care practice, *J Fam Pract* 46(4):293, 1998.

7a. Pickles WN: *Epidemiology in country practice,* Bristol, UK, 1949 (reissue), John Wright & Sons.

8. Reif C: Personal communication, May 1998.
9. Rivo ML: It's time to start practicing population-based health care, *Fam Pract Man* June 1998.
10. Taplin S, et al: Putting population-based care into practice: real option or rhetoric? *J Am Board Fam Pract* 11:116-126, 1998.
11. White RL, Connelly JE: *The medical schools' mission and the population's health,* New York, 1992, Springer-Verlag.

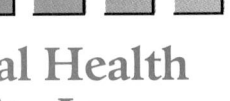

CHAPTER 11

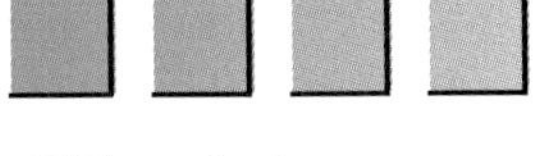

Occupational Health and Disability Issues in Primary Care

John W. Burress
David C. Christiani

What is your occupation?

The above question should be routinely incorporated into the primary care data base (see Chapter 4). Box 11-1 provides a sample occupational history and evaluation form. When an occupational history suggests a potential hazard, further questions should detail the extent and character of exposure. When a correlation between past or current exposures and an adverse health effect is suspected, additional measures or appropriate referrals can confirm or rule out that initial clinical impression. Table 11-1 lists occupations, pertinent toxicants, and possible diseases or adverse effects; Table 11-2 matches presenting conditions with toxicants and potential exposures.

Disability issues inevitably arise in primary care patients and are discussed later in this chapter. The primary care physician has several potential roles in occupational health and disability determination. The initial patient history, recorded accurately with sufficient detail including key direct quotes by the patient, gets heavy consideration during any future record review. Other potential roles of the primary care physician include: (1) advocating for appropriate resources for injured or ill workers, (2) performing preplacement evaluations that establish baseline data and distinguish whether accommodations are necessary, (3) providi

Box 11-1. Occupational Health History and Evaluation

Worker's name ______________________________

Social Security # __________ Age _____ Principal occupation (for most of working life) ______________________

Agenda: major concerns of worker and who need copy (e.g., lawyer)

Occupational history in chronologic order*

(This section includes the following factors: years, job title, employer, job description, notable hazards, exposure severity,† protective equipment, and injuries or lost time.)

Specific questions related to possible exposures

(The above open-ended questioning is preferable, but memory may be stimulated further with direct questions.)

During any of the above jobs, have you missed work or lost time because of a work-related injury or illness?

Have you ever changed jobs or transferred to another work area because of health problems or symptoms you relate to work?

Have you or any of your co-workers ever experienced health problems that you or someone else related to work?

Have you ever noticed a pattern in which a symptom (e.g., cough, headache, rash) would go away over a weekend or holiday, only to return on resumption of any of the above jobs?

While at work, have you ever experienced shortness of breath or trouble breathing that was not from exertion?

At work or later that night, have you ever experienced cough, wheezing, or trouble breathing that you related to dust or fumes?

Have you ever developed a rash, burn, or severe itching from a substance you came in contact with at work?

During any of the above jobs, did you ever notice consistently becoming nauseated when exposed to certain substances or fumes?

Did co-workers, your family, or you ever notice a consistent alteration in thinking, speech, or ability to focus on a task during or after work at any of the above jobs?

At work or while enjoying a hobby, have you been exposed to any of the following chemicals or substances?
Check box if yes:

- ▫ Acids
- ▫ Alcohols (industrial)
- ▫ Alkalis
- ▫ Ammonia
- ▫ Arsenic
- ▫ Asbestos
- ▫ Benzene
- ▫ Beryllium
- ▫ Cadmium
- ▫ Carbon tetrachloride
- ▫ Chlorinated naphthalenes
- ▫ Chloroform
- ▫ Chloroprene
- ▫ Chromates
- ▫ Coal dust
- ▫ Cold (severe)
- ▫ Dichlorobenzene
- ▫ Ethylene dibromide
- ▫ Ethylene dichloride
- ▫ Fiberglass
- ▫ Halothane
- ▫ Heat (severe)
- ▫ Isocyanates
- ▫ Ketones
- ▫ Lead
- ▫ Manganese
- ▫ Mercury
- ▫ Methylene chloride
- ▫ Nickel
- ▫ Noise (loud)
- ▫ PBBs
- ▫ PCBs
- ▫ Perchloroethylene
- ▫ Pesticides
- ▫ Phenol
- ▫ Phosgene
- ▫ Radiation
- ▫ Rock dust
- ▫ Silica powder
- ▫ Solvents
- ▫ Styrene
- ▫ Talc
- ▫ Toluene
- ▫ TDI or MDI
- ▫ Trichloroethylene
- ▫ Trinitrotoluene
- ▫ Vibration
- ▫ Vinyl chloride
- ▫ Welding fumes
- ▫ X-rays

Environmental exposure

Where do you live? ______________ For how long? ______________ ▫ House ▫ Apartment ▫ Other (specify) ______________ How many people live with you? ______________ Do you have any of the following? ▫ Pets (specify) ______________ ▫ Humidifier ▫ Air conditioner

What type of heat? ______________ Type of stove? ______________

What hobbies do you enjoy?

Have you ever noticed any associated health problems or symptoms?

Have you ever moved because of a health concern, bad smell, or hazard?

Have people in your neighborhood had complaints about health problems related to pollution?

Do you live next to a factory?

Do you have a garden? Do you use pesticides on your garden or lawn? What household chemicals do you use?

History of present illness

(Write *he reports pain* instead of *he has pain.* Document key points in patient's own words.)

Past medical history

(Ask about allergies, organ pathology, hospital stays, etc. Consider if any disease is associated with organ system toxicity from any of the above exposures.)

Medications

Smoking and substance abuse history

Family history

Social history

Review of systems

(This especially includes respiratory, skin, musculoskeletal, and nervous systems.)

Physical examination

Diagnostic testing

(Include laboratory tests, imaging studies, physiologic testing, and pulmonary function tests.)

Assessment

(Inform worker of your opinion about the severity of exposures and whether a relationship may exist among symptoms, health problem[s], and work.)

Plan

(Discuss with worker your level of certainty, the need for further testing to confirm diagnoses, or your inclination to refer for consultation.)

*Appropriate space would be provided on actual form.

†Estimate time (hours per day, days per week) and include markers of exposure severity (e.g., "dust so thick we couldn't see 10 feet" or "noise so loud we had to shout into each other's ears to communicate").

Table 11-1. Representative Job Categories, Toxicants, and Possible Diseases to Consider When Taking an Occupational History

Job category	Toxicants	Possible diseases
Agricultural worker	Pesticides, pathogens, gases, sunlight	Pesticide poisoning, farmer's lung, skin cancer
Anesthetist	Anesthetic gases, infectious agents	Reproductive effects, cancer, HIV, TB
Animal handler	Infectious agents, allergens	Asthma
Automobile worker	Asbestos, plastics, lead, solvents	Asbestosis, dermatitis
Baker	Flour	Asthma
Battery maker	Lead, arsenic	Lead poisoning, cancer
Butcher	Vinyl plastic fumes	"Meat wrapper's asthma"
Caisson worker	Pressurized work environments	Caisson disease
Carpenter	Wood dust, wood preservatives, adhesives	Nasopharyngeal cancer, dermatitis
Cement worker	Cement dust, metals	Dermatitis, bronchitis
Ceramic worker	Talc, clays	Pneumoconiosis
Demolition worker	Asbestos, wood dust	Asbestosis
Drug manufacturer	Hormones, nitroglycerin, etc.	Reproductive effects
Dry cleaner	Solvents	Liver disease, dermatitis
Dye worker	Dyestuffs, metals, solvents	Bladder cancer, dermatitis
Embalmer	Formaldehyde, pathogens	Dermatitis
Felt maker	Mercury, polycyclic hydrocarbons	Mercurialism
Foundry worker	Silica, molten metals	Silicosis
Glass worker	Heat, solvents, metal powders	Cataracts
Hospital worker	Infectious agents, cleansers, lifting	TB, HIV, hepatitis, back pain
Insulator	Asbestos, fibrous glass	Asbestosis, lung cancer, mesothelioma
Jackhammer operator	Vibration	Raynaud's phenomenon
Lathe operator	Metal dust, cutting oils	Lung disease, cancers, dermatitis
Laundry worker	Bleaches, soaps, alkalis	Dermatitis
Lead burner	Lead	Lead poisoning
Miner (coal, hard rock, metals, etc.)	Talc, radiation, metals, coal dust, silica	Pneumoconiosis, lung cancer
Natural gas worker	Polycyclic hydrocarbons	Lung cancer
Nuclear worker	Radiation, plutonium	Metal poisoning, cancer
Office worker	Poor lighting, poorly designed equipment	Eye problems, cumulative trauma
Painter	Solvents, isocyanates, lead	Neurologic problems, asthma, lead poisoning
Paper maker	Acids, alkalis, solvents, metals	Lung disease, dermatitis
Petroleum worker	Polycyclic hydrocarbons, catalysts, zeolites	Cancer, pneumoconiosis
Plumber	Lead, solvents, asbestos	Lead poisoning
Railroad worker	Creosote, sunlight, oils, solvents, asbestos	Cancer, dermatitis
Seaman	Sunlight, asbestos	Cancer, accidents
Smelter worker	Metals, heat, sulfur dioxide, arsenic, lead, carbon monoxide	Cancer, lead and carbon monoxide poisoning
Steelworker	Heat, metals, silica	Cataracts, heatstroke
Stone cutter	Silica	Silicosis
Textile worker	Cotton dust, finishers, dyes, carbon disulfide	Byssinosis, dermatitis, psychosis
Varnish maker	Solvents, waxes	Dermatitis
Vineyard worker	Arsenic, pesticides	Cancer, dermatitis
Welder	Fumes, nonionizing radiation	Lead poisoning, cataracts, metal fume fever

Modified from Rom WN, editor: *Environmental and occupational medicine*, ed 3, Philadelphia, 1998, Lippincott-Raven.
HIV, Human immunodeficiency virus; *TB*, tuberculosis.

consultation to companies and assisting in the education of employees and employers, (4) performing return-to-work or fitness-for-duty evaluations, (5) providing acute injury management, (6) performing impairment evaluations, and (7) assisting with surveillance programs. Primary care physicians should be familiar with the major workplaces in their communities, as well as agencies and experts involved in occupational health and safety (Box 11-2).

Occupational exposures can affect any organ system. The most common occupational problems include those of the skin, respiratory tract, and musculoskeletal system. Although primary care physicians focus on individual patients, recognizing a sentinel health problem in one worker in company or an industry can help protect others. I occupational medicine, medical surveillance programs a implemented to pick up adversely affected individua (screening) or assess groups to look for significant tren (surveillance) using either biomarkers of exposure (e.g blood lead level) or biomarkers of effect (e.g., pulmona function tests). See Box 11-2 for information on k regulations protecting workers such as the Right to Kno Laws that ensure an employee's physician access information on potential hazards (e.g., Material Safety Da Sheets [MSDSs]).

Table 11-2. Examples of Occupational Health Conditions

Condition	Agent	Potential exposures
Intermediate or short-term effects		
Dermatoses (allergic or irritant)	Metals (chromium, nickel), fibrous glass, epoxy resins, cutting oils, solvents, caustic alkali, soaps	Electroplating, metal cleaning, plastics, machining, leather tanning, housekeeping
Headache	Carbon monoxide, solvents	Firefighting, automobile exhaust, foundry, wood finishing, dry cleaning
Acute psychoses	Lead, mercury, carbon disulfide	Handling gasoline, seed handling, fungicide, wood preserving, viscose rayon industry
Asthma or dry cough	Formaldehyde, toluene diisocyanate, animal dander	Textiles, plastics, polyurethane kits, lacquer use, animal handler
Pulmonary edema, pneumonitis	Nitrogen oxides, phosgene, halogen gases, cadmium	Welding, farming ("silo filler's disease"), chemical operations, smelting
Cardiac dysrhythmias	Solvents, fluorocarbons	Metal cleaning, solvent use, refrigerator maintenance
Angina	Carbon monoxide	Car repair, traffic exhaust, foundry, wood finishing
Abdominal pain	Lead	Battery making, enameling, smelting, painting, welding, ceramics, plumbing
Hepatitis (may become a long-term effect)	Halogenated hydrocarbons (e.g., carbon tetrachloride), viral hepatitis	Solvent use, lacquer use, hospital workers
Latent or long-term effects		
Chronic dyspnea		
Pulmonary fibrosis	Asbestos, silica, beryllium, coal, aluminum	Mining, insulation, pipefitting, sandblasting, quarrying, metal alloy work, aircraft or electrical parts
Chronic bronchitis emphysema	Cotton dust, cadmium coal dust, organic solvents, cigarettes	Textile industry, battery production, soldering, mining, solvent use
Lung cancer	Asbestos, arsenic, uranium, coke oven emissions	Insulation, pipefitting, smelting, coke ovens, shipyard workers, nickel refining, uranium mining
Bladder cancer	β-Naphthylamine, benzidine dyes	Dye industry, leather, rubber-working chemists
Peripheral neuropathy	Lead, arsenic, *n*-hexane, methyl n-butyl ketone, acrylamide	Battery production, plumbing, smelting, painting, shoemaking, solvent use, insecticides
Behavioral changes	Lead, carbon disulfide, solvents, mercury, manganese	Battery makers, smelting, viscose rayon industry, degreasing, manufacturing/repair of scientific instruments, dental amalgam workers
Extrapyramidal syndrome	Carbon disulfide, manganese	Viscose rayon industry, steel production, battery production foundry
Aplastic anemia, leukemia	Benzene, ionizing radiation	Chemists, furniture refinishing, cleaning, degreasing, radiation workers

rom Goldman RH, Peters JM: The occupational and environmental health history, *JAMA* 246:2831, 1981.

MEDICAL PRESENTATIONS OF OCCUPATIONAL DISEASE

Respiratory Disease

ewer than 5% of occupational respiratory disease cases are rrectly identified as being associated with work. When sessed at a one-time clinical visit, symptoms are often distinguishable from those caused by the myriad of noccupational etiologies. Primary care physicians should utinely ask about occupational and environmental expo- res whenever a patient has respiratory symptoms. Further- re, most work-related respiratory diseases are not curable d must be discovered early in their course to avoid future ability. Airborne pollutants at work can interact, additively synergistically, with smoking to produce disease (e.g., nchitis).[4]

The clinical evaluation for an occupational respiratory disease entails at least four elements: (1) complete history, including occupational and environmental exposures; cigarette-smoking history; and a careful review of respiratory symptoms focusing on cough, sputum production, dyspnea, wheezing, chest discomfort, and allergic responses to work or nonwork environments. Attention to a temporal relation to occupational exposure is very important (e.g., symptoms are worse at the end of a workday, better when on vacation); (2) physical examination, with special attention to breath sounds, although patients with significant disease may have normal examinations; (3) chest x-ray (CXR), with attention to parenchymal and pleural disease. For example, linear irregular opacities in the lower fields may suggest asbestosis, whereas rounded opacities in upper fields may suggest

Box 11-2. Key Occupational Health Agencies, Standards, and Legal References

Agencies and Organizations

Occupational Safety and Health (OSHA)

The Occupational Safety and Health Act (OSHAct) provides some general protection under specific standards and its "general duty clause" of Section 5(a)(1): "Each employer shall furnish to each of his employees employment and a place of employment which are free from recognized hazards that are causing or are likely to cause death or serious physical harm to his employee." Enforcement stems from inspections, citations, and fines that can be initiated by a complaint from a worker or a health care provider. The limitations of OSHA are significant and vary, depending on resources allowed for enforcement and resistance to setting new standards. For example, only about 25 hazardous substances and five hazardous situations have specific standards. Also, large segments of workers are not covered by OSHA including federal government employees, self-employed persons, workers on family farms, and workers at workplaces covered by other agencies or federal statutes, such as mining, fishing, railroad, and nuclear industries. Office of Information and Public Affairs: 202-523-8151; OSHA Home Page: http://www.osha.gov or OSHA Technical Center: http://www.osha-slc.gov/SLTC/.

National Institute for Occupational Safety and Health (NIOSH)

Research and education agency that investigates workplace illness and injuries to determine nature and extent of hazards; does not have enforcement powers. For information and free literature searches: 800-35N-IOSH or http://www.cdc.gov/niosh/homepage.html.

Environmental Protection Agency (EPA)

Agency responsible for the assessment and control of environmental problems, including pesticides, noise, toxic substances, radiation, and air, water, and solid waste pollution. 202-260-2090 or http://www.epa.gov.

Centers for Disease Control and Prevention (CDC)

This agency provides information, does research, and investigates outbreaks of infectious disease; it has broadened its scope to address prevention of noninfectious disease issues as well. Call 888-329-4232 or visit CDC Home Page: http://www.cdc.gov.

Department of Transportation (DOT)

This department has oversight responsibilities for the nation's highways and other modes of transportation. Questions about a DOT examination can be directed to this administration at 800-526-1144 or visit DOT Home Page: http//www.dot.gov.

Agency for Toxic Substances Registry (ATSDR)

This agency produces excellent booklets on various toxins and does investigative work regarding environmental concerns. Visit http://atsdr1.atsdr.cdc.gov:8080/atsdrhome.html.

American Conference of Governmental Industrial Hygienists (ACGIH)

This organization publishes threshold limit values (TLVs) for chemical substances and physical agents as well as biologic exposure indices (BEIs). Updated periodically, this reference contains a broader scope of chemicals and is much more current than most of the OSHA standards. Try http://www.aiha.org/.

Selected Standards and Legal References

Americans with Disabilities Act (ADAct)

Important legislation whose goal is to help those with disabilities mainstream into the U.S. workforce. The implications and practical implementations for occupational health are discussed in latter part of this chapter, or see ADA Document Center http://janweb.icdi.wvu.edu/kinder/.

Family Medical Leave Act (FMLA)

Important legislation allowing up to 12 weeks unpaid leave for those with personal or family needs. A worker must invoke this to obtain job security benefit. Try http://www.osha.gov.oshpubs/employee.html or www.law.cornell.edu.

Right to Know Law

Hazard Communication Standard (HAZCOM, 29 CFR 1910.1200[a]; final rule 59 FR 6126) stipulates the employer inform workers of potential exposures. Material Safety Data Sheets (MSDSs) must be available. Primary care providers should request pertinent MSDSs to facilitate the evaluation of workers with chemical or other exposures. Toxicologists can usually be accessed via listed emergency numbers on the MSDSs. The MSDS contains first aid information, the properties of the chemical(s) (e.g. pH), and the Chemical Abstract Number (CAS), which can facilitate further research. Many MSDSs are now available online; try http://research.nwfsc.noaa.gov/msds.html.

Another standard (29 CFR 1910.20) provides the right to access exposure information previously compiled by the employer, including biologic monitoring. Medical Records Generated by Employer (e.g., as part of surveillance program) HAZCOM 29 CFR 1910.20(e)(2) provides an employee unrestricted access to his or her medical records as well as, upon written consent, access to an analysis of a co-worker's medical records. The employer is obligated to retain records of any "adverse reactions to health" based on HAZCOM 29 CFR 1910.1200[d][1]; for companies dealing with chemicals, access is stipulated under the Toxic Substance Control Act (section 8[c]); visit http://www.hammock.ifas.ufl.edu/txt/fairs/26242.

Hearing Conservation

OSHA standard CFG 1910.95 provides an "action" level of 85 db, above which an employer is required to provide baseline audiograms, workplace monitoring, employee notification, audiometric testing, and hearing protection.

silicosis. A NIOSH-certified "B reader" can provide a semiquantitative interpretation of the CXR through comparison with a standardized set of films that focuses on size, shape, concentration, and distribution of parenchymal opacities and pleural thickening or calcification; and (4) pulmonary function tests (PFTs), which help distinguish among variou respiratory diseases. Comparing spirometry done before an after work shifts can also be informative (e.g., occupation asthma). Table 11-3 provides a brief summary of work-relat respiratory disease.[4,5]

Table 11-3. Major Types of Occupational Respiratory Disease

Pathologic process	Occupational disease examples	Clinical history	Physical examination	Chest x-ray	Pulmonary function pattern*
Fibrosis	Silicosis	Dyspnea on exertion, shortness of breath	Clubbing, cyanosis	Nodules	Restrictive or mixed obstructive and restrictive
	Asbestosis	Dyspnea on exertion, shortness of breath	Clubbing, cyanosis, rales	Linear densities, pleural plaques, calcifications	Normal or ↓ DLCO†
Reversible airways obstruction (mucus plugging, asthma)	Byssinosis, isocyanate poisoning, asthma	Cough, chest tightness, shortness of breath, asthma attacks	↑ Respiratory rate Wheeze	Usually normal	Normal or obstructive with bronchodilator improvement Normal or high DLCO
Emphysema	Cadmium poisoning (chronic)	Cough, sputum, dyspnea	↑ Respiratory rate ↑ Expiratory phase	Hyperaeration bullae	Obstructive Low DLCO
Granulomata	Beryllium disease	Cough, weight loss, shortness of breath	↑ Respiratory rate	Small nodules	Usually restrictive with low DLCO
Pulmonary edema	Smoke inhalation	Frothy, bloody sputum production	Coarse bubbly rales	Hazy, diffuse; air space disease	Usually restrictive with ↓ DLCO Hypoxemia at rest

↑, Increased; ↓, decreased.
*Restrictive PFTs: ↓ FEV_1, ↓ FVC, FEV_1/FVC may be normal. Obstructive PFTs: ↓ FEV_1, ↓ FEV_1/FVC, FVC may be normal.
† Diffusion capacity (level) for carbon monoxide.

Acute Irritant Responses. Workplace exposures usually elicit specific regional inflammatory effects that depend on characteristics of the irritant, including the concentration of the agent in respired air, its solubility, the duration of exposure, the presence of a carrier aerosol, and the level of physical activity and physical fitness of the worker. These combine to determine the regional site, severity, and timing of irritant response. In general, highly water-soluble agents irritate the upper respiratory tract. They tend to act quickly, causing burning of the eyes, nasal congestion, frontal headache, and runny nose. A dry cough may be seen with throat involvement or, with severe exposure, epiglottic edema; very high exposures can produce bronchospasm and pulmonary edema. Ammonia, hydrogen chloride, and hydrogen fluoride are examples of water-soluble irritants. Odor and immediate symptoms often alert the worker and limit duration of exposure unless the worker inadvertently becomes trapped (e.g., in a confined space). Moderately water-soluble irritants affect the midrespiratory tract to cause bronchoconstriction. Insoluble agents can induce delayed (6 to 24 hours) pulmonary edema via direct toxicity to capillary walls. Bronchospasm may precede effects at the alveolar level. Ozone, phosgene, and oxides of nitrogen are common examples. Persisting sequelae are possible from either single high-dose exposure or episodic low-dose exposures causing irritant asthma (reactive airways dysfunction syndrome).[4]

Occupational Asthma. Asthma is a common clinical entity in the general population. An estimated 2% to 15% of cases are thought to be caused or aggravated by work exposures, but this may grossly underestimate the true prevalence because of both underdiagnosis and employees leaving work settings with exposures that they associate with adverse health effects. A variety of materials have proved to be asthmogenic (Table 11-4). These differ greatly as to period of sensitization required, latency, pattern of asthmatic response, duration of symptoms, and progression. All these factors may differ among individuals, adding to the complexity of the diagnosis.

Three general patterns of asthmatic response to challenge tests are immediate (onset within minutes, maximal symptoms at 20 minutes, recovery in 1 to 2 hours), late (onset in several hours, peak at 4 to 8 hours, recovery in 24 hours), and dual (a combination of immediate and late). In the workplace these patterns may manifest as (1) maximal deterioration on first working day, (2) daily similar deterioration with overnight recovery, or (3) progressive deterioration throughout the workweek. The intensity as well as duration of exposure may be important for sensitization.

Atopy is a risk factor for occupational asthma from exposure to high-molecular-weight exposures, but not from exposure to low molecular weight (see Table 11-4). For example, isocyanate-induced asthma is as common among nonatopic as atopic workers (5% to 15% of all workers significantly exposed will be sensitized). Major or minor constituents and accidental by-products of substances may be inciting agents. Thus an appropriate clinical suspicion and subsequent history (temporal association with workplace exposure) are crucial in making the diagnosis. The physician should document intermittent respiratory symptoms (cough, chest tightness, dyspnea, wheezing, decreased exercise tolerance) and, if possible, physiologic evidence of reversible or variable airways obstruction (i.e., a peak expiratory flow rate diary pattern showing a consistent 20% drop or cross-shift PFTs with 10% variability in forced expiratory volume in 1 second [FEV_1] temporally related to work). The necessity of these and other measures, including bronchoprovocation with methacholine or dilute aerosols of workplace substances, depends on the strength of the history, whether others have been affected, and knowledge of exposure levels at the workplace. Objective evidence is desired because history alone may not be reliable. It is important to

Table 11-4. Selected Causes of Occupational Asthma*

Agents	Workers at risk
High-molecular-weight compounds	
Animal products: dander, excreta, serum, secretions	Animal handlers, laboratory workers, veterinarians
Plants: grain, dust, flour, tobacco, tea, hops, latex	Grain handlers, tea workers, bakers and workers in natural oil manufacturing and tobacco and food processing, health care workers
Enzymes: *Bacillus subtilis,* pancreatic extracts, papain, trypsin, fungal amylase	Bakers and workers in detergent, pharmaceutical, and plastic industries
Vegetable: gum acacia, gum tragacanth	Printers, gum-manufacturing workers
Other: crab, prawn	Crab and prawn processors
Low-molecular-weight compounds	
Diisocyanates: toluene diisocyanate (TDI), methylene diphenyldiisocyanate (MDI)	Polyurethane industry workers, plastics workers, workers using varnish, foundry workers
Anhydrides: phthalic and trimellitic anhydrides	Epoxy resin and plastics workers
Wood dust: oak, mahogany, California redwood, Western red cedar	Carpenters, sawmill workers, furniture makers
Metals: platinum, nickel, chromium, cobalt, vanadium, tungsten carbide	Platinum- and nickel-refining workers, hard metal workers
Soldering fluxes	Solderers
Drugs: penicillin, methyldopa, tetracyclines, cephalosporins, psyllium	Pharmaceutical and health care workers
Other organic chemicals: urea formaldehyde, dyes, formalin, azodicarbonamide, hexachlorophene, ethylene diamine, dimethyl ethanolamine, polyvinyl chloride pyrolysates	Workers in chemical, plastic, and rubber industries; hospitals; laboratories; foam insulation manufacture; food wrapping; and spray painting

Modified from Chan-Yeung M, Lam S: Occupational asthma, *Am Rev Respir Dis* 133:686, 1986.

*Mechanism believed to be immunoglobulin E (IgE), mediated for high-molecular-weight compounds and for some low-molecular-weight compounds. The immunologic mechanism for asthma from many low-molecular-weight substances remains undefined.

realize, however, that no definitive diagnostic criteria exist. Eosinophil elevation in sputum or blood may help distinguish allergic asthma from nonallergic asthma and bronchitis; skin testing or other immunologic tests for allergens indicate sensitization but may not correlate well with the actual airways exposure and may not even be available for many workplace agents.

Acute care of workers with occupational asthma exacerbations does not differ from that of nonoccupational attacks (see Chapter 72). However, further management is required, including cessation of workplace exposure, assessment of risk to other workers, and follow-up to document resolution or lack thereof. Once an individual is sensitized to an agent, even low levels of that agent can trigger an attack. If return to a suspected exposure is anticipated, personal protective devices such as a respirator, along with close monitoring of symptoms and lung function, are certainly warranted but may not prevent exacerbations. Continued exposure may indeed result in generalized airway hyperresponsiveness (i.e., workers become sensitive to exposures outside the workplace to which they had not previously been sensitive) that fails to resolve on cessation of exposure.[4]

Byssinosis and Other Illnesses Related to Vegetable Dust. Unlike occupational asthma, byssinosis (Greek for "white thread") may produce bronchoconstriction without prior exposure. The mechanism is thought to occur through direct toxicity and to involve endotoxin from gram-negative bacterial contaminants of cotton dust that produce acute symptoms and a decrease in lung function. Workers involved in the initial processing of (in decreasing order of potency) soft hemp, flax, cotton, jute, and sisal are at greatest risk. With cotton, higher "trash" or impurity content material generates more inhalable dust. Ginning and the early stages of yarn preparation, which involve breaking open bales of cotton to separate impurities and then "carding" (aligning fibers into parallel threads), historically have been associated with the greatest prevalence of byssinosis. Engineering controls to reduce dust exposure, such as enclosed and automated carding machines, have greatly improved textile mill conditions in the United States. Processing of cloth, or finishing, is practically free of dust, especially after the cloth has been washed. The diagnosis of byssinosis is based mainly on symptoms of shortness of breath and chest tightness, with or without cough and sputum production. The pattern of symptoms is characteristic, being more pronounced on the first day of the workweek or after a vacation ("Monday morning tightness"). A decrease in FEV_1 may be seen with these symptoms. Further investigation is warranted if the FEV_1 decreases 3% or 75 ml in a group of 20 or more workers. A decrease of 10% or 200 ml or more may be significant for an individual. OSHA standards mandate medical surveillance of preshift and postshift lung function. CXR and skin tests have no characteristic findings. Mild cases probably are reversible, but prolonged exposure to high dust levels may lead to irreversible disease. The advanced stage is characterized by fixed airways obstruction with hyperinflation and air trapping; chronic bronchitis increases the severity. Cigarette smokers also exposed to cotton dust are at particular risk of irreversible airways obstruction.

Also associated with the cotton industry are two conditions known as mill fever and weaver's cough. Mill fever is self-limited, occurs on first exposure to cotton dust environment, and lasts 2 to 3 days. It is a flulike illness, and symptoms include headache, malaise, and fever similar to metal and polymer fume fever. Weaver's cough occurs in

Table 11-5. Examples of Hypersensitivity Pneumonitis

Disease	Antigenic material	Antigen
Farmer's lung	Moldy hay or grain	Thermophilic actinomycetes
Bagassosis	Moldy sugar cane	
Mushroom worker's lung	Mushroom compost	
Humidifier fever	Dust from contaminated air conditioners or furnaces	
Maple bark disease	Moldy maple bark	*Cryptostroma* species
Sequoiosis	Redwood dust	*Graphium* species, Pullularia
Bird-breeder's lung	Avian droppings or feathers	Avian proteins
Pituitary snuff user's lung	Pituitary powder	Bovine or porcine proteins
Suberosis	Moldy cork dust	*Penicillium* species
Paprika splitter's lung	Paprika dust	*Mucor stolonifer*
Malt worker's lung	Malt dust	*Aspergillus clavatus* or *A. fumigatus*
Fish meal worker's lung	Fish meal	Fish meal dust
Miller's lung	Infested wheat flour	*Sitophilus granarius* (wheat weevil)
Furrier's lung	Animal pelts	Animal fur dust
Coffee worker's lung	Coffee beans	Coffee bean dust
Chemical worker's lung	Urethane foam and finish	Isocyanates (TDI, HDI), anhydrides

outbreaks of acute respiratory illness characterized by a dry cough. It may be associated with mildewed yarn.[4]

Hypersensitivity Pneumonitis. Also known as extrinsic allergic alveolitis, hypersensitivity pneumonitis (HP) is characterized by an interstitial and infiltrative process after exposure to certain organic dusts and chemicals in predisposed individuals. As opposed to bronchoconstriction in asthma with immunoglobulin E (IgE)-mediated (type I) immediate reactions, HP appears to be caused by inadequate control or regulation of cellular (type IV) immune function. Although most individuals exposed to inhaled antigen develop an immune response, only a small percentage develop clinical disease. In one study, for example, only the 10% of pigeon breeders who developed HP had defective suppressor lymphocytes. HP occurs most often in workers exposed to fungi or bacteria found in thermophilic material; however, it is also seen with longstanding exposure to some animal antigens and inorganic haptens (Table 11-5). Atopy is not a risk factor. For unclear reasons, nonsmokers may be more susceptible than smokers.

Clinical features vary along a spectrum of acute, subacute, and chronic forms of HP. Acute disease symptoms occur 4 to 8 hours after exposure and include headache, fever, sweating, rigors, anorexia, nausea, vomiting, dry cough, chest tightness, and dyspnea on exertion. On physical examination, there may be fine basilar rales on inspiration without wheezing along with fever and tachycardia. Symptoms generally subside in 48 hours, but repetitive acute episodes may cloud the history. CXR may reveal patchy infiltrates or diffuse micronodular shadowing. PFTs often reveal a restrictive pattern, with FEV_1 reduced in proportion to forced vital capacity (FVC). In an acute attack of HP, there may be decreased diffusion capacity (DLCO) and lung compliance, as well as hypoxemia accentuated with exercise.

With very few exceptions, therapy for HP includes lifelong avoidance of the inciting agent. A trial of systemic corticosteroids while monitoring blood gases and PFTs may be indicated. Full or partial reversal of the lung disease may be possible. The chronic form may be preceded by bouts of acute symptoms or may arise insidiously from repeated low-level exposures, yielding persistent flulike symptoms. Progressive dyspnea associated with cough, malaise, lethargy, and weight loss may develop. Chronic HP may result in restrictive, obstructive, or mixed ventilatory defects with decreased diffusion capacity. CXR suggests interstitial fibrosis; continued exposure may yield a honeycomb appearance on the CXR in end-stage disease.

Prevention of HP includes workplace controls, such as exhaust ventilation or the elimination of conditions that foster bacterial or fungal growth, and early avoidance through medically mandated removal of workers who develop symptoms.[4,6]

Inhalation Fever. Certain inhalation exposures can result in acute self-limited flu-like illness. Symptoms begin within hours after an exposure. Welding galvanized steel can release zinc oxide, producing metallic taste at first, and then throat irritation followed by fever, chills, myalgia, malaise, and a nonproductive cough; occasionally headache, nausea, and vomiting occur. The pathogenesis differs from HP; instead of an allergic mechanism, leukocyte recruitment to the lungs with release of cytokines thought to cause the systemic symptoms has been postulated. In addition to zinc, copper and magnesium can produce "metal fume fever." Inhalation of combustion products of polytetrafluoroethylene (Teflon) can yield "polymer fume fever." Several bioaerosols can impart a similar clinical syndrome. Examples include contaminated humidifier mist ("humidifier fever") and inhalation of products from moldy silage, compost, or wood chips ("organic dust toxic syndrome"). Although the reason is unclear, repeated attacks of inhalation fevers may lead to long-term sequelae.[3,4,6]

Pneumoconiosis. Respirable inorganic dust is a causal agent in silicosis, asbestosis, and coal workers' pneumoconiosis. Although the epidemiology and pathology differ, the clinical features are similar, including nonproductive cough initially, followed by progressive shortness of breath with perhaps distant heart sounds, distant breath sounds, and if severe enough, signs and symptoms of right-sided heart failure. Dust less than 5 microns in aerodynamic diameter can reach terminal bronchioles and alveoli; when suspended in air, dust of this size is not visible and can lead to a potentially unrecognized hazard. Secondary prevention to avoid further loss of reserve lung function is of paramount concern, given the lack of cure. Workers should be removed from exposure on finding evidence of pneumoconiosis. However, progression may still continue even after removal from exposure.

Coal workers' pneumoconiosis (CWP) is caused by coal dust, principally carbon, and affects a defined group of workers in an industry. Simple CWP is distinguished from complicated CWP (also called progressive massive fibrous [PMF] and involving about 1% of cases) by the relative size and confluence of nodular opacities on CXR. The pathogenesis of PMF is controversial. Continued reduction in exercise tolerance may be seen. Unlike asbestosis or silicosis, simple CWP generally does not progress after the worker is removed from exposure, although PMF may progress. An upper lobe predominance is seen, similar to silicosis. Coal dust can also produce chronic bronchitis and centrolobular emphysema independent of smoking, but smokers have additional risk when working with coal because of a combined effect. The associated chronic bronchitis can contribute to disability and is dose related to coal dust exposure in both smokers and nonsmokers. Federal mandates provide CXR screening together with a protection program that allows a miner to work in a reduced-dust environment with increased monitoring.

In contrast, silica and asbestos are encountered in multiple industries (see Table 11-1) by a greater number of workers who produce a diverse range of products, making control and surveillance more difficult. Of the two basic types, silicosis exemplifies typically localized and nodular peribronchial fibrosis, in contrast to the diffuse interstitial fibrosis of asbestosis.

The amount of fibrosis in silicosis appears proportional to the free silica content and duration of exposure. For example, acute silicosis stems from an intense exposure that leads to onset of symptoms within weeks and death within a year. A chronic form of silicosis is more common; this form entails CXR findings 15 years after exposure and symptoms even later. Accelerated silicosis falls between these two extremes, with findings within 5 to 15 years. Typically, nodules on CXR show an upper lobe predominance. Silicosis imparts an increased risk of *Mycobacterium tuberculosis* and atypical mycobacteria infection.

Asbestos exposure leads to several distinct manifestations of lung disease. The most common are benign pleural plagues. Asbestosis refers to the diffuse interstitial pneumoconiosis. Lung cancer and mesothelioma are also associated with asbestos exposure.

Asbestosis results from lung inflammation and fibrosis caused by persisting activation of alveolar macrophages, creating patchy, linear, and irregular fibrosis with a lower lobe predominance. Important to the diagnosis are a history of exposure, somewhat dose related, with an appropriate latency period of about 15 years; a CXR suggesting interstitial fibrosis; PFTs with a restrictive pattern (although obstructive or mixed patterns can be seen); and decreased diffusion capacity, which may be the first sign of early disease. Occasionally, open-lung biopsy is needed for definitive diagnosis. Rales are present in only about 20% of those affected; clubbing is rare and seen in advanced cases only. There is a fivefold increased incidence of lung cancer associated with asbestos exposure alone, a tenfold to twentyfold increase in smokers, but a fiftyfold to ninetyfold increase with both exposures together. Two scientific controversies remaining are (1) whether lung cancer caused by asbestos occurs only in those with the interstitial fibrosis of asbestosis (currently a minority stance) and (2) whether asbestos-related pleural disease alone, without interstitial fibrosis of lung parenchyma, conveys any increased risk of lung cancer.

Pleural calcifications and plaques seen incidentally on CXR suggest asbestos-related disease. These pleural plaques are generally asymptomatic until extensive and severe, when pleuritic chest pain or tightness may be found. When plaques are present, it is appropriate to do follow-up CXR and PFTs every 3 years. If a decrement in PFTs is found and CXR findings suggest parenchymal disease, yearly follow-up is warranted. It is important that patients understand the difference between benign plaques and lung cancer or mesothelioma. Mesothelioma may occur in persons with only a distant, brief exposure to asbestos and no asbestos-related pleural disease or pulmonary fibrosis. A pleural effusion is often the presenting finding of mesothelioma. Some increased risk of gastrointestinal tract cancer secondary to asbestosis exposure has been noted, thus warranting screening.

Exposure to respirable synthetic vitreous fibers (SVFs) (e.g., fibrous glass, mineral wool, ceramic fiber) has been associated with irregular opacities consistent with pneumoconiosis in some studies but not in others. A twofold elevation in lung cancer risk was found in one large study of exposure to SVFs on 30-year follow-up. Current levels of exposure are much less, and studies are ongoing to ascertain a health effect, if any.[4-6]

Granulomatous Disease. Exposure to beryllium, talc, and some synthetic fibers can result in granuloma formation clinically similar to sarcoidosis. Beryllium is a metal with very desirable characteristics for many high-tech and space applications (e.g., lightweight, high tensile strength, high melting point, ability to stop neutrons). The pulmonary reaction in berylliosis is out of proportion to the amount of metal dust in the lungs. CXR may reveal an interstitial pattern of ground-glass appearance or more discrete, small, rounded opacities; hilar adenopathy is present in 30% to 40% of patients with chronic berylliosis. PFT findings relate to the distribution of granulomas and can be restrictive, obstructive, or normal with reduced diffusion capacity from interstitial involvement. The lymphocyte proliferative test (LPT) from blood and/or bronchoalveolar lavage fluid is both sensitive and specific for berylliosis. Before 1949, fluorescent light manufacturing was the origin of most cases. Machining of beryllium for various high-tech applications is increasing. Of interest, bystander cases or disease in individuals not directly involved in machining but sharing air space has been documented, warranting strict adherence to prevention (e.g., local exhaust).[4,5]

Industrial Bronchitis. Many work exposures can cause chronic bronchitis, including mineral dusts and fumes such as coal and metals, organic dusts such as cotton and grain, plastic compounds such as phenolics and isocyanates, acids and smoke inhalation. Although smoking is the most common cause of bronchitis, there may be a superimposed occupationally related component.[4]

Emphysema. Emphysema can be the late manifestation of such occupational exposures as coal dust in PMF cadmium, and isocyanates. However, emphysema does not appear to occur in workers chronically exposed to cotton dust more frequently than would be attributable to cigarette smoking. Whether this response occurs after other occupational exposures is unclear at present.[4]

Skin Disorders

Skin disorders account for 20% to 30% of all new cases of occupational illness. Of these cases, 90% are contact dermatitis. Four fifths of contact dermatitis cases are from acute or chronic exposure to an irritant, and one fifth are allergic cases caused by a specific sensitizer (Box 11-3). These dermatoses may be induced or aggravated by the work environment. It is very useful for the primary care physician to determine the occupational cause of the dermatitis both to facilitate management decisions (e.g., when the patient can return to work, whether it is necessary to perform a patch test) and to prevent further illness in that worker or similarly exposed co-workers. The pattern of eruption and type of lesion, together with a thorough occupational and medical history, are therefore crucial. Work-related illness is more plausible if a temporal relationship and an exposure capable of causing the dermatosis exist.

The ability of an irritant to cause dermatitis depends both on the agent, including its concentration and duration of exposure to the skin, and the skin itself, including the skin thickness, the presence of hair follicles, existing skin disruption, and underlying skin conditions. Of note, the area of a healed lesion is at greater risk of recurrence of dermatitis for at least 3 months. Also, some agents are particularly toxic in synergy with sun exposure, yielding a phototoxic dermatitis. Certain preexisting skin conditions predispose workers to develop other skin problems more easily. For example, patients with psoriasis may develop additional lesions at the site of mechanical trauma (Koebner's phenomenon), those with atopic dermatitis may experience a flare-up when exposed to an irritant, and those with vitiligo may develop depigmentation at the site of mechanical trauma.

In acute irritant contact dermatitis, there is typically a sharp demarcation of the affected skin areas at the site of the exposure. Then, erythema or vesiculation usually follows. The irritant should be irrigated immediately with water if the agent is water soluble or with mineral or olive oil if it is hydrophobic. Local therapy such as wet dressings may help remove remaining traces of the irritant and ease the discomfort.

In contrast, chronic irritant dermatitis stems from longer exposure to a mildly irritating chemical. Erythema, scaling, pruritus, fissuring, and lichenification of a less well delineated area are characteristic. Chronic irritant dermatitis is the most common occupational skin disease. Aggressive therapy includes high-dose topical or in some instances oral corticosteroids. The prognosis is guarded for some patients with chronic hand dermatitis; the condition may not abate even with a job change, reinforcing the need for early detection.

Chemical burns as a form of contact irritant dermatitis are distinct in that substantial skin necrosis and inflammation result from a one-time, usually brief exposure. Acids coagulate protein through oxidation, reduction, desiccation, or salt formation. Alkalis coagulate protein but also saponify fats and cause liquefaction necrosis. In all cases, copious irrigation with water is warranted initially. Most authorities consider pH neutralization after lavage to be unnecessary. Therapy is similar to burn care, with topical sulfadiazine, nonadherent surgical dressings, and cautious debridement as needed.

Some specific concerns relate to problematic agents. Hydrofluoric acid, used as a rust remover, an etching agent in the semiconductor industry, and a reagent in fluorination processes, produces intense pain and erythema. If the concentration is less than 20%, symptoms may be delayed by several hours. A worker can use a dilute solution without

Box 11-3. Contact Dermatitis: Four Types, Possible Causes, and Examples of Occupations at Risk

Irritant Contact Dermatitis

Acids, alkalis, solvents, surfactants, enzymes, oxidants, foods: custodian, construction, food service

Allergic Contact Dermatitis

Nickel* and other metals: electronics assemblers, hairdressers,† metal alloy workers, jewelry makers, silver workers
Potassium dichromate*: cement and leather work, cleaning with bleaches and household cleansers
Paraphenylenediamine* and related dyes: hairdressers,† rubber workers, furriers, film developers
Epoxy resins: electronics workers, construction, aircraft assembly, electrical utility workers, painters
Rubber accelerators (thiram, mercaptobenzothiazole): tire makers and repairmen, rubber products, fungicides
Acrylic monomers: dental technicians, printers, acrylic ink manufacturing
Formaldehyde: embalmers, insulation workers, woodworkers, resin manufacturers
Pharmaceuticals (penicillin, neomycin, glutaraldehyde, chlorpromazine): health care workers, veterinarians, pharmacists
Plants (Rhus, tulips, exotic woods, chrysanthemums): outdoor workers, florists
Latex via Type IV or cellular immune reaction (gloves, catheters, balloons, condoms): health care workers, rubber industry workers

Phototoxic Dermatitis

Psoralens, sulfonamides: pharmaceutical workers
Citrus, celery, parsnips: agricultural workers, grocery clerks
Creosote, tars: roofers, railway workers, construction workers
Wild carrot, Queen Anne's lace: forestry workers, cleanup workers, utility workers
Oil of bergamot: cosmetic industry workers

Contact Urticaria

Saliva, urine, danders: small animal handlers
Foods, especially shellfish: food handlers
Ammonium persulfate: hairdressers
Pharmaceuticals (penicillin, streptomycin, neomycin, others)
Sodium benzoate (nonimmunologic)
Latex via Type I or immediate hypersensitivity reaction involving IgE: health care workers, rubber industry workers

Modified from LaDou J, editor: *Occupational medicine*, East Norwalk, Conn, 1990, Appleton & Lange.
*Most common in United States.
†Most frequently abandoned job because of dermatitis.

gloves for a prolonged period and then seek medical attention for mild discomfort and redness, only to return later when symptoms peak. Fluoride's affinity for calcium can lead to extensive underlying bone destruction and, most important, life-threatening systemic toxicity from hypocalcemia. If the burn area is greater than 4 cm, admission for cardiac monitoring is indicated. Local calcium gluconate injections and even arterial infusion may be necessary for pain control and management. Calcium gluconate gel (10%) applied topically, preferably at the workplace, can be tried initially. Alkyl mercury compounds, which are used as disinfectants, wood preservatives, and fungicides, are extremely toxic to the central nervous system. If alkyl mercury causes blistering, the necrotic skin should be debrided as soon as possible to avoid continued absorption. Phenol or carbolic acid burns can cause depigmentation but also systemic toxicity. Water irrigation is less effective, and polyethylene glycol diluted with alcohol is recommended to help remove residual phenol. Chromic acid, used in electroplating, etching, and glass cleaning, oxidizes tissue to produce small, painless ulcers called "chrome holes."

Allergic contact dermatitis may mimic chronic irritant dermatitis in its presentation. Often the work history identifies exposure to a known sensitizer (see Box 11-3). A latent period of about 2 weeks is required after initial exposure. The allergenic chemical binds to a skin protein to become a complete antigen, eliciting a Type IV or cell-mediated immune response. One approach is to prescribe topical steroid therapy along with avoidance of suspected allergen(s). If the worker returns to work and redevelops the dermatitis, the diagnosis is clear. However, workplace exposures are often complex, and effective management, including recommending appropriate restrictions, process modification, personal protective equipment, or job transfer, may be difficult. Patch testing may be necessary and should be performed in a standard manner and interpreted with caution.

Contact urticaria also requires a latency period of weeks to years but differs in that histamine and other vasoactive substances are liberated by the principal mediator IgE and onset is more rapid (see Box 11-3).

Exposure to the protein allergens in natural rubber latex can induce both a Type IV or cell-mediated response producing contact dermatitis and a Type I or IgE immediate hypersensitivity response producing urticaria. The latter can involve respiratory (asthma) and even anaphylactic reactions. Cornstarch powder in gloves can absorb latex allergen and become airborne. Thus exposure routes include inhalation in addition to cutaneous, mucosal, and visceral. Hospitals therefore make efforts to limit latex use to prevent sensitization in health care workers.

Other skin manifestations of occupational exposures include depigmentation from phenols and hydroquinone, chloracne from polychlorinated biphenyls (PCBs), and occupational Raynaud's disease from vibration. Skin cancer, as from exposure to ultraviolet (UV) light, and skin infections, as from herpes simplex, also may result from exposure at work.

Primary and secondary prevention consists of engineering controls, industrial and personal hygiene, gloves, and protective clothing. The type of glove and its resistance to the offending agent should be considered (Box 11-4). Despite these efforts, assiduous avoidance may still be necessary.[3,6]

Box 11-4. Preferred Gloves for Use with Specific Irritant Chemicals

Heavy rubber: inorganic acids, organic acids, soaps and detergents
Nitrile: aromatic solvents, chlorinated solvents
Neoprene: aliphatic solvents, vegetable oils

Low Back Pain Case Management

Work-related low back pain occurs frequently, roughly 20% of work injuries that present for care, and accounts for more than 30% of the cost of all claims. The disproportion is typically due to the high cost of a minority of cases that experience prolonged or indefinite disability. Chapter 127 covers the diagnosis and care of low back pain. When considered work-related, the physician should be attentive to aspects of management that can prevent a worker from becoming "disabled." First, it is important to have the initial history carefully documented. Second, the physician should consider more frequent follow-up (e.g., weekly) to deal with workplace issues, refine modified duty restrictions, and document progress. Third, it is important to elicit the worker's own perception of his or her low back pain, correct misconceptions, and provide realistic information as to the prognosis. Fourth, if progress is slower than anticipated, it is useful to document inconsistent objective signs, positive Waddell's signs (suggesting symptom magnification or malingering as noted in Chapter 127), and poor cooperation with therapies. When recovery is delayed, the physician should assess the patient for an underlying depression. Appropriate referrals, judicious diagnostics, and communication with the employer and/or case manager are prudent steps. A fine line can exist between being supportive and enabling disability or the "sick role." It is important to assess any ergonomic hazards that might lead to recurrence or similar injury in co-workers (Box 11-5). When appropriate and with the worker's consent, it can be very constructive to engage the employer in discussion as to the worker's condition and potential modified duty assignments. Doing so can greatly facilitate successful transition back to work. See the section on "Disability Issues" for more details.[3]

Musculoskeletal Cumulative Trauma or Repetitive Motion Injury

Cumulative trauma or repetitive motion injury results from microtears to soft tissues and an inflammatory response. Depending on both the demands of the work setting and an individual's healing capacity, these lesions frequently are not allowed to heal properly and may progress.

Cumulative trauma disorders (CTDs) account for about 3% of the total workers' compensation claims. The focus on CTDs stems from an increasing prevalence, especially in some industries such as meatpacking, with an estimated 15% of workers affected. Table 11-6 shows the types of CTDs associated with different jobs. Work-related factors that increase the likelihood of CTDs include repetition, forceful exertion, incentive- and machine-paced work, awkward joint posture, mechanical pressure, vibration, cold, and job

Box 11-5. Factors Associated With Low Back Pain

Related to Job

Manual handling tasks (almost two thirds of compensated cases)
Lifting (about one half of claims; most often from floor)
Twisting (about one fifth of cases)
Bending (one tenth of cases)
Falling (one tenth of cases)
Reaching
Excessive weights
Prolonged sitting
Vibration

Related to Individual

Prior episode (threefold risk if occurred within 3 years)
Job dissatisfaction (very important; based on longitudinal questionnaire data)
Smoking (accelerates disk degeneration)
Obesity and genetic factors

dissatisfaction. The primary care physician should make a specific and accurate diagnosis (Table 11-7). The history should include questions aimed at substantiating a work-related cause, if one exists, including a temporal relationship between the onset of symptoms and performing a predisposing job task, as well as the absence of alternative explanations such as a fall or a sports-related injury. Especially with recurrent or recalcitrant CTDs, a systemic medical condition causing increased vulnerability should be considered (e.g., hypothyroidism). The overall goal is to prevent progression and permanent loss of function. See the individual chapters in Part Two, Section IX for specific diagnoses and therapies. Sometimes the patient can return to work on "modified duty." However, if symptoms persist, a trial of "active rest" away from work for at least 2 weeks may be necessary. See Disability Issues for more details, including return-to-work issues.[2-4]

Cardiovascular Disease

The extent of cardiovascular disease attributable to workplace exposure is unknown. Several toxic agents have been shown to affect the heart adversely through several different mechanisms (Table 11-8). Acute overwhelming exposures to carbon monoxide (CO), halogenated solvents, and organophosphate pesticides can result in death. However, today's primary care physicians are much more likely to encounter patients with chronic low-level exposures, such as those with exacerbation of coronary heart disease by CO exposure. A young worker with an unusual presentation of cardiovascular disease should prompt a detailed occupational history, with emphasis on those toxins known to cause heart disease. If the influence of a cardiotoxin is suspected, an exposure measurement at work may be necessary. Other workers may also be similarly exposed and affected. Some workplace cardiotoxins can act through more than one mechanism. For example, chronic CO exposure may accelerate atherosclerosis; induce carboxyhemoglobin formation, which can burden existing heart and lung disease via decreased tissue oxygenation; and cause congestive cardiomyopathy from chronic high-level exposure. Nitrates from explosive and certain pharmaceutical manufacturing processes exert their effects on withdrawal because of rebound vasospasm of the coronary arteries. A worker with an occupational exposure to nitrates might experience headaches temporally associated with work. Heart disease in certain professions (e.g., firefighting) may be compensable on the basis of special laws in some states.[3,6]

Table 11-6. Partial List of Cumulative Trauma Disorders and Associated Occupations

Disorder	Occupation
Tenosynovitis	Food packer Buffing/grinding worker Cashier Data entry clerk Musician
Wrist tendinitis	Small parts assembler Package assembler Butcher/meat packer Reporter/editor Espresso maker
De Quervain's tenosynovitis	Sewer/cutter Packer Electronic assembly worker
Trigger finger	Labeler
Epicondylitis	Musician Construction worker Electrician Butcher/meat packer
Carpal tunnel syndrome	Butcher/meat packer Cake decorator Postal worker Assembly worker Garment/sewing worker Rock driller Grocery checker
Ulnar nerve entrapment	Glass cutter Telephone operator
Shoulder tendinitis	Overhead assembly worker Punch press operator Butcher/meat packer
Hand-arm vibration syndrome	Forest worker Chipper/grinder Rock driller

Rempel DM: Work-related cumulative trauma: disorders of the upper extremity, *JAMA* 267:838, 1992.

Renal and Urinary Tract Disorders

The heightened susceptibility of the kidney to toxic agents stems from its enormous blood flow, concentrating function, high metabolic rate, vast glomerular endothelial surface, and conversion of conjugated substances back into their toxic form. The physician is at a disadvantage in identifying early kidney injury given the lack of sensitivity of blood urea nitrogen (BUN) and creatinine testing and the lack of early warning symptoms. Much research is underway to establish more

Table 11-7. Tests for Common Cumulative Trauma Disorders

Disorder	Diagnostic tests/indicators
De Quervain's tenosynovitis	Finkelstein test
Tendinitis	Localized tenderness Pain with passive stretching Pain with contraction of associated muscles
Carpal tunnel syndrome	Percussion test (Tinel's sign) Wrist flexion test (Phalen test) Von Frey pressure test* Electrodiagnostic study
Tenosynovitis	Localized pain with tendon motion or stretching
Cubital tunnel syndrome	Elbow flexion test Percussion test (Tinel's sign) Electrodiagnostic study
Lateral epicondylitis	Cozen test†
Neck tension syndrome	Muscle spasm of trapezius Pain with active resistance of neck motion
Cervical root syndrome	Spurling test‡

Rempel DM: Work-related cumulative trauma: disorders of the upper extremity, *JAMA* 267:838, 1992.

*Semmes-Weinstein monofilaments.

†Pain at lateral epicondyle with resisted wrist extension and radial deviation while forearm is pronated.

‡Compression on top of head with neck in 20 degrees at extension.

Table 11-8. Classification of Cardiovascular Diseases and Possible Toxic Causes

Condition	Toxic agents
Cardiac dysrhythmia	Arsenic Chlorofluorocarbon propellants Hydrocarbon solvents (e.g., 1,1,1-trichloroethane, trichloroethylene) Organophosphate and carbamate insecticides
Coronary artery disease	Carbon disulfide Carbon monoxide ?Lead
Hypertension	Cadmium Carbon disulfide Lead
Myocardial injury	Antimony Arsenic Arsine Cobalt Lead
Nonatheromatous ischemic heart disease	Organic nitrates (e.g., nitroglycerin, ethylene glycol dinitrate)
Peripheral arterial occlusive disease	Arsenic Lead
Cardiomyopathy	Arsenic, lead (from hypertension renal symptoms), cobalt, carbon monoxide, solvents

Modified from LaDou J, editor: *Occupational and environmental medicine*, Stamford, Conn, 1997, Appleton & Lange.

effective methods of early detection. At present, functional abnormalities must be extrapolated from abnormal urinalysis findings, 24-hour urine test for protein and creatinine clearance, and ultrasound; additional tests include fractional sodium excretion, urine chemistry, β_2-microglobulin, and renal biopsy (see Chapter 144). Very high short-term exposures can cause acute renal failure (e.g., high level exposure to carbon tetrachloride or inorganic mercury). However, the unknown extent of chronic renal failure and hypertension caused by occupational and environmental toxins has potentially greater impact. In general, lower and more long-term exposure to toxins may lead to accelerated loss of renal function and possible chronic renal failure. Table 11-9 groups toxins according to site of action. Some toxins such as cadmium and mercury bioaccumulate in the kidney. Several mechanisms (direct, indirect, immunologic) and exposure routes (ingestion, inhalation, dermal) are possible. Bladder cancer can result from aromatic amines such as aniline dye, presumably related to the concentration of such chemicals in the trigone area.

Hepatic Disorders

The primary care physician should be alert to possible hepatoxic interactions involving different workplace chemicals, ethanol ingestion, medications, drugs, and infections (see Chapter 104). Common occupational liver disease includes acute toxic hepatitis from chlorinated hydrocarbon solvents, halogenated aromatics, and epoxy resins. Table 11-10 lists toxicants according to type of hepatic injury.[3]

Neurologic Problems

Work-related neurotoxicity can be peripheral, central, or both. It is important to assess the patient for (1) workplace chemicals or substances used, (2) circumstances of use, (3) duration of exposure (i.e., brief from a spill or long term), and (4) other disease processes or nonoccupational exposures that might explain the problem. Findings are often nonspecific. Box 11-6 lists symptomatic presentations of common neurotoxins.

Peripheral nerve dysfunction usually manifests itself first as numbness or tingling of the distal lower extremities, then the upper extremities. A progression to weakness is seen next, from distal to proximal. In the most severe cases, muscle atrophy and fasciculation occur. The symmetric, distal, and graded neurologic loss extending proximally often results from axonal degeneration secondary to presumed metabolic derangement within the neuron, with the longest fibers affected first. However, new study techniques have revealed that peripheral nerves are vulnerable at multiple sites (e.g., altered vasa nervorum from lead, defective slow axoplasmic transport with acrylamide).

Variations in the onset and course depend on the exposure characteristics. Acute exposure to a toxin may have a delayed onset (e.g., acrylamide in 2 to 3 weeks from accumulation of microfilament, organophosphates in 1 to 2 weeks from the "aging" of a specific esterase enzyme), which then presents in an acute manner and follows a monophasic course.

Chronic low concentrations of toxic exposure may yield an insidious, progressive neuropathy with a slow recovery

Table 11-9. Renal Toxicants Grouped by Site of Action and Associated Occupations

Site of action	Toxicant	Occupations
Glomerulus	Silica	Stone cutting, sandblasting
	Solvents	Use of paints, degreasers, and fuels
Proximal tubule	Lead (inorganic)	Battery manufacture, smelting, lead abaters
	Cadmium	Manufacture of alloys, glass, paints, and electrical equipment, smelting
	Mercury (inorganic)	Manufacture of mirrors, batteries, alloys, and scientific equipment, mining; dental office work
	Halogenated aliphatic hydrocarbons (e.g., CCl_4)	Solvent use, dry cleaning, work with fumigants
Interstitium	Uranium	Mining, refining
Acute tubular necrosis	Cadmium	Welding of cadmium-plated metal (other heavy metals are possible toxicants, including chromium, mercury, and vanadium)
	Arsine gas	Coal or metal processing, semiconductor manufacturing (secondary to hemoglobinuria)
Accelerated atherosclerosis (prerenal)	Carbon disulfide	Manufacture of rayon and neoprene tires
Bladder (cancer)	Aromatic amines	Manufacture and use of synthetic dyes

Table 11-10. Chemical Toxicants Associated with Occupational Liver Disease

Toxicant	Type of injury	Occupation or use
Arsenic	Cirrhosis, hepatocellular carcinoma, angiosarcoma	Pesticides
Beryllium	Granulomatous disease	Ceramics workers
Carbon tetrachloride	Acute hepatocellular injury, cirrhosis	Dry cleaning
Dimethylformamide	Acute hepatocellular injury	Solvent and chemical manufacture
Dimethylnitrosamine	Hepatocellular carcinoma	Rocket manufacture
Dioxin	Porphyria cutanea tarda	Pesticides
Halothane	Acute hepatocellular injury	Anesthesiology
Hydrazine	Steatosis	Rocket manufacture
Methylene dianiline (MDA)	Cholestasis	MDA production workers
2-Nitropropane	Acute hepatocellular injury	Painters
Phosphorus	Acute hepatocellular injury	Munitions workers
Polychlorinated biphenyls (PCBs)	Subacute liver injury	Electrical utility and PCB production workers
Tetrachloroethane	Acute or subacute hepatocellular injury	Aircraft manufacture
Trichloroethylene	Acute hepatocellular injury	Cleaning solvent sniffing
Trinitrotoluene (TNT)	Acute or subacute hepatocellular injury	Munitions workers
Vinyl chloride	Angiosarcoma	Rubber workers

Modified from LaDou J, editor: *Occupational and environmental medicine*, Stamford, Conn, 1997, Appleton & Lange.

once exposure is stopped. Peripheral neuropathies caused by *n*-hexane, methyl n-butyl ketone (MBK), and acrylamide may progress for 3 to 4 weeks after cessation of exposure. In general, most toxic peripheral neuropathies are mixed sensorimotor, and most resolve if identified early and if further exposure is avoided. Examples of exceptions include lead-induced neuropathy, which affects the motor system primarily, and acrylamide-induced injury, which may not resolve. Along with physical examination findings, sensory and motor nerve conduction velocity (NCV) tests, electromyography (EMG), and even nerve biopsy may be of assistance. Subtle neurologic loss may only be detected by serial examinations over time. Other causes of peripheral neuropathy should also be considered (see Chapter 167).

Central nervous system (CNS) dysfunction most often results from a high concentration of a toxin in an acute exposure. Often the offending agent is readily known, and other workers may be similarly affected. CNS depression or narcosis may be entirely nonspecific. Recovery is usually rapid and complete, but permanent damage or death does occur in severe cases (e.g., when a worker is trapped in a confined space).

Chronic low-level exposure causing CNS dysfunction, as with organic solvents and chronic toxic encephalopathy, is more challenging diagnostically. Reported symptoms may include headache, vertigo, blurred vision, tremor, decreased coordination, irritability, and fatigue. Clinical findings may include difficulty with concentration, memory, reasoning, and complex concept formation. Depression may occur secondary to the toxic effects or as a reaction to the resultant

Box 11-6. Symptomatic Presentations of Some Common Neurotoxins

Lead: impaired CNS functioning is manifested by fatigue, irritability, and difficulty concentrating; peripheral motor neuropathy affects upper (e.g., wristdrop) more than lower extremities; classic abdominal colic also present.

Mercury: elemental form causes shyness, anxiety, inability to concentrate, irritability, and tremor (coarse, rapid); organic form causes severe neurologic effects, including sensorimotor neuropathy, ataxia, tremor, deafness, visual field constriction, and mental disturbances.

Organophosphate insecticides: anticholinesterase inhibition leads to autonomic overactivity acutely, with nausea, vomiting, and diarrhea (mild exposure), versus cholinergic crisis, with convulsions, miosis, and involuntary defecation/urination (severe exposure); delayed neuropathy and CNS dysfunction out of proportion to initial symptoms occur with acute high level.

Organic solvents: CNS depression or anesthesia on acute inhalation; propensity to affect frontal cortex (e.g., decreased attentiveness); chronic exposure may yield encephalopathy, characterized by irritability, impaired mentation, impaired attentiveness, headache, possible ataxia, and depression abating over months; also, possible irreversible toxic encephalopathy.

CNS, Central nervous system.

impairment. Formal neuropsychologic testing may pinpoint deficits and can be repeated to document recovery while the patient is not exposed to toxins. In general, chronic CNS toxic exposures do not result in radiologically or pathologically identifiable structural lesions, except with CO and toluene, which create multiple, small, white matter lesions, as identified on computed tomography (CT) scanning.

Examples of other neurologic disorders stemming from an occupational exposure include a parkinsonian disorder in workers exposed to carbon disulfide, CO, and manganese; facial weakness and numbness in trichloroethylene exposure; and bladder neuropathy and sexual dysfunction from the catalyst dimethylaminopropionitrile (DMAPN).[3-6]

Hematologic Disorders

Workplace exposure to hematotoxins can lead to one or more abnormalities (Box 11-7). The classic example is benzene. Benzene previously was used frequently as an effective solvent. Chronic low-level exposure through inhalation was found to cause blood dyscrasias, such as aplastic anemia, leukopenia, and thrombocytopenia. Benzene is now considered a leukemogen by NIOSH and the International Agency for Research on Cancer (IARC), a program of the World Health Organization (WHO). NIOSH has recommended that use of benzene as a solvent or diluent in open operations be prohibited, and in 1987 OSHA set a permissible exposure limit (PEL) of 1 ppm. Benzene is a good example of how cycles of toxicity have occurred since the 1800s; new chemicals are introduced and their industrial advantages exploited before full appreciation of the human toxicity is realized.

Differences in individual susceptibility to specific toxins clearly exist. For example, people with glucose-6-phosphate dehydrogenase (G6PD) deficiency who are exposed to chemicals that produce an oxidative stress develop cyanosis and a life-threatening hemolytic anemia.[3]

Box 11-7. Hematotoxins Grouped According to Effect With Associated Agents and Occupations

Red Blood Cell Survival

Hemolysis and methemoglobinemia

Oxidative chemicals (e.g., aniline, toluidine); nitrates; trinitrotoluene (TNT); naphthalene: rubber, dyes; fertilizer/explosives manufacturing; fumigants in clothing industry

Hemolysis (altered red cell membrane suspected)

Heavy metals (e.g., arsine); lead; copper: semiconductor, smelting, refining, plus chemical industries; lead abaters, painting, construction, battery manufacturing; leather industry (India)

Metabolism of Red Blood Cell (Porphyria)

Herbicides and fungicides (e.g., hexachlorobenzene; 2,4-dichlorophenol; 2,3,7,8-tetrachlorodibenzo-*p*-dioxin [a herbicide contaminant]): manufacturing and use

Others (e.g., *o*-benzyl-*p*-chlorophenol, vinyl chloride, lead, cleanser and disinfectant use, plastics industry)

Formation of Red Blood Cell (Aplasia)

Aplastic anemia (e.g., benzene); ionizing radiation; arsenic; TNT: rubber and shoe manufacturing; petroleum and chemical production; nuclear power plant workers; glass, herbicide, and paint manufacturing

Morphology and function (Myelodysplasia, Leukemia)

Benzene, ionizing radiation (see above for occupations)

Coagulation (Thrombocytopenia)

Pyrethrin, lethane, DDT; turpentine; toluene diisocyanate: use of insecticides, organic solvents, and hardeners (e.g., autobody painters)

Decreased Oxygen Saturation

CO and methylene chloride (breaks down to CO): forklift operators, use of combustion engines indoors, firefighters, auto mechanics

Reproductive Hazards

This section emphasizes providing the primary care physician with an approach using clinical risk assessment for this complex topic. One difficulty in attributing adverse reproductive outcomes to a specific occupational hazard is the high rates of background infertility (one in eight couples), spontaneous abortion (20% of pregnancies between 4 and 28 weeks, as high as 75% of all conceptions), major birth defects (3%), and low birth weight (7%). There is differential vulnerability of the reproductive process, both male and female, at the different stages, reflecting the precisely regulated hormonal milieu in which the progressive sequence of gametogenesis, transport, fertilization, implantation, and embryo-fetal growth and development occurs. Further-

Table 11-11. Human Evidence for Adverse Reproduction or Developmental Effects of Selected Agents

Agent	Human outcomes*	Strength of data
Female		
Anesthetic gases	Subfertility, SAB, BDs	+/?
Antineoplastic drugs	SAB, BDs	++
Arsenic	SAB, LBW	+
Carbon disulfide	SAB/menstrual disorders	+/?
Carbon monoxide	SAB, LBW	+
DDT	Menstrual disorders	?
Dioxins	Menstrual disorders, SAB, BDs	?
Electromagnetic fields (EMF)	SAB/childhood cancer	?/+
Ethylene glycol ethers	SAB	++
Ethylene oxide	SAB	+
Lead	Infertility, SAB, preterm, neurologic	++
Mercury	Menstrual disorders, SAB/LBW, CNS malformation, cerebral palsy	+/++
Physical stress	Preterm, LBW/SAB	+/?
PCBs	LBW, hyperpigmentation/menstrual disorders	++/?
Radiation, ionizing	Infertility, menstrual disorders, SAB, BDs, childhood cancer	++
Solvents, organic	Menstrual disorders, SAB/BDs	–/?
Tobacco smoke	Fetal loss/LBW	+/++
Video display terminals (VDT)	SAB, BDs	–
Male		
Alcohol	Azoospermia, testicular atrophy	+
Boron	Oligospermia	+
Cadmium	Reduced fertility	+
Carbon disulfide	Oligospermia, asthenospermia, and teratospermia	++
Carbaryl	Teratospermia	+
Chlordecone	Oligospermia, asthenospermia, and teratospermia	++
Chloroprene	Asthenospermia, teratospermia, and decreased libido	++
Dibromochloropropane	Azoospermia, oligospermia, and hormonal changes	++
2,4-Dichlorophenoxyacetic acid (2,4-D)	Oligospermia and teratospermia	+
DDT	Detected in semen of infertile men	+
Estrogens	Oligospermia	++
2-Ethoxyethanol	Oligospermia and teratospermia	+
Ethylene dibromide	Oligospermia, asthenospermia, and teratospermia	+
Ethylene glycol ethers	Oligospermia	+
Excessive heat	Oligospermia	++
Lead	Oligospermia, teratospermia, and asthenospermia	++
Manganese	Decreased libido and impotence	+
Mercury, inorganic	Decreased libido and impotence	+
Radiation, ionizing	Oligospermia	++
Radiation, microwave	Oligospermia and asthenospermia	+
Vinyl chloride	Decreased libido and impotence	+

*All have shown at least limited positive effects in animals.
SAB, Spontaneous abortion; *LBW*, low birth weight or decreased weight; *BDs*, birth defects; ++, strong evidence; +, limited evidence; ?, preliminary or conflicting evidence; –, no association.
Modified from LaDou J, editor: *Occupational and environmental medicine*, Stamford, Conn, 1997, Appleton & Lange.

more, breast milk concentrates many lipophilic toxins that may adversely affect infants. Knowledge of the physical, chemical, and infectious agents hazardous to human beings of both genders is growing but remains limited (Table 11-11). Animal reproductive toxins are generally considered probable reproductive toxins in humans; regulatory agencies apply "safety factors" of 100 to 1000 to animal data to establish arbitrary allowable levels.

Specific issues should be addressed for the pregnant worker. In particular, the altered physiology of pregnancy should be considered (Table 11-12). In some cases, removal of the worker from exposure may be indicated; for example, some toxins such as lead are regulated for the worker's protection. In general, the goal is to inform the worker of potential problems so that decisions can be made rationally. The degree of uncertainty should be conveyed so that the worker can decide on what is an "acceptable risk."[3,4,6]

Infectious Diseases

Illness from infectious agents of all categories can occur in the workplace. The jobs at risk include those involving contact with infected persons; laboratory workers in contact with infected human or animal tissue, secretions, or excretions; business travelers in contact with endemic disease; and workers in contact with infected animals. The occupational history may help reveal the origin of a puzzling

Table 11-12. Hypothesized Occupational Health Impact Physiologic Changes in Pregnancy

Some known physiologic changes	Agent or condition	Example of possible impact	Suggested occupational accommodations
General			
↑ Fatigue or stress	Inflexible hours Shift work	May be aggravated	Scheduling flexibility Frequent rest breaks
↑ Nausea	Ketones or acrylates Exhaust fumes	↑ Sensitivity to chemicals with strong, unpleasant odors	Improve ventilation ↑ Respiratory protection
↑ Metabolic rate	Carbon tetrachloride Protective gear	↑ Hepatotoxicity (especially if metabolically activated) ↑ Discomfort or heat intolerance	Minimize exposure
Cardiovascular			
↑ Uteroplacental flow	Hemolytic agents (e.g., arsine)	↓ Maternal oxygen-carrying capacity	Minimize exposure
	Asphyxiants (e.g., CO or agents metabolized to CO [e.g., methylene chloride])	↓ Fetal oxygenation leading to hypoxia	
↑ Myocardial irritability	Chlorinated hydrocarbons (e.g., tetrachloroethylene)	↑ Dysrhythmias or myocardial infarction	Minimize exposure
↑ Autonomic control of vasomotor tone	Anesthetic agents Organic solvents	↑ Arterial pressure Preeclampsia	Minimize exposure
↑ Renal blood flow	Cadmium	↑ Renal toxicity	Minimize exposure
Respiratory			
↑ Respiratory rate ↑ Tidal volume	All airborne chemicals	↑ Absorbed dose per unit time	Minimize exposure
↑ Hyperemic engorgement, capillary dilation	Formaldehyde Sulfur dioxide	↑ Sensitivity to irritants and allergens	Minimize exposure
Musculoskeletal			
↑ Lower back pain ↑ Lumbar lordosis, symphyseal and sacroiliac loosening Shifted center of gravity	Heavy lifting Ergonomically poor chairs and workstations	Difficulty lifting Aggravation of pain	↑ Mobility for postural changes ↓ Maximum lifting: 20%-25% in last trimester Well-designed chairs and workstations

Modified from LaDou J, editor: *Occupational medicine,* East Norwalk, Conn, 1990, Appleton & Lange.

infectious disease. Table 11-13 provides a selected list of infectious diseases by occupation.

The Bloodborne Pathogen Standard mandates a risk assessment discussion with a qualified provider after an exposure. Triple drug prophylaxis for those human immunodeficiency virus (HIV) exposures of greatest risk (e.g., large bore deep needle stick from a patient with high viral load) warrants immediate attention. The CDC updates recommendations periodically. Currently baseline labs should be performed on the worker exposed (HIV, hepatitis B virus [HBV] surface antigen, HBV antibody titer, hepatitis C, alanine aminotransferase [ALT]) and the source patient if possible. Hepatitis B passive immunization (HBIG) should be considered in high-risk exposures to workers without immunity; otherwise active immunity is checked and updated. No prophylaxis is available for hepatitis C, which carries an intermediate infection risk per needle stick exposure (3.5%) compared with HIV (0.3%) and hepatitis B (30%). Labs on the exposed worker are repeated at 6 weeks and 3 months. Safe sex practices should be recommended through the 3-month period.

Health care workers should not become complacent, since the degree of protection offered by universal precautions and other procedural and engineering controls is not absolute. Studies have found that during surgery, approximately one needle stick occurs in 2% to 5% of cases despite universal precautions. It may be helpful to consider total career risk of contracting a bloodborne pathogen when planning control strategies. In addition to the exposure rate from injury, other factors may affect career risk including seroprevalence of patients served, cases or tasks with potential exposure per year, frequency of extenuating circumstances (e.g., emergencies or combative patients), and efficacy of transmission (e.g., 30% for HBV, 0.3% for HIV-infected patients but transmission higher as CD4 count decreases and viral burden increases). Thus maximizing engineering and procedural controls is warranted.

Other potential infectious agents that pose occupational risks for health care workers are listed in Box 11-8. Pregnancy may be a contraindication to care for HIV-infected patients because of cytomegalovirus risk. Tuberculosis (TB) prevalence is increasing again; multidrug-resistant strains pose considerable risk where endemic, such as in New York City. Many countries have epidemic multidrug-resistant TB (e.g., the Philippines). Therefore immigrants and those traveling from such areas of the world require careful

Table 11-13. Selected Work-Related Infectious Diseases by Occupation

Occupation	Selected work-related infectious diseases
Bulldozer operator	Coccidioidomycosis, histoplasmosis
Butcher	Anthrax, erysipeloid, tularemia
Cat and dog handler	*Bartonella henselae, Pasteurella multocida* cellulitis, rabies
Cave explorer	Rabies, histoplasmosis
Construction worker	Rocky Mountain spotted fever, coccidioidomycosis, histoplasmosis
Cook, food-processing worker	Tularemia, salmonellosis, trichinosis
Cotton mill worker	Coccidioidomycosis
Dairy farmer	Milker's nodules, Q fever, brucellosis, tinea barbae
Day care center worker	Hepatitis A, rubella, cytomegalovirus, other childhood infectious diseases
Delivery person	Rabies
Dentist	Hepatitis B, hepatitis C, AIDS
Ditch digger	Creeping eruption (cutaneous larva migrans), hookworm disease, ascariasis
Diver	Swimming pool granuloma *(Mycobacterium marinum)*
Dock worker	Leptospirosis, swimmers' itch (*Schistosoma* species)
Farmer	Rabies, anthrax, brucellosis, Rocky Mountain spotted fever, tetanus, plague, leptospirosis, tularemia, coccidioidomycosis, ascariasis, histoplasmosis, sporotrichosis, hookworm disease
Fisherman, fish handler	Erysipeloid, swimming pool granuloma
Florist, nursery worker	Sporotrichosis
Forestry worker	California encephalitis, Lyme disease, Rocky Mountain spotted fever, tularemia, ehrlichiosis
Fur handler	Tularemia
Gardener	Sporotrichosis, creeping eruption (cutaneous larva migrans)
Geologist	Plague, California encephalitis
Granary and warehouse worker	Murine typhus (endemic)
Hide, goat hair, and wool handler	Q fever, anthrax, dermatophytoses
Hunter	Lyme disease, Rocky Mountain spotted fever, plague, tularemia, trichinosis, ehrlichiosis
Laboratory worker	Hepatitis B, tuberculosis, salmonellosis
Livestock worker	Brucellosis, leptospirosis
Meat packer/slaughterhouse (abattoir) worker	Brucellosis, leptospirosis, Q fever, salmonellosis, *Staphylococcus aureus*
Mental retardation institute worker	Hepatitis A and B
Miner	Tuberculosis*
Nurse	Hepatitis B, rubella, tuberculosis, hepatitis C, AIDS, herpes simplex
Pet shop worker	*P. multocida* cellulitis, psittacosis, dermatophytoses
Physician	Hepatitis B, rubella, tuberculosis, hepatitis C, AIDS, bacille Calmette-Guérin
Pigeon breeder	Psittacosis
Poultry handler	Newcastle disease, erysipeloid, psittacosis
Prison guard	Tuberculosis
Rancher	Lyme disease, rabies, Rocky Mountain spotted fever, Q fever, tetanus, plague, tularemia, trichinosis, ehrlichiosis
Rendering plant worker	Brucellosis, Q fever
Sewer worker	Leptospirosis, hookworm disease, ascariasis
Shearer	Orf, tularemia
Shepherd	Anthrax, brucellosis, orf, plague
Soldier	Tularemia and other infectious diseases
Trapper, wild animal handler	Leptospirosis, Lyme disease, tularemia, rabies, Rocky Mountain spotted fever, ehrlichiosis
Veterinarian	Anthrax, brucellosis, erysipeloid, rabies, leptospirosis, *P. multocida* cellulitis, tularemia, salmonellosis, orf, psittacosis, *B. henselae*
Zoo worker	Psittacosis, tuberculosis

AIDS, Acquired immunodeficiency syndrome.
*Silicotuberculosis occurs among quarry workers, sandblasters, other silica processing workers, and workers in mining, metal foundries, and the ceramics industry.
From Gantz NM: Infectious agents. In Levy BS, Wegman DH, editors: *Occupational health: recognizing and preventing work-related disease and injury,* ed 4, Philadelphia, 2000, Lippincott Williams & Wilkins.

assessment and management (see Chapter 74). The Centers for Disease Control and Prevention (CDC) has published guidelines that emphasize point-of-contact identification of those with suggestive symptoms. If TB is suspected, the patient should wear a mask and be taken immediately to a negative-pressure room. Health care facilities are categorized according to the number of TB skin test conversions in their health care workers and the prevalence of TB in the community served. Engineering controls, such as UV light and use of special filters in the ventilation system, are recommended to decrease the bioaerosol content of waiting areas. It is recommended that health care workers use respirators during high-risk procedures, such as administering nebulizers, which might induce coughing, or performing a bronchoscopy or intubation in a patient suspected of having TB.

Box 11-8. Some Infectious Agents That Are Occupational Risks for Health Care Workers

Virus

Adenovirus
B virus
Creutzfeldt-Jakob agent
Cytomegalovirus
Ebola virus
Hepatitis B
Hepatitis C
Herpes simplex
Human immunodeficiency virus
Influenza
Lassa fever
Measles
Mumps
Parainfluenza
Parvovirus B19
Poliovirus
Respiratory syncytial virus
Rotavirus
Rubella
Rubeola
Varicella-zoster

Bacteria

Bordetella species
Campylobacter species
Corynebacterium diphtheriae
Mycobacterium tuberculosis
Neisseria meningitidis
Salmonella species
Shigella species
Yersinia pestis

Others

Chlamydia psittaci
Coxiella burnetii
Cryptosporidium species
Mycoplasma pneumoniae
Sarcoptes scabiei

From Gantz NM: Infectious agents. In Levy BS, Wegman DH, editors: *Occupational health: recognizing and preventing work-related disease and injury,* ed 4, Philadelphia, 2000, Lippincott Williams & Wilkins.

Many occupations require international travel. Traveler's diarrhea is the most common health problem in those who visit developing countries. Dietary precautions remain the most important preventive measures, but the development of resistance to some antibiotics and the advent of the fluoroquinolones as new first-line therapy have changed the management. See Chapter 111 for the indications of prophylaxis and more information.

Workers exposed to animals are at risk of developing zoonoses, diseases primarily of animals that are transmitted to humans. Examples include leptospirosis, plague, tularemia, rabies, murine typhus, and psittacosis. Workers involved in earth-moving jobs are at risk of deep fungal infections (e.g., blastomycosis, histoplasmosis, coccidioidomycosis) resulting from inhalation of spore-containing dust in endemic areas. Superficial candidal infection may be a hazard in bakers and other workers whose hands are often wet.

In patients with flulike symptoms, physicians should consider the inhalation fevers such as metal fume fever and polymer fume fever, which can masquerade as an infectious disease (see Respiratory Disease).[4,6]

Stress in the Workplace

The influence of occupational stress on health appears to be substantial. In the workplace, individual and environmental factors interact to produce circumstances that may elicit stress responses (Box 11-9).

The ability to predict a stress response in an individual remains poor. Efforts to minimize the influence of this occupational hazard are more successfully directed at recognizing early manifestations and at primary and secondary prevention by addressing the offending factor(s).

Ideally, a workplace should provide sufficient flexibility to allow workers to change their job description through redesign or transfer as necessary. Often this is not the case, however, and job security may be threatened, adding further stress. Violence in the workplace often represents a failure to address stressful issues.

Box 11-9. Workplace Stress

Stressors

Factors related to individual

Conflicting nonoccupational demands
Inadequate communication skills
Moral or ideologic conflict with goals of organization
Insufficient social support mechanisms
Emotionally laden life events
Extreme personality traits

Factors related to work environment

Organizational change within company
Relationship to supervisors
Conflictive corporate atmosphere
Poor communication within company
Promotion or lack thereof
Underloading or overloading of job demand, mental or physical
Excessive expectations of functional level
Lack of control or decision latitude
Role conflict or ambiguity
Inadequate resources to accomplish job
Inadequate authority to accomplish job
Responsibility for others
Rotating shift work
Machine-paced work
Boring, repetitive work
Noise and vibration
Ergonomic problems
Poor aesthetics
Odors, temperature extremes, bad lighting
Obvious safety hazards

Manifestations of Stress

Early

Decreased satisfaction, absenteeism, anxiety, tension, irritability, trouble concentrating, decreased family participation, marital discord, altered social activity, decreased stamina, increased time required to recover from physical demands, increased accidents

Late

Clinical depression, cumulative trauma disorders, adjustment disorders, substance abuse, somatic symptoms, exacerbation of existing medical and psychiatric conditions, cardiovascular disease, gastrointestinal distress (especially peptic ulcer), accidents, increased workers' compensation claims, violence

Courtesy of Stover Snook, PhD, Liberty Mutual Insurance, ergonomic research; lecturer, Harvard School of Public Health.

Physical Hazards

Physical conditions such as temperature, noise, vibration, high pressure, and radiation at the workplace can adversely affect the worker. The physician concerned about prevention of a suspected physical hazard is encouraged to refer to the recommended threshold limit values (TLVs) published by the American Conference of Governmental Industrial Hygienists (ACGIH).

Noise. Noise is a common physical hazard, affecting about 10 million U.S. workers. An estimated 17% of production workers have at least some hearing impairment. The 90 dB time-weighted average (TWA) limit of the 1983 OSHA standard may not be sufficiently protective. The primary care physician should be aware that an "action" level of 85 db TWA exists (Section 1910.95 amendment) that mandates both a baseline audiogram and a hearing conservation program (see Box 11-2). Prevention is important because the greatest damage is done in the first 10 years of exposure, typically when the worker is young and has enough hearing reserve to allow the hearing loss to go unnoticed. The impact of a hearing impairment may be greatest in the retirement years, when conversational difficulty may lead to decreased socialization and to depression. There also may be an association between chronic noise exposure and the development of hypertension from a stress response.

A patient may present to the primary care physician with complaints of tinnitus, difficulty hearing the telephone ring, and inability to hear conversation in a crowded room or distinguish words, such as "six" from "sit" (consonants have a higher frequency than vowels). Often a family member first notes the hearing change. It is useful to differentiate acute from chronic and conductive from sensorineural hearing loss. Conductive hearing loss may result, for example, from a slag burn of the tympanic membrane of a welder.

This discussion focuses on noise-induced hearing loss (NIHL). Especially in chronic, bilateral sensorineural hearing loss, it is important to inquire about environmental and occupational noise exposure. The noise source can be continuous or from recurring short impulses. The decibel scale is logarithmic, with loudness doubling every 3 dB; sound at 90 dB is actually 10 times louder than at 80 dB. The evaluation of the worker includes a thorough head and neck physical examination, with attention to hearing, including the ability to distinguish whisper, Weber's and Rinne tests with a 512-Hz tuning fork, and audiometry.

Typical NIHL reveals a "notch" between 3000 and 6000 Hz. Interestingly, the anatomy of the cochlea is such that the first turn occurs at the 4000-Hz level. Two possible explanations for temporary threshold shift (TTS) include the cochlea hair cells being "knocked over" or metabolically exhausted by noise trauma. A TTS should delay testing or should be repeated after at least 16 hours without further noise insult. If the deficit persists, it is considered a permanent threshold shift (PTS).

A basic audiogram quantitates hearing thresholds at the proper frequencies (with hearing loss graded as mild, 20 to 40 dB; moderate, 40 to 60 dB; severe, 60 to 80 dB; profound, greater than 80 dB). An audiologist can assess speech discrimination (expressed in percentage of words repeated correctly; normal, 88% to 100%) and other tests as appropriate. The physician addressing a possible occupational etiology should look for a standard threshold shift (STS), meaning a greater than 10-dB average change relative to a baseline audiogram over the 500-, 1000-, 2000-, and 3000-Hz ranges in either ear after adjusting for aging using the appropriate tables (available in the OSHA regulation). This should be placed on the company's OSHA 200 log and should mandate hearing protection. To ensure compliance, the physician may refer to the OSHA standard (Section 1910.95) or request consultation. The ACGIH TLVs for noise, both continuous and impulse noise exposure, offer a more protective guideline for workers. Although it varies with the frequency, the ideal attenuation efficacy of personal protective devices is approximately 25 dB for waxed cotton, 35 dB for earmuffs, and 45 dB when combined.[1,3]

Cold Stress. Workers at risk of cold injury, whether systemic or localized, include meatpackers (refrigerated work areas) and those with outdoor jobs in winter cold. Elderly employees, intoxicated workers, those taking certain medications, or those with such chronic diseases as diabetes, adrenal insufficiency, and cardiovascular disease may be at increased risk. Cold also predisposes people to cumulative musculoskeletal trauma when repetitive, forceful movements are used. The ACGIH TLVs take into consideration windchill, physical exertion, task, and contacted surfaces. Early warning signs of cold stress include extremity pain. Systemic hypothermia can occur in water that is 72° F (22.2° C) and lower and with air temperatures of 65° F (18.3° C) and lower. The diagnosis requires a core body temperature less than 95° F (35° C).[1,3]

Heat Stress. Workers at risk of hyperthermia include smelters, steel workers, blast furnace operators, glassblowers, and those with outdoor summer jobs, especially farmers, ranchers, fishermen, and construction workers. Predisposing factors include health conditions or medications that inhibit the sweating mechanism, such as obesity, dehydration, cardiac disease, and anticholinergics (e.g., tricyclic antidepressants). There are four clinical states of progressive heat stress: heat cramps, heat syncope, heat exhaustion, and life-threatening heatstroke. Several dermatologic problems caused by heat are also possible. ACGIH TLVs take into consideration solar load, relative humidity, air velocity, protective clothing requirements, caloric expenditure, and task. The TLVs apply to acclimatized workers who are physically fit, and work/rest schedules are recommended for the various conditions and temperatures. Extra caution is advised for workers who are unacclimatized, which requires about 1 week, and for those in poor health, such as those with reduced circulatory response. A core temperature greater than 102.2° F (39° C) in the first trimester of pregnancy should be avoided (e.g., more than about 10 minutes in a sauna for an otherwise active woman); core temperature greater than 100.4° F (38° C) may be associated with temporary infertility in either gender. It may be advisable to have medical clearance for occupations known to involve significant heat stress.[1,3]

Vibration. An oscillating source imparts mechanical energy to another structure to produce a vibration. Every structure has an inherent vibration level at which resonance, or amplification, occurs, including the human body and its specific parts. The vibration frequency determines the effect on the exposed individual. Motion sickness develops at 0.2

Hz; whole-body vibration in the 1- to 30-Hz range, although worst at about 5 Hz; hand, arm, and shoulder involvement in the 30- to 100-Hz range; and hand involvement above 100 Hz. In general, the higher the frequency, the more absorbed by the contacting body part. Other characteristics, such as peak acceleration and direction relative to the body, play important roles and also lead to overlap among the categories just listed. Vibration is considered an ergonomic stress along with force and repetition. Effects from whole-body vibration may include circulatory and internal organ problems, persistent anemia, low back pain, and disk calcification.

Hand-arm vibration syndrome (HAVS), a vibration-induced Raynaud's phenomenon, occurs in workers using tools (e.g., pneumatic impact tools such as jackhammers) that impart local vibration within the resonance frequency of the hands and arms; cold stress can increase the likelihood and severity of HAVS. Early stages usually are reversible, but advanced cases can progress to permanent loss of hand function. In general, workers should avoid continuous exposure, use minimal hand grip force, keep hands warm and dry, avoid smoking, and use antivibration tools and gloves.[1,3,6]

Decompression Sickness (Caisson Disease). Decompression sickness can occur when the body moves from a higher-pressure environment (where nitrogen is more concentrated in tissues) to one of normal atmospheric pressure. Mechanical and physiologic effects of expanding gases cause damage unless sufficient time is allowed for their gradual dissolution. Caisson workers who work in a pressurized enclosure for underwater construction and divers are at risk. It is recommended that workers have preplacement examinations, looking for predisposing conditions such as obesity, vascular disorders, chronic lung disease, dehydration, or recent bone fractures. Three types of decompression illness are distinguished: type 1 involves the large joints (the "bends"), leading to a stooped posture from pain, and may be immediate or delayed up to 12 hours; type 2 involves pulmonary (the "chokes") as well as CNS manifestations and with possible permanent sequelae from tissue infarction or massive air emboli; and type 3 is characterized by aseptic necrosis of bone, especially the head or shaft of the humerus, and often has associated CNS manifestations. Treatment of types 1 and 2 consists of placing the patient in Trendelenburg's position with a slight left tilt to minimize risk of cerebral embolism, giving 100% oxygen, and providing hyperbaric chamber oxygenation. Contact the National Diving Accident Network for further assistance at 919-684-8111.[5,6]

Radiation Exposure. Ionizing radiation imparts sufficient energy when absorbed to produce ions and free radicals. Exposure to ionizing radiation occurs in many occupations, such as nuclear power plant and submarine industries, cathode ray and vacuum tube manufacturing, health care professions, and uranium mining. The average amount of energy deposited per unit length of path is called the linear energy transfer (LET) of radiation. Radiobiologists distinguish high-LET radiation (e.g., neutron, alpha) from low-LET radiation (e.g., gamma, x-ray) by determining the relative potency that causes damage to tissues, cells, and chromosomes. Effects are categorized as acute radiation syndrome, acute localized radiation injuries, delayed effects (e.g., radiodermatitis, atrophy), and low-dose effects, which include an increased risk of some cancers. For example, the association between ionizing radiation and an increase in leukemia (latency of 5 years) is well accepted, and a 15% increase in the risk of brain cancer (latency of 10 years) with ionizing radiation has been reported. Lifetime and yearly limits of 5 and 2 rem, respectively, are regulated and measured with a badge that quantifies cumulative low-LET (principally gamma) radiation. Thus far, tests cannot readily measure personal exposure to neutrons and ingested particles; their contribution to the risk of cancer is not well defined.[5]

Occupational Cancer

An estimated 30% to 40% of people in the industrialized world will develop a malignancy during their lifetime. Occupational and environmental exposures play an important role, although estimates vary widely regarding the proportion attributable to these exposures. Table 11-14 lists workplace substances known or suspected to cause cancer. The signs, symptoms, and course of occupational cancer are indistinct from non–work-related tumors of the same type. However, a few otherwise very rare tumors are considered sentinel or almost pathognomonic for specific occupational exposures, such as mesothelioma from asbestos exposure and angiosarcoma of the liver from vinyl chloride.

Latency is the time from first exposure to the occurrence of cancer and varies greatly among carcinogens (e.g., as short as 4 to 5 years for leukemia, as long as 40 years for mesothelioma). Knowledge of a specific cancer's anticipated latency allows (1) more focused inquiries as to past exposures during a primary care patient's medical history and (2) more appropriate design of surveillance strategies for workers who have been exposed. Latency also helps to determine the biologic plausibility of whether a cancer is "more likely than not" attributable to a prior workplace exposure.

A reasonable course of action for any health provider faced with an anxious worker concerned about a chemical exposure is to review the MSDS, then obtain current information from available sources, such as computer databases (e.g., Toxline, Registry of Toxic Effects of Chemical Substances [RTECS], Hazardous Substance Data Bank [HSDB]), government agencies (see Box 11-2), or a regional poison control center. Consultation with an occupational physician might also be considered. Providing a summary of an imperfect information base is often all that is possible.

When a patient presents with cancer, determination of a work relationship depends mainly on the history and exposure information, including the types of occupational and nonoccupational exposures as well as their duration and intensity. Then the available information must be analyzed in view of what is known about that cancer's epidemiology, such as the anticipated latency. The histopathology may also yield insight, as in lung cancer with fibrosis and asbestos bodies.[3-5]

DISABILITY ISSUES

The concept of disability evokes different thoughts and feelings in each of us, just as any other highly stigmatized subject. Personal philosophy aside, it should be realized that the physician rarely makes a final determination, but is one part of a complex process. The physician's role is to

Table 11-14. Established Human Occupational Carcinogens (IARC Group 1)*

Exposures	Examples of occurrence	Target organ/comment
Aflatoxins	Grains, peanuts (farm workers)	Liver
4-Aminobiphenyl	Rubber industry	Bladder
Arsenic and its compounds	Insecticides	Lung, skin, hemangiosarcoma
Asbestos	Insulation, friction products	Lung, mesothelioma, respiratory tract, gastrointestinal system
Benzene	Chemical industry	Leukemia
Benzidine	Rubber and dye industries	Bladder
Beryllium and its compounds	Aerospace, nuclear, electric and electronics industries	Lung
bis-Chloromethyl ether and chloromethyl methyl ether	Chemical industry	Lung
Cadmium and its compounds	Metalworking industry, batteries, soldering, coatings	Prostate
Chromium (IV) compounds	Metal plating, pigments	Lung
Coal tar pitches	Coal distillation	Skin, scrotum, lung bladder
Coal tars	Coal distillation	Skin, lung
Dioxin (2,3,7,8-tetrachlorodibenzo-*p*-dioxin)	Herbicide production and application	All sites combined, lung
Erionite	Environmental (Turkey)	*See* asbestos
Ethylene oxide	Sterilant in health care settings; chemical component	Lymphoma, leukemia
Hepatitis B and C virus	Health care settings	Liver
Human immunodeficiency virus	Health care settings	Sarcoma
Mineral oils	Machining, jute processing	Skin
Mustard gas	Production, war gas	Lung
2-Naphthylamine	Rubber and dye industries	Bladder
Nickel compounds	Nickel refining and smelting	Nose, lung
Radon and its decay products	Indoor environments, mining	Lung
Schistosoma hematobium infection	Farming and other outdoor work in endemic areas	Bladder
Shale oils	Energy production	Skin
Silica, crystalline	Hard rock mining, sandblasting, glass and porcelain manufacturing	Lung
Solar radiation	Outdoor work	Skin
Soots	Chimneys, furnaces	Skin, lung
Sulfuric acid—containing strong inorganic acid mists	Metal, fertilizer, battery, and petro-chemical industries	Larynx, lung, ? nasal sinus
Talc (with asbestiform fibers)	Talc mining, pottery manufacturing	*See* Asbestos
Vinyl chloride	Plastic industry	Hemangiosarcoma
Wood dust	Wood and furniture industries	Nose, sinuses

From Frumkin H, Thun M: Carcinogens. In Levy BS, Wegman DH, (eds): *Occupational health: recognizing and preventing work-related disease and injury*, ed 4, Philadelphia, 2000, Lippincott Williams & Wilkins.
*Other carcinogens, including medications (especially cancer chemotherapeutic agents, a risk for health care workers), foods, tobacco, and viruses, and classified in Group 1 are not listed here.

communicate key pieces of information and the clinical rationale for any opinions rendered. This input typically helps others make informed decisions. Good information from the primary care physician can be persuasive if it is objective and well substantiated by the medical record.

The primary care physician is confronted with disability issues daily (e.g., forms regarding medical absences from work or whether a patient is suitable for a particular job). The questions asked may vary, but addressing issues of disability begins with an objective assessment of functional capabilities. An individual's function, as relevant to establishing disability, involves (1) activities of daily living (ADLs), (2) social functioning, (3) ability to concentrate on tasks, to persist in finishing tasks, and to perform tasks with appropriate speed or pace, and (4) endurance (i.e., whether deterioration of clinical and functional status occurs in work settings). The intellectual challenge is to quickly ascertain the patient's real or perceived key limitations. Observing movements and using simple assessments of lifting and positional tolerance can be very helpful. The primary care physician's insight into how that person performs other life tasks may be very helpful in gauging any emotional or cognitive limitations.[2,5]

Preplacement Evaluation

When patients ask their physician to fill out a form attesting to their readiness for a particular job, the physician should act in accordance with Americans with Disabilities Act (Title I) (see Box 11-2). The ADAct prohibits preemployment medical examinations and allows postoffer examinations. The goal of the ADA legislation is to "mainstream" individuals with disabilities. Understanding key aspects of the ADAct provides a useful framework for preplacement questions as well as many other disability issues. An occupational and environmental health questionnaire (see Box 11-1) and a form suitable for communicating the results of an evaluation (Box 11-10) are included.

During a preplacement evaluation the physician should look for (1) primary care concerns that may affect the worker's performance, (2) problems with performing essen-

Box 11-10. Assessment of Functional Capacity

Purpose of evaluation (circle one):

Return to work/fitness for duty/preplacement/case management update

Worker's name ____________________

Social security # ____________________

Employer __________ Contact person __________

Phone/fax ____________________

Sponsor: ▫ Workers' compensation ▫ Private insurance ▫ Self-pay

Evaluation date ____________________

Date of injury or recognition of illness ____________

Is written job description available from employer?
▫ Yes ▫ No

If a workers' compensation claim has been filed, please provide the following information pertinent to the case:

Diagnoses ____________________

Principal therapies (include frequency and duration) ____________________

Are sedating effects of medications anticipated?
▫ Yes ▫ No Until when? ____________

Diagnostic tests ____________________

Significant findings ____________________

Was worker's injury or illness more likely than not to have resulted from or been aggravated by employment?
▫ Yes ▫ No

Recommended exertion level this worker may tolerate?*

- ▫ Sedentary work: mostly sitting with minimal physical activity; intermittent standing and slow walking that do not substantially increase heart rate or lead to shortness of breath (e.g., sorting)
- ▫ Light work: sitting and standing as tolerated with slow walking and activities using a few muscle groups that do not result in shortness of breath if performed consistently for more than 1 hour (e.g., filing)
- ▫ Moderate work: standing and walking with activities using several muscle groups that, if performed consistently, would lead to increased heart rate, shortness of breath, and slight fatigue after 1 hour (e.g., assembling at moderate pace)
- ▫ Vigorous work: movements and tool use requiring most muscle groups that, if performed consistently for 20 minutes, would result in shortness of breath, rapid heart rate, and fatigue (e.g., digging)

Recommended restrictions and/or accommodations*

Worker should not perform or may be adversely affected by:

- ▫ Lifting over (circle 5-lb range)
  3-5-10-15-20-25-30-35-40-45-50
- ▫ Repetitive or frequent lifting over (circle 5-lb range)
  3-5-10-15-20-25-30-35-40
- ▫ Bending from waist, stooping, or twisting trunk
- ▫ Prolonged standing
- ▫ Prolonged sitting
- ▫ Squatting, kneeling, or crawling into tight spaces
- ▫ Using stairs, up or down
- ▫ Climbing ladders
- ▫ Reaching above shoulders or head
- ▫ Pushing or pulling with more than very light force (about 10 lb)
- ▫ Grasping with hand (circle one or both): left right
- ▫ Fine manipulation with fingers
- ▫ Flexion or extension of wrist (circle one or both): left right
- ▫ Repetitive wrist or hand movements (circle one or both): left right
- ▫ Keyboard use
- ▫ Rotating shift work
- ▫ Other ____________________

Worker may benefit from the following:

- ▫ More frequent than usual rest and stretch breaks
- ▫ More flexible work schedule (e.g., start 1 hour later)
- ▫ Alternating sitting and standing positions
- ▫ Improving accessibility to work; specify __________
- ▫ Assistive devices; specify __________
- ▫ Work station or equipment modification; specify __________
- ▫ Other ____________________

Safety-sensitive restrictions; worker should not:

- ▫ Operate heavy machinery or vehicles (e.g., forklift)
- ▫ Work at heights
- ▫ Drive passenger vehicle
- ▫ Drive personnel vehicle
- ▫ Other ____________________

Current capacity status*

- ▫ May return to full duty without restrictions
- ▫ May return on a part-time basis of ____ hours per day, ____ days per week as tolerated on a trial basis (assess tolerance, allow gradual reconditioning and/or acclimation to work setting)
- ▫ Qualified to perform essential functions without accommodations
- ▫ May return or be placed in the described job at the designated exertion level and with recommended restrictions and/or accommodations (modified duty)
- ▫ Totally incapacitated at this time

Exertion level, restrictions, and/or accommodations are more likely than not ▫ temporary ▫ indefinite

Recommended date of reevaluation ____________

Name, signature, and title of evaluator ____________

*These recommendations are based on clinical judgment and should be implemented on a trial basis and observed for effect.

tial functions of the job with or without accommodations (i.e., appropriate job modifications), and (3) potential "direct threat" concerns (i.e., significant risk of substantial harm to the health or safety of self, co-workers, or the public that cannot be eliminated by reasonable accommodation). The latter two require the primary care physician to make a assessment of risk.

The physician may need additional information to perform this risk assessment. A written or at least verbal job description can often be obtained from the employer; a adequate description can help one determine which tasks are essential and which ones might be assumed by others (e.g., marginal functions). One can also communicate directly with the company to further clarify exactly what the patient will be doing and/or what exposures would be involved. To be covered under the ADAct an individual must have or be perceived to have physical or mental impairment that substantially limits one or more of the major ADLs. The employer is responsible for determining whether a reasonable accommodation is feasible. Accommodations can entail physical changes in the workplace, such as increased accessibility via a ramp and modification of equipment, or administrative changes, such as a modified work schedule and the provision of a reader.

Companies should help preserve confidentiality through separate filing of medical and personnel records. However, an emphasis of the Equal Employment Opportunity Commission (EEOC) is to reinforce communication between the company, the medical provider, and the employee in implementing the ultimate goal of the ADAct. To achieve the goal of mainstreaming individuals with disabilities, the primary care physician should be aware that detailed medical information, including specific diagnoses, can be relayed to the proper official of the employer on a need-to-know basis (per page 21 of the ADA Enforcement Guidance: Preemployment Disability-Related Questions and Medical Examinations; EEOC; 10-10-95). The employer has the responsibility for making decisions as to hiring and whether or not the company can accommodate the worker. One pragmatic approach is to ask the preplacement candidate for his or her permission to call the proper company official in the presence of the patient and discuss pertinent information. This approach allows the physician to address additional questions on the spot and sends a clear message that the physician is interested in advocating for placement with accommodations when prudent based on accurate information. (For further information call the EEOC, 1-800-669-EEOC, or The President's Committee's Job Accommodation Network, 1-800-ADA-WORK).[2,5,6]

Return to Work

The worker's employers and their human resource personnel rely on and need information from the treating physician in order to fairly administrate various benefits. Using a preprinted form can save time and facilitate communication (see Box 11-10). If there is inadequate communication, then the company may request the worker to see another physician. It is important to know that, as a condition of obtaining wage loss and medical benefits under the workers' compensation system, the worker forfeits medical confidentiality as it pertains to a claim. To save time and help advocate for the worker, it is very useful to have a clear, concise, and legible note that is specific to the injury (e.g., does not contain other general health information). If questions arise, then this note can be faxed to the requesting agent. Many states mandate utilization review, and frequently a case manager will be assigned to the case; your note, preferably dictated, should allow these individuals to do their job, thus obviating the need for a phone conference or additional forms.

The decision as to the timing of when the patient can return to work can be a difficult one. The physician should acknowledge and respect the worker's intimate knowledge of his or her workplace and elicit the worker's input. However, the physician should develop his or her own opinion regarding readiness for modified or full duty.

If questions remain as to whether modified duty is available or exactly what the job entails, one can call the proper company official in the presence of the patient. This sends a powerful message to all those concerned that your goal is to assimilate information and make prudent management decisions. More and more companies are providing modified duty for injured workers during their recovery period. This presents a win-win option when it works (i.e., recovery is not impeded). More frequent follow-up is often justified to refine modified duty assignments and ensure its success.

There are several techniques to qualify and roughly quantitate the worker's ability so that appropriate modified duty can be prescribed. One approach in performing a quick functional assessment consists of having the patient hold an examination room stool (about 15 pounds) against his or her stomach at waist height. If this is tolerated, then the patient can carefully extend his or her arms, stopping if discomfort is experienced; raising the stool to shoulder height can also be observed as well as lowering the stool to the floor. Observing these efforts takes only a few seconds but can afford a wealth of information. In addition, lifting technique and basic body mechanics can be reviewed with the patient during this quick exercise. To the extent possible, it is useful to simulate key job tasks in the examination room. For example, if it is unclear whether a certified nursing assistant is ready to return to modified or full duty, one might have the worker assist you from sitting to standing (e.g., simulate a transfer). Alternatively, the physician can use his or her own upper body to assess the worker's tolerance to pulling, pushing, gripping, holding, and twisting. Such common sense efforts increase the accuracy of the physician's determination and the confidence of workers in themselves and in the physician's judgment. If additional questions remain, one can request that a physical or occupational therapist perform a formal job simulation.[2,5]

Workers' Compensation

Historically, workers' compensation laws developed as a compromise between labor and industry. Industry's common-law defenses from liability for workers' injuries operated too harshly on the claims of disabled workers. Nevertheless, the risk of expensive suits against industry eventually led to discussions with labor. The resulting compromise offered important benefits to both labor and industry. Industry reduced its liability; labor achieved a "no fault" system that would expeditiously provide for injured or ill workers and their families, while accepting legal limitations in the worker's right to sue the employer (Box 11-11). Employers have a financial incentive to maintain a safe and healthy workplace, since insurance premiums to cover workers' compensation costs are rated according to a company's experience; also, many companies and towns are self-insured.

The direct and indirect costs of workers' compensation in the United States (amounting to about 2% of the U.S. gross national product) are substantial, although several states have reformed their systems and realized a decrease in costs over the last few years. Nevertheless, the burden of these direct and indirect costs reduces global competitiveness. The medical community can contribute by cooperating with requests for the required paperwork, becoming familiar with

Box 11-11. Basic Components of Workers' Compensation Systems

Limited liability without fault
Compulsory insurance
Guaranteed benefits
Medical care
Indemnity (replacement of percentage of lost wages)
Death benefits
Expeditious resolution of disputes

legal aspects of workplace issues, increasing its comfort level with caring for workers, promoting functional healing, and facilitating employees' return to work.

The physician caring for an injured worker should encourage the worker to fill out an injury report, a necessary first step that initiates a claim. As opposed to injuries, the worker may not relate the symptoms of an illness (e.g., wheeze of occupational asthma at night) to a work exposure. Thus the physician should inform the worker of a suspected relationship to work and encourage notification so that indemnity coverage (lost wages) and medical benefits can be obtained. If the treating physician requests a test or other resource and coverage is denied by a utilization review (UR) person or an adjuster, that decision can be appealed. Typically, a physician will review the treating physician's records and rationale for the test; the reviewer may contact the treating physician by phone to discuss the case prior to making a final decision. The treating physician should be aware that the guidelines used by the UR agent cover 90% of cases at most. In addition, there may or may not be a guideline for what the treating physician has requested. Therefore, the treating physician's rationale for the test or resource is of critical importance and should be explicitly stated.

Disability benefits are also provided by other federal and state agencies, as well as private disability insurers. Compensation systems differ from state to state; Box 11-11 lists some basic features in common, although it is important to be familiar with the requirements and processes specific to one's state. A listing of features by state, including a directory of workers' compensation administrators, is available (Domestic Policy Publications, U.S. Chamber of Commerce, 1615 H Street NW, Washington, D.C., 20062).

Physicians can provide the worker with timely, invaluable insights regarding workers' rights and also limitations under workers' compensation. Specifically, each worker should understand exclusive remedy, which means that he or she cannot sue the company (with very rare exceptions) and that only 60% to 65% of base pay up to a predetermined maximum is allowed. Even though this compensation is tax free, many workers incur a sharp loss of income (e.g., no overtime pay). Unfortunately, delays in the initiation of payments are common. Pragmatically, there may be ramifications in terms of future insurability (e.g., the worker may be asked to sign a waiver releasing obligation for the affected body part[s] or be flatly denied coverage), future employability, and even present job security. The worker's long-term best interest may be to minimize the length of temporary disability and avoid permanent disability through workplace modification or job transfer.

Nevertheless, if a relationship between illness or injury and work is suspected, the physician should document precise historic data, including time and date, objective findings, and concise opinions. In this way the physician will best serve the worker and the company by allowing expedient review by those who will make the final determination of compensability. When stating a medical opinion that may be used later for legal purposes, attention to wording is important. For example, phrases such as "more likely than not" establish a legally sufficient basis for a "medically probable" opinion, whereas qualifying terms suggesting speculation, such as "could be," do not.

More frequent follow-up, weekly instead of every 2 weeks, may be justified to expedite the worker's recovery, given the cost of replacing wages. Continuation of benefits may hinge on the physician's periodic reports indicating partial or total temporary disability. When progress stalls or maximal medical improvement has been reached, referral for an independent medical examination to determine fitness for work or level of impairment may be in order (see following sections). The primary care physician's records will be reviewed, with assessment of pertinent data such as mechanism of injury, active range of motion, impact on ADLs, inconsistencies on physical examination, and assessment of function. Vocational rehabilitation should be considered and is a covered benefit in many states. The physician should identify the proper resources of referral, such as company human resource personnel, workers' compensation administrators, responsible legal counsel, and a physician board certified in occupational medicine. Disputes over claims are common. If the claim is denied, there are statutes of time limitations, typically 1 year, to initiate proceedings; the case is then reviewed by a compensation board or commission. Dispute resolution mechanisms were designed in theory not to require legal representation. The worker must weigh the risk of losing a claim against the legal fee, typically 15% to 30%, although some states set a maximum. A physician's input usually is limited to review of medical records, but sometimes a legal deposition is taken, which can be done in the physician's office.[3,5,6]

Short- or Long-Term Disability Due to a Non–Work-Related Medical Problem

Increasingly, many companies and municipalities serve as their own insurance company for group health and workers' compensation. Hence these employers are interested in managing funds spent on various benefits. The primary care physician should cooperate with requests for information so that benefits can be administrated fairly. Often, employees are treated harshly simply due to the lack of adequate information to substantiate their claim. The policies and benefits offered vary widely. The physician should be aware that if wage loss benefits are not available or have been exhausted, the Family Medical Leave Act (FMLAct) (see Box 11-2) may represent an important option that can provide job security for up to 12 months with certain stipulations. The FMLAct requires pertinent medical information be transferred to the employer so that it can be ascertained whether that employee should be covered.[5]

Fitness for Duty

Primary care physicians may be asked to perform an evaluation of the relationship between a worker's health and the demands of a specific job (see sample result form in box 11-10). Currently, adequate and appropriate communication between the patient, the treating physician, and the decision-making authorities represents an explicit goal in implementing the ADAct as directed by the EEOC. If a workplace injury or illness has been claimed, then information pertinent to that claim is no longer confidential. However, non–work-related medical problems that result in difficulties with essential functions or raise the question of direct threat to self or others can present a challenge.

The ADAct limits disclosure of diagnostic information to the employer. The American College of Occupational and Environmental Medicine code of ethics suggests employers are entitled to input from the physician about a person's fitness but not, "diagnoses on specific details, except in compliance with laws and regulations." For instance an assessment of fitness such as "worker is fit for duty with the following restrictions" would be preferable to "worker has cirrhosis of the liver and should avoid solvent exposure." However, the health and safety of the worker, co-workers, and the public still must be considered. Decisions regarding continued employment and allocation of benefits require adequate information. One should consider discussing with patients what may be in their best interest to disclose to enhance the likelihood of their case being adequately understood by others.

When considering whether a worker is fit for duty, an appreciation for the workplace in general and the specific task(s) is crucial. The physician needs a detailed job description from the employer. Ideally, this information should be corroborated by the worker. The physician's role includes (1) providing a critical assessment of the available medical information as to completeness and validity, (2) identifying impairments that can "reasonably be anticipated" to affect performance of essential functions, (3) determining if impairments are permanent, and (4) identifying impairments that may result in a sudden or gradual adverse consequence (e.g., incapacitation in a safety-sensitive job, communicable disease) or a "direct threat" (i.e., significant risk of substantial harm to the health or safety of self, co-workers, or the public that cannot be eliminated by reasonable accommodation). When the evaluation is performed because of a deficiency in job performance, the physician should determine whether or not a medical condition contributed to that deficiency. The physician may want to comment on whether the information available supports a worker's capacity to travel to and from work, be at work for the specified time, and perform the assigned task(s). The physician's limitations in predicting the likelihood of an untoward occurrence should be stated clearly. One approach that can increase the worker's confidence in the quality of the evaluation is to dictate the report in the presence of the worker and request a copy of the final report be sent to the worker. The physician should remind the worker that management decides employability.[5]

The Determination of Impairment and Independent Medical Examinations

An independent medical examination (IME) typically entails an evaluation by a physician who has not been involved in the management of that injury or illness and who will not be assuming a treating role. The IME evaluator acts as a consultant for the requesting party who sometimes advances specific questions (e.g., whether the workplace caused the injury or illness). Ideally, the IME evaluator should make every effort to deliver opinions without consideration of the requesting party. Unfortunately, this is not always the case, and the quality of reports varies widely. Some states have dealt with this problem through establishing a list of "impartial" evaluators. Such evaluations are performed according to a specific outline and the opinions rendered can be binding after being considered by the judges who requested them. However, the majority of IMEs performed are requested by insurance agencies and other parties who are faced with questions of whether or not to allow or continue coverage. If an adverse decision is rendered based on an IME, then the treating provider should request a copy of the report. An appeals process usually exists. The following section should help the primary care physician be a better advocate for his or her own patient during the process of impairment determination.

Few concerns are as emotionally laden as disability in a worker who perceives that a condition has been caused or aggravated in the workplace. Providers of occupational health care need to be knowledgeable about their role with respect to impairment evaluation and disability determination in order to strike a balance between worker advocacy and better management of the resources in society.

An understanding of the definitions of frequently used terms should be helpful (Box 11-12). Intimate knowledge of the interface between the worker and the workplace, such as the environmental, exertional, ergonomic, psychologic, and cognitive demands specific to the site and job tasks, may allow the health care physician to convey useful insights and express an opinion on an impairment's possible impact on an individual's capacity. However, the employee must be made aware that a workers' compensation board or administrative law judge makes the determination of disability, not the health care physician. Understandably, such detailed and

Box 11-12. Definitions of Terms Used to Discuss Disability

Impairment: loss or reduced use of a body part, function, or system; medically determined alteration in health status.

Disability: result of a combination of medical and nonmedical factors that conveys a limitation or absence of capacity to meet occupational, personal, or social demands; how an impairment affects the person.

Handicap or *physical challenge:* when an impairment is associated with an obstacle to an activity or task; if that obstacle cannot be overcome by an assistive device or accommodation, that person is considered both handicapped and disabled for that activity or task.

Temporary disability indemnity: payment to replace wages during a healing period; may be partial or total.

Permanent disability: when capacity is static without hope of further improvement despite medical or rehabilitative measures; may be partial or total and is compensable either on a scheduled basis for the remainder of the worker's life or as a settlement.

Box 11-13. Medical Record Data That May Facilitate Impairment Evaluation

Mechanism of injury
Type and duration of exposure
Any inconsistencies on history or physical examination
Diagnostic tests performed and their results
Radiographic findings
Recovery progress, including ranges of motion, therapies used, and patient's response
Functional level
Recreational pursuits
Activities of daily living (ADLs) assessment
Underlying behavioral and psychosocial stressors
Suicidal or homicidal ideation

intimate knowledge of the workplace may be beyond the scope and time constraints of a primary care physician.

A medical determination of impairment is required to establish a disability. What is the primary care physician's role? Certainly, medical records that contain pertinent data greatly facilitate the process (Box 11-13). An independent medical examination involves reviewing these records. The physician should strive to avoid two pitfalls: (1) raising unrealistic expectations in the worker and (2) enabling prolonged, ineffective, or inappropriate care. Some familiarity with the *AMA Guides to the Evaluation of Permanent Impairment* (the *Guides*) can assist in avoiding these pitfalls. Explaining how the *Guides* is used and showing workers the criteria listed may give them valuable perspective.

The *Guides* represents a process or method for collecting, recording, and communicating information about human impairment. The *Guides* is not a standard or a law, but its use in assessing impairment is mandatory in 19 states; an additional 18 states refer, by law, to using the *Guides*. The *Guides* is a consensus document that has been refined empirically over the years. Scientifically derived and medically accepted data on many organ systems have been incorporated and referenced in the *Guides*. However, minimal evidence exists to confirm that tests of these systems predict work capability. No normative data on musculoskeletal, nervous, reproductive, integumentary, or behavioral systems exist; thus the clinical experience, judgment, and consensus of the contributors to the *Guides* were drawn on to estimate normal functioning. The evaluator is therefore expected to go beyond the *Guides* if clinical circumstances warrant. Further limitations on the validity of using the *Guides* include the variability among evaluators, which at best is still 15%; the reliability of laboratory tests and clinical procedures; psychosocial factors; and the dynamic nature of ADLs.

The *Guides* acknowledges that ADLs are the basis and determining factor in the design of whole-body ratings. In addition, all physical and mental impairments affect the whole person and should be combined (i.e., different areas of impairment put together according to a specific chart in the *Guides*). Three main steps are involved in evaluating impairment: (1) medical evaluation, including history of the case, current status, and clinical impressions; (2) analysis of findings, including impact on ADLs, whether maximal medical improvement (MMI) has been reached (i.e., when comfort, functioning, or impairment cannot reasonably be anticipated to change by more than 3%), prognosis, and restrictions; and (3) interpretation of the findings in the context of the *Guides* criteria, including an explanation to justify appropriate impairment ratings. The *Guides* uses active, not passive, motion when assessing range of motion. The 4th edition of the *Guides* deemphasizes spinal range of motion in favor of a new "injury model" that categorizes levels of impairment into one of eight diagnosis-related estimates. If feasible, prostheses are removed for an evaluation. The *Guides* glossary section provides working definitions for terms. The evaluating physician is given latitude through ranges of percentages for each impairment category. An explanation of why the physician chose one extreme or the other is generally included in the final report.[2,5]

REFERENCES

1. American Conference of Governmental Industrial Hygienists: *1992-1993 threshold limit values,* Cincinnati, 1992, ACGIH.
2. American Medical Association Committee on the Rating of Mental and Physical Impairments: *Guides to the evaluation of permanent impairment,* ed 4, Chicago, 1994, AMA.
3. LaDou J, editor: *Occupational & environmental medicine,* ed 2, East Norwalk, Conn, 1997, Appleton & Lange.
4. Levy BS, Wegmen DH, editors: *Occupational health: recognizing and preventing work-related disease,* Boston, 1995, Little, Brown.
5. Rom WN, editor: *Environmental and occupational medicine,* ed 3, Philadelphia, 1998, Lippincott-Raven.
6. Zenz C, Dickerson OB, Horvath EP, editors: *Occupational medicine,* St Louis, 1994, Mosby.

CHAPTER 12

Complementary and Alternative Medicine

Wadie Najm

Prior to the development of the current biomedical model of health care, people received the majority of their health care from folk healers and home remedies. As time progressed, immigrants relied on home remedies and Native American healing modalities for much of their health care. Today, a large portion of the population in developing countries rely on traditional healers, herbalists, birth attendants, and others for their primary health care needs. The World Health Organization (WHO) estimates that 95% of all rural births and 70% of urban births in developing countries are assisted by birth attendants. These therapeutic modalities are used either alone or in combination with other healing systems. In the United States, 100 million Americans supplement their diets with vitamins, minerals, herbs, and amino acids.

DEFINITION

The terminology and definition of complementary and alternative medicine (CAM) are constantly changing. Several terms have been used over the past decades, including *unorthodox, traditional, folk, natural, quack, holistic alternative, complementary,* and most recently *complementary and alternative medicine.*

The definition of CAM has been increasingly debated, and several definitions have been advanced, including:

1. Modalities used in addition to what is currently known as Western medicine
2. Modalities neither widely taught in U.S. medical schools nor generally available in U.S. hospitals
3. Ways of protecting and restoring health that existed before the arrival of modern medicine
4. Modalities usually outside the official health sector

As our understanding and acceptance of CAM evolves, so does its definition.

In April 1995, the National Institutes of Health's (NIH) Office of Alternative Medicine (OAM) assembled a panel of experts to define CAM. The panel defined CAM as a "broad domain of healing resources that encompasses all health systems, modalities, and practices and their accompanying theories and beliefs, other than those intrinsic to the politically dominant health system of a particular society or culture in a given historical period. CAM includes all such practices and ideas self-defined by their users as preventing or treating illness or promoting health and well being. Boundaries within CAM and between CAM domains of the dominant system are not sharp or fixed."[15]

Although the definition of CAM is comprehensive and intended to be applicable in all situations, it is too complex. This chapter defines CAM as healing practices and modalities not taught, practiced, or integrated in the current Western biomedical model of medicine.

CAM covers a number of health care modalities and practices. Table 12-1 presents the CAM classification system devised by the ad hoc Advisory Panel to the NIH's National Center for Complementary and Alternative Medicine (NCCAM).

EPIDEMIOLOGY

Use of CAM is on the rise. Studies looking at the use of CAM in different clinics reported rates between 9% and 50%.[6a,18] In a 1997 national survey, Eisenberg et al reported that 42.1% of the adult population used CAM. Some 46.3% of CAM users visited an alternative medicine practitioner. The estimated number of visits to CAM providers in 1997 exceeded by 243 million the projected number of visits to all primary care physicians. Visits to chiropractors and massage therapists accounted for half of those visits. The out-of-pocket expenditure for alternative medicine was estimated at $34.4 billion, which is comparable to the 1997 out-of-pocket expenditure for all physicians' services. These results show a gradual increase in users and out-of-pocket expenditure compared with a similar survey in 1990. About 96% of individuals who saw a CAM provider for a principal medical condition saw a physician for the same condition. Few CAM users (38.5%) discussed these therapies with their physician.[7]

CAM users are generally between 35 and 49 years old, well educated, in a higher-income bracket, and living in the west. Women are more likely to use CAM. African-Americans (33.1%) are less likely than other racial groups (44.5%) to use CAM. Users were found tohave a higher prevalence of chronic medical conditions, chronic pain, anxiety, and belief in holistic practices.[3]

Over the last decades, the increase in consumer interest and demand of CAM prompted the medical community to develop an interest in this field. Several U.S. medical schools have incorporated CAM into their curriculum.[5] The NIH established the NCCAM to evaluate these therapies.

Table 12-1. Complementary and Alternative Medicine Classifications and Therapies

System	Therapy
Alternative health care systems	Traditional Oriental medicine Acupuncture Ayurveda Homeopathy Naturopathy Tibetan medicine Native American practices Shamanism
Bioelectromagnetic applications	
Diet, nutrition, lifestyle changes	Nutritional supplements Alternative diets Macrobiotics Orthomolecular medicine
Herbal medicine	
Manual healing	Acupressure Alexander technique* Biofield therapeutics Chiropractic Massage therapy Osteopathy Reflexology† Rolfing‡ Therapeutic touch§
Mind/body control	Art therapy Biofeedback Guided imagery Humor therapy Hypnosis Imagery Meditation Music therapy Prayer and mental healing Relaxation techniques Yoga
Pharmacologic and biologic treatments	Antioxidizing agents Antineoplastons Cell treatment Chelation therapy Neural therapy Oxidizing agents

*Alexander technique: releasing muscle tension and correcting posture through gentle touch and verbal instructions.

†Reflexology: manipulating specific points on feet, hands, or limbs that correspond to different parts of the body to reestablish homeostasis.

‡Rolfing: a form of deep massage and postural retraining.

§Therapeutic touch: practitioners place hands over the body to detect energy field flow and blockage, and work to correct and replenish energy.

NATIONAL CENTER FOR COMPLEMENTARY AND ALTERNATIVE MEDICINE

Based on increased public and professional demand, a congressional mandate established the OAM in 1992. The office was given a minimal budget of $2 million dollars and a mandate to facilitate research in CAM, to act as an information clearinghouse, and to facilitate research training programs. As a result of the increased interest in and explosion of information about CAM, the office earned

Table 12-2. Centers of Research in CAM Supported by the NCCAM

Focus/specialty	Principal investigator	Institution
Addictions	Thomas Kiresuk	Minneapolis Medical Research Foundation *www.mmrfweb.org/caamrpages/caamrcover.html*
Aging and women's health	Fredi Kronenberg	Center for CAM Research in Aging Columbia University 630 West 168th Street New York, NY 10032
Arthritis	Brian Berman	Center for Alternative Medicine Research on Arthritis University of Maryland School of Medicine *www.compmed.ummc.umaryland.edu/*
Cardiovascular disease	Steven Bolling	Center for Complementary and Alternative Medicine Research in CVD The University of Michigan Taubman Health Care Center (734) 936-4984
Cardiovascular disease and aging in African-Americans	Robert Schneider	Center for Natural Medicine and Prevention Maharishi University of Management Fairfield, IA 52557
Chiropractic	William Meeker	Consortial Center for Chiropractic Research Palmer Center for Chiropractic Research *www.palmer.edu*
Craniofacial disorders	B. Alexander White	Center for Health Research Kaiser Foundation Hospitals 3800 N. Interstate Avenue Portland, OR 97227-1110
Neurologic disorders	Barry Oken	Oregon Center for Complementary and Alternative Medicine in Neurological Disorders Oregon Health Sciences University 3181 SW Sam Jackson Park Road Portland, OR 97201
Pediatrics	Fayez Ghishan	University of Arizona Health Sciences Center Department of Pediatrics 1501 N. Campbell Avenue Tucson, AZ 85724-5073 (520) 626-5170

Modified from the National Center for Complementary and Alternative Medicine.

increased authority and status and was elevated to a "center" (NCCAM), with its 1999 budget increased to $50 million. Since its inception, the NCCAM has supported the development of 13 centers of research in CAM. These centers cover different aspects of medical care (Table 12-2). In addition, the center has funded several small and large grants to obtain preliminary data and experience in CAM research areas.

The NCCAM receives more than 1300 public inquiries per month covering a variety of topics, including nonspecific medical conditions (56%), general variety (32%), cancer (8%), chronic pain (3%), and the human immunodeficiency virus (HIV) and acquired immunodeficiency syndrome (AIDS) (1%). The center has accumulated an impressive database of more than 180,000 citations in coordination with the National Library of Medicine.

MODALITIES

Ayurveda

The word ayurveda is derived from the Sanskrit *ayur,* meaning long life, and *veda,* knowledge. One of the world's oldest traditional healing systems, it has been documented and practiced in India for thousands of years. Ayurveda is a holistic system that deals with every aspect of life: the mind, body, and spirit.

A basic theory states that everything in the material world is a manifestation of the unseen universe of energy or life force. The world was created from the unseen universe when the primordial sound created the five fundamental elements responsible for the material world: space, air, fire, water, and earth. These five elements manifest in the human physiology as three life energies called *doshas*. The three doshas are *vata* (space and air), *pitta* (fire and water), and *kapha* (water and earth). Each dosha, its subdivision, and underlying structures confer a particular characteristic and quality to each person. Each person is believed to be a unique combination of these three doshas, hence a unique entity.

Health is a state of balance between the mind, body, and consciousness. Several factors can disturb this balance including congenital and genetic factors, natural tendencies habits, seasonal factors, and internal and external traumas. The imbalance produced in the doshas disturbs the life force producing the disease state.

Diagnosis is based on identifying the exact quality and

nature of the imbalance and correcting it. This is accomplished through a detailed history, inspection, and examination. Radial pulses (three superficial and three deep pulses, bilaterally) and tongue, nail, and eye examinations, among others, are important parts of the ayurvedic diagnostic examination. Treatment consists of strengthening or reestablishing the body's balance through a combination of interventions, including lifestyle changes, diet modifications, meditation, yoga, breathing exercises, massage, aromatherapy, herbs, and detoxification.

Although the primary aim of ayurvedic medicine is prevention and health maintenance, it also helps in several acute and chronic medical conditions. Limitations include situations involving acute traumatic conditions, advanced disease, acute pain, and surgery.

Studies have documented the beneficial effects of regular meditation on reducing cardiovascular risk factors and stress. Studies investigating the effects of the herbal products on a wide variety of conditions including cancer, aging, and health promotion are encouraging.

Several CAM disciplines have origins in ayurvedic medicine. These include aromatherapy, homeopathy, and massage. There is no national standardization of training and credentialing of ayurvedic providers. A wide variance of training and experience exists among providers. Physicians interested in referring patients need to inquire about the extent of training, certification, and expertise of ayurvedic providers.

Traditional Chinese Medicine

Traditional Chinese medicine (TCM) is a comprehensive system of health care developed and refined over thousands of years. It operates on the notion that health is a dynamic process of perpetual balance and counterbalance between different forces. Man is represented as a union between heaven and earth. The laws of nature are used to help understand the inner functioning of the human body. It recognizes the influence of the mind, body, and spirit and their interaction with nature, nutrition, and the environment on the person's health. The focus of Oriental medicine is on health promotion and preventative care at every stage of the person's life.

Interaction between heaven and earth results in a life force called *qi* (pronounced chee). Several forms of qi exist. Blood *(xue)*, mind *(shen)*, essence *(jing)*, and body fluids *(jing-ye)* are all part of vital energy. Health is present if vital energy flows freely and equitably among the different organs and along specific channels, called *meridians*. There are 14 meridian channels, 11 organs (six yang organs, five yin organs). In addition to the free flow of vital energy, health is the result of balance between opposed forces described as yin and yang. Yin and yang forces are seen everywhere and may apply to any topic. Disease is described as an imbalance between the yin and yang and in the flow of vital energy through the meridians.

Wood, fire, metal, water, and earth are five basic elements thought to be important to man; they are important constituents of the universe. Properties of these elements were assigned to everything in the material world. These elements are constantly interacting.

Evaluation is done through inspection of the tongue, palpating the pulse, listening to the voice, smelling the body, and taking a history. Once a diagnosis is reached, several therapeutic modalities are prescribed. These include diet, lifestyle changes, herbals, acupuncture, moxibustion, manipulative therapy, massage, exercise, bone setting, and bloodletting. Exercises include tai-chi (balances energy) and qi gong (builds energy).

Table 12-3. Medical Conditions Helped by Acupuncture and Type of Research Available

Conditions	Evidence
Postoperative nausea and vomiting Postchemotherapy nausea Postoperative dental pain	Good research data
Postoperative pain Myofascial pain Low back pain	Good clinical experience; some research data
Addiction Stroke rehabilitation Carpal tunnel syndrome Osteoarthritis Headache	Positive clinical experience; less convincing research data

Modified from the National Center for Complementary and Alternative Medicine.

Acupuncture. Acupuncture was initially publicized in 1972, after President Nixon's visit to China. Over the last few decades, several studies have investigated the mechanism of action and the efficacy of acupuncture. Activation of endogenous opioids, cortisol, neurotransmitters, and afferent fibers through the nervous system have all been advanced as possible mechanisms of action.

Although acupuncture is part of the TCM therapeutic arsenal, it is currently being used as a stand-alone modality. Evaluations should be based on the recognition of imbalance using the TCM diagnostic method described above. Once the imbalance is recognized, a treatment plan is devised, and needles are placed in acupuncture points along the appropriate meridians to help restore the balance.

An NIH consensus panel assembled in 1997 to review the literature on acupuncture concluded that the quality and value of acupuncture studies are variable. Of great concern is the validity of controlled studies using sham-points. After review the panel reported that current scientific evidence indicates that acupuncture is helpful in certain conditions (Table 12-3). Research into the efficacy of acupuncture in the treatment of other medical conditions is in progress.[1]

Adverse Effects. In the hands of qualified providers, acupuncture is a very safe and effective therapy. Possible side effects include syncope, drowsiness, organ puncture, and infection. Although rare, pneumothorax is the most common organ puncture reported. Infection from acupuncture needles is a major concern. Use of unsterilized needles has been responsible for reports of hepatitis B transmission. Although HIV infection is a major concern, there is no documented report of HIV transmission as a result of acupuncture.

Identifying anatomic structures, judicious clinical judgment, and use of disposable needles can greatly assist in avoiding many complications.[16]

Requirements for providing acupuncture treatment vary greatly between states. Few states require licensed physicians to complete formal training in acupuncture. For nonphysicians, licensing requirements and the scope of practice also vary between states. In certain states, practice is limited to acupuncture itself, whereas others include herbalism.

Acupuncture is currently recognized and included as a benefit or as a rider to the health plan by several health insurance policies. Coverage and reimbursement vary between insurance companies and in different states.

Homeopathy

The word homeopathy is derived from the Greek *homios,* meaning like, and *pathos,* suffering. Descriptions of homeopathy have been found in the ancient Hippocratic writings, as well as in early Arab and Inca writings. The current principles of homeopathy are ascribed to Samuel Hahneman, a physician in the eighteenth century. Having become despondent with the practice of medicine, Hahneman concentrated his efforts in 1796 on research and translation of medical literature.

It was during his translation of Cullen's *Materia Medica* that Hahneman tested the effects of Peruvian bark on himself, developing symptoms consistent with malaria. Subsequent experiments confirmed his suspicion that quinine caused the same symptoms it was supposed to treat in malaria. After repeat testing using other products, he eventually came to the conclusion that the symptoms of an illness can be regarded as nature's way to healing, rather than fighting an illness. Hence the first doctrine of homeopathy: *Simlia similbus curentar* or *Let like be treated by like.*

In his experiments, Hahneman used simple, uncompounded substances from herbs, minerals, and snake venom. He found that diluting the amount used in a dose seemed to increase the potency, even when diluted to almost infinitesimal dilution. He was not able to explain why this system worked in a biomedically accepted model, other than to suggest that it rallied the body's defensive forces. He believed that diluted doses avoided the risk of stronger medications, which could affect both healthy and sick organs/tissues. This led him to the second doctrine: *Microdose potentization.*

Hahneman thought that a physician should build up the patient's strength and trust the life force to do the rest. Hence, in treating any kind of illness, the nature of the patient, as well as the disease, must be considered, so that the treatment could be regulated according to his or her needs. Since each patient has a different constitution, or temperament, knowledge of that person is a prerequisite of a successful handling of his or her disease. This led to the third doctrine: *Treat the patient* (rather than the disease).

From these three doctrines, the current system of homeopathy arose.

Dane Hans Graham introduced homeopathy in the United States in the 1820s. The first Hahneman society was founded in Philadelphia in 1833, and the American Institute of Homeopathy was founded in 1844. Soon after, homeopathic medical schools and hospitals began to appear and flourish by the end of the nineteenth century.

Opinions are divided on the merits of homeopathy. Much of the controversy arises from the difficulty in explaining its effects in conventional terms. A great number of studies have looked at the effects of homeopathic remedies. The quality of these studies is variable. Three meta-analyses of homeopathic trials have been published[10,11,14] (Table 12-4). The quality of these studies and the methodology used for each are different. Although the overall results were slightly in favor of homeopathic remedies, because of the limited quality of the studies, no clear conclusions could be drawn about the effectiveness of homeopathy for any single medical problem or for any single remedy.

Table 12-4. Three Meta-Analyses of Homeopathic Trials

Trial	Trials reviewed	Results
Hill C, Doyon F[10]	40 Randomized controlled trials	19 Positive 19 No efficiency 2 Not assessable
Kleijnen J, et al[11]	107 Controlled trials (68 Randomized)	81 Positive 24 Negative 2 Not assessable
Linde K, et al[14]	Review 186 trials 89 Adequate data for meta-analysis	26 Good quality studies Odds ratio 1.66

Chiropractic

The word chiropractic derives from the Greek words *chier,* meaning hands, and *practicikos,* meaning practitioner. Chiropractic care has its origins in the manipulative health care modalities. It was developed in 1895 by Daniel D. Palmer, a lay healer who established a successful practice and eventually a school centered on achieving health through manipulation of the spine. Chiropractic care struggled to establish its place in health care over the last 100 years. Over the last decade, chiropractic care has gained gradual acceptance and developed into a treatment and wellness modality that is practiced by 55,000 licensed practitioners and used by roughly 10% of the U.S. population. Chiropractic care is licensed in all 50 states, with 45 requiring insurers to include it in their plans. There is a wide variation in the scope of practice; certain states limit the practice to spinal manipulation, whereas others permit different procedures to be performed, such as acupuncture, electromyography, and laboratory diagnosis.

Education is provided at 16 accredited colleges. Since 1974 chiropractic education has been established with a 4-year curriculum monitored by the Council on Chiropractic Education (CCE). Admission requirements vary from school to school, although a minimum of 2 years of college education and specific science courses are required by all.

A chiropractic system of health is based on two principles: a testable principle, which suggests that the structure and condition of the body influence how the body functions and heals, and the untestable principle, which indicates that the mind-body relationship is instrumental in maintaining health and affects the healing processes. Hence the focus is on the body's ability to self-heal, on the nervous system's role in overall health, and on the interaction between body structure and the functioning of the nervous system.

Evaluation consists of taking a comprehensive history and physical examination. X-rays are taken as needed. Treatment plans consist of manual manipulation of the spine extremities to correct the underlying problem and allow the body to heal.

The most common condition evaluated by chiropractors is low back pain. A 1992 meta-analysis by Shekelle[17] included 9 studies looking at acute and subacute low back pain uncomplicated by sciatica. The study indicated that spinal manipulation is more efficacious than comparison treatments. However, data were insufficient to reach a conclusion for chronic low back pain or patients with sciatica. Review of 36 randomized clinical trials of spinal manipulation for low back pain[12,13] concluded that it is not statistically proven that spinal manipulation is beneficial for any low back pain syndrome.

Fewer randomized controlled studies have looked at the efficacy of spinal manipulation for neck pain. Quality of these studies is variable. A recent meta-analysis[2] looking at a variety of manual therapies for neck pain found a benefit for the manual therapy–treated group; however, because of the heterogeneity among treatment modalities and patients, direct conclusions cannot be extrapolated.

There are a small number of published studies looking at chiropractic care and nonmusculoskeletal health conditions such as asthma, hypertension, otitis media, dizziness, headaches, and infantile colic. Current data do not support the benefit of chiropractic care for any of these conditions (Box 12-1).

Box 12-1. Contraindications for Manipulative Therapy

Acute fracture
Acute inflammatory joint disease
Osteoporosis
Active neurologic symptoms
Bleeding tendencies/disorder
Underlying bone/joint infection, tumor, metastasis

Naturopathic Medicine

The history of naturopathic medicine is not concise. Similar to other therapeutic modalities, elements of naturopathy can be found in the Hippocratic principle of *life force*. The recent history of naturopathy can be attributed to V. Priessnitz, a farmer in Austria, who used water and air treatments to enhance the healing power of nature. Benedict Lust, a German physician, introduced naturopathy to the United States. He used the term *naturopathy* (from *natur,* to indicate nature, and *pathy* from homeopathy) to encompass all the natural approaches to healing. Since then, several healing modalities have been added to the healing module to arrive at modern naturopathy.

Naturopathic medicine is far from being a single scientific discipline. The basic principle is that healing comes from within more than from without, and that medicine depends on the healing power of nature to cure. Naturopathy employs various natural means to empower the individual to reach the ability to self-heal. The tools include lifestyle modifications, nutrition, dietetics, herbs, education, and hydrotherapy. In addition, naturopaths may elect to use a variety of healing modalities, including acupuncture, botanicals, homeopathy, massage, Oriental medicine, and minor surgery.

Training includes undergraduate premedical coursework and completion of a 4-year curriculum in an accredited school. Currently only three schools are accredited in the United States. More than a dozen states license naturopaths. The scope of practice in each of those states is variable and state-specific. In general, naturopaths function as primary care providers. The emphasis of their practice is on prevention, education, and health maintenance.

Herbalism

General Considerations. Herbs have been used for medicinal purposes for thousands of years. Almost one quarter of the current pharmacopoeia is derived from botanicals. Digoxin is derived from foxglove, aspirin is derived from willow bark, narcotics are derived from opium poppy, and birth control pills were developed from the Mexican yam. Current herbal preparations are sold mainly as nutritional products. They are sold over-the-counter (OTC), and are not subject to the same quality control process as pharmaceutical products. Producers are exempt from the Food and Drug Administration (FDA) regulations imposed on medicinal products, provided that the labels do not make any medicinal claims. Preparations can be found in a variety of forms: crude plants, freeze-dried, tea, dry powdered extracts, soft extracts, fluid extracts, and tinctures. Herbal medicines could utilize any part of the plant. As such, several variables could interfere with production.

The FDA regulates products considered as drugs. To market a product as a treatment, the manufacturer has to submit an Investigational New Drug (IND) application for FDA approval. This process goes through multiple stages requiring several years of testing at high cost before approval. Since nutritional therapies cannot be patented, companies do not invest time and resources into the FDA approval process. Hence these manufacturers cannot make health claims or market them as intended to treat or cure.

The Nutrition Labeling and Education Act (NLEA) was enacted by Congress in 1990 to provide a clear relationship of nutrition to disease. Under this act, disease-related health claims could be used on labeling of nutritional products, provided that there is agreement among qualified scientists that the claim made is valid. In 1994, Congress enacted the Dietary Supplement Health and Education Act (DSHEA). Dietary supplements include products that contain vitamins, minerals, herbs, amino acids, or other dietary products either alone or in combination. This act reaffirms that dietary supplements are foods, thus exempting them from the requirements of new drugs. However, the FDA can remove misbranded products from the market. For detailed information and a review of the other herbal products see Table 12-5.

SPECIFIC DISEASES

Increasing interest in the use of CAM for the treatment of a wide variety of medical conditions exists. Current evidence to support the efficacy of these modalities is mostly anecdotal. Studies to evaluate and validate these therapies are ongoing. The following is an overview of some of the therapies used in these medical conditions.

Cancer

Cancer is the major reason people inquire about CAM. Several surveys have demonstrated that approximately 22%

Table 12-5. Outline of Current Knowledge about Commonly Used Herbs

Name	Species	Parts used	Proposed action	Common use	Proposed dose	Side effects	Contraindication
Echinacea	*E. purpurea* *E. angustifolia* *E. pallida*	Root & above-ground part	Increases phagocytosis; promotes activity of lymphocytes and leukocytes; releases tumor necrosis factor; promotes induction of interferon activity; inhibits activity of hyaluronidase	Common cold; upper respiratory tract infections; topical wound healing; acute and chronic infections	6-9 ml expressed juice; dry powder: 150-300 mg; freeze-dried: 325-650 mg	Allergic reaction	Progressive systemic disorder; HIV infection; tuberculosis; multiple sclerosis
Feverfew	*Tanacetum parthenium*	Aboveground	Lactone and parthenolide active against phospholipase A_2; limits IgE-induced histamine release	Headaches; arthritis; premenstrual syndrome		Mouth ulcers; allergic reactions	Pregnancy; lactating mothers; children less than 2 years
Garlic	*Allium sativum*	Bulbs	Allicin increases the level of antioxidant; sulfur compounds inhibit lipid peroxidation in the liver	Supportive measure to lower lipids; prevention of age-dependent vascular changes; may have antibacterial activity	4 gm fresh garlic, 8 mg essential oil	Gastrointestinal symptoms	None reported
Bilberry	*Vacinium myrtillus*	Ripe fruit	Tannins, anthocyanins, and flavonoid glycosides are active ingredients	Externally for mild inflammation of mucous membrane of mouth and throat; orally for acute nonspecific diarrhea; night vision	80-160 mg three times daily; 10% topical decoction	None reported	None reported
Valerian	*Valeriana officinalis*	Root	Mono and sesquiterpenes influence serotonin and stimulate release of γ-aminobutyric acid (GABA) and inhibit its reuptake	Restlessness; sleep disorder	Tincture: 1-3 ml/dose; infusion: 2-3 gm/cup; extracts: 2-3 gm equivalent/dose	Headache and restless state; liver damage with prolonged use in people with liver problems	None reported
Ginkgo biloba		Leaves	Ginkoflavoglycosides and terpenoids as free radical scavengers; enhances cerebral and peripheral circulation; reduces capillary fragility and inhibits platelet activating factor (PAF)	Peripheral vascular disease; intermittent claudication; cerebral circulatory disorder; mild to moderate memory impairment	40 mg TID or 60 mg BID	Gastrointestinal disturbances; headache; allergic skin reaction	Avoid with anticoagulants
St. John's Wort	*Hypericum perforatum*	Dried above-ground	Inhibition of serotonin uptake by postsynaptic receptors; monoamine oxidase (MAO) inhibitor	Antidepressant; antiviral and topical wound healing	2-4 gm (0.2-1 mg total hypericin)	Allergic reaction; photosensitivity	With prescription antidepressants
Saw Palmetto	*Serenoa repens*	Berry	Antiandrogenic and antiexudative	Urinary problems in mild to moderate benign prostate hypertrophy	1-2 gm of berry or 320 mg lipophilic ingredients	Stomach problems	None known
Korean ginseng	*Panax ginseng*	Root and root hair	Divers effect depending on species, dose; analgesic, antiinflammatory activity and papaverine-like action on smooth muscle; CNS activity and antistress activity through the adrenal glands have been	Tonic, adaptogenic effect	0.6-3 gm of root or equivalent TID eaten or as tea	May potentiate the effect of caffeine: sleeplessness, nervousness, diarrhea with prolonged high-dose use	Pregnancy (controversial)

of patients with cancer use CAM treatments. Dietary and psychologic therapies are most commonly used. Younger patients and being married were positive indicators of CAM use. About 75% of patients tried more than one therapy. The majority of patients learned about these therapies through family, friends, and personal research. Approximately 40% of patients did not discuss CAM therapies with their physician.[4]

The current cancer therapies have limited efficacy in the majority of cancers and great side effects. Given these limitations and uncertainties, people are willing to try other therapeutic options. There has been a myriad of formulations, therapies, and claims made; however, to date scientific evidence does not exist to confirm those claims. More recently, studies have been undertaken to evaluate the effectiveness of shark cartilage on angiogenesis in tumor cells and the effect of antineoplastons in treatment of brain cancer in pediatric patients.

Antineoplastons. Developed by Dr. S. Burzynkis, antineoplastons cause cancer cells to undergo differentiation and eventually cause them to die through programmed cell death. Current research does not support these claims.

Essiac. Essiac is a combination of several herbs promoted initially by R.M. Caisse, a Canadian nurse. Since her death, several companies have marketed this product. The exact formulation is not clear and varies between producers. Research looking into its antitumor activity has been disappointing.

Hoxsey Treatment. Hoxsey therapy consisted of an external application of a paste or powder and the oral intake of tonic formulated on a case-by-case basis. This product and its constituents have undergone review by the National Cancer Institute (NCI) and were not found to have antitumor activity.

Immunoaugmentative Therapy. Developed by L. Burton, PhD, immunoaugmentative therapy consisted of injection of protein extracts that manipulates the immune defense system. Little or no data exist to allow a clear review and evaluation of this product. Analysis of some of the material given to patients showed no evidence of the effects claimed by Dr. Burton.

Laetrile. Laetrile, a relative of amygdalin, also referred to as "vitamin B_{17}," was first used in California in the 1950s as a selective antitumor treatment. Data from several animal models did not support its claims as antitumor treatment. A 1982 multicenter study sponsored by the NCI failed to demonstrate any benefit.

Shark Cartilage. Shark cartilage received wide publicity, particularly after the publication of *Sharks Don't Get Cancer.* Research at MIT (1983)[13a] and in Japan (1990)[14a] on ocular tumor sites in rabbit models showed antiangiogenesis effect. Research conducted at the NCI showed some antiinflammatory response. The response depended on the cancer site and the dose used. Further studies are still pending to evaluate its benefits and use.

Vitamins such as B_6, C, E, folic acid, and coenzyme Q_{10} have been used for cancer treatment. The proposed mechanism of action is variable, but in general includes an antioxidant effect. Investigational studies looking into the effects of vitamins and minerals for treatment of cancer are pending. Some studies have demonstrated the benefit of acupuncture to alleviate postchemotherapy nausea.

AIDS

In many respects, patients with AIDS have been at the forefront of CAM. Studies looking at the use of CAM by patients with HIV indicate that approximately 70% of patients with HIV were using CAM therapies. The majority started using these therapies after learning that they were HIV-positive. Vitamins, herbal therapies, and dietary supplements were the most common therapies used. The major reasons CAM therapies were used were to boost immunity, fight infections, and treat nausea, diarrhea, and weight loss. Acupuncturists and massage therapists were the most common CAM providers visited. Pain relief, neuropathy, and stress relief were the major reasons for those visits. In addition to CAM therapies, 23.9% of patients with HIV reported using marijuana for nausea and weight loss. Patients learned about these therapies from friends, family, special organizations, newsletters, publications, and their physicians. Contrary to the general population, approximately 64% of patients with HIV infection informed their physicians about the visits and use of CAM therapies.[9]

Several clinics, universities, and organizations across the United States have been pioneering CAM treatment for patients with AIDS. Evidence to validate these therapies is still sparse and controversial. These therapies include:

1. Acetylcarnitine (2 to 3 gm/day) is used to treat lipodystrophy, a side effect of protease inhibitors.
2. Glutamine (20 to 40 gm/day) has been used to treat "leaky gut" associated with the damage to intestinal tissue. Several herbs have been used alone or in combination to control viral load: bitter melon, curcumin extract of tumeric plant, glycyrrhiza, and boxwood extract SPV-30. Initial data showed some promises of antiretroviral effect; however, follow-up studies were nonconclusive.
3. Meditation, yoga, and prayer have been used to decrease stress. Vitamins A, C, E, B_6, and B_{12}, zinc, selenium, coenzyme Q_{10}, L-carnitine, and dehydroepiandrosterone (DHEA) have been used to enhance the immune system and fight against oxidative stress. Evidence to support their use is controversial.
4. Low glutathione and thiol levels have been noted in patients with HIV. Supplementation with N-acetylcysteine (NAC) and sulfur amino acids has been used to restore the levels of reduced glutathione (GSH). An increase in the levels of T cells and inhibition of tumor necrosis factor (TNF) have also been proposed. Vitamin C in high doses has been used to treat HIV patients. The mechanism of action proposed is an increase in intracellular glutathione, which protects the immune system function from oxidative damage and inhibits viral replication.

Asthma

Current observer blinded crossover studies looking at the efficacy of chiropractic manipulation in the treatment of asthma do not show any difference in the pulmonary function tests between sham manipulation and chiropractic care. New studies looking at chiropractic manipulation and asthma are in progress, and data are pending.

Box 12-2. Guidelines for Choosing a CAM Provider

Graduate of an accredited college
Licensed, and in good standing
Limits practice to health problems within his or her scope of practice
Does not extend duration of care inappropriately
Communicates and collaborates with primary care physician

Studies looking at yoga suffer from several methodologic flaws and biases. Available studies show variable outcomes in respiratory function (peak expiratory flow rate [PEFR], forced expiratory volume in 1 second [FEV_1]) and decrease in heart and respiratory rates. Use of yoga, meditation, and biofeedback in stress-exacerbated mild to moderate asthma may be beneficial.

In Oriental medicine, asthma is due to a deficiency in lung, kidney, or spleen energy. The difference is based on the symptoms. In the majority of cases, acupuncture and herbal treatments (e.g., ma huang *[Ephedra herba],* astragalus, *Ginkgo biloba,* American ginseng, saiboko-to [herbal mixture]) are used. Information to support these therapies is minimal and controversial. The NIH consensus panel reviewing the world literature on acupuncture concluded that acupuncture is an acceptable adjunct treatment or could be helpful in a comprehensive treatment plan for asthma.

Naturopathic medicine considers that in addition to allergies, several factors impact chronic asthmatic conditions. These include hypoglycemia, hypothyroidism, hypochlorohydria, increased toxic load, decreased adrenal function, maldigestion, and inability to eliminate toxins. Treatment is directed toward addressing these factors. In addition to dietary and lifestyle changes, breathing exercises, stress reduction, aromatherapy, hydrotherapy, and supplements are used.

Antioxidants (vitamins A, C, and E, carotenes, and selenium) are also used to inhibit bronchial constriction and decrease the inflammatory response in asthma.

ETHICAL CONSIDERATION

CAM modalities derive from different cultures, health care principles, and paradigms. The therapeutics of many CAM modalities are not based on the biomedical principles but on several centuries of observations, trials, and errors. Until recently, most of the CAM modalities were practiced mainly by specific cultures, ethnic groups, and geographic areas. Incorporating these therapeutic modalities into the prevailing medical paradigm of a new culture and belief system may require a period of adaptation and modification.

The health care benefits of these different modalities may not be easily evaluated by the current scientific methods and principles. Certain modalities such as music therapy, imagery, and biofeedback are subject to personal attitudes, beliefs, and interpretation, and hence are very difficult to evaluate on the basis of the current biomedical and statistical methods.

Health care is regulated by the states. The definition of medical practice may differ between states. States license practitioners and define the scope of practice for different health care providers. Medical licensing offers a means of control by forcing providers to fulfill certain requirements before receiving a license to practice. By requiring a minimum level of competence, licensing provides some degree of quality control and protects consumers from charlatans. It also entails several risks, the groups involved in risk being (1) unlicensed providers, (2) physicians who refer patients to or employ unlicensed providers, and (3) licensed providers working outside the scope of their practice.

Patients have the right to quality-verified care. The patient's bill of rights states that patients have the right to receive information about the risks, benefits, costs, and alternative treatment modalities appropriate for their condition. In addition patients should receive guidance from their physician about the optimal treatment plan. Because the majority of CAM are not accepted as standards of car

Box 12-3. Resources for Providers

National Center for Complementary and Alternative Medicine (NCCAM)
Box 8218
Silver Springs, MD 20907
(888) 644-6226 Clearing House
http://altmed.od.nih.gov

American Botanical Council
P.O. Box 144345
Austin, TX 78714-4345
(512) 926-4900
http://www.herbalgram.org

The American Association of Naturopathic Physicians
2366 Eastlake Ave., Suite 322
Seattle, WA 98102
(206) 323-7610
http://www.infinite.org/naturopathic.physician

American Association of Oriental Medicine
433 Front St.
Catasauqua, PA 18032
http://www.aaom.org

The Council for Homeopathic Certification
1709 Seabright Ave.
Santa Cruz, CA 95062
(408) 421-0565

American Chiropractic Association
1701 Clarendon Blvd.
Arlington, VA 22209
(703) 761-2682
http://www.americhiro.com

Food and Drug Administration
5800 Fishers Lane
Rockville, MD 20857
(800) 332-1088
http://www.fda.gov

Office of Dietary Supplements
http://ods.od.nih.gov

physicians have no duty to inform their patients about therapy that is not generally recognized or accepted by the medical community. This opinion has been rendered by the courts in the case of Moore vs. Baker in 1992.

Recently some insurance companies included certain CAM modalities in their covered benefits. Chiropractic care and acupuncture are covered benefits in some plans.

What are the liabilities of physicians referring to a CAM provider? The same considerations applicable to all referrals apply to referral to CAM. Physicians may be held liable (1) if they refer patients to CAM therapies that they know, or should know, have limited or no benefit to the patient, or (2) when the CAM therapist provides negligent or harmful care while practicing under the supervision of the physician.

State legislatures often look to professional organizations for guidance and oversight of licensing and accreditation. When recognized and licensed in a state, the courts apply the standards of care guided by standards from experts in that field of practice. If unlicensed by that state, the courts will tend to judge CAM practitioners according to the conventional standard of care. For guidelines for choosing a CAM provider see Box 12-2.

SUMMARY

The popularity and use of CAM is on the rise. WHO estimates that 80% of the world's population use traditional medicine for their care. In the United States 40% of the population use CAM as part of their health care. Over the last decade an increasing number of patients, physicians, and insurance carriers have embraced aspects of CAM. The current scientific literature is limited and controversial. The NCCAM at the NIH has funded several research centers across the United States to evaluate and review the merits of CAM. Research that provides sound scientific evidence to support or refute the therapeutic effectiveness of CAM is necessary. Until more scientific evidence is available, physicians should proceed with caution, as they would do with any new therapy or treatment. It is important to keep an open mind, being willing to learn and review scientific evidence about CAM. Several CAM therapies have been accepted and integrated into the current standards of care. As research and experience with CAM blossom, new modalities will be included for specific medical problems. The future of medicine will include an integrated health care system where scientifically proven CAM will be practiced and provided alongside the current dominant medical system. For information about resources for providers see Box 12-3.

REFERENCES

1. Acupuncture: NIH Consensus Conference, *JAMA* 280:1518-1524, 1998. And Statement Online 1997 November 3-5; *http://odp.od.nih.gov/consensus/cons/107/107 statement.htm*
2. Aker PD, Gross AR, Goldsmith CH, et al: Conservative management of mechanical neck pain: systematic overview and meta-analysis, *BMJ* 313(7068):1291-1296, 1996.
3. Astin JA: *Why patients use alternative medicine: results of a national study, JAMA* 279(19):1548-1553, 1998.
4. Begbie SD, Kerestes ZK, Bell DR: Patterns of alternative medicine use by cancer patients, *MJA* 165:545-548, 1996.
5. Carlston M, Stuart M, Jonas W: Alternative medicine instruction in medical schools and family practice residency programs, *Fam Med* 29(8):559-562, 1997.
6. Cherkin D, Mootz R: Chiropractic in the United States: training, practice and research, *AHCPR,* Pub. No. 98-N002, 1997.

6a. Elder NC, Gillcrist A, Minz R: Use of alternative health care by family practice patients, *Arch Fam Med* 6(2):181-184, 1997.

7. Eisenberg DM, Davis RB, Ettner SL, et al: Trends in alternative medicine use in the United States, 1990-1997: results of a follow-up national survey, *JAMA* 280:1569-1575, 1998.
8. Elion RA, Cohen C: Complementary medicine and HIV infection, *Prim Care,* 24(4):905-919, 1997.
9. Fairfield KM, Eisenberg DM, Davis RB, et al: Patterns of use, expenditures, and perceived efficacy of complementary and alternative therapies in HIV-infected patients, *Arch Intern Med* 158:2257-2264, 1998.
10. Hill C, Doyen F: *Rev Epidemiol Sante Publique* 38(2):139-147, 1990.
11. Kleijnen J, et al: *BMJ* 302:316-323, 1991.
12. Koes BW, Assendelft WJ, van der Heijden GJ, et al: Spinal manipulation and mobilisation for back and neck pain: a blinded review, *BMJ* 303(6813):1298-1303, 1991.
13. Koes BW, Assendelft WJ, van der Heijden GJ, et al: Spinal manipulation for low back pain: an updated systematic review of randomized clinical trials, *Spine* 21(24):2860-2871, 2872-2873, 1996.

13a. Lee A, Langer R: Shark cartilage contains inhibitors of tumor angiogenesis, *Science* 221(4616):1185-1187, 1983.

14. Linde K, et al: *Lancet* 350:834-843, 1997.

14a. Oikawa T, Ashino-Fuse H, Shimamura M, et al: A novel angiogenic inhibitor derived from Japanese shark cartilage. I. Extraction and estimation of inhibitory activities toward tumor and embryonic angiogenesis, *Cancer Letters* 51(3):181-186, 1990.

15. Panel on Definition and Description, CAM Research Methodology Conference, April 1995: Defining and describing complementary and alternative medicine, *Altern Ther* 3(2):49-57, 1997.
16. Rampes H, James R: Complications of acupuncture, *Acupunct Med13(1):26-33, 1995.*
17. Shekelle PG, Adams AH, Chassin MR, et al: Spinal manipulation for low-back pain, *Ann Intern Med,* 117(7):590-598, 1992.
18. Verhoef MJ, Sutherland LR, Brkich L: Use of alternative medicine by patients attending a gastroenterology clinic, *CMAJ* 142(2):121-125, 1990.

ADDITIONAL READINGS

General

Jonas WB, Levin JS, editors: *Essentials of complementary and alternative medicine*, Baltimord, 1999, Williams & Wilkins.

Micozzi MS: *Fundamentals of complementary and alternative medicine,* New York, 1996, Churchill-Livingstone.

Spencer JW, Jacobs JJ: *Complementary/alternative medicine: an evidence-based approach,* St Louis, 1998, Mosby.

Vincent C, Furham A: *Complementary medicine: a research perspective,* New York, 1997, Wiley.

Herbals/Nutrition

Blumenthal M, Buse WR, Goldberg A, et al: *The complete German Commission E monographs: therapeutic guide to herbal medicines,* Austin, TX, 1998, American Botanical Council.

Lawson LD, Bauer R, editors: *Phytomedicines of Europe: chemistry and biology activity,* Washington, DC, 1998, American Chemical Society.

McGuffin M, Hobbs C, Upton R, Goldberg A: *American Herbal Products Association's botanical safety handbook,* Boca Raton, Fla, 1997, CRC.

The review of natural products, St Louis, 1999, Facts and Comparisons, (800) 223-0554.

Homeopathy

Ernst E, Hahn EG, editors: *Homeopathy: a critical appraisal,* Oxford, 1998, Butterworth Heinemann.

Leckridge B: *Homeopathy in primary care,* New York, 1997, Churchill-Livingstone.

Manual

Phillips RB, Mootz RD, Hadelman S, editors: *Contemporary chiropractic philosophy: principles and practice of chiropractic,* ed 2, Norwalk, Conn, 1992, Appleton & Lang.

Ethics/Legal

Cohen MH: *Complementary and alternative medicine: legal boundaries and regulatory perspectives,* Baltimore, 1998, Johns Hopkins.

Humber JH, Almeder RF: *Alternative medicine and ethics*, Totowa, NJ, 1998, Humana Press.

Others

Benson H: *Timeless healing: the power and biology of belief*, New York, 1996, Fireside.

Boik J: *Cancer and natural medicine: a textbook of basic science and clinical research*, Princeton, Minn, 1996, Oregan Medical.

Dossey L: *Healing words: the power of prayer and the practice of medicine*, San Francisco, 1993, Harper Collins.

Gordon JS: *Manifesto for a new medicine: your guide to healing partnerships and the wise use of alternative therapies*, Reading, Ma, 1996, Addison-Wesely.

CHAPTER 13

Medical Evaluation of the Patient Undergoing Surgery

James J. Heffernan
Robert A. Witzburg
Gerald W. Smetana

Consultation practice is an important component of many physicians' professional activity. Up to 30% of the clinical activity of general internists and up to 50% of the patient care activities of selected medical subspecialists may be devoted to consultation. The continued growth of managed care may increase the role of primary care physicians on surgical services. Denial of preoperative hospital days by health insurers has already shifted preoperative evaluation of patients undergoing elective surgery to the outpatient setting, sometimes to specialized preoperative clinics and sometimes to the clinical practice sites of primary care physicians.

Effective interaction with colleagues in other specialties requires a thorough grounding in the language and science of these other disciplines, as well as an awareness of basic guidelines for consultation (Box 13-1). The consultant's role in perioperative care focuses on those medical factors that may increase the risks of anesthesia and surgery, with the formulation of a management plan to minimize risk.

Continued advances in the techniques of anesthesia and surgery have made surgical death very uncommon. In the United States, expected perioperative mortality (during surgery or within the first 48 hours postoperatively) is less than 0.03% in healthy adults younger than 70 years undergoing elective surgery. Of all perioperative deaths, 10% to 15% occur during anesthesia induction, 30% to 40% during surgery, and the remaining 45% to 60% during the subsequent 48 hours. This broad temporal distribution of perioperative mortality dictates the need for medical vigilance well into the recovery phase.

Systematic assessment of surgical risk requires the identification of anesthesia-related, procedure-related, practitioner-related, and, especially, patient-related factors. No one method of anesthesia appropriate for major procedures is inherently safer than another. The selection of anesthetic technique for a given patient, procedure, surgeon, and anesthetist is highly individualized and remains the primary responsibility of the anesthesiologist rather than of the consultant.

Certain procedures carry a higher risk, such as craniotomy and cardiovascular surgery, whereas others carry a lower risk, such as herniorrhaphy, cystoscopy, cervical dilation and curettage, and ophthalmologic surgery. The importance of comorbid disease in determining surgical risk may outweigh the nature of the procedure in predicting outcome. Any procedure conducted as an emergency carries an increased risk—as much as twice the expected mortality for similar surgery performed electively.

Several protocols have been developed for estimating an overall, integrated risk profile for patients subjected to general anesthesia and surgery. The traditional and most widely utilized classification system is that of the American Society of Anesthesiologists (ASA), which can assist in risk stratification (Table 13-1). This schema is predicated on a global assessment of the patient's medical problems and functional status. Clinical studies have demonstrated that a patient's functional status, especially exercise capacity, is an excellent and independent predictor of surgical outcome, most likely as a reflection of overall cardiopulmonary reserve. Patients in higher risk classes generally require more intensive preoperative evaluation and more vigilant perioperative management.

PREOPERATIVE EVALUATION OF THE HEALTHY PATIENT

Healthy patients may undergo surgery with an extremely low risk of morbidity and mortality. Patient- and procedure-related factors contribute more to risk than anesthetic considerations. Perioperative mortality in ASA class I patients is less than 0.03%. Recent surveys suggest an even lower risk. In a study of patients undergoing ambulatory surgery, there were no deaths among 14,609 ASA class I patients.[18] Since the risk is extremely low in healthy patients, extensive preoperative evaluation does not often bring to light factors that increase risk. Furthermore, most abnormal findings are false-positives. One may identify a higher risk subset of healthy patients through the use of a screening questionnaire, a focused clinical evaluation, and selective laboratory testing.

The primary goal of preoperative evaluation is to identify previously unrecognized illness that may have an impact on surgical risk. Preoperative screening questionnaires correctly identify most patients who are at higher than average risk. With one such questionnaire, negative answers to all questions predicted fitness for surgery in 96% of cases, as determined by the clinical evaluation of 10 staff anesthesiologists (Box 13-2).

Poor exercise capacity identifies patients at higher risk for overall morbidity, as well as cardiac and pulmonary complications. Patients who are unable to walk at least two blocks on level ground are at higher risk.

Screening Blood Tests

Most routine preoperative laboratory tests are performed out of habit and are not justified by evidence in the medical literature. These tests are costly in the aggregate and may lead to patient worry and unnecessary delay of surgery. Physicians can usually predict abnormal results based on a patient's known medical problems; routine preoperative laboratory testing rarely influences management. In a study of 20

Box 13-1. Guidelines for Consultation Practice

Complete a prompt, thorough, generalist-oriented evaluation.
Respond specifically to the question(s) posed.
Indicate clearly the perioperative importance of any observations and recommendations outside the area of initial concern.
Provide focused, detailed, and precise diagnostic and therapeutic guidance.
Communicate verbally with the anesthesiologist and surgeon, particularly to resolve complex issues.
Avoid chart notations that unnecessarily create or exacerbate regulatory or medicolegal risk.
Employ frequent follow-up visits in difficult cases to monitor clinical status and compliance with recommendations.

Modified from Witzburg RA: In *Medical knowledge self-assessment program IX*, Philadelphia, 1991, American College of Physicians.

patients, only 0.22% of routine preoperative blood tests were of potential surgical significance.[9] None of these abnormalities were recognized and acted on prior to surgery and there were no adverse consequences. Other authors have reported similar results.

Suggested routine blood tests include a pregnancy test for women who may be pregnant, hematocrit if expected major blood loss, and a serum creatinine measurement if hypotension is likely or the patient is over age 50 years. One should not obtain serum glucose, urinalysis, liver function tests, electrolytes, or tests of hemostasis routinely in the preoperative evaluation of the healthy patient.

Other preoperative laboratory screenings should be driven by the history of underlying illness, with directed laboratory evaluation in the setting of known or suspected renal impairment; liver disease; metabolic disease, especially diabetes mellitus; hemorrhagic or thromboembolic diatheses; or treatment with medications known to cause metabolic derangements, especially diuretics.

Results of tests performed in the preceding 4 months may be safely substituted for preoperative screening tests if the previous results were normal and there is no obvious clinical indication for retesting.

Electrocardiogram

Patients with certain abnormal findings on electrocardiogram (ECG) have an increased risk of postoperative cardiac complications. These abnormalities include Q waves of indeterminate age, more than 5 premature ventricular contractions per minute, atrial ectopy, and a rhythm other than sinus. These findings are more often present in patients who are older, have known cardiac disease, or have diabetes. Clinically important ECG findings in patients under age 45 are rare. We support the recommendations first proposed by Goldberger and O'Konski (Box 13-3).

Chest Radiograph

The frequency of abnormal chest radiographs increases with age. The reported rates of abnormal preoperative chest radiographs vary from 1.2% to 52.9% among patients in different clinical series. Most abnormal studies, however, do not influence perioperative management. In a meta-analysis including a total of 14,390 routine chest radiographs, there were only 140 unexpected abnormal studies and only 14 studies that influenced management.[3] Recent data suggest that patients undergoing abdominal surgery who have abnormal chest radiographs have a higher likelihood of postoperative pulmonary complications. Reasonable criteria for obtaining a preoperative chest radiograph include age greater than 60 years or suspicion of cardiac or pulmonary disease on the basis of history and examination.

Table 13-1. Physical Status Scale of the American Society of Anesthesiologists

Class	Physical status
I	Normal healthy person under age 80
II	Mild systemic disease or healthy person 80 or older
III	Severe but not incapacitating systemic disease
IV	Incapacitating systemic disease that is a constant threat to life
V	Moribund patient not expected to survive 24 hours despite surgery
E	Suffix to any class indicating emergency surgery

Box 13-2. Questionnaire to Identify Potential Risk Among Healthy Surgical Patients

Do you feel unwell?
Have you had any serious illnesses in the past?
Do you get more short of breath on exertion than other people of your own age?
Do you have any cough?
Do you have any wheeze?
Do you have any chest pain on exertion?
Do you have any ankle swelling?
Have you taken any medications or pills in the last 3 months (including excess alcohol)?
Have you any allergies?
Have you had an anesthetic in the last 2 months?
Have you or your relatives had any problems with a previous anesthetic?
Observation of serious abnormality from "end of bed" (which might affect anesthetic)
Date of last menstrual period

Modified from Wilson ME, Williams NB, Baskett PJF, et al: Assessment of fitness for surgical procedures and the variability of anaesthetists' judgments, *Br Med J* 1:509-512, 1980.

CARDIOVASCULAR RISK ASSESSMENT AND MODIFICATION

Risk Assessment

Cardiac complications are the leading cause of morbidity and mortality in the perioperative period. All requests for preoperative medical evaluation should include an assessment of cardiac risk. In most cases, a careful history and physical examination are sufficient to assess risk.

Box 13-3. Clinical Indications for Selective Ordering of Preoperative ECGs

Men older than 45 years, women older than 55 years
History of clinically important heart disease, including dysrhythmias
Conditions associated with heart disease, especially peripheral vascular disease
Conditions predisposing to heart disease, such as diabetes mellitus
Potentially cardiotoxic medications
Intrathoracic, intraperitoneal, aortic, or emergency surgery
Predisposition toward electrolyte abnormalities

Modified from Goldberger AL, O'Konski M: Utility of the routine electrocardiogram before surgery and on general hospital admission, *Ann Intern Med* 105:552-557, 1986.

In 1977, Goldman and colleagues first outlined the principal cardiac risk factors in their groundbreaking report of a multifactorial cardiac risk index.[8] This study demonstrated that a myocardial infarction within the previous 6 months and congestive heart failure at the time of surgery were the two most important predictors of cardiac risk. Among possible findings of congestive heart failure, only jugular venous distention and an S3 were correlated with an increased risk. Other independent risk factors in the multivariate analysis included age greater than 70 years, rhythm other than sinus, frequent premature ventricular beats, significant aortic stenosis, and poor general medical status as defined by several metabolic parameters. In addition, there was a higher risk with thoracic, abdominal, aortic, and all emergency procedures. One can assign a total number of points based on the strength of each factor in the multivariate analysis. Patients are grouped into one of four risk categories. This index has been repeatedly validated prospectively and correctly estimates risk among patients undergoing nonvascular surgery. Factors that do not increase risk in the Goldman analysis include stable hypertension, stable angina, diabetes, elevated cholesterol, and cigarette smoking.

Limitations of the Goldman index include an underestimation of risk in vascular surgical procedures, absence of unstable angina or angina at low workload as risk factors, and an underappreciation of the risk associated with significant aortic stenosis. Detsky and colleagues developed a modified index that addresses the last two of these concerns (Table 13-2).

In general, patients who are able to perform at least Canadian Cardiovascular Society class II activities without limitation or cardiac symptoms have an average risk of postoperative cardiac complications. Examples of class II activities include the ability to walk two blocks on level ground or to carry two bags of groceries up one flight of stairs. Exercise testing is no more predictive of cardiac complications than a reliable history of exercise tolerance and should not be a routine preoperative test.

Recently the American College of Cardiology (ACC) and the American Heart Association (AHA) proposed a new cardiac risk assessment guideline grounded in an evidence-

Table 13-2. Modified Cardiac Risk Index*

Variable	Points, *n*
Coronary artery disease	
Myocardial infarction < 6 months earlier	10
Myocardial infarction > 6 months earlier	5
Canadian Cardiovascular Society angina classification†	
Class III	10
Class IV	20
Unstable angina within 6 months	10
Alveolar pulmonary edema	
Within 1 week	10
Ever	5
Suspected critical aortic stenosis	20
Dysrhythmias	
Rhythm other than sinus or sinus plus atrial premature beats on ECG	5
> Five premature ventricular contractions on ECG	5
Poor general medical status, defined as any of the following:	
Po_2 < 60 mm Hg, pCO_2 > 50 mm Hg, K^+ level < 3 mEq/l, HCO_3 < 20 mEq/l, blood urea nitrogen > 50 mg/dl, creatinine level > 3 mg/dl, abnormal SGOT, signs of chronic liver disease, bedridden	5
Age > 70 years	5
Emergency surgery	10

*Class I = 0 to 15 points; class II = 20 to 30 points; class III = more than 30 points.
†Canadian Cardiovascular Society classification of angina: 0 = asymptomatic; I = angina with strenuous exercise; II = angina with moderate exertion; III = angina with walking one to two level blocks or climbing one flight of stairs or less at a normal pace; IV = inability to perform any physical activity without development of angina.
Modified from Detsky AS et al: Predicting cardiac complications in patients undergoing non-cardiac surgery, *J Gen Intern Med* 1:211-219, 1986.

based review of the available medical literature.[1] This guideline includes an assessment of functional capacity, clinical predictors of risk, and procedure-related risks. These factors are incorporated into a complex algorithm designed to identify those patients who may proceed directly to surgery and those who will benefit from preoperative cardiac testing. This algorithm has been validated in a prospective study of high-risk patients.

In 1997, the American College of Physicians (ACP) published a cardiac risk assessment guideline, also developed after evidence-based review of the literature[2,15] (Figs. 13-1 and 13-2). Practicing physicians will likely find this guideline easier to use than the ACC/AHA proposal. According to the ACP guideline, all patients are stratified by the Detsky modified risk index. For risk class II or III patients, strategies for risk reduction are individualized based on the nature of the risk. For risk class I patients undergoing vascular surgery, one applies additional clinical risk variables to identify patients who would benefit from further study (Table 13-3). Low-risk patients may proceed directly to surgery. We recommend the use of this guideline for preoperative cardiac risk stratification.

In 1999, Lee and colleagues proposed a revised cardiac index based on a prospective study of 4315 patients undergoing elective major noncardiac procedures.[10a] In their multivariate analysis of derivation and validation cohorts different risk factors emerged than in previous analyses. Si

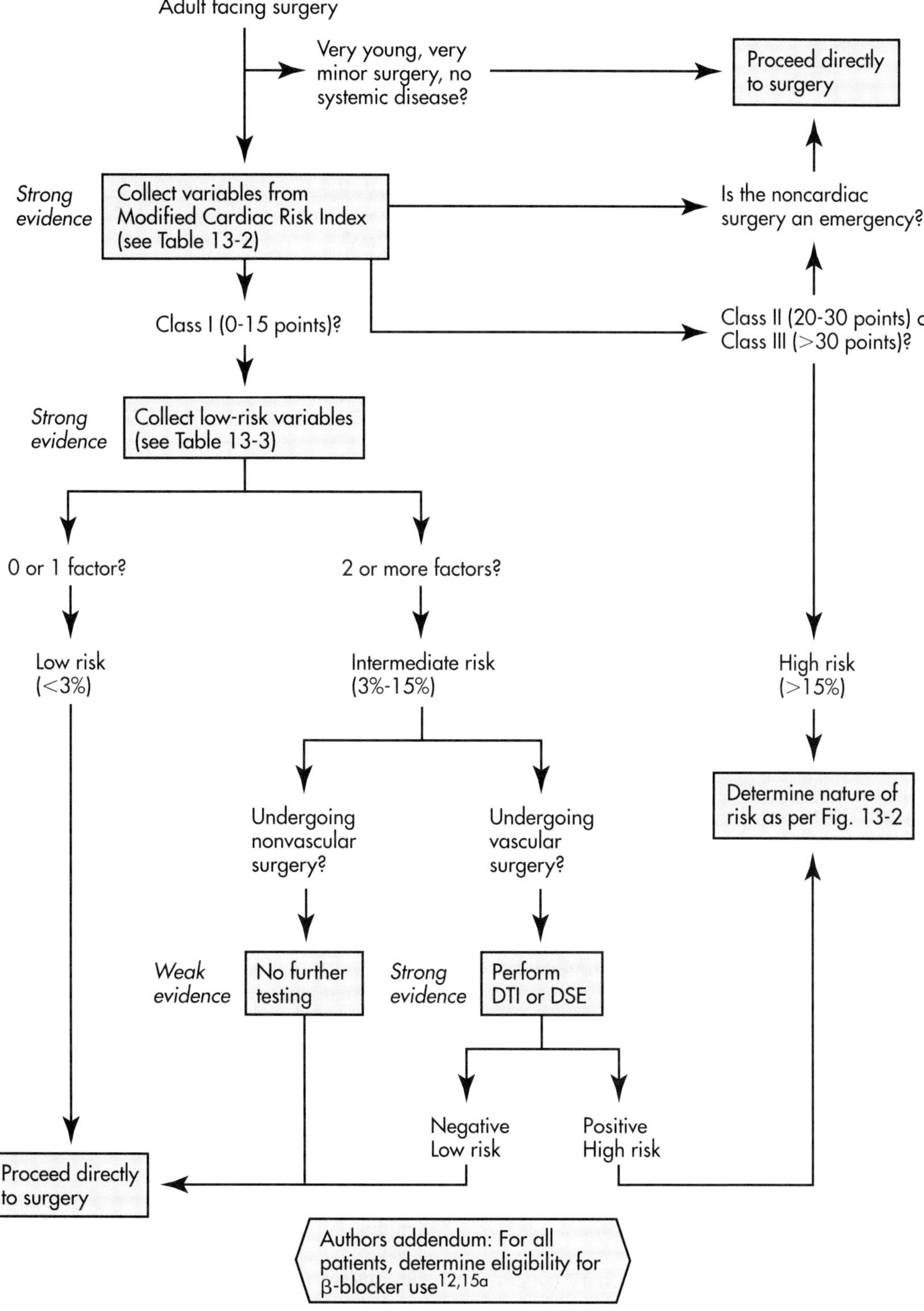

Fig. 13-1. Suggested algorithm for the risk assessment and management of patients at low or intermediate risk for perioperative cardiac events, usually myocardial infarction and death. Boxed phrases indicate recommended actions. The italicized words beside the boxes indicate the level of evidence supporting the recommendation. If no italicized word is present, no evidence exists for or against use. *DTI,* Dipyridamole thallium imaging; *DSE,* dobutamine stress echocardiography. (Modified from American College of Physicians: Guidelines for assessing and managing the perioperative risk from coronary artery disease associated with major noncardiac surgery, *Ann Intern Med* 127:309-312, 1997.)

factors equally predicted risk and were assigned one point each in the revised index. These factors included high-risk surgery (intraperitoneal, intrathoracic, or suprainguinal vascular), ischemic heart disease, history of congestive heart failure, history of cerebrovascular disease, insulin therapy for diabetes, or preoperative serum creatinine > 2 mg/dl. Postoperative cardiac complication rates were 0.4%, 0.9%, 7%, and 11% among patients with no, one, two, or ≥ three factors, respectively. The revised cardiac risk index outperformed the original Goldman index, the Detsky modified

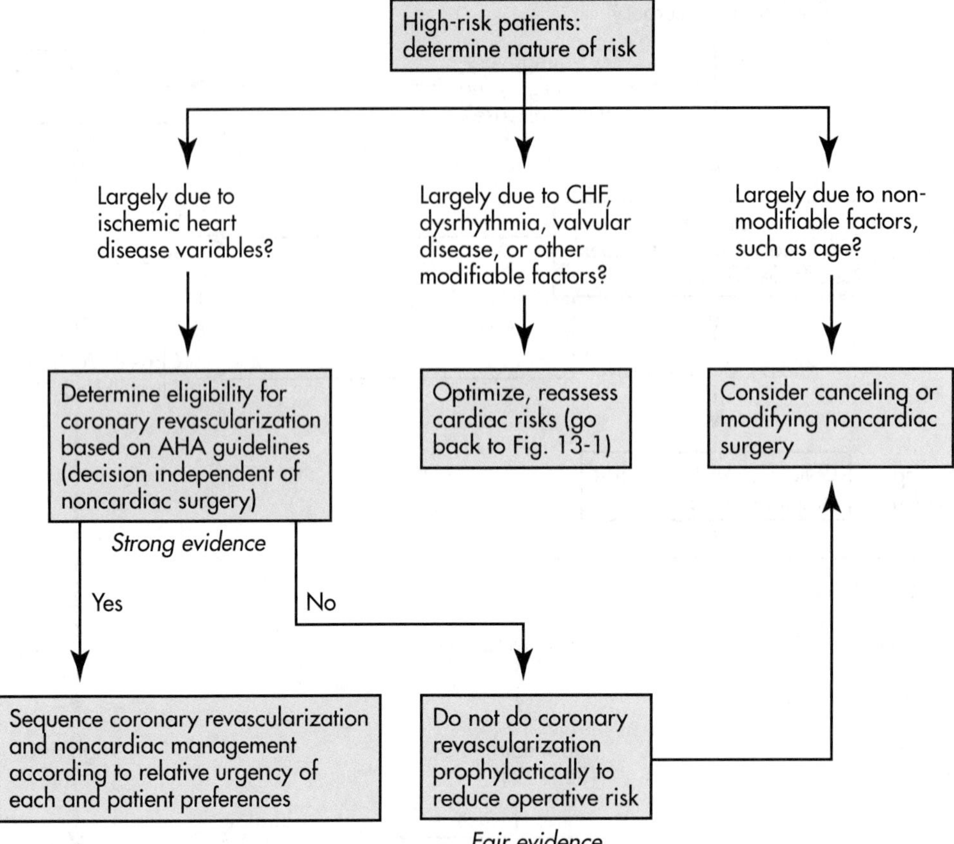

Fig. 13-2. Suggested algorithm for the management of patients at high risk for perioperative cardiac events. Boxed phrases indicate recommended actions. The italicized words below the boxes indicate the level of evidence supporting the recommendation. If no italicized word is present, no evidence exists for or against use. *AHA*, American Heart Association; *CHF*, congestive heart failure. (Modified from American College of Physicians: Guidelines for assessing and managing the perioperative risk from coronary artery disease associated with major noncardiac surgery, *Ann Intern Med* 127:309-312, 1997.)

index, and the ASA classification in the prediction of cardiac risk in the validation cohort. Whether physicians will use this index in lieu of other established indices in the initial estimation of cardiac risk remains to be determined.

Strategies to Reduce Perioperative Cardiac Risk

Risk reduction strategies follow logically from the well-known risk factors. Physicians should delay elective surgery until at least 6 months after a myocardial infarction. Six to 12 weeks following myocardial infarction, semielective surgery may be considered after a cardiac functional assessment such as an exercise test. One should diurese patients in congestive heart failure until there is no pulmonary congestion but not so aggressively as to lead to orthostasis. There is no evidence to support routine antidysrhythmic therapy for patients whose risk is based on the presence of atrial or ventricular ectopy. One should evaluate all patients with aortic stenosis that is severe on physical examination or symptomatic. Each metabolic abnormality in the general medical status risk category should be corrected if possible. Finally, one may consider a less ambitious procedure for patients at high risk with few other opportunities for risk reduction.

The most important recent observation in this field is that the perioperative use of atenolol reduces risk among patients at high risk.[12] Eligible patients were those with known coronary artery disease or with at least two of the following risk factors: age greater than 65 years, hypertension, current smoking, cholesterol greater than 240 mg/dl, and diabetes. The authors excluded patients with congestive heart failure, bronchospasm, or third-degree heart block. Thirty minutes before surgery and again immediately after surgery, the study group received 5-mg intravenous atenolol, followed in 5 minutes by a second infusion if tolerated clinically by the systolic blood pressure (>100 mm Hg) and the pulse (>55). Similarly as tolerated, the patient received 50- to 100-mg oral atenolol daily until discharge, up to a maximum of 7 days. One-year all-cause mortality was 3% in the atenolol group and 14% in the placebo group. The ACP guideline recommends perioperative atenolol for patients who meet the criteria of this study.

Recently, another study confirmed the benefit of perioperative β-blockers in high-risk patients undergoing major vascular surgery.[15a] Eligible patients had at least one cardiac risk factor and a positive dobutamine echocardiogram. Study patients received oral bisoprolol beginning at least 1 week before surgery and continuing for 30 days after surgery. If unable to take oral medications in the immediate perioperative period, intravenous metoprolol was used instead to keep the heart rate below 80 beats per minute. The combined incidence of cardiac death and nonfatal myocardial infarction was 34% in the standard-care group and 3.4% in the

Table 13-3. Low-Risk Variables

Criteria of Eagle et al*	Criteria of Vanzetto et al†
Age > 70 years	Age > 70 years
History of angina	History of angina
Diabetes mellitus	Diabetes mellitus
Q waves on ECG	Q waves on ECG
History of ventricular ectopy	History of myocardial infarction
	ST-segment ischemic abnormalities during resting ECG
	Hypertension with severe left ventricular hypertrophy
	History of congestive heart failure

*Eagle KA, et al: Combining clinical and thallium data optimizes preoperative assessment of cardiac risk before major vascular surgery, *Ann Intern Med* 110:859-866, 1989.

†Vanzetto G, et al: Additive value of thallium single-photon emission computed tomography myocardial imaging for prediction of perioperative events in clinically selected high risk patients having abdominal aortic surgery, *Am J Cardiol* 77:143-148, 1996.

bisoprolol group. This dramatic risk reduction was similar in magnitude to that previously reported in the atenolol study.

No prospective trials have evaluated the potential benefit of coronary revascularization prior to noncardiac surgery. In a retrospective review of the Coronary Artery Surgery Study (CASS) experience, the risk of coronary bypass surgery among patients with stable angina approximately equaled the reduction of risk in subsequent noncardiac surgery. There are no studies of percutaneous transluminal coronary angioplasty (PTCA) prior to noncardiac surgery. Both the ACP and AHA/ACC guidelines recommend preoperative coronary revascularization only for those patients who have an indication independent of the need for noncardiac surgery. The data suggest that perioperative β-blockade is more likely to reduce cardiac morbidity than preoperative coronary revascularization.

PULMONARY RISK ASSESSMENT AND MODIFICATION

Postoperative pulmonary complications are as frequent as cardiac complications and are an important component of overall perioperative risk. Important complications include prolonged mechanical ventilation, pneumonia, atelectasis, bronchospasm, and exacerbation of chronic lung disease. In recent years, studies have identified the principal risk factors for pulmonary complications. These may be divided into patient-related and procedure-related risk factors. (Pulmonary embolism, which has different risk factors, is discussed later.)

Patient-related risk factors include smoking, poor general health status, and chronic obstructive pulmonary disease (COPD). Current cigarette smokers have a twofold to sixfold higher risk of pulmonary complications than nonsmokers. Patients who stop smoking for less than 8 weeks prior to surgery have an unexpectedly higher risk of pulmonary complications than current smokers. Physicians should therefore encourage patients to stop smoking for at least 8 weeks prior to elective surgery.

Patients with poorer general health and functional capacity are at higher risk. A high Goldman cardiac-risk index, ASA class greater than 2, and poor exercise capacity are all predictors of higher risk. Advanced age and obesity are not significant risk factors when one controls for comorbid conditions.

Well-controlled asthma does not increase the risk of postoperative pulmonary complications significantly. Patients with asthma should be treated aggressively to reduce airflow obstruction. Patients should achieve a peak flow of at least 80% of predicted or of their personal best. Corticosteroids, if necessary, may be safely used to achieve this goal without an increase in the risk of surgical site infections.

Patients with COPD have a threefold to fivefold increase in postoperative pulmonary complications. This risk may be reduced by the same treatment one would use for an exacerbation of COPD in the nonoperative setting. Studies support a beneficial effect of multimodality treatment including bronchodilators, chest physical therapy, smoking cessation, and corticosteroids. Patients with symptomatic COPD should receive inhaled ipratropium and supplemental inhaled β-agonists. Although not all patients with COPD respond to systemic corticosteroids, one should consider this treatment if the patient is not at his or her best personal baseline and symptoms are not reduced optimally with other therapies. Physicians should use antibiotics only if respiratory infection is suspected; they do not reduce risk in unselected patients with COPD prior to surgery.

The most important predictor of risk of pulmonary complications is the surgical site. Upper abdominal and thoracic procedures carry the highest risk as a result of splinting and diaphragmatic dysfunction. The average risk of pulmonary complications in upper abdominal, lower abdominal, and thoracic surgeries is 25%, 10%, and 20%, respectively. Pulmonary complications occur in fewer than 1% of patients undergoing laparoscopic cholecystectomy. There is a low risk for all surgeries outside of the chest and abdomen. Other surgical risk factors include surgery lasting longer than 3 hours, the use of general anesthesia, and the use of the long-acting neuromuscular blocker pancuronium.

Physical examination findings that identify patients at higher risk include decreased breath sounds, dullness to percussion, wheezes, rhonchi, and a prolonged expiratory phase.

Despite decades of study, the role of pulmonary function testing prior to surgery remains controversial. Although these studies are clearly valuable prior to lung resection, their predictive value prior to other surgeries is debated. Authors who support the routine use of spirometry suggest a higher risk for patients with a forced expiratory volume in one second (FEV_1) or forced vital capacity (FVC) of less than 70% of the predicted value, or an FEV_1 to FVC ratio of less than 65%.

Several recent studies have shown no increased risk of postoperative pulmonary complications among patients with abnormal spirometry. A recent case-control study found clinical variables to be more predictive of pulmonary complications than spirometry.[10] These variables were abnormal chest examination, abnormal chest radiograph, a high Goldman score, and a high score on the Charlson comorbidity index. There was no difference in the frequency of abnormal spirometry between the complication and control groups.

Other authors have reported acceptable risks of perioperative morbidity in patients with COPD and abnormal spirometry. Because clinical evaluation may be more

Box 13-4. Strategies to Reduce the Risk of Postoperative Pulmonary Complications

Preoperative

Encourage cessation of cigarette smoking for at least 8 weeks
Treat airflow obstruction in patients with COPD or asthma
Administer antibiotics and delay surgery if respiratory infection is present
Begin patient education regarding lung expansion maneuvers

Intraoperative

Limit duration of surgery to less than 3 hours
Use spinal or epidural anesthesia*
Avoid use of pancuronium
Use laparoscopic procedures when possible
Substitute less ambitious procedure for upper abdominal or thoracic surgery when possible

Postoperative

Use deep-breathing exercises or incentive spirometry
Use continuous positive airway pressure
Use epidural analgesia*
Use intercostal nerve blocks*

*This strategy is recommended, although variable efficacy has been reported in the literature.

Modified from Smetana GW: Preoperative pulmonary evaluation, *N Engl J Med* 340:937-944, 1999.

predictive of complications than spirometry, and risks are acceptable even in high-risk patients as defined by spirometry, spirometric results should not be used to deny surgery.

Physicians should employ risk reduction strategies for patients undergoing upper abdominal or thoracic surgery who have other risk factors for complications. Postoperative strategies include lung expansion maneuvers, such as chest physical therapy or deep-breathing exercises, and pain control by either postoperative epidural analgesia or intercostal nerve blocks. Lung expansion maneuvers reduce the risk by one half. There have been mixed reports of the benefit of pain control. Strategies to reduce the risk of postoperative pulmonary complications are summarized in Box 13-4.

PREVENTION OF BACTERIAL ENDOCARDITIS

Patients with valvular heart disease, hypertrophic cardiomyopathy, most congenital cardiac lesions, and systemic-pulmonary shunts should receive endocarditis prophylaxis before certain surgical or dental procedures. The risk of endocarditis in a given patient depends on the type and severity of the underlying cardiac condition, the specific nature of the surgical or dental procedure to be performed, and its association, if any, with bacteremia (Box 13-5). α-Hemolytic streptococci *(Streptococcus viridans)* and related organisms are the leading cause of endocarditis following dental and respiratory tract procedures, whereas enterococci pose the greatest risk of endocarditis in patients undergoing genitourinary, gynecologic, or gastrointestinal procedures. The standard of care has shifted toward a single preoperative dose of one or two clinically appropriate antibiotics (Table 13-4).

HEMODYNAMIC MONITORING

Substantial reductions in perioperative cardiovascular complications and mortality have been noted among patients undergoing noncardiac surgery over the past 40 years. Perioperative mortality among patients over 80 years of age has dropped from 20% in 1960 to approximately 6%,[5] and perioperative cardiac reinfarction within 3 months of initial myocardial infarction has dropped from 30% to 5.8%.[16] These reductions are probably due in part to pulmonary artery catheter monitoring, although there are no prospective, randomized trials assessing the benefit of pulmonary artery catheter monitoring among general surgery patients. Several trials have demonstrated significant benefit among peripheral vascular surgery patients. Reasonable criteria for selecting patients in whom perioperative central hemodynamic monitoring appears warranted include recent (within 6 months) myocardial infarction; clinically apparent congestive heart failure, or suspected congestive heart failure in a patient requiring emergency surgery; severe aortic or mitral stenosis; planned major vascular surgical procedure in the setting of coronary heart disease; pulmonary edema of unknown etiology; and patients scheduled for coronary revascularization if they have any of the following: (1) recent myocardial infarction, (2) poor left ventricular function, (3) severe/unstable angina, or (4) high-grade left main coronary artery stenosis.

PERIOPERATIVE DRUG THERAPY

Questions regarding the manipulation of ongoing drug treatment constitute some of the most common and difficult issues in perioperative consultation. Often, the literature does not support clear, forceful articulation of guidelines, and the internist must tailor management to individual circumstances. In general, three factors must be considered in managing each situation: (1) Have the indications and dosages for the specific drug been clearly defined? (2) What are the likely anesthetic and surgical complications/interactions? (3) Is a clinically important withdrawal syndrome likely, and how can it be safely managed?

Most drugs used in the management of chronic medical illness should be continued through the perioperative period. For minor procedures the patient can receive an oral dose with sips of water on the morning of surgery and another dose later in the day as indicated. For more difficult surgery with a prolonged recovery period, long-acting or parenteral substitutes for chronic therapy may be needed.

PROPHYLACTIC ANTIMICROBIAL THERAPY

Elective surgery should be delayed until preexisting bacterial infections are treated. Bacterial colonization or infection of the urinary tract is relatively common, especially among individuals with a history of urinary tract infection, in those with indwelling catheters, in those with atonic bladders or obstructive uropathy, and among the elderly. A preoperative screening urinalysis and, when the urinalysis is abnormal, a culture with antibiotic sensitivities, are appropriate in such patients. To reduce the likelihood of perioperative urosepsis, treatment should be initiated with an appropriate antibiotic

Box 13-5. Endocarditis Prophylaxis Guidelines

Cardiac Condition

Prophylaxis recommended

High risk

Prosthetic cardiac valves
Previous bacterial endocarditis
Complex cyanotic congenital heart disease
Surgically constructed systemic pulmonary shunts or conduits

Moderate risk

Most other congenital cardiac malformations
Rheumatic and other acquired valvular dysfunction
Hypertrophic cardiomyopathy
Mitral valve prolapse with regurgitation and/or thickened leaflets

Prophylaxis not recommended

Isolated secundum atrial septal defect
Surgical repair, without residua beyond 6 months, of atrial septal defect, ventricular septal defect, or patent ductus arteriosus
Previous coronary artery bypass graft surgery
Mitral valve prolapse without regurgitation
Physiologic, functional, or innocent heart murmurs
Previous Kawasaki disease without valvular dysfunction
Previous rheumatic fever without valvular dysfunction
Cardiac pacemakers and implanted defibrillators

Dental, Surgical, and Other Procedures

Prophylaxis recommended

Dental or periodontal procedures known to induce gingival or mucosal bleeding, including professional cleaning
Intraligamentary oral anesthetic injections
Tonsillectomy/adenoidectomy
Surgery involving intestinal or respiratory mucosae*
Bronchoscopy with rigid bronchoscope
Sclerotherapy for esophageal varices*
Esophageal dilation*
Endoscopic retrograde cholangiography with biliary obstruction*
Biliary tract surgery*
Prostatic surgery
Cystoscopy
Urethral dilation

Prophylaxis not recommended

Dental procedures not likely to induce gingival or mucosal bleeding
Local oral anesthetic injections (nonintraligamentary)
Endotracheal intubation
Bronchoscopy with a flexible bronchoscope, with or without biopsy†
Tympanostomy tube insertion
Transesophageal echocardiography†
Endoscopy with or without gastrointestinal biopsy†
Vaginal hysterectomy†
Vaginal delivery†
Cesarean section
In uninfected tissue:
- Urethral catheterization
- Uterine dilation and curettage
- Therapeutic abortion
- Sterilization procedures
- Insertion/removal of intrauterine devices

Cardiac catheterization, including balloon angioplasty
Implanted cardiac pacemakers, defibrillators, or stents
Incision or biopsy of surgically scrubbed skin
Circumcision

*Prophylaxis recommended for high-risk patients, optional for medium-risk patients.
†Prophylaxis is optional for high-risk patients.

before surgery in patients with evidence of bacterial colonization or infection of the urinary tract, especially if urinary tract instrumentation is necessary.

Acute exacerbations of chronic bronchitis should be treated to the point of resolution or substantial improvement before surgery. Subsequent perioperative flares must be assumed to be caused by bacteria resistant to whatever antibiotic might have been employed preoperatively.

Antimicrobial agents may be given perioperatively to prevent infection of normally sterile tissues by direct contamination during a surgical procedure. Such therapy is appropriate when the likelihood of infection is great or the sequelae of infection are severe, when relatively well-tolerated drugs are effective against the likely organisms, and when available evidence demonstrates a reduction in perioperative morbidity as a result of prophylaxis.

Most clinical trials have focused on clean-contaminated procedures such as vaginal hysterectomy and colorectal surgery or unusual and extensive clean surgery such as cardiothoracic procedures and hip arthroplasty. However, limited recent data suggest that antibiotic prophylaxis may also be cost-effective for some commonly performed, relatively simple clean procedures such as inguinal herniorrhaphy and certain types of breast surgery. Recent trials have also highlighted the efficacy of very short courses of therapy; a single dose of antibiotic immediately before surgery, followed by no more than one dose postoperatively, is as effective as longer regimens and less likely to be associated with toxicity or the development of resistant organisms.

Table 13-5 lists the common surgical procedures for which antibiotic prophylaxis is recommended. The specific regimen must be individualized to the patient and the local microbial environment.

THROMBOEMBOLISM PROPHYLAXIS

The surgical environment often presents circumstances that fulfill Virchow's triad: stasis, intimal injury, and a hypercoagulable state. However, some patients and procedures present a particularly high risk. Specific factors predisposing patients to thromboembolic complications include advanced age, prolonged anesthesia or surgery, extended perioperative immobilization, paralysis, malignancy, history of venous disease or thromboembolism, and premenopausal exogenous estrogen use (Table 13-6).

Table 13-4. Endocarditis Prophylaxis Regimens

Clinical setting	Special issues	Antibiotics and dosages
Dental, oral, and upper respiratory tract procedures	Standard	Amoxicillin 2 gm PO 1 hr before procedure
	Penicillin-allergic, immediate hypersensitivity	Clindamycin 600 mg PO 1 hr before procedure, or azithromycin or clarithromycin 500 mg PO 1 hr before procedure
	Penicillin-allergic, not immediate hypersensitivity	Cephalexin or cefadroxil 2 gm PO 1 hr before procedure
	Unable to take PO	Ampicillin 2 gm IV/IM within 30 min before procedure
	Unable to take PO and penicillin-allergic (immediate hypersensitivity)	Clindamycin 600 mg IV within 30 min before procedure
	Unable to take PO and penicillin-allergic (not immediate hypersensitivity)	Cefazolin 1 gm IV within 30 min before procedure
Genitourinary/gastrointestinal (excluding esophageal) procedures	High risk	Ampicillin 2 gm IV/IM plus gentamicin 1.5 mg/kg (not to exceed 120 mg) within 30 min of starting procedure; then ampicillin 1 gm IV/IM or amoxicillin 1 gm PO 6 hr later
	High risk and allergic to ampicillin/amoxicillin	Vancomycin 1 gm IV over 1 to 2 hr plus gentamicin 1.5 mg/kg (not to exceed 120 mg) within 30 min of starting procedure
	Moderate risk	Amoxicillin 2 gm PO 1 hr before procedure or ampicillin 2 gm IV/IM within 30 min of starting procedure
	Moderate risk and allergic to ampicillin/amoxicillin	Vancomycin 1 gm IV over 1 to 2 hr; complete infusion within 30 min of starting procedure

There is general agreement that patients at moderate or high risk for perioperative thromboembolism should receive prophylaxis. Available data from a number of well-conducted clinical studies have demonstrated substantial reductions in thromboembolic complications with a variety of regimens in different surgical settings. The American College of Chest Physicians (ACCP) publishes evidence-based recommendations for treating and preventing thromboembolic disease every 3 years.[4] Guidelines, by category of surgery and perceived underlying risk, for thromboembolism prophylaxis in the surgical patient are summarized in Box 13-6. Although there are convincing data supporting an independent risk of thromboembolic disease from postmenopausal estrogens, the ACCP does not include this as a specific predisposing risk factor.

MANAGEMENT OF SELECTED CLINICAL PROBLEMS IN PATIENTS UNDERGOING SURGERY

Hypertension

Patients with hypertension experience greater blood pressure lability during anesthesia, surgery, and the perioperative period than do normotensive individuals. This lability manifests primarily in hypertensive episodes, although interventions to support blood pressure (fluid challenge or adrenergic agents) are more common among hypertensive patients than those with normal blood pressure taking no medications. Among hypertensive patients this lability is largely independent of preoperative blood pressure control and appears to be mediated primarily by transient sympathetic overactivity following noxious stimuli, such as laryngoscopy before endotracheal intubation.[11] Sympathetic overactivity may also occur on reversal of anesthesia as a result of pain, hypoxia, or hypercarbia. Acute elevations in blood pressure may occur intraoperatively from reflex vasoconstriction as a result of vascular or visceral traction. Blood pressure elevations 2 to 3 days postoperatively may result from recruitment of third-spaced fluid. Perioperative hemorrhagic complications, generally within the operative field, are believed to be more common among patients with poor preoperative blood pressure control (diastolic blood pressure 110 mm Hg or higher). Available data suggest no increase in risk for stable preoperative diastolic blood pressure values <110 mm Hg.[7] Of note, perioperative use of β-blockers among patients at increased risk for cardiovascular complications has been associated with decreased mortality.[12,15a] On the other hand, an unexpected finding in a randomized trial of cardiac valve replacement patients receiving a dihydropyridine Ca^{++} channel blocker vs. placebo was an excess in major postoperative bleeding among those treated with nimodipine.[17] See Box 13-7 for management points on hypertension.

Diabetes Mellitus

Diabetes mellitus is the most common endocrine problem encountered among surgical patients. Patients with diabetes require surgery more often than do nondiabetic individuals, and surgery among diabetic patients is more often associated with complications, especially adverse cardiovascular events and perioperative infections. As many as half the diabetic individuals in the United States are undiagnosed, and it is not uncommon for a patient's diabetes to first come to medical attention when he or she presents for evaluation of a surgical problem. Although surgical and perioperative mortality and morbidity are increased in patients with diabetes, most such patients fare extremely well when appropriately supported

Table 13-5. Perioperative Wound Infection Prophylaxis

Procedure	Regimen
Cardiothoracic and vascular	1
Median sternotomy	
Coronary artery bypass*	
Prosthetic valve	
Pacemaker insertion	
Lobectomy/pneumonectomy	
Peripheral vascular	
General surgery	
Breast surgery†	3
Colorectal procedures	4 or 5
Biliary tract‡	1
Herniorrhaphy†	3
Appendectomy (primary)	5
Gastroduodenal/small bowel‡	1
Penetrating abdominal trauma	5
Gynecologic surgery	1
Cesarean section§	
Hysterectomy	
Orthopedic surgery	1 or 2
Arthroplasty/joint replacement	
Internal fixation	
Amputation of lower limb	
Neurosurgery	
Craniotomy‖	6 or 7
Cerebrospinal fluid shunt¶	8
Head and neck surgery	
Mucous membranes crossed	1

1, Cefazolin, 1 gm IM or IV immediately before surgery and 6-8 hr later; *2*, vancomycin, 1 gm IV immediately before surgery; *3*, cefonicid, 1 gm IV immediately before surgery; *4*, neomycin and erythromycin, 1 gm each by mouth at 1 PM, 2 PM, and 11 PM the day before surgery, with mechanical bowel preparation; *5*, cefoxitin, 2 gm IV immediately before surgery, *6*, clindamycin, 300 mg IV immediately before surgery and 4 hr after; *7*, vancomycin, 1 gm IV, and gentamicin, 80 mg IV, immediately before surgery; *8*, trimethoprim, 160 mg, sulfamethoxazole, 800 mg, IV immediately before surgery and every 12 hr for three doses.

*Poorly substantiated by literature, but the standard practice.

†Based on recent data; no uniform practice yet established.

‡High risk; advanced age, infection or inflammation, biliary tract obstruction, jaundice.

§High risk; emergency, premature rupture of membranes, obesity.

‖High risk; open wound, reexploration, microsurgery.

¶May be beneficial in centers with high infection rates.

through surgery. Several clinical series have demonstrated a modest advantage of intravenously infused insulin over the use of intermediate-acting insulin injected subcutaneously in patients undergoing surgery. In practice, insulin infusion is generally reserved for surgical patients perceived to be at unusually high risk or those who are in ketoacidosis and require emergent surgery. Diabetic patients undergoing coronary artery bypass surgery, however, generally require an insulin infusion to achieve reasonable glucose control intraoperatively and in the immediate postoperative period.

Objectives in the management of the diabetic patient undergoing surgery include (1) characterization of the status of the patient's diabetes, (2) preoperative optimization of glucose control, (3) identification of preexisting complications, treating those amenable to immediate intervention and anticipating problems with others, (4) provision of adequate insulin and substrate for cellular function during surgery, striving for smooth, moderate blood glucose control (150 to 250 mg/dl) and avoiding hypoglycemic and hyperglycemic peaks and ketoacidosis, (5) resumption of appropriate diabetic maintenance therapy and nutritional support postoperatively, and (6) aggressive postoperative monitoring of potential problems arising from the chronic complications of diabetes. See Box 13-8 for management points on diabetes mellitus.

Thyroid Disease

Hypothyroidism is quite prevalent in the general population, especially among older individuals. Patients who are euthyroid when taking replacement L-thyroxine are at no increased surgical risk. Patients with mild to moderate hypothyroidism who have not been treated should generally be made euthyroid before elective surgery. These patients, however, and even those who are severely myxedematous, can be safely managed throughout urgently required surgery. Special attention must be paid to (1) the mode and rate of treatment of the underlying hypothyroidism, (2) monitoring for hypoglycemia and hyponatremia, (3) exaggerated responses to anesthetic and other agents in the setting of an often profound hypometabolic rate, (4) avoidance of cold stress and hypothermia in the operative and postoperative setting, and (5) anticipated hypoventilation and its implications for assisted ventilation.

Untreated hyperthyroidism poses a more serious risk to the operative patient than does either treated or untreated hypothyroidism. The predominant risks of general anesthesia and surgery in thyrotoxic patients are (1) the predisposition toward dysrhythmias and high-output cardiac failure engendered by striking increases in metabolic rate, (2) the unpredictable level and duration of response to various medications, including anesthetic agents, and (3) the induction of thyroid storm, with its substantial associated morbidity and 5% to 10% mortality. Although the symptoms and signs of hyperthyroidism can be ameliorated in thyrotoxic patients, thyroid storm cannot be prevented until the patient is rendered euthyroid for several months. Indeed, in older clinical reviews surgery was the most common precipitant of this endocrine emergency. Accordingly, elective surgery should be postponed until a known hyperthyroid patient has been made and maintained euthyroid for 3 months.

Thyrotoxic patients who need urgent or emergent surgery require extremely close monitoring and aggressive management. A combination of thyroid-blocking agents, sympatholytics, and stress-dose corticosteroids is generally employed. See Box 13-9 for management points on thyroid disease.

The Patient Taking Corticosteroids

Primary adrenal insufficiency (Addison's disease) is quite uncommon, as is secondary adrenal insufficiency on the basis of an intrinsic deficit of corticotropin. Adrenal suppression by exogenous corticosteroid administration is, on the other hand, quite prevalent. Patients who receive potentially suppressive doses of exogenous corticosteroids are most often those with severe dermatoses, inflammatory rheumatologic conditions,

Table 13-6. Classification of Level of Risk of Venous Thromboembolism (VTE)

	Low*	Moderate†	High‡	Highest§
Calf vein thrombosis	2%	10% to 20%	20% to 40%	40% to 80%
Proximal vein thrombosis	0.4%	2% to 4%	4% to 8%	10% to 20%
Clinical pulmonary embolism	0.2%	1% to 2%	2% to 4%	4% to 10%
Fatal pulmonary embolism	0.002%	0.1%-0.4%	0.4% to 1.0%	1% to 5%
Successful preventive strategies	No specific measures	LDUH (q12h), LMWH, IPC, ES	LDUH (q8h), LMWH, IPC	LMWH, oral anticoagulants, IPC (& LDUH or LMWH), ADH

LDUH, Low-dose unfractionated heparin; *LMWH,* low-molecular-weight heparin; *IPC,* intermittent pneumatic compression; *ES,* elastic stockings; *ADH,* adjusted dose (unfractionated) heparin.

Modified from Clagett GP et al: Prevention of venous thromboembolism, *Chest* 114:531S-560S, 1998.

*Example: uncomplicated minor surgery in patients < 40 yr with no clinical risk factors.

†Examples: any surgery (major and minor) in patients 40 to 60 yr but no additional risk factors; major surgery in patients < 40 yr but no additional risk factors; minor surgery in patients with risk factors.

‡Examples: major surgery in patients > 60 yr without additional risk factors; major surgery in patients 40 to 60 yr who have additional risk factors; patients with MI and medical patients with risk factors.

§Examples: major surgery in patients > 40 yr plus prior VTE or malignant disease or hypercoagulable state; patients with elective major lower extremity orthopedic surgery, or hip fracture, or stroke, or multiple trauma, or spinal cord injury.

Box 13-6. Recommended Venous Thromboembolism (VTE) Prophylaxis for Patients Undergoing Surgery

General Surgery

Low risk: early ambulation
Moderate risk: LDUH, LMWH, IPC, ES
High risk:
—With additional risk factors: LDUH, LMWH
—Prone to wound complications: IPC
Highest risk:
—With multiple risk factors: (LDUH or LMWH) plus IPC
—Selected very high risk: warfarin (INR 2.0-3.0)
Aspirin is not recommended in general surgery patients

Orthopedic Surgery

Elective total hip replacement (THR): LMWH, warfarin, ADH
—Adjuvant ES or IPC may provide additional efficacy
—LDUH, aspirin, dextran, IPC (alone) are all less effective
Elective total knee replacement (TKR): LMWH, warfarin, IPC
Optimal duration of prophylaxis after THR or TKR is uncertain
—At least 7 to 10 days for LMWH or warfarin
—Emerging data suggest benefit from 29 to 35 days with LMWH
Routine screening with duplex ultrasonography in asymptomatic patients after THR and TKR is not recommended
Hip fracture surgery: preoperative LMWH or warfarin, begun either preoperatively or immediately after surgery
Prophylactic IVC filter limited to high-risk patients with active bleeding

Elective Neurosurgery, Acute Spinal Cord Injury, and Trauma

Intracranial neurosurgery: IPC +/– ES
—LMWH or LDUH may be acceptable alternatives
—Combination of physical (IPC or ES) and pharmacologic (LMWH or LDUH) modalities may be more effective
Acute spinal cord injury: LMWH
—LDUH, ES, IPC are ineffective when used alone
—ES and IPC might have benefit in combination with LMWH or if anticoagulation is contraindicated
—LMWH or oral anticoagulation may provide protection during rehabilitation
Trauma patients: LMWH as soon as it is considered safe to do so
—IPC if LMWH will be delayed or is contraindicated
—In patients with high risk for VTE and suboptimal prophylaxis, consider screening with duplex ultrasound
—In patients with proximal DVT and contraindication to anticoagulation, consider IVC filter

Other

Long-term indwelling central venous catheters: warfarin 1 mg daily
Patients having spinal puncture or epidural catheter placement: LMWH should be used with caution

LDUH, Low-dose unfractionated heparin; *LMWH,* low-molecular-weight heparin; *IPC,* intermittent pneumatic compression; *ES,* elastic stockings; *ADH,* adjusted dose (unfractionated) heparin; *INR,* international normalized ratio; *DVT,* deep vein thrombophlebitis; *IVC,* inferior vena cava.
Modified from Clagett GP et al: Prevention of venous thromboembolism, *Chest* 114:531S-560S, 1998.

Box 13-7. Management Points: Hypertension

Maintain usual antihypertensive medications throughout surgery and the perioperative period in the patient whose blood pressure is in reasonable control.
- Administer with a sip of water on the morning of surgery; continue usual regimen postoperatively.
- For a patient unable to take oral medications postoperatively, substitute appropriate parenteral forms of β-blockers, methyldopa, enalaprilat, calcium blockers, or diuretics.
- To preclude rebound hypertension in a patient taking clonidine expected to be unable to take oral medications postoperatively, wean from clonidine and/or substitute a β-blocker or methyldopa preoperatively. A parenteral β-blocker or methyldopa can be administered perioperatively. Transdermal clonidine is an alternative, but cutaneous absorption may be unpredictable intraoperatively.

For a newly identified hypertensive patient who requires surgery, consider a β-blocker preferentially if preoperative treatment is necessary.
- Avoid new use of diuretics in the several weeks before surgery to preclude volume depletion and electrolyte disturbances.

Elevated blood pressure in the postoperative period often responds to analgesia or optimization of respiratory status and oxygenation.
- Persistent moderate or severe elevation of blood pressure, without evidence of acute end-organ damage, generally responds to initiation of a maintenance dose of an oral agent (or the appropriate parenteral form in patients unable to take oral medications).

Because of the documented risk of extreme blood pressure lability, worsening tachycardia, cardiac ischemic events, and possible increased perioperative bleeding, sublingual nifedipine should not be used to treat perioperative hypertension.

Treat true perioperative hypertensive crises (defined by end-organ damage) with appropriate parenteral agents, generally sodium nitroprusside or labetalol.

hematologic or lymphoproliferative disorders, or asthma or other forms of COPD. Individuals who have received more than 40-mg prednisone per day, or its equivalent, for more than 1 week in the preceding year are at risk of adrenal suppression. Smaller doses of oral corticosteroids administered for longer periods, and even the inhaled corticosteroids employed now as mainline therapy in the management of reactive airways disease, may also result in adrenal suppression. Of note in this regard is the recent report of a small randomized trial of preoperative patients maintained on oral prednisone with evidence of adrenal suppression on cosyntropin stimulation test. Patients all received their usual prednisone dose and were randomized to either supplemental stress doses of hydrocortisone in saline, or saline alone. No differences were noted in perioperative hypotension or tachycardia.[6] Due to small sample size, the power of this study is limited. Alternate-day administration of relatively low doses of oral corticosteroids (less than 20-mg prednisone equivalent) reduces the risk of suppression. Long-term treatment with very low doses of corticosteroids (less than 5 mg per day prednisone equivalent) is also associated with a low likelihood of adrenal suppression.

Box 13-8. Management Points: Diabetes Mellitus

Diabetic patients should have a preoperative determination of serum creatinine and a urinalysis to exclude pyuria, bacteriuria, and substantial proteinuria.

All adult diabetic patients should have an ECG preoperatively, as well as for any episode of postoperative chest discomfort or of global or otherwise unexplained deterioration.

Diabetic patients who are maintained on diet with moderate or tight glycemic control may be managed operatively without insulin and with non–dextrose-containing intravenous fluids.
- Close monitoring of blood glucose and acid-base status is necessary.
- Initiate insulin therapy for blood glucose values over 250 mg/dl or for incipient ketoacidosis.
- Operative and postoperative patients who are receiving no alimentation may develop ketoacidosis at low blood glucose levels and may require concurrent glucose and insulin infusions.

Diabetic patients maintained on oral hypoglycemic agents should hold these medications for 24 hours (tolbutamide or glipizide) or 36 to 72 hours (tolazamide, glyburide, or chlorpropamide) preoperatively. Metformin should be held for 48 hours preoperatively to preclude the development of perioperative lactic acidosis.
- Operative management is as described for the diet-maintained diabetic patient, with very close monitoring of blood glucose, especially in patients who had been using long-acting oral hypoglycemic agents.

Patients maintained preoperatively on insulin with good glycemic control can generally be managed throughout surgery with half to two thirds of their usual intermediate-acting insulin administered subcutaneously **and** provision of adequate substrate, generally 100-mg glucose per kilogram of body weight per hour (equivalent to a 5% dextrose-containing intravenous infusate at 2 ml/kg/hour).
- Where close operative glucose monitoring is available, insulin infusion to start at 1 to 2 U per hour, concurrent with adequate substrate delivery as above, is an appropriate alternative and should be employed as a routine for coronary artery bypass surgery in insulin-requiring diabetic patients.

Patients in diabetic ketoacidosis who require emergent surgery should receive aggressive volume resuscitation, intravenous insulin (bolus followed by infusion), and correction of major metabolic derangements in whatever preoperative period is available.

Postoperative screening of the surgical wound, vascular access sites, and the urinary tract is essential to identify incipient infection.

Until more data are available, the goal of perioperative management for patients with known or suspected adrenal suppression remains the provision of sufficient exogenous corticosteroid to match the maximal physiologic output caused by the stress of surgery and anesthesia. This has been established at 300- to 400-mg cortisol equivalent in the first 24 hours after general anesthesia and major surgery. Hydrocortisone sodium succinate or hydrocortisone sodium phosphate should be employed preferentially to achieve combined glucocorticoid and mineralocorticoid effects. Protocols using the intramuscular route of administration

Box 13-9. Management Points: Thyroid Disease

Hypothyroid and hyperthyroid patients should be rendered euthyroid before elective surgery.
- The effects of hypothyroidism can be largely corrected over a period of 3 to 4 weeks.
- Hyperthyroidism generally requires several months to achieve control.

Hypothyroid patients who require urgent or emergent surgery may be managed safely with special attention to the following:
- Propensity to develop hypoglycemia and hyponatremia
- Exaggerated response to anesthetics and other medications
- Sensitivity to cold stress
- Hypoventilation

Initiate thyroid replacement therapy as soon as possible in hypothyroid patients who need urgent or emergent surgery with the exception of those undergoing coronary revascularization in whom thyroid replacement should be initiated only following revascularization.

Thyrotoxic patients who need urgent or emergent surgery require close preoperative, intraoperative, and postoperative monitoring and management, consisting of the following:
- Intensive care unit level of monitoring.
- Initiation of thyroid blockade, preferably with propylthiouracil, 100 to 300 mg orally or per nasogastric tube every 8 hours. Methimazole may be employed alternatively (at a dosage of 30 to 60 mg daily) but does not block peripheral conversion of thyroxine (T_4) to triiodothyronine (T_3).
- Sodium iodide (250 mg intravenously every 6 hours or 500 to 1000 mg intravenously every 12 hours) may be an appropriate adjunct to block thyroid hormone secretion and reduce gland vascularity.
- Sympathetic overactivity may be controlled with propranolol (initial dosage 10 to 40 mg orally or 1 to 2 mg intravenously every 4 to 6 hours) titrated to achieve a pulse less than 90. Parenteral esmolol or labetalol may be substituted, especially in refractory cases.

Patients with significant hyperthyroidism or hypothyroidism who require emergent or urgent surgery should receive stress-dose steroid coverage.

Box 13-10. Management Points: Patient Taking Corticosteroids

Suspected adrenal suppression may be excluded by a normal response to a cosyntropin stimulation test performed preoperatively (see Chapter 98). If adrenal suppression is confirmed or is suspected in a patient who requires surgery urgently or in whom a cosyntropin stimulation test has not been performed, the following apply:
- When possible, a priming dose of hydrocortisone (100 mg) may be administered orally, intramuscularly, or intravenously at midnight before the patient's surgery.
- Administer hydrocortisone sodium succinate or hydrocortisone sodium phosphate, 100 mg, intravenously on call to the operating room and every 6 to 8 hours thereafter for 24 hours. After initial bolus, an infusion of hydrocortisone at 10 mg per hour may be substituted for repeated boluses.
- After complicated or prolonged surgery, consider extending stress-dose steroid coverage with hydrocortisone, 50 mg, every 6 to 8 hours on postoperative day 1 and hydrocortisone, 25 mg, every 6 to 8 hours on postoperative day 2.
- For intraoperative or postoperative hypotension include intravenous bolus administration of hydrocortisone, 50 to 100 mg, in the treatment regimen.

have demonstrated variable effectiveness. Repeated intravenous boluses or combined bolus and infusion protocols are the most reliable means of supporting patients through surgery. Up to 40% of bolus-administered hydrocortisone may be lost in the urine. See Box 13-10 for management points on the patient taking corticosteroids

The Elderly Patient

Changing demographics combined with advances in anesthetic and surgical technique have led to a steady increase in minor and major surgery for elderly patients. Although the elderly currently constitute less than 15% of the population, they account for 20% to 40% of all surgery, 50% of emergency procedures, and 75% of overall surgical mortality. Age itself appears to account for little, if any, of the excess mortality seen in elderly surgical patients. More important variables include the nature and severity of underlying disease(s), and the type of surgery, especially if performed as an emergency procedure. Age is, however, an independent risk factor for cardiovascular morbidity, including congestive heart failure, myocardial infarction, and stroke. Therefore the commonly utilized schema for quantifying perioperative risk, described earlier, includes an adjustment for age alone. There are no data to support the routine use of perioperative invasive hemodynamic monitoring in the elderly, although such monitoring can be carried out safely when indicated on the basis of underlying disease. As in younger patients, an inadequate cardiovascular response to exercise is an important predictor of risk and constitutes an indication for additional evaluation, aggressive perioperative management, and/or reconsideration of the surgical decision. A recent systematic review of medical issues related to the management of hip fracture has broad applicability.[14]

Delirium is a special risk among seniors undergoing general anesthesia and major surgery, and may occur in as many as 30% to 50% of older surgical patients. Individuals with preexisting cognitive impairment are at special risk, as are those over age 70, or those with a history of alcohol or other substance abuse and those undergoing certain categories of operation.[13] Many medications employed in the perioperative setting are associated with delirium, especially anticholinergics, sedatives, and narcotics, especially meperidine. Delirium may also be the mode of presentation of major medical insults, such as myocardial infarction or sepsis. See Box 13-11 for management points on the elderly patient.

Liver Disease

Patients with serious underlying liver disease tolerate general anesthesia and surgery poorly. All anesthetic regimens, including epidural and spinal anesthesia, reduce hepatic blood flow. Older halogenated hydrocarbon anesthetic gases (halothane and methoxyflurane) carry an independent risk of hepatic toxicity. Isoflurane, in wide use at present, is not a direct hepatotoxin but does cause systemic vasodilatation and

Box 13-11. Management Points: The Elderly Patient

Preoperative evaluation should include explicit estimation of functional status and rehabilitation goals.
Supplement history and physical examination with baseline renal function tests, glucose determination, a screening test for thyroid function, and other studies as indicated clinically.
In cases where cardiovascular reserve is uncertain, and in patients undergoing high-risk procedures, preoperative exercise testing or dipyridamole radionuclide imaging may provide guidance.
Meticulous attention to drug selection and dosing is necessary.
Establish resuscitation wishes and a health care proxy preoperatively in all patients, including elderly operative candidates.
Postoperative delirium should be anticipated and sought; if identified, one should focus efforts on suspect medications, toxic/withdrawal states, and treatable medical complications.

a reduction in cardiac output, with resultant risk of impaired hepatic blood flow.

The quantifiable risk of surgery in patients with underlying liver disease correlates with the extent of hepatic functional impairment. This is generally manifested by readily identifiable factors: encephalopathy, cutaneous stigmata of chronic hepatic dysfunction, the presence and severity of ascites, elevation in serum bilirubin, hypoalbuminemia, and coagulopathy. Hepatic synthetic dysfunction may complicate acute processes (viral, alcoholic, or drug-induced hepatitis, shock liver) or chronic liver diseases (cirrhosis, chronic viral or autoimmune hepatitis). Surgical and perioperative mortality among patients with cirrhosis undergoing major vascular surgery (excluding portal-systemic shunt surgery) ranges from less than 10% in those with well-compensated livers to greater than 75% in those with evidence of severe derangements in hepatic function. Elevations in hepatic transaminases alone do not predict an adverse outcome from anesthesia and surgery, but must be interpreted in context, and may be an early marker of severe hepatic injury after shock, trauma, or toxic insult, or in severe viral hepatitis.

Preoperative efforts for a patient with evidence of hepatic dysfunction must be directed at optimizing nutritional and volume status, including reduction of significant ascites, correcting coagulopathy, anticipating and treating encephalopathy, and correcting electrolyte disturbances. Common operative complications include excessive hemorrhage and exaggerated responses to sedatives, narcotic analgesics, intravenous induction agents, and neuromuscular blocking agents. Postoperative complications include worsening of hepatic function, hemorrhage in the operative field and from the gastrointestinal tract, encephalopathy, impaired wound healing, pneumonia, volume and electrolyte derangements, acute tubular necrosis, and hepatorenal syndrome. See Box 13-12 for management points on liver disease.

Box 13-12. Management Points: Liver Disease

Quantify risk by profiling clinical features (encephalopathy, ascites, cutaneous stigmata) and biochemical markers (albumin, bilirubin, coagulation studies) of hepatic dysfunction in patients with known or suspected liver disease.
Perform noninvasive imaging studies preoperatively to identify an obstructive basis for jaundice.
Consider alternatives to surgery for patients with severe, irremediable hepatic dysfunction.
Temporize to allow correction of remediable derangements in patients where surgery is necessary.
Administer vitamin K, fresh frozen plasma, and occasionally plasmapheresis combined with plasma infusion for coagulopathy. DDAVP at a dose of 0.3 mg/kg SC may reduce the bleeding time.
Manage edema/ascites with the following:
- Bed rest in lateral decubitus position and lower extremity elevation
- Rigid salt restriction (250- to 500-mg sodium per day) and moderate fluid restriction (less than 1.5 L per day)
- Escalating doses of spironolactone, beginning at 100 mg per day, increasing by 100 mg per day every 3 days, to a total of 600 mg per day, in divided doses, monitoring serum potassium, blood urea nitrogen (BUN), and creatinine closely
- Occasional supplementation with a loop diuretic, beginning at furosemide, 40 mg per day, or equivalent
- Large-volume paracenteses (up to 5 L), generally with intravenous albumin infusion, to achieve control of refractory ascites

Treat or prevent hepatic encephalopathy with dietary protein restriction and lactulose (30 ml three times daily).

Renal Disease

Special precautions are necessary in patients with acute renal failure (ARF), chronic renal failure (CRF), or the nephrotic syndrome. Among such patients physiologic derangements relevant to surgery include impairment of fluid and electrolyte balance, acidosis, increased risk from hypotension and potential nephrotoxins, exaggerated responses to neuromuscular blocking agents eliminated through renal means, anemia, a hemorrhagic diathesis from platelet dysfunction, hypercoagulability in the setting of the nephrotic syndrome, increased risk of infection, and impaired wound healing.

Azotemic patients handle volume loads poorly, and such patients are at risk for both dehydration and volume overload with perioperative stresses that would be well compensated in individuals with normal renal function. Volume overload, in particular, may result in the rapid development of hypertension, pulmonary edema, or peripheral edema despite normal cardiac function. Hypoalbuminemia from the nephrotic syndrome enhances the risk of total body volume overload and confounds estimation of intravascular volume status.

Potassium handling is impaired in patients with severe renal dysfunction but may also be quite deranged among those with only modest degrees of azotemia in the clinical setting of distal tubulointerstitial disease or the hyporenin-hypoaldosterone syndrome, most commonly noted in diabetic patients. Operative stresses, muscle injuries, burns, gastrointestinal or traumatic hemorrhage, and perioperative infections markedly enhance catabolism, with the production of enormous endogenous potassium loads, whereas transfused blood contributes an added exogenous potassium burden. Metabolic acidoses and further derangements in calcium-phosphate balance may also be engendered by the same processes that promote perioperative hyperkalemia.

A variety of diagnostic pharmaceuticals and medications may compound preexisting renal abnormalities in the perioperative setting. Those that pose the greatest risk to azotemic surgical patients include iodinated radiocontrast agents and aminoglycoside antibiotics. Other medications that carry substantial nephrotoxic risk, but which are less often indicated perioperatively, include nonsteroidal antiinflammatory drugs, chemotherapeutic agents, amphotericin B, and angiotensin-converting enzyme inhibitors. Substitution of interventions with less potential nephrotoxicity should be considered when feasible; if a potential nephrotoxin is strongly indicated on clinical grounds, pretreatment optimization of volume status and close monitoring of renal function are necessary.

Human recombinant erythropoietin improves the anemia associated with renal failure, but in the setting of surgery such patients often require transfusion to achieve or maintain an optimal hematocrit, generally above 30%. Dialysis itself may also improve the anemia somewhat. Clinically significant platelet dysfunction associated with uremia is generally manifested by an abnormal bleeding time. This disorder often does not fully correct despite dialysis but generally responds promptly to some combination of arginine vasopressin, cryoprecipitate, and red cell transfusion. Estrogens have also been found to be effective in controlling the bleeding that is associated with uremia.

Hemodialysis provides the means of optimizing volume, electrolyte balance, acid-base status, and to some extent the hemostasis defect associated with renal failure. Dialysis is generally best timed to occur on the days preceding and following surgery. Patients with the nephrotic syndrome have an increased risk of venous thromboembolism, which is compounded by surgery, and require appropriate prophylaxis (see Table 13-6). See Box 13-13 for management points on renal disease.

Box 13-13. Management Points: Renal Disease

Where hemodialysis is indicated to correct volume, electrolyte, acid-base, and hemostasis defects, perform preferentially at least 12 hours before and 12 to 24 hours after planned surgery.

For a patient not on dialysis, salt and fluid requirements may be estimated from results of a 24-hour urine collection when patient is in balance.

Correct mild overhydration by fluid restriction and administration of loop diuretics.

Consider hemodynamic monitoring to determine intravascular volume status in patients with severe renal failure with or without hypoalbuminemia and pulmonary edema.

Emergency dialysis may be necessary to correct serious refractory volume derangements.

Treat clinically significant hyperkalemia (generally over 6 mEq/L with ECG abnormalities) emergently with calcium chloride, dextrose and insulin infusion, and/or sodium bicarbonate infusion (see Chapter 145).

Definitive treatment generally requires diuresis, generally effective only in the setting of mild renal dysfunction, ion exchange resins, or dialysis.

Optimize intravascular volume status before administration of iodinated radiocontrast administration in the setting of renal failure; avoid such studies if possible.

Atracurium or vercuronium should be employed preferentially to achieve operative neuromuscular blockade.

Restrict use of aminoglycoside antibiotics, nonsteroidal antiinflammatory drugs, angiotensin converting enzyme inhibitors, and other potential nephrotoxins or, when strongly indicated, monitor closely in the perioperative setting.

Employ dialysis, recombinant erythropoietin, and transfusion to achieve and maintain hematocrit at 30% or greater.

Correct defects in hemostasis with dialysis, arginine vasopressin, cryoprecipitate, or red cell infusion.

The Pregnant Patient

Pregnant women generally tolerate nonobstetric surgery without significantly increased morbidity or mortality. Putative risks from exposure of the fetus to general anesthetic agents can be minimized by avoiding all but emergent surgery during the periods of organogenesis (first trimester) and central nervous system myelination (third trimester); indeed, the risk to the fetus of nonemergent maternal surgery performed in the second trimester has been shown to be extremely low. The risk of fetal loss or of premature delivery increases substantially with increasing severity of the underlying surgical problem, with intraoperative shock, hypoxemia, or acidosis, and with postoperative complications. Trauma and acute abdominal processes, such as appendicitis and cholecystitis, are the most common clinical conditions necessitating urgent or emergent surgery among pregnant women. Abdominal processes may confound or be confounded by obstetric complications. The possibility of pregnancy must be considered in any woman of childbearing potential who requires surgery.

Evaluation and management of the pregnant woman undergoing nonobstetric surgery require knowledge of the major physiologic changes associated with pregnancy. Blood pressure drops in early to midgestation; relatively modest blood pressure elevations near term, especially after the twenty-eighth week, may presage the obstetric emergency of preeclampsia. Dyspnea, pedal edema, and a third heart sound are common findings in late stages of normal pregnancies. Also late in gestation, uterine compression of the vena cava and aorta may compromise both maternal cardiac output and placental perfusion when a pregnant woman is maintained in supine recumbency, a position also associated with arterial hypoxemia. The normal respiratory pattern of pregnancy is one of hyperventilation (Pco_2 25 to 30 mm Hg) with metabolic compensation (HCO_3 17 to 22 mEq/L), factors that must be considered in pregnant patients who require intubation and mechanical ventilation. In normal pregnancies blood and plasma volumes increase substantially, generally with little clinical consequence, although the volume of distribution of many medications may be affected. Venous stasis, from increased filling of capacitance vessels and extrinsic compression of pelvic veins by the uterine contents, and the hypercoagulability associated with pregnancy result in a marked increase in the risk of thromboembolic disease, a situation compounded by trauma or surgery. Delayed gastric emptying and relaxation of the lower esophageal sphincter

Box 13-14. Management Points: The Pregnant Patient

Avoid all but urgent or emergent surgery during pregnancy.
Optimal time for *necessary* surgery is second trimester.
Limit adjunctive medication usage to agents that are safe in pregnancy and clearly indicated on strong clinical grounds (see above).
Anticipate increased volume of distribution and accelerated renal excretion of medications.
Position the pregnant patient who requires surgery in lateral decubitus position or supine with the right hip tilted up at least 15 degrees from the horizontal.
For patients who require ventilatory support, maintain Pco_2 in range normal for pregnant state (30 mm Hg).
Anticipate increased risk of aspiration of gastric contents and treat expectantly by delay of procedures after feedings, head-of-bed elevation, and antacids.
Survey for urinary retention and infection.
Conduct aggressive prophylaxis and treatment for thromboembolic disease with an appropriate heparin regimen supplemented by venous compression (see Chapter 80).

during pregnancy lead to an increased perioperative risk of aspiration pneumonitis. Dilation of the urinary collecting system predisposes to retention, bacterial colonization, and infection. The glomerular filtration rate increases 30% to 50% in normal pregnancies, with an associated increase in the clearance of many drugs.

Pregnant women undergoing nonobstetric surgery often require adjunctive medications, such as antibiotics, in the perioperative period. Many medications can be safely administered to a pregnant woman without adversely affecting the fetus: heparin, most β-lactam antibiotics, erythromycin, methyldopa, hydralazine, most asthma medications, and others. In many instances, especially with newer drugs, the fetal risk is unknown. A moderate number of common medications are known to be fetotoxic or result in malformations; these should be employed during pregnancy only when strongly indicated and when suitable alternatives do not exist or cannot be used because of other reasons, such as drug allergy. Medications that are problematic in pregnancy include aminoglycoside, tetracycline, quinolone, and sulfonamide antimicrobials; warfarin; angiotensin-converting enzyme inhibitors; phenytoin; barbiturates; high-dose aspirin; histamine$_2$-blockers; and a wide range of chemotherapeutic agents. See Box 13-14 for management points on the pregnant patient.

Seizure Disorders

New-onset seizures in the perioperative setting generally relate to metabolic derangements, such as hypoglycemia, severe hyponatremia, and malignant hyperthermia; unanticipated alcohol or sedative-hypnotic withdrawal; toxic medication effects, as with enflurane, high doses of local anesthetic agents, or meperidine against a backdrop of monoamine oxidase inhibitor use; or a structural problem, such as an intracranial tumor or abscess, but especially after trauma, with central nervous system hemorrhage, cerebral contusion, or penetrating brain injury. Patients with established seizure disorders that are well controlled with anticonvulsant medications generally tolerate surgery well, without neurologic sequelae. Indeed, although inhalation induction of anesthesia and emergence are risk periods for increased seizure activity, barbiturate coma and general anesthesia are accepted therapies for refractory status epilepticus. Maintenance of oral anticonvulsant therapy in the perioperative period may not be possible, and alternate dosage forms or different agents may be necessary. Prophylaxis of seizure activity in the neurologically injured patient is somewhat controversial, although there is consensus on treating certain categories of such patients (see below). See Box 13-15 for management points on seizure disorders.

Box 13-15. Management Points: Seizure Disorders

Delay elective surgery until clinical control of underlying epilepsy is achieved and appropriate blood levels of anticonvulsants are confirmed.
Maintain phenytoin (orally or intravenously) or phenobarbital (orally, intramuscularly, or intravenously) through the perioperative period. Fosphenytoin sodium, the prodrug of phenytoin in a water-soluble form, may be administered intravenously or intramuscularly.
Substitute phenytoin or phenobarbital for carbamazepine in patients unable to receive medications enterally in the perioperative period who require maintenance therapy.
Valproic acid syrup may be administered rectally in special situations, but substitution of phenytoin or phenobarbital, as for carbamazepine, is generally more appropriate in patients unable to continue oral valproate. Valproate sodium is also now available for parenteral use.
Identify metabolic, toxic, withdrawal, and anatomic causes of new-onset seizures in perioperative patients and treat accordingly.
Consider seizure prophylaxis in patients with the following:
- Intracranial abscess or subdural empyema
- Intracranial trauma patients with a history of acute hematoma, early posttraumatic seizures, penetrating head wounds, or depressed skull fractures
- Tumors at or near the motor cortex
- Planned surgery where seizure activity would be catastrophic

The Alcoholic Patient

There are 10 million to 20 million alcoholics and problem drinkers in the United States. These individuals require surgery at a greater rate than the nondrinking public on the basis of the medical complications of alcohol (and usually concurrent tobacco abuse), but especially as a result of trauma associated with alcohol use—motor vehicle and other accidents, burns, and interpersonal violence. Complications of surgery in alcohol-abusing patients may relate to (1) metabolic derangements, especially of intermediary metabolism and of potassium, calcium, and magnesium homeostasis, (2) organ system dysfunction, especially of the cardiac, hematologic, hepatic, and central nervous systems, and (3) the withdrawal state. Treatment is predicated on rapid identification and treatment of correctable derangements and anticipatory treatment of alcohol withdrawal states. See Box 13-16 for management points on the alcoholic patient.

Box 13-16. Management Points: The Alcoholic Patient

Elicit history of alcohol, tobacco, and other drug use in all preoperative patients.
- Use CAGE questionnaire or an alternative in alcohol-using patients to further estimate severity of use (see Chapter 51).

Preoperative examination should include testing for fecal blood loss.

For patients suspected of significant recent or sustained alcohol use, preoperative laboratory screen should include complete blood count, glucose, sodium, bicarbonate, potassium, magnesium, BUN, creatinine, calcium, phosphate, bilirubin, albumin, transaminases, prothrombin and partial thromboplastin times, and urine dipstick for ketones.

Administer thiamine, 100 mg intravenously or intramuscularly, to all acutely ill alcoholic patients undergoing urgent surgery.

Alcohol-induced thrombocytopenia is rarely profound and generally responds to abstinence with appropriate vitamin supplementation, especially folate.

Alcoholic ketoacidosis generally responds promptly to dextrose infusion.

One should anticipate a drop in serum phosphate with dextrose administration and treat severe hypophosphatemia (less than 1 mg/dl) cautiously with intravenous potassium phosphate.

Modest elevations in serum transaminases among alcoholics are common and do not carry an independent risk of adverse outcome but may serve as markers of a higher likelihood of alcohol withdrawal.

Hepatic synthetic dysfunction, manifested by encephalopathy, physical stigmata of chronic liver disease (e.g., ascites, spider angiomata, palmar erythema), coagulopathy, hyperbilirubinemia, and hypoalbuminemia, presages significant surgical mortality.
- Delay all but life-saving emergent surgery until remediable defects are corrected.
- Coagulopathy rarely responds to vitamin K and often requires support with plasma or clotting factor concentrates.

Treat early symptoms of alcohol withdrawal aggressively to minimize the likelihood of progression in perioperative patients.
- Diazepam, 20 mg orally every hour for 3 to 6 hours or until control of symptoms in patients able to take oral medication with mild to moderate withdrawal symptoms.
- Lorazepam, 1 to 4 mg intramuscularly every 1 or 2 hours in patients unable to use the alimentary tract with symptoms of mild to moderate withdrawal.
- β-Blockers are reasonable adjuncts for patients with uncontrolled tachycardia or hypertension, if benzodiazepine administration does not result in acceptable control.
- Employ intravenous diazepam in a monitored setting for patients in frank delirium tremens.
- Intravenous haloperidol is a reasonable adjunct for patients whose alcoholic delirium or hallucinosis fails to respond fully to benzodiazepines.

Narcotic-, Sedative-Hypnotic–, and Cocaine-addicted Patients

Patients addicted to narcotics require special attention to analgesics and other medications in the perioperative period. Narcotic tolerance and metabolism are generally enhanced in such patients. Those addicted at the time of surgery require administration of narcotic agents sufficient to suppress withdrawal and control pain, most often achieved by the administration of an appropriate methadone regimen to suppress withdrawal supplemented by appropriate narcotic agonists. Narcotic antagonists and mixed agonist-antagonists must be avoided to preclude precipitating acute narcotic withdrawal. Coordination of this aspect of care with the anesthesiologist is clearly important, since administration of narcotic antagonists and mixed agonist-antagonists in the operative setting is common. Narcotic-addicted patients scheduled to undergo elective surgery may be offered a withdrawal regimen before surgery.

Patients who have been maintained on long-term sedative hypnotics, most commonly benzodiazepines, may experience a withdrawal reaction similar to that associated with withdrawal from alcohol, including seizures and frank delirium, in the postoperative setting. Onset of symptoms may be quite delayed in patients addicted to agents with longer half-lives. Treatment is predicated on identification of the risk of withdrawal, observation for minor symptoms, and administration of appropriate cross-tolerant agents.

Box 13-17. Management Points: Narcotic-, Sedative-Hypnotic–, and Cocaine-Addicted Patients

Offer addicted individuals the opportunity for detoxification, whenever possible, before elective surgery.

For a patient maintained on methadone up to the time of surgery, administer the usual oral dose daily and provide appropriate analgesia with narcotic agonists or nonsteroidal antiinflammatory drugs as clinically indicated.
- Intramuscular or subcutaneous methadone, two thirds the usual oral maintenance dose every 12 hours, may be substituted for oral methadone in patients unable to take oral medications in the perioperative period.

For a narcotic-addicted patient who requires surgery and is not on a methadone maintenance regimen, achieve immediate analgesia and suppression of withdrawal with an appropriate potent narcotic agonist.
- In the postoperative period titrate a methadone maintenance regimen or withdrawal regimen as wished by the patient.

Coordinate perioperative analgesic use with the anesthesiologist.
- Consider epidural or other regional analgesic techniques.
- Avoid narcotic antagonists or mixed agonist-antagonists.

Anticipate shorter duration of action of narcotic analgesics among narcotic addicts than among nonaddicted patients with similar surgical pain.

Anticipate a withdrawal reaction in patients habituated to sedative-hypnotic drugs.
- Observe for symptoms similar to those seen with alcohol withdrawal.
- Provide patient's maintenance medication or an appropriate cross-tolerant agent (e.g., clonazepam or diazepam orally or lorazepam intramuscularly) to suppress withdrawal.

Defer surgery, when possible, until 2 weeks after last cocaine or amphetamine use.

Treat cocaine-associated cardiovascular instability with standard agents but with a preference for labetalol.

Cocaine-addicted individuals carry to surgery an enhanced risk of cardiovascular complications, including blood pressure lability, cardiac ischemic events, dysrhythmias, stroke, and vascular compromise of other organs. This risk appears to persist for at least 2 weeks after last use of cocaine. Elective surgery should be delayed accordingly. Optimum prophylaxis and treatment of these complications in cocaine-addicted individuals who require emergency surgery are not known, but α- and β-adrenergic blockers, labetalol, and chlorpromazine have been used in individual cases. Individuals abusing amphetamines in the preoperative period may experience reactions similar to those associated with cocaine as well as frank psychosis perioperatively. See Box 13-17 for management points on narcotic-, sedative-, hypnotic-, and cocaine-addicted patients.

REFERENCES

1. American College of Cardiology/American Heart Association Task Force on Practice Guidelines: Guidelines for perioperative cardiovascular evaluation for noncardiac surgery, *Circulation* 93:1278-1317, 1996.
2. American College of Physicians: Guidelines for assessing and managing the perioperative risk from coronary artery disease associated with major noncardiac surgery, *Ann Intern Med* 127:309-312, 1997.
3. Archer C, Levy AR, McGregor M: Value of routine preoperative chest x-rays: a meta-analysis, *Can J Anaesth* 40:1022-1027, 1993.
4. Clagett GP, et al: Prevention of venous thromboembolism, *Chest* 114:531S-560S, 1998.
5. Djokovic JL, Hedley-White J: Prediction of outcome of surgery and anesthesia in patients over 80, *JAMA* 242:2301-2306, 1979.
6. Glowniak JV, Loriaux DL: A double-blind study of perioperative steroid requirements in secondary adrenal insufficiency, *Surgery* 121:123-129, 1997.
7. Goldman L, Caldera DL: Risks of general anesthesia and elective operation in the hypertensive patient, *Anesthesiology* 50:285-292, 1979.
8. Goldman L, et al: Multifactorial index of cardiac risk in noncardiac surgical procedures, *N Engl J Med* 297:845-850, 1977.
9. Kaplan EB, et al: The usefulness of preoperative laboratory screening, *JAMA* 253:3576-3581, 1985.
10. Lawrence VA, Dhanda R, Hilsenbeck SG, et al: Risk of pulmonary complications after elective abdominal surgery, *Chest* 110:744-750, 1996.

10a. Lee TH, Marcantonio ER, Mangione CM, et al: Derivation and prospective validation of a simple index for prediction of cardiac risk of major noncardiac surgery, *Circulation* 100:1043-1049, 1999.

11. Low JM, Harvey JT, Prys-Roberts C, et al: Studies of anesthesia in relation to hypertension, *Br J Anaesth* 58:471-477, 1986.
12. Mangano DT, Layug EL, Wallace A, et al, for the Multicenter Study of Perioperative Ischemia Research Group: Effect of atenolol on mortality and cardiovascular morbidity after noncardiac surgery, *N Engl J Med* 335:1713-1720, 1996.
13. Marcantonio ER, et al: A clinical prediction rule for delirium after elective noncardiac surgery, *JAMA* 271:134-139, 1994.
14. Morrison RS, Chassin MR, Siu AL: The medical consultant's role in caring for patients with hip fracture, *Ann Intern Med* 128:1010-1020, 1998.
15. Palda VA, Detsky AS: Perioperative assessment and management of risk from coronary artery disease, *Ann Intern Med* 127:313-328, 1997.

15a. Poldermans D, Boersma E. Bax JJ, et al. The effect of bisoprolol on perioperative mortality and myocardial infarction in high-risk patients undergoing vascular surgery, *N Engl J Med* 341:1789-1794, 1999.

16. Rao TLK, Jacobs KH, El-Etr AA: Reinfarction following anesthesia in patients with myocardial infarction, *Anesthesiology* 59:499-505, 1983.
17. Wagenknecht LE, Furberg CD, Hammon JW, et al: Surgical bleeding; unexpected effect of a calcium antagonist, *Br Med J* 310:776-777, 1995.
18. Warner MA, Shields SE, Chute CG: Major morbidity and mortality within 1 month of ambulatory surgery and anesthesia, *JAMA* 270:1437, 1993.

PRESENTING SIGNS AND SYMPTOMS II

Abdominal Pain, Chronic

Leonor Fernandez

Chronic abdominal pain is defined as intermittent or continuous abdominal pain or discomfort for longer than 3 to 6 months. It is a difficult disorder to manage; its persistence often leaves the patient and physician unsure of how much diagnostic certainty to pursue. This quandary reflects concern about missing a treatable disorder and diagnosing a functional gastrointestinal (GI) disorder. The functional disorders, by definition, lack any clear physiologic or structural markers, although recent studies about increased nociception are challenging traditional notions of organic vs. functional illnesses (see Chapter 50). Many patients with chronic abdominal pain undergo repeated surgery and its accompanying risks because other gynecologic and surgical problems were wrongly attributed to functional disorders. Given the high prevalence of these functional disorders, an emerging consensus is that physicians should seek a positive diagnosis rather than rely only on a diagnosis of exclusion. This approach can help avoid the cascade of tests and procedures that otherwise may occur, with associated financial and medical costs.[5] Data are limited, however, to guide the primary care physician to the most helpful tests. This chapter outlines a general diagnostic approach to patients with chronic abdominal pain; further studies are needed to evaluate diagnostic tests in the primary care setting.

(A) *History.* The differential diagnosis for chronic abdominal pain includes chronic pancreatitis, intestinal angina, inflammatory bowel disease, pancreatic cancer, porphyria, Addison's disease, abdominal adhesions, small and large bowel cancer, and peritoneal metastases (see Chapter 107). It also includes several functional GI disorders, such as functional abdominal pain syndrome, functional abdominal bloating, and irritable bowel syndrome (IBS) (see Chapter 110). The physician should routinely inquire about the chronology, severity, pattern and location of pain, exacerbating and alleviating factors, change in stool quality or caliber, hematochezia, weight loss, family history, medication and drug use, and travel history. A psychosocial history is very important, since prior trauma or sexual abuse may predispose to chronic pain.

When patients describe chronic intermittent pain with complete lack of pain between episodes, the physician should assess for features of biliary colic, intermittent intestinal obstruction, metabolic disorders (e.g., porphyria, lead intoxication), endometriosis, intestinal angina, and IBS.

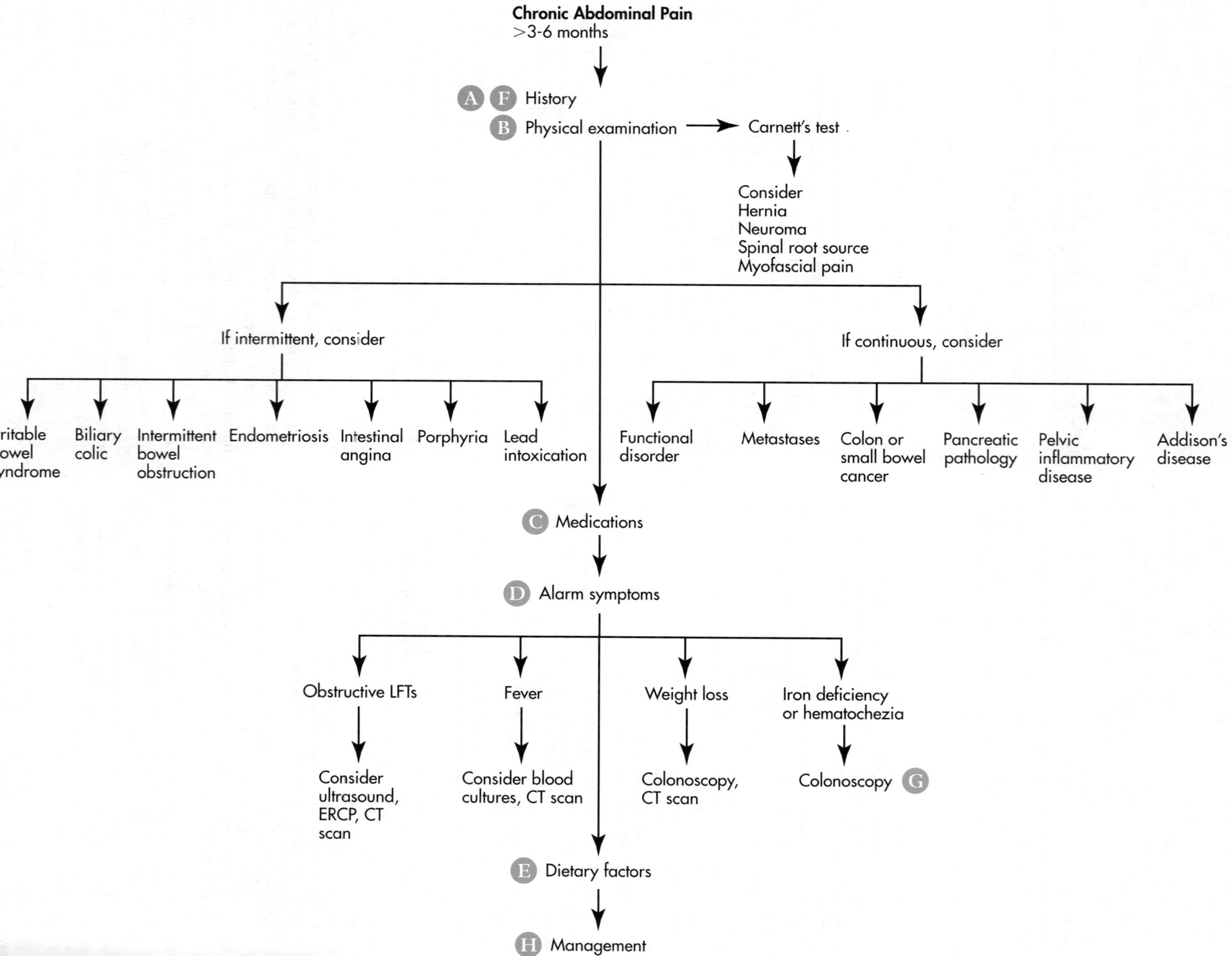
Chronic Abdominal Pain
>3-6 months
A F History
B Physical examination
Carnett's test
Consider
Hernia
Neuroma
Spinal root source
Myofascial pain
If intermittent, consider
Irritable bowel syndrome
Biliary colic
Intermittent bowel obstruction
Endometriosis
Intestinal angina
Porphyria
Lead intoxication
If continuous, consider
Functional disorder
Metastases
Colon or small bowel cancer
Pancreatic pathology
Pelvic inflammatory disease
Addison's disease
C Medications
D Alarm symptoms
Obstructive LFTs
Consider ultrasound, ERCP, CT scan
Fever
Consider blood cultures, CT scan
Weight loss
Colonoscopy, CT scan
Iron deficiency or hematochezia
Colonoscopy G
E Dietary factors
H Management

Continuous pain may suggest functional syndromes, metastases, pelvic inflammatory disease (PID), colon or small bowel cancer, pancreatic pathology, or adrenal insufficiency. A prior history of hematochezia, excess alcohol use, or the triad of diabetes, steatorrhea, and weight loss may suggest pancreatitis as a cause of abdominal pain (although the triad is not a sensitive indicator).

The pain of chronic pancreatitis may differ from typical acute pancreatitis and may be in the right or left upper quadrants or in the back. It is often deep, persistent, and unresponsive to antacids. A family history of episodic abdominal pain, especially if accompanied by neurologic symptoms, suggests porphyria. Women with lower abdominal and pelvic pain should be evaluated for possible PID, endometriosis, and other gynecologic disorders (see Chapter 37). Dull or cramping abdominal pain 15 to 30 minutes after a meal and lasting for several hours may suggest chronic mesenteric insufficiency or intestinal angina, particularly in patients with risk factors for atherosclerosis.

Many patients with chronic abdominal pain have IBS, especially of the bloating type. From 10% to 20% of the U.S. adult population reports symptoms compatible with IBS, although only 15% to 50% of those affected seek medical attention.[3,4] The pain is often described as crampy, variable in intensity, and generally on the left side, although location may vary. Emotional stress and eating may exacerbate the pain, and defecation typically relieves it. A longer duration of symptoms generally favors IBS over "organic" disease. Most patients with IBS develop symptoms in early adulthood or even younger; therefore the new onset of IBS in a patient over 50 should prompt a more rigorous evaluation (colonoscopy, computed tomography [CT] scan). Many women (48% to 79%) with chronic pelvic pain, dyspareunia, and dysmenorrhea also have symptoms that meet the criteria for IBS.[3]

B *Physical Examination.* After being weighed, the patient is assessed for location of tenderness and presence of any organ enlargement, masses, jaundice, or ascites. Many patients have abdominal scars because of the predisposition to undergo abdominal surgery. The usefulness of a stool guaiac test is controversial,[4] especially if obtained by digital rectal examination. Patients over age 50 or with risks for colon cancer should probably undergo a structural colon examination (colonoscopy, sigmoidoscopy, or barium enema) even with a negative guaiac test. Patients with IBS will often have tenderness over the sigmoid colon. Patients with functional abdominal pain syndrome usually have a pattern of diffuse tenderness with no clear localization. A complete pelvic and bimanual examination is important in the evaluation of women. *Carnett's test* involves palpating the supine patient's abdomen to elicit the area of tenderness. The examiner keeps the palpating fingers over the tender spot while the patient lifts the head, contracting the abdominal wall muscles. When the source of the pain is in the abdominal wall, the pain is as severe or increased; when the source is intraabdominal, the tensed muscles protect the viscera, and pain should decrease.[2]

C *Medications.* Chronic narcotic use may result in a narcotic constipation syndrome with abdominal pain. Several medications (e.g., exogenous gonadal steroids, barbiturates, sulfonamide antibiotics, anticonvulsants) can trigger abdominal pain in porphyria. Chronic steroid use may predispose to secondary adrenal insufficiency, leading to abdominal pain.

D *Alarm Symptoms.* Anorexia, weight loss, or malnutrition should prompt further workup. These are not features of IBS and may be caused by psychiatric comorbidity (e.g., depression). Pancreatic cancer may also present with depression. New onset of IBS in an older patient is unusual (see A). Anemia and unexplained low albumin should be evaluated further. Hematochezia and hematemesis also require further workup, although rectal bleeding from hemorrhoids is common.[7] Fever requires further evaluation for infectious, neoplastic, or other etiologies (e.g., abscess, lymphoma, familial Mediterranean fever, rheumatologic conditions). Pain that awakens the patient at night also suggests a more serious pathology, although it may be difficult to distinguish between pain-induced awakening and poor sleep for other reasons (e.g., depression).[1]

E *Dietary Factors.* Lactose, fructose, and sorbitol intake may aggravate diarrhea-predominant IBS. A trial of dietary exclusion of dairy products may be considered when lactose intolerance is suspected. Given the high efficacy of any intervention in patients with IBS, dairy products should probably be reintroduced eventually even if the trial is successful. Indeed, self-reported lactose intolerance and actual lactose malabsorption seem to be poorly correlated. In one study, one third of patients who reported severe lactose intolerance absorbed lactose normally.[6]

F *Psychosocial History.* This should be elicited in the initial evaluation and then again over time as the patient's trust in the physician increases. Depression, generalized anxiety disorder, and a history of sexual abuse are more common in patients with functional GI disease. Their identification may enable treatment, and their mere acknowledgment may strengthen the physician-patient relationship. Understanding the symptom's meaning and cultural context is important.

G *Laboratory and Other Studies.* Few data are available on the cost-effectiveness of studies on patients presenting to a primary care physician (vs. the more selected population presenting to a gastroenterologist). Most agree that a limited laboratory and structural evaluation is sufficient for many patients. The patient's age, predominant symptom, and its duration and severity may help physicians to select tests. A complete blood count (CBC) should be done to check for anemia and leukocytosis. Some authors suggest blood chemistry, including liver function tests (LFTs) and amylase, erythrocyte sedimentation rate (ESR), and thyroid-stimulating hormone (TSH). In patients with typical IBS symptoms, more blood tests may not be helpful. Stool ova and parasites may be considered, especially in patients with predominant diarrhea, and in those with a relevant travel history or possible exposure to *Giardia* organisms or in immunosuppressed patients.

The presence of alarm symptoms should indicate imaging studies such as a CT scan and colonoscopy. A flexible sigmoidoscopy or colonoscopy is reasonable for many patients with chronic abdominal pain and is essential in those over age 50 or with risk factors for colon cancer. In a young patient with typical IBS symptoms, however, the structural examination has a low yield. If diarrhea predominates as a symptom, it may be necessary to rule out inflammatory bowel disease. A rectal biopsy (e.g., to rule out collagenous proctitis) is not routinely necessary, especially in patients who fulfilled symptom criteria for IBS.[4] A CT scan may be helpful with suspected pancreatic pathology, with alarm symptoms and an unrevealing colon evaluation, or with a suspected hernia not obvious on examination. The role for laparoscopy is controversial; often it is suggested to rule out adhesions in patients with prior surgery. One study found a high prevalence of asymptomatic adhesions in an autopsy study of women (50% in women with no prior history of surgery, 69% in those with prior surgery).[8] This may suggest that adhesions are common and nonspecific. Endoscopic retrograde cholangiopancreatography (ERCP) is used to investigate biliary tract pathology; some authors question its utility in the absence of structural abnormalities.

H *Management.* Alarm symptoms should prompt a referral and further investigations, as described. If no alarm symptoms are present and the diagnostic criteria for a functional disorder are met, the patient can be managed with a drug regimen targeting the specific symptom (see Chapter 110). An exacerbation of symptoms without an alarm symptom does not require reinvestigation with multiple tests.

These patients often benefit from a multidisciplinary approach, with the input of gynecologists, gastroenterologists, pain specialists, and social workers working with the primary care physician. This approach may help avoid fragmentation of care (e.g., through emergency room use) and unnecessary tests and surgeries. As with other chronic illnesses, setting realistic goals, providing reassurance, and involving patients in their care reduces the burden of the disorder[1] (see Chapter 142).

REFERENCES

1. Camilleri M, Prather CM: The irritable bowel syndrome: mechanisms and a practical approach to management, *Ann Intern Med* 116:1001-1008, 1992.
2. Gallegos NC, Hobsley M: Abdominal wall pain: an alternative diagnosis, *Br J Surg* 77:1167, 1990.
3. Kruis W, Thieme CH, Weinzierl M, et al: A diagnostic score for the irritable bowel syndrome: its value in the exclusion of organic disease, *Gastroenterology* 87:1, 1984.
4. Longstreth GF: Irritable bowel syndrome: diagnosis in the managed care era, *Dig Dis Sci* 42:1105, 1997.
5. Mold JW, Stein HF: The cascade effect in the clinical care of patients, *N Engl J Med* 314:512, 1986.
6. Suarez FL, Savaiano DA, Levitt MD: A comparison of symptoms after the consumption of milk or lactose-hydrolyzed milk by people with self-reported severe lactose intolerance, *N Engl J Med* 333:1, 1995.
7. Talley NJ, Phillips SF, Melton LF, et al: Diagnostic value of the Manning criteria in the irritable bowel syndrome, *Gut* 31:77, 1990.
8. Weibel MA: Peritoneal adhesions and their relation to abdominal surgery, *Am J Surg* 126:345, 1973.

CHAPTER 15

Anorexia

Leonor Fernandez

Anorexia is a loss or decrease in appetite. The symptom of anorexia has been studied in the context of cancer, aging, and the human immunodeficiency virus (HIV), but most epidemiologic studies have focused on the clinical entity of *weight loss* rather than anorexia. It is therefore difficult to give an estimate of the prevalence of anorexia. In practice, anorexia is often associated with unintentional weight loss, and the evaluation may be approached similarly (see Chapter 25). This chapter highlights some unique aspects of the evaluation of anorexia.

The pathophysiology of anorexia is complex and incompletely understood. Several cytokines (e.g., interleukins 1 and 6, tumor necrosis factor-α) may mediate anorexia in cancer, HIV disease, and rheumatoid arthritis by acting on the hypothalamic feeding-associated sites.[1,5] Some evidence indicates that anorexia may be adaptive in the short term with certain infections because it may serve to "starve" pathogens of nutrients.[2] The *anorexia-cachexia syndrome* is associated with a variety of conditions, such as chronic pain, depression, anxiety, hypogeusia, hyposmia, early satiety, and iatrogenic factors (e.g., chemotherapy, radiotherapy).[6] Aging often leads to a gradual decrease in appetite. This physiologic anorexia of aging is thought to result from a decrease in an opioid responsible for the feeding drive and an increase in the satiating effect of cholecystokinin.[3]

A *History.* When taking a history, the examiner should screen for several common conditions that may cause anorexia, including depression, anxiety, substance abuse (alcohol, intravenous drugs, and cocaine may lead to decreased appetite), and eating disorders, particularly in young women, athletes, dancers, and models, all known to be at increased risk for anorexia nervosa (see Chapter 55). Eliciting a fear of gaining weight or excessive worry about body fat may provide clues to eating disorders. A menstrual history is important in all women because amenorrhea often accompanies eating disorders and substantial weight loss. It is reasonable to assess HIV risk in all patients with anorexia.

Social factors that affect ability to eat should be evaluated, such as social isolation, lack of money, and physical impairments, since the patient or family may not always express the reasons for not eating. A thorough review of symptoms may be helpful, such as inquiring about fever, sweats, symptoms of hyperthyroidism and hypothyroidism, change in bowel habits or other gastrointestinal (GI) functions, and symptoms suggesting malignancy or neurologic disease. A travel history should be obtained to consider a variety of chronic infections. Medication use should be evaluated.

B *Physical Examination.* The patient's weight and body mass index (BMI) enable the physician and patient to document weight loss over time. The examiner should assess the most common sites of malignancy: lungs, breast, skin,

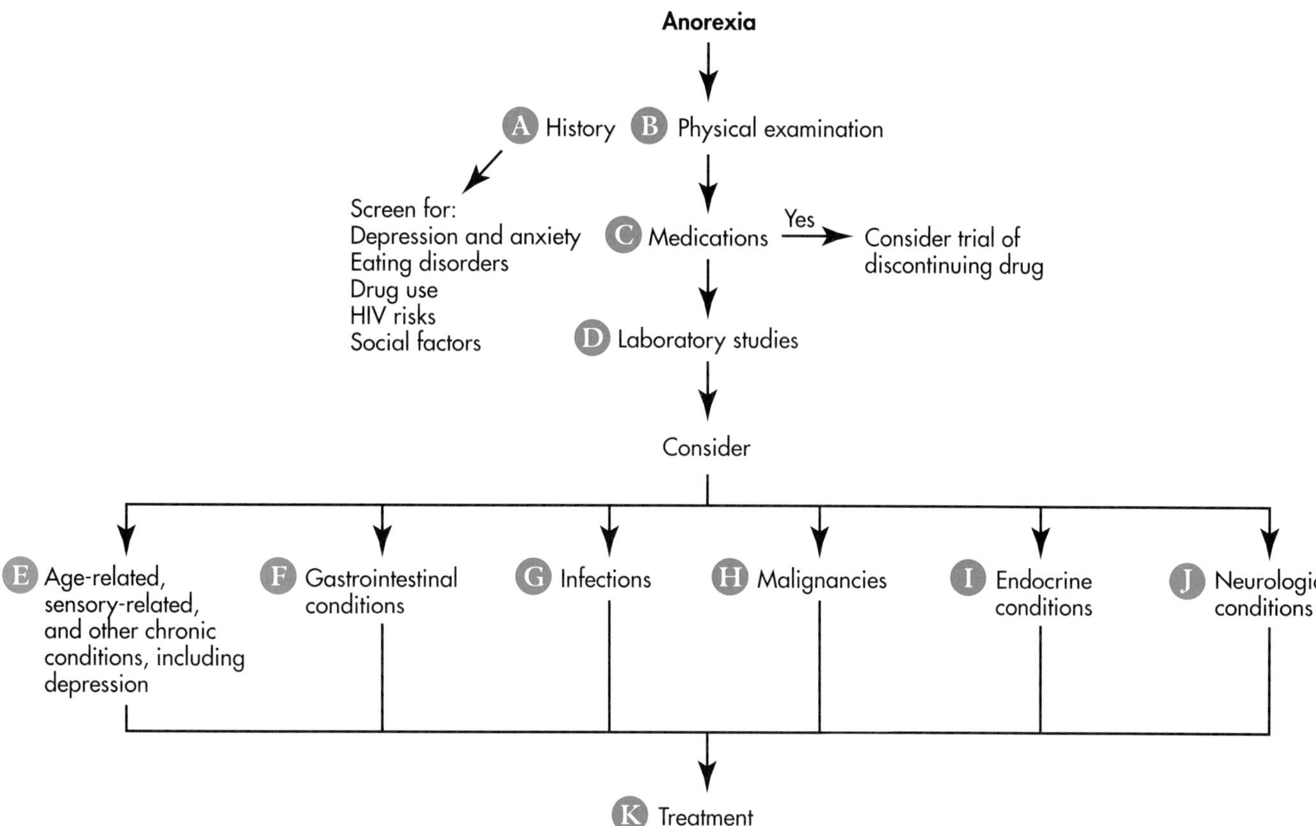

prostate, and colon. The lymph nodes and thyroid should also be assessed, with a check for hepatosplenomegaly, jaundice, or signs of central nervous system (CNS) dysfunction, including papilledema and dementia. The oral cavity should be examined to make sure no lesions or denture problems are causing difficulty eating. Patients with bulimia may have loss of tooth enamel.

C *Medications.* Drugs are a common cause of anorexia or dysgeusia (parageusia), and a trial of discontinuation should be considered. Culprits include sedatives, psychotropics, digoxin, appetite suppressants, interferon, thiazide diuretics, levodopa, narcotics, antibiotics, and chemotherapeutics.

D *Laboratory and Other Studies.* These are determined by the history but may reasonably include electrolytes, glucose, thyroid-stimulating hormone (TSH), calcium, liver function tests (LFTs, particularly albumin), and complete blood count (CBC). All these may not be necessary, however, if the anorexia is minimal or of recent onset. Few data indicate which studies are best. The patient with epidemiologic risk factors may have HIV serology. A Mini Nutritional Assessment may be used as a screening tool for early malnutrition in patients[7] (Fig. 15-1). A chest radiograph may be considered to evaluate the possibility of lung cancer, tuberculosis, and abscess. All applicable screening tests (e.g., mammogram, Papanicolaou smear, sigmoidoscopy, colonoscopy) should be updated, especially if no cause is readily identified for the anorexia.

E *Age-related Symptoms.* The physiologic (mild) anorexia of aging is partly related to the hypogeusia experienced with increasing age. The sense of smell is an integral part of the taste experience, and thus the decreased olfaction associated with chronic allergic rhinitis, smoking, advanced age, and rare neurologic problems may make food less desirable. Other chronic conditions, such as chronic pain, severe congestive heart failure, uremia, and respiratory failure, may also decrease interest in food.

F *Gastrointestinal Conditions.* GI malignancy may present with anorexia because of gastric outlet obstruction, intestinal obstruction, esophageal mass, or distant metastases. Other GI conditions that may cause anorexia include peptic ulcer disease, malabsorption, hepatitis, biliary disease, dysmotility, and oral cavity disease. Symptoms may guide the need for tests, such as stool for fat or parasites, sigmoidoscopy, endoscopy, radionuclide emptying scan, or upper GI series with small bowel follow-through. Hepatitis often causes dysgeusia in addition to decreased appetite.

G *Infections.* Patients with anorexia should be screened for HIV risk factors. Other infections to consider include tuberculosis, subacute bacterial endocarditis, parasitic infection, and abscess. Anorexia may occur in many acute infections, such as pneumonia, mononucleosis, and endocarditis, and is particularly common in viral hepatitis.

H *Malignancies.* Many malignancies may present with anorexia, especially those involving the GI tract. Renal cancer also may accompany this condition.

I *Endocrine Conditions.* Both hyperthyroidism and hypothyroidism may cause anorexia. One study on Graves' disease found that appetite decreased in 27% of hyperthyroid patients in their 70s.[4] Other causes include marked

NESTLÉ NUTRITION SERVICES

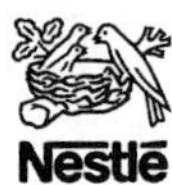

Mini Nutritional Assessment MNA®

Last name: First name: Sex: Date:

Age: Weight, kg: Height, cm: I.D. Number:

Complete the screen by filling in the boxes with the appropriate numbers.
Add the numbers for the screen. If score is 11 or less, continue with the assessment to gain a Malnutrition Indicator Score.

Screening

A Has food intake declined over the past 3 months due to loss of appetite, digestive problems, chewing or swallowing difficulties?
0 = severe loss of appetite
1 = moderate loss of appetite
2 = no loss of appetite ☐

B Weight loss during last months
0 = weight loss greater than 3 kg (6.6 lbs)
1 = does not know
2 = weight loss between 1 and 3 kg (2.2 and 6.6 lbs)
3 = no weight loss ☐

C Mobility
0 = bed or chair bound
1 = able to get out of bed/chair but does not go out
2 = goes out ☐

D Has suffered psychological stress or acute disease in the past 3 months
0 = yes 2 = no ☐

E Neuropsychological problems
0 = severe dementia or depression
1 = mild dementia
2 = no psychological problems ☐

F Body Mass Index (BMI) (weight in kg) / (height in m)^2
0 = BMI less than 19
1 = BMI 19 to less than 21
2 = BMI 21 to less than 23
3 = BMI 23 or greater ☐

Screening score (subtotal max. 14 points) ☐ ☐

12 points or greater Normal – not at risk – no need to complete assessment
11 points or below Possible malnutrition – continue assessment

Assessment

G Lives independently (not in a nursing home or hospital)
0 = no 1 = yes ☐

H Takes more than 3 prescription drugs per day
0 = yes 1 = no ☐

I Pressure sores or skin ulcers
0 = yes 1 = no ☐

J How many full meals does the patient eat daily?
0 = 1 meal
1 = 2 meals
2 = 3 meals ☐

K Selected consumption markers for protein intake
- At least one serving of dairy products (milk, cheese, yogurt) per day? yes ☐ no ☐
- Two or more servings of legumes or eggs per week? yes ☐ no ☐
- Meat, fish or poultry every day yes ☐ no ☐

0.0 = if 0 or 1 yes
0.5 = if 2 yes
1.0 = if 3 yes ☐.☐

L Consumes two or more servings of fruits or vegetables per day?
0 = no 1 = yes ☐

M How much fluid (water, juice, coffee, tea, milk...) is consumed per day?
0.0 = less than 3 cups
0.5 = 3 to 5 cups
1.0 = more than 5 cups ☐.☐

N Mode of feeding
0 = unable to eat without assistance
1 = self-fed with some difficulty
2 = self-fed without any problem ☐

O Self view of nutritional status
0 = view self as being malnourished
1 = is uncertain of nutritional state
2 = views self as having no nutritional problem ☐

P In comparison with other people of the same age, how does the patient consider his/her health status?
0.0 = not as good
0.5 = does not know
1.0 = as good
2.0 = better ☐.☐

Q Mid-arm circumference (MAC) in cm
0.0 = MAC less than 21
0.5 = MAC 21 to 22
1.0 = MAC 22 or greater ☐.☐

R Calf circumference (CC) in cm
0 = CC less than 31 1 = CC 31 or greater ☐

Assessment (max. 16 points) ☐ ☐.☐

Screening score ☐ ☐

Total Assessment (max. 30 points) ☐ ☐.☐

Malnutrition Indicator Score

17 to 23.5 points at risk of malnutrition ☐

Less than 17 points malnourished ☐

Ref.: Guigoz Y, Vellas B and Garry PJ. 1994. Mini Nutritional Assessment: A practical assessment tool for grading the nutritional state of elderly patients. *Facts and Research in Gerontology.* Supplement #2:15-59.
Rubenstein LZ, Harker J, Guigoz Y and Vellas B. Comprehensive Geriatric Assessment (CGA) and the MNA: An Overview of CGA, Nutritional Assessment, and Development of a Shortened Version of the MNA. In: "Mini Nutritional Assessment (MNA): Research and Practice in the Elderly". Vellas B, Garry PJ and Guigoz Y, editors. Nestlé Nutrition Workshop Series. Clinical & Performance Programme, vol. 1. Karger, Bâle, in press.

Fig. 15-1. Mini Nutritional Assessment (MNA) form. (Courtesy Societé des Produits Nestlé SA, 1998.)

hypercalcemia, uncontrolled diabetes, hyperparathyroidism, adrenal insufficiency, and panhypopituitarism. Diabetes may also cause delayed gastric emptying, which may occur with early satiety.

J *Neurologic Conditions.* Dementia and Parkinson's disease are often accompanied by decreased appetite. CNS tumors, especially those involving the hypothalamus, may present with anorexia.

K *Treatment.* Referral to a nutritionist may be helpful. Caloric supplements, enteral feeding, peripheral nutrition, and a variety of drugs (e.g., growth hormone, megestrol, cyproheptadine, tetrahydrocannabinol, anabolic steroids, prokinetic agents, antidepressants) are used with variable success (see Chapters 32 and 118). Contributing social and economic factors need to be addressed.

REFERENCES

1. Albrecht JT, Canada TW: Cachexia and anorexia in malignancy, *Hematol Oncol Clin North Am* 10:791, 1996.
2. Exton MS: Infection-induced anorexia: active host defense strategy, *Appetite* 29:369, 1997.
3. Morley JE: Anorexia in older persons: epidemiology and optimal treatment, *Drugs Aging*, 8(2):134, 1996.
4. Nordyke RA, Gilbert FI, Harada ASM: Graves' disease: influence of age on clinical findings, *Arch Intern Med* 148:626, 1988.
5. Plata-Salaman CR: Anorexia during acute and chronic disease, Nutrition 12:69, 1996.
6. Plata-Salaman CR: Cytokines and anorexia: a brief overview, *Semin Oncol* 25(suppl 1):64, 1998.
7. Vellas B, Guigoz Y, Garry PJ, et al: The Mini Nutritional Assessment and its use in grading the nutritional state of elderly patients, *Nutrition* 15:116, 1999.

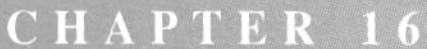

CHAPTER 16

Chest Pain

Charles Telfer Williams

Pains or discomfort in the chest can be caused by a multitude of ailments encompassing the psychiatric, neurologic, respiratory, cardiovascular, musculoskeletal, gastrointestinal (GI), and dermatologic systems. Increasingly good studies delineate guidelines for the assessment of chest pain in the emergency department setting.[2,5,6] Less is known about chest pain in the ambulatory setting (Table 16-1).[1,3,4] The STARNET study, which screened for anxiety and panic in ambulatory patients presenting with chest pain, before the physician interview, found that half the patients (25 of 51) had either infrequent panic or panic disorder and that physicians frequently missed these symptoms.[3]

Although the diseases that present with chest pain are well described, precise diagnosis is complicated by cultural differences in disease presentation, physiology of pain perception in the chest area, and coexistence of other disease. Given these confounding factors, a simple algorithmic approach to the diagnosis of chest pain is at best a guideline. A careful history and physical examination are essential and can help the physician prioritize disease risks. The first task is to rule out the potentially life-threatening causes: myocardial infarction (MI), unstable angina, dissecting aneurysm, pulmonary embolism (PE), pneumothorax, or the depressed patient with suicidal intent.

Table 16-1. Causes of Chest Pain in Ambulatory Setting

	ASPN[1] (1990)	MIRNET[4] (1994)	STARNET[3] (1997)
Musculoskeletal	239 (28%)	36.2%	9 (17%)
Cardiovascular	287 (34%)	16.1%	4 (7%)
Psychiatric	62 (7%)	7.5%	19 (35%)
Gastrointestinal	114 (14%)	18.9%	5 (9%)
Respiratory	36 (4%)	5.1%	2 (4%)
Other	94 (11%)	16.1%	12 (22%)
TOTAL PATIENTS	832		51

A *History.* The history starts with a good knowledge of the characteristic symptoms of the different diseases that present with chest pain (Table 16-2). Psychiatric disorders can mimic many of these symptoms, in particular cardiac symptoms. Any evaluation of chest pain should consider anxiety disorders, especially panic attacks, because of their frequency in primary care settings. Panic symptoms include (1) shortness of breath or a smothering sensation; (2) dizziness, unsteady feelings, or faintness; (3) palpitations or accelerated heart rate; (4) trembling or shaking; (5) sweating; (6) choking; (7) nausea or abdominal distress; (8) depersonalization or derealization; (9) paresthesias; (10) flushes or chills; (11) chest pain or discomfort; (12) fear of dying; and (13) fear of "going crazy" or losing control (see Chapter 49). Chronic chest pains are unlikely to result from panic but can be caused by other psychiatric illnesses, including anxiety, somatiform disorder, and depression. Patients with recurring or chronic chest pain should be screened for these disorders (see Chapters 48 and 50).

The history should include the patient's risk factors for atherosclerotic disease: personal history of coronary artery disease (angina or prior MI), gender (males are more likely to have disease at a younger age), hypertension, diabetes, high LDL (low-density lipoprotein) or total cholesterol, low HDL (high-density lipoprotein) cholesterol, smoking, family history of premature coronary artery disease (male under age 55, female under 65), and obesity. Many patients with angina or MI, however, have none of these risk factors.* Finally, asking about substance use, particularly cocaine, is necessary because cocaine use may cause angina or MI.

B *Physical Examination.* The examination can help clarify the differential diagnoses generated by the history. The general appearance of the patient is nonspecific but often is revealing. Cyanosis indicates hypoxemia from abnormal respiratory function (e.g., ventilation/perfusion mismatch) or

*For calculation of risk based on Framingham Study data, visit http://www.biostat.washington.edu/~thomas/CHS/framol.html.

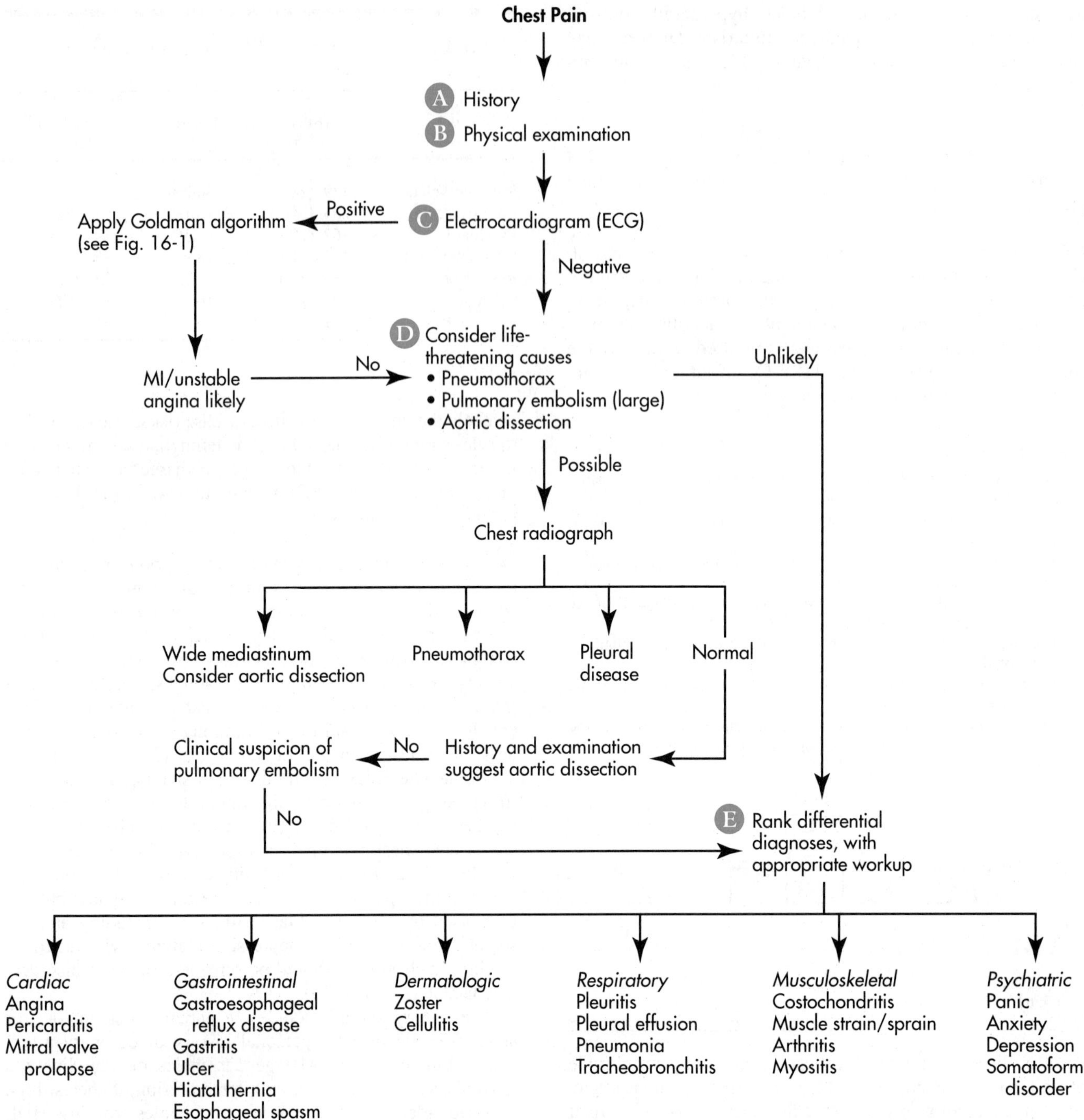

low cardiac output. Severe pain is unlikely to signify mild disease. Sweating is often associated with MI. High anxiety levels may be seen in any chest pain presentation but may suggest panic or anxiety disorder.

The vital signs are important in determining the patient's stability. Tachycardia can be associated with anxiety, MI, PE, and pneumothorax. Bradycardia may be seen in healthy normal patients or those with MI. Hypertension may be an underlying or acute condition and is unlikely to help clarify the diagnosis; hypotension is more suggestive of MI (likelihood ratio [LR] 3.1) but may also be seen in patients with PE.[7] Blood pressures in both arms and a leg should be performed to rule out aortic dissection.

Respirations can be increased in any cause of chest pain but are most likely in pulmonary processes. Respiratory examination may reveal absent breath sounds or a deviated trachea consistent with pneumothorax or tension pneumothorax. Pulmonary friction rubs may indicate a pleural process. Dullness to percussion or increased tactile fremitus may indicate consolidation, as in pulmonary infarction. Fine crackles may indicate heart failure. Tachypnea may be seen with anxiety, MI, PE, pneumothorax, pleural irritation, or "splinting" from musculoskeletal injury.

The cardiac examination may be entirely normal in a patient having an acute MI, but a third heart sound is somewhat predictive (LR 3.2).[7] A new mitral regurgita-

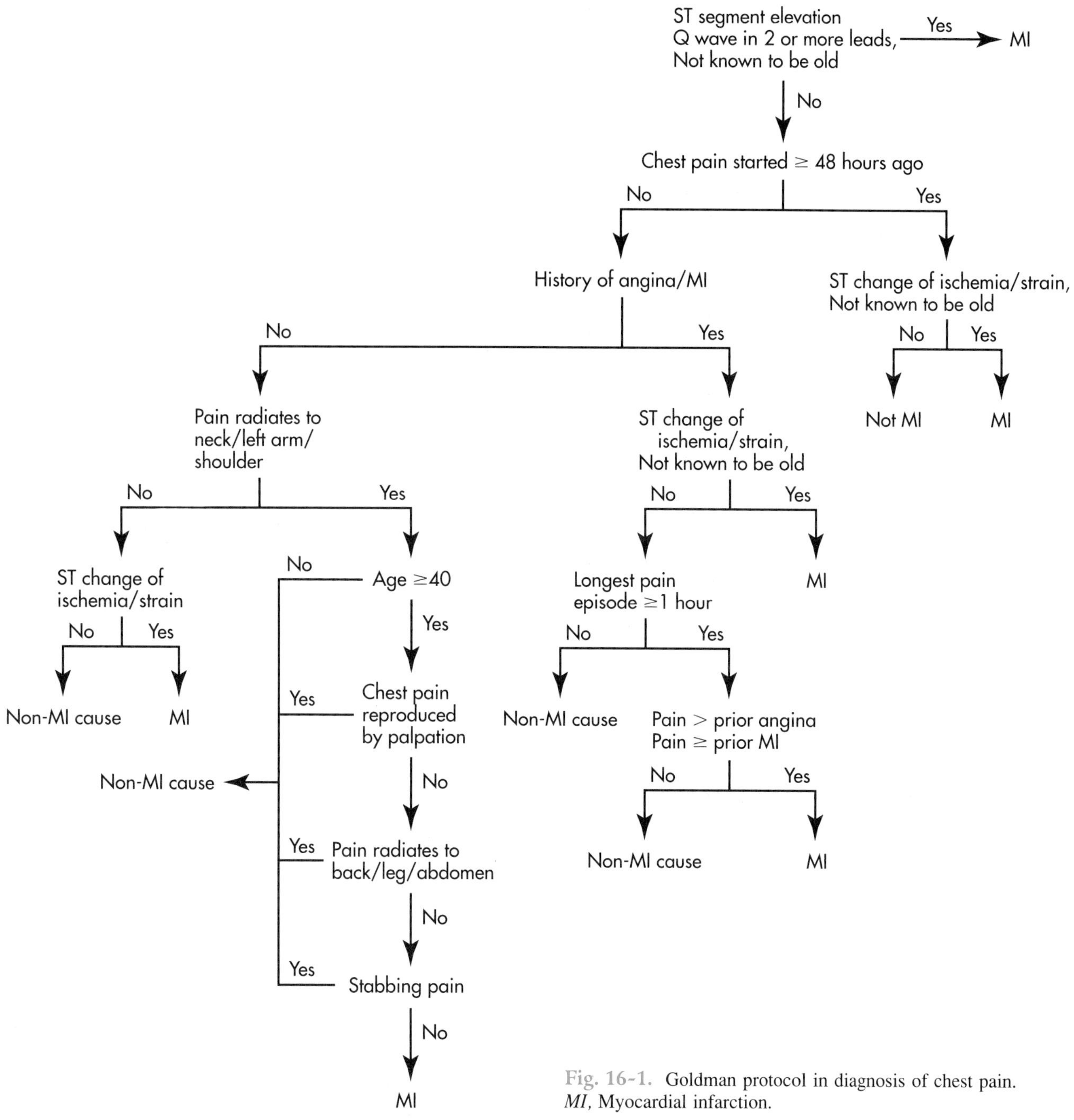

Fig. 16-1. Goldman protocol in diagnosis of chest pain. *MI*, Myocardial infarction.

tion murmur may be noted with papillary muscle dysfunction from an MI. A cardiac friction rub suggests pericarditis.

Palpation of the chest wall, shoulders, and abdomen is crucial. If this palpation reproduces the chest pain syndrome, it is likely to be musculoskeletal. The examiner must ensure that palpation is reproducing the pain symptoms, not just causing pain. A way to test this is to inject anesthetic into the pain site; if the pain is alleviated, it is likely musculoskeletal. Likewise, if nitroglycerin eliminates the pain, a cardiac etiology is much more likely. If reproduced by palpation (LR 0.2 to 0.4) or positional (LR 0.3), pain is unlikely to be from an MI. Extremity examination reveals signs of deep venous thrombosis in 50% of patients with PE.

C *Electrocardiogram (ECG).* This relatively inexpensive and easily obtained test may be helpful for identifying cardiac disease as well as some pulmonary pathologies (e.g., massive embolism). In a stable patient in whom the pretest probability of cardiac ischemia is low, the physician may consider *not* obtaining an ECG. Lee et al[5] identified three criteria that predicted a low probability of MI or unstable angina: (1) sharp or stabbing pain, (2) no history of angina or MI, and (3) pleuritic or positional pain, or pain reproduced by palpation of the chest wall. In patients who met all three criteria (48 of 596), none had MI or unstable angina, and the ECG in 30 (63%) was potentially misleading. Even if these criteria are met, however, an ECG may still be helpful in clarifying other diagnoses.

Table 16-2. Diseases that Present with Chest Pain

Etiology	Quality and associated symptoms	Region and distribution	Severity	Timing	Provocative activities	Palliative interventions
Angina	Heaviness, pressure, or squeezing, (occasionally burning) or deep dull ache; accompanied by nausea, diaphoresis, or hypotension	Substernal or anterior chest; may radiate to upper back, neck, teeth, shoulder, or arm	Variable: mild to severe	Gradual onset and resolution; continuous pain typically 1-10 minutes; lag after precipitating events before it starts	Exercise, emotional stress, food, increased heart rate, cold, hypoglycemia, cocaine	Rest, nitroglycerine; not relieved in a few seconds of rest; pain that vanishes immediately on ceasing exercise unlikely to be angina
Variant angina (Prinzmetal's)	As with angina; often a history of migraine or Raynaud's phenomenon	As with angina	Variable: mild to severe		Often at rest or awakening patient from sleep; can be exercise related	
Myocardial infarction (MI)	As with angina	As with angina	Generally more severe	Similar onset; duration exceeds 20-30 minutes	As with angina	Not relieved by rest or nitroglycerine
Pericarditis	Most often pleuritic (see Pleural pain) but can resemble angina	May be felt in top of shoulder (when irritation near central diaphragm) or in lateral chest and back in dermatomal distribution; occasionally substernal or radiating to neck	Variable	Gradual onset lasts longer than angina; often associated with connective tissue disease or following MI or viral illness	Often increased by lying down or swallowing	Sitting up
Aortic dissection	True pain not vague as with angina	Center of chest, radiating to back	Usually severe	Abrupt onset in 80%; pain rapidly increases over hours and does not diminish	Not affected by position	None
Pulmonary infarction from pulmonary embolism	Ranges from deep crushing pain similar to MI or more pleuritic; may be accompanied by weakness, [illegible] vomiting, and	Substernal, if massive; lesser pulmonary infarction pain in chest area	Variable	Sudden onset	None; 50% have signs or symptoms of deep venous thrombosis peripherally	None

			[illegible]	Sudden onset	Trauma, sports, spontaneous and occasionally heavy lifting	None
Pleural pain	Sharp, knifelike; dull ache possible between sharp pains	Superficial chest wall	Mild to severe	Generally occurs with provocative maneuvers	Deep breath, cough, laugh, and movements	Splinting or positional changes
Tracheobronchitis	Burning or ache after prolonged coughing	Substernal; middle or upper	Mild to moderate	Accompanies or follows respiratory tract infection	Cough	
Esophagitis, esophageal pain, gastroesophageal reflux disease	Deep burning, may be indistinguishable from MI or angina	Epigastrium or substernal; as with angina	Variable	Generally gradual onset and more chronic with fluctuating course	Alcohol, NSAIDs, foods, large meals	Food, water, antacids
Esophageal spasm	Indistinguishable from MI					
Gastric/peptic ulcer	Deep burning/dull ache	Epigastric or substernal	Variable	60-90 minutes after eating	Anything that increases gastric or duodenal acidity	Milk, antacids
Cholecystitis	Ache or crampy pain	Epigastric, right upper quadrant, or substernal	Variable	After meals, minutes to hours; may be constant or fluctuating (colicky)	Fatty or rich foods	Time
Mediastinal emphysema	Intense, sharp pain	Substernal or shoulders	Severe	After trauma or coughing		None
Mediastinitis, tumors	Similar to pleuritis	Greatest in substernal region				
Costochondritis	Ranges from sharp (seconds) to dull (days to weeks) ache to tightness	Substernal, costal margins or lower ribs	Variable but rarely severe	Variable	May be worsened by motion or exercise	
Shoulder and muscle pain	Variable	Shoulder with radiation to anterior or posterior chest	Variable		Motion of arms, but not general exertion	Rest

NSAIDs, Nonsteroidal antiinflammatory drugs.

When reading an ECG, the physician should especially note signs suggestive of MI (ST segment elevation, new Q wave, dysrhythmias), pericarditis (diffuse ST elevation, PR depression), embolism (S1Q3T3, right bundle branch block, R axis, hyperacute P waves), or pneumothorax (change in axis). A normal ECG is fairly reassuring, although 20% of patients with MI have normal ECGs.

D *Life-threatening Causes.* The next step is to stratify the patient according to risk and rule out the potentially life-threatening causes of chest pain: MI, unstable angina, pneumothorax, PE, and aortic dissection. The physician first must determine whether the patient is having an acute MI or unstable angina, which would likely require admission to an intensive care setting; this is more likely than the other diagnoses. After the history and ECG have been obtained, apply the Goldman protocol or modifications of this protocol (see Chapter 13) (Fig. 16-1).[2] This sorts out MI/unstable angina with fairly good accuracy (sensitivity 88.0%, specificity 74.0%) and recommends monitoring in a cardiac care unit (CCU). In a prospective trial this protocol was equal to clinicians in detecting MI (88.0 vs. 87.8%) and superior to clinicians in ruling out MI (74.0 vs. 71.0%). Although the Goldman model identifies the patients needing admission to a CCU, it does not help determine which patients to send home or which to monitor in the hospital. Clinical judgment may still lead the physician to monitor the patient in an inpatient setting and should not be ignored.

Diagnosing aortic dissection, PE, and pneumothorax is usually aided by a chest radiograph, which can help rule out a pneumothorax and may indicate aortic dissection or pulmonary infarction. Aortic dissection should be suspected in patients with arm/arm or arm/leg blood pressures differences, pain radiating to the back, or a radiograph that shows a widened aorta. A high suspicion for the diagnosis of PE or pulmonary infarction is always required because classic signs (hemoptysis, tachypnea, tachycardia, fever) are not always present. Pneumothorax can often be diagnosed by physical examination, but a chest film during expiration rarely misses significant pneumothorax on careful review.

E *Differential Diagnosis and Workup.* Once illnesses requiring the most acute attention have been excluded, the physician should differentiate the other causes of chest pain: cardiac (angina, pericarditis, mitral valve prolapse), GI (gastroesophageal reflux disease [GERD], gastritis, ulcer, hiatal hernia, esophageal spasm), dermatologic (herpes zoster, cellulitis), respiratory (tracheobronchitis, pleuritis, pneumonia, pleural effusion), psychiatric (panic, anxiety, depression, other somatoform disorders), and musculoskeletal (costochondritis, strains, sprains, arthritis, myositis). A physical examination may indicate a musculoskeletal cause. Differentiating angina and GI causes of chest pain may be difficult. Evaluation of overall atherosclerotic risk factors helps to determine whether a cardiac workup should take precedence. In a young patient with few risk factors and atypical chest pain, therapy for GERD or gastritis should probably be done before a cardiac workup. Anxiety may be difficult to sort out but should be kept in the differential diagnosis to prevent misdiagnosis and prolonged workup (Table 16-2).

REFERENCES

1. Ambulatory Sentinel Practice Network: An exploratory report of chest pain in primary care, *J Am Board Fam Pract* 3:13, 1990.
2. Goldman L, Cook EF, Brand DA, et al: A computer protocol to predict myocardial infarction in emergency department patients with chest pain, *N Engl J Med* 318:797, 1988.
3. Katerndahl DA, Trammell C: Prevalence and recognition of panic states in STARNET patient presenting with chest pain, *J Fam Pract* 45:54, 1997.
4. Klinkman MS, Stevens D, Gorenflo DW: Episodes of care for chest pain: a preliminary report from MIRNET, *J Fam Pract* 38:345, 1994.
5. Lee TH, Cook EF, Weisberg M, et al: Acute chest pain in the emergency room: identification and examination of low-risk patients, *Arch Intern Med* 145:65, 1985.
6. Nichol G, Walls R, Goldman L, et al: A critical pathway for management of patients with acute chest pain who are at low risk for myocardial ischemia: recommendations and potential impact, *Ann Intern Med* 127: 996, 1997.
7. Panju AA, Hemmeigarn BR, Guyatt GH, Simel DL: Is this patient having a myocardial infarction? *JAMA* 280:1256, 1998.

CHAPTER 17

Cough

J. Mark Madison
Richard S. Irwin

Cough is a reflex that serves as a clearance mechanism when tracheobronchial mucociliary clearance is inadequate. Airflow generated during cough is normally sufficient to expel secretions or foreign bodies from the respiratory tract. Even in their absence, however, cough still can be precipitated by disease processes that directly or indirectly stimulate the sensory nerve fibers of the vagus nerve that serve as cough receptors.

Normal people without an illness rarely cough. Cough is a very common clinical problem. In a national ambulatory medical care survey in the United States in 1991, cough was the most common complaint for which patients sought medical attention and the second most frequent reason for a general medical examination.[9] The common cold is almost always associated with cough and accounts for many of these patient evaluations.

Cough can be a debilitating symptom. It is inappropriate to minimize a complaint of cough and advise the patient to "live with it." Referrals of patients with persistently troublesome cough of unknown etiology account for up to 38% of a pulmonologist's outpatient practice.[4] Relatively few conditions, however, account for most cases of persistently troublesome cough.[2-4] In prospective studies that included smokers, chronic cough is caused by postnasal drip syndrome (PNDS), asthma, gastroesophageal reflux disease (GERD), chronic bronchitis, or bronchiectasis in 91% to 94% of cases. Among nonsmokers who are not taking an angiotensin-converting enzyme inhibitor (ACEI) drug and who have a normal chest radiograph, persistently troublesome cough is almost always caused by PNDS, asthma, or GERD. Multiple causes may contribute simultaneously to the cough in at least 25% of these patients.[4]

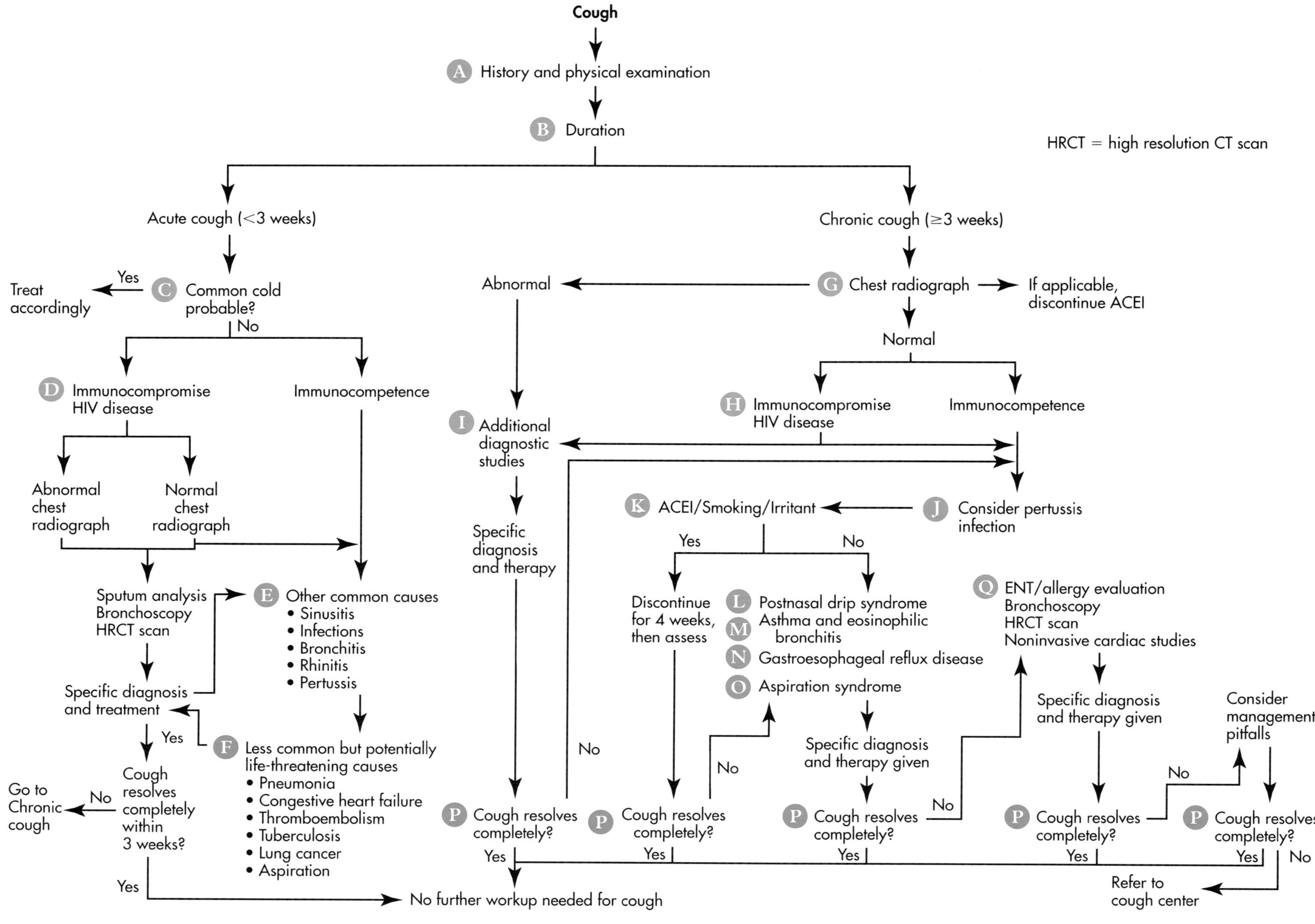
Cough
A History and physical examination
B Duration
HRCT = high resolution CT scan
Acute cough (<3 weeks)
Chronic cough (≥3 weeks)
Yes
Treat accordingly
C Common cold probable?
No
D Immunocompromise HIV disease
Immunocompetence
Abnormal chest radiograph
Normal chest radiograph
Sputum analysis Bronchoscopy HRCT scan
E Other common causes
• Sinusitis
• Infections
• Bronchitis
• Rhinitis
• Pertussis
Specific diagnosis and treatment
Yes
F Less common but potentially life-threatening causes
• Pneumonia
• Congestive heart failure
• Thromboembolism
• Tuberculosis
• Lung cancer
• Aspiration
Go to Chronic cough
No
Cough resolves completely within 3 weeks?
Yes
No further workup needed for cough
Abnormal
G Chest radiograph
If applicable, discontinue ACEI
Normal
H Immunocompromise HIV disease
Immunocompetence
I Additional diagnostic studies
Specific diagnosis and therapy
J Consider pertussis infection
K ACEI/Smoking/Irritant
Yes
No
Discontinue for 4 weeks, then assess
L Postnasal drip syndrome
M Asthma and eosinophilic bronchitis
N Gastroesophageal reflux disease
O Aspiration syndrome
Q ENT/allergy evaluation
Bronchoscopy
HRCT scan
Noninvasive cardiac studies
Specific diagnosis and therapy given
Specific diagnosis and therapy given
Consider management pitfalls
No
P Cough resolves completely?
Yes
P Cough resolves completely?
Yes
No
P Cough resolves completely?
Yes
No
P Cough resolves completely?
Yes
No
P Cough resolves completely?
Yes
No
Refer to cough center

A *History and Physical Examination.* The character and timing of cough are not helpful diagnostically.[8] A comprehensive history should be taken seeking evidence for uncommon but potentially life-threatening causes of cough, such as congestive heart failure and pulmonary thromboembolism. The history should also specifically identify symptoms suggestive of asthma or GERD.

Examination of the nasopharynges and oropharynges may reveal mucopurulent secretions or a cobblestoned mucosa when PNDS occurs from rhinosinus conditions. A cobblestoned mucosa may also be caused by GERD with reflux of gastric contents into the posterior oropharynx. Wheezing heard on auscultation of the chest suggests but is not diagnostic of asthma.

B *Duration.* The differential diagnosis of cough depends on the duration of symptoms.[3,4] Cough of less than 3 weeks' duration is defined as acute, whereas chronic cough is present for longer than 3 weeks and is persistently troublesome.

Acute Cough

C *Common Cold.* The common cold is the most common cause of acute cough (see Chapter 33). The diagnosis is usually certain when an acute upper respiratory illness predominantly affects the nasal passages (rhinorrhea, sneezing, nasal obstruction, postnasal drip). Patients may also have fever, lacrimation, and irritation of the throat, with a normal chest examination. Since cough from the common cold is mainly caused by postnasal drip, its treatment relieves the cough (see L).[1,3]

D *Immunocompromise.* For the patient who may be immunocompromised, acute cough should be evaluated further when the common cold seems unlikely clinically. An abnormal chest radiograph or a normal chest radiograph with a CD4 count less than 200 cells/mm^3, a CD4 count of 200 to 499 cells/mm^3 when the patient is clinically ill, and oxygen desaturation on exercise are indications for additional diagnostic studies to exclude intrathoracic opportunistic infection[10] (see Chapter 32).

E *Other Causes.* Other common causes of acute cough are acute bacterial sinusitis, acute lower respiratory tract infections, exacerbation of chronic bronchitis, allergic rhinitis, environmental irritant rhinitis, and pertussis.[2,3] When acute bronchitis causes cough in patients without underlying lung disease, it is most often caused by a virus, and antibiotics should not be given.

Pertussis needs to be considered in the evaluations of both acute and chronic cough.[3] Adult patients may not have the characteristic inspiratory whoop at the end of a coughing paroxysm, but they often vomit and usually have a catarrhal stage followed by paroxysmal and convalescent stages. The physician should consider diagnostic testing and treatment for pertussis infection in patients with cough-vomit syndrome, characteristic whoop, recent close contacts, or particularly severe cough in a high endemic area. If taken early in the course of the illness, a nasopharyngeal smear for culture, direct fluorescent antibody (DFA), or more recently polymerase chain reaction (PCR) for *Bordetella pertussis* will confirm the diagnosis. Beginning treatment with a macrolide antibiotic within 8 days of infection is effective in decreasing the severity of infection and transmission. Because pertussis is contagious, prophylaxis for exposed persons is important.

F *Life-threatening Conditions.* Acute cough can also be the presenting symptom of serious illnesses such as pneumonia, asthma, congestive heart failure, pulmonary thromboembolism, tuberculosis, lung cancer, and aspiration.[2] About 50% of patients with pulmonary embolism have cough, which may be the only respiratory complaint. Further workup (e.g., chest radiograph ventilation-perfusion scan) may be appropriate at this stage in patients at high risk for or with compelling clinical reasons to suggest a serious illness.

Chronic Cough

G *Chest Radiograph.* After the history and physical examination, a chest radiograph is the first step in the evaluation of almost all patients with chronic cough.[2-4] The chest radiograph is extremely useful in initially ranking diagnostic possibilities. A normal or near-normal radiograph makes PNDS, asthma, and GERD likely but makes bronchogenic carcinoma, interstitial disease of the lung parenchyma, and bronchiectasis unlikely. For a young nonsmoker without underlying cardiopulmonary disease who is taking an ACEI, the physician should consider stopping the ACEI before proceeding with radiographic evaluation.

H *HIV Disease.* If the patient is or may be immunocompromised by HIV disease and the chest radiograph is normal, a CD4 count and oximetry during exercise should be ordered (see D).

I *Diagnostic Studies.* For the immunocompetent host, chest radiograph abnormalities should be pursued with sputum analysis, bronchoscopy, high-resolution computed tomography (HRCT), and noninvasive cardiac studies according to the most likely diagnostic possibility.[2] For the immunocompromised host, sputum analysis and bronchoscopy are used to identify opportunistic lung infections.

J *Pertussis.* Since the cough caused by pertussis infection can last more than 4 to 6 weeks, pertussis needs to be considered in the evaluations of both acute and chronic cough (see E).

K *Other Causes.* Diagnostic studies in current smokers or patients taking ACEIs should not be done until the response to smoking cessation or ACEI discontinuation for 4 weeks can be assessed.[2,3] ACEI-induced cough has been reported to appear within a few hours of taking a first dose in many patients but may not become apparent for months. In general, cough from ACEIs should improve significantly within 4 weeks of stopping the medication. Cough appears to be a class effect of these drugs and is not dose related. Losartan, an angiotensin II receptor antagonist, is a different class of drug that has not been associated with cough and can be substituted for an ACEI.[7]

Chronic bronchitis typically causes chronic cough, but smokers do not usually seek medical attention for cough. When evaluating a smoker with chronic cough, it is important to eliminate smoking for at least 4 weeks to see if this alone resolves the cough. A careful environmental and work history also should be taken to identify and eliminate other environmental irritants that could be triggering the cough (see Chapter 11).

L *Postnasal Drip Syndrome.* PNDS secondary to rhinosinus diseases refers to symptoms such as cough, dyspnea, and wheeze arising from the drainage of excessive secretions into the hypopharynx and larynx. Patients with PNDS often describe a dripping sensation in their throats, nasal discharge, and the frequent need to clear the throat. PNDS is the most common cause of chronic cough in adults.[4] For adults with chronic cough from PNDS, *sinusitis* is the cause of the PNDS in 30% to 60% of patients.

The other major cause of PNDS is *rhinitis* of any cause. Rhinitis (e.g., allergic, perennial nonallergic, postinfectious, environmental irritant, vasomotor) leading to PNDS is treated with an antihistamine-decongestant combination and, when feasible, avoidance of environmental precipitating factors. For the initial therapy of rhinitis, our preference is to prescribe combination therapy that includes dexbrompheniramine as a first-generation H_1 antagonist plus pseudoephedrine as a decongestant, or equivalent drug. All forms of rhinitis generally respond to therapy that includes first-generation antihistamines. For patients with allergic rhinitis who do not tolerate the sedating effects, the newer nonsedating H_1 antagonists also are effective. Nonallergic rhinitis, which is not histamine mediated, does not respond to these H_1 antagonists because they lack significant anticholinergic activity. When antihistamine-decongestant combination therapy cannot be tolerated, rhinitis may respond to intranasal corticosteroids or intranasal ipratropium. These nasal medications should be used rather than older-generation antihistamine-decongestant combination therapy when the patient has glaucoma, benign prostatic hypertrophy, or poorly controlled hypertension.

If PNDS does not improve after 1 week of treatment for rhinitis, sinusitis may be the cause of the PNDS. Sinus radiographs should be ordered to confirm the diagnosis rather than prescribing antibiotics empirically. Treatment of cough caused by chronic sinusitis includes antibiotics, antihistamines, and decongestants that facilitate sinus drainage.[3] Antibiotics should cover *Haemophilus influenzae, Streptococcus pneumoniae,* and upper respiratory tract anaerobes. The physician may also prescribe a first-generation antihistamine-decongestant oral medication for 3 weeks and a decongestant nasal spray for a maximum of 5 days.

M *Asthma.* Asthma is the second most common cause of chronic cough in adults.[4] Patients with asthma complain of episodic wheezing, shortness of breath, and cough and may wheeze on examination. The examiner should recognize, however, that cough may be the only manifestation of asthma (i.e., cough-variant asthma). Nonspecific pharmacologic bronchoprovocation challenge testing with methacholine or histamine is extremely helpful in ruling out asthma as a cause of cough.[6]

Uncomplicated cough-variant asthma responds to standard asthma medications.[3] Cough begins to improve within 1 week of beginning inhaled β_2-adrenergic agonists and resolves within 6 to 8 weeks of beginning inhaled corticosteroids. Combination therapy with inhaled β_2-adrenergic agonists plus inhaled corticosteroids or inhaled nedocromil is recommended. If these agents themselves provoke cough, different proprietary formulations, spacer devices, and oral therapy are helpful.

A related, newly described cause of chronic cough is eosinophilic bronchitis.[3] The prevalence of this disease as a cause of chronic cough is not yet established. Patients have sputum eosinophilia, negative bronchoprovocation challenge testing, and rapid improvement with corticosteroids.

N *Gastroesophageal Reflux Disease.* GERD is the third most common cause of chronic cough.[1,5] GERD should be suspected as a cause of cough when patients complain of frequent heartburn, regurgitation, or sour taste. These symptoms are sufficient to make a diagnosis of GERD without resorting to barium esophagography or 24-hour esophageal pH monitoring. In the evaluation of cough, these diagnostic techniques are reserved for identifying "silent" GERD, or GERD producing cough without other symptoms.

Prolonged, 24-hour esophageal pH monitoring is helpful in linking silent GERD and cough in a cause-and-effect relationship. Cough and reflux events can be correlated when patients keep a symptom diary during the monitoring session. The session can be considered consistent with GERD as a cause of chronic cough when reflux events (acid or alkaline) are temporally correlated with cough and when any reflux parameter slips from the normal range (e.g., percentage of time that pH is less than 4.0). Although a less sensitive and less specific test for diagnosing GERD, barium esophagography may reveal reflux to the midesophagus or higher, even when not detected by pH probe testing.

For cough, maximal medical therapy for GERD is recommended initially: a high-protein, low-fat antireflux diet; acid suppression with H_2 antagonists or proton pump inhibitors; a prokinetic agent; treatment of obstructive sleep apnea; and when possible, elimination of medications for comorbid diseases that worsen GERD (see Chapter 24). If cough is not at least partially improved in 3 months, 24-hour esophageal pH monitoring can determine whether GERD is still the likely cause of cough but has failed to respond to therapy. In that case, surgery may be considered[3] (see Chapter 101).

O *Aspiration Syndrome.* In the appropriate clinical context (e.g., patient with cerebrovascular accident) an aspiration syndrome should also be considered in the differential diagnosis of chronic cough. A modified barium swallow study is useful in evaluating this possibility.

P *Diagnoses and Therapies.* Diagnostic studies only suggest the cause(s) of chronic cough.[2] The definitive diagnosis always depends on observing a favorable response to a specific treatment of the suspected cause. The general aproach to treating chronic cough is to begin specific therapy and observe for a clinical response. If at least partial resolution of cough occurs with the treatment regimen, the specific diagnosis is confirmed. After additional evaluation, other potential causes of cough may be identified, and then specific treatments are added to the existing regimen. This sequential addition of specific therapy is highly effective.[2,4] Nonspecific antitussive therapy is indicated when specific therapy cannot be given, either because the cause of cough is not known or because specific therapy has not had a chance to work or will not work (e.g., inoperable lung cancer). Nonspecific therapies shown to be clinically effective are codeine, dextromethorphan, and ipratropium in chronic bronchitis.[3]

Q *Additional Studies.* Less common causes of chronic cough are bronchiectasis, bronchogenic carcinoma, chronic interstitial pneumonia (e.g., idiopathic pulmonary fibrosis), metastatic carcinoma, left ventricular failure, and psychogenic cough. The latter is a diagnosis of exclusion and, in our experience, rare.

The following additional testing may be useful if cough persists after evaluation and treatment for PNDS, asthma, and GERD[2,3]: (1) ear, nose, and throat (ENT) consultation when sinusitis fails to respond to medical therapy; (2) allergy consultation when PNDS fails to respond to therapy but suspicion of allergic disease remains high; (3) bronchoscopy to check for endobronchial abnormalities; (4) HRCT scan to assess for interstitial lung disease and bronchiectasis; and (5) noninvasive cardiac studies.

R *Management Pitfalls.* The most common management pitfalls are (1) failure to consider common causes of cough when one diagnosis seems obvious on clinical or radiographic grounds; (2) failure to consider that cough may have more than one cause; (3) failure to consider ACEI as a cause of cough; (4) use of newer nonsedating H_1 antagonists to treat nonallergic inflammatory disease; (5) assumption that a positive methacholine challenge test is diagnostic of asthma as the cause of cough; (6) failure to recognize that inhaled asthma medications may cause cough; (7) failure to use prolonged esophageal pH monitoring and to assess the response to medical therapy; (8) failure to consider that treatment for GERD may require 2 to 3 months before being even partially effective; and (9) failure to consider that maximal medical treatment for GERD may fail.

REFERENCES

1. Harding SM, Richter JE: The role of gastroesophageal reflux in chronic cough and asthma, *Chest* 111:1389, 1997.
2. Irwin RS: Cough. In Irwin RS, Curley FJ, Grossman RF, editors: *Diagnosis and treatment of symptoms of the respiratory tract,* Armonk, NY, 1997, Futura.
3. Irwin RS, Boulet L-P, Cloutier MM, et al: Managing cough as a defense mechanism and as a symptom: a consensus panel report of the American College of Chest Physicians, *Chest* 114(suppl):133S, 1998.
4. Irwin RS, Curley FJ, French CL: Chronic cough: the spectrum and frequency of causes, key components of the diagnostic evaluation, and outcome of specific therapy, *Am Rev Respir Dis* 141:640, 1990.
5. Irwin RS, French CL, Curley FJ, et al: Chronic cough due to gastroesophageal reflux: clinical, diagnostic, and pathogenetic aspects, *Chest* 104:1511, 1993.
6. Irwin RS, French CL, Smyrnios NA, et al: Interpretation of positive results of a methacholine challenge and 1 week of inhaled bronchodilator use in diagnosing and treating cough-variant asthma, *Arch Intern Med* 157:1981, 1997.
7. Lacourciere Y, Brunner H, Irwin RS, et al: Effects of modulators of the renin-angiotensin-aldosterone system on cough, *J Hypertension* 12: 1387, 1994.
8. Mello CJ, Irwin RS, Curley FJ: Predictive values of the character, timing, and complications of chronic cough in diagnosing its cause, *Arch Intern Med* 156:997, 1996.
9. Schappert SM: National Ambulatory Medical Care Survey, 1991: summary. In *Vital and health statistics,* no 230, Rockville, Md, 1993, US Department of Health and Human Services.
10. Wallace JM, Hansen NI, Lavange L, et al: Respiratory disease trends in the pulmonary complications of HIV infection study cohort, *Am J Respir Crit Care Med* 155:72, 1997.

CHAPTER 18

Constipation

Charles Telfer Williams

Constipation is difficult to define. A strictly quantitative measure can be used, such as the number of bowel movements, but reports of perceived constipation (including straining, painful bowel movements, or sense of incomplete evacuation) have little relation to the number of bowel movements. For this reason a better definition of constipation is a perceived change in bowel habits, which leads to more difficult or less frequent bowel movements. Using a self-report of constipation, the incidence of disease is 12.8%.[6] Clinically this self-report is the most useful definition, since it more accurately reflects patient's presenting symptoms.

General factors contributing to constipation are mechanical blockage, relative dehydration of the colonic feces, decreased intestinal transit time, and suppression of the natural urge to defecate. Many of these factors relate to diet (fluid and fiber intake) and physical activity. Mechanical blockages can be purely obstructive, can contribute to decreased transit time, or can lead to suppression of defecation in painful conditions such as hemorrhoids. The hydration of the colonic contents is crucial to the passage of stool by ensuring lubrication, bulk, and consistency of the stool. Decreased intestinal transit time leads to increased time for water absorption in the colon and thus relative dehydration of the fecal matter. Similarly, suppression of the natural defecation urge leads to increased colonic time; if habitual, it can cause rectal distention and megacolon, which may damage the nerves and muscles, leading to decreased colonic motility. The interrelation of these factors is complex, making the treatment of chronic constipation a challenge.

A *History.* The history is the key to the correct diagnosis and treatment of the vast majority of patients with constipation. Differentiating between chronic and acute constipation is a useful first step. *Acute constipation* may be defined as a persistent change in bowel habits for less than 3 months. Acute constipation is often caused by a change in only one of the general factors that lead to constipation and is therefore often easier to treat. *Chronic constipation* is change in bowel habits longer than 3 months, is more frequent as people age, and tends to result from a more complex interplay of the general factors that lead to constipation. Defining what was "normal" for the patient and what has changed is important. Quantifying the number of bowel movements, consistency (loose, soft, normal, hard, rocklike), pattern, and volume can be useful, especially for tracking improvement after starting treatment. It is important to assess fluid and fiber intake and physical activity levels and note any changes that might be associated with the constipation.

The age of the patient is relevant; not only does the incidence of constipation increase with age,[2] but the etiology of constipation in older patients is more frequently multifactorial as well.[5] Young patients are more likely to have a single, common problem (e.g., irritable bowel syndrome, pregnancy) or an unusual etiology (e.g., Hirschsprung's disease).

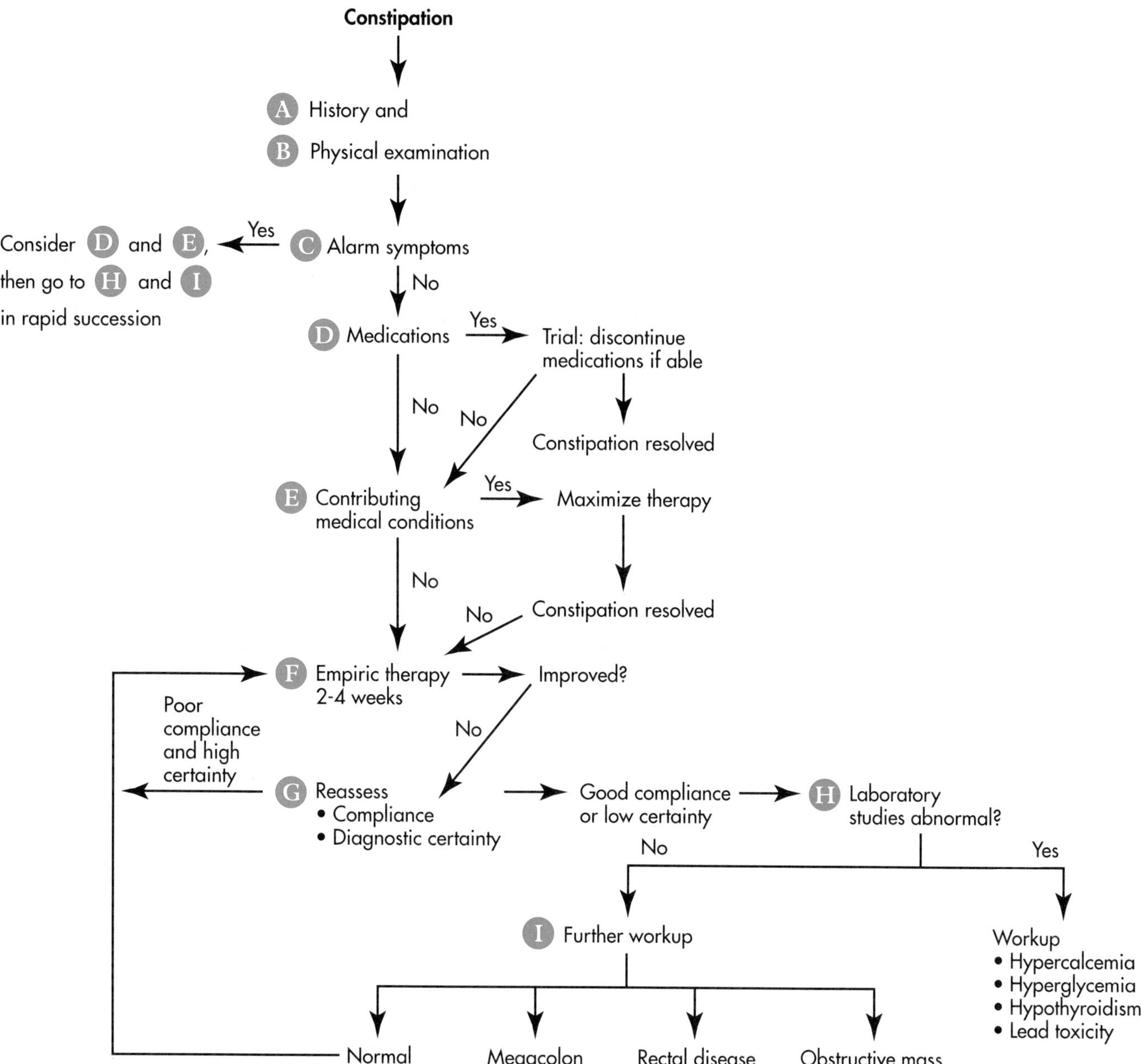

Associated symptoms of distention or bloating, abdominal pain, anorexia, hematochezia, painful movements, tenesmus, straining, urgency, and presence of flatus or grease can help clarify the etiology. Obtaining evidence of other medical conditions contributing to constipation, including a past medical history or current symptoms of hypothyroidism, scleroderma, CREST syndrome, and other diseases associated with autonomic neuropathies (e.g., diabetes mellitus), is necessary. Psychiatric assessment for depression and other mental disorders can be helpful.

Finally, the physician should assess the patient's efforts at self-treatment. Chronic laxative use may lead to distention of the bowels and actually exacerbate constipation.

B *Physical Examination.* The examination should be aimed at confirming or disproving possible causes raised by the history. Hydration status should be assessed by evaluation of the oral mucosa, skin turgor, tears, and color or specific gravity of the urine. Examination of the thyroid should be done on all patients to rule out enlargement or nodules. An abdominal examination evaluates for surgical scars, distention, masses (stool or other), and tenderness. An anorectal examination looks for fissures, hemorrhoids, strictures, masses, rectal prolapse, prostatic hypertrophy, stool consistency, and size and muscle tone of the rectum. A guaiac test for occult blood is controversial, since a vigorous rectal examination can cause bleeding. Anal fissures can result from constipation as well as perpetuate it because of painful defecation and suppression of the evacuative urge. Hemorrhoids can block normal defecation, or their pain can lead to suppression of the normal urge. Anorectal strictures can be a mechanical barrier to normal bowel movements. In female patients, bimanual examination of the pelvic organs can rule out masses or enlarged organs not palpable by abdominal examination. The patient should strain to allow an adequate assessment for rectal prolapse or rectocele. A general neurologic examination assesses for spinal cord injuries, spina bifida occulta, cerebral palsy, multiple sclerosis, Parkinson's disease, and specifically, perianal sensation and rectal tone.

C *Alarm Symptoms.* Although serious illnesses (e.g., carcinoma) as causes of constipation are rare, several alarm symptoms may trigger an expedited evaluation: (1) persons over 40 (due to the increasing incidence of colorectal carcinoma), (2) unexplained constipation of recent onset, (3) worsening constipation with abdominal pain accompanied by blood or mucus, (4) progressively decreasing number of bowel movements, (5) symptoms of obstipation (acute constipation, nausea, vomiting, abdominal pain and distention, inability to defecate, hard stool in rectum), (6) rectal bleeding, and (7) unexplained weight loss.[7] In the absence of acute severe signs, a symptomatic approach to the evaluation and treatment may be justified initially, even without a clearly identified diagnosis. Most constipation will respond to this approach, and if it does not, further evaluation is warranted.

D *Medications.* Drugs are one of the most common causes of constipation. Functional intestinal hydration is decreased by cholestyramine and diuretics, leading to harder stools and difficult passage. Intestinal motility is decreased by medications with anticholinergic properties, including anti-Parkinson's agents (benztropine, trihexyphenidyl, biperiden, ethopropazine), tricyclic antidepressants, monoamine oxygenase inhibitors, and neuroleptics. Other medications often associated with constipation are iron preparations, aluminum, opiates, phenytoin, sympathomimetics (cold medications), calcium channel blockers, and oral contraceptives.

E *Medical Conditions.* Medical illnesses can lead to constipation. Irritable bowel syndrome is probably the most common of these, affecting an estimated 17% of the population,[3] and can vary in presentation from intermittent diarrhea to constipation and often a combination of the two (see Chapter 110). Psychiatric illness, particularly new depression, is often associated with constipation. Even with a quantitative measure of bowel movements in the normal range, persons with psychiatric illnesses are five times more likely to report constipation.[1] These patients should be reoriented as to what constitutes "normal." Uncontrolled diabetes can lead to dehydration and enteropathy, which leads to decreased transit time. Hyperparathyroidism and other causes of hypercalcemia may similarly be associated with dehydration and constipation. Constipation is seen in more than 50% of patients with hypothyroidism.

F *Empiric Therapy.* After assessment, consideration of treatment begins. Since life-threatening pathology as yet undetected is relatively uncommon, an empiric trial of lifestyle modification is usually a safe and productive course. Empiric therapy is also indicated when patients are taking essential medications that tend to constipate or if an underlying disease causing constipation is not fully treatable. The usual empiric trial includes increasing three elements: fluids, fiber, and activity (FFA), because the lack of these three is associated with constipation.[6] Generally, consumption of 2 to 3 L of liquid a day or a 30% increase above the current level should be adequate. Two simple ways to aid compliance are to have the patient fill a 2-L soda bottle with water or to drink enough water so that the urine is clear (not yellow). Decreasing caffeine may also be useful in improving hydration. Stool hydration can also be improved by the use of nonabsorbable sugars; naturally occurring sorbitol is found at high levels in fruits (e.g., apples, prunes, their juice forms). Dietary fiber may be increased through food (fruits, vegetables, whole grains, beans) or fiber additives (e.g., psyllium, bran). A high-fiber diet of 20 to 30 gm a day is recommended.[4] Increased activity for most patients involves changing habits rather than inability. Walking 30 minutes a day for at least 5 days a week is a good start. Activities that promote inactivity (e.g., TV watching) should be limited. A 2- to 4-week trial of these changes should result in some improvement.

If FFA are insufficient to improve constipation, it may be necessary to initiate stooling with enemas or suppositories with or without the judicious use of cathartics. In general, however, these should be avoided.

G *Reassessment.* If a trial of FFA does not produce the desired effect, it is necessary to assess the patient's compliance and the physician's diagnostic certainty. If the diagnostic certainty is high and patient compliance was poor, it is reasonable to give another trial of FFA while trying to improve compliance. If compliance was good or diagnostic certainty is low, the physician should consider further workup.

H *Laboratory Studies.* The next step is to rule out underlying diseases by blood tests: calcium, glucose, thyroid-stimulating hormone (TSH), and lead, since hypercalcemia, hyperglycemia, hypothyroidism, and lead toxicity can all cause constipation. If an abnormality is found, efforts should be directed to clarify the cause and treat the underlying illness. If no abnormality is found, the physician should strongly consider proceeding to further diagnostic tests before returning to empiric therapy.

I *Further Workup.* Abdominal radiography is a relatively inexpensive test and may reveal some causes of constipation. If an abnormality is found, further workup is indicated. If the abdominal radiograph is normal, the physician should proceed with further evaluation, which could include flexible sigmoidoscopy and barium enema. Obtaining stool for fecal occult blood is inexpensive and should be done. Colonoscopy could substitute for flexible sigmoidoscopy and barium enema in some patients, especially those with symptoms suggestive of carcinoma or with a strong family history. If the patient recently immigrated from or traveled to lesser developed regions, evaluation of stool for ova and parasites may be warranted. Intestinal motility studies can also be done in treatment- resistant cases with a normal workup. Biofeedback may be helpful in patients with decreased intestinal motility.

REFERENCES

1. Ashraf W, Park F, Lof J, Quigley E: An examination of the reliability of reported stool frequency in the diagnosis of idiopathic constipation, *Am J Gastroenterol* 91:26, 1996.
2. Campbell AJ, Busby WJ, Horwath CC: Factors associated with constipation in a community based sample of people aged 70 years and over, *J Epidemiol Community Health* 47:23, 1993.

3. Goldfinger SE: Constipation and diarrhea. In Wilson JD, Braunwald E, Isselbacher KJ, et al, editors: *Harrison's principles of internal medicine,* ed 12, New York, 1991, McGraw-Hill.
4. Krevsky B: A practical approach to managing constipation, *Fam Pract Recert* 17:41, 1995.
5. Read NW, Celik AF, Katsinelos P: Constipation and incontinence in the elderly, *J Clin Gastroenterol* 20:61, 1995.
6. Sandler RS, Jordan MC, Shelton BJ: Demographic and dietary determinants of constipation in the US population, *Am J Public Health* 80:185, 1990.
7. Seller RH: *Differential diagnosis of common complaints,* ed 4, Philadelphia, 2000, Saunders.

CHAPTER 19

Dyspnea

John J.W. Fangman
David H. Roberts

Dyspnea, an uncomfortable awareness of breathing, is a common problem in primary care. Although the exact frequency of dyspnea complaints is not known, it is the presenting complaint in many common disorders such as congestive heart failure (CHF), acute myocardial ischemia, chronic obstructive pulmonary disease (COPD), and asthma. The sensation of dyspnea may result from activation of the cerebral cortex, from central and peripheral chemoreceptors, or from an array of mechanoreceptors in the upper airway, lung, and chest wall.[2] Afferent traffic is processed in higher brain centers and is influenced by context and behavior. The pathophysiology of dyspnea may involve dissociation of incoming afferent information and central respiratory motor activation. This mismatch may heighten or even produce the sensation of dyspnea. Dyspnea may also result when the level of ventilation and O_2 consumption is increased (e.g., exercise). It is important to note that behavioral style and emotional state can contribute markedly to the sensation of dyspnea.

Dyspnea resulting from cardiac disease is characterized by inadequate cardiac output to meet cellular oxygen demand. Although most often the result of decreased cardiac output and elevated pulmonary capillary wedge pressure, dyspnea can also result from high-output states (e.g., anemia, hyperthyroidism) and normal output states (e.g., diastolic dysfunction). Dyspnea secondary to pulmonary disease may result from a sensation of increased respiratory drive, chest wall movement, hyperinflation, bronchoconstriction, or impaired gas exchange.

A History

Timing and Setting. Even when not disabling or life threatening, rapidly progressive dyspnea demands aggressive evaluation (see C). A sudden increase in severity of chronic dyspnea should also prompt a search for additional causes of shortness of breath.[4] The setting in which dyspnea occurs often provides important clues to its etiology. Shortness of breath in a young person after exercise, exposure to cold or dry air, or inhalation of irritants suggests bronchospasm. Although anxiety often accompanies dyspnea of any cause, agoraphobia, peripheral paresthesias, and hyperventilation suggest panic attacks or other anxiety disorders. Dyspnea associated with cough that is more prominent at night or worse after meals suggests reflux. Dyspnea after surgery may indicate diaphragmatic injury, pneumonia, or pulmonary embolism. Although a nonspecific complaint, severe exertional dyspnea most often results from pulmonary vascular disease, severe obstructive disease, or left ventricular (LV) dysfunction. *Orthopnea* (shortness of breath when lying flat) and paroxysmal nocturnal dyspnea are also signs of left-sided heart failure. *Platypnea* (shortness of breath when upright) suggests intracardiac, vascular, or pulmonary shunt.

Risk Factors. It is important to quantify tobacco use and assess for other risk factors for coronary artery disease when evaluating the patient with dyspnea. Risk factors include occupational exposures, environmental exposures or allergens, and a family history of congenital heart disease or hereditary pulmonary diseases (e.g., cystic fibrosis).

Description. Careful attention should be paid to the patient's description of dyspnea. Patients with bronchospasm or myocardial ischemia often complain of chest tightness or constriction. Patients with interstitial lung disease or conditions that result in excessive load on the respiratory muscles (e.g., neuromuscular disease, severe airway obstruction) often describe an increased work of breathing. *Air hunger,* the exaggerated urge to breathe, may signal the increased respiratory drive associated with conditions such as acute hypercapnia, pregnancy, anemia, pulmonary embolism, acidosis, or CHF. Finally, patients who have normal cardiac and respiratory function but who are deconditioned often complain of heavy or rapid breathing with exertion. Patients whose dyspnea is multifactorial may complain of several different types of dyspnea.

Medical Conditions. A detailed review of the patient's history of cardiac or pulmonary disease is an important first step. Pregnancy, malignancy, and anemia also are often associated with dyspnea. The patient's current medication list and medical record should be reviewed for exposure to drugs that produce acute or chronic lung disease (see D). Psychiatric disease, especially panic attacks and other anxiety disorders, are associated with dyspnea. In dyspneic immunocompromised patients, evaluation focuses on infectious and toxic risk factors particular to the immunodeficiency and its treatment. Finally, it is important to assess the patient's cardiovascular conditioning by clarifying both baseline level of activity and ability to perform activities of daily living (ADLs).

B Physical Examination

General. The physical examination should first establish the severity of respiratory distress.[5] Measurement of vital signs, including temperature, heart rate, blood pressure, respiratory rate, and oxygen saturation, is the first step. The respiratory pattern (e.g., muscle use, chest wall movement, pursed-lip breathing) and the degree of cyanosis should be assessed. The patient's level of anxiety, affect, mobility, respiratory effort, and use of supplemental oxygen are noted.

Respiratory. Examination of the upper airway should rule out obstruction (e.g., nasal or pharyngeal obstruction, neck mass, stridor). Similarly, the patient should be examined for chest wall deformities (e.g., kyphoscoliosis, pectus excavatam, increased anteroposterior diameter, traumatic injury)

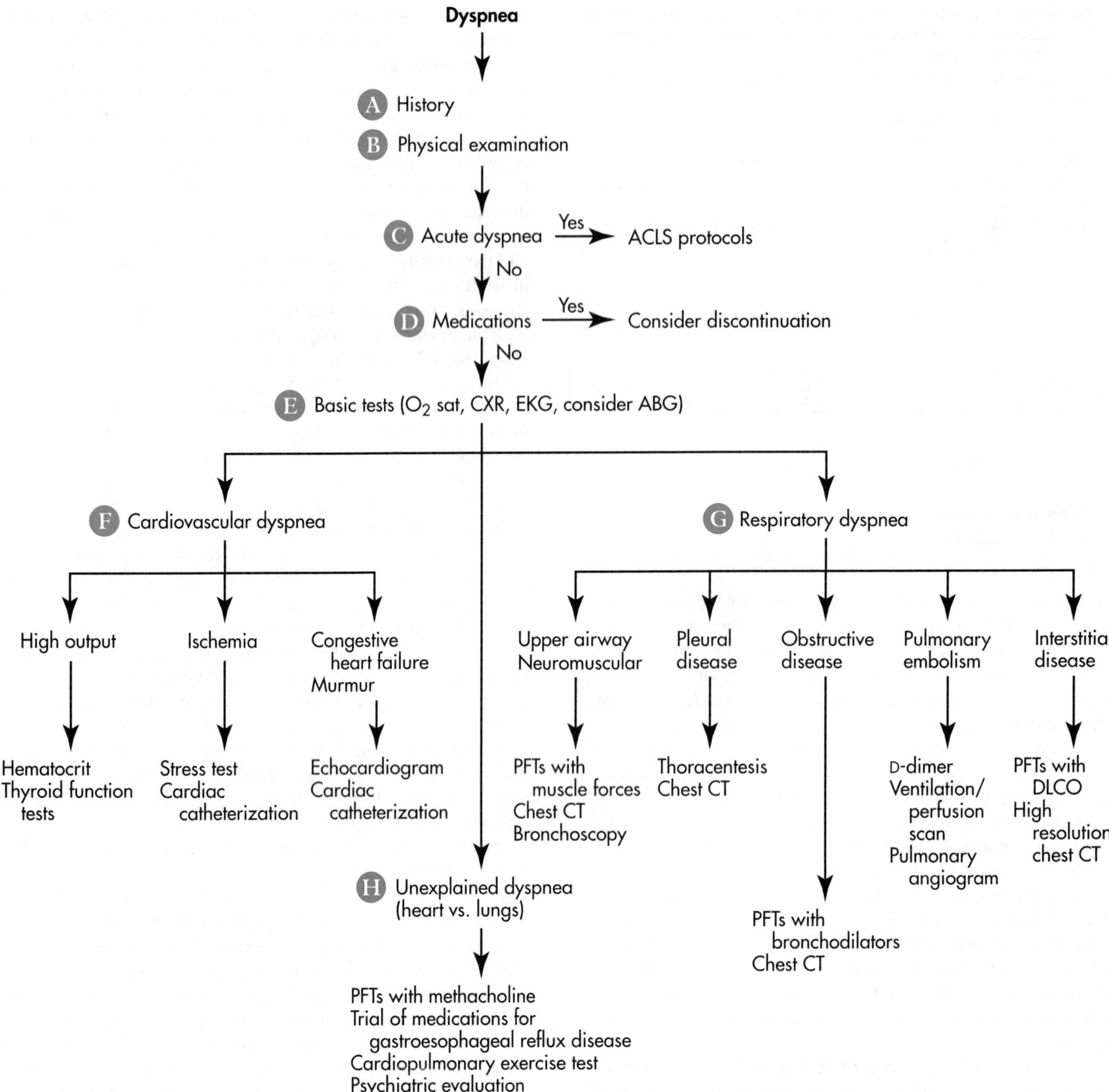

PFTs, Pulmonary function tests; *DLCO,* carbon monoxide diffusing capacity.

that may affect ventilation. Percussion of the back may reveal hyperinflation (low-lying diaphragm with minimal expansion), whereas dullness to percussion of the lung fields suggests pleural disease or parenchymal consolidation. Auscultation helps assess the focality of any pulmonary process and the volume of air movement. *Rales,* the short high-pitched sounds that result from the rapid opening of collapsed alveoli, may indicate interstitial lung disease, pneumonia, or CHF. Whispered pectoriloquy and egophony suggest consolidation. *Rhonchi,* the result of turbulent flow in large airways, often indicate increased mucus production associated with such disorders as chronic bronchitis. Although classically associated with diseases such as asthma and COPD, wheezing may also indicate LV dysfunction.

Cardiac. Auscultation of the heart may reveal murmurs, rhythm disturbances, or evidence of reduced LV compliance or overload (S_4 and S_3, respectively). Palpation of the precordium should identify both the point of maximum impulse (PMI) and abnormalities of cardiac impulses that suggest right ventricular (RV) or LV dysfunction (e.g., RV heave, pulmonary artery tap, and loud pulmonic component of S_2 suggesting pulmonary hypertension; diffuse, laterally displaced PMI suggesting LV dilation). Examination of peripheral and carotid pulses may reveal vascular disease or suggest valvular abnormalities, dysrhythmia, shunt, or heart failure. Jugular venous distention suggests right-sided or left-sided heart failure, pericardial disease, or restrictive heart disease.

Additional Findings. Other findings that suggest an etiology for dyspnea include abnormalities in the neck, abdomen, and extremities. A large goiter with a bruit suggests hyperthyroidism. Tense ascites may limit movement of the diaphragm and, along with hepatomegaly and peripheral edema, may suggest right-sided heart failure. Painful unilateral limb swelling should prompt evaluation for deep venous thrombosis and pulmonary embolus. Examination of the nail beds may reveal signs of decreased perfusion, cyanosis, or even clubbing. Since anemia may both mask significant hypoxemia and produce significant dyspnea, pallor is also important to note.

C *Acute Dyspnea.* The differential diagnosis of acute dyspnea includes hyperventilation secondary to anxiety, bronchospasm, pulmonary edema, pulmonary embolism, and pleural/chest wall injury (e.g., rib fracture, hemothorax/pneumothorax, pulmonary contusion).[3] Pneumonia, pleural effusion, fibrosing lung disease, and toxic inhalation can also produce rapidly progressive dyspnea. When confronted with the patient with acute dyspnea, the evaluation should include a focused history and examination with chest radiograph, electrocardiogram (ECG), and arterial blood gases (ABGs). Patients with severe or rapidly progressive dyspnea should be treated according to the American Heart Association Advanced Cardiac Life Support (ACLS) protocol for acute dyspnea. Acute hyperventilation occurs as both a primary manifestation of anxiety and an appropriate response to cardiorespiratory pathology. The evaluation of an initial episode of acute dyspnea should usually occur in a monitored setting (e.g., emergency department).

D *Medications.* A broad array of medications may trigger anaphylaxis, but the list of drugs that typically produce isolated dyspnea is limited. β-Blockers, adenosine, nonsteroidal antiinflammatory drugs (NSAIDs), and aspirin may trigger wheezing in patients predisposed to bronchospasm. Amiodarone, a commonly used antidysrhythmic, can produce a dose-related interstitial lung disease. Many chemotherapeutic agents produce pulmonary toxicity; bleomycin is the most common offender, but cyclophosphamide, chlorambucil, melphalan, nitrosoureas, and methotrexate all can produce lung disease. The effects of these agents are often magnified when administered with radiation therapy.

E *Basic Diagnostic Testing.* Data collected in the history, physical examination, and basic laboratory evaluation may allow the physician to categorize the patient's shortness of breath as either cardiovascular or respiratory. Recognizing that some individuals experience a multifactorial dyspnea, this division allows the physician to focus further evaluation and to limit unnecessary testing.

Desaturation while performing limited exercise, such as walking down the office hall, suggests severely limited respiratory reserve and should prompt aggressive evaluation and treatment. If acute in onset or rapidly progressive, such a workup is often best accomplished in the hospital. Dyspnea secondary to anemia is rare when the hemoglobin is more than 10 gm/dl. Indirect measurement of hemoglobin saturation with a pulse oximeter is an important screening tool. Its utility is limited, however, because it is an insensitive tool for detecting subtle changes in arterial oxygenation. In cases of unexplained dyspnea, it is important to calculate the alveolar-arterial gradient using the alveolar gas equation. ABGs identify patients with COPD who retain carbon dioxide and those with significant acidosis.

Radiographic examination should assess abnormalities of the ribs and chest wall, large airways, lung parenchyma, pulmonary vasculature, pleura, diaphragm, and cardiac silhouette. If possible, previous films should be examined to assess for interval change. ECG analysis demonstrates abnormalities of cardiac rhythm, evidence of ischemia or past injury, and abnormalities of voltage that suggest ventricular hypertrophy or pericardial disease. Again, a review of previous tracings can provide insight into a patient's changing cardiorespiratory status. Simple office spirometry evaluates basic flow rates (FEV_1) and forced vital capacity (FVC) and can document obstructive lung disease when FEV_1/FVC is less than 70%. Full pulmonary function tests (PFTs), including measurement of the lung diffusing capacity for carbon monoxide (D_LCO), are necessary when spirometry is nondiagnostic.

F *Cardiovascular Dyspnea.* Dyspneic patients with chest pain, significant cardiac risk factors, or suggestive ECG changes should be evaluated for ischemic heart disease (see Chapter 63). The patient with a murmur or evidence of CHF should receive an echocardiogram to rule out heart failure, valvular disease, or pericardial disease (see Chapters 65, 66, and 68). Patients with documented CHF and either normal cardiac output or a dilated, diffusely hypokinetic left ventricle may require cardiac catheterization to define the etiology of their cardiomyopathy. Dyspnea secondary to intracardiac shunt may be confirmed with echocardiography (with or without agitated saline or "bubble study") and cardiac catheterization. Shortness of breath secondary to dysrhythmia (arrhythmia) often requires correlation with symptoms during ambulatory monitoring (see Chapter 61).

G *Respiratory Dyspnea.* Dyspneic patients with or without chest pain and with nondiagnostic studies should be evaluated for pulmonary embolus using D-dimer, ventilation/perfusion scan, and pulmonary angiography (see Chapter 80). Upper airway obstruction is suggested by the contour of the flow volume loop seen during PFTs and can be confirmed by high-resolution computed tomography (HRCT) of the chest and bronchoscopy. Chest wall abnormalities are generally apparent on examination and radiographs, and neuromuscular disease is characterized by decreased respiratory muscle forces and normal gas exchange/D_LCO. Pleural disease is often identified in the initial evaluation and confirmed with further imaging and thoracentesis (see Chapter 79). Both asthma and COPD are characterized by wheezing, hyperinflation, and an obstructive pattern on PFTs and can be distinguished by D_LCO and chest imaging (see Chapters 72 and 75). When bronchospasm is suspected but FEV_1 is normal, bronchial provocation testing (methacholine challenge) may establish the diagnosis. Pneumonia is suggested by cough, fever, and sputum production and is confirmed by microbiologic evaluation and imaging (see Chapter 73). Although patients with interstitial lung disease may have only subtle radiographic findings, PFTs demonstrate decreased FEV_1, FVC, and D_LCO. HRCT often reveals parenchymal or mediastinal abnormalities as well (see Chapter 76).

H *Unexplained Dyspnea.* When a dyspneic patient's initial evaluation does not suggest an etiology or produces inconsistent results, further evaluation is indicated. In studies of patients referred to pulmonary clinics for evaluation of unexplained dyspnea, occult bronchospasm is diagnosed most often.[1] If not done previously, PFTs with bronchial provocation should be performed. In such referral populations, gastroesophageal reflux disease is another common cause of dyspnea, and some experts recommend an empiric trial of acid suppression with or without motility agents (see Chapter 24). If an etiology for a patient's dyspnea still has not emerged, referral to a pulmonologist for cardiopulmonary exercise testing (CPEX) is indicated. Such testing can both clarify a patient's functional status and assess the relative contribution of coexisting cardiovascular and respiratory disease.

After evaluation fails to disclose a convincing cardiac or respiratory etiology for a patient's dyspnea, psychiatric causes must be considered. Generalized anxiety disorder, panic attacks, obsessive-compulsive disorder, and hyperventilation syndromes all may produce significant dyspnea (see Chapter 49).

REFERENCES

1. DePaso WJ, Winterbauer RH, Lusk JA, et al: Chronic dyspnea unexplained by history, physical examination, and spirometry: analysis of a seven year experience, *Chest* 100:1293, 1991.
2. Manning HL, Schwartzstein RM: Pathophysiology of dyspnea, *N Engl J Med* 333:1547, 1995.
3. Meek PM, Schwartzstein RM, Adams L, et al: Dyspnea: mechanisms, assessment, and management: a consensus statement. *Am J Respir Crit Care Med* 159:321, 1999.
4. Michelson E. Hollrah S: Evaluation of the patient with shortness of breath: an evidence-based approach, *Emerg Med Clin North Am* 17:221, 1999.
5. Schwartzstein RM, Thibault GE: Approach to the patient with dyspnea. In Goldman L, Braunwald E, editors: *Primary cardiology,* Philadelphia, 1998, Saunders.

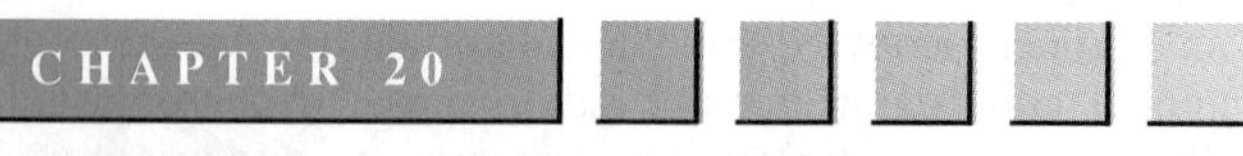

Edema

Geoffrey A. Modest

Edema typically results from either an increase in fluid pressure (e.g., from obstruction, congestive heart failure), decrease in oncotic pressure (e.g., from nephrotic syndrome, chronic hepatic insufficiency), or increased capillary permeability (from medications such as calcium channel blockers or idiopathic cyclic edema). In an average-sized person, edema is clinically detectable after 5 to 10 lbs of excess fluid. The algorithm for edema is divided into patients presenting with generalized, typically symmetric edema vs. those with regional, asymmetric edema (e.g., edema of one arm or leg).

Generalized/Symmetric

A *History.* There are several clues in the pattern of edema that might suggest different etiologies: monthly edema in menstruating women suggests idiopathic cyclic edema (probably estrogen-mediated), the development of ascites before peripheral edema suggests cirrhosis as the etiology, the development of edema prior to ascites suggests cardiac or renal etiologies, and the association with emotional stress or allergens suggests angioedema. Edema preferentially of the face or eyes suggests a renal etiology (acute glomerulonephritis, nephrotic syndrome), angioedema, myxedema, or protein malnutrition. Nonpitting edema suggests either chronic lymphedema, lipedema (lipodystrophy of the lower legs, typically sparing the feet), chronic venous stasis edema, myxedema (typically pretibial, either diffuse or in well-circumscribed areas, and associated with Graves' disease), and angioedema. See the algorithm for generalized pitting edema.

B *Physical Examination.* It is important to check the jugular venous pressure (JVP), preferably using the right side of the neck, since the right innominate and jugular veins form a straight line. Isolated clinical examination findings are, however, of limited utility.[2] Increases in JVP can occur without cardiorespiratory etiology, and JVP can be normal even in patients with severe systolic dysfunction.

C *Medications.* Medications can be associated with edema; some may be mediated through worsening congestive heart failure (e.g., β-blockers) and others perhaps by direct vascular effects (e.g., dihydropyridine calcium channel blockers such as nifedipine have associated edema up to 10% of the time). Steroids and estrogen are also associated with edema.

D *Laboratory.* A chest x-ray may be helpful at this point. However, if the history and physical examination are highly suggestive of a heart failure (see E), the chest x-ray may not be necessary because the sensitivity (51%) and specificity (79%) for an ejection fraction of less than 40% are not sufficiently informative in most clinic situations, especially as an isolated finding.[2]

E *Cardiac or Pulmonary.* Cardiac or pulmonary etiologies are likely if there is a known history of cardiac or pulmonary disease, or if specific symptoms or signs are present that are related to decreased ejection fraction (e.g., systolic dysfunction) and/or increased filling pressure (e.g., diastolic dysfunction, valvular or pericardial disease, or pulmonary disease). The clinical predictors[2] for increased filling pressure are radiographic vascular redistribution, JVP elevation, dyspnea, orthopnea, tachycardia, decreased systolic or pulse pressure, S_3, rales, and abdominal-jugular reflux; the clinical predictors for decreased ejection fraction are radiographic cardiomegaly or vascular redistribution, anterior Q waves on electrocardiogram (ECG), left bundle branch block, sustained apical impulse, pulse greater than 90, systolic blood pressure less than 90, S_3, rales, dyspnea, prior myocardial infarction (MI), or high creatine kinase (CK) elevation in post-MI patients. More than three of the above predictors are usually present if edema is due to a cardiac/pulmonary etiology (high probability). If a ches

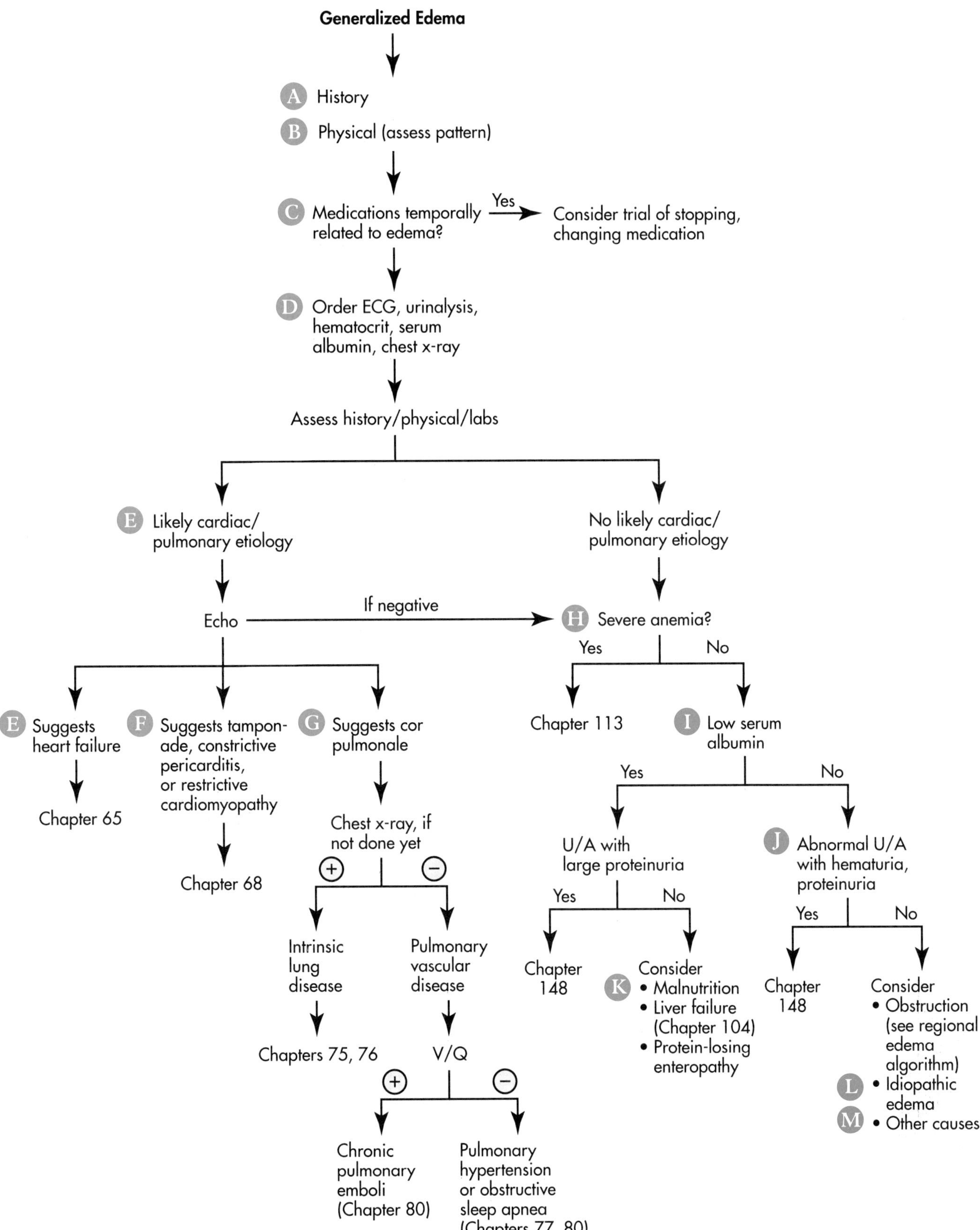
Generalized Edema
A History
B Physical (assess pattern)
C Medications temporally related to edema?
Yes
Consider trial of stopping, changing medication
D Order ECG, urinalysis, hematocrit, serum albumin, chest x-ray
Assess history/physical/labs
E Likely cardiac/ pulmonary etiology
No likely cardiac/ pulmonary etiology
Echo
If negative
H Severe anemia?
Yes
No
E Suggests heart failure
Chapter 65
F Suggests tamponade, constrictive pericarditis, or restrictive cardiomyopathy
Chapter 68
G Suggests cor pulmonale
Chest x-ray, if not done yet
+
−
Intrinsic lung disease
Chapters 75, 76
Pulmonary vascular disease
V/Q
+
−
Chronic pulmonary emboli (Chapter 80)
Pulmonary hypertension or obstructive sleep apnea (Chapters 77, 80)
Chapter 113
I Low serum albumin
Yes
No
U/A with large proteinuria
Yes
No
Chapter 148
K Consider
• Malnutrition
• Liver failure (Chapter 104)
• Protein-losing enteropathy
J Abnormal U/A with hematuria, proteinuria
Yes
No
Chapter 148
Consider
• Obstruction (see regional edema algorithm)
L • Idiopathic edema
M • Other causes

x-ray had not been done previously (and it may not be useful in patients with a high probability of heart disease based on clinical grounds solely), it may provide useful information in the group of patients with an intermediate probability (i.e., between one and three of the above clinical predictors).

(F) *Cardiac Tamponade and Constrictive Pericarditis.* Cardiac tamponade most typically occurs in the setting of uremia, neoplastic disease, and idiopathic pericarditis. In diagnosing cardiac tamponade, a study of 56 patients[4] found the frequency of specific signs was increased cardiac silhouette on chest x-ray in 95%, respiratory rate >20/min in 80%, tachycardia in 77%, paradoxical pulse in 77%, systolic blood pressure >100 mm Hg in 64%, hepatomegaly in 55%, and decreased heart sounds in 34%. A normal echocardiogram effectively rules out this diagnosis. Constrictive pericarditis typically occurs in the setting of a preexisting disorder (e.g., tuberculosis [TB], amyloid, uremia, cardiac surgery, acute pericarditis, rheumatoid arthritis, lupus). The examination often is similar to hepatic cirrhosis with hepatomegaly and development of ascites disproportionate to peripheral edema, but with the additional findings of increased JVP, which may be associated with Kussmaul's sign (failure of neck veins to decline during inspiration), and paradoxical pulse (in 30%). Restrictive cardiomyopathies (e.g., secondary to amyloid, sarcoid, hemochromatosis) present similarly. The echocardiogram may not be abnormal in these settings, and in patients with a high likelihood of either constrictive pericarditis or restrictive cardiomyopathy further testing may be required.

(G) *Cor Pulmonale.* Cor pulmonale typically presents as dyspnea not relieved by sitting upright and tachypnea. A pronounced right ventricular heave and loud pulmonary component of the second heart sound may be appreciated. Cor pulmonale may be associated with pulmonary vascular disease (chronic pulmonary emboli, primary pulmonary hypertension), parenchymal pulmonary disease (chronic obstructive pulmonary disease [COPD], interstitial lung disease), or obstructive sleep apnea. The echocardiogram is a very sensitive test in the setting of cor pulmonale associated with peripheral edema.

(H) *Severe Anemia.* Severe anemia can be associated with high-output heart failure. The echocardiogram may not be sensitive enough to rule out this diagnosis. Even moderate degrees of anemia (hemoglobin below 7.5 gm/dl) may cause heart failure in a patient with reduced myocardial reserve.

(I) *Severe Hypoalbuminemia.* Severe hypoalbuminemia, with serum albumin less that 2 gm/dl, is typically necessary to cause edema. This low level of albumin is usually secondary to nephrotic syndrome (with marked proteinuria on urinalysis), advanced cirrhosis (although typically disproportionately more ascites to edema from portal hypertension), protein-losing enteropathy, or severe malnutrition.

(J) *Acute Glomerulonephritis.* In acute glomerulonephritis, edema is predominantly in the periorbital areas, although it may exist elsewhere (dependent edema, ascites). The urinalysis is abnormal, with red cells and protein (usually nonnephrotic range). Red cell casts (frequently diagnostic) may be intermittent.

(K) *Malnutrition.* Malnutrition from severe protein-energy restriction may be accompanied by loss of subcutaneous fat and muscle mass, serum transferrin level <1 gm/L, lymphocyte counts <800, and impaired delayed hypersensitivity.

(L) *Idiopathic Edema.* Idiopathic edema is a diagnosis of exclusion, typically in women of childbearing age, associated with several pound changes in weight over the course of the day and followed by fluid mobilization upon recumbency and diuresis. These patients when given a water load will excrete the excess water when recumbent and not when upright.

(M) *Preeclampsia and Cushing's Syndrome.* Preeclampsia should be considered in a pregnant woman with edema, especially with proteinuria and hypertension. Also, 62% of patients with Cushing's syndrome have edema, although the typical body habitus, hypertension, hirsutism, and purple striae suggest the diagnosis (see Chapter 98).

Regional/Asymmetric

(A) *History and Physical Examination.* There are several items in the history and physical examination that help guide the workup and diagnosis of regional edema. The time course of the edema is useful. Sudden onset of regional edema would suggest a traumatic origin, a ruptured Baker's cyst, or acute thrombophlebitis. Edema after leg trauma or after prolonged sitting, especially on a hard bench, suggests deep venous thrombosis (DVT). Erythema and warmth suggest an inflammatory etiology (e.g., cellulitis, gout, DVT), and accompanying tender nodularity suggests erythema nodosum. Enlarged adenopathy suggests an infectious etiology (cat-scratch, filariasis). Varicose veins can be associated with mild edema. Chronic venous insufficiency from incompetent venous valves and/or DVT can result in a dull aching in the legs and edema, especially after prolonged standing, which resolve on leg elevation. Brown discoloration of the skin often accompanies long-term chronic venous insufficiency. Of note, bilateral, apparently generalized leg edema can be associated with either bilateral regional causes (e.g., bilateral DVTs or venous insufficiency) or a more proximal regional cause (e.g., DVT obstruction in the inferior vena cava).

(B) *Trauma.* Trauma can be associated with a variety of conditions leading to regional edema, including a ruptured muscle or tendon (e.g., gastrocnemius tear), local hematoma, and compartment syndrome.

(C) *Venous Stasis Disease.* Venous stasis disease typically presents with chronic edema and brown skin discoloration, related to the breakdown of red blood cells. Sometimes there can be stasis dermatitis, where this background pigment can have a superimposed erythema and warmth, occasionally difficult to differentiate from cellulitis.

(D) *Acute Inflammation.* Acute inflammation may cause edema, commonly associated with gout, cellulitis (which may be associated with an underlying osteomyelitis), or stasis dermatitis. It is frequently difficult to distinguish these entities, since gout may be associated with significant periarticular erythema and edema (and appear as cellulitis), and stasis dermatitis (with its underlying brown discoloration and superimposed erythema) may be associated with a cellulitis

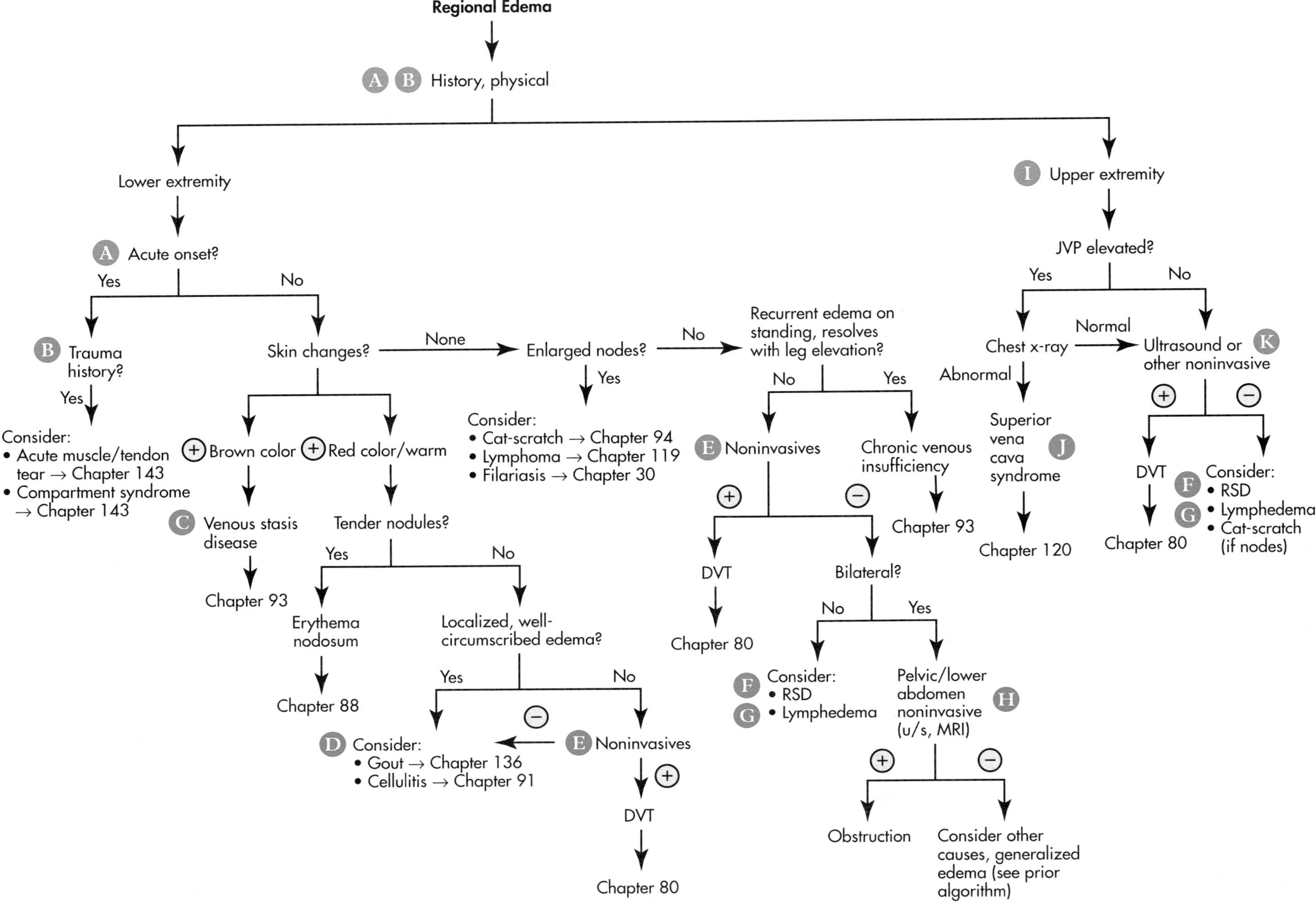
Regional Edema
A B History, physical
Lower extremity
A Acute onset?
Yes
No
B Trauma history?
Yes
Consider:
• Acute muscle/tendon tear → Chapter 143
• Compartment syndrome → Chapter 143
Skin changes?
None
+ Brown color
+ Red color/warm
C Venous stasis disease
Chapter 93
Tender nodules?
Yes
No
Erythema nodosum
Chapter 88
Localized, well-circumscribed edema?
Yes
No
D Consider:
• Gout → Chapter 136
• Cellulitis → Chapter 91
−
E Noninvasives
+
DVT
Chapter 80
Enlarged nodes?
Yes
Consider:
• Cat-scratch → Chapter 94
• Lymphoma → Chapter 119
• Filariasis → Chapter 30
No
Recurrent edema on standing, resolves with leg elevation?
No
Yes
E Noninvasives
Chronic venous insufficiency
Chapter 93
+
−
DVT
Chapter 80
Bilateral?
No
Yes
F Consider:
• RSD
G • Lymphedema
Pelvic/lower abdomen noninvasive (u/s, MRI) H
+
−
Obstruction
Consider other causes, generalized edema (see prior algorithm)
I Upper extremity
JVP elevated?
Yes
No
Chest x-ray
Normal
Abnormal
Superior vena cava syndrome J
Chapter 120
Ultrasound or other noninvasive K
+
−
DVT
Chapter 80
Consider:
F • RSD
G • Lymphedema
• Cat-scratch (if nodes)

E *Acute Venous Thrombosis.* Acute venous thrombosis, either superficial or deep, typically presents with unilateral edema, calf pain, and erythema. The clinical predictors of DVT[1] include active cancer, paralysis or recent plaster immobilization, recently bedridden more than 3 days and/or major surgery, localized tenderness along the deep venous system distribution, swelling of the entire leg, calf swelling more than 3 cm when compared to the opposite leg, collateral superficial vein dilation (excluding varices), and the lack of other likely alternative diagnoses. There is high probability of DVT when three or more of these criteria are present. Other predisposing factors include hypercoagulable states, recent pregnancy, and lupus. Although contrast venography is the gold standard for diagnosis, serial compression ultrasonography (days 1, 2, and 8) has a positive predictive value of 94%.[5] Recent studies suggest a role for magnetic resonance imaging as a sensitive test for proximal DVT, with the additional benefit of providing excellent resolution of the inferior vena cava, pelvic veins, and pulmonary emboli.[3]

F *Reflex Sympathetic Dystrophy.* In reflex sympathetic dystrophy (RSD) edema can be a prominent feature, along with pain (typically burning or aching, and increased with dependency of extremity), in early RSD. Later, RSD can be associated with autonomic dysfunction, increased reflexes, spasm, and trophic changes. Precipitating events are found in two thirds of cases: assess history of trauma (most common etiology), MI (now less than 1%), cerebrovascular accident (CVA), tendinitis/bursitis, and certain medications (antituberculous medications, barbiturates, cyclosporin A).

G *Lymphedema.* Lymphedema can be bilateral/symmetric or regional. Initially, there is soft, pitting edema, which becomes nonpitting and "woody" after years, as tissues become indurated and fibrotic. Lymphedema is rarely primary; however, when lymphedema is primary, it often appears before age 20, with a "tarda" form beginning after age 35. Usually, lymphedema is secondary to infection (thrombosis and fibrosis after recurrent bacterial lymphangitis), tumor (most often prostate in men and lymphoma in women), filariasis, trauma, rheumatoid arthritis, and chronic contact dermatitis. Lymphedema should be differentiated from lipedema, where there is lipodystrophy with accumulation of fatty tissue, typically sparing the feet.

H *Obstruction.* Obstruction can cause bilateral peripheral edema if obstruction of venous return is above the legs, including use of a tight girdle, retroperitoneal fibrosis, proximal DVT (i.e., pelvic or higher), fibroids or ovarian pathology in women, or prostate cancer in men.

I *Upper Extremity Edema.* Upper extremity edema is unusual, but it is often associated with superior vena cava syndrome or trauma (including postsurgical, intravenous catheter).

J *Superior Vena Cava Syndrome.* Superior vena cava (SVC) syndrome typically presents as rapid progression of facial and upper body edema. SVC syndrome may be associated with dyspnea and stridor, especially when the patient is supine, as the syndrome becomes more severe. SVC syndrome is typically associated with an increased JVP. There may be prominent cutaneous veins of upper chest and abdomen. The vast majority of cases are associated with cancer, typically lung cancer or lymphoma.

K *Noninvasive Studies.* Noninvasive studies are reliable in detecting obstruction at the point that the obstruction is complete enough to cause distal edema.

REFERENCES

1. Anand SS, Wells PS, Hunt D, et al: Does the patient have deep venous thrombosis? *JAMA* 279:1094-1099, 1998.
2. Badgett RG, Lucey CR, Mulrow CD: Can the clinical examination diagnose left-sided heart failure in adults? *JAMA* 277:1712-1719, 1997.
3. Evans AJ, Sostman HD, Knelson MH, et al: Detection of deep venous thrombosis: prospective comparison of MR imaging with contrast venography, *Am J Roentgenol* 161:131-139, 1993.
4. Guberman BA, Fowler NO, Engel PJ, et al: Cardiac tamponade in medical patients, *Circulation* 64:633-640, 1981.
5. Heijboer H, Buller HR, et al: A comparison of real-time compression ultrasonography with impedance plethysmography for the diagnosis of deep-vein thrombosis in symptomatic outpatients, *N Engl J Med* 329:1365, 1993.

ADDITIONAL READINGS

Alexander DW, Schlant RC, Fuster V: *Hurst's the heart,* ed 9, New York, 1998, McGraw-Hill.

Isselbacher KJ, et al: *Harrison's principles of internal medicine,* ed 13, New York, 1994, McGraw-Hill.

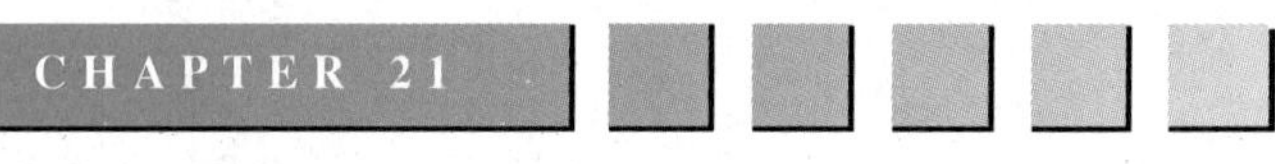

Fatigue

Geoffrey A. Modest

Fatigue is a remarkably common problem that affects individuals of all socioeconomic strata, although patients commonly do not identify fatigue as their chief complaint. The algorithm is for patients with chronic fatigue, defined as fatigue of at least 30 days, although some studies define it as 6 months. A large British community survey found that 38% of those surveyed had substantial fatigue, with 18% symptomatic for more than 6 months.[5] Similar numbers have been found in U.S. primary care studies. Fatigue is a major public health problem, similar to other chronic disabilities, interfering with family life and occupation. The pathophysiology of fatigue is not well characterized, although a wide variety of medical and psychologic conditions (see below) are associated with fatigue. One note of caution: although fatigue is associated with many medical diagnoses, it may be erroneous to attribute the fatigue to one of those diagnoses, since there may be a concomitant (perhaps associated) and treatable psychologic cause.

In one study,[4] approximately 25% of 1159 consecutive patients complained of fatigue as a major problem (fatigue that interferes with work or home responsibilities), with fatigue being somewhat more common in women than men (28% vs. 19%). After excluding suspected medical conditions, 80% of the remaining patients (vs. 12% of controls) had underlying depression or anxiety. Laboratory examination in patients without suspected medical causes of fatigue was remarkably unuseful, with only four (4%) having subclinical hypothyroidism (none of whose fatigue improved with thyroxine therapy), four with newly discovered diabetes, and

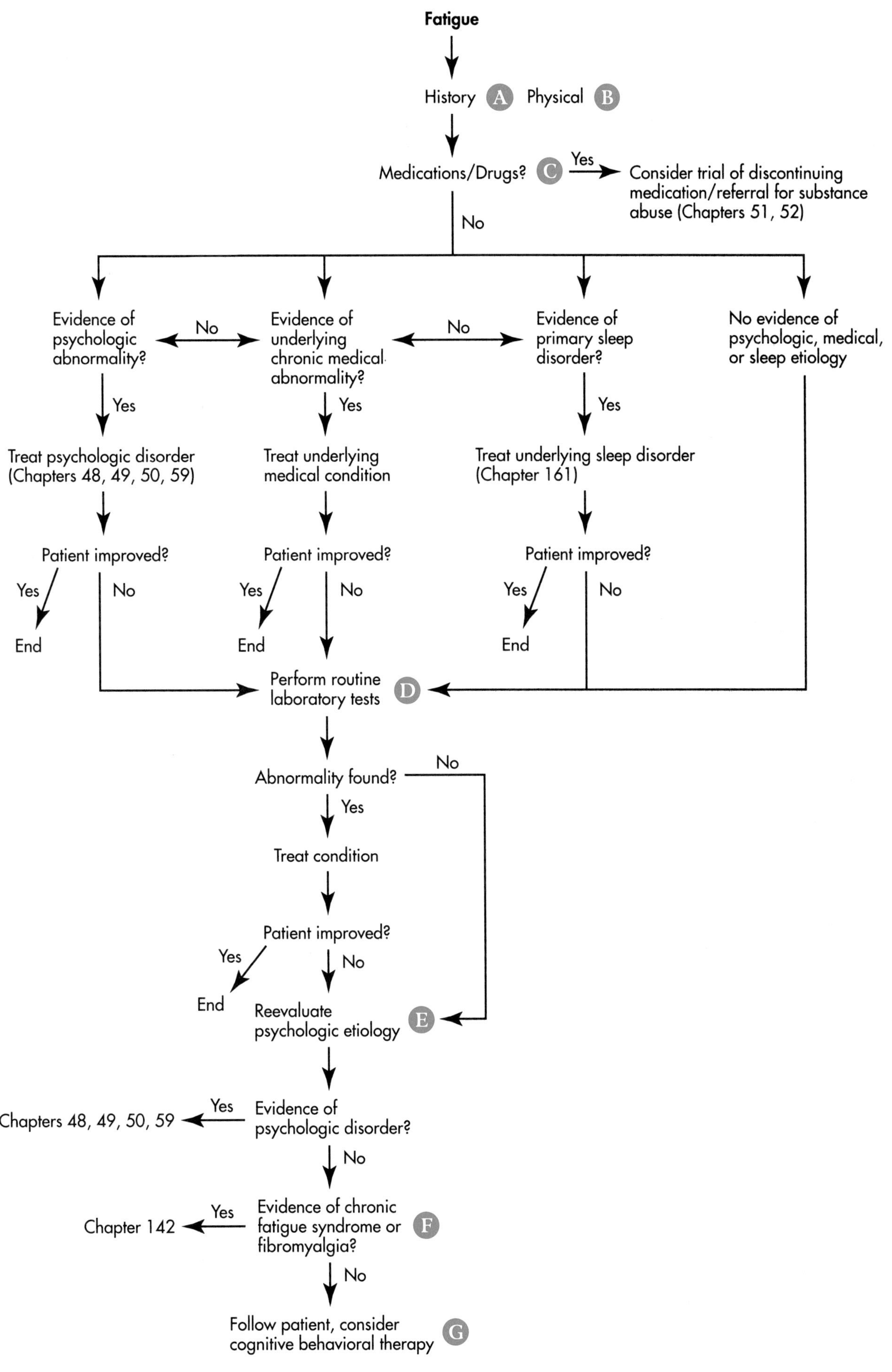
Fatigue
History A
Physical B
Medications/Drugs? C
Yes
Consider trial of discontinuing medication/referral for substance abuse (Chapters 51, 52)
No
Evidence of psychologic abnormality?
No
Evidence of underlying chronic medical abnormality?
No
Evidence of primary sleep disorder?
No evidence of psychologic, medical, or sleep etiology
Yes
Treat psychologic disorder (Chapters 48, 49, 50, 59)
Yes
Treat underlying medical condition
Yes
Treat underlying sleep disorder (Chapter 161)
Patient improved?
Yes
End
No
Patient improved?
Yes
End
No
Patient improved?
Yes
End
No
Perform routine laboratory tests D
Abnormality found?
No
Yes
Treat condition
Patient improved?
Yes
End
No
Reevaluate psychologic etiology E
Yes
Chapters 48, 49, 50, 59
Evidence of psychologic disorder?
No
Yes
Chapter 142
Evidence of chronic fatigue syndrome or fibromyalgia? F
No
Follow patient, consider cognitive behavioral therapy G

one with mild anemia. No new illnesses were found on 1-year follow-up in the cohort. Other studies have found similar conclusions.

A *History.* There are several components to the history of the chronically fatigued patient. First, it is important to assess the patient for any medical conditions[2] that might cause chronic fatigue. Any chronic organ system dysfunction can be associated with chronic fatigue, including infectious diseases (e.g., tuberculosis, fungal, parasitic, occult bacterial, viral, human immunodeficiency virus [HIV]), endocrinopathy (hyperthyroidism, hypothyroidism, diabetes, Cushing's syndrome, Addison's disease), malignancy, anemia, connective tissue disorder, chronic pulmonary disease (restrictive or obstructive), chronic liver disease, chronic heart disease (congestive heart failure, coronary artery disease), inflammatory bowel disease, and chronic granulomatous diseases (sarcoid). In addition, pregnancy, menopause, and surgery (especially within the previous 3 months) can feature fatigue as a prominent symptom. Second, a detailed sleep history is important to rule out a primary sleep disorder (see Chapter 161), obstructive sleep apnea, other causes of disturbed sleep (e.g., asthma, menopausal symptoms, nocturnal limb movements), or psychiatric causes. Third, a detailed assessment of medications and drug use should be sought (see C). Fourth, a screen should be done for depression, anxiety disorder (including posttraumatic stress disorder), domestic violence, and sexual abuse; even in the presence of a medical condition or medication that might cause chronic fatigue, an underlying and treatable psychiatric condition might exist and should still be investigated.

B *Physical Examination.* The physical examination should target specific issues uncovered in the history (see A). In addition, it is important to distinguish fatigue from weakness, which may be attributable to neurologic, muscular, or psychiatric disorders (e.g., conversion reaction) (see Chapters 50, 167, and 168).

C *Medications/Drugs.* Chronic fatigue can be associated with the use of several different substances (e.g., alcohol, opiates, cocaine), as well as a variety of medications. See Chapters 51 and 52 for patients identified with substance abuse. Although a large percentage of medications have been associated with fatigue, the major classes clearly associated include β-blockers, centrally acting α-blockers, anticholinergics, antihistamines, antipsychotics, and antidepressants.

D *Laboratory Tests.* Although there are very few data to confirm the utility of an extensive laboratory investigation without either abnormalities suggested by history or physical examination, or the use of medications that might cause laboratory test abnormalities, the general workup suggested by several different investigators includes a complete blood count, electrolytes, blood sugar, liver enzymes, renal function, thyroid stimulating hormone, erythrocyte sedimentation rate, and urinalysis.[3]

E *Psychologic Etiology.* A psychologic etiology may still account for the chronic fatigue, since patients may be reluctant to discuss depression, anxiety, or physical or sexual abuse, especially on the first encounter. Since psychologic issues are the predominant cause of fatigue, a subsequent reexploration is appropriate.

F *Chronic Fatigue Syndrome.* Chronic fatigue syndrome is differentiated from chronic fatigue by a variety of accompanying symptoms as defined by the Centers for Disease Control and Prevention (CDC) (see Chapter 142). Of note, in several large studies of chronically fatigued patients, only 1% to 4% met the CDC case definition. A recent community-based study in Kansas,[1] however, found a markedly higher prevalence of chronic fatigue syndrome than expected (303 cases per 100,000 women, instead of the 4 to 9 per 100,000 suggested in prior studies), notably with only 16% previously diagnosed using the strict CDC definition. Fibromyalgia is a condition associated with fatigue, sleep disturbance, and tender "trigger points" (see Chapter 142).

G *Follow-up.* In general, there is a low likelihood of uncovering an etiology for the fatigue if none has become apparent so far. In one study[4] if no etiology had been apparent initially, no important new diagnoses were found after 1 year of follow-up, and only 28% of the patients without diagnosis or therapy improved spontaneously in 1 year. Some success has been reported with cognitive behavioral therapy,[6] wherein patients receive 16 weekly sessions geared to helping patients reevaluate their beliefs about their illness, including the role of social and psychologic factors, coupled with a gradual increase in activity.

REFERENCES

1. Bates DW, Schmitt W, Buchwald D, et al: Prevalence of fatigue and chronic fatigue syndrome in primary care, *Arch Intern Med* 153:2759-2765, 1993.
2. Elnicki DM, Shockcor WT, Brick JE, et al: Evaluating the complaint of fatigue in primary care: diagnoses and outcomes, *Am J Med* 93:303-306, 1992.
3. Epstein KR: The chronically fatigued patient, *Med Clin North Am* 79:315-325, 1995.
4. Kroenke K, Wood DR, Mangelsdorff AD, et al: Chronic fatigue in primary care: prevalence, patient characteristics, and outcome, *JAMA* 260:929-934, 1988.
5. Pawlikowska T, Chalder T, Hirsch SR, et al: Population-based study of fatigue and psychological distress, *Br Med J* 308:763-766, 1994.
6. Sharpe M, Hawton K, Simkin S, et al: Cognitive behavior therapy for the chronic fatigue syndrome: a randomised controlled trial, *BMJ* 312:22-26, 1996.

CHAPTER 22

Gynecomastia

Geoffrey A. Modest

Male gynecomastia is remarkably common, occurring in about one half of adolescent males and one third to one half of postpubertal males. The occurrence of postpubertal gynecomastia increases with age and body mass index. In general, the development of gynecomastia is related to the ratio of estrogens to androgens and is typically found in the following settings: increased estrogen (e.g., from tumors); increased aromatization of androgens—either testicular testosterone or adrenal androstenedione—in fat, muscle, and liver cells (e.g., from hyperthyroidism, obesity, liver disease); increased sex hormone binding globulin, which binds testosterone more avidly than estrogen and causes a relatively higher free estrogen level (e.g., from liver disease, hyperthyroidism); or decreased androgens (e.g., from aging, liver disease, hypogonadism). Although high prolactin levels are most typically associated with galactorrhea, there is also an associated suppression of testosterone, which can also cause gynecomastia. Different medications can lead to gynecomastia through any of the above mechanisms (see D.) It is important to note that all of the causes of bilateral gynecomastia can initially present with unilateral or markedly asymmetrical gynecomastia. Also, because of the high prevalence of gynecomastia, it may well coexist with other medical conditions without a causal relationship.

In general, approximately 25% of patients presenting to a physician for gynecomastia have idiopathic gynecomastia, 25% have persistence of pubertal gynecomastia, 10% to 20% are secondary to drugs, 8% to cirrhosis or malnutrition, 8% to hypogonadism, 3% to testicular tumors, 2% to secondary hypogonadism, 1.5% to hyperthyroidism, and 1% to renal disease.[1]

A *History.* Important historical clues can help elucidate both the etiology and appropriate workup of gynecomastia. The history should focus on medication/drug use (see D), symptoms of associated medical problems (liver or renal disease, hyperthyroidism, underlying malignancy, Cushing's disease, human immunodeficiency virus [HIV] infection), history of testicular problems (trauma, torsion, cryptorchidism, mumps orchitis, radiation), and symptoms of hypogonadism (decreased libido, erectile dysfunction, or infertility), as well as specific characteristics of the gynecomastia (acute vs. chronic, and whether or not it is painful or rapidly increasing in size). Painful, rapidly expanding gynecomastia is more likely to be pathologic.

B *Physical Examination.* Gynecomastia (true glandular tissue) needs to be differentiated from pseudogynecomastia (adipose tissue), which can usually be reliably done through the physical examination. True glandular tissue feels rubbery and is subareolar when grasped between the thumb and index finger. If there is a question, compare this tissue with tissue in the axillary fold. When necessary, mammography can be used to differentiate gynecomastia from pseudogynecomastia. Most studies have defined gynecomastia as more than 2 cm of glandular tissue. Gynecomastia of greater than 5 cm is more likely to be pathologic. In addition to performing a standard physical examination, it is important to do a detailed breast examination (noting position, texture, and mobility of the breast tissue, as well as the presence of skin changes or discharge), and a detailed testicular examination, noting size (testes less than 3 cm suggest hypogonadism), and consistency (a nodule could represent an estrogen-secreting tumor). Also, it is useful to assess the patient for concurrent feminization, specifically for female hair pattern, small testes, and a eunuchoid body habitus. An abnormal physical finding (e.g., testicular mass, feminization) can lead directly to the appropriate branch on the algorithm.

C *Male Breast Cancer.* Male breast cancer, which constitutes less than 1% of all male cancers and less than 1% of all breast cancers, usually presents as unilateral, eccentric breast tissue enlargement that is firm, irregular, and fixed to the underlying tissue. This enlargement may be accompanied by axillary adenopathy, nipple discharge, and skin dimpling. Mammography is often helpful, although as with suspicious lesions in females, biopsy is often necessary even with a negative mammogram. Other conditions can cause eccentric, asymmetric breast tissue, including lipomas, neurofibromas, and dermoid cysts.

D *Medications.* A complete medication history is extremely important because many different medications can be associated with gynecomastia. Since gynecomastia is so common in older men, and since the use of medications for chronic diseases also increases with age, it is useful to formally assess men for gynecomastia before beginning any of the following medications, which have been associated with gynecomastia[3]: estrogens, antiandrogens (cyproterone, flutamide, finasteride, leuprolide), calcium channel blockers (especially verapamil, although also reported with nifedipine and diltiazem), cancer chemotherapy agents (especially alkylating agents), digitalis preparations, H_2-receptor blockers (especially cimetidine, but also reported with much lower frequency with ranitidine), phenothiazines (mostly associated with hyperprolactinemia and galactorrhea, but case reports of gynecomastia), ketoconazole, reserpine, spironolactone, marijuana and other substances of abuse (alcohol, amphetamines, heroin, methadone), and a variety of medications with a few case reports, including angiotensin-converting enzyme (ACE) inhibitors (captopril, enalapril), amiodarone, auranofin, clomiphene, diazepam, etretinate, isoniazid, methyldopa, metoclopramide, metronidazole, omeprazole, penicillamine, phenytoin, sulindac, theophylline, and tricyclic antidepressants. Discontinuation of the potentially offending medication should lead to decreasing gynecomastia within 1 month, if that medication is the culprit.

E *Underlying Medical Conditions.* Gynecomastia is found in men with *renal failure,* as well as in 50% of men on dialysis. *Cirrhosis* has been one of the classical settings for gynecomastia; however, one recent small study did confirm the anticipated hormonal changes in cirrhotic men, but without confirming an increased prevalence of gynecomastia.[2] Gynecomastia can occasionally be the presenting symptom of *hyperthyroidism.* Some, but not all, authorities consider laboratory screening for these conditions (e.g., renal, liver, and thyroid function tests) in all cases of postpubertal gynecomastia even in the absence of specific symptoms or signs. In addition, gynecomastia has been reported with *HIV infection, Cushing's syndrome,* and *refeeding* after starvation (e.g., prisoners of war). It has been postulated that gynecomastia associated with therapy for some cancer, tuberculosis, diabetes, or other chronic disorders may be related to regaining weight after the nutritional insult of these diseases.

F *Further Endocrinologic Workup.* Further endocrinologic workup is appropriate (blood for free testosterone, human chorionic gonadotropin, luteinizing hormone, and estradiol) when investigation shows no systemic disease or potentially offending medication usage, especially if the patient is non-obese, or the gynecomastia is increasing and painful.

G *Adolescents.* Adolescents typically have gynecomastia approximately 6 months after pubertal development (development of pubic hair, testicular enlargement). If gynecomastia occurs before puberty or later than 6 months after,

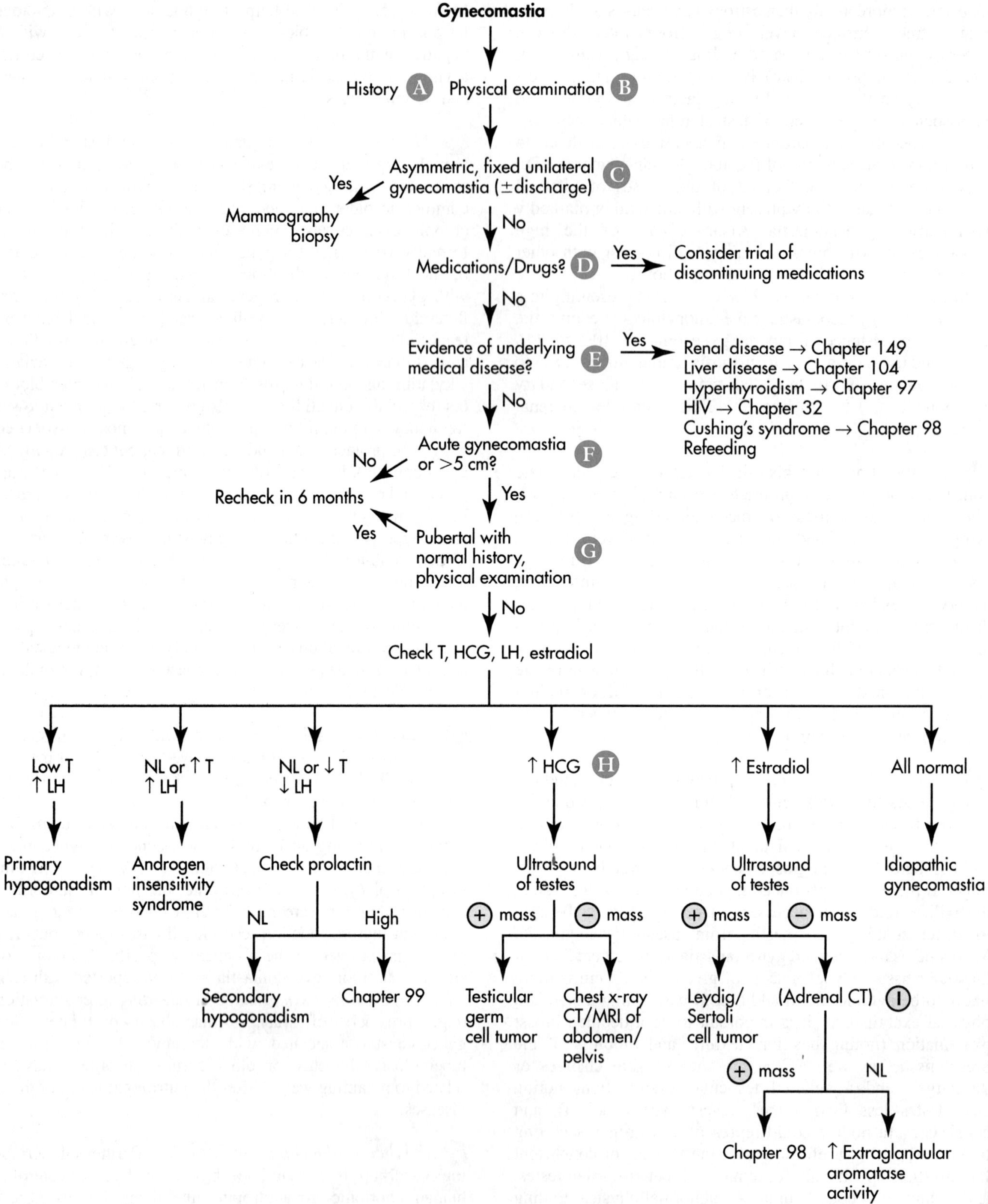
Gynecomastia
History A
Physical examination B
Asymmetric, fixed unilateral gynecomastia (±discharge) C
Yes
Mammography biopsy
No
Medications/Drugs? D
Yes
Consider trial of discontinuing medications
No
Evidence of underlying medical disease? E
Yes
Renal disease → Chapter 149
Liver disease → Chapter 104
Hyperthyroidism → Chapter 97
HIV → Chapter 32
Cushing's syndrome → Chapter 98
Refeeding
No
Acute gynecomastia or >5 cm? F
No
Recheck in 6 months
Yes
Pubertal with normal history, physical examination G
Yes
No
Check T, HCG, LH, estradiol
Low T ↑ LH
Primary hypogonadism
NL or ↑ T ↑ LH
Androgen insensitivity syndrome
NL or ↓ T ↓ LH
Check prolactin
NL
High
Secondary hypogonadism
Chapter 99
↑ HCG H
Ultrasound of testes
⊕ mass
⊖ mass
Testicular germ cell tumor
Chest x-ray CT/MRI of abdomen/ pelvis
↑ Estradiol
Ultrasound of testes
⊕ mass
⊖ mass
Leydig/ Sertoli cell tumor
(Adrenal CT) I
⊕ mass
NL
Chapter 98
↑ Extraglandular aromatase activity
All normal
Idiopathic gynecomastia

T, Testosterone; *HCG*, human chorionic gonadotropin; *LH*, luteinizing hormone; *NL*, normal limits.

further workup is appropriate. Pubertal gynecomastia often resolves spontaneously within 6 months, 75% regressing within 2 years and 90% within 3 years.

H *High Human Chorionic Gonadotropin Levels.* High human chorionic gonadotropin (hCG) levels are found with testicular and extragonadal germ cell tumors, as well as non-trophoblastic tumors of the lung, stomach, liver, or kidney.

I *Adrenal Tumors.* Adrenal tumors that are capable of causing gynecomastia should be large enough to be visualized by computed tomography (CT) scan.

TREAT OR REFER

It is probably best to refer the patient to an endocrinologist for therapy when no underlying, correctable cause can be found. In patients with recent onset gynecomastia, some success has been reported with injectable dihydrotestosterone, danazol, clomiphene, tamoxifen, and testolactone (an aromatase inhibitor) and with surgery.

REFERENCES

1. Braunstein GD: Gynecomastia, *N Engl J Med* 328:490-495, 1993.
2. Cavanaugh J, Niewoehner CB, Nuttall FQ: Gynecomastia and cirrhosis of the liver, *Arch Intern Med* 150:563-565, 1990.
3. Thompson DF, Carter JR: Drug-induced gynecomastia, *Pharmacotherapy* 13(1):37-45, 1993.

ADDITIONAL READINGS

DeGroot LJ, et al: *Endocrinology*, ed 3, Philadelphia, 1995, WB Saunders.

CHAPTER 23

Hiccup

John Noble

Hiccup is a complex reflex action. The hiccup reflex appears to be generated from a locus in the medullary reticular formation, the hiccup-evoking site, where stimuli produce both a powerful diaphragmatic contraction and a temporal suppression of the posterior cricoarytenoid muscles, causing closure of the glottis. Spasms may occur 40 to 100 times per minute. The majority occur unilaterally involving the left hemidiaphragm. Afferent impulses are carried by the vagus nerves and the dorsal afferent sympathetic nerves (T10-T12) from the diaphragm to the hiccup center. Efferent impulses are believed to be carried from the center to the diaphragm by the phrenic nerve, formed by branches from the fourth cervical segment and smaller branches from the third, fifth, and sixth segments. Hiccups may be produced by stimuli applied at any site located along the phrenic nerve or diaphragm. The reflex pathways are similar to pathways that produce coughing, sneezing, swallowing, and vomiting.

A *History and Physical Examination.* Hiccups occur commonly and, in the vast majority of cases, are transient. Cessation occurs spontaneously or may be facilitated by mechanical or medical treatments. Etiologic factors in 220

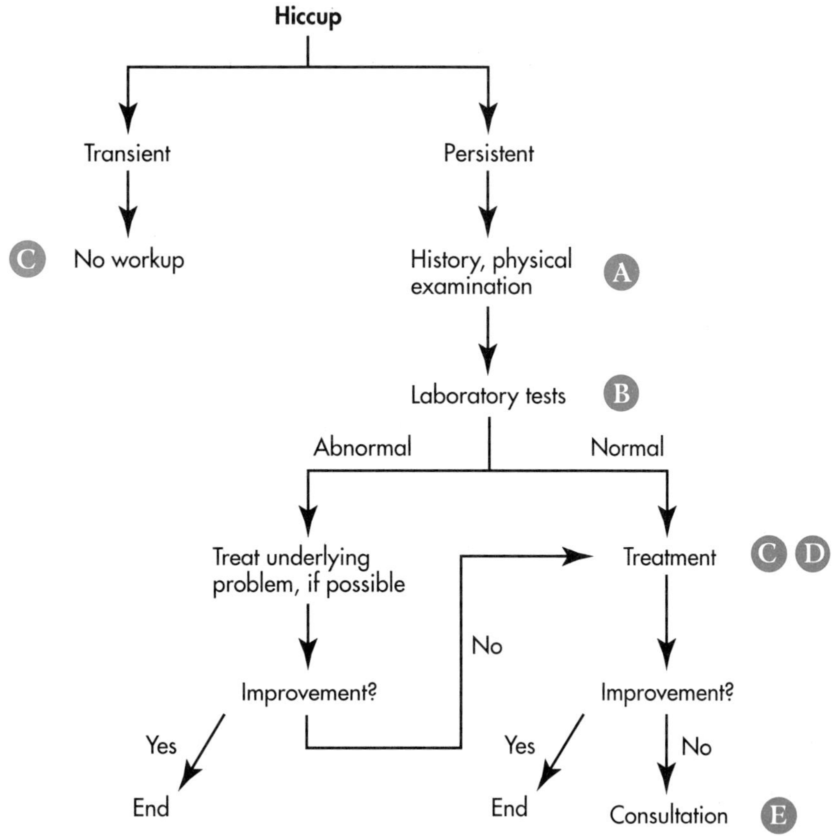

hiccup patients reported from the Mayo Clinic revealed that five times as many men were afflicted as women, and a large proportion of the men had associated medical or surgical problems.[6] In this study, transient hiccup in women and in a smaller percentage of men appeared to be caused by (or were associated with) psychologic or stress-related factors.

A medical history should include history of stroke; recent neurologic, chest, or abdominal surgery; renal failure; dialysis; or ingestion of new medications. The history must be detailed, including dietary and medication histories. For example, a small number of patients on renal hemodialysis have been reported to develop persistent hiccup after eating star fruit, which is reported to contain a hiccup-producing excitatory neurotoxin.[4] Treatment with dexamethasone has also been reported to cause untreatable hiccups.[1] Hiccups are also commonly encountered among older adults during rehabilitation following a stroke.

The history and physical examination should be focused on identifying any potential abnormalities that could interfere with normal neural transmissions along the complex pathways that are part of the hiccup reflex. Lesions of the tympanic membrane, pharynx, neck, chest, diaphragm, pericardium, gallbladder, esophagus, and stomach must all be suspected (Box 23-1).

B *Laboratory.* Laboratory examinations are not indicated for patients with transient hiccups. If hiccups are recurrent or intractable, however, a careful laboratory evaluation is critically important unless the probable etiology is evident (see A). Tests should include electrolytes, blood urea nitrogen (BUN), creatinine, and chest x-ray. A computed tomography (CT) scan of the abdomen and chest should be obtained to identify possible lesions that may be compressing the diaphragm or neural pathways connecting it with the medulla. If hiccups are intractable, a magnetic resonance imaging (MRI) scan may reveal occult neuropathology. In patients with strokes, MRI scans of the brain have identified lesions in the pons and other locations that have contributed to hiccups, aspiration pneumonia, malnutrition, and respiratory arrest.[3]

C *Nonpharmacologic Treatment.* Treatment for hiccup may be divided between traditional methods for terminating transient hiccup and various therapies, including pharmacologic and nonpharmacologic, for persistent or intractable hiccup. These treatments are appropriate for transient hiccup and may be tried in patients with intractable hiccup. Many physicians, however, will use pharmacologic therapy as a first choice for treating intractable hiccup. A few of the many nonpharmacologic treatments include breath holding; breathing into a paper bag; stimulating gagging by swallowing dry granulated sugar, lifting the uvula with a spoon, or drinking water from the wrong side of a cup; gargling; and passing a nasopharyngeal catheter.

D *Medical Therapy.* Persistent, intractable hiccup may present a major therapeutic challenge. Many different medications have been prescribed for the control and termination of this condition.[2] Recent best evidence suggests that a majority of patients will respond to one or combinations of the following three regimens[5]:

1. Cisapride (Propulsid) and/or omeprazole (Prilosec) to reduce gastric acid production and facilitate gastric emptying through blocking afferent input. Dosage: cisapride 10 mg po 15 min before meals and hs, or omeprazole 20 to 40 mg po qd.
2. Baclofen (Lioresal), an antispasmodic, reduces excitability as a γ-aminobutyric acid agonist and depresses reflex activity. Dosage: 5 to 20 mg po q6-12h.
3. Chlorpromazine (Thorazine), a major tranquilizer, is often effective in treating hiccup. Dosage: 25 to 50 mg IV q6h; if successful, switch to po route with same dose.

E *Consultation.* Intractable hiccup is a complex and difficult disorder. Consultation based on the individual medical circumstances is in order when initial medical therapy is not effective or when complex drug regimens and interventions designed to modulate, stimulate, or oblate the phrenic or vagus nerve are being considered. Neurologic consultation is most often engaged unless intraabdominal problems are present, in which case gastroenterology consultation may be helpful.

Box 23-1. Conditions Contributing to Hiccup

Central Nervous System
Cerebrovascular accident
Trauma
Tumor
Infection
Neurologic surgery
Demyelinating or other neurodegenerative disorders

Metabolic
Chronic renal failure
Toxins
Diabetes mellitus
Alcoholism
Electrolyte imbalance

Pharmacologic Preparations
Steroids
Barbiturates
Tranquilizers
α-Methyldopa

Peripheral Nerve
Esophageal irritation or dilation
Gastric dilation
Hiatus hernia
Gallbladder disease
Hepatitis
Subdiaphragmatic abscess
Pancreatitis
Pericarditis
Pneumonia
Pleurisy
Neoplasm
Tympanic membrane irritation

REFERENCES

1. Cersosimo RJ, Brophy MT: Hiccups with high dose dexamethasone administration, *Cancer* 82:412-414, 1998.
2. Friedman NL: Hiccups: a treatment review, *Pharmacotherapy* 16:986-995, 1996.
3. Marsot-Dupach K, Bousson V, et al: Intractable hiccups: the role of MR in cases without systemic cause, *Am J Neuroradiol* 16:2093-2100, 1995.
4. Neto MM, Robl F, Netto JC: Intoxication by star fruit in six dialysis patients, *Nephrol Dial Transplant* 13:570-572, 1998.
5. Petroianu G, Hein G, Petroiana A, et al: Idiopathic chronic hiccup: combination therapy with cisapride, omeprazole and baclofen, *Clin Ther* 19:1031-1038, 1997.
6. Souadjian JV, et al: Intractable hiccups: etiologic factors in 220 patients, *Postgrad Med* 43:72, 1968.

CHAPTER 24

Indigestion and Heartburn

Leonor Fernandez

Indigestion and *heartburn* are terms patients sometimes use when referring to a variety of symptoms that involve the upper gastrointestinal (GI) tract. *Dyspepsia,* as defined by the medical profession, refers to persistent or recurrent pain or discomfort centered in the upper abdomen for greater than 1 month with symptoms more than 25% of the time.[1] The prevalence of dyspepsia is very high, up to 20% to 40% of adults in some studies, and accounts for up to 2% to 5% of primary care visits.[7]

Clinically it is difficult to distinguish between the various causes of dyspepsia. The subclassification of types of dyspepsia into "dysmotility-like," "refluxlike," and "ulcer-like," which had been proposed in the past, has poor discriminant value for each disease.[7] The current consensus is to treat patients having "classic" reflux symptoms (see A) with a strategy that targets the reflux physiology. The remaining patients are considered dyspeptic. When these dyspeptic patients are studied by endoscopy, approximately 15% to 25% have peptic ulcer disease, 5% to 15% have gastroesophageal reflux disease (GERD), less than 2% have gastric cancer, and 50% to 60% have no endoscopic abnormalities (with their clinical picture then termed *nonulcer dyspepsia*).[1,7] The algorithm describes the features that help the physician evaluate reflux and dyspepsia, and then outlines a management strategy for each.

A *History.* Although dyspepsia is centered in the upper abdomen, many patients report symptoms elsewhere in the abdomen as well. Indeed, there is considerable overlap between patients who experience dyspepsia and those who experience irritable bowel syndrome, and many patients who start out with symptoms centered in the upper abdomen may describe a change in the primary location over time to the lower abdomen, or vice versa. The location and quality of discomfort may be even more difficult to ascertain when the patient is of a different cultural or linguistic background than the physician.

Classic gastroesophageal reflux symptoms, in contrast, include epigastric or substernal burning, belching, and regurgitation. The pain often radiates to the back. It usually occurs postprandially, and is aggravated by certain foods (see H), by certain drugs (see C), and by bending over or lying down. The extent of reflux does not appear to correlate well with symptoms: many patients with extensive acid reflux as documented by endoscopy or pH monitoring do not report current symptoms.[13]

Biliary colic should be considered, but this is usually manifested by more prolonged episodes of pain, lasting hours, accompanied often by nausea. There have been reports of Oddi's sphincter dysfunction causing similar symptoms. Less common diagnoses to consider include gastroparesis (often diabetic), ischemic heart disease, metabolic disorders (e.g., hypercalcemia), pancreatitis, and others (see Chapter 103).

B *Physical.* The physical examination should include attention to the patient's weight, presence of jaundice, and presence of any abdominal masses, organ enlargement, or lymphadenopathy.

C *Medications.* Several medications may worsen dyspepsia or GERD. These include antibiotics, nonsteroidal antiinflammatory drugs (NSAIDs), niacin, potassium chloride, iron, corticosteroids, quinidine, colchicine, narcotics, estrogen, progestins, aminophylline, calcium channel blockers, and even acetaminophen according to a recent report.

D *Laboratory Tests.* Laboratory tests that may be considered include a complete blood count (CBC) and amylase. Liver function tests may occasionally be useful. Since both dyspepsia and asymptomatic gallstones are common, there may be many patients with both. Therefore it is not recommended to look for gallstones (e.g., with ultrasound) unless the history is suggestive of biliary colic.

E *Alarm Symptoms.* Weight loss, hematemesis, odynophagia, dysphagia, anemia, and melena are considered *alarm symptoms* that suggest more serious pathology, such as complications from GERD, gastric cancer, and duodenal ulcer.[1,9] Complications from GERD include esophagitis of various degrees, peptic esophageal strictures, and intestinal metaplasia of the esophagus (Barrett's esophagus).[8]

Dysphagia often suggests the presence of erosive esophagitis or strictures. Odynophagia usually signifies severe esophagitis. The majority of patients with GERD do not have endoscopic evidence of esophagitis.[13] The prevalence of complications is associated with increasing age, male sex, duration of symptoms (>5 years), and conditions such as Zollinger-Ellison syndrome and scleroderma. The presence of gastric cancer is associated with a family history of gastric cancer, and positive *Helicobacter pylori* serology.

F *Age.* Gastroenterologists generally agree that referral for endoscopy is indicated in older patients with new onset dyspepsia. In the United States and western Europe, the incidence of gastric cancer is less than 1 per 100,000 before the age of 45 but then increases significantly, so this is the recommended age threshold. A lower age threshold is recommended in Japanese and other populations where gastric cancer is more common in younger age groups, or in patients with a family history of gastric cancer or other risk factors, such as pernicious anemia or known gastric polyps.

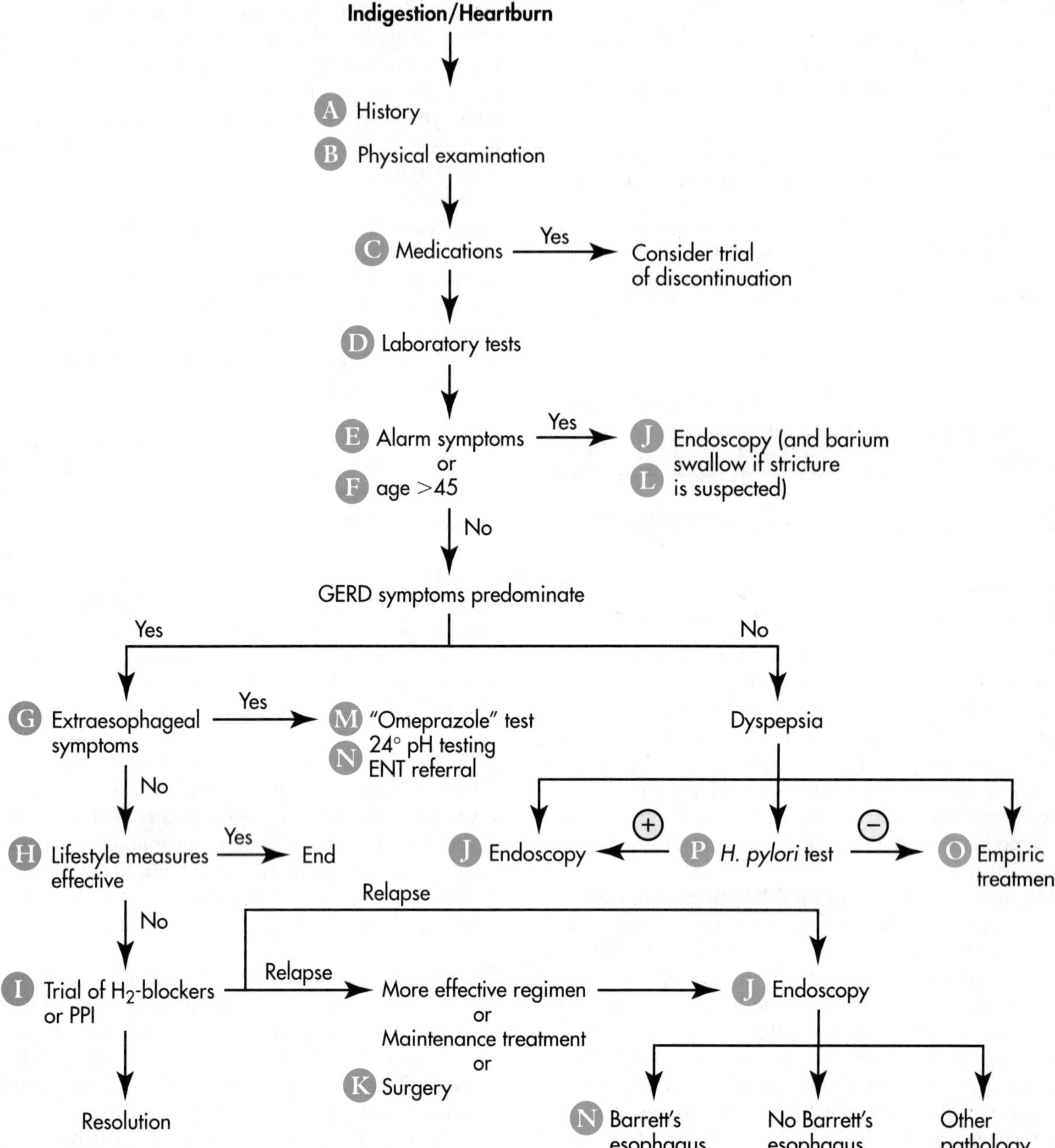

GERD

G *Extraesophageal or "Atypical" Symptoms.* Extraesophageal or "atypical" symptoms may include chest pain simulating angina, hoarseness, sore throat, asthma, and cough, especially nighttime cough (see Chapter 72). Patients may not necessarily report heartburn symptoms at all with these conditions. The association between GERD and asthma is complex, since it is not necessarily causal. Antireflux treatment improved asthma symptoms in 69% of subjects, reduced asthma medication use in 62%, but did not improve spirometry in a recent review that combined data from several studies.[6]

H *Lifestyle Changes.* Lifestyle changes or nonpharmacologic measures may have a modest benefit. These include raising the head of the bed 6 inches, avoidance of precipitating agents (alcohol, spicy foods, citrus, chocolate, peppermint, coffee, fatty meals, tobacco), avoidance of meals for 3 hours prior to recumbency, and withdrawal of medications that may exacerbate symptoms. Antacids are not effective agents to heal esophagitis, but do help symptoms quickly. Alginic acid forms a viscous solution that floats over the gastric pool and acts as a mechanical barrier. It is not effective when the patient is lying down.

I *Treatment (see Chapter 101).* H_2-blockers are all equally effective but often require very high doses to heal esophagitis; mild esophagitis heals in 75% to 90% of cases whereas severe heals in only 40% to 50%.[4] Proton pump inhibitors (PPIs) are potent long-acting inhibitors of acid secretion and are highly efficacious in the healing of all grades of esophagitis. PPIs may promote gastric atrophy in patients who are infected with *H. pylori,* and this atrophy may be a precursor to gastric cancer.[10] The clinical significance of this finding is unclear, however, since the use of PPIs has not been associated with an increase in stomach cancer

Nonetheless, for this reason some have advocated the testing and treatment of all patients with *H. pylori* who are maintained on PPIs for more than a short time. Prokinetic agents are generally viewed as second line and used as a complement to H_2-blockers or PPI or when dysmotility is suspected. Cisapride interacts with several medications and may result in QT prolongation and risk of torsades. *Step-down* therapy may be considered when symptoms stabilize: consider discontinuation of medications, or lower doses, and change from PPIs to H_2-blockers. In general, the symptoms should guide pharmacologic therapy unless severe asymptomatic esophagitis or Barrett's esophagus has been documented.

J *Endoscopy.* Endoscopy is the best method to determine the presence of any mucosal damage and to rule out Barrett's esophagus. Biopsies are necessary, since areas that look like columnar epithelium may not in fact always represent the histologic precursor for adenocarcinoma.[13] A recent study suggests that the *frequency of symptoms* (of heartburn and reflux), their *occurrence at night* (relative risk of 11 compared with asymptomatic persons), and their *duration* were all highly associated with risk of esophageal adenocarcinoma.[11] Endoscopy is very dependent on operator skill; according to some studies it is preferred by patients to barium swallow (see D and E). It is more expensive, but allows direct tissue sampling and therapy such as stricture dilation.

K *Antireflux Surgery.* Antireflux surgery may be considered in younger patients with severe GERD who would require lifelong medical treatment, and in those patients with strictures or recurrent symptoms on therapy. In expert hands surgery has an efficacy of approximately 90%.[9] Manometry is important preoperatively to confirm normal esophageal peristalsis. Several other tests are used less frequently than in the past (e.g., the acid infusion [Bernstein] test, scintigraphy) because of their lower sensitivity and specificity, and are best ordered, if necessary, by the GI specialist.

L *Barium Swallow.* Barium swallow is especially useful in patients with dysphagia. It is more sensitive for subtle strictures and rings than endoscopy, but its sensitivity for mild reflux esophagitis was only 24% in one study.[4] Moreover, it does not allow for any histologic diagnosis or grading.

M *Esophageal pH Monitoring.* Esophageal pH monitoring (24 hour) is considered the gold standard for the diagnosis of GERD, although this has been questioned recently. A pH monitor is placed at the lower esophagus, and pH is recorded over 24 hours. It is probably most helpful in patients who have persistent symptoms despite treatment and a normal endoscopy, as a way to correlate symptoms with episodes of reflux. It is also used by some to diagnose reflux as the cause of non-cardiac chest pain, although some advocate that an empiric 1-week trial of treatment with high-dose PPI (60 mg per day) may be less costly and less invasive. This "omeprazole test" had 78% sensitivity and 86% specificity in one study.[5]

N *Barrett's Esophagus.* Recent practice guidelines[14] on the diagnosis, surveillance, and treatment of Barrett's esophagus suggested that follow-up should be based on the histologic grade seen in the multiple biopsy samples that should be obtained. As with any guideline, these need to be interpreted in light of the individual patient's situation, such as the potential to prolong life expectancy and the patient's eligibility for therapy. The cost-effectiveness and the efficacy of this surveillance have not yet been determined.

Dyspepsia

O *Empiric Treatment.* Empiric treatment of dyspepsia is perhaps the most common management strategy followed by primary care physicians, usually with H_2-blockers or prokinetic agents. Prokinetic agents may in fact be more effective for dyspepsia.[7] There is some limited evidence[3] that empiric treatment of dyspepsia with H_2-blockers in younger patients may be as expensive as early endoscopy and result in lesser patient satisfaction (in part because of a high recurrence rate of symptoms requiring subsequent visits and endoscopy.) The empiric treatment strategy has also been criticized because it may promote long-term use of an ineffective medication and mask the symptoms of malignant ulcers.

P Helicobacter pylori. *H. pylori* has been found to be an etiologic agent for gastric cancer, gastritis, and duodenal ulcer (DU), although its role in nonulcer dyspepsia remains uncertain. Recent guidelines by the American Gastroenterological Association[1] suggest a "test and treat" strategy, where all patients with dyspepsia and positive *H. pylori* test should be treated. In this way all those who had dyspepsia as a presentation of their ulcer diathesis would be treated, but at the cost of also treating others with infection but without peptic ulcer disease (PUD). Two large recent studies on the efficacy of treating *H. pylori* infection in this setting have yielded mixed results. One study[12] found that dyspepsia symptoms resolved at 1 year in 21% of patients who received a metronidazole-based eradication regimen and in only 7% of those treated with omeprazole alone, while the other study[2] found no significant difference between similarly randomized patients.[8] In both studies, however, more than 70% of the patients did *not* get significant relief with eradication of *H. pylori.* Some authors advocate the use of *H. pylori* testing for the purpose of risk stratification in patients under 45 years of age with dyspeptic symptoms (excluding those with classic GERD). They suggest that an endoscopy is not warranted when the *H. pylori* is negative and the young patient does not use NSAIDs; the likelihood of significant findings on endoscopy in such circumstances is extremely low. In those that are positive for *H. pylori,* they believe treatment may benefit the 15% to 25% who have ulcers (or are destined to develop them).[1]

When to Refer

Patients should be referred to a gastroenterologist if they have "alarm" symptoms (as defined above). If a patient above the age of 45 or with risk factors for gastric cancer experiences new onset of dyspepsia, a referral should be considered as well. There is controversy regarding the need to refer patients with reflux symptoms for greater than 5 years, although physicians should be mindful of their increased risk for esophageal cancer. The benefit of surveillance, however, remains unproven. Patients with extraesophageal symptoms consistent with GERD may benefit from an otolaryngology referral. Any patient with Barrett's esophagus should be followed by a GI specialist. There is controversy regarding the cost-effectiveness and utility of referring a young patient with dyspepsia and no alarm symptoms. A more prompt referral is in order if the patient would benefit a lot from the reassurance value of an endoscopy. As the cost of endoscopy declines, the cost-effectiveness of prompt endoscopy increases.

REFERENCES

1. American Gastroenterological Association Medical Position Statement: Evaluation of dyspepsia, *Gast* 114:579-581, 1998.
2. Blum AL, et al: Lack of effect of treating *Helicobacter pylori* infection in patients with nonulcer dyspepsia, *N Engl J Med* 339:1875-1881, 1998.
3. Bytzer PB, Hansen JM, Schaffalitzky de Muckadell OB: Empirical H_2-blocker therapy or prompt endoscopy in the management of dyspepsia, *Lancet* 343:811-816, 1994.
4. DeVault KR, Castell DO: Guidelines for the diagnosis and treatment of gastroesophageal reflux disease, *Arch Intern Med* 155:2165-2173, 1995.
5. Fass R, Fennerty MB, Ofman JJ, et al: The clinical and economic value of a short course of omeprazole in patients with non-cardiac chest pain, *Gastroenterology* 115:42-49, 1998.
6. Field SK, Sutherland LR: Does medical antireflux therapy improve asthma in asthmatics with GERD? A critical review of the literature, *Chest* 114(1):275-283, 1998.
7. Fisher RS, Parkman HP: Management of nonulcer dyspepsia, *N Engl J Med* 339:1376-1381, 1998.
8. Friedman LS: *Helicobacter pylori* and nonulcer dyspepsia, *N Engl J Med* 339:1930-1932, 1998.
9. Kahrilas PJ: Gastroesophageal reflux disease, *JAMA,* 276:983-988, 1996.
10. Kuipers EJ, et al: Atrophic gastritis and *Helicobacter pylori* infection in patients with reflux esophagitis treated with omeprazole or fundoplication, *N Engl J Med* 334:1018-1022, 1996.
11. Lagergren J, Bergström R, Lindgren A, et al: Symptomatic gastroesophageal reflux as a risk factor for esophageal adenocarcinoma, *N Engl J Med* 340:825-831, 1999.
12. McColl K, et al: Symptomatic benefit from eradicating *Helicobacter pylori* infection in patients with nonulcer dyspepsia, *N Engl J Med* 339:1869-1874, 1998.
13. Richter JE: Long-term management of GERD and its complications, *Am J Gastroenterol* 92(4 Suppl):30S-35S, 1997.
14. Sampliner RE: Practice guidelines on the diagnosis, surveillance, and therapy of Barrett's esophagus, *Am J Gastroenterol* 93 (7):1028-1032, 1998.

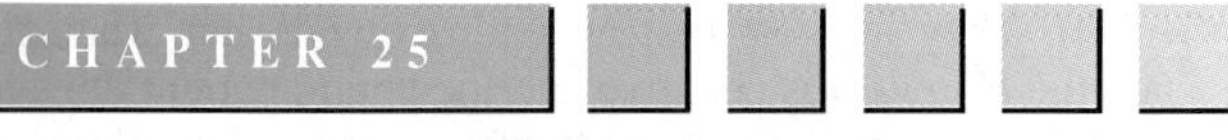

Unintentional Weight Loss

Glennon O'Grady

Unintentional weight loss (UWL) is defined as a documented 5% or more weight loss without a specific goal to lose weight. Self-reported weight loss is often unreliable. Weight loss can be verified by documenting clothes-size change or photographs, if the weight is not documented in the medical record. The medical literature is limited, with relatively few studies done on specific age groups of patients and minimal follow-up, making it difficult to define an evidence-based approach for a workup of UWL. The difficulty for physicians is clear: 25% to 30% of cases have no easily identifiable cause, and yet some of the causes are life threatening. Since failure to diagnose cancer is the most frequent cause for malpractice cases, the lack of applicable studies makes it difficult for the primary care physician to develop a cost-effective approach. Given the literature, it makes sense to stratify different risks of certain diseases and tailor the diagnostic workup by the prevalence of disease, taking into account the patient's age and risk factors. For example, in older age groups the risk of malignancy and Alzheimer's disease increases, whereas in younger groups depression and eating disorders are more frequent. Studies done in 1981[2] and 1986[4] found significantly different frequencies for the etiology of UWL. One study[2] followed a younger all-male veteran population and had relatively fewer neurologic and adverse drug reactions as etiologies (Table 25-1). These studies were done prior to the human immunodeficiency virus (HIV) epidemic or in populations that were not at increased risk for HIV.

A *History and Physical Examination.* History and physical examination can help differentiate the various etiologies for UWL and further refine the use of laboratory tests, x-rays, or procedures. The history should screen for depression, anxiety, and eating disorders. It should include a family history and a risk assessment for lung, gastrointestinal (GI), breast, prostate, and hematologic cancers. Symptoms of endocrine disorders should be elicited, especially thyroid disease and diabetes, which are the most common. A history of symptoms of malabsorption, vomiting, or difficulty chewing or swallowing is important, as well as detailed dietary and social histories that can identify nutritional deficiencies that may be related to financial or adverse living situations. The history should include symptoms or risk factors for any chronic disease, HIV, tuberculosis (TB), and parasites.

In addition to the general physical examination, there should be a specific focus on areas identified by the history. The examination should include screening for cancer, with breast, colorectal, lung, skin, and prostate being the most common. The mouth should be examined, with attention to dentition. A neurologic and mental status examination should assess for neurologic problems that might lead to poor swallowing mechanics and for Alzheimer's disease.

B *Medications.* Medications can cause anorexia, nausea, and vomiting or increased metabolism leading to UWL. Patients should be asked about erythromycin, tetracycline, nonsteroidal antiinflammatory medications, theophylline preparations, selective serotonin reuptake inhibitors, digoxin, amantadine, potassium, corticosteroids, oral contraceptives, metformin, amphetamines, decongestants, over-the-counter diet medications, and thyroid medications. Patients should be screened for substance use, including alcohol, cocaine, and narcotics.

C *Laboratory Tests.* Initial laboratory testing should include a complete blood count (CBC), thyroid-stimulating hormone (TSH), glucose, stool for guaiac, and urinalysis. If the history and physical examination point in a particular direction, appropriate testing should be considered. For example, diarrhea will lead to stool testing for signs of malabsorption or infection.

D *Infectious Diseases.* Any chronic infectious disease can be associated with UWL. The workup needs to be guided by

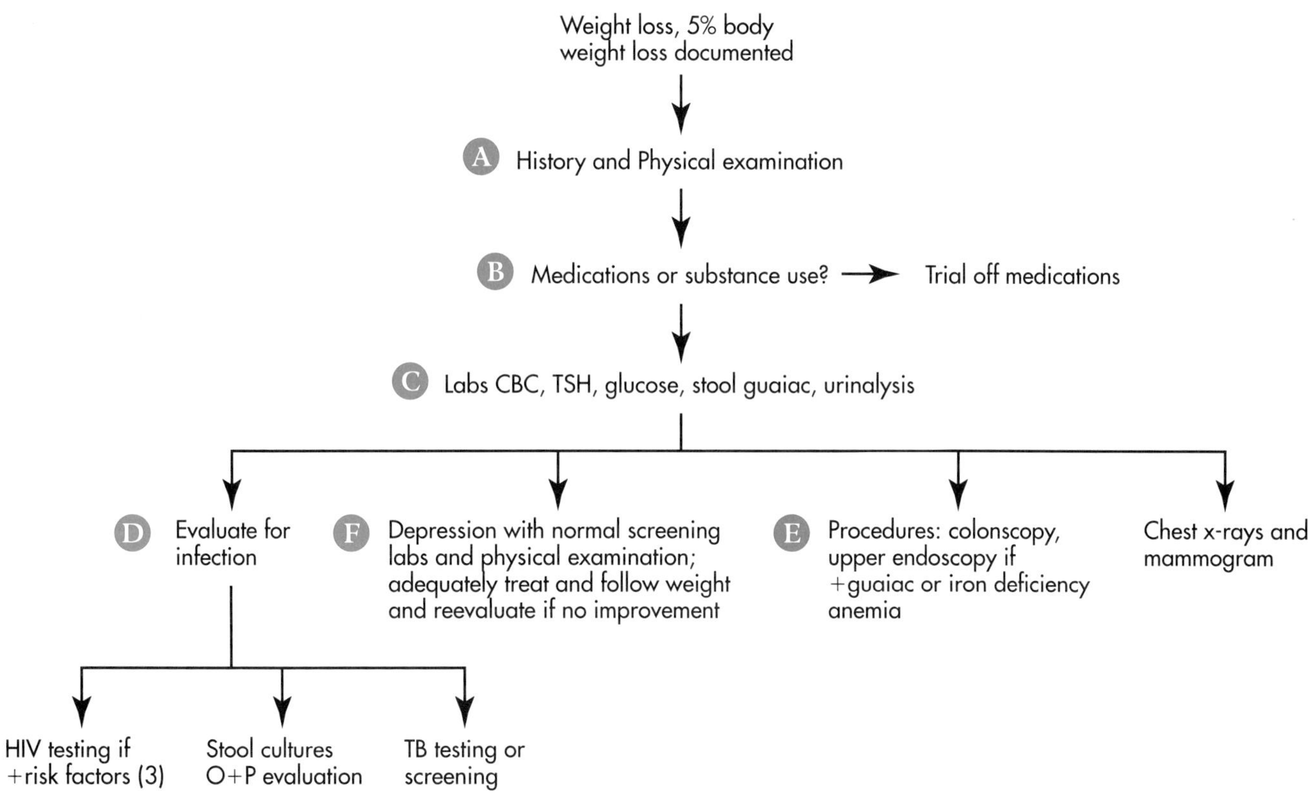

Table 25-1. Etiologies of Unintentional Weight Loss

	Marton[1]	Thompson and Morris[4]	Rabinovitz et al[3]	Morley and Kraenzle[2]
Design	Prospective	Retrospective	Retrospective	Retrospective
Sample	91 Male veterans, both inpatient and outpatient	45 Family practice center patients >63 years	154 Internal medicine inpatients	185 Nursing home patients
Mean age	59	72	64	80
Body weight lost	>5% in 6 mo	>7.5% in 6 mo	>5% (time not specified)	>5 lbs in 3 mo
Mortality/time	25%/18 mo	9%/24 mo	38%/30 mo	Unspecified
Diagnosis (%)				
Cancer	19	16	36	7
Nonmalignant GI	14	11	17	3
Psychiatric	17	18	8	58
Neurologic	2	7	5	15
Adverse drug reactions	2	9	NA	14
Other	20	15	11	NA
Unknown	26	24	23	3

From Gazewood J, Mehr D: Diagnosis and management of weight loss in the elderly, *J Fam Pract* 47:19-24, 1998.

the history of travel and other risk factors. HIV is associated with a wasting syndrome and should be tested for if a patient has identifiable or suspected risk factors. The wasting syndrome is often associated with specific GI symptoms such as swallowing troubles, decreased appetite, or diarrhea. TB is also associated with weight loss as well as night sweats and is reasonable to screen for in high-risk populations.

E *Additional Tests.* Further workup may include chest x-ray and mammogram, which can help diagnose two of the most common cancers. Colonoscopy or upper endoscopy is indicated when labs show iron deficiency anemia or guaiac + stool. It should be noted that iron deficiency anemia is common in menstruating women. Although many physicians consider ruling out colon cancer in patients older than 40, colon cancer can occur in younger people as well.

F *Psychologic Evaluation.* If the history points toward depression and the physical examination and initial labs are normal, adequately treating the depression and following the weight are appropriate management. If there is no improvement or weight loss continues, *consider further evaluation.* It is appropriate to *rescreen for psychosocial causes* that may have been missed in the initial evaluation.

REFERENCES

1. Marton KI: Involuntary weight loss: diagnostic and prognostic significance, *Ann Intern Med* 95:568-574, 1981.
2. Morley JE, Kraenzle D: Causes of weight loss in a community nursing home, *J Am Geriatr Soc* 42:583-585, 1994.
3. Rabinovitz M, et al: Unintentional weight loss: a retrospective review of 154 cases, *Arch Intern Med* 146:186-197, 1986.
4. Thompson MP, Morris LK: Unexplained weight loss in ambulatory elderly, *J Am Geriatr Soc* 39:497-500, 1991.

III INFECTIOUS DISEASE

CHAPTER 26

Fever of Undetermined Origin

Howard Libman
Sharon B. Brodie

Fever is a common presenting problem in primary care practice. Often its cause is determined by the presence of associated localized symptoms, and its course is self-limited. Examples include upper respiratory tract infection manifesting as fever and nasal congestion and acute gastroenteritis presenting with fever and diarrhea. Less frequently, fever occurs without localization of symptoms and is persistent. The concern with these patients is the possibility of occult disease, and diagnostic evaluation is warranted.

Febrile illnesses of less than 2 weeks' duration are often infectious in etiology, most frequently viral, or secondary to drug toxicity, and a specific diagnosis is sometimes not established. For an immunocompetent patient who does not appear particularly ill and has a normal physical examination, the diagnostic evaluation should be limited. Many systemic disorders begin with a prodrome characterized by fever, and observation ultimately leads to identification of the illness.

Fevers lasting longer than 2 weeks are generally associated with localized symptoms or signs that suggest an appropriate diagnostic evaluation. For patients without localized complaints, occult bacterial infection is more likely if they are age 50 or older or have diabetes mellitus, a complete blood count (CBC) characterized by leukocytosis or a leftward shift in the white cell count, or an erythrocyte sedimentation rate (ESR) of 30 or above. The physician should consider a hospital setting for evaluating such patients, as well as ill-appearing individuals, immunocompromised hosts, and patients with a history of valvular heart disease or injection drug use.[12]

In 1961, Petersdorf and Beeson[14] defined fever of undetermined origin (FUO) as a febrile illness of more than 3 weeks' duration in which temperatures exceed 38.3° C (101° F) on several determinations and no diagnosis is reached after 1 week of intensive evaluation.[14] The purpose of these restrictive criteria is to eliminate most self-limited conditions. The differential diagnosis of FUO includes infections (approximately 30% of cases), neoplastic diseases (30%), inflammatory disorders (15%), and miscellaneous conditions (15% to 20%)[6] (Box 26-1). FUO is less often related to central nervous system (CNS) diseases that affect the thermoregulatory center of the hypothalamus directly. Because the medical literature predominantly describes hospitalized patients, however, the prevalence of specific diagnoses in an outpatient population with undifferentiated febrile illness may be different.[8]

In a comparison of the two major studies of patients with FUO in 1961 and 1980,[11,14] tuberculosis, subacute bacterial endocarditis (SBE), rheumatic fever, systemic lupus erythematosus (SLE), and familial Mediterranean fever were much less common in the latter series. Conditions that increased in frequency included cytomegalovirus (CMV) infection, osteomyelitis, sinusitis, malignant histiocytosis, juvenile rheumatoid arthritis of the adult (Still's disease), regional enteritis, and occult hematomas.

Technologic advances have permitted detection of many diseases without hospitalization, including infections by more sensitive culturing methods and serologic tests, neoplasms by radiologic techniques, and rheumatologic conditions by serologic testing. Durack and Street[5] updated the definition of FUO to include etiologies detected in outpatient settings and classified FUOs in four categories: (1) classic, (2) nosocomial, (3) neutropenic, and (4) human immunodeficiency virus (HIV)–associated FUO.

Classic FUO is based on the original definition by Petersdorf and Beeson but only requires an evaluation of 3 days in the hospital, three outpatient visits, or 1 week of intensive outpatient testing without determination of the cause of fever. This is in contrast to the previous requirement of 1 week of intensive inpatient evaluation. *Nosocomial FUO* is limited to hospitalized patients who develop new fever after admission. The minimum evaluation required for diagnosis is 3 days, including 2 days for incubation of cultures. *Neutropenic FUO* encompasses febrile patients with a neutrophil count less than 500/μl with no specific cause identified after 3 days, including 2 days of culture incubation. *HIV-associated FUO* describes patients with documented HIV infection whose fevers persist for 4 weeks in the outpatient setting or 3 days in a tertiary care center with no source found after 3 days, including 2 days of incubation of cultures.

This classification scheme also suggests a tailored approach to diagnosis. For example, in patients with nosocomial FUO, potential etiologies of fever to be explored would include occult sites of hospital-acquired infections (e.g., sinusitis) and complications of medical treatment (e.g., *Clostridium difficile* diarrhea). This chapter focuses on the category of classic FUO, unless otherwise specified.

Etiologies of FUO to be considered differ according to patient country of origin and travel history. Even within the United States the prevalence of certain diseases varies dramatically among some subpopulations, such as elderly persons,[10] injection drug users, and HIV-infected patients (see Chapter 32).

PATHOPHYSIOLOGY OF FEVER

Normal body temperatures taken orally in the basal state range between 36° and 37.8° C, with rectal temperatures generally 0.6° higher. Accurate oral temperatures may be

Box 26-1. Differential Diagnosis of Fever of Undetermined Origin

Infections

Bacterial

Dental abscess
Sinusitis/mastoiditis
Endocarditis
Intraabdominal/pelvic abscess
Biliary tract infection
Prostatitis
Septic pelvic vein thrombophlebitis
Osteomyelitis
Prosthetic device infection
Systemic infections
- Tuberculosis
- Atypical mycobacterial infection
- Salmonellosis
- Disseminated gonococcal infection
- Syphilis
- Lyme disease
- Leptospirosis
- Brucellosis

Viral

Cytomegalovirus
Epstein-Barr virus
Human immunodeficiency virus

Chlamydial

Psittacosis

Rickettsial

Q fever
Rocky Mountain spotted fever

Fungal

Cryptococcosis
Histoplasmosis

Parasitic

Malaria
Amebiasis
Toxoplasmosis
Pneumocystosis

Neoplasia

Lymphoma
Leukemia
Renal cell carcinoma
Hepatoma
Metastatic carcinoma to bone, liver, or central nervous system
Atrial myxoma
Malignant histiocytosis

Inflammatory Diseases

Rheumatic fever
Systemic lupus erythematosus
Juvenile rheumatoid arthritis
Mixed connective tissue disease
Vasculitis

Miscellaneous Conditions

Drug fever
Sarcoidosis
Multiple pulmonary emboli
Regional enteritis
Whipple's disease
Alcoholic hepatitis
Hemolysis
Occult hematoma
Tissue infarction
Metabolic disorders
Familial Mediterranean fever
Thermoregulatory disorders
Factitious fever

difficult to obtain in patients with CNS impairment or hyperventilation, and rectal, axillary, or tympanic membrane temperatures are preferred. Diurnal variation in body temperature is usual in healthy individuals, with the lowest reading in the early morning and the highest in the late afternoon and early evening.

Fever, defined as a sustained abnormally high body temperature, occurs when heat production exceeds heat loss for an extended period. Chills, which may be experienced by the patient at the onset of fever, are characterized physiologically by muscular contraction, cutaneous vasoconstriction, and piloerection. Other associated symptoms include fatigue, sweats, arthralgias, and myalgias. Altered mental status may occur in chronically ill and elderly patients, especially with underlying cardiopulmonary or CNS disease. Although fevers above 41° C are uncommon, sustained higher temperatures are frequently associated with neurologic dysfunction and death.

Heat production occurs from energy-producing biologic reactions, and under normal circumstances, heat dissipation is accomplished through loss of water vapor during respiration and by insensible cutaneous evaporation. When a transient increase occurs in heat production (e.g., with vigorous exercise), sweating, hyperventilation, and cutaneous vasodilation provide additional heat loss.

The hypothalamus, or specifically, its thermoregulatory center located anteriorly near the base of the third ventricle, is important in the control of body temperature. This region serves to regulate the temperature set point and is susceptible to stimulation by cytokines known as *endogenous pyrogens*. These polypeptides are released by monocytes and tissue macrophages in response to a variety of stimuli, including exogenous pyrogens (e.g., viruses, bacterial products such as endotoxin, yeast, protozoa), phagocytosis, immune complexes, and tissue injury. The major endogenous pyrogens include interleukin-1 and tumor necrosis factor (cachectin). Interferons are also thought to be pyrogenic, although their pathophysiologic mechanism is as yet undefined. Endogenous pyrogens act on the hypothalamus by inducing phospholipases, which make arachidonic acid available for prostaglandin synthesis. Prostaglandin E_2, through the generation of cyclic adenosine monophosphate (cAMP), serves to increase the thermal set point of the hypothalamus. Aspirin and nonsteroidal antiinflammatory drugs (NSAIDs) such as ibuprofen lower body temperature by inhibiting cyclooxygenase activity, thereby blocking prostaglandin synthesis.[4]

PATIENT EVALUATION

The general diagnostic approach to FUO begins with a careful history and physical examination, followed by a selective laboratory evaluation. Initial diagnostic efforts are directed at the early identification of potentially serious illnesses that are amenable to specific treatment. Common causes of FUO in young adults include CMV infection, lymphoma, SLE, and regional enteritis. In elderly patients, SBE, tuberculosis, lymphoma, and temporal arteritis should be considered. An atypical presentation of a common disease is more frequent than uncommon conditions. In immunocompromised patients the differential diagnosis is expanded to include opportunistic as well as common diseases (Table 26-1).

History

A careful history of the present illness is essential in focusing the differential diagnosis and determining an appropriate laboratory evaluation of the patient with FUO. An inaccurate or incomplete history may lead to inappropriate diagnostic tests and increased morbidity. The physician should consider the onset of symptoms and any localization over time. The history should include chronic or immunocompromising disorders, recent hospitalizations or surgeries, and medications. Travel history, exposure to tuberculosis, wild and domestic animal exposure, drug use, work environment, avocations, geographic origins, and HIV risk factors should be reviewed in detail. The patient should be questioned about similar symptoms in close contacts or other associates.

Physical Examination

A careful physical examination should be performed and repeated at periodic intervals. The physician should assess

Table 26-1. Differential Diagnosis of Fever in Immunocompromised Patients

Underlying condition	Compromising factor(s)
Solid tumor	D, E
Acute leukemia	A, D
Chronic lymphocytic leukemia	B
Lymphoma	C, E
Multiple myeloma	B
Asplenism	B
Organ transplantation	C, D
HIV disease	C, D
Injection drug use	D, F
Corticosteroid therapy	C

Compromising factor	Pathogens	Sites of infection
A. Granulocytopenia	Enteric bacteria *Staphylococcus* *Candida* *Aspergillus*	Skin Oropharynx Esophagus Lungs Perianal region
B. Defective humoral immunity	*Pneumococcus* *Haemophilus*	Lungs
C. Defective cellular immunity	Tuberculosis Atypical mycobacteria Cytomegalovirus, herpes simplex virus, varicella-zoster virus *Listeria* *Nocardia* *Candida* *Cryptococcus* Cytomegalovirus *Pneumocystis* Toxoplasmosis	Depends on pathogen
D. Disruption of skin or mucosa	Regional flora	Skin Lungs Gastrointestinal tract Urinary tract
E. Anatomic obstruction	Regional flora	Lungs Biliary tract Urinary tract
F. Altered consciousness	Pharyngeal flora	Lungs

whether the patient appears acutely or chronically ill and describe any fever pattern. The skin may reveal peripheral stigmata of SBE, malar rash of SLE, maculopapular rash of drug eruption, generalized rash of secondary syphilis, or evidence of vasculitis. Lymphadenopathy may indicate CMV, Epstein-Barr virus (EBV), HIV infection, syphilis, or lymphoma. Funduscopic examination may reveal evidence of retinitis secondary to CMV infection or toxoplasmosis or Roth's spots suggestive of SBE. Percussion and transillumination of the sinuses may indicate sinusitis. Examination of the mouth and pharynx may show occult dental infection, pharyngitis or tonsillitis, or manifestations of HIV disease (e.g., thrush, oral hairy leukoplakia).

The presence of new or changing cardiac murmurs may indicate endocarditis or atrial myxoma. Cardiopulmonary auscultation may also establish the diagnosis of pneumonia, pericarditis, or pleuritis. Abdominal palpation may reveal hepatomegaly, splenomegaly, abscess, or a mass. Digital rectal examination may suggest prostatitis or show evidence of occult blood. Bimanual pelvic examination may indicate pelvic inflammatory disease. Musculoskeletal examination may show arthritis, bursitis, or localized bony tenderness suggesting osteomyelitis. Neurologic examination may reveal evidence of meningismus or occult focal deficits indicative of pyogenic CNS disease.

Fever Patterns. Although fever patterns are generally nonspecific, the following patterns are sometimes useful in the differential diagnosis[13]:

1. *Intermittent:* characterized by an exaggeration of normal diurnal variation of temperature. This pattern is most often associated with irregular use of antipyretic drugs and with pyogenic abscesses, tuberculosis, and lymphoma.
2. *Sustained:* characterized by little variation in temperature and is often related to significant systemic infections (e.g., SBE, pneumococcal pneumonia).
3. *Relapsing:* characterized by alternating extended periods of fever and normal temperature and frequently occurs with malaria, lymphoma, and some unusual infections.
4. *Temperature-pulse disparity:* characterized by high temperature with a disproportionately slow pulse. This pattern is typically described with salmonellosis, chlamydial and rickettsial infections, legionnaires' disease, drug fever, and factitious fever.

Febrile response to disease may be attenuated or absent in elderly patients, uremic and diabetic individuals, and persons receiving corticosteroid or antipyretic therapy.

Box 26-2. Laboratory Evaluation of Patient with Occult Febrile Illness

Initial Evaluation

Complete blood count
Differential white blood cell count
Kidney and liver function tests
Blood cultures
Syphilis serology
Serum protein electrophoresis
Skin test for tuberculosis with controls
Chest radiograph
Urinalysis
Acute-phase serum sample

Additional Studies Based on Clinical Presentation

Viral hepatitis serologies
Serologies for EBV, CMV, HIV, Lyme disease, toxoplasmosis, or other infectious diseases
Antinuclear antibody
Rheumatoid factor
Antistreptolysin O test

Radiologic Imaging Studies

Sinus radiographs
CT or MRI scan of head
Echocardiography
Doppler studies of extremities
Ventilation/perfusion lung scan
Upper gastrointestinal series/barium enema
CT or MRI scan or ultrasound of abdomen and pelvis
Intravenous pyelogram
Bone radiographs/scan

Invasive Studies

Skin biopsy
Liver biopsy
Bone marrow biopsy
Lymph node biopsy
Aspiration of abnormal fluid collections
Lumbar puncture
Exploratory laparotomy

DIAGNOSIS

Laboratory Evaluation

The initial laboratory evaluation of all patients with an occult febrile illness should consist of a CBC with differential count, kidney and liver function tests, blood cultures, syphilis serology, serum protein electrophoresis, skin test for tuberculosis (PPD), chest radiograph, and urinalysis (Box 26-2). An acute-phase serum sample should also be obtained. Additional diagnostic testing should be individualized based on findings from the history and physical examination.[15]

The CBC may show (1) lymphocytosis, suggestive of viral infection; (2) leukocytosis or leftward shift of white cells, indicative of bacterial infection; or (3) evidence of leukemia. Monocytosis is described with tuberculosis, CMV infection, lymphoma, and metastatic carcinoma. Eosinophilia is often associated with lymphoma, drug fever, and vasculitis. Anemia and thrombocytosis are described with many acute and chronic infections and neoplastic and inflammatory diseases. Thrombocytopenia may indicate an acute infection or immune-mediated disorder. Liver function test abnormalities may suggest hepatitis or infiltrative disease of the liver or biliary tract disease, both of which are generally associated with a disproportionate increase in serum alkaline phosphatase. The ESR and C-reactive protein, nonspecific markers of acute and chronic diseases, are not sufficiently sensitive or specific to be clinically useful in most patients.

Three sets of blood cultures obtained through separate venipunctures are generally sufficient to diagnose conditions associated with continuous bacteremia (e.g., SBE). Infections with intermittent bacteremia (e.g., pneumonia, visceral abscess) may require repeated blood cultures over time. The microbiology laboratory should be notified if an atypical or slow-growing organism is suspected. The serum protein electrophoresis may show nonspecific hypergammaglobulinemia or a monoclonal spike characteristic of a plasma cell dyscrasia. Chest radiograph may reveal hilar adenopathy, diffuse or localized infiltrates, or pleural effusion suggestive of infectious, neoplastic, or connective tissue diseases. Urinalysis may show proteinuria, microscopic hematuria, or evidence of infection.

A positive screening test for syphilis should always be confirmed by specific serology. Hepatitis A, B, and C viral serologies are indicated with unexplained liver function test abnormalities. Serologies for EBV, CMV, HIV infection, Lyme disease, toxoplasmosis, and other infectious diseases should be considered in the appropriate clinical settings. The antinuclear antibody (ANA) test and rheumatoid factor are reserved for patients with suspected SLE and rheumatoid arthritis. An antistreptolysin O titer to establish antecedent streptococcal infection is indicated if rheumatic fever is a diagnostic consideration.

Radiologic Imaging Studies

Radiologic imaging studies are useful in establishing specific diagnoses suggested by history, physical examination, and initial laboratory evaluation. Sinus films may indicate the presence of sinusitis, and computed tomography (CT) or magnetic resonance imaging (MRI) scans of the head may show occult brain abscesses. Echocardiography may reveal valvular vegetations indicative of endocarditis or atrial myxoma. Doppler studies of the lower extremities or ventilation/perfusion lung scan may suggest multiple pulmonary emboli.

The diagnosis of inflammatory bowel disease may be supported by findings on upper gastrointestinal series or barium enema. Abdominal/pelvic ultrasound or CT or MRI scan may show biliary tract disease, pelvic inflammatory disease, or occult abscess. Renal ultrasound or intravenous pyelogram with nephrotomogram may be useful in diagnosing renal cell carcinoma or abscess. Plain radiographs or radionuclide scans of the bone may suggest osteomyelitis. Gallium and indium scan findings are generally nonspecific but sometimes helpful in localizing an occult disease process.[3,9]

Invasive Studies

Invasive studies and biopsy procedures should only be used (1) when the initial clinical assessment suggests systemic or localized disease but is insufficient to establish a definitive diagnosis and (2) when findings from the procedure may significantly alter clinical management.

Skin biopsy may be useful in establishing the diagnosis of vasculitis or drug toxicity. Lymph node biopsy is indicated if lymphoma or adenitis secondary to disseminated infection such as tuberculosis is suspected. In general an excisional biopsy is preferred; the inguinal region should be avoided, if possible, because of an increased rate of nonspecific findings. Liver biopsy should be considered with evidence of chronic hepatitis or infiltrative disease. In the context of pancytopenia, bone marrow biopsy may be useful in establishing the diagnosis of hematologic malignancy or disseminated infection. Abnormal fluid collections involving the pericardial, pleural, abdominal, or joint spaces should be aspirated and sent for cell count, chemistries, culture, and cytology. A lumbar puncture is indicated with meningismus or CNS dysfunction. Exploratory laparotomy is reserved for patients with compelling evidence of significant, undiagnosed intraabdominal disease.

DIFFERENTIAL DIAGNOSIS

Infections

Tuberculosis, SBE from slowly growing or difficult-to-grow organisms, biliary tract infection, intraabdominal abscess, septic pelvic vein thrombophlebitis, and viral infections (e.g., CMV, EBV, HIV) are frequent causes of FUO. Abscesses, the most common type of bacterial infection presenting as an FUO, are often localized in the abdomen or pelvis. Renal abscess with obstruction, perinephric abscess, or prostatic abscess in males may not be associated with any abnormalities on urinalysis. Diagnosis of these conditions is generally established with a radiologic imaging study (e.g., ultrasound, CT or MRI scan).

With the widespread use of blood cultures in recent years, intravascular infection is now a relatively infrequent cause of FUO, although atypical causes of endocarditis (e.g., *Haemophilus* species, fungi) and infections that cause intermittent bacteremia (e.g., salmonellosis, disseminated gonococcal infection, brucellosis) are still described. Culture-negative endocarditis is suggested by the presence of vegetations on echocardiogram. Diagnosis of other bacteremic infections may require multiple or special blood cultures, aspiration of fluid from affected body sites (e.g., bone marrow, joints), or specific serologic tests. Other occult bacterial infections that may cause FUO include sinusitis, mastoiditis, and chronic osteomyelitis. Iatrogenic infections should be considered in patients with prosthetic joints, vascular devices, or other implanted synthetic materials.

Tuberculosis, particularly extrapulmonary disease, and atypical mycobacterial infection, especially *Mycobacterium avium* complex in patients with advanced HIV disease, are important causes of FUO. After decades of decreasing prevalence, tuberculosis has increased in frequency in the United States, with urban areas affected disproportionately. Symptoms of extrapulmonary tuberculosis are variable and depend on the site(s) of involvement. Diagnosis is made by isolator blood culture or tissue biopsy. Symptoms of *M. avium* complex infection are generally nonspecific, but diagnostic evaluation may reveal evidence of bone marrow or liver involvement. Diagnosis is most often established by isolator blood culture.

EBV and CMV infections may be prolonged and have few, if any, localizing signs. Generalized lymphadenopathy, splenomegaly, and rash may be present. Diagnosis is made by serology or culture. Primary HIV infection may present in a similar manner, and patients with advanced HIV disease sometimes have persistent fever and constitutional symptoms not attributable to a specific opportunistic infection or neoplasm. Diagnosis of primary HIV infection is established serologically, and fever related to advanced HIV disease is determined by the exclusion of other conditions.

The chlamydial and rickettsial infections, psittacosis and Q fever, sometimes present with fever and constitutional symptoms. Their diagnosis is often suggested by history of contact with birds or farm animals and can be confirmed serologically. Parasitic infections that may cause FUO include malaria, amebic liver abscess, and toxoplasmosis in patients with advanced HIV disease. Diagnosis is made by appropriate serologic, imaging, and cytologic or histologic studies. Spirochete diseases, including secondary syphilis, Lyme disease, and leptospirosis, may also present with fever, but localized symptoms often suggest the etiology. Diagnosis of each condition is made serologically.

Neoplasms

Lymphoma, leukemia, renal cell carcinoma, hepatoma, and metastatic carcinoma to the bone, liver, or CNS are the most frequent neoplastic causes of FUO.[2] Hodgkin's disease, especially early in its course, may present with fever alone, and lymphadenopathy may be limited to the abdomen or retroperitoneal space. Non-Hodgkin's lymphoma is generally associated with palpable lymphadenopathy, hepatosplenomegaly, or both. Diagnosis of lymphoma is made by excisional biopsy of affected lymph nodes or less often by bone marrow biopsy. Acute leukemia may present with high-grade fever in conjunction with anemia and leukopenia or leukocytosis. Bone marrow aspiration and biopsy are usually diagnostic. In patients with chronic lymphocytic or granulocytic leukemia, fever often indicates accompanying infection.

Most solid tumors are not associated with fever in the absence of obstruction or tissue necrosis. Notable exceptions include renal cell carcinoma, which may present with flank pain and hematuria, and hepatoma, which generally occurs in the context of chronic hepatitis B infection. Presumptive diagnosis is most often made by radiologic imaging study. Metastatic gastrointestinal and ovarian tumors to the bone, liver, or CNS may also be associated with fever. Atrial myxoma, an infrequent cause of FUO, may be clinically confused with bacterial endocarditis, presenting with fever, changing heart murmurs, and peripheral embolic phenomena. Diagnosis is suggested by echocardiography.

Inflammatory Diseases

Rheumatic fever, SLE, juvenile rheumatoid arthritis, mixed connective tissue disease, and vasculitis are the most common inflammatory disorders responsible for FUO. Rheumatic fever generally occurs during childhood or in a young adult, with the diagnosis established by specific clinical and laboratory criteria in the context of serologic evidence of recent streptococcal infection. The diagnosis of SLE is also established by specific clinical, laboratory, and serologic findings. Fever associated with SLE may represent a manifestation of the disease or of a complicating infection in patients receiving immunosuppressive therapy. The diagnosis of rheumatoid arthritis is generally established by the presence of polyarthritis and a positive rheumatoid factor. However, Still's disease, which manifests with fever, polyarthritis, generalized lymphadenopathy, organomegaly, and rash, is a diagnosis of exclusion.

Vasculitic conditions, including periarteritis nodosa, Wegener's granulomatosis, and temporal arteritis, may also present with fever. Diagnosis is made by angiography and biopsy. Polymyalgia rheumatica is a disease of elderly persons manifested by fever, headache, myalgias, and arthralgias. It may occur with or without temporal arteritis and is often associated with a very high ESR.

Miscellaneous Conditions

Drug fever, sarcoidosis and other granulomatous diseases, multiple pulmonary emboli, regional enteritis, Whipple's disease, alcoholic hepatitis, hemolytic episodes, occult hematomas, metabolic diseases, familial Mediterranean fever, factitious fever, and thermoregulatory disorders constitute the miscellaneous causes of FUO.

Box 26-3. Agents Associated with Drug Fever

Allopurinol	Meperidine
Amphotericin B	Methyldopa*
Antihistamines	Nifedipine
Antituberculosis medications	Nitrofurantoin
Atropine	Penicillin*
Barbiturates*	Phenolphthalein
Bleomycin	Phenytoin*†
Cephalosporins	Procainamide†
Clofibrate	Quinidine
Heparin	Sulfonamides*
Hydralazine†	Thiouracils

*May be associated with serum sickness–like syndrome.
†May be associated with SLE-like syndrome.

Drug Fever. Drugs are a relatively common cause of fever, and drug fever should be considered in the differential diagnosis of all febrile illnesses. Although fever has been attributed to many different medications, it is usually associated with a relatively small number of agents (Box 26-3). Fever related to drug treatment may also be the result of endotoxin release in response to antibiotic therapy (e.g., Jarisch-Herxheimer reaction) or the lysis of tumor cells after chemotherapy. Self-limited fever is also common after administration of many vaccines.

Drug fever may be low or high grade and sustained or intermittent and sometimes is disproportionate to the degree of systemic toxicity. Its onset often immediately follows initial use of a medication but may be delayed weeks, months, or even years. Clinical improvement is generally noted within 24 to 48 hours of discontinuation of the causative agent. Drug fever may present with rash, hemolysis, bone marrow suppression, or eosinophilia. Certain drugs, especially barbiturates, methyldopa, penicillin, phenytoin, and sulfonamides, have been associated with a serum sickness–like syndrome, manifested by rash, lymphadenopathy, arthritis, nephritis, and edema. An SLE-like syndrome, characterized by fever, arthralgias, and positive ANA test, has been described with hydralazine, phenytoin, procainamide, and other agents.[7]

Granulomatous Diseases. Sarcoidosis is a systemic granulomatous disease of unknown etiology. Fever has been described in association with hilar lymphadenopathy, arthritis, or hepatic involvement. Diagnosis is made through biopsy of an affected organ, with the characteristic finding of noncaseating granuloma. Infectious causes of granulomatous disease must be ruled out. Granulomatous hepatitis manifests as fever, hepatomegaly, and increased serum alkaline phosphatase. Diagnosis is made by liver biopsy, with the differential diagnosis including tuberculosis, syphilis, histoplasmosis, lymphoma, sarcoidosis, drug reactions, and other conditions.

Table 26-2. Management of Fever

Intervention	Adult dosage	Comments
Acetaminophen therapy	650 mg every 3 to 4 hours	Avoid high dose in patients with significant hepatic dysfunction
Aspirin therapy	650 mg every 3 to 4 hours	Avoid in children because of association with Reye's syndrome May induce gastritis and platelet dysfunction
Ibuprofen* therapy	200 mg every 6 hours	Appears useful in controlling fever associated with malignancy May induce gastritis and platelet dysfunction
Cool compresses or baths	As needed	No advantage to use of alcohol over water
Cooling blanket	As needed for hyperpyrexia	Reduce temperature to 39.5° C and then use traditional measures May induce cutaneous vasoconstriction

From Gartner JC Jr: *Adv Pediatr Infect Dis* 7:6, 1992.
*Other nonsteroidal antiinflammatory agents can be used in equipotent dosages.

Other Disorders. Multiple pulmonary emboli, generally the result of asymptomatic deep venous thrombosis of the lower extremities, typically present with recurrent respiratory symptoms associated with low-grade fever. Diagnostic evaluation includes Doppler studies of the legs, ventilation/perfusion lung scan, or pulmonary angiography. Myocardial infarction is also sometimes associated with a low-grade fever secondary to tissue necrosis.

Gastrointestinal disorders presenting with fever include regional enteritis and Whipple's disease (recently attributed to *Tropheryma whippelii*), which are usually characterized by weight loss, abdominal pain, and malabsorption syndrome. Alcoholic hepatitis may manifest as fever with unexplained abnormalities in liver function tests. Hemolysis from a hematologic disorder, systemic disease, or drug toxicity may present as fever without localizing symptoms, as may occult hematomas secondary to trauma or bleeding dyscrasia. Rarely, FUO is the result of metabolic diseases such as gout, hyperthyroidism, thyroiditis, hyperparathyroidism, or pheochromocytoma.

Familial Mediterranean fever, also known as periodic disease, is an uncommon autosomal recessive disease characterized by periodic fevers associated with atypical chest and abdominal pain in persons of Mediterranean background. Arthritis and skin lesions have also been described. Diagnosis is established clinically.

Thermoregulatory disorders caused by hypothalamic dysfunction secondary to encephalitis, stroke, or hemorrhage occur infrequently. Diagnosis may be suggested by CT or MRI scan of the brain. Fever secondary to hypothalamic disease may respond to chlorpromazine therapy.

Factitious Fever. Factitious fever, most often described in young women and persons with medical training or experience, is a fever that has been artificially produced by the patient. Clinical clues to the diagnosis include lack of constitutional symptoms and systemic toxicity and presence of a temperature-pulse disparity. Diagnosis is established by supervised temperature measurements. Rarely, fraudulent fever may result from self-inoculation of pyogenic substances or ingestion of foreign material.

MANAGEMENT

Except for extreme hyperpyrexia, defined as temperature greater than 41° C, which can cause CNS dysfunction, no information suggests that fever is deleterious in humans. In addition, indirect evidence implies that fever may be beneficial to patients through the activation of specific host defense mechanisms. Indiscriminate treatment of fever could theoretically interfere with immune responsiveness. It could also obscure the natural history of an undiagnosed condition and the response to specific therapy of an identified disease. Despite these concerns, many physicians choose to initiate antipyretic therapy in febrile patients in an effort to alleviate their physical discomfort.

Definite indications for treatment of fever include avoidance of tachycardia in persons with a history of or at increased risk for congestive heart failure, hyperventilation in those with pulmonary decompensation or dehydration, encephalopathy in those with underlying CNS disease, and febrile convulsions in predisposed younger children. Antipyretic agents include acetaminophen, aspirin, and NSAIDs such as ibuprofen (Table 26-2). Each appears to be effective when given in adequate dosage. Aspirin is contraindicated for the management of fever related to viral illness in children because of its association with Reye's syndrome. Because intermittent antipyretic therapy usually results in alternating fever, chills, and sweats, continuous treatment is generally preferable. Alternative methods for fever control include sponging the body with tepid water and using cooling blankets, although the latter sometimes induces cutaneous vasoconstriction and shivering. Alcohol baths have no particular advantage. Extreme hyperpyrexia should be managed by immersing the patient in an ice water bath until fever is reduced to 39.5° C, followed by traditional measures.

More than 90% of adults with FUO are diagnosed with a specific disorder over time, and with few exceptions, blind therapeutic trials should be avoided. Empiric antimicrobial therapy increases the risk of superinfection and drug toxicity. Antituberculous therapy is indicated for high-risk patients diagnosed with granulomatous disease pending culture results. The combination of penicillin G and an aminoglycoside is recommended if the working diagnosis is culture-negative SBE. Empiric corticosteroid therapy should be reserved for suspected connective tissue disease; it may mask the clinical symptoms of other disorders without affecting their natural history. A trial of NSAIDs has been suggested as a means of distinguishing infectious from neoplastic causes of fever in patients with preexisting cancer.

EBM EVIDENCE-BASED MEDICINE

The primary source for this chapter was a MEDLINE electronic search dating back to 1990 conducted in January

1999. It focused on identifying systematic reviews, meta-analyses, and large prospective studies with clinical endpoints.

REFERENCES

1. Armstrong WS, Katz JT, Kazanjian PH: Human immunodeficiency virus–associated fever of unknown origin: a study of 70 patients in the United States and review, *Clin Infect Dis* 28:341, 1999.
2. Chang JC: Neoplastic fever: a proposal for diagnosis, *Arch Intern Med* 149:1728, 1989.
3. De Kleijn EMHA, Oyen WJG, Claessens RAMJ, et al: Utility of scintigraphic methods in patients with fever of unknown origin, *Clin Infect Dis* 18:601, 1994.
4. Dinarello CA, Cannon JG, Wolff SM: New concepts in the pathogenesis of fever, *Rev Infect Dis* 10:168, 1988.
5. Durack DT, Street AC: Fever of unknown origin: reexamined and redefined. In Remington JS, Swartz MN, editors: *Current clinical topics in infectious diseases,* Cambridge, Mass, 1991, Blackwell.
6. Hirschmann JV: Fever of unknown origin in adults, *Clin Infect Dis* 24:291, 1997.
7. Johnson DH, Cunha BA: Drug fever, *Infect Dis Clin North Am* 10:85, 1996.
8. Kazanjian PH: Fever of unknown origin: review of 86 patients treated in community hospitals, *Clin Infect Dis* 15:968, 1992.
9. Knockaert DC, Mortelmans LA, De Roo MC, et al: Clinical value of gallium-67 scintigraphy in evaluation of fever of unknown origin, *Clin Infect Dis* 18:601, 1994.
10. Knockaert DC, Vanneste LJ, Bobbaers HJ: Fever of unknown origin in elderly patients, *J Am Geriatr Soc* 41:1187, 1993.
11. Larson EB, Featherstone HJ, Petersdorf RG: Fever of undetermined origin: diagnosis and follow-up of 105 cases, 1970-1980, *Medicine* 61:269, 1982.
12. Mellors JW, Horwitz RI, Harvey MR, et al: A simple index to identify occult bacterial infection in adults with acute unexplained fever, *Arch Intern Med* 147:666, 1987.
13. Musher DM, Fainstein V, Young EJ, et al: Fever patterns: their lack of clinical significance, *Arch Intern Med* 139:1225, 1979.
14. Petersdorf RG, Beeson PB: Fever of unexplained origin: report on 100 cases, *Medicine* 40:1, 1961.
15. Vickery DM, Quinnell RK: Fever of unknown origin: an algorithmic approach, *JAMA* 238:2183, 1977.

CHAPTER 27

Guidelines for Antimicrobial Therapy and Prophylaxis

Matthew E. Levison

The goal of antimicrobial therapy is to clear the tissues of the infecting organisms. This requires that (1) the organism be susceptible to concentrations of the antimicrobial agent at the site of infection, (2) the dose and route of administration result in adequate levels at the site of infection for a sufficient time, (3) local factors at the site of infection not interfere with the activity of the antimicrobial agent, (4) the presence of host defenses to facilitate microbial clearance, and (5) adjunctive therapies be used, when necessary, such as drainage of abscesses or relief of obstructed excretory sites.

ANTIMICROBIAL DRUG EFFECTS

Spectrum of Antimicrobial Activity

Table 27-1 provides the antimicrobial spectrum of selected drugs. The beta-lactams all have a β-lactam ring either with an attached five-member ring that contains a sulfur (penams, penems), oxygen (clavams, clavems), or carbon (carbapenams, carbapenems) molecule or with an attached six-member ring that contains a sulfur (cephem), oxygen (oxacephem), or carbon (carbacephem) (Fig. 27-1). Two penams, sulbactam and tazobactam, and the clavam, clavulanic acid, are inferior antimicrobial agents but do irreversibly bind some common β-lactamases, such as those of *Staphylococcus aureus, Haemophilus influenzae, Escherichia coli, Klebsiella pneumoniae,* and *Bacteroides fragilis.* Therefore they are marketed in combination with the β-lactam antibiotics, ampicillin, ticarcillin, piperacillin, and amoxicillin. This allows the β-lactam antibiotics to be active against these bacteria, which would otherwise destroy the antibiotics because of β-lactamase production.

The cephems are either cephalosporins, produced by a *Cephalosporium* species, or cephamycins, produced by a *Streptomyces* species. The various cephalosporins are classified into four "generations," based loosely on spectrum of activity; the first-generation drugs have the greatest activity against methicillin-sensitive *S. aureus,* and the fourth-generation cefepime has the greatest activity against gram-negative bacilli. Cefoxitin and cefotetan, the two cephamycins, are classified with the second-generation cephalosporins, but unlike most, they have some activity against *Bacteroides.* Ceftriaxone and cefotaxime, third-generation cephalosporins, and cefepime are the most potent β-lactams against *Streptococcus pneumoniae,* including those strains with some degree of penicillin resistance.

All fluoroquinolones have a similar basic structure; structural modifications have resulted in the fluoroquinolones being categorized into generations, as with the cephalosporins. All the fluoroquinolones have excellent activity against most gram-negative bacillary pathogens, although *Pseudomonas aeruginosa* is the least susceptible among these microorganisms. Ciprofloxacin has the greatest potency against *P. aeruginosa.* The fluoroquinolones also are active against staphylococci, although less so against methicillin-resistant strains. The newer fluoroquinolones, sparfloxacin, grepafloxacin, trovafloxacin, and levofloxacin, have greater activity against *S. pneumoniae.* Trovafloxacin is active against obligate anaerobes, although its usefulness is greatly diminished by its hepatotoxicity. Aminoglycosides have an antimicrobial spectrum similar to that of the older fluoroquinolones.

The macrolides are active against many gram-positive cocci and bacilli, such as *Corynebacterium diphtheriae, Streptococcus pyogenes, S. pneumoniae,* and *S. aureus,* although resistance has emerged among some of these species, especially penicillin-resistant *S. pneumoniae* and methicillin-resistant *S. aureus.* The macrolides are also active against *Neisseria meningitidis, N. gonorrhoeae, Campylobacter jejuni, Borrelia burgdorferi, Mycoplasma pneumoniae, Legionella pneumophila, Chlamydia* species, and *Bordetella pertussis.* Both clarithromycin and azithromycin are active against *Mycobacterium avium* complex and *H. influenzae.* Clindamycin is active against gram-positive cocci (except enterococci) and many obligate anaerobes. Unlike the macrolides, clindamycin is not active against *Mycoplasma.*

Table 27-1. Antimicrobial Activity of Selected Drugs

Organism	Ampicillin	Broad-spectrum penicillins	Cefazolin	Cefamandole	Cefoxitin	Third-generation cephem	Ceftazidime	Cefepime	Aztreonam	Amoxicillin/clavulanic acid Ampicillin/sulbactam	Ticarcillin/clavulanic acid Piperacillin/tazobactam	Meropenem, Imipenem	Aminoglycosides	Fluoroquinolones
Escherichia coli	R	S*	R	S*	S*	S*	S*	S*	S*	S*	S*	S	S	S*
Proteus mirabilis	S	S	S	S	S	S	S	S	S	S	S	S	S	S
Klebsiella pneumoniae	R	R	S*	S*	S*	S*	S*	S*	S*	S*	S*	S	S*	S*
Proteus vulgarus	R	S*	R	R	S*	S*	S*	S	S*	R	S*	S	S*	S*
Enterobacter	R	S*	R	S*	R	S*	S*	S	S*	R	S*	S	S*	S*
Serratia	R	S*	R	R	R	S*	S*	S	S*	R	S*	S	S*	S*
Pseudomonas aeruginosa	R	S*	R	R	R	R	S*	S	S*	R	S*	S*	S*	S*
Staphylococcal aureus	R	R	S†	S†	S†	S†	S†	S†	R	S†	S†	S†	S†	S†
Streptococci	S	S	S‡	S‡	S‡	S‡	S‡	S‡	R	S	S	S	R	R/S§
Bacteroides fragilis	R	S*	R	R	S*	R	R	R	R	S	S	S	R	R

R, ≥5-10% of strains resistant; *S*, susceptible.
*Emerging resistance.
†Except methicillin-resistant staphylococci.
‡Enterococci are resistant.
§Newer fluoroquinolones, levofloxacin, gatifloxacin, and moxifloxacin are active against streptococci.

Tetracyclines have broad-spectrum activity, but the development of resistance has limited their use generally to treatment of infections caused by rickettsiae, chlamydiae, mycoplasmas, *Treponema pallidum,* and *B. burgdorferi.* Trimethoprim-sulfamethoxazole (TMP-SMX) has broad-spectrum activity, but the development of resistance has limited also its use, although it remains the drug of choice for *Pneumocystis carinii* infection. The glycopeptides (vancomycin, teicoplanin) are generally active against gram-positive cocci and metronidazole against obligate anaerobes. Rifampin has broad-spectrum activity. Because resistance develops rapidly if used alone, however, rifampin is usually administered in combination with another antibiotic, such as an another antistaphylococcal agent, usually for staphylococcal infection involving a foreign body or bone.

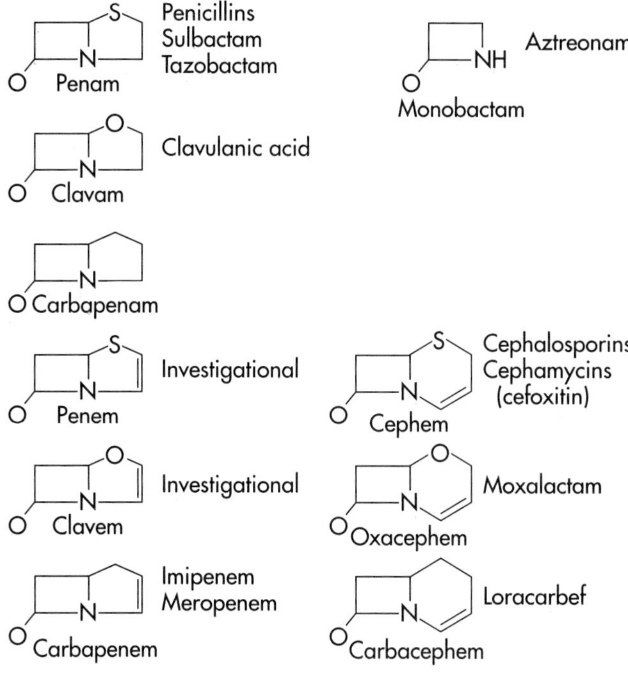

Fig. 27-1. Schematic representation of β-lactam structures.

Mechanisms of Action

The number of targets for the antimicrobial effects of currently available drugs are limited (Table 27-2). The β-lactams bind to penicillin-binding proteins (PBPs), which are enzymes in the cell membrane that the microorganisms require for synthesis of the peptidoglycan component of the cell wall. When bound to β-lactams, these enzymes fail to synthesize cell wall, and the organisms die. The type and number of PBPs vary among species. Gram-negative bacilli have at least six types of PBPs. Inhibition of specific PBPs results in different morphologic changes in the bacterial cell. Most β-lactams bind to PBP-3 of gram-negative bacilli, an enzyme required for cell wall synthesis between newly formed bacilli (i.e., for septation to occur), and as a result of its inhibition, long filaments are formed that die slowly. The carbapenems imipenem and meropenem and the cephalosporin cefepime bind to PBP-2 and result in aggregated cells that burst relatively rapidly. The glycopeptides vancomycin and teicoplanin also interfere with synthesis of peptidoglycan.

Table 27-2. Mechanisms of Action and Resistance of Selected Drugs

Class of drug	Mechanisms of action	Mechanisms of resistance	Resistant pathogens
β-Lactams	Inhibit cell wall synthesis by binding to enzymes (penicillin-binding proteins, PBPs)	Decreased permeability (loss of porin channels)	*Pseudomonas aeruginosa*
		Enzyme inactivation (β-lactamases)	*Staphylococcus aureus, Enterobacter, Serratia, Escherichia coli, Klebsiella, Haemophilus influenzae, Neisseria gonorrhoeae, Bacteroides*
		Altered PBP target	Enterococci, *Streptococcus pneumoniae,* MRSA, β-lactamase-negative-*H. influenzae* and *N. gonorrhoeae*
Aminoglycosides	Inhibit protein synthesis by 30S ribosomal binding plus additional unknown mechanisms	Decreased permeability	*P. aeruginosa, Enterobacter, Serratia*
		Enzyme inactivation	*E. coli, Klebsiella,* enterococci, MRSA
		Altered ribosomal target	
Fluoroquinolones	Inhibit DNA gyrase and topoisomerase IV	Altered target	*P. aeruginosa, Enterobacter, Serratia, E. coli, Klebsiella,* enterococci, MRSA
Glycopeptides	Inhibit cell wall synthesis by binding to d-ala-d-ala	Altered cell wall precursor target (d-ala-d-lac)	Enterococci
Tetracyclines	Inhibit ribosomal function by binding to 30S subunit	Increased efflux	MRSA, *N. gonorrhoeae*
		Altered ribosomal target (methylation enzymes)	*Mycoplasma, Ureaplasma*
Macrolides	Inhibit ribosomal function by binding to 50S subunit	Altered ribosomal target (methylation enzymes; cross-resistance with clindamycin and streptogramin)	MRSA, *S. pneumoniae,* enterococci
		Increased efflux	*S. pneumoniae*
Clindamycin	Inhibit ribosomal function by binding to 50S subunit	Altered ribosomal target (methylation enzymes)	MRSA, *S. pneumoniae*

MRSA, Methicillin-resistant *Staphylococcus aureus.*

The macrolides (e.g., erythromycin, clarithromycin, azithromycin, dirithromycin), clindamycin, streptogramins (e.g., Synercid), chloramphenicol, tetracyclines (e.g., tetracycline, doxycycline, minocycline), and aminoglycosides interfere with protein synthesis at the ribosomal level. Trimethoprim and sulfonamides interfere with purine synthesis. Rifampin inhibits ribonucleic acid (RNA) synthesis by binding to deoxyribonucleic acid (DNA)–dependent RNA polymerase. The fluoroquinolones interfere with DNA folding by binding to DNA gyrase and topoisomerases.

Mechanisms of Resistance

Microorganisms are inherently resistant to some of the antimicrobial agents; the resistance is a characteristic of the species. In addition, because of selective pressure from exposure to specific agents, microorganisms can acquire resistance to the antimicrobial agent. Resistance develops by mutation, with different genes having different spontaneous mutation rates, or by acquisition of DNA from other microorganisms.

Antimicrobial agents have been produced by microorganisms for many millennia. Microorganisms have survived because of their ability to evolve mechanisms to resist these agents' activity. Humans have produced these drugs for less than 50 years. As a result of the selective pressure of increasing massive exposure of microorganisms to antimicrobial agents that are used in clinical practice, animal husbandry, and agriculture, the emergence of multidrug resistance among human pathogens has become a major problem. Multidrug resistance is now frequently found in the following pathogens: pneumococci, gonococci, enterococci, staphylococci, salmonellae, shigellae, *Campylobacter,* tubercle bacillus, and nosocomial gram-negative bacilli.

A decrease in the use of specific antimicrobial drugs may lower selective pressure and may be associated with loss of the acquired resistance. Since acquired antimicrobial resistance is an evolving process, selection of appropriate antimicrobial therapy requires knowledge of current antimicrobial susceptibilities of the community-acquired and nosocomial pathogens. Such data should be published regularly by the local hospital's clinical microbiology laboratory. As a corollary, antimicrobial recommendations for many infections must be revised frequently as acquired resistance patterns change. Table 27-2 lists some common mechanisms of resistance.

In vitro susceptibility testing can usually detect microbial resistance. Routine testing may fail to detect some types of resistance, however, because of low concentrations of enzymes capable of inactivating the antimicrobial agent (e.g., β-lactamase) or low numbers of a resistant subpopulation of a mutant in vitro. Nevertheless, their presence is sufficient in the infected patient to result in clinical resistance. For example, antibiotic resistance in *Serratia marcescens, Enterobacter cloacae, Citrobacter freundii, Morganella morganii, P. aeruginosa,* and *Acinetobacter calcoaceticus* has been attributed to two related mechanisms: inducible production of chromosomal-encoded β-lactamases and selection of mutants that have lost the genes that control expression of β-lactamase production. This group of organisms has a relatively high mutation rate for loss of the genes that repress β-lactamase production in the absence of a β-lactam agent and that allow β-lactamase production in the presence of a β-lactam agent. The mutation results in continuous production of large amounts of β-lactamase *(stable derepression).* The derepressed mutants are resistant to third-generation cephalosporins, aztreonam, and broad-spectrum penicillins. In addition, these chromosomal-encoded, inducible β-lactamases are not inhibited by clavulanic acid, sulbactam, or tazobactam, the so-called β-lactamase inhibitors.

Derepressed mutants are present in the dense bacterial populations of infected tissue at the initiation of antibiotic therapy. Selection of the derepressed mutants in the presence of the β-lactam antibiotic is especially a problem in severely immunocompromised patients, whose defective host defenses are unable to control the growth of the few resistant mutants; this apparently accounts for emergence of resistance during therapy in these patients. The only β-lactams that maintain activity against the derepressed mutants are the carbapenems (imipenem, meropenem) and fourth-generation cephalosporin (cefepime). The fluoroquinolones and aminoglycosides may retain activity against these mutants. TMP-SMX may also remain active against these gram-negative bacilli, except *P. aeruginosa,* which is inherently resistant to TMP-SMX.

Another example in which in vitro testing may fail to predict in vivo resistance is production of plasmid-encoded, extended-spectrum β-lactamases (ESBLs). Nosocomial strains of *K. pneumoniae* and to a lesser extent *E. coli* have acquired these ESBLs that inactivate all third-generation cephalosporins, especially ceftazidime, and the monobactam aztreonam. These strains are also frequently resistant to the fluoroquinolones and TMP-SMX. ESBLs are inactivated to a variable extent by sulbactam, clavulanic acid, and tazobactam. Imipenem, meropenem, and to a lesser degree cefepime are most reliable antimicrobial agents against these strains.

Bacteriostatic vs. Bactericidal Activity

Antimicrobial agents are classified into two major groups: bacteriostatic (i.e., inhibit growth of but do not kill microorganisms) and bactericidal (Box 27-1). Bacteriostatic agents are sufficient to treat most infections, but infections in patients with impaired host defenses (e.g., neutropenia) and at sites of impaired host defenses (e.g., endocarditis, meningitis) require therapy with bactericidal agents to clear pathogens from the site of infection. Bactericidal agents are capable of clearing pathogens from tissues in the absence of host defenses, whereas the residual organisms regrow once bacteriostatic therapy is stopped.

The type of antimicrobial activity of some agents may be microorganism specific. For example, the macrolides, clindamycin, streptogramins, chloramphenicol, and tetracyclines are generally bacteriostatic, although bactericidal activity may occur under certain conditions or against specific microorganisms. Although generally bactericidal, the penicillins are bacteriostatic against enterococci. The activity may also vary with the concentration of an antimicrobial agent that is, the agent may be bacteriostatic at low concentration and bactericidal at higher concentrations. The β-lactam antibiotics have a bactericidal effect on only exponentially growing bacteria, which express PBPs, whereas the fluoroquinolones have a bactericidal effect on both exponentially growing and nongrowing microorganisms. Growing microorganisms are found in young cultures and early infection. The majority of microorganisms in most well-established infections are nongrowing. The rapidity and extent of bactericidal activity for the aminoglycosides, fluoroquino-

Box 27-1. Bactericidal and Bacteriostatic Agents

Bacteriocidal

β-Lactams:
Penams (penicillin, ampicillin, amoxicillin, nafcillin, ticarcillin, piperacillin)
Penems (none as yet marketed)
Carbapenem (imipenem, meropenem)
Cephems (cephalosporins, cefoxitin)
Carbacephems (loracarbef)
Monobactam (aztreonam)
Aminoglycosides: gentamicin, tobramycin, amikacin, netilmicin, streptomycin
Quinolones: ciprofloxacin, ofloxacin, norfloxacin, enoxacin, lomefloxacin, levofloxacin, sparfloxacin, gatifloxacin, moxifloxacin
Glycopeptides: vancomycin, telcoplanin
Others: trimethoprim-sulfamethoxazole, metronidazole, rifampin

Bacteriostatic

Macrolides: erythromycin, clarithromycin, azithromycin, dirithromycin
Clindamycin
Streptogramins (Synercid)
Chloramphenicol
Tetracyclines: tetracycline, minocycline, doxycycline

lones, and metronidazole are concentration dependent; that is, the higher the concentration, the greater the rate of bactericidal activity. The bactericidal activity of the β-lactams and vancomycin is slow, and the rate of bactericidal activity is minimally enhanced with increasing drug concentrations.

Postantibiotic Effect

Drugs may also exhibit persistent suppression of microbial growth as a result of transient drug exposure after removal of the drug, the so-called postantibiotic effect (PAE). Drugs that exhibit concentration-dependent bactericidal activity, (aminoglycosides, fluoroquinolones, metronidazole) also exhibit PAE against susceptible organisms, and the duration of their PAE is also concentration dependent. In contrast, most β-lactams, except the carbapenems and cefepime, exhibit no PAE against gram-negative bacilli and relatively short PAEs against gram-positive cocci. Consequently, the bactericidal activity of β-lactams and vancomycin depends on the time the drug concentration exceeds the minimal concentration that inhibits microbial growth (i.e., time-dependent bactericidal activity).

Inoculum Effect

Activity of certain antimicrobial agents may also depend on the bacterial density, being reduced by dense bacterial populations or enhanced by sparse bacterial populations, the so-called inoculum effect. Dense populations can be less susceptible to antimicrobial agents because of (1) the predominance of nongrowing organisms in dense populations, (2) the high concentration of certain bacterial products in dense populations that inactivate the antimicrobial agents (e.g., β-lactamases), or (3) a greater likelihood that subpopulations of resistant mutants will be present in dense populations that can emerge with antimicrobial therapy.

Synergy and Antagonism

A greater rate and extent of bactericidal activity seen with combinations of two antimicrobial agents, in contrast to the activity exhibited by each agent alone, are called *synergy*. For example, a combination of bacterial cell wall active agents (e.g., penicillin, ampicillin, vancomycin) alone is at best only slowly bactericidal against enterococci, and an aminoglycoside alone exhibits only inhibitory activity; the combination of the cell wall active agent with an aminoglycoside, however, results in rapid bactericidal activity. This results from enhanced bacterial penetration of the aminoglycoside in the presence of the cell wall active agent. Similarly, synergy has been shown with cell wall active agents/aminoglycoside combinations against hemolytic streptococci, *S. aureus*, and many gram-negative bacilli. Synergy has been defined as a 2 log 10 or greater or 99% reduction in bacterial count after overnight incubation with the combination vs. that with each of the agents alone.

Combinations of some agents have been found to be antagonistic. For example, β-lactam's bactericidal effect, which requires growing organisms, may be converted to a bacteriostatic effect when combined with another agent that prevents microbial growth.

Minimum Inhibitory and Bactericidal Concentrations

Antimicrobial activity is measured routinely in vitro in terms of the (1) lowest concentration of the drug that inhibits the growth of 10^5 colony-forming units (CFUs)/ml of broth of a specific microorganism in the exponential phase of growth after overnight incubation, or *minimum inhibitory concentration* (MIC), and (2) the lowest concentration that lowers the inoculum by 99.9% (a 3 $\log_{10}$ fall in bacterial count) after overnight incubation, or *minimum bactericidal concentration* (MBC). The MIC and MBC determinations are performed in serial twofold dilutions of the drug in broth and have an error of plus/minus one dilution. In practice the MIC requires only inspection of the broth culture for the development of turbidity. The lowest drug concentration that prevents visible growth (i.e., turbidity) of an initially clear bacterial suspension (i.e., growth of at least 1 $\log_{10}$, from 10^5 to 10^6 CFU/ml) is the MIC. MBC determination requires the more laborious quantification of bacteria remaining in the visibly clear suspension in broth after overnight incubation.

The in vitro conditions of the MIC and MBC determination do not necessarily mimic in vivo conditions. For example, MIC and MBC, which are determined after overnight incubation, reflect a specific time point and do not provide information on the time course of antimicrobial activity. In addition, the in vitro drug concentrations remain constant throughout the incubation period, unlike the varying drug concentrations in vivo. MIC and MBC are measured against a standard inoculum (10^5/ml) that does not necessarily correspond to bacterial densities at the site of infection (10^{8-10}/gm). Also, the inoculum is in the exponential phase of growth, unlike the majority of organisms in an established infection, which are nongrowing.

Antimicrobial susceptibility testing is done for most clinical isolates, unless the organism has predictable susceptibility to drugs of choice. The National Committee for Clinical Laboratory Standards (NCCLS) has provided guidelines for performance of susceptibility tests and interpretation of the results. Microorganisms are considered *sensitive* if their MICs are below a breakpoint concentration and *resistant* if the MICs are above this concentration. *Breakpoint concentrations* are related to serum levels achieved with standard dosing, except for the few antimicrobial agents used exclusively for treatment of lower urinary tract infection, when breakpoint concentrations are related to urinary levels. Determination of breakpoint concentrations is complicated, and results of in vitro testing may not adequately predict clinical outcome, which also depends on pharmacokinetic and pharmacodynamic factors. For example, the peak drug concentration relative to the MIC for concentration-dependent drugs and time the serum drug concentrations exceed the MIC for time-dependent drugs have been correlated with drug efficacy in clinical trials.

THERAPEUTIC APPROACHES

Use of antimicrobial agents may be empiric, pathogen directed, or prophylactic.

Empiric Therapy

Empiric therapy is usually the initial use of an antimicrobial agent, when the patient is first seen and judged to be critically ill. Patients who require immediate antimicrobial therapy include elderly persons, moderately to severely ill patients with a focal infection, septic patients, febrile neutropenic patients, and those with acute endocarditis or meningitis. At this time the pathogen has not been identified, but any delay in initiation of appropriate antimicrobial therapy would be life threatening. In such patients the antimicrobial regimen should be broad in spectrum, that is, active against all the possible pathogens causing the patient's illness, especially those likely to be rapidly fatal if untreated. The antimicrobial regimen should also be bactericidal because (1) bacteriostatic agents require host defenses to clear the pathogen from tissues, and (2) host defense in critically ill patients may be not adequate to clear the tissues of the pathogens.

Clues to possible pathogens may be present. For example, the presence of focal infection (e.g., pneumonia, urinary or biliary tract, secondary intraabdominal, meningitis) may suggest certain possible pathogens that cause infection more often at the specific site. A history of prior antibiotic use may indicate that the infection is caused by pathogens resistant to the previous antimicrobial regimen. Institutional-acquired infections are more likely to be caused by multidrug-resistant staphylococci or gram-negative bacilli.

Before starting antimicrobial therapy, blood should be cultured and exudates and appropriate body fluids examined microscopically and cultured to determine the causative pathogen. Gram's stain of exudate or body fluid may quickly indicate the causative pathogen. Cultures obtained after initiation of antimicrobial therapy may not reliably yield the causative pathogen, and because of subsequent alteration of bacterial flora of mucosal surfaces and wounds, growth from posttreatment cultures of sputum or exudates may actually be misleading.

Selection of appropriate antimicrobial agents for empiric therapy requires consulting the antimicrobial susceptibility patterns of community-acquired and nosocomial pathogens regularly published by the local hospital's clinical microbiology laboratory. Once results of pretreatment cultures are available, the empiric regimen can be altered according to results of susceptibility tests to the narrowest spectrum, least toxic, and least costly agent among those of comparable efficacy available for the particular type of infection.

Pathogen-directed Therapy

Pathogen-directed therapy is used when the pathogen is known and laboratory testing has determined its antimicrobial susceptibility.

Prophylactic Use

Prophylaxis may be primary or secondary. *Primary prophylaxis* attempts to prevent a pathogen from causing disease in a patient who has never been infected by that pathogen. Examples include perioperative antibiotic administration to prevent surgical wound infection and antibiotic administration immediately before procedures likely to induce bacteremia with microorganisms that cause endocarditis in patients with certain cardiac conditions. *Secondary prophylaxis* attempts to prevent a reinfection or relapse. For example, antibiotics can be used to prevent reinfection with group A streptococcal pharyngitis and consequent recurrence of rheumatic carditis in a patient with a history of rheumatic carditis. Antibiotics can also be used to prevent clinical relapse of a pathogen by eradication of clinically latent infection (e.g., isoniazid to prevent tuberculosis in a patient who has a positive tuberculin skin test) or only to suppress the clinical emergence of latent infection (e.g., recurrence of *P. carinii* pneumonia in patients with AIDS).

Combination Therapy

An antimicrobial regimen may either involve a single agent or a combination of two or more agents. Combinations are used (1) to broaden the spectrum in an empiric regimen, (2) to treat polymicrobial infection, (3) to prevent emergence of antimicrobial resistance (because emergence of mutants resistant to one of the antimicrobial agents is more likely than emergence of a doubly resistant mutant), and (4) to improve the rate and extent of bactericidal activity (i.e., synergy). Therapy with an agent active against *E. coli,* combined with another agent that is active against anaerobes (e.g., *B. fragilis*), is required for treatment of secondary intraabdominal infection, although monotherapy is now possible with the development of single agents with activity against both *E. coli* and anaerobes. Combination therapy with an antienterococcal β-lactam plus an aminoglycoside is required to achieve bactericidal activity for treatment of enterococcal endocarditis. An antistreptococcal β-lactam/aminoglycoside combination has been used to shorten the duration of antimicrobial therapy of streptococcal endocarditis. Similarly, an anti–*P. aeruginosa* β-lactam/aminoglycoside combination has been used to treat severe *P. aeruginosa* infections. Rifampin is frequently used in combination with an antistaphylococcal agent for staphylococcal infection involving a foreign body (e.g., prosthetic joint, cardiac valve) or vascular graft.

Duration of Therapy

The optimal duration for many infections is unknown but should be the shortest time necessary to eradicate the pathogen from the site of infection and prevent relapse. Duration will vary with (1) the rate of clearance, which i characteristic for the specific antimicrobial agent; (2) the presence of effective host defenses at the site of infection, which may enhance antimicrobial efficacy; (3) the age of the infection, which determines the number of growing organisms and the bacterial density; and (4) the ability to eliminate local conditions at the site of infection that favor microbial survival (e.g., foreign bodies, renal or biliary stones, dead bone and other necrotic tissue, continued contamination) or that interfere with the activity of the antimicrobial agents used. For example, only a short course of antimicrobial therapy (about 24 hours) is required for sterile peritonitis that occurs around an infected but resected intraabdominal organ (e.g., appendix, gallbladder) or after adequate surgical early debridement and closure of traumatic perforation of the bowel, whereas weeks of antimicrobial therapy combined with drainage and debridement may be required once intraperitoneal abscesses have formed.

The duration of antimicrobial therapy depends on severity of infection, clinical response to therapy, and normalization of the white blood cell count. Once the patient can tolerate oral therapy, well-absorbed antimicrobial agents can be given orally rather than intravenously, if oral agents are available that have antimicrobial efficacy comparable to that of the intravenous (IV) regimen.

Adjunctive Therapy

Additional management includes drainage, debridement, relief of obstruction, removal of foreign bodies, and restoration of host defenses. Closed-space infections such as abscesses are difficult to eradicate with antimicrobial therapy without drainage. The poor drug entry and the presence of antimicrobial-inactivating enzymes and other substances, an acidic anaerobic environment, and high microbial density with predominantly nongrowing organisms in abscesses impair the therapeutic efficacy of many antimicrobial drugs. The presence of foreign bodies, stones, dead bone, and other nonviable tissue favors persistence of organisms.

Cost

Antibiotics constitute 20% to 30% of hospital pharmacy costs. Cost of these drugs includes not only the purchase price, but also the costs of pharmacy and nursing time, supplies required for drug preparation and administration, untoward consequences of their use (e.g., emergence of antimicrobial resistance), and other adverse drug reactions. Costs can be reduced by switching from IV to oral therapy, decreasing the frequency of dosing, switching from multidrug to single-drug therapy, and using drugs or drug combinations with less potential adverse reactions. Oral antimicrobial therapy at home is least costly, but outpatient IV therapy is still less costly than receiving antimicrobial therapy in the hospital. Outpatient infusion therapy can be delivered at an infusion center, by a visiting nurse at home, or by self-administration at home. Outpatient infusion ideally should be with agents requiring infrequent dosing; antibiotics that require frequent dosing should be given by more expensive electronic infusion pumps, if drug stability and solubility are not problems.

PHARMACOKINETICS

Pharmacokinetics is the study of the time course of a drug's disposition in the body, which is usually described in terms of the drug's concentration in serum because of the relative ease of measurement in this body fluid. The therapeutic effect, however, depends on the time course of the drug concentration at the site of infection.

Absorption

Most antimicrobial agents are administered intermittently at fixed dosing intervals. The extent of absorption from the site of drug administration is measured by the fraction of the dose absorbed *(bioavailability)*, the maximum serum concentration (C_{max}), and the time to reach the maximum concentration after administration (T_{max}). For most drugs the bioavailability and T_{max} are independent of dose, whereas C_{max} is dose dependent. After IV bolus administration, absorption is assumed to be rapid and complete. In contrast, absorption after oral or intramuscular (IM) administration is variably slower and incomplete, and the T_{max} is delayed (usually 1 to 2 hours) and the C_{max} is lower, because the drug is being eliminated before absorption from the gastrointestinal (GI) tract or from the IM site is complete. Bioavailability after oral absorption can be compromised by GI dysfunction, such as hypochlorhydria (gastric acidity is required for effective absorption of cefuroxime axetil, cefpodoxime proxetil, itraconazole, and ketoconazole), vomiting, rapid intestinal motility, short-gut syndrome, and ileus. Food may interfere with GI absorption of some antimicrobial agents, and divalent and trivalent cations may interfere with absorption of several fluoroquinolones and tetracyclines by chelation. However, the bioavailability after proper oral administration of fluoroquinolones, doxycycline, TMP-SMX, fluconazole, rifampin, and metronidazole is excellent, and their C_{max} after oral administration approximates that achieved after IV administration. IV administration is used for life-threatening infection because GI function is likely to be impaired in this situation. Many mild infections can be treated entirely with oral agents, or their course of antimicrobial therapy can be completed with oral agents once the patient's condition is no longer critical and the GI tract is functional, if oral agents are available to which the pathogen is sufficiently susceptible. Otherwise, the course of antimicrobial therapy can be completed with IV administration at home once the patient is stabilized.

Maximum Serum Concentration. C_{max} occurs at the completion of an IV infusion or absorption from the GI tract or IM site. The C_{max} depends on the size of the dose administered, the amount of the drug eliminated during infusion or absorption, and its volume of distribution (V_d). C_{max} is higher if the dose is larger, if the rate of infusion or absorption is faster, or the V_d is smaller. Too rapid IV infusion (i.e., less than 1 to 2 hours) is not used for certain drugs to avoid toxic reactions, such as chills and fever with amphotericin B and "red-man's" syndrome with vancomycin. Otherwise, IV infusions of antimicrobials are usually given over 20 to 30 minutes.

Volume of Distribution. V_d is a proportionality constant that relates the total amount of drug in the body to the serum concentration (e.g., V_d = IV bolus dose + C_{max}), as if the drug were present throughout the body at the same concentration as found in serum. It is a theoretic value and does not correspond to any actual body compartment. V_d is useful to compare distribution characteristics of different drugs. Drugs that distribute primarily in extracellular fluid

(ECF) (e.g., β-lactams, aminoglycosides) will have a relatively small V_d (20% to 30% of lean body weight, or about 15 to 20 L), although patients with an expanded ECF volume (e.g., congestive heart failure, fluid overload, extensive burns, abundant ascites, sepsis) will have a larger V_d and require higher doses to achieve desired serum levels. Drugs that distribute intracellularly (e.g., azithromycin, clarithromycin, fluoroquinolones, rifampin, clindamycin) will have a large V_d (40 L or greater).

Distribution

A drug is initially distributed after administration throughout the blood volume and tissues in rapid equilibrium with blood, such as highly perfused tissues of the heart, lungs, liver, and kidneys. Active transport pumps from the systemic circulation are present only at excretory sites, such as the liver or kidneys. Otherwise, antimicrobial drugs move from blood to the ECF of tissues by passive diffusion along a concentration gradient. Levels of antimicrobial drugs in interstitial fluid are at best equal to or lower than peak serum levels. Factors that favor transfer of drug from the blood into interstitial fluid include (1) high blood flow and large surface area of the vascular bed of the tissue, (2) absence of endothelial tight junctions and presence of capillary pores in the tissue's vascular bed, (3) high serum drug levels, and (4) low serum protein binding. In tissues such as lung that are well perfused by capillary beds fenestrated by pores, the level of drug in the ECF is similar to free drug levels in serum. Diffusion of drug into closed-space infection (e.g., abscess, empyema) is impaired because the ratio of surface area of the vascular bed to volume of the space is low.

Drugs have difficulty diffusing into tissues that have tight junctions and the absence of capillary pores, such as the eye, prostate, and brain. These sites have an endothelial lipid membrane barrier that limits passive diffusion of hydrophilic drugs such as the β-lactams, although these drugs are able to penetrate the cerebrospinal fluid (CSF) to some extent in the presence of intense inflammation. In addition, the continual formation of CSF lowers CSF drug levels by dilution, and active pumps of organic acids, such as β-lactams, in the eye and choroid plexus lower drug levels in vitreous fluid and CSF, respectively. Lipophilic drugs (e.g., doxycycline, metronidazole, rifampin, trimethoprim, chloramphenicol) readily cross lipid membranes. Lipophilic drugs also enter the prostate and the intracellular fluid (ICF) by another related mechanism, *ion trapping,* which depends on the pK_a of the drug and ionic charge of the drug molecule at the different pH values of the fluid on either side of the lipid membrane. Weak bases (e.g., macrolides, fluoroquinolones, trimethoprim, clindamycin) are unionized (nonionized) at the pH of serum, and being lipid soluble, the unionized drug diffuses into the cell. Once within the cell, the drug becomes charged at the more acid pH of ICF and is less able to diffuse out. Most β-lactams are weak acids and thus are unionized in the acidic ICF and diffuse more readily out of the cell.

Because capillary pores do not permit passage of serum protein into extravascular sites, only that portion of a drug not bound to serum protein is free to diffuse into tissues. Highly serum protein-bound drugs (generally defined as being 90% or greater protein bound), such as nafcillin, cefazolin, and ceftriaxone, have less free drug to diffuse into tissues than drugs with lower serum protein binding. Protein binding also decreases the antimicrobial activity of drugs in serum. Only the drug's free, unbound portion in serum is active against bacteria. In general, for highly protein-bound drugs, C_{max} will overestimate antimicrobial activity that is based on MIC testing in a protein-free system, such as broth. The presence of certain serum factors, however, may enhance the antimicrobial effect with some drug-bacteria combinations.

Tissue is mainly cellular, and intracellular water accounts for most of its volume. Only a small portion of tissue volume is ECF. For drugs distributed only in ECF (e.g., β-lactams, aminoglycosides), total tissue levels (ICF plus ECF levels) may be only a small fraction of the drug's free serum levels, although ECF levels actually may be similar to free serum levels. For drugs distributed in both ICF and ECF (e.g., fluoroquinolones, rifampin, clindamycin), tissue levels approach or exceed the drug's free serum levels. Bacteria in tissues may be located in ECF, phagocytes, or both. However, ICF location of the pathogen may not correspond exactly to the ICF location of the drug, or the intracellular conditions may interfere with the drug's antimicrobial activity, in which case the desired antimicrobial effect may not necessarily occur.

Time Course of Serum Levels

Serum levels decline after the peak concentration, and when plotted vs. time on semilog scale, the rate of decline may have one or more phases (Fig. 27-2). The initial rapid portion, called the *α-phase,* results from mixing with blood and diffusion into those tissues in rapid equilibration with blood. The rate of decline of the subsequent portion, called the *β-phase*, is slower and is mainly caused by elimination from the body through metabolism or excretion. An additional slower decline, or γ-phase, is seen with some drugs at low serum levels and is mainly caused by slow release of drug from secluded tissue foci.

The rate of elimination, or β-phase, is constant for most antimicrobial agents. The elimination of these drugs is described by their *elimination half-life* ($T_{½}$, or the time required to eliminate 50% of the drug present (equals 0.693/slope of β-phase serum level curve, or elimination rate

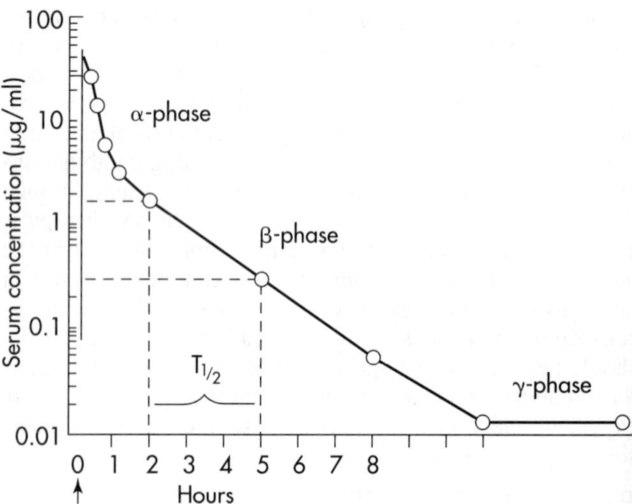

Fig. 27-2. Concentrations of drug in serum after administration *(arrow)* showing α-, β-, and γ-phases of serum concentration curve and β-phase serum half-life ($T_{½}$).

constant). Elimination is almost complete in four to five half-lives. Most β-lactams have serum $T_{1/2}$ of 2 hours or less and are usually given every 4 to 8 hours. The exception is ceftriaxone, with a $T_{1/2}$ of 6 to 8 hours, which is usually dosed every 24 hours. The older quinolones (e.g., norfloxacin, ciprofloxacin, enoxacin) have serum $T_{1/2}$ of 4 hours and are dosed every 12 hours. Structural modifications have resulted in a longer serum $T_{1/2}$ for sparfloxacin, levofloxacin, gatifloxacin, and moxifloxacin, which allows dosing every 24 hours, and decreased renal excretion for moxifloxacin.

In contrast to most antimicrobial agents, the rate of elimination for the ureidopenicillins (e.g., piperacillin, azlocillin, mezlocillin) is dose dependent; the larger the dose (e.g., 5 rather than 3 gm), the longer is the $T_{1/2}$, and the less frequently these drugs need to be administered (e.g., every 8 rather than every 4 hours, respectively).

Area Under Curve. Another important pharmacokinetic parameter is the area under the concentration curve (AUC) over the dosing interval. AUC integrates both time and intensity of drug concentrations. AUC depends on the dose, the elimination rate constant *(k)*, and the V_d:AUC = Dose/ $V_d \times k$, or Dose $\times T_{1/2}/V_d \times 0.693$.

Elimination

Renal excretion may be through glomerular filtration, tubular secretion, or both. Elimination by glomerular filtration is passive diffusion of the portion of the drug not bound to serum protein. Glomerular clearance is equal to the percentage of free drug times glomerular filtration rate (GFR). Estimated GFR equals (140 − age in years) (ideal body weight in kg)/(serum creatinine in mg/dl) × 72 in males or 0.85 × male value in females. Tubular secretion is an active transport process. Probenecid inhibits the tubular secretion of organic acids, such as many of the β-lactams, and prolongs their $T_{1/2}$. Although hemodialysis removes variable amounts of many antimicrobial agents, peritoneal dialysis removes very little of most antimicrobial agents. Drugs instilled into the peritoneal cavity, however, are rapidly absorbed over the large expanse of the peritoneal surface into the systemic circulation, so that serum levels achieved will be equal to the concentration of the drug added to the peritoneal dialysis fluid.

Some relatively lipid-soluble antimicrobial agents (e.g., rifampin, macrolides, imidazole antifungals) are metabolized to more polar, less lipid-soluble, and more readily excreted products that also often have reduced antimicrobial effects and toxicity. The enzyme systems involved with metabolism of many of these antimicrobial drugs are located in the liver microsomal, smooth endoplasmic reticulum. A drug may enhance its own metabolism by stimulating the activity of these enzymes, or the activity can be induced by other drugs. The rate of metabolism may also be influenced by competing endogenous and exogenous substances. Induction and competition may result in complex interactions with other drugs and endogenous substances. For example, rifampin, which competes with bilirubin for biliary excretion, initially will elevate serum bilirubin levels, until bilirubin glucuronide production and its excretion in bile increase, as a result of enzyme induction during the first 6 days of treatment, and serum bilirubin levels return to normal. Similarly, rifampin enhances the metabolism of several other drugs, such as prednisone, the sulfonylureas, warfarin, and ketoconazole.

Loading Doses

Therapy of critically ill patients requires that antimicrobial levels be established at the site of infection as quickly as possible. If the dosing interval is less than four to five half-lives, a progressive increase in serum levels occurs until a steady state is reached (Fig. 27-3). *Steady state* occurs when the amount of drug administered during the dosing interval equals the amount eliminated. The time required to reach a steady state is also about four to five half-lives. If a drug is given by continuous infusion rather than by intermittent administration, the serum levels rise slowly until equilibration is reached. As with intermittent administration, equilibration occurs between four and five half-lives. If therapeutic levels will only be reached at steady state (i.e., in four to five half-lives), a larger-than-usual dose (a loading dose) of the antimicrobial agent must be administered to achieve therapeutic serum levels with the first dose (Fig. 27-3). A loading dose is recommended for a few of the antimicrobial agents for which the dosing interval is less four to five half-lives (Table 27-3). As with most antimicrobial agents, if the drug is administered at dosing intervals equal to or greater than four half-lives, subsequent doses result in little or no

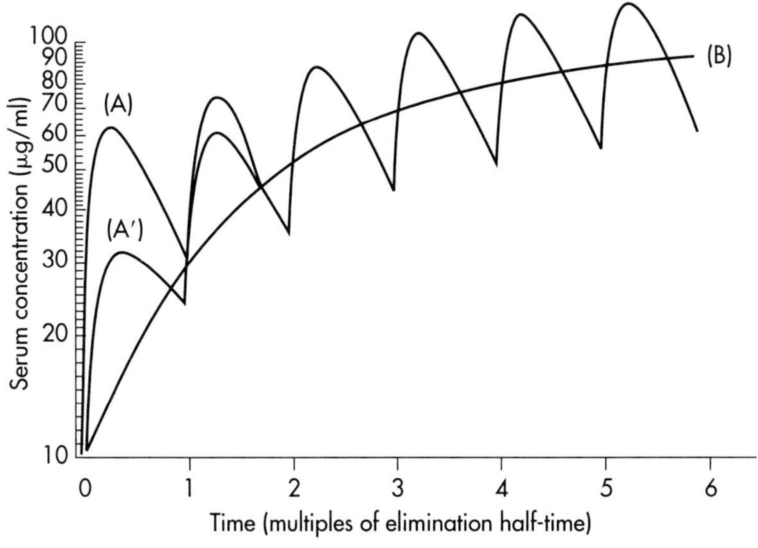

Fig. 27-3. Concentration of drug in serum during administration by intermittent infusion every $T_{1/2}$ with **(A)** and without **(A′)** a loading dose or by continuous infusion **(B)**.

Table 27-3. Recommended Loading Doses for Antimicrobial Agents

Agent	Serum half-life (hours)	Dosing interval (hours)	Recommended loading dose
Sparfloxacin	15-20	24	Double maintenance dose
Metronidazole	6-14	6-12	Double maintenance dose†
Sulfadiazine	10	6	2-4 gm, followed by 1 gm
Sulfisoxazole	4-7	4-6	2-4 gm, followed by 1 gm
Trimethoprim-sulfamethoxazole	11/10	6-12	None
Vancomycin	6	12	None
Azithromycin	68	24	Double maintenance dose
Tetracycline	6-10	6	None
Doxycycline	16-18	24	Double maintenance dose
Minocycline	16-18	12	Double maintenance dose
Amphotericin B	24	24	None
Fluconazole	25	24	Double maintenance dose
Itraconazole	21	24	None
Pentamidine	29	24	None

*When trovafloxacin is used to treat nosocomial pneumonia, gynecologic and pelvic infections, and complicated intraabdominal infections, including postsurgical infections.
†When metronidazole is used to treat serious infections caused by anaerobic microorganisms.

accumulation between doses (i.e., each dose results in serum levels that are identical with those obtained after the initial dose). In this case, each dose should be sufficient to achieve therapeutic serum levels, and no loading dose is necessary.

Dose Modification. A loading dose is also necessary when doses are reduced to compensate for reduced elimination (e.g., renal failure). The loading dose is equal to the usual dose given to a patient with normal drug elimination in order to achieve an initial C_{max} and trough level that fall within the therapeutic range. The size of the maintenance dose, the dosing interval, or both can be altered to prevent drug accumulation in these patients. The pharmacodynamic properties of the drug to be used will influence which modification is preferable. Extension of the dosing interval to about four to five half-lives, while maintaining the size of subsequent doses equal to the loading dose, results in the desired C_{max} but possibly prolonged periods with subtherapeutic levels; this is the preferred option for drugs exhibiting concentration-dependent pharmacodynamics, such as aminoglycosides and fluoroquinolones. Alternatively, lowering the maintenance dose, while maintaining the normal dosing interval, results in more constant levels with less fluctuation between C_{max} and trough concentrations; this is the preferred option for drugs exhibiting time-dependent pharmacodynamics, such as β-lactams and vancomycin (see next section).

Although with renal failure the creatinine clearance can be used to judge dose modification for drugs excreted by the kidney, with impairment of hepatic function no such measure of hepatic function exists for drugs excreted by the liver. Drug levels should be determined in serum at peak and trough concentrations at steady state (four to five half-lives), if possible, when doses are reduced for renal failure and should be repeated when the dose or renal function has changed, because recommendations for dose reduction are approximations. Determination of levels is also important in patients with normal elimination for drugs with therapeutic levels that are close to the toxic levels or with individual variability in pharmacokinetics (e.g., aminoglycosides, vancomycin). For example, vancomycin and teicoplanin have more rapid drug elimination and may have larger volumes of distribution in IV drug users, which necessitate determination of peak and trough serum levels of these drugs to ensure a therapeutic effect.

PHARMACODYNAMICS

Pharmacodynamics describes the antimicrobial effect at the site of infection in relation to the concentrations of the antimicrobial agent during therapy. After a limited exposure of microorganisms to an antibacterial agent, such as after intermittent drug administration, a variable portion of the microbial population persists. The size of this population when the next dose is given will depend on (1) the size of the initial population, (2) the potency (MIC and MBC) and pharmacokinetic characteristics of the antimicrobial agent, (3) the rate and extent of any bactericidal effect, (4) the presence of a postantibiotic effect, and (5) the rate of regrowth of persistent organisms. If doses are spaced too far apart, the residual bacterial count may increase in the later portion of each dosing interval; thus the bacterial count could equal or exceed the count at the beginning of the dosing interval. The factors that allow infrequent dosing without loss of efficacy involve pharmacokinetic variables in relation to antimicrobial effects.

Time-dependent Bactericidal Action

Bacterial killing by β-lactam antibiotics and vancomycin is not enhanced by increasing drug concentrations above the MBC, and the bactericidal action of these drugs is relatively slow. Consequently, there will be a relatively large residual population when levels fall below the MBC. Once the levels fall below the MIC, persistent suppression of growth may occur either from inhibitory activity of sub-MIC residual drug levels against low bacterial densities (i.e., inoculum effect at both low drug and bacterial levels) or local host defenses. After levels at the site of infection fall below the MIC, the residual population can regrow quickly, because there is either no PAE for most β-lactams against gram-negative bacilli or relatively short PAE against gram-positive cocci. The rate of regrowth depends on many factors, including the inherent doubling time of the microorganism, the availability of nutrients in the infected tissues, and the adequacy of host defense mechanisms. In the absence of host defenses, microorganisms can increase in vivo exponentially at a rate similar to that which occurs in vitro.

Some regrowth may restore susceptibility of the bacterial population to the bactericidal effect of β-lactam antibiotics. Ideally, the next dose is given before significant regrowth occurs. For drugs such as the β-lactams and vancomycin, with concentration-independent bactericidal activity and no or small PAEs, dosing strategies that maximize duration of exposure, such as smaller fractions of the total daily dose given at frequent intervals or use of β-lactams with long serum $T_{1/2}$ (e.g., ceftriaxone, with $T_{1/2}$ of 6 to 8 hours), would be efficacious. An effective dosing regimen for time-dependent antibiotics requires that serum drug concentrations exceed the MIC of the causative pathogen for at least 40% to 50% of the dosing interval. The time above the MIC can be used to compare the effectiveness of different time-dependent antibiotics. As a corollary, drugs within a class having the greater potency (i.e., a lower MIC) will be anticipated to have longer time above MIC ratios and therefore greater effectiveness.

Concentration-dependent Bactericidal Action

For drugs with concentration-dependent bactericidal action, such as aminoglycosides, fluoroquinolones, and metronidazole, the rate of bactericidal activity will be greatest at the C_{max}. As drug concentration decreases, bactericidal activity will decrease. Higher doses will increase not only the rate of reduction of bacteria, but also the length of time of drug exposure to bactericidal concentrations. This dependence on both the magnitude and the duration of exposure of bactericidal concentrations implies that concentration-dependent drugs are influenced by the C_{max} and the AUC for a particular dose. For drugs with time-dependent activity, however, the rate of reduction of bacteria is constant, and the extent of bactericidal activity will depend solely on the duration of drug exposure.

After drug levels at the site of infection fall below the MBC but still exceed the MIC, bacterial counts may continue to fall because of local host defenses (e.g., phagocytes, antibody, complement), or the residual population may remain stable because of the inhibitory effect of the antimicrobial agent. Once residual drug is entirely eliminated from tissues, suppression of growth may persist because of a PAE, the duration of which is also concentration dependent for aminoglycosides and fluoroquinolones; the higher the drug concentration, the longer the PAE. Eventually the PAE will wane, and the residual organisms will begin to regrow.

For concentration-dependent drugs, dosing strategies that maximize the intensity of drug exposure (e.g., giving total daily dose as single dose every 24 hours rather than giving smaller divided doses) would increase the C_{max} and allow for comparable efficacy at greater convenience and lower cost if adverse effects were not also concentration dependent. Dose-dependent toxicity was once thought to limit giving the total daily dose of an aminoglycoside as a single dose every 24 hours. Data from both animal models and human trials, however, suggest dosing regimens that provide very high peak aminoglycoside concentrations relative to the MIC and prolonged periods of subinhibitory aminoglycoside concentrations may be equally or more effective, without excessive toxicity, than regimens that provide lower peaks but more persistent inhibitory concentrations. These clinical studies, however, have primarily involved combination therapy with other antimicrobial agents or treatment of less severely ill patients or less virulent pathogens.

An effective dosing regimen for concentration-dependent antibiotics requires that either the 24h-AUC/MIC be at least 125 for gram-negative bacilli and probably 25 to 50 for *S. aureus* and *S. pneumoniae* or the C_{max}/MIC of the causative pathogen be at least 10. These ratios can be used to compare the effectiveness of different concentration-dependent antibiotics. As a corollary, drugs within a class having the greater potency (i.e., lower MIC) will have higher AUC/MIC or C_{max}/MIC ratios and therefore will be anticipated to have greater effectiveness. It will be clear that an infection from susceptible pathogens with relatively high MICs may not be adequately treated with standard dosing of the antimicrobial agent. For example, gentamicin-susceptible strains of *P. aeruginosa* with gentamicin MICs of 1 to 4 μg/ml may respond suboptimally to standard dosing regimens that provide mean peak serum gentamicin levels of 6 μg/ml. Similarly, ciprofloxacin- susceptible strains of *P. aeruginosa* with ciprofloxacin MICs of 0.5 to 1 μg/ml may respond suboptimally to standard dosing regimens that provide peak serum ciprofloxacin levels of about 3 to 4 μg/ml. Levofloxacin-susceptible strains of *S. pneumoniae* with levofloxacin MICs of 1 to 2 μg/ml may respond suboptimally to standard dosing regimens that provide peak serum levofloxacin levels of about 5 μg/ml.

Bacteriostatic Activity

The macrolides, clindamycin, and the tetracyclines exhibit little if any concentration-dependent killing. These drugs produce prolonged PAE, however, which allows them to be efficacious when concentrations exceed the MIC for less than 50% of the dosing interval.

Rate and Extent of Bactericidal Effect

Higher rates of bactericidal action result in lower residual bacterial counts and longer intervals before significant regrowth occurs. With concentration-dependent drugs, maximizing the AUC/MIC or C_{max}/MIC ratio will maximize the rate and extent of bactericidal activity. Similar considerations occur with the use of synergistic drug combinations (i.e., use of two drugs that exert significantly more rapid and extensive bactericidal action in combination than if used alone). Synergistic combinations to clear more rapidly the tissues of the infecting microorganism have been used to shorten the course of therapy for α-hemolytic streptococcal endocarditis (i.e., penicillin or ceftriaxone plus gentamicin for 2 weeks vs. penicillin or ceftriaxone alone for 4 weeks) and for uncomplicated methicillin-sensitive *S. aureus*, right-sided endocarditis (nafcillin plus gentamicin for 2 weeks vs. nafcillin alone for 4 weeks).

Prevention of Resistance

Dense populations of bacteria in tissue likely contain subpopulations of bacteria with relatively higher MICs. The likelihood that resistant subpopulations will emerge on antimicrobial therapy depends on (1) the propensity for resistance within the population, (2) the ability of host defenses to control the resistant microorganisms, and (3) the magnitude of the antimicrobial drug levels at the site of infection. Drug levels should be at least eight times the MIC to prevent emergence of resistant subpopulations. This can be accomplished by using a single daily aminoglycoside dose, the most potent fluoroquinolone, or high doses of a β-lactam.

ADDITIONAL READINGS

Alvarez-Elcoro S, Enzler MJ: The macrolides: erythromycin, clarithromycin and azithromycin, *Mayo Clin Proc* 74:613, 1999.

Barza M: Pharmacologic principles. In Gorbach SL, Bartlett JG, Blacklow NR, editors: *Infectious diseases*, Philadelphia, 1992, Saunders.

Carbon C: Pharmacodynamics of macrolides, azalides, and streptogramins: effects on extracellular pathogens, *Clin Infect Dis* 27:28, 1998.

Craig WA: Pharmacokinetic/pharmacodynamic parameters: rationale for antimicrobial dosing in mice and men, *Clin Infect Dis* 26:1, 1998.

Drusano GL: Human pharmacodynamics of beta-lactams, aminoglycosides and their combination, *Scand J Infect Dis Suppl* 74:235, 1991.

Edson RS, Terrell CL: The aminoglycosides, *Mayo Clin Proc* 74:519, 1999.

Estes L: Review of pharmacokinetics and pharmacodynamics of antimicrobial agents, *Mayo Clin Proc* 73:1114, 1998.

Hellinger WC, Brewer NS: Carbapenems and monobactams: imipenem, meropenem, and aztreonam, *Mayo Clin Proc* 74:420, 1999.

Ingerman MJ, Pitsakis PG, Rosenberg AF, et al: The importance of pharmacodynamics in determining the dosing interval in therapy for experimental *Pseudomonas* endocarditis in the rat, *J Infect Dis* 153:707, 1986.

Lacy MK, Nicolau DP, Nightingale CH, Quintiliani R: The pharmacodynamics of aminoglycosides, *Clin Infect Dis* 27:23, 1998.

Levison ME: Pharmacodynamics of antimicrobial agents: bactericidal and post-antibiotic effects, *Infect Dis Clin North Am* 15:518, 1995.

Lode H, Borner K, Koeppe P: Pharmacodynamics of fluoroquinolones, *Clin Infect Dis* 27:33, 1998.

Marshall WF, Blair JE: The cephalosporins, *Mayo Clin Proc* 74:187, 1999.

Preston SL et al: Pharmacodynamics of levofloxacin: a new paradigm for early clinical trials, *JAMA* 279:125, 1998.

Turnidge JD: The pharmacodynamics of β-lactams, *Clin Infect Dis* 27:10, 1998.

Wright AJ: The penicillins, *Mayo Clin Proc* 74:290, 1999.

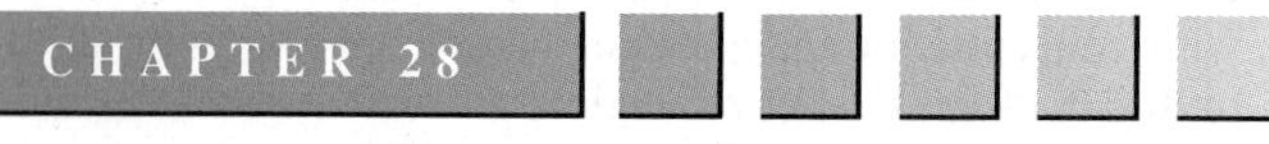

Antivirals

Michael Katzman

A chapter devoted to antivirals was unnecessary in early textbooks of primary care medicine because few antiviral agents were available. Viral infections were diagnosed clinically, patients were told they "had a virus," and symptomatic treatment was provided. Often, antibacterial agents were prescribed to treat possible bacterial infection, in hopes of preventing superinfection, or to appease the patient. Clinicians now have the tools, however, to diagnose and treat many viral infections. The number of antiviral agents increases each year, and indications for established agents continue to expand (Fig. 28-1 and Table 28-1). This chapter discusses antiviral drugs that primary care physicians are most likely to use, with a focus on typical outpatient

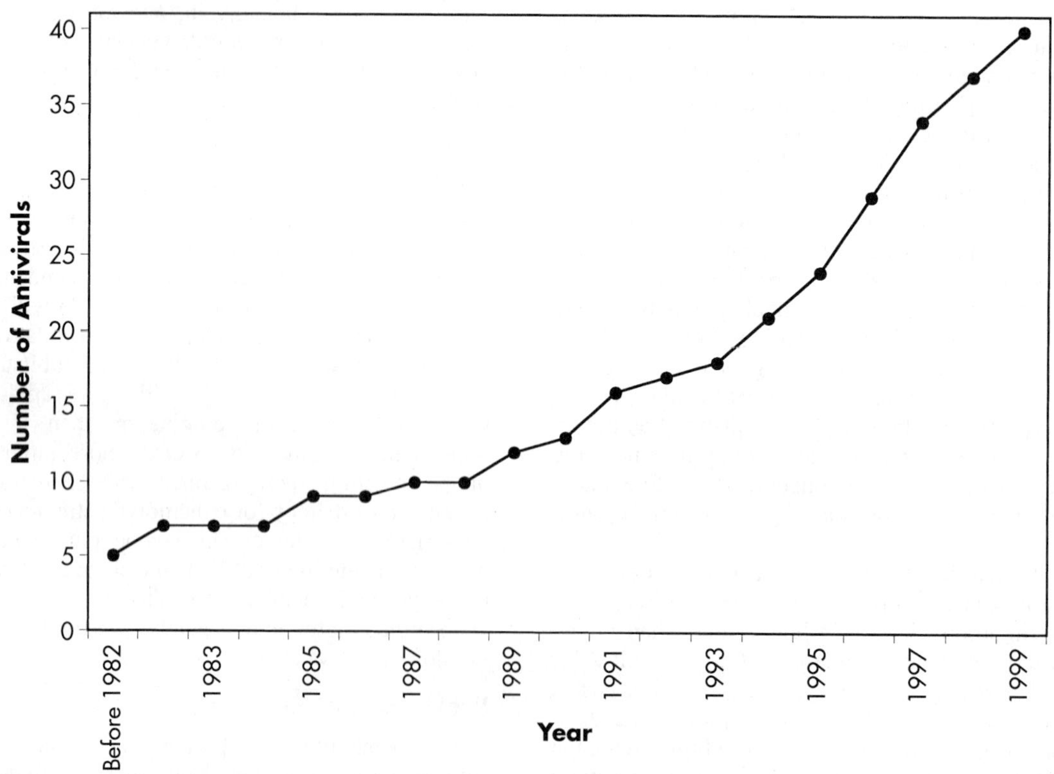

Fig. 28-1. Cumulative number of antiviral agents. Data were derived from drug-approval dates obtained from the U.S. Food and Drug Administration (FDA) and other sources. An anti-HIV drug available by an expanded-access program was included in 1999 data. Each major new formulation (e.g., topical, oral, intravenous, subcutaneous/intramuscular) was counted separately; thus the final number differs from that in Table 28-1.

situations. Comprehensive reviews and package inserts should be consulted for more details.[11]

GENERAL PRINCIPLES

Role of Primary Care Physician

The decision to begin therapy with an antiviral drug often must be made quickly (e.g., within hours for influenza virus or herpesvirus), and the primary care physician is in the best position to determine and initiate such therapy. In other situations the physician may manage patients with chronic viral infections (e.g., hepatitis, human immunodeficiency virus [HIV]), sometimes following an initial referral to a specialist. Even when the physician is not directly responsible for the long-term management of a chronic infection, patients may ask about possible adverse reactions or may seek general advice. In practice, simply knowing the names of the various antiviral agents is helpful (and often sufficient), whereas a working familiarity is required only for a limited number of drugs.

Goals of Therapy

Prevention is the most important way to limit morbidity and mortality from viral infections, through public health measures, infection control practices, personal hygiene, appropriate sexual practices, or vaccination. Viruses will continue to infect humans, however, and physicians will need to prescribe pharmacologic agents to treat such infections. Because infections with most ribonucleic acid (RNA) viruses (e.g., influenza) are acute and self-limited, the goal of a short course of antiviral therapy in these patients is to speed recovery and limit complications.

In contrast, the herpesviruses cause lifelong infections that intermittently reactivate. Although many of the manifestations of herpes infections also are self-limited, short courses of therapy can hasten recovery, such as for initial or recurrent episodes of genital herpes. With herpes encephalitis, recovery is unlikely without antiviral therapy. Immunocompromised patients are at risk for dissemination and death from herpes infections unless treatment is provided. Antiviral agents may

Table 28-1. Currently Available Antiviral Agents

Generic name	Brand name	Route or form*	FDA approved against†
1. Abacavir (ABC)	Ziagen	Oral	HIV
2. Acyclovir	Zovirax	Ointment, IV, oral	HSV, VZV
3. Adefovir‡	Preveon	Oral	HIV
4. Amantadine	Symmetrel	Oral	Influenza A
5. Amprenavir	Agenerase	Oral	HIV
6. Cidofovir	Vistide	IV	CMV
7. Delavirdine	Rescriptor	Oral	HIV
8. Didanosine (ddI)	Videx	Oral	HIV
9. Efavirenz	Sustiva	Oral	HIV
10. Famciclovir	Famvir	Oral	HSV, VZV
11. Foscarnet (PFA)	Foscavir	IV	CMV, HSV
12. Ganciclovir (DHPG)	Cytovene	IV, oral	CMV
13. Idoxuridine	Herplex	Ophthalmic drops	HSV
14. Indinavir	Crixivan	Oral	HIV
15. Interferon alfa-2a	Roferon-a	SC, IM	Hep C, KS
16. Interferon alfa-2b	Intron-a	SC, IM, IL	Hep B or C, KS, CA
17. Interferon alfa-n1	Wellferon	SC, IM	Hep C
18. Interferon alfa-n3	Alferon N	IL	CA
19. Interferon alfacon-1	Infergen	SC	Hep C
20. Lamivudine (3TC)	Epivir	Oral	HIV, Hep B
21. Nelfinavir	Viracept	Oral	HIV
22. Nevirapine	Viramune	Oral	HIV
23. Penciclovir	Denavir	Cream	HSV
24. Ribavirin	Virazole	Aerosol	RSV
25. Ribavirin	Rebetol	Oral	Hep C
26. Rimantadine	Flumadine	Oral	Influenza A
27. Ritonavir	Norvir	Oral	HIV
28. Saquinavir	Invirase	Oral (hard GCs)	HIV
29. Saquinavir	Fortovase	Oral (soft GCs)	HIV
30. Stavudine (d4T)	Zerit	Oral	HIV
31. Trifluridine	Viroptic	Ophthalmic drops	HSV
32. Valacyclovir	Valtrex	Oral	HSV, VZV
33. Vidarabine (Ara-A)	Vira-A	Ophthalmic ointment	HSV
34. Zalcitabine (ddC)	Hivid	Oral	HIV
35. Zidovudine (AZT, ZDV)	Retrovir	Oral, IV	HIV

**IV*, Intravenous; *SC*, subcutaneous; *IM*, intramuscular; *IL*, intralesional; *GCs*, gelatin capsules.

†Not all forms are active for all types of infection. *FDA*, U.S. Food and Drug Administration; *HIV*, human immunodeficiency virus; *HSV*, herpes simplex virus; *VZV*, varicella-zoster virus; *CMV*, cytomegalovirus; *Hep*, hepatitis; *KS*, Kaposi's sarcoma (due to human herpes virus-8); *CA*, condylomata acuminata (due to human papillomavirus); *RSV*, respiratory syncytial virus.

‡Not FDA approved but available by expanded access program.

be used chronically to prevent clinical recurrences, such as for genital herpes. With HIV infection, combinations of antiviral drugs are given indefinitely to suppress virus replication and thereby protect the patient's immune system from deterioration. Physicians must be aware that some approved therapies offer only marginal benefits, which must be weighed against the cost and toxicity of particular regimens.

Mechanisms and Resistance

Successful antiviral agents must target specific steps in virus replication while limiting toxicity to human cells. This ideal is difficult to achieve because viruses, as intracellular parasites, depend on cellular machinery for replication. Viruses vary tremendously in size and shape, may or may not have a surrounding envelope, and may have a single-stranded or double-stranded RNA or deoxyribonucleic acid (DNA) genome. The replication of *all* viruses at the cellular level, however, depends on three basic steps: (1) entry of viral genetic information into the infected cell, (2) replication of that genetic information, and (3) assembly and release of new infectious viral particles. Only two antiviral drugs (amantadine and rimantadine) act at the first step. The vast majority of antiviral agents resemble the building blocks of nucleic acid and interfere with the second step, whereas interferon alfa and inhibitors of the HIV protease enzyme act later in replication.

When antiviral agents are used repeatedly or for long times, the development of drug resistance must be considered. Sensitivity testing is not generally available for antiviral agents but will likely play a role in the management of viral infections in the future.

INFLUENZA

Influenza is a major public health problem responsible for tens of thousands of unnecessary deaths and significant morbidity during most winters. The role of vaccination in the prevention of influenza and associated deaths cannot be overemphasized.[4] Antiviral drugs have an important role when vaccination has not been provided or is inadequate. Amantadine and rimantadine are inexpensive agents that are effective for the prevention and treatment of influenza type A. Neither has activity against influenza B. Amantadine is approved for the treatment and prophylaxis of adults and children aged 1 year and older. Rimantadine currently is approved for the treatment and prophylaxis of adults, but only for prophylaxis in children (Table 28-2). The major differences between these drugs are the route of elimination, incidence of side effects, and cost. Oral or inhaled neuraminidase inhibitors, which are active against influenza A and influenza B, will likely be available in the future.

Table 28-2. Treatment and Prophylaxis of Influenza A

Drug	Age group (years)	Dose for treatment or prophylaxis*
Amantadine	1-9	5 mg/kg/day, up to 150 mg, in two doses
	10-13	100 mg bid if ≥40 kg; otherwise 5 mg/kg/day
	14-64	100 mg bid†
	≥65	≤100 mg qd
Rimantadine	1-9	5 mg/kg/day, up to 150 mg, in one or two doses‡
	10-13	200 mg qd if ≥ 40 kg; otherwise 5 mg/kg/day‡
	14-64	200 mg qd§
	≥65	100 or 200 mg qd§‖

Modified from *MMWR* 48:1, 1999.

bid, Twice a day; *qd,* every day.

*Doses are oral. Single or twice-daily doses with either agent are reasonable. Treatment should be started within 48 hours and limited to 3-5 days; see text for duration of prophylaxis.

†Reduce dose for impaired renal function as follows: for creatinine clearance 30-50 ml/min/1.73m^2: 200 mg then 100 mg qd; 15-29 ml/min/1.73m^2: 200 mg, then 100 mg every other day; <15 ml/min/1.73m^2: 200 mg once a week.

‡Rimantadine is FDA approved for prophylaxis but not treatment in children.

§Reduce dose to 100 mg qd if severe hepatic dysfunction or creatinine clearance ≤10 ml/min.

‖Use 100 mg qd in elderly nursing home residents or if side effects develop at 200 mg qd.

Amantadine and Rimantadine

Amantadine (Symmetrel) and rimantadine (Flumadine) are symmetric tricyclic amines that interfere with an early step in virus replication. They act to block uncoating of the influenza virus genome, perhaps by increasing the pH within the lysosomes of cells. The target of this action is the M2 matrix protein of influenza A. Resistance to either of these agents is caused by single amino acid substitutions in the transmembrane portion of the M2 protein. These oral agents are well absorbed and achieve good levels within nasal secretions. They have relatively long half-lives (about 12 to 18 hours for amantadine and 24 to 36 hours for rimantadine), permitting once-daily dosing,[7] although some sources recommend two doses per day.[8] Amantadine is not significantly metabolized and is highly dependent on renal excretion. In contrast, rimantadine is extensively metabolized in the liver and is not as renal dependent.

The most common side effects are nausea and anorexia (3% of patients), insomnia, nervousness, anxiety, difficulty concentrating, and lightheadedness. The central nervous system effects are more common with amantadine (13%) than rimantadine (6%), compared with a 4% incidence in placebo recipients.[4] Both drugs are relatively free of serious adverse effects, except for seizures in patients with a seizure history, delirium in those with psychiatric disorders, or delirium in association with high drug levels when dosage adjustments are not made for renal function or age. Both drugs are teratogenic in animals and should not be used during pregnancy.[8]

The cost of a 5-day course of amantadine is less than $10, and the cost of a similar regimen of rimantadine is less than $30. This price difference is likely to be significant only in institutional settings or when the drugs are used prophylactically for several weeks.

Prophylactic Use. Both amantadine and rimantadine are 70% to 90% effective in preventing clinical disease from influenza A when taken by healthy adults or children before and during an epidemic period.[4,7] After influenza A has entered a community, unvaccinated individuals at high risk for complications of influenza or caring for high-risk persons can begin either drug. Chemoprophylaxis should be continued for 2 weeks if concomitant vaccination is performed, by which time healthy adults should have a protective antibody response to the vaccine. Children who are receiving influenza vaccine for the first time (and who thus require a second dose of vaccine) should receive prophylaxis until 2 weeks after the second vaccination. Chemoprophylaxis can be continued for the duration of peak influenza A activity (typically 4 to 8 weeks) if vaccine is not administered because of patient refusal or allergy to vaccine components or if the vaccine is known to lack effectiveness against the circulating strain. Chemoprophylaxis can also be continued in individuals expected to have a poor antibody response to vaccination because of immunodeficiency.

When outbreaks occur in institutions with patients at high risk for complications from influenza, either of these drugs should be given to all residents, whether or not they were vaccinated that season, and offered to unvaccinated staff. Prophylaxis in this setting should be continued until 1 week after the outbreak ends.[4] Postexposure prophylaxis in household settings has not been effective when the index case was treated concurrently. In one study approximately 35% of households had secondary cases whether rimantadine or placebo was used, and drug-resistant viruses were recovered from cases in treated households.[12] This fact emphasizes the need to limit contact between influenza patients and susceptible individuals. Dosing recommendations are provided in Table 28-2.

Therapeutic Use. Many studies have shown that amantadine and rimantadine decrease the duration of fever and symptoms from influenza A by 1 to 2 days if started within 48 hours of symptom onset.[7] Institution of empiric antiviral therapy is appropriate when a patient has a compatible clinical illness and influenza A is documented in the community; it is not appropriate for undocumented influenza or for influenza B. Because studies generally excluded patients with symptoms longer than 48 hours, it may be incorrect to conclude that these drugs are ineffective if started after 48 hours; however, a major benefit is unlikely to occur by that point in such a self-limiting illness.

Although no data show that treatment prevents the complications of influenza, the benefits of these drugs on the usual course of the flu are sufficient to justify wider use. Because resistant viruses have spread within households of treated patients,[12] however, therapy should be limited to 3 to 5 days or 24 to 48 hours after the disappearance of signs and symptoms.[4] Although the effectiveness of these drugs for infections of the lower respiratory tract is unproved, instituting therapy with either agent may be appropriate for any hospitalized patient who may have primary influenza pneumonia. Dosing recommendations are provided in Table 28-2.

HERPES SIMPLEX AND VARICELLA-ZOSTER

Herpes simplex virus (HSV) and varicella-zoster virus (VZV) cause a wide range of clinical syndromes, many of which respond to timely administration of antiviral therapy. Intravenous (IV) acyclovir is the drug of choice for treatment of serious infections caused by HSV or VZV. Three other antivirals (valacyclovir, penciclovir, famciclovir) are also available for outpatient therapy of clinical problems. Acyclovir or related drugs may be the most important antiviral agents available to primary care physicians. Antivirals that are active against cytomegalovirus are also effective for some HSV and VZV infections (see later discussion).

Acyclovir

Acyclovir (Zovirax) is a deoxyguanosine analog that blocks viral DNA synthesis. Within infected cells, the drug is phosphorylated to a monophosphate by the viral thymidine kinase enzyme and further phosphorylated by cellular enzymes to the active triphosphate form, which inhibits the viral DNA polymerase and acts as a chain terminator when incorporated into viral DNA. The most common type of resistance results from loss of viral thymidine kinase activity so that acyclovir monophosphate is not produced. Although thymidine kinase–deficient viruses are less virulent in animal models, such viruses have caused severe mucocutaneous disease, especially in patients with acquired immunodeficiency syndrome (AIDS).

Acyclovir is most active against HSV types 1 and 2, slightly less active against VZV, less active against Epstein-Barr virus, and only minimally active against cytomegalovirus. Acyclovir is available for topical, oral, and IV use. Given its poor bioavailability (only 10% to 20% of an oral dose), plasma levels from oral formulations are much lower than those achieved by the IV route. The drug distributes throughout body water, including cerebrospinal fluid and vaginal secretions, but levels in saliva are only about 10% of those in plasma. The plasma half-life is approximately 3 hours in patients with normal renal function. Acyclovir is minimally metabolized and is excreted by the kidneys. IV dosing should be reduced if the creatinine clearance is 50 ml/min/1.73 m^2 or less; oral doses do not need adjustment unless renal function is severely impaired.

Acyclovir is generally well tolerated but can cause nausea, diarrhea, rash, or headache. Renal toxicity can occur from crystallization within the kidneys if patients are dehydrated, and neurotoxicity (including encephalopathy and seizures) can occur in patients with renal insufficiency and high plasma levels, which is rare after oral administration. High levels of acyclovir cause chromosomal damage in some in vitro assays; however, a pregnancy registry has not revealed any increase in the incidence of birth defects from exposure during the first trimester.[8]

The cost of oral acyclovir ranges from approximately $30 for a 5-day course of 200 mg five times a day (e.g., recurrent genital herpes) to more than $100 for a 7-day course of 800 mg five times a day (e.g., shingles).

Acyclovir as a 5% ointment is approved for limited non-life-threatening mucocutaneous HSV disease in immunocompromised patients and for initial episodes of herpes genitalis. It is not useful for orolabial herpes in nonimmunocompromised persons or for recurrent genital herpes. The oral form of acyclovir is approved for acute treatment of chickenpox, herpes zoster, and initial and recurrent episodes of genital herpes and for suppression of recurrent genital herpes. IV acyclovir is approved for initial and recurrent mucosal and cutaneous HSV or VZV infections in immunocompromised patients, for herpes encephalitis in patients over 6 months of age, and for severe initial episodes of herpes genitalis (although the oral form is most often used). In practice, acyclovir is used for an even larger spectrum of herpes infections (Tables 28-3 and 28-4).

Table 28-3. Treatment for Herpes Simplex Virus Infections

Indication	Options for adults*
Immunocompetent patients with orolabial herpes	No treatment, or penciclovir cream applied q2h for 4 days†
Immunocompromised patients with mucocutaneous disease	Acyclovir, 400 mg 5 times/day or 5 mg/kg IV q8h for 7-14 days For limited disease, can apply acyclovir ointment 4-6 times/day
Orolabial herpes, suppression	Acyclovir, 400 mg bid‡
Genital herpes	
First episode	Acyclovir, 400 mg tid or 200 mg 5 times/day for 7-10 days Valacyclovir, 1 gm bid for 7-10 days Famciclovir, 250 mg tid for 5-10 days‡
Recurrence§	Acyclovir, 400 mg tid or 200 mg 5 times/day for 5 days Valacyclovir, 500 mg bid for 5 days Famciclovir, 125 mg bid for 5 days
Suppression	Acyclovir, 400 mg bid Valacyclovir, 500 or 1000 mg daily Famciclovir, 250 mg bid
Herpetic whitlow	Acyclovir, 400 mg tid†
Herpes encephalitis	Acyclovir, 10 mg/kg IV q8h for 10-21 days
Keratoconjunctivitis‖	Trifluridine, 1 drop q2h, up to 9 drops/day, for 10 days¶
Ocular disease, suppression‖	No treatment, or acyclovir, 400 mg bid‡
Pneumonia or hepatitis	Acyclovir, 5 mg/kg IV q8h (optimal duration unknown)‡
Acyclovir-resistant infections	If treatment indicated, foscarnet, 40 mg/kg IV q8h for 14-21 days

Modified from *Med Lett Drugs Ther* 39:69, 1997.
q2h, Every 2 hours; *IV,* intravenously; *bid,* twice a day; *tid,* three times a day.
*Doses are oral unless indicated otherwise; see text for dosing in renal dysfunction.
†Should be started within 1 hour of onset.
‡Not FDA approved for this indication.
§Should be started within 24 hours of onset and as soon as possible to maximize benefits.
‖An ophthalmologist should be consulted.
¶Trifluridine (Viroptic) is preferred to idoxuridine (Herplex) or vidarabine (Vira-A).

Table 28-4. Treatment for Varicella-Zoster Virus Infections

Indication	Options for adults*
Chickenpox (primary varicella)†	No treatment, or if within 24 hours: Acyclovir, 20 mg/kg (800 mg maximum) qid for 5 days; if immunocompromised, 10 mg/kg IV q8h for 7 days
Shingles (zoster)‡	
Normal hosts	No treatment, or if within 72 hours: Acyclovir, 800 mg 5 times/day for 7-10 days Valacyclovir, 1 gm tid for 7 days Famciclovir, 500 mg tid for 7 days
Immunocompromised patients	Acyclovir, 10 mg/kg IV q8h for 7 days§
Varicella pneumonia	Acyclovir, 10 mg/kg IV q8h for 7 days‖
Acyclovir-resistant infections	If treatment indicated, foscarnet, 40 mg/kg IV q8h for 10 days‖

Modified from *Med Lett Drugs Ther* 39:69, 1997.
qid, Four times a day; *IV,* intravenously; *q8h,* every 8 hours; *tid,* three times a day.
*Doses are oral unless indicated otherwise; see text for comments on dosing in renal dysfunction.
†See Box 28-1 for treatment recommendations.
‡See Box 28-2 for treatment recommendations and the text for the role of steroids.
§Some physicians would use one of the oral regimens in AIDS patients with localized zoster.
‖Not FDA approved for this indication.

Valacyclovir

Valacyclovir (Valtrex) is an oral prodrug (the *l*-valyl ester) of acyclovir. After oral administration, valacyclovir is rapidly absorbed and almost completely converted to acyclovir in the intestinal wall and liver, yielding a bioavailability greater than 50%. The resulting serum levels of acyclovir are several times higher than with oral acyclovir and approach those obtained with IV acyclovir. Dosage does not need to be adjusted unless renal function is severely impaired (creatinine clearance less than 30 ml/min) or the maximum dose of 3 gm/day is indicated and renal function is moderately impaired (creatinine clearance less than 50 ml/min). Valacyclovir carries a warning that thrombotic thrombocytopenic purpura/hemolytic uremic syndrome, sometimes fatal, has occurred in bone marrow or renal transplant recipients or patients with advanced AIDS who received 8 gm/day, suggesting a unique toxicity for the prodrug. That dose, however, is more than twice the currently recommended maximum dose. The price of valacyclovir is comparable to that of acyclovir. Valacyclovir is approved for treatment of herpes zoster and treatment and suppression of genital herpes, including initial episodes (see Tables 28-3 and 28-4).

Penciclovir

Penciclovir (Denavir) is structurally related to acyclovir and has a similar spectrum of activity. As with acyclovir, it must be phosphorylated by viral thymidine kinase and host enzymes. Although penciclovir triphosphate is less potent than acyclovir triphosphate in inhibiting viral DNA polymerase, it is present at higher concentrations and for longer times in infected cells. Penciclovir is available as a 1% cream and is approved for topical treatment of recurrent herpes labialis (cold sores). The cost to the pharmacist for a 2-gm tube is $21.[22]

Famciclovir

Famciclovir (Famvir) is an oral prodrug of penciclovir. After oral administration it is rapidly absorbed and almost completely converted to penciclovir in the intestinal wall and liver, yielding a bioavailability greater than 70%. Because penciclovir has a longer intracellular half-life than acyclovir, it can be dosed less frequently. Doses must be adjusted if the creatinine clearance is less than 40 ml/min (when the typical regimen is indicated) or less than 60 ml/min (when the high-dose regimen is indicated for herpes zoster). Famciclovir is generally well tolerated but can cause headache, nausea, and diarrhea. The price of low-dose regimens of famciclovir is comparable to that of acyclovir, but high dose or long-term regimens can be almost twice as expensive. Famciclovir is approved for treatment of herpes zoster and treatment or suppression of recurrent genital herpes, as well as for treatment of recurrent mucocutaneous HSV infections in HIV-infected patients (Tables 28-3 and 28-4).

Antiherpes Agents in Specific Clinical Situations

Herpes Labialis. In healthy individuals, orolabial infections with HSV, often referred to as cold sores or fever blisters, are self-limited. Although topical acyclovir ointment may diminish viral shedding, it offers no clinical benefit in terms of duration, pain relief, or size of the lesion.[20] Recently, topical penciclovir was approved for recurrent oral herpes, based on statistically significant but marginal clinical benefits. In two large studies of patients with frequent herpes labialis, patients were instructed to begin application within 1 hour of the first sign of a recurrence and to repeat the application every 2 hours while awake (about nine times per day) for 4 days. Compared with placebo, the time to pain resolution was decreased from 4 days to 3.3 days and the time to healing from 5.4 days to 4.6 days.[22]

No oral agents are approved for treatment of recurrent oral herpes in healthy individuals, although one group reported that oral acyclovir at 400 mg five times daily had a minor benefit in pain resolution and loss of hard crusts (by about 1 day compared with placebo) when started within 1 hour of symptom onset.[21] In contrast, oral acyclovir can suppress frequent recurrences (six or more episodes per year) of herpes labialis by about 50% and can prevent sun-induced outbreaks.[18] In addition, topical, oral, or IV acyclovir (see Table 28-3) speeds recovery in immunocompromised patients with mucocutaneous HSV infections. In particular, oral acyclovir reduced the duration of various clinical end points by 5 to 13 days in bone marrow transplant recipients.[19]

Herpes Genitalis. Initial episodes of genital herpes may be associated with severe local and systemic symptoms, and antiviral therapy can provide significant benefit (see Table 28-3). Treatment with oral acyclovir or valacyclovir (and probably famciclovir) can reduce symptoms and time to healing by several days; treatment also decreases viral shedding but not recurrences. Although prompt institution of therapy is most effective, the benefit for acyclovir was demonstrated when patients started treatment at a mean of 3½ days (and up to 6 days) from onset.[3] Recurrent episodes of genital herpes, although often troublesome, are associated with less severe symptoms. Rapid institution of therapy with acyclovir, valacyclovir, or famciclovir can decrease duration of symptoms and time to healing by ½ to 2 days. These benefits can be maximized by institution of therapy during the prodromal symptoms heralding an outbreak of lesions. When any of the three antivirals is used for chronic suppression, frequent recurrences (six or more episodes per year) can be significantly reduced; 80% or more of patients will benefit, with 50% of patients free of recurrences at 1 year.[10]

Herpes Encephalitis and Other HSV Infections. Encephalitis from HSV is the most common cause of fatal sporadic encephalitis in the United States, and high-dose IV acyclovir dramatically reduces mortality.[27] Primary care physicians must be aware of the benefits of therapy, since the patient's level of consciousness and prompt initiation of treatment influence the outcome. Similarly, it is important to know that herpetic keratitis can be treated with topical agents. Moreover, one study showed that long-term acyclovir therapy reduced recurrent ocular disease (including sight-threatening deep infections) from 32% to 19% at 1 year.[13] Anecdotal evi dence also supports use of acyclovir for herpetic whitlow (see Table 28-3).

Chickenpox (Primary Varicella). When started within 24 hours of onset of rash, acyclovir can shorten the duration of fever by about 1 day and reduce new lesions and total lesions in children, adolescents, and adults.[9,26] Treatment has not been shown to affect the rate of complications, spread of infection, or duration of absence from school, although adults can be expected to return to work sooner. The clinical significance of some benefits may be marginal (e.g., reduction in median lesion number from 386 to 277), and theoretic and economic concerns surround treating millions of young children with acyclovir. Thus the American Academy of Pediatrics[5] recommends treatment of chickenpox only in certain situations (Box 28-1). Universal childhood vaccination against varicella should diminish the need to face this clinical decision.

Although treatment of adults within 24 hours of onset of lesions is reasonable, some guidelines do not recommend routine treatment even in this setting.[29] Significantly, no benefit of treatment was noted when adults started treatment 25 to 72 hours from onset.[26] Some guidelines do not recommend treatment of uncomplicated varicella during pregnancy,[5] whereas others suggest that the risk of pneumonitis during the latter half of pregnancy justifies treatment of women beyond the twentieth week who present within 24 hours of onset of chickenpox.[16] Data are limited on the efficacy of treatment for viral-mediated complications of primary varicella, such as pneumonia or encephalitis, but high-dose IV acyclovir is recommended for such patients, even pregnant women.

Shingles (Herpes Zoster). The use of pharmacologic agents, including antivirals and steroids, in the treatment of zoster has long been a controversial topic. Conflicting results have been published, both for effects on acute symptoms and

Box 28-1. Recommendations for Treatment of Chickenpox*

1. Treatment is not routinely recommended in otherwise healthy children with uncomplicated varicella.
2. Consider oral acyclovir if it can be started within 24 hours for:
   a. Children over 12 months old
      (1) Chronic cutaneous or pulmonary disorders
      (2) Short course of aerosolized steroids
      (3) Chronic salicylate therapy (theoretically to decrease risk of Reye syndrome)
      (4) Infected from household contact because of the risk of more severe disease
   b. Nonpregnant individuals older than 12 years (some guidelines recommend treating women beyond week 20 of pregnancy who present within 24 hours)
3. Use IV acyclovir for immunocompromised patients, which would include those receiving high-dose steroids.
4. Use IV acyclovir for serious viral-mediated complications in normal hosts, regardless of pregnancy status.

*See Table 28-4 for drug doses.

Box 28-2. Recommendations for Treatment of Zoster in Immunocompetent Patients*

1. Antiviral drug therapy is not routinely recommended if rash is present longer than 72 hours.
2. Antiviral drug therapy is optional if rash is present 72 hours or less, patient is under 50 years old, and rash and pain are mild.
3. Antiviral drug therapy is recommended if rash is present 72 hours or less and with any of the following:
   a. Patient is 50 years or older.
   b. Rash or pain is moderate or severe.
   c. Patient has ophthalmic involvement (i.e., V^1 distribution of trigeminal nerve).
4. Consider antiviral drug therapy for ophthalmic involvement regardless of duration of rash (referral to an ophthalmologist is encouraged).
5. For patients prescribed antiviral therapy, consider addition of prednisone (60 mg daily for 7 days, then 30 mg daily for 7 days, then 15 mg daily for 7 days) if the patient is age 50 or older and has no contraindications (diabetes, hypertension, glaucoma, osteoporosis).

Modified from Kost RG, Straus SE: Postherpetic neuralgia: pathogenesis, treatment, and prevention, *N Engl J Med* 335:32, 1996.
*See Table 28-4 for antiviral drug options.

for influencing postherpetic neuralgia; the latter complication is a common and at times debilitating problem that is especially frequent in those over age 50. Acyclovir started within 72 hours of onset of rash has been shown to shorten the time to full crusting by 1 to 2 days and to decrease the severity of acute pain. Valacyclovir appears at least as effective for these end points, and famciclovir was shown to accelerate lesion healing but not to affect duration of acute pain before healing.[2,24] A recent meta-analysis concluded that treatment with acyclovir can reduce the number of patients who have any pain in the distribution of the rash at 6 months by 46%.[14] Famciclovir was reported to shorten the duration (but not reduce the incidence) of postherpetic neuralgia in those over age 50.[24] Another study found a lower incidence of postherpetic neuralgia when famciclovir, as compared with acyclovir, was started within 48 hours of rash onset.[6] A different study reported that the incidence of neuralgia at 6 months was reduced to 20% in those treated with valacyclovir for 7 days, compared with 26% for those who received acyclovir (p=0.08).[2] Overall the three oral antiherpes drugs are unlikely to be dramatically different for acute or long-term end points. For some patients the less frequent dosing required for the newer agents may be an advantage.

The role of steroids in preventing postherpetic neuralgia is even more controversial. In an attempt to settle the issue, a large study of more than 300 patients compared 7 vs. 21 days of acyclovir, with or without oral prednisolone (starting at 40 mg/day and tapered over 3 weeks). Only minor differences were found acutely, with no difference in the incidence of postherpetic neuralgia.[30] The authors concluded that treatment should consist of 7 days of acyclovir without steroids. Interestingly, they thought that a true placebo group was unethical given the previously reported benefits of acyclovir during the acute phase. A subsequent report compared 21 days of acyclovir alone, prednisone alone (60 mg daily for the first week, 30 mg daily for the second week, 15 mg daily for the third week), acyclovir plus prednisone, or neither drug in the treatment of zoster.[28] Notably, the incidence of postherpetic neuralgia was no different at 3 to 6 months between any of the four groups. However, the combined treatment group had accelerated time to total crusting and healing and an improved quality of life (return of uninterrupted sleep, return to usual activities, discontinuation of analgesic agents) compared with the double-placebo group. Both drugs contributed to the beneficial effects. Assessing the safety of this relatively expensive regimen is limited by the exclusion of patients with osteoporosis, diabetes, or hypertension from the study. The data also demonstrated that the severity of pain at baseline and the number of lesions at enrollment were predictive of outcome. Box 28-2 summarizes recommendations on these issues.[15]

OTHER VIRAL INFECTIONS

Epstein-Barr Virus

Infectious mononucleosis is most often caused by Epstein-Barr virus (EBV), a herpesvirus. In a small trial of IV acyclovir (10 mg/kg every 8 hours) for young adults with infectious mononucleosis and respiratory obstruction or dehydration severe enough to warrant hospitalization, modest benefit was demonstrated only when several parameters (fever, weight loss, sore throat, tonsillar swelling, self-assessment) were combined.[1] Benefit in mild cases or with an oral regimen is even less likely; a placebo-controlled study with 120 patients failed to demonstrate any clinical benefit from oral acyclovir.[25] Thus antiviral therapy is not recommended for this EBV syndrome. The routine use of steroids also is not recommended, since no clinical benefit was found in a double-blind study that compared acyclovir plus prednisolone with placebo.[23] However, many would prescribe steroids for certain complications, such as respiratory obstruction, thrombocytopenia, hemolytic anemia, myocarditis, pericarditis, or neurologic involvement. One infection associated with EBV infection does seem to respond to antiviral treatment. Oral acyclovir often causes resolution of oral hairy leukoplakia in AIDS patients, although relapse can be expected after treatment.[17]

Cytomegalovirus

Cytomegalovirus (CMV) can cause a self-limited mononucleosis syndrome in healthy adults but is most significant for the variety of illnesses it causes in immunocompromised patients. Ganciclovir (Cytovene), foscarnet (Foscavir), and cidofovir (Vistide) are IV drugs used to treat the CMV-related retinitis or gastrointestinal inflammation that is common in such patients. An oral form of ganciclovir is also available and is approved for prevention of CMV disease in patients with advanced HIV infection, for maintenance treatment of CMV retinitis in immunocompromised patients (although not as effective as the IV form), and for prevention of CMV disease in solid organ transplant recipients. Although the drug has very poor bioavailability (less than 10%), it can cause significant neutropenia or thrombocytopenia and is carcinogenic, mutagenic, and teratogenic. The usual dose is 1000 mg three times daily with food, with a reduction in dose if creatinine clearance is less than 70 ml/min.

Respiratory Viruses

Ribavirin (Virazole) administered as a continuous aerosol for 12 to 18 hours daily is approved for treatment of high-risk infants and hospitalized young children with respiratory syncytial virus (RSV) infection. The benefits of therapy in these patients (now considered questionable), however, are not relevant to adult patients. Because oral ribavirin (Rebetol) has become available for therapy of hepatitis C, future controlled studies may describe use of this toxic but broad-spectrum antiviral for adults with serious respiratory infections from RSV and other viruses.

Viral Hepatitis

Intramuscular or subcutaneous administration of recombinant interferon alfa-2b (Intron-a) can induce remissions in some patients with chronic hepatitis B infection. Oral lamivudine (Epivir), which was originally approved for HIV infection, was also recently approved for treatment of chronic hepatitis B. In addition, recombinant interferon alfa-2b, alfa-2a (Roferon-a), or alfacon-1 (Infergen) and lymphoblastoid interferon alfa-n1 (Wellferon) can be used to treat chronic hepatitis C infection, although the combination of interferon alfa-2b and oral ribavirin (packaged together as Rebetron) is more effective (see Chapter 104). Interferons typically cause a flulike syndrome. Depression and suicidal behavior, cardiovascular toxicity, and other serious side effects may also occur. Table 28-5 lists antiviral uses of interferon.

Human Immunodeficiency Virus

Many antiviral drugs are now available to treat HIV infection. When used in combination regimens referred to as *highly active antiretroviral therapy* (HAART), these drugs can have a dramatic clinical effect on morbidity and mortality (Table 28-6; see Chapter 32).

Table 28-5. FDA-Approved Antiviral Uses for Interferon

Indication	Virus	Interferon*
Chronic hepatitis B	Hepatitis B	Alfa-2b
Chronic hepatitis C	Hepatitis C	Alfa-2a, alfa-2b, alfa-n1, alfacon-1, or alfa-2b combined with oral ribavirin
Kaposi's sarcoma	Human herpes virus type 8	Alfa-2a or alfa-2b
Condylomata acuminata	Papillomavirus	Intralesional alfa-2b or alfa-n3

*Administered by the subcutaneous or intramuscular route unless stated otherwise.

Table 28-6. Anti-HIV Drugs

Generic name	Brand name	Dose
Nucleoside reverse transcriptase inhibitors (NRTIs)		
Zidovudine (AZT)	Retrovir	200 mg tid or 300 mg bid
Didanosine (ddI)	Videx	200 mg bid or 400 mg qd
Zalcitabine (ddC)	Hivid	0.75 mg tid
Stavudine (d4T)	Zerit	40 mg bid
Lamivudine (3TC)	Epivir	150 mg bid
Abacavir (ABC)	Ziagen	300 mg bid
Lamivudine/zidovudine	Combivir	150 mg/300 mg bid
Nucleotide reverse transcriptase inhibitor		
Adefovir (not yet approved)	Preveon	120 mg qd
Non–nucleoside reverse transcriptase inhibitors (NNRTIs)		
Nevirapine	Viramune	200 mg bid
Delavirdine	Rescriptor	400 mg tid
Efavirenz	Sustiva	600 mg qd
Protease inhibitors		
Saquinavir	Invirase	600 mg tid
	Fortovase	1200 mg tid or 1600 mg bid
Ritonavir	Norvir	600 mg bid
Indinavir	Crixivan	800 mg tid
Nelfinavir	Viracept	750 mg tid or 1250 mg bid
Amprenavir	Agenerase	1200 mg bid

tid, Three times a day; *bid*, twice a day; *qd*, every day.

EBM EVIDENCE-BASED MEDICINE

Medline entries from 1991 to early 1999 were searched by using a strategy that identified systematic reviews, practice guidelines, and controlled clinical trials for influenza, herpes labialis, herpes genitalis, chickenpox, zoster, and mononucleosis. All entries since 1996 related to therapy or drug therapy for these syndromes also were identified.

REFERENCES

1. Andersson J et al: Effect of acyclovir on infectious mononucleosis: a double-blind, placebo-controlled study, *J Infect Dis* 153:283, 1986.
2. Beutner KR et al: Valaciclovir compared with acyclovir for improved therapy for herpes zoster in immunocompetent adults, *Antimicrob Agents Chemother* 39:1546, 1995.
3. Bryson YJ et al: Treatment of first episodes of genital herpes simplex virus infection with oral acyclovir, *N Engl J Med* 308:916, 1983.
4. Centers for Disease Control and Prevention: Prevention and control of influenza: recommendations of the Advisory Committee on Immunization Practices (ACIP), *MMWR* 48:1, 1999.
5. Varicella-zoster infections. In Peter G, editor: *1997 Red Book: Report of the Committee on Infectious Diseases,* ed 24, Elk Grove Village, Ill, 1997, American Academy of Pediatrics, pp 573-585.
6. deGreef H: Famciclovir, a new oral antiherpes drug: results of the first controlled clinical study demonstrating its efficacy and safety in the treatment of uncomplicated herpes zoster in immunocompetent patients, *Int J Antimicrob Agents* 4:241, 1995.
7. Douglas RG Jr: Prophylaxis and treatment of influenza, *N Engl J Med* 322:443, 1990.
8. Drugs for non-HIV viral infections, *Med Lett Drugs Ther* 39:69, 1997.
9. Dunkle LM et al: A controlled trial of acyclovir for chickenpox in normal children, *N Engl J Med* 325:1539, 1991.
10. Engel JP: Long-term suppression of genital herpes, *JAMA* 280:928, 1998.
11. Hayden FG: Antiviral agents. In Mandell GL, Bennett JE, Dolin R, editors: *Principles and practice of infectious diseases,* ed 4, New York, 1995, Churchill Livingstone.
12. Hayden FG et al: Emergence and apparent transmission of rimantadine-resistant influenza A virus in families, *N Engl J Med* 321:1696, 1989.
13. Herpetic Eye Disease Study Group: Acyclovir for the prevention of recurrent herpes simplex virus eye disease, *N Engl J Med* 339:300, 1998.
14. Jackson JL et al: The effect of treating herpes zoster with oral acyclovir in preventing postherpetic neuralgia: a meta-analysis, *Arch Intern Med 157:909, 1997.*
15. Kost RG, Straus SE: Postherpetic neuralgia: pathogenesis, treatment, and prevention, *N Engl J Med* 335:32, 1996.
16. Nathwani D et al: Varicella infections in pregnancy and the newborn: a review prepared for the UK Advisory Group on Chickenpox on behalf of the British Society for the Study of Infection, *J Infect* 36(suppl 1):59, 1998.
17. Resnick L et al: Regression of oral hairy leukoplakia after orally administered acyclovir therapy, *JAMA* 259:384, 1988.
18. Rooney JF et al: Oral acyclovir to suppress frequently recurrent herpes labialis: a double-blind, placebo-controlled trial, *Ann Intern Med* 118:268, 1993.
19. Shepp DH et al: Oral acyclovir therapy for mucocutaneous herpes simplex virus infections in immunocompromised marrow transplant recipients, *Ann Intern Med* 102:783, 1985.
20. Spruance SL et al: Treatment of herpes simplex labialis with topical acyclovir in polyethylene glycol, *J Infect Dis* 146:85, 1982.
21. Spruance SL et al: Treatment of recurrent herpes simplex labialis with oral acyclovir, *J Infect Dis* 161:185, 1990.
22. Topical penciclovir for herpes labialis, *Med Lett Drugs Ther* 39:57, 1997.
23. Tynell E et al: Acyclovir and prednisolone treatment of acute infectious mononucleosis: a multicenter, double-blind, placebo-controlled study, *J Infect Dis* 174:324, 1996.
24. Tyring S et al: Famciclovir for the treatment of acute herpes zoster: effects on acute disease and postherpetic neuralgia: a randomized, double-blind, placebo-controlled study, *Ann Intern Med* 123:89, 1995.
25. van der Horst C et al: Lack of effect of peroral acyclovir for the treatment of acute infectious mononucleosis, *J Infect Dis* 164:788, 1991.
26. Wallace MR et al: Treatment of adult varicella with oral acyclovir: a randomized, placebo-controlled trial, *Ann Intern Med* 117:358, 1992.
27. Whitley RJ, Lakeman F: Herpes simplex virus infections of the central nervous system: therapeutic and diagnostic considerations, *Clin Infect Dis* 20:414, 1995.
28. Whitley RJ et al: Acyclovir with and without prednisone for the treatment of herpes zoster, *Ann Intern Med* 125:376, 1996.
29. Wilkins EGL et al: Management of chickenpox in the adult: a review prepared for the UK Advisory Group on Chickenpox on behalf of the British Society for the Study of Infection, *J Infect* 36(suppl 1):49, 1998.
30. Wood MJ et al: A randomized trial of acyclovir for 7 days or 21 days with and without prednisolone for treatment of acute herpes zoster, *N Engl J Med* 330:896, 1994.

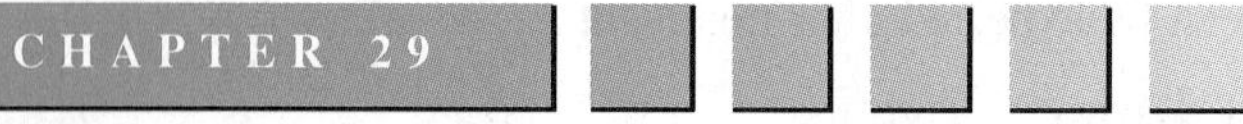

Sexually Transmitted Diseases

Robin R. Ingalls
Peter A. Rice

Sexually transmitted diseases (STDs) are a continuing public health problem, and the "traditional" venereal diseases, including syphilis, gonorrhea, chancroid, lymphogranuloma venereum, and granuloma inguinale, account for only a part of STDs in industrialized societies. Whether the measure of the problem is the number of infections and accompanying physical and psychologic morbidity or the resulting complications such as pelvic inflammatory disease (PID), infertility, and perinatal morbidity, most infections are caused by microorganisms outside the traditional sphere of venereology. Primary care physicians and other health care providers must understand the increased scope of the etiology, epidemiology, prevention, and pathogenesis of STDs if these conditions are to be recognized and managed in individual patients and controlled in populations. Although a syndromic approach may serve as a useful initial guide to a differential diagnosis, most STDs have overlapping modes of presentation, and individual infections may produce several complaints. Further evaluation, including physical and laboratory examinations, is usually necessary to make a specific diagnosis and to formulate a plan for management.

This chapter focuses primarily on men; Chapter 46 discusses vaginitis, mucopurulent cervicitis, and PID.

EVALUATION

Any person who engages in unprotected sexual activity is at risk for acquiring an STD, so screening is sound preventive medicine. Although the optimal frequency of STD screening visits is not well established, we recommend annual visits. In high-risk groups, such as sexually active adolescent females, testing for STDs should be offered twice a year.[2,3] Indications for more frequent testing include a new partner and a history of sexually acquired infections.

Patient History. A detailed sexual history is necessary, although time may be limited in a screening setting because of the extensive agenda. The physician should inquire about any history of sexual intercourse (frequency, last occurrence), gender preference, contraceptive or condom use, number of sexual partners within past 30 to 60 days and over patient's lifetime, and route of penetration (i.e., penile-vaginal, penile-anal, oral-genital). The normal review of systems should include asking about any symptoms of pain, discharge, dysuria, pruritus, or skin rashes. Female patients should describe their menstrual cycle, including timing of last menstrual period and symptoms of dysmenorrhea, amenorrhea, and spotting.

Physical Examination. A routine examination should include inspection of the external genitalia and a general skin examination. The patient at risk for STDs should have a complete physical and genital examination.

The male examination should include inspection of the inguinal region, pubic hair, scrotum, and penile shaft for any skin lesions. The testes in the scrotal sac should be palpated for a mass or tenderness, and the patient should be taught testicular self-examination. A rectal examination should be done if the patient reports any symptoms or a history of receptive anal intercourse. A urethral swab for Gram's stain and specific testing for *Chlamydia* and gonorrhea should be obtained if history or examination warrants.

Females should have a breast examination, inspection of pubic hair and inguinal area, external genital assessment for discharge or lesions, and bimanual examination for evaluation of uterine size, cervical motion tenderness, and adnexal swelling or tenderness. At least once a year, sexually active females should have a speculum examination with a Papanicolaou (Pap) smear. The cervix should be examined for friability and discharge, and if warranted by history, endocervical specimens should be tested for gonorrhea and *Chlamydia* at least once a year, even in the absence of symptoms.

Laboratory Examination. Clinical data alone are inaccurate predictors of most STDs, so diagnostic testing is routinely used to confirm any clinical suspicion. In addition to diagnostic testing, laboratory screening is especially useful when used to diagnose infections associated with few or no symptoms. Screening implies that a diagnostic test in an asymptomatic person will lead to early diagnosis of a disease and will improve the outcome, as with Pap smear screening of cervical cancer and early diagnosis of *Chlamydia* to prevent the complications of PID. A useful screening tool has been the development of an inexpensive, highly sensitive urine-based test for *Chlamydia* based on detection of plasmid deoxyribonucleic acid (DNA) by the polymerase chain reaction (PCR) or ligase chain reaction (LCR). Infections with generally asymptomatic pathogens, such as *Chlamydia,* syphilis, hepatitis B, and human immunodeficiency virus (HIV), are all useful targets for screening purposes.

Counseling and Contact Tracing. All sexually active persons need to be educated about reducing risk factors for STDs and HIV infection. If an STD is diagnosed, sexual partners must be identified and treated as part of the patient's management. Because many infections are not reportable to the Centers for Disease Control and Prevention (CDC), the provider cannot rely on the partners being contacted by public health authorities. Voluntary notification of all partners must be judiciously emphasized to the patient as a mature and necessary action. In most states the health department will assist in partner notification, allowing the index case to remain anonymous; the patient is usually interviewed by a trained staff member, who obtains the names and location of sexual partners. Sexual partners at least should be brought to medical attention for examination. Treatment is often administered, even without symptoms or confirmatory laboratory tests, especially when the diagnosis of a treatable STD appears likely. Syphilis, gonorrhea, and acquired immunodeficiency syndrome (AIDS) are reportable diseases throughout the United States. The requirement for reporting other STDs, such as *Chlamydia* infection, varies from state to state.

MALE URETHRITIS

Urethritis, or inflammation of the urethra, is the most frequent STD found in men in developed countries. It is caused by an infection that leads to the discharge of mucopurulent or purulent material from the urethra and burning during urination. The only bacterial pathogens of proven clinical importance in men with urethritis are *Neisseria gonorrhoeae* and *Chlamydia trachomatis.*[4] *Ureaplasma urealyticum* has also been associated with some cases of urethritis. Currently in the United States, most cases of sexually acquired urethritis do not have an established etiology. Although most of these have an epidemiologic pattern that is consistent with a recently acquired STD, they may have a waxing and waning course, and not all cases will respond to antibiotic therapy.

N. gonorrhoeae is a small, gram-negative diplococcus. During the course of infection in males, invasion of urethral epithelial cells by gonococci has been documented, thus explaining the usual clinical manifestation of acute anterior urethritis.[1] Typically the incubation period is 2 to 5 days, followed by rapid onset of dysuria and purulent urethral discharge.[11] Compared with other causes of urethritis discussed next, gonorrhea usually has a shorter incubation period and produces more intense symptoms of dysuria and discharge (Fig. 29-1, *A*). Although more than 95% of men infected with gonorrhea will develop overt urethritis and come to medical attention, a small proportion may remain asymptomatic.[10] In the general population an estimated 2% to 10% of infected men never become symptomatic, accumulate in number over time, and constitute about two thirds of all infected men at any point in time.

Nongonococcal urethritis (NGU) includes all cases from which *N. gonorrhoeae* is not isolated. Many organisms have been associated with NGU, but the only clinically important bacterial pathogen in men with urethritis is *C. trachomatis. Chlamydia* is an obligate intracellular organism estimated to account for 23% to 55% of NGU cases in men.[4] Many men infected with gonorrhea are also coinfected with *Chlamydia.* NGU is now the most common bacterial STD in industrialized countries, and asymptomatic urethral carriage in men may be an even more important epidemiologic problem than urethritis with *N. gonorrhoeae.* The symptoms of NGU are similar to those of gonorrhea but are less intense and develop more slowly after a longer incubation period. Dysuria and urethral discharge occur in only about a third of men with NGU, and NGU is more likely to present with a single symptom than is gonococcal urethritis.[12] When present, the discharge in NGU usually appears only after penile stripping. In contrast to gonococcal urethritis, NGU discharge is sparse, with a mucoid rather than a purulent appearance (Fig. 29-1, *B*).

Evaluation of History and Symptoms. The symptoms of urethral infection in men may vary from vague discomfort to dysuria, or urinary frequency without a discharge to frank dysuria accompanied by a thick purulent discharge. The major historic features to be elicited from the patient are (1) recent sexual exposure; (2) estimate of the incubation

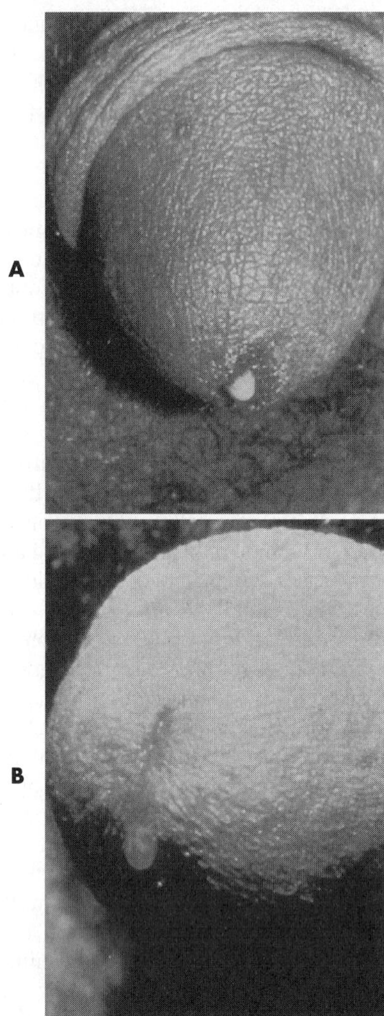

Fig. 29-1. Urethritis in men. **A,** Gonococcal urethritis classically produces profuse, purulent discharge. **B,** Nongonococcal urethritis (NGU) more often results in scant, mucoid discharge.

period, if possible (i.e., last sexual contact); (3) recently acquired and treated STD, since the current event may represent a treatment failure or a reinfection with an untreated sexual partner; (4) drug allergies, particularly to penicillin; and (5) identification of sexual contacts. Urethritis may occur in association with urinary tract infections, bacterial prostatitis, urethral stricture, and phimosis and secondary to catheterization or other instrumentation of the urethra.

Physical and Laboratory Examinations. If the patient is not circumcised, the foreskin should be retracted to examine the glans completely. Inability to retract the foreskin may indicate adhesion to the glans or phimosis. Edema of the foreskin may result from vigorous sexual activity or infection. For example, *balanitis* can occur from urethral discharge being trapped, resulting in an inflammatory reaction of the glans and the overlying foreskin. *Hypospadias,* or displacement of the urethral meatus to the underside of the shaft, is common and usually causes no problem. The examiner should carefully inspect for the presence and characteristics of a urethral discharge, which may be seen only as staining of the underwear. Unfortunately, the presence of a visibly clear urethral discharge or even small amounts of mucoid discharge does not always indicate urethritis. Other lesions on the penile shaft and at the base of the shaft and the presence or absence of inguinal lymphadenopathy should also be determined.

If a discharge is not present, the penis should be milked or stripped by applying gentle pressure over the ventral and dorsal surfaces of the base and moving the fingers toward the meatus to bring forward small amounts of discharge. Gonococcal urethritis usually results in a profuse and purulent discharge, in contrast to NGU, which is more often associated with a scant mucoid discharge (see Fig. 29-1). A dacron or rayon swab mounted on wire (not the routine wooden or nylon cotton swab) should be inserted 2 cm into the urethra to obtain a specimen for microscopic examination and culture. If sufficient moist material is obtained, the swab first is rolled on a glass slide for Gram's stain. If facilities are available for culture of gonorrhea, the remaining sample should then be transferred onto a modified Thayer-Martin plate for culture by rolling the swab in a large Z pattern. Because *N. gonorrhoeae* grows best in relatively anaerobic conditions, culture plates should be incubated at 37° C in a 2% to 10% carbon dioxide (CO_2) environment within 30 minutes of being plated. A candle jar is a simple and convenient way to achieve a CO_2 environment for growing gonorrhea. Culture media transport systems are also available if longer holding periods are required.

Although culture is considered the gold standard, it is not always practical. Alternate testing methods include a DNA probe, which can test for both gonorrhea and *Chlamydia* infection. PCR and LCR, which have become the mainstay of *Chlamydia* testing, are also available for diagnosis of gonorrhea. In a review of 21 studies on two nucleic acid–based tests, Gen-Probe and Amplicor LCR, for the diagnosis of gonorrhea, sensitivity was 85% and 98% and specificity 95% and 99%, respectively. When the proficient performance of culture is available, these tests offer no advantage over culture.[13]

For diagnosis of *Chlamydia* infection, a second swab should be obtained, with particular attention paid to rolling the swab against the walls of the urethra so as to obtain sloughing cells where the *Chlamydia* organisms reside intracellularly. Obtaining discharge alone is not sufficient either for *C. trachomatis* antigen detection assays or for culture. In many settings, culture is impractical because *Chlamydia* must be grown intracellularly in a tissue culture facility. Rapid antigen tests are available (e.g., DFA, EIA), but most lack sufficient sensitivity and specificity, especially in asymptomatic men. The techniques of PCR and LCR have become the new gold standard of *Chlamydia* testing. They are highly sensitive and specific and can also be done with urine samples if urethral (or cervical) samples cannot be obtained (Box 29-1). Thus they are quite useful for screening populations at risk, such as adolescents. A recent study compared the cost- effectiveness of pelvic examination and culture with urine testing by LCR to prevent PID in sexually active, asymptomatic adolescent females.[18] Urine-based LCR screening was the most cost-effective strategy to detect chlamydial and gonococcal infections in this population, and given the ease of implementation, it would likely prevent the greatest number of PID cases.

Gram's stain is often overlooked for diagnosis of STDs but is a sensitive test for the diagnosis of gonococcal urethritis in

Box 29-1. Comparison of Diagnostic Tests for *Chlamydia Trachomatis*

DNA probes: sensitivity about 75%, specificity greater than 99%
Immunologic assays (e.g., EIA): sensitivity about 70%-75%, specificity greater than 99%
DNA amplification (e.g., PCR, LCR): sensitivity about 90%-95%, specificity 100%

symptomatic men. We recommend that a Gram's stain be performed on any discharge and the stained smear examined under oil-immersion microscopy for polymorphonuclear neutrophils (PMNs) as well as for gram-negative intracellular diplococci (Fig. 29-2). The examiner should record exactly what is seen on the slide. To avoid counting superimposed cells, an area of the slide consisting of a monolayer of separate cells should be found. The presence of five or more white blood cells (WBCs) per field in five oil-immersion fields indicates an inflammatory discharge in a male. These criteria are analogous to those employed in men without apparent urethral discharge who are undergoing evaluation for signs and symptoms of urethritis.

The urinary dipstick leukocyte esterase test (LET) is also used to predict culture-verified urethral infections with *C. trachomatis* and *N. gonorrhoeae* in men.[16] Although the sensitivity of this test varies with the status of clinical symptoms and the overall prevalence of infections in the population being tested, the specificity for either of these infections may be greater than 90%. Unfortunately, some men will have *N. gonorrhoeae* or *C. trachomatis* isolated when the urethral Gram's stain and first-voided urine sediment do not contain PMNs or when the LET is negative.

Confirmation of Urethritis. According to the CDC guidelines, physicians should document that urethritis is present before treatment by any of the following signs: (1) mucopurulent or purulent discharge, (2) positive Gram's stain of urethral secretions demonstrating five or more WBCs per oil-immersion field, or (3) positive LET on first-voided urine, or microscopic examination of first-voided urine demonstrating 10 or more WBCs per high-power field. If none of these criteria is present, treatment should be deferred pending documentation of *N. gonorrhoeae* or *C. trachomatis* or appropriate clinical follow-up.[4]

Treatment. The following treatment recommendations are based on 1998 CDC guidelines.[4] Options for the treatment of gonococcal urethritis include ceftriaxone, 125 mg intramuscularly (IM) in a single dose, or cefixime, 400 mg orally as a single dose. The spectra of activity for cefixime and ceftriaxone are quite similar, but ceftriaxone provides a higher and more sustained level of drug and is slightly better than cefixime (99.1% vs. 97.1%) in clinical trials.[4] Other single-dose regimens include ciprofloxacin, 500 mg, or ofloxacin, 400 mg. For patients who cannot tolerate cephalosporins or quinolones, spectinomycin, 2 gm IM in a single dose, is an option. Because coinfection with

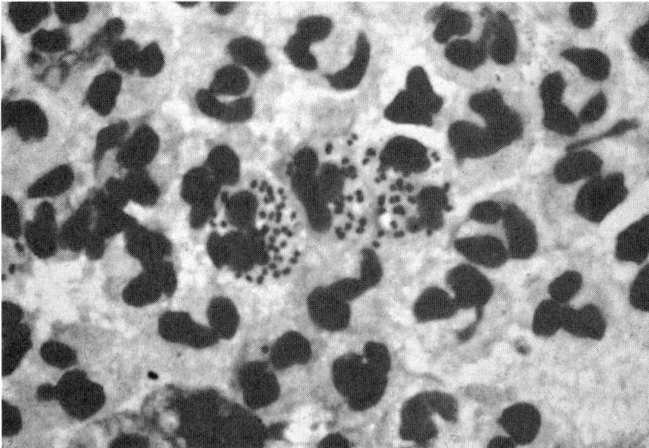

Fig. 29-2. Gram's stain of urethral discharge from patient with gonococcal urethritis. Note extensive number of neutrophils in discharge, as well as gram-negative intracellular diplococci in center of field.

C. trachomatis occurs in about 40% of patients with gonorrhea, treatment for *Chlamydia* is also recommended.

For treatment of NGU or chlamydial infection, two options are available: azithromycin, 1 gm orally as a single dose, or doxycycline, 100 mg orally twice a day for 7 days. Although some formulations are more expensive than doxycycline, azithromycin is the preferred agent because of patient compliance. For patients who cannot tolerate either regimen or for whom the drugs are contraindicated, erythromycin base, 500 mg four times a day for 7 days, is an alternative. Although single-dose therapy with 2 gm of azithromycin is effective against both gonorrhea and *Chlamydia,* it is generally not used because this increased dose is associated with significant gastrointestinal distress.

Follow-up. Patients should be instructed to abstain from sexual intercourse until therapy is completed. All sexual partners within the previous 2 months should be referred for evaluation and treatment. Sexual contacts of symptomatic patients should be treated if their last sexual contact was within 30 days of the onset of symptoms; if the patient was asymptomatic, contacts should be treated if they were within 60 days. In the case of gonorrhea, partners should also be treated for *Chlamydia* infection.

Medical follow-up for urethritis is not routinely recommended. Increasingly, however, repeat DNA amplification assays performed 1 month after treatment in persons at high risk for STDs have resulted in a 10% positive (relapse or reinfection) rate. Patients should be instructed to return for evaluation if symptoms persist or recur after completion of therapy. Symptoms alone, without documentation of signs or laboratory evidence of urethral inflammation, or suspicions of reinfection are not sufficient cause for re-treatment.

Recurrent or Persistent Urethritis

The management of persistent or recurrent symptoms of dysuria and discharge can be challenging. The physician must look for objective signs of urethritis before initiating another course of antimicrobial therapy. Because effective regimens have not been identified for treating patients with persistent symptoms or frequent recurrences after initial treatment, no set guidelines exist.

The evaluation should include a wet-mount examination and culture of an intraurethral swab specimen for *Trichomonas vaginalis*. Urologic examinations usually do not reveal a specific etiology. The simple cases show clear evidence of noncompliance or reexposure, and re-treatment should be offered. Often, re-treatment is attempted with the opposite drug than originally chosen (i.e., azithromycin or doxycycline), but it is not necessary to change agents. For the remainder of the cases, the differential diagnosis of dysuria should be expanded to include trichomoniasis or herpes simplex virus. Reiter's syndrome should also be considered.

If the patient was compliant with the initial regimen and reexposure can be excluded, the following regimen is recommended by the CDC.[4] Metronidazole, 2 gm orally in a single dose, *plus* erythromycin base, 500 mg orally four times a day for 7 days, or erythromycin ethylsuccinate, 800 mg orally four times a day for 7 days.

EPIDIDYMITIS

Acute epididymitis is characterized by pain and swelling of the epididymis. Among sexually active men under age 35, epididymitis is most often caused by a *C. trachomatis* or *N. gonorrhoeae*. Epididymitis caused by sexually transmitted *Escherichia coli* infection can also occur among homosexual men who are the insertive partners during anal intercourse. Sexually transmitted epididymitis is usually accompanied by asymptomatic urethritis. Nonsexually transmitted epididymitis associated with urinary tract infections caused by gram-negative enteric organisms occurs more frequently among men over 35 years old, men who have recently undergone urinary tract instrumentation or surgery, and men with anatomic abnormalities.

The treatment for epididymitis is similar to that outlined earlier for urethritis, except doxycycline should be administered for 10 days, not 7; single-dose azithromycin is not recommended. For epididymitis most likely caused by enteric organisms or for patients allergic to cephalosporins or tetracyclines, the recommendation is for ofloxacin, 300 mg orally twice a day for 10 days. Although most patients can be treated on an outpatient basis, hospitalization should be considered when severe pain suggests other diagnoses (e.g., torsion, testicular infarction, abscess) or when patients are febrile or might be noncompliant with an antimicrobial regimen. Epididymitis is often associated with urethritis.

Follow-up. Most patients should be reexamined 2 to 4 days after starting therapy. Failure to improve should prompt reconsideration of the diagnosis. The differential diagnosis includes tumor, abscess, infarction, testicular cancer, and tuberculous or fungal epididymitis. Partners should be treated for possible gonorrhea and chlamydial infection.

EVALUATION OF GENITAL SKIN LESIONS

Genital skin lesions can be classified broadly as ulcerative or nonulcerative. They may or may not have an infectious etiology, and not all infections are sexually transmitted. Numerous lesions are related to trauma; some are secondary to a dermatologic disorder or a neoplastic process. Even when all available tests are used by experienced physicians, as many as 40% of ulcerative lesions do not yield a specific diagnosis.

Evaluation of History and Symptoms. Initially the patient should be questioned to determine if trauma is the cause of the genital lesion, particularly with an ulcerative lesion. If trauma is implicated, the onset of the lesion should have been noted shortly after the trauma, and the traumatic event should have been noticeably painful at the time. The patient should provide a complete history of sexual activity and uncommon sexual exposure. A history of vesicular lesions in a patient with genital erosion, particularly if the lesions are recurrent, suggests herpes simplex infection. Patients infected with pediculosis pubis or scabies may complain of significant pruritus, and erosions may be secondary to excoriation.

Physical and Laboratory Examinations. In the assessment of patients with genital lesions, simple and careful clinical observations are essential in evaluating potential causes and in establishing priorities for the implementation of laboratory methods to assist and confirm the clinical impression. More than one STD may coexist, and thus ulcerative and nonulcerative patterns may be mixed. Clinical findings are sometimes diagnostic (e.g., herpetic vesicles) and with epidemiologic considerations may help guide initial therapy. Many genital ulcerations, however, cannot be diagnosed on examination alone. Syphilis must be excluded by appropriate serology in all patients. When possible, darkfield or direct immunofluorescent microscopy should be performed by experienced technologists on lesions that suggest primary (usually ulcerative) or secondary (usually nonulcerative) syphilis.

ULCERATIVE GENITAL LESIONS

The infectious causes of genital ulcers include HSV, *Treponema pallidum, Haemophilus ducreyi,* three specific serotypes of *C. trachomatis,* and *Calymmatobacterium granulomatis.* The incidence and etiology of sexually transmitted infectious causes of genital ulceration vary according to geographic area. In certain parts of Asia and Africa, genital ulceration is the usual reason for a patient to attend a clinic, and both syphilis and chancroid are very common. In Western industrial societies, urethritis and vaginitis are much more frequent reasons to visit clinics, herpes simplex infection is the most common form of ulceration, followed by syphilis and chancroid. Lymphogranuloma venereum and granuloma inguinale (formerly known as donovanosis) are rare causes of genital infections in the United States but are endemic in parts of Africa, South America, Asia, the Caribbean, Australia, and New Guinea. Thus it is important to obtain a travel history along with a sexual history, since casual sexual encounters during overseas travel may result in unusual causes of genital ulceration.

Patient Evaluation. Although clinical features can often help differentiate between the various causes of genital ulcers, a diagnosis based only on the history and physical examination often is inaccurate. Therefore the evaluation of all patients with genital ulcers should include a serologic test for syphilis and an evaluation for herpes. Table 29-1 broadly classifies the differential diagnosis of genital ulcer disease, and Table 29-2 describes laboratory procedures that assist in the diagnosis of ulcerative lesions.

Table 29-1. Genital Ulcers

Clinical observation	Herpes simplex virus	Syphilis	Chancroid	Lymphogranuloma venereum	Granuloma inguinale
Incubation period	2-7 days	10-90 (mean 21) days	1-14 (mean 3-5) days	Initial lesion rarely noticed, 1-4 weeks (mean 10-14 days)	Unknown, probably 1-12 weeks
Location of ulcer	Male: glans, prepuce, shaft of penis Female: cervix, vagina, labia	Male: coronal sulcus, glans, shaft of penis, perianal area Female: cervix, vagina	Male: frenulum, prepuce, coronal sulcus, glans, shaft of penis Female: cervix, vagina, fourchette, labia, perianal area	Male: glans, shaft of penis Female, vagina, labia	Male: glans, prepuce, shaft of penis, perianal area Female: labia, fourchette
Number of lesions	Multiple, at times confluent; more lesions with first infection than with recurrences	Usually one, multiple not rare	Usually 1 to 3, may be up to 10	Usually single	Single or multiple
Initial appearance of lesion	Vesicle	Papule	Inflamed macule/papule/pustule	Papule/vesicle/pustule	Papule
Shape of typical ulcer	Small, grouped, variable border	Round, oval; if irregular, symmetrically so	Irregular ragged, variable size	Discrete	Sharply defined, but irregular
Depth of ulcer	Superficial	Superficial cup or saucer shape, elevated edges	Hollow, excavated, undermined	Superficial	Elevated
Surface of ulcer	Bright red	Smooth, shiny, glazed, crust	Rough, uneven, grayish		Clean, friable, beefy granulation, depigmentation
Secretion	Moderate, serous	Scanty, serous	Abundant, purulent, and frequently necrotic	Variable	Rare
Induration	None	Firm, parchmentlike, movable, circumscribed, does not change shape with pressure	Rarely present, changes shape with pressure, boggy	None	Firm granulation tissue
Pain	Often; more pain with initial infection than with recurrences	Rarely	Often	Variable	Rare
Inguinal adenopathy	Tender; bilateral in approximately 50% of primary disease	Bilateral, multiple, constant, and painless	Usually single, unilateral, tender, and unilocular; overlying erythema; bilateral involvement can occur; suppuration and rupture of fluctuant nodes in 5-8 days may occur, leaving single large ulcer	Cause of usual presentation; initally firm, tender, discrete, moveable, later indolent fixed, matted, occasionally leading to suppuration and fistulas, sign of groove; unilateral (60%) and bilateral (40%) involvement	Rare
Constitutional symptoms	Common in primary, less common in recurrences	Rare in primary	Rare	Frequent	Rare
Course	Recurrence is the rule; reinfection occurs	Slowly resolves to latency without treatment; relapse and reinfection possible	Frequently progresses to erosive lesions; relapses or reinfections reported	Local lesion heals without scars; systemic disease proceeds	Worsens slowly; deep ulcers occasionally develop

Modified from Wiesner P et al: Genital ulcers. In Holmes KK, Mardh P-A, editors; *International perspectives in neglected sexually transmitted diseases,* New York, 1983, McGraw-Hill.

Table 29-2. Laboratory Procedures for Diagnosis of Sexually Acquired Genital Ulcerative Lesions

Procedure	Specific technique	Specimen	Criteria	Diagnosis
Reagin test	RPR-CT (rapid plasma reagin card test) or VDRL test	Serum	Reactive titer	Probable syphilis
Direct immunofluorescopy	Reaction with fluorescein-conjugated specific monoclonal antibody	Exudate from lesion or aspirate of bubo	Yellow-green fluorescence of elementary bodies	LGV
Darkfield microscopy	Unstained preparation	Exudate from lesion or aspirate of bubo	Motile spirochetes, *Treponema pallidum*	Syphilis
Bacteriologic cultures	Chocolate agar enriched with 1% Isovitalex and vancomycin (3μg/ml) added	Exudate from lesion or aspirate of bubo	Normucoid, yellow-gray, translucent, movable colonies containing pleomorphic clumps of gram-negative bacilli, *Haemophilus ducreyi*	Chancroid
Light microscopy	Papanicolaou smear (or other specially stained preparation)	Exudate from lesion	Intranuclear inclusions in multinucleated giant cells	HSV
	Gram-stained preparation	Exudate from ulcer or aspirate of bubo	Gram-negative bacilli in chains	Possible chancroid
	Wright-Giemsa stain	Crushed tissue from biopsy	*Calymmatobacterium granulomatis*	Granuloma inguinale
Basic serology	LGV complement fixation assay	Serum	Reactive titer ≥1:64	Probable LGV
Tissue culture	*Chlamydia* culture	Exudate or aspirate of bubo	Typical stains and cytopathic effects	LGV
	HSV culture	Exudate from lesion	Typical stains and cytopathic effects	HSV
Advanced serology	Microimmunofluorescence	Sera	Reactive titer ≥1:256	LGV
	Serologic typing	Agent isolated by culture	*N. gonorrhoeae, C. trachomatis*	Research tools

Modified from Wiesner P et al: Genital ulcers. In Holmes KK, Mardh P-A, editors: *International perspectives in neglected sexually transmitted diseases,* New York, 1983, McGraw-Hill.
VDRL, Venereal Disease Research Laboratories; *LGV,* Lymphogranuloma venereum; *HSV,* herpes simplex virus.

Genital Herpes

Genital herpes is caused by herpes simplex virus (HSV), a DNA virus with two serotypes. Type 1 is usually found in oral lesions but also causes 10% to 20% of genital herpes. In contrast, type 2 occurs predominantly in genital infections. The two types can be distinguished by various laboratory techniques, including differing cytopathic effects, neutralization, and immunofluorescence. In general, genital infection with HSV-1 is associated with less severe disease and fewer recurrences than with HSV-2.

Clinical Manifestations. After skin inoculation, HSV replicates locally, producing the characteristic thin-walled vesicle on an inflammatory base. The incubation period of primary genital herpes is typically 3 to 5 days but can range from 2 to 7 days. At the onset, prodromal burning of the skin occurs, usually followed by the appearance of grouped vesicles. These vesicles rupture to form multiple shallow painful ulcers, which may coalesce into one or more larger ulcers (Fig. 29-3). In men, herpetic lesions typically occur on the glans, prepuce, or shaft of the penis; in women the labia minora and majora and the fourchette are often affected. In 90% of women with primary genital herpes, HSV can be recovered from the cervix, even without clinically apparent lesions. Homosexual men often have perianal herpetic lesions, making defecation intensely painful.

The predominant symptom in primary HSV is pain. In addition, tender bilateral inguinal lymphadenopathy, dysuria,

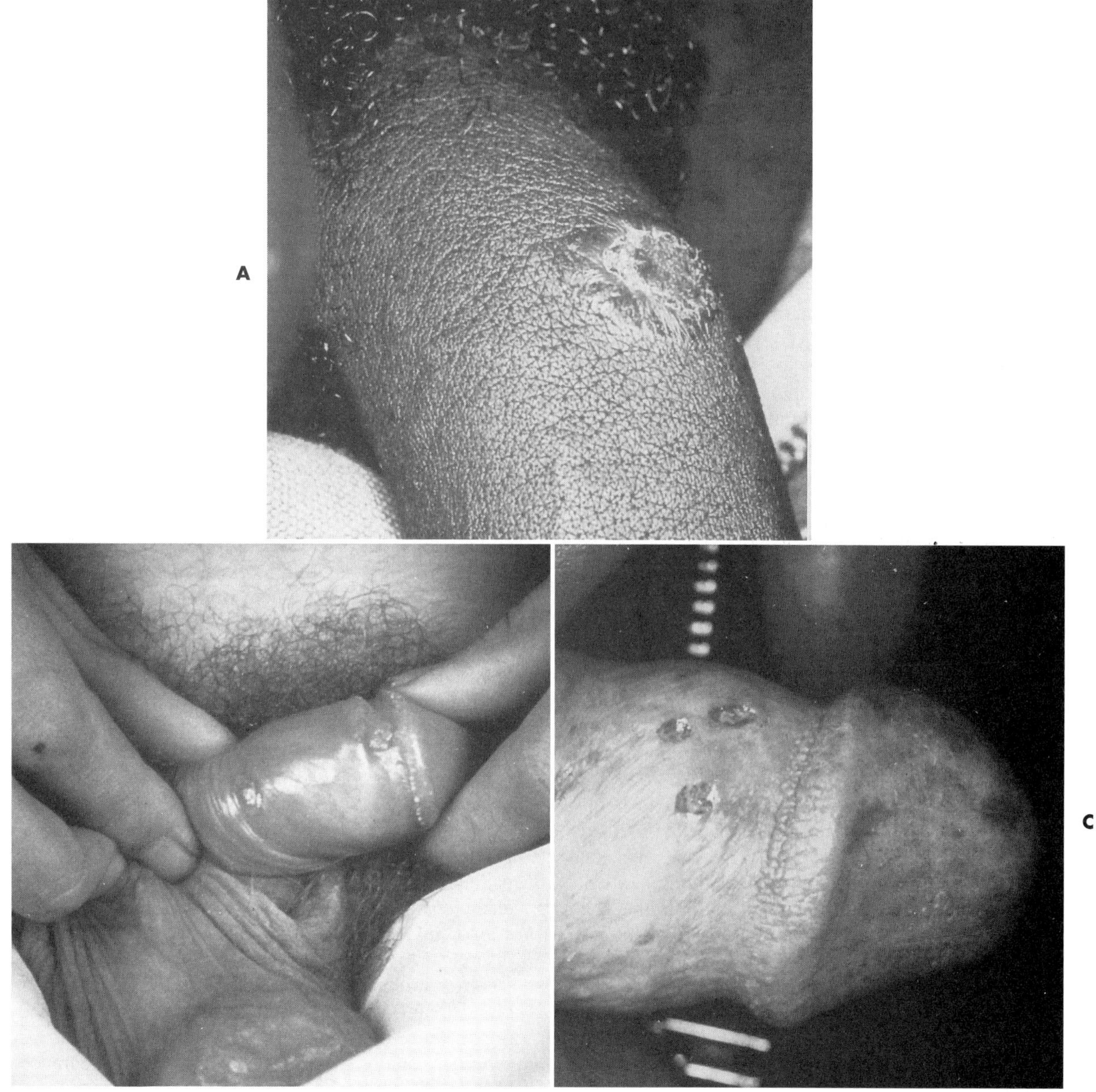

Fig. 29-3. Genital ulcerative lesions in men. **A,** Primary syphilis is associated with solitary, round ulcers that are usually superficial with raised edges. **B,** Chancre associated with chancroid may be multiple, with irregular shape, rough surface, and undermined edges. **C,** Herpetic ulcers initially appear as vesicles that evolve into multiple, painful, superficial ulcers. (**A** and **C** from Meheus A, Ursi JP: *Sexually transmitted diseases,* Kalamazoo, Mich, 1982, Upjohn.)

and constitutional symptoms (e.g., malaise, fever, headache) are also common. Complications include the development of extragenital lesions, which may occur in up to 20% of patients, and aseptic meningitis. In some patients, HSV may cause a sacral radiculitis, leading to constipation, urinary retention, and perigenital anesthesia.[6] Without bacterial superinfection the course is usually self-limited, and healing occurs in 1 to 3 weeks. Concurrent HIV infection, however, may lead to a more severe, prolonged course of disease.

In recurrent genital herpes the ulceration is often milder, and the associated constitutional symptoms are slight or absent. A prodrome of itching, burning, or tingling often precedes the appearance of lesions. Lesions are usually less painful and fewer in number than with the primary episode and heal in 6 to 10 days. Viral shedding is possible between recurrences, and even without visible lesions, viral transmission can occur. In addition, autoinoculation from genital to extragenital sites (or vice versa) can occur, and patients should be cautioned about developing genital herpes from an oral lesion.

Diagnosis. At present the most sensitive laboratory method for HSV diagnosis is tissue culture isolation. Recovery of virus is easier from an intact vesicle or early ulcer than from a late ulcer and is easier from primary than recurrent lesions. The sample should be collected in virus transport medium, held at 4° C, and sent to the laboratory within 12 hours. Although smear tests (immunofluorescence, immunoperoxidase, Pap) are specific for HSV, their sensitivity may be as low as 50%.[4] The serology test demonstrates a fourfold rise in titer of antibodies to HSV, as detected by complement fixation or neutralization tests; however, the difficulties in collecting acute and convalescent sera and the delay in obtaining results make this an inferior method of diagnosis.

Treatment. For the treatment of first clinical episodes of genital herpes, several options are available: acyclovir, 400 mg orally three times a day for 7 to 10 days; acyclovir, 200 mg orally five times a day for 7 to 10 days; famciclovir, 250 mg orally three times a day for 7 to 10 days; or valacyclovir, 1 gm orally twice a day for 7 to 10 days.[4] The treatment can be extended if healing is incomplete after 10 days of therapy. Treatment of initial episodes of genital herpes generally prevents development of new lesions, hastens the period of crusting and healing, and shortens the time of viral shedding.

The physician must discuss the natural history of herpes infection with the patient during the initial episode, especially the potential for recurrent episodes, and the risk of sexual transmission during asymptomatic viral shedding. Patients should be encouraged to inform their sex partners that they have genital herpes and should be advised to abstain from sexual activity when lesions or prodromal symptoms are present. Condoms should be used during all sexual exposures with new or uninfected sex partners. The risk for neonatal infection should be explained to all patients, including men.

Because most patients with genital herpes will experience recurrent lesions, episodic or suppressive therapy should be discussed. If treatment can be instituted during the prodrome or within the first day of onset, episodic therapy can be beneficial. If patients experience frequent recurrences (e.g., more than six episodes per year), however, daily suppressive therapy may be preferable.

Treatment for recurrent episodes includes acyclovir, 400 mg orally three times a day for 5 days, 200 mg orally five times a day for 5 days, or 800 mg orally twice a day for 5 days; famciclovir, 125 mg orally twice a day for 5 days; or valacyclovir, 500 mg orally twice a day for 5 days.[4]

For patients with frequent or severe recurrences, daily suppressive therapy is an option. The original studies done with acyclovir found the drug to be well tolerated and effective.[9,19] Development of resistant virus while receiving long-term therapy, even after 6 years, has not been encountered, at least in immunocompetent individuals.[7,8] Although suppressive therapy will reduce viral shedding, it will not eliminate it completely, and patients should be encouraged to discuss this with their sexual partners. Suppressive regimens include acyclovir, 400 mg orally twice a day; famciclovir, 250 mg orally twice a day; valacyclovir, 250 mg orally twice a day; or valacyclovir, 500 or 1000 mg orally once a day.[4]

Syphilis

Syphilis is a systemic infection caused by *T. pallidum* subspecies *pallidum,* a slender, close-coiled, spiral organism that is motile and multiplies by binary fission every 30 hours. Although too slender to be seen by ordinary light microscopy, it is visible by darkfield or direct immunofluorescent microscopy. It has never been propagated in artificial media or in tissue culture but will grow in rabbit testicle tissue. The recent sequencing of the *T. pallidum* genome has disproved earlier reports that the organism contained endotoxin or lipopolysaccharide in the outer membrane.[4]

Clinical Manifestations. Clinically, syphilis can be divided into five stages: incubating, primary, secondary, latent, and late (or tertiary) syphilis. *Incubating syphilis* refers to the period between exposure and onset of symptoms. *Primary syphilis* has an incubation period of 9 to 90 days and is characterized by an ulcer or chancre at the site of inoculation (see Fig. 29-3). In men the primary chancre develops at the frenulum, coronal sulcus, urinary meatus, or shaft of the penis. In women primary chancres occur on the labia, at the fourchette, near the clitoris, or sometimes on the cervix. In anoreceptive homosexual men, chancres may appear at the anus or in the anal canal, although they may easily escape diagnosis because they are often inconspicuous.

A primary chancre first appears as a papule that soon becomes eroded, forming a well-defined, hardened ulcer with a sloughing or granulating floor. Although slow to heal, the ulcer is painless, unless it becomes secondarily infected. This is in contrast to HSV ulcers, which are typically painful. Primary chancres are usually single, but about 15% of patients have multiple chancres. Within a week or so of chancre appearance, inguinal lymphadenopathy, either unilateral or bilateral, develops in most patients. The nodes are discrete, rubbery in consistency, and usually painless.

After infection with *T. pallidum,* the organism enters the bloodstream and disseminates throughout the body; any organ can be invaded. This marks the beginning of *secondary syphilis,* usually 2 to 8 weeks after the appearance of the chancre. Secondary syphilis has many manifestations, but the classic and most common presentation is a rash. The appearance can be macular, papular, maculopapular, and pustular. Except for congenital syphilis, however, the rash is never vesicular. The location is typically the truncal and proximal extremities, but any site can be involved. Other skin manifestations include papular cutaneous lesions on the genitals or near the anus, which may erode to form shallow ulcers, and mucous patches that may appear on the oral or genital mucosa. In addition, diffuse or patchy alopecia can occur, as well as the loss of eyelashes and lateral eyebrows.

Because the rash of secondary syphilis can mimic almost any dermatologic condition, it is often prudent to obtain a sexual history from a patient with a rash and send tests when appropriate. Patients with secondary syphilis often have other systemic signs and symptoms, including lymphadenopathy, constitutional symptoms (e.g., fever, malaise, pharyngitis), and central nervous system symptoms (e.g., headache, meningismus). Hepatitis, glomerulonephritis, and arthritis have also been reported. Because of the variety of presentations, secondary syphilis has been called "the great imitator."

Latent syphilis is defined as the stage at which the serologic test is positive but the patient has no clinical manifestations. Latent syphilis is termed *early latent syphilis* during the period when clinical relapses resembling secondary syphilis occur, usually within the first 1 to 2 years after primary infection; beyond this period all other cases of latent syphilis are either *late* latent syphilis or syphilis of unknown duration. In theory the treatment for late latent syphilis, as well as tertiary syphilis, requires a longer duration of therapy because organisms are dividing more slowly, but this has never been proved.

Late syphilis, or tertiary syphilis, is a slowly progressive disease that can affect any organ system in the body and produce illness years after the initial infection. Depending on the site involved, it is referred to as *neurosyphilis, cardiovascular syphilis,* or *gummatous syphilis.*

Diagnosis. The following recommendations are based on current CDC guidelines.[4] The definitive diagnosis of early syphilis requires the detection of *T. pallidum,* usually by darkfield or direct immunofluorescent microscopy, in fluid obtained from lesions or from aspirated lymph nodes. This technique requires a specialized microscope and experienced reader. PCR has recently been studied to detect *T. pallidum* in ulcer swabs, and a multiplex-PCR reaction is available that can simultaneously amplify for *H. ducreyi, T. pallidum,* and HSV-1 and HSV-2.[15] A presumptive diagnosis of syphilis can be made using serologic tests, although serology is less reliable in early disease (i.e., when the patient presents with an ulcer), and should be repeated a week later when serologic tests are negative and a diagnosis of primary syphilis is suspected.

The two types of serologic tests for syphilis are (1) nontreponemal, Venereal Disease Research Laboratories (VDRL), or rapid plasma reagin (RPR) tests and (2) specific treponemal tests; fluorescent treponemal antigen-absorbed (FTA-ABS) or microhemagglutination assay (MHA-TP). Both tests are clinically useful, and together they are used to plan diagnosis and treatment. The nontreponemal tests are usually obtained first as a screening test. Because false-positive nontreponemal test results can occasionally occur, usually secondary to concurrent medical conditions, all positive nontreponemal tests must be confirmed with one of the specific tests (Box 29-2). Nontreponemal tests should be reported quantitatively, as a titer, which usually correlates with disease activity and should be used to assess response to therapy. Because of test variability, a fourfold change in titer, equivalent to a change of two dilutions (e.g., from 1:16 to 1:4 or from 1:8 to 1:32), is considered a clinically significant difference between two test results. Nontreponemal tests should become negative following therapy, although in some patients the test can remain positive with a low titer. In these cases the patients are considered serofast, and the test will remain positive for the remainder of their lives, regardless of treatment or disease activity.

The diagnosis of neurosyphilis can be more complicated (see Chapter 165).

Box 29-2. Approach to Patient with Positive Rapid Plasma Reagin (RPR) Test

1. Confirm result with specific treponemal test (FTA-ABS or MHA-TP). False-positive RPR tests can occur with a number of medical conditions.
2. Determine if patient has had unprotected sexual exposures within past year, has a history of documented seroconversion, or has received treatment for STDs.
3. If history and examination do not suggest infection within past year, treat for late latent syphilis.
4. Consider cerebrospinal fluid examination in any patient with neurologic symptoms or known HIV.

Treatment. The CDC[4] recommends the following therapies for syphilis in nonimmunocompromised patients.[4] Penicillin G is the drug of choice for treatment of all stages of syphilis. The tetracyclines are also effective and can be used in nonpregnant, penicillin-allergic patients. Penicillin is the only therapy with documented efficacy for neurosyphilis. The *Jarisch-Herxheimer reaction* may occur within the first 24 hours after therapy for syphilis. This reaction consists of an acute febrile illness accompanied by headache and myalgias. Patients should be warned about this acute illness, and antipyretics may be used as needed.

For cure, serum levels of penicillin must reach at least 0.03 μg/ml for a minimum of 7 days. The treatment for primary and secondary syphilis, 2.4 million U of benzathine penicillin G administered IM in a single dose, will ensure that these levels are reached. Patients who are allergic to penicillin should be treated for 2 weeks with oral doxycycline, 100 mg twice a day, or tetracycline, 500 mg four times a day. With no proven alternatives to penicillin, the pregnant woman with penicillin allergy should be treated with penicillin after undergoing desensitization. Erythromycin should not be used because it does not reliably cure an infected fetus. Some physicians treat secondary syphilis with longer regimens, reasoning that the duration of therapy must increase as the disease progresses. Such prolonged regimens include a second injection of benzathine penicillin G, 2.4 million U administered 1 week after the first. Some physicians prescribe the second dose of benzathine penicillin G for primary syphilis as well.

Patients who have latent syphilis should be evaluated for evidence of tertiary disease. If no evidence of neurosyphilis is found on cerebrospinal fluid (CSF) examination, treatment consists of benzathine penicillin G, 7.2 million U total, administered IM as three doses of 2.4 million U at 1-week intervals. Patients with neurosyphilis or syphilitic eye disease should be treated with 18 to 24 million U of aqueous penicillin G, administered as 3 to 4 million U IV every 4 hours for 10 to 14 days.

Follow-up. Response to therapy should be monitored by clinical examination and a quantitative reagin test (VDRL or RPR) at 3 and 6 months after treatment. Patients being treated for neurosyphilis should also have CSF examination repeated every 6 months until it is normal. Successful treatment of seropositive early syphilis reduces the reagin titer. The FTA-ABS test often remains reactive indefinitely and is therefore not useful for follow-up. Persistent or recurrent symptoms and a sustained fourfold rise in the nontreponemal test titer suggest treatment failure or reinfection. If the titer does not decline by fourfold at 3 months, the patient also is at risk for treatment failure. In a pregnant woman this titer should decrease at 1 month, and if not, she should be re-treated. After 1 year, all adequately treated patients with seropositive primary syphilis have become seronegative; after 2 years, 95% to 100% of patients with secondary syphilis are seronegative. If, after 2 years, reagin tests are either negative or stabilized at a low titer, further follow-up is not needed. Homosexual men and members of other high-risk groups, however, should be urged to undergo serologic testing every 6 months indefinitely.

Sexual transmission of *T. pallidum* occurs only when mucocutaneous syphilitic lesions are present, but persons exposed sexually to a patient with syphilis in any stage should be evaluated clinically and serologically. Again, persons who were exposed within the 90 days preceding the diagnosis of primary, secondary, or early latent syphilis in a sex partner might be infected even if seronegative.

Human Immunodeficiency Virus and Syphilis. Concurrent HIV disease is a special situation that requires rather close patient follow-up. First, HIV-infected patients can have abnormal serologic test results (i.e., unusually high, unusually low, and fluctuating titers), making it difficult to determine response to therapy. Second, minor CSF abnormalities are not uncommon in HIV disease even without other central nervous system infections. Often this leads to confusion about the diagnosis of possible neurosyphilis. Thus it is important that HIV-infected patients be evaluated clinically and serologically for treatment failure at 3, 6, 9, 12, and 24 months after therapy. Although unproved, many experts also recommend a CSF examination after therapy (i.e., at 6 months). HIV- infected patients who meet the criteria for treatment failure should be managed the same as those without concurrent HIV. Also, penicillin regimens should be used to treat all stages of syphilis in HIV-infected patients; those with penicillin allergy should be considered candidates for desensitization, especially if being treated for latent syphilis.

Chancroid

The etiologic agent of chancroid is *Haemophilus ducreyi,* a short, gram-negative rod with rounded ends. In stained clinical specimens it is usually obscured by other organisms. *H. ducreyi* is fastidious, requiring special enriched media for culture. Improved culture techniques have shown that chancroid is a more common cause of genital ulcer disease than previously thought. A recent study found the prevalence of chancroid in genital ulcers on culture to range from 12% in Chicago to 20% in Memphis.[14] In addition, coinfection with HIV, *T. pallidum,* or HSV may occur.

Clinical Manifestations. The incubation period of chancroid is 1 to 5 days. The lesions are papular at first but soon form superficial ulcers that are multiple, ragged, and painful, but not indurated (see Fig. 29-3). The granulation tissue at the ulcer base may be covered with a necrotic exudate and easily bleeds with manipulation. In men, ulcers occur at the meatus (where they may cause phimosis or paraphimosis) or on the glans or shaft of the penis. Homosexual men often develop perineal or anal ulceration. In women, ulcers often affect the introitus, labia, and vagina; perianal ulcers in women are often small and may not be painful. Thus a careful examination is important in recognizing these lesions. Genital and perianal chancroid heals slowly. More than 50% of patients develop regional inguinal lymphadenopathy. Lymph nodes become painful and tender, and suppuration may cause a fluctuant inguinal abscess (see Table 29-1).

Diagnosis. A definitive diagnosis of chancroid requires identification of *H. ducreyi* on special culture media not widely available commercially. If culture is an option, a swab from the ulcer should be plated directly onto enriched chocolate agar, which is then incubated in a 5% to 10% CO_2 environment at 33° C. Colonies may not appear for a week or longer. Even with the appropriate media, sensitivity is 80% or less. In areas with infrequent cases, results of culture are correspondingly less satisfactory. PCR has recently emerged as a sensitive diagnostic assay for chancroid.[5] Also, multiplex-PCR reaction can simultaneously amplify for *H. ducreyi, T. pallidum,* and HSV-1 and HSV-2.[15] No reliable serologic test exists for chancroid. Thus the diagnosis is most often a clinical one. The combination of a painful ulcer and tender inguinal adenopathy, which occurs among one third of patients, suggests chancroid; when accompanied by suppurative inguinal adenopathy, these signs are almost pathognomonic. According to CDC guidelines,[4] probable diagnosis, for both clinical and surveillance purposes, may be made if certain criteria are met (Box 29-3).

Treatment. The CDC currently recommends three regimens for treatment of chancroid: (1) single-dose therapy with azithromycin, 1 g orally, or ceftriaxone, 250 mg IM; (2) ciprofloxacin, 500 mg orally twice a day for 3 days; or (3) erythromycin base, 500 mg orally four times a day for

Box 29-3. CDC Guidelines for Diagnosis of Chancroid

- Patient has one or more painful genital ulcers.
- Patient has no evidence of *T. pallidum* infection by darkfield examination of ulcer exudate or by serologic test for syphilis performed at least 7 days after onset of ulcers.
- Clinical presentation, appearance of genital ulcers, and regional lymphadenopathy, if present, are typical for chancroid, and test for herpes simplex virus (HSV) is negative.

7 days. Because its safety has not been established, azithromycin should not be administered to pregnant or lactating women. Ciprofloxacin is contraindicated in pregnancy. Patients should be reexamined 3 to 7 days after starting therapy. If there is no clinical improvement, the physician should reconsider the diagnosis or the patient's compliance.

After successful treatment, prolonged follow-up of chancroid is not necessary. However, if nontreponemicidal drugs were used in the treatment, the patient should undergo a final serologic test for syphilis 3 months after the original exposure to infection.

Lymphogranuloma Venereum

Lymphogranuloma venereum (LGV) is a rare disease in the United States caused by *C. trachomatis* serovars L1, L2, and L3. These strains are immunologically distinct from the *C. trachomatis* strains associated with ocular disease and urethritis/cervicitis.

Clinical Manifestations. The incubation period of LGV is typically less than a week. The initial lesion, a small papule or painless herpetiform ulcer, is transient and inconspicuous. The patient and physician often fail to notice these lesions, which may be seen in women; in men they appear on the glans or shaft of the penis. The most prominent feature of early LGV is inguinal adenitis, which follows the primary lesion by a few days to several weeks. Both inguinal and femoral lymph nodes may be affected. Large, tender masses of nodes appear, sometimes grooved by the inguinal ligament. Lymphadenopathy may be unilateral or bilateral. Abscesses form, causing fluctuant swellings that can discharge spontaneously. Women and homosexual men may have proctocolitis or inflammatory involvement of perirectal or perianal lymphatic tissues, which can result in fistulas and strictures. The inflammation is chronic, with extensive fibrosis, and clinically may be confused with anal carcinomas. Recovery from lymphadenitis is slow, especially without prompt treatment.

Diagnosis. The diagnosis usually is made serologically and by exclusion of other causes of inguinal lymphadenopathy and genital ulcers, such as syphilis, herpes, chancroid, bacterial lymphadenitis, and lymphoproliferative disorders. The most common diagnostic test is a complement fixation test, which uses either LGV or psittacosis antigens; a microimmunofluorescence test is somewhat less widely available. In a patient with LGV the complement fixation test becomes positive a week or two after the infection is acquired, usually with a titer of 1:64 or higher. It is usually impractical to demonstrate a rising titer of antibodies, since in clinical practice, serology is often limited to a single test.

If chlamydial culture facilities are available, LGV may be conclusively diagnosed by isolation of the agent from aspirated buboes. Although the *Chlamydia* detection can probably be accomplished with PCR, the use of this test on aspirated pus has not been rigorously studied.

Treatment. The preferred agent for treatment of LGV is doxycycline, 100 mg by mouth twice a day for 3 weeks. Erythromycin base, 500 mg orally four times a day, is an alternative. Pregnant women should be treated with erythromycin. Azithromycin may be effective in multiple doses over 2 to 3 weeks, but clinical data are lacking.[4] Patients should have follow-up until symptoms have resolved. If the chosen regimen has not resulted in a good clinical response, it may need to be repeated. The stage of the disease when treatment is begun appears to be the most important predictor of success. Inguinal abscesses should undergo aspiration rather than incision.

Granuloma Inguinale

Granuloma inguinale is a poorly understood disease caused by the intracellular gram-negative bacterium, *Calymmatobacterium granulomatis*. A rare disease in the United States, it is endemic in certain tropical and developing areas, including India, Papua New Guinea, central Australia, and southern Africa. The causative organism cannot be cultured on standard microbiologic media, and diagnosis requires visualization on tissue crush preparation or biopsy of dark-staining *C. granulomatis* (Donovan bodies) within the cytoplasm of macrophages. Because this organism cannot be readily cultured and has not been thoroughly characterized, the Koch's postulates have not been fulfilled.

Clinical Manifestations. Granuloma inguinale presents clinically as painless papules on the genitals. These lesions ulcerate and slowly develop into granulation tissue, which spreads over large areas of the genitals without regional lymphadenopathy. The lesions are highly vascular (i.e., beefy red in appearance) and bleed easily on contact. Although inguinal adenitis does not occur, *pseudobuboes* (subcutaneous granulations in the inguinal region) may appear. In anoreceptive homosexuals, granulating lesions develop at the anus and may spread to surrounding areas.

Diagnosis. Microscopy of lesion specimens can confirm a clinical diagnosis. The examiner removes a small fragment of granulomatous tissue from the lesion's edge and smears the undersurface on a glass slide. The specimen is then dried, fixed with methanol, and stained with Wright-Giemsa. Microscopic viewing reveals Donovan bodies within large mononuclear tissue cells; these pink, ovoid bodies are surrounded by two capsules and exhibit bipolar staining. This may be the only aid to diagnosis; culture for *C. granulomatis* is not routinely available, and no serologic test exists.

Treatment. Treatment recommendations include trimethoprim-sulfamethoxazole, one double-strength tablet twice a day for 3 weeks, or doxycycline, 100 mg twice a day for 3 weeks. Patients should be seen for monthly follow-ups until all lesions are healed.[4]

NONULCERATIVE GENITAL LESIONS

Nonulcerative lesions may also appear on the genital surfaces. Some may be infected but not sexually acquired; others are caused by STDs. With the exception of syphilis, the diagnosis of nonulcerative genital lesions is predominantly clinical. However, this clinical diagnosis must be supplemented by biopsy if the diagnosis is unclear or if a premalignant condition is suspected. Genital warts are the most common nonulcerative genital lesion seen, and their appearance is familiar but varied. Condylomata acuminata, genital warts, must be distinguished from warts seen in secondary syphilis, condylomata lata. Often this is only possible with darkfield analysis and serologic testing for syphilis. Again, the two diseases may coexist, so inclusion of one does not always exclude the other. The presence of a smooth rounded umbilicated papule varying in size from barely visible to 3 to 4 mm in diameter suggests a diagnosis of molluscum contagiosum. Sexually transmitted pruritic lesions are usually caused by either scabies or crab lice. Specific diagnostic features, including laboratory investigations, are described later under each condition.

Biopsy for anogenital warts is problematic. Although most are benign, malignancy does develop in some; warts that fail to respond to treatment or that are atypical in any way should be excised for histopathologic examination. Previous podophyllin therapy may make the histology difficult to interpret.

Pruritic lesions should be evaluated for scabies or crab lice. Some nonulcerative genital or anal lesions are caused by STDs. Others are infective but are caused by organisms not sexually transmitted. Others are noninfective, but since they enter into the differential diagnosis of STDs, the physician needs to be familiar with them.

Anogenital Warts

Human papillomavirus (HPV) is the etiologic agent of genital warts. Infection with HPV has increased tenfold over the past 15 years, making anogenital warts the most frequently diagnosed STD in the United States. More than 30 types of HPV infect the anogenital skin and mucosa, causing condylomata and intraepithelial neoplasia of varying severity. HPV types 6 and 11 are associated most often with anogenital warts. HPV types 16, 18, and 45 are distinguished from the others by their strong association with high-grade intraepithelial neoplasia and anogenital malignancy. The oncogenic activity of HPV appears to be related to the expression of three proteins, E6, E7, and E5, which disrupt the normal control of the cell cycle.[17]

HPV has a specific cell tropism and infects the basal layer of squamous or transitional epithelium. As a result of HPV infection, epithelial cells are stimulated to grow, producing hyperplastic proliferation of the epidermis *(acanthosis)* often associated with increased superficial keratin *(hyperkeratosis)*. The host response to HPV infection is poorly understood, but an intact immune system is clearly important in the control of infection. Patients with immune deficiencies, such as HIV infection or transplant recipients, have much more frequent and severe disease.

Clinical Manifestations. Genital warts often result from intercourse with individuals who already have warts. The incubation period is 2 to 3 months. On moist surfaces these lesions appear as sessile or pedunculated exophytic lesions, known as *condylomata acuminata.* Condylomata begin as minute swellings, rapidly growing into fleshy exophytic lesions with pointed surfaces and sometimes fusing into large, irregular masses. In men, condylomata often develop on the glans penis, prepuce, coronal sulcus, or within the urethral meatus (Fig. 29-4, *B*). Typical sites in women include the labia, vaginal introitus, and perianal region. Condylomata may also occur internally on the cervix or vagina and should be suspected in women with vulvar warts.

Other clinical manifestations of HPV infection include papular warts, which are usually small, multiple, keratotic, and less papillary. These usually occur on nonmucosal surfaces such as the penile shaft in men or the labia majora in women. More often, however, HPV infection is subclinical.

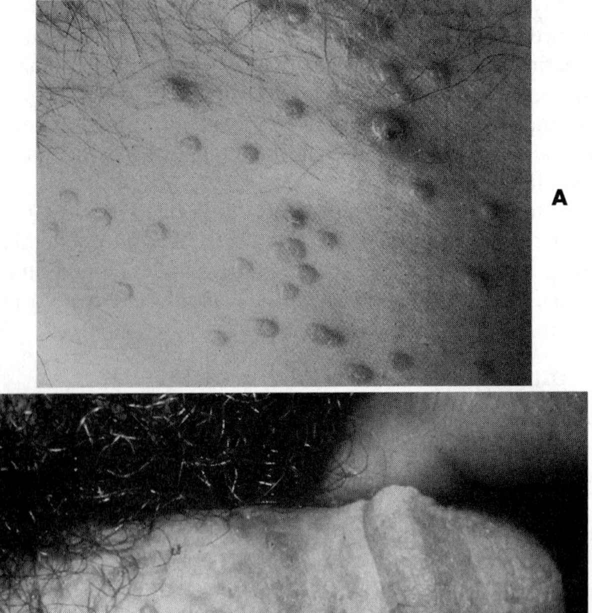

Fig. 29-4. Nonulcerative genital lesions. **A,** Molluscum contagiosum of suprapubic area. Note flesh-colored papules with central umbilication. **B,** Typical condylomata of penile warts, most often associated with human papillomavirus type 6 or 11. (**A** from Holmes KK et al, editors: *Sexually transmitted diseases,* New York, 1984, McGraw-Hill; **B,** from Bingham JS: *Pocket picture guides: sexually transmitted diseases,* London, 1994, Gower.)

Diagnosis. The diagnosis of genital warts is usually clinical. For subclinical infections with HPV, detection can be accomplished only by soaking the area with 3% to 5% acetic acid for 2 to 5 minutes and examining either directly or under magnification for shiny, aceto-whitened areas. Aceto- whitening is not specific for HPV, however, and false-positive tests are common. Colposcopy has been the traditional method of detecting HPV infection in women, but it has recently been advocated for use in male patients as well.

Cytologic and histopathologic examination is helpful in establishing a diagnosis of HPV infection, but its accuracy is difficult to determine without a gold standard for comparison. The classic cytologic findings of HPV infection include squamous cells with hyperchromatic nuclei surrounded by a perinuclear clear zone (koilocytes), multinucleated giant cells, acanthosis, and papillomatosis. Newer methods of detecting HPV infection include nucleic acid hybridization techniques, Southern blot analysis, immunohistochemical techniques, and PCR. The accuracy of Pap smears is variable and depends on the sampling method and the pathologic criteria used. About 10% or more of tissue specimens from women with normal Pap smears may contain HPV DNA, as determined by these other methods, but the clinical significance of this viral DNA is unclear.

Treatment. HPV infection is treated for a variety of reasons, including cosmetic purposes, symptomatic improvement, reduction of viral transmission, and prevention of neoplasia. No current data, however, prove that treatment affects either the transmission or the natural history of the disease. The usual treatment for warts is cytotoxic therapy or ablative therapy.

For provider-administered treatment, several options are available.[4] Cryotherapy with liquid nitrogen or cryoprobe can be applied every 1 to 2 weeks. Podophyllin resin (10% to 25%), an antimitotic agent, can also be applied to the lesions once or twice a week. A single application should not exceed 0.5 ml of a 25% solution because of the risk of absorption and ensuing toxic symptoms. Podophyllin should remain in contact with the lesions for 4 hours before being washed off. Trichloroacetic acid (TCA) or bichloroacetic acid (BCA) 80% to 90% can also be applied weekly. Finally, surgical removal is an option for large warts.

For patient-applied treatment, two options are recommended: podofilox 0.5% solution or imiquimod 5% cream. Patients apply podofilox daily for 3 days, followed by 4 days of no therapy, and repeat this cycle three more times if necessary. Imiquimod cream should be applied at bedtime three times a week for as long as 6 weeks.

The CDC currently recommends cryotherapy as first-line management for anogenital warts. Early studies on BCA and TCA cryotherapy are promising. Unlike podophyllin, TCA can be used in pregnant women and for cervical warts. Liquid nitrogen cryotherapy usually can be swabbed or sprayed onto a lesion. Each individual lesion is frozen down to its base with some adjacent epithelium. Unfortunately, depth of tissue destruction cannot be controlled, and cervical lesions extending into the endocervical canal cannot be reached. Ablative therapy can also be done by specialists with surgical excision, electrocautery/electrodissection, CO_2 laser therapy, and the loop electroexcisional procedure. Although laser therapy does not seem to impart any significant advantage over electrocautery and is costly, cautery is more effective than topical therapies, with recurrence rates of about 25%. Cautery and laser fumes, however, contain bioactive HPV particles, which can contaminate the mucous membranes of the surgical team.

Immunotherapy is probably based more on humoral responses than cell-mediated mechanisms. The direct injection of interferon-α into condylomata has been approved for refractory lesions, although it may have systemic side effects. Immunotherapy is probably most efficacious in an adjuvant setting. For example, trials have demonstrated significantly decreased recurrence rates of condylomata among patients treated with surgical ablation plus intralesional interferon compared with those treated with surgery alone.

All women with external anogenital warts or contacts of patients with anogenital warts should have a Pap smear. Any evidence of atypical cervical cytology is an indication for colposcopy. Patients with condylomata on the urethral meatus or perianal area should also undergo urethroscopic or proctoscopic examination, respectively. In the absence of coexisting dysplasia, treatment of subclinical HPV infection, as detected by Pap smear, colposcopy, biopsy, acetowhitening, or nucleic acid detection, is not recommended (see Chapter 46).

Genital Molluscum Contagiosum

Genital molluscum contagiosum is caused by a poxvirus that has not yet been cultured in vitro. Thus virologic techniques are not used for diagnosis. Although lesions can occur anywhere on the body, in adults they are particularly common on the genitals. The incubation period lasts from 2 to 8 weeks, after which lesions appear. These are raised, flesh-colored, umbilicated papules, 2 to 5 mm in diameter, each with a central depression containing a white plug made up of degenerated epithelial cells and viral inclusion bodies (Fig. 29-4, *A*). The lesions are found on the penis or scrotum in men, on the labia majora in women, and on the inner thighs and pubic area of both sexes.

The lesions are benign and usually resolve spontaneously without significant associated symptoms. In patients coinfected with HIV, however, molluscum can have a severe and unremitting course and may be found in areas outside the genital tract (see Chapter 32).

Scabies

Scabies are caused by the itch mite. The adult female, a round-bodied, eight-legged mite measuring 400 μm in length, travels across human skin at the rate of 2.5 cm (1 inch) per minute. The mite chooses a suitable location and burrows into the horny layer to the boundary of the stratum granulosum, remaining there for the rest of its approximately 30-day life. Within hours of burrowing it begins laying huge eggs, which develop into adult mites in 10 days. The average infested patient hosts about 11 adult female mites.

Clinical Manifestations. The mites tend to settle in specific areas, especially the hands and wrists. Because the eruption is partially caused by immature stages of the mite and by sensitization, the distribution of scabietic lesions does not correspond to that of the adult females. In primary infestation, itching and eruption occur only after sensitization, which takes several weeks. Itching characteristically occurs at night.

The hands are frequently the first areas infested; the lesions, often eczematous, appear primarily on the finger webs and the sides of the digits. Lesions often develop on the flexor surfaces of the wrists, as well as on the extensor surfaces of the elbows (where lesions may be nodular but are usually dry and eczematous) and the anterior axillary folds. In women, eczematic lesions may develop on the breasts. Papular lesions often occur on the abdomen, frequently arranged in a spokelike pattern around the umbilicus. The penis is typically involved; here the lesions may take the form of nodules, pyoderma, or chancriform changes. The infestation may spread to the crease where the buttocks join the upper part of the thighs, causing impetiginous crusting in this area. In adults the palms, soles, scalp, face, neck, and upper back are usually not involved.

The pathognomonic burrow is a short wavy line, dirty in appearance, which often crosses skin lines. It appears most frequently on the finger webs, volar wrists, elbows, and penis. Most infested areas have small, erythematous, often excoriated papules, many of which are larval sites. Secondary eczematization and infection may obscure other features and make diagnosis more difficult. In general, scabies causes polymorphic lesions, although occasionally a patient has urticaria as the only cutaneous feature.

Diagnosis. Diagnosis of scabies requires a specimen from freshly developed, unexcoriated papules or burrows; these can be located with the aid of a hand lens or head loupe.

The physician places mineral oil on a sterile scalpel blade and allows the oil to trickle onto the lesions. Six or seven vigorous scrapes of the scalpel remove the surface of the burrows or papules, along with the oil. The specimen is placed on a glass slide, covered by a coverslip, and viewed under the microscope. The presence of any stage of the mite, or the more numerous fecal pellets, confirms the diagnosis.

Treatment. The CDC-recommended treatment is 5% permethrin cream (Elimite), applied to all areas of the body from the neck down and washed off after 8 to 14 hours.[4] Alternatives include 1% lindane (Kwell) lotion (1 oz) or cream (30 gm), applied thinly from the neck down and washed off thoroughly after 8 hours, or 6% sulfur ointment, applied nightly for 3 nights with thorough washing after the third night. Lindane should not be used after a bath, and it is not recommended for persons with extensive dermatitis, pregnant or lactating women, and children under 2 years of age. An alternative is pyrethrins with piperonyl butoxide, applied and washed off after 10 minutes. Bedding and clothing should be decontaminated as well, but decontamination of the living areas is not necessary. Pruritus can persist for several weeks, but some experts recommend re-treatment if patients are still symptomatic after 1 week. Sexual and close household contacts should be evaluated and treated if necessary.

Pediculosis Pubis (Pubic Lice)

Lice are wingless insects that are obligate parasites. Two species parasitize humans: *pediculus humanus* (which is subdivided into two populations, the head louse and the body louse) and *Phthirus pubis,* the pubic or crab louse, which causes pediculosis pubis. The pubic louse ranges from 0.8 to 1.2 mm in length and is broader than it is long. Powerful claws on the second and third pairs of legs enable the louse to latch onto the pubic hair. From egg to egg, the life cycle of the pubic louse is about 25 days.

Clinical Manifestations. The pubic area is the most common site of infestation. Although the lice tend to remain at the initial site of contact, they occasionally spread to the hairs of the thighs and trunk, especially in hairy individuals, and even to the beard and mustache. Involvement of the eyelashes and periphery of the scalp occurs mainly in children and is probably acquired by close contact with an infested mother.

Pruritus, the most common symptom, begins about 30 days after exposure. Initiated by the louse inserting its mouthparts into a cutaneous cavity and sucking blood, the itching may be immunologic rather than mechanical. Excoriations may lead to pyoderma, which may obscure the organisms. Lymphadenitis and febrile episodes may ensue, although these secondary symptoms are probably less common in developed countries because of early diagnosis and prompt, effective therapy.

Diagnosis. Although not common, the maculae ceruleae are characteristic of pubic lice infestation. These asymptomatic, bluish or slate-colored macules appear on the trunk and thighs and fade shortly thereafter. Two likely causes of the macules are hemoglobin breakdown products of the host and secretions from the parasite's salivary gland.

Involvement of areas other than the pubic region may complicate the diagnosis. Any pruritic eruption of a hairy area should suggest crab lice. In some cases, examination of other areas (e.g., axillae) may be more readily diagnostic, since the patient may have already eradicated the pubic infestation by self-treatment. Eyelash infestation is especially troublesome to diagnose because it may simulate seborrheic, infectious, or eczematous blepharitis; however, careful examination shows that the crusts consist of the parasites.

Pediculosis pubis is rare among STDs in that it can be diagnosed by physical examination alone. The adult lice can be identified with a magnifying lens, especially after feeding, when they become rust colored. Particles of rust-colored excreta may be visible at sites of infestation. Usually, however, the disease is diagnosed by recognizing the numerous nits or ova, which the parasites attach to the pubic hair with a cementlike secretion. Since the nits are initially affixed to the hair at skin level, then grow out with the hair, the length of the infestation can be estimated by the distance of the nits from the skin surface. Although the nits are visible to the naked eye, they can be confused with kinks and knots in the hair or flakes of seborrheic dermatitis. The diagnosis should be confirmed by plucking the hair and identifying the nit under the microscope.

Treatment. The two CDC-recommended regimens are 1% permethrin cream rinse (Elimite), applied to all body areas from the neck down and washed off after 8 to 14 hours, or 1% lindane (Kwell) shampoo, applied thinly from the neck down and washed off thoroughly after 8 hours.[4] Lindane should not be used after a bath, and it is not recommended for persons with extensive dermatitis, pregnant or lactating women, and children under 2 years of age. An alternative is pyrethrins with piperonyl butoxide, applied and washed off after 10 minutes. Bedding and clothing should be decontaminated as well, but decontamination of the living areas is unnecessary. Although pruritus can persist for several weeks, some experts recommend re-treatment if patients are still symptomatic after 1 week. Although corticosteroids may reduce the pruritus associated with pediculosis, they should be avoided. If used before diagnosis, corticosteroids potentiate the infestation, allowing it to become generalized.

Sexual contacts of pediculosis patients should be treated simultaneously to prevent reinfection; other noninfested household members need not be treated. Once the parasites have been eradicated, the patients and sexual partners should wash and dry all used underwear, pajamas, sheets, and pillowcases by machine (hot cycle) or have them dry-cleaned.

REFERENCES

1. Apicella MA, Ketterer M, Lee FK, et al: The pathogenesis of gonococcal urethritis in men: confocal and immunoelectron microscopic analysis of urethral exudates from men infected with *Neisseria gonorrhoeae, J Infect Dis* 173:636, 1996.
2. Burstein GR, Gaydos CA, Diener-West M, et al: Incident *Chlamydia trachomatis* infections among inner-city adolescent females, *JAMA* 280:521, 1998.
3. Burstein GR, Waterfield G, Joffe A, et al: Screening for gonorrhea and chlamydia by DNA amplification in adolescents attending middle school health centers: opportunity for early intervention, *Sex Transm Dis* 25:395, 1998.
4. Centers for Disease Control and Prevention: 1998 Guidelines for treatment of sexually transmitted diseases, *MMWR* RR-01, 1998.

5. Chui L, Albritton W, Paster B, et al: Development of the polymerase chain reaction for diagnosis of chancroid, *J Clin Microbiol* 31:659, 1993.
6. Corey L, Adams HG, Brown ZA, et al: Genital herpes simplex virus infections: clinical manifestations, course, and complications, *Ann Intern Med* 98:958, 1983.
7. Fife KH, Crumpacker CS, Mertz GJ, et al: Recurrence and resistance patterns of herpes simplex virus following cessation of $6 years of chronic suppression with acyclovir: Acyclovir Study Group, *J Infect Dis* 169:1338, 1994.
8. Fraser CM, Norris SJ, Weinstock GM, et al: Complete genome sequence of *Treponema pallidum,* the syphilis spirochete, *Science* 281:375, 1998.
9. Gold D, Corey L: Acyclovir prophylaxis for herpes simplex virus infection, *Antimicrob Agents Chemother* 31:361, 1987.
10. Handsfield HH, Lipman TO, Harnisch JP, et al: Asymptomatic gonorrhea in men: diagnosis, natural course, prevalence and significance, *N Engl J Med* 290:117, 1974.
11. Harrison WO, Hooper RR, Wiesner PJ, et al: A trial of minocycline given after exposure to prevent gonorrhea, *N Engl J Med* 300:1074, 1979.
12. Jacobs NF, Kraus SJ: Gonococcal and nongonococcal urethritis in men: clinical and laboratory differentiation, *Ann Intern Med* 82:7, 1975.
13. Koumans EH, Johnson RE, Knapp JS, et al: Laboratory testing for *Neisseria gonorrhoeae* by recently introduced nonculture tests: a performance review with clinical and public health considerations, *Clin Infect Dis* 27:1171, 1998.
14. Mertz KJ, Trees D, Levine WC, et al: Etiology of genital ulcers and prevalence of human immunodeficiency virus coinfection in 10 U.S. cities: the Genital Ulcer Disease Surveillance Group, *J Infect Dis* 178:1795, 1998.
15. Orle KA, Gates CA, Martin DH, et al: Simultaneous PCR detection of *Haemophilus ducreyi, Treponema pallidum,* and herpes simplex virus types 1 and 2 from genital ulcers, *J Clin Microbiol* 34:49, 1996.
16. Perera SA, Jones C, Srikantha V, et al: Leucocyte esterase test as rapid screen for non-gonococcal urethritis, *Genitourin Med* 63:380, 1987.
17. Pfister H: The role of human papillomavirus in anogenital cancer, *Obstet Gynecol Clin North Am* 23:579, 1996.
18. Shafer MA, Pantell RH, Schachter J: Is the routine pelvic examination needed with the advent of urine-based screening for sexually transmitted diseases? *Arch Pediatr Adolesc Med* 153:119, 1999.
19. Straus SE, Takiff HE, Seidlin M, et al: Suppression of frequently recurring genital herpes: a placebo-controlled double-blind trial of oral acyclovir, *N Engl J Med* 310:1545, 1984.

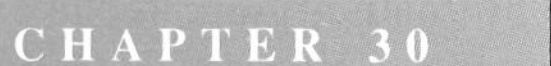

Common Parasitic Diseases

Manoj Jain

PARASITIC AND TROPICAL DISEASES

Parasitic diseases occur worldwide. Tropical diseases are only "tropical" because of climatologic factors affecting vectors and intermediate hosts. Tropical and parasitic diseases can be imported readily into nonendemic areas in an age of rapid air travel and mass migration. An individual acquiring Lassa fever in West Africa may fly to Paris, then to New York, and on to Kansas City within 24 hours, with the evolution of symptoms and the potential for spread throughout the trip. This may lead to secondary cases in persons who are in transit to dozens of other destinations.

This chapter is designed as an overview for the primary care physician to suggest diagnostic possibilities in a limited number of settings. The reader is referred to detailed textbooks of parasitic and/or tropical diseases and geographic medicine for more comprehensive coverage of particular diseases.

Many parasitic diseases are easily diagnosed and treated by well-established routine procedures and management options. The diagnosis and management of other parasitic diseases may be challenging and may require special expertise, uncommon tests, and unusual drugs. The practitioner should be aware of the services provided by the appropriate departments in medical and public health schools and by local public health agencies. The U.S. Centers for Disease Control and Prevention (CDC) provides advice in the diagnosis and management of parasitic diseases and telephone health advice for travelers. (The website for the CDC is www.cdc.com.) It is a source of unreleased and investigational drugs. The CDC also publishes information about parasitic and tropical diseases in the *Morbidity and Mortality Weekly Reports* and its supplements. Periodic supplements review recommendations for health aspects of world travel. Similar services are available through public health ministries and agencies in other countries, as well as from the World Health Organization (WHO).

Parasites of the Alimentary Tract

Parasitic worms of the alimentary tract are highly adapted to existence in the human gastrointestinal tract, its vasculature, and the biliary tract. Table 30-1 lists the parasitic worms that commonly infest and infect the alimentary tract and related structures. The successful parasite causes limited morbidity in its host. The vast majority of people infested with the common worm parasites are asymptomatic. In fact, symptoms are usually the result of a larger than usual number of parasites, or a heavy "worm load." Asymptomatic infestation, however, may have chronic effects on the host that are not immediately apparent. Symptomatic bearers of worms usually have nonspecific complaints, except for peculiar clinical syndromes discussed later. Many times alimentary tract worms are discovered incidentally when stool is examined in the course of a diagnostic workup for complaints that may or may not be related to the infestation. Diarrhea caused by the protozoan parasites is discussed later.

The worm or metazoan (multicellular) parasites of the human alimentary tract and associated organs are divided between two phyla: the flatworms or Platyhelminthes and the roundworms or Nematoda. The worms of both major groups have complex life cycles involving varied intermediate and definitive hosts and larval stages.

Roundworms of the Alimentary Tract. The intestinal nematodes, or roundworms, have a worldwide distribution and infest hundreds of millions of individuals. The human intestinal roundworms include *Strongyloides stercoralis,* the hookworms (*Ancylostoma duodenale* and *Necator americanus*), *Ascaris lumbricoides,* the whipworm *(Trichuris trichiura),* and the pinworm *(Enterobius vermicularis).* Over one billion persons worldwide are estimated to be carriers of *Ascaris,* at least 500 million carry *Trichuris,* and an estimated 42 million in the United States are infested with pinworms. Other worms include *Capillaria philippinensis,* which is an intestinal nematode that causes a severe disease in humans, mostly limited in distribution to parts of the Philippines, but

Table 30-1. Parasitic Worms That Commonly Infest or Infect the Alimentary Tract and Associated Structures

Parasite	Common name
Roundworms	
Ascaris lumbricoides	Large roundworm
Ancylostoma duodenale	Old World hookworm
Necator americanus	New World hookworm
Strongyloides stercoralis	Threadworm
Trichuris trichiura	Whipworm
Enterobius vermicularis	Pinworm
Capillaria philippinensis	
Flatworms	
Tapeworms	
Taenia solium	Pork tapeworm
Taenia saginata	Beef tapeworm
Diphyllobothrium latum	Broad fish tapeworm
Hymenolepis nana	Dwarf tapeworm
Hymenolepis diminuta	Rat tapeworm
Dipylidium caninum	Dog tapeworm
Blood flukes	
Schistosoma mansoni	
Schistosoma japonicum	
Schistosoma mekongi	
Schistosoma malayensis	
Schistosoma haematobium	
Schistosoma intercalatum	
Intestinal flukes	
Fasciolopsis buski	
Heterophyes heterophyes	
Metagonimus yokogawai	
Liver flukes	
Clonorchis sinensis	Chinese liver fluke
Opisthorchis felineus	
Opisthorchis viverrini	
Fasciola hepatica	Sheep liver fluke
Fasciola gigantica	

rarely reported in other parts of the world as well. These worms live in the mucosa of the small bowel and are occasionally invasive. They are acquired by ingesting freshwater fish containing larvae. The intestinal nematodes have host dependence of varying degree. *S. stercoralis* can live and reproduce in soil as a free-living organism. The larvae of hookworms feed in soil but require a host for maturation and reproduction. The larvae of *Ascaris, T. trichiura,* and *E. vermicularis* develop in excreted eggs and hatch when the eggs are ingested by another host.

Strongyloides Stercoralis. The life cycle of *S. stercoralis* is summarized in Fig. 30-1. Eggs hatch in the host intestine, giving rise to free-living rhabditiform larvae that are passed in the stool. In warm, moist soil the rhabditiform larvae may go on to mature to free-living adult forms or develop into filariform larvae that are capable of invading human skin. Larvae migrate from the skin to the bloodstream and are carried to the lung, where they penetrate the airway, climb the trachea, and are subsequently swallowed. In the proximal small bowel the larvae mature to the adult forms that invade the mucosa. The rhabditiform larvae also may develop into filariform larvae in the gut lumen, leading to autoinfection and maintenance of the disease despite removal of the host from an endemic area. In immunosuppressed and debilitated patients, patients with human immunodeficiency virus (HIV) infection, and patients on corticosteroids, this cycle of autoinfection may lead to a syndrome of hyperinfection with *S. stercoralis*.

Most patients with strongyloidiasis are asymptomatic. A heavy worm load can lead to epigastric pain, weakness, malaise, and watery diarrhea, perhaps due to an absorptive defect. Upper gastrointestinal radiographic studies may show duodenal and jejunal mucosal edema. Ulceration and even intestinal perforation may occur. The hyperinfective syndrome can be an overwhelming systemic disease that is often fatal. Extensive migration of larvae can lead to derangement of multiple organs, abscesses in the liver and other organs, and development of adult worms in the bronchial tree. The diagnosis of strongyloidiasis is made by demonstrating larval forms in the stool (Fig. 30-2) or parasites in duodenal aspirates or biopsies.

Hookworm. Hookworm disease is transmitted by passage of eggs in the stool, which hatch in warm, moist soil, forming rhabditiform larvae that develop within a few days into filariform larvae. There are no free-living adult forms. Filariform larvae invade the skin and migrate in the same way as the larvae of *S. stercoralis*. The life cycle of the hookworm is summarized in Fig. 30-3. Once the larvae reach the small intestine, they mature to adults that attach to the duodenal and jejunal mucosa and suck blood. An adult *A. duodenale* is capable of sucking up to 0.1 to 0.3 ml of blood per day; *N. americanus* removes somewhat less. The worms produce an anticoagulant that causes blood to ooze around the feeding worm, leading to blood in the stool and more blood loss. Worm load can be in the thousands, and the life span of adult hookworms may be several years. Humans may develop infestation with other species of hookworm that have animals, such as dogs and cats, as primary hosts.

The most important clinical manifestation of hookworm disease is anemia. The degree of anemia is a function of the worm load. This iron deficiency anemia is due to chronic blood loss and is compounded by malnutrition; it may be severe enough to lead to cardiomegaly. Varying degrees of malabsorption are a concomitant of the infestation and further complicate the disease. Children with significant worm loads may experience growth retardation and inanition. Individuals with hookworm disease may also complain of hunger and nondescript abdominal pain. The diagnosis is made by demonstrating the hookworm ova in the stool (see Fig. 30-2). Hookworm should be suspected in any patient with hypochromic, microcytic anemia who is living in a warm climate with direct exposure to moist soil.

The filariform larvae of *S. stercoralis* and the hookworms can cause a localized dermatitis, called ground itch, when they invade the skin. The usual setting is warm, moist soil and bare feet. Likewise, larval migration through tissues may lead to systemic and pulmonary symptomatology. Skin and systemic syndromes produced by migrating nematode larvae are discussed later.

Ascaris Lumbricoides. *A. lumbricoides* is the largest intestinal roundworm, reaching lengths of up to 30 cm. The life cycle of the worm is presented in Fig. 30-4. The infestation is acquired when embryonated eggs, which are passed in the stool and mature in soil, are ingested. The larvae hatch in the bowel, invade the bowel wall, and are carried to

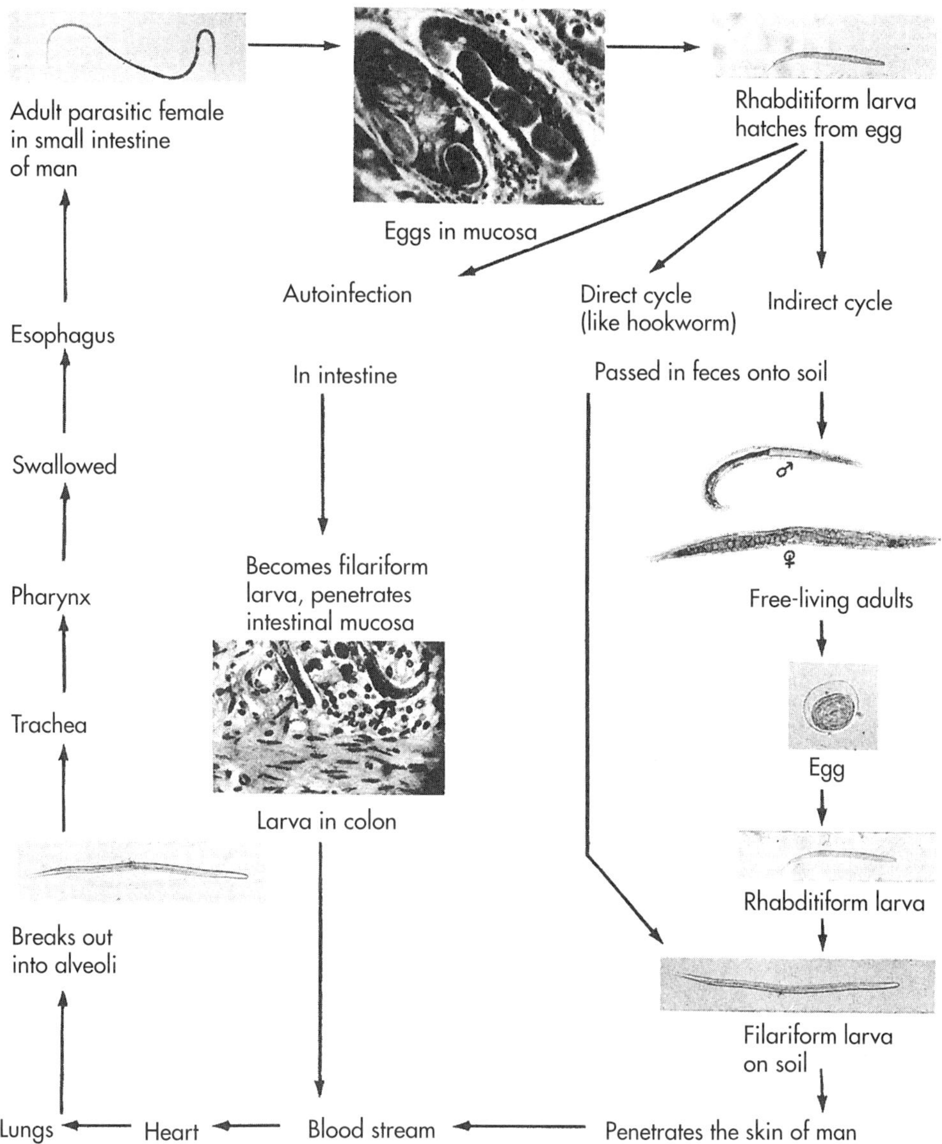

Fig. 30-1. Life of cycle of *Strongyloides stercoralis*. (From Brown HW, Neva FA: *Basic clinical parasitology*, ed 5, Norwalk, Conn, 1983, Appleton-Century-Crofts.)

the lungs, where they penetrate the alveoli, climb the trachea, and are swallowed. This migration can lead to marked peripheral eosinophilia and pulmonary infiltrates. The adult worms mature in the small intestinal lumen, and the mature female worm can produce more than 200,000 eggs a day.

The major symptoms of ascariasis are due to the migrating larvae. These systemic symptoms are discussed later in the chapter. Individuals carrying adult worms are usually asymptomatic. Symptoms, when they occur, are related to the worm load. With light to moderate infestation, vague abdominal pain may occur. With heavy infestation, especially in children, the major complication is mechanical obstruction of the intestine caused by the mass of worms. Worms may migrate to aberrant locations causing biliary tract obstruction, pancreatitis, or appendicitis. Occasionally bowel perforation and peritonitis occur. Diagnosis of ascariasis is made by demonstrating fertilized and unfertilized eggs in stool (see Fig. 30-2). Adult worms in the bowel lumen may appear on intestinal radiographic contrast studies.

Trichuris Trichiura. The adult *T. trichiura*, the whipworm, attaches to the colonic mucosa. Eggs passed in the stool mature in the soil. Ingested eggs hatch in the small bowel, and the larvae pass into the colon where they mature. The larvae do not invade tissue. Most patients with whipworm are asymptomatic. Heavy infestation may lead to dysentery-like symptoms and occasionally hemorrhage and anemia. Rectal prolapse may occur, and the small white worms may be seen attached to the prolapsed mucosa ("coconut cake" rectum). Diagnosis is made by demonstrating the typical eggs in the stool (see Fig. 30-2).

Enterobius Vermicularis. The pinworm, *E. vermicularis*, also inhabits the colon. Adult female worms migrate through the anus at night and deposit eggs on the perianal and perineal skin. The migration causes intense pruritus. The eggs become infective within hours and are resistant to drying. They can disseminate widely, similar to dust particles, leading to autoinfection as well as family and institutional outbreaks (Fig. 30-5). Whole families typically become infested. After

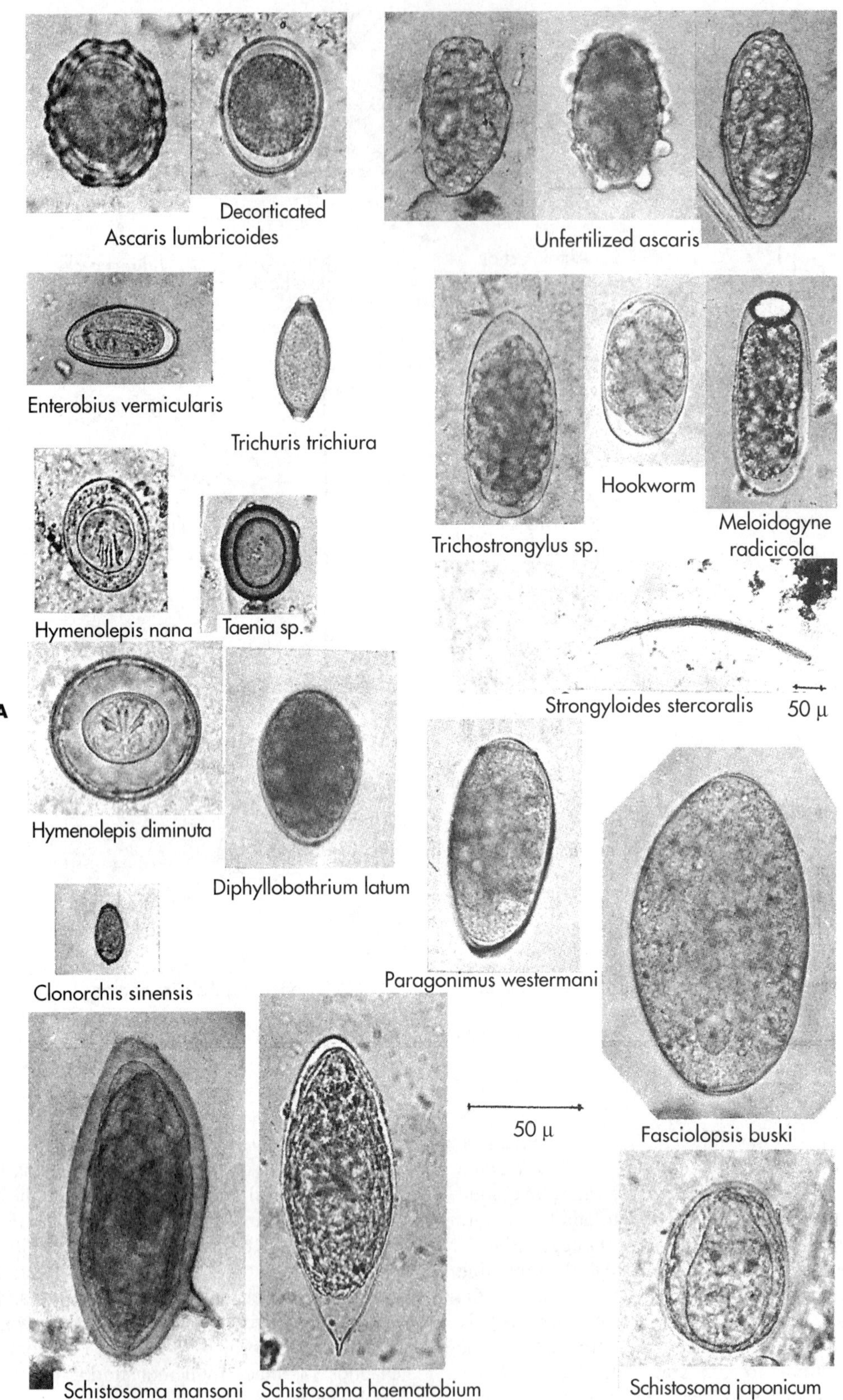

Fig. 30-2. Worm eggs (**A**) encountered during microscopic examination of stool. (From Brown HW, Neva FA: *Basic clinical parasitology,* ed 6, Norwalk, Conn, 1994, Appleton-Century-Crofts.)

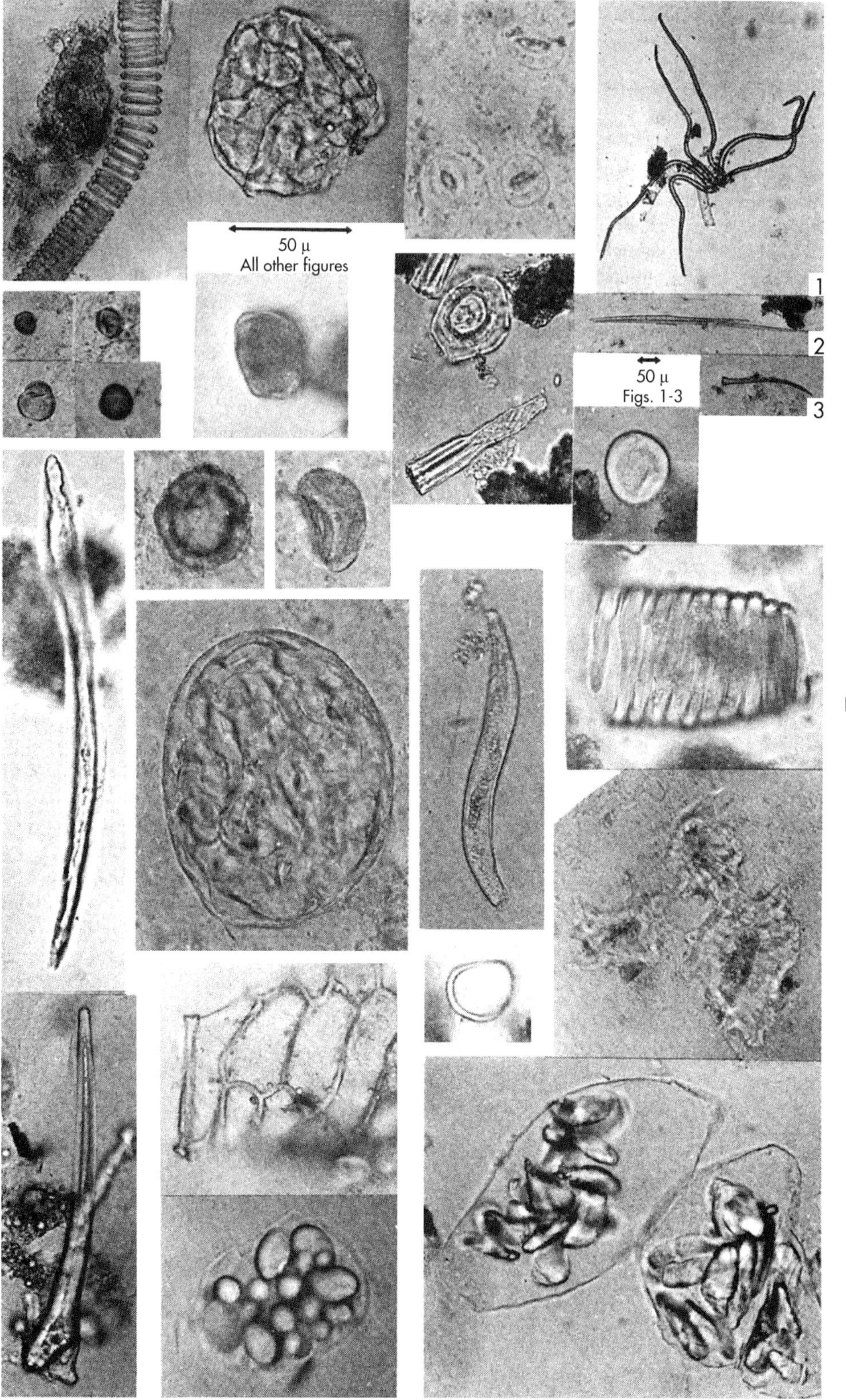

Fig. 30-2, cont'd. Fecal vegetable artifacts (**B**) that may be confused with ova and parasites.

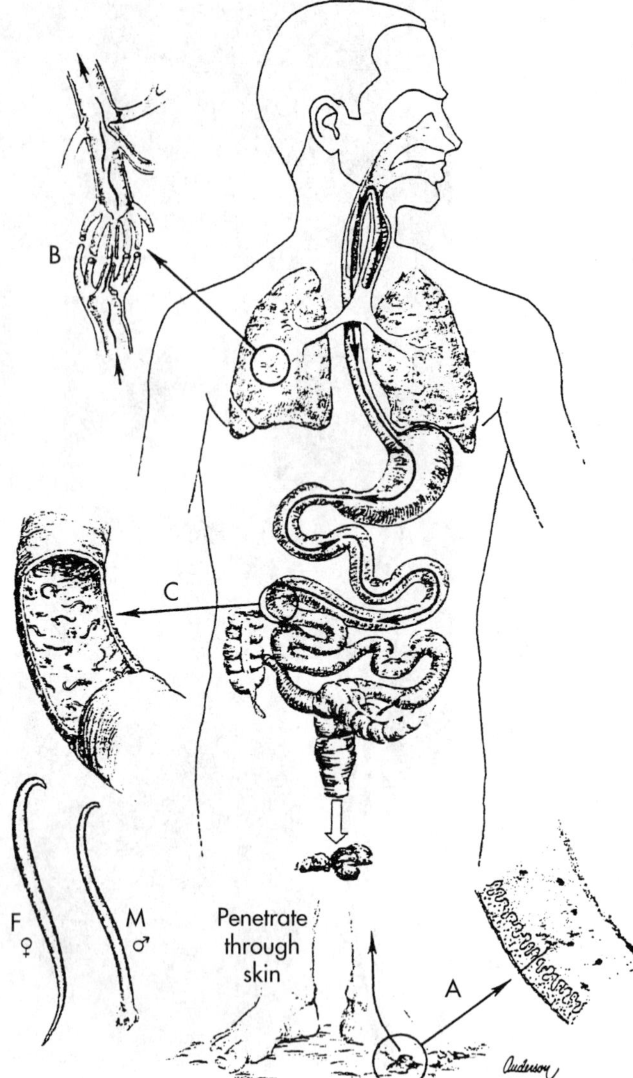

Fig. 30-3. Life cycle of the hookworm. Filariform larvae in *(A)* the soil penetrate the skin and are carried in the circulation to the lungs *(B)* where they break out of the capillary bed into the alveolar spaces, are swept up the bronchial tree, are swallowed, and become adult worms *(C)* in the small intestine. (From Beck JW, Davies JE: *Medical parasitology,* ed 3, St Louis, 1981, Mosby.)

ingestion, the eggs hatch in the small bowel and migrate to the colon, where they mature. There is no tissue invasion.

The primary symptoms of pinworm infestation are related to the nocturnal migration of the gravid female worms. Moderate to severe perianal pruritus occurs, and excoriation from scratching results. Migration to the vagina may cause vaginitis. The diagnosis may be made by demonstrating eggs or worms in the stool, but it is more easily established by microscopic examination of transparent (Scotch) tape, the adhesive side of which has been pressed to the anus and perianal skin (see Fig. 30-5). The highest yield is obtained during the night or early morning. Adult female worms are captured on the adhesive tape.

The treatment for intestinal nematodes has been made simpler by the availability of mebendazole (Vermox). This agent can be used for all the worms except *S. stercoralis.* Asymptomatic, light infestation with hookworms, without anemia, need not be treated. In the case of mixed infestations, including *Ascaris,* treatment is directed against *Ascaris* first, since inadequate treatment of these worms may result in their aberrant migration. Entire families of patients with pinworm should be treated to prevent recurrence. *S. stercoralis* infestations are treated with thiabendazole. Current recommendations for the treatment of persons with intestinal roundworms are summarized in Table 30-2. Mebendazole is teratogenic in animals and should not be used during pregnancy (albendazole is a related benzimidazole), although the alternative, pyrantel pamoate, has not been established as safe in pregnant women and the fetus.

Tapeworms. The tapeworms, or cestodes, are hermaphroditic flatworms. Adults live in the gut lumen of the definitive host. These worms have no gut and absorb nutrients across their integument. Larval forms encyst in the tissues of intermediate hosts.

Four tapeworms are important human intestinal parasites: *Taenia saginata* (beef tapeworm), *T. solium* (pork tapeworm), *Diphyllobothrium latum* (broad or fish tapeworm), and *Hymenolepis nana* (dwarf tapeworm). The first three are named after the usual food source from which people acquire the parasite. Larval forms, encysted in meat or fish (the cysticercus or plerocercoid, respectively), are ingested and develop into adult forms in the gut lumen. *H. nana* uses the human as both definitive and intermediate host. Cysticerci of this species develop in the bowel wall, and larvae are released into the lumen to form more adults. *H. nana* is transmitted through ingestion of ova passed in stool. *T. solium* (Fig. 30-6) also is capable of using humans as its intermediate host. Ova may be ingested with material contaminated with stool from an affected person, or ova may reach the stomach or

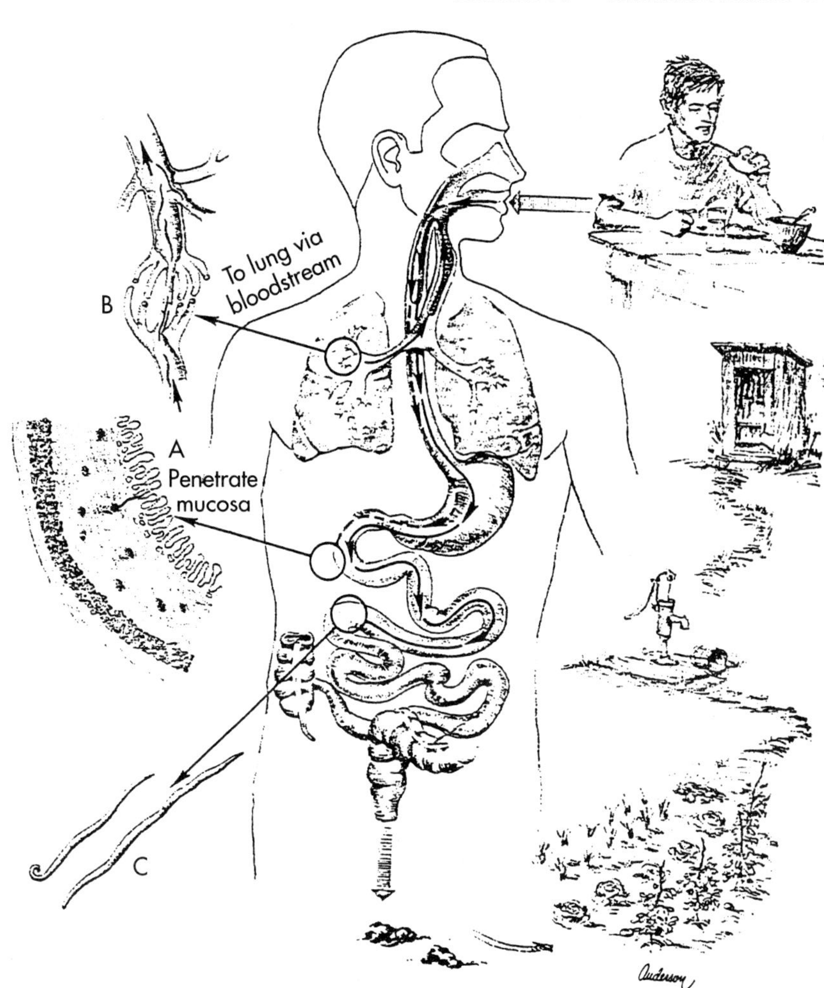

Fig. 30-4. Life cycle of *Ascaris lumbricoides*. Infective eggs, ingested in contaminated food and water, hatch in the small intestine where *penetration of the mucosa (A)* results in invasion of the bloodstream by the larvae, which are carried to the lungs. The larvae, too large to cross the capillary bed, break out into the alveolar spaces *(B)*, are carried up the bronchial tree, are swallowed, and reach the small intestine where they become adult worms *(C)*. (From Beck JW, Davies JE: *Medical parasitology*, ed 3, St Louis, 1981, Mosby.)

duodenum by reverse peristalsis. The ova hatch, producing larvae that invade tissue, leading to cysticercosis, a disease discussed below in the section dealing with parasites that cause mass lesions in tissue.

Several tapeworms, which are primarily parasites of other animals, are occasionally found in the human gut. Of note are *Dipylidium caninum* (dog or cat tapeworm) and *H. diminuta* (rat tapeworm), which infect humans when the intermediate host, the flea, is inadvertently ingested.

Tapeworms are composed of a scolex, or head, that attaches to the intestinal mucosa, and a chain of progressively mature segments (proglottids) that contain the reproductive parts and produce ova. Gravid proglottids and eggs are shed in the stool. These ova may then reinfect in the case of *H. nana* or are ingested by intermediate hosts, hatch, invade, and form tissue cysts. Tapeworms are cosmopolitan parasites. Epidemics of *D. latum* in the United States have been associated with eating certain types of fish from Midwestern lakes. Control measures for tapeworms include adequate cooking of meat and fish, sanitary hygiene practices, and assurance of safe feed for hogs and cattle.

Most patients with tapeworms are asymptomatic. Worms may be harbored in the gut for many years. Symptoms, when they occur, may be related to heavy worm load and are usually nondescript; they include mild abdominal pain, diarrhea, malaise, and occasionally constipation. The motile proglottids of *Taenia* sometime force their way through the anus. *D. latum* can successfully compete with the host for vitamin B_{12} and infestation with this tapeworm can lead to megaloblastic anemia. The ability of *H. nana* to autoinoculate may lead to heavy worm loads and cramping pain, diarrhea, nausea and vomiting, and headache. Intestinal erosions may occur. In children, heavy *H. nana* infestation may be associated with irritability and rarely seizures. These neurologic manifestations have been ascribed to absorption of toxic substances produced by the worms. The diagnosis of tapeworm infestation is made by demonstrating eggs (see Fig. 30-2) or proglottids in the stool.

Praziquantel is the drug of choice for tapeworm disease. The oral dose is 5 to 10 mg/kg in one dose for *T. solium, T. saginata,* and *D. latum* and 25 mg/kg in one dose for *H. nana*. The alternative agent for tapeworms is niclosamide in an adult dose of 2 gm once for all the tapeworms except for *H. nana,* which is treated with 2 gm as one dose, then 1 gm/day for 6 days, as the drug is inactive against the cysticerci in the bowel wall that erupt after 4 days. The pediatric doses of niclosamide are adjusted to 1.0 or 1.5 gm.

Flukes

Schistosomiasis (Blood Flukes). Acute schistosomiasis may present as a febrile, systemic process. It occurs 1 to 2 months after exposure to cercariae, at a time corresponding to the onset of egg production by the parasite. It is characterized by fever, weight loss, diarrhea, cough, abdominal pain, and headache. Acute disease may be especially severe with *Schistosoma japonicum* infection and is called Katayama fever. Peripheral blood eosinophilia is often of marked degree.

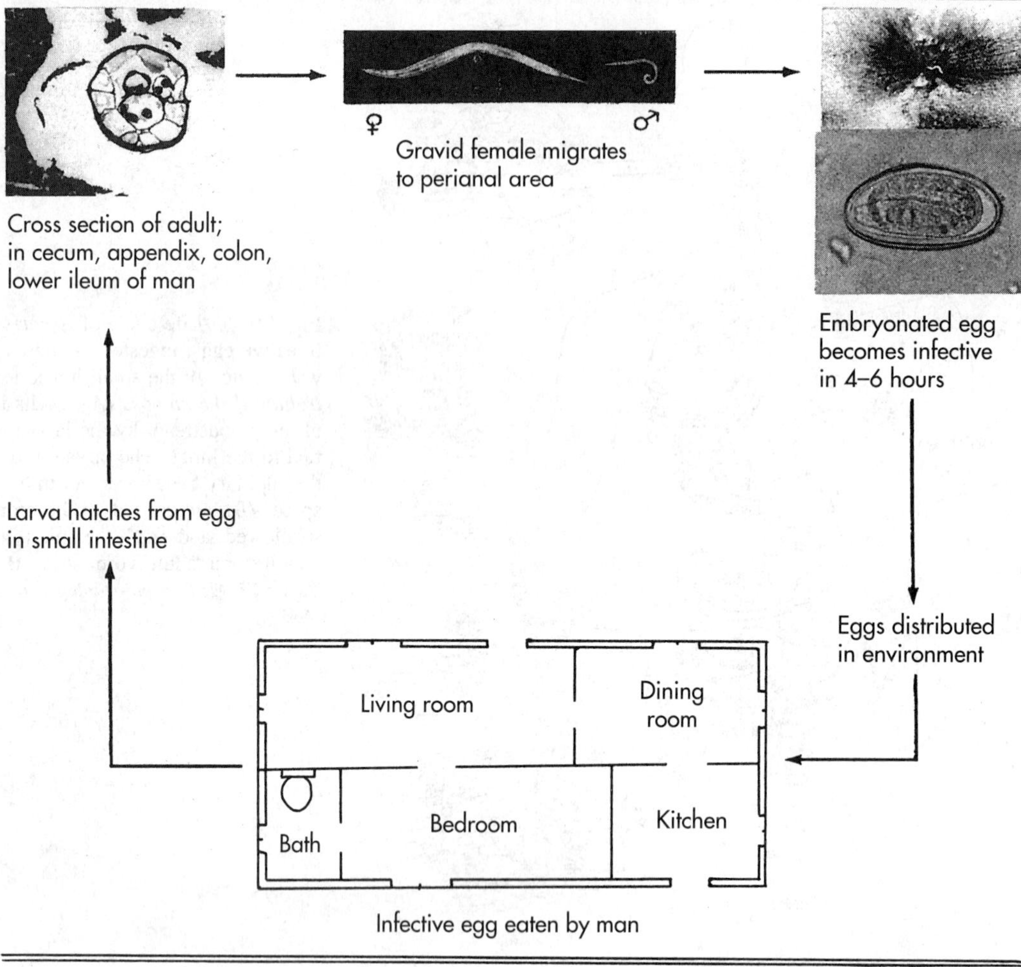

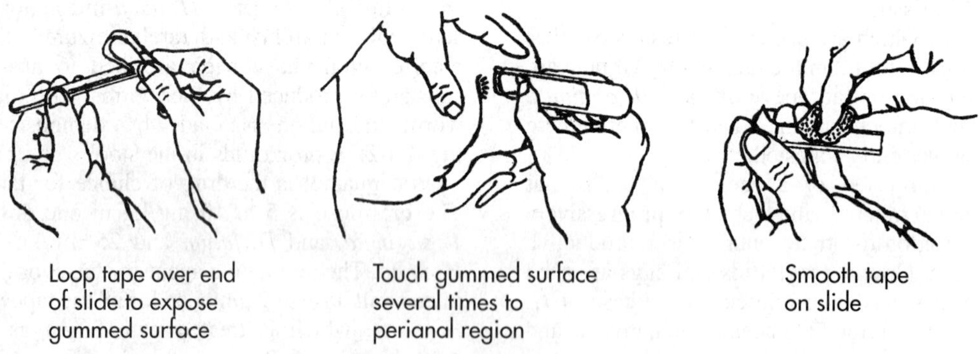

Fig. 30-5. Life cycle of *Enterobius vermicularis* and the procedure for the adhesive tape test to reveal migrating worms. (From Brown HW, Neva FA: *Basic clinical parasitology,* ed 5, Norwalk, Conn, 1983, Appleton-Century-Crofts.)

Several trematode worms, or flukes, are capable of infecting humans. The most important human flukes are in the genus *Schistosoma*. More than 200 million people worldwide have schistosomiasis. The predominant species that infect humans are *S. mansoni, S. japonicum, S. mekongi,* and *S. haematobium. S. malayensis* occurs in Southeast Asia and resembles *S. japonicum* and *S. mekongi. S. intercalatum* is closely related to *S. haematobium* and is an increasing problem in Africa.

Schistosomes have complex life cycles (Fig. 30-7), which involve specific snails as intermediate hosts. The disease occurs in many parts of the world. Its distribution depends on the distribution of particular species of snail. The disease is acquired by exposure to fresh water containing the fork-tailed larvae, called cercariae, which are released from the intermediate host. Cercariae are capable of penetrating the skin, where they lose their tails and become schistosomula. Schistosomulae migrate to the lung, then the liver, where they

Table 30-2. Treatment for Intestinal Roundworms

Parasite	Drug of choice	Alternative agent	Comment
Strongyloides stercoralis	Thiabendazole, 25 mg/kg, by mouth, bid for 2 days (maximum dose 3 g/day)	Ivermectin, 200 μg/kg/day, by mouth for 1 to 2 days	Hyperinfection syndrome requires longer therapy or other agents.
Hookworms *Ancylostoma duodenale* *Necator americanus*	Mebendazole, 100 mg, by mouth, bid for 3 days	Albendazole, 400 mg, by mouth, once	Doses are the same for children >2 years old. Pyrantel is considered investigational in the treatment of hookworm.
		Pyrantel pamoate, 11 mg/kg, by mouth, as a single dose (maximum 1 gram)	Nutritional support and iron supplements are important. Blood loss may continue after worms are shed.
Ascaris lumbricoides	Mebendazole, 100 mg, by mouth, bid for 3 days	Pyrantel pamoate, as above Albendazole, 400 mg by mouth, once	Pediatric (>2 years) doses are the same.
Trichuris trichiura	Mebendazole, 100 mg, by mouth, bid for 3 days	Albendazole, 400 mg, by mouth, once	Heavy infestation may require 3 days of albendazole. Pediatric (>2 years) doses are the same.
Enterobius vermicularis	Mebendazole, 100 mg, by mouth, one dose; repeat in 2 weeks	Pyrantel pamoate, as above, as one dose; repeat in 2 weeks Albendazole, 400 mg, by mouth, once, repeat in 2 weeks	Family and household contacts should be treated. Pediatric doses are the same.

mature to adult forms. The adult forms then join in permanent sexual coupling and migrate to their final intravascular location, the mesenteric veins in the case of *S. mansoni, S. japonicum, S. mekongi,* and *S. malayensis;* the perirectal venules in the case of *S. intercalatum;* and the venous plexus of the urinary bladder in the case of *S. haematobium.* The mating pair of adult worms produce hundreds to thousands of eggs daily over several years. These eggs make their way across the intestinal and bladder mucosae and are excreted. In fresh water the eggs hatch larvae, called miracidia, which invade snails and continue the cycle.

The signs and symptoms of schistosomiasis depend on the worm load. An acute illness usually occurs about 1 month (2 weeks to 2 months) after exposure to the cercariae and correlates with the time of initial egg production. This syndrome is characterized by fever, abdominal pain, diarrhea, and pulmonary complaints associated with marked peripheral blood eosinophilia. *S. japonicum* is the most prodigious egg producer, and the syndrome it produces, Katayama fever, usually occurs with the most severe infection due to other species, but it may occur with heavy infection due to other species. Most of the morbidity of schistosomiasis is seen with chronic infection. Chronically affected individuals may have systemic complaints, diarrhea, and abdominal pain. Presinusoidal portal hypertension may result from eggs lodging in the sinusoids of the liver with resultant chronic inflammation. Eggs may be shunted to the systemic circulation with deposition in the lungs, central nervous system (CNS), and other organs. Involvement of the urinary tract with *S. haematobium* can lead to structural abnormalities due to granuloma formation with obstruction, secondary infection, and uremia.

The diagnosis of schistosomiasis is made by demonstrating the characteristic eggs in stool or urine (see Fig. 30-2). Urine is best collected between noon and 2 PM. Because eggs may continue to make their way into excreta for a prolonged period, a count of viable eggs, allowed to hatch in vitro, is a better indicator of live worm load than simple stool examination. Rectal biopsy with demonstration of eggs in the mucosa may be used to diagnose all species.

Praziquantel is the drug of choice for the treatment of schistosomiasis. Recommended doses vary depending on the species of schistosome. Oxamniquine also is effective in the treatment of *S. mansoni* infection. Metriphonate is an alternative drug for the treatment of *S. haematobium.* The latter drugs and advice about their use are available through the CDC. Current recommendations for the treatment of schistosomiasis are summarized in Table 30-3. Many patients with schistosomiasis have a small worm burden and do not require therapy. The decision to treat should be based on the severity of symptoms, clinical activity, and worm load.

Intestinal Flukes. The intestinal flukes, *Fasciolopsis buski, Heterophyes heterophyes,* and *Metagonimus yokogawai,* inhabit the small bowel. These worms have a complex life cycle involving snails and aquatic plants or fish as intermediate hosts. They occur primarily in Asia, but *H. heterophyes* also is seen in Egypt. Most affected individuals are symptomatic, although abdominal pain and diarrhea are occasionally associated with infestation. Diagnosis is made by demonstrating eggs in stool (see Fig. 30-2). Praziquantel in doses of 25 mg/kg three times in 1 day is effective for the treatment of intestinal flukes.

Liver Flukes. Five species of liver fluke are most likely to infect humans: *Clonorchis sinensis, Opisthorchis felineus, O. viverrini, Fasciola hepatica,* and *F. gigantica.* The first three occur primarily in Asia and Eastern Europe, whereas *Fasciola* species are common parasites of sheep and cattle and are distributed widely. The liver flukes have a complex life cycle, with snails as primary intermediate hosts; secondary intermediate hosts include fish and aquatic plants. The

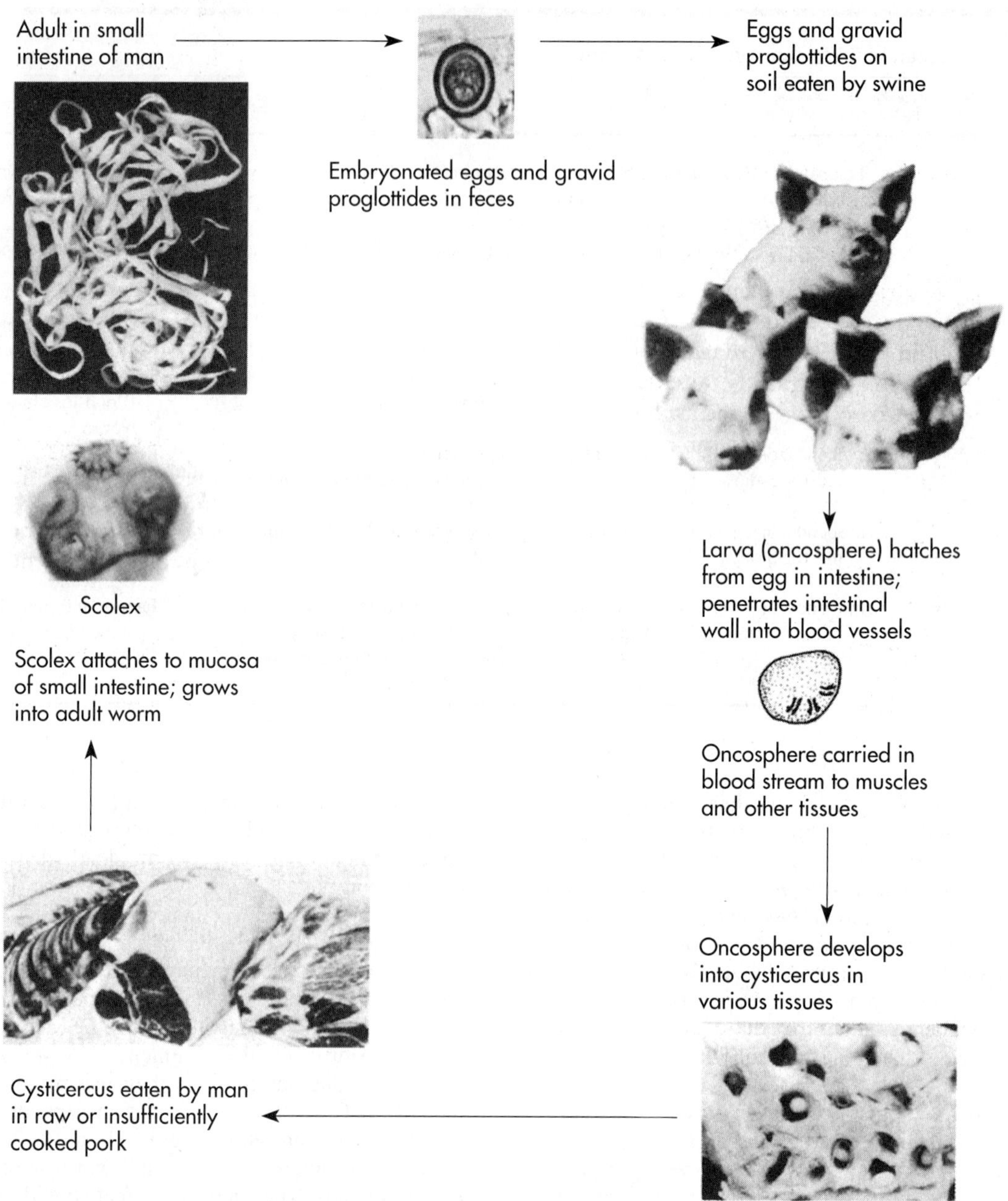

Fig. 30-6. Life cycle of *Taenia solium*. (From Brown HW, Neva FA: *Basic clinical parasitology*, ed 5, Norwalk, Conn, 1983, Appleton-Century- Crofts.)

adult worms live in the biliary tract. The vast majority of individuals with liver flukes are asymptomatic, but early in *F. hepatica* infection the migration of worms into the biliary tract may be associated with fever, hepatomegaly, right upper quadrant pain, and eosinophilia. Occasionally, biliary obstruction and cholangitis occur. Eggs appear in bile and stool.

Praziquantel in a dose of 25 mg/kg three times in 1 day is effective therapy for *Opisthorchis* species and *C. sinensis*. Bithionol (available from the CDC) in a dose of 20 mg/kg twice a day, every other day, for 10 to 15 doses is currently recommended for *F. hepatica*. Triclabendazole, a veterinary drug that may have fewer side effects, also has been used to treat sheep liver flukes.

Protozoan Infections

Protozoa are single cell organisms that cause a wide range of infections. Protozoa invade various organs of the body causing infection of the intestine, blood, or deep tissues. Some protozoa, such as *Pneumocystis carinii, Toxoplasma gondii,* and *Cryptosporidium* have become significant causes of morbidity and mortality among acquired immunodeficiency syndrome (AIDS) patients.

Intestinal Protozoan Infections

Entamoeba Histolytica (see Chapter 111). The diagnosis of amebiasis is made by demonstrating trophozoites or cysts in the stool of the affected individual (Fig. 30-8). These are best demonstrated in a fresh stool sample. Several other amebae that are of little or no pathogenic significance may be found in the stool, so that examination of the stool requires an experienced observer.

Effective treatment of symptomatic intestinal amebiasis must be directed toward eradication of both invasive organisms and luminal trophozoites and cysts. Metronidazole

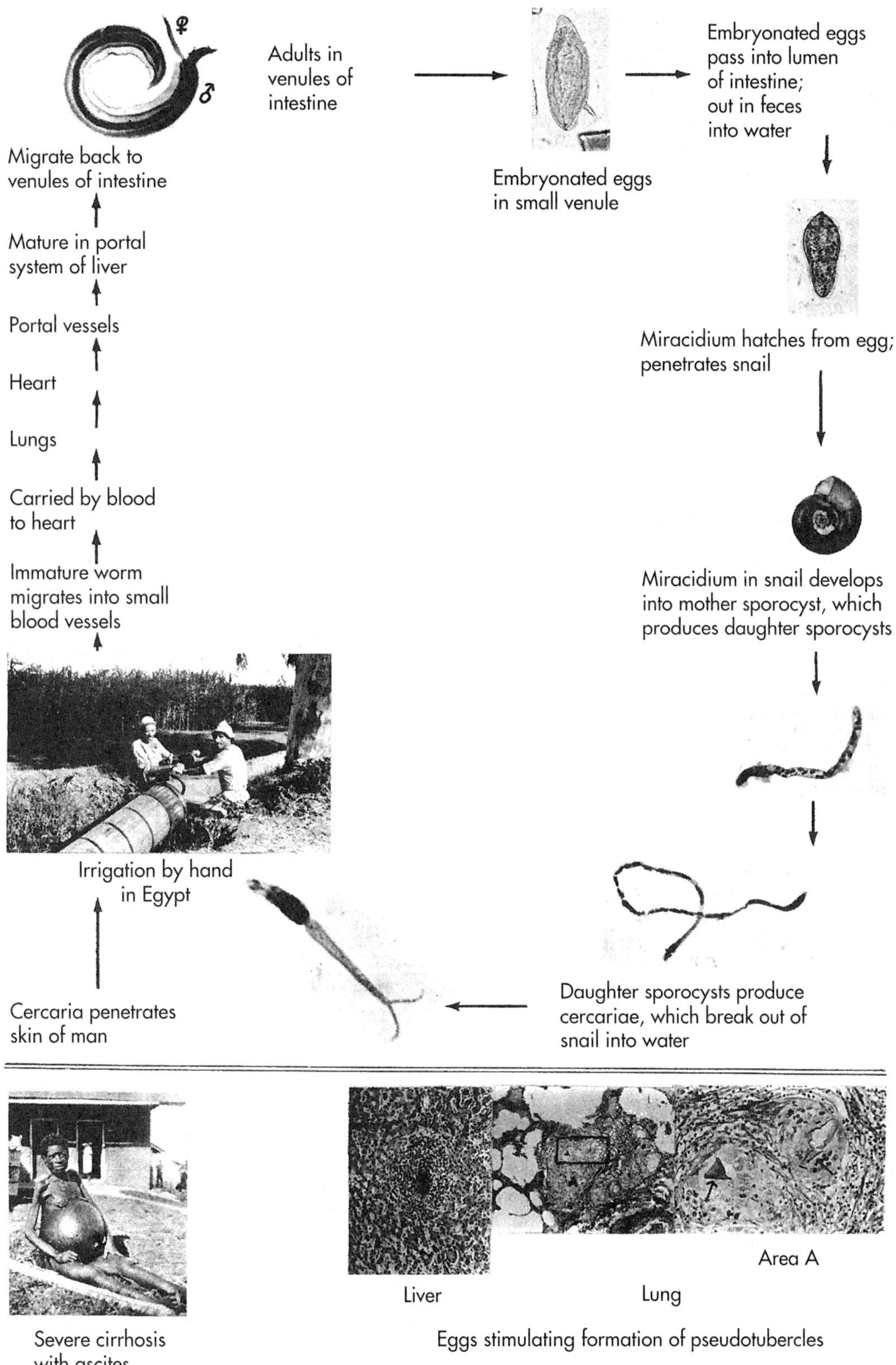

Fig. 30-7. Life cycle of *Schistosoma mansoni*. (From Brown HW, Neva FA: *Basic clinical parasitology*, ed 5, Norwalk, Conn, 1983, Appleton-Century-Crofts.)

(750 mg, by mouth, three times a day for 10 days) is the drug of choice for the former, followed by iodoquinol (650 mg, by mouth, three times a day for 20 days; exceeding the dose carries the risk of optic neuritis) or diloxanide furoate (500 mg, by mouth, three times a day for 10 days; available only through the CDC) for the latter. Tinidazole, a drug closely related to metronidazole, may replace metronidazole as the drug of choice. Asymptomatic carriers of cysts and/or trophozoites may be treated with diloxanide furoate to prevent evolution of invasive disease and transmission of the

agent. Iodoquinol (650 mg, by mouth, three times a day for 20 days) is an alternative to diloxanide, but doses in excess of those recommended have been associated with optic neuritis.

Giardia Lamblia. *G. lamblia* is a flagellate protozoan parasite of the intestine that is being increasingly recognized as a cause of diarrhea. The parasite attaches to the epithelium of the proximal small bowel and causes abdominal cramps, bloating, and diarrhea. Symptoms may be remittent. Cyst forms passed in the stool transmit the infection.

The natural history of the parasite is poorly elucidated, and several primary animal hosts have been proposed. Most outbreaks of giardiasis have been associated with waterborne transmission, although the fecal-oral route is clearly important in households, family day care, and institutional transmission. Sporadic cases of giardiasis occur throughout the world, and it is a frequent cause of diarrhea in travelers.

The diagnosis of giardiasis depends on demonstrating the trophozoite or cyst in stool or other specimens. If stool is negative, and if the diagnosis is strongly suspected on clinical and epidemiologic grounds, aspiration of duodenal contents or the "string test" may be undertaken. The string test is accomplished by having the patient swallow a commercially available gelatin capsule containing 140 cm of nylon string, the free end of which is secured to the face. The string usually passes to the duodenum and may be gently removed after several hours. Examination of material expressed from the distal end of the string is examined for parasites.

Treatment of giardiasis is with quinacrine (100 mg, by mouth, three times a day for 5 days) or metronidazole (250 to 750 mg, by mouth, three times a day for 5 to 10 days). Metronidazole appears to be safe and effective, but larger than usual doses may be required in some cases. Treatment of asymptomatic as well as symptomatic household contacts may be indicated.

Blastocystis Hominis. *B. hominis* is a protozoan parasite first described in the early part of this century. It has been associated with diarrhea for many years, but its role as a cause of diarrheal illness has not been clearly established. Diarrhea with *B. hominis* in the stool in large numbers (>5 per oil immersion field) has been linked epidemiologically with travel and with drinking of untreated water. The drug of choice has not been determined. Metronidazole is usually selected because of its efficacy in other similar infections, and iodoquinol or trimethoprim-sulfamethoxazole has been used as an alternative.

Other Intestinal Protozoan Infections. Recently a newly recognized protozoan parasite has been described in association with outbreaks of diarrhea in widespread parts of the world. This organism is thought to be either a cyanobacterium or a coccidian parasite and has been named *Cyclospora cayetanensis*. The disease has an abrupt onset of watery diarrhea, nausea, and anorexia with a waxing and waning prolonged course of 2 to 12 weeks. Resolution is also abrupt, but may be followed by prolonged fatigue. Organisms have

Table 30-3. Treatment for Schistosomiasis

Schistosome parasite	Drug	Dose
Schistosoma mansoni	Praziquantel	20 mg/kg × 2 *doses,* 4 to 6 hours apart in 1 day, with meals
	Oxamniquine	15 mg/kg, once
S. japonicum *S. mekongi* *S. malayensis* *S. intercalatum*	Praziquantel	20 mg/kg × 3 *doses,* 4 to 6 hours apart in 1 day, with meals
S. haematobium	Praziquantel	20 mg/kg × 2 *doses,* 4 to 6 hours apart in 1 day, with meals

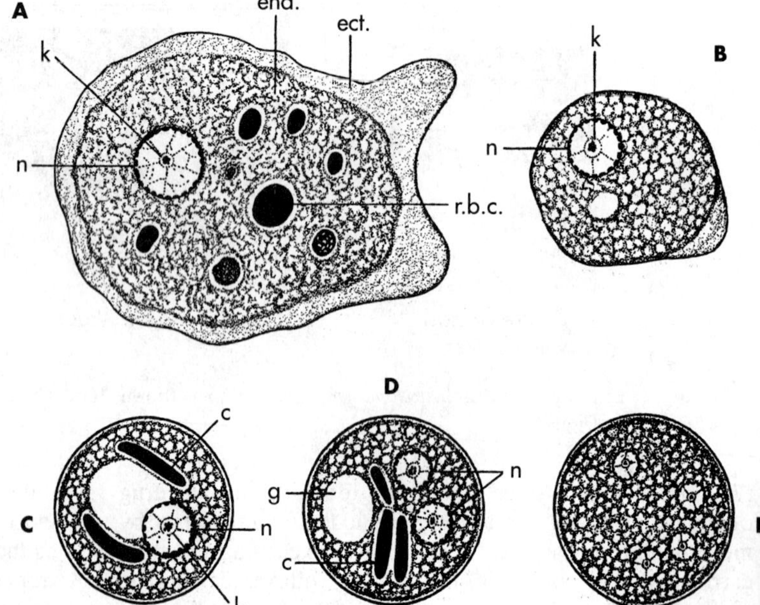

Fig. 30-8. *Entamoeba histolytica.* **A,** Trophozoite containing phagocytized red blood cells. **B,** Precystic ameba. **C,** Young cyst. **D,** Binucleate cyst. **E,** Mature cyst (with four nuclei). *c,* Chromatoid bodies; *ect.,* ectoplasm; *end.,* endoplasm; *g,* glycogen acuole; *k,* karyosome; *n,* nucleus; *r.b.c.,* red blood cells. (From Brown HW, Neva FA: *Basic clinical parasitology,* ed 6, Norwalk, Conn, 1994, Appleton-Century-Crofts.)

been seen in duodenal aspirates, as well as in stool. The disease tends to occur during warm and wet seasons. Transmission seems to be predominantly waterborne. Sporadic cases may occur in the absence of a recognized outbreak. Successive infections in the same individual have been documented. Treatment options are under investigation, but trimethoprim-sulfamethoxazole appears to be promising.

Human infection with protozoal parasites of the gastrointestinal tract of domesticated animals is becoming recognized in widespread parts of the world. In immunocompetent hosts, symptomatic disease related to these parasites appears to be confined to a self-limited episode of gastroenteritis, although asymptomatic carriage of organisms may be prolonged. Severe, intractable diarrhea has been observed in patients with AIDS due to *C. parvum, Isospora belli,* and other protozoa. Effective drugs against these parasites that are safe for use in humans, are not available. Recently, a large epidemic of *C. parvum* infection that was related to contamination of drinking water with cysts occurred in Milwaukee. *C. parvum* is commonly found in surface waters and probably causes a number of sporadic diarrheal illnesses in persons with altered immune function due to underlying disease or age. Vigorous pursuit of more effective water treatment methods is underway.

Blood and Tissue Protozoan Infections

Malaria. The first known description of malaria is that of Hippocrates during the fourth century BC. It was only during the late nineteenth and early twentieth centuries that the etiology and natural history of malaria were elucidated. Great strides were made in the control and treatment of malaria during the first half of this century. Whereas in many areas, such as Europe and the United States, the disease has been eradicated, in other areas of the world the parasite is making new gains. The emergence of mosquitoes resistant to pesticides has contributed to this increase, as have sociopolitical setbacks. These factors and others have led to a resurgence of the disease in the tropics. The ability of the parasite to develop resistance to antimalarial drugs has made treatment and prevention more difficult. Thus malaria is an increasing world health problem. The effect of this disease on the health and economy of the world is immeasurable. In the United States most cases of malaria are imported. Failure to diagnose and treat early results in a more than tenfold increase in mortality rate over that observed when the diagnosis is considered at clinical presentation.

Human malaria is caused by four species of the protozoan genus *Plasmodium: P. falciparum, P. vivax, P. ovale,* and *P. malariae.* Disease is transmitted by infection of the sporozoite form through the bite of an anopheline mosquito. Sporozoites invade liver parenchymal cells, and after 2 weeks merozoites are released into the bloodstream. Merozoites invade erythrocytes and the parasite develops into a trophozoite. Trophozoites differentiate in erythrocytes to produce either more merozoites or gametocytes. Merozoites continue the cycle of erythrocyte parasitism.

Male and female gametocytes, taken up by mosquitoes during a blood meal, initiate a phase of sexual reproduction, and development ultimately produces sporozoites. The life cycle of *Plasmodium* is summarized in Fig. 30-9. *P. vivax* and *P. ovale* are capable of latent infection of liver cells, which may give rise to merozoites and therefore clinical disease at times distant from exposure. *P. falciparum* does not have an exoerythrocytic phase. Malaria also may be transmitted by blood transfusion and intravenous injection using contaminated needles.

Clinical signs and symptoms of malaria relate directly to red blood cell parasitism. Erythrocytes parasitized with developing parasites lodge in the microvasculature, causing tissue ischemia with resultant dysfunction and damage. Such tissue ischemia contributes to the dangerous process of cerebral malaria. The malarial paroxysm consists of chills and headache progressing to high fever, severe headache, myalgia, abdominal pain, delirium, nausea, and vomiting. The classic paroxysm of malaria occurs every 2 days, or in the case of *P. malariae* every 3 days, during the early evening at the time when the vectors, anopheline mosquitoes, usually feed. With acute malaria and malaria in the nonimmune person, the classic paroxysm with regular periodicity usually is not seen. Patients are often persistently febrile and symptomatic or have irregularly intermittent fever and symptoms. The paroxysm is associated with the lysis of parasitized erythrocytes with release of merozoites and other parasite products. The release of these products leads to fever and other systemic effects.

Another important pathophysiologic consequence is the hemolytic anemia resulting from destruction of red blood cells and the sequestration of parasitized erythrocytes in the spleen. Anemia may vary from mild to severe. Severe hemolysis may lead to hemoglobinuria and renal failure. Symptoms and anemia are usually most severe with *P. falciparum* infection, as this organism tends to cause the heaviest parasitemia because of its ability to invade erythrocytes of all ages (the other species have a predilection for young or old cells). Splenomegaly is frequent and splenic rupture is a dangerous but uncommon complication. Severe *P. falciparum* infection may be complicated by encephalopathy, "cerebral malaria," due to hypoxia resulting from deep vascular sequestration of parasitized erythrocytes. Nephrotic syndrome occurs only with *P. malariae* infection. This is probably related to the chronic, low-grade, subclinical parasitism that occurs with this species. Such subclinical parasitism accounts for the observation that most transfusion-related cases of malaria are caused by *P. malariae.*

The diagnosis of malaria is made by examining stained smears of the peripheral blood. In a patient with unexplained fever, suspicion of malaria should be aroused by a history of residence in an endemic area. Blood smears may show ring forms, trophozoites, schizonts, and gametocytes. Interpretation of smears as to species usually requires expert consultation. Simultaneous infection with more than one species may occur.

The therapy of malaria is complicated by the widespread emergence of chloroquine resistance by *P. falciparum,* the species that causes the most severe disease. Chloroquine has been an effective, relatively inexpensive, and safe therapy for all forms of malaria. *P. falciparum,* probably related to the high levels of parasitemia it achieves, is capable of evolving mechanisms of drug resistance through pressure of natural selection. The widespread use of chloroquine provided this selective pressure. Chloroquine-resistant strains of this species are present, and new treatment strategies have been developed and are under investigation. Unfortunately, *P. falciparum* is becoming more resistant to other agents as well.

Treatment of choice for uncomplicated malaria caused by *P. vivax, P. ovale,* and *P. malariae* is chloroquine phosphate,

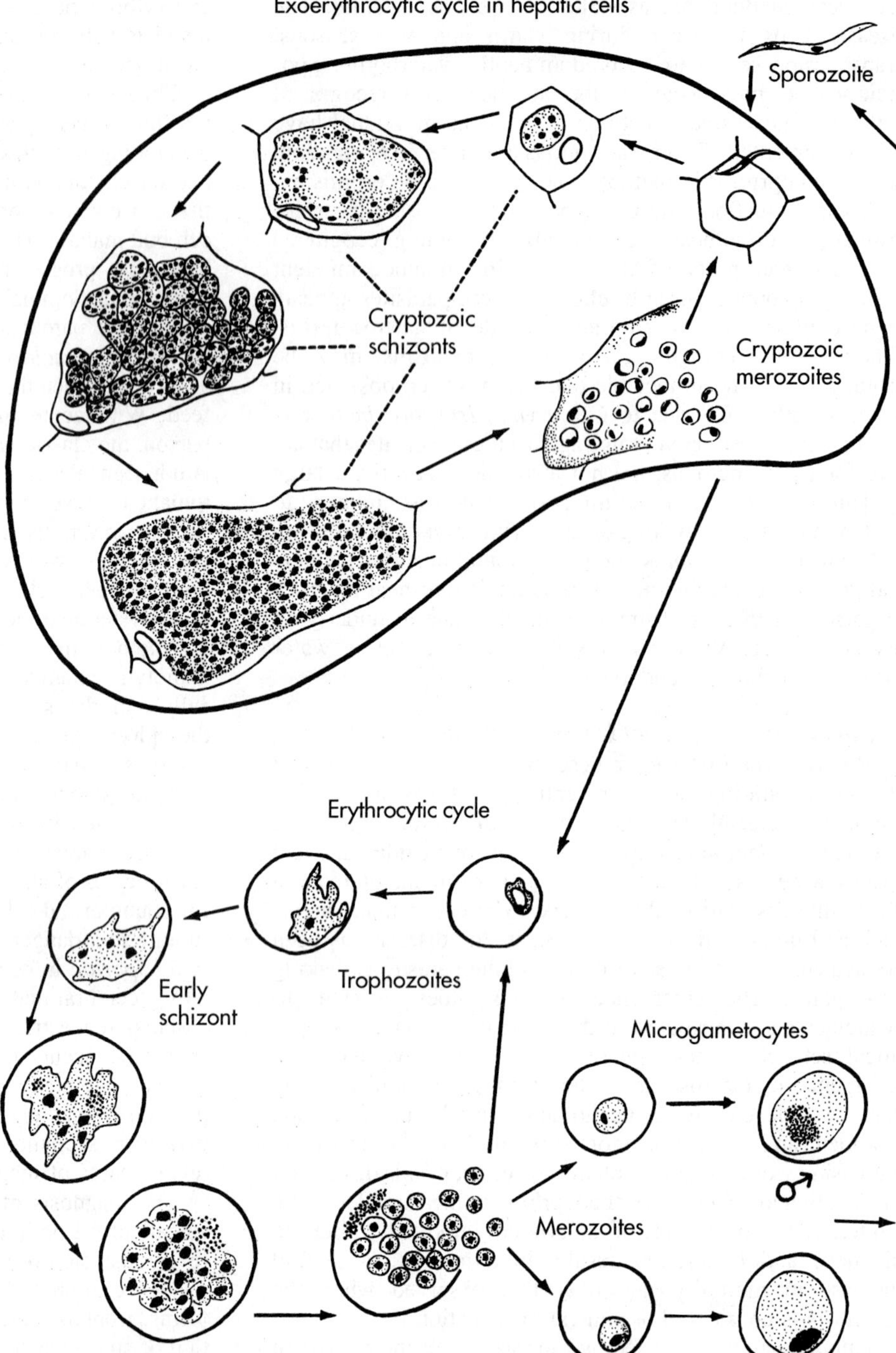

Fig. 30-9. Life cycle of the malaria *Plasmodium* in humans. The sporozoite is introduced in the saliva of the biting mosquito. (From Brown HW, Neva FA: *Basic clinical parasitology,* ed 5, Norwalk, Conn, 1983, Appleton-Century-Crofts.)

1 gram (600 mg base) orally, followed by half this dose at 6 hours and then once a day for 2 days. The equivalent initial pediatric dose would be 10 mg base/kg. Severe illness is treated with intravenous quinidine gluconate (with electrocardiographic [ECG] monitoring) followed by oral therapy if possible. Treatment of *P. vivax* and *P. ovale* must include primaquine phosphate, 15 mg base daily for 14 days or 45 mg base weekly for 8 weeks (0.3 mg base/kg/day for 14 days in children) for "radical" cure with elimination of exoerythrocytic forms. Glucose-6-phosphate dehydrogenase deficiency must be ruled out before initiating primaquine therapy, because the drug may precipitate hemolysis. Chloroquine-resistant *P. falciparum* is treated with quinine sulfate (650 mg, by mouth, every 8 hours for 3 to 7 days) combined with pyrimethamine/sulfadoxine (three tablets on the last day of quinine), tetracycline, or clindamycin. Mefloquine and halofantrine are alternative agents. Intravenous quinidine gluconate is used for severe disease or if oral therapy is not possible. Suspected or documented *P. falciparum* acquired in areas where chloroquine resistance is known to occur is

treated as if it were chloroquine-resistant. Suppressive and chemoprophylactic therapy of malaria is discussed later (see Advice to Travelers).

Babesiosis. Babesiosis is a zoonosis caused by protozoa of the genus *Babesia,* which are transmitted by ticks. The parasite infects a number of mammals but is rarely transmitted to humans. The disease is not tropical. It occurs in a number of regions, but most cases have been reported from the United States, especially on Nantucket Island and Martha's Vineyard. Asplenic individuals are particularly susceptible to severe infection.

Signs and symptoms are similar to those of malaria: fever, splenomegaly, and anemia. Significant complications include massive hemolysis and renal failure. Diagnosis is made by demonstrating intraerythrocytic parasites on blood smears. Effective therapy has not been established. Chloroquine may cause symptomatic relief without eradication of the parasites. Clindamycin plus quinine are often used to treat babesiosis, but this therapy is considered investigational. Babesiosis also has been treated with exchange transfusion.

Toxoplasmosis. Toxoplasmosis is a disease of animals and people, widely distributed throughout the world. The protozoan *T. gondii* is an intracellular parasite capable of invading virtually all mammalian cell types. The definitive host is the cat. In the cat the parasite undergoes sexual reproduction, producing oocysts that are passed in the stool. In tissue the parasite is capable of multiplying asexually, leading either to the release of invasive trophozoites after cell lysis or the formation of tissue cysts. Toxoplasmosis is transmitted by ingestion of oocysts, ingestion of undercooked meat containing tissue cysts, or transplacentally. Undercooked meat is the most common means of transmission. Most cases of toxoplasmosis are subclinical. Serologic evidence of past infection increases in prevalence with increasing age. In some parts of the United States, as many as 70% of adults have antibody to *Toxoplasma.* Tissue cysts cause latent disease that may reactivate long after the initial exposure.

Clinically evident toxoplasmosis may present in several different forms of illness. In normal immunocompetent adults and children, the disease is typically a generalized febrile illness with lymphadenopathy, malaise, myalgia, sore throat, and hepatosplenomegaly. This syndrome is similar to infectious mononucleosis, and atypical lymphocytes may appear in the peripheral blood. Occasionally, a maculopapular rash occurs. The disease also may present predominantly as a localized process involving the CNS, liver, heart, or other organ. Of special importance is ocular toxoplasmosis, which is usually the result of congenital infection, but occasionally is acquired after birth. Characteristic lesions of chorioretinitis may be seen on funduscopic examination. These lesions may remain latent or reactivate with increasing damage to vision.

Congenital toxoplasmosis occurs after primary infection during pregnancy. Congenital infection has protean manifestations ranging from asymptomatic infection to severe multisystem involvement with retardation. Chorioretinitis is common with congenital infection.

Toxoplasmosis has become an important problem in immunocompromised patients because of the ubiquitous distribution of the parasite and its ability to exist in a latent form. Severe, newly acquired, or reactivated latent disease occurs in association with AIDS, in transplant recipients, in patients with neoplastic diseases, and others receiving immunosuppressive therapy. These patients may present with severe systemic illness or disease located predominantly in one organ or organ system, especially the CNS. CNS toxoplasmosis is an important AIDS-related opportunistic infection. Toxoplasmosis is among several diseases presenting with pneumonitis and encephalitis in the immunocompromised patient.

The diagnosis of toxoplasmosis may be made by isolating the parasite or demonstrating it in histologic sections, but usually is made on the basis of serologic testing. Several serologic tests are available, including the Sabin-Feldman dye test and the indirect fluorescent antibody (IFA) test. Because of the high prevalence of positive serology in many populations, the presence of a single significant titer in these tests cannot differentiate acute from old infection. Rising titers imply recent infection. Acute toxoplasmosis may be diagnosed by the immunoglobulin M (IgM)-IFA test. A single titer of 1:80 or greater, or a rising titer on two or more observations, signifies acute infection.

Acute toxoplasmosis is usually self-limited. Treatment is limited to patients with severe disease or those who are immunocompromised. The therapy of choice is pyrimethamine combined with sulfadiazine. The dose of pyrimethamine for adults is 25 to 100 mg/day for 1 month. The dose of sulfadiazine is 1 to 1.5 gm qid for the same period. Pyrimethamine is a potent bone marrow suppressant, and patients should receive 10 mg folinic acid a day to support the marrow. Folic acid must not be given, since it inhibits the activity of pyrimethamine against *T. gondii.* Steroids are usually used in the treatment of ocular toxoplasmosis in addition to specific therapy, since the inflammatory response to *T. gondii* increases retinal damage. In patients with AIDS, suppressive therapy should be maintained indefinitely after therapy of acute disease.

Leishmaniasis. Visceral leishmaniasis, or "kala-azar," is a systemic disease caused by the intracellular protozoan parasite *Leishmania donovani.* Other species of the genus *Leishmania* cause cutaneous and mucocutaneous leishmaniasis. Kala-azar occurs in many parts of the world but primarily in tropical and semitropical regions. The parasite has many animal reservoirs and is transmitted by the bite of sandflies of the genus *Phlebotomus.* The parasites invade reticuloendothelial cells throughout the body, leading to marked proliferation and hyperplasia. Hyperglobulinemia and antigen-antibody complexes further complicate the disease and glomerulonephritis may occur. The onset may be insidious or acute and is associated with high fever. Chills and diarrhea frequently are present. The disease then has a progressive course of prolonged fever, weight loss, organomegaly (which is often of a marked degree), anemia, hypoalbuminemia, and peripheral edema. Visceral leishmaniasis may complicate HIV infection and other causes of immunocompromise.

The diagnosis is made on the basis of typical clinical findings in the right epidemiologic setting or the demonstration of parasites in tissue.

The disease is treated with stibogluconate (antimony) 20 mg/kg per day (up to 800 mg/day) intramuscularly or intravenously for 20 to 28 days. The dose in children is 10 mg/kg per day (up to 600 mg). Stibogluconate resistance has been seen in some areas of the world. Pentamidine and amphotericin B are alternative therapeutic agents when stibogluconate cannot be used or resistance is encountered. The combination of interferon-γ and stibogluconate may be superior to stibogluconate alone. Untreated, symptomatic disease is usually fatal.

Trypanosomiasis. Trypanosomes are hemoflagellate protozoans that cause African trypanosomiasis, or sleeping sickness, and American trypanosomiasis, or Chagas' disease. *Trypanosoma brucei gambiense* (West African) and *T. brucei rhodesiense* (East African) are the etiologic agents of sleeping sickness and are transmitted by various strains of the tsetse fly. After the bite of an infected fly, a skin lesion appears at the site. The parasites reproduce in the skin lesion. Dissemination from the initial lesion leads to fever, severe headache, rash, and localized areas of edema. Lymphadenopathy then becomes prominent, especially of the posterior cervical chain. Hepatomegaly and splenomegaly may occur. The disease spreads to the CNS where cerebral damage occurs, leading to the characteristic signs of somnolence, headache, and other neurologic manifestations that eventually lead to continuous sleep. *T. brucei rhodesiense* tends to cause a fulminant disease over months, whereas *T. brucei gambiense* causes a disease that progresses over years. Inapparent infection has been described with the latter.

Diagnosis usually is made by demonstrating parasites in the blood or lymph node aspirates, although serologic tests also are available. Early disease, characterized by a predominance of systemic signs and lymphadenopathy, is treatable with suramin, eflornithine, or pentamidine, whereas CNS disease is treated with melarsoprol or eflornithine. These drugs are available through the CDC and should be used only with the guidance of the Parasitic Diseases Division of the CDC.

Chagas' disease is caused by *T. cruzi* and is transmitted through the feces of biting insects of the reduviid group. These insects defecate while taking their blood meal, and parasites in the feces make their way into small wounds, conjunctivae, and mucous membranes. The disease is limited to the Western Hemisphere and has occurred as far north as Texas. Reduviid bugs capable of transmitting *T. cruzi* are found in large parts of North America; therefore the potential for spread of infection in the United States exists wherever small mammals live in close proximity to humans. Transmission of trypanosomiasis by blood transfusion from asymptomatic, chronically infected donors also is a concern.

Among infected individuals, 10% to 30% eventually develop symptomatic disease. The morbidity of American trypanosomiasis is primarily related to chronic infection. In endemic areas, Chagas' disease is a major cause of myocarditis and cardiomyopathy, as well as alimentary tract dysfunction manifested by megaesophagus and megacolon. Acute Chagas' disease is a febrile illness that appears 1 to 2 weeks after exposure to the parasite. It is characterized by systemic toxicity, variable fever, lymphadenopathy, hepatosplenomegaly, and signs of myocarditis. A chagoma (a macular, desquamating lesion) may be seen at the site of inoculation. Romaña's sign, unilateral ophthalmia with palpebral edema, may occur. In most cases the acute disease lasts approximately 2 weeks. Acute Chagas' disease in the immunocompromised host can follow a fulminant course. This development has been observed in patients immunosuppressed from cancer chemotherapy. It can be presumed that similar severe disease may occur in patients with immunosuppression due to HIV infection.

The classic means of diagnosing acute Chagas' disease is by xenodiagnosis (i.e., allowing laboratory-bred bugs to bite the patient and examining the bugs for parasites after 1 to 2 months). Parasites also may be demonstrated directly in peripheral smears or by injection of blood into mice. Several serologic tests are available including an enzyme-linked immunosorbent assay (ELISA) that are useful in screening for chronic infection.

Acute Chagas' disease is treatable with two agents, nifurtimox and benznidazole, but the required treatment is prolonged and associated with a high rate of adverse reactions. All cases are not cured. Chronic disease is treated supportively.

Tissue-Invasive Roundworms

Filariasis. Filarial infections are caused by a number of tissue-dwelling nematodes. These diseases occur primarily in tropical and semitropical regions and are transmitted by biting insects. The sexually mature filarial worms live in various tissues and produce microfilarial larvae that migrate in blood and tissues. Clinical manifestations of these infections result from the residence of adult forms in tissue, migration of the adult worms, and the release and migration of the larvae. Much of the morbidity results from hypersensitivity to the parasites. Filarial infections are summarized in Table 30-4.

The major filarial infections, due to *Wuchereria bancrofti, Brugia malayi, Loa loa,* and *Onchocerca volvulus,* affect millions of people in endemic areas, but only a small proportion of those affected develop overt clinical disease. The adult worms cause most of the signs and symptoms of these infections, except for *O. volvulus* infection, in which the microfilariae cause eye damage leading to "river blindness." Hypersensitivity reactions to microfilariae cause most of the systemic manifestations of these diseases, and eosinophilia is usually prominent (see later). Several animal filaria have been described in humans, almost all cases of which have been recognized in the United States. Human zoonotic filarial disease is basically the result of the host reaction to parasites that find themselves in an incompatible host.

Diethylcarbamazine is effective against most of the human filariae, but the adult forms of *O. volvulus* are not killed and go on to produce more microfilariae unless excised or treated with an effective drug such as ivermectin. Ivermectin has become the drug of choice for the treatment of *O. volvulus.* Diethylcarbamazine can produce an encephalopathy in patients who have a heavy infection with *L. loa.* Relatively severe allergic reactions can result from the breakdown of killed microfilariae of *L. loa* and *O. volvulus* when diethylcarbamazine is used. Such reactions may require treatment with steroids and antihistamines.

Trichinosis. Trichinella spiralis is an intestinal roundworm, the invasive larvae of which encyst in muscle tissue and produce the systemic disease trichinosis. The life cycle of *T. spiralis* is presented in Fig. 30-10. The disease is acquired by ingestion of poorly cooked meat, especially pork, that contains encysted larvae. Outbreaks in the United States also have been associated with bear meat. The ingested larvae become sexually mature in the small intestine, and the adults attach to the mucosa and produce offspring; these larvae invade the gut, migrate to muscle tissue, and encyst. The adult worms are shed in the stool after 2 to 4 weeks. The severity of trichinosis depends on the number of invading larvae and ranges from asymptomatic to fatal.

Table 30-4. Filarial Infections in Humans

Agent	Distribution	Vector	Clinical manifestations related to: Residence of adult worms	Clinical manifestations related to: Migration of microfilariae	Diagnostic procedure	Treatment
Wuchereria bancrofti	Asia Latin America Pacific islands	Mosquitoes	Lymphatic tissue Lymphadenitis Lymphadenopathy Elephantiasis Hydrocele Chyluria	Blood Eosinophilia Allergic reactions Usually nocturnal periodicity	Membrane filtration of blood	Diethylcarbamazine [DEC] PO Day 1: 50 mg, once Day 2: 50 mg, tid
Brugia malayi *B. timori*	Southeast Asia India China, Korea Indonesia	Mosquitoes		Some subperiodicity		Day 3: 100 mg, tid Days 4-21: 2 mg/kg, tid
Loa loa	West Africa Central Africa	Tabanid horseflies (*Chrysops* sp.)	Migratory in subcutaneous tissue Erythematous "Calabar" swellings Visible subconjunctival migration	Blood (eosinophils) Diurnal periodicity	(At peak microfilaria parasitemia, when periodicity presents)	DEC, PO Days 1-3: as above Days 4-21: 3 mg/kg, tid
Mansonella perstans	Africa South America	Midges	Body cavities Asymptomatic to mild abdominal pain and swellings	Blood Minimal to no symptoms Nonperiodic		Mebendazole, PO 100 mg, bid for 30 days
M. ozzardi	South America Central America	Midges	Body cavities Mild systemic symptoms	Blood Nonperiodic		Ivermectin, PO 150 µg/kg, once
M. streptocerca	Central Africa West Africa	Midges	Skin	Skin, lymph nodes Dermatitis	Skin biopsy	? DEC (see above)
Onchocerca volvulus	Africa Central America South America Yemen	Black flies (*Simulium* sp.)	Soft tissue Subcutaneous nodules	Skin and subcutaneous tissue Rash Keratitis, iritis Blindness	Skin snips (larvae) Biopsy of nodule (adult)	Ivermectin 150 µg/kg once Repeat every 6 to 12 months

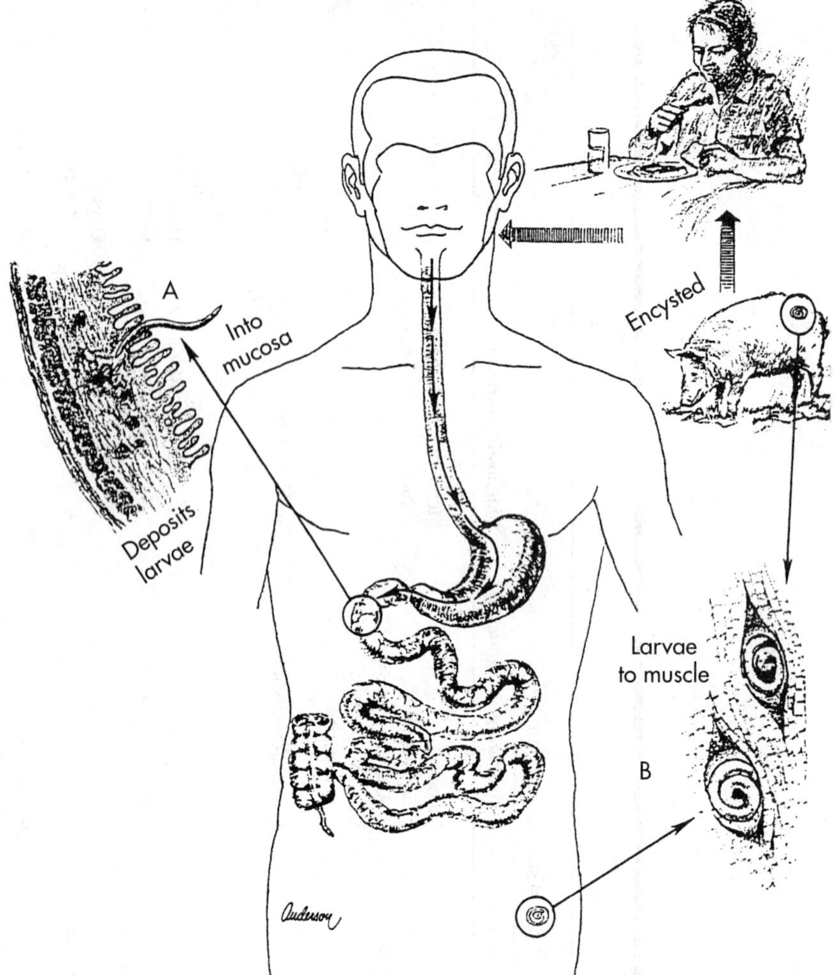

Fig. 30-10. Life cycle of *Trichinella spiralis*. Infective larvae, encysted in pork and other meat, when ingested, become adult worms in the small intestine. The female burrows into the mucosa and deposits larvae into lacteals and blood vessels. Circulating larvae eventually penetrate skeletal muscle and become encysted *(A)*. In humans these larvae are at a dead end, but in the pig and other animals, they become a source of infection *(B)*. (From Beck JW, Davies JE: *Medical parasitology,* ed 3, St Louis, 1981, Mosby.)

The disease manifests as an early phase of diarrhea and abdominal pain followed by characteristic periorbital edema, myalgia, fever, sweats, weakness, and eosinophilia. Myocarditis is an important cause of death, and the disease may affect the CNS.

The diagnosis is usually made on clinical grounds, especially when there is a history of ingestion of suspect meat. Diagnosis is made definitively by biopsy of muscle. Several serologic tests also are available, the simplest and most rapid being the bentonite flocculation test.

Specific therapy for muscle disease is not available. Mebendazole and steroids are usually used in severe disease. Control of this disease depends on adequate cooking of meat (freezing for 3 weeks or more is also effective) and safe food sources for swine.

Visceral Larva Migrans. Visceral larva migrans is a systemic disease, usually occurring in children, that is caused by tissue migration of the larvae of nonhuman ascarid parasites of the genus *Toxocara*. The usual host of *T. canis* is the dog and of *T. cati* the cat. Eggs are shed in the feces of young dogs and cats. Children become infected by ingesting contaminated soil. The eggs hatch in the intestine, and larvae invade the bowel and begin a persistent migration through the liver, CNS, muscle, and other organs. This migration may persist for weeks to months to years.

Most patients with visceral larva migrans are asymptomatic but may have pronounced peripheral blood eosinophilia. Symptomatic disease is primarily due to the host response to the parasite and is characterized by fever, cough, bronchospasm, hepatomegaly, and abdominal pain. CNS abnormalities and seizures may predominate. Endophthalmitis also may occur, usually in older children and often without significant systemic signs.

The diagnosis is made by association of the clinical picture with eosinophilia and a history of pica. These larval parasites share A and B blood group antigens with humans, and elevated titers of isoagglutinins may be helpful in diagnosis.

The disease is usually self-limited, and symptoms usually resolve despite continued eosinophilia. Severe disease is treated with diethylcarbamazine, 2 mg/kg, three times a day for 7 to 10 days; alternatives are mebendazole and albendazole. Endophthalmitis is treated with adjunctive steroids.

Enteric Bacterial Infections

Vibrio Cholerae. Cholera due to *Vibrio cholerae* still occurs in many parts of the world. The seventh pandemic caused by the *eltor* strain began in 1961 in southern Asia and has spread to central Asia, Africa, and South America, with occasional outbreaks in southern Europe and the South Pacific. Cases resulting from earlier strains of the organism surviving in natural habitats for long periods have occurred along the Gulf Coast of the United States.

When sufficient numbers of *V. cholerae* are ingested to provide an infective dose, they multiply in the small intestine lumen and adhere to epithelial cells without damaging them. They then produce cholera toxin, which stimulates epithelial cell adenylate cyclase. This produces elevated levels of cyclic adenosine monophosphate (AMP), blocking sodium uptake by the cells and causing massive flux of water, bicarbonate, and chloride into the lumen. The organisms do not invade tissue. The severe watery diarrhea produced by the physiologic derangement resulting from cholera toxin is abrupt in onset and may lead to severe dehydration, nausea, muscle cramps, and shock. The disease state is the product of the water and electrolyte loss.

Diagnosis is based on the epidemiologic circumstances and the severe, watery diarrhea. Microscopic examination of stained stool smears may show a monotonous flora of curved gram-negative rods. Treatment is designed to compensate for the water and electrolyte losses with intravenous fluids. Oral replacement fluid composed of sodium and potassium chloride, glucose, and bicarbonate is used. This solution provides sodium in the presence of glucose. The glucose-linked uptake of sodium by the intestinal epithelium is a system independent of the sodium uptake system blocked by the effect of cholera toxin. Preparations of oral rehydration solution ingredients are available for use in cases of diarrhea of any cause and are the mainstay of supportive treatment of moderate to severe diarrhea. Tetracycline and other antimicrobial agents are used to eradicate organisms.

Some strains of *V. Cholerae* are not of the 01 serotype (which includes the classic and *eltor* strains). These so-called nonagglutinable or non-01 strains occasionally have been implicated in small outbreaks of diarrheal illness and cases of invasive diarrhea similar to shigellosis. In 1992, a non-01 *V. cholerae* of the 0139 serotype caused epidemics of cholera-like illness in Bangladesh and India. *V. cholerae* 0139 produces cholera toxin and causes illness indistinguishable from cholera. It has continued to spread and cause epidemic disease and may be on its way to causing the eighth pandemic of cholera. The management of infection and disease with *V. cholerae* 0139 is the same for *V. cholerae* 01 of both the classic and *eltor* varieties.

Typhoid Fever. Typhoid fever is the systemic infection caused by the gram-negative bacillus *Salmonella typhi.* Although all the salmonellae that are pathogenic for humans are capable of causing disseminated infection after gastrointestinal invasion (i.e., enteric fever), such disease is the rule with *S. typhi.* This organism has a special virulence for humans, and people are its only natural hosts. The disease is still a major health problem in parts of the developing world. Approximately 400 to 500 cases are reported in the United States each year, with about half occurring in recent travelers.

Typhoid is transmitted by the fecal-oral route. Chronic carriers are important sources of disease in areas where the disease occurs sporadically. In places where there are many cases and sanitation is poor, sewage contamination of water and foodstuffs is important. The organisms reproduce in the small intestine and, like all the salmonellae, are capable of penetrating the intestinal mucosa. The organisms are then phagocytosed by macrophages, but are resistant to killing, so they reproduce intracellularly and eventually cause bacteremia and disseminated foci of viable bacteria in the reticuloendothelial system. The incubation period from ingestion to clinical disease is usually 1 to 2 weeks; however, it may be as long as 1 month.

Patients with typhoid fever may present with severe toxemia or relatively mild fever and systemic complaints of headache and myalgia. They then go on to develop increasing abdominal pain, constipation, and abdominal distention. Rose spots, the maculopapular rash that is classic for typhoid fever, may appear, usually on the trunk, during the full-blown evolution of the disease. Bleeding in the rectum may occur. The disease is characterized by persistent bacteremia. Complications include bowel perforation, hemorrhage, and metastatic foci (e.g., osteomyelitis, meningitis, and pyelonephritis). Most patients have peripheral leukopenia during the disease. Overwhelming disease may lead to hepatic and renal damage. The untreated disease may progress for weeks with increasing fever and debilitation, or it may remit after 2 to 3 weeks (with the possibility of relapse). Some patients (about 3%) retain a focus of gallbladder infection after acute disease and remain chronic asymptomatic carriers of the organism and potential sources of new infection.

The diagnosis of typhoid fever is made in a patient who has the characteristic signs and symptoms of the illness with a history of possible exposure consistent with the epidemiology of the disease. Blood cultures provide the definitive diagnosis. During the first 1 to 2 weeks of illness, blood cultures are almost always positive. Later these cultures may be negative, but they usually become positive with relapse. Stool and urine cultures are more likely to be positive late in the disease. Serologic tests are available and a fourfold rise in agglutination (Widal's test) titer is consistent with disease, although cross-reactions with other salmonellae may occur.

Ciprofloxacin and third-generation cephalosporin antibiotics, such as ceftriaxone and cefoperazone, have become drugs of choice for the treatment of typhoid fever. Although chloramphenicol, trimethoprim-sulfamethoxazole, and ampicillin have remained effective for susceptible strains of *S. typhi,* many multidrug-resistant strains that are resistant to some or all of these agents are being isolated in developing countries. Ciprofloxacin in a dose of 400 mg, intravenously, every 12 hours for 10 to 14 days and orally, 500 mg, twice a day for an additional 7 to 11 days should be effective in most cases. In patients with mild illness who are capable of oral therapy, ciprofloxacin 500 to 750 mg orally twice a day for 14 to 21 days may be used. Neither ciprofloxacin nor any other fluoroquinolone should be given to children or pregnant women because of interference with cartilage formation and possible teratogenic effects. Ceftriaxone may be given in a dose of 2 gm intravenously once a day and cefoperazone as 2 gm intravenously twice a day, both for 14 days. Ampicillin and trimethoprim-sulfamethoxazole, parenterally and orally, are satisfactory and less costly alternatives when the infecting strain is known to be sensitive. Corticosteroid therapy with dexamethasone is beneficial as adjunctive therapy in severe typhoid fever.

Typhoid vaccine affords some protection against acquisition of *S. typhi* infection, but is no substitute for caution (see Advice for Travelers). Parenteral heat-phenol-inactivated vaccine has been available for many years. It is administered in two doses, 4 weeks apart with a booster every 3 years. A more recently developed oral, live-attenuated vaccine of the Ty21a strain of *S. typhi* also has efficacy. The oral vaccine is given with cool liquids, 1 hour before meals, every other day, for four doses.

The best preventive measures for typhoid are good sanitation, good personal hygiene, identification of carriers, and careful follow-up of cases.

Systemic Bacterial Diseases (Including Plague)

Many bacterial diseases have a higher prevalence in tropical regions. Diseases such as cholera, typhoid fever, and meningococcal, staphylococcal, and streptococcal infections are discussed elsewhere in the text. Certain febrile diseases caused by bacteria have particular geographic distributions and are associated with tropical and semitropical areas. The following discussion is limited to bacterial diseases that cause systemic, febrile illness and that are not discussed in sections dealing with particular organ systems.

Brucellosis. Brucellosis is a disease of worldwide distribution, but is especially prevalent along the Mediterranean Sea (where it is known as Mediterranean fever) and in Mexico and South America. The disease is primarily a zoonosis affecting many domestic and wild animals. Four species of gram-negative bacilli of the genus *Brucella* infecting humans have been described: *B. abortus* (usually from a bovine source), *B. melitensis* (goats), *B. suis* (swine), and *B. canis* (dogs). People acquire disease through close exposure to infected animals, meat, and dairy products. Most cases in the United States are related to occupational exposures (e.g., meat packing and farming).

The spectrum of the disease can range from mild inapparent infection, to localized abscess formation, to severe systemic disease. Onset of disease is usually insidious with nonspecific symptoms of fatigue, sweats, chills, myalgia, arthralgia, and headache. Fever ranges from hectic to intermittent to absent. Axillary and cervical lymphadenopathy may occur, and splenomegaly has been observed in about 50% of patients with bacteremia. Fatality is rare with brucellosis, but some patients develop chronic infection with persistent malaise, anorexia, depression, and visceral or skeletal abscesses. The course of brucellosis may be complicated by mycotic aneurysm, encephalitis, meningitis, endocarditis, pneumonia, renal disease, and osteomyelitis.

Diagnosis of brucellosis is made by isolating the organism from blood or tissues or serodiagnosis, usually using agglutination tests. Treatment is with tetracycline for 3 to 4 weeks, combined with streptomycin for severe disease. Relapses after therapy are common.

Bartonellosis. *Bartonella bacilliformis* is a gram- negative bacillus that is the causative agent of bartonellosis, or Oroya fever, and the skin disease verruga peruana. The organism is transmitted from person to person through the bites of sandflies of the genus *Phlebotomus*. The disease occurs naturally in only one part of the world, the Andean mountain valleys of Peru, Ecuador, and Colombia. Asymptomatic carrier rates approach 5% in this area.

The bacilli are capable of invading endothelial cells and erythrocytes. Hemolytic anemia results from destruction of parasitized erythrocytes. The clinical disease is associated with irregular fever, anemia, headache, myalgia, arthralgia, bone pain, and lymphadenopathy. Fatality rates in untreated cases approach 40%, and patients with bartonellosis have a peculiar susceptibility to invasive salmonellosis that commonly complicates the disease. Survivors of Oroya fever may go on to develop the cutaneous phase of the disease, verruga peruana, which consists of pathognomonic skin lesions and nodular hemangiomas.

The diagnosis is made on clinical grounds by the association of fever and hemolytic anemia in a person exposed to the endemic area. The organism may be isolated in blood cultures or demonstrated on the surface of erythrocytes on a blood smear. The drug of choice for treatment is chloramphenicol.

Plague. Plague is an ancient disease of enormous historical significance that still warrants fear and concern. The etiologic agent is the gram-negative bacillus, *Yersinia pestis*. Sylvatic plague is a zoonosis of wild rodents that is prevalent in large parts of the world including South America, South and Central Africa, Central Asia, the Near East, and the southwestern United States. The disease is maintained in wild, burrowing rodents as a relatively mild illness. Sylvatic plague may be passed to people by the bite of a flea from an infected wild rodent, and sporadic cases of human plague occur in endemic areas. The great plague epidemics resulted from a domestic cycle of infection involving rats and their fleas. Domestic rats with plague usually die and their fleas go to other rats or people, thereby spreading the epizootic and epidemic.

Plague occurs in several forms in humans. Bubonic plague is usually the result of flea-transmitted infection. The incubation period is 2 to 7 days. Bubonic plague begins as a febrile illness associated with the development of painful, swollen lymph nodes, or buboes. After evolution of the lymphadenitis, a secondary septicemia occurs with severe toxicity, prostration, and shock. Pestis minor is a clinical variant of bubonic plague characterized by the presence of a bubo with less severe systemic signs. Primary septicemic plague without evident localized infection occurs in few cases during epidemics. Approximately 5% of patients with plague develop pneumonia, usually as a preterminal event. Primary pneumonic plague results from person-to-person transmission of plague via droplets or as the result of inhalation of other material contaminated by plague bacilli. Pneumonic plague may be maintained in a cycle of person-to-person transmission.

Patients with plague often develop hemodynamic instability, staggering gait, confusion, and delirium. The course of plague may be complicated by meningitis, pneumonia, and disseminated intravascular coagulation. The fatality rate of untreated bubonic plague is 50% and higher, and pneumonic and primary septicemic plague are almost always fatal.

Diagnosis of plague is made by demonstrating organisms in smears of bubo aspirates, blood, or spinal fluid. It is confirmed by culture.

Treatment must begin before culture results are known, since delays result in failure of clinical cure despite bacteriologic response, and the patient may die of irreversible toxic effects of infection. The drug of choice is streptomycin, and it is often combined with chloramphenicol or tetracycline. Persons closely exposed to wild rodents in plague-endemic areas or who have potential laboratory exposure to plague should receive plague vaccine. Case contacts are handled by defleaing, surveillance, quarantine, and chemoprophylaxis.

In the American Southwest, sporadic cases of human plague occur as the result of exposure to prairie dogs, squirrels, chipmunks, and other burrowing rodents. The disease frequently is seen in hunters. Because the plague bacillus is endemic in most of the Southwest United States, it must always be considered in the diagnosis of severe febrile illness or lymphadenopathy in that area, be diagnosed as rapidly as possible, and be treated early. Proper isolation precautions must be taken to prevent spread.

Tularemia. Tularemia is an infection of rodents and rabbits caused by the gram-negative bacillus *Francisella tularensis,* which is transmitted to people by exposure to infected tissues, by inhalation of contaminated material, and by biting arthropods. The disease occurs only in the northern temperate zones.

Tularemia in humans appears as several clinical syndromes that might be confused with plague. Ulceroglandular tularemia is characterized by an ulcerative skin lesion with regional lymphadenitis. Glandular tularemia refers to the presence of bubolike lymphadenitis without a skin lesion. Oculoglandular disease results from conjunctival inoculation and involves the periorbital tissues and lymph nodes of the head and neck. Septicemic tularemia is similar to primary septicemic plague in that localized lymph node or skin involvement may not be apparent. Ingestion tularemia is characterized by gastrointestinal symptoms with or without pharyngitis. Pulmonary tularemia may be primary, but more commonly occurs as a complication of septicemic disease.

Tularemia in the United States occurs primarily as the result of occupational exposure to animal materials (e.g., pelts) or in hunters similarly exposed. Fleas are important vectors. An epidemic of tularemia pneumonia occurred in New England that was related to inhalation of drafts from a chimney containing a dead animal. Tularemia should be suspected in any case of relatively severe systemic disease (especially with skin lesions) or pneumonia in an individual exposed to wild animals.

Diagnosis of tularemia is confirmed by culture or serology. Streptomycin is the drug of choice for therapy; however gentamicin, tetracycline, and chloramphenicol are also effective.

Rat-Bite Fever. The term *rat-bite fever* is used to describe two diseases. Rat-bite fevers occur in areas of crowding and poor socioeconomic conditions where close exposure to rats leads to bites or other contacts. One rat-bite disease is caused by the gram-negative rod *Streptobacillus moniliformis* and is called Haverhill fever. The disease is characterized by edema, ulceration, and abscess formation at the rat-bite site, which is associated with intermittent fever paroxysms, a maculopapular to petechial rash, and polyarthritis. The rash frequently involves the palms and soles. Diagnosis is made by the clinical history and the course of the disease, by serologic studies, or by animal inoculation.

The other disease, sodoku, is caused by *Spirillum minus,* a gram-negative organism that is transmitted primarily by rat bite. The disease is characterized by inflammation at the bite site, lymphadenitis, paroxysmal fever, and a dark red, macular rash. Arthritis is absent. The diagnosis is made by darkfield examination of exudates or animal inoculation.

Haverhill fever has been described primarily in the United States, whereas sodoku is the prevalent rat-bite fever in Japan and Asia. A fatality rate of 10% is reported in untreated cases of both diseases. The treatment of choice for both is penicillin, with tetracycline and streptomycin as alternatives.

Rickettsial Diseases

Rickettsiae are obligate, intracellular bacteria that infect a variety of mammals and arthropod vectors. The organisms invade endothelial cells and cause vasculitis. Most diseases caused by rickettsiae can be categorized into two groups: the spotted fevers and the typhus group. Other rickettsial diseases are Q fever, trench fever, and ehrlichiosis.

Among the rickettsial spotted fevers are Rocky Mountain spotted fever (caused by *Rickettsia richettsii*); boutonneuse fever, South African tick bite fever, and Indian and Kenyan tick typhus (all caused by *R. conorii*); Queensland tick typhus *(R. australis);* and North Asian tick typhus *(R. sibirica).* All of these diseases are transmitted by ticks and have wild rodent and other animal reservoirs.

The spotted fevers are characterized by an acute febrile illness with chills and headache, followed in several days by the eruption of a maculopapular rash often involving the palms and soles. The rash may become petechial to purpuric. A primary ulcerative lesion with an eschar at the site of the tick bite usually occurs with *R. conorii* and *R. sibirica* infections, occasionally in Queensland tick typhus, but never in Rocky Mountain spotted fever. Rocky Mountain spotted fever occurs in North and South America. Boutonneuse fever and the other *R. conorii* infections occur along the Mediterranean Sea and in Africa and India. The geographic distribution of the other rickettsial spotted fevers are indicated by their name.

Rickettsialpox is another member of the spotted fever group and is caused by *R. akari,* which has the house mouse as reservoir and a mite as vector. The course is usually mild. This disease is characterized by a primary papule followed by a febrile illness and a maculopapular rash that becomes vesicular. The primary papule becomes vesicular and then evolves into an eschar. Rickettsialpox has been described primarily in the United States and Russia in urban settings, but sporadic cases from tropical areas also have been reported.

Rocky Mountain spotted fever is the most important of the rickettsial spotted fevers in the United States. The name of the disease derives from where it was first studied. Most cases now occur along the East Coast of the United States, especially in suburban areas of Virginia and Maryland, and places such as Cape Cod. The disease occurs in any area in which the tick vector, usually of the genus *Dermacentor,* is prevalent. The most important preventive measure is avoidance of ticks.

Rocky Mountain spotted fever should be suspected in any patient who has a febrile illness with severe headache that progresses in association with the development of a petechial or purpuric rash. In Rocky Mountain spotted fever, prodromal symptoms usually occur for several days before the rash, whereas in meningococcal disease the rash usually appears shortly after the onset of illness. Obviously the differential diagnosis of these two diseases is critical. Treatment must be prompt in either case.

The typhus group of rickettsial diseases includes epidemic typhus *(R. prowazekii).* Epidemic typhus appears to have humans as its only reservoir, although flying squirrels have been implicated; it is transmitted by the body louse. Epidemic typhus may occur anywhere in the world under situations of deprivation, crowding, and pediculosis. Recurrent typhus, known as Brill-Zinsser disease, may occur many years after initial infection and may appear in immigrants to areas where practitioners are unfamiliar with epidemic typhus. Murine typhus occurs worldwide in domestic cycles involving rats and their fleas. Scrub typhus, which occurs in the South Pacific and Asia, is transmitted by chigger bites from a natural reservoir in small mammals.

Epidemic typhus and murine typhus are characterized by fever, headache, myalgia, and a macular rash. Murine typhus is a milder disease than epidemic typhus, with the fatality rate among untreated cases being 2% in the former and 10% to 40% in the latter. Brill-Zinsser disease is typically milder than primary disease, and the rash may be absent. Scrub typhus is associated with an ulcer that has an eschar at the site of the chigger bite, febrile illness, a maculopapular rash, lymphadenopathy, and often pulmonary signs and symptoms.

Coxiella burnetii, a rickettsial organism, is the etiologic agent of Q fever. *C. burnetti* differs from organisms of the genus *Rickettsia* in several ways, including the ability to invade a wider variety of cells and a relative resistance to desiccation and heat. The organism has a number of wild and domestic animal reservoirs and has been found in several varieties of tick. It occurs worldwide. The usual transmission to humans is through the air via dusts contaminated by animal tissues, placental material, and birth fluids. Outbreaks in the United States have been associated with the handling of cattle, abattoirs, and aerosolized material emanating from slaughterhouses. Cases also have occurred in laboratory workers handling the organism.

The disease is characterized by a sudden onset of febrile illness with chills, myalgia, and prominent headache that lasts 1 to 2 weeks and occasionally longer. Multiple areas of pneumonitis may be apparent on chest radiograph, and the patient may complain of nonproductive cough and pleuritic chest pain. Abnormal liver function tests are frequent, but clinical jaundice is unusual. Rash and lymphadenopathy are absent. *C. burnetti* also can cause a chronic syndrome that is essentially Q fever endocarditis. Q fever endocarditis should be suspected in patients with "culture-negative" endocarditis with possible environmental exposure to *C. burnetii* and associated active liver disease.

Trench fever is caused by *Rochalimaea quintana* and is transmitted by lice. The reservoir is human and the disease occurs under conditions of crowding and pediculosis. It is usually a mild systemic febrile illness, frequently with characteristic shin pain. Occasionally, chronic or relapsing infections occur.

Ehrlichia sennetsu is the etiologic agent of sennetsu fever. The organism was formerly assigned to the genus *Rickettsia.* The mode of transmission has not been clearly established, but ticks are suspected. Sennetsu fever is a systemic febrile illness associated with lymphadenopathy and hepatosplenomegaly that occurs in Japan and other parts of Asia. In the 1980s, human ehrlichiosis was recognized in the United States. The organism is now identified as *E. chaffeensis,* closely related to the dog pathogen *E. canis.* The vector of human disease has not been established, but canine ehrlichiosis is transmitted by ticks. Human ehrlichiosis is generally a mild, nondescript systemic illness that, in some instances, is associated with macular or petechial rash. Severe illness is complicated by shock and multisystem organ failure and, in some cases, a toxic shock–like syndrome.

The diagnosis of rickettsial disease depends on the recognition of acute febrile illness associated with rash. Important diagnostic clues derive from the epidemiology of the diseases, geographic distribution, history of arthropod bites, and animal exposures. The character of the rash, or its absence, and the presence or absence of an eschar also help make the diagnosis.

The Weil-Felix reaction, which is based on the agglutination of three strains of *Proteus vulgaris* (Ox-19, Ox-2, Ox-K) by serum from patients with various rickettsial diseases, is the classic serologic test for infection due to rickettsiae. Agglutinin titers against Ox-19 and Ox-2 typically rise in all the diseases of the spotted fever group, except rickettsialpox. Agglutinin to Ox-19 usually rises in epidemic and murine typhus, whereas the antibody response to Ox-2 is variable in these. The Ox-K, but not the Ox-19 and Ox-2, agglutinins are elevated in scrub typhus. None of the agglutinins rise in rickettsialpox or Q fever, and titers may not change in Brill-Zinsser disease.

The Weil-Felix reactions generally have been supplanted by specific serologic tests for confirmation of diagnosis. All of the serologic tests show titer changes late in disease and usually are not useful for acute diagnosis. Serologic tests for various Q fever antigens can help in the diagnosis of Q fever endocarditis. Demonstration of rickettsia in skin biopsies from patients with rashes can be accomplished by direct immunofluorescent staining. In vitro isolation of rickettsiae and in vivo isolation by injection of patient material into laboratory animals are occasionally performed, but the techniques required are available only in special research laboratories, and such isolations are dangerous to laboratory personnel. The differential diagnosis of rickettsial diseases is summarized in Table 30-5.

Tetracycline and chloramphenicol are the drugs of choice for the treatment of rickettsial infections. These drugs are equally effective in the treatment of the spotted fevers and diseases of the typhus group. Tetracycline is usually preferred because of the potential toxicity of chloramphenicol. Response to therapy is prompt, except for Q fever, which is much less responsive, especially in the endocarditis form. Relapses of rickettsial infections may occur after treatment; they are usually related to therapy being initiated early in the course of disease and respond to retreatment. Treatment, however, must not be delayed to avoid relapse and complications. The morbidity and mortality associated with Rocky Mountain spotted fever, typhus, and scrub typhus are substantial in untreated patients.

Spirochetoses

Spirochetes are the cause of several human diseases. Nonpathogenic spirochetes are ubiquitous members of the normal oral flora. Syphilis is discussed in Chapter 29 and the other diseases caused by spirochetes of the genus *Treponema* are discussed under Skin Lesions. *Leptospira* species and *Borrelia* species are spirochetes that cause systemic, febrile illnesses.

The various serotypes of *Leptospira* causing human infection were previously given individual species names but are now considered varieties of one species, *Leptospira interrogans.* Leptospirosis is a zoonosis that affects many animals worldwide. The disease is present in rural and urban parts of the developing world. Humans acquire leptospirosis by contact with infected animals or their urine, or contaminated water or soil. The organisms are capable of penetrating damaged skin and mucous membranes.

Table 30-5. Epidemiologic, Clinical, and Laboratory Characteristics of Diseases Caused by Rickettsia

Disease	Organism	Vector	Reservoir	Occurrence	Rash/eschar	Serology* (Weil-Felix)
Spotted fever group						
Rocky Mountain spotted fever	*Rickettsia rickettsii*	Tick	Rodents	North America South America	+/–	Ox-19, Ox-2
Boutonneuse fever	*R. conorii*	Tick	Rodents	Mediterranean Africa, Southeast Asia	+/+	Ox-19, Ox-2
North Asian tick typhus	*R. sibirica*	Tick	Rodents	North Asia	+/+	Ox-19, Ox-2
Queensland tick typhus	*R. australis*	Tick	Rodents, marsupials	Australia	+/+	Ox-19, Ox-2
Rickettsialpox	*R. akari*	Mite	Mice	Temperate zones	+/+	0
Typhus group						
Epidemic typhus	*R. prowazekii*	Louse	Humans	Worldwide	+/–	Ox-19, +/–Ox-2
Murine typhus	*R. typhi*	Flea	Rodents	Worldwide	+/–	Ox-19, +/–Ox-2
Scrub typhus	*R. tsutsugamushi*	Chigger	Rodents	Asia, South Pacific	+/+	Ox-K
Other						
Trench fever	*Rochalimaea quintana*	Louse	Humans	North and South America, Africa, Europe	+/–	0
Q fever	*Coxiella burnetii*	None	Domestic animals	Worldwide	–/–	0
Sennetsu fever	*Ehrlichia sennetsu*	?Tick		Asia	–/–	0
Ehrlichiosis	*E. chaffeensis*	?Tick	?Domestic animals	North America	+/–	0

*Specific serologic diagnostic tests are available for each infection.

Evidence suggests subclinical infection occurs. The clinical disease is usually biphasic. Mild disease, referred to as anicteric, manifests as a septicemic phase (characterized by fever, myalgia, headache, malaise, and gastrointestinal complaints lasting several days to 1 week) and an "immune" phase (that may overlap the initial phase and primarily manifests as meningitis, rash, and uveitis). Severe disease—icteric hemorrhagic fever or Weil's disease—composes 10% or fewer clinical leptospirosis infections and is characterized by jaundice, renal functional impairment, and vasculitis with bleeding.

The diagnosis of leptospirosis is made by recognizing the characteristic clinical features, with or without a history of exposure to animals or to water likely to contain animal urine. Leptospires may be isolated in culture using special techniques. Blood cultures may be positive early in the disease, and later the organism may be isolated from cerebrospinal fluid and urine. Serologic tests also are available.

It is unclear whether antibiotics significantly alter the course of leptospirosis. Penicillin or tetracycline may be beneficial if therapy is started early in the course of disease. Doxycycline has been used as a prophylactic agent to prevent leptospirosis in situations in which unavoidable exposure is expected.

Relapsing fever is caused by spirochetes of the genus *Borrelia*. The disease occurs as two epidemiologic types, louse-borne and tick-borne. Although the disease may occur in virtually any area of the world, the epidemic louse-borne infection occurs under socioeconomic conditions associated with the presence of lice and is seen primarily in the higher elevations of Africa and South America. Endemic tick-borne disease occurs in widespread geographic foci (including areas of North America) where ticks and the small animals that serve as the reservoir reside. The clinical disease is related to the cyclic appearance of the spirochetes in the bloodstream.

The organisms, which reappear in the blood after sequestration in tissue, are capable of changing their surface antigens to overcome specific antibody. This results in relapses with fever, chills, myalgia, headache, and cough (lasting 3 to 6 days); about 1 week elapses between episodes. The febrile periods usually end in a crisis. Hepatosplenomegaly, bleeding, and a papular, petechial, or macular rash may occur. Louse-borne infection usually results in one relapse, whereas multiple relapses with higher fever are typical of the tick-borne infection. CNS involvement may present as "aseptic" meningitis.

The diagnosis of relapsing fever is made by demonstrating blood-borne spirochetes during febrile episodes by darkfield examination or on stained smears. Animal inoculation also is used, but serologic tests are of limited value because of the antigenic variability of the organism.

Tetracycline is the drug of choice for treatment, although chloramphenicol, penicillin, and erythromycin also are effective. A Jarisch-Herxheimer reaction (fever, chills, myalgia) typically occurs with therapy. Untreated epidemic disease has a mortality rate of up to 40%, but with treatment the mortality rate is low.

Arbovirus Diseases and Hemorrhagic Fevers

Several acute viral illnesses are transmitted by arthropod vectors, and the viruses that cause these diseases are often referred to as arboviruses (for arthropod-borne). Approximately 80 to 100 of these viruses infect humans. Diseases occur primarily in tropical and semitropical regions, although some arboviruses cause summer epidemics in the temperate zones. The arboviruses belong to several distinct families of viruses, but all are RNA viruses. Arboviruses cause three disease syndromes—nondescript febrile illnesses, hemorrhagic fevers, and encephalitis—although there is overlap in many cases.

Many arboviruses cause acute, relatively benign, nondescript febrile illnesses often with arthralgia, myalgia, and rash. An example of this group is dengue, or breakbone fever. This disease is widespread in tropical areas and is transmitted by mosquitoes. Its endemic areas are currently enlarging, especially in the Caribbean and Gulf of Mexico. Dengue has been acquired in Texas. Large parts of the southern United States are at potential risk of dengue activity. The disease is characterized by sudden onset of fever, chills, severe headache, retroorbital pain, conjunctivitis, lymphadenopathy, and severe myalgia and arthralgia. The acute disease lasts about 1 week, often with saddleback fever, with a fall and then a rise of daily fever spikes over the week. A diffuse, scarlet fever–type maculopapular rash occurs in the midst of the acute disease. Leukopenia is typical. Recovery is often followed by a prolonged period of depression and fatigue. Similar diseases occur in various parts of the world and are often marked by more severe joint pain with or without rash. These include such exotically named diseases as chikungunya, o'nyong-nyong, Rift Valley fever, and Colorado tick fever. These diseases are transmitted by mosquitoes, ticks, and sandflies.

More severe systemic arbovirus diseases are referred to as hemorrhagic fevers. The classic example is yellow fever, although dengue and chikungunya viruses also cause hemorrhagic fever, especially in Asia. The pathophysiology of hemorrhagic fevers is not well defined and is under intense investigation. Dengue hemorrhagic fever and the dengue shock syndrome appear to have an immunologic basis and occur with subsequent episodes of dengue. The hemorrhagic fevers are characterized by leukopenia, thrombocytopenia, ecchymoses, and gross bleeding. In severe cases, shock and death result. Yellow fever is a hemorrhagic fever so named because of the hepatitis and jaundice it produces. It has an important history in the United States, with epidemics occurring as far north as Philadelphia up to 150 to 200 years ago. The conquest of yellow fever contributed to the success of the effort to build the Panama Canal. Nephritis also may occur in patients with yellow fever. Severe yellow fever is associated with profound jaundice, hemorrhage, and hypotension, with a peculiar relative bradycardia. Mortality rates in arbovirus hemorrhagic fevers are approximately 5% to 10%. Other examples are Omsk hemorrhagic fever, Kyasanur Forest disease, and Crimean-Congo fever.

The third disease syndrome associated with arboviruses is encephalitis. The arbovirus encephalitides include eastern equine, western equine, Venezuelan equine, St. Louis, Japanese, California, West Nile, Russian spring-summer, Powassan, and others. These diseases have several animal reservoirs and are transmitted by mosquitoes and ticks. The diseases begin with fever, headache, and systemic viral symptoms; the patients then become somnolent, develop meningeal signs, and may go on to seizures, paralysis, coma, and death. Aseptic meningitis is common. The diseases have a spectrum of severity, and fatality rates range from 50% to 60% for Japanese and eastern equine encephalitis to 5% and less for others, with California encephalitis usually being the least severe. Long-term neurologic sequelae may result, especially in young survivors.

Japanese B encephalitis is transmitted by mosquito throughout large parts of Eastern and Southern Asia. Pigs are important reservoirs of the virus. Whereas mild infections are more common than severe and are associated with myalgia, fever, and headache, severe disease with life-threatening acute illness and neurologic sequelae in survivors also occurs. Incubation period is approximately 1 week. An inactivated vaccine recently was licensed in the United States and is recommended for anyone who will be spending a month or longer in Asia during the warm season, especially if there is to be exposure to rural areas. Three doses of vaccine are given over 1 month, but an accelerated 2-week schedule may be used if necessary. The last dose should be given at least 10 days before travel commences.

Several non–arthropod-borne viruses cause hemorrhagic fevers, often with renal impairment or other systemic and organ-specific complications. These viruses belong to several taxonomic groups and include the Junin and Machupo viruses, which cause Argentine and Bolivian hemorrhagic fever, respectively; the Lassa fever virus, which occurs in West Africa; and the *Hantavirus,* which causes Korean hemorrhagic fever in Asia and *Hantavirus* pulmonary syndrome in the United States. These viruses have rodent reservoirs and are transmitted through exposure to the excreta of infected mice and rats. Mortality rates are high, and Lassa fever is highly communicable. A related virus with a worldwide distribution and the house mouse as a reservoir is lymphocytic choriomeningitis (LCM) virus, which causes a nonspecific, systemic viral syndrome with or without meningoencephalitis. Two additional viruses, the Marburg and Ebola viruses, cause hemorrhagic fever in Africa. The reservoirs and modes of transmission of these viruses are not established. Mortality rates during outbreaks have been high (30% to 70%).

There are no specific therapies for the viral fevers, hemorrhagic fevers, and viral encephalitides. Ribavirin, active against RNA viruses, is being investigated as a specific therapy through several protocols. Serum from survivors of Lassa fever and Ebola virus infection has been used to treat these diseases with some success.

Ectoparasites

Detailed information about pediculosis, lice, and scabies is presented in Chapter 29.

Chiggers are trombiculid mites, the larvae of which attach to the skin and feed on tissue fluid and necrotic debris. Chiggers occur worldwide in areas of scrub vegetation. They are the vector of scrub typhus in the South Pacific and Asia. The area of chigger skin attachment develops a macular lesion that may evolve into a papular, then vesicular, and then hemorrhagic lesion. Pruritus leads to removal of the parasites by scratching. A systemic reaction may occur in the very young and very old. Chiggers of the skin are treated with a variety of alcoholic solutions and other topical agents such as fingernail polish.

Myiasis is the infestation of the skin with fly larvae or maggots. Maggots may be present in preexisting traumatic lesions and, in fact, have been purposely used for debridement of wounds in the past. Certain species of fly are capable of injecting eggs into undamaged skin, causing furuncular myiasis. Several such species occur in South America, North America, and Africa. Furuncular myiasis results in painful, furuncle-like lesions that may be secondarily infected. Furuncular maggots may be removed by means of forceps or by excision. Maggots of colonizing superficial lesions may be treated with chloroform dressings or by pouring ether over the lesions.

Ticks are arachnid parasites that bury their mouth parts in the skin and take a blood meal (see Chapter 94).

DISEASE SYNDROMES IN TRAVELERS

Fever

Fever in a traveler from the tropics is often a cause of anxiety in the traveler and the primary care physician. The traveler may be terrified about an exotic infectious disease acquired overseas. The primary care physician may be anxious about recalling numerous parasite syndromes, shapes, and life cycles learned in medical school.

The differential diagnosis of fever in a returned traveler or an immigrant is extensive, but can be quickly narrowed by a good history, physical examination, and appropriate laboratory data. Box 30-1 presents the relative risk for several infections, diseases, and injuries for international travelers. Initially, the "nontropical" causes of fever such as community acquired respiratory diseases and urinary tract infection must be ruled out, because they account for over half of fevers among returned travelers. A detailed travel history, food exposure, and animal contact history can narrow the list of diagnoses. A physical examination to look specifically for rash, lymphadenopathy, and hepatosplenomegaly is essential. Distinctive clues in the laboratory findings such as anemia or eosinophilia are extremely helpful. A list of diseases to be considered in the differential diagnosis of febrile illness in travelers and immigrants with some of the clues leading to those diagnoses is provided in Box 30-1.

The physician must then order specific diagnostic tests unique in the diagnosis of parasitic diseases such as thick and thin blood smears for malaria and examination for ova and parasites in the stool. If the diagnosis is still not evident, often the case, the physician must make a decision to treat empirically and consider consultation with an infectious diseases or a tropical medicine specialist.

Common Causes of Fever. Common causes of difficult-to-diagnose fever in travelers are malaria, hepatitis, and upper respiratory infection. Other causes of fever include enteric fever, arboviral infection (dengue), and tuberculosis.

Malaria must be suspected in every patient who returns from the tropics without a localized source for fever. Even if the traveler reports compliance with chemoprophylaxis, malaria can occur due to the resistant *P. falciparum* and possible inadvertent noncompliance. Failure of chemoprophylaxis may occur in the compliant individual. Eighty percent of the malaria cases reported in the United States from 1980 to 1988 were acquired in sub-Sahara Africa. Even with appropriate prophylaxis, *P. vivax* and *P. ovale* can cause relapse months after the traveler returns, with the persistence of the extraerythrocytic (hepatic) stage.

Enteric fever may be due to *S. typhi* or nontyphoidal *Salmonella* species. Typhoid fever and enteric fever must be considered in returning travelers even if immunized, especially if at risk for hypochlorhydria due to age, blockers of gastric acid secretion, or previous surgical procedure. Blood and stool cultures are usually positive.

Box 30-1. A Differential Diagnosis of Some Selected Systemic Febrile Illnesses to Consider in Returned Travelers and Immigrants*

Common

Acute respiratory tract infection (worldwide)
Gastroenteritis (worldwide) [food-borne, water-borne, fecal-oral]
Enteric fever, including typhoid (worldwide) [food, water]
Urinary tract infection (worldwide) [sexual contact]
Drug reactions [antibiotics, prophylactic agents, other] {rash frequent}
Malaria (tropics, limited areas of temperate zones) [mosquitoes]
Arboviruses (Africa; tropics) [mosquitoes, ticks, mites]
Dengue (Asia, Caribbean, Africa) [mosquitoes]
Viral hepatitis (worldwide)
Hepatitis A (worldwide) [food, fecal-oral]
Hepatitis B (worldwide, esp. Asia, sub-Sahara Africa) [sexual contact] {long incubation period}
Hepatitis C (worldwide) [blood or sexual contact]
Hepatitis E (Asia, North Africa, Mexico, ?others) [food, water]
Tuberculosis (worldwide) [airborne, milk] {long period to symptomatic infection}
Sexually transmitted diseases (worldwide) [sexual contact]

Less Common

Filariasis (see Table 30-4) (Asia, Africa, South America) [biting insects] {long incubation period, eosinophilia}
Measles (developing world) [airborne] {in susceptible individual}
Amebic abscess (worldwide) [food]
Brucellosis (worldwide) [milk, cheese, food, animal contact]
Listeriosis (worldwide) [food-borne] {meningitis}
Leptospirosis (worldwide) [animal contact, open fresh water] {jaundice, meningitis}
Strongyloidiasis (warm and tropical areas) [soil contact] {eosinophilia}
Toxoplasmosis (worldwide) [undercooked meat]

Rare

Relapsing fever (western Americas, Asia, northern Africa) [ticks, lice]
Hemorrhagic fevers (worldwide) [arthropod and nonarthropod transmitted]
Yellow fever (tropics) [mosquitoes] {hepatitis}
Hemorrhagic fever with renal syndrome (Europe, Asia, North America) [rodent urine] {renal impairment}
Hantavirus pulmonary syndrome (western North America, ?other) [rodent urine] {respiratory distress syndrome}
Lassa fever (Africa) [Rodent excreta, person to person] {high mortality rate}
Other-chikungunya, Rift Valley, Ebola-Marburg, etc. (various) [insect bites, rodent excreta, aerosols, person to person] {often severe}
Rickettsial infections (see Table 30-5) {Rashes and eschars}
Leishmaniasis, visceral (Middle East, Mediterranean, Africa, Asia, South America) [biting flies] {long incubation period}
Acute schistosomiasis (Africa, Asia, South America, Caribbean) [fresh water]
Chagas' disease (South and Central America) [reduviid bug bites] {often asymptomatic}
African trypanosomiasis (Africa) [Tsetse fly bite] {neurologic syndromes, sleeping sickness}
Bartonellosis (South America) [sandfly bite; cb {skin nodules}
HIV infection/AIDS (worldwide) [sexual and blood contact]
Trichinosis (worldwide) [undercooked meat] {eosinophilia}
Plague (temperate and tropical plains) [animal exposures and fleas]
Tularemia (worldwide) [animal contact, fleas, aerosols] {ulcers, lymph nodes}
Anthrax (worldwide) [animal, animal product contact] {ulcers}
Lyme disease (North America, Europe) [tick bites] {arthritis, meningitis, cardiac abnormalities}

*Diagnoses for which particular symptoms are indicative are in *italics*. Exposure to regions of the world that are most likely to be significant to the diagnosis are presented in (parentheses). Vectors, risk behaviors, and sources associated with acquisition are presented in [brackets]. Special clinical characteristics are listed within.

Arboviruses are capable of causing flulike illness, hemorrhagic fever, or encephalitis. Dengue is a classic example in which the patient presents 1 to 2 weeks after returning with fever, chills, myalgia, arthralgia, and in some instances rash. Recovery is characterized by prolonged fatigue. Hemorrhagic fever caused by viruses such as the Lassa fever virus must be considered in patients with leukopenia, thrombocytopenia, ecchymoses, and gross bleeding. Immediate strict isolation and public health consolation are necessary. Encephalitis due to arboviruses needs to be considered if a history of headache, meningeal signs, and mental status changes present after a nonspecific prodrome.

Fever patterns in general are unreliable guides to diagnosis. Fever-pulse dichotomy may occur in typhoid fever or brucellosis. Relapsing fever presents classically as febrile episodes of 3 days followed by afebrile periods of 6 to 7 days in patients returning from western South America. Dengue fever may have saddleback pattern with relapse after 2 to 3 weeks.

Region Traveled. Travel history is essential for appropriate differential diagnosis. Activity, length of stay, and site of stay help include or exclude specific diagnoses. A traveler who has ventured into rural areas, or lived for a prolonged time with native populations, is at a much greater risk of tropical diseases, such as dengue or typhoid fever, than businessmen who go for short visits and stay in western-style hotels. In addition, a disease such as bartonellosis need only be considered in a traveler returning from Peru, Ecuador, or Colombia with possible exposure to sandflies. African trypanosomiasis should be considered in patients who present with fever 2 to 4 weeks after returning from a rural site in East or West Africa with a history of remembered or potential fly bite.

Onset of Fever After Return. Incubation periods for tropical diseases vary greatly and are important indicators of possible diagnoses. Arboviral infection, spotted fevers, and plague have short incubation periods and occur within 1 or 2 weeks of return from the tropics, whereas malaria, acute schistosomiasis, and leishmaniasis can occur up to 1 month or more after return.

Acute schistosomiasis can present 4 to 6 weeks after return from an endemic area such as Egypt with fever, weight loss, diarrhea, and marked peripheral eosinophilia. Visceral leishmaniasis may present 2 to 4 months or longer after return from endemic areas such as India, with high fever and organomegaly associated with a history of exposure to sandflies.

Exposures. Specific exposure to animals, flies, ticks, foods, or fresh water adds a new set of diagnoses to be considered in the febrile patient. The traveler often does not volunteer the information because he or she does not realize its significance. For example, brucellosis usually requires exposure to animals, meat, or dairy products and presents with hectic fevers, myalgia, adenopathy, and positive blood cultures. Plague must be considered in patients with potential exposure to rodents presenting with fever and painful and swollen lymph nodes (buboes) within a week after return from an endemic area.

Empiric Therapy. Indiscriminate use of antibiotics should be avoided; however, when patients are critically ill or malaria is suspected, empiric treatment is required. Empiric treatment for malaria should be considered in persons who return from endemic regions, with or without history of prophylaxis, who are systemically ill with no focal signs of infection, even if initial thick or thin blood smears are negative.

Broad-spectrum antibiotics used for empiric therapy of bacterial and rickettsial infections include chloramphenicol and the tetracyclines. Chloramphenicol or tetracyclines are often effective for many potentially lethal diseases that are difficult to diagnose on presentation including typhoid fever, brucellosis, relapsing fever, bartonellosis, glanders, melioidosis, anthrax, plague, tularemia, Rocky Mountain spotted fever, epidemic typhus, and scrub typhus. In such diseases empiric therapy is the rule rather than the exception.

Of course, fever may not be the only sign of illness. Rash, diarrhea, lymphadenopathy, or respiratory symptoms can point to diagnoses. The differential diagnoses of illness with these findings is presented in the designated sections of this chapter and in other parts of this book under specific organ systems.

Traveler's diarrhea is described in Chapter 111.

Respiratory Infections

Respiratory illness is among the most common causes of morbidity and mortality in the tropics, largely due to crowded living conditions and socioeconomic deprivation. The causes of illness are quite similar to those in the developed countries with additional organisms specific to the tropics. Travelers who acquire respiratory tract pathogens in the tropics may present special diagnostic problems. A list of unusual infections with pulmonary infiltrates that may be encountered in returning international travelers is presented in Box 30-2.

Box 30-2. Infections Associated with Pulmonary Infiltrates that may be Encountered in Returning International Travelers

Bacterial
Tuberculosis
Legionellosis
Q fever
Melioidosis
Tularemia
Glanders
Psittacosis
Plague
Brucellosis
Typhoid
Rickettsiosis

Fungal
Blastomycosis
Coccidioidomycosis
Histoplasmosis

Viral
Measles
Hemorrhagic fevers
Influenza
Adenovirus

Parasitic
Amebiasis
Toxoplasmosis
Ascariasis
Hookworm
Strongyloidiasis
Filariasis
Paragonimiasis
Schistosomiasis (Katayama fever)
Echinococcosis
Toxocariasis
Trichinosis

Other causes of pneumonia that commonly occur in the United States are not listed, but should always be ruled out because they are common causes of pneumonia worldwide.

Several organisms that cause systemic infection may cause pulmonary illness. *S. typhi* frequently causes bronchitis or nonspecific bronchopneumonia. *Yersinia pestis*, the etiologic agent of plague, is infectious through the respiratory route and causes a rapidly progressive pneumonia. If the patient has been exposed to rabbits or slaughtered animals, tularemic pneumonia should be considered. Half of leptospirosis cases have nonspecific pulmonary involvement. Several etiologic agents that cause pneumonia and that are not discussed in other sections of the text are included below.

Melioidosis is an infection caused by the gram-negative bacillus *Pseudomonas pseudomallei*. The organisms live in water and soil and are capable of infecting several animals in addition to people. The disease is uncommon and occurs primarily in Southeast Asia and the Pacific, with sporadic cases occurring in various other areas. It is acquired through close contact with soil and water. The disease is usually pulmonary, although inapparent infection, skin infection, lymphadenitis, septicemia, and visceral abscesses have been encountered. Acute pulmonary disease is characterized by fever, pleuritic chest pain, myalgia, and headache. Consolidation in the upper lobes, often with cavitation, is the typical radiographic finding. Septicemia and metastatic suppurative infection may complicate pneumonia. Chronic pulmonary infection, with recrudescence at a later time, may occur, and the disease may resemble tuberculosis. Diagnosis is made on the basis of Gram's stain and culture. Serologic tests also are available. Treatment is with tetracycline, chloramphenicol, or a sulfonamide, alone or in combination depending on susceptibility tests, for 30 to 60 days or longer depending on the location of infection and chronicity. Ceftazidime also has been used successfully.

Glanders, a disease of horses and other equine animals, has a worldwide distribution and is caused by *Pseudomonas mallei*. It occasionally occurs in humans, causing syndromes similar to melioidosis. The disease is differentiated from melioidosis by culture. Treatment is usually with streptomycin combined with tetracycline or a sulfonamide.

Psittacosis is a systemic disease caused by *Chlamydia psittaci* that usually presents in humans as a respiratory disease. *C. psittaci* is primarily a pathogen of birds, especially psittacine birds (e.g., parrots, parakeets). People acquire the disease by exposure to sick or well birds that are shedding the organism. The disease is characterized by fever, severe headache, myalgia, lethargy, cough productive of scant sputum, dyspnea, splenomegaly, and occasionally a macular rash similar to the rose spots of typhoid. Chest radiograph may show diffuse, patchy infiltrates or nodular or miliary lesions. The diagnosis is usually made on the basis of clinical signs and symptoms in a patient with a history of avian exposure and is confirmed serologically or, less commonly, by isolating the organism from blood or sputum. Treatment is with tetracycline, to which there is usually a prompt response, although relapses may occur.

Paragonimus westermani, the lung fluke, is a trematode that infects the lung. The disease occurs primarily in Asia, especially Korea, although foci of infection are present in other parts of the world. Other species of *Paragonimus* also infect humans. The disease is acquired by ingestion of larvae encysted in the secondary intermediate hosts, freshwater crabs and crayfish. Snails are primary intermediate hosts. Encysted larvae migrate through the intestinal wall and make their way to the lung and other organs. Fibrous cysts form around adult worms in the lung and other tissues. Chronic cough productive of copious sputum and hemoptysis are the usual symptoms. A variety of neurologic symptoms and signs results from cerebral involvement.

Chest radiograph shows small nodular infiltrates or larger lesions that are seen with heavy pulmonary worm loads. The diagnosis is suspected on the basis of residence in an endemic area, productive cough, hemoptysis, eosinophilia, and chest radiographic findings. The diagnosis is confirmed by demonstrating the characteristic operculated eggs in sputum (see Fig. 30-2). Treatment with praziquantel in a dose of 75 mg/kg per day in three divided doses for 2 days is safe and effective. Bithionol is an alternative agent.

Among viral causes of pneumonia, measles-associated pneumonia still accounts for 25% of pneumonia among children in developing countries. Several parasitic diseases can cause primary or associated respiratory illness. Hepatic abscess due to *Entamoeba histolytica* can lead to sympathetic pleural effusion or secondary pneumonitis. Worms can cause pulmonary disease as they migrate through the lung alveoli (ascaris or hookworm) or as they pass through the pulmonary vasculature (schistosomiasis or filariasis) or as they lodge in the lung tissue (paragonimiasis or echinococcosis). Pulmonary infiltrates with eosinophilia are discussed under eosinophilia.

A traveler who presents with a respiratory illness is most likely to be infected with a cosmopolitan organism. Several diagnoses, however, need to be kept in mind. *Mycobacterium tuberculosis* infection is present in 50% to 60% of people in developing countries and is a particular threat to travelers returning from prolonged stays in the tropics. Epidemiologic clues of animal exposure are often essential to reach the diagnosis of Q fever, psittacosis, or tularemia. Workup must include the standard sputum Gram's stain and culture, along with acid-fast stain and mycobacterial culture. Blood count with differential count to check for eosinophilia is important. Examination of sputum and stool for ova and parasites may be helpful.

Eosinophilia

The eosinophilic granulocyte is a cell that participates in hypersensitivity reactions and plays a role in host defenses, particularly against multicellular parasites. Peripheral blood eosinophilia, usually defined as more than 450 eosinophils/mm^3, occurs with a number of allergic reactions and disease processes, but on a worldwide basis the most common cause is parasitic infection.

Peripheral blood eosinophilia is associated with helminthic parasites, not single cell protozoa such as *E. histolytica* or *Giardia* species. Tissue-invasive or tissue-dwelling worms or those that have invasive larvae are most commonly associated with eosinophilia. Among the intestinal roundworms, the larval migration stages of *Ascaris,* the hookworms, and *S. stercoralis* are associated with eosinophilia, whereas pinworm and *Trichuris trichiura,* which do not have invasive larvae, are not. *S. stercoralis,* which has the potential for autoinfection, may cause persistent eosinophilia in affected individuals. High degrees of eosinophilia are seen with trichinosis, and eosinophilia is observed with all forms of filariasis.

Several parasites with nonhuman usual hosts may infect humans and cause tissue infection associated with eosinophilia. These include *Echinococcus granulosus* and *E. multilocularis,* which cause hydatid cysts; *Toxocara* species, which cause visceral larva migrans; and animal hookworms, the invasive larvae of which cause cutaneous larva migrans. The rodent parasite *Angiostrongylus cantonensis* causes the syndrome eosinophilic meningitis with an eosinophilic pleocytosis in the cerebrospinal fluid. *Gnathostoma spinigerum,* a dog and cat nematode, can cause a similar syndrome. Eosinophilic gastritis is associated with the fish-borne, sea mammal ascarid *Anisakis*. The early phase of infection with the liver fluke *F. hepatica* is associated with marked eosinophilia, as in infection with the lung fluke *(P. westermani).* Severe scabies may be associated with eosinophilia.

Tropical eosinophilia is a syndrome seen in all parts of the tropics but most commonly in Asia. It is due to unidentified microfilariae. The disease is characterized by dyspnea, cough, wheezing, systemic complaints, and peripheral blood eosinophilia. The diagnosis is usually presumptive and the syndrome is treated with diethylcarbamazine.

The syndrome of pulmonary infiltrates with eosinophilia (PIE) is closely related to tropical eosinophilia. PIE is seen in some cases of asthma, polyarteritis nodosa, infections with nematodes that migrate through the lung (e.g., *Ascaris, S. stercoralis,* hookworms, trichinosis), and ectopic migration of *F. hepatica* larvae. When idiopathic and self-limited, the PIE syndrome is referred to as Loeffler's syndrome.

Several noninfectious conditions may be associated with peripheral blood eosinophilia. These conditions, the infections already discussed, and some other infections associated with eosinophilia are listed in Box 30-3.

Patients with eosinophilia should have a careful history taken for geographic exposure and other contacts that might cause one to suspect helminthic disease. A thorough physical examination may be helpful in distinguishing parasitic from nonparasitic causes. A stool specimen for ova and parasite examination is of obvious importance, and duodenal aspiration for *S. stercoralis* may be required. The blood should be examined for microfilariae depending on the history of travel and residence. A negative history and the absence of evidence of parasitic infection should lead to a more extensive workup for the other causes of eosinophilia. The differential diagnosis indicated by the conditions listed in Box 30-3 can serve as a guide to other diagnostic tests and procedures.

Box 30-3. Causes of Significant Peripheral Blood Eosinophilia

Helminthic Parasites

Ascaris lumbricoides (invasive larval stage)
Hookworms (invasive larval stage)
Strongyloides stercoralis (initial infection and autoinfection)
Trichinosis
Filariasis
Echinococcus granulosus and *E. multilocularis*
Toxocara species
Animal hookworms
Angiostrongylus cantonensis and *A. costaricensis*
Schistosomiasis
Liver flukes
Fasciolopsis buski
Anisakiasis
Capillaria philippinensis
Paragonimus westermani
"Tropical eosinophilia" (unidentified microfilariae)

Other Infections/Infestations

Pulmonary aspergillosis
Severe scabies

Allergies

Asthma
Hay fever
Drug reactions
Atopic dermatitis

Autoimmune and Related Disorders

Polyarteritis nodosa
Necrotizing vasculitis
Eosinophilic fasciitis
Pemphigus

Neoplastic Diseases

Hodgkin's disease
Mycosis fungoides
Chronic myelocytic leukemia
Eosinophilic leukemia
Polycythemia vera
Mucin-secreting adenocarcinomas

Immunodeficiency States

Hyperimmunoglobulin E with recurrent infection
Wiskott-Aldrich syndrome

Other

Addison's disease
Inflammatory bowel disease
Dermatitis herpetiformis
Toxic/chemical syndrome
(Eosinophilic myalgia syndrome-tryptophan, toxic oil syndrome)
"Hypereosinophilic syndrome" (unknown etiology)

Mass Lesions

Several parasites of humans and other animals and a variety of other infectious agents cause diseases that result in mass lesions of the soft tissue and organs.

Extraintestinal amebiasis results when trophozoites of *E. histolytica* invade the bowel wall, are carried in the bloodstream, and settle in tissue. Lesions usually occur in the liver via seeding of the portal blood. Amebic liver abscesses typically occur in the setting of asymptomatic bowel infection, most commonly as single in the right lobe. They are characterized by liquefaction necrosis centrally, with invasive amebae in the wall of the lesion. Patients may have insidious development of symptoms or abrupt systemic signs. A tender mass may be palpated through the abdominal wall. Rarely, amebic abscesses occur in the brain, lung, or spleen. Liver abscess may be complicated by rupture into the peritoneal cavity and extension into the pleural space, lung, or pericardial sac.

Diagnosis is made on clinical grounds, or the lesion may be demonstrated on radionuclide scan. Needle aspiration of liver abscesses reveals necrotic material that may resemble anchovy paste. Serologic tests are usually positive in patients with invasive amebiasis.

Amebic liver abscess may be treated with oral metronidazole, 750 mg, three times a day (35 to 50 mg/kg per day in children) for 10 days. Needle aspiration also may have therapeutic benefit in some cases. Diloxanide furoate or iodoquinol is often used in conjunction with metronidazole to ensure eradication of amebae in the intestinal lumen.

Migrating adults of the filarial worm *L. loa* cause localized areas of inflammation in subcutaneous tissue, resulting in characteristic "calabar swellings." *Dracunculus medinensis,* the guinea worm, is a tissue-invasive nematode that causes characteristic serpiginous lesions in the subcutaneous tissue of the lower extremities. Dracunculosis occurs in Africa, the Middle East, and southern Asia. The parasite is acquired by ingesting the intermediate host, copepods (small crustaceans), with drinking water. Larvae penetrate the intestinal wall, mature, and mate in the retroperitoneum. Adult female worms migrate to the lower extremities and may reach lengths of up to 80 cm in the subcutaneous tissue. Motile larvae are released through a blister in the skin. Worms may be removed by incising the skin or by gradual extraction by winding the worm on a stick. Niridazole, thiabendazole, and metronidazole have been used and the result is extrusion of the worm.

Humans are both definitive and intermediate hosts of the pork tapeworm *T. solium.* The larvae of *T. solium* invade the intestinal wall and migrate to tissue, where they encyst as cysticerci, causing cysticercosis. Infection may result from ingestion of eggs or by autoinfection from eggs shed by adult tapeworms in the intestine. Cysticerci may be widely distributed in many tissues, but of most significance are lesions in the eye and brain. Cerebral cysticercosis may result in recurrent seizures or increased intracranial pressure secondary to obstruction of cerebrospinal fluid flow. Cysticerci remain viable for several years.

Lesions containing dead *T. solium* cysticerci may calcify and diagnosis may be made by radiographic demonstration of calcified lesions in soft tissue that have a characteristic "puffed rice" appearance or by biopsy of accessible lesions. Computed tomography (CT) of the head is useful in diagnosing cerebral cysticercosis. Surgical resection of lesions, especially in the case of anatomic compromise, is indicated. Praziquantel is useful in treatment of cysticercosis in a dose of 50 to 100 mg/kg per day in three divided doses for 30 days. Albendazole is an alternative agent. Steroids are usually used in conjunction with treatment to limit tissue damage.

Hydatid cysts are mass lesions caused by the larvae of the canine tapeworms *E. granulosus* and *E. multilocularis*. The disease occurs primarily in areas where dogs are used for herding. Humans become intermediate hosts after ingesting eggs with material contaminated by canine feces. Larvae invade the intestinal wall and migrate to tissue where they produce progressively enlarging cysts. Lesions usually occur in the liver and lung and may involve any tissue. Invasion of blood vessels may result in dissemination. Symptoms are related to the mass effect of lesions. Rupture of cysts, either spontaneously or at surgery, may result in anaphylactic reactions and seeding of new lesions. Cysts may calcify and thus be demonstrable radiographically. Eosinophilia may be present. Serologic tests are available, but cross-reactions with other parasites exist. Treatment is limited to careful surgical excision of symptomatic lesions or careful drainage of cysts previously sterilized with formalin or silver nitrate. Albendazole is effective adjunctive therapy for *E. granulosus*.

Actinomycosis is caused by the anaerobic gram-positive filamentous bacterium *Actinomyces israelii* and related species. *Actinomyces* species are normal inhabitants of the human oral cavity. Disease due to these organisms usually manifests as suppurative and/or granulomatous lesions, often in the jaw and occasionally in the thorax, abdomen, or skin. Lesions are firm and slowly spreading, and they develop draining sinuses that may contain macroscopic colonies of the organism with the appearance of "sulfur granules." The diagnosis is suggested by the characteristic lesions and confirmed by culture. Treatment is usually with penicillin for a prolonged period, with tetracycline as an alternative agent.

Nocardia asteroides is an aerobic actinomycete that causes pulmonary and disseminated infection. The organism is a ubiquitous saprophyte in soil. Infection of the skin can produce abscesses with draining sinuses. Treatment is with sulfonamides.

Mycetoma is an infection of the skin, subcutaneous tissue, and often bone that is characterized by mass swelling with draining sinuses and extensive tissue destruction. Lesions usually occur in the feet (i.e., Madura foot), but also occur on the legs and hands. The disease is caused by a variety of actinomycetes (e.g., *N. asteroides* and *Streptomyces* species), as well as several fungi, including *Madurella* and *Cephalosporium* species. These organisms are soil saprophytes. The disease occurs in tropical and semitropical areas worldwide. It is acquired through abrasions and puncture wounds. Lesions of the shoulder and back have been described in burden bearers. Treatment depends on the causative agents, but cure with chemotherapy alone is difficult.

Pyomyositis, or tropical pyomyositis, is a bacterial abscess of striated muscle, virtually always due to *Staphylococcus aureus*. The disease is common in several tropical areas, including Asia, Africa, and the West Indies; it occurs only rarely in temperate areas. Patients present with complaints of fever, chills, and malaise, as well as pain and swelling in the muscle involved, usually in the thigh and buttocks. The pathogenesis of this disease is unclear, as muscle tissue is normally resistant to bacterial infection. One suggestion as to the etiology of pyomyositis is that migrating helminth larvae damage tissue, making it susceptible to bacteria of hematogenous origin or organisms carried by the worm. Treatment involves surgical drainage and antistaphylococcal agents.

Skin Lesions

A new skin lesion in a traveler can be a cause of concern. Among the most common skin disorders for which returned travelers are seen by their primary care physician are secondarily infected insect bites, pyodermas, cutaneous larva migrans, and nonspecific dermatitis. Short-term travelers are unlikely to acquire diseases such as leprosy, yaws, or filariasis. As in other diseases in travelers, the exposure history is crucial in reaching a diagnosis and workup is greatly dependent on suspected diagnoses.

Viral exanthems, purpuric lesions from viral and bacterial infections, rickettsial diseases, syphilis, and fungal infections are all causes of skin lesions in developed countries. Several skin lesions that occur primarily in the tropics or are caused by parasites are discussed here.

Orf is a disease caused by a pox virus of sheep. It is seen in areas where sheep are raised. Lesions usually occur on the hand, but any area of skin may be involved. Lesions may be single or multiple and begin as reddish blue papules that progress to bullous lesions that rupture, leaving ulcers covered by gray-white crusts. The disease is self-limited; significant systemic signs are absent, but it is occasionally associated with a transient maculopapular rash of the trunk. A similar lesion, called milker's nodule, is caused by a bovine pox virus.

Anthrax is a zoonosis of several domesticated animals caused by *Bacillus anthracis*. The disease usually begins as a cutaneous lesion at an inoculation site. The lesion is initially a vesicle and then becomes a painless ulcer covered by a black eschar surrounded by erythema and edema. Patients may go on to develop lymphadenitis and septicemia, and the fatality rate in untreated disease is 5% to 20%. Treatment is with penicillin. Ulcerative lesions with lymphadenopathy also occur with tularemia, bubonic plague, glanders, and rat-bite fever (see earlier discussion).

Several spirochetal diseases are endemic in the tropics and are caused by organisms that are similar to or identical with *Treponema pallidum* of syphilis. Pinta is a disease of the skin alone caused by *T. carateum;* it occurs in Central and South America and is transmitted by close contact and perhaps biting insects. The initial lesion is a papule that enlarges and develops satellite papules. Secondary pinta occurs after 1 to several months. The lesions of secondary pinta, called pintids, are scaly macular lesions that develop blue pigmentation. The bluish lesions gradually progress to depigmentation and late lesions are white.

Yaws is caused by *T. pertenue* and is usually a childhood disease. It has a widespread distribution in the tropics. This disease involves bone as well as skin. The initial lesion at the inoculation site is a pruritic papilloma, called the mother yaw. Secondary lesions include scaly macules, papules, and small papillomas. Painful papules occur on the palms and soles. Late lesions are destructive gummas of the skin and bones.

Bejel, or nonvenereal syphilis, usually occurs in children, mostly in the desert regions of Asia and Africa. Initial lesions appear on mucous membranes or in mucocutaneous areas. They are usually papules or condylomas. Later manifestations are similar to those of secondary and late syphilis. All these treponematoses are associated with positive serologic tests for syphilis. Spirochetes are demonstrable in skin lesions at various times, and the diseases can be spread by contact. Treatment is with penicillin or, in the penicillin-allergic patient, tetracycline.

Leprosy, or Hansen's disease, is a chronic infection due to *M. leprae,* a bacterium that has not been cultured in artificial media. Currently the disease occurs primarily in tropical and subtropical regions, but sporadic cases occur worldwide. Lesions of the skin and peripheral nerves are the most notable manifestations. Two forms of the disease occur—lepromatous and tuberculoid leprosy—but there is considerable overlap. The lepromatous form is characterized by enormous numbers of organisms in lesions without a significant delayed hypersensitivity response. The tuberculoid form is characterized by more limited lesions, a cellular reaction, and few organisms in tissue.

With all types of leprosy, peripheral nerve involvement leads to varying degrees of denervation. Palpable thickening of superficial nerves is often noted. The skin lesions of tuberculoid leprosy are well demarcated, hypopigmented macules with hypesthesia that tend to develop circular borders. The lesions of lepromatous leprosy may be macules, papules, or nodules. There is also marked thickening of the skin leading to the typical leonine facies and pendulous ear lobes. Skin lesions of leprosy preferentially occur on the coolest portions of the skin (e.g., face [especially the cheek, nose, and brow], elbows, knees, buttocks). The midline of the back is usually spared, and in lepromatous leprosy loss of the lateral eyebrows is typical. An immune reaction, erythema nodosum leprosum, occurs in lepromatous leprosy and is characterized by tender, erythematous, subcutaneous nodules associated with fever and lymphadenopathy. Lucio's phenomenon is seen in lepromatous leprosy, especially in Mexico, and is characterized by angular dermal ulcers secondary to arteritis.

The diagnosis of leprosy is based on clinical appearance and demonstration of acid-fast organisms in skin biopsies. Treatment is with sulfones (e.g., dapsone). Several other drugs are being evaluated for efficacy, especially since the emergence of dapsone resistance. Thalidomide is curiously effective in the treatment of erythema nodosum leprosum.

M. marinum, a saprophytic water organism, causes a localized skin lesion called swimming pool granuloma. The lesion is papular to nodular and often ulcerates. The disease occurs sporadically in many parts of the world. It is treated with minocycline or antituberculous agents. Primary cutaneous tuberculosis may result in a similar lesion.

Visceral leishmaniasis has been discussed. Severe, progressive, diffuse leishmaniasis can occur with any form of cutaneous disease and appears to be related to immune compromise. There are several forms of cutaneous leishmaniasis. Old World cutaneous leishmaniasis, or oriental sore, occurs along the Mediterranean Sea, in the Middle East, and in southern Asia; it is caused by *Leishmania tropica.* The protozoan parasites are transmitted by the bite of sandflies of the *Phlebotomus* species. Two types of lesion occur at the site of the bite. In the rural, or moist, type an ulcer forms after a period of weeks to months and is associated with regional lymphadenopathy. In the dry, or urban, form a purple, pruritic nodule forms and breaks down to form an ulcer. These ulcers heal after several months to a year, leaving hypopigmented scars.

Three species of *Leishmania* occur in Central and South America. *L. mexicana* causes chiclero ulcer in Central America. Ulcers that heal within several months occur on exposed surfaces, usually the hands or face of forest workers, especially chicle harvesters. *L. peruviana* causes uta, which occurs at high altitude and is characterized by single or multiple ulcers that heal. The most significant form of American leishmaniasis is caused by *L. brasiliensis.* It is transmitted by sandflies in jungle areas. A primary skin ulcer is followed by disseminated lesions to the mucous membranes. The disease is thus called American mucocutaneous leishmaniasis, or espundia. The mucous membrane lesions can be destructive or hypertrophic, leading to deformity of the nose, palate, and larynx, as well as obstruction of the airway. Systemic signs and symptoms of fever, anorexia, and anemia are frequent.

The diagnosis of all forms of cutaneous leishmaniasis is usually made on clinical grounds. It is confirmed by demonstrating organisms in lesions or by culture. Several drugs are used for treatment, stibogluconate being the usual one. Amphotericin B has also been used in cases of severe American mucocutaneous leishmaniasis.

Helminthic parasites of humans and other animals that have skin-invasive larvae can cause dermatitis. Human hookworm larvae may cause a pruritic, edematous, maculopapular rash, usually on the feet, called ground itch. Larvae of cat and dog hookworms of the genus *Ancylostoma* cause a comparable rash called creeping eruption, or cutaneous larva migrans. Similar dermatitis from larvae of *S. stercoralis* occasionally occurs. Autoinfection with this worm can lead to erythematous and urticarial skin lesions. Pruritus and urticaria may appear at the time of invasion of the skin by the cercariae of *Schistosoma* species. Schistosome dermatitis may result from exposure to nonhuman, especially avian, schistosome larvae after sensitization. This dermatitis is called swimmers' itch.

Systemic fungal infections such as blastomycosis, cryptococcosis, and histoplasmosis occasionally cause skin lesions. African histoplasmosis caused by *Histoplasma duboisii* is primarily a skin disease characterized by granulomas. *Sporotrichum schenckii* is a saprophytic fungus that causes ulcerative skin lesions along lymph channels, usually after contact with rose thorns or sphagnum moss. Chromoblastomycosis is a fungal disease of the skin caused by *Phialophora* species that occurs mostly in the rural tropics; the disease is characterized by spreading cauliflower-like lesions. Rhinosporidiosis is a rare destructive skin and mucous membrane disease of the tropics caused by the fungus *Rhinosporidium seeberi.*

GENERAL ADVICE

It is important to remind travelers of some basic common sense tips about their travel.

- Plan ahead. If planning travel, ask early about potential health concerns. Immunization is most effective when given at the appropriate time. Information gathering may take time.
- Review general health status regarding underlying conditions and medication requirements that may be affected by foreign destinations (e.g., insulin supply, needles and syringes, transport of medications, allergies, air travel, and pulmonary disease). Persons with conditions that may require emergency care should carry appropriate health status identification. Persons who wear glasses should carry a copy of their prescription.
- Travelers should be counseled as to the risk of blood-borne infection from nonsterile needles, syringes, and transfusions in the developing world.
- The risk of sexually transmitted infections, including HIV and infections caused by antibiotic-resistant organisms, is higher in many other parts of the world than in the United States. Vacationing travelers and lone travelers may be especially vulnerable to unsafe sex. Sexual contact with persons who may be infected should be avoided, and persons choosing to have sexual contact may reduce their risk of acquiring a sexually transmitted disease by always using a latex condom and avoiding anal intercourse.
- Activities should be modified for conditions of heat, humidity, and altitude.
- Adequately chlorinated pools are generally safe for swimming. Salt water is generally safe, but sea water and beaches may be contaminated with human sewage or animal feces. Swimming or wading in freshwater streams, ponds, or lakes may present risk for diseases such as schistosomiasis, leptospirosis, and giardiasis.
- Patients should be reminded that illnesses developing even months after return from a trip may be related to travel, and travel history should be reported to health care providers from whom treatment is sought.
- For diarrhea prevention, see Chapter 111.

VACCINE RECOMMENDATIONS

Chapter 5 discusses routine and travel-specific immunizations that must be considered for travelers and reviews special considerations for use of vaccines in travelers.

MALARIA PREVENTION

Malaria is an important problem in many tropical countries and occurs in up to 2% of travelers who visit West Africa without prophylaxis. The only areas considered not to have risk of malaria are the United States, Canada, Europe, and Japan. Risk in other areas varies from country to country, and place to place within countries, as do the recommendations. Specific details about areas of risk are available.

Avoiding contact with arthropods is an important method of preventing malaria; this fact must be emphasized by the health care provider. The best defenses against arthropod bites are avoidance of outdoor activities at dawn, dusk, and evening; use of insect repellent; and appropriate use of screens and bednetting. Such precautions also are helpful against other arthropod-borne diseases such as dengue fever.

Chloroquine-resistant *P. falciparum* has now spread to most areas with malaria. Chloroquine phosphate is still recommended for prevention of malaria for travel to areas where chloroquine-resistant *P. falciparum* has not been reported. The dose is 300 mg base (500 mg salt) once a week beginning 1 to 2 weeks before and continuing for 4 weeks after exposure to an area of low or no risk for chloroquine-resistant malaria. Travelers to areas where chloroquine-resistant *P. falciparum* malaria has been reported should take mefloquine alone. The adult dose is 228 mg base (250 mg salt) per week starting 1 week before travel and continuing weekly during stay in the area of risk and for 4 weeks after leaving the area. Doxycycline alone is an alternative agent for short-term travelers who cannot take mefloquine; however, doxycycline failure has been well documented. Mefloquine is not approved for pregnant women, and an approved pediatric dose has not been established. Mefloquine is contraindicated in travelers on β-blockers, those with a history of seizures, or those whose occupation requires fine coordination. Chloroquine alone is an alternative for pregnant women and children, but travelers who take chloroquine alone in areas at risk for chloroquine-resistant *P. falciparum* should be provided with and counseled about pyrimethamine-sulfadoxine (Fansidar) self-treatment for febrile illness occurring when professional medical care is not available. Mefloquine in therapeutic dose is associated with a high frequency of side effects and is not recommended for self-treatment. There are also mefloquine-resistant *P. falciparum* on the Thailand-Myanmar border; hence daily doxycycline is recommended for travelers in this region.

ADDITIONAL READINGS

American College of Physicians Task Force on Adult Immunization and Infectious Diseases Society of America: *Guide for adult immunization,* ed 2, Philadelphia, 1990, American College of Physicians.

Ash LR, Orihel TC: *Atlas of human parasitology,* ed 3, Chicago, 1990, American Society of Clinical Pathologists.

Beck JW, Davies JE: *Medical parasitology,* ed 3, St Louis, 1981, Mosby.

Benenson AS, editor: *Control of communicable diseases in man,* ed 15, Washington, DC, 1990, American Public Health Association.

Centers for Disease Control and Prevention: *Health information for international travel,* Washington, DC, yearly, Government Printing Office.

Garcia LS, Bruckner DA: *Diagnostic medical parasitology,* ed 2, Washington, DC, 1993, American Society for Microbiology.

Lederberg J, Shope RE, Oaks SC Jr, editors: *Emerging infections: microbial threats to health in the United States,* Washington, DC, 1992, National Academy.

Neva FA, Brown HW: *Basic clinical parasitology,* ed 6, Norwalk, Conn, 1994, Appleton & Lange.

Rosenblatt JE: Antiparasitic agents, Mayo Clinc Proc 74:1161-1175, 1999.

Strickland GT, editor: *Hunter's tropical medicine,* ed 7, Philadelphia, 1991, WB Saunders.

The Medical Letter: Drugs for parasitic infections, *Med Lett Drugs Ther* March 2000.

Warren KS, Mahmoud AAF, editors: *Tropical and geographical medicine,* ed 2, New York, 1990, McGraw-Hill.

Wilson ME: *A world guide to infections: disease, distributions, diagnosis,* New York, 1991, Oxford University.

CHAPTER 31

Infectious Mononucleosis and Mononucleosis-like Disorders

Nelson M. Gantz

A 19-year-old man presenting with malaise, fever, sore throat, and cervical lymphadenopathy should suggest the diagnosis of acute infectious mononucleosis. Supporting this diagnosis is a white blood cell count showing a lymphocytosis with atypical lymphocytes and a positive monospot test, which measures the presence of heterophile antibodies. In addition to the positive monospot test, this patient will develop virus-specific antibodies to the Epstein-Barr virus (EBV). In most cases, the diagnosis of EBV infectious mononucleosis is not difficult. Problems occur for the physician when the clinical findings are not classic and the monospot test is negative. Several disorders can cause a monospot-negative, mononucleosis-like illness including cytomegalovirus (CMV), EBV, toxoplasmosis, group A β-hemolytic streptococci, and human immunodeficiency virus (HIV).

This chapter reviews the epidemiology, clinical manifestations, diagnosis, complications, clinical course, and management of acute EBV infectious mononucleosis. The disorders that clinically mimic infectious mononucleosis are also discussed.

EBV is one of nine herpesviruses. The other viruses in this group include herpes simplex virus-1, herpes simplex virus-2, varicella-zoster virus, CMV, human herpesvirus-6A, human herpesvirus-6B, human herpesvirus-7, and human herpesvirus-8. EBV is a DNA virus that infects B lymphocytes and nasopharyngeal epithelial cells. The virus does not produce cytopathic changes in the infected cells. In response to EBV infection, numerous antibodies are produced including heterophile antibodies and virus-specific EBV antibodies.

EPIDEMIOLOGY

Antibodies to EBV are found in persons all over the world, and their prevalence is highest in lower socioeconomic groups. For example, in China by age 5 years, about 95% of persons have EBV antibodies, whereas in the United States and Great Britain the seropositive rate for EBV antibodies is about 50% by that age. Acute infectious mononucleosis is diagnosed most frequently in adolescents in higher socioeconomic groups.[11] The incidence of acute infectious mononucleosis is highest in persons 15 to 24 years of age. The symptoms of acute EBV infection depend on the age during which the infection is acquired. Those acquiring an acute EBV infection before age 15 years usually have an asymptomatic infection or a mild "flulike" illness. Persons acquiring EBV infection after age 15 years usually have the typical acute infectious mononucleosis illness with fever, pharyngitis, malaise, and cervical and axillary lymphadenopathy.

METHODS OF TRANSMISSION

Using special techniques, EBV can be demonstrated in the pharynx of patients with acute infectious mononucleosis for up to 18 months after recovery from an acute illness. The virus also can be identified in throat washings from patients with leukemia or lymphoma, as well as renal transplant recipients. The virus is not highly contagious, and most cases probably are acquired from asymptomatic shedders after close contact. Exchange of saliva with kissing may be responsible for viral transmission; the disease has been called the "kissing disease." The paradox of a high seroprevalence rate and low degree of contagion results because infected persons shed the virus for prolonged periods after an acute illness. Documented cases of intrafamilial transmission are unusual as are clusters of acute infectious mononucleosis. In experimental studies, the usual incubation period is 35 to 50 days in the adult. No precautions are required once an index case is identified. Acute infectious mononucleosis also can spread by a blood transfusion and is a cause for the *postpump perfusion syndrome;* however, most cases of postpump perfusion syndrome are caused by CMV.

CLINICAL MANIFESTATIONS

Classic acute infectious mononucleosis is an illness characterized by fever, sore throat, malaise, and lymphadenopathy. The clue to the diagnosis is a young adult with a "toxic" appearance with a pharyngitis of more than 3 days' duration with posterior cervical lymphadenopathy. Pharyngeal exudates are often present (50%) and palatal petechiae may be seen. Other complaints include headache, anorexia, myalgias, chills, nausea, and abdominal discomfort. On physical examination, in addition to the lymphadenopathy, fever, pharyngitis, and splenomegaly occur in 50% of patients. Other findings include hepatomegaly, jaundice, periorbital edema, and a rash. The skin rash does not have a characteristic pattern and may be erythematous, maculopapular, or petechial. Interestingly, when a patient with acute infectious mononucleosis is given the antibiotic ampicillin, a nonallergic skin rash occurs in about 90% of patients. A skin rash also occurs in patients with CMV mononucleosis who have been given ampicillin, although less often than in patients with acute EBV infectious mononucleosis. However, this difference is not the way to establish the diagnosis of acute EBV mononucleosis. Table 31-1 lists the symptoms and signs of acute infectious mononucleosis. In addition to posterior cervical adenopathy, patients may have submandibular, anterior cervical, axillary, and inguinal lymphadenopathy. Splenomegaly is present in 50% of patients and is usually maximal in size during the second week of illness. Splenic rupture is a rare complication of infectious mononucleosis, and trauma such as contact sports should be avoided during the first few weeks after diagnosis.[5,8,10]

DIAGNOSIS

Laboratory features of acute infectious mononucleosis include the presence of more than 50% lymphocytes with at least 10% atypical lymphocytes. Other causes of atypical lymphocytes include CMV infections, toxoplasmosis, viral hepatitis, rubella, roseola, mumps, and drug reactions. The total white blood cell count is usually in the range of 10,000 to 20,000 cells/mm^3. A characteristic laboratory abnormality is the presence of heterophile antibodies. The term *heterophile antibody* refers to an antibody that reacts with an antigen of another species. These antibodies in patients with acute infectious mononucleosis react with sheep or horse red blood cells, but not guinea pig kidney cells. In contrast, heterophile antibodies found in patients with serum sickness react with guinea pig kidney cells. The heterophile antibody is detected in 90% of patients with acute infectious mononucleosis, but may require 3 weeks to become positive.[4]

Most laboratories use the monospot test to detect heterophile antibodies. The heterophile antibody is an immunoglobulin M (IgM) antibody and is not directed against the EBV. The heterophile antibody usually disappears in most patients by 3 months, but rarely may persist longer. Thus the presence of a positive monospot test indicates an acute infection. There is no need to follow or repeat the monospot test because the titer or duration of the heterophile antibody response does not correlate with the clinical course of the illness. Rarely, false-positive monospot tests occur in patients with varicella, influenza, or lymphoma. The most frequent cause of a false-positive monospot test is laboratory error.

Approximately 80% to 90% of patients with EBV mononucleosis have a positive monospot test by the third week of illness. In the other 10% to 20% of patients, the diagnosis can be established by obtaining EBV antibody titers. EBV antibodies are listed in Table 31-2. There is usually no need to follow EBV serology by repeating the test because most of the antibody levels persist for life. However, the appearance of antibody to Epstein-Barr nuclear antigen (EBNA) in a patient with a prior negative EBNA antibody test is suggestive of a recent infection.[14,15] Other laboratory abnormalities include mild liver function test dysfunction, mild thrombocytopenia, positive cold agglutinins, and the presence of cryoglobulins.

Table 31-1. Clinical Features of Acute Infectious Mononucleosis

Symptoms and signs	Frequency (%)
Symptoms	
Sore throat	80
Malaise	60
Headache	50
Anorexia	20
Myalgias	20
Chills	15
Nausea	10
Abdominal pain	10
Signs	
Lymphadenopathy	95
Pharyngitis	85
Fever	75
Splenomegaly	50
Periorbital edema	30
Hepatomegaly	10
Palatal exanthem	10
Jaundice	10
Skin rash	5

COMPLICATIONS

The majority of patients with an acute EBV infection recover spontaneously in 3 to 4 weeks. Rarely, complications occur (Box 31-1). Splenic rupture, especially during the second or third week, can be life-threatening. Thrombocytopenia is common but severe thrombocytopenia with an intracerebral bleed has been reported only rarely. Neurologic complications occur in less than 1% of patients but can dominate the clinical picture. At the time of presentation in patients with central nervous system (CNS) disease, the monospot test can be negative, and the numbers of atypical lymphocytes are low or absent. Rarely, neurologic complications, splenic rupture, or upper airway obstruction results in death.

MANAGEMENT

Treatment of acute infectious mononucleosis is mainly supportive. Contact sports should be avoided during the initial 3 weeks of the illness to avoid splenic rupture. Corticosteroids may be useful in patients with impending airway obstruction, severe thrombocytopenia, or hemolytic anemia. A 1- to 2-week course of corticosteroid therapy usually is administered. For normal hosts, acyclovir or other antiviral agents are not appropriate therapies for this disorder. In a placebo-controlled study in normal hosts,[17] the combination of acyclovir and corticosteroid therapy decreased oral EBV shedding but did not affect the clinical symptoms such as duration of illness or sore throat. If a throat culture reveals group A β-hemolytic streptococci, however, then antibiotic therapy should be given.

DIFFERENTIAL DIAGNOSIS OF MONONUCLEOSIS-LIKE SYNDROMES

Heterophile-negative and EBV-negative infectious mononucleosis can be caused by several disorders. The various disorders are listed in Box 31-2.[2,7]

Table 31-2. Antibodies to Epstein-Barr Virus

Antibody	Time of appearance	Persistence	Comments
Viral capsid antigens (VCA)			
VCA IgM	At presentation	2 months	Indicates an acute infection
VCA IgG	At presentation	Lifelong	Not helpful for acute diagnosis
Early antigens (EA)			
Anti EA	At presentation	Lifelong	—
Anti EBNA	1 month after presentation	Lifelong	A positive test on presentation usually indicates past infection. A negative test followed by a positive test 1 month later suggests a recent infection.

Cytomegalovirus

In most studies, CMV is the most frequent cause of this syndrome. Patients with CMV are usually older (mean age 28 years) than those with EBV infectious mononucleosis (peak age 17 years). Fever tends to be more prolonged in patients with CMV mononucleosis compared with that seen in patients with EBV infectious mononucleosis. Pharyngitis and lymphadenopathy occur more often in patients with EBV infectious mononucleosis, and are noted in only 20% of patients with CMV infectious mononucleosis. A rash occurs in about one third of patients with CMV mononucleosis. Atypical lymphocytes also can be present. The diagnosis of acute CMV can be established by demonstrating CMV IgM antibodies. However, this test is associated with both false-positive and false-negative results. A diagnosis by serology also can be made by showing a fourfold rise in CMV IgG antibody titers.[3] Other methods of diagnosis include detection of CMV antigens in the blood using a shell vial assay or using the polymerase chain reaction (PCR) to identify CMV DNA. Isolation of CMV from saliva or urine is not proof of acute infection, since prolonged viral secretion often occurs for months or years.

Box 31-1. Complications of Acute Epstein-Barr Virus Infection

Hematologic
Hemolytic anemia
Thrombocytopenia
Neutropenia

Gastrointestinal
Liver function test abnormalities
Jaundice
Splenic rupture

Neurologic
Aseptic meningitis
Guillain-Barré syndrome
Transverse myelitis
Bell's palsy
Seizures

Dermatologic
Maculopapular rashes

Cardiac
Myocarditis

Other
Postanginal sepsis
Renal failure

Box 31-2. Mononucleosis-Like Disorders

EBV
Hepatitis
CMV
HIV
Trichinosis
Malaria
Toxoplasmosis
Lymphogranuloma venereum
Secondary syphilis
Lyme disease
Cat-scratch disease
Subacute bacterial endocarditis
Yersinia enterocolitica
Brucellosis
Tularemia
Salmonella bacteremia
Miliary tuberculosis
Leptospirosis
Systemic lupus erythematosus
Drug-induced mononucleosis syndrome
Juvenile rheumatoid arthritis
Lymphoma
Chronic fatigue syndrome

Modified from Gleckman RA, Czachor JS. In Gleckman RA, Gantz NM, Brown RB, editors: *Infections in outpatient practice: recognition and management*, New York, 1988, Plenum Press.

Hepatitis

The prodrome of acute viral hepatitis can mimic acute EBV infection, although pharyngitis and lymphadenopathy are absent. Fever, malaise, myalgias, arthralgias, and a rash may occur. Atypical lymphadenopathy may be present. The diagnosis is suggested by the marked elevation in liver function tests. Diagnosis is established by obtaining the serologic tests for the hepatitis viruses.

Human Immunodeficiency Virus

HIV can produce a self-limited infectious mononucleosis-like illness 2 to 4 weeks after the virus is acquired. The illness is characterized by fever, sore throat, headache, anorexia, malaise, arthralgias, myalgias, and weight loss. A diffuse erythematous rash may occur. Symmetric lymphadenopathy is common.[12] Laboratory abnormalities most often include leukopenia, lymphopenia, and thrombocytopenia. Atypical lymphocytes also may occur. Detection of HIV antibody by enzyme-linked immunosorbent assay (ELISA) may be negative during the first few weeks of an acute primary infection. HIV seroconversion usually occurs 3 months after the virus is acquired. During the acute primary HIV infection, which mimics EBV infectious mononucleosis, a transient decline in the CD 4 cell count may occur. Determination of serum p24 HIV antigen levels or use of the PCR to detect HIV virus may be useful to establish the diagnosis of HIV disease. Otherwise, if there is a suspicion of HIV infection, the HIV antibody test should be repeated over time.[13]

Trichinosis

Trichinosis is acquired by eating raw or poorly cooked meat containing the viable larvae of *Trichinella spiralis*. The protean manifestations of trichinosis—fever, myalgias, malaise, and rash—may mimic the symptoms of infectious mononucleosis. Pharyngitis and lymphadenopathy are absent. Clues that suggest the diagnosis of trichinosis include diarrhea, periorbital edema, subconjunctival hemorrhages, eosinophilia, and a low or normal erythrocyte sedimentation rate. The diagnosis can be established by demonstrating antibodies 3 weeks after the infection using the bentonite flocculation test. A muscle biopsy is usually unnecessary, but when obtained from a tender muscle reveals the characteristic worm (see Chapter 30).

Malaria

A history of travel should alert the physician to the possibility of malaria. Features that suggest acute infectious mononucleosis include fever, chills, fatigue, myalgias, and arthralgias. Pharyngitis and lymphadenopathy are absent (see Chapter 30).

Toxoplasmosis

Acute toxoplasmosis can mimic EBV or CMV infectious mononucleosis in the normal host. Toxoplasmosis, however, causes less than 1% of mononucleosis syndromes. Clinical features include fever, malaise, myalgias, and sore throat. Cervical lymphadenopathy is a prominent feature. Atypical lymphocytes may be present. The diagnosis of toxoplasmosis is made by demonstrating IgM antibody to *Toxoplasma*. Acute toxoplasmosis in the normal host is a self-limited illness, and specific acute toxoplasmosis therapy is not indicated.[9]

Lymphogranuloma Venereum

Lymphogranuloma venereum (LGV) is caused by a type of *Chlamydia trachomatis* designated as types L1, L2, and L3. The initial stage is characterized by a small, asymptomatic ulcerative lesion. In the secondary stage, lymphadenopathy and prominent constitutional symptoms may mimic infectious mononucleosis. The constitutional symptoms include fever, chills, anorexia, myalgias, and arthralgias. Inguinal lymphadenopathy occurs, but enlarged cervical lymph nodes and pharyngitis are lacking. Diagnosis of LGV usually is established by demonstrating an antibody rise to one of the LGV-specific types (see Chapter 29).

Secondary Syphilis

Constitutional symptoms such as fever, malaise, anorexia, pharyngitis, arthralgias, and painless lymphadenopathy occur in patients with secondary syphilis. A macular, maculopapular, and/or pustular rash, especially involving the palms and soles, strongly suggests the diagnosis. A characteristic feature is enlargement of the epitrochlear lymph nodes. The serologic tests for syphilis (rapid plasma reagin, Venereal Disease Research Laboratory, and fluorescent treponemal antibody absorption) are always positive in patients with secondary syphilis and will establish the diagnosis (see Chapter 29).

Lyme Disease

Lyme disease caused by *Borrelia burgdorferi* may resemble infectious mononucleosis in the early stages. Early symptoms include malaise, fatigue, headache, fever, arthralgias, myalgias, and sore throat. These constitutional symptoms may occur before and persist after the characteristic rash of erythema chronicum migrans (ECM) disappears. Lymphadenopathy also occurs and is usually regional but may be generalized. The diagnosis of Lyme disease in the presence of the rash of ECM is not difficult. In the absence of the rash, the diagnosis is based on the epidemiologic findings and correlating the clinical features of the illness with the serologic results (see Chapter 141).

Cat-Scratch Disease

Cat-scratch disease can resemble acute infectious mononucleosis. The infection is caused by a fastidious gram-negative bacillus identified as *Bartonella henselae*. The disease is characterized by a primary lesion, a papule or pustule, which develops 3 to 10 days after a cat scratch. The hallmark of the illness is chronic regional lymphadenopathy, which develops about 2 weeks after the cat scratch. Constitutional symptoms that mimic infectious mononucleosis include fever, fatigue, sore throat, headache, and anorexia. The diagnosis is suggested by the history of localized lymphadenopathy in a patient with cat contact or a scratch. The organism can be identified on a lymph node biopsy. A serologic test also may be helpful in establishing the diagnosis.

Subacute Bacterial Endocarditis

The clinical features of subacute bacterial endocarditis (SBE) can mimic several disorders such as malignancy, cerebrovascular accident, rheumatic disease, and infectious mononucleosis. Patients with SBE can present with fever, fatigue, anorexia, myalgias, and arthralgias. Pharyngitis and lymphadenopathy are absent. The diagnosis of SBE is made by obtaining three sets of blood cultures.

Yersinia Enterocolitica

Yersinia is a gram-negative bacillus that usually causes diarrhea and abdominal pain. The organism also can cause acute pharyngitis with fever not associated with diarrhea. The diagnosis can be established by cultures.[16]

Brucellosis

Acute brucellosis can mimic infectious mononucleosis. Symptoms include malaise, headache, anorexia, myalgias, arthralgias, and fever. Lymphadenopathy and splenomegaly may occur. Because patients with brucellosis present with nonspecific symptoms, a history of an epidemiologic exposure to animals or dairy products is key to suspect the diagnosis. Cases are diagnosed by serology or culture.

Tularemia

Tularemia is caused by *Francisella tularensis,* a small, gram-negative rod. Most infections are acquired from the bite of an infected animal such as a rabbit. The illness can mimic acute infectious mononucleosis, with patients having fever, chills, malaise, fatigue, and sore throat. On examination, pharyngitis and cervical lymphadenopathy may be present. Although the organism can be identified by culture, most infections are diagnosed serologically.

Leptospirosis

Leptospirosis is a zoonosis with clinical features that can mimic acute infectious mononucleosis. Fever, headache, and myalgias may occur. A rash, lymphadenopathy, and hepatosplenomegaly may be present. Pharyngitis is present in about 20% of patients. A history of exposure to animals such as rats or dogs is an important clue to the diagnosis (see Chapter 30). Most infections are diagnosed serologically.[6]

Other Disorders

Several other disorders, including human herpesvirus-6 infection, salmonella bacteremia, miliary tuberculosis, systemic lupus erythematosus, juvenile rheumatoid arthritis, and lymphoma, may at times mimic acute infectious mononucleosis.[1] Drugs such as procainamide, isoniazid, and phenytoin also can be associated with a mononucleosis-like illness.

Chronic Fatigue Syndrome

Chronic fatigue syndrome (CFS) is a disorder characterized by fatigue for at least 6 months and a complex or other symptoms. The illness is not new but has attracted increased attention and controversy since the late 1980s. The cause of the syndrome is unknown. In addition to the presence of chronic relapsing fatigue present for at least 6 months, clinical features include low-grade fever, chills, sore throat, lymphadenopathy, myalgias, arthralgias, headache, sleep disturbances, decreased ability to concentrate, and decreased memory (see Chapter 142).

REFERENCES

1. Akashi K, et al: Severe infectious mononucleosis-like syndrome and primary human herpesvirus 6 infection in an adult, *N Engl J Med* 325:168, 1993.
2. Bergman MM, Gleckman RA: Heterophile negative infectious mononucleosis-like syndrome, *Postgrad Med* 81:313, 1987.
3. Cohen JE, Corey GR: Cytomegalovirus infection in the normal host, *Medicine* 64:100, 1985.
4. Davidsohn I, Walker PH: The nature of the heterophilic antibodies in infectious mononucleosis, *Am J Clin Pathol* 5:455, 1935.
5. Evans AS: Infectious mononucleosis and related syndromes, *Am J Med Sci* 276:325, 1978.
6. Evans ME, et al: Tularemia: a 30-year experience with 88 cases, *Medicine* 64:251-269, 1985.
7. Gleckman RA, Czachor JS: Mononucleosis and mononucleosis-like syndromes. In Gleckman RA, Gantz NM, Brown RB, editors: *Infections in outpatient practice: recognition and management,* New York, 1988, Plenum, pp 125-146.
8. Hoagland RJ: Infectious mononucleosis, *Am J Med* 13:158-171, 1952.
9. McCabe RE, et al: Clinical spectrum of 107 cases of toxoplasmic lymphadenopathy, *Rev Infect Dis* 9:754, 1987.
10. Niederman JC, et al: Infectious mononucleosis: clinical manifestations in relation to EB virus antibodies, *JAMA* 204:203, 1968.
11. Porter DD, et al: Prevalence of antibodies to EB virus and other herpesviruses, *JAMA* 208:1675-1679, 1969.
12. Schacker T, Collier AC, Hughes J, et al: Clinical and epidemiologic features of primary HIV infection, *Ann Intern Med* 125:257-264, 1996.
13. Schacker TW, Hughes JP, Shea T, et al: Biological and virologic characteristics of primary HIV infection, *Ann Intern Med* 128:613-620, 1998.
14. Sumaya CV, Ench Y: Epstein-Barr virus infectious mononucleosis in children: I. Clinical and general laboratory findings, *Pediatrics* 75:1003-1010, 1985.
15. Sumaya CV, Ench Y: Epstein-Barr virus infectious mononucleosis in children: II. Heterophile antibody and viral specific responses, *Pediatrics* 75:1011-1019, 1985.
16. Tacket CO, et al: *Yersinia enterocolitica* pharyngitis, *Ann Intern Med* 99:40-42, 1983.
17. Tynell E, et al: Acyclovir and prednisolone treatment of acute infectious mononucleosis: a multicenter, double-blind, placebo-controlled study, *J Infect Dis* 174:324-331, 1996.

CHAPTER 32

Primary Care of the HIV-infected Patient

Cynthia J. Whitener
John J. Zurlo

Before the era of acquired immunodeficiency syndrome (AIDS), immunodeficiency disorders were rare, typically congenital diseases. Comparatively little was known about the immune system, its specialized cells, complex web of interactions, and unique chemical messengers, the cytokines. Care of affected patients typically was relegated to specialized physicians at tertiary care centers. With early recognition that profound immune dysfunction defined the nature of AIDS, medical care was provided by the same specialists at the outset. As the epidemic unfolded through the early and middle 1980s, however, two facts became obvious. First, the numbers of infected patients would quickly outstrip the numbers of available specialists. Second, with both the explosion of scientific information about the immune system and the increased familiarity with the clinical course of AIDS patients, the nonspecialist could play a significant role in management. Since those early days and with the advent of highly active antiretroviral therapy (HAART), which has resulted in a dramatic decrease in hospitalization rates, human immunodeficiency virus (HIV) infection has become an integral part of the outpatient practices of many primary care physicians throughout the United States.

PATHOPHYSIOLOGY

HIV is a retrovirus and possesses the unique ability to convert its own single-stranded ribonucleic acid (RNA) to double-stranded deoxyribonucleic acid (DNA) for incorporation into the host cell genome. This reaction is catalyzed by the enzyme *reverse transcriptase,* the major target for two of the three classes of licensed anti-HIV drugs. Two types of HIV, HIV-1 and HIV-2, cause immunodeficiency in humans. *HIV-1* is the predominant viral species infecting patients in the United States and throughout most of the developed world. *HIV-2* is found almost exclusively in western Africa, where it is the predominant viral type. HIV-1 is divided into distinct subtypes, termed *clades.* Clades A through I are the M (major) subtypes; a different subtype O (outlier) also has been described. Clade B is by far the predominant type in the United States and Western Europe. Detailed descriptions of HIV structure, life cycle, and molecular pathophysiology can be found in major AIDS textbooks and reviews.

Host Response and Viral Replication

Immediately after infection with HIV, rapid viral replication occurs (Fig. 32-1).[9] High levels of viremia can be measured early in the plasma. During this period an estimated 50% to 70% of patients develop symptomatic illness (primary HIV infection). Symptoms often include fever, chills, malaise, diffuse lymph node swelling, diarrhea, skin rash, headache, and sore throat. This syndrome typically lasts 1 to 3 weeks and then resolves. The initial host immune response to HIV infection is brisk and aggressive. High antibody levels can be measured to virtually all viral proteins. Cytotoxic T cells appear that specifically target virally infected cells. After acute infection, levels of plasma viremia drop precipitously. The T-helper lymphocyte (CD4) count drops transiently during primary HIV infection, occasionally to very low levels. Along with the development of antiviral antibodies, the CD4 count rises, although not completely back to baseline levels.

After the initial viremic phase of infection, the virus invades its target organs, principally the lymphoid organs. Soon thereafter and continuously over the course of the infection, HIV replicates usually at a high rate, which varies from individual to individual. The rate of replication is determined by a complex interplay between virulence of the particular virus strain and adequacy of host immune response. This replication rate can be estimated by measurement of viral messenger RNA (mRNA, *viral load*) in plasma. For each infected individual, a unique viral load set-point is reached within a few months after primary infection. Symptomatic primary HIV infection has been associated with

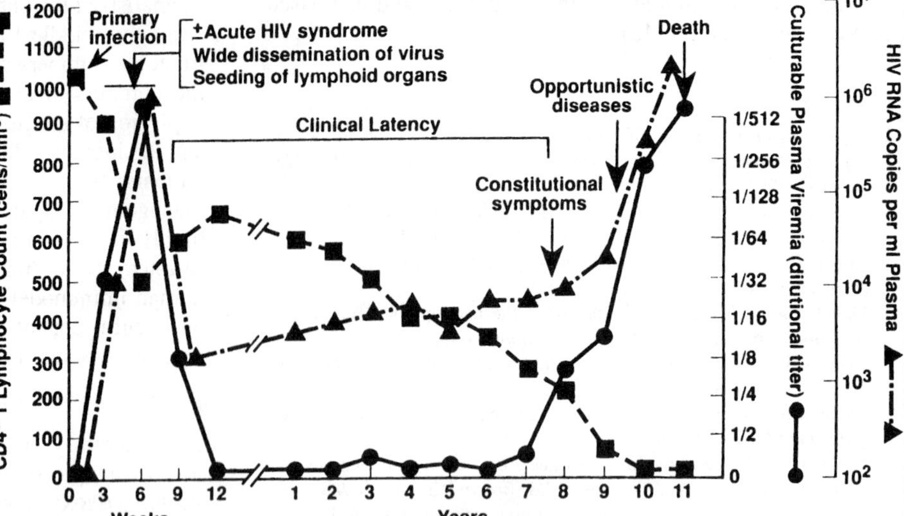

Fig. 32-1. Multifactorial, multiphasic, and overlapping factors of immunopathogenic mechanisms of HIV disease. (From Fauci AS, Pantaleo G, Stanley S, Weissman D: *Ann Intern Med* 124:654, 1996.)

a higher viral load set-point compared with asymptomatic infection. The viral load for any given CD4 count has great prognostic value in predicting long-term clinical outcomes. The higher the viral load, the more rapid the clinical decline (Fig. 32-2).[12] The viral load also serves as a measure of response to antiviral therapy. It has therefore become an invaluable prognostic and therapeutic management tool.

With each replication cycle, new virions are produced, which in turn infect and destroy other CD4 cells. The rate of CD4 cell destruction is nearly matched by the host's ability to replace lost cells. Over time the vast majority of patients experience a progressive decline in CD4 cell number, resulting in profound immunodeficiency.

In addition to its high replication rate the virus has a high mutation rate. Over time this combination of high replication and mutation rates results in the generation of multiple viral strains *(quasispecies)* in a given individual. This potential for wide genetic variability has great implications for the host, since suboptimal antiretroviral therapy selects for the generation of quasispecies with reduced susceptibility to antiretroviral agents.

Immunologic Abnormalities

The primary target cell for HIV is the CD4 cell, which has a pivotal role in orchestration of the immune response; not surprisingly, therefore, virtually all arms of the immune system are damaged during progressive infection. Qualitative and quantitative CD4 cell defects induced by the virus impair overall T-helper cell function. CD4 cells do not proliferate normally when stimulated, nor do they elaborate the proper complement of cytokines necessary to generate appropriate responses from other arms of the immune system. Cells of the macrophage/monocyte lineage become dysfunctional in antigen presentation. The humoral immune response is impaired and worsens with advancing disease. As a result, patients develop an inadequate antibody response when exposed to neoantigens. All these immune system defects ultimately lead to the host becoming susceptible to a large group of opportunistic pathogens that are common to other cellular immunodeficiency states. Abnormalities in immune surveillance of neoplastic clonal expansion may be one important mechanism by which HIV-infected patients develop neoplasms such as non-Hodgkin's lymphoma.

Cellular Targets

In addition to lymphocytes and macrophages, HIV can infect several other cells, although the mechanisms of attachment and viral entry may differ. In particular, virus has been isolated from several types of cells in the central nervous system (CNS). CNS invasion probably occurs early in the course of infection, with lymphoid organ seeding during and after primary HIV infection. The clinical implications of CNS infection for the host are great; patients have CNS manifestations ranging from benign aseptic meningitis to encephalopathy and myelopathy. Infection of gut epithelial cells may be important in the diarrhea and weight loss so common in infected patients.

ACQUISITION AND TRANSMISSION

Although HIV has been isolated from a variety of body fluids, the only fluids recognized to transmit disease are blood and blood products, semen, vaginal fluid, and breast milk (Box 32-1). Other fluids, such as saliva and tears, which contain low concentrations of viral particles, and cerebrospinal fluid, which can have high viral titers, have not been shown to transmit infection. Any body fluid can be rendered infectious if contaminated with blood. The major means of HIV transmission worldwide is by heterosexual intercourse. Other recognized modes of transmission include anal-receptive intercourse among gay men, sharing of contaminated needles among injection drug users (IDUs), transfusion of infected blood products, and vertical transmission (in utero, the intrapartum, or breast-feeding).

Heterosexual Transmission

During vaginal intercourse, either partner can infect the other, although male-to-female transmission is more efficient than the reverse. In the case of semen, inflammatory cells, which are found in seminal secretions, probably represent the major means by which virus is transmitted. Virus then infects macrophages and lymphocytes within the cervix or higher up in the uterine body, with subsequent dissemination of

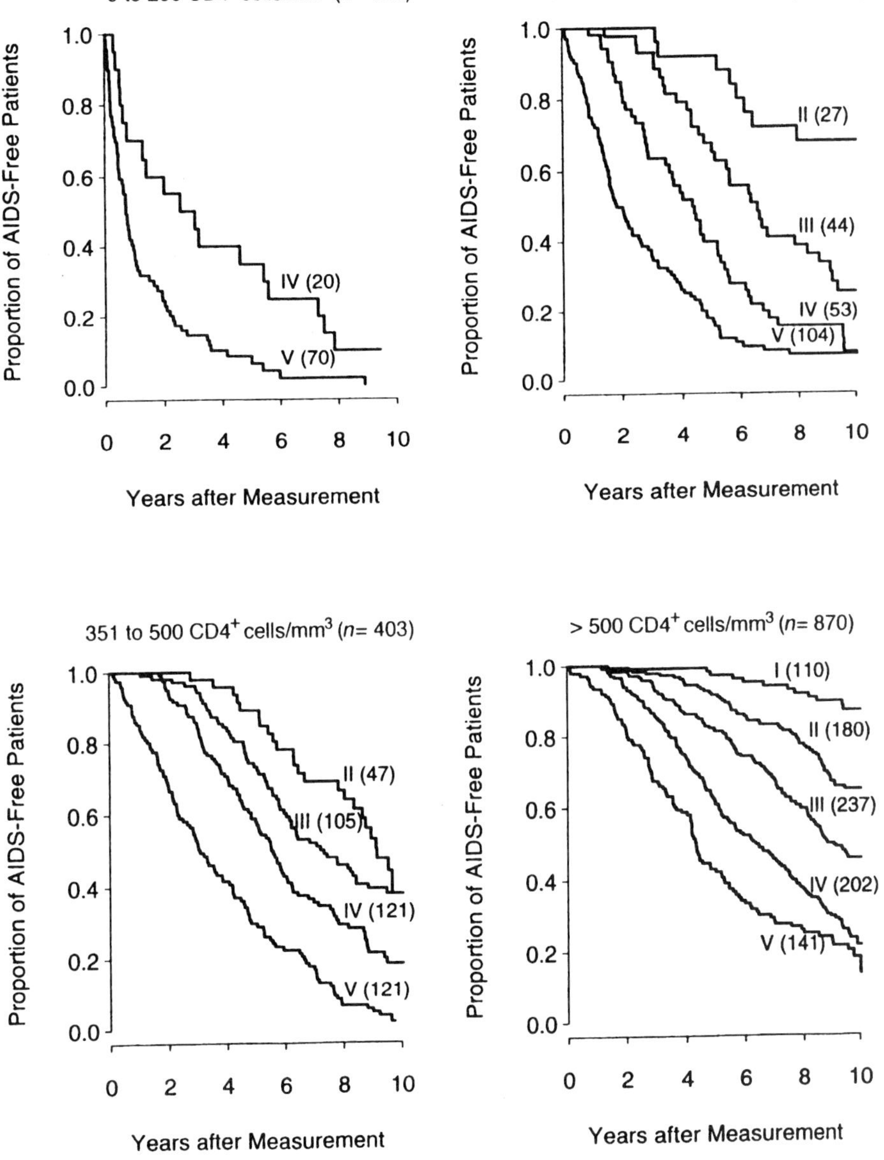

Fig. 32-2. AIDS-free survival by HIV-1 RNA category among groups with different baseline CD4+ lymphocyte counts. Five categories were *I*, 500 copies/ml or less; *II*, 501 to 3000 copies/ml; *III*, 3001 to 10,000; *IV*, 10,001 to 30,000 copies/ml; and *V*, more than 30,000 copies/ml. Numbers in parentheses are sample sizes of groups at baseline. Groups that were too small to provide estimates were omitted. (From Mellors JW, Munoz A, Giorgi JV, et al: *Ann Intern Med* 126:946, 1997.)

infection. For HIV-infected women, vaginal secretions also contain cell-associated and cell-free virus, which probably infects macrophages within the male urethra, leading to disseminated infection. The presence of an active sexually transmitted disease (STD) clearly increases the efficiency of transmission. Whether the lesions are ulcerative (e.g., syphilis, chancroid) or nonulcerative (e.g., gonorrhea), the common feature among STDs is the preponderance of inflammatory cells, which from the infected partner can increase the infectivity of the fluid or in the noninfected partner can increase the number of exposed susceptible targets.

Transmission Among Men Who Have Sex with Men

Among gay men, anal-receptive intercourse has the highest likelihood of HIV transmission. It was originally believed that small tears in the rectal mucosa provided a portal for viral

Box 32-1. HIV Infectivity of Various Body Fluids

Fluids Known to Transmit Infection

Blood
Blood products
Semen
Vaginal fluid
Breast milk

Fluids Not Known to Transmit Infection

Saliva
Tears
Urine
Cerebrospinal fluid
Amniotic fluid

entry. It is now believed that virus attaches to and infects mucosal epithelial cells, from which virus spreads to underlying tissue macrophages, leading to widespread dissemination. As with heterosexual transmission, active STDs increase the efficiency of transmission.

Transmission Secondary to Infected Blood Products

Within the blood compartment, virus can be isolated in both the cellular compartment (mononuclear cells) and the plasma. Infected cells are probably the more important vehicles of infection because of the absolute number of viral particles that can be detected intracellularly compared with plasma. In the United States, before universal testing of blood products for HIV in 1985, many patients were infected after receiving blood components, including packed red cells, platelets, and fresh-frozen plasma. Patients who received transfusions from donors with late-stage HIV infection tended to progress more quickly than those transfused with blood products from early-stage, asymptomatic donors. This probably reflects the higher viral inoculum transmitted from the blood of patients with late-stage disease and the greater virulence of HIV associated with advanced disease. Patients with hemophilia A and other clotting disorders also have been infected from contaminated blood products pooled from many donors. At present, all blood products in the United States are tested for HIV antibodies and are considered safe. The chance of HIV transmission from a single unit of transfused blood now is estimated to be 1 in 500,000.

Injection Drug Users

The sharing of needles without sterilization between IDUs results in parenteral exposure to HIV-infected blood. The efficiency of transmission is not clear. The use of a syringe/needle contaminated with blood from an individual with late-stage HIV infection probably imparts the highest risk of transmission.

Vertical Transmission

An HIV-infected mother can transmit infection in utero, during delivery, or by breast-feeding. In utero and intrapartum transmissions account for the vast majority of vertical infections. In utero transmission occurs transplacentally, most likely during the third trimester. Intrapartum transmission probably takes place as the fetus is exposed to infected body fluids while passing through the birth canal. Strong evidence suggests that many more infections occur intrapartum than in utero, making the intrapartum period an attractive target for infant prevention modalities. Infection of an infant from exposure to infected breast milk is a comparatively uncommon means of transmission in the developed world but remains a significant risk among individuals in such developing regions as Africa and southeastern Asia.

Other Modes of Transmission

With the exception of a few rare reports, the transmission of HIV by casual contact is extremely unlikely. Family members and close friends who care for sick and dying patients have no appreciable risk of contracting HIV infection provided that they follow standard infection control procedures.

Transmission in the Health Care Setting

The occupational risk of transmission of HIV to health care workers (HCWs) from infected patients is extremely low but is still a source of great concern. Of the reported cases of work-related HIV transmission, percutaneous exposures from HIV-contaminated needle-stick injuries have been the most common mode of infection. HCWs also have become infected by mucous membrane or nonintact skin exposure, but such events have been extremely rare. The risk of seroconversion after percutaneous exposure to HIV-infected fluid is approximately 0.25% to 0.3%.[4] The seroconversion rate from mucocutaneous exposure to contaminated blood is considerably lower than for percutaneous exposure, probably less than 0.1%. Injuries that impart the highest risk of transmission include deep sticks involving hollow-bore needles contaminated with freshly drawn blood. The risk of transmission of virus from HCW to patient has received much attention in light of infection of a group of six patients by an infected dentist in Florida by unknown means. A possible case of transmission to a patient from an orthopedic surgeon during a procedure was also reported. In the usual health care setting, HCW-to-patient transmission would most likely happen during an invasive procedure, although specific risk factors for this type of transmission have not been identified clearly. Although it cannot be established reliably, the HCW-to-patient rate is likely to be several orders of magnitude less than that for patient-to-HCW transmission.

COURSE AND NATURAL HISTORY

Course of Disease

After primary HIV infection, during which a transient fall occurs in the CD4 count, patients typically become asymptomatic (Fig. 32-3). Immune thrombocytopenia, herpes zoster (shingles), and persistent generalized lymphadenopathy (PGL) are among the earliest manifestations. Herpes zoster can be recurrent and involve more than one dermatome

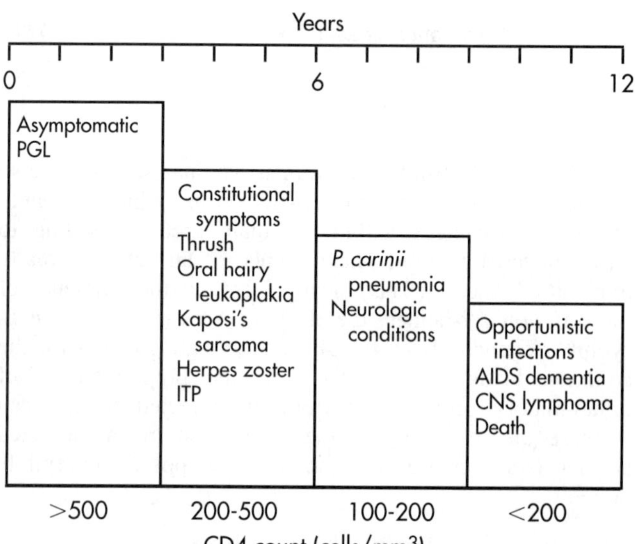

Fig. 32-3. Clinical course of HIV infection. Diagram shows disease progression associated with CD4 count over approximately 12 years. *PGL,* Persistent generalized lymphadenopathy; *ITP,* immune thrombocytopenia purpura; *CNS,* central nervous system.

during a single outbreak. With PGL, lymph nodes in multiple locations, especially the occipital, posterior cervical, and axillary regions, become enlarged, firm, nontender, and unattached to the underlying tissue. Although some patients note a waxing and waning of lymph node size, the adenopathy generally persists for many months or longer. During this "asymptomatic" period the CD4 count remains at or near the normal range (500 cells/mm^3 or higher).

With further CD4 count decline, various constitutional symptoms begin to appear, including fatigue, intermittent unexplained fevers, diarrhea, and night sweats. For the first time, patients feel ill. By now the CD4 count has typically dropped to between 200 and 500 cells/mm^3. Pulmonary tuberculosis and bacterial pneumonia can occur during this early stage of HIV infection, as can lymphoma and Kaposi's sarcoma, although all these conditions occur more often with lower CD4 counts.

At a CD4 count of about 200 cells/mm^3, patients are at risk for developing *Pneumocystis carinii* pneumonia (PCP), which, until the widespread use of prophylaxis, was the most common opportunistic infection seen in patients with AIDS in the developed world. With a CD4 count of 100 to 200 cells/mm^3, other conditions may include the early peripheral and central nervous system complications of infection. Once the CD4 count has dropped below 50 to 100 cells/mm^3, patients become susceptible to the remaining AIDS-related conditions, including cryptococcal meningitis, cytomegalovirus retinitis, toxoplasmic encephalitis, disseminated *Mycobacterium avium* complex infection, AIDS wasting syndrome, primary CNS lymphoma, and AIDS dementia complex.

In 1993 the Centers for Disease Control and Prevention (CDC) revised its surveillance case definition for AIDS, which was first proposed in 1986 (Box 32-2).[2] Two important changes were made. First, the definition of AIDS was expanded to include all HIV-infected patients with CD4 counts below 200 cells/mm^3, whether or not they had a recognized complication. Second, pulmonary tuberculosis, recurrent bacterial pneumonia, and invasive cervical cancer in women were added to the list of AIDS-defining conditions.

The preceding account is a stylized description of the typical course of an HIV-infected patient. Unfortunately, there are many exceptions to this course of events. For example, symptomatic primary HIV infection is not recognized in 30% to 50% of patients. Also, the rate of decline of CD4 cells varies considerably among individuals, as largely determined by the viral load set-point (see Fig. 32-2). More important, many patients remain completely asymptomatic, even as their CD4 counts drop to very low levels. Therefore a clinician cannot reliably predict the CD4 count in an asymptomatic HIV-infected patient. In contrast, the CD4 count is predictably low in symptomatic patients, particularly if they have been diagnosed with one of the late-stage, AIDS-defining conditions. As a result, some of the early staging systems used in HIV infection that were based on symptoms alone inaccurately reflected the true stage of disease in many cases. Similarly, staging systems based on the CD4 count alone also are inaccurate because symptoms clearly influence prognosis. Finally, CD4 count recovery as a result of HAART has further complicated the efforts to devise a useful staging system for HIV infection. Table 32-1 lists the current CDC staging system, which is the one used most extensively.[2]

Natural History of Infection

HIV infection causes disease that is measured not in weeks or months but in years. Several studies have examined the time course of infection in selected populations. The Multicentered AIDS Cohort Study (MACS), a study of gay men in four major cities originally begun in the late 1970s to study hepatitis B, was adapted to study HIV. Only 2% of patients developed AIDS within 2 years of seroconversion, and 10 years were required for slightly more than 50% of patients to develop AIDS. Interestingly, a small percentage of patients (less than 5%) remained symptom free with normal CD4 counts for more than 15 years.

The natural history of HIV infection also has been studied for hemophiliac patients and transfusion recipients. Hemophiliacs appear to progress less rapidly than gay men, with one study reporting that only 27% had progressed to AIDS by 7 years from the time of seroconversion. The rate of progression to AIDS correlated inversely with age; younger patients, particularly those less than 17 years of age, had a much slower progression than those over age 35. In contrast, transfusion recipients as a group appear to progress more rapidly than either gay men or hemophiliacs, with approximately 50% of patients developing AIDS by 7 years. Natural history data for HIV-infected IDUs are limited but probably similar to data for gay men.[1] The prognosis for active users with HIV is generally poor because of the lack of ongoing medical care, nonadherence to treatment plans, poor

Box 32-2. 1993 CDC Expanded Surveillance Case Definition for AIDS

HIV seropositivity
and CD4 count less than 200/mm^3
or one or more of the following conditions:

- Candidiasis, esophageal, bronchial, or pulmonary
- Cervical cancer, invasive
- Coccidioidomycosis, disseminated or extrapulmonary
- Cryptococcosis, extrapulmonary
- Cryptosporidiosis, chronic intestinal
- Cytomegalovirus, retinitis or nonlymphoid
- Encephalopathy, HIV related
- Herpes simplex, esophagitis, pneumonitis, or chronic ulcerative
- Histoplasmosis, disseminated or extrapulmonary
- Isosporiasis, chronic intestinal
- Kaposi's sarcoma
- Lymphoma, primary central nervous system, immunoblastic, or Burkitt's
- *Mycobacterium avium* complex or *M. kansasii*, disseminated
- *Mycobacterium tuberculosis*, pulmonary or extrapulmonary
- *Mycobacterium* species (other), disseminated or extrapulmonary
- *Pneumocystis carinii* pneumonia
- Pneumonia, recurrent
- Progressive multifocal leukoencephalopathy
- *Salmonella* septicemia, recurrent
- *Toxoplasma* encephalopathy
- Wasting, HIV related

From Centers for Disease Control and Prevention: *MMWR 41(RR-17):1, 1992.*

Table 32-1. 1993 CDC Classification System for HIV Infection

	Clinical categories		
CD4 count	(A) Asymptomatic, first-degree HIV infection or PGL	(B) Symptomatic, not (A) or (C) conditions	(C) AIDS-indicator conditions
(1) >500/mm^3	A1	B1	C1
(2) 200-499/mm^3	A2	B2	C2
(3) <200/mm^3	A3	B3	C3

From Centers for Disease Control and Prevention: *MMWR* 41(RR-17):1, 1992.
PGL, Persistent generalized lymphadenopathy.

nutrition, and greater exposure to tuberculosis and other infectious agents.

EPIDEMIOLOGY

North America

As of December 1999 an estimated 920,000 adults and children were living with HIV/AIDS in North America.[11] In the United States a total of 393,045 adults and children living with HIV/AIDS were reported to the CDC as of June 1999 (Table 32-2).[5] Therefore the majority of patients living with the infection are not reported and presumably undiagnosed. The major recent changes in epidemiology in the developed world have involved a large decline in mortality and in the incidence of new AIDS cases, primarily because of the widespread use of HAART (Fig. 32-4).[7] The rate of decline in the incidence of AIDS has slowed somewhat from 1996-97 (18%) to 1997-98 (11%). In contrast to AIDS cases, new cases of HIV infection, while declining during the middle to late 1980s, have remained relatively unchanged in the 1990s. The World Health Organization (WHO) estimates that 44,000 new cases of HIV infection occurred in North America in 1998-99. Given the declining death rate and stable incidence, the proportion of the population living with HIV infection has increased during the middle to late 1990s.

Table 32-3 shows the AIDS cases among adults and adolescents (male and female) by exposure category through June 1999, both cumulative and for the previous 12-month reporting period.[5] For American men, transmission by men having sex with men (MSM) remains the largest cumulative risk category. The percentage of reported cases among gay men decreased from July 1998 to June 1999. Unfortunately, some large cities report that the safe-sex guidelines instituted in the 1980s in the gay community are being ignored by the next generation of gay men now that HAART has been introduced. For women, heterosexual transmission, usually from a past or active IDU, overtook direct injection drug use in the early 1990s as the principal means of HIV transmission.

Fig. 32-5 shows the cumulative AIDS cases according to race and ethnicity as of June 1999. The trend of overrepresentation by minority communities has worsened during the 1990s. Africans and Hispanics now account for more than 50% of reported cases. This disproportionate overrepresentation likely results from poverty, greater risk of exposure in inner-city environments, and poor access to preventive health care services.

Table 32-2. Vital Statistics of HIV and AIDS in United States* Through June 1999

Cases/group	Cumulative total
Cases of AIDS reported*	711,344
Patients living with HIV infection†	104,784
Patients living with AIDS	288,261
Patients living with HIV/AIDS	393,045

From Centers for Disease Control and Prevention: *HIV/AIDS Surv Rep* 11:1, 1999.
*Adults and children since beginning of epidemic in 1981.
†HIV infection without AIDS. Note that as of June 1999, at least 20 states or dependencies/possessions were not yet reporting cases of HIV infection.

Worldwide Perspective

WHO estimates that approximately 33.6 million adults and children were living worldwide with HIV/AIDS as of December 1999 (Table 32-4).[11] The majority of cases are in sub-Saharan Africa, where in some large urban areas, up to one quarter of adults between ages 18 and 45 are HIV infected. Areas that show the largest number of new cases include sub-Saharan Africa, southern and southeastern Asia, central Asia, and Latin America. An estimated 16,000 new infections occur daily, meaning that 5.6 million people were newly infected in 1999 alone. WHO estimates that more than 16 million people already have died from HIV infection.

PATIENT EVALUATION

Since it is presumed that the majority of Americans infected with HIV are unaware of their infection, such patients are not benefiting from early intervention. The role of the primary care physician in diagnosing HIV disease is critical. During the early years of the AIDS epidemic, surveillance focused on members of "high-risk groups" (gay and bisexual men, IDUs, hemophiliacs, individuals from Haiti); however, that approach is less useful today. A growing number of HIV-infected individuals contract their infection through heterosexual contact or are unaware of their mode of transmission. It has become more accurate therefore to think in terms of *risk behaviors* rather than risk groups. As a result, a thorough history, including nonjudgmental but specific questioning about sexual activity and drug use, has become even more important in identifying patients at risk for HIV infection.

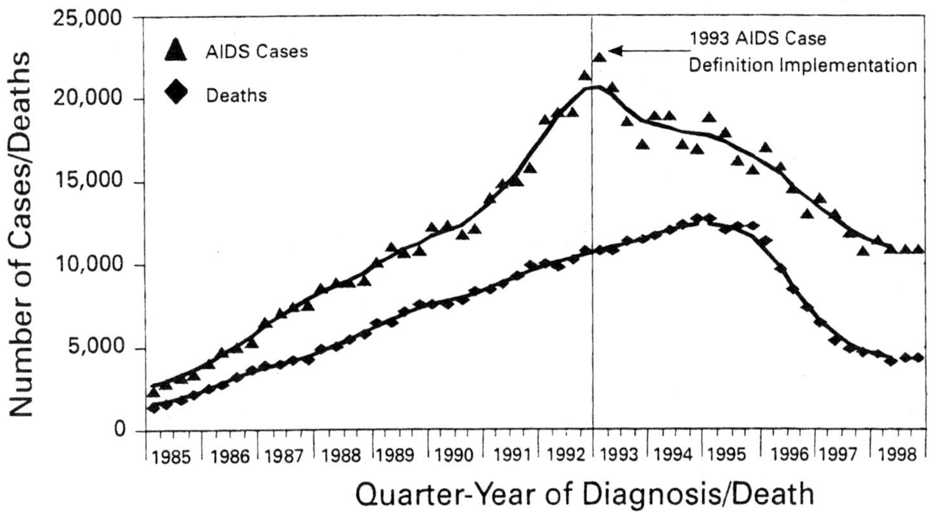

Fig. 32-4. Estimated incidence of AIDS and number of deaths among adults (age 13 and older) with AIDS in the United States, 1985 to 1998. (From Centers for Disease Control and Prevention: *MMWR* 48(RR-13):1, 1999.)

Table 32-3. AIDS Cases Among Adults and Adolescents Age 13 and Older by Exposure Category Through June 1999

Risk category	July 1998–June 1999 number (%)	Cumulative total (%)
Men who have sex with men (MSM)	15,999 (34)	334,073 (48)
Injection drug user (IDU)	10,536 (23)	179,228 (26)
MSM and IDU	1940 (4)	45,266 (6)
Coagulation disorder	171 (0)	5010 (1)
Heterosexual contact	7051 (15)	70,582 (10)
Blood component recipient	266 (1)	8430 (1)
Other risk (not reported or identified)	10,798 (23)	60,159 (9)
TOTAL	46,761 (100)	702,748 (100)

From Centers for Disease Control and Prevention: *HIV/AIDS Surv Rep* 11:1, 1999.

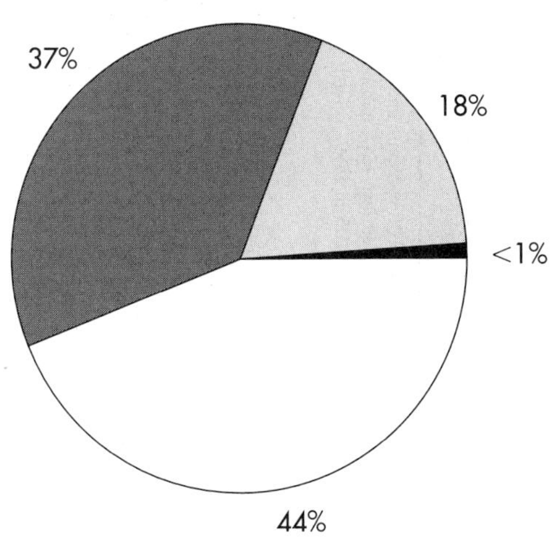

Fig. 32-5. Cumulative AIDS cases by race/ethnicity through June 1999 in United States. (From Centers for Disease Control and Prevention: *HIV/AIDS Surv Rep* 11:1, 1999.)

Table 32-4. Worldwide HIV/AIDS Statistics and Features, December 1999

Region	Epidemic started	Adults and children living with HIV/AIDS	Adults and children newly infected with HIV	Adult prevalence rate*	HIV-positive adults who are women	Main mode(s) of transmission for adults living with HIV/AIDS
Sub-Saharan Africa	Late 1970s-early 1980s	23.3 million	3.8 million	8.0%	55%	Hetero
North Africa and Mideast	Late 1980s	220,000	19,000	0.13%	20%	IDU, Hetero
South and Southeast Asia	Late 1980s	6 million	1.3 million	0.69%	30%	Hetero
East Asia and Pacific	Late 1980s	530,000	120,000	0.068%	15%	IDU, Hetero, MSM
Latin America	Late 1970s-early 1980s	1.3 million	150,000	0.57%	20%	MSM, IDU, Hetero
Caribbean	Late 1970s-early 1980s	360,000	57,000	1.96%	35%	Hetero, MSM
Eastern Europe and central Asia	Early 1990s	360,000	95,000	0.14%	20%	IDU, MSM
Western Europe	Late 1970s-early 1980s	520,000	30,000	0.25%	20%	MSM, IDU
North America	Late 1970s-early 1980s	920,000	44,000	0.56%	20%	MSM, IDU, Hetero
Australia and New Zealand	Late 1970s-early 1980s	12,000	500	0.1%	10%	MSM, IDU
TOTAL		33.6 million	5.6 million	1.1%	46%	

From Joint United Nations Programme on HIV/AIDS: AIDS epidemic update, December 1999.
MSM, Sexual transmission among men who have sex with men; *IDU,* transmission through injection drug use; *Hetero,* heterosexual transmission.
*Proportion of adults (ages 15 to 49) living with HIV/AIDS in 1999, using 1998 population numbers.

Indications for testing also include STDs, pregnancy, and active tuberculosis. HIV testing should be considered in patients with PGL, unexplained dementia, aseptic meningitis, or peripheral neuropathy; chronic, unexplained fever, diarrhea, or weight loss; generalized herpes simplex or multidermatomal herpes zoster infection; unexplained cytopenias; B-cell lymphoma; or other opportunistic conditions suggestive of cell-mediated immunodeficiency.

Diagnosis

Unfortunately, the diagnosis of HIV disease may still lead to social stigmatization, loss of health insurance, and discrimination in employment and housing. Because of the potential consequences to the patient, informed consent is recommended and in most states required before HIV testing can be initiated. In addition, HIV testing should be accompanied by pretest and posttest counseling, which should include discussion of the purpose of the test, prognosis and natural history of HIV infection, value of early intervention, transmission of HIV and risk reduction, partner notification, and other medical and social issues related to the diagnosis.

The criteria for a positive HIV test are a repeatedly positive enzyme-linked immunosorbent assay (ELISA) followed by a positive Western blot. The accuracy of testing is extremely high. False-negative results are uncommon and usually occur during the window period between infection and seroconversion, a period with a maximum duration of 6 months. False-negative results also have been described in patients infected with subtype O and those with late-stage HIV infection whose serostatus paradoxically becomes negative in the face of very advanced infection. False-positive results are rare. Patients with a positive ELISA and one or two bands on Western blot are reported as indeterminate. Indeterminate tests may occur in seroconverting patients, those with advanced HIV disease, and patients with alloantibodies (pregnancy, transfusions, organ transplantation) or autoantibodies (autoimmune diseases, malignancy).[1] Although patients in low-risk categories with indeterminate tests are unlikely to be infected, repeat tests in 3 and 6 months are usually performed for confirmation. If the indeterminate test is caused by seroconversion, it will usually become positive within 1 month.

Other methods to detect HIV infection include viral isolation, polymerase chain reaction (PCR), and standard HIV viral load testing. Because of the accuracy of the standard HIV test, however, these techniques are rarely necessary. Rapid tests for HIV antibodies are available and comparable in accuracy to the ELISA. They are highly sensitive; a negative result is definitive and can be reported in several minutes. Specificity is lower, however, and all positive results must be confirmed with standard tests.

Box 32-3. Initial and Follow-up Evaluations of HIV-infected Patient

Initial Evaluation

Complete history and physical examination
Confirmation of HIV seropositivity
CD4 count and CD4 percent
HIV mRNA (viral load)
CBC, differential, and chemistries (electrolytes, renal and liver profiles, fasting lipids)
Urinalysis
Chest radiograph
Toxoplasma and cytomegalovirus serologies (IgG)
Syphilis screen (RPR or VDRL)
Hepatitis screen (hepatitis A antibody, HBsAg, HBsAb, HBcAb, hepatitis C antibody)*
Tuberculin skin test (PPD) and tuberculosis exposure history
Pap test and screening for *Chlamydia* and gonorrhea
G6PD screen*
Vaccinations (pneumococcal, influenza, hepatitis A and B)*

Follow-up Evaluations

History and physical examination
Chemistries, repeated periodically (e.g., liver profile, lipid panel)
CD4 count and percent (every 3 to 6 months)
Viral load (every 3 to 4 months; also 3 to 4 weeks after any change in antiviral regimen)
Tuberculin skin test (PPD) and syphilis screen (annually)
Pap test (at least annually)
Vaccinations (influenza yearly; pneumococcal at 5 years)*

*See text.

Initial Evaluation

Physicians evaluating patients with HIV infection who are new to their practice should take a careful history (Box 32-3). Some patients may be newly diagnosed by the primary care physician doing the evaluation. Other patients have been previously diagnosed and treated by one or more physicians in the past. For either group the physician must ascertain when the patient was likely infected, by what means (if known), and when the patient was diagnosed. Patients should be questioned about their past medical history, including HIV-related opportunistic infections and malignancies, STDs, chickenpox, hepatitis, gynecologic problems (particularly Pap testing), vaccinations, and tuberculosis, both tuberculin skin testing and possible close contacts with individuals with active tuberculosis. Additional questions should focus on common HIV-related symptoms, including fevers, night sweats, weight loss, diarrhea, cough, skin rashes or lesions, oral thrush or ulcerations, headache, and changes in neurologic function or mental status. For the patient previously diagnosed with HIV and treated with antiretroviral agents, the physician should obtain a detailed antiviral history, including start and stop dates, reasons for medication discontinuation, drug failures, and results of genotype and phenotype testing, if available. Records of prior CD4 counts and viral load determinations are also important. In practice, obtaining an accurate antiretroviral history and accompanying test results is often difficult and the historic profile incomplete.

Physical Examination. A complete physical examination should be performed, with special attention to the evaluation of lymph nodes, funduscopic examination, oropharynx and skin, abdominal examination to detect enlargement of the liver or spleen, genital examination, and neuropsychologic screening to evaluate cognitive function and detect early dementia. Patients who are cachectic or who report significant weight loss require medical evaluation to look for reversible causes.

Laboratory Studies. Several initial laboratory studies are appropriate in patients with HIV infection. Patients who have no documentation of their HIV serology results or who were tested anonymously should have a repeat HIV test. Anemia, leukopenia, and thrombocytopenia are common in HIV-infected individuals and are readily detected with a complete blood count (CBC) with differential, which also is used to calculate the total CD4 lymphocyte count. A chemistry panel also should be performed, including electrolytes, renal and liver profiles, urinalysis, and fasting lipid panel, because of the alterations in lipid metabolism caused by the virus and secondary to antiretroviral therapy. A nontreponemal test for syphilis, such as Venereal Disease Research Laboratories (VDRL) or rapid plasma reagin (RPR), and a tuberculin skin test (purified protein derivative, PPD) should be performed at baseline and repeated yearly.

Serologic testing for prior exposure to *Toxoplasma gondii* using the anti-*Toxoplasma immunoglobulin G* (IgG) is useful in determining the need for *Toxoplasma* prophylaxis. Seronegative patients should probably be retested when their CD4 count approaches 100/mm^3. Although the *Toxoplasma* serology has limited utility diagnostically, a seronegative patient with a CNS space-occupying lesion is less likely to have toxoplasmosis than a seropositive patient.[6]

Because of the high incidence of hepatitis B and C coinfection, all HIV-infected patients should be screened with hepatitis B surface antigen (HBsAg), core antibody (HBcAb), and surface antibody (HBsAb), and hepatitis C antibody. Hepatitis A serostatus also should be ascertained, since a negative result in a hepatitis C–infected patient should prompt consideration for hepatitis A vaccination.[6] Serologic testing for prior cytomegalovirus (CMV) infection is advocated, since those who are seronegative should receive only CMV-negative blood products. Furthermore, although routine prophylaxis against CMV disease is not currently recommended, it may be indicated in the future for seropositive individuals with advanced HIV disease. Serologic testing for varicella should be performed in patients who are unable to give a history of chickenpox. This baseline test helps determine the need for postexposure prophylaxis with varicella-zoster immune globulin (VZIG) in patients exposed to chickenpox or shingles.

Routine screening for glucose-6-phosphate dehydrogenase (G6PD) deficiency is sometimes recommended, especially in black patients and patients of Mediterranean descent. Several oxidant drugs, such as dapsone, primaquine, and sulfonamides, are often used in HIV-infected patients and may lead to hemolysis in G6PD-deficient patients.

Because HIV-infected patients are highly susceptible to a variety of pulmonary complications and infections, a baseline chest radiograph may be useful. Furthermore, the chest radiograph may be helpful in screening for occult tuberculosis.

HIV-infected women are at increased risk for several gynecologic problems, including pelvic inflammatory disease and tuboovarian abscesses, candidal vaginitis, cervical dysplasia, and invasive cervical carcinoma. All HIV-infected women should have a baseline pelvic examination with Pap smear. Screening for clinically silent chlamydial and gonococcal cervicitis is recommended. The use of routine colposcopy is controversial, but the test is indicated in women with abnormal Pap smears or a history of vaginal condylomata. Pap smears should be repeated at least annually in women with normal results and every 6 months in women with a previously abnormal Pap smear.

The CD4 count, CD4 percentage, and HIV mRNA (viral load) are measured during the initial evaluation of a newly HIV-infected individual. The CD4 count and percentage provide the best available clinical data on the relative health of the immune system. The CD4 count is used in (1) staging HIV infection, (2) determining the need for antiretroviral therapy and for prophylaxis of opportunistic infections, (3) assessing the risk of specific HIV-related conditions, and (4) making and reporting the diagnosis of AIDS. The physician and patient must be aware of the substantial variation in the results of CD4 counts. Because in most laboratories the absolute CD4 count is determined by multiplying the white blood cell (WBC) count, percentage of lymphocytes, and percentage of CD4 lymphocytes, variation in any of these components can affect the total CD4 count. Because the CD4 percentage is not subject to variation based on the WBC count and lymphocyte count, it may provide a less variable and more accurate reflection of the patient's immunologic status. Total CD4 counts of 200 and 500/mm^3 generally correspond to CD4 percentages of 14% and 29%, respectively.

HIV viral load is the other key measure of the status of HIV-infected patients. Viral load complements the CD4 count. Although the CD4 count provides information on immune system function, viral load indirectly measures the rate of viral replication. Three assays for the measurement of viral load are currently approved in the United States: Roche Amplicor RT-PCR assay, Chiron bDNA assay, and Organon Teknika Nuclisens HIV-1 QT assay.[1] All are accurate and fairly reproducible. Results with the Roche and the Organon Teknika assays are about double those of the Chiron assay. Each assay can measure down to a level of 40 to 50 mRNA copies/ml. The initial viral load measurement should be done twice over 1 to 2 weeks to ensure an adequate baseline, since intercurrent illnesses and even vaccinations can cause significant transient rises in the viral load.

Vaccinations Specific to HIV-infected Patients. Advancing HIV infection impairs the host's ability to form specific antibodies with infection or immunization. Therefore vaccinations must be given as early in the course of HIV infection as possible. Although its efficacy is not well established in this population, the pneumococcal polysaccharide vaccine is indicated for all HIV-infected patients with CD4 counts greater than 200/mm^3 because of the high incidence of pneumococcal pneumonia and bacteremia associated with HIV disease. It is given as a single dose, with revaccination after 5 years. Patients with lower counts are unlikely to respond but probably should also be vaccinated. For patients vaccinated in this low CD4 count range, the physician should consider revaccination before 5 years after they have had a significant CD4 count response (greater than 200/mm^3) to HAART.[6]

The influenza vaccine should be given yearly to prevent influenza and its potential complications, primarily bacterial pneumonia. Because of the high risk of hepatitis B among many HIV-infected patients, hepatitis B vaccination should be offered to all patients who are HBcAb negative.[6] Vaccination is given at 0, 1, and 6 months. A postvaccination titer should be performed 1 to 6 months after the final dose to ensure vaccine efficacy. Hepatitis A vaccine is now recommended for all HIV-infected patients with chronic hepatitis C, since the acute hepatic insult associated with hepatitis A infection in such patients carries substantial morbidity and risk of death. Two doses of vaccine are given at 6-month intervals.[6]

Follow-up Evaluations

Frequency of follow-up visits depends on stage of disease, stability of the antiviral response, comorbid conditions, and the patient's psychosocial stability. In general, patients with late-stage disease are seen more frequently than those with early-stage disease. For patients just starting antiviral therapy, a follow-up visit should take place in 3 to 4 weeks; adherence to treatment and possible side effects should be discussed in detail, and viral load should be tested to determine the magnitude of the initial drop. Patients should be seen 1 to 2 months later and then at least every 3 months. Viral load measurements should be repeated every 3 to 4 months; the CD4 count should be repeated every 3 to 6 months.[8]

In addition to following response to antiviral therapy, patients need to be followed carefully for both their standard adult preventive care as well as HIV-related preventive care. The standard adult preventive care plan should be similar to the standard plan of age-matched, non-HIV-infected patients (e.g., screening for cardiovascular risk factors, mammograms for women, counseling for smoking cessation). HIV-specific preventive care has many facets. Vaccination status must be continually updated, as discussed. Patients should undergo annual PPD screening and testing for syphilis with a VDRL or RPR. For women, Pap smears need to be performed at least yearly. The CD4 count must be closely watched to determine the need for opportunistic infection prophylaxis. For patients with CD4 counts less than 100 to 150/mm^3, an opthalmologist should perform a yearly retinal examination to screen for CMV retinitis. For patients with hepatitis B and C coinfection, liver enzymes should be periodically rechecked. Similarly, given the lipid profile abnormalities associated with some antiretroviral agents, repeat lipid studies should also be performed.

With the complexity of current antiretroviral therapy and the urgent need to keep up with the general health maintenance of this patient group, most physicians prefer to track information in a paper or computed flowsheet. A detailed record of the antiretroviral history is essential, including start and stop dates of medications, reasons for medication and dose changes, and some subjective estimate of patient adherence. Chronologic listing of CD4 counts, CD4 percentages, and HIV viral load measurements should be kept. Ideally these data should be recorded to allow easy comparisons between the antiretroviral regimen and the viral load and CD4 response to facilitate future decisions regarding medication changes. The flowsheet should also contain a record of initial screening results and annual screenings for HIV-related preventive care.

Mental Health Considerations

In addition to medical management, HIV health care providers must be able to recognize and treat many of the psychiatric complications common in HIV-infected patients. As a group these patients have an increased lifetime risk of major mental illness.

Persistent signs or symptoms of emotional distress in any HIV-infected patient are indications for a thorough psychiatric evaluation. History should focus on any family history of mental illness, substance abuse, present medications, and any previous psychiatric disorders. Laboratory studies to rule out organic etiologies include RPR, thyroid-stimulating hormone (TSH), folate and B_{12} levels, and CNS imaging in selected patients.

Major depression is the most frequent diagnosed psychiatric disorder in this population. In addition to depressed mood, patients manifest social withdrawal, fatigue, loss of self-esteem, feelings of helplessness, and vegetative features (sleep disturbances, anorexia, weight loss, psychomotor retardation). The incidence of depression appears to increase with advancing HIV infection and declining CD4 counts. Risk assessment for suicidal ideation is an important consideration in any depressed patient. Many patients will benefit from antidepressant therapy.

Anxiety also is common in the HIV-infected population, and providers should attempt to identify specific stressors in the patient's environment. Psychotherapy and the judicious use of anxiolytics may be helpful. Obsessive behavior in the form of fixation with health-related issues is not unusual. Overt psychotic disorders (schizophrenia, mania) may be related to a premorbid condition or a medication or may be secondary to another psychiatric disorder. Conventional treatment with psychotherapy and antipsychotic medications is indicated.

Because a high proportion of HIV-infected patients have a history of substance abuse, the primary care physician often becomes integral in formulating and perpetuating an effective treatment plan. Important components include (1) detoxification and management of withdrawal, (2) continued abstinence (maintenance), and (3) diagnosis and treatment of conditions predisposing to substance abuse. Community programs such as Alcoholics Anonymous, Narcotics Anonymous, and AIDS support organizations are excellent resources.

Special Management Issues

Although HIV infection shares many features of other chronic diseases, caring for HIV-infected patients also entails certain unique responsibilities. Frequent discussion of the avoidance of transmission is important. Although laws regarding sexual and drug-use contact notification vary from state to state, primary caregivers often play a role in encouraging or assisting with the disclosure of the patient's HIV status. In many communities, physicians care for patients with more immediate concerns of substance abuse, mental illness, homelessness, child care, lack of medical insurance, and poverty. Physicians must be aware of community resources that can assist their patients with these obstacles so that their medical problems can be addressed. Physicians also may become involved in issues of employment or housing discrimination. They may have patients who are rejected by their families or friends because of their disease, leaving them without the support so crucial in maintaining their health. Understanding and management of HIV disease progress rapidly, and patients expect their caregivers to maintain up-to-date knowledge. Patients may ask for unapproved or experimental treatment or may take alternative therapies with or instead of standard drugs. Physicians must be aware of experimental protocols and make them available to their patients, when appropriate. They also must be familiar with the potential risks and benefits of the alternative therapies being advocated in the community so that they can counsel their patients about the use of these therapies and monitor them appropriately if they choose to take them.

As with any chronic disease, physicians caring for HIV-infected patients interact frequently with families and support networks. HIV disease is unique, however, because the patient's spouse, partner, friends, or family members may also be infected. Physicians must recognize the importance of nontraditional families. Among gay couples, for example, the patient's partner is usually a more appropriate decision maker than the next of kin, if the patient is unable to speak for himself. For this role to be legally recognized, however, the partner must have been designated as the "health care proxy" or "durable power of attorney for health." Despite the major improvement in the prognosis imparted by HAART, patients should be encouraged as early as possible in the course of the disease to make their wishes known to their physician and family regarding their proxy for health care decisions, their wishes regarding terminal care and its aggressiveness, and the disposition of their property after death. Whenever possible, their wishes should be formalized with the legal arrangements appropriate to their particular state.

ANTIRETROVIRAL THERAPY

Specific antiretroviral therapy for HIV infection was made available 5 years after the first descriptions of AIDS and 3 years after the identification of the responsible virus. The unprecedented acceleration of the drug approval and availability process beginning in the 1980s continued through the 1990s. The appropriate use of the growing number of new drugs, however, has been confusing and controversial. Before fall 1995, therapy of HIV infection was generally restricted to persons with advanced disease, those who were symptomatic or who had AIDS. Treatment of asymptomatic individuals with CD4 counts between 200 and 500 cells/mm^3 was controversial, and therapy of those patients with over 500 cells/mm^3 was discouraged. Decisions regarding initiation or changes of antiretroviral therapy were based on CD4 count trends and patient symptoms. Plasma viral load testing was not available. Zidovudine (AZT, ZDV) monotherapy was the mainstay of therapy. The other three available licensed nucleoside analogs, stavudine (d4T), didanosine (ddI), and zalcitabine (ddC), were used alternatively as monotherapy agents if a patient failed or was intolerant to AZT therapy. Although combination therapy was being considered, it was not employed routinely because early studies, including a large multicenter trial (ACTG 155) that compared AZT alone, ddC alone, and the combination, showed no differences in overall efficacy.

Therapeutic approaches were altered in late 1995 and early 1996 when three large clinical trials demonstrated that combination nucleoside analog therapy delayed HIV progression and improved survival. In addition, the rapid development and availability of new and more potent drugs, such as the protease inhibitors (PIs) and nonnucleoside reverse transcriptase inhibitors (NNRTIs), as well as tests to measure plasma viral burden, led to dramatic changes and increasing complexity of the clinical treatment of HIV-infected persons. Viral load testing, now routinely performed, enables the physician to determine better the optimal time to initiate or change therapy, before declining CD4 counts.

In 2000 a typical antiretroviral regimen, HAART, consists of at least three agents: two nucleoside reverse transcriptase inhibitors (NRTIs) combined with one or two PIs or one NNRTI. The goal of therapy is to reduce measurable plasma viral burden to very low levels and restore or preserve immunologic function. The clinical impact of these therapies has been dramatic, with a sharp drop in the incidence of opportunistic infections and other complications, a marked decrease in hospitalization rates for HIV-related disease, and a lower mortality from AIDS nationwide (see Fig. 32-4). HAART has offered substantial hope to many patients.

Initiation

Before prescribing medications, the physician should factor the patient's prognosis, as predicted by the CD4 counts and plasma HIV RNA levels, into the decision. Prognosis is based on MACS data, which demonstrated a correlation between risk of progression to an AIDS-defining illness and the plasma viral load when stratified according to CD4 count (see earlier discussion and Fig. 32-2).[12]

The Panel on Clinical Practices for Treatment of HIV Infection convened by the U.S. Department of Health and Human Services (DHHS) and the Henry J. Kaiser Family Foundation publishes regularly updated guidelines on the internet for the use of antiretroviral agents.[8] Therapy should be offered to patients with primary HIV infection, those within 6 months of HIV seroconversion, and all patients with symptoms caused by HIV infection. Asymptomatic chronically infected persons are considered for treatment based on virologic and immunologic factors. Those patients with less than 500 CD4 cells/mm^3 or plasma HIV RNA levels exceeding 10,000 copies/ml (bDNA assay) or 20,000 copies/ml (RT-PCR assay) should be offered therapy (Table 32-5).[8]

The antiviral drug regimens can be complex, cause numerous potential side effects and drug interactions, and require rigid adherence, so an assessment of the patient's interest and willingness to accept the treatment is essential. Despite the clear benefits of therapy for most patients, others may benefit most from deferring therapy, particularly when poor adherence is likely. Compliance of less than 95% of medication doses increases the likelihood of viral resistance and cross-resistance within the drug classes, compromising the effectiveness of future therapies. Thus the potential benefits and risks must be considered carefully before initiating therapy (Box 32-4).

The goals of therapy are to (1) suppress viral load completely for a prolonged duration, (2) restore or at least maintain immunologic function, (3) minimize HIV-related morbidity and mortality, and (4) improve quality of life. These goals can be achieved by maximizing adherence to the drug regimen, sequencing drugs rationally, preserving future treatment options, and using resistance testing in certain clinical settings.[8] At this time, therapy is suppressive, not curative, and is lifelong.

Drugs and Regimens

Combination therapy is superior to monotherapy because of additive antiviral effects, delay in the emergence of resistance, and possibly a decrease in viral fitness. Nucleoside analog combinations are generally more effective when used with NNRTIs or PIs. Table 32-6 lists suggested antiretroviral agents for initial treatment of established HIV infection. Priority is given to regimens for which clinical trials data suggest sustained suppression of HIV RNA and sustained

Table 32-5. Indications for Initiation of Antiretroviral therapy in Chronically HIV-infected Patients

Clinical category	CD4+ T cell count and HIV RNA	Recommendation
Symptomatic (AIDS, thrush, unexplained fever)	Any value	Treat
Asymptomatic	CD4+ T cells <500/mm^3 *or* HIV RNA >10,000 (bDNA) or >20,000 (RT-PCR)	Treatment should be offered. Strength of recommendation is based on prognosis for disease-free survival and willingness of patient to accept therapy.*
Asymptomatic	CD4+ T cells >500/mm^3 *and* HIV RNA <10,000 (bDNA) or >20,000 (RT-PCR)	Many experts would delay therapy and observe; others would treat.

From DHHS Panel on Clinical Practices for Treatment of HIV Infection: Guidelines for the use of antiretroviral agents in HIV-infected adults and adolescents, http://www.hivatis.org.
*Some experts would observe patients with CD4+ counts of 350-500/mm^3 and HIV RNA levels <10,000 (bDNA) or <20,000 (RT-PCR).

Box 32-4. Risks and Benefits of Antiretroviral Therapy in Asymptomatic HIV-infected Patients

Possible Benefits

Control of viral replication and mutation with reduction of viral burden
Prevention of progressive immunodeficiency; potential preservation or restoration of normal immune system
Delayed progression to AIDS and prolonged survival
Decreased risk of selection of resistant virus
Decreased risk of drug toxicity
Possible decreased risk of viral transmission

Potential Risks

Reduction in quality of life from adverse drug effects and inconvenience of maximally suppressive regimens
Earlier development of drug resistance
Transmission of drug-resistant virus
Limited choices of antiretroviral drugs in future because of development of resistance
Unknown long-term toxicity of antiretroviral agents
Unknown duration of effectiveness of current antiretroviral treatments

From DHHS Panel on Clinical Practices for Treatment of HIV Infection: Guidelines for the use of antiretroviral agents in HIV-infected adults and adolescents, http://www.hivatis.org.

increases in CD4 count, along with favorable clinical outcome. Regimens that have been compared directly with other regimens are emphasized. Additional consideration is given to the regimen's pill burden, dosing frequency, food requirements, convenience, toxicity, and drug interaction profile. Because of the rapidly evolving and complex nature of antiretroviral therapies, HIV clinical expert advice is necessary to determine the appropriate regimen for most patients.[8]

Nucleoside Analog Reverse Transcriptase Inhibitors. The NRTIs bind to viral DNA and inhibit HIV reverse transcriptase, the enzyme essential for transcribing RNA into DNA. Six NRTIs are currently licensed for use: zidovudine (AZT, ZDV, Retrovir), didanosine (ddI, Videx), zalcitabine (ddC, Hivid), stavudine (d4T, Zerit), lamivudine (3TC, Epivir), and abacavir (ABC, Ziagen) (Table 32-7).[8] Serious potential adverse effects are bone marrow suppression from zidovudine; fatal and nonfatal pancreatitis with didanosine alone or in combination with other drugs, particularly stavudine and hydroxyurea; and severe hypersensitivity reaction from abacavir, which could cause death if abacavir is restarted after discontinuance.

Nonnucleoside Reverse Transcriptase Inhibitors. Similar to the NRTIs, the NNRTIs inhibit HIV reverse transcriptase, but by a different noncompetitive mechanism. The NNRTIs directly bind to the reverse transcriptase and prevent effective transcriptional activity. The three NNRTIs currently available are nevirapine (NVP, Viramune), delavirdine (DLV, Rescriptor), and efavirenz (EFV, DMP 266, Sustiva). Based on in vitro and in vivo data, efavirenz may be the most potent of the three, and recent evidence suggests efavirenz plus two NRTIs is as effective as PI plus NRTI regimens (Table 32-8).[8] Rash is most common with nevirapine. Efavirenz is unique in the class with regard to its potential for CNS symptoms, such as lightheadedness, abnormal dreams, impaired concentration, agitation, hallucinations, and euphoria. Cross-resistance is great among the three NNRTIs.

Protease Inhibitors. Inhibition of HIV protease stops effective production of infectious virions. HIV protease cleaves protein precursors that eventually comprise the core proteins and enzymes of mature virions. Thus, even if a virion buds through the host cell membrane, the particle will be incapable of infecting new cells. Five PIs are licensed for use: saquinavir (Invirase, Fortovase), indinavir (Crixivan), ritonavir (Norvir), nelfinavir (Viracept), and amprenavir (Agenerase). Their effects have been dramatic when used in combination with NRTIs. The limitations to their use have been the development of resistance, drug-specific intolerance, and more recently the link with some unique potential metabolic adverse effects, including lipid abnormalities, fat redistribution, and hyperglycemia (Table 32-9).[8] Dual-PI combinations often are used as part of an aggressive initial regimen and in salvage therapy. Substantial cross-resistance occurs among the PIs.

Table 32-6. Recommended Antiretroviral Agents for Initial Treatment of Established HIV Infection

Recommendation	Column A	Column B
Strongly recommended: one choice each from columns A and B	Efavirenz Indinavir Nelfinavir Ritonavir + Saquinavir [soft gel capsule (SGC) or hard gel capsule (HGC)]	Stavudine + lamivudine Stavudine + didanosine Zidovudine + lamivudine Zidovudine + didanosine
Recommended as alternative: one choice each from columns A and B	Abacavir Amprenavir Delavirdine Nelfinavir + saquinavir SGC Nevirapine Ritonavir Saquinavir SGC	Didanosine + lamivudine Zidovudine + zalcitabine
Not recommended	Saquinavir HGC	Stavudine + zidovudine Zalcitabine + lamivudine Zalcitabine + stavudine Zalcitabine + didanosine
Not recommended: all monotherapies, whether from column A or B	—	—
No recommendation: insufficient data	Hydroxyurea in combination with other antiretroviral drugs Ritonavir + indinavir Ritonavir + nelfinavir	

From DHHS Panel on Clinical Practices for Treatment of HIV Infection: Guidelines for the use of antiretroviral agents in HIV-infected adults and adolescents, http://www.hivatis.org.

Table 32-7. Characteristics of Nucleoside Reverse Transcriptase Inhibitors (NRTIs)

Zidovudine (AZT, ZDV, Retrovir)	Didanosine (ddI, Videx)	Zalcitabine (ddC, HIVID)	Stavudine (d4T, Zerit)	Lamivudine (3TC, Epivir)	Abacavir (ABC, Ziagen)
Dosing					
200 mg tid *or* 300 mg bid *or* with 3TC as Combivir, 1 bid	>60 kg: 200 mg bid *or* 400 mg qd <60 kg: 125 mg bid *or* 250 mg qd	0.75 mg tid	>60 kg: 40 mg bid <60 mg: 30 mg bid	150 mg bid <50 kg: 2 mg/kg bid *or* with ZDV as Combivir, 1 bid	300 mg bid
Food effect					
No significant effect	Levels decrease 55% with food. Take ½ hour before or 1 hour after meal.	No significant effect	No significant effect	No significant effect	No significant effect
Adverse effects*					
Bone marrow suppression: anemia, neutropenia Gastrointestinal intolerance Headache, insomnia Asthenia	Pancreatitis Peripheral neuropathy Nausea, diarrhea	Peripheral neuropathy Stomatitis	Peripheral neuropathy	Minimal toxicity Nausea	Hypersensitivity reaction, potentially fatal if drug reintroduced after discontinuation Fever, rash, nausea, vomiting, malaise, fatigue, loss of appetite

From DHHS Panel on Clinical Practices for Treatment of HIV Infection: Guidelines for the use of antiretroviral agents in HIV-infected adults and adolescents, http://www.hivatis.org.
tid, Three times daily; *bid,* twice daily; *qd,* daily.
*For all NRTIs, lactic acidosis with hepatic steatosis is a rare but potentially life-threatening toxicity.

Table 32-8. Characteristics of Nonnucleoside Reverse Transcriptase Inhibitors (NNRTIs)

	Nevirapine (Viramune)	Delavirdine (Rescriptor)	Efavirenz (Sustiva)
Dosing	200 mg daily for 14 days, then 200 mg twice daily	400 mg three times daily Separate dosing with ddI or antacids by 1 hour	600 mg daily at bedtime
Food effect	No significant effect	No significant effect	Avoid taking after high fat meal; levels increase by 50%.
Adverse effects	Rash Increased transaminase levels Hepatitis	Rash Increased transaminase levels Headaches	Rash Central nervous system symptoms Increased transaminase levels False-positive cannabinoid test Teratogenic in monkeys

From DHHS Panel on Clinical Practices for Treatment of HIV Infection: Guidelines for the use of antiretroviral agents in HIV-infected adults and adolescents, http://www.hivatis.org.

Table 32-9. Characteristics of Protease Inhibitors (PIs)

	Indinavir (Crixivan)	Ritonavir (Norvir)	Nelfinavir (Viracept)	Saquinavir SGC (Fortovase)	Amprenavir (Agenerase)
Dosing	800 mg q8h Separate dosing with ddI by 1 hour	2-week dose escalation to 600 mg bid Separate dosing with ddI by 2 hours	750 mg tid *or* 1250 mg bid	1200 mg tid	1200 mg bid
Food effect	Levels decrease 77%. Take 1 hour before or 2 hours after meals; may take with skim milk or low-fat meal.	Levels increase 15%. Take with food, which also may improve tolerance.	Levels increase 2-3 times. Take with meal or snack.	Levels increase sixfold. Take with large meal.	Can be taken with or without food, but avoid high-fat meal.
Adverse effects*	Nephrolithiasis GI intolerance, nausea Elevated indirect bilirubin Headache, asthenia, dizziness, rash, metallic taste, thrombocytopenia Hyperglycemia	GI intolerance, nausea, vomiting, diarrhea Paresthesias (circumoral, extremities) Hepatitis Asthenia, taste perversion Increased triglycerides, transaminases, creatine kinase, and uric acid Hyperglycemia	Diarrhea Hyperglycemia	GI intolerance, nausea, diarrhea, abdominal pain, dyspepsia Headache Elevated transaminases Hyperglycemia	GI intolerance, nausea, vomiting, diarrhea Rash Oral paresthesias Elevated liver function tests Hyperglycemia

From DHHS Panel on Clinical Practices for Treatment of HIV Infection: Guidelines for the use of antiretroviral agents in HIV-infected adults and adolescents, http://www.hivatis.org.
q8h, Every 8 hours; *bid*, twice daily; *tid*, three times daily; *GI*, gastrointestinal.
*For all PIs, fat redistribution and lipid abnormalities.

Hydroxyurea. Hydroxyurea inhibits cellular ribonucleotide reductase, leading to a lower intracellular store of deoxynucleoside triphosphates (dNTPs), thus increasing the uptake of nucleoside analogs. Hydroxyurea has been used investigationally in combination with antiretroviral agents such as didanosine and stavudine for treatment of HIV infection. Its utility has not been established because of conflicting efficacy data and potential serious toxicities, such as persistent cytopenias, hepatotoxicity, neuropathy, and teratogenic potential.

Monitoring Therapeutic Response

The impact of effective antiretroviral therapy can be detected quickly. Results of therapy are evaluated primarily with plasma HIV mRNA levels (viral load). At a minimum the HIV mRNA level is expected to decrease by 10-fold (1 log) at 8 weeks and to no detectable virus (less than 50 copies/ml) at 4 to 6 months after initiation of treatment. More than 90% of patients who eventually achieve undetectable viral loads accomplish this within 12 weeks of therapy. The CD4 count change with therapy is variable. The counts may gradually rise during a period of months to years if suppression of the viral load continues. Patients with a stable clinical course and adequate laboratory values can be monitored with viral load measurements every 3 to 4 months and CD4 counts every 3 to 6 months. Persistently detectable virus after 16 to 24 weeks of therapy and repeatedly detectable virus in a patient who previously achieved an undetectable viral load are criteria for drug failure. The recent use of "third-generation" or "ultrasensitive" viral load assays, which can detect HIV RNA to a level of 20 to 50 copies/ml, has led to the identification of a greater number of "virologic failures" at an earlier stage.

Changing Therapy

Specific criteria that suggest a need to change antiretroviral medications include the following[8]:

1. Less than a 0.5-log to 0.75-log reduction in plasma HIV RNA by 4 weeks or less than a 1-log reduction by 8 weeks
2. Failure to suppress plasma HIV RNA to undetectable levels within 4 to 6 months
3. Repeated detection of virus in plasma after initial suppression to undetectable levels, suggesting the development of resistance
4. Any reproducible significant increase, defined as threefold or greater, from the nadir of plasma HIV RNA that is not attributable to intercurrent infection, vaccination, or test methodology
5. Undetectable viremia in the patient receiving double nucleoside therapy to decrease the risk of virologic failure
6. Persistently declining $CD4^+$ T-cell numbers
7. Clinical deterioration
8. Regimen intolerance

If therapy has led to virologic suppression but the patient has intolerance or toxicity, a single drug can be substituted to replace the offending drug. When therapy requires alteration because of therapeutic failure, the regimen options are more complex but generally require changing at least two drugs. Before altering therapy, the physician must recognize that the choice of available agents is limited and that new drug regimens may reduce future treatment options. Thus it is preferable for some patients to continue a regimen that has not achieved complete viral suppression. Referral or consultation with an experienced HIV clinician is strongly encouraged when considering a change in therapy.

Regimen changes also are guided by a thorough drug treatment history and more recently by the results of drug resistance testing. *Phenotypic* resistance assays measure an HIV isolate's ability to grow in the presence of specific drugs in varying concentrations. The assays are time-consuming, labor intensive, and expensive. Currently, *genotypic* assays are more available and widely used. These assays detect drug resistance mutations that are present in the viral genes. Each mutation identified must be present in at least 20% of circulating viral particles to be detected. Thus mutations that developed in the past but are not predominant at testing may be missed. Interpretation of resistance testing results requires knowledge regarding the range of mutations that antiretroviral drugs select for and the potential of mutations for cross-resistance to other drugs. Again, an expert in HIV care should be consulted.

Drug Interactions

Many drugs should not be used with certain antiretroviral agents, and many drug interactions can occur between antiretrovirals and other drugs. All PIs are substrates and inhibitors of the hepatic cytochrome P-450 enzyme system with varying degrees of potency; for example, rifampin levels increase and PI levels decrease with coadministration, so these agents should not be used together. Other drug groups whose levels may be altered by antiretrovirals include antifungals (ketoconazole), antihistamines (astemizole, terfenadine), gastrointestinal motility agents (cisapride), oral contraceptives, anticonvulsants, psychotropics, antidepressants, antiarrhythmic agents, ergot alkaloids, analgesics, lipid-lowering agents, and methadone. Some of these drugs may alter antiretroviral drug levels as well. Certain combinations require dosing adjustments, whereas other combinations are contraindicated and should not be prescribed.

Interactions also occur between some antiretroviral agents; for example, coadministration of saquinavir and efavirenz is not recommended because levels of both drugs decrease, especially saquinavir. Higher doses of indinavir are prescribed when used concomitantly with efavirenz because of lower levels of indinavir in this combination. Because of such potential interactions, all prescription and nonprescription medications coadministered with antiretroviral drugs should be evaluated for potential interactions.[1,8]

Occupational Exposure

HCWs occupationally exposed to HIV by a needle-stick injury or other exposure should receive immediate prophylaxis, preferably within 1 hour. Postexposure prophylaxis with zidovudine may result in an 80% reduction in the risk of infection. The decision to use postexposure prophylaxis depends on the likelihood of HIV infection in the source patient and the nature of the exposure.[4]

FEMALE AND PREGNANT PATIENTS

Men constituted most cases early in the U.S. HIV epidemic, but throughout the 1990s the numbers of new cases in women increased dramatically. Between July 1998 and July 1999, 32% of new adult cases of HIV infection in the United States were women.[5] Also, the vast majority of HIV-infected women during this period (77%) were black or Hispanic. A large proportion of these women are poor and have inadequate access to health care. Although HIV infection likely progresses at similar rates in women and men, delays in the recognition of a woman's risk of HIV infection may lead to a relatively late diagnosis. Women, particularly adolescents, infected through heterosexual sex often are unaware of the HIV infection status of their male partner and do not think they are at increased risk.

The first HIV-related clinical manifestations in women often involve the reproductive tract. Nearly one third of women have an active gynecologic problem at their first HIV clinic visit, most often (1) recurrent vaginal candidiasis,

(2) severe genital HSV-2 infection, (3) cervical dysplasia and neoplasia, and (4) recurrent or severe pelvic inflammatory disease (PID). Recurrent vaginal candidiasis is the most common initial manifestation of HIV, as well as one of the most frequent opportunistic infections during HIV infection in women, which may not be recognized as HIV related. Perineal herpetic infections may be more severe and persistent with HIV infection. Women are at increased risk for cervical dysplasia from human papillomavirus. In general for this population, Pap smears are more often abnormal, cervical dysplasia more severe and extensive, and progression to invasive cancer more common, with poor response to conventional therapy. A high-grade cervical lesion on routine Pap screening should alert the physician to possible HIV infection. PID, as with many other STDs, is common in HIV-infected patients, who may have an increased rate of complications (e.g., tuboovarian abscess) and require surgical intervention more often than HIV-negative women.

The social impact of HIV infection in women has yet to be fully appreciated. No longer a problem predominantly of substance abusers, heterosexually acquired HIV infection will likely continue to expand. Many HIV-infected women are mothers, with tremendous implications for their role as primary caregiver of their families. By the early part of the millennium, millions of children worldwide will be orphaned as a result of the HIV epidemic. Child care and other family-related concerns may drive many women to obtain and comply with medical care. As the numbers continue to increase, the primary care physician needs to assume an integral role in the diagnosis, treatment, and education of women with HIV infection.

Antiretroviral Therapy

Zidovudine significantly reduces the incidence of perinatal transmission, by 66% in one study. Furthermore, combination antiretroviral therapy (HAART) further reduces the transmission rate. Pregnant women should doubly benefit from HAART: improved maternal health and prognosis and decreased risk of perinatal transmission. Besides zidovudine, however, experience with most antiretrovirals during pregnancy is limited. The physician and patient should make treatment decisions carefully, preferably with the guidance of experts in accordance with the following principles:

1. All HIV-infected pregnant women should be treated with antiretroviral therapy during pregnancy, instituted no later than the second trimester if possible. Treatment of the mother should be based on the currently accepted treatment guidelines (see earlier), taking into account the latest data on drug safety in pregnancy.
2. Zidovudine should probably be a part of any antiretroviral regimen because it has proven safety and efficacy in pregnancy.
3. The therapeutic goal should be reduction in viral load to as low a level as can be achieved, since the nadir viral load predicts durability of response for the mother and since viral load correlates with risk of perinatal transmission.
4. Consideration should be given to delaying institution of antiretroviral therapy during the first trimester (the period of organogenesis) if possible.
5. Patients on stable therapy before pregnancy should probably continue their medications; if treatment is to be discontinued, all antiviral medications should be discontinued.

Zidovudine monotherapy can be considered for patients with well-maintained CD4 counts (greater than 500/mm^3) and viral loads less than 10,000 to 20,000 copies/ml because the development of resistance to ZDV has been observed to be low. Regardless of regimen, the newborn needs to receive ZDV for the first 6 weeks of life.[8]

Modes of Delivery

Most perinatal transmissions of HIV presumably occur during delivery as the newborn is exposed to infected fluids during transit through the birth canal. Consequently, many studies have examined the influence of mode of delivery on the infection rate. A meta-analysis of multiple studies concluded that cesarean birth performed before rupture of membranes reduced vertical transmission by approximately 50%.[10] Combined with antiretroviral therapy during pregnancy, the risk of transmission is reduced to less than 5%. Elective cesarean delivery for HIV-infected women however, has some important pros and cons. First, greater morbidity is associated with cesarean than vaginal delivery. Most important, the risk of perinatal transmission with combination antiretroviral therapy is likely to be very low regardless of mode of delivery. The additional benefit from cesarean birth may not be worth the risk for many pregnant women, particularly those with greatly suppressed viral loads. Therefore pregnant women must be counseled carefully to ensure a guided, informed decision.

Breast-Feeding

Although most vertical transmission of HIV infection is thought to occur during the perinatal period, the risk of a child uninfected at birth acquiring HIV through breast milk is estimated at 14% to 29%. HIV-infected women in the developed world should be strongly discouraged from breast-feeding. In the developing world, where access to clean water may be difficult and the cost of infant formula prohibitive, decisions on the relative risks of breast-feeding vs. formula feeding are more controversial.

Antiretroviral Pregnancy Registry

Primary care physicians are encouraged to report cases of prenatal exposure to antiretroviral drugs in order to accumulate information that will help refine the approach to the pregnant HIV-infected woman. A registry has been established to track this information:

Antiretroviral Pregnancy Registry, 115 North Third Ave, Suite 306, Wilmington, NC 28401; 1-800-258-4263 (tel), 1-800-800-1052 (fax).

COMPLICATIONS

The introduction of HAART in late 1995 has resulted in major declines in mortality and in frequency of AIDS-related opportunistic infections (OIs) (see Fig. 37-4).[7] For example, results of the HIV Outpatient Study (HOPS) revealed a decline in the incidence of three major OIs—*Pneumocystis carinii* pneumonia (PCP), *Mycobacterium avium* complex disease, and CMV retinitis—from 21.9 in 1994 to 3.7 per 100 person-years by mid-1997.[13] Despite this decrease, AIDS- related complications continue to occur, primarily in three groups: (1) newly diagnosed HIV-infected patients with late-stage infection, (2) late-stage patients who are not receiving or who are poorly compliant with antiretroviral therapy, and (3) late-stage patients who are refractory to antiretroviral therapy.

When approaching the HIV-infected patient with symptoms that may suggest an acute complication, the primary care physician must consider several factors, including the state of immunodeficiency, as determined by the best characterized immune marker, the CD4 count (see Fig. 32-3). The lower the CD4 count, the higher the level of concern should be that a given symptom or set of symptoms may indicate a serious complication. The physician must also know the patient's antiviral medication history, likely adherence, length of treatment, and response to therapy. Incidence of the major AIDS-related OIs is substantially lower in patients with low or unmeasurable viral loads, particularly those patients whose CD4 counts have rebounded to or remained above 200/mm^3. Incidence of OIs is also low for patients whose viral loads have significantly decreased, even without a commensurate increase in CD4 count. In general, occurrence of OIs drops significantly within 3 to 6 months of beginning an effective antiviral regimen. The physician must know the patient's current maintenance treatment for previously diagnosed OIs, as well as medications taken for primary and secondary prophylaxis.

This section reviews the diagnosis and management of the major complications associated with HIV infection and AIDS that the primary care physician is likely to encounter. Prevention of infectious complications is addressed in the section on prophylaxis.

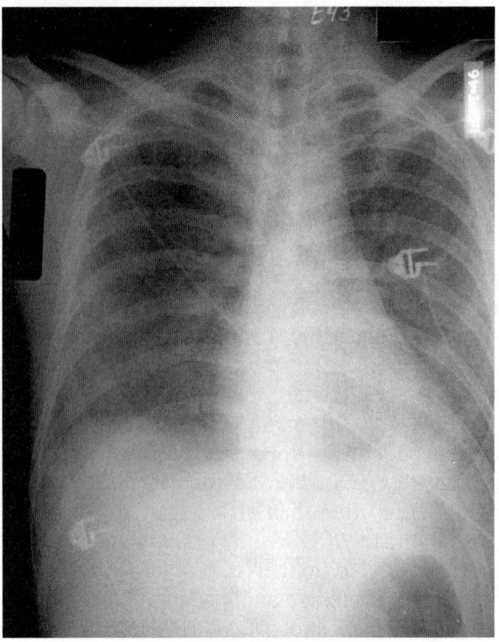

Fig. 32-6. Chest radiograph of patient with late-stage HIV infection and classic *Pneumocystis carinii* pneumonia demonstrating diffuse bilateral interstitial infiltrates.

Respiratory Tract Infections

Pneumocystis carinii *Pneumonia*. Although antiretroviral therapy and Pneumocystis prophylaxis have reduced the morbidity and mortality from PCP, it is still one of the most common OIs in AIDS patients. Disease most likely results from reactivation of latent infection acquired through the respiratory route early in life. PCP is often insidious in onset, with progression of symptoms over several weeks. The patient typically has fever, dyspnea, nonproductive cough, and chest tightness with inspiration. Fatigue and weight loss also may be present. Physical examination may reveal fever and tachypnea, but findings on chest examination are often normal. The chest radiograph typically reveals diffuse, bilateral, interstitial or alveolar infiltrates (Fig. 32-6). However, PCP also may present with focal infiltrates, consolidation, cavitary or cystic lesions, nodular densities, or a normal radiograph.

PCP is unusual in patients with a CD4 lymphocyte count less than 200 to 250/mm^3. Laboratory abnormalities are nonspecific. Although the serum lactate dehydrogenase (LDH) level is elevated in most patients with PCP, LDH elevations are also seen in other AIDS-related respiratory illnesses. Arterial blood gases (ABGs) may demonstrate hypoxemia, an elevated alveolar-arterial oxygen gradient, or respiratory alkalosis, but normal ABGs do not exclude PCP. Oxygen desaturation with exercise suggests PCP.

Because many other HIV-related conditions can mimic PCP and because therapy is prolonged and associated with significant toxicity, diagnostic confirmation is usually necessary. The initial diagnostic procedure in patients with suspected PCP is an examination of sputum induced by nebulized hypertonic saline. With proper induction techniques and appropriate monoclonal antibody stains, this test's sensitivity can exceed 90%, approaching that of bronchoscopy. When examination is negative, fiberoptic bronchoscopy should be performed. The sensitivity of bronchoalveolar lavage alone ranges from 79% to 98%, and when combined with transbronchial biopsy, the sensitivity of bronchoscopy is between 94% and 100%. Repeat bronchoscopy or open lung biopsy should be considered in patients who have had nondiagnostic bronchoscopy and who are clinically deteriorating.

A number of acceptable treatment options are available for patients with PCP. Trimethoprim-sulfamethoxazole (TMP-SMX, 15 to 20 mg/kg/day of trimethoprim), given orally or intravenously in three to four divided doses for 21 days, is effective in the treatment of *P. carinii* infection and is the drug of choice for initial therapy in most cases. Adverse reactions are common and include fever, rash, leukopenia, and hepatic dysfunction. The traditional alternative to TMP-SMX is pentamidine (4 mg/kg/day), given intravenously over 1 hour. Pentamidine also is associated with frequent adverse reactions, including renal dysfunction, hypoglycemia and hyperglycemia, hypotension, fever, and neutropenia. Intravenous administration is preferred because intramuscular administration is painful and associated with sterile abscesses.

The combination of oral trimethoprim (15 to 20 mg/kg/ day in three or four divided doses) and dapsone (100 mg/day) is an alternative to TMP-SMX and appears to be as effective and better tolerated in patients with mild to moderate PCP. Toxicities of dapsone include hemolytic anemia in patients with G6PD deficiency and rash, nausea, and methemoglobinemia.

A regimen of oral or intravenous clindamycin (1800 to 2400 mg/day in three or four divided doses) and oral primaquine (15 mg primaquine base/day) also is effective in treating PCP. Side effects include rash, diarrhea, leukopenia, and methemoglobinemia. Primaquine should be avoided in G6PD-deficient patients.

Atovaquone is approved for use in patients intolerant to

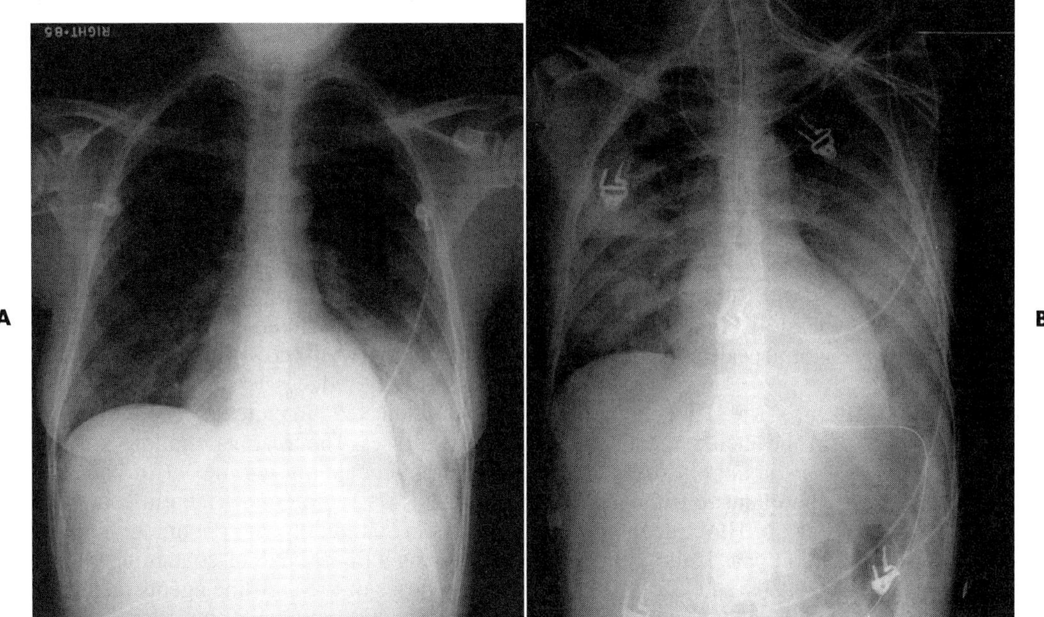

Fig. 32-7. Chest radiographs of patient with late-stage HIV infection and pneumococcal pneumonia. **A,** Left lower lobe infiltrate at presentation. **B,** Multilobar involvement 1 day later. Patient was bacteremic and expired within 48 hours of admission.

TMP-SMX. Although it is somewhat less effective than TMP-SMX, it is associated with fewer treatment-limiting adverse reactions. The recommended dose is 750 mg orally twice a day. Absorption of atovaquone is variable and improved by administering the drug with fatty foods.

Trimetrexate, a folate antagonist, is approved for use in patients with moderate-to-severe PCP failing therapy or intolerant of the first line regimens. It is given as a daily intravenous infusion of 45 mg/m^2 over 60 to 90 minutes. As with atovaquone, it is less effective but better tolerated than TMP-SMX. Patients taking trimetrexate also should be given folinic acid to minimize bone marrow toxicity. The most common adverse effects are neutropenia and thrombocytopenia.

Adjunctive corticosteroids reduce short-term mortality and respiratory deterioration in patients with moderate to severe PCP. Steroids are recommended for PCP patients with an oxygen pressure less than 70 mm Hg or an alveolar-arterial oxygen gradient greater than 35 mm Hg on room air at presentation. The recommended regimen is prednisone, 40 mg twice a day for 5 days, then 20 mg twice a day for 5 days, followed by 20 mg a day for the remaining 11 days of therapy.

Bacterial Pneumonia

Common Community-acquired Infections. The association of community-acquired pneumonia with HIV infection was recognized early in the AIDS epidemic. The most common causative organisms are *Streptococcus pneumoniae* and *Haemophilus influenzae*. IDUs are at greater risk than homosexual men, and individuals who smoke tobacco or other drugs also are at increased risk. Because profound immunosuppression is not required, pyogenic bacterial infections, including pneumonia, may be one of the earliest manifestations of HIV disease and should prompt consideration of HIV testing.

The clinical presentation of bacterial pneumonia is similar in patients with and without HIV infection. The onset of symptoms is more abrupt than with PCP, and the patient is more likely to experience a productive cough and pleuritic chest pain and to have localized findings on chest examination. A relative leukocytosis and left shift are common. Radiographic features typically include localized segmental or lobar consolidation, especially with pneumococcal pneumonia (Fig. 32-7). Radiographic manifestations of *H. influenzae* pneumonia are more variable and include diffuse bilateral infiltrates resembling PCP. Bacterial pneumonia in HIV-infected patients may be associated with a more severe course, higher incidence of multilobar involvement and bacteremia, less rapid response to antibiotics, and higher rates of mortality and recurrence.

Patients with CD4 counts less than 200/mm^3 and clinical and radiographic features of pneumonia should have bacterial cultures of blood and sputum performed. Gram's stain of the sputum is helpful in making a presumptive diagnosis, particularly when the sputum is purulent. The diagnosis of concurrent PCP is difficult when purulence is present. In the past, TMP-SMX was considered adequate as a single agent when suspected pathogens included both *P. carinii* and pyogenic bacteria; because of the increasing incidence of TMP-SMX resistance by *S. pneumoniae,* however, a β-lactam antibiotic such as cefuroxime or ceftriaxone also should be included initially. When PCP is less likely, as in a patient with a focal infiltrate or a CD4 count greater than 200/mm^3, options for empiric treatment include second- or third-generation cephalosporins or amoxicillin–clavulanic acid. If culture confirms the diagnosis of pneumococcal pneumonia, specific therapy should be adjusted according to sensitivity testing.

Other Infections. Other bacterial pathogens reported to cause pneumonia in patients with HIV infection include other streptococcal and *Haemophilus* species, *Moraxella catarrha-*

lis, and gram-negative bacilli. *Pseudomonas aeruginosa* has been described as a cause of fulminant community-acquired pneumonia, typically in patients with low CD4 counts. The frequency of pneumonia caused by *Mycoplasma pneumoniae* and *Chlamydia pneumoniae* in this patient population is largely unknown. Pneumonia caused by *Legionella* species has been described in patients with HIV infection, causing cavitation in some cases.

Nosocomial pneumonia in patients with AIDS is usually caused by gram-negative bacilli, including enteric organisms, and by *Staphylococcus aureus.* As with other hospitalized patients, risk factors include general debilitation, use of broad-spectrum antibiotics, and endotracheal intubation.

Mycobacterium tuberculosis. The HIV epidemic has resulted in a worldwide rise in the incidence of tuberculosis (TB). Because *M. tuberculosis* is more virulent than many of the other HIV-associated opportunistic pathogens, it often causes disease at an earlier stage of HIV infection and is frequently the initial manifestation, particularly in the developing world. During the late 1980s and early 1990s, new cases of TB increased in the United States, largely because of HIV infection and lapses in the public health infrastructure. Multidrug-resistant TB (MDR-TB), defined as infection with organisms resistant to at least isoniazid and rifampin, also became widespread, with major outbreaks in prisons, hospitals, and homeless shelters. By the late 1990s, with improvements in public health and infection control, the upsurge in TB cases has been significantly reduced along with TB incidence.

The natural history of TB is altered dramatically by HIV infection. In individuals with latent *M. tuberculosis* infection who acquire HIV infection, the annual rate of reactivation is 1.7% to 7.9% per 100 patient-years, a rate considerably higher than for non-HIV-infected controls. HIV-infected persons who acquire new *M. tuberculosis* infection have a high risk of developing primary TB. TB also accelerates the clinical course of HIV infection.

The clinical presentation of TB in HIV-infected patients varies depending on the degree of immunosuppression. Patients with mild to moderate depression of the CD4 count who present with reactivation TB usually have isolated pulmonary disease with typical radiographic features. In patients who develop TB at a more advanced stage of HIV infection, however, radiographic findings may be atypical or may mimic those of primary TB. Cavitary disease is unusual in these patients, and lower lobe infiltrates or miliary patterns occur frequently. Thus, for any HIV-infected patient, particularly with a low CD4 count, who presents with an undiagnosed pneumonia, TB must be considered at the initial presentation and appropriate infection control measures instituted, especially respiratory isolation. Intrathoracic adenopathy, extrapulmonary dissemination, and bacteremia also are more common in patients with advanced HIV disease.

Diagnosis of pulmonary TB is made by examination of sputum for acid-fast bacilli (AFB), followed by mycobacterial culture. The diagnostic yield of the sputum smear may be lower in patients with more advanced HIV disease. The sensitivity of smear and culture is increased by bronchoalveolar lavage. Because bacteremia occurs in many patients, blood cultures for AFB should be performed on all patients with suspected TB. A positive tuberculin skin test with intradermal PPD may provide supportive diagnostic evidence, but a negative skin test should never be used to exclude TB, since patients typically become anergic with progressive depression of cellular immunity.

Patients with AFB on smear or culture of respiratory specimens should be treated for presumed TB until the species has been identified. For drug-sensitive TB, any of the standard treatment regimens are effective, and long-term maintenance therapy or prophylaxis is unnecessary. Rates of treatment failure and relapse do not appear to be significantly higher than in patients without HIV infection. The patient's antiretroviral regimen must be taken into consideration. Rifampin, a well-known inducer of hepatic P-450 enzymes, significantly reduces levels of both NNRTIs and PIs and is contraindicated in patients receiving any of the agents in these classes. The treatment options are divided into 6-month rifampin-containing regimens (for patients not receiving PIs or NNRTIs), 6-month rifabutin-containing regimens, and 9-month streptomycin-containing regimens (for patients receiving a PI- or NNRTI-containing regimen). In general the daily doses of the first-line agents include isoniazid, 300 mg; rifampin, 600 mg (or 450 mg for patients weighing less than 50 kg); rifabutin, 150 to 450 mg; pyrazinamide, 20 to 30 mg/kg; ethambutol, 25 mg/kg; and streptomycin, 15 mg/kg.[3]

Adverse reactions to antituberculous agents occur more frequently in HIV-infected patients than in their noninfected counterparts. When initiated concurrently with antiretroviral therapy, a paradoxic response to antituberculous therapy also has been described. Patients with this syndrome develop symptoms that suggest worsening TB, including fevers, lymphadenopathy, and pleural effusions, thought to be related to improving delayed hypersensitivity response to the organism in association with recovery of T-cell function. Judicious treatment with corticosteroids has been advocated during severe reactions.

Satisfactory therapy for MDR-TB is not currently available, and the mortality from disease caused by these strains in late-stage HIV-infected patients is very high. If multidrug resistance is suspected, patients should be treated with a standard four-drug regimen consisting of isoniazid, rifampin, pyrazinamide, and ethambutol, plus at least two other agents to which local MDR-TB strains are susceptible. The regimen should be modified when susceptibility test results become available. Because of the poor response to treatment, appropriate isolation procedures for hospitalized patients must be maintained to reduce the risk of nosocomial transmission.

Atypical Mycobacteria. *Mycobacterium kansasii* is a cause of serious pulmonary disease in patients with advanced HIV disease. Although only disseminated *M. kansasii* infection is an AIDS-indicator condition, pulmonary disease appears to be the most common. The clinical manifestations of *M. kansasii* pneumonia are similar to those of pulmonary TB. Radiographic features vary considerably, but diffuse interstitial or apical infiltrates and thin-walled cavities are characteristic. Treatment with a regimen of isoniazid, rifampin, and ethambutol is usually effective.

Although *Mycobacterium avium* complex (MAC) is a common cause of disseminated infection in advanced HIV disease, it has only rarely been reported to cause isolated pulmonary disease. Although it may predict dissemination and be an indication for prophylaxis, growth of MAC from respiratory specimens without histopathologic evidence of disease is not an indication for treatment. The same is true for many other nontuberculous mycobacterial species (e.g., *haemophilum, genavense, xenopi*), although on occasion they have been associated with true pneumonia.

Fungi. Although most patients with disease from *Cryptococcus neoformans* have meningitis, it also is the most common cause of fungal pneumonia in AIDS patients. The portal of entry of *C. neoformans* is the lung, and clinically silent pulmonary infection is probably more common than overt pneumonitis. Cryptococcal pneumonia may be an indolent or rapidly progressive disease. The most common radiographic findings are focal or diffuse interstitial infiltrates; other findings include nodular or miliary infiltrates, alveolar infiltrates, mass lesions, cavitation, pleural effusion, and mediastinal adenopathy. Detection of cryptococcal antigen in the serum is a rapid and highly sensitive screening test for invasive cryptococcal disease such as meningitis, but it may be negative when disease is confined to the lungs. Definitive diagnosis of cryptococcal pneumonia requires a culture of *C. neoformans* from a respiratory specimen. Most data about the treatment of cryptococcosis come from studies of patients with meningitis. Amphotericin B is the preferred agent to be used initially, particularly for patients who are very ill or septic. Fluconazole has been used successfully for long-term maintenance or as initial therapy in more stable patients.

The filamentous fungus *Aspergillus* is an uncommon cause of pneumonia in AIDS patients. However, both invasive aspergillosis and obstructing bronchial aspergillosis have been described as late-stage complications of AIDS. *Histoplasma capsulatum* and *Coccidioides immitis* are important causes of pneumonia and disseminated disease in AIDS patients from endemic areas (see section on endemic mycoses).

Viruses. Although CMV is an important cause of retinal and gastrointestinal disease in HIV-infected patients, the isolation of CMV from pulmonary secretions usually represents infection without true pneumonitis. Patients with both *P. carinii* and CMV isolated from respiratory specimens do not appear to have a worse prognosis than patients with PCP alone. In the rare cases when CMV does cause pneumonitis, clinical features are similar to those seen in PCP: nonproductive cough, progressive dyspnea, hypoxemia, and diffuse interstitial infiltrates. The definitive diagnosis of CMV pneumonitis requires a compatible clinical picture, as well as (1) positive cultures for CMV from lung tissue or bronchoalveolar lavage, (2) the presence of typical intranuclear inclusion bodies in pulmonary tissue, and (3) the absence of other pathogenic organisms, such as *P. carinii*. Treatment options include ganciclovir, foscarnet, or cidofovir.

Varicella pneumonia may complicate both primary varicella-zoster virus (VZV) infection or disseminated secondary infection in patients with HIV infection. Patients may present with mild respiratory symptoms or may develop severe hypoxia and respiratory failure. Clinical findings may be minimal despite extremely abnormal radiographic findings. Patients should be treated with intravenous acyclovir, 10 mg/kg every 8 hours for at least 7 days.

Sinusitis. Sinusitis is extremely common in HIV-infected patients, but relatively little is known about its pathogenesis, microbiologic etiology, or treatment. Sinusitis occurs more often in patients with late-stage disease, at which time it can be recurrent and refractory to therapy. Multiple sinus involvement is the rule, with the maxillary and ethmoid sinuses most frequently involved. The bacterial pathogens most associated with sinusitis are *S. pneumoniae* and *H. influenzae*. Initial treatment of sinusitis, particularly for patients with frequent relapses, should include an antibacterial agent with activity against β-lactamase-producing *H. influenzae,* a decongestant combined with guaifenesin, and inhaled nasal steroids. For patients who fail initial antibiotic therapy, alternate antibacterial agents include clindamycin to treat anaerobes, amoxicillin/clavulanate, or a fluoroquinolone to treat *P. aeruginosa*. For patients with truly refractory disease, antral puncture for microbiologic culture may be helpful, although many such patients likely will require surgical drainage.

Neurologic Complications

The neurologic manifestations of AIDS are protean and cause significant morbidity and mortality. HIV infection affects the central, peripheral, and autonomic nervous systems and causes neuromuscular disease. In addition to the disease caused by HIV itself, the nervous system is subjected to a variety of OIs because of the depressed immune state. Drugs used to treat AIDS are frequently neurotoxic, and their use confounds the complicated clinical picture. The clinical picture, natural history, and response to treatment of many neurologic complications of HIV infection are dramatically different from the same diseases in patients without HIV infection.

Mass Lesions of Central Nervous System

Toxoplasmosis. Encephalitis caused by the obligate intracellular parasite *Toxoplasma gondii* is the most common mass lesion of the CNS in adult patients with AIDS. More than 95% of cases in the United States are caused by reactivation of latent infection in patients with AIDS and advanced immune dysfunction (CD4 count less than $100/mm^3$). In the United States, 10% to 70% of AIDS patients are latently infected (positive *Toxoplasma* IgG). Cats are the definitive host and reservoir for the oocyst form of *T. gondii;* other mammals serve as incidental hosts for the tachyzoites and cyst forms. All three forms are potentially infectious to humans, and transmission may occur by oral and congenital routes. Ingestion of undercooked meat and foods contaminated with oocysts is the most common mechanism. Reactivation of latent organisms encysted within the brain results in the multifocal, necrotic, and inflammatory abscesses characteristic of toxoplasmic encephalitis.

The clinical presentation is variable, with headache, altered mentation, seizures, and lethargy the most common symptoms. Fever, focal neurologic deficits, and abnormal level of consciousness are the most common signs. Analysis of cerebrospinal fluid (CSF) may be entirely normal or may reveal only a mild pleocytosis and elevated protein. Serum and CSF anti-*Toxoplasma* IgG antibodies are positive in more than 80% of patients. Immunoglobulin M (IgM) antibodies to *Toxoplasma* are rarely positive, as expected in a reactivated infection. Contrast computed tomography (CT) scan typically shows multiple, bilateral, ring-enhancing lesions with edema or mass effect and a predilection for the frontal lobes, basal ganglia, and corticomedullary junction. Single lesions are

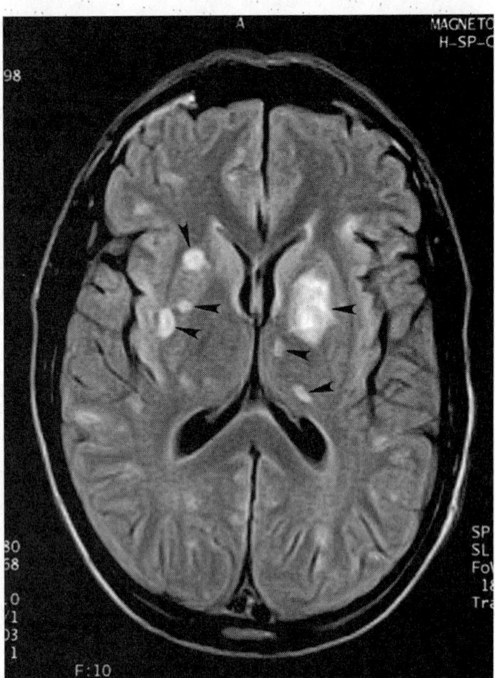

Fig. 32-8. Magnetic resonance image of patient with late-stage HIV infection and toxoplasmosis showing multiple enhancing lesions involving basal ganglia *(arrows)*. Patient had excellent response to anti-*Toxoplasma* therapy.

seen in approximately 25% and nonenhancing lesions in 5% to 10% of patients. Magnetic resonance imaging (MRI) with enhancement is more sensitive than CT (especially if the patient has a nonfocal neurologic examination) and frequently demonstrates lesions not evident on contrast CT (Fig. 32-8).

The diagnosis of toxoplasmosis is usually made presumptively with the appropriate clinical and neuroradiologic presentation. In this setting, empiric therapy is indicated. Seronegative patients with a single lesion on MRI, an atypical clinical presentation, or refractoriness to empiric therapy are candidates for a stereotactic CT-guided brain biopsy. A clinical response to therapy occurs within 2 weeks in about 85% of affected patients, whereas the radiographic response may lag over 4 to 6 weeks. Less than 5% of patients die during the initial episode of infection. Because of the high response rates to empiric therapy, failure to respond to initial therapy generally suggests another diagnosis, usually lymphoma.

Primary therapy for toxoplasmosis consists of oral pyrimethamine (200 mg loading dose followed by 50 to 100 mg/day), sulfadiazine (4 to 6 gm/day in four divided doses), and folinic acid (10 to 50 mg/day). The CBC should be monitored frequently during initial therapy because pyrimethamine may cause bone marrow toxicity. Adjunctive corticosteroids should be considered only in patients with significant edema and mass effect. Anticonvulsants may be required to control seizure activity. About 40% of AIDS patients treated with this combination manifest drug toxicity (usually rash or cytopenia) severe enough to warrant discontinuation of drug(s). Therapy with pyrimethamine and clindamycin (2700 to 3600 mg/day in three or four divided doses) seems almost as effective and is associated with less hematologic toxicity and cutaneous eruptions. Primary therapy is continued until a complete or marked clinical and radiographic improvement is achieved, usually 6 to 8 weeks. Because the currently available drugs are unable to eradicate the infection, relapse occurs routinely if therapy is withdrawn. It is uncertain whether HAART-induced immune reconstitution reduces the risk of reactivation. Therefore lifelong suppressive therapy is required using pyrimethamine (50 mg/day) and either sulfadiazine (500 mg four times a day) or clindamycin (300 to 450 mg three or four times a day).[6]

Prophylaxis in patients at risk for toxoplasmosis is discussed later. Avoidance of cat litter and undercooked meat is recommended for seronegative patients.

Primary Lymphoma. Primary CNS lymphoma is the second leading cause of CNS mass lesions in patients with AIDS. Affected patients typically have CD4 counts less than 50/mm^3. These tumors are high-grade B-cell malignancies of the non-Hodgkin's type. Focal findings may be absent in up to 50% of patients, and the radiographic appearance can be indistinguishable from toxoplasmosis. Lymphoma is more likely if a single lesion is present on MRI or located centrally at the corpus callosum. Unfortunately, none of these indicators is completely reliable, and up to 40% of patients with CNS lymphoma have multiple lesions. The diagnosis is usually made presumptively in patients seronegative for *Toxoplasma* with atypical MRI findings or unresponsive to empiric anti-*Toxoplasma* therapy. Definitive diagnosis requires brain biopsy. Cranial radiation with or without chemotherapy is standard therapy, with steroids given for edema or increased intracranial pressure. Response rates are poor, with a median survival of less than 6 months.

Progressive Multifocal Leukoencephalopathy. PML is an OI caused by a human papovavirus, JC virus. PML typically is seen in patients with CD4 counts less than 200/mm^3. Viral infection of oligodendrocytes causes progressive demyelination. There is no associated brain edema, and patients are rarely obtunded. The clinical course is subacute, with focal neurologic deficits, most often aphasia, visual field deficits, sensory loss, and ataxia. MRI is the imaging modality of choice and demonstrates single or multiple, nonenhancing, white matter lesions situated at the gray-white junction. Characteristic MRI findings combined with a slowly progressive clinical course are generally sufficient for the diagnosis, although brain biopsy for histologic examination is occasionally needed. Adequate therapy for this infection is not available. Reports are conflicting about the effectiveness of HAART in treating PML; it helps some patients and therefore should be optimized.

Meningitis

Cryptococcal Meningitis. Cryptococcal meningitis is the most common CNS infection in patients with AIDS. *C. neoformans* is an encapsulated yeast with global distribution. Infection occurs through the respiratory route, but meningitis is the most frequent clinical presentation. Because *C. neoformans* is a pathogen of relatively low virulence, profound immunosuppression (CD4 lymphocyte counts less than 50 to 100/mm^3) is required for disease to occur.

The clinical presentation of cryptococcal meningitis is often nonspecific. Patients may present with a prolonged febrile illness with or without headache. Overt signs of meningeal irritation, such as meningismus and photophobia, frequently are absent. Fortunately, the serum cryptococcal antigen test is highly sensitive for invasive cryptococcal disease. Patients with a positive test should undergo lumbar puncture to confirm the diagnosis of meningitis. The CSF cryptococcal antigen and India ink preparations are much more useful than routine CSF studies. The CSF WBC count is generally low, with a predominance of lymphocytes. The low or absent CSF pleocytosis is associated with a poor prognosis. Other poor prognosticators include a high cryptococcal antigen titer, a positive India ink test, cryptococcemia, and altered mental status at presentation. Culture of *C. neoformans* from CSF is the gold standard for the diagnosis of cryptococcal meningitis.

Treatment of choice for cryptococcal meningitis is amphotericin B, with or without 5-flucytosine (5-FC). Traditionally, amphotericin B has been given at doses of 0.7 to 1.0 mg/kg/day during the first 1 to 2 weeks, when mortality is highest. The optimal total dose is unknown. After an adequate clinical response, amphotericin B can be discontinued and fluconazole substituted at 400 mg daily for 6 to 10 weeks. The dose can then be reduced to 200 mg daily and continued lifelong.[1] As with toxoplasmosis, it is not yet clear whether immune reconstitution associated with a successful HAART regimen will obviate the need for long-term maintenance therapy.[6]

Aseptic Meningitis. A syndrome of aseptic meningitis may occur in a small percentage of patients after HIV seroconversion, representing the initial CNS response to viral invasion. Presenting features are headache and meningismus and occasionally include cranial neuropathies, encephalitis, or myelopathy. The illness is self-limited, and patients improve over several weeks. CSF analysis shows a mild lymphocytic pleocytosis and elevated protein. A second form of HIV-related aseptic meningitis occurs most often during the transition from asymptomatic to symptomatic HIV infection (CD4 count, 200 to 500/mm^3) and affects up to 60% of patients. Acute symptoms include headache, photophobia, and meningeal signs. CSF typically demonstrates mild pleocytosis and mild abnormalities of glucose and protein.

Encephalopathies and Myelopathies

AIDS Dementia Complex. Subcortical dementia caused by HIV, or AIDS dementia complex (ADC), refers to a constellation of disturbances believed to result from HIV infection of the brain. This AIDS-indicator condition is usually found in patients with late-stage infection. Approximately 90% of patients dying of AIDS have pathologic correlates of ADC at autopsy.

Cognitive impairment, altered motor performance, and abnormal behavior define the clinical triad of ADC. It is useful to divide ADC into progressive stages, from subclinical or mild involvement to severe dementia. Early symptoms reflect difficulties in memory and concentration. Patients describe a generalized "slowness" of the thought process. Routine neuropsychologic testing may be essentially normal at this time, although response times on tests of attention (serial 7s) often are delayed. With disease progression, difficulty in managing daily affairs is followed by a more general and debilitating confusion. Behavioral changes resulting in indifference and apathy are frequently misinterpreted as signs of depression. Judgment tends to be retained until the later stages, but a small number of patients may become agitated or overtly manic. On examination, subtle evidence of motor dysfunction can be detected before symptoms are obvious. Motor performance gradually deteriorates as the patient becomes clumsy, unsteady, and finally too weak to ambulate. Frontal release signs and bowel/bladder incontinence often are present in the late stages of disease. The final phase of ADC is a near-vegetative state characterized by global dementia, mutism, and paraplegia or quadriplegia, although the patient usually remains arousable.

Box 32-5. Diagnostic Criteria for AIDS Dementia Complex

Confirmed HIV seropositivity
History of progressive cognitive and behavioral decline with apathy, memory loss, and slowed mental processing
Neuropsychiatric assessment: deterioration on serial testing in at least two areas, including frontal lobe, motor, speech, and nonverbal memory
Absence of major affective disorder or active substance abuse
Absence of metabolic derangement (i.e., hypoxia, sepsis)
Absence of central nervous system opportunistic infections or neoplasms
CT/MRI: normal cranial atrophy or white matter rarefaction
CSF: negative VDRL and cryptococcal antigen

CT/MRI, Computed tomography/magnetic resonance imaging; *CSF,* cerebrospinal fluid; *VDRL,* Venereal Disease Research Laboratories.
Modified from McArthur JC: In Asbury AK, McKhann GM, McDonald WI, editors: *Diseases of the central nervous system,* Philadelphia, 1992, Saunders.

Accurate diagnosis of ADC is particularly important because of the prognostic and legal implications. Evaluation for other potentially reversible causes of dementia should include CSF analysis, VDRL, drug history, and metabolic profile. Neuroradiologic imaging also is useful to rule out other conditions and to visualize the typical (but not pathognomonic) changes consistent with brain atrophy. Neuropsychologic tests for psychomotor speed, attention, and memory are fairly sensitive for early ADC and should be monitored serially. Box 32-5 outlines the basic criteria for diagnosis of ADC.

Anecdotal evidence suggests that HAART may be beneficial in treating ADC. Zidovudine has shown clear clinical benefit long before the advent of PIs and NNRTIs and probably should be included in the antiretroviral regimen. Other CNS-penetrating antiviral agents that should be considered include stavudine, didanosine, abacavir, and nevirapine.

HIV-associated Myelopathy. Subacute vacuolar myelopathy is the most common spinal cord syndrome associated with HIV infection and closely resembles the subacute combined spinal cord degeneration of the posterior and lateral columns seen with vitamin B_{12} deficiency. The clinical presentation consists of progressive spastic paraparesis, sensory ataxia, and dementia. This condition is probably a variant form of ADC in which motor abnormalities predominate over cognitive impairment. Vitamin B_{12} deficiency, spinal cord compression, and HTLV-1 infection should be ruled out. The role of HAART in the treatment of HIV-associated myelopathy is unknown, but antiretroviral therapy should be optimized. Antispasticity agents may be palliative. Rarely, an acute myelopathy (transverse myelitis) may be caused by VZV, CMV, toxoplasmosis, or TB. Patients have rapid onset of paraparesis, bowel and bladder incontinence, and a distinct sensory level (unlike HIV-associated myelopathy) on examination.

Peripheral Neuropathies

Predominantly Sensory Neuropathy. A distal symmetric polyneuropathy caused by nerve fiber degeneration develops in as many as 30% of AIDS patients. Patients experience numbness, tingling, burning, and contact hypersensitivity involving the distal lower extremities. Physical examination reveals depressed or absent ankle jerks, loss of vibration sense, and hyperalgesia. The diagnosis is made clinically; electrophysiologic studies and nerve biopsy are rarely needed for confirmation. The differential diagnosis includes drugs, especially antiretroviral agents (e.g., didanosine, zalcitabine, stavudine), entrapment neuropathies, and vitamin B_{12} deficiency. Treatment of this often painful and occasionally debilitating condition is mainly symptomatic. Pain-modifying tricyclic antidepressants (e.g., amitriptyline, nortriptyline) in modest doses and other centrally acting analgesics (e.g., gabapentin) may be helpful. Patients with severe cases often require narcotic analgesics.

Inflammatory Demyelinating Polyneuropathies. This group of possibly immune-mediated polyneuropathies occurs in association with primary or early HIV infection. The acute form (Guillain-Barré syndrome) presents as an ascending motor paralysis with a mononuclear pleocytosis on CSF analysis. The chronic form develops over several months with a tendency for a relapsing course. Plasmapheresis is the treatment of choice.

Other Neuropathies. Less common neuropathies described in association with HIV infection include mononeuritis multiplex, entrapment syndromes, and autonomic neuropathy. *Mononeuritis multiplex* develops over days to weeks to involve several cranial, limb, and truncal nerves in a scattered distribution. The condition may progress into a chronic inflammatory demyelinating polyneuropathy, may stabilize, or may improve spontaneously. Bedridden patients are prone to entrapment neuropathies involving the ulnar and peroneal nerve compartments. Autonomic neuropathies may be present asymptomatically in AIDS patients or manifest as orthostasis, gastrointestinal dysfunction, or urinary incontinence.

Oral and Cutaneous Complications

Oral lesions are often found in HIV-infected patients. Except for the higher incidence of Kaposi's sarcoma in gay men, few differences in the prevalence of oral lesions are based on risk group, geography, or ethnic origin. Diagnosis is usually made clinically and may be confirmed with culture and biopsy.

Oral Complications

Oropharyngeal Candidiasis (Thrush). Oropharyngeal candidiasis is a common manifestation of HIV infection. It usually occurs before the development of other OIs and is predictive of progression to AIDS, independent of the CD4 lymphocyte count. The most common form, pseudomembranous candidiasis, is easily recognized as removable white plaques on the oral mucosa. Oropharyngeal candidiasis also can present in an erythematous form, with smooth red patches on the palate, buccal mucosa, or tongue; as angular cheilitis, with cracks and fissures at the corners of the mouth; and as candidal leukoplakia, with nonremovable white lesions resembling oral hairy leukoplakia (OHL). Although oropharyngeal candidiasis can be diagnosed by potassium hydroxide (KOH) preparation or fungal culture, the diagnosis usually is made clinically. Therapy with topical antifungal agents, such as clotrimazole oral tablets or nystatin solution, is preferred. Although the azole antifungal drugs are effective, they are expensive and may increase the risk of resistant candidiasis.

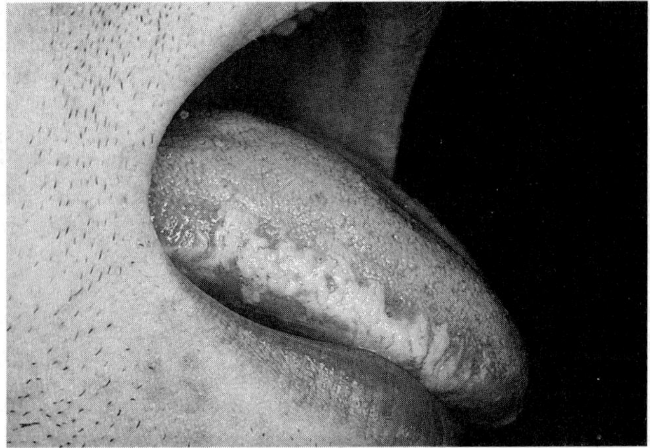

Fig. 32-9. Oral hairy leukoplakia. Note white verrucoid plaques on lateral aspect of tongue.

Oral Hairy Leukoplakia. OHL caused by the Epstein-Barr virus involves the lateral aspects of the tongue. Asymptomatic verrucous white patches that cannot be scraped off are the typical presentation (Fig. 32-9). Hairlike projections may be visualized macroscopically or microscopically. OHL is generally asymptomatic. The differential diagnosis is candidiasis (thrush), which is similar to OHL in appearance but can be diagnosed by KOH examination. Treatment with acyclovir (800 mg five times daily) is often effective for symptomatic disease, although recurrences are common.

Periodontal Disease. Periodontal disease is the most common bacterial infection of the oral cavity associated with HIV infection. The high prevalence is probably related to virally induced immunosuppression but is clearly exacerbated by the poor dental care of many HIV-infected patients. Patients with gingivitis may have the typically mild gum line erythema seen in immunocompetent individuals or a necrotizing ulcerative gingivitis in severe cases. HIV-related periodontitis is a painful condition distinguished by severe soft tissue necrosis and rapid loss of supporting bone and periodontal attachments. A necrotizing stomatitis may occur, with spread to adjoining soft tissue and intraseptal sequestration of alveolar bone. Organisms implicated in the pathogenesis of these conditions include a mixture of aerobic and anaerobic gram-negative bacteria, spirochetes, and yeast. Therapy is difficult and involves debridement of necrotic tissue, irrigation with povidone-iodine/chlorhexidine oral solutions, and antibiotics (e.g., clindamycin, metronidazole).

Aphthous Ulcers. Recurrent aphthous ulcers develop with increased frequency and severity in HIV-infected patients. Three lesions have been described: (1) "herpetiform" crops of tiny (1 to 2 mm) ulcers, (2) small (3 to 5 mm) often persistent ulcers, and (3) large (1 to 2 cm) painful ulcers that occur singly or in groups. Before initiating therapy for symptomatic lesions, it is reasonable to culture and treat empirically for herpes simplex infection. Treatment options directed at idiopathic lesions include (1) multiagent oral suspensions consisting of various concentrations of diphenhydramine, viscous lidocaine, tetracycline, and dexamethasone; (2) topical steroids; (3) systemic steroids; and (4) thalidomide. Thalidomide prescription in the United States requires physician registration and strict guidelines for use, especially in women of childbearing age.

Cutaneous Complications. Skin disease occurs in almost all patients infected with HIV. Some dermatoses are characteristic of HIV infection, whereas others simply occur more often or with atypical features when associated with HIV infection. Examination of the entire skin surface and mucous membranes is essential to making an accurate diagnosis.

Diseases Characteristic of HIV

Bacillary angiomatosis. Bacillary angiomatosis (BA) was first observed in patients with AIDS. Two species of bacilli, *Bartonella quintana* (the agent of trench fever) and *B. henselae,* have been isolated from skin lesions and are the causative agents of BA. Epidemiologic evidence suggests that both cat scratches and cat bites are strong risk factors for the development of BA.

The mechanism of disease in BA is not known. Angiomatous proliferation in skin and viscera is most common, but a spectrum of disease, including bacteremia with fever, lymphadenitis, and bone lesions, also may be present. BA typically develops over several months; tender skin lesions are the usual presentation. Other symptoms may include fevers, bone pain, focal cutaneous swelling, and abdominal pain. The typical skin manifestations are raised nodules with a friable or eroded surface and an erythematous base. The lesions can resemble pyogenic granulomas or Kaposi's sarcoma. They can appear anywhere on the skin or mucosal surfaces and number from one to hundreds. Less often a cellulitic plaque or a subcutaneous mass is the initial finding. Biopsy for histologic confirmation is essential for diagnosis. Characteristic histologic findings are usually evident with light microscopy using routine and special stains. Electron microscopy is occasionally helpful.

Erythromycin (2 gm/day) or doxycycline (100 mg twice daily) are considered the agents of choice and may result in complete resolution of BA.[1] Duration of treatment is unknown, but minimum courses of 6 to 8 weeks are generally recommended. With extensive disseminated infection, longer courses may be necessary to ensure response. An immunologic reaction similar to the Jarisch-Herxheimer reaction in syphilis can occur during the first 48 hours of treatment, and pretreatment with antipyretics should be considered.

Molluscum contagiosum. Mollusca contagiosa are caused by a poxvirus and in healthy individuals consist of small, dome-shaped papules with a central punctum or umbilication. In HIV-infected patients the lesions are usually on the face and are frequently large (1 to 2 cm) compared with those in healthy hosts (0.5 cm). The surface may be hyperkeratotic, resembling verrucae, or smooth, resembling basal cell carcinomas (Fig. 32-10). Patients usually are asymptomatic, and the goal of treatment is to correct the disfigurement. Cryotherapy and other destructive measures (e.g., curettage, excision) are effective. Periodic re-treatment is usually required because recurrence is the norm and eradication is not possible.

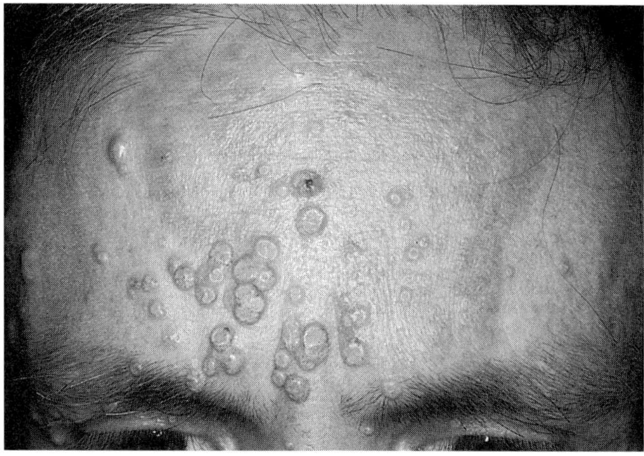

Fig. 32-10. Molluscum contagiosum may appear atypically in HIV-positive patients. Note large size, varicoid appearance, and central keratin plugging.

HIV-associated eosinophilic folliculitis. Eosinophilic folliculitis is a characteristic dermatosis of HIV infection. It consists of intensely pruritic urticarial follicular papules on the head and neck, trunk, and proximal extremities. Lesions tend to be individual and can resemble arthropod bites. Patients have significant reductions in total CD4 counts (less than 250 to 300 cells/mm^3), making the disease a marker of advanced HIV disease. Eosinophilia and elevated levels of immunoglobulin E (IgE) may be present. The differential diagnosis includes staphylococcal folliculitis, which can be excluded by culture or Gram's stain of biopsy material. Treatments include ultraviolet light (UVB) therapy, antihistamines, and topical corticosteroids. Most cases resolve gradually with treatment.

Diseases with Atypical Presentations in HIV Infection

Herpes simplex. Infection with herpes simplex virus (HSV type 1 or 2) in HIV-infected individuals usually presents with ulcerative lesions or erosions. Common sites include anogenital (Fig. 32-11), oral, and digital (Fig. 32-12) areas. Vesicles are frequently absent. Diagnosis is by culture and occasionally by skin biopsy. A hyperkeratotic papular form of chronic HSV infection is seen in patients with AIDS.

Treatment of HSV is with acyclovir (400 mg three times daily), famciclovir (250 mg three times daily), or valacyclovir (1 gm twice daily) for 7 to 10 days. Intravenous acyclovir or foscarnet may be required for refractory cases. Chronic oral, perianal, or genital ulceration secondary to HSV is often seen in patients with low CD4 counts. These ulcers are extremely painful and may be debilitating. Chronic maintenance therapy (e.g., acyclovir 400 mg twice daily) often is required to prevent recurrences once the ulcers are fully healed. Long-term foscarnet may be necessary for viral disease resistant to first-line oral agents.

Herpes zoster. Herpes zoster may be the first sign of HIV infection. It is important to assess HIV risk factors in patients with herpes zoster and to serotest those at risk. Herpes zoster usually presents in its typical form in HIV disease, although severe forms involving more than one dermatome may be seen. Recommended treatments vary and usually are based on severity. Most use oral acyclovir, famciclovir, or valacyclovir for 7 days and reserve intravenous treatment for established dissemination.

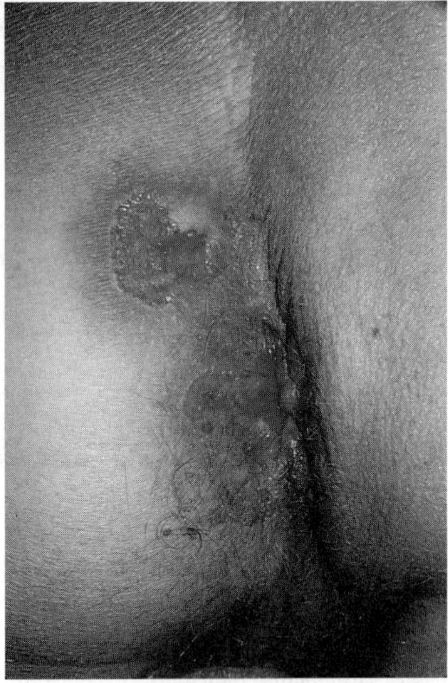

Fig. 32-11. Atypical herpes simplex in HIV-positive patient. Note deep, often chronic, erosive lesions.

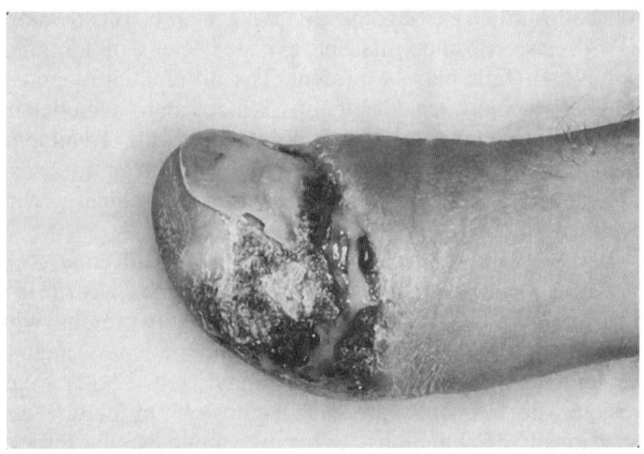

Fig. 32-12. Herpes simplex infection of thumb (herpetic whitlow). Note atypical presentation resembling bacterial cellulitis.

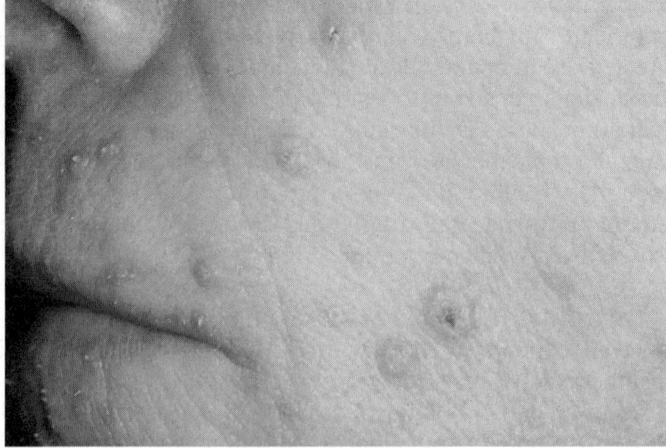

Fig. 32-13. Hyperkeratotic herpes zoster. Note papular (nonvesicular) and hyperkeratotic lesions distributed on facial dermatome.

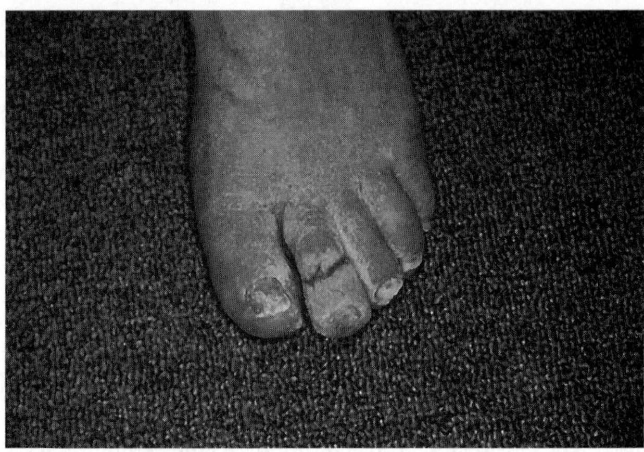

Fig. 32-14. Hyperkeratotic scabies in patient with AIDS. Note localized hyperkeratotic patch containing large numbers of mites.

Patients with advanced HIV disease may have an atypical form of herpes zoster in which persistent hyperkeratotic papules develop in a dermatomal or disseminated distribution (Fig. 32-13). These usually occur after treatment with acyclovir and are thought to be caused by the development of a thymidine kinase–negative strain resistant to acyclovir. The lesions are fixed and tend to be painful. Diagnosis of hyperkeratotic herpes zoster usually requires biopsy confirmation or culture. Treatments include prolonged use of acyclovir or foscarnet.

Scabies. In the setting of HIV disease, scabies can present in a hyperkeratotic form similar to the type described in neurologically impaired patients (Norwegian scabies). Hyperkeratotic plaques located anywhere on the body are characteristic of this form of scabies (Fig. 32-14). Pruritus is frequently less severe than with scabies in healthy individuals. The large amount of mites in the plaques makes these patients able to transmit the disease through fomites such as linens, clothing, and furniture. Diagnosis is easily made by KOH examination of skin scrapings, which demonstrates numerous mites and eggs. Patients should be treated with applications of permethrin 5% cream (Elimite) or γ-benzene hexachloride (lindane, Kwell). Repeated applications may be required. An alternative inexpensive treatment in recurrent cases is with the use of 6% precipitated sulfur in petrolatum for 12 hours, 3 days in a row, then weekly as needed. Attention to subungual areas is important because these areas can be a source of reinfestation if not adequately treated.

Diseases with Increased Frequency in HIV Infection

Seborrheic dermatitis. HIV-associated seborrheic dermatitis frequently precedes other signs of HIV infection and can be considered a possible marker of HIV infection. The cause is not known, but evidence implicates overgrowth of the yeast *Pityrosporum* as a causative factor. Typical signs are patches of erythema with scaling on the sides of the nose, central forehead, and hair-bearing areas of the scalp and beard region. In more severe cases the ears, chest, axillae, and pubic area are involved. Symptoms are usually minimal. Diagnosis usually can be made by inspection; biopsy is helpful in difficult cases. Treatment choices include medicated shampoos containing zinc, tar, or selenium sulfide, plus topical preparations containing corticosteroids or imidazole antifungal agents. Maintenance therapy is usually required.

Pruritus. Many HIV-associated skin diseases present with pruritus. Most patients with pruritus have an identifiable dermatosis (Box 32-6). Generalized pruritus without skin disease requires determination of an underlying cause.

Gastrointestinal Manifestations

Esophagitis. Odynophagia and dysphagia are the primary symptoms related to esophageal involvement in HIV-infected patients. Although candidal esophagitis is the most common etiology, other infectious and noninfectious causes are possible. Esophageal candidiasis, which requires a much greater degree of immunosuppression than oropharyngeal candidiasis, is an AIDS-indicator condition according to the CDC case definition. Patients typically have odynophagia and dysphagia and usually fewer than 200 CD4 cells/mm^3. Differential diagnosis includes CMV, HSV, and aphthous esophagitis. Because esophageal candidiasis is so common and easily treatable, diagnosis based on symptoms is appropriate, and an empiric 14-day to 21-day course of fluconazole (100 to 200 mg/day) should be initiated. Patients who do not respond to therapy should undergo upper endoscopy to rule out other causes. Patients who develop recurrent esophageal candidiasis are candidates for suppressive therapy with daily fluconazole.

Patients with herpes esophagitis often have concurrent oral ulcers. Endoscopic examination with biopsies is necessary for definitive diagnosis. Oral acyclovir (400 mg three times daily) for 7 to 14 days is effective for mild symptoms, whereas intravenous acyclovir (15 mg/kg/day) is needed for severe cases or to overcome partial viral resistance. Relapses may follow discontinuation of therapy. The presentation and endoscopic appearance of CMV esophagitis are similar to those of HSV. Intravenous ganciclovir or foscarnet for 2 to 3 weeks is effective. The need for maintenance therapy has not been established.

Intestinal Disorders. Intestinal disease is one of the most common HIV-related manifestations, with 30% to 80% of patients experiencing some form of diarrhea during their illness. The CDC defines AIDS-associated diarrhea as three or more liquid stools per day persisting for longer than 1 month. The incidence of chronic diarrhea correlates with advancing HIV infection and may lead to an AIDS-defining diagnosis. Enteric infection as a cause of diarrhea occurs in 30% to 50% of HIV-infected patients in the United States, with a higher prevalence in homosexual men, and in more than 90% of patients in developing countries. Patients with diarrhea that is predominantly related to the small bowel present with malabsorption, voluminous stools, dehydration, weight loss, and periumbilical pain. Distinguishing features of large-bowel diarrhea include small-volume stools, relatively intact absorption, lower quadrant pain, and WBCs in the stool.

Box 32-7 outlines a recommended diagnostic evaluation for AIDS-associated diarrhea. A complete evaluation is costly, ranging from several hundred dollars for stool cultures to several thousand dollars if endoscopy is needed. Specific pathogens can be identified in 40% to 60% of patients using only stool studies and in 70% to 85% when combined with aggressive endoscopy and biopsy. Multiple pathogens are present in up to 30% of patients. Several unidentified pathogens, viruses, and HIV enteropathy are likely responsible for cases in patients with a negative evaluation. Unfortunately, a treatable pathogen is identified in only 30% to 40% of evaluated patients.

Bacteria. Enteric bacterial infections are more common, severe, and prolonged in HIV-infected patients. Diagnosis is usually established by stool culture. *Salmonella* infection is 20 to 100 times more common than in the general population and is associated with a higher incidence of bacteremia and recurrence. Patients present with abdominal pain, high fever,

Box 32-6. Pruritic Dermatoses in HIV Disease

Eosinophilic folliculitis
Bacterial folliculitis
Tinea corporis
Tinea versicolor
Granuloma annulare
Insect bite reactions
Hyperkeratotic scabies
Drug reactions
Photosensitivity
Xerosis

Box 32-7. Diagnostic Evaluation of Patients with AIDS Who Have Diarrhea

Step 1

Stool cultured for *Salmonella* and *Shigella* species and *Campylobacter jejuni* at least three times and assayed for *Clostridium difficile* toxin

Stool specimens (direct, concentrated, or both) examined for parasites using saline, iodine, trichrome, and acid-fast preparations

Step 2

Gastroduodenoscopy and colonoscopy to inspect tissue and to obtain biopsy specimens and luminal material

Duodenal biopsy specimens cultured for cytomegalovirus and mycobacteria

Colonic biopsy specimens cultured for cytomegalovirus, adenovirus, mycobacteria, and herpes simplex virus

Biopsy specimens stained with hematoxylin-eosin for protozoa and viral inclusion cells, with methenamine silver or Giemsa for fungi, and with other stains for mycobacteria

Duodenal fluid specimens examined as for parasites

Step 3

Biopsy specimens examined by electron microscopy for Microsporida (duodenal tissue) and adenovirus (colonic tissue)

From Smith PD et al: *Ann Intern Med* 116:63, 1992.

and bloody or nonbloody stools. Antibiotics (e.g., ciprofloxacin, ceftriaxone) are usually required, and oral suppressive therapy may be needed after the acute episode. The presentation of *Campylobacter* gastroenteritis is similar. A quinolone or erythromycin is the preferred therapy. *Shigella* infects the large bowel and causes abdominal pain, tenesmus, fever, and bloody diarrhea. Treatment is the same as for *Salmonella*. *Clostridium difficile* may occur even without a history of recent antimicrobial therapy. Fever and profuse watery diarrhea are observed. Toxin assays of the stool are highly sensitive. Oral vancomycin or metronidazole may be less effective than in patients without HIV. Diarrhea may be a major manifestation of disseminated MAC infection. The small bowel is often involved, resulting in fever, abdominal pain, chronic diarrhea, and malabsorption. Diagnosis requires evidence of invasive disease on small-bowel biopsy. Treatment for disseminated disease involves multidrug therapy.

Protozoa. Cryptosporidiosis has historically been an AIDS-indicator condition in 2% to 4% of patients, although its incidence has declined with the introduction of HAART. Persistent large-volume diarrhea, abdominal pain, and malabsorption are typical. Fever is uncommon and symptoms may be intermittent. Diagnosis is made by modified AFB stain or by antibody testing of the stool. Treatment to date has been poor, although paromomycin (1000 mg twice daily) with or without azithromycin (500 to 600 mg/day) for the first month appears to be effective in some patients. The small intestinal parasite, *Isospora belli,* is an uncommon cause of diarrhea in U.S. patients. Diagnosis is made by visualization of the characteristic oocyst in Kinyoun-stained stool specimens. TMP-SMX is effective therapy. Microsporidians are intracellular parasites of the small bowel that are a likely (although controversial) pathogen in patients with AIDS. Diagnosis is made by electron microscopy of a small-bowel biopsy specimen. Albendazole (400 to 800 mg twice daily) has been effective in some patients. *Giardia lamblia* and *Entamoeba histolytica* are encountered infrequently, and the manifestations and response to therapy do not appear to be affected by HIV infection. Diagnosis is made by ova and parasite examination of the stool or by immunofluorescent antibody (giardiasis). Symptomatic patients are treated with metronidazole or other luminacidal agents.

Viruses. Evidence of disseminated CMV infection is demonstrated at autopsy in 90% of AIDS patients. Colonic manifestations include diarrhea, abdominal pain, and occasionally hemorrhagic ulcers. Colonoscopy shows focal inflammation with hemorrhagic plaques and ulcerations secondary to vasculitis. Therapy with foscarnet or ganciclovir is beneficial, but the relapse rate is high. Direct invasion by HIV (HIV enteropathy) may be associated with villous atrophy and malabsorption in the absence of identifiable pathogens.

Hepatitis. Liver involvement secondary to a number of opportunistic pathogens has been a well-described part of the spectrum of HIV-related complications. Although seldom the cause of substantial morbidity or mortality in the early part of the AIDS epidemic, hepatobiliary disease has become increasingly common in the HAART era. The high incidence of chronic viral hepatitis in this population, compounded by the hepatotoxic effects of antiretroviral agents, has contributed to the increasing frequency of the problem.

Intrahepatic and extrahepatic causes of biliary tract obstruction have been described in patients with AIDS. Patients generally have right upper quadrant pain, fever, increased serum alkaline phosphatase, and jaundice. Acute acalculous cholecystitis, papillary stenosis, and sclerosing cholangitis are the most common syndromes. Infection with *Cryptosporidium,* microsporidians, or CMV may be the cause of cholangitis. Diagnosis is made by nuclear scan (acalculous cholecystitis) or by endoscopic retrograde cholangiopancreatography (ERCP) (papillary stenosis, cholangitis). Urgent surgery or endoscopic improvement of biliary drainage (sphincterotomy or stent) may be required.

Parenchymal disease of the liver may be caused by infection, neoplasm, or drug effect. Disseminated TB and MAC are the most common OIs affecting the liver. Patients present with fever, hepatomegaly, elevated transaminases, and elevated alkaline phosphatase or γ-glutamyl transpeptidase. Diagnosis can be made by biopsy unless the organism can be demonstrated in blood or in other tissue. Cryptococcosis, histoplasmosis, coccidioidomycosis, CMV, and HSV infection of the liver occur rarely. Lymphoma and Kaposi's sarcoma also can involve the liver. Medications implicated as causes of liver toxicity in HIV-infected patients include many antiretroviral agents, sulfonamides, ketoconazole, isoniazid, and pentamidine. Varying degrees of transaminase elevation can be seen with drug-induced hepatic injury.

Serologic evidence of hepatitis B virus (HBV) infection can be seen in approximately 10% to 15% of HIV-infected persons, depending on the specific population studied. Although there appear to be no clinical or biochemical differences in the HIV-infected patients with acute HBV, the risk of becoming a chronic carrier is significantly increased. The impairment of cell-mediated immunity in this population seems to result in milder chronic HBV infection with less hepatocellular destruction. Unfortunately, hepatitis B viral load and infectivity increase accordingly. Vaccination of seronegative individuals to prevent this complication is able to confer immunity in only 30% to 50% of HIV-infected patients and varies with the CD4 count. Response to interferon therapy is poor.

The majority of HIV-positive individuals who acquired HIV parenterally are hepatitis C seropositive. Progression to chronic hepatitis C infection occurs in more than 50% of infected patients and carries a significant risk of cirrhosis. Exacerbation of hepatitis has been associated with the use of antiretroviral agents. Ritonavir appears to be the most hepatotoxic agent in this setting, with an incidence of severe hepatotoxicity of approximately 30%.[14] Treatment with interferon-α (3 million units three times a week) plus ribavirin (1000 to 1200 mg/day, divided twice daily) has proved the most effective therapy in non-HIV-infected patients and is probably the most effective for HIV-infected patients as well. Candidates for treatment include patients with intact immune function and evidence of fibrosis as well as those who experience hepatotoxic reactions when antiretroviral agents are instituted. Patients should be carefully screened for depression before deciding on therapy, since interferon carries the risk of severe exacerbation, including suicidal ideation.

Anorectal Disorders. Diseases involving the rectum are significantly increased in gay men. Typical symptoms include pain, discharge, ulceration, and bleeding. HSV infection and lesions related to human papillomavirus (HPV) infection (warts, squamous cell cancer) are most often encountered. Syphilis, gonorrhea, CMV, and chlamydia also may be diagnostic considerations.

An increased incidence of HPV-associated anal neoplasia is recognized in gay men with HIV infection and chronic immunodeficiency. Screening with routine anoscopy and possible anal Pap smears are recommended for high-risk men. The threshold for biopsy and follow-up examinations should be low. Treatment with electrocautery or cryotherapy is effective.

Nutrition and AIDS Wasting

Malnutrition is common in HIV-infected patients and is frequently associated with anorexia and weight loss. Primary mechanisms of malnutrition include (1) inadequate dietary intake resulting from depression, fatigue, drugs, and systemic infection, as well as from conditions affecting the CNS or gastrointestinal tract; (2) enteropathies from OIs or HIV leading to malabsorption with nutrient depletion; and (3) hypermetabolism during the late stages of HIV infection. Before HAART, AIDS wasting was a common complication of late-stage HIV infection. The syndrome is defined as a loss of at least 10% of usual body weight. Although the loss primarily is lean body mass, loss of adipose tissue also occurs, particularly for obese men. Loss of body fat is proportionally greater in women than men.

A comprehensive nutritional assessment includes evaluation of gastrointestinal function, serum albumin level, calculation of calorie intake, estimation of protein and energy requirements, and documentation of the degree of lean body mass loss. Counseling allows specific dietary deficiencies to be addressed, vitamin and mineral supplements prescribed, and high-calorie protein-containing foods to be recommended. Continued or severe malnutrition should prompt a more aggressive therapeutic approach. Evaluation for underlying conditions (e.g., hypogonadism) should be undertaken. Chronic diarrhea from a variety of etiologies may be reduced with the judicious use of antidiarrheal agents (e.g., loperamide). Treatment options for AIDS wasting include appetite stimulants for anorectic patients (dronabinol 2.5 to 5 mg/day, megestrol acetate 800 mg/day) and testosterone and its analogs for patients who are concomitantly hypogonadal. Human growth hormone has been shown beneficial in rebuilding lean body mass, but its high cost and potential side effects are significant, and decisions on its use should be made judiciously.

Hematologic Complications

The hematologic system may be affected during any stage of HIV infection. The peripheral cell lines, bone marrow, and coagulation system may be involved singly or in combination. Multifactorial etiologies include myelosuppressive drugs (e.g., ZDV, ganciclovir), direct suppression by HIV, bone marrow infiltration by infections (e.g., disseminated MAC) and neoplasms, and nutritional disorders.

Anemia occurs in more than 60% of AIDS patients. The usual pattern is a normochromic, normocytic anemia, with increased iron stores, that worsens over time. Macrocytosis is observed with ZDV therapy. Gastrointestinal bleeding, bone marrow infiltration, and drugs (e.g., AZT, dapsone) should be considered in the differential diagnosis of anemia. Treatment strategies include discontinuation of the offending agents, treatment of underlying processes, and erythropoietin (rEPO) with careful monitoring of response.

Leukopenia is found in 75% of symptomatic HIV patients and 20% of asymptomatic patients. Drug-induced neutropenia often results from ZDV, high-dose TMP-SMX, ganciclovir, interferon-α, and antineoplastic therapy. Granulocyte colony-stimulating factor (G-CSF) is effective in reversing neutropenia from a variety of HIV-related causes.

HIV-induced thrombocytopenia was recognized early in the AIDS epidemic. The mechanism appears to be an autoimmune IgG-mediated peripheral destruction of platelets that occurs early in symptomatic HIV infection (CD4 greater than 200/mm^3). Normalization of the platelet count often precedes progression to AIDS. Significant hemorrhage is rare. The CBC shows an isolated thrombocytopenia, and increased megakaryocytes are present on bone marrow studies. ZDV (as part of the antiviral regimen) can reverse the thrombocytopenia early in infection with sustained effects. Fifty percent of patients respond initially to oral prednisone, but the risks of further immunosuppression may outweigh the benefits. Despite an initial response rate of 75%, intravenous immune globulin is expensive and associated with a high incidence of relapse. Splenectomy for refractory cases may be considered.

Cardiac and Renal Complications

Cardiac disease may occur secondary to OIs or malignancies or from HIV itself. An HIV-related cardiomyopathy presumably results from direct effects of the virus or viral proteins on cardiac muscle. It is generally a complication seen in patients with low CD4 counts and in its late stages is indistinguishable from other causes of dilated cardiomyopathy.

HIV-related renal disease may develop secondary to an AIDS-related complication, as a consequence of nephrotoxic medications, or from the virus in association with injection drug use (HIV nephropathy). HIV nephropathy is a glomerular disease, typically focal sclerosing glomerulonephritis that presents with azotemia and marked proteinuria. The syndrome has a rapidly progressive course to end-stage renal disease.

Disseminated Infections

Mycobacterium avium *Complex.* MAC includes a group of related species that cause serious, disseminated infection in AIDS patients. Disseminated MAC infection occurs almost exclusively in patients with profoundly depressed CD4 counts (typically less than 50/mm^3). The organism is ubiquitous in the environment and is easily culturable in soil and water. Patients likely become infected by ingestion or inhalation of the organism, which then is engulfed by macrophages. Lacking the capacity to kill the organism, infected macrophages subsequently disseminate the organism widely to lymph nodes in the gastrointestinal tract and to the liver, spleen, and bone marrow. Patients typically present with the insidious onset of fevers, night sweats, chills, weight loss, anorexia, and diarrhea. Examination often reveals hepatosplenomegaly but is otherwise nondiagnostic. Associated laboratory abnormalities include anemia and granulocytopenia resulting from bone marrow infiltration and elevated liver enzymes, especially alkaline phosphatase. Mycobacterial blood cultures are positive in the majority of cases. The diagnosis also can be made by bone marrow biopsy or by culture and biopsy of other involved organs. Positive cultures from sputum and stool specimens may reflect colonization and have only weak predictive value for the development of disseminated disease. The organism load in tissue is typically overwhelming, in excess of 10^{10} organisms per gram of tissue. If patients are untreated, the median survival with disseminated MAC infection is 4 to 7 months.

Treatment of disseminated MAC infection has improved greatly with the introduction of the broad-spectrum, long-acting macrolide antibiotics, clarithromycin and azithromycin. Both agents have significant activity against MAC and are orally active. The use of either clarithromycin (500 mg twice daily) or azithromycin (500 mg daily) plus ethambutol (15 to 20 mg/kg/day) with or without rifabutin (300 mg/day) improves symptoms and reduces the level of bacteremia in a high proportion of patients.[6] Other agents that should be considered in severe or refractory cases are amikacin and ciprofloxacin. With the introduction of HAART the incidence of disseminated MAC infection has greatly decreased. As with TB, initiation of HAART in patients with low CD4 counts and untreated clinical or subclinical MAC infection may result in focal suppurative reactions in lymph nodes, bones, and joints. Treatment consists of drainage of the infected site(s) for symptomatic relief and continuation of antimycobacterial and antiretroviral therapy. It is not yet clear whether anti-MAC therapy can be discontinued in patients who have successfully responded to antiretroviral therapy. Small series suggest that the relapse rate is probably low.

Treponema pallidum *(Syphilis).* Transmission and pathogenesis of HIV and *T. pallidum* are intimately intertwined. As an ulcerative STD, the presence of active cutaneous or mucosal syphilitic lesions increases the efficiency of HIV transmission. In turn, the cell-mediated immunodeficiency induced by HIV appears to increase the virulence of T. pallidum.

Several features about syphilis in HIV-infected patients appear to be unique. First, the course of syphilis may be accelerated in HIV-infected patients. In particular, symptomatic CNS involvement occurs earlier and with greater frequency. Second, treatment for all stages of syphilis may need to be more intensive than what is generally accepted for normal immune hosts. Finally, the standard serologic tests used in the diagnosis may be unreliable. Therefore the primary care physician should maintain a high clinical suspicion for syphilis and a low threshold to biopsy-suspicious lesions.

The clinical presentation of syphilis in the setting of HIV infection is often similar to that observed in noninfected patients. Chancres and maculopapular rashes are common, with unusual nodular or ulcerative lesions described less often. Ocular infection can result in keratitis, retinitis, and optic neuritis. Patients may occasionally present with sensorineural hearing loss. Symptoms of neurologic disease are variable, ranging from isolated cranial nerve abnormalities to aseptic meningitis to significant behavioral changes.

Diagnosis of syphilis can be made using the standard nontreponemal serologic tests (RPR or VDRL), followed by confirmatory treponemal tests (FTA-ABS). In seronegative patients with a high clinical suspicion of active syphilis, biopsy of potential lesions should be considered. Lumbar puncture (LP) is required for all patients who have neurologic signs or symptoms, including behavioral changes or visual or auditory symptoms or signs. LP also should be considered in any patient with disease of greater than 1 year's duration, a positive RPR for longer than 1 year, or an RPR or VDRL titer that does not fall with standard treatment.

Penicillin is the agent of choice for the treatment of all forms of syphilis. For disease of less than 1 year's duration, a single intramuscular dose of benzathine penicillin G (2.4 million units) is adequate. For the treatment of disease greater than 1 year's duration in the absence of proven or likely CNS involvement, intramuscular benzathine penicillin G (2.4 million units) is given weekly for three doses. Treatment of patients with proven or suspected neurosyphilis consists of 10 to 14 days of aqueous intravenous penicillin G (12 to 24 million units/day). Symptoms and quantitative serologic titers should be followed to determine response to treatment.

Endemic Mycoses

Histoplasma capsulatum. *H. capsulatum* is an important cause of pneumonia and disseminated disease in AIDS patients living in endemic areas. In the United States the principal endemic regions are the central and south-central states. Disease results from exogenous exposure and reactivation of latent infection. The presentation is often chronic or subacute, and progressive constitutional symptoms are more common than pulmonary complaints. Isolated pulmonary disease is uncommon in patients with advanced HIV disease; the vast majority of patients present with disseminated disease. Radiographic abnormalities occur in approximately half of patients and typically consist of diffuse infiltrates, which usually are interstitial but may be reticulonodular or alveolar. Localized infiltrates occur but are less common. Mediastinal adenopathy and calcification, hallmarks of pulmonary histoplasmosis in patients with normal immune function, rarely are seen in HIV-infected patients with disseminated disease.

A septicemia-like syndrome, with hypotension, coagulopathy, and multiorgan system failure, is seen in 10% to 20% of cases. Neurologic manifestations, including encephalopathy, meningitis, and focal brain lesions, occur in 5% to 20% of patients. Patients with CNS involvement are less responsive to treatment and have a higher mortality than other patients with disseminated disease.

Histoplasmosis is diagnosed definitively by culture. Diagnostic evaluation should include fungal cultures of blood and bone marrow and of respiratory specimens in those with pulmonary manifestations. Growth of *H. capsulatum* may take 1 to 2 weeks, however, so a presumptive diagnosis must be made by histopathology or serology. Smears of peripheral blood, bone marrow, respiratory specimens, or tissue stained with periodic acid–Schiff (PAS) or Grocott-Gomori methenamine–silver nitrate may demonstrate the typical yeast forms. Biopsy of skin lesions may be especially useful in making a rapid diagnosis of disseminated histoplasmosis. Demonstration of *Histoplasma* polysaccharide antigen (HPA) in serum or urine allows for the strong presumptive diagnosis of both new infection and relapse. More widely available serologic tests for anti–*H. capsulatum* antibodies, such as immunodiffusion and complement fixation, are less sensitive and specific but may provide clues to the diagnosis.

Patients with disseminated histoplasmosis should be treated with amphotericin B (0.5 to 1.0 mg/kg) for 1 to 2 weeks, followed by itraconazole (200 mg twice daily). Itraconazole also can be used for treatment of mild to moderate histoplasmosis. As with many other OIs in patients with AIDS, histoplasmosis cannot be eradicated, and effective treatment requires lifelong maintenance. The effects of HAART on the need for lifelong maintenance therapy are unknown.

Coccidioides immitis. *C. immitis* is a soil fungus found primarily in the deserts of the U.S. Southwest. Infection is acquired through inhalation of arthroconidia, and disease usually results from reactivation of latent infection. In patients with AIDS, pulmonary involvement is the most common clinical manifestation, although disseminated or extrapulmonary disease occurs more frequently than in patients without HIV infection. In patients with early-stage HIV infection and intact cellular immunity, disease is similar to that seen in patients without HIV infection. In patients with more advanced immunosuppression, however, disease is more severe and more often disseminated or extrapulmonary. As with histoplasmosis, patients present with slowly progressive constitutional symptoms, although respiratory symptoms (e.g., dyspnea, dry or productive cough, pleuritic chest pain) occur more frequently. Radiographic findings often are much more extensive than those seen in patients without HIV infection. Diffuse interstitial or nodular infiltrates are common, although miliary infiltrates, adenopathy, and nodular and cavitary lesions have been described.

The diagnosis of coccidioidomycosis should be considered in any HIV-infected patient with pulmonary disease who has spent time in an endemic area. Although serology (tube precipitin or complement fixation) may be helpful, false-negative tests may occur, and the definitive diagnosis is made either by visualization of the coccidioidal spherule on a KOH mount of sputum or by culture. Patients should be treated with 2 to 2.5 gm of amphotericin B, followed by chronic maintenance therapy with an oral triazole agent. Fluconazole (400 mg/day) is probably the best agent; itraconazole (200 mg twice daily) also is active.

Neoplastic Complications

Non-Hodgkin's Lymphoma. Non-Hodgkin's lymphoma has been the AIDS-defining condition in 3% of U.S. cases and occurs in all risk groups. About 25% of all cases occur in patients with HIV infection. Nonprimary CNS lymphoma can occur with any CD4 count, although cases tend to predominate in patients with low counts. In contrast, primary CNS lymphoma is seen almost exclusively in patients with severely depressed counts (less than 100/mm^3). Unlike non-HIV-related cases, these lymphomas are intermediate-grade or high-grade neoplasms of the immunoblastic or small noncleaved cell type (Burkitt's or non-Burkitt's) with prominent extranodal involvement. The incidence has been shown to increase with prolonged survival in HIV, but that trend may change during the HAART era. The etiology is unclear but may be related to polyclonal B-cell stimulation and to Epstein-Barr virus coinfection in the case of primary CNS lymphoma.

Constitutional symptoms are present in 80% of patients at diagnosis, and many have extranodal disease involving the gastrointestinal tract (4% to 28%), bone marrow (21% to 33%), and liver (9% to 26%). Staging evaluation should include a body CT scan, bone marrow biopsy, and LP to rule out meningeal disease. As discussed in the section on CNS lesions, non-Hodgkin's lymphoma may be confined to the brain. Factors associated with decreased survival include bone marrow involvement, prior diagnosis of AIDS, Karnofsky score less than 70%, and primary CNS lymphoma.

Therapy is complicated by toxicity, poor bone marrow reserve, and infection. Treatment options range from low-dose combination therapy (e.g., M-BACOD) to high-dose chemotherapy with colony-stimulating factor support (e.g., MACOP-B). Multiagent regimens can achieve a complete response in 30% to 50% of patients depending on the tumor's histologic grade. Early indications are that effective HAART may reduce the frequency of relapse and prolong survival.

Kaposi's Sarcoma. Before the AIDS epidemic was recognized in 1981, Kaposi's sarcoma (KS) was observed in three forms: (1) classic KS seen on the legs of elderly men, (2) African KS seen in a variety of forms in African children and adults, and (3) KS associated with immunosuppressive therapy. The form now called *AIDS-associated KS* (AIDS-KS) was first seen in the early 1980s in homosexual men who showed other signs of immunosuppression. It was observed to be a rapidly progressive form of KS, frequently with a fatal outcome.

The etiology of KS has been related to a novel herpesvirus (HHV-8), consistent with the epidemiology of an STD. Evidence suggests that factors other than HIV may play a role in the development and growth of AIDS-KS. In recent years the proportion of patients with AIDS diagnosed with AIDS-KS has declined, possibly reflecting a change in high-risk sexual behaviors as well as the beneficial effects of HAART.

KS typically affects the oral cavity, nasal mucosa, genitalia, and feet in addition to the trunk; careful examination of these areas is important. Early lesions may start as macular areas of discoloration that enlarge to form papules, nodules, and large plaques (Figs. 32-15 and 32-16). Initially the color may be a red-brown, and as the tumor enlarges, a violaceous color becomes more prominent. Early lesions usually are asymptomatic, but extensive large areas may become ulcerated and painful, and lymphatic involvement can lead to lymphedema. Oral involvement most often affects the hard and soft palate. Histologic confirmation by skin biopsy is indicated, even when the diagnosis appears evident clinically. The pathology is usually diagnostic, although there is a wide spectrum of histologic variation. Visceral involvement with KS usually is confined to individuals with low CD4 counts. Gastrointestinal effects and

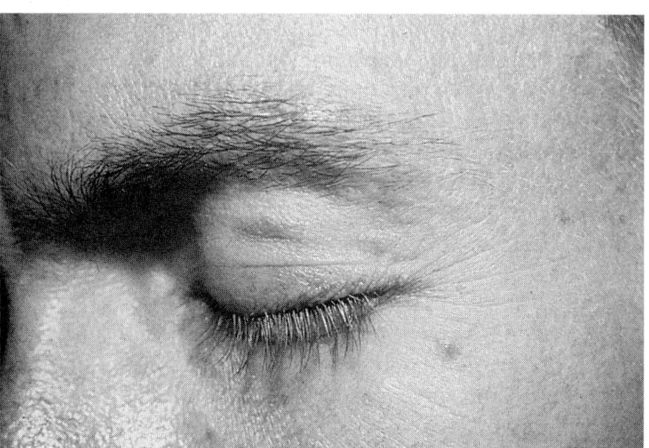

Fig. 32-15. Kaposi's sarcoma (early lesion). Note erythematous violaceous plaque on eyelid.

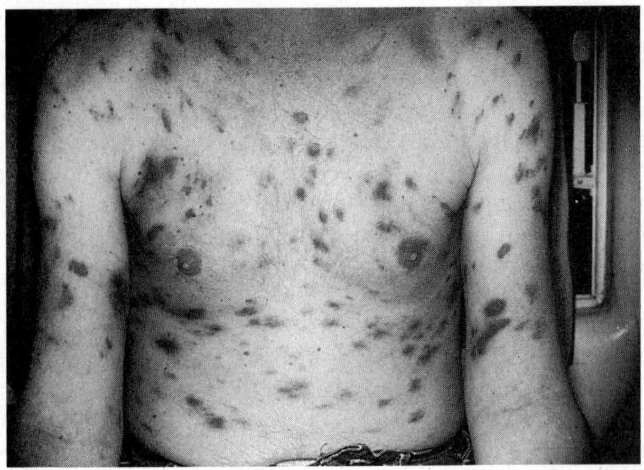

Fig. 32-16. Kaposi's sarcoma (more advanced lesions). Note widespread hemorrhagic plaques and nodules.

pulmonary involvement often occur, and the latter is associated with a particularly poor prognosis.

None of the existing treatments for AIDS-KS is curative, but several treatments for both local and widespread disease effectively reduce the extent of disease and provide palliation. The goals of therapy should be based on patient needs and may include correction of cosmetic disfigurement, size reduction of oral lesions to allow normal eating and speaking, and correction of lymphedema, pain, or symptomatic visceral involvement.

Excision, cryotherapy, intralesional chemotherapy, and radiation are all effective local treatments for KS. Liquid nitrogen-cryotherapy, although incomplete histologically, results in clinical improvement of small lesions for up to 6 months. Intralesional injection with vinblastine or vincristine provides an acceptable clinical response in more than 60% of patients. Radiation therapy is indicated in large oral lesions or cutaneous plaques not amenable to other treatments; radiation dermatitis or mucositis are common side effects. Excision successfully removes small lesions. Systemic chemotherapy may be offered to patients with aggressive cutaneous disease, symptomatic visceral disease, pulmonary involvement, or lymphedema. Response rates range from 30% to 70% with active single agents and from 45% to 88% with combination therapy.

Ophthalmologic Complications

Before HAART, as many as 80% of HIV-infected patients developed clinically apparent ophthalmic lesions. Most ophthalmologic complications fall into one of three categories: opportunistic infections, microvascular abnormalities, and neoplasms. In addition to these major categories, neuroophthalmologic signs indicative of CNS diseases also may be seen. Other complications that do not fall under these general categories include retinal vasculitis and closed-angle glaucoma.

Cytomegalovirus Retinitis. CMV retinitis from reactivation of latent virus is one of the most common AIDS-related OIs in patients with CD4 counts lower than $100/mm^3$. Symptoms of CMV retinitis can be insidious in onset, developing over several weeks. Patients complain of seeing flashes, spots, "floaters," or visual field defects. CMV retinitis develops unilaterally in most cases, although untreated it inexorably spreads to the unaffected eye. Within the retina, disease can begin either peripherally or centrally. With peripheral disease, retinal involvement may be quite extensive at presentation because patients may not notice visual symptoms until the central areas become affected.

The primary care physician must always be attentive to the retinal examination in patients with low CD4 counts. CMV retinal lesions appear as areas of fluffy exudate intermixed with hemorrhage. Disease can be recognized readily if the pupils are dilated before the funduscopic examination.

For all the available systemic agents (ganciclovir, foscarnet, cidofovir) used to treat CMV retinitis, dose adjustments must be made for renal dysfunction (Table 32-10).[15] All regimens have pros and cons and significant toxicities. Ganciclovir often causes neutropenia, especially when combined with zidovudine; blood counts should be followed closely, especially when the IV form is used. Foscarnet is well-known to cause renal dysfunction, electrolyte abnormalities, anemia, and seizures; patients should be kept well hydrated, with electrolytes, renal function, and blood counts monitored closely. Cidofovir causes neutropenia and is significantly nephrotoxic, requiring oral probenecid and IV hydration to reduce the toxicity; renal function and blood counts should be monitored.

None of the regimens provides long-term antiviral effect; in the absence of additional interventions, virtually all patients will relapse if they do not succumb to another HIV-related complication. Antiretroviral therapy is the most effective means of improving the durability of the anti-CMV response. Patients achieving good results with HAART (CD4 count greater than $100/mm^3$ with a marked viral load reduction) have a very low rate of relapse, even with discontinuation of anti-CMV maintenance therapy. It is now considered acceptable to discontinue anti-CMV therapy in patients with sustained CD4 count increases (greater than 100 to $150/mm^3$), assuming close ophthalmologic and medical follow-up.[6]

Vitritis may be caused by CMV in association with newly administered HAART. Presumably, immune reconstitution results in an acute inflammatory reaction to CMV in the vitreous, similar to the reactions seen with treatment of mycobacterial infections, as described earlier. Periocular or systemic corticosteroids have been advocated for such reactions once other OIs have been excluded.

Other Herpesvirus Infections. Herpes simplex and herpes zoster have rarely been implicated in causing retinal disease. Their more common ocular manifestations include keratitis and conjunctivitis. Herpes zoster keratitis occurs during outbreaks of disease involving the trigeminal nerve. The diagnosis should be considered for any patient who has dermatomal zoster with ophthalmic trigeminal distribution. HSV occasionally causes keratitis in this patient group. For HSV keratitis, treatment with trifluridine ophthalmic solution should be initiated. For both types of herpesvirus infection, treatment with acyclovir may ameliorate the course of disease and, particularly with HSV, prevent recurrence.

Microvascular Abnormalities. Cotton-wool spots may be the most common ocular abnormality in HIV-infected patients, most frequently in those with low CD4 counts but occurring at any stage of disease. On examination they appear similar to the cotton-wool spots seen in diabetic patients.

Table 32-10. Treatment of Cytomegalovirus (CMV) Retinitis

Regimen	Induction	Maintenance	Reinduction
IV ganciclovir	5 mg/kg q12h for 14-21 days	5 mg/kg qd	7.5 mg/kg q12h 14-21 days, then 10 mg/kg qd thereafter
IV foscarnet	90 mg/kg q12h 14-21 days	90-120 mg/kg qd	
Combination IV ganciclovir and foscarnet	*Prior ganciclovir:* ganciclovir 5 mg/kg qd plus foscarnet 90 mg/kg q12h for 14-21 days *Prior foscarnet:* ganciclovir 5 mg/kg q12h plus foscarnet 90-120 mg/kg q12h for 14-21 days	Ganciclovir 5 mg/kg qd plus foscarnet 90-120 mg/kg qd	Ganciclovir 5 mg/kg q12h plus foscarnet 90 mg/kg q12h for 14-21 days, then ganciclovir 5 mg/kg qd plus foscarnet 90-120 mg/kg qd
IV then oral ganciclovir	Same as IV ganciclovir	Oral ganciclovir 1 g tid with food	—
Intraocular ganciclovir implant	4.5 mg	Replacement every 5-8 months Concomitant oral ganciclovir 1 g tid	—
IV cidofovir	5 mg/kg weekly for 2 weeks	5 mg/kg every 2 weeks	—

From Whitley RJ, Jacobson MA, Friedberg DN, et al: *Arch Intern Med* 158:957, 1998.
IV, Intravenous; *q12h*, every 12 hours; *qd*, every day, once daily; *tid*, three times daily.

Their presence is a reflection of focal retinal ischemia. Cotton-wool spots are typically asymptomatic and require no treatment. They often resolve spontaneously even as new lesions appear elsewhere in the retina. Microaneurysms and retinal hemorrhages also are seen frequently in HIV-infected patients.

PROPHYLAXIS FOR OPPORTUNISTIC INFECTIONS

Pneumocystis carinii

From the outset of the AIDS epidemic, *P. carinii* pneumonia (PCP) was recognized as one of the most common OIs, typically affecting patients with CD4 counts less than 200 to 250/mm^3. One of the earliest therapies found to prolong survival in patients with AIDS was prophylaxis against PCP. Primary prophylaxis is indicated for all HIV-infected patients with CD4 counts less than 200/mm^3 or with thrush, regardless of CD4 count. Although most patients who develop PCP respond to treatment and survive, often without sequelae, the incidence of recurrence is high. Therefore long-term secondary prophylaxis is indicated for all patients with a history of PCP.[6]

TMP-SMX is the most effective agent for both primary and secondary prophylaxis. For patients with sulfa intolerance, several alternative regimens are available (Table 32-11).[6] The combination of dapsone and pyrimethamine offers additional prophylaxis against toxoplasmosis. Aerosolized pentamidine was widely used immediately after its approval, but its use has declined because of its relative ineffectiveness. Pentamidine remains advantageous, however, since the aerosol form avoids most of the systemic side effects. Pentamidine must be administered with a Respirgard II nebulizer. Many patients taking pentamidine also require bronchodilators.

For patients receiving primary prophylaxis who have had good response to HAART, with CD4 counts rebounding above 200/mm^3 for more than 3 to 6 months, the incidence of PCP is extremely low. PCP prophylaxis can be safely discontinued in such patients (Table 32-12).[6] For patients with prior PCP and a similarly good response to HAART, their incidence of recurrence is also low. Until sufficient data are accumulated, however, such patients should continue PCP prophylaxis.

Toxoplasma gondii

Before the HAART era, toxoplasmosis was one of the common AIDS-related complications. Since the vast majority of cases probably develop from reactivation of latent infection, and since *Toxoplasma* seroprevalence is much less common in the United States than elsewhere, the most appropriate strategy is to reserve prophylaxis for patients at highest risk for toxoplasmic encephalitis: anti-*Toxoplasma* IgG–seropositive patients with advanced HIV disease.

The physician should consider specific prophylaxis in patients with a positive anti-*Toxoplasma* IgG and a CD4 count less than 100/mm^3. Seronegative patients should be counseled on preventing infection by avoiding ingestion of undercooked meat and using proper precautions when handling cat feces. In patients already taking TMP-SMX for PCP prophylaxis, no further intervention is necessary. Patients who cannot tolerate TMP-SMX should receive the combination of dapsone and pyrimethamine with folinic acid, which also is effective in preventing PCP (see Table 32-11). *Toxoplasma* seropositivity should be considered in patients responsive to HAART who are being evaluated for discontinuation of PCP prophylaxis.[6] Limited clinical experience does not allow recommendations to discontinue primary prophylaxis for toxoplasmosis.

Mycobacterial Infections

Disseminated infection with MAC is seen as a late-stage complication when the CD4 cell count has fallen below 50/mm^3. Both azithromycin (1200 mg/week) and clarithromycin (500 mg twice daily) are effective in reducing the incidence of infection, with benefits in both morbidity and survival.[6] Rifabutin combined with azithromycin was shown

Table 32-11. Primary Prophylaxis for Opportunistic Infections in Adults and Adolescents with HIV Infection

Pathogen	Indication	First choice	Alternatives
Pneumocystis carinii	CD4 count <200/mm^3 or thrush	TMP-SMX 1 DS po qd TMP-SMX 1 SS po qd	Dapsone 50 mg po qd plus pyrimethamine 50 mg po qw plus leukovorin 25 mg po qw Dapsone 50 mg po bid or 100 mg po qd Dapsone 200 mg po plus pyrimethamine 75 mg po plus leukovorin 25 mg po qw Aerosolized pentamidine 300 mg every month Atovaquone 1500 mg po qd TMP-SMX 1 DS po three times a week
Toxoplasma gondii	Positive IgG serology and CD4 count <100/mm^3	TMP-SMX 1 DS po qd	TMP-SMX 1 SS po qd Dapsone 50 mg po qd plus pyrimethamine 50 mg po qw plus leukovorin 25 mg po qw Atovaquone 1500 mg po qd +/– pyrimethamine 25 mg po qd plus leukovorin 10 mg po qd
Mycobacterium avium complex	CD4 count <50/mm^3	Azithromycin 1200 mg po qw Clarithromycin 500 mg po bid	Rifabutin 300 mg po qd Rifabutin 300 mg po qd plus azithromycin 1200 mg po qw
Mycobacterium tuberculosis			
Isoniazid (INH) sensitive	TST reaction ≥5 mm or prior positive TST without treatment or contact with active tuberculosis	INH 300 mg plus pyridoxine 50 mg po qd for 9 months INH 900 mg plus pyridoxine 100 mg po twice weekly for 9 months RMP 600 mg plus PZA 20 mg/kg po qd for 2 months	Rifabutin 300 mg plus PZA 20 mg/kg po qd for 2 months. RMP 600 mg po qd for 4 months
Isoniazid resistant	Same as above; high probability of INH-resistant strain	RMP 600 mg plus PZA 20 mg/kg po qd for 2 months	Rifabutin 300 mg plus PZA 20 mg/kg po qd for 2 months RMP 600 mg po qd for 4 months Rifabutin 300 mg po qd for 4 months
Multidrug resistant (MDR)	Same as above; high probability of exposure to MDR strain	Consult public health authorities	None
Varicella-zoster virus (VZV)	Significant exposure to chickenpox or shingles and no history of prior VZV infection or seropositivity	VZIG, five vials (1.25 ml each) intramuscularly within 96 hours of exposure (preferably within 48 hours)	None

From Centers for Disease Control and Prevention: *MMWR* 48(RR-10):1, 1999.
TMP-SMX, Trimethoprim-sulfamethoxazole; *DS*, double-strength tablet; *SS*, single-strength tablet; *po*, orally; *qd*, everyday; *qw*, every week; *bid*, twice daily; *TST*, tuberculin skin test; *RMP*, rifampin; *PZA*, pyrazinamide; *VZIG*, varicella-zoster immune globulin.

to be even more effective but also more toxic. Currently, because of its favorable pharmacokinetics, which allow for once-weekly dosing, azithromycin has become the favored agent. Rifabutin alone is not as effective as either of the macrolides and can affect the metabolism of many common medications; it therefore should be considered an alternative agent. Prophylaxis should be started for all patients with CD4 counts below 50/mm^3. With immune reconstitution secondary to HAART, MAC incidence is sufficiently low that prophylaxis can safely be discontinued for patients whose CD4 counts rebound above 100/mm^3 and who achieve sustained antiviral suppression (see Table 32-12).[6]

HIV-infected patients with latent *M. tuberculosis* infection are at high risk for the development of reactivation TB and should be given prophylaxis regardless of age. Candidates for prophylaxis include patients with a PPD reaction of at least 5 mm of induration, a history of a positive PPD and never previously treated, or a recent history of close contact with a person with infectious TB.[6] The predictive value of anergy testing is poor in HIV-infected patients, and these tests are no longer thought to be helpful in determining the need for prophylaxis.

Isoniazid, once daily or twice weekly for 9 months, is as effective in HIV-infected persons as in nonimmunosuppressed patients (see Table 32-11).[6] The addition of pyridoxine, 50 mg daily, is recommended to reduce the

Table 32-12. Criteria for Discontinuing and Restarting Opportunistic Prophylaxis for Adults with HIV Infection

Opportunistic illness	Criteria for discontinuing prophylaxis: Primary	Criteria for discontinuing prophylaxis: Secondary	Criteria for restarting prophylaxis
Pneumocystis carinii pneumonia (PCP)	CD4 >200/mm^3 for >3-6 months	NC	Same as for initiating
Disseminated *Mycobacterium avium* complex	CD4 >100/mm^3 for >3-6 months; sustained suppression of HIV viral load	NC	Same as for initiating
Toxoplasmosis	NC	NC	NA
Cryptococcosis	NA	NC	NA
Histoplasmosis	NA	NC	NA
Coccidioidomycosis	NA	NC	NA
Cytomegalovirus (CMV) retinitis	NA	CD4 >100-150/mm^3 for >3-6 months Durable viral load suppression Non-sight-threatening lesion Adequate vision in contralateral eye Regular ophthalmologic exams	Restart maintenance when CD4 drops to <50-100/mm^3

From Centers for Disease Control and Prevention: *MMWR* 48(RR-10):1 1999.
NC, No criteria recommended for stopping; *NA*, not applicable.

incidence of peripheral neuropathy. A 2-month regimen of rifampin plus pyrazinamide is as effective as longer regimens. Because of the effects of rifampin on the metabolism of NNRTIs and PIs, however, decisions on its use should be made carefully, preferably in consultation with experts.

For patients likely infected with isoniazid-resistant strains, rifampin or rifabutin with pyrazinamide or rifampin or rifabutin alone are used for prophylaxis. HIV-infected individuals likely infected with multidrug-resistant strains have fewer options, and experts should be consulted.[6]

Viral Infections

VZV is the only virus strongly recommended as requiring primary prophylaxis.[6] HIV-infected patients without a history of clinical varicella or those who are VZV seronegative should receive varicella-zoster immune globulin (VZIG) after significant exposure to active viral infection, either varicella or shingles. VZIG preferably should be given within 48 hours of the exposure but certainly within 96 hours (see Table 32-11).

CMV is the most common cause of serious opportunistic viral disease in patients with HIV infection. Patients with CD4 count less than 50/mm^3 have a high risk of developing end-organ disease, especially retinitis. The high incidence, significant morbidity, and high cost and toxicity of therapy make CMV disease an appropriate target for prophylaxis. Oral ganciclovir (1 gm three times daily) is effective in preventing CMV disease, but its use is not recommended because of its toxicity, cost, and potential for selecting ganciclovir resistance.[6]

Fungal Infections

Although fungal infections are common complications of HIV disease, enthusiasm for routine antifungal prophylaxis has been tempered by the lack of data, the high cost of oral antifungal agents, and the potential for promotion of resistance. At present, prophylaxis for invasive fungal infections (e.g., itraconazole for histoplasmosis, fluconazole for cryptococcosis) is not routinely indicated but should be considered in special cases for patients with low CD4 counts (less than 50 to 100/mm^3) at high risk of infection.

Bacterial Infections

HIV-infected patients are at increased risk for bacterial infections with common community-acquired pathogens such as *S. pneumoniae* and *H. influenzae*. Not surprisingly, the use of TMP-SMX for PCP prophylaxis reduces the risk of bacterial infections. The pneumococcal polysaccharide vaccine is indicated for all HIV-infected adults and should be given as early as possible in the course of HIV infection. Conjugated *H. influenzae* type B vaccine is not recommended, since the incidence of type B infection is low and the vaccine's efficacy in this population has not been well established.

REFERENCES

1. Bartlett JG: *Medical management of HIV infection*, Baltimore, 1999, Johns Hopkins University Press.
2. Centers for Disease Control and Prevention: 1993 Revised classification system for HIV infection and expanded surveillance case definition for AIDS among adolescents and adults, *MMWR* 41(RR-17):1, 1992.
3. Centers for Disease Control and Prevention: Prevention and treatment of tuberculosis among patients infected with human immunodeficiency virus: principles of therapy and revised recommendations, *MMWR* 47(RR-20):1, 1998.
4. Centers for Disease Control and Prevention: Public Health Service guidelines for the management of health-care worker exposures to HIV and recommendations for postexposure prophylaxis, *MMWR* 47(RR-7):1, 1998.
5. Centers for Disease Control and Prevention: *HIV/AIDS Surv Rep* 11:1, 1999.
6. Centers for Disease Control and Prevention: 1999 USPHS/IDSA guidelines for the prevention of opportunistic infections in persons infected with human immunodeficiency virus, *MMWR* 48(RR-10):1, 1999.

7. Centers for Disease Control and Prevention: Guidelines for national human immunodeficiency virus case surveillance, including monitoring for human immunodeficiency virus infection and acquired immunodeficiency syndrome, *MMWR* 48(RR-13):1, 1999.
8. DHHS Panel on Clinical Practices for Treatment of HIV Infection: Guidelines for the use of antiretroviral agents in HIV-infected adults and adolescents, http://www.hivatis.org.
9. Fauci AS, Pantaleo G, Stanley S, Weissman D: Immunopathogenic mechanisms of HIV infection, *Ann Intern Med* 124:654, 1996.
10. International Perinatal HIV Group: The mode of delivery and the risk of vertical transmission of human immunodeficiency virus type 1, *N Engl J Med* 340:977, 1999.
11. Joint United Nations Programme on HIV/AIDS: *AIDS epidemic update,* December 1999.
12. Mellors JW, Munoz A, Giorgi JV, et al: Plasma viral load and CD4$^+$ lymphocytes as prognostic markers of HIV-1 infection, *Ann Intern Med*126:946, 1997.
13. Palella FJ, Delaney KM, Moorman AC, et al: Declining morbidity and mortality among patients with advanced human immunodeficiency virus infection, *N Engl J Med* 338:853, 1998.
14. Sulkowski MS, Thomas DL, Chaisson RE, Moore RD: Hepatotoxicity associated with antiretroviral therapy in adults infected with human immunodeficiency virus and the role of hepatitis C or B virus infection, *JAMA* 283:74, 2000.
15. Whitley RJ, Jacobson MA, Friedberg DN, et al: Guidelines for the treatment of cytomegalovirus diseases in patients with AIDS in the era of potent antiretroviral therapy, *Arch Intern Med* 158:957, 1998.

CHAPTER 33

Common Cold

Thomas A. O'Bryan
Nirmal Joshi

The term *common cold* generally refers to self-limited viral illnesses causing acute inflammation in the nasopharynx, resulting in typical symptoms of rhinorrhea, sore throat, coughing, and sneezing. In the United States the common cold is the leading cause of physician visits and a major reason for work and school absenteeism. Treatment of colds is often frustrating to both patient and physician. Almost $2 billion is spent each year for over-the-counter products to remedy cold symptoms. Use of home-based and alternative therapy may be increasing. Primary care physicians frequently feel pressure from patient expectations to inappropriately prescribe antibiotics. Health care providers should be prepared to provide education to patients with cold symptoms to dispel common misconceptions, provide realistic expectations, and discuss publicized treatment claims. This chapter reviews current concepts in epidemiology, pathogenesis, clinical characteristics, and evidence-based treatment of this all-too-familiar malady.

EPIDEMIOLOGY

Prevalence and Environmental Factors

The common cold is not a single clinical entity but rather a group of diseases with overlapping symptoms caused mainly by several families of viruses (Box 33-1). *Rhinovirus* is the most common pathogen associated with the common cold, accounting for 30% to 40% of colds in most population studies. *Coronavirus* is another important etiologic agent, causing an estimated 10% of common colds. Less is known about this organism due to lack of culture and diagnostic techniques. About 25% to 40% of colds are presumably caused by undiscovered viruses. In addition to many viral pathogens, multiple distinct immunotypes of specific viruses exist, such as the more than 100 known antigenic types of rhinovirus. Furthermore, reinfection, particularly with coronavirus, is known to occur. For these reasons the "cure for the common cold" remains unrealistic.

Box 33-1. Viruses Identified with Common Cold

Rhinovirus
Coronavirus
Respiratory syncytial virus
Parainfluenza virus
Influenza virus
Adenovirus
Enteroviruses

Colds occur worldwide. In temperate climates, illnesses from respiratory viruses are present throughout the year but peak in the cooler months. The seasonal nature may be related to increased indoor crowding and low relative humidity favored by some viruses. Certain viruses follow a seasonal pattern. Rhinovirus infections peak in the early fall and late spring, whereas coronavirus infections are more common during the winter months. Psychologic stress has been implicated as predisposing to cold symptoms. Cold temperature, damp environments, and presence or absence of tonsils do not appear to be independent risk factors in the development of colds (Box 33-2).[3-7,9,12,15,16]

Colds are most common in early childhood but occur throughout life. One study reported a frequency of six acute respiratory illnesses per year in children under age 3, with boys having a higher rate than girls.[23] Infection rates generally fell with increasing age, but increased somewhat in young adult females, most likely because of exposure to young children. Adults experienced a mean of two to three respiratory illnesses per year, declining to about 1.3 per year after age 60.

Young children are the main reservoir for respiratory viruses. Among adults, colds occur more frequently in those with children in the home. Colds are most often transmitted in the home, school, or day care. Studies suggest children in day-care facilities have a higher rate of respiratory illnesses during ages up to 36 months.[16] The incidence may be lower in later years for children who remain in day care from infancy through the preschool years.

Transmission

Our understanding of the transmission of the common cold is incomplete. Most knowledge of spread is based on experimental data of rhinovirus. The extent to which this information is applicable to the natural environment or to other etiologic agents of the common cold is unclear.

Rhinovirus appears to require close contact for transmission. In a study of married childless couples in whom

Box 33-2. Epidemiologic Factors Associated with Common Cold Viral Infection

Strong Association

Seasonality
Close contact with infected individuals
Close contact with young children
Hand-to-hand transmission
Self-inoculation into nose or eye
Contaminated objects
Day-care facilities

Weaker Association

Transmission by aerosols
Transmission by kissing
Psychologic stress

No Association

Exposure to cold environment
Tonsillectomy

one partner was experimentally infected with rhinovirus, transmission occurred in 38% of susceptible spouses.[5] Volunteer studies have demonstrated a linear relationship between transmission rate to susceptible individuals and donor-hours of exposure (number of infected donors times hours of confinement). Of recipients, 44% were infected after 150 donor-hours of exposure. None of five recipients was infected after 45 donor-hours of exposure. Similarly, brief contact (3 to 36 hours) with infected persons resulted in a transmission rate of less than 10%.[4,22]

Experimental data suggest that direct contact with infectious secretions is the likely means of transmission in most rhinovirus infections. Viral transfer occurred in a majority of exposures after 10 seconds of hand contact with infected individuals.[12] Rhinovirus has been recovered on 40% of hands but less than 10% of cough or sneeze samples from persons with colds. Virus has been shown to survive on hands and environmental surfaces for several hours. Experimental infections have been acquired by hand contact with contaminated objects such as coffee cup handles and plastic tiles.[11] Furthermore, cold transmission in the home setting was significantly reduced when individuals with natural colds treated their hands with a virucidal solution, implying the importance of hand contact in the spread of natural colds.[14]

The risk of infection clearly depends on the site of inoculation. The amount of viral inoculum needed for a 50% infection rate is about 8000-fold less by the nasal mucosa route than by the oral route. Prolonged kissing has been shown to be an inefficient means of rhinoviral spread, with a transmission rate of 8% in one study.[4] Most symptomatic subjects do not have detectable virus in their saliva. Inoculation into the conjunctiva, however, results in transmission rates similar to the nasal mucosa.[14] Rather than infecting conjunctival tissue, the virus presumably passes down the tear duct into the nasal mucosa.

Thus the accumulated data support the hypothesis that most common colds under natural conditions spread from hand-to-hand contact, followed by autoinoculation into the nasal mucosa or eye. Observational studies suggest that children and adults place themselves at risk for autoinoculation into their eyes or nose from their fingers several times a day.[15]

Experimental rhinoviral transmission by aerosols has been demonstrated[6] but appears to be a less efficient means of transmission.[6] The extent to which this occurs in the natural setting is not known. Finally, viral pathogens other than rhinovirus may behave differently. For example, influenza and adenovirus seem to spread by small-particle aerosols.

PATHOGENESIS

As with our knowledge of transmission of common colds, most information on the pathogenesis comes from experimental studies of rhinovirus infection in volunteers. After intranasal inoculation, the rhinovirus gains entry into host cells by binding to intercellular adhesion molecule 1 (ICAM-1). Infection appears to begin in the posterior nasopharynx, progressing anteriorly to the turbinates 1 or 2 days later. Predominantly cilial epithelial cells are infected, although nonciliated cells may also be involved. Interestingly, biopsies of the nasal mucosa during experimental infection reveal focal infection of relatively few cells. Examination of specimens of the nasal epithelium by light or electron microscopy reveals no consistent lesions.[29] Thus cytotoxicity does not appear to be a major component of rhinovirus upper respiratory infection.

Recent evidence suggests that chemical mediators play an important role in the pathogenesis of the common cold. The interleukins IL-1, IL-6, and IL-8 have been demonstrated in the nasal secretions of symptomatic subjects within 24 hours of experimental rhinovirus inoculation.[24,27,30] The concentrations of these proteins appear to correlate with severity and duration of symptoms. Polymorphonuclear neutrophil leukocytes (PMNs), kinins, and albumin are also found in nasal lavage specimens of subjects with rhinovirus infections. As with interleukins, their concentrations seem to match the time course and degree of symptoms. The interrelationships among these mediators and their role in the disease process are unclear. The interleukins are potent chemoattractants for PMNs. IL-1 may increase the responsiveness of some cells to bradykinin and may increase vascular permeability, resulting in a transudate of increased albumin and kinin in the nasal passage. Intranasal challenges with bradykinin, IL-8, and certain prostaglandins have each produced rhinorrhea in normal volunteers. Corticosteroids, pentoxyfylline, and a bradykinin antagonist have failed to alleviate common cold symptoms. Further understanding of the role of mediators will require the availability of specific inhibitors.

Neutralizing antibody in serum is present 2 to 3 weeks after infection, although nonspecific immunoglobulins may be found in nasal secretions within a few days. Symptomatic individuals with experimental rhinovirus infection have demonstrated peripheral increases in PMNs and decreases in T lymphocytes. Increased PMN and T-lymphocyte concentrations are seen in the nasal mucosa and nasal secretions.[18,19] These leukocyte migrations likely reflect the release of cytokines and suggest that the cellular immune response plays a role in rhinoviral pathogenesis. Other observations imply that the host's neurologic response, particularly cholinergic and α-adrenergic pathways, may also play a role in the development of rhinorrhea during rhinovirus colds.

CLINICAL MANIFESTATIONS

The typical clinical manifestations of the common cold are well known and are most frequently associated with infections from rhinoviruses and coronaviruses. Most individuals infected with rhinovirus become symptomatic. Rhinovirus infections typically present after an incubation period of 1 to 4 days. Symptoms usually begin with rhinorrhea and sneezing accompanied by nasal congestion. Sore throat is often present and may be the initial complaint. Significant systemic symptoms, such as headache and malaise, are relatively mild, and fever is usually absent. In most patients the illness resolves spontaneously without significant adverse consequences in 5 to 9 days (mean 7.4 days). In about 25% of patients, symptoms may last up to 2 weeks. Children may develop lower respiratory infection. Persistent cough has been noted, particularly in smokers. Also, rhinovirus infection may acutely exacerbate respiratory symptoms in patients with chronic obstructive lung disease.

The clinical manifestations of coronavirus infection are similar, with the exception of a slightly longer incubation period and a slightly shorter duration of illness (mean 6 to 7 days). In some studies the amount of nasal discharge in patients with common colds from coronaviruses is greater than in those from rhinoviruses. The prevalence of coronavirus infection is particularly high in late fall, winter, and early spring, when rhinovirus infections are somewhat less common.

Symptoms caused by other viruses may overlap those from the common cold but usually have clinically distinguishing features. Influenza virus, for example, is typically associated with marked constitutional symptoms, such as headache, myalgias, fever, and malaise. Infections from respiratory syncytial virus and parainfluenza virus are particularly prevalent in children and tend to cause lower respiratory tract illness.

DIAGNOSIS

The diagnosis of the common cold is made almost exclusively on clinical grounds. The typical constellation of symptoms, including rhinorrhea, sore throat, cough, and low-grade fever, in the absence of severe constitutional symptoms is usually sufficient. A more important issue to the physician may be to consider coexisting or complicating conditions that may require specific therapy, such as streptococcal pharyngitis or sinusitis. In the patient with pharyngeal exudate and fever, definitive diagnosis of a bacterial etiology is difficult on clinical grounds alone, and a throat culture or rapid antigen testing is usually required.

TREATMENT

Several medications have been used, primarily directed at symptoms of the common cold. Consistently effective therapy directed toward the causative organism is still lacking. Unfortunately, clinical studies on treatment are difficult to perform and interpret because of the highly subjective and variable reports of symptoms.

Antihistamines and Anticholinergic Agents

Luks and Anderson[20] reviewed clinical studies on antihistamines for the common cold, including terfenadine, chlorpheniramine, astemizole, and clemastine. The outcome measures included total symptom scores and nasal symptoms (sneezing and nasal discharge). Although some studies showed a statistically significant improvement in specific nasal symptoms, no study was able to demonstrate a statistically significant ($p < 0.05$) improvement in total symptom scores. In addition, the authors noted several flaws in study design and also questioned the *clinical* significance of the modest improvement in symptoms. They concluded that little data supported the use of antihistamines in the treatment of the common cold. An earlier review, however, reported that the antihistamine chlorpheniramine and the anticholinergic agents atropine and ipratropium improved nasal symptoms in adults with common cold. More recently, the antihistamine clemastine was found to improve sneezing and rhinorrhea.[28] Again, it is difficult to quantify the clinical significance of this finding. Also, sedation was noted in 14% of clemastine recipients.

Terfenadine (no longer commercially available), a second-generation, nonsedating, selective H_1-receptor antihistamine, is ineffective in the treatment of symptoms of common cold. Although loratadine inhibits histamine-induced expression of ICAM-1 in cultured respiratory epithelial cells in vitro, the results of clinical efficacy trials are currently not available. In one study, the anticholinergic nasal spray ipratropium bromide was used at a dose of two sprays three times daily in each nostril. Compared with controls, rhinorrhea and sneezing were reduced by 30% in the treatment group. Patient assessment of overall effectiveness of treatment was more favorable for ipratropium than for control spray. Nasal dryness was noted as a side effect in 12% of ipratropium recipients.[13]

Decongestants

Through the sympathomimetic effect, decongestants result in vasoconstriction of the nasal mucosa, reducing discharge and blockage. Smith and Feldman[25] reviewed studies using these agents. Oral pseudoephedrine resulted in a substantial decrease in nasal symptoms, including congestion and sneezing. Oxymetazoline and phenylpropanolamine improved nasal patency and symptom scores. At least one study, however, reported medication side effects in 30% of recipients, including tachycardia, palpitations, and elevated blood pressure. Smith and Feldman's review also reported the lack of efficacy of expectorants such as guaifenesin.

Antiinflammatory Agents

A placebo-controlled trial using sodium chromoglycate nasal spray for acute respiratory illness of undefined primary etiology showed improvement in cough and voice disturbances in the treatment group.[1] A related compound, nedocromil sodium, reduced colds' severity and nasal mucous secretion in experimental rhinovirus infection.[2] These agents, in addition to preventing the release of inflammatory mediators from mast cells, may also affect neurogenic reflexes, which may contribute to cold symptoms.

Oral corticosteroids have not been found to be beneficial in the treatment of the common cold. Since prostaglandins can induce some symptoms of common colds when administered intranasally to healthy subjects, nonsteroidal antiinflammatory drugs (NSAIDs) have been tried clinically. In experimental rhinovirus-induced colds, early treatment with naproxen was effective in reducing headache, malaise, myalgia, and cough.[26] Aspirin and acetaminophen have been found to impair antibody response and increase symptoms of nasal congestion and discharge; no effect on viral shedding was noted.[8]

Other Agents

The use of *zinc* in the form of lozenges has been extensively studied recently. Of 11 double-blind, placebo-controlled trials, five reported benefit and six did not, and several flaws were highlighted for each study.[21] For studies reporting benefit, inadequate blinding remains a concern because of the distinctive taste of zinc lozenges. For those studies reporting no benefit, certain formulations may result in inactivation of zinc salts before absorption. A meta-analysis of available studies concluded that there is insufficient evidence of zinc's efficacy in reducing the duration of common colds.[17] Clearly, better studies are needed to ensure adequate blinding and intake of adequate doses of bioavailable zinc and to make more definite clinical recommendations.

Encouraging initial results have been reported with specific antiviral therapy using *interferon-α* as prophylaxis against rhinovirus infection. Combination therapy using this agent with ipratropium and naproxen within 24 hours of experimental rhinovirus infection may be useful in reducing symptoms and viral shedding. Cost and potential toxicity will likely limit the use of such therapy.[10]

REFERENCES

1. Aberg N, Aberg B, Alestig K: The effect of inhaled and intranasal sodium chromoglycate on symptoms of upper respiratory tract infections, *Clin Exp Allergy* 26:1045, 1996.
2. Barrow GI, Higgins PG, Al-Nakib W, et al: The effect of intranasal nedochromil sodium on viral upper respiratory tract infections in human volunteers, *Clin Exp Allergy* 20:45, 1990.
3. Cohen S, Tyrrell DAJ, Smith AP: Psychological stress and susceptibility to the common cold, *N Engl J Med* 325:606, 1991.
4. D'Alessio DJ, Meschievitz CK, Peterson JA, et al: Short-duration exposure and the transmission of rhinoviral colds, *J Infect Dis* 150:189, 1984.
5. D'Alessio DJ, Peterson JA, Dick CR, et al: Transmission of experimental rhinovirus colds in volunteer married couples, *J Infect Dis* 133:28, 1976.
6. Dick EC, Jennings LC, Mink KA, et al: Aerosol transmission of rhinovirus colds, *J Infect Dis* 156:442, 1987.
7. Douglas RG, Lindgren KM, Couch RB: Exposure to cold environment and rhinovirus common cold: failure to demonstrate effect, *N Engl J Med* 279:742, 1968.
8. Graham NMH, Burrel CJ, Douglas RA, et al: Adverse effects of aspirin, acetaminophen and ibuprofen on immune function, viral shedding and clinical status in rhinovirus-infected volunteers, *J Infect Dis* 62:1277, 1990.
9. Gwaltney JM Jr: The common cold. In *Principles and practice of infectious diseases*, ed 4, New York, 1995, Churchill Livingstone.
10. Gwaltney JM Jr: Combined antiviral and antimediator treatment of rhinovirus colds, *J infect Dis* 166:776, 1992.
11. Gwaltney JM Jr, Hendley JO: Transmission of experimental rhinovirus infection by contaminated surfaces, *Am J Epidemiol* 116:828, 1982.
12. Gwaltney JM Jr, Moskalski PB, Hendley JO: Hand-to-hand transmission of rhinovirus colds, *Ann Intern Med* 88:463, 1978.
13. Hayden FG, Diamond L, Wood PB, et al: Effectiveness and safety of intranasal ipratropium bromide in common colds: a randomized, double-blind, placebo-controlled trial, *Ann Intern Med* 125:89, 1996.
14. Hendley JO, Gwaltney JM Jr: Mechanism of transmission of rhinovirus infections, *Epidemiol Rev* 10:242, 1988.
15. Hendley JO, Wenzel RP, Gwaltney JM Jr: Transmission of rhinovirus colds by self-inoculation, *N Engl J Med* 288:1361, 1973.
16. Hurwitz ES, Gunn WJ, Pinsky PF, et al: Risk of respiratory illness associated with day-care attendance: a nationwide study, *Pediatrics* 87:62, 1991.
17. Jackson JL, Peterson C, Lesko E: A meta-analysis of zinc salt lozenges and the common cold, *Arch Intern Med* 157:2373, 1997.
18. Levandowski RA, Ou DW, Jackson GG: Acute-phase decrease of T lymphocyte subsets in rhinovirus infection, *J Infect Dis* 153:743, 1986.
19. Levandowski RA, Weaver CW, Jackson GG: Nasal-secretion leukocyte populations determined by flow cytometry during acute rhinovirus infection, *J Med Virol* 25:423, 1988.
20. Luks D, Anderson MR: Antihistamines and the common cold: a review and critique of the literature, *J Gen Intern Med* 11:240, 1996.
21. Macknin ML: Zinc lozenges for the common cold, *Cleveland Clin J Med* 66:27, 1999.
22. Meschievitz CK, Schultz SB, Dick EC: A model for obtaining predictable natural transmission of rhinoviruses in human volunteers, *J Infect Dis* 150:195, 1984.
23. Monto AS: Studies of the community and family: acute respiratory illness and infection, *Epidemiol Rev* 16:351, 1994.
24. Proud D, Gwaltney JM Jr, Hendley JO, et al: Increased levels of interleukin-1 are detected in nasal secretions of volunteers during experimental rhinovirus colds, *J Infect Dis* 169:1007, 1994.
25. Smith MB, Feldman W: Over-the-counter cold medications: a critical review of clinical trials between 1950 and 1991, *JAMA* 269:2258, 1993.
26. Sperber SJ, Hendley JO, Hayden FG, et al: Effects of naproxen on experimental rhinovirus colds: a randomized, double-blind, controlled trial, *Ann Intern Med* 117:37, 1992.
27. Turner RB, Weingand KW, Yeh C: Association between interleukin-8 concentration in nasal secretions and severity of symptoms of experimental rhinovirus colds, *Clin Infect Dis* 26:840, 1998.
28. Turner RB, Sperber SJ, Sorrentino JV, et al: Effectiveness of clemastine fumarate for treatment of rhinorrhea and sneezing associated with the common cold, *Clin Infect Dis* 25:824, 1997.
29. Winther B: Effects on the nasal mucosa of upper respiratory viruses (common cold), *Dan Med Bull* 41:193, 1994.
30. Zhu Z, Tang W, Anuradha R, et al: Rhinovirus stimulation of interleukin-6 in vivo and in vitro: evidence for nuclear factor κB-dependent transcriptional activation, *J Clin Invest* 97:421, 1996.

PART TWO

Disease State Management by Organ System

I Women's Health

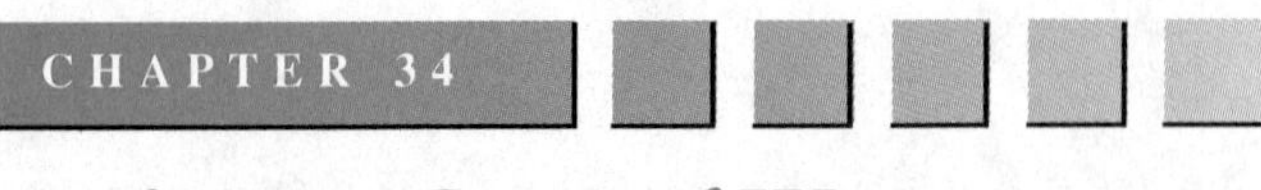

Primary Care of Women

Janet B. Henrich

Over the past decade, women's health has emerged as a rapidly expanding field of scientific inquiry and knowledge with important implications for clinical practice and for the education and training of physicians. The increasing scientific information about the influence of gender differences on health and disease has expanded our concept of women's health beyond the traditional focus on reproductive organs and their function. Women's health can be viewed broadly as the study of the effect of sex and gender on health and disease that occurs across the spectrum of the biologic, behavioral, and social sciences. This broader interdisciplinary perspective of women's health has created an area of new knowledge and scholarship that is distinct from or more detailed than the knowledge base of existing disciplines. It has provided a new model to study the interactions among biologic mechanisms and psychosocial and environmental factors, as well as their influence on human growth and development and on women's response to health challenges. The clinical application of this information to women across all age groups highlights the interdisciplinary nature of this field.

BASIC PRINCIPLES

The concept of women's health requires a reassessment of the importance of gender differences on health and disease. Complex interactions exist among sex hormones, normal and abnormal physiology, and the physical and emotional well-being of women. As early as the embryonic period, there are structural differences between female and male brains. Many of these differences are programmed during fetal life by hormones. During the reproductive years the influence of sex hormones on sexual development and reproductive function differentiates a category of health issues that are unique to women. As women age and sex hormones decrease during the menopause, women's risk factors for disease change dramatically and become more similar to men's risks. Although women develop the diseases that affect men, biologic mechanisms and psychosocial factors influence the course of disease differently in women.

Until recently, most of the information used to make clinical decisions in women was based on studies conducted primarily in men. Women were excluded from research on diseases that are important to both sexes because of misconceptions about women's health, legal and ethical issues, and cultural biases. Because women, on average, live longer than men and are affected by major diseases at a later age, it was often perceived incorrectly that women were healthier than men. In fact, throughout life, women experience poorer health than men, especially in the advanced years. The lack of information concerning women had important implications. Information based primarily on studies done in men was often applied inappropriately to women or resulted in different standards of care.

Efforts to increase our knowledge about women's health issues require an integrated approach that acknowledges the diversity among women and considers the social factors that influence their lives. One of the important social trends over the past 50 years has been the increasing participation of women in the work force. Since World War II the number of women who work has more than doubled and now exceeds 80%. The full effects of multiple roles, work stress, and new environmental exposures on women's health and reproductive status are largely unknown but are certain to have important health and social ramifications. Paralleling the growing numbers of women in the work force is the increasing number of single-parent families headed by women, especially minority women. Many of these families live in poverty. Increasing evidence indicates that socioeconomic factors are major indicators of health and that, for some health outcomes, poverty and lack of education are more important determinants of health than ethnicity. However, important ethnic and racial differences remain in women's susceptibility and response to certain diseases that cannot be explained completely by socioeconomic status. For example, mortality rates for coronary heart disease, stroke, and breast cancer are higher in black than in white women, whereas death rates from lung cancer are higher in white women.

The increasing diversity of the population will affect health trends in the United States and the health status of women specifically. Regardless of their minority group, ethnic minority women have a lower life expectancy than white women and experience greater health problems. These differences are most pronounced in areas related to reproductive issues and childbearing, the occurrence and course of chronic disease, the incidence and outcome of cancer, and acts of interpersonal violence. Along with changes in society, human immunodeficiency virus (HIV) infection and homelessness have recently become additional special health concerns of minority women.

One of the most important factors underlying the current interest in women's health is the increasing number of women entering the health professions, especially medicine. Since the early 1900s the proportion of women represented in the physician population increased threefold, from 6% to 17%. According to projections, this proportion will increase to 30% early in this century. Already, women represent more than 40% of entering medical students and 50% of minority graduates from medical schools. Although significant barriers remain to their attaining equal professional and academic status, the potential for women to influence the structure of their profession, the delivery of health care, and the direction of medical research is considerable.

MORBIDITY AND MORTALITY

At the turn of the twentieth century the average life span of women in the United States was 48 years, compared with 46 years in men. Life expectancy is now 79 years for women and 73 years for men. Because of the gender gap in life expectancy, women currently constitute almost two thirds of the population over age 65 and three fourths of the population over age 85. The fastest growing age group in the United States is the population aged 85 years and older. As a result, it is estimated that women outnumber men by 2:1 in the age groups over 65 and 3:1 in the population over 85. The reasons for the dramatic increase in overall life expectancy are thought to be related to the control of infectious diseases and progress in the treatment of chronic diseases such as diabetes and cardiovascular disease. The reasons for the disparity in life expectancy between women and men are less well established but are thought to be primarily biologic.

Table 34-1 shows the leading causes of death in women of all ages and races. Despite a dramatic decline in mortality rates for heart disease in both sexes over the past two decades, *cardiovascular disease* remains the leading cause of death for women and accounts for one third of all deaths in women. Heart disease occurs about 10 years later in women than in men. This delayed onset is thought to result primarily from the protective effect of estrogens in premenopausal women and accounts for 90% of heart disease mortality in women occurring after the menopause. Significant racial and ethnic differences are associated with mortality among women. Black women are more likely to die from heart disease than white women up to age 75; thereafter, death rates are higher in white women. In contrast, Hispanic and Native American women have significantly lower rates of death from heart disease. Evidence suggests that heart disease, once it develops, is more serious in women than in men, resulting in higher mortality rates. In addition to biologic factors, the poorer survival of women may result from the older age and increased prevalence of comorbid conditions in women at diagnosis, as well as less well-defined social factors that influence the diagnosis and treatment of heart disease in women.

Cancer is the second leading cause of death in women and is the most common cause of premature death. The mortality rate for all cancers combined in women has changed little during the last part of the twentieth century. Major advances in the diagnosis and treatment of cervical and uterine cancers in women have been offset by increased mortality rates for lung and breast cancer. Although breast cancer is still the most common cancer diagnosed in women, *lung cancer* is now the leading cause of cancer deaths. Unfortunately, most of these deaths can be attributed to cigarette smoking. Whereas deaths from lung cancer in men have begun to decline because of a decrease in male cigarette use, death rates for women increased between 1990 and 1995 and probably will continue to rise.

Breast cancer is the second leading cause of cancer deaths in women. Although the incidence of breast cancer has risen over the past decade, mortality rates have remained relatively stable. This disparity is thought to be caused partly by the widespread use of screening mammography and the detection of earlier-stage cancers that have a more favorable prognosis. Significant age and racial differences are associated with breast cancer mortality. Declining mortality rates in younger women have been offset by an increase in older women. Although breast cancer incidence rates are 12% lower in black than in white women, mortality rates are 15% higher in black women. Reasons for racial differences in breast cancer incidence and mortality are unclear but may be related to socioeconomic and biologic factors as well as certain health behaviors, such as participation in screening mammography. Although breast cancer screening with mammography and clinical breast examination decrease mortality from breast cancer in women over age 50 by approximately 30%, less than 50% of American women 50 years and older receive regular screening, and this figure is considerably lower in poor, minority, and elderly women.

Table 34-1. Age-adjusted Mortality Rates From Leading Causes of Death in U.S. Females, 1995

Cause of death	Rate (per 100,000 population)	Percent of total deaths
All causes	847.3	100.0
Cardiovascular disease	278.8	32.9
Malignant neoplasms (cancer)	191.0	22.5
Cerebrovascular disease (stroke)	71.7	8.5
Chronic lung (pulmonary) disease	36.4	4.3
Pneumonia/influenza	33.6	4.0
Diabetes	24.6	2.9
Accidents and adverse effects	23.7	2.8
Alzheimer's disease	10.1	1.2
All other causes	177.2	20.9

From Anderson RN, Kochanek KD, Murphy SL: Report of final mortality statistics, 1995, *Mon Vital Stat Rep* 45(11, suppl 2), 1997.

Although stroke-related deaths have declined by almost 60% in the United States over the past 25 years, deaths from *stroke (cerebrovascular disease)* still account for approximately 6% of all deaths in women and rank third as a cause of mortality. Striking racial differences exist in stroke mortality: death rates in black women are almost twice those for white women. Most stroke deaths in women result from thromboembolic disease and occur in older women. However, subarachnoid hemorrhage, the least common form of stroke, is more common in women than in men and contributes to stroke mortality, particularly in younger women.

Death rates from *chronic pulmonary diseases* have increased steadily for both women and men during the past 25 years, but with a greater increase in women. Because this increase has been linked to patterns in cigarette smoking, death rates in women for pulmonary disease, as well as for lung cancer, will probably continue to rise. Death rates from pneumonia and influenza closely parallel pulmonary-related deaths and vary over time based on the epidemiology of these acute illnesses.

Diabetes has consistently ranked as a leading cause of death in women. Moreover, the reported death rate from diabetes most likely underestimates the impact of this disease on mortality because of its strong association with other life-threatening medical conditions, such as cardiovascular disease, stroke, and kidney failure. It is estimated that diabetes affects one in six women over age 45; however, prevalence rates are higher in black, Hispanic, and Native American women. Separate from disease-related death rates, diabetes is a significant cause of morbidity and, in women of childbearing age, has important adverse effects on pregnancy outcome, resulting in an increased risk of fetal and perinatal mortality as well as congenital malformations.

Although *HIV infection* is not one of the 10 leading causes of death in women overall, it is responsible for the largest percent increase in death rates of all the major causes of mortality. HIV-related mortality rates are nine times higher for black than for white women. As a result, HIV infection ranks third in leading causes of death in black women ages 15 to 24 and first in the age group 25 to 44 and, in some geographic areas, has become the number-one cause of death. As the epidemiology of this epidemic changes, with heterosexual transmission accounting for an increasing proportion of HIV infection in women, these rates are expected to continue to rise.

Mortality rates alone do not provide a complete picture of women's health status. Although women live longer than men, overall measures of health status are worse in women (Table 34-2). Based on estimates from the National Health Interview Survey (NHIS), more women than men report symptoms or seek care for acute medical conditions, such as respiratory and digestive disorders, and are more disabled by these self-limited illnesses, as measured by number of bed days or days lost from work. In addition, several chronic conditions occur more frequently in women and cause significant disability, such as arthritis, thyroid disease, migraine, bladder disorders, gastritis, colitis, and chronic constipation. Data from other sources show that affective disorders, especially major depressive episodes, and the anxiety disorders are significantly more prevalent in women. Most importantly, women have a lower perception of their health status than men. According to estimates from the NHIS, only 36% of women describe their health as excellent, compared with 41% of men.

Table 34-2. Selected Age-adjusted Indicators of Health Status and Medical Care Utilization, 1991

Indicator	Female	Male	Female/male
Physician contacts (per person)	6.6	4.9	1.3
Acute conditions (per 100 persons)	204.7	178.1	1.2
Restricted activity days (per person)	8.2	6.4	1.3
Work loss days (per person age 18 or older)	3.7	2.8	1.3
Hospitalization (excluding births)	5.4%	4.8%	1.1
Excellent health (self-report)	35.8%	41.4%	0.9

From *Current estimates from the National Health Interview Survey, 1991,* DHHS Pub No (PHS) 93-1512, 1992, Centers for Disease Control, National Center for Health Statistics.

LIFE SPAN GROUPS

Many of the important health issues in women have their onset or greatest impact at certain ages and are intricately linked with women's psychosocial and sexual development. To develop a more integrated concept of women's health, it is instructive to look at the important health issues in women within the major life span groups. Several governmental and institutional sources were used to compile this information. Of these, the themes developed by the *Report of the National Institutes of Health: Opportunities for Research on Women's Health,* known as the Hunt Valley Report, form the basis of this section.

Birth to Young Adulthood

As young women reach puberty, health issues are related primarily to developmental changes involving physical and sexual growth and changing relationships within and outside the family. Central to the psychosocial development of young women is the process of gender identification and orientation and the development of self-esteem. Intentional and unintentional injuries, including increasingly frequent acts of physical and sexual violence, are the primary cause of death and disability in young women and account for half of all deaths in this age group. A small proportion of girls develop a chronic disease or disability. Most of these conditions are related to autoimmune disorders, such as lupus erythematosus, juvenile rheumatoid arthritis, and thyroid disease. Because of hormonal influences, many of these conditions first occur or are exacerbated during puberty.

Ages 15 to 44 Years

During young adulthood, mortality rates in women are relatively low, and deaths from injury predominate. As women progress through this age group, cancers of the breast and reproductive tract emerge as the leading cause of death, followed by unintentional injury and heart disease. Among the unintentional and intentional injuries in this age group, motor vehicle accidents, homicide, and suicide account for three fourths of all injury deaths. The death rate from motor vehicle accidents is highest in women ages 15 to 24; more than half these deaths are alcohol related. A major tragedy in the United States is the rapidly increasing death rate from homicide and suicide in young women. Black women, similar to black men, are most likely to be homicide victims, and firearms are used in more than half these deaths. Because 30% of murders in women are perpetrated by a family member or acquaintance, the contribution of ongoing family violence to these fatal events is probably substantial.

The most dramatic trend in this age group has been the emergence and rapid rise of *HIV infection* as a major cause of death. Poor and minority women have experienced the greatest increase in death rates from this disease. The biologic and social aspects of HIV infection are difficult to separate; however, evidence suggests that HIV infection in women may have a different presentation and clinical course and worse prognosis than in men. The consequences of this disease for gynecologic care and reproductive counseling in women are unique. Because of the potential interrelationship among HIV disease, human papillomavirus infection, and cervical neoplasia, as well as recent questions about the accuracy of the Papanicolaou (Pap) test in women with HIV disease, the Centers for Disease Control and Prevention (CDC) recommends that HIV-infected women have a Pap smear annually. As a result of HIV transmission during pregnancy, HIV infection is the fourth leading cause of death among black children. The social consequences of this disease are enormous and result in loss of productive life, disruption of family structure, and premature death. The challenge to primary care physicians to help control the transmission of HIV infection is an essential part of national prevention efforts.

An important role of physicians in the care of young women is to recognize and reduce risk taking and other unhealthy behaviors. Health habits become established during early adulthood. Unhealthy behaviors not only place women at risk for life-threatening events but also have important implications for the development of illness later in life. For example, early or unprotected sexual activity increases women's risk for sexually transmitted diseases. Not only are these diseases transmitted more easily from men to women, but women are disproportionately affected because of infectious complications that can lead to disorders of reproductive function, such as pelvic inflammatory disease, ectopic pregnancy, and infertility. Unfortunately, efforts at risk reduction, particularly in the use of harmful substances, are hampered by industry and market forces and other social factors that influence women's lives. For example, the adverse effects of cigarette smoking on lung cancer and other respiratory diseases, heart disease, osteoporosis, and reproductive function are well documented, but women become established smokers at an earlier age and have longer lifetime smoking histories than men. The effect of recent advertising restrictions on women's tobacco use is as yet unclear. Social values and cultural pressures have also contributed to the increasing prevalence of dieting and eating disorders. Using strict criteria, an estimated 5% of adolescent girls and young women have bulimia or anorexia. These disorders are often refractory to treatment and can be life threatening.

This life span group delineates women's reproductive years. In addition to traditional childbearing and family responsibilities, women are increasingly assuming new roles. The effect of multiple and often conflicting roles on women's mental and physical health remains to be determined but is closely linked to reproductive freedom and health. Thus physicians need to understand the safety, effectiveness, and acceptability of current methods of contraception in culturally diverse women. Because of an increased understanding of many other common disorders of reproductive function, primary care physicians can no longer view these disorders as exclusively gynecologic problems. The association of polycystic ovary disease with insulin resistance and the hyperandrogenic state and the contribution of nonreproductive causes to chronic pelvic pain highlight the general medical nature of these disorders.

Autoimmunity links many medical disorders with highest prevalence in women ages 15 to 44. Most of the autoimmune diseases are more common in women than in men and cause greater morbidity. Many are influenced by changes in estrogen levels, particularly during pregnancy. Among the collagen vascular diseases, rheumatoid arthritis, systemic lupus erythematosus, and scleroderma have prevalence rates that are three to nine times higher in women. Many autoimmune-related endocrinopathies, such as Hashimoto's thyroiditis and Graves' disease, have a female/male ratio as high as 15:1. Other autoimmune diseases that are more prevalent in women are type 1 diabetes mellitus, idiopathic adrenal failure, multiple sclerosis, and myasthenia gravis. Less well recognized is the role of autoimmunity in recurrent pregnancy loss and infertility in women.

Among the mental disorders, *depressive illnesses* are twice as common in women as men. An estimated 6% of women will experience a major depressive episode sometime during their lifetime, and twice that many will have chronic low-grade symptoms of depression. The greater risk of depression in women increases from childhood to adolescence and extends throughout life; however, the genetic, biologic, and environmental contributions to this gender effect are not fully understood. Women are also three times as likely as men to be diagnosed with an anxiety disorder, including agoraphobia, simple phobia, and panic disorder, as well as with somatization disorders. In addition, many women experience mood, cognitive, or behavioral changes associated with cyclic changes in hormone levels during the menstrual cycle or with marked changes in levels during the postpartum period or at the menopause.

A major cause of psychosocial morbidity in women is sexual and physical *abuse*. It is reported that 20% of adult women, 15% of college-age women, and 12% of adolescent girls have experienced sexual abuse and assault, and one of eight women in an ongoing relationship with a man has been assaulted by her partner. Pregnancy is a particularly high risk factor for assault. Unfortunately, due to lack of knowledge and training and misconceptions about domestic violence, physicians often fail to recognize or address symptoms of abuse. Adequate screening tools are especially crucial in the emergency department, where up to 30% of abused women may seek care. To ensure widespread detection of abuse, screening should become a regular part of the medical history in any setting.

Ages 45 to 64 Years

Death rates for women in this age group have declined by 30% in the past 25 years. Previously the leading cause of death was heart disease; however, cancer is now ranked number one, with lung cancer emerging as the leading cause of cancer deaths. These shifts in rates reflect primarily the decline in mortality from heart disease in both sexes attributed to lifestyle changes, such as better control of hypertension and lower blood cholesterol levels.

Many of the important chronic conditions in women first appear between ages 45 and 64, with the prevalence of some increasing greatly during this period. Significant racial and ethnic differences are associated with the prevalence of many of these conditions. The prevalence of obesity especially is disproportionately high in minority women; 52% of black and 50% of Hispanic women are overweight, compared with 33% of white women. Because obesity is a major risk factor for diabetes, heart disease, stroke, gallbladder disease, and some cancers and may be a factor in osteoarthritis, weight control in women is an important public health issue.

The emergence of many of these conditions is inextricably linked to the *menopause* and the marked decline in estrogen levels that occur during this age period. Decreased estrogen levels contribute to the development or progression of many disorders central to the aging process in women, such as heart disease, osteoporosis and cancer. Since hormonal replacement therapy (HRT) decreases the risk of developing some of these disorders, a woman's decision to use HRT should consider the beneficial effects of HRT on menopausal symptoms, osteoporosis, and cardiovascular disease, as well as the reported risks associated with HRT, specifically an increased risk of uterine and breast cancer.

Although the menopause encompasses many of the physiologic changes that define this period, women also experience major transitions in social roles and life circumstances that profoundly affect their physical and mental health. Children leave home, many women become widowed or divorced, parenting roles change as women care for aging parents, and disabilities increase, making it difficult for some women to function within and outside the home. Not surprisingly, 3% of women will experience a major depressive episode during this period. An understanding of these life events is essential to the comprehensive care of mature women.

Ages 65 Years and Older

Cardiovascular disease is the leading cause of death in older women, followed by cancer and cerebrovascular disease (stroke). Mortality rates for all three disorders rise steeply after age 65 and begin to approach the rates for men. Chronic pulmonary disease and pneumonia continue to cause high death rates because of the increase and severity of infections associated with an age-related decline in immune function. Injury is the sixth leading cause of death in older women; most of these deaths are related to falls.

After age 65, many other chronic illnesses, such as hypertension, diabetes, the arthritides, most digestive disorders, and thyroid disease, are more common in women than men of the same age and cause significant morbidity. As women's longevity increases, they bear the burden of illnesses that are seen primarily in very old persons. Of these, the neurologic degenerative diseases, such as dementia, sleep disorders, and neurosensory and movement disorders, are particularly common in women. Unfortunately, the added years of life in women are often spent in a frail or dependent state and often result in institutionalization. Currently, women residing in nursing homes outnumber men by 3:1. In particular, urinary incontinence and osteoporosis put women at high risk for institutionalization. Prevalence rates of *urinary incontinence* are twice as high in women as in men and affect up to one half of community-dwelling women. *Osteoporosis* is associated with deformity and pain secondary to vertebral fractures; however, hip fracture, usually the result of a fall, is the most serious consequence of osteoporosis in older women. According to the National Osteoporosis Foundation, one half of older women with a hip fracture will never walk independently, one third will never live independently, and one fifth will die within a year of the fracture.

The social and psychologic changes that women experience as they age add to the burden of illness. Social isolation increases with the death of loved ones, loss of financial stability, and increasing physical disabilities. In addition to an increasing incidence of dementia with age, mental health problems become more prevalent or serious. The role of the primary care physician is to recognize and help reduce the impact of these accumulated conditions on women's ability to function and on their quality of life.

EDUCATION AND TRAINING

Academic medical institutions are increasingly aware of the importance of women's health. Questions remain, however, concerning the domain of women's health, and the best way to train physicians, and which discipline(s) should be primarily responsible for curriculum development, clinical care, and training in this area.

Data from the National Ambulatory Medical Care Survey (NAMCS) provide insight into the complex nature of women's health care. Family practitioners provide most nonobstetric care to women ages 15 and older (57%), and internists and gynecologists provide decreasing amounts of the remaining services (25% and 18%, respectively). As women age, the proportion of care delivered by gynecologists decreases, whereas care provided by internists increases. Gynecologists provide few services to women over 65. Family practitioners and internists deliver services for both acute and chronic nongynecologic disorders, whereas gynecologists provide little of this care. In contrast, gynecologists provide more than half of general medical examinations and two thirds of routine gynecologic services.

Considerable overlap exists between the practice parameters of family practice and general internal medicine and those of obstetrics and gynecology. In addition, many physicians in medical subspecialties provide some generalist care to women outside their subspecialty focus. Female patients seek care from one or a range of these providers over their lifetime, and the patterns of care vary depending on the age and the social, economic, and health status of each woman. Where women fall in this health care matrix determines to a large extent the type and comprehensiveness of care received.

These findings have important implications for the health care of women. The lack of uniform standards of care, especially regarding preventive services, and the splintering of routine care among disciplines may result in poorly coordinated and incomplete care. The multiprovider approach fostered by this system does not necessarily mean improved services to women and is antithetic to the concept of primary care. Faced with overlapping but often inadequate services, women must increasingly take responsibility for directing and monitoring their health care.

In response to these findings, the Council on Graduate Medical Education recommends that all physicians, regardless of their educational level and specialty interest, be educated in the fundamentals of women's health and demonstrate competence in providing care to women. To implement these recommendations, women's health must have a form and a structure, a source of funding, and a recognized place in the medical community. Many of these objectives can be achieved by the establishment of collaborative interdisciplinary centers or programs in women's health within academic health centers. The U.S. Department of Health and Human Services, through the Public Health Service Office on Women's Health, funded six such vanguard centers in 1996, six in 1997, and an additional six in 1998. These centers are designed to facilitate the development of innovative clinical models, integrated curricula, and interdisciplinary research in women's health and to foster the development of women faculty.

Some disciplines are also expanding residency training to address new national residency training requirements in women's comprehensive health care. In internal medicine, training programs must now include women's health topics as part of their core curricula; some offer additional clinical experience through multidisciplinary women's health centers. A few programs have developed separate residency tracks within sections of general internal medicine that focus on women's health. At the fellowship level, scattered programs in women's health exist as separate tracks in general medicine fellowship programs.

Recommendations for Core Curriculum

As a foundation for addressing women's health conditions, physicians must understand basic female physiology and reproductive biology. In addition, they need to appreciate the complex interaction between the environment and the biology and psychosocial development of women. Among the conditions not specific to women, physicians must be aware of those aspects of disease that are different in women or have important gender implications. The ability to apply this information requires that physicians adopt attitudes and behavior that are culturally and gender sensitive. Women's relationship to the medical system is also changing and requires physicians to understand women's patterns of health seeking and forms of communication and interaction, as well as to appreciate gender differences in clinical decision making.

To assist academic medical institutions in implementing curricular changes, the Public Health Service Office on Women's Health, in collaboration with the National Institutes of Health Office of Research on Women's Health and the Health Resources and Services Administration, published a report in 1996 that provides the rationale for the development of a women's health curriculum and outlines the educational philosophy, scope, and content of a core curriculum. The report's recommendations are designed to augment and enhance rather than duplicate or replace existing curricula in the traditional disciplines. Although the report is directed at undergraduate medical education, its concepts and content can be applied broadly across the educational spectrum and may be helpful in modifying and updating residency training in the traditional medical disciplines.

ADDITIONAL READINGS

Anderson RN, Kochanek KD, Murphy SL: Report of final mortality statistics, 1995, *Mon Vital Stat Rep* 45(11, suppl 2), 1997.

Council on Graduate Medical Education: *Fifth report: women and medicine*, Pub No HRSA-P-DM-91-1, 1995, US Department of Health and Human Services.

National Institutes of Health: *Opportunities for research on women's health*, NIH Pub No 92-3457, 1992, US Department of Health and Human Services, Public Health Service, National Institutes of Health.

Wingo PA, Ries LA, Rosenberg HM, et al: Cancer incidence and mortality, 1973-1995: a report card for the U.S., *Cancer* 82:1197, 1998.

Women's Health in the medical curriculum: report of a survey and recommendations, 1996, US Department of Health and Human Services, Health Resources and Services Administration, National Institutes of Health.

CHAPTER 35

Abnormal Menstruation

Ru-fong Cheng
Steven Sondheimer

Abnormal uterine bleeding has varying significance. It can represent a harmless disruption in the estrogen/progesterone ratio, a complication of pregnancy, or a warning sign of cancer. It can disrupt a woman's lifestyle and is alarming to the patient. Historically the term *dysfunctional uterine bleeding* was used to describe an event of acute bleeding. Now, with a better understanding of the sequence of hormonal events leading to menstrual bleeding and other functional etiologies of heavy uterine bleeding, dysfunctional uterine bleeding is usually reserved to describe anovulatory uterine bleeding.

Many ways exist to quantify uterine bleeding. The simplest method is by patient history, specifically, information about number of days of bleeding, passage of blood clots, and number of pads used. *Menorrhagia* is defined as profuse bleeding with flooding of clots or repetitive periods lasting more than 8 days. Because the history is poorly correlated with amount of blood lost, an objective approach would be documentation of anemia caused by chronic blood loss. Ultimately the best measure of menstrual blood loss is the degree of lifestyle disruption and change from a previous bleeding pattern. If the patient is unable to leave her house on days of menses due to fear of an embarrassing menstrual accident, that patient has abnormal uterine bleeding.

To understand abnormal menstruation, normal menstruation must first be defined. Normal menstrual cycles are remarkably consistent in ovulating women, with a similar pattern of flow from menses to menses and frequently an accompanying sense of premenstrual awareness. Cycle length is defined as the time from the first day of bleeding from one cycle to the first day of bleeding in the next cycle. Normal cycle length is 28 ± 7 days. Normal duration of flow is 4 ± 2 days, and normal quantity of blood flow is 40 ± 20 ml per cycle.[3]

PATHOPHYSIOLOGY

The menstrual cycle consists of two distinct phases, each with characteristic physiologic and hormonal events. The *proliferative phase*, usually days 1 through 14, is characterized by the endometrium preparing to receive the egg. Ovulation occurs in conjunction with the luteinizing hormone (LH) surge on day 14. The corpus luteum that persists from the ovarian follicle secretes progesterone, which then stimulates the endometrium to become inactive secretory endometrium. This marks the beginning of the *luteal phase*. Without pregnancy the corpus luteum regresses, and the subsequent decrease in estrogen and progesterone levels prepares the endometrium for orderly sloughing. Prostaglandins are released, leading to vasospasm and cellular necrosis. Cellular death, bleeding, and shedding of the functional endometrium ensue.

PATIENT EVALUATION

The first step is to obtain a complete medical history, with special attention to the menstrual history: age of menarche, frequency of menses, duration of bleeding, severity, cyclicity, and any changes from the previous pattern. Additional important information includes prior pregnancies and contraceptive method, medications, social history (including domestic violence and assault), and review of systems (general well-being, gastrointestinal and genitourinary symptoms). The physical examination should include vital signs and abdominopelvic evaluation. Tests should include a urine pregnancy test, Pap smear, and gonorrhea and chlamydial cultures. In addition, endometrial biopsy should be performed on women over age 35 with abnormal bleeding to rule out endometrial hyperplasia. Serum testing should include complete blood count, prothrombin/partial thromboplastin times, thyroid-stimulating hormone, prolactin, follicle-stimulating hormone, LH, and liver function tests.

Additional studies may include a pelvic ultrasound to rule out fibroids or structural abnormalities. Sonohysterography is a similar study in which the uterus is instilled with sterile saline to separate the uterine walls while ultrasound is employed to visualize the uterus. This study is especially helpful to delineate submucous myomas or endometrial polyps. In dilation and curettage (D&C) with hysteroscopy the endometrium is sampled and the endometrial cavity visualized with a fiberoptic hysteroscope while the uterine walls are distended with carbon dioxide or liquid medium. Magnetic resonance imaging (MRI) can be used to identify uterine anomalies or fibroids, but cost limits its use.[5]

DIFFERENTIAL DIAGNOSIS

The approach to the differential diagnosis of abnormal uterine bleeding may be directed by the patient's age and reproductive status (Table 35-1). Menarcheal patients are usually in the teen years; the two etiologies of abnormal uterine bleeding common to this age group are anovulation and bleeding disorders. Anovulation may result from immaturity of the hypothalamic-pituitary axis and lack of appropriate feedback response to circulating estradiol.[4] Unopposed estrogen action on endometrium leads to irregular shedding. Bleeding disorders should be suspected if patients give a history of easy bruising and nosebleeds. Platelet deficiencies, defects in platelet activity (e.g., von Willebrand's disease), and prothrombin deficiency can be associated with abnormal uterine bleeding.

Ovulatory patients, from teenage girls to women in their 40s, have the most possible reasons for abnormal uterine bleeding. Pregnancy is the most obvious etiology and may be a normal intrauterine pregnancy or a threatened, incomplete, or complete abortion. Because of life-threatening implications, ectopic pregnancy must also be considered. Trophoblastic disease is a variant of pregnancy in which malignant trophoblastic tissue produces human chorionic gonadotropin (hCG) and may cause bleeding. After recent pregnancy the woman may have retained placental tissue, a placental polyp, or subinvolution of the placental implantation site. Infection of the vagina, cervix, endometrium, and fallopian tubes may present with abnormal bleeding. Anovulation may also occur sporadically in menstruating women. If anovulation is chronic, it is called *polycystic ovarian syndrome* (PCOS). Initially characterized by Stein-Leventhal syndrome, PCOS involves androgen excess, with small ovarian follicles visualized on ultrasound.[3] Fibroids (leiomyomata, myomas) are benign smooth muscle tumors of the uterine muscle that can disrupt normal menstrual patterns by altering the endometrial vasculature, impairing normal hemostatic mechanisms (e.g., platelet adherence, fibrin plug formation). Endometriosis, characterized by growth of endometrial glands and stroma outside the uterus, and adenomyosis, characterized by endometrial glands and stroma in the myometrium, can also cause abnormal uterine bleeding. Thyroid disease, especially hypothyroidism, can cause heavy menses. Hypothalamic etiologies of heavy menses may be caused by stress and changes in weight. Lesions on the cervix and vagina caused by dysplasia, cancer, or trauma can cause bleeding. Iatrogenic causes of bleeding include use of oral contraceptives (OCs), Depo-Provera, Norplant, and intrauterine device (IUD). Other medications associated with abnormal bleeding include phenytoin, antidepressants, digitalis, anticoagulants, corticosteroids, and tranquilizers. Finally, disease in other organ systems can result in abnormal bleeding. Liver cirrhosis causes decreased metabolism of estrogen; decreased conjugation leads to increased circulating estrogen levels, which stimulate the endometrium and cause irregular bleeding.[3]

In perimenopausal women in their 40s and 50s, abnormal bleeding is caused by malignancy until proved otherwise.

Table 35-1. Diagnosis of Uterine Bleeding Based on Patient's Age and Reproductive Status

Reproductive status	Age group	Diagnosis
Menarcheal	Teens	Anovulation: Immaturity of hypothalamic-pituitary-ovarian axis, PCOS Bleeding disorder: von Willebrand's disease
Ovulatory	Teens to 40s	Pregnancy: normal, abortion, trophoblastic disease, postpregnancy placental abnormality Infection: cervix, vagina, endometrium, tubes; PID; tuboovarian abscessses Chronic anovulation: PCOS (Stein-Leventhal) Fibroids Endometriosis or adenomyosis Thyroid disease Hypothalamic: stress, weight change, excess exercise Lesions of cervix or vagina: dysplasia, trauma Iatrogenic: hormonal contraception (OCs, Depo-Provera, Norplant, progesterone IUD), psychotropic medications, antidepressants, digitalis, anticoagulants, corticosteroids, tranquilizers, phenytoin Systemic disease: liver cirrhosis
Perimenopause	40s to 50s	Rule out malignancy: cervical dysplasia, endometrial hyperplasia

PCOS, Polycystic ovarian syndrome (disease); *PID*, pelvic inflammatory disease; *OCs*, oral contraceptives; *IUD*, intrauterine device.

Endometrial hyperplasia is a particular concern in chronic anovulatory women and is characterized as simple or complex and with or without atypia. Hyperplasia with atypia can progress to endometrial cancer. The incidence of endometrial cancer increases with increasing age, although malignant transformation may also occur in younger women. Polyps of endometrial or cervical origin can also be a cause of abnormal uterine bleeding.

MANAGEMENT

Treat Condition

Treatment of abnormal uterine bleeding is directed toward the underlying etiology. For menarcheal patients with anovulation, withdrawal bleeding may be induced with cyclic medroxyprogesterone acetate, 10 mg/day for 10 days, or cyclic OCs. Patients with abnormal bleeding but no anatomic lesions who do not respond to medical treatments should be evaluated for bleeding disorders. *Von Willebrand's disease* is a heterogenous disorder with defective functioning of von Willebrand's factor (vWF). Its estimated prevalence is 1% of the population. Treatment is with desmopressin (a synthetic analog of vasopressin) nasal spray or intravenous injection, which promotes the release of vWF from storage sites. Treatment is effective in achieving hemostasis in 75% of those affected.[4]

Pregnancy can be confirmed with a urine hCG test. Normal intrauterine pregnancies can be documented with ultrasound as early as 5 to 6 weeks, after quantitative serum β-hCG level reaches 1000 to 2000 mIU/ml, although this number may vary from center to center. Abortions are marked by vaginal bleeding. *Threatened abortions* usually present with vaginal bleeding and a closed cervical os on examination. *Incomplete abortions* are preceded by vaginal bleeding, followed by partially extruded products of conception at the dilated cervical os. *Missed abortions* are classically described as findings of a nonviable fetus and a closed cervical os. In the current age of high-resolution ultrasound, this term may be used for the detection of early fetal demise (absence of cardiac activity). Types of abortion can be differentiated by physical examination and by following serial β-hCG levels. In normal pregnancy, quantitative β-hCG values double every 48 to 72 hours. If levels do not rise as expected, the pregnancy is not normal, and the patient may need a D&C to evacuate the uterus if bleeding persists. If bleeding ceases, the abortion may have completed on its own, and serial quantitative β-hCG levels should be followed until they fall to zero. *Ectopic pregnancies* may also present with abnormal uterine bleeding (see later discussion). Quantitative β-hCG levels do not rise as expected, and no intrauterine pregnancy is seen on ultrasound. If patients have abdominal pain and acute peritoneal signs, tubal rupture may have occurred, which requires acute surgical intervention with either laparoscopy or laparotomy. *Trophoblastic disease* is another variant of pregnancy that may present with bleeding. This entity is quite rare and is treated with chemotherapy under the supervision of a gynecologic oncologist.

Abnormal bleeding resulting from trauma may require intervention. If the bleeding is acute, surgical therapy may be necessary. Otherwise, documentation of findings and inquiries about domestic violence are appropriate. If domestic violence is an issue, child abuse may also be occurring. Referrals to local police and support agencies should be offered. Most major cities have counseling resources available.

With infection of the pelvic organs, the physical examination may demonstrate purulent discharge, cervical motion tenderness, or uterine fundal tenderness. *Cervicitis* is diagnosed by gonorrheal and chlamydial culture and *endometritis* by endometrial biopsy. Cervicitis is treated with antibiotics and appropriate counseling regarding treatment of sexual partners and use of barrier contraceptives. Endometritis is also treated with antibiotics. If infection of the fallopian tubes or pelvic inflammatory disease (PID) is suspected, inpatient antibiotic therapy is given if the patient is unable to tolerate oral medications, has never been pregnant, is positive for human immunodeficiency virus (HIV), or is unable to comply with outpatient follow-up. Otherwise, outpatient antibiotic treatment is appropriate.

In women with thyroid disease, correction of the underlying disorder will correct the menstrual disturbance. If the etiology of abnormal bleeding is hypothalamic (e.g., stress, recent weight change), efforts should correct the underlying problem. If this is not possible or resumption of regular menses is desired, combination OCs may be used to regulate bleeding. For iatrogenic causes of bleeding, the risks and benefits of continuing the medication responsible for bleeding must be assessed. If the patient cannot discontinue the medication and control of menses is desired, cyclic OCs may be prescribed.

Fibroids may be palpable on examination or identified by ultrasound. Medical treatment of fibroids is with gonadotropin-releasing hormone (GnRH) analogs, which provide only temporary relief. Surgical treatment is technically easier and associated with less blood loss if GnRH agonists are used preoperatively to shrink the size of the myomas and thin the endometrium. Endometrial ablation may be performed with the laser or the resectoscope or roller ball. Interventional radiologists can perform uterine artery embolization for poor surgical candidates or patients who want to maintain their uteri. Myomectomy, which shells out the myomas while leaving the remainder of the myometrium as intact as possible, preserves fertility, but myomas may recur. Myomectomy may be approached hysteroscopically with the resectoscope or abdominally. Hysterectomy definitively treats uterine bleeding.

Adenomyosis and *endometriosis* are similar entities in which endometrial glands and stroma are found outside the endometrium. Diagnosis is primarily made by the patient history; treatment options are similar to those for fibroids. *Endometrial hyperplasia* is evaluated with hysteroscopy and D&C and then treated with progestational agents or hysterectomy. *Cervical dysplasia* is managed with colposcopy and biopsy. *Endometrial cancer* warrants referral to a gynecologic oncologist and most often results in hysterectomy and staging. *Polyps,* whether endometrial or cervical, should be removed by hysteroscopically directed D&C.

Control Bleeding

Once structural abnormalities have been excluded, the management of anovulatory bleeding is aimed at controlling bleeding and preventing recurrence. Historically, D&Cs were performed for treatment. Modern treatment is medical and involves high-dose estrogen to promote rapid endometrial growth, clotting, and healing of denuded epithelial surfaces. Estrogen administration is followed by progesterone to prevent subsequent bleeding. Sometimes progesterone can be used alone to stop bleeding, but if sloughing has already occurred, it may make bleeding worse by creating more decidualized atrophic endometrium. Specific regimens to treat anovulatory bleeding include conjugated equine estrogen and OCs (Box 35-1).[4] If the patient is hypovolemic or anemic (hemoglobin less than 7.0 mg/dl), hospitalization or prolonged observation in the emergency department should be considered. If the patient does not respond to acute medical treatment, surgical treatment with D&C and concomitant hysteroscopy should be pursued to visualize any anatomic abnormalities (e.g., polyps, submucous fibroids, potential hyperplasia). The exact mechanism of bleeding cessation after D&C is unknown. Theoretically, curettage removes functional endometrial tissue and allows the basal layer to regenerate, which leads to cessation of bleeding. Curettage also stimulates release of prostaglandins, causing vasoconstriction.[2]

For less acute medical treatment of anovulatory bleeding, the goal is to control blood loss. Treatment is with cyclic combination OCs; nonsteroidal antiinflammatory drugs (NSAIDs) may be used the first 3 days of menses or

Box 35-1. Medical Management of Abnormal Uterine Bleeding

Acute

1. High-dose estrogen, then progesterone
   a. Conjugated equine estrogen, 25 mg intravenously every 4-6 hours
   b. *or* Conjugated equine estrogen, 2.5 mg orally every 8 hours
   c. *or* OCs with 50 μg ethinyl estradiol tid
2. If no response in 24-48 hours, perform dilation and curettage (D&C).
3. If bleeding slows down, use combination OCs with 35-50 μg ethinyl estradiol, one tablet daily for 7 days.
4. After withdrawal bleeding occurs, start combination OC (any type) for 3-4 normal cycles.

Less Acute

1. Cyclic combination OCs *plus*
2. Nonsteroidal antiinflammatory drugs (NSDAIDs)
   a. Mefenamic acid, 500 mg tid
   b. *or* Ibuprofen, 600 mg tid
   c. *or* Meclofenamate, 100 mg tid
   d. *or* Naproxen, 550-mg loading dose, then 275 mg every 6 hours

OCs, Oral contraceptives; *tid,* three times a day.

throughout menses (see Box 35-1).[4] NSAIDs are effective in reducing menstrual blood loss by blocking the formation of prostacyclin, a vasodilator that inhibits platelet aggregation.

Less acute surgical treatment may be accomplished with endometrial ablation; 80% of patients have good long-term results, and about 50% report complete amenorrhea.[2] Ablation may be performed with the laser or the resectoscope or coagulating roller ball. Another technique involves use of an intrauterine balloon for thermal treatment and ablation of the endometrium. Results are best if (1) the endometrium has been thinned with concomitant use of a GnRH agonist or danazol or (2) suction curettage is done at ablation. This is a good option for patients considering hysterectomy but is not recommended for those interested in future childbearing.

Long-term medical management of patients with anovulatory bleeding is with progestins, which stop endometrial growth and support and organize endometrium that has been primed by estrogen. After progesterone is withdrawn, the endometrium sloughs and bleeding ceases when adequate estrogen is present. This can be accomplished with medroxyprogesterone acetate, 10 mg orally on days 1 to 10 of each month or days 16 to 25 of each cycle. The same effect can be achieved with combination OCs. An IUD that releases progesterone or levonorgestrel may also be an effective treatment for heavy menses.[4]

Perimenopausal abnormal uterine bleeding can be managed with cyclic conjugated equine estrogen, 0.625 to 1.25 mg/day on days 1 to 25 of each month, along with medroxyprogesterone acetate, 10 mg/day on days 15 to 25 of each month. Alternatively, these patients may be given combination OCs if they are not tobacco users.

Hysterectomy is reserved for patients whose bleeding does not respond to the previous measures or whose frustration with persistent bleeding necessitates definitive treatment.

ECTOPIC PREGNANCY

Patients at risk for ectopic pregnancy, defined as a pregnancy found outside the uterine cavity, include women with a history of chlamydial infection; previous ectopic pregnancy; tobacco use, which decreases ciliary motility in the fallopian tubes; prior tubal surgery for fertility or tubal reanastomosis; previous diethylstilbestrol (DES) exposure; and increasing maternal age. The rate of ectopic pregnancies has increased, with 4.5:1000 reported pregnancies in 1970 vs. 20:1000 in 1992. The diagnosis is made by documenting inadequately rising β-hCG levels (less than 100% increase in 48 to 72 hours) with no intrauterine gestational sac on ultrasound. A gestational sac is usually visible with transvaginal ultrasound when the β-hCG level reaches 1000 to 2000 mIU/ml, although this value may vary from center to center. An ectopic pregnancy should be also be suspected when a D&C has been performed for a suspected miscarriage and the pathology does not reveal products of conception.

In the past, all patients with suspected ectopic pregnancy underwent surgery, either laparoscopically or by laparotomy, and a *salpingostomy* (removal of pregnancy tissue while sparing the tube) or *salpingectomy* (removal of the entire tube) was done. Both procedures have similar postoperative fertility rates of about 60%, with a subsequent ectopic pregnancy rate of 10% to 30%.[7] Women without a history of surgery for ectopic pregnancy have a 90% fertility rate.[6]

With the advent of sensitive assays for β-hCG and increasingly high-resolution ultrasound, the diagnosis of ectopic pregnancy can be made before the patient becomes symptomatic and before a life-threatening emergency exists. Currently, patients can be offered medical treatment with methotrexate, a folic acid antagonist that inhibits dihydrofolic acid reductase and interferes with DNA synthesis, repair, and cellular reproduction.[1] Posttreatment fertility rates are the same as those for surgical treatment.

REFERENCES

1. American College of Obstetricians and Gynecologists: *Medical management of tubal pregnancy,* Practice bulletin no 3, December 1998.
2. Benrubi GI, editor: *Obstetric and gynecologic emergencies,* Philadelphia, 1994, Lippincott.
3. Brenner PF: Differential diagnosis of abnormal uterine bleeding, *Am J Obstet Gynecol* 175:766, 1996.
4. Chuong CJ, Brenner PF: Management of abnormal uterine bleeding, *Am J Obstet Gynecol* 175:787, 1996.
5. Long CA: Evaluation of patients with abnormal uterine bleeding, *Am J Obstet Gynecol* 175:784, 1996.
6. Menken J, Trussel IJ, et al: Age and infertility, *Science* 23:1389, 1986.
7. Sherman D, Langer R, et al: Improved fertility following ectopic pregnancy, *Fertil Steril* 37:497, 1982.

CHAPTER 36

Hirsutism and Hyperandrogenism

James C. Shaw

In both men and women, hair growth on the face and other androgen-sensitive areas is a clinical marker for androgen effect. In the absence of androgens, terminal hair does not develop in these areas. Lifetime patterns of hair growth in women are highly variable, are influenced by genetic factors, and may or may not be considered abnormal depending on social custom. Some increase in the quantity and coarseness of hair typically occurs with aging.

Idiopathic hirsutism refers to increased androgen-mediated hair growth without an identifiable disease. Clinical presentations within the idiopathic category also include acne, androgenic alopecia, and menstrual irregularities. Since advances in hirsutism research have identified *hyperandrogenism* in most cases, the designation idiopathic hirsutism will likely become less useful.

ETIOLOGY AND PATHOPHYSIOLOGY

Androgen-mediated hair growth is a complex process that is influenced primarily by circulating levels of testosterone and its precursors or metabolites. Sources of androgens in women are the ovaries, adrenal glands, and those from target tissue metabolism of androgen precursors. In adult women, ovaries are most often the source of androgens. Anovulation with loss of cyclic menstrual function leads to increased androgen production by the ovaries, a condition called *functional ovarian hyperandrogenism;* the most severe form is full-blown polycystic ovary syndrome. Adrenal hyperandrogenism is much less common and occurs in the setting of late-onset adrenal hyperplasia.

PATIENT EVALUATION

History. The most common clinical history in hirsute women is irregular menses, onset of hirsutism during the teenage years or early 20s, and gradual worsening of the condition. Acne is frequently associated with worsening hirsutism. The rapidity of development of hirsutism is important. A woman who develops hirsutism after age 25 and demonstrates rapid progression of masculinization over several months may have an androgen-producing tumor. Other less common causes that may be addressed in the history include Cushing's syndrome, acromegaly, and pregnancy. Drugs can stimulate hair growth by both androgen-mediated and non-androgen-mediated mechanisms (e.g., methyltestosterone, anabolic steroids, danazol, phenytoin, diazoxide). *Hypertrichosis* refers to increased nonsexual hair and may be associated with porphyrias and environmental factors that produce chronic irritation or reactive hyperemia of the skin.

Physical Examination. Increased hair growth in patients with hirsutism and hyperandrogenemia ranges from fine vellus hair on the face to marked terminal (full-sized) hair on the face, breasts, genitalia, lower abdomen, and extremities. Other physical findings that suggest hyperandrogenemia include acne, increased oiliness of the skin, and androgenic alopecia. Masculinizing features such as clitorimegaly, android muscle distribution, and a deep voice are only seen in women with severe hyperandrogenemia.

DIAGNOSIS

Women with normal menses and mild hirsutism require little or no hormonal evaluation. Women with hirsutism, obesity, and menstrual irregularities may benefit from an endocrinologic evaluation for polycystic ovary syndrome, diabetes, or Cushing's syndrome. In women with rapid onset of hirsutism and in those with oligomenorrhea, hormonal evaluation is indicated to rule out androgen-secreting tumors and other endocrine causes. A basic evaluation to screen for androgen-secreting tumors includes plasma total testosterone, dehydroepiandrosterone sulfate (DHEAS), and 17-hydroxyprogesterone (17-OHP), which is used optionally to diagnose late-onset adrenal hyperplasia. An expanded evaluation for women with more severe disease usually includes total testosterone, free testosterone, DHEAS, luteinizing hormone (LH), follicle-stimulating hormone (FSH), prolactin, adrenocorticotropic hormone (ACTH) stimulation, and glucose tolerance tests.

Testosterone Level. Plasma testosterone levels (normal 20 to 80 ng/dl [0.69 to 2.8 nmol/L]) are primarily a measure of ovarian testosterone production and are elevated in the majority of women (70%) with anovulation and hirsutism. Individual variation is great, largely because of the changes in the testosterone-binding capacity of sex hormone–binding globulin (SHBG) in the blood. Measuring the free testosterone (a technically difficult and expensive assay) is not necessary. A routine testosterone assay adequately screens for testosterone-secreting tumors because these tumors are associated with testosterone levels in the male range and do not rely on fine discrimination of the free testosterone level. If the testosterone level exceeds 200 ng/dl (7 nmol/L), an androgen-producing tumor must be suspected.

DHEAS Level. DHEAS is derived almost exclusively from the adrenal gland. It is a direct measure of adrenal androgen activity and correlates clinically with urinary 17-ketosteroid levels. The upper limit of normal in most laboratories is 350 μg/dl (9.5 μmol/L). A random sample of DHEAS is sufficient for the evaluation of hirsutism because a slow turnover rate results in a large and stable pool in the blood with insignificant variation. Elevated levels of DHEAS contribute to the clinical problem of hirsutism because DHEAS is a prehormone in hair follicles, providing substrate for the hair follicle synthesis of androgens.

When the DHEAS level is normal, adrenal disease is unlikely, and the source of excess androgen production is most likely the ovaries. Rare cases of adrenal tumors with normal DHEAS levels have been reported; testosterone levels are elevated in these patients. Late-onset adrenal hyperplasia is not usually associated with increased DHEAS. Moderately elevated DHEAS levels are frequently found in patients with anovulation and polycystic ovaries.

17-OHP Level. 17-OHP is elevated in the setting of late-onset adrenal hyperplasia. The normal baseline 17-OHP level is less than 200 ng/dl (6 nmol/L). Levels greater than

800 ng/dl are diagnostic of 21-hydroxylase deficiency. Levels between 200 and 800 ng/dl require ACTH testing to determine the degree of 21-hydroxylase deficiency (see Chapter 98).

Differential Diagnosis

Several conditions can cause hirsutism associated with hyperandrogenemia. Idiopathic hirsutism and polycystic ovary syndrome account for more than 90% of cases, and because of the heterogenous nature of polycystic ovary syndrome, functional ovarian hyperandrogenism is used to describe these patients' condition. Less common causes of hirsutism include congenital adrenal hyperplasia, late-onset adrenal hyperplasia, Cushing's syndrome, androgen-producing tumors of the ovary or adrenal gland, and luteoma associated with pregnancy.

MANAGEMENT

Treatment options for hirsutism are mechanical hair removal and medical therapy, including androgen receptor blockers and suppression of ovaries and adrenal glands (Box 36-1). Frequently a combination of mechanical and medical therapy is used.

Mechanical Therapy

Hair removal by shaving, plucking, waxing, or electrolysis temporarily reduces hirsutism. Most patients experience a recurrence and require ongoing use of these modalities. A new approach uses lasers of several types, with longer-lasting results. It is not clear which wavelength of laser will produce the best results.

Pharmacologic Therapy

Systemic Therapy. All systemic therapies are hormonal and are designed (1) to suppress the production of androgens in either the ovaries or the adrenals or (2) to block the end-organ effect of androgens. Hirsutism responds slowly to treatment. Because the hair growth cycle is long, change takes time. Patients should be informed that at least 6 months of hormonal suppression is necessary before reduced hair growth can be observed. Some patients return after a period of treatment expressing disappointment because hair is still present. The effect of treatment (prevention of new hair growth) may not be apparent unless previously established hair is removed. Ovarian suppression to prevent new hair growth combined with electrolysis or laser therapy to remove the old hair may be most effective.

Box 36-1. Treatment of Hirsutism

- Ovarian suppression
  - Oral contraceptives
  - Gonadotropin-releasing hormone (GnRH) agonists
- Adrenal suppression
  - Corticosteroids
- Antiandrogens (androgen receptor blockers)
  - Spironolactone
  - Flutamide

After 1 to 2 years the medication should be stopped and the patient observed for a return of ovulatory cycles. Even in patients who continue to be anovulatory, testosterone suppression continues for 6 months to 2 years after discontinuing treatment. If anovulation is still present, hirsutism will eventually return.

Ovarian Suppression

Oral Contraceptives. Suppression of ovarian androgens is usually accomplished with oral contraceptives (OCs). In addition to suppressing ovarian activity, OCs increase SHBG levels, thus decreasing circulating testosterone. The progestins in OCs also inhibit the activity of 5α-reductase, the enzyme that converts testosterone to the more active dihydrotestosterone (DHT). Low-dose OCs are as effective as the higher-dose formulations in treating hirsutism and suppressing free testosterone levels. Multiphasic formulations appear to be equally effective. Well-designed studies are needed to determine whether the newer OCs with less androgenic progestins (norgestimate, desogestrel) have more effect on hirsutism than other OCs.

When OCs are contraindicated or unwanted, good results can be achieved with *medroxyprogesterone acetate,* either 150 mg intramuscularly every 3 months or 30 mg orally every day. The mechanism of action of medroxyprogesterone acetate is slightly different from that of the combination OC. Since suppression of gonadotropins is less intense, ovarian follicular activity continues. LH suppression is significant, however, and testosterone production is decreased, although to a lesser degree than with combined OCs. In addition, testosterone clearance from the circulation is increased. This latter effect is caused by induction of liver enzyme activity. Although medroxyprogesterone acetate decreases SHBG, resulting in a relative increase in free testosterone, suppression of total testosterone production is so great that the net amount of free testosterone is decreased. The overall effect yields a clinical result comparable to that achieved with the combination OC.

Cyproterone Acetate. Cyproterone acetate has been successfully used worldwide to treat hirsutism and acne. It is a steroidal progestin with androgen receptor–blocking activity that is used alone or as the progestin in OCs. Cyproterone acetate is not available in the United States.

Gonadotropin-releasing Hormone (GnRH) Agonists. Because ovarian androgen production is LH dependent, suppression of the pituitary with chronic GnRH agonist treatment improves hirsutism. A higher dose of GnRH agonist is required to suppress ovarian androgen production than to suppress estradiol secretion. Therefore treatment should be monitored with testosterone levels. *Leuprolide,* 3.75 mg/month, is effective. To avoid problems associated with estrogen deficiency, therapy with an OC containing estrogen and progestin should be initiated after the GnRH agonist maintenance dose has been established. This method of treatment is relatively complicated and expensive and should be reserved for severe cases of ovarian hyperandrogenism.

Adrenal Suppression. Suppression of endogenous ACTH secretion is used in women who have an adrenal enzyme deficiency with resultant adrenal hyperplasia. *Dexamethasone* is given nightly (to achieve maximal suppression of the central nervous system adrenal axis, which peaks during sleep) at a dose of 0.5 mg. The equivalent dose of prednisone is 5 to 7.5 mg. If this treatment suppresses the morning plasma cortisol level below 2.0 μg/dl (56 nmol/L), the dose should be reduced to avoid an inability to react to stress. Fortunately, adrenal androgen secretion is more sensitive to suppression by dexamethasone than is cortisol secretion. Patients with classic (congenital) adrenal hyperplasia may require higher doses to normalize the steroid blood levels. With higher doses, alternative day therapy can still accomplish significant adrenal androgen suppression without affecting cortisol secretion.

Antiandrogens (Androgen Receptor Blockers)

Spironolactone. Although spironolactone is well known for its use as an aldosterone-antagonist diuretic in hypervolemic states, it also produces hormonal effects, including competitive androgen receptor blockade, inhibition of ovarian and adrenal steroidogenesis, and inhibition of 5α-reductase activity. The peripheral receptor blockade is responsible for most of the clinical antiandrogen effect. Spironolactone has been successful in the treatment of hirsutism in doses ranging from 50 to 200 mg/day. Usually some response is noted within 3 months, but longer treatment may be required before change is evident. Side effects are usually minimal and dose related. Potential side effects include a diuresis in the first few days of use, occasional complaints of fatigue, dysfunctional uterine bleeding, and breast tenderness. Spironolactone is contraindicated in pregnancy because of a potential feminizing effect on a developing male fetus. Concomitant OC use prevents this potential complication, prevents menstrual irregularities, and corrects the common underlying steady state of anovulation.

Flutamide. Flutamide is a nonsteroidal antiandrogen that blocks androgen receptors at peripheral tissue. Although its primary use is treatment of prostate cancer, flutamide has been used successfully in women with hirsutism. Doses range from 125 mg twice a day to 250 mg three times a day. Flutamide is generally well tolerated, but fatal hepatotoxicity has been reported with its use in men in doses of 750 mg or more per day, and close monitoring of liver function is important.

Finasteride. Finasteride inhibits 5α-reductase and is indicated for use in benign prostatic hypertrophy and androgenetic alopecia in men. Finasteride is somewhat effective in women with hirsutism, but less so than spironolactone and cyproterone acetate. Because of potential effects on developing male fetuses, finasteride is not recommended for women of childbearing age.

ADDITIONAL READINGS

Barth JH, Cherry CA, Wojnarowaka F, Dawber RP: Spironolactone is an effective and well tolerated systemic anti-androgen therapy for hirsute women, *J Clin Endocrinol Metab* 68:966, 1989.

Carmina E, Lobo RA: The addition of dexamethasone to antiandrogen therapy for hirsutism prolongs the duration of remission, *Fertil Steril* 69:1075, 1998.

Erenus M, Yucelten D, Durmusoglu F, et al: Comparison of finasteride versus spironolactone in the treatment of idiopathic hirsutism, *Fertil Steril* 68:1000, 1997.

Kohn B et al: New MI, late-onset steroid 21-hydroxylase deficiency: a variant of classical congenital adrenal hyperplasia, *J Clin Endocrinol Metab* 55:817, 1982.

Lobo RA: Hirsutism in polycystic ovary syndrome: current concepts, *Clin Obstet Gynecol* 34:817, 1991.

Marcondes JAM et al: Treatment of hirsutism in women with flutamide, *Fertil Steril* 57:543, 1992.

Rittmaster RS: Differential suppression of testosterone and estradiol in hirsute women with the superactive gonadotropin-releasing hormone agonist leuprolide, *J Clin Endocrinol Metab* 67:651, 1988.

Rittmaster RS: Hirsutism, *Lancet* 349:191, 1997.

Rittmaster RS: Hyperandrogenism—what is normal? *N Engl J Med* 327:194, 1992 (editorial).

Shaw JC: Spironolactone in dermatologic therapy, *J Am Acad Dermatol* 24:236, 1991.

Shaw JC: Antiandrogen therapy in dermatology, *Int J Dermatol* 85:770, 1996.

White PC, New MI, Dupont B: Congenital adrenal hyperplasia, *N Engl J Med* 316:1519, 1987.

CHAPTER 37

Pelvic Pain

Sharon K. Knight
Gary H. Lipscomb
Frank W. Ling

Pelvic pain is a common complaint among women seeking medical care. Pain that persists for longer than 6 months' duration is defined as chronic. After a prolonged period, patients often develop characteristics consistent with a *chronic pain syndrome,* including pain refractory to medical management or out of proportion to identified pathology; impaired physical function, including recreational, work, or sexual activity; signs of depression, such as sleep disturbance; or a change in family role.

The diagnostic and therapeutic approach to a patient with chronic pain is different than that for a patient with acute symptoms. Although rarely life threatening, chronic pelvic pain is potentially debilitating and can be a source of frustration for both patient and physician. A multidisciplinary or integrated approach is most appropriate.

EPIDEMIOLOGY AND PATHOPHYSIOLOGY

The prevalence of chronic pelvic pain is uncertain because of difficulties in obtaining such information, but an estimated 40% of women seeking primary care and 15% of all reproductive-age women have complaints of chronic pelvic pain. More than 50% of women with pelvic pain report not knowing the etiology of their pain. Pelvic pain is a frequent indication for gynecologic surgery, accounting for 12% of hysterectomies and up to 40% of laparoscopies. Thus this diagnosis may have a significant social and economic impact.

The pathophysiology of chronic pain is not completely understood, and several theories have been proposed. In the traditional *somatic model* of pain perception, tissue damage at the periphery causes stimulation of pain receptors, resulting in the perception of pain. This model explains acute pain well but is not appropriate for chronic pain. The *biopsychosocial model* postulates that a complex interaction of somatic symptoms with various psychosocial factors creates an outcome such as chronic pain. Potential contributing factors include the patient's response to pain, psychologic diagnoses and mood states, family patterns of pain response, and personal history of physical or sexual abuse.

Recent research has implicated a neurologic explanation for chronic pain. An afferent stimulus, such as pain, may cause permanent alterations to neurologic pathways at the level of the spinal cord, leading to altered responses to future stimuli that result in hyperalgesia, decreased pain threshold, or altered muscle response. Clinically these changes may be associated with chronic pain, recurrence of pain at previous sites of injury, resistance to therapy, or muscle spasm.

PATIENT EVALUATION

History

A complete history is essential for the proper evaluation of chronic pelvic pain. Initial questions should concern the basic qualities of the pain, including location, character, duration, frequency, patterns of radiation, and alleviating or aggravating factors. The physician notes the chronology of pain with changes over time and any relationship to menstrual cycle, sexual activity, bladder or bowel function, and emotional state. An extensive medical, gynecologic, obstetric, surgical, social, and family history includes previous diagnoses such as pelvic inflammatory disease (PID). The pain's effect on the patient's lifestyle and personal interactions should be determined; a pain or symptom diary may be helpful.

Box 37-1 lists the differential diagnoses of chronic pelvic pain using the classic gynecologic approach of dividing the pain into cyclic and noncyclic categories. The two lists are not mutually exclusive because conditions that generally produce cyclic pain may present with noncyclic pain, and vice versa. If the pain is cyclic, the physician obtains a detailed menstrual history, including age at menarche, quantification of amount of bleeding and interval, and regularity and number of days of bleeding. The physician should determine if the pain has been present since menarche or is a new phenomenon. A positive gastrointestinal, urologic, or musculoskeletal review of systems may provide insight into the etiology of pain or help guide the workup or management.

Box 37-1. Differential Diagnosis of Chronic Pelvic Pain

Cyclic

- Primary dysmenorrhea
- Secondary dysmenorrhea
  - Endometriosis
  - Adenomyosis
  - Endometritis
  - Cervical stenosis
  - Leiomyoma
- Premenstrual syndrome
- Ovarian remnant syndrome
- Pelvic congestion syndrome

Noncyclic

- Pelvic inflammatory disease
- Pelvic adhesions
- Symptomatic pelvic organ prolapse
- Pelvic pain without organic cause
- Musculoskeletal disorders
- Gastrointestinal disorders
- Urinary tract disorders
- Psychogenic factors

Physical Examination

A detailed and systematic physical examination should first note the patient's gait and sitting posture on the table. Poor posture, standing with weight mainly on one leg, or sitting primarily on one side may indicate a musculoskeletal cause.

Before the abdominal examination the patient should be asked to indicate the site of the pain with one finger. Gentle abdominal palpation begins at a site distant from the primary location of the pain while checking for masses or areas of tenderness. If an area of tenderness is located, the patient should be questioned about its similarity to the primary pain. Superficial palpation is critical to identifying musculoskeletal pain. During voluntary contraction of the abdominal musculature the patient is asked to place her chin on her chest and lift her legs slightly off the table. Pain that increases is typically musculoskeletal in origin, whereas pain that decreases is usually deep or visceral in origin; no change is equivocal.

Neurologic examination of the lower extremities may reveal abnormal reflexes, muscle weakness, or sensory findings. These may indicate a herniated disk or other neurologic cause, and more extensive neurologic evaluation may be necessary.

The pelvic examination should begin with visual inspection of the external genitalia. Gentle palpation with a moistened cotton-tip swab at the introitus and hymenal region may aid in identifying vulvar vestibulitis, a variant of pelvic pain that often presents as new-onset dyspareunia. A systematic one-handed (monomanual) pelvic examination should precede the traditional bimanual examination to help differentiate pelvic pain from abdominal wall pain. Initially the anterior vaginal wall should be palpated to assess for tenderness at the bladder base or urethra. The physician should also attempt to express discharge from the urethra. The examining fingers should then be turned posteriorly to palpate the levator ani muscles at approximately the 5 and 7 o'clock positions. Further palpation lateral and anterior to this area as well as cephalad and slightly lateral to the ischial spine aids in evaluation of the obturator internus and piriformis muscles, respectively. Systematic examination of these muscle groups aids in the diagnosis of pelvic floor muscle spasm, which may be a primary source of pain or a contributing factor to pain caused by other etiologies. The patient's ability to perform a voluntary pelvic floor contraction should be evaluated.

Pain caused by palpation of the cervix and adnexal regions or the presence of cervical motion tenderness should be assessed monomanually, followed by the traditional bimanual examination. Uterine size, mobility, and tenderness and the reproducibility of the primary complaint by uterine palpation provide important information if hysterectomy is subsequently considered. Similar information should be obtained regarding both adnexa. Rectovaginal examination is necessary to assess the uterosacral ligaments adequately and may delineate findings not obtained from vaginal examination alone. Visual inspection with a speculum should be done at the end so that other aspects are not altered by potential discomfort.

CYCLIC PAIN

An estimated 30% to 50% of reproductive-age women have cyclic pelvic pain, 10% to 15% of whom have symptoms severe enough to interfere with normal activities. Although the cyclic nature of pain implies a causal relationship with the female reproductive system, care must be taken to differentiate true menstrual-related symptoms from symptoms aggravated by body changes occurring during the menstrual cycle. The physician must also differentiate cyclic pain unrelated to the menstrual cycle from true dysmenorrhea.

Dysmenorrhea is broadly divided into two categories: primary and secondary. Secondary dysmenorrhea has a readily identifiable cause (e.g., fibroids, endometriosis), whereas primary dysmenorrhea has no identifiable cause.

Primary Dysmenorrhea

Most menstrual women experience some degree of primary dysmenorrhea at some time in their lives. The pain is characteristically sharp or cramplike and generally occurs in the first 3 days of menstruation. Pain is generally suprapubic but may radiate to the back, inner thighs, or deep pelvis. Nausea, with or without vomiting, and diarrhea may also occur. Dyspareunia, even during menstruation, is uncommon and should suggest other pathology. The diagnosis of primary dysmenorrhea is one of exclusion (i.e., no other abnormalities should suggest the cause of dysmenorrhea).

Patients with secondary dysmenorrhea often have other symptoms in addition to cyclic pain that suggest the underlying etiology. Heavy menstrual flow with dysmenorrhea suggests a diagnosis of uterine leiomyoma, adenomyosis, or endometrial polyps. Likewise, cyclic pain in a patient with primary amenorrhea suggests outflow obstruction. Gastrointestinal, urinary, or musculoskeletal complaints should raise the possibility of a nongynecologic process (see later discussions).

Laboratory studies are of limited use in the evaluation of patients with dysmenorrhea. Blood counts to assess blood loss in patients with excessive bleeding and sedimentation rates to identify a chronic inflammatory process are occasionally helpful. Ultrasound and other radiologic modalities rarely provide additional helpful information except when the physical examination is inadequate or is suspicious but not conclusive of a particular condition. Imaging techniques may even further confuse the diagnosis by identifying a small physiologic ovarian cyst or other benign process, which may result in additional unnecessary tests and, occasionally, unnecessary surgery.

Because the underlying pathophysiology in patients with primary dysmenorrhea is related to prostaglandin synthesis, the mainstay of treatment is nonsteroidal antiinflammatory drugs (NSAIDs). Although the chemical structures of the NSAIDs are similar, patients who have poor or partial response to one NSAID may respond well to a different agent.

Hormonal agents are frequently prescribed for dysmenorrhea. Oral contraceptives (OCs) are widely used for relief of primary dysmenorrhea in patients not desiring pregnancy. Since none appears to be superior to the others, physicians should use the OCs with which they are most familiar. Although OCs are generally prescribed on a 28-day cycle (21 days of hormone followed by 7 hormone-free days), they can be used continuously (no hormone-free days) in an attempt to produce amenorrhea if patients still have dysmenorrhea during withdrawal bleeding. Unfortunately, breakthrough bleeding is common and often limits the use of this regimen. Depo-Provera may also be used to induce hypomenorrhea or amenorrhea in these patients, but only 50% can be expected to become totally amenorrheic in the first year of use. Likewise, gonadotropin-releasing hormone (GnRH) agonists have been used to obtain amenorrhea, but their use is limited by the high cost of therapy and associated bone loss with long-term use. GnRH agonists for dysmenorrhea should probably be reserved for therapy of symptomatic endometriosis.

Although all these treatment modalities for primary dysmenorrhea may also be used for secondary dysmenorrhea, results are less satisfactory. Only specific therapy for the cause of secondary dysmenorrhea provides satisfactory results.

Secondary Dysmenorrhea

Endometriosis is one of the most common diagnoses for women with complaints of chronic pelvic pain. The classic symptoms associated with this condition include a longstanding history of dysmenorrhea, deep dyspareunia, and infertility. The dysmenorrhea often becomes progressively worse, lasts throughout menses, and begins premenstrually. Many women with endometriosis are asymptomatic. In women undergoing laparoscopic sterilization, one study found an equal incidence of endometriosis among those with and those without chronic pain.[2] Also, severity of pain correlates inconsistently with degree of endometriosis and may have an inverse relationship. Physical findings that suggest endometriosis include a fixed, poorly mobile uterus and tenderness, induration, or nodularity of uterosacral ligaments.

Adenomyosis is diagnosed histologically by the finding of endometrial glands and stroma infiltrating myometrial tissue. When symptomatic, adenomyosis typically presents as dysmenorrhea, menorrhagia, and central deep dyspareunia; it is a common incidental finding after hysterectomy. Pelvic examination may reveal a mildly enlarged, tender, globular, symmetric uterus. Similar symptoms may be associated with uterine leiomyoma; however, examination may differ with a greatly enlarged or asymmetrically enlarged uterus.

Pelvic congestion is another proposed etiology of chronic pain, with overdistention of pelvic vasculature causing pelvic discomfort. Clinical presentation includes secondary dysmenorrhea, which may worsen as the day progresses and with prolonged standing, menorrhagia, dyspareunia, and back pain. Varicosities may be visualized at surgery. Ultrasound and venography are suggested diagnostic tools.

Ovarian Remnant Syndrome

Ovarian remnant syndrome[4a,8] has been described in young women who have underdone surgical removal of both ovaries. This syndrome may occur when residual ovary is unintentionally left at the time of surgery, typically when the procedure required extensive or difficult dissection such as with endometriosis or pelvic inflammatory disease. The primary symptom is cyclic or constant chronic pelvic pain with or without a pelvic mass. Dyspareunia, urinary symptoms secondary to urethral obstruction, and dyschezia have been described. The patient may also report lack of menopausal symptoms. Examination may aid in the identification of a mass. FSH and LH levels are typically in a premenopausal range. Surgical excision of all functional ovarian tissue is the treatment of choice.

NONCYCLIC PAIN

Gynecologic Etiologies

In patients with a history of PID or pelvic surgery, adhesions are a potential source of chronic pain. Their role, however, is controversial; patients with chronic pelvic pain and pain-free controls have a comparable incidence of adhesions. Adhesions may be suspected with decreased mobility of pelvic organs or a sense of thickening, but adequate evaluation of adhesive disease severity by physical examination is difficult.

Pelvic organ prolapse may be associated with chronic pain. Patients with prolapse often report a sensation of pelvic pressure or heaviness ("something falling out") that increases as the day progresses and with standing. Discomfort may limit the patient's ability to perform normal daily activities and is often relieved by the supine position. Pelvic examination should include an assessment of the position of the cervix or vaginal vault as well as the anterior and posterior vagina during Valsalva's maneuver. Placement of a pessary may be a therapeutic as well as a diagnostic measure to determine if the pain improves when the prolapse is reduced. Surgical therapy may also be corrective.

Nongynecologic Etiologies

Musculoskeletal Causes. The musculoskeletal system is the most common source of nongynecologic chronic pelvic pain. Unfortunately, the musculoskeletal evaluation is also the most frequently overlooked component in the patient evaluation. Factors that suggest a musculoskeletal source of chronic pelvic pain include poor posture, scoliosis, unilateral standing habits, marked lumbar lordosis, leg length discrepancy, abnormal gait, abdominal wall trigger points or tenderness, history of low back trauma, and a previous, normal laparoscopy. A thorough examination is especially important in diagnosing a potential musculoskeletal cause.

Slocumb[6] suggested that hypersensitive areas of the abdominal wall (trigger points) are the most common cause of pelvic pain. These trigger points are hyperirritable areas that are tender when compressed and may generate referred pain and tenderness. Trigger points typically develop after some muscle strain and can often be found within a taut band of skeletal muscle. Trigger points can respond dramatically to specific therapy. In his classic study, Slocumb[6] used trigger point injections of local anesthetic agents to treat 122 patients with chronic pelvic pain. More than 50% of patients became pain free, only 13 had surgery, and all those with only abdominal wall injections had a successful response. Those with vaginal trigger points had an 84.6% response rate to injections.

In the patient with demonstrable trigger points, injection with local anesthetic may be a useful therapeutic and diagnostic aid. A 1-inch to 1½-inch, 22-gauge needle is recommended for superficial musculature. Although smaller needles cause less discomfort on skin penetration, they are less able to disrupt a trigger point mechanically. Smaller needles may also be too flexible, sliding around taut muscle bands and masking tactile clues. Trigger points are injected using aseptic technique. The patient may feel a muscle twitch or flash of referred pain during insertion. The palpating finger should maintain tension on the skin as various injection tracts are made. If a trigger point is not identified directly, the injection may be less effective but still useful diagnostically. Successful injection results in loss of tenderness and, if originally present, relaxation of the tight muscle band.

Although any local anesthetic may be used for trigger point injections, bupivacaine 0.25% is our agent of choice. Volumes of 10 ml or less are usually adequate to produce a clear diagnostic test. Interestingly, pain relief often extends far beyond the drug's normal duration of action and is frequently longer with subsequent injections, which may indicate recovery of normal muscle and nerve function. Relief of pain after trigger point injection shows the patient her pain is at least partially musculoskeletal and not necessarily from gynecologic causes. Trigger point injections can be diagnostic and also therapeutic, either alone or as a series of injections.[6] Trigger point injections should be viewed as helpful adjuncts in an overall management plan.

Levator ani and pelvic floor muscle spasms are other frequently overlooked causes of pelvic pain. Careful monomanual examination may reveal evidence of this syndrome. Patients with other sources of pelvic pain in turn may develop spasm of pelvic floor musculature as an additional source of pain.

Physical therapy, when included in a multidisciplinary approach, has been very successful in managing patients with chronic pelvic pain due to musculoskeletal causes. Referral to a physical therapist for further evaluation or more intensive physical therapy instruction is frequently helpful. If referral is unavailable or not practical, NSAIDs, muscle relaxants, and heat application may be effective. Initial use of these agents on a scheduled rather than an as-needed basis for the first 1 to 2 weeks of treatment is recommended. These medications may also be used in conjunction with physical therapy. Newer nerve stimulation therapies have shown promise as potential therapeutic options.

Gastrointestinal Causes. Up to 60% of patients referred for chronic pelvic pain may have gastrointestinal (GI) symptoms, particularly irritable bowel syndrome. Because of the visceral innervation of the bowel, it is often difficult to differentiate lower abdominal pain of gynecologic origin from that of GI origin. A careful history, especially bowel habits, may reveal details that suggest a GI etiology. Abdominal pain associated with irritable bowel syndrome characteristically improves after a bowel movement and is often worse with eating. Other common symptoms include a sense of rectal fullness or incomplete rectal evacuation, passage of pelletlike stools, and exacerbation of pain during stress. Although dyspareunia is frequently gynecologic in origin, many women with an irritable bowel also have dyspareunia.

The physical examination should always include a rectal examination and testing for occult blood. Tenderness localized over the sigmoid colon in the absence of inflammatory signs is frequently present in patients with irritable bowel syndrome, whereas a tender mass in the left lower quadrant in a febrile patient suggests diverticulitis. No known detectable structural or biochemical abnormality is associated with irritable bowel syndrome, but activation of hypersensitive receptors in the bowel wall due to physiologic distention or contraction may be responsible for the pain. The conscious threshold for perception of visceral sensation in the form of pain may be altered in patients with irritable bowel syndrome. Many women have coexisting psychopathology, such as somatization disorders, anxiety disorders, depression, and other psychologic syndromes.

Current medical treatment for irritable bowel syndrome is generally unsatisfactory; 30% to 70% of patients have continued symptoms even after long-term treatment. Treatment consists primarily of reassurance, education, stress reduction, bulk-forming agents, anxiolytics, and low-dose tricyclic antidepressants; bulk formers are the most effective therapy. Anticholinergics are generally ineffective. Multidisciplinary pain management is often appropriate for these patients, as for any patient with chronic pelvic pain.

Urinary Tract Causes. Because the urinary and gynecologic tracts share a complex neurologic system, pain originating from the urinary tract may be difficult to differentiate from gynecologic pain. Thus questions regarding urinary frequency, urgency, nocturia, dysuria, hematuria, incontinence, voiding difficulty, and previous urologic workup are important, particularly if the gynecologic evaluation is inconclusive. Potential urinary tract causes of chronic pelvic pain include interstitial cystitis, urethral syndrome, urethral diverticulum, urolithiasis of the bladder or lower ureter, radiation cystitis, urethral caruncle, and neoplasm. Initial tests should include a urinalysis with culture and sensitivity to rule out microbiologic sources. A 24-hour voiding diary may provide more accurate assessment of the patient's symptoms.

Generally, cystourethroscopy should be performed in patients with irritative voiding symptoms (urgency, frequency) or hematuria. This procedure allows evaluation of the urethra and the bladder mucosa for evidence of chronic infection, bladder stones, tumors, or diverticula. These diagnoses must be ruled out before the chronic pain syndromes, interstitial cystitis and urethral syndrome, are considered.

Interstitial cystitis is a chronic idiopathic bladder syndrome characterized by irritative voiding symptoms, no objective evidence for another disease process (diagnosis of exclusion), and a characteristic cystoscopic appearance. Significant findings at the time of cystoscopy include the classic Hunner's ulcer (velvety red patch, present in only 6% to 8% of cases), linear submucosal hemorrhages (glomerulations), and a reduced bladder capacity under anesthesia. Prevalence estimates range from 10 to 500/100,000. The majority of patients are Caucasian females between the ages of 40 and 48 years. Examination may reveal tenderness at the bladder base, urethra, or suprapubic region. However, no findings are pathognomonic. When this diagnosis is suspected by history and office evaluation, a double fill cystoscopy may be helpful. This involves passive hydrodistention of the bladder under anesthesia. After 2 to 5 minutes, the bladder is drained and once again hydrodistention is performed to maximum capacity. The bladder is then inspected for the characteristic findings previously discussed. Hydrodistention may be therapeutic in up to 60% of patients. Proposed etiologies and attempted therapies are numerous. Therapies targeted at the level of the glycosaminoglycan layer have been used most frequently. This layer forms a protective "blood-urine" barrier at the bladder mucosa, which prevents adherence of bacteria and crystals, as well as transfer of solutes into the urine. Dimethylsulfoxide (DMSO) is an intravesical therapy targeted at this level, with success rates ranging from 34% to 40%. Pentosanpolysulfate (elmiron) is an oral heparin analog also targeted to this level. Initial success with elmiron was promising; however, long-term success has been disappointing, ranging from 6% to 19%. Currently neuromodulation-based therapies are under study and may represent the direction of future therapy.

Urethral syndrome is also a diagnosis of exclusion. Although good epidemiologic data are lacking, it is thought primarily to affect reproductive-age females. Dysuria, voiding dysfunction, and particularly, postcoital voiding dysfunction are common complaints in addition to irritative voiding symptoms. Multiple etiologies have been proposed, including chronic urethritis with inflammation of the urethral glands, hypoestrogenism, and urethral spasm. Cystourethroscopy and urodynamic testing may contribute to the diagnosis. Therapies are aimed at these proposed causes and include suppressive antibiotic therapy, urethral dilation, local estrogen therapy, skeletal muscle relaxants, α-blockers, biofeedback, and nerve stimulation therapy.

Because these patients with interstitial cystitis or urethral syndrome present a confusing or changing clinical picture, consultation with a urologist or urogynecologist may be extremely helpful.

History of Abuse. Multiple studies have attempted to evaluate the relationship between chronic pelvic pain and sexual or physical abuse. It is difficult to compare these results because of differences in study design and definition of abuse. Most studies, however, show an overall increased rate of abuse among women with chronic pelvic pain compared with pain-free controls. One study reported that women with chronic pelvic pain had significantly higher rates of previous sexual abuse compared with pain-free subjects or women with chronic pain at other sites.[3] In general, abuse prevalence rates are approximately 50% in chronic pelvic pain patients vs. 20% in control groups.

Evaluation of a patient with chronic pelvic pain should include a physical and sexual abuse history. Even if the patient is unable to discuss such issues at the first interview, disclosure may take place in the future. Knowledge of an abuse history enables the physician to guide the patient to appropriate counseling or support services.

Psychiatric Issues. Depression coexists with chronic pain in up to 50% of patients. The cause-and-effect relationship of these conditions has been debated; some even suggest that these diagnoses should be considered a single entity. Regardless, it is important to recognize and treat depression when present. Such therapy, although not curative, is an important adjunct to other therapies. After treatment for depression, the patient may feel better overall and respond better to other attempted therapies.

Multiple pharmacologic choices for therapy are available. Selective serotonin reuptake inhibitors (SSRIs) have gained popularity because of their favorable side effect profile. Antidepressants such as imipramine (a tricyclic antidepressant) and amitriptyline (a MAO inhibitor), however, have the added effect of pain relief through a neurologic mechanism. One common side effect of many antidepressant medications is sexual dysfunction, which may already be an issue for many women with chronic pelvic pain.

Psychiatric consultation should be considered if the patient has a history of inadequately treated depression, other psychiatric conditions, suicidal ideation, or failure of single-drug treatment regimens. A common psychiatric manifestation in patients with chronic pelvic pain is *somatization,* in which emotional problems are expressed as physical symptoms[1] (see Chapter 50). These symptoms may cause significant distress but are not fully explained by clinical findings. Principles of management of somatizing patients are based on their ongoing needs for sanctioned caregiving and include the following:

1. Schedule set amounts of time and intervals for physician visits. Do not vary time of visits or make contact contingent on symptoms.
2. Accept the patient's need to be considered ill, realizing that some patients may be threatened by the prospect of complete cure or relief.
3. Ask open-ended questions to allow the patient to structure the discussion.
4. Minimize secondary gain (e.g., time off work, disability pay).
5. Recognize and control personal reactions (frustration, anger) toward patients.
6. Remain alert for intercurrent illness.

MANAGEMENT

Nonsurgical treatments for potential etiologies of chronic pelvic pain are discussed earlier (Box 37-2); this section focuses on surgical options. Surgery is often a logical extension of a thorough diagnostic and therapeutic management scheme in patients who have chronic pelvic pain. For the nonsurgically trained physician, this requires referral to a specialist.

Box 37-2. First-line Therapies For Chronic Pelvic Pain

- General measures
  - Multidisciplinary management
  - Antidepressants
- Primary dysmenorrhea
  - NSAIDs
  - OCs
- Secondary dysmenorrhea
  - NSAIDs
  - OCs
  - Specific therapy for cause
- Irritable bowel syndrome
  - Bulk-forming agents
- Musculoskeletal pain
  - Physical therapy
  - Trigger point injections
  - NSAIDs
- Urinary tract
  - Interstitial cystitis
    - Hydrodistention
    - Intravesical therapies
  - Urethral syndrome
    - Suppressive antibiotics
    - Local estrogen therapy
    - Urethral dilation
    - Skeletal muscle relaxants, α-blockers

NSAIDs, Nonsteroidal antiinflammatory drugs; *OCs,* oral contraceptives.

Diagnostic Laparoscopy

The traditional gynecologic approach to chronic pelvic pain has included diagnostic laparoscopy for all patients. The need for this procedure is debated. A prospective randomized study showed no benefit of laparoscopy in diagnosis or success of therapy compared with a multidisciplinary approach that did not include laparoscopy.[4] Several studies have shown similar rates of pathology (e.g., adhesive disease, endometriosis) in patients with chronic pelvic pain and pain-free patients undergoing laparoscopy for other indications. Therefore the decision to proceed with diagnostic laparoscopy is the physician's choice. Since approximately 30% of patients with chronic pelvic pain will have normal findings at laparoscopy, a plan for further management of these patients must be developed.

Adhesiolysis

Surgical lysis of adhesions either through the laparoscope or by laparotomy appears to be the logical therapy for patients with documented adhesive disease from PID. Unfortunately, no evidence indicates that adhesions are always a cause of such pelvic pain. Only a small percentage of patients with chronic pelvic pain have documented adhesive disease, and as noted, studies show a comparable incidence of adhesions in patients and controls. Success rates range from almost no success (except in subsets of patients with significant bowel involvement) to 65% complete or partial improvement. Patients considering adhesiolysis should be informed that (1) adhesions are present but may not be the cause of pain; (2) they may not obtain relief with the procedure, or the pain may become worse; and (3) adhesions may re-form and result in further pain. The patient should also know the risks associated with the surgery.

Nerve Ablation Procedures

Uterosacral nerve ablation has a limited role in the treatment of chronic pelvic pain and is only indicated as a second line of therapy for dysmenorrhea. The purpose is transection of afferent fibers within the uterosacral ligaments. Assessment of pain relief with injection of local anesthetic at the uterosacral ligaments should be performed before ablation. The procedure can potentially be performed at laparoscopy if no other pathology is found. Long-term complications are not defined.

Presacral neurectomy has been proposed as a potential therapy for dysmenorrhea, dyspareunia, chronic central pelvic pain, and sacral backache. The primary indication is unsuccessful medical management of primary dysmenorrhea; success rates are 70% to 80%.

Uterine Suspension

Uterine retrodisplacement may be associated with pelvic pain. Since up to one third of all women may have a retroverted uterus, this finding in itself is not an indication for uterine suspension. Typical symptoms include pelvic pressure, low back pain, and deep dyspareunia. If pain related to retrodisplacement is suspected, a trial of therapy with a Smith-Hodge pessary to antevert the uterus should be undertaken. If pain is relieved, a uterine suspension is a potential therapeutic option. In a patient who no longer desires fertility, vaginal hysterectomy is another option.

Ovarian Remnant Removal

After surgical removal of the uterus and ovaries, cyclic pain from an ovarian remnant may develop (ovarian remnant syndrome). This typically occurs after oophorectomy during difficult surgeries for endometriosis or adhesive disease. In younger patients this diagnosis may be suspected if follicle-stimulating hormone levels are not elevated. Radiologic procedures (e.g., computed tomography scan, ultrasound) may be helpful in making the diagnosis. Patients may obtain relief with surgical removal of the remnant, but the procedure may be technically challenging.

Hysterectomy

Chronic pelvic pain is the third most common indication for hysterectomy and accounts for approximately 15% of all hysterectomies performed. Hysterectomy should be reserved for patients who have failed conservative therapy. Although no randomized prospective studies have assessed success rates of hysterectomy for chronic pelvic pain, one study[9] reported a 75% cure rate at 6 months in women who had a hysterectomy for central pelvic pain.

Integrated Approach

A multidisciplinary approach that includes gynecology, gastroenterology, urology/urogynecology, anesthesiology, psychiatry, and physiotherapy in a single geographic site, such as a pain clinic, is ideal for management of patients with chronic pelvic pain. Multiple studies have noted increased success rates with such an approach. If these resources are not available, an integrated approach using appropriate consultants is acceptable. Certain aspects of an integrated approach, such as psychiatric consultation, are more likely to be accepted by patients when introduced at an early time and as a routine part of management.[5,7]

REFERENCES

1. Badura AS et al: Dissociation, somatization, substance abuse, and coping in women with chronic pelvic pain, *Obstet Gynecol* 90:405, 1997.
2. Balasch J, Creus M, Fabregues F, et al: Visible and nonvisible endometriosis at laparoscopy in fertile and infertile women and in patients with chronic pelvic pain: a prospective study, *Hum Reprod* 11(2):387-391, 1996.
3. Collet BJ, Cordle CJ, Stewart CR, et al: A comparative study of women with chronic pelvic pain, chronic nonpelvic pain, and those with no history of pain attending general practitioners, *Br J Obstet Gynecol* 105(12):1338-1339, 1998.
4. Peters AAW et al: A randomized clinical trial to compare two different approaches in women with chronic pelvic pain, *Obstet Gynecol* 77:740, 1991.

4a. Price FV, et al: Ovarian remnant syndrome: difficulties in diagnosis and management, *Obstet Gynecol Surv* 45(3):151-156, 1990.

5. Reiter RC: Evidence-based management of chronic pelvic pain, *Clin Obstet Gynecol* 41:422, 1998.
6. Slocumb J: Neurologic factors in chronic pelvic pain: trigger points and the abdominal pelvic pain syndrome, *Am J Obstet Gynecol* 149:536, 1984.
7. Steege JF et al: *Chronic pelvic pain: an integrated approach*, Philadelphia, 1998, Saunders.
8. Steege JF: Ovarian remnant syndrome, *Obstet Gynecol* 70:64, 1987.
9. Stovall TG, Ling FW, Crawford DA: Hysterectomy for chronic pelvic pain of presumed uterine etiology, *Obstet Gynecol* 75(4):676-679, 1990.

CHAPTER 38

Contraceptive Choices

Andrew M. Kaunitz

Half of all pregnancies in the United States are unintended, and about 1.4 million induced abortions are performed annually in U.S. women.[1] Primary care physicians can play an important role in encouraging their patients to use effective methods of contraception. Unfortunately, no single method is ideal for all patients. Therefore physicians must consider such factors as overall effectiveness, patient compliance, and side effects as they help their patients make prudent contraceptive choices. This chapter reviews oral, injectable, implantable, intrauterine, barrier, and periodic abstinence contraception, focusing on approaches that help candidates select appropriate methods and management measures that maximize contraceptive efficacy and patient satisfaction.

Among U.S. women of reproductive age, approximately 64% used some form of contraception in 1995 (Fig. 38-1).[8] The most popular method, used by 27.7% of women practicing contraception, was female sterilization. The next most common method was combination oral contraceptives (OCs), used by 26.9%. Approximately 21% used condoms for contraception, 3% used depot medroxyprogesterone acetate injections, 1.3% implants, and 0.8% intrauterine devices. Table 38-1 lists rates for first-year contraceptive failure and continuation.

ORAL CONTRACEPTIVES

Since they first were marketed in the 1960s, the dose of sex steroids in combination OCs has dramatically declined. The highest-dose formulations now available contain 50 μg of ethinyl estradiol, and most currently prescribed OCs contain 30 or 35 μg. Formulations with 20 μg of estrogen represent the lowest-dose estrogen combination OCs currently available (Table 38-2). Monophasic OCs contain a constant dose of both estrogen and progestin in each of the 21 active tablets. Phasic OCs alter the progestin and/or estrogen dose among the 21 active tablets in an effort to minimize total steroid dose, as well as metabolic and side effects, while maintaining contraceptive efficacy.

Most contraindications to combination OCs relate to their estrogen component (Box 38-1). Progestin-only OCs ("minipills," POPs) do not contain estrogen, with all the 28 tablets in each pack containing hormone. Because POPs contain progestins in even lower doses than combination OCs, failure rates with POPs are somewhat higher than with combination OCs.[10] POPs, along with progestin-only injections and implants (see later sections), are well suited for use by lactating and older reproductive-age women with cardiovascular risk factors, two relatively less fertile groups for whom contraceptive doses of estrogen are contraindicated (Box 38-2). Contraceptive recommendations for women with medical problems are available.[6]

Mechanism of Action. Combination OCs prevent ovulation by inhibiting gonadotropin secretion. The progestin

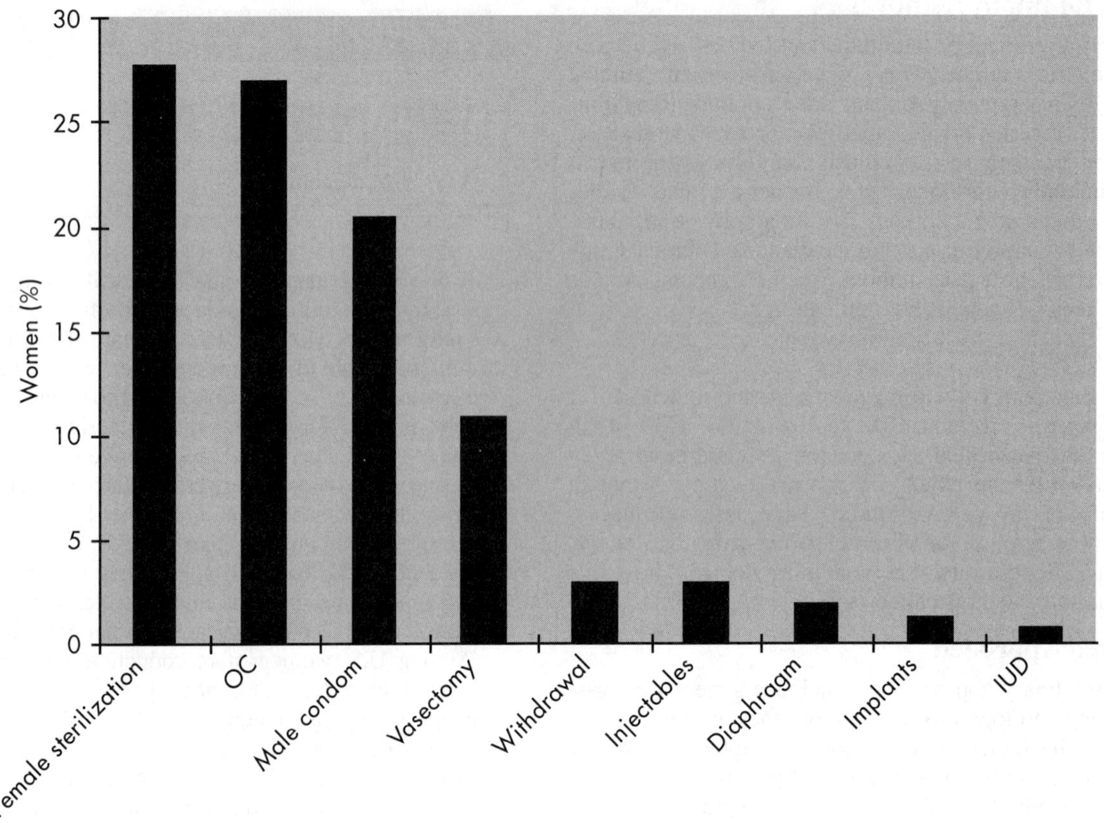

Fig. 38-1. Contraceptive use by U.S. women, ages 15-44. *OCs,* Oral contraceptives; *IUD,* intrauterine device. (Modified from Piccinino LJ, Mosher WD: *Fam Plann Perspect* 30;4, 1998.)

Table 38-1. First-year Contraceptive Failure (Unintended Pregnancy) and Continuation Rates in U.S. Women (%)

Method	Lowest expected rate	Typical rate	Continuation rate
None	85	85	
Spermicides	6	26	40
Periodic abstinence	1 to 9	25	63
Withdrawal	4	19	
Cervical cap			
Parous	26	40	42
Nulliparous	9	20	56
Diaphragm	6	20	56
Condom			
Female (Reality)	5	21	56
Male	3	14	61
Combination OCs	0.1	3	71
Progestin-only OCs	0.5	3	71
Progesterone T IUD	1.5	2	81
Copper T 380A IUD	0.6	0.8	78
Depo-Provera	0.3	0.3	70
Norplant (6 capsules)	0.05	0.05	88
Female sterilization	0.5	0.5	100
Male sterilization	0.1	0.15	100

Modified from Trussel J: Contraceptive efficacy. In Hatcher RA, Stewart F, Trussel J, et al, editors: *Contraceptive technology,* ed 17, New York, 1998, Ardent Media.
OCs, Oral contraceptives; *IUD,* intrauterine device.

suppresses luteinizing hormone (LH) secretion, and the estrogen component suppresses follicle-stimulating hormone (FSH) secretion, preventing selection of a dominant follicle. The estrogen component also stabilizes the endometrium, thereby minimizing breakthrough bleeding. The progestin component also thickens the cervical mucus, minimizing entry of sperm into the endometrial cavity.

The substantially lower progestin doses of POPs blunt but do not totally eliminate midcycle LH peaks, with ovulation sometimes occurring in POP users. The effects of the POP on cervical mucus last about 20 hours, so meticulous pill taking is crucial to ensure high contraceptive efficacy. When a woman takes her POP more than 3 hours late, a backup method of contraception, such as condoms or a spermicide, should be used for the next 48 hours.

Initiation and Use. When OCs are initiated on either the first day of menses or the first Sunday after menses starts, backup contraception is unnecessary. Associating pill taking with a daily ritual, such as tooth brushing, may enhance compliance. If one or two tablets are missed, the patient should take one tablet as soon as possible, then one tablet twice a day until all the missed tablets are taken. If three or more tablets have been missed, backup contraception should be used until the current pack is completed.

Side Effects. As with all hormonal contraceptives, OC side effects represent the major cause of noncompliance and discontinuation. Because breast tenderness and nausea are common estrogen-related side effects, physicians may

Table 38-2. Oral Contraceptive Formulations Available in the United States

	Name	Estrogen	Progestin	Mg
50 μg estrogen				
Monophasic	Norlestrin 1/50	EE	Norethindrone acetate	1.0
	Norlestrin 2.5/50	EE	Norethindrone acetate	2.5
	Ovcon 50*	EE	Norethindrone	1.0
	Ortho-Novum 1/50	Mestranol	Norethindrone	1.0
	Norinyl 1 + 50	Mestranol	Norethindrone	1.0
	Demulen	EE	Ethynodiol diacetate	1.0
	Ovral	EE	Norgestrel	0.5
35 μg EE				
Monophasic	Modicon*	EE	Norethindrone	0.5
	Brevicon*	EE	Norethindrone	0.5
	Ovcon 35*	EE	Norethindrone	0.4
	Ortho-Cyclen	EE	Norgestimate	0.25
	Demulen 1/35*	EE	Ethynodiol diacetate	1.0
	Ortho-Novum 1/35*	EE	Norethindrone	1.0
	Norinyl 1 + 35*	EE	Norethindrone	1.0
Biphasic	Ortho-Novum 10/11*	EE	Norethindrone	0.5/1.0
Triphasic	Ortho-Novum 7/7/7	EE	Norethindrone	0.5/0.75/1.0
	Ortho-Tri-cyclen†	EE	Norgestimate	0.18/0.215/0.25
	Trinorinyl	EE	Norethindrone	0.5/1.0/0.5
	Estrostep	EE 20/30/35	Norethindrone acetate	1.0
30 μg EE				
	Loestrin 1.5/30	EE	Norethindrone acetate	1.5
Monophasic	Ortho-Cept	EE	Desogestrel	0.15
	Desogen	EE	Desogestrel	0.15
	Lo-Ovral	EE	Norgestrel	0.15
	Nordette*	EE	Levonorgestrel	0.15
	Levlen*	EE	Levonorgestrel	0.15
Triphasic	Triphasil*	EE 30/40/30	Levonorgestrel	0.05/0.075/0.125
	Tri-Levlen*	EE 30/40/30	Levonorgestrel	0.05/0.075/0.125
20 μg EE				
Monophasic	Loestrin 1/20	EE	Norethindrone acetate	1.0
	Levlite	EE	Levonorgestrel	0.1
	Alesse	EE	Levonorgestrel	0.1
	Mircette‡	EE	Desogestrel	0.15
Progestin-only OCs				
Monophasic	Micronor	—	Norethindrone	0.35
	Nor-QD	—	Norethindrone	0.35
	Ovrette	—	Norgestrel	0.075

EE, Ethinyl estradiol.
*Generic versions also available.
†Indicated for treatment of acne as well as contraception.
‡Also includes 5 tablets containing 10 μg EE.

consider prescribing 20-μg estrogen OCs when these side effects persist for more than several months. Breakthrough bleeding occurs in up to one third of women during their first 3 months of OC use, subsequently becoming less common. Rates of breakthrough bleeding are higher among women using 20-μg estrogen than those using 30- or 35-μg formulations.[3] The new onset of intermenstrual bleeding after 3 months of OC use should alert physicians to noniatrogenic causes, such as cervical infection or neoplasia. Once these conditions are excluded, oral estrogen (e.g., 1.25 mg of conjugated estrogen, esterified estrogen, or estropipate; 1 to 2 mg of estradiol) can be taken with each active OC tablet to minimize breakthrough bleeding caused by progestin-induced changes.

Amenorrhea caused by progestin-induced endometrial changes may result after long-term OC use, with resulting patient anxiety about possible pregnancy. Many physicians and users believe that OC use causes weight gain and

Box 38-1. Contraindications to Use of Combination Oral Contraceptives

Smokers over age 35 years
Thrombophlebitis, thromboembolic disorders, cerebrovascular disease, coronary artery disease
Greatly impaired liver function
Known or suspected breast cancer
Undiagnosed abnormal vaginal bleeding
Known or suspected pregnancy

Box 38-2. Clinical Settings for Progestin-only Contraceptives

Smokers older than age 35
Vascular disease associated with diabetes or lupus
Coronary artery disease
Congestive heart failure
Cerebrovascular disease
Complicated migraine headaches
- With focal neurologic phenomena
- Intensified during combination OC use

Increased risk of thromboembolism
Diabetes
Lipid disorders, including hypertriglyceridemia
Postpartum (partially or not breast-feeding within 3 weeks postpartum)
Fully breast-feeding (begin 6 weeks postpartum)
When combination OCs cause persistent estrogen-related side effects

headaches. A recent randomized placebo-controlled trial, however, found that rates of these "side effects" among women using an OC containing 35 μg of ethinyl estradiol combined with the new progestin norgestimate were nearly identical to those taking placebos.[8a]

Health Risks. The estrogen component of combination OCs increases hepatic production of serum clotting factors, particularly factors I (fibrinogen), VII, and X. With use of OCs formulated with less than 50 μg of ethinyl estradiol, the risk of venous thromboembolism (VTE) is three to four times that of nonusers. Accordingly, women with a history of thromboembolism should not use combination OCs. To place this risk in perspective, pregnancy is associated with a VTE risk six times higher than in nonpregnant, non-OC-using women. Epidemiologic data do not suggest that VTE risk is lower with 20-μg estrogen formulations compared with 30 to 35 μg. Although initial data suggested that VTE risk was higher with OCs containing the newer progestin desogestrel, subsequent studies have not confirmed such differential risk.

Box 38-3. Hepatic Enzyme–inducing Medications that May Impair Efficacy of Oral and Implantable Contraceptives

Carbamazepine
Felbamate
Phenobarbital
Phenytoin
Primidone
Rifampin
Topiramate

Combination OC use, even long term, does not cause atherosclerosis. Likewise, the risk of myocardial infarction or stroke does not appear increased among healthy, nonsmoking women using OCs formulated with less than 50 μg of estrogen.[3] Because OC use and smoking synergistically increase myocardial infarction risk, women age 35 and older who smoke should not use combination OCs.

Fears regarding breast cancer prevent many women from using OCs. A massive reanalysis has clarified associations between OC use and breast cancer. Ten or more years after discontinuing OCs, breast cancer risk is the same in ever-users and never-users of OCs. A modestly increased breast cancer risk noted in current and recent OC users may reflect increased screening in this population of women.[3] Although OCs may increase risk of cervical adenocarcinoma, well-controlled studies have not found an increased risk of the more common squamous cell cervical cancer among OC users. Likewise, OC use has not been noted to impact the natural history of cervical human papillomavirus infection. As with all sexually active women, regular cytology screening is appropriate in women using hormonal contraception. A history of cervical intraepithelial neoplasia does not contraindicate OC use.

Concomitant Medications. Certain anticonvulsants, as well as the antibiotic rifampin, may reduce the efficacy of OCs, particularly POPs (Box 38-3). The anticonvulsant valproic acid and the antibiotics doxycycline, tetracycline, metronidazole, and ampicillin do not appear to reduce OC efficacy.

Noncontraceptive Benefits and Therapeutic Uses. Prevention of endometrial and ovarian cancer represents the most important noncontraceptive benefit of OC use. Because this protection persists for at least two decades after discontinuing pills, OC users in their late 30s and 40s can reduce their risk of being diagnosed with these malignancies during those decades of life when they would otherwise experience their highest lifetime risk of these cancers (Boxes 38-4 and 38-5).[3]

Use in Perimenopausal Women. Use of combination OCs is safe in healthy nonsmoking women of any reproductive age. U.S. women in their 40s are increasingly taking advantage of the effective contraceptive protection offered by OCs. In addition, perimenopausal women benefit

Box 38-4. Noncontraceptive Health Benefits of Oral Contraceptives

Prevention

Endometrial cancer
Ovarian cancer
Ovulatory pain
Functional ovarian cysts
Ectopic pregnancy
Pelvic inflammatory disease
Loss of bone mineral density

Menstrual Improvement

Regular cycles
Less flow
Less dysmenorrhea

Box 38-5. Therapeutic Uses* of Oral Contraceptives

Hypothalamic amenorrhea
Premature ovarian failure
Functional ovarian cysts
Chronic anovulation
Hirsutism
Acne?
Endometriosis
Control of bleeding in women with blood dyscrasias
Menorrhagia and dysmenorrhea (including when associated with uterine leiomyomata)

*Use of OCs for indications other than contraception represents off-label use not approved by the U.S. Food and Drug Administration (FDA).
†Triphasic norgestimate/ethinyl estradiol (Ortho-Tri-cyclen) is approved for treatment of acne.

from the regularization of menses, relief from vasomotor symptoms, and positive impact on bone mineral density offered by combination OCs. Because gonadotropin levels fluctuate in perimenopausal women, assessment of FSH levels to determine when older OC users no longer need contraception is expensive and may be misleading. A preferable approach is to continue having healthy nonsmoking women take combination OCs into their middle 50s. At this time, the likelihood of ovulation is low; hormonal replacement therapy can be initiated in such women on an individualized basis.

POSTCOITAL OR EMERGENCY CONTRACEPTION

About half the unintended pregnancies in the United States occur in women not using contraception. Emergency contraception (EC), commonly referred to as the "morning-after pill" or postcoital contraception, is a method of preventing pregnancy after unprotected sexual intercourse. The best studied and most commonly used EC method in the United States is the *Yuzpe regimen,* consisting of 0.1 mg of ethinyl estradiol and 1.0 mg of DL-norgestrel (two Ovral tablets; see Table 38-2) taken within 72 hours of unprotected intercourse, with a second dose taken 12 hours later. Recent U.S. Food and Drug Administration (FDA) approval of an EC kit containing a urine pregnancy test and four tablets (Preven) facilitates use of the Yuzpe regimen. The most common side effect of EC is nausea and vomiting; an antiemetic taken 1 hour before each dose may reduce this side effect. Use of POPs can provide effective EC without estrogen-induced nausea; this approach utilizes one Plan B tablet or 20 75-μg norgestrel tablets (Ovrette), with this dose then repeated in 12 hours.

INJECTABLE CONTRACEPTIVES

Depot medroxyprogesterone acetate (DMPA) is marketed in the United States as Depo-Provera, a 150-mg solution of aqueous microcrystals administered by deep intramuscular injection every 3 months.[2] A new drug application has been filed with the FDA for a monthly contraceptive injection combining 25 mg of medroxyprogesterone acetate with 5 mg of estradiol cypionate (Lunelle).[5]

Mechanism of Action. DMPA provides highly effective contraception by blocking the LH surge and preventing ovulation.

Initiation and Use. When DMPA is initiated within 5 days of the onset of menses, backup contraception is unnecessary. After initial or subsequent injections, ovulation does not occur for at least 14 weeks, allowing a 2-week grace period when 3-month injection intervals are followed. For women more than 2 weeks late for their reinjection, pregnancy should be ruled out before reinjection and backup contraception used for 1 week subsequently.[2] Depo-Provera package labeling states that pregnancy should be excluded in women more than 1 week late for reinjection. Fortunately, contraceptive doses of DMPA inadvertently administered during pregnancy do not appear to result in increased risk of congenital anomalies.

Side Effects. Menstrual changes occur in all women using DMPA. Episodes of unpredictable, irregular bleeding and spotting lasting 7 or more days typically occur in the first months of use. With increasing duration of use, frequency and duration of these episodes decrease, and amenorrhea becomes common. After four injections of DMPA, half of women report amenorrhea, with this percentage increasing to more than three fourths with longer use. Based on unrealistic expectations of immediate amenorrhea, users may prematurely discontinue their contraceptive injections after experiencing unpredictable spotting and bleeding. Candid counseling before the first injection, as well as supportive follow-up measures, can enhance injectable contraceptive continuation. If reassurance is not sufficient to encourage women experiencing menstrual changes to continue DMPA, persistent, irregular bleeding can be treated with continuous daily oral estrogen supplementation (as described earlier for OC breakthrough bleeding). After the discontinuation of supplemental estrogen, however, the bleeding may return. Possible side effects from DMPA include bloating, alopecia, and reduced libido. Although anecdotal observations had suggested that DMPA use might cause weight gain and depressive symptoms, recently published well-controlled studies have not confirmed this.

Return to Fertility. Return to fertility can be delayed after discontinuing DMPA. Within 10 months of the last injection, half of women who have discontinued DMPA to become pregnant will have conceived. Fertility does not return in some women for up to 18 months after the last injection, however, underscoring that DMPA is not an appropriate choice for women who may want to conceive in the next 1 or 2 years.

Health Risks. Use of DMPA is associated with modest suppression of ovarian estradiol production. Although earlier studies suggested that users experience a reversible decline in bone mineral density, larger recent studies have not consistently confirmed this concern. As in all reproductive-age women, appropriate calcium intake should be encouraged. Because adolescent DMPA users and women who use DMPA for more than 5 years continuously may be at increased risk for low bone mineral density, estrogen supplementation (i.e., conjugated estrogen 1.25 mg daily or its equivalent) can be used along with DMPA. Levels of high-density lipoproteins have been found to be lower in DMPA users. World Health Organization studies have found that DMPA does not affect cervical or ovarian cancer risk but greatly reduces endometrial cancer risk. DMPA's impact on breast cancer risk appears similar to that of OCs.[2]

Noncontraceptive Benefits and Therapeutic Uses. Boxes 38-6 and 38-7 list noncontraceptive benefits and therapeutic uses of DMPA. Concomitant use of liver enzyme–inducing medications has not been demonstrated to impair DMPA effectiveness (see Box 38-3). Since DMPA has intrinsic anticonvulsant properties, some believe it should be the contraceptive of choice for women with seizure disorders.

Box 38-6. Preventive Benefits of Depot Medroxyprogesterone Acetate

Iron deficiency anemia
Pelvic inflammatory disease
Ectopic pregnancy
Endometrial cancer
Hysterectomy in women with uterine leiomyomata

Box 38-7. Therapeutic Uses* of Depot Medroxyprogesterone Acetate

Menorrhagia and dysmenorrhea (including when associated with uterine leiomyomata)
Premenstrual syndrome
Pain in women with endometriosis
Seizures refractory to conventional anticonvulsants
Painful crises in women with hemoglobinopathy
Menstrual hygiene problems in handicapped women
Vasomotor symptoms in menopausal women
Pelvic pain and dyspareunia of ovarian origin; posthysterectomy
Ovulatory pain
Endometrial hyperplasia
Metastatic endometrial cancer
Metastatic breast cancer

*Use of DMPA for indications other than contraception or endometrial cancer represents off-label use not approved by the FDA.

CONTRACEPTIVE IMPLANTS

The *Norplant* subdermal contraceptive system consists of six 34 × 2.4–mm Silastic tubes, each containing 36 mg of crystalline levonorgestrel. The six implants release a total of 85 μg/day initially, with the levels dropping to 30 μg/day by the fifth year of use. The 5-year cumulative failure rate is 1.3 per 100 users, comparable to the failure rate of tubal sterilization.[7,9] Failure rates slowly rise as the levonorgestrel release rates gradually decline. Because failure rates rise above 2 per 100 woman-years in the sixth year of use, implants should be replaced after 5 years. The risk of congenital anomalies does not appear to be increased among offspring born to women with implants who have conceived.

Mechanism of Action. Circulating progestin levels are sufficient to prevent ovulation in most women using implants. However, approximately one third of implant users do experience cyclic luteal activity in the first year. This luteal activity becomes more frequent in subsequent years and is associated with regular withdrawal bleeding episodes. In these ovulatory implant users, fertilization is prevented by progestin-induced luteal insufficiency, impaired oocyte maturation, and progestin-induced cervical mucus. Implant users with cyclic menses are at higher risk of pregnancy and should be counseled about the importance of pregnancy testing if their regular menses abruptly cease.

Medications that induce hepatic enzymes can decrease implant efficacy (see Box 38-3). Some physicians have successfully placed two sets of implants (12 total implants) in women taking concomitant hepatic enzyme inducers. A two-implant levonorgestrel system that provides at least 3 years of contraception has been FDA approved but is not currently marketed in the United States.

Initiation, Use, and Return to Fertility. Insertion of the implants within 7 days of the onset of menses avoids the need for backup contraception. Insertion and removal of implants are minor office procedures performed under local anesthesia. Removal takes longer and is associated with more discomfort than insertion. Appropriate insertion technique facilitates removal. Because serum progestin levels fall rapidly after removal, fertility returns within days or weeks of removal. This observation underscores that women having their implants removed need to initiate an alternate method of contraception immediately if they want to avoid conceiving.

Side Effects. Irregular bleeding is the most common side effect leading to implant discontinuation and can be treated with estrogen supplementation (e.g., DMPA). Headache (nonmigraine), mood changes, and weight gain are the most common nonmenstrual side effects leading to implant discontinuation in U.S. women.[9] Some women using implants have reported hair loss, a side effect that appears to diminish during implant use.

Health Risks. No epidemiologic data have assessed risk of reproductive tract cancers in implant users. Functional ovarian cysts arising from persistent dominant follicles develop in some implant users but rarely require surgical intervention.

INTRAUTERINE DEVICES

Intrauterine devices (IUDs) offer convenient, highly effective, and safe contraception. Low use of IUDs among U.S. women likely reflects myths that IUDs act as abortifacients and cause pelvic inflammatory disease (PID), infertility, and ectopic pregnancies. By educating women and dispelling myths, primary care physicians can encourage appropriate candidates to take advantage of this underused contraceptive.[4]

The two IUDs currently available in the United States are the Copper T 380A (Paragard) and the progesterone-releasing IUD (Progestasert). Paragard is a polyethylene device covered with 380 mm^2 of copper. Two white monofilament threads are tied to the device's bulbous stem. Progestasert is a T-shaped ethylene/vinyl acetate copolymer device whose stem is filled with 38 mg of progesterone, released at a rate of 65 μg per day. Two blue-black monofilament strings are attached to the stem base. Barium sulfate is incorporated into the frame of these IUDs, making them radiopaque.

Mechanism of Action. IUDs prevent fertilization by creating a sterile, inflammatory foreign body response in the endometrial cavity that is hostile to sperm. Copper causes local prostaglandin production and inhibits endometrial enzymes, intensifying the spermicidal impact of the copper IUDs. Paragard is approved for 10 years of use, with first-year failure rates of 0.5 to 0.8 per 100 woman-years and a cumulative 10-year failure rate of 2.1 per 100 woman-years, comparable to tubal sterilization.[7] Recent data suggest this IUD remains effective for at least 12 years.

Progestasert not only inhibits sperm survival but also may prevent implantation by creating an atrophic decidualized endometrium. The progesterone-releasing IUD also thickens the cervical mucus, preventing sperm entry into the endometrium. Approved for 1 year of use, the first-year failure rate is a reported 2 per 100 woman-years.[10]

Initiation and Use. Many physicians believe that IUDs are best inserted during menses, when insertion-related bleeding is masked, discomfort may be minimized by increased cervical dilation, and pregnancy is ruled out. IUDs, however, may be inserted any time during the cycle as long as pregnancy can be reliably excluded. Although uterine perforation can occur during insertion, this complication rarely occurs with the copper or progesterone-releasing IUDs. Skilled physicians who perform a careful preinsertion bimanual examination have perforation rates of approximately one per 1000 insertions. Appropriate sterile technique and patient selection (i.e., avoiding insertion in patients with current genital infections or at increased risk for sexually transmitted diseases) preclude the necessity for prophylactic antibiotics. Expulsion rates are approximately 5% in the first year of copper IUD use. Vaginal discharge, cramping, a lengthening string, and plastic protruding from the cervix suggest partial expulsion, and barrier backup contraception should be used until the patient can be evaluated. Partially expelled IUDs should be removed. A new device can be inserted after infection and pregnancy are excluded.

Side Effects. Copper IUDs increase both menstrual flow and cramping. Careful screening of candidates to avoid insertion in women with preexisting menorrhagia or dysmenorrhea will reduce patient discontinuation resulting from these problems. Use of nonsteroidal antiinflammatory drugs (NSAIDs) is appropriate for women using copper IUDs and experiencing dysmenorrhea. Because the progesterone-releasing IUD reduces menstrual flow and cramps, women with underlying heavy flow or dysmenorrhea may be good candidates for or may even benefit from its use.

Health Risks. In contrast with barrier and hormonal contraception, IUDs do not prevent sexually transmitted diseases (STDs) or PID. Selection of mutually monogamous candidates with no evidence of genital tract infection and use of good insertion technique should result in little if any increased risk of pelvic infection after IUD insertion. Because copper IUDs reduce the overall risk of ectopic pregnancy, a history of ectopic pregnancy does not contraindicate their use. Conditions no longer considered contraindications to IUD use include nulliparity, diabetes mellitus, valvular heart disease, treated cervical dysplasia, anovulatory cycles, lactation, and corticosteroid use without immunocompromise.

Uncomplicated vaginitis or cervicitis encountered in IUD users should be treated as in any other patient. Simple endometritis can be treated with doxycycline and metronidazole (or ampicillin/clavulanate) for 14 days without IUD removal if the patient responds appropriately. Although no controlled study has addressed this issue, many authorities believe PID requires removal of the IUD after initiation of antibiotics. *Actinomyces* has been found on Papanicolaou smears in up to one third of women with plastic IUDs and in almost 1% of copper IUD users with long duration of use. In women with *Actinomyces* infection and either uterine tenderness or an associated pelvic mass, appropriate treatment includes removal of the device and oral penicillin for 1 month.

Although the copper-T IUD does not increase ectopic pregnancy risk, when contraceptive failures occur in IUD users, a high percentage of such pregnancies are ectopic. Accordingly, physicians diagnosing pregnancy in an IUD user should promptly arrange sonography to determine the implantation site. The risk of spontaneous abortion is increased if an IUD remains in place with an intrauterine pregnancy. If the string is visible, the IUD should be gently removed, regardless of the woman's pregnancy intentions. Once the IUD is removed, the increased risk of abortion resolves. If the string is not visible, some experts recommend sonographically guided removal by a physician skilled in such procedures. If the IUD cannot be retrieved, the risk for congenital anomalies has not been shown to be increased, but the risk of preterm labor or intrauterine infection is greater.

BARRIER AND SPERMICIDAL METHODS

Paralleling increased awareness of human immunodeficiency virus (HIV) infection and other STDs, the use of male condoms among U.S. couples has become more common.

Barrier methods can be relatively effective when used consistently and correctly. Younger age, lower socioeconomic class, and less education correlate with higher barrier and spermicide failure rates. Vaginal foams, jellies, suppositories, creams, and films containing the spermicidal detergent nonoxynol 9 kill or immobilize sperm on contact. Combining these spermicidal methods with barriers may increase contraceptive efficacy, but many couples perceive spermicides as messy or having an unpleasant flavor.

Initiation and Use. Diaphragms and spermicides used alone require proper placement before penile-vaginal contact, with additional spermicide placed with each subsequent sex act. *Diaphragms* should be left in place for at least 6 hours after sexual relations. Arcing-spring diaphragms are used most often and can be used by women with pelvic relaxation or an anterior cervix associated with a posterior uterus. Flat-spring diaphragms are also available.

In contrast with diaphragms, cavity rim *cervical caps* have the advantages of (1) allowing longer use, up to 36 hours at a time; (2) not requiring concomitant spermicide use with each coitus; and (3) maintaining appropriate placement in women with pelvic relaxation by means of the suction created. Failure rates with the cap are higher in parous than nulliparous women, with rates as high as 20% reported among parous women consistently using this device.

Diaphragms and cervical caps are available in different sizes, must be professionally fitted, and require users knowledgeable about and comfortable manipulating their genital anatomy. Male and female condoms can be used effectively without spermicides.

Side Effects. Vaginal pain or ulceration is rare with a properly fitted diaphragm or cervical cap. Diaphragm users should be reevaluated for correct fit annually, after any 4.5-kg (10-pound) or greater weight change, after an abortion, and postpartum.

Health Risks. Urinary tract infections are approximately twice as common among women using diaphragms as among those using OCs. Some individuals are allergic to latex condoms, diaphragms, or cervical caps.

Noncontraceptive Benefits and Therapeutic Uses. Use of barriers and spermicides reduces the transmission of bacterial and viral STDs.

PERIODIC ABSTINENCE

The *rhythm (calendar) method, cervical mucus method,* and *symptothermal method* are approaches to contraception that rely on observation of signs and symptoms of the "fertile" period during the menstrual cycle. Accordingly, women with irregular menses, vaginitis, or cervicitis are not appropriate candidates for use of periodic abstinence. Periodic abstinence is the only method of contraception allowed by some religions. The need to abstain from sex for many days each menstrual cycle and the high failure rate limit this approach to fertility regulation.

SUMMARY

Hormonal and intrauterine contraception offer women safe, effective, and reversible contraception. Use of oral and injectable contraceptives also confers a number of important noncontraceptive benefits. Barrier and spermicidal methods are readily accessible and offer women protection against unintended pregnancy and STDs. By individualizing counseling and recommendations based on relevant behavioral and medical considerations, primary care physicians can maximize their patients' success with contraceptives.

REFERENCES

1. Henshaw SK: Unintended pregnancy in the United States, *Fam Plann Perspect* 30:24, 1998.
2. Kaunitz AM: Injectable depot medroxyprogesterone acetate contraception: an update for U.S. clinicians, *Int J Fertil* 43:73, 1998.
3. Kaunitz AM: Oral contraceptive estrogen dose considerations, *Contraception* 58:15S, 1998.
4. Kaunitz AM: Intrauterine devices: safe, effective and underutilized, *Women's Health Prim Care* 2:39, 1999.
5. Kaunitz AM, Mishell DR Jr, editors: Meeting contraceptive needs worldwide: the role of monthly combined contraceptives, *Int J Gynecol Obstet* 62(suppl 1):S1, 1998.
6. Kaunitz AM, Illions EH, Jones JL, Sang LA: Contraception: a clinical review for the internist, *Med Clin North Am* 79:1377, 1995.
7. Peterson H, Xia Z, Hughes J, et al: The risk of pregnancy after tubal sterilization: findings from the U.S. Collaborative Review of Sterilization, *Am J Obstet Gynecol* 174:1161, 1996.
8. Piccinino LJ, Mosher WD: Trends in contraceptive use in the United States: 1982-1995, *Fam Plann Perspect* 30:4, 1998.

8a. Redmond G, et al: Use of placebo controls in an oral contraceptive trial, *Contraception* 60:81-85, 1999.

9. Sivin I, Mishell DR Jr, Darney P, et al: Levonorgestrel capsule implants in the United States: a 5 year study, *Obstet Gynecol* 92:337, 1998.
10. Trussel J: Contraceptive efficacy. In Hatcher RA, Stewart F, Trussel J, et al, editors: *Contraceptive technology,* ed 17, New York, 1998, Ardent Media.

CHAPTER 39

Primary Care of Lesbians

Jocelyn C. White

The care of lesbians and women who have sex with women (WSWs) has received little attention, and medical literature rarely addresses the needs of this group. Lesbians and WSWs may compose up to 15% or more of the female population depending on demographic characteristics such as geographic area, religion, and education.[3] These women are a large group of patients with unique medical, psychologic, and social needs.[10] According to current theories, sexual orientation is most likely determined by a combination of biologic and environmental factors.[1] Contemporary researchers define "lesbian" in ways that include self-definition, women as sexual partners, and sexual attraction to or desire of women. For primary care purposes the aspects of self-identification and sexual partners are most relevant. Identification as a lesbian is based on emotions and psychologic responses, societal expectations, and the individual's own choices in identity formation. Therefore some women call themselves lesbians but are not sexually active with women or exclusively with women; conversely, some are sexually active with women but do not identify as lesbians. The specific identity and sexual practices of an individual patient determine her risks of particular conditions and are important in developing individual medical recommendations.

Lesbians and WSWs are a diverse group of women from all racial, economic, geographic, religious, cultural, and age populations. Despite this diversity, lesbians have formed a culture and community of their own that often provides an alternative family or kin group to its members. Many older women who developed their lesbian identity before the modern gay and lesbian era feel less connected to this culture and community. These older women may be more reluctant to reveal their identity because of experiences with or fears of discrimination. Community resources may be helpful to physicians looking for lesbian-sensitive referrals for social services, counseling, or peer support.

Although the body of research is growing, scientific information is limited about the lesbian and WSW populations. The studies available are often methodologically flawed by sample bias or small sample size, and physicians may not be able to generalize from these results. In other areas, such as cancer risks and screening, specific information about lesbians and WSWs is unavailable, but inferences can be drawn from larger epidemiologic studies of women.

PHYSICIAN-PATIENT INTERACTION

Many lesbians are reluctant to share their sexual orientation with physicians for fear of negative judgments and homophobic responses. Some lesbians do not share this information even when asked. Negative experiences with health care professionals make lesbian patients more likely to terminate care and avoid routine screening and other care. On the other hand, physicians may feel inexperienced in dealing with lesbian health issues or uncomfortable deciding what language to use to elicit information sensitively. Because of both patient and physician discomfort, important information is often not shared.

An effective physician-patient interaction has three functions: information gathering, rapport building, and patient education. The physician needs to communicate with all women in ways that will (1) elicit information needed to identify lesbian and WSW patients and provide appropriate medical care, (2) demonstrate a nonjudgmental attitude that conveys a sense of acceptance, and (3) provide educational information, resources, and referrals sensitive to the needs of lesbians and WSWs.

Gathering information from female patients about sexual orientation and sexual practices may be the first pitfall. Typical patient interview questions often lead to inaccurate or incomplete information and set up barriers for the lesbian and WSW patient because they assume she is heterosexual; "What form of birth control do you use?" is a common example. Questions that facilitate communication include "Have you ever had sex with men, women, or both?" and "How do you identify your sexual orientation?" (Box 39-1). Physicians should ask these questions of all women from adolescence through old age. It is important to recognize elderly lesbians because of their risk of social isolation. Physicians may be a significant source of support to these patients.

Sensitivity to important concerns of the lesbian patient improves rapport (Box 39-2). For example, offering to include a partner in discussions and ensuring that she has access to patient care areas (e.g., delivery room, intensive care unit) demonstrate acceptance. The physician also builds rapport by discussing the stresses of homophobia and exploring the patient's perceptions of the health care system. In addition, physicians can ensure that all next-of-kin policies and discussions of advance directives include the possibility of a female partner and that office and hospital forms use wording that recognizes alternative family structures, such as "living with a partner" or "living as a couple" in addition to "spouse."

Providing education for lesbian patients involves physician self-education and access to reference materials and brochures with information specific to lesbians. Verbal instruction in preventing the transmission of sexually transmitted diseases (STDs), including human immunodeficiency virus (HIV), should be clear and specific to sexual practices between women. Physicians should be able to counsel or refer patients for counseling about such issues as parenting, coming out, battery, and hate crimes. Referrals should include other providers and community-based resources sensitive to

Box 39-1. Helpful Questions in Taking a History

When a Woman's Sexual Orientation Is Unknown

Who do you consider to be in your immediate family?
Are you single, partnered, or married?
Are you in an intimate relationship with a man or woman?
Are your sex partners men, women, or both?
Do you have a need for contraception?
If you become ill, is there someone important to you whom I should involve in your care?

When a Woman Is Identified as a Lesbian

Have you told your family and friends that you are a lesbian?
Are you "out" at work?
Who do you consider part of your support system?
Do you have any questions about having or raising children?
Do you experience any stress because you're a lesbian?
Have you ever been harassed because you're lesbian?

Box 39-2. How to Indicate Acceptance of Lesbian Patients

Include *living with a partner* or *living as a couple* along with *married* and *single* as options on office forms.
Use the term *spouse* or *partner* on office forms.
Include the possibility that a partner may want to be included in next-of-kin and advance directive discussions.
Train staff not to use "Mrs." to address all women patients.
Display brochures on lesbian health issues.
Compile and use lesbian-sensitive educational materials and community resources.
Ask patients about their preferences for documenting sexual orientation in the chart, and discuss options.
Ask patients if they want their partner to participate in the medical visit.

the needs of lesbians.* Hotlines, book stores, and bibliographies can help educate. Youth groups and senior groups, community centers, lesbian and gay religious organizations and retirement centers, substance abuse support groups, and counselors who deal with lesbian issues can provide support.

Finally, it is important for physicians to discuss explicitly with lesbians the documentation of sexual orientation and sexual partners in the chart. Because the information is integral to providing high-quality health care, physicians may consider using a coded entry in the chart if a patient does not want her lesbian identity documented. This provides physicians with a record to remind them about the patient's sexual orientation but prevents inadvertent breaches of confidentiality through use of the chart.

SEXUALLY TRANSMITTED DISEASES

STDs, except for HIV, appear to be less common in lesbians and WSWs than in other populations. Sexual practices between women include kissing, breast stimulation, manual and oral stimulation of the genitals and anus, friction of the clitoris against the partner's body, and penetration of the vagina and anus with fingers and devices. No gynecologic problems are unique to lesbians or WSWs, and none occurs more often than in other populations. Human papillomavirus (HPV), the cause of genital warts and cervical dysplasia, has been shown to be sexually transmitted between women.[4] Therefore female partners of infected women should also be evaluated.

Nonspecific vaginitis, more recently called *bacterial vaginosis,* often occurs in lesbians. According to recent research the female partners of infected women are most likely infected. Physicians should inquire about vaginal discharge in lesbians and evaluate those partners of infected patients who have symptoms. Although bisexual women report vaginal candidiasis more often than do lesbians, probably because of heterosexual contact, transmission between women is possible. Partners of lesbians with vaginal candidiasis should be evaluated.

Trichomonas vaginalis bacteria have been found in women sexually active exclusively with women, women with no sexual contact at all, and lesbians with a bisexual woman as contact. Physicians should include *T. vaginalis* infection in the differential diagnosis of vaginal discharge in lesbians. Sexual partners of lesbians diagnosed with *Trichomonas* infection should also be evaluated.

Screening and testing for STDs is appropriate in the setting of risk factors based on specific sexual history. Chlamydial and herpes organisms are found infrequently in lesbians who have been sexually active exclusively with women. Herpes can be transmitted between women, but the prevalence in the lesbian population seems to be low. Pelvic inflammatory disease (PID) also appears to be rare among lesbians. Unlike in the gay male population, enteric infections caused by hepatitis A, *Amoeba, Shigella,* and helminths have a low prevalence in lesbians. Hepatitis B and C occur when risk factors are present.

Human Immunodeficiency Virus

Of the Centers for Disease Control and Prevention (CDC) reported cases of acquired immunodeficiency syndrome (AIDS) in lesbians, about 93% were intravenous drug users. To date, transmission of HIV between women as a result of sexual contact only may have occurred in up to nine cases, likely related to exposure to menstrual and traumatic bleeding. However, HIV has been cultured from cervical and vaginal secretions and cervical biopsies taken throughout the menstrual cycle and may theoretically be transmitted by infected women who are not bleeding.[2] Because of the low rate of transmission from infected women to men in the general population, however, the rate of transmission between women is probably also low.

Physicians should counsel lesbians to avoid contact with cervical and vaginal secretions, menstrual blood, and blood from vaginal and rectal trauma in partners whose HIV status is unknown.[9] Methods believed to protect against transmission for oral-genital contact include latex squares known as dental dams, latex condoms or gloves cut open and laid flat, and odor-impermeable brand-name plastic wrap. For vaginal penetration, latex gloves used on hands and condoms on sexual toys are appropriate. Recommendations for HIV testing should be based on individual risk factors.

Lesbians who undergo artificial insemination with either fresh semen from donors in the community or frozen semen from sperm banks are also at risk for HIV infection. Sperm banks routinely test donors for HIV infection at the time of donation and 6 months later before releasing the sample for use. Because of delays in seroconversion, however, it is possible for lesbians to be exposed to HIV through fresh semen from a seronegative donor. Lesbians should avoid using fresh semen for insemination.

CANCER

There are no population-based studies of gynecologic and breast cancer risk in lesbians. As a result, cancer screening decisions in lesbians should be based on individual risk factors using standard screening guidelines for women. Based on their sexual and reproductive histories, however, the incidence of certain cancers in lesbians may differ.

Cervical cancer appears less common among lesbians than other women, as suggested by lower rates of dysplasia. HPV is transmissible between women, however, and cervical cancer occurs in women sexually active exclusively with women. Current American Cancer Society (ACS) recommendations and other preventive health guidelines give no guidance for cervical cancer screening in women who are sexually active with women only. Physicians need to screen these women according to current guidelines.

Little information exists on breast cancer in lesbians.[7] However, many lesbians are nulliparous, older with the first birth, have never breastfed, or have a higher body mass index. Physicians should adhere to current guidelines for breast examination and mammography.

Ovarian cancer has been reported to occur more frequently in women who have not used oral contraception and those who have not given birth. Endometrial cancer is also more common in nulliparous women. Based on these risk factors, some lesbians may be at a slightly higher risk for ovarian and endometrial cancers, and physicians should follow current guidelines on screening for these cancers where available.

*For further information and referral sources for lesbian and gay health issues, contact Gay and Lesbian Medical Association, 273 Church St, San Francisco, CA 94114; 415-255-4547.

SPECIAL ISSUES

Parenting and Reproduction

Lesbians may have children from previous heterosexual relationships, from adoption, by artificial insemination, or by being a foster parent. Although some members of society oppose motherhood for lesbians, studies have not demonstrated differences between children raised by lesbians and those raised by heterosexuals.[6] Open communication with children about parents' lesbianism appears important in family function.

Most lesbians who want to conceive find artificial insemination, also called *alternative insemination* or *therapeutic insemination,* the preferred method. Some physicians are uncomfortable performing artificial insemination for lesbians, whereas others believe it is ethically justifiable but should not be mandated. A physician who is unable to comply with a patient's wishes should refer the patient to another provider for the service.

A pregnant lesbian may find it more difficult than other women to find social or family support for her pregnancy. The development of her identity as a mother may also be more complex. Primary care physicians can support the pregnant lesbian by demonstrating nonjudgmental attitudes, encouraging acceptance of lesbian motherhood among members of the obstetric team and childbearing classes, and including partners in the process of conception, prenatal care, and delivery.

Psychosocial and Psychologic Issues

In general, psychologic illness is no more common in lesbians than in heterosexual women. Lesbians do experience unique psychosocial stressors, however, that often affect their physical and emotional health. The issues most relevant for primary care physicians include homophobia, coming out, alcohol and substance abuse, suicide, lesbian battery, and hate crimes.

Stress experienced by lesbians may result from a conflict between their chosen identity and the identity they express to the outside world. Although lesbians' self-esteem is similar to that of heterosexual women, lesbians often find it difficult to act in accordance with their identity because of society's negative attitudes, known as *homophobia.* Societal attitudes may be compounded by the lesbian's own internal homophobia developed from years of living in an intolerant society.

Evaluation of a lesbian patient's support network is necessary to determine her ability to cope with these and other stressful life events. Lesbians most often derive support from partners, friends, and lesbian and gay community organizations. The quality of the relationship with a partner can be particularly important to a lesbian's psychologic well-being. Discord in a lesbian couple can be even more stressful than for a married heterosexual couple because of a lack of traditional social support.

The process of discovering one's sexual orientation and revealing it to others, known as *coming out,* may begin at any age and may be associated with significant emotional distress. The process of coming out has been well described. It involves a shift in core identity that takes place in four stages: (1) awareness of homosexual feelings, (2) testing and exploration, (3) identity acceptance, and (4) identity integration and disclosure to others. Internalized and societal homophobia cause the lesbian to perform a fatiguing cost-benefit analysis for each situation in which she considers coming out. If the costs are high, she may ultimately become socially isolated or deny the identity.[5] Lesbian adolescents are particularly vulnerable to the emotional distress of coming out, and this distress often confounds their developmental tasks. Parental acceptance during this process, especially maternal, may be the primary determinant of the development of healthy self-esteem in adolescent lesbians. Signs of sexual orientation confusion in adolescents may include diminished school performance, alcohol and substance abuse, acting out, depression, and suicidal ideation and attempt. It is important for the primary care physician to screen adolescents for these signs and to consider sexual orientation confusion in the differential diagnosis of depression and substance use.[8]

As part of a comprehensive clinical evaluation, primary care physicians should screen all women, including their lesbian patients, for alcohol and substance abuse, depression, and violence. Lesbians are less likely to abstain from alcohol than other women, more likely to be moderate drinkers, especially in middle decades of life, equally likely to be heavy drinkers, and more likely to report an alcohol problem. A recent national mail survey from a lesbian publication reported that 59% of subjects had used alcohol to cope with stress and 42% had considered suicide. Marijuana and cocaine use also appear to be higher in lesbians. Violence is an issue in lesbian as well as heterosexual relationships. One small study reported that among lesbians aged 22 to 52 years, about 38% had experienced battery by a partner, and alcohol or drug use was involved in 64% of these incidents.

Hate crimes against lesbians, including verbal abuse, threats of violence, property damage, physical violence, and murder, are increasing each year. Lesbians at universities report being victims of sexual assault twice as frequently as heterosexual women. According to a study for the U.S. Department of Justice, lesbians and gay men may be the most victimized group in the nation. About 25% of lesbians in a Philadelphia study reported being the victim of a crime committed by a family member. Many gay and lesbian adolescents may leave home because of abuse related to their sexual orientation. The primary care provider should be aware of the possibility that a patient has been a victim of violence, particularly when patients present with symptoms of depression or anxiety.

End of Life

Advance directives are necessary for lesbians who want to appoint their partners as surrogate health care decision makers. Completing this document is the best way to avoid a tragic conflict between a partner and a legal next of kin in a time of crisis. As with all patients, a discussion of advance directives should be included in the preventive care evaluation.

Caregiving issues for lesbians can be different than those for other women. Lesbians caring for partners with breast cancer report unique considerations that are best addressed in support groups for lesbian caregivers. Physicians should refer caregivers to local lesbian cancer projects or cancer centers with groups for lesbians.

SUMMARY

Many primary care physicians are caring for lesbian patients without recognizing their sexual orientation or their unique medical and psychologic needs. Enhanced knowledge and skills allow these physicians to provide optimal and sensitive patient care for lesbians. Clearly, much more research on this group is needed to provide appropriate guidelines for physicians.[8a]

REFERENCES

1. Byne W, Parsons B: Human sexual orientation, *Arch Gen Psychiatry* 50:228, 1993.
2. Kennedy MB, Scarlett MI, Duerr AC, Chu SY: Assessing HIV risk among women who have sex with women: scientific and communication issues, *J Am Med Women's Assoc* 50:103, 1995.
3. Laumann EO, Gagnon JH, Michael RT, Michales S: *The social organization of sexuality: sexual practices in the United States*, Chicago, 1994, University of Chicago Press.
4. Marrazzo JM, Koutsky LA, Stine KL, et al: Genital human papillomavirus in women who have sex with women, *J Infect Dis* 178:1604, 1998.
5. O'Hanlan KA, Cabaj RP, Schatz B, et al: A review of the medical consequences of homophobia with suggestions for resolution, *J Gay Lesbian Med Assoc* 1:25, 1997.
6. Patterson CJ: Children of lesbian and gay parents, *Child Dev* 63:1025, 1992.
7. Roberts SA, Dibble SL, Scanlon JL, et al: Differences in risk factors for breast cancer: lesbian and heterosexual women, *J Gay Lesbian Med Assoc* 2:93, 1998.
8. Ryan C, Futterman D: Lesbian and gay youth: care and counseling, *Adolesc Med* 8:207, 1997.

8a. Solarz AL, editor: *Lesbian health: current assessment and directions for the future*, Washington, DC, 1999, National Academy Press.

9. White J: HIV risk assessment and prevention for lesbians and women who have sex with women: practical information for clinicians, *Health Care Women Int* 18:127, 1997.
10. White J, Levinson W: Primary care of lesbian patients, *J Gen Intern Med* 8:41, 1993.

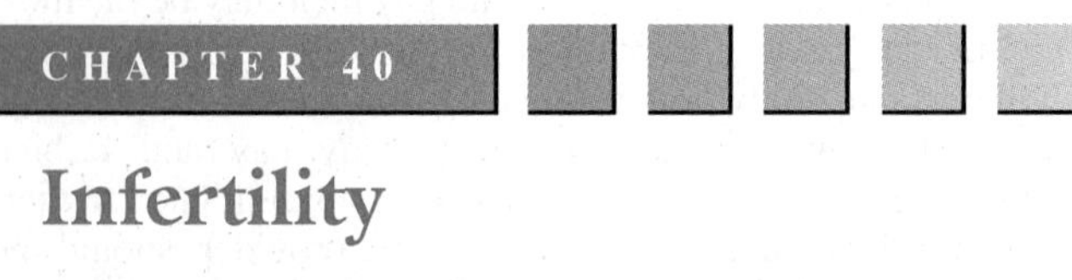

CHAPTER 40

Infertility

Edward H. Illions

Infertility is a relatively common disorder in the United States affecting 12% to 15% of married couples, many of whom seek medical care through their primary care physicians in their attempts to achieve a successful pregnancy outcome. The majority of managed care systems and insurance companies fail to provide adequate coverage for infertility evaluation and treatment, thereby placing undue financial and emotional stress on both the infertile couple and the physician. Although the percentage of infertile couples has not changed, the actual number of infertile patients seeking care has greatly increased in the last three decades, from 600,000 visits in 1968 to 1.35 million in 1988.[20] Increased demand for infertility services mandates that primary care physicians develop an understanding of infertility tests and treatments.

Infertile couples are characterized by their inability to conceive within 1 year in the absence of contraception. *Primary infertility* reflects couples never having conceived, whereas couples with at least one successful conception are considered to have *secondary infertility.* The infertility evaluation commences after 1 year of unprotected coitus because approximately 50% of couples will conceive in 3 months, 75% at 6 months, and 88% to 90% will achieve a viable pregnancy after 1 year. Approximately 20% to 25% of couples will achieve a conception within a given menstrual cycle, referred to as *fecundity.* An increasing number of women over age 35 are seeking infertility services. In fact, one of every five U.S. women is having her first child after age 35, which reflects postponement of childbearing secondary to career and monetary issues. This aging infertile population represents a unique problem to infertility specialists and primary care physicians, given the well-documented age-related decline in fecundity. Tables 40-1 and 40-2 outline women's patient history and physical examination associated with fertility evaluation and infertility management.

ETIOLOGIES

The reproductive potential of a female begins to decline in the early to middle 30s, with a marked reduction in fecundity beyond age 40. Career and financial considerations have prompted a delay in childbearing, along with associated factors, such as increased contraceptive use and increased prevalence of myoma and endometriosis in this age group. Ovarian function begins to diminish well in advance of the natural menopause and is the principal reason for diminished reproductive potential in this age group.[21] Waning ovarian function is often indicated by progressive rise in serum follicle-stimulating hormone (FSH) levels obtained in the early proliferative phase of the menstrual cycle.[14] Estrogen levels vary greatly in this age group and may be elevated. Collectively, these biochemical changes reflect ovarian reserve and provide indirect evidence of the functional capacity of the ovarian follicular apparatus.

An FSH value early in the proliferative phase is a useful screening test for ovarian reserve. FSH values are inversely related to successful pregnancy outcome. FSH values in excess of 20 mIU/ml indicate poor ovarian reserve, manifested by low clinical pregnancy rates with in vitro fertilization cycles.[32] Determinations of both FSH and estradiol after the administration of Clomid (clomiphene citrate challenge test) provide a more expanded assessment of ovarian reserve.[28]

Pelvic Infections

Postinfection tubal infertility accounts for approximately 30% to 40% of all female infertility. A steep rise in the incidence of sexually transmitted diseases (STDs) in the last 20 to 30 years has contributed greatly to both the risk of tubal infertility and the associated rise in ectopic pregnancies. Risk factors for pelvic inflammatory disease (PID) include young age, single marital status, multiple sexual partners, prior STD history, and illicit drug use. *Chlamydia* infection and gonorrhea are the two primary offending agents; however, many cases of PID involve polymicrobial infection. Prompt recognition and treatment are mandated because tubal factor infertility rises with subsequent tubal infections.

Lifestyle Factors

Lifestyle issues are associated with cigarette smoking, athletic activity and weight loss, alcohol, and illicit drugs. The detrimental effects on fetal development from cigarette smoking are well known. Despite a growing public awareness campaign linking these agents to adverse reproductive out-

Table 40-1. Female History and Fertility

Category	Findings	Impact on fertility
General medical	Significant weight change Decreased energy level Cold intolerance	Hypothyroidism*
	Body hair distribution (hirsutism)	Androgen excess*
	Headaches Visual complaints Galactorrhea	Pituitary adenoma (hyperprolactinemia)*
Infertility	Maternal age	Advanced maternal age: decreased fecundity, increased rate of spontaneous abortions, increased risk of chromosomal anomalies
	Infertility duration	More than 3 years, more refractory to treatment
Menstrual	Age of menarche	Abnormal pubertal development
	Cycle characteristics: frequency, duration, presence of molimina	Ovulation in 95%-98% of women with normal cyclic menses and molimina
	Dysmenorrhea Dyspareunia	Endometriosis, pelvic adhesions
Gynecologic	Sexually transmitted disease Pelvic inflammatory disease	Tubal factor infertility
	Abnormal Pap smears, LEEP, or cone biopsy of cervix	Abnormal cervical mucus
	Diethylstilbestrol (DES) exposure	Structural abnormalities of cervix and uterus
Sexual	Coital frequency and technique	Inadequate exposure
	Use of lubricants/postcoital douching	Spermicidal
Past medical	Chronic medical illness: thyroid, diabetes mellitus, renal, human immunodeficiency virus, seizure disorders	Ovulatory dysfunction
Obstetric	Antepartum complications	Risk of recurrence
	Pregnancy terminations	Cervical stenosis or Asherman's syndrome
	Second-trimester losses Postpartum complications	Müllerian anomalies
Past surgical	Abdominal surgery (complications, previous tubal surgery)	Tubal factor (e.g., ruptured appendix yields 4.8 relative risk for tubal factor infertility)
Social/occupational	Work environment (toxins, chemicals), cigarettes, alcohol, illicit drug use	Gametotoxic Effects on cervical mucus, tubal function, and ovulation
Medication	Type, duration, trimester exposed	Isotretinoin (Accutane): teratogenic Androgens: virilization Tetracyclines: skeletal and dental effects Heavy metals: stillborn, central nervous system effects

Modified from Illions EH, Valley MT, Kaunitz AM: *Med Clin North Am* 82(2):271, 1998.
*Disrupts ovulation.

come, approximately 20% to 30% of young women continue to smoke. Cigarette smokers often experience early menopause because of oocyte depletion with a subsequent reduction in estradiol levels.[11] Smoking cessation programs offer some promise; however, long-term compliance remains a significant health problem.

Significant data exist linking alcohol consumption to adverse reproductive outcome in both sexes. In utero fetal exposure to alcohol increases the incidence of growth retardation, craniofacial abnormalities, and developmental delay, collectively known as *fetal alcohol syndrome*. Males experience decreased testosterone levels, abnormal spermatogenesis, and subnormal sexual performance.[12]

Strenuous exercising and low body weight (alterations in percentage of body fat) are independent risk factors for ovulatory dysfunction in young women.[1] Major hypothalamic-pituitary-gonadal dysfunction with diminished gonadotropin and estradiol levels can occur when both risk factors are combined.

Anorexia nervosa represents an extreme example of hypothalamic-pituitary dysfunction. Serum gonadotropin levels are frequently undetectable in this setting. Intense psychologic counseling aimed at lifestyle changes may restore ovulatory function.

Ovulatory Dysfunction

Ovulatory dysfunction accounts for 25% to 30% of all female infertility. Ovulatory status should be assessed early in the infertility evaluation (Fig. 40-1). Ovulatory dysfunction may be clinically obvious (e.g., anovulation) or subtle (e.g., luteal-phase defect). Often a combination of ovulation tests is necessary to precisely delineate the nature of the disorder. Table 40-3 lists various tests available to physicians to monitor ovulation.

Ovulation. The normal menstrual cycle in a female is divided into three distinct phases: follicular, periovulatory, and luteal. Follicle selection and growth commences in the

Table 40-2. Female Physical Examination and Fertility

System	Findings	Impact on fertility
General	Body habitus eunuchoid	Hypogonadism
	Increased body mass index	Obesity
	Short stature	Genetic abnormalities
	Body hair distribution*	Androgen excess (ovulatory dysfunction)
Thyroid	Nodules, masses, tenderness, enlarged (diffusely)	Thyroiditis, autoimmune thyroid dysfunction
		Hypothyroidism leading to anovulation
Breasts	Tanner stage (stages I-IV)	Abnormal pubertal development
	Galactorrhea	Hyperprolactinemia (ovulation disruption)
Abdomen	Surgical incisions	Prior surgery: tubal factor
	Truncal obesity	Hypercortisolism affecting ovulation
	Abdominal striae	
	Tenderness, masses	Infection, endometriosis
Genitalia	Clitoromegaly	Androgen excess (anovulation)
	Fusion of labioscrotal folds	Congenital adrenal hyperplasia
	Hypospadias	
	Blind vaginal pouch	Complete androgen insensitivity or Müllerian agenesis
	Structural abnormalities of cervix	DES exposure or prior surgery on cervix
	Broad uterine fundus	Müllerian anomalies
	Enlarged uterus	Nodular (asymmetric): fibroids
		Symmetric: adenomyosis
	Adnexal tenderness, masses	Infection, endometriosis, or polycystic ovarian syndrome
	Uterosacral nodularity	Endometriosis

Modified from Illions EH, Valley MT, Kaunitz AM: *Med Clin North Am* 82(2):271, 1998.
*Excess coarse terminal hair in midline distribution indicates increased androgen effects.

late luteal phase of the preceding cycle, when a new cohort of follicles are recruited. The follicle growth continues in the early proliferative phase of the cycle, directed through a complex interplay of hypothalamic-releasing factors and peptides secreted from the anterior pituitary. Hypothalamic release of gonadotropin-releasing hormone (GnRH) directs both synthesis and release of FSH and luteinizing hormone (LH) from the anterior pituitary. FSH action on the ovary is crucial for follicle development (folliculogenesis), and LH augments FSH-directed follicle development, directs the periovulatory events, and stimulates gonadal steroid production. Through unclear mechanisms a dominant follicle is selected by cycle day 5 or 6. With continued growth of this dominant follicle, estrogen levels rise, prompting a midcycle LH surge culminating in ovulation.

The midcycle gonadotropin surge causes resumption of meiosis, luteinization of theca and granulosa cells within the ovary, and activation of certain proteolytic enzymes vital to follicle extrusion. Follicle release results in the formation of a corpus luteum, with subsequent production of progesterone and 17-hydroxyprogesterone. Corpus luteum formation marks the onset of the *luteal phase,* characterized by progestational support of the endometrium in preparation for implantation of a fertilized oocyte. The length of the luteal phase in primates is constant (10 to 16 days) in the absence of conception. A new cohort of follicles is recruited when gonadal steroid levels abruptly drop in the late luteal phase. The dissolution of the corpus luteum (luteolysis) marks the end of the luteal phase as endometrial vascular changes ensue, resulting in menstruation.

Luteal-phase Defect. Luteal-phase defect (LPD) is a relatively uncommon disorder and arises from either subnormal progesterone levels (inadequate luteal phase) or a shortened duration of action of progesterone on the endometrium (shortened luteal phase). A shortened or inadequate luteal phase often results from inadequate folliculogenesis. Treatment is therefore directed toward improving the follicular phase of the menstrual cycle. Specifically, prolactin and androgen excess as well as a variety of hypothalamic disorders may impair follicular function, leading to LPD.

LPD is confirmed when two late luteal endometrial biopsies performed 10 to 12 days after ovulation demonstrate at least a 2-day histologic lag in endometrial development. Basal body temperatures and midluteal progesterone levels are less sensitive indicators of luteal-phase dysfunction. Luteal-phase temperature elevations of less than 11 days suggest LPD, as does subnormal progesterone levels (less than 10 ng/ml). Recent data demonstrate that transvaginal sonography and urinary LH kits most consistently agree with late luteal histologic dating. Basal body temperature charting and chronologic dating of the next menstrual cycle predicted ovulation only 77% and 65% of the time, respectively.[29] Therefore ultrasound monitoring of follicular development and use of commercially available LH kits more precisely predict ovulation compared with all other ovulatory testing.

Treatment for LPD is directed toward the underlying disorder. Clomiphene, 50 to 100 mg/day from cycle days 5 to 9, augments follicular development. Progesterone therapy yields similar results, and recent U.S. Food and Drug Administration (FDA) approval of a new locally administered vaginal progesterone gel (Crinone) offers additional treatment routes. Crinone's success rates parallel more traditional routes of progesterone administration even in the absence of systemic absorption.[6] Patients with LPD from androgen

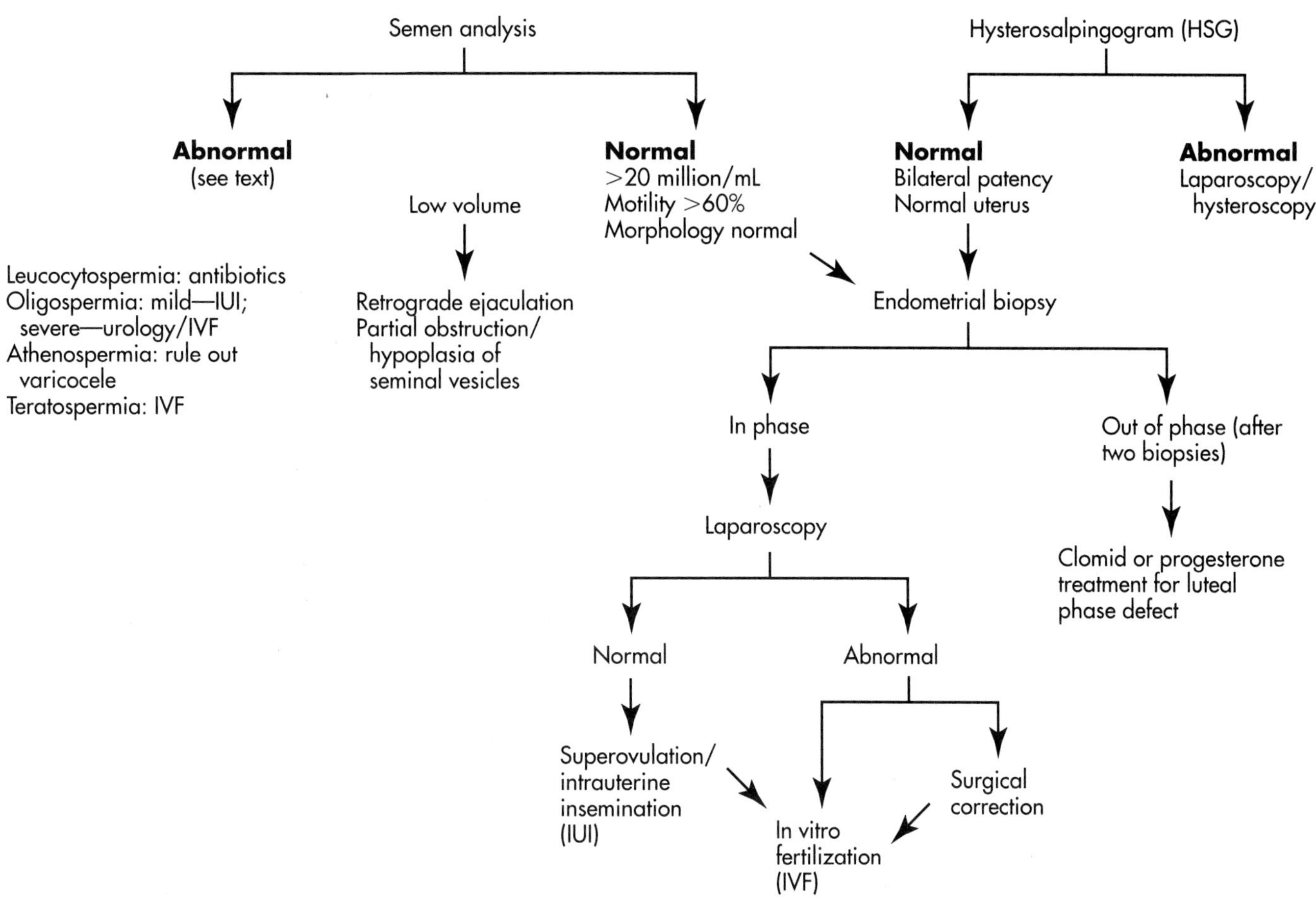

Referral Pattern

Hysterosalpingogram: performed by gynecologist or radiologist
Semen analysis: performed by gynecologist or primary care physician
Endometrial biopsy: performed by gynecologist or primary care physician
Surgery (laparoscopy, hysteroscopy, laparotomy): performed by gynecologist
Assisted reproductive technology (ART): performed by reproductive endocrinologist

Fig. 40-1. Infertility evaluation.

excess or hyperprolactinemia should receive treatment for these disorders.

Hyperprolactinemia. Prolactin excess disrupts hypothalamic function with clinical presentation ranging from complete anovulation to LPD. A variety of physiologic and pathologic conditions increase anterior pituitary production and secretion of prolactin (Box 40-1). Clinically, patients with hyperprolactinemia demonstrate both ovulatory dysfunction (anovulation or oligoovulation) and galactorrhea.

Most patients with hyperprolactinemia have physiologic or pharmacologic etiologies. Pituitary microadenomas (prolactinomas) are the most common pathologic cause of prolactin excess. Women with prolactin-producing tumors often have prolactin levels in excess of 150 or 200 ng/ml and require detailed radiographic imaging of the pituitary and surrounding areas. Treatment of anovulation and galactorrhea secondary to hyperprolactinemia is directed toward the underling etiology. Pharmacologic causes are best treated

Table 40-3. Tests to Determine Ovulation

Test	Criteria
Basal body temperature	Luteal elevation (0.5° F) for at least 11 days
Cervical mucus	Abundant watery discharge, ferning pattern on glass slide, distensibility of mucus
Endometrial biopsy (late luteal phase)	Histology within 2 days of chronologic-cycle day based on luteinizing hormone (LH) surge
Menstrual history	Most cycles 26-40 days (range 23-35 days)
Midluteal progesterone	Values >10 ng/ml
Urinary LH kits	Values ≥40 mIU/ml

From Illions EH, Valley MT, Kaunitz AM: *Med Clin North Am* 82:271, 1998.

Box 40-1. Causes of Hyperprolactinemia

Physiologic

Sleep-associated elevation
High protein content at lunch
Exercise
Stress
Coitus
Late follicular and luteal phase of menstrual cycle
Pregnancy

Pharmacologic

Ovarian steroids
Tricyclic antidepressants
Metoclopramide
Cimetidine
Opiates
Phenothiazines
α-Methyldopa
Anesthesia
Reserpine

Pathologic

Prolactinoma
Acromegaly
Nonsecreting pituitary tumor
Craniopharyngioma
Nelson's syndrome
Empty-sella syndrome
Primary hypothyroidism
Chest wall lesions
Trauma to pituitary stalk
Renal failure
Pseudocyesis (false pregnancy)
Cushing's disease
Infiltrative disorders: tuberculosis, sarcoidosis, histiocytosis

with discontinuation of the medication, if clinically indicated. Most other causes respond favorably to medical management. Since prolactin production and secretion are controlled through tonic inhibition by central nervous system (CNS)–derived dopamine, contemporary medical regimens restore this inhibition through activation of the dopamine receptor.

Dopamine agonists are frequently used to lower prolactin levels and shrink prolactinomas. Recurrence rates are exceedingly high when medication is discontinued. In addition, approximately 30% of patients experience side effects from dopamine agonists, including nausea, vomiting, and orthostatic hypotension. Fortunately, most patients with idiopathic hyperprolactinemia and microadenomas have indolent courses; 30% of untreated patients regain ovulatory function.[17] Patients with macroadenomas (tumor size in excess of 10 mm) present a special challenge, especially during pregnancy. Approximately 15% to 20% of macroadenomas increase in size during pregnancy, risking suprasellar extension and subsequent compression of the optic chasm. Some researchers recommend continuation of dopamine agonists during pregnancy for patients with macroadenomas, whereas others suggest transsphenoidal resection before conception. Patients with longstanding hyperprolactinemia from any cause are often hypoestrogenic due to suppression of hypothalamic GnRH. Estrogen supplementation often preserves bone mineral density in these patients and prevents additional sequelae of hypoestrogenism.

Hyperandrogenism. Patients with androgen excess often present with ovulatory dysfunction and hirsutism. Ovarian and adrenal androgens as well as peripheral conversion of other gonadal steroids constitute the total androgen pool in females.

Ovarian and adrenal androgen production rates are best screened by obtaining total testosterone and dehydroepiandrosterone sulfate (DHEAS) levels. Total testosterone in excess of 200 ng/dl or DHEAS over 600 μg/dl raise clinical suspicion for an androgen-producing tumor and mandate radiographic imaging. Androgen-producing tumors often cause virilization (temporal balding, clitorimegaly, deepening of voice, increased muscle mass) from the rapid rise in serum androgen levels. Free testosterone levels are increased in most hirsute patients and therefore offer limited clinical utility in the evaluation of hyperandrogenism.

Many clinically hirsute patients with or without ovulatory dysfunction have normal circulating androgen levels and are considered to have idiopathic hirsutism. Increased androgen receptor sensitivity within the hair follicle and increased enzymatic conversion of testosterone to more active metabolites (dihydrotestosterone) account for the clinical expression in these individuals. Clinically hirsute patients with ovulatory dysfunction and elevated serum testosterone levels have ovarian hyperandrogenism, also known as *polycystic ovarian syndrome* (PCOS). These individuals experience elevated ovarian androgen production, presumably from abnormal feedback within the hypothalamic-pituitary-ovarian axis.[34] Tonic increases in pituitary-derived LH directly stimulate the ovarian stromal compartment, with a subsequent rise in total testosterone levels. Increased intraovarian androgen levels prompt early follicular destruction (atresia) and subsequent anovulation.

Recent studies demonstrate that most patients with ovarian hyperandrogenism have hyperinsulinism secondary to peripheral insulin resistance.[9] Despite hyperinsulinism, most patients with PCOS demonstrate normal carbohydrate metabolism. Recent evidence suggests, however, that 30% will eventually demonstrate glucose intolerance, and 7% to 10% will develop type II diabetes.[5] Ovulation induction using clomiphene (Clomid) effectively induces ovulation in approximately 70% of patients. Clomid, 50 mg daily, is administered from cycle days 5 to 9, with ovulation typically occurring 7 to 10 days after completing therapy. Clomiphene-resistant patients are best treated with parenteral gonadotropin therapy. Recently, insulin-sensitizing agents used to reduce hyperinsulinism have proved clinically effective in reducing serum androgen levels and promoting ovulation.[33] Metformin (Glucophage) and troglitazone (Rezulin) are two such agents and ostensibly either promote gluconeogenesis or increase the intracellular response to insulin, respectively.

Endocrine Disorders. Certain untreated endocrine disorders disrupt ovulation, resulting in infertility. Thyroid dysfunction, hypercortisolism, and diabetes mellitus are three such disorders for which prompt recognition and intervention favorably impact pregnancy rates and obstetric outcome.[26] *Hypothyroidism* accounts for only 1% of all cases of secondary amenorrhea, but prompt thyroid replacement restores normal cyclic menses. Hypothyroid individuals often present with weight gain, increased lethargy, decreased energy level, and cold intolerance. Hypothyroidism disrupts ovulation by elevating prolactin levels and lowering sex hormone–binding globulin levels, with subsequent alterations in circulating free gonadal steroids.

Patients with *hypercortisolism* often present to the gynecologist or primary care physician complaining of anovulation and hirsutism. Other common physical signs include dorsocervical hump, supraclavicular fat pads, truncal obesity, facial plethora, moon facies, hypertension, glucose intolerance, abdominal striae, and proximal muscle wasting. Initial screening tests (e.g., 24-hour urinary free cortisol level, overnight dexamethasone suppression) are needed to confirm hypercortisolism, with additional tests to localize the source. Treatment is directed toward the underlying etiology, with pituitary-producing adrenocorticotropic hormone (ACTH) adenomas most frequently encountered. Exceedingly high cure rates occur with transsphenoidal resection of pituitary ACTH-producing adenomas.[15]

Approximately 1% to 5% of reproductive-age hirsute women have *late-onset congenital adrenal hyperplasia* (LOCAH). Although relatively common, this autosomal recessive condition is frequently misdiagnosed as PCOS. Proliferative-phase elevations of 17-hydroxyprogesterone in excess of 800 ng/dl confirm the diagnosis; whereas values greater than 200 ng/dl prompt confirmatory testing with a 1-hour ACTH stimulation test. Glucocorticoid treatment often normalizes the elevated androgen levels, thereby restoring ovulation. Prenatal diagnosis is available to at-risk couples; however, the vast majority of affected offspring arise de novo without any antecedent family history. Patients at high risk for LOCAH should be treated during pregnancy with glucocorticoids to minimize or prevent virilization of a potentially affected female fetus in utero. Glucocorticoid therapy is initiated preferably before 5 weeks' gestation and is discontinued when antenatal testing (amniocentesis, chorionic villus sampling) identifies either a male or unaffected female fetus in utero.

Diabetes mellitus exists when fasting glucose levels exceed 126 mg/dl. Marked derangements in glucose metabolism disrupt ovulation, but even modest preconceptual glucose elevations increase the risk of major congenital malformations by threefold. Meticulous glucose control often prevents these adverse events.[26]

A variety of lifestyle situations, such as extreme weight loss, exercise, and stress, disrupt ovulation by altering GnRH pulsatility. Individuals manifesting ovulatory dysfunction secondary to CNS aberration in GnRH release have *hypothalamic amenorrhea*. Anorexia nervosa represents an extreme variant, and many patients are refractory to conventional therapy. Intense counseling that successfully alters lifestyle habits may restore ovulation. Since these patients are often hypoestrogenic, treatment is directed at either ovulation induction or long-term estrogen replacement to prevent osteoporosis and cardiovascular disease. The intense hypoestrogenic state often precludes successful ovulation induction with clomiphene, so patients often require parenteral gonadotropin therapy. Untreated patients with hypothalamic amenorrhea typically fail to bleed to a progestin challenge, thereby distinguishing them from most other anovulatory individuals.

Uterine, Tubal, and Peritoneal Disorders

The 30% incidence of tubal dysfunction in the infertile population parallels a 20-year rise in STDs. Ascending infections from the lower genital tract can affect the uterine lining (endometrium) and fallopian tubes. Although acute and/or chronic endometritis is a rare cause of infertility, significant endometrial scarring, as seen in Asherman's syndrome, may impede sperm motility and disrupt implantation of a fertilized oocyte. Postpartum instrumentation of an infected uterus represents a significant risk factor for the development of intrauterine scarring. Affected patients often present with amenorrhea, oligomenorrhea, and infertility.

Ascending pathogens destroy tubal mucosa, affect intraluminal cilia function, and eventually obliterate the tubal fimbria. Untreated cases of salpingitis may result in significant peritoneal involvement (PID). Clinical presentations often include significant abdominal pain, leukocytosis, and fever with an eventual perihepatitis (Fitz-Hugh–Curtis syndrome). Infertility is common secondary to occluded fallopian tubes and peritubal adhesions restricting tubal mobility. Prompt and aggressive multiagent antibiotic therapy eradicates existing PID but cannot reverse significant tubal and peritoneal scarring.

Endometriosis is characterized by the ectopic location of endometrial glands and stroma and most often involves dependent pelvic structures. Endometriosis arises from either retrograde tubal menstruation or coelomic metaplasia.[31] As in PID, endometriosis-related infertility may result from disruption of ovum selection and reduced embryo transport caused by peritubal disease. Decreased fertility in patients with mild and minimal endometriosis results from subtle defects in ovulation and alterations in the peritoneal fluid environment.[7]

Treatment is based on the severity and stage of endometriosis. Significant disease disrupting pelvic anatomy requires surgical correction either by laparoscopy or laparotomy. Successful surgical treatment of endometriosis-related infertility correlates with the surgeon's ability to normalize pelvic anatomy. Whereas 70% of patients with stage I or II disease conceive within 2 years of surgery, only 30% to 40% with severe endometriosis conceive.[3] Patients unable to conceive after surgery often require in vitro fertilization (IVF). Infertile women with minimal endometriosis have essentially normal pelvic anatomy. Expectant management is often warranted, whereas superovulation combined with intrauterine insemination (IUI) is reserved for refractory cases.

Hysterosalpingography (HSG) evaluates the uterine cavity and documents fallopian tube patency. HSG is performed early in the infertility evaluation, along with the semen analysis and determination of ovulatory status. This fluoroscopic evaluation, performed in the early proliferative phase of the menstrual cycle, involves introduction of a water-soluble radiopaque dye into the uterine cavity. Patients with previous reactions to iodine are better assessed initially with a combined laparoscopic-hysteroscopic approach. A similar diagnostic approach is recommended for individuals at risk for PID. Post-HSG infections are uncommon (1% to 3%), and prophylactic antibiotics may reduce their occurrence. HSG readily identifies myomas, polyps, müllerian anomalies, and Asherman's syndrome. Except for Asherman's syndrome, intrauterine pathology rarely causes infertility. Abnormal findings should be confirmed by hysteroscopy. Hysteroscopic resection of Asherman's syndrome corrects amenorrhea in 70% of patients while improving fertility rates.[16]

Instillation of sterile saline into the uterine cavity under ultrasound guidance *(sonohysterography)* is an attractive alternative to HSG. Compared with HSG, sonohysterography is less expensive, avoids ionizing radiation, and has similar sensitivity and specificity for detecting intrauterine pathology.

Both proximal and distal tubal pathology is readily identified with HSG. Abnormal fallopian tubes are best evaluated laparoscopically. The laparoscopic identification of peritubal adhesions and endometriosis increases diagnostic acumen beyond that of HSG alone. Laparoscopic adhesiolysis with restoration of tubal patency increases pregnancy rates in select individuals. Those with extensive pelvic adhesions, thick-walled fallopian tubes, and lack of normal tubal mucosa often fail to respond to laparoscopic surgery and require IVF. Patients with both proximal and distal tubal disease (bipolar tubal disease) should similarly be referred for IVF.

MALE FACTOR INFERTILITY

Abnormalities in sperm production or transit account for 30% to 40% of all cases of infertility. These data mandate early evaluation of the male and underscore that infertility is truly a couple's disorder. Tables 40-4 and 40-5 outline men's patient history and physical examination associated with fertility evaluation and infertility management.

A *semen analysis* is performed on all males as an initial screening test. Multiple semen analyses are often required because of marked variability in spermatogenesis and in collection technique. Proper collection and abstinence techniques are crucial when evaluating semen analyses. A masturbated specimen is collected into a wide-mouth jar after 48 to 72 hours of abstinence. Prompt laboratory evaluation is

Table 40-4. Male History and Fertility

Category	Findings	Impact on fertility
Sexual	Coital techniques/frequency Erectile/ejaculatory dysfunction	Inadequate gamete exposure
Pubertal development	Cryptorchidism, decreased libido, decreased shaving, impotence	Defects in androgen production (hypogonadal)
Injections	Mumps	Abnormal spermatogenesis
Medications	Sulfasalazine, nitrofurantoin, chemotherapy	Abnormal spermatogenesis
Environmental	Cigarettes, alcohol, illicit drugs, heavy metals, organic solvents, ionizing radiation, excessive heat	Abnormal spermatogenesis
Chronic medical conditions	Chronic sinusitis Chronic respiratory disorders	Sperm motility disorders (Immotile cilia syndrome)
	Chronic renal failure	Abnormal spermatogenesis
	Liver dysfunction	Abnormal spermatogenesis, Leydig cell dysfunction (decreased testosterone)
Prior surgery	Inguinal hernia	Altered spermatogenesis
	Varicocele	Diminished sperm motility

Modified from Illions EH, Valley MT, Kaunitz AM: *Med Clin North Am* 82(2):271, 1998.

Table 40-5. Male Physical Examination and Fertility

System	Findings	Impact on fertility
General	Eunuchoid body habitus Body hair distribution (sparse or absent)	Hypogonadism
	Short stature	Genetic disorder
Thyroid	Nodules, masses, tenderness, diffusely enlarged	Thyroiditis Hypothyroidism
Breast	Gynecomastia	Hypogonadism, androgen resistance syndrome, medications
Genitalia	Cryptorchidism Hypospadias Ambiguous genitalia Infantile (underdevelopment)	Androgen resistance syndrome; defect in testosterone biosynthesis leading to hypogonadism
	Absent vas deferens	Cystic fibrosis
	Epididymal tenderness	Infection
	Prostate tender or enlarged	Infection
	Prostate nonpalpable	Androgen resistance syndrome (5α-reductase deficiency)

Modified from Illions EH, Valley MT, Kaunitz AM: *Med Clin North Am* 82(2):271, 1998.

necessary, and Table 40-6 delineates normal semen parameters as suggested by the World Health Organization (WHO). Low semen volumes may indicate retrograde ejaculation, ductal obstruction, or absence of the seminal vesicles. Rectal probe ultrasound evaluates both the prostate and the seminal vesicles. Absence of fructose in the semen specimen suggests either obstruction or congenital absence of seminal vesicles. A vasogram will confirm partial or total ductal obstruction in the male. Retrograde ejaculation is confirmed when sperm are found in a postejaculate urine specimen.

Individuals with sperm counts between 10 and 20 million/ml are classified as having mild oligospermia. Pregnancies in this group frequently occur, and as such, these individuals are classified as subfertile rather than infertile. Males with sperm counts below 5 million/ml have severe oligospermia. Such individuals, as well as azoospermic males, require an endocrine evaluation. FSH, LH, thyroid-stimulating hormone (TSH), prolactin, testosterone, and estradiol levels should be obtained. FSH and LH values in excess of 40 mIU/ml indicate primary testicular failure, which is refractory to treatment. Donor sperm or adoption should be recommended to these couples. Low FSH, LH, and testosterone levels indicate a hypothalamic-pituitary disorder, requiring radiographic imaging of the sella turcica.

A variety of conditions, such as genital infections and varicoceles, adversely affect sperm motility. Most varicoceles are readily diagnosed on physical examination, whereas ultrasound-directed Doppler studies of the scrotum identify subclinical varicoceles. Significant numbers of white blood cells in semen (greater than 1 million/ml) constitute leukocytospermia by WHO criteria. Antibiotic therapy is indicated for these males as presumptive treatment for infection, since seminal fluid cultures prove unreliable and are expensive. Antisperm antibodies, especially when bound to the sperm tail, may adversely affect sperm motility. Diminished fertilization rates occur when significant numbers of antisperm antibodies bind to the sperm head.

With the advent of new IVF laboratory techniques, sperm morphology may be considered the most important seminal parameter. Strict morphologic criteria more accurately assess and predict sperm function compared with traditional WHO criteria. Under this system, adequate IVF fertilization rates occur when at least 14% of sperm have normal strict morphology.[13] Males with extremely abnormal semen, including those with severe oligospermia, poor motility, and a high percentage of abnormally shaped sperm, benefit from IVF. The recent advent of intracytoplasmic sperm injection (ICSI) allows treatment for males who have no motile sperm and less than 4% normal strict morphology.[25]

Table 40-6. Normal Semen Analysis

Test parameter	Value
Volume	2-6 ml
Concentration	20 million/ml or greater
Vicosity	Liquefaction in less than 30 minutes
Motility	50% or more with forward progression; 25% or greater with rapid progression; within 60 minutes of ejaculation
Morphology	More than 50%-60% oval (normal forms)
Cellularity (leukocytes)	Less than 1 million/ml

Modified from Illions EH, Valley MT, Kaunitz AM: *Med Clin North Am* 82(2):271, 1998.

CERVICAL FACTOR INFERTILITY

Infertility secondary to cervical factor abnormalities is rare, accounting for approximately 3% to 5% of all etiologies. Normal cervical mucus production is vital to filter bacteria and debris from seminal fluid and to assist sperm transport to the upper genital tract. At midcycle, cervical mucus is abundant, acellular, and nonviscous, thereby facilitating sperm transport to coincide with ovulation. Cervical mucus quality and sperm-mucus interaction are initially assessed with a postcoital test (PCT). Patients with prior histories of cervical cone biopsies, loop excisions of the transformation zone, and multiple dilation and curettage procedures are at risk for poor cervical mucus production. Also, antisperm antibodies bound to sperm membranes decrease sperm motility, thereby adversely affecting sperm-mucus interaction.

PCTs must be performed in the periovulatory phase of the menstrual cycle. Commercially available ovulation predictor kits enable precise timing, increasing test reliability. Couples should have intercourse the evening of the LH surge. A PCT is performed early the next morning, when the examining physician can evaluate cervical mucus using appropriate guidelines.[10] Part two of the PCT assesses the number of motile sperm per high-power field of cervical mucus, which indirectly measures cervical mucus competency. However, poorly designed studies, inconsistent methodology, and variable interpretation have largely invalidated PCT results, which also fail to correlate with pregnancy rates.[8]

Intrauterine insemination involves placement of washed sperm into the uterine cavity, bypassing the cervix. Pregnancy rates are acceptable when IUI is used to treat cervical factor infertility and unexplained infertility.

UNEXPLAINED INFERTILITY

Unexplained infertility identifies about 10% of infertile couples having no identifiable cause. This diagnosis is one of exclusion and mandates completion of a detailed and accurate infertility assessment. Subtle defects in ovulation, poor sperm function, and altered ovum selection may escape detection by currently available infertility testing. IVF has identified defective gametes and fertilization failure in some couples with unexplained infertility.[22] Some physicians use secondary testing (e.g., antisperm antibodies, specialized sperm function tests, transvaginal sonography) to evaluate infertility when initial testing remains normal.

Without an identifiable cause, treatments are largely empiric. Three to five cycles of controlled ovarian hyperstimulation with fertility drugs combined with IUI increase conception rates.[4] Ovarian stimulation with clomiphene yields an 8% to 10% per cycle pregnancy rate when combined with IUI, and parenteral gonadotropin therapy increases success to 12% to 15% per cycle. Approximately 23% to 25% of couples with unexplained infertility will conceive after three cycles of superovulation and IUI with gonadotropins, which equals the success seen after one IVF cycle.[27] Although superovulation with IUI remains the initial treatment for couples with unexplained infertility, those who

Table 40-7. Genetic Disorders and Carrier Status

Genetic disorder	At-risk population	Carrier frequency
Tay-Sachs disease	Eastern European Jews, French Canadian	1:27 Eastern European Jews
β-Thalassemia	Mediterranean, Southeast Asian Indian, Pakistani, African	Variable: 1:70 in African Americans, 1:6-1:50 in Indians, 1:10-1:50 in Italians
α-Thalassemia	Southeast Asian, African	25% of African Americans and 5%-8% of Thais are heterozygotes for α-thalassemia type 2
Sickle cell anemia	African, Mediterranean, Middle Eastern, Latin American, Indian	8% of African Americans
Fragile X syndrome	Mental impairment, microorchidism	Females 1:1000
Down syndrome	Advanced maternal age, affected family member	1:35,000 if one parent has translocation involving chromosome 21;2:100 (2%) if previously affected child with Down syndrome and parental karyotype *not* known

fail often benefit from more advanced reproductive technology (e.g., IVF).

ASSISTED REPRODUCTIVE TECHNOLOGIES

Assisted reproductive technology (ART) includes all procedures in which male and female gametes are artificially combined. IVF is indicated for couples with severe tubal disease, advanced endometriosis, severe male factor, refractory ovulatory dysfunction, and those patients with unexplained infertility failing to conceive with controlled ovarian hyperstimulation and IUI. Patients with unexplained infertility, because of their normal pelvic anatomy, are also candidates for a variety of tubal transfer procedures, such as gamete intrafallopian transfer (GIFT) and zygote intrafallopian transfer (ZIFT). Current data from the Society for Assisted Reproductive Technology (SART) delineate success rates for various ART procedures expressed in terms of delivery rates per retrieval: IVF, 22.5%; GIFT, 27%; and ZIFT, 27.9%.[30]

PRECONCEPTUAL COUNSELING

The primary care physician may uncover various risk factors for future pregnancies by obtaining a detailed history of reproductive performance, significant medical conditions, and familial disorders. Obstetric complications such as first-trimester miscarriages, second- and third-trimester fetal losses, postpartum hemorrhage, and premature labor may indicate a recurrent disorder. Prompt identification and treatment may ultimately reduce the risk of recurrence. A detailed family history may reveal certain genetic disorders and identify the need for carrier testing. Carrier screening can be offered based on ethnicity, racial background, and gender. All genetic disorders are uniformly noncorrectable, but their identification by carrier testing allows for adequate patient education and preparation before delivery (Table 40-7).

A variety of medical problems may pose significant risks during pregnancy. Some chronic illnesses exacerbate either during pregnancy or immediately postpartum. Alternatively, others adversely affect pregnancy outcome (Table 40-8).

A detailed social evaluation may identify couples at risk for domestic abuse, a situation likely to exacerbate during pregnancy and increase the risk of placental separation, bleeding, and premature labor and delivery. The marked prevalence of cigarette smoking and alcohol consumption represents significant social concerns, negatively impacts reproductive function, and poses significant risk to a developing fetus. Alcohol, tobacco, cocaine, and other drugs are well-described fetal teratogens.[35] Persistent use of these agents may adversely affect spermatogenesis in men as well as ovulatory and fallopian tube function in women. Effective preconceptual counseling may reduce their use. Less common environmental toxins, such as heavy metals, pesticides, and organic solvents, also pose significant risk to a developing fetus, and obtaining an adequate occupational history in the infertile couple is important.

Patients who significantly restrict their caloric intake by following unusual diets place the fetus at risk for developmental delay and growth retardation. The American College of Obstetrics and Gynecology has established guidelines for caloric intake and calcium supplementation in reproductive-age females. At least 0.4 mg (400 μg) of folic acid daily is necessary to reduce the risk of neural tube defects in patients contemplating pregnancy. These requirements are increased to 4 mg daily in women with a previously affected offspring. Folic acid supplementation should be initiated at least 1 month before conception.

Certain infectious disorders pose significant risks to a developing fetus. Susceptible individuals should be vaccinated when possible to reduce perinatal transmission and congenital birth defects. Rubella screening is mandatory in reproductive-age women because significant birth defects occur in 50% to 80% of fetuses in first-trimester maternal infection. Health care workers and child care attendants, including teachers, are at increased risk for hepatitis B, tuberculosis, and cytomegalovirus. At-risk women should be screened and counseled when indicated. Women susceptible to toxoplasmosis infection should be counseled to avoid handling cat feces and consuming raw meat. Reproductive-age women should be offered human immunodeficiency virus (HIV) screening; approximately 30% to 50% of offspring born to untreated HIV-infected women are seropositive.[18,19] Prompt identification of HIV-positive pregnant women is vital because retroviral therapy may reduce vertical transmission to the fetus.[2] Screening for other STDs (e.g., *Chlamydia,* syphilis, gonorrhea) are indicated in the appropriate clinical setting.

Table 40-8. Selected Medical Conditions and Preconception Recommendations

Medical problems	Effects and recommendations
Acne	*Isotretinoin (Accutane)* highly teratogenic; almost 25% of fetuses exposed in first trimester have major anomalies.
Androgens	Virilization of females
Bipolar disorder	*Lithium* associated with congenital heart disease (Ebstein's anomaly) and should be avoided if possible.
Diabetes	Tight glucose control before conception decreases incidence of congenital anomalies.
Folic acid antagonists (e.g., methotrexate)	Increased risk of spontaneous abortions; 30% fetal malformation rate with first-trimester exposure.
Hypertension	*Angiotensin-converting enzyme inhibitors* associated with fetal renal morbidity; patient should be converted to other antihypertensives.
Lead	Increased abortion rates and stillbirths; central nervous system effects noted; preconceptual lead levels may be helpful.
Organic mercury	Microcephaly, mental impairment, seizures, blindness, cerebral atrophy
Phenylketonuria	Dietary regimens that result in lower maternal phenylalanine levels are associated with a lower risk of fetal malformations.
Primary pulmonary hypertension	Maternal mortality approaches 50% with pregnancy; fetal mortality exceeds 40%.
Seizure disorders	Whether disease process, anticonvulsants, or both cause increase in congenital anomalies is debated. Need for medication should be reassessed, and if medication is required, a single agent typically used in pregnancy, such as *carbamazepine, phenobarbital,* or *phenytoin,* should be used. *Trimethadone* and *paramethadione* are no longer used in pregnancy because less toxic agents are available; both associated with 60% to 80% risk of spontaneous abortion or birth defects with first-trimester exposure.
Tetracycline	Hypoplasia of tooth enamel; incorporation of tetracycline into teeth and bone (usually only associated with second- and third-trimester exposure)
Thromboembolism prophylaxis	*Coumadin* associated with warfarin embryopathy; patients should be converted to *heparin.*

SUMMARY

Infertility affects 12% to 15% of married couples in the United States, underscoring the need for systematic and thorough evaluation. Treatment should be etiology based; however, some couples with normal testing (unexplained infertility) benefit from empiric therapy with superovulation and IUI. Indications for ART continue to expand as innovations occur. The recent advent of ICSI enables reproductive specialists to treat previously refractory male factor. Adoption, psychologic counseling, and infertility support groups benefit many infertile couples. An integrated approach to infertility effectively treats a large number of infertile couples.

REFERENCES

1. Bullen BA, Skrinar GS, Beitins IZ, et al: Induction of menstrual disorders by strenuous exercise in untrained women, *N Engl J Med* 312:1349, 1985.
2. Centers for Disease Control and Prevention: Recommendations of the US Public Health Service task force on the use of zidovudine to reduce perinatal transmission of human immunodeficiency virus, *MMWR* 43:1, 1994.
3. Cook AS, Rock JA: Surgical management of endometriosis, *Semin Reprod Endocrinol* 9:138, 1991.
4. Dodson WC, Whitesides DB, Hughes CL Jr, et al: Superovulation with intrauterine insemination in the treatment of infertility: a possible alternative to gamete intrafallopian transfer and in vitro fertilization, *Fertil Steril* 48:441, 1987.
5. Dunaif A: Insulin resistance and the polycystic ovary syndrome: mechanisms and implications for pathogenesis, *Endocr Rev* 18:774, 1997.
6. Gibbons WE, Toner JP, Hamacher P, Kolm P: Experience with a novel vaginal progesterone preparation in a donor oocyte program, *Fertil Steril* 69:96, 1998.
7. Gleicher N, El-Roeiy A, Confino E, et al: Is endometriosis an autoimmune disease? *Obstet Gynecol* 70:115, 1987.
8. Griffith CS, Grimes DA: The validity of the postcoital test, *Am J Obstet Gynecol* 162:615, 1990.
9. Guzick DS: Cardiovascular risk in women with polycystic ovarian syndrome, *Semin Reprod Endocrinol* 14:45, 1996.
10. Insler V, Melmed I, Echenbrenner I, et al: The cervical score: a simple semiquantitative method for monitoring of the menstrual cycle, *Int J Gynaecol Obstet* 10:23, 1972.
11. Jick H, Parker R, Morrison AS: Relationship between smoking and age of natural menopause, *Lancet* 1:1354, 1977.
12. Johnston DE, Chiao Y, Gavaler JS, et al: Inhibition of testosterone synthesis by ethanol and acetaldehyde, *Biochem Pharmacol* 30:1827, 1981.
13. Kruger TF, Acosta AA, Simmons KF, et al: Predictive value of abnormal sperm morphology in in vitro fertilization, *Fertil Steril* 49:112, 1988.
14. Lee SJ, Lenton EA, Sexton L, et al: The effect of age on the cyclical patterns of plasma LH, FSH, oestradiol and progesterone in women with regular menstrual cycles, *Hum Reprod* 3:851, 1988.
15. Mampalam TJ, Tyrrell JB, Wilson CB: Transsphenoidal microsurgery for Cushing's disease: a report of 216 cases, *Ann Intern Med* 109:487, 1988.
16. March CM: Hysteroscopy for infertility. In Baggish MS, Barbot J, Valle RF, editors: *Diagnostic and operative hysteroscopy: a test and atlas,* Chicago, 1989, Year Book.
17. Martin TL, Kim M, Malarkey WB: The natural history of idiopathic hyperprolactinemia, *J Clin Endocrinol Metab* 60:855, 1985.
18. Minkoff H, Nanda D, Menez R, Fikrig S: Pregnancies resulting in infants with acquired immunodeficiency syndrome or AIDS-related complex: follow up of mothers, children, and subsequently born siblings, *Obstet Gynecol* 69:288, 1987.
19. Minkoff HL, Henderson C, Mendez H, et al: Pregnancy outcomes among mothers infected with human immunodeficiency virus and uninfected control subject, *Am J Obstet Gynecol* 163:1598, 1990.
20. Mosher WD, Pratt WF: The demography of infertility in the United States. In Asch RH, Studd JW, editors: *Annual progress in reproductive medicine,* Pearl River, NY, 1993, Parthenon.

21. Navot D, Bergh PA, Williams MA, et al: Poor oocyte quality rather than implantation failure as a cause of age related decline in female infertility, *Lancet* 337:1375, 1991.
22. Navot D, Muasher SJ, Oehninger S, et al: The value of in vitro fertilization for the treatment of unexplained infertility, *Fertil Steril* 49:854, 1988.
23. New MI, Lorenzen F, Lerner AJ, et al: Genotyping steroid 21-hydroxylase deficiency: hormonal reference data, *J Clin Endocrinol Metab* 57:320, 1983.
24. Olive DL, Henderson DY: Endometriosis and mullerian anomalies, *Obstet Gynecol* 69:412, 1987.
25. Palermo G, Joris H, Derde MP, et al: Sperm characteristics and outcome of human assisted fertilization by subzonal insemination and intracytoplasmic sperm injection, *Fertil Steril* 59:826, 1993.
26. Reece EA, Hobbins JC: Diabetic embryopathy: pathogenesis, prenatal diagnosis and prevention, *Obstet Gynecol Surv* 41:325, 1986.
27. Rice RP, Karasick S, Goldfarb AF: Peritoneal adhesions in infertile women: diagnosis with hysterosalpingography, *Am J Roentgenol* 152:111, 1989.
28. Scott RT, Leonardi MR, Hofmann GE, et al: A prospective evaluation of clomiphene citrate challenge test screening in the general infertility population, *Obstet Gynecol* 82:539, 1993.
29. Shoupe D, Mishell DR, Lacarra M, et al: Correlation of endometrial maturation with four methods of estimating day of ovulation, *Obstet Gynecol* 73:88, 1989.
30. Society for Assisted Reproductive Technology and the American Society for Reproductive Medicine: Assisted reproductive technology in the United States and Canada: 1995 results, *Fertil Steril* 69:389, 1998.
31. Suginami H: A reappraisal of the coelomic metaplasia theory by reviewing endometriosis occurring in unusual sites and instances, *Am J Obstet Gynecol* 165:214, 1991.
32. Van Kooij RF, Looman CWN, Habberna JDF, et al: Age-dependent decrease in embryo implantation rate after in vitro fertilization, *Fertil Steril* 66:769, 1996.
33. Velazquez EM, Mendoza S, Hamer T, et al: Metformin therapy in polycystic ovarian syndrome reduces hyperinsulinemia, insulin resistance, hyperandrogenemia, and systolic blood pressure while facilitating normal menses and pregnancy, *Metabolism* 43:647, 1994.
34. Yen SSC: Chronic anovulation caused by peripheral endocrine disorders. In Yen SSC, Jaffe RB, editors: *Reproductive endocrinology,* ed 3, Philadelphia, 1991, Saunders.
35. Zuckerman B, Frank DA, Hinson R: Effects of maternal marijuana and cocaine use on fetal growth, *N Engl J Med* 320:762, 1989.

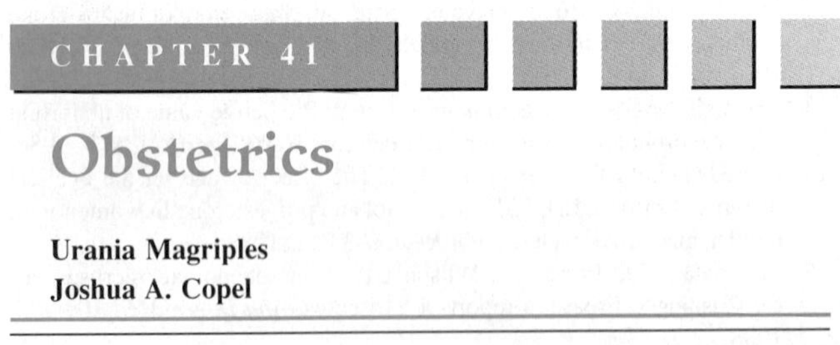

CHAPTER 41

Obstetrics

Urania Magriples
Joshua A. Copel

EPIDEMIOLOGY AND HIGH-RISK GROUPS

The physician delivering obstetric care has the unique opportunity to provide general medical treatment and screening to a large portion of the population that might not otherwise gain access to the health care system. There are over 7 million pregnancies in the United States yearly, with over 4.1 million live births (Fig. 41-1). Although rates of infant mortality and morbidity have been drastically reduced in this century, the United States still has one of the highest rates among industrialized countries, ranking twenty-first.

Certain demographic groups are at higher risk for poor outcomes. For example, the United States has one of the highest teenage pregnancy rates, with 1 million teenagers, or 5% to 8% of the teenage population, becoming pregnant each year. Teenagers are more likely to register late for prenatal care, be unmarried, and have less education, and they have more than twice the risk of low-birth-weight infants, neonatal mortality, and maternal mortality compared with older mothers. Racial differences persist in both maternal and infant morbidity and mortality. Currently, the infant mortality rate of African-Americans is higher than that of impoverished nations such as Cuba. As more women and children fall below the poverty line in the United States, a concerted effort is needed to expand access to prenatal care and thereby entry into the medical system.

PHYSIOLOGIC CHANGES OF PREGNANCY

The emerging concept that reproductive changes are a physiologic adaptation rather than a pathologic state has led internists and obstetricians to redefine their approach to the primary care of women. Although the physiologic changes during pregnancy are profound, most occur within a short period of time and are completely reversible. Those that are of primary interest to generalists are reviewed in Table 41-1.

HISTORY AND PHYSICAL EXAMINATION

The presence of pregnancy must be considered in every woman of reproductive age. Common signs and symptoms of pregnancy include amenorrhea, breast fullness and tenderness, fatigue, nausea and/or vomiting, increased appetite, and increased abdominal girth. On physical examination, the cervix appears bluish, and on bimanual palpation it is soft and flexible. The uterus increases in size with advancing gestational age and fills the pelvis at around 12 weeks. It is palpated above the pubic bone after that point and reaches the umbilicus at 20 weeks. After 20 weeks, the fundal height correlates roughly with centimeters above the pubic bone.

LABORATORY STUDIES

Pregnancy can be rapidly ruled out using commonly available sensitive serum or urinary pregnancy tests. Human chorionic gonadotropin (hCG) is a specific marker for viable trophoblast tissue and is directly correlated with gestational age. Most urinary tests are enzyme-linked immunosorbent assays (ELISA), which use a color reaction produced by an enzyme that is linked to an antibody. They vary in sensitivity with the lower limits of the assays, ranging from 200 to 800 IU/ml. Urine tests are available that are positive by day 25 after the last menstrual period. Serum radioimmunoassays are sensitive and accurate if directed to the β-subunit of the hCG molecule. In early pregnancy, hCG concentrations double approximately every 2 days, and an inadequate rise should raise the question of either a nonviable gestation or an ectopic pregnancy.

DIFFERENTIAL DIAGNOSIS

Vaginal bleeding in the first trimester is not uncommon and occurs in about 25% of pregnancies. Implantation bleeding is common and consists of minimal bleeding around the time of the first missed menstrual period. Flow may vary from mere spotting to bleeding that is similar to a period, but is rarely heavier than a period. If bleeding is observed from a closed

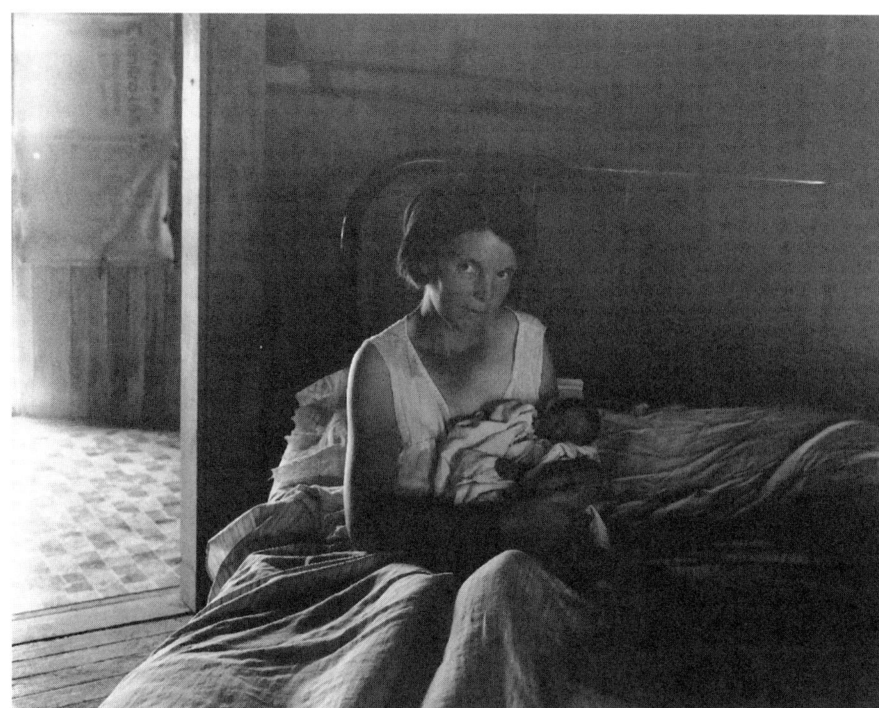

Fig. 41-1. Mother and her youngest child, 1937. (From Collections of the Library of Congress.)

cervical os and there is a documented intrauterine pregnancy, the diagnosis of a threatened abortion can be made. The uterus is generally appropriate in size but may be tender to examination. Once the cervix is dilated or the bleeding is profuse, the diagnosis of an inevitable abortion is made. An incomplete abortion signifies that there is tissue still within the uterus. Incomplete abortions become more common after 6 weeks of gestation. In an anembryonic gestation, formerly referred to as a missed abortion, the pregnancy has partially resorbed but there is still viable trophoblast-secreting hCG.

Ectopic pregnancy should be suspected in any woman of reproductive age presenting with abdominal pain or vaginal bleeding. Because approximately 2% of pregnancies are ectopic, constant vigilance is necessary to make the diagnosis. Ectopic pregnancies are the most common cause of maternal mortality in the first half of pregnancy and account for up to 50 maternal deaths annually. The rates of ectopic pregnancy are two times higher for nonwhite females than white females; however, mortality rates are six times higher for African-American women, making ectopic pregnancy the single most common cause of all maternal deaths in this population. Risk factors for ectopic pregnancy include multiparity, pelvic inflammatory disease, tubal surgery, previous pelvic surgery, previous ectopic, and intrauterine device (IUD) use.

The most common presenting signs are abdominal and adnexal tenderness, which are present in nearly all patients. Vaginal bleeding is present in 90% of cases. A pelvic mass is palpable in over half of patients, and the uterus is usually not appropriately enlarged. Tachycardia, orthostasis, and shock may follow rupture. Levels of hCG over 2000 IU/ml without the presence of an intrauterine pregnancy by vaginal ultrasonography suggest an ectopic pregnancy. Ultrasonographic detection of a pelvic mass is not definitive in the diagnosis of an ectopic pregnancy, since a corpus luteum or other benign ovarian tumor may be present; therefore correlation with the quantitative hCG level is recommended. Medical intervention with methotrexate is a treatment option for early ectopic pregnancies.

MANAGEMENT

Prenatal Care

The physician taking care of women has the opportunity to have an impact not only on the lives of women, but on the lives of their children and future generations. Preconceptual care is essential in minimizing exposure to drugs and teratogens, maximizing nutritional status, and identifying medical conditions that may either affect pregnancy or be influenced by it. Primary care physicians play an important role in the care of women of reproductive age who are considering pregnancy.

In the United States, 200,000 birth defects and over a half million infant deaths, spontaneous abortions, stillbirths, and miscarriages occur each year from defective fetal development. It is estimated that 1% to 5% of congenital anomalies may be drug or chemical related. Factors that determine a drug's effect on the fetus include dosage, duration, and time of exposure, as well as drug metabolism, concurrent use of other drugs, genetic susceptibility, and placental transfer. There is a critical period of embryonic development from the third through the twelfth week when the embryo is undergoing organogenesis. Before this time, exposures tend either to cause abortion or to have no effect at all (known as the all-or-none phenomenon). Beyond the twelfth week, effects are generally limited to growth and neural development. Primary care physicians often care for women in the crucial weeks of fetal organogenesis and therefore need to be aware of the effects of drugs on fetal development. Examples of recognized teratogens and their associated malformations are listed in Table 41-2.

Infectious agents also cause maldevelopment in the human (Table 41-3). The lethal or developmental effects are the

Table 41-1. Physiologic Changes of Pregnancy by System

Organ System	Change	Effect
Hematologic		
Blood volume	Increases by 1200 cc (45%)	"Dilutional anemia"
Plasma volume	Increases	
Red cell volume	Increases by 250-450 cc (25%)	
Iron requirements	Increase	Iron deficiency common
White blood cell count	Increases to 12,000 cells/mm^3 (higher in stress or labor)	Diagnosis of infection difficult
Fibrinogen, plasminogen, factors VII, VIII, and X	Increase	Increased risk of venous thrombosis
Platelets	Decrease (normal >100,000)	
Cardiovascular		
ECG	Left axis deviation	Nonspecific T wave changes
CXR	Superior, lateral, and anterior displacement of heart by enlarging uterus	Enlarged cardiac silhouette, straightened left border
Cardiac output	Increases by 30% to 50% Increased end-diastolic dimensions Myocardial hypertrophy	Systolic ejection murmurs common
Stroke volume	Increases	Increased cardiac work
Heart rate	Increases	Palpitations common; increase in premature atrial contractions
Blood pressure	Decreases in first and second trimester Increases to baseline in third trimester	Difficulty in distinguishing chronic hypertension from preeclampsia
Renal		
Kidney length	Increases by 1.5 cm	
Ureters	Dilate	Right > left
Bladder	Relaxes	Increased dead space, increased risk of urinary tract infections and pyelonephritis
Renal plasma flow	Increases by 50%	
Glomerular filtration	Increases by 50% (normal 120-160 ml/min)	Increased clearance of medications, difficulty attaining therapeutic dosing
Proteinuria	Increases	Underlying proteinuria; worsens with pregnancy
Glycosuria	Increases	Poor indicator of diabetes in pregnancy
Alimentary		
Gastric emptying	Delayed	Heartburn, reflux
Sphincter tone	Decreases	
Motility	Decreases	Constipation
Gallbladder	Increase in residual volume	Increase sludge and stone formation
Cholesterol	Doubles	
Binding proteins	Increase	Increase in thyroid requirements
Transferrin	Increases	
Albumin	Decreases	
Alkaline phosphatase	Increases (placental origin)	Unreliable test of liver disease
Transaminases	Unchanged	
Drug metabolism	Increases	Close monitoring of drug levels necessary
Pulmonary		
Minute ventilation	Increases	Subjective shortness of breath, mild respiratory alkalosis
Total lung capacity	Decreases by 5%	
Expiratory reserve volume	Decreases by 20%	
Tidal volume	Increases by 40%	
Vital capacity	Unchanged	
Inspiratory reserve volume	Unchanged	
FEV_1	Unchanged	Decrease not explained by pregnancy
PaO_2	Unchanged	Hypoxemia abnormal

Table 41-2. Teratogenic and Fetopathic Therapies and Environmental Agents

Agent	Reported effects
Alcohol	FAS, IUGR, microcephaly, mental retardation, cardiac anomalies, maxillary hypoplasia, characteristic facies. (Data based on chronic, heavy use [10 to 12 drinks/day], which is associated with 30% incidence of FAS. Less known about lower amounts.)
Aminopterin, methotrexate (antifolates)	Microcephaly, hydrocephaly, cleft palate, meningomyelocele, IUGR, abnormal cranial ossification, reduction in derivatives of first branchial arch, mental retardation, postnatal growth retardation.
Androgens	Masculinization of the female embyro, clitoromegaly.
Angiotensin-converting enzyme inhibitors	Oligohydramnios, pulmonary hypoplasia, neonatal anuria, IUGR, skull hypoplasia, fetal and neonatal death (second and third trimester exposure).
Carbamazepine	Minor craniofacial defects, fingernail hypoplasia, developmental delay.
Cocaine	Genitourinary malformations.
Cyclophosphamide	IUGR, ectrodactyly, syndactyly, cardiovascular anomalies.
Diethylstilbestrol	Cervical and uterine anomalies.
Diphenylhydantoin	Microcephaly, IUGR, mental retardation, cleft lip/palate, hypoplastic nails and distal phalanges.
Indomethacin	Prenatal ductus arteriosus closure (reversible), oligohydramnios.
Iodine deficiency	Mental retardation, spastic diplegia, deafness, fetal goiter.
Isotretinoin	CNS, cardiovascular and ear anomalies, cleft lip/palate, branchial arch abnormalities.
Lead	CNS abnormalities, microcephaly.
Lithium carbonate	Ebstein's anomaly of the tricuspid valve and other cardiovascular anomalies.
Methimazole	Aplasia cutis.
Methyl mercury	Growth deficiency, microcephaly, poor muscle tone, deafness, blindness.
Nicotine	IUGR, increased incidence of sudden infant death syndrome.
Penicillamine	Cutis laxa, hyperflexibility of joints.
Quinine	Ototoxicity and vestibular damage (high dose).
Radiation (external)	Microcephaly, mental retardation, eye anomalies, IUGR, visceral anomalies. (No effect seen at 5 rads or less; all-or-none phenomenon seen early in gestation.)
Tetracycline	Bone and tooth staining. High doses can cause hypoplastic tooth enamel.
Thalidomide	Limb reduction defects, facial hemangioma, esophageal or duodenal atresia, cardiovascular, renal, and ear anomalies.
Trimethadione	IUGR, V-shaped eyebrows, low set ears, high-arched palate, irregular teeth, CNS anomalies, severe developmental delay.
Valproic acid	Neural tube defects, dysmorphic facies, IUGR, cardiac abnormalities.
Warfarin	Nasal hypoplasia, stippling of secondary epiphysis, IUGR, anomalies of eyes, hands, and neck, CNS anomalies.

Modified from Brent RL, Beckman DA: Prescribed drugs, therapeutic agents, and fetal teratogenesis, *Clin Perinatol* 13:649, 1986.
FAS, Fetal alcohol syndrome; *IUGR*, Intrauterine growth retardation.

Table 41-3. Infection-induced Fetopathy

Agent	Reported effects
Cytomegalovirus	Microcephaly, chorioretinitis, deafness, mental retardation, hepatosplenomegaly, hydrocephalus, epilepsy, cerebral palsy, death.
Herpes simplex	Encephalitis, seizures, conjunctivitis, pulmonary disease, vesicular lesions, hepatitis, hemolytic anemia, thrombocytopenia.
Parvovirus B19	Hydrops secondary to anemia, death.
Rubella	IUGR, microcephaly, mental retardation, deafness, cataracts, glaucoma, cardiovascular abnormalities, hepatosplenomegaly, neonatal bleeding, purpura.
Syphilis	Skin rash, hepatosplenomegaly, hypotonia, rhinorrhea, periostitis.
Toxoplasmosis	Microcephaly, hydrocephaly, anencephaly, cerebral calcifications, hydrops, chorioretinitis, seizures, hepatosplenomegaly, growth retardation.
Varicella	Mental retardation, seizures, cataracts, microphthalmia, optic atrophy, chorioretinitis, growth retardation, limb hypoplasia, cutaneous scars.
Venezuelan equine encephalitis	Hydrocephalus, porencephaly, cataracts, microphthalmia.

IUGR, Intrauterine growth retardation.

result of mitotic inhibition, direct cytotoxicity, or necrosis. Inflammatory responses to infection can lead to metaplasia, scarring, or calcification, which further damages normal development.

Chronic maternal conditions also are associated with an increased risk of teratogenicity. For example diabetic mothers with hemoglobin A_{1C} levels greater than 7.5 have a twofold increased risk of congenital malformations, and the risk is greater with increasing levels. Levels of phenylalanine greater than 20 mg/dl in mothers with phenylketonuria are associated with a 90% incidence of congenital malformations, whereas levels less than 16 mg/dl are associated with a 20% incidence. Women with seizures have a twofold to threefold increased incidence of congenital anomalies regardless of whether they are on medications. Folate requirements increase in pregnancy and in women on antiepileptic medications. Therefore folate supplementation is recommended.

Nutrition. Current recommendations for nutrition in pregnancy are based on the pregnant woman's pregravid weight. For women who are within the optimal weight range for their height, the recommended weight gain is 20 to 35 pounds, with 5 pounds gained in the first trimester and approximately 1 pound per week in the second and third trimesters. For women who are overweight (20% or more above ideal body weight) the total weight gain should be about 15 to 25 pounds, with 2 pounds gained in the first trimester and about two thirds of a pound gained per week in the second and third trimesters. For women who are underweight (10% or more below ideal body weight), the total weight gain should be 28 to 40 pounds, with 5 pounds gained in the first trimester and at least a pound a week gained in the second and third trimesters, depending on the pregravid weight.

Protein, iron, and calcium requirements increase during pregnancy; however, the need for supplementation depends on the pregravid nutritional status. Women with short interpregnancy intervals, teenagers, grand multiparae, and patients of low socioeconomic status are at highest risk for nutritional deficiencies. Protein requirements increase in pregnancy from 50 to 90 gm/day. Iron needs average about 3.5 mg/day. Total iron demands during a singleton pregnancy average 1000 to 1100 mg and are higher for gestations with more than one fetus. Calcium requirements increase to 1200 mg/day, 50% higher than the nonpregnant recommendation. Folate requirements increase to 800 mg, and periconceptual folate supplementation decreases the incidence of neural tube defects.

Prenatal Visits. The basic laboratory tests recommended for all pregnant women are listed in Box 41-1. Routine visits are scheduled monthly until 30 weeks, every 2 weeks until 36 weeks, and then weekly. At each visit, weight, blood pressure, urine screening for protein and glucose, and measurement of the fundal height and auscultation of the fetal heart are performed.

Genetic testing by amniocentesis or chorionic villus sampling (CVS) is routinely offered to women who will be 35 years old at the time of delivery because they are at increased risk for fetal aneuploidy. Thorough patient and family histories will reveal other risk factors for genetically transmissible diseases. A stillborn fetus has a 6% to 11% risk of having a chromosomal abnormality; therefore women with a history of stillborn births should be counseled. Couples with a history of three or more pregnancy losses or prolonged infertility have up to a 6% risk of a chromosomal abnormality. A previous child with a chromosomal abnormality or congenital malformation likewise puts the parents in a high-risk group with future pregnancies.

Ethnicity is also important, since certain groups carry a higher risk for genetic diseases. Whites have a 1 in 20 risk of carrying the recessive gene for cystic fibrosis. Individuals of Mediterranean descent have a 1 in 12 risk of being carriers of the β-thalassemia gene. (The mean corpuscular volume [MCV] is useful as a screening test for thalassemia trait.) Ashkenazi Jews, who have a 1 in 30 risk of carrying the gene for Tay-Sachs disease and a 1 in 40 risk of carrying the gene for Canavan's disease, should be offered testing for these carrier states. The carrier rate for sickle-cell disease is 1 in 12 in African-Americans. The chance of having an affected child when both parents are carriers of any of these autosomal recessive diseases is 25%, and prenatal testing should be offered.

Although the risk of Down syndrome (trisomy 21) is greatest in women aged 35 or over, the majority of affected infants are born to women younger than 35, since they represent a larger percentage of the childbearing population. Prenatal diagnosis on the basis of age alone detects only 20% to 30% of these infants; thus screening for maternal serum markers has been used to increase detection. Alpha-fetoprotein (AFP) is the major early fetal serum protein. It enters the amniotic fluid via fetal renal excretion, transudation through skin, and open lesions such as spina bifida and ventral wall defects. An elevated level is found with open neural tube and ventral wall defects, twin gestations, intrauterine fetal demise, as well as pregnancies at risk for

Box 41-1. Basic Laboratory Tests

Complete blood count
Blood type and antibody screen (indirect Coombs')
Hepatitis surface antigen
VDRL or RPR
Rubella
HIV
Pap smear
Cervical cultures for gonorrhea and chlamydia
Urinalysis (culture of >3 to 5 WBC/HPF)
Glucose tolerance test (at 28 weeks)
Triple screen (maternal serum alpha-fetoprotein, estriol, and human chorionic gonadotropin)*
Genetic testing*
Ultrasound*

Routine Visit

Weight
Blood pressure
Urine dipstick
Estimation of fetal size by fundal height
Auscultation of fetal heart
Brief physical examination including reflexes and edema
Determination of symptoms of preterm labor (contractions, rupture of membranes, and bleeding)

*Requires counseling before implementation.

growth retardation and fetal death. In contrast, a low level of maternal serum AFP (MSAFP) has been associated with an increased risk of trisomy 21 and other trisomies. MSAFP testing in women under the age of 35 will detect an additional 25% of pregnancies affected by Down syndrome, with a 5% false-positive rate. Recent studies have shown that maternal serum concentrations of hCG are at least two times higher than normal, and those of unconjugated estriol are 25% lower in the presence of fetal Down syndrome. The additional use of these markers improves the detection rate to 67%, with a 7.2% false-positive rate.

Ultrasound has been used as a screening tool in the detection of neural tube and ventral wall defects in women with elevated MSAFP, and in experienced hands has a very high sensitivity and specificity. Unfortunately, the detection rate of trisomies by ultrasound is variable, and therefore ultrasound is not expected to replace amniocentesis in women at high risk. Routine ultrasound in all obstetric patients is a controversial issue, but certainly if the couple desires information on prenatal diagnosis of congenital anomalies, then second trimester ultrasound at a tertiary center is advisable.

A fetal karyotype can be obtained by CVS or amniocentesis. An advantage of CVS is that it can be performed in the first trimester (10 to 12 weeks), with results obtained in less than a week. Thus pregnancy termination, if desired, is a less complicated procedure. CVS has a procedure-related miscarriage rate of 0.5% to 1%. Amniocentesis can be performed after 15 weeks' gestation with a procedure-related miscarriage rate of 0.5%. Amniocytes take 10 days to 2 weeks to grow in culture. Because of these delays, termination of pregnancy requires either a dilation and evacuation, a more complex procedure than in the first trimester, or induction of labor with prostaglandin.

Medical Complications of Pregnancy

The primary care physician may intervene at two points in a high-risk pregnancy (Table 41-4). In the preconceptual patient, the physician has the opportunity to control disease and plan for its management during pregnancy. The primary

Table 41-4. Medical Complications of Pregnancy

Disease	Effect of pregnancy	Therapeutic considerations
Asthma	Unpredictable	Increased dosage of theophylline; side effects of steroids (hypertension, gestational diabetes).
Deep venous thrombosis	Increased risk (present in all trimesters)	Most commonly left leg thrombosis; right leg is rare. Coumadin contraindicated secondary to teratogenicity. (Can be used in breastfeeding.)
Diabetes	Insulin resistance increases Pregnancy does not accelerate retinopathy or nephropathy	Congenital anomalies two to three times general population; correlated with Hgb A_{1C} >7.5. Oral hypoglycemics contraindicated. Poor control correlated with fetal morbidity/mortality, macrosomia, and increased risk of C-section. Increased risk of preeclampsia.
Hypertension	Improvement in first trimester 30% risk of preeclampsia	Angiotensin converting enzyme inhibitors and diuretics contraindicated (except in heart failure).
Nephropathy	Moderate renal insufficiency (20%-40% have decline in CrCl) Proteinuria may worsen	Poor prognosis with Cr >1.5 mg/dl, proteinuria >3 gm in 24 hours in first trimester or poorly controlled hypertension.
Rheumatoid arthritis	75% remission (90% flare postpartum)	See systemic lupus erythematosus; teratogenicity of penicillamine; gold salts do not cross placenta.
Systemic lupus erythematosus	Remission 6 months before conception best prognosis. Increased risk of flare postpartum	Teratogenicity of antimalarials, nonsteroidals and alkylating agents. Main treatment steroids. Anti-Ro and La antibodies associated with congenital heart block. Lupus anticoagulant and anticardiolipin antibodies associated with recurrent abortions, IUGR, and fetal death.
Seizures	50% no change 25% improve 25% worsen	Baseline malformation rate twice normal (regardless of medications). Teratogenicity of Dilantin, valproic acid, Tegretol, trimethadione. Depletion of folate and vitamin K–dependent factors. Preconceptual folate recommended to decrease risk of neural tube defects.
Ulcerative colitis	Increased risk of flares first trimester and postpartum	If disease active at time of conception, higher risk of miscarriage, intrauterine growth retardation, and fetal death. If quiescent, same as general population.
von Willebrand's disease	Improvement	Increased risk of bleeding with first trimester miscarriages and postpartum.

IUGR, Intrauterine growth retardation.

care physician also may be involved in managing women who develop medical complications after conception. These patients are best cared for in close consultation with a perinatologist.

Diabetes. Previously diagnosed diabetes complicates 0.5% of pregnancies in the United States; gestational diabetes affects an additional 4% and is predominantly diet controlled.

The hormonal changes of pregnancy cause an increased insulin response to a glucose load in normal pregnant women and worsening of control in the diabetic pregnancy. Estrogen and progesterone induce pancreatic β-cell hyperplasia and increased insulin secretion, as well as increased glycogen storage, peripheral glucose utilization, and decreased hepatic glucose production. In the late second and third trimesters, human placental lactogen, prolactin, and cortisol combine to increase insulin resistance and decrease glucose tolerance and ensure adequate levels of glucose and amino acids for fetal growth. Because of these changes, patients with insulin-dependent diabetes will commonly have frequent episodes of hypoglycemia and ketonuria in the first trimester and are more prone to ketoacidosis in the second and third trimesters.

Gestational Diabetes. Gestational diabetes is defined as the onset or recognition of glucose intolerance during pregnancy. This definition includes patients with preexisting diabetes that is first detected in pregnancy and those who develop glucose intolerance only in pregnancy. The latter group is not prone to hyperglycemia or ketosis in the first trimester and the associated increased incidence of congenital malformations.

All pregnant women should routinely be screened at 28 weeks of gestation with a 50 gm oral glucose tolerance test. Those with strong risk factors (e.g., obesity, a history of gestational diabetes, or an infant with a congenital anomaly, macrosomia, or fetal demise) should be screened earlier. Women who have an abnormal screening test (1 hour serum glucose greater than 145 mg/dl) undergo a 3-hour 100 gm glucose test. Criteria for diagnosing gestational diabetes vary. Many physicians follow the guidelines developed by the National Diabetes Data Group (NDDG) in which two elevated blood glucose values greater than 105, 190, 165, and 145 mg/dl for the fasting, 1-, 2-, and 3-hour tests, respectively, are considered abnormal. Although these criteria have been criticized as being too high, the current recommendations are that the NDDG data be used until an international consensus can be obtained.

The mainstay of therapy in gestational diabetes is diet. Current recommendations call for individualized caloric intake according to the patient's weight and a dietary composition containing 50% to 60% carbohydrate, 12% to 20% protein, and approximately 25% fat, with less than 10% as saturated fatty acids, up to 10% as polyunsaturated fatty acids, and the remainder of ingested fat derived from monosaturated forms. Glucose monitoring is accomplished with daily home blood glucose monitoring of fasting and 2-hour postprandial glucose assessment. The use of insulin is recommended for those with fasting glucose values consistently greater than 100 mg/dl, or 2-hour postprandial levels greater than 120 mg/dl. Oral hypoglycemics are not recommended for use in pregnancy, as the sulfonylureas are known to cross the placenta and stimulate the fetal pancreas to secrete insulin. (Hyperinsulinemia is one of the postulated mechanisms for adverse fetal outcomes such as macrosomia.) Oral hypoglycemics also cause prolonged neonatal hypoglycemia due to slower hepatic elimination of these drugs by the neonate.

Infants of gestational and overt diabetics are at an increased risk of perinatal complications, including hypoglycemia, hyperbilirubinemia, hypocalcemia, polycythemia, respiratory distress syndrome, macrosomia, and fetal trauma. Fetal demise due to poor control of gestational diabetics is rarely seen today since the implementation of glucose monitoring, diet, and antenatal testing.

Debate continues about the long-term maternal consequences of gestational diabetes. Women who have gestational diabetes are at increased risk for diabetes later in life. Longitudinal studies of women followed up to 20 years after the diagnosis of gestational diabetes report prevalence rates of diabetes requiring therapy as high as 21% and of diabetes not requiring therapy up to 54%. Individuals with persistent obesity are at highest risk for developing subsequent diabetes.

Insulin-dependent Diabetes. The leading cause of perinatal mortality in infants of mothers with insulin-dependent diabetes is congenital malformations. Major anomalies are two to three times more common and are correlated with an elevated hemoglobin A_{1C} (glycosylated hemoglobin). Malformations are most common in the central nervous system, cardiovascular, gastrointestinal, genitourinary, and skeletal systems. Preconceptual control is advocated to decrease the incidence of these malformations, as they occur in the first few weeks after conception, often before a patient presents for prenatal care. Because of these risks, a targeted ultrasound, maternal serum triple screen determination, and fetal echocardiogram are indicated.

Infants of diabetic mothers are at increased risk of developing diabetes later in life. Insulin-dependent diabetes is transmitted less frequently to the offspring of diabetic women than diabetic men. Offspring with two diabetic parents have the highest risk (30%) of developing diabetes. Type II diabetes is probably inherited as an autosomal dominant trait; thus 50% of offspring with one affected parent will inherit the tendency for the disease, although other factors, such as obesity and diet, influence penetrance.

Glucose control is accomplished by one to three daily injections of insulin and glucose monitoring to maintain fasting and two hour postprandial glucose levels less than 90 and 120 mg/dl, respectively. The addition of long-acting insulin at bedtime is often necessary to obtain euglycemia. The first trimester is characterized by episodes of hypoglycemia, whereas the second and third trimesters are characterized by increasing glucose and insulin resistance; therefore close monitoring is necessary. Poor control, frequent insulin reactions, and new onset diabetes require hospitalization for management and education.

Pregnancies complicated by diabetes are monitored closely by ultrasound for abnormalities in fetal growth and for polyhydramnios. All diabetic pregnancies have a higher incidence of preeclampsia, pyelonephritis, and worsening of hypertension and need to be monitored closely. Patients should be seen every 2 weeks until 30 weeks, then weekly. Pregnancies with good control are allowed to progress to term, whereas pregnancies with poor control, worsening hypertension, or fetal growth derangements are delivered before term after documentation of fetal lung maturity by amniocentesis.

In addition to a careful history and physical examination, all pregnant diabetic women should be screened for end-organ complications with a baseline ophthalmologic examination, 24-hour urine collection for creatinine and protein determinations, serum electrolytes, cholesterol, and electrocardiogram. Pregnant diabetic women with preexisting nephropathy, who have a creatinine level greater than 1.5 mg/dl, proteinuria greater than 3 gm in 24 hours in the first trimester, or poorly controlled hypertension have a poor prognosis in terms of pregnancy outcome. Renal function may remain stable after the pregnancy; however, in 20% to 40% of patients it declines. Pregnancy-induced hypertension occurs in 25% of diabetic pregnancies and is associated with worsening of renal function; therefore close monitoring is warranted. Proteinuria commonly increases along with the glomerular filtration rate (GFR), but returns to baseline after pregnancy in the majority of patients. Elevated blood pressure and a rapid decrease in creatinine clearance are the most common events leading to preterm delivery; therefore strict blood pressure control is necessary.

Most women with nephropathy have evidence of microvascular disease and atherosclerosis. The influence of pregnancy on diabetic retinopathy is not well understood. Initially, there was concern that pregnancy accelerated the process, particularly with rapid normalization of serum glucose; however, these changes may reflect the natural progression of disease and its identification in pregnancy. Close ophthalmologic follow-up is warranted. Maternal mortality rate may be as high as 67% in women with diabetes and ischemic heart disease; therefore pregnancy termination for maternal indications should be considered in these patients.

Hypertension. Hypertension complicates 10% of pregnancies and causes significant fetal and maternal mortality and morbidity. Preeclampsia accounts for 70% of cases of hypertension in pregnancy, with chronic hypertension accounting for most of the remaining 30% of cases. The American College of Obstetrics and Gynecology defines hypertension in pregnancy as either a systolic pressure of 140 mm Hg or an increment of 30 mm Hg from the first prenatal value, or a diastolic pressure of 90 mm Hg or an increment of 15 mm Hg. The decrease in peripheral vascular resistance during pregnancy can make the diagnosis of hypertension difficult, since blood pressure normally drops in the first and second trimesters only to increase in the third trimester.

Preeclampsia is classically described as the triad of edema, proteinuria, and hypertension. Unfortunately, edema is present in up to 80% of normotensive pregnancies and is not always present in eclampsia. Mild preeclampsia is diagnosed by a blood pressure reading of 140/90 taken on two occasions 6 hours apart in the presence of proteinuria. Severe preeclampsia is diagnosed when one of the following is present: (1) blood pressure ≥160 mm Hg systolic or ≥110 mm Hg diastolic on two occasions at least 6 hours apart with the patient at bed rest, (2) proteinuria ≥5 gm in a 24-hour urine collection or +3 on dipstick in at least two random clean catch samples 4 hours apart, (3) oliguria (urine output <30 cc/hour), (4) cerebral or visual disturbances, (5) epigastric pain, or (6) pulmonary edema or cyanosis. The appearance of preeclampsia in the first and second trimesters raises the suspicion of a molar pregnancy or maternal systemic lupus erythematosus.

Risk factors for preeclampsia include preexisting hypertension, renal disease, diabetes, multiple gestations, nulliparity, family history of preeclampsia, and a fetus with hydrops. Treatment of preeclampsia is delivery of the fetus and placenta. If the pregnancy is at or near term, delivery can be accomplished by cervical ripening and induction of labor. If the pregnancy is remote from term, then management depends on the severity of disease. Mild preeclampsia can be managed as an outpatient or inpatient, depending on patient reliability and compliance with bed rest and follow-up. Severe preeclampsia warrants admission and careful monitoring of maternal renal, hepatic, and hematologic parameters, as well as treatment of diastolic blood pressures ≥105 mm Hg. If fetal pulmonary maturity is documented, then delivery is warranted. If fetal pulmonary maturity is not present, conservative management can be considered if fetal well-being can be monitored. Steroids are given to accelerate lung maturation. These pregnancies are at high risk for intrauterine growth retardation (IUGR), fetal distress, and stillbirth; therefore close fetal monitoring and consultation with maternal-fetal medicine and neonatal teams are mandatory for conservative management of severe preeclampsia.

The reported incidence of HELLP syndrome (*h*emolysis, *e*levated *l*iver enzymes, *l*ow *p*latelets) in preeclampsia ranges from 2% to 12%. A severe form of preeclampsia, it can be confused with other disorders associated with liver dysfunction or hemolytic anemia.

Eclampsia is defined as the development of seizures or coma in a patient with signs and symptoms of preeclampsia. The reported incidence is up to 0.5% of all deliveries. Only about 50% of cases occur antepartum.

Magnesium sulfate is widely used in the United States in preeclampsia to prevent and control seizures. The drug is administered by continuous intravenous infusion with a 6 gm load over 20 minutes followed by a maintenance rate of 2 gm/hour. Serum magnesium levels are followed, and the rate of the infusion is adjusted to maintain a level between 4.8 and 9.6 mg/dl. Magnesium is excreted by the kidneys; therefore close monitoring of urine output is necessary and dose adjustment is warranted in the face of persistent oliguria. In the therapeutic range, magnesium slows neuromuscular conduction. Suppression of deep tendon reflexes, respiration, and eventually coma and asystole are seen in overdoses. Overdose can be reversed with the administration of intravenous calcium gluconate. Magnesium sulfate therapy is continued for 24 hours postpartum or after an eclamptic episode. Other anticonvulsants have been used including phenobarbital, diphenylhydantoin and valium, but there are studies to support that magnesium sulfate is more effective at both prevention and recurrence of eclampsia.

Antihypertensive drug therapy in pregnancy is limited by concerns of teratogenicity and fetal side effects. Methyldopa has been used for many years with no adverse fetal side effects. Calcium channel blockers are now widely used in pregnancy for both the treatment of hypertension and preterm labor with minimal side effects. β-Blockers also have been used widely, and although initially they were thought to cause frequent fetal side effects, it is now established that side effects are due to maternal condition rather than drug effect. Angiotensin-converting enzyme inhibitors have been associated with oligohydramnios, IUGR, fetal renal failure, and intrauterine demise and are contraindicated in pregnancy. Diuretics are contraindicated for treatment of hypertension in pregnancy, as they decrease intravascular volume and therefore placental perfusion. Diuretics are used only in patients with congestive heart failure and pulmonary edema. Neither low-dose (80 mg) aspirin nor calcium supplementation has been shown to be effective in reducing the risk of preeclampsia or growth restriction in pregnancy and therefore are not indicated as treatment modalities.

Treatment of hypertension has significant maternal benefit, but there has been no proven fetal benefit in prolonging gestation, increasing birthweight, or reducing the risk of placental abruption or preeclampsia.

Thyroid Disease. Several physiologic changes occur in the thyroid gland during pregnancy to maintain a euthyroid state. The thyroid increases iodine uptake and production of thyroid hormone in response to a decline in plasma iodine concentration that results from an increase in GFR and iodine clearance. Estrogen stimulates production of thyroid-binding globulin (TBG), and because 85% of circulating thyroid hormone is bound to TBG, levels of thyroxine (T_4) and triiodothyronine (T_3) increase. The T_3 uptake (T_3U), which is inversely related to thyroid hormone-binding capacity in serum, is reduced due to elevated TBG concentrations. Levels of free thyroid hormone (free thyroxine index) are in the normal range. Thyroid-stimulating hormone (TSH) levels are slightly suppressed in the first trimester and subsequently normalize; therefore they are an accurate marker for hypothyroidism.

Hypothyroidism. Although hypothyroidism is common in reproductive-aged women, untreated hypothyroidism is not commonly seen in pregnancy, probably because of the inability of hypothyroid patients to ovulate.

Untreated hypothyroidism during pregnancy is associated with an increased incidence of spontaneous abortion, IUGR, stillbirth, and congenital anomalies, as well as preeclampsia and abruption. Autoimmune thyroiditis usually improves during pregnancy and relapses postpartum. Antimicrosomal and antithyroglobulin antibodies, if present, are rarely associated with any fetal side effects.

Treatment of hypothyroidism is with oral L-thyroxine at a starting dose of 125 to 150 mg, with follow-up determinations of serum TSH and T_4 levels every 3 weeks. If TSH levels remain elevated, the dose of L-thyroxine is increased by 50-mg increments. The increase in TBG may necessitate higher doses than in the nonpregnant state.

Hyperthyroidism. Hyperthyroidism occurs in about 2 of every 1000 pregnancies. Graves' disease or autoimmune thyrotoxicosis is the most common cause. Subclinical hyperthyroidism may be difficult to distinguish in early pregnancy, as an increase in heart rate, heat intolerance, skin warmth, nausea, and poor weight gain are common symptoms in the first trimester. Tachycardia, thyromegaly, exophthalmos, and failure to gain weight with normal or increased caloric intake are not normal and can be helpful clues. Thyrotoxicosis can be associated with severe vomiting and may be the cause of hyperemesis gravidarum, or result from molar gestations and choriocarcinoma. In the latter two conditions, elevated hCG levels, which stimulate thyroid hormone, and the thyroid dysfunction are completely reversible with uterine evacuation.

Hyperthyroidism is diagnosed by elevated free T_4 level and values of TSH below 0.1 mU/ml. Occasionally, the free T_4 is normal and the T_3 is elevated. Determination of the presence of autoantibodies (thyroid-stimulating immunoglobulins or long-acting thyroid stimulator) is necessary because they are IgG and can cross the placenta. Fetal or neonatal hyperthyroidism secondary to transfer of maternal antibodies complicates approximately 1% of pregnancies in women with a history of Graves' disease or Hashimoto's thyroiditis. In women who have undergone thyroid ablation, the presence of antibodies still must be determined.

In pregnancy, treatment of hyperthyroidism is most commonly medical. The thiourea derivatives propylthiouracil (PTU), methimazole, and carbamazole are all used. PTU is the most commonly used medication and is not associated with fetal abnormalities. The objective is to maintain the mother in the high normal range to avoid fetal hypothyroidism. Initially, thyroid function tests are followed every 2 weeks, but when a stable dosage is obtained, they can be followed monthly. If a drug reaction occurs, therapy is changed to methimazole (Tapazole). Methimazole is associated with reversible aplasia cutis in the fetus and therefore is kept as the second-line drug. Although both drugs are secreted in breast milk, less PTU is secreted because it is more protein-bound. Thyroidectomy is reserved for women who cannot adhere to medical therapy or who have toxic side effects to it. Radioactive iodine is contraindicated in pregnancy, since iodine is concentrated in the fetal thyroid after 10 weeks and can result in fetal goiter.

Maternal complications of hyperthyroidism in pregnancy include hyperemesis, poor weight gain, preterm labor, thyroid storm, and high-output cardiac failure. Fetal complications include fetal tachydysrhythmias, high output cardiac failure, hydrops, IUGR, and goiter.

Cardiac Disease. The physiologic changes of pregnancy, delivery, and the puerperium cause significant alteration in the maternal cardiovascular system. Increase in the myocardial workload is related to increased blood volume, metabolic demands, cardiac output, and heart rate. Increases in blood pressure and anemia also can affect cardiac output. Patients with well-compensated heart disease may thus have heart failure for the first time during pregnancy. The goal of medical management is to optimize maternal hemodynamics by changing preload, afterload, and contractility once symptomatology is present. Diuretics are reserved for pulmonary edema or right-sided heart failure. Digoxin is used to control atrial fibrillation. Afterload reduction may be beneficial in improving cardiac output.

Labor and delivery are a crucial time, with increased hemodynamic load associated with contractions, pain, anesthesia, possible surgery, blood loss, and intravenous therapy. Therefore complete hemodynamic monitoring optimizes fluid management and pharmacologic manipulation of cardiac output. In labor, epidural anesthesia is recommended to relieve pain and to avoid Valsalva maneuvers. Use of the lateral position is important, since it minimizes hypotension and increases preload and cardiac output. Cesarean delivery is undertaken for obstetric indications, as vaginal delivery avoids the stress and blood loss of surgery. Instrumental delivery by low forceps or vacuum extraction is recommended to avoid Valsalva's maneuvers. Postpartum, intensive monitoring in the first 48 hours is necessary, since this is the period of highest risk for fluid shifts secondary to autotransfusion with placental delivery and uterine involution.

Classification of maternal mortality for various types of cardiac disease is useful in counseling patients. Mitral stenosis with atrial fibrillation or New York Heart Association classes III and IV aortic stenosis, uncorrected tetralogy of Fallot, previous myocardial infarction, and Marfan syndrome with a normal aorta are associated with a maternal mortality rate of 5% to 15%. Pulmonary hypertension, aortic coarctation, and Marfan syndrome with aortic root dilation greater than 4 cm carry a 25% to 50% maternal mortality rate and can be considered a contraindication to pregnancy.

Peripartum cardiomyopathy is characterized by the development of cardiac failure in the third trimester or within 5 months of delivery for which no other cause can be determined. The incidence of peripartum cardiomyopathy is 1 in 3000 to 4000 pregnancies. In the United States, it is more frequent among older, multiparous African-American women, twins, and patients with preeclampsia. It has a tendency to recur with subsequent pregnancies. Some investigators have implicated inadequate nutrition, viral agents, preeclampsia, or immunologic factors in its pathogenesis. Another theory suggests that viral myocarditis may be the primary inciting factor. The prognosis for dilated cardiomyopathy is poor, with progressive deterioration once symptoms occur. The mortality rate for peripartum cardiomyopathy in the United States ranges from 25% to 50%. There may be a subset of patients in whom the heart size returns to normal who have a significantly better prognosis. This group also may include patients who had stable cardiac disease before conception.

ADDITIONAL READINGS

Briggs GG, Freeman RK, Yaffe SJ: *Drugs in pregnancy and lactation: a reference guide to fetal and neonatal risk,* ed 5, Baltimore, 1998, Williams & Wilkins.

Burrow GN, Duffy TP: *Medical complications during pregnancy,* ed 5, Philadelphia, 1999, WB Saunders.

Creasy RK, Resnik R, editors: *Maternal-fetal medicine: principles and practice,* ed 4, Philadelphia, 1999, WB Saunders.

Geronimus AT, Bound J: Black/white differences in women's reproductive-related health status: evidence from vital statistics, *Demography* 27:457, 1990.

Gleicher N, editor: *Principles and practice of medical therapy in pregnancy,* ed 3, Connecticut, 1998, Appleton & Lange.

Milunsky A, editor: *Genetic disorders and the fetus,* Baltimore, 1992, Johns Hopkins University.

Nyberg DA, et al, editors: *Transvaginal sonography,* St Louis, 1992, Mosby.

Reece EA, Coustan DR, editors: *Diabetes mellitus in pregnancy: principles and practice,* ed 2, New York, 1995, Churchill Livingstone.

Reece EA et al, editors: *Medicine of the mother and fetus,* ed 2, Philadelphia, 1999, Lippincott-Raven.

Wegman ME: Annual summary of vital statistics—1991, *Pediatrics* 90:835, 1992.

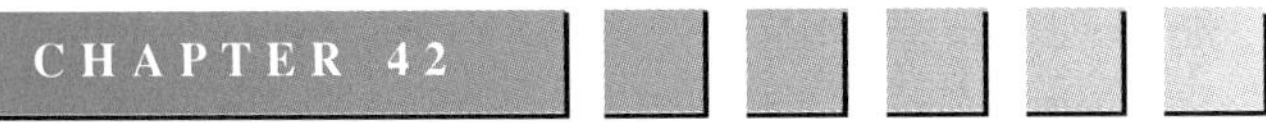

CHAPTER 42

Menopause

David L. Keefe

More than one third of the women in the United States have reached menopause, and with female life expectancy approaching 80 years, many will spend more than a third of their lives in a postmenopausal state.[8] The first born of the baby boom generation are approaching their fifth decade, so the number of menopausal women is expected to increase further over the next 20 years. Although menopause is a natural phenomenon, the loss of ovarian estrogen production can evoke symptoms and exacerbate a number of age-related diseases, including coronary heart disease and osteoporosis. Hormone therapy alleviates menopausal symptoms and reduces the risks of coronary heart disease and osteoporosis, but may induce side effects. Thus menopausal women constitute a large and growing portion of physicians' practices for whom recognition and treatment of hypoestrogenism may improve the quality and duration of life. The physician must help the menopausal woman to weigh potential benefits against risks of hormone therapy in order to decide whether hormone therapy is the right choice for her.

DEFINITIONS

Menopause is the woman's final menstrual period. Usually defined retrospectively after 6 to 12 months of amenorrhea, menopause occurs at an average age of 51. Loss of ovarian function before age 40 is termed *premature ovarian failure.* The transition from reproductive to nonreproductive ovarian function, a period that spans over 10 years in most women, is the *climacteric.* The association of estrogen deficiency symptoms with decline in ovarian function is the *menopausal syndrome.*

ETIOLOGY

Natural menopause arises as a consequence of follicular depletion, a process that begins before birth and progresses throughout the life of the woman. Oocyte mitosis ceases, and oocyte and follicle atresia begins while the female herself is still in utero. At birth, oocyte number declines from over 8 million to fewer than 2 million. Most follicles degenerate before ovulating, which explains why decreasing or increasing the number of ovulations by oral contraceptive pills, pregnancy, lactation, or fertility drugs does not influence appreciably the onset of menopause. During the decade preceding the menopause (roughly corresponding to the climacteric), the rate of follicular loss accelerates. Nonetheless, some oocytes remain, even after the cessation of menstruation. Follicular atresia probably involves apoptosis. Neuroendocrine changes precede follicular exhaustion in rodents, although neuroendocrine contributions to reproductive aging in women have been less studied.

Premature ovarian failure may result from oophorectomy, radiation, chemotherapy, autoimmune disease, chromosomal abnormalities (especially Turner mosaic), infection, metabolic abnormalities or trauma. Menopause may begin at an earlier age in smokers. Often the cause of premature ovarian failure remains unclear. In some cases, ovarian biopsy can clarify the etiology of premature ovarian failure, but the associated risk and cost rarely justify its use, because the results usually do not alter clinical management.

Psychosocial Perspectives

Women from every population exhibit physiologic changes with menopause. Indeed, references to the menopause in ancient and classical texts resemble modern clinical reports.[8] Yet, the incidence of menopause-associated symptoms varies greatly among cultures. Women from cultures that confer prestige and dignity on menopausal women report fewer symptoms than women from cultures that perceive the menopause in a more negative light. The role of menopausal women in Western culture is complex. On the one hand, Western culture increasingly deemphasizes the reproductive role of women; on the other hand, it remains emphatically youth-oriented. Not surprisingly, reactions of Western women to menopause vary according to the meaning it holds for them. Most women accept menopause as a normal stage in the cycle of life, one that they share with their mothers, sisters, and friends. Indeed, in the Massachusetts Women's Health Study, a large community survey showed that 70% of menopausal women expressed relief or neutral feelings about the cessation of menses. For many women, the menopause years are a time of personal satisfaction and professional productivity.

The physician may encounter women experiencing difficulty with menopause. For example, those who have struggled with long-term infertility may find that the finality of menopause removes their last hope of having their own child. Others see menopause as a sign of aging. Since menopause occurs at a stage of life when children leave home, partners take sick, or parents die, its meaning may become entangled with grief associated with such losses. For these women the physical nature of menopausal symptoms may be less painful to face and easier to understand than the underlying emotional turmoil. Even though physicians can offer hormone therapy to alleviate symptoms and protect against some potentially fatal diseases, the universality of the menopause and the variability of reactions to it prompt some to caution against "medicalization" of such a natural event. Because of this great diversity of reactions to the menopause, the physician must help the individual woman place menopause within the broader context of her own life, and make her a partner in every aspect of clinical decision making related to it.

EPIDEMIOLOGY

Cessation of ovarian function by the fifth or sixth decade is a universal phenomenon among women. Indeed, females of most mammalian species undergo reproductive failure by midlife, leading some sociobiologists to hypothesize that midlife loss of reproductive capacity among aging females confers survival value to species. Because of the aging world population, the number of menopausal women is increasing. Almost 60% of the U.S. population aged 65 or older, and over 70% of the population aged 85 or older, are women. Improved public health and health care in developing countries have ensured survival of increasingly large numbers of women into the menopausal years, so globally more than 470 million women are menopausal. Since hypoestrogenism contributes to debilitating chronic diseases, such as coronary heart disease and osteoporosis, the evaluation and treatment of the menopause have enormous public health and clinical implications.

Although menopause is a universal experience, only about 40% of menopausal women seek treatment for symptoms related to estrogen deficiency. As discussed above, reporting of menopausal symptoms depends on complex psychosociobiologic interactions. Differences in the incidence of menopausal symptoms reflect not only cultural influences on symptom reporting, but also genetic variation in body habitus, which directly affects estrogen levels by influencing rates of aromatization. Variation in dietary consumption of plant estrogens (phytoestrogens) also may influence development of symptoms, although evidence in support of this hypothesis is still preliminary.

PATHOPHYSIOLOGY

After menopause the ovary becomes small and fibrotic, and takes on a pitted surface.[8] Microscopically, decreased numbers of primordial follicles and increased numbers of fibroblasts, interstitial cells, and connective tissue appear, reflecting atrophy of the ovarian cortex and hyperplasia of the medulla. Considerable variation in the degree of interstitial hyperplasia exists, which explains in part the variation in levels of ovarian steroidogenesis reported in menopausal women.

The pattern of steroidogenesis changes after the menopause. Before menopause steroidogenesis is cyclical; during the follicular phase the graafian follicle secretes estradiol-17β; then during the luteal phase the corpus luteum secretes progesterone and estradiol-17β. After menopause, production of ovarian estrogen and progesterone virtually ceases. Less potent estrogens, principally estrone, are produced from androgens by the enzyme aromatase, located in adipose, muscle, and brain. Considerable differences in the extent of extraovarian estrogen formation exist among menopausal women, which may explain in part differences in the incidence of estrogen-related symptoms. High circulating levels of luteinizing hormone maintain androgen secretion from interstitial and hilar cells within the ovary, which is why oophorectomy of menopausal women reduces circulating testosterone by 50% and androstenedione by 30%, but barely affects estrogen production.

Although absolute levels of androgens also decrease, estrogen levels decrease so significantly at menopause that the ratio of circulating androgens to estrogens actually increases after menopause. Since androgens and estrogens interact at a number of levels (e.g., they down-regulate each other's receptors and reciprocally influence sex hormone binding globulin levels), an increased androgen/estrogen ratio unmasks androgenic activity in some women. Women undergoing surgical menopause experience much greater decline in androgen levels.

The manifold effects of estrogen deprivation on menopausal women should come as no surprise, since estrogen receptors appear throughout the body, where they regulate many critical functions. Estrogen receptors appear in highest concentrations in reproductive tissues, such as breast and urogenital tract, and in phylogenetically ancient parts of the brain involved in regulation of the neuroendocrine and autonomic nervous systems. Measurable levels of estrogen receptor also appear in many other tissues, including liver, blood vessels, and bone.

Estrogen receptors are part of the steroid hormone receptor superfamily. When bound to hormone, steroid receptors attach to specific DNA sequences, called hormone response elements, to regulate transcription of steroid-sensitive genes. Some products of steroid receptor–induced transcription themselves regulate transcription, which creates a cascade of regulatory events within the cell. Extremely rapid effects of estrogens, especially on some tissues that lack detectable levels of estrogen receptor, suggest that sex steroids also may act independently of their receptors.

PATIENT EVALUATION

Symptomatology

Estrogen deficiency symptoms usually begin during the climacteric, at first interspersed with symptom-free periods. As menopause approaches, they may become increasingly frequent and severe. Most symptoms associated with menopause can be explained by the effects of estrogen deprivation on sensitive tissues. Hot flushes and sleep disturbance, the most common symptoms of the menopause, arise from the effects of estrogen deprivation on those parts of the brain that regulate body temperature and sleep, respectively. Hot flushes typically begin in the chest, spread to the face, and last seconds to minutes. They may be associated with anxiety and palpitations, and are followed by profuse sweating and shaking. Some women experience up to 20 episodes per 24-hour period, and most women find hot flushes increase in frequency at night. Eating, stress, or alcohol may trigger hot flushes. In at least 50% of women they abate spontaneously within 5 years after the menopause, even without hormone therapy. Women who develop premature ovarian failure before attaining adult levels of estrogen (e.g., Turner's syndrome patients) do not report hot flushes. Sleep disturbance is characterized by frequent nocturnal awakenings, which may be associated with hot flushes. Sleep apnea also has its onset after the menopause in some women.

Urogenital atrophy, manifesting as urinary frequency, dysuria, dyspareunia, genital bleeding, and occasionally stress urinary incontinence, results from the effects of estrogen deprivation on the bladder, urethra, and associated pelvic supports. Amenorrhea, which may be preceded by luteal phase defects, shortening of menstrual cycle length, or menstrual irregularity, results from loss of cyclic estrogen and progesterone effects on the endometrium. Decreased estrogen/androgen ratio contributes to mild hirsutism and breast atrophy in some women.

Decreased sex drive may arise from urogenital atrophy or psychodynamic reactions to menopause. Women who have undergone oophorectomy may experience decreased libido because of loss of ovarian androgen production. More controversial is the role of estrogen deprivation on mood and cognitive function.

Declining fertility and fecundity, which begin more than a decade before the menopause, even before detectable alterations in menstrual cyclicity, result largely from declining oocyte developmental potential, and possibly from abnormal endometrial receptivity.

Some menopausal women present with symptoms associated with osteoporosis, such as back pain, kyphoscoliosis, and decreased height (revealed earliest by changing dress hem length). Coronary heart disease in menopausal women may present with classic angina, but atypical angina may be more common. Early detection of coronary heart disease symptoms is especially critical in menopausal women, because their outcome after myocardial infarction may be worse than men (see Chapter 45). Osteoporosis and heart symptoms typically appear in women only several years past menopause.

Physical Examination

Physical examination of the menopausal woman reveals atrophy of sex steroid–dependent tissues. Skin on the vulva thins, vaginal epithelium becomes dry and loses rugations, the cervix and uterus decrease in size, and the portio of the cervix becomes friable. Breasts decrease in size and fullness. Such observations provide more reliable assessment of the state of estrogenization than measurement of circulating estradiol-17β because these tissues reflect overall estrogen effects, whereas the estradiol-17β level measures only one of many bioactive estrogens. Some women develop mild hirsutism in response to declining estrogen/androgen ratio. Older postmenopausal women may have kyphoscoliosis and spinous tenderness from osteoporotic vertebral fractures.

Physical examination of the menopausal woman should include careful examination of the breasts and associated lymph nodes, and of the cervix, vagina, uterus, adnexa, vulva, and rectum to screen for evidence of malignancy. A Pap smear and stool guaiac should be obtained.

DIAGNOSIS

Diagnostic Procedures

Although the physical examination provides a sensitive "bioassay" for the state of estrogenization, a number of laboratory assays can confirm the presence of hypoestrogenism. Levels of estradiol-17β less than 40 pg/ml, follicle stimulating hormone (FSH) greater than 20 mIU, and vaginal cytology exhibiting parabasal cells signal ovarian failure. A number of accurate and reliable methods exist to quantify bone density. Standard x-rays reflect only late-stage osteoporosis, but quantitative bone densitometry using single or dual photon absorptiometry or other methods measures bone demineralization with greater sensitivity. The role of broad-based radiographic screening for osteoporosis is controversial at present, but most physicians agree that bone densitometry should include women who need osteoporosis risk assessment in order to weigh potential risks against benefits of hormone therapy.

Risks for a number of life-threatening diseases, such as coronary heart disease, stroke, breast cancer, and osteoporosis, increase after the menopause. Most risks for these conditions can be determined by interview and physical examination, but cholesterol screening, mammography, and occasionally bone densitometry studies may provide additional information.

Women experiencing premature menopause should have a cosyntropin (Cortrosyn) stimulation test. Thyroid stimulating hormone (TSH), calcium, and phosphorus levels should be evaluated for associated hypoadrenal, hypothyroid, and hypoparathyroid states, respectively.

Differential Diagnosis

The interview and physical examination must search for evidence of conditions that mimic menopause, especially in young women with premature ovarian failure. Carcinoid, pheochromocytoma, or systemic mastocytosis can present with flushing, but usually can be differentiated by concomitant attacks of diarrhea, hypertension, or hypotension, and the absence of other signs of hypoestrogenism.

Hyperprolactinemia lowers estrogen levels, usually does not cause vasomotor instability, but does cause galactorrhea. Hyperandrogenic states arising from functioning adrenal or ovarian tumors produce more marked virilization with more rapid progression than the mild and insidious hirsutism that appears in some menopausal women. Hypothalamic amenorrhea differs from menopause by its lack of hot flushes and decreased rather than increased FSH levels. Patients with osteoporosis should be evaluated for primary hyperparathyroidism, hyperthyroidism, or hypercortisolism.

Vulvar dermatoses or neoplasia may be mistaken for menopausal urogenital atrophy, and excoriations on atrophic vulva menopausal women may be mistaken for neoplasia. Only biopsy can distinguish these. Any white, erythematous or raised vulvar lesions should be biopsied in women of all ages.

Sleep disturbance, decreased sex drive, and hot flushes associated with hypoestrogenism may resemble anxiety and mood disorders. A history of anxiety and mood disorders antedating the menopause may suggest a functional etiology for these symptoms. However, many physicians will prescribe hormone therapy if other signs and symptoms suggest hypoestrogenism. Symptoms remaining after hormonal treatment of the hypoestrogenic state may require additional psychotherapeutic and/or psychopharmacologic intervention.

MANAGEMENT

Hormone replacement therapy (HRT) effectively treats most symptoms associated with menopause, and prevents disease and prolongs life even in asymptomatic women. In women who cannot tolerate HRT, a number of nonhormonal alternatives exist that provide some symptomatic relief and/or disease prevention.

A major potential benefit of hormone therapy is reduced risk of cardiovascular disease.[1,6,9,10] Cardiovascular disease is the leading cause of death among women in developed countries, accounting for 50% of all deaths in women over age 50. The incidence of cardiovascular disease increases fiftyfold after menopause. Consistent evidence from observational studies demonstrates that unopposed estrogen reduces the risk for coronary heart disease by 35% to 50%, although only randomized, controlled clinical trials, which are still underway, can demonstrate conclusively cardioprotective effects of estrogen. The mechanisms underlying hormone therapy's cardioprotective effects remain incompletely understood. Hormone therapy induces favorable changes in lipid factors, but recent evidence indicates that changes in lipids account for only 20% of its cardioprotective effects.

Addition of progestin to estrogen also probably reduces the risk of coronary heart disease, although the magnitude of risk reduction cannot be estimated with current data. Indeed, the cardioprotective effects of combined regimens may depend on the dose and chemical structure of the specific progestin employed. Since progestins that structurally resemble androgens induce androgenic side effects, they can abrogate some of the beneficial effects of estrogen.

Hormone therapy with estrogen or estrogen/progestin also reduces the risk for osteoporosis-related hip fracture by 25% and for vertebral fractures by over 50% (see Chapter 45).[4]

Estrogen deprivation increases osteoporosis because it increases bone turnover. Since estrogen deficiency increases bone resorption more than formation, it causes a net decrease in bone density. Hormone therapy rapidly restores normal levels of bone resorption and formation. Progestins do not counteract estrogen's protective effect on bone. The protective effects of hormone therapy are greatest when they are initiated before menopause, but even women with advanced osteoporosis may experience improvement.

These potential benefits must be weighed against possible risks and side effects of hormone therapy. The risks of hormone therapy have been overestimated by studies based on oral contraceptive pills and on unopposed estrogen. Hormone therapy provides levels of estrogenic activity close to that encountered in premenopausal women, whereas even the lowest-dose oral contraceptive pills contain estrogenic activity many times greater than that provided by hormone therapy. Furthermore, the addition of progestin to estrogen lowers the risk of endometrial cancer associated with estrogen replacement therapy to below that of women who take no hormone therapy at all.[5] Other side effects attributed to sex steroids based on studies of oral contraceptive pill users, such as hypertension and thromboembolic disease, also generally do not apply to hormone therapy.

The most troubling, but at the same time most controversial, risk attributed to hormone therapy is increased lifetime probability of breast cancer.[2,3,7] Data are extensive, but conclusions are inconsistent concerning the risk of developing breast cancer in women taking estrogen. The fact that men almost never get breast cancer and the fact that early menarche and late menopause increase risk for breast cancer are consistent with the hypothesis that extending the duration of the exposure to estrogens by hormone therapy may increase breast cancer risk. However, data suggest that women who use estrogen therapy for less than 5 years probably do not increase their risk of breast cancer. The risk for breast cancer may increase slightly among women who take estrogen for longer than 15 years, and may be concentrated among those with other risk factors, but here the data are less conclusive.

Contrary to early reports, progestins do not protect against breast cancer. Indeed, fundamental studies on the effects of sex steroids on breast tissue predict that combination therapy may increase risk for breast cancer, and some preliminary clinical studies corroborate this.

For most women the most annoying side effect of hormone therapy is vaginal bleeding. In women with a uterus, estrogen therapy produces unpredictable vaginal bleeding in up to 40% of treated women per year. The addition of progestins on a monthly basis synchronizes bleeding, but often replaces it with symptoms of weight gain, irritability, and depression attributable to the progestin. Other side effects associated with estrogen therapy include breast tenderness, bloating, and headache. However, in most women these symptoms are mild. Often they improve after several months of therapy.

Before prescribing hormone therapy, the physician should explain these risks and benefits. Although public health considerations dictate that most menopausal women at least consider hormone therapy, the decision to begin it ultimately must be reached only after balancing potential risks and benefits for the individual. The physician should uncover pertinent risk factors, then discuss feelings and beliefs the woman has regarding menopause and hormone therapy in order to help her make a rational decision about hormone therapy. For example, the physician may counsel a woman that five times more women die of heart disease each year than from breast cancer, and that hormone therapy reduces the risk of heart attack by 30% to 50%, while its effect on breast cancer is still controversial. Yet, the woman who has a strong family history of breast cancer and minimal risk factors for heart disease very reasonably may elect to refuse hormone therapy and pursue alternatives, such as bisphosphonates or selective estrogen receptor modulators (SERMS). Conversely, women who have coronary heart disease risks are likely to benefit from hormone therapy, even if they are also at increased risk for breast cancer.

Hormone therapy can be given as unopposed estrogen, unopposed progestin, or estrogen/progestin combination regimens. Women who have undergone hysterectomy do not need progestin therapy. Women who have a uterus require combined estrogen/progestin therapy. Combined regimens include estrogen plus cyclic progestin and estrogen plus continuous progestin. The continuous combined regimen may eliminate vaginal bleeding if the uterus becomes atrophic. However, usually months of irregular bleeding ensue before this goal is attained. A wide variety of hormone preparations are available (Box 42-1).

Women presenting with symptoms of hypoestrogenism and prolonged amenorrhea electing continuous estrogen and cyclic progestin should take an estrogen alone until symptoms abate. The estrogen is then titrated to achieve the minimal effective dose, a process that may take up to 2 months. Such a short course of unopposed estrogen carries minimal risk for the endometrium in such patients and enables the physician to adjust one hormone at a time. Furthermore, for many women the progestin creates the biggest barrier to compliance. Delaying progestin therapy until the abatement of menopausal symptoms enhances trust in the physician-patient relationship, and increases patient motivation to work through the optimization of the progestin dose. Progestin is added at a low dose for at least 12 days, beginning the first of each month (a schedule that helps the woman remember when to take progestin). If bleeding begins before day 10 of the progestin, the progestin dose is increased.

Women presenting with irregular menses, even in association with evidence of hypoestrogenism, and women who develop vaginal bleeding on hormone therapy must undergo evaluation to exclude endometrial cancer. The ease and accuracy of office biopsy largely has supplanted operative dilation and curettage, but suspicious histology, inadequate tissue, technical difficulty (especially in older women with a stenotic cervical os), and persistently irregular bleeding are all indications for operative fractional curettage. Some physicians perform a transvaginal ultrasound at the first sign of unexpected bleeding. An endometrial stripe less than or equal to 5 mm nearly excludes the risk of endometrial hyperplasia and allows the patient to avoid a painful endometrial biopsy. After exclusion of neoplasia, perimenopausal dysfunctional uterine bleeding should be treated by monthly progestin therapy.

Contraindications to hormone therapy include breast cancer; other estrogen-dependent malignancies; acute liver, pancreatic, or gallbladder disease; chronically impaired liver function; or undiagnosed vaginal bleeding (Box 42-2). Relative contraindications include previous venous thrombophlebitis, strong family history of breast cancer, or other estrogen-dependent malignancy. For these women, clonidine

Box 42-1. Estrogen and Progestin Regimens

Common Doses Used

Estrogens

0.3 mg conjugated estrogen
0.625 mg conjugated estrogen
0.9 mg conjugated estrogen
1.25 mg conjugated estrogen
0.05 mg transdermal estrogen
0.10 mg transdermal estrogen
1 mg micronized estradiol-17β
2 mg micronized estradiol-17β

Progestins

2.5 mg medroxyprogesterone acetate
5 mg medroxyprogesterone acetate
10 mg medroxyprogesterone acetate
5 mg norethindrone acetate
5 mg norethindrone

Typical Regimens

Continuous estrogen plus cyclic progestin

Estrogen: (0.625 mg conjugated estrogen, 1 mg micronized estradiol-17β daily or transdermal patch changed two times/week)

Progestin: first 12 days of every month (5 or 10 mg)

OR

Continuous/combined

Estrogen and progestin daily (0.625 mg conjugated estrogen, 1 mg micronized estradiol-17β daily or transdermal patch changed two times/week; progestin—2.5 mg daily).

Box 42-2. Contraindications to Estrogen Use

Absolute Contraindications

Stroke
Recent myocardial infarction
Breast cancer
Endometrial adenocarcinoma
Other estrogen-dependent tumors
Acute liver disease
Pancreatic disease
Gallbladder disease
Chronic impaired liver function
Recent venous thromboembolic event
Chronic thrombophlebitis
Undiagnosed vaginal bleeding

Relative Contraindications

Cigarette smoking/significant nicotine abuse
Fibrocystic breast disease
Familial hyperlipidemia
Hypertension aggravated by estrogen therapy
Pancreatitis
Hepatic porphyria
Endometrial hyperplasia
Leiomyomata uteri
Endometriosis
Migraine headache
Thrombophlebitis

Modified from Young RL, Kumar NS, Goldzieher JW: Management of menopause when estrogen cannot be used, *Drugs* 40(2):220-230, 1990.

Table 42-1. Alternatives to Estrogen Therapy

Therapy	Dose/frequency	Benefits	Side effects/risks
Medroxyprogesterone acetate	10 mg po qd	Relieves hot flushes, prevents osteoporosis	Worsening symptoms of urogenital atrophy, depression/sedation, decreased libido, decreased HDL, effect on breast cancer not known
SERMS (e.g., raloxifene)	60 mg/day	Prevents osteoporosis, may lower cardiac risk factors, may lower risk of breast cancer, may not cause endometrial hyperplasia	May worsen hot flushes, more expensive than estrogen, no effect on HDL cholesterol, no cardioprotective effects
Bisphosphonate (e.g., Alendronate)	10 mg/day	Prevents osteoporosis	Esophageal irritation
Calcium supplementation	1500 mg po qd	Minimal effect on osteoporosis prevention	Unmask asymptomatic hyperparathyroidism
Clonidine	0.1 mg po qd or bid	Moderate relief of hot flushes	Dry mouth, sedation
Bellergal	1 tablet bid	Relieves hot flushes	Drowsiness, paresthesias (rare)
Low-fat diet		Lower cardiac risk factors	
Exercise	As tolerated	Lower cardiac risk factors Prevent osteoporosis	

or ergot preparations reduce hot flushes. Dietary supplementation with calcium reduces osteoporosis risk, although not as completely as estrogen, and exercise and restriction of dietary cholesterol and fat consumption reduce coronary heart disease risk (Table 42-1). SERMS act as estrogen receptor agonists in some tissues, but as antagonists in other tissues. Tamoxifen and raloxifene, two currently available SERMS, spare bone and protect the heart, although not as well as estrogen, and protect the breast from the proliferative effects of estrogen. They also can exacerbate hot flushes. Such "designer estrogens" some day may provide patients with the advantages of estrogen without the side effects or risks. However, for the present they provide only partial protection against the effects of estrogen deprivation. Bisphosphonates, such as Alendronate, reduce the risk of osteoporosis, but do not provide the cardioprotection nor the symptom relief provided by estrogens.

REFERENCES

1. Bush TL, et al: Cardiovascular mortality and noncontraceptive use of estrogen in women: results from the lipid research clinics program follow-up study, *Circulation* 75:1102-1109, 1987.
2. Delmas PD, Bjarnason NH, Mitlak BH, et al: Effects of raloxifene on bone mineral density, serum cholesterol concentrations, and uterine endometrium in postmenopausal women, *N Engl J Med* 337:1641-1647, 1997.
3. Grady D, et al: Guidelines for counseling postmenopausal women about preventive hormone therapy, *Ann Intern Med* 117:1038-1041, 1992.
4. Grady D, et al: Hormone therapy to prevent disease and prolong life in postmenopausal women, *Ann Intern Med* 117:1016-1037, 1992.
5. Kiel DP, et al: Hip fracture and the use of estrogens in postmenopausal women: the Framingham Study, *N Engl J Med* 317:1169-1174, 1987.
6. Persson I, et al: Risk of endometrial cancer after treatment with oestrogens alone or in conjunction with progesterones: results of a prospective study, *BMJ* 298:147-151, 1989.
7. Stampfer MJ, et al: Postmenopausal estrogen therapy and cardiovascular disease: ten-year follow-up from the Nurse's Health Study, *N Engl J Med* 325:756-762, 1991.
8. Steinberg KK, et al: A meta-analysis of the effect of estrogen replacement therapy on the risk of breast cancer, *JAMA* 265:1985-1990, 1991.
9. U.S. Congress, Office of Technology Assessment, *The menopause, hormone therapy, and women's health,* OTA-BP-BA-88, Washington, DC, 1992, US Government Printing Office.
10. Wilson PWF, Garrison RJ, Castelli WP: Postmenopausal estrogen use, cigarette smoking, and cardiovascular morbidity in women over 50: the Framingham Study, *N Engl J Med* 313:1038-1043, 1985.

CHAPTER 43

Breast Diseases

Barbara A. Ward
Michael Reiss

Breast cancer afflicts one of every eight to nine American women, an alarming statistic. Among women in the United States, it is the most often diagnosed malignancy and follows only lung cancer as the leading cause of cancer death. Given the high incidence of this disease, a working knowledge of breast anatomy, diagnostic procedures, and breast cancer treatment is essential. Moreover, issues of breast cancer risk assessment and prevention are becoming increasingly relevant to the primary care physician. In addition, benign conditions that affect the breast are quite common and often perplexing. This chapter outlines the basic steps regarding breast evaluation and describes the options in the management of breast masses and breast cancer.

OVERVIEW

Common Benign Conditions

Fibrocystic disease, or *mastopathy,* refers to breast lumpiness accompanied by pain and tenderness that is most severe in the premenstrual phase of the cycle. Although the term *fibrocystic* is nonspecific, most physicians can identify the clinical picture it represents. It is most accurate to describe fibrocystic changes based on the specific microscopic entity involved, including fibroadenomas, macrocysts, periductal mastitis, papillomatosis, apocrine metaplasia, sclerosing adenosis, and hyperplastic lesions of the duct and lobule.

Fibroadenomas typically present during the second and third decades but may be found at any age. Excision is generally advised because the lesions may continue to grow and may be confused with cystosarcoma phyllodes or a carcinoma. *Cysts* tend to appear suddenly and are much more common in the premenopausal age group. They are often tender and may be aspirated to relieve symptoms and to confirm the diagnosis. Although ultrasound is helpful in differentiating a cyst from a solid mass, needle aspiration with complete resolution of a palpable mass is the gold standard. *Macrocysts* generally diminish after menopause but may persist in the patient receiving hormonal replacement therapy (HRT). *Periductal mastitis* is a chronic condition characterized by repetitive infections that are difficult to treat. Excision of the involved duct system is the recommended treatment. Although antibiotics may temper the inflammation, they are not curative, because nests of purulent fluid remain in undrained recesses.

Breast Cancer

In 2000, an estimated 182,800 new breast cancers will be diagnosed in the United States, and an estimated 40,800 women will die from this disease. Over her lifetime an American woman has a 12.5% risk of developing breast cancer and a 3.5% risk of dying from it. The incidence and risk of developing breast cancer increase with age, and the majority of cases occur in postmenopausal women (Fig. 43-1). Nonetheless, even though 80% of women who die are over 55, breast cancer is the second most common cause of death in younger women between ages 35 and 55.

Breast cancer incidence in females increased from 88.6 per 100,000 in the early 1970s to 109.8 in 1990. Since 1990 the incidence has remained stable. Changes in lifestyle may have contributed to the increased incidence of breast cancer in the 1970s and 1980s. Earlier menarche, delayed childbearing, and pharmacologic uses of estrogens have increased the total period in a woman's life that her breast epithelium is exposed to and stimulated by estrogens and progestins. Changes in nutrition and other environmental factors yet to be identified may have also played a role. For example, population studies have suggested a direct correlation between dietary fat consumption and breast cancer incidence around the world, although case-controlled studies have been unable to confirm this association. Furthermore, the evidence that modifying dietary fat intake reduces breast cancer risk remains inconclusive. The relationship between alcohol consumption and breast cancer risk remains equally controversial.

The relative incidence of in situ and lymph node–negative invasive cancer increased rapidly from 1982 through 1987 and has since leveled off, whereas the relative incidence of lymph node–positive invasive breast cancer has decreased since 1987. These recent fluctuations in stage at diagnosis of breast cancer likely reflect the introduction and large-scale application of screening mammography since the early 1980s.

Between 1973 and 1990 the age-adjusted breast cancer *mortality* rate for U.S. women rose steadily at a rate of approximately 0.2% per year. Since 1990, however, breast

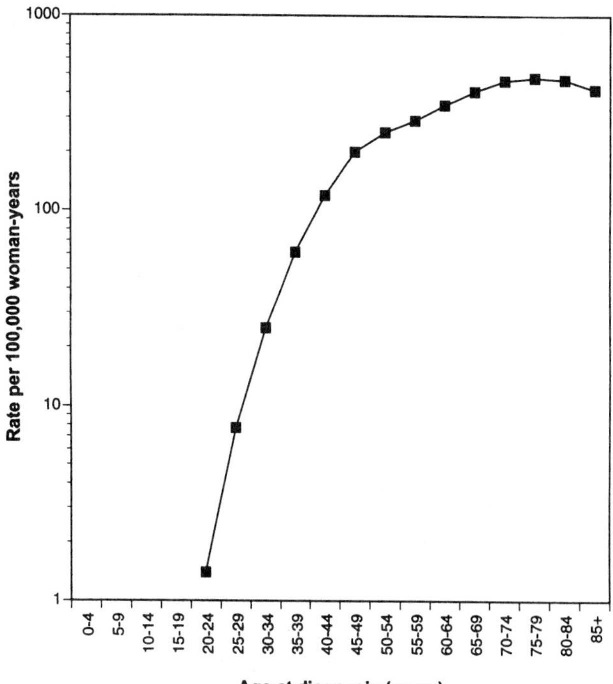

Fig. 43-1. Age-specific breast cancer incidence in women (SEER Program), 1991 to 1995. Rates are per 100,000 women and are age adjusted to standard world population. (From Ries LAG, Kosary CL, Hankey BF, et al, editors: *SEER cancer statistics review, 1973-1995*, Bethesda, Md, 1998, National Cancer Institute.)

cancer mortality has greatly decreased, by approximately 2% per year, in all age groups. Statistical modeling indicates that this recent drop in breast cancer mortality is too rapid to be explained solely by the increased use of mammography but almost certainly reflects the impact of improvements in systemic adjuvant therapy (see later discussion).

PATHOPHYSIOLOGY

Growth and Development

Anatomically the breast is a hormonally sensitive gland that develops and regresses with each menstrual cycle and with age. The adult breast is composed of epithelial and stromal elements. The stroma contains adipose tissue and fibrous connective tissue, both of which predominate in the nonlactating breast (Fig. 43-2). The epithelial component consists of 15 to 20 branching ducts that originate from the nipple and terminate in lobules with clusters of small acini. During pregnancy this glandular component increases so that the breast is composed mainly of epithelial elements, which persist throughout lactation. After lactation, breasts undergo a process of involution and return almost completely to the virginal state. After menopause, stromal adipose tissue increases, whereas all other stromal and epithelial elements diminish in size.

Variations in breast anatomy are common. The majority of women have a slight asymmetry to their external breast appearance; this difference may be marked in some individuals. Accessory nipples, which are apparent at birth, are generally but not necessarily bilateral and are found along the midclavicular line. Breast tissue extending to the axilla

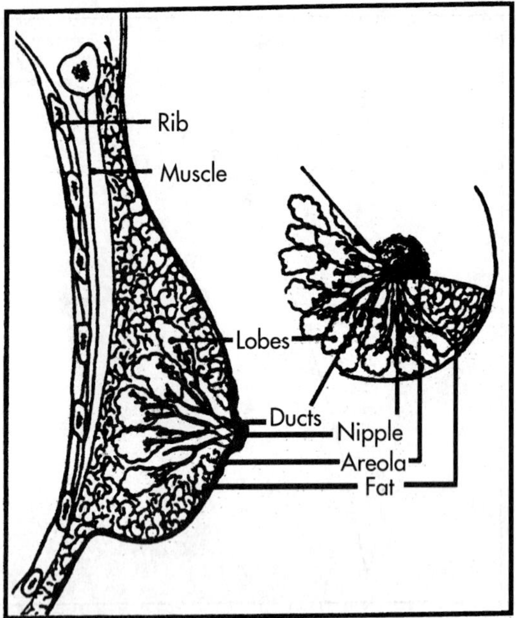

Fig. 43-2. Anatomy of female breast. (Redrawn from NIH Pub No 91-1556, October 1990.)

may not be clinically apparent until pregnancy occurs and the area becomes swollen and tender. If symptoms are marked, the areas may be excised postpartum in anticipation of future pregnancies. The syndromes of virginal breast hypertrophy and Poland's syndrome, the congenital absence of the breast, nipple, and pectoralis muscles, are rare. Male gynecomastia is usually seen in the prepubertal male and is generally transient (see Chapter 7). Surgery can be performed if the patient finds significant enlargement embarrassing or painful. Gynecomastia is also common in the aging male and is exacerbated by certain medications or hepatic dysfunction. It is characterized by classic findings on mammography.

Histopathology of Breast Cancer

Most invasive breast cancers are *adenocarcinomas,* which can be quite heterogenous in histologic appearance and can be classified into several different subtypes with varying prognostic implications. Approximately 80% of adenocarcinomas are of the infiltrating (i.e., invasive) ductal type. Although they vary in degree of differentiation, infiltrating ductal carcinomas have a common natural history and metastasize predominantly to the skeleton, lungs, liver, and brain. Infiltrating lobular carcinomas account for approximately 10% of adenocarcinomas. Although the overall prognosis is similar to that for invasive ductal carcinoma, invasive lobular carcinomas tend to spread to the meninges rather than the brain parenchyma; to serosal surfaces such as the pleura, the peritoneum, and the surface of the ovaries; and to mediastinal and retroperitoneal lymph nodes. Less common variants of breast carcinoma, including tubular, medullary, mucinous, and papillary carcinomas, are well differentiated and carry a relatively favorable prognosis.

Noninvasive cancer that is confined to the ducts without penetration of the basement membrane is termed *ductal carcinoma in situ* (DCIS), or intraductal carcinoma. DCIS is the earliest form of breast cancer and is often detected only by screening mammography. In contrast, *lobular carcinoma in situ* (LCIS) is not a malignant lesion but a histopathologic entity that confers an increased risk for developing invasive breast cancer in either the ipsilateral or the contralateral breast.

Table 43-1. Diagnostic Approaches to Palpable Breast Masses

Age group	Most common lesion	Diagnostic evaluation
15-25	Fibroadenoma	Ultrasound and/or aspiration Mammogram not necessary
25-35	Fibroadenoma (cyst or cancer possible but uncommon)	Ultrasound and/or aspiration Mammogram if clinically suspicious
35-50	Fibrocystic changes, cancer, cyst	Mammogram Ultrasound if recommended by mammographer
Over 50	Cancer unless proved otherwise	Mammogram Ultrasound if recommended by mammographer
Pregnant or lactating	Lactating adenoma, cyst, mastitis, cancer	Ultrasound Unilateral mammogram if requested by surgeon Magnetic resonance imaging (MRI)

EVALUATION OF BREAST MASS

The differential diagnosis of a breast mass includes primary breast cancer; fibrocystic changes, cyst, fibroadenoma, or an associated benign mass; abscess or mastitis; phyllodes tumor; lipoma; fat necrosis; duct ectasia; sarcoma; sarcoidosis; lymphoma; metastatic cancer; skin conditions such as sebaceous cysts; costochondritis; superficial thrombophlebitis or Mondor's disease; and tumors of the chest wall. Certain lesions are most common in different age groups (Table 43-1). A new breast mass in a woman older than 50 years should be considered cancerous until proved otherwise. In contrast, cancer is uncommon in women under age 35 and highly uncommon in those under 25. The history and physical examination generally narrow down the differential diagnosis, but ultimately, pathologic examination is required for the definitive diagnosis.

Patient History

The patient's age is critical in the assessment of new breast masses and helps to categorize risk. *A family history of breast cancer should be noted, but because the majority of women who develop breast cancer do not have a family history of this disease, a negative family history cannot be assumed to be protective.* A complete history should include assessment of duration, growth pattern, relation to menstrual cycle, spontaneous nipple discharge, pain, and tenderness. Cumulative estrogen exposure should be estimated by noting age at menarche and menopause, use of oral contraceptives and

HRT, number of pregnancies and live births, and duration of breast-feeding. Previous breast biopsies, timing of mammograms, and previous ultrasounds need to be ascertained as well.

Past medical history may be relevant. A previous diagnosis of colon or endometrial cancer places the patient in a higher risk category for breast cancer. Other diseases that may involve the breast include sarcoidosis, lymphoma, and metastatic melanoma. Past surgery, such as oophorectomy, is important, as are certain medications, such as antidepressants, which may be associated with nipple discharge.

Nipple discharge is a fairly common complaint and is generally related to a benign condition. Concern increases if the discharge is unilateral, spontaneous, and bloody; emanates from one duct system alone; or occurs in a postmenopausal patient. Even with these concerns, the most common source for nipple discharge is an intraductal papilloma, a benign condition treated by excision alone. Cytologic examination of the nipple discharge may reveal malignant cells, but a negative cytologic examination does not confirm benignity. Mammography should be performed to identify any occult mass or source for the discharge, followed by nipple exploration and duct excision. Some surgeons find ductograms helpful in delineating the anatomy of the duct system and intraluminal defects.

Physical Examination

The breast is a pear-shaped structure, with the tail of Spence angled toward the axilla. Most active breast tissue is located in the upper outer quadrant, where most benign and malignant masses occur. Glandular breast tissue resembles a bunch of grapes, with the grapes representing the lobules and the branches coalescing as the ducts at the nipple. The outer breast tissue has a normal "lumpy" consistency, similar to the outer periphery of a bunch of grapes. A true mass, however, is distinct from the bunch and possesses three dimensions. Firm masses with irregular borders are suspicious for malignancy. Normal ridges of tissue are palpable medially, where breast tissue may be accentuated by the underlying rib structure; inferiorly, where a ptotic breast forms an inframammary fold; and centrally around the edge of the nipple, where a "rim" effect may be felt. These variations should be bilateral unless surgery has altered breast symmetry.

Because of normal cyclic changes of the breast throughout menses, the best time for examination is generally 10 to 14 days after menstruation. Immediately before the onset of menses, the breasts are most engorged and tender; cysts may be largest at this time and recede after menstruation. Pregnancy produces a more sustained engorgement, which is ultimately relieved with lactation. A lumpy texture results as milk is temporarily sequestered in lobules. A persistent, new mass that presents during lactation should be evaluated, however, beginning with an ultrasound. Solid masses should be biopsied, although this procedure may require that breast feeding be interrupted. As the patient approaches menopause, the breast may be affected by fluctuations in hormonal levels, resulting in increased tenderness and enlarging cysts. Because the aging breast is at increased risk for cancer, these new masses should be evaluated, aspirated if appropriate, and followed. After menopause, cysts are uncommon unless the patient is maintained on HRT. The difficulties of follow-up in the cystic breast must then be weighed against the potential benefits of HRT for a given patient.

The examination should begin with the patient disrobed in the upright position. The examiner checks for symmetry, skin thickening, nipple changes, and skin dimpling, particularly with the patient's arms raised. One breast may be slightly larger than the other, and most patients will confirm that this condition has been longstanding. The patient is then asked to lie down and raise her arm laterally above her head as each breast is examined. This maneuver is most helpful in women with large breasts. In a woman with smaller breasts, the skin may be too taut with the arm raised, and examination is easier with the patient's arm at her side. If a patient has noted a mass, she should point it out. The examination should then proceed, covering all four quadrants of the breast in a uniform, thorough manner. If a patient is not familiar with breast self-examination (BSE), this is a good time to repeat these steps with her hand (Fig. 43-3). Although some women find BSE awkward, it is a shared responsibility, and most patients improve with encouragement, coaching, and instructional materials.

The physical examination proceeds with an examination of the supraclavicular and axillary lymph nodes. Small axillary lymph nodes are typically felt in a thin person; however, a palpable node becomes more relevant when a coincident breast mass is also palpated. The axillary node is best examined with the patient in the upright position and the arm relaxed, resting on the examiner's forearm. The node examination may be slightly uncomfortable because this is often a tender area in a totally benign axilla. Palpation for axillary nodes from the posterior may make the axillary examination less uncomfortable for the patient. In the unfortunate patient with a highly suspicious mass, the physical examination should include a search for metastatic disease, such as hepatomegaly and points of bony tenderness.

When a breast mass is present, its physical characteristics may be helpful in determining a diagnosis. A suspicious mass is three dimensional and firm with indistinct margins. Fibroadenomas classically are slippery, smooth, and easily movable within the breast. Although cysts are also smooth, they are not significantly mobile. Cysts may feel ballotable, as a water-filled balloon, or hard when they are tense with fluid. Although these characteristics are "classic," a diagnosis should not be made exclusively based on clinical characteristics. Every physician has been fooled by a cancer that presents as a "nonsuspicious" smooth mass. Given this dilemma, it is generally safe to recommend a biopsy, which provides a definitive microscopic diagnosis.

Given the high frequency of breast cancer, every woman should be instructed regarding the three tools to early diagnosis: BSE, mammography, and periodic examination by a health care professional. Because mammography is least helpful in the dense, lumpy breast, physical examination is an essential tool.

Diagnostic Procedures

Screening mammography has led to the detection of breast cancers at earlier stages than those detected without screening. The American Cancer Society (ACS) recommends that mammograms be performed every year to every other year between ages 40 and 50 and every year after age 50. The benefit of screening mammography is greatest in women ages 50 to 69; several studies have demonstrated a reduction of breast cancer mortality in this population. Currently the value of screening mammography in women ages 40 to 49 remains

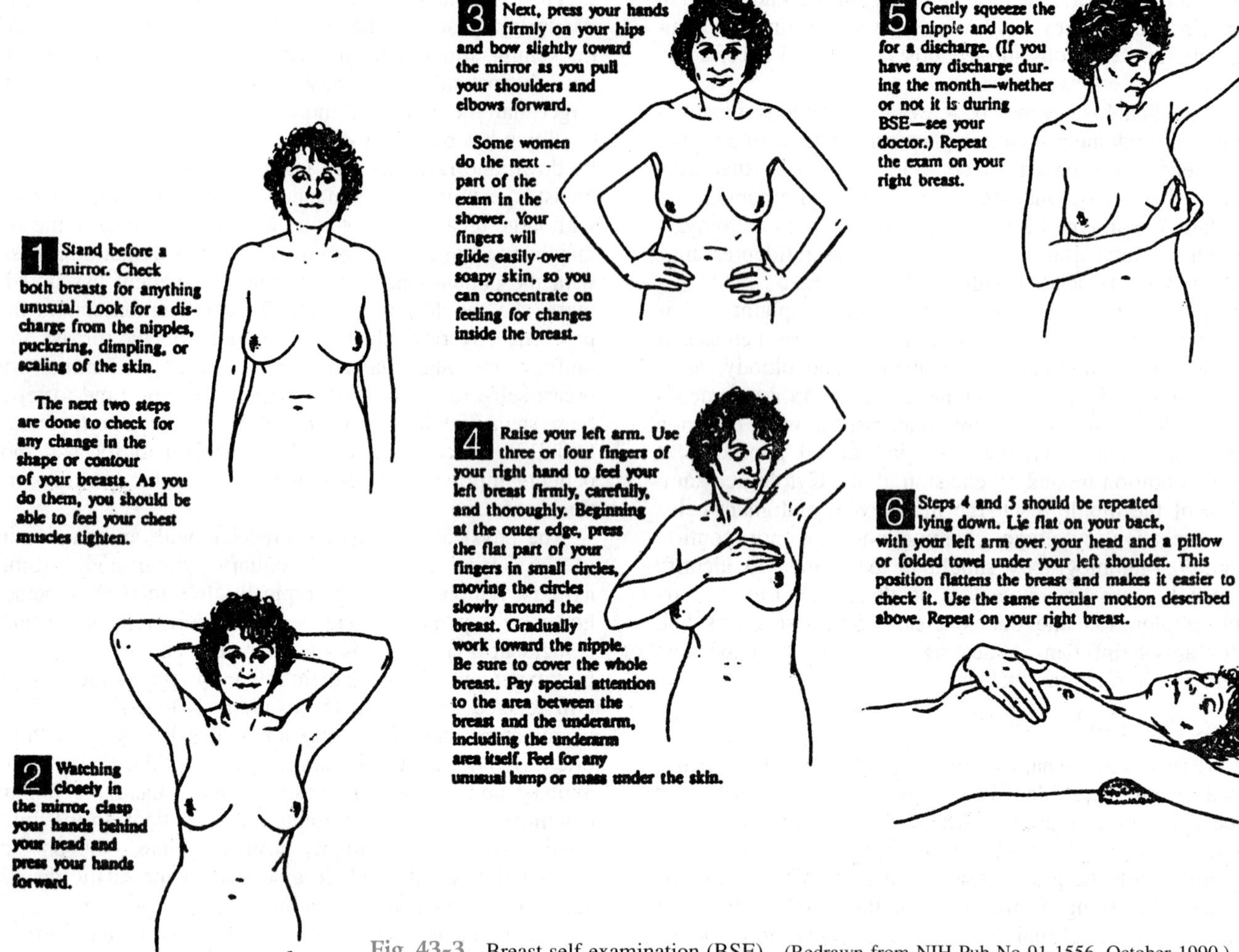

1 Stand before a mirror. Check both breasts for anything unusual. Look for a discharge from the nipples, puckering, dimpling, or scaling of the skin.
The next two steps are done to check for any change in the shape or contour of your breasts. As you do them, you should be able to feel your chest muscles tighten.
2 Watching closely in the mirror, clasp your hands behind your head and press your hands forward.
3 Next, press your hands firmly on your hips and bow slightly toward the mirror as you pull your shoulders and elbows forward.
Some women do the next part of the exam in the shower. Your fingers will glide easily over soapy skin, so you can concentrate on feeling for changes inside the breast.
4 Raise your left arm. Use three or four fingers of your right hand to feel your left breast firmly, carefully, and thoroughly. Beginning at the outer edge, press the flat part of your fingers in small circles, moving the circles slowly around the breast. Gradually work toward the nipple. Be sure to cover the whole breast. Pay special attention to the area between the breast and the underarm, including the underarm area itself. Feel for any unusual lump or mass under the skin.
5 Gently squeeze the nipple and look for a discharge. (If you have any discharge during the month—whether or not it is during BSE—see your doctor.) Repeat the exam on your right breast.
6 Steps 4 and 5 should be repeated lying down. Lie flat on your back, with your left arm over your head and a pillow or folded towel under your left shoulder. This position flattens the breast and makes it easier to check it. Use the same circular motion described above. Repeat on your right breast.

Fig. 43-3. Breast self-examination (BSE). (Redrawn from NIH Pub No 91-1556, October 1990.)

controversial. Results from the Canadian National Breast Screening Study showed no survival benefit from screening in this age group after 5 to 7 years. However, these results have been refuted by other studies, leading the U.S. National Cancer Institute (NCI) to suggest screening in this age group. Most physicians believe that it is reasonable to continue to follow the recognized guidelines until sufficient evidence results in a change. Furthermore, if a patient has a mother or sister with premenopausal breast cancer, the screening recommendations are moved up by 10 years before the age at cancer diagnosis in the first-degree relative; at a minimum, yearly mammograms are performed after age 40. Issues about screening should not be confused with the importance of mammography in the workup of symptomatic patients.

When mammographic abnormalities are seen on a screening study, patients may be asked to return for magnification or compression views to clarify a problem. With a cancer, compression may accentuate the finding, whereas in normal dense parenchyma the abnormality is dispersed. Macrocalcifications are not related to cancers, but clustered microcalcifications, which are laid down within a lobule or duct, can herald an early malignant lesion. An increase in the number and density of microcalcifications is a common reason for biopsy, even though only 25% to 30% of biopsies performed for microcalcifications yield a diagnosis of cancer. If possible, it is often reassuring to show patients their mammographic abnormality. This approach gives them a real estimate of the minute size of the lesion being addressed.

Biopsies can be performed using several different methods. If a mass is palpable, a *needle biopsy* may be performed in the surgeon's office. This procedure is generally reserved for a mass that is suspicious for cancer. A negative result, in this instance, would still require an excisional biopsy to remove the entire mass. *Excisional biopsies* are usually performed in the outpatient setting, with treatment decisions based on the final pathologic finding.

New techniques have been developed for nonpalpable masses seen only by mammography. Biopsy using *needle localization* requires placement of a barbed wire or contrast dye in proximity to the lesion, followed by two mammographic views demonstrating the relationship of the lesion to the wire or contrast dye. The surgeon then removes the designated tissue surrounding the wire. Because the surgeon usually cannot see the "lesion" even after making the incision, the specimen is subjected to radiography to confirm removal of the abnormality. *Stereotactic biopsy* is a relatively new technique that uses a specialized mammographic machine to localize precisely the area of breast abnormality. Approximately five to eight large-core needle biopsies are taken, which provide samples of tissue for pathologic examination. The technique is valuable in diagnosing a finding highly suspicious for cancer on mammography as well as lesions thought to be consistent with a fibroadenoma or intramammary lymph node. A core biopsy that confirms a benign lesion (e.g., fibroadenoma) negates the need for an open biopsy. If the biopsy yields only normal breast tissue, however, an *open biopsy* is recommended if the lesion is highly suspicious mammographically for cancer; alternatively, a 6-month follow-up mammogram may be recommended for less suspicious lesions. The *advanced breast biopsy instrumentation* (ABBI) technique combines stereotactic localization with an excisional biopsy device that removes a 5-mm to 20-mm core of breast tissue. In many diagnostic centers, stereotactic or ABBI biopsies have largely replaced the open biopsy method with needle localization.

The role of magnetic resonance imaging (MRI), Doppler ultrasound, Sestamibi scans, and other modalities in the diagnosis of breast cancer are currently being investigated. These techniques may differentiate malignancy from benign disease based on differences in enhancement and vascular signals. More proof of clinical efficacy is needed before these techniques become part of the routine evaluation of breast disorders. Currently they are used to assist with the interpretation of complex mammograms and to differentiate between malignant changes and scar tissue.

BREAST CANCER MANAGEMENT

Staging

The purpose of staging is to provide an estimate of tumor burden, which is the most important predictor of prognosis (Table 43-2). Patients with DCIS (Stage 0) have the best outcome, with nearly universal cure; patients with distant metastases (stage IV) have the worst prognosis, with essentially no chance for cure. Women with early-stage or localized breast cancer are at varying risk of developing metastatic disease, depending primarily on involvement of axillary lymph nodes with metastatic cancer. Thus nodal status is most often used to discriminate between stage I (lymph node–negative) and stage II (lymph node–positive) early-stage breast cancer. Women with locally advanced (stage III) breast cancer require an aggressive combined-modality approach to therapy because of an exceedingly high risk of systemic disease.

Sentinel lymph node identification is a novel technique for staging of regional lymph nodes. Using a radioisotope (technetium 99) or a vital dye (isosulphan blue), the flow of lymph from a breast cancer to the lymph node basin can be mapped. A complete axillary lymph node dissection may be avoided when the sentinel node is identified and histologically free of tumor.

Table 43-2. Incidence and Outcome of Breast Cancer by Stage

Stage	Clinical presentation	Total cases (%)	5-year survival (%)	10-year survival (%)
0	Noninvasive*	5-10	99	98
I	Early/node negative	40-45	85-95	70
II	Early/node positive	35-40	65-75	40-50
III	Locally advanced	10-15	45-50	5-20
IV	Metastatic	About 7	20-30	0.2

*Ductal carcinoma in situ (DCIS).

Table 43-3. Prognostic Indicators of Early-stage Breast Cancer

Indicator	Favorable	Unfavorable
Metastatic potential	Lymph node negative	Lymph node positive
Hormone dependency*	ER and/or PR positive	ER and PR negative
Tumor size	≤1 cm	>1 cm
Proliferative rate	Low S-phase fraction	High S-phase fraction

**ER*, Estrogen receptor; *PR*, progesterone receptor.

Prognostic Indicators

The prognosis of cancer is directly related to the presence of micrometastases and their propensity to develop into clinically important metastases. In the absence of direct assays for the presence of subclinical metastases, other factors are used to predict which patients with early-stage breast cancer are more or less likely to develop recurrent disease. This information is particularly useful for patients with stage I disease, for whom the relatively low risk of recurrence must be balanced against inherent risks of systemic adjuvant therapy.

The two most important prognostic factors are (1) the presence or absence of metastases in regional lymph nodes and (2) the expression of hormone receptors in the primary tumor (Table 43-3). Patients without lymph node metastases (stage I) have a significantly lower risk of developing and dying from recurrent breast cancer than patients with nodal metastases detected at diagnosis (stage II). Furthermore, the risk of recurrence and mortality increases with the number of lymph nodes containing metastatic deposits. Tumors that express either estrogen receptors (ER-positive tumors) or progesterone receptors (PR-positive tumors) have an improved prognosis and are more likely to benefit from adjuvant hormonal therapy and to respond to endocrine therapy for metastatic disease.

In patients with lymph node–negative disease, indices such as the size of the primary tumor, ER and PR expression, proliferative rate, and deoxyribonucleic acid (DNA) content are important independent determinants of outcome and are helpful in making recommendations for adjuvant systemic therapy. Generally, patients with tumors less than 1 cm in diameter have an extremely low risk of recurrence and do not require adjuvant therapy. Laboratory analysis by flow cytometry detects tumors that contain a high fraction of cells in S phase and therefore are rapidly proliferating. Such tumors carry a worse prognosis than those that divide more slowly (low S-phase fraction).

Ductal Carcinoma In Situ

The use of mammography has led to a dramatic proportional increase in the number of women diagnosed with DCIS over the past 15 years. These lesions are most often identified on mammograms as clustered microcalcifications with or without a palpable mass. Although these lesions are traditionally treated by mastectomy, recent data support the efficacy of lumpectomy and radiation for women with localized DCIS. Treatment decisions are tailored to the clinical scenario. For example, when a minute focus of DCIS is discovered, lumpectomy alone may be used. Alternatively, when mammography demonstrates extensive microcalcifications involving a large segment of the breast, simple mastectomy is the treatment of choice. Generally, axillary lymph node dissection is not required in the treatment of DCIS. Exceptions to this approach include (1) involvement of a large area of breast in which an area of microinvasion may be missed on histology and (2) the diagnosis of comedo carcinoma, which is known to have a low but recognized risk of lymph node metastases. After excision and radiation therapy, treatment of DCIS with the antiestrogen tamoxifen may further reduce the incidence of local recurrence and second primary cancers.

Early-Stage Invasive Disease

Local Treatment. The standard options for the primary treatment of invasive breast cancer are wide local excision (lumpectomy) and axillary lymph node dissection, combined with radiation therapy, or modified radical mastectomy, which includes a lymph node dissection. Multiple studies have shown that the survival of women treated with either of these two approaches is identical. Survival rates ultimately reflect spread to distant organ sites, which is not affected by type of treatment.

The primary goal of *lumpectomy* is to excise the tumor with negative microscopic margins. If the initial biopsy demonstrates that the cancer extends beyond the margins of resection, a reexcision is performed at the time of lymph node dissection. Radiation therapy is given over 6 weeks in divided doses, sometimes supplemented by a "boost" to the lumpectomy site with x-rays, electron beam, or brachytherapy. The patient is followed by interval mammography of the treated breast and the contralateral breast. Approximately 10% to 15% of women will develop a local recurrence after lumpectomy and radiation therapy and generally are treated by mastectomy.

Indications for *modified radical mastectomy,* which spares the chest wall muscles, include large tumors in a relatively small breast. If a lumpectomy would result in a distorted appearance or positive margins, mastectomy is also preferable. Traditionally, subareolar lesions were treated by mastectomy, but many patients prefer lumpectomy, even if this results in a breast without a nipple, to breast reconstruction. These options must be discussed with the patient. Patients with multifocal disease, a history of prior chest irradiation, collagen vascular disease, or inability to travel for radiation treatments are better served with mastectomy.

Breast reconstruction can be accomplished at the time of the primary treatment or after chemotherapy. If the physician and patient are concerned about the apparent aggressiveness of a tumor with suspicious palpable axillary nodes at presentation, reconstruction should be delayed because wound healing or implant infections could prolong the postoperative convalescent period and delay further treatment. Other than this consideration, reconstruction at mastectomy has multiple benefits, including a single operative procedure and hospitalization and a superior cosmetic result. The choice of reconstruction is decided by the patient and plastic surgeon, based on body habitus and personal choice. Common options currently include saline implant placement or myocutaneous flaps that use the rectus abdominis or latissimus dorsi muscles.

Adjuvant Therapy. Adjuvant systemic therapy is administered to patients with early-stage invasive breast cancer when a strong potential exists for relapse from subclinical micrometastases. Because approximately 60% to 70% of patients with node-positive and 30% of patients with node-negative malignancies eventually develop metastatic breast cancer, a large cohort of women may benefit from adjuvant chemotherapy. All women who harbor micrometastatic disease likely derive some benefit from adjuvant therapy even if micrometastases are not eradicated, because the treatment delays the onset of metastatic disease.

Polychemotherapy. An analysis of almost 50 randomized clinical trials of systemic adjuvant chemotherapy involving about 18,000 women worldwide has provided clear evidence that adjuvant combination chemotherapy (polychemotherapy) significantly improves the survival of women with early-stage breast cancer (Table 43-4). Overall, adjuvant chemotherapy reduces the risk of recurrence (i.e., metastatic disease) by 35% in women under 50 and by 20% in women over 50. This has resulted in significant improvements in overall survival at 10 years in all age groups, although the impact of chemotherapy is clearly greatest in younger women. Adjuvant chemotherapy also has been shown to improve the outcome of women regardless of involvement of axillary lymph nodes; however, the magnitude of this benefit is generally greater for women with node-positive than those with node-negative breast cancer.

Table 43-4. Impact of Adjuvant Polychemotherapy in Early-stage Breast Cancer at 10 Years

	Tumor recurrence (%)		Overall survival (%)	
	Proportional risk reduction	Absolute risk reduction	Proportional risk reduction	Absolute risk reduction
Women <50	35 ± 4		27 ± 5	
Negative nodes		58 → 68 (10)		72 → 78 (6)
Positive nodes		32 → 48 (16)		41 → 54 (13)
Women 50-69	20 ± 3		11 ± 3	
Negative nodes		60 → 66 (6)		67 → 69 (2)
Positive nodes		38 → 43 (5)		46 → 49 (3)

Combination chemotherapy regimens such as cyclophosphamide, methotrexate, and 5-fluorouracil (CMF) administered for 6 months or doxorubicin (Adriamycin) administered for 3 months are often recommended for women with a significant risk of recurrent disease. The addition of paclitaxel (Taxol) may further improve the outcome of women with node-positive disease. High-dose chemotherapy with autologous or peripheral blood stem cell support is under active investigation for women who are at extremely high risk of recurrence (i.e., those with four or more positive lymph nodes). Using this approach, 65% of patients with 10 or more involved lymph nodes have remained free of disease after 10 years, compared with only 30% of historic controls treated with conventional chemotherapy. Recently a regimen of sequential administration of dose-intense Adriamycin, Taxol, and cyclophosphamide (ATC regimen) that does not require stem cell support has similar efficacy with greatly reduced toxicity and cost.

Endocrine Therapy. *Oophorectomy,* which removes the principal source of estrogen, is a highly effective way to improve survival of premenopausal women with early-stage breast cancer. Similarly, adjuvant therapy with the antiestrogen tamoxifen prolongs disease-free and overall survival. Based on a meta-analysis of 55 randomized trials involving 37,000 women, adjuvant tamoxifen administered for at least 5 years reduces the risk of recurrence by almost 50% and the risk of death by more than 25% (Table 43-5). The risk of developing a contralateral second primary breast cancer is also reduced by 50%. All women diagnosed with ER-positive or PR-positive cancer derive the same proportional benefit from adjuvant tamoxifen, regardless of their age and involvement of axillary lymph nodes. The benefits of adjuvant chemotherapy and tamoxifen appear to be independent and additive. Thus, whenever chemotherapy is indicated, patients derive significant incremental benefit from the addition of tamoxifen if the tumor is ER or PR positive. Furthermore, because tamoxifen displays estrogen agonist properties in the cardiovascular and skeletal systems, the risk of death from cardiovascular disease may be reduced, and loss of bone mineral density is slowed. Table 43-6 summarizes current recommendations for adjuvant systemic therapy in breast cancer.

Toxicity. The benefits of adjuvant endocrine therapy and chemotherapy must be weighed against the risks of immediate and delayed toxicity. Table 43-7 lists the most common acute and long-term side effects associated with adjuvant endocrine therapy and chemotherapy. Leukopenia occurs more frequently with doxorubicin-containing regimens, but life-threatening infections are rare. Fatigue occurs in more than 50% of patients, regardless of the regimen. Marked alopecia is rare with CMF but occurs in virtually 100% of patients receiving doxorubicin. Weight gain of 4 to 5 kg within 1 year is typical. Premature menopause occurs in 95% of patients over age 40 who receive

Table 43-5. Impact of 5 Years of Adjuvant Tamoxifen in Early-stage Breast Cancer at 10 Years*

	Tumor recurrence (%)		Overall survival (%)	
	Proportional risk reduction	**Absolute risk reduction**	**Proportional risk reduction**	**Absolute risk reduction**
All women	47 ± 3		26 ± 4	
Negative nodes		64 → 79 (15)		73 → 79 (6)
Positive nodes		45 → 60 (15)		51 → 61 (10)

*Excluding estrogen receptor–negative cancers.

Table 43-6. Current Recommendations for Adjuvant Systemic Therapy in Breast Cancer

Tumor stage	Subset	Recommended adjuvant treatment
Lymph node negative (stage I)	Low risk All tumors <1 cm	No adjuvant therapy (consider tamoxifen for prophylaxis)
	Intermediate risk 1-2 cm ER and/or PR positive Age >50	Tamoxifen for 5 years or longer
	High risk >2 cm High S-phase fraction	Chemotherapy for 3-6 months, followed by tamoxifen if tumor is ER and/or PR positive
Lymph node positive (stage II)	1-3 positive nodes	Chemotherapy for 3-6 months, followed by tamoxifen if tumor is ER and/or PR positive
	4 or more positive nodes	Intensive, paclitaxel-containing chemotherapy for 3-6 months, followed by tamoxifen if tumor is ER and/or PR positive

ER, Estrogen receptor; *PR,* progesterone receptor.

Table 43-7. Toxicity Associated with Adjuvant Systemic Therapy

	Common	Infrequent
Polychemotherapy	Bone marrow suppression Alopecia Fatigue Premature menopause Weight gain	Nausea, vomiting Mucositis Sepsis Hemorrhagic cystitis Conjunctivitis Congestive heart failure Depression
Tamoxifen	Hot flashes Irregular menses Vaginal discharge or dryness Dyspareunia	Venous thrombosis Pulmonary emboli Endometrial cancer

CMF-based adjuvant chemotherapy regimens but is significantly less frequent after the shorter doxorubicin regimen. Early menopause is associated with all the symptoms of physiologic menopause, including hot flashes, atrophic vaginitis, decreased libido, infertility, osteoporosis, and increased risk of cardiovascular disease. Periodic measurements of bone mineral density should be performed and treatment of osteopenia and/or osteoporosis with calcium supplementation, exercise, and biphosphonates may be required.

Tamoxifen is well tolerated in most patients and is associated with few side effects. The major toxic effects occur in premenopausal patients and are limited to hot flashes (55%) and irregular menses (40% to 60%). One fourth of both premenopausal and postmenopausal women experience increased vaginal discharge. Phlebitis and early-stage endometrial carcinoma occur infrequently. Tamoxifen has additional long-term side effects that are beneficial rather than detrimental, such as improvement in bone mineral density and serum lipid profile and a reduction in ischemic heart disease. Because tamoxifen and raloxifene have similar antiresorptive properties, women being treated with adjuvant tamoxifen are unlikely to benefit from the addition of raloxifene.

Follow-up. All breast cancer patients should undergo lifetime surveillance for second primary breast cancers, as well as for recurrent disease. Although the majority of metastases occur within 5 years of diagnosis, relapses may be delayed for as long as two or three decades. Furthermore, these women have a lifelong risk of developing secondary breast cancers of approximately ½% to 1% per year. Follow-up evaluations should include a history and complete physical examination, complete blood count (CBC), liver function tests, and yearly mammography. Patients are typically seen every 3 to 4 months for the first 3 years, twice a year for the next 2 years, and yearly thereafter. No definitive evidence shows that early detection of asymptomatic metastases improves survival or palliation. Thus, although symptoms should be investigated to rule out metastatic disease, routine screening of asymptomatic patients, using chest radiographs, bone scans, and computed tomography (CT) scans, is not cost-effective.

Locally Advanced Disease (Stage III)

The term *locally advanced breast cancer* (LABC) has been applied to a heterogenous group of large tumors with extensive regional lymph node metastases and involvement of the skin or chest wall. This group composes 10% to 15% of breast cancer patients in the United States. The majority of patients with LABC will eventually develop distant metastases and thus have a uniformly poor prognosis.

Current management of LABC includes so-called neoadjuvant or induction chemotherapy before definitive local treatment of the primary lesion with surgery or radiation. This strategy improves both local and distant control, with more than 90% of patients rendered free of all gross disease. Dose-intense postoperative adjuvant regimens of chemotherapy with peripheral blood stem cell support are currently under investigation, particularly for women found to harbor large numbers of metastatic lymph nodes at surgery. Combined-modality therapy appears to have substantially improved survival of patients with LABC, with up to 50% of patients currently surviving for 5 years or more.

Inflammatory breast carcinoma (IBC) is often distinguished from other forms of LABC because of its aggressive natural history, with almost uniform mortality within 2 years due to the rapid development of disseminated disease. Clinical diagnosis is based on diffuse enlargement of the breast with erythema and induration or peau d'orange appearance of the skin. Because there is often no discrete underlying mass, this entity is often confused with acute mastitis. The latter, however, rarely occurs in nonlactating women. Involvement of dermal lymphatics with tumor emboli is the pathologic hallmark of IBC. The treatment strategy for IBC is similar to that for other forms of LABC.

Recurrent Disease

Local. Locoregional recurrence after mastectomy often heralds systemic disease. For an isolated chest wall recurrence, complete surgical resection followed by radiotherapy is the treatment of choice. Local therapy may be all that is warranted, particularly if the time between primary therapy and recurrence (disease-free interval, DFI) is prolonged. Radiotherapy is indicated for the palliation of localized pain from inoperable metastases to the chest wall, axilla, or brachial plexus. HRT and chemotherapy can be effective in controlling local disease that is not amenable to surgery and radiation or that occurs coincident with systemic disease. In addition to local therapy, most patients eventually require systemic therapy, because they develop distant metastases that lead ultimately to death.

A recurrence within the breast after lumpectomy and radiation therapy does not confer the same dire prognosis as recurrence after mastectomy. Salvage mastectomy leads to prolonged survival in more than 50% of patients.

Metastatic. Most patients with metastatic breast cancer (MBC) present with specific symptoms related to organ damage. MBC is a diverse disease. Its course ranges from indolent progression with a high quality of life to rapidly disabling symptoms that result in early death. From 20% to 30% of patients with MBC survive for 5 years, and up to 10% of patients survive for more than 10 years. The median survival is 2 to 3 years.

In general, MBC is highly treatable but rarely curable. Although most patients are responsive to initial systemic therapy, only a minority achieve complete remission (i.e., resolution of all evidence of disease). The primary goal of systemic therapy is the relief of symptoms and improvement or maintenance of a high quality of life. In many patients, even a toxic regimen that is effective in inducing tumor shrinkage is more likely to improve quality of life than a less toxic treatment with a low likelihood of response.

The success of MBC treatment depends on three main variables: tumor burden, tumor responsiveness to treatment, and patient performance status. Therefore patients should first undergo a staging workup to determine disease extent. Treatment is administered for a given period, usually 2 to 4 months, followed by restaging to assess response. A decision is then made whether to continue with the same therapy, change to a different therapy, or discontinue therapy altogether.

Staging and Treatment. Breast cancers can metastasize to virtually any organ, leading to a variety of symptoms and complications. At autopsy, 50% to 70% of patients who die of breast cancer have widespread disease to lung, liver, and bone. Once MBC has been documented, a staging workup is performed to determine the sites and extent of metastases. Staging typically includes laboratory evaluation (CBC, liver enzymes, calcium, tumor markers such as carcinoembryonic antigen [CEA] and CA15-3), CT scans of the chest and abdomen, and a radionuclide bone scan. Documentation of MBC extent not only helps determine prognosis and the most appropriate approach to therapy, but also provides an objective way to measure the response to therapy.

The selection of systemic therapy is determined by MBC sites, hormone receptor status of tumor, patient age, and DFI. In general, patients with disease confined to soft tissue or bone are more likely to respond to endocrine therapy and survive longer than those with visceral disease. Patients with metastases involving the liver or with lymphangitic spread to the lungs are poor candidates for endocrine therapy and should be offered chemotherapy. In addition, patients with ER-positive or PR-positive tumors have a better prognosis, and more than 60% respond to hormonal manipulation. Patients with a DFI longer than 2 years have a significantly longer survival and a higher probability of responding to endocrine therapy than those with a shorter DFI.

Endocrine Therapy. Pharmacologic doses of estrogens, antiestrogens, progestins, androgens, or corticosteroids, as well as pituitary, adrenal, and ovarian blockade, have been used to treat MBC with nearly equivalent response rates. Tamoxifen is currently the hormonal treatment of choice because of its low toxicity profile (see Table 43-7). Approximately two thirds of hormone receptor–positive patients respond to tamoxifen therapy. Up to half of hormone-sensitive patients who eventually fail tamoxifen therapy subsequently respond to second-line endocrine therapy. Two novel nonsteroidal inhibitors of *aromatase,* the enzyme that catalyzes the final step in the biosynthesis of estradiol and estrone outside the ovary, *anastrozole* and *letrozole,* are currently the drugs of choice in this setting because of their favorable toxicity profile. Alternatively, *megestrol* (Megace) a progestational agent, is often used in the United States. Its principal toxicity, which occurs in 20% to 50% of patients, is weight gain due to appetite stimulation. Fluid retention may be prohibitive in patients with cardiac dysfunction. Androgens, high doses of estrogens, and corticosteroids are rarely used because of undue toxicity.

Five percent to 10% of patients who embark on endocrine therapy experience a *tumor flare,* a transient worsening of pain at sites of bone metastases, within hours to weeks of treatment onset. Hypercalcemia may be induced or may worsen during this period but usually can be managed with supportive care without discontinuing treatment.

Chemotherapy. Chemotherapy results in an objective (measurable) response in approximately two thirds of patients with MBC. Complete remission, however, is observed in only about 20%, and the median duration of response is about 1 year. Objective response rates to secondary regimens are 20% to 35%. The median survival after initiation of chemotherapy is approximately 3 years, but some patients may survive as long as 10 years. Chemotherapy is indicated for symptomatic relief for patients who are not good candidates for endocrine therapy. This group includes patients who have failed to respond to hormonal manipulation, are ER negative, have had a short DFI, or have liver lesions or lymphangitic spread to the lungs.

Combinations of cyclophosphamide and fluorouracil with either methotrexate (CMF) or doxorubicin (CAF) are often used as the primary regimens for most patients. The taxanes, which include paclitaxel (Taxol) and docetaxel (Taxotere), are highly active drugs for breast cancer and are often used as single agents, as is doxorubicin. The most active second-line regimens include other alkylating agents (e.g., thiotepa, melphalan), vinorelbine, 5-fluorouracil as prolonged infusion (or the oral equivalent, capecitabine), and mitomycin C. The most frequent toxicities observed with these chemotherapeutic agents are myelosuppression, nausea, vomiting, mucositis, and alopecia (see Table 43-7). Toxicities specific to individual agents include cardiotoxicity (doxorubicin), hemorrhagic cystitis (cyclophosphamide), neuropathy (paclitaxel), capillary leak syndrome (docetaxel), diarrhea (5-fluorouracil, capecitabine), ileus (vinorelbine), and pulmonary toxicity or hemolytic uremic syndrome (mitomycin C).

An exciting new agent for MBC treatment, Herceptin, is a humanized monoclonal antibody directed at the HER2/neu/erbB2 growth factor receptor. This relatively nontoxic agent dramatically potentiates the efficacy of cytotoxic agents such as paclitaxel in patients whose breast cancers overexpress HER2.

Unlike hormonal agents administered continuously for as long as response persists, there is probably no advantage to continuing the administration of chemotherapy beyond the time necessary to induce the best possible response (usually, approximately 6 months). Patients may then be followed off therapy until symptomatic progression occurs.

High-dose Therapy. In recent years the focus of clinical research for MBC has shifted from palliation to cure for selected patients. Early findings indicate that high-dose chemotherapy followed by autologous bone marrow transplant or peripheral blood stem cell support may improve both disease-free survival and overall survival of MBC patients. The best candidates for this approach appear to be patients previously untreated for metastatic disease who have chemosensitive disease, with minimal residual tumor burden after induction chemotherapy. In early clinical trials, 15% to 20% of patients have remained free of disease off therapy for up to 3½ years. Longer follow-up is needed to determine how long these patients will remain in remission. Attempts to prolong these remissions by using antitumor vaccines or other biologic agents (e.g., Herceptin) are under investigation.

Specific Metastatic Sites. The most common initial site of metastasis in breast cancer is bone. Radionuclide bone scanning is the most sensitive method for diagnosing skeletal metastases. Bone metastases can cause significant morbidity because of pain, pathologic fractures with resultant loss of function, and hypercalcemia. Expansion of vertebral metastases is the most common route of entry into the epidural space, leading to spinal cord compression with resultant paralysis. Abnormalities in weight-bearing bones should be further evaluated to rule out impending fractures that may require prophylactic orthopedic intervention. Monthly intravenous administration of a biphosphonate, such as pamidronate, significantly reduces the incidence of pathologic fractures and the need for radiation therapy to skeletal metastases for pain control.

Besides the bony skeleton, the lungs and pleurae are the most common sites of MBC. The major manifestations of pulmonary metastases include dry, irrepressible cough and dyspnea, whether from parenchymal disease, endobronchial metastases, or malignant pleural effusions. Although systemic therapy is indicated, highly symptomatic patients may require interventions that provide more rapid palliation. Chest tube drainage of large pleural effusions followed by pleurodesis produces symptomatic responses lasting longer than 1 month in 80% to 90% of patients. Endobronchial lesions that cause proximal airway obstruction can be effectively treated with laser ablation in most patients. High-dose corticosteroids may provide symptomatic relief of dyspnea in patients with lymphangitic carcinomatosis refractory to chemotherapy.

The incidence of clinically manifest brain metastases is approximately 10%. Presenting symptoms include headaches, behavioral changes, seizures, and focal neurologic deficits. After diagnosis with CT or MRI scans, symptomatic brain metastases are treated with high-dose dexamethasone and whole-brain irradiation. Surgery should be considered for the minority of patients with solitary metastases and well-controlled systemic disease. Patients who are able to undergo resection of solitary brain metastases followed by radiotherapy have a prolonged survival and better functional status than those who undergo radiotherapy alone.

Leptomeningeal metastasis (carcinomatous meningitis) presents with cranial nerve palsies and spinal or nerve root symptoms, along with the less specific findings of headache, nausea, vomiting, and mental status changes. Diagnosis is made by cytologic evaluation of the cerebrospinal fluid, although meningeal enhancement on gadolinium-enhanced MRI scans is highly suggestive. Localized irradiation may be administered for symptomatic cranial nerve palsies or other focal findings, followed by treatment with intrathecal chemotherapy. Although the majority of patients improve with therapy, fewer than 10% of patients survive for more than 1 year.

Breast cancer is the most common cause of epidural spinal cord compression. Rapid diagnosis and treatment are crucial to prevent permanent paralysis and sphincter dysfunction. Progressive back pain is the heralding symptom and is often accompanied by radicular pain. Signs of myelopathy, weakness, and sensory loss ensue and may progress rapidly. Total-spine MRI scans have supplanted myelography for rapid diagnosis and should be obtained at the first suspicion of cord compression. High doses of dexamethasone should be instituted immediately on diagnosis, followed by spinal irradiation. Most patients experience pain relief with treatment, but impaired ambulation or sphincter function is often irreversible and depends on the time of cord compromise. Neurosurgical intervention should be considered for rapidly progressive neurologic dysfunction despite radiation therapy.

PREVENTION OF BREAST CANCER

After the discovery of cytotoxic and endocrine agents active against breast cancer in the 1940s and 1950s, clinical research focused primarily on MBC treatment (Fig. 43-4). In the early 1970s, investigations focused on adjuvant systemic therapy, which successfully treats many women and significantly decreases overall breast cancer mortality. Results of the first large-scale intervention studies aimed at preventing the onset of breast cancer women at high risk have recently been reported. In the twenty-first century the main focus of research is likely to shift to primary prevention, affecting the lives of the estimated 29 million healthy women at increased risk. Primary care physicians must understand how to assess breast cancer risk in healthy women and how best to apply the available treatment modalities.

Risk Factors

Although most women with breast cancer have no known genetic predisposition, definite risk factors for the development of breast cancer include genetic factors (family history, breast histopathology), hormonal factors (early menarche, late menopause, reproductive history, use of exogenous hormones), and environmental factors (high dietary fat intake, alcohol consumption, exposure to ionizing radiation). Table 43-8 summarizes the relative risks associated with various factors.

Family History. A family history of breast cancer is among the strongest risk factors, particularly for women with first-degree relatives who have had breast cancer. The risk of developing breast cancer for patients with a second-degree relative who has had breast cancer is only slightly higher than the risk in the general population. A family history that includes both first-degree and second-degree relatives with breast cancer, however, particularly if the family members were diagnosed at a young age, constitutes strong evidence for autosomal dominant inheritance of a genetic predisposition for breast cancer. Such familial cases are more often bilateral and are often diagnosed at a younger age than sporadic cases. The inheritance of inactivating mutations in two genes, BRCA1 and BRCA2, may be directly involved in the development of most familial forms of breast cancer. Women who have inherited a mutant allele have an 80% lifetime risk of developing breast cancer, tenfold higher than women without the allele. Truly hereditary breast cancers constitute fewer than 5% of all cases.

Personal History. Women with a past diagnosis of breast cancer are at high risk for the development of second primary breast cancer at an estimated rate of ½% to 1% per year. For example, a woman with early-stage breast cancer at age 30 and a remaining expected life span of 50 years has a 25% to 50% risk of developing a secondary cancer in either breast. As breast cancers are diagnosed earlier and their prognosis improves, the issue of preventing secondary primary cancers will become increasingly important.

Benign Breast Disease. Epidemiologic analysis of benign (fibrocystic) breast disease has shown that nonprolifera-

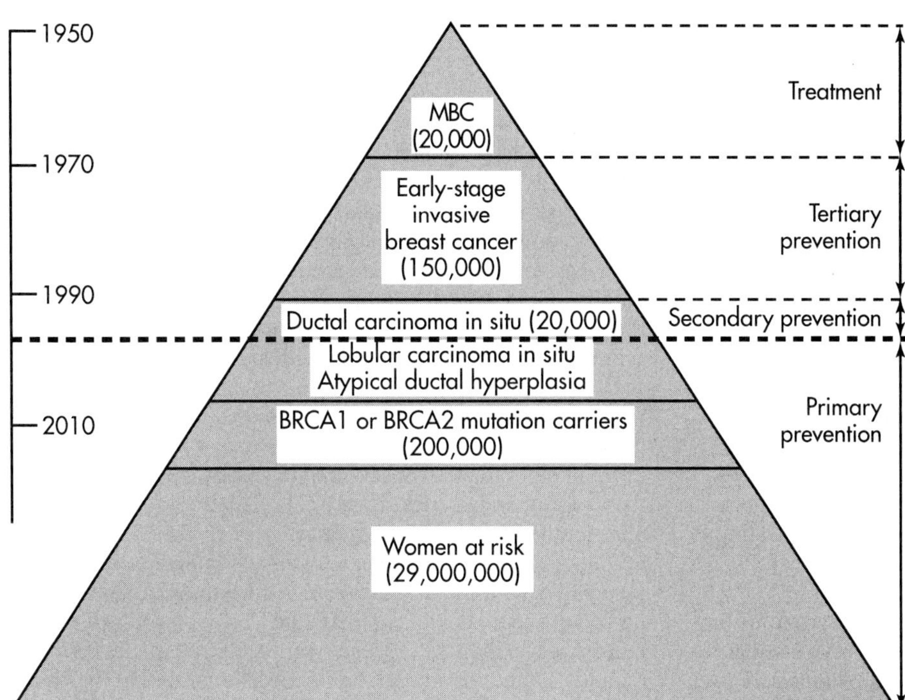

Fig. 43-4. Treatment and prevention pyramid for women at risk for breast cancer, 1950-2010. *MBC,* Metastatic breast cancer.

tive lesions, including cysts, fibroadenoma, duct ectasia, fibrosis, and metaplasia, are not associated with an increased risk for breast cancer. Hyperproliferative epithelia without atypia, including ductal hyperplasia, sclerosing adenosis, and papilloma, are associated with a minimal increase in risk. Two histopathologic entities, atypical ductal hyperplasia and LCIS, are associated with a strong increase in risk for both the involved breast and the contralateral breast (approximately 0.2% per year), independent of family history (see Table 43-8).

Hormonal Factors. Estrogens promote growth and development of breast cancer. Thus prolonged exposure of the breast epithelium to endogenous estrogens, as manifested by early menarche, late menopause, delayed childbearing, or postmenopausal obesity, increases breast cancer risk, whereas early menopause (without estrogen replacement) and multiple pregnancies have the opposite effect. The association between oral contraceptive use and breast cancer risk remains controversial. Prolonged use may mildly increase risk, but the risk level returns to baseline soon after the drug is discontinued. Moreover, most of the available data were derived from studies of women treated with higher doses of contraceptive estrogen than currently prescribed. Current evidence does not support the avoidance of oral contraceptive use (see Chapter 38). Postmenopausal HRT is extremely beneficial in terms of preventing bone loss and cardiovascular events. Beyond approximately 10 years, however, the risks of HRT in terms of promoting breast cancer development probably outweigh their beneficial effects on other organ systems (see Chapter 42).

Table 43-8. Estimated Relative Risks of Developing Breast Cancer by Risk Factor

Risk factor	Relative risk
Family history	
First-degree relative, premenopausal	2-3
First-degree relative, postmenopausal	1.5-2.5
First-degree relative, premenopausal, bilateral breast cancer	9.5
First-degree relative, postmenopausal, bilateral breast cancer	4
Two first-degree relatives	5.6
Second-degree relative	1-1.5
History of breast disease	
Atypical hyperplasia	4-5
Atypical hyperplasia and first-degree relative	9-11
Lobular carcinoma in situ (LCIS)	7-10
History of breast cancer	4
Hormonal factors	
Early menarche	1.3
Late menopause (after age 55)	1.5
Late age at first live birth (≥30 vs <20)	1.9
Environmental factors	
Alcohol (3 oz/day vs none)	2
Ionizing radiation	10-75

Environmental Factors. Exposure of the breast to therapeutic doses of ionizing radiation (typically about 40 Gy, e.g., in treatment of Hodgkin's disease), particularly during breast development (ages 10 to 19 years), dramatically increases cancer risk. Breast cancers become manifest after a lag period of approximately 15 years and with a frequency 10 to 75 times as high as in the general population. Thus 6-month clinical breast examinations and yearly mammograms are recommended for this group of women, beginning 10 to 15 years after the radiation exposure.

Risk Assessment Tools

A simple computerized interactive breast cancer risk assessment tool developed by Gail and others is distributed free by the NCI.* A computer algorithm is used to calculate an individual's 5-year or lifetime risk for the development of breast cancer, based on age at menarche, age at first live birth, history of breast cancer in first-degree relatives, and history of past breast biopsies, particularly if these revealed atypical ductal hyperplasia or LCIS. The Gail model is a useful and reliable tool in most patients but is poorly suited to identify women with hereditary breast cancer, who have a much higher lifetime risk. Thus the physician should obtain a detailed family history to identify women who are likely carriers of a BRCA1 or BRCA2 gene mutation. These include women with a first-degree relative with breast or ovarian cancer diagnosed under age 50 or those with multiple first-degree or second-degree relatives with breast cancer. These should then be referred for genetic counseling and testing.

Preventive Interventions

Prophylactic Mastectomy. Prophylactic mastectomy is reserved for highly selected patients in a high-risk category. The indications for prophylactic mastectomy supported by the Society of Surgical Oncology include atypical hyperplasia of lobular or ductal origin, particularly if it is bilateral and multifocal; family history of premenopausal bilateral breast cancer in a mother or sister (family cancer syndrome); and fibronodular, dense breasts that are mammographically and clinically difficult to follow, coupled with either of the preceding problems.

Chemoprevention. The high mortality rate of breast cancer despite advances in early diagnosis and treatment has prompted investigations into preventive measures using hormonal, dietary, and vitamin manipulations. Two nationwide clinical trials have been designed to study interventions that may reduce the incidence of breast cancers: the Breast Cancer Prevention Trial, conducted by the National Surgical Adjuvant Breast and Bowel Project (NSABP P-1 trial), and the Women's Health Initiative (WHI), sponsored by the National Institutes of Health. The WHI is designed to test the overlapping effects of a low-fat diet, HRT, and calcium supplements on the incidence of cardiovascular disease, breast cancer, colon cancer, and osteoporosis. Results of this study will likely become available during the next decade.

The Breast Cancer Prevention Trial was designed to determine whether 5 years of therapy with tamoxifen can prevent breast cancer in women at increased risk. More than 13,000 women were enrolled in this trial. At a median follow-up of 69 months the incidence of new in situ and invasive breast cancers among women receiving tamoxifen was 50% lower than in the control group. In a second study of the same magnitude (P-2 or STAR trial) the preventive effect of tamoxifen will be compared to that of a novel estrogen receptor modulator, raloxifene, which may have a more favorable toxicity profile.

*The Breast Cancer Risk Assessment software can be ordered by calling 1-800-4-CANCER or by visiting NCI's cancer Trials Web site at http://cancertrials.nci.nih.gov.

SPECIAL PATIENT POPULATIONS

Pregnant Patients

Gestational breast cancer complicates approximately 1 : 1000 pregnancies, accounting for about 3% of all breast cancers and 7% to 14% of breast cancers in women under age 40. Historically, breast cancer diagnosed during pregnancy was thought to carry a particularly poor prognosis. More recent studies, however, in which pregnant patients were compared with age-matched and stage-matched controls, have not demonstrated any difference in prognosis. Nonetheless, pregnant patients generally have more advanced disease at presentation, presumably from a delay in diagnosis of up to several months.

Modified radical mastectomy is the local treatment of choice for gestational breast cancer unless the pregnancy is terminated or the diagnosis is made close to delivery, because the radiotherapy necessary for breast preservation is contraindicated during pregnancy.

Pregnancy after treatment for breast cancer has not been associated with increased risk of recurrence. Patients should be counseled, however, that the risk of breast cancer recurrence continues for several years after the primary diagnosis, and family planning decisions should be made accordingly.

Patients Receiving Hormonal Replacement Therapy

HRT decreases the morbidity and mortality associated with cardiovascular disease and osteoporosis in postmenopausal women. Because premature menopause is a common side effect of adjuvant therapy for early-stage breast cancer, many young women face the risks of premature heart and bone disease and other conditions related to estrogen deficiency. Although the addition of progestins to estrogen protects against the development of estrogen-dependent endometrial carcinomas, the safety of HRT with respect to breast cancer has not been established. Therefore HRT is not advised for patients with a history of breast cancer. Adjuvant therapy with tamoxifen, however, has been shown to decrease bone loss because of its estrogen agonist effect on osteoclasts.

Elderly Patients

Breast cancer in elderly persons generally follows a more indolent course, often presenting as a well-circumscribed mass in this unscreened population. Mammography is helpful in estimating the amount of breast involvement and thus in planning treatment. Lumpectomy followed by tamoxifen alone can be substituted for more aggressive forms of treatment, particularly when extreme old age or other medical illnesses complicate the use of conventional therapy.

Male Patients

Approximately 1000 men are diagnosed with breast cancer in the United States every year, resulting in about 300 deaths a year. The mean age of men diagnosed with breast cancer is 60 to 70 years, approximately a decade older than that of women with breast cancer. Risk factors are similar to those in women: family history, exposure to radiation, high endogenous estrogen levels (secondary to liver disease or Klinefelter's syndrome), or exposure to exogenous estrogens. Stage for stage, survival rates are similar for men and women.

Management of male breast cancer parallels that for

female breast cancer. Local treatment generally consists of mastectomy, followed by radiotherapy for LABC. The efficacy of adjuvant chemotherapy or tamoxifen for node-positive cancer in men has not been evaluated in randomized trials because of the small number of patients, but retrospective studies indicate that it is similar to that in women.

ADDITIONAL READINGS

American Cancer Society: *Cancer facts and figures, 2000*, Atlanta, 2000, American Cancer Society.

Claus EB, Risch N, Thompson WD: Autosomal dominant inheritance of breast cancer, *Cancer* 73:643, 1994.

Early Breast Cancer Trialists' Collaborative Group: Tamoxifen for early breast cancer: an overview of the randomised trials, *Lancet* 351:1451, 1998.

Early Breast Cancer Trialists' Collaborative Group: Polychemotherapy for early breast cancer: an overview of the randomised trials, *Lancet* 352:930, 1998.

Fisher B, Costantino JP, Wickerham DL, et al: Tamoxifen for prevention of breast cancer: report of the National Surgical Adjuvant Breast and Bowel Project P-1 Study, *J Natl Cancer Inst* 90:1371, 1998.

Harris JR, Lippman ME, Morrow M, Hellman S: *Diseases of the breast*, New York, 1996, Lippincott-Raven.

Wingo PA, Ries LA, Rosenberg HM, et al: Cancer incidence and mortality, 1973-1995: a report card for the U.S., *Cancer* 82:1197, 1998.

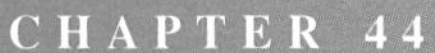

CHAPTER 44

Gynecologic Neoplasms

Joseph T. Chambers
Setsuko K. Chambers

The most common gynecologic cancer in the United States is endometrial cancer, followed by ovarian and cervical cancers (Table 44-1).[1] In general, the peak age for invasive gynecologic cancers is between 55 and 65 years (Fig. 44-1); however, for carcinoma in situ (CIS) of the cervix it is between 25 and 35 years. The mortality rate for ovarian cancer exceeds that for cancers of the cervix and endometrium combined (Fig. 44-2). Since the survival rates for these cancers decrease with increasing extent of disease at diagnosis, early detection offers the best chance for cure. Unfortunately, except for Pap smear screening for squamous cervical cancer, effective screening does not exist.

CERVICAL CANCER

Epidemiology

Although invasive cervical cancer ranks as the third most common form of gynecologic cancer, it is the second most common cause of gynecologic cancer death. Every year 1.2 million new cases of cervical intraepithelial neoplasia (CIN), the preinvasive lesion, are detected, including 55,000 new CIS cases. Sexual activity is thought to be a prerequisite for the development of cervical cancer. Multiple sexual partners and an early age of first intercourse increase the risk. Sexually transmitted diseases, such as human papillomavirus (HPV), human immunodeficiency virus (HIV), or herpes simplex virus (HSV), have been associated with the development of cervical cancer. Although there is strong evidence for an etiologic role for HPV, this infection alone does not appear to constitute sufficient cause for cervical neoplasia and requires a cocarcinogen for its actions. The importance of immunosuppression in the development of malignancies is demonstrated by the association between HIV infections and CIN; nearly half of HIV-infected women demonstrate CIN on routine colposcopy, with the majority coinfected with HPV. Smoking, with its propensity for DNA damage, carries a fourfold increased risk for the development of cervical cancer. Infrequently, an unusual form of cervical cancer, such as diethylstilbestrol (DES)-associated clear cell carcinoma, may develop in a woman who has never been sexually active.

Table 44-1. Gynecologic Cancers in the United States, 2000

Site	New cases	Annual cancer deaths
Invasive cervix	12,800	4600
Corpus uteri	36,100	6500
Ovary	23,100	14,000
Other gynecologic	5500	1400

From American Cancer Society: *CA Cancer J Clin* 50(1):12-13, 2000.

An increased risk in the lower socioeconomic populations has been associated with poor access to the health care preventive services and excessive risk-taking behavior. Lack of education and compliance of the general population add to the problems. Approximately 40% of the general population do not receive annual Pap smears; older and low-income women are least likely to have ever had a Pap smear.

Pathophysiology

Although 36% of CIS cases progress to invasive cervical cancer, 75% of lower grade dysplasias regress or persist without treatment, with the remaining progressing over protracted time intervals. Studies report that the average transit time from the diagnosis of CIN to CIS is between 3.8 to 5.7 years.[12] Reports of cancers arising in the setting of negative Pap smears suggest that transit times from a normal cervix to the diagnosis of cancer may be getting shorter. However, observations may be due to false-negative Pap smears.

HPV has long been known to cause benign anogenital infections resulting in condylomata; however, the majority of CIN and cervical cancers also contain HPV DNA. Of the many HPV subtypes that have been identified, oncogenic subtypes are more likely to be associated with CIS and invasive cancers. The finding of HPV DNA in cervical cancer is not only an association but also causal in part. The DNA of the oncogenic subtypes is integrated into the host (patient) genome, and early viral proteins are actively expressed. The significance of the proteins lies in their ability to bind to and functionally eliminate tumor suppressor genes, allowing for the formation of cancer.

Pap Smear Screening

The Pap smear has been shown to be a successful screening test around the world, reducing mortality from squamous cell cancers of the cervix. Its purpose is to detect premalignant conditions of the cervix. Screening may reduce the risk of

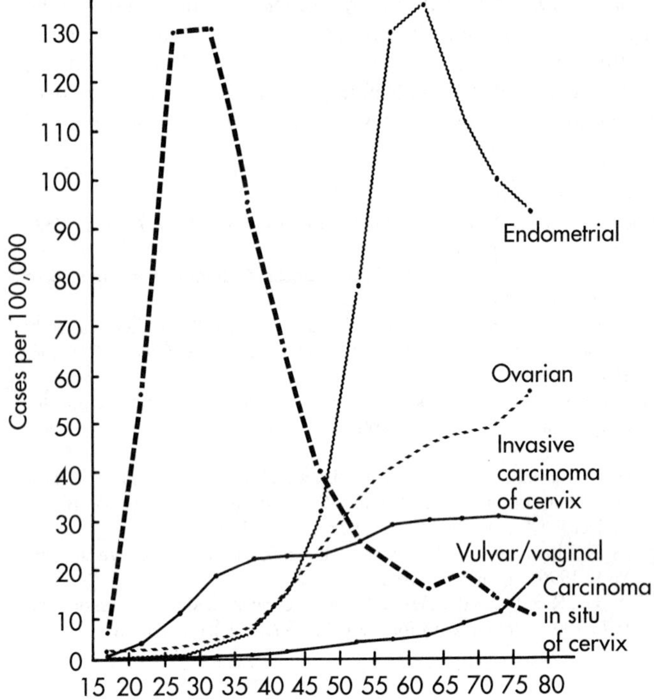

Fig. 44-1. Age-specific incidence curves for gynecologic cancers in the United States. (From Knapp RC, Berkowitz RS, editors: *Gynecologic oncology,* New York, 1986, Macmillan.)

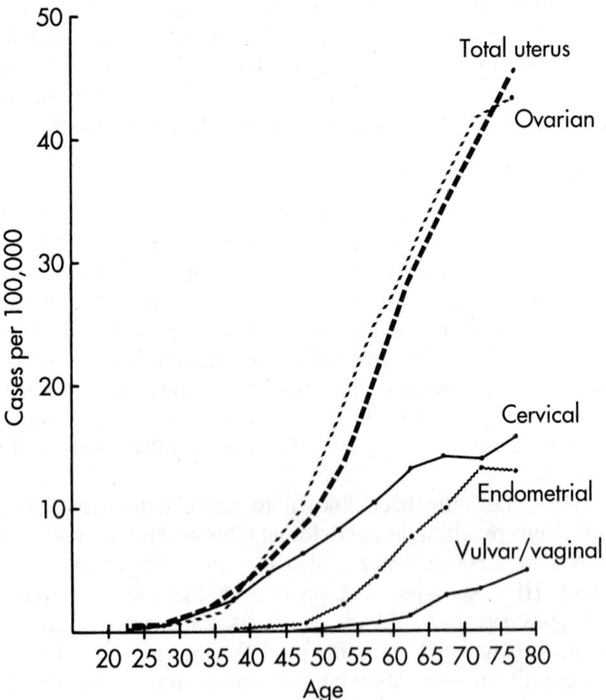

Fig. 44-2. Age-specific mortality curves for gynecologic cancers in the United States. (From Knapp RC, Berkowitz RS, editors: *Gynecologic oncology,* New York, 1986, Macmillan.)

death from cervical cancer by as much as 80%.[8] CIN, which is asymptomatic, develops at the squamocolumnar junction (SCJ) of the cervix. The SCJ undergoes a process of repair and formation of squamous metaplasia with aging and sexual activity, gradually receding into the endocervical canal and becoming invisible in the postmenopausal woman. This process of continual repair increases the opportunity for DNA mutations and the formation of dysplasia. Therefore efforts to obtain an adequate Pap smear that contains endocervical cells and to investigate an abnormal smear should be directed at the SCJ.

Although the Pap smear is a specific test, it is only 50% sensitive. Some authors have reported false-negative rates for CIN as high as 40% and for cervical cancer as high as 60%. The false-negative rates are due to quality-control problems in cytology laboratories, as well as to errors in sampling technique and interpretation. An endocervical brush should be used to increase the yield of endocervical cells. The Pap smear can detect abnormal changes associated with squamous dysplasia more easily than those associated with glandular dysplasia. Adenocarcinoma, which constitutes at least 20% of cervical cancers and is increasing in incidence, arises in the endocervical canal and is unfortunately not routinely detected by the Pap smear. This problem is magnified by the introduction of automated fluid-based methods for preparation of the Pap smear (such as the Thin Prep). Although numerous studies have testified to the increased ability of the Thin Prep Pap test to detect low-grade squamous intraepithelial lesion (LGSIL) and high-grade squamous intraepithelial lesion (HGSIL), with improved specimen quality due to homogeneous sampling of cells during preparation of the smear, the yield of endocervical cells is lower with this technique, as is the percentage of glandular abnormalities detected. At the current time, there is no good screening test for detection of glandular dysplasia, adenocarcinoma in situ, or adenocarcinoma of the endocervix.

The Bethesda system is currently used for Pap smear classification (Box 44-1). The major advantage of this system is that it distinguishes benign cellular changes (infection, reactive, or reparative) from truly atypical changes (atypical squamous cells or atypical glandular cells of undetermined significance [ASCUS or AGUS]). The Bethesda system also replaces the categories of CIN 2 and 3 with HGSIL, and

Box 44-1. The 1991 Bethesda System

Statement on specimen adequacy
General categorization
- Within normal limits
- Benign cellular changes
- Epithelial cell abnormality

Descriptive diagnosis
- Benign cellular changes
  - Infection
  - Reactive
- Epithelial cell abnormalities
  - Squamous cell
    - ASCUS
    - Low-grade SIL
    - High-grade SIL
    - Squamous cell carcinoma
  - Glandular cell
    - Benign endometrial cells
    - AGUS
    - Adenocarcinoma

Other malignant neoplasm
Hormonal evaluation

ASCUS, Atypical squamous cells of undetermined significance; *SIL*, squamous intraepithelial lesion; *AGUS*, atypical glandular cells of undetermined significance.

Table 44-2. Classification of Preinvasive Cervical Disease

Dysplasia	Cervical intraepithelial neoplasm	Bethesda
Normal	Normal	Normal
Atypia	Atypia	Atypical squamous cells of undetermined significance (ASCUS)
Mild dysplasia	CIN 1	Low-grade squamous intraepithelial lesion
Moderate dysplasia	CIN 2	High-grade squamous intraepithelial lesion
Severe dysplasia	CIN 3	High-grade squamous intraepithelial lesion
Carcinoma in situ	Carcinoma in situ	High-grade squamous intraepithelial lesion
Cancer	Cancer	Cancer

CIN, Cervical intraepithelial neoplasia.

morphologic changes that occur with HPV infection and CIN 1 with LGSIL, in the belief that the behavior of those lesions grouped together is similar (Table 44-2).

The causes of an abnormal Pap smear are not limited to pathologies of the cervix. Lower genital tract dysplasias and cancer, upper genital tract lesions, and, rarely, urologic malignancies all have been implicated as causes of an abnormal Pap smear.

Workup of an Abnormal Pap Smear

The flow chart (Fig. 44-3) depicted outlines the steps in the workup of an abnormal Pap smear. The first step is to distinguish those Pap smears that require prompt workup (true ASCUS or AGUS, or suggestive of dysplasia or cancer) from those related to benign changes. If the Pap smear indicates a benign inflammatory change, it may also identify an infectious agent. Appropriate treatment usually results in resolution of the mild inflammatory or reactive abnormality. Other reparative atypical changes may not resolve (e.g., those associated with radiation therapy). A follow-up Pap smear at 3 months is important to assess the efficacy of the treatment and to rule out more serious underlying causes.

Workup of an abnormal Pap smear requires the use of colposcopy, unless there is a visible lesion. Colposcopy is then unnecessary, and prompt biopsy should be performed. Colposcopy is an office procedure that uses a microscope to magnify the cervical epithelium after the application of a 3% acetic acid solution. The acetic acid highlights areas of abnormal vascular patterns or thickened epithelium. After careful visualization, biopsies are performed, along with an endocervical curettage (ECC) in the nonpregnant patient.

Management of Cervical Intraepithelial Neoplasia

The modality of treatment of CIN depends on several factors, including the desire to preserve the SCJ for ease of future follow-up, to preserve fertility, and to have an additional pathologic specimen. For patients with unequivocal CIN (negative ECC, SCJ visualized in its entirety on colposcopy, and Pap smears congruous with the biopsy) a recent randomized trial has shown equal efficacy for ablative (cryocauterization, laser vaporization) and excisional (loop electrosurgical excision) techniques.[10] Uncertainty about the pathologic diagnosis or suspicion of invasive cancer dictates the use of an excisional technique such as conization of the cervix using either a cold knife or laser technique, rather than an ablative technique or loop electrosurgical excision. These approaches must include a separate endocervical evaluation above the excisional biopsy. Whatever the treatment modality, follow-up Pap smears are crucial to assess success. In general, a hysterectomy should be reserved for women who have completed childbearing and for those in whom other procedures have failed (e.g., prior cone biopsy with positive margins, or a positive ECC).

Evaluation of the Patient with Invasive Cervical Cancer

If Pap smear screening fails, or if the cancer is not detected by the Pap smear (such as adenocarcinoma), the patient with invasive cervical cancer usually presents with symptoms of abnormal vaginal discharge, bleeding, or pelvic pain in more advanced cases.

On physical examination, the cervix may have an erosion or ulcer or may be partially replaced by a fungating tumor. If the tumor has arisen in the endocervix, the exocervix may occasionally appear normal; however, on palpation, it will feel indurated and may balloon out. Both bimanual and rectovaginal examinations should be performed to assess the local extent of spread into the parametria and uterosacral ligaments.

Workup of Invasive Cervical Cancer

Cervical cancer spreads by direct penetration into the lateral parametria or by lymphatic spread to the pelvic lymph nodes. Once the diagnosis is confirmed by cervical biopsy, a chest radiograph and an abdominal/pelvic computed tomography

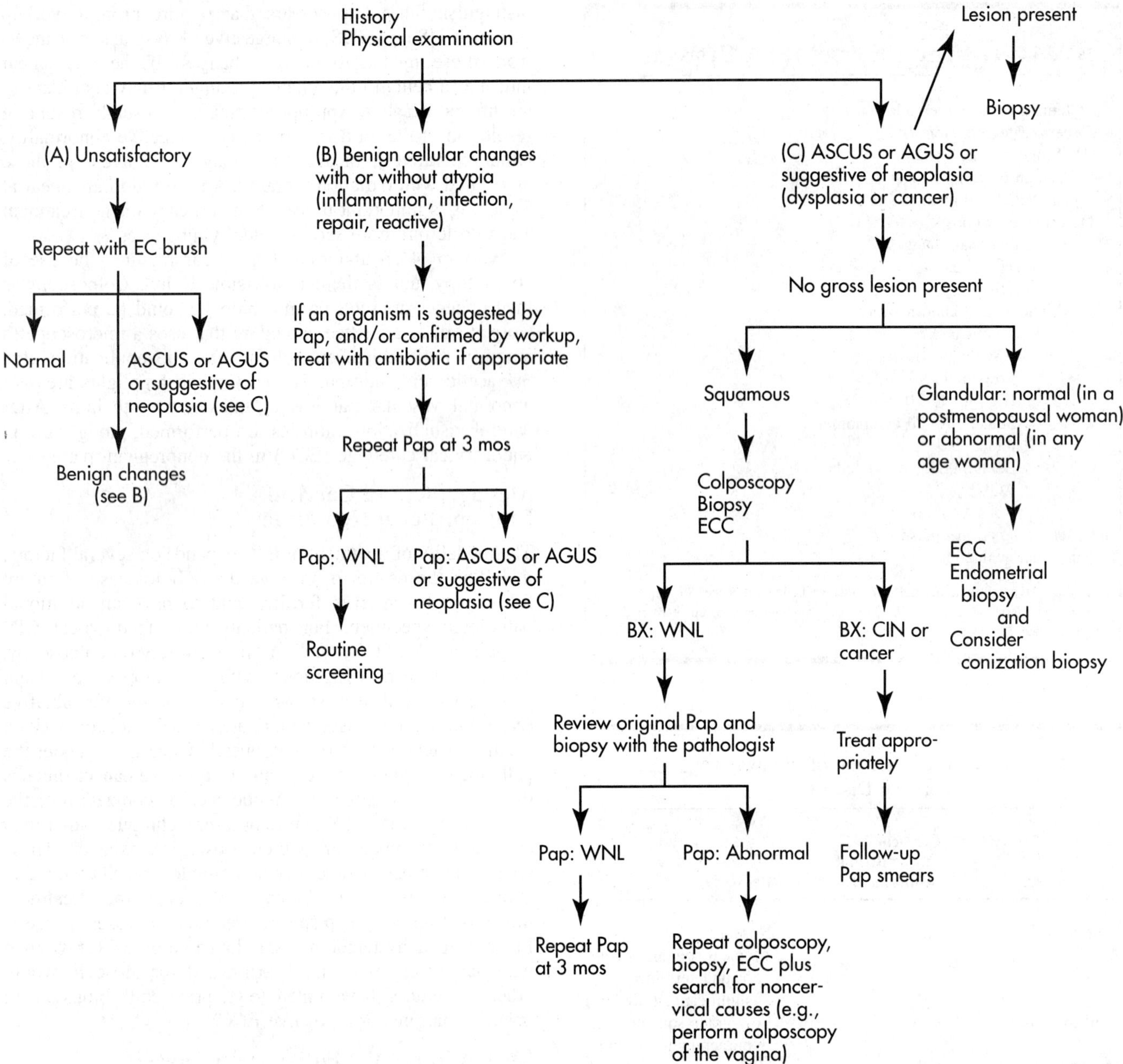

Fig. 44-3. Algorithm for the workup of an abnormal Pap smear. *ECC,* Endocervical curettage; *WNL,* within normal limits; *ASCUS or AGUS,* atypical squamous cells or atypical glandular cells of undetermined significance.

(CT) scan should be obtained. Other diagnostic imaging studies, such as nuclear scans or barium enemas, are not routinely indicated unless dictated by clinical findings. Cystoscopy, with or without proctoscopy, is usually performed for staging purposes. Because accurate pretreatment clinical staging is important, the patient should be referred for formal staging by a gynecologic oncologist in conjunction with a radiation oncologist.

Management of Cervical Cancer

Cervical cancer is staged clinically. Stage IB (involvement of the cervix alone) or early stage IIA (involvement also of upper vagina) disease is treated by radical hysterectomy or radiation therapy. Radiation therapy results in castration of the premenopausal patient, and in the possibility (usually less than 5%) of severe long-term effects on the vagina, bladder, and rectum. Mild changes, such as a decreased bladder capacity with urinary urgency and dyspareunia, are more common. The use of vaginal dilators or sexual activity during and after radiation therapy and estrogen replacement, if appropriate, help prevent dyspareunia. Alternatively, radical hysterectomy can be performed with translocation of the ovaries in the event postoperative radiation therapy is necessary. There is a small (less than 1%) acute operative complication rate and larger (up to 30% in some studies) long-term bladder and/or rectal dysfunction rates. These problems can be obviated in most cases with careful attention during postoperative regimens to restore bladder and rectal functions.

Five-year survival rates correlate with stage and range,

from 85% for stage IB disease to minimal survival for disease that has spread beyond the pelvis. Fortunately, 50% of cervical cancers present as stage IB disease.[5] Adenocarcinomas tend to have a worse prognosis than squamous cell cancers, stage for stage. Increased tumor size, a measure of tumor bulk, and lymph node involvement impart a significantly worse prognosis. Primary radiation therapy with chemotherapy has become the standard treatment for advanced disease.[10a]

ENDOMETRIAL CANCER

Epidemiology

Endometrial cancer is the most common gynecologic malignancy and can be associated with prolonged or excessive estrogen states. Exogenous estrogens in postmenopausal women are firmly established as a risk factor for endometrial cancer, with a risk increased twofold to fourfold in estrogen users compared with nonusers. The use of combination oral contraceptive pills (OCPs) for at least 12 months has been associated with a 0.60 relative risk (95% confidence interval 0.3-0.9)[3] of developing endometrial cancer compared with women who never used OCPs. The protection persists for at least 5 years after OCP use is discontinued.

Other conditions that can be associated with excessive estrogen states include chronic anovulation, as seen in polycystic ovarian or thyroid diseases, delayed menopause, and hormone-producing ovarian tumors (e.g., granulosa cell tumors).

Obesity is a constitutional factor that frequently has been associated with the development of endometrial cancer, presumably a result of the increased production of estrone from the peripheral aromatization of androstenedione (of adrenal origin) in adipose tissue.

Pathophysiology

During the normal menstrual cycle, the endometrium is exposed to an ordered changing of levels of hormones. The mitogenic effects of estradiol that predominate during the early proliferative phase of the cycle are down-regulated by the opposing effect of progesterone during the late secretory phase. Disruptions in these cyclic influences on the endometrium may lead to a hyperplastic state, and subsequent unknown factors may cause the development of atypical hyperplasia and, eventually, endometrial carcinoma. Because hyperplasia develops in women who have had prolonged exposure to unopposed estrogen and is frequently associated with cancer, estrogen is considered to be a causative agent in the development of endometrial cancer. In a recent study, 29% of women with complex glandular patterns and cytologic atypia developed endometrial cancer, whereas only 1% with simple glandular patterns and no atypia developed cancer.[6] Thus the finding of complex atypical hyperplasia must be considered a premalignant state.

Differential Diagnosis and Workup of Abnormal Vaginal Bleeding

Abnormal vaginal bleeding could stem from pathology of any of the reproductive organs or from the gastrointestinal or urologic tracts (Fig. 44-4). Involvement of the latter two can generally be excluded by the lack of supporting symptoms and a negative stool or catheterized urine specimen. An ectopic or molar pregnancy or miscarriage must be considered in the premenopausal patient, and a serum pregnancy test should be performed. Thyroid or liver function tests, or coagulation studies to rule out blood dyscrasias, may be indicated. In addition to these conditions, abnormal bleeding frequently signals a benign endometrial or myometrial cause (e.g., fibroids or dysfunctional uterine bleeding). In perimenopausal and postmenopausal women, an evaluation of the endometrial cavity is imperative to rule out a malignancy.

Evaluation of Patient with Endometrial Cancer

Endometrial cancer is generally associated with abnormal vaginal bleeding. Although only 20% of all women who present with vaginal bleeding have a gynecologic malignancy, this risk increases with age. Premenopausal women diagnosed with endometrial cancer often have a history of heavy irregular menstrual bleeding. During the perimenopausal period, the pattern of bleeding should become lighter and less frequent. Significant deviations from this pattern suggest underlying pathology. Symptoms related to pelvic pressure, uterine enlargement, or extrauterine spread may be part of the initial presentation in patients with advanced disease.

Examination should begin with inspection of the vulva, vagina, and cervix. If gross lesions are seen, a biopsy should be obtained. If no lesion is apparent, a Pap smear of the cervix should be performed. The uterus may be normal sized or enlarged, irregular, firm, or even soft. The presence of an adnexal mass is less likely to represent a metastasis from an endometrial primary than a benign condition, such as a pedunculated fibroid or a functional ovarian cyst.

An office endometrial biopsy using a flexible plastic tube curet is the starting point for the evaluation of abnormal uterine bleeding. The indications and few contraindications for this procedure are listed in Box 44-2. When bacterial endocarditis is a risk, antibiotic prophylaxis is indicated. Complications from endometrial sampling are rare. Perforation of the uterus can occur in patients with cervical stenosis, severely flexed uteri, or a necrotic uterus caused by endometrial cancer.

Several series have shown that the diagnostic accuracy of an office biopsy is 80% to 95%.[2] If the biopsy specimen shows atypical cells or is insufficient for diagnosis (6% incidence in symptomatic patients), a dilation and curettage (D&C) should be performed. A review of a large number of patients with perimenopausal bleeding demonstrates that the diagnosis of endometrial cancer or its precursor, complex atypical hyperplasia, is made 8% to 9% of the time. In contrast, the likelihood that malignant or premalignant changes are the cause of abnormal bleeding in patients with postmenopausal bleeding is more than 20%.

Although several studies have indicated that one third to one half of patients with endometrial cancer will have abnormal cervical cytology, the routine use of a Pap smear to evaluate the endometrium is inappropriate. However, endometrial cells found on a Pap smear in a postmenopausal woman, even if normal, should alert the physician to the possibility of underlying endometrial pathology.

Newer modalities used in the evaluation of the endometrium include hysteroscopy and transvaginal ultrasound (TVS). Ultrasound findings in a postmenopausal woman that warrant further workup with endometrial sampling include a fluid-filled endometrial cavity or a thickened endometrial stripe.

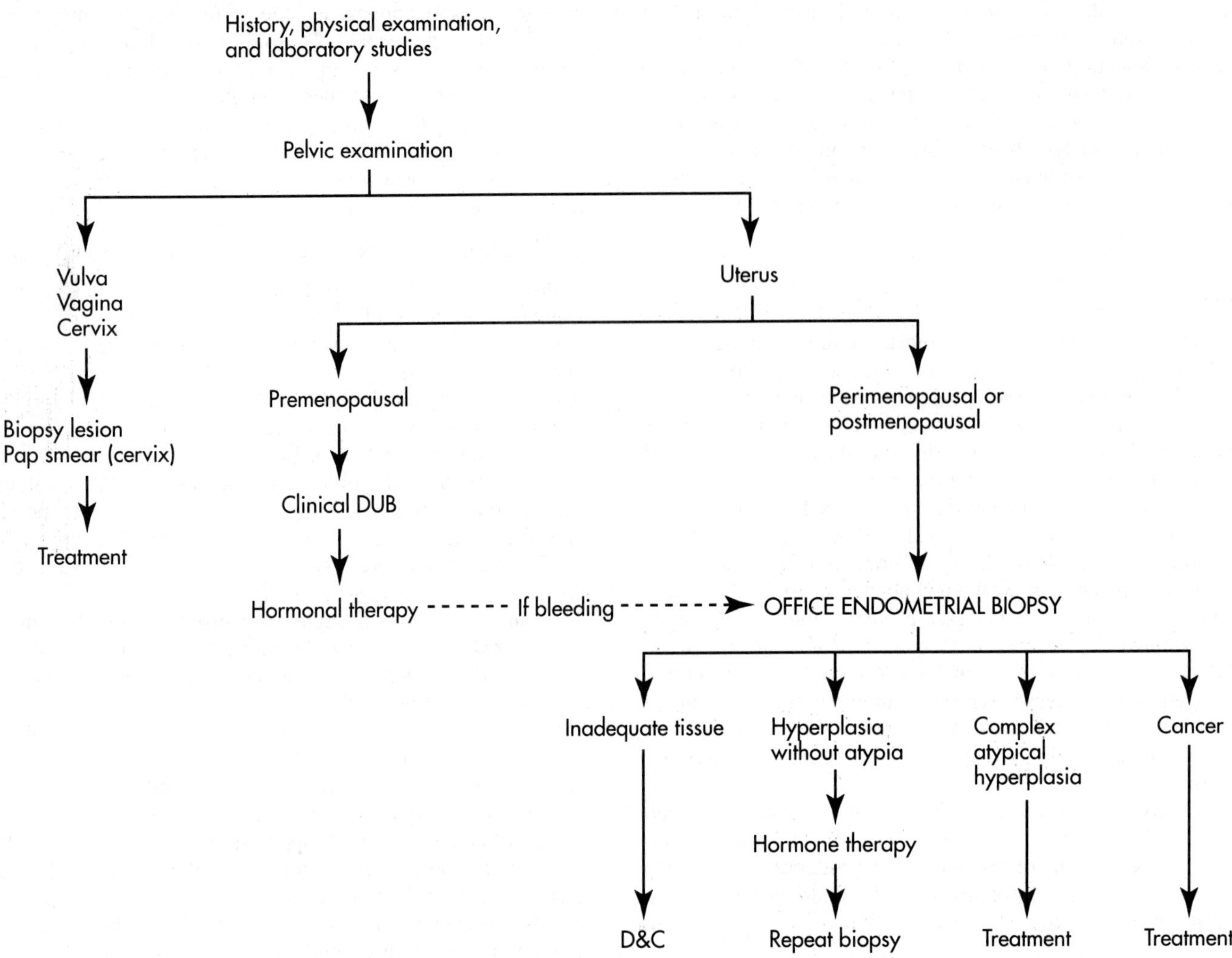

Fig. 44-4. Algorithm for the workup of abnormal vaginal bleeding.

> **Box 44-2. Endometrial Sampling**
>
> **Indications**
>
> Dysfunctional uterine bleeding
> Postmenopausal bleeding
> Unanticipated bleeding on hormonal replacement therapy
> Tamoxifen therapy
> Abnormal endometrial cytology
> Normal endometrial cytology in a postmenopausal woman
> Follow-up of medical therapy for endometrial hyperplasia
> Evaluation of infertility
>
> **Contraindications**
>
> Pregnancy
> Acute pelvic inflammatory disease
> Coagulopathy
> Cervical stenosis

Hysteroscopy provides a direct visualization of the endometrial cavity. Although hysteroscopy can consistently identify endometrial polyps and submucosal fibroids better than an endometrial biopsy, the necessity of this approach to workup abnormal uterine bleeding in all patients has not been documented. However, in a woman who has persistent uterine bleeding and who has undergone a D&C that is negative for a malignancy, or in a woman who has failed to respond to medical therapy for a hyperplastic state, a hysteroscopic evaluation may help identify the source of the problem.

Management of Patient with Endometrial Cancer

Endometrial cancer is treated surgically with total abdominal hysterectomy and bilateral salpingo-oophorectomy, pelvic cytology, and pelvic and paraaortic nodal samplings. Use of adjuvant radiation therapy to the vaginal apex, pelvic external beam radiation therapy, or a combination of both depends on the final pathologic staging.

About 90% of endometrial carcinomas are adenocarcinomas; the degree of histologic differentiation of endometrial cancer is an important prognostic feature; well-differentiated (grade 1) types have a significantly better prognosis than poorly differentiated types (grade 3). Deep myometrial tumor invasion or the presence of tumor outside the uterus, including lymph node metastases, and older age at diagnosis are poor prognostic factors. For example, 5-year survival rates approach 97% in women less than age 60 with low-grade histologic lesions confined to the uterus. In contrast, 5-year survival rates may be as low as 7.5% in older patients with undifferentiated carcinomas, or with aggressive variants including clear cell, papillary serous, and adenosquamous carcinoma.

A significant decrease in vaginal apex recurrence has been documented with the use of radiation therapy. Pelvic external beam radiation therapy decreases pelvic recurrence in those who are at risk (e.g., deep myometrial invasion, positive lymph nodes, or endocervical involvement). Patients who are unacceptable anesthetic risks or refuse surgery may be treated with radiation therapy alone. Survival rates, however, are lower than surgery and radiation therapy combined.

The management of advanced disease spread outside the pelvis is individualized. Radiation therapy often is used to palliate symptoms. Cytotoxic chemotherapy in patients with metastatic disease has response rates of 15% to 35%. Unfortunately, complete responses are uncommon and disease-free intervals are short, although occasional patients with low-grade tumors have prolonged responses.

Special Issues

Hormonal Replacement Therapy and Endometrial Sampling. Approximately one third of postmenopausal women in the United States use some type of hormone replacement. Because the risk of endometrial hyperplasia and/or endometrial cancer is increased in women receiving unopposed estrogen replacement therapy, it is recommended that women receive both estrogen and progestin (given sequentially or low-dose continuously) if the uterus is present. Physicians often sample the endometrium before initiating hormonal therapy. In asymptomatic, postmenopausal women, the prevalence rate for abnormal endometrial findings (hyperplasia or cancer) is approximately 5%. The need for a baseline biopsy depends on the patient's pattern of bleeding. If she has been amenorrheic for several months, a baseline biopsy may be optional.

In postmenopausal women receiving daily estrogen and at least 12 days of progestins (medroxyprogesterone [Provera], 10 mg) monthly, withdrawal bleeding on day 11 or later after the addition of progestins is associated with a predominantly secretory endometrium or lack of endometrial tissue, and routine sampling is not necessary. Endometrial sampling is recommended for those women whose bleeding occurs earlier than day 11.[11] Many women cannot tolerate the side effects that occur with this dose of Provera and receive lower doses for a shorter duration. In these circumstances, the subsequent bleeding pattern may not reliably correlate with endometrial histology, and routine sampling on a yearly basis is reasonable. TVS has been recommended as an alternative or adjunct to endometrial biopsy in screening asymptomatic women on hormonal replacement therapy (HRT). However, a recent study showed that although TVS is sensitive for detection of endometrial hyperplasia (in particular simple hyperplasia in women on unopposed estrogen), an increase in endometrial stripe does not correlate with an increase in severity of disease, and TVS appears to have poor positive predictive value overall for detecting endometrial abnormalities.[9] In general, a low cut-off of <5 mm for the endometrial stripe is associated with a high negative predictive value, whereas a high cut-off of >10 mm can signal endometrial pathology.

Continuous low-dose estrogen and progestin therapy frequently results in endometrial atrophy and amenorrhea after 3 to 6 months, and routine endometrial sampling is not recommended for amenorrheic women. Any unanticipated or heavy bleeding, however, signals the need for endometrial sampling. Tamoxifen treatment of breast cancer leads to a 2.3-fold increased risk for endometrial cancer due to its selective estrogenic agonistic effects.[13] The optimal screening method for endocarcinoma for patients on tamoxifen has not been defined; the TVS may be falsely positive using conventional endometrial stripe cut-offs defined for postmenopausal women, a result of the association of tamoxifen with endometrial polyps.

Estrogen Replacement Therapy After Successful Endometrial Cancer Treatment. Prospective, randomized studies to guide recommendations for estrogen replacement therapy (ERT) in women with a history of endometrial cancer are not available. Estrogens are contraindicated in those with a hormonally sensitive cancer. The American College of Obstetrics and Gynecology (ACOG) recommended that in selected women with a history of endometrial cancer, estrogens could be used for the usual indications. Eligible women should be completely informed about alternatives and the potential risks involved. If the patient is truly free of cancer, ERT should not increase the likelihood of recurrent disease. On the other hand, estrogen can be a potential mitogen for patients whose cancer cells are viable but quiescent after treatment. In general, it would be prudent to wait approximately 3 years after treatment before considering ERT for women who would benefit. Studies of the safety of newly designed selective estrogen receptor modulators, such as raloxifene, on the endometrium are ongoing. Although the endometrial thickness of normal postmenopausal women does not appear to be increased by raloxifene on TVS, studies of the safety of these drugs in patients with endometrial cancer have not been performed.[4]

OVARIAN CANCER

Epidemiology

Epithelial ovarian cancer accounts for 90% of all ovarian cancers and is responsible for more deaths than all other gynecologic cancers combined (Fig. 44-2). It is a disease of industrialized nations, and environmental and dietary factors likely play a role. The lifetime risk in the general population for the development of epithelial ovarian cancer is 1 in 70 (1.4%). Genetic factors are an important risk factor; the lifetime risk increases to 39% in the presence of two first-degree relatives with ovarian cancer. These familial ovarian cancer patients constitute a recognized high-risk group, which accounts for approximately 5% of all cases. Mutations in the BrCA1 or BrCA2 gene have been found to account for the majority of familial ovarian cancer cases, with BrCA2 having a lower penetrance for ovarian cancer than BrCA1. Other risk factors, such as nulliparity, infertility, and prior history of breast cancer, increase the lifetime risk to approximately 2%.

Pathophysiology

Whether epithelial ovarian cancer arises from cells derived from the ovarian surface epithelium and/or the peritoneal mesothelium is unclear; however, more than 70% of women present with tumor involving multiple peritoneal surfaces, suggesting the presence of metachronous peritoneal tumors. In particular, primary peritoneal carcinoma appears to be one of the familial ovarian cancer phenotypes.

The association of ovarian cancer with incessant ovulation and elevated circulating gonadotropins points to an ovarian origin. Ovulation results in disruption of the ovarian surface, which, on repair by growth and invasion of the ovarian surface epithelium, results in the formation of inclusion cysts. The observed protective effect of OCPs on ovarian cancer risk (RR = 0.64 [CI 0.57-0.83]) and the reduced risk in multiparous women may be due to suppression of ovulation and to the decreased potential for DNA mutations (and thus initiation of neoplasia) that arise during repair of the surface of the ovulating ovary.[3] The observed protective effect of tubal ligation (RR = 0.64 [CI 0.42-0.96]) may be due to disruption of ovarian circulation with local imbalance of gonadotropins.[3]

Ovarian Cancer Screening

Although it has been suggested that early detection by screening may improve the prognosis for ovarian cancer, the benefits of screening in the general population have not been established. Studies are underway to assess the efficacy of screening in high-risk women, but clear benefits to date have not been shown even in this population.

TVS is used to detect early morphologic changes associated with ovarian cancer. The ultrasonographic characteristics of an ovarian mass that are reported to correlate with malignancy include overall increased size or wall thickness, or the presence of intracystic papillary formations, septation, or solid areas. In a recent study, TVS had sensitivities of 87.5% and 82.6% for premenopausal and postmenopausal patients for detection of ovarian cancer among women undergoing surgery for an adnexal mass, while specificity was 75.4% and 64.7%, respectively.[7] In populations prospectively screened for ovarian cancer by TVS, low specificity and poor positive predictive values have precluded a clear benefit. The addition of color Doppler flow studies has not had an impact on either the ability to discriminate between benign and malignant pelvic masses or the accuracy of screening patients for ovarian cancer.

CA-125 is a widely used serum tumor marker that is valuable in detecting small tumor burdens in patients with a known history of ovarian cancer. Although more than 80% of women with clinically apparent ovarian cancer have an elevated CA-125, the CA-125 is elevated in only 50% of women with stage I disease (disease confined to the ovary).[5] In addition, 0.5% to 1% of normal women, as well as those with a variety of physiologic conditions, including endometriosis, salpingitis, pregnancy, fibroids, and menstruation, have an elevated level. The calculated positive predictive value for the detection of ovarian cancer by this modality alone is only 2.3%. Thus isolated CA-125 screening in the general population is not appropriate.

Combined use of CA-125 and TVS has increased the specificity for detection of ovarian cancer in postmenopausal women; however, guidelines for screening premenopausal women at high risk are not yet available. Because women with a family history of ovarian cancer develop the disease at a younger average age than those with the sporadic form (49 vs. 59 years) and those with the Lynch II syndrome (a rare hereditary disorder in which family members are at increased risk for endometrial, colon, and ovarian cancer) develop disease at an average age of 45 years, it would seem prudent to start screening family members at risk in their reproductive years. It has been suggested that patients with known mutations in BrCA1 or BrCA2 commence CA-125 and TVS screening every 6 to 12 months starting at age 25 to 35, although data proving benefit of screening in high-risk families are lacking.[3] OCP usage may be beneficial in these high-risk patients, and consideration given to prophylactic oophorectomy after completion of childbearing. Unfortunately, prophylactic oophorectomy does not protect against primary peritoneal carcinoma.

Evaluation of Patient With an Adnexal Mass

The symptoms of an adnexal mass depend on patient age. Since most neoplasms in the premenarchal age group are benign or malignant germ cell tumors, pain from a rapidly growing cyst or neoplasm or adnexal torsion is the most common presenting symptom. Frequently, the preoperative diagnosis is appendicitis. The diagnosis of an adnexal mass is usually made by palpation of an abdominal mass or by imaging studies rather than by pelvic examination.

Most adnexal masses are diagnosed in women of reproductive age and are usually benign. They are found frequently on routine pelvic examination, as well as during the workup of a specific symptom. The presentation includes acute abdominal/pelvic pain or chronic discomfort, fever, abnormal menses, dysmenorrhea, symptoms of pregnancy, change in bowel or urinary habits, or back pain. The majority of early ovarian cancers are asymptomatic. The most common symptom of advanced ovarian cancer is vague abdominal swelling or discomfort. Findings of bilaterality, firmness, fixation, nodularity, and lack of tenderness on pelvic examination suggest a malignant process, as does the concomitant presence of ascites or cul-de-sac nodules. In the postmenopausal patient, any pelvic mass (other than known stable fibroids) is cause for concern and dictates further workup.

Differential Diagnosis of an Adnexal Mass

The adnexa consist of the ovaries, fallopian tubes, and embryologic remnants in the broad ligament. Masses that are palpated or imaged in this area, however, may arise from many other organs (Table 44-3). The differential diagnosis of an adnexal mass varies considerably with age.

Fibroids, the most common uterine neoplasm, are usually clearly related to the body of the uterus. However, they may be located in the broad ligament or attached to the uterus by a thin stalk and feel like an adnexal mass. They are generally solid, but may become partially cystic with degeneration, infarction, or torsion. In the United States, at least 10% of Caucasian and 30% to 40% of African-American women over the age of 35 have fibroids. These estrogen-dependent neoplasms should shrink in the absence of hormonal replacement after the menopause. Sarcomatous elements are associated with fibroids only 0.1% of the time. Thus fibroids should be considered benign unless they are solitary and rapidly growing.

Functional ovarian cysts are the most common cause of ovarian enlargement in the reproductive age group and include both follicular and corpus luteum cysts, theca-lutein cysts, pregnancy luteomas, sclerocystic ovaries, and endometriotic cysts. These cysts are usually asymptomatic and are a result of normal ovarian activity. They can cause pain and abnormal menses. Some will respond to OCP suppression; others will regress without intervention.

Endometriosis results from implantation of endometrial glands and stroma outside the endometrial cavity. The diagnosis is most common in Caucasian and infertile women aged 35 to 45 years. The most common presenting symptom is pelvic pain. When the ectopic location of the implants

Table 44-3. Differential Diagnosis of an Adnexal Mass

Site	Mass
Ovary	Functional cyst
	Benign neoplasm
	Malignant neoplasm
	Endometriosis
Fallopian tube	Tuboovarian abscess
	Hydrosalpinx
	Paratubal cyst
	Ectopic pregnancy
	Benign neoplasm (rare)
	Malignant neoplasm
Uterus	Fibroid (pedunculated, interligamentous)
Gastrointestinal tract	Bowel loops with feces
	Diverticular disease
	Appendicitis
	Inflammatory bowel disease
	Benign small bowel neoplasm (leiomyoma)
	Colon cancer
Urinary tract	Distended bladder
	Pelvic kidney
	Urachal cyst
Retroperitoneum	Benign neoplasm (myxoid tumor)
	Sarcoma, lymphoma, or teratoma
	Abdominal wall hematoma or abscess

includes the uterosacral ligaments, nodularity and tenderness can be found on rectovaginal examination.

Tuboovarian abscess can occur with prior or concomitant pelvic inflammatory disease. Symptoms of acute pelvic infection such as pelvic pain, fever, vaginal discharge, and abnormal bleeding, along with findings of an exquisitely tender pelvic mass, suggest this diagnosis. These findings may be absent with a chronic tuboovarian abscess. Shrinkage and resolution of the mass with intense antibiotic treatment confirm the clinical impression.

The most common ovarian neoplasms are benign: the serous and mucinous cystadenomas and the dermoids (mature cystic teratomas). They are usually asymptomatic, as are early-stage epithelial ovarian cancers. In contrast to functional cysts, these neoplasms do not regress with observation or use of OCP suppression. Patients with advanced epithelial ovarian cancers usually present with abdominal swelling or bloating, generalized abdominal discomfort, dyspepsia and early satiety, lack of appetite, malaise, urinary frequency, and weight change (either gain or loss). A fixed nodular pelvic mass may be found on pelvic examination. Diffuse peritoneal implants are readily seen on ultrasound and almost always involve the omentum, which becomes enlarged and firm and presents as a large ballotable mass (omental cake). Ovarian cancer should be considered foremost in women with unexplained ascites, with or without confirmation of a pelvic mass.

Workup of Patient with an Adnexal Mass

The workup depends on patient age, clinical presentation, and physical findings. Directed blood work includes a complete blood count (CBC) and erythrocyte sedimentation rate (ESR) for an inflammatory process, CA-125 for a malignancy, and a serum pregnancy test if indicated. Pelvic ultrasound should be used as the screening imaging modality. Magnetic resonance imaging (MRI) scans can help differentiate fibroids or endometriosis from ovarian neoplasms or simple functional cysts but are very expensive.

The use of laparoscopy for diagnosis and for surgical extirpation of pelvic masses has increased; however, strict criteria for safety and appropriateness have not been developed, especially if malignancy is suspected.

If the presentation, physical examination, and initial imaging studies suggest an ovarian neoplasm, a CT scan is used to evaluate the retroperitoneum, urologic structures, rectum, pancreas, and liver. This information is important in determining treatment approach and prognosis. Paracentesis is not indicated in the usual workup of women with suspected ovarian cancer because of the risk of rupture of a large encapsulated early-stage neoplasm.

Management of Patient with Ovarian Cancer

Ovarian cancer is staged surgically through a midline abdominal incision. Ascites or washings are taken for cytologic analysis. A thorough exploration of the entire peritoneal cavity is undertaken with removal of the primary neoplasm and resection of all metastases. In addition, a generous sampling of the omentum, retroperitoneal lymph nodes, and peritoneal and diaphragmatic surfaces is performed, even if these structures appear normal. With a few exceptions in a reproductive-aged woman who wishes to preserve childbearing potential, the procedure includes removal of the contralateral ovary and hysterectomy. If conservative surgery is planned, complete staging includes a biopsy of the normal contralateral ovary, because some neoplasms, such as serous tumors, are frequently bilateral.

The prognosis of invasive epithelial ovarian cancer is dismal and relates to stage and residual disease after completion of initial debulking surgery. The 5-year survival of stage III and IV disease (extrapelvic spread) is 18%; unfortunately, 70% of patients have extrapelvic spread.[5] They usually die from progressive inanition resulting from small bowel entrapment by tumor. The prognosis of early-stage invasive ovarian cancers, as well as the borderline malignant tumors of all stages, is significantly better. The prognosis of germ cell tumors, if treated promptly with aggressive chemotherapy in a cancer referral center, is excellent. Similarly, sex-cord stromal tumors, which usually present when confined to a single ovary, are responsive to chemotherapy.

The primary treatment of epithelial ovarian cancer is aggressive surgical tumor debulking. Treatment of remaining small or microscopic tumor burden depends on the sensitivity of these tumors to platinum-based combination chemotherapy or, in selected cases, to whole abdominal radiation therapy. Currently, the usual first-line treatment is a platinum compound and paclitaxel. Although the original response to chemotherapy is 80%, the majority of patients relapse and go on to receive multiple regimens, which inevitably fail.

Support for terminal care in the community with the establishment of effective hospice networks and team approaches, including home nursing services, is necessary. Moreover, the placement of a percutaneous gastrostomy for palliation of refractory nausea and vomiting and the use of transdermal approaches and continuous infusion pumps for the administration of narcotics for effective pain control have helped improve care.

VULVAR DISEASE

Differential Diagnosis of Vulvar Pruritus

Vulvar and perineal pruritus are common symptoms in women. It is important to remember that pruritus is a symptom, not a disease, and the underlying cause must be determined to treat it effectively.

Pruritus of the vulva may be caused by epithelial changes in the vulvar skin or by irritation of the nerve endings that richly supply the genital area. The primary causes of the condition include nonneoplastic epithelial diseases (squamous cell hyperplasia or lichen sclerosus), vulvar intraepithelial neoplasms (VIN), candidiasis, and dermatologic conditions (e.g., psoriasis, seborrheic or contact dermatitis).

Techniques of Evaluation

Careful inspection of the vulva and vagina, using either a magnifying glass or colposcope, followed by an office biopsy, is the best method to establish a specific diagnosis. The glabrous skin must also be inspected because many of the dermatoses (e.g., psoriasis or lichen planus) that affect the vulva also affect this area. The evaluation for possible systemic causes, such as diabetes mellitus in a woman with recurrent vulvar candidiasis, must be considered.

Management of Nonneoplastic Epithelial Diseases

The nonneoplastic epithelial diseases (squamous cell hyperplasia or lichen sclerosus) are a benign set of conditions with similar symptoms and signs. The patient usually complains of severe vulvar pruritus, and on physical examination the vulva has irregular patches of thinned or thickened skin. The skin color is white, red, or darker gray and may be a combination of these. In addition, the lesion may be multiple or single and raised or flat. The progression of these lesions to malignancy is rare. Treatment is usually with very high–potency topical corticosteroids (e.g., clobetasol propionate) for up to 4 weeks, followed by maintenance with a lower potency corticosteroid given less frequently.

VIN and Vulvar Cancer

VIN is increasing in incidence, especially in younger women, and may be HPV-related. The presenting symptom is usually pruritus of varying intensity. The multicentric lesions are flat, with mild to moderate changes in pigmentation; 20% to 40% of patients with VIN have had or will have similar lesions at other sites of the anogenital tract. Multiple condylomata may be associated with VIN in some cases. Because the invasive potential of VIN has not been established, conservative management is appropriate. Wide, local excision of the specific areas involved is usually performed. For extensive and multifocal lesions, a partial skinning vulvectomy may be necessary. Laser ablation or ultrasonic surgical aspiration may also be used. The use of topical chemotherapy with 5% 5-fluorouracil cream can produce responses in 50% of patients, but is associated with significant morbidity due to local irritation. Unfortunately, because the area at risk is extensive and cannot be treated adequately with any of these modalities, recurrences are frequent.

Vulvar cancer is uncommon and accounts for only 1% to 5% of all female cancers. Over 75% of all patients with this disease are age 55 or older. The etiology remains unknown, but the association of squamous cell cancer of the vulva with other premalignant neoplasms of the anogenital mucosa suggests a role for HPV.

Invasive squamous cell cancer accounts for 85% to 90% of vulvar malignancies and usually presents as a vulvar mass causing discomfort after a long history of vulvar pruritus. On gross examination the lesion is raised, fleshy, ulcerative, or warty; multiple sites are involved in 5% of cases. The importance of a biopsy with appropriate early referral for surgery must be stressed. The disease spreads through lymphatic pathways; hence the inguinal nodes should be palpated. Radical surgery is the treatment of choice and includes removal of the primary lesion with adequate margins. A unilateral or bilateral inguinal lymphadenectomy is indicated depending on the location and size of the primary lesion. Small lesions with minimal stromal invasion have led to the use of more conservative surgical approaches, but these must be highly individualized.

GESTATIONAL TROPHOBLASTIC NEOPLASIA

Gestational trophoblastic disease is a rare gynecologic malignancy that may present after a normal, ectopic, or molar pregnancy or a miscarriage. Any reproductive-aged woman with abnormal vaginal bleeding, even without a recognized antecedent pregnancy, should be considered a candidate for this entity. A sensitive tumor marker produced by the tumor, human chorionic gonadotropin (hCG), correlates with the number of viable cells present and can be measured simply by obtaining a sensitive serum pregnancy test. The malignancy is exquisitely sensitive to chemotherapeutic regimens and is curable if recognized promptly, even when metastatic. These rare tumors should be treated by a gynecologic oncologist.

REFERENCES

1. American Cancer Society: Cancer statistics 1998, *CA Cancer J Clin* 48(1):6, 1998.
2. Chambers JT, Chambers SK: Endometrial sampling: When? Where? Why? With what? *Clin Obstet Gynecol* 35(1):28, 1992.
3. Chen L-M, Karlan BY: Early detection and risk reduction for familial gynecologic cancers, *Clin Obstet Gynecol* 41(1):200-214, 1998.
4. Delmas PD, Bjarnason NH, Mitlak BH, et al: Effects of raloxifene on bone mineral density, serum cholesterol concentrations, and uterine endometrium in postmenopausal women, *N Engl J Med* 337(23):1641-1647, 1997.
5. Hoskins WJ, Perez CA, Young RC, editors: *Principles and practice of gynecologic oncology,* ed 2, Philadelphia, 1997, Lippincott-Raven.
6. Kurman RJ, Kaminski PF, Norris HJ: The behavior of endometrial hyperplasia: a long-term study of "untreated" hyperplasia in 170 patients, *Cancer* 56:403, 1985.
7. Kusnetzoff D, Gnochi D, Damonte C, et al: Differential diagnosis of pelvic masses: usefulness of CA125, transvaginal sonography, and echo-Doppler, *Int J Gynecol Cancer* 8:315-321, 1998.
8. Laara E, Day NE, Hakama M: Trends in mortality from cervical cancer in the Nordic countries: association with organized screening programs, *Lancet* 1247-1249, 1987.
9. Langer RD, Pierce JJ, O'Hanlan KA, et al: Transvaginal ultrasonography compared with endometrial biopsy for the detection of endometrial disease, *N Engl J Med* 337(25):1792-1839, 1997.
10. Mitchell MF, Tortolero-Luna G, Cook E, et al: A randomized clinical trial of cryotherapy, laser vaporization, and loop electrosurgical excision for treatment of squamous intraepithelial lesions of the cervix, *Obstet Gynecol* 92(5):737-744, 1998.

10a. Morris M, Eifel PJ, Lu J, et al: Pelvic radiation with concurrent chemotherapy compared with pelvic and para-aortic radiation for

high-risk cervical cancer, *New Engl J Med* 340(15)1137-1143, 1999.
11. Padwick M, Prysc-Davies J, Whitehead M: A simple method for determining the optimal dosage of progestin in postmenopausal women receiving estrogens, *N Engl J Med* 315(15):930, 1986.
12. Rubin SC, Hoskin NJ, editors: *Cervical cancer and preinvasive neoplasia,* Philadelphia, 1996, Lippincott-Raven.
13. van Leeuwen FE, Benraadt J, Coebergh JWW, et al: Risk of endometrial cancer after tamoxifen treatment of breast cancer, *Lancet* 343:448-452, 1994.

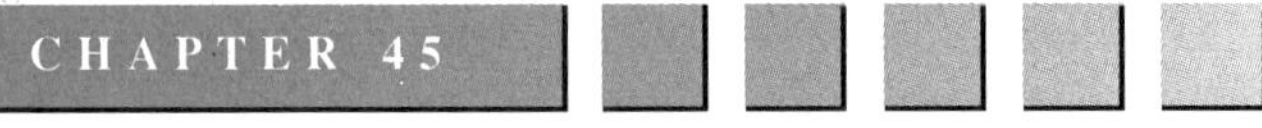

CHAPTER 45

Metabolic Bone Disease

Michael F. Holick

Metabolic bone disease is a general term that includes diversity of bone diseases caused by a metabolic abnormality or pathology, such as renal failure, liver disease, endocrinopathies, vitamin D deficiency, estrogen deficiency, and Paget's disease. This chapter discusses osteoporosis, which affects four times as many women as men, and Paget's disease (see Chapter 100).[7]

OSTEOPOROSIS

Osteoporosis is the most common metabolic bone disease and afflicts approximately 20 million women and 5 million men in the United States. The simplest definition of osteoporosis is porotic bone or holes in the bone (Fig. 45-1). This is an important distinction because porosity of bone does not cause bone pain. The consequence of osteoporosis (i.e., decrease in both bone matrix and bone mineral content), however, leads to compromised bone structure and strength, increasing the risk of fracture. Skeletal fracture in turn leads to acute and chronic bone and muscle pain.

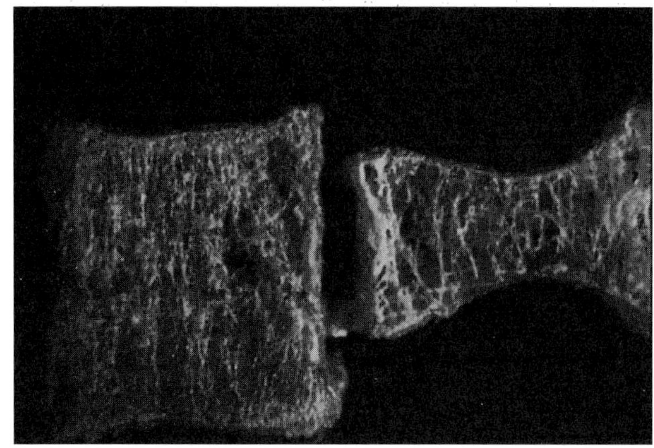

Fig. 45-1. Vertebral bodies from young woman *(left)* and elderly osteoporotic woman *(right)*. Note marked loss of horizontal and vertical struts (trabeculae), wide spaces (holes), and severe compression of vertebral body on right.

Epidemiology and Risk Factors

Classically, osteoporosis is associated with a thin, white female who has been menopausal for 10 to 15 years. Both men and women of all races, however, are at risk of developing osteoporosis in their lifetime. The prevalence of osteoporosis increases progressively with age; by age 80, an estimated 25% of women and 15% of men have had a hip fracture. Although osteoporosis is often considered a benign disease of little consequence, osteoporotic fractures cause chronic debilitating pain, diminished quality of life, and even death. About 1.5 million skeletal fractures and 250,000 hip fractures occur annually because of this disease. Of patients with a hip fracture, 10% to 15% die within the first year from complications, 50% never regain their previous quality of life, and many require chronic care in a nursing home. Approximately $8 billion is spent annually for the acute care of patients with hip fractures. As the U.S. population grows older, by 2020 an estimated $120 billion dollars a year will be spent for the acute and chronic care of these patients.[3]

Risk factors for osteoporosis include early age of onset for menopause, family history, history of amenorrhea or oligomenorrhea during the second and third decades, and poor lifetime intake of calcium (Box 45-1). Genetically, blacks have "stronger" bones (higher bone mineral density), but they are still at risk for osteoporosis because of poor calcium nutrition, often from lactase deficiency. Blacks also have decreased ability to make vitamin D_3 in their skin because of increased skin melanin, which leads to chronic vitamin D deficiency and secondary hyperparathyroidism.[1]

Box 45-1. Risk Factors for Development of Osteoporosis

Caucasian or Asian heritage
Early menopause (natural or surgical)
Amenorrhea or oligomenorrhea in second and third decades
Thin body habitus
Family history
Inadequate lifelong calcium intake (<800 mg/day)
Chronic vitamin D deficiency
Hypogonadism
Cigarette smoking
Premature graying (50% of hair turns gray before age 40)
Steroid therapy
Excessive thyroid hormone replacement
Immobilization

Pathophysiology

Causes of osteoporosis include loss of ovarian function, calcium and vitamin D deficiency, and aging (Box 45-2). Osteoporosis is classified as two types: *type I* is caused by estrogen deficiency after menopause or ovariectomy (oophorectomy), and *type II* is associated with aging. These designations, however, are not particularly helpful in either diagnosis or treatment because osteoporosis is a multifactorial disease.[10]

In women, estrogen plays an essential role in the bone-remodeling process. Osteoblasts, which lay down the collagen matrix for bone mineralization, have receptors for estrogen. Estrogen regulates bone mineralization and demineralization by coupling osteoblastic with osteoclastic activity. Without estrogen, this process uncouples, leading to de-

Box 45-2. Causes of Osteoporosis and Osteopenia

Common

Estrogen deficiency
Testosterone deficiency
Vitamin D deficiency
Calcium deficiency
Thyrotoxicosis (natural or TSH-suppressive doses of thyroxine)
Chronic glucocorticoid use
Hyperadrenocorticism (Cushing's syndrome)
Immobilization
Hyperparathyroidism

Less Common

Malabsorption
Vitamin C deficiency (scurvy)
Chronic heparin administration
Systemic mastocytosis
Adult hypophosphatasia
Chronic renal failure
Primary biliary cirrhosis
Cancer
Chronic obstructive lung disease
Rheumatoid arthritis

Inherited

Osteogenesis imperfecta
Ehlers-Danlos syndrome
Marfan syndrome
Homocystinuria

TSH, Thyroid-stimulating hormone.

creased osteoblastic function and increased osteoclastic destruction of both the matrix and the mineral. This uncoupling can lead to rapid bone loss. As women enter menopause, they can lose 2% to 3% of their bone mass each year. This is usually unrelenting and continues for at least a decade, with up to a 30% to 50% reduction in skeletal density. Both men and women have an age-related decrease in bone of approximately ½% to 1% a year after age 50 years. Although the exact cause is unknown, this loss may result from the kidney's inability to produce an adequate amount of activated vitamin D_3 (1,25-dihydroxyvitamin D_3, [1,25(OH_2)D_3]), resulting in a decrease in intestinal calcium absorption. Steroids also can decrease the efficiency of intestinal calcium absorption and alter the bone-remodeling process, causing rapid loss of bone mineral content even in children and young adults.

Chronic calcium and vitamin D deficiency leads to an increase in serum levels of parathyroid hormone (PTH), which increases the mobilization of calcium stores from the bone, leading to or exacerbating osteoporosis. In addition, vitamin D deficiency causes a mineralization defect of the bone matrix *(osteomalacia)*, resulting in decreased bone mineral content and increased risk of fracture. *Primary hyperparathyroidism*, which affects approximately 0.1% of the adult U.S. population, can lead to osteoporosis.[6] Because hyperparathyroid disease enhances cortical bone loss more than trabecular bone loss, these patients are at increased risk of wrist and hip fractures.

Patient History

Although women are more likely to develop osteoporosis at an earlier age than men, it is important to document lifetime intake of calcium for both men and women. A low intake of calcium during the formative teenage and young adult years results in a decrease in attainable peak bone mass, which occurs between ages 20 and 30. An estimated 50% of the calcium in an adult skeleton is deposited during the formative ages of 13 to 17 years. To evaluate vitamin D status, the physician should ask about multivitamin use, sun exposure, and sunscreen use. A sunscreen with a sun protection factor (SPF) of 15 may reduce the cutaneous production of vitamin D_3 by more than 95%.[5] Vitamin D_3 production is greatly reduced or halted in the winter at latitudes above Washington, D.C. A family history of osteoporosis, especially maternal grandmother, mother, and sister(s); heavy alcohol use; cigarette smoking; early menopause; and premature graying (i.e., 50% of hair has turned gray by age 40) are associated with increased risk of osteoporosis. Steroid treatment with doses greater than 5 mg of prednisone or 25 mg of hydrocortisone daily for only 3 to 6 months contributes to significant bone loss in some patients. Prolonged hyperthyroidism or suppressive doses of thyroxine for treating goiter or suppressing recurrence of thyroid cancer can increase bone turnover, leading to osteoporosis.[7] Severe chronic liver disease and chronic renal failure can cause severe metabolic bone disease, which contains a component of osteoporosis. Prolonged anticoagulant therapy with heparin is associated with increasing risk of osteoporosis. Institutionalized patients taking multiple antiseizure medications are at risk for vitamin D deficiency, osteomalacia, and osteoporosis.

A useful tool to evaluate for osteoporosis is to ask patients how tall they are (verified by measuring their height) and how tall they were as a young adult. A loss of an inch or more in height suggests the possibility of one or more spinal fractures caused by osteoporosis. Increased flexibility of joints (double jointed) or increased skin elasticity may be consistent with genetic disorders of collagen cross-linking, such as osteogenesis imperfecta and Ehlers-Danlos syndrome, which are associated with a decrease in bone mineral content. Regional bone pain over the rib cage or spine may be caused by a new fracture. Isolated or more generalized, aching bone pain may be caused by osteomalacia. Osteoporosis does not cause bone pain unless there is an acute fracture.

Patient Evaluation

A careful measurement of a patient's height could be the first indication of osteoporosis. The body habitus is also helpful because multiple compression fractures of the spine result in the classic hunched-over appearance (dowager's hump) (Fig. 45-2). Exophthalmos may be an indicator of hyperthyroidism or previous Graves' disease. Blue sclera is a classic finding in patients with osteogenesis imperfecta. An increase in skin elasticity or a doughy skin texture and increased flexibility of finger joints are evidence of a collagen–cross-linking genetic disease. Warm, velvety, moist skin, brisk reflexes, or tachycardia are consistent with hyperthyroidism. Thin, transparent, frail skin is often caused by chronic estrogen deficiency or chronic topical or oral steroid use. Black and blue marks, centripetal obesity, and proximal muscle wasting and weakness are consistent with either excess exogenous or endogenous steroids. For males a testicular examination to rule out hypogonadism is warranted.

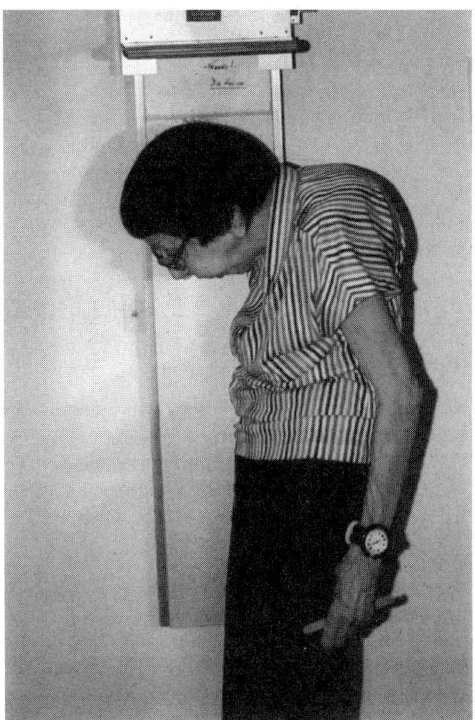

Fig. 45-2. Elderly woman next to stadiometer used to measure her height accurately. She has severe osteoporosis with multiple vertebral compression fractures and classic dowager's hump.

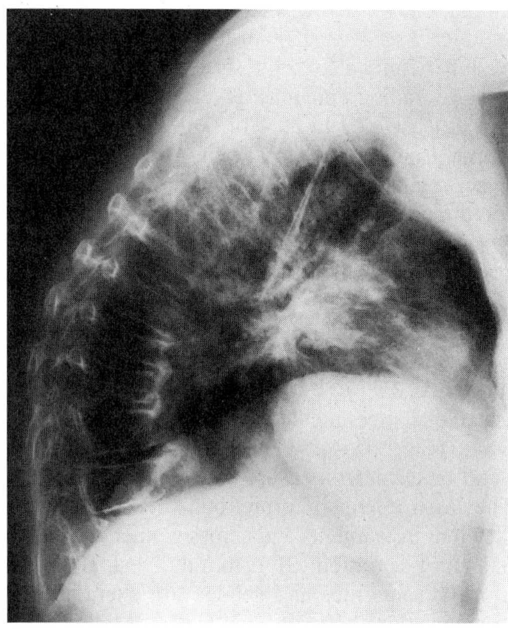

Fig. 45-3. Lateral radiograph of 81-year-old female with lower back pain radiating down left leg to knee. Note severe osteopenia of thoracic and lumbar vertebral bodies with multiple wedge compression fractures. Marked osteopenia of trabecular bone with preservation of rim of cortical bone gives rise to classic fish-mouth appearance between two vertebral bodies, evidence of trabecular collapse and compression fractures.

Lower back pain with sciatic symptoms or a positive straight-leg test exacerbating sciatic symptoms may be consistent with lumbar and sacral spinal fractures and nerve compression (Fig. 45-3). Palpation of the vertebral bodies eliciting point tenderness may indicate a recent compression fracture, whereas point tenderness on the rib cage may be a rib fracture. Palpation with mild thumb pressure on the upper sternum or on periosteum of the radius or tibia that causes pain may indicate osteomalacia.

Goals. The major goals of the initial evaluation are to (1) document the patient's present height (see Fig. 45-2); (2) rule out endocrinopathies, including hyperthyroidism, hypogonadism, and hypercortisolism, or a genetic defect in collagen cross-linking; and (3) determine if bone pain is associated with osteomalacia.

Assessing Individual Risk. Assessment of individual risk is necessary to optimize treatment decisions. For example, a white female with a strong family history of osteoporosis should consider hormonal replacement therapy (HRT) at the first signs of menopause. A premenopausal black woman who is genetically programmed to have a higher bone mineral density (BMD) would benefit from counseling to increase her calcium and vitamin D intake. Patients with asthma, collagen vascular disease, or an autoimmune disorder who will receive long-term steroid therapy should increase their calcium and vitamin D intake and may receive an antiresorptive agent (e.g., bisphosphonate).[4]

The increased risk of skeletal fractures with decreased BMD must be evaluated in relation to the patient's gender, age, and other considerations. For example, a 30-year-old white female in her childbearing years who has a low BMD based on screening densitometry should not necessarily receive a bone-active drug such as a bisphosphonate. The half-life of these drugs in the skeleton is about ½ year. The physician should determine whether the patient has low bone mass because of genetics, environmental factors, premature graying, anorexia, or ovarian dysfunction in her second or third decade of life. Measurement of a urine bone resorption marker helps identify increased bone resorption. A repeat BMD test in 1 year may also be helpful. No significant change in 1 to 2 years indicates that the patient's low BMD, from whatever cause, is not becoming worse.

Determining Secondary Causes. The most common cause of secondary osteoporosis in both men and women is steroid therapy (see Box 45-2). The second most common cause is an endocrinopathy, such as hyperthyroidism, primary hyperparathyroidism, and hypercortisolism. Chronic renal failure leads to severe secondary hyperparathyroidism, causing renal osteodystrophy, which can exacerbate osteoporosis. Severe parenchymal and cholestatic liver disease causes intestinal malabsorption of vitamin D and decreases the production of 25-hydroxyvitamin D [25(OH)D]. In addition, toxins not cleared by the liver likely decrease osteoblastic activity, which can lead to unrelenting osteoporosis, as typically seen in patients with chronic primary biliary cirrhosis.

Laboratory Evaluation and Diagnostic Procedures

Osteoporosis is usually asymptomatic unless a fracture (e.g., acute spinal) causes severe localized bone pain that gradually resolves over 2 to 4 weeks. An inch or more decrease from young adult height also suggests osteoporosis. Although a routine chest radiograph may reveal osteopenia and spinal fractures, at least 30% to 50% of skeletal mass has been lost by this time. Lumbar and sacral films evaluating patients with lower back pain often reveal compression fractures and a fish-mouth appearance of vertebral bodies, demonstrating severe wasting of tubercular bone with concave compression fractures and preservation of cortical bone (see Fig. 45-3).

The gold standard for determining the presence of osteoporosis is measuring BMD. A dual-energy x-ray absorptiometer (DXA) has a single x-ray beam that can determine with 1% to 2% precision the mineral content of various skeletal sites, including the lumbar spine, hip region, and wrist (Fig. 45-4). Other screening techniques use ultrasound or DXA to measure BMD in the wrist, finger, or heel. The *T score* helps interpret bone densitometry readings from different instruments and across gender, age, and race; it is the standard deviation (SD) from the peak bone mass of a person of the same race and gender. For example, a T score of −1.5 means that the individual has a BMD that is 1.5 SD below the mean for a person of the same race and gender at their peak bone mass. The World Health Organization (WHO) has defined a T score of −1 to −2.5 as decreased BMD (i.e., osteopenia). T scores greater than −2.5 indicate osteoporosis with increased risk of fracture.

Quantitative computed tomography (QCT) of the lumbar spine is another method to assess for osteoporosis. This procedure exposes the patient to a large amount of radiation, however, and therefore is no longer used for this purpose. The amount of radiation exposure from DXA is equal to about 10% of a chest radiograph (less than 5 mrem), whereas radiation exposure from QCT can be as much as a barium enema (300 mrem). Health maintenance organization (HMO) and Medicare guidelines for DXA reimbursement include (1) estrogen-deficient women at clinical risk for osteoporosis, (2) patients with radiographically demonstrable vertebral abnormalities indicative of low bone mass (osteopenia) or vertebral fracture, (3) patients receiving glucocorticoid (steroid) therapy equivalent to 7.5 mg of prednisone per day for more than 3 months or if the expected duration is greater than 3 months, (4) patients with primary hyperparathyroidism, and (5) those being monitored to assess response to or efficacy of Food and Drug Administration (FDA)–approved osteoporosis drug therapy. These groups often only reimburse for one skeletal site; the usual choice is a spinal bone density. Unfortunately, if the patient has had compression fractures, osteoarthritis, osteophytes, or sclerosis of the region being measured, the reading will be falsely evaluated (Fig. 45-5). If one site only will be reimbursed, the hip is a better choice because these artifacts are usually absent.

Women approaching menopause should know their bone density. A follow-up measurement in 1 to 2 years can identify women losing 2% to 3% of their bone mass a year and at increased risk of osteoporosis. Bone density also documents the effectiveness of therapy and therefore can increase patient compliance (see Fig. 45-4).

The blood tests to evaluate a patient identified as having osteopenia or osteoporosis include calcium, phosphorus, albumin, alkaline phosphatase, liver function tests, creatinine, 25(OH)D (for determining vitamin D status), and TSH. 1,25(OH)D should *not* be measured because it can be low, normal, or even elevated depending on the patient's vitamin D status and the degree of secondary hyperparathyroidism. For males, free testosterone should be measured if hypogonadism is suspected. These tests will rule out more than 95% of the metabolic causes for osteoporosis. PTH is not routinely obtained. If the serum calcium is normal and serum PTH is elevated, it could falsely indicate that the patient has early primary hyperparathyroidism, when the patient more likely has secondary hyperparathyroidism caused by vitamin D deficiency. An intact PTH is worthwhile to obtain only when the serum calcium is elevated. This assists in the differential diagnosis of hypercalcemia, that is, primary hyperparathyroidism when it is inappropriately normal (when it should be suppressed) or elevated. The second most likely cause of

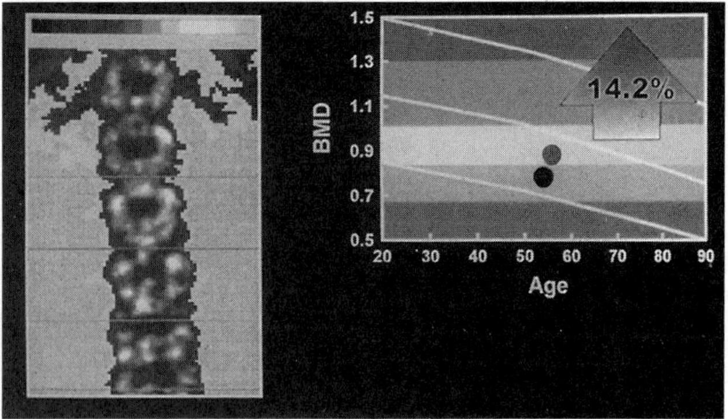

Fig. 45-4. Bone mineral density *(BMD)* printout of 55-year-old woman's lumbar spine showing density of vertebral bodies *(left)* and plot of BMD relative to age *(right)*. Initial average BMD for L2-L4 *(lower dot)* showed patient had severe osteopenia. After 2 years of calcium and vitamin D therapy, BMD increased by 14.2% *(upper dot)*.

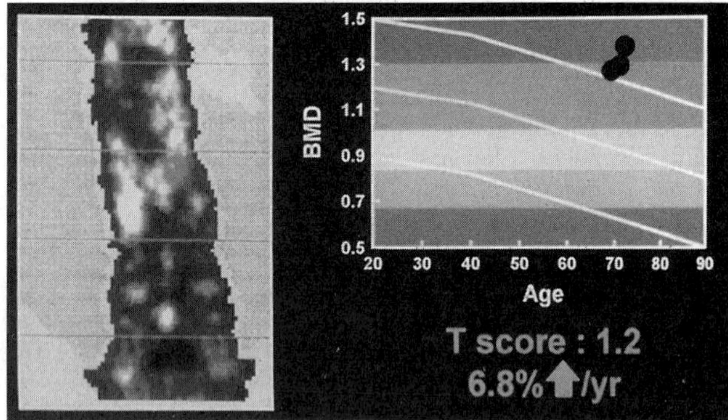

Fig. 45-5. Bone mineral density *(BMD)* of 72-year-old woman who had lost 4 inches in height *(right)*. T score of 1.2 suggests normal BMD, even increasing by 6.8% each year during subsequent 2 years. Examination of printout on left, however, shows white areas (signifying increased density) that are not uniform, indicative of osteoarthritis, osteophytes, or compression fractures. Patient was continuing to lose height, suggesting that BMD increase resulted from new compression fractures in lumbar spine.

hypercalcemia in menopausal women is malignancy. A thorough workup is needed, including a bone scan to evaluate for bone metastasis and PTH-related peptide, which is elevated in about 50% of patients with hypercalcemic malignancy, often caused by squamous cell tumors, especially of the lung.

It is especially important to measure 25(OH)D to rule out vitamin D deficiency; adults over age 50 are at risk.[9] Vitamin D deficiency results in secondary hyperparathyroidism, which can cause and exacerbate osteoporosis. Normal serum calcium provides no information about the patient's vitamin D status; most patients with vitamin D deficiency have a normal serum calcium level. However, a fasting serum phosphorus level is often in the low-normal or low range because of secondary hyperparathyroidism. Serum alkaline phosphatase is elevated.

Measurement of a marker for bone collagen breakdown also helps to determine if increased bone remodeling is resulting in bone loss. The 24-hour urine hydroxyproline test has been replaced with assays that measure the hydroxylysine component of collagen, the pyridinium cross-links in the urine (*N*-telopeptide or Pyralinks assays). They are often found to be high normal or elevated in postmenopausal women not receiving HRT. These assays are also elevated in patients with vitamin D deficiency and secondary hyperparathyroidism, primary hyperparathyroidism, and other metabolic bone diseases (e.g., Paget's disease).

Management

Nonpharmacologic Therapy. The aims of preventing and treating osteoporosis are to decrease rate of bone loss and increase bone mineral content (Box 45-3). Both men and women should increase their calcium and vitamin D intakes to the new recommended adequate intake (AI) levels recommended by the Institute of Medicine in 1997 (Table 45-1). In addition, weight- bearing exercise helps to maintain and may even increase BMD, as well as muscle mass and muscle tone, thereby decreasing their risk of falling and fracture. Once the exercise has stopped, however, any bone gain is lost. Osteoporosis cannot be addressed simply with exercise; every muscle cannot be exercised to influence the BMD of every bone in the body. The best recommendation for adults is to walk 3 to 5 miles a week. This helps to maintain and marginally increase BMD of the lumbar and sacral spine and hip regions.

Exercise. Patients with spinal cord injury can lose 30% to 50% of the skeletal calcium content of the affected limbs within 6 months to 1 year after injury. Astronauts in a weightless environment have complete unloading of their skeleton in microgravity and lose an average 1% to 2% of their bone mass per month. Patients on strict bed rest can have a substantial increase of calcium mobilization from their skeletons, similar to what astronauts experience. The goal is to mobilize invalid patients as soon as possible so that gravity can interact with muscles and bone and thus maintain bone mass. Weightlifting or other exercises (e.g., volleyball, tennis) that involve a loading stress on the skeleton temporarily increase BMD as long as they are continued. Swimming is good for the cardiovascular system and for muscle tone; the buoyancy causes an unloading on the skeleton, however, and therefore swimming does not increase BMD. Again, the best and easiest exercise program to help maintain spinal and hip BMD is walking 3 to 5 miles a week.

Box 45-3. Recommendations to Maximize Bone Health

- Increase dietary calcium intake.
- Receive some exposure to sunlight, or take vitamin D supplement.
- Perform weight-bearing exercises (e.g., walking 3 to 5 miles a week).
- Quit cigarette smoking.
- Decrease alcohol consumption.

Table 45-1. Recommended Adequate Intakes for Calcium and Vitamin D

Age	Calcium (mg/day)	Vitamin D IU (μg/day)
0-6 months	210	200 (5)
6-12 months	270	200 (5)
1-3 years	500	200 (5)
4-8 years	800	200 (5)
9-18 years	1300	200 (5)
19-50 years	1000	200 (5)
51-70 years	1200	400 (10)
>70 years	1200	600 (15)
Pregnancy		
≤18 years	1300	200 (5)
19-50 years	1000	200 (5)

*Courtesy Institute of Medicine, 1997.

Diet. It is often stated that increasing calcium intake prevents and treats osteoporosis. After men and women have reached their peak bone mass, they can lose 0.25% to 0.5% of their bone mass a year if they are not receiving adequate calcium in their diet (see Table 45-1). Thus 20 years of inadequate calcium intake can lead to as much as a 5% to 15% reduction in BMD before age 50. The easiest method to obtain an AI of calcium is by drinking skim milk; since 8 ounces of skim milk has 300 mg of calcium, drinking one glass with each meal approaches the recommended AI for calcium in adults up to age 50.

When deciding which calcium supplement to recommend, cost and bioavailability are important (Table 45-2). Patients who have achlorhydria and chew or swallow their calcium carbonate supplement (e.g., Tums) with their meals are able to absorb the calcium adequately. If they swallow a calcium carbonate pill, however, they are often unable to dissolve it due to lack of stomach acid; therefore the tablet is not broken down or absorbed in the small intestine. Calcium citrate products have a small advantage by increasing the efficiency of calcium absorption by about 10% to 15%. When considering the cost, however, a cheaper chewable form of calcium carbonate may be better. If the patient shows no evidence of magnesium deficiency, magnesium supplementation or a magnesium- containing calcium product is unnecessary; magnesium does not enhance the bioavailability of calcium.

Table 45-2. Calcium Supplements

Brand	Calcium type	Calcium content (mg)
Tums	Carbonate	200
Tums Ex	Carbonate	300
Tums Ultra	Carbonate	400
Tums 500	Carbonate	500
OsCal 250	Carbonate	250
OsCal 500	Carbonate	500
Caltrate	Carbonate	500
Citracal	Citrate	325
GNC calcium supplement	Citrate	250

Most young and middle-aged adults have adequate exposure to sunlight and therefore no need for concern about vitamin D deficiency. Vitamin D deficiency is common in adults over age 50, however, especially those living in northern latitudes and not exposed to sunlight without a sunscreen. For adults up to age 50, 200 IU/day of vitamin D is recommended; for adults ages 50 to 70 and 71% years, however, the AI is 400 and 600 IU daily, respectively. The only foods that naturally contain vitamin D are fatty fish, but one must eat it two or three times a week to receive sufficient vitamin D. To treat vitamin D deficiency quickly, 50,000 IU of vitamin D_2 once a week for 8 weeks is effective.[9] A daily multivitamin containing 400 IU of vitamin D provides AI for adults up to 70 years.

Pharmacologic Therapy

Prevention. Women approaching or initiating menopause should be counseled about AI of 1000 to 1200 mg of calcium daily, weight-bearing exercise program such as walking, and exposure to some sunlight, along with a multivitamin containing 400 IU of vitamin D. This approach helps guarantee maximum bone health as estrogen deficiency ensues. Most women with decreased blood estrogen levels have a significant increase in bone calcium mobilization, resulting in 1% to 3% BMD loss per year. Intervention with HRT should be the first pharmacologic course of action to preserve bone health in women at risk for osteoporosis.

There are two approaches to therapy (Table 45-3). *Cyclic therapy,* which has lost favor because it causes a monthly menstrual cycle, includes Premarin (0.625 mg) on days 1 to 25 and Provera (5 or 10 mg) on days 14 to 25; the cycle is resumed on day 1. *Combination therapy* with Premarin (0.625 mg) and Provera (2.5 mg) daily benefits bone health as well as the cardiovascular system but causes cessation of the menstrual cycle. For women who develop breakthrough bleeding, Provera is increased to 5 to 10 mg a day for 6 to 12 months. Combination products are available for either cycling (Premphase) or combination therapy (Prempro containing 2.5 or 5 mg of Provera). Women entering menopause who no longer want to continue menstruating and still have an active endometrium should use Premphase (5 mg) since the higher daily dose of Provera (progestin) in the combined medication will shut down endometrial growth and result in less breakthrough bleeding. For women still bleeding an additional 5 mg of Provera is helpful to promote endometrial atrophy. Since women who have been menopausal for at least 10 years have an atrophied endometrium, Prempro (2.5 mg) provides the needed estrogen (Premarin) and the low-dose Provera (2.5 mg) to prevent endometrial hyperplasia that can lead to breakthrough bleeding. This is a convenient way for women to take these medications.

For women with a history, strong family history, or fear of breast cancer who refuse to consider HRT, there are two alternative approaches. A *selective estrogen receptor modulator* (SERM) is a reasonable choice for women with a history or strong family history of breast cancer. Raloxifene is the newest SERM and is given at 60 mg a day. For women who want an alternative to HRT or SERM therapy, a low dose of alendronate (Fosamax, 5 mg a day) helps preserve bone mass to the same extent as HRT.

Treatment. The major class of drugs that will increase BMD and decrease risk of skeletal fractures are known as *antiresorptive agents* (see Table 45-3). The *bisphosphonates* are prescribed most often and structurally resemble pyrophosphate. The oxygen between the two phosphoruses has been replaced with a carbon, however, making the compound essentially indestructible. The various attachments on this carbon give rise to a wide variety of bisphosphonates, which are used to treat hypercalcemia of malignancy and metabolic bone diseases, including osteoporosis and Paget's disease. Bisphosphonates are deposited on the surface of new bone, which decreases osteoclastic bone resorption, allowing osteoblasts to lay down new bone not only to replace what was lost but also to add a small amount, thus increasing bone matrix and mineral. Therefore patients receiving bisphosphonate therapy often have increased BMD of 2% to 5% per year over at least 5 years of therapy.

The most popular bisphosphonate prescribed worldwide for the treatment and prevention of osteoporosis is *alendronate* (Fosamax).[8] This medication may increase BMD of both the hip and the spine by 2% to 5% a year and may decrease the risk for fractures of the hip and spine by 51% and 63%, respectively (Fig. 45-6). The advantage of alendronate over the first-generation bisphosphonate etidronate (Didronel) is that daily use will not cause the mineralization defect of osteomalacia. For patients unable to tolerate alendronate because of the strict dosing regimen (10 mg once a day or 70 mg once a week with 8 ounces of water and waiting ½ hour before eating) or the gastrointestinal (GI) discomfort, an alternative is etidronate, 400 mg at night for 2 weeks followed by a free period of 13 weeks. The 15-week cycle is repeated for up to 5 years. These drugs are effective only if the patient is vitamin D sufficient and receiving adequate calcium. Third-generation bisphosphonates being developed may have the same skeletal benefits and reduced risk of fracture but with fewer GI effects. If the patient cannot tolerate oral bisphosphonates, an alternative is *pamidronate* (Aredia), 30 mg intravenously over 4 hours once every 3 months.

Another class of antiresorptive drugs is the calcitonins (see Table 45-3). *Calcitonin* is a polypeptide made by the C cells in the thyroid gland that inhibits osteoclastic activity. Calcitonin is available by subcutaneous (50 IU every other day) and intranasal (200 IU/day) routes of administration. However, this drug has marginal, if any, long-term benefit for treatment or prevention of osteoporosis. Calcitonin may help decrease bone resorptive activity, especially in patients with high-turnover osteoporosis. Calcitonin may also marginally increase BMD by 1% to 2% for the first 12 to 24 months, but

Table 45-3. Pharmacologic Management for Preventing and Treating Osteoporosis and Osteopenia

Medication	Indication	Dose	Dosage schedule	Side effects
Calcium	Prevention	<50 years: 1000 mg/day >50 years: 1200 mg/day	250-500 mg with meals to attain adequate intake	Bloating, constipation
Vitamin D	Prevention	<50 years: 200 IU/day 50-70 years: 400 IU/day >70 years: 600 IU/day	400-IU multivitamin once daily >70 years: 2 tablets acceptable	None
	Vitamin D deficiency	50,000 IU	Once weekly for 8 weeks (total 8 pills)	None
Premphase	Prevention	Premarin 0.625 mg, Provera 5 mg days 15-28 only	1 tablet/day	Menstrual cycle restored
Prempro	Prevention	Premarin 0.625 mg, Provera 2.5 or 5 mg	1 tablet/day	Breakthrough bleeding
Alendronate (Fosamax)	Osteoporosis	10 mg/day or 70 mg once a week	Once daily in morning on empty stomach with 8 oz water; patient waits 30 minutes before eating breakfast and is not in reclining position	Upset stomach, nausea, gastritis, diarrhea, esophagitis
Alendronate (Fosamax)	Prevention	5 mg	Once daily in morning on empty stomach with 8 oz water; patient waits 30 minutes before eating breakfast and is not in reclining position	Upset stomach, nausea, gastritis, diarrhea, esophagitis
Etidronate (Didronel)	Osteoporosis	400 mg	Once at bedtime and at least 1 hour after last meal for 14 days; patient stops for 13 weeks and repeats cycle	Upset stomach, arthralgia
Pamidronate (Aredia)	Steroid-induced osteoporosis	90 mg	Intravenously (IV) over 2-4 hours for initial dose, then 30 mg IV once every 3 months	Arthralgia, myalgia, fever, flulike symptoms
Calcitonin	Prevention*	50 units	Subcutaneously every other day	Facial flushing, nausea, dermatitis, immediate hypersensitivity response, anaphylaxis
		200 IU	Intranasal daily	Nasal problems, adverse events, possible allergic reaction, flushing, nausea, respiratory irritation

*No evidence indicates that calcitonin prevents fractures.

with little effect thereafter. Most patients develop tachyphylaxis to the medication in a relatively short time.

Box 45-4 lists specific drug therapy recommendations.

Adverse Effects. The major side effects of alendronate therapy are esophagitis and gastritis, which can be minimized by ensuring the patient is taking the medication on an empty stomach with 8 ounces of water. The patient should not lie down or be in a reclining position for at least ½ hour to prevent the symptoms. Some evidence indicates that the aminobisphosphonates such as alendronate decrease esophageal motility and increase the transit time of the medication in the esophagus, causing lower esophageal irritation. Etidronate is not an aminobisphosphonate and usually does not cause GI distress. Taking the medication for only 2 weeks will not cause osteomalacia.

Estimating Benefits. HRT prevents bone loss from estrogen deficiency, decreases risk of cardiovascular disease by about 44%, and may prevent or delay the onset of Alzheimer's disease. Alendronate therapy (10 mg/day or 70 mg once a week) is effective in increasing BMD in the hip and spine, decreasing the risk of height loss and new spinal and hip fractures. Cyclic etridonate therapy also increases BMD and decreases the risk of hip and spinal fractures. Calcitonin decreases bone resorptive activity and may

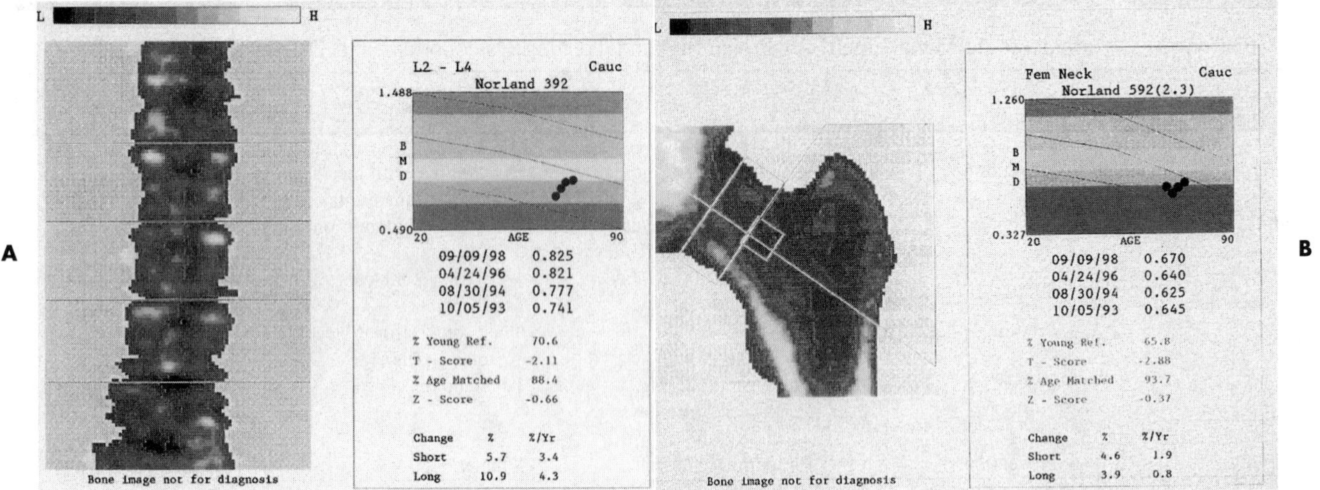

Fig. 45-6. Effect of alendronate therapy on bone mineral density (BMD) of lumbar spine (**A**) and hip (**B**) in 62-year-old woman with osteoporosis who received 1200 mg of calcium, 400 IU of vitamin D, and 10 mg of alendronate daily for 5 years. Annual increase in BMD of hip and spine averaged 3.4% and 1.9%, respectively.

Box 45-4. Managed Care Guide: Recommendations for Pharmacologic Prevention and Treatment of Osteoporosis

- All men and women over age 50 should have adequate calcium and vitamin D intake (see Table 45-1).
- Perimenopausal and postmenopausal women may receive HRT to maintain osteoblastic function and bone mass. These women can sustain their normal BMD with HRT or with raloxifene or low-dose alendronate (5 mg/day).
- Women postmenopausal for longer than 10 years with osteoporosis still benefit from HRT to maintain and marginally increase BMD.
- Because of all its other beneficial effects, HRT is highly recommended.
- Patients with demonstrable osteoporosis should receive an antiresorptive medication such as alendronate (10 mg/day or 70 mg once a week) to prevent risk of fractures.
- Men with osteoporosis benefit from testosterone replace-
- ment if deficient and treatment with alendronate therapy
- (10 mg/day).
- Men and women receiving long-term prednisone therapy should increase calcium intake to 1.2-1.5 gm/day and vitamin D intake to 400-800 IU/day. Alendronate (5 or 10 mg/day) can help decrease bone resorptive activity.

HRT, Hormonal replacement therapy; *BMD,* bone mineral density.

marginally increase BMD for a short duration. No evidence indicates that bisphosphonate or calcitonin therapy alters the healing of hip or spinal fractures, and therefore therapy can continue when a patient sustains a bone fracture.

Special Issues. Although nutritional and pharmacologic approaches can prevent and treat osteoporosis, it may continue to be a major health problem in the twenty-first century, with staggering health care costs to treat acute fractures and manage chronic lower back pain and hip fractures. Physicians should evaluate patients for dietary calcium and vitamin D intake, exposure to sunlight, exercise, and HRT and then institute appropriate pharmacologic osteoporosis treatment and prevention programs.

Poor Adherence to Drug Regimen. Only about 30% of women prescribed HRT are taking the medication after 1 year. The physician should explain the consequences of HRT, including breakthrough bleeding and breast tenderness so that the patient is not surprised by the symptoms and does not stop the medication without further consultation with the physician. HRT is so important for women's health that every effort should be made to encourage women to consider this first line of preventive therapy as they are entering menopause. Less than 50% of patients who initiate alendronate therapy remain on therapy after 1 year, partly because of the rigorous regimen. To encourage compliance, the physician can show the patient the significant BMD benefit from the therapy.

Other Treatments. The active form of vitamin D [$1,25(OH)_2D_3$] and its 25-deoxy analog [$1\alpha(OH)D_3$] are routinely prescribed in Europe and Japan for the treatment of osteoporosis. This medication increases the efficiency of intestinal calcium absorption and stimulates osteoblastic activity to increase BMD. It is especially effective for women who are unable to tolerate, for whatever reason, the recommended AI for calcium. $1,25(OH_2)D_3$ has not been approved to treat osteoporosis in the United States and has a very narrow window of therapeutic efficacy and safety. Active vitamin D can easily cause hypercalciuria and even hypercalcemia.

Another medication that greatly increases BMD is *fluoride;* however, high doses cause bone fluorosis, which increases the risk of skeletal fractures. Although new forms of slow-release fluoride are being developed, none is currently available or FDA approved for treatment or prevention of osteoporosis.

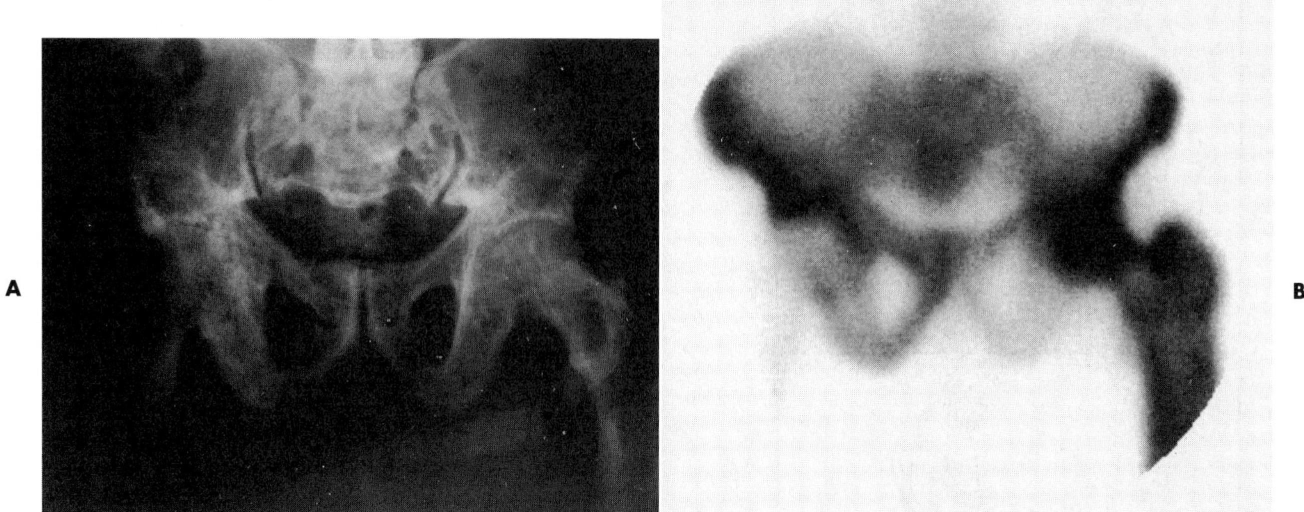

Fig. 45-7. **A,** Radiograph of pelvis in 82-year-old black male complaining of left hip pain. Note mottled appearance of left and right hemipelves and left femoral head, which is classic for Paget's disease. **B,** Bone scan of pelvis and femur of same patient showing greatly increased uptake in left and right hemipelves and left femoral head.

PAGET'S DISEASE

The first indication of Paget's disease is often a routine pelvic radiograph for ruling out spinal fractures that is found incidentally to have a mottled area in the pelvis consistent with the disease. Paget's disease is characterized by an increase in the bone-remodeling process and in both osteoblastic and osteoclastic activity. As a result, the collagen laid down by the osteoblasts is disorganized in a woven fashion, which causes the classic mottled appearance on radiographs (Fig. 45-7).

Epidemiology and Pathophysiology

Paget's disease occurs with equal frequency in both men and women; 3% of patients over age 55 may have manifestations of the disease. The cause of Paget's disease is uncertain. Some suggest a viral infection similar to the measles virus, and others suggest a genetic disorder, but neither has been substantiated.

High turnover and haphazard formation result in a woven bone that has little architectural integrity or strength. Thus the pagetic bone is weaker and more susceptible to fracture. The bones most often affected, in order of frequency, are sacrum, spine, femur, skull, sternum, and pelvis. Involvement of the long bones is less common; however, the disease can occur at any skeletal site involving one or many bones. Patients with Paget's disease have an increased risk of osteogenic sarcoma associated with lytic lesions in the bone on radiographs and rapidly increasing alkaline phosphatase levels. Increased bone-remodeling activity causes increased vascularity in the affected area. When the disease is widespread, affecting more than 30% of the skeleton, it can substantially increase cardiac output, with up to 10% of output shunted to perfuse the pagetic bone. This can increase the risk of congestive heart failure (CHF) in compromised cardiac patients. Increased warmth in the area from the increased vascularity is often noted on physical examination, especially if the skull or long bones are involved. A decrease in warmth over the area after treatment is an effective way to evaluate therapeutic efficacy.

Although usually not painful, pagetic bone can cause chronic pain if a joint such as the hip is affected. Pagetic involvement of the spine can cause nerve impingement, leading to spinal stenosis, neuropathy, muscle wasting, and sciatica. Paget's disease of the skull, especially involving the small bones of the middle ear, can lead to deafness. Pagetic involvement of the auditory canal and surrounding areas can also lead to eighth cranial nerve dysfunction, including the vestibular manifestations of dizziness, vertigo, and tinnitus.

The increased remodeling process mobilizes calcium and may cause mild hypercalciuria. Significant hypercalciuria and hypercalcemia may occur, however, when patients are immobilized because of decreased bone formation from skeletal unloading. Hypercalcemia in patients with Paget's disease who are not immobilized suggests another cause for hypercalcemia, including malignancy, hyperparathyroidism, or diuretic (hydrochlorothiazide) therapy.

Patient Evaluation

As noted, Paget's disease is usually discovered as an incidental finding on a radiograph of the pelvis, chest, or skull. If the site (e.g., pelvis) does not put the patient at risk for complications, further therapeutic intervention is unnecessary. A bone scan can help determine whether the patient has pagetic involvement elsewhere in the skeleton. Increased uptake of the radioactive marker indicates increased bone turnover, as seen in Paget's disease (see Fig. 45-7).

Goals. The two goals for the initial evaluation are to assess the patient's risk of (1) developing a complication from Paget's disease or (2) developing high-output CHF.

Assessing Individual Risk. Patients who have pagetic involvement of their skull, long bones, and hip joint require aggressive antiresorptive therapy. Involvement of long bones can lead to bone deformation and may cause a bowing of the leg, increasing the risk of fracture and causing degenerative joint disease in the ipsilateral hip. Early intervention for

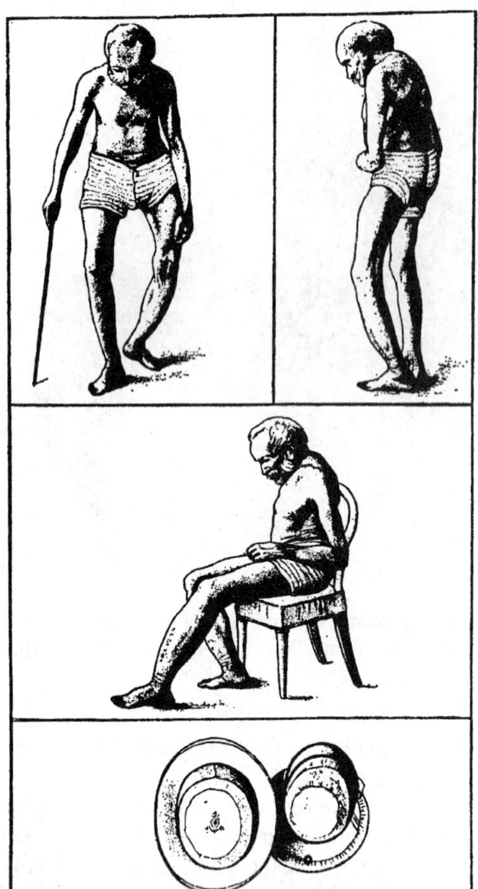

Fig. 45-8. Classic appearance of bony deformities associated with pagetic involvement of left leg and skull. Note cap size *(right)* from same patient worn in 1844 and increased hat size *(left)* in 1867. (From Sir James Paget, before the Royal Medical Chirurgical Society of London, Nov. 14, 1876.)

Pagetic skull involvement can prevent serious hearing loss and vestibular abnormalities. Identification of hip joint involvement (femoral head or hip socket) reduces the risk of severe degenerative joint disease.

Clinical and Laboratory Evaluation

Most patients with Paget's disease are asymptomatic. Patients with skull involvement, however, may note an increase in hat size, increased frequency and intensity of headaches, tinnitus, hearing loss, dizziness, and vertigo. Involvement of the extremities can lead to bone deformities, especially of weight-bearing bones such as the femur and tibia (Fig. 45-8).

Touching the affected area (e.g., skull, long bone) with the back of the hand may suggest pagetic involvement by increased warmth compared with surrounding areas. Full neurologic evaluation of the cranial nerves, especially the eighth nerve, is indicated for pagetic skull involvement. Spinal involvement requires an evaluation of sensory and motor neuron functions of the affected area.

Markers for osteoblastic and osteoclastic activity are used to assess disease activity. Serum alkaline phosphatase is a reliable indicator of Paget's disease, but not all patients with the disease have greatly elevated levels. A measure of increased bone remodeling is the 24-hour urine excretion of hydroxyproline or a spot urine test for determining pyridinium cross-links. To determine if more than one skeletal site are involved with Paget's disease, a radionuclide bone scan is valuable (see Fig. 45-7). Radiographs of suspected sites are useful for differentiating pagetic bone and metastatic bone disease. For patients with skull involvement, audiologic evaluation should be considered.

Management

Most patients with incidental Paget's disease of the pelvis do not require therapeutic intervention. If pain is associated with pagetic involvement, however, therapy should be considered. An alkaline phosphatase level more than two to three times the upper limit of normal; active disease of a long bone, the skull, or hip joints; or involvement of one or more vertebral bodies is often an indication for aggressive therapy to prevent potentially serious consequences. Surgical intervention is often required if nerve impingement is observed with sudden neurologic impairment, such as weakness of an extremity.

Bisphosphonate Therapy. Bisphosphonates are effective in about 85% to 90% of patients with Paget's disease. Etidronate (Didronel), 200 to 400 mg/day (up to 20 mg/kg body weight), is usually given for 4 to 6 months, then stopped for 2 to 4 months, and reinstituted again. Because continual use causes osteomalacia and because of its low efficacy, etidronate is rarely used. Two second-generation bisphosphonates approved for treatment of Paget's disease are alendronate (40 mg/day) and risedronate (20 mg/day).[2] These medications can be taken daily continuously and do not increase the risk of osteomalacia.

Pamidronate. An effective alternative is intravenous (IV) pamidronate, with the advantage of therapy only once a week for 4 weeks. Pamidronate has been approved for treating hypercalcemia of malignancy. It is usually administered as an IV test dose of 30 mg over 4 hours in the physician's office. If the patient has no side effects, such as severe myalgias or arthralgias (flulike symptoms and fever may occur but usually resolve rapidly), the patient returns 1 week later to receive 60 mg over 2 to 4 hours. This is repeated once a week for an additional 3 weeks. An alternative is to give 30 mg/day for 3 successive days. In most patients the serum alkaline phosphatase level and urinary pyridinium cross-links will substantially decline within a few weeks and remain in the normal range. If Paget's disease recurs, however, a repeat of the IV regimen of 60 mg/week for 4 weeks often puts the patient into remission. This may be much easier for the patient than taking a medication every day.

Plicamycin. Formerly called mithramycin, plicamycin is a cytotoxic antibiotic and potent inhibitor of osteoblastic activity. It is administered intravenously over 4 hours at 10 μg/kg body weight. Side effects include bone marrow toxicity and liver abnormalities, and thus this drug is no longer used for Paget's disease.

Calcitonin. Once considered the treatment of choice for Paget's disease, calcitonin has been largely replaced by the second-generation bisphosphonates. The mode of administration, subcutaneous or intranasal, can be problematic, and only about 50% to 60% of patients respond to calcitonin therapy. Often they develop a resistance to therapy over time due to the development of antibodies or a down-regulation of the calcitonin receptor. The usual dose is 50 to 100 IU/day subcutaneously or 200 IU/day intranasally.

Nonsteroidal Antiinflammatory Drugs. NSAIDs do not treat Paget's disease but may help relieve the pain associated with pagetic involvement of joint spaces (e.g., hip). Indomethacin, 25 mg three or four times daily, or NSAID such as Motrin may help relieve the pain.

REFERENCES

1. Aloia JF, Yeh JK, Flaster E: Risk for osteoporosis in black women, *Calcif Tissue Int* 59:415, 1996.
2. Brown JP, Hosking DJ, Ste-Marie LG, et al: Risedronate, a highly effective, short-term oral treatment for Paget's disease: a dose-response study, *Calcif Tissue Int* 64:93, 1999.
3. Cummings SR, Kelsey JL, Nevitt MC, O'Dowd KJ: Epidemiology of osteoporosis and osteoporotic fractures, *Epidemiol Rev* 7:178, 1985.
4. Disla E, Tamayo B, Fahmy A: Intermittent etidronate and corticosteroid-induced osteoporosis, *N Engl J Med* 337:1921, 1997.
5. Holick MF: Vitamin D: new horizons for the 21st century, *Am J Clin Nutr* 60:619, 1994.
6. Holick MF, Krane SM, Potts JT: Calcium, phosphorus, and bone metabolism: calcium-regulating hormones. In Fuaci AS, Braunwald E, Isselbacher KJ, et al, editors: *Harrison's principles of internal medicine,* ed 14, New York, 1998, McGraw-Hill.
7. Krane SM, Holick MF: Metabolic bone disease. In Fauci AS, Braunwald E, Isselbacher KJ, et al, editors: *Harrison's principles of internal medicine,* ed 14, New York, 1998, McGraw-Hill.
8. Liberman VA, Weiss SR, Broll J, et al: Effect of oral alendronate on bone mineral density and incidence of fractures in postmenopausal osteoporosis, *N Engl J Med* 333:1437, 1995.
9. Malabanan A, Veronikis IE, Holick MF: Redefining vitamin D insufficiency, *Lancet* 351:805, 1998.
10. Riggs BL, Khosla S, Melton LJ: A unitary model for involutional osteoporosis: estrogen deficiency causes both type I and type II osteoporosis in postmenopausal women and contributes to bone loss in aging men, *J Bone Miner Res* 13:763, 1998.

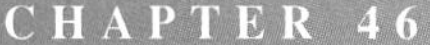
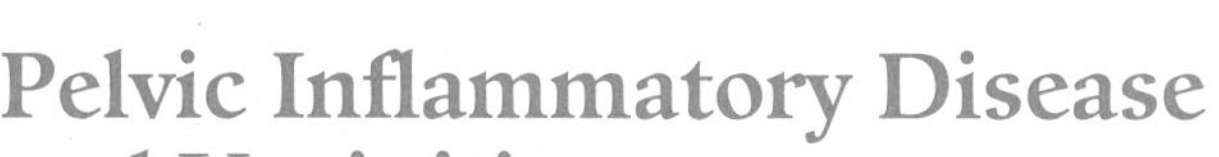

CHAPTER 46

Pelvic Inflammatory Disease and Vaginitis

J. Chris Carey

PELVIC INFLAMMATORY DISEASE

Epidemiology

Pelvic inflammatory disease (PID) is estimated to be responsible for 2.5 million outpatient visits each year, as well as 275,000 hospitalizations. The disease is more common in younger reproductive-age women, single women, women with multiple sexual partners or a new partner in the last 6 months, and nonwhite women. Women who use barrier contraceptives are at lower risk. Use of an intrauterine device has been associated with an increased risk of PID, mainly related to the risk of insertion and to acquisition of a sexually transmitted disease (STD).

Table 46-1. Essential Elements of History in Suspected Pelvic Inflammatory Disease (PID)

History	Elements
Present illness	Lower abdominal and pelvic pain (duration, location, quality, severity, relation to menses, dyspareunia), vaginal discharge, fever
Past medical	Prior episodes of PID, previous sexually transmitted diseases, prior episodes of lower abdominal pain, previous evaluations and therapies
Menstrual	Last menstrual period, postmenopausal, intermenstrual bleeding
Sexual	Last intercourse, use of barrier methods with recent intercourse, frequency of recent intercourse, number of partners in last year and lifetime, new sexual partner
Contraceptive	Current contraceptive method, prior methods, use of barrier methods

Pathophysiology

PID results from an ascending infection by organisms that have colonized the endocervix. The syndrome includes nonpuerperal endometritis, salpingitis, oophoritis, and adnexitis. *Neisseria gonorrhoeae* and *Chlamydia trachomatis* are the most common etiologic agents, but secondary infection with a variety of anaerobic and aerobic agents also occurs. A polymicrobial infection with aerobic and anaerobic bacteria is found in up to 40% of women who have laparoscopically proven acute salpingitis. Many of these organisms found in the upper tract are the same organisms found in increased numbers in the vagina of women with bacterial vaginosis, which is more common in women with PID. It is not known, however, whether bacterial vaginosis is a risk factor for development of PID, or develops concurrently with PID, or develops as a result of PID.

Retrograde menstruation is thought to play a role in the development of PID. Sexually transmitted organisms that inhabit the endocervix may be spread to the fallopian tubes by retrograde menstruation. Secondary infection of the fallopian tubes by aerobic and anaerobic organisms may lead to abscess formation or overt sepsis. Tuboovarian abscesses usually contain anaerobic bacteria.

Infertility is an important sequela of PID. The risk of tubal factor infertility roughly doubles after each episode of PID. After one, two, and three episodes of PID the risk of infertility is 8%, 19.5%, and 40%, respectively. The risk of ectopic pregnancy is increased fourfold after documented salpingitis.

Patient Evaluation

History. PID may present with a wide variety of symptoms and signs. The classic history is of acute lower abdominal pain, usually after menstruation, with fever and a foul or purulent vaginal discharge (Table 46-1). Many women with PID, however, have subtle or mild symptoms. Pelvic and lower abdominal pain is the most common symptom, is usually bilateral, and may not be severe. Endocervicitis may lead to a complaint of vaginal discharge. Persistent spotting while taking oral contraceptives (OCs) or after pregnancy termination may be a symptom of PID. Nausea and vomiting may result from peritonitis with or without fever. Inflammation of the liver by peritoneal spread can lead to acute hepatitis (Fitz-Hugh–Curtis syndrome).

Physical Examination. The triad of lower abdominal tenderness, adnexal tenderness, and cervical motion tenderness is considered sufficient to make the diagnosis of PID if no other cause for the illness can be found. Other physical findings consistent with the diagnosis of PID include mucopurulent cervicitis, which can be diagnosed by a marked increase of inflammatory cells on a saline preparation of the endocervical mucus. A palpable adnexal mass suggests a tuboovarian abscess. An elevated temperature is further evidence of PID.

Diagnosis

Acute PID is difficult to diagnose because of the wide variation in symptoms and signs. Many cases of PID go unrecognized. On the other hand, many women who have other conditions are treated for PID. No single historic, physical, or laboratory finding is both sensitive and specific for the diagnosis of PID. Combinations of diagnostic findings that improve either sensitivity or specificity do so at the expense of the other. Therefore the diagnosis of PID is usually based on clinical findings. The clinical diagnosis of acute PID is also imprecise. A clinical diagnosis of symptomatic PID has a positive predictive value (PPV) for salpingitis of 65% to 90% compared with laparoscopy. The PPV of a clinical diagnosis of acute PID differs depending on epidemiologic characteristics and the clinical setting, with higher PPVs among sexually active young (especially teenage) women and among patients attending STD clinics or from settings where rates of gonorrhea or chlamydial infection are high.

Because of the difficulty in diagnosis and the potential for infertility after even mild PID, primary care physicians should maintain a high suspicion for PID and a low threshold for its diagnosis (Box 46-1). Empiric therapy for PID can be instituted based on minimum criteria in patients with initial episodes. Initiation of antibiotic therapy for PID is unlikely to interfere with the diagnosis and management of other causes of lower abdominal pain. Women with repeated episodes, failed initial therapy, or questionable diagnosis of PID should have additional diagnostic studies.

Box 46-1. Criteria for Diagnosis of Pelvic Inflammatory Disease (PID)

Minimum Criteria

1. Lower abdominal tenderness
2. Adnexal tenderness
3. Cervical motion tenderness
4. (All three must be present, and no other cause can be identified.)

Additional Criteria

1. Oral temperature greater than 101° F (38.3° C)
2. Abnormal cervical or vaginal discharge
3. Elevated erythrocyte sedimentation rate
4. Elevated C-reactive protein
5. Laboratory documentation of cervical infection with *N. gonorrhoeae* or *C. trachomatis*

Definitive Criteria

1. Histopathologic evidence of endometritis on endometrial biopsy
2. Transvaginal sonography or other imaging techniques showing thickened fluid-filled tubes with or without free pelvic fluid or tuboovarian complex
3. Laparoscopic abnormalities consistent with PID

Data from Centers for Disease Control and Prevention: 1998 Guidelines for treatment of sexually transmitted diseases, *MMWR* 47(RR-1), 1998.

Diagnostic Procedures

Cultures. Cultures or other screening methods for *N. gonorrhoeae* and *C. trachomatis* should be obtained from every woman with suspected PID. A positive culture not only supports the diagnosis of PID but emphasizes the need to treat sex partners. Screening tests for other STDs, such as human immunodeficiency virus (HIV) and syphilis, are also recommended.

Ultrasound. Ultrasound is indicated if an adnexal mass is suspected, if the diagnosis is in question, or if a patient does not respond to initial therapy. Ultrasound is both sensitive and specific for the presence of a tuboovarian abscess. The presence of tubal edema and fluid is highly suggestive of PID, but a nondiagnostic ultrasound does not exclude PID.

Laparoscopy. Although it can be used to obtain a more accurate diagnosis of PID and a more complete specimen for culture, laparoscopy is not always available for immediate diagnosis. The expense and risk of laparoscopy are difficult to justify for routine diagnosis of PID. Laparoscopy may not detect endometritis or subtle salpingitis. Laparoscopy should be considered in women with an uncertain diagnosis, particularly if an ectopic pregnancy is suspected, and women with a history of multiple outpatient treatments for PID to exclude other causes of pain (e.g., endometriosis). Laparoscopy may also be useful in preserving fertility by lysis of adhesions.

Endometrial Biopsy. Acute or chronic inflammation on an endometrial biopsy offers an alternative, objective method of diagnosing upper tract inflammation. Endometrial biopsy is useful in patients with subtle signs, including abnormal bleeding.

Differential Diagnosis. Ectopic pregnancy should be considered in every woman with signs suggestive of PID. A negative serum pregnancy test should exclude ectopic pregnancy. In any woman who is thought to be pregnant and have PID, it is imperative to exclude an ectopic pregnancy. Ultrasound to localize the pregnancy should be the first step. If ectopic pregnancy cannot be excluded by ultrasound, laparoscopy should be considered.

Appendicitis can be difficult to distinguish from PID. Appendicitis more often presents with unilateral pain, nausea, vomiting, and peritoneal signs. Physical examination and ultrasound can sometimes distinguish appendicitis and PID. If appendicitis is suspected, a laparoscopy may be indicated. *Endometriosis* typically presents with cyclic pain and dysmenorrhea and can be difficult to distinguish from PID. The definitive diagnosis of endometriosis can be made only by laparoscopy. *Ovarian cysts* may present with acute symptoms similar to PID. Midcycle onset of pain, unilateral pain, palpation of a cyst, and absence of mucopurulent cervicitis suggest an ovarian cyst. Ultrasound is useful in this diagnosis.

Management

Nonpharmacologic Therapy. Prevention of STDs is the mainstay of nonpharmacologic management of PID. Counseling of patients about safe sexual practices and the risks of acquiring STDs should be part of contraceptive counseling. Women at risk for acquisition of an STD who use OCs should be counseled to use condoms as well. Screening for asymptomatic *N. gonorrhoeae* and *C. trachomatis* is indicated for at-risk populations (e.g., women under age 25 with new partner in last year, populations with high incidence of STDs). Women with clinically apparent mucopurulent cervicitis should also be screened for these organisms.

Pharmacologic Therapy. Antibiotic therapy for PID must provide empiric, broad-spectrum coverage of likely pathogens. Antimicrobial coverage should include *N. gonorrhoeae, C. trachomatis,* anaerobes, gram-negative facultative bacteria, and streptococci. Several antimicrobial regimens have been effective in achieving clinical and microbiologic cure in randomized clinical trials with short-term follow-up (Box 46-2). However, few investigations have assessed and compared these regimens with regard to elimination of infection in the endometrium and fallopian tubes or have determined the incidence of long-term complications, such as infertility or ectopic pregnancy. Oral ofloxacin is effective against both *N. gonorrhoeae* and *C. trachomatis* and as a single agent. The addition of metronidazole provides ofloxacin's lack of anaerobic coverage. Amoxicillin/clavulanate plus doxycycline has obtained short-term clinical response, but gastrointestinal symptoms might limit the overall success of this regimen.

Consultation and Hospitalization. Some authorities recommend intravenous therapy for all PID patients or for women with PID who have not completed childbearing (Box 46-3). The physician should decide whether hospitalization is necessary (Box 46-4). No currently available data compare the efficacy of parenteral with oral therapy or inpatient with outpatient treatment settings. Until the results from ongoing trials comparing parenteral inpatient therapy with oral outpatient therapy for women with mild PID are available, such decisions must be based on observational data and consensus opinion.

Patients receiving oral or parenteral therapy should show substantial clinical improvement in 3 days. Defervescence usually precedes subsidence of pain. Patients who do not show improvement in 3 days usually require additional therapy or surgery. Women treated as outpatients should be reexamined in 3 days and evaluated for improvement. Some authorities recommend repeat screening in 4 to 6 weeks for patients who had positive tests for *N. gonorrhoeae* or *C. trachomatis.* If a polymerase or ligase chain reaction (PCR, LCR) was used as a screening test, at least 4 weeks should elapse to prevent false-positive repeat screens.

Special Issues

Sexual Partners. Sexual partners of women with PID should be screened for *N. gonorrhoeae* and *C. trachomatis* if they have had intercourse within the last 60 days. Negative cervical cultures or other screens do not exclude carriage of these organisms by sexual partners. Screening and treatment of sexual partners are important to prevent reacquisition of STDs and recurrent PID.

Box 46-2. Outpatient Regimens for Pelvic Inflammatory Disease

Regimen A

Ofloxacin, 400 mg orally twice a day for 14 days, *plus* metronidazole, 500 mg orally twice a day for 14 days

Regimen B

Ceftriaxone, 250 mg intramuscularly (IM) once
or Cefoxitin, 2 gm IM, *plus* probenecid, 1 gm orally in single dose concurrently once
or Other parenteral third-generation cephalosporin (e.g., ceftizoxime, cefotaxime)
plus
Doxycycline, 100 mg orally twice a day for 14 days

Data from Centers for Disease Control and Prevention: 1998 Guidelines for treatment of sexually transmitted diseases, *MMWR* 47(RR-1), 1998.

Box 46-3. Parenteral Regimens for Pelvic Inflammatory Disease

Parenteral Regimen A

Cefotetan 2 gm intravenously (IV) every 12 hours
or Cefoxitin, 2 gm IV every 6 hours
plus
Doxycycline, 100 mg IV or orally every 12 hours

Parenteral Regimen B

Clindamycin, 900 mg IV every 8 hours, *plus* gentamicin loading dose IV or IM (2 mg/kg), followed by maintenance dose (1.5 mg/kg) every 8 hours (Single daily dosing may be substituted.)

Data from Centers for Disease Control and Prevention: 1998 Guidelines for treatment of sexually transmitted diseases, *MMWR* 47(RR-1), 1998.

Box 46-4. Indications for Hospitalization for Pelvic Inflammatory Disease

- Surgical emergencies (e.g., appendicitis) cannot be excluded
- Pregnancy
- Failure to respond clinically to oral antimicrobial therapy
- Unable to follow or tolerate outpatient oral regimen
- Severe illness, nausea and vomiting, or high fever
- Tuboovarian abscess
- Immunodeficiency (e.g., HIV infection with low CD4 counts, immunosuppressive therapy, other disease)

Pregnancy. Because of the high risk for maternal morbidity, fetal wastage, and preterm delivery, pregnant women with suspected PID should be hospitalized and treated with parenteral antibiotics. Ectopic pregnancy must be excluded in every pregnant woman who may have PID. Disseminated gonococcal infection is more common in pregnant women than nonpregnant women, and women with suspected infection should be treated with parenteral therapy. Doxycycline and ofloxacin are contraindicated in pregnancy, as is erythromycin estolate. Pregnant patients with PID must receive a sufficiently long course of an agent against *C. trachomatis*. Erythromycin base, 500 mg four times a day for 7 days, is recommended. The safety and efficacy of azithromycin has not been established in pregnant or lactating women.

HIV Infection. It is not clear whether PID has different clinical manifestations in HIV-infected women and HIV-negative women. Early observational studies found that HIV-infected women with PID were more likely to require surgical intervention. In a subsequent and more comprehensive observational study, HIV-infected women with PID had more severe symptoms than HIV-negative women but responded equally well to standard parenteral antibiotic regimens. Immunosuppressed HIV-infected women with PID should be managed aggressively using parenteral antimicrobial regimens.

Box 46-5. Flora Isolated from Normal Vaginas

Lactobacilli (60-80%)
Group B streptococci (10-20%)
Mycoplasma hominis (20-35%)
Ureaplasma urealyticum (35-85%)
Gardnerella vaginalis (40-60%)
Bacteroides species (10-20%)
Peptococcus/Peptostreptococcus (6-10%)
Anaerobic gram-positive rods (4-10%)
Gram-negative aerobes (1-2%)

Box 46-6. Common Causes of Vaginitis

Bacterial vaginosis
Fungal vaginitis
Trichomoniasis
Atrophic vaginitis

VAGINITIS

Epidemiology

Vaginitis is one of the most common reasons for physician visits by women, accounting for approximately 10 million office visits per year. No reliable figures define the incidence of vaginitis in the United States. Its prevalence is difficult to estimate because (1) many women with abnormal flora may have minimal symptoms and may not complain of vaginitis, and (2) many women self-medicate with over-the-counter medications. The largest studies of prevalence of vaginitis were performed in pregnant women. The Vaginal Infections and Prematurity study screened 13,914 pregnant women for vaginal and cervical pathogens. *Candida albicans* was isolated from 8.2%, *Trichomonas vaginalis* was isolated by culture from 12.5%, and bacterial vaginosis was diagnosed by Gram's stain in 16.2%. Data from Great Britain indicate that the incidence of symptomatic vulvovaginal candidiasis increased from 118 to 200 per 100,000 from 1980 to 1990. Sales of antifungal medications in the United States have also increased, indicating a greater incidence of vaginitis.

The prevalence and type of vaginitis vary greatly by age and race. Bacterial vaginosis and *T. vaginalis* are more common in reproductive-age women and in black women, whereas candidiasis is more common in white women. Atrophic vaginitis is more common in postmenopausal women.

Pathophysiology

Lactobacilli are the predominant organisms in the normal vagina. Because lactobacilli produce lactic acid and hydrogen peroxide, the vagina normally has a pH of 3.8 to 4.4 and has a high oxidative potential. The combination of these two factors helps prevent growth of other organisms, such as anaerobic bacteria. Each gram of vaginal discharge usually has about 10^4 organisms. Five to 15 different organisms can usually be cultured from the vagina of a normal woman (Box 46-5). The normal vaginal discharge consists primarily of desquamated epithelial cells and is white to gray, flocculent, and not malodorous.

Infectious vaginitis results from an alteration of normal vaginal flora and has several common causes (Box 46-6). Becauseto other organisms almost never cause vaginitis, their treatment is rarely if ever indicated.

In bacterial vaginosis the lactobacilli decrease in number with an overgrowth of other organisms, such as *Gardnerella vaginalis,* anaerobic bacteria, and mycoplasmas. The total number of bacteria increase from 10^4 to 10^{11} per gram of vaginal discharge. Symbiotic metabolism produces aromatic amines such as putrescine, cadaverine, and trimethylamine, which cause the characteristic "dead fish" or "dead mouse" malodorous discharge. Bacterial vaginosis is a noninflammatory condition; patients rarely have significant pain or burning but may have some itching. Approximately half of patients with bacterial vaginosis are asymptomatic.

Patient Evaluation

History. Symptoms of vaginitis include vaginal discharge, itching, burning, and dyspareunia. Symptoms help delineate different forms of vaginitis. Women with *C. albicans* typically have a white, clumpy discharge that may have a yeastlike odor. Itching and to a lesser degree burning are the primary complaints. Women with a noncandidal fungal infection often have less discharge and have more burning than itching. Women with bacterial vaginosis have an increased or different discharge that is gray and malodorous. Because bacterial vaginosis is noninflammatory, patients usually do not have the degree of itching seen with candidal infections. *T. vaginalis* causes an intense inflammatory response with pain, edema, and purulent discharge. Symptoms overlap greatly, however, and the diagnosis of vaginitis cannot be made from symptoms alone.

Other important elements of the history include duration of symptoms, prior episodes, including prior therapies and results; associated conditions and other illnesses or infections; antibiotic use or other medications; and any conditions or medications that could cause immunosuppression. Prior therapies should include prescription, over-the-counter (OTC), alternative, and home remedies. Many patients will have used OTC or alternative therapies. Patients with vaginitis may have developed a secondary inhibited sexual desire from dyspareunia. Although this complication is uncommon with acute vaginitis, it is common in women with chronic vaginitis. Patients with chronic or recurrent vaginitis should be asked about inhibited sexual desire.

Physical Examination. The general examination should document any dermatitis or signs of other infections. Pelvic examination should document any skin changes of the external genitalia and the amount and character of any vaginal discharge. The cervix should be examined for discharge. The remainder of the pelvic examination is completed as usual.

Diagnosis

Diagnostic Procedures. Microscopy is the cornerstone of diagnosis. A wet mount can be prepared by taking a swab from the junction of the upper third and lower two thirds of the vaginal side wall and placing the swab in a small test tube containing three drops of normal saline. The swab is then rotated to obtain a uniform suspension. A wet mount and a 10% potassium hydroxide (KOH) preparation can then be made at microscopy. The vaginal pH can be measured by using narrow-range pH paper from the swab. The wet mount and KOH prep should be examined under both low and high power. The saline mount should be examined for motile trichomonads and for *clue cells,* epithelial cells coated with coccobacilli. The KOH prep is examined for hyphae and buds. Gram's stain of the vaginal smear is easily prepared in the office, with the types of bacteria quantified to make the diagnosis of bacterial vaginosis.

Vaginal cultures are rarely indicated. Cultures are used only if the appropriate transport media are available, if the laboratory can isolate the organisms of interest, and if qualitative culture results are available. Fungal cultures may be indicated for recurrent or persistent infections.

Vulvar biopsy should be performed if the vulvar skin has visible lesions. Postmenopausal women who are diagnosed with atrophic vaginitis but do not respond to estrogen should have a vulvar biopsy if another cause cannot be determined.

Differential Diagnosis. The diagnosis of *bacterial vaginosis* can be made by meeting three of the following four criteria: (1) thin, gray, malodorous discharge that adheres to vaginal wall, (2) elevated vaginal pH (over 4.5), (3) clue cells and decreased lactobacilli, and (4) positive "whiff" test (release of amine odor with addition of KOH).

Fungal vaginitis presents with itching and burning and a thick, white, "cottage cheese" discharge. Microscopy shows the presence of hyphae or buds. The pH is usually normal (3.8 to 4.4).

Trichomoniasis presents with a copious, purulent discharge that may have an amine or foul odor. The patient usually has erythema and edema of the vagina and vulva. The pH is usually elevated (over 4.5). Microscopy reveals the presence of motile trichomonads.

Atrophic vaginitis may present with a reddened, inflamed vagina or with a pale, thin mucosa. Patients may have pain or itching. The pH is usually elevated. Microscopy reveals intermediate and parabasal epithelial cells that have a round shape and large nuclei.

Vulvar dystrophies may present with itching or burning. Symptoms are usually limited to the vulva, and the vulvar skin appears abnormal. Vaginal discharge is normal.

Vulvar vestibulitis is a rare condition characterized by inflammation of the minor vestibular glands. Physical findings are erythema of the vestibule and extreme tenderness to light touch of the vestibule.

Vulvodynia is a symptom and means "painful vulva." Conditions that cause vulvodynia include chronic fungal infections, vestibulitis, and neuropathic (essential) vulvodynia.

Management

The key step in management of vaginitis is establishing a correct diagnosis (Table 46-2). Management of uncomplicated vaginitis is usually straightforward.

Bacterial Vaginosis. Bacterial vaginosis is treated with either oral or vaginal metronidazole or clindamycin. Women who do not respond to these therapies may be treated with other oral antibiotics active against anaerobes or with intravaginal sulfas. Treatment of sexual partners has not been shown to increase the success of therapy or decrease the risk of recurrence of bacterial vaginosis. *Gardnerella vaginalis* can be isolated from the prostatic secretions of sexual contacts of women with bacterial vaginosis, however, and some advocate treatment of sexual partners in cases of recurrent bacterial vaginosis.

Fungal Vaginitis. Initial therapy of fungal vaginitis is vaginal imidazoles or triazoles. One-day, 3-day, or 7-day therapies appear to be equally effective, and symptom resolution occurs at approximately the same rate, 3 to 5 days after beginning therapy. Oral fluconazole, 150 mg as a single dose, seems as effective as vaginal preparations.

The treatment of women who do not respond to initial therapy or who have recurrent cyclic candidal vaginitis has not been established. Some of these patients may respond to intravaginal boric acid (600 mg for 10 nights). The boric acid can be compounded into a water-based suppository or placed in a number-three gelatin capsule. Noncandidal strains are often resistant to imidazoles and may respond to boric acid, high-dose triazoles (e.g., itraconazole, 200 to 400 mg/day for 14 days), intravaginal gentian violet, oral terbinafine (Lamisil), oral ketaconozole (200 mg/day for 14 days), or rarely, intravaginal 5% amphotericin B cream. These latter therapies are not approved by the U.S. Food and Drug Administration (FDA) and should be used only after consultation.

Table 46-2. Recommended Treatment for Various Types of Vaginitis

Type	Initial therapy	Secondary therapy
Bacterial vaginosis	Metronidazole, 500 mg orally twice a day for 7 days *or* Clindamycin cream 2%, one full applicator (5 gm) intravaginally at bedtime for 7 days *or* Metronidazole gel 0.75%, one full applicator (5 gm) intravaginally twice a day for 5 days	Metronidazole, 2 gm orally in a single dose *or* Clindamycin, 300 mg orally twice a day for 7 days
Fungal vaginitis	Butoconazole 2% cream, 5 gm intravaginally for 3 days *or* Clotrimazole 1% cream, 5 gm intravaginally for 7-14 days *or* Clotrimazole, 100-mg vaginal tablet for 7 days or two tablets for 3 days *or* Clotrimazole, 500-mg vaginal tablet *or* Miconazole 2% cream, 5 gm intravaginally for 7 days *or* Miconazole, 200-mg vaginal suppository for 3 days *or* Miconazole, 100-mg vaginal suppository for 7 days *or* Nystatin 100,000-unit vaginal tablet for 14 days *or* Tioconazole 6.5% ointment, 5 gm intravaginally in single application *or* Terconazole 0.4% cream, 5 gm intravaginally for 7 days *or* Terconazole 0.8% cream, 5 gm intravaginally for 3 days *or* Terconazole, 80-mg vaginal suppository for 3 days *or* *Oral agent:* Fluconazole, 150-mg oral tablet	Boric acid, 600 mg intravaginally for 10 nights *or* Ketoconazole 200 mg orally for 10 nights *or* Itraconazole 200-400 mg orally for 10 nights
Trichomoniasis	Metronidazole, 2 gm in single dose	Metronidazole, 500 twice a day for 7 days
Atrophic vaginitis	Vaginal estrogen	Oral estrogen

Trichomoniasis. Metronidazole is the only FDA-approved drug that is active against *T. vaginalis.* Various regimens have been recommended, and all appear to have 90% to 95% efficacy. It is important to treat all sexual partners to prevent reacquisition of the organism.

Atrophic Vaginitis. The primary treatment of atrophic vaginitis is oral or vaginal estrogen. Women who develop atrophic vaginitis progress from a normal, pink vaginal epithelium to a red, inflamed epithelium and then a pale, thin vaginal mucosa. With treatment the process reverses; women with a pale, thin epithelium develop a red epithelium that may itch because of increased blood supply to the vagina. Because patients may interpret this process as an allergy or irritation and stop the medication, they should be told to continue the treatment and that the process will continue to a normal, pink vagina.

Consultation and Hospitalization. Hospitalization is rarely indicated for vaginitis. Consultation should be considered for women who (1) fail initial therapy, (2) do not have a clear diagnosis, (3) have repeated recurrences, (4) have vulvar dystrophies or vulvar vestibulitis, and (5) have associated sexual dysfunctions.

Special Issues

Pregnancy. A variety of vaginal and cervical infections have been associated with preterm birth or low birth weight. Studies have shown an association between bacterial vaginosis and preterm birth, but randomized clinical trials have failed to show that treatment prevents preterm birth. *T. vaginalis* has also been associated with preterm birth, but no data show a reduced risk of preterm birth after treating trichomoniasis. Programs to screen and treat women for vaginal infections should not be undertaken until data from randomized clinical trials show a benefit of treatment.

HIV Infection. Recurrent fungal vaginitis can be the first symptom of HIV infection. Women with HIV infection are more likely to have fungal vaginitis and to be infected with noncandidal strains and are less likely to respond to standard antifungal agents. Fungal vaginitis does not appear to increase the risk of mother-to-infant transmission of HIV or of heterosexual transmission of HIV.

Bacterial vaginosis is also associated with HIV infection in both pregnant and nonpregnant women. It is not clear whether HIV leads to increased risk for bacterial vaginosis, or vice versa, or if both are associated with other STDs.

ADDITIONAL READINGS

American College of Obstetricians and Gynecologists: *Vaginitis,* Technical bulletin 226, Washington, DC, 1996, The College.

American College of Obstetricians and Gynecologists: *Antibiotics and gynecologic infections,* Educational bulletin 237, Washington, DC, 1997, The College.

Centers for Disease Control and Prevention: 1998 Guidelines for treatment of sexually transmitted diseases, *MMWR* 47(RR-1), 1998.

II Psychiatric, Psychosocial, and Behavioral Issues

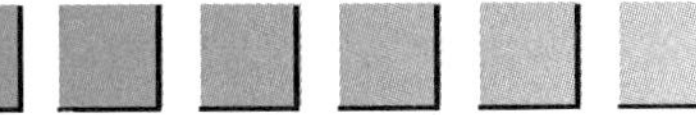

CHAPTER 47

Mental and Behavioral Disorders in Primary Care: Bridging the Gap

Steven A. Cole

Mental disorders in primary care are common, the source of significant suffering and disability, and often unrecognized or undertreated. Furthermore, primary care physicians often find that patients with mental or behavioral disorders can be personally troubling to them and emotionally difficult to manage. This section of the text focuses on these common conditions, with particular emphasis on the basic principles of assessment and management for the primary care practitioner.

Although each of the other chapters in the section reviews a particular problem in depth, this introductory chapter takes a broader perspective. Regardless of the specific psychiatric diagnosis, most patients with mental and behavioral disorders in primary care present the following difficulties for the practitioner:

- Somatic presentation
- Difficulty understanding and accepting that mental disorders usually cause physical suffering
- Reluctance to accept a psychiatric diagnosis because of stigma
- Reluctance to accept psychiatric consultation/referral/collaboration because of stigma
- Emotional reactivity (anger, sadness, anxiety)

This chapter explores pragmatic strategies to address these problems on a generic rather than a case or disease-specific level. Because the common denominator of difficulty rests on the somatic presentation of mental and behavioral disorders, the assessment and management of unexplained physical complaints will be discussed. These skills function to bridge the gap between disabling and unexplained physical symptoms and the accurate diagnosis and effective treatment for underlying mental or behavioral disorders.

Unexplained physical symptoms account for the vast majority of the presenting complaints in primary care.[5] Many of these complaints are short-lived and are probably the result of multiple biologic and psychosocial etiologies. However, when these unexplained physical symptoms are recurrent, do not fit into recognizable pathophysiologic patterns, and refer to multiple organ systems, the likelihood that the patient suffers from a mental disorder increases dramatically.[4]

Mental disorders in primary care practice represent significant sources of reversible suffering and disability. Depression alone has been noted by the World Health Organization as the fourth leading cause of medical disability in all ages worldwide. Among individuals aged 15 to 44, it is the single leading cause of medical disability.[6]

In addition, poorly recognized and inadequately treated psychiatric disorders contribute to excess general medical utilization. Early recognition and treatment of mental disorders in primary care can lead to significant improvement in patients' well being and to decreased spending on unnecessary utilization. In addition, patients with mental disorders often present significant frustration for physicians; the physicians struggle with the interpersonal demands of patients who experience the physical discomforts associated with psychiatric disorders, but who do not understand or accept the psychiatric explanation for their distress.

Because of the stigma associated with mental illness, patients with mental disorders often get their only health care from nonpsychiatric physicians. Only about 50% of individuals with mental disorders will get any help at all for their disorders. About 18% of all these individuals go only to primary care physicians for help for their problems and 17% to mental health specialists. Only 3% of the individuals with mental disorders get help from both primary care physicians and mental health specialists.[7] It is likely that this small percentage will increase dramatically as comanagement and collaborative care strategies between primary care and behavioral health specialists increase in the era of managed care and disease management.[3]

Epidemiologic research now documents that many of these disorders are overlooked in busy office practices. Even when they are recognized, the disorders are often inadequately treated or the outcome is suboptimal. The public health message is clear. Medical schools, medical societies, and health care organizations are now devoting increasing resources toward appropriate identification and treatment of medical patients with psychiatric disorders. The barriers to effective integration, unfortunately, remain considerable.[2]

Whether these mental disorders occur alone or in the context of other comorbid physical illnesses, the current health care environment now expects primary care physicians to accrue the knowledge and to master the skills necessary to treat uncomplicated mental disorders or to successfully refer more complicated disorders to behavioral health specialists. This section of the text covers the knowledge base necessary for physicians to diagnose and treat the most common and uncomplicated mental disorders in their medical practices:

depression, anxiety, alcohol and substance abuse, somatoform disorders, and eating disorders.

Unfortunately, although "book" knowledge of these disorders is certainly necessary, it is not sufficient for the primary care physician to take adequate care of his or her patients. Improved care for psychiatric disorders in primary care depends on the development of certain patient management skills, including the ability to:

1. Obtain relevant psychosocial data on all patients
2. Observe and appropriately respond to a patient's verbal and nonverbal cues of emotional distress
3. Transition the data-collection process from the biologic domain to the psychosocial
4. Collect sufficient data to make accurate psychiatric diagnoses
5. Educate the patient to accept a paradigm shift from a general biomedical to biopsychosocial frame of reference
6. Deliver care in a complex biopsychosocial frame of reference for patients who suffer from both general medical and psychiatric morbidity
7. Refer, consult, and collaborate effectively with behavioral health specialists when needed

The rest of this chapter will briefly discuss these seven skills necessary to efficiently assess and manage mental disorders in busy primary care practices. Physicians who desire further training may develop these skills by attending workshops and courses on interviewing skills that are discussed more fully in Chapter 2.

PATIENT MANAGEMENT SKILLS

Obtain Psychosocial Background Data on All Patients

Psychosocial data relating to current life stresses and supports are essential for the effective management of all chronic conditions in primary care (see Chapter 2). In the assessment and management of persistent unexplained physical symptoms, one of the very first objectives of the physician should be to ascertain background psychosocial data (e.g., "Tell me a little about what's happening now in your life, at home and at work" or "What kind of stresses are you under lately?").

Observe Patients Closely and Respond to Verbal and Nonverbal Cues of Emotional Distress

Verbal and nonverbal signals of emotional distress often go unacknowledged in the busy practice of primary care. In the face of unexplained physical symptoms, however, these cues become especially important. When the physician observes, for example, that a patient's head and eyes are downcast, shoulders shrugged, and words punctuated by increased sighing, or if there are tears in the eyes, the physician should use skills of reflection and legitimation, through such comments as "I can see that you feel distressed" (reflection) or "I understand why you feel so distressed. Most people would feel the same way" (legitimation).[1]

Sometimes physicians observe these signs, but are reluctant to acknowledge the feelings because they fear unlocking a Pandora's box of emotions. Acknowledging the patient's emotional distress may lead to the expression of more feelings (e.g., crying) or to more data about life stresses. In the busy office practice, physicians may sometimes consciously avoid this type of inquiry.

The avoidance of these emotional issues is generally a strategic, as well as humanistic, mistake. From the humanistic point of view, patients generally want to be heard and understood by their physicians. Ignoring signs of emotional turmoil leads patients to feel that they are neither understood nor cared about. This leads to patient dissatisfaction, poor partnership, and poor adherence.

From a strategic point of view, addressing emotional concerns early increases overall interviewing efficiency. Skillful attention to the emotional domain of the physician-patient encounter saves time—always in the long run, and almost always in the short-term. The alliance with the patient is secured and less time is wasted on unproductive exploration of other complaints. When emotional cues are ignored, Pandora's box rarely stays closed—it usually builds up pressure from the lack of understanding and explodes in dysfunctional, unpredictable, and inefficient ways. The bane of many physicians mercilessly emerges: the end-of-the-interview, hand-on-the doorknob "Oh, by the way, doctor . . ." comment occurs in at least 20% of all interviews and always causes physicians time and emotional distraction.

In contrast, the skilled interviewer moves gracefully from the physical realm of discourse to the psychosocial and emotional domain, without the catastrophe of unlocking Pandora's box. Focusing the discussion on emotional and psychosocial problems in an empathic way is as important an interviewing skill for the primary care physician as focusing the discussion on physical symptoms.

Move the Data-Collection Process from the Biologic Domain to the Psychosocial

Inquiry about the impact of symptoms on the patient's quality of life can provide a graceful transition. If and when patients with unexplained physical complaints acknowledge distress, it becomes important for physicians to collect information that can rule in or out mental disorders. Transition statements can be helpful in this regard (e.g., "I understand that your stomach pain is your central problem. However, I think I can also help you better if I find out a little more about other symptoms you may be having" or "How has your stomach pain affected your life in general? How are you sleeping . . . how is your energy . . . how is your mood . . . how are things going at home and at work?").

Collect Sufficient Information to Make an Accurate Psychiatric Diagnosis

The disorders described in this section represent medical syndromes that can be diagnosed with relatively clear-cut inclusion and exclusion criteria. It is important that primary care physicians understand the importance of accurate diagnosis in order to implement effective treatment strategies. Because some disorders have labels that are the same as some of their symptoms (e.g., depression causing a depressed mood), it is not hard to confuse the presence of symptoms with the presence of a treatable disorder. Better outcomes will be achieved if rigorous attention is paid to understanding and applying evidence-based diagnostic criteria.

Educate the Patient to Accept a Paradigm Shift From a General Biomedical to Biopsychosocial Frame of Reference

This is the most difficult transition skill that primary care physicians must possess to function efficiently and effectively with patients who present with psychiatric disorders and unexplained physical complaints. These physical complaints are experienced as true physical discomfort; hence if a physician is perceived as trying to "explain away" the physical complaints as secondary to mental disorders, the patient generally and understandably feels discounted and angry, telling the physician that the problem is "not in my head!"

Since the patient does, in fact, experience the problem physically, the physician needs to fully understand and empathize with the patient's frustration. The physician can usually improve the alliance by emphasizing his or her recognition of this experience. It is also often easier to avoid the mind/body dualistic split (i.e., viewing the problem in either the body or mind). Rather, when the physician explains that the problem is in both domains (the body and the emotions), patient acceptance of psychosocial assessment and management usually increases. For example, the following might be said to the patient who suffers from stomach pain and a major depression:

> I certainly understand that you are suffering with these stomach pains. They are certainly not "in your head." At the moment, unfortunately, I do not have a definite answer and all your lab tests and other studies are normal at the present time. I am not concerned at the present time that I am missing an important physical problem. I will watch you closely, prescribe appropriate symptomatic treatment, and send you for other medical tests as necessary.
>
> In the meantime, however, I also think you are suffering from a lot of stress and a related depression. I would like for you to work with me in thinking about appropriate treatment for that condition as well. In my experience, when we find effective treatment for the depression, the stomach pain often becomes more manageable and somewhat less troubling.

This approach often works better than arguing that the stomach pain is caused by a depression. For patients who experience actual physical pain, accepting the possibility that treatment of a mental disorder can actually cure a distant physical pain requires an extraordinary leap of faith because it flies in the face of the patient's own bodily experience and interpretation of reality. From a strategic point of view, it is usually better to maintain an agnostic wait-and-see approach concerning the possible relationship between an unexplained physical symptom and a treatable mental disorder such as depression.

Operate in a Complex Biopsychosocial Frame of Reference for Patients Who Suffer From Both General Medical and Psychiatric Morbidity

Many patients with chronic medical problems also suffer from comorbid mental disorders (e.g., many patients with coronary artery disease and Parkinson's disease also have depression). It is essential that physicians avoid colluding in or promoting the "fallacy of good reasons." That is, physicians should not reinforce the maladaptive point of view that their patients may have "good reasons to be depressed." The good reasons argument misserves patients who might otherwise receive effective treatment to reduce suffering, increase quality of life, and quite possibly decrease morbidity and mortality. Patients in severe life stress or with severe physical illness may indeed have good reasons to be sad, but do not have good reasons to explain away and avoid effective treatment for a clinically significant psychiatric disorder (e.g., depression or anxiety).

Refer, Consult, or Collaborate Effectively with Behavioral Health Specialists in the Treatment of Mental Disorders

Disease management studies now suggest that patient outcome improves when primary care patients receive some collaborative care from mental health specialists.[8] Thus, although many patients with uncomplicated mental disorders can be effectively treated in the primary care setting, patients with significant psychiatric and medical comorbidity may need referral, consultation, or collaboration with mental health specialists.

Many patients, unfortunately, do not readily accept referral, consultation, or collaboration with behavioral health specialists. Consultation involves a one-session assessment that has limited impact on patient outcome. Collaborative care, or comanagement, on the other hand, involves serial consultation or ongoing specialty input, which facilitates the shaping of a treatment plan, over time, consistent with the patient's developing need and individual response to treatment. Collaborative care does improve outcome.

Effective and increased collaboration, however, will require overcoming many barriers to integrated care. Therefore, in the interest of developing collaborative care models, it is important that primary care physicians help decrease the stigma and reluctance of patients to accept appropriate help, when needed. Empathy, reassurance, and offers of continued support can be helpful in this regard. For example, a physician might say:

> As you know, I am interested in helping you feel better and overcome this depression. However, I will need some help in making sure that I am treating the correct condition with the correct management strategy and medications. I understand your reluctance, but I really think I can treat you better if you would accept a consultation from a psychiatrist (psychologist/social worker/nurse) colleague of mine who has seen many of my patients. After you see him, I will talk to him about how we can treat you most effectively.

BRIDGING THE GAP

Mental disorders in primary care are common, disabling, and often unrecognized and undertreated. Patients with these disorders are complex and often frustrating for physicians to manage. Much of this difficulty stems from problems related to shifting the frame of reference from the physical/biomedical realm of discourse to a biopsychosocial one. This chapter presents seven basic skills that can help a physician bridge this gap, in the interest of improving the alliance with the patient, to improve assessment, treatment planning, and, ultimately, outcome.

REFERENCES

1. Cole S, Bird J: *The medical interview: the three function approach,* ed 2, St Louis, Mosby. (In Press.)
2. Cole S, Raju M: Overcoming barriers to integration of primary care and behavioral healthcare: focus on knowledge and skills, *Behavioral Healthcare Tomorrow* 5(5):30-37, 1996.
3. Katon W, Von Korff M, Lin E, et al: Stepped collaborative care for primary care patients with persistent symptoms of depression: a randomized trial, *Arch Gen Psychiatry,* 56:1109-1115, 1999.
4. Kroenke K, Jackson JL, Chamberlin J: Depressive and anxiety disorders in patients presenting with physical complaints: clinical predictors and outcome, *Am J Med* 103(5):339-347, 1997.

5. Marple RL, Kroenke K, Lucey CR, et al: Concerns and expectations in patients presenting with physical complaints: frequency, physician perceptions and actions, and 2-week outcome, *Arch Intern Med* 157(13):1482-1488, 1997.
6. Murray C, Lopez A: The global burden of disease: Harvard School of Public Health, World Health Organization, and the World Bank, Boston, 1996, Harvard University.
7. Regier D, Narrow W, Rae R, et al: The de facto US mental and addictive disorders service system, *Arch General Psychiatry* 50:85-94, 1993.
8. Von Korff M, Gruman J, Schaefer J, et al: Essential elements for collaborative management of chronic illness, *Ann Intern Med* 127:1097-1102, 1997.

CHAPTER 48

Mood Disorders

Steven A. Cole

Five mood disorders are of importance to primary care physicians: major depression, dysthymia, adjustment disorder with depressed mood, depression caused by a general medical condition (or substance), and bipolar disorder. Depression is one of the most painful conditions that can afflict an individual. Depressed persons generally report that their depression has caused more suffering than any other problem. Depression is common, disabling, and often unrecognized and untreated in primary care practices. This chapter reviews the epidemiology, diagnosis, and treatment of major depression in detail and briefly discusses other mood disorders.

Major depression (MD) is the most severe form of depression and is associated with considerable disability, morbidity, and mortality. In several careful epidemiologic studies, MD has been associated with as much disability (days in bed; days absent from work; impaired social, role, and interpersonal functioning) as other chronic illnesses, including arthritis and coronary artery disease. In addition, MD is also associated with considerable physical morbidity and mortality, most specifically related to the risk of suicide, but also as a risk factor for poor outcome and death in nursing home patients and those with general medical conditions (e.g., coronary artery disease, traumatic brain injury).

Dysthymia, or "chronic" depression, represents a milder form of depressive illness that does not meet the severity criteria of MD but is marked by considerable chronicity. Dysthymia is diagnosed when a depressed mood and at least two other symptoms of depression are present "most days" during the previous 2 years. Dysthymia can be considered a form of "minor depression" but is itself associated with significant pain and impaired functioning and may not remit spontaneously.

Adjustment disorder with depressed mood describes a psychiatric condition resulting from an identifiable stressor (e.g., divorce, job loss) that represents a level of impairment greater than what could normally be expected for most individuals. It can only be diagnosed within the first 6 months after a stressor has occurred. If the condition lasts longer than 6 months, the diagnosis would change to depressive disorder, NOS (not otherwise specified). A "normal" reaction to a distressing life event should not be diagnosed as an adjustment disorder. If an identifiable stressor precipitates a depressive syndrome that meets the severity criteria for MD, the diagnosis of MD is made (and not adjustment disorder).

Mood disorder caused by a general medical condition (or substance) refers to a psychiatric syndrome that the physician judges to result from the direct physiologic consequence of a general medical condition or medication (e.g., hypothyroidism or reserpine). The treatment should focus on resolution of the underlying general medical problem or withdrawal of the causative medication, but specific psychiatric treatment is also usually needed and recommended.

Bipolar disorder, previously called "manic-depressive" illness, occurs in about 1% of the population and represents a common and quite severe form of mental illness that has a very strong biologic and genetic substrate. About 10% of children who have one parent with bipolar disorder will develop the illness.

EPIDEMIOLOGY AND ETIOLOGY

Most epidemiologic studies indicate that the lifetime prevalence of MD is 5% to 10% in men and 10% to 20% in women. The reasons for these gender differences are unclear; numerous factors point to endocrine and biologic factors, whereas others attribute the differences to sociocultural factors. The 1-year prevalence of MD in the community is 2% to 4% for men and 4% to 8% for women. Studies of medical outpatients demonstrate similar rates, whereas studies of medical inpatients and studies in some diseases thought to predispose biologically (e.g., cerebrovascular accident [CVA, stroke], Parkinson's disease, traumatic brain injury) or psychologically (cancer) indicate much higher rates (10% to 50%). Although clinical lore has long suggested depression is more common in elderly persons, recent epidemiologic findings demonstrate lower 1-year prevalence rates of depression in elderly persons (1% to 2%).

Many patients and physicians consider depression to be "expected" in the face of significant stress. Stressful life events certainly predispose to major depression, but MD is not the uniform outcome (either clinically or statistically) of any stressful event. In fact, studies of individuals under stress (e.g., from terminal cancer, natural disaster) show rates of MD greater than the general population rate, but almost always less than 50%. That is, despite the seriousness of the circumstance, most individuals do not develop an MD syndrome under stress. Sad or depressed affect is an expected accompaniment of a stressful event, but the full syndrome of MD does not uniformly emerge. In this sense, no "good reasons" exist for MD. When such a syndrome develops, it is best considered a major (clinical) depression and not a "reactive depression."

Historically, the term *reactive depression* suggested (1) a mild version of the syndrome; (2) one that resulted entirely from a psychologic precipitant; (3) one that did not have a biologic substrate; and (4) one that should be treated with psychotherapy. None of these four assumptions is true about depressive syndromes precipitated by life events or physical illness. A very severe depressive syndrome can result from a stressful event (just as a myocardial infarction [MI] can result from a stress); a biologically predisposed individual may have MD in response to a life event; a MD resulting from a life stress may develop a biologic substrate; and a MD resulting from a life stress may respond as well or better to biologic therapy than to psychotherapy.

Thus the presence or absence of identifiable precipitants (stressors) is irrelevant to the diagnosis of MD. MD may be precipitated by stressful life events, but the diagnosis should be based only on the presentation of the signs and symptoms of MD. When MD results from a life stress or general medical illness, it is best to consider the MD a dread complication of the stress (or illness) and to diagnose aggressively and treat the depression as a comorbid condition.

Many physical symptoms of MD (see following discussion), such as fatigue, anorexia, and psychomotor retardation, can often be attributed to a comorbid general medical condition such as cancer or Parkinson's disease. This contribution of a general medical illness to the symptom profile of depression often leads physicians to discount their relevance and thus overlook the possibility of a treatable depression. Emerging data and the revised *Diagnostic and Statistical Manual of Mental Disorders,* fourth edition (DSM- IV) criteria for MD point to the importance of including these symptoms in the diagnostic approach to depression in medically ill patients. Although this inclusive approach might tend to overdiagnose MD, studies of CVA, Parkinson's disease, and traumatic brain injury indicate that the problem of overdiagnosis, if it exists, is quite low (about 2%).

PATHOPHYSIOLOGY: BIOPSYCHOSOCIAL MODEL OF DEPRESSION

Because MD is still a syndromal diagnosis, the illness itself probably represents a heterogenous group of disorders, many of which include a variable array of etiologic determinants. No clear anatomic, physiologic, or biochemical lesion has been found that can explain MD. Most investigators agree that MD is a complex biopsychosocial syndrome that, at present, can only be diagnosed on clinical criteria. Many promising studies point to possible etiologic dimensions and suggest future therapeutic interventions.

Research to date indicates mixtures of environmental and biologic factors underlying severe mood disorders. Genetic and family experiences certainly play a role, but not a determining one. Even for bipolar disorder, monozygotic twins share less than a 50% concordance and dizygotic twins about 10% concordance (about the same as siblings). With respect to MD in women, recent data indicate that negative life events also play a significant etiologic role. Animal studies demonstrate that early environmental stress predisposes to biologic and behavioral abnormalities associated with depression that may not emerge until adult life.

Numerous biologic "markers" of depression may underlie MD but do not necessarily "cause" it. An environmental stress may lead to psychic distress, which then precipitates a biologic cascade leading to MD. Although no marker is specific enough for diagnostic use, several markers reliably and statistically differentiate groups with and without MD. Some of these markers include endocrine factors: elevated cortisol, failure to suppress cortisol after the administration of exogenous dexamethasone (DST), blunted response of thyroid-stimulating hormone (TSH) to challenge with thyroglobulin-releasing factor (TRF), and increased growth hormone (GH) response to prolactin. Neurotransmitter levels such as norepinephrine (NE) and serotonin (5-HT) may be altered, but more likely, NE or 5-HT receptor function or number is altered during depression. One marker of altered central nervous system (CNS) 5-HT receptor function is platelet imipramine or platelet paroxetine binding. Sleep physiology is also changed in MD, with an early induction of rapid eye movement (REM) sleep and an overall increase of REM density during sleep. Finally, neuroimaging studies using positron emission tomography (PET) have demonstrated anatomically specific metabolic differences between depressed individuals and control subjects.

Loss of a parent (especially mother) is weakly predictive of future depression, whereas a low level of perceived social support (especially a wife's perception of an unsupportive husband) is predictive of future depression. Recent interpersonal, behavioral, and cognitive approaches to understanding depressive etiology and pathology have also generated important and promising therapeutic approaches, some of which are as effective as medication for the treatment of mild but not severe depression.

PATIENT HISTORY

DSM-IV criteria for MD requires five of nine symptoms for a 2-week period (Box 48-1). One of the nine symptoms must be either a persistent depressed mood or a pervasive anhedonia (loss of interest or pleasure in living). "Persistent" is defined as "present most of the day, nearly every day." Four hallmarks of MD for the purpose of clinical evaluation are (1) depressed mood, (2) anhedonia, (3) physical symptoms (sleep disorder, appetite problem, fatigue, psychomotor changes), and (4) psychologic symptoms (trouble concentrating or indecisiveness, guilt or low self-esteem, and hopelessness). The physical symptoms are important because they are predictive of a good response to biologic treatments. In particular, when middle insomnia is present (awaking at 3 or 4 AM with inability to return to sleep) and when a diurnal variation in mood is present (feeling more depressed in AM), patients are more likely to respond to biologic intervention. The psychologic symptoms are helpful in recognizing MD in patients with general medical illnesses.

Medical Interview

The medical interview is the key to making the diagnosis of MD. Although MD is diagnosed by a positive response to five

Box 48-1. Diagnosis of Major Depression (MD)

Five symptoms from the following list lead to the diagnosis of MD. The symptoms must all have been present most of the time for the last 2 weeks.

1. Depressed mood
2. Anhedonia (lack of interest or pleasure in all or almost all activities)
3. Sleep disorder (insomnia or hypersomnia)
4. Appetite loss, weight loss, appetite gain, or weight gain
5. Fatigue or loss of energy
6. Psychomotor retardation or agitation
7. Trouble concentrating or difficulty making decisions
8. Low self-esteem or guilt
9. Recurrent thoughts of death or suicidal ideation

of nine symptoms, physicians often miss the diagnosis if they do not routinely screen for depression. About 50% of depressed patients are not recognized because of time limitations for the interview, lack of knowledge and skill, fear of "opening Pandora's box," and the stigma associated with psychiatric illness.

Often, nonverbal cues can suggest depression to the busy physician. Downcast eyes, slow speech, wrinkled brow, and tearful looks all express a sad mood. However, a depressed mood is not synonymous with MD. Physicians interested in screening for MD can focus on anhedonia ("What do you do for a good time?") and sleep ("How is your sleep?"). When MD is present, these questions often yield positive responses, despite the patient's focus on other complaints and a tendency to deny depressed mood.

When physicians suspect a psychiatric disorder underlying a presenting physical problem, an open-ended questioning style may help reveal important data early in the interview. When patients indicate emotional distress surrounding a stressful life situation or distress related to a physical symptom, the physician should investigate the emotional issue immediately. Recognizing and treating a major depression early in the course of a general medical evaluation can save much time and expense.

Somatic Presentations

The depressed patient in primary care does not say, "I have a major depression, doctor; please prescribe proper treatment." More often, the patient experiences a somatic problem such as pain (headache, backache), fatigue, insomnia, or spells. The physician should attempt to rule out significant general medical problems and assess depression simultaneously. Developing these skills to evaluate both general medical and psychiatric problems simultaneously can save much time and expense and decrease frustration of both physician and patient.

Resistance (Stigma)

Many patients are reluctant to accept the diagnosis of depression. They do not experience this illness as a psychologic problem, and they often resist their physicians' explanation of a psychiatric problem. There is a stigma to having depression, and patients often think they are to blame. Physicians can help overcome this stigma by explaining that depression is an illness with a biochemical derangement, as in diabetes, and that proper treatment is necessary to restore function. For severe depression, proper treatment is usually biologic. Patients should be told that depression is not their fault and is a common condition. Severe depression does not usually remit on its own, but proper treatment usually ensures a good outcome.

"Pandora's Box"

Many physicians often are reluctant to pursue psychiatric or emotional problems for fear this will open Pandora's box and take an unreasonable amount of time. In fact, when physicians are able to respond appropriately to patients' emotions and recognize psychiatric disorders, the overall amount of time can be decreased. Extended workups for nonspecific physical complaints can be avoided.

Suicide

Suicidal ideation needs to be evaluated in all patients with symptoms of depression. Suicide is one of the top 10 causes of death in all age groups and one of the top three causes in young adults and teenagers. Besides depression, risk factors for suicide include gender (elderly white males are the highest-risk group), alcoholism, psychosis, chronic physical illness, and lack of social support. Clinically, suicidal intent, hopelessness, and a well-formulated plan all indicate high risk. Many patients who eventually commit suicide visit a primary care physician in the months before they take their lives.

The topic of suicidal ideation can be approached gradually with nonspecific questions such as, "Do you ever feel so discouraged that life does not seem worth living?" (Box 48-2). Patients can be asked to elaborate on their answers. Ultimately the physician should ask a very direct question, "Do you ever feel like taking your own life?" Physicians need to be aware that asking about suicide will not increase a patient's risk. To the contrary, inquiries about suicide can reassure the patient and enable the physician and patient together to make a plan to prevent suicide.

Once a patient has admitted to any suicidal ideation, the primary care physician must decide whether emergency psychiatric consultation and hospitalization are necessary. This is a clinical judgment for which no absolute guidelines can be set. Risk factors should be kept in mind, but the clinical evaluation should be primary. If this assessment suggests outpatient management, physicians should consider using a "no suicide contract." Although data on the effectiveness of this technique are not available, it does represent a standard clinical practice that has a high degree of face validity. Patients are simply asked to promise the physician that they will contact the physician (or alternative covering caregiver) if they think they are losing control of a suicidal impulse.

PHYSICAL EXAMINATION

No specific signs on physical examinations indicate depression. Nonverbal cues can be helpful, however, such as furrowed brow, downcast eyes, slow speech, psychomotor retardation or agitation, hand wringing, frequent sighing, and frequent shoulder shrugging. Some general medical conditions may also present with depression or depressive symptoms, such as endocrine problems (hypothyroidism, Cushing's syndrome), Parkinson's disease, and cerebrovascular disease.

Box 48-2. Questions for Suicidal Patient

1. How does the future look to you?
2. Do you ever feel that life is not worth living?
3. Do you sometimes feel it doesn't matter whether you live or die?
4. Have you ever considered taking your own life?
5. Have you developed a plan about how you might kill yourself?
6. Are you willing to promise me that you will call me (or this number) if you feel you cannot control an impulse to take your own life?

LABORATORY STUDIES AND DIAGNOSTIC PROCEDURES

A routine laboratory screen, including complete blood count (CBC), chemistry profile, and urinalysis, should be part of the workup of depression because many general medical illnesses present with the symptoms of depression (e.g., fatigue, poor sleep). Thyroid studies (including TSH) and vitamin B_{12} levels should also be completed on depressed patients to ensure that a metabolic derangement is not leading to depressive symptoms. Unfortunately, these studies only rule out other conditions that may mimic or exacerbate depression. No laboratory studies are yet available to "rule in" MD. In treatment of refractory cases or when indicated by medical history or physical examination, computed tomography (CT), magnetic resonance imaging (MRI), electroencephalography (EEG), or lumbar puncture can be considered, but these studies do not need to be part of the standard workup. In patients over age 40, however, an electrocardiogram (ECG) is usually necessary to rule out conduction disturbances or bradycardia, although this does not usually add to the differential diagnosis.

Screening instruments for depressive symptoms (e.g., Zung Depression Scale, Beck Depression Scale) can be helpful to recognize potential patients and monitor changes. However, these tools rate the severity of symptoms and do not yield diagnoses. A new scale, PHQ-9, is the first paper-and-pencil instrument that yields valid diagnoses as well as provides quantitative severity measures to monitor response to treatment.

DIFFERENTIAL DIAGNOSIS

Psychiatric Disorders

Many other psychiatric disorders present with symptoms similar to depression and can lead to misdiagnosis. Furthermore, depression often presents in addition to another psychiatric disorder. Thus an awareness of the other psychiatric disorders common in primary care is essential. The best way to avoid problems is to evaluate and treat MD if it is present. When another psychiatric condition is also present, treatment must be adapted to account for this comorbidity.

Anxiety Disorders

Anxiety is a ubiquitous symptom in primary care practices. Anxiety is common in MD, and depressive symptoms are common in anxiety disorders. Primary care physicians should be especially aware of generalized anxiety disorder (GAD), panic disorder, and obsessive-compulsive disorder (OCD). Key symptoms of these disorders include long-lasting and pervasive anxiety (GAD), discrete panic attacks, and the presence of unreasonable and disabling behaviors or thoughts (OCD). When MD occurs with GAD, panic, or OCD, a psychiatric referral is generally indicated. Treatment of MD, however, often helps to resolve or improve these other conditions.

Somatoform Disorders

Some patients are "addicted" to their physical problems. For unclear reasons, they focus on body ailments, and reassurance from the physician often does not help. Because depression also presents frequently with unexplained body complaints, the differentiation between a depressive illness and a somatoform disorder (SD) can be quite difficult. Primary care physicians will do best by focusing on the symptoms of MD. When MD is present, despite symptoms of an SD, appropriate treatment of the MD often significantly improves the SD.

Substance Abuse

Alcoholism or other substance abuse problems are common and often disabling conditions that can present with MD. Unlike anxiety disorders or SD, treatment of the MD that is comorbid with alcoholism does not usually relieve the substance abuse problem. Physicians need to evaluate patients for substance abuse and design separate treatment programs when substance abuse is present, whether or not MD is present and treated. In general, physicians should be cautious about treating only MD in the patient with a substance abuse problem. Such an action can be enabling to the substance abuser. Rather, the substance abuse needs aggressive confrontation and treatment.

Personality Disorders

Personality disorders can complicate the diagnosis and treatment of a mood disorder. Because patients with personality disorders can be difficult and demanding, physicians (as with others) often minimize their contacts with such individuals. This may lead to avoiding emotional issues and missing the diagnosis of depression. When MD coexists with a personality disorder, however, effective treatment of the MD often improves functioning, in general, even if the underlying personality disorder is not fundamentally changed. Thus physicians should evaluate the basic symptoms of depression in all distressed individuals, whether or not they have a comorbid personality disorder.

Depression Caused by Condition or Substance

The DSM-IV diagnosis of "depression due to a general medical condition" implies a psychiatric condition that the physician considers to be the direct physiologic result of a condition such as hypothyroidism or hyperthyroidism, pancreatic cancer, Parkinson's disease, and left-sided CVAs (Table 48-1). Because the prevalence of MD is not 100% in any physical illness, the final diagnosis of "depression due to a general medical condition" ultimately must be made on

Table 48-1. General Medical Conditions with High Prevalence Rates of Major Depression

Condition	Prevalence (%)
Alzheimer's disease	0-27
End-stage renal failure	5-30
Parkinson's disease	17-29
Cerebrovascular accident	5-34
Cancer/acquired immunodeficiency syndrome	0-50
Chronic fatigue	10-77
General outpatient	2-16
General inpatient	5-22
Chronic pain	8-57

From Cohen-Cole SA, Kaufman K: *Depression* 1:181, 1993.

clinical inference alone. Unfortunately, no clear criteria can help guide clinicians in this endeavor. When five of nine of the symptoms of MD are present, however, the diagnosis becomes "depression due to a general medical condition, with major depressive episode." Thus, when this diagnosis is made, physicians should indicate the presence of a major depressive episode, whether or not it is presumably caused by another general medical condition. Furthermore, when this severity criterion is reached, data seem to indicate that standard treatments for MD should be used and are effective.

Similarly, DSM-IV recognizes that depression can be caused by exogenous medications (Box 48-3). The prototype of this condition is reserpine, which has long been known to cause a severe depressive condition in 15% of patients. No medication has been noted to "cause" depression in all patients. The most important clinical factors are evaluating the history and linking the initiation of depressive symptoms to starting a new medication or changing the dosage.

MANAGEMENT

Patient/Family Education: Overcoming Stigma/Resistance

The stigma associated with depression is so common that primary care physicians should routinely assume that patients and families will resist the diagnosis and its treatment. Most resistance can be managed by clarifying that MD (1) is common, (2) is not the patient's fault, (3) reflects a biologic disorder, (4) causes great suffering, (5) can exacerbate other physical complaints or illnesses, and (6) is treatable. Also, the medication to treat MD corrects biologic disorders and is not addictive.

Enlistment of family or other supports can also be extremely important in gaining patient acceptance of the diagnosis and adherence to treatment. Patients and families can be educated about the relative benefits and costs of medication vs. psychotherapy. For mild MD, psychotherapy (including office counseling by the physician) may be effective. Mild MD may also remit on its own; if the MD has not improved in 2 to 3 months after "watchful waiting" or after formal psychotherapy, however, antidepressant medication is clearly indicated. On the other hand, severe MD responds much more effectively to medication than to psychotherapy. The distinction between mild and severe MD is relative, with no clear-cut criteria. The physician can make this clinical distinction, however, through clinical judgment based primarily on the patient's level of functioning. If functioning remains high and suffering mild, the MD can be considered relatively mild. If suffering is great and functioning impaired, the MD should be considered severe. Often, family, friends, or colleagues are needed to help the physician evaluate the extent of impairment. Patients are often reluctant to admit changes in functioning and may even be unaware of such changes.

Box 48-3. Medications That Can Cause Depression

- Antihypertensives
- Hormones
- Anticonvulsants
- Steroids
- Digitalis
- Antiparkinsonian agents
- Antineoplastic agents
- Antibiotics

Treatment Efficacy

Treatment is usually effective in more than 90% of patients. If the first treatment attempt (psychotherapy, medication, or combination) is not effective, switching medications, changing psychotherapy, or initiating another treatment (e.g., electroconvulsive therapy [ECT]) is almost always effective. Patients should be told that (1) they deserve to feel better; (2) they will probably continue to suffer the same symptoms without treatment; and (3) underlying conditions may also have a worse outcome.

Length of Treatment and Prophylaxis

Biologic treatment of an MD episode should last 6 to 9 months after it has fully remitted. Because approximately 50% of patients with one episode of MD have a recurrence, many should receive prophylactic medication probably should not decrease the chances of recurrence. Patients probably should not receive medication for life after a first depressive episode. Thus, 6 to 9 months after the first episode abates, the physician can begin gradually withdrawing the patient from the medication. Slow tapering over 6 to 8 weeks is preferred.

Once it is recognized that a patient clearly has recurrent major depression (i.e., at least three episodes), research now supports the concept of prophylactic antidepressant treatment to decrease the likelihood of recurrence. The data support chronic use of the full treatment dosage of antidepressant medication.

Role of Physician Support

The importance of the physician-patient relationship cannot be overemphasized. The physician must convey a feeling of concern for the patient to be willing to discuss personal and distressing life issues, including suicidal feelings. The effective physician also must be skilled at the recognition and management of emotional distress in patients. Many physicians possess some of these skills, and literature and workshops are available for further training.

Regular visits are essential for the proper care of the depressed patient. Brief weekly visits (or biweekly) are usually indicated at the start of treatment to evaluate dosage, side effects, and changes in condition. Instead of weekly visits, weekly phone contacts can be substituted. Patients should generally not receive more than 1 week's supply of a medication that can be lethal in overdose. Once the patient has stabilized on a medication, monthly visits are important for support. If chronic prophylactic treatment is necessary, quarterly visits are usually appropriate, if the depression itself has remitted.

Role of Psychotherapy

Short-term (12 to 16 weeks) interpersonal, cognitive, and behavioral therapies have demonstrated efficacy for the treatment and prophylaxis of depression. Short-term "problem-solving" therapy (four sessions of 30 minutes each) has shown promise for depressed patients in primary care settings. Such treatment is as effective as medication for patients with mild MD but generally not as effective as medication for severe MD. Psychotherapy may also help prevent recurrences.

Office counseling by the primary care physician may be helpful to many patients. The physician should clarify that the patient is not being offered formal psychotherapy (unless the physician has such training). Physicians who become involved in complex interpersonal issues or notice that strong feelings (positive or negative) emerge in either the patient or themselves during office counseling should consider supervision or consultation. Psychotherapeutic situations invariably arouse strong emotions in both patients and physicians, and sensitivity to these issues is often essential to good outcomes.

Antidepressant Medications

About two thirds of patients with MD respond to an antidepressant medication within 3 weeks after reaching a therapeutic plasma level. This two-thirds proportion of responders can be increased to 90% by switching initial nonresponders to another class of antidepressants or by using augmentation strategies (e.g., addition of lithium or triiodothyronine). About one third of patients with MD (usually milder forms) improve with a placebo or general support.

Patients treated for MD should keep taking medication for 4 to 9 months after full remission of the syndrome. Patients with recurrent MD should be considered for long-term prophylaxis. When stopping antidepressants, medications should be tapered over 1 to 2 months or more slowly and the dose raised if prodromal symptoms of depression reappear.

Some uncertainty surrounds antidepressant treatment of dysthymia or adjustment disorders (including grief). Data from randomized clinical trials increasingly point to the efficacy of antidepressant medication for the acute treatment and long-term prophylaxis of dysthymia. No good outcome studies, however, have evaluated the treatment of minor depressive episodes, such as adjustment disorders with depressed mood. Emotional support by the physician may be sufficient to resolve an adjustment disorder, but when a patient experiences significant impairment in function (e.g., poor work performance, poor sleep, distressed relationships), an antidepressant may be helpful.

Numerous medications are available to treat depression (Table 48-2). All the agents are equally efficacious, and no particular agent or class has been shown to be more effective in ameliorating certain symptoms of depression, such as agitation or insomnia. No agent has been shown to improve depressive symptoms at a faster rate than other medications. Thus the choice of antidepressant can only be made on issues other than efficacy (e.g., side effects, costs, compliance).

Heterocyclic Medications

The heterocyclic medications include the tricyclics, which have been available since the 1950s, and several other agents that are similar in structure, including maprotiline, amoxapine, and trazodone. The heterocyclic antidepressants are similar in side effects, dosing strategies, and efficacy. Their major advantage over newer agents is their lower cost per unit dosage. Recent pharmacoeconomic studies, however, indicate that total health system expenditures (e.g., total psychiatric and nonpsychiatric outpatient visits, laboratory expenditures) for patients taking tricyclics and for those taking the newer

Table 48-2. Antidepressants: Side Effects, Mechanisms of Action, and Dosages

Antidepressant	Sedation	ACh blockade	Orthostasis	SRI	NRI	Other activity	Dosage
Tricyclics							
Amitriptyline (Elavil)	+++	+++	+++	++	+	0	75-300 mg
Desipramine (Norpramin)	+	+	+	0	+++	0	75-250 mg
Doxepin (Sinequan)	+++	+++	+++	++	+	0	75-300 mg
Imipramine (Tofranil)	++	+++	++	+	++	0	75-300 mg
Nortriptyline (Pamelor)	++	++	++	+	++	0	50-150 mg
SSRIs							
Citalopram (Celexa)	0	0	0	+++	0	0	20-40 mg
Fluoxetine (Prozac)	0	0	0	+++	0	0	20-80 mg
Paroxetine (Paxil)	+	+	0	+++	0	0	20-50 mg
Sertraline (Zoloft)	0	0	0	+++	0	0	50-200 mg
Other new agents							
Bupropion (Wellbutrin)	0	0	0	0	+	DA/NE	150-450 mg
Mirtazapine (Remeron)	+++	0	0	0	0	*	15-45 mg
Nefazodone (Serzone)	++	0	0	+	0/+	$5\text{-}HT_{2A}$†	300-600 mg
Reboxetine (Vestra)	0	0	+	0	+++	0	8-10 mg
Venlafaxine (Effexor)	0	0	0	+++	++	0	75-375 mg

0, None; +, slight; ++, moderate; +++, marked.

SRI, Serotonin reuptake inhibition; *NRI,* norepinephrine reuptake inhibition; *DA/NE,* dopaminergic/noradrenergic activity; *SSRIs,* selective serotonin reuptake inhibitors.

*Blockade of α_2NE, $5\text{-}HT_{2A}$, $5\text{-}HT_{2C}$, and $5\text{-}HT_3$ receptors.

†Blockade of $5\text{-}HT_{2A}$ receptors.

From the John D. and Catherine T. MacArthur Foundation, 1998.

agents are about the same. The newer agents are more expensive, but patients taking tricyclics incur extra costs related to more office visits and more general medical expenditures.

Use of heterocyclic medications requires starting at low doses and gradually building up doses to a therapeutic level. Plasma levels can be followed, but with the exception of nortriptyline, which has a therapeutic window (i.e., levels below and above the window are less likely to lead to remission of depression), blood levels function primarily as crude indicators of whether or not the patient is taking the medication. More importantly, physicians should treat the patient and not the blood level. Many patients with high or low blood levels may do very well clinically. For problematic situations, consultation with psychiatrists expert in psychopharmacology may be advisable. Patients may require up to 3 weeks at a therapeutic blood level to respond fully, so they should be informed that it may take time before they begin to notice any positive effects.

The heterocyclic antidepressants are characterized by varying degrees of problematic side effects. The *anticholinergic* effects include dry mouth, constipation, urinary retention, tachycardia, increased ocular pressure, and confusion. The primary *antihistaminic* effects are sedation and inhibition of gastric acid secretion. These effects have led to use of some antidepressants for urticaria, especially doxepin, which seems to be the most potent. The *antiadrenergic* effects cause postural hypotension, which can be quite dangerous in medically ill or elderly patients. Nortriptyline seems to be the safest of the heterocyclics in this regard. All the heterocyclics (except trazodone) have *quinidine-like* effects, delaying conduction across the bundle of His and increasing the QT interval on the ECG. Patients with bundle branch block and increased conduction from other causes are at risk of higher degrees of heart block when given these medications. This side effect is probably responsible for the high lethality of these drugs in overdose. A corrected QT interval of 0.44 differentiates between low-risk and high-risk patients.

Among the tricyclics, desipramine (a metabolite of imipramine) and nortriptyline (a metabolite of amitriptyline) are the least anticholinergic, the least sedating, and the least likely to cause postural hypotension. Among the heterocyclic medications, trazodone does not cause anticholinergic or conduction problems and has very low lethality in overdose. Trazodone, however, is quite sedating and also causes postural hypotension.

Newer Agents

New agents have revolutionized psychiatric practice, especially for the treatment of depression in patients with comorbid general medical illnesses and in elderly persons. The side effects are so much less toxic and the medication so well tolerated that many patients who were too physically ill to be safely treated in the 1970s and 1980s can now receive antidepressant medication without fear of dangerous side effects. These newer agents seem safe from the standpoint of overdose, with a very low therapeutic index.

The newer agents include four selective serotonin reuptake inhibitors (SSRIs: citalopram, fluoxetine, paroxetine, and sertraline) and four others: bupropion, mirtazapine, nefazodone, and venlafaxine. These agents are remarkably safe for use in elderly patients and those with comorbid general medical illnesses. They do not cause postural hypotension or cardiac conduction delay; antihistaminic and anticholinergic side effects are minimal. Choosing among these agents can be difficult because they are all so well tolerated and effective (see Table 48-2).

Fluoxetine has the longest half-life (24 to 27 hours) and has a long-acting, active metabolite (half-life of 7 days). Doses can be given every other day, and when the drug is being withdrawn, the doses can eventually be given once or twice a week to allow for very smooth tapering. The other SSRIs have half-lives of about 24 hours and have no active metabolites with longer half-lives. This allows once-a-day dosing and rapid washout. The other new agents have shorter half-lives and must be given more than once a day, except for the slow-release form of venlafaxine.

The starting dose of the SSRIs may also be the effective treatment dose, as with fluoxetine (20 mg) and possibly with paroxetine (20 mg) and sertraline (50 mg). Patients not responding to the starting doses of SSRIs after 1 month should be given increased doses. Frail elderly persons and patients with liver disease or other general medical illness require smaller starting doses. One-half the recommended starting dose in this population is usually preferred. The SSRIs inhibit various isoenzymes of the cytochrome P-450 system in the liver, thus potentially leading to the buildup of other medications metabolized in the liver, such as anticonvulsants, digitalis, and coumadin. To avoid potentially dangerous pharmacokinetic interactions, it may be necessary to monitor blood levels or clinical indicators of toxicity.

The SSRIs sometimes cause side effects such as anxiety, insomnia, gastrointestinal distress, agitation, and sexual difficulties. With the exception of sexual difficulties, which may occur in 30% to 50% of patients, these side effects occur in less than 20% of patients, are usually mild, and do not lead to discontinuation of medication. Adjunctive use of a sedating antihistamine (diphenhydramine, hydroxyzine), a sedating antidepressant (trazodone, doxepin), or an anxiolytic (lorazepam, clonazepam) can be helpful. These adjuncts can usually be discontinued after a short time, although continued treatment with two agents may be indicated. If a long-acting benzodiazepine (clonazepam) is used in elderly persons, care must be exercised to avoid buildup of medication over time, which can lead to confusion, sedation, or falls after several weeks of treatment.

Among the newer agents, *venlafaxine* and *bupropion* have effects similar to those of the SSRIs. In doses greater than 300 mg, venlafaxine can cause persistent blood pressure elevation in about 10% of patients. Bupropion also has been associated with a 1% to 4% prevalence of seizures, which is a very low overall risk but probably slightly more common than with other antidepressant medications. The medication must be given in divided doses because of its short half-life, should not be given to individuals at risk for seizures (e.g., head trauma), and should never be administered in any single dose greater than 150 mg. The starting dose (75 mg two or three times a day) should be increased slowly (once a week) to therapeutic levels of 300 to 450 mg/day to minimize the risk of seizures. The medication should also not be given to bulimic patients (patients who gorge food and often induce vomiting) because of a possible increased seizure risk.

Nefazodone is a new serotonergic agent that blocks a postsynaptic serotonin receptor, in addition to being a weak inhibitor of serotonin reuptake. It is more sedating than pure SSRIs, but it does not cause sexual side effects and may be more effective than SSRIs and other newer agents in preserving normal sleep architecture. Because of its anxiolytic properties, nefazodone can often be used as monotherapy for patients with depression and coexisting anxiety. *Mirtazapine* blocks several serotonin receptions and adrenergic receptors. It shares the benefits of a favorable side effect profile, with the exception of causing sedation and weight gain. All four newer non-SSRI agents can be used as alternatives to the SSRIs for patients who develop sexual side effects. Nefazodone and mirtazapine can be useful for patients with anxiety.

Elderly and Medically Ill Patients

As noted, the newer agents have generally become the drugs of choice in elderly and medically ill patients. Among the heterocyclics, the safest agents are nortriptyline and desipramine, which are still widely used in these patients. They also seem to have a role in the treatment of refractory depression.

Dosing strategies in elderly and medically ill patients need to "start low and go slow." From the pharmacokinetic point of view (i.e., absorption, metabolism, and elimination; the effect of the body on medication), these agents are metabolized more slowly in these two groups. Accumulation and toxicity can become a problem. Protein binding is also lower in these patients because albumin levels are lower; this can lead to toxic effects. Similarly, lower doses may lead to efficacious treatment. Pharmacodynamic differences (i.e., impact of the medication on the body) in elderly persons can also lead to toxicity or efficacy at lower-than-expected doses.

Electroconvulsive Therapy

ECT is still the most effective treatment available for the treatment of depression. Although many patients and physicians have prejudices and fears about ECT, new methodologies of administration have shown ECT to be a safe and effective treatment modality. In frail elderly persons, ECT can be safer than antidepressants. Some reversible short-term memory loss is a common side effect, but this reverts to normal in virtually all patients. ECT can be lifesaving and should not be denied to patients because of lack of understanding or unrealistic fear.

ECT does not lead to permanent remission of depression in patients susceptible to recurrence. Patients with recurrent depression who receive ECT should receive either prophylactic medication or maintenance ECT, about once a month on an outpatient basis.

Referral

The clinical criteria for referral to a psychiatrist or other mental health specialist depend greatly on the experience and expertise of the primary care physician. In general the most common reasons for referral are lack of response to initial treatment, suicidal ideation, or psychosis. Physicians can inform patients early that referral to a mental health specialist is sometimes needed; this can make referral at a later stage much more acceptable. Because partial remission often occurs, physicians should establish clear indications of predepression functioning, and the patient who does not return to baseline functioning should be referred to a specialist.

ADDITIONAL READINGS

Cole S, Bird J: *The medical interview: the three function approach, ed 2,* St Louis, 2000, Mosby.

Cohen-Cole SA, Kaufman K: Major depression in physical illness: diagnosis, prevalence, and antidepressant treatment (a ten-year review: 1982-1992), *Depression* 1:181, 1993.

Depression Guideline Panel: *Depression in primary care,* vol 1, Detection and diagnosis, Clinical practice guideline no 5, Rockville, Md, 1993, US Department of Health and Human Services.

Depression Guideline Panel: *Depression in primary care,* vol 2, Treatment of major depression, Clinical practice guideline no 5, Rockville, Md, 1993, US Department of Health and Human Services.

Spitzer RL, Kroenke K, Williams JBW: Validation and utility of a self-report version of PRIME-MD: the PHQ primary care study, *JAMA* 282:1737-1744, 1999.

Stahl S: Selecting an antidepressant by using mechanism of action to enhance efficacy and avoid side effects, *J Clin Psychiatry* 59(suppl 18):23, 1998.

Wulson LR, Vaillant GE, Wells VE: A systematic review of the mortality of depression, *Psychosom Med* 61:6, 1999.

CHAPTER 49

Anxiety and Anxiety Disorders

David M. Benedek

Charles C. Engel, Jr.

Anxiety may be defined as a diffuse and unpleasant sense of apprehension and restlessness. Often the main symptoms of anxiety are physical, such as headache, tremor, chest tightness, palpitations, stomach discomfort, or perspiration (Table 49-1). When overlooked, minimized, misdiagnosed, or mismanaged, these symptoms can become enigmatic, frustrating, costly, and disabling. *Normal anxiety* is a universal experience, an adaptive response to new or threatening situations that allows a person to take appropriate preventive measures. Less often, anxiety becomes pathologic, interfering with social, occupational, or interpersonal functioning because of its timing, intensity, or duration. If anxiety assumes certain disabling patterns for an individual, it may be diagnosed as a disorder. *Disabling anxiety* may also be a manifestation of other problems, such as another psychiatric disorder, a general medical condition mimicking a psychiatric disorder (see Table 49-3), or the undesired effects of a medication or drug of abuse.

Disabling anxiety, although less common than normal anxiety, is surprisingly prevalent among people seeking health care. A basic understanding of its natural history, differential diagnosis, clinical features, and primary care management can improve the physician's effectiveness when addressing anxiety-related complaints or determining the need for specialist collaboration or referral.

EPIDEMIOLOGY

Anxiety disorders are among the most common psychiatric disorders in the general population (Box 49-1). The National Comorbidity Study reported that one in four people meets diagnostic criteria for at least one anxiety disorder during

The views expressed in this article are those of the authors and do not reflect the official policy or position of Walter Reed Army Medical Center, the Department of the Army, Uniformed Services University, the Department of Defense, or the U.S. Government.

Table 49-1. Physical Manifestations of Anxiety and Anxiety Disorders

Symptom	Manifestations
Muscular tension	Trembling or twitching
	Muscle aches or soreness
	Feeling "shaky," "tense," or "restless"
Autonomic stimulation	Palpitations or accelerated heart rate
	Diaphoresis, including cold or clammy hands
	Flushing, chills
	Dizziness, lightheadedness
	Dry mouth
	Difficulty swallowing
	Nausea, stool changes, stomach discomfort
	Urge to urinate
Cognitive arousal	Feeling "keyed up" or "on edge"
	Easily startled
	Difficulty concentrating, "blanking out"
	Irritability
	Difficulty falling asleep or maintaining sleep

Box 49-1. DSM-IV* Anxiety Disorders

Generalized anxiety disorder
Panic disorder
Panic disorder with agoraphobia
Agoraphobia without panic attacks
Obsessive-compulsive disorder
Acute stress disorder
Posttraumatic stress disorder
Social phobia
Simple phobia
Anxiety disorder not otherwise specified

**Diagnostic and statistical manual of mental disorders*, ed 4.

Box 49-2. Screening Questions for Anxiety Disorders

1. *Generalized anxiety disorder:* Would you describe yourself generally as a nervous person? Are you a worrier? Do you feel nervous or tense?
2. *Panic disorder:* Have you ever had a sudden attack of rapid heartbeat or rush of intense fear, anxiety, or nervousness? Did anything seem to trigger it?
3. *Agoraphobia:* Have you ever avoided important activities because you are afraid you will have a sudden attack like the one I just asked you about?
4. *Social phobia:* Some people have strong fears of being watched or evaluated by others. For example, some people seldom eat, speak, or write in front of people for fear they will embarrass themselves. Is anything like this a problem for you?
5. *Specific phobia:* Some people have strong fears or phobias about things like heights, flying, bugs, and snakes. Do you have any strong fears or phobias?
6. *Obsessions:* Some people are bothered by intrusive, silly, unpleasant, or horrible thoughts that keep repeating over and over. For example, some people have repeated thoughts that they will hurt someone they love even though they don't want to; that a loved one has been seriously hurt; that they will yell obscenities in public; or that they are contaminated by germs. Has anything like this troubled you?
7. *Compulsions:* Some people are bothered by doing something over and over that they cannot resist, even when they try. They might wash their hands every few minutes, or repeatedly check to see that the stove is off or the door is locked, or count things excessively. Has anything like this been a problem for you?
8. *Acute stress and posttraumatic stress disorder:* Have you ever seen or experienced a traumatic event when you thought your life was in danger? What happened?

Modified from Zimmerman M: *Diagnosing DSM-IV psychiatric disorders in primary care settings: an interview guide for the nonpsychiatrist physician*, Philadelphia, 1994, Psych Products Press, pp 4-7.

their lifetime and that the 12-month prevalence of anxiety disorder is 17.7%. The PRIME-MD 1000 study found that 18% of patients presenting to primary care physicians meet criteria for at least one anxiety disorder. In general, women are twice as likely to experience anxiety disorders as men. Anxiety disorders, particularly panic disorder, are strongly associated with frightening physical symptoms and heightened patient concerns regarding physical illness. Despite physician reassurances, patients with anxiety frequently attribute autonomic symptoms to catastrophic medical problems and make multiple visits to emergency or ambulatory care settings. Anxiety disorders frequently go unrecognized, and patients may see numerous physicians and receive many unnecessary diagnostic tests before the correct diagnosis is made. Physicians must actively poll patients for prototypical anxiety symptoms to make the appropriate diagnosis (Box 49-2). When an anxiety disorder is present, treatment is usually best initiated empirically and without delay, since it can be easily discontinued if another medical problem is uncovered.

PATHOPHYSIOLOGY

Regardless of diagnostic category or classification, the etiology of anxiety symptoms is complex and stems from multiple factors. Contributors include biologic abnormalities and genetic predisposition, behaviorally conditioned or learned responses, and both conscious and unconscious psychosocial stressors.

Psychologic Theories

Freud originally posited that anxiety stemmed from unconscious sexual tension. Later he viewed anxiety as a "signal" communicating the presence of danger in the unconscious. This is similar to current behavioral or social-learning theories that view anxiety as a conditioned response to environmental stimuli. For example, a passenger may escape from a serious automobile accident with minor injuries but experience tremendous fear, anxiety, and autonomic hyperactivity during the event. Consequently, this person may develop mistrust for the driving of others or suffer panic attacks when riding in a car. Cognitive psychology might

Table 49-2. Substances and Medications Associated with Anxiety

Class	Examples	Comments
Vitamins or "foodstuffs"	Niacin	Causes flushing
	Ginseng	Contains ephedrine
Over-the-counter preparations	Alcohol	Associated with withdrawal
	Diet pills	Contain stimulants
	Cough/cold preparations	
	Laxatives	
	Caffeine	
Prescription medications	Thyroid preparations	
	Theophylline preparations	
	Hypoglycemic agents	Hypoglycemia may mimic anxiety.
	β-Agonists	
	Antidepressants	Paradoxic responses
Controlled prescription medicines	Stimulants (methylphenidate, dextroamphetamine)	Typically during intoxication or immediately after intoxication
	Benzodiazepines, other central nervous system (CNS) depressants	Typically during withdrawal (as with alcohol)
	Narcotic analgesics	Withdrawal more than intoxication
Illicit substances	Ketamine	Occasionally used as preanesthetic
	MDMA ("ecstasy")	Intoxication with most illicit substances (except CNS depressants) may present as anxiety.
	Cocaine	
	Phencyclidine (PCP)	
	Inhalants	
	LSD ("acid"), mescaline, psilocybin (mushrooms), other hallucinogens	Flashbacks and "bad trips" result in symptoms.

view this as an example of *cognitive distortion*. Because of the recent and traumatic nature of the accident, the victim overestimates (distorts) the likelihood of another accident occurring and consequently overreacts to the possibility with disabling anxiety symptoms when driving.

Biologic Theories

The observation that anxiety is frequently accompanied by observable signs of autonomic nervous system (ANS) hyperactivity (e.g., tremor, diaphoresis) has led to theories relating ANS dysregulation to the pathogenesis of anxiety disorders. Subsequent studies have demonstrated that ablation of the locus ceruleus (a brainstem site where noradrenergic cell bodies are localized) inhibits the ability of primates to form a fear response. Studies also show that β-adrenergic and α_2-adrenergic antagonists increase firing rates of neurons in the locus ceruleus and provoke panic attacks in some individuals, providing further support for such theories. Infusions of sodium lactate may also precipitate panic attacks, leading to the hypothesis that panic involves an excessive centrally mediated respiratory response to hypoxia. Observations that serotonergic and noradrenergic neurons project to similar locations within the limbic system and cerebral cortex and that serotonergic antidepressant medications help in anxiety disorders have prompted investigation into the role of serotonin in the genesis of anxiety. Studies using brain scans suggest abnormalities in regional cerebral blood flow among people with anxiety disorders. Finally, the role of the inhibitory neurotransmitter γ-aminobutyric acid (GABA) in anxiety disorders is strongly supported by the anxiolytic effects of benzodiazepines. These drugs probably decrease anxiety by increasing the activity of the GABA-A receptor.

Studies indicate that heredity contributes to the onset of anxiety disorders by both genetic and environmental mechanisms. Although only about 1% of the general population suffers from panic disorder, approximately half of all patients with panic disorder have at least one affected relative. Other anxiety disorders show similar but less dramatic familial associations.

SPECIFIC DISORDERS

Substance-induced Anxiety Disorder

After phobias, substance use disorders are the most common mental disorders. Virtually all substances of abuse, as well as many prescription medications and over-the-counter preparations, may result in clinically significant anxiety as a result of cumulative effect, intoxication, or withdrawal (Table 49-2). Substance-induced anxiety may take the form of generalized anxiety, panic attacks, obsessive-compulsive symptoms, or phobias. Many patients with anxiety disorders "self-medicate" with drugs of abuse in misguided attempts to feel better. Obtaining a longitudinal history in patients with substance misuse and anxiety can offer clinical evidence regarding which problem is primary.

Anxiety Disorder Due to General Medical Condition

A variety of medical conditions can present with symptoms of anxiety (Table 49-3). Hypothyroidism, hyperthyroidism, hypoglycemia, and vitamin B_{12} deficiencies are among the most common conditions associated with anxiety. Cardiac dysrhythmia or endocrine tumors (e.g., pheochromocytoma) less frequently produce episodic anxiety symptoms. Careful attention to patient history, physical examination, and focused diagnostic testing directed by clinical suspicion is imperative

Table 49-3. Common Medical Conditions Associated with Anxiety

Condition	Comments
Ischemic heart disease	Panic attacks may mimic. Differentiating factors: (1) absence of cardiac risk factors, negative electrocardiogram (ECG), negative exercise stress test; (2) presence of subjective symptoms of anxiety (e.g., "lump in the throat," "feel like I'm going crazy")
Dysrhythmias	ECG or Holter monitoring may differentiate. Dysrhythmia may decrease after anxiety treated.
Mitral valve prolapse	Auscultation and echocardiogram differentiate.
Thyroid disease	Tests for thyroid-stimulating hormone and thyroxine differentiate. Hyperthyroidism or hypothyroidism may present with subjective symptoms of anxiety. Hyperthyroidism may cause panic attacks and persistent anxiety between attacks. Heat intolerance, brittle hair, and hyperreflexia suggest hyperthyroidism.
Pulmonary embolism	Consider in patients with first panic attack, especially those with history of peripheral vascular disease, smokers, and women taking oral contraceptives. Screen with pulse oximetry, chest radiograph, and ECG.
Reactive airway disease	Cough and wheezing on examination differentiates. β-Agonist treatment worsens anxiety.
Bowel/bladder disorders	Gastrointestinal or genitourinary complaints may be caused by anxiety. Tricyclic antidepressants often relieve urinary frequency and loose stools through anticholinergic effects.
Pheochromocytoma (PC)	Headaches, flushing, tachycardia, and sweating more often result from anxiety than PC (i.e., PC very rare, anxiety common). Malignant hypertension, tachycardia, and orthostatic hypotension should prompt laboratory evaluation. Urinary catecholamine metabolites are highly elevated in patients with PC.
Meniere's syndrome and other inner ear diseases	Differentiate true vertigo (spinning sensation) from giddy sensation. Vertigo is common in inner ear disease (lateral nystagmus on examination). Giddiness is typical with anxiety disorders (no nystagmus on examination). Bedside maneuvers sometimes reproduce symptoms and signs of inner ear disease.
Partial complex seizures (temporal lobe epilepsy)	Aura before episode or clouded cognition afterward suggests seizure disorder. Electroencephalogram confirms seizures but is not sensitive.
Excessive caffeine intake or caffeinism	Chronic or heavy consumption of coffee, tea, chocolate, or soda; abstinence syndrome

for anxious patients, especially those with disease risk factors. Treatment of anxiety may proceed as the diagnostic evaluation is undertaken.

Panic Disorder

Panic disorder is diagnosed when a patient experiences one or more panic attacks that occur without environmental provocation (i.e., are "uncued") and are accompanied by at least a month of fear about further attacks or worry about the implications of the attack (e.g., worry about having a heart attack or "going crazy"). One of the most debilitating aspects of panic disorder is the impact of subsequent worry that another panic attack will occur in a public or open space. This fear is called *agoraphobia* and occurs in varying degrees for most people with panic disorder. In extreme cases, patients are so fearful of having an attack they refuse to leave their own homes.

Generalized Anxiety Disorder

Generalized anxiety disorder (GAD) is often chronic; 25% of patients relapse within 1 month of discontinuing a 6- to 12-month course of treatment, and 60% to 80% of patients relapse within a year. Excessive worry or anxiety about several events or activities (e.g., school or work) characterizes GAD. Symptoms occur most days over 6 months or longer and result in significantly impaired functioning. Three of the following six symptoms are necessary: (1) restlessness or feeling "keyed up" or on edge, (2) easy fatigability, (3) difficulty concentrating or mind going "blank," (4) irritability, (5) muscle tension or a feeling of weakness, and (6) sleep disturbance (difficulty falling or staying asleep, restless sleep).

Adjustment Disorder with Anxious Mood

Disabling anxiety within 3 months of an identifiable stressful event suggests an adjustment disorder with anxious mood. If symptoms persist for 6 months or longer after resolution of the stressor, another disorder should be considered. A careful patient history often elicits one or more recent stressful events (e.g., newly diagnosed chronic or terminal illness, job change, divorce, relocation). The temporal association between an event and symptoms as well as the patient's sense that the event contributed to distress help confirm the diagnosis.

Acute Stress Disorder and Posttraumatic Stress Disorder

When a person is involved in an extremely traumatic or catastrophic event (e.g., natural disaster, motor vehicle accident, sexual assault), flashbacks, nightmares, hypervigilance, heightened startle response, and other signs of autonomic arousal may accompany anxiety symptoms. When these symptoms occur within a month of the event and symptoms are not yet persistent beyond 4 weeks, acute stress disorder is diagnosed. When symptoms start more than 4 weeks after the stressful event or persist for more than a month, posttraumatic stress disorder (PTSD) is diagnosed. Chronically poor coping, poor functioning, and substance misuse are often present, frequently predate the traumatic event, and may complicate the diagnosis and management of PTSD.

Obsessive-Compulsive Disorder

Recurrent intrusive thoughts, feelings, or ideas are *obsessions*. Repetitive rituals such as checking, handwashing, or counting are termed *compulsions*. When obsessions and compulsions are extensive and cause marked distress, consume large amounts of time, or create other disability, obsessive-compulsive disorder (OCD) is diagnosed. In persons with OCD, obsessions result in increased anxiety, whereas compulsions are maladaptive attempts to reduce anxiety. Most OCD patients recognize at some point that their obsessions and compulsions are unreasonable or irrational. Because obsessions often manifest violent or sexual themes, and because the compulsions that reduce them have social consequences (e.g., fighting, masturbation), patients may be reluctant to share these symptoms with their physicians. In patients with undiagnosed anxiety symptoms, screening questions regarding obsessions or compulsions may provide the patient "permission" to disclose these symptoms (see Box 49-2).

The Phobias (Social Phobia, Specific Phobia, Agoraphobia)

A *phobia* is an irrational fear that causes the person to avoid the feared object or situation or that produces marked anxiety or panic attacks when the feared object or situation cannot be avoided. Persons with social phobias have excessive fears of humiliation or embarrassment in social settings (e.g., speaking in public, attending a party). Small animals or insects, heights, needles, dentists, and airplane flights are among the more common foci for specific phobias. Persons with panic disorder often develop agoraphobia, the fear of open spaces or public places, as a result of worry that an uncontrollable panic attack will occur in such a location. Agoraphobia may also occur in the absence of panic disorder. Epidemiologic studies have demonstrated that phobias are the most common mental disorder in the U.S. population, 15% of whom acknowledge having one or more phobias during their lifetime. Although phobias are extremely common, on average they are the least disabling of the anxiety disorders. Most persons with phobias either choose to live with them or overcome them without medical attention. For some, however, social or specific phobias may have severe occupational or social consequences.

Mixed Mild Anxiety and Depression

Perhaps the most common primary care presentation associated with anxiety does not meet the formal criteria for any psychiatric disorder. Anxiety occurs along a spectrum of severity and disability, and much recent attention has focused on *subsyndromal* forms of anxiety and depression. The level of disability associated with subsyndromal anxiety is usually less than that associated with the more characteristic anxiety syndromes just described. Because most anxiety encountered in primary care is not associated with a psychiatric disorder, however, the prevalence of subsyndromal anxiety is high, accounts for a large portion of the primary care physician's clinical time, and is associated with the largest proportion of population disability due to anxiety. Similarly, consistently effective management of subsyndromal symptoms and associated psychosocial stressors can have a substantial impact on the average health of the physician's patient panel. The treatment of subsyndromal anxiety and depression is currently the focus of intense, primary care–oriented clinical research.

DIFFERENTIAL DIAGNOSIS

As described, anxiety symptoms often occur normally or as a manifestation of one of the anxiety disorders. In addition, anxiety symptoms may be caused by other psychiatric disorders (e.g., substance use, mood, psychotic personality) or medical illnesses. Fig. 49-1 diagrams a differential diagnostic approach to anxiety. The first step is to determine whether anxiety symptoms are caused by illicit or prescription substance use. The following questions help discriminate a causal from a coincidental relationship:

1. Is there an association between the substance of concern and anxiety symptoms? Is the association consistent over time? Is it consistent across methods of estimating the severity of substance use (e.g., laboratory vs. reported use)? The more consistent and striking the association between symptoms and substance use, the more likely a causal link exists.
2. Is there a dose-response relationship between the substance of concern and anxiety symptoms? Does the history suggest that periods of more extensive substance use are marked by more severe anxiety symptoms? If so, a substance-induced disorder is more likely.
3. Which comes first, the anxiety symptoms or use of the substance of concern? If anxiety typically precedes substance use, a substance-induced disorder is less likely.
4. Is a causal relationship between the substance and anxiety biologically plausible? For example, stimulant intoxication and alcohol withdrawal are more plausible causes of anxiety than is alcohol intoxication.

The only clinically reliable method of diagnosing a substance-induced anxiety disorder is to observe reduced anxiety after an extended period without the substance of concern. Often, however, significant anxiety symptoms persist despite discontinuation of the suspected substance, or discontinuation of the suspected substance is not possible or feasible.

Next the physician should consider the physiologic relationship between anxiety symptoms and any coexisting medical illness. The same clinical clues used to determine the relationship between substances and anxiety (plausibility, timing, consistency and strength of association, dose-response relationship) are useful for determining whether a given medical condition is causally related to anxiety symptoms. As with substance-induced anxiety, anxiety due to a general medical condition is confirmed if improving the status of the condition consistently reduces anxiety. If no comorbid medical problems exist, if significant anxiety symptoms persist despite the improved status of coexisting conditions, or if improvement of the medical condition is not possible or feasible, the physician should manage the anxiety as a symptom of a primary psychiatric disorder.

Before considering an anxiety disorder as the primary cause of symptoms, the physician should consider other

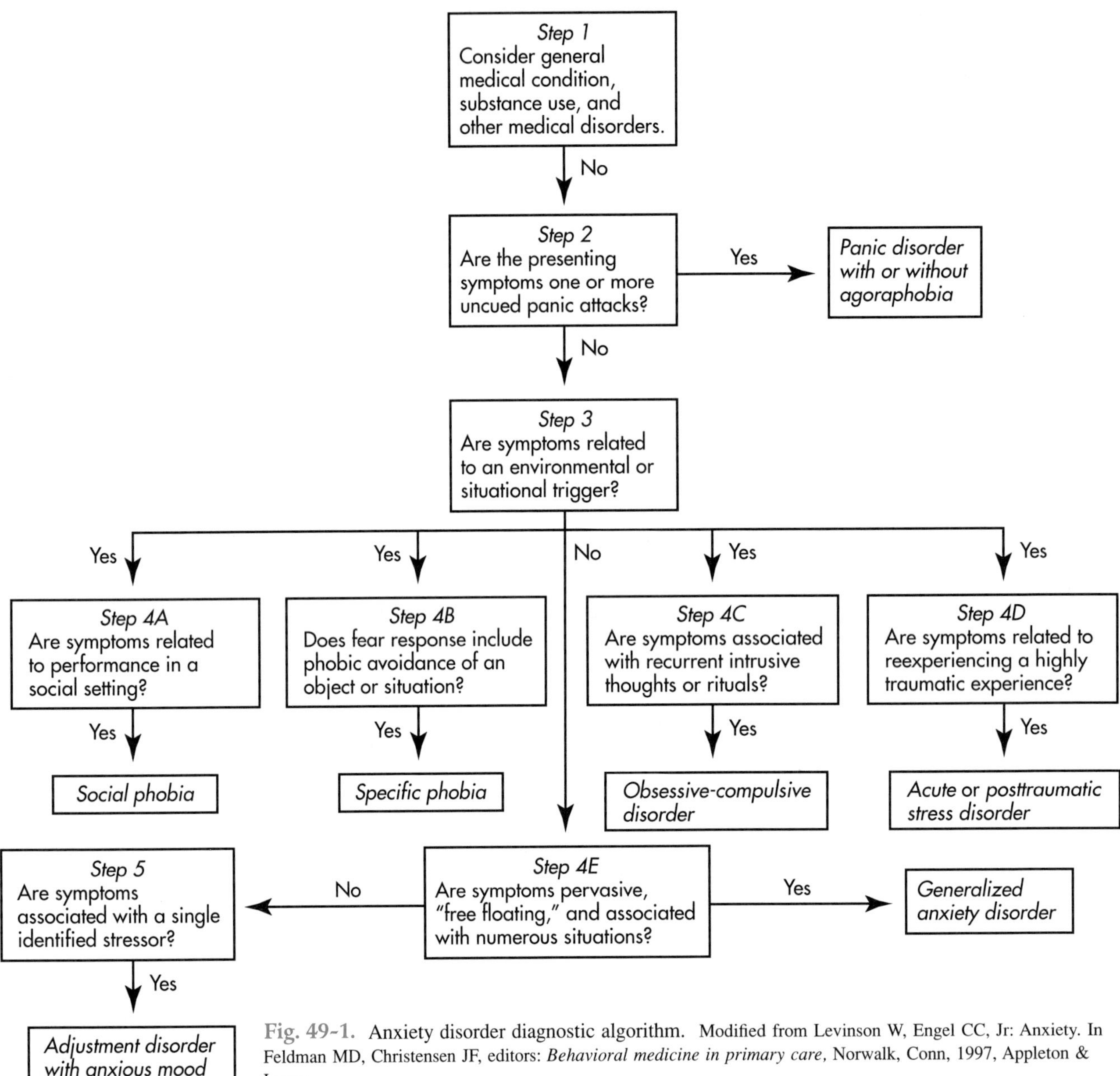

Fig. 49-1. Anxiety disorder diagnostic algorithm. Modified from Levinson W, Engel CC, Jr: Anxiety. In Feldman MD, Christensen JF, editors: *Behavioral medicine in primary care,* Norwalk, Conn, 1997, Appleton & Lange.

psychiatric disorders that can cause anxiety symptoms. For example, psychosis typically causes anxiety symptoms because patients who are psychotic experience frightening hallucinations or delusions. Depressive disorders are more common and subtle causes of anxiety symptoms than psychosis, especially in primary care settings.

Determining whether a patient's anxiety occurs in discrete episodes, is environmentally or behaviorally cued or relieved, or persists in a "free-floating" manner is a quick and practical way to focus the differential diagnosis (see Fig. 49-1). The physician first determines whether the patient has panic attacks. Panic attacks are sudden, discrete episodes of anxiety that last from minutes to hours. If panic attacks are present, can the patient identify any environmental triggers or "cues"? If panic attacks occur without specific cues, panic disorder is likely. If cues are present, the nature of the cue may suggest the diagnosis. If the cue is a specific event, object, place, person, or situation, one or more of the phobias may be present (social phobia, specific phobia, or agoraphobia). If the cue is a chronic stressor or an event or situation resembling a past traumatic event, adjustment disorder with anxious mood or acute stress disorder or PTSD may be present. If the cue is the interruption of a compulsive ritual or the exacerbation of an obsessive fear (e.g., contamination), OCD is the most likely diagnosis. If panic attacks are not present, panic disorder and the phobias are unlikely. Persistent, free-floating anxiety characterized by worry over several life concerns suggests GAD but may be a prominent feature of any of the anxiety disorders. For example, panic disorder sometimes generalizes from episodic attacks to persistent anxiety.

MANAGEMENT

The management of anxiety parallels its differential diagnosis. Principal treatment of substance-induced anxiety is discontinuation of the offending substance. This may require

Table 49-4. Medications Indicated for Anxiety Disorder Treatment

Common agents	Starting dose	Daily maintenance dose	Contraindications	Comments
Selective serotonin uptake inhibitors (SSRIs)				
Fluoxetine	10-20 mg qAM	20-80 mg	Prior allergy	Increase TCA levels
Paroxetine	20 mg qd	20-60 mg	Sexual dysfunction	Interacts with many agents metabolized in hepatic cytochrome P-450 system
Sertraline	50 mg qd	50-200 mg		
Fluvoxamine	50 mg hs	100-300 mg		
Tricyclic antidepressants (TCAs)				
Desipramine	10-25 mg hs	150-300 mg	History of acute (angle-closure) glaucoma	Anticholinergic, orthostatic, and histaminic (weight gain, sedation) side effects
Nortriptyline	10-25 mg hs	50-150 mg	Cardiac conduction abnormalities	Overdose highly toxic
Clomipramine*	25 mg hs	100-250 mg	History of suicide attempts	
Benzodiazepines (BZPs)				
Alprazolam	0.25 mg tid	0.5-6 mg	History of substance abuse	Efficacy of long-term use not established
Clonazepam	0.5 mg bid	1-4 mg	Chronic depression (may exacerbate)	Rapid onset of action
Lorazepam	0.5 mg tid	2-6 mg	Chronic obstructive pulmonary disease (respiratory depression)	Dependence possible without tolerance
Diazepam	2 mg bid	4-40 mg		Withdrawal from high-dose or short-acting agents associated with seizures
Other anxiolytic				
Buspirone	5 mg tid	15-50 mg		Safe, well tolerated; Effective for generalized anxiety only; Latent onset of action; Less effective for those who have taken BZPs

qAM, Every morning; *qd*, every day; *hs*, at bedtime; *bid*, twice a day; *tid*, three times a day.
*Approved by U.S. Food and Drug Administration for obsessive-compulsive disorder only.

a gradual taper (e.g., benzodiazepine-induced anxiety) or cross-treatment with other pharmacologic agents (e.g., alcohol withdrawal) to reduce anxiety symptoms and prevent other complications. Similarly, the primary treatment for anxiety due to a general medical condition is treatment of the underlying condition. If there are no medical or substance-related treatment considerations, or if anxiety symptoms persist even after substance and medical factors are fully addressed, pharmacologic and psychosocial options should be considered.

Psychopharmacologic Approaches

Medications used for the treatment of anxiety disorders are becoming increasingly safe, tolerable, and effective (Table 49-4; see Chapter 48). Primary care physicians should develop skill and experience with one or two agents within each drug class. This section discusses general approaches pertaining only to the treatment of anxiety and anxiety disorders.

Short-term use of benzodiazepines (8 weeks or less) to reduce incapacitating anxiety and treat insomnia often bolsters coping, improves functioning, and enhances the therapeutic alliance when patients have an adjustment disorder or acute stress disorder. No single medication is highly effective for PTSD, so medication management is usually determined by the presence or absence of various associated disorders, such as major depressive disorder, dysthymic disorder, panic disorder, or a substance use disorder.

Psychopharmacologic treatment of panic disorder generally relies on antidepressants, typically the selective serotonin reuptake inhibitors (SSRIs) or tricyclic agents, with or without benzodiazepine therapy. The different antidepressants are equally efficacious and should be chosen by side effect profile, past patient experience, and current patient preference. The favorable side effect profile of the SSRIs and their ease of administration have increasingly made them the medications of first choice in primary care. Antidepressant therapy, however, is typically not effective until several weeks after therapeutic doses are achieved. The benzodiazepines are rapidly effective and may be used early in a panic attack to abort it. Benzodiazepines may also help to reduce panic attacks in the first weeks of antidepressant therapy and then can be discontinued later to avoid the adverse effects of chronic benzodiazepine use. Unfortunately, tolerance, rebound anxiety symptoms, and potential for misuse often limit the long-term usefulness of benzodiazepines. A few patients with panic disorder require long-term administration of benzodiazepines, however, and collaboration with a psychiatrist may help the primary care physician intermittently reassess the appropriateness of this approach.

Duration of therapy for panic disorder is based on several considerations. Panic disorder is frequently chronic, and duration of therapy is usually 6 to 12 months even when the disorder is mild, uncomplicated, and of recent onset. If symptoms are chronic or seriously disabling, or if previous exacerbation was associated with suicidal ideation or suicide attempts, pharmacologic treatment may be required indefinitely.

Buspirone is effective for GAD but is not effective for other anxiety disorders. Buspirone therapy requires a 3- to 4-week latent period before onset of effectiveness, and it is relatively less effective among patients who have been previously treated with benzodiazepines. Antidepressants do not reduce anxiety for patients with GAD but may reduce the depression that frequently complicates GAD.

OCD is responsive to relatively high doses of SSRIs or clomipramine (a predominantly serotonergic tricyclic agent). As with panic disorder, OCD tends to be chronic, and relapse is frequent even after extended (6 months or more) trials of medication.

Low doses of β-blocking agents such as atenolol or propranolol are often helpful for phobias when exposure to the focus of fear can be anticipated and medication administered in advance. These agents block many of the autonomic manifestations of anxiety but do not reduce the subjective sense of fear or worry. Care must be taken to avoid the adverse effects of these agents (e.g., hypotension, lethargy). These agents are not effective for anxiety symptoms unrelated to a phobic stimulus.

Antipsychotic (neuroleptic) agents are seldom if ever indicated as maintenance therapy for anxiety in the absence of psychosis. These agents are not habit forming and will reduce anxiety, but they are associated with an unacceptably high risk of *tardive dyskinesia,* an iatrogenic and treatment-resistant movement disorder that can be extremely disabling.

Psychosocial Approaches

Primary care physicians vary in the amount of time, skill, and motivation they bring to the care of patients with anxiety. Physicians should maximize, however, their awareness and level of comfort with using a number of primary care–based strategies for ameliorating anxiety symptoms and related disability. These strategies include patient education, reassurance, behavioral modification, problem solving, physical reactivation, relapse prevention, support groups, and self-help tools.

Patient Education. All patients benefit from a clear understanding of their problems. Primary care physicians should equip their waiting rooms with take-home literature on the basic anxiety disorders. The stigma associated with psychiatric disorders may prevent many patients from asking for literature unless it is readily accessible. Clinics should equip their patient libraries with more intensive education materials, such as self-help books, videotapes, and fact sheets, that can be made available to patients as indicated.

Physicians should develop, practice, and memorize a few simple and direct explanations for patients with various anxiety disorders. This eases stigma, increases patient trust and hope, and enhances patient adherence to treatment. It is essential to emphasize the biologic nature of anxiety disorders and the availability of effective therapies. For example, patients with panic disorder may be told the disorder is caused by a malfunctioning "fight-or-flight" switch in the brain that causes it to switch "on" without warning at inappropriate times, and medicines can help "recalibrate" the switch. Explaining the biologic nature of symptoms reduces the guilt, shame, and self-doubt that many people with panic disorder experience.

Reassurance. Reassurance is critical for patients with anxiety, especially those with prominent physical health concerns. Panic disorder involves the rapid and unexpected onset of protean physical symptoms. Consequently, many patients with panic disorder seek urgent medical care and not psychiatric care. Before the patient can be reassured, it is typically necessary to evaluate worrisome physical symptoms (e.g., chest tightness, shortness of breath). Once an appropriate evaluation is completed, the physician should avoid repeating diagnostic tests unless new objective findings are present, since unnecessary testing is costly, increases the likelihood of false-positive results, and leads patients to think they have an undiagnosed illness.

Reassurance is also important for patients who have suffered stressors or traumatic life events that are driving anxiety symptoms. Patients with acute stress disorder should be reassured that nightmares, flashbacks, and autonomic arousal in the immediate posttraumatic period do not necessarily indicate a chronic mental illness. Empathic comments help patients feel understood (e.g., "The symptoms you describe are common and normal when people go through an awful experience like the one you had.").

Problem Solving and Physical Reactivation. Physicians often underestimate the value of offering their anxious patients brief assistance with problem-solving strategies during the visit. Anxious patients, especially those with adjustment disorder or subsyndromal anxiety, will benefit from efforts to help them identify and troubleshoot their problems. Anxiety can prevent normally high-functioning people from thinking clearly and coping effectively with a life circumstance. Often patients find they have overlooked simple strategies, such as writing out a problem and listing some initial steps to address it. Other patients may not connect their symptoms to a clearly stressful life event, and direct, nonjudgmental questioning may help them connect transient physical symptoms such as fatigue to important stressors.

Simple suggestions to promote physical reactivation, including instructions on light exercise or encouragement to consider leisure activities, can help patients refocus their attention and energy. Patients can track the time they spend in these activities using charts or a diary and review these during follow-up visits.

Behavioral Modification. Phobic anxiety symptoms can be blocked with medications, but avoidance of past phobic foci will persist until extinguished using behavioral modification. For example, in panic disorder, medication will reduce the intensity and frequency of panic symptoms, but agoraphobia-related avoidance behavior (e.g., reluctance to go shopping) will continue even in the absence of panic attacks until behavioral strategies are employed. Primary care physicians can help (alone or in collaboration with a nonphysician provider) phobic patients develop and implement a plan for behavioral modification using *systematic desensitization.* For example, a person with social phobia might be taught to rehearse social speaking in a series of progressively more threatening situations. The patient might first learn and practice relaxation and visual imaging to rehearse speaking before a series of progressively larger and more frightening imaginary audiences. The patient can then practice speaking before a few real but familiar people in a comfortable setting about a safe topic. Later the setting, topic, and size and composition of the audience may be altered gradually to become more threatening as the patient masters the tendency to avoid frightening situations. Desensitization continues as a series of homework assignments until avoidance is overcome and confidence is regained. The key to this approach is gradual and controlled exposure to whatever was previously avoided.

Similar behavioral approaches are also useful for patients with OCD. For example, a patient with compulsive handwashing might be instructed to count the times handwashing occurs each day and eliminate one episode of handwashing every few days. The patient can graph this progress and bring graphs to follow-up appointments. The physician can offer encouragement and reassurance until handwashing occurs normally.

Relapse Prevention. Prevention of relapse is especially important for patients with an established history of anxiety problems. Patients with GAD, panic disorder, or PTSD must be reminded of the cyclic nature of their anxiety symptoms. They can be taught to attend to the early physical and social manifestations of anxiety (e.g., increased muscle tension, increased sleep latency, avoidance of certain situations or people) and encouraged to seek early assistance rather than wait until symptoms are severe, disabling, or treatment resistant. Relapse prevention strategies are particularly important to emphasize for people with substance-induced anxiety when the substance is a drug of abuse.

Support and Self-help. Often, community support groups are available for people experiencing common situational stressors (e.g., cancer, single parenting, sexual assault, family member with a chronic disease) that give rise to anxiety or exacerbate a chronic anxiety disorder. Support groups help ill patients to realize they are not alone with their problems and to obtain satisfaction helping others encountering similar challenges. For patients with complicating substance problems, Alcoholics Anonymous, Narcotics Anonymous, or similar 12-step support programs have become an important standard of care. The local veterans affairs medical center lists service organizations that offer support groups and resources for military veterans with PTSD. Assistance in finding these and similar groups may be obtained through the clinic's social worker.

Primary care physicians should be able to refer anxious patients to appropriate self-help literature. These books can help patients implement their own self-therapy programs, including cognitive therapies, self-hypnosis, and relaxation techniques for panic disorder, OCD, and coping with stressful situations. A brief bibliography of such books should be maintained and updated in the patient library.

SPECIALIST COLLABORATION, CONSULTATION, AND REFERRAL

Primary care physicians can effectively treat most patients with anxiety disorders, who may prefer one modality to another. Unfortunately, some disabled patients will reject all treatment unless the physician speaks directly, hopefully, and candidly about the anxiety disorders and the available treatment options. Collaboration, consultation, or referral may be necessary when a patient expresses a preference for a psychosocial treatment the primary care physician is uncomfortable with or unskilled at performing.

Epidemiologic studies have shown that panic disorder is associated with an increased risk of suicide. Patients with suicidal thoughts or a history of suicidal or other forms of risk-taking behavior (e.g., violence) should prompt the primary care physician to consider specialist collaboration or consultation. Erratic behavior (e.g., frequent missed appointments, unstable interpersonal relationships, impulsive actions, criminal charges, aggressive acts) or poor adherence with recommended treatment suggests a personality or substance use disorder. Specialist consultation may help clarify factors complicating effective treatment and may result in recommendations for augmenting strategies or adjunctive treatments.

Incomplete symptom response to feasible primary care intervention in an appropriate time frame should prompt additional referral, particularly with complicating issues such as coexisting medical or psychiatric illnesses. Consultation or collaboration is also suggested for patients with an apparent adjustment disorder if symptoms or related disabilities persist beyond the stressor.

ADDITIONAL READINGS

Cassem EH: Depression and anxiety secondary to medical illness, *Psychiatr Clin North Am* 13:597, 1990.

Gabbard GO: *Psychodynamic psychiatry in clinical practice: the DSM-IV edition,* Washington, DC, 1994, American Psychiatric Press.

Hales R, Yudofsky S, editors: Anxiety disorders. In *Textbook of psychiatry,* Washington, DC, 1995, American Psychiatric Press.

Kaplan HI, Sadock BJ, editors: Anxiety disorders. In *Synopsis of psychiatry,* ed 8, Baltimore, 1998, Williams & Wilkins.

Kessler RC et al: Lifetime and 12-month prevalence of DSM-III-R psychiatric disorder in the United States: results from the National Comorbidity Survey, *Arch Gen Psychiatry* 51:8, 1994.

Spitzer RL et al: Utility of a new procedure for diagnosing mental disorders in primary care: the PRIME-MD 1000 study, *JAMA* 272:22, 1994.

Self-Help Literature

Bourne EJ: *Anxiety and phobia workbook,* New York, 1997, Fine Communications.

Peurifoy RZ: *Anxiety, phobias, and panic: a step-by-step program for regaining control of your life,* New York, 1995, Warner Books.

CHAPTER 50

Somatization

Charles C. Engel, Jr.
Wayne J. Katon

Mention somatization, and many physicians respond with animated tales about their most frustrating patients. Physicians' frustration over somatization occurs for a number of reasons. Somatization contradicts most physicians' professional sense that people with psychiatric disorders present

The views expressed by Dr. Engel in this article are his own and do not reflect the official policy or position of the Uniformed Services University Department of the Army, Department of Defense, or the U.S. Government.

with emotional symptoms. Similarly, physicians often believe that physical symptoms in the absence of "hard" supporting evidence (examination or test findings) are less serious or debilitating than symptoms occurring in the context of an identifiable disease. Instead, somatizing patients may minimize the extent of their psychologic distress and describe high levels of disability, even though accompanying diagnostic evaluations offer few satisfying leads. Disability often persists in spite of reasonable physician reassurances. Requests for time off work or to fill out disability forms often add to physician discomfort. The somatizing patient may further alienate physicians by challenging their reassurances or even questioning their competence.

Fortunately, troublesome patients with puzzling chronic physical symptoms are not the rule for somatization. This chapter emphasizes that somatization is:

- Ubiquitous in medical practice and human experience
- Associated with substantial unrecognized morbidity and high health care costs
- Shaped by predisposing, precipitating, and perpetuating factors into a continuum of severity and duration that includes acute, subacute, and chronic types

Somatization has been defined as a psychologic defense mechanism, a physical symptom caused by a psychiatric disorder, or a physical expression of psychosocial distress. This chapter considers somatization broadly, as *any physical symptom that prompts the sufferer to seek health care but remains unexplained after an appropriate medical evaluation.* Somatization is therefore perceptual (a person feels symptoms), cognitive (the person experiencing symptoms decides they are ominous), and behavioral (the person with symptoms seeks health care for them). Physician-patient conflict often occurs because of the mismatch between the patient's view (the symptom is ominous) and the physician's view (the symptom has no biomedical basis).

The purpose of this chapter is to help primary care physicians recognize, diagnose, and manage the spectrum of somatization. *Chronic somatization,* a relatively unusual and disabling form of somatization, lies at one end of the spectrum. People with chronic somatization have long histories of unexplained physical symptoms with associated episodes of high health care use, and often present for care of many simultaneous physical symptoms spanning multiple body systems. They typically deny or minimize their distress despite its obvious clinical manifestations and its frequent associations with extensive childhood and adulthood adversity. At the other end of the spectrum is *acute somatization.* Acute somatization is very common in clinical practice and is marked by the absence of a significant history of unexplained symptoms, fewer numbers of physical symptoms on presentation, the usual presence of a precipitating stressful life event, and a more transient course (depending on the duration of the stressful event). In the middle of the spectrum lies *subacute somatization.* This is characterized by recurrent bouts of several unexplained physical symptoms interspersed with asymptomatic periods. Symptomatic periods are usually associated with treatable anxiety or depressive disorders.

EPIDEMIOLOGY

Symptom diaries show that primary care patients record an average of one new symptom every 7 days, the most common being headaches, fatigue, muscle aches, and gastrointestinal (GI) or respiratory symptoms. One community study found that more than 4% of people had multiple, chronic, unexplained physical complaints. Only about 5% of symptoms experienced by community respondents are reported to physicians. Studies of medical patients with unexplained symptoms reveal high rates of major depression and panic disorder (Tables 50-1 and 50-2). Individuals with unexplained

Table 50-1. Prevalence of Major Depressive Disorder Among Patients With Medically Unexplained Physical Symptoms vs. Control Patients With Clearly Explained Physical Symptoms

	Major depression		Depressive episodes	
Symptom	Current	Lifetime	Lifetime	Associated features
Chest pain without CAD	35%	64%	5	Panic disorder
Chest pain with CAD	3%	16%		
Pelvic pain	34%	66%	5	Substance abuse
No pain laparoscopy	10%	16%		Sexual abuse
Tinnitus	60%	75%	3.5	Mild high-frequency hearing loss
Sensorineural hearing loss	7%	15%		
Fatigue	15%	77%	2	Somatization disorder
Rheumatoid arthritis	3%	42%		
Irritable bowel syndrome	21%	61%	2.5	Panic disorder
Inflammatory bowel disease	6%	17%		Somatization disorder
Fibromyalgia	14%	86%		Past abuse (sexual, physical)
Rheumatoid arthritis	6%	31%		Somatization disorder
Idiopathic dizziness	12%	42%	2	Panic disorder
Controls	5%	18%		

CAD, Coronary artery disease on arteriogram.

physical complaints and coexisting psychiatric disorders tend to use inordinate amounts of medical care at great cost to society. In a 3-year retrospective study of 1000 ambulatory care patients, 38% had new complaints of at least 1 of 14 common symptoms. Two thirds of symptoms were evaluated diagnostically, but only 10% to 15% of evaluations yielded a physical explanation not apparent at the initial visit. This 1988 study also found that the average cost per physical explanation was then $2252. An estimated 25% to 35% of primary care patients have current psychiatric disorders, but these are missed 50% to 80% of the time, largely because of inaccurate diagnosis in those patients who complain of medical illness or physical symptoms rather than emotional concerns.

There is a strong relationship between unexplained physical symptoms and psychiatric disorders, especially anxiety and depression. One study of the general population showed that 49% of subjects reporting five or more functional symptoms (vs. 6% of control subjects with no symptoms) had at least one current psychiatric disorder. Seventeen percent of the group with five or more symptoms had current panic disorder (vs. 0.1% of controls), and 15% had current major depression (vs. 1% of controls). Research suggests a similar relationship between the number of pain complaints a person has and his or her level of anxiety and depression.

PATHOPHYSIOLOGY

Hereditary Factors

Family studies have been completed for only the most severe forms of somatization. Patients with somatization disorder, a prototypical chronic somatization problem (Box 50-1), have an increased prevalence of somatization disorder among first-degree female relatives and antisocial personality disorder, alcohol abuse, and possibly attention deficit disorder among first-degree male relatives. Adoption and twin studies are inconclusive regarding the relative genetic and environmental contributions to these associations.

Neurophysiologic Explanations

Neurobiologic theories propose central nervous system (CNS) modulation of peripheral physical sensations. For example, chronic pain perception is dampened centrally via the endogenous opioid system. Monoamine neurotransmitters serotonin and norepinephrine may interact to alter chronic pain perception. Research suggests that CNS alterations in monoamines also occur among patients with anxiety and mood disorders, disorders often associated with somatization. Tricyclic antidepressants reduce presynaptic reuptake of these neurotransmitters, have documented analgesic effects in both depressed and nondepressed patients with chronic pain, and reduce other physical symptoms among patients with panic disorder and major depression.

Stress and emotions appear related to body symptoms via altered physiologic arousal. Autonomic arousal increases smooth muscle contractions and skeletal muscle tone. Smooth muscle contractions in the GI tract are temporally related to physical discomfort. Painful skeletal muscles often have higher electromyographic potentials than do control muscles, and evidence suggests that skeletal muscle contractions may coincide with back and myofascial pain syndromes.

One study observed that fibromyalgia patients have alpha-wave intrusion into slow-wave sleep. The demonstration that experimental disruption of stage IV sleep in normal subjects results in musculoskeletal and mood symptoms led to postulation that fibromyalgia is a nonrestorative sleep disorder. Over half of chronic pain patients report a sleep disturbance. Disruption of sleep patterns by anxiety and depressive disorders, as well as psychosocial stressors, may also cause physical symptoms.

Studies of patients with somatization disorder have revealed abnormal auditory-evoked potentials, abnormal right frontal electroencephalographic (EEG) frequencies, and bifrontal impairment and nondominant hemispheric dysfunction on neuropsychologic testing. Most unilateral conversion

Table 50-2. Panic Disorder Among Various Samples With and Without Medically Unexplained Physical Symptoms

Sample source	Prevalence of panic disorder (%)
Community	0.6-1.0
Primary care	7
Chest pain without CAD	33-43
Hypertensives tested for pheochromocytoma	35
Irritable bowel syndrome	29
Unexplained dizziness	13
Migraine headaches	5-15
Chronic fatigue	11-30
Chronic pelvic pain	8

Box 50-1. Diagnostic Criteria for Somatization Disorder

A. A history of many physical complaints beginning before age 30 years that occur over several years and result in treatment being sought or significant impairment in social, occupational, or other important areas of functioning
B. Each of the following criteria must have been met, with individual symptoms occurring at any time during the course of the disturbance:
   1. Four pain symptoms in at least four different sites or functions
   2. Two gastrointestinal symptoms other than pain
   3. One sexual or reproductive symptom other than pain
   4. One pseudoneurologic symptom (a symptom or deficit suggestive of a neurologic condition not limited to pain)
C. Either of the following must occur:
   1. After appropriate investigation, each of the symptoms in criterion B cannot be fully explained by a known general medical condition or the direct effects of a substance
   2. When there is a related general medical condition, the physical complaints or resulting social or occupational impairments are in excess of what would be expected from the history, physical examination, or laboratory findings
D. The symptoms are not intentionally produced or feigned (as in factitious disorder or malingering)

Modified from DSM-IV.

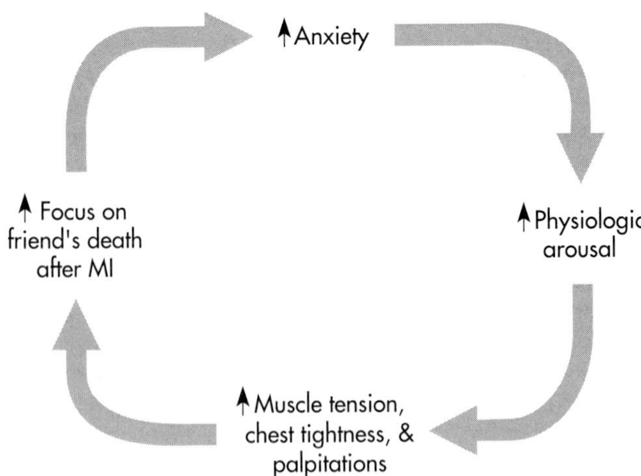

Fig. 50-1. Cycle of anxiety, physiologic arousal, and somatic symptoms in a person with chest pain whose friend recently suffered a fatal myocardial infarction (MI).

symptoms involve the left side of the body in right-handed individuals, and nondominant hemispheric dysfunction is one possible explanation.

Psychologic Explanations

Cognitive-behavioral, behavioral, and psychodynamic theories offer ways of understanding and treating somatization. Cognitive-behavioral psychology (CBP) postulates that perceived symptoms are linked to emotions, care seeking, and disability via underlying beliefs regarding cause (sometimes called *explanatory illness beliefs*). Fig. 50-1 shows how one's beliefs regarding the cause of a physical symptom can result in an escalating cycle of anxiety, physiologic arousal, and physical symptoms. The figure depicts this cycle for a man with recurrent musculoskeletal chest discomfort who has recently lost a close friend from an acute myocardial infarction. Previously unnoticed chest pain prompts worry and fears of sudden death. Worry and fear promote psychophysiologic arousal, manifesting as sweating, shortness of breath, and more chest discomfort. Cognitive-behavioral therapy (CBT) helps patients assess potentially harmful illness beliefs and replace them with more appropriate ones.

Behavioral psychology posits that behaviors are learned. Two ways of learning relevant to somatization are modeling (learning by imitating) and operant conditioning (learning by rewards and punishments). Modeling may explain why disabled or chronically ill family members are common among somatizing patients. Operant conditioning explains why patients receiving illness "rewards" (e.g., workers' compensation or relief from aversive responsibilities) may be prone to chronic disability.

Psychodynamic psychology views somatization as a defense against conscious awareness of (or an unconscious solution to) conflicting psychologic needs or fears. A woman who has always subordinated her emotional needs and fears being alone may, for example, develop sudden paralysis of her legs as she prepares to leave an abusive husband. This "conversion" of psychologic conflict to physical symptoms is the historical reason that neurologic symptoms occurring in relation to identifiable stressors were usually diagnosed as conversion disorder.

Table 50-3. Duration and Severity of Somatization (Acute, Recurrent, Chronic) and the Likelihood of Potentially Coexisting Psychiatric Disorders

Disorders	Acute	Recurrent	Chronic
Adjustment	+++	+	0
Anxiety	+	++	+++
Depressive	+	++	+++
Substance	+	++	+++
Psychotic	0	+	+
Personality	0	+	+++
Somatoform	0	+	+++
Factitious/malingering	0	+	++

Rated from +++ for most likely to 0 for least likely.

Sociocultural Theories

Mentally ill patients are too often ostracized and viewed by society as irresponsible and unworthy of social assistance. Patients with physical illness, however, are usually seen as victims who are sick and deserving of sympathy, care, and relief from work and other taxing responsibilities. This undoubtedly causes some distressed patients to preferentially report their physical rather than their emotional concerns to their physicians. Families are another social system that can affect symptom reporting. For example, a child may develop abdominal pain to distract parents from arguing, violence, or other family strife.

DIFFERENTIAL DIAGNOSIS

Differential diagnosis varies according to the severity and duration of functional symptoms. Table 50-3 outlines the relative importance of various psychiatric disorders to acute, subacute, and chronic forms of somatization.

Undiagnosed Medical Illness

Somatization, distress, and physical illness frequently coexist, so evaluation for one should not come at the expense of the others. Physicians should carefully consider illnesses that can present in vague, unusual, or multisystem patterns. Multiple sclerosis, collagen vascular diseases, endocrine diseases, and other conditions should be weighed against the patient's presentation.

Psychiatric Disorders Associated with Unexplained Physical Symptoms

Most, if not all, psychiatric disorders are associated with unexplained physical symptoms. Most somatization is associated with common treatable anxiety and depressive disorders or precipitating psychosocial stressors. Physicians must be alert to recognize and treat these disorders. Chapters 48 and 49 describe them in detail, and only issues pertaining to somatization are discussed here.

Anxiety Disorders. Criteria for a panic attack include sudden bouts of palpitations, sweating, shaking, shortness of breath, choking, chest pain, nausea or other GI distress, dizziness, numbness or tingling, or chills. Criteria for generalized anxiety disorder (GAD) include muscular tension, sleep disturbance, fatigue, and concentration and memory problems. The link between anxiety and physical symptoms exists, however, even when anxiety is measured without using these physical symptom criteria. Anxiety can increase attention to and worry about any coexisting physical symptoms. Panic disorder occurs in 6% to 8% of primary care patients, and in addition to physical symptoms, is strongly associated with amplified physical health concerns and high medical care use. If undiagnosed, the protean physical manifestations of panic disorder may cause affected patients to visit many doctors and emergency rooms. Appropriate pharmacologic treatment can ameliorate disabling panic attacks, physical symptoms, and health concerns.

Depressive Disorders. Depression has been shown to be associated with increased physical symptoms in multiple research studies. Physical symptoms in depressed patients may result from vegetative symptoms such as fatigue; increased symptom sensitivity; pessimistic symptom interpretations; a mode of communicating distress; a mood-state-dependent memory of prior physical illness; and somatic delusions (e.g., fixed, false belief one's "insides are rotting") from major depression with psychotic features. Major depression and dysthymic disorder are easily overlooked when patients describe only physical symptoms or describe depressive symptoms as secondary to their pain or somatic discomfort. Physicians must have a high index of suspicion to look past physical manifestations to assess vegetative and emotional symptoms of depression. Past or family history of depression, antidepressant treatment, or psychiatric hospitalization can provide diagnostic clues.

Somatoform Disorders

Somatoform disorders are psychiatric disorders in which one or more unexplained physical symptoms are the central defining feature. The physical manifestations of somatoform disorders do not involve conscious intent by the patient.

Conversion Disorder. Conversion disorder is similar to a somatically expressed adjustment disorder. It is characteristically acute, is associated with a precipitating life event or conflict, and has a good prognosis (passing of the precipitating event is usually associated with symptom resolution). Classic conversion symptoms have become less common over time. Most people with conversion disorder describe characteristic neurologic symptoms such as paralysis, numbness, or blindness in association with a significant psychosocial stressor. Past or coexisting mood, anxiety, or substance use disorders are risk factors for conversion disorder, and conversion disorder is a risk factor for somatization disorder (a lifetime pattern of multisystem conversion symptoms). Women are most often affected, but men with acute, severe stressors (e.g., war or natural disaster) or occupational injuries may be at elevated risk.

Anatomic, physiologic, or other inconsistencies in the symptom presentation may cause the physician to suspect conversion. In many cases, conversion causes amplification of a symptom caused by a neurologic or other physical illness. For example, many patients with epilepsy also have intermittent pseudoseizures.

Pain Disorder with Psychologic Features. Pain disorders include pain in one or more anatomic sites that requires clinical attention, causes significant distress or impairment, and is initiated, exacerbated, or perpetuated by psychologic factors. Common anatomic sites for pain include low back, head, pelvis (in women), abdomen, and chest. General medical conditions or injuries are often present in conjunction with psychosocial factors. Psychosocial factors should be investigated if pain persists beyond the normal tissue healing time (3 months is generally adequate) or if the patient's disability exceeds that expected by objective findings. Excessive use of the health care system, failure of the patient to accept physician reassurance, or prolonged or excessive use of narcotic analgesics, sedative-hypnotics, or alcohol suggests psychiatric complications. Symptoms of anxiety or depression are typically disabling, and routine assessment of chronic pain patients for these conditions is recommended.

Somatization Disorder. Patients with somatization disorder manifest a pattern of significant impairment due to multiple unexplained physical symptoms that prompt medical visits beginning before age 30 and lasting for several years. Individuals with somatization disorder tend to view themselves as having been in poor health their entire life. To be diagnosed with somatization disorder, a patient must have had at any time during the course of the disorder: four pain symptoms, two GI symptoms, one sexual symptom, and one symptom the patient interprets as neurologic. If a medical explanation is present, then physical symptoms or disabilities are in excess of what is expected.

Somatization disorder is unusual in the general population (0.1%) but overrepresented in primary care practice (0.4% to 5%). Studies show it occurs frequently among psychosocially distressed persons with high use of ambulatory care (20%), women undergoing hysterectomy for a reason besides cancer (27%), and patients with chronic pain (12%), irritable bowel (17% to 28%), fibromyalgia (70%), chronic fatigue syndrome (10% to 20%), and multiple chemical sensitivity (27%). Coexisting psychiatric disorders are the rule. Recurrent major depression or anxiety disorders are present in the majority. As the number of physical symptoms increases, so does the likelihood of coexisting alcohol problems, prescription drug misuse, early life adversity, and chronic maladaptive coping. Patients with somatization disorder often relate destructively to health care systems. Their lengthy medical records often reveal "doctor shopping," prescription drug dependence, multiple unrevealing invasive procedures or surgeries, and iatrogenic injuries.

Hypochondriasis. Hypochondriasis is the nonpsychotic but persistent concern that one has a serious disease, despite medical evidence and reassurance to the contrary. Hypochondriasis is closely associated with depression, anxiety, and psychosocial stressors, leading some to doubt if hypochondriasis ever occurs independently. Patients with panic disorder often think they are dying during attacks and are difficult to reassure. Depressed patients may manifest pessimism about their health or obsessive ruminations about imagined disease. Transient hypochondriasis sometimes occurs after an acute stressor. For instance, after myocardial infarction, patients may become excessively preoccupied with minor physical symptoms such as GI discomfort or palpitations. About 4% to 6% of medical outpatients have hypochondriasis, independent of the severity of their medical illness. Hypochondriasis usually starts in the third decade of life, and males and females are equally affected.

Malingering and Factitious Disorder

Perhaps the most important difference between the somatoform disorders and malingering or factitious disorder is that the latter disorders involve conscious patient attempts to misrepresent or even manufacture physical illness.

In malingering, an external incentive drives the deceit over illness. Malingering is often suspected but seldom "proved." It should be considered when clear incentives exist, such as pending litigation or avoidance of military conscription; when severe disability and symptoms occur without objective findings; or when the patient is uncooperative with diagnostic evaluations or treatment efforts. Patients with a history of criminal acts, lying, stealing, cheating, gambling, or substance abuse may malinger to avoid the adverse consequences of their previous actions.

Deceit over illness in factitious disorder may be quite driven and self-destructive. In contrast to malingering, external illness incentives are typically absent. The medical literature contains many colorful but morbid descriptions of this rare psychiatric disorder. Factitious fever may be most common; other types include factitious diarrhea, acquired immune deficiency syndrome (AIDS), urinary tract infection, skin rash, anemia, hypoglycemia, thyrotoxicosis, pheochromocytoma, asthma, psychosis, and dementia. "Münchausen's by proxy" occurs when a mother feigns illness in her child. Most patients with factitious disorder are women less than 40 years old. Many have worked in medical settings, allowing them to achieve an unusual level of medical sophistication. There may be a range of associated psychopathology from mild depression or hypochondriasis to severe personality problems characterized by poor tolerance of minor stress, erratic behavior, impulsive relationships, substance misuse, and early life adversity leading to intense anger at authority figures and themselves. Some with factitious disorder have gained the medical sophistication to alter diagnostic tests through a background as a patient, nurse, physician, or technician. Diagnosis involves medical staff detective work and can result in difficult ethical dilemmas.

Other Disorders

Bereavement, the normal reaction to the loss of a loved one, can precipitate a "lump in the throat" or other physical symptoms. Substance misuse may cause minor physical complaints during intoxication, "hangovers," or withdrawal. Less commonly, somatization is an easily recognizable feature of psychosis from schizophrenia, mania, depression, delusional disorder, or delirium or dementia.

HISTORY

Chart Review

Chronic somatization often leads to long, confusing medical records bearing witness to doctor shopping, repeated visits to medical specialists for ambiguous symptom clusters, equivocal diagnostic tests, and negative trials of empiric treatment. The chart must be carefully reviewed to avoid overlooking progressive or catastrophic disease and to find clues to a psychiatric disorder. Symptoms may relate temporally to psychosocial stressors, and potential symptom incentives may be discovered. Recurrent urgent or emergent care for sudden, ominous, episodic symptoms followed by negative evaluations suggests panic disorder. Excessive prescription drug use, elevated blood alcohol levels, macrocytic anemia, or elevated liver enzymes may suggest substance abuse.

Present Illness

Focus first on the patient's chief concern: physical symptoms. Vague, multiple, or inconsistently presented symptoms suggest somatization. While listening to the history, strive to assume the patient's perspective of the symptoms to secure his or her cooperation and enhance empathy and rapport. Understanding the patient's symptoms in a biopsychosocial framework is essential. Many patients troubled by physical symptoms reveal feelings of being trapped by their life situation or powerless over personal circumstances. Several visits will pass before many patients entrust their psychosocial concerns to their physician, and some never do, especially if they feel the physician is minimizing or belittling of their health concerns. Some patients will only (but readily) discuss their psychosocial issues if they are asked, so early and direct questioning regarding these issues, as well as anxiety, depression, and substance misuse, is important for all patients in whom somatization is suspected. If the patient is unreceptive, then delay the issue without persistence, since confrontation early in the physician-patient relationship almost always leads to unfavorable results. Depressed patients who are defensive often minimize or deny a depressed or anxious mood but will relate vegetative symptoms. Those with panic disorder will often minimize anxiety but will acknowledge sudden and recognizable physical symptom spells. Consider whether stressors and changes in functioning are temporally related to vegetative symptoms or symptom spells. Impairment out of proportion to symptom severity suggests psychiatric illness. Investigate the extent and quality of patients' support systems. Supporters may perpetuate disability by relieving patients of responsibilities that are undesirable to either the patient or their supporters. Look also for financial, legal, or other factors that may perpetuate symptoms.

Past Medical History

Determine levels and types of health care used over the previous 5 years including number of visits, number of physicians, surgical procedures and indications, and chronic pain or psychophysiologic problems (e.g., GI distress, palpitations). Listen to patients' descriptions: those with chronic somatization often view previous physicians with exaggerated scorn but are overly optimistic about their new physician's abilities. Clarify patients' past psychiatric history (substance abuse, hospitalizations, medications, suicide attempts, violence, criminal acts, or psychotherapy) and assess indicators of early life adversity such as childhood abuse, neglect, parental death, or chronic illness. Inquire about family history of depression, anxiety, substance abuse, suicide, crime, violence, and somatization. Chronic illness or physical disability in the nuclear family may serve as learning models for the patient.

PHYSICAL EXAMINATION

A thorough initial physical examination including mental status assessment is necessary, with a brief examination performed at subsequent visits. This serves as a cost-effective screening device and reassures and validates patients' concerns. Physical stigmata of alcoholism and intravenous or intranasal substance use can confirm substance misuse. Musculoskeletal injuries, scars, burns, lacerations, bruises, and abrasions may be clues to undisclosed abuse, violence, suicide attempts, or self-injury and should always result in direct, respectful questioning about how they were obtained.

LABORATORY AND DIAGNOSTIC ASSESSMENT

The main benefit of testing is additional information regarding patients' physiologic status. However, the costs associated with diagnostic testing for patients suspected of somatization are often subtle but high. The likelihood of a false-positive result increases with the number of tests performed. The false-positive rate also increases when testing is used to rule out clinically unlikely diagnoses. Testing is expensive, and it often wrongly suggests to the patient that the physician suspects serious undiagnosed disease. Therefore a conservative approach to testing is advised. Objective examination findings or classic symptom constellations are the main indications for laboratory assessment, and normal or equivocal test results should seldom be repeated. Sometimes, reviewing the medical record or talking with past practitioners provides enough information to dispel current medical concerns. When tests or imaging studies must be done, reduce iatrogenic worries by diligently reviewing them with the patient, emphasizing normal findings when appropriate.

MANAGEMENT OF THE SOMATIZATION SPECTRUM

A stepped care approach to somatization management aims to match the intensity of treatment to the severity of somatization. For most patients, somatization is acute, mild, and self-limited. For a relatively few patients, somatization is chronic, disabling, and relatively unremitting. It is not possible to know which patients will progress from acute to chronic somatization, even though it is possible to identify patients at relatively high risk. Instead, it is prudent to monitor patients for persistence of symptoms and progression of disability and increase the intensity of care accordingly. The basic elements of stepped care for somatization include routine primary care, collaborative primary care, and intensive specialty care.

Routine Primary Care Management

Routine primary care is most appropriate for patients with acute somatization. In routine primary care, the physician is the primary provider and care is delivered in the context of the usual office visit. The success of psychosocial intervention depends on development of a supportive, caring, respectful, and empathetic physician-patient relationship. It is important to inquire about patient fears of illness (e.g., "I'm afraid I have cancer"). Important psychosocial elements of care are physician-initiated reassurance, education, problem solving, patient activation, and bolstering of support. Education typically focuses on information about physiologic effects of stressors, anxiety, and mood and reassurance about specific illness fears. Especially in the setting of some acute stressor, the physician should convey optimism regarding unexplained physical symptoms, allow time for patients to ventilate frustrations, help them delineate problems, and suggest simple, action-oriented solutions for them to try. Emphasize the importance of maintaining usual life routines and roles to the maximum extent possible. Recommendations for rest or time away from work are seldom necessary; the relief from potentially undesirable responsibilities that rest affords may eventually reinforce patterns of disability. Encourage significant others to join the patient in the office because they often have questions regarding the nature of acute somatization symptoms and may encourage the patient to rest and break from routines unless advised otherwise.

Ask patients undergoing a stressor or crisis if they would prefer discussing their problems with a mental health professional. Defensive patients can be reassured that such suggestions are routine for unexplained physical symptoms because they are often distressing for the sufferer, not because symptoms are imaginary. A brief course of a sedative-hypnotic can improve sleep and bolster patient coping during or immediately after an acute stressor (e.g., rape, abuse, assault, unexpected loss) precipitates physical symptoms. Either an antihistamine like diphenhydramine or a short-acting sedative can reduce transient stress-related insomnia. Courses of sedative-hypnotics longer than 5 weeks are rarely appropriate, since these drugs can set up harmful illness incentives and their side effects can impair function.

Collaborative Primary Care Management

If a patient's somatization is more intermittently relapsing or subacute in nature, then a collaborative multidisciplinary intervention based in the primary care setting is frequently indicated. Patients with subacute somatization most often have a coexisting anxiety or mood disorder creating or compounding episodic physical symptoms. Increasingly, many primary care practices are integrating on-site mental health professionals within their clinics, an arrangement that supports primary care physician efforts to reduce the likelihood of refractory symptoms and impaired functioning. Implementing mental health care in the primary care setting normalizes the experience for patients, increases the likelihood of completed mental health referral, and creates opportunities for "curbside" dialogue between mental health care providers and the primary care physician.

The more persistent the unexplained symptoms, the more frustrating the primary care physician's experience, especially in the absence of on-site collaboration. If symptom eradication is the goal, this will further strain the physician-patient relationship. Rather than targeting physical symptoms per se, it is usually more rewarding and clinically useful to focus on patient functioning as the outcome of interest. The importance of an empathic physician-patient relationship is even greater for subacute than acute somatization. On-site collaboration can assuage the daunting task of achieving a psychotherapeutic posture while addressing biomedical concerns, all during the usual 15-minute primary care visit. The collaborative care plan should call for time-contingent rather than symptom-contingent visits to the physician. In between these physician visits, patients meet with mental health care specialists who can clarify the psychosocial history, evaluate for treatable anxiety or depressive disorders, monitor adherence to treatment while helping patients implement activation strategies, identify problems, and implement practical solutions. Collaborating providers can also engage patients' significant others and help teach patients and supporters about anxiety and depression.

On-site collaboration affords primary care physicians with

rewarding opportunities to improve their somatization management skills, something they generally prefer to simply referring interesting patients to an outside specialist. Reassurance in the setting of subacute and chronic somatization involves more than simply assuring patients that their symptoms are not serious, an approach they may find belittling. Instead patients should be reassured of the physical reality of their symptoms. Illness beliefs must be elucidated and assurances directed at those concerns through counseling, education, prognostication, and treatment recommendation. Examples of some common but harmful illness beliefs are: (1) "My symptoms are a sign of disease"; (2) "When I hurt it means I am seriously injuring myself" (e.g., pinching a nerve); and (3) "When I have symptoms, I can't make it without rest and a break from my responsibilities." Physicians should refine their ability to offer one or two simple medical explanations for the common psychiatric disorders complicating somatization. Patients with panic disorder, for example, can be told that the disorder involves dysregulation of the "stress thermostat" that controls their "fight-or-flight" mechanism. Such explanations destigmatize anxiety and depression, leading to improved rapport and treatment adherence. It helps to tell some patients that physical symptoms often are distressing and that this distress, in turn, can impair their ability to cope effectively with the symptoms. Self-help materials such as audiotapes and books about stress reduction, relaxation techniques, depression, and anxiety are widely available.

Psychopharmacologic interventions are an essential aspect of the management of subacute somatization. Antidepressants can reduce unexplained physical symptoms and physical health concerns among patients with chronic pain, panic disorder, and major depression. Doses should start low and increase slowly, since somatically focused patients are more sensitive to side effects. Before starting medication, offer patients a complete explanation of common side effects. Then, if side effects occur, the physician's expertise and trustworthiness are reinforced rather than diminished. Routinely instructing somatizing patients to call before they discontinue treatment on their own often avoids the situation in which the patient is seen some weeks later and has made little progress. Inform patients that it takes 3 to 5 weeks for full antidepressant effects to occur while side effects lessen during the period. Weekly follow-up visits during the first month of treatment (either in-person or via telephone) optimize patient education and adherence for the depressed or anxious somatizing patient.

Intensive Multidisciplinary Care

Chronic somatization is the most severe, yet least common, form of somatization and requires the most intensive collaboration to manage effectively. As the duration and number of unexplained physical symptoms increase, so does the likelihood that patients will manifest persistent coping deficits, erratic behavior, relapsing mental disorders, and personality problems. Primary care management of chronic somatization requires careful physician adherence to the following strategies:

- The patient should have only one primary care physician.
- Appointments should occur at regular, time-contingent intervals of about every 4 to 6 weeks.
- A brief physical examination is performed at each visit to address new physical concerns.
- Diagnostic evaluations should be done only for classic symptom constellations or acute objective signs.
- Gradually shift the focus of care from rehashes of "old" symptoms to discussions of current functioning, psychosocial stressors, and support structures.
- Corroborate interval history, disability, treatment adherence, substance use, and health care use by integrating family and other available support resources into the care plan.

This level of structure and emphasis on physician-patient rapport and trust is difficult but essential. Consistency requires limit-setting on patient-initiated visits or those precipitated by an exacerbation of chronic symptoms, so it is important to negotiate an advanced plan with the patient regarding how these visits will be handled. Empathic but direct reminders of the plan can quell patient concerns about rejection when limit-setting becomes necessary.

Other intensive strategies can bolster primary care management. Physical therapy programs of paced and gradually increasing exercise can help patients discharge stress, increase stamina, improve function, and reverse weight gain that has occurred after chronic avoidance of significant physical activity. A vocational counselor can help unemployed patients return to work, reducing dependence on disability compensation, improving morale and self- confidence, and maximizing ability to meet financial obligations and other role expectations.

Suggestions for Specialty Consultation

Coordination of specialty care is an essential aspect of managing somatizing patients. Chronic somatization often requires intensive collaboration with specialists to reduce doctor shopping and avoid unnecessary diagnostic tests and invasive procedures. It is best to know a consultant in each specialty who orders tests conservatively and understands the management of somatization. If possible, refer a somatizing patient to a specialist only after informing the specialist of the patient's propensity to report medically unexplained symptoms. Some consultants typically initiate lengthy diagnostic evaluations, tend to assume the care of patients rather than collaborate in their management with primary care physicians, or rely on prescriptions for narcotics or sedative-hypnotics for management. The best somatization consultants recommend care rather than assume it, because multiple providers increase the opportunity for uncoordinated care and unnecessary or iatrogenic services.

Most somatizing patients are best managed in primary care settings; indeed, many will actively resist psychiatric consultation. Some, however, require or request direct psychiatric assistance. The best psychiatric consultants usually have a subspecialty interest or training in consultation-liaison psychiatry. Unfortunately, many general psychiatrists have only infrequent exposure to somatizing patients and often do not readily appreciate the need to collaborate carefully with primary care. Psychiatric consultation often helps to:

- Suggest ways of improving treatment adherence.
- Elucidate stressors in defensive patients.
- Confirm diagnoses of anxiety, depressive, somatoform, or other psychiatric disorders.
- Decide about psychopharmacologic treatment for pa-

tients with many past treatment failures or complicating medical problems.
- Answer questions about suicide or violence potential in those with past attempts or current ideation.
- Evaluate for involuntary treatment or hospitalization.

Patient defensiveness, erratic style, and excessive rejection fears, as well as social stigmas associated with psychiatric care, are among the obstacles to effective psychiatric consultation for somatization. When somatization is suspected, mention psychiatric consultation early rather than waiting for the completion of an exhaustive negative diagnostic evaluation. Reassure patients that you respect their struggle with real and debilitating symptoms, and explain that the suffering their symptoms cause is often reduced through proper mental health assistance. The patient may be less than receptive at first, but over time they may be less prone to viewing psychiatric referral as rejection. Another strategy to minimize rejection concerns is to routinely schedule patients for a return primary care visit after psychiatric consultation.

ADDITIONAL READINGS

Katon WJ: *Panic disorder in the medical setting,* Washington, DC, 1991, American Psychiatric Press.

Katon WJ, Sullivan M: Antidepressant treatment of functional somatic symptoms. In Mayou RA, Bass C, Sharpe M, editors: *Treatment of functional somatic symptoms,* New York, 1995, Oxford University.

Katon W, Walker E: Medically unexplained symptoms in primary care, *J Clin Psychiatry* 59(suppl 20):15-21, 1999.

Kirmayer LJ, Robbins JM, editors: *Current concepts of somatization: research and clinical perspectives,* Washington, DC, 1991, American Psychiatric Press.

Kroenke K: Symptoms in medical patients: an untended field, *Am J Med* 92(suppl 1A):1A-3S, 1A6S, 1992.

Kroenke K, Spitzer RL, Williams JBW, et al: Physical symptoms in primary care, *Arch Fam Med* 3:774-779, 1994.

Lipowski ZJ: Somatization: the concept and its clinical application, *Am J Psychiatry* 145:1358, 1988.

Simon GE, Von Korff M: Somatization and psychiatric disorder in the NIMH Epidemiologic Catchment Area Study, *Am J Psychiatry* 148:1494, 1991.

Smith GR: *Somatization disorder in the medical setting,* Washington, DC, 1991, American Psychiatric Press.

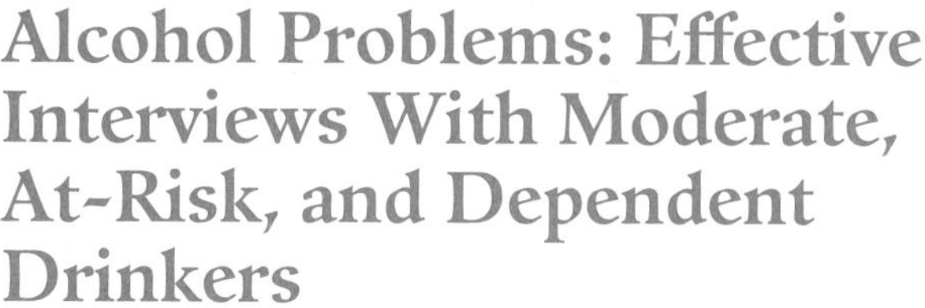

Alcohol Problems: Effective Interviews With Moderate, At-Risk, and Dependent Drinkers

William D. Clark

People with alcohol problems act irresponsibly despite sanctions, and are therefore heavily stigmatized. Physicians report that conversations about drinking are stressful and conflict-laden, and that patients are unmotivated and do not change. Physicians' negative feelings derive also from family experiences or from encounters with intoxicated patients who are hostile, uncooperative, and often violent. These dynamics, in combination with the sense that drinking is not a "medical" issue, silence physicians, patients, and families. However, conclusive evidence demonstrates that physicians who intervene with drinkers succeed in reducing harm caused by alcohol. Not only do physicians lower morbidity for patients and family members, but they also strengthen family and social relationships, self-esteem, and emotional stability.

EPIDEMIOLOGY

Alcohol problems exist on a continuum, and in an individual case, diagnosis may be elusive because of scant or imprecise information. Nevertheless, experts agree on an evidence-based classification system that is useful in guiding physician actions[9] (Table 51-1). People with the prototype syndrome, *alcohol dependence* (often called *alcoholism*), suffer medical and social consequences from uncontrolled drinking. A striking 5% to 10% of adults develop this syndrome. People with alcohol dependence are recognizable across cultures (and countries) because a distinctive, defensive interactive style develops in conjunction with typical medical and social complications. They hide important facts, defend their "right" to drink, and respond with hostility and reticence to attempts to talk about drinking.

People with problems of lower severity have *alcohol abuse,* a "maladaptive pattern that leads to impairment or distress." Expert consensus holds that *moderate drinking* is defined by low quantity of intake (<14 drinks per week for men, <seven for women), a social setting for drinking, and little intoxication (not more than four drinks per occasion for men, three for women)[8,9,12] (see Table 51-1). Drinking above these limits is variously called *at-risk* or *hazardous,* and is likely to cause harm, according to long-term studies. The neurologic complications of alcohol are reviewed extensively in Chapter 166.

Prevalence of alcohol problems is high, with a lifetime prevalence of alcohol abuse and alcohol dependence of 10% to 20%. A population-based study in British physicians' offices found that 10% of men were CAGE-positive (see Box 51-2), 7.6% averaged more than 3.5 daily drinks, and 3.2% thought they had problems with drinking. A Wisconsin primary care study found 17% of primary care patients in several sites were drinking above the moderate level. Women consistently show 30% to 50% fewer problems. Yearly health care costs for people with alcohol dependence average 100% higher than for comparable nonalcoholic people. Total medical costs directly attributable to alcohol are estimated at $10.5 billion, only a fraction of the more than $100 billion total alcohol-abuse costs.

ETIOLOGY AND PATHOPHYSIOLOGY

No one asks to develop alcoholism, nor is any person immune to nervous tissue actions of alcohol. Most people drink to have good times in the company of others, modulating their drinking according to feedback from internal states such as shame or hangover, and external cues such as reprimands, criticism, and sanctions. People succeed or fail in limiting drinking because of the interplay of physiologic, psychologic, and social/cultural factors. Data that confirm a physiologic and genetic influence include, for example, the dysphoria (flushing, nausea) that prevents many Asians from drinking; the finding that sons of alcoholic fathers predict their alcohol

Table 51-1. Terms and Criteria for Patterns of Alcohol Use

Term	Criterion
Moderate drinking (NIAAA)	Men: ≤2 drinks/day Women: ≤1 drink/day Over 65: ≤1 drink/day
At-risk drinking (NIAAA)	Men: >14 drinks/wk or >4 drinks/occasion Women: >7 drinks/wk or >3 drinks/occasion
Alcohol abuse (APA)	Maladaptive pattern of alcohol use leading to clinically significant impairment or distress, manifested within a 12-mo period by one or more of the following: Failure to fulfill role obligations at work, school, or home Recurrent use in hazardous situations Legal problems related to alcohol Continued use despite alcohol-related social or interpersonal problems Symptoms have never met criteria for alcohol dependence
Alcohol dependence (APA)	Maladaptive pattern of alcohol use leading to clinically significant impairment or distress, manifested within a 12-mo period by three or more of the following: Tolerance (either increasing amounts used or diminished effects with the same amount) Withdrawal (withdrawal symptoms or use to relieve or avoid symptoms) Use of larger amounts over a longer period than intended Persistent desire or unsuccessful attempts to cut down or control use Great deal of time spent obtaining or using or recovering from use Important social, occupational, or recreational activities given up or reduced Use despite knowledge of alcohol-related physical or psychologic problems
Hazardous use (WHO)	Person at risk for adverse consequences
Harmful use (WHO)	Use resulting in physical or psychologic harm

NIAAA, National Institute on Alcohol Abuse and Alcoholism; *APA,* American Psychiatric Association; *WHO,* World Health Organization.
From O'Connor P, Schottenfeld R: Patients with alcohol problems, *N Engl J Med* 338:593, 1998.

level less accurately than men from nonalcoholic backgrounds; and the finding that intensity of anxiety under the influence of alcohol varies with familial alcoholism. Twin and adopted sibling investigations implicate genetic factors, and extensive animal studies are confirmatory.

The predictable, inevitable, and multitudinous brain effects of heavy drinking facilitate a vicious circle of drinking more, developing problems, and discounting the role of alcohol. The insidious development of tolerance to intoxication, the cognitive deficits, and the dysphoric aspects of related states (e.g., hangover) engender unhealthy social dynamics. These relationship problems are exaggerated because friends and family resent the (apparently) voluntary "having fun and being irresponsible" nature of overindulgence. People become adept at ignoring reality and suppressing negative feelings. Longer time spent in brain- altered states results in the dramatic neurophysiologic changes of addiction. Furthermore, emotional isolation develops because people make excuses for their behavior, direct blame onto others, and show hostility whenever sensible limits are discussed. They select friends and partners who tolerate drinking and tacitly agree to overlook consequences. Higher problem rates are found among homeless persons, those with a major psychiatric disorder, and people in the criminal justice system. Which comes first remains uncertain.

PATIENT EVALUATION

Physicians were urged to screen for alcohol dependence, but substantial costs derive from overindulgence by at-risk drinkers who are not "alcoholic." The prior focus on *screening for alcoholism* is too narrow according to research and consensus panels. New studies on costs and effectiveness of brief interventions suggest that physicians can help at-risk drinkers avoid complications. This is analogous to working with the patient with angina or high cholesterol, rather than waiting for the heart attack. Current recommendations urge physicians to expand their interventions to all drinkers.

Research indicates that physicians should look for three types of patients with whom to talk about drinking. One group drinks in a moderate manner and will benefit from discussion of potential benefits and hazards. A second group is at risk (drinking too heavily), and needs information and advice about why to cut down, and how to do so. Finally, those who drink in a poorly controlled fashion (alcohol abuse or dependence) need action recommendations and referral for more expert professional treatment. Physicians require a combination of reminders, incentives, and skill building to succeed at making alcohol-related inquiry and intervention the routine matters that they should be. We suggest simple strategies that separate healthy drinkers from potentially problematic ones. Subsequent sections advise physicians about what to do in each case.

HISTORY

Because drinking is not an illness, but a behavior that carries with it societal myths and stigmas, talking with any person about drinking is a sensitive matter. The history-taking style and techniques strongly affect patients' subsequent willingness to participate in treatment activities. Many studies suggest that a structured, stepped approach is both efficient in practice and effective with patients.

Step One

In *step one* (Box 51-1), the physician asks about alcohol use in the past year. If the patient has had no beer, wine, or hard liquor in the past year, nothing else need be done. The

Box 51-1. Three Steps to Diagnosis

Step one: Any alcohol in past year?
Step two: CAGE (or other screen)
Step three: NIAAA quantity and frequency questions

Box 51-2. CAGE Screening Test for Dependence Symptoms

C: "Have you ever felt the need to *C*ut down on your drinking?"
A: "Have people *A*nnoyed you by criticizing your drinking?"
G: "Have you ever felt bad or *G*uilty about your drinking?"
E: "Have you ever had a drink first thing in the morning to steady your nerves or get rid of a hangover? (*E*ye opener)"

Box 51-3. NIAAA Questions on Quantity and Frequency of Drinking[8]

On average, how many days per week do you drink?
On a typical day when you drink, how many drinks do you have?
What is the maximum number of drinks you had on any given occasion during the last month?

Box 51-4. Standard Drinks[8]

A drink is 12 oz. beer, 5 oz. wine, or 1.5 oz. (bar shot) of hard liquor

Box 51-5. Safe Limits

Men: 14 drinks per week, and not more than four per occasion.
Women: seven drinks per week, and not more than three per occasion.

abstinent subgroup with past alcohol problems usually discloses this spontaneously.

Step Two

In *step two,* the physician seeks to identify current drinkers who deserve substantial attention.[3] We favor a screen for alcohol dependence as the next step. As with hypertension or cervical cancer, lives can be saved by screening. Because the typical defensive interactive style of people with alcohol dependence promotes minimization and cover-up rather than exposure, there may be no discernible clue unless a screening strategy is used. At present, physicians miss 60% to 80% of cases. A good option is the CAGE test (Box 51-2), a thoroughly studied simple screen. It is less accurate for women and African-Americans. The two questions ("In the last year, have you ever drunk or used drugs more than you meant to?" and "Have you felt you wanted or needed to cut down on your drinking or drug use in the last year?") assess drug use at the same time as alcohol.[4] A single question from the Alcohol Use Disorders Inventory Test (AUDIT) was effective in one study. Consistent application of a validated strategy is a more powerful determinant of clinical effectiveness than which strategy a physician chooses for routine use.

We recommend that physicians avoid using the natural question, "How much do you drink?" as step two. Asking "How much?" not only reminds people of shameful overindulgence and fails to encourage reflection, but also limits patients' responses to subsequent questioning if asked too early, as research demonstrates.

Step Three

If step two is negative, ask the National Institute on Alcohol and Alcoholism (NIAAA) recommended questions about quantity and frequency (Boxes 51-3 and 51-4).[8] According to the NIAAA expert panel, the "safe limits" for men are 14 or fewer drinks a week, with no more than four on any one occasion, and for women are seven or fewer per week, and no more than three per occasion (Box 51-5). If a person drinks below these limits, *and* step two shows no positive response, *and* no other hints exist that the patient has alcohol problems, no urgent intervention is needed.

Of course, when withdrawal symptoms are apparent, liver disease is accompanied by odor of alcohol, or the spouse confides about problems, physicians do not need screening strategies.

If any CAGE question is positive, if intake exceeds safe limits, or if another clue from examination or the family suggests a drinking problem, the physician needs more detail. A search for characteristic elements of alcohol problems is warranted and not time-consuming if thoughtfully structured. Box 51-6 provides ample data for the primary care assessment. Interviews with others, including family, nurses, and social workers, enlarge the inquiry if the patient furnishes insufficient data. Records from other physicians or hospitals may contain unanticipated information that establishes a diagnosis.

Obtaining a thorough evaluation allows the physician to discuss impressions in a compassionate manner. In fact, experimental data show that thoughtful diagnostic conversation itself produces beneficial therapeutic effects.

PHYSICAL EXAMINATION AND LABORATORY STUDIES

Physical and laboratory examinations are useful adjuncts to structured interviewing and help doctors set priorities for the pacing and vigor of subsequent discussions. Odor of alcohol is alarming, and distinctly abnormal in medical encounters. If

Box 51-6. Symptoms of Alcohol Problems

Somatic

Gastritis
Trauma
Hypertension
History of liver trouble
New-onset seizure

Psychosocial

Symptoms of anxiety or depression
Insomnia
Overdose
Requests for psychotrophic medication

Alcohol-specific

Spontaneous mention of drinking, such as "partying," hangover, family history, AA attendance, arrests for driving under the influence, blackouts, tolerance, withdrawal symptoms

one easily smells alcohol in the room, the blood alcohol level (BAL) is likely greater than 125 mg/dl; a less dramatic odor indicates a BAL between 75 and 125 mg/dl. The nose is a good breath analyzer. Alcohol on the breath is a convincing sign, and always signals a serious alcohol disorder.

Intoxication in any encounter is worrisome, and means a high likelihood of alcohol disorder, even in the emergency situation. To underscore this important point, assume that the alcoholic 10% of the population are drunk once a week, and assume that the 60% who are moderate drinkers are intoxicated once yearly. Thus, in a year, from a population of 100, 30 abstainers yield no episodes of intoxication, 60 moderate drinkers yield 60, and 10 alcohol-dependent people yield 520! Furthermore, moderate drinkers seldom become as intoxicated and are more likely to drink in controlled environments (e.g., where someone else can drive). Intoxicated people in the emergency situation are not healthy drinkers who "have had one too many."

If the odor of alcohol is apparent, and if the patient manifests no evidence of intoxication (slurred speech, incoordination, and emotional lability), tolerance to alcohol effect is present. Tolerance indicates brain adjustment to intoxicating alcohol levels, which is caused by heavy drinking, is inevitably toxic, and means alcohol dependence is present. Withdrawal syndromes (see next section) indicate additional brain dysfunction, and are easier to discern than tolerance.

Other physical and laboratory findings are poor screening tests (low sensitivity and specificity). Because of alcohol's broad toxicity, however, an abnormality may prove useful in context. First, an unexplained finding may begin a fruitful investigatory process. For example, despite a negative CAGE test, the concerned physician of a young woman with palmar erythema continues the assessment, allowing the patient to reveal her alcohol problem. Second, in the presence of a clue, physical or laboratory findings substantially raise the posttest probability. Physicians should order a mean corpuscular volume (MCV) and liver enzymes (include a γ-glutamyltransferase [GGT] the most sensitive to alcohol intake). For example, a 55-year-old man with chronic pulmonary disease is admitted for atrial fibrillation. His wife complained about his drinking, and elevated MCV and aspartate aminotransferase (AST) confirmed not only alcoholism, but also "holiday heart."

Box 51-7. Physical and Laboratory Manifestations of High Utility to Detect Alcohol Problems

General

High blood pressure
Intoxication
Tolerance
Odor of alcohol

Hepatic

Icterus
Palmar erythema
Spider angiomata
Bruising
Hepatomegaly
AST (SGOT), γ-glutamyltransferase (GGT), or other enzyme elevation

Hematopoietic

Elevation of MCV
Anemia
Low platelets

Skin

Facial telangiectases
Seborrheic dermatitis
Rosacea
Skin atrophy
Distal extremity hair loss
Superficial infections

Neuromuscular

Agitation
Tremor
Emotional lability
Poor tandem gait (or wide-based gait)
Ankle, wrist weakness
Atrophy of shoulder, pelvic girdle muscles

Cardiac

Tachycardia
Atrial fibrillation
Cardiomyopathy

Genitalia

Testicular atrophy

Box 51-7 presents findings of high utility and underscores the value of thorough examination.

MANAGEMENT OF WITHDRAWAL AND MEDICAL COMPLICATIONS

Treatment of alcohol withdrawal is of special concern to the primary care physician. Other urgent complications such as dysrhythmia, hepatic failure, bleeding, gastritis, and pancreatitis are covered in specialty chapters.

As physical dependence develops, initial manifestations of anxiety, sleep disorder, tremor, and vague discomforts are mild, sometimes not attributed to alcohol, but easily relieved by drinking. As months pass, however, alcohol less reliably controls symptoms, and intoxication is fleeting, occurring only at high BAL (greater than 250 mg/dl). Withdrawal is not an all-or-nothing state, and addicted patients experience symptoms whenever their BAL falls. The altered neurophysiology in the brain perceives a drop in BAL as disruptive to the new steady state condition of addiction, and expresses the disruption through withdrawal symptoms. Soon the person drinks steadily to alleviate withdrawal, but relief is brief. The range of BAL at which the person feels "not sick" diminishes, and severe symptoms, even delirium tremens, may develop despite a BAL of 300 mg/dl or more.

Severity of an episode of withdrawal is hard to predict. Outpatient treatment is sensible in mild cases, but inpatient support is required for severe ones. Physicians should hospitalize patients with clouded sensorium, fever, hyperventilation, or a concomitant medical problem (e.g., hepatic failure, pancreatitis). In addition, the presence of three factors from Box 51-8 suggests inpatient management. Degree of tremor, anxiety, tachycardia, and stomach symptoms are poor predictors of need for inpatient care (see Chapter 166).

When outpatient management is feasible, pharmacologic support helps with symptom relief (Box 51-9) and should be integrated with patient education and referral options designed to help patients change entrenched behaviors.

Box 51-8. Risk Factors for Severe Alcohol Withdrawal

Drinking around the clock
Daily consumption of a fifth of liquor, a case of beer, or more than a half gallon of wine
Heavy drinking more than 5 years
Poor nutrition
Concomitant heavy sedative, cocaine, or narcotic use
Past history of severe withdrawal

Box 51-9. Outpatient Withdrawal Regimen

50-100 mg chlordiazepoxide PO (IM unreliably absorbed) in office; initiate referral to counseling or structured program.
Day 1: take 25-50 mg PO every 4-6 hours as needed.
Day 2: take 25 mg PO every 4-6 hours as needed; visit the office.
Day 3: take 25 mg PO once or twice as needed.
NOTE:
Give patient not more than 250 mg to take away.
Expect 200-300 mg total for average severity.
Do not exceed 250 mg day 1, 150 mg day 2, 50 mg day 3.
Lethal dose of chlordiazepoxide uncertain; exceeds 2 gm.
If patient drinks, admit for detoxification.

CHANGING DRINKING PATTERNS: LIFESTYLE CHANGE

Prochaska and colleagues[10a] have found that people progress through a series of stages on the way to successful lifestyle change. This is true across studies of at least a dozen behaviors. In the first stage, *precontemplation,* a person is not thinking that the behavior (e.g., drinking) is a problem, and naturally has no interest in changing. People thinking about changing are in *contemplation.* Ambivalence is the hallmark of this stage, and people find reasons to stay the same as well as reasons to change. As the balance tips toward change, people enter *preparation* and imagine change strategies or new behaviors (e.g., wondering where to find an Alcoholics Anonymous [AA] meeting). In the *action* stage, people take action and try out new behaviors (e.g., changing from liquor to beer, or quitting for a time). When persistently successful and no longer sliding back to old behaviors, people are in the *maintenance* stage.

Experienced physicians find the concept of stages intuitively useful. Tracking whether a preponderance of patient conversation suggests progression through stages is useful for physicians, as they evaluate readiness to change and consider potential interventions. However, this advance in thinking has some important limitations. First, a patient's stage is neither fixed nor all inclusive. Patients may say, "I'll go to AA, but I'm not going to stop drinking" (or vice versa), "My liver is sick, so I'll cut back for a time," or "I'd like to stop drinking to improve my family relationships, but I have to drink with my professional clients." The patient may take action to dry out and relieve withdrawal symptoms but fail to understand the need for continued treatment. In a single interview, a patient may display aspects of many stages, and move frequently between stages. Also, the skills that researchers have described that help people effect change overlap the stages, so the functional aspects of helping people change are not linked directly to the stages.

Physicians complain that patients are not motivated. Researchers have developed new perspectives about motivation.[7] Motivation is not a unitary phenomenon, nor is it entirely an individual phenomenon. Successful lifestyle change is blocked by myriad inner pressures, both psychologic and physiologic (neuronal adaptation), as well as by external forces committed to the status quo, such as drinking partners, social needs, and dysfunctional family dynamics. The thoughts and questions that hold patients back are familiar to physicians: "Do I have a problem? What is the nature of the problem? I don't know what to do for this problem. The work of changing is too hard. I'm not strong enough or good enough to do this. No one cares if I change. Will it make a difference if I try?" Physicians' ability to help patients express these doubts and physicians' responses to them can either facilitate movement toward successful change or contribute to a patient's demoralization and discouragement, thereby increasing resistance to change. As researchers untangle the threads of effective interventions, they have shifted emphasis from description of patients (e.g., are they strong or weak, compliant or not, motivated or not) to enhancement of physicians' skills.

Because only the patient can effect change, the physician's task is to trigger change. The general mechanism is to create a discrepancy between patients' perception of their current status and their desired short- or long-term goals. The specific strategies and skills vary according to patients' readiness to address important questions. Evidence shows that empathic, trusted physicians who build a sense of autonomy, optimism, and confidence help trigger change, if they are willing to intervene.

Physicians should initiate dialog whenever they perceive a potential problem with alcohol. Patients who drink too heavily have high levels of ambivalence and resistance. Physicians do not have to be certain how serious problems are (except to recognize and treat withdrawal or other medical problems), since their initial interventions need to address similar dynamics about the change process. As the work continues, physicians obtain more data, improve the accuracy of their diagnoses, and fine-tune their interventions. Studies show that recurrent brief encounters using the style and skills discussed in the following sections are more critical to success than getting any one encounter "exactly right." People and lifestyle are too complex and entrenched to expect that one "right answer" or "correct" conversation can accomplish the goals of change.

AN INDISPENSABLE INTERVENTION STRATEGY

Reflection, also called *active listening,* is a basic interview skill that helps increase motivation in all types of drinkers (Box 51-10). Reflection, especially when the patient seems negative or hostile, is not an intuitive response. Physicians usually prefer asking questions (getting more data), giving advice, or shifting the interview focus. When physicians reflect back the message they receive from patients, they generate an atmosphere of alliance and partnership because reflection shows a desire to understand the speaker and lets the speaker choose where to go next (unlike, for example, questions, advice, agreement or disagreement, or statements of values). Reflection demonstrates acceptance of the person, and a willingness to listen more. Because it is neither aggressive nor defensive, reflection helps minimize arguing, fighting, hostility, and negativity. Studies demonstrate that physicians who reflect negative, resistant, or reluctant statements help patients to voice the more positive view. (For example, if the patient says, "I drink a lot because of the neuropathy and pain in my feet, so that I can sleep," the physician might respond, "So, alcohol helps you a lot." This might prompt the patient to say, "Well, it's probably not so good for my internal organs.") This is one aspect of helping patients find a discrepancy between their current status and what they might desire. Physicians can reflect a person's statements about feeling, thinking, attribute, choice, action, or behavior.

Reflection encourages the patient to share more of his or her perspectives, feelings, and thoughts, and thus engenders more trust and a feeling of safety in both persons. As patients who initially show disinterest, hostility, sullenness, or confusion reveal more of themselves, physicians become less judgmental and critical, becoming more inclined to join patients and to support them in their struggles with life. Patients who feel joined become better able to listen to their physicians, and have more strength to take responsibility for attempting change that might at first seem unimaginable.

The following section discusses use of *autonomy supportive* skills in working with alcohol-dependent drinkers, who must abstain from alcohol to regain health, and whose difficulty doing so is dramatic.

Box 51-10. Reflection

Description: Tell the patient the message you heard or nonverbally perceived. Always statements, not questions, agreement or disagreement, judgment, etc. Always brief: reflector may have to choose among several messages in order to be brief.

Examples: "I see, you think that none of your problems are related to drinking." "Alcohol really helps you to sleep." "That I think these abnormal liver tests are from alcohol is confusing to you, because you drink so little." "You seem upset with my continuing to talk about drinking."

GIVING ADVICE TO ALCOHOL-DEPENDENT DRINKERS

The section on pathophysiology emphasizes the deep roots of alcohol dependence. It is sustained by alcohol-induced brain changes, unhealthy social dynamics, and emotional isolation, as well as by the intense feeling that the "devil you know" must be better than changing. People in recovery say that asking the dependent drinker to stop drinking is tantamount to asking the unimaginable, to confront obstacles as insurmountable as learning to fly (without airplanes). Change seems like jumping into a black, featureless abyss. This illness dynamic ensures that patients will ignore reality, suppress negative feelings, and so flawlessly, as if by second nature, reject sound advice. The challenge for physicians is correspondingly great, and finding the motivation and developing discrepancy are complex tasks.

Patients' behaviors are negative, confusing, and hurtful. Often, roles are reversed, and the physician, directly or unwittingly, rejects and humiliates the patient. This fundamental distortion in physicians' experience of caring for patients is painful and profoundly unsatisfying. So, it is no surprise that physicians fail to intervene, and mirror patients' lack of awareness, reluctance, and often hopelessness. Physicians come to believe that any intervention is unwarranted interference in the patient's life. The situation becomes framed as, "Shall I now confront the patient and waste valuable time for unlikely gain, or address the patient's high blood pressure?" Drinking remains unaddressed.

Studies of interventions show that effective interviewers enhance motivation and discrepancy by using the following skills: create dialog; create an objective, scientific climate; develop options and choices; and create commitment. These are important elements of the autonomy supportive style.[14]

Create Dialog

True dialog is difficult in conversations that involve differentials in perspectives, expertise, and/or power. Patients tend to defend a point of view or to be passive and silent. Physicians can encourage dialog by consciously employing a format of "tell, ask, tell, ask," which supports taking turns in talking. Briefly tell bits of information or feedback (Box 51-11) and then ask the patient what he or she thinks about it, or how it feels to hear it, or what he or she intends to do about it. Keeping the "telling" brief helps clarity, and "asking" allows the patient to choose a *change-enhancing* or *change-obstructing* response. The manner in which patients

Box 51-11. Autonomy Support

Description: Tell bits of information, feedback, or advice. Keep bits short. Give facts, not opinions or conclusions. Be scientific, not personal. Be tentative and conditional. *Ask* the patient what he or she thinks about this, or how it feels to hear this, or what he or she intends to do about this. *Tell* another bit. *Ask* the patient for his or her reaction.

Examples: "Steady drinking changes brain function, How does that strike you?" "Three of your liver tests are abnormal. What do you think of that?" "One option is that you stop drinking all alcohol. What do you want to do about this?" "Of course, this might not work for you. How do you feel, hearing me say this?" "No one can be certain what will happen to your liver if you stop drinking. How does that sound to you?"

respond to being asked also suggests to the physician which steps to use next. Change-enhancing responses include statements of agreement, commitment, or optimism, and suggest that exploring the facts might be helpful. Change-obstructing responses, such as statements of disagreement, reservation, pessimism, defensiveness, and noncommitment, as well as all questions that do not ask for clarification of meaning, suggest that the physician should reflect back the response as the next step in the conversation. Reflection invites patients to look inside themselves, and encourages motivation and discrepancy. "Asking" thus fosters exploration and choice.

Create an Objective, Scientific Climate for Educating Patients

Create a climate of fact, not opinion, by giving all information, feedback, and advice/recommendations in an objective or scientific way, with the cautions that apply to science (today's truth is tomorrow's fiction, and every case is unique). In short, start with the facts, not conclusions or opinions about meaning. Then, when giving advice, do so tentatively and conditionally, as part of a search for options or alternatives. "Wagging one's finger," actually or figuratively, pushes patients into a corner, highlights any feelings of shame or stigma, and generally inhibits discussion. The following paragraphs give examples as well as more details.

Tell information about what is known about alcohol problems[2] in an impersonal way, scrupulously avoiding reference to the patient (Box 51-12). This might sound like: "Research shows that treatment helps"; "Steady drinking changes brain function"; "Having a high tolerance for alcohol means that a person is deprived of the early warning system that tells him to stop drinking before the alcohol level gets so high as to be dangerous"; "90% of men drink less than 35 drinks per week"; "Many people are terrified to imagine stopping drinking"; or "Generally, being sick in the morning until after a drink means a person's brain has become hooked on alcohol." Next, *ask* the patient what he or she thinks of this information.

Tell feedback about the patient's situation as a fact, a number, or score, rather than a conclusion (Box 51-13). You might say, "Three of your liver tests are abnormal," rather

Box 51-12. Information for Patients About Pathophysiology

Drinking is voluntary, but no one asks for trouble, especially for alcohol dependence.

No one is immune to the negative effects of alcohol.

Many people develop serious problems without noticing how serious they are, because alcohol affects judgment and thinking.

Experts have extensively researched the question of amount, and set safe limits (see Box 51-5).

Drinking more than this puts one at risk, and major risks include the following:

- Accidents at home or work, or while driving (or arrest for driving intoxicated).
- Poor judgment or impulsive behaviors, leading to arguments, unsafe sex, overspending, driving under the influence, operating a boat or machinery, etc.
- Relationship problems with family and others who love you.
- Health problems, mainly liver and brain damage, some cancers, pancreatitis.
- Gradual increase in intake and/or loss of control, which catches people by surprise.

Some people should not drink at all, or should have one drink at most, for example:

- Pregnant women.
- People who are driving a vehicle or operating machines.
- People with alcohol-related medical problems (e.g., liver trouble, pancreatitis).
- People with important mental health problems (e.g., bipolar depression, schizophrenia).
- People with illnesses potentially affected by alcohol (e.g., diabetes, liver trouble, IV disease, other substance dependence, and as advised by physicians).

For those who are uncertain what to do, or what they think, help is readily available.

Counseling and treatment are effective.

Box 51-13. Feedback to Patients About Their Risks

Write down the average daily and weekly intake, in standard drinks (see Box 51-4).

Tell specific risks for this patient, which may include the following:

- Patient's demonstration of tolerance (takes more than two drinks to feel any alcohol effect)
- Patient's family history of alcohol problems
- Patient's medical or psychiatric conditions potentially worsened by alcohol
- Alcohol incidents in this patient's life (e.g., accidents, arrests, relationship problems, concerns expressed by others, unwillingness to discuss safe limits or adhere to them)
- Patient's abnormal laboratory findings (MCV, GGT, or other liver tests or other labs)

than "Alcohol has damaged your liver"; "Your alcohol level when you arrived in the ED was .160," rather than "You were drinking heavily before you came into the ED"; "You have a broken arm and stitches in your face," rather than "You were injured because of your drinking"; "You mentioned three important things—that your relationship with your wife is going poorly, that you are having a lot of stomach trouble, and that you lost your license to drive," rather than "Alcohol is wrecking your marriage, your career, and your body"; or "You are very shaky and sick until you have your first drink each morning," rather than "You are addicted to alcohol." Next, *ask* the patient what he or she thinks of this information. The patient's response to the "ask" indicates whether motivation and discrepancy are enhanced, and gives the physician ideas about the next steps.

Tell advice and explicit *recommendations* with two characteristics. First, give an objective rationale derived from a broader data base than simply this case, and second, give advice tentatively and conditionally. This might sound like: "One option that I recommend, based on data in the medical literature, and my experience with experts who have advised me about similar patients, is that you stop drinking all alcohol. Of course, no one can be certain that this is the right thing for you to do, or that it will work for you," or "Most people find that talking with people in Alcoholics Anonymous is helpful. AA might or might not be right for you. I recommend you go there." Next, *ask* the patient what he or she thinks of this advice (Box 51-14).

Patients will not do things that they themselves do not choose to do—commanding or ordering rather than checking the results of giving advice and making recommendations ensures lack of adherence. If physicians push ahead and try persuading patients in spite of reluctance, they foster continued ambivalence, raise resistance to change, and begin an enervating downward spiral in which both participants become further demoralized and discouraged.

Box 51-14. Advice/Recommendations for All Patients Who Meet Criteria for Abuse and for Most Who Drink Above Safe Limits

Compare patient's intake with safe limits, and advise cutting down to safe limits
Advise a period of abstinence to get information about living without alcohol
Advise attending six different meetings of Alcoholics Anonymous to get information and to have opportunity to reflect on patient's own drinking outside the office
Advise patient to listen to what loved ones tell him or her because they care.
If patient's family and good friends are not talking about patient's drinking, patient should ask them what they think
Advise patient to make a return visit to the physician to discuss patient's findings and thinking
Advise referral to an expert, since they can help explore the issues and decide which action option is best

Create Commitment and Confidence About Change

Commitment can only be augmented in an atmosphere that tolerates a genuine and full expression of ambivalence, and of negatives as well as positives, including both facts and feelings. Using reflection and emphasizing autonomy and choice create and support such an atmosphere. People develop commitment when credible, trusted, reliable advisors explicitly witness the special and unique strengths of those persons. People also develop commitment when they find a new chance to explicitly witness their own strengths and successes. Two skills that might achieve the goal of generating a discrepancy by suggesting to the patient a different aspect of reality or a new framing of reality follow, the first more direct, the second more subtle.

First, at a suitable moment when the conversation is going well (a true dialog, and not argumentative or discouraging), the patient should be told why he or she has a chance of success, based on facts the physician knows about the patient's unique characteristics, past successes, attitude, and other attributes. For example, the physician might say, "You've told me how independent, even stubborn, you can be, and that may mean that when you decide to do something difficult, you can stick to it"; "You quit drinking for 5 years once before, so you know it is possible"; or "You said you are pretty depressed, and I also see that you have come through similar moments in the past by getting involved with people in AA." Experts call this action *supporting self-efficacy.*

Another, sometimes more effective method is to help people express their own commitment, especially if they can do so emphatically. Again, find a suitable moment when the conversation is going well. Then, when the patient makes a statement that is positive, or hopeful, or promises success, the physician expresses the patient's previously stated skepticism, doubt, or ambivalence. This reminder (a reflection) of earlier patient statements encourages the patient to take the other side in the dialog. The patient can emphatically state a commitment, perhaps even claim strength, or cite a new reason for hope. For example, if a physician says, "From what you said earlier, it does not seem to me that you are quite ready to attempt quitting," the patient might respond, "I feel my only good choice is to get to AA!" The physician can then build on this discrepancy between prior and current expectations.

TREATMENT OPTIONS FOR ALCOHOL-DEPENDENT PATIENTS

Available options depend on competing priorities (e.g., pancreatitis, homelessness) and previous treatment experience. A list of options often includes those shown in Box 51-15. Patients entrenched in precontemplation may limit action to a return visit. Observing the consequences of future drinking and generating a list of pros and cons about change represent more active steps.[1]

Physicians should recommend abstinence as the preferred option and refer people for treatment; research data show that attempted referral is helpful, whether or not the referral is completed. This finding reflects the dynamics previously discussed regarding exploring ambivalence, giving choices, not rushing decisions, and clearly expressing support and concern. Physicians must know local resources in order to

Box 51-15. Referral Options

Alcoholics Anonymous
Physician specialist in addiction medicine (preferably certified by the American Society of Addiction Medicine [ASAM])
Licensed or certified substance abuse counselor
Family therapist specifically experienced in substance abuse
Substance abuse treatment agency (for inpatient or outpatient treatment)

provide quality referrals. Patients who are cognitively impaired (intoxicated or in withdrawal) need to "dry out" before treatment referral is attempted. Patients should be referred to outpatient treatment unless they are medically ill, psychotic, or homeless or have previously failed outpatient counseling. Most communities have specialized services available in both public and private sectors. Community mental health centers employ substance abuse specialists. Specialized licensing in substance abuse is available in all states for credentialed therapists, such as social workers and psychologists.

AA should be part of the referral for each patient, whether the perceived problem is early or late, mild or severe; all patients can benefit. The experienced physician presents AA attendance as a joint educational effort and suggests that talking over experiences at meetings will help the physician and patient more fully understand the situation. Recovery from dependence is facilitated by participation because patients identify with others who have faced the abyss and are now doing well. Patients can learn the "how to" as well as the "why" for being sober. For patients without dependence, meetings provide nonverbal, intuitive opportunities to discover that their "alcoholic" stereotype is too narrow. Participating with recovering people who seem otherwise like themselves enables patients to witness the discrepancy between what they thought and what they experience, and provides motivation.[5]

GIVING ADVICE TO MODERATE DRINKERS

Patients who drink within safe limits (see Box 51-5) need advice and reassurance. The advice might acknowledge the health benefits of 6 to 10 drinks per week,[11] and clearly state the safe limits. People drinking less should not be encouraged to drink up to the limits, since the benefits are small, and the risks of adverse effects (primarily brain effects that facilitate loss of control) increase with amount. Alcohol is always a sensitive topic, so physicians should use reflection and autonomy support strategies to promote a healthy physician-patient relationship.

GIVING ADVICE TO AT-RISK DRINKERS (HAZARDOUS DRINKERS)

People who drink more than the safe limits and those who abuse alcohol are reluctant to discuss drinking at any length. They want to keep drinking as they do, but have a lot to gain from their physicians' concern and advice.[10,13] What is pertinent for this group, not yet in deep trouble, to hear and heed? Like dependent drinkers, they need information about pathophysiology, feedback about their own condition, and advice to change. Patients need to know what research has shown. Studies show that some patients remain stable over long periods, and others progress to more serious problems. People who succeed at moderating their drinking to the safe limits or below usually do so after a period of abstinence (a minimum of about 3 months but often several years); statistically they are more often women, young, and not using other mood-altering drugs (prescribed or illicit), and they have had relatively few adverse consequences. Most have never met criteria for alcohol dependence. Patients who have already encountered problems from drinking only rarely succeed in avoiding further consequences if they continue to drink above safe limits. Patients who wish to cut back to safe limits can be encouraged to do so and referred to substance abuse professionals who can teach skills and monitor effectiveness. This particular lifestyle change is complex and troublesome for most people.

For this mixed group of heavy drinkers, some with no apparent problems and others with relatively minor problems, the safest option is to abstain, and physicians should recommend abstinence, at least for a few weeks. These patients are especially difficult for physicians, since they are reluctant to abstain or cut back. Negotiations may carry on for months or years in pursuit of continuing good health. Physicians are frustrated by the difficulty in convincing patients to see the same reality that the physician does concerning the nature of the problem. Persuasion, threats, a mountain of facts, and excellent suggestions for action steps seem only to harden the patient's resistance, maddeningly so. In fact, slogans from the self-help community such as, "No one but the patient can make a diagnosis" or "He won't do anything until he hits bottom," reflect lay wisdom derived from the frustration of pressing for change when people are not ready.

Effective physicians tolerate ambivalence and minimize resistance through use of reflection. They continue to explore drinking and its consequences with patients, and to provide feedback and new information. Standing by autonomy principles is precisely the proper course. Giving clear recommendations, but also helping patients make their own decisions and supporting any effort to change, is effective.

PHARMACOLOGIC CONSIDERATIONS IN PRIMARY CARE MANAGEMENT

One option that a primary care physician might suggest is disulfiram or naltrexone. Each has been shown effective in certain circumstances. Disulfiram provokes acetaldehyde accumulation after the ingestion of alcohol, producing a toxic state manifest by nausea, headache, unpleasant flushing, and respiratory distress. Severity depends on dose of alcohol and blood level of disulfiram. It takes several days without medication to avoid a toxic reaction, and it takes several doses of disulfiram to produce an appropriate blood level. Randomized studies of disulfiram use are negative. However, physicians who are using the skills discussed earlier and who present disulfiram as one option to patients not doing well find patients who clearly benefit from disulfiram. The recommended prescription is two 250-mg tablets daily for 4 days, then one daily. Anticipate use in 3-month blocks.

Randomized studies show naltrexone, an opioid antagonist, has beneficial effects in treatment of alcohol problems. Naltrexone diminishes craving, and treated patients who drank did not move into full relapse as often as control subjects did. Naltrexone may be a useful addition to the menu of treatment options. Referral for professional treatment is always appropriate when physicians prescribe naltrexone.

SUMMARY

This chapter presents guidelines for physician action regarding the broad spectrum of alcohol problems. Conversations about drinking are painful. Successful intervention requires that physicians value patient autonomy and use skills that encourage patients' reflection, dialog, the choice for change, confidence, and help seeking. When patients express little motivation for change, physicians who attend to their own frustration and reframe it as an incentive to better witness patients' ambivalence and resistance will improve patients' outcomes.

REFERENCES

1. Adams A, Ockene J, Wheeler E, et al: Alcohol counseling: physicians will do it, *J Gen Int Med* 13:692-698, 1998.
2. Bradley K, Badrinath S, Bush K, et al: Medical risks for women who drink alcohol, *J Gen Intern Med* 13:627-639, 1998.
3. Bradley K, Bush K, McDonell M, et al: Screening for problem drinking: comparison of CAGE and AUDIT, *J Gen Intern Med* 13:379-388, 1998.
4. Brown R, Leonard T, Saunders L, et al: A two-item screening test for alcohol and other drug problems, *J Fam Pract* 44:151-160, 1997.
5. Friedman P, Saitz R, Samet J: Management of adults recovering from alcohol or other drug problems: relapse prevention in primary care, *JAMA* 279:1227-1231, 1998.
6. Mayo-Smith M: Pharmacological management of alcohol withdrawal: a meta-analysis and evidence-based practice guideline, *JAMA* 278:144-151, 1997.
7. Miller W: Motivational interviewing: research, practice, and puzzles, *Addict Behav* 21:838-842, 1996.
8. NIAAA: The physicians' guide to helping patients with alcohol problems, Washington, DC, 1995, Government Printing Office, NIH publication #95-3769.
9. O'Connor P, Schottenfeld R: Patients with alcohol problems, *N Engl J Med* 338:592-602, 1998.
10. Peters C, Wilson D, Bruneau A, et al: Alcohol risk assessment and intervention for family physicians, *Can Fam Physician* 42:681-689, 1996.

10a. Prochaska J, Di Clemente C, Norcross J: In search of how people change: applications to addictive behaviors, *Am Psychol* 47:1102-1114, 1992.

11. Sacco R, Elkind M, Boden-Albala B, et al: Protective effect of moderate alcohol consumption on ischemic stroke, *JAMA* 281:53-60, 1999.
12. Sanchez-Craig M, Wilkinson D, Davila R: Empirically based guidelines for moderate drinking: 1-year results from three studies with problem drinkers, *Am J Pub Health* 85:823-828, 1995.
13. Wilk A, Jensen N, Havighurst T: Meta-analysis of randomized control trials addressing brief interventions in heavy alcohol drinkers, *J Gen Intern Med* 12:274-283, 1997.
14. Williams G, Deci E, Ryan R: Building healthcare partnerships by supporting autonomy: promoting maintained behavior change and positive health outcomes. In Suchman A, Bothelo R, Hinton-Walker P, editors: *Partnerships in health care* U of Rochester, Rochester, NY, 1998, University of Rochester, pp 67-87.

CHAPTER 52

Drug Abuse and Dependence

Robert M. Swift

APPROACH TO THE DRUG-ABUSING PATIENT

Drug abuse and dependence are common problems and therefore are encountered regularly by primary care physicians. The Epidemiological Catchment Area Study, a survey of mental health and substance abuse disorders in nearly 20,000 adult Americans, identified a 7% lifetime prevalence of drug dependence. The high prevalence of drug use is associated with considerable morbidity and mortality. Drugs are strongly associated with violent crime and are responsible for both work-related and non–work-related accidents. Each year, alcoholism is estimated to cause 100,000 excess deaths; illicit drug abuse, 19,000 excess deaths; and tobacco, 400,000 excess deaths. Drug abuse and dependence are major causes of psychologic and social problems including family dysfunction, family violence, and child abuse. The total yearly costs to the U.S. economy from drug abuse and dependence are estimated at $98 billion. Of this, almost $10 billion is attributed to direct health care costs of hospitals, treatment centers, nursing homes, and professional services. Alcoholism and drug dependence are associated with 25% to 50% of all general hospital admissions and 50% to 75% of psychiatric admissions, and contribute to complications and increased costs in those patients admitted to hospitals for other reasons.

Clinical treatment outcome studies have demonstrated that treatment for drug addiction can be effective. However, since drug abuse and dependence are chronic relapsing disorders, treatment for these conditions may not be completely effective or may require multiple treatment episodes. The optimal goal of treatment should be abstinence from drugs. With proper diagnosis, intervention, and treatment, 1-year abstinence rates of 30% to 70% can be achieved. Even patients who are unable to achieve long-term abstinence may still benefit from treatment by having their lives prolonged, their morbidity minimized, and their quality of life improved. Controlled research studies, such as the California Drug and Alcohol Treatment Assessment (CALDATA) Study have demonstrated that addiction treatment is also cost-effective. In this study, approximately seven dollars was saved for every dollar invested in treatment. Reviews of published studies on health care utilization find significant savings in total health care costs when drug abuse treatment is available.

It is therefore important for primary care physicians to properly assess and diagnose substance abuse and dependence, to possess knowledge about therapies for the acute management of intoxicated or withdrawing patients, and to possess knowledge regarding long-term treatment and rehabilitation. An overall biopsychosocial approach to addiction treatment is preferred. A treatment plan that is practical, economical, and based on well-established principles should be utilized. In addition, treatment should be individualized: the patient should be matched to the best modality of treatment for the type and severity of the problems. Substance abuse treatment is complex, since it often involves other family members, legal and forensic systems, public assistance services, schools, and child protection agencies. The ability of the primary care physician to work with professionals from these disciplines is important. This chapter discusses the diagnosis and treatment of drug abuse and dependence in the primary care setting.

Definitions

Historically, clinical thinking about addictive disorders has been clouded by questions of whether use of addictive psychoactive substances constitutes a medical or a moral problem. The situation is further complicated by ambiguities over the legal status of some drugs. Some governmental authorities consider any use of certain drugs illegal, whereas in other localities, use of the same drugs is permitted for medicinal, recreational, and religious purposes. Thus it may be difficult to ascertain exactly where medically acceptable use ends and problem use begins. An example is marijuana. This substance, illegal in most locations, is now approved for medicinal use in California and Arizona and is also used for religious purposes by at least one religious order.

Language used to describe addictive disorders can be misleading because the words describe other conditions. Commonly used, *abuse* is a pejorative term that implies voluntary unlawful conduct and does not necessarily connote a disease state, as such. *Dependence* is a term derived from pharmacology and describes a physiologic state of adaptation that occurs after chronic use of a drug. *Tolerance* refers to the state in which the physical or behavioral effects of a constant dose of a drug decrease over time, or when a greater amount of the substance is required to produce the same effect. Dependence and tolerance occur with many pharmacologic agents, besides addictive substances. The word *addiction* is commonly used to describe a repertoire of pathologic behaviors that serve to maintain drug use (e.g., lying, stealing, purchase of illegal drugs).

The American Psychiatric Association (APA) and the World Health Organization (WHO) have declared problem use of psychoactive substances to be medical disorders and have defined these disorders using specific diagnostic criteria. The criteria for Substance-Related Disorders in the Diagnostic and Statistical Manual, Version IV (DSM-IV) of the APA, and the International Classification of Diseases, Version 10 (ICD-10) of the WHO, represent the manifestations of addictive use of alcohol/drugs and include psychologic and social dysfunction, in addition to tolerance and dependence. A special version of the DSM-IV has been adapted for use by primary care physicians. However, the medical definition for substance-use disorders does not rule out the role of personal responsibility for seeking and complying with treatment, and does not excuse patients for crime or damages to others as a consequence of alcohol/substance use.

Classification of Addictive Disorders

According to the DSM-IV, the acute and chronic effects of psychoactive substances are classified under two major categories: *substance-use disorders* and *substance-induced disorders*. The two substance-use disorders are *substance-dependence* and *substance-abuse*. Substance-induced disorders include the behavioral and neurologic effects of acute and chronic drug use. These are substance intoxication, substance withdrawal, substance-induced psychotic disorder, substance-induced mood disorder, substance-induced anxiety, substance-induced sleep disorder, substance-induced persisting dementia (and amnestic) disorders, and substance-induced sexual dysfunction. The various disorders are described in Boxes 52-1 and 52-2.

Substance-Dependence. Substance-dependence is a maladaptive pattern of substance use with adverse clinical consequences. This includes substance use that is uncontrolled and substance use in spite of adverse consequences. In the DSM-IV nomenclature, *abuse* is a residual category that describes patterns of drug use that do not meet the criteria for dependence.

Substance Abuse. Substance abuse is a residual category that describes patterns of drug use that do not meet the criteria for dependence. Substance abuse is a maladaptive pattern of substance use that causes clinically significant impairment. This may include impairments in social, family or occupational functioning; use in the presence of psychologic or physical problems; or use in hazardous situations, such as driving while intoxicated.

DSM-IV designates 11 distinct classes of psychoactive substances: alcohol; amphetamine or related substances; caffeine; cannabis; cocaine; hallucinogens; inhalants; opioids; nicotine; phencyclidine or related substances; and sedatives, hypnotics, or anxiolytics. Each class is associated with both an organic mental disorder and a substance-use disorder. Under the category of *substance-use disorders*, 10 classes (all but nicotine) are associated with abuse and

Box 52-1. Classification of Addictive Disorders

Diagnosing substance dependence requires at least three of the following conditions occurring over a 12-month period:

- *Tolerance*, that is, the need for increased amounts of the substance in order to achieve intoxication or other desired effect, or markedly diminished effect with use of the same amount of substance
- Characteristic *withdrawal* symptoms (may not apply to cannabis, hallucinogens or PCP), or the use of the substance (or a closely related substitute) to relieve or avoid withdrawal
- Substance often taken in larger amounts or over a longer period of time than intended
- Persistent desire or one or more unsuccessful attempts to cut down or to control substance use
- A great deal of time spent in activities necessary to get the substance (e.g., theft), taking the substance (e.g., chain-smoking), or recovering from its effects
- Important social, occupational, or recreational activities given up or reduced because of substance use
- Continued substance use despite knowledge of having a persistent or recurrent social, psychologic, or physical problem that is caused by or exacerbated by use of the substance

Modified in part from American Psychiatric Association DSM-IV, 1995.

Box 52-2. Classification of Substance-Induced Disorders

Substance intoxication: reversible, substance-specific physiologic and behavioral changes resulting from recent exposure to a psychoactive substance. Produced by all substances.

Substance withdrawal: a substance-specific syndrome that develops following cessation of, or reduction in, dosage of a regularly used substance. Occurs with chronic use of all substances, except perhaps cannabis and hallucinogens.

Substance-induced delirium (confusion, psychosis): occurs with overdose of many substances.

Substance-induced psychotic disorder (psychosis): may occur with PCP and hallucinogens, stimulants, cannabis, and alcohol.

Substance-induced mood disorder (depression, mania), also anxiety: common with many substances, especially stimulants. Disorder must be distinguished from primary psychiatric disorder that preceded drug use.

Substance-induced sleep disorder: a sleep disturbance attributable to acute or chronic substance use. Common with sedatives and stimulants.

Substance-induced persisting dementia (and amnestic) disorders: a substance-specific syndrome of cognitive dysfunction that persists after acute intoxication or withdrawal abates.

Substance-induced sexual dysfunction: alcohol, benzodiazepines, and opioids commonly reduce sexual responsiveness and performance.

dependence; dependence only is defined for nicotine. Polysubstance dependence is defined as using three or more categories of substances. A category for *other substance-use disorders* includes use of anabolic steroids, nitrate inhalants, anticholinergic agents, and other psychoactive substances.

Extent of Drug Abuse

The Federal government, researchers, and clinicians utilize national surveys of drug use to determine current incidence and prevalence and to track patterns over time. Each of these survey methods targets different population groups, but the data are generally concordant. Unfortunately, systematic studies of drug abuse prevalence have not been conducted in primary care patient populations; however, the trends are probably similar. Two of the most commonly cited surveys are described below.

The National Household Survey on Drug Abuse is an annual survey of selected households regarding recent, remote, and lifetime drug use. Results of this survey may be biased, since it may miss nontraditional households or those who live on the streets. During 1992, data indicated that approximately 22.9 million persons consumed illicit drugs during the previous year. Marijuana in its various forms was the most commonly used illicit drug, used by 17.4 million persons in 1992. About 7.8 million persons used psychotherapeutic drugs, such as stimulants, sedatives, tranquilizers, and analgesics, for nonmedical reasons. Cocaine in all forms, including crack, was used by almost 5 million persons, and 2 million and 2.4 million persons used inhalants and hallucinogens, respectively. There are estimated to be 1 million regular users of heroin, of whom 15% are in some form of treatment, most commonly methadone maintenance. Trends in substance use are shown in Fig. 52-1.

The Drug Abuse Warning Network (DAWN) surveys hospitals throughout the United States to obtain reports on drug-related emergency room visits. The data are biased, because the information is based on persons seeking emergency treatment in hospitals. Although it underestimates total use and overrepresents more intensive use leading to acute complications, it provides objective data, rather than data based on self-reports.

Data from these two surveys indicate that casual drug use has declined dramatically since the late 1970s, while intensive use has significantly increased since that time. According to 1993 DAWN data, an estimated 466,900 drug abuse–related emergency room episodes occurred in the United States. This is a 16% increase from the 403,600 episodes found in the 1988 DAWN survey. The rate of drug-related episodes per 100,000 persons age 6 and older increased from 186 in 1988 to 204 in 1993. Of concern is the trend for increased illicit drug and alcohol use—including use of marijuana, cocaine, and inhalants—among the 12 to 17 year olds in the United States. Nearly twice as many adolescents took drugs in the month before being interviewed in 1995 than was the case 2 years before. Heroin use among young adults has also increased, rising from 0.3% among 18 to 25 year olds in 1988 to 1.3% in 1992. Multiple drug use appears to be increasing and is common among opiate, sedative, and stimulant abusers.

The Causes of Addictive Disorders

Studies of individuals with addictive disorders or at risk for developing substance abuse and dependence have identified many factors that foster the development and continuance of substance use. Genetic, familial, environmental, occupational, socioeconomic, cultural, personality, life stress, psychiatric comorbidity, biologic, social learning, behavioral, and conditioning factors have all been proposed to influence the development of addictive disorders. The relative contributions of any of these factors vary from individual to individual and no single factor accounts for all of the risk.

The influence of genetic factors in addictive disorders has been primarily studied in alcohol dependence; less is known about genetic influences in drug dependence. However, a recent study of 1934 female twins found higher concordance rates for abuse and dependence of cocaine and marijuana in identical twins than fraternal twins, suggesting that genetic factors are important. Similar results were found in a study of male twin pairs. The identification of specific genes that predispose one to drug abuse is an active area of investigation.

Advances in neurobiology have led to an increased understanding of the neurochemistry of drug and alcohol dependence. It is hypothesized that the pleasurable, stimulating, and positively reinforcing effects of alcohol and other drugs of abuse are mediated by a brain dopaminergic pathway that projects from the ventral tegmental area to the nucleus accumbens. Repeated drug use sensitizes the system and leads to the development of dependence.

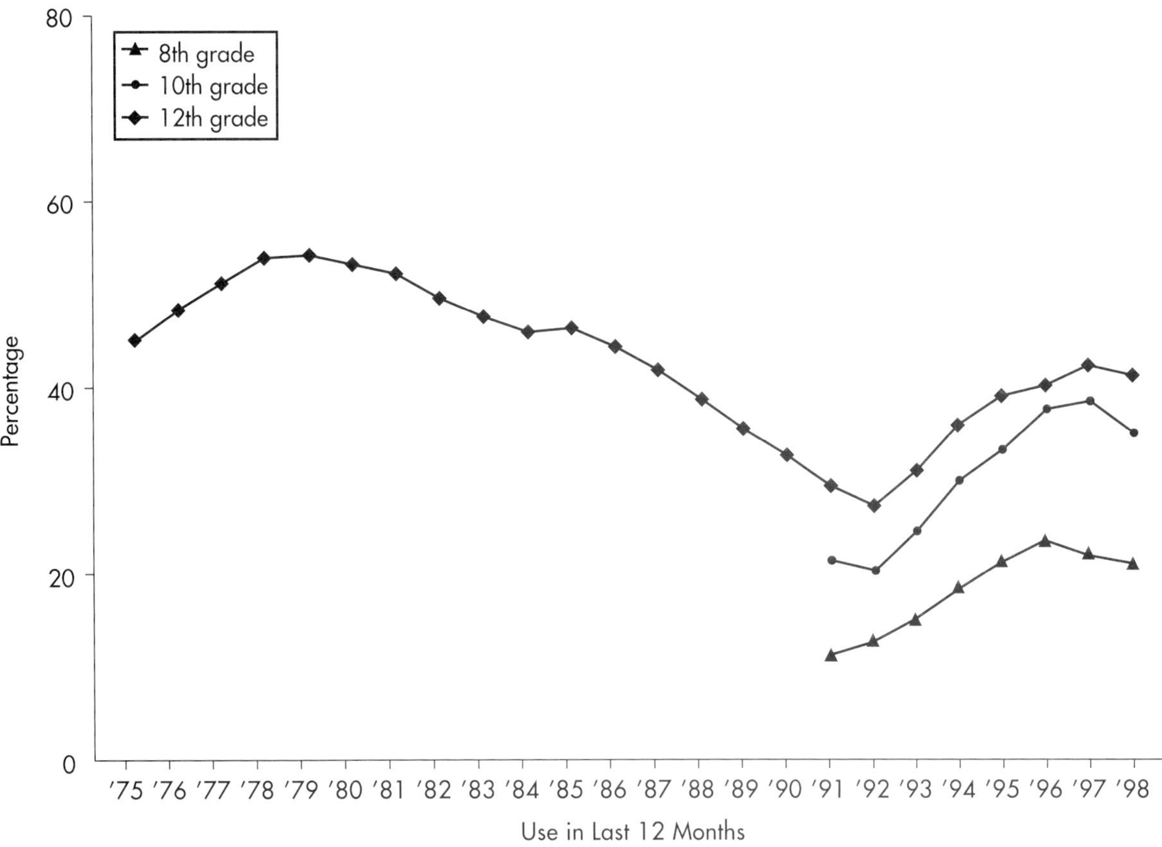

Fig. 52-1. Trends in annual prevalence of an illicit drug use index for eighth, tenth, and twelfth graders. (From *Monitoring the future study*, University of Michigan.)

ASSESSMENT AND DIAGNOSIS

History

All patients should be screened for alcohol, drug, and tobacco use as part of the routine medical history and examination. Although some patients present with drug use as a chief complaint, others present with medical or surgical problems and only later reveal a substance-use disorder through physical or laboratory findings or incidental discovery. Often, patients may be reluctant to report the extent of their drug use out of shame or fear of social or legal consequences. Inherent in addictive illness is resistance by the addict and significant others to consider that drugs are a problem. This minimization and rationalization of the problem is usually referred to as denial; denial permits the continued propagation of the addiction.

The best way to elicit accurate information is through a supportive, therapeutic relationship. In the context of this relationship, the physician should conduct a detailed drug and alcohol history, conduct a physical and mental status examination, order and interpret necessary laboratory tests, and meet with family or significant others to obtain additional information. If the presence of drug use is not recognized, the addictive disease will continue unabated.

To obtain information about the patient's drug and alcohol use, many physicians routinely ask quantity and frequency questions about psychoactive substances, such as "How much?" and "How often?" These types of questions are most useful in low to moderate drug users. Heavy users tend to underreport their use and quantity, and frequency questions can be unreliable in this group. It is more effective to explore whether the heavy user has experienced deleterious social or behavioral consequences from drug use, or has poor control of use.

Several formalized interviews have been developed that discriminate alcoholism using these criteria. The CAGE questionnaire is a simple four-item test that uses the letters *C*, *A*, *G*, and *E* as a mnemonic for questions about alcohol use (Box 52-3). A positive answer on more than two questions is considered suspicious for alcohol abuse. The CAGE may be a better predictor of alcoholism in medical patients than laboratory tests. The CAGE is often adapted to drug use, as well.

Two interviews that effectively address the behavioral consequences of drug abuse are the Drug Abuse Screening Test (DAST) and the Addiction Severity Index (ASI). These instruments have been primarily utilized in clinical research and have not been widely used in clinical practice.

Other items in the medical history that should increase suspicion about substance use include divorce, problems at work (job loss, tardiness, absenteeism, work-related injuries), injuries (falls, auto accidents, fights), arrests, driving while intoxicated, leisure activities involving drugs or alcohol, and financial problems. Having a drug- or alcohol-abusing parent or spouse increases the risk for substance use.

Box 52-3. The CAGE Interview

C: "Have you ever felt the need to *C*ut down on your drinking (or drugs)?"
A: "Have people *A*nnoyed you by criticizing your drinking (or drug use)?"
G: "Have you felt bad or *G*uilty about your drinking (or using drugs)?"
E: "Have you ever had a drink first thing in the morning to steady your nerves or get rid of a hangover (*E*ye opener) (or used drugs to get going in the morning)?"

Other Drugs and Medications. The propensity to freely exchange one drug for another, or to use them simultaneously, is common. Studies indicate that a high percentage of problem drug users, particularly those under the age of 30, use at least one other drug regularly, including nicotine. Some 50% to 75% of heroin addicts, 80% of cocaine addicts, and 40% of cannabis addicts are addicted to alcohol. Over 80% of drug users are also nicotine-dependent. In obtaining a history of drug use and related consequences, a careful screen for alcohol, tobacco, and other drugs is mandatory.

Physical Examination

During the routine physical examination, the examining physician needs to be alert for findings indicative of drug abuse or dependence. A physical examination can provide important information about the presence of substance use and its medical complications. Physical stigmata of substance use can be due to the drug used or can be associated with the route of administration. Route-specific problems include the presence of a necrotic nasal septum from cocaine nasal insufflation, as well as respiratory and oropharyngeal problems in smokers of cocaine, cannabis, heroin, or nicotine; intravenous drug users may show track marks of intravenous injection and signs and symptoms of human immunodeficiency virus (HIV)-related illnesses and hepatitis B or C regardless of the drug injected. Medical consequences specific to each organ system are discussed below.

Constitutional Symptoms. Heavy users of any drug may show general physical debilitation, including weight loss and malnutrition, or evidence of repeated trauma, especially to the head. Fatigue, fevers, night sweats, and chills of unknown significance occur commonly in intravenous drug users; however, such symptoms can be signs of more serious systemic infections, including endocarditis, tuberculosis, and HIV.

Skin. The examination of the skin can provide evidence of intravenous drug use and its duration. The examination must be complete and include skin on unexposed areas. Fresh abscesses, cellulitis, and tissue necrosis are all signs of recent drug use. Injection trauma is usually more common with cocaine, resulting from tissue vasoconstriction produced by the drug; however, this can occur with any drug. Parallel needle marks, a single row of scars, hyperpigmentation overlying a vein, and palpably sclerotic veins are all signs of chronic intravenous use. In those patients with absent peripheral veins, the axillary, penile, internal jugular, and femoral veins should be observed for signs of injection. Such patients are at risk for venous and lymphatic insufficiency, leading to lymphedema and systemic infection. Trauma to the skin, including abrasions, lacerations, and cigarette burns, is often observed in drug users. Excoriations can result from opiate-induced pruritus, poor hygiene, or cocaine-induced tactile hallucinations. Although Kaposi's sarcoma is uncommon in heterosexual drug abusers with acquired immunodeficiency syndrome (AIDS), other skin infections including herpes zoster are observed.

Head and Neck. Perforation of the nasal septum is often found in nasal drug users, particularly those using stimulants. Poor dentition is extremely common among opiate and stimulant users. Jaundice and scleral icterus usually indicate the presence of acute hepatitis of viral or toxic etiology. Ophthalmoscopic examination of the retina may disclose emboli, ischemia, and central nervous system (CNS) disease associated with AIDS. Infections of the mucous membranes, especially oral candidiasis, are also common in AIDS patients.

Chest. Drug users of all types may develop cardiac disease. Cocaine and other sympathomimetic stimulants can induce tachycardia, dysrhythmias, and myocardial ischemia. Congestive heart failure involving the right or left ventricles can have multiple etiologies, including pulmonary disease from injection emboli, and heart valve disease from infection, infarction, or cardiomyopathy. Cardiomyopathy is associated with heroin, cocaine, alcohol, and organic solvent use.

Pulmonary disease is common in drug users. Most drug users are also heavy tobacco users. Smokers of marijuana, cocaine, or other drugs are at greater risk for the development of lung disease, including pneumonias. Opiate and sedative abusers are at particular risk because of suppression of their respiration and cough reflexes, and HIV-positive patients because of immune impairment. In HIV-positive patients, the possibility of tuberculosis, atypical mycobacterium infection, or *Pneumocystis carinii* or other opportunistic infection should be considered on the development of dyspnea and cough.

Male users of marijuana or methadone may present with drug-induced gynecomastia. Chronic alcohol use or other liver disease should also be considered in such patients.

Abdomen. Hepatitis is common in drug users and a complete examination of the liver should be performed to assess tenderness to palpation and hepatomegaly. Splenomegaly is a relatively common finding in otherwise healthy parenteral drug users. Enlargement of the spleen should, however, prompt closer examination of the lymph nodes to rule out other systemic diseases including HIV.

Prostitution is common in both male and female users of illicit drugs. Genital/pelvic and rectal examinations should be conducted to exclude venereal disease and cervical cancer. Blood in the stool may be due to anal sex, chronic constipation from opiates, and gastritis due to alcohol or consumption of drugs containing aspirin.

Lymphatic System. Adenopathy is common in injection drug users; its presence, particularly in the groin and axillae, is likely related to repeated injection of antigenic and infectious materials into the extremities. However, adenopathy may indicate more serious illness such as systemic infections and lymphomas. Lymphedema of the extremities due to chronic venous obstruction is commonly observed in injection drug users.

Nervous System. Peripheral neuropathies are commonly observed in alcohol and drug users. Brachial plexus neuropathy (so-called "Saturday night palsy") is seen with drugs producing obtundation, including opiates, alcohol, and sedatives. Peripheral neuropathies can occur secondary to tissue necrosis from drug injection, associated infections, or inflammatory response. CNS conditions are also common. Cerebral infarction or bleeding due to stimulants and cocaine may produce a variety of focal neurologic findings. Chronic solvent use can induce cerebellar ataxia and cerebral atrophy. HIV-positive patients are subject to bacterial, viral, and fungal infections of the CNS.

Mental Status Examination

All patients should receive a screening mental status examination to assess cognitive and psychiatric function. Psychiatric disorders such as mood disorders, anxiety disorders, attention deficit disorder, and personality disorders frequently coexist with substance use disorders. Drug use is also associated with head trauma. The screening mental status examination should at minimum include an assessment of orientation (person, place, and time), memory (recent and remote), and speech and thought processes. Slurred speech or speech that is not normal in form or content suggests drug intoxication or the presence of other mental disorders. If abnormalities are found on the mental status examination, a more extensive psychologic and psychiatric assessment should be conducted to formally assess attention, cognition, and mood.

Laboratory and Toxicologic Screening for Substance Use

As part of the physical assessment, patients should receive routine laboratory testing, including complete blood count, tests of kidney and liver function, and a urinalysis. If intravenous drug use is suspected, serologic testing for hepatitis B and C and HIV should be considered. All patients tested for viral hepatitides and HIV, regardless of whether the results are positive or negative, should receive both pretest and posttest counseling about the meaning of the results and about the dangers of needle sharing and unprotected sex. Patients with positive hepatitis C serology should be referred for follow-up liver function tests, viral load, possible liver biopsy, and treatment with interferon-α or other antiviral agents. Patients with positive HIV serology should be referred for T lymphocyte subset testing and antiretroviral therapy.

Serum and urine toxicologic screens have an important role in the assessment and treatment of patients with substance-use disorders. However, it is important that physicians be aware of how to properly conduct such testing and how to interpret the results. Optimally, informed consent should be obtained for all drug testing unless the patient is unable to give consent or testing is required by law. Most toxicologic analyses are conducted on urine, although analyses are sometimes conducted on blood, amniotic fluid, saliva, and hair. To minimize errors and adulteration of the sample, all samples should be obtained while the patient is directly observed. Positive test results should be confirmed with a second test using a different analytic method, since compounds in foods or medications that are chemically similar to drugs can yield false-positive results under certain analytic methods. A positive test suggests use of a psychoactive substance, but it may not indicate the extent of use, when it occurred, or whether there was behavioral impairment.

TREATMENT

Overview

The most effective way to reduce the medical, social, and psychologic impact of drugs is through effective treatment. Addiction treatment may be defined as medical, psychologic, and social interventions to reduce or eliminate the harmful effects of drugs on the individual, his or her family and associates, and others in society. Although abstinence is the goal of most treatments, reductions in quantity and frequency of drug use can still bring about "harm reduction." Treatment usually consists of the following components:

1. *Intervention:* initiation of treatment and/or referral
2. *Detoxification:* removal of drug from the body and the treatment of withdrawal
3. *Rehabilitation:* medical, psychologic, and social measures to help avoid the use of psychoactive substances in the future
4. *Aftercare:* processes to assist in maintaining a drug-free state

Treatment for substance abuse and dependence ranges from very low cost, less intensive methods (e.g., brief advice to stop drug use, information on self-help programs) to higher cost, more intensive methods (e.g., inpatient detoxification, residential rehabilitation programs). There are also many different orientations toward treatment, ranging from the medical/biologic to the spiritual/religious, and from total abstinence to substitution therapies (such as methadone maintenance), which are utilized to different extents by different programs.

At any given time, a large number of individuals are undergoing treatment for drug and alcohol problems. One government survey of treatment programs found more than 800,000 clients are in active alcohol or drug treatment in specialized treatment programs on any given day: 29% are in treatment for drug addiction, 45% for alcoholism, and 26% for combined drug addiction and alcoholism. However, studies indicate that a far greater number of individuals require intervention and treatment.

For patients with *substance dependence,* the goals of treatment usually include the establishment of a drug-free state. If total abstinence is not obtainable, a significant reduction in harmful drug or alcohol use will still be of some benefit. For patients with *substance abuse,* the goal should be a reduction in harmful drug or alcohol use. All physicians should be able to assist patients who are identified as having potential drug disorders by using a number of treatment strategies that include brief interventions, counseling, pharmacotherapy, and referral to specialized treatment and other community programs.

For all patients, treatment goals should include psychologic, medical, family, and social interventions to reduce or eliminate the harmful effects of drugs. Changes in living situation, work situation, or friendships may be necessary to decrease drug availability and to reduce social pressure to use drugs. Individual and group psychotherapy is necessary for understanding the role of the drug in the individual's life, improving self-esteem, and relieving psychologic distress. The treatment of underlying psychiatric illness and pain is important, since this may reduce the need for self-medication. Although most treatment can be provided in an outpatient setting, halfway houses, therapeutic communities, and other residential treatment situations may be necessary to ensure a drug-free environment. Self-help groups, such as Narcotics Anonymous (NA), Cocaine Anonymous (CA), Alcoholics Anonymous (AA), ALANON, and Rational Recovery, provide effective treatment, education, emotional support, and hope to patients and their families.

When a patient is referred to a specialized addiction treatment program or an addiction treatment professional, it is important for the primary care physician to remain in contact with the patient, the family, and the other clinicians, so as to maintain continuity of care and to help coordinate treatment.

Legal Aspects of Addiction Treatment

State and federal laws can influence drug treatment in several ways. First, the possession and use of many drugs or drug paraphernalia are often criminal offenses. Persons arrested for drug use or possession may be remanded to involuntary treatment for a specified duration by criminal courts or drug courts. Such patients may enter treatment to avoid incarceration or to maintain a driver's license or other professional license. Because these patients do not voluntarily choose to enter treatment, they may see treatment as a punishment and present resistance to treatment. Indeed, the physician may be placed in the position of having to inform the court or other authorities should the patient leave treatment or relapse to drug use. Optimally, treatment should proceed according to a written plan, so that each party understands his or her respective responsibilities and options and so that misunderstandings do not occur later. Physicians should educate themselves about federal and state confidentiality laws pertaining to substance abuse treatment, as well as institutional policies on confidentiality and patient rights.

Law or rules of regulatory agencies may determine the format of certain treatments. Methadone maintenance is an example of such a treatment. The guidelines for methadone maintenance were instituted by an act of Congress that established treatment eligibility, methadone dosages that may be used, the frequency of service delivery, and the ancillary psychologic, social, and medical services that must be provided for patients. The Food and Drug Administration (FDA) and the Drug Enforcement Administration (DEA) tightly regulate methadone maintenance treatment.

Intervention

After identification of drug abuse or dependence, the physician needs to provide feedback on diagnosis and treatment options and to assess the individual's readiness to engage in treatment. Surveys of physicians demonstrate a lack of confidence in treating substance abuse and dependence. However, in the past decade, several methods have been developed to help primary care physicians successfully intervene with patients. *The Physician's Guide to Helping Patients With Alcohol Problems,* recently released by the National Institute on Alcohol Abuse and Alcoholism (NIAAA), presents useful intervention methods.

A model of human behavior that has been widely accepted to explain the process of behavioral change in addictive behaviors is the *transtheoretic model* of behavioral change. The transtheoretic model posits that behavioral change is a series of stages: the *precontemplative* stage (not even thinking about changing); the *contemplative* stage (thinking about changing); the *action* stage (making efforts toward change); and the *maintenance* stage (maintaining the changes). Understanding the stage that the patient is in at the time of intervention can assist with optimizing the intervention. For example, a patient in the precontemplative stage would benefit most from basic education about his or her disorder and its consequences; a patient in the action phase would benefit most from receiving skills to help with avoiding addictive substances. The goal of the intervention is to move the patient from precontemplation into contemplation or from contemplation into action (treatment).

Brief interventions conducted in a supportive manner have proven extremely effective in enhancing entrance into alcoholism treatment. Brief interventions can consist of one or more sessions in the physician's office, during which education about substance use and dependence is provided and a plan for cutting down or eliminating substance use is negotiated. The patient and physician together should develop a contract, preferably written, defining the treatment and intervention plan. A formal means of assessment of effectiveness and follow-up should be part of the plan. Motivational interviewing, a technique that identifies and motivates the patient to utilize his or her own treatment resources, has been shown to be effective in engaging patients in treatment and reducing use of addictive substances.

Unfortunately, drug users are frequently uninterested in substance abuse treatment or medical treatment for associated problems. The denial of problems or the rejection of necessary medical treatment on the part of the patient can produce frustration, anger, and discouragement in the clinical personnel who are attempting to help the patient. The physician needs to keep a clinical and nonjudgmental perspective, and to recognize that rejection of treatment is part of the behavior associated with addiction.

Detoxification and Treatment of Withdrawal

Many patients entering treatment require detoxification to achieve a drug-free state and to minimize morbidity associated with withdrawal. Ideally, detoxification should be closely supervised. This may be accomplished in an outpatient, inpatient, or residential setting depending on the drug used, the level of dependence, and the presence of coexisting medical and psychiatric problems. Several methods for drug detoxification are described in Box 52-4.

Withdrawal. Withdrawal is a distinct physiologic and behavioral state that follows cessation or reduction in the amount of drug used. In general, the signs and symptoms of withdrawal are the opposite of those that the drug produces (e.g., withdrawal from depressants produces excitation). The proposed neurobiologic mechanism for withdrawal is a change in the number of postsynaptic neurotransmitter receptors or in receptor sensitivity that occurs with chronic drug use. It should be emphasized that withdrawal is not specific to addictive substances, chronic use of medications such as β-adrenergic blockers, antihistamines, antidysrhyth-

Box 52-4. General Methods of Drug Detoxification

1. Controlled administration of the drug, with a slow taper in the daily drug dose (e.g., tapering pentobarbital over time in pentobarbital dependence).
2. Administration of a similar or cross-tolerant agent that is slowly tapered over time (e.g., methadone taper in opioid withdrawal; chlordiazepoxide in alcohol withdrawal).
3. Administration of an alternate agent to suppress signs and symptoms of withdrawal (e.g., clonidine in opioid withdrawal, anticonvulsants in sedative withdrawal).
4. Nonpharmacologic detoxification, with supportive care (e.g., social-setting detoxification in alcohol dependence).

mics, and antidepressants may be associated with a withdrawal syndrome following drug discontinuation.

SPECIFIC DRUGS

The following section describes the pharmacology and treatment of drug intoxication and dependence induced by specific drugs.

Sedatives and Hypnotics

Intoxication. Sedatives and hypnotic drugs (e.g., benzodiazepines, barbiturates), sometimes referred to as *downers* or *minor tranquilizers*, consist of drugs that have depressant effects on the CNS. This class of drugs includes barbiturates, benzodiazepines, ethchlorvynol, glutethimide, meprobamate, and γ-hydroxybutyrate. Sedative medications are a major source of drug emergencies including overdose. Yet, they are among the most prescribed drugs, and are routinely used for their anxiolytic and hypnotic effects. Patients may obtain these medications illicitly from the street or from physicians who unwittingly (or purposely) may be contributing to abuse or dependence. Most of the medications in this group augment the activity of the inhibitory brain neurotransmitter, γ-aminobutyric acid (GABA). Specific binding sites at the chloride channel–GABA receptor complex in neurons exist for benzodiazepines, barbiturates, and other drugs. When these sites are occupied by drug, increased chloride conductance leads to hyperpolarization and inhibition of neurons.

Manifestations of intoxication from sedatives and tranquilizers include initial euphoria, followed by sedation, slowed mention and coordination, confusion, and loss of consciousness. At higher doses, depressants can cause hypotension, bradycardia, and slowed respiratory rate and coma. Impaired respiration can lead to acidosis, dysrhythmias, arrest, and death. Many sedative overdoses involve multiple medications, including psychotropic medications (antidepressants, antipsychotics) and alcohol that can potentiate respiratory and CNS suppression. The length of sedative intoxication depends on the medication dose, the medication half-life, and whether use is acute or chronic. Chronic users show increased tolerance and more rapid metabolism.

The treatment of sedative intoxication is generally supportive. For patients presenting within an hour of intoxication, induction of vomiting or gastric lavage followed by activated charcoal administration may prevent absorption of pill fragments remaining in the stomach. Obtunded patients require close monitoring and respiratory support if respiratory distress is noted. Alert patients need monitoring and protection from harm.

Sedative Withdrawal. Chronic sedative use leads to tolerance, physical dependence, and withdrawal when medication is stopped or the dose is reduced. Signs of withdrawal are agitation; increased psychomotor activity; tremulousness; fever; sweating; delirium; convulsions; tachycardia; hypertension; coarse tremor of tongue, eyelids, and hands; and seizures. Symptoms of withdrawal are anxiety, euphoria, depression, incoherent thoughts, hostility, grandiosity, disorientation, and tactile, auditory, and visual hallucinations. Typically, the period of withdrawal depends on the half-life of the medication. For short-acting medications such as triazolam, withdrawal can begin within hours of stopping the medication and may persist for 2 to 3 days. For intermediate-acting sedatives (e.g., pentobarbital, alprazolam) the peak of withdrawal is 2 to 4 days, and the typical duration of withdrawal is 4 to 7 days; for long-acting sedatives (e.g., diazepam, phenobarbital) peak period of withdrawal is 4 to 7 days, and duration 7 to 14 days.

Treatment. Sedative-dependence treatment occurs in two stages, detoxification and long-term rehabilitation. Detoxification can be accomplished by gradually tapering the drug, substituting another depressant drug that shares pharmacologic cross-tolerance, or administering another agent to suppress withdrawal symptoms. Benzodiazepines show cross-tolerance with each other and with most other sedative/hypnotic drugs and alcohol. Therefore benzodiazepines can be substituted for other benzodiazepines and barbiturates and vice versa. The conversion for equivalent doses can be calculated if doses are actually known prior to taper. A long half-life medication is usually more effective than short-acting preparations in suppressing withdrawal symptoms, in producing a gradual and smooth transition to the abstinent state, and in enhancing patient compliance.

The duration of the tapering schedule is determined by the half-life of the sedative drug that is being withdrawn. (1) For intermediate-acting sedatives such as alprazolam or pentobarbital, 7 to 10 days of a gradual taper with a long-acting benzodiazepine or barbiturate is often sufficient: 7 days for low-dose and short duration of use and 10 days for high-dose and long duration of benzodiazepine use. In the case of alprazolam, because of higher rates of withdrawal seizures, the use of phenobarbital substitution is recommended for the taper. (2) For the long-acting benzodiazepines, 10 to 14 days of a gradual taper with a long-acting benzodiazepine or barbiturate is often sufficient: 10 days for low-dose and short duration and 14 days for high-dose and long duration of use. The doses can be given in qid or tid intervals. The long-acting preparations accumulate during the taper to result in a self-leveling effect of the blood level of the benzodiazepine or barbiturates over time.

Antiepileptic medications, such as carbamazepine or valproic acid, have also been used for the treatment of sedative and benzodiazepine withdrawal. Patients receive rapidly escalating doses of the anticonvulsant to produce therapeutic blood levels over 1 to 2 days. These blood levels are maintained for 7 to 14 days and then tapered. The advantage of using antiepileptic medications is that patients do not receive potentially addictive substances as part of their treatment. This is particularly advantageous for outpatient detoxification, where the patients may be likely to abuse medications.

Following detoxification, the patient should be engaged in long-term treatment. Treatments should be individualized to the patient, but may include residential drug-free programs, outpatient counseling, and self-help groups such as AA or NA.

Cannabis

Cannabis sativa, also called marijuana or hemp, is a plant indigenous to India but now grown worldwide. The leaves, flowers, and seeds of the plant contain many biologically active compounds, the most important of which is Δ^9-tetrahydrocannabinol (THC). The biologically active substances are administered by smoking or ingesting dried plant parts (marijuana, bhang, ganja), the resin from the plant (hashish), or extracts of the resin (THC or hash oil). Much of the American population has used marijuana. In 1996, an estimated 10.1 million Americans were regular users of marijuana. The percentage of youth (12 to 17) who have used marijuana appears to be increasing and has doubled from 1992 to 1995 to 7.1% of this population group.

After inhalation or ingestion, THC rapidly enters the CNS. It has biphasic elimination, with a short initial half-life (1 to 2 hours) reflecting redistribution and a second half-life of days to weeks. THC is hydroxylated and excreted in bile and urine. Recent research has demonstrated the presence of cannabinoid receptors on brain cells. The receptor is linked to a G protein and inhibits adenylate cyclase in neurons. THC receptors are widely distributed throughout the brain, and an endogenous neurotransmitter for these receptors is hypothesized.

Cannabis intoxication is characterized by tachycardia, muscle relaxation, euphoria, and a sense of well being. Time sense is altered and emotional lability, particularly inappropriate laughter, may be seen. Performance on psychomotor tasks, including driving, is impaired. Depersonalization, paranoia, and anxiety reactions occur with high doses. Although tolerance to the effects of cannabis occurs with chronic use, cessation of use does not produce significant withdrawal phenomena. Chronic cannabis use has been associated with an amotivational state and a feminization syndrome in men that improves on drug discontinuation. Marijuana has antiemetic and analgesic effects; it stimulates appetite in wasting illness such as AIDS and cancer. It reduces intraocular pressure in glaucoma. Δ^9-THC is now available by prescription as dronabinol for the medical treatment of these conditions. In Arizona and California, the marijuana leaf is available legally by physician prescription for "medical use," although the U.S. government has challenged its distribution in this manner.

Treatment. Treatment of cannabis dependence is similar to treatment of other drug dependencies. As part of the initial assessment, all patients should undergo complete medical and psychiatric evaluations. Short-term goals should focus on reducing or stopping cannabis use. Inpatient treatment may be necessary to achieve an abstinent state. Since many patients with cannabis dependence are adolescents or young adults, family involvement in assessment and treatment is important. Long-term treatment should involve addictive disorder specialists. Often, a change in social situation is necessary to decrease drug availability and reduce peer pressure. Individual and group psychotherapy may be useful for understanding the role of the drug in the individual's life, improving self-esteem, and providing alternate methods of relieving psychosocial distress. Self-help groups can provide group and individual support and are most effective when patients are matched with an appropriate peer group.

Opioids

Opioid abuse and dependence are significant social and medical problems in the United States, with an estimated opioid addict population of greater than 500,000. These patients are frequent users of medical and surgical services because of the multiple medical sequelae of intravenous drug use, and the crime and violence associated with the addict lifestyle. Psychiatric disorders, particularly anxiety disorders and affective disorders, are also common in opioid-dependent patients. Most opioid users are at least occasional intravenous injectors, which places them at risk for infectious hepatitis, HIV, and other infections. Over the past decade, there has been an increasing trend toward smoking or "snorting" heroin, as users have become aware of the risks of HIV infection associated with intravenous drug use.

Opiate drugs have effects on many organ systems. Their action is due to stimulation of receptors for endogenous hormones, enkephalins, endorphins, and dynorphins. There exist at least three distinct opioid receptors, which are designated by the Greek letters μ, κ, and δ. Drugs that act primarily through μ-receptor effects include heroin, morphine, and methadone; such drugs produce analgesia, euphoria, and respiratory depression. Drugs that are mediated through the κ-receptor include the so-called mixed agonist-antagonists, buprenorphine, butorphanol, and pentazocine, which produce analgesia, but less respiratory depression. The δ-receptor appears to bind endogenous opioid peptides.

Treatment of Opioid Intoxication. During opiate intoxication, drugs cause a suppression of central and peripheral nervous system activity. Important diagnostically, pupils are constricted and poorly reactive. Hypotension and constipation are common findings. Effects of severe intoxication include seizures, pulmonary edema, respiratory suppression, and cardiovascular arrest.

Opiate overdose is life-threatening and should be suspected in any patient presenting with coma and respiratory suppression. Treatment of overdose includes support of cardiovascular and respiratory functions. Opiate intoxication can be reversed with the opiate antagonists naloxone (Narcan) or nalmefene. Naloxone is given intravenously in doses of 0.4 to 0.8 mg every 20 minutes as required. The dose is titrated by response until an upper limit of 24 mg is attained over a 12-hour period. Opioid antagonists rapidly reverse coma and respiratory suppression caused by opioids, but do not reverse CNS depression caused by other sedative drugs, including alcohol. Naloxone and nalmefene will precipitate withdrawal in any patient who is dependent on opioids, causing the patient whose life was just saved to be most ungrateful.

Diagnosis and Treatment of Opioid Withdrawal. Opiate withdrawal, although rarely life-threatening, is subjectively distressing and is marked by an intense drive to use more opiates. The period of peak withdrawal depends on the opiate used: for short-acting opiates such as morphine, heroin, or meperidine, the peak withdrawal is 1 to 3 days and duration is 5 to 7 days. For longer acting opiates, such as methadone, the peak is 3 to 5 days and the duration 10 to 14 days. When opiate receptors are no longer stimulated by opiates (e.g., morphine or heroin), a rebound excitation of norepinephrine occurs mediated through α_2-receptors and contributes to the signs and symptoms of withdrawal.

Signs of opiate withdrawal are: (1) pulse 10 beats per minute or more over baseline or over 90 if there is no history of tachycardia and the baseline is unknown; systolic blood pressure 10 mm Hg or more above baseline or over 160/90 in patients without hypertension; (2) dilated pupils; (3) gooseflesh, diaphoresis, rhinorrhea, lacrimation, diarrhea; (4) agitation, insomnia, mood lability; and (5) drug seeking. Symptoms of opiate withdrawal are intense muscular cramps, anxiety, arthralgias, nausea, malaise, and compelling desire to use opiates.

Opiate withdrawal can be minimized with an opiate taper or with clonidine. A gradually decreasing dose of any opioid can be used for detoxification. Methadone is most commonly used due to its long half-life and once-daily oral administration. Those patients for whom an opiate taper is indicated include intravenous users, inpatients, users of methadone, and those who have medical and psychiatric complications and poor compliance with withdrawal from opiates. Those patients for whom clonidine is indicated are intranasal users, outpatients, and those who are motivated for a drug-free state.

Methadone detoxifications are performed by substituting the abused opioid with methadone and then gradually decreasing the dose of methadone over a period of up to 21 days, as specified by federal law. Initially, patients should be given 10 to 20 mg methadone orally every 2 to 4 hours until withdrawal symptoms are suppressed. The total daily dose received is typically 20 to 40 mg for heroin addicts. This dose is then decreased by approximately 10% daily. For patients unable to receive oral medications, the same dose of intramuscular methadone may be administered twice daily in divided doses.

The α_2-adrenergic agonist, clonidine hydrochloride, suppresses many autonomic signs and symptoms of opioid withdrawal. Clonidine acts at presynaptic noradrenergic nerve endings in the locus ceruleus of the brain, and blocks the adrenergic discharge produced by opioid withdrawal. Clonidine has been reported as clinically effective for suppressing opioid withdrawal following opioid discontinuation. Its main side effects include orthostatic hypotension, sedation, and dry mouth.

Clonidine detoxification is performed as follows: On the day before beginning clonidine, the usual dose of opioid is received. On day 1, the opioid is stopped completely, and instead, clonidine is given at a dose of 0.1 mg each 8 hours. From day 2 to day 4 the dose of clonidine is gradually increased to suppress withdrawal signs and symptoms, but without allowing blood pressure to decrease below 80 mm systolic and 60 mm diastolic. Typically, a dose of 0.6 to 1.2 mg clonidine is required by day 4, but the dose will depend on the quantity of opioid used. This dose continues until day 7 for patients using short-acting opioids, such as heroin, morphine, or meperidine, and until day 10 to 12 for those using longer acting methadone. The clonidine dose is then reduced by 0.2 to 0.3 mg per day until discontinued. Outpatient clonidine detoxification has been performed without significant morbidity but requires close monitoring with daily blood pressure determinations. Clonidine is less effective in attenuating drug craving, insomnia, and arthralgias and myalgias. Insomnia is best treated with a hypnotic such as chloral hydrate or a benzodiazepine. Muscle and joint pains respond to acetaminophen or ibuprofen.

Ultrarapid Opioid Detoxification. Because the opioid withdrawal syndrome is so physically and emotionally distressing, it often leads patients to reinstitute their opioid use. The administration of opioid antagonists, such as naloxone or naltrexone, during the withdrawal period reduces the duration of withdrawal, but significantly increases withdrawal intensity. Recently, a number of physicians have combined opioid antagonists and clonidine with conscious sedation or general anesthesia in a technique called ultrarapid opioid detoxification (UROD). Using this technique, opioid-dependent patients may be detoxified in less than 24 hours. Proponents of the technique claim that the detoxification is safe and results in long-term abstinence. However, there are few controlled studies to compare the efficacy and safety of UROD with more traditional detoxification methods.

Maintenance Treatment of Opioid Dependence. The most widely used pharmacologic treatments for opioid-dependent individuals include pharmacologic maintenance (substitution) treatments with the opiate agonists methadone and L-α-acetylmethadol (LAAM); maintenance with the partial opiate agonist buprenorphine; and opiate antagonist therapy with naltrexone. All of these medications are best used in the setting of a structured, maintenance treatment program, which includes monitored medication administration, periodic random urine toxicologic screening, and intensive psychologic, medical, and vocational services. Maintenance treatments reduce use of illicit opiates by increasing drug tolerance, thereby decreasing the subjective effects of administered illicit opiates, and by stabilizing mood, thereby decreasing self-medication. Maintenance treatments also provide an incentive for treatment so that patients can be exposed to other therapies.

Methadone Maintenance. Methadone is a synthetic opiate that is orally active, possesses a long-duration of action, produces minimal sedation or "high," and has few side effects at therapeutic doses. Since its introduction in 1965, methadone maintenance has become a major modality of long-term treatment of opioid abuse and dependence. Currently, over 100,000 individuals are maintained on methadone in the United States. Although some programs may have waiting lists for treatment, patients who are pregnant or who have significant problems, such as renal failure, heart disease, or AIDS, are usually accepted directly without a waiting period.

Many studies have shown the efficacy of methadone maintenance in the treatment of addicts who are dependent on heroin and other opiates. Methadone-treated patients show increased treatment retention, improved physical health, decreased criminal activity, increased employment, and decreased chance of becoming HIV-positive. Methadone is most effective in the context of a program that provides intensive psychosocial and medical services and adequate methadone dosing. As mentioned above, the use of methadone for maintenance is highly regulated by government agencies. Maintenance programs must be licensed and follow regulations regarding treatment eligibility, allowable methadone dosages, frequency of urine toxicologic monitoring, and provision of psychosocial and medical services.

Methadone is dissolved in a flavored liquid that is administered to patients daily, under observation. Long-standing program participants are allowed "take-home" doses of methadone, which patients may self-administer. Methadone doses usually range from 20 mg per day to over 100 mg per day. Higher doses are shown to be associated with better treatment retention. Urine toxicologic screening is performed randomly and periodically to assess treatment compliance. Counseling, medical care, and other social services are provided to patients on a regular basis.

If patients receiving methadone maintenance are hospitalized, their usual daily dose of methadone should be continued in the hospital. It is important to maintain frequent communication with the methadone program, particularly regarding changes in methadone dosage and discharge planning. If opioid pain medication is necessary, patients should receive additional short to intermediate acting opioids, such as meperidine or oxycodone, besides their usual dose of methadone, rather than increasing the methadone dose (see below). Certain mixed agonist-antagonist medications, such as pentazocine and butorphanol, should be avoided, since they may precipitate withdrawal.

L-α-Acetylmethadol Acetate. LAAM is a long-acting, orally active opiate with pharmacologic properties that are similar to methadone. Studies on LAAM have shown it to be equal or superior to methadone maintenance in reducing IV drug use, when used in the context of a structured treatment program. The advantages of LAAM include a slower onset of effects and a longer duration of action than methadone. This allows LAAM to be administered only three times per week, and eliminates the need for take-home medications that may be diverted to illegal uses. However, some patients dislike the inability to get take-home medication and reject LAAM in favor of methadone. Patients treated with LAAM should be started on 20 mg administered three times weekly, with the dose increased weekly in 10 mg increments as necessary. Doses up to 80 mg three times weekly are safe and effective.

Buprenorphine. Buprenorphine is a partial agonist opiate medication (mixed agonist-antagonist), originally used medically as an analgesic. The drug has both agonist and antagonist properties—agonist properties predominate at lower doses and antagonist properties predominate at higher doses. Buprenorphine has two major advantages over methadone: it is less likely to be abused and the withdrawal syndrome is much milder. At the time of publication of this book, buprenorphine has not yet been approved for opioid dependence by regulatory agencies; however, its use is widespread in research settings and approval is expected shortly.

A structured treatment program combining counseling and daily dosing with buprenorphine has been shown to be effective in the maintenance treatment of narcotics addicts. Buprenorphine may also reduce cocaine use. Buprenorphine doses usually range from 4 mg per day to up to 16 mg per day, administered sublingually, since the medication is not effective orally. Advantages of buprenorphine include a milder withdrawal syndrome on discontinuation and less potential for abuse, as agonist effects diminish at higher doses. Opioid-dependent patients may be started on 2 to 4 mg buprenorphine immediately after opiates are discontinued, and the dose of buprenorphine titrated to 8 to 16 mg over several days.

Opioid Antagonist Therapy. Opioid antagonist therapy reduces the use of illicit drugs by blocking the effect of the drugs at opioid receptors, leading to decreased use. There is some evidence that opiate antagonists may also block craving. Naltrexone is an orally active opioid antagonist approved for the treatment of opiate dependence and narcotic addiction. Naltrexone blocks the intoxicating effects of opioids and has few effects in individuals not dependent on opioids. The usual dose of naltrexone is 50 mg per day, administered orally, although three times weekly dosing with 100, 100, and 150 mg has also been shown to be effective. High doses of naltrexone have been associated with hepatotoxicity; however, deleterious hepatic effects are rarely observed with 50 mg per daily dosing. Other common side effects include anxiety, sedation, and nausea. Naltrexone therapy has been shown to be most effective in motivated individuals with good social supports (such as health care professionals and federal probationers) and appears less helpful for street heroin addicts. Although any physician may prescribe naltrexone, the medication is most effective when part of a comprehensive rehabilitative program.

Drug-Free Treatment. Nonpharmacologic and behavioral treatment modalities are quite efficacious in the treatment of opioid dependence. Such treatments include individual and group counseling, residential treatment, and self-help programs. Long-term residential treatment may be most useful for the chronic opioid abuser who requires a change in lifestyle and vocational and psychologic rehabilitation. Residential programs may differ in lengths of stay, treatment intensity, and theoretic orientation. Attending NA is helpful for many patients. Recently, needle-exchange programs have become common. Although these programs do not provide treatment, per se, they reduce the risks of acquiring infectious hepatitis and HIV by providing clean syringes and needles to addicts in exchange for used injection equipment.

Pain and Addiction. A particularly difficult clinical problem is the treatment of pain in patients with addiction. Patients with addictive disorders are prone to conditions that produce pain and require analgesic treatment. Drug and alcohol use are major causes of injuries due to accidents and violence. The medical consequences of drug and alcohol use include painful conditions such as pancreatitis, cancers, infections, and HIV-related illnesses. Important issues in treating patients with combined addictive disorders and pain include the type of drug producing dependence (e.g., alcohol, opiates), whether or not the patient is in addiction treatment, and the type of addiction treatment (drug-free, substitution, or antagonist therapy).

All such patients should be entered into an addiction program that coordinates treatment with the physicians providing the treatment for pain. When analgesic medications are required, nonnarcotic substances should be used, if possible. If narcotic analgesics are required, the type of addiction treatment that the patient is receiving will influence analgesic therapy. Patients receiving drug-free, abstinence-oriented therapy will respond to opioids, but require careful monitoring to reduce the chances of abuse and dependence. Those receiving substitution therapy with methadone, LAAM, or buprenorphine may require higher doses of narcotic analgesics because of their increased tolerance. A different opioid medication, such as meperidine or oxycodone, should be utilized. This differentiates the use of opioids for analgesia from the use of opioids for maintenance and does not change the dose of the agent used for substitution therapy. For patients receiving antagonist therapy with naltrexone, the effect of opioids is blocked during the period of antagonist therapy and for 24 to 72 hours after therapy. Stopping the antagonist 1 to 3 days prior to scheduled surgery or dental procedures will remove the opioid blockade. If opioids are needed emergently, higher doses of opioids can overcome the blockade, since naltrexone is a competitive antagonist. However, the opioid administration must be performed with careful monitoring.

Cocaine and Other Stimulants

The use of CNS stimulants, such as cocaine and amphetamines, is extremely common. The prevalence of cocaine use peaked in the mid-1980s and has slowly declined since. Based on the 1996 National Survey of Drug Abuse, over 20 million Americans tried cocaine at least once and 2.6 million used it during the preceding year. Cocaine and amphetamines are administered by intranasal "snorting" of powder, smoking, or intravenous injection. Amphetamines may also be used orally. Freebase cocaine base is now widely available as *crack,* which is potent, inexpensive, and easily distributed. Crack vapor is inhaled through heated pipes or by adding a small piece to a burning cigarette.

Cocaine has major physiologic and behavioral effects: (1) it is a local anesthetic of high potency that blocks the initiation and propagation of nerve impulses by affecting the sodium conductance of cell membranes; (2) it is a potent sympathomimetic agent that potentiates the actions of catecholamines in the autonomic nervous system and a potent vasoconstrictor; and (3) it is a potent stimulant of the CNS, potentiating the action of central catecholamine neurotransmitters, norepinephrine, and dopamine. Amphetamines have similar actions to cocaine, although they are not local anesthetics. Stimulants block the reuptake of dopamine and other catecholamines and increase their effects on postsynaptic receptors. However, after prolonged use, stimulants deplete the presynaptic supplies of these neurotransmitters.

Signs and symptoms of cocaine and amphetamine intoxication are sympathomimetic:dilated and reactive pupils, tachycardia, elevated temperature, elevated blood pressure, dry mouth, perspiration or chills, nausea and vomiting, tremulousness, hyperactive reflexes, repetitious compulsive behavior, stereotypic biting or self-mutilation, cardiac dysrhythmias, and flushed skin. Particularly common and serious psychiatric symptoms during intoxication are depression and suicidal and homicidal ideation. Chronic users have poor self-care, weight loss, and wasting. Cocaine overdose produces hyperpyrexia, hyperreflexia, and seizures, which may progress to coma and respiratory arrest.

The plasma half-life of cocaine following oral nasal or intravenous administration is approximately 1 to 2 hours, which correlates with its behavioral effects. With the decline in plasma levels, most users experience a period of dysphoria or "crash," which often leads to additional cocaine use within a short period. The dysphoria is intensified and prolonged following repeated use.

Treatment. The treatment of acute stimulant intoxication is essentially supportive. Patients with mild intoxication should be monitored in a supportive, protected environment that minimizes sensory stimulation. Those with severe anxiety or paranoia may benefit from benzodiazepines and low-dose neuroleptics. Patients with severe intoxication, coma, seizures, and hyperpyrexia require intensive care treatment with respiratory and circulatory system support.

The optimal treatment of the chronic cocaine user is still not established. Cessation of stimulant use is not followed by a physiologic withdrawal syndrome of the magnitude of that seen with opioids or alcohol; however, intense dysphoria, depression, and drug craving often occur and make abstinence difficult. Psychotherapy, group therapy, and behavior modification are useful in maintaining abstinence.

Some psychiatric and drug hospitals offer short-term inpatient cocaine treatment, although managed care generally does not support inpatient treatment of cocaine. For recidivists, long-term residential drug-free programs, including therapeutic communities, may be helpful, providing intensive psychologic treatment and drug education in a drug-free environment. Self-help groups such as NA may be useful both as a primary treatment modality for cocaine dependence and as an adjunct to other treatment. An innovative, behaviorally oriented treatment program using payment vouchers to provide positive reinforcement for cocaine abstinence has shown considerable success in reducing cocaine use in research settings.

There is interest in pharmacologic agents as adjunctive treatments for cocaine dependence. Several reports have shown efficacy of antidepressant agents such as imipramine, desipramine, fluoxetine, or trazodone in reducing cocaine craving and decreasing use. The medication doses used were similar to those used for antidepressant therapy. Although there have been reports that carbamazepine, amantadine, and bromocriptine may partially block cocaine craving, controlled clinical trials have not shown them to be effective. At the present time, no pharmacologic agent has been proven effective as a treatment for cocaine dependence.

Certain psychiatric disorders such as depression and attention deficit disorder may be common in stimulant users. Recognition and treatment of these underlying disorders may be necessary to stop cocaine use. In addition, many stimulant users also use alcohol or other drugs, particularly sedatives and heroin, and may require treatment for these substances as well.

Caffeine

Caffeine and the related methylxanthines theophylline and theobromine are consumed by more than 80% of the population. These drugs are found in coffee, tea, cola and other carbonated drinks, chocolate, and many prescribed and over-the-counter medications, including stimulants (NoDoze), appetite suppressants (Dexatrim), analgesics (Anacin, APC tablets), and cold and sinus preparations (Dristan, Contac).

Knowledge of the extent of the patient's use of caffeine and other methylxanthines is important in the overall assessment and treatment of the primary care patient. CNS effects of caffeine include psychomotor stimulation, increased attention and concentration, and suppression of the need for sleep. Low to moderate doses of caffeine can produce sleep disturbances and anxiety, and may increase requirements for neuroleptic or sedative medications. At high doses and in sensitive individuals, caffeine and other methylxanthines produce tremor and agitation. Cardiac effects include a mild tachycardia, premature ventricular contractions (PVCs), and a slight increase in systolic blood pressure.

Clinically significant caffeine withdrawal is commonly observed in even low to moderate regular caffeine users following reduced caffeine intake. Lethargy, hypersomnia, irritability, and severe headache characterize the caffeine withdrawal syndrome. The duration of withdrawal is usually 24 to 72 hours. The signs and symptoms of caffeine intoxication or caffeine withdrawal may complicate medical or psychiatric treatment by increasing patient distress and by leading to an unnecessary workup for other disorders.

Methylxanthines produce physiologic effects through actions at the cellular level. They produce cardiac stimulation, diuresis, bronchodilation, and CNS stimulation through several mechanisms. They inhibit the enzyme cyclic adenosine monophosphate (AMP) phosphodiesterase and increase intracellular levels of this cyclic AMP, thereby augmenting the action of many hormones and neurotransmitters. Methylxanthines also have a direct inhibitory effect on adenosine receptors.

Treatment of caffeine dependence limits consumption of caffeine-containing foods, medications, and beverages. Beverages such as coffee or cola may be substituted with decaffeinated forms. Often, patients are unaware of the extent of their caffeine consumption. They require education about the caffeine content of their diet and medications. Withdrawal symptoms such as headache and lethargy are best treated with slow caffeine taper and with analgesics and rest.

Hallucinogens and Phencyclidine (PCP)

Many drugs are used for their psychotomimetic or hallucinogenic effects. These include the psychedelics lysergic acid diethylamide (LSD), mescaline, psilocybin, and dimethyltryptamine; hallucinogenic amphetamines such as methylenedioxyamphetamine (MDA) and methylenedioxymethamphetamine (MDMA, or ecstasy); PCP, ketamine and similarly acting arylcyclohexylamines; and anticholinergics, such as scopolamine. All cause a state of intoxication characterized by hallucinosis, affective changes, and delusions. The mechanism of action of hallucinogens is not well understood and varies according to the drug. LSD and amphetamines are thought to act on dopaminergic and/or serotonergic brain systems, especially the 5HT-2 receptor. PCP and ketamine act at sigma sites on glutamate receptors. Anticholinergics act at muscarinic cholinergic receptors.

Diagnosis and Treatment of Hallucinogen Intoxication. Cognitive or memory impairment, disorientation, and confusion often occur in intoxication from psychedelic use. Psychedelic agents also produce electroencephalogram (EEG) changes similar to those seen during rapid eye movement (REM) sleep, which may account for the dreamlike quality of the high reported by those using this class of drugs. Most cases of hallucinogen intoxication are short-lived (lasting several hours) and resolve without incident; however, occasionally, prolonged drug-induced psychoses may occur. Also, some users may report persistent visual *trails* and *flashbacks* of the hallucinogen experience. Hallucinogens may precipitate mania or psychosis in individuals with a previous personal history or a family history of these psychiatric disorders.

PCP and the related drug ketamine are particularly dangerous drugs. Those under the influence show impaired judgment and impulsiveness that place users and others at risk for harm. Symptoms of PCP intoxication are hyperactivity, insensitivity to pain, hallucinations, paranoid delusions, and memory loss. Signs include hypertension, tachycardia, eyelid retraction (producing a wide-eyed stare), dry flushed skin, dilated pupils, nystagmus, and an excitable, angry affect. The analgesic and anesthetic action of PCP reduces pain perception and imparts the user with the capability of great motor strength not limited by pain (e.g., breaking out of restraints and overpowering staff). Ketamine, used clinically as a dissociative anesthetic in pediatric surgery, has become increasingly popular as a party drug ("Special K").

The differential diagnosis of hallucinogen- or PCP-induced psychosis includes schizophrenia, bipolar affective disorder, delusional disorder, and organic mental disorders such as encephalitis, brain tumors, and toxic encephalopathies.

Treatment of Hallucinogen Intoxication. Treatment includes supportive measures in a quiet setting to prevent patients from harming themselves or others, to maintain cardiovascular and respiratory functions, and to ameliorate agitation and psychotic symptoms until the effects of the drug subside. Pharmacologic treatment for the management of behavioral symptoms is sometimes required. Lorazepam (Ativan) 1 to 2 mg po or IV q 1 to 2 hours prn or diazepam (Valium) 5 to 10 mg po q 2 to 4 hours prn can be given to calm and sedate. For PCP, symptoms of intoxication are diminished or reversed by haloperidol 5 to 10 mg intramuscularly or orally every 1 to 6 hours as needed for behavioral control. Lorazepam 1 to 2 mg IV or diazepam 5 to 10 mg po q 1 to 6 hours can also be given. Following detoxification, the patient should be engaged in long-term treatment, which may include residential programs, outpatient counseling, and self-help groups such as NA.

Inhalants

Inhalants are volatile organic compounds that are inhaled for their psychotropic effects. Substances in this class include organic solvents (gasoline, toluene, ethyl ether, fluorocarbons) and volatile nitrates (nitrous oxide, amyl and butyl nitrate). Inhalants are readily available in households, stores, and worksites. At low doses, inhalants induce mood changes (especially euphoria), hallucinosis, and ataxia; at high doses they induce dissociative states and sedation. A main danger of inhalants is suffocation, since inhalant substances can displace oxygen and can reduce respiratory drive. Consequences of organic solvent use include bone marrow suppression, hepatotoxicity, and both central and peripheral neuropathies. Cardiac dysrhythmias may occur, leading to sudden death. Inhaled nitrates may produce hypotension and methemoglobinemia. The typical user of inhalants is a male adolescent. According to the National Household Survey on Drug Abuse, 9.1% of 12 to 17 year olds and 12.8% of 18 to 25 year olds have tried an inhalant at least once.

The optimal treatment of the inhalant user is similar to that for any substance dependence. Patients need comprehensive medical and psychiatric assessments, as well as addiction treatment. Since inhalant users are usually adolescents, treatment should involve the family. Long-term residential treatment may be helpful in the treatment of heavy users.

Anabolic Steroids

The use of anabolic steroids, once predominantly a problem in fanatic athletes, has now become a relatively common problem in adolescents. A recent study found 6.5% of adolescent boys and 1.9% of adolescent girls reported using anabolic steroids without a physician's prescription. The use of anabolic steroids is associated with the use of other substances, including cocaine, alcohol, injectable drugs, marijuana, and cigarettes.

Medical complications of anabolic steroid use include myocardial infarction, stroke, and hepatic disease. Users are usually completely naïve or deny the medical hazards of anabolic steroid use. HIV infection has been associated with shared needle use in steroid injectors. Psychiatric symptoms associated with anabolic steroid use include severe depression, psychotic (paranoid) symptoms, aggressive behavior, homicidal impulses, euphoria, irritability, anxiety, and hyperactivity. Although these symptoms gradually abate with drug discontinuation, depression, fatigue, decreased sex drive, insomnia, anorexia, and body image dissatisfaction may continue.

The treatment of anabolic steroid dependence should be within the same general model of other addictions, with due consideration to the high likelihood of dependency on other drugs, particularly in adolescents. Psychiatric management of drug-induced mood and paranoid syndromes is necessary. Issues regarding narcissistic body image are often present in certain athletes and body builders and should be considered in the psychotherapy of such individuals.

ADDITIONAL READINGS

American Psychiatric Association: *Diagnostic and statistical manual of mental disorders,* primary care version, ed 4, Washington, DC, 1995, American Psychiatric Association.

Annas GJ: Reefer madness: the federal response to California's medical marijuana law, *N Engl J Med* 337(6):435-439, 1997.

Compton PA, Wesson DR, Charuvastra VC, et al: Buprenorphine as a pharmacotherapy for opiate addiction, *Am J Addict* 5:220-230, 1996.

Cornish JW, Metzger D, Woody GE, et al: Naltrexone pharmacotherapy for opioid dependent federal probationers, *J Subst Abuse Treat* 14(6):529-534, 1997.

D'Aunno T, Vaughn TE: Variations in methadone treatment practices, *J Am Med Assoc* 267:253-258, 1992.

Dinwiddie S: Abuse of inhalants: a review, *Addiction* 89:925, 1994.

DuRant RH, Rickert VI, Ashworth CS, et al: The use of multiple drugs among adolescents who use anabolic steroids, *N Engl J Med* 328:922-926, 1993.

Fletcher JM, Page JB, Francis DJ, et al: Cognitive correlates of long-term cannabis use in Costa Rican men, *Arch Gen Psychiatry* 53:1051-1057, 1996.

Fultz JM Jr, Senay EC: Guidelines for the management of hospitalized narcotics addicts, *Ann Intern Med* 82:815-818, 1975.

Gastfriend DR, McLellan AT: Treatment matching: theoretic basis and practical implications, *Med Clin North Am* 81(4):945-966, 1997.

Gawin FH, Ellinwood EH Jr: Cocaine and other stimulants: actions, abuse and treatment, *N Engl J Med* 318(18):1173-1182, 1988.

Gerstein DR, et al: Evaluating recovery services: the California Drug and Alcohol Treatment Assessment (CALDATA), *California Department of Alcohol and Drug Programs,* 1994.

Hoffmann NG, DeHart SS, Fulkerson JA: Medical care utilization as a function of recovery status following chemical addictions treatment, *J Addict Dis* 12:97-108, 1993.

Hughes JR, Higgins ST, Bickel WK, et al: Caffeine self-administration, withdrawal and adverse effects among coffee drinkers, *Arch Gen Psychiatry* 48(7):611-617, 1991.

Kendler K, Prescott C: Cocaine use, abuse and dependence in a population-based sample of female twins, *Br J Psychiatry* 173:345-350, 1998.

Kidd KK: Trials and tribulations in the search for genes causing neuropsychiatric disorders, *Soc Biol* 38:163-178, 1992.

Koob GF, Sanna PP, Bloom FE: Neuroscience of addiction, *Neuron* 21(3):467-476, 1998.

Levin FR, Lehman AF: Meta-analysis of desipramine as an adjunct in the treatment of cocaine addiction, *J Clin Psychopharmacol* 11:374-378, 1991.

Ling W, Rawson RA, Compton PA: Substitution pharmacotherapies for opioid addiction: from methadone to LAAM and buprenorphine, *J Psychoactive Drugs* 26:119-128, 1994.

Martin CS, Clifford PR, Maisto SA, et al: Polydrug use in an inpatient sample of problem drinkers, *Alcohol Clin Exp Res* 20(3):413-417, 1996.

McCarron M, Schulze B, Thompson G: Acute phencyclidine intoxication: incidence of clinical findings in 1,000 cases, *Ann Emerg Med* 10:237, 1981.

McGinnis JM, Foege WH: Actual causes of death in the United States, *J Am Med Assoc* 270:2201-2212, 1993.

Milby JB, Sims MK, Khuder S, et al: Psychiatric comorbidity: prevalence in methadone maintenance treatment, *Am J Drug Alcohol Abuse* 22(1):95-107, 1996.

Miller WR, Rollnick S: *Motivational interviewing: preparing people to change addictive behavior,* New York, 1991, Guilford Press.

Mirin SM, Weiss RD, Michael J, et al: Psychopathology in substance abusers: diagnosis and treatment, *J Drug Alcohol Abuse* 14:139-157, 1988.

Musty RE, Reggio P, Consroe P: A review of recent advances in cannabinoid research and the 1994 International Symposium on Cannabis and the Cannabinoids, *Life Sci* 56(23-24):1933-1940, 1995.

National Consensus Development Panel on Effective Medical Treatment of Opiate Addiction, *J Am Med Assoc* 280:1936-1943, 1998.

National Survey on Drug Abuse, 1996. (1998). Rockville, MD, 1998, Institute of Drug Abuse.

NIAAA: *The physician's guide to helping patients with alcohol problems,* NIH Publication No. 95-3769, 1995.

O'Brien CP, McLellan AT: Addiction medicine, *J Am Med Assoc* 18:277(23):1840-1841, 1997.

O'Connor PG, Kosten TR: Rapid and ultrarapid opioid detoxification techniques, *J Am Med Assoc* 279:229-234, 1998.

O'Malley SS: Integration of opioid antagonists and psychosocial therapy in the treatment of narcotic and alcohol dependence, *J Clin Psych* 56(suppl 7):30-38, 1995.

Pope HG, Katz DA: Affective and psychotic symptoms associated with anabolic steroid use, *Am J Psychiatry* 145:487-490, 1988.

Prochaska JO, DiClemente CC, Norcross JC: In search of how people change: applications to the addictive behaviors, *Am Psychol* 47:1102-1114, 1992.

Robinson TE, Berridge KC: The neural basis of drug craving: an incentive-sensitization theory of addiction, *Brain Res Rev* 18:247-291, 1993.

Samet JH, Rollnick S, Barnes H: Beyond CAGE: a brief clinical approach after detection of substance abuse, *Arch Intern Med* 156:2287-2293, 1996.

SAMHSA: *Highlights from the 1991 NDATUS survey,* Rockville, MD, 1992.

Skinner HA: The drug abuse screening test, *Addict Behav* 7(4):363-371, 1982.

Skinner HA, Holt S, Schuller R, et al: Identification of alcohol abuse using laboratory tests and a history of trauma, *Ann Intern Med* 101:847-851, 1984.

Smith D, Wesson D: Phenobarbital technique for treatment of barbiturate dependence, *Arch Gen Psychiatry* 24:56, 1971.

Stein M: Medical consequences of intravenous drug abuse, *J Gen Intern Medicine* 5:249-257, 1990.

Swift RM, Griffiths W, Camara P: Special technical considerations in laboratory testing for illicit drugs. In Stoudemire A, Fogel BS, editors: *Medical psychiatric practice, vol 1,* Washington, 1991, APA Press.

Young T, Lawson GW, Gacocn CB: Clinical aspects of phencyclidine (PCP), *Int J Addict* 22:1-15, 1987.

CHAPTER 53

Psychotic Disorders

Frank W. Brown

Although often used to describe states of confusion, disorientation, or delirium, *psychosis* is best viewed as a state of brain dysfunction characterized by delusions, hallucinations, and formal thought disorder (e.g., derailment, thought blocking, thought insertion) (Box 53-1). Psychosis should not be viewed as a disease but as a dynamic state induced by a neurochemical dysfunction that leads to the specific clinical presentation.[3] Psychosis may be transient, intermittent, or continuous.

ETIOLOGY

Etiologies of psychosis may be described in terms of neurobiologic, genetic, environmental, and sociocultural factors. Brain structural and neuropathologic factors are thought to increase the risk of psychosis. The greatest risk factor for late-life psychosis appears to be progressive dementia. Three primary neurochemical systems (dopamine, neurotensin, and serine metabolism) are implicated in the development of a psychotic state.[3]

Stressful life events tend to occur before an episode of psychosis but are not causes of psychosis; rather, they can be viewed as destabilizing factors that exacerbate a preexisting tendency to develop psychosis. People with prolonged psychosis tend to experience *social drift;* that is, their impairment causes a downward shift in social class. Whether this change in social class is causative or is an effect of a prolonged psychotic state is not always clear. Most current data suggest that lower social class is a consequence of the psychosis.

EPIDEMIOLOGY AND PATHOPHYSIOLOGY

The 1-year prevalence rate of psychosis in the United States is less than 2.5%. Schizophrenic-related disorders have a 1.1%, severe cognitive impairment with superimposed psychosis approximately a 1%, and other causes (e.g., medical illness, drug/alcohol-induced psychosis) a 0.5% 1-year prevalence.[7] Psychosis resulting from a schizophrenic disorder has strong genetic influences, as shown from adoption, family, and twin studies. No simple pattern of inheritance has been isolated. Historic data have indicated that the risk of a person developing schizophrenia (1% throughout the population) increases if other relatives have the disorder, up to 10% with a schizophrenic sibling, 12% with a schizophrenic parent, and 40% to 45% if both parents have schizophrenia.

Theories on the *neurobiology of psychosis* implicate neurochemical, structural, or functional factors.[4] Most likely, multiple events (e.g., drugs, brain injury, morphologic changes) cause impairment in neurochemical pathways, producing the expression of psychosis. Dopamine modulation through dysfunctional serine metabolism, brain regional neurotensin levels, and increased activity of dopamine or selected dopamine receptors in certain areas of the brain are important in the etiology of psychosis. Trigger events may be different, but the final common pathway involves altered thalamic filtering.

Box 53-1. Symptoms of Psychosis

Delusions: beliefs or situations not based on reality
Hallucinations: visual, auditory, olfactory, or tactile perceptions without external stimuli
Thought insertion: placement of thoughts into one's brain by an outside force (e.g., belief that neighbor is putting images into patient's head)
Derailment: process in which one's thought processes suddenly go astray without apparent reason (patient talking about one subject, then suddenly shifts to unrelated topic)
Thought blocking: process in which one's thoughts appear to be stalled (patient talking about a subject, then suddenly is unable to collect thoughts and "goes mentally blank")

PATIENT EVALUATION

Psychiatric History

The description of the current episode of psychosis is crucial in establishing a differential diagnosis. The knowledge that a psychosis is present does little in determining the etiology and appropriate management. Causes of psychosis can be divided into *primary* (psychoses with psychiatric illness) and *secondary* (induced psychosis). These categories overlap because a fundamental impairment remains in neurochemical pathways of the brain.

Duration of the psychotic symptoms needs to be established. An acute onset of visual hallucinations indicates a medical illness or drug-induced psychotic process. In contrast, a 2- to 4-week history of increasing auditory and visual hallucinations suggests a schizophrenia-related disorder. *Prodromal development* of psychosis refers to more subtle manifestations of an early psychotic process. Before the actual psychosis, the patient may have displayed social withdrawal, decreased attention to personal hygiene, or gradual difficulty with school or work performance. These symptoms would support psychosis of gradual onset. Prodromal development is most often seen in schizophrenia-related disorders and rarely in acute psychosis caused by medical illness or medications.

Hallucinations. Visual hallucinations can occur in patients with schizophrenia; however, organic causes must be closely evaluated, such as in drug and alcohol intoxication and withdrawal. Olfactory hallucinations, which are less common in schizophrenia, require careful assessment to rule out sella turcica tumors. Auditory hallucinations are often a feature of a schizophrenic type of disorder. Auditory hallucinations should be assessed as to whether the voices command the patient to perform some act (self-harm or violence), how often the hallucinations occur, and whether the patient perceives them as threatening or frightening. When auditory hallucinations and delusions are present, it is important to assess the patient for suicidal risk.

Prior Episodes. Previous episodes and treatment history of psychotic symptoms provide invaluable information as to diagnosis and management techniques that will likely benefit the patient. Primary psychiatric disorders with recurrent features of psychosis include schizophrenia-related disorders, major depression with psychosis, bipolar disorder, and dementia with psychosis. If similar psychotic features recur, the physician should explore the previous diagnosis and treatment. The patient with a chronic psychosis may respond well to a prior treatment plan. The patient who has a major depression with psychosis requires treatment directed at the depression as well as the psychosis; attempting to treat only the psychosis without antidepressants or electroconvulsive therapy will likely fail or delay adequate response.

Family History. Because of the genetic "loading" of many of the primary psychiatric illnesses, a family history of similar psychotic symptoms or other psychiatric history provides valuable information. Effective management techniques used in the past to treat a family member will often be effective in the patient who has a similar psychotic presentation. This is especially important with a family history of schizophrenia, major depression, or bipolar disorder.

Substance Abuse. Substance abuse is known to predispose a person to develop psychosis especially with acute ingestion of substances such as alcohol, lysergic acid diethylamide (LSD), phencyclidine (PCP), and cocaine or with acute withdrawal. Psychotic states from drugs generally have an acute onset and generally can remit with appropriate removal of the substance unless functional brain impairment occurs, as with use of LSD or PCP.

Examination and Testing

Although a routine physical examination is appropriate for the patient with psychosis, a few areas should be emphasized. Possible sources of infection need to be identified, such as pneumonia or urinary tract infection. Evidence of a low-grade temperature and slight tachycardia in a patient with recent onset of untreated psychosis should prompt evaluation for an induced psychosis. Drug intoxication with illicit or prescription drugs may present with symptoms similar to a schizophrenic disorder.

The office or bedside examination should include a screening mental status examination. Hallucinations may be described as to *type, complexity* (single voice or image vs. multiple voices or complex visual images), and *duration.* Other psychotic symptoms should be described as to first onset, when they occur, and whether they ever occurred in the past. The patient's mood and affect (depressed, normal, or elevated) should be noted. Many schizophrenic patients have a flat or blunted affect with limited range of expression. A minimal assessment for violence or suicide is necessary. Prior episodes of violence, current threats of violence, impaired judgment, and drug-seeking behavior are risk factors for recurrence of violence. If patients are hearing commanding voices, they will generally acknowledge this if asked directly but rarely volunteer this information. Suspicion of psychosis should increase if the patient appears distracted or seems to be looking or responding to one part of the room, since this could indicate that the patient is responding to hallucinations. Guardedness and hyperalertness can indicate paranoia. Directed questions (e.g., "Do you feel safe here?" "Are there voices that are bothering you?") may elicit the patient's acknowledgement of the psychosis.

Most routine laboratory tests ordered are appropriate for the patient with acute-onset or chronic psychosis (Table 53-1). The goal of these evaluations is to uncover secondary causes of psychosis. Urine drug screens are most valuable in evaluating recent illicit drug use or inappropriate prescription drug use. A urine drug screen should be considered especially for acute onset of psychosis or the reemergence of a previously controlled psychosis when visual hallucinations are prominent.

Psychologic Testing. Psychologic tests are often misunderstood and ordered too infrequently. Comprehensive psychologic testing can be useful in evaluating selected psychotic patients who are stable enough to participate in testing. Many acutely psychotic patients simply cannot focus on this task long enough to make these tests worthwhile. The tests may be beneficial in determining degree of paranoia or delusional thinking, especially if the patient does not volunteer information to directed questions.

Other Studies. Chest radiographs may identify a pneumonia or congestive heart failure, which could aggravate a psychotic state. An electrocardiogram (ECG) is recommended in at-risk patients to evaluate for recent but silent myocardial infarction and dysrhythmias. A lumbar puncture is not part of a normal evaluation but should be considered if infection or subarachnoid hemorrhage is suspected. An electroencephalogram (EEG) is appropriate if temporal lobe seizures are suspected. Systemic lupus erythematosus (SLE) may first present as psychosis. Neuroimaging in the workup of psychosis should only be ordered when a specific reason exists, that is, signs of trauma or focal neurologic deficits. The acute onset of psychosis in a young person with a negative psychiatric history and negative family psychiatric history or new-onset psychosis in an elderly person should suggest neuroimaging. With microvascular brain disease, neurologic signs and symptoms may not always be elicited. Microvascular insults to deep white matter and the caudate may be

Table 53-1. Laboratory Tests in Evaluating Psychosis

Laboratory test	Indication
Complete blood count with differential	Infection
Urinalysis	Infection
Liver enzymes	Hepatic encephalopathy
Serum creatine	Uremia
Blood urea nitrogen	Uremia
Thyroid function tests	Hypothyroidism, hyperthyroidism
VDRL (FTA-ABS)*	Syphilis
Arterial blood gases (pulse oximeter)	Hypoxia
Electrolytes	Hyponatremia, hypernatremia
Glucose	Hypoglycemia
Urine drug screen	Drug ingestion, especially cocaine, phencyclidine, and marijuana

*Venereal Disease Research Laboratories (fluorescent treponemal antibody absorption).

predisposing factors in the development of psychosis in elderly persons.

DIFFERENTIAL DIAGNOSIS

Greater urgency is shown the patient with a relatively recent onset of psychosis, the presence of a clouded sensorium, or onset of a psychotic process later in life. The patient with a recurrence of psychosis associated with a history of a schizophrenic disorder may not need to be as aggressively evaluated. Psychosis occurring with a clouded sensorium, as in delirium, signals a nonschizophrenic process; medical illnesses, metabolic abnormalities, and drug intoxication are major causes. Although onset in later life is often associated with dementia, the absence of memory impairment with psychosis requires close evaluation of medication side effects, vascular disease, and other physical illnesses (e.g., hypothyroidism, visual impairment, hypoxia).

Primary Causes

The most common presentation of psychosis in psychiatric illness occurs in schizophrenia-related disorders, major depression with psychotic features, bipolar disorder, and dementing disorders (Box 53-2). A detailed description of each is available in the *Diagnostic and Statistical Manual of Mental Disorders,* fourth edition (DSM-IV).[2]

Schizophrenia normally is associated with bizarre delusions, prominent auditory hallucinations, incoherence, inappropriate or flat affect, looseness of association, or catatonia. Associated features include a decrease in social or work performance. The patient may show prominent changes in activities of daily living (e.g., poor grooming), lack of drive, social withdrawal, or unusual behaviors (e.g., talking to oneself while walking down the street).

Box 53-2. Causes of Psychosis

Primary

Schizophrenia related*
Major depression
Dementia
Bipolar disorder

Secondary

Drug use†	Hypomagnesemia
Drug withdrawal‡	Epilepsy
Drug toxicity§	Meningitis
Charles Bonnet syndrome	Encephalitis
Infections (pneumonia)	Brain abscess
Electrolyte imbalance	Herpes encephalopathy
Syphilis	Hypoxia
Congestive heart failure	Hypercarbia
Parkinson's disease	Hypoglycemia
Trauma to temporal lobe	Thiamine deficiency
Postpartum psychosis	Postoperative states
Hypothyroidism/ hyperthyroidism	

*Includes schizophrenia, schizophreniaform disorder, brief reactive psychosis.
†Includes hypnotics, glucocorticoids, marijuana, phencyclidine, atropine, dopaminergic agents (e.g., amantadine, bromocriptine, L-dopa), immunosuppressants.
‡Includes alcohol, barbiturates, benzodiazepines.
§Includes digitalis, theophylline, cimetidine, anticholinergics, glucocorticoids, catecholaminergic agents.

Secondary Causes

When psychosis results from a secondary cause, the presentation may vary. Most secondary causes are seen in the context of a delirium or altered mental status. Important secondary causes of psychosis are infections, electrolyte imbalance, and drug/medication use, withdrawal, and toxicity. In susceptible people, hyponatremia can induce a mild psychosis before the occurrence of seizures. This is most often seen during a mild delirium and slowly clears once the hyponatremia is corrected. Infections, especially pneumonia and urinary tract infections in elderly persons, often are associated with patients having visual hallucinations or mild delusions. After the infection has been successfully treated, these psychotic symptoms may linger for days to weeks and may require low-dose neuroleptics.

Substance abuse and drug/medication use, withdrawal, and toxicity are prime causes of delirium (see Box 53-2). Key features include an inability to maintain attention to a task (e.g., conversation), disorganized thought processes, visual hallucinations, labile affect, alteration in sleep-wake cycle, and impaired short-term memory. Effects of drugs and medications are more pronounced on the aging or immature brain and the previously injured brain (e.g., cerebrovascular accident, head trauma). One review noted that 83% of 177 medications had psychosis as a potential side effect.[1]

MANAGEMENT

Management of psychotic patients incorporates nonpharmacologic and pharmacologic interventions. Choice of treatment depends on the severity, type, and presumed etiology of the psychosis. Chronic psychotic patients (e.g., with schizophrenia) generally require only minor changes in their neuroleptics unless an acute exacerbation of the psychosis occurs. Then aggressive treatment with psychotropic drugs usually is required, along with nonpharmacologic interventions. Patients with acute onset of psychosis should always have the cause of the psychosis actively treated.

Nonpharmacologic Treatment

Any factor that could cause or potentiate a psychotic process should be eliminated, including suspected medications, illicit drugs, and potential environmental stressors. A schizophrenic patient who decompensates on entering the workplace may benefit from a more structured work environment (e.g., set work hours, specific work task).[6]

Most mild forms of psychosis do not require hospitalization if no major medical illness is present. Keeping the mildly psychotic patient at home in familiar surroundings may prevent further psychotic decomposition compared with hospitalization in unfamiliar surroundings. The family should be educated about the illness, associated symptoms, treatment and management options, and prognosis so that they can provide a home environment with minimal change and maximal routine, with fewer behavioral problems. Community programs provide structured activities or employment and are especially important because they assist the family while monitoring psychotic patients for evidence of relapse, medication compliance, or side effects. These programs are generally developed for patients with chronic psychosis but can be beneficial for those recovering from an acute psychotic episode. State associations for mentally ill persons can provide a listing of resources in a specific community.

Behavioral intervention and *reality orientation* are necessary for some patients. Acutely psychotic patients need to be oriented to reality (e.g., calendars and clocks in room, reassurance from staff or family as to who they are, where they are, and the date, time, and situation). Interactions with psychotic individuals are best done by one individual at a time; psychotic patients do poorly when they must shift attention between two or more people. A better approach is having one physician or staff member talk to and examine the patient while others remain at the side (not back) of the patient. Soft background music (no words) may also decrease the risk of physical agitation. Calm reassurance may be offered to the patient, and the physician or staff can redirect the patient to nonpsychotic themes. Health care professionals must be alert to protect themselves from a patient who strikes out or feels threatened.

Electroconvulsive therapy (ECT) is appropriate in select patients: depression with psychotic features, manic disorder with psychosis, psychosis with catatonia, ECT used with success previously, and psychosis with strong affective component. ECT may also benefit patients with psychosis resulting from hypopituitarism or Parkinson's disease.

Pharmacologic Treatment

Neuroleptics. Neuroleptics are the main treatment for psychosis. They generally have very similar efficacy, and thus the choice of neuroleptic generally depends on the side effect profile best suited for the patient (Table 53-2). Schizophrenic patients not treated with antipsychotic drugs will likely relapse within 3 years, with greater intensity of psychosis and more frequency than patients treated with antipsychotic medication.[5] Except for some atypical neuroleptics, all these medications can cause extrapyramidal side effects, tardive dyskinesia, and other anticholinergic side effects.[6] Neuroleptic malignant syndrome (fever, muscle rigidity, altered mental status, autonomic instability) occurs rarely with neuroleptics but must be considered.

Neuroleptics with lower potency (e.g., chlorpromazine, thioridazine) tend to have greater anticholinergic side effects and thus increase the risk of falls and orthostatic blood

Table 53-2. Antipsychotic Medications

Class/medication	Equivalent to 1 mg haloperidol (approx. mg)	Average daily dosage range (mg)	Route*	Relative cumulative side effect profile†
Butyrophenones‡				
Haloperidol (Haldol)	1	1-25	PO, IM, IV	1
Haloperidol decanoate	1	25-200	IM	1
Thioxanthene‡				
Thiothixene (Navane)	2.5	15-30	PO, IM	1
Phenothiazines				
Aliphatic				
Chlorpromazine (Thorazine)	50	200-1000	PO, IM§	4
Piperidine				
Thioridazine (Mellaril)	50	100-600	PO	3
Phenazines				
Fluphenazine (Prolixin)‡	1	2-20	PO, IM	1
Fluphenazine decanoate‡	1	25-100	IM, SC	1
Piperazine				
Trifluoperazine (Stelazine)	2.5	2-20	PO, IM	2
Dibenzoxazepine				
Loxapine (Loxitane)	5	60-100	PO, IM	2
Atypical agents				
Clozapine (Clozaril)‖	75	25-700	PO	1
Risperidone (Risperdal)	0.5	1-8	PO	1
Olanzapine (Zyprexa)	—	5-20	PO	1
Quetiapine (Seroquel)	—	150-400	PO	1

**PO,* Oral; *IM,* intramuscular; *IV,* intravenous; *SC,* subcutaneous.
†*1,* Minimal; *4,* greatest. Lower score reflects higher potency and lower anticholinergic side effects.
‡Acute extrapyramidal reactions more common.
§Also available as suppositories.
‖1% to 2% incidence of agranulocytosis. A weekly complete blood count is required. Other side effects include orthostatic blood pressure changes and lowered seizure threshold.

pressure changes, especially in elderly patients. These agents are more sedating, which is a benefit in younger agitated patients. Neuroleptics can also lower the seizure threshold. When prescribing a neuroleptic for a psychotic patient, the physician should obtain informed consent from the family or guardian to treat with this class of medication. Two long-acting depot intramuscular neuroleptics, haloperidol decanoate given every 4 to 5 weeks and fluphenazine decanoate every 3 to 4 weeks, are useful for the noncompliant patient or the chronic psychotic patient who will not take or is sporadic in taking oral medications. Other newer atypical neuroleptics (olanzapine, risperidone, and quetiapine) are excellent choices as first-line neuroleptics.

Other Medications. Carbamazepine and valproic acid may be effective if an ictal focus is contributing to the psychosis. Benzodiazepines, when combined with a neuroleptic in the severely agitated psychotic patient, are very effective in achieving more rapid control of the agitation and psychosis. For the young to middle-aged psychotic patient, oral or intramuscular haloperidol (3 to 5 mg) and lorazepam (1 to 2 mg) may be given every 30 to 60 minutes until control is achieved. This combination can be more effective than a neuroleptic alone.

Consultation or Hospitalization

Consultation with a psychiatric colleague for a patient with psychosis usually is recommended if there is any concern about the etiology, diagnosis, or management. Although the primary care physician is able to diagnose accurately the presence of a psychosis, evaluating the etiology of psychosis may be difficult. Psychiatric consultation can assist in determining the optimal pharmacologic and nonpharmacologic interventions.

Actively psychotic patients may present such a risk of harm to themselves and others that hospitalization should be strongly considered. Disadvantages to hospitalization include (1) removing patients from a potentially safe and structured environment and (2) placing them on a rapidly changing hospital ward where they may become more psychotic. Psychosis itself does not require hospitalization, but other features often seen with psychosis may require it; psychotic patients often have impaired judgment and impulse control. Hospitalization is highly recommended, however, for certain patients. If the psychotic patient is suicidal or is hearing voices that command self-harm, or if a delusion is present that mandates self-mutilation, hospitalization with aggressive treatment is advised.

Violence or physical agitation is often a major concern of family or health care providers. Most episodes of physical agitation are nondirected and defensive in nature, except for the delusional person with focused paranoia who may attack a specific person.[8] These patients are often noncompliant with outpatient management. Hospitalization provides safety as well as a means to gain better control of the psychosis.

Psychosis with other major mental illness (e.g., major depression, mania) is very difficult to manage on an outpatient basis and places the patient at high risk from impaired judgment and impulse control. Outpatient management of these patients should only be considered if trained 24-hour sitters are available.

SPECIAL PATIENT POPULATIONS

Suicidal Patients

Approximately 15% of schizophrenic patients end their life by suicide. Most psychotic patients who commit suicide are young unemployed males with a high level of social functioning before the onset of psychosis. The early detection and treatment of psychosis, especially with depressive features, represent a major strategy to prevent suicide. The physician assessing a psychotic patient for suicide risk at a minimum should address the following questions: (1) Is there a history of prior suicide attempts? (2) Is there a plan and means to commit suicide? (3) Does the patient have feelings of hopelessness or that life is not worth living? and (4) Are there thoughts of death? The presence of command hallucinations needs to be determined because the commands are often for self-injury. A psychotic patient who fears mental disintegration or has not been compliant with treatment is at higher risk for completed suicide.

When a psychotic patient is identified at moderate to high suicide risk (a subjective decision), hospitalization and psychiatric consultation are indicated. A patient with only occasional transient suicidal ideations may be managed as an outpatient; however, the clinician must be knowledgeable about the treatment of psychosis as well as affective disorders, while realizing that a psychotic patient's judgment is generally impaired. Outpatients should be provided community services that combine treatment with recreational and occupational activities.

Adolescents

When psychosis occurs in the adolescent, the physician must evaluate for primary vs. secondary psychosis. Brief reactive psychosis generally is time limited and may only require supportive care and a structured environment. The use of neuroleptics in this age group requires careful consideration of whether the benefits outweigh the risks for development of tardive dyskinesia. If the psychosis necessitates a medication because of auditory or visual hallucinations, commanding voices, or delusions, one of the atypical antipsychotics may be useful.

Adolescents require special concern regarding suicide potential. An acutely psychotic adolescent is at increased risk of self-harm because of impaired impulse control, impaired judgment, and commanding voices. This patient should be hospitalized; unless experienced in managing young psychotic patients, the physician should consult with a trusted psychiatrist.

Pregnant and Postpartum Patients

Psychosis during pregnancy places mother and fetus at risk from its sequelae. The physician must consider the risks and benefits of any treatment. Potential causes of the psychosis must be excluded and environmental control maximized. If the pregnant patient is taking a neuroleptic, the dosage should be kept as low as possible to control the psychosis. Any use of a neuroleptic requires the patient's informed consent. Although the risk for an increased rate of physical malformation from neuroleptic use is minimal, even during the first trimester, the potential effects of neuroleptics on the developing fetal brain for future behavior are not known. If a psychosis must be treated during pregnancy and other treatable causes of the psychosis have been excluded, the physician should consider a low-dose neuroleptic therapy (e.g., haloperidol, 2 mg daily increased by 1 to 2 mg every other day, up to a maximum of 10 mg). A chronic psychotic process may best be treated with a low-dose maintenance neuroleptic. Because of the potential teratogenic effect of pharmacotherapy, ECT should be considered, especially if affective or catatonic symptoms are present.

A small subset (less than 1%) of postpartum women will develop a psychosis within the first weeks after delivery. These psychotic episodes may occur during a postpartum depression. Aggressive treatment to control the primary illnesses (antidepressants for the depression, neuroleptics for the psychosis) should be undertaken to maintain maternal-infant bonding and to reduce the overall disruption from the psychosis. If the mother is taking neuroleptics, she must be cautioned against breast-feeding because the newborn would be exposed to potentially significant levels of the neuroleptic. Low doses of a neuroleptic (e.g., haloperidol, 2 to 5 mg/day) should be used until the psychosis is controlled. After the psychosis is under control for 4 to 8 weeks, the neuroleptic can be decreased by 1 mg each week until discontinued, with careful attention to psychotic recurrence. ECT is useful in postpartum psychosis with an affective component.

Elderly Patients

Geriatric patients with psychosis fall into four broad diagnostic groups: (1) delirium related or drug/illness induced, (2) continuation of lifelong or chronic psychotic illness, (3) affective disorders with psychosis, and (4) dementia-related syndromes with psychosis. The first group, although likely requiring neuroleptics, should have aggressive intervention to correct the underlying deficits (e.g., hypoxia, infection, decreased cerebral blood flow) causing the delirium. Neuroleptics in elderly patients should be started at low doses and slowly titrated (e.g., risperidone, 0.25 to 0.50 mg increased by 0.25 to 0.50 mg every 1 to 2 days). Faster titration may be needed but requires greater attention to orthostatic blood pressure monitoring. Acute episodes of psychosis with agitation may require higher initial doses (e.g., 1.0 to 1.5 mg of risperidone). Elderly patients show the greatest sensitivity to neuroleptic side effects, especially orthostasis, increased risk of falls, and extrapyramidal symptoms, and therefore require lower doses and slower titration. The newer atypical agents (risperidone, olanzapine, quetiapine) are ideally suited for this age group. Cumulative effects of neuroleptics may require that the dose be decreased after about 3 to 4 weeks, since some patients become more sedated as the psychosis is controlled.

Perioperative Patients

Psychotic patients awaiting surgery must have individualized treatment recommendations. An actively psychotic patient may receive a high-potency oral or intramuscular neuroleptic 2 hours before anesthesia as long as the anesthesiologist notes potential side effects. Stable patients with a chronic psychotic illness may safely have their neuroleptics stopped 12 to 24 hours before surgery; psychosis generally does not reemerge immediately, usually taking weeks to reappear. Neuroleptics can then be safely restarted 24 to 48 hours postoperatively.

Hospitalized Medical Patients

Hospitalized patients are more at risk to develop a psychotic reaction than the general population. The stress of the medical illness, a different environment, and the interaction of medications (e.g., Sinemet and Parlodel) can precipitate a psychosis. The medical patient with a history of psychosis and reemergence of psychotic symptoms can generally be treated with the same neuroleptic regimen effective in the past. Medical patients with no previous psychotic symptoms require careful evaluation so that the causative agent(s) may be removed or reduced, if possible. Short-term use of high-potency neuroleptics (e.g., haloperidol, 1 to 8 mg/day) is appropriate for control of hallucinations, delusions, and agitation. Besides neuroleptics, management should incorporate a structured environment with a reduction in external disrupting noise. Potential for suicide must be assessed, and the patient at risk should receive one-to-one care until consultation is obtained.

Stable Compensated Patients

Stable compensated patients with a prior history of psychosis should be maintained with a similar treatment plan that has kept them stable in the past. The primary care physician should realize that neuroleptics are generally only one part of this treatment approach. The patient may have been in a structured home setting or group home environment, and maintaining these nonpharmacologic interventions should not be overlooked.

Neuroleptic-induced side effects (e.g., akathisia, stiffness, cogwheel rigidity) are a major reason for medication noncompliance. For patients with evidence of cogwheel rigidity or extrapyramidal symptoms, benztropine (1 to 2 mg orally twice a day for 2 to 4 weeks) is generally effective. Decreasing the neuroleptic can reduce these side effects and is especially helpful in decreasing or eliminating akathisia. Tapering an antipsychotic in a patient with a history of chronic psychosis to the lowest effective dosage should be attempted slowly and in small increments over several months. Recent hallucinations, delusions, bizarre behaviors, and decreased attention to grooming are concerns for the reemergence of psychosis. If these symptoms emerge, the physician should consider increasing the neuroleptic dose by 10% to 20%. If the patient is still stable at 6 months, the neuroleptic can be decreased by 10% to 20%, with close follow-up to ensure that psychosis does not recur.

SUMMARY

Psychosis is a state of brain dysfunction characterized by delusions, hallucinations, and formal thought disorder. It can often be managed very effectively, and in many patients with secondary induction, sustained remission can be achieved. Neuroleptic treatment remains the cornerstone of care for the psychotic patient. Neuroleptics have similar efficacy, and thus the choice of neuroleptic should be based on the most desired side effect profile. Pharmacologic developments will pursue the reduction of troublesome side effects, resulting in more effective treatment and better compliance.

EBM EVIDENCE-BASED MEDICINE

Primary sources for the revision of this chapter were MEDLINE. Electronic searches dating back to 1995 were conducted. Areas of focus included psychosis and psychotic disorders.

REFERENCES

1. Abramowicz MA, editor: Drugs that cause psychiatric symptoms, *Med Lett* 35:65, 1993.
2. American Psychiatric Association: *Diagnostic and statistical manual of mental disorders,* ed 4, Washington, DC, 1994, American Psychiatric Association.
3. Brown FW: The neurobiology of late-life psychosis, *Crit Rev Neurobiol* 7:275, 1993.
4. Carlsson A: The current status of the dopamine hypothesis of schizophrenia, *Neuropsychopharmacology* 1:179, 1988.
5. Davis JM et al: Dose response of prophylactic antipsychotics, *J Clin Psychiatry* 54(suppl):24, 1993.
6. Herz MI, Liberman RP, Lieberman JA, et al: *Practice guidelines for the treatment of patients with schizophrenia,* Washington, DC, 1997, American Psychiatric Association.
7. Regier DA et al: The de facto U.S. mental and addictive disorders service system: epidemiologic catchment area 1-year prevalence rates of disorders and services, *Arch Gen Psychiatry* 50:85, 1993.
8. Wessely S: Acting on delusions. I. Prevalence, *Br J Psychiatry* 163:69, 1993.

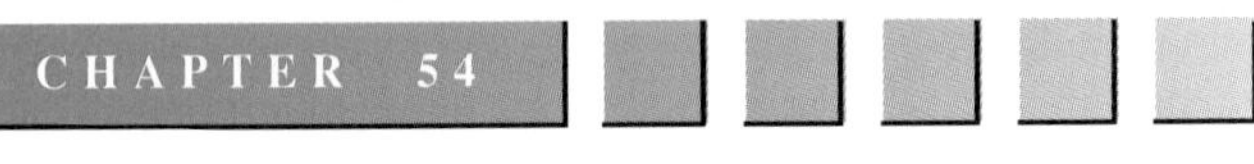

Personality Disorders

Philip R. Muskin
Elizabeth Haase

The term *personality* refers to an individual's habitual and pervasive patterns of thinking, feeling, and acting. Personality has two main components: temperament and character. *Temperament* is "hard-wired," is not influenced by sociocultural learning, and includes the automatic elements of individual emotional response. In genetic and adopted twin studies, temperament has been shown to be 50% heritable, with the remainder encoded and fixed by random repetitive environmental experience. In contrast, *character* refers to elements of personality that mature over the life span and are 85% to 90% determined by nongenetic factors. These include advanced intellectual functions (e.g., abstract thinking), self-concept, typical fantasies, characteristic defenses and coping styles, repeating but individualized patterns of interpersonal interaction, values, and ideals.

The term *personality disorder* is used when the person's style of behavior "deviates markedly from the expectations of the individual's culture, is pervasive and inflexible . . . and leads to distress and impairment."[1] The lifetime prevalence of personality disorders in a community sample is approximately 10% to 13%.[13] However, 42% of patients referred from a primary care setting for a behavioral health assessment are found to have a personality disorder.[2] The rates of personality disorders vary depending on the clinical population studied[4] (Table 54-1). What patients with personality disorders think about themselves and how they deal with others cause difficulties at work and in relationships. They are poorly equipped to handle the complex situations and increased stress created by the sick role and the demands of medical care.

CLASSIFICATION

The classification of personality disorders is controversial, with two major models: categorical and dimensional. The *Diagnostic and Statistical Manual of Mental Disorders* (DSM-IV) uses a *categorical model,* in which personality disorders are diagnosed by the presence of a minimum number of prototypical features. This model establishes a "threshold" above which recognizable pathologic types are defined, in the same way hypertension is defined with consistent measurements above a certain number.

The *dimensional model* defines personality disorders as extremes of normal personality traits. Traits are identified on a continuum, using various conceptual schemas. For example, paranoia is seen as a pathologic form of a normally adaptive trait (i.e., vigilance toward the possibility of an external threat). The dimensional approach to personality is useful to the primary care physician for two reasons. First, under the stress of medical illness, a normal personality trait may appear suddenly dysfunctional, just as a normotensive patient may show "white-coat hypertension" on office visits. Recognizing that a normal trait is being expressed in an extreme form, then responding appropriately to these changes in the patient's behavior, helps the physician to work effectively with a distressed patient during a crisis. Second, since all patients have a personality but few have personality disorders, patients need their physicians to understand and respond to their personality style. A physician who notes "emotionally intense," "anxious," or "impulsive tendencies" can anticipate how these traits might require management under stress, for example, allowing the emotionally

Table 54-1. Personality Disorder Rates in Various Clinical Populations

Population	Diagnostic instrument	DSM-IV axis II diagnosis* (%)	Most frequent disorder
Somatizers referred for psychiatric consultation	Clinical	32	Compulsive/histrionic
Outpatient cocaine abusers	SCID-II	58	Antisocial/passive-aggressive
Anabolic steroid users	PDQ	85	Antisocial/paranoid Histrionic/borderline
Normal-weight bulimic outpatients	PDQ	75	Schizotypal/borderline
Repetitive self-injurers	Clinical	88	Borderline
Male alcoholic Veterans Administration inpatients	DIS	34	Antisocial

Modified from Fogel B, Stoudemire A, editors: *Psychiatric care of the medical patient,* New York, 1993, Oxford University Press.
*Axis II is for the personality disorders and mental retardation, and for noting maladaptive features of personality. All other psychiatric diagnoses are coded on Axis I.

labile patient time for tears or stating to the impulsive patient, "You may want to terminate the chemotherapy when you get discouraged. How can we anticipate this?" Such approaches derive from knowledge about the dimensions of normal personality (Table 54-2).

Psychologic Defenses

A third way of understanding patients with personality disorders, which is critical in working with medically ill patients, is by their typical level of psychologic defenses. A *defense* is an automatic psychologic mechanism used to handle "psychic danger," that is, anxiety arising when a person experiences a conflict between inner wishes or drives and the demands of reality. Defenses are most adaptive when they allow maximal expression of wishes and needs with a minimum of negative consequences. Four levels of defenses are grouped by how effectively they allow a patient to express needs and wishes without causing negative external consequences.[3] Many people employ a mixture of these levels at various times. An otherwise stable individual may use lower level defenses when confronted with a serious medical illness; this is called *regression*. The levels of defense are mature, neurotic, borderline, and psychotic (Box 54-1).

Mature defenses allow the person to deal most effectively with the demands of real life and inner psychologic conflicts. This level of defense allows for flexibility and adaptability in people. *Neurotic defenses* are less adaptable because the person's psychologic conflicts limit the emotional options. When stressed, patients who use neurotic defenses primarily can become problem patients. Their anxiety, need for information, depression, or need for attention can block the physician's delivery of care. *Borderline defenses* are based on a psychologic process known as *splitting*. Patients who rely on splitting see themselves and others in totally black or white terms, and they may rapidly change their perceptions from one to the other. Because this prevents them from having an integrated and modulated view of events, they are prone to transient episodes of misperception, derealization, depersonalization, and moments of temporary psychosis that severely limit their ability to respond to medically challenging situations. These patients are often classified as "difficult" by their physicians.

For patients using *psychotic defenses*, reality is too painful to be experienced. Patients may deny that they are ill at all, although not every patient who does so or who refuses treatment is psychotic.[11,12] Psychotic patients may accept that they are ill but have delusions about the etiology (e.g., voodoo curse). Some psychotic patients function well during a medical illness, but many require extra attention, need pharmacologic treatment of their psychiatric symptoms, and benefit greatly from a psychiatric consultation.

Table 54-2. Personality Style–Personality Disorder Continuum

Style →	Disorder
Conscientious →	Obsessive-compulsive
Self-confident →	Narcissistic
Dramatic →	Histrionic
Vigilant →	Paranoid
Mercurial →	Borderline
Devoted →	Dependent
Solitary →	Schizoid
Leisurely →	Passive-aggressive
Sensitive →	Avoidant
Idiosyncratic →	Schizotypal
Adventurous →	Antisocial
Self-sacrificing →	Self-defeating
Aggressive →	Sadistic

Courtesy J Oldham, MD.

Box 54-1. Defense Mechanisms

Mature Defenses

Suppression: consciously putting a disturbing experience out of mind.
Altruism: vicarious but instinctively gratifying service to others.
Humor: overt expression of normally unacceptable feeling without unpleasant effect.
Anticipation: realistic planning for inevitable discomfort.
Sublimation: attenuated expression of instinct in alternative fields without adverse consequence.

Neurotic Defenses

Repression: involuntary forgetting of a painful feeling or experience.
Controlling: manipulation of external events to avoid unconscious anxiety.
Displacement: transferring an experienced feeling from one person to another.
Reaction-formation: expression of unacceptable impulses as directly opposite attitudes and behaviors.
Intellectualization: replacing feelings with facts and details.
Ambivalence: coexistence of opposite feelings.
Distortion: reorganization of external reality to fit inner needs.
Inhibition: restricting thoughts or behaviors because of fear that unacceptable feelings will erupt.
Isolation: recall of memories and experiences without emotion.

Borderline Defenses

Splitting: experiencing self and others as all good or all bad.
Idealization: seeing self or others as all powerful, ideal, or godlike.
Devaluation: depreciating others.
Projection: attributing unacceptable impulses to others.
Projective identification: causing others to experience one's unacceptable feelings; one then fears or tries to control the unacceptable behavior in the other person.
Denial: refusal to acknowledge painful realities.

Psychotic Defenses

Extreme splitting
Acting out: expression of intolerable ideas through behavior.
Somatization: expression of impulses or feelings through medical illness.
Schizoid fantasy: withdrawal from conflict into social isolation and fantasizing.

Modified from Feinstein RE, Vanderberg S: Personality disorders in office practice. In Rakel RE, editor: *Textbook of family practice*, Philadelphia, 1995, Saunders.

A strong correlation exists between the level of defenses used by the person and global measures of mental health. In primary medical practice this assessment is crucial because it guides the physician in predicting how a patient will cope with medical illness, what measures will support the patient psychologically, and what issues may arise that turn the person into a "difficult patient."

ETIOLOGY

Psychoanalytic theory contends that personality structure arises from a child's drives and wishes interacting with the environmental feedback received from parents, siblings, and others. Freud believed that the child was born with certain temperamental dispositions that developed in discrete stages: oral, anal, and genital. Stressful life experiences at these early stages were seen to have a permanent impact on personality formation.

This view is remarkably consistent with current scientific consensus about the etiology of personality disorders. Certain personality traits are clearly genetically determined. The environment can have a protective or a destabilizing effect on patients with these biologic vulnerabilities. Environment and genetics can interact; an individual's psychologic perception of external events is modulated from birth by temperament, so a "shared environment" does not have the same impact on every member of a family. An anxious child may experience parents as more aggressive than a relaxed child. Also, because genes appear to turn on and off during different stages of development, these genetic predispositions may increase or decrease as the child grows up.

People with personality disorders report more experiences of physical and sexual abuse than those without disorders. Their histories are notable for sustained deficits in care; an isolated incident of severe abuse is much less predictive of personality disorder than chronic moderate neglect. The incidence of abuse is highest for patients with borderline and antisocial personality disorders, approaching 60% in borderline patients.[8]

PATIENT EVALUATION

Patients with personality disorders are often viewed as difficult patients.[5,7] Their distorted views, maladaptive defenses, and interpersonal abrasiveness thwart effective care. Such patients frustrate physicians by noncompliance and self-destructive health behavior. They communicate their needs poorly through repeated and vague complaints, which consume time and waste resources. They are simultaneously clinging and hostile, or "hateful patients."[6] Physicians dread their visits, hope they will not return, and are reluctant to schedule return visits. The physician often feels inadequate, helpless, rageful, and guilty or feels "tricked" after patient encounters. Finding a patient "difficult" is usually the physician's first clue to the presence of a personality disorder. Many problems in the physician-patient relationship, however, are not caused by personality disorders. Patients' reactions to the fear of illness, the differing expectations of the social role of the patient and physician, and sociocultural pressures influencing the humane practice of medicine all can have a negative impact on the patient-physician relationship.

Initial Assessment

The medical encounter evokes within patients many aspects of the parent-child relationship. Physicians touch, care for, sometimes hurt, and often tell their patients what to do. As with children, patients occasionally depend on the physician for functions they normally perform independently. The stimulation of childhood fears in the patient and the parental functions of the physician in the medical encounter leads to regression. In regression, patients stop using more mature behavior and defenses and fall back on earlier coping skills. A common example of regression is a child's return to bed-wetting or thumb-sucking after the birth of a sibling. A patient's ability to relinquish control temporarily when ill may facilitate medical care; however, the person's overall function may be more childlike, less reality oriented, less stable, and less able to respond efficiently to others' needs. This behavior may surprise the physician. When regressed, a patient uses *primitive defenses.* In every setting, people unconsciously expect and recreate patterns of behavior with former caregivers. This phenomenon is known as *transference* because early relationships are transferred into a new, often inappropriate, situation.

The limitations on confidentiality, reimbursement, and flexibility in medical care have resulted in new difficulties in the physician-patient relationship that do not reflect personality disorders. Patients are more vigilant and suspicious; physicians are more frustrated, and their time, authority, and ability to evaluate and treat patients seem compromised. Such issues are best addressed with open acknowledgment of the realities affecting each party.

Assessment for Medical Causes

The next step in the assessment of difficult or unusual behavior is an evaluation for medical and psychiatric illness that may exacerbate underlying personality traits or mimic traits of a personality disorder. A medical illness that is responsible for a change in the patient's behavior may respond to pharmacologic treatment, whereas personality disorders require management in the primary care setting.

An axis I DSM-IV psychiatric disorder is likely in more than 60% of patients labeled as difficult, especially somatoform disorders, major depression, dysthymia, alcohol abuse, generalized anxiety disorder, and panic disorder. Axis I psychiatric illness influences personality in two ways. First, apparent personality traits may be symptoms of a psychiatric illness (Table 54-3). Seductive dress may be an expression of mania; pill noncompliance may be an expression of a specific phobia of choking. Such patients may seek medical care at times of greater mental, not physical, disturbance. Treating the psychiatric disorder may curtail the acute dramatic expressions of personality disturbance. For example, an untreated major depressive disorder in a patient with borderline personality disorder and bulimia could present as increased self-induced vomiting, with the resultant medical complications.

It cannot be overemphasized how often medical illnesses and medications used in medical practice disturb personality (Box 54-2). Prominent among these are the dementias, vascular diseases of the brain, bulbar diseases, seizure disorders, and other chronic neurologic illnesses. Generally, such disorders cause existing personality traits to become more rigid and extreme, although many patients develop de novo changes in personality or new features. For example, temporal lobe epilepsy may lead to the development of schizotypal features (e.g., stereotyped interests) or parapsychotic experiences (e.g., derealization).

Table 54-3. DSM-IV Axis I Disorders That May Simulate Personality Problems

Disorder	Interpersonal problems
Depression	Dependency, irritability, poor compliance, insecurity
Mania	Irritability, seductiveness, depreciation or grandiosity, antisocial behaviors
Panic disorder	Dependency, reassurance seeking, avoidance
Obsessive-compulsive disorder	Demanding, requests for facts, details, and time
Posttraumatic stress disorder	Irritability, hostility, impulsivity
Paranoid schizophrenia	Hostility, suspiciousness, demanding

Modified from Goldman L, Wise T, and Brody D, editors: *Psychiatry for primary care physicians,* Chicago, 1998, AMA Press.

Physician Responses

Recognition of an underlying personality disorder often starts with a physician's awareness of uncharacteristic responses to a patient. These patients are often difficult, draining, or unrewarding. Patients with personality disorders evoke three patterns of unusual subjective response. First, *emotional responses* to such patients tend to be stronger than usual and intrude into professional reasoning. Feelings of love or sexual arousal, or feelings of wanting to rescue a patient or give special care, may alternate rapidly with feelings of hate or betrayal. Physicians may have unusual *fantasies* about a patient in free hours, dream of a patient, or worry about the patient excessively. The feelings elicited by patients with personality disorders often compel physicians to *atypical behaviors.* Physicians may order extra tests to placate a patient and may offer free services or unreasonable availability. Such thoughts and behaviors reflect the physician's response to the intensity of the patient's emotional needs. Because they arise in reaction to, or counter to, the patient's transferred expectations of interpersonal relationships, these expressions are known as *countertransference.* These experiences are the cue to a physician that the patient's personality dynamics are impacting on the professional relationship.

MANAGEMENT

Primary care physicians frequently see and must adeptly manage the common personality types in medical practice, but they rarely need to make formal DSM-IV personality diagnoses. Awareness of a problem is typically more useful than a DSM-IV personality diagnosis. A general management approach for patients with more severe personality disorders can prevent many disruptive explosions in the physician's office. General techniques that diffuse conflict include the following:

1. *Consistency.* Strategies that help difficult patients manage medical care include minimizing changes in plans, medications, schedules, and personnel; making sure all staff respond to a patient with the same information; clarifying the length and time of visits in advance; and anticipating and planning for vacations and future events explicitly. Consistency is particularly important for dependent and borderline patients.
2. *Clarifying the treatment contract.* Exploring the patient's hopes regarding treatment and explaining the rationale, method, limits, and objectives of treatment can prevent disappointments and misunderstandings, to which such patients may react dramatically. Paranoid, obsessive-compulsive, and narcissistic patients may especially benefit from this approach.
3. *Limit setting.* Explaining which behaviors and requests will or will not be allowed forms the foundation of management techniques. The physician must not be manipulated or intimidated by the patient or be punitive or rejecting of the patient. Both are overreactions to patients' behavior, often their aggression. A confident, balanced, and supportive approach works best, allowing unimportant behaviors to go unchallenged while standing firm on disruptive or dangerous outbursts. Examples include providing physical therapy, but not narcotics, for patients

Box 54-2. Common Medical Causes of Personality Change

Diseases

Neurosyphilis
AIDS and other viral encephalitides
Alzheimer's disease and other dementias
Pseudobulbar palsy
Head injury
Central nervous system tumors, especially frontal and temporal
Arteriovenous malformations
Hydrocephalus
Multiple sclerosis
Epilepsy, especially temporal lobe
Lupus erythematosus
Pernicious anemia
Hypothyroidism
Diabetes mellitus
Pituitary endocrinopathies (e.g., Turner's syndrome)
Mercury, magnesium, or other metallic intoxication

Medications

Herbal drugs
Steroids
Narcotics, especially meperidine and pentazocine
Benzodiazepines
Stimulants, including theophylline
Antiparkinsonian agents (dopa agonists)
Anticholinergics (including topical)
Antineoplastics
Barbiturates
Antiretrovirals
Cimetidine
Metoclopramide
Yohimbine
Metrizamide
Cardiac drugs, especially propranolol, captopril, clonidine, digitalis, lidocaine, methyldopa, mexiletine, reserpine, and disopyramide

with a history of addiction, and hearing out a patient's anger, but clarifying that throwing things will not be accepted.

Beyond general strategies, particular character styles can generate extreme reactions in physicians. Groves[6] identifies four common "hateful" personality types: dependent clingers, entitled demanders, manipulative help-rejecters, and self-destructive deniers. These patients always seem to be entitled and dependent while simultaneously hopelessly filled with rejecting self-hatred. They are destructive of care, which can provoke punishment, attack, or withdrawal from their physicians. Kahana and Bibring[9] list seven categories of difficult medical patients (with approximately corresponding DSM-IV diagnoses): (1) *dependent/needy* (borderline, dependent), (2) *orderly/controlled* (obsessive-compulsive), (3) *dramatizing/captivating* (histrionic), (4) *long suffering/self-sacrificing* (self-defeating), (5) *guarded/querulous* (paranoid), (6) *superior* (narcissistic), and (7) *uninvolved/aloof* (schizoid, avoidant). Table 54-4 outlines interventions for these particular styles.

The following sections focus on the five most common and most troublesome behaviors—anger, anxiety, sadness, seductiveness, and suspiciousness—and ways for the physician to address these behaviors productively. The key is to (1) understand why the patient is responding in a particular manner, (2) attempt to demonstrate that understanding to the patient, and (3) legitimize or validate the emotion as understandable given what the patient is experiencing. This is an operationalized definition of *empathy,* which will solve these problems. Inappropriate responses can then be gently confronted as not in keeping with the reality of the situation as experienced by the physician.

Anger

Although any of the personality types may respond with anger when confronted with frightening medical news, antisocial, borderline, and paranoid personalities are most likely to respond this way. People who rely on facts to control their world (i.e., obsessional people) may also respond with anger if they feel they are not being given adequate information. The anger may be overtly or subtly expressed. Anger frightens other people, including physicians; the initial response is to engage the "flight-or-fight" mechanisms. One approach is not to *react* to the patient but to think for a moment and then *respond.* During that moment the physician understands that anger is an emotion that substitutes for fear. Telling patients that what they experience as the "real" emotion is *not* real will be heard as invalidating and will be rejected. Saying instead, "I see that you are angry, but I am not sure I understand what is causing you to feel this way," may be more successful than presenting psychologic interpretation. Once the patient has explained the feelings, the physician can follow up with, "It is understandable that you would feel angry given what you have said. I think we can work this out together." The physician then outlines a plan to deal with the issues; not retaliating with more anger reassures the patient of good intentions. At times the only approach may be to suggest that some time elapse before talking again,

Table 54-4. Personality Types and Management Recommendations

Style	Reaction to illness	Problematic caregiver reactions	Recommendations
Paranoid	Fears exploitation, hurt, invasion	Feels accused, defensive Counterattacks, proving patient right	Avoid excess warmth. Provide clear detailed explanations. Accept irrational fears.
Schizoid/schizotypal	Feels threat to self-integrity Withdraws, delays care	Feels rejected Tries to overcome patient aloofness with excess warmth	Accept privacy and distance. Stress technical and mechanical elements of care. Encourage daily routines to preserve fragile sense of self.
Antisocial	Fears vulnerability Lies for secondary gain	Anger; desire to uncover lies and punish	Empathize with feeling "had" or deprived. Explain that lies lead to poor care; give just care.
Histrionic	Believes illness threatens love and attractiveness	Seduced, flattered, embarrassed Poor care from undertreatment	Provide friendly interactions. Appreciate courage and strengths.
Borderline/dependent	Fears abandonment Rage/panic/suicide Rejects help, devalues, demands attention	Feels manipulated Wants alternately to rescue or be rid of patient Burnout	Plan for absences. Give reality test; interpret splitting. Set firm limits; stop care if patient breaks agreements.
Narcissistic	Loss of self-worth Acts entitled, "special" Devalues care	Feels inferior Wants to put patient in caregiver's place Avoids patient	Support entitlement. Acknowledge mistakes; offer consultation.
Obsessive-compulsive	Shame over loss of bodily control	Impatience; tries to control treatment	Be thorough and methodical. Make patient a partner. Use homework, lists, and details.

Modified from Feinstein RE, Vanderburg S: *Personality disorders in office practice.* In Rakel RE, editor: *Textbook of family practice,* Philadelphia, 1995, WB Saunders.

then schedule the next conversation. The physician can disagree with the anger but still respect the person's need to feel angry.

Anxiety

Anxious responses may take several forms, some of which may not appear as anxiety to the physician. The overtly anxious person is most helped by the physician identifying that the anxiety is understandable. Understandable does not mean the physician shares the patient's anxiety and cannot face a realistic appraisal of the situation. "You are much too anxious given what I have told you," is less effective than, "I appreciate that what we are discussing is making you anxious, but I want you to know I see this as something we can deal with together effectively." By adding the word "together," the physician establishes partnership with the patient, which is calming.

Patients who have an obsessional personality style may demonstrate their anxiety by asking many questions, often repeatedly. Their demand on time will be frustrating to the physician. In this situation the empathic response is first to identify the behavior (i.e., the repetitive questions or the need to know more and more). The physician might say, "I realize that we have been over this before. Perhaps I have not done an adequate job of explaining this to you, so let me review it now. Sometimes, when people are anxious about hearing bad news, they miss the facts and then don't feel that they know enough. I want you to understand thoroughly what is going on." Obsessional people do best when they have information with which they can control their anxiety. Giving pamphlets to patients, suggesting appropriate research literature, or suggesting websites help the patient to contain the emotions. Acknowledging that the patient is "distressed" or that the illness has caused anxiety helps the patient consider the repeated questioning as anxiety rather than as necessary information seeking. This also helps when patients blame physicians for not providing enough information.

Sadness

An important moment in a patient-physician relationship occurs when the physician comments, "You look sad." Tears may come but are typically brief. If the physician fails to recognize and validate these feelings, the patient may regard the physician as insensitive and cold. Ignoring the sadness is most likely to result in noncompliance, missed follow-up visits, or a search for a new physician. Identifying and empathizing with the patient's sadness form the core of physician support. Any patient can feel sad, but this should alert the physician that this patient could be at risk for a mood disorder. Once identified as sadness appropriate to the condition, the physician can inquire at future visits about the patient's mood, sleep, appetite, and interest in activities. This brief assessment can be rapidly diagnostic for a major depressive disorder. When patients experience their physicians as compassionate and empathic, they are more likely to reveal important information. This allows the physician to understand the patient better, which leads to greater compliance and better overall health care. If left unidentified, the patient who becomes depressed may present with a variety of physical complaints that do not respond well to "medical" treatment. By acknowledging the patient's emotions, the physician can connect the emotions to physical symptoms, diagnose the depression, and offer effective treatment.

Seductiveness

Patients with antisocial, borderline, histrionic, and narcissistic personality styles may use seductive behavior with the physician. Seduction can vary from minimal to overtly sexual, but much of what constitutes seduction is not sexual in nature. The seductive behavior is the patient's attempt to feel in control of the situation; to ensure that the patient is admired, respected, or acceptable; and to control anxiety. Sexually seductive behavior makes most physicians uncomfortable because it threatens their professional identity with inappropriate impulses. A natural response is chastising the patient or becoming angry or rejecting. Patients who need to act seductively will then increase their seductive efforts to receive attention, or they will feel angry because they are not actually seeking sex. The behavior should not be ignored, however, since this is likely to yield the same result as chastisement. Having a nurse in the room during a physical examination may be a practical solution, but this is not appropriate in other situations. The patient may need to be told that the physician is uncomfortable, even though the patient may feel rejected. These patients need the reassurance that their illness does not make them less attractive, appealing, interesting, important, or powerful. Comments on these issues address the patient's psychologic needs and reduce the motivation to use seductive behavior to assuage underlying fears.

Seduction may occur in nonsexual ways, such as offering the physician favors, tickets, or gifts. All patients do this to some extent; the physician's psychologic reaction determines the seductive potential. If the physician feels uncomfortable with the type of gift, the expense, or the feeling of being beholden; feels envy for the patient's power, importance, or wealth; or feels incapable of saying no to an inappropriate request, the physician probably has been seduced. Similar to the handling of sexual behavior, prevention works quite well. Gifts can be gently refused, with the recommendation that the "grateful" patient make a charitable contribution. Acknowledging the patient's "specialness" is what the patient desires; accepting anything from the patient is not necessary to accomplish this goal.

Suspiciousness

Physicians assume they are trusted and dislike the experience of a patient who confronts them with, "I don't think you are doing the best for me," or, "I don't believe you are telling me the truth." Although antisocial, borderline, paranoid, and schizoid personality styles are most likely to take this approach, narcissistic and obsessive patients are also suspicious. The patient may be responding to the physician's discomfort with telling the patient about the illness. Patients deserve to hear the truth about their condition but do not need to be robbed of hope. In an attempt to find the right balance, the physician may convey an attitude of withholding information. Finding out what the patient already knows, what the patient thinks is occurring, and how much the patient wants to know helps guide information disclosure and prevent naturally suspicious patients from becoming more suspicious.

When patients fear they may not recover, when they find it difficult to cope with the demands of physical illness, and when the illness destabilizes their psychologic equilibrium, patients with antisocial, borderline, paranoid, and schizoid personality styles may handle their fears by regarding others as harming them. This maladaptive way of coping is psychologically easier. The suspiciousness makes the physician the enemy, an enemy who can be controlled (or so the patient believes). This replaces the fear that the illness cannot be controlled, a fear that is overwhelming for the person. Prevention is extremely useful in these situations. Recognizing which patients constantly question, never seem satisfied, and always act cheated or mistreated is a crucial preventive step for the physician. Informing these patients about tests in advance, reporting test results, and explaining the need for a procedure or treatment take extra time but are preferable to an unpleasant confrontation by the suspicious patient. The language of "entitlement" is also of great benefit when speaking with these patients. They respond to statements such as, "You deserve the best, which is why I want to do this test, to be sure we know what is going on. However, the procedure may cause you some discomfort."

TREATMENT

Referral

In general, patients with personality disorders serious enough to disrupt their lives or interfere with their health and medical care should receive careful referral to a mental health professional. Some patients will experience this referral as a rejection or as an abandonment by the physician. Reiterating the physician's intent to continue to provide medical care and providing psychologic support will aid in alleviating the patient's concerns. When patient behavior exceeds the limits of acceptability, the patient must be told that continued medical care is not possible under such circumstances. In these situations the physician should arrange a psychiatric consultation to understand the patient's behavior, and should attempt to control the behavior.

Psychotherapy

Personality disorders comprise diverse symptom clusters and ways of relating to others, and thus varied treatments can effectively target aspects of disturbance. Psychotherapy is the preferred treatment for personality disorders. Psychotherapy can be cognitive behavioral, family, or psychoanalytic in approach. Generally, psychodynamic and cognitive behavioral psychotherapy is highly effective for anxious, narcissistic, histrionic, and borderline personality disorders but less effective for paranoid, schizoid, and antisocial disorders. Dialectic behavioral therapy for borderline personality disorder is an example of specific psychotherapy. Short-term psychotherapy interventions may help patients handle specific acute stressors. Patients with personality disorders benefit most and permanently from psychotherapies lasting several years. Respectfully supporting the patient's courage in continuing such self-exploration can be invaluable to a long-term primary care relationship. The acute psychotherapeutic interventions may augment the physician's recommendation for a psychotherapy referral.

Psychopharmacology

Some aspects of personality disorders respond to psychopharmacologic treatment. Psychopharmacology is targeted to specific symptom clusters. The perceptual and cognitive distortions seen in borderline, schizotypal, and paranoid personalities may respond to low doses of neuroleptics such as haloperidol (Haldol), risperidone (Risperdal), or olanzapine (Zyprexa). Atypical presentations of depression, as well as more typical forms, can be treated with antidepressants. The decision regarding which medication to use is often dictated by side effects or drug interactions.[10] The impulsive behavior seen in antisocial and borderline personalities often responds to anticonvulsants (e.g., carbamazepine, gabapentin, valproic acid). Benzodiazepines are not recommended for long-term treatment but may be useful in acutely stressful situations. Care should be taken in prescribing benzodiazepines to borderline and antisocial patients due to the risk of substance abuse. Buspirone is useful for patients with persistent anxiety, without the addiction concerns associated with the benzodiazepines. The antianxiety effect does not develop for several weeks. Pharmacologic treatment is best undertaken in consultation with a psychiatrist.

SUMMARY

The "difficult" patient may have a personality disorder that intrudes into all aspects of life, including the medical relationship. The person's typical style of behavior may not be an everyday problem but is causing a problem in the patient-physician relationship. The vast majority of these problem patients are dealt with effectively in the primary care setting by knowledgeable and compassionate physicians with the routine skills needed to deliver effective medical care.

REFERENCES

1. *Diagnostic and statistical manual of mental disorders,* ed 4, Washington, DC, 1994, American Psychiatric Association.
2. Emerson J, Pankratz L, Joos S, et al: Personality disorders in problematic medical patients, *Psychosomatics* 35:469, 1994.
3. Feinstein R, Vanderberg S: Personality disorders in office practice. In Rakel RE, editor: *Textbook of family practice,* Philadelphia, 1995, Saunders.
4. Fogel B: *Personality disorders in the medical setting.* In Fogel B, Stoudemire A, editors: *Psychiatric care of the medical patient,* London, 1993, Oxford University Press.
5. Goldman L, Hahn S: Difficult patient situations. In Goldman L, Wise T, Brody D, editors: *Psychiatry for primary care physicians,* Chicago, 1998, AMA Press.
6. Groves J: Taking care of the hateful patient, *N Engl J Med* 298:883, 1978.
7. Hahn SR, Kroenke K, Spitzer RL, et al: The difficult patient: prevalence, psychopathology, and functional impairment, *J Gen Intern Med* 11:1, 1996.
8. Herman JL et al: Childhood trauma and borderline personality disorder, *Am J Psychiatry* 146:490, 1989.
9. Kahana RJ, Bibring GL: Personality types in medical management. In Zinberg N, editor: *Psychiatry and medical practice in a general hospital,* Madison, Conn, 1964, International University Press, pp 108-123.
10. Muskin PR: Depression in medically ill patients, *Postgrad Med,* suppl:3, 1998.
11. Muskin PR, Feldhammer T, Gelfand JL, Strauss DH: Maladaptive denial of physical illness: a useful new "diagnosis," *Int J Psychiatry Med* 28:503-517, 1998.
12. Strauss DH, Spitzer RL, Muskin PR: Maladaptive denial of physical illness: a proposal for DSM-IV, *Am J Psychiatry* 147:1168, 1990.
13. Weissman MM et al: Psychiatric disorders in a U.S. urban community, 1975-1976, *Am J Psychiatry* 135:459, 1978.

ADDITIONAL READINGS

Karasu T, Bellak L: Brief psychotherapy of stress response syndromes. In Karasu T, editor: *Specialized techniques in individualized psychotherapy,* New York, 1980, Brunner/Mazel.

Kass F, Skodol A, Charles E, et al: Scaled ratings of DSM-III personality disorder, *Am J Psychiatry* 142:627, 1985.
Oldham JM: Personality disorders: current perspectives, *JAMA* 272:1770, 1994.
Perry JC, Cooper SH: Empirical studies of psychological defense mechanisms. In Michels R et al, editors: *Psychiatry*, New York, 1997, Lippincott-Raven.
Sansone RA, Wiederman MW, Sansone LA, et al: Early onset dysthymia and personality disturbance in a primary care setting, *J Nerv Ment Dis* 186:57, 1998.
Silk KR: Biology of personality disorders. In Oldham JM, Riba MD, editors: *Review of psychiatry series*, Chicago, 1998, American Psychiatric Press.
Sparr LF, Boehnlein JK, Cooney TG: The medical management of the paranoid patient, *Gen Hosp Psychiatry* 8:49, 1996.

CHAPTER 55

Eating Disorders

Jarol B. Knowles

The eating disorders—anorexia nervosa, bulimia nervosa, rumination syndrome, binge eating disorder, and anorexia athletica—are relatively common maladies. Once believed to be problems largely among young women, the disorders are being found increasingly among children, young athletes, men, and elderly women. Primary care physicians may be the first to suspect potential problems, including a patient's fixation on food, weight, dieting, physique, and exercise. Patients who have struggled in silence for years may turn to their trusted physician for support and understanding. Primary care physicians can encounter eating disorders when patients seek help with medical or psychiatric complications of malnutrition or illness-related behaviors or when family members bring them to the physician's attention (often against the patient's wishes). Eating disorders are complex and involve two sets of issues and behaviors: those directly relating to food and weight and those involving the relationships with self and others. The phrase "eating disorder" is somewhat misleading in that it implies that the essence of the problem is disordered eating and suggests that the solution is to learn to eat normally again. Often accompanied by depression, anxiety, and personality disorders, eating disorders may be difficult to diagnose.

ANOREXIA NERVOSA

Definition and Epidemiology

Anorexia nervosa is characterized by prominent behavioral, psychologic, and physiologic disturbances, including refusal to maintain a minimally healthy body weight (85% of that expected), dramatic weight loss, fear of gaining weight even though underweight, preoccupation with food, and abnormal food consumption patterns.[5] Biologic indicators of anorexia nervosa include reductions in heart rate, blood pressure, and metabolic rate; increased cortisol production; and a profound decrease in the production of estrogen (or, in males, testosterone).[12,13,15] Anorexia is not the result of a single biologic factor or psychologic aberration, but rather the product of a dynamic interaction of biologic, psychologic, and social influences.

Anorexia nervosa primarily affects women (about 95% of cases). In the United States, 27% of adolescent girls who view themselves as being at the "right weight" still attempt to lose weight, compared with less than 10% of adolescent boys.[10] The prevalence of anorexia nervosa is an estimated 0.7% among randomly selected females, although it is higher among those in the uppermost socioeconomic strata (1% of a group of British private-school students). Both American and European studies imply that the incidence may be increasing, although these data may be skewed by increased media attention.

Pathogenesis and Pathophysiology

Sociocultural Factors. In both anorexia nervosa and bulimia nervosa the modern cultural value for females to be thin plays a role in the pathogenesis. The increased prevalence of eating disorders among women who engage in certain activities and occupations (e.g., professional models, ballet dancers) is evidence of the strong influence of sociocultural phenomena in the genesis of anorexia nervosa. The higher prevalence of eating disorders among Western societies (and the development of these disorders among individuals of Eastern heritage transplanted to Western societies) is further evidence of a strong cultural influence on eating disorder pathogenesis. Social pressures from peers, particularly during adolescence, seem to influence young women and girls to engage in anorectic behaviors. Since anorexia nervosa has been described for more than 300 years, however, modern sociocultural ideals are not the sole cause of this disease but create the environment for the expression of an eating disorder in the predisposed individual.

Psychologic Factors. Anorectic patients may have an incompletely developed personal identity and struggle to maintain a sense of control over their environment. These individuals often describe growing up with the sense that they are expected to excel, but they lack the sense that they are valued and loved for themselves. Low self-esteem has been cited as the most important predictor of future anorexia nervosa among several risk factors for the disease. In response to parental expectations, the preanorectic child learns to be hard working, eager to please, and attentive to family needs. In turn the parents may support and indulge their child's behaviors. These mutually reinforced actions produce interdependence among the family members (i.e., enmeshment). Rather than developing a sense of self-worth based on internal standards, the preanorectic girl becomes engaged in an obsessive quest for external approval; she has a difficult time separating her goals and desires from those of her environment. Furthermore, if the external environment values thinness, the preanorectic female is validated in her quest for thinness.

More than 80% of anorectic patients develop symptoms within 7 years of menarche. In a normal child, biologic and psychologic events (e.g., menarche, growth spurt, school, adolescent peer pressure) encourage individuation and separation from the family. The biologic and emotional changes associated with menarche lead to a feeling of being out of control. In the predisposed individual the conflicts and loss of control are resolved by the pursuit of thinness, which allows the person to control one aspect of life absolutely. The sensation of a loss of control is heightened by the major life changes (leaving home to start school, marriage, death of a parent) that may occur at this time of life. One of these events often precipitates the onset of symptoms.

Data indicate a high prevalence of sexual abuse among anorectic patients and, more frequently, among bulimic patients. In one study of 158 patients admitted to an eating disorder unit, 50% of the anorectic and bulimic patients reported sexual abuse, compared with 28% of the patients with other eating disorder diagnoses.[7] The relation of this traumatic psychologic experience to the development of an eating disorder is uncertain. Abusive experiences may not be causative but may affect the clinical expression of the disorder.

Amenorrhea and loss of body fat may maintain the anorectic female in a prepubertal childlike state, thereby reducing the psychosocial pressures related to her developing sexuality.

Biologic Factors. Biologic factors may increase susceptibility to developing anorexia nervosa. Anorexia nervosa has a 6% prevalence in siblings, and in one study of twin pairs, 9 of 12 monozygotic and 1 of 14 dizygotic pairs were concordant for the disorder.[8] Also, anorexia nervosa and depressive disorder may coexist in first-degree relatives of anorectic patients.

Recent studies of serotonin and leptin in patients with anorexia nervosa suggest that physiologic abnormalities may play a role. Increases in brain serotonin function lead to reductions in food intake, and decreases in brain serotonin function are associated with depression. Cerebrospinal fluid (CSF) levels of the major serotonin metabolite, 5-hydroxyindoleacetic acid (5-HIAA), are low in underweight individuals with anorexia nervosa but then rise to above-normal levels in those with longstanding recovery.[17] Low CSF levels of 5-HIAA are associated with impulsive behavior, such as suicide attempts. High levels of 5-HIAA in recovered patients may indicate perfectionism and rigidity, characteristics seen in many individuals with anorexia nervosa before the illness develops. Thus a premorbid disturbance in serotonergic function might be a risk factor for the development of this disorder.

Leptin is a hormone secreted by fat cells that plays a role in the regulation of body fat stores and appetite. Serum leptin levels correlate with fat mass and tend to be low in underweight anorexic patients. These levels increase with weight gain but appear to precede normalization of body weight. The negative feedback effect of serum leptin on the appetite center in the brain may explain patients' difficulties with attaining and maintaining normal weights.[6]

Natural History. Typically, patients with anorexia nervosa present in the teenage years. Some have described a bimodal incidence curve, with one peak at 13 to 14 years and another at 17 to 18 years. Many individuals who develop anorexia nervosa during adolescence eventually make full recoveries. For approximately 50% of patients the long-term outcome is variable, with a significant number reaching adulthood with irrational concerns about weight gain. The mortality, from complications of starvation or from suicide, is substantial, approximately 5% per decade of follow-up.[11] The degree of social integration (with parents and friends) is a stronger predictor of a favorable outcome than either medical treatment or psychotherapy.

Patient History

Suspected anorexia nervosa demands a careful patient history with assessment of eating attitudes. Anorectic patients are often preoccupied with food and may exhibit bizarre food preferences or elaborately prepare food for others. Most lose weight through dietary restriction and exercise (i.e., restrictor subgroup), but up to 50% also self-induce vomiting or take purgatives (i.e., bulimic subgroup). Obtaining a history of these disorders requires sensitivity and recognition of the patient's reluctance to disclose "shameful" information. The primary care physician must establish a sense of trust and ask questions in a caring and nonjudgmental manner.

Patients are often brought to the physician's attention by friends or relatives. Recent media attention focusing on the dangers of anorexia nervosa has led to a generation of adolescents who deny their problem, creating a treatment challenge. Anorectic patients may also have constipation, crampy abdominal pain, abdominal bloating, or amenorrhea; a high index of suspicion is needed in such patients.

Physical Examination

A complete physical examination is important in patients with suspected anorexia nervosa and should include a nutritional assessment. Height and weight are usually sufficient screening parameters. Two methods can determine the degree of malnutrition: measurement of body mass index (BMI) or comparison to standardized weight tables for percentage of ideal body weight (% IBW). A BMI less than 18 is abnormal, but a % IBW less than 85% is more often used to diagnose anorexia nervosa.

Findings may include a thin body habitus, increased amounts of fine, downy body hair (lanugo), and acrocyanosis (Box 55-1). Subcutaneous fat may be greatly decreased. The skin of anorectic patients is often dry and scaly and may have a slightly yellow cast due to carotenemia. Mild peripheral edema, without associated hypoproteinemia, may be noted. Vital signs are frequently notable for decreased core body temperature, bradycardia, and mild hypotension. If symptoms develop before puberty, secondary sex characteristics may not have developed. Unlike patients with involuntary starvation, anorectic patients do not usually manifest signs and symptoms of vitamin deficiency, although scurvy and pellagra have been reported.

Psychologic and Behavioral Findings. Anorectic patients frequently overestimate their body width and insist that they are overweight despite objective evidence to the contrary; however, their perception of others' body size is unimpaired. Abnormalities in perception of enteroceptive stimuli are also present; the sensation of satiety is altered, and patients often deny fatigue. Frequently they work or exercise to the point of exhaustion. Recognition of emotional states (e.g., anger, depression) is blunted. Disturbances in mood, primarily depression, are common, and on clinical presentation, major affective disorder is seen in approximately 50% of patients. Defects in conceptual thought and abstract reasoning are evidenced by the patient's sense of being controlled by the environment and resultant feelings of ineffectiveness. Anorectic patients tend to view situations in extremes; they have difficulty perceiving the "grays" in life and interpret the actions of others in a rigid and highly personalized form.

Box 55-1. Medical Findings in Anorexia Nervosa

Physical Examination
Thin body habitus
Increased lanugo hair
Acrocyanosis
Decreased subcutaneous fat
Dry, scaly skin
Decreased body temperature
Bradycardia
Mild hypotension
Delayed development of secondary sex characteristics

Endocrine
Amenorrhea
Hypoestrogenemia
Mild hypothyroid symptoms (without biochemical evidence of hypothyroidism)
Decreased plasma norepinephrine levels
Increased human growth hormone levels
Decreased somatomedin C levels

Cardiovascular
Left ventricular wall thinning
Decreased cardiac output
Arrhythmias (dysrhythmias)
Electrocardiographic abnormalities
Refeeding congestive heart failure

Gastrointestinal
Delayed gastric emptying
Increased gastrointestinal transit times
Constipation
Crampy abdominal pain
Elevated serum transaminases and alkaline phosphatase
Hepatic steatosis
Acute gastric dilation, acute pancreatitis, malabsorptive diarrhea with refeeding

Renal
Prerenal azotemia
Decreased glomerular filtration rate
Refeeding peripheral edema

Miscellaneous
Elevated serum carotene, cholesterol, and vitamin A
Mildly decreased serum albumin and total protein
Mild leukopenia, anemia, and thrombocytopenia
Hypocomplementemia

Box 55-2. DSM-IV Criteria for Anorexia Nervosa

Refusal to maintain body weight over a minimal normal weight for age and height, e.g., weight loss leading to maintenance of body weight 15% below that expected; or failure to make expected weight gain during period of growth, leading to body weight 15% below that expected
Intense fear of gaining weight or becoming fat, even though underweight
Disturbance in the way in which one's body weight, size, or shape is experienced, e.g., claiming to feel fat even when obviously underweight
In females, absence of at least three consecutive menstrual cycles when otherwise expected to occur (primary or secondary amenorrhea)

From *Diagnostic and statistical manual of mental disorders*, ed 4, Washington, DC, 1994, American Psychiatric Association.

Medical Findings. The medical findings of anorexia nervosa are primarily the result of starvation (see Box 55-1). The progression of complications correlates with the severity of malnutrition.

Endocrine abnormalities are among the most consistent medical findings among anorectic patients. *Amenorrhea* is part of the *Diagnostic and Statistical Manual of Mental Disorders* (DSM-IV) diagnostic criteria; its onset may precede weight loss (Box 55-2). Amenorrhea in anorexia nervosa is caused by hypothalamic-pituitary dysfunction. Serum estradiol levels in anorectic patients are uniformly lower than in normal controls, as are serum follicle-stimulating hormone (FSH) and luteinizing hormone (LH) levels. The patterns of LH secretion in anorectic patients are similar to those seen in pubescent or prepubescent females. Patients who recover normal weight often have resumption of menses; amenorrhea may persist in up to 38% of these patients. Studies have shown that a body fat content of 17% is required for the initiation of gonadotropin cycling. Weight loss below this level before menarche results in *primary* amenorrhea; weight loss below this level after menarche results in *secondary* amenorrhea. Resumption of menses after a weight loss cessation usually requires a higher body fat content (about 22%). *Psychogenic* amenorrhea (amenorrhea in times of severe psychologic stress in the absence of weight loss) is a well-recognized phenomenon and may account for some of the menstrual irregularities observed in anorectic patients. Hypoestrogenemia, along with nutritional deficiencies, contributes to the osteoporosis sometimes seen in anorexia nervosa.

Neuroimaging in anorexic patients has revealed morphologic and functional alterations in the brain, most of which are currently interpreted as consequences of the anorectic state that are reversible, at least partially, after weight gain. Enlargement of CSF spaces, mainly of cortical sulci, is evident on computed tomography (CT) and magnetic resonance imaging (MRI). This reversible shrinkage of brain tissue (pseudoatrophy) also affects the pituitary gland. Positron emission tomography (PET) has revealed caudate hyperactivity during the anorectic state; several mild right-left asymmetries, possibly related to alterations of mental state (e.g., vigilance, depression), have also been reported in bulimia nervosa.

Starvation-induced alterations of neuropeptide activity probably contribute to neuroendocrine dysfunction in anorexia nervosa. For example, corticotropin-releasing hormone (CRH) alterations contribute to hypercortisolemia, and neuropeptide Y alterations may contribute to amenorrhea. Alterations of these peptides and in opioid, vasopressin, and oxytocin activity could contribute to other characteristic psychophysiologic disturbances (e.g., reduced feeding) in acutely ill patients. Such neuropeptide disturbances may contribute to the vicious cycle hypothesized to occur in anorexia nervosa; that is, the consequences of malnutrition perpetuate pathologic behavior.

Findings consistent with hypothyroidism (dry skin, brittle nails, coarse hair, cold intolerance, bradycardia, delayed deep tendon reflex relaxation, and constipation) are often seen; however, clinically significant hypothyroidism does not occur in anorexia nervosa, and thyroid supplementation is not indicated. Thyroid-stimulating hormone (TSH) and free thyroxine levels are usually normal. Reverse triiodothyronine (rT_3) is elevated in response to starvation and is responsible for a decreased metabolic rate as an adaptive response to starvation. Increasing weight results in a reversal of the relative hypothyroid state.

Adrenal hormone abnormalities include normal or slightly increased plasma cortisol and decreased levels of urinary 17-hydroxycorticosteroids. These changes probably result from decreased clearance of cortisol from the plasma and an increase in cortisol-binding capacity, since 24-hour cortisol production rate and basal adrenocorticotropic hormone (ACTH) secretion are normal. Plasma norepinephrine levels are diminished, a finding also seen in starvation; these values return to normal with weight increase.

Cardiovascular findings include left ventricular wall thinning, decreased left ventricular chamber size, and consequent decreased cardiac output. These are adaptive changes to decreases in circulating catecholamine levels and can lead to decreased blood pressure and peripheral edema. Electrocardiographic (ECG) abnormalities (e.g., decreased QRS amplitude, prolongation of QT interval, nonspecific ST segment changes, U waves) may be related to electrolyte abnormalities. Arrhythmias (dysrhythmias) may occur, especially in patients with electrolyte abnormalities, and sudden death has occurred in severely malnourished patients. Refeeding may precipitate acute congestive heart failure.

Changes in gastrointestinal function are common in anorectic patients, who typically complain of early satiety, bloating, belching, vomiting, and constipation. Evidence indicates gastric electrical dysrhythmias, impaired antral contraction, and delayed emptying of a solid meal. Improvement in gastric emptying with domperidone suggests dysfunction of dopaminergic peptides or their receptors in the central and enteric nervous systems. Chronic constipation results from decreased oral intake, decreased intestinal transit, laxative or diuretic abuse, or any combination. Fecal impaction should be considered if constipation suddenly develops. With or without laxative abuse, barium enema studies may show a dilated, atonic, and ahaustral colon. Rapid refeeding in anorectic patients can result in acute gastric dilation, acute pancreatitis, and malabsorptive diarrhea (which may be caused by deficiencies in pancreatic and intestinal brush border digestive enzymes). Elevations in serum transaminases and alkaline phosphatase are caused by starvation-induced hepatic steatosis. Most of the gastrointestinal manifestations resolve with careful refeeding.

Renal complications include prerenal azotemia, which is caused by increased protein catabolism and intravascular volume depletion, resulting in decreased glomerular filtration rate (GFR). Decreased GFR may result in an increased tendency toward nephrolithiasis. Refeeding may cause volume overload secondary to aldosterone-induced sodium retention; such changes may take months to reverse completely.

Other miscellaneous findings include increases in serum carotene, cholesterol, and vitamin A levels, in contrast to most patients with starvation where these are decreased. The reason for these differences in the anorectic population is unknown, although the increased intake of vegetables high in β-carotene and thus vitamin A value may account for their elevated levels, and shifts in adrenocortical or thyroid metabolism may cause the elevated cholesterol. Mild decreases in serum albumin and other serum proteins may be seen in anorexia nervosa; these findings are less pronounced relative to similar abnormalities seen in other starved patients. Finally, anorectic patients may manifest hematologic abnormalities, including leukopenia, mild anemia, and thrombocytopenia. Hypocomplementemia has been reported. However, these patients do not have a substantially increased risk of infectious complications.

Differential Diagnosis

The diagnosis of anorexia nervosa is made using the DSM-IV diagnostic criteria (see Box 55-2). Although definitive diagnosis must exclude specific diseases that produce malnutrition, such considerations should include only those with a reasonable index of suspicion because of historic or physical examination data. The differential diagnosis includes Addison's disease, diabetes mellitus, panhypopituitarism, hyperparathyroidism, hypothyroidism or hyperthyroidism, celiac disease, Crohn's disease, intestinal parasitosis, tuberculosis, acquired immunodeficiency syndrome (AIDS), lymphoma (or other neoplastic processes), hypothalamic tumor, schizophrenia, and primary major depression. Laboratory tests should be individualized and obtained only if the diagnosis is in question or to assess metabolic derangements (Box 55-3). Some patients require minimal tests, whereas others, particularly extremely malnourished patients, require more diagnostic testing.

Management

The treatment of anorexia nervosa must address the nutritional and medical consequences of the disorder and the psychologic and environmental factors that maintain the anorectic behavior. A multidisciplinary approach, with medical, psychologic, and nutritional support, is therefore crucial.

The primary care physician is usually responsible for medical and nutritional care as well as psychologic support. Factors in the effectiveness of this ongoing care include fostering a sense of autonomy in the patient by encouraging her to take responsibility in the treatment, remaining objective and honest to maintain the patient's sense of trust, working with the family, and serving as the liaison (and patient's advocate) with consultants and counselors. The physician must help the patient to acknowledge and relate thoughts and feelings and should strive to encourage behaviors that reinforce the patient's status as a fully differentiated individual. It is essential to inform the patient that she may see treatments as undesirable, that she may feel that her control is threatened by them, and that a return to better health is in her best interest. The methods and goals of treatment and any later changes should be explained, with ample time for the patient to express thoughts and feelings. Any lack of consistency, evasiveness, or judgmental behavior

Box 55-3. Laboratory Tests for Differential Diagnosis in Eating Disorders*

Complete blood count, sedimentation rate
Serum electrolytes, blood urea nitrogen, creatinine, liver enzymes, serum amylase
Total protein, albumin
Serum cholesterol, vitamin A levels
Serum carotene
Thyroid function tests
Fasting plasma cortisol level
Sigmoidoscopy
Stool examination for occult blood, fecal fat, and parasites
CT scan of brain (or MRI)
Upper gastrointestinal series with small-bowel follow-through
Stool and urine cathartic screens

*The decision to obtain specific tests should be guided by historic data, physical examination results, and other clinical findings that suggest metabolic abnormalities or underlying organic disease.

will undermine the patient's sense of trust; such a loss of trust substantially impedes the treatment process. Family involvement is encouraged. Initially, therapy should be directed toward modifying the dysfunctional pattern within the family that helps maintain the patient's anorectic behavior. Later, family members can be used to aid the patient in weight gain through positive reinforcement. The primary care physician, with the input of appropriate consultants, should make all long-term treatment decisions.

Correction of Nutritional Deficits. Nutritional repletion is usually accomplished on an outpatient basis, unless a life-threatening condition (e.g., cardiac dysrhythmias, severe electrolyte and mineral deficiencies) requires hospital admission. Adaptation to a lower energy intake over time usually results in normal serum chemistries. Hospitalization should be considered for abnormal serum chemistries (low serum albumin, potassium, phosphorus, or magnesium). Postural hypotension is an indication for intravenous fluid replacement. Fluid and electrolyte replacement can be accomplished in the emergency room, with careful measurement of electrolyte abnormalities; electrolyte and mineral deficiencies are often seen after fluid replacement. Careful monitoring for electrolyte imbalance, especially potassium, phosphorus, and magnesium, is important during fluid replacement. *Refeeding syndrome* is a common complication of rapid repletion of energy deficits and is avoided by a judicious rate of replacement. Care should be taken during refeeding to observe for congestive heart failure, acute gastric dilation, and pancreatitis. A follow-up plan should be provided to the patient before discharge from the hospital.

Encouraging oral intake can be extremely difficult. The anorectic patient often survives on 250 kcal per day and has adapted to this low energy intake. Oral nutritional supplements can be helpful because real food is often shunned. The patient should be told that the supplements are like prescription medicine that needs to be taken three or four times daily. Addition of a prokinetic agent (domperidone, metoclopramide) may help with gastric emptying. An initial goal of 750 to 1000 kcal per day (three or four cans of a nutritional supplement) is reasonable. This level of feeding provides the recommended nutrition intake (RNI) for vitamins. A multivitamin may be added and is rarely refused. Forced feedings may worsen the patient's sense of a loss of control; focusing on the medical consequences of continued weight loss helps to involve the patient in the therapy without forced feedings. The oral intake should be maintained above starvation levels.

If the patient refuses to comply with this approach, the physician should consider initiation of tube feedings, which most anorectic patients try to avoid. Rarely, parenteral nutrition is necessary, especially with a noncompliant patient or multiple complications of malnutrition. When parenteral supplements are used, caloric delivery should start at half the daily requirement on day 1 to three fourths on day 2, with full repletion on day 3 and thereafter. This is to minimize the possible complications from rapid infusion of hyperosmolar solutions. Refeeding peripheral edema is common. Elevated transaminases associated with tender hepatomegaly may result from fatty infiltration of the liver during refeeding; this responds to decreasing the infusion rate.

When considering involuntary feeding measures in anorectic patients, a balance must be struck between the patient's willingness to undergo such feedings and their medical necessity. Forced feedings may exacerbate psychologic symptoms of the illness, but if the patient understands the medical need for such feedings and actively participates in the decision to initiate them, these effects may be minimized. Nutrition intervention strategies designed to correct specific medical concerns are effective if the patient can see a direct relationship between food intake and health.

Some patients with anorexia nervosa are refractory to outpatient treatment and may require referral to a residential treatment center. A hospital or residential setting provides a safe, controlled environment for initiating or reestablishing medical, psychologic, and nutritional rehabilitation. A defined nutrition care plan establishes the daily caloric intake, rate of weight gain, weight range goal for discharge, limitations in food choices, and need for supervision during and immediately after meals. In addition, limits on activity may be useful in ensuring weight gain in patients with low body weight. Unfortunately, most residential treatment centers operate on a for-profit basis and are financially inaccessible for some families.

The goals of supplemental nutrition in anorexia nervosa are (1) to achieve a weight that removes the patient from acute medical danger and (2) to correct overt metabolic derangements. Supplemental feedings should be discontinued when the medical and nutritional goals are achieved. This period often allows for mobilization of a multidisciplinary team or referral to a specialized facility. Since each patient's recovery process is unique, treatment plans need to be highly individualized. The key to success in nutrition intervention for outpatients is a very gradual change in food intake patterns and related behaviors.

Psychotherapy. It is essential to separate food-related and weight-related behaviors from feelings and psychologic issues. This process involves helping patients separate their identity, feelings, and unresolved issues from the focus on food, hunger, and weight so that the two problems can be addressed separately. The drive to be thin can be put in the context of societal expectations about weight and body issues.

Psychotherapy has met with variable success. Behavioral therapy uses operant conditioning to promote weight gain and may include cognitive methods and social skills training. Coming to terms with the need for control, the need for perfection, and external factors that influence behavior can be useful in some patients. Family therapy has also been used and appears to have some success in the long term, especially in younger patients with a shorter duration of illness. Combined behavioral modification and family therapy approaches have demonstrated impressive long-term positive results. No current consensus exists on a uniform method of psychotherapy in anorexia nervosa.

Pharmacotherapy. Drugs have no proven benefit in anorexic patients, although the selective serotonin reuptake inhibitors (SSRIs) may be helpful in certain patients. Patients with anorexia nervosa often exhibit symptoms of other psychiatric disorders. Many are depressed, and many are obsessed with thoughts about weight and eating and engage in compulsive rituals suggestive of obsessive-compulsive disorder (OCD). The SSRIs are useful in the treatment of depression and OCD but have limited value during the weight gain phase of treatment.[3,16] One study reported that patients receiving fluoxetine after weight restoration in a hospital had a lower rate of relapse during the succeeding year than did patients receiving placebo.[9]

BULIMIA NERVOSA

Definition and Epidemiology

Bulimia (from the Greek terms for "ox hunger") is a compulsive behavior defined by episodic bouts of overeating (binge eating) usually followed by acts designed to avert weight gain (self-induced vomiting, cathartic or diuretic use). This behavior can be seen in anorexia nervosa, but patients with bulimia nervosa are distinguished by their normal body size. Bulimia nervosa also typically affects young (under 30 years) white women (90% to 95%). Although the point prevalence using the DSM-IV criteria is about 1% of the general population, studies of female high-school and college students report that 4.5% to 18% have had bulimia and that 19.6% of college women had binge-purge behaviors consistent with bulimia. The prevalence of bulimic behaviors among men is less than among women, although the estimated prevalence of such behaviors among college-age men is 10%. Most patients exercise their bulimic behaviors in secret; one British survey revealed that only a third of a group of about 500 women who met diagnostic criteria for bulimia had ever discussed their eating problems with a physician.[14] As with anorexia nervosa, bulimia nervosa is believed to have a multifaceted origin; biologic predisposition combines with psychologic and sociobehavioral determinants to yield the integrated syndrome.

Pathogenesis and Pathophysiology

Biologic Factors. Evidence of an underlying biologic defect in bulimia nervosa is circumstantial but compelling. As noted in patients with anorexia nervosa, bulimic patients have a higher familial incidence of affective disorders than the general population. Alcoholism and major depression have the strongest correlations. Bulimic patients, even those of normal weight, frequently have menstrual abnormalities; a significant proportion have amenorrhea. The strongest evidence of a biologic aberration may be the neurotransmitter abnormalities noted with bulimia nervosa. Evidence exists for a defect in serotonin-mediated satiety regulation; serotonin metabolism in bulimic patients is abnormal. Norepinephrine metabolism is persistently altered in bulimic patients as well. Cholecystokinin (CCK), a gut peptide secreted in response to food intake, is also a neurotransmitter in the central nervous system (CNS) involved in the regulation of the satiety response. One study found that postprandial serum CCK levels in bulimic patients were blunted compared with normal controls.[4] Satiety sensation was also blunted in the bulimic group. A subgroup of bulimic patients treated with anti-depressants had a significant increase in both CCK response to eating and satiety sensation. These data imply that bulimic behaviors are related to CNS neurotransmitter and receptor dysregulation, supporting the use of psychopharmacologic agents in treatment.

Psychologic Factors. The psychologic underpinnings of bulimia nervosa are similar to those of anorexia nervosa. Bulimic patients also tend to come from families with conflict resolution problems and express similar feelings of a loss of control, low self-esteem, and use of external sources (e.g., parents) for validation of self-worth. Childhood sexual abuse, as mentioned earlier, is emerging as a risk factor for the development of bulimia nervosa.

Sociocultural Factors. The same social pressures to be thin noted in the discussion of anorexia nervosa apply to the genesis of bulimia nervosa. Purging behavior becomes a prominent manner in which the bulimic patient attempts to control weight to attain a perceived ideal body habitus in the face of a periodic uncontrollable urge to have an eating binge.

Natural History. Bulimia nervosa classically begins later in life than anorexia nervosa (usually ages 17 to 25) and may occur in an individual with a history of anorexia. The prebulimic patient is typically mildly overweight and has attempted to lose weight by dieting without success. She may be introduced to purging as a means of weight control by a friend or relative; often, purging behaviors precede binge eating. At some point the hallmark of the disorder appears: the uncontrollable urge to eat and the inability to stop. Subsequently, repeated cycles of binge-purge behavior ensue; the patient's sense of a lack of control intensifies after each binge episode, with reduced self-esteem. Because of the secretive nature of their behaviors and their usually normal weight, patients often do not present for treatment until their 30s or 40s. Bulimic patients may be diagnosed because of a medical complication or major psychologic distress. By this time most bulimic patients are clinically depressed, and 5% have attempted suicide. They are more likely to exhibit impulsive behaviors (e.g., kleptomania, substance abuse, sexual promiscuity) than anorectic patients. The risk of drug and alcohol use among bulimic patients is three to five times greater than in nonbulimic women in the general population. Bulimia is often characterized as having an irregular course, with frequent relapses and remissions. In general, bulimic outpatients with at least 1-year follow-up demonstrate recovery rates of 30% to 70% (average 50%). Most recoveries have been noted within 1 year of presentation; those who fail to recover by that point are unlikely to do so. Relapse rates are high (40% to 63%). Factors predictive of a poor outcome include a history of ethanol abuse, suicide attempts, and increased depressive symptoms. Mortality is not increased over the rate in the general female population.

Patient History

Although bulimic patients are more distressed by their behaviors than anorectic patients (and therefore are more likely to seek medical attention), they also are often embarrassed by their binge-purge activities and may not be willing to reveal these activities to their primary care physician. Again, a careful history with assessment of eating attitudes is essential (Box 55-4). As with anorectics, bulimics may have constipation, crampy abdominal pain, and amenorrhea; they may also have complications from their binge-purge activity.

Physical Examination

As with anorexia nervosa patients, a complete physical examination is important in bulimia nervosa patients and may provide clues to the diagnosis in patients with suspected bulimia. Physical findings associated with bulimia include painless parotid or salivary gland swelling, bruised or abraded knuckles secondary to self-induced vomiting (Russell sign), and facial ecchymoses, conjunctival hemorrhages, pharyngitis, and dental enamel erosions caused by repeated emesis (Box 55-5).

Psychologic and Behavioral Findings. The characteristic behavioral manifestation of bulimia nervosa is the *binge-purge cycle.* This is typified by episodes of compulsive eating with a failure to respond to or achieve normal satiety. Patients typically binge on high-calorie foods rich in carbohydrates that require little chewing. Binge episodes, during which the bulimic individual consumes between 1000 and 55,000 kcal during a relatively brief interval, usually occur in secret after extensive planning. The binge is usually terminated by feelings of guilt or physical discomfort (nausea, abdominal pain). At this point most patients self-induce vomiting or take laxatives. Although patients report feelings of excitement and anticipation while planning a binge, most feel shame afterward. Bulimic patients are typically embarrassed by their symptoms and are reluctant to reveal details of their illness to family members and health care providers. Their obsession with food-related and binge-related activities can interfere with social interactions. Unlike anorectics, however, bulimics are usually outgoing and engage in heterosexual relationships.

Bulimic patients view their behavior as an uncontrollable compulsion and thus are more willing to try and stop. By contrast, anorectic patients hide their behavior from friends and co-workers because they are unwilling to change.

Affective disorders are common; estimates of depression in bulimic patients range from 20% to 80%. They also have a higher incidence of anxiety disorders (45%) than either anorectic patients or the general population. The presence of bulimia has been correlated with personality disorders, particularly borderline personality disorder. Obese bulimic patients are less likely to use purgatives than normal-weight patients and are more prone to have affective disorders (91% vs. 70%), especially major depression.

Box 55-4. Screening Questions for Patients with Suspected Eating Disorders

1. Have you had any difficulties or concerns with controlling your weight?
2. Do others see your body size as different than you do?
3. How would you estimate your body size? Too heavy? Too thin? Too light?
4. At what weight would you feel most comfortable?
5. Have you had experiences with binge eating, that is, having an uncontrollable desire to overeat?
6. Are you satisfied with your eating patterns?*
7. Do you ever eat in secret?*

From Freund KM et al: *J Gen Intern Med* 8:236, 1993.
*These questions have been shown to have a positive predictive value of 0.36 in screening patients with suspected bulimia, based on a 5% prevalence of disease. The sensitivity and specificity of these questions were 1.00 and 0.90 for bulimic patients, respectively.

Box 55-5. Medical Findings and Complications of Bulimia

Physical Examination Findings

Parotid and salivary gland swelling
Bruised or abraded knuckles (Russell sign)
Facial ecchymoses
Conjunctival hemorrhages
Pharyngitis
Dental enamel erosions

Endocrine

Menstrual irregularity (including amenorrhea)

Gastrointestinal

Esophagitis
Esophageal erosions and ulcerations
Mallory-Weiss tears
Esophageal rupture
Delayed gastric emptying
Crampy abdominal pain
Acute gastric dilation (with binge)
Constipation
Pancreatitis
Asymptomatic elevations in serum amylase

Miscellaneous

Ipecac cardiotoxicity
Dysrhythmias
Pneumomediastinum
Aspiration pneumonia
Metabolic alkalosis or acidosis
Hypochloremia
Hypokalemia
Hypomagnesemia
Hypocalcemia
Hyponatremia
Hypophosphatemia

Medical Findings. Endocrine abnormalities may include menstrual irregularities (40% to 50%), and 20% of bulimic women without a history of anorexia have amenorrhea for at least 3 months at some point during their illness. Approximately 50% have abnormal dexamethasone suppression tests. Serum cortisol levels and secretion patterns are normal.

Gastrointestinal effects of bulimia primarily related to repeated emesis may include oropharyngeal complications (dental erosions, pharyngitis, parotid enlargement), esophagitis, esophageal erosions and ulcerations, Mallory-Weiss tears, and esophageal rupture (see Box 55-5). Peptic acid esophageal injury has a higher incidence in bulimic patients than in the general population. Delayed gastric emptying and prolonged whole-gut transit times in bulimic patients may explain the symptoms of bloating and crampy abdominal pain. Acute gastric dilation has been described, usually in relation to the ingestion of large meals, as has gastric rupture. Constipation is a common complaint. Degeneration of Auerbach's plexus results from chronic stimulant laxative use (cathartic colon). With asymptomatic elevations in serum amylase, the salivary isoenzyme fraction is predominant in most cases. Acute pancreatitis may be caused by alcohol abuse or abrupt pancreatic stimulation during binge eating.

Cardiovascular effects of bulimia may include ipecac cardiotoxicity from alkaloid poisoning and dysrhythmias from hypokalemia, a common electrolyte abnormality in bulimic patients. Pulmonary findings may include pneumomediastinum, resulting from pulmonary rupture caused by vigorous emesis, and aspiration pneumonia, often from vomiting while under the influence of alcohol. Metabolic complications may include metabolic alkalosis from repeated emesis (the most common finding), metabolic acidosis from laxative abuse, hypochloremia, hypokalemia, hypomagnesemia, hypocalcemia, hyponatremia, and hypophosphatemia. Dehydration may also occur, leading to secondary hyperaldosteronism and to reflex peripheral edema, which may be pronounced with cessation of the abused diuretics or laxatives.

Differential Diagnosis

The DSM-IV diagnosis of bulimia nervosa is based on the presence of the binge eating pattern, the persistent overconcern about body shape and size, and the exclusion of other medical conditions (Box 55-6). The differential diagnosis is limited and includes schizophrenia, seizure disorders, and rare neurologic disorders (e.g., Kleine-Levin syndrome, Klüver-Bucy syndrome). Diagnostic testing is usually not necessary, except as indicated by historic and physical examination data and as needed to monitor complications.

Management

Because bulimic patients are cognizant of the maladaptive nature of their behaviors, they are often willing to work with their physician in therapy. The patient can usually interpret symptoms in terms of current and past emotional issues, so psychologic concerns and establishment of better coping methods should be discussed. The family may need to be involved. Generally, inpatient therapy is not recommended.

Psychotherapy. The psychotherapeutic approach to bulimia usually emphasizes controlling the abnormal behaviors. Cognitive behavioral therapy is often used; the patient recognizes the specific abnormal behaviors and uses behavior modification techniques to control them. This technique uses a three-stage approach, beginning with a *self-monitoring* period, during which the patient is taught to become more aware of her eating behavior and to establish a regular pattern of eating, with conscious avoidance of binge behavior by decreasing available food. This is followed by a *recognition* period (patient recognizes association between binges and stress, achieving greater control over eating pattern) and a *maintenance* period (patient records tactics used to avert bingeing and purging during stress to reinforce learned behavioral adaptations). Both individual and group approaches have been used successfully.[1]

Box 55-6. DSM-IV Criteria for Bulimia Nervosa

Recurrent episodes of binge eating (rapid consumption of a large amount of food in a discrete period of time)

A feeling of lack of control over eating behavior during the eating binges

Self-induced vomiting, use of laxatives or diuretics, strict dieting or fasting, or rigorous exercise to prevent weight gain

A minimum of two binge eating episodes per week for at least 3 months

Persistent overconcern with body shape and weight

From *Diagnostic and statistical manual of mental disorders,* ed 4, Washington, DC, 1994, American Psychiatric Association.

Pharmacotherapy. Antidepressants can successfully treat bulimia, with striking reductions (average 50%) in binge frequency compared with placebo in both depressed and nondepressed bulimic patients. Most studies have been short term (6 to 8 weeks' duration), however, and some reports indicate that long-term efficacy is not as high for all medications tested. Notably, patients taking fluoxetine seem to maintain their response as long as they take the medication, although higher doses (e.g., 60 mg/day) may be needed in some patients. The usual tricyclic antidepressant dose (e.g., 100 to 250 mg/day of desipramine) seems to be effective. The best candidates for pharmacotherapy are those who have failed cognitive behavioral therapy, severely depressed patients, and responsible patients capable of communicating potential beneficial and adverse drug effects to the physician. Patients with a partial response to cognitive behavioral therapy or pharmacotherapy may benefit from combined therapy.[18]

RUMINATION SYNDROME

Rumination syndrome *(merycism),* considered a medical curiosity for more than 300 years, is infrequently diagnosed because physician recognition is lacking. The patient with this eating disorder repetitively regurgitates small amounts of food from the stomach, rechews the food, and reswallows it. The three subgroups with rumination disorder are (1) emotionally deprived or mentally impaired children and adults; (2) persons in whom the behavior develops as a maladaptive habit, worsening in times of stress; and (3) persons in whom rumination is associated with bulimia.

The prevalence of rumination in adults is unknown. Patients who seek treatment report symptoms of weight loss, regurgitation, or vomiting and may express concern of an underlying medical disorder. The diagnosis is made by manometric or radiographic studies, which reveal that episodes are initiated by a belch or a swallow. The lower esophageal sphincter pressure is lowered to allow creation of a common channel between the stomach and esophagus.[2] At the same time, diaphragmatic and rectus muscle contractions raise intraabdominal pressure, leading to regurgitation. Diagnosis is based on identifying the typical clinical features and excluding other medical or psychiatric disease. Extensive diagnostic testing is usually not needed. Since the disorder appears to be a learned maladaptive habit, behavioral modification and biofeedback techniques are recommended as treatment approaches.

EATING DISORDER NOT OTHERWISE SPECIFIED

The DSM-IV classification of eating disorder not otherwise specified is reserved for disorders of eating that do not meet the criteria for anorexia nervosa or bulimia nervosa. If the primary symptom is recurrent episodes of binge eating without the regular use of inappropriate compensatory behaviors (e.g., self-induced vomiting, fasting), the diagnosis of *binge eating disorder* can be applied. The typical patient is overweight and consults the primary care physician for help with weight loss. In weight loss clinics about one quarter to one third of patients meet criteria for binge eating disorder. The arbitrary choice of two episodes of bingeing per week suggests the diagnosis.

Binge eating also appears to be associated, independent of weight, with a greater frequency of psychiatric problems, such as depression, larger and more frequent weight fluctuations, and more severe weight-related distress. These findings suggest a meaningful distinction between obese binge eaters and nonbinge eaters. Some of these individuals may initially resist psychotherapy because they do not understand the relationship between underlying emotional or psychologic issues and the inability to cease binge eating.

Starvation and self-imposed dieting may result in eating binges (once food is available) and psychologic manifestations (preoccupation with food and eating, increased emotional responsiveness, dysphoria, distractibility). Caution is thus advisable in counseling patients to restrict their eating to lose weight, since the negative sequelae may outweigh the benefits of restrained eating. Instead, healthful, balanced eating without specific food restrictions should be recommended as a long-term strategy to avoid the perils of restrictive dieting.

ANOREXIA ATHLETICA

Evidence suggests an increasing prevalence of eating disorders and body weight obsessions in certain subpopulations of female athletes. The pressure on female athletes to improve their performances and physiques, coupled with the general sociocultural demand placed on all women to be thin, often results in attempts to achieve unrealistic body size and body weight goals. For some female athletes the pressure to achieve and maintain a low body weight leads to potentially harmful patterns of restrictive eating or chronic dieting. The interrelationships among menstrual dysfunction, athletic training, and disordered eating are not fully understood. The high incidence of menstrual abnormalities in female athletes has critical health consequences, however, because amenorrheic athletes are at greater risk of developing osteopenia and bone injury compared with normally menstruating athletes or nonathletic, normally cycling females.

Body weight should be monitored frequently to check calorie intake. Athletes with low caloric intakes who train for more than 90 minutes a day should consume 45 to 50 kcal/kg body weight/day, as well as foods with high contents of iron, calcium, magnesium, zinc, and vitamin B_{12}. Fluid, electrolyte, and energy supplementation supports circulatory, metabolic, and thermoregulatory functions. No special food will help elite athletes perform better; the most important aspect of athletes' diet is that it follows the basic guidelines for healthy eating.

REFERENCES

1. Agras WS: Nonpharmacologic treatments of bulimia nervosa, *J Clin Psychol* 52(suppl):29, 1991.
2. Amarnath RP, Abell TL, Malagelada JR: The rumination syndrome in adults: a characteristic manometric pattern, *Ann Intern Med* 105:513, 1986.
3. Attia E, Haiman C, Walsh BT, et al: Does fluoxetine augment the inpatient treatment of anorexia nervosa? *Am J Psychiatry* 155:548-551, 1998.
4. Devlin MJ, Walsh BT, Guss JL, et al: Postprandial cholecystokinin release and gastric emptying in patients with bulimia nervosa, *Am J Clin Nutr* 65(1):114-120, 1997.
5. *Diagnostic and statistical manual of mental disorders*, ed 4, Washington, DC, 1994, American Psychiatric Association.
6. Friedman JM, Halaas JL: Leptin and the regulation of body weight in mammals, *Nature* 395:763, 1998.
7. Hall RC, Tice L, Beresford TP, et al: Sexual abuse in patients with anorexia nervosa and bulimia, *Psychosomatics* 30:73, 1989.
8. Holland AG: Anorexia nervosa: a study of 34 twin pairs and one set of triplets, *Br J Psychiatry* 145:414, 1984.
9. Kaye WH: Persistent alterations in behavior and serotonin activity after recovery from anorexia and bulimia nervosa (review), Ann N Y Acad Sci 817:162-178, 1997.
10. Siegel PZ, Brackbill RM, Frazier EL, et al: Behavioral risk factor surveillance, 1986-1990, *MMWR CDC Surveill Summ* 40(4):1-23, 1991.
11. Sullivan PF: Mortality in anorexia nervosa, *Am J Psychiatry* 152(7):1073-1074, 1995.
12. Thomas MA, Rebar RW: The endocrinology of anorexia nervosa and bulimia nervosa (review), *Curr Opin Obstet Gynecol* 2(6):831-836, 1990.
13. Tomova A, Kumanov P: Sex differences and similarities of hormonal alterations in patients with anorexia nervosa, *Andrologia* 31(3):143-147, 1999.
14. Turnbull S, Ward A, Treasure J, et al: The demand for eating disorder care: an epidemiological study using the general practice research database, *Br J Psychiatry* 169(6):705-712, 1996.
15. Walsh BT: Eating disorders. In Tasman A, Kay J, Lieberman JA, editors: *Psychiatry*, Philadelphia, 1997, Saunders, pp 1202-1216.
16. Walsh BT, Devlin M: Psychopharmacology of anorexia nervosa, bulimia nervosa and binge eating. In Bloom FE, Kupfer DJ, editors: *Psychopharmacology: the fourth generation of progress*, New York, 1995, Raven, pp1581-1589.
17. Walsh BT, Devlin MJ: Eating disorders: progress and problems, *Science* 280:1387, 1998.
18. Walsh BT, Devlin MJ: The pharmacologic treatment of eating disorders, *Psychiatr Clin North Am* 15:149, 1992.

CHAPTER 56

Sexual Disorders

Thomas N. Wise

Sexual behavior is not simply a biologic function for procreation but also a fundamental human experience that brings pleasure and interpersonal intimacy. Sexuality is no longer a taboo topic. The "sexual revolution" fostered a freedom that has been countered by the risk of unsafe sexual practices with possible human immunodeficiency virus (HIV) infection. Furthermore, sexual issues continue to be anxiety provoking for many people, with wide variation in attitudes. People are increasingly aware, however, that sexual difficulties can be acknowledged and often effectively treated with newer psychotherapeutic and pharmacologic interventions.

The *Diagnostic and Statistical Manual of Mental Disorders* (DSM-IV) categorizes sexuality conditions into dysfunctions and disorders.[2] *Sexual dysfunctions* are difficulties in sexual performance as it relates to libido, arousal, and orgasm. *Sexual disorders* refer to unusual sexual stimuli that are preferred or necessary for erotic arousal. Sexual dysfunctions are common in the general population, and the individual often turns to the primary care physician first for counseling and treatment.

The diagnosis and management of sexual dysfunctions in primary care may be as simple as changing the medication that is causing the dysfunction or may be extremely complex, mandating attention to biologic, psychologic, and social issues. The primary care physician must identify the dysfunction within the sexual response cycle and not minimize its importance to the patient. Once the dysfunction is identified, etiologic issues should be investigated, with attention to pathophysiologic causes, psychiatric factors, and social issues that either cause or maintain the problem. Referral to the appropriate specialist is often necessary to best manage these dysfunctions, which can cause personal and interpersonal pain for both patient and sexual partner.

BIOLOGIC BASIS OF HUMAN SEXUALITY

The human sexual response cycle consists of four phases: drive (desire), arousal, release (orgasm), and resolution (refractory period) (Fig. 56-1). The biologic underpinnings of the sexual response cycle are the end product of contributions from the endocrine, nervous, and vascular systems.[4]

The *desire phase* of sexual response appears to be mediated by endocrine factors, especially androgens in both men and women. Testosterone may foster sexual drive in both men and women, and thus low levels of testosterone may impair sexual desire but not necessarily sexual functioning. Conversely, administration of testosterone may increase libido but generally will not restore impaired sexual function. The lower levels of androgen in perimenopausal women may also diminish libido.[8] Elevated levels of prolactin decrease sexual interest. Hyperprolactinemia may reflect central dopaminergic activity and is often found in individuals treated with phenothiazines. The role of estrogen and progesterone is less well understood in modulating sexual drive. The central nervous system contribution to sexual drive appears to be related to the limbic system and hypothalamus. Thus frontal lobe disease may foster disinhibition but also may lower libido.

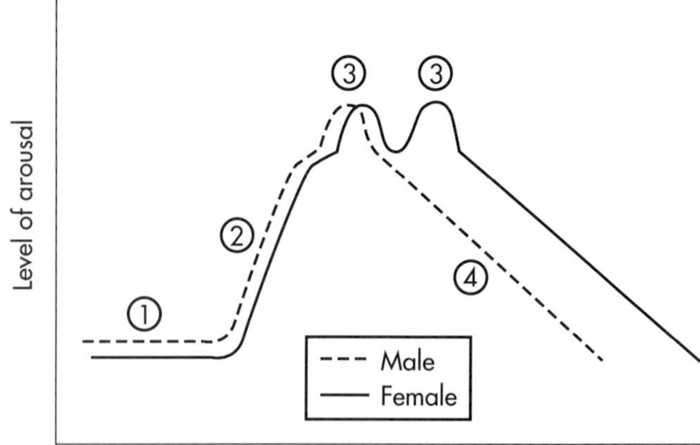

Fig. 56-1. Sexual response cycle. *1,* Drive (desire) phase; *2,* arousal phase; *3,* orgasm (release); *4,* refractory (resolution) phase.

The second phase of the sexual response cycle, *sexual arousal,* is characterized by erectile tumescence in the male and vaginal ballooning and labial engorgement in the female. Its biologic basis resides in the autonomic nervous system, where the parasympathetic system stimulates erection through relaxation of the smooth muscles, which allows increased blood flow in the penile corpora cavernosa, and tumescence results. A parallel mechanism is thought to be responsible for labial engorgement and vaginal lubrication. Autonomic arousal also occurs in this phase and is characterized by rapid heart rate, increased respiration, and hardening of the nipples. Recent studies implicate the sympathetic nervous system in activating sexual arousal in women. The vascular system is necessary during the arousal phase, and thus obstructions to blood flow, as in peripheral vascular disease or venous leakage, can inhibit erection in the male.

The third phase of the sexual response cycle is release, or *orgasm.* In the male, sympathetic discharge fosters ejaculation after emission of the ejaculate into the urethra. For the female, orgastic release is characterized by vaginal contractions that she may or may not perceive. The major difference between male and female orgastic release is that women are able to have multiple orgasms; in the male a single orgasm is followed by a refractory period.

The final phase, *resolution,* or the refractory period, changes as the individual ages. In males over age 65 the resolution is prolonged up to 8 to 12 hours between orgastic experiences. Aging causes other phenomena in the sexual response cycle. Postmenopausal women may experience a decline in libidinal drive due to loss of circulating androgens, particularly those with oophorectomies, since the ovaries are a major source of circulating androgens. Estrogen deprivation in postmenopausal women may result in vaginal thinning, which can cause dyspareunia. For the aging male the perception of ejaculatory inevitability is less specific.

SEXUAL HISTORY

The primary care physician should be able to pinpoint the sexual difficulties of patients within the sexual response

Table 56-1. Sexual Response Cycle

Phase of sexual cycle	Characteristics	Causes of dysfunction
Drive	Libidinal urge for erotic experience	Depression, anxiety, malaise Medical illness Medications
Arousal	Erection in male Vaginal ballooning, labial enlargement, and lubrication in female General autonomic arousal	Performance anxiety Sexual abuse Diabetes, vascular disease, neurologic disorders (e.g., spinal cord trauma, multiple sclerosis) Medications
Orgasm	Premature in male Inability to achieve orgasm (anorgasmy) in female or male	Anxiety Idiopathic Medications
Resolution	Inability to become aroused physically for a time (refractory period)	Aging

cycle. This demands a careful sexual history. The sexual history is often omitted from primary care evaluations because of the fear that patients will react negatively to such inquiries. Patients respond favorably to questions about their sexual lives, however, and report that physicians who take such histories are more interested in them as people.

The physician should start with general questions regarding patients' satisfaction with their sexual life. Initiating such a history with global, open-ended questions such as, "Are you experiencing any problems with sexuality?" allows the patient to either acknowledge or deny any difficulties. Often a response may indicate that the patient's spouse is the source of difficulties or that the patient has experienced some problems in this area. An open-ended approach allows patients to respond in a manner consistent with their comfort level. If a problem is acknowledged, the physician should plot the dysfunction along the sexual response cycle by designating it as a drive difficulty, arousal dysfunction, or orgastic problem, such as premature ejaculation or inability to achieve an orgasm (Table 56-1). Frequently, individuals have concurrent sexual difficulties, such as an arousal-phase disorder, erectile problem, and a secondary libidinal decline.

The physician also must determine the time course of the difficulty: sudden occurrence, gradual development, or lifelong problem. This often helps differentiate organic from psychogenic difficulties. Specifically, erectile problems that result from an acute personal problem or situational experience differ from organic phenomena that occur over time. The physician can quantify erectile capacity by asking the patient on a scale of 1 to 10, with 10 the best erection ever experienced and 1 no erection, what has been the best erection during the most recent sexual experience. This often helps patients talk more freely about their dysfunction.

Situations in which dysfunctions occur are also important. Do they occur with one partner and not another, or is fear of pregnancy an issue? To determine the general frequency of sexual activity and the individual's baseline, the patient should carefully review the last sexual encounter and how difficulties relate to prior functioning. Who initiated the relationship? Did foreplay occur? The partner's reactions to the dysfunction are also important.

To organize the data obtained in the sexual history, the physician can partition information using a *biopsychosocial model*. What are the disease states or medications that could contribute to the dysfunction (*biologic elements*)? Common disease states such as diabetes or coronary artery disease may impede sexual functioning. Could a psychiatric disorder such as anxiety or depression explain the problem (*psychologic factors*)? Depressed patients often have a decreased sexual drive, whereas manic patients have an increased drive. It is unusual for a manic individual to complain of increased sexual drive, but their partners frequently do. What relationship issues with sexual partners inhibit sexual comfort or activity (*social issues*)? Relationship problems often manifest in sexual difficulties. An ongoing relationship with a sexual partner must be evaluated. Do difficulties occur in other areas with the sexual partner? How comfortable is the patient with sexuality and the partner? The sexual history should include the patient's ideas about why the sexual dysfunction is occurring, taken in the context of the patient's stage in life, nature of the partner, and history of their sexual education and experience.

DESIRE-PHASE DISORDERS

Sexual desire is a motivated behavior with a subjective craving for sexual release. This tension dissipates after orgastic release but can be modified by a variety of factors, including fatigue, malaise, anxiety, depression, and distraction. Married adults report having sexual activity one or two times per week, but the actual level of sexual drive varies greatly.[5] Thus normal discrepancies in sexual drive between partners can create interpersonal difficulties without any clearly defined drive disorder. In such situations, education and communication between the couple to better understand mutual needs may suffice.

Hypoactive sexual desire disorders denote a basic absence or unusually low level of libidinal desire. Such a deficiency must be considered in the context of the patient's life, medical status, and social situation. The disturbance must cause marked distress or interpersonal difficulty to be properly designated as a disorder. The physician must ascertain whether this is a lifelong or acquired dysfunction. Primary lifelong low sexual desire is an unusual disorder that may be associated with low to low-normal free testosterone levels in males. In females, such disorders may also be linked to early childhood sexual abuse. The perimenopausal woman may also complain of lowered libido, which can be secondary to decreased androgen levels. Some clinicians suggest addition of androgens to estrogenic hormonal replacement. The physician must look for both psychologic and medical comorbid conditions to define better the etiology of such drive disorders. Depressed or anxious patients may report low sexual desire. Direct treatment of the psychologic disorder may improve the drive deficiency. Organic conditions, such as malaise caused by a serious systemic illness or nausea and pain after chemotherapy, may also result in lower sexual drive.

In patients with systemic disease states the physician must assess the patient's physiologic capacity for sexual performance. The cardiovascular demands for intercourse are equivalent to a brisk walk around a block or being able to walk up two flights of stairs. If patients have such a capacity, they generally are capable of sexual intercourse. In patients with severe congestive heart failure or obstructive lung disease, limited cardiopulmonary function may make intercourse difficult and lead to lowered drive. Shame and embarrassment after a mastectomy or colostomy also can lower drive; sexual partners must understand this. A variety of medications inhibit sexual drive, including the frequently used selective serotonin reuptake inhibitors (SSRIs)[1] (Box 56-1). Another common cause of lower drive disorder is a reaction to another sexual dysfunction. Men with premature ejaculation or women with anorgasmy may become sufficiently frustrated by their primary sexual dysfunction to react with a secondary drive disorder.

Another sexual dysfunction during the drive phase is *sexual aversion disorder.* These patients present with lower sexual drive. The dysfunction is aversion and repulsion to all or part of the sexual act with one or all partners. These individuals may report sexual fantasies and daydreams about sexual relations with other individuals. They may enjoy autoerotic activity but also may be globally aversive to all erotic activities. Aversion disorder is more common in women than men. Psychotherapy is the main form of treatment, although patients with a phobic aversion to sexual activity may benefit from monoamine oxidase inhibitors.

Box 56-1. Drugs That Inhibit Sexual Functioning

Diminished Desire

Antiandrogens: medroxyprogesterone acetate, Depo-Provera, leuprolide
- Phenothiazines, risperidone
- Tricyclic antidepressants
- Selective serotonin reuptake inhibitors (SSRIs)
- Digoxin
- Antihypertensives: spironolactone, methyldopa, guanethidine

Impaired Arousal

Antidepressants: tertiary amines, monoamine oxidase inhibitors (MAOIs), trazodone*
- Phenothiazines, lithium
- Antihypertensives: propranolol, hydrochlorothiazide, clonidine, atenolol
- Alcohol, cocaine
- Phenytoin (Dilantin), carbamazepine (Tegretol)
- Cimetidine
- Disulfiram

Orgastic Dysfunction

Antidepressants: tricyclics, SSRIs, MAOIs
- Phenothiazines
- α-Methyldopa
- Alcohol
- Alprazolam, lorazepam

*Trazodone may also cause priapism.

AROUSAL-PHASE DISORDERS

Arousal-phase disorders are dysfunctions that occur during male tumescence and female sexual arousal. As with all sexual dysfunctions, the physician must partition psychologic from organic etiologic factors.

Male erectile disorders are quite common and increase throughout the life cycle because of comorbid medical disorders.[7] The male arousal-phase disorder, *erectile dysfunction* (ED), is defined as the inability to obtain and maintain a penile erection sufficient for satisfactory sexual intercourse. The incidence of ED is not fully defined but may affect more than 20% of men over age 50. The patient's sexual partner should confirm the dysfunction, since many men tend to overestimate their erectile ability. The initial challenge for the physician is to differentiate psychogenic from organic ED. The acute onset of ED, with the ability to develop a firm and full erection during masturbation and full erections during the night, suggests psychogenic etiologies. Gradual onset of ED, with inability to develop a firm erection through masturbation as well as a comorbid systemic illness or medication use that affects sexuality, may indicate organic factors. The presence of substance abuse also suggests organic etiologies. Alcoholism and illicit substances can impair sexual arousal and lower drive. Despite such historic elements, it is often difficult to partition etiologic factors clearly. Nocturnal penile tumescence (NPT) testing may better define causes. This test documents the presence or absence of turgid erections during deep stages of sleep. Less expensive but much less reliable tests include the use of penile rings that break during full nocturnal erections. Unfortunately, circumferential change is not the only indicator of a fully functional erection, since buckling capacity must be measured as well. Major mood disorders may also foster ED and may diminish full erections during NPT testing. Thus the etiologic elements of such ED may remain imprecisely defined, and the designation of mixed causes (organic and psychologic) is common.

Treatment of ED depends on the etiologic factors. Psychogenic factors often include performance anxiety; initial failures become reinforced by increasing concerns about performance, and ED becomes self-fulfilling. This dynamic can occur in patients with a high baseline of anxiety, low self-esteem, or inhibitions and fears about sexual performance. Behavioral therapy focuses on symptoms and is best done with the patient's ongoing sexual partner. For patients without a partner, individual psychotherapy must be directed toward issues that have limited such relationships. Combined behavioral therapy and dynamic psychotherapy are often indicated to examine deeper causes, such as unconscious conflicts.

For organic causes of ED, the physician must determine whether a disease state (e.g., peripheral vascular disease, diabetes) or a medication (e.g., antidepressant, H_2 blocker, antihypertensive) is the cause. Switching to a different medication without the side effect of diminished erectile capacity often improves functioning. One of the most common classes of medications responsible for ED is the antidepressants. Introduction of the SSRIs alerted clinicians to this common side effect, which was also found in tricyclic antidepressants. Three antidepressants—mirtazapine, nefazodone, and bupropion—have minimal sexual side effects.

The introduction of sildenafil (Viagra) has added a new approach to the treatment of ED.[3] This medication inhibits type V cyclic guanosine monophate (GMP) phosphodiesterase enzyme, which potentiates smooth muscle relaxation in the corpus cavernosum and allows tumescence. The medication is indicated for patients with ED caused by organic factors but clinically is effective in psychogenic disorders as well. Sildenafil is contraindicated in patients taking any form of nitrate because of the hypotensive effects. The medication is used once per day and is initiated with a 50-mg dose, which may be increased to 100 mg per day and used approximately 2 hours before intercourse. Sildenafil enhances the ability for full tumescence but depends on sexual drive. Meals rich in fat delay absorption. Side effects include transient headache and abdominal discomfort, as well as a visual disturbance with a bluish hue, which is transitory. The medication is well tolerated in males. A potential problem exists for patients with serious cardiovascular disease who have not participated in any form of physical exertion. The use of sildenafil in women is not yet indicated.

DISORDERS OF ORGASM

Male

Orgasmic disorders among men may be divided into premature ejaculation and retarded ejaculation. *Premature ejaculation* is defined as the persistence of rapid ejaculation with minimal sexual stimulation before or shortly after vaginal penetration or before ejaculation is desired. This definition demands clinical assessment of arousal-phase duration and situation. Anxiety or a new partner may reduce the ability to control ejaculatory inevitability. The disorder is quite common and has been linked to penile sensitivity and anxiety. Behavioral treatment may focus on prolonging the excitement phase using systematic desensitization or SSRIs, which can prolong ejaculatory inevitability. Initial dosing (e.g., 25 mg of sertraline, 10 mg of paroxetine) may be increased, depending on the clinical effects. Chlorimipramine, a tricyclic antidepressant with serotonin reuptake inhibition, may be effective in premature ejaculation but has many more side effects than the usual SSRIs.

Male orgasmic disorder, formerly known as inhibited male orgasm or retarded ejaculation, is the inability to achieve an orgasm after sexual excitement.[8] The etiology of this dysfunction is not well understood, although interpersonal difficulties with the sexual partner may be a cause. Treatment is difficult but includes behavioral desensitization therapies coupled with relaxation.

Female

Female orgasmic disorder, formerly known as inhibited orgasm or anorgasmy, is the persistent inability to achieve orgasm after sexual excitement. The disorder may be primary (patient has never had orgasm) or secondary (after emotional, medical, or therapeutic events). Etiologic factors include psychologic issues (e.g., fear of loss of control) or potentially organic issues (e.g., higher physiologic thresholds). Interpersonal issues such as psychologic attitudes toward the partner have also been cited. Medical conditions involving malaise or nervous system traumas (e.g., spinal cord injuries, multiple sclerosis) can also cause orgasmic disorders. Medications may also modify orgastic potential. SSRIs, antipsychotics, and drugs of abuse (e.g., alcohol) may cause such difficulties. Behavioral interventions include the sensate focus approach with the sexual partner or individual behavioral paradigms such as orgasmic retraining, in which generalized relaxation is coupled with the patient's self-stimulation. If medication is causing the dysfunction, changing to another agent is usually recommended.

VAGINAL PAIN SYNDROMES

The final dysfunctions delineated in the DSM-IV are the vaginal pain syndromes, dyspareunia and vaginismus.[6]

Dyspareunia may occur in males or females but is more common in women. It is characterized by persistent pain associated with intercourse but has a wide variety of presentations. It may occur only on deep penile thrusting or with any penile penetration. Dyspareunia is differentiated from *vaginismus,* which is the presence of involuntary contractions of the perineal muscles surrounding the outer third of the vaginal canal when any digital object (tampon, finger, penis) is inserted. Vaginismus may be diagnosed during the gynecologic examination by observation of these muscular contractions and pain. Dyspareunia, however, may be more difficult to evaluate; etiologic factors remain problematic, with increasing interest in organic etiologies. Psychologic causation has linked painful intercourse to an earlier traumatic experience, such as rape.

Vulvar vestibulitis, characterized by hyperesthesia and erythema at the vaginal introitus, is increasingly recognized as a common cause of vaginal pain. This inflammatory condition causes burning and soreness on penetration. The etiology is not clear, but human papillomavirus is found in many patients with vestibulitis. Treatment approaches include low-oxalate diets, interferon therapy, and biofeedback of the lower pelvic musculature. Surgery is often done when these approaches are unsuccessful. Excision of the inflammatory tissue and more aggressive excision of Bartholin's glands have been reported.

The treatment for vaginismus is behavioral desensitization; the woman is taught generalized relaxation therapy and combines this with gradual vaginal insertion of either fingers or cylinders of increasing diameter. These specialized techniques are best used by a therapist trained in behavioral medicine.

OTHER DISORDERS

Sexual disorders such as fetishistic behaviors, pedophilias, and transvestism are seen infrequently in primary care settings. A spouse or parent, however, may seek advice regarding such sexual preferences. The physician must refer the person to a mental health professional with experience in such disorders.

HOMOSEXUALITY ISSUES

Sexual orientation toward the same gender is not a psychiatric disorder, but the reactions of family members may cause emotional pain to gay or lesbian individuals. The primary

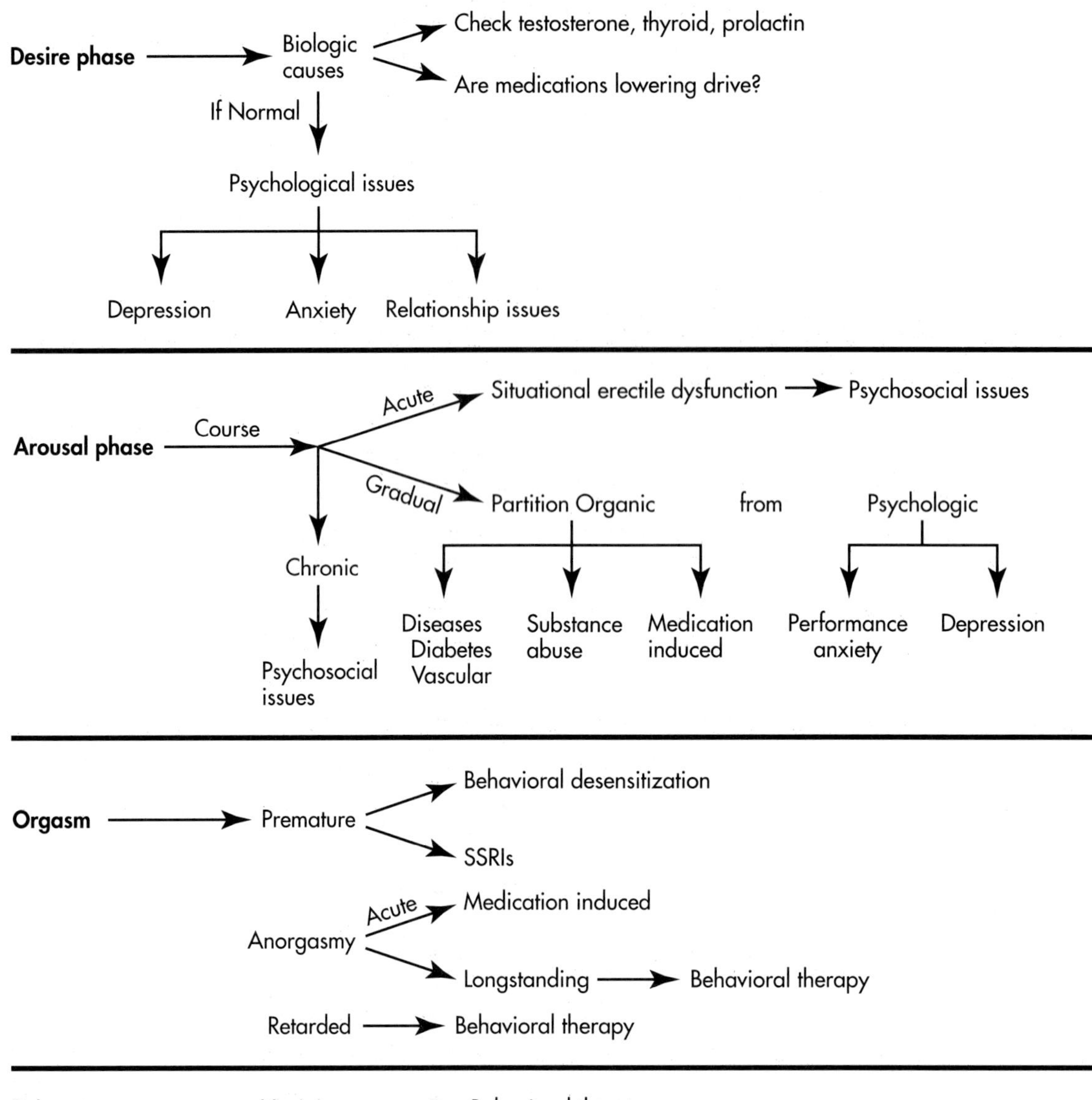

Fig. 56-2. Algorithm for treatment of sexual dysfunctions. *SSRIs,* Selective serotonin reuptake inhibitors.

care physician can educate patients and refer them to community resources for better understanding of such orientations. One important clinical situation includes the gay adolescent who reveals his or her sexual orientation to the physician or family members. Such individuals often experience loneliness, confusion, and despair. The physician must assess the level of depression and whether suicidal ideation is present. The gay adolescent or young adult must also be educated about safe sex practices regarding HIV and other sexually transmitted diseases.

SUMMARY

The primary care physician must be comfortable with taking a sexual history, understanding the biologic and psychologic underpinnings of sexual functioning. From this framework a careful evaluation can lead to specific diagnoses to delineate etiologic factors. Optimal rational treatment can then proceed (Fig. 56-2). To avoid this important area is to suggest covertly that sexual dysfunctions are not important. The primary care physician is also an important educator about safe sexual practices for all patients.

REFERENCES

1. Crenshaw TL, Goldberg JP: *Sexual pharmacology: drugs that affect sexual function,* New York, 1996, Norton.
2. *Diagnostic and statistical manual of mental disorders,* ed 4, Washington, DC, 1994, American Psychiatric Association.
3. Goldstein I, Lue TF, Padma-Nathan H, et al: Oral sildenafil in the treatment of erectile dysfunction, *N Engl J Med* 338:1397, 1998.
4. Kaplan HS: *The sexual desire disorders: dysfunctional regulation of sexual motivation,* New York, 1995, Brunner-Mazel.
5. Laumann EO, Gagnon JH, Michael RT, Michaels S: *The social organization of sexuality: sexual practices in the United States,* Chicago, 1994, University of Chicago Press.
6. Meana M, Binik YM: Painful coitus: a review of female dyspareunia, *J Nerv Ment Dis* 182:264, 1994.
7. National Institutes of Health, Consensus Development Panel on Impotence: Impotence, *JAMA* 270:83, 1993.
8. Zgourides GD, Warren R: Retarded ejaculation: overview and treatment implications, *J Psychol Hum Sexuality* 2:139, 1989.

CHAPTER 57

Behavior Change: The Example of Smoking Cessation

Barrie J. Guise
Michael G. Goldstein

Lifestyle factors significantly contribute to more than half of the annual deaths in the United States. In addition, medical goals are closely linked to behavioral goals. Nevertheless, facilitating desired health behavior change among patients remains a challenging aspect of primary care.

Human behavior change has traditionally been the bailiwick only of behavioral scientists. In the early 1970s as human health problems became increasingly linked to behavior, collaborations among theorists and investigators in both behavioral psychology and medicine produced the interdisciplinary field of behavioral medicine.

Behavioral medicine's mandate is to apply the knowledge and techniques of behavioral and biomedical science to the prevention, diagnosis, and treatment of medical illness. Although they are critical to effective medical practice and compatible with the practical aspects of medical care, knowledge and skill in the formulation and treatment of health behavior problems have unfortunately been slow to find a prominent place in medical training, resulting in feelings of frustration and incompetence among many primary care physicians.

This chapter introduces the reader to the fundamental principles and techniques of behavioral medicine and then elaborates in detail, using smoking cessation treatment as an example.

FUNDAMENTALS OF BEHAVIOR CHANGE

Behavior changes that promote health range from increasing the frequency of some behaviors (e.g., exercise) to decreasing the frequency of others (e.g., cigarette smoking) to introducing new behaviors (e.g., home blood glucose monitoring). To accomplish behavior change, it is necessary to systematically formulate behavior as a target for intervention. Early behavioral scientists first described paradigms that applied the experimental method to the study of observable behavior, explained behavior in terms of controlled operations, and permitted the reliable prediction of behavior given particular environmental conditions.

The following very basic principles of operant and then classical conditioning are derived from that extensive literature and are borne out in everyday experience: (1) if behavior persists, it is being reinforced (e.g., eating tasty high-fat foods); (2) if behavior ceases, it either has not been reinforced or has been punished (e.g., noncompliance with ineffective medications or those with troublesome side effects); and reinforcement and punishment are defined by the effect each has on behavior, and not by whether each seems positive or negative to an outside observer. For example, although frequent hospitalizations due to noncompliance with an asthma regimen seem negative or like punishment, the avoidance of medication side effects operates on this behavior and acts as a reinforcer, although it is not "positive" per se. Classical conditioning consists of repeated pairings between unrelated experiences or stimuli, such that one thereafter cues the other. This principle accounts for most specific urges to smoke in habitual situations, for instance, with a cup of coffee or in a favorite chair.

In more recent years it has been asserted that cognitions (thoughts and beliefs) can be governed by the same principles as observable behavior and that motivation is an important mediating variable for human behavior. The health belief model[3] asserts that an individual's beliefs about his or her vulnerability to the consequences of disease and about the likelihood that intervention will be protective are important factors in determining health behavior. More recently, the transtheoretic model of change[14] proposes that an individual's motivation or readiness to change is an important factor in predicting the response to strategies designed to modify behavior and that individuals move through a series of stages of readiness to change: *precontemplation* (not yet willing to consider change), *contemplation* (ambivalent but considering change), *preparation* (intending to change imminently), *action* (actively attempting to change), and *maintenance* (attempting to maintain a change).

These models have important implications for the selection of interventions. For example, it stands to reason that an individual who is not yet willing to consider starting an exercise program might not make much use of specific instructions on how to begin exercising. This individual may benefit more from efforts to move him or her along to the contemplation stage, such as an effort to personalize a rationale for exercise. This implies that low motivation need not be an intractable barrier to change, but rather a legitimate target for change. Indeed, traditional learning paradigms are combined with motivational and often pharmacologic interventions to facilitate desired health outcomes.

BEHAVIOR CHANGE: CIGARETTE SMOKING

The beginning of this chapter has presented a brief exposure to the principles by which behavior may be formulated systematically in the day-to-day practice of medicine. The remainder of this chapter is devoted to integrating behavioral and biomedical principles and techniques to address perhaps the most important behavioral challenge in primary care: cigarette smoking. It is helpful to keep in mind that, with the exception of the specific pharmacologic therapies discussed in the upcoming sections, similar general ideas and approaches are applicable to other lifestyle challenges, such as diet and low physical activity.

Scope of the Problem

The Surgeon General has stated that smoking is the chief avoidable cause of death in our society. Annually, 3 million deaths are attributed to smoking worldwide. It is estimated that this number will rise to 10 million by the year 2025. Cigarette smokers have greater overall morbidity than nonsmokers, more restricted activity days, more bed disability days, more school and work absenteeism, and higher utilization of inpatient and outpatient services. An additional 53,000 nonsmoker deaths per year are attributed to the effects of environmental tobacco smoke.

Because the majority of smokers visit a physician at least once each year, primary care physicians can play a central role in reducing the morbidity and mortality associated with cigarette smoking. Although most primary care physicians report that they provide smoking cessation advice to all or almost all of their smoking patients,[13a] a recent population-based survey of patients reported that 51% of smokers were talked to about their smoking; 45.5% were advised to quit; 14.9% were offered help; 3% had a follow-up appointment arranged; and 8.5% were prescribed medication.

In a recent survey, more physicians rated smokers' lack of motivation as the most important barrier to smoking cessation.[8] More than two thirds of this sample also reported that counseling about smoking is frustrating. These findings suggest that physicians feel especially unprepared and ineffective when faced with patients who are not yet ready to quit smoking. For some physicians these negative feelings are fueled by unrealistic expectations. Because even the most effective physician-delivered intervention results in 1-year abstinence rates of less than 25%, physicians become increasingly frustrated if they expect their efforts to produce abstinence rates of greater magnitude.[13] This barrier may be overcome by helping physicians to develop more realistic expectations, by providing specific training in motivational and behavioral techniques, and by encouraging physicians to focus on intermediate outcomes, such as moving a patient who is not interested in quitting to the point of considering it. Strategies to address these barriers are discussed in both Assessment and Management.

Assessment

Biologic, behavioral, and psychologic factors all contribute to the initiation and maintenance of cigarette smoking. Therefore assessment must be designed to identify the specific elements corresponding to these areas for each smoker.

The principal goals of this assessment process are to (1) characterize the patient's level of motivation or readiness to quit smoking, (2) assess the severity of nicotine dependence, (3) assess the architecture of an individual's smoking habit, and (4) identify the psychiatric comorbidity that is likely to complicate treatment.

Assessing the Patient's Motivation to Quit. Much of the frustration and time expenditure physicians experience in counseling smokers is due to a mismatch between the intervention used and the patient's level of motivation. The transtheoretic model of change described earlier can help physicians to assess and intervene more effectively and time-efficiently with their smoking patients. This model provides a way of characterizing different levels of motivation such that treatment can be stage-matched. Staging a smoker's readiness is accomplished by applying the answers to three questions in a simple algorithm (Fig. 57-1).

Individuals at the precontemplation and contemplation stages, who may represent as many as 80% of current smokers seen in a typical medical practice, are not likely to respond to exhortations to quit smoking or interventions that are oriented to quitting, such as nicotine replacement. These patients need motivational interventions that increase awareness and help the individual to recognize the negative aspects of smoking (the cons) (see Management). Only about 20% of smokers who seek medical care are in the preparation stage and have taken steps toward quitting, such as making recent attempts to quit, delaying their first cigarette in the morning, or cutting down on the number of cigarettes that they smoke. These individuals are most likely to respond to interventions that will help them to successfully manage a subsequent attempt to quit, such as nicotine replacement, self-help manuals, behavioral skill training, and referral to a formal treatment program or group.

After individuals have quit smoking, a single question assesses their current stage: "How long ago did you quit smoking?" If the answer is less than 6 months, the patient is in the action stage. If the answer is more than 6 months, the patient is in the maintenance stage. Because smokers are very likely to relapse during the action stage, especially during the first few days and weeks after quitting, these individuals benefit from interventions that are designed to prevent slips and relapses (see Management).

Assessing the Level of Nicotine Dependence. Smoking leads to the development of physical dependence on nicotine in the vast majority of smokers. Nicotine, the major psychoactive substance in cigarettes, has a wide variety of

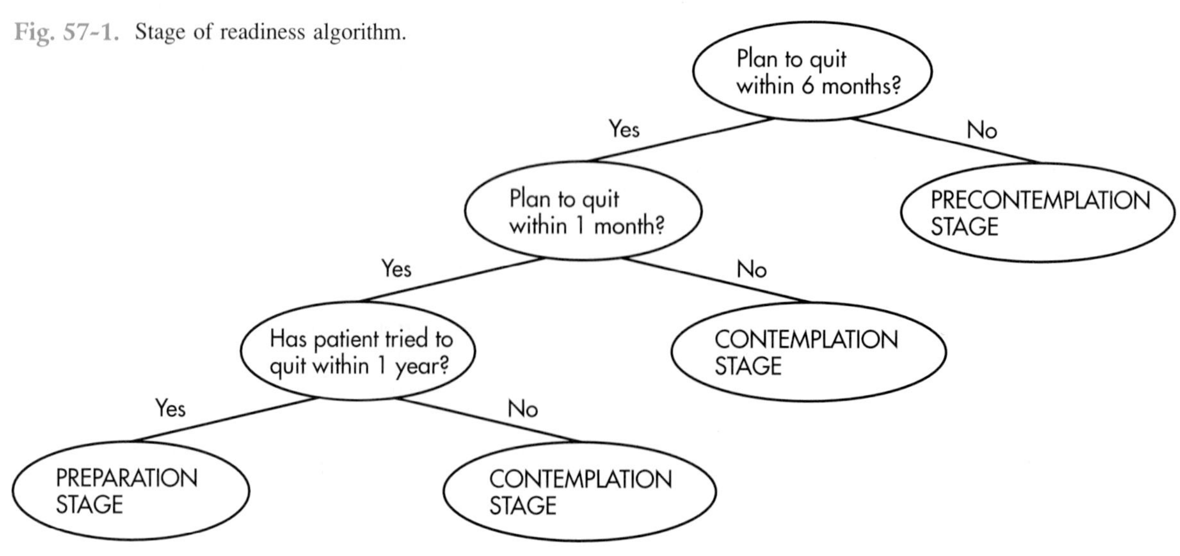

Fig. 57-1. Stage of readiness algorithm.

euphoriant, stimulant, anxiolytic, and antinociceptive effects involving multiple physiologic systems.[16] Each of these effects contributes to nicotine's power as a reinforcer of smoking behavior. Moreover, nicotine produces a well-defined abstinence or withdrawal syndrome (Box 57-1),[1] the avoidance of which maintains smoking.

Several strategies can assess a patient's level of nicotine dependence (see Box 57-2). Perhaps the most common measure of nicotine dependence is the Fagerstrom tolerance questionnaire (FTQ),[5] a seven-item, self-administered form that identifies behaviors thought to reflect nicotine dependence (e.g., high smoking rate and brand nicotine level, smoking when ill or soon after awakening). Scores on the FTQ are related to withdrawal symptoms and the success of smoking cessation. The scale can be administered within several minutes and is easily scored. The time to the first cigarette in the morning, a specific item on the FTQ, appears to be an independent predictor of smoking cessation outcome. A response of "less than 30 minutes" suggests that the patient is smoking to control the withdrawal that results from overnight abstinence. In addition, individuals who smoke more than 25 cigarettes per day may be more likely to report withdrawal symptoms during abstinence than smokers consuming fewer cigarettes, although the evidence for this relationship is limited. The physician should ask about withdrawal signs and symptoms during abstinence in previous attempts to quit. Symptoms may also have occurred when the patient switched to a low-nicotine cigarette, or after the patient stopped using smokeless tobacco products or nicotine-replacement medication.

Although biologic tests of nicotine exposure (i.e., cotinine assays or expired alveolar carbon monoxide) provide objective measure of nicotine dependence, they are costly and time-consuming. These assays are neither feasible nor necessary for effective smoking cessation treatment in the clinical setting.

Assessing Smoking Architecture. The fundamental principles of behavior change described earlier guide the physician's understanding of and then approach to the variables maintaining smoking for a given individual. Recalling that the effects of inhaled nicotine are reinforcing and immediate, and repeatedly paired with a wide range of situations, provides the key to long-term abstinence from cigarettes.

Box 57-1. Summary of DSM-IV Nicotine Withdrawal Symptoms

Craving
Anxiety
Irritability, frustration, or anger
Difficulty concentrating
Restlessness
Increased appetite or weight gain
Decreased heart rate
Disrupted sleep
Depressed mood

A useful assessment strategy is to make a detailed functional analysis of the situations and circumstances in which an individual patient smokes. Patients are simply instructed to monitor their smoking for a few days, keeping a log of the time of each cigarette, the situation in which smoking took place, their mood or affect, and their thoughts about the cigarette. The physician and patient review the self-monitoring record to make note of patterns that easily reveal frequent or powerful cues for smoking.

Assessment of Comorbidity. A crucial step in assessment is to determine whether there is any evidence for psychiatric comorbidity. There is a strong association between smoking and other psychiatric disorders, especially depression, other substance-use disorders, schizophrenia, and anxiety disorders. The current existence or a history of any of these disorders is likely to make smoking cessation more difficult. Moreover, smoking cessation may precipitate the development of depressive symptoms in patients with a history of depression and may even precipitate a relapse of depression in susceptible patients. Smoking cessation does not appear to increase the risk of relapse of alcohol abuse or dependence.

The identification of psychiatric comorbidity has important implications for treatment. Although there are few research-based data on the treatment of nicotine dependence of patients with psychiatric comorbidity, identification, monitoring, and treatment of psychiatric comorbidity are important components of the management of such patients (Box 57-2) (see Management).

Management

After assessment is completed, interventions can be tailored to match each patient's needs. A step-care approach has been advocated for matching patients and treatments. The first step in management is to provide an intervention that is matched to the patient's stage of readiness to change. Since most patients are not ready for action, motivational interventions are usually most beneficial.[12]

Once patients are ready to quit, a decision is made regarding the level, type, and intensity of smoking cessation treatment. This decision should be based on the patient's preferences, the level of nicotine dependence, the presence or absence of psychiatric comorbidity, the history of previous attempts to quit, and relevant behavioral parameters. Patients with low levels of nicotine dependence and little experience with quitting are most likely to respond to the lowest level of care: low-cost, minimal interventions, such as self-help, advice, and follow-up in the primary care setting. Those who

Box 57-2. Assessment of Smokers

Stage of readiness to quit
Level of nicotine dependence
- Smoking rate >25 q day
- Smoking within 30 minutes of awakening
- Previous quit attempts

Smoking architecture
Psychiatric comorbidity

Box 57-3. Summary of Recommendations of the AHCPR Smoking Cessation Clinical Practice Guideline

1. Effective smoking cessation treatments are available, and every patient who smokes should be offered one or more of these treatments.
2. It is essential that physicians determine and document the tobacco-use status of every patient treated in a health care setting.
3. Brief cessation treatments are effective, and at least a minimal intervention should be provided to every patient who uses tobacco.
4. A dose-response relation exists between the intensity and duration of a treatment and its effectiveness. In general, the more intense the treatment, the more effective it is in producing long-term abstinence from tobacco.
5. Three treatment elements, in particular, are effective, and one or more of these elements should be included in smoking cessation treatment:
   - Nicotine replacement therapy
   - Social support (physician-provided encouragement and assistance)
   - Skills training/problem solving (techniques on achieving and maintaining abstinence)
6. Effective reduction of tobacco use requires that health care systems make institutional changes that result in systematic identification of, and intervention with, all tobacco users at every visit.

From Fiore M, Bailey W, et al: *Smoking cessation: clinical practice guideline no. 18,* Agency for Health Care Policy and Research, Public Health Service, U.S. Department of Health and Human Services, 1996.

have failed self-help approaches and those with high levels of nicotine dependence should be considered for the next level in care: brief face-to-face counseling and follow-up in the primary care setting or elsewhere (see Quitting Strategies).[7]

In 1996, the Agency for Health Care Policy and Research (AHCPR) published an evidence-based clinical practice guideline[6] for smoking cessation. See Box 57-3 for a summary of the recommendations of the AHCPR expert panel.

The AHCPR guideline stresses the pivotal role of primary care physicians and strongly recommends the implementation of office systems to identify and document smoking, the delivery of brief advice or counseling to all smokers at every visit, and the offer of nicotine replacement to all smokers who are committed to making a quit attempt. The recommendation to offer nicotine replacement therapy (NRT) to all smokers was based on evidence for the effectiveness of NRT when provided with only minimal adjuvant behavioral treatment and even when the smokers' levels of nicotine dependence were low.

The AHCPR panel also noted a dose-response relationship between the intensity of smoking cessation counseling and cessation outcome; brief advice increased quit rates by 20% (over no advice), 3 to 10 minutes of counseling increased rates by 40%, while 10 or more minutes of counseling more than doubled quit rates (Table 57-1). Counseling that utilized

Table 57-1. Smoking Cessation Rates for Various Intensity Levels of Person-to-Person Contact

Level of contact	Estimated odds ratio (95% C.I.)	Estimated cessation rate (95% C.I.)
No contact (reference group)	1.0	8.8
Minimal contact (≤ 3 min)	1.2 (1.0-1.15)*	10.7 (8.9-12.5)
Brief counseling (> 3 min to ≤ 10 min)	1.4 (1.2-1.7)	12.1 (10.0-14.3)
Counseling (> 10 min)	2.4 (2.1-2.7)	18.7 (16.8-20.6)

From Fiore M, Bailey W, et al: *Smoking cessation: clinical practice guideline no. 18,* Agency for Health Care Policy and Research, Public Health Service, U.S. Department of Health and Human Services, 1996.
*Actual 95% lower confidence estimate equals 1.03.

a problem-solving approach and provided personal support was found to be particularly effective.

Patients with psychiatric comorbidity, including other substance abuse, may require a specific treatment for their associated problem before, or concurrent with, treatment for nicotine dependence. These patients, as well as those who have failed despite repeated attempts to quit, are also candidates for more intensive, formal treatment programs.

Because practitioners of primary care have an opportunity to intervene with smokers repeatedly over time, results of the initial intervention can be reviewed at subsequent visits. During follow-up, patients who have not successfully quit smoking can be reassessed, can be provided with another intervention at the same level, or can be advanced to a more intensive intervention. The discussion on the management of smoking cessation concludes with a section on organizational resources and aids available to primary care physicians.

Matching Interventions to the Patient's Stage of Change.

Motivational Interventions. It is important to remember that successful counseling of smokers often results in changes in level of readiness or motivation to quit and not imminent quitting. Nicotine dependence is a stubborn problem that often requires persistent yet empathic efforts to increase motivation before actual behavior change occurs.

As discussed earlier, motivation is an important mediator of behavior change. Patients in the precontemplation stage respond best to motivational interventions that help them begin to think about quitting smoking.[15] Personalized information and feedback can raise smokers' awareness of the ways in which smoking is affecting their health, thus raising the cons of smoking. Pulmonary function tests and other direct physiologic evidence of smoking's health effects are useful components to feedback. Asking patients in the precontemplation stage to reflect on their feelings about smoking is another useful intervention. It helps to make empathic statements, such as "I know it may be hard to quit smoking," and supportive statements, such as "When you are ready to quit, I'm willing to help." Feelings of demoralization can be addressed by informing the patient that most smokers make several attempts to quit before they are finally successful.

For patients in the contemplation stage it is especially useful to explore the reasons for smoking (the pros), as well as other barriers to quitting, so that potential solutions for overcoming barriers can be discussed. For example, if a patient reports that she depends on smoking to help her to manage her weight, the offer and provision of alternative weight-management strategies may tip the balance of pros and cons toward a decision to quit smoking. If a smoking patient's spouse or other family member smokes, an offer to help both of them to quit may remove another barrier to taking action.

Providing a menu of options from which the patient may choose is another effective motivational tool. Patients who become chronically stuck in the contemplation stage may benefit from encouragement to take small steps toward action, such as cutting down the number of cigarettes they smoke, delaying their first cigarette of the day, or trying to quit for only 24 hours. These patients may also be willing to monitor their smoking to identify important barriers and triggers that can be reviewed at a subsequent visit.

Patients in the contemplation stage may express negative feelings or fears about quitting. Clarification and legitimization of their feelings and expressions of support and respect may help these patients to feel heard and understood. Statements such as "I'm glad that you're thinking about quitting" are especially useful, since they reinforce patients' interest in quitting. Even if patients do not decide to quit in the near future, these interventions may help them to feel more comfortable when talking to their physicians about smoking and to feel more receptive to future interventions.

Quitting Strategies. When the patient is finally in the preparation stage, or ready for action, appropriate action-oriented strategies can be advised or prescribed (Box 57-4). Several reviews have described strategies in considerable detail for patients in the action or the maintenance stage.[4,9] Useful interventions for patients in the action stage are listed in Box 57-4 and include setting a specific date with the patient to quit; writing a contract; providing self-help materials; suggesting use of over-the-counter (OTC) NRT; prescribing NRT, bupropion, or other pharmacologic adjuncts; teaching behavioral skills (e.g., self-monitoring, setting goals, self-reward, stimulus control, substituting alternative behaviors, relaxation exercises, coping skills training); and enhancing social support. Individuals are most successful when multiple cognitive and behavioral strategies are used when attempting to quit smoking. Encouraging patients to begin or to continue a program of regular exercise is another useful intervention for patients in the action or maintenance stage.

Box 57-4. Interventions for Patients in Preparation, Action, or Maintenance Stages of Change

Set a specific date to quit
Write a contract
Provide self-help materials
Prescribe nicotine replacement (when appropriate)
Teach behavioral skills
- Self-monitoring
- Setting goals
- Self-reward
- Stimulus control
- Substituting alternative behaviors
- Relaxation exercises
- Coping skills training
- Relapse prevention skills

Identify and treat psychiatric comorbidity
Recommend an exercise program
Refer to formal treatment programs
Enhance social support

Follow-up. Follow-up visits become especially important when patients are in the action or maintenance stage. Since the vast majority of patients relapse after attempted abstinence, follow-up visits can help patients to use relapse as an opportunity for learning. By exploring the circumstances that led to a return to smoking, the physician and patient can develop a revised plan that includes specific strategies to address the triggers that led to the relapse. It may become apparent that the patient experienced the development or exacerbation of an underlying psychiatric disorder. These disorders may require specific treatment or referral before the patient is able to successfully quit smoking.

At the follow-up visit the health care provider can praise the patient's efforts and reinforce the strategies that the patient used effectively. Praise and reinforcement are also useful to patients who are abstinent at follow-up. Anticipation of and planning for future problem situations and triggers for relapse are also beneficial.

Pharmacologic Interventions. Pharmacologic agents are effective as interventions for smoking cessation, especially when used in conjunction with behavioral interventions. Although long-term abstinence depends ultimately on behavior change, pharmacologic agents are important because they minimize withdrawal and craving, making the time needed to decay the various learned aspects of the habit of smoking pass more easily. Our recommendations for use of pharmacotherapy are based on the AHCPR 1996 clinical practice guideline,[6] the American Psychiatric Association's 1996 nicotine dependence guideline,[2] and a recent review article that focused on advances in pharmacotherapy for smoking cessation since the publication of these guidelines.[9] Use of NRT and bupropion, the only pharmacologic agents approved by the Food and Drug Administration (FDA) for smoking cessation, will be discussed here. The reader is referred to recent reviews for more detailed information about NRT and bupropion and for information about other pharmacologic interventions.[9,10] Four forms of NRT have been approved by the FDA for use as aids to smoking cessation: nicotine gum, transdermal nicotine, nicotine nasal spray, and nicotine inhaler. Nicotine gum and transdermal nicotine are both available OTC and increase quit rates by 50% to 100%, even when administered with minimal or no adjuvant behavioral treatment. However, absolute smoking cessation rates are clearly enhanced when more intensive behavioral treatment is provided with transdermal nicotine and nicotine gum. There is limited information available regarding the efficacy of nicotine nasal spray and nicotine inhaler when these agents are administered with minimal behavioral treatment. Nicotine inhaler and spray are available by prescription only.

Choosing the form of NRT for an individual patient is based primarily on patient preference. This conclusion is based on the following evidence: (1) three of the four forms of NRT (transdermal patches, nasal spray, and inhaler) have very similar efficacies; (2) although the efficacy of nicotine gum is somewhat lower than the other three, this may be due to decreased compliance as well as improper chewing technique; (3) we are not aware of any published studies that have directly compared smoking cessation outcomes for different forms of NRT; and (4) there is no evidence to suggest that specific forms of NRT are more effective with subgroups of smokers. However, highly dependent smokers, as measured by the FTQ, benefit more from the 4 mg dosage form than the 2 mg gum.[17]

Patient preferences for different forms of NRT relate to ease of administration (e.g., once-a-day administration for patch), differing side effect profiles (e.g., patch more likely to produce sleep disturbances; gum more likely to produce dyspepsia and dental problems; nasal spray more likely to cause rhinitis), onset of action (e.g., fastest for spray, slowest for patch), and sense of personal control over craving (e.g., least for patch). Recent evidence suggests that combined transdermal nicotine and nicotine gum may be more effective than either alone. See Boxes 57-5 and 57-6 for nicotine patch and gum guidelines.

Bupropion, an antidepressant with noradrenergic and dopaminergic activity, is the first FDA-approved nonnicotine drug treatment for smoking cessation and the only smoking cessation treatment available in pill. Results of clinical trials have demonstrated that bupropion is effective in promoting long-term smoking cessation when combined with brief counseling and is at least as effective as nicotine replacement. The dose of bupropion that is most effective for smoking cessation is 150 mg (of the sustained release [SR] preparation) twice-a-day. Medication is started 2 weeks before the quit day at 150 mg per day and is increased to 300 mg per day after 3 days. Recommended duration of therapy is 7 to 12 weeks after quitting. Longer term trials are currently being evaluated. Bupropion and transdermal nicotine may be used in concert, although the long-term benefit is not clear. The most common side effects of bupropion are tremor, rash, headache, and urticaria. Because bupropion may lower the threshold for seizures, it is contraindicated in patients with a history of seizures and should be used with caution in patients with a personal or family history of seizures, active alcohol or other substance abuse, or a history of head injury. However, no seizures were reported in any of the bupropion SR smoking cessation trials, which included a total of 1828 patients.

Referral to Formal Treatment Programs. Referral to a formal treatment program is indicated only when the patient is highly motivated to quit and is willing to attend such a treatment program. Patients with high levels of nicotine dependence, those who have repeatedly failed to quit using self-help methods and brief counseling, and patients with psychiatric comorbidity are most likely to benefit from formal treatment. Formal treatment programs range from volunteer-led programs that combine group support with an introduction to behavioral quitting strategies, to multidisciplinary

Box 57-5. Suggestions for Use of Nicotine Gum

Selection of patients: Avoid during pregnancy and breastfeeding, in the presence of unstable angina or other unstable vascular disease. Patients with jaw pain, gum disease, poor dentition, or peptic ulcer disease may be unable to use due to side effects.

Dosage and duration: Patients with high levels of nicotine dependence (more than 25 cigarettes per day, smoking within 30 minutes after awakening) should use 4 mg gum. Initially, patients should chew at least one piece per hour for several weeks, then taper gradually. Maximum is 30 pieces per day for 2 mg, 20 pieces per day for 4 mg.

Instructions for use: Instruct patient not to smoke while using gum. Gum must be chewed properly to get benefit and avoid side effects. Chew slowly until taste emerges, then "park" between gum and cheek to facilitate absorption. Alternate chewing and parking for 20-30 minutes. Acidic beverages must be avoided before and during gum use.

From Fiore M, Bailey W, et al: *Smoking cessation: clinical practice guideline no. 18,* Agency for Health Care Policy and Research, Public Health Service, U.S. Department of Health and Human Services, 1996.

Box 57-6. Suggestions for Use of Nicotine Transdermal Patches

Selection of patients: Avoid during pregnancy and breast-feeding, in the presence of unstable angina or other unstable vascular disease. Patients with an allergy to adhesive or generalized skin diseases may be unable to use patches.

Dosage and duration: Initially, use highest dose patch *unless* smoking less than 10 cigarettes per day or if the patient weighs less than 100 pounds. After 4 weeks at initial dose, taper to intermediate dose for 2 weeks and lowest dose for 2 weeks. Consider supplementing with nicotine gum if breakthrough craving or withdrawal occurs. Use of more than one patch at a time can be considered for patients with significant withdrawal symptoms on single patch.

16- vs. 24-hour patches: Base on patient preference. 24-hour patch is more likely to cause sleep disturbance or vivid dreams, whereas 16-hour patch may be associated with early morning withdrawal symptoms.

Instructions for use: Apply first patch after awakening on quit day. Apply patches to a relatively hairless, although unshaven, clean, and dry skin location, preferably above the waist. Apply new patches at the same time each day. Rotate patch sites to limit skin irritation. Instruct patients not to smoke while on patch and to discontinue patch if the patient smokes more than five cigarettes/day for several consecutive days.

From Fiore M, Bailey W, et al: *Smoking cessation: clinical practice guideline no. 18,* Agency for Health Care Policy and Research, Public Health Service, U.S. Department of Health and Human Services, 1996.

outpatient and inpatient treatment centers that can provide intensive behavioral and pharmacologic treatment. The success of formal treatment programs with carefully selected, motivated smokers ranges from 15% to 40%.

Organizational Resources and Aids. Kottke, Solberg, and Brekke[11] described the organizational components and systems that are essential to the delivery of effective and consistent counseling in primary care office settings. Because research has demonstrated that physician-delivered smoking cessation interventions are most likely to be effective when physicians are routinely reminded to intervene with all smoking patients with the use of chart stickers or similar reminder systems, these systems should be integrated into all office practices.

Resources for patients, physicians, and office staff members are important tools that enhance the capacity of health care providers to provide information and advice. Self-help manuals for smoking cessation are effective and are available through voluntary agencies.

REFERENCES

1. American Psychiatric Association: *Diagnostic and statistical manual of mental disorders (DSM-IV),* ed 3, Washington, DC, 1994, American Psychiatric Association.
2. American Psychiatric Association: Practice guideline for the treatment of patients with nicotine dependence, *Am J Psychiatry* 153(10):1-31, 1996.
3. Becker MH: The health belief model and sick role behavior, *Health Educ Monograph,* 2:409-419, 1974.
4. Brown RA, et al: Nicotine dependence: assessment and management. In *Principles of medical psychiatry,* ed 2, New York, 1993, Oxford University Press.
5. Fagerstrom KO, Schneider NG: Measuring nicotine dependence: a review of the Fagerstrom tolerance questionnaire, *J Behav Med* 12(2):159, 1989.
6. Fiore M, Bailey W, et al: *Smoking cessation: clinical practice guideline no. 18,* Agency for Health Care Policy and Research, Public Health Service, U.S. Department of Health and Human Services, 1996.
7. Goldstein MG, et al: Behavioral medicine strategies for medical patients. In Stoudemire A, editor: *Clinical psychiatry for medical patients,* Philadelphia, 1990, JB Lippincott.
8. Goldstein MG, Niaura R, Willey-Lessne C, et al: Physicians counseling smokers: a population-based survey of patients' perceptions of health care provider–delivered smoking cessation interventions, *Arch Intern Med* 157(12):1313-1319, 1997.
9. Hughes JM, Goldstein M, et al: Recent advances in pharmacotherapy of smoking cessation, *JAMA* 281(1):72-76, 1999.
10. Hurt R, Sachs D, et al: A comparison of sustained-release bupropion and placebo for smoking cessation, *N Engl J Med* 337:1195-1202, 1997.
11. Kottke TE, et al: Smoking cessation strategies and evaluation, *J Am Coll Cardiol* 12(4):1105, 1988.
12. Miller WR, Rolnick S: *Motivational interviewing: preparing people to change addictive behavior,* New York, 1991, Guilford.
13. Ockene JK: Physician-delivered interventions for smoking cessation: strategies for increasing effectiveness, *Prev Med* 16(5):723, 1987.

13a. Orleans CT, George LK, Houpt JL, et al: Health promotion in primary care: a survey of US family practitioners, *Prev Med* 14:636-637, 1985.

14. Prochaska JO, DiClemente CC: Towards a comprehensive model of change. In Miller WR, Heather N, editors: *Treating addictive disorders: processes of change,* New York, 1986, Plenum.
15. Prochaska JO, Goldstein MG: Process of smoking cessation: implications for clinicians, *Clin Chest Med* 12(4):727, 1991.
16. Redd WH: Management of anticipatory nausea and vomiting. In Holland JC, Rowland JH, editors: *Handbook of psychooncology,* New York, 1990, Oxford University.
17. Sachs DPL, Leischow SJ: Pharmacologic approaches to smoking cessation, *Clin Chest Med* 12(4):769, 1991.

CHAPTER 58

Obesity and Weight Management

Louis J. Aronne

OBESITY

Obesity is an accumulation of excess adipose tissue that leads to impairment of health. This chronic disease is increasingly impacting the health of people around the world.[17] Studies examining metabolic and genetic causes of obesity have proved that this disease arises from an excess of energy intake compared to expenditure.[9] Each individual inherits a set of genes that control appetite and metabolism. A wide variety of environmental factors, such as food availability, level of physical activity, and individual psychology and culture, may exacerbate prevalent genetic tendencies to gain weight.[8] Thus obesity is not simply the result of gluttony and a lack of willpower.

Data from the National Health and Nutrition Examination Survey (NHANES) suggest that more than two-thirds of individuals with a body mass index (BMI) greater than 27 (Table 58-1) have at least one additional complicating condition such as diabetes, hypertension, hyperlipidemia, sleep apnea, or arthritis of the lower extremities. Despite this positive relationship between obesity and these conditions, the treatment of obesity by physicians in the office setting has been largely ignored. As the understanding of the weight regulating mechanisms progresses, however, obesity appears to be a neuroendocrine disorder rather than a disorder of willpower.[13,16] The successful treatment of obesity will play an important role in improving the health care of adults and children in the coming years.[6]

Epidemiology

The prevalence of overweight and obesity is increasing worldwide in adults and children at a rapid rate. The World Health Organization (WHO) is investigating the scope of the problem, which occurs in developed, as well as developing, countries.

When obesity is defined as a BMI greater than or equal to 30 (see Table 58-1), 19.9% of men and 24.9% of women are obese compared with 10.4% of men and 15.1% of women in 1960. The prevalence of overweight, which is defined as a BMI of 25 to 29.9, has increased only slightly over the same period of time (Fig. 58-1). In the United States, obesity affects minority populations more than whites. Women but not men of low socioeconomic status are more likely to be obese. Obesity is less common in the elderly, possibly because of greater mortality associated with a higher BMI or because of a decrease in BMI after age 60.

The direct health care cost of treating the proportion of diseases (such as diabetes, hypertension, and cardiovascular disease) directly attributable to obesity was estimated at $51.6 billion, representing 5.7% of the national health care expenditure in 1995. The indirect cost of obesity, which includes lost productivity as a result of these comorbidities and other associated disabilities, is $47.6 billion; this is

Table 58-1. Calculation of Body Mass Index for Overweight/Obesity

	Normal							Overweight					Obesity (class I)					Obesity (class II)					Extreme obesity (class III)									
BMI	19	20	21	22	23	24	25	26	27	28	29	30	31	32	33	34	35	36	37	38	39	40	41	42	43	44	45	46	47	48	49	50
Height (inches)	**Body weight (pounds)**																															
58	91	96	100	105	110	115	119	124	129	134	138	143	148	153	158	162	167	172	177	181	186	191	196	201	205	210	215	220	224	229	234	239
59	94	99	104	109	114	119	124	128	133	138	143	148	153	158	163	168	173	178	183	188	193	198	203	208	212	217	222	227	232	237	242	247
60	97	102	107	112	118	123	128	133	138	143	148	153	158	163	168	174	179	184	189	194	199	204	209	215	220	225	230	235	240	245	250	255
61	100	106	111	116	122	127	132	137	143	148	153	158	164	169	174	180	185	190	195	201	206	211	217	222	227	232	238	243	248	254	259	264
62	104	109	115	120	126	131	136	142	147	153	158	164	169	175	180	186	191	196	202	207	213	218	224	229	235	240	246	251	256	262	267	273
63	107	113	118	124	130	135	141	146	152	158	163	169	175	180	186	191	197	203	208	214	220	225	231	237	242	248	254	259	265	270	278	282
64	110	116	122	128	134	140	145	151	157	163	169	174	180	186	192	197	204	209	215	221	227	232	238	244	250	256	262	267	273	279	285	291
65	114	120	126	132	138	144	150	156	162	168	174	180	186	192	198	204	210	216	222	228	234	240	246	252	258	264	270	276	282	288	294	300
66	118	124	130	136	142	148	155	161	167	173	179	186	192	198	204	210	216	223	229	235	241	247	253	260	266	272	278	284	291	297	303	309
67	121	127	134	140	146	153	159	166	172	178	185	191	198	204	211	217	223	230	236	242	249	255	261	268	274	280	287	293	299	306	312	319
68	125	131	138	144	151	158	164	171	177	184	190	197	203	210	216	223	230	236	243	249	256	262	269	276	282	289	295	302	308	315	322	328
69	128	135	142	149	155	162	169	176	182	189	196	203	209	216	223	230	236	243	250	257	263	270	277	284	291	297	304	311	318	324	331	338
70	132	139	146	153	160	167	174	181	188	195	202	209	216	222	229	236	243	250	257	264	271	278	285	292	299	306	313	320	327	334	341	348
71	136	143	150	157	165	172	179	186	193	200	208	215	222	229	236	243	250	257	265	272	279	286	293	301	308	315	322	329	338	343	351	358
72	140	147	154	162	169	177	184	191	199	206	213	221	228	235	242	250	258	265	272	279	287	294	302	309	316	324	331	338	346	353	361	368
73	144	151	159	166	174	182	189	197	204	212	219	227	235	242	250	257	265	272	280	288	295	302	310	318	325	333	340	348	355	363	371	378
74	148	155	163	171	179	186	194	202	210	218	225	233	241	249	256	264	272	280	287	295	303	311	319	326	334	342	350	358	365	373	381	389
75	152	160	168	176	184	192	200	208	216	224	232	240	248	256	264	272	279	287	295	303	311	319	327	335	343	351	359	367	375	383	391	399
76	156	164	172	180	189	197	205	213	221	230	238	246	254	263	271	279	287	295	304	312	320	328	336	344	353	361	369	377	385	394	402	410

Instructions:

Find the appropriate height in the left-hand column. Move across to a given weight. The number at the top of the column is the BMI at that height and weight. Pounds have been rounded off.

Calculating BMI

BMI can be calculated as follows:

$$\text{BMI} = \frac{\text{weight (kg)}}{\text{height squared (m}^2\text{)}}$$

If pounds and inches are used:

$$\text{BMI} = \frac{\text{weight (pounds)} \times 703}{\text{height squared (inches}^2\text{)}}$$

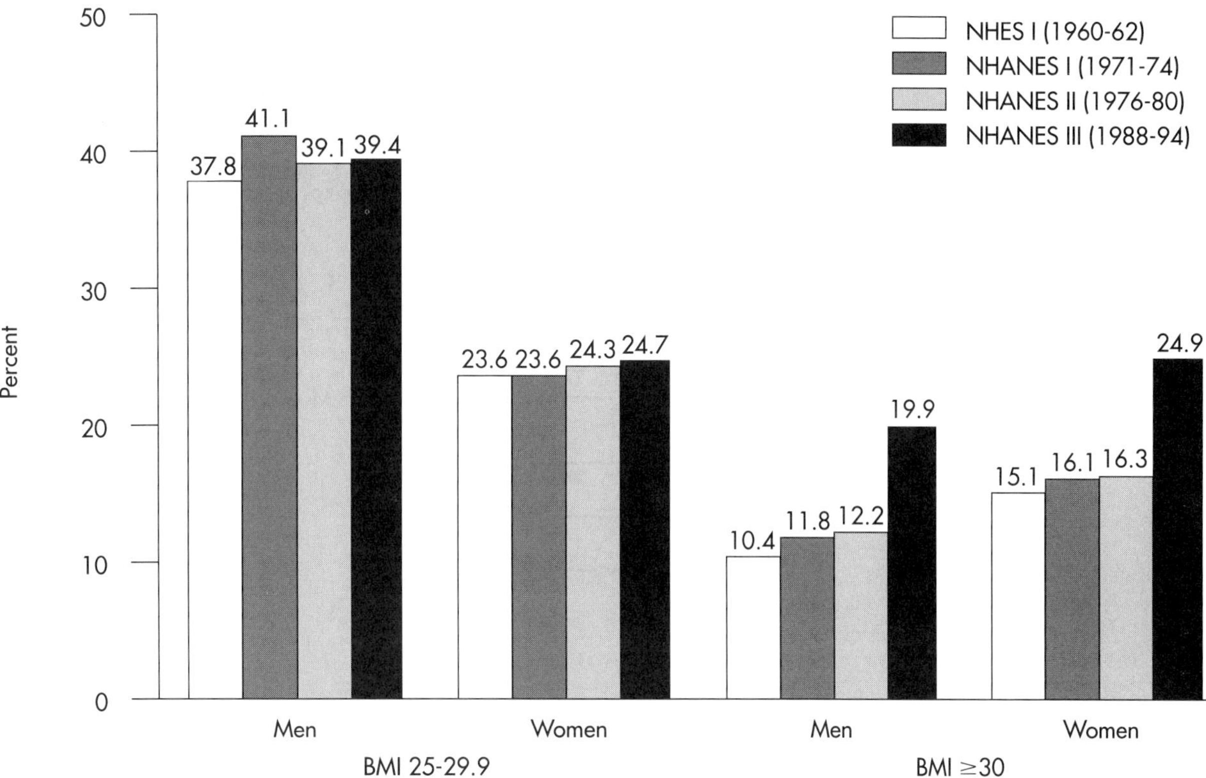

Fig. 58-1. Age-adjusted prevalence of overweight (BMI 25-29.9) and obesity (BMI >30). CDC/NCHS, United States, 1960-1994 (ages 20 to 74 years). (From *Obes Res* 6(S2)51S-210S, 1998.)

comparable with the economic losses due to cigarette smoking.[6,17]

Pathophysiology

Like essential hypertension, obesity results from a genetic predisposition combined with environmental factors. Both are necessary for obesity to occur, but the genetic predisposition seems to be quite common based on the high prevalence of the disorder. The increasing prevalence of obesity around the world is likely the result of a changing environment, which now requires less physical activity and favors overconsumption of food.[6,8,17]

Enormous strides have been made in our understanding of the weight regulating mechanisms of the body over the past few years. The discovery of the *ob* gene in 1994 and its product, *leptin,* a 146-amino acid protein hormone produced primarily by adipose tissue, galvanized the field of obesity research by providing concrete evidence that the body contains a classic negative feedback system that regulates body weight[10,13,16] (Fig. 58-2). Mice with a homozygous mutation of the *ob* gene develop massive obesity as a result of increased food intake and decreased metabolic rate leading to diabetes. The syndrome, which includes impaired reproduction, is rapidly reversed by administration of recombinant leptin. While several extremely obese children around the world have been found to have similar mutations (and are now losing weight on leptin replacement therapy), defects in leptin and its production appear to be a rare cause of obesity. While not as rare, defects of the leptin receptor and other single gene defects of receptors and other components of the weight-regulating mechanism have not proved to be common causes of obesity thus far.

Obesity seems to result from minor gains in energy, which lead to gradual weight gain over a long period of time. External factors leading to the increase in obesity are the ready availability of inexpensive, high-fat, calorie-dense, good-tasting food, and a reduction in the need to exercise combined with a weight-regulating mechanism designed to prevent weight loss more forcefully than weight gain. Once weight is gained, physiologic mechanisms that developed over time to prevent starvation defend the new, higher body weight. The result is a "ratcheting up" of body weight—it can be gained easily but not easily lost. The body must "allow" this weight gain to occur; short-term experiments in which volunteers are overfed the same number of calories demonstrate wide variability in the amount of weight gained. This process appears to be controlled by the energy expended by muscle. However, the weight gained during these experiments is invariably lost soon after the experiment ends, in marked contrast to what the average obese patient experiences; this indicates that those who gain weight have some inherent tendency to do so. Box 58-1 contains eight key points about the energy balance system.

Regional Distribution of Fat. The regional distribution of fat plays an important role in determining the risk of a given level of obesity.[6,14,17] Abdominal or "apple-shaped" obesity is more common in men and is associated with a greater risk of most of the complications of obesity. An accumulation of excess intraabdominal or visceral fat is believed to account for most of the increased risk. Intraabdominal adipose tissue is more cellular, has greater blood flow, has more cortisol and testosterone receptors, and has greater lipolysis in response to catecholamines when

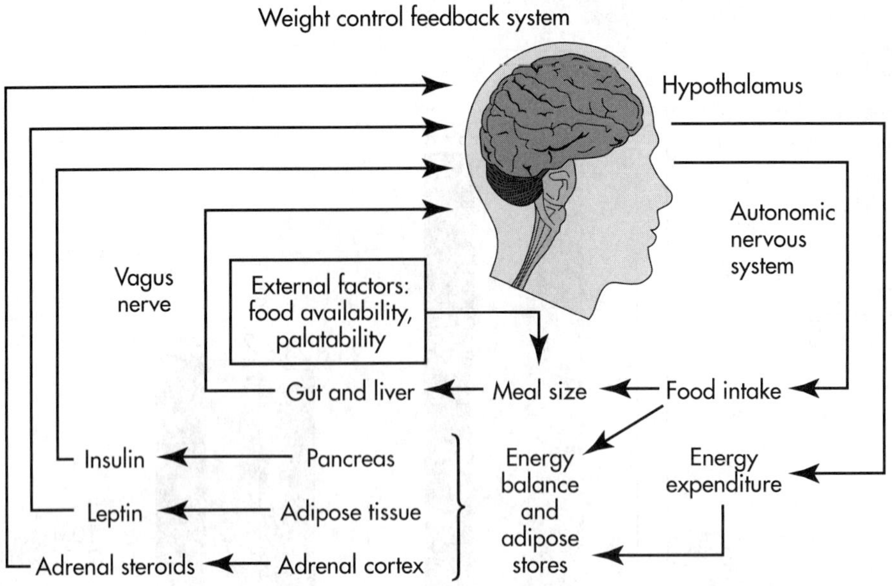

Fig. 58-2. Model of the weight control feedback system. The weight regulating mechanism appears to resemble a highly integrated and redundant homeostatic mechanism for defending body weight. (Adapted from Campfield LA et al: *Science* 280:1383-1387, 1998; Porte D et al: *Diabetologia* 41:863-881, 1998.)

Box 58-1. Key Points of the Energy Balance System

1. Body weight (adiposity) is regulated by a classic negative feedback system involving the central nervous system (CNS).
2. The defended level of fuel stored in the form of adipose tissue is determined by the sum total of all of the genetic and environmental influences interacting on the system; therefore there is no "set-point" for adiposity that is "hard-wired."
3. Afferent circulating signals originate in the endocrine pancreas, adipose tissue, and the adrenal cortex, are hormones sensitive to energy balance, and regulate adipose tissue mass. They include insulin, leptin, and adrenal steroids.
4. Each of the circulating adiposity signals is regulated by factors in addition to body fat stores. Thus there is no primary system that determines fat-store size, and there is no apparent essential minimum or maximum adipose mass that can be maintained.
5. Afferent neural signals originate in the gut and liver in response to nutrients, are carried in the vagus, and regulate meal size, not adipose tissue mass.
6. CNS systems integrate the afferent neural and circulating information by modulating the activity of neuronal efferent pathways that utilize amines (including serotonin and catecholamines) and neuropeptides (including neuropeptideY(NPY), corticotropin-releasing hormone (CRH), α-melanocyte-stimulating hormone (α-MSH), and their receptors.
7. Effectors that determine energy balance include food intake, largely by modifying meal size, and energy expenditure in brown fat, liver, and muscle.
8. Obesity and cachexia are disorders of this regulatory system.

From Porte D, Seely RJ, Woods SC, et al: *Diabetologia* 41:863-881, 1998.

Box 58-2. Metabolic Abnormalities and Disorders Associated with Abdominal Obesity

Insulin resistance
Hyperinsulinemia
Glucose intolerance
Type 2 diabetes mellitus
Hypertension
Elevated VLDL
Elevated LDL
Reduced HDL
Increase in small dense LDL particles (reflected in an increased level of Apo B)
Elevated fibrinogen
Osteoarthritis
Menstrual irregularities
Gallbladder disease

compared with subcutaneous adipose tissue. Most importantly, intraabdominal adipose tissue is in the portal circulation; as a result, the liver is exposed to more free fatty acids, which may contribute to insulin resistance and other manifestations of "the metabolic syndrome." Metabolic abnormalities associated with abdominal obesity include insulin resistance, hyperinsulinemia, glucose intolerance, adult-onset diabetes mellitus, hypertension, high very low-density lipoprotein (VLDL), high low-density lipoprotein (LDL), with an increase in small dense LDL particles reflected in an increased level of Apo B, low high-density lipoprotein (HDL), high fibrinogen, arthritis, menstrual irregularities, and gallbladder disease (Box 58-2).

Premenopausal women tend to accumulate more fat in

the gluteofemoral region. This "pear-shaped" distribution may explain why women are at proportionately less risk than men of the same degree of obesity. While the tendency to develop abdominal obesity is genetically determined, as with total body weight, external factors play a role. For example, women who develop abdominal obesity are more likely to smoke cigarettes and use alcoholic beverages, have socioeconomic disadvantages, psychosomatic diseases, and more psychiatric and psychologic problems than women with a gluteofemoral predominance. They may be anovulatory and hyperandrogenic, with increased cortisol and insulin secretion.

Assessment of Fat Distribution. The most precise methods of measuring fat distribution are computed tomography (CT) scanning and magnetic resonance imaging (MRI), but these are too expensive and cumbersome for routine use. Waist measurement is useful in estimating abdominal adiposity, although it obviously cannot distinguish visceral adipose tissue from overlying subcutaneous adiposity. However, measurement of waist circumference has become the accepted form of risk assessment for the regional distribution of obesity (Box 58-3 and Table 58-2).

Box 58-3. Measuring Waist Circumference

Place a measuring tape in a horizontal plane at the level of the iliac crest, without compressing the skin, and read the value at the end of a normal expiration. Men with a waist circumference greater than 40 inches and women with a waist circumferences greater than 35 inches are at higher risk because of excess abdominal fat and should be considered one risk category above that defined by their BMI.

From *Obes Res* 6(2):51S-210S, 1998.

Complications

Diabetes Mellitus. The positive relationship between obesity and type 2, or noninsulin–dependent, diabetes mellitus has been demonstrated in many studies. The duration and magnitude of increased body weight, predominance of abdominal distribution of fat, and further weight gain all increase the risk of developing type 2 diabetes. The risk begins at a BMI of about 22 and rises strikingly, about 25% for each BMI unit. For example, in the Nurses Health Study, the age-adjusted relative risk of developing diabetes in women with a BMI greater than 35 was 60 *times* that of the lowest risk group. In addition, a history of childhood obesity, steady weight gain as an adult, abdominal fat distribution, lack of physical activity, and poor diet are important risk factors. In some ethnic groups, abdominal fat distribution is an even greater risk factor for diabetes than BMI. Such patients may be at risk from excess accumulation of visceral fat even though their BMI is in the normal range. Weight reduction of 10% to 20% is associated with marked improvement in glucose and insulin sensitivity in obese, diabetic patients even before much weight is lost. Individuals who have been diabetic for longer and have lower insulin levels do not fare as well.

Hypertension. Obesity is a well-established risk factor for developing hypertension. The prevalence of hypertension is at least 2 to 3 times greater in the overweight and obese population. The risk of developing hypertension is greater in younger individuals and increases with duration of obesity, particularly in women. The increase in sodium retention, blood volume, cardiac output, and systemic vascular resistance seen in the obese is believed to underlie the relationship. Blood pressure is reduced by weight reduction, probably because of a reduction in sympathetic nervous system activity and suppression of the renin-angiotensin system. About one-half of hypertension in whites and one-quarter of hypertension in blacks is weight-related.

Cardiovascular Disease and Lipid Disorders. Obesity is an independent risk factor for cardiovascular disease,

Table 58-2. Classification of Overweight and Obesity by BMI and Waist Circumference and the Associated Disease Risk

			Disease risk* (relative to normal weight and waist circumference)	
	BMI (kg/m^2)	Obesity class	Men ≤40 in (≤102 cm) Women ≤35 in (≤88 cm)	>40 in (>102 cm) >35 in (>88 cm)
Underweight	<18.5	—	—	—
Normal†	18.5-24.9	—	—	—
Overweight	>25.0	—	Increased	Increased
Pre-obese	25.0-29.9	—	Increased	High
Obesity	30.0-34.9	I	High	Very high
	35.0-39.9	II	Very high	Very high
Extreme obesity	≥40	III	Extremely high	Extremely high

Modified from WHO: Obesity: preventing and managing the global epidemic. Report of a WHO consultation of obesity, Geneva, 1997, World Health Organization; *Obes Res* 6(suppl 2): 51S-210S, 1998.

*Disease risk for type 2 diabetes mellitus, hypertension, and cardiovascular disease.

†Increased waist circumference can also be a marker for increased risk even in persons of normal weight.

including coronary heart disease (CHD), stroke, and peripheral vascular disease. Increased body weight and abdominal obesity predispose individuals to cardiovascular risk factors, including elevated levels of total cholesterol, LDL cholesterol, triglycerides, apo-B (a marker for small dense LDL), insulin, plasminogen activator-1 (PAI-1), and a reduction in HDL cholesterol. Not uncommonly, obese individuals develop multiple cardiovascular risk factors. The cluster of hypercholesterolemia, hypertriglyceridemia, hyperuricemia, impaired glucose tolerance, diabetes, and hypertension in various combinations is known as "the metabolic syndrome" or "syndrome X." The clustering of these disorders is related to hyperinsulinemia and insulin resistance, a result of visceral fat. Data from the Framingham Study placed obesity as the third most important risk factor for CHD in men after age and dyslipidemia. Risk is greater in younger age groups and in those with abdominal obesity. Weight gain as an adult further increases CHD risk.

Sleep Apnea. The clinician should be alert to the possible presence of obstructive sleep apnea, which is a disorder that is often overlooked in obese patients. Proper diagnosis of this disorder is important because sleep apnea places the patient at even higher risk of cardiovascular morbidity and it improves with specific treatment. Evaluation of the patient for sleep apnea is contained in the section on medical history.

Gastrointestinal Disorders. The prevalence of symptomatic gallstones increases sharply above a BMI of 30; for example, women with a BMI of 35 are at 4 times the risk of women with a BMI less than 24. An increased production of cholesterol by the liver with increasing body weight is a contributing cause. During weight loss, the risk of cholelithiasis increases because of an increase in cholesterol flux. A slower rate of weight loss, as well as the use of ursodiol, minimizes the possibility of stone formation. Finally, hepatic steatosis, fatty liver in nonalcoholic and nondiabetic patients, and gastroesophageal reflux are increased in the overweight and obese and respond well to weight reduction.

Osteoarthritis. While the role of overweight and obesity in the more rapid deterioration of weight-bearing joints, such as the knees, ankles, and hips, is clearly mechanical, there is a small increase in osteoarthritis in nonweight-bearing joints as well.

Cancer. Cancer of the prostate, colon, and rectum is more common in men who are overweight, while women are at risk for cancers associated with elevated levels of estrogen, including endometrial, breast, cervical, and ovarian cancer, as well as cancer of the gallbladder.

Gynecologic Disorders. Irregular menstrual periods, menometrorrhagia, and reduced fertility are associated with increased body weight.

Patient Evaluation

A history, physical examination, and laboratory evaluation should be performed on an obese patient starting a weight loss regimen. The medical history and physical examination should focus on causes and complications of obesity to assess the risk of obesity in each case, guide treatment, and assist with prognosis. BMI should be calculated and waist circumference measured to assess risk, as well as to offer a measure of outcome in addition to weight loss (Box 58-4).

Box 58-4. Steps in Evaluating and Treating the Overweight and Obese Patient

Calculate BMI.
Measure waist circumference.
Review the patient's medical condition:
- Look for causes of obesity, including the use of medications known to cause weight gain.
- Assess comorbidities: how many are present, and how severe are they? Do they need to be treated in addition to the effort at weight loss?

Does the patient want to lose weight? If not, urge weight maintenance and manage comorbidities.
If yes, work with the patient to set reasonable goals.
Develop a treatment plan based on Table 58-3.

History. The history is important for evaluating risk and deciding on treatment. Family history is important because of the strong heritability of obesity. Questions should address age of onset of obesity, minimum weight as an adult, events associated with weight gain, recent weight loss attempts, and previous weight loss modalities used successfully and unsuccessfully, and their complications. Loss of weight to below adult minimum weight is unusual, for example, and an earlier age of onset of obesity often but not always predicts a less successful outcome. A treatment modality that was previously unsuccessful or during which the patient experienced complications should generally be avoided. A history of eating disorders, bingeing, and purging by vomiting or laxative abuse are relative contraindications to treatment, and referral to a specialist in these areas is indicated. Alcohol and substance abuse require specific treatment that should take precedence over obesity treatment. Cigarette smoking can complicate treatment history, since weight is often gained when the patient stops smoking. While smoking cessation should be urged, implementing a diet and exercise program upon or before stopping can minimize weight gain.

The patient's current level of physical activity is important to determine the starting point for exercise recommendations. Some individuals may be completely sedentary, while others are vigorously active, and the same recommendation to both would be inappropriate. Similarly, the patient's understanding of nutrition will determine whether a basic or a more sophisticated level of nutrition education should be taught. This evaluation is crucial toward helping the patient get the most out of each session. Material that is too advanced won't be retained, and material that is too basic will be boring.

Although the causes of obesity are not fully known, certain factors clearly play a role. Diseases such as polycystic ovarian disease and hypothyroidism are known causes of weight gain and require specific treatment (even though that treatment alone may not result in weight loss). Patients may also exhibit substantial weight gain in the year before developing type 2 diabetes mellitus.

The clinician should search for complications of obesity, such as hypertension, type 2 diabetes, hyperlipidemia, CHD, osteoarthritis of the lower extremities, gallbladder disease, gout, and certain cancers. As previously mentioned, obesity in men is associated with colorectal and prostate cancer; in women, it is associated with endometrial, gallbladder, cervical, ovarian, and breast cancer. Signs and symptoms of these disorders, such as vaginal or rectal bleeding, may have been overlooked by the patient and should be carefully reviewed by the physician.

The clinician should also be alert to the possible presence of obstructive sleep apnea, which is a disorder that is often overlooked in obese patients. Symptoms and signs include very loud snoring or cessation of breathing during sleep that is often followed by a loud clearing breath then brief awakening. The patient may be a restless sleeper; some persons find that they can only sleep comfortably in the sitting position. The patient's partner may best describe these symptoms. Daytime fatigue, with episodes of sleepiness at inappropriate times, and morning headaches also occur. On examination, hypertension, narrowing of the upper airway, scleral infection, and leg edema, secondary to pulmonary hypertension, may be observed. Laboratory studies may show polycythemia. If signs of sleep apnea are present, referral to a pulmonologist or sleep specialist is appropriate.

The use of medications that may cause weight gain (Box 58-5) is important. In some cases, it may be possible to change medications in favor of those that do not cause weight gain. The use of medications that may interact with planned treatment, such as monoamine oxidase (MAO) inhibitors and other antidepressants should be elicited. In addition, some patients take over-the-counter (OTC) weight control products and cold remedies that the clinician must be aware of because of side effects and possible interactions with medications that may be prescribed. Examples include pseudoephedrine and phenylpropanolamine, which may be found in cold remedies and diet products, and ephedra (ma huang), which is a nonspecific β-agonist found in diet products. Both are contraindicated if prescribing a sympathomimetic appetite suppressant.

Physical Examination. The clinical manifestations of the complications of obesity are the major targets of the physical examination. Height and weight should be measured and the BMI calculated. Waist circumference should be assessed with a tape measure (see Box 58-3). Blood pressure should be checked with an appropriately-sized cuff. Examine the thyroid and look for manifestations of hypothyroidism (although important to find because it requires specific treatment, thyroid hormone supplementation does not result in weight loss in most patients). In addition, acanthosis nigricans, which suggests hyperinsulinemia, leg edema, cellulitis, and intertriginous rashes with signs of skin breakdown are often seen in the very obese.

Recall the other disorders associated with obesity and look for their signs and symptoms: type 2 diabetes, hyperlipidemia, CHD, osteoarthritis of the lower extremities, gallbladder disease, gout, and colorectal and prostate cancer in men and endometrial, gallbladder, cervical, ovarian, and breast cancer in women.

Laboratory Tests. Laboratory evaluations should focus on risk assessment and the discovery of the causes and complications of obesity, such as type 2 diabetes, gout, hyperlipidemia, and hepatic steatosis. Other laboratory tests may indicate disorders, such as hypothyroidism and hyperinsulinemia, that may be involved in the induction of obesity and require specific treatment. Complete evaluation might include laboratory tests for glucose, uric acid, BUN, creatinine, uric acid, ALT, AST, total and direct bilirubin, alkaline phosphatase, total cholesterol, HDL, LDL, triglycerides, complete blood count, TSH, and urinalysis. In some cases, a 2-hour postprandial insulin level is valuable in diagnosing hyperinsulinemia. At present, serum leptin levels and genetic studies are research tools. Measurements of body composition, using bioelectrical impedance, while motivating to some patients, are not necessary for treating the average patient.

Box 58-5. Drugs That May Promote Weight Gain

Phenothiazines
Antidepressants
Lithium
Neuroleptics
Hormonal contraceptives
Corticosteroids
Progestational steroids
Insulin
Sulfonylureas
Thiazolidinediones
Antihistamines
β-Adrenergic blockers

NOTE: While these drugs may cause weight gain in some patients, they will not affect weight in others. Consideration should be given to changing a patient's regimen if possible, if weight gain is noted in concordance with the use of a medication.

WEIGHT MANAGEMENT

Patient Selection

While healthy eating and the performance of behaviors that prevent weight gain should be encouraged in every patient, the primary target for treatment should be those individuals at risk because of their excess weight. This includes overweight and obese patients with a BMI greater than 25, particularly in the presence of comorbidities. Table 58-3 outlines a guide to selecting the appropriate treatment based on BMI.

Contraindications to Treatment

In general, obesity treatment is contraindicated during pregnancy, in patients with anorexia nervosa, or in patients in the terminal stage of an illness. Medical or psychiatric illnesses should be stable before weight reduction is initiated. Patients with cholelithiasis and osteoporosis must be warned that these conditions may be aggravated by weight loss. Weight loss during lactation is possible, provided milk production is well-established, and less aggressive treatment, such as a mildly hypocaloric diet, is utilized and monitored by a dietitian.

Assessing the Patient's Readiness to Lose Weight

The physician should assess the patient's readiness to lose weight before attempting to treat obesity, because an unwilling patient rarely if ever succeeds, which frustrates both the

Table 58-3. Guide to Selecting Treatment

	BMI category					
	<24.9	25-26.9	27-29.9	30-35	35-39.9	>40
Treatment						
Diet, exercise, behavior therapy	–	With comorbidities	With comorbidities	+	+	+
Pharmacotherapy	–	–	With comorbidities	+	+	+
Surgery	–	–	–	–	With comorbidities	+

From *Practical guide to the identification, evaluation, and treatment of overweight and obesity in adults* (preprint), Bethesda, Md, September, 1998, National Institutes of Health and the North American Association for the Study of Obesity.

patient and the practitioner. If the patient does not wish to lose and is not at high risk, weight maintenance should be encouraged. If the patient is at high risk, the clinician should make an effort to motivate the patient by discussing the medical consequences related to the patient's case.

Goals of Obesity Treatment

Given the current state of knowledge and technology, the goal of obesity treatment should be the lowest weight the patient can comfortably maintain, which in the average patient is about 5% to 10% of total body weight or 2 BMI units. Attaining "ideal" body weight or a loss of 20% or 30% or more of total body weight is not possible for the vast majority of overweight individuals. Loss of as little as 5% to 10% of body weight can improve risk factors associated with obesity.[2,6] Unfortunately, most patients are disappointed with not achieving their personal goal, or "dream" weight, which may contribute to the poor long-term results of obesity treatment.

To prevent disappointment, the patient should be counseled that his or her body might not allow the magnitude of weight loss sought and that cosmetic goals should be discouraged. Alternative goals may include improvement in comorbidities, mobility, and feelings of well-being, a reduction in waist circumference, and simple adherence to a diet and exercise regimen. Remind the patient that research indicates that overweight men who exercise ½-hour per day have a lower risk of dying than thin ones who are completely sedentary. These alternative goals are achievable, while a cosmetic ideal is often not achieved.

Prevention of weight gain is another important treatment goal that is often minimized, but which may have an enormous positive impact on health. Many obese patients come for treatment as a result of recent weight gain. The fact that they have gained weight puts them at risk for further weight gain, and prevention must be stressed.

TREATMENT

Calorie-Restricted Diets

To induce weight loss, a calorie deficit must be created. Dieting, or a change in eating habits that results in a reduction of body weight, is the most widely used approach and is appropriate as a first-line treatment in patients seeking an appropriate BMI.[6,14] Caloric restriction may be achieved in one of two ways. First, general guidelines for healthy eating, such as a reduction in fat, sugar, and alcohol intake, may be emphasized without calorie guidelines. This method is recommended in patients with a BMI < 25 but may also be utilized in patients with a greater BMI. Second, intentional caloric restriction with a food or formula diet may be tried. Compliance is enhanced by structure, which may include attendance at an organized program, a daily meal plan, a regular exercise regimen, and record-keeping. Results at 6 months to 1 year show 2% to 7% mean body weight loss over this period, depending on the intensity of the program. Most weight is lost over the first 4 months with a plateau of weight loss thereafter.[6,15]

Many primary care providers feel uncomfortable prescribing a diet because of lack of formal training and time constraints. Dietitians in the community or hospital setting can provide customized diet and support that can help the patient to succeed. Balanced diets should contain a minimum of 1000 to 1200 kcal/day and have adequate amounts of all essential nutrients. Support for the clinician treating obesity in the office, including sample diets and other patient education material, may be found in the NIH publications, *Clinical Guidelines on the Identification, Evaluation and Treatment of Overweight and Obesity in Adults—The Evidence Report,*[6] the *Practical Guide to the Identification, Evaluation, and Treatment of Overweight and Obesity in Adults (preprint),*[14] or on the NIH website at www.nhlbi.nih.gov/nhlbi/cardio/obes/prof/guidelns/ob_home.htm.

Sweet, fatty foods, such as ice cream, cakes, and chocolate, are highly palatable and calorie dense. Consumption of foods such as these can increase body weight over time in susceptible individuals and can be difficult to fit into a weight loss program. Calories consumed as fat are easier to overeat because they are "denser" (9 cal/gm vs. 4 cal/gm for protein and carbohydrate), easily hidden in foods, and increase food palatability. When compared with carbohydrate, fat may have a delayed effect on satiety that makes it more likely to be overeaten. Despite an apparent decrease in fat intake over the past decade, the weight of Americans continues to rise. Among other possibilities, it seems clear that total calorie intake rather than fat content alone is of primary importance and that eating too many calories of low-fat foods may prevent weight loss or lead to weight gain.

Behavioral Therapy

Behavioral techniques are not used alone but in conjunction with all other approaches, including diet and exercise, medication, or surgery.[4,6,14] The goal of behavior therapy is to overcome barriers to compliance with a diet and physical activity regimen. Behavior therapy assumes that patterns of eating and physical activity are learned behaviors and can be modified and that the environment must be changed to change these patterns over the long term. In some cases, behavioral therapy is administered on an individual basis and in other cases as group sessions. Professionals with training in psychology or a related area who can engage a group in a cohesive manner are optimal for leading such groups. Many commercial weight loss programs and self-help groups use lay leaders or successful patients; in some cases, these individuals are not prepared for the complexity of dealing with the problems that arise. More than 100 controlled trials have been published demonstrating the effectiveness of behavioral techniques, which have become more sophisticated over time.

Although dozens of behavioral techniques are used as part of the behavioral treatment of obesity, the following have been shown to enhance compliance with a program of diet and exercise.

Self-monitoring is a component of all behavioral interventions. It involves recording behaviors, including time and place of eating, associated thoughts and feelings, feeling of control, and who else was present; food consumed, including portion sizes and calorie content; and exercise, including length of sessions and intensity. By reviewing this diary with a member of the treatment team, the patient can get specific feedback about situations that are high risk and interventions that may help. In many cases a simple food and exercise diary is effective.

Stimulus control helps the patient to identify and change cues that are associated with eating too much and exercising too little. For example, limiting exposure to food by keeping it out of sight and avoiding food handling, preparation, or purchase, particularly of problem foods, may be helpful in some individuals. Eating may be limited to specific times and places separated from other activities such as reading or watching television. Efforts are made to break routine eating, which results from a long-term and ingrained "automatic" chain of behavior.

Stress management helps the patient to cope with stressful events by developing better *problem-solving skills* and having outlets other than eating, like meditation, for reducing stress. Problem solving (identifying problem areas and generating solutions) is important for evaluating setbacks, determining how to do better next time, and breaking the chain of negative thinking ("I blew my diet with that donut, I may as well eat the whole box") and self-punishment.

Reinforcement is used to enhance the perceived benefit of positive behaviors, such as dietary compliance and exercise, often in the face of physical discomfort experienced as part of that compliance. Reinforcement can come from the therapist, friends and family as part of *social support,* or the patient alone may utilize getting nonfood rewards for reaching goals.

Cognitive change addresses potentially self-defeating negative thoughts, beliefs, and attitudes to increase the chances of success.

Relapse prevention skills recognize that obesity is a chronic disease requiring chronic treatment and are aimed at teaching patients coping skills so that when lapses occur (an almost predictable sequence of events leading to "collapse"), the patient's willful discontinuation of efforts at weight control can be averted.

Crisis intervention, a more intensive, structured program than is usually utilized in weight maintenance might be indicated at such a point.

A summary of recent studies[15] combining behavioral treatment with moderate dietary restriction and exercise as part of a comprehensive program showed 8.5 kg average weight loss from an initial average weight of 91.9 kg over 21 weeks of treatment with a 22% rate of attrition. A 5.6 kg loss was maintained after 1 year of follow-up. Behavior therapy, a structured diet, nutrition education, and increased physical activity constitute the first-line approach for the vast majority of patients, and perhaps the only approach suggested for those with a BMI less than 30 who have no comorbid conditions. Longer periods of treatment yield better results, and continued intermittent treatment is appropriate.

Exercise

Physical activity plays an important role in increasing energy expenditure and is a key component of any weight maintenance program.[12,14] Weight loss is accompanied by a striking reduction in total energy expenditure, seemingly as part of the body's effort to halt weight loss and facilitate the regain of lost weight. Recent evidence suggests that variations in energy expenditure during daily activities aside from exercise (Non-Exercise Activity Thermogenesis [NEAT]) determines how much weight is gained during a prolonged period of experimental overeating in humans. This result may be due to an increase in "fidgeting" or an intrinsic property of muscle. Clinical studies, however, suggest that the effect of exercise appears to be greater on preventing weight regain than it is in facilitating weight loss. In effect, it is possible that exercise prevents a compensatory mechanism that reduces energy expenditure with weight loss from functioning as effectively.

Cardiovascular training, or aerobic activity, is most often utilized for weight management because of the large number of calories expended during its performance and because fat is burned once a certain threshold is reached. Anaerobic strength training, or resistance exercise such as circuit weight training, is now being recommended as well because it builds lean body mass and may induce changes in body composition that favor a lower body fat mass. Most importantly, the overweight patient can achieve health benefits from regular exercise even if he or she remains overweight, mainly by improving cardiovascular risk factors. Regular adherence to an exercise program may also promote dietary compliance or be a marker of better dietary compliance and improve quality of life by enhancing self-esteem, reducing stress, and relieving depression.

Any physical activity that the patient enjoys and is willing to perform is recommended. For the completely sedentary patient, walking is often the best way to get started. Patients with physical limitations secondary to arthritis or size may start with water exercises, bedside stretching, seated activities, or a program designed by an exercise physiologist or physical therapist. In general, 30 to 45 minutes of exercise 3 to 5 days per week is recommended, although more is better and greater intensity may be better. No maximum has been suggested, but generally up to 1 hour daily, with 1 day off is reasonable. Three 10-minute periods of activity yield about the same benefit as a single 30-minute period, and compliance with such a program is better. Increasing physical activity during daily life, such as climbing stairs instead of taking an elevator; walking or cycling rather than taking a car; and parking further away from the entrance to the mall, can be simple ways to add small periods of physical activity to a busy lifestyle.

Formula Diets

Liquid formula diets of 800 calories given as 4 or 5 (or more) "shakes" per day are also known as supplemented fasts. At present, there is no evidence that using less than 800 calories per day is of any benefit, and the use of such a diet is not recommended. Starvation diets or "water fasting" is not recommended because of the excessive loss of lean body mass and the risk of cardiac arrhythmias. Examples of liquid formula diets include Optifast, HMR, and Medifast.

These diets are only appropriate for well-informed patients with a BMI greater than 30 who have not been successful with other methods. They are contraindicated during pregnancy and breastfeeding and in patients with bulimia and anorexia nervosa and relatively contraindicated in patients with type 1 diabetes, renal or liver disease, unstable angina, and malignant dysrhythmias and in patients with systemic infections and protein-wasting disorders that include use of corticosteroids. Formula diets provide superior weight loss (1.5 to 2.5 kg/week) and rapidly reduce the severity of a number of complications of obesity, including diabetes, hypertension, hyperlipidemia, and sleep apnea. Under careful medical supervision, a 90-day formula diet has been shown to be safe in patients with more than 50 lbs to lose. Common side effects include fatigue, weakness, dizziness, constipation or diarrhea, dry skin, irregular menses, brittle nails, and nausea. Electrolyte abnormalities are rare with modern, properly-used formula diets, but hyperuricemia and gout, which respond to liberalization of calories and carbohydrate, can occur. Gallstones develop in about 11% of patients and 25% become symptomatic, although patients on traditional diets have also been noted to develop gallstones. The use of ursodiol can prevent gallstone formation. Cardiac risk, initially a concern in the late 1970s, has been shown to be as low as expected in similarly obese individuals not dieting.

These diets *must* be combined with support and behavior, nutrition, and exercise education.[4,6,15] If used alone, rapid weight regain is almost certain, even if the diet is "medically supervised." Even if a comprehensive program is used, long-term follow-up shows no difference when compared with a balanced diet. In the short-term, however, since compliance is higher and if losing weight is medically important, formula diets can be considered.

Fad Diets

Fad diets and other diet methods often promise a quick, easy way to lose weight. Unfortunately, these methods distract the patient from the real task at hand. While many methods of unhealthy dieting can reduce weight in the short run, the true test comes in long-term weight loss. Diets that are too drastic are difficult to follow long-term: unfortunately, the patient too often bears the blame for the lack of success, adding to a vicious cycle of failure.

Medication

The concept of using medication for the treatment of obesity has undergone radical changes over the past few years.[1,3] The new understanding of obesity makes it appear as much a metabolic, endocrine disorder as diabetes; therefore obesity also deserves a medical treatment when indicated. The side effect profile of early amphetamine-based appetite suppressants was severe, and their use led to addiction and habituation because escalating doses were often needed to maintain lost weight. As a result, medications were used in the short-term to induce weight loss and were then discontinued, leaving the patient to maintain the weight loss. When patients inevitably regained weight, they were blamed for not having enough motivation. Later appetite suppressants, such as phentermine, diethylpropion, and phendimetrazine, had fewer side effects but had limited impact since only short-term studies were performed in which weight loss, rather than improvement in comorbidity, was usually the only outcome measured. As a result, most states limited prescriptions to a maximum of 3 months.

In 1992, the publication of a small 4 year-long trial of phentermine and fenfluramine by Weintraub popularized the notion of chronic treatment. Dexfenfluramine was approved for long-term use in 1996 after 10 years of use around the world. However, concerns about unacceptable side effects, primarily regurgitant valvular lesions of the heart and pulmonary hypertension, led to the withdrawal of fenfluramine and dexfenfluramine in September 1997. In November 1997, the FDA approved sibutramine for long-term use in obesity, and in April 1999, orlistat was approved for long-term use.

In general, medication helps patients to comply with a reduced calorie regimen (Table 58-4). Not every patient responds to a given medicine. If a patient loses more than 4 pounds during the first month, the prognosis for losing more than 5% of body weight is good. If not, consideration should be given to changing medication after another month of treatment.

Drugs Approved for Long-term Use. Sibutramine (Meridia), a norepinephrine and serotonin reuptake inhibitor (SNRI), was originally developed as an antidepressant but was more effective at reducing weight.[3] Although a schedule IV compound, sibutramine demonstrated little or no evidence for abuse or habituation like the other drugs in the SNRI category. A 1-year placebo-controlled trial demonstrated that 65% of patients who received 15 mg sibutramine daily lost more than 5% of body weight compared with only 29% of patients taking placebo; and 39% lost more than 10% of their body weight compared with 8% reaching the same mean weight loss in the placebo-treated group. Health benefits demonstrated with the use of sibutramine include reductions in triglycerides, uric acid, total cholesterol, and LDL cholesterol and an increase in HDL cholesterol. Adverse events seen during randomized trials included dry mouth, constipation, insomnia, increased appetite, dizziness, and nausea. A mean increase in blood pressure of 4 mm Hg was also seen in trials. The increase is less in patients who lose more than 5% of body weight and who would be most likely to continue treatment. About 12% of patients have an increase in systolic blood pressure of 15 mm Hg or more; however, less than 1% of patients treated had to be withdrawn from trials as a result of an increase in blood pressure. Blood pressure and pulse should be checked 2 to 4 weeks after starting the drug and then monthly for the first 6 months, then every 2 months or more often if indicated. If a patient with hypertension is getting good weight loss, you may consider treating the blood pressure more aggressively for a period to see if it drops with continued weight loss. The majority of patients who lose weight experience a drop in blood pressure.

Orlistat (Xenical), an inhibitor of pancreatic lipases, prevents the absorption of 30% of fat consumed, thus reducing caloric intake.[7] Analysis of patients completing a

Table 58-4. Weight Loss Drugs

Drug	Dose	Action
Long-term use		
Sibutramine (Meridia)	5, 10, 15 mg 10 mg PO daily to start, may be increased to 15 mg or decreased to 5 mg	Norepinephrine, dopamine, and serotonin reuptake inhibitor; reduces appetite, increases thermogenesis
Orlistat (Xenical)	120 mg 120 mg PO tid before meals	Inhibits pancreatic lipase, decreases fat absorption
Short-term use*		
Phentermine (Ionamin, Adipex, Fastin)	15, 30 mg 15 mg to start	Norepinephrine and dopamine release; reduces appetite
Diethylpropion (Tenuate)	25 mg, 75 mg long acting 25 mg PO tid before meals	Norepinephrine and dopamine release; reduces appetite

*Short-term use is 3 months or less.

1-year placebo-controlled trial demonstrated that 55% of patients treated with orlistat lost more than 5%, and 25% lost more than 10% of their body weight compared with 33% and 15%, respectively, achieving the same mean weight loss in the placebo-treated group. In addition, orlistat slowed down the rate of weight regain in the second year of treatment. Health benefits demonstrated in clinical trials of orlistat include a reduction in LDL and increase in HDL cholesterol, reduction in blood pressure and fasting insulin levels, improvement in oral glucose tolerance test outcomes, and improved glycemic control in obese diabetics. The gastrointestinal side effects associated with orlistat use were usually mild in intensity and occurred early in treatment. Dropout rates due to side effects have been low in controlled trials. No effect on mineral balance, gallstone, or renal stone formation was seen. A mild reduction in the levels of vitamin D and beta-carotene was noted in some treated patients during trials. Supplementation with a multivitamin taken remotely from a dose of orlistat has been recommended.

Drugs Approved for Short-term Use. Noradrenergic agents, such as the schedule IV drugs phentermine (Ionamin, Fastin, Adipex) and diethylpropion (Tenuate), and the over-the-counter (OTC) drug phenylpropanolamine (Dexatrim, Accutrim) have been shown to be better than placebo in short-term studies. No long-term studies of weight loss or health benefit have been performed. As a result, if these drugs are used for longer than 3 months, the patient must be informed that such use is "off-label" and has not been studied.

Drugs Not Approved for Obesity Treatment. Selective serotonin reuptake inhibitors (SSRI), such as fluoxetine and sertraline, have not been found to be useful in long-term obesity treatment. Studies suggest that weight regain may occur after 6 months of treatment despite ongoing use of the drugs. These drugs have, however, been shown to be beneficial as an adjunct to the behavioral management of binge eating disorder.

Over-the-counter Products. A wide variety of products are available to the public. Some, like chromium picolinate, which is a trace mineral, and chitosan, which is a fiber product, L-carnitine, and hydroxycitric acid, show insufficient efficacy to recommend their use. These products are marketed as "nutritional supplements" with insufficient testing or proof that they work as advertised. Others, like the combination of ephedrine (ephedra, ma huang, herbal "fen/phen") and caffeine (guarana, kola nut) often seen in "fat burning products," have been shown to be effective but are not safe for unsupervised use because of the risk of side effects like tachycardia and hypertension and are not approved for treatment of obesity. Phenylpropanolamine, a sympathomimetic also used widely in OTC decongestants, is also available as an OTC appetite suppressant for short-term use only.

Future Pharmacologic Treatment. The future of the pharmacologic treatment of obesity is particularly promising, with more than fifty new drugs in the early stages of development.[5] Human trials of recombinant leptin are currently underway. Like insulin, leptin and its analogs will be administered either subcutaneously or intravenously, thus limiting its use. Preliminary clinical trials have shown only modest weight loss in a subset of patients.

Other drugs under development include compounds that activate central melanocortin receptors, unbind corticotropin-releasing factor from its binding protein, and β-agonists, which act selectively on skeletal muscle or adipose tissue to increase metabolic rate and lipolysis.

Medical Management of the Obese Diabetic

Drugs that do not cause weight gain should be considered as first-line therapy in the treatment of the obese type 2 diabetic. Metformin (Glucophage), which inhibits intestinal glucose transport, reduces hepatic gluconeogenesis, enhances peripheral glucose uptake by muscle and adipose tissue, and tends to cause weight loss rather the weight gain usually seen with the use of insulin and sulfonylureas. In addition, an increase in HDL, reduction in triglycerides, and even a reduction in blood pressure have been reported. Despite the rare but potentially serious side effect of lactic acidosis, metformin should be considered first-line treatment for overweight type 2 diabetics. Acarbose (Precose), an α-glucosidase inhibitor that slows down the absorption of carbohydrate, is also valuable in minimizing the demand for insulin in an obese type 2 diabetic.

Surgery

Surgery should be considered in obese patients with a BMI greater than 40 or between 35 and 40 who fail other methods of treatment if serious obesity-related complications are present.[6,11] Careful screening of candidates is required if the patient is to benefit from the procedure. Surgical candidates must be motivated and well-informed about the risks of the procedure, as well as the change in their lives that will occur as a result of the procedure and its long-term effects. These changes may be relatively minor, such as the need for long-term treatment with vitamin and mineral supplements, or may include chronic vomiting or diarrhea after meals. In general, weight loss of 60% to 80% of the excess is achieved. Weight loss reaches a maximum at 18 months to 2 years, with some weight regain up to the fifth year postoperatively and weight stability thereafter. Unfortunately, in some surgical series up to 20% of patients ultimately regain all lost weight.

The *vertical-banded gastroplasty* (gastric stapling) is the most commonly performed procedure. A 30 cc pouch with a restricted outlet is constructed along the lesser curvature of the stomach. A Silastic ring or band of Marlex mesh restricts the outlet size, and four rows of staples reinforce the free wall to prevent breakdown. The amount of weight lost is correlated with the volume of the pouch and diameter of the outlet, with larger volume and diameter yielding less weight loss, but fewer side effects. In general, 70% of patients maintain a loss of 20% of total body weight on 5-year follow-up. It is not as effective as the gastric bypass in carbohydrate cravers because of the "soft-calorie syndrome," in which highly caloric liquid or meltable foods are consumed to excess, leading to weight regain.

The *gastric bypass* involves constructing a small proximal gastric pouch as with the gastroplasty, whose outlet is a limb of small bowel of varying lengths, as in a Roux-en-Y gastrojejunostomy. Increasing the length of the loop increases weight loss, as well as long-term side effects and nutrient malabsorption. The procedure produces malabsorption of food and the dumping syndrome; it is effective in patients who might not respond to gastroplasty because of carbohydrate craving. Because of the malabsorption of vitamins and minerals, these patients need careful nutritional instruction and follow-up, as well as behavioral training. More weight is lost with this procedure than with gastroplasty, but the risk of complications is greater.

Mortality associated with obesity surgery is about 1% in the hands of surgeons experienced with these procedures and the perioperative management of the severely obese patient. Early morbidity of both procedures that occur in about 10% of cases include perioperative complications such as wound infection, dehiscence, leaks from staple-line breakdown, stomal stenosis, marginal ulcers, deep vein thrombophlebitis, and other pulmonary problems. Longer-term complications, which occur with both procedures, include cholecystitis and failure to lose weight. Complications of the gastroplasty include pouch and distal esophageal dilation with esophageal reflux and persistent vomiting, with or without stomal obstruction. Additional complications that may occur with the bypass include vitamin and mineral deficiencies, including calcium, B-12, folate, and iron, and dumping syndrome, in which meals are followed by gastrointestinal discomfort, diarrhea, and other symptoms.

In women of childbearing age, the effects of the particular nutrient deficiencies noted with gastric bypass are of concern because of the risk of their known association with fetal damage. In general, women who have had either procedure should be on birth control during the weight loss phase because of the uncertainty and the risks of fetal development in the setting of weight loss and maternal undernutrition. Women who have had these procedures and are at a stable weight may become pregnant, but they must be carefully monitored during pregnancy to prevent such deficiencies. The increased calorie, protein, and nutrient demands must be emphasized along with the usual weight gain of pregnancy.

Despite these risks and complications a large, multicenter study comparing surgery with diet alone has been ongoing in Sweden. The Swedish Obese Subjects (SOS) trial enrolled approximately 4000 patients considered appropriate for obesity surgery. Obesity surgery was performed on 2000 and 2000 have been treated with diet alone. After 4 years of follow-up, surgery has produced substantial weight loss and an improvement in all variables monitored, including new cases of diabetes and hypertension, mortality, time lost from work, mood, and disability, in both men and women.

REFERENCES

1. Aronne LJ: Modern medical management of obesity: the role of pharmaceutical intervention, *J Am Diet Assoc* 2:S23-26, 1998.
2. Blackburn G: Effect of degree of weight loss on health benefits, *Obes Res* 3:211-216S, 1995.
3. Bray G: *Contemporary diagnosis and management of obesity,* Newtown, Penn, 1998, Handbooks in Health Care.
4. Brownell KD, Wadden TA: *The LEARN program for weight control—medication edition,* Dallas, 1998, American Health Publishing.
5. Campfield LA, Smith FJ, Burn P: Strategies and potential molecular targets for obesity treatment, *Science* 280:1383-1387, 1998.
6. Clinical guidelines on the identification, evaluation, and treatment of overweight and obesity in adults—the evidence report, *Obes Res* 6(2):51S-210S, 1998. Available at http://www.nhibi.nih.gov/nhibi/cardio/obes/prof/guideins/ob_home.htm
7. Davidson MH, et al: Weight control and risk factor reduction in obese subjects treated for 2 years with orlistat: a randomized controlled trial, *JAMA* 281(3):235-42, 1999.
8. Hill JO, Peters JC: Environmental contributions to the obesity epidemic, *Science* 280:1371-1374, 1998.
9. Leibel RL, Rosenbaum M, Hirsch J: Changes in energy expenditure resulting from altered body weight, *N Engl J Med* 332:621-628, 1995.
10. Mantzoros CS: The role of leptin in human obesity and disease: a review of current evidence, *Ann Int Med* 130:651-657, 1999.
11. National Institutes of Health: Gastrointestinal surgery for severe obesity, NIH consensus development conference consensus statement March 25-27, 1991, *Am J Clin Nutr* 55:615S-619S, 1992.
12. Pavlou KN, Krey S, Steffe WP: Exercise as an adjunct to weight loss and maintenance in moderately obese subjects, *Am J Clin Nutr* 49:1115-1123, 1989.
13. Porte D, Seely RJ, Woods SC, et al: Obesity, diabetes and the central nervous system, *Diabetologia* 41:863-881, 1998.
14. Practical guide to the identification, evaluation, and treatment of overweight and obesity in adults (preprint), Bethesda, Md, September, 1998, National Institutes of Health and the North American Association for the Study of Obesity.
15. Wadden TA: Treatment of obesity by moderate and severe caloric restriction: results of clinical research trials, *Ann Int Med* 119:688-693, 1993.
16. Woods SC, Seely RJ, Porte D, et al: Signals that regulate food intake and energy homeostasis, *Science* 280:1378-1383, 1998.
17. World Health Organization: Obesity: preventing and managing the global epidemic. Report of a WHO consultation on obesity, Geneva, 1997, World Health Organization.

CHAPTER 59

Domestic Violence

Carole Warshaw
Kim Riordan

In response to the growing recognition of domestic violence as a major public health problem, new standards of care have evolved for addressing intimate partner abuse within the health care setting. The Joint Commission for the Accreditation of Health Care Organizations now requires that hospitals and clinics have protocols and training for identification, assessment, intervention, and referral for victims of abuse and violence. For many victims, the health care setting is the only place they will seek help, and health care providers play a critical role in creating a safe atmosphere for patients to discuss the abuse and violence they have experienced. Yet, many physicians still have difficulty integrating routine inquiry about domestic violence into their day-to-day practice.

Because domestic violence is a complex social problem rather than a strictly biomedical one, addressing it requires more than adding new diagnostic categories to differential diagnoses or new technical skills to clinical repertoires. This complexity obliges physicians to step beyond traditional medical paradigms to confront the personal beliefs and feelings that shape their responses to patients, to consider larger social issues while treating symptoms, and to work in partnership with community groups committed to ending domestic violence. This chapter addresses the challenges faced by clinicians and patients in raising these issues and describes the identification, assessment, and intervention skills that primary care physicians need to respond effectively and sensitively to domestic violence.

BACKGROUND AND EPIDEMIOLOGY

The term *domestic violence,* although sometimes used more broadly, is generally considered synonymous with intimate partner abuse, a phenomenon that is largely directed toward adult women and adolescent girls.* Domestic violence is an ongoing pattern of domination and control perpetrated against a current or former intimate partner through a combination of actual or threatened physical violence, sexual assault, and psychologic abuse. This violence occurs in adult and adolescent dating, married, or separating relationships in gay, lesbian, and heterosexual couples. Random population surveys estimate that 10% to 12% of women experience physical or sexual assault at the hands of an intimate partner each year. Lifetime prevalence rates range from 21% to 34%.[5,6,18]

While a small percentage of victims of partner abuse are male, the US Department of Justice estimates that women are up to eight times more likely than men to be victimized by an intimate partner.[19] When women do assault male partners, it is more likely to be in self-defense and rarely as part of an ongoing pattern of coercion and control. Domestic violence is also a significant problem in same-sex relationships, and initial research indicates that prevalence rates may be similar to those found among heterosexual couples. Disabled women face additional risks for physical and sexual violation by caretakers and attendants and are likely to be trapped for longer periods of time. Elder abuse, too, may reflect longstanding domestic violence rather than more recent caregiver stress.

Physical violence is only one of many tactics batterers use to harm their victims, to undermine their autonomy and sense of self, and to keep them isolated and entrapped. Sexual violation is particularly degrading and often the most difficult to discuss. Whenever there is physical or sexual abuse, however, psychologic abuse is invariably present and may be quite severe. This often takes the form of verbal intimidation and threats, ridicule and humiliation, stalking and monitoring the victim's activities, isolating the victim from friends and family, and controlling their access to money, education, and jobs. Emotional withdrawal, threats of abandonment, and threats to harm or take away children are also powerful tactics of coercion and control.[11] Abuse survivors describe this as the most devastating aspect of their experience.

Medical Consequences

Over the past 2 decades, research has begun to document the impact of abuse and violence on women's health. Prevalence studies indicate that approximately 5% to 27% of women seen in a range of clinical settings are currently being abused by their partners. Between 21.4% and 54.2% of women seen in emergency departments or primary care clinics have reported physical or emotional abuse by a partner in adulthood, and at least one in three have experienced some form of abuse during their lives.[1,5,11] While, almost any type of injury can result from domestic violence, primary care providers often see the later consequences of these assaults. In addition to visible injuries and scars, physical abuse may present as chronic pain, complications of head and neck trauma (e.g., seizures, difficulties with performance and concentration), or deprivation of basic needs (e.g., food, water, shelter, medication, and sleep).

The majority of abused women, however, seek help for medical problems rather than physical injuries.[12,17] Although acute injuries may be the most obvious manifestation of domestic violence, the long-term medical and psychologic consequences of living with ongoing abuse tend to be more debilitating over time. For example, there are significant differences in health status between abused and nonabused women, even when the abuse is emotional and not physical, and psychologic abuse is more predictive of low self-esteem, depression, and posttraumatic stress disorder (PTSD) than physical abuse. Health and mental health status are further diminished in women who were subjected to victimization in childhood as well.[9]

Women who are being abused frequently present with exacerbations or poor control of chronic medical conditions, such as diabetes, hypertension, asthma, or angina, or develop

This chapter was adapted in part from Warshaw C: Identification, assessment and intervention with victims of domestic violence. In Warshaw C, Ganley A, Salber P: *Improving the health care response to domestic violence: a resource manual for health care providers,* San Francisco, 1998, The Family Violence Prevention Fund.

*Male pronouns are generally used in referring to perpetrators of domestic violence, while feminine pronouns are generally used to reference victims. This is not meant to detract from those cases where the victim is male or the perpetrator is female. This pronoun use reflects the fact that the majority of domestic violence victims are female.

sleep and appetite disturbances, fatigue, dizziness, weight change, and other physical symptoms associated with depression, anxiety, or posttraumatic stress. Other illnesses, such as gastrointestinal and autoimmune disorders, have also been associated with abuse.[7,20] Sometimes, however, women seek help for problems that are seemingly unrelated to abuse—a blood pressure check, a routine physical, treatment of allergies, or an upper respiratory infection.

Complications of pregnancy, prolonged labor, preterm deliveries, low-birth-weight infants, and postpartum difficulties are also found at higher rates among women who are abused.[15] Battered women, particularly when subject to sexual abuse, may experience dyspareunia, chronic pelvic pain, sexual dysfunction, and frequent vaginal and urinary tract infections. Sexual coercion increases women's risks for exposure to any of the complications of unprotected sex, such as human immunodeficiency virus/acquired immunodeficiency syndrome (HIV/AIDS), sexually transmitted diseases (STDs), and unplanned pregnancies, and must be addressed during safe sex counseling.

Mental Health Consequences of Abuse and Violence

At a time when primary care providers are encouraged to diagnose and treat common psychiatric disorders, it is important to recognize that many of these disorders are more prevalent among patients who have been abused. Studies of battered women indicate that 37% to 63% meet criteria for depression,[3] 46% for anxiety disorders, and 33% to 58% for posttraumatic stress responses or PTSD.[5,12] Somatoform disorders, eating disorders, sexual difficulties, and psychotic episodes have also been correlated with adult and childhood abuse. Partner abuse is a significant risk factor for suicide attempts as well.[17]

Strong correlations also exist between battering and substance abuse among both victims and perpetrators. This relationship is a complex one. Alcohol consumption may contribute to violent behavior in already abusive men, but there is no evidence that substance abuse actually causes violence against women and children. Research also indicates that alcohol and drug use among abuse survivors is more likely to result from the victimization itself (e.g., self-medication or coercion into consuming alcohol and other drugs).[8]

A diagnosis of PTSD is often used to describe the psychophysiologic sequelae that follow sexual assault, battering, and child sexual abuse.[5] People who have been assaulted develop responses similar to victims of other types of trauma: shock, confusion, helplessness, and betrayal, as well as dissociation, intrusive recollections, increased reactivity to reminders of the trauma, avoidance of possible triggers, and continuing hypervigilance. Research on the neurobiology of trauma indicates that alterations in physiologic reactivity and stress hormone secretion contribute to these responses.[20] However, when abuse is chronic and severe, involves betrayal by someone trusted and loved, and is deliberately intended to control and undermine the victim's sense of self, a more complex set of responses may ensue. In fact, the frequency of comorbidity associated with PTSD has led a number of authors to conceptualize comorbidity as a misnomer and to propose that a more complex form of PTSD may be found among those who experience longstanding abuse.[2] Disorders of extreme stress not otherwise specified (DESNOS) incorporates a broader spectrum of the axis I and axis II sequelae of chronic abuse and is listed as an associated feature of PTSD.

Yet, even these diagnoses do not fully capture patients' psychologic responses to abuse, the perpetrator behaviors that generate them, or the larger contexts in which they emerge. For women who are still at risk, the "stress" is not "post," the trauma is ongoing—symptoms may be an adaptive response to danger and entrapment, and heightened sensitivity can be a necessity for survival.[17] Women often exhibit considerable strength and ingenuity, attempting to remedy their situations through talking, seeking help, fighting back, and trying to change the conditions either that they perceive or are told cause the abuse. When those attempts fail, however, they then may retreat into a mode that appears more passive and "compliant," but which actually reflects how they have learned to reduce their immediate danger. Dissociation, denial, and avoidance may be used to protect against feelings that have become unbearable in the face of limited options for leaving or stopping the violence. For some women, substance abuse becomes another way of "coping" or "leaving." When a person becomes increasingly isolated from outside resources, suicide or homicide may seem like the only way to end the abuse. These responses, while making it possible to survive intolerable conditions, may constrict a person's capacity to reach out for help. In addition, the ongoing trauma of social discrimination, lack of basic resources, and revictimizing experiences within systems a woman turns to for help not only affect her ability to psychically "heal" from the abuse but also to mobilize the resources necessary to build a safe, independent life.

Some patients present with PTSD initially, while others do not develop symptoms until years after they have left. Although avoidant responses may predominate at that time, treatment is still likely to be beneficial. In addition, avoidant posttraumatic stress responses may interfere with taking medication, having regular pap smears or mammograms, or agreeing to invasive medical procedures that may again evoke the experience of physical violation and loss of control.

IDENTIFICATION

Addressing Barriers

Despite the frequency with which battered women present to health practitioners, the abuse itself often goes unrecognized. Early studies indicate that only 6% of battered women were accurately identified in emergency departments.[14] Health care providers give many reasons for not asking about domestic violence—lack of awareness, lack of time, thinking abuse is not that prevalent in their practice, not knowing what to do if abuse is identified, fear of being intrusive, and fear of being overwhelmed. Physicians may avoid asking because they find it difficult to tolerate the pain and helplessness they feel in hearing patients talk about abuse or having their own traumatic experiences evoked by listening to another's. In addition, when professional competence is tied to one's sense of mastery and control, it is harder to deal with situations that require an empathic presence rather than the ability to "fix" or cure. Clinician attitudes toward gender roles and family privacy may also prevent them from asking. Physicians, nonetheless, do overcome discomfort about other "private" matters, when they know it will improve clinical care. These barriers can largely be addressed through education, self-reflection, support from colleagues, and knowledge of community resources.[21]

Patients also face numerous barriers to discussing abuse, accessing services, and leaving abusive partners. For example, threats of retaliation are common and abusers often try to prevent their partners from seeking help. In addition, patients may feel shame about the abuse and not want to risk being judged or blamed. Not trusting that a provider will understand their situation—loving a partner, hoping he'll change, wanting their children to grow up in an intact home, or not being able to survive financially on their own—can also prevent disclosure. Gay men and lesbians may be particularly reluctant to discuss abuse if they do not know how their provider feels about same-sex relationships. Immigrant women are frequently threatened with deportation and not aware of laws that can protect them. Cultural or religious constraints can also make it harder for a woman to discuss the abuse with someone outside her community, and she may face social isolation and ostracism if she leaves. A person's attitudes toward revealing personal information to outsiders and feelings of loyalty toward a partner, family, or community will play a role in how they feel about discussing the abuse and with whom they feel comfortable discussing it. Despite these concerns, studies consistently show that most women are relieved when a physician asks them about abuse.

Universal Screening

One of "the most important contributions physicians can make to ending abuse and protecting the health of its victims is to identify and acknowledge the abuse."[4] Because presentations of domestic violence are so varied, inquiring only when abuse is suspected is no longer considered adequate. Current guidelines for domestic violence recommend routine inquiry of all women patients and although less studied, men who may be at risk—men with disabilities, elderly men, and men in gay relationships.[10] Because the field is new, interventions are only beginning to be evaluated. Recent studies, however, demonstrate that advocacy and counseling significantly reduce violence, increase quality of life, and help women expand their networks of support.[16]

Before inquiring about domestic violence, it is essential to create an environment in which it is safe for patients to talk freely. Visibly displayed posters and brochures can help create this kind of atmosphere. A battered woman may be afraid to disclose information if she thinks the batterer will learn she has talked about the abuse or she may fear losing her children to protective services. Patients should be told that the information they give is confidential and within the confines of the law will not be revealed to the batterer or anyone else without their permission. For those physicians who practice in states with mandatory reporting laws, it is essential to inform the patient of this requirement in the beginning of the evaluation, preferably before she or he has discussed the abuse. It is also important to discuss reporting obligations before inquiring about child abuse.

All patients should be interviewed in private until abuse is ruled out, because any accompanying individual could be an abuser. This includes male or female friends, family, personal attendants, and nonprofessional translators who may be sympathetic to the perpetrator. Assailants may appear solicitous and concerned about the patient's well being, impersonate relatives, or insist on being present during the examination. It is helpful to inform accompanying parties that policy requires all patients to be seen alone. Self-report forms should not be mailed to the home before a visit or administered in waiting rooms where the batterer may be present. Strategies should be developed for safely separating patients from abusers should that become necessary. If there appears to be an immediate threat from the abuser, be prepared to notify the police or security, outlining any potential risk (e.g., husband is in waiting room intimidating staff).

Inquiring about domestic violence is the first stage of intervention. Asking about abuse helps to reduce the isolation abused patients experience and lets them know resources are available if and when they feel they can use them. Many women will readily talk about the violence if they feel safe and supported. All women patients seen in primary care settings should be asked at initial visits and at periodic intervals. Inquiry should also take place when a woman's relationship status changes, she is pregnant or contemplating pregnancy, her symptoms suggest abuse, or there are frequent unexplained appointment changes. Screening questions on domestic violence can be easily incorporated into the current and past medical history, social history, and review of systems.

Sometimes it feels awkward to suddenly introduce the subject of abuse, particularly if there are no obvious indications a patient is being abused. Clinicians can help decrease discomfort by framing questions in ways that let patients know that they are not alone and that the clinician is comfortable hearing about domestic violence. Possible questions include: "I don't know if this is happening to you, but many of the women I see as patients are involved with someone who threatens them or tries to control them. Some are too afraid or uncomfortable to bring it up themselves, so I've started asking about it routinely." or "Many of the lesbians and gay men I see are being hurt by their partners. Has your partner ever threatened you or tried to hurt you?"

Because patients may not define themselves as battered, the medical practitioner should always ask direct, specific questions. For example, asking, "Has your partner ever punched or kicked you?" or "Are you ever afraid of your partner?" will be more effective than asking "Are you being battered?" Questions about emotional and sexual abuse should also be included in the assessment (Box 59-1). Sexual histories should always incorporate questions about abuse, for example, "Does your partner ever pressure you to engage in sexual activities that make you uncomfortable or force you to have sex against your will?"

If a patient denies abuse but the clinician is still concerned, he or she can gently voice those concerns, address potential fears about disclosure (e.g., deportation, child custody), and offer information about abuse. Sometimes, a woman will listen silently, without overtly acknowledging what is being said. Clinicians should provide the patient with a referral sheet or telephone numbers and encourage her to let them know if she has any problems in the future and to contact any of the resources provided. Concerns should be documented in the medical record.

ASSESSMENT

Although it usually takes less than a minute to ask initial questions about abuse, listening to the patient and providing adequate assessment and intervention can take somewhat longer. This time can be reduced when a domestic violence advocate or social worker is available to complete the

Box 59-1. Asking About Abuse

Sample Opening Questions

- "Because violence is so common in many women's lives, I've started to ask about it routinely."
- "I'm concerned that some of your medical problems might be the result of someone hurting you. Is that happening?"
- "You mentioned your partner's problem with . . . drinking/temper/stress. When that happens, has he ever threatened you or hurt you?"

Sample Screening Questions

- "Has your partner ever physically hurt you? Has he (or she) ever threatened to hurt you or someone you care about?"
- "Do you feel safe in your current relationship? Are you ever afraid of your partner?" "What kinds of things does he or she do that make you afraid?"
- "Has your partner ever humiliated you, controlled you, or tried to keep you from doing things you want to do?"
- "When you are with your partner, do you feel like you are walking on eggshells?"
- "Has your partner ever forced or pressured you into engaging in sexual activities that made you uncomfortable or into having sex when you didn't want to?"
- "Do you feel you can say no if you don't want to have sex?"

Box 59-2. Validation and Information

Let patients know the following:

- Abuse experiences are common.
- You are glad she (or he) decided to discuss this with you.
- You believe her and are concerned about her safety and well-being.
- You understand how difficult it is for her to change her situation.
- She is not alone in figuring this out, and you will support her through this process.
- The abuse is not her fault, and the perpetrator is solely responsible for stopping his abusive behavior.
- She does not deserve to be treated that way; no one does.
- There are options and resources available. With assistance and support, many women are able to increase their safety and the safety of their children.
- She will not be judged or stigmatized as a result of what she has said to you.
- All information will be confidential within the confines of mandatory reporting laws.

evaluation. At a minimum, providers should let patients know they were glad to be told and address safety, document the abuse and its impact, and make referrals to community agencies.

In the primary care setting, a more detailed history of abuse is warranted. If a patient is being seen for an injury or other symptoms related to an acute battering event, ask in detail about what happened. Inquire specifically as to when the episode started, who inflicted the injuries, and whether there have been prior incidents. Patients should also be asked to describe both current and prior patterns of abuse and the relationship between abuse and the onset or exacerbation of symptoms. When time allows, a complete social history can be obtained, including any history of previous abuse in childhood or adulthood. The following issues are also important to discuss: how the abuse has affected the patient and her children, how she protects her children and herself, what she does to cope, her degree of isolation vs. support, what has she tried in the past, her assessment of the situation, what she would like to see happen, and what issues she faces in achieving those goals.

Safety Assessment

Many abused women are still in danger at the time they seek help and if they decide to leave, the danger may increase significantly. Anyone who is battered should be assessed for risk of serious injury or homicide before discharge. The process of inquiry itself can help clarify the danger the victim faces. Risk factors commonly associated with escalating danger include evidence of violence outside the home, threats of homicide or suicide, and imminent plans to leave (Box 59-2). If, after reviewing all her risk factors, the patient feels she is in danger of being seriously injured or killed, take this very seriously. If she says no, but there is reason to believe she is in danger, discuss this frankly. If she is at high risk and planning to leave the relationship, advise her to seriously consider leaving without telling her partner. Try to assist her in finding a safe place to go.

Mental Health Assessment

While it appears that many battered women do well without mental health intervention because symptoms resolve once they are safe, others need help in managing symptoms before they can mobilize the resources necessary for change. Psychiatric problems including major depression, panic disorder, PTSD, psychosis, suicidality, or substance abuse may hinder a battered woman's ability to assess her situation or take appropriate action. When serious psychiatric conditions are present, an appropriate plan includes psychiatric evaluation and treatment. On the other hand, emotional, behavioral, and cognitive responses to abuse can be misinterpreted as psychiatric in origin.

In either case, assessing and treating the psychiatric manifestations of domestic violence present a number of challenges. Once a woman is given a psychiatric diagnosis, she risks having it used against her in court by the abuser to gain custody of her children or to impugn her credibility. It can also reinforce the abuser's ability to make her feel that she is crazy. If a psychiatric diagnosis is made, discuss these issues with the patient and clearly document the abuse, its relationship to her psychiatric symptoms, and the efforts she has made to protect and care for herself and her children.

Treatment presents its own set of issues. In a busy primary care setting, prescribing medication can easily take the place of time spent with patients. Interventions that focus solely on the victim's symptoms without addressing the abuse itself, however, are not acceptable forms of care. Also, some medications can impair the ability to assess and respond to danger and should be prescribed with caution. If indicated, medication should be offered as a tool to help patients regain their sense of autonomy and control, as well as to manage their symptoms.

Women with psychotic disorders can also be victims of domestic violence. In fact, they are at even greater risk. Physicians must be cautious to take allegations of abuse seriously, even if the patient appears to be delusional. Women with serious mental illness are more vulnerable to repeat victimization, and symptoms may be aggravated by the abuse or by the abuser's control of her medications. Providers must take care not to assume that a partner's history is accurate and never ask him to confirm what a woman has said about the abuse.

Evaluating a woman's safety includes assessing for potential suicide or homicide. Victims of abuse should be asked about suicidal ideation. If there is significant risk, the patient should be kept safe at least until an emergency psychiatric evaluation can be obtained. Homicidal ideation also warrants emergency evaluation. In the majority of cases, women who kill their partners have been severely abused for long periods of time and see no other way out. They kill in self-defense or to prevent themselves or their children from being murdered or seriously injured. If homicide is a possible scenario, the patient should be asked directly if she has plans to kill or harm her partner. Psychiatric hospitalization can be initiated as a way to protect her and the potential victim until safe alternatives can be developed. However, providing her with safe alternatives may obviate this need.

Physical Examination and Preservation of Evidence

Physical examinations and medical procedures can be retraumatizing for patients who have been abused. Care must be taken to explain all procedures, obtain consent, maintain verbal and eye contact, ask what the patient needs to feel safer, and when possible, allow her to control the pace of the examination. Patients should be asked to disrobe and gown so hidden injuries can be seen. A thorough examination should be performed, including neurologic and mental status examinations when indicated.

Injuries should be described specifically (e.g., multiple bilateral contusions to the neck consistent with manual strangulation-like mechanism of injury will support allegations of attempted strangling). Include other details such as areas of tenderness, broken fingernails, smeared makeup, and disheveled or torn hair. If a patient indicates there has been a recent sexual assault, assess for evidence of forced sexual activity, including injuries to the genitalia and restraint marks on the skin. Also, assess the patient's emotional state and her risk for exposure to STDs, HIV, and pregnancy. Record nonbodily evidence of torn clothing and broken jewelry. Preserve as evidence bloodied clothing, foreign objects, or objects used as weapons. Obtain permission from the patient to preserve these items after explaining that evidence may be necessary for legal documentation now or in the future. Have her sign a release of information form and explain the conditions under which the evidence can be released. The clinician's opinion as to whether the injuries are consistent with the explanation given should also be noted.

In cases where there is concern that abuse may be occurring, but the woman does not acknowledge it, be sure to note in the chart whether the injuries are compatible with her explanation. This may provide documentation in the event that she decides to pursue legal action in the future. The names of all personnel who examined or talked with the patient about the abuse should be documented.

Box 59-3. Danger Assessment

- Escalation of threats.
- Obsession with victim (cannot live without her, is stalking or harassing victim).
- Threats of homicide or suicide (e.g., "If I can't have you, no one else will" or "If you leave me I'll kill myself!").
- Weapons, especially firearms, are present in the home or readily accessible.
- Violence outside of the home.
- Violence against the children.
- Abuse during pregnancy.
- Sexual assault.
- Batterer abuses drugs, especially those known to increase violence (amphetamines, PCP, crack cocaine).
- Victim has sought outside intervention to end the abuse.
- Victim has recently left or intends to leave her partner in the near future.
- Batterer has threatened friends or family members.
- Batterer has seriously injured victim in the past.
- Victim states she is afraid for her life.

INTERVENTION

Validation and Empowerment

Intervention begins by letting a battered woman know that she is not alone, that she does not deserve to be abused, that assistance is available, and that this is a place she can continue to come for help whatever she decides to do (Box 59-3). Success should not be measured by whether or not a woman is able to leave an abusive partner. What women describe as most beneficial is being listened to and believed and taken seriously, rather than being judged or given advice they cannot use. Supporting a woman's choices despite fears for her safety is one of the most difficult tasks clinicians face. In addition, the time constraints under which most physicians practice can foster behavior that is controlling and directive—behavior that is particularly disempowering to victims of abuse. Compassionate interactions, however, need not take a lot of time. Respect and concern can be communicated through eye contact and tone of voice and by avoiding body language that conveys one is not interested in hearing about abuse.

Providing Information

It is important to discuss the patterns of abuse in violent relationships. Describing the typical controlling behaviors used by perpetrators and emphasizing that the perpetrator is solely responsibility for stopping the abuse—not the victim—can help patients gain perspective on their own situations. Most violence continues, and isolation, fear, entrapment, and lethality risk tend to increase over time. Many batterers enter counseling solely to keep their partners from leaving. If a woman is seeking help for her abusive partner, discuss what is known about perpetrator interventions. Perpetrators are likely to continue their controlling behaviors even if they stop the physical abuse and many are not willing to make the long-term commitment necessary to change. For a percentage of those who do, approved batterer intervention programs can be effective in reducing re-assault. In addition, women often want their children to grow up in intact homes, yet are deeply concerned for their children's safety. They may wish to stay if the children are not being abused and their partner appears to be a good father. Discussing the long-term traumatic effects of witnessing parental violence can help women weigh these painful alternatives. Finally, it is important to let a woman know that while she faces many difficult choices, there are options available should she decide to leave and that many women are able to find safety and rebuild their lives.

Safety Planning

Women currently in danger should be encouraged to develop safety and escape plans if they are staying with an abusive partner or he has access to them and to explore their options if leaving. Safety planning with a battered woman depends on her situation, her priorities, and the options she decides will work best for her. Many battered women choose to return home after an abusive incident. Sometimes they feel it is their safest option given the nature of the abuser's threats and the realities of the legal protection available to them. Others do not feel they can survive on their own or provide their children with the same resources if they leave. There are a number of things women can do in addition to calling the police or a crisis line or getting a protective order from the courts. If a domestic violence advocate or social worker is not available, clinicians should help patients develop safety plans that are practical and doable (Boxes 59-4 and 59-5). Other women do need to leave their homes and stay somewhere else temporarily, and physicians can explore possible alternatives with their patients. Establishing a working relationship with local domestic violence programs can make this process easier for clinicians. Women often decide to stay with family or friends, but if there are no other options, temporary hospitalization under an assumed name can provide immediate safety.

Contacting the Police

Patients identified as victims of domestic violence should be informed that battering is a crime and that help from the legal system is available. Physicians should ask patients if they want the police to be called and inform them about what to expect when that happens. Clinicians can offer to call themselves or assist the patient in doing so. Domestic violence programs can usually provide information about police and legal system responses within their communities. Patients should be asked if they want someone present during the police report, and if so, efforts should be made for that to happen. The name of the investigating officer and any actions taken should be documented in the patient's record. If the patient is unsure about filing a report, let her know that a paper trail may be beneficial for future court actions and about what protective orders can provide (e.g., eviction, prohibition of contact, financial support). Discuss the possible benefits and dangers of arrest and short-term detention of the abuser. It is important not to pressure patients into filing police reports that may increase their danger. They are usually in the best position to judge their own safety.

Referrals

Providers should maintain an updated list of local domestic violence agencies and other community resources to give to patients who are battered. Numbers can be written on the back of an appointment card or disguised in a list of other services. Many community organizations (e.g., serving lesbians and gay men, immigrant or indigenous communities, and people with disabilities) also have expertise in domestic violence. Domestic violence advocacy programs and shelters provide a wide range of services for battered women and their children, as well as public education and training for service providers (Box 59-6). Most of these services are confidential and either free or available for a nominal fee. While most women do not actually stay in shelters, they do utilize many of the other available services. In addition, domestic violence agencies generally are experienced in dealing with the legal system, the child protective service system, and immigration laws. Many programs also have informational materials that can be adapted for use in the health care setting. These should

Box 59-4. Safety Planning

- Review previous episodes for information that identifies predictable patterns and locations that may be dangerous.
- Anticipate and reduce danger if possible.
- Make provisions for children (rehearse escape strategies, places to stay, numbers to call, how to make credit card calls).
- Locate a safe place to go in an emergency.
- Make provisions for leaving quickly; have necessary items and papers packed, accessible, and hidden from the abuser.
  Police can escort a woman back to the scene if she needs to gather belongings. If an abuser suspects his partner is leaving, however, he may destroy valuable items and papers.
- Open a personal bank account and keep change or phone cards available at all times.
- Keep in touch with friends and get to know neighbors. Reduce isolation as much as possible.
- Develop and rehearse an escape plan.
- Develop a plan for getting help when escape is not possible (e.g., signal to neighbors, teach children to dial 911).

Box 59-5. Safety After a Woman Has Left the Relationship

- Change the locks.
- Install security features.
- Obtain a restraining order.
- Inform neighbors that former partner should not be near your premises.
- Make sure teachers and others who care for the children know who does and does not have permission to pick them up.
- Let co-workers and supervisors know about the situation. Ask them to warn you if the abuser shows up at work.
- Avoid following same routine and utilizing same business as when you lived with the abuser.
- Get counseling and develop a support network.

Box 59-6. Domestic Violence Advocacy Services

- 24-hour hotline and crisis intervention counseling.
- Assistance in evaluating options, resources, safety planning, and referrals.
- Information about legal remedies and legal and court advocacy (e.g., assistance with protective orders).
- Emergency shelter, hotel vouchers, safe homes.
- Counseling, support groups, and referrals for therapy.
- Immigrant rights information (in some areas).
- Advocacy with child protective services.
- Special programs and counseling for children (in some shelters).
- Literacy programs, job training, and transitional housing.
- Appropriate referrals for abusers in some communities.

be made available for women to read during their visits and to take with them if it is safe.

Whenever possible, clinicians should refer to mental health providers who are knowledgeable and sensitive to abuse-related issues and their legal ramifications. Providers should emphasize that a referral does not mean the patient is crazy, but that symptoms are an understandable response to overwhelming trauma. Abuse survivors may benefit from trauma-focused support groups, individual and group psychotherapy, and medication. Although there is some support in the literature for couples counseling when the level of violence is low and the perpetrator has demonstrated a commitment to change, couples therapy is generally contraindicated in cases of domestic violence as it may actually increase the risk of harm to the victim.[5] Many women report serious assaults during or after couples sessions when abuse was discussed. Only if the abuse has ceased for many months to years, the abuser has taken full responsibility for his behavior, and both partners want to rebuild the relationship should this modality be considered.[5,12]

LEGAL OBLIGATIONS

Duty to Report

Because health care providers in some states are required by law to report injuries they suspect resulted from a battering incident, it is important to become familiar with state reporting laws. Statutory reporting mandates vary greatly from state to state based on who is required to report, what kind of injuries need to be reported, penalties for failure to report, and immunity from liability. Clinicians can potentially be held liable for subsequent injuries sustained by a patient who returns to an abusive situation if no inquiries about abuse were made when they initially presented.

While clinicians must be frank about the potential consequences of involving child protective services (inquiry, retaliation by the abuser, losing children to foster care), it is important to discuss the hazards of children continuing to live in a home where they are abused. Let women know there is help available for them and their children. If a woman feels that reporting will provoke immediate retaliation from her partner, help arrange a safe place for her and her children to go.

Duty to Warn

If a medical care provider is aware of a patient's intent to harm a third party, such as the patient's spouse or partner, the provider may have a legal duty to breach the patient's confidence and to warn the third party of the impending danger. In cases of domestic violence, one must intervene in a way that protects both the victim and batterer. The victim must be told of your intention and offered protective services. If commitment to a psychiatric facility is planned, the third party is thus protected and does not have to be warned.

DOCUMENTATION

Medical Record

Thorough, well-documented medical records can be essential for the prevention of further abuse. They provide concrete evidence of abuse and violence that can be crucial in any legal case. For example, if at trial the medical record and the abuser's testimony are in conflict, the record is usually considered more credible. Old records may also be helpful in uncovering and documenting past abuse.

Record the chief complaint and detail the specific descriptions of the abuse, including the identity of the perpetrator, his or her relationship and access to the patient, and the time, date, and location of abusive episodes. Use the victim's own words in quotes whenever possible. For example, "My husband hit me with a bat" is better than "Patient has been battered." Use neutral language, such as "Mrs. Smith says . . ." rather than "the patient alleges." Do not include information that is extraneous to medical facts, such as "It was my fault he hit me because . . ." or "I deserved to be hit because I was . . ." (Box 59-7). If a woman is concerned that documentation may jeopardize her safety, keep separate records in a safe place.

Photographs and Body Maps

Photographs are particularly valuable as evidence and should be offered to all patients with visible injuries. Even if they are not planning to file a case against the assailant at this time, photographs will be very helpful should they decide to do so in the future. Physicians should ask patients for permission and obtain written consent to take photographs. Explain that the photos will become part of the medical record and can only be released to the police or prosecutor with her written permission or by court order. At least one photo should contain the patient's face and something (e.g., coin or ruler) to measure the size of the injuries. Photos should be signed and dated by the patient, photographer, and a witness and placed in a sealed envelope in the patient's record.

A preprinted or hand-drawn body map can be very useful to document injuries that may not show up well in photographs. Each site on the body map should be labeled with the description of the patient's complaint, e.g., mark the area of the scalp and draw a line to a statement, such as, "My scalp hurts when you touch me because last night my husband kept slamming my head against the wall."

Laboratory Tests, X-Rays, and Imaging

X-rays showing old injuries can support a past history of abuse. Laboratory abnormalities can also reflect abuse (e.g., blood sugar level is consistently elevated after episodes of abuse). Reports of computed tomography (CT) scans and other imaging procedures should be documented to provide additional concrete evidence of abuse-related trauma.

Box 59-7. Essential Elements of Documentation

History

- *Chief complaint/history of present illness:* Precise details of the abuse and its relationship to presenting problem. Include relevant trauma history and relationship of abuse to current medical symptoms.
- Use patient's own words: "Jimmy, my husband, hit me in the eye."
- *Past medical history/review of systems:* Any medical, trauma, obstetric, gynecologic, psychiatric, or substance abuse histories that are related to domestic violence or conditions that will affect the patient's safety or ability to deal with the abuse.
- *Sexual history:* Sexual assaults, lack of barrier protection, STDs, unplanned pregnancy, abortions, miscarriages, and ability to use birth control.
- *Medication history:* Relationship between the abuse and the use of psychoactive, analgesic, or other medications.
- *Relevant social history:* Relationship to abuser, living arrangement, abuser's access to victim.

Physical Examination

- Precise details of findings related to abuse, including a neurologic and mental status examination.
- Body map and photographs to supplement written descriptions.
- Standard evidence collection techniques for acute injury or sexual assault.

Laboratory and Other Diagnostic Procedures

- Results of any laboratory tests, x-rays, or diagnostic procedures and their relationship to the abuse.

Safety Assessment

- Information pertaining to the patient's risk for suicide or homicide and potential for serious harm or injury.
- Whether it is safe for patient to go home.
- Safety of children or other dependents.
- Degree of entrapment and level of fear.

Police Report

- Whether report was filed, name of investigating officer, and actions taken.

Options Discussed and Referrals Offered

- Safety plan if returning home or abuser has access.
- Options for staying elsewhere.
- Do not document where she will be if that could endanger her.
- Referrals for patient, children, abuser.

Arrangements for Follow-up/Discharge Information

- Safe number to call her or leave messages.
- Next appointment.
- Information given.

DISCHARGE

When discharging patients, providers should discuss what written material will be safe to take home. Try to avoid writing information about abuse on the discharge instructions if this will increase the likelihood of retaliation, and be sure the patient knows what is written on papers the abuser may see so that she can take precautions (Box 59-8).

Box 59-8. Discharge Review

Have the following been provided?

- Screening for possible abuse.
- Treatment of acute medical and psychiatric problems.
- Assessment and treatment of mental health problems.
- Assessment of pattern and impact of abuse.
- Validation and concern.
- Safety assessment and plan.
- Information about domestic violence in verbal and written form.
- Options for shelter, legal assistance, and counseling.
- Appropriate documentation and evidence collection.
- Appropriate follow-up care (or referral) for her medical, psychologic, and advocacy needs.
- Assurance of confidentiality to extent legally possible.

CONTROVERSIAL ISSUES

Currently, much less is known about how to approach patients who may be batterers. Routine screening of male patients also remains controversial. Screening for perpetration can potentially increase a woman's danger and restrict her ability to return for care, particularly when the physician is treating both members of a couple. Confidentiality must be carefully preserved and physicians should not confront a perpetrator whose partner has revealed abuse. In addition, men who present as "victims" with injuries inflicted by a female partner often turn out to be perpetrators who were injured in self-defense or retaliation. Perpetrators tend to minimize, rationalize, or deny their abusive behavior and may be likeable and charming. Many clinicians find it difficult to knowingly care for an abuser without either colluding with his denial and rationalization or becoming critical and judgmental. Before providers consider asking about perpetration, they should be well grounded in understanding the dynamics of abuse and connected to established advocacy programs in their communities. If a patient does reveal that he engages in abusive behavior, it is important to let him know that persisting in this behavior compromises his own health and safety, as well as that of those he says he cares about. The physician should also make it clear that this behavior is both dangerous and unacceptable. Let the patient know that resources are available in most communities, and encourage him to accept and follow through with a referral to an approved batterers' intervention program. Individual treatment of batterers by physicians is unstudied and, given the current state of expertise in this area, should not be attempted.

SUMMARY

Providing quality health care involves integrating routine inquiry about domestic violence into ongoing clinical practice. This means asking all women patients, as well as others who may be at risk, about abuse in their lives. Whether or not a woman chooses to use services or leave her partner, intervention by health care providers is important. Some women return to violent partners numerous times before they feel safe enough to leave, feel they can survive on their own, or are able to mobilize the resources they will need to do so.

When clinicians fail to ask about abuse, they further isolate patients who are living in great danger. Asking questions can build bridges, decrease isolation, and create hope. Providing a safe place for patients to talk about abuse and consider their options is supportive, fostering their ability to end the violence in their lives. Through their interventions, primary care providers can play a significant role in reducing and preventing domestic violence.

REFERENCES

1. Abbott J, Johnson R, Koziol-McLain J, et al: Domestic violence against women: incidence and prevalence in an emergency room population, *JAMA* 273(22):1763, 1995.
2. Brady KT: Posttraumatic stress disorder and comorbidity: recognizing the many faces of PTSD, *J Clin Psychiatry* 9:12-15, 1997.
3. Campbell J, Kubb J: Depression in battered women, *J Am Med Women's Assoc* 51(3):1996.
4. Council on Ethical and Judicial Affairs, AMA physicians and domestic violence: Ethical considerations, JAMA 14(2):16-21, 1992.
5. Crowell NA, Burgess AW: Understanding violence against women, Washington, 1996, National Academy Press.
6. Dearwater SR, Coben JH, Campbell JC, et al: Prevalence of intimate partner abuse in women treated at community hospital emergency departments, *JAMA* 280(5):433-438, 1998.
7. Drossman DA, Talley NJ, Leserman J, et al: Sexual and physical abuse and gastrointestinal illness. Review and recommendations, *Ann Intern Med* 123(10):774, 1995.
8. Fazzone PA, Holton JK, Reed BG: Substance abuse treatment and domestic violence treatment improvement protocol, Rockville, Md, 1997, US Department of Health and Human Services, Center for Substance Abuse Treatment.
9. Felitti VJ, Anda R, Nordenberg D, et al: Relationship of childhood abuse and household dysfunction to many of the leading causes of death in adults. The adverse childhood experiences (ACE) study, *Am J Prev Med* 13(4):245-258, 1998.
10. Flitcraft A, Hadley S, Hendricks-Mathews MB, et al, eds: Diagnostic and treatment guidelines on domestic violence, Chicago, 1992, American Medical Association.
11. Ganley A: Understanding domestic violence. In Warshaw C, Ganley AL: *Improving the health care response to domestic violence: a resource manual for health care providers,* San Francisco, 1995b, Family Violence Prevention Fund, Pennsylvania Coalition Against Domestic Violence.
12. Koss M, Goodman A, Browne L, et al: No safe haven: male violence against women at home, at work and in the community, Washington, 1994, American Psychological Association.
13. McCauley JM, Kern DE, Kolodner K, et al: The battering syndrome: prevalence and clinical characteristics of domestic violence in primary care internal medicine practices, *Ann Intern Med* 123(10):737-46, 1995.
14. McLeer SV, Anwar R: A study of battered women presenting in an emergency department, *Am J Public Health* 79:65-66, 1989.
15. Parker B, McFarlane J, Soeken K: Abuse during pregnancy: effects on maternal complications and birth weight in adult and teenage women, *Obstet Gynecol* 84(3):323-328, 1994.
16. Parker B, McFarlane J, Soeken K, et al: Testing and intervention to prevent further abuse to pregnant women, *Res Nurs Health* 22:59-66, 1999.
17. Stark E, Flitcraft A: *Women at risk: domestic violence and women's health,* Thousand Oaks, Calif, 1996, Sage Publications.
18. Tjaden P, Thoennes N: Prevalence, incidence and consequences of violence against women: findings from the national violence against women survey, Washington, 1998, US Dept. of Justice, National Institute of Justice and Centers for Disease Control.
19. US Department of Justice: Violence by intimates: analysis of data on crimes by current or former spouses, boyfriends and girlfriends, Washington, 1997, US Department of Justice.
20. van der Kolk BA, McFarlane AC, Weisaeth L: *Traumatic stress: the effects of overwhelming experience on mind, body, and society,* New York, 1996, Guilford.
21. Warshaw C: Domestic violence and medical education: creating a framework for change, *Acad Med* 72(1): January, 1997.

ADDITIONAL RESOURCES

National Domestic Violence Hotline, 800-799-7233.
National Resource Center on Domestic Violence, 800-537-2238.

CARDIOVASCULAR DISEASE III

CHAPTER 60

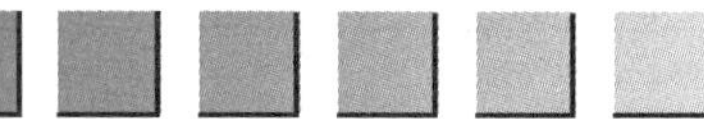

Hypertension

Cynthia Mulrow
Richard M. Hoffman
Harry L. Greene, II
Curtis Kapsner

The upper limit of normal adult blood pressure has been defined as 140/90 mm Hg. The Joint National Committee (JNC-VI) on Detection, Evaluation, and Treatment of High Blood Pressure further classifies hypertension into three stages based on systolic and diastolic blood pressures (Table 60-1).

Nearly 60 million Americans have high blood pressure or are being treated with antihypertensive medications. The annual cost for hypertension, including medications, office visits, and laboratory visits, is estimated to be more than $10 billion. Although these direct costs alone are substantial, hypertension also contributes to hundreds of thousands of premature deaths each year, and is a leading risk factor for congestive heart failure, renal failure, stroke, coronary artery disease, and retinopathy.

Recognition of the public health burden from high blood pressure led to the creation of the National High Blood Pressure Education Program in 1972. Ongoing educational efforts, including publication of consensus guidelines, have considerably improved the detection, treatment, and control of hypertension. In 1972, National Health and Nutrition Examination Survey (NHANES II) data showed that only half of hypertensive patients were aware of their condition and only one in six cases was adequately controlled. By 1991, 73% of hypertensive patients were aware of their high blood pressure and nearly 30% of all cases were adequately controlled. This trend toward increased awareness and control has not been maintained, however. NHANES III (Phase 2) data collected from 1991 to 1994 showed that only 68% of hypertensive patients were aware of their high blood pressure and only 27% were controlled to a systolic pressure below 140 mm Hg and a diastolic pressure below 90 mm Hg.

EPIDEMIOLOGY

Hypertension is more prevalent with increasing age and in African-Americans, among the less educated, and in lower socioeconomic classes. Most diastolic hypertension develops in the second and third decades, although it can occur at any age. In young adulthood and early middle age, hypertension is more prevalent in men than in women, but this reverses

Table 60-1. Classification of Blood Pressure for Adults Age 18 and Older*

Category	Systolic (mm Hg)		Diastolic (mm Hg)
Optimal†	<120	and	<80
Normal	<130	and	<85
High-normal	130-139	or	85-89
Hypertension‡			
Stage 1	140-159	or	90-99
Stage 2	160-179	or	100-109
Stage 3	≥180	or	≥110

From JNC-VI.

*Not taking antihypertensive drugs and not acutely ill. When systolic and diastolic blood pressures fall into different categories, the higher category should be selected to classify the individual's blood pressure status. For example, 160/92 mm Hg should be classified as stage 2 hypertension, and 174/120 mm Hg should be classified as stage 3 hypertension. Isolated systolic hypertension is defined as SBP of 140 mm Hg or greater and DBP below 90 mm Hg and staged appropriately (e.g., 170/82 mm Hg is defined as stage 2 isolated systolic hypertension). In addition to classifying stages of hypertension on the basis of average blood pressure levels, physicians should specify presence or absence of target organ disease and additional risk factors. This specificity is important for risk classification and treatment (Table 60-2).

†Optimal blood pressure with respect to cardiovascular risk is below 120/80 mm Hg. However, unusually low readings should be evaluated for clinical significance.

‡Based on the average of two or more readings taken at each of two or more visits after an initial screening.

after age 60. Isolated systolic hypertension is seen most often in the elderly.

Between 1972 and 1994, age-adjusted mortality from coronary heart disease decreased approximately 53%, and mortality from stroke decreased by nearly 60%. These declines have been observed for men and women, and for African-Americans and whites. Part of the decline is attributable to decreases in cigarette smoking and fat intake, but improved control of high blood pressure has also been an important factor. There is convincing evidence from randomized, placebo-controlled intervention trials that antihypertensive therapy reduces the risk of cardiovascular disease. A consistent finding has been a substantial decrease in the risk of stroke, with a more modest effect on coronary artery disease. Psaty et al's 1997 meta-analysis of 18 placebo-controlled trials estimated a 36% to 51% reduction in the incidence of strokes and a 1% to 28% decrease in the incidence of coronary heart disease (CHD) events.[21]

PATHOPHYSIOLOGY

Although the exact mechanism remains elusive, many steps in the regulation of blood pressure have been discovered and a number of pathogenic mechanisms have been suggested. Blood pressure (BP) is related to cardiac output (CO) and peripheral vascular resistance (PVR). Cardiac output, in turn, is related to stroke volume and heart rate. These formulas are shown below:

$$BP = CO \times PVR$$

$$CO = \text{Stroke Volume} \times \text{Heart Rate}$$

Stroke volume is largely related to the venous return of blood to the heart and to cardiac contractility. A number of other organs interact through feedback loops to maintain an adequate blood pressure. Any change in blood pressure is sensed by baroreceptors located throughout the circulatory system. The receptors send afferent signals to the central nervous system (CNS), which sends efferent output to the adrenal glands that is relayed through the autonomic nervous system to the heart and blood vessels. These feedback mechanisms can increase or decrease heart rate. Catecholamine secretion may increase or decrease, leading to either vasoconstriction or vasodilatation, respectively.

Additionally, the renin-angiotensin-aldosterone system allows the kidney to play a major role in blood pressure control. Renin, a proteolytic enzyme produced by smooth muscle cells in the juxtaglomerular apparatus of the afferent arteriole in the kidney, is released in response to decreased renal perfusion pressures, low sodium concentration, and β-adrenergic stimulation.

In the liver, an α-globulin, called renin substrate, is synthesized and released into the circulation. Renin acts on this substrate to produce a decapeptide called angiotensin I, which is converted to angiotensin II after exposure to a converting enzyme in the lungs and other organs, including the heart, and blood vessels. Angiotensin II regulates renal sodium uptake, acts as a powerful vasoconstrictor, and stimulates the adrenal cortex to produce aldosterone. These effects are mediated through the binding of angiotensin II to the angiotensin II type I receptor in the various target tissues. Aldosterone acts on the renal tubules to promote the reabsorption of sodium and water. Plasma volume is increased through this reabsorption, thus increasing cardiac output. The combination of aldosterone (increasing volume) and angiotensin II (producing vasoconstriction) increases blood pressure. This process is turned off when the juxtaglomerular apparatus in the kidney decreases renin production after fluid volume, blood pressure, and angiotensin II reach threshold levels.

A number of other factors that affect blood pressure have been identified, including factors from vascular endothelial cells, the atrial natriuretic factor, calcium-regulating hormones, the kallikrein system, and vasopressin. Vascular endothelial cells produce both endothelin, a vasoconstrictor, and nitric oxide, a relaxing factor. The interplay of these substances may control vascular pressure at the local level. Another peptide, atrial natriuretic factor, is produced by atrial tissue in response to atrial dilation. This hormone causes vasodilatation, increases the glomerular filtration rate, and enhances sodium excretion. Atrial natriuretic factor release is associated with decreased renin and aldosterone secretion.

Kininogen is a plasma substrate synthesized in the liver and acted on by kallikrein (from the kidney) to produce bradykinin. Bradykinin is converted into inactive bradykinin by angiotensin-converting enzyme (ACE), the same enzyme that converts angiotensin I to angiotensin II. The calcium-controlling hormones, calcitriol (vasoconstrictor) and parathyroid hormone (vasodilator), also have vascular effects on blood pressure. Finally, antidiuretic hormone (ADH), or vasopressin, is produced by the pituitary and released in response to major hemorrhage, severe stress, or head injury. ADH is a potent vasoconstrictor and causes increased sodium and water reabsorption.

DETECTING HYPERTENSION

Hypertension control begins by routinely detecting and confirming high blood pressure. In the office, three separate

Box 60-1. Guidelines for Measuring Blood Pressure

I. Conditions for the patient.
  A. Posture
    1. Some prefer readings after the patient has been supine for 5 minutes. Sitting pressures usually adequate.
    2. Patient should sit quietly with back supported for 5 minutes and the arm supported at the level of the heart.
    3. For patients who are over age 65, diabetic, or receiving antihypertensive therapy, check for postural changes by taking readings immediately and 2 minutes after the patient stands.
  B. Circumstances
    1. No caffeine for the preceding hour.
    2. No smoking for the preceding 15 minutes.
    3. No exogenous adrenergic stimulants (e.g., phenylephrine in nasal decongestants or eyedrops for pupillary dilation).
    4. A quiet warm setting.
    5. Home readings taken under varying circumstances: 24-hour ambulatory recordings may be preferable and more accurate in predicting subsequent cardiovascular disease.

II. Equipment
  A. Cuff size: The bladder should encircle and cover two thirds of the length of the arm. If not, place the bladder over the brachial artery. If the bladder is too small, spuriously high readings may result.
  B. Manometer: Aneroid gauges should be calibrated every 6 months against a mercury manometer. (Do not use finger monitors.)

III. Technique
  A. Number of readings
    1. On each occasion, take at least two readings, separated by as much time as is practical. If readings vary by more than 5 mm Hg, take additional readings until two are close.
    2. For diagnosis, obtain three sets of readings at least a week apart.
    3. Initially, take pressure in both arms; if pressure differs, use arm with higher pressure.
    4. If arm pressure is elevated, take pressure in one leg, particularly in patients below age 30.
  B. Performance
    1. Inflate the bladder quickly to a pressure of 20 mm Hg above the systolic, as recognized by the disappearance of the radial pulse.
    2. Deflate the bladder 3 mm Hg every second.
    3. Record the Korotkoff's phase V (disappearance) except in children, in whom use of phase IV (muffling) is advocated.
    4. If Korotkoff's sounds are weak, have the patient raise the arm and open and close the hand five to ten times, after which the bladder should be inflated quickly.

Modified from Kaplan NM: Arterial hypertension. In Stein JH et al, editor: *Internal medicine,* ed 4, St Louis. 1994, Mosby.

Table 60-2. Rechecking Blood Pressures

Systolic	Diastolic	Follow-up frequency
<130	<85	2 years
130-139	85-89	1 year
140-159	90-99	2 months
160-179	100-109	Evaluate or refer ≤1 month
≥180	≥110	Evaluate or refer immediately

readings should be taken and averaged. Kaplan has provided useful guidelines for measuring blood pressure (Box 60-1). Hypertension should not be diagnosed or treated on the basis of initial readings unless the patient has evidence of acute target-organ damage (hypertensive crisis or urgency). Table 60-2 shows recommended intervals for following elevated blood pressures.

Ambulatory readings may help to assess blood pressure. "White-coat" hypertension or elevated blood pressure readings occurring only in the office setting may occur in as many as 10% to 25% of subjects. Studies have shown that ambulatory blood pressures correlate better with target-organ damage, particularly left ventricular hypertrophy, and with cardiovascular complications. Regression to the mean also occurs in measuring blood pressure; high pressures tend to be lower when repeated. Readings taken during emergency room visits for trauma or painful complaints should be interpreted cautiously since they are known to be misleadingly high. Conversely, hypertensive patients hospitalized with bed rest often have misleadingly low pressures. These patients may be discharged without adequate blood pressure medication, only to remanifest their hypertension soon after leaving the hospital.

Physicians should also be aware of pseudohypertension, although exact age-specific prevalences are unknown. Some elderly patients have stiff, noncompliant atheromatous arteries that can be occluded only with very high sphygmomanometric pressures, leading to falsely elevated blood pressure readings. In these patients, an intraarterial pressure reading is the only way to truly determine the blood pressure; Osler's maneuver is inaccurate. Unfortunately, determining intraarterial pressure is impractical for most patients. Pseudohypertension should be suspected in elderly patients with chronically elevated blood pressures, widened pulse pressures, orthostatic hypotension on medication, and no evidence of target-organ damage.

PATIENT EVALUATION

Goals of Initial Evaluation

The goals of initial evaluation are assessing the patient's individual risk of cardiovascular disease, the presence of target-organ damage, and whether secondary causes of hypertension warrant consideration.

Table 60-3. Risk Stratification and Treatment*

	Risk group A	Risk group B	Risk group C
Blood pressure stages (mm Hg)	No risk factors; no TOD/CCD†	At least one risk factor, not including diabetes; no TOD/CCD†	TOD/CCD† and/or diabetes, with or without other risk factors
High-normal (130-139/85-89)	Lifestyle modification	Lifestyle modification	Drug therapy§
Stage 1 (140-159/90-99)	Lifestyle modification (up to 12 months)	Lifestyle modification‡ (up to 6 months)	Drug therapy
Stages 2 and 3 (≥160/≥100)	Drug therapy	Drug therapy	Drug therapy

From JNC-VI.

For example, a patient with diabetes and a blood pressure of 142/94 mm Hg plus left ventricular hypertrophy should be classified as having stage 1 hypertension with target-organ disease (left ventricular hypertrophy) and with another major risk factor (diabetes). This patient would be categorized as Stage 1, Risk Group C, and recommended for immediate initiation of pharmacologic treatment.

*Lifestyle modification should be adjunctive therapy for all patients recommended for pharmacologic therapy.

†TOD/CCD indicates target-organ disease/clinical cardiovascular disease.

‡For patients with multiple risk factors, physicians should consider drugs as initial therapy plus lifestyle modifications.

§For those with heart failure, renal insufficiency, or diabetes.

Box 60-2. Components of Cardiovascular Risk Stratification in Patients with Hypertension

Major Risk Factors

Smoking
Dyslipidemia
Diabetes mellitus
Age older than 60 years
Sex (men and postmenopausal women)
Family history of cardiovascular disease: women under age 65 or men under age 55

Target-Organ Damage/Clinical Cardiovascular Disease

Heart diseases
- Left ventricular hypertrophy
- Angina/prior myocardial infarction
- Prior coronary revascularization
- Heart failure

Stroke or transient ischemic attack
Nephropathy
Peripheral arterial disease
Retinopathy

Assessing Individual Risk

Assessment of individual risk is necessary to optimize decisions about whom to treat with what therapy (Table 60-3). It also identifies important comorbid cardiovascular risk factors that warrant treatment. The risk for cardiovascular morbidity and mortality increases with higher levels of systolic and diastolic pressures, and is synergistically related to the presence of other cardiovascular risk factors and target-organ damage (Box 60-2). For example, Framingham data showed that the 8-year cardiovascular risk from diastolic hypertension for 40-year-old men increased tenfold in the presence of high cholesterol, cigarette smoking, and diabetes mellitus. Simple risk equations and tables based on level of blood pressure and the presence of other risk factors (Figs. 60-1 and 60-2) are used to estimate a patient's pretreatment risk and the likely benefit of therapy.

CLINICAL AND LABORATORY EXAMINATION

History

Hypertension is usually asymptomatic, and is often detected only during routine screening. Patients with elevated pressures should be questioned about symptoms of cardiovascular, cerebrovascular, and renal disease and about family history of high blood pressure, cardiovascular disease, or diabetes. If hypertension has already been diagnosed, the patient should be asked about the duration and levels of blood pressure, any complications of hypertension, and the types and results of previous treatments. The history should also identify other cardiovascular risk factors, such as smoking, hyperlipidemia, inactivity, obesity, and diabetes mellitus. Other important factors to ask about include drug use and dietary intake of salt, cholesterol, and saturated fats.

A quick review of systems may suggest possible causes of secondary hypertension. Suggestive symptom clusters of uncommon secondary causes include episodic headaches, palpitations, orthostatic hypotension, pallor, and sweating (pheochromocytoma), and weight gain, central obesity, striae, hirsutism, myopathy, and amenorrhea (Cushing's syndrome).

Physical Examination

A rational physical examination in the hypertensive patient ideally includes checking for evidence of increased cardiovascular disease risk factors and target-organ damage, and for findings that may suggest secondary causes of hypertension. The most efficient and accurate examination for these checks is unknown. Many experts recommend measuring blood pressure in both arms and using the arm with the higher reading for subsequent monitoring. In patients less than age 30 years, blood pressure differences between arms and legs may be measured if coarctation of the aorta is being considered. In older patients and those with orthostatic symptoms, postural changes in blood pressures are important. Weight and height should be checked to estimate body mass index. Waist-to-hip circumference ratios may be measured to help establish risk of cardiovascular disease: ratios greater

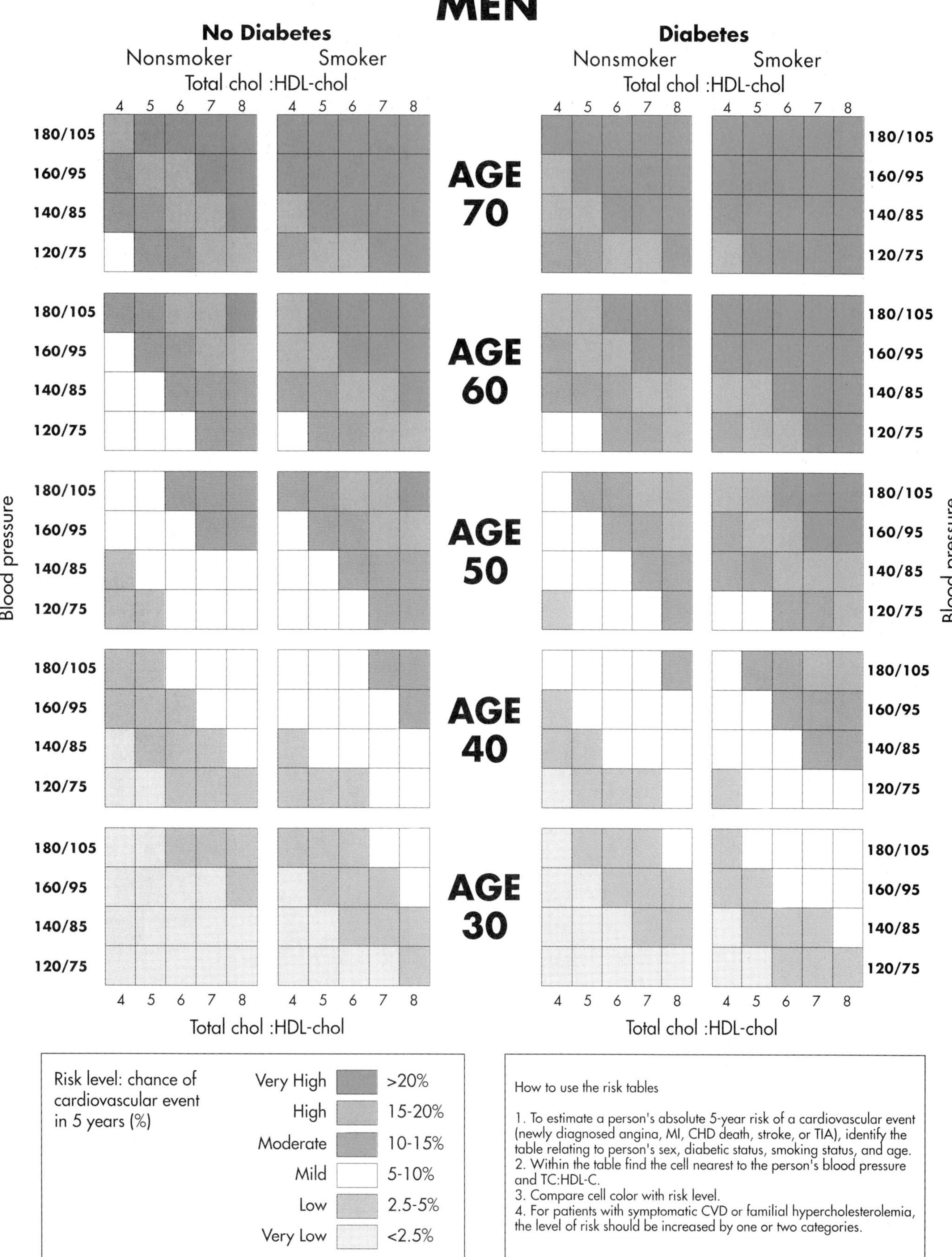

Fig. 60-1. Absolute 5-year risk of a cardiovascular event for men.

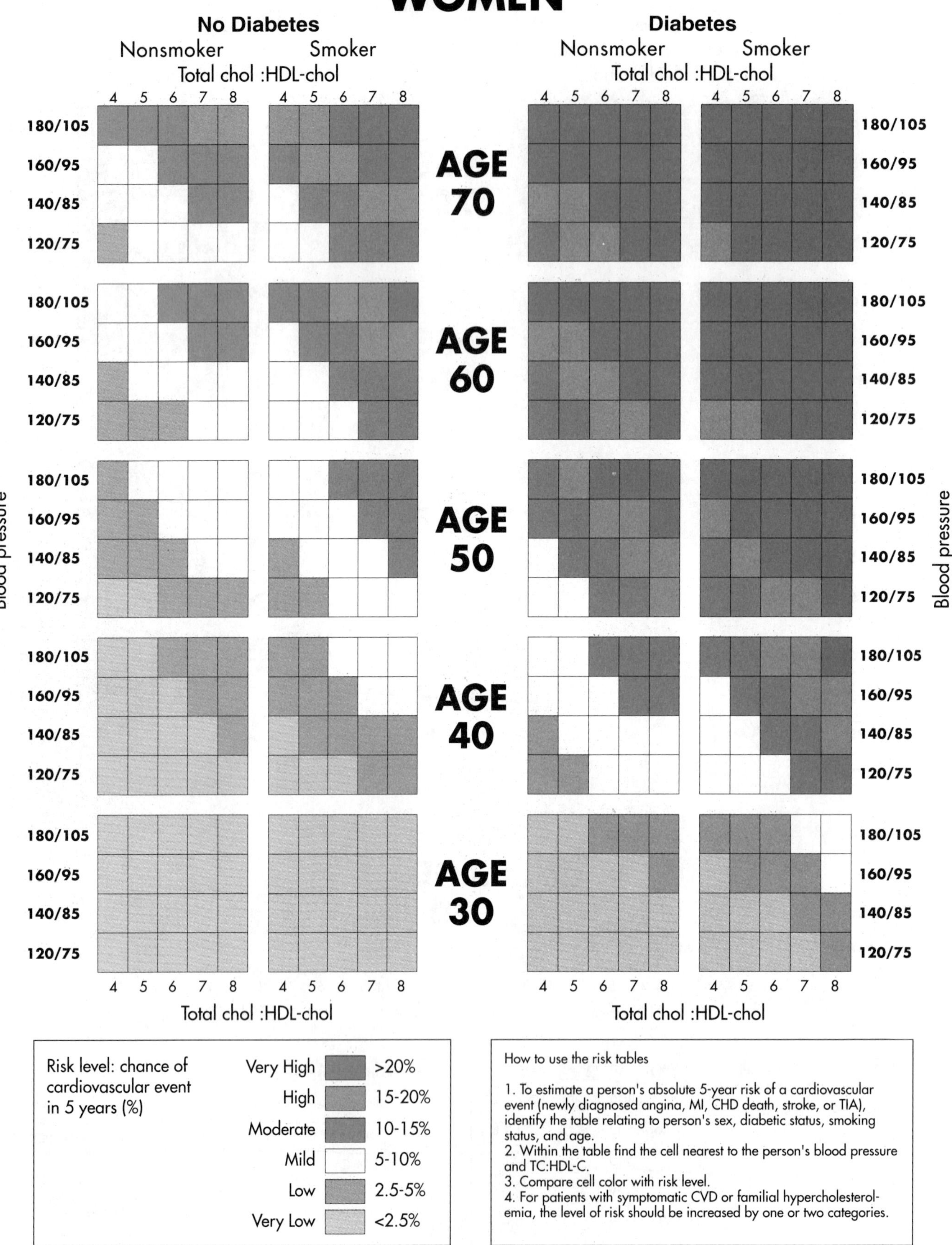

Fig. 60-2. Absolute 5-year risk of a cardiovascular event for women.

than 0.8 in women and greater than 1.0 in men correlate with higher risks.

Some experts recommend examining the optic fundus for evidence of retinopathy, although the accuracy of this examination in undilated eyes is likely to be low. Quickly examining the neck for thyroid abnormalities, elevated jugular pressure, and carotid bruits may be useful. Cardiovascular examination should focus on detection of dysrhythmias (atrial fibrillation is common in older hypertensive patients); S3 gallops, which may indicate systolic dysfunction; and murmurs. The presence or absence of rales and edema should be noted. Abdominal bruits, especially those that lateralize or have a diastolic component, may suggest renovascular disease. In some instances, abdominal aortic aneurysms may be palpable. Diminished peripheral pulses may suggest atherosclerosis. A neurologic examination including a cognitive status screen may help establish target-organ damage.

Laboratory Evaluation

Routine laboratory testing should include urinalysis, fasting blood sugar, potassium, urea nitrogen, creatinine, total cholesterol, high-density lipoprotein (HDL), and an electrocardiogram (ECG). The ECG, urinalysis, and renal panel help to determine the extent of hypertensive target-organ damage; fasting blood sugar and lipids identify other cardiovascular risk factors, and potassium levels provide baseline values for following the biochemical effects of therapy. Some experts also recommend complete blood count, 24-hour protein, low-density lipoprotein (LDL), glycosylated hemoglobin, and uric acid levels.

Determining Secondary Causes

Essential (primary) hypertension affects more than 90% of hypertensive patients and has no identifiable cause. Secondary causes are present in less than 10% of hypertensive patients, and many secondary causes are very uncommon (Box 60-3). Demographic, historical, symptomatic, physical, and laboratory findings may increase suspicion of secondary causes, although the actual sensitivity, specificity, and utility of using particular clusters of findings to guide workup for secondary hypertension is not well studied. Fig. 60-3 shows examples of clusters of findings that may suggest particular workups.

Briefly, secondary hypertension, by definition, has an identifiable underlying cause. Secondary hypertension should be suspected in patients presenting with sudden onset or worsening of hypertension, refractory hypertension, onset before age 20 or after age 50, malignant or accelerated hypertension, or suggestive features on initial clinical examination. Although less than 5% of hypertensive patients have secondary hypertension, this accounts for nearly 3

Box 60-3. Possible Causes of Hypertension

Most Common (>90% prevalence)

Essential or primary hypertension

Less Common (1-10% prevalence)

Renal parenchymal disease (e.g., glomerulonephritis, chronic nephritis, diabetic nephropathy, hydronephrosis, connective tissue disease, polycystic disease)
Renovascular disease
Acute stress (e.g., alcohol withdrawal, surgery, acute illness)
Drugs (e.g., nonsteroidal antiinflammatory drugs [NSAIDs], estrogen, appetite suppressants, corticosteroids, sympathomimetics)
Primary aldosteronism

Uncommon (<1% Prevalence)

Renal

Renin-producing tumors
Renoprival
Primary sodium retention (Liddle syndrome, Gordon syndrome)

Endocrine

Acromegaly
Hypothyroidism
Hyperthyroidism
Hypercalcemia (hyperparathyroidism)
Cushing's syndrome
Congenital adrenal hyperplasia
Pheochromocytoma
Extra-adrenal chromaffin tumors
Carcinoid
Mineralocorticoids: licorice
Tyramine-containing foods and monoamine oxidase inhibitors

Vascular

Coarctation of the aorta

Neurologic disorders

Brain tumor
Encephalitis
Respiratory acidosis
Quadriplegia
Acute porphyria
Familial dysautonomia
Lead poisoning
Guillain-Barré syndrome

Increased cardiac output

Aortic valvular regurgitation
Arteriovenous fistula, patent ductus
Thyrotoxicosis
Paget's disease of bone
Beriberi
Hyperkinetic circulation

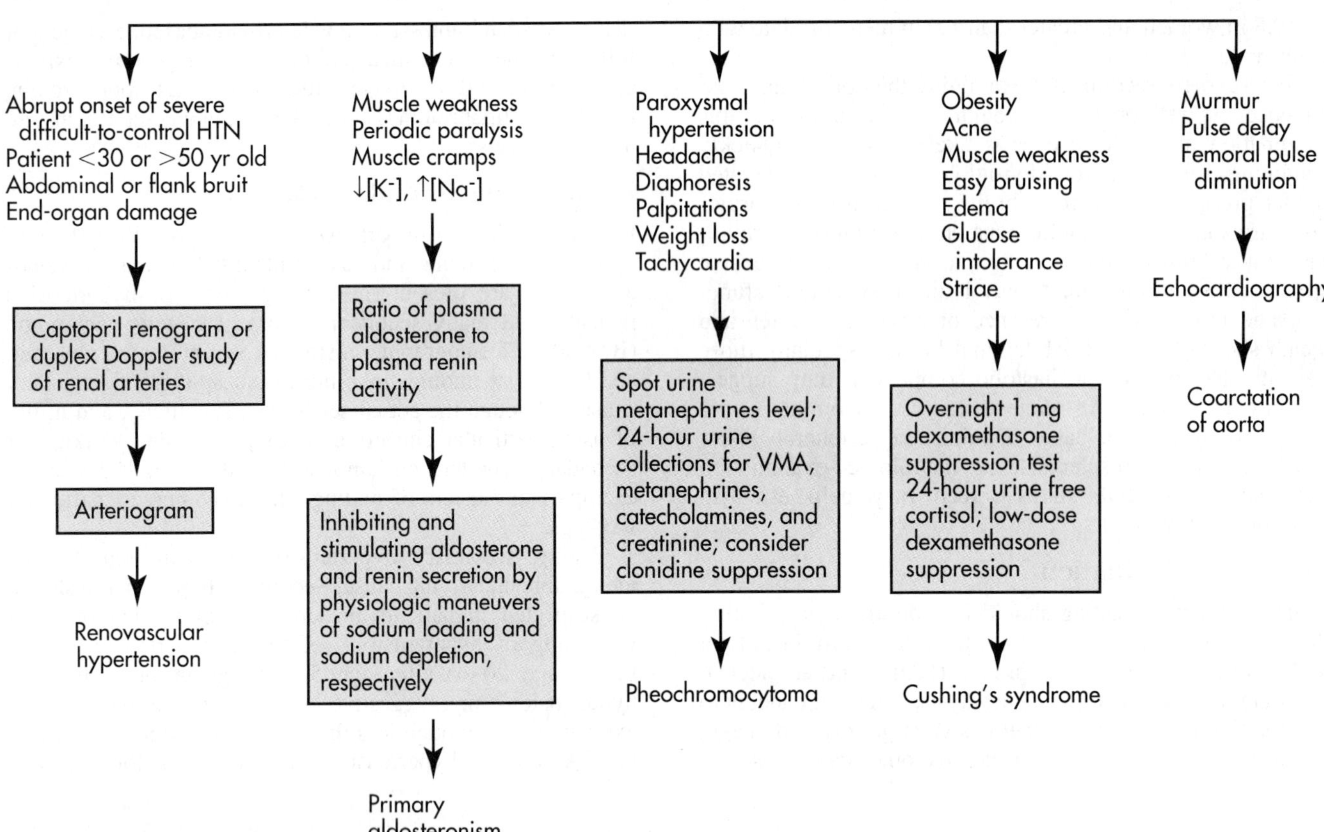

Fig. 60-3. Algorithm for the evaluation of secondary causes of hypertension based on clusters of findings. (Modified from Greene HL, Johnson WP, Maricie MJ, editors: *Decision making in medicine,* St Louis, 1993, Mosby and JNC-VI.)

million people in the United States. Searching for a secondary cause is important because the hypertension may be curable.

The most common cause of secondary hypertension is renal parenchymal disease, which is responsible for 2% to 3% of all hypertension. The diagnosis is based on finding elevated blood urea nitrogen (BUN) and creatinine, decreased creatinine clearance, and an abnormal urinalysis.

Renovascular disease (RVD) accounts for approximately 1% of hypertension and is suggested by severe or resistant hypertension (diastolic blood pressure greater than or equal to 125 mm Hg), other evidence of vascular disease, a suggestive abdominal bruit (up to 50% of RVD patients in contrast to 9% of those with essential hypertension), worsening renal function (especially after being placed on an ACE-inhibitor), occurrence in younger women or older men, and asymmetric renal size. Although renal vascular disease can be caused by cholesterol or clot emboli, aortic dissection, compression of the arteries, or vasculitis, the most frequent etiologies are fibromuscular dysplasia and atherosclerosis. Fibromuscular dysplasia occurs principally in young, white women, whereas the more common atherosclerosis is often seen in elderly men.

Workup for renovascular disease should only be initiated in patients who are candidates for either angioplasty or surgical revascularization. Renal arteriography may be the initial step in the evaluation of patients in whom there is a high degree of suspicion for RVD because it is the gold standard for imaging the renal arteries. Also, arteriography should be considered in patients with possible ischemic nephropathy because the nephrogram phase of the arteriogram can help estimate the amount of remaining viable kidney tissue. Patients in whom there is a moderate degree of suspicion for RVD should undergo either captopril renography or duplex sonography and then proceed to arteriography if either of those tests are positive.

A number of exogenous drugs and chemicals can lead to hypertension. Physicians should always query patients about using nasal decongestants, which contain sympathomimetics, and nonsteroidal antiinflammatory drugs (NSAIDs), which cause fluid retention and interfere with antihypertensive agents. Most women who take oral contraceptives have an increase in blood pressure, usually within the normal range. After prescribing birth control pills, the physician should recheck the blood pressure within the first 2 to 4 weeks and at 3- to 6-month intervals thereafter. Low-dose postmenopausal hormone replacement is not a cause of hypertension. Other drugs to consider include corticosteroids, thyroid supplements, diet pills, caffeine, cyclosporine, erythropoietin, antidepressants, amphetamines, and cocaine.

The various medullary and cortical adrenal hyperfunctions account for approximately 0.5% of hypertension. Pheochromocytoma is associated with sustained or intermittent episodes of tachycardia, tremor, sweating, pallor, headache, and orthostatic hypotension. A spot urine test for metanephrine is the initial screening test. Values greater than 1 mg per mg of creatinine should be followed by a 24-hour urine collection for vanillylmandelic acid, metanephrines, and catecholamines. These urine assays have a sensitivity of 84% to 96% and a specificity of 99% for detecting pheochromocytomas. If the urine assays are borderline, plasma

Table 60-4. Estimate of Antihypertensive Treatment Effect by Sex

Variable	Total mortality	Cardiovascular-related death	Fatal strokes	All strokes	Fatal coronary events	All major coronary events	Main cardio-vascular events
Women							
Odds ratio (95% CI)	0.91 (0.81-1.01)	0.86 (0.74-1.01)	0.71 (0.53-0.96)	0.62 (0.52-0.73)	0.92 (0.74-1.16)	0.85 (0.72-1.01)	0.74 (0.66-0.83)
Men							
Odds ratio	0.88 (0.80-0.97)	0.80 (0.70-0.91)	0.57 (0.41-0.78)	0.66 (0.56-0.78)	0.83 (0.71-0.97)	0.82 (0.73-0.92)	0.78 (0.71-0.86)

Modified from Queyffier F et al: *Ann Intern Med* 126:761-767, 1997.

epinephrine and norepinephrine levels can be measured following a clonidine suppression test; levels remain high in patients with a pheochromocytoma.

Nearly 80% of patients with Cushing's syndrome have elevated blood pressure because the high levels of cortisol have mineralocorticoid activity. Cushing's syndrome is suggested by moon facies, truncal obesity, proximal muscle weakness, and hirsutism. The initial diagnostic test is a morning plasma cortisol after suppression with 1 mg of dexamethasone at bedtime the night before. A cortisol level under 5 μg/dl excludes Cushing's syndrome with 98% certainty. Patients with highly suggestive features should undergo both a 24-hour urine free cortisol measurement and low-dose (0.5 mg every 6 hours for 2 days) dexamethasone suppression test. Normal urine cortisol levels exclude cortisol hypersecretion.

Primary aldosteronism induces hypertension and potassium wasting, although hypokalemia is not always present. Patients with unprovoked hypokalemia or those who become severely hypokalemic on minimal diuretic therapy may have hyperaldosteronism. The most useful screening test for primary aldosteronism is measuring the plasma aldosterone/plasma renin activity ratio. A ratio of greater than 20:1 with an absolute plasma aldosterone concentration of greater than 15 ng/dl suggests primary hyperaldosteronism. A positive screening test needs to be confirmed by demonstrating inappropriate aldosterone secretion by measuring urinary aldosterone after oral sodium chloride administration or measuring plasma aldosterone after giving intravenous sodium chloride. If hyperaldosteronism is confirmed, computed tomography (CT) scanning and adrenal venous sampling can localize pathology. Bilaterally elevated aldosterone levels suggest idiopathic hyperaldosteronism, which is treated medically. Conn's syndrome is characterized by a unilateral secretion of aldosterone and an adrenal adenoma that, if removed surgically, usually results in improvement of both the hypertension and the hypokalemia. Other endocrine causes of secondary hypertension include acromegaly, hypothyroidism, hyperthyroidism, and hypercalcemia (hyperparathyroidism). These diagnoses are suggested by characteristic clinical findings (gigantism, thyromegaly, or thyroid nodules) or abnormal laboratory studies (serum calcium, thyroid function tests).

Coarctation of the aorta is suggested by delayed or absent femoral pulses and decreased lower extremity blood pressure. A chest x-ray may show the "E" sign, formed by the abnormal contour of the aortic knob and the uppermost portion of the descending aorta. Notching of rib may be noted. An aortogram confirms the diagnosis, but coarctation may also be demonstrated on CT scan or on magnetic resonance angiogram (MRA).

Other miscellaneous causes of hypertension are shown in Box 60-3.

ESTIMATING BENEFITS OF TREATMENT FOR THE INDIVIDUAL

Benefits of treating individuals vary depending on their baseline risks for cardiovascular disease and their competing risks of dying from noncardiovascular-related causes. An example of high competing risks that may minimize or negate the benefits of treating hypertension is a patient with multiple serious conditions such as Alzheimer's disease, obstructive lung disease, frequent falls, urinary incontinence, and gout.

Estimates of benefits for individuals depend on the magnitude of relative treatment benefits and the patient's baseline risks for cardiovascular disease. The relative efficacy for preventing mortality and cardiovascular events is presented as odds ratios in Table 60-4; estimates of baseline cardiovascular risks for patients with different risk factors are given in Figs. 60-1 and 60-2. Table 60-5 can be used to calculate the number of patients who would need to be treated (NNTs) for 5 years to prevent cardiovascular events. For example, the odds ratio associated with preventing a cardiovascular event in men is 0.78 (see Table 60-4). A 60-year-old diabetic man who smokes, has a total cholesterol to HDL-cholesterol ratio of 4, and a blood pressure of 160/100 would have a greater than 20% chance of experiencing a cardiovascular event in the next 5 years (see Fig. 60-1). Crossing this patient expected event rate with the corresponding odds ratio yields an approximate NNT of 30 (see Table 60-5). Conversely, if the patient was 34 and neither a smoker nor diabetic, his 5-year risk of a cardiovascular event is less than 2.5%. Crossing this expected event rate with the same odds ratio (0.78) yields an approximate NNT of 204.

MANAGEMENT

The aim of treating high blood pressure is to prevent premature death and disease by reducing the risk of coronary heart disease and stroke, with minimum adverse effects. Treatment options for hypertension include lifestyle modifications, dietary supplementations, and pharmacologic therapy.

Nonpharmacologic Therapy

Lifestyle Interventions. Numerous studies have shown that lifestyle changes, such as weight reduction, salt restriction, regular aerobic exercise, and decreased alcohol consumption, can lower blood pressure (Table 60-6). Although there are no long-term studies proving that using these modalities prevents the morbidity and mortality of hypertension, the interventions are generally harmless, may reduce other risk factors for cardiovascular disease, and avoid the costs and side effects of medication. Behavioral science studies show that a physician's advice alone can affect behavior, and the chance of bringing about a true lifestyle change may be increased by combining frequent follow-up visits with client-centered counseling, contracting, and setting achievable goals.

Exercise. Exercising aerobically at least three times a week for 30 to 45 minutes lowers blood pressure.[13] Exercise is also a valuable adjunct to weight control. The key is to begin gradually with a realistic program that fits the patient's lifestyle. A useful start may be a simple walking program, which is easily achievable and has minimal risk of injury.

Diet. Saturated fat increases blood pressure, independent of obesity, and a switch to polyunsaturated and monounsaturated fats may reduce blood pressure. This dietary change may impact two cardiovascular risk factors—hypertension and cholesterol. A high potassium and magnesium diet rich in fruits, vegetables, and low-fat dairy products and reduced in saturated and total fat can substantially reduce blood pressure—5.5/3.0 mm Hg—compared with the typical American diet.[2]

Table 60-5. Calculation of the NNT from Odds Ratios

	Odds ratio		
PEER	**0.50**	**0.55**	**0.90**
0.001	2001	2223	10009
0.025	81	90	409
0.05	41	46	209
0.10	21	24	110
0.20	11	13	61
0.30	8	9	46
0.40	7	8	40
0.50	6	7	38

Modified from McQuay HJ, Moore RA: *Ann Intern Med* 712-720, 1997.
The formula for determining the NNT for preventive interventions is $\{1 - [PEER \times (1 - OR)]\}/[(1 - PEER) \times PEER \times (1 - OR)]$.
PEER, Patient expected event rate.

Weight Loss. Modest weight reductions of 3% to 9% of body weight can effectively reduce blood pressure in obese, hypertensive people who are sufficiently motivated to follow a long-term weight loss regimen. The effect of weight loss is independent of sodium restriction or increased exercise.

Reducing Alcohol Intake. Daily alcohol consumption greater than 2 oz has been associated with hypertension in multiple epidemiologic studies. The relationship is generally linear, although some studies show threshold effects at two to three drinks daily. A small randomized trial in treated hypertensive men (initial blood pressures 142/85 mm Hg) who were moderate to heavy drinkers showed that reducing alcohol consumption from 452 to 64 ml of ethanol per week lowered systolic blood pressure 5 mm Hg and diastolic 3 mm Hg.[22] People with raised blood pressure should reduce alcohol consumption to two drinks or less daily.

Salt Restriction. Salt restriction may lead to modest reductions in blood pressure.[9] Effects vary depending on baseline amounts of salt consumption, amount of reduction that is achievable, and age. For motivated persons older than age 45 who consume more than 3 gm of salt daily, reduction of 1 gm or more can lead to sustained reductions of approximately 6/2 mm Hg (systolic/diastolic). Practically speaking, patients could refrain from salting food at the table and while cooking, and could avoid processed foods with a high salt content. Of note, there is no direct evidence that low-salt diets are harmful, but epidemiologic data conflict, with one observational study suggesting very low salt intakes may be associated with increased myocardial infarction in men.[1]

Dietary Supplementation (Table 60-7). There is no direct evidence of the effect of dietary supplementation on mortality or morbidity in people with hypertension.

Potassium Supplementation. Several small randomized trials showed an increase in potassium intake of about 60 mmol/day (60 mEq or 2000 mg) on top of typical consumption of dietary potassium produces a reduction in

Table 60-6. Evidence of Effectiveness of Lifestyle Interventions for Essential Hypertension

Intervention	No. of RTCs (patients)	Trial participants	Change in targeted factor	Decrease in BP mm Hg
Exercise	29 (1533)	80% male, age 28-72	50 mins aerobic 3/week	5/3
Low-fat, high fruit and vegetable diet	1 (459)	50% male, mean age 44		5.5/3
Weight loss	18 (2611)	55% male, mean age 50	3.9% of body weight	3/3
Salt restriction	58 (2161)	Mean age 49	118 mmol/day	4/1
	28 (1131)	Mean age 47	60 mmol/day	2/0.5
Alcohol restriction	1 (44)	100% male, mean age 50	From 452- to 64-ml ethanol per week	5/3

blood pressure of approximately 4 mm Hg systolic and 2.5 mm Hg diastolic.[26] Greater reductions may be seen in persons with higher urinary sodium excretion and in African-Americans compared with white persons. About 2% to 10% of persons taking potassium supplementation have gastrointestinal adverse effects such as belching, flatulence, diarrhea, and abdominal discomfort.

Fish Oil Supplementation. Large daily intakes of fish oil (200 gm/day of fish high in v_2 polyunsaturated fatty acids or 6 to 10 capsules/day) reduced blood pressure by approximately 4.5 mm Hg systolic and 2.5 mm Hg diastolic.[18] Such high intake may be difficult to maintain. There is no evidence of beneficial effect on blood pressure at lower intakes. Belching, bad breath, fishy taste, and/or abdominal pain may occur in approximately 30% of persons taking high doses of fish oil.

Calcium and Magnesium Intake. Calcium supplementation has minimal effects on blood pressure in people with hypertension and normal calcium levels.[10] There is no evidence that magnesium supplementation reduces blood pressure in people with hypertension and normal magnesium levels.

Relaxation and Biofeedback. Evidence concerning effects of relaxation and biofeedback therapies on blood pressure is equivocal. Some trials show minimal reductions, but others with sham control groups show no effects.

Smoking Cessation. Smoking cigarettes raises blood pressure slightly and may attenuate the cardiovascular protective effect of antihypertensive therapy. Smoking cessation is strongly encouraged because it is a major risk factor for cardiovascular disease that interacts synergistically with hypertension.

Pharmacologic Therapy

Pharmacologic therapy reduces blood pressure more than lifestyle interventions.[19] Average blood pressure reductions are approximately 12 to 16/5 to 10 mm Hg (systolic/diastolic). Randomized controlled trials involving more than 37,000 patients show particular regimens reduce stroke in people under 65 years and reduce total mortality and fatal and nonfatal cardiovascular events in older people up to 80 years of age. Trials in middle-aged adults usually compared thiazide diuretics, β-blockers, or reserpine with placebo. Drug therapy in middle-aged adults prevented one stroke (CI 0 to 2; NNT = 833) for every 1000 patient years of treatment, and did not significantly affect coronary events or mortality. Trials in older persons greater than age 60 often compared placebo with diuretics (usually thiazides with the addition of amiloride or triamterene) and β-blockers (usually atenolol or metoprolol) in a stepped-care approach. On average, treating 1000 older adults for 1 year prevented five strokes (CI 2 to 8; NNT = 197), three coronary events (CI 1 to 4; NNT = 225), and four cardiovascular deaths (CI 1 to 8; NNT = 225) (Table 60-8). Of note, trials, especially in older adults, have included people healthier than in the general population, with lower rates of cardiovascular risk factors, cardiovascular disease, and comorbidity. Patients with higher cardiovascular risk can expect greater short-term benefits than seen in the trials, whereas patients with major competing risks such as terminal cancer or end-stage Alzheimer's disease can expect lesser benefits.

Specific Drug Treatment Choices. Ideal antihypertensive treatment should be inexpensive, be simple to take, be in long-acting formulation, and have proven mortality and morbidity benefits and minimal side effects. Initial therapy with diuretics (thiazide or combination thiazide and potassium sparing agent) or β-blockers (atenolol or metoprolol) comes closest to meeting ideal criteria. According to

Table 60-7. Effectiveness of Dietary Supplementation for Essential Hypertension

Intervention	No. of RTCs (patients)	Trial participants	Change in targeted factor	Decrease in BP mm Hg
Potassium supplementation	21 (1560)	Age 19-79	60-100 mmol/day	4/2.5
Fish oil supplementation	7 (339)	Mean age 50	3 gm or more	4.5/2.5
Calcium supplementation	42 (4560)	Not clear	800-1500 mg/day	1.5/1

Table 60-8. Benefits of Pharmacologic Treatments for Hypertension

Patients	Stroke	Coronary events
Middle-aged adults	Prevents 1/1000 pt yr tx (CI 0 to 2) (NNT = 833)	No significant effects
Adults older than 60 years	Prevents 5/1000 pt yr tx (CI 2 to 8) (NNT = 197)	Prevents 3/1000 pt yr tx (CI 1 to 4) (NNT = 362)

From Gueyffier F: *J Hum Hypertens* 10:1-8, 1996.

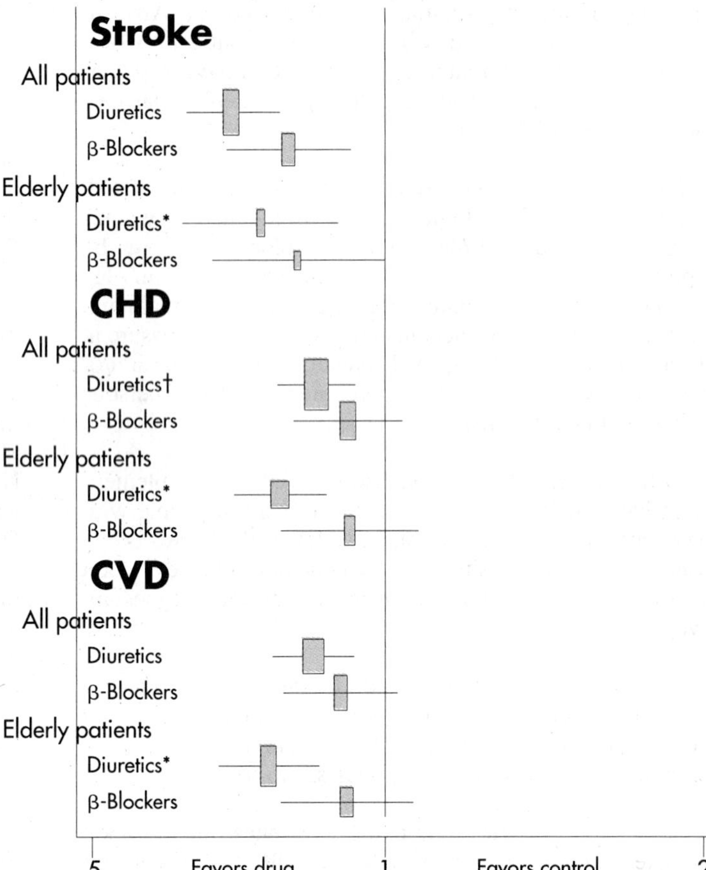

Fig. 60-4. Summary of trial outcomes that used either diuretics or β-blockers as first-line agents. (Modified from *JAMA* 277:739-745, 1997; *JAMA* 279:1903-1907, 1998.)

one large randomized controlled trial, a long-acting dihydropyridine calcium channel blocker, nitrendipine, also meets these criteria for older persons with isolated systolic hypertension.[23]

The relative efficacy of different agents is largely unknown. Systematic reviews have compared results of trials that used diuretics as first-line agents with results of trials that used β-blockers as first-line agents.[17,21] The findings suggest but do not prove that diuretics are superior to β-blockers as first-line therapy, particularly for older adults, and are summarized in Fig. 60-4.

As of 1999, there was no direct placebo-controlled, randomized controlled trial evidence of the effects of ACE inhibitors, α-blockers, and angiotensin II receptor antagonists on morbidity and mortality in the treatment of hypertension and only limited evidence for calcium channel blockers. In 380 hypertensive non–insulin-dependent diabetic patients, an ACE-inhibitor, fosinopril, significantly lowered risk of major vascular events compared with a long-acting dihydropyridine calcium channel blocker, amlodipine (hazards ratio = 0.49; CI 0.26 to 0.95; NNT = 15).[24] A second trial involving 470 hypertensive non–insulin-dependent diabetic patients found a long-acting dihydropyridine calcium channel blocker, nisoldipine, controlled blood pressure as well as an ACE inhibitor, enalapril.[8] However, nisoldipine was associated with a higher incidence of fatal and nonfatal myocardial infarctions than enalapril (adjusted risk ratio 7; CI 2.3 to 21.4; NNT = 12). Whether the ACE inhibitors were improving outcomes, the calcium channel blockers were worsening outcomes, or both effects were occurring in these two trials was not clear.

There are comorbid conditions where particular antihypertensive drugs improve clinical outcomes. Patients and physicians may preferentially opt for these drugs. The conditions, preferred drug, and outcomes are outlined in Table 60-9.

Harms and Adverse Effects of Pharmacotherapy. Systematic reviews of randomized trials of pharmacotherapy show no increase in noncardiovascular mortality in treated hypertensive patients.[12] Comparable data on noncardiovascular morbidity are not available, although trials and case-control studies suggest no increase in cancer incidence with antihypertensive therapy. Case-control, cohort, and randomized studies suggest short- and intermediate-acting dihydropyridine calcium channel blockers, such as nifedipine and isradipine, may increase cardiovascular morbidity and mortality.[7] Unfortunately, as of 1998, there was only one published large, well-designed, placebo-controlled trial of a long-acting dihydropyridine calcium channel blocker in hypertensive patients.[23] This study showed a significant reduction in cardiovascular events with active treatment. Ongoing studies with different calcium channel blockers

Table 60-9. Examples of Improved Clinical Outcomes with Particular Antihypertensives

Condition	Agent	Outcome
Left ventricular systolic dysfunction	ACE inhibitors, angiotensin II receptor blockers	Improves survival, functional status; decreases morbidity
Diabetes mellitus with proteinuria (Type I)	ACE inhibitors	Retards renal deterioration
Myocardial infarction	Nonintrinsic sympathomimetic β-blockers	Improves survival
Diabetes mellitus (Type 2)	Diuretics	Reduces cardiovascular morbidity and mortality

will help clarify which ones are appropriate for which patients.

Symptomatic adverse effects vary by drug class and by agents within classes. Examples of specific adverse effects as well as costs of therapies are given in Table 60-10. A significant proportion of patients have been reported to change or discontinue treatment because of adverse effects. More recent studies of lower dose drugs show good tolerance. Over 4 years of double-blind therapy with placebo or one of five antihypertensive agents, 59% of patients on placebo and 72% assigned to pharmacotherapy remained on their initially assigned treatment.[19] Moreover a systematic review and several recent trials show quality of life is not adversely affected and may be improved in those who remain on treatment.[4,5] In the three long-term double-blind comparisons of low-dose diuretics, β-blockers, ACE inhibitors, and calcium channel blockers, tolerability and overall quality of life indicators tended to be more favorable for diuretics and β-blockers than for newer drugs.[10,15,20]

A large number of studies have reported adverse effects of diuretics and β-blockers on blood lipids (both drug groups), blood glucose, potassium, and uric acid (diuretics). Most of these studies either were of short duration or used high doses; when diuretics and β-blockers are used in low doses, long-term follow-up indicates only minor metabolic effects that are unlikely to be clinically significant.[3,11,25] For example, secondary analysis of results from a large diuretics treatment trial of elderly patients with isolated systolic hypertension showed similar cardiovascular relative risk reductions in diabetic and nondiabetic patients.[6]

Specific Oral Antihypertensive Agents. The drug treatment of hypertension is the single greatest indication for medication use in the United States. A vast array of drugs are available: diuretics, sympatholytics, ACE inhibitors, peripheral inhibitors, calcium channel blockers, angiotensin II receptor blockers, and vasodilators. Specific drugs, their doses, costs, and adverse effects are given in Table 60-10.

Diuretics

Thiazide diuretics. Thiazide diuretics promote the excretion of sodium and water primarily by inhibiting their reabsorption in the distal renal tubule. Thiazides cause a slight fall in serum potassium in most patients, although only a few develop symptoms of severe hypokalemia. The importance of diuretic-induced hypokalemia is controversial. For patients on digitalis (where hypokalemia may exacerbate toxicity) or patients with a history of ischemic heart disease or ventricular dysrhythmias, the serum potassium is closely monitored and the potassium is replaced if hypokalemia develops. Hypokalemia can be treated with potassium replacement or with the addition of a potassium-sparing diuretic. Longer acting diuretics, such as chlorthalidone and metolazone, may produce more severe hypokalemia. Serum uric acid increases approximately 1 mg/dl in all patients started on diuretics. Unless clinical gout develops, modest hyperuricemia need not be treated. If diuretic therapy is essential for the patient with frequent gouty attacks, a uric acid–lowering agent may be added.

Loop diuretics: ethacrynic acid, furosemide, bumetanide. Ethacrynic acid and furosemide block sodium absorption in the loop of Henle. These short-acting agents, which need to be administered twice daily, are more potent diuretics than the thiazides but have no greater antihypertensive effect. Because loop diuretics are more expensive than thiazides and have a propensity for causing large fluid shifts, they should be used as second-line drugs. In general, they are used for patients with renal failure (serum creatinine greater than 2.5 mg/dl) or for patients with fluid retention and congestive heart failure.

Potassium-sparing diuretics: triamterene, amiloride, spironolactone. Potassium-sparing diuretics promote sodium excretion and potassium retention by preventing sodium/potassium exchange in the distal nephron. These drugs are rarely used as the sole diuretic for treating hypertension unless the patient has thiazide sensitivity, diet-controlled glucose intolerance, or gout. They are particularly useful in combination with other diuretics for patients at risk for hypokalemia. Because these drugs can cause hyperkalemia, they are best avoided for patients with impaired renal function, diabetic patients with type IV renal tubular acidosis, or those receiving a converting enzyme inhibitor.

Sympatholytic Agents. Sympatholytic agents include β-blockers, α-blockers, and α- and β-adrenergic blockers. Blood pressure is lowered through β-adrenergic blockade and, at higher dosages, through a CNS mechanism. β-Blockers are ideal for hypertensive patients with angina, myocardial infarction, migraine headaches, and essential tremor.

There are a large number of β-blockers available. From a pharmacologic standpoint, these agents can be grouped into the nonspecific β-antagonists, the selective β-antagonists, and those with and without intrinsic sympathomimetic activity (ISA). At low dosages, β-blockers, such as atenolol and metoprolol, should not induce bronchospasm in patients with reactive airway disease. Agents like acebutolol and pindolol have intrinsic sympathomimetic activity and may not lower the heart rate as much as agents without sympathomimetic activity. Agents with ISA are not recommended for postmyocardial infarction patients; cardioselective agents are preferred.

Table 60-10. Dose, Cost, and Adverse Effects of Specific Drugs

Generic name	Brand name	Initial dose (frequency)	Maintenance dose (frequency)	Monthly cost in $ (based on AWP)	Adverse effects
Diuretics: thiazide type					
Hydrochlorothiazide	Esidrix, HydroDiuril, others	25 mg qd	12.5-25 mg qd	0.59-1.50	Hyperuricemia, hypokalemia, hypomagnesemia, hyperglycemia, hyponatremia, hypercalcemia, hypercholesterolemia, hypertriglyceridemia, pancreatitis, rashes, weakness, sexual dysfunction
Chlorthalidone	Hygroton	25 mg qd	12.5-100 mg qd	1.65-3.12	
Indapamide	Lozol	1.25 mg qd	1.25-5 mg qd	9.09-20.62	
Metolazone	Zaroxolyn	2.5 mg qd	2.5-10 mg qd	14.60-19.87	
	Mykrox	0.5 mg qd	0.5-1 mg qd	22.09-44.18	
Diuretics: loop					
Bumetanide	Bumex, others	0.5-2 mg qd	0.5-5 mg qd-bid	5.15-36.22	Dehydration, circulatory collapse, hypokalemia, hyponatremia, hypomagnesemia, hypocalcemia, hyperglycemia, metabolic alkalosis, hyperuricemia, blood dyscrasias, rashes, lipid changes as with thiazide diuretics
Ethacrynic acid	Edecrin	12.5-50 mg qd	25-100 mg qd-bid	9.66-27.54	
Furosemide	Lasix	20-40 mg qd-bid	40-320 mg qd-bid	1.26-5.68	
Torsemide	Demadox	5 mg qd	5-10 mg qd-bid	15.09-16.71	
Diuretics: potassium-sparing					
Amiloride	Midamor, others	5 mg qd	5-10 mg qd	11.07-22.14	Hyperkalemia, gastrointestinal disturbances; amiloride: rash, headache; spironolactone: hyponatremia, mastodynia, gynecomastia, agranulocytosis, menstrual abnormalities, rash; triamterene: nephrolithiasis
Spironolactone	Aldactone, others	25-50 mg qd-bid	25-100 mg qd-bid	2.24-9.41	
Triamterene	Dyrenium, others	50-200 qd-bid	100-300 mg qd-bid	14.52-43.56	
Diuretics: combination					
HCTZ 25, spironolactone 25	Aldactazide, others	1 tablet qd	1-4 tablets qd	2.88-11.52	Same as individual components
HCTZ 50 mg, spironolactone 50 mg	Aldactazide, others	1 tablet qd	1-2 tablets qd	14.30-28.60	
HCTZ 25 mg, triamterene 37.5 mg	Dyazide	1 capsule qd	1-2 capsules qd	11.26-22.52	
HCTZ 25 mg, triamterene 37.5 mg	Maxzide-25	1 tablet qd	½-2 tablets qd	3.14-12.54	
HCTZ 25 mg, triamterene 50 mg	Others	1 capsule qd	1-2 capsules qd	5.10-8.87	
HCTZ 50 mg, triamterene 75 mg	Maxzide, others	1 tablet qd	1 tablet qd	3.53	
HCTZ 50 mg, amiloride	Moduretic	½-1 tablet qd	½-2 tablets qd	2.19-5.44	

β-Adrenergic blocking drugs					
Atenolol	Tenormin	25-50 mg qd	25-100 mg qd	3.99-4.04	Fatigue, depression, bradycardia, decreased exercise tolerance, congestive heart failure, aggravation of peripheral arterial insufficiency, GI disturbances, bronchospasm, masking of symptoms of hypoglycemia, Raynaud's phenomenon, insomnia, vivid dreams or hallucinations, organic brain syndrome, rare blood dyscrasias and other allergic disorders, increased serum triglycerides, decreased HDL cholesterol, generalized pustular psoriasis, transient hearing loss, sudden withdraw can lead to exacerbation of angina and myocardial infarction
Betaxolol	Kerlone	5-10 mg qd	5-40 mg qd	12.51-75.06	
Bisoprolol	Zebeta	2.5-5 mg qd	2.5-20 mg qd	15.57-62.26	
Metoprolol	Lopressor	50-100 mg bid	50-300 mg bid	3.96-12.79	
Metoprolol sustained release	Toprol XL	50-100 mg qd	50-300 mg qd	15.90-71.82	
Nadolol	Corgard	20-40 mg qd	20-320 mg qd	25.60-101.22	
Propranolol	Inderal	80 mg bid	40-240 mg bid-tid	5.36-7.80	
Propranolol sustained release	Inderal LA	80 mg qd	80-160 mg qd	23.76-40.59	
Timolol	Blocadren	20 mg bid	10-40 mg bid	19.08-39.06	
β-Adrenergic blocking drugs with intrinsic sympathomimetic activity					
Acebutolol	Sectral	200-400 mg qd-bid	200-1200 mg qd-bid	25.23-90.90	Similar to other β-adrenergic blocking drugs but with less bradycardia and lipid changes; acebutolol is cardioselective at low dosages and can be associated with a positive antinuclear antibody test and occasional drug-induced lupus
Carteolol	Cartrol	2.5 mg qd	2.5-10 mg qd	31.80-63.60	
Penbutolol	Levatol	20 mg qd	10-20 mg qd	19.62-37.23	
Pindolol	Visken	10 mg bid	10-60 mg bid	36.96-143.10	
α-β Adrenergic blocking drugs					
Carvedilol	Coreg	12.5 mg bid	50 mg bid	90.00	Similar to other β-adrenergic blocking drugs but has intrinsic sympathomimetic activity and more orthostatic hypotension, fever, and hepatotoxicity
Labetalol	Normodyne, Trandate	200 mg bid	200-1200 mg bid	31.98-120.84	
α-Adrenergic blocking drugs					
Doxazosin	Cardura	1 mg qhs	1-16 mg qhs	29.13-64.20	Syncope with first dose (prazosin, terazosin), dizziness and vertigo, nasal congestion, palpitations, fluid retention, headache, drowsiness, weakness, priapism, urinary incontinence
Prazosin	Minipress	2-3 mg bid	2-30 mg bid	3.98-38.70	
Terazosin	Hytrin	1 mg qhs	1-20 mg qhs-bid	43.50-92.40	
Peripheral adrenergic inhibitors					
Guanadrel	Hylorel	10 mg qd-bid	10-75 mg qd-bid	11.24-168.53	Guanethidine: orthostatic hypotension, exercise hypotension, diarrhea, may aggravate bronchial asthma, bradycardia, sodium and water retention, retrograde ejaculation; reserpine: depression, nightmares, nasal stuffiness, drowsiness, GI disturbances, bradycardia
Guanethidine	Ismelin	10 mg qd	10-100 mg qd	18.09-118.20	
Reserpine	Serpasil	0.5 mg qd × 2 weeks	0.1-0.25 mg qd-bid	0.89-1.05	

HCTZ, Hydrochlorothiazide; *AWP*, average wholesale price from the *1998 Drug Topics Red Book*. The lowest priced generic was used when available. Table courtesy of David Green, PharmD.

Continued

Table 60-10. Dose, Cost, and Adverse Effects of Specific Drugs—cont'd

Generic name	Brand name	Initial dose (frequency)	Maintenance dose (frequency)	Monthly cost in $ (based on AWP)	Adverse effects
Central sympatholytic drugs					
Clonidine	Catapres	0.1-0.2 mg bid	0.1-0.6 mg bid	2.25-2.85	Clonidine: drowsiness, sedation, dry mouth, bradycardia, heart block, rebound hypertension; guanabenz: similar to clonidine; guanfacine: similar to clonidine but milder; methyldopa: similar to clonidine, also fatigue, orthostatic hypotension. GI disturbances including colitis, hepatitis, cirrhosis, hepatic necrosis; fever; Coombs' positive hemolytic anemia, lupus-like syndrome, immune thrombocytopenia, red cell aplasia
Guanabenz	Wytensin	8 mg bid	8-64 mg bid	31.92-190.08	
Guanfacine	Tenex	1 mg qhs	1-2 mg qhs	21.18-29.04	
Methyldopa	Aldomet	500 mg bid	500-2000 mg bid	9.01-14.52	
Angiotensin-converting enzyme (ACE) inhibitors					
Benazepril	Lotensin	10 mg qd	5-40 mg qd-bid	22.76-45.51	Cough, hypotension—particularly with a diuretic or volume depletion, loss of taste with anorexia, rash, acute renal failure with bilateral renal artery stenosis or stenosis of the artery to a single kidney, cholestatic jaundice, pancreatitis, angioedema, hyperkalemia, blood dyscrasias, may increase fetal mortality and should not be used during second and third trimesters of pregnancy
Captopril	Capoten	25-75 mg bid-tid	12.5-150 mg qd-tid	2.66-11.64	
Enalapril	Vasotec	2.5-5 mg qd	2.5-40 mg qd-bid	24.06-91.20	
Fosinopril	Monopril	10 mg qd	10-80 mg qd-bid	24.87-49.74	
Lisinopril	Prinivil, Zestril	5-10 mg qd	5-40 mg qd	25.29-40.89	
Moexipril	Univasc	7.5 mg qd	7.5-30 mg qd-bid	15.81-31.62	
Quinapril	Accupril	5-10 mg qd	5-80 mg qd-bid	28.50-57.00	
Ramipril	Altace	1.25-2.5 mg qd	1.25-20 mg qd-bid	19.89-57.90	
Trandolapril	Mavik	1-2 mg qd	1-4 mg qd-bid	18.75-37.50	
Angiotensin II receptor antagonists					
Candesartan	Atacand	16 mg qd	8-32 mg qd-bid	36.00-50.40	Hyperkalemia, hypotension, acute renal failure with bilateral renal artery stenosis or stenosis of the artery to a single kidney
Irbesartan	Avapro	150 mg qd	75-300 mg qd	36.15-63.26	
Losartan	Cozaar	50 mg qd	25-100 mg qd	36.30-72.60	
Valsartan	Diovan	80 mg qd	80-320 mg qd	35.10-70.20	
Calcium channel blockers					
Nondihydropyridines					
Diltiazem					Dizziness, headache, edema, constipation (especially verapamil), heart block, bradycardia, heart failure, gingival hyperplasia
Capsules (sustained release)	Cardizem SR	60-120 mg bid	120-360 mg bid	51.52-81.27	
	Cardizem CD	180-240 mg qd	120-360 mg qd	34.20-84.72	
	Dilacor-XR	180-240 mg qd	120-480 mg qd	30.30-80.40	
	Tiazac	120-240 mg qd	120-540 mg qd	26.01-86.09	

Capsules (sustained release)	Verelan	120-180 mg qd	120-480 mg qd-bid	37.50-88.80	
Tablets (sustained release)	Isoptin SR	120-180 mg qd	120-480 mg qd-bid	26.01-70.34	
	Calan SR	120-180 mg qd	120-480 mg qd-bid	26.01-70.34	
	Covera-HS	180 mg qhs	180-480 mg qhs	33.60-92.40	
Tablets (intermediate release)	Calan, Isoptin	120-240 mg tid	120-480 mg tid	24.53-35.04	
Dihydropyridines					Dizziness, headache, peripheral edema, flushing, tachycardia, rash, gingival hyperplasia
Amlodipine	Norvasc	5 mg qd	2.5-10 mg qd	38.70-65.23	
Felodipine	Plendil	5 mg qd	2.5-10 mg qd	28.19-50.62	
Isradipine (sustained release)	DynaCirc CR	5 mg qd	5-20 mg qd	35.79-113.78	
Isradipine (intermediate release)	DynaCirc	5 mg bid	5-20 mg bid	41.43-120.72	
Nicardipine (sustained release)	Cardene SR	60 mg bid	60-120 mg bid	41.92-79.68	
Nicardipine (intermediate release)	Cardene	60 mg tid	60-120 mg tid	35.32-70.64	
Nifedipine (sustained release)	Adalat CC	30 mg qd	30-120 mg qd	28.65-88.35	
	Procardia XL	30 mg qd	30-120 mg qd	40.50-121.20	
Nisoldipine (sustained release)	Sular	10-20 mg qd	10-60 mg qd	26.73-53.46	
Direct vasodilators					
Hydralazine	Apresoline	25 mg bid	50-200 mg qd-qid	1.13-2.57	Hydralazine: GI disturbances, tachycardia, aggravation of angina, headache, dizziness, fluid retention, nasal congestion, rashes and other allergic reactions, lupus-like syndrome, hepatitis; minoxidil: tachycardia, aggravation of angina, marked fluid retention, possible pericardial effusion, hirsutism, thrombocytopenia, leukopenia
Minoxidil	Loniten	5 mg qd	5-40 mg qd	5.84-17.24	

Central Inhibition of Sympathetic Drive

Clonidine, guanabenz, and guanfacine. Clonidine, guanabenz, and guanfacine are centrally adrenergic acting α_2-adrenergic agonists that decrease sympathetic output in the CNS. Clonidine is usually added to a diuretic or another agent when single therapy proves unsatisfactory. Occasionally, clonidine is a useful single-drug treatment for patients who cannot be managed with diuretics or β-blockers, but it should be given twice daily. Rebound hypertension, often accompanied by tachycardia, may occur with sudden withdrawal of clonidine or guanabenz. Readministration of the drug is usually sufficient treatment. Patients should be advised not to run out of medicine and doses should be tapered over 2 or 3 weeks when stopping the drug. These drugs should probably be avoided in patients with a history of intermittent or poor compliance.

Methyldopa. Methyldopa is also a central-acting adrenergic agonist. It may act by a mechanism that is similar to clonidine or by forming a false neurotransmitter. Methyldopa has been used safely for more than 20 years in the treatment of mild to moderate hypertension, usually in combination with a diuretic and/or other therapeutic agents. Some physicians believe that methyldopa's side effects, such as drowsiness, fatigue, and impotence, may limit its effectiveness. Methyldopa may be safely used in pregnancy.

Peripheral Adrenergic Inhibitors. Reserpine decreases the availability of norepinephrine, lowering sympathetic tone and peripheral vascular resistance. Reserpine also depletes catecholamines in the brain, potentially leading to sedation and depression, and in the myocardium, potentially decreasing cardiac output and slowing the heart rate. Guanethidine and guanadrel reduce peripheral resistance by decreasing the amount of norepinephrine released by stimulated adrenergic nerves. These medications blunt the normal vasoconstrictive response to assuming an upright posture and may lead to orthostatic hypotension.

α-Adrenergic Blockers. Prazosin, terazosin, and doxazosin block the smooth muscle postsynaptic α_1-receptors, dilating arteries without causing reflex tachycardia. In general, α-adrenergic blockers are not used as initial therapy, but rather in combination with a diuretic or another sympatholytic medication. α-Adrenergic blockers may be particularly beneficial for hypertensive patients with benign prostatic hypertrophy or peripheral arterial disease.

Combination α- and β-blockers. Labetalol has both properties, with the α effect being roughly one third of the β effect. Labetalol causes some slowing of the heart rate; however, in contrast to pure β-blockers, it does not decrease cardiac output or increase peripheral vascular resistance. For these reasons, labetalol offers some theoretic advantages over β-blockers, but its current place in the treatment of hypertension has not been clearly defined. The drug is relatively expensive and requires dosing twice daily.

Vasodilating agents. Direct-acting vasodilators are usually added as a third drug for patients who cannot be controlled with two drugs. The medications available in this class are hydralazine and minoxidil. Hydralazine is a direct-acting vasodilator that causes decreased arterial resistance, a reflex increase in heart rate, and a secondary increase in plasma renin. It has been used for years in the therapy of hypertension. Because hydralazine induces reflex tachycardia and fluid retention, it is most often used in combination with a diuretic and a β-blocker, clonidine, or nondihydropyridine calcium antagonist.

Minoxidil is a direct-acting vasodilator that also causes reflex tachycardia and fluid retention. It is a potent antihypertensive agent used in severe resistant hypertension and may be especially effective for patients with renal failure. Cardiovascular side effects, including congestive heart failure, hypotension, and angina, can be severe, and its associated hypertrichosis and coarsening of facial features may be unacceptable to women and adolescents, although balding men may be pleased.

Angiotensin-Converting Enzyme Inhibitors. ACE inhibitors inhibit the enzyme that converts angiotensin I (inactive) to angiotensin II, a potent vasoconstrictor that causes aldosterone secretion from the adrenal gland. Peripheral resistance is lowered without decreasing cardiac output or decreasing the glomerular filtration rate. ACE inhibitors reduce mortality for patients who have congestive heart failure and slow the progression of renal failure in diabetic patients.

Because ACE inhibitors can cause hyperkalemia, they should not be used concomitantly with potassium-sparing agents or for patients with diabetes and potassium retention. ACE inhibitors can cause serious nephrotoxicity by dramatically decreasing renal blood flow in patients with bilateral renal artery stenosis or unilateral stenosis with a solitary kidney.

Angiotensin II–Receptor Blockers. Angiotensin II (AII)-receptor blockers prevent the binding of angiotensin II to receptors in the kidney, brain, heart, and arterial walls, thus inhibiting the renin-angiotensin system and causing a dose-dependent fall in peripheral resistance. The AII-receptor blockers inhibit the action of angiotensin II synthesized independently of ACE and do not increase kinin levels, the presumed mediator of the ACE inhibitor–induced cough. Since bradykinin stimulates the release of the vasodilator nitric oxide from the endothelium, an effect which is believed to account in part for the vasodilator effects of the ACE inhibitors, AII-receptor blockers may prove to be less effective in the long term than ACE inhibitors. AII-receptor blockers are effective in lowering blood pressure, but whether they affect morbidity and mortality from cardiovascular disease is unknown.

Calcium Channel Blockers. Calcium is essential for muscle contraction, and increased levels of calcium may play a role in the development, if not the maintenance, of hypertension. By excluding the influx of calcium into smooth muscle cells, blood pressure can be reduced. From a functional standpoint, calcium channel blockers act as vasodilators. They come in two chemical forms: (1) the dihydropyridines (e.g., nifedipine, amlodipine, felodipine, isradipine, and nicardipine) and (2) the nondihydropyridines (e.g., verapamil and diltiazem). Although both classes of drugs lower blood pressure, verapamil and diltiazem have a substantial negative chronotropic effect and need to be used carefully in patients using β-blockers or with conduction defects. As previously mentioned, some of the dihydropyridines have been associated with possible increased morbidity and mortality. In 1998, their use in specific patients was still unclear.

Combination Drugs. Combinations of diuretics and potassium-sparing agents have been available for many years. Recently, other combinations have been formulated, including adrenergic blockers and diuretics, ACE inhibitors and diuretics, angiotensin II receptor antagonists and diuretics, and calcium channel blockers and diuretics. Reducing the number of pills can improve compliance. Combination drugs can be synergistic, allowing lower doses of the component drugs and reducing the risk of adverse effects.

Combined Lifestyle Modifications and Pharmacologic Treatment

There is no direct evidence of the effect of combined treatment on mortality or morbidity in people with hypertension. Compared with nonpharmacologic treatment alone, the addition of drug treatment produces greater decreases in blood pressure, especially when the nonpharmacologic treatment is weight loss. Compared with drug treatment alone, the addition of salt restriction appears to be no more effective in reducing blood pressure and may reduce quality of life.

Target Blood Pressures and Therapy Titration

Although the aim of antihypertensive therapy is to reduce risk of cardiovascular events and mortality, it is not possible to titrate therapy in individual patients using these outcomes. Most physicians monitor therapy based on blood pressure level and symptomatic adverse effects. A trial involving 18,790 patients with average age of 62 years and diastolic blood pressures between 100 to 115 mm Hg evaluated target diastolic blood pressures of ≤ 90 mm Hg, ≤ 85 mm Hg, and ≤ 80 mm Hg.[14] Most patients received a long-acting dihydropyridine calcium antagonist, felodipine (78%), and an ACE inhibitor (41%). There were no differences in major cardiovascular events among the three groups. The subset of diabetic patients randomized to the ≤ 80 group had half the rate of major cardiovascular events than those randomized to the ≤ 90 group (RR,90 vs. 80, 2.1; CI 1.2 to 3.4).

Strategies for titrating and changing particular drug regimens are largely opinion-based. JNC-VI recommends considering combinations of low-dose drugs rather than maximizing doses of one agent and then adding another. Their suggested algorithm for drug management is shown in Fig. 60-5.

Antithrombotic Treatment in Hypertensive Patients

Benefits and risks of treating hypertensive patients with antithrombotic treatment are finely balanced. The HOT trial showed approximately 200 older hypertensive patients would need to be treated for about 4 years with 75-mg aspirin daily to prevent one myocardial infarction. Numbers needed to harm for major or fatal bleeds were about 160.[14] Another large placebo-controlled trial, the thrombosis prevention trial (TPT), showed low-intensity anticoagulation with warfarin (target international normalized ratio 1.5) reduced the rate of fatal and nonfatal ischemic events by 20% (95% CI 1% to 35%) in high-risk patients who were in the top 20% to 25% of a cardiovascular risk score distribution.[16] Statistically nonsignificant excess intracranial and extracranial bleeds occurred at a rate of approximately 0.5 per 1000 individuals treated per year.

SPECIAL ISSUES

Resistant Hypertension

Almost all patients with hypertension can achieve good blood pressure control with minimal side effects, although a few patients may persistently have unacceptably high diastolic pressures (diastolic blood pressure greater than 105 mm Hg). For these patients, consider the following:

Poor Adherence to Drug Regimen. Nonadherence to drug therapy is probably the major cause of poor blood pressure control. An estimated 50% of patients take less than 80% of their prescribed antihypertensive pills (see below).

Sodium Retention. Patients who take one or more nondiuretic antihypertensive agents often have reflex sodium retention. Adding a diuretic (or using a more potent one) and reemphasizing the need for a low-sodium diet may improve blood pressure control.

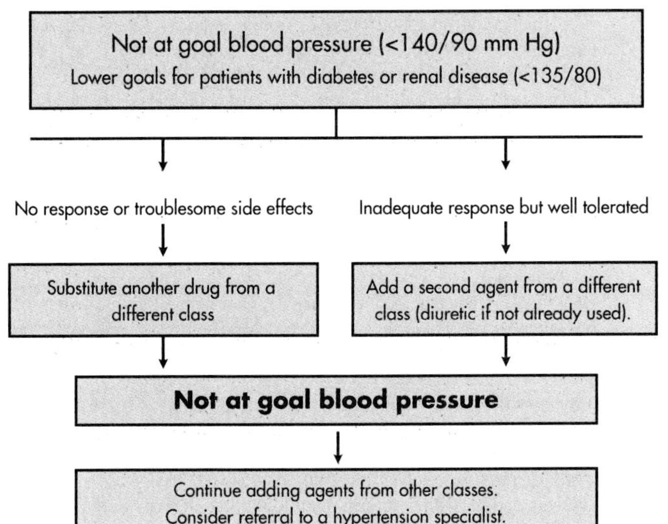

Fig. 60-5. Algorithm for drug management of hypertension. (Modified from JNC-VI.)

Excessive Alcohol Intake. If the hypertensive patient has a substantial alcohol intake, physicians should encourage total abstention from alcohol for 4 to 6 weeks while monitoring changes in blood pressure.

Secondary Hypertension. Refer to the previous section on secondary hypertension for screening evaluations and taking a medication history.

Substitute More Potent Antihypertensive Agents. For example, substitute minoxidil or an ACE inhibitor for hydralazine.

Close observation is essential for patients with resistant hypertension. Physicians should evaluate these patients for causes of secondary hypertension and carefully monitor the drug regimen and diet. A few patients may require hospitalization to control their blood pressure. Most patients experience a fall of 5 to 15 mm Hg in diastolic blood pressure during hospitalization, but this does not necessarily reflect increased drug effect. Occasionally, poor adherence can be diagnosed if there is a substantial blood pressure fall to almost hypotensive levels when the patient is hospitalized and continued on the prescribed medication.

Noncompliance with Treatment

Diagnosing poor compliance can be difficult and requires a frank, nonjudgmental exploration with the patient about pill-taking habits. Physicians may preface this discussion by acknowledging that pills are expensive, symbolic of illness, sometimes accompanied by unpleasant side effects, and, for many people, including physicians, difficult to take as prescribed. Another helpful approach is to identify the time of day when the patient takes medications and to review the exact number of pills taken during the previous 24 hours. Compliance occasionally may be assessed clinically or biochemically because some antihypertensive agents cause predictable physiologic effects. For example, β-blockers consistently decrease pulse, and thiazide diuretics consistently increase uric acid and usually decrease serum potassium.

Some methods that may improve adherence include:

1. Educating patients. Communicate clear target goals for blood pressure and discuss in a nonthreatening way the consequences of high blood pressure and the benefits of treatment. Emphasize that treating high blood pressure does not generally make patients feel better but, rather, is designed to prevent morbidity and mortality.

2. Encouraging patients to report side effects. Acknowledge that unpleasant side effects can occur during drug therapy and select an acceptable treatment regimen. Ask patients specifically about side effects they may be reluctant to voluntarily discuss, such as sexual dysfunction or the expense of treatment.

3. Simplifying drug regimens. Ask if once-a-day therapy would be easier than twice-a-day therapy. If so, use long-acting preparations that provide adequate 24-hour control.

4. Providing simple, written instructions about dosage and side effects. Review pill-taking habits with the patient. Recommend keeping pill bottles in a convenient location and emphasize the need to take pills at set times.

5. Improving the convenience of office visits and using other health care providers (e.g., nurses, physicians' assistants) to help with case management if feasible. Sending appointment reminders, having flexible scheduling hours, and contacting patients who have missed appointments help to improve adherence. Emphasize that high blood pressure may be a lifelong problem and that patients are responsible for returning for follow-up appointments and promptly refilling their medication. Give the patient shared responsibility for treatment and monitoring.

EBM EVIDENCE-BASED MEDICINE

Primary sources for this chapter were MEDLINE, Embase, and Joint National Committee VI guidelines. Electronic searches dating back to 1995 were conducted in June 1999. They focused on identifying systematic reviews, meta-analyses, and large randomized trials with clinical endpoints. Acknowledgments: Materials for drug tables were provided by David Green, PharmD.

REFERENCES

1. Alderman MH, Madhavan S, Cohen H, et al: Low urinary sodium associated with greater risk of myocardial infarction among treated hypertensive men, *Hypertension* 25:1144-1152, 1995.
2. Appel LJ, Moore TJ, Obarzanek E, et al: A clinical trial of the effects of dietary patterns on blood pressure, *N Engl J Med* 336:1117-1124, 1997.
3. Berglund G, Andersson OK, Widgren BR: Low-dose antihypertensive treatment with a thiazide diuretic is not diabetogenic: a ten-year controlled trial with bendroflumethiazide, *J Hum Hypertens* 4(suppl 5):S525-S527, 1986.
4. Beto JA, Bansal VK: Quality of life in treatment of hypertension: a meta-analysis of clinical trials, *Am J Hypertens* 5:125-133, 1992.
5. Croog SH, Levine S, Testa MA: The effects of antihypertensive therapy on quality of life, *N Engl J Med* 314:1657-1664, 1986.
6. Curb JD, Pressel SL, Cutler JA, et al: Effect of diuretic-based antihypertensive treatment on cardiovascular disease risk in older diabetic patients with isolated systolic hypertension, *JAMA* 276:1886-1892, 1996.
7. Cutler JA: Calcium channel blockers for hypertension—uncertainty continues, *N Engl J Med* 338:679-680, 1998.
8. Estacio RO, Jeffers BW, Hiatt WR, et al: The effect of nisoldipine as compared with enalapril on cardiovascular outcomes in patients with non–insulin-dependent diabetes and hypertension, *N Engl J Med* 338:645-652, 1998.
9. Graudal NA, Galloe AM, Garred P: Effects of sodium restriction on blood pressure, renin, aldosterone, catecholamines, cholesterols, and triglyceride, *JAMA* 279:1383-1391, 1998.
10. Griffith LE, Guyatt GH, Cook RJ, et al: Effects of dietary calcium supplementation on blood pressure, *Am J Hypertens* 12:84-92, 1999.
11. Grimm RH, Flack JM, Grandits GA, et al: Long-term effects on plasma lipids of drugs to treat hypertension, *JAMA* 275:1549-1556, 1996.
12. Gueyffier F, Froment A, Gouton M: New meta-analysis of treatment trials of hypertension: improving the estimate of therapeutic benefit, *J Hum Hypertens* 10:1-8, 1996.
13. Halbert JA, Silagy CA, Finucane P, et al: The effectiveness of exercise training in lowering blood pressure: a meta-analysis of randomised controlled trials of 4 weeks or longer, *J Hum Hypertens* 11:641-649, 1997. Search date 1996; Primary sources MEDLINE, Embase, Science Citation Index.
14. Hansson L, Zanchetti AZ, Carruthers SG, et al: Effects of intensive blood pressure lowering and low-dose aspirin in patients with hypertension: principal results of the Hypertension Optimal Treatment (HOT) trial, *Lancet* 351:1755-1762, 1998.
15. Materson BJ, Reda DJ, Cushman WC, et al: Single drug therapy for hypertension in men, *N Engl J Med* 328:914-921, 1993.
16. The Medical Research Council's General Practice Research Framework: Thrombosis prevention trial: randomised trial of low-intensity anticoagulation with warfarin and low-dose aspirin in the primary prevention of ischaemic heart disease in men at increased risk, *Lancet* 351:233-241, 1998.

17. Messerli FH, Grossman E, Goldbourt U: Are beta blockers efficacious as first-line therapy for hypertension in the elderly? A systematic review, *JAMA* 279:1903-1907, 1998.
18. Morris MC, Sacks F, Rosner B: Does fish oil lower blood pressure? A meta-analysis of controlled clinical trials, *Circulation* 88:523-533, 1993.
19. Neaton JD, Grimm RH, Prineas RJ, et al: Treatment of mild hypertension study: final results, *JAMA* 270:713-724, 1993.
20. Philipp T, Anlauf M, Distler A, et al: Randomised, double blind, multicentre comparison of hydrochlorothiazide, atenolol, nitrendipine, and enalapril in antihypertensive treatment: results of the HANE study, *Br Med J* 315:154-159, 1997.
21. Psaty BM, Smith NS, Siscovick DS, et al: Health outcomes associated with antihypertensive therapies used as first line agents: a systematic review and meta-analysis, *JAMA* 277:739-745, 1997.
22. Puddey IB, Beilin LJ, Vandongen R: Regular alcohol use raises blood pressure in treated hypertensive subjects, *Lancet* I:647-651, 1987.
23. Staessen JA, Fagard R, Thijs L, et al: Randomised double-blind comparison of placebo and active treatment for older patients with isolated systolic hypertension, *Lancet* 350:757-764, 1997.
24. Tatti P, Pahor M, Byington RP, et al: Outcome results of the fosinopril versus amlodipine cardiovascular events randomized trial (FACET) in patients with hypertension and NIDDM, *Diabetes Care* 21:597-603, 1998.
25. Weir MR, Flack JM, Applegate WB: Tolerability, safety, and quality of life and hypertensive therapy: the case for low-dose diuretics, *Am J Med* 101 (suppl 3A):83S-92S, 1996.
26. Whelton PK, He J, Cutler JA, et al: Effects of oral potassium on blood pressure: meta-analysis of randomized controlled clinical trials, *JAMA* 277:1624-1632, 1997.

Arrhythmias

David T. Martin

The term *arrhythmia* is used to describe any disorder of cardiac impulse formation or conduction, whether it be for a single beat or sustained for minutes, days, or decades. A healthy adult heart beats approximately 100,000 times a day, and the proportion of irregular or premature beats increases gradually with increasing age. This chapter will describe the general and specific mechanisms of arrhythmias, their clinical presentation and evaluation, and the range of therapies currently available. In addition, this chapter will provide guidelines for specialist referral.

PATHOPHYSIOLOGY

Cardiac myocytes are excitable cells and have intrinsic pacemaker activity. The rate of depolarization is dependent on the location and autonomic, pharmacologic, and pathologic state of these cells within the heart; in the normal heart the sinus node drives cardiac activation because these cells depolarize more rapidly than those cells in subsidiary pacemakers such as the atrioventricular (AV) node or intraventricular conduction (His-Purkinje) system. Enhanced automaticity of subsidiary pacemaker tissue causes premature beats and other arrhythmias (Fig. 61-1); this mechanism is probably responsible for atrial and ventricular premature beats and therefore is the most common arrhythmia mechanism in clinical practice, being responsible both for single premature beats and for the initiation of many sustained tachycardias. Reentry is an arrhythmia mechanism of both healthy and diseased cardiac cells; it requires unidirectional conduction block (usually caused by a premature beat) and an anatomic barrier that permits the formation of a circuit for the wavefront of cardiac activation to become self-perpetuating. Almost all sustained tachycardias observed in clinical practice are mediated by a reentrant mechanism; there may be a single (macro-reentrant) wavefront of activation as in ventricular tachycardia, atrial flutter, or those tachycardias associated with accessory pathways, or there may be multiple wavefronts as in atrial or ventricular fibrillation. Finally, disorders of action potential repolarization leading to "triggered" automaticity are responsible for arrhythmias associated with the congenital or acquired long QT syndrome, quinidine use, and digoxin toxicity.[2]

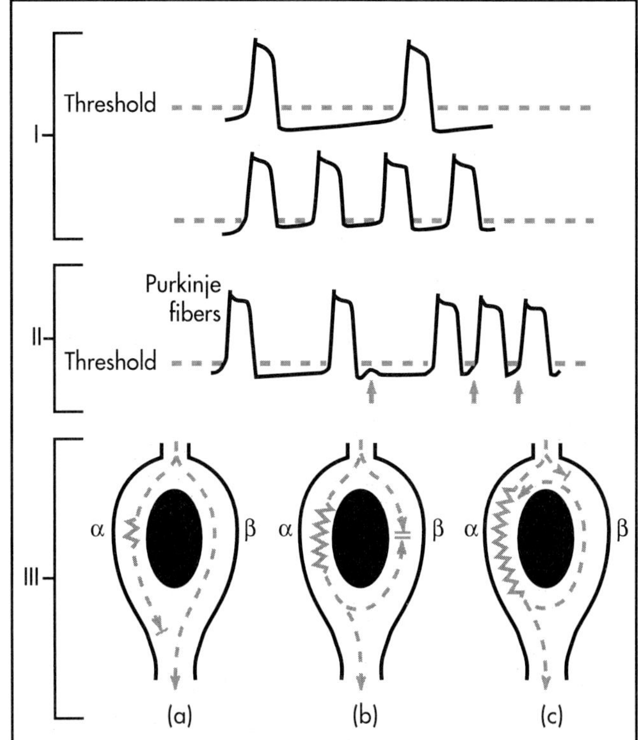

Fig. 61-1. Arrhythmia mechanisms. *Panel I,* Enhanced automaticity. This shows a normal rate of depolarization in phase 4 of the action potential in the upper portion. In contrast, the lower portion shows inadequate repolarization of the action potential during phase 3, which, given that the rate of depolarization in phase 4 is unchanged, leads to more rapid heart rates due to more rapid achievement of threshold voltage for cellular depolarization. *Panel II,* Triggered activity. This shows abnormal membrane depolarization during phase 3 of the action potential, which causes rapid and irregular heart rates when these brief oscillations in voltage reach cellular threshold. *Panel III,* Reentry. This is the most common clinical mechanism of tachycardia, and both an anatomic (or functional) barrier and unidirectional block are required to initiate and sustain such arrhythmias. *(a)* Cardiac impulse conducts via pathway β since the α pathway has a longer conduction time. *(b)* A premature beat finds the β pathway blocked (due to refractoriness) and therefore conducts down the slower α pathway, which has a shorter refractory period. Retrograde penetration of this impulse into the β pathway renders it refractory for antegrade conduction and *(c)* allows for continuous reentry of the impulse down the α pathway and up the β pathway.

CLINICAL PRESENTATION AND PATIENT EVALUATION

The various manifestations of arrhythmias are protean and often highly challenging for the physician (Box 61-1). Patients with the potential for life-threatening arrhythmias may have no symptoms; conversely, patients with benign arrhythmias caused by atrial premature beats may be disabled by palpitations. In general the degree of concern about the patient's symptoms or arrhythmia is more dependent on the context in which the symptoms occur than on the phenomenology of the symptoms themselves.[48] The presence or absence of heart disease is often the key determinant of the pace and location of the evaluation of the arrhythmia patient; prompt hospitalization is essential for the patient with a history of heart failure who presents with near-syncope, but would be inappropriate for a patient without clinical evidence of heart disease presenting with a hemodynamically stable episode of atrial fibrillation.

History

The specific history of palpitations is often revealing; the patient should be asked to indicate the rate and regularity of the heart during symptoms, as well as any subjectively apparent provoking or relieving characteristics. Are episodes abrupt in onset? Are they more likely to occur during exercise or rest? Are they affected by vagal maneuvers? Associated symptoms during episodes of palpitations may also be helpful in determining the mechanism of tachycardia: the sensation of throbbing in the neck during regular tachycardia has been associated with AV nodal reentry presumably because of the simultaneous atrial and ventricular activation during this arrhythmia leading to atrial contraction against a closed tricuspid valve. A careful medical history for evidence of cardiac disease (particularly coronary artery disease with left ventricular dysfunction, which predisposes to ventricular tachycardia), pulmonary disease (which predisposes to atrial fibrillation, atrial flutter, and atrial tachycardia), and thyroid disease (which predisposes to atrial fibrillation) is essential. A family history of sudden cardiac death should raise concern about hypertrophic cardiomyopathy or long QT syndrome, but is also relevant in the patient with coronary artery disease.

Use of medications and nonprescription remedies that may be arrhythmogenic is also an important component of the history (Table 61-1); similarly, alcohol and other recreational substance consumption, particularly cocaine, may predispose to both cardiac structural disease and arrhythmia. Alcohol is a well-recognized cause of atrial fibrillation, even in the absence of an associated cardiomyopathy, and long-term abstinence may be sufficient to eliminate recurrences of this arrhythmia.

Physical Examination

Although such opportunities are rare, the physical examination may be most helpful during the arrhythmia: a tachycardia is present when the heart rate exceeds 100 beats per minute. Marked irregularity suggests atrial fibrillation. Inspection of the venous pulse may reveal intermittent cannon waves indicative of AV dissociation (most commonly caused by ventricular tachycardia). The neck veins may exhibit regular rapid flutter waves, which are suggestive of atrial flutter, particularly if the heart rate is approximately 150 beats per minute.

Box 61-1. Clinical Manifestations of Arrhythmias

Palpitations	Heart failure
Dizzy spells	Confusion
Dyspnea	"Failure to thrive"
Lethargy	Syncope
Angina	Sudden death

Table 61-1. Potentially Arrhythmogenic Drugs

Compounds/class	Associated arrhythmia
Class 1A antiarrhythmic drugs (quinidine, disopyramide, procainamide)	Bradycardia Torsades de pointes*
Class IC antiarrhythmic drugs (flecainide, encainide, propafenone)	Monomorphic (VT) ventricular tachycardia Atrial flutter or tachycardia with 1:1 conduction
Sotalol	Bradycardia Torsades de pointes
Amiodarone	Sinus bradycardia AV block
Digoxin	Atrial tachycardia Ventricular premature beats AV block
Diuretics	Sinus tachycardia Polymorphic VT
Haloperidol	Torsades de pointes
Erythromycin	Torsades de pointes
Tricyclic antidepressants	Sinus tachycardia Ventricular tachycardia
Any anticholinergic agent	Sinus tachycardia Atrial fibrillation
Theophylline	Sinus tachycardia Multifocal atrial tachycardia

*Torsades de pointes is a polymorphic ventricular tachycardia associated with prolonged QT interval that usually occurs in the context of an underlying bradycardia.

DIAGNOSIS

It is a helpful exercise for the evaluating physician to classify each patient after obtaining the history, physical examination, and surface electrocardiogram (ECG) into one of three clinical categories:

1. *Definite arrhythmia:* The symptoms and ECG are recorded together and the diagnosis is not in doubt; all that remains is for appropriate therapy to be selected.
2. *Potential arrhythmia:* Specific symptoms of arrhythmia are not present, but significant structural heart disease or other arrhythmia substrates such as Wolff-Parkinson-White pattern on the ECG raise the question of arrhythmia potential. Such patients may be at high risk despite the apparent absence of symptoms, and ambulatory (Holter) monitoring or electrophysiologic evaluation may be advisable.
3. *Possible arrhythmia:* The patient may have symptoms

suggestive of arrhythmia but will require further investigation to correlate the symptom(s) with the cardiac rhythm. The evaluation of such patients is often expedited by ambulatory patient-activated event monitoring.

Diagnostic Procedures

For the last hundred years the gold standard in arrhythmia diagnosis has been the 12-lead ECG, and despite the advent of intracardiac electrophysiologic recording techniques, this simple noninvasive tool remains central to the investigation of arrhythmias. The key features of the ECG that are relevant in arrhythmia interpretation are given in Box 61-2. In many patients it may not be possible to obtain an ECG recording of all 12 leads during an arrhythmia; this difficulty in capturing brief episodes of arrhythmia led to the development of monitoring techniques, including Holter monitoring in which the patient wears the recording unit attached to skin electrodes for at least a 24-hour period and keeps a diary of symptoms during that time. The recording is analyzed later and provides a quantitative evaluation of the cardiac rhythm during the recording period. This quantitative report is useful in defining the frequency and grade of atrial (particularly atrial fibrillation) and ventricular arrhythmia, which may be asymptomatic. However, because this technique does not easily allow for correlation of symptoms with cardiac rhythm, and is likely to yield little in the patient with infrequent symptoms, this test has in many cases been superseded by event monitoring in which the patient wears the monitoring equipment for 30 days (changing skin electrodes daily) and activates the device only when symptoms are present; the monitor records continuously for a programmable period prior to patient activation (continuous loop), as well as for some minutes after activation. The captured rhythm is then transmitted transtelephonically by the patient to a central monitoring station where the technician is able to provide immediate advice to the patient as well as notify the physician if necessary.[49]

Other noninvasive techniques have recently been developed for evaluation of arrhythmia risk, particularly regarding ventricular tachycardias and sudden death. The earliest of these to gain widespread use in clinical practice was the signal-averaged electrocardiogram; this technique records, averages, and amplifies a few hundred beats of a resting ECG, with the focus on the terminal portion of the QRS complex where "late potentials" may be found. This subtle widening of the QRS complex represents the slowed conduction of the cardiac impulse that occurs around the border zone of the scar that is present after myocardial infarction. The presence of a late potential indicates that the substrate for ventricular tachycardia exists. However, it does not necessarily suggest that ventricular tachycardia will actually occur clinically, and studies of this technique indicate that the sensitivity for ventricular tachycardia is quite low. The specificity, however, is high, suggesting that a patient with a negative test after myocardial infarction would not be expected to have inducible ventricular tachycardia at electrophysiologic study.[41] It should be noted that signal averaging of the ECG cannot be interpreted in the presence of an intraventricular conduction defect or bundle branch block, significantly limiting its clinical application.

Prediction of arrhythmic events in patients with heart disease (usually after myocardial infarction) has been studied using other noninvasive techniques including heart rate variability analysis and T wave alternans testing.[31,37] These tests provide information about autonomic function in the heart and electrical stability regarding the risk of ventricular fibrillation, respectively, but neither has gained wide currency in the United States. All of the noninvasive tests used for risk stratification regarding sudden death have the significant limitation of relatively low sensitivity; integrating such test data with the clinical context and most importantly with the ejection fraction provides more clinically useful information to aid decision making in patients who may be candidates for prophylactic defibrillator implantation.

Box 61-2. ECG Features in Tachycardia Diagnosis

Is it regular or irregular?
- Irregular tachycardias are almost always atrial fibrillation

Is the QRS complex narrow or broad (>120 ms)?
- QRS complex < 120 ms is a supraventricular tachycardia (SVT)
- QRS complex > 120 ms is usually ventricular tachycardia (VT), but old ECG in sinus rhythm is helpful to confirm. Note that aberrantly conducted SVT exhibits typical bundle branch block pattern, which VT often does not

Are there any P waves?
- 1:1 P-QRS relationship suggests SVT (evaluate R-P interval)
- AV dissociation or ventriculo-atrial block confirms VT

Is the rate 150 beats per minute?
- Atrial flutter should be suspected

Are there capture or fusion beats?
- Confirms VT

What is the QRS axis?
- Normal axis does not exclude VT
- Bizarre axis suggests VT

MANAGEMENT

General Principles

In the last 10 years clinical cardiac electrophysiology has evolved from a predominantly academic enterprise of little practical benefit to patients, to a recognized subspecialty of cardiology in which effective therapies can be offered for management of both atrial and ventricular arrhythmias. Referral for electrophysiologic evaluation and possible definitive therapy should be considered for many patients (Table 61-2).

Management strategies for tachycardias include suppression or rate control using drugs or implantable devices, repeated termination using implantable antitachycardia devices, and ablation (destruction) of the tachycardia substrate using catheter or surgical techniques (Table 61-3).

The treatment of tachycardias may be considered in two phases: acute management and long-term therapies. The acute termination of any tachycardia in which the patient is hemodynamically unstable should be performed using cardioversion or defibrillation. This procedure requires intimate familiarity with the functioning of the defibrillator and the

Table 61-2. Rationale for Electrophysiologic Referral: Common Clinical Scenarios

Indication	Clinical scenarios	Likely outcome(s)
Arrhythmia diagnosis	Recurrent syncope in context of structural heart disease	EPS showing inducible ventricular tachycardia or (less likely) conduction disease indicating risk of bradycardia
Risk stratification	Asymptomatic nonsustained ventricular tachycardia in context of significant left ventricular dysfunction and coronary artery disease	EPS showing inducible ventricular tachycardia; noninducibility of ventricular tachycardia suggests lower risk for sudden death
	Syncope in context of Wolff-Parkinson-White ECG pattern	Characterization of accessory pathway conduction properties provides prognostically useful information
Therapy selection	Sustained ventricular tachycardia	EPS guides ICD programming; occasionally EPS reveals a tachycardia that is curable by ablation
Curative therapy	Recurrent paroxysmal supraventricular tachycardia	Catheter ablation provides >95% cure for all common forms of SVT
	Atrial flutter	Catheter ablation provides >80% cure for common flutter
Palliative therapy	Aborted sudden cardiac death	ICD "rescue" therapy for recurrent cardiac arrest provides clear survival advantage over drug treatment
	Drug refractory rapid atrial fibrillation	AV junction ablation and permanent pacing provide long-term improvement in functional status and quality of life

EPS, Electrophysiologic study; *ICD*, implantable cardioverter-defibrillator; *SVT*, supraventricular tachycardia; *AV*, atrioventricular.

Table 61-3. Established and Evolving Indications for Radiofrequency Catheter Ablation

Arrhythmia	Target
Established Indications	
AV nodal reentrant tachycardia	"Slow" Pathway
AV reentrant tachycardia	Accessory pathway
Atrial fibrillation	AV junction
Atrial flutter	Right atrium, subeustachian isthmus
Ectopic atrial tachycardia	Right or left atrium
Idiopathic ventricular tachycardia	RV outflow tract, left ventricle
Bundle branch reentrant tachycardia	Right bundle branch
Evolving Indications	
"Focal" atrial fibrillation	Pulmonary veins
Atrial fibrillation	Left atrium (linear lesions)
Ventricular tachycardia (CAD)	Left ventricle

CAD, Coronary artery disease.

need to synchronize energy discharge to the QRS complex. Intravenous sedation or anesthesia is often required, and it should never be necessary to deliver a transthoracic shock to a patient who is alert. This procedure is effective for termination of all reentrant arrhythmias, but often needs to be supplemented with agents designed to prevent recurrence.

In the diagnosis and termination of tachycardias in the emergency setting, the use of the endogenous nucleoside adenosine has recently gained popularity because of its favorable safety profile when compared with verapamil; both agents safely terminate narrow QRS complex regular tachycardias about 90% of the time.[14] Adenosine has a half-life of only a few seconds, and although it may produce complete AV block, such effect is transient and permits safe arrhythmia diagnosis even when a wide complex tachycardia is present; the use of verapamil under such circumstances is absolutely contraindicated because of its hypotensive effects and the risk that a relatively stable ventricular tachycardia will degenerate to ventricular fibrillation.

Intravenous lidocaine is indicated for the acute treatment of the stable patient with ongoing ventricular tachycardia, and intravenous procainamide may be used as a second-line agent for this indication also, although intravenous amiodarone is probably more efficacious. Procainamide has also been used for the acute termination of atrial fibrillation, and in particular for treatment of preexcited atrial fibrillation complicating the Wolff-Parkinson-White syndrome. However, the recently marketed agent, ibutilide, may have more utility for the acute termination of both atrial fibrillation and flutter in the emergency setting; this short half-life agent prolongs action potential repolarization and appears to have about 30% efficacy in restoring sinus rhythm, with a risk of proarrhythmia (polymorphic ventricular tachycardia) of about 2%.[30]

Catheter ablation using radiofrequency energy has revolutionized the treatment of supraventricular tachycardias and other less common arrhythmias.[28] In the treatment of ventricular arrhythmias, automatic defibrillator implantation has become the standard of care for patients who have suffered a life-threatening arrhythmic event or who are at high risk for such an event.[29,42]

Atrial and Ventricular Premature Beats

Premature beats are ubiquitous; more than 60% of healthy adults undergoing ambulatory (Holter) monitoring for a single 24-hour period exhibit asymptomatic atrial or ventricular premature beats, and because of the unpredictability and inherent variation of such events, it is thought that they are more widely present in the general population. The frequency of both atrial and ventricular premature beats is increased in the presence of heart disease; over 80% of postinfarction patients exhibit ventricular premature beats, and when more than 10 are present per hour the mortality risk is elevated. However, the Cardiac Arrhythmia Suppression Trial (CAST) clearly demonstrated that adequate suppression of such arrhythmia with the class Ic drugs flecainide and encainide does not reduce the risk of death but actually increases it.[43,44] Therefore specific treatment of premature beats with antiarrhythmic agents is not indicated; the risk that such beats confer in the postinfarct patient is related more to the presence of associated ventricular dysfunction and ongoing ischemia than to the arrhythmia itself.

Atrial premature beats are identified on the ECG by the occurrence of an early P wave, which often has a configuration different from the sinus node P wave. Atrial premature beats may originate in the left or right atrium, and may be multifocal in origin; they usually conduct to the ventricle normally, but very early premature beats may conduct aberrantly (with a widened QRS complex) or not at all. Such blocked atrial premature beats are often misinterpreted as second-degree heart block, and it is important to emphasize that the normal physiology of the AV node in these circumstances is to delay or block conduction in a fashion that is directly related to the degree of prematurity of the early P wave. The presence of AV nodal blocking drugs increases the likelihood that atrial premature beats will be nonconducted.

The management of atrial and ventricular premature beats in asymptomatic patients consists of reassurance alone that no specific treatment is required. In a significant minority of patients premature beats cause disabling symptoms, usually palpitations described as "thumping," "fluttering," or "flip flop" in the chest. Occasionally a patient complains of a sensation that the heart is stopping. Again, once the symptoms have been correlated with premature beats (since up to 40% of patients with such complaints have no arrhythmia whatsoever during their symptoms), it is important to reassure the patient that these symptoms reflect a benign ubiquitous condition and that elimination of alcohol and adrenergic stimulants may be sufficient to abolish the palpitations. However, if such simple alterations in lifestyle are ineffective, then the use of β-blockers is recommended; these agents do not abolish premature beats but reduce cardiac contractility and thereby eliminate the vigorous postextrasystolic beat that causes the symptom of palpitations.

Tachycardias

Tachycardia is the occurrence of three or more consecutive complexes faster than 100 beats per minute. If the patient is hemodynamically stable, an attempt should be made to determine the arrhythmia mechanism because this will usually lead to appropriate therapy. Narrow QRS complex tachycardias are supraventricular in origin, and wide QRS complex tachycardias may be either supraventricular or ventricular, although in the absence of data to suggest otherwise, it is best to assume that the arrhythmia is ventricular tachycardia.

The availability of a sinus rhythm ECG for comparison with that recorded during the tachycardia often aids prompt arrhythmia diagnosis. Bedside techniques that facilitate identification of the arrhythmia mechanism include carotid massage and other vagal maneuvers and the administration

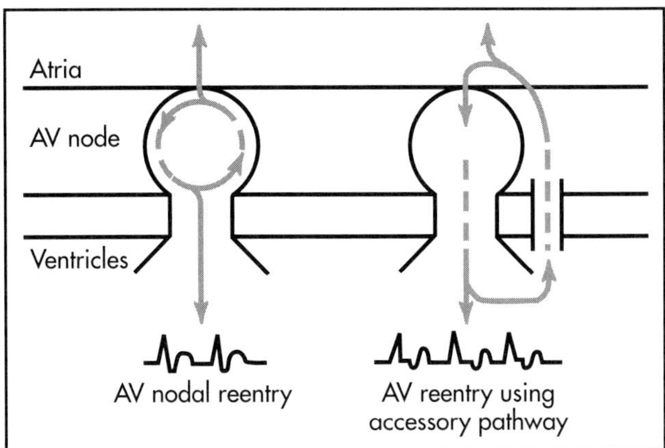

Fig. 61-2. Common mechanisms of paroxysmal supraventricular tachycardia. The left panel shows a reentrant circuit within the region of the atrioventricular (AV) node. Because the circuit is short and conduction is rapid within it, impulses exit to activate atria and ventricles virtually simultaneously, thus producing the typical ECG appearance where the P wave is buried within the QRS complex during such tachycardias. The right panel shows a reentrant circuit involving activation of the ventricles via the normal AV nodal pathway, but retrograde activation of the atria via an accessory pathway, which is often some distance from the AV node. Therefore the reentrant circuit is relatively long, and there is a significant difference in the timing of activation of the atria and ventricles, causing the typical ECG appearance where the P wave is visible between QRS complexes.

of intravenous adenosine. Neither intervention should be performed without the ready availability of continuous ECG monitoring and emergency resuscitation equipment, including a defibrillator. Carotid massage should not be performed in patients with neck bruits.

Sinus Tachycardia. In the adult, sinus tachycardia rarely exceeds 200 beats per minute and is not considered a primary arrhythmia; it is characterized by gradual increases and decreases in rate, with typical sinus P waves preceding each QRS complex. The PR interval is usually not prolonged, reflecting the enhanced adrenergic tone, and carotid massage has little or no effect on the rate or PR interval. The presence of sinus tachycardia should prompt a search for the underlying cause, on which diagnosis the management should be based. Occasionally an apparent sinus tachycardia is observed to begin and terminate abruptly; this arrhythmia is seen in patients with sinus node disease and is referred to as sinus node reentrant tachycardia. It is exquisitely sensitive to vagal maneuvers, which abruptly terminate it, and it has been successfully treated with verapamil.[16] Patients with sinus node reentry may also have significant bradycardias due to sinus node disease and may require permanent pacing.

Paroxysmal Supraventricular Tachycardia. There are two reentrant mechanisms that account for over 80% of the arrhythmias with this common presentation (Fig. 61-2).[13] AV nodal reentrant tachycardia (AVNRT) is the most common and is more likely to occur in older patients with paroxysmal supraventricular tachycardia (Fig. 61-3). The ECG during this arrhythmia usually shows a narrow complex tachycardia that may be very rapid (up to 260 beats per minute) and in which P waves are not visible because there is

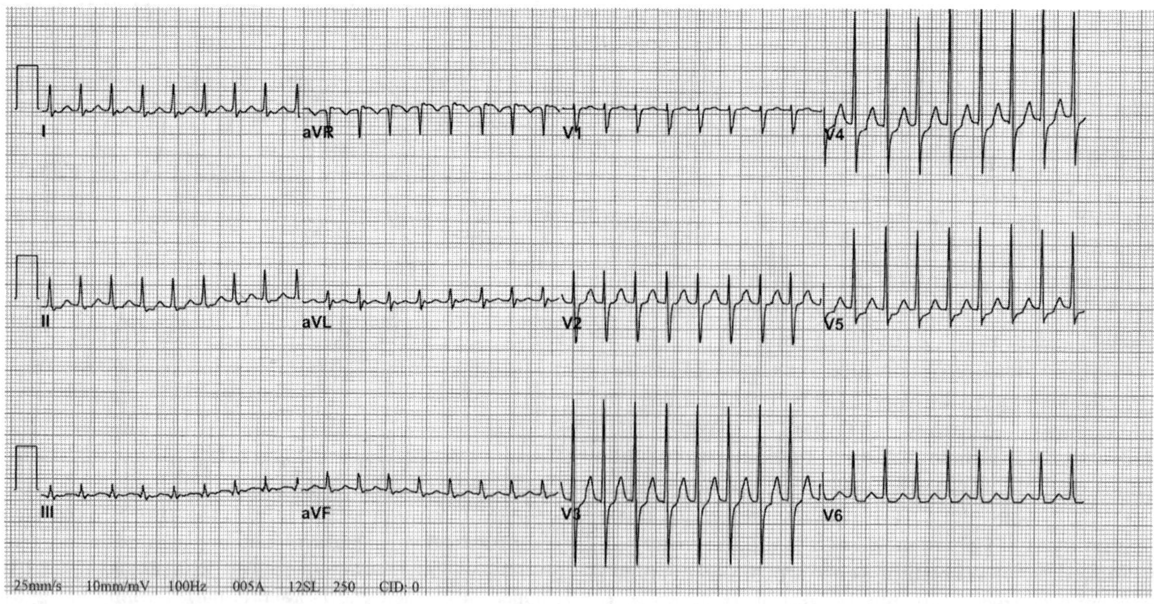

Fig. 61-3. ECG example of atrioventricular nodal reentrant tachycardia. This ECG shows a regular narrow QRS complex tachycardia at 200 bpm. There is a 1 : 1 relationship between P waves and QRS complexes; P waves are visible in the terminal portion of the S wave in the inferior leads, particularly lead II.

simultaneous atrial and ventricular activation and P waves are buried within the QRS complex. Orthodromic AV reentrant tachycardia (AVRT) is mediated by an accessory pathway and is one of the arrhythmias that occurs in the Wolff-Parkinson-White syndrome. Most patients with this form of supraventricular tachycardia, however, do not evidence the Wolff-Parkinson-White pattern on the ECG during sinus rhythm, suggesting that the pathway conducts only retrogradely. During tachycardia the P waves may or may not be visible, depending on the rate of the arrhythmia and the location of the accessory pathway; however, since most pathways are located laterally on the mitral annulus and the ventriculoatrial conduction time is therefore relatively long, inverted P waves are often seen in the inferior and lateral ECG leads between QRS complexes (Fig. 61-4). Since the AV node participates in the tachycardia circuit in both these mechanisms, the response to vagal maneuvers and adenosine is usually abrupt termination of the arrhythmia.

Typically, the patient is aware of sudden onset of rapid palpitations with or without concomitant symptoms of chest discomfort, dizziness, or syncope. Episodes may be brief and self-terminating or may last for hours until terminated in an emergency department. The degree to which these symptoms cause anxiety and interfere with lifestyle varies widely and reflects the wider variation in arrhythmia frequency. Where episodes are infrequent and symptoms are well tolerated, treatment may consist merely of advice about how to perform Valsalva's maneuver at home; alternatively drug or ablation therapy is appropriate for many patients with frequent or bothersome symptoms. Commonly used drugs include β-blockers, digoxin, and calcium channel blockers such as verapamil or diltiazem. Drug selection should be empiric, but it is important to note that neither digoxin nor calcium channel blockers should be used if there is any possibility of Wolff-Parkinson-White syndrome, since these agents may enhance anterograde conduction in the accessory pathway and predispose the patient to ventricular fibrillation should atrial fibrillation occur. In general, patients with recurrent tachycardia after a single drug trial should be offered catheter ablation early in the management of this condition, since it has a salutary effect on quality of life and has been shown to be more cost-effective than lifelong drug therapy.[22,27]

Catheter ablation of these tachycardias is a safe and effective procedure and is advised by many authorities as first-line therapy.[38] The target site for ablation in AVNRT is the slow pathway, which is in the floor of the right atrium between the orifice of the coronary sinus and the annulus of the tricuspid valve; this area is relatively remote from the compact AV node, and therefore the risk of heart block complicating the procedure is low (1% to 2% at most) compared with the previously used technique targeting the fast pathway following which the risk of heart block was reported to be up to 8%. In AVRT the target for ablation is the accessory pathway itself, either at its atrial or ventricular insertion point around the mitral or tricuspid annulus. The risk of heart block is present in these cases only where the pathway itself is close to the AV node, a rare occurrence. For both arrhythmias ablation is successful in approximately 98% of cases.[19,20]

Atrial Fibrillation. Atrial fibrillation is the most common sustained cardiac arrhythmia (Fig. 61-5).[34,47] It is a major public health problem in the United States, afflicting approximately 1.7% of the population aged 60 to 64 and up to 12% of those over the age of 75; as the general population ages, and appears to be surviving other cardiac conditions due possibly to improved therapies for coronary artery disease, the frequency of atrial fibrillation is increasing markedly. Although atrial fibrillation is regarded by some physicians as an acceptable alternative to sinus rhythm, it must be remembered that this arrhythmia is a major cause of thromboembolism and is responsible for both impaired left ventricular function (due probably to uncontrolled ventricular rates) as well as poor quality of life. Many of the symptoms

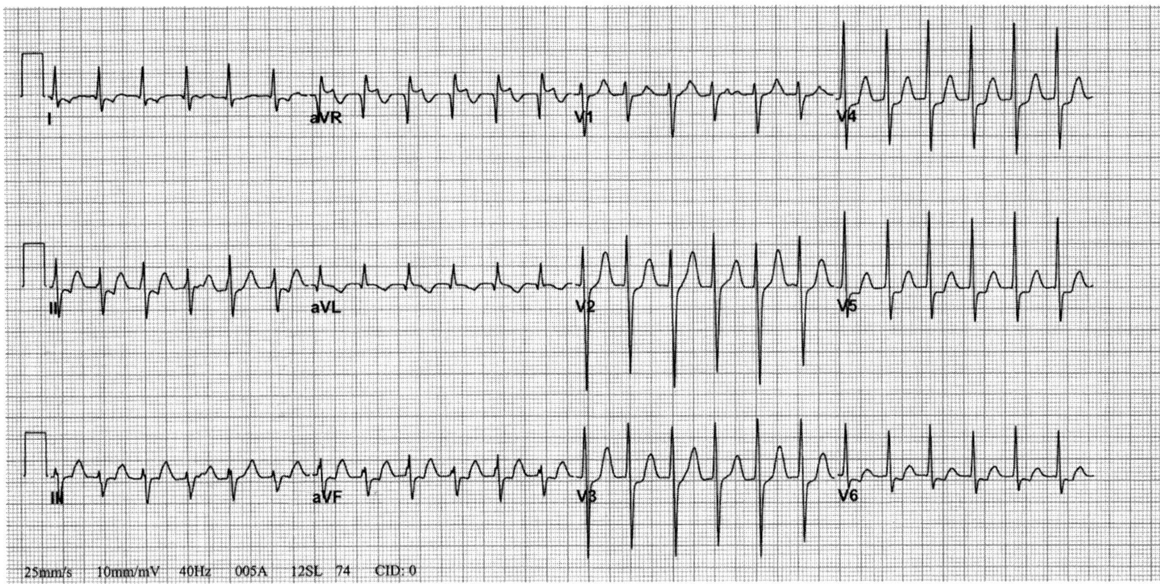

Fig. 61-4. ECG example of atrioventricular reentrant tachycardia. This ECG shows a regular narrow QRS complex tachycardia at 145 bpm. The P waves deform the T waves in the inferior leads and leads I and V1. In addition, there is QRS alternans where the amplitude of the R and S waves varies beat-by-beat in most leads.

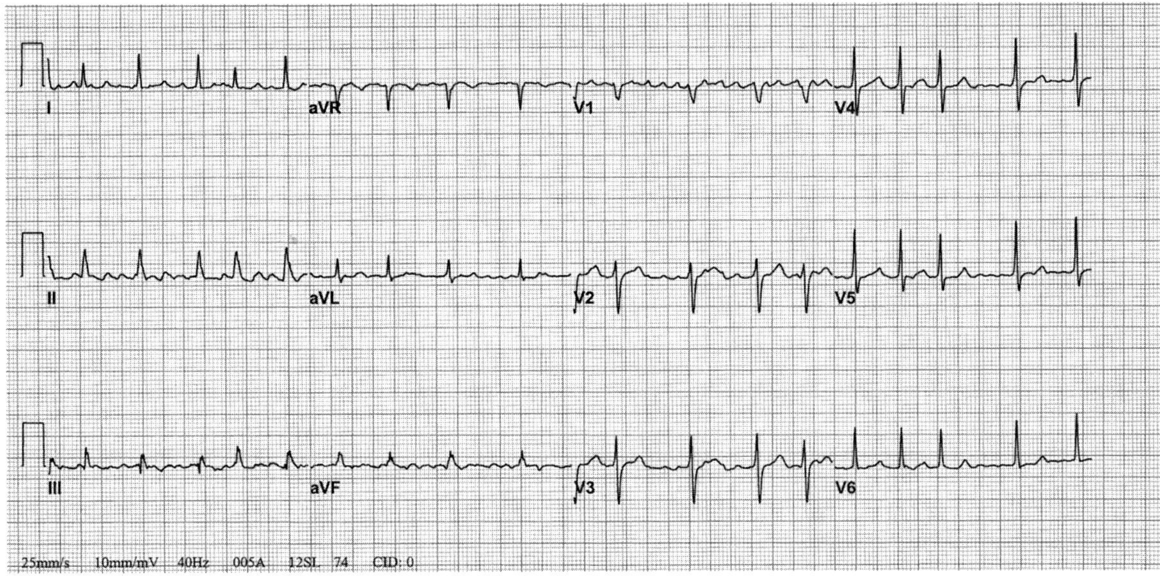

Fig. 61-5. ECG example of atrial fibrillation. The ECG shows complete irregularity in timing of the QRS complexes in association with a baseline reflective of disorganized atrial activity.

are subtle and nonspecific; the effects of sustained atrial fibrillation may be insidious, suggesting this condition be compared more with hypertension than with acute disorders such as ventricular tachycardia or unstable angina. Most patients complain of fatigue and exertional shortness of breath, palpitations being surprisingly uncommon; in one study the initial quality of life of patients with atrial fibrillation undergoing AV junction ablation was less than that of patients recovering from myocardial infarction or with severe rheumatoid arthritis.

The importance of atrial fibrillation as a cause of stroke is well known. The annual risk of stroke ranges from about 1.5% in the 40 to 50 age group to >20% in patients older than 70; the Framingham data suggest that atrial fibrillation is an independent risk factor for stroke[47] (risk ratio 5.6 compared with matched controls in sinus rhythm) and that this risk is increased significantly in the presence of hypertension (risk ratio 12), heart failure (risk ratio 12), or mitral stenosis (risk ratio 17). It has been estimated that atrial fibrillation accounts for 15% of all symptomatic cerebral emboli, and studies of computed tomographic (CT) scanning in asymptomatic patients with nonrheumatic atrial fibrillation have shown silent cerebral infarctions in up to 26%.[9,33] Prospective trials have shown repeatedly that the risk of stroke can be essentially eliminated by warfarin anticoagulation targeted to an international normalized ratio (INR) of 2 to 3; as the INR falls below 2 the risk of stroke progressively and steeply rises[18]; above an INR of 4 the risks of bleeding increase significantly.[5] Unfortunately, precise anticoagulant control within the 2 to 3 range is not always possible, and warfarin is considered contraindicated in many patients; moreover, anticoagulation is a lifelong undertaking that is associated with substantial costs and restriction of activities. Therefore, although warfarin anticoagulation should generally be employed in patients with atrial fibrillation, it may be forgone in some patients considered at low risk for stroke; such patients include younger individuals (<65) with *lone atrial fibrillation* (i.e., no known heart disease, hypertension, or alcoholism) or infrequent paroxysmal atrial fibrillation.

It has recently been recognized that atrial fibrillation may be responsible for a reversible dilated cardiomyopathy, and that left ventricular function can be normalized by either cardioversion or rate control achieved by AV junction ablation[17,36]; atrial fibrillation frequently coexists with heart failure since it is the quintessential arrhythmia of patients with significant left ventricular dysfunction. Often there may be a "chicken and egg" situation in which rapidly conducting atrial fibrillation leads to worsening heart failure but it may not be clear which is primarily responsible for the patient's deterioration. It is often unclear whether rapid ventricular rates (and consequent impaired cardiac filling), loss of atrial transport (which in heart failure may be responsible for up to 30% of cardiac output), or the irregular ventricular response is responsible alone or in combination for decompensated heart failure. It is certainly a common paradox that those patients who most need to have sinus rhythm (and atrial transport) restored are those in whom the use of antiarrhythmic drugs presents most risk. Generally, however, vigorous attempts at cardioversion (usually using adjunctive amiodarone) or heart rate control (often by AV junction ablation) are rewarded by marked symptomatic improvement as well as by objectively demonstrable increases in ventricular function.

The goals of treatment in atrial fibrillation are to control ventricular rate, to prevent thromboembolism, and to both convert to and maintain sinus rhythm. The order and urgency with which these goals are achieved vary widely according to clinical circumstances. It is likely that the tacit acceptance of atrial fibrillation by many physicians is contributed to by the lack of effective therapies. Although external direct current (DC) cardioversion is about 90% effective, atrial fibrillation recurs in a majority of patients within a year. Even in those treated with antiarrhythmic drugs such as quinidine or sotalol the recurrence rate is approximately 50% at 1 year, and with these agents the risk of proarrhythmia and sudden death may be up to 15% per year in patients with structural heart disease.[3,6] Amiodarone may be associated with a greater success rate, but this agent has other significant toxicities that limit its long-term use and its applicability to younger patients.

Cardioversion may be achieved by pharmacologic or electrical means. Oral quinidine loading has been used for over 40 years for cardioversion but has only a 20% efficacy rate at best. Ibutilide has the advantage of a shorter half-life and probably greater efficacy than these other agents; in addition, there is evidence from a randomized trial of ibutilide pretreatment prior to transthoracic electrical cardioversion that this drug may also reduce the energy requirement and thereby facilitate the restoration of sinus rhythm.[32] However, there remains a need to further define the optimal management strategy for conversion to sinus rhythm since the relative cost-effectiveness of ibutilide versus (or in combination with) DC cardioversion is unknown.

Internal cardioversion has a higher success rate than external cardioversion, and has led to the concept of the automatic implantable atrial defibrillator, a device currently in clinical development; this notion has been supported by recent data from a goat model suggesting that the ease of cardioversion is directly related to the duration of the arrhythmia and that "atrial fibrillation begets atrial fibrillation."[46] Therefore longer term maintenance of sinus rhythm may be possible by repeated and early cardioversion; however, this theory remains to be validated by clinical data.

Of the drugs available for ventricular rate control, β-blockers have become first-line agents since it has been shown that digoxin is neither effective in restoring nor maintaining sinus rhythm; rate control with digoxin is difficult to achieve under circumstances of heightened sympathetic tone such as with exercise or after surgery.

In patients who receive pacemakers for the treatment of sinus node disease, the incidence of atrial fibrillation is lower in those who receive dual chamber or atrial-based systems compared with those who receive ventricular pacemakers.[25] In addition, there is retrospective data suggesting that the frequency of preexisting paroxysmal atrial fibrillation in patients receiving dual chamber or atrial-based pacemakers is reduced after implantation. In some patients it is clearly important to prevent sinus bradycardia in order to reduce the frequency of atrial fibrillation, and there is an additional subgroup of patients with "vagally mediated" atrial fibrillation who seem to benefit from atrial-based pacing.[7] In conditions associated with sinus bradycardia, pacing is thought to have a salutary effect by overdrive suppression of atrial ectopy and by decreasing dispersion of atrial refractoriness.

Radiofrequency ablation of the AV junction combined with permanent pacing has now become an accepted approach. There is strong evidence of a marked improvement in both quality of life and functional status of patients who have undergone this procedure.[12] Although there remains a need for anticoagulation, and patients are often highly dependent on pacing for survival, this procedure offers the opportunity to avoid treatment with drugs that are usually associated with significant adverse effects. With the advent of pacemakers that can automatically alter the mode of pacing when atrial arrhythmias appear, the use of dual chamber pacing in patients with paroxysmal atrial fibrillation now offers the benefits of AV synchrony between arrhythmia episodes.

Finally, the use of catheter ablation has been explored for the definitive cure of atrial fibrillation. The surgical experience with a range of procedures designed to abolish atrial fibrillation has led to the use of specially designed catheters to create linear atrial lesions that reduce the mass of left and right atrial myocardium in continuity and prevent the propagation of reentrant wavelets.[8] This catheter-based maze procedure is still experimental and is likely to remain restricted in its application until better catheters are available. Such approaches are predicated on the conventional notion that atrial fibrillation is a generalized phenomenon of both atria in which there are multiple circulating wavelets of reentry. However, in a selected group of generally younger patients with lone atrial fibrillation it may be the case that a single focus is responsible for paroxysmal atrial fibrillation; recent reports suggest that such foci of atrial fibrillation in or around the orifices of the pulmonary veins may be identified and successfully ablated using radiofrequency current.

Atrial Flutter. Atrial flutter is common and usually occurs in patients with structural heart disease or pulmonary disease, or after cardiothoracic surgery. Atrial flutter is characterized by rapid atrial rates of approximately 280 to 340 beats per minute; the ventricular response is often rapid, since it is constrained to a fixed ratio of the atrial rate. The ECG typically shows prominent atrial activity with a "saw-tooth" pattern in the inferior leads and no evidence of an isoelectric period during the cardiac cycle (Fig. 61-6).[45] The most common clinical presentation is with a regular tachycardia of 150 beats per minute, and any tachycardia that is fixed at this rate should raise the clinical suspicion of atrial flutter. Although the ratio of atrial to ventricular events during flutter may vary, the ventricular response is often rapid and difficult to control medically. Prolonged periods of sustained rapidly conducting atrial flutter may cause a tachycardia-induced cardiomyopathy, and elimination of the arrhythmia has been associated with normalization of ventricular function in some patients. The use of AV nodal blocking drugs is commonly ineffective and poorly tolerated; antiarrhythmic agents such as quinidine or flecainide have been used with some efficacy, but these drugs are associated with significant slowing of the atrial rate that may lead to paradoxical increase in ventricular rate with the development of 1 : 1 AV conduction.[35]

In the intensive care or postoperative setting cardioversion is the preferred management approach for termination of atrial flutter. Although very low electrical energies (10 J or less) can often be used successfully, it is well recognized that such low energy discharges may convert atrial flutter to atrial fibrillation because the discharge (synchronized to ventricular activation) may be delivered during the vulnerable period of atrial repolarization. Therefore an initial energy of 50 J or higher is generally recommended.

The reentrant circuit in atrial flutter is now well characterized[11]; typically the activation wavefront circles the right atrium, activating the left atrium passively. Activation proceeds up the interatrial septum and down the lateral atrial wall anterior to the crista terminalis before entering the narrow isthmus in the floor of the right atrium between the tricuspid annulus and the orifice of the inferior vena cava. It is in this compact area of right atrial tissue that the zone of slow conduction is localized; catheter ablation designed to create a line of bidirectional conduction block in this subeustachian isthmus has been successfully employed for the long-term elimination of atrial flutter.[40] This procedure is effective in approximately 80% of cases, and offers safe control of an arrhythmia that is not easily treated medically. Because atrial flutter may be the primary arrhythmia in some patients with atrial fibrillation, elimination of this tachycardia may also be effective in preventing recurrences of atrial fibrillation.

Some patients manifest primarily atrial fibrillation, although atrial flutter may also occur from time to time; in these patients antiarrhythmic drugs may effectively eliminate fibrillation and organize reentry within the atria such that atrial flutter is the dominant tachycardia. In such circumstances catheter ablation of the flutter circuit combined with long-term antiarrhythmic drug treatment of atrial fibrillation (so-called *hybrid therapy*) may be salutary.[26]

Following cardiac surgery in which an atrial incision is made there is a risk of reentrant arrhythmias occurring around the fibrous scar; these tachycardias often appear decades after surgery. Such atrial flutters are also successfully treated with catheter ablation, as are many other apparently atypical atrial flutters in which the usual ECG appearances discussed above are absent.[39]

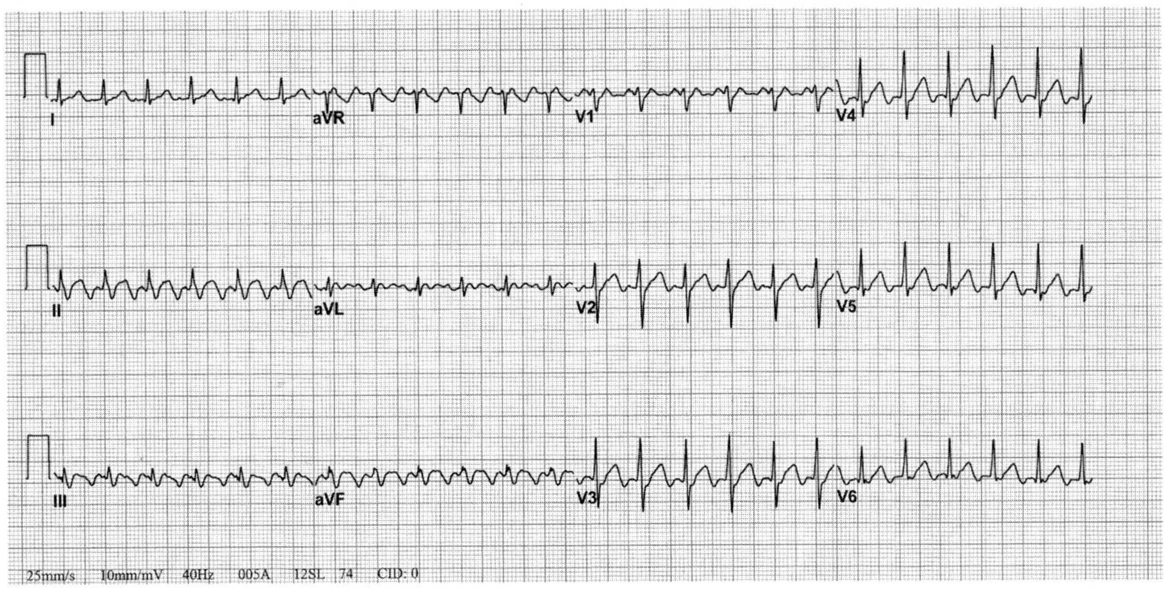

Fig. 61-6. ECG example of atrial flutter. This ECG shows a regular narrow QRS complex tachycardia at approximately 150 bpm. There is no isoelectric period in the baseline between QRS complexes, and there is a clear saw-tooth pattern in the inferior leads suggestive of common or type I atrial flutter.

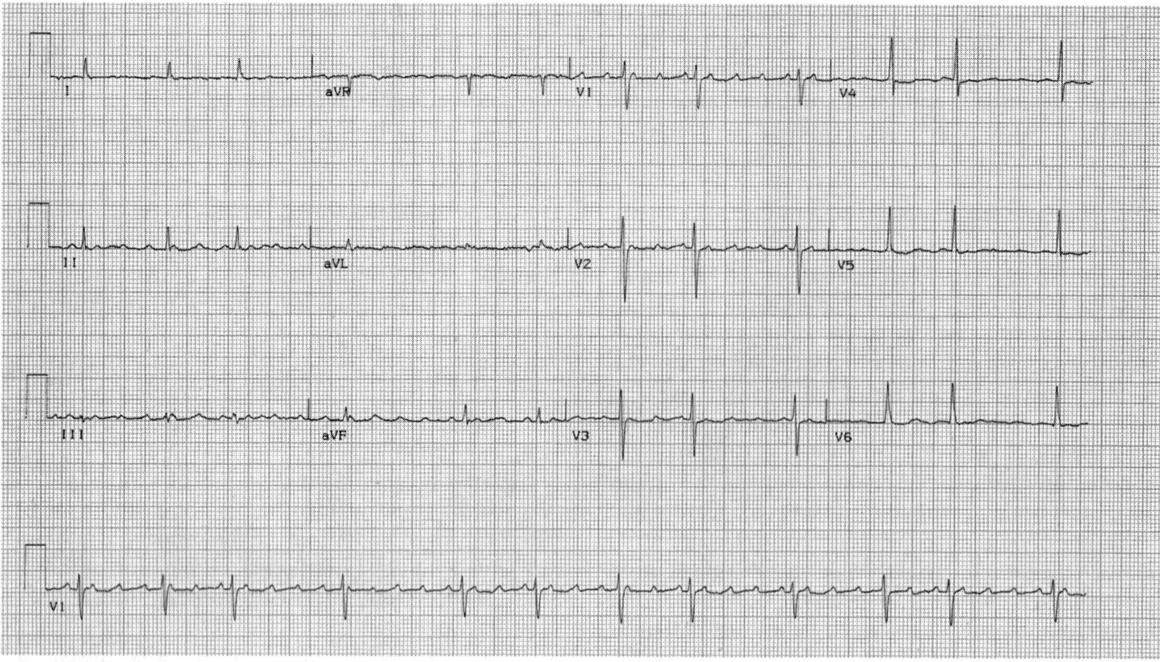

Fig. 61-7. ECG example of atrial tachycardia. This ECG shows an irregular rhythm where the R-R intervals are not random as in atrial fibrillation, but are somewhat consistent during the recording. The atrial activity is rapid and regular, with discrete P waves particularly prominent in lead V1.

Atrial Tachycardias. There are a variety of tachycardias of atrial origin that have varying mechanisms and are of importance in clinical practice. These tachycardias are associated with rapid atrial rates, usually with consistent P wave morphology and an isoelectric period between P waves. The ventricular response may be rapid or there may be varying degrees of AV block (Fig. 61-7). Atrial tachycardias are often associated with advanced atrial disease such as that found in severe heart failure; such patients may also be digoxin toxic (occasionally with normal blood levels of digoxin) with or without hypokalemia and the arrhythmia is truly an ectopic atrial tachycardia. In approximately 70% of such cases the arrhythmia can be treated by merely normalizing the metabolic abnormalities. In other patients, particularly those with pulmonary disease, the tachycardia may be reentrant in mechanism (intraatrial reentry) or ectopic with multiple foci of activation (multifocal atrial tachycardia [MAT]). In MAT the P wave morphology is variable with at least three different P waves and PR intervals identifiable on the ECG; this arrhythmia is closely associated with severe chronic lung disease and theophylline therapy but may occur in other chronically ill patients; verapamil has been recommended as the treatment of choice. It is important to recognize that atrial tachycardias in general exist on a spectrum of atrial arrhythmias with atrial flutter and fibrillation; many patients with advanced atrial disease may exhibit all of these arrhythmias in an evanescent fashion that precludes specific ablation therapy. However, when these tachycardias are difficult to control and are hemodynamically significant, catheter ablation of the AV junction may be appropriate if a specific target is not identifiable at electrophysiologic study.[10]

Preexcitation Syndromes. The Wolff-Parkinson-White syndrome is the most common example of the rare preexcitation syndromes; during sinus rhythm part of the ventricle is prematurely activated by an accessory pathway that bypasses the normal conduction route via the AV node. The ECG during sinus rhythm therefore shows a short PR interval and a widened QRS complex with a slurred upstroke known as the delta wave (Fig. 61-8). The frequency of such congenital anomalies is thought to be about 1:10,000 live births but it is important to note that most patients probably never experience tachycardia even though the ECG may demonstrate that the substrate exists.

The most common form of tachycardia in Wolff-Parkinson-White syndrome is orthodromic AVRT (described earlier). This is typically a regular narrow complex QRS tachycardia, although the QRS complex may be wide if bundle branch block occurs during the arrhythmia. It is important to recognize the Wolff-Parkinson-White pattern on the ECG in a patient with symptoms of arrhythmia because of the potential risk of sudden death if atrial fibrillation occurs (Fig. 61-9). In a minority of patients the accessory pathway may be capable of such rapid conduction during atrial fibrillation that ventricular fibrillation may supervene. Although rare, this is a well-described mechanism of sudden death in otherwise healthy patients, and can be prevented by catheter ablation.

Ventricular Tachycardia and Sudden Cardiac Death. Sudden death strikes approximately 300,000 individuals in the United States every year; the resuscitation rate varies greatly according to the geographic setting and sophistication of local rescue services, but the overall survival is no better than 20%. Most deaths (>80%) are related to coronary artery disease and the final event is thought to be ventricular fibrillation in approximately 90%.[15] In many of these cases there is preexisting left ventricular dysfunction due to previous myocardial infarction and the inciting event is

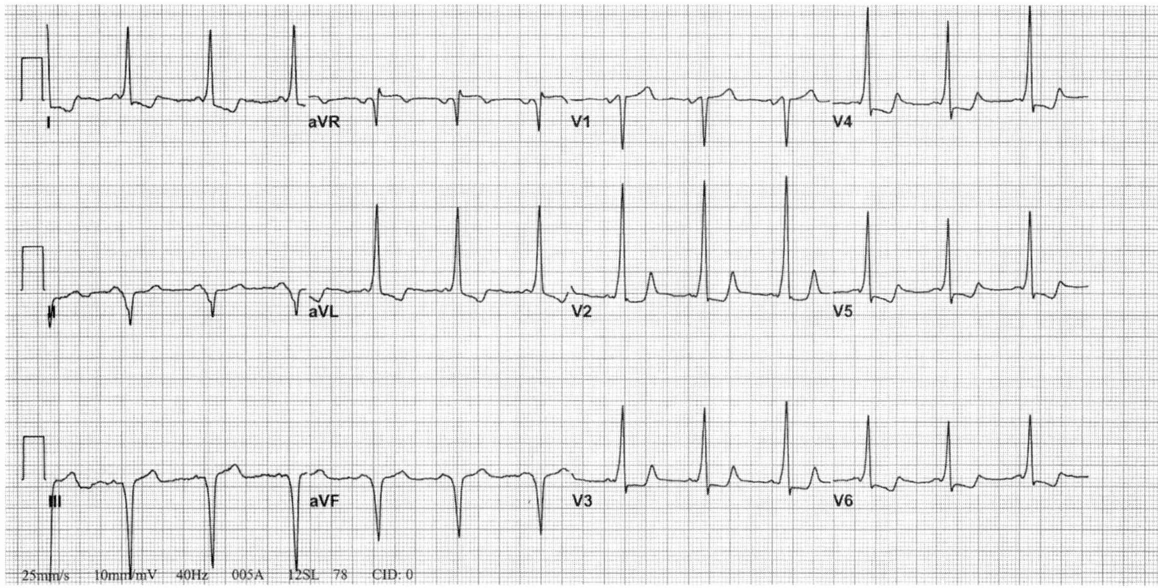

Fig. 61-8. ECG example of Wolff-Parkinson-White pattern. This ECG shows sinus rhythm with a short PR interval and a wide QRS complex due to delay in the upstroke of the R wave. This slurred upstroke is referred to as a delta wave. Note that in the inferior leads the delta wave polarity is negative and this often leads to inappropriate diagnosis of inferior myocardial infarction. This pseudo-inferior infarct pattern is typical of a manifest posteroseptal accessory pathway.

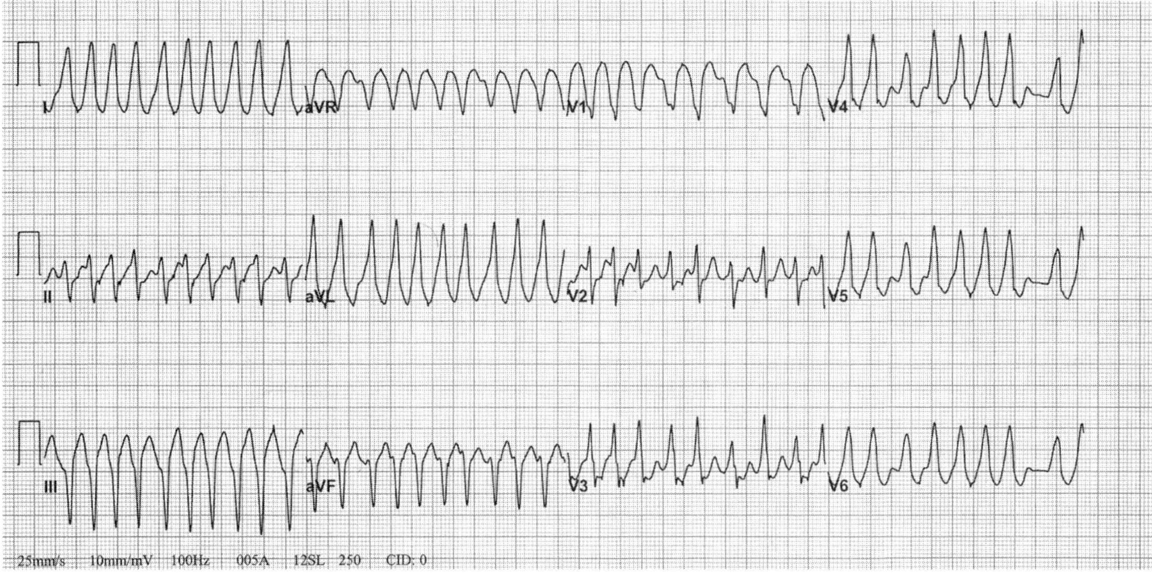

Fig. 61-9. ECG example of atrial fibrillation in a patient with Wolff-Parkinson-White syndrome. This ECG shows a completely irregular wide complex tachycardia that is very rapid and associated with a bizarre appearance and leftward axis of the QRS complex. This arrhythmia may degenerate to ventricular fibrillation and therefore requires prompt termination followed by catheter ablation of the accessory pathway.

ventricular tachycardia, which then degenerates to ventricular fibrillation. Acute ischemic events also play a significant role in the etiology of sudden cardiac death and are important to identify and treat aggressively in resuscitated patients as for other patients with acute myocardial infarction. The clinical setting in which cardiac arrest occurs is relevant in that patients with primary ventricular fibrillation associated with acute myocardial infarction have a good long-term prognosis, whereas those patients who experience ventricular fibrillation unassociated with an acute ischemic event have a recurrence rate of up to 30% in the year following the event; these patients therefore require ongoing protective therapy, usually an implantable cardioverter-defibrillator (ICD).

Sustained ventricular tachycardia may be monomorphic or polymorphic in ECG characteristics; in the former, the QRS complexes are uniform beat-by-beat with a fixed appearance often from one episode to another (Fig. 61-10). This reflects the abnormal cardiac activation in this reentrant arrhythmia originating in the border zone at the margin of a (usually chronic) infarct. The ECG appearances of polymorphic ventricular tachycardia show a constantly shifting QRS axis and amplitude in each ECG lead, and the ECG may not be

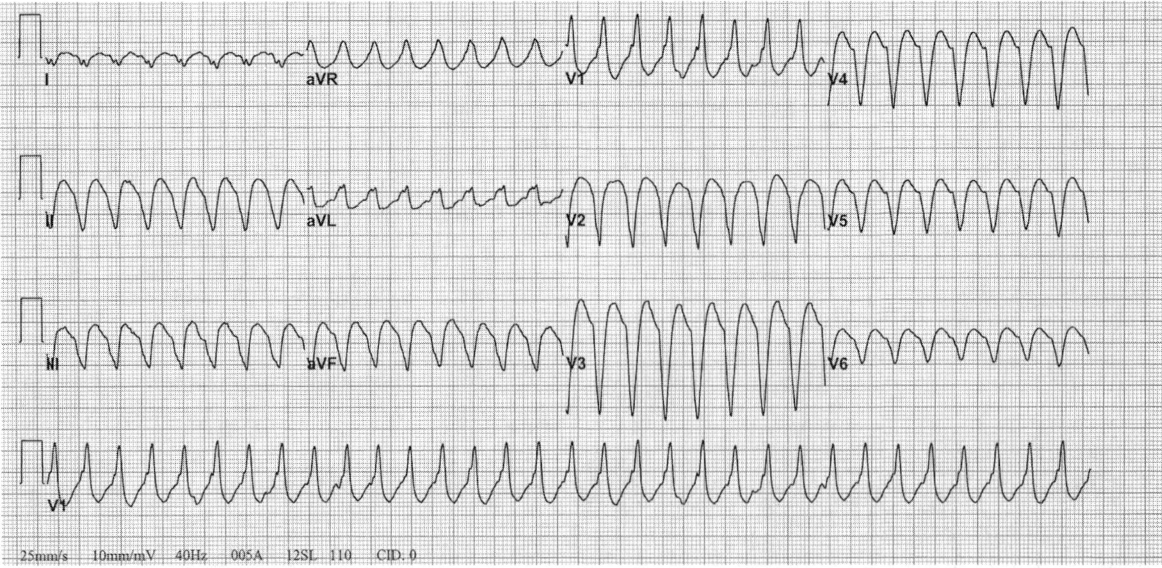

Fig. 61-10. ECG example of monomorphic ventricular tachycardia. This ECG shows a regular wide complex tachycardia at 190 bpm in which P waves are intermittently visible in the inferior leads and V1. This lack of a relationship between P waves and QRS complexes is diagnostic of ventricular tachycardia.

distinguishable from ventricular fibrillation, both of which arrhythmias are thought to be caused by multiple circulating reentrant wavelets in ventricular myocardium.

Ventricular tachycardia occurring in the context of structural heart disease with left or right ventricular dysfunction is a life-threatening arrhythmia and must be treated aggressively. Historically, treatment of such tachycardias relied on the use of antiarrhythmic drugs, but recent data from such large trials as AVID (Antiarrhythmics Versus Implantable Defibrillators) demonstrate that the ICD offers a clear survival advantage in such patients.[42]

Data from the CAST study and others suggested that certain antiarrhythmic drugs may adversely affect survival, and the results of two large trials of the most efficacious agent, amiodarone, demonstrate that although this drug may reduce arrhythmic events, the overall survival of patients treated after myocardial infarction is not improved.[4,21] In current U.S. practice, the majority of patients with ventricular tachycardia or fibrillation that is not caused by a reversible factor receive an ICD; antiarrhythmic agents are used to supplement such therapy in order to reduce the frequency of device discharges as necessary.

Occasionally ventricular tachycardia is amenable to definitive therapy and it is important to recognize such arrhythmias.[1] Such tachycardias include bundle branch reentrant tachycardia in which the reentrant circuit involves the left and right bundle branches of the His-Purkinje system; this circuit can be readily abolished by ablation of the right bundle branch, but such patients usually have extensively diseased and dilated hearts and therefore often require ICD therapy for other ventricular tachycardias. Patients without evidence of structural heart disease using conventional clinical and imaging techniques who present with recurrent ventricular tachycardia represent a small but important group of patients, since these arrhythmias are usually curable by ablation. Repetitive monomorphic idiopathic ventricular tachycardia is usually suggested by one of two ECG appearances; the more common exhibits a left bundle branch block configuration with markedly positive QRS complex in the inferior leads (II, III, aVF) and originates in the outflow tract of the right ventricle. A less common idiopathic ventricular tachycardia exhibits a QRS morphology of right bundle branch block with left axis deviation and originates in the posterior fascicle of the left bundle branch; it may also be sensitive to verapamil, which may be an effective long-term treatment alternative to ablation.

Bradycardias

Traditionally, a bradycardia has been defined as a heart rate lower than 60 beats per minute; however, with the widespread use of β-blockers and other negatively chronotropic agents this definition has now been revised to include only heart rates that are below 50 beats per minute. Irrespective of the mechanism of bradycardia, obvious pauses in heart rhythm not due to a reversible factor that lead to syncope or dizziness require pacing, as do most pauses of greater than 3 seconds that are apparently asymptomatic. It is, however, important to consider the relationship between symptoms and heart rate, since a heart rate of 60 beats per minute in the face of fever or heart failure may reveal underlying pathology that justifies long-term pacing in a patient who has no overt symptoms of bradycardia. Often such symptoms of bradycardia are recognized only in retrospect after pacemaker implantation.

Sinus node disease or *sick sinus syndrome* is a heterogeneous entity in which various bradycardias and tachycardias may coexist at different times; common to all is that the origin of the rhythm disturbance is in or surrounding the sinus node. Sinus bradycardia is common but probably underrecognized and must be evaluated in the context of the patient's physiologic state and drug history; it is often associated with chronotropic incompetence, an inability of the sinus node to respond to the usual stimuli that increase heart rate during exercise or other stressful physiologic states. Such patients complain of fatigue and an inability to exercise, which may be difficult to assess clinically; exercise testing may reveal blunted heart rate response, with typical peak

Box 61-3. Classification of AV Block

First Degree

PR interval > 200 ms
(no blocked P waves)

Second Degree

Mobitz type I (Wenckebach)
- Common, related to AV nodal pathology
- Characterized by gradual lengthening of PR intervals and shortening of RR intervals prior to blocked P wave

Mobitz type II
- Rare, usually seen in acute ischemia
- Nonconducted P wave occurs without preceding lengthening of PR intervals

2:1 AV block

AV nodal: conducted PR interval usually long
Infranodal: conducted PR usually <200 ms

Complete AV Block

No relationship between P waves and QRS complexes

Advanced (High-Grade) Block

Consecutively nonconducted P waves

exercise heart rates of less than 100 beats per minute. Rate-modulated pacing in which the implanted pacemaker has a biosensor that permits physiologic heart rates with daily activity usually has a beneficial impact on the quality of life of these patients.[24] Sinus pauses, exit block, and sinus arrest are common indications for permanent pacing; identification of these often intermittent problems may be difficult, but the use of long-term event monitoring has enhanced diagnostic yield. Bradycardias related to sinus node disease may be secondary to tachycardias originating in the sinus node region. These tachycardias suppress sinus node automaticity such that when the tachycardia terminates there is a long offset pause that provokes syncope, which may be the only overt symptom. Adequate treatment of the tachycardia with β-blocker or other negatively chronotropic agents will require concomitant pacemaker therapy in most of these patients.

AV block is common and represents the most common indication for cardiac pacing worldwide. The classification of AV block is given in Box 61-3; it is important to emphasize that the goal of the clinical and ECG evaluation of AV block is to identify those patients at risk for progression to high-grade, third-degree AV block in which the escape mechanism is likely to be unstable. Localizing the site of block to the AV node or the His-Purkinje system is key to this process of defining risk, since AV nodal block is associated with a stable junctional escape of 40 to 50 beats per minute, whereas infranodal block is often associated with a slow and erratic ventricular escape of only 20 to 30 beats per minute. Localizing the site of block cannot be done reliably using noninvasive tools, but the presence of a wide QRS complex and/or Mobitz type II second-degree AV block both suggest a tenuous conduction system; conversely, a long PR interval and Wenckebach's periodicity with a narrow QRS complex all suggest AV nodal disease with a more stable escape mechanism.

Current pacemaker technology permits the implantation of sophisticated small devices with an expected longevity of 6 to 8 years on average.[23] Both single and dual chamber pacemakers feature flexible programming of multiple parameters and additional memory storage for internal diagnostic data and arrhythmic events. Rate-responsive pacemakers incorporate a sensor, based usually on body activity or minute ventilation, that accelerates the paced rate according to a predetermined algorithm when triggered. Although data on the mortality benefit (if any) are lacking, it is clear that cardiac pacing improves quality of life and functional status of patients who have sinus and AV node disease. Pacing therapy is cost-effective at any age, an important consideration given that most patients requiring pacemakers are of advanced age.

REFERENCES

1. Akhtar M: Clinical spectrum of ventricular tachycardia, *Circulation* 82:1561-1573, 1990.
2. Akhtar M, Tchou PJ, Jazayeri M: Mechanisms of clinical tachycardias, *Am J Cardiol* 61:9A-19A, 1988.
3. Antman EM, Beamer AD, Cantillon C, et al: Therapy of refractory symptomatic atrial fibrillation and atrial flutter: a staged care approach with new antiarrhythmic drugs, *J Am Coll Cardiol* 15:698-707, 1990.
4. Cairns JA, Connolly SJ, Roberts R, et al: Randomised trial of outcome after myocardial infarction in patients with frequent or repetitive ventricular premature depolarisations: CAMIAT, Canadian Amiodarone Myocardial Infarction Arrhythmia Trial Investigators, *Lancet* 349:675-682, 1997.
5. Cannegieter SC, Rosendaal FR, Wintzen AR, et al: Optimal oral anticoagulant therapy in patients with mechanical heart valves, *N Engl J Med* 333:11-17, 1995.
6. Coplen SE, Antman EM, Berlin JA, et al: Efficacy and safety of quinidine therapy for maintenance of sinus rhythm after cardioversion: a meta-analysis of randomized control trials, *Circulation* 82:1106-1116, 1990.
7. Coumel P: Paroxysmal atrial fibrillation: a disorder of autonomic tone? *Eur Heart J* 15 Suppl A:9-16, 1994.
8. Cox JL, Boineau JP, Schuessler RB, et al: Five-year experience with the maze procedure for atrial fibrillation, *Ann Thorac Surg* 56:814-814, 1993.
9. Feinberg WM, Seeger JF, Carmody RF, et al: Epidemiologic features of asymptomatic cerebral infarction in patients with nonvalvular atrial fibrillation, *Arch Intern Med* 150:2340-2344, 1990.
10. Feld GK: Catheter ablation for the treatment of atrial tachycardia, *Prog Cardiovasc Dis* 37:205-224, 1995.
11. Feld GK, Fleck RP, Chen PS, et al: Radiofrequency catheter ablation for the treatment of human type 1 atrial flutter: identification of a critical zone in the reentrant circuit by endocardial mapping techniques, *Circulation* 86:1233-1240, 1992.
12. Fitzpatrick AP, Kourouyan HD, Siu A, et al: Quality of life and outcomes after radiofrequency His-bundle catheter ablation and permanent pacemaker implantation: impact of treatment in paroxysmal and established atrial fibrillation, *Am Heart J* 131:499-507, 1996.
13. Ganz LI, Friedman PL: Supraventricular tachycardia, *N Engl J Med* 332:162-173, 1995.
14. Garratt C, Linker N, Griffith M, et al: Comparison of adenosine and verapamil for termination of paroxysmal junctional tachycardia, *Am J Cardiol* 64:1310-1316, 1989.
15. Goldstein S: Toward a new understanding of the mechanism and prevention of sudden death in coronary heart disease, *Circulation* 82:284-288, 1990.
16. Gomes JA, Mehta D, Langan MN: Sinus node reentrant tachycardia, *Pacing Clin Electrophysiol* 18:1045-1057, 1995.
17. Grogan M, Smith HC, Gersh BJ, et al: Left ventricular dysfunction due to atrial fibrillation in patients initially believed to have idiopathic dilated cardiomyopathy, *Am J Cardiol* 69:1570-1573, 1992.
18. Hylek EM, Skates SJ, Sheehan MA, et al: An analysis of the lowest effective intensity of prophylactic anticoagulation for patients with nonrheumatic atrial fibrillation, *N Engl J Med* 335:540-546, 1996.

19. Jackman WM, Beckman KJ, McClelland JH, et al: Treatment of supraventricular tachycardia due to atrioventricular nodal reentry, by radiofrequency catheter ablation of slow-pathway conduction, *N Engl J Med* 327:313-318, 1992.
20. Jackman WM, Wang X, Friday KJ, et al: Catheter ablation of accessory atrioventricular pathways (Wolff-Parkinson-White syndrome) by radiofrequency current, *N Engl J Med* 324:1605-1611, 1991.
21. Julian DG, Camm AJ, Frangin G, et al: Randomised trial of effect of amiodarone on mortality in patients with left-ventricular dysfunction after recent myocardial infarction: EMIAT, European Myocardial Infarct Amiodarone Trial Investigators, *Lancet* 349:667-674, 1997.
22. Kalbfleisch SJ, El-Atassi R, Calkins H, et al: Safety, feasibility and cost of outpatient radiofrequency catheter ablation of accessory atrioventricular connections, *J Am Coll Cardiol* 21:567-570, 1993.
23. Kusumoto FM, Goldschlager N: Cardiac pacing, *N Engl J Med* 334:89-97, 1996.
24. Lamas GA, Orav EJ, Stambler BS, et al: Quality of life and clinical outcomes in elderly patients treated with ventricular pacing as compared with dual-chamber pacing, Pacemaker Selection in the Elderly Investigators, *N Engl J Med* 338:1097-1104, 1998.
25. Langenfeld H, Grimm W, Maisch B, et al: Atrial fibrillation and embolic complications in paced patients, *Pacing Clin Electrophysiol* 11:1667-1672, 1988.
26. Lesh MD, Kalman JM, Olgin JE: New approaches to treatment of atrial flutter and tachycardia, *J Cardiovasc Electrophysiol* 7:368-381, 1996.
27. Man KC, Kalbfleisch SJ, Hummel JD, et al: Safety and cost of outpatient radiofrequency ablation of the slow pathway in patients with atrioventricular nodal reentrant tachycardia, *Am J Cardiol* 72:1323-1324, 1993.
28. Manolis AS, Wang PJ, Estes NA: Radiofrequency catheter ablation for cardiac tachyarrhythmias, *Ann Intern Med* 121:452-461, 1994.
29. Moss AJ, Hall J, Cannom DS, et al: Improved survival with an implanted defibrillator in patients with coronary disease at high risk for ventricular arrhythmia, *N Engl J Med* 335:1933-1940, 1996.
30. Naccarelli GV, Lee KS, Gibson JK, et al: Electrophysiology and pharmacology of ibutilide, *Am J Cardiol* 78:12-16, 1996.
31. Odemuyiwa O, Malik M, Farrell T, et al: Comparison of the predictive characteristics of heart rate variability index and left ventricular ejection fraction for all-cause mortality, arrhythmic events and sudden death after acute myocardial infarction, *Am J Cardiol* 68:434-439, 1991.
32. Oral H, Souza JJ, Michaud GF, et al: Facilitating transthoracic cardioversion of atrial fibrillation with ibutilide pretreatment, *N Engl J Med* 340:1849-1854, 1999.
33. Petersen P, Madsen EB, Brun B, et al: Silent cerebral infarction in chronic atrial fibrillation, *Stroke* 18:1098-1100, 1987.
34. Pritchett EL: Management of atrial fibrillation, *N Engl J Med* 326:1264-1271, 1992.
35. Randazzo DN, Schweitzer P, Stein E, et al: Flecainide induced atrial tachycardia with 1:1 ventricular conduction during exercise testing, *Pacing Clin Electrophysiol* 17:1509-1514, 1994.
36. Rodriguez LM, Smeets JL, Xie B, et al: Improvement in left ventricular function by ablation of atrioventricular nodal conduction in selected patients with lone atrial fibrillation, *Am J Cardiol* 72:1137-1141, 1993.
37. Rosenbaum DS, Jackson LE, Smith JM, et al: Electrical alternans and vulnerability to ventricular arrhythmias, *N Engl J Med* 330:235-241, 1994.
38. Ruskin JN: Catheter ablation for supraventricular tachycardia, *N Engl J Med* 324:1660-1662, 1991.
39. Saul JP, Triedman JK: Radiofrequency ablation of intraatrial reentrant tachycardia after surgery for congenital heart disease, *Pacing Clin Electrophysiol* 20:2112-2117, 1997.
40. Saxon LA, Kalman JM, Olgin JE, et al: Results of radiofrequency catheter ablation for atrial flutter, *Am J Cardiol* 77:1014-1016, 1996.
41. Shenasa M, Fetsch T, Martinez-Rubio A, et al: Signal averaging in patients with coronary artery disease: how helpful is it? *J Cardiovasc Electrophysiol* 4:609-626, 1993.
42. The Antiarrhythmics versus Implantable Defibrillators (AVID) Investigators: A comparison of antiarrhythmic-drug therapy with implantable defibrillators in patients resuscitated from near-fatal ventricular arrhythmias, *N Engl J Med* 337:1576-1583, 1997.
43. The CAST Investigators: Preliminary report: effect of encainide and flecainide on mortality in a randomized trial of arrhythmia suppression after myocardial infarction, The Cardiac Arrhythmia Suppression Trial (CAST) Investigators, *N Engl J Med* 321:406-412, 1989.
44. The CAST Investigators: Effect of the antiarrhythmic agent moricizine on survival after myocardial infarction. The Cardiac Arrhythmia Suppression Trial II Investigators, *N Engl J Med* 327:227-233, 1992.
45. Waldo AL: Mechanisms of atrial fibrillation, atrial flutter, and ectopic atrial tachycardia—a brief review, *Circulation* 75:III37-III40, 1987.
46. Wijffels MC, Kirchhof CJ, Dorland R, et al: Atrial fibrillation begets atrial fibrillation: a study in awake chronically instrumented goats, *Circulation* 92:1954-1968, 1995.
47. Wolf PA, Abbott RD, Kannel WB: Atrial fibrillation as an independent risk factor for stroke: the Framingham Study, *Stroke* 22:983-988, 1991.
48. Zimetbaum P, Josephson ME: Evaluation of patients with palpitations, *N Engl J Med* 338:1369-1373, 1998.
49. Zimetbaum PJ, Kim KY, Josephson ME, et al: Diagnostic yield and optimal duration of continuous-loop event monitoring for the diagnosis of palpitations: a cost-effectiveness analysis, *Ann Intern Med* 128:890-895, 1998.

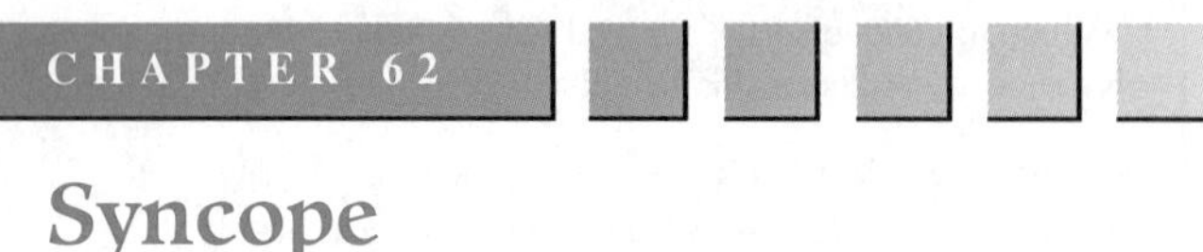

Syncope

Wishwa N. Kapoor

EPIDEMIOLOGY AND ETIOLOGY

Syncope is defined as a sudden transient loss of consciousness associated with loss of postural tone with spontaneous recovery not requiring cardioversion. Syncope must be separated from seizures and other states of altered consciousness such as dizziness, vertigo, coma, and narcolepsy (see Chapter 50).

Syncope is a common problem. Loss of consciousness is reported by 12% to 30% of young adults. This symptom accounts for 1% to 6% of hospital admissions and up to 3% of emergency department visits. Syncope is also common in the elderly. In one study of residents of a long-term care institution (older than 75 years of age), the annual incidence was 6%, and 23% had previous lifetime episodes.

Syncope can be a prelude to sudden death in certain subgroups. Patients with cardiac causes of syncope have higher 1-year mortality and sudden death rates than patients with noncardiac or unknown causes. Patients with underlying structural heart disease also have higher mortality regardless of the cause of syncope.

Syncope has a large differential diagnosis from benign problems to life-threatening illnesses (Box 62-1). A detailed description of these entities is beyond the scope of this review; see Additional Readings for further sources.

In studies that evaluated patients presenting with syncope, there has been a wide variation in the proportion of patients diagnosed with various etiologies. This variation is largely due to patient selection (differences ranging from emergency room to intensive care unit [ICU] patients) and lack of uniform criteria for assigning causes of syncope. The most common etiologies include vasovagal syncope diagnosed clinically and orthostatic hypotension. In approximately one third of patients a cause could not be determined. Since that time, tilt testing has become more widely used. Additionally, greater attention has been paid to psychiatric illnesses as causes of syncope. Comorbid illness and medications may be

Box 62-1. Etiologies of Syncope

Vasomotor Instability and Hypotension

Vasovagal
Situational
  Micturition
  Cough
  Swallow
  Defecation
Orthostasis
Postprandial hypotension
Drugs
Neuralgias
Psychiatric illness

Focal Decreased Cerebral Blood Flow

TIA

Decreased Cardiac Output

Obstruction to LV outflow
  Aortic stenosis, IHSS
  Mitral stenosis, myxoma
Obstruction to RV outflow
  Pulmonic stenosis
  PE, pulmonary hypertension
  Myxoma
Pump failure
  MI, CAD, coronary spasm
Tamponade, dissection
Dysrhythmias

TIA, Transient ischemic attack; *IHSS*, idiopathic hypertrophic subaortic stenosis; *LV*, left ventricle; *RV*, right ventricle; *PE*, pulmonary embolism; *MI*, myocardial infarction; *CAD*, coronary artery disease.

responsible for syncope in the elderly without the ability to assign a single etiology as the cause. Taking this recent information into account, it appears that unexplained syncope is much less frequent, constituting less than 10% of the cases. More specifically, studies noted above diagnosed vasovagal syncope on a clinical basis (e.g., syncope in the setting of various precipitating factors such as pain and instrumentation) or using associated autonomic symptoms. Recent studies using upright tilt testing to provoke vasovagal syncope have shown that symptoms can be induced on tilt testing in 26% to 87% of selected patients with unexplained syncope, suggesting that vasovagal syncope may be a very common cause of syncope.

A subgroup of patients with unexplained syncope may have psychiatric diseases (15% to 20%) that are not recognized as a possible cause of syncope. These illnesses include generalized anxiety disorder, panic disorder, major depression, and somatization disorder.

A third group of patients are those in whom new diagnoses, which caused their initial syncopal episode, become apparent in follow-up. This group composes less than 5% of patients with unexplained syncope and includes patients with dysrhythmias (e.g., supraventricular tachycardia) and seizures.

PATHOPHYSIOLOGY

The vast majority of causes of syncope result from transient reduction of cerebral blood flow to those parts of the brain subserving consciousness (brainstem, reticular activating system). There are four broad categories of mechanisms that may result in a sudden decrease in cerebral blood flow (see Box 62-1): (1) vasomotor instability associated with disorders that decrease systemic vascular resistance, venous return, or both; (2) severe reduction of cardiac output owing to obstruction of blood flow within the heart or pulmonary circulation; (3) cardiac dysrhythmias leading to a transient decline in cardiac output; and (4) transient ischemia due to cerebrovascular disease with focal or generalized decreased cerebral perfusion.

Rarely, normal or even increased cerebral blood flow may be associated with loss or alteration of consciousness because of a lack of essential nutrients necessary for cerebral metabolism. These states include hypoglycemia and hypoxemia; however, these disorders more frequently lead to somnolence and coma than syncope. Additionally, seizures may present as syncope; in this instance cerebral blood flow is generally normal.

PATIENT EVALUATION

History

The evaluation of syncope begins with defining the episode and associated symptoms. Once the patient is found to have had syncope, a workup can be initiated to determine the etiology.

A detailed history of the episode (from the patient and a witness, if present) is needed to separate syncope from other states of altered consciousness such as dizziness, vertigo, drop attacks, coma, and seizure. A particularly difficult distinction is between syncope and seizure. One study comparing the symptoms of syncope and seizure showed that seizures were associated with blue face (or not pale), frothing at the mouth, tongue biting, disorientation, aching muscles, sleepiness after the event, and duration of unconsciousness of more than 5 minutes. By contrast, symptoms associated with syncope were sweating or nausea before the event and being oriented after the event. The best discriminatory symptom is disorientation after the episode, which often signifies a seizure.

Once it has been determined that the patient had syncope, a history is crucial in choosing diagnostic tests selectively to arrive at an etiology. Emphasis is placed on the details of the events leading to the episode, the characteristics of the loss of consciousness, and symptoms immediately after the patient regains consciousness (Table 62-1). For example, in diagnosing vasovagal syncope a history of a particular precipitating factor or the presence of autonomic symptoms is useful. Micturition, cough, defecation, and swallowing may be associated with sudden loss of consciousness. These disorders, termed *situational syncope,* are diagnosed by history from the patient. Brainstem ischemia due to transient ischemic attacks, basilar artery migraines, and subclavian steal syndrome may lead to drop attacks or syncope, but loss of consciousness is generally associated with other neurologic symptoms and signs referable to the brainstem. A detailed drug history may uncover a potential etiology for syncope. The most common drugs causing syncope include nitrates, vasodilators, and β-blockers (Box 62-2).

History may suggest specific entities that can be further evaluated by directed testing (see Table 62-1). For example, syncope with arm exercise suggests subclavian steal syndrome; loss of consciousness in a deaf child with effort or emotional distress may be due to ventricular

Table 62-1. Clinical Features Suggestive of Specific Causes

Symptom or finding	Diagnostic consideration
After sudden unexpected pain, unpleasant sight, sound, or smell	Vasovagal syncope
During or immediately after micturition, cough, swallow, or defecation	Situational syncope
With neuralgia (glossopharyngeal or trigeminal)	Bradycardia or vasodepressor reaction
Upon standing	Orthostatic hypotension
Prolonged standing at attention	Vasovagal
Well-trained athlete after exertion	Vasovagal
Changing position (from sitting to lying, bending, turning over in bed)	Atrial myxoma, thrombus
Syncope with exertion	Aortic stenosis, pulmonary hypertension, mitral stenosis, IHSS, coronary artery disease
With head rotation, pressure on carotid sinus (as in tumors, shaving, tight collars)	Carotid sinus syncope
Associated with vertigo, dysarthria, diplopia, and other motor and sensory symptoms of brainstem ischemia	TIA, subclavian steal
With arm exercise	Subclavian steal

IHSS, Idiopathic hypertrophic subaortic stenosis; *TIA,* transient ischemic attack.

Box 62-2. Common Drugs Causing Syncope

Vasodilators

Nitrates
Calcium channel blockers
ACE inhibitors
Others (e.g., prazosin, hydralazine)

Drugs Associated with Torsades de Pointes

Quinidine
Procainamide
Disopyramide
Flecainide
Encainide
Amiodarone
Sotalol

Diuretics

Psychoactive Drugs

Phenothiazines
Antidepressants (e.g., tricyclic agents, MAO inhibitors)
CNS depressants (e.g., barbiturates)

β-Blockers

Other Mechanisms

Vincristine and other neuropathic drugs
Digitalis
Insulin
Marijuana
Alcohol
Cocaine

Reprinted from Kapoor WN: Diagnostic evaluation of syncope, *Am J Med* 90:91-106, 1991.
ACE, Angiotensin-converting enzyme; *CNS,* central nervous system; *MAO,* monoamine oxidase.

tachydysrhythmias associated with congenital long QT syndromes; and fainting in a patient with flushing and itching may be a manifestation of systemic mastocytosis. Box 62-1 shows specific features from the history that suggest various diagnoses.

Physical Examination

A detailed physical examination may provide information needed to establish specific entities as a cause of syncope and exclude others. Findings on examination of particular importance are orthostatic hypotension, cardiovascular abnormalities, and neurologic signs.

Syncope due to orthostatic hypotension can be difficult to diagnose, since 5% to 55% of patients with other etiologies of syncope have orthostatic hypotension (defined as a systolic blood pressure decline of 20 mm Hg or more), and postural hypotension is reported in up to 24% of the elderly. Thus the development of syncope or presyncope upon standing, in association with orthostatic blood pressure decline, is important in the diagnosis of the etiology of loss of consciousness. Blood pressure measurements should be performed upon standing after a supine period of 5 to 10 minutes. Lack of a blood pressure drop upon sitting does not exclude orthostatic hypotension. Several blood pressure determinations upon standing during a 2-minute period are sufficient to detect orthostatic hypotension in most patients. Repeated orthostatic blood pressure measurements are needed when there is high clinical suspicion for orthostatic hypotension, since postural hypotension can be episodic. Orthostatic hypotension may be worse upon arising in the morning or after meals.

Cardiovascular findings may be important clues to the etiology of syncope. For example, aortic dissection and subclavian steal syndrome are associated with differences in the pulse intensity and blood pressure (generally less than 20 mm Hg) in the two arms. Many organic heart diseases that cause syncope have specific cardiovascular findings. These entities include aortic stenosis, idiopathic hypertrophic subaortic stenosis, pulmonary hypertension, myxomas, and aortic dissection.

When a cause of syncope can be found, the history and physical examination lead to the etiology in approximately 45% of patients. Furthermore, organic cardiac diseases and neurologic diseases (e.g., subclavian steal syndrome) are strongly suspected by the history and physical examination. Testing for these diseases should be selective and based on findings from the history and physical examination. Suggestive findings on the history and physical examination are helpful in assigning the ultimate cause of syncope by directed testing in approximately 8% of additional patients.

DIAGNOSIS

Diagnostic Testing

Results of blood tests are generally not helpful in assigning an etiology for syncope. Hypoglycemia, hyponatremia, hypocalcemia, and renal failure have been found in 2% to 3% of patients, but primarily in those with seizures. These disorders were often clinically suspected; in one study only one unexpected finding was discovered (hyponatremia with seizures). Syncope due to bleeding has been diagnosed clinically with confirmation by Hemoccult tests or complete blood counts.

When the history and physical examination do not lead to an etiology or provide clues for directed testing, further evaluation focuses on dysrhythmia detection, search for vasovagal syncope, and, less commonly, psychiatric illnesses.

Dysrhythmia Detection. Dysrhythmias are primarily of concern in patients with structural heart disease or abnormal electrocardiogram (ECG). If symptoms are consistent with dysrhythmic syncope, efforts should be directed first to rule out dysrhythmias as the cause of syncope. The following means are available for diagnosis of dysrhythmias.

ECG/Rhythm Strip. An ECG or a rhythm strip is useful in three ways. First, an ECG may show severe abnormalities that are diagnostic of the cause of syncope (2% to 11% of patients). Examples include complete heart block, symptomatic supraventricular tachydysrhythmias, and ventricular tachycardias. Second, an ECG may show abnormalities that increase the likelihood of dysrhythmic syncope but are not diagnostic of the cause of syncope (e.g., bundle branch block, Wolff-Parkinson-White syndrome). Third, an ECG may be normal, which markedly decreases the probability of dysrhythmias as the cause of syncope.

Treadmill testing can be used to provoke exercise-induced tachydysrhythmias when they are suspected clinically (e.g., patients with exertional syncope) or to look for ischemia. However, this test is rarely useful in establishing a cause of syncope.

Carotid Massage. Less than 1% of patients presenting with syncope are assigned the diagnosis of carotid sinus syncope. Carotid sinus hypersensitivity is found in 5% to 25% of asymptomatic populations, but only 5% to 20% of these individuals have spontaneous symptoms consistent with carotid sinus syncope. Consider carotid sinus syncope in (1) those who have spontaneous symptoms suggestive of carotid sinus syncope (e.g., syncope while shaving, wearing tight collars, or turning the head), and (2) in elderly patients with recurrent syncope with a negative diagnostic evaluation. Carotid sinus syncope is diagnosed when carotid massage reproduces the patient's spontaneous symptoms. To diagnose carotid hypersensitivity, carotid massage can be performed for 5 to 15 seconds on each side with concurrent ECG and blood pressure monitoring. A cardioinhibitory response is defined as cardiac asystole of greater than 3 seconds. A vasodepressor response is diagnosed when there is a systolic blood pressure decline of 50 mm Hg or more that is not associated with bradycardia or occurs after bradycardia has been abolished with atropine or atrioventricular sequential pacing.

Prolonged ECG Monitoring. The sensitivity and specificity of ECG monitoring for diagnosis of dysrhythmic syncope are not known because of the lack of criteria for abnormal results or a gold standard that is independent of dysrhythmias diagnosed by monitoring. The only certain means of diagnosing dysrhythmias as a cause of syncope is to document dysrhythmias at the time of symptoms. The results of ambulatory monitoring have been disappointing, since symptom correlation is found in only 4% of patients. In an additional 17% no dysrhythmias are found during symptoms, thus potentially excluding dysrhythmias as the etiology. In the remaining patients (approximately 80%) either asymptomatic dysrhythmias or no dysrhythmias are found. Since dysrhythmias may be episodic, finding asymptomatic brief dysrhythmias or no dysrhythmias does not exclude a rhythm disturbance as a cause of syncope.

Monitoring longer than 24 hours is not likely to increase the yield of symptomatic dysrhythmias. In one study, although there was an increased yield of brief dysrhythmias after the first 24 hours (14.7% were abnormal during the first 24 hours, 11% during the second 24 hours, and 4.2% during the third 24 hours), none of the dysrhythmias during the second and third 24 hours were associated with symptoms.

More prolonged monitoring for weeks to months is also possible using patient-activated intermittent loop recorders. This type of recorder can capture dysrhythmias during a syncopal episode if the patient activates it after regaining consciousness. Studies of loop monitoring have included patients referred because of frequent recurrences (median events exceeding 10 per patient). In these highly selected patients, true-positive results (dysrhythmias detected during syncope) were found in 8% to 20% and true-negative results (no dysrhythmias during syncope) in 12% to 27%.

Electrophysiologic Studies. In patients with structural heart disease or abnormal ECG (e.g., bundle branch block, accessory pathway, old myocardial infarction), electrophysiologic studies (EPS) should be considered if dysrhythmias are not excluded by noninvasive tests (ECG and ambulatory or loop monitoring). These tests are generally not indicated in patients without heart disease and normal ECG. The diagnostic yield of EPS is approximately 50% (ventricular tachycardia and bradycardias) in patients with organic heart disease and 10% in patients with a normal heart.

Some centers have used the detection of low-amplitude signals in the terminal portion of QRS complex by signal-averaged ECG as a screening test for selecting patients for EPS. The sensitivity of low-amplitude signals (late potentials) is reported to be 73% to 89%, with a specificity of 89% to 100% for detection of inducible sustained ventricular tachycardia in patients with syncope. However, this test is not generally useful to eliminate further consideration of EPS; complete studies are often needed in patients with organic heart disease and syncope because other abnormalities (conduction system disease and supraventricular tachycardia) are relatively common findings on these tests.

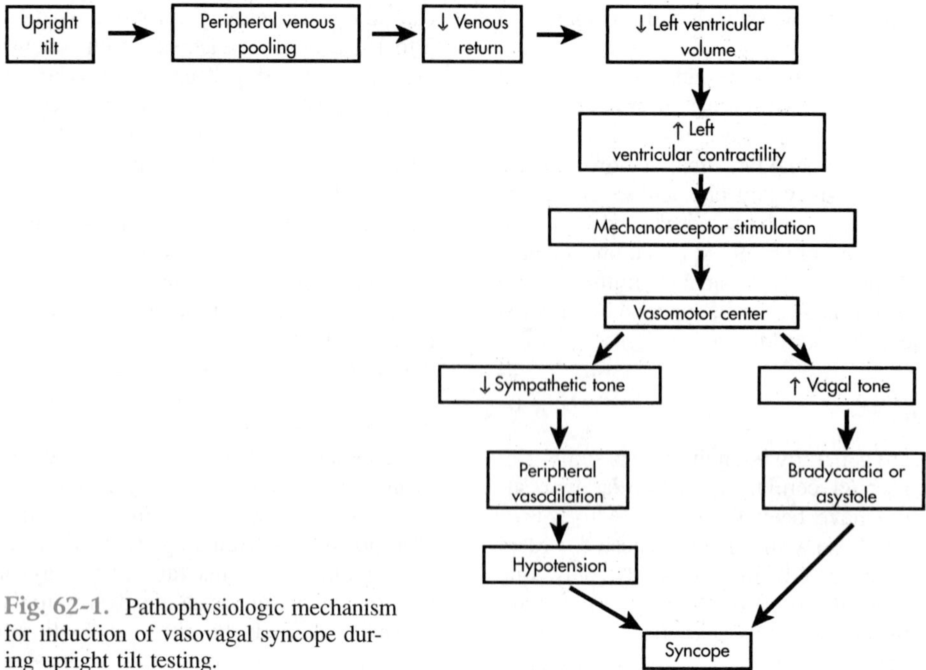

Fig. 62-1. Pathophysiologic mechanism for induction of vasovagal syncope during upright tilt testing.

Upright Tilt Testing. Vasovagal syncope (also known as neurally mediated or neurocardiogenic syncope) can be induced by keeping susceptible individuals upright on a tilt table with or without stimulation with adrenergic agents such as isoproterenol. The mechanism of tilt-induced syncope is not entirely understood (Fig. 62-1). Inhibitory reflexes originating from the heart are widely believed to be responsible for this type of syncope. This reflex originates in the cardiac sensory receptors (mechanoreceptors) located primarily in the inferior and posterior wall of the left ventricle. These receptors may be stimulated by stretch; cardiac distention; forceful, rapid systolic contraction; or chemical substances. The stimulation of receptors leads to increased neural discharges through unmyelinated C fibers to the medulla (vasomotor center), leading to enhanced parasympathetic and decreased sympathetic activity. The result is sudden hypotension and/or bradycardia.

Upright posture leads to pooling of blood in the lower limbs, resulting in decreased venous return (see Fig. 62-1). Normal compensatory response to orthostatic stress is reflex tachycardia, more forceful contraction of the ventricles, and vasoconstriction. However, in individuals susceptible to vasovagal syncope, this forceful ventricular contraction, in the setting of a relatively empty ventricle, may activate the cardiac mechanoreceptors, triggering reflex hypotension and/or bradycardia. Catecholamine release (as may occur with anxiety, fear, and panic), by increasing ventricular contraction, may also activate the nerve endings responsible for triggering this reflex.

A large number of studies have been reported using many different tilt testing protocols. Most of the protocols in the United States use isoproterenol after a period of drug-free tilt testing. Table 62-2 summarizes some of the performance characteristics of tilt testing without considering the heterogeneity in testing protocols.

What is the role of tilt table testing in evaluating syncope? In patients without heart disease in whom the history, physical examination, and initial ECG do not lead to an etiology of syncope, upright tilt testing may define a potential diagnosis. Furthermore, in patients who have underlying heart disease and do not have evidence of dysrhythmias based on ECG monitoring and EPS, this test may provide a specific diagnosis. However, because of problems with the specificity of the test, only symptom reproduction during testing should be considered a positive response. Furthermore, tilt testing should generally be limited to patients who have had multiple recurrences of syncope, since treatment is the major issue in this group.

Table 62-2. Tilt Testing in Syncope

Characteristic	%
Sensitivity	67-83
Specificity	75-100
Positive response in unexplained syncope	49-64
Reproducibility	35-85

Psychiatric Assessment. Several psychiatric illnesses can result in syncope. Generalized anxiety disorder may produce hyperventilation and vasodepressor reaction. In panic disorder, up to 9% of the patients have faintness as a somatic complaint. Patients with somatization disorders have multiple physical symptoms including loss of consciousness, which is reported in 4.5% of patients with this disorder. Medical patients with major depression often have nonspecific physical complaints, and syncope may be one of the manifestations. Patients with syncope due to psychiatric disorders are generally younger and have multiple episodes. They have lower prevalence of heart disease and may have other nonspecific complaints associated with syncope such as headache, fatigue, dizziness, and palpitations.

Low-yield Tests. Other tests are rarely helpful in assigning an etiology for syncope. Skull films, lumbar puncture, radionuclide brain scan, and cerebral angiography have not yielded diagnostic information for a cause of syncope in the absence of clinical findings suggestive of a specific neurologic process. Glucose tolerance testing has not led to a diagnosis of hypoglycemia in patients with syncope. Electroencephalogram (EEG) and head computed tomography (CT) scans have shown diagnostic abnormalities in 2% to 4% of patients when these tests are performed. These abnormalities are almost always suspected clinically (history of seizure, symptoms suggestive of seizure or abnormal neurologic examination). Head CT scan is needed if subdural bleeding due to head injury is suspected.

Summary of Diagnostic Approach. Fig. 62-2 is a flow diagram that summarizes the diagnostic approach to syncope. A detailed clinical assessment (by history and physical examination) of patients with syncope is crucial and leads to the assignment of the vast majority of the causes of syncope. Additionally, in a smaller proportion of patients, clinical assessment suggests specific entities such as aortic stenosis or neurologic signs and symptoms suggestive of a seizure disorder. These findings should be used to guide further testing to arrive at a diagnosis and initiate treatment.

An ECG is needed in most patients with syncope, except when the etiology by the history and physical examination is clearly not cardiac. As noted previously, a normal ECG may help decrease the probability of cardiac etiologies.

When a cause of syncope is not established by the history, physical examination, and initial ECG, the following approach can be used to proceed with the diagnostic evaluation.

Tests for Dysrhythmia Detection. Dysrhythmic syncope is a major concern in patients with structural heart disease or abnormal ECG. The first step in the evaluation of these patients is prolonged ECG monitoring, since this is a noninvasive test. If a diagnosis is made by finding dysrhythmias and correlating symptoms, invasive tests such as EPS may be avoided. In patients with negative or unclear findings on ECG monitoring (e.g., asymptomatic brief nonsustained ventricular tachycardia) who have recurrent syncope, event recorders are recommended. If ambulatory and event recorders are nondiagnostic, EPS should be considered for selection of therapy. In patients with structural heart disease who have one episode of syncope suggestive of cardiac etiology, EPS is recommended for evaluation of dysrhythmic syncope.

Since the prognosis of patients with negative EPS is favorable, empiric therapy (with a pacemaker or antidysrhythmic drugs) is not justified. Upright tilt testing is recommended in patients with recurrent or disabling symptoms who have negative EPS to define a potential etiology and initiate treatment.

In patients with structural heart disease and syncope, evaluation of the extent and severity of heart disease is needed in order to plan treatment. Thus stress testing and echocardiography may allow better definition of the extent of coronary artery disease and ventricular function in patients with possible ischemic heart disease. These tests are recommended prior to the consideration of EPS and tilt testing, which can result in hypotension that is best avoided in patients with coronary artery disease.

Patients Without Heart Disease. Prognosis of syncope patients without heart disease is excellent with regard to the outcome of mortality. In young patients with a normal ECG, the likelihood of dysrhythmias is low. In this group, prolonged ECG monitoring or EPS is generally negative and not needed. Vasovagal syncope and psychiatric disorders are the major diagnostic considerations and should be pursued as the initial step in the evaluation. A similar diagnostic approach can be taken with older patients without heart disease and a normal ECG, but further studies are needed to define better the role of prolonged ECG monitoring in these patients. The yield of EPS is low in this group, and so it is not justified in the vast majority of the patients.

Recurrent Syncope. In patients with recurrent syncope, the diagnostic considerations are large, but these patients are less likely to have dysrhythmias and are more likely to have psychiatric illnesses and vasovagal syncope. The initial approach to diagnostic testing should be based on the presence or absence of heart disease (as noted above). In this group of patients, if a cause of syncope is not established, patient-activated intermittent ECG loop recorders may be useful for the evaluation of brief episodic dysrhythmias.

Although studies in the 1980s have shown that a cause of syncope was not established in up to 45% of patients, by using the approach outlined here with the availability of newer diagnostic modalities a cause of syncope can be assigned in the vast majority of patients presenting with this symptom. Patients without a diagnosis have a low incidence of mortality and sudden death but should be followed closely and reevaluated on recurrence.

MANAGEMENT

Treatment decisions are based on the etiology of syncope. A detailed discussion of the treatments of all of the etiologies is covered in specific chapters. General considerations for treatments are as follows.

Vasovagal Syncope

The severity and natural history of vasovagal syncope are variable. Patients may have a large number of events at one time that diminish or resolve spontaneously. There are rare patients who continue to have episodes over many years. Thus the frequency and severity of events are important in devising treatment plans for the patient. Because treatments may have potential side effects, they should be reserved for patients who have frequent or disabling symptoms. Treatment should be avoided in those with one or rare lifetime episodes.

Many patients with vasovagal syncope have precipitating factors or situations. These situations should be identified by a careful history, and the patient instructed to avoid them. Common triggers include prolonged standing, venipuncture, large meals, and heat (such as hot baths or sunbathing). Additionally, fasting, lack of sleep, and alcohol intake may predispose to vasovagal syncope and should be avoided. Since psychiatric illnesses probably lead to vasovagal reactions, screening for the psychiatric illnesses noted above should be performed. Treatment of the psychiatric illness often resolves the recurrent syncope.

Several types of drug therapies have been tried for patients with vasovagal syncope (Table 62-3). β-Blockers (e.g., metoprolol, atenolol) are the most commonly used drugs. The

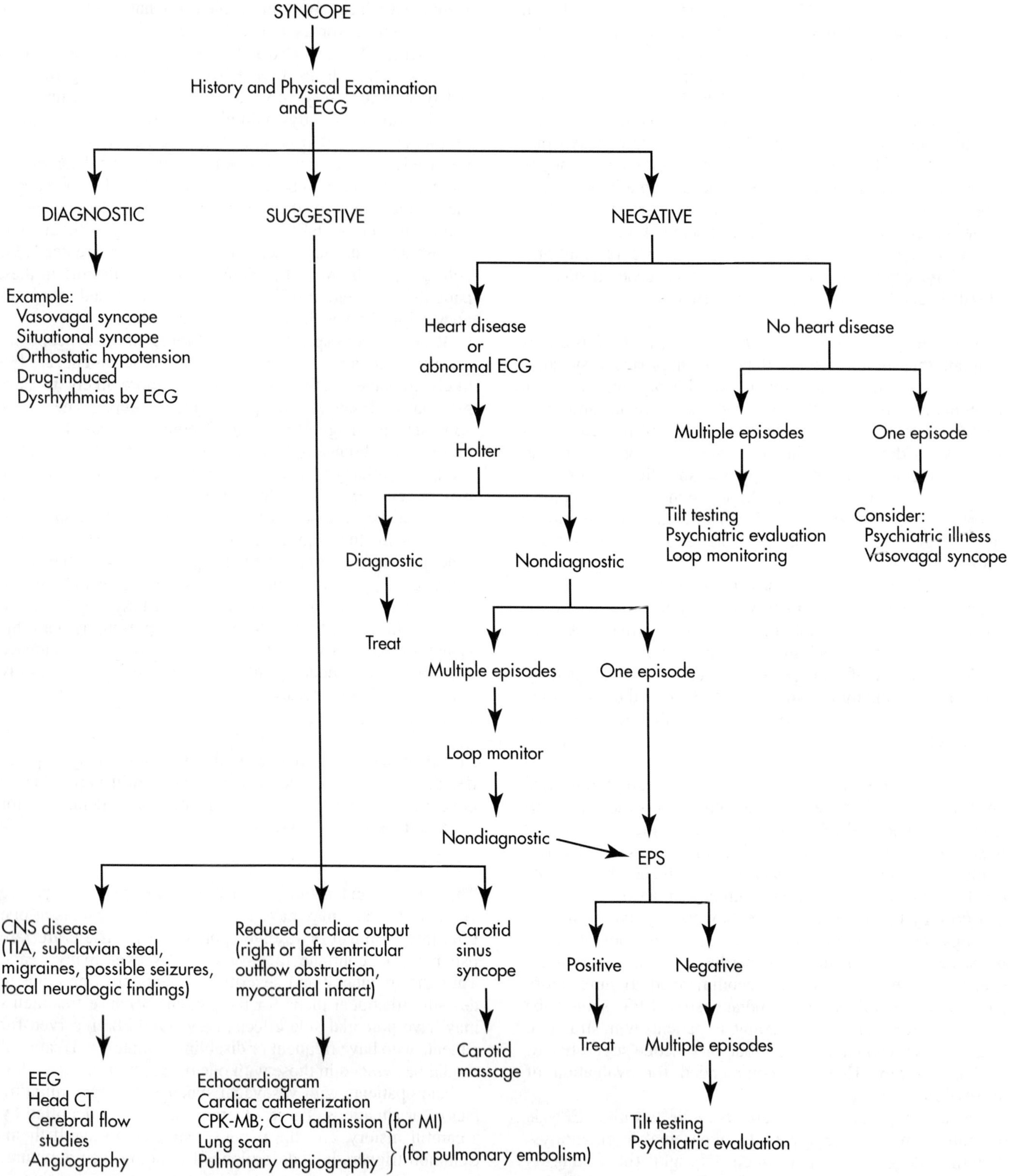

Fig. 62-2. Algorithm summarizing the diagnostic approach to syncope.

mechanism of action of β-blockers is not fully understood, but they can diminish cardiac contractility, inhibiting the activation of cardiac mechanoreceptors. Anticholinergic agents such as transdermal scopolamine (one patch every 3 days) are particularly useful in patients with profound bradycardia during upright tilt testing. Disopyramide has also been reported to decrease recurrence of syncope. This drug has anticholinergic and negative inotropic effects, which may inhibit activation of cardiac mechanoreceptors. Theophylline has rarely been used at doses as low as 6 to 12 mg/kg/day. The mechanism of action of theophylline in the treatment of vasovagal syncope is not known, but a blockade of the effects

Table 62-3. Commonly Used Therapies for Recurrent Vasovagal Syncope

Therapies	Dosage
β-Blockers	
Atenolol	25-200 mg/day
Metoprolol	50-200 mg/day
Propranolol	40-160 mg/day
Disopyramide	200-600 mg/day
Fludrocortisone	0.1-1 mg/day
Fluoxetine	40 mg/day
Scopolamine patch	1 patch every 2-3 days
Theophylline	6-12 mg/kg/day

of adenosine, which has vasodilatory effects, is postulated. Measures to expand volume have been used and include increased salt intake, custom-fitted counterpressure support garments from ankle to waist, and fludrocortisone acetate. Potential side effects include recumbent hypertension, hypokalemia, fluid retention, and congestive heart failure. Finally, atrioventricular pacing may be considered in patients with significant bradycardia in response to upright tilt testing. Even in these patients, the initial treatment of choice is pharmacologic. Pacemaker therapy should be reserved for those who have disabling symptoms and fail drug therapy.

Orthostatic Hypotension

The initial approach to treatment of orthostatic hypotension is to ensure adequate salt and volume intake and to avoid or discontinue drugs that cause orthostatic hypotension. Patients with orthostatic hypotension should be advised to raise the head of the bed at night, to rise from bed or chair slowly, and to avoid prolonged standing. Compressive stockings applied up to thigh levels may help decrease venous pooling. Frequent small feedings may be helpful in patients with marked postprandial orthostatic hypotension.

Pharmacologic agents of potential benefit include fludrocortisone (0.1 to 1 mg/day) in conjunction with increased salt intake. Various adrenergic agents have been used, including ephedrine, phenylephrine, and others. A more detailed discussion of pharmacologic treatment of orthostatic hypotension is found elsewhere.

SYNCOPE IN THE ELDERLY

The elderly often have multiple chronic diseases and physiologic impairments that can predispose to syncope. Thus in the elderly, several seemingly mild abnormalities may contribute to a sudden reduction of cerebral blood flow and syncope. As an example, mild volume depletion with upper respiratory tract infection in a patient with chronic renal insufficiency and systolic hypertension may be sufficient to cause syncope, whereas any one problem alone is not severe enough to cause loss of consciousness.

The initial approach to the management of the elderly should be to search for a single disease as a cause of syncope. If a single disease is found (such as severe aortic stenosis, symptomatic bradycardia, or symptomatic orthostatic hypotension), treatment of that disease can be planned. However, a single disease as the cause of syncope is often not apparent. In these patients, inability to compensate for common situational stresses may be a factor in the setting of multiple medical problems, medications, and physiologic impairments. A careful assessment of the effect of underlying pathologic conditions and medications is important to determine whether multiple pathologic processes could have led to syncope. Once these potential processes are identified, treatment should be directed to correcting these factors. As an example, consider an elderly patient presenting with syncope, who has taken enalapril, 10 mg/day, and has anemia (hemoglobin 9.0), mild orthostatic hypotension, and a recent upper respiratory tract infection. In this patient, if no other etiology of syncope is apparent based on clinical findings and selective use of laboratory tests, volume repletion, treatment of anemia, and adjustment or change of antihypertensive medication may help prevent further episodes of syncope.

ADDITIONAL READINGS

Abboud FM: Neurocardiogenic syncope, *N Engl J Med* 328:1117, 1993.

Benditt DG, Ferguson DW, Grubb BP, et al: Tilt table testing for assessing syncope, *J Am Coll Cardiol* 28:263-275, 1996.

Benditt DG, Remole S, Bailin S, et al: Tilt table testing for evaluations of neurally-mediated (cardioneurogenic) syncope: rational and proposed protocols, *Pacing Clin Electrophysiol* 14:1528-1537, 1991.

DiMarco JP, Philbrick JT: Use of ambulatory electrocardiographic (Holter) monitoring, *Ann Intern Med* 113:53, 1990.

Guidelines for clinical intracardiac electrophysiological and catheter ablation procedures: A report of the American College of Cardiology/American Heart Association Task Force on practice guidelines. (Committee on clinical intracardiac electrophysiologic and catheter ablation procedures). Developed in collaboration with the North American Society of Pacing and Electrophysiology, *Circulation* 92:673-691, 1995.

Kapoor WN: Evaluation and outcome of patients with syncope, *Medicine* 69:160, 1990.

Kapoor WN, Brant NL: Evaluation of syncope by upright tilt testing with isoproterenol: a nonspecific test, *Ann Intern Med* 116:358, 1992.

Kapoor WN, Fortunato M, Hanusa BH, et al: Psychiatric illnesses in patients with syncope, *Am J Med* 99:505-512, 1995.

Kapoor WN, Smith MA, Miller NL: Upright tilt testing in evaluating syncope: a comprehensive literature review, *Am J Med* 97:78-88, 1994.

Lipsitz L: Orthostatic hypotension in the elderly, *N Engl J Med* 321:952, 1989.

Linzer M, Yang EH, Estes NA, et al: Diagnosing syncope: Part 1: Value of history, physical examination, and electrocardiography: the clinical efficacy assessment project of the American College of Physicians, *Ann Intern Med* 126:989-996, 1997.

Linzer M, Yang EH, Estes NA, et al: Diagnosing syncope: Part 2: Unexplained syncope, *Ann Intern Med* 127:76-86, 1997.

Ischemic Heart Disease

Leonard S. Lilly

Ischemic heart disease (IHD) is the leading cause of mortality in industrialized societies. This condition afflicts 11 million individuals in the United States and is responsible for more than 500,000 deaths annually. Despite these daunting numbers, during the past 3 decades there has been a gradual decline in IHD-related deaths, which likely reflects the recognition and correction of cardiac risk factors and

Table 63-1. Clinical Definitions

Syndrome	Description
Ischemic heart disease	Condition in which all imbalance between myocardial oxygen supply and demand results in myocardial hypoxia and accumulation of waste metabolites; most often due to atherosclerotic disease of the coronary arteries
Angina pectoris	Uncomfortable sensation in the chest or neighboring anatomic structures produced by myocardial ischemia
Stable angina	Chronic pattern of transient angina pectoris, precipitated by physical activity or emotional upset, relieved by rest within a few minutes; episodes often associated with temporary depression of the ST segment, but permanent myocardial damage does not result
Variant angina	Typical anginal discomfort, usually at rest, which develops because of coronary artery spasm, rather than an increase of myocardial oxygen demand: episodes often associated with transient shifts of the ST segment (usually ST elevation)
Unstable angina	Pattern of increased frequency and duration of angina episodes, produced by less exertion, or at rest; high frequency of progression to myocardial infarction if untreated
Silent ischemia	Asymptomatic episodes of myocardial ischemia; can be detected by ECG and other laboratory techniques
Myocardial infarction	Region of myocardial necrosis due to prolonged cessation of blood supply; most often results from acute thrombus at site of coronary atherosclerotic stenosis; may be first clinical manifestation of ischemic heart disease, or there may be a history of angina pectoris

Modified from Lilly LS, editor: *Pathophysiology of heart disease,* Philadelphia, 1993, Lea & Febiger.

dramatic improvements in medical and surgical therapies. The primary care physician plays a pivotal role in the prevention, diagnosis, and long-term management of individuals with this condition.

The clinical presentation of patients with IHD is highly variable (Table 63-1). It may be manifest by classic exertional angina, but in other cases myocardial ischemia may occur without any symptoms (silent ischemia). Sometimes the first manifestation is an acute myocardial infarction (MI) or sudden death.

PATHOPHYSIOLOGY OF MYOCARDIAL ISCHEMIA

Myocardial ischemia results when there is an imbalance between myocardial oxygen supply and demand. This most often occurs because of the presence of atherosclerotic plaque within one or more coronary arteries, which limits the normal rise in coronary blood flow in response to increases in myocardial oxygen demand.

The major determinants of myocardial oxygen demand are heart rate, the force of ventricular contraction, and ventricular wall tension. The latter is proportional to ventricular volume and pressure. Conditions that increase myocardial oxygen consumption, such as physical exertion and emotional stress, result in myocardial ischemia unless there is a concomitant rise in oxygen supply.

Myocardial oxygen supply depends on the oxygen-carrying capacity of the blood, coronary blood flow, and the ability of the heart muscle to extract oxygen from circulating blood. The oxygen-carrying capacity relates to the content of hemoglobin and systemic oxygenation, and in the absence of anemia or lung disease it is fairly constant. Unlike other organs, the extraction of oxygen from the blood by heart muscle is nearly maximal in the resting state and cannot be significantly increased during periods of increased demand. Therefore it is primarily the increase in coronary blood flow that adjusts myocardial supply when oxygen demands increase. During periods of increased myocardial work, the local accumulation of vasoactive metabolites stimulates coronary arteriolar dilation and causes the coronary blood flow to rise several-fold. However, when atherosclerotic disease is present, the artery lumen is narrowed and vasodilation is impaired, such that coronary blood flow cannot increase in the face of increased demands, and ischemia may result. When ischemia occurs, it is frequently accompanied by the chest discomfort known as angina pectoris. The predictable pattern of intermittent symptoms of myocardial ischemia during exertion or emotional stress is known as *chronic stable angina.*

The degree of narrowing in an atherosclerotic vessel is not constant; it can vary from moment to moment because of alterations in coronary vascular tone and vasospasm, which may further reduce blood flow. The mechanism of coronary vasospasm is not known but may relate to endothelial dysfunction in the setting of atherosclerotic disease, with impaired release of natural vasodilators including nitric oxide and prostacyclin. In some patients, alterations of vascular tone play a minor role in narrowing the coronary lumen, but in other individuals the degree of vasospasm may be even more important than the degree of fixed atherosclerotic stenosis itself. In the majority of patients with angina the development of myocardial ischemia results from a combination of fixed and vasospastic stenosis. The variation in vascular tone may explain the variable threshold of angina: one day exertion might not produce any angina at all, but on another day similar effort does result in symptoms of ischemia.

A small number of patients experience episodes of intense focal coronary artery spasm in the absence of underlying atherosclerotic disease. In that situation angina can occur at rest (i.e., not provoked by increased myocardial oxygen demand) because of the marked reduction in coronary blood flow. This form of ischemia, known as *variant* or *Prinzmetal's angina,* is rare.

A patient with chronic stable angina may develop a sudden increase in the frequency and duration of ischemic episodes, occurring at lower workloads than previously or even at rest. This acceleration is known as *unstable angina,* and up to 20% of such patients sustain an MI over the ensuing 3 months. Although the majority of such patients have severe atherosclerotic coronary disease, unstable angina can also arise in patients with only mildly obstructive coronary lesions. Catheterization and angioscopy studies have shown that the pathogenesis of unstable angina is multifactorial, often involving rupture of an atherosclerotic plaque with subsequent platelet aggregation and local thrombus formation. In other cases transient periods of intense coronary vasospasm at sites of atherosclerotic plaque play a role. Similar mechanisms also appear responsible for the development of MI: more than 90% of acute MIs result from an acute thrombus obstructing a coronary artery with resultant prolonged ischemia and tissue necrosis. This summary of the pathophysiology of IHD has therapeutic consequences: the treatment of chronic angina is directed at minimizing myocardial oxygen demand and increasing coronary flow, whereas in the acute syndromes of unstable angina or MI primary therapy is also directed against platelet aggregation and thrombosis.

EPIDEMIOLOGY OF ISCHEMIC HEART DISEASE

Many large epidemiologic studies have implicated certain habits and predisposing conditions in the development of atherosclerosis and IHD. The Framingham Heart Study, for example, identified four major potentially modifiable risk factors: hyperlipidemia (elevated low-density lipoprotein [LDL] cholesterol or reduced high-density lipoprotein [HDL] cholesterol [see Chapter 71]), hypertension, cigarette smoking, and diabetes mellitus (Box 63-1). Recently, the American Heart Association has added obesity (a body mass index > 30) to the list of major modifiable risk factors. Several nonmodifiable risk factors include advanced age, male sex, and a family history of premature coronary disease (i.e., coronary disease in related males age 55 or less or females age 65 or less). Other potential risk factors of unproven magnitude include a sedentary lifestyle and stressful emotional states.

Correction of the modifiable risk factors is critical to the long-term management of IHD to prevent disease progression and resulting complications. For example, clinical trials discussed in Chapter 71 show that control of abnormal cholesterol levels can substantially slow, and possibly reverse, the development of atherosclerotic plaque, as well as substantially reduce cardiac events and mortality.

In addition to these traditional risk factors, certain blood constituents correlate with the development of atherosclerosis and cardiac events. For example, epidemiologic studies have related the concentration of the amino acid homocysteine to the incidence of coronary, cerebral, and peripheral vascular disease. The risk of MI is three times greater in patients with the highest levels of homocysteine compared with those with the lowest levels. Supplementation of the diet with folate and other B vitamins reduces the level of homocysteine, but it is not yet known whether such therapy improves the coronary risk.

Circulating thrombogenic factors are also related to the development of IHD. For example, an elevated level of plasma fibrinogen is an independent risk factor for coronary artery disease in both men and women. Recent epidemiologic studies have confirmed that individuals with the highest fibrinogen levels are several times more likely to suffer a coronary event than cohorts with the lowest levels. Similarly, elevated levels of coagulation factor VII have been shown to be a risk factor for MI. In one recent report, an elevated factor VII level, in the presence of either smoking or hypertension, increased the relative risk of an MI up to fiftyfold.

Box 63-1. Major Risk Factors for Coronary Artery Disease

- Hypercholesterolemia (↑ LDL, ↓ HDL)
- Hypertension
- Cigarette smoking
- Diabetes mellitus
- Advanced age
- Male sex
- Family history of premature CAD
- Obesity

LDL, Low-density lipoprotein; *HDL*, high-density lipoprotein.

CLINICAL FEATURES OF ANGINA PECTORIS

History

The most common manifestation of myocardial ischemia is the intermittent discomfort of angina pectoris. Although many laboratory tests can identify the presence of ischemia, the most important aspect of the clinical evaluation remains a careful history to evaluate for anginal symptoms. Several characteristics derived from the history can aid in the differentiation between myocardial ischemia and other causes of chest discomfort (Table 63-2). Features of angina relate to the quality of the discomfort, its location and radiation, precipitating factors, and frequency.

Quality of Discomfort. Most often angina is described as a tightness, squeezing, heaviness, pressure, burning, indigestion, or aching sensation. It is only rarely described as a pain, and patients sometimes correct the physician who refers to it as such. It is *never* sharp, stabbing, prickly, spasmodic, or pleuritic. It is usually a steady discomfort that lasts a few minutes, rarely more than 10, unless unstable angina or an MI is evolving. It *always* lasts more than a few seconds, which helps differentiate it from some types of musculoskeletal pain. Angina is usually relieved quickly by sublingual nitroglycerin (in less than 5 minutes), which can be a useful distinguishing feature. Sometimes, while describing angina, a patient raises a clenched fist to the sternum (Levine sign) as if to indicate the constrictive sensation by that tight grip.

Symptoms that frequently accompany angina include dyspnea, diaphoresis, and nausea, which resolve quickly with cessation of the chest discomfort.

Location and Radiation. Angina is usually a diffuse sensation rather than located at a discrete spot. If the patient can localize the discomfort with a single finger, myocardial ischemia is an unlikely cause. Generally, the discomfort is most intense retrosternally or in the anterior left chest but may occur anywhere between the jaw and the upper abdomen. It frequently radiates to the shoulders, upper back, neck, or inner aspect of the arms, particularly on the left side.

Table 63-2. Differential Diagnosis of Recurrent Chest Pain

Condition	Helpful distinguishing features
Myocardial ischemia	Diffuse tightness/constriction/heaviness; not sharp or pleuritic Brought on by exertion or emotional upset
Pericarditis	Sharp, pleuritic, positional Friction rub Diffuse ST elevation, PR depression on ECG
Chest wall pain	Sharp, localized pain Reproduced by palpation over painful area
Cervical or thoracic spine pain	Shooting pain or ache worsened by movement of neck or back Pain may be in dermatomal distribution
Esophageal or gastric pains	Nonexertional pains Often associated with dysphagia or gastric reflux Worsened by certain foods, aspirin, lying supine May be relieved by antacids
Biliary pain	Right upper quadrant tenderness Fatty food intolerance

Although the location of angina may vary between individuals, it is usually the same sensation in a given patient with each attack, unless an MI is in progress, at which time it is generally more diffuse and severe.

Precipitants. Angina, except when due to pure vasospasm, is caused by factors that increase myocardial demand. Typically it is provoked by exertion, such as climbing stairs, walking up an inclined surface,vigorous work using the arms, or sexual activity. Other factors that increase myocardial oxygen demand and can result in angina include emotional excitement, eating a large meal, and physical activities in cold weather. The latter results in vasoconstriction of the extremities, an increase in systemic vascular resistance, and therefore an increase in myocardial wall tension and oxygen requirements. In addition, myocardial ischemia displays a circadian rhythm, such that the threshold for angina is usually lower in the morning hours.

Patients who primarily experience coronary vasospasm most often have symptoms at rest, independent of activities that increase myocardial oxygen demand. Chest discomfort that awakens a patient from sleep may be precipitated by this mechanism, or because of the emotional stress (and therefore increased myocardial oxygen demand) of a bad dream.

Frequency. For an individual with IHD the level of exertion needed to precipitate angina and therefore its frequency remains fairly constant (depending on superimposed vascular tone). However, the patient may quickly realize what activities produce angina and avoid them. Therefore it is important to ask about any recent reduction in exertion levels when taking the history.

Physical Examination

The general examination of patients with suspected IHD should address the manifestations of atherosclerosis as well as transient findings during episodes of angina. External signs of hypercholesterolemia may be present, including arcus senilis and tendinous xanthomas. Funduscopic examination may show evidence of chronic hypertension or diabetes. Also look for signs of hyperthyroidism, which can contribute to increased myocardial oxygen demand.

A general vascular examination should assess for the equality of blood pressure between the two arms (to rule out atherosclerotic narrowings), as well as palpation and auscultation of the carotid and peripheral arteries and examination of the abdomen for evidence of an aortic aneurysm.

On cardiac examination an S_4 is common in patients with coronary artery disease (CAD) because of atrial contraction into a "stiffened" left ventricle. This sign is not diagnostic for IHD, however, since it is present in many healthy elderly patients. The cardiac examination may be otherwise normal while the patient is asymptomatic, but during an episode of angina, several transient physical findings may appear. Increased sympathetic tone during chest pain may result in an increase in heart rate and blood pressure. Myocardial ischemia may result in papillary muscle dysfunction with a transient systolic murmur of mitral regurgitation. Ischemia-induced left ventricular wall motion abnormalities may be detected as an abnormal precordial bulge on chest palpation. A transient S_3 gallop and pulmonary rales may appear if ischemia-induced left ventricular dysfunction occurs.

DIAGNOSTIC TESTS

Blood tests to evaluate for underlying risk factors include measurement of the serum lipids (see Chapter 71) and fasting serum glucose. The hematocrit and thyroid function tests should be measured if clinically appropriate, since anemia and hyperthyroidism can exacerbate myocardial ischemia.

Noninvasive cardiac testing is useful to confirm the diagnosis of IHD, to help stratify patients into categories of risk, and to guide therapy. Many of these tests are expensive, and it is therefore important to choose the appropriate study for each patient. Beyond the resting electrocardiogram (ECG) they include exercise testing, with or without nuclear scintigraphy, exercise radionuclide ventriculography or echocardiography, pharmacologic stress testing, and ambulatory ECG monitoring.

Resting ECG

Many patients with CAD have normal baseline ECGs, or may demonstrate pathologic Q waves indicative of previous infarction. In many patients minor ST and T wave abnormalities are present but are not specific for CAD. However, the ECG can be diagnostically useful if recorded during an episode of chest pain, whereupon ischemia often results in transient horizontal or downsloping ST segments or T wave inversions, which normalize following resolution of the pain. Less often, transient ST elevation may be observed, which suggests severe transmural ischemia or coronary artery spasm.

Exercise Stress Testing

The most useful noninvasive studies in the evaluation of angina involve exercise testing. In patients without resting ST or T wave abnormalities the standard treadmill (or bicycle) exercise test, without additional imaging modalities, should be the initial procedure, since it is the most convenient and cost-effective. For patients whose presentation strongly suggests myocardial ischemia, the exercise test has a sensitivity and specificity greater than 85%. However, when the probability of significant coronary disease is low (e.g., a young woman with prickly chest pains), the test is less specific, and false-positive results are more common.

Exercise testing is most commonly used (1) to confirm the diagnosis of angina, (2) to identify IHD patients at high risk of complications, (3) to assess the response of antianginal therapy, and (4) as a screening procedure for certain asymptomatic populations, such as individuals with strong cardiac risk factors, older patients about to begin exercise programs, and individuals whose well being could affect public safety (e.g., airline pilots).

Different protocols may be used for exercise testing, but in each the intensity of exercise is incrementally augmented (e.g., increased grade and speed on the treadmill) to raise myocardial oxygen consumption. During the test the ECG and heart rate are monitored continuously and the blood pressure measured every few minutes. The product of heart rate and systolic blood pressure (known as the double product) correlates with myocardial oxygen demand and is useful in describing a patient's anginal threshold.

Exercise is continued until a target heart rate (usually 85% of the maximal predicted heart rate based on the patient's age) or symptom-limited end points (e.g., precipitation of anginal pain) are achieved. However, the test should be terminated immediately if hypotension, high-grade ventricular dysrhythmias, or more than 3 mm ST segment depression develop. The complications of exercise testing are few, and death and MI are extremely uncommon. However, the risks are increased and the test should not be performed in individuals with unstable angina or advanced aortic stenosis.

Exercise testing suggests the presence of IHD if the patient's typical chest discomfort is reproduced, or if specific ECG abnormalities develop (Box 63-2). The ECG criteria for a positive test is 1 mm (0.1 mV) horizontal or downsloping ST depression, measured 0.08 second after the termination of the QRS complex. The degree and location of ST segment abnormalities are not always a reliable indication of the extent and anatomic localization of CAD. However, taken together, the magnitude, time of onset, duration, and number of ECG leads that develop abnormal ST segments can predict the severity of CAD. For example, individuals who develop ST depression in multiple leads during the first 3 minutes of exercise are very likely to have left main or severe three-vessel disease. Other criteria for a markedly positive test that are indicative of such severe coronary artery disease and a poor cardiac prognosis are listed in Box 63-2.

Conversely a negative test or one that becomes positive only after 9 minutes of exercise or at a heart rate greater than 160 beats/min correlates with a very optimistic prognosis, even if angina or ST segment depressions develop during the test.

The diagnostic value of an exercise test may be limited by medications, especially β-blockers, which can blunt the achieved heart rate or rise in blood pressure. If the purpose of the stress test is to confirm the presence of angina, such medications should be withheld for 1 to 2 days before the test, and if necessary sublingual nitroglycerin can be used as needed during that time. However, if the purpose is to judge the effects of and gauge medical therapy, then the usual drug regimen should be continued on the day of testing.

Box 63-2. Interpretation of Exercise Treadmill Test

Positive Test

- Reproduction of chest pain
- ST depression (horizontal or downsloping at 0.08 second after termination of QRS)

Markedly Positive Test (Predictors of Severe Coronary Disease)

- Chest pain or ST changes in first 3 minutes of test
- ≥3 mm ST depression during test
- Persistence of ST changes > 5 minutes after exercise stopped
- Decline in systolic BP during test
- Multifocal ventricular ectopy or ventricular tachycardia during or after exercise, if accompanied by ST segment changes
- Poor duration of exercise (≤2 minutes) due to cardiopulmonary limitations

Radionuclide Studies

Two types of nuclear studies are used to enhance the diagnostic value of standard exercise tests: myocardial perfusion imaging and radionuclide ventriculography. These tests can provide additional information regarding the location and extent of CAD, and their interpretations are not hampered by resting ECG abnormalities. However, they are more expensive than standard treadmill tests and should be used judiciously (Boxes 63-3 and 63-4).

Myocardial Perfusion Scintigraphy. Myocardial perfusion scintigraphy is generally more sensitive and specific than conventional stress testing. During this test a radionuclide (e.g., ^{201}Tl or ^{99m}Tc sestamibi) is used, which after peripheral venous injection distributes to the myocardium in proportion to coronary blood flow. The radionuclide is injected at peak exercise, and immediate imaging is performed. Perfusion defects (cold spots) indicate regions of prior infarction or exercise-induced ischemia. Repeat imaging at rest several hours later shows filling in of the zones that were ischemic, differentiating them from regions of previous infarction. The location of perfusion abnormalities correlates with coronary disease in the respective territory (e.g., left anterior descending artery disease results in perfusion abnormalities within the anterior wall). Multiple large perfusion defects correlate with left main or severe three-vessel disease.

In experienced departments of nuclear medicine, thallium scintigraphy has a sensitivity of 75% to 90% but may be positive in up to 20% of normal individuals. In women, attenuation due to breast tissue artifact is a common cause of false-positive studies. In addition to previous MIs, other conditions that may produce persistent myocardial defects

Box 63-3. Commonly Used Forms of Stress Testing

Standard Tests
- Exercise treadmill
- Stationary bicycle
- Arm ergometry (if arms are better conditioned than legs)

If Baseline ECG Precludes Interpretation of Exercise-Induced Ischemia, or if Greater Sensitivity and Specificity Required*
- Exercise perfusion scintigraphy (^{201}TI or other radionuclides)
- Exercise radionuclide ventriculogram (^{99m}Tc)
- Exercise echocardiography

If Unable to Exercise*
- Dipyridamole (or adenosine) perfusion scintigraphy (^{201} TI or other radionuclides)
- Dobutamine perfusion scintigraphy
- Dipyridamole or dobutamine echocardiography

*Choice of study should be dictated by local expertise.

Box 63-4. Criteria for Use of Perfusion Scintigraphy

- An abnormal baseline ECG that precludes interpretation of the standard ETT (left bundle branch block, baseline ST-T wave abnormalities, WPW syndrome)
- To confirm exercise test results that conflict with the clinical impression (unexpected ST shifts during exercise in an asymptomatic patient)
- To increase the sensitivity of CAD detection in an individual with a negative exercise test, but strongly suspected coronary disease
- To localize regions of ischemia (to identify culprit lesions responsible for ischemia in patients with multi-vessel CAD).

ETT, Exercise tolerance test; *WPW*, Wolff-Parkinson-White.

include infiltrative disease (e.g., sarcoidosis) and dilated cardiomyopathy.

For patients who are unable to exercise, pharmacologic stress testing in conjunction with myocardial perfusion imaging can be undertaken. IV adenosine (or dipyridamole) produces vasodilation and increases flow to the myocardium perfused by healthy coronaries. This effect steals blood away from stenotic coronaries, creating regional ischemia that can be detected following injection of radionuclides such as ^{201}T1. This type of non-exercise stress test has proven useful in predicting cardiac ischemic events in patients with chronic stable angina and in those about to undergo noncardiac surgery. Another form of pharmacologic stress testing utilizes the adrenergic-stimulating drug dobutamine to artificially increase heart rate and systolic blood pressure.

Exercise Radionuclide Ventriculography. Exercise radionuclide ventriculography entails imaging blood flow through the left ventricle during the cardiac cycle at rest and then with exercise. Two commonly used techniques are (1) the first-pass technique, in which a large bolus of radionuclide (e.g., ^{99m}Tc) is injected and the tracer is imaged as it flows through the heart as it is quickly cleared from the circulation; and (2) the multigated equilibrium technique (MUGA) in which red blood cells are labeled and several minutes of transventricular flow are analyzed as a composite image.

In normal individuals, contractile function of the left ventricle increases with exercise. Myocardial ischemia is suggested if the ejection fraction falls with exercise or if segmental left ventricular wall motion abnormalities develop. Exercise radionuclide ventriculography has a sensitivity similar to that of ^{201}T1 perfusion imaging, but it is less specific because other etiologies of left ventricular dysfunction can produce similar results.

Echocardiography

Imaging of the left ventricle by ultrasound can reveal segmental wall motion abnormalities indicative of ischemia or previous infarction. In exercise echocardiography, left ventricular function is assessed before and during vigorous exercise (supine bicycle or treadmill); exercise-induced segmental regional wall motion abnormalities are an indication of ischemia. Exercise echocardiography is therefore analogous to exercise radionuclide ventriculography and has similar sensitivity and specificity for the presence of significant coronary disease.

For patients who are unable to exercise, pharmacologic stress testing with echocardiography can be performed in one of two fashions: (1) using potent vasodilators such as adenosine or dipyridamole (analogous to pharmacologic ^{201}T1 scintigraphy described above), or (2) using an adrenergic stimulating drug (e.g., dobutamine). Either of these techniques signifies the presence of myocardial ischemia by drug-induced left ventricular wall motion abnormalities.

Ambulatory ECG Monitoring

Frequency-modulated ambulatory ECG monitors detect shifts in the ST segments indicative of ischemia. Approximately 40% of patients with known stable CAD display such transient shifts, and in most cases, asymptomatic silent episodes (described below) are even more common than symptomatic events. The role of this technique in documenting the presence of CAD has not yet been defined; however, some studies have shown its usefulness as a prognostic guide. For example, the absence of ST segment shifts on ambulatory monitoring predicts a low risk of cardiac complications in patients undergoing noncardiac surgery.

Coronary Arteriography

Coronary arteriography allows selective visualization of the coronary arteries and their major branches and is the most accurate means to detect the presence and extent of CAD. In experienced laboratories it is performed with low mortality (approximately 0.2%) or severe vascular complications (0.7%). However, this technique is costly, is not risk-free, and is seldom needed to simply establish the diagnosis of significant coronary disease. The decision to proceed with arteriography should be dictated by the patient's clinical presentation and only when a change in therapeutic

Box 63-5. Common Indications for Coronary Arteriography in Ambulatory Patients

- Chronic angina with limiting symptoms refractory to medical therapy
- Markedly positive exercise test
- Chronic angina with left ventricular dysfunction (ejection fraction less than 40%)
- Angina soon after myocardial infarction (spontaneous or exercise test–induced)
- Cardiomyopathy in which coronary disease is suspected cause
- Patients with chest pain who are diagnostic dilemmas

plan is under consideration. Commonly accepted indications for coronary angiography are presented in Box 63-5 and Fig. 63-1.

Note that an individual with mild to moderate angina that is reasonably controlled with medical therapy does not generally require cardiac catheterization, since the long-term prognosis and quality of life may not be significantly affected. However, if that individual has other markers of a poor prognosis by exercise testing or impaired left ventricular function, then catheterization should be performed (see Fig. 63-1).

At catheterization, coronary narrowings of greater than 70% are considered significant (i.e., the ones most likely to produce angina). Natural history studies have shown that the mortality of patients with CAD correlates with the number of significantly narrowed vessels, and those with left main disease (defined as a stenosis > 50%) have the highest mortality. Outcomes are correspondingly worse in patients with decreased left ventricular contractile function.

Left ventriculography can be performed at the time of cardiac catheterization to measure global and regional left ventricular function and assess the presence of mitral regurgitation. However, such information can often be derived by noninvasive techniques (echocardiography or radionuclide ventriculography), sparing the patient from additional intravenous contrast material.

MANAGEMENT OF PATIENTS WITH SUSPECTED ANGINA

General Principles

Fig. 63-1 summarizes the approach to the evaluation and management of patients with suspected IHD. Once angina is suggested by the clinical history, stress testing is useful to confirm the diagnosis and stratify patients into high- and low-risk groups. The standard form of stress testing is the graded treadmill test, but for those patients with abnormal baseline ECGs or those unable to exercise, the alternative forms of testing are appropriate. Patients with markedly positive stress tests should undergo coronary arteriography because of the high likelihood of left main or three-vessel coronary disease, conditions that could warrant mechanical revascularization. For patients with only mildly positive stress tests or those with nondiagnostic studies, a trial of pharmacologic management is recommended, with further evaluation dictated by the response to therapy. An alternative approach in inactive or elderly patients is to begin a trial of medical therapy based on the clinical history of angina, without stress testing. The early response to therapy would determine whether further evaluation is needed.

The management goals for IHD are to reduce anginal symptoms, prevent complications such as MI, and prolong life. General measures begin with a discussion of the disease and the importance of eliminating risk factors that have led to it. Patients should be encouraged to stop smoking, lose excess weight, and control hypertension and diabetes. Lipid-lowering in appropriate patients is a critical aspect of management. Patients with CAD and an elevated LDL-cholesterol should achieve lower levels (generally <100 mg/dl). HMG-CoA reductase inhibitors are particularly effective in achieving this goal, and such therapy has been shown to reduce the risk of both primary and secondary coronary events (see Chapter 71).

There are often psychosocial issues faced by individuals who are diagnosed with angina for the first time. Many patients may be unnecessarily pessimistic about their prognosis, so a frank discussion should stress the common nature of IHD and the advanced therapeutic options available that often allow the quality of life to be unimpaired. Similarly, it is important to inform the patient that transient anginal attacks do not result in permanent heart damage.

Angina is particularly likely to occur during bursts of activity, particularly after periods of rest (e.g., walking up a flight of stairs after watching TV for several hours). Therefore a period of warming up (e.g., walking around the house a few times before mowing the lawn) is often a useful way to prevent angina. In addition, the prophylactic use of nitroglycerin should be encouraged before activities likely to bring on chest discomfort. Angina often exhibits a circadian pattern, with episodes more common in the hours shortly after arising, so the use of prophylactic nitroglycerin before dressing and shaving can be particularly beneficial. If a patient notes that angina is frequently precipitated by emotional upset, attempts should be made to minimize these; counseling or antianxiety medications may be useful.

Patients with stable angina should be encouraged to participate in a regular exercise program, most often walking. Such activity can have a beneficial conditioning effect on skeletal muscles and may contribute to raising the anginal threshold. Patients who exercise are also less likely to smoke and more likely to watch their diet and weight.

Pharmacologic Therapy

In the prevention or treatment of angina, pharmacologic therapy is aimed at restoring the balance between myocardial oxygen supply and demand. The agents most useful in this regard are the nitrates, β-blockers, and calcium channel blockers.

Nitrates. The major antianginal effect of nitrates is to reduce myocardial oxygen demand. These agents relax vascular smooth muscle, particularly in the venous circulation at usual dosages. Since this action reduces venous return to the heart, there is a corresponding decline in left ventricular volume (a determinant of wall stress), which causes myocardial oxygen consumption to fall. To a lesser extent the nitrates act as arteriolar dilators, an action that beneficially reduces the resistance against which the left ventricle contracts, further reducing wall tension and oxygen

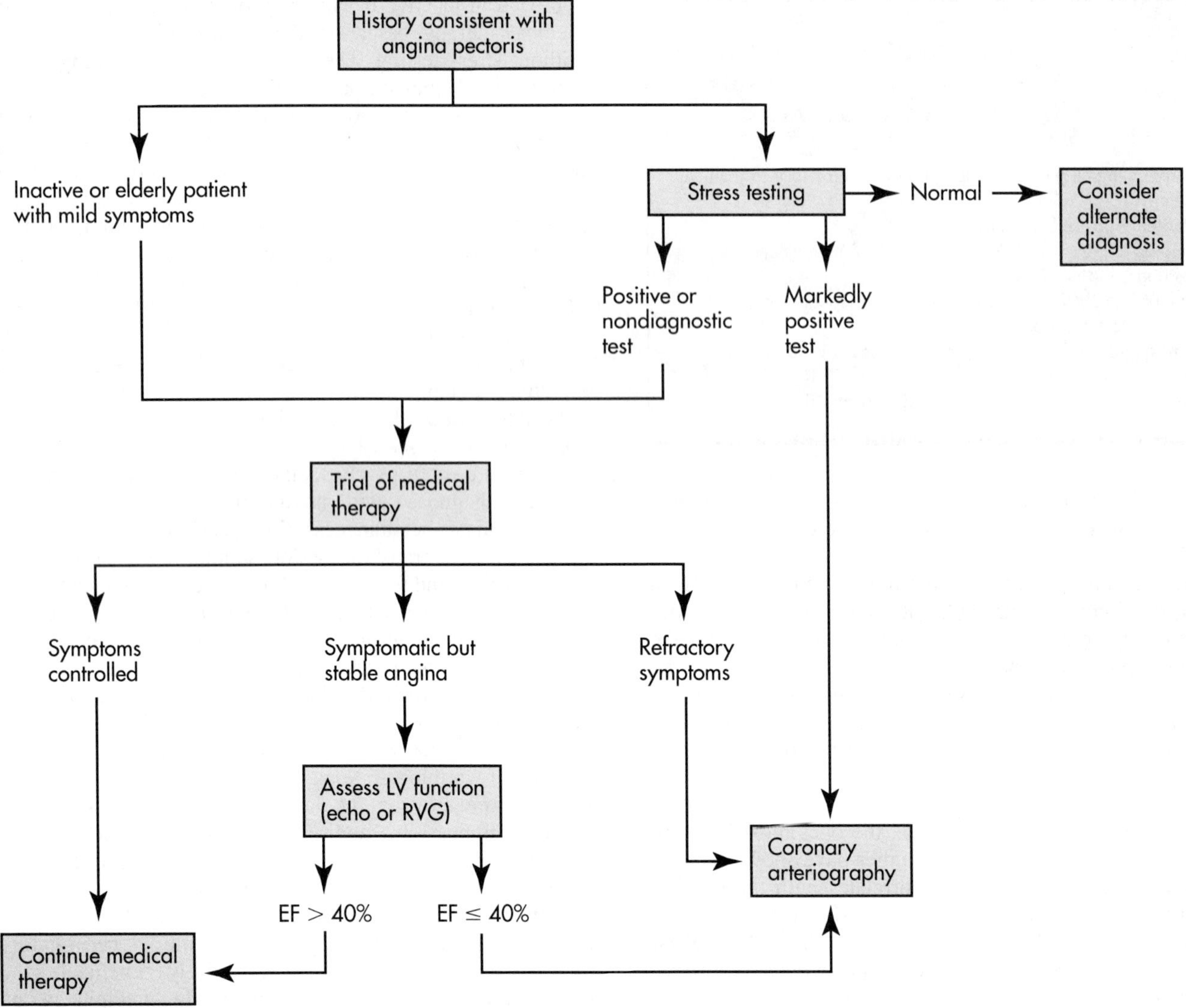

Fig. 63-1. Suggested approach to patients with suspected angina. Recommended forms of stress testing are listed in the text. *ECHO,* Echocardiogram; *RVG,* radionuclide ventriculogram.

demand. A third action of the nitrates is to dilate the coronary arteries with augmentation of coronary blood flow. This action increases myocardial oxygen supply and may be particularly important in the prevention and treatment of coronary artery vasospasm. Experimental animal studies have shown that nitroglycerin redistributes blood flow from normal to ischemic regions of the myocardium, especially in the subendocardial muscle, which may be mediated by increased collateral blood flow.

Rapidly acting nitroglycerin remains the drug of choice to treat acute anginal attacks. Sublingual or aerosol nitroglycerin spray (Table 63-3) typically relieves angina in less than 5 minutes, although sometimes repeated doses are necessary, and can be administered at 5-minute intervals.

Some clinical tips on the use of nitroglycerin are indicated in Box 63-6. For many patients the use of nitrates is accompanied by a feeling of generalized warmth and a transient throbbing headache or lightheadedness. This can be quite frightening if not expected, and patients should be warned about these effects. Even better is to stand by as the patient administers the first nitroglycerin in your office, so as to explain these reactions and instill confidence. The patient should also be instructed to sit down before using nitroglycerin the first few times, to avoid the potential of symptomatic hypotension. In addition, advice should be given that, if an anginal episode persists longer than usual or is unresponsive to two nitroglycerin tablets, then the appropriate course is to proceed to the closest emergency department for evaluation of possible unstable angina or MI.

Long-acting nitrates (see Table 63-3) are useful in the chronic prevention of anginal episodes and are available in oral and transdermal preparations. Low initial dosages should be used to avoid headache and lightheadedness and can be augmented over time. Side effects are similar to, but often less pronounced than, those associated with rapidly acting nitroglycerin administration. If a headache occurs, acetaminophen can be prescribed concurrently during the first few days of therapy, after which side effect tends to wane. An important problem associated with chronic nitrate therapy is the development of drug tolerance (i.e., continued administration of the drug leads to decreased effectiveness over time). It can be prevented by allowing an 8- to 10-hour nitrate-free

Table 63-3. Commonly Used Nitrates

	Usual dosage	Onset of action (min)	Duration of action	Recommended dosing frequency
Short-acting agents				
Sublingual TNG	0.15-0.6 mg (usual dose 0.4 mg)	2-5	10-30 min	As needed
Aerosol TNG	0.4 mg (1 inhalation)	2-5	10-30 min	As needed
Sublingual ISDN	2.5-10 mg	5-20	1-2 hr	As needed
Long-acting agents				
Oral ISDN	5-30 mg	15-30	4-6 hr	tid (mealtimes)
Sustained-action	40 mg	30-60	6-10 hr	bid (once in AM, then 7 hours later)
Oral PET	10-40 mg	30-60	3-6 hr	tid (mealtimes)
Sustained-action	30-80 mg	Slow	6-10 hr	bid (once in AM. then 7 hours later)
TNG ointment (2%)	0.5-2 in	15-60	3-8 hr	qid (with one 7- to 10-hr nitrate-free interval)
TNG skin patches	0.1-0.6 mg/hr	30-60	Up to 24 hr	Apply in morning, remove in evening
Oral ISMO	20-40 mg	30-60	12-14 hr	bid (once in AM, then 7 hours later)
Extended-release	30-240 mg	30-60	>12 hr	qd

TNG, Nitroglycerin; *ISDN*, isosorbide dinitrate; *PET*, pentaerythritol tetranitrate; *ISMO*, isosorbide mononitrate.

Box 63-6. Clinical Tips for Successful Nitroglycerin (TNG) Use

1. Observe patient in your office during first test dose of sublingual TNG and guide through expected reaction: burning under tongue, diffuse warmth or flushing, brief head-throbbing.
2. Instruct patient to sit down when using TNG for first few times to avoid hypotension.
3. Teach prophylactic use of TNG before activities likely to precipitate angina.
4. Usual dose is 0.3 or 0.4 mg sublingual, but elderly patients may not tolerate more than 0.15 mg.
5. Tablets should be kept in the provided darkened glass bottle to minimize decomposition by light. After a bottle of TNG is opened, it should be discarded after 6 months, since potency wanes after exposure to air (patient may notice lack of normal sublingual burning during use). TNG spray does not have this limitation and may be preferred for patients who have only occasional angina.
6. Assure patient that TNG has no long-term side effects, and liberal use should be encouraged.

Table 63-4. β-Blockers Approved for Use in the United States

	Usual oral dosage	β-Agonist activity
Nonselective agents		
Carteolol	2.5-10 mg qd	+
Labetalol*	100-600 mg bid	
Nadolol†	40-80 mg qd	
Penbutolol	20 mg qd	+
Pindolol	5-30 mg bid	+
Propranolol†	20-60 mg qid	
Sustained-action†	80-160 mg qd	
Timolol†	20 mg bid	
β_1-selective agents		
Acebutolol	200-1200 mg qd	+
Atenolol†	50-100 mg qd	
Betaxolol	10-20 mg qd	
Bisoprolol	2.5-20 mg/d	
Metoprolol†	50-100 mg bid	
Sustained-action†	50-100 mg qd	
Esmolol	50-200 μg/kg/min IV	

*Also has α_1-blocking properties.
†Approved by FDA for use in coronary artery disease.

interval each day, and effective dosage schedules to accomplish this are indicated in Table 63-3.

For elderly or inactive patients, long-acting nitrates may alone suffice as chronic antianginal therapy. However, for many physically active individuals additional drugs are usually required.

β-Blockers. β-Adrenergic antagonists have become the mainstay of therapy to prevent effort-induced angina and also have been shown to reduce mortality following MI. The main antianginal effect of β-blockers is to reduce myocardial oxygen demand by slowing the heart rate, reducing the force of ventricular contraction, and lowering blood pressure. In the United States only a handful of β-blockers have been approved for the treatment of angina, although most are probably effective and have been used for this purpose (Table 63-4). β-Blockers differ from one another by several properties that influence their choice in certain patient groups, based on their duration of action, selectivity for the β_1-receptor, partial β-agonist activity, and α-adrenergic blocking properties. The goal of β_1-selectivity is to block myocardial receptors with less effect on bronchial and vascular smooth muscle, of theoretic benefit to those with asthma or intermittent claudication. However, at the high doses used to treat angina, β_1-selectivity is often lost.

β-Blockers with partial β-agonist activity (also termed *intrinsic sympathomimetic activity* [ISA]) have the unusual property of mild direct stimulation of the β-receptor while blocking the receptor against circulating catecholamines. Thus the resting heart rate tends not to fall as much as with other drugs of this class, but the chronotropic response to exercise is blunted. Agents with ISA may be less desirable in patients with angina, since the comparatively higher heart rates during their use may exacerbate angina, and, unlike β-blockers without this property, they have not reliably reduced mortality following acute MI.

The duration of action of β-blockers largely depends on their lipid solubility and accounts for the different dosage schedules listed in Table 63-4. Esmolol is a very short-acting agent administered intravenously. Its effectiveness and any adverse reactions disappear within minutes of its discontinuation; thus it can be used to test the tolerability of β-blockade. It is used most commonly in the treatment of acute tachydysrhythmias and as a continuous infusion in unstable angina.

Several randomized trials have shown that, following MI, cardiovascular mortality and nonfatal secondary MIs are reduced by β-blocker therapy (see below). Some, but not all, primary prevention trials have shown that β-blockers may reduce the incidence of first MIs among patients with hypertension. These attributes, combined with the β-blockers' ability to raise the anginal threshold at least as well as other antianginal drugs, place them at the forefront of chronic antianginal therapy.

Contraindications to the use of β-blockers include symptomatic congestive heart failure, a history of bronchospasm, marked resting bradycardia or AV block, and peripheral vascular disease with symptoms of claudication. In patients without such contraindications, β-blockers are started at the lower range of doses listed in Table 63-4 and advanced until the resting heart rate falls to 50 to 60 beats/min or side effects occur.

Common side effects of β-blockers include bronchoconstriction in patients with reactive airways disease, the precipitation of congestive heart failure in some patients with left ventricular systolic dysfunction, depression, sexual dysfunction, AV block, exacerbation of claudication, and potential masking of hypoglycemia in insulin-dependent diabetic patients. Rarely, the abrupt cessation of β-blocker therapy can lead to tachycardia, angina, or MI. In addition, β-blockers have the theoretic potential of decreasing coronary blood flow in patients with predominant coronary artery vasospasm (by inhibiting vasodilatory β_2-receptors) and should be avoided in such patients. Another long-term adverse effect of β-blocker therapy relates to the serum lipids, since they may result in the reduction of HDL cholesterol and an increase in triglycerides. These values should be monitored in patients with adverse baseline lipid profiles. This effect does not occur with β-blockers that have β-agonist activity (see Table 63-4) or α-blocking properties (i.e., labetalol).

Calcium Channel Blockers. The calcium channel blockers are effective antianginal agents when used alone or in combination with β-blockers or nitrates. They can prevent exertional angina and are also helpful in patients with episodes of coronary vasospasm. Each drug in this class can reduce myocardial oxygen requirements and increase myocardial oxygen supply. However, the available agents (Table 63-5) differ in their structure and specific actions. Nifedipine and the other dihydropyridine calcium blockers are potent arterial vasodilators that reduce systemic vascular resistance, blood pressure, and therefore left ventricular wall stress with a decrease in myocardial oxygen consumption. The resultant fall in blood pressure may trigger an increase in the heart rate, an undesired effect that can be blunted by concomitant use of a β-blocker. Diltiazem and verapamil are also arteriolar dilators but are less potent than the dihydropyridines. However, they demonstrate additional properties that decrease myocardial oxygen demand: they slow the resting heart rate and decrease the left ventricular force of contraction, so concomitant β-blocker therapy is not necessary and in many cases is not desirable.

Recent reports have questioned the safety of short-acting dihydropyridine calcium channel antagonists as they have been associated with an *increased* frequency of MI and mortality. Thus calcium channel blockers should be considered secondary agents in the management of stable angina, to be prescribed only after β-blocker and nitrate therapy has been considered. When dihydropyridine calcium channel blockers are used, only the long-acting formulations should be prescribed.

All of the calcium channel blockers have the potential to adversely reduce left ventricular contractility and should be used cautiously in patients with underlying left ventricular dysfunction. Newer dihydropyridines (e.g., amlodipine, felodipine) have the least negative inotropic effects. One study has demonstrated that amlodipine is tolerated in patients with advanced heart failure without causing hemodynamic deterioration or increased mortality when added to a regimen of an ACE inhibitor, diuretic, and digoxin. Other common side effects of the calcium channel blockers are listed in Table 63-5.

Antiplatelet Therapy. Coronary thrombosis has been implicated in the majority of patients with MIs and in unstable angina. Aspirin, as an antiplatelet antithrombotic agent, has demonstrated a beneficial role in secondary prevention of coronary events post-MI (see below). Furthermore, a meta-analysis of 300 studies, including 140,000 patients, has shown improved cardiovascular outcomes among patients with angina, with prior MI, and following coronary artery bypass graft (CABG) surgery. In the absence of contraindications (bleeding, gastritis, or drug allergy) aspirin (81 to 325 mg every day) is recommended as part of the routine antianginal regimen. A newer (and costlier) antiplatelet agent, clopidogrel, was recently approved by the FDA for prevention of atherosclerotic events in patients with recent MI, stroke, or peripheral vascular disease. In one large study, this drug was modestly superior to aspirin for prevention of ischemic events. Unlike the closely related drug ticlopidine, it has not been associated with neutropenia or thrombotic thrombocytopenic purpura. At present, we reserve the use of clopidogrel in chronic CAD for patients who are intolerant of aspirin.

Antioxidant Therapy. LDL cholesterol undergoes oxidation in proximity to the arterial wall and in that form is

Table 63-5. Calcium Channel Antagonists

	Usual oral dose	Vasodilatation	↓ Inotropy	↓ Heart rate and AV conduction	Adverse effects
Verapamil*	40-120 mg tid-qid	Moderate	↓↓↓	↓↓↓	Hypotension Bradycardia
SR formulation	120-240 mg qd-bid				AV block Heart failure Constipation
Diltiazem*	30-120 mg tid-qid	Moderate	↓↓	↓↓	Hypotension Peripheral edema
SR formulation	60-180 mg bid				Bradycardia
CD formulation*	180-360 mg qd				AV block Heart failure
Dihydropyridines					
		Marked	0 to ↓	0	Hypotension
Nifedipine*	10-30 mg tid-qid				Peripheral edema
XL formulation*	30-120 mg qd				Headache
Nicardipine*	20-40 mg tid		†		Flushing
SR formulation	30-60 mg bid		†		
Isradipine	2.5-10 mg bid		†		
Felodipine	5-20 mg qd		†		
Amlodipine*	2.5-10 mg qd		†		

*Approved by FDA for use in coronary artery disease.
†Least negatively inotropic agents.

particularly prone to contribute to the atherosclerotic process. In the Cambridge Heart Antioxidant Study, the antioxidant vitamin E was compared with placebo in 2002 patients with angiographically documented CAD. After an average of 17 months vitamin E reduced the rate of nonfatal MI, but cardiovascular and total mortality were not reduced. A recent prospective study of 34,486 postmenopausal women without CAD showed that an increased dietary intake of Vitamin E (i.e., from food, not supplements) was associated with lower coronary death rates over a 7-year follow-up period. Although the lack of firm data precludes definite guidelines, some cardiologists recommend that their patients with CAD take 200-400 IU of vitamin E daily. Studies of β-carotene and vitamin C thus far have not shown a reduction in cardiac events.

Approach to Antianginal Drug Selection

The use of the above antianginal drugs alone, or in combination, depends on the severity of symptoms, concomitant illnesses, and the patient's activity level (Box 63-7). All patients with angina should be taught the proper use of nitroglycerin for acute attacks. For chronic suppression of angina in elderly or inactive patients one can choose a long-acting nitrate (e.g., isosorbide mononitrate extended-release once daily, or nitroglycerin applied each morning and removed at bedtime) plus aspirin, 81 to 325 mg daily.

For active individuals with chronic stable exertional angina, consider a β-blocker, and if symptoms persist add a long-acting nitrate or calcium channel blocker (not verapamil, to avoid the additive bradycardic effect), or both. For those with contraindications to β-blockade, a calcium channel blocker is recommended. If the contraindication to β-blockade is the presence of bronchospasm, insulin-dependent diabetes, or claudication, any of the calcium channel blockers approved for angina are appropriate. However, verapamil or diltiazem is preferred because of the effect on slowing the heart rate. For patients with resting bradycardia or AV block, a dihydropyridine calcium blocker is a better choice. In patients with symptomatic congestive heart failure, nitrates are the preferred initial antianginal agents; if additional therapy is needed, amlodipine should be considered.

Patients suspected of having primarily coronary vasospasm should not be treated with β-blockers, which could aggravate coronary constriction; rather nitrates and calcium channel blockers are preferred. In patients with concomitant hypertension, β-blocker or calcium channel blockers are useful in treating both conditions. Similarly, patients with IHD and atrial fibrillation would benefit from a β-blocker, verapamil, or diltiazem, each of which can slow the ventricular rate.

For patients who do not respond to initial antianginal therapy, the drug dosages should be increased unless side effects occur. Combination therapy often allows the successful use of lower dosages of each agent while minimizing individual drug side effects. Typical beneficial combinations include the following:

1. A nitrate plus a β-blocker, as the latter blunts the nitrate-associated tachycardia.
2. A nitrate plus verapamil or diltiazem for similar reasons.
3. A long-acting dihydropyridine calcium channel blocker plus a β-blocker is similarly beneficial, but a dihydropyridine plus nitrate is often not tolerated without concomitant β-blockade because of marked vasodilation, with resultant headache and increased heart rate. As indicated above, a β-blocker should be combined only very cautiously with verapamil or diltiazem because of the potential of excessive bradycardia or precipitation of congestive heart failure in patients with left ventricular dysfunction.

Box 63-7. Medical Management of Chronic Stable Angina

1. Correct cardiac risk factors.
2. Identify reversible contributors (e.g., anemia, hyperthyroidism, hypertension).
3. Initiate pharmacologic therapy.
   a. Nitroglycerin (sublingual, spray) as needed
   b. Aspirin, 80-325 mg/day
   c. Long-acting agents (consider concomitant diseases):
      (1) Sedentary, elderly patients: long-acting nitrates (Table 63-3)
      (2) Active, otherwise healthy patients: β-blocker (or verapamil or diltiazem)
      (3) Bronchospastic disease: calcium channel blocker* or nitrates
      (4) Insulin-dependent diabetes: calcium channel blocker* or nitrates
      (5) Intermittent claudication: calcium channel blocker* or nitrates
      (6) Resting bradycardia or AV block: calcium channel blocker (NOT verapamil or diltiazem) or nitrates
      (7) CHF: nitrates ± dihydropyridine calcium channel blocker (especially amlodipine)
      (8) Atrial fibrillation: β-blocker, verapamil, or diltiazem

*Verapamil or diltiazem preferred for negative chronotropic effect, especially if combined with nitrates.

As illustrated in Fig. 63-1, patients with angina who become asymptomatic on medical therapy can be followed clinically without additional interventions. Those individuals with frequent angina refractory to multidrug therapy should be referred for cardiac catheterization and consideration of mechanical revascularization. The approach to patients with diminished but persistent symptoms on medical therapy depends on whether left ventricular contractile function is compromised. Many studies indicate that patients with impaired left ventricular function (e.g., ejection fraction less than 40%) have a worse cardiac prognosis than those with similar coronary disease but preserved left ventricular function. Therefore our policy in patients with even mildly persistent angina is to obtain an assessment of left ventricular function (echocardiography or radionuclide ventriculography); if the ejection fraction is less than 40%, the patient is considered for coronary arteriography to identify those whose prognosis would improve by mechanical revascularization.

Mechanical Revascularization

As indicated above, many patients with chronic stable angina can be successfully managed by pharmacologic therapy alone. However, for those with refractory symptoms or in certain high-risk subgroups, revascularization procedures, including CABG surgery and percutaneous transluminal coronary angioplasty (PTCA), are recommended.

Coronary Artery Bypass Graft Surgery. CABG consists of suturing segments of saphenous vein between the ascending aorta and to the coronary arteries distal to their stenotic narrowings (see Chapter 64). At present, in most routine cases surgeons attempt to bypass at least one diseased vessel (normally the left anterior descending coronary artery [LAD]) with an internal mammary artery, since the latter results in a higher long-term patency rate (80% to 90% at 10 years) compared with venous bypasses (10% occlusion in the first year, 2% per year for the next 6 years, 5% per year thereafter). Antiplatelet therapy with aspirin has been shown to improve long-term graft patency rates, and aggressive lipid-lowering to achieve an LDL cholesterol < 100 mg/dl has been shown to slow the development of atherosclerosis within bypass grafts.

After CABG anginal symptoms usually are relieved, exercise capacity is improved, and the need for pharmacologic therapy diminishes. The mortality of CABG is low (1% to 3% in otherwise healthy individuals) with an incidence of perioperative MI of 2% to 6%. The risk increases in patients with impaired left ventricular function, those requiring other cardiac procedures (e.g., valve replacement), elderly patients, and those undergoing repeat CABG. In addition the recuperation of elderly or frail patients can be quite slow and accompanied by postoperative reductions of cognitive function. Therefore it is incumbent upon the physician to weigh the potential benefits of surgery against the risks of the procedure and its impact on a patient's total quality of life before recommending bypass surgery. The insight of the patient's long-term primary care physician is of great importance in rendering this decision.

CABG has been shown to prolong survival in patients with (1) greater than 50% obstruction of the left main coronary artery and (2) three-vessel disease and impaired left ventricular contractile function (ejection fraction less than 40%). Patients with one- or two-vessel disease could be expected to have symptomatic improvement with CABG but no increase in longevity compared with medical therapy alone. Many patients with one- or two-vessel disease refractory to medical therapy can be managed by PTCA. In patients with three-vessel disease and preserved left ventricular function the evidence for improved survival with CABG is less clear, and we operate on such patients only if they display persistent symptoms while undergoing medical therapy, they have severe proximal disease (especially of the LAD), or extensive ischemia is demonstrated by noninvasive testing. One recent study demonstrated that in diabetic patients with three-vessel disease, CABG offers a better prognosis than catheter-based interventions (see below).

Percutaneous Transluminal Coronary Angioplasty and Intracoronary Stents. With increased experience and improved technology the range of coronary lesions amenable to PTCA has expanded over recent years. It can be successfully performed in multivessel coronary disease as well as in stenoses of coronary bypass grafts. The lesions most likely to benefit are short and are located proximally within a coronary artery away from vessel branch points. Although patients with left main or severe three-vessel disease are usually best-suited for CABG, PTCA is now widely successful in relieving ischemia in patients with one- and two-vessel lesions and selected patients with three-vessel disease. The major complication of the procedure is dissection of the vessel intima with subsequent occlusion of the vessel requiring repeat PTCA or emergent coronary bypass graft surgery. Even after successful PTCA approximately one third of dilated vessels redevelop significant stenosis within the following 6 months. In more than 60% of angioplasty procedures today, metal tubular stents are permanently deployed in the vessel, leaving no, or minimal, residual stenosis and a much improved rate of occlusion or restenosis, using antiplatelet protocols that include aspirin plus ticlopidine. Preliminary results of trials using even more potent antiplatelet agents (glycoprotein IIb/IIIa inhibitors) at the time of stent placement suggest even better long-term cardiac outcomes. As discussed in Chapter 64, the benefits of stent implantation in each case must be weighed against potential drawbacks, including a higher cost of the procedure and the potential development of in-stent stenosis.

Patients who undergo angioplasty procedures have much shorter hospital stays and easier recuperation compared with those who undergo CABG. This has contributed to the explosive popularity of this technique, but there is concern about its overuse. Although one study has shown that PTCA is superior to medical therapy for symptomatic relief of angina, it did not reduce the risk of infarction or mortality.

Randomized trials have compared the outcome of PTCA versus CABG in patients with coronary lesions in multiple vessels that could be suitably approached by either technique. In 5-year follow-up the risks of MI or death are similar, although patients who underwent PTCA had more frequent recurrence of angina and need for repeat revascularization procedures. In addition, patients with diabetes and two- and three-vessel disease achieved better cardiovascular outcomes with CABG. Thus our general recommendations for patients with refractory angina on medical therapy are as follows: (1) patients with one- and two-vessel disease with normal left ventricular function are referred for catheter-based procedures, and (2) patients with two- and three-vessel disease with widespread ischemia, left ventricular dysfunction, or diabetes, and those with lesions not amenable to catheter-based techniques, are referred for CABG.

UNSTABLE ANGINA

Patients with CAD may show a stable pattern of symptoms for many years. Unstable angina refers to an acceleration of symptoms in which ischemic episodes occur more frequently, are more intense, last longer, and are precipitated by less activity than previously, or even by rest. A large number of such patients progress to acute MI due to the presence of complicated coronary lesions with ulceration, hemorrhage, or thrombosis at the site of atherosclerotic plaque. In other cases the lesions responsible for unstable angina may heal and the patient's symptoms return to a more stable pattern.

Unstable angina is a medical emergency. The patient should be hospitalized in an ECG-monitored unit and confined to bed (Box 63-8). During episodes of angina transient ST segment shifts or T wave flattening or inversion is likely. In addition, signs of left ventricular dysfunction (pulmonary rales, S_3, mitral regurgitation) may accompany ischemic episodes. Contributing factors to the imbalance between myocardial oxygen supply and demand should be considered and corrected, including hypoxemia, anemia, hypertension, thyrotoxicosis, and tachydysrhythmias.

Therapy of unstable angina consists of measures to reduce myocardial oxygen demand and increase coronary flow. In addition, since intravascular thrombosis appears to play such an important role in the pathogenesis of unstable angina, antiplatelet and anticoagulant agents are a mainstay of therapy. Both aspirin and intravenous heparin have been shown to decrease the incidence of MI and cardiac death in unstable angina, whether used alone or together. Our policy is to begin aspirin (160 to 325 mg daily) immediately on presentation (the oral antiplatelet drug ticlopidine has also been shown to reduce complications of unstable angina and is a reasonable alternative in aspirin-intolerant individuals). At present, we use full-dose intravenous heparin to achieve an activated partial thromboplastin time (aPTT) of two times control. Low-molecular-weight heparin (i.e. enoxaparin) was recently studied in unstable angina and was found to be even more effective at preventing ischemic events and death (at 30 days and 1-year after administration) than standardized intravenous heparin, although minor bleeding complications were more frequent. Its use is likely to increase in this syndrome. Thrombolytic therapy has *not* been shown to reduce morbidity or mortality in the setting of unstable angina in the absence of an acute MI.

Box 63-8. Initial Management of Unstable Angina

1. Admit to monitored bed, prescribe supplemental oxygen, mild sedation
2. Consider contributing factors: anemia, hypoxemia, hypertension, thyrotoxicosis
3. Anticoagulant and antiplatelet therapy:
   a. Aspirin, 160-325 mg on admission, then daily
   b. IV heparin to maintain aPTT at two times control
   c. Consider IV glycoprotein IIb/IIIa inhibitor in consultation with cardiologist
4. Nitrates: oral, transcutaneous paste, or IV (start at 10 μg/min and titrate upward)
5. β-Blocker (to attain heart rate 60-70) (e.g., IV metoprolol, 5 mg every 5 minutes for 3 doses, then switch to oral)
6. If symptoms persist, add calcium channel blocker (if β-blocker contraindicated, use verapamil or diltiazem; if added in conjunction with β-blocker, use nifedipine or other dihydropyridine calcium channel blocker)

Drugs that inhibit the platelet glycoprotein IIb/IIIa receptor are an important recent advance in the pharmacologic management of unstable angina, since they further reduce the risk of MI and death. The FDA has approved two intravenous drugs of this class (tirofiban and eptifibatide) for patients with unstable angina, and a third (abciximab) for patients with unstable angina when angioplasty techniques are planned within 24 hours. Consultation with a cardiologist would be appropriate when considering this type of therapy since many patients will subsequently proceed to cardiac catheterization and revascularization procedures.

For patients who are refractory to medical therapy, coronary arteriography should be performed urgently (Fig. 63-2) followed by mechanical revascularization (CABG or percutaneous catheter-based interventions). If facilities for these procedures are not available, an intraaortic balloon pump may be placed transcutaneously to improve diastolic perfusion of coronary arteries and to provide afterload reduction to the left ventricle while the patient is transferred to an institution where revascularization procedures can be undertaken.

For patients who do stabilize on medical therapy, there remains a risk of recurrent unstable angina or MI, and

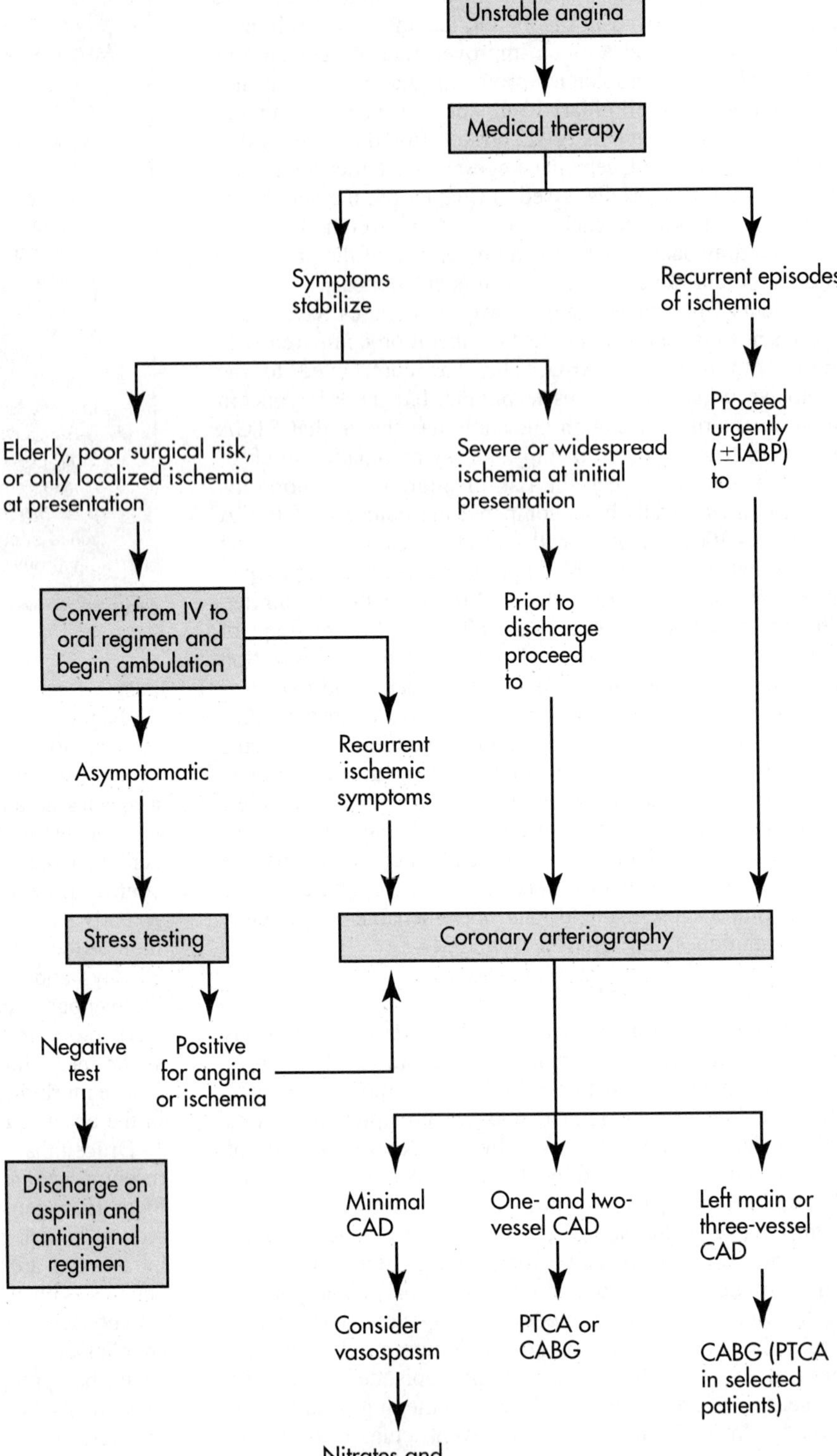

Fig. 63-2. Management decisions in unstable angina. *IABP,* Intraaortic balloon pump; *CAD,* coronary artery disease; *PTCA,* percutaneous transluminal coronary angioplasty; *CABG,* coronary artery bypass graft surgery.

additional evaluation is necessary (see Fig. 63-2). For active patients who were admitted to the hospital with severe symptoms and marked, diffuse ECG evidence of ischemia, elective cardiac catheterization is recommended before discharge to determine whether revascularization procedures are warranted. In selected patients, such as the elderly, those at poor surgical risk, or those with less severe presentations and more limited ECG evidence of ischemia, a less invasive approach is reasonable. That is, after 2 to 3 days, if symptoms of angina have responded to therapy, the intravenous agents can be replaced by oral drugs and gentle ambulation begun. Before discharge, exercise or pharmacologic stress testing should be performed. If spontaneous or exercise-induced ischemia is demonstrated, coronary angiography would be recommended. However, those who do well on exercise testing could be discharged on the oral antianginal regimen with further interventions guided by their symptoms.

Sometimes the recent onset of angina in a previously asymptomatic individual is also termed unstable angina. However, if symptoms occur only on exertion and are quickly relieved by rest or medical therapy, the need for hospitalization and the aggressive therapy indicated in Box 63-8 are often not necessary.

TYPICAL ANGINA PECTORIS WITH NORMAL CORONARY ARTERIOGRAM

This condition, often referred to as *syndrome X,* is characterized by classic exertional angina in individuals found to have no significant coronary stenoses at cardiac catheterization. Yet such patients may have convincing evidence of myocardial ischemia at exercise testing and nuclear scintigraphy. Some of these patients have coronary artery spasm, but most do not. Rather, many patients with this syndrome have evidence of inadequate coronary vasodilator reserve: small branches of the coronaries (the resistance vessels not visible by angiography) do not dilate appropriately during periods of increased myocardial oxygen demand, resulting in ischemia. The underlying mechanism is unknown, but the prognosis of such patients is excellent. Symptoms often respond to nitrate or calcium channel blocker therapy.

This syndrome is to be distinguished from other forms of cardiac pathology that produce ischemia in the absence of coronary disease, due to increased myocardial oxygen demand, such as advanced aortic stenosis. In addition, some patients with classic symptoms of angina and normal coronary arteries do not have organic illness at all. They have no evidence of ischemia by exercise scintigraphy or other testing and may suffer from anxiety disorders. An understanding attitude by the physician, reassurance of an excellent prognosis, and psychologic counseling may be of great benefit.

SILENT ISCHEMIA

When patients with chronic stable angina undergo ambulatory ECG monitoring, ST segment shifts usually occur during anginal episodes. But many patients demonstrate similar ischemic ST shifts during the day in the absence of symptoms, and this is termed *silent* or *painless ischemia.* Why some episodes are symptomatic and others silent is not known, but the presence of ST shifts on ambulatory monitoring, whether accompanied by symptoms or not, portends increased risk of MI and cardiac death.

In addition, among patients with severe coronary artery disease there is a subset who demonstrate ST shifts with activity, but *never* experience anginal discomfort. Such individuals have abnormal ST shifts during exercise tests but no accompanying chest pain. These patients are believed to have a defective anginal warning system, the mechanism of which is not known, but this syndrome is more common in diabetics. Despite the lack of symptoms, patients with totally silent ischemia are at risk for acute MI or cardiac death. Indeed, it is estimated that approximately 20% of acute MIs are clinically silent.

The proper management of patients with silent ischemia is the subject of ongoing clinical trials. Although the incidence of asymptomatic shifts can be reduced by antianginal medical therapy, angioplasty techniques, or CABG, it has not been conclusively shown that such treatment alters a patient's prognosis. Thus the management of patients with silent ischemia must be individualized and often depends on the degree of positivity of exercise testing. For example, our policy is that patients with severe or diffuse ischemia on exercise or pharmacologic stress testing are prescribed antianginal medications (e.g., β-blocker or calcium channel blocker plus aspirin) and undergo cardiac catheterization. If significant left main or three-vessel disease with left ventricular dysfunction is demonstrated, mechanical revascularization is usually recommended.

ACUTE MYOCARDIAL INFARCTION

Acute MI is a dreaded outcome in patients with ischemic heart disease. Nearly 1.5 million people sustain an MI in the United States each year, with a mortality rate of 25%. Nearly 60% of MI-related deaths occur before medical facilities are reached, mostly of the basis of lethal dysrhythmias. The location and extent of myocardial damage determine the acute presentation as well as early and long-term complications of MI. As such, early detection and reperfusion to limit the size of an acute infarct is of paramount clinical importance.

Etiology

MI is the result of prolonged myocardial ischemia that leads to irreversible necrosis of heart muscle. In more than 90% of cases the causal event is the development of an acute thrombus at the site of underlying coronary atherosclerosis. Although the exact mechanism is not known, such thrombosis appears to be the result of interactions between disturbed atherosclerotic plaque, the coronary endothelium, circulating platelets, and dynamic vasomotor tone of the coronary arterial wall. "Vulnerable" plaques, those most likely to rupture and incite coronary thrombosis, tend to be lipid-laden, with a thin fibrous cap separating the atheroma from circulating blood. These lesions often appear quite minor angiographically, in distinction to chronic, stable plaques with thick fibrous caps that cause more vessel narrowing but are less susceptible to rupture.

Rarely, MI may be due to nonatherosclerotic causes, examples of which are indicated in Box 63-9. These should be suspected particularly in young individuals and those without underlying coronary risk factors. Cocaine use is a rare and unfortunate cause of infarction. It is likely due to the ability of cocaine to increase myocardial oxygen demand, induce coronary vasospasm, and promote coronary thrombosis, in association with platelet activation and endothelial cell dysfunction.

Clinical Presentation

The initial diagnosis of MI relies on the presenting history, physical examination, and ECG. The most common symptom is severe crushing chest pain, the location of which may be similar to previous angina, but it lasts longer, is more intense, and is often accompanied by nausea, diaphoresis, dyspnea, and the feeling of impending doom. There is a circadian variability to the development of MI, occurring most commonly in the morning hours, soon after awakening. Symptoms of MI usually begin while at rest, and only occasionally are brought on by physical exertion that may have resulted in anginal episodes previously. Rather than severe chest pain,

Box 63-9. Nonatherosclerotic Causes of Myocardial Infarction

Coronary emboli
- Endocarditis
- Prosthetic heart valve thromboemboli

Congenital anomalies
- Abnormal origin of the left anterior descending coronary artery, allowing it to be physically compressed

Acquired coronary abnormalities
- Coronary artery aneurysm or dissection

Severe coronary artery spasm
- Prinzmetal's
- Cocaine-induced

Vasculitis
- Systemic lupus erythematosus
- Takayasu's arteritis

Increased blood viscosity
- Polycythemia vera
- Thrombocytosis

Marked increase in myocardial oxygen demand
- Severe aortic stenosis

Box 63-10. Major Physical Signs in Acute Myocardial Infarction

General appearance
- Diaphoresis, anxious
- Cool, clammy skin

Vital signs
- Mild tachycardia and hypertension frequent, but bradycardia and hypotension common in inferior wall MI (increased vagal tone)

Jugular veins
- Distended if biventricular heart failure or right ventricular infarction present

Pulmonary
- Rales if LV heart failure present

Cardiac
- Precordial bulge if large anterior MI
- S_4 common, also S_3 if heart failure present
- Mitral regurgitation murmur if papillary muscle ischemia/infarction present

some patients with acute MI present with less pronounced symptoms, including generalized weakness, dyspnea, and indigestion. In up to 20% of cases an acute MI is free of any symptoms and is detected only in retrospect by changes on a routine ECG.

Common physical findings in MI (Box 63-10) relate to impaired left ventricular systolic and diastolic function, associated inflammatory responses, and stimulation of the sympathetic and parasympathetic nervous systems.

Certain other causes of substernal chest pain may resemble that of acute MI (Table 63-6) and must be considered to avoid inappropriate initial therapy. In particular, aortic dissection or pulmonary emboli may be fatal if not quickly recognized. If confused with MI, inappropriate administration of thrombolytic therapy to patients with pericarditis or aortic dissection could result in severe complications or death.

Electrocardiogram

Typically, ECG changes occur during an acute MI in a characteristic, sequential fashion. As shown in Fig. 63-3, in *Q wave infarction,* initial hyperacute T waves and ST elevation are present in the leads overlying the involved myocardium. Over the next several hours, as cell death occurs, there is loss of the R wave and progressive Q wave development. The T wave begins to invert, followed by return of the ST segment to its baseline over subsequent days. The T wave may remain inverted for weeks to months before returning to its baseline, but the new Q wave persists as a permanent marker of the infarction. The anatomic site of infarction is determined by the ECG leads affected by these sequential changes (Table 63-7). Note that posterior wall infarctions produce a mirror image pattern in the anterior chest leads, with initial ST segment *depression,* T wave inversion, and development of tall R waves in leads V1 and V2.

In *non–Q wave infarction,* the ECG evolution is more subtle: new ST depression and/or T wave inversions persist for 48 hours or longer in the leads overlying the infarcting segments. The ST segments later normalize, but pathologic Q waves do not appear. Such patients may otherwise have typical symptoms and enzyme abnormalities indicative of acute MI, and the natural history and therapeutic implications of this type of infarct are described below.

In patients with markedly abnormal baseline ECGs (e.g., left bundle branch block) diagnostic ECG evolution may not occur, and the diagnosis of MI relies on the presence of serum markers and other laboratory modalities.

Serum Markers of Infarction

Certain proteins are released into the circulation in a predictable temporal fashion during acute MI, and are therefore diagnostically helpful.

Creatine kinase (CK) rises in the plasma within 4 to 8 hours, peaks at 24 hours, and returns to normal by 48 to 72 hours. The peak rise is greater and occurs earlier (less than 12 hours) following thrombolytic therapy. The total CK is not specific for myocardial damage; it can also rise after skeletal muscle trauma, and intramuscular injections, and in hypothyroidism.

The CK-MB isoenzyme is more specific for the diagnosis of acute MI. It is present in only tiny quantities in noncardiac tissues and is not greatly influenced by skeletal muscle injuries. The serum CK-MB rises and peaks slightly earlier than the total CK and returns to normal within 36 to 72 hours. Serum CK-MB levels may be elevated in other conditions such as myocarditis, following cardiac surgery, after repetitive cardioversions, and in hypothyroidism. However, in these conditions the temporal sequence of release seen in MI does not occur. In acute MI, the CK-MB (mass assay) is usually greater than 2.5% of the total serum CK. The serum CK and CK-MB isoenzyme should be measured on admission, then 12 and 24 hours later in the diagnostic evaluation of an acute MI.

Isoforms of CK-MB exist in the plasma after an MI and are very sensitive for the detection of infarction. For example, a ratio of $CK\text{-}MB_2/CK\text{-}MB_1$ of >1.5 is more than 90% sensitive for detection of an MI when measured 4 to 6 hours after the onset of coronary occlusion.

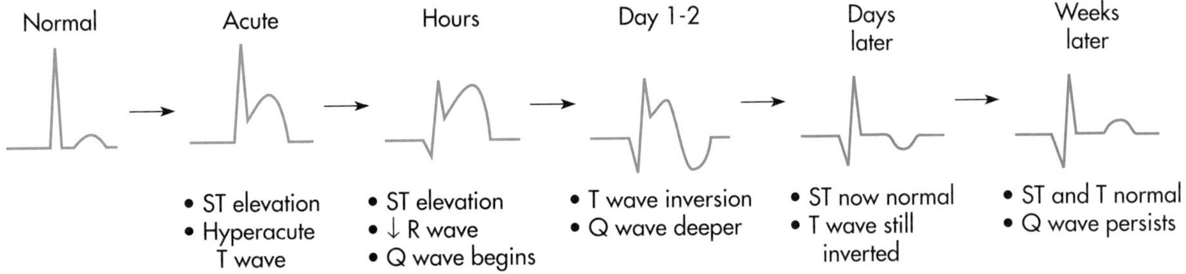

Fig. 63-3. ECG evolution of acute Q wave infarction. (Modified from Lilly LS, editor: *Pathophysiology of heart disease*, Philadelphia, 1993, Lea & Febiger.)

Table 63-6. Conditions That May Mimic Pain of Acute Myocardial Infarction

Condition	Clues to diagnosis	Confirmatory studies
Aortic dissection	Sharp, ripping pain that migrates Asymmetry of arterial pulses	Transesophageal echo, MRI, CT, angiography
Acute pericarditis	Sharp, pleuritic, positional pain Pericardial friction rub Diffuse ST elevation on ECG	Pericardial effusion on echocardiogram
Pulmonary embolism	Dyspnea, pleuritic chest pain Predisposing factors for venous thrombosis	Ventilation/perfusion scan Pulmonary angiography
Pneumothorax	Sudden dyspnea, very sharp pain Absent breath sounds over affected region	Chest x-ray
Esophageal spasm	Worse upon swallowing History of dysphagia, especially to cold liquids	Barium swallow Esophageal manometry
Acute cholecystitis	Right upper quadrant tenderness Nausea, vomiting History of fatty food intolerance	Abdominal ultrasound

Table 63-7. Myocardial Infarction Localization

Anatomic site	Leads with acute changes	Coronary artery likely involved
Inferior	II, III, aVF	RCA
Anteroseptal	V1-V2	LAD (proximal)
Anteroapical	V3-V4	LAD or its branches
Anterolateral	V5-V6, I, aVL	Mid-LAD or CFX
High lateral	I, aVL	CFX
Extensive anterior	V1-V6	LAD (proximal)
Posterior	V1-V2*	PDA

RCA, Right coronary; *LAD,* left anterior descending; *CFX,* left circumflex; *PDA,* posterior descending.
*Mirror-image changes in these leads, (i.e., ST depression and tall R waves in Q wave posterior MI).

Cardiac forms of troponin subunits (cardiac troponin I and T) are also sensitive and highly specific markers of acute myocardial infarction. Their levels begin to rise within 3 hours after the onset of infarction and remain elevated for several days, permitting detection of infarction even in those individuals who present later than 48 hours after the onset of chest discomfort. At many hospitals these are now the preferred markers for detection of acute infarction. Furthermore, the presence and magnitude of these serum markers are of prognostic value in patients with acute coronary syndromes. Studies completed over the past 5 years have shown that higher troponin I levels, or early positivity of a bedside troponin T assay, correlate with greater short-term mortality.

Myoglobin is released into the circulation very early after myocardial injury and can be detected within 2 hours of infarction. However, its rapid renal clearance and low specificity limit its diagnostic role.

Lactate dehydrogenase (LDH) rises within 24 to 48 hours of MI, peaks at 3 to 5 days, and returns to baseline by 7 to 10 days. Historically, its usefulness has been greatest in patients who are admitted to the hospital 2 to 3 days after the onset of symptoms, at which time the CK evolution has already passed; the advent of troponin assays has largely supplanted the need for LDH measurements in that setting. LDH is present in many tissues, but of its five isoenzymes, LDH_1 is most specific for the heart. A level of LDH_1 greater than LDH_2 suggests myocardial necrosis in the appropriate clinical setting.

Other Laboratory Studies

In some cases the history, ECG, and serum markers are not sufficient to confirm the diagnosis of MI, and other laboratory tests can be useful. For example, acute infarct scintigraphy using ^{99m}Tc pyrophosphate is highly sensitive for imaging large transmural infarcts. This type of hot spot scan is positive

2 to 7 days after MI, so is most useful for patients who are seen a few days after the onset of symptoms. In addition, echocardiography and radionuclide ventriculography can identify wall motion abnormalities indicative of infarction, but unless a previous study is available, they do not specify when the injury occurred.

Management

The in-hospital mortality for acute MI has fallen substantially in the past 30 years thanks to marked improvements in therapy. The primary goals of hospitalization are to achieve rapid reperfusion of the obstructed vessel, to limit the infarct size, and to promptly recognize and manage complications.

Thrombolytic Therapy. As indicated above, most MIs result from the formation of an acute thrombus that obstructs a coronary artery. Thrombolytic therapy activates the natural fibrinolytic system to dissolve the responsible thrombus. Large studies have demonstrated that contemporary thrombolytic regimes restore patency in 65% to 85% of infarct-related coronary arteries at 90 minutes after infusion. Such therapy has been conclusively demonstrated to reduce mortality and improve recovery of left ventricular function following acute MI. The greatest benefit occurs when there is early reperfusion with substantial and sustained patency of the obstructed coronary artery.

Thrombolytic Agents. The FDA-approved agents are streptokinase (SK), anisoylated plasminogen-SK activator complex (APSAC), tissue plasminogen activator (alteplase or t-PA), and modified plasminogen activator (reteplase or r-PA). Whereas t-PA and SK require continuous intravenous infusions, APSAC and r-PA are administered as short bolus injections, simplifying their delivery. Each of these drugs results in the conversion of the proenzyme plasminogen to active plasmin, which dissolves fibrin clots. However, different mechanisms of action and pharmacology of these drugs result in varying specificity for the thrombus responsible for the MI (Table 63-8). For example, t-PA attaches preferentially to a formed thrombus and lyses it without substantially activating fibrinolysis in the general circulation, in contrast to SK. Nonetheless, bleeding is the most important risk of each of these agents and their adjunctive therapies.

Successful reperfusion is heralded by the relief of chest pain, and an early peak of serum CK (within 12 hours). Reperfusion dysrhythmias, especially accelerated idioventricular rhythm, are common and do not usually require therapy (see below). To maintain patency of the coronary vessel following thrombolysis, antiplatelet and anticoagulant therapies are used. Aspirin inhibits platelet function and reduces reocclusion following thrombolysis, so it is administered at the time of admission, and each day thereafter (160 to 325 mg/day). With use of t-PA or r-PA, intravenous heparin is needed to maintain vessel patency after initial thrombolysis, and is administered to achieve an activated PTT of 50 to 75 seconds, for 48 hours. Intravenous heparin may also be beneficial for patients receiving SK or APSAC who are at high risk for systemic emboli (e.g., in the presence of atrial fibrillation, large anterior MI, or left ventricular thrombus). However, if there is a low risk for thromboembolism, patients treated with SK or APSAC do not require IV heparin therapy.

Several trials have compared the efficacy of thrombolytic agents. In 1993, the international GUSTO-1 trial found a small survival advantage of t-PA compared with SK following an MI. In that study, the greatest benefit of t-PA occurred in patients with anterior MI and when treatment was administered within 4 hours after the onset of symptoms. Intracranial hemorrhage was higher with t-PA than SK, but did not negate the net clinical advantage of t-PA. In the TIMI-4 trial, t-PA was also found to be superior to APSAC at achieving early coronary artery patency and clinical outcomes. Thus use of the latter drug has waned. The GUSTO-III trial compared r-PA to t-PA and found similar clinical efficacy of these two agents. Perhaps the most important message from the thrombolytic trials is that early and sustained patency of an infarct-related coronary artery improves survival. No matter which thrombolytic agent is used, it is crucial that patients receive such therapy as quickly

Table 63-8. Thrombolytic Agents

	Streptokinase	APSAC	t-PA (alteplase)	r-PA (reteplase)
Fibrin clot specificity	None	Mild	Moderate	Moderate
Patency rate (partial or complete at 90 min)	50-60%	60-75%	75-85%	80-85%
Major advantage	Least expensive	Ease of administration	Survival advantage in certain subgroups Limited systemic lytic state	Ease of administration Efficacy and other benefits similar to t-PA
Major complications	Bleeding and antigenic reactions	Bleeding and antigenic reactions	Bleeding	Bleeding
Dose	1.5 Million units IV over 1 hour	30 Units IV over 5 min	(Preferred accelerated regimen): 15 mg bolus, then 0.75 mg/kg over 30 min (not to exceed 50 mg), then 0.5 mg/kg over 60 min (not to exceed 35 mg)	Two 10 U boluses, 30 min apart
Approximate cost ($)	300	1700	2200	2200

as possible. A reasonable goal is a target "door-to-drug" time of 30 minutes in the emergency department.

Patient Selection. The criteria for selecting patients for thrombolytic therapy include evidence of an evolving Q wave MI and the ability to administer the thrombolytic drug within a period likely to result in an improved outcome (Fig. 63-4). The greatest survival benefit occurs when thrombolytic therapy is administered less than 6 hours after the onset of chest pain. Nonetheless, several studies have shown that treatment as late as 24 hours into the course of an MI can reduce the mortality rate. Therefore in certain situations, such as a stuttering course of chest pain during an evolving MI, it is reasonable to undertake thrombolytic therapy up to 24 hours after the onset of symptoms.

The major contraindications to thrombolytic therapy are situations that increase the likelihood of bleeding (see Fig. 63-4). In addition, patients who have received SK or APSAC previously should not be rechallenged with either agent because of the potential of allergic reactions. Advanced age is not a contraindication to thrombolytic therapy; although most often administered to those under 75 years old, it should also be considered in older patients who are otherwise healthy and do not have specific contraindications.

Direct PTCA (often with stent deployment) is an alternative to thrombolytic therapy in centers in which it can be performed rapidly by highly skilled cardiologists. Those most likely to benefit from primary PTCA in place of thrombolysis include patients with a contraindication to thrombolytic therapy, with cardiogenic shock, and in the setting of a large anterior MI.

Studies have shown that routine coronary angiography and revascularization following successful thrombolytic therapy offer no advantage, but should be pursued in patients with recurrent spontaneous ischemia, or if ischemia is provoked by a predischarge exercise test (see below).

Routine MI Management. Whether or not thrombolytic therapy is administered, MI management is aimed at restoring the balance between myocardial oxygen demand and supply and at relieving ischemic pain (Box 63-11).

General Measures. The patient should be admitted to a monitored coronary care unit bed for 24 to 48 hours where

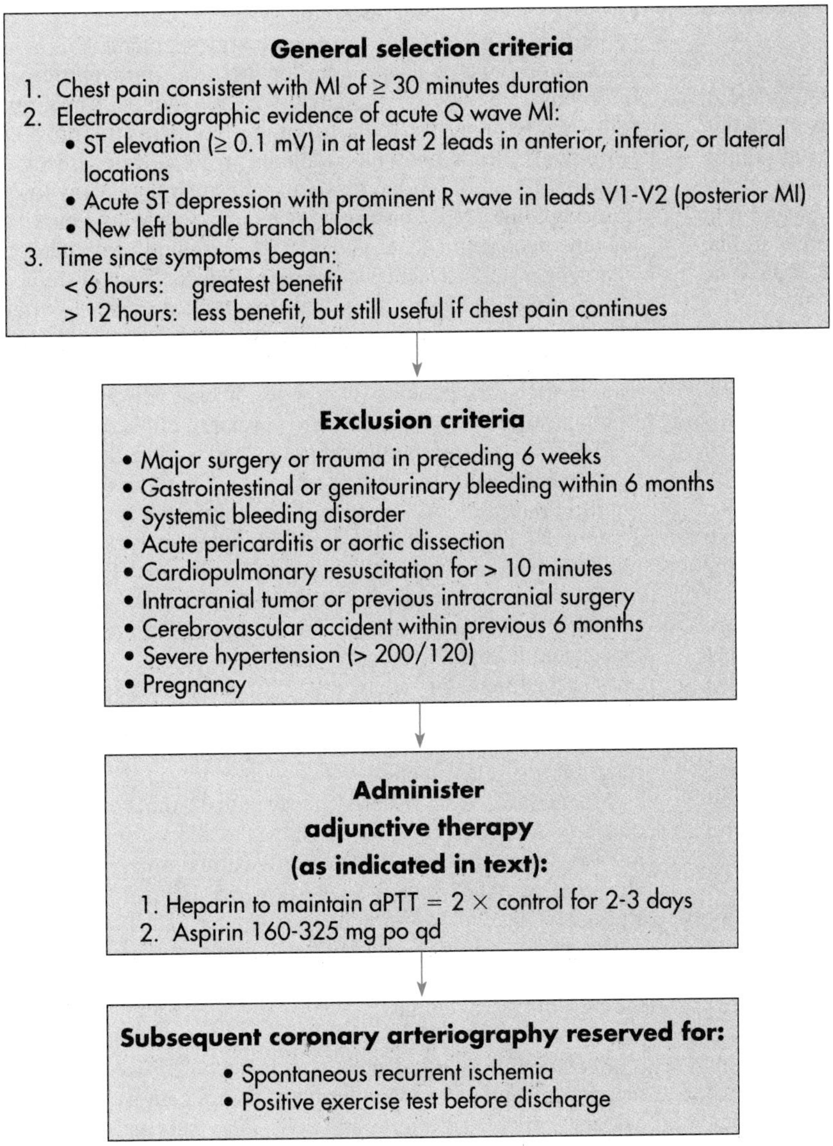

General selection criteria

1. Chest pain consistent with MI of ≥ 30 minutes duration
2. Electrocardiographic evidence of acute Q wave MI:
   - ST elevation (≥ 0.1 mV) in at least 2 leads in anterior, inferior, or lateral locations
   - Acute ST depression with prominent R wave in leads V1-V2 (posterior MI)
   - New left bundle branch block
3. Time since symptoms began:
   < 6 hours: greatest benefit
   > 12 hours: less benefit, but still useful if chest pain continues

↓

Exclusion criteria

- Major surgery or trauma in preceding 6 weeks
- Gastrointestinal or genitourinary bleeding within 6 months
- Systemic bleeding disorder
- Acute pericarditis or aortic dissection
- Cardiopulmonary resuscitation for > 10 minutes
- Intracranial tumor or previous intracranial surgery
- Cerebrovascular accident within previous 6 months
- Severe hypertension (> 200/120)
- Pregnancy

↓

Administer adjunctive therapy (as indicated in text):

1. Heparin to maintain aPTT = 2 × control for 2-3 days
2. Aspirin 160-325 mg po qd

↓

Subsequent coronary arteriography reserved for:

- Spontaneous recurrent ischemia
- Positive exercise test before discharge

Fig. 63-4. Approach to thrombolytic therapy in acute Q wave MI.

Box 63-11. Initial Routine Management of Acute Myocardial Infarction

Admit to monitored bed, supplemental oxygen, soft diet, mild sedation
Pain relief:
Nitroglycerin, 0.4 mg sublingual every 5 minutes for 3 doses (if not hypotensive)
Morphine sulfate, 1-4 mg IV every 5 to 10 minutes
IV nitroglycerin, start at 10 Fg/min (see text)
β-Blocker (e.g., metoprolol, 5 mg IV every 2 to 5 minutes for 3 doses)
Aspirin, 160-325 mg (chewed or swallowed) on admission and every day thereafter
ACE inhibitor (e.g., captopril 6.25-50 mg po tid) for Q wave infarction or signs of CHF
Heparin:
Administer IV (to achieve a PTT 2 times control) if patient receives thrombolytic therapy or has large akinetic segment or intraventricular thrombus (see text)
OTHERWISE
7500 U subcutaneous every 12 hours

activities should be minimized, mild sedation administered, a soft diet and stool softener prescribed, and an intravenous line placed for emergency access, should a sudden dysrhythmia appear. Supplemental oxygen (2 to 4 L/min via nasal cannula) is often useful, since mild hypoxemia is common in acute MI. The hemoglobin oxygen saturation can be measured noninvasively by pulse oximetry and should be maintained at greater than 90%.

Pain Relief. Sublingual nitroglycerin (0.3 to 0.4 mg) can be administered every 5 minutes in the absence of hypotension. If pain persists for more than three doses, morphine sulfate should be used, 1 to 4 mg every 5 to 10 minutes. Side effects of morphine include nausea, dizziness, hypotension, and respiratory depression (reversible by naloxone, 0.4 mg IV). Morphine may also produce bradycardia via a vagal effect, which responds to atropine (0.6 to 1.0 mg IV). Intravenous nitroglycerin can be added for patients with persistent ischemia and for patients with severe hypertension or signs of congestive heart failure. Although early intravenous nitroglycerin may have a beneficial effect on limitation of infarct size in selected patients, it may also result in detrimental hypotension or reflex tachycardia, and must be carefully titrated.

β-Blockers. Pooled analyses from randomized clinical trials in the prethrombolytic era demonstrated reduced mortality and reinfarction rates among MI patients who received early intravenous, followed later by oral, β-blocker therapy. A study in the thrombolytic era, the TIMI-IIb trial, revealed a significant reduction of recurrent ischemia and reinfarction in patients who received β-blockers. Thus β-blockers should be administered routinely in acute MI if contraindications (i.e., heart rate < 55, systolic blood pressure < 100 mm Hg, bronchospasm, uncontrolled congestive heart failure, high-grade AV block) are absent. β-Blockers are particularly useful in patients with sympathetic hyperactivity manifest as hypertension or tachycardia, to reduce myocardial oxygen demand. Our standard regimen is to administer three doses of metoprolol, 5 mg IV, 2 to 5 minutes apart, followed by oral doses of 25 to 100 mg every 8 to 12 hours. For patients at potential risk of β-blocker complications, the ultra–short-acting agent esmolol HCl is preferred, since its side effects resolve quickly upon its discontinuation. It is administered as a 250- to 500-μg/kg bolus over 1 minute, followed by 50 μg/kg/min titrated to a heart rate of 55 to 60 beats/min.

Aspirin. Aspirin is an essential drug in acute MI management. In the Second International Study of Infarct Survival (ISIS-2) aspirin decreased mortality by 23% at 35 days following acute MI; its benefit was additive to that of thrombolytic therapy. In the absence of contraindications, 160 to 325 mg should be administered (swallowed, or chewed for more rapid absorption) at the time of admission and continued orally each day thereafter.

Heparin. Heparin should be administered intravenously to patients who receive t-PA or r-PA thrombolytic therapy, and to those who receive SK or APSAC who are at increased thromboembolic risk, as indicated above. It should be initiated with a weight-adjusted bolus (70 U/kg) followed by a continuous infusion of approximately 15 mg/kg per hour, adjusted to maintain an aPTT of 1.5 to 2.0 times control (50 to 75 seconds), for 48 hours.

Patients who develop large akinetic segments (e.g., in association with a large anterior MI) or intraventricular thrombus are also candidates for intravenous heparin, followed by oral warfarin for 3 to 6 months to prevent peripheral thromboemboli. Patients who do not receive intravenous anticoagulation should be maintained on low-dose heparin, 7500 units subcutaneously every 12 hours to prevent deep venous thrombosis, at least until ambulatory.

Angiotensin-Converting Enzyme Inhibitors. Several studies of oral ACE inhibitors show that they reduce mortality after MI. These agents improve left ventricular dysfunction and adverse ventricular remodeling and their greatest benefit is seen in high-risk patients (e.g., anterior wall MI or evidence of congestive heart failure). Based on large clinical trials, an oral ACE inhibitor should be prescribed within the first 24 hours of an acute MI in patients with ST elevation or left bundle branch block, or those with congestive heart failure symptoms. Therapy should continue indefinitely in patients with reduced left ventricular contractile function (EF < 40%) at the time of discharge.

Calcium Channel Blockers. No studies to date have found that calcium channel blockers serve a beneficial role in the initial treatment of acute MI and they should *not* be prescribed routinely in this setting. Their early use should be confined to the management of hypertension or angina refractory to other agents.

Magnesium. Administered intravenously during the early phase of MI, magnesium was shown to reduce mortality in retrospective and small prospective randomized studies. However, a more recent trial known as ISIS-4 found no significant benefit in the acute MI setting. Thus at present, magnesium therapy should not be administered routinely, but reserved for patients with decreased serum levels to reduce the risk of dysrhythmias.

Recognition and Treatment of Complications. The recognition and prompt resolution of complications following MI are critical for short- and long-term survival. Most of

Table 63-9. Common Rhythm Disorders in Acute Myocardial Infarction

Disorder	Etiology	Initial treatment
Sinus bradycardia	Increased vagal tone	Atropine 0.6-1.0 mg IV Temporary pacemaker rarely needed
	Effects of drugs (β-blockers, verapamil, diltiazem)	Reduce dosage
Sinus tachycardia	Pain, anxiety, fever, anemia, hypovolemia, congestive heart failure	Correct underlying cause Treat hypovolemia and congestive heart failure (see Tables 63-10 and 63-11)
Supraventricular premature beats	Metabolic (hypoxia, hypokalemia, hypomagnesemia)	Correct underlying disorder
Atrial fibrillation	Congestive heart failure or atrial ischemia	If unstable: cardioversion If no CHF: slow rate with diltiazem, verapamil, or β-blocker If congestive heart failure present: slow rate with digoxin
Ventricular premature beats (VPBs)	Ischemia, congestive heart failure, or metabolic (hypoxia, hypokalemia, hypomagnesemia)	Treat underlying cause If ≥6 VPBs/min, couplets, or R-on-T VPBs: IV lidocaine* or procainamide† If no congestive heart failure: consider β-blocker therapy
Ventricular tachycardia (VT)	Same as for VPBs	If unstable: defibrillation If stable: IV lidocaine* or procainamide† For refractory VT: bretylium‡ or amiodarone§
Ventricular fibrillation	Same as for VPBs	Defibrillation
Accelerated idioventricular rhythm	Often benign rhythm during acute MI Common reperfusion rhythm after thrombolytic therapy	No therapy usually needed If symptomatic: atropine 0.6-1.0 mg IV

*IV lidocaine 1 mg/kg bolus, then 2-4 mg/min (a second bolus, 0.5 mg/kg 10 min, after the first is recommended).
†IV procainamide 500-1000 mg load (no faster than 50 mg/min), then 2-5 mg/min.
‡IV bretylium tosylate 5 mg/kg over 5 min, then 1-2 mg/min.
§IV amiodarone 150 mg over 10 min, followed by infusion at 1 mg/min for 6 hours, then 0.5 mg/min.

these conditions are best approached in consultation with a cardiologist.

Recurrent Ischemia and Reinfarction. Approximately 30% of patients develop recurrent ischemia during the early phase of hospitalization, which is associated with increased mortality. Prompt referral for coronary arteriography should be performed to assess which patients would benefit from PTCA or CABG. If cardiac catheterization facilities are not immediately available, aggressive therapy with nitrates, β-blockade, and intravenous heparin should be undertaken as arrangements are made to transfer the patient to an institution where such procedures can be performed.

Dysrhythmias. Dysrhythmias are common in the acute MI period and usually require immediate attention. Potential contributors to the development of dysrhythmias include electrolyte disorders (e.g., hypokalemia, hypomagnesemia), hypoxemia, acidosis, congestive heart failure, and certain drugs (e.g., digitalis, dopamine). Table 63-9 lists the most common rhythm disturbances following MI, their likely causes, and recommended initial therapies.

The *prophylactic* use of lidocaine is not recommended because ventricular dysrhythmias can be rapidly recognized and treated in coronary care units, and potential side effects of lidocaine administration include respiratory arrest, seizures, and suppression of sinus node activity. When lidocaine *is* used, dosage should be reduced in the elderly and those with congestive heart failure or hepatic disease, since these conditions can slow the drug's metabolism and increase its toxicity.

Conduction Blocks. Atrioventricular block is common during acute MI. First-degree atrioventricular block does not require therapy. Second-degree block is most often of Wenckebach's type (Mobitz type I) and requires treatment only if it results in a symptomatically slow heart rate. If so, it usually responds to atropine, 0.6 to 1.0 mg IV.

The prognostic significance of third-degree (complete) atrioventricular block depends on whether it occurs in the setting of an acute inferior (IMI) or anterior (AMI) infarction. In IMI complete heart block is usually transient and occurs because of heightened vagal tone or temporary ischemia of the atrioventricular node. The ventricular escape rhythm usually consists of narrow (i.e., normal) QRS complexes, since the block is high within the conduction system. Often atrioventricular conduction can be restored in this situation by IV atropine (0.6 to 1 mg), but if not, a temporary pacemaker is required.

Conversely, when atrioventricular block develops in the setting of an acute AMI, the site of block is usually more distal and widespread within the conduction pathway, due to extensive tissue destruction. Mobitz type II and complete heart block in AMI are ominous prognostic signs, and emergency placement of a temporary pacemaker is required, followed by permanent pacemaker placement later. Patients who develop complete heart block in the setting of AMI have a high mortality rate due to the severe underlying myocardial damage.

Other conduction defects that portend progression to complete heart block include (1) new left bundle branch block and (2) new right bundle branch block with left anterior or left posterior hemiblock. Prophylactic transvenous pacemakers should generally be placed in such individuals. External pacing units can be placed temporarily and sometimes reduce the need for prophylactic transvenous wires in these settings, but are useful only for short periods because of the discomfort associated with their use.

Hypertension. During an acute MI hypertension may result from chest pain or anxiety or simply reflect chronic blood pressure elevation. It often improves during routine MI management, resolution of pain, and mild sedation. However, persistent hypertension can be deleterious since it increases the afterload against which the left ventricle contracts and therefore increases myocardial oxygen demand. Several therapeutic options exist, including (1) mild diuresis with IV furosemide if congestive heart failure is also present, (2) transcutaneous or oral nitrates (see Table 63-3); (3) IV or oral β-blockers (see Table 63-4), and (4) for severe hypertension IV nitroprusside or nitroglycerin (see below). If intravenous therapy is used, an arterial line should be placed for careful blood pressure monitoring.

Hemodynamic Complications. Hemodynamic complications include the development of congestive heart failure, hypotension, and shock. Left ventricular failure in the setting of an MI can result from both reduced systolic contractile function and decreased diastolic compliance of the myocardium. The severity of congestive heart failure depends on the extent of infarcted tissue and whether superimposed mechanical complications have occurred.

Mild congestive heart failure, manifest by basilar rales and a third heart sound is very common during early hospitalization. Therapy is similar to that for congestive heart failure in other conditions (see Chapter 65), including diuretic and ACE inhibitor therapy. Digitalis is not usually beneficial acutely in the absence of atrial fibrillation.

In patients with more advanced heart failure or those with hypotension that does not quickly respond to fluid administration, invasive hemodynamic monitoring (with a balloon-tipped pulmonary artery catheter and arterial line) can greatly aid in diagnosis and therapy. Measurements of pulmonary capillary wedge pressure and the cardiac index can categorize the hemodynamic abnormality and guide an appropriate course of action (Table 63-10). Because the left ventricle is often stiff due to diminished compliance in the setting of a large MI, the optimal pulmonary capillary wedge pressure is higher than normal, at approximately 15 to 18 mm Hg. Echocardiography is very useful in the evaluation of patients with congestive heart failure or hypotension in acute MI, to determine the degree of contractile dysfunction and to assess for complications such as mitral regurgitation, ventricular septal defect, cardiac tamponade, or right ventricular infarction (Table 63-11).

Right ventricular infarction should be considered when a patient with an IMI shows signs of diminished cardiac output and jugular venous distention out of proportion to left ventricular failure. The pulmonary capillary wedge pressure is commonly low in this situation, but the right atrial pressure is elevated (greater than 10 mm Hg). The diagnosis is further suggested by the presence of ST segment elevation in ECG leads placed over the right parasternal region, and right ventricular dysfunction can be confirmed by echocardiography. As a result of impeded flow through the poorly contractile right ventricle, hypotension may result and can be worsened by diuretic therapy, which further reduces filling of the heart. Appropriate therapy of right ventricular infarction consists of fluid administration to achieve a pulmonary

Table 63-10. Hemodynamic Categories in Acute Myocardial Infarction

Condition	Cardiac index (L/min/m²)	PCWP (mm Hg)	Systolic BP (mm Hg)	Treatment
Normal in acute MI	>2.5	≤18	>100	
Hypovolemia	<2.5	<15	<100	Successive boluses of 100 ml normal saline If inferior MI in evolution and right atrial pressure >10: consider RV infarction
Volume overload	>2.5	>18	>100	Diuretic (e.g., furosemide 10-20 mg IV) Nitroglycerin, topical paste or IV (see Table 63-3)
LV failure	<2.5	>18	>100	Diuretic (e.g., furosemide 10-20 mg IV) IV nitroglycerin, or if markedly hypertensive use IV sodium nitroprusside
Severe LV failure	<2.5	>18	<100	If BP ≥90: IV dobutamine ± IV nitroglycerin or sodium nitroprusside If BP <90: IV dopamine If accompanied by pulmonary edema: attempt diuresis with IV furosemide; may be limited by hypotension May require intraaortic balloon pump
Cardiogenic shock	<1.8	>18	<90 with oliguria and confusion	IV dopamine Intraaortic balloon pump Emergency coronary angioplasty may be life-saving

PCWP, Pulmonary capillary wedge pressure; *RV*, right ventricle; *LV*, left ventricle.

capillary wedge pressure of 15 to 18 mm Hg, to ensure optimal left ventricular filling.

Mechanical Defects. Mechanical defects include full or partial *rupture of a papillary muscle,* or the development of a *ventricular septal defect* (VSD) due to focal weakening of the infarcting myocardium. Although these complications occur rarely, they may result in pulmonary edema, cardiogenic shock, or death. They typically present 3 to 7 days following acute AMI or IMI, and each results in a new systolic murmur. The location of the murmur is at the cardiac apex in mitral regurgitation and at the left parasternal region in the case of a VSD. Both conditions can be readily identified by Doppler echocardiography. Invasive hemodynamic monitoring confirms the presence of a VSD by demonstrating a rise in the oxygen saturation in the pulmonary artery compared with the right atrium. In acute mitral regurgitation, the pulmonary capillary wedge tracing shows a large systolic v wave, although that sign is not specific for this disorder. The initial treatment of these mechanical defects includes IV vasodilators (nitroprusside or nitroglycerin) (Table 63-12), inotropic support (dobutamine or dopamine), and if cardiogenic shock supervenes, the placement of an intraaortic balloon pump. Unstable patients require urgent surgical repair.

Rupture of the left ventricular free wall due to ischemic necrosis occurs in less than 1% of acute MIs and is nearly always fatal because of the development of cardiac tamponade and shock. It occurs within the first week following MI and is most common in older women, those with a history of hypertension, and patients treated in the early postinfarct period with steroids or nonsteroidal

Table 63-11. Differential Diagnosis of Hemodynamic Complications Following Myocardial Infarction

Complication	Clinical findings	Doppler echocardiography	Right heart catheter findings
Hypovolemia	Hypotension without jugular venous distention Absence of pulmonary rales	LV contractile dysfunction not sufficiently severe to explain hypotension	PCWP ≤18 mm Hg
Severe LV contractile dysfunction	Left- and right-sided CHF; pulmonary rales, S_3 jugular venous distention	Marked LV contractile dysfunction	PCWP >18 mm Hg
Cardiac tamponade (due to pericarditis of LV free-wall rupture)	Hypotension with pulsus paradoxus Jugular venous distention Pericardial rub	Pericardial effusion with right-sided chamber compression	Elevated and equal PCWP and RA pressures
Mitral regurgitation	New apical systolic murmur Acute pulmonary edema common	Abnormal systolic blood flow from LV into LA	Large v wave on PCWP tracing
Ventricular septal defect	New left parasternal systolic murmur Acute pulmonary edema common	Abnormal systolic blood flow from LV into RV	Increascd oxygen saturation in pulmonary artery compared with RA
Right ventricular infarction	In setting of inferior MI Jugular venous distention without pulmonary rates ST elevation in *right* parasternal chest leads	RV contractile dysfunction with relatively preserved LV contraction	Elevated RA pressure (>10 mm Hg) but usually normal PCWP (<18 mm Hg)

LV, Left ventricle; *RV,* right ventricle; *RA,* right atrium; *LA,* left atrium; *PCWP,* pulmonary capillary wedge pressure; *CHF,* congestive heart failure.

Table 63-12. Intravenous Vasodilators and Inotropic Drugs Used in Acute Myocardial Infarction

Drug	Starting dose	Dosage range	Comment
Nitroglycerin	10 μg/min	Up to 10 μg/kg/min	May improve coronary blood flow to ischemic myocardium
Sodium nitroprusside	0.25 μg/kg/min	Up to 10 μg/kg/min	More potent vasodilator than nitroglycerin; less beneficial for improving coronary blood flow Thiocyanate toxicity (blurred vision, tinnitus, delirium) can occur during prolonged therapy or in renal failure
Dobutamine	2.5 μg/kg/min	Up to 20 μg/kg/min	Promotes ↑ cardiac output, ↓ PCWP, but does not raise blood pressure
Dopamine	2 μg/kg/min	10 μg/kg/min or higher	More useful than dobutamine if hypotensive Effects vary by dosage: <5 μg/kg/min ↑ renal blood flow 2.5-10 μg/kg/min positive inotrope >10 μg/kg/min vasoconstriction

antiinflammatory drugs. If the rupture is incomplete, the leak may be held in check by localized thrombus that plugs the defect. This unstable condition is termed a *pseudoaneurysm* and surgical repair is indicated to prevent delayed rupture.

A *true left ventricular aneurysm* is a late complication of Q wave infarctions and consists of a scarred area of myocardium that bulges outward during systole. It can be suspected by persistent ST elevation on the patient's ECG many weeks following an acute MI and can be confirmed by echocardiography or left ventricular angiography. This type of aneurysm does not usually rupture, but it can lead to heart failure, ventricular dysrhythmias, or thromboemboli. Surgical repair of the aneurysm is indicated if these complications are refractory to standard medical therapy.

Pericarditis. Manifest by pleuritic chest pain, low-grade fever, and a pericardial friction rub, pericarditis has been reported in 10% to 15% of patients within the first week following MI. Its incidence has been declining in the thrombolytic era, likely due to reperfusion-associated limitation of infarct size. Aspirin (up to 650 mg every 4 to 6 hours) is the recommended therapy for pain relief, but steroids and nonsteroidal antiinflammatory agents should be avoided because they can delay healing of the infarcting myocardium. Anticoagulation with heparin or Coumadin is relatively contraindicated in patients with pericarditis to avoid hemorrhagic tamponade.

A late form of pericarditis occurring 2 to 10 weeks following MI is known as Dressler's syndrome. It develops in less than 5% of post-MI patients and is thought to be of autoimmune origin. It, too, responds to aspirin, but since the myocardium has already substantially healed by the time of its occurrence, other nonsteroidal antiinflammatory agents are also used. Glucocorticoids (prednisone, 1 mg/kg/day) should be considered only as a last resort, since such therapy can be very difficult to taper without recurrence of pain and long-term steroid dependence may result.

REHABILITATION, RISK STRATIFICATION, AND SECONDARY PREVENTION OF RECURRENT MI

The average length of hospitalization for uncomplicated MIs in the late 1990s is 5 days but can be prolonged by the superimposed conditions described above. The patient usually remains in the coronary care unit for 24 to 48 hours. Activities are limited to near total bed rest for the first 12 hours, but progress to sitting in a chair within the first 24 hours. By day 3 the patient is usually allowed to walk within the hospital room and may shower if stable.

The long-term prognosis following acute MI depends on three main factors: the degree of residual myocardium at ischemic risk, the extent of left ventricular dysfunction, and the presence of ventricular dysrhythmias. Assessment of these variables should be part of routine post-MI management (Table 63-13). A submaximal exercise test aiming for 70% of the maximal predicted heart rate (with radionuclide perfusion scintigraphy only if needed for accurate interpretation, or a pharmacologic [e.g., adenosine or dipyridamole] imaging study if the patient is unable to exercise) should be performed before or soon after discharge. This level of exercise exceeds the energy expended in climbing a flight of stairs and is useful to gauge activities at home. Patients with positive stress tests (development of angina, significant ST segment shifts, or hypotension) should undergo cardiac catheterization to assess subsequent prognosis and need for revascularization. Standard exercise testing, achieving 85% of the maximal predicted heart rate, can be performed 4 to 6 weeks after MI and is useful to guide further physical activities in the rehabilitation process.

Assessment of left ventricular function by echocardiography or radionuclide ventriculography is also recommended before discharge, since left ventricular dysfunction is a strong predictor of outcomes after infarction. Several studies have shown that patients with a left ventricular ejection fraction < 40% after infarction benefit from long-term angiotensin-

Table 63-13. Evaluation and Long-term Therapy After Myocardial Infarction

Therapy or procedure	Comments
Submaximal exercise test	Target heart rate = 70% maximal, using low-level protocol
	If positive for angina or evidence of ischemia then proceed to cardiac catheterization
	If negative, prescribe medical therapy as indicated below and perform full exercise test (85% maximal heart rate) 4-6 weeks post-MI
Evaluate left ventricular contractile function (echocardiography or radionuclide ventriculography)	If LV ejection fraction ≤40%, add ACE inhibitor (e.g., captopril titrated to 50 mg po tid)
	If intraventricular thrombus or large anterior akinetic segment present (by echo), prescribe warfarin for 3-6 months (achieve INR 2-3), then replace with aspirin
Ambulatory ECG monitoring	Not recommended for patients without symptomatic dysrhythmias
	If symptomatic ventricular dysrhythmias present, add β-blocker as indicated below, and obtain cardiology consultation to determine whether electrophysiologic testing or empiric antidysrhythmic therapy appropriate
β-Blocker	If no contraindications (e.g., timolol 10 mg, bid or metoprolol 50-100 mg bid)
	If β-blocker contraindicated (e.g., asthma) and no evidence of CHF, consider verapamil
	In non–Q wave infarction without CHF consider diltiazem in place of β-blocker
Aspirin	160-325 mg po qd (withhold if on warfarin therapy)
Correct predisposing risk factors	Target LDL cholesterol ≤100 mg/dl
	Control hypertension, diabetes
	Eliminate cigarette smoking

LV, Left ventricular; *ACE,* angiotensin-converting enzyme; *CHF,* congestive heart failure; *LDL,* low-density lipoprotein.

converting enzyme inhibitor therapy (e.g., captopril, titrated to 50 mg three times a day), even if such a patient is free of congestive heart failure symptoms. Treated patients have demonstrated a significant decline in mortality, development of congestive heart failure, or reinfarction.

The presence of ventricular dysrhythmias (more than 10 ventricular premature beats per hour or repetitive forms) correlates with decreased survival following MI. However, routine ambulatory ECG monitoring and signal-averaged ECG measurements are not recommended, because in recent studies, antiarrhythmic therapy for *asymptomatic* ventricular ectopy following an MI has not been shown to reduce, and in some cases has increased, post-MI mortality. Patients with symptomatic ventricular dysrhythmias, or patients with asymptomatic ventricular dysrhythmias and left ventricular dysfunction, do require interventions, however, and should be referred to a cardiologist to determine whether electrophysiologic testing or drug therapy is appropriate.

Routine pharmacologic therapy following hospital discharge for acute MI includes aspirin, a β-blocker, and an angiotensin-converting enzyme inhibitor (if left ventricular dysfunction is present, as indicated above). The long-term use of aspirin, in dosages of 325 mg daily or less, has been conclusively shown in placebo-controlled trials to reduce subsequent mortality by 10% to 15% and reinfarction rates by 20% to 30%. Chronic β-blocker therapy also reduces mortality and reinfarction rates. In the absence of contraindications typical regimens include the following: timolol, 10 mg twice a day; atenolol, 50 to 100 mg daily; or metoprolol, 50 to 100 mg twice a day. If β-blockers are contraindicated, verapamil may be a reasonable alternative, since limited data have shown it to reduce death and reinfarction rates in patients *without significant left ventricular dysfunction* after MI.

Pharmacologic therapy of patients who have sustained a non–Q wave infarction needs to be considered separately. This type of infarct represents an incomplete process such that viable myocardium may remain at ischemic risk. Although the early prognosis in non–Q wave MI is good, subsequent reinfarction and the need for mechanical revascularization *exceeds* that of Q wave infarcts. Nonetheless, a recently completed Veterans Administration trial (known as VANQWISH) demonstrated that not all patients with this syndrome should undergo invasive approaches. In this trial, patients with non–Q wave MI were randomized to either an early invasive strategy (cardiac catheterization followed by revascularization if needed) versus a conservative approach (pharmacologic therapy and noninvasive testing with subsequent invasive management only if spontaneous or induced ischemia was demonstrated). The mortality rate was lower in the conservatively treated patients over 1 year of follow-up.

In other studies following non–Q wave MI, β-blockers have not consistently reduced cardiac morbidity. However, the calcium channel blocker diltiazem has been shown to reduce the rate of reinfarction in this setting, *if* there is no evidence of congestive heart failure. Therefore our approach to stable patients following non–Q wave MI is to proceed with exercise testing; if ischemia is induced, cardiac catheterization is undertaken. Otherwise, aspirin and diltiazem (if congestive heart failure is absent) are prescribed.

Finally, the risk factors that lead to the development of atherosclerosis should be addressed. Sustaining an acute MI can be a powerful motivator for the patient to improve harmful lifestyle attributes such as smoking or obesity. Patients who stop smoking reduce the risk of reinfarction and death within a year of quitting. The treatment of hypertension and diabetes should also be strongly reinforced by the patient's primary care physician and cardiologist. Several recent large randomized trials have firmly established that pharmacologic reduction of LDL cholesterol post-MI using HMG-CoA reductase inhibitors greatly reduces reinfarction rates, subsequent stroke rates, and mortality (see Chapter 71). The goal for serum LDL cholesterol over the long-term is <100 mg/dl by both dietary and pharmacologic means. Note that serum lipid levels drawn within 24 to 48 hours of acute infarction accurately represent a patient's profile, whereas such levels may be misleadingly low if drawn over the subsequent 2 months.

Following discharge from the hospital, the patient can perform limited activities at home but should avoid isometric activities such as lifting objects heavier than 10 pounds. Two to 4 weeks after discharge, patients should walk ½ to 1½ miles a day, depending on the results of exercise testing; normal sexual activity can resume during this time. Additional activities can be gauged by supervised rehabilitation programs, and most patients can return to work 4 to 12 weeks following discharge. It is an important role of the patient's primary care physician to reinforce a positive outlook during this period and encourage progressive activity to aid in the rehabilitation process. The emotional stress and uncertainties that follow an MI can weigh heavily on the patient and the family. An understanding, compassionate attitude by physicians and other health care providers can greatly facilitate emotional recuperation.

ISCHEMIC HEART DISEASE IN WOMEN

CAD has historically been considered a disease of men, but the magnitude of this condition and its complications in women has become increasingly clear. IHD accounts for 23% of mortality among women and is the leading cause of death in women over the age of 50, resulting in 250,000 deaths per year in the United States. The manifestations of coronary disease in women may differ from those in men, in terms of its onset and outcome. For example, on average, women develop symptoms of coronary disease 10 years later than men, after the menopause, associated with the fall in serum estrogen levels. Although the rate of CAD-related mortality in men is constant after age 60, it continues to rise in women until age 70. Furthermore, women experience a greater proportion of silent MIs than men, and when an MI is symptomatic, women generally come to the hospital after a greater time delay than men with comparable symptoms. In the setting of an acute MI, the outcome for women is worse than male counterparts: there are more complications, longer hospital stays, and a greater likelihood of mortality during hospitalization and during the first post-MI year.

Nonetheless, studies have shown that the evaluation of chest pain, invasive testing, CABG, and PTCA are all performed less often in women than in men with similar symptoms. When they are referred for revascularization procedures, women are usually at more advanced stages of disease, when morbidity and mortality would be expected to be greater.

It is not known whether the comparably adverse outcome in women reflects their older age at presentation, more severe concurrent illnesses, or less intensive therapies prescribed by physicians. However, chest pain symptoms in a woman should not be downplayed, and female patients with documented angina should be educated to respond promptly to symptoms of MI to increase the likelihood of receiving beneficial early interventions.

As in men, it is crucial to reduce risk factors for coronary disease in the female population, particularly cigarette smoking, hypertension, hypercholesterolemia, and diabetes. In postmenopausal women hormone administration *may* also play an important role, but this is controversial. Observational studies have suggested lower cardiovascular event rates in postmenopausal women who take estrogen supplements. However, a recently completed randomized, placebo-controlled study (the Heart and Estrogen/Progestin Replacement Study) has cast doubt on previous conclusions. In this trial, 2763 postmenopausal women with established coronary disease and an intact uterus were treated with either estrogen plus progesterone or placebo for an average of 4.1 years. At the end of the trial there was no difference in nonfatal MI or coronary death between the two groups. Of concern, the hormone-treated group experienced more thromboembolic events and gallbladder disease than the placebo-treated patients. Although it is not known if these results can be generalized to patients without CAD (i.e., for primary prevention) or to those who do not require progesterone therapy (i.e., patients who have undergone hysterectomy), hormone replacement therapy cannot be considered a standard approach to reduce cardiac risk at this time. The decision to prescribe such therapy requires careful consideration by the physician and patient, who must also weigh the other beneficial effects (e.g., osteoporosis prevention and for menopausal symptoms) versus the potential adverse risks of hormonal replacement.

Pooled analyses of secondary prevention studies following an MI in women have shown that aspirin significantly reduces mortality, reinfarction rates, and stroke, similar to the results in men. β-Blockers also have comparable effectiveness in both sexes in preventing reinfarction.

As indicated above, aspirin therapy contributes to primary prevention of MI in men. However, in women, primary prevention studies have been limited to observational data rather than randomized, prospective trials, and the results have been mixed. For example, in the Nurses' Health Study, women who used one to six aspirins per week had a 25% reduction in the incidence of MI compared with those who did not use aspirin. However, no benefit was seen in those taking more than seven aspirins per week. Future results from large prospective randomized trials will be necessary for clarification of the benefits of aspirin in women.

ADDITIONAL READINGS

Braunwald E: Unstable angina: an etiologic approach to management. *Circulation* 98:2219-2222, 1998.

Bypass Angioplasty Revascularization Investigation (BARI) Investigators: Comparison of coronary bypass surgery with angioplasty in patients with multivessel disease, *N Engl J Med* 335:217-225, 1996.

Cannon CP: Management of acute coronary syndromes, Totowa, NJ, 1998, Humana.

Deedwania PC, Amsterdam EA, Vagelos RH: Evidence-based, cost- effective risk stratification and management after myocardial infarction, California Cardiology Working Group on Post-MI Management, *Arch Intern Med* 157:273-280, 1997.

Hennekens CH, Albert CM, Godfried SL, et al: Adjunctive drug therapy of acute myocardial infarction—evidence from clinical trials, *N Engl J Med* 335:1660-1667, 1996.

Hsia JA: Cardiovascular diseases in women, *Med Clin North Am* 82:1-19, 1998.

Madan M, Berkowitz SD, Tcheng JE: Glycoprotein IIb/IIIa integrin blockade, *Circulation* 98:2629-2635, 1998.

Miller DB: Secondary prevention for ischemic heart disease, *Arch Intern Med* 157:2045-2052, 1997.

Peterson ED, Shaw LJ, Califf RM: Risk stratification after myocardial infarction, *Ann Intern Med* 126:561-582, 1997.

Ryan TJ, Anderson JL, Antman EM, et al: American College of Cardiology/American Heart Association guidelines for the management of patients with acute myocardial infarction, *J Am Coll Cardiol* 28:1328-1428, 1996.

Scanlon PJ, Faxon DP, Audet AM, et al: ACC/AHA guidelines for coronary angiography. A report of the American College of Cardiology/American Heart Association Task Force on practice guidelines (Committee on Coronary Angiography). Developed in collaboration with the Society for Cardiac Angiography and Interventions, *J Am Coll Cardiol* 33:1756-1824, 1999.

Solomon AJ, Gersh BJ: Management of chronic stable angina: medical therapy, percutaneous transluminal coronary angioplasty, and coronary artery bypass graft surgery: lessons from the randomized trials, *Ann Intern Med* 128:216-223, 1998.

Theroux P, Fuster V: Acute coronary syndromes: unstable angina and non–Q wave myocardial infarction, *Circulation* 97:1195-1206, 1997.

CHAPTER 64

Myocardial Revascularization

Eric H. Lieberman

Jaime Burkle

Symptomatic coronary artery disease is present in more than 6 million people in the United States. Despite the availability of effective medical therapy, a significant proportion of patients are candidates for a revascularization procedure because of unacceptable symptoms or potentially life-threatening lesions.[44] An estimated 300,000 coronary artery bypass operations and 500,000 coronary angioplasty procedures were performed in 1996, a more than tenfold increase over the past decade.

Direct myocardial revascularization began in 1958 with Sones and collaborators at the Cleveland Clinic, when selective coronary angiography was introduced. In January of 1962, Effler was able to repair a severe obstruction of the left main coronary artery by the patch graft technique developed by Senning. Shortly thereafter, Sones demonstrated for the first time that by means of collateral circulation, coronary bypass could ameliorate the myocardial perfusion deficit of the anterolateral wall of the left ventricle due to a severe obstruction of the left anterior descending branch of the left coronary artery.

Although Sabiston and then Garret and DeBakey performed aortosaphenous vein coronary artery bypass in 1962 and 1964, respectively, Favaloro and Effler established this procedure as a reliable and effective treatment for patients with severe coronary atherosclerosis. Since 1969 the coronary artery bypass graft (CABG) operation has become the most completely studied operation in the history of surgery. It is highly effective in the relief of severe angina, and under some circumstances has the capability for considerably prolonging useful life. The CABG operation consists of the construction of new pathways (conduits) between the aorta (or other major arteries) and segments of coronary arteries beyond obstructive lesions for the purpose of bringing blood to myocardium made ischemic by these lesions. Since the early years of the operation, reversed segments of autologous saphenous vein have been used as the conduit. In 1968 Green used the left internal mammary artery to bypass the left anterior descending coronary artery, leading to better and longer graft patency rates. Segments of radial artery, arm veins, allograft arteries, and veins and synthetic tubes are now being used with variable results.[36]

Coronary angioplasty was first introduced by Gruentzig in 1977 as an alternative form of revascularization and led to a revolution in the management of patients with coronary artery disease.[26] During the early years of its application, Gruentzig and others used the procedure predominantly to treat patients with discrete, proximal, noncalcified, subtotal occlusive lesions in a single coronary artery. Although the early experience with angioplasty was limited to patients with stable symptoms, normal left ventricular function, and proximal, discrete stenoses, technologic development and operator experience have greatly widened the indications for percutaneous coronary intervention (PCI). In subsequent years the technique has been used successfully in patients with multivessel disease, multiple subtotal stenoses in the same vessel, certain complete occlusions, partial occlusion of saphenous vein or internal mammary artery grafts, or recent total thrombotic occlusions associated with acute myocardial infarction. Acute complications resulting from the angioplasty procedure itself and the occurrence of late restenosis following the procedure have motivated cardiologists to seek alternative methods of improving flow through obstructed arteries. Directional and rotational coronary atherectomy, laser angioplasty, and coronary stenting have improved initial results in certain anatomic situations.

INDICATIONS FOR MYOCARDIAL REVASCULARIZATION IN CHRONIC ISCHEMIC HEART DISEASE

Medical vs. Surgical Therapy

When evaluating a patient with chronic stable angina for the best possible therapy to achieve relief of symptoms as well as survival benefit, special consideration should be made of the following factors: left ventricular function (i.e., ejection fraction), number of diseased vessels, location of stenotic lesions, severity of angina, age, sex, presence of peripheral vascular disease, abnormal electrocardiogram (ECG), and hypertension. An effective clinical strategy in managing patients with chronic stable angina should seek to identify patients whose lives would likely be prolonged by CABG. Based on a retrospective analysis of the three largest clinical trials of coronary artery bypass grafting, the Veterans Administration Cooperative Study of coronary artery surgery (VACS),[54] the European Coronary Surgery Study (ECSS),[53] and the Coronary Artery Surgery Study (CASS),[2] the sicker the patient, as gauged by relevant measures of coronary disease and cardiovascular morbidity, the more likely CABG will prolong life. The VACS included 686 male patients younger than 67 years of age, with chronic stable (predominantly class II and III) angina for >6 months, left ventricular dysfunction in more than half of them (ejection fraction [EF] <50%), and at least 6 months since the last acute coronary event. The ECSS randomized 768 male patients younger than 65, with chronic class I to III angina for >3 months but no evidence of left ventricular dysfunction (EF >50% in all patients). Finally the CASS trial included 780 patients (90% male) younger than 65, with no worse than class II angina for at least 2 months (or 3 weeks after acute myocardial infarction), and ejection fractions of at least 35. The patient population underrepresented or excluded certain categories of patients with high incidence of coronary disease, including women, patients over 65 years of age, patients with moderate and severe angina, those with new onset angina or recent myocardial infarction, and patients with severely impaired left ventricular function. In summary, a CABG-related improvement in survival is therefore more likely to occur if there is left ventricular dysfunction, multivessel disease, proximal coronary lesions (more muscle is threatened by such lesions), high-grade lesions as determined by angiography, more severe angina, or low-level inducible ischemia.

Thus, patients are likely to live longer after CABG if they have:

1. Left main disease (see Special Considerations)
2. Three-vessel disease with left ventricular dysfunction (ejection fraction less than 50%); class III or IV angina; provokable ischemia; or disease in the proximal left anterior descending coronary artery
3. Two-vessel disease with proximal left anterior descending coronary artery involvement
4. Two-vessel disease with class III or IV angina and either severe left ventricular dysfunction alone or moderate left ventricular dysfunction together with at least one proximal lesion

When it is less clear whether to do CABG, the presence of peripheral vascular disease, female sex, baseline electrocardiographic ST-segment and T wave changes, or older age (over 60) should weigh in favor of doing CABG.[41]

Surgical vs. Percutaneous Coronary Intervention

Coronary angioplasty and coronary bypass grafting are both intended to improve myocardial blood flow. Both are palliative rather than curative and should be seen as complementary rather than competitive procedures and are associated with potential risks including stroke, myocardial injury, and death. The major advantage of coronary angioplasty is its relative ease of use, making unnecessary general anesthesia, thoracotomy, extracorporeal circulation, mechanical ventilation, and prolonged convalescence. Repeat angioplasty can be performed more easily than repeat bypass surgery and revascularization can be achieved more quickly in emergency situations. The disadvantages of angioplasty are high early restenosis rates (especially in the pre-stent era) and the inability to relieve many stenoses because of the nature and extent of the coronary lesions.

The preferred method of revascularization (i.e., CABG vs. PTCA) remains controversial. Several randomized studies comparing PTCA with CABG have recently been completed. The Randomized Intervention Treatment of Angina trial (RITA), an Argentine trial of PTCA and CABG (ERACI), the

German Angioplasty Bypass Surgery Investigation (GABI), the Emory Angioplasty versus Surgery Trial (EAST), the Coronary Angioplasty Bypass Revascularization Investigation (CABRI), and the Bypass Angioplasty Revascularization Investigation (BARI) together enrolled almost 4800 patients. The EAST trial was the first of the randomized trials of angioplasty vs. CABG.[33] It consisted of 392 patients with multivessel disease; 40% had three-vessel disease and 60% had two-vessel disease. Three-year survival data from the EAST trial demonstrate no significant difference between those patients initially randomized to PTCA or CABG.[34] The BARI trial, designed to test a primary endpoint of total mortality at 5 years, randomized 1829 patients.[5] There was no significant difference between the PTCA and CABG groups (86.3% vs. 89.3%, $p = 0.19$). Patients randomized to an initial strategy of PTCA in both the EAST and the BARI trial had a significantly higher rate of repeat revascularization. It is worth noting that the diabetic subgroup in the BARI trial demonstrated that those randomized to CABG had an 80% 5-year survival compared with 65% for the PTCA group.[6]

It is important to note that the patients randomized represent only a small proportion of the entire population, and this raises the issue of selection bias. Coronary bypass surgery has the advantages of greater durability (graft patency rates exceeding 90% at 10 years with arterial conduits) and more complete revascularization irrespective of the morphology of the obstructing atherosclerotic lesion. Generally speaking, the greater the extent of coronary atherosclerosis and its diffuseness through the vessel wall, the more compelling the choice of coronary artery bypass surgery, particularly if the left ventricular function is depressed. Patients with lesser extent of disease and localized lesions are good candidates for percutaneous coronary intervention.

Medical Therapy vs. Percutaneous Coronary Intervention

The development of PTCA led to significant questions about the appropriate treatment of patients with stable angina. The widespread use of PTCA had no impact on the incidence of coronary artery bypass surgery, suggesting that PTCA primarily replaced medical therapy for a large number of patients.[40] A number of randomized studies of PTCA have been performed in an effort to define the appropriate use of these techniques. The first randomized trial was the Angioplasty Compared to Medicine (ACME) trial.[42] This study randomized 212 patients with stable angina and one-vessel disease, an abnormal stress test, or a recent myocardial infarction to either PTCA or medical therapy. The primary endpoints were exercise tolerance and symptoms at 6 months. PTCA was associated with better symptom relief and improved performance on an exercise test compared with medical therapy. There was no difference in the frequency of MI or death between the two groups. A follow-up ACME trial involved 101 patients with two-vessel disease, stable angina, and evidence of ischemia on stress testing.[23] This study failed to show any difference in exercise duration, relief of symptoms, and overall quality of life. RITA-2 randomized 1018 patients with stable angina to either PTCA or medical therapy. This study included patients with multivessel disease and left ventricular dysfunction. The primary endpoint was the combination of all-cause mortality and nonfatal myocardial infarction. Although patients randomized to PTCA had greater reductions in anginal symptoms, the risk of death and nonfatal myocardial infarction was increased to 6.3% of PTCA patients vs. 3.3% of medically treated patients ($p = 0.02$).[43] In reviewing these studies, the following conclusions can be made: (1) PTCA affords better relief of angina than medical therapy, especially for those patients with more severe angina, and (2) the improvement in symptomatic relief comes at the expense of increased risk of morbidity and mortality.

SURGICAL REVASCULARIZATION

There are a variety of risk factors that affect morbidity and mortality in patients undergoing coronary artery surgery. Recent acute myocardial infarction, hemodynamic instability, left ventricular dysfunction, the presence of left main coronary disease, and severe or unstable angina adversely affect surgical outcome. In addition, factors related to the aggressiveness of the atherosclerotic process, as reflected in associated carotid peripheral vascular disease, impact on risk. Biologic factors, including age at operation, diabetes mellitus, and female gender, increase the perioperative risk of surgery. Intraoperative factors that impact on outcome include ischemic damage and type of graft used; use of internal mammary grafts favorably impacts on long-term outcome.[12,37]

A number of complications can occur in patients undergoing CABG. Perioperative myocardial infarctions are more likely to occur in women and in patients with severe perioperative angina pectoris, severe stenosis of the left main coronary artery, and three-vessel disease. Unstable angina and prolonged cardiopulmonary bypass times are also risk factors for perioperative myocardial infarction. Perioperative myocardial infarction, particularly if it is associated with hemodynamic or dysrhythmic complications or preexisting left ventricular dysfunction, has a major adverse effect on early and late prognosis. The diagnosis of perioperative myocardial infarction is hampered by the lack of specificity of repolarization abnormalities and enzyme changes during the perioperative period.[46]

Postoperative changes in pulmonary function after CABG are frequent and troublesome, but rarely serious, except in patients with preexisting chronic lung disease or the elderly. Impaired hemostasis and bleeding complications are an inherent risk of coronary bypass surgery. Reoperation for bleeding is required in 2% to 5% of patients.[50] Cardiopulmonary bypass causes derangements of the intrinsic coagulation and fibrinolytic systems in addition to platelet function. The risk of bleeding is increased with age, a smaller body surface area, reoperation, bilateral internal thoracic artery grafts, and the preoperative use of heparin, aspirin, and thrombolytic agents. Major perioperative wound complications, especially mediastinitis and/or wound dehiscence, occur in approximately 1% of patients. These are associated with markedly increased in-hospital mortality, morbidity, and length of stay. This risk is substantially increased by the use of double internal mammary artery grafts, particularly in diabetic patients.[39]

The incidence of stroke is 1% to 5% and is age-related. The return of a normal level of consciousness is delayed in approximately 3% of patients; intellectual dysfunction in the early postoperative period, as assessed by a battery of neurocognitive tests, has been noted in approximately 75% of patients. Transient mild visual deficits are common. Fortunately, major long-term sequelae are uncommon. Mild degrees of confusion, agitation, and delusional behavior are frequent and usually transient.[30]

Atrial fibrillation is one of the most frequent complications of coronary bypass surgery, occurring in up to 40% of patients. Preoperative and postoperative administration of β-blockers has been shown to reduce the risk of postoperative atrial fibrillation.[24] In the early postoperative period, rapid ventricular rates and loss of atrial transport may compromise systemic hemodynamics and increase the risk of embolization. Administration of β-blockers, calcium antagonists, digoxin, or a combination of these medications is indicated to control the ventricular response. Occasionally rate control alone will facilitate conversion back to normal sinus rhythm (NSR). When restoration of NSR is not achieved within 24 hours, antidysrhythmic therapy (i.e., procainamide, ibutilide, or sotalol) may be instituted. If chemical cardioversion is unsuccessful, then direct current (DC) cardioversion can be attempted in an effort to restore NSR. If conversion to NSR is unsuccessful within 48 to 72 hours, full anticoagulation is indicated to prevent risk of systemic embolization. Chronic requirement of antidysrhythmic therapy for postoperative atrial fibrillation is extremely rare, unless the patient was taking the medication before surgery. Differences of opinion remain as to whether efforts should be made to actively restore NSR in the immediate postoperative period or if anticoagulation should be instituted and cardioversion attempted at a later time if atrial fibrillation does not spontaneously revert to NSR.

The incidence of postoperative bradydysrhythmias requiring permanent pacemaker implantation was 0.8% in a series of 1614 consecutive patients discharged from the hospital after CABG.[18] Predictive factors were preoperative left bundle branch block, concomitant left ventricular aneurysmectomy, and older age. Patients with coronary disease who develop fascicular conduction disturbances often have diffuse myocardial disease and unfavorable prognosis. The causes of death are ventricular dysrhythmias and cardiac failure.

In-hospital mortality after isolated coronary bypass surgery was characterized by a steady decline from 1967 to the early 1980s. Overall mortality for elective first bypass procedures in the United States from 1980 to 1990 was 2.2% in 58,384 patients in the Society of Thoracic Surgeons database. It was 2.6% in elective patients without internal mammary artery grafts and 1.3% in patients receiving such an implant.[13] More recently there has been a stabilization or even a slight overall increase in morbidity and mortality, which reflects the changing characteristics toward an older and sicker population of patients undergoing operation.

The CABG operation has a favorable effect on symptoms and useful life expectancy in many patients. However, it does not cure atherosclerotic heart disease, and in most patients, usually many years after operation, clinical evidence of myocardial ischemia returns and is followed by death, which in more than half the patients is related to recurrent myocardial ischemia. Death from any cause is a secure endpoint with which to judge the efficacy of CABG, and to compare it with alternative forms of therapy. In general, about 96.5% of heterogeneous groups of patients survive at least 1 month after the operation, and 95%, 88%, 75%, and 60% respectively, survive 1, 5, 10, or > 15 years after the operation.

The evidence, both symptomatic and from graded exercise testing, is complete that the coronary artery bypass operation relieves angina in most patients. However, the return of angina is the most prevalent of the postoperative ischemic events. The return of angina shortly after coronary bypass, typically recognized with resumption of activity, usually is due to incomplete revascularization or early closure of grafts. Angina occurring later usually is a reflection of narrowing or closure of one or more grafts or progression of native vessel disease, or both.

In general, sudden cardiac death is uncommon after CABG. By 10 years after undergoing the operation, 95% of patients are alive, as are about 90% by 15 years. Only 5% to 10% of deaths after CABG occur in patients with the syndrome of chronic heart failure. In part, this is because patients with ischemic heart disease and important chronic heart failure usually have severe left ventricular dysfunction as a result of extensive myocardial scarring, and are not advised to undergo bypass surgery.

It is nearly impossible to quantify an unsatisfactory quality of life after CABG, even though it is one of the most important unfavorable outcome events. This relates in part to the fact that a satisfactory quality of life is a composite of at least freedom from limiting angina or heart failure, the preservation of a reasonable exercise capacity, and reasonable freedom from the need for medication, rehospitalization, and reintervention. Most surviving patients have a satisfactory quality of life early after bypass operation, but the probability of retaining this quality begins gradually to decline after about 5 years. The rate of decline in the quality of life is probably similar to that of the freedom from angina.[1]

Conduits

Since the early years of the operation, reversed segments of autologous saphenous vein have been used as the conduit. Greater saphenous vein is expendable, generally available in sufficient length, appropriately sized to match the coronary arteries, capable of reaching beyond the stenoses of all diseased arteries, pliable enough to allow easy suturing, and autologous. When a greater saphenous vein is not available, the lesser saphenous vein can be used. Saphenous veins are used as free grafts, anastomosed proximally to the ascending aorta and distally to one or more coronary arteries.

The time-dependent diminution of patency in saphenous vein bypass grafts has led to the wide use of the left internal mammary artery (LIMA), particularly for revascularization of the left anterior descending (LAD) coronary artery system. The LIMA is left attached to its origin from the left subclavian artery, mobilized from the chest wall, and anastomosed distal to the LAD stenosis. The right internal mammary artery (RIMA) can often be used in a similar fashion. The highest patency rates for coronary bypass grafts are associated with the use of the LIMAs to bypass important proximal stenoses of the LAD coronary artery. These patency rates are approximately 95% at 10 years after operation, and failure to use the mammary arteries in this matter has been demonstrated to be a risk factor for premature late death after the operation.[48]

The use of LIMA or RIMA as a free graft from the ascending aorta to the LAD provides almost comparable results. Currently available information indicates that the LIMA should be used almost routinely for revascularizing the LAD system in the coronary bypass operation. Use of bilateral internal mammary artery grafting has become popular, but as yet the available evidence does not support the hypothesis that long-term survival is increased by its use, and the risk of sternal wound complications is increased by the double internal mammary artery procedure in obese or diabetic patients. The patency advantage of the internal mammary artery when anastomosed to vessels other than the LAD is uncertain.

When neither the LIMA nor the RIMA can be used, the right gastroepiploic artery, the inferior mesenteric artery, or the inferior epigastric artery may be used, although long-term advantages of these arteries over saphenous vein grafts have not been demonstrated. Segments of radial artery, upper extremity veins, allograft arteries and veins, and synthetic tubes (polytetrafluoroethylene) have been less satisfactory as conduits and should be used only as a last resort.

Minimally Invasive Direct Coronary Artery Bypass (MIDCAB) Grafting

The morbidity and mortality of CABG is largely attributed to the use of cardiopulmonary bypass, global cardiac arrest, hypothermia, and median sternotomy. A major limitation appears to be a 6.1% incidence of neurologic events observed in retrospective studies. These neurologic events are attributed to plaque emboli that are dislodged by manipulating the ascending aorta and to low perfusion pressure or microemboli due to the extracorporeal circulation. The trend to operate on progressively older patients is expected to exacerbate the problem of adverse cerebral outcome. The "invasive" nature of cardiopulmonary bypass implies that obviating the need for it is likely to be of major benefit to the patient. CABG on the beating heart, however, requires temporary interruption of the coronary flow in the recipient artery and anastomosis site stabilization. If only a LIMA to LAD graft is needed, a limited anterolateral thoracotomy *(minithoracotomy)* is aesthetically attractive, reduces bleeding, and prevents sternal infection and dehiscence, a rare but serious complication of median sternotomy. The results warrant further exploration of beating-heart coronary surgery.

Recent reports of cumulative experience in MIDCAB in more than 14 different countries have revealed promising results. As expected, the approaches vary and the numbers vary widely. With few exceptions, beating-heart coronary operation is associated with arterial grafting. About 49% of patients had one-vessel disease and 28% and 13% had two- and three-vessel disease, respectively. The average number of anastomoses per patient ranges from one to two. CABG without cardiopulmonary bypass constitutes 1% to 43% of the current bypass procedures performed in specialized centers. CABG on the beating heart may reduce the hospital length of stay from a median of 8 days after conventional CABG to about 4 days, or even less in the case of minithoracotomy LIMA-LAD grafting. Work and social activities may be resumed after 2 to 3 weeks rather than after 2 to 3 months. In selected patients, the costs of coronary revascularization will be reduced substantially. The ultimate value of the currently evolving, less invasive surgical treatment strategies for coronary artery disease remains to be established.[4]

PERCUTANEOUS CORONARY INTERVENTION

In general the procedural success rate for PTCA is estimated to be 92% to 98%; 1% to 3% of patients require emergent coronary artery bypass surgery, myocardial infarction occurs in 1% to 3%, and death in less than 1%.[29] Despite the early success rate, it has been estimated that 25% to 50% of patients require repeat coronary intervention due to restenosis, incomplete revascularization, or disease progression.[56] Perhaps the greatest limitation of angioplasty has been the threat of restenosis. Depending on a number of factors, restenosis occurs in 10% to 50% of lesions. The mechanisms accounting for restenosis include elastic recoil, accelerated atherosclerosis, and neointimal hyperplasia. This neointimal hyperplasia results from the response to the injury of the intima that is a necessary component of the angioplasty.

A number of situations are associated with increased risk of restenosis. These include coronary spasm, lesion location (left anterior descending greater than right or circumflex artery), serum lipid concentrations, presence of unstable angina, previous angioplasty, and multivessel disease. In addition, saphenous vein grafts have been shown to have the highest rate of restenosis.[57] A variety of pharmacologic regimens were studied in an effort to alleviate the threat of restenosis. The studies included trials of anticoagulation, antiplatelet agents, steroids, antimitotic agents such as colchicine, vasoactive agents (calcium channel blockers and angiotensin-converting enzyme [ACE] inhibitors), and lipid-lowering agents. None of these trials demonstrated any significant reductions in the risk of restenosis. Due to the disappointing results associated with systemic administration of these pharmacologic agents, interest has developed in the potential of local drug delivery to limit the rate of restenosis. To date there are no studies demonstrating efficacy to this approach. The recent proliferation of stent appears to have had a favorable effect on the incidence of restenosis; however, the problem has not been eliminated. Efforts continue to develop mechanical and biologic solutions to the problem of restenosis.

Factors Affecting Risk

There are a number of clinical factors that appear to affect the risk of complications occurring with angioplasty. Patients undergoing percutaneous intervention in the setting of an acute ischemic syndrome (unstable angina, myocardial infarction) are at increased risk of abrupt vessel closure and thrombosis.[7-9,25,35,45] The development of platelet IIb/IIIa inhibitors has significantly lowered this risk, allowing complication rates similar to those for patients with stable angina.[20] Older patients also appear to be at increased risk of complications.[10,32] The higher incidence of calcified lesion and more diffuse disease may account for this increased risk.[14] In addition patients who have either low (<25 kg/m^2) or high (>35 kg/m^2) body mass index are at increased risk.[16]

There are a number of anatomic features that affect the procedural success of angioplasty. A scoring system was codified by the American College of Cardiology and subsequently modified by Ellis that defined the expected success and risk of intervening on a particular lesion. Variables included lesion length and morphology, tortuosity of the vessel, presence or absence of thrombus, and a number of other variables.[15] This classification system, however, appears to be becoming outdated with the advent of new techniques, pharmacologic agents, and increased operator experience. Certain factors remain important in evaluating a lesion for percutaneous interventions. These factors include the ability to access the lesion, ability to cross the lesion with the interventional device (e.g., balloon, atherectomy catheter, stents), and the characteristics of the lesion. The characteristics of the lesion that affect intervention include the presence and severity of calcification, presence of thrombus, proximity to side branches or bifurcation, and the presence or absence of collateral vessels supplying or being supplied by the target vessel. The presence of significant calcium at the site of intervention interferes with the ability to successfully perform the intervention and often necessitates the use of adjuvant devices (i.e., rotational atherectomy). Branch vessels increase the complexity of the intervention as well as the risk of complications due to the potential of closure of these side branches. If the target vessel is supplied by collateral, the risk of the procedure is diminished. However, if the target vessel supplies collaterals to other vessels, the risk of the procedure is increased.

Operator experience also appears to impact on both procedural success and the treatment of complications associated with PTCA.[17,31] A number of reports have shown a direct correlation between operator caseload and lower complication rates.[27] The risk of death in association with angioplasty is related to the amount of myocardium that is jeopardized by an abrupt vessel closure. The risk of death is significantly increased when there is a large amount of ischemic or nonfunctional myocardium. A successful angioplasty procedure is likely to occur if the following factors are present:

1. Experienced operator at a high-volume institution
2. Patient-related factors include younger age, male gender, and no history of diabetes mellitus, prior myocardial infarction, prior bypass surgery, or impaired left ventricular function
3. Favorable angiographic appearance defined as a discrete (<10 mm length), concentric, readily accessible, nonangulated segment with smooth contour, little or no calcification, less than totally occlusive, not ostial in location, without major side branch involvement, and with absence of thrombus.

Newer Technology

Simpson developed directional coronary atherectomy (DCA), which was first used in the peripheral circulation in 1985, and was subsequently extended to the coronary circulation. DCA was designed to remove atheromatous tissue and improve the angiographic results relative to PTCA. Initially the device was targeted for those lesions that were not effectively treated with balloon angioplasty, including aortoostial lesions, bifurcation lesions, and lesions with a large amount of atheromatous material. The first randomized trial of DCA, the CAVEAT trial, compared the technique with balloon angioplasty in native coronary arteries. In this trial, no significant benefit in terms of restenosis was found, and there was an increase in the risk for non–Q wave myocardial infarction in the DCA group.[52] One-year follow-up showed an excess mortality in the DCA group. CAVEAT 2 tested DCA in saphenous vein grafts; however, no benefit of DCA compared with balloon angioplasty was found.[28] The BOAT trial attempted to optimize the use of DCA by more vigorous removal of tissue. The investigators found that by utilizing this technique, incidence of restenosis was 32% in the DCA group compared with 40% in the balloon group.[3] Nevertheless, DCA has fallen out of favor, especially with the advent and widespread use of stents. Although DCA provides excellent angiographic results when used by experienced operators, no significant improvement in clinical outcome has been demonstrated. Furthermore the technique is more tedious and time-consuming, and fails to achieve the same clinical benefits as stenting.

The transluminal endarterectomy atherectomy catheter (TEC) was designed by Stack to cut and aspirate atheroma. The role of TEC in percutaneous interventions remains controversial; however, it may have a role in degenerating saphenous vein bypass grafts and/or thrombotic lesions. In contrast to DCA and TEC, rotational atherectomy removes plaque by abrading it and dispersing the debris into the distal vessels. The major indication for rotational atherectomy is in calcified lesions. It also appears to have a role in "pretreating" lesions that cannot be crossed with an angioplasty balloon, ostial lesions, bifurcation lesions, and distal lesions.

The rotational atherectomy device (Rotoblator) spins at a speed of 150,000 to 200,000 rpm and ablates tissue. The ablated tissues are sent downstream and removed in the microcirculation. Overly vigorous advancement of the device can result in the generation of larger particles that can lead to obstruction of the microcirculation or to dissection of the vessel. It is targeted for patients with calcific lesions and those who cannot be successfully dilated with balloon angioplasty. The device does not improve the risk of restenosis.

Despite initial enthusiasm, laser angioplasty has been disappointing. The laser ablates tissue by vaporization and shock waves. The ERBAC demonstrated no advantage in terms of restenosis. When compared with the NACI registry, lasers appear to have a higher complication risk. The lesions most suitable for laser therapy include aortoostial lesions, undilatable lesions, total occlusions, calcified lesions, and long lesions. Lesions that are contraindicated for use of the laser include those in tortuous segments, those containing thrombus, and those at the site of bifurcation. Ongoing research efforts with laser angioplasty include investigating its use in stent restenosis and the use of a "laser wire" to cross total chronic occlusions. In addition, lasers may have applicability in treated diffuse stent restenosis.

The greatest advances in percutaneous intervention since the development of balloon angioplasty have come from application of stents. Stents provide a scaffold that is designed to enlarge the lumen and seal dissections associated with coronary angioplasty. Stent design varies considerably and includes meshes, slotted tubes, coils, and rings. They can be made of stainless steel, nitinol, tantalum, or a number of other materials. Newer stent designs included heparin-coated stents and radioactive stents, both designed to further reduce the risk of restenosis. The Belgium Netherlands Stent Trial (BENESTENT) and the Stent Restenosis Trial (STENT) demonstrated that intracoronary stents reduced the incidence of angiographic restenosis in patients undergoing an initial percutaneous coronary intervention.[22,49] Restenosis rates for those patients treated with stents were lowered from 42% to 32% in STRESS and from 32% to 22% in BENESTENT. The initial limitation to stenting was the risk of stent thrombosis; subsequently efforts were aimed at reducing the risk of thrombosis. Vigorous anticoagulation regimens were developed that led to marked reductions in stent thrombosis; however, there was a significant excess risk of bleeding due to these regimens.

Positive clinical results increased with the improvements in achieving complete stent deployment and the discovery that antiplatelet therapy with ticlopidine and aspirin would effectively prevent subacute thrombosis. The ISAR trial demonstrated that ticlopidine effectively prevented subacute stent thrombosis while reducing the risk of bleeding that was associated with more vigorous anticoagulation regimens that included warfarin.[47] Aspirin alone was shown to be inadequate in the prevention of stent thrombosis in the STARS trial.[38] Clopidogel is the subject of a number of ongoing trials; earlier results suggest that it is likely to be a safe alternative (in addition to aspirin) to ticlopidine for patients undergoing revascularization with a stent. These interventions led to reductions in subacute thrombosis, bleeding complications, and hospital length of stay. As a result of these studies, stent deployment is rapidly growing, with many centers utilizing stents in the majority of their percutaneous interventions. Further economic analyses are necessary to determine the cost-effectiveness of stenting relative to balloon angioplasty. The greatest question remains the overall impact of stenting on clinical outcome in patients with multivessel disease relative to surgical revascularization. Two ongoing trials, ARTS and SOS, are evaluating the impact of an initial strategy of multivessel stenting vs. surgical revascularization on death, myocardial infarction, and need for revascularization.

There has been a tremendous proliferation in the design and availability of new stents. Currently over 40 stents are being used worldwide. These newer stents broaden the applicability of the device to other lesions and locations. Despite the enthusiasm for stenting, problems do remain. Although the rate of restenosis is reduced with stenting, stent restenosis is more difficult to treat and less likely to respond to redilation.

Coronary Revascularization and Acute Coronary Syndromes

The overall success rate for percutaneous intervention for patients with unstable angina is somewhat lower than patients undergoing the procedure for stable angina. Patients with unstable angina have a higher mortality, risk of myocardial infarction, and need for emergency coronary artery bypass surgery. It is thought that the increased risk of complications is due to increased thrombotic milieu that accompanies acute ischemic syndromes. These patients have increased platelet reactivity and vasospasm, putting them at increased risk of acute vessel closure. The risk associated with percutaneous intervention for unstable angina appears to diminish if there is an initial period of "stabilization" prior to the intervention.

New pharmacologic intervention has had an impact on the risk of PCI in the setting of acute ischemic syndromes. Platelet aggregation occurs as a consequence of fibrinogen binding to platelets and allowing for cross bridging of platelets, resulting in a platelet plug. The glycoprotein IIb/IIIa receptor mediates the binding of fibrinogen to the platelet surface. This receptor is expressed once platelets are activated; it is the final common step in platelet activation regardless of the stimulus for platelet activation. The first randomized control trial of a IIb/IIIa receptor inhibitor was the Evaluation of 7E3 in Preventing Acute Ischemic Complications Trial (EPIC).[19] EPIC studied abciximab, a monoclonal antibody to the IIb/IIIa receptor, in patients with unstable angina or high-risk lesion who were to undergo angioplasty. It demonstrated that this IIb/IIIa receptor blockade results in a clinically and statistically significant reduction in the risk of acute complications. Furthermore, the benefits achieved have been maintained over a 3-year follow-up. In this study, however, patients treated with abciximab had a significantly increased risk of bleeding. Follow-up studies, including EPILOGUE, demonstrated that similar efficacy could be achieved with lower risk of bleeding by adjusting the dose of the heparin that was used concomitantly.[200]

EXPERIMENTAL TECHNIQUES

Transmyocardial Laser Revascularization

Transmyocardial laser revascularization (TMR) has been introduced for the treatment of refractory angina (class IV) in patients who are not candidates for CABG or catheter-based revascularization. Clinical trials of TMR have demonstrated significant improvements in angina class, decreased need for antianginal medications, and fewer hospitalizations for angina. Operative mortality in stable patients with class IV angina has been acceptable. The procedure consists of a standard left anterolateral thoracotomy, and dissection of the pericardium, creating a cradle. Using a laser system with variable output, frequency, and pulse width, transmural channels are made beginning in the area of reversible ischemia on the basis of preoperative thallium studies or coronary artery anatomy and clinical judgment if the patient had not been able to tolerate a preoperative thallium perfusion study. Laser channels are placed about 1 cm apart to provide a distribution of 1 laser channel per cm^2. A mean of 30 to 40 laser channels is made. Bleeding from the channels is controlled with digital pressure or, rarely, an epicardial suture. After creation of the transmural channels, a pericardial chest tube is placed and standard wound closure is performed.[11]

Brachytherapy

The effect of radiation therapy for the prevention of restenosis was tested initially using external beam radiation. Early reports suggested the effectiveness of this treatment in reducing neointimal formation postvascular injury in experimental models, but the findings of accelerated atherosclerosis and vascular injury following radiation therapy for patients undergoing cancer treatment further delayed investigation of radiation as a mode of therapy with potential for vascular applications.

In 1965 Friedman described the potential of endovascular radiation to prevent restenosis in an injured atherosclerotic rabbit aorta that inhibited smooth muscle cell proliferation. Liermann and Schoppol in 1991 started using endovascular radiation to prevent restenosis in the peripheral vascular system. These investigators have recently reported an 80% patency rate at 5-year follow-up using endovascular gamma radiation with 192-iridium.

In 1992, Waksman, Weinberger, and Raizner initiated studies to determine the effectiveness of intracoronary radiation therapy against restenosis following balloon overstretch injury with and without stenting in animal models. These animal models utilized both γ- and β-isotopes, demonstrating nearly complete inhibition of neointimal formation at 2 and 4 weeks following vascular injury. Hehrlein and Fischell began utilizing endovascular brachytherapy using radioactive stents. This concept was tested and found to be effective and safe in animal models. Clinical studies have subsequently been initiated to determine the effectiveness of this therapy in humans. In 1994 the first patient was treated with intracoronary radiation after balloon angioplasty utilizing a wire that hand-delivered 192-iridium into a close-end lumen catheter. The BERT study utilized 90-Sr/Y as a pure β-emitter. The SCRIPPS trial was a randomized double-blind trial that studied 55 patients with restenosis, demonstrating a significant reduction of restenosis rates by angiographic findings, intravascular ultrasound (IVUS), and clinical events. The BETA WRIST trial demonstrated that patients with in-stent restenosis treated with β-radiation utilizing a 90-yttrium source had lower than expected rates of angiographic and clinical restenosis.[55] Additional trials of brachytherapy are ongoing.

Growth Factors

Delivering treatment directly to the myocardium and the coronary arteries promises a revolution in the management of serious and life-threatening cardiac diseases. The pericardial sac provides the route for a variety of treatments aimed directly at the subepicardial structures, essentially within the epicardium. This technique utilizes therapeutic agents in concentrations that could not be tolerated systemically, as well as angiogenic factors to increase vascularity in patients with subacute and chronic coronary artery disease who are not good candidates for other types of revascularization. The elevated levels of various angiogenic cytokines in patients with myocardial ischemia indicate a potential role of the pericardium in ischemia-induced angiogenesis. Intrapericardial or epicardial administration of these cytokines appears to result in functionally significant angiogenesis in animal models of chronic myocardial ischemia. In a recent study, Laham and collaborators demonstrated the ability of a single bolus injection of basic-fibroblast growth factor (bFGF) into the pericardial space to induce myocardial angiogenesis and improve regional perfusion, regional left ventricular function, and microvascular reactivity, and to increase angiographically visible collaterals and magnetic resonance-detected collaterals. Thus the pericardial space offers an attractive drug delivery reservoir that might be used to deliver therapeutic substances to the heart.[51]

REFERENCES

1. ACC/AHA Task Force Report: Guidelines and indications for coronary artery bypass graft surgery, *J Am Coll Cardiol* 17:543-589, 1991.
2. Alderman EL, et al: Ten-year follow-up of survival and myocardial infarction in the randomized coronary artery surgery study, *Circulation* 82:1629-1646, 1990.
3. Baim DS, et al: Final results of the Balloon vs. Optimal Atherectomy Trial (BOAT), *Circulation* 97:322-331, 1998.
4. Borst C, et al: Minimally invasive coronary artery bypass grafting: on the beating heart and via limited access, *Ann Thorac Surg* 63:S1-S5, 1997.
5. Bourassa MG, et al: Bypass Angioplasty Revascularization Investigation: patient screening, selection, and recruitment, *Am J Cardiol* 75:3C, 1995.
6. Bypass Angioplasty Revascularization Investigation (BARI) Investigators: Comparison of coronary bypass surgery with angioplasty in patients with multivessel disease, *N Engl J Med* 331:1179, 1994.
7. DeFeyter PJ, et al: Coronary angioplasty for early post-infarction unstable angina, *Circulation* 74:1365-1370, 1986.
8. De Feyter PJ, Serruys PW, Wijns W, et al: Emergency PTCA in unstable angina pectoris refractory to optimal medical treatment, *N Engl J Med* 313:342-346, 1985.
9. De Feyter PJ, Surypranta H, Serruys PW, et al: Coronary angioplasty for unstable angina: immediate and late results in 200 consecutive patients with identification of risk factors for unfavorable early and late outcome, *J Am Coll Cardiol* 12:324-333, 1988.
10. de Jaegere P, et al: Immediate and long-term results of percutaneous coronary angioplasty in patients aged 70 and over, *Br Heart J* 67:138-143, 1992.
11. Dowling RD, et al: Transmyocardial revascularization in patients with refractory unstable angina, *Circulation* 98:73-76, 1998.
12. Edwards FH, Clark RE, Schwartz M: Impact of internal mammary artery conduits and operative mortality in coronary revascularization, *Ann Thorac Surg* 56:27, 1994.
13. Edwards FH, Clark RE, Schwartz M: Coronary artery bypass grafting: The Society of Thoracic Surgeons National Database Experience, *Ann Thorac Surg* 57:12, 1994.
14. Ellis SG, et al: Angiographic and clinical predictors of acute closure after native vessel coronary angioplasty, *Circulation* 77:372-379, 1988.
15. Ellis SG, et al: Coronary morphologic and clinical determinants of procedural outcome with angioplasty for multivessel coronary disease: implications for patient selection, *Circulation* 82:1193-1202, 1990.
16. Ellis SG, et al: Low-normal or excessive body mass index: newly identified and powerful risk factors for death and other complications with percutaneous coronary intervention, *Am J Cardiol* 78:642-646, 1996.
17. Ellis SG, Weintraub W, Holmes D, et al: Relation of operator coronary revascularization at hospitals with high interventional volumes, *Circulation* 95:2479-2484, 1997.
18. Emlein G, et al: Prolonged bradyarrhythmias after isolated coronary artery bypass graft surgery, *Am Heart J* 126:1084, 1993.
19. EPIC Investigators: Use of a monoclonal antibody directed against the platelet glycoprotein IIb/IIIa receptor in high-risk coronary angioplasty, *N Engl J Med* 330:956-961, 1994.
20. EPILOGUE Investigators: Platelet glycoprotein IIb/IIIa receptor blockade and low-dose heparin during percutaneous coronary revascularization, *N Engl J Med* 336:1689-1696, 1997.
21. Reference deleted in pages.
22. Fischman DL, et al, for the Stent Restenosis Study investigators: A randomized comparison of coronary-stent placement and balloon angioplasty in the treatment of coronary artery disease, *N Engl J Med* 331:496-501, 1994.
23. Folland ED, Hartigan PM, Parisi AF, for the Veterans Affairs ACME Investigators: Percutaneous transluminal coronary angioplasty versus medical therapy for stable angina pectoris: outcomes for patients with double-vessel versus single-vessel coronary artery disease in a Veterans Affairs cooperative randomized trial, *J Am Coll Cardiol* 29:1505, 1997.
24. Frost L, et al: Atrial fibrillation and flutter after coronary artery bypass surgery: epidemiology, risk factors and preventive trials, *Int J Cardiol* 36:253, 1992.
25. Gottlieb SO, Walford GD, Ouyang P, et al: Initial and late results of coronary angioplasty for early postinfarction unstable angina, *Cathet Cardiovasc Diagn* 13:93-99, 1987.
26. Gruentzig AR: Transluminal dilation of coronary artery stenosis (letter), *Lancet* 1:263, 1978.
27. Hannan EL, et al: Coronary angioplasty volume-outcome relationships for hospitals and cardiologists, *JAMA* 279:892-898, 1997.
28. Holmes D, et al: A multicenter, randomized trial of coronary angioplasty versus directional atherectomy for patients with saphenous vein bypass graft lesions, *Circulation* 91:1966-1974, 1995.
29. Holmes DR Jr, et al: Co-investigators of the National Heart, Lung, and Blood Institute Angioplasty Registry: Comparison of complications during percutaneous transluminal angioplasty from 1977-1981 and from 1985-1986: The National Heart, Lung, and Blood Institute Angioplasty Registry, *J Am Coll Cardiol* 12:1149-1155, 1988.
30. Hornick P, Smith PL, Taylor KM: Cerebral complications after coronary bypass grafting, *Curr Opin Cardiol* 9:670, 1994.
31. Jollis JG, et al: Relationship between physician and hospital coronary angioplasty volume and outcome in elderly patients, *Circulation* 95:2485-2491, 1997.
32. Kern MJ, et al: Percutaneous transluminal coronary angioplasty in octogenarians, *Am J Cardiol* 61:457-458, 1988.
33. King SB III, et al: Emory Angioplasty versus Surgery Trial (EAST): Design, recruitment, and baseline description of patients, *Am J Cardiol* 75:42C, 1995.

34. King SB III, et al: Randomized trial comparing coronary angioplasty with coronary bypass surgery, *N Engl J Med* 331:1044, 1994.
35. King SB III, Douglas JS Jr: Coronary plaque morphology in postinfarction patients: implications for early versus deferred coronary angioplasty, *J Am Coll Cardiol* 16:1807-1088, 1990.
36. Kirklin JW, et al: ACC/AHA Task Force Report: Guidelines and indications for coronary artery bypass graft surgery, *J Am Coll Cardiol* 17:543-589, 1991.
37. Kirklin JW, Naftel DC, Blackstone EH, et al: Summary of a consensus concerning death and ischemic events after coronary artery bypass grafting, *Circulation* 79(Suppl):81, 1989.
38. Leon MB, et al: Clinical and angiographic results from the stent anticoagulation regimen study (STARS) (abstract), *Circulation* 94(suppl I):I-685, 1996.
39. Loop FD, et al: Sternal wound complications after isolated coronary bypass grafting: early and late mortality, morbidity and cost of care, *Ann Thorac Surg* 49:179, 1990.
40. Lyte BW, Cosgrove D, Loop FD: Future implications of current trends in bypass surgery, *Cardiovasc Clin* 21:265, 1991.
41. Nwasokwa ON, et al: Bypass surgery for chronic stable angina: predictors of survival benefit and strategy for patient selection, *Ann Intern Med* 114:1035-1049, 1991.
42. Parisi AF, Folland ED, Hartigan P, for the Veterans Affairs ACME Investigators: A comparison of angioplasty with medical therapy in the treatment of single vessel coronary artery disease, *N Engl J Med* 326:10, 1992.
43. RITA-2 Trial Participants: Coronary angioplasty versus medical therapy for angina: The second Randomized Intervention Treatment of Angina (RITA-2) trial, *Lancet* 350:461, 1997.
44. Ryan TJ, et al: ACC/AHA Task Force Report: Guidelines for percutaneous transluminal coronary angioplasty, *J Am Coll Cardiol* 22:2033-2054, 1993.
45. Safian RD, Synder LD, Synder BA, et al: Usefulness of percutaneous transluminal coronary angioplasty for unstable angina pectoris after non–Q wave acute myocardial infarction, *Am J Cardiol* 59:263-266, 1987.
46. Schaff HV, Gersh BJ, Fisher LD: Detrimental effect of perioperative myocardial infarction on late survival after coronary artery bypass, *J Thorac Cardiovasc Surg* 88:972, 1984.
47. Schomig A, et al: A randomized comparison of antiplatelet and anticoagulant therapy after the placement of coronary-artery stents, *N Engl J Med* 334:1084-1089, 1996.
48. Sergeant P, Lessafre E, Flameng W, et al: Internal mammary artery: methods of use and their effect in survival, *Eur J Cardiothorac Surg* 4:72-78, 1990.
49. Serruys PW, et al, for the BENESTENT Study Group: A comparison of balloon-expandable-stent implantation with balloon angioplasty in patients with coronary artery disease, *N Engl J Med* 331:489-495, 1994.
50. Shainoff JR, et al: Low factor XIIIA levels are associated with increased blood loss after coronary artery bypass grafting, *J Thorac Cardiovasc Surg* 108:437, 1994.
51. Spodick DH, et al: Intrapericardial therapeutic and diagnostics, *Clin Cardiol* 22(Suppl I):I-1, I-8, 1999.
52. Topol E, et al: A comparison of directional atherectomy with coronary angioplasty in patients with coronary artery disease, *N Engl J Med* 329:221-227, 1993.
53. Varnauskas E: Twelve-year follow-up of survival in the randomized European Coronary Surgery Study, *N Engl J Med* 319:332-337, 1988.
54. Veterans Administration Coronary Artery Bypass Surgery Cooperative Study Group: Eleven-year survival in the Veterans Administration Randomized Trial of Coronary Bypass Surgery for Stable Angina, *N Engl J Med* 311:1333-1339, 1984.
55. Waksman R, Bhargava B, White L, et al: Intracoronary β-radiation therapy inhibits recurrence of in-stent restenosis, *Circulation* 101:1895-1898, 2000.
56. Webb JG, et al: Bidirectional crossover and late outcome after coronary angioplasty and bypass surgery: 8 to 11 year follow-up, *J Am Coll Cardiol* 16:57, 1990.
57. Wong SC, et al: Stents improve late clinical outcomes: results from the combined (I%II) Stress Restenosis Study, *Circulation* 92(Suppl):I-281, 1995.

CHAPTER 65

Heart Failure

Michael M. Givertz
Wilson S. Colucci

DEFINITION

Heart failure, often referred to as congestive heart failure, is a clinical syndrome resulting from cardiac decompensation and characterized by signs and symptoms of interstitial volume overload and/or inadequate tissue perfusion. In pathophysiologic terms, heart failure occurs when the heart is unable to pump blood at a rate sufficient to meet the metabolic needs of the body or when it can do so only with an elevated filling pressure. The contractile performance of the heart may be preserved when impairment of cardiac filling or emptying leads to symptoms and signs of heart failure. Myocardial failure, a term used to denote abnormal systolic or diastolic function, may be asymptomatic or progress to heart failure. Circulatory failure is not synonymous with heart failure, since a variety of noncardiac conditions (e.g., hemorrhagic shock) can lead to circulatory collapse while cardiac function is preserved.

EPIDEMIOLOGY

Incidence and Prevalence

Heart failure is a major cause of morbidity and mortality in the United States. It is estimated that 4.8 million Americans suffer from heart failure (~2% of the population), with greater than 400,000 new cases diagnosed each year. The prevalence of heart failure increases dramatically with age, occurring in 1% to 2% of patients aged 50 to 59, and up to 10% of patients over the age of 75[10] (Fig. 65-1). Heart failure is the leading discharge diagnosis in Medicare patients. Despite a steady decrease in the incidence of coronary artery disease and stroke, the prevalence of heart failure continues to rise. This may be due in part to the aging of the population and the improved survival of patients with cardiovascular disease. Heart failure has an enormous economic impact on the U.S. health care system due to direct medical costs, disability, and loss of employment. Estimated treatment costs in 1994 were $38 billion, of which $23 billion was spent on hospitalizations.

Prognosis

Once heart failure is diagnosed, the prognosis is poor. The overall 5-year mortality for all patients with heart failure is approximately 50%, and the 1-year mortality in patients with severe heart failure may be as high as 35% to 40%. In the United States alone, approximately 250,000 patients die of heart failure each year. Recent data from the Framingham Heart Study showed a median survival of 1.7 years for men and 3.2 years for women[9] (Fig. 65-2). Over 90% of deaths are due to cardiovascular causes, most commonly progressive heart failure or sudden cardiac death. Several clinical and laboratory parameters have been shown to be important independent predictors of mortality in heart failure (Box 65-1).

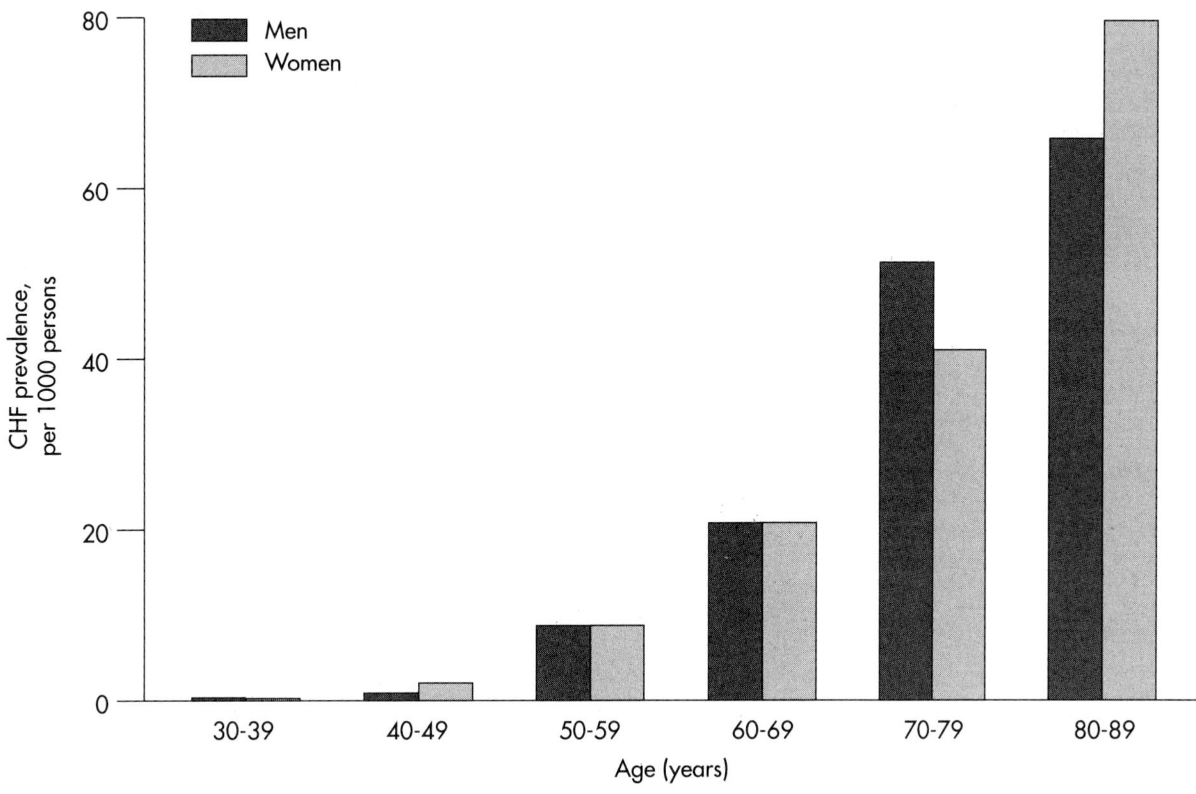

Fig. 65-1. Prevalence rates of congestive heart failure (CHF) among Framingham Heart Study subjects, by gender and age. Among men, the prevalence increased from 8 cases/1000 in those aged 50-59 years to 66 cases/1000 in those aged 80-89 years. Among women, the prevalence increased from 8 cases/1000 in those aged 50-59 years to 79 cases/1000 in those aged 80-89 years. (Modified from Ho KK, Pinsky JL, Kannel WB, et al: *J Am Coll Cardiol* 22:6A-13A, 1993.)

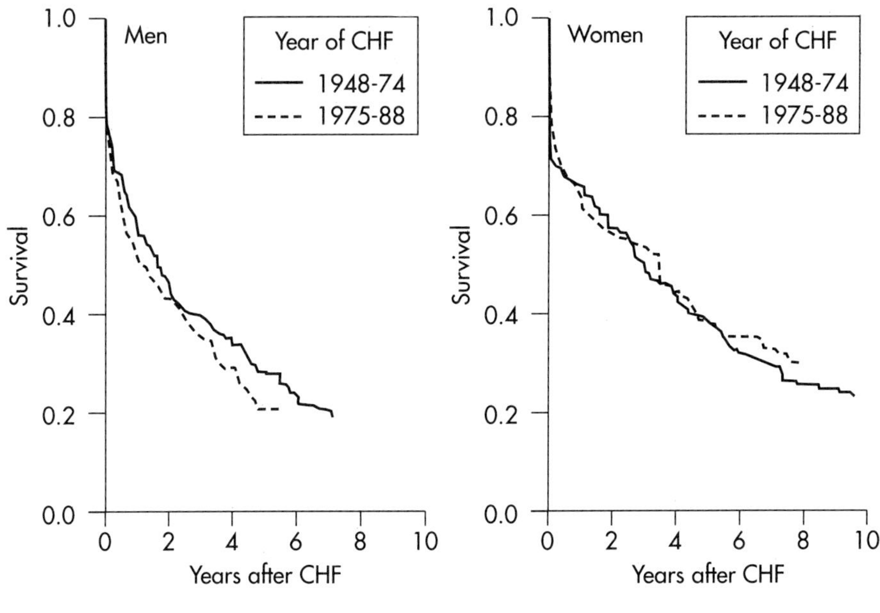

Fig. 65-2. Survival after the onset of heart failure in Framingham Heart Study subjects. Graphs show age-adjusted survival rates after congestive heart failure (CHF) by calendar year of first diagnosis of CHF for men and women developing CHF during the calendar years 1948-1988. (Modified from Ho KK, Anderson KM, Kannel WB, et al: *Circulation* 88:107-115, 1993.)

Box 65-1. Negative Prognostic Factors

Clinical

Increasing age
Diabetes
Smoking or alcohol use
Increased NYHA class

Laboratory

Hyponatremia
Elevated plasma neurohormones (e.g., norepinephrine, renin, endothelin-1)

Hemodynamic

Reduced left and/or right ventricular ejection fraction
Increased pulmonary capillary wedge pressure
Decreased cardiac index
Reduced peak oxygen consumption

Electrophysiologic

Atrial fibrillation or flutter
Ventricular ectopic activity
Ventricular tachycardia or sudden death

NYHA, New York Heart Association.

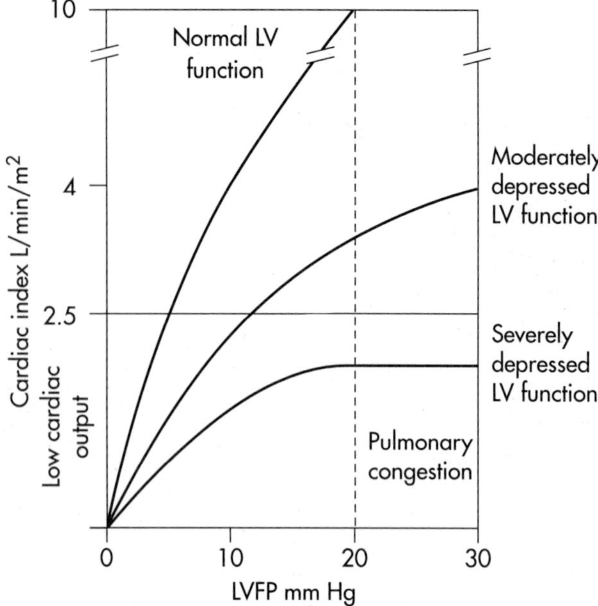

Fig. 65-3. Ventricular function curves depicting the relation between left ventricular filling pressure (LVFP) and cardiac index based on the Frank-Starling mechanism for normal and moderately and severely decompensated hearts. Values for cardiac index below 2.5 L/min/m^2 are associated with low cardiac output and diminished tissue perfusion. Values for LVFP greater than 20 mm Hg are associated with pulmonary congestion.

PATHOPHYSIOLOGY

Ventricular performance may be quantified by the amount of blood that the heart is able to pump each minute, also termed the *cardiac output*. Cardiac output (liters per minute) is equal to the stroke volume (liters/beat) times the heart rate (beats/min). In the intact human heart, the three main determinants of stroke volume are preload, afterload, and cardiac contractility.

Preload

Preload refers to the passive stretch on the myocardium just prior to contraction, or the ventricular wall tension at the end of diastole. In the intact heart, preload corresponds to the end-diastolic volume or end-diastolic pressure. In clinical terms, left ventricular end-diastolic pressure may be approximated by the pulmonary capillary wedge pressure, whereas right ventricular filling pressure is reflected by central venous or right atrial pressure. According to Starling's law, the higher the preload, the greater the force of ventricular contraction and the greater the stroke volume. When heart failure develops, cardiac output may be maintained within normal limits by an increase in preload. Diastolic filling increases in part due to an increase in venous return resulting from vasoconstriction and intravascular volume expansion. However, in severe heart failure, the ventricular function curve may be flat at higher end-diastolic volumes; thus cardiac output may not be augmented by an increase in filling, and a marked increase in end-diastolic pressure causes pulmonary venous congestion (Fig. 65-3).

Afterload

Afterload refers to the ventricular wall stress during systole or the force that the ventricle must overcome to eject its contents. According to Laplace's law, systolic wall stress is directly proportional to ventricular pressure and chamber radius and inversely proportional to ventricular wall thickness. The major determinant of left ventricular afterload is systemic vascular resistance. Afterload is typically increased in systemic hypertension and aortic stenosis. Additionally, in patients with heart failure and reduced left ventricular (LV) systolic function, systemic vascular resistance may be increased secondary to neurohormonal activation (see below).

Contractility

Contractility or inotropic state is a fundamental property of the myocardium that determines the strength of contraction. At a constant preload and afterload, an increase in contractility results in an increase in the extent and velocity of fiber shortening. Circulating catecholamines or positive inotropic agents such as digoxin may increase contractility. By contrast, negative inotropic agents such as calcium channel blockers, myocyte loss, or acidosis may decrease contractility. In the clinical setting, contractility is difficult to measure. Commonly used measures of LV performance such as ejection fraction may be altered by changes in preload and afterload and thus do not necessarily reflect changes in contractility. Isovolumic indices of cardiac performance, such as the peak rate of rise of LV pressure (peak % dP/dt), are not used clinically because of the need for invasive measurements and their dependence on cardiac loading conditions. Recently, use of the pressure-volume relationship to determine end-systolic elastance has been suggested as a load-independent method of assessing myocardial contractility.

Systolic and Diastolic Dysfunction

Most commonly, heart failure reflects an abnormality of ventricular contractile function (Fig. 65-4). End-systolic

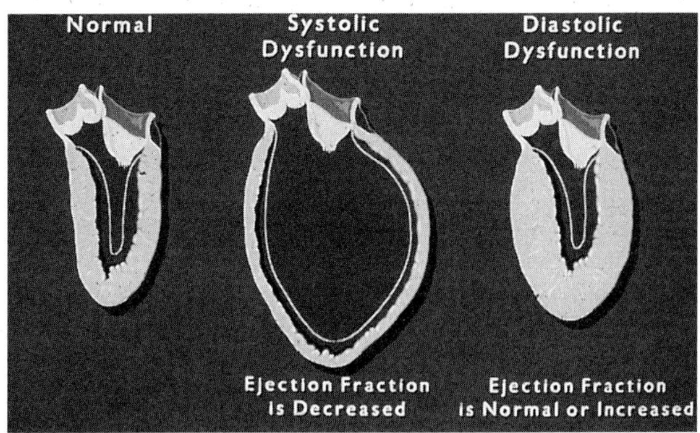

Fig. 65-4. Systolic and diastolic LV dysfunction compared with normal left ventricular function. Solid lines indicate the extent of ventricular contraction during systole.

Table 65-1. Systolic vs. Diastolic Dysfunction

Parameter	Systolic	Diastolic
History		
Coronary artery disease	++++	++
Hypertension	++	++++
Diabetes	+++	++
Physical Examination		
Cardiomegaly	+++	+
S_3 gallop	+++	+
S_4 gallop	+	+++
Rales	++	++
Peripheral edema	+++	+
Electrocardiogram		
Low voltage	+++	–
Left ventricular hypertrophy	++	++++
Echocardiogram		
Low ejection fraction	++++	–
Left ventricular hypertrophy	++	++++

Modified from Young JB: Assessment of heart failure. In Colucci WS, editor: *Heart failure: cardiac function and dysfunction.* In Braunwald E, series editor: *Atlas of heart disease,* ed 2, Philadelphia, 1999, Current Medicine, pp 7.1-7.19.

volume, end-diastolic volume, and end-diastolic pressure are increased, and stroke volume falls. Symptoms of reduced cardiac output (e.g., fatigue) develop. In addition, increased LV end-diastolic pressure is transmitted back to the pulmonary veins, resulting in transudation of fluid into the pulmonary interstitium and symptoms of pulmonary congestion. The most common cause of contractile dysfunction is loss of myocytes due to myocardial infarction. Other causes of systolic heart failure include dilated cardiomyopathy, myocarditis, and chronic alcohol use.

One third to one half of patients with heart failure have normal ventricular contractile function, and are said to have diastolic heart failure[1] (Table 65-1). Abnormal diastolic function may be due to impaired early relaxation, increased stiffness of the ventricle, or both. Diastolic dysfunction results in impairment in ventricular filling. LV end-diastolic pressures are elevated, leading to pulmonary venous congestion. Diastolic dysfunction is most commonly associated with left ventricular hypertrophy (LVH) due to hypertension, and occurs frequently in elderly women. Increased resistance to filling results from the increased LV mass itself, and also from interstitial fibrosis and subendocardial ischemia. Diastolic dysfunction can occur in the absence of LVH due to ischemia, myocardial infiltration (e.g., amyloidosis), or pericardial constriction.

The most common form of heart failure, that due to coronary artery disease, often reflects a combination of systolic and diastolic dysfunction. Systolic dysfunction is due to prior infarction and ischemia-induced decrease in contractility. Diastolic dysfunction is due to chronic replacement fibrosis and ischemia-induced decrease in distensibility.

Myocardial Hypertrophy and Remodeling

Increased ventricular wall stress due to LV dilation or increased afterload stimulates the development of myocardial hypertrophy. Increased wall thickness, in turn, normalizes wall stress and helps to maintain normal contractile function. When the primary stimulus to remodeling is chronic volume overload, the radius of the ventricle enlarges in proportion to a mild increase in wall thickness. By contrast, chronic pressure overload results in a moderate to severe increase in wall thickness. If additional chamber dilation occurs or the increase in wall thickness is insufficient, systolic and diastolic wall stresses remain abnormally elevated, and hemodynamic failure ensues.

Cellular events contributing to ventricular remodeling include increases in mitochondrial and myofibrillar mass and myocyte size, and alterations in the quantity and composition of the extracellular matrix. Molecular events include the regression to a molecular phenotype characterized by the expression of fetal genes and the production of abnormal contractile proteins. In addition to mechanical stress, other factors that contribute to myocardial hypertrophy and remodeling in heart failure include neurohormones such as angiotensin and norepinephrine, ischemia, and inflammatory cytokines. These mediators also cause loss of myocytes due to both necrosis and apoptosis (programmed cell death)[3] (Fig. 65-5).

Neurohormonal Activation

Reduced cardiac output and increased filling pressures cause activation of several important neurohormonal systems, including the sympathetic nervous system and the renin-angiotensin system. Primary consequences of neurohormonal activation include an increase in systemic vascular resistance and sodium and water retention. During an initial compensatory phase, cardiac output, blood pressure, and vital organ perfusion are maintained. If chronic, neurohormonal activation may lead to decompensation due to excessive vasoconstriction and volume retention, electrolyte abnormalities, direct myocardial toxicity, and cardiac arrhythmias.

Autonomic Nervous System. Decreased perfusion pressure sensed by carotid sinus and aortic arch receptors results in increased sympathetic and decreased parasympathetic tone. Circulating catecholamines are elevated, and direct sympathetic outflow to the heart, peripheral vasculature, and

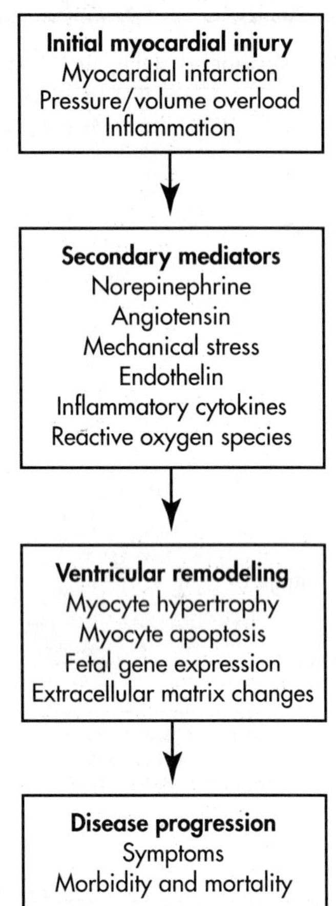

Fig. 65-5. Proposed sequence of events in the progression of myocardial failure. After an initial injury, various secondary mediators such as norepinephrine, angiotensin, and mechanical stress act on the myocardium to cause ventricular remodeling. Recent studies suggest that additional mediators, including endothelin, cytokines, and reactive oxygen species, are up-regulated in human heart failure. Since these factors have the ability to cause growth and apoptosis in cardiac myocytes, and alter the extracellular matrix, they may also play an important role in remodeling. (Modified from Colucci WS: *Am J Cardiol* 80:15L-25L, 1997.)

muscles is increased. Short-term consequences include increased contractility and heart rate to augment cardiac output, systemic vasoconstriction to increase preload and maintain blood pressure, and redistribution of blood flow away from the skin, muscles, and kidneys to vital organs. The long-term cardiovascular effects of sympathetic activation, however, are deleterious.[4] These include myocyte necrosis and apoptosis, and interstitial fibrosis causing further impairment in systolic and diastolic function; cardiac norepinephrine depletion and β-receptor down-regulation, resulting in inotropic and chronotropic incompetence; calcium overload and proarrhythmia; and activation of the renin-angiotensin system (see below).

Baroreflex control of adrenergic outflow from the central nervous system is also impaired in heart failure. Examples include blunted reflex tachycardia in response to vasodilators and orthostatic hypotension. In addition, desensitization of atrial stretch receptors results in a reduced ability to excrete salt and water in response to increased atrial pressures and release of natriuretic peptides.

Renin-Angiotensin System. Reduced cardiac output results in activation of the renin-angiotensin system, which acts in concert with increased sympathetic activity to maintain arterial pressure. Stimuli for renin secretion by the kidney include decreased renal perfusion, increased sympathetic activity, and a reduction in serum sodium. Angiotensin II, formed by the action of angiotensin-converting enzyme (ACE) on angiotensin I, is a potent vasoconstrictor. Elevated levels in heart failure result in systemic vasoconstriction and intravascular volume expansion. Release of angiotensin also results in increased levels of aldosterone, which has potent sodium-retaining properties. Vasoconstriction and volume retention may initially be compensatory in helping to maintain arterial pressure and stroke volume, but over time contribute to the clinical manifestations of heart failure.

Greater than 90% of ACE in the body is found in tissues (e.g., heart and kidney), and less than 10% is in the circulation. Myocardial production of ACE is increased in heart failure, and stimulation of local angiotensin receptors leads to myocardial hypertrophy and fibrosis. As with systemic responses to circulating angiotensin II, cellular remodeling may be compensatory at first, but ultimately results in progressive myocardial dysfunction.

Arginine Vasopressin. Circulating levels of the pituitary hormone arginine vasopressin (AVP) are elevated in patients with LV dysfunction. In heart failure, AVP levels are hyperresponsive to reductions in plasma osmolality or increases in atrial stretch, and thus contribute to the inadequate ability to excrete free water. The increase in intravascular volume serves to augment preload and cardiac output, but ultimately contributes to clinical decompensation. Increased aldosterone and AVP levels are both responsible for hyponatremia in advanced heart failure. In addition to its antidiuretic effects, AVP is a vasoconstrictor.

Natriuretic Peptides. Circulating levels of atrial natriuretic peptide (ANP) and b-type or brain natriuretic peptide (BNP) are elevated in patients with heart failure. ANP is stored mainly in the right atrium and released in response to increased atrial stretch or pressure, whereas BNP is stored and secreted mainly by the cardiac ventricles. In contrast to norepinephrine and angiotensin II, ANP and BNP are potent vasodilators and thus serve as counterregulatory hormones in heart failure. Other beneficial actions include increased sodium and water excretion, inhibition of the renin-angiotensin system, and a reduction in heart rate via baroreceptor modulation and/or a direct effect on the sinus node.

Endothelin, Inflammatory Cytokines, and Oxidative Stress. Whereas systemic vasoconstriction and volume retention contribute to the progression of LV failure, increased pulmonary vascular tone may contribute to right ventricular failure and reduced exercise tolerance. Endothelin (ET)-1 is a potent vasoconstrictor peptide with growth-promoting effects that may play an important role in pulmonary hypertension associated with heart failure. ET-1 also mediates hypertrophy and fibrosis in failing myocardium. Other factors that have the potential to cause or contribute to myocardial remodeling in heart failure include inflammatory cytokines such as tumor necrosis factor-α, nitric oxide, and other reactive oxygen species.[8]

ETIOLOGY

Classification

Heart failure has been described by various terms. Some such as backward or forward heart failure are of historical significance only. In current practice, one or more categories may be used to try and describe a pathophysiologic state. Treatment, however, may be similar regardless of the type of heart failure.

Systolic vs. Diastolic Heart Failure. For the heart to eject blood commensurate with metabolic requirements during systole, it first has to receive blood during diastole. As stated, heart failure is deemed to be present if the heart is unable to receive blood without an increase in ventricular filling pressure. Symptoms and signs of systemic or pulmonary venous congestion result from diastolic impairment. Symptoms of systolic impairment generally result from inadequate cardiac output with weakness, fatigue, and other symptoms of hypoperfusion. Although isolated diastolic dysfunction is being increasingly recognized as the cause of heart failure with normal systolic function, in chronic heart failure, both forms often coexist.

Acute vs. Chronic Heart Failure. The clinical manifestations of heart failure depend on the rate at which the syndrome develops, and specifically on whether enough time has elapsed for compensatory mechanisms to become operative and interstitial fluid to accumulate (Table 65-2). In acute heart failure, symptoms are due to the sudden reduction in cardiac output with poor organ perfusion and/or marked pulmonary congestion. Examples include acute myocardial infarction, sustained tachyarrhythmia, and valve rupture due to infective endocarditis. When the reduction in cardiac output occurs gradually (e.g., due to chronic valvular regurgitation or remodeling postmyocardial infarction), compensatory mechanisms become operative and allow the patient to tolerate hemodynamic abnormalities with few or no signs and symptoms. However, an intercurrent event such as infection, myocardial ischemia, or medication noncompliance may precipitate manifestations of acute heart failure.

Table 65-2. Acute vs. Chronic Heart Failure

Feature	Acute heart failure	Chronic heart failure
Symptom severity	Marked	Mild to moderate
Pulmonary edema	Frequent	Infrequent
Peripheral edema	Rare	Frequent
Total body fluid	No change or mild increase	Increased
Cardiomegaly	Uncommon	Common
Sympathetic activation	Marked	Mild to marked
Repairable lesion	Common	Occasional

Modified from Leier CV: Unstable heart failure. In Colucci WS, editor: *Heart failure: cardiac function and dysfunction.* In Braunwald E, series editor: *Atlas of heart disease,* ed 2, Philadelphia, 1999, Current Medicine, pp 9.1-9.17.

Left-sided vs. Right-sided Heart Failure. According to the "backward failure" hypothesis, fluid accumulates behind the ventricle that is initially affected. Thus patients with left-sided heart failure (e.g., due to anterior myocardial infarction or mitral regurgitation) initially develop pulmonary venous congestion. Elevated pulmonary venous pressures in turn lead to pulmonary hypertension and subsequent right-sided heart failure. Fluid accumulation becomes generalized and patients develop signs of right-sided failure including lower extremity edema, tender hepatomegaly, and pleural effusions. Pure right-sided failure may occur secondary to primary pulmonary hypertension or chronic pulmonary emboli.

Low-output vs. High-output Heart Failure. Low cardiac output at rest, or in milder cases during exercise or stress, characterizes most etiologies of heart failure. Peripheral vasoconstriction may result in cold, pale extremities, a narrow pulse pressure, and a widened arterial-venous oxygen (A-V-O_2) gradient. High-output states in which the pumping function of the heart is unable to meet the abnormally high metabolic demands of the body less commonly lead to heart failure. Examples include thyrotoxicosis, anemia, arteriovenous fistula, thiamine deficiency (beriberi), and Paget's disease. The extremities are often warm and flushed, the pulse pressure normal or widened, and the A-V-O_2 difference narrowed.

Underlying Causes

Many structural or functional abnormalities of the cardiovascular system can result in heart failure. These include loss of contractility, volume or pressure overload, abnormal cardiac filling, and increased metabolic demand (Table 65-3). The underlying causes of heart failure may vary depending on the demographics of the study population. In a 1971 report from the Framingham Study, 75% of patients with heart failure had hypertension, with coronary artery disease present alone in only 10%. In more recent data from the Studies of Left Ventricular Dysfunction (SOLVD), nearly three quarters of patients had ischemic heart failure, with hypertension considered to be the primary etiology in less than 5%.

Precipitating Factors

Patients with heart failure may be asymptomatic or mildly symptomatic either because the cardiac impairment is mild or because compensatory mechanisms help to normalize cardiac function. However, symptoms of heart failure may develop when precipitating factors increase cardiac workload and disrupt the balance in favor of decompensation. Precipitants may be identified in 50% to 90% of hospital admissions and can be divided into patient-related factors, physician-related factors, heart failure–related disease states, and other causes (Box 65-2). Inability to recognize and correct these factors promptly may lead to persistent heart failure despite adequate treatment.

PATIENT EVALUATION

History

Symptoms of Pulmonary Venous Congestion. ***Dyspnea*** or breathlessness is a cardinal manifestation of left-sided heart failure. Mechanisms of dyspnea include pulmonary venous congestion and transudation of fluid into the interstitium, leading to decreased lung compliance, increased airway resistance, hypoxemia, and ventilation/perfusion mismatch. Stimulation of J receptors leading to an

Table 65-3. Etiology of Heart Failure

Contractile dysfunction	Pressure overload	Volume overload	Impaired filling: Valvular dysfunction	Impaired filling: Diastolic dysfunction	Increased demand
Ischemic heart disease	Hypertension	Aortic regurgitation	Mitral stenosis	Hypertrophic cardiomyopathy	Anemia
Dilated Cardiomyopathy	Aortic stenosis	Mitral regurgitation	Tricuspid stenosis	Amyloidosis	Thyrotoxicosis
Myocarditis	Aortic coarctation	Left-to-right shunt	Atrial myxoma	Constrictive pericarditis	Arteriovenous fistula
Toxins (alcohol, doxorubicin)					Thiamine deficiency
Infection (HIV, sepsis)					Paget's disease

Box 65-2. Precipitating Factors

Patient-Related Factors

Excess exertion or emotional stress
Excess fluid and/or sodium intake
Noncompliance with prescribed medications
Moderate to heavy alcohol consumption

Physician-Related Factors

Use of medications that cause salt and water retention (e.g., nonsteroidal antiinflammatory agents)
Use of negative inotropic agents (e.g., calcium channel blockers)

Heart Failure–Related Disease States

Uncontrolled hypertension
Unstable angina or acute myocardial infarction
Atrial or ventricular arrhythmias
Pulmonary emboli
Infective endocarditis

Other Disease States

Systemic infection
Renal or hepatic failure
High-output states (e.g., anemia, hyperthyroidism, pregnancy)

Box 65-3. New York Heart Association Classification

Class I

No limitations. Ordinary physical activity does not cause undue fatigue, dyspnea, palpitations, or angina.

Class II

Slight limitation of physical activity. Comfortable at rest. Ordinary physical activity (e.g., carrying heavy packages) may result in fatigue, dyspnea, palpitations, or angina.

Class III

Marked limitation of physical activity. Comfortable at rest. Less than ordinary physical activity (e.g., getting dressed) leads to symptoms.

Class IV

Severe limitation of physical activity. Symptoms of heart failure or angina are present at rest and worsen with any activity.

increased ventilatory drive and reduced blood flow to respiratory muscles may cause lactic acidosis and the sensation of dyspnea.

In the early stages of heart failure, dyspnea occurs primarily on effort. As the disease progresses, the extent of effort required to provoke dyspnea decreases. Finally, the patient becomes dyspneic at rest. The New York Heart Association (NYHA) classification may be used to categorize patients based on the relation between symptoms and the amount of effort required to provoke them (Box 65-3). Although NYHA class has been used to stratify patients in clinical studies and provides prognostic information, its accuracy and reproducibility are limited. In addition, there is a poor correlation between NYHA class and other, more objective functional measures of heart failure severity such as exercise duration and peak oxygen consumption.

Orthopnea refers to dyspnea that occurs in the recumbent position. It is due to redistribution of fluid from the abdomen and the lower body into the chest, an increase in the work of breathing when a patient with decreased lung compliance lies flat, and elevation of the diaphragm by ascites and hepatomegaly. Orthopnea usually occurs within a minute or two of assuming recumbency, and develops when the patient is awake. Initially, breathing at night is made easier by elevating the head on two or more pillows. As heart failure progresses, the patient may have to sleep sitting up.

Two symptoms related to orthopnea are *nocturnal cough* and *trepopnea* (or dyspnea limited to one lateral decubitus position). The exact mechanism for trepopnea is unclear but may be related to distortions of the great vessels or alterations in coronary perfusion pressure. With advanced biventricular failure, orthopnea may diminish as symptoms of right-sided failure supervene (see below).

Paroxysmal nocturnal dyspnea is a form of orthopnea, and may occur with further progression of LV failure. The patient awakens suddenly with a feeling of severe anxiety and suffocation, and has to sit bolt upright for relief. In contrast to orthopnea, paroxysmal nocturnal dyspnea usually occurs after prolonged recumbency, is less predictable in its occurrence, and may require 30 minutes or longer in the upright position for relief. Episodes are often accompanied by coughing and wheezing and may be extremely frightening to the patient and family.

When significant wheezing is associated with paroxysmal nocturnal dyspnea, it resembles an acute asthmatic attack and may be referred to as *cardiac asthma*. Bronchospasm, which is caused by congestion of the bronchial mucosa and by interstitial pulmonary edema compressing small airways, increases the work of breathing. *Acute pulmonary edema* can be a further extension of paroxysmal nocturnal dyspnea. Alternatively, acute pulmonary edema may occur as a primary manifestation of acute myocardial infarction or accelerated hypertension. The patient is extremely short of breath and coughs up pink, frothy sputum. Acute pulmonary edema occurs when there is marked elevation of the pulmonary capillary wedge pressure leading to alveolar edema. Untreated, it can be fatal.

Symptoms of Decreased Cardiac Output. Symptoms related to decreased cardiac output can occur with right-sided or left-sided heart failure but more commonly occur in patients with chronic biventricular failure. Fatigue and weakness, particularly in the lower extremities, are nonspecific symptoms thought to be due to decreased cardiac output to exercising muscles. Impaired flow-mediated vasodilation, autonomic imbalance, and altered skeletal muscle metabolism may also play contributory roles. Mental dullness and confusion, especially in older patients with cerebrovascular disease, may result from decreased cerebral perfusion. Other causes of fatigue in patients with heart failure include hyponatremia, volume depletion, and medications (e.g., β-blockers).

Symptoms of Systemic Venous Congestion. Whereas symptoms of left-sided heart failure are related to pulmonary venous congestion and fluid accumulation in the lungs, symptoms of right-sided heart failure result from systemic venous congestion. One of the earliest symptoms of right heart failure may be an inappropriate weight gain. In ambulatory patients, this is followed by swelling in the feet or ankles at the end of the day, which generally resolves overnight. In bedridden patients, edema first develops in the presacral region. With progressive right heart failure, dependent edema becomes persistent. Finally, the development of massive edema involving the entire body is termed *anasarca*.

Elevated systemic venous pressures may result in right upper quadrant abdominal pain as the liver becomes engorged with fluid and its capsule is stretched. Other symptoms associated with edema of the gastrointestinal tract include nausea, vomiting, anorexia, early satiety, and constipation. These symptoms are nonspecific, and digoxin toxicity should be ruled out. Ascites results in an increase in abdominal girth, and unilateral or bilateral pleural effusions can contribute to the sensation of dyspnea.

Cardiac Cachexia. Longstanding, severe heart failure may lead to chronic weight loss. Factors contributing to cardiac cachexia include poor oral intake due to anorexia, and impaired fat absorption due to bowel wall edema. Metabolic pathways that cause catabolic/anabolic imbalance have also been implicated in this syndrome including the growth hormone–insulin-like growth factor-1 system and the pituitary-thyroid hormone axis. Circulating levels of tumor necrosis factor-α, a proinflammatory cytokine, are elevated in patients with severe heart failure and contribute to cardiac cachexia.

Nocturia and Oliguria. Urinary symptoms are common in heart failure. Nocturia may occur early in the course of disease. During daytime activities, urine output is reduced due to the redistribution of blood flow away from the kidneys. When the patient lies down at night, improved cardiac output and renal vasodilation lead to increased urine formation. With biventricular failure, insomnia due to nocturia may be exacerbated by orthopnea and paroxysmal nocturnal dyspnea. Oliguria is a sign of end-stage heart failure and is due to severe reductions in cardiac output and renal blood flow.

Physical Examination

The physical signs of left-sided heart failure relate to pulmonary venous congestion, whereas signs of right-sided heart failure relate to systemic venous congestion. In the discussion that follows, physical signs are presented in the order in which they are typically assessed. Rigorous criteria for identifying heart failure based on both the clinical history and physical findings were developed for the Framingham Study (Box 65-4). However, heart failure may not be recognized in up to 40% of patients due to the limited reliability of these findings.[14]

General Appearance. Patients with compensated chronic heart failure often appear well nourished and comfortable at rest. Even patients with moderate heart failure may appear to be in no distress after resting for several minutes, but become dyspneic during or immediately after activity. By contrast, patients with decompensated heart failure may appear anxious, dusky, and diaphoretic, and are often dyspneic at rest or on lying down. Other findings suggestive of severe heart failure include cool extremities and peripheral cyanosis resulting from low cardiac output and systemic vasoconstriction. As noted, chronic biventricular failure can result in cardiac cachexia. In severe right heart failure, hepatic congestion can cause scleral icterus and jaundice. Patients with recent onset of heart failure often appear acutely ill but are usually well nourished.

Vital Signs. Resting sinus tachycardia is common, and is due to increased adrenergic tone. In mild heart failure, the heart rate at rest may be normal, but increases excessively with exercise and is slow to normalize with rest. The pulse may be irregular if atrial fibrillation is present or in the presence of frequent premature ventricular complexes. In severe LV failure, the peripheral pulse may be alternatingly strong and weak and is referred to as *pulsus alternans*. Pulsus alternans is attributed to reduced LV contraction in every other cardiac cycle due to incomplete recovery causing alternation in the LV stroke volume. Rarely, weaker beats may fail to open the aortic valve, resulting in an apparent halving of the pulse rate, a condition termed *total alternans*.

Box 65-4. Framingham Study Criteria for Congestive Heart Failure

Major Criteria

Paroxysmal nocturnal dyspnea
Neck vein distention
Rales
Radiographic cardiomegaly
Acute pulmonary edema
S_3 gallop
Increased central venous pressure
Circulation time ≥25 sec
Hepatojugular reflux
Visceral congestion or cardiomegaly at autopsy
Weight loss ≥4.5 kg in 5 days in response to treatment

Minor Criteria

Bilateral ankle edema
Nocturnal cough
Dyspnea on ordinary exertion
Hepatomegaly
Pleural effusion
Decrease in vital capacity by ⅓ from maximum value recorded
Tachycardia (rate ≥120/min)

Tachypnea may be present in patients with severe LV failure and dyspnea at rest, or secondary to pleural effusions or ascites in patients with right heart failure. The respiratory rate may be normal in the sitting position, but increase in the patient with pulmonary venous congestion on lying down. Advanced heart failure may be associated with *Cheyne-Stokes respiration,* also called periodic breathing. Cheyne-Stokes respiration consists of periods of hyperpnea alternating with apnea, and is probably caused by prolonged circulation time from the heart to the brain, which affects the normal regulation of breathing. In addition, there is diminished sensitivity of the respiratory center to the arterial carbon dioxide pressure, which waxes and wanes during periods of hyperpnea and apnea. The fall in oxygen pressure and rise in carbon dioxide pressure during the apneic phase stimulate the respiratory center and result in hyperpnea, and the cycle continues. Cheyne-Stokes respiration is common among elderly patients with LV failure in whom the presence of cerebral arteriosclerosis and use of hypnotics may be contributory. The patient is usually unaware of the altered breathing pattern, but other family members may notice it and become alarmed. Cheyne-Stokes respiration may contribute to daytime somnolence in patients who are awakened frequently during periods of hyperpnea.

The systolic blood pressure may be elevated in diastolic heart failure due to chronic hypertension, normal in compensated systolic heart failure, or low in advanced heart failure. Diastolic blood pressure may be slightly elevated due to increased adrenergic activity. A significant reduction in cardiac output is reflected by a narrow pulse pressure, which is defined as the difference between the systolic and diastolic blood pressures. For example, when the pulse pressure is less than 25% of the systolic pressure, the cardiac index is generally less than 2.2 L/min/m^2. When the volume status is unclear in a patient with dyspnea, a bedside Valsalva's maneuver may be used to detect elevated left ventricular filling pressures.

A low-grade fever resulting from cutaneous vasoconstriction may occur in severe heart failure, and subside when compensation is restored. Temperatures greater than 101°F should suggest infection.

Jugular Venous Pulse. Elevation of the jugular venous pressure is a hallmark of elevated systemic venous pressure. The upper limit of normal is approximately 4 cm above the sternal angle when the patient is examined at a 45-degree angle, corresponding to a right atrial pressure of less than 10 cm of water. Higher levels of venous pressure, approaching the angle of the jaw, are common in right sided failure. When tricuspid regurgitation is present, the descending limb of the a wave is attenuated, and the height of the v wave increases with a rapid y descent. Rarely, venous pressure is so high that veins under the tongue or on the dorsum of the hand are dilated. Kussmaul's sign is present when jugular venous pressure increases with inspiration.

In patients with mild right heart failure, jugular venous pressure may be normal at rest but increase with compression of the right upper quadrant. *Hepatojugular reflux* may be elicited by gently applying firm, continuous pressure over the liver for up to 1 minute while observing the neck veins. The patient must breathe normally and not strain during this maneuver. Normally, abdominal or hepatic compression leads to a transient increase in jugular venous pressure. In heart failure, the abnormal right ventricle is unable to accept an increase in venous return and jugular venous pressure remains elevated. In biventricular failure, elevated jugular venous pressure at rest or after hepatic or abdominal compression is a moderately sensitive and highly specific marker of increased pulmonary capillary wedge pressure.

Examination of the Heart

Precordial Palpation. Chronic heart failure is accompanied by cardiac enlargement. Commonly, the apical impulse is displaced downward and to the left, and may be either diffuse (in dilated cardiomyopathy) or sustained (in pressure-overloaded states such as aortic stenosis). In biventricular heart failure or severe right-sided heart failure, a right ventricular impulse may be palpated along the lower sternal edge. A palpable third heart sound may also be present. In acute heart failure or heart failure secondary to constrictive pericarditis or restrictive cardiomyopathy, cardiac enlargement is usually not present.

Auscultation. Although the presence of a third heart sound is common in healthy children and young adults, in adults over age 40, an S_3 gallop generally implies ventricular dysfunction. In patients with mitral or tricuspid regurgitation or left-to-right shunts, excessive flow into the ventricles can also cause a third heart sound without ventricular dysfunction. In heart failure, the presence of a third heart sound is probably related to a sudden deceleration of ventricular inflow that takes place after the early filling phase. Abnormal compliance or diastolic dysfunction may also contribute to a gallop rhythm.

Ventricular remodeling in heart failure may lead to incompetence of the atrioventricular (AV) valves. Thus holosystolic murmurs of mitral or tricuspid regurgitation may be present in the absence of structural valvular abnormalities, especially in advanced heart failure. These murmurs typically decrease in intensity or disappear after successful treatment of decompensation. In biventricular failure or isolated right heart failure, pulmonary hypertension is reflected in a loud pulmonary component of the second heart sound.

Examination of the Lungs. Rales result from the transudation of fluid into the alveoli and airways. In general, rales are heard at the lung bases; but in severe heart failure, they may be heard throughout the lung fields. Wheezing and rhonchi can occur with congestion of the bronchial mucosa, and can lead to the misdiagnosis of reactive airways disease. In biventricular failure, bilateral pleural effusions can occur, and are recognized as dullness to percussion and decreased breath sounds at the bases. When rales or pleural effusion is limited to one side, the right side of the chest is typically involved. Importantly, the absence of pulmonary rales does not exclude significant elevation of the pulmonary capillary wedge pressure in patients with chronic LV systolic failure.

Examination of the Abdomen and Extremities. Hepatomegaly is an early sign of systemic venous congestion. In the early stages of right heart failure, the liver may be tender due to stretching of its capsule, but with progression of disease, tenderness may disappear. In patients with tricuspid regurgitation, the liver may be pulsatile due to transmission of the v wave. Longstanding hepatic congestion may lead to cardiac cirrhosis with portal hypertension and congestive splenomegaly. Ascites results from increased pressure in the hepatic veins and the veins draining the peritoneum. In most patients with heart failure, ascites is minimal. With massive ascites, the physician should suspect constrictive pericarditis or primary liver failure.

Dependent lower extremity edema is common in biventricular or isolated right heart failure, and is typically symmetrical and pitting. In chronic heart failure, the amount of edema does not correlate well with systemic venous pressure; in acute heart failure, edema may be absent despite marked systemic venous hypertension. With advanced heart failure, edema may become massive and generalized (anasarca). Chronic edema of the distal lower extremities may cause reddening and induration of the skin.

DIAGNOSIS

Diagnostic Procedures

Laboratory Studies. Anemia is not diagnostic of heart failure, but when present may exacerbate underlying ischemic heart disease and should be corrected. Rarely, severe anemia may cause high-output failure. The erythrocyte sedimentation rate often decreases in heart failure because of impaired fibrinogen synthesis and decreased fibrinogen concentration. A marked increase in sedimentation rate may suggest infective endocarditis.

Serum Electrolytes. Dilutional *hyponatremia* is common in severe heart failure and is the result of prolonged sodium restriction, diuretic therapy, and expansion of extracellular volume. Increased vasopressin levels may also contribute to hyponatremia. Hyponatremia is a negative prognostic indicator at the time of hospital admission for heart failure, and predicts decreased long-term survival.

Hypokalemia is most often due to thiazide or loop diuretics given without oral potassium supplementation, but may also result from increased aldosterone levels due to activation of the renin-angiotensin system. If uncorrected, hypokalemia may lead to ventricular arrhythmias, especially in the presence of digoxin. *Hyperkalemia* may result from marked reductions in glomerular filtration rate and inadequate delivery of sodium to the distal renal tubule. Excess total body potassium may be exacerbated by the use of potassium-sparing diuretics or angiotensin-converting enzyme inhibitors, and in particular, their concurrent use. During hospitalization for heart failure, hyperkalemia is a common cause of iatrogenic morbidity, and even mortality. Other electrolyte abnormalities seen in heart failure include hypophosphatemia and hypomagnesemia, both of which are commonly associated with chronic alcohol use.

Renal and Hepatic Function. Blood urea nitrogen and creatinine levels are often moderately elevated in severe heart failure because of a reduction in renal blood flow and glomerular filtration rate. Proteinuria may also be present, especially in the setting of longstanding hypertension or diabetes. Chronic right-sided heart failure with congestive hepatomegaly leads to abnormal liver function. Serum aminotransferase, lactic dehydrogenase, and alkaline phosphatase levels are elevated, typically 2 to 3 times normal. Marked elevation in transaminases suggesting "shock liver" can be associated with severe low output states. Hyperbilirubinemia is common in heart failure, and in severe cases of acute heart failure jaundice may occur. In patients with cardiac cirrhosis, hypoalbuminemia may exacerbate fluid accumulation.

Chest Radiograph. The size and shape of the cardiac silhouette provide important information regarding the nature of the underlying heart disease. A cardiothoracic ratio greater than 0.5, for example, is a good indicator of increased LV volume. The other major radiographic abnormality associated with left heart failure is pulmonary venous congestion. The degree of pulmonary venous congestion often parallels increases in the pulmonary capillary wedge pressure. Early radiologic signs of pulmonary venous hypertension and interstitial edema include distention of the pulmonary veins extending upward from the hila, haziness of hilar shadows, and thickening of interlobular septa (Kerley's B lines). When the pulmonary capillary wedge pressure is moderate to severely elevated, often greater than 25 mm Hg, alveolar edema is present as diffuse haziness extending downward toward the lower portions of the lung fields (so-called butterfly pattern). In patients with chronic LV failure, higher pressures can be accommodated with fewer radiologic signs due to enhanced lymphatic drainage. Pleural effusions of varying size and distribution are common in biventricular failure.

Electrocardiogram. No specific electrocardiographic pattern is diagnostic of heart failure. However, the ECG may provide important information regarding the nature of the underlying cardiac disease. For example, LVH and left atrial enlargement suggest left heart failure resulting from antecedent hypertension or aortic stenosis. Pathologic Q waves in ischemic heart disease indicate the presence and location of myocardial infarction, while nonpathologic Q waves (pseudoinfarction) may be seen with restrictive or dilated cardiomyopathy. Abnormal cardiac rhythms such as atrial fibrillation may be secondary to heart failure or may represent inadequacy of therapy if the ventricular response is uncontrolled. If present, ventricular ectopic activity may indicate increased risk of sudden cardiac death, or reflect digoxin toxicity or electrolyte imbalance (e.g., hypokalemia).

Cardiopulmonary Exercise Testing. Treadmill or bicycle exercise testing with continuous gas-exchange analysis provides a safe, objective, and reproducible measure of functional capacity in patients with LV failure. In advanced heart failure, peak oxygen consumption carries important prognostic information, and is used to decide on the timing of cardiac transplantation. Cardiopulmonary exercise testing may also be used to differentiate cardiac from pulmonary causes of dyspnea.

Noninvasive Studies. Echocardiography is commonly performed in the evaluation and management of heart failure. Two-dimensional echocardiographic imaging provides an accurate and rapid determination of ventricular size and function, and valvular morphology and function, and can detect intracavitary thrombi and pericardial effusions. Important hemodynamic data including cardiac output, pulmonary artery pressures, and valve areas can be obtained using Doppler echocardiographic techniques. Diastolic function is more difficult to assess, although newer techniques may provide accurate, load-independent measures of LV relaxation. The advent of transesophageal echocardiography has made it possible to obtain reliable information when transthoracic "windows" are inadequate.

Two other noninvasive techniques commonly used in the assessment of cardiac function are *radionuclide ventriculography* (RVG) and *cardiac magnetic resonance imaging* (MRI). RVG provides a reliable quantification of right and left ventricular ejection fraction, and can characterize wall motion abnormalities in ischemic heart disease. Recently, cardiac MRI has emerged as a highly accurate and quantitative tool for the evaluation of ventricular function and myocardial mass. Serial MRI studies can assess ventricular remodeling in response to therapy.

Invasive Studies. In the intensive care setting, assessment of volume status and/or cardiac output may be necessary to differentiate cardiogenic from noncardiogenic pulmonary edema, and manage hemodynamic instability. The gold standard for evaluating cardiac hemodynamics is *right heart* (or Swan-Ganz) *catheterization* using a balloon-tipped flotation catheter. This procedure may be performed safely at the bedside, and is used primarily to determine response to parenteral inotropic and/or vasodilator therapy in severe heart failure. Simultaneous measurement of right and left heart filling pressures in the cardiac catheterization laboratory can be used to distinguish restrictive cardiomyopathy from constrictive pericarditis.

Coronary angiography is indicated to exclude ischemic heart disease as an underlying, potentially reversible cause of left ventricular dysfunction. The presence of multivessel or left main disease with viable myocardium and adequate distal vessels may be an indication for surgical revascularization. Diagnostic angiography is also used to guide percutaneous revascularization (e.g., percutaneous transluminal coronary angioplasty [PTCA] or stent) in the treatment of angina or acute myocardial infarction. Complications associated with routine coronary angiography include local vascular complications, myocardial infarction, stroke, and death. *Left ventriculography* provides an assessment of LV size, function, and the severity of mitral regurgitation.

The role of right ventricular *endomyocardial biopsy* in the management of heart failure and cardiomyopathy remains controversial. Proposed clinical indications include detection and monitoring of myocarditis, and differentiation of restrictive cardiomyopathy (e.g., cardiac amyloidosis) from constrictive pericarditis. Following cardiac transplantation, endomyocardial biopsy is used to diagnose cardiac allograft rejection. Although the overall complication rate from endomyocardial biopsy is low (2% to 6%), cardiac perforation and death may rarely occur.

Differential Diagnosis

Many symptoms and physical findings suggesting heart failure may be caused by other conditions (Table 65-4). In a patient with dyspnea, the physician must distinguish cardiac from pulmonary causes. Sometimes, this differentiation is difficult. For example, orthopnea may be a well-established symptom in some patients with severe chronic obstructive pulmonary disease. Patients with underlying pulmonary disease may also experience episodic dyspnea during sleep that mimics paroxysmal nocturnal dyspnea. In pulmonary disease, this is usually due to accumulation of tracheobronchial secretions and is relieved by coughing and expectoration, but in cardiac disease, the patient has to sit upright. Wheezing caused by bronchoconstriction may be a prominent symptom when left-sided heart failure supervenes in individuals with reactive airways disease. Patients with cardiac asthma more frequently exhibit diaphoresis and varying degrees of cyanosis than those with bronchial asthma. Differentiating dyspnea related to heart disease from that related to pulmonary disease may be impossible when the diseases coexist, a situation common in chronically ill elderly patients. Pulmonary function studies may help distinguish whether pulmonary or cardiac disease is the predominant condition causing dyspnea. In ambulatory patients, cardiopulmonary exercise testing can help to make this distinction.

MANAGEMENT

The overall goals in the management of heart failure are to prevent or eliminate symptoms, improve quality of life, and prolong survival. The relative importance of these goals varies depending on the clinical stage of disease and on patient preference. For example, although delay of disease progression is central to the management of asymptomatic LV dysfunction, improvement in quality of life may be the primary aim of therapy for advanced heart failure. Three

Table 65-4. Differential Diagnosis

Symptom or sign	Differential diagnosis
Dyspnea	Pulmonary disease
	Anxiety
	Anemia
Edema	Venous insufficiency
	Nephrotic syndrome
	Deep vein thrombosis
Ascites	Hepatic cirrhosis
	Portal vein thrombosis
Distended neck veins	Superior vena cava syndrome
	Constrictive pericarditis
	Pericardial effusion

general approaches to achieving therapeutic goals include recognition and treatment of underlying cardiac disease, removal of precipitating factors, and management of heart failure symptoms:

1. *Remove Underlying Cause.* All patients with heart failure should undergo evaluation for treatable causes. This includes but is not limited to improvement in coronary blood flow with coronary artery bypass grafting (CABG) or percutaneous revascularization, repair or replacement of dysfunctional cardiac valves, surgical correction of hypertrophic cardiomyopathy or congenital heart disease, control of severe hypertension, and removal of cardiac toxins (e.g., alcohol). If heart failure is due to impaired relaxation with preserved systolic function, treatment of hypertension and/or ischemia may be indicated.
2. *Remove Precipitating Factors.* The prompt recognition, treatment, and, if possible, prevention of exacerbating factors (see Box 65-2) are crucial to the successful management of heart failure.[7] Examples include the treatment of acute ischemia or infection, pharmacologic control or cardioversion of arrhythmias, discontinuation of negative inotropic agents, and anticoagulation for pulmonary emboli. Other important precipitants to address when present include excessive alcohol use and medication noncompliance.
3. *Control Symptoms.* Symptoms of heart failure reflect the hemodynamic abnormalities of elevated cardiac filling pressures and reduced cardiac output. Less commonly, symptoms may be secondary to arrhythmias (e.g., atrial fibrillation with rapid ventricular response), thromboembolic events, or adverse drug effects. As discussed below, ACE inhibitors can prevent the development of symptoms, while digoxin and diuretics decrease symptoms once they occur.

Nonpharmacologic Therapy

Rest vs. Exercise. Appropriate restriction of physical activity is essential in the treatment of patients with heart failure. Physical rest reduces metabolic demands and thus the overall work of the failing heart. Bed rest in the hospital is usually necessary in the management of acute heart failure and other forms of severe cardiac decompensation. Progressive mobilization is initiated when the patient's condition permits and is encouraged as further clinical improvement results. Explicit instructions regarding physical activity are discussed before discharge. Patients who work full-time may need to reduce their hours or stop working altogether, depending on the physical and mental demands of the job. It may be beneficial to avoid emotional stress and use relaxation techniques.

Exercise is not contraindicated in patients with heart failure. Supervised cardiac rehabilitation in selected patients may increase exercise tolerance, reduce symptoms, and improve quality of life. Reduction in morbidity and mortality has been reported. These clinical benefits are associated with important physiologic changes including improved vascular endothelial function and skeletal muscle metabolism and decreased sympathetic tone. Thus a program of regular, aerobic exercise for patients with heart failure is recommended.

Diet. Expanded extracellular volume, due in part to avid sodium retention by the kidney, may be treated in most patients with diuretics (see below) and reduction in the dietary intake of sodium. The average American diet without salt restriction contains as much as 10 gm/day of salt. Prohibiting the addition of salt to cooked food and eliminating some salty foods (e.g., potato chips) often reduce salt intake to about 4 to 5 gm/day (Table 65-5). A salt substitute or herbs and spices may be used to flavor food. Removal of salt from cooking altogether reduces intake to about 2 gm of salt per day but often results in unpalatable food and poor compliance. This degree of salt restriction is often unnecessary unless edema persists after vigorous diuretic therapy. Further reduction of salt intake requires elimination of most processed foods and when possible, substitution with low-sodium foods (e.g., fresh vegetables, low-sodium milk, cheese, and bread).

In obese patients with heart failure, supervised weight reduction is of critical importance in reducing the workload of the heart. Specific advice regarding caloric restriction is given, and the therapeutic goal of weight loss is reinforced during follow-up.

Risk Factor Management. For all patients with cardiovascular disease, control of modifiable risk factors should be emphasized. Treatment of hypertension and hyperlipidemia, as well as smoking cessation, have all been shown to have favorable effects on the primary and secondary prevention of ischemic heart disease and cerebrovascular disease. In patients with ischemic heart disease, antihypertensive therapy reduces the risk of developing heart failure.

Pharmacologic Therapy

Therapy for LV dysfunction is generally escalated in relation to severity of symptoms and hemodynamic compromise[12] (Fig. 65-6). ACE inhibitors have been shown to improve survival in all patients with heart failure, including those with asymptomatic LV dysfunction, and β-blockers improve survival in patients with mild to moderate heart failure. Digoxin and diuretics decrease symptoms once they have developed. For patients who remain severely symptomatic despite conventional therapy, including parenteral inotropes and/or vasodilators, mechanical assist and cardiac transplantation may be indicated.

An important goal of combination therapy is to maximally restore a normal relationship between stroke volume and LV

Table 65-5. Salt Content of Foods

Food	Portion	Sodium (mg)
Dill pickle	1	928
McDonald's Big Mac	1	980
Corn chips	1 oz	231
Chicken noodle soup	1 cup	1107
Spaghetti sauce	7 oz	1054
Hot dog	1	639
Pepperoni pizza	½ pie	813
Ham	3 oz	1114
Canned corn or beans	1 cup	350
Frozen corn or beans	1 cup	5

Modified from Kubo SH, Cohn JN: Long-term management of the ambulatory patient with heart failure. In Smith TW, editor: *Cardiovascular therapeutics: a companion to Braunwald's heart disease*, ed 1, Philadelphia, 1996, WB Saunders, p 212. Source U.S. Department of Agriculture.

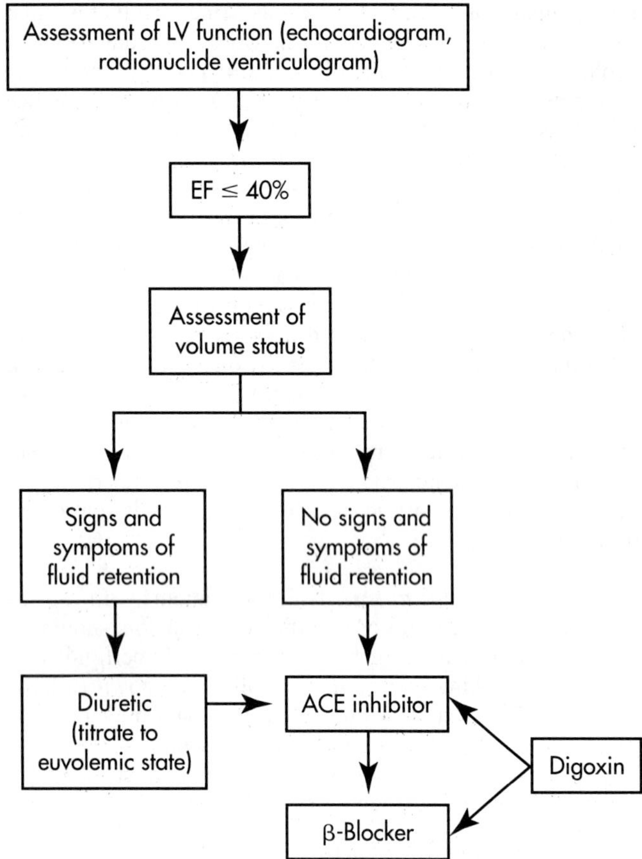

Fig. 65-6. Approach to the patient with heart failure. LV function should be assessed in all patients with heart failure to detect those with systolic dysfunction (EF ≤ 40%). Patients with evidence of fluid retention should receive a diuretic until euvolemia is achieved, and diuretic therapy should be continued to prevent recurrence of fluid retention. An ACE inhibitor should be initiated in all patients, unless it is not tolerated or contraindicated, and a β-blocker should be added in mild to moderate heart failure. Digoxin may be added at any time to reduce symptoms or slow the ventricular response in atrial fibrillation. (Modified from Packer M, Cohn JN: *Am J Cardiol* 83:1A-38A, 1999.)

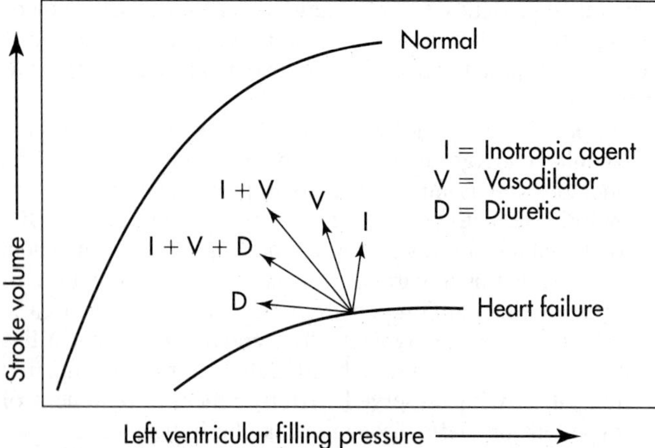

Fig. 65-7. Directional shifts in the relationship between left ventricular filling pressure and stroke volume produced by various pharmacologic interventions designed to reduce preload and/or afterload and to increase cardiac contractility in the severely decompensated heart. Endpoints indicate improved hemodynamic status.

filling pressure (Fig. 65-7). The combination of an inotropic agent and a vasodilator with or without a diuretic may achieve more normal LV function than does the administration of an inotrope, vasodilator, or diuretic alone.

Diuretics. Diuretic therapy is an important element in the treatment of edema associated with heart failure. By reducing the reabsorption of sodium and water by the renal tubule, diuretics improve symptoms related to excess volume and may prevent ventricular remodeling by reducing cardiac filling pressures. Current recommendations are to reserve diuretic therapy for patients with signs and symptoms of fluid retention on an ACE inhibitor (or other vasodilator) and moderate salt restriction, with or without digoxin. Commonly used diuretics in heart failure are thiazides, loop diuretics, and potassium-sparing diuretics (Table 65-6).

Thiazides and Related Compounds. Thiazides, including chlorothiazide and hydrochlorothiazide, exert their diuretic effects primarily by inhibiting sodium and chloride reabsorption in the distal convoluted tubule. They are well absorbed orally and may be used in the management of mild to moderate heart failure, or in combination with loop diuretics to treat refractory edema. However, their utility may be limited by avid solute reabsorption in the more proximal nephron (diuretic resistance), especially when renal function is impaired. Also, because thiazides enhance the secretion of potassium, hypokalemia and potassium depletion can result. Metabolic alkalosis, hyperglycemia, hyperuricemia, and dilutional hyponatremia are other complications of thiazide use.

Although chemically different from thiazides, chlorthalidone, metolazone, and indapamide have similar sites of action and potency. Metolazone has a long duration of action (24 to 48 hours) because of serum protein binding and retains its diuretic properties even when renal function is compromised. Indapamide has vasodilatory and diuretic effects, and does not significantly alter serum cholesterol and triglyceride levels.

Loop Diuretics. These agents, which include furosemide, bumetanide, and ethacrynic acid, are potent inhibitors of sodium and chloride reabsorption in the thick ascending limb of the loop of Henle. Because their initial action augments renal blood flow, loop diuretics, unlike the thiazides, generally retain their diuretic potency when glomerular filtration rates are reduced. Once- or twice-daily oral administration is recommended in the outpatient management of moderate to severe heart failure, while IV administration is reserved for hospitalized patients with acute pulmonary edema or decompensated heart failure. Because of their potent diuretic effects, high doses may result in a severe reduction in intravascular volume and hypotension. Other side effects include hypokalemia, azotemia, metabolic alkalosis, hyperuricemia, ototoxicity (particularly with ethacrynic acid), and neurohormonal activation. Efficacy of loop diuretics may be diminished by nonsteroidal antiinflammatory agents or by decreased gastrointestinal absorption due to bowel wall edema. Torsemide, a new loop diuretic with improved bioavailability, may be used to treat right heart failure resistant to oral furosemide.

Potassium-Sparing Diuretics. The potassium-sparing drugs include spironolactone, triamterene, and amiloride. All three

Table 65-6. Diuretic Therapy in Heart Failure

Generic name	Trade name	Usual dose	Duration of action (h)
Thiazides			
Chlorothiazide	Diuril	500-1000 mg/day	6-12 hours
Hydrochlorothiazide	HydroDIURIL	50-100 mg/day	>12
Metolazone	Zaroxolyn	5-10 mg/day	24-48
Chlorthalidone	Hygroton	100 mg/day	24
Indapamide	Lozol	1.25-5 mg/day	24
Loop diuretics			
Furosemide	Lasix	40-160 mg/day po 20-80 mg IV	6-8 (po)
Bumetanide	Bumex	0.5-4 mg/day po 0.5-2 mg IV	4-6 (po)
Ethacrynic acid	Edecrin Sodium Edecrin	50-150 mg/day po 50-100 mg IV	6-8 (po)
Torsemide	Demadex	5-20 mg/day po 5-20 mg IV	1-4 (po)
Potassium-sparing diuretics			
Spironolactone	Aldactone	25-100 mg/day	3 days after starting
Triamterene	Dyrenium	100-200 mg/day	12-16
Amiloride	Midamor	5-10 mg/day	24

have relatively mild diuretic potency when used alone. However, when used with a thiazide or loop diuretic, they enhance sodium excretion and counteract the potassium-wasting properties of these drugs. Therefore combination therapy may be of particular use in patients with refractory edema and hypokalemia. Potassium-sparing diuretics are contraindicated in renal failure because they may result in life-threatening hyperkalemia.

A recent study (RALES) demonstrated a survival benefit of spironolactone in patients with severe heart failure, and favorable effects on LV remodeling have been suggested. Newer selective aldosterone receptor antagonists (SARAs) are being developed for the treatment of heart failure.

Mechanical Fluid Removal. In patients with massive edema resistant to high-dose or combination diuretics, cautious mechanical removal of fluid from the pleural or peritoneal spaces occasionally results in marked improvement of symptoms. In heart failure associated with compromised renal function, isolated ultrafiltration without hemodialysis has been used successfully to remove excess fluid and has resulted in sustained clinical benefits.

Vasodilators. An important advance in the treatment of heart failure was the recognition that pump function was critically dependent on afterload.[2] Agents that preferentially dilate arteriolar resistance vessels (e.g., hydralazine) shift the ventricular function curve upward and to the left, resulting in an increase in cardiac output often with little or no change in blood pressure. Agents that preferentially increase capacitance in the venous system (e.g., nitrates) redistribute blood volume from the central to peripheral reservoirs and decrease the signs and symptoms of elevated filling pressures. ACE inhibitors, which have a balanced effect on the arterial and venous system, also slow the progression of heart failure by interfering with the renin-angiotensin system. The dosage and characteristics of vasodilators commonly used in the treatment of heart failure are shown in Table 65-7.

Several large, prospective, controlled trials have demonstrated the beneficial effects of ACE inhibitors and other vasodilators on exercise tolerance, clinical signs and symptoms, neurohormonal activation, quality of life, and survival in patients with chronic heart failure (Table 65-8).

ACE Inhibitors. By inhibiting the enzyme that converts angiotensin I to angiotensin II, ACE inhibitors exert several important hemodynamic and neurohormonal effects in heart failure. A decrease in circulating angiotensin II causes balanced vasodilation and inhibition of aldosterone secretion; inhibition of tissue angiotensin II prevents myocardial hypertrophy and fibrosis; and reduced bradykinin metabolism stimulates prostaglandin and nitric oxide synthesis. Cardiovascular effects include reduction in right and left ventricular filling pressures and increases in stroke volume and cardiac output.

All patients with heart failure due to left ventricular systolic dysfunction should receive an ACE inhibitor, unless contraindicated. Similar mortality benefits are observed with several different agents, including captopril, enalapril, and lisinopril, and in a broad range of patients,[6] and a recent study (ATLAS) demonstrated the superiority of high-dose therapy. ACE inhibitors are generally added to diuretics and may be used together with β-blockers or digoxin. In clinical practice, the choice of an ACE inhibitor may be dictated more by cost and frequency of administration.

Hypotension and lightheadedness are common side effects of ACE inhibitors, particularly in patients with marked activation of the renin-angiotensin system (identified by the presence of hyponatremia or the recent occurrence of rapid diuresis). Symptomatic hypotension can be avoided by holding diuretic therapy on the first day of treatment, and by starting with low doses and titrating slowly to target doses.

Table 65-7. Vasodilator Therapy in Heart Failure

Generic name	Trade names	Route of administration	Usual dose
ACE inhibitors			
Captopril	Capoten	Oral	6.25-50 mg tid
Enalapril	Vasotec	Oral	2.5-20 mg bid
Lisinopril	Zestril, Prinivil	Oral	5-40 mg qd
Fosinopril	Monopril	Oral	10-40 mg qd
Nitrates			
Nitroglycerin	Nitrostat	Sublingual	0.3-0.4 mg initial
Nitroglycerin	Nitro-Dur, Nitrodisc	Transdermal	0.1-0.6 mg patch 12 h/day
Isosorbide dinitrate	Isordil	Oral	10-40 mg tid
Isosorbide mononitrate	Imdur	Oral	30-120 mg qd
Other vasodilators			
Hydralazine	Apresoline	Oral	25-100 mg tid-qid
Losartan	Cozaar	Oral	25-100 mg qd
Amlodipine	Norvasc	Oral	2.5-10 mg qd

Table 65-8. Randomized Controlled Trials of Vasodilators in Heart Failure

Study	Drug(s) studied	Number enrolled	NYHA class (%)	Patients with IDC (%)	Key findings
CONSENSUS I	Enalapril	253	IV (100)	15	Enalapril reduced symptoms and mortality in severe heart failure
V-HeFT I	Hydralazine plus isosorbide dinitrate, prazosin	642	II (NA) III (NA)	NA	Hydralazine-isosorbide dinitrate reduced mortality in mild-moderate heart failure
V-HeFT II	Hydralazine plus isosorbide dinitrate, enalapril	804	I (6) II (51) III (43)	NA	Enalapril was superior to hydralazine-isosorbide in reducing mortality in mild-moderate heart failure
SOLVD Treatment	Enalapril	2569	I (11) II (57) III (30)	18	Enalapril reduced mortality and hospitalizations in mild-moderate heart failure
SOLVD Prevention	Enalapril	4228	I (67) II (33)	10	Enalapril reduced heart failure and hospitalizations in patients with asymptomatic LV dysfunction
SAVE	Captopril	2231	I (100)	0	Captopril reduced mortality in patients with asymptomatic LV dysfunction postmyocardial infarction
ATLAS	Lisinopril	3164	II (16) III (77) IV (7)	35	High-dose Lisinopril was superior to low-dose Lisinopril in reducing death or hospitalization in mild-moderate heart failure
ELITE II	Captopril, losartan	3152	II (52) III (43) IV (5)	21	Losartan was not superior to captopril in improving survival in elderly heart failure patients

IDC, Idiopathic dilated cardiomyopathy.

Hyperkalemia may occur with ACE inhibitors, and potassium supplementation should be carefully monitored. Nonproductive cough occurs in 5% to 15% of patients and is the most common reason for drug discontinuation. Major adverse effects include anuric renal failure, especially in the presence of bilateral renal artery stenosis, and angioedema. ACE inhibitors are contraindicated in pregnancy.

Other Vasodilators. In patients who are intolerant of ACE inhibitors, the combination of hydralazine and isosorbide dinitrate should be considered as a therapeutic option. These agents may also be used in advanced heart failure in addition to ACE inhibition. Hydralazine reduces systemic vascular resistance by preferentially dilating arterioles. Reductions in pulmonary and renal vascular resistance also occur. Reflex tachycardia, typically seen in patients without cardiomegaly, is uncommon in heart failure. As with ACE inhibitors, treatment with hydralazine should be started at a low dose (10 to 25 mg orally four times daily) and slowly titrated over days to weeks to a target dose of ≥200 mg/day. Side effects include flushing, headaches, and gastrointestinal upset. Patients treated with high doses for prolonged periods frequently develop positive ANA titers. Less commonly, a lupus-like syndrome develops, which usually resolves with drug withdrawal.

Due to their preferential venodilator effects, nitrates reduce ventricular filling pressures and may be used to treat pulmonary congestion without significantly affecting cardiac output or blood pressure. In patients with underlying ischemic heart disease, nitrates can reduce myocardial ischemia via coronary vasodilation. Nitroglycerin can be given sublingually, topically, or intravenously. Isosorbide dinitrate is typically given by mouth three to four times daily in a dose of 20 to 60 mg, although longer-acting oral formulations are now available. A daily nitrate-free interval is recommended to avoid the development of nitrate tolerance. The most common adverse effects of nitrate therapy include hypotension, flushing, and headaches.

Although the use of angiotensin receptor antagonists in ACE inhibitor–intolerant patients remains unproved, increasing evidence suggests that these agents may prevent ventricular remodeling and reduce symptoms in heart failure. The recently completed ELITE II study failed to demonstrate superiority of losartan over captopril in elderly patients with heart failure. Several other large, randomized trials (CHARM, Val-HeFT, Valiant) are currently underway to test whether ACE inhibition, angiotensin receptor blockade, or the combination is more effective at slowing disease progression. Long-acting calcium channel blockers such as amlodipine may be used safely in heart failure patients on ACE inhibitors to treat angina or hypertension.

Digitalis Glycosides. Although digoxin and related compounds have been used for over 200 years to treat heart failure, debate continues regarding their safety and efficacy. Multicenter trials have shown that digoxin increases ejection fraction and exercise tolerance, and decreases symptoms in patients with systolic heart failure, and withdrawal of digoxin leads to increased symptoms and hospitalizations (Table 65-9). The recently completed DIG trial showed no difference in survival with digoxin compared with placebo when given with an ACE inhibitor and diuretic.[5] In the digoxin-treated group, fewer deaths attributable to the progression of heart failure were offset by an increase in deaths due to other causes.

Digoxin increases cardiac contractility by inhibiting sacrolemmal Na-K-ATPase, thereby increasing the amount of intracellular calcium available to the contractile apparatus. Cardiac output increases and diuresis ensues. Digoxin also increases baroreceptor sensitivity, attenuates neurohormonal activation, slows heart rate, and decreases systemic vasoconstriction. Finally, digoxin decreases AV nodal conduction velocity, which makes it a useful agent for treating heart failure in patients with atrial fibrillation or flutter with rapid ventricular response.

Digoxin is given to outpatients as a maintenance oral dose of 0.125 to 0.25 mg per day. In the presence of normal renal function, full digitalization occurs within 5 to 7 days. If rapid digitalization is required (e.g., in a hospitalized patient with rapid atrial fibrillation), an initial dose of 0.25 to 0.5 mg is given intravenously, followed by 0.125 to 0.25 mg every 2 to 4 hours up to a total of 1 mg. The peak effect is usually achieved between 1.5 and 6 hours. Electrocardiographic monitoring should be used to monitor for proarrhythmia, with the knowledge that some changes (e.g., shortening of the QT interval, flattening or inversion of the T wave) reflect drug effect rather than drug toxicity.

Digoxin has a low toxic to therapeutic ratio. However, there is little evidence to support using serum levels to guide dose selection. Hypokalemia, renal insufficiency, and hypoxia commonly predispose patients to the toxic effects of digoxin. Digoxin should also be used with caution in older patients with slower renal excretion; in patients with acute myocardial infarction, myocarditis, or hypothyroidism; and in patients treated with drugs such as quinidine, verapamil, and amiodarone that increase serum digoxin levels. Digoxin is contraindicated in patients with second- or third-degree AV block unless a temporary pacemaker has been inserted.

Toxic manifestations of digoxin include gastrointestinal upset, visual disturbances, and a wide range of cardiac arrhythmias. The new occurrence, or increased frequency, of ventricular premature beats is the most common rhythm disturbance related to excess digoxin. Other cardiac arrhythmias include second-degree AV block, paroxysmal atrial tachycardia with block, and life-threatening ventricular tachycardia and fibrillation. Digoxin toxicity is usually reversed by simply withdrawing the drug. Hypokalemia, if present, should be corrected. High-grade AV block may require temporary pacing, while significant ventricular arrhythmias are treated with lidocaine, phenytoin, and propranolol. Severe digoxin toxicity associated with recurrent ventricular arrhythmias (e.g., following massive overdose) can be treated with purified Fab fragments of digoxin-specific antibodies. The digoxin antibody complex is excreted in the urine.

β-Adrenergic Antagonists. Historically, β-blockers were contraindicated in the treatment of heart failure because of concern for negative inotropic effects precipitating clinical deterioration. It is now recognized that chronic overactivity of the sympathetic nervous system plays an important role in the pathophysiology of heart failure, and drugs that interfere with this system can prevent disease progression. In the 1970s and early 1980s, small uncontrolled trials suggested beneficial effects of β-blockers in dilated cardiomyopathy. A large body of evidence now indicates that β-blockers improve LV function, reduce hospitalizations, and prolong survival in patients with chronic systolic heart failure (Table 65-10). β-Blockers also cause reverse remodeling of the left ventricle.

Carvedilol, a combination α- and β-blocker with in vitro antioxidant properties, has been approved for the treatment of mild to moderate heart failure.[11] Large, prospective trials of bisoprolol (CIBIS II) and metoprolol (MERIT-HF) were stopped early due to a 34% reduction in all-cause mortality. Recent consensus guidelines recommend β-blockers, in addition to ACE inhibitors and diuretics, for the long-term management of patients with mild to moderate heart failure. In ischemic heart failure, β-blockers may also be used to treat hypertension, prevent recurrent myocardial

Table 65-9. Randomized Controlled Trials of Digoxin in Heart Failure

Study	Drug(s) studied	Number enrolled	NYHA class (%)	Patients with IDC (%)	Key findings
Captopril-Digoxin Multicenter Research Group	Captopril, digoxin	300	I (26) II (50) III (24)	32	Digoxin improved ejection fraction and decreased hospitalizations for heart failure
PROVED	Digoxin withdrawal	88	II (84) III (16)	36	Withdrawal of digoxin worsened exercise tolerance and increased hospitalizations in patients not on ACE inhibitor
RADIANCE	Digoxin withdrawal	178	II (73) III (27)	37	Withdrawal of digoxin worsened heart failure, exercise tolerance, and ejection fraction in patients on ACE inhibitor
Digitalis Investigation Group (DIG)	Digoxin	6800	I (13) II (54) III (31)	15	Digoxin decreased hospitalizations for heart failure, but did not reduce overall mortality in LV dysfunction

Table 65-10. Randomized Controlled Trials of β-Blockers in Heart Failure

Study	Drug studied	Number enrolled	NYHA class (%)	Patients with IDC (%)	Key findings
MDC	Metoprolol	383	II (45) III (49) IV (4)	100	Metoprolol tended to reduce the risk of death or transplant listing in idiopathic dilated cardiomyopathy
CIBIS I	Bisoprolol	641	III (95) IV (5)	36	Bisoprolol reduced hospitalizations and symptoms in moderate-severe heart failure
U.S. Carvedilol Heart Failure Study	Carvedilol	1094	II (53) III (44) IV (3)	52	Carvedilol reduced mortality in mild-moderate heart failure
CIBIS II	Bisoprolol	2647	III (83) IV (17)	12	Bisoprolol reduced mortality in moderate-severe heart failure
MERIT-HF	Metoprolol CR/XL	3991	II (40) III (56) IV (4)	NA	Metoprolol reduced mortality in mild-moderate heart failure
BEST	Bucindolol	2708	III (92) IV (8)	NA	Bucindolol did not reduce mortality in moderate-severe heart failure

infarction or ventricular arrhythmias, and control ventricular response in atrial fibrillation.

β-Blockers may have variable actions related in part to their non–β-blocking effects (e.g., direct vasodilation). Adverse effects include lightheadedness, worsening heart failure, and bradycardia or heart block. β-Blockers must be started at very low doses (e.g., carvedilol 3.125 mg orally twice daily, metoprolol XL 12.5 mg orally once daily), and titrated slowly in symptomatic patients. Antiadrenergic therapy should not be started in patients who are hospitalized for heart failure, hypotensive or bradycardic, or in a fluid overloaded state. Bronchospasm due to asthma or chronic obstructive pulmonary disease is a contraindication to β-blocker use.

Anticoagulation and Antiarrhythmic Therapy. Heart failure due to LV systolic dysfunction increases the risk of thromboembolic events, and chronic anticoagulation with warfarin has been recommended. However, in the absence of definitive clinical trials, anticoagulation appears to be most justified in heart failure patients with atrial fibrillation and in those with a history of thromboembolism or mobile intracavitary thrombus. Anticoagulants may also be given to patients with severe LV systolic dysfunction (EF ≤20%) and moderate-severe LV dilation, in the absence of contraindications. Amiodarone may be used to manage symptomatic ventricular or atrial arrhythmias that complicate heart failure, while its role in the treatment of heart failure per se is unproved. For refractory ventricular tachycardia or ventricular fibrillation, an implantable cardioverter-defibrillator is indicated for the prevention of sudden cardiac death. Radiofrequency catheter ablation of ventricular tachycardia may be curative, but more often is palliative. Permanent pacing is indicated for treatment of symptomatic bradyarrhythmias, and has been used with limited success in hypertrophic cardiomyopathy to reduce the intracavitary gradient, and in patients with dilated cardiomyopathy and prolonged AV nodal conduction to improve exercise tolerance.

Management of Diastolic Heart Failure. The management of diastolic heart failure differs from that of systolic heart failure.[1] Principles of therapy include blood pressure control, prevention or treatment of ischemia, and reduction in cardiac filling pressures (Table 65-11). In diastolic heart failure due to hypertension and LVH, blood pressure control is important to prevent progression of LVH and possibly to promote its regression. In addition, effective antihypertensive therapy may improve diastolic filling properties, relieve the load on the left atrium, and help preserve sinus rhythm. Calcium channel blockers may reduce symptoms of diastolic heart failure not only by lowering blood pressure, but also by improving ventricular relaxation. Antagonists of the renin-angiotensin system (e.g., ACE inhibitors and angiotensin receptor blockers) have also been suggested as positive lusitropic agents for diastolic dysfunction, and may slow or reverse myocardial fibrosis. However, there is no evidence that either calcium channel blockers or ACE inhibitors improve survival in diastolic heart failure.

Patients with LVH are prone to subendocardial ischemia, even in the absence of coronary artery disease. Ischemia increases myocardial diastolic stiffness and exacerbates diastolic dysfunction. Since most coronary flow occurs in diastole, tachycardia with reduced diastolic filling time compromises subendocardial perfusion. Therefore heart rate control is central to preventing or treating ischemia associated with diastolic heart failure. β-Blockers and calcium channel blockers (e.g., verapamil and diltiazem) are useful negative chronotropic agents. In patients with obstructive coronary artery disease, percutaneous or surgical revascularization may be indicated to treat ischemia.

Pulmonary venous congestion associated with diastolic dysfunction usually responds rapidly to preload reduction with diuretics and/or nitrates. However, because of increased myocardial stiffness, a small decrease in LV volume can cause a marked decrease in LV filling pressure, stroke volume, and cardiac output. Therefore it is important to avoid excessive preload reduction, which can cause symptomatic hypotension.

Because of increased LV diastolic stiffness, patients with diastolic dysfunction have reduced passive LV filling in early and mid-diastole and depend on an active atrial contribution to late ventricular filling. Maintenance of sinus rhythm is important for achieving adequate stroke volume and cardiac output. Electrical or chemical cardioversion should be considered for all patients with diastolic dysfunction and atrial fibrillation. While awaiting therapeutic anticoagulation, β-blockers, calcium blockers, or digoxin may be used to control the ventricular response.

Table 65-11. Management of Diastolic Heart Failure

Goal of treatment	Method of treatment
Regression of LVH	Antihypertensive therapy Surgery (e.g., valve replacement for aortic stenosis)
Improve ventricular relaxation	Decrease afterload Antiischemic therapy Calcium channel blockers (?)
Prevent and/or treat ischemia	β-Blockers Nitrates Coronary artery bypass grafting, PTCA or stent
Decrease venous pressures	Diuretics Nitrates ACE inhibitors Sodium restriction
Decrease heart rate	β-Blockers Verapamil Digoxin in atrial fibrillation
Maintain atrial contraction	Cardioversion of atrial fibrillation

Modified from Smith TW, Kelly RA, Stevenson LW, et al: Management of heart failure. In Braunwald E, editor: *Heart disease: a textbook of cardiovascular medicine*, ed 5, Philadelphia, 1997, WB Saunders, p 504.

Box 65-5. Disease Management Strategies

- Early evaluation and aggressive intervention
- Nurse-based case management
- Home health services
- Patient and family education
- Dietary counseling
- Risk factor modification
- Exercise programs
- Referral to transplant center

Disease Management. Many emergency room visits and hospitalizations for heart failure can be prevented by a comprehensive, disease-oriented approach to patient care.[13] Important components of a heart failure disease management program are listed in Box 65-5. Patients enrolled in a heart failure program report decreased symptoms and improved quality of life. Overall health care costs are reduced.

EBM EVIDENCE-BASED MEDICINE

Primary sources for this chapter were MEDLINE, and Consensus Recommendations of the Advisory Council To Improve Outcomes Nationwide in Heart Failure (see reference 12). Electronic searches dating back to 1977 were conducted in February 1999, using the keywords *Heart Failure, Congestive* and *Myocardial Diseases*. They focused on identifying large, randomized controlled trials with prespecified morbidity and mortality endpoints, and systematic reviews.

REFERENCES

1. Bonow RO, Udelson JE: Left ventricular diastolic dysfunction as a cause of congestive heart failure: mechanisms and management, *Ann Intern Med* 117:502-510, 1992.
2. Cohn JN, Franciosa JA: Vasodilator therapy of cardiac failure (first of two parts), *N Engl J Med* 297:27-31, 1977.
3. Colucci WS: Molecular and cellular mechanisms of myocardial failure, *Am J Cardiol* 80:15L-25L, 1997.
4. Colucci WS, Braunwald E: Pathophysiology of heart failure. In Braunwald E, editor: *Heart disease: a textbook of cardiovascular medicine*, Philadelphia, 1997, WB Saunders, pp 394-420.
5. Digitalis Investigation Group: The effect of digoxin on mortality and morbidity in patients with heart failure, *N Engl J Med* 336:525-533, 1997.
6. Garg R, Yusuf S: Overview of randomized trials of angiotensin-converting enzyme inhibitors on mortality and morbidity in patients with heart failure: Collaborative Group on ACE Inhibitor Trials, *JAMA* 273:1450-1456, 1995.
7. Ghali JK, Kadakia S, Cooper R, et al: Precipitating factors leading to decompensation of heart failure: traits among urban blacks, *Arch Intern Med* 148:2013-2016, 1988.
8. Givertz MM, Colucci WS: New targets for heart-failure therapy: endothelin, inflammatory cytokines, and oxidative stress, *Lancet* 352 Suppl 1:S134-S138, 1998.
9. Ho KK, Anderson KM, Kannel WB, et al: Survival after the onset of congestive heart failure in Framingham Heart Study subjects, *Circulation* 88:107-115, 1993.
10. Ho KK, Pinsky JL, Kannel WB, et al: The epidemiology of heart failure: the Framingham Study, *J Am Coll Cardiol* 22:6A-13A, 1993.
11. Packer M, Bristow MR, Cohn JN, et al: The effect of carvedilol on morbidity and mortality in patients with chronic heart failure. U.S. Carvedilol Heart Failure Study Group, *N Engl J Med* 334:1349-1355, 1996.
12. Packer M, Cohn JN, on behalf of the membership of the Advisory Council to Improve Outcomes Nationwide in Heart Failure: Consensus recommendations for the management of chronic heart failure, *Am J Cardiol* 83:1A-38A, 1999.
13. Rich MW, Beckham V, Wittenberg C, et al: A multidisciplinary intervention to prevent the readmission of elderly patients with congestive heart failure, *N Engl J Med* 333:1190-1195, 1995.
14. Stevenson LW, Perloff JK: The limited reliability of physical signs for estimating hemodynamics in chronic heart failure, *JAMA* 261:884-888, 1989.

CHAPTER 66

Valvular Heart Disease

Edgar C. Schick, Jr.

Significant valvular heart disease is likely to be found in only a small proportion of patients in the average primary care practice. The primary physician, however, has much to contribute to the detection of valvular disease and the initial management of these patients. Despite the growth of noninvasive diagnostic technology, the answers to many important questions about possible valvular pathology remain the prerogative of the bedside physician. Diligent auscultatory characterization of heart murmurs and pursuit of cogent ancillary physical findings often provide adequate basis for a diagnosis and obviate the need for additional, more expensive studies. Evaluation of the patient with valvular disease offers the physician a gratifying opportunity to exercise cardiovascular diagnostic skills but also poses challenging questions related to such matters as drug therapy, referral for a cardiologist's opinion, cardiac catheterization, anticoagulation, and prophylactic antibiotic use. This chapter focuses specifically on these aspects and attempts to provide the busy physician with a capsular overview of management for the valvular heart disease patient.

AORTIC STENOSIS

Aortic stenosis is the most common acquired valvular disease. After adolescence but before the seventh decade, stenosis of the aortic orifice develops as a consequence of congenital bicuspid valvular anatomy in two of every three cases. Idiopathic sclerocalcific degeneration of a normal tricuspid aortic valve predominates among older patients. Rheumatic fever may also cause aortic stenosis but seldom without evidence of mitral valvular involvement.

Pathophysiology

When the stenotic process has contracted the aortic orifice, normally between 2 and 4 cm^2, by about half (Fig. 66-1), the left ventricle is presented with a progressively increasing pressure burden. This challenge is adaptively matched by ventricular hypertrophy, which maintains the systolic stress on the myocardium within the normal range. Significant ventricular dilation is not a feature of uncomplicated aortic stenosis; when present it indicates failure of the primary compensatory mechanism or superimposition of a new problem, such as coronary artery disease. Systolic wall stress increases as a result, and the ejection fraction declines. In the

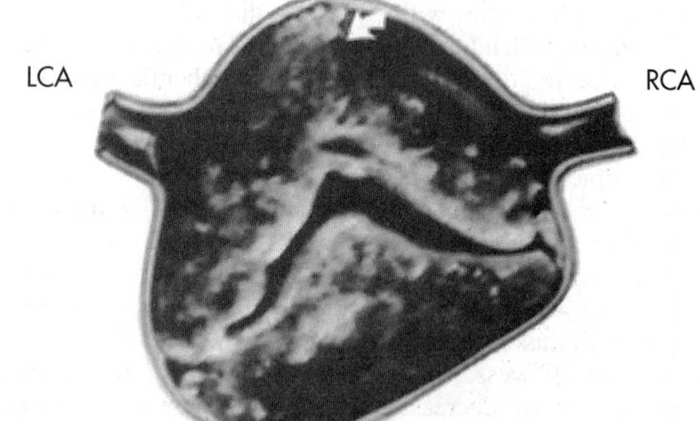

Fig. 66-1. Calcific stenosis of a congenitally bicuspid aortic valve. The effective orifice is reduced to a V-shaped slit, less than 10% of the area available for opening under normal circumstances. The arrow points to a raphe at the site of what would have been the commissure between the right and left coronary cusps. *RCA*, Right coronary artery; *LCA*, left coronary artery. (From Edwards JE: *Pract Cardiol* 8:117, 1982.)

majority of patients these abnormalities reverse after surgery; a depressed ejection fraction improves, but may not fully normalize.

History and Physical Examination

Patients with evolving aortic stenosis may remain free of symptoms for extended periods. The cardinal symptoms are dyspnea, angina, and exertional syncope. Dyspnea initially reflects the development of abnormal diastolic function in the hypertrophied ventricle. Despite maintenance of normal diastolic volumes and ejection fraction, resting diastolic pressures become elevated and may rise dramatically during exercise. Systolic dysfunction may also develop. Exertional angina occurs in the absence of coronary artery disease. Ischemic symptoms result from insufficiency of coronary flow reserve to meet markedly increased demand. Significant coronary lesions are seldom present in patients with aortic stenosis who do not report angina and occur in about 50% of patients with angina. The traditional teaching that syncope in aortic stenosis develops as a consequence of exertional muscular vasodilation in the presence of a cardiac output response that is limited by the stenosis seems at best only a partial explanation. Abnormal vasodepressor responses to exercise or transient dysrhythmias are other likely possibilities.

Innocent Murmur. Aortic flow murmurs are very common among adolescents and young adults. These murmurs are usually harsh in quality, crescendo-decrescendo in profile, and best appreciated along the middle to lower left sternal border. Uncertainty about the significance of murmurs with these features presents a common clinical problem. How can the so-called innocent, functional, or normal flow murmur be distinguished from that which either connotes the presence or portends the development of important valvular pathology?

Although a completely satisfactory distinction cannot always be made, several features of the examination may be helpful. Typically, aortic murmurs radiate to the upper right parasternal area and the neck in contrast to the innocent pulmonic flow murmur, which, although often prominent along the lower sternal margin, radiates to the upper left parasternal region. Pulmonic flow murmurs are characteristically associated with high-output states (e.g., pregnancy, fever, or anemia), although similar conditions may induce or augment aortic murmurs as well. Innocent flow murmurs are generally grade II/VI or less in intensity, reach their peak amplitude during early systole, are relatively brief, and diminish greatly in prominence or disappear altogether during the strain phase of Valsalva's maneuver.

Although an aortic murmur with these characteristics may bespeak a completely normal valve in the adolescent and young adult, it may also represent developing but hemodynamically inconsequential aortic sclerosis in the middle-aged adult. Findings that may be dismissed as innocuous in the young assume a different significance if discovered for the first time in an adult, particularly during the fifth and sixth decades. Several studies have demonstrated that, once established, the stenotic process may progress from insignificant to severe over spans as brief as 2 years, but the majority of patients show little or no progression over a span of several years.

Physical Findings. The peripheral manifestations of critical aortic stenosis are a reduced pulse volume and delayed upstroke, usually best appreciated on carotid artery palpation, which may also reveal systolic vibration or shudder, palpable evidence of stenotic jet-related turbulence (Fig. 66-2). The cardiac apex impulse is not displaced in uncomplicated aortic stenosis but is forceful and sustained. An exaggerated presystolic excursion somewhat medial to the apex may represent exaggerated atrial kick. A systolic thrill is often palpable at the base. A normal first sound is followed, usually after a brief gap, by a harsh, but occasionally musical murmur that radiates to the right base and neck, as mentioned above. The second heart sound is most often single in older adults, as a result of prolongation of ejection time and attenuation of A_2 by the immobility of the rigid aortic cusps.

Milder degrees of aortic stenosis are indicated by an earlier peak of the systolic murmur and preservation of the aortic closure sound in the adult. A murmur that peaks in mid to late systole usually corresponds with moderate or severe stenosis. A systolic ejection click is the hallmark of the bicuspid aortic valve, but this may be absent with advanced scarring and calcification of the leaflets. Aortic ejection sounds may indicate bicuspid valvular anatomy even in the absence of a systolic murmur.

Diagnosis

Further evaluation of a basal ejection murmur is obligatory whenever aortic valve pathology is suggested. This applies to all adults with ejection murmurs of grade III/VI or greater intensity, particularly when accompanied by any additional signs of significant stenosis. Adolescents or adults with less prominent murmurs are referred for noninvasive study if an early systolic sound compatible with an aortic ejection click is detected. Although confirmation of an abnormal aortic valve may not lead to immediate corrective therapy, the noninvasive studies may prove very useful in reassuring patients in whom valvular disease can be excluded, identifying individuals who are at risk and require closer follow-up, and establishing the diagnosis of bicuspid valvular anatomy, which has other therapeutic implications. Noninvasive studies also help to identify the muscular and discrete subvalvular membranous variants of left ventricular outflow obstruction, which are the most common entities to be differentiated from valvular stenosis in the adult.

Echocardiography with Doppler provides accurate assessment of the severity of stenosis, approximation of aortic valve area, and recognition of complicating features. Exercise testing may provide useful information about functional limitation in patients with mild or vague symptoms, but should be performed with extreme caution under close supervision.

Management

Once the diagnosis of aortic stenosis has been established, management has been aptly characterized as "masterly inactivity but cat-like observation." Morbidity and mortality risk is negligible during the asymptomatic phase, and serial noninvasive studies are unnecessary. Although the individual symptoms carry slightly different prognostic implications, it is the presence of any cardiac symptom in conjunction with physical evidence of aortic stenosis that is of paramount importance. Coincident with the advent of symptoms is a sharp downward turn in life expectancy, with an average

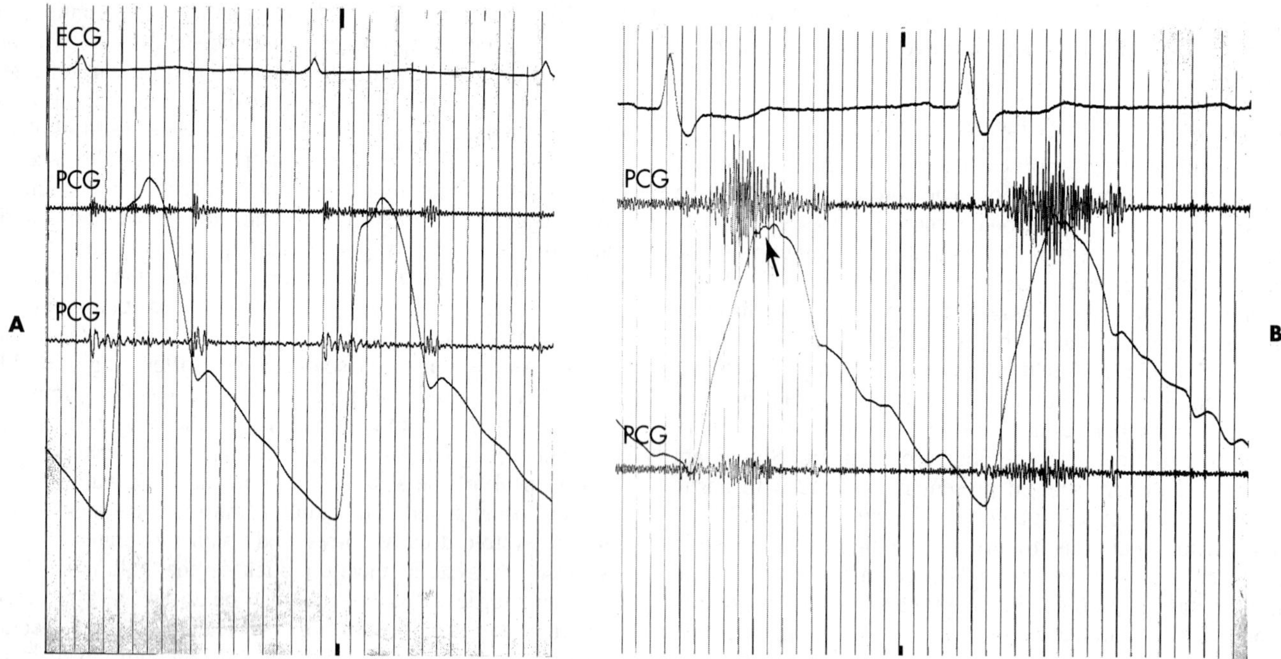

Fig. 66-2. Comparison of a normal carotid pulse (**A**) and the pulse tracing of a patient with aortic stenosis (**B**). Note the delay in upstroke with aortic stenosis and the vibration or shudder evident at the pulse peak *(arrow)*. A prominent systolic murmur, which peaks in midsystole, is evident on the phonocardiogram *(PCG)*.

survival thereafter of approximately 3 years. Thus the occurrence of angina, syncope, or congestive heart failure in the presence of a reasonable suspicion of aortic stenosis should always prompt referral for specialized evaluation.

Surgical replacement of the aortic valve is the only effective remedy currently available. Because of discouraging clinical results, balloon valvuloplasty has been relegated to a palliative role. Except for antibiotic prophylaxis, there is no medical treatment for aortic stenosis.

Only recently has the natural course of the bicuspid aortic valve become susceptible to prospective study. Older pathology studies suggested that about two thirds of these patients develop clinical evidence of some degree of aortic stenosis or insufficiency beyond age 40. A recent prospective echocardiographic study found that within 15 years of the diagnosis one quarter of the patients required aortic valve replacement. Because of the risk of endocarditis in these patients, antibiotic prophylaxis is a foremost consideration. For this reason, all young patients with suspected aortic ejection sounds (even if a murmur is not heard) should undergo echocardiography (Fig. 66-3) to elucidate aortic valve anatomy.

AORTIC REGURGITATION

Aortic regurgitation is encountered in clinical practice in acute, severe, and chronic forms. The hemodynamic differences are summarized in Fig. 66-4.

Chronic Aortic Regurgitation

Although the etiologic list is long, the most likely basis for chronic aortic regurgitation is a congenitally bicuspid aortic valve. Other causes include endocarditis, connective tissue disorders (e.g., Marfan syndrome), aortic aneurysm, myxomatous valvular degeneration, rheumatic fever, syphilis, and aortic involvement by rheumatoid arthritis or one of its variants.

History and Physical Examination. Most often, patients with chronic aortic regurgitation are asymptomatic at the time of diagnosis. The essential features of the physical examination are the bounding, collapsing (water-hammer) peripheral pulses with a widened pulse pressure; a downward, laterally displaced, hyperdynamic apex impulse; and the characteristic murmur. The high-pitched, blowing diastolic murmur is usually best heard along the left sternal margin; audibility to the right of the sternum suggests an aortic aneurysm. Of the plethora of eponymic designations assigned to the many peripheral manifestations of dynamic ejection of an abnormally large stroke volume, none contribute significantly to assessment of severity or management.

Diagnosis and Management. Echocardiography is indicated in all patients with aortic regurgitation and is used to establish the etiology, assess the severity of regurgitation, evaluate left ventricular size and function, and provide a basis for serial comparison.

Although severe aortic regurgitation can be tolerated for many years without symptoms, the adaptive reserve of the left ventricle is eventually exhausted. Ventricular function then declines, and symptoms of congestive heart failure or, rarely, angina appear. The latter symptom has been attributed to the increased left ventricular muscle mass and low diastolic (coronary perfusion) pressure.

Contemporary management is predicated on the repeatedly confirmed observation that replacement of the aortic valve prior to the onset of left ventricular dysfunction, even in asymptomatic patients, achieves better outcomes.[1,2] The most recent recommendations for management of chronic aortic

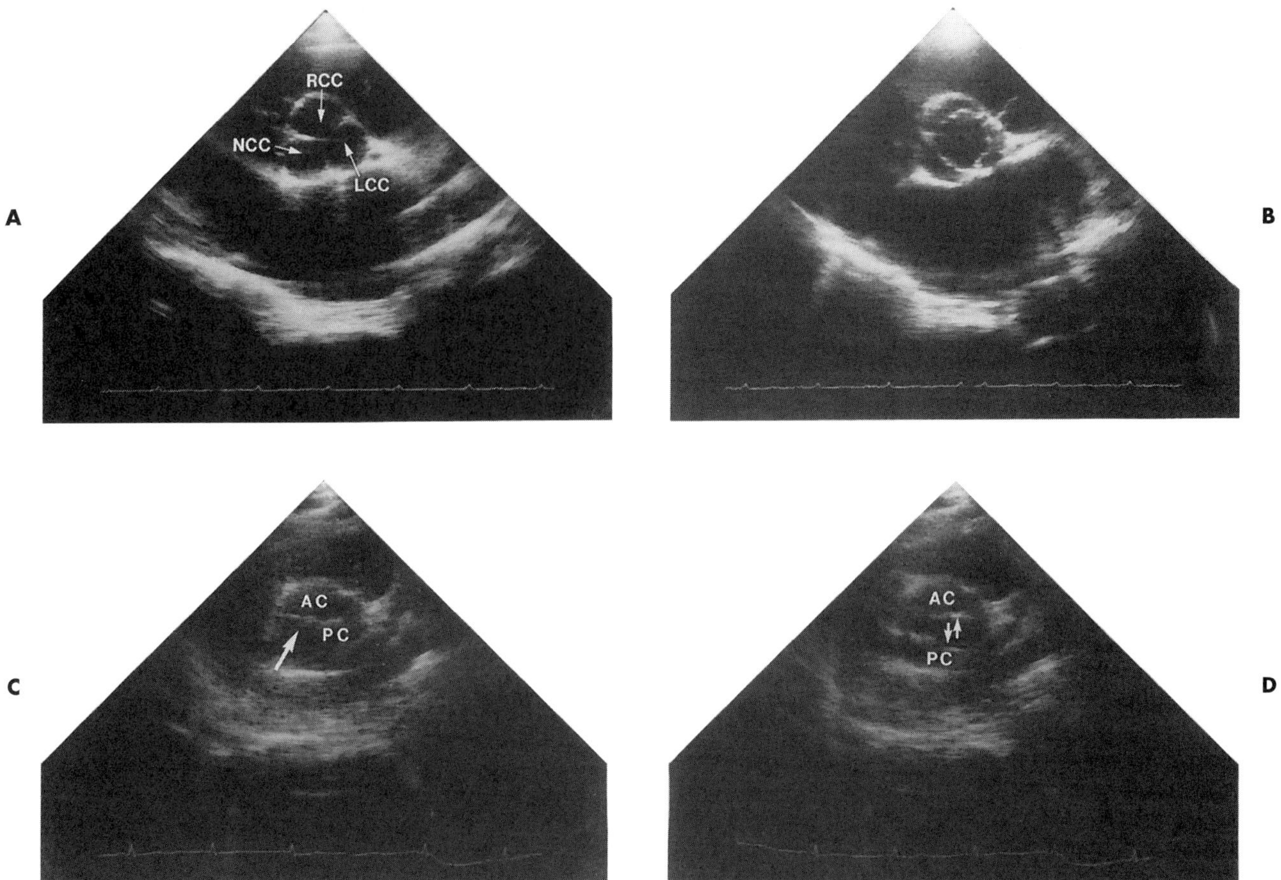

Fig. 66-3. Two-dimensional echocardiogram of a normal tricuspid aortic valve (**A** and **B**) and a bicuspid valve (**C** and **D**). Diastole is to the left and systole to the right. Three aortic cusps are clearly seen in the normal recording. A single horizontal commissure is evident during diastole in the bicuspid valve *(arrow)* with restricted opening during systole *(arrow)*. *RCC,* Right coronary cusp; *LCC,* left coronary cusp; *NCC,* noncoronary cusp; *AC,* anterior cusp; *PC,* posterior cusp.

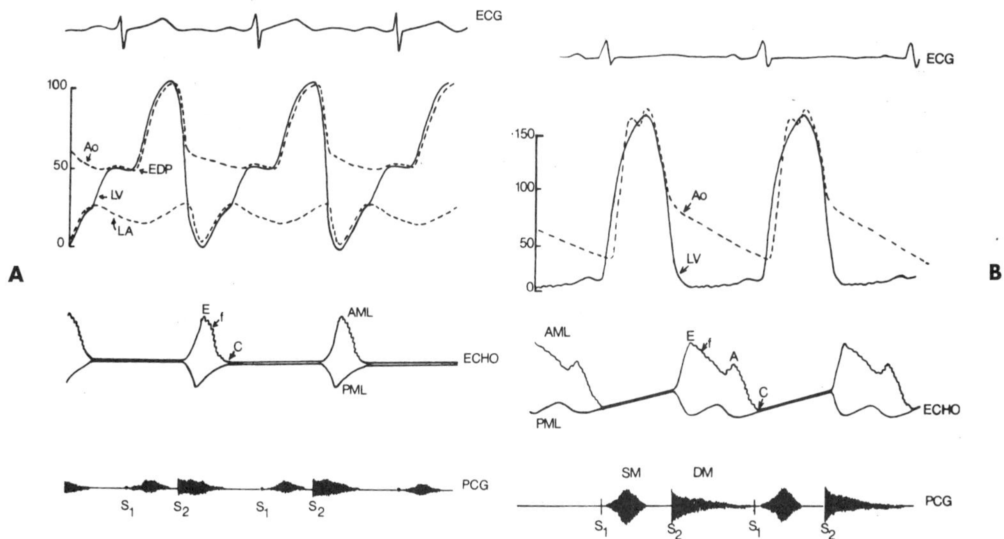

Fig. 66-4. Hemodynamic, echocardiographic *(ECHO),* and phonocardiographic *(PCG)* differences between acute severe (**A**) and chronic severe (**B**) aortic regurgitation. Left ventricular end diastolic pressure *(EDP)* is much higher in **A** with a narrower pulse pressure and preclosure of the mitral valve. *Ao,* Aorta; *LV,* left ventricle; *LA,* left atrium; *AML,* anterior mitral leaflet; *PML,* posterior mitral leaflet; *f,* flutter of the anterior mitral leaflet; *C,* mitral closure; *SM,* systolic murmur; *DM,* diastolic murmur. (From Morganroth J, et al: *Ann Intern Med* 87:223, 1977.)

Table 66-1. Guidelines for Management of Chronic Aortic Regurgitation

Severity	Left ventricular size and function	Symptoms	Management
Mild-Moderate	Normal	No	Annual clinical evaluation, antibiotic prophylaxis Echocardiogram every 2-3 years
Moderate-Severe	Enlarged (>60 mm) Normal Function	No	Clinical evaluation every 6 months Echocardiogram every 6-12 months depending on severity and stability* Vasodilator therapy
		Yes	Referral for consideration of aortic valve replacement Vasodilator therapy
	Abnormal (LVEF <0.50)†	Yes or No	Referral for aortic valve replacement Vasodilator therapy

*Serial echocardiography is recommended at 4-6 month intervals in those with advanced LV dilation (end-diastolic dimension >70, end-systolic >50).
†Valve replacement is recommended for all patients with severe LV dilation (end-diastolic dimension >75 mm, or end-systolic dimension >55 mm).

regurgitation are summarized in Table 66-1. Vasodilator therapy theoretically reduces regurgitant volume; slows, stabilizes, or reverses left ventricular dilation; and preserves left ventricular function. Salutary effects have been demonstrated with hydralazine and nifedipine in the short term (1 to 2 years) and with sustained-release nifedipine in the longer term (up to 6 years). Results with converting enzyme inhibition have been less compelling. Vasodilator therapy is indicated in all patients with severe aortic regurgitation accompanied by hypertension.

Acute Aortic Regurgitation

Pathophysiology. Most commonly, infective endocarditis causes acute aortic regurgitation. Less often, aortic trauma, prolapse, or rupture of a myxomatous valve, aortic dissection, or rupture of one of the sinuses of Valsalva, which may result in regurgitation into the right heart, is responsible. In contrast to the slowly progressive regurgitation dealt with above, sudden, massive aortic valvular incompetence precludes effective adaptive compensation. In the chronic situation, the left ventricle gradually dilates to accommodate the necessarily larger end-diastolic volume while maintaining a normal end-diastolic pressure (i.e., improved compliance). Following the Frank-Starling relationship, total stroke volume increases. The abrupt increase in diastolic volume with acute regurgitation into a nondilated ventricle produces a sharp increase in end-diastolic pressure. The contractile response is overwhelmed, and stroke volume decreases; increases in left atrial pressure and pulmonary arterial pressure ensue, aggravated by tachycardia and premature closure of the mitral valve.

Physical Examination. The characteristic bounding pulse and low diastolic pressure of the chronic counterpart are absent. Furthermore, lowered aortic pressure and tachycardia conspire to obscure the diastolic murmur, which often assumes a lower-pitched, coarser quality and may evade detection. More often, however, a to-and-fro auscultatory impression is imparted along the left sternal edge (see Fig. 66-4).

Diagnosis and Management. Echocardiography establishes the diagnosis, and transesophageal study provides superior definition of etiology (e.g., vegetations, aortic dissection).

Severe regurgitation of this type, apart from considerations pertinent to the primary cause (e.g., aortic dissection), is best managed by prompt replacement of the aortic valve. Interim support is frequently necessary, since these patients often verge on shock. Infusion of dobutamine or dopamine, with or without nitroprusside, as circumstances may allow, usually helps temporarily. When endocarditis presents in this fashion, the risk of mortality outweighs that of subsequent infection of the replacement valve, and surgery should not be deferred.

MITRAL STENOSIS

Etiology and Pathophysiology

Classic rheumatic mitral stenosis has virtually disappeared from practice in this country over the last 2 decades, and is now encountered most often in late evolution among the elderly or as a recurrent problem in patients who have previously undergone surgical or percutaneous palliation. Significant stenosis may occasionally be related to extensive calcification of the mitral annulus, and is infrequently simulated by an atrial tumor or a supravalvular membrane (cor triatriatum).

When the original mitral valve orifice has been reduced by about half, atrial pressure must increase to maintain normal diastolic flow into the left ventricle; tachycardia (reduced time for atrial emptying) or an increase in cardiac output raises atrial pressures further. Atrial pressures may reach 20 to 25 mm Hg at rest when the orifice is reduced to about 1 cm^2 or during exertion with less severe stenosis. This pressure is transmitted to the pulmonary capillary bed, tipping the normal transcapillary balance and producing interstitial edema. This mechanism is counterpoised to some extent by the development of pulmonary arteriolar vasoconstriction, pulmonary hypertension, and the decline in cardiac output that is characteristic of mitral stenosis.

History and Physical Examination

The course of rheumatic mitral stenosis, as elucidated by the now classic observations of Wood, includes a prolonged asymptomatic latency, a span of 20 years or more after the episode of rheumatic fever. Typically, this phase is punctuated by symptoms during periods of cardiovascular stress, particularly pregnancy, before sustained manifestations materialize. Once established, symptoms progress to disabling proportions over roughly a decade. Wide individual

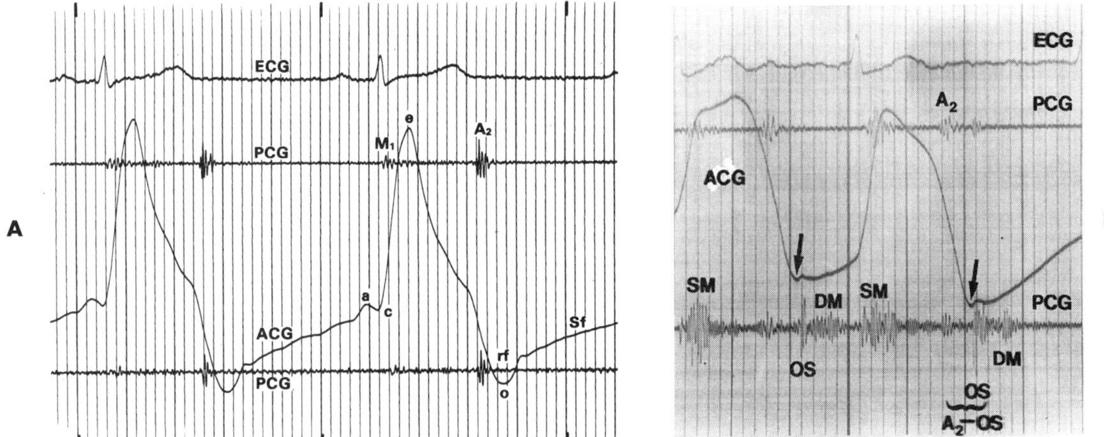

Fig. 66-5. A normal apexcardiogram *(ACG)* and phonocardiogram *(PCG)* (**A**) contrasted with that from a patient with mild mitral stenosis in atrial fibrillation (**B**). A mitral opening snap *(OS)* occurs shortly after the O point and is followed by a murmur *(DM)* that extends through only half of diastole with longer cycles. The A_2-OS stenosis interval of 125 ms is consistent with mild mitral stenosis. The rapid filling deflection *(rf)*, normally corresponding to rapid early diastolic filling, is notably attenuated *(arrow)*. A brief systolic murmur *(SM)* is also present. The normal a wave (a) is absent with atrial fibrillation. *A_2*, Aortic second sound.

variability, however, applies, and although progression of stenosis usually leads to symptoms during the fourth and fifth decades, a significant proportion of patients remain asymptomatic for much longer periods, some for a lifetime.

From the hemodynamic considerations cited above, the primacy of dyspnea as a manifestation of mitral stenosis, as well as the basis for the exacerbations of pulmonary congestion that accompany febrile conditions, anemia, and pregnancy, is readily apparent. Asymptomatic or mildly symptomatic patients may decompensate precipitously with the onset of atrial fibrillation, which occasions an abrupt rise in left atrial pressure. When querying patients with mitral stenosis, it is important to consider the dilatory pace of the symptoms, which affords the opportunity for both physiologic and psychologic adaptation.

On examination, the left ventricular apex impulse, which may elude palpation because of posterior rotation by an enlarged right ventricle, is normal in diameter, tapping, and nearly always accompanied by a systolic lift along the lower sternal edge. Emblematic of mitral stenosis are accentuation of S_1; the opening snap, a high frequency sound heard during early diastole and widely transmitted across the precordium caused by an abrupt halt to opening of the pliable though tethered anterior mitral leaflet (Fig. 66-5); and the low-pitched diastolic rumble. The diastolic murmur, as underscored by Sir William Osler, "may be concealed under a quarter of a dollar." It is thus essential to listen with the bell of the stethoscope applied immediately over the apex impulse.

Diagnosis and Management

Echocardiographic imaging and Doppler study confirm the diagnosis and accurately categorize the severity. Valuable additional information provided includes atrial dimension, the extent and severity of leaflet thickening and calcification, the presence and degree of subvalvular chordal involvement, semiquantitation of any associated mitral regurgitation, and assessment of right ventricular function and pulmonary artery pressure (Fig. 66-6). All of these factors contribute to management decisions. Doppler evaluation with exercise may be useful when symptoms seem disproportionately more or less severe than resting hemodynamics imply.

Mindful of the tendency for these patients to view behavioral adjustments, restrictions, and omissions as normal, symptoms that limit routine daily activities should prompt referral for evaluation and possible percutaneous or surgical intervention. Patients with evidence of NYHA class II symptoms and more than moderate stenosis (mitral valve area ≤ 1.5 cm^2) should be considered for valvuloplasty if valve morphology is suitable, and all patients with more advanced symptoms should be referred for intervention. In general, the results of percutaneous balloon valvulotomy are equivalent to those achieved with open surgical commissurotomy when performed by experienced operators, establishing this technique as the initial modality of choice when valvular morphology and related considerations are favorable.[3]

Atrial fibrillation commonly develops in patients with mitral stenosis, and often marks the onset of the progressive symptomatic phase. Digitalis is used for control of the ventricular response rate. Addition of low-dose calcium channel blocker or β-blocker may be necessary in some instances. Systemic embolization, most commonly cerebral, complicates the course of mitral stenosis in about 10% to 20% of cases and is usually associated with atrial fibrillation. All patients with atrial fibrillation and any patient with a history of embolization, regardless of rhythm, should be anticoagulated with warfarin.

Subacute bacterial endocarditis is seldom encountered as a complication of pure mitral stenosis. Nevertheless, antibiotic prophylaxis is recommended for dental and other procedures in the presence of rheumatic valvular disease.

MITRAL REGURGITATION

Pathophysiology and Natural History

Competence of the mitral valve during ventricular systole requires precisely coordinated interaction of the principal components of the mitral valve complex: valve leaflets, chordae tendineae, papillary muscles, and mitral annulus. Mitral regurgitation may be caused by dysfunction of any of

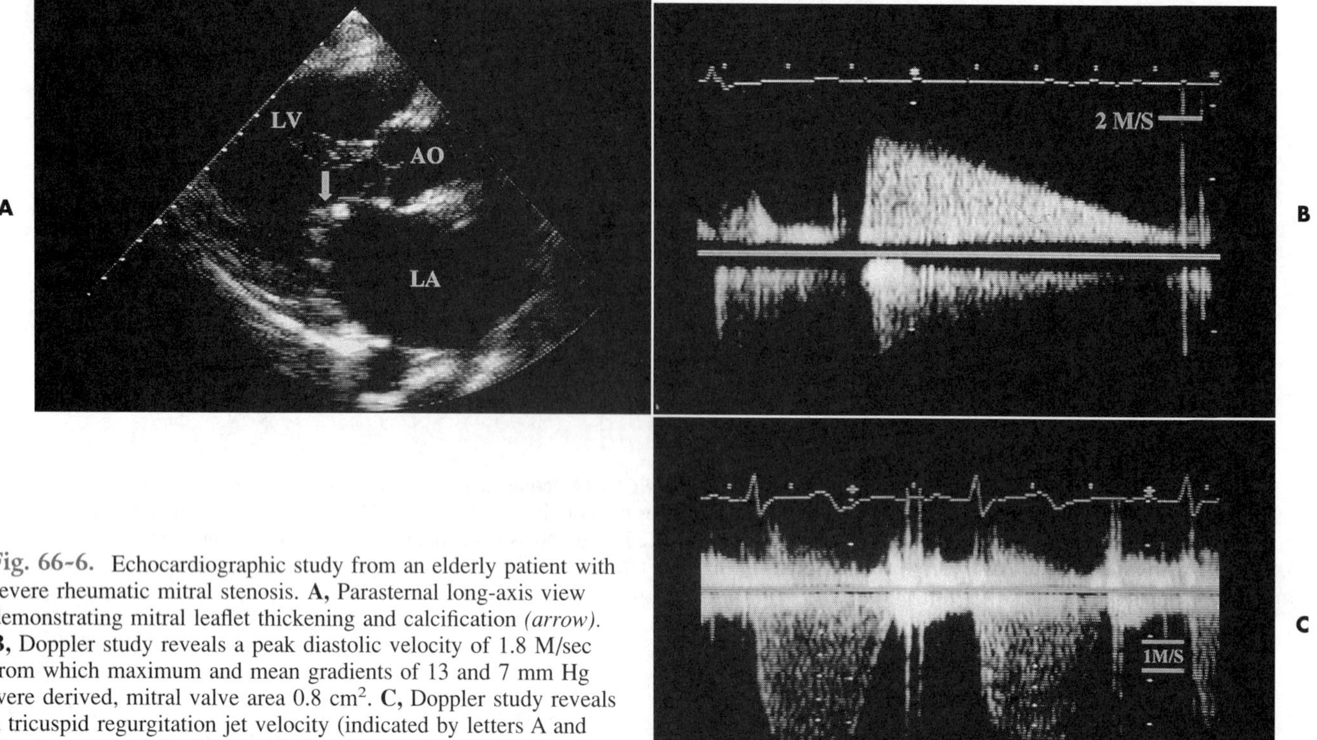

Fig. 66-6. Echocardiographic study from an elderly patient with severe rheumatic mitral stenosis. **A,** Parasternal long-axis view demonstrating mitral leaflet thickening and calcification *(arrow).* **B,** Doppler study reveals a peak diastolic velocity of 1.8 M/sec from which maximum and mean gradients of 13 and 7 mm Hg were derived, mitral valve area 0.8 cm^2. **C,** Doppler study reveals a tricuspid regurgitation jet velocity (indicated by letters A and B) of approximately 4 M/sec, indicating a pulmonary artery systolic pressure of nearly 75 mm Hg. *AO,* Aorta; *LA,* left atrium; *LV,* left ventricle.

these components. Common causes of mitral incompetence are mitral valve prolapse (myxomatous degeneration of the mitral valve), ruptured chordae tendineae, rheumatic fever, papillary muscle ischemia or infarction, tissue erosion related to endocarditis, and calcification of the mitral annulus. The term *functional mitral regurgitation* applies when regurgitation develops as a consequence of left ventricular dilation.

The natural history of this disorder is highly variable and depends on the etiology, acuity, and severity of the regurgitation, as well as the ability to mount and sustain an adaptive response. As an extreme example, the severe acute mitral regurgitation occasioned by papillary muscle rupture or endocarditic valvular disruption is immediately associated with pulmonary edema and often rapidly fatal if uncorrected. On the other hand, some patients with clinically severe mitral regurgitation may maintain functional class I status for over 20 years.

The left ventricle's ability to withstand the often massive volume overload imposed by mitral incompetence apparently results from the rapid decline in systolic wall tension (related to the product of systolic pressure and radius) permitted by left atrial decompression. Ventricular radius shortens more rapidly than normal in the presence of regurgitation. Because development of tension is a much more important determinant of myocardial oxygen demand than an actual decrease in muscle length, this compensation limits the energy cost and allows prolonged stability. Ventricular compensatory reserve, however, may eventually be exhausted; elevated diastolic pressures and progressive congestive symptoms follow. The left atrium also contributes importantly to the adaptive response. In chronic mitral regurgitation the left atrium dilates and may provide a cushion for the pulmonary circuit by absorbing a large regurgitant volume with minimal increases in pressure. Massive acute regurgitation into a small, noncompliant atrium, however, often results in marked pulmonary venous hypertension and pulmonary edema (Fig. 66-7).

Physical Examination

A briskly rising and somewhat collapsing arterial pulse termed *little water hammer* (an allusion to similar but much more pronounced findings in aortic regurgitation) is typical of compensated chronic severe mitral regurgitation. The apical impulse is enlarged, displaced downward to the left, and is a rapidly retracted or dynamic impulse. A systolic lift appreciated along the lower left sternal edge may suggest right ventricular overload but is as likely to reflect anterior displacement of the entire heart by left atrial expansion in systole. An attenuated S_1 coincides with the onset of a high-pitched, holosystolic murmur, which may radiate to the axilla and extend beyond A_2. Because A_2 occurs prematurely due to the inability to sustain ventricular pressure, splitting of the second sound may be noted during expiration. Rapid, early diastolic filling of the left ventricle produces a prominent S_3 gallop, which may be followed by a brief flow rumble. The presence of an S_4 gallop is indicative of a small, noncompliant, forcefully contracting left atrium and implies regurgitation of recent onset (within approximately 18 months) (e.g., chordal rupture).

Diagnosis and Management

Echocardiographic imaging with Doppler is indicated to confirm the diagnosis, determine the etiology, and establish baseline values for left ventricular dimensions and systolic function for serial comparison.

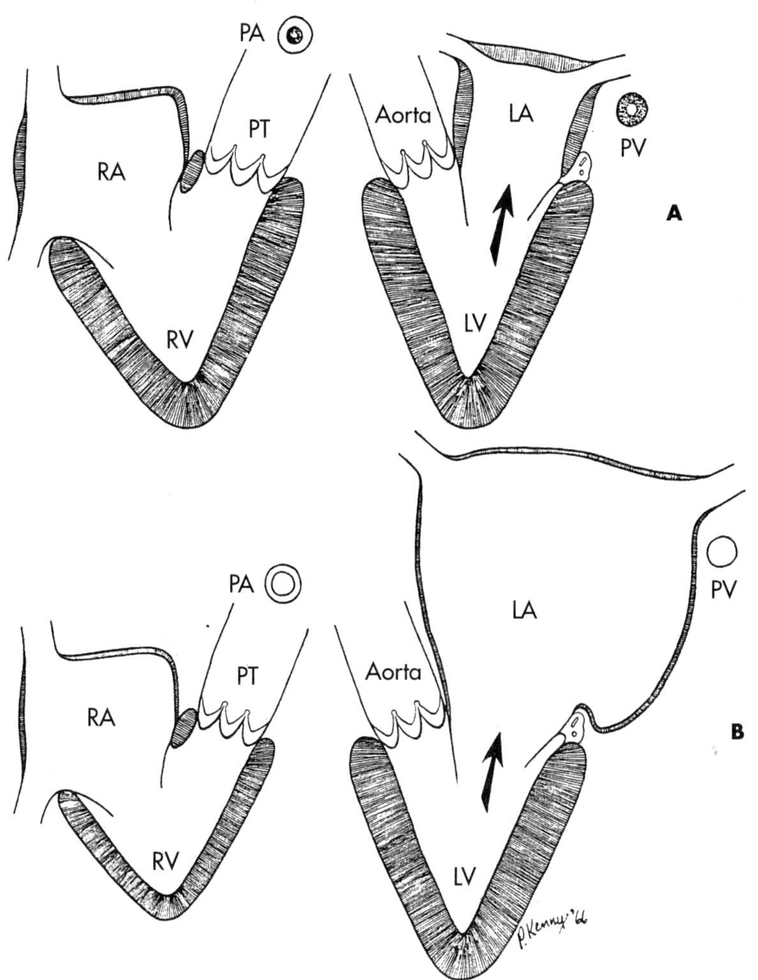

Fig. 66-7. The two extremes of pure mitral regurgitation *(MR)*. **A,** In acute severe MR, the left atrium *(LA)* is small and not compliant. As a result, high pressures are transmitted to the pulmonary venous *(PV)* and arterial *(PA)* system, resulting in medial hypertrophy in these vessels as well as hypertrophy of the right ventricle *(RV)*. **B,** With chronic severe MR, the LA dilates and is able to "absorb" regurgitant volume without marked pressure elevation, thereby sparing the pulmonary circulation. *PT,* Pulmonary trumk; *RA,* right atrium; *LV,* left ventricle. (From Roberts WC, Perloff JK: *Ann Intern Med* 77:939, 1972.)

The goal of medical therapy for acute, severe regurgitation is stabilization prior to surgery. Nitroprusside, alone or in combination with an inotropic agent, such as dobutamine, and aortic balloon counterpulsation are most commonly employed.

Management of chronic mitral regurgitation has been somewhat more controversial, particularly the indications for and timing of surgery. The most current recommendations are summarized in Table 66-2. The aim is to intervene prior to the development of left ventricular decompensation that may lead to suboptimal outcomes after valve repair or replacement. Although vasodilator therapy has some intuitive appeal, it is of no proven benefit in nonhypertensive patients with mitral regurgitation.[4]

MITRAL VALVE PROLAPSE

The observations of Reid and Barlow just over 3 decades ago established the relationship between systolic prolapse of the mitral valve leaflets and the auscultatory findings of midsystolic click with or without a late systolic murmur. This disorder has now emerged as the most prevalent and problematic concern of the medical practitioner, affecting approximately 5% of the general population. Prolapse is encountered at all ages, and, contrary to popular belief, involvement appears to be approximately equal in men and women.

Pathophysiology

The term *primary mitral prolapse* is used to distinguish inherent abnormalities in the mitral valve apparatus from prolapse secondary to other conditions. The primary abnormality is myxomatous degeneration that disrupts the normal connective tissue architecture of the valve leaflets, chordae, or annulus. Myxomatous tissue, consisting of an abundant mucopolysaccharide matrix within which collagen fibers are sparsely and haphazardly arrayed, is ultimately responsible for the characteristic redundancy or hooding of the valve leaflets on gross inspection and for the propensity to chordal rupture associated with mitral prolapse. Cohort studies indicate that primary prolapse is hereditary and transmitted as an autosomal dominant trait with variable expression. The causes of secondary mitral prolapse are numerous, but connective tissue disorders, notably Marfan syndrome, secundum atrial septal defect, coronary artery disease, and mitral valvuloplasty, are commonly cited.

History and Physical Examination

Population studies indicate that the vast majority of affected individuals are asymptomatic. Furthermore, several symptoms traditionally ascribed to prolapse (e.g., dyspnea in the absence of significant mitral regurgitation, fatigue, dizziness, and neurosis) seem to bear no direct relation to the valvular abnormality and may be only coincidentally associated.

Table 66-2. Guidelines for Management of Chronic Mitral Regurgitation

Severity	Left ventricular size and function	Symptoms	Management
Mild-Moderate	Normal	No	Annual clinical evaluation, antibiotic prophylaxis Echocardiography only with evidence of significant clinical changes Patients instructed to report symptoms of dyspnea or palpitations immediately
Moderate-Severe	Enlarged (>60 mm) LV ejection fraction >0.60 End-systolic dimension <45 mm	No	Refer for cardiology evaluation and consideration of early repair (versus continued medical management) based on etiology and suitability
		Yes	Refer for surgery
	LV ejection fraction <0.60 End-systolic dimension >45 mm	Yes or No	Refer for surgery

The two most common complaints from patients with mitral prolapse are chest pain and palpitations. Chest pain usually differs from typical angina in several respects; specifically, the character is usually sharp or stabbing, the duration is often protracted, a relationship to exertion is absent, and nitroglycerin seldom affords relief. Very rarely the pain closely mimics angina.

Thoracic cage abnormalities, such as pectus excavatum or straight back, are associated with mitral prolapse. The hallmark of prolapse is the mid to late systolic click, which is the only detectable manifestation in more than half the cases. Aortic or pulmonic ejection clicks are frequently mistaken as a manifestation of prolapse but are distinguishable by their timing with the upstroke of the carotid pulse and by typical respiratory variation in the case of the pulmonic click. Rarely, a prolapsing mitral leaflet generates an early systolic click. Estimates vary, but in approximately 15% of cases the click is followed by a brief midsystolic or late systolic murmur. Occasionally the murmur is pansystolic in duration or honking in quality.

The timing of mitral prolapse has been demonstrated to occur reproducibly at a critical systolic volume, thereby accounting for the effects of various maneuvers in evoking characteristic responses in this condition (Fig. 66-8). Measures that decrease cardiac filling (e.g., standing, Valsalva's strain, amyl nitrite administration) reduce ventricular end-diastolic volume. As a result the critical systolic volume and the click/murmur occur earlier. Conversely, passive leg elevation or a deep knee bend increases ventricular filling, delays attainment of the prolapse volume, and either displaces the click/murmur into later systole or eradicates the findings altogether. The variability in auscultation from one examination to another may be striking. Some patients exhibit only a click on occasion, no evidence of prolapse at times, and both click and murmur in other instances.

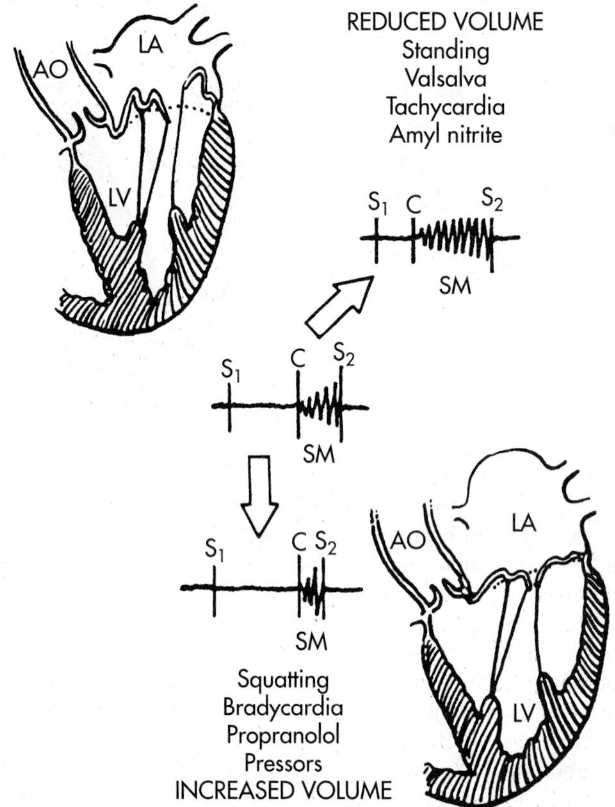

Fig. 66-8. Effects of various maneuvers that influence diastolic ventricular volume on the timing of the click *(C)* and murmur *(SM)* in mitral valve prolapse. *AO*, Aorta; *LA*, left atrium; *LV*, left ventricle. (From Devereux RB et al: *Circulation* 54:3, 1976.)

Diagnosis

Echocardiography corroborates clinical findings and may identify the estimated 20% of patients in whom auscultatory evidence is lacking. Echocardiography also provides important prognostic information, such as the presence or absence of leaflet thickening, left atrial or ventricular enlargement, and mitral regurgitation.

Somewhat more than one third of patients display ECG repolarization abnormalities. These usually consist of T wave flattening or inversion in the inferior leads; variable ST-segment changes accompany these changes, which frequently are noted in the lateral precordial leads as well.

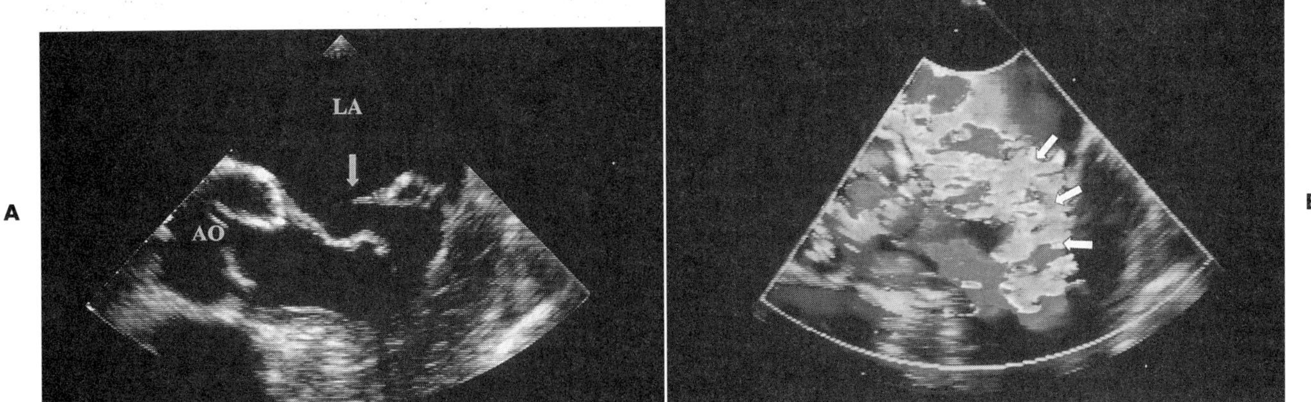

Fig. 66-9. Transesophageal echocardiographic study of a patient with mitral valve prolapse, chordal rupture, and severe mitral regurgitation. **A,** Partially flail segment of the posterior leaflet with detached chordal remnant at its tip *(arrow)*. **B,** Color Doppler reveals a large area of regurgitant jet flow *(arrows)*. *LA,* left atrium, *AO,* aorta.

The occurrence of falsely positive exercise ECG in patients with mitral prolapse should be recalled when exercise testing is considered.

Management

The outlook for most patients with mitral prolapse is favorable, and this aspect deserves the strongest emphasis in discussions of the diagnosis with patients. Because of selection bias, relevant literature includes a disproportion of symptomatic patients. This complicates projection of progression to chordal rupture or significant mitral regurgitation, reported at about 15%, to the asymptomatic patient seen in the office. The presence of a systolic murmur at diagnosis and the presence of significant leaflet thickening or mitral regurgitation on echocardiography confer a higher risk for subsequent complications (Fig. 66-9), and these individuals warrant more cautious observation. As a rule, annual follow-up with echocardiograms when changes are suspected suffices for those with mild regurgitation. Significant mitral regurgitation is managed as previously outlined.

Although it is widely conceded that prolapse poses a hazard for endocarditis in patients with a systolic murmur, there is no firm evidence that an isolated click imparts the same liability. Currently, it is recommended that patients with a murmur and those with features implying a higher risk for endocarditis (e.g., leaflet thickening, left atrial or ventricular enlargement) receive prophylaxis.

All varieties of dysrhythmia have been associated with mitral prolapse, but the actual prevalence is substantially less than case reports imply. It has been suggested that supraventricular premature beats and tachydysrhythmias in mitral valve prolapse may be caused by depolarization of smooth muscle cells that have been identified in excised mitral valve tissue. Alternatively, concealed atrioventricular (AV) nodal bypass tracts, so-called because they permit any retrograde conduction (ventricle to atrium), may foster reentry. Regardless of the substrate, therapy is necessary only for symptomatic and distressing dysrhythmias, and a β-blocker is a good first choice.

Sudden death occurs in a very small proportion of patients with prolapse. Reported cases occurred predominantly in women, age 40 or older, usually with evidence of advanced mitral regurgitation. Ventricular ectopy was evident in more than three fourths of those for whom relevant information was available, and more than half of those described in sufficient detail had previously experienced syncope. Patients with recurrent syncope and symptomatic ventricular dysrhythmias should be referred for electrophysiologic evaluation.

Both transient and permanent neurologic impairment have been observed in patients with mitral valve prolapse. An excessive prevalence of mitral prolapse has also been noted among patients under 40 years of age who incur a stroke. The inference that cerebral embolism explains these observations derives from the identification of macroscopic coalescence of platelets and fibrin on the atrial surface of the abnormal mitral leaflets in some patients. Attractive as this hypothesis may seem, it is far from firmly established. The role played by atrial rhythm disturbances requires further clarification, and an association of migraine headache with prolapse suggests another possible basis (i.e., vasospasm). Conclusive data notwithstanding, warfarin is usually utilized in patients with transient ischemia or stroke. Aspirin may be of benefit for patients in sinus rhythm and high-risk prolapse by echocardiography.

TRICUSPID VALVE DISEASE

Tricuspid Stenosis

Tricuspid stenosis is nearly always a consequence of rheumatic fever and is invariably accompanied by left heart valvular involvement. The pathology resembles mitral stenosis. Fatigue, a consequence of low cardiac output, is a prominent symptom, as are the other signs of right atrial hypertension including edema or anasarca, ascites, and hepatomegaly.

Diagnostic physical findings include large jugular a waves with sinus rhythm and sluggish y descent, which may be more palpable than visible if atrial fibrillation is present. The most helpful auscultatory finding is the diastolic decrescendo murmur to the left of the lower sternum, which is relatively high-pitched and easily misconstrued as aortic regurgitation. Echocardiography reveals leaflet thickening with reduced mobility and provides accurate assessment of the valvular gradient.

Tricuspid Regurgitation

Tricuspid regurgitation most often develops as a late consequence of left ventricular failure, regardless of etiology, as a result of sustained reactive pulmonary hypertension. Chronic right ventricular volume overload and dilation in atrial septal defect may induce secondary or "functional" tricuspid incompetence. Other primary causes of tricuspid regurgitation include trauma, carcinoid syndrome, endocarditis, rheumatic fever, myxomatous degeneration, and Ebstein's anomaly.

History and Physical Examination

Primary tricuspid regurgitation may be tolerated well for an indefinite period in the absence of pulmonary hypertension. Secondary regurgitation, however, serves only to exacerbate the manifestations of right ventricular failure. Examination discloses sustained ascent instead of descent of the jugular meniscus during systole and palpable hepatic pulsation. Echocardiography with Doppler confirms the diagnosis and clarifies etiology.

Management

Secondary tricuspid regurgitation usually responds to therapeutic measures directed at the principal offender (i.e., diuretics, and vasodilators in left ventricular failure), surgical correction of aortic or mitral valve disease, and measures intended to lower pulmonary pressures in the presence of lung disease. Indications for referral to a cardiologist include those previously indicated for any associated valvular disease, symptomatic primary tricuspid regurgitation, or recalcitrance to the medical therapy. Surgical tricuspid annuloplasty is the treatment of choice in refractory cases; valve replacement is reserved for circumstances in which satisfactory annular plication cannot be achieved.

Surgery for tricuspid stenosis is usually undertaken simultaneously with correction of the mitral and aortic valve abnormalities and most often consists of bioprosthetic valve replacement. Selected patients may be candidates for percutaneous commissurotomy.

VALVULAR DISEASE ASSOCIATED WITH APPETITE-SUPPRESSANT DRUGS

Recognition that the use of the anorectic agents phentermine, fenfluramine, and dexfenfluramine might produce a form of fibrosclerotic heart valve damage similar to that associated with ergotamine and methysergide has provoked a level of concern proportionate to the inordinate use of these agents. Published estimates vary considerably, but abnormalities of the aortic, mitral, or tricuspid valves may be detected in up to one third of patients who have received these agents alone or in combination for more than 4 months. The incidence of clinically significant valvular insufficiency is substantially lower, but the natural course of mild abnormalities awaits definition.

Routine echocardiographic screening of patients who have received these anorectic drugs is not recommended, but diagnostic evaluation is appropriate when a murmur, particularly a new murmur of aortic or mitral insufficiency, is detected on examination.

ENDOCARDITIS

Clinical features, bacteriologic aspects, and antibiotic therapy are discussed in detail in Chapter 69. The combination of antibiotic therapy and timely surgical intervention has substantially reduced mortality with infective endocarditis. Questions regarding the need for and the timing of surgery, however, are often problematic because of the wide-ranging variability in the complexity and severity of the cardiac manifestations and the difficulty in balancing benefit-risk considerations. Relevant factors include valve type, heart failure, persistent infection, embolization, infecting organism, extravalvular extension, and other complications. Generally a cardiologist should be involved in the management of these patients.

Consideration of surgery in endocarditis must include a decision analysis that balances the risks of medical treatment with those of surgical intervention, which include not only operative mortality and morbidity, but the long-term complications of valvular prostheses and anticoagulation. Absolute indications for surgical intervention are advanced heart failure that is directly related to valve dysfunction and uncontrolled infection, including evidence of serious perivalvular extension. Relative indications for surgery include (1) perivalvular infection, (2) recurrent embolization, especially in the presence of large, mobile vegetations, (3) *Staphylococcus aureus* endocarditis, (4) infection with fungal or other resistant organisms, and (5) relapse after appropriate treatment.

Moderate to severe heart failure caused by infective endocarditis and valve dysfunction confers a high mortality risk without corrective surgery. Medical therapy alone is associated with mortality rates of approximately 75% and can be reduced to about 25% with surgery. Thus patients with advanced heart failure should undergo operation before extreme or refractory hemodynamic deterioration develops. Failure to clear bacteremia after 3 to 5 days of appropriate antibiotic therapy or other clinical evidence that treatment has failed to control the infective process constitutes a strong indication for surgery.

Infection extends beyond the valve leaflets in 10% to 20% of patients with native valve endocarditis, and infections complicated by the formation of perivalvular abscesses and fistulas are notoriously resistant to antibiotic therapy. For this reason, evidence of such a complication is a strong indication for surgical intervention. Transesophageal echocardiography (TEE) is required in all instances where such complications are suspected (Fig. 66-10).

In older literature, the finding of vegetations on echocardiography was associated with a higher risk of death, congestive failure, or need for surgery during the course of endocarditis. Many, but not all, published reports on vegetation size indicate an increased probability of complications when vegetations measuring one centimeter or more in diameter are detected by echocardiography. Recent reports relating to vegetation size are not uniform: some suggest that large vegetations correlate with systemic emboli but not heart failure or mortality, others that size alone is a poor predictor of embolization. The decision to proceed to surgery should not be based solely on vegetation size. Other features of a vegetation may help to identify those more likely to produce embolization. Clearly, large vegetations combined with recurrent embolization in the treated patient present a strong indication for surgery.

Patients with severe valve dysfunction who respond to antibiotic therapy and who manifest evidence of no more than mild, nonprogressive heart failure should complete a full

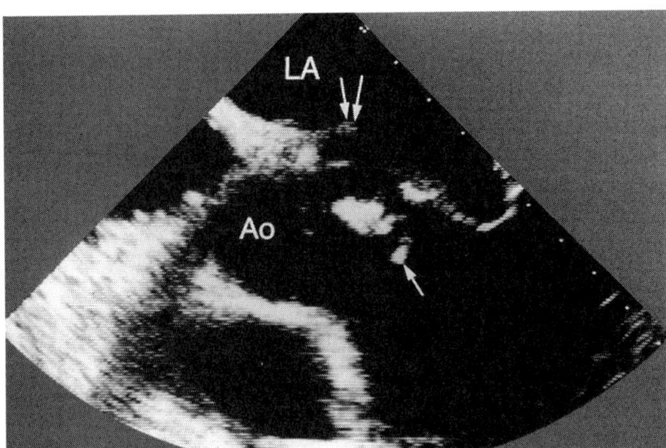

Fig. 66-10. Transesophageal echocardiogram from a patient with a bicuspid aortic valve and *S. aureus* endocarditis. The frame shows an aortic ring abscess *(double arrow)* bulging into the left atrium *(LA),* as well as a large mobile vegetation in the left ventricular outflow tract *(single arrow). Ao,* Aorta.

course of antibiotics before surgery is undertaken. If progressive heart failure occurs or evidence of other complications develops, surgery should be performed as soon as possible. An exception to this general guideline is the patient with cerebral embolization. Cardiac surgery and related anticoagulation increase the risk of additional neurologic damage. For this reason, surgery should be delayed 5 to 10 days in patients who have had an embolic stroke and at least twice that interval in those with evidence of intracranial hemorrhage.

POSTOPERATIVE VALVULAR PATIENTS

Current estimates place the number of heart valve operations above 50,000 annually, which cumulatively projects to a large population of patients who require vigilant follow-up care. Obviously, it is impractical to expect the physician to command the minute details of individual artificial valves, but design features allow manageable grouping, and the long-term complications are similar among all prostheses. Familiarity with fundamental aspects is essential, considering the high probability that postoperative valvular patients will be encountered in any practice.

Replacement heart valves are categorized by components as either mechanical or bioprosthetic. Two types of mechanical prostheses are currently available in the United States, caged-ball (Starr Edwards) valves, now seldom used, and tilting disk valves, which may have one (Medtronic Hall, Omniscience) or two (St. Jude, Carbomedics) pivoting disks. Bioprostheses include porcine valves, bovine pericardial valves, and homografts.

After successful surgery, complications may be grouped into three major categories: (1) prosthetic valve failure, (2) thromboembolism and the hazards of anticoagulation, and (3) prosthetic endocarditis.

Prosthetic Valve Dysfunction

Prosthetic valve dysfunction is usually not a consequence of structural failure of currently available mechanical prostheses. Thus the term most often implies prosthetic obstruction or regurgitation; the former usually results from pannus ingrowth or thrombosis, and the latter is actually periprosthetic. Bioprosthetic tissue is obviously subject to dysfunction by erosion or scarring. The current literature suggests an annual failure rate of about 1% over the first 5 years, with cumulative incidence of 20% for homografts and 30% for porcine heterografts by 10 to 15 years. Studies suggest lower failure rates for the newer bovine pericardial valves, approximately 5% at 10 years.

Auscultatory expectations vary with the type of prosthesis. More important than any a priori findings specified for a particular valve is a thorough and meticulous documentation of auscultation in the early postreplacement interval. Valvular dysfunction is typically heralded by the disappearance of previously audible clicks or the development of new murmurs that cannot be accounted for by changes in hemodynamic state, such as variable intensity of opening and closure sounds with atrial fibrillation or enhancement of murmurs by anemia. It is well recognized, however, that even severe prosthetic abnormalities may develop without detectable auscultatory evidence. When sinus rhythm is present, beat-to-beat alteration in prosthetic sound intensity always suggests dysfunction. Patients suspected to have prosthetic valvular dysfunction require referral for specialized evaluation.

Echocardiography plays an important role in follow-up of postoperative valvular patients, and a baseline study should be obtained prior to hospital discharge or soon thereafter without exception. Imaging and Doppler evaluation are very helpful when valvular dysfunction is suspected, and the superior resolution of transesophageal study may provide important additional information, particularly when mitral prosthetic function is at issue. Although some hemolysis occurs with all mechanical prostheses, an increase in the degree of hemolysis may occur with valve dysfunction. Determination of lactic dehydrogenase (LDH) and haptoglobin levels once patients have fully recovered from surgery establishes a potentially useful reference base.

Thromboembolism

For anticoagulated patients, the risk of thromboembolism from a mechanical aortic prosthesis averages 1% per year or less; the risk is about double this for a mitral prosthesis. Patients with bioprostheses in normal sinus rhythm do not require anticoagulation beyond the immediate postoperative period, and this is the most attractive feature of these valves. However, atrial fibrillation and severe left ventricular dysfunction remain as indications for long-term anticoagulation in patients with bioprosthetic valves. An isolated thromboembolic event need not occasion extensive evaluation in the absence of other indications of valve dysfunction. Recurrent embolization in the presence of a therapeutic INR may be managed by addition of aspirin or other antiplatelet agents. Although advocated by some, routine use of low-dose aspirin in addition to warfarin for mechanical prostheses is not the practice of most authorities.[5] Estimates of significant hemorrhage in anticoagulated patients range as high as about 6% annually, with severe episodes in 2% and related fatality in about 0.5%.

Anticoagulation should be temporarily withheld following embolic stroke until the possibility of a hemorrhagic component can be clarified. For major surgery, dental extractions, gynecologic procedures, or diagnostic procedures that may eventuate in surgery, anticoagulation is usually discontinued 3 to 5 days beforehand and resumed as soon as possible thereafter. The administration of vitamin K is discouraged. Relevant literature neither strongly supports nor refutes the interim use of intravenous or low-molecular-weight heparin for these short terms, but parenteral anticoagulation is indicated when the INR falls below 2 for 5 days. The potential for embryopathy and the unpredictable need for restitution of normal coagulation at delivery provides the rationale for the substitution of subcutaneous heparin for warfarin during the first trimester and again immediately before term in pregnant women with prostheses.

Prosthetic Endocarditis

The annual rate of prosthetic valvular infection approaches 1%. Infection that develops within 2 months of valve replacement (early PVE) is most often caused by coagulase-negative staphylococci, *S. aureus,* or gram-negative bacilli. The mortality rate, despite antibiotic therapy, remains high (50% to 75%). Late PVE is more often of streptococcal etiology and carries a lower mortality risk (40% to 50%). Antibiotic cures may be achieved with PVE, and are most likely when there is evidence of bioprosthetic leaflet involvement and maintenance of perivalvular integrity. Infection of mechanical prostheses is perivalvular, and the probability of successful eradication with antibiotics, except with an organism displaying high antibiotic susceptibility, is low. Most patients will require surgery, which is usually preceded by a period of drug therapy. Removal of an infected prosthesis is indicated if there is persistent bacteremia despite appropriate therapy, evidence of valve dehiscence or dysfunction, and relapse after treatment.

Patients with prosthetic valves share a higher risk of endocarditis following bacteremia and should be imbued with a strong sense of the need for antibiotic prophylaxis for dental and other procedures (see Chapter 69). Embolization may be an indication of prosthetic infection, and this possibility should always be considered. The limited data available suggest that cerebrovascular morbidity is higher if anticoagulation is stopped during the course of prosthetic endocarditis; thus warfarin should be continued unless another specific contraindication arises.

REFERENCES

1. Bonow RO, Carabello B, de Leon AC Jr, et al: ACC/AHA guidelines for the management of patients with valvular heart disease: executive summary. A report of the American College of Cardiology/American Heart Association Task Force on Practice Guidelines (Committee on Management of Patients with Valvular Heart Disease), *Circulation* 98:1949-1986, 1993.
2. Carabello BA, Crawford FA: Valvular heart disease, *N Engl J Med* 337:32-41, 1997.
3. Glazier JJ, Turi ZG: Percutaneous balloon mitral valvuloplasty, *Prog Cardiovasc Dis* 40:5-26, 1997.
4. Levine HJ, Gaasch WH: Vasoactive drugs in chronic regurgitant lesions of the mitral and aortic valves, *J Am Coll Cardiol* 28:1083-1091, 1996.
5. Tiede DJ, Nishimura RA, Gastineau DA, et al: Modern management of prosthetic valve anticoagulation, *Mayo Clin Proc* 73:665-680, 1998.

CHAPTER 67

Adult Manifestations of Congenital Heart Disease

Edgar C. Schick, Jr.

Congenital heart disease comprises unusual fare for the adult practitioner. Even among major adult cardiology referral centers, congenital defects seldom constitute more than 5% of all cases; of those, atrial septal defects account for about half, and coarctation of aorta, patent ductus arteriosus, and pulmonic stenosis the bulk of the remainder. Unmodified cyanotic congenital disease has all but vanished from adult practice as a result of advances in surgical correction or palliation. The survivors of these procedures often present complex combinations of persistent anatomic abnormalities, as well as a spectrum of iatrogenic problems almost invariably requiring follow-up at specialized centers. The following considerations are limited to those problems most likely to be encountered in the adult.

ACYANOTIC CONGENITAL DISEASE WITHOUT SHUNT

Pulmonic Stenosis

Valvular pulmonic stenosis imposes a systolic pressure burden on the right ventricle that leads to right ventricular hypertrophy. Symptoms, when present, reflect limitation of cardiac output because of increased afterload on the right ventricle and the right heart failure that may ensue. Exertional fatigue and dyspnea are common; chest pain and syncope are encountered less frequently. Patients with mild to moderate degrees of obstruction, usually defined as a peak transvalvular gradient of 40 mm Hg or less, may remain asymptomatic through adult life. Those with more severe obstruction are candidates for intervention.

The clinical findings generally correlate well with the hemodynamic measurements. A crescendo-decrescendo murmur most prominent at the upper left sternal edge that ends well before aortic valve closure indicates mild stenosis. A prolonged systolic murmur, which may extend beyond and obscure the sound of aortic closure, suggests more severe obstruction. A pulmonic ejection click is typically present, and with increasingly severe stenosis the click migrates toward the first heart sound. The pulmonic component of the second heart sound, when audible, is delayed; as a result, the second sound is widely split (Fig. 67-1). Further markers of severe stenosis include a prominent jugular a wave, a right ventricular lift, a systolic thrill along the left sternal edge, and an S_4 gallop that intensifies on inspiration.

The electrocardiogram (ECG) is usually normal with mild pulmonic stenosis and exhibits evidence of right ventricular hypertrophy and right atrial enlargement with increasing severity. The x-ray may show poststenotic dilation of the main pulmonary artery. Echocardiography provides precise identification of the level of obstruction, accurate characterization of hemodynamic severity, and assessment of right ventricular wall thickness and function (Fig. 67-2).

Mild pulmonary stenosis carries an excellent prognosis.[3] Patients with evidence of mild stenosis (peak systolic

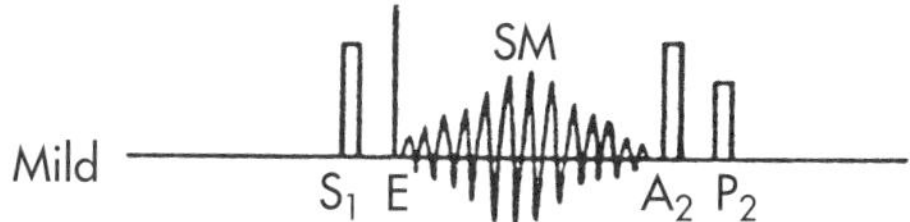

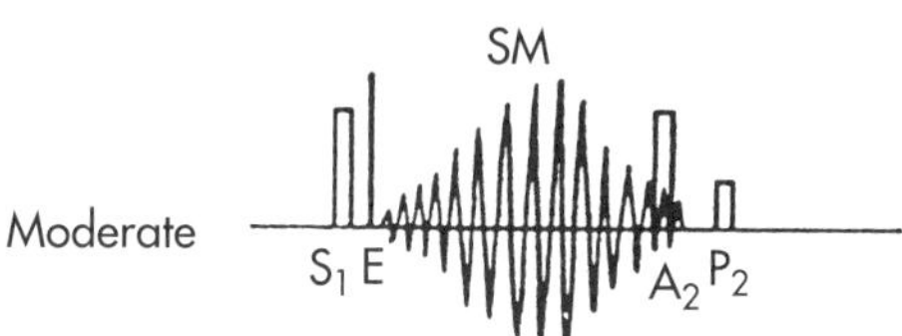

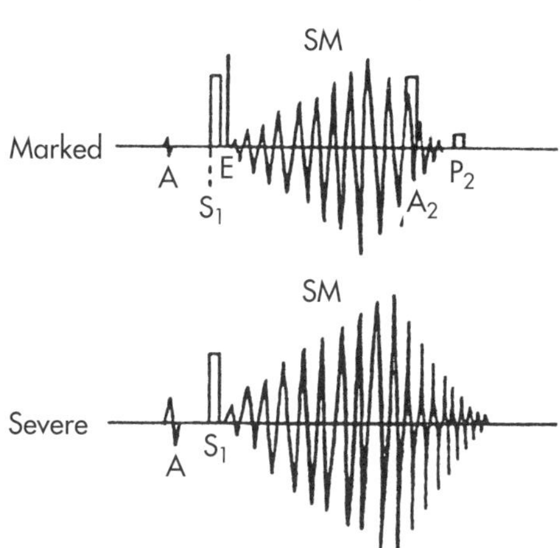

Fig. 67-1. Auscultatory findings in congenital pulmonic stenosis. With increasing severity, the duration of the murmur *(SM)* is prolonged and the intensity of the pulmonic closure *(P_2)* diminishes. *S_1*, First heart sound; *E*, pulmonic ejection click; *A_2*, aortic closure. (From Perloff JK: *The clinical recognition of congenital heart disease*, Philadelphia, 1970, WB Saunders.)

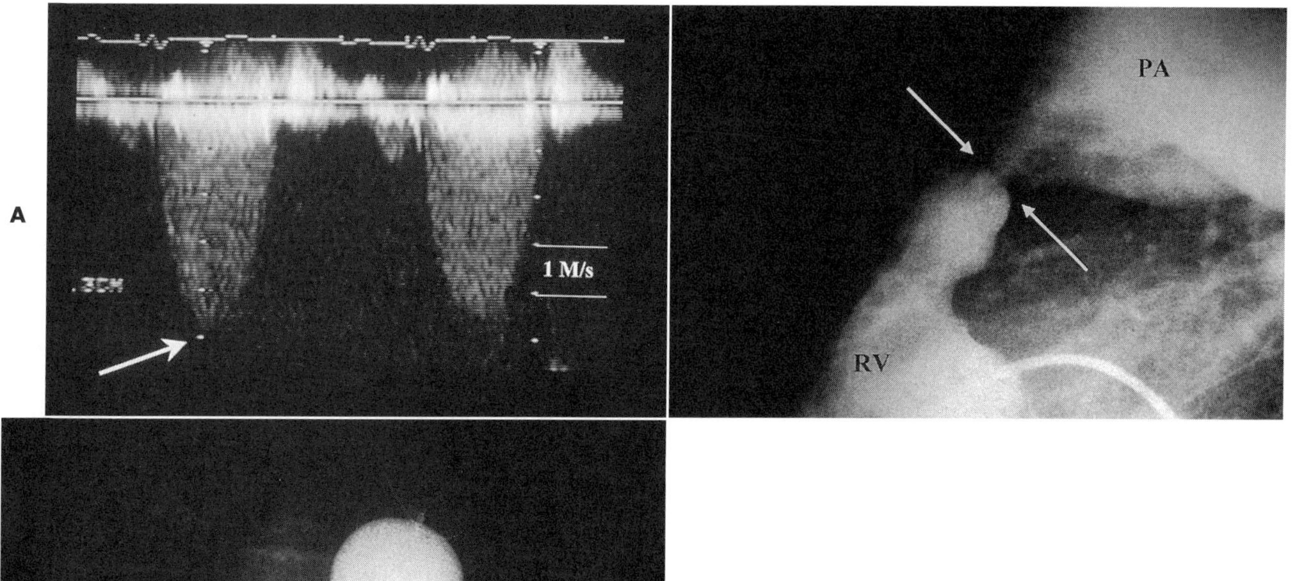

Fig. 67-2. **A,** Continuous-wave Doppler recording of pulmonic ejection velocity from a patient with pulmonic stenosis. The arrow indicates a peak velocity of nearly 5 M/s, corresponding to a gradient approaching 100 mm Hg. **B,** An angiographic frame from the same patient. The arrows point to the thickened valve leaflets and the narrow stenotic flow jet. Poststenotic dilation of the pulmonary artery *(PA)* is also evident. **C,** Cine frame showing a balloon catheter positioned across the stenotic valve during valvuloplasty.

gradient under 40 mm Hg) during adolescence are unlikely to develop problems later and require only periodic clinical reevaluation and antibiotic prophylaxis. Patients in whom the measured gradient falls in the moderate range (i.e., between 40 and 80 mm Hg) may do well for extended periods; however, natural history studies indicate that most will eventually require intervention, and cardiology evaluation is appropriate, particularly if symptoms are present. Systolic gradients above 80 mm Hg warrant early intervention.

Balloon pulmonary valvuloplasty, now the procedure of choice, has a high success rate[4] in reducing the valvular gradient to acceptable levels. Surgical valvotomy is reserved for those with suboptimal results. The pulmonic insufficiency resulting from these procedures is usually mild and well tolerated. Postoperatively, a systolic murmur almost invariably persists, and a low-pitched, rumbling pulmonary regurgitant murmur is common.

Coarctation of Aorta

Aortic coarctation, a correctable cause of hypertension, refers to a narrowing of the aorta by a fibrous dorsal invagination most often at or just beyond the origin of the left subclavian artery (Fig. 67-3). Coarctation is more common in men and is occasionally associated with Turner's syndrome. Although heart failure may occur during infancy, the condition is frequently well tolerated into adult life. Because of the sustained left ventricular pressure burden, however, symptoms of congestive failure become the rule beyond age 40. In those undetected until adulthood, the most common associated abnormality is a bicuspid aortic valve (see Chapter 66). Other complications encountered with coarctation include bacterial endarteritis at the site of the coarctation or endocarditis involving the bicuspid aortic valve, stroke from cerebral aneurysms, aortic dissection, and rupture.

Physical examination reveals upper torso hypertension in most patients with coarctation, but this may not be evident in the left arm if the narrowed segment includes the left subclavian artery. Rarely, arm hypertension may be absent altogether if the right subclavian artery arises aberrantly distal to the coarctation. The carotid pulses are bounding, and a prominent suprasternal pulse may be present. Femoral pulses may be reduced or absent, but comparatively delayed arrival of the femoral pulse on simultaneous palpation of the radial artery is the most diagnostically specific characteristic. Additional systolic or diastolic murmurs arising from associated aortic valve disease are common.

The ECG is likely to manifest evidence of left ventricular hypertrophy in adults. On chest x-ray, a dilated transverse aorta and the poststenotic dilation of the descending aorta may create a "figure-three" sign along the upper left cardiac margin (Fig. 67-4). Rib notching related to intercostal collateral development may become apparent after childhood,

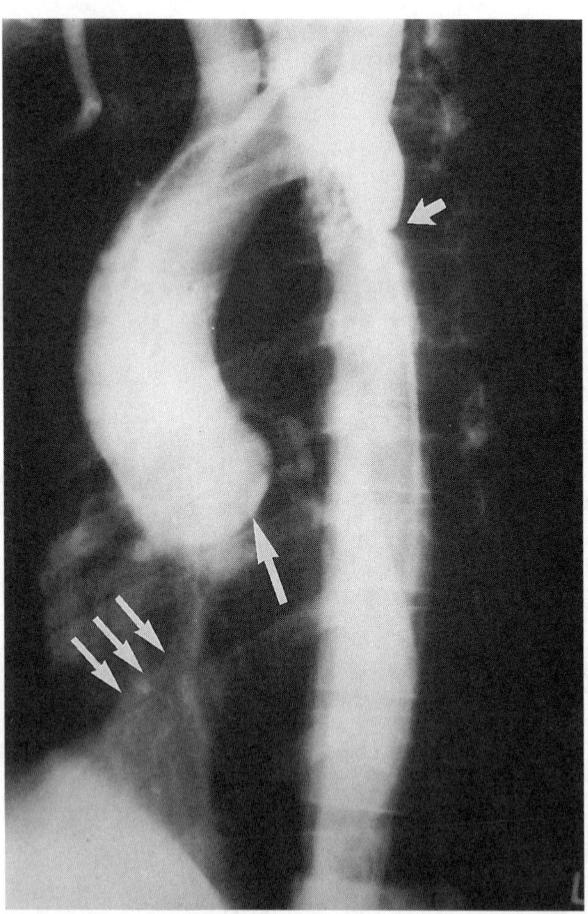

Fig. 67-3. Aortogram from a patient with coarctation. The coarctation is well visualized *(upper arrow)* beyond the origin of the left subclavian artery. A bicuspid aortic valve is also present *(lower arrow)* with a faint blush of aortic regurgitation *(arrows)*.

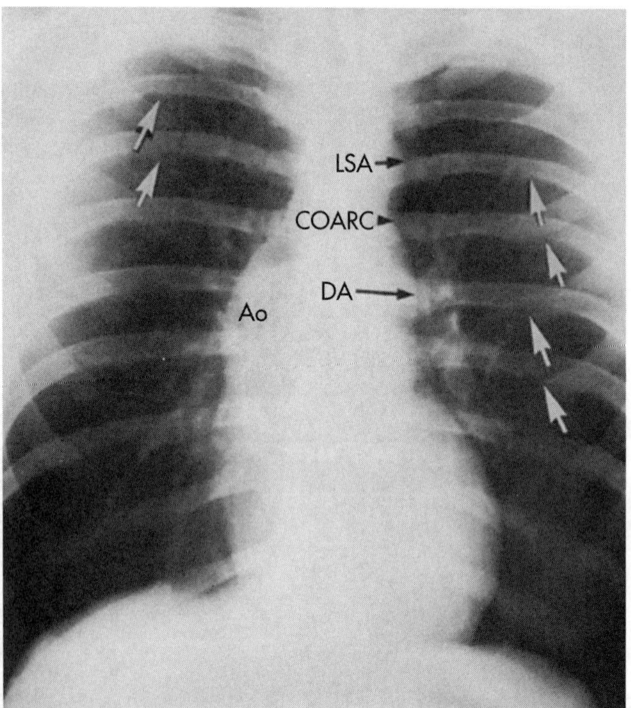

Fig. 67-4. Chest film from a patient with aortic coarctation illustrating the components that contribute to the "figure-three" sign. The convexity of the left subclavian artery *(LSA)* and the descending aorta *(DA)* separated by the indentation of the coarctation create the "3." The dilated ascending aorta *(Ao)* is also notable, as well as rib notching *(arrows)*. (From Perloff JK: *The clinical recognition of congenital heart disease,* 1970, Philadelphia, WB Saunders.)

usually involving the third to eighth ribs posteriorly. Echocardiographic study from a suprasternal transducer position may directly visualize the coarctation, particularly in younger patients; despite difficulty with imaging in older patients, measurement of the gradient is usually possible by Doppler.

Since patients with uncorrected coarctation are at risk for serious complications, suspicion of the diagnosis always warrants cardiology evaluation. Currently, repair is recommended when the gradient exceeds 20 mm Hg or when angiography demonstrates severe coarctation with extensive collateralization. Correction during childhood is preferred, but the optimal mode of treatment is controversial. Operative approaches continue to be favored at some centers, but successful use of balloon angioplasty and stenting is increasingly reported, and balloon angioplasty is generally considered to be the approach of choice for recoarctation.

After childhood, because of a progressive increase in the incidence of residual hypertension with age, the earlier the correction the more favorable the results. Studies suggest a 25% incidence of hypertension after correction if performed before age 10 and about 50% thereafter.[2] Despite correction, coarctation patients remain subject to such problems as cerebral aneurysm rupture, progression of aortic valve disease, and infective endocarditis.

ACYANOTIC CONGENITAL DISEASE WITH SHUNT

Atrial Septal Defect

Atrial septal defect (ASD), the most common intracardiac shunt diagnosed in the adult, frequently eludes early diagnosis because its characteristic features are absent at birth and subtle enough to escape recognition in childhood. Symptoms frequently do not emerge until mid-adult life or later. Defects of the atrial septum occur more frequently in women, and may be hereditary in some instances, notably in conjunction with hypoplastic abnormalities of the thumb and forearm as part of Holt-Oram syndrome.

Of the several types of ASD, the septum secundum defect is most common (Fig. 67-5). It is located in the mid-atrial septum, circumscribing the usual site of the fossa ovalis, the landmark corresponding to the fetal foramen ovale. Even in the absence of detectable shunting, the limbs of the foramen frequently fail to fuse and may provide a potential interatrial communication in up to 30% of adults. Defects in the low atrial septum (ostium primum defect) are a form of endocardial cushion defect, and are accompanied by clefts in the atrioventricular valves. Sinus venosus defects, located high in the atrial septum, are associated with both anomalous pulmonary venous return to the right atrium and abnormalities of the sinus node.

Diversion of flow from the left to the right atrium via the ASD produces volume overload of the right heart and the pulmonary circuit. Commensurate with the course of other chronic volume overload states, this burden is usually well tolerated throughout young adult life, but thereafter complications begin to appear. Symptoms predominantly reflect right ventricular decompensation, and are occasionally abetted by development of pulmonary hypertension. Left-to-right shunting may worsen with age, particularly if other conditions, such as hypertension or coronary disease, lead to elevation of filling pressures in the left heart.

Exertional dyspnea, probably caused by the increased lung blood volume, is a frequent complaint of patients with ASD. Overt right heart failure begins to appear after age 30. Supraventricular dysrhythmias, facilitated by atrial enlargement (most importantly atrial fibrillation), contribute substantially to morbidity. Although the incidence of pulmonary hypertension increases with age, obliterative pulmonary vascular disease sufficient to result in shunt reversal (Eisenmenger's syndrome) develops in fewer than 5% of patients. The association between secundum ASD and mitral valve prolapse has received considerable attention, with an incidence in excess of 50% reported in some series. Mitral regurgitation severe enough to warrant consideration of valve repair or replacement is, however, unusual.

On physical examination, a dynamic systolic impulse immediately to the left of the sternum should direct attention to the possibility of increased volume flow through the right heart. A brief, flow-related systolic ejection murmur is usually audible in the pulmonic area. The two components of the second heart sound are widely split during expiration with imperceptible variation on inspiration. This phenomenon, referred to as fixed splitting, constitutes the single most important and most frequently overlooked or misinterpreted clue to the presence of a shunt. Wide, fixed splitting of S_2, a nearly universal finding with ASD in younger patients, may become less consistent in older adults and when pulmonary hypertension develops. However, any expiratory splitting of the second sound in adults unexplained by right bundle branch block should bring suspicion of ASD to the fore. An audible diastolic rumble at the lower left sternal edge, created by torrential flow across the tricuspid valve, almost invariably indicates a significant left-to-right shunt. A midsystolic click may be audible over the apex if mitral valve prolapse coincides, and a murmur of mitral regurgitation may represent either mitral prolapse or a mitral valve cleft in the case of an ostium primum defect.

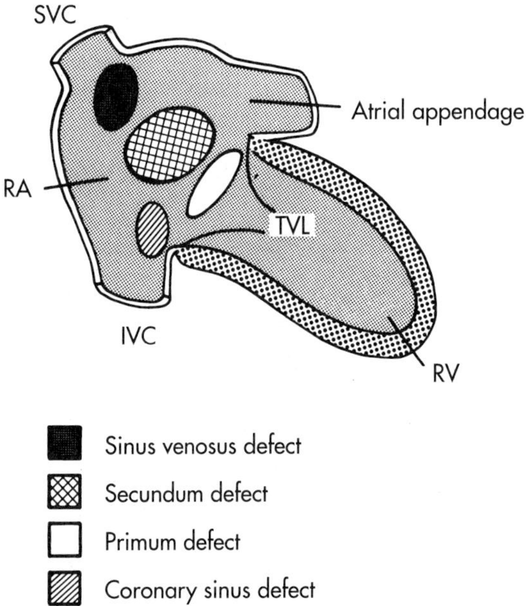

Fig. 67-5. Location of the four types of atrial septal defect. *SVC*, Superior vena cava; *RA*, right atrium; *IVC*, inferior vena cava; *RV*, right ventricle; *TVL*, tricuspid valve leaflet.

The ECG pattern of incomplete right bundle branch is present in about 90% of patients with ASD. Associated left axis deviation connotes a defect of the endocardial cushion and predicts the presence of a primum ASD. Marked right axis deviation implies the presence of pulmonary hypertension. The chest x-ray reveals variable enlargement of the right heart chambers, dilation of the central pulmonary arteries, and a pattern of peripheral pulmonary vascular plethora (Fig. 67-6).

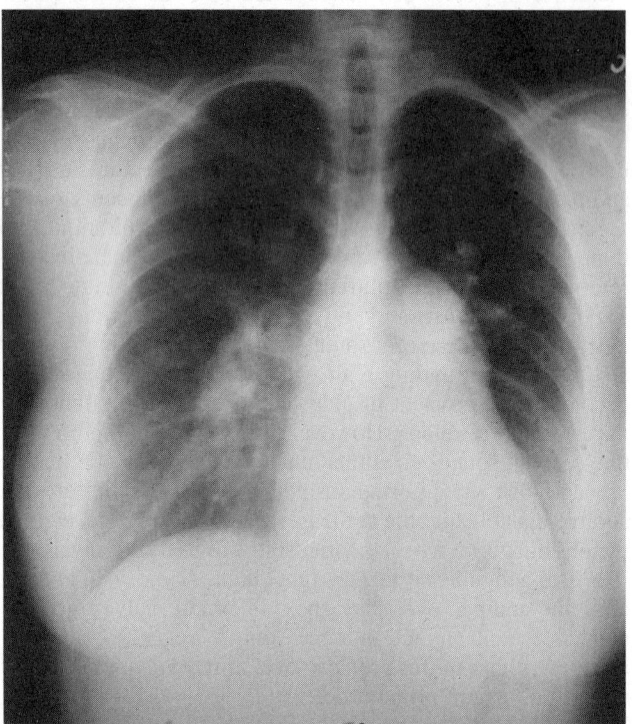

Fig. 67-6. Posteroanterior chest film from a patient with a secundum atrial septal defect (3.7 : 1 pulmonary-systemic flow ratio) and normal pulmonary artery pressures. Note the dilation of the main pulmonary artery segment, which obscures the left pulmonary artery, and the prominent right pulmonary artery and branches.

Thanks to recent advances in color flow and transesophageal imaging, echocardiography provides for complete anatomic and hemodynamic characterization of ASD in most patients (Fig. 67-7). These advances have eliminated the need for catheterization in most younger patients with a straightforward anomaly.

To deter late complications of ASD, repair is recommended for all patients with evidence of a physiologically significant shunt (e.g., right atrial and right ventricular enlargement). Recent studies indicate that ASDs may be safely corrected in patients over age 60 even when pulmonary resistance is markedly elevated, as long as a net left-to-right shunt is present; shunt reversal, however, is a contraindication to closure. Despite evidence that normal right ventricular function is unlikely to be fully restored and that atrial fibrillation may not be prevented, overt right ventricular failure should not deter surgery, which arrests an otherwise progressive process.[1,5]

Increasingly, attention in the literature has focused on the use of percutaneous devices for closure of secundum ASDs. Although a number of devices are currently under investigation, none have been approved for routine clinical use in the United States.

Ventricular Septal Defect

The ventricular septum may be divided into inlet, membranous, trabecular, and outlet (infundibular) regions. Perimembranous septal defects, either directly involving or immediately adjacent to the membranous septum, are by far the most common. They are found at the base of the interventricular septum immediately behind the septal leaflet of the tricuspid valve and below the crista supraventricularis, a muscular bar that separates the right ventricular inflow and outflow tracts. Typically, these defects lie subjacent to the right coronary cusp on the left side of the septum. Muscular defects, the second most common ventricular septal defect (VSD), may involve any of the other three segments and are often multiple.

A spectrum of physiologic derangement is possible with a defect in the interventricular septum, ranging from pure volume overload of both ventricles to pure pressure overload of the right ventricle (Eisenmenger's syndrome). The

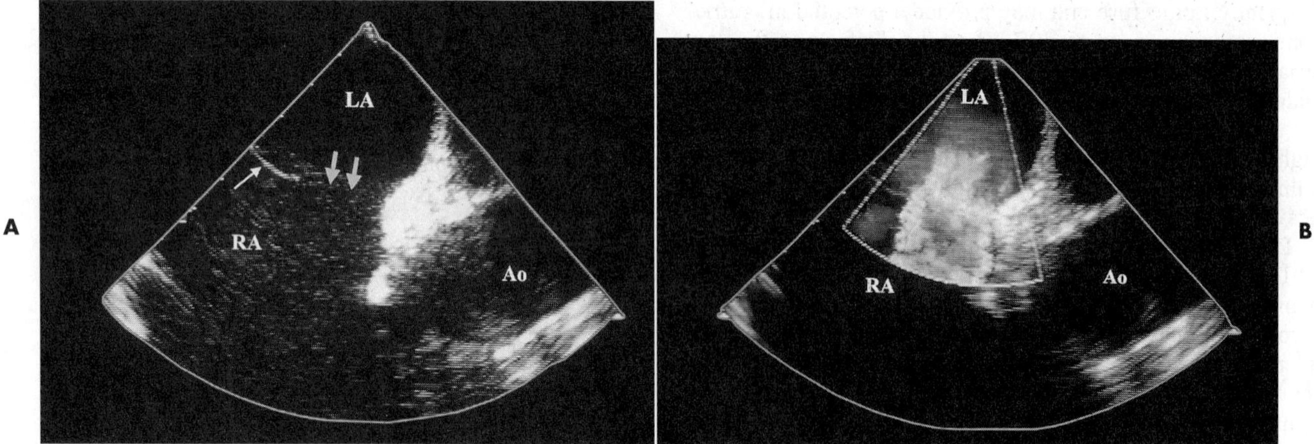

Fig. 67-7. **A,** Transesophageal echocardiogram from a patient with a secundum atrial septal defect. The large arrows indicate a large defect in the atrial septum *(small arrow).* **B,** Doppler recording demonstrating left-to-right flow through the ASD. *LA,* Left atrium; *RA,* right atrium; *Ao,* aorta.

governing features are the size of the defect and pulmonary outflow (vascular) resistance. Volume effects predominate when large defects concur with low pulmonary resistance, whereas both pressure and volume overload of the right ventricle ensue if pulmonary resistance increases.

As a result of improved diagnosis and emphasis on correction of significant defects during childhood, experience with VSD in adult practice is generally limited to patients with small, hemodynamically insignificant shunts (maladie de Roger) or those with minor residual shunting following surgical correction. Physical examination may reveal a harsh holosystolic murmur along the left sternal border radiating to the right; rarely, a systolic thrill may be evident in the same region. Echocardiography provides complete physiologic characterization in most instances (Fig. 67-8). Patients in whom findings suggest a significant left-to-right shunt or pulmonary hypertension should always be referred for cardiology evaluation.

The asymptomatic patient with the murmur of VSD without symptoms, evidence of significant volume overload, or pulmonary hypertension requires only endocarditis prophylaxis. The risk of endocarditis is low, as indicated by the 1.9 cases per 1000 patient-years found in a large cooperative study.[3] About 5% of VSD patients develop aortic regurgitation, partly because of abnormal tissue support for the aortic cusps. The regurgitation may progress irrespective of VSD closure; in fact, the regurgitation may first appear after repair of the defect. Successful aortic valvuloplasty has been combined with VSD repair, but the management of aortic regurgitation in combination with a small VSD is the same as aortic regurgitation alone.

ECG abnormalities are common after VSD repair. Complete heart block, once a frequent manifestation of surgical trauma to the conduction system, which courses in proximity to the inferior margins of the perimembranous defect, now occurs only rarely. Right bundle branch block is common following right ventriculotomy for surgical closure and is less common following repair via the right atrium, the preferred approach. Ventricular dysrhythmias, which are evident in 40% to 50% of patients after surgical repair, are more likely after ventriculotomy. Late sudden death occurs in approximately 4% of the patients. Management of these dysrhythmias is identical to that for ventricular dysrhythmias of other etiologies in the adult (see Chapter 61).

Patent Ductus Arteriosus

The ductus arteriosus, which shunts blood from the pulmonary to the systemic circuit during fetal development, closes functionally within 24 hours of birth in the normal situation. Anatomic obliteration usually follows within the first 2 months, and patency of the ductus beyond this is abnormal. As with VSD, improved detection and treatment have virtually eliminated encounters with patent ductus arteriosus (PDA) and a significant shunt from adult practice. The finding of a continuous murmur to the left of the upper sternum is the distinctive feature on examination (Fig. 67-9).

All patients suspected to have ductal patency should be referred for cardiology evaluation. Closure, increasingly accomplished by percutaneous techniques, is the preferred treatment of PDA, regardless of shunt magnitude, because of the risk of endocarditis. The patient with a tiny flow jet consistent with ductal patency discovered incidentally on

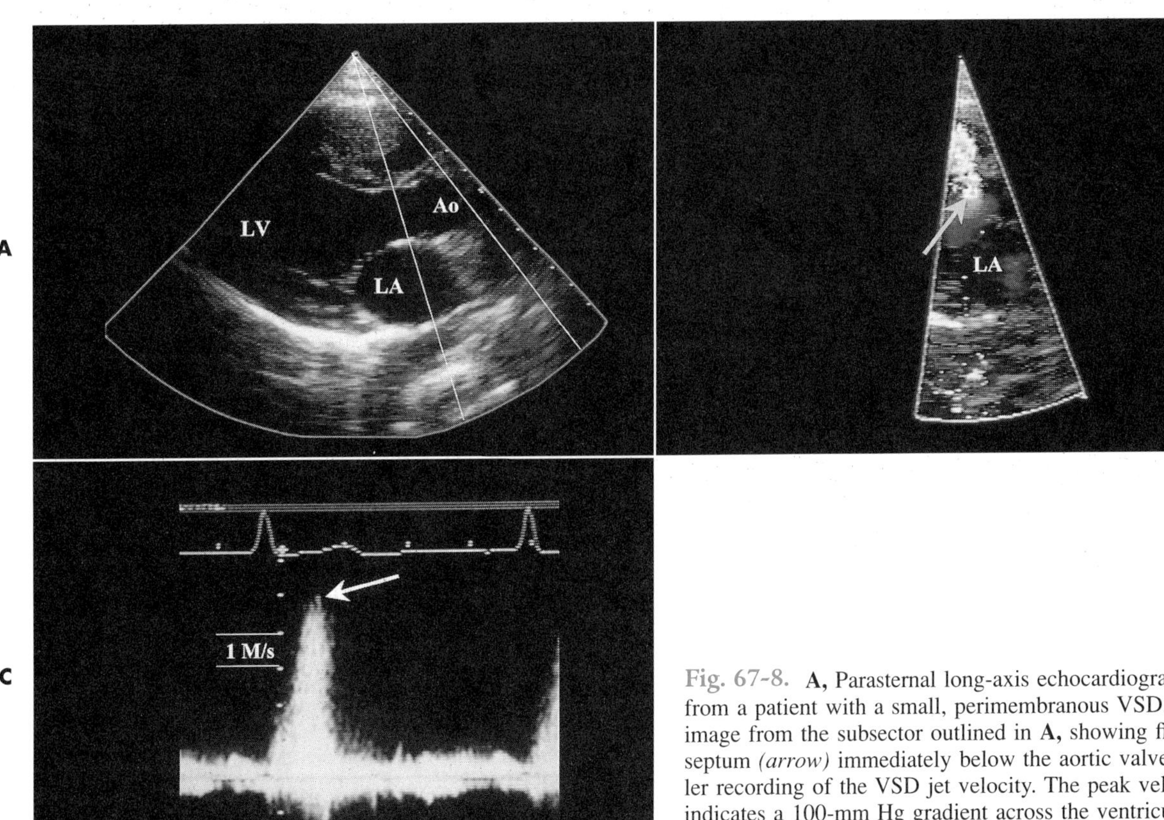

Fig. 67-8. **A,** Parasternal long-axis echocardiographic image from a patient with a small, perimembranous VSD. **B,** Doppler image from the subsector outlined in **A,** showing flow across the septum *(arrow)* immediately below the aortic valve. **C,** Doppler recording of the VSD jet velocity. The peak velocity of 5 M/s indicates a 100-mm Hg gradient across the ventricular septum and implies normal right ventricular and pulmonary artery pressures. *LV,* Left ventricle; *LA,* left atrium; *Ao,* aorta.

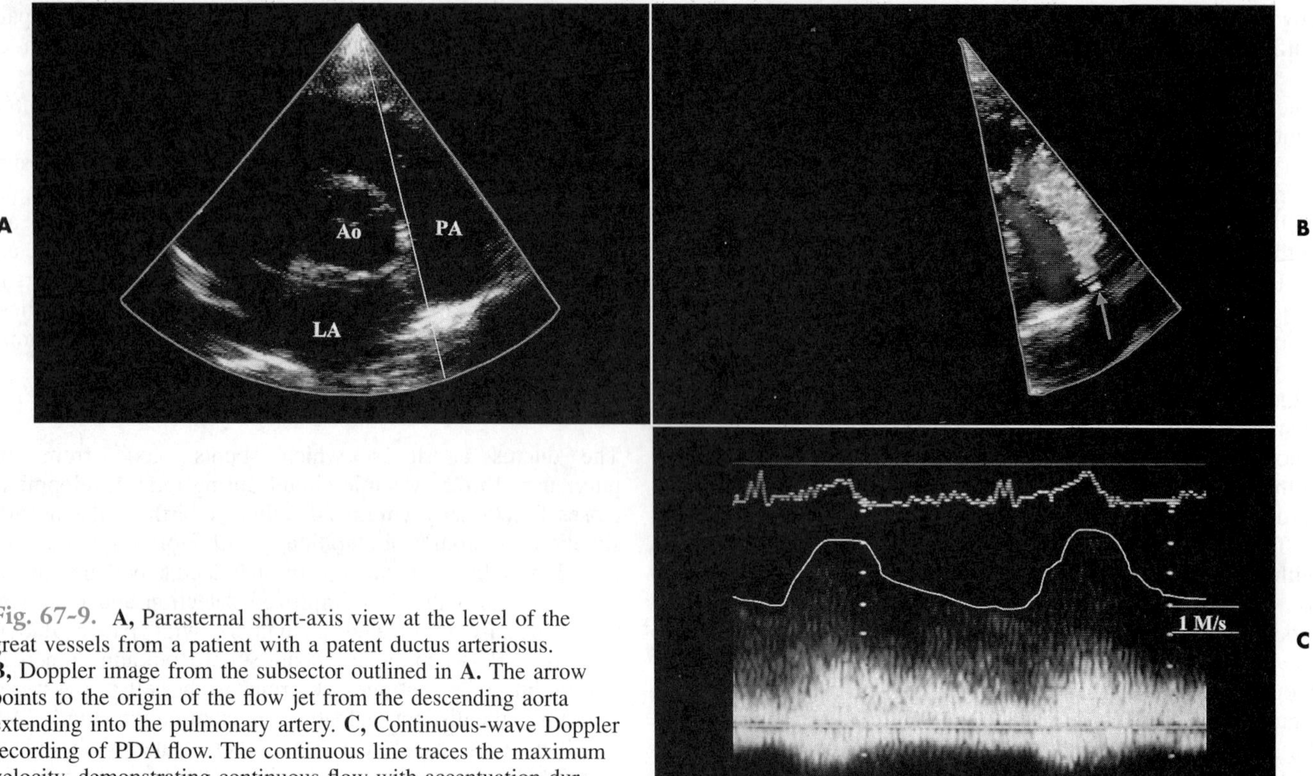

Fig. 67-9. **A,** Parasternal short-axis view at the level of the great vessels from a patient with a patent ductus arteriosus. **B,** Doppler image from the subsector outlined in **A.** The arrow points to the origin of the flow jet from the descending aorta extending into the pulmonary artery. **C,** Continuous-wave Doppler recording of PDA flow. The continuous line traces the maximum velocity, demonstrating continuous flow with accentuation during systole, which corresponds to the features of the characteristic murmur. *Ao,* Aorta; *LA,* Left atrium; *PA,* pulmonary artery.

echocardiography is an exception to this rule and requires only endocarditis prophylaxis. Advanced age may also temper the therapeutic approach to the asymptomatic patient with a small shunt in whom ductal tortuosity and calcification may increase the technical difficulty and risks of catheter closure or ligation; preprocedural angiographic definition is a must in these cases. Antibiotic prophylaxis is not required after closure if there is no echocardiographic evidence of a shunt.

CYANOTIC CONGENITAL DISEASE

Cyanotic congenital disease in the adult is a rarity. Most often, patients with a history of cyanotic heart disease in infancy or childhood will have undergone previous evaluation and either a palliative or corrective procedure. With few exceptions, these patients remain subject to a variety of potential problems and complications that require follow-up at subspecialized centers familiar with their management. Although declining in incidence, Eisenmenger's syndrome remains a not uncommon cardiac cause of cyanosis in the adult. In these patients, a congenital lesion with a left-to-right shunt, often undetected in childhood, leads to the development of irreversible pulmonary hypertension and shunt reversal, which precludes correction of the primary defect. Despite this, many of these patients survive well into adult life, and aspects of their medical management deserve some consideration.

Patients with Eisenmenger's syndrome demonstrate central cyanosis and clubbing on physical examination as well as cardiac findings associated with pulmonary hypertension. Management of patients with mild symptoms is conservative, since prognosis in this group is better than lung or heart-lung transplantation, and consists of avoidance of, or meticulous monitoring during, situations presenting an increased risk of morbidity for these patients. Patients who develop more severe symptoms as a consequence of right heart failure should be considered for transplantation.

Problematic situations in these patients include those associated with vasodilation and volume depletion (e.g., infection, hemorrhage, surgery, angiography), which may intensify the right-to-left shunt, resulting in precipitous deterioration.[6] Pregnancy is contraindicated by the high risk of both maternal mortality and fetal loss; modes of contraception not associated with an increase in thromboembolic risk are preferred. These patients are particularly at risk for paradoxical embolization, and meticulous attention to intravenous lines is necessary to minimize the chances of air embolization or cerebral abscess. Erythrocytosis is common, and if excessive (e.g., hemoglobin > 20 gm %), symptoms of hyperviscosity may occur. Routine phlebotomy, however, is not recommended, since this may be associated with the development of microcytosis, which has been associated with an increased thromboembolic risk. Additional common problems include hyperuricemia and gout related to increased red cell turnover. A number of coagulation abnormalities and renal dysfunction may also occur. In this regard nonsteroidal antiinflammatory agents are problematic and should be avoided in these patients.

REFERENCES

1. Allen HD, Beekman RH, Garson AJ, et al: Pediatric therapeutic cardiac catheterization: a statement for healthcare professionals from the council on cardiovascular disease in the young, *Circulation* 97:609, 1998.

2. Gatzoulis MA, Freeman MA, Siu SC, et al: Atrial arrhythmia after closure of atrial septal defect in adults, *N Engl J Med* 340:839, 1999.
3. Konstantinides S, Geibel A, Olschewski M, et al: A comparison of surgical and medical therapy for atrial septal defect in adults, *N Engl J Med* 333:469, 1995.
4. O'Fallon WM, Weidman WH, editors: Long-term follow-up of congenital aortic stenosis, pulmonary stenosis, and ventricular septal defect. Report from the Second Joint Study on the Natural History of Congenital Heart Defects (NHS-2), *Circulation* 87 (suppl I): I1, 1993.
5. Stewart AB, et al: Coarctation of the aorta life and health 20-44 years after surgical correction, *Br Heart J* 69:65, 1993.
6. Vongpatanasin W, Brickner E, Hillis LD, et al: The Eisenmenger syndrome in adults, *Ann Intern Med* 128:745, 1998.

CHAPTER 68

Myocardial and Pericardial Disease

Edward K. Kasper
Kenneth L. Baughman

EPIDEMIOLOGY AND ETIOLOGY

Cardiomyopathies are diseases of the heart muscle. The three categories of cardiomyopathy are dilated, hypertrophic, and restrictive.[14] Ventricular enlargement and contractile dysfunction characterize dilated cardiomyopathy, the most common type. Hypertrophic cardiomyopathy is characterized by ventricular hypertrophy, often asymmetric and involving the left ventricular septum. Systolic left ventricular outflow tract gradients are common. Only 4% of patients with cardiomyopathy have the hypertrophic form. Restrictive cardiomyopathy is characterized by restricted ventricular filling with normal ventricular systolic function and wall thickness. Restrictive cardiomyopathy is the least common form in the developed world, but may account for 15% to 25% of the deaths due to heart disease in equatorial Africa.[9] These functional categories are not absolute and overlap may exist. Reliable incidence and prevalence data on restrictive cardiomyopathy do not exist. The prevalence of dilated cardiomyopathy in 1984 was 36.5/100,000 person-years, and that of hypertrophic cardiomyopathy was 19.7/100,000 person-years.[3] As with heart failure, the prevalence of dilated cardiomyopathy increases with age and is more common in males.

The most common cause of dilated cardiomyopathy is coronary artery disease with prior myocardial infarction. A partial listing of the possible causes of dilated cardiomyopathy in the absence of coronary artery disease is found in Box 68-1. In evaluating patients with dilated cardiomyopathy, one must exclude "look-alikes" not due to primary muscle disease, including focal coronary artery disease (left ventricular aneurysm), primary valvular disease (aortic stenosis and aortic or mitral regurgitation), and pericardial disease (pericardial tamponade or constrictive pericarditis). The etiologies of dilated cardiomyopathy that may be reversible include myocarditis, metabolic disorders (thyroid disease or pheochromocytoma), toxicity (alcohol or drugs), tachycardia-induced, infiltrative diseases (hemochromatosis or sarcoidosis), septic shock, carnitine deficiency, and peripartum.

Hypertrophic cardiomyopathy is recognized as an autosomal dominant disease in approximately 50% of the patients. Multiple genes on several chromosomes are associated with familial hypertrophic cardiomyopathy. All these genes code for proteins of the contractile apparatus, of which cardiac myosin heavy chain seems to be the most frequently mutated.[10] Some patients with hypertrophic cardiomyopathy have no family history due to variable penetrance or spontaneous mutations. Patients with hypertension may develop a hypertensive hypertrophic cardiomyopathy. These patients, presumably in response to longstanding hypertension, develop significant concentric hypertrophy. Other causes of hypertrophic cardiomyopathy are listed in Box 68-1.

Restrictive cardiomyopathy is commonly due to the infiltration of a foreign substance in or around the myocardial cells. Etiologies include amyloidosis, hemochromatosis, and sarcoidosis. Virtually all patients with these disorders display evidence of systemic illness, making the diagnosis more obvious. Noninfiltrative forms also exist and are listed in Box 68-1.

Pericardial disease may cause congestive heart failure due to restriction of ventricular diastolic filling. Potential forms of

Box 68-1. Causes of Cardiomyopathy

Dilated
- Idiopathic
- Ischemic
- Inflammatory (infectious)
  - Viral
  - Bacterial
  - Fungal
  - Parasitic
  - Rickettsial
- Inflammatory (noninfectious)
  - Collagen diseases
  - Sarcoidosis
- Metabolic
  - Thiamine
  - Carnitine deficiency
  - Obesity
  - Thyroid
  - Acromegaly
  - Cushing's syndrome
  - Pheochromocytoma
  - Diabetes
  - Hypocalcemia
- Toxic
  - Alcohol
  - Adriamycin
  - Cocaine
- Drug sensitivity
  - Sulfa
  - Penicillin
- Infiltrative
  - Amyloid
  - Hemochromatosis
- Muscular dystrophy
- Physical agents
  - Heat stroke
  - Hypothermia
  - Tachycardia
- Peripartum
- Sepsis

Hypertrophic
- Hypertensive
- Familial
  - With gradient
  - Without gradient
- Renal disease

Restrictive
- Idiopathic
- Infiltrative
  - Amyloid
  - Sarcoidosis
  - Hemochromatosis
  - Glycogen storage diseases
- Endomyocardial
  - Fibrosis
  - Hypereosinophilic syndrome
  - Carcinoid
  - Radiation

involvement include pericarditis, pericardial effusion possibly resulting in tamponade, and pericardial constriction. Acute pericarditis, or inflammation of the pericardium, is the most common form of pericardial involvement. It is most often idiopathic or caused by viral infection or acute myocardial infarction. Other causes are listed in Box 68-2. It is more common in men than women and adults than children. Pericardial effusion develops as a response to pericardial injury, often inflammatory pericarditis. Pericardial constriction occurs when a fibrotic, thickened, and adherent pericardium restricts diastolic filling of the heart.[6] It usually begins with an episode of acute pericarditis resulting in pericardial effusion followed by pericardial fibrosis and thickening. Most cases of acute pericarditis do not result in constriction. Constrictive pericarditis may be difficult to differentiate from restrictive cardiomyopathy.

Box 68-2. Pericardial Disease

Acute Pericarditis

- Idiopathic
- Inflammatory (infectious)
  - Viral
  - Bacterial
  - Fungal
  - Tuberculosis
- Inflammatory (noninfectious)
  - Collagen disease
  - Sarcoidosis
- Myocardial infarction
- Dressler's syndrome
- Postpericardiotomy syndrome
- Chest trauma
- Uremia
- Cancer
  - Lung
  - Breast
  - Leukemia
  - Lymphoma
- Radiation
- Drugs
  - Hydralazine
  - Procainamide
  - Phenytoin

Pericardial Effusion

- Most common causes
  - Cancer
  - Idiopathic
  - Uremia
  - Myocardial infarction
  - Postpericardiotomy
- Other
  - See acute pericarditis

Constrictive Pericarditis

- Most common causes
  - Idiopathic
  - Viral
  - Postpericardiotomy
  - Radiation
  - Tuberculosis
- Other
  - See acute pericarditis

PATHOPHYSIOLOGY

Dilated cardiomyopathy is initiated by an insult that decreases left ventricular contractility. This insult may be coronary disease, a viral illness, alcohol, or the toxic effect of a medication. The decrease in contractility reduces stroke volume and results in activation of the renin-angiotensin system, adrenergic system, and other neurohormones as mentioned in Chapter 65. Neurohormonal activation leads directly and indirectly to the syndrome of congestive heart failure and the progressive worsening of ventricular function. Dilated cardiomyopathy is associated with a poor prognosis, with only 50% survival 5 years after diagnosis.[4]

In hypertrophic cardiomyopathy, the ventricle is characterized by abnormalities of diastolic relaxation and increased contractility with hyperdynamic ejection of ventricular volume.[16] Because of dramatic hypertrophy, the left ventricular cavity is small and diastolic filling is incomplete, resulting in elevated ventricular diastolic pressure. Although this is the antithesis of dilated cardiomyopathy, the end result is the same, with elevated filling pressures and a low stroke volume. Dynamic left ventricular outflow tract gradients are commonly seen and probably result from the anterior leaflet of the mitral valve contacting the ventricular septum in the outflow tract. The gradient may be labile, increasing with increased contractility as well as decreased preload or afterload. A gradient from the left ventricular apex to just below the aortic valve of 50 to 150 mm Hg is not uncommon. Abnormalities of diastolic filling are always present whether or not a pressure gradient is present. Late in the course of the disease, a picture of dilated cardiomyopathy may develop most likely due to repeated episodes of ischemia with resulting fibrosis. The natural history of hypertrophic cardiomyopathy is variable, with some patients remaining stable for years. The risk of sudden death is highest in children and young adults and occurs especially during or right after vigorous physical exertion.

Restrictive cardiomyopathy is characterized by an infiltration in and around the myocardial cells of a substance that alters myocardial relaxation. Diastolic compliance is much more dramatically influenced than systolic contractility until late in the course of the disease. Like patients with hypertrophic cardiomyopathy, these patients have markedly elevated filling pressures and a low stroke volume. Unlike patients with hypertrophic cardiomyopathy, patients with restrictive cardiomyopathy may have normal ventricular wall thickness. Filling pressures are usually equal in both ventricles, and diastolic pressure tracings demonstrate a "dip and plateau" configuration also seen in constrictive pericarditis. The prognosis in restrictive cardiomyopathy is variable. Restrictive cardiomyopathy due to amyloidosis is associated with an especially poor prognosis. Treatment of the primary disorder associated with restrictive cardiomyopathy only rarely improves the patient's overall prognosis.

Injury, infection, or inflammation of the pericardium may result in fluid accumulation. If the fluid accumulates rapidly, even small amounts may dramatically decrease ventricular filling due to the inability of the pericardium to stretch abruptly and the subsequent compression of the heart. Pericardial effusions accumulated over long periods, however, may result in massive accumulations of fluid before symptoms occur. As the pericardium surrounds the right and left ventricle, pressure in the pericardial space is equally distributed to both ventricles. Pericardial pressure elevation will increase both left and right ventricular end-diastolic pressures. Therefore, when the pressure in the pericardial space is higher than the intrinsic ventricular diastolic pressure, the diastolic ventricular pressures will rise to the pericardial pressure. Additionally, pericardial fluid or constriction may limit ventricular filling. When the mitral and tricuspid valves are open, diastolic pressures in all chambers of the heart are equivalent and are also equal to the pericardial pressure. As with the cardiomyopathies, the end result of pericardial disease may be an increase in diastolic filling pressures and a decrease in stroke volume. The natural history of pericardial constriction is progressive hemodynamic compromise. However, all forms of pericardial disease are treatable and, in fact, virtually curable. The primary mission of the treating physician is to differentiate pericardial disease, which is curable, from restrictive cardiomyopathy, which is terminal. Pericardial effusions can be drained, regardless of their etiology, and the patient's hemodynamics normalized. Pericardial constriction can be prevented by appropriately treating the cause of the pericardial effusion. Pericardial constriction demands surgical pericardiectomy, which is usually curative.

Since all forms of cardiomyopathy, pericardial effusion, and constrictive pericarditis may result in the heart failure syndrome, it is important to identify the underlying pathophysiology so that appropriate treatment can be initiated.

PATIENT EVALUATION

History

Patients with cardiomyopathy, pericardial effusion, or constrictive pericarditis may present with the signs and symptoms of heart failure as outlined in Chapter 65. In addition, patients with dilated cardiomyopathy may have embolic events originating from the heart. Ventricular dysrhythmias are common in all forms of cardiomyopathy and may result in palpitations, lightheadedness, dizziness, presyncope, syncope, and sudden death. Supraventricular dysrhythmias, particularly atrial fibrillation, are also common and may result in symptomatic deterioration.

Some specific historical features may help distinguish the form of cardiomyopathy present. Patients with hypertrophic cardiomyopathy more frequently complain of ischemic chest pain and often have dizziness following exercise or with Valsalva's maneuver. Patients with restrictive cardiomyopathy, pericardial effusion, or constrictive pericarditis often display right-sided signs and symptoms of congestion much in excess of left-sided. Dramatic elevation of the right atrial pressure, commonly seen in restrictive cardiomyopathy and constrictive pericarditis, results in massive jugular venous distention, hepatomegaly, ascites, anorexia, abdominal pain, and peripheral edema.

A commonly encountered error in the management of patients with cardiomyopathy is the misdiagnosis of a patient presenting with cough, congestion, and breathlessness. Such patients are usually thought to have bronchitis and are treated with antibiotics before the myocardial or pericardial etiology is recognized. Orthopnea and paroxysmal nocturnal dyspnea are clues to a cardiac cause of the presenting symptoms and indicate the need for echocardiography. Patients may also present with asymptomatic cardiomyopathy or pericardial disease. All family members of a patient with hypertrophic cardiomyopathy should be screened for the disorder.

Patients with pericardial effusion or constriction often begin with acute pericarditis. These patients present with precordial discomfort, which is usually more omnipresent than angina and is position-dependent, being exacerbated by lying down and eased by sitting up and leaning forward. The pain is usually retrosternal and sharp, and may radiate to the neck or shoulder. Unlike angina, the pain lasts for hours or days and is not exacerbated by exertion. Pericarditis may be associated with pleural inflammation as well, resulting in a pleuropericardial syndrome with exacerbation of the pain with deep inspiration or cough. These symptoms may be confused with the symptoms of acute myocardial infarction, pulmonary emboli, or aortic dissection. Acute pericarditis may also present with dyspnea, at least partly caused by the need to breathe shallowly in order to avoid chest pain.

Physical Examination

Jugular Venous Pressure. Patients with congestive heart failure have elevations of the right atrial pressure and therefore distended jugular veins. Patients with dilated cardiomyopathy have modest distention of the jugular veins and often large v waves due to tricuspid regurgitation. In these cases the regurgitation is due to dilation of the tricuspid annulus secondary to myocardial disease. Patients with hypertrophic cardiomyopathy display prominent A waves in the venous pulse. This is due to the increased right atrial pressure necessary to force blood into the stiff right ventricle. Patients with restrictive cardiomyopathy display even greater elevations of the A waves for similar reasons. Patients with pericardial tamponade or constriction display dramatic abnormalities of the venous pressure. These patients have equally prominent A and v waves. Patients with pericardial constriction have dominant x and y descents after the A and v waves, whereas patients with pericardial tamponade display only a prominent x descent.

Carotid Pulse. In dilated and restrictive cardiomyopathy, as well as pericardial disease, the carotid volumes are diminished due to the low stroke volume of the left ventricle. In dilated cardiomyopathy, the rate of rise of the carotid pulse is diminished. The carotid upstroke in patients with restrictive cardiomyopathy is usually maintained until late in the course of the disease. In pericardial disease the carotid upstroke is normal, although decreased in volume. Patients with hypertrophic cardiomyopathy have a hyperdynamic carotid upstroke due to the ejection of blood from the ventricle. A bifid contour of the peak of the carotid upstroke is associated with hypertrophic cardiomyopathy and left ventricular outflow tract obstruction. It is due to the early rapid ejection of blood from the ventricle followed by outflow tract obstruction and then a later secondary peak of ejection. The peripheral pulses are relatively indistinguishable in these disorders, with the exception of the paradoxical pulse seen in pericardial tamponade and constrictive pericarditis. Pulsus paradoxus is an inspiratory decrease in the amplitude of the arterial pulse greater than 10 mm Hg. Other disorders, such as chronic obstructive pulmonary disease (COPD), restrictive cardiomyopathy, and massive pulmonary embolism, may also cause pulsus paradoxus.

Lung. When the left atrial pressure is elevated, it is transmitted to the pulmonary veins. This results in exudation of fluid into the alveoli, producing crackles. Patients may also have peribronchial edema, resulting in wheezing. Not infrequently, patients with severe disease have absolutely clear lung fields, particularly if the left atrial hypertension has occurred over a long period. Patients with restrictive cardiomyopathy may display lung involvement with a primary process such as sarcoidosis or amyloidosis.

Heart. The point of maximal impulse in patients with dilated cardiomyopathy is markedly displaced and weak, often with a palpable S_3 gallop. Patients with hypertrophic cardiomyopathy have a dynamic, forceful, heaving left-ventricular point of maximal impulse. Those with restrictive cardiomyopathy have a weakened but usually minimally displaced point of maximal impulse. Patients with pericardial disease have a quiet precordium. Heart sounds are also variable. Patients with dilated cardiomyopathy usually have soft heart sounds and S_3 gallops. Hypertrophic cardiomyopathies usually have brisk heart sounds and S_4 gallops, depending on the degree of compliance abnormality in the left ventricle and the rate of deceleration of blood entering the cavity. Restrictive cardiomyopathy patients often have S_4 gallops. Patients with pericardial constriction may have an early diastolic pericardial knock, which must be differentiated from an S_3 gallop. The pericardial knock usually occurs earlier and has a higher frequency than the typical S_3.

Patients with dilated cardiomyopathy develop murmurs of mitral and tricuspid regurgitation as a result of annular dilation and malalignment of the chordae tendineae. Patients with hypertrophic cardiomyopathy often have an outflow murmur, which is typically harsh, diamond-shaped, and heard best in the aortic region. It is similar to aortic stenosis and often associated with a blowing murmur at the apex of the heart compatible with mitral regurgitation. Patients with restrictive cardiomyopathy frequently have no murmurs whatsoever. Patients with acute pericarditis usually have a one-, two-, or three-component friction rub. The components of the rub are usually described as presystolic, ventricular systolic, and rapid ventricular filling. There are therefore two diastolic components and one systolic component to the typical three-component friction rub. The ventricular systolic component is the loudest and is present in almost all cases. The rub is a scratchy, grating, high-frequency sound that may be evanescent. Finally, a friction rub may be heard in patients with small or large pericardial effusions.

Abdomen. The liver may be enlarged in any patient with right atrial hypertension. Since pericardial effusion and constrictive pericarditis, as well as restrictive cardiomyopathy, more often have higher right-sided pressures than dilated or hypertrophic cardiomyopathy, the liver is frequently more congested in these diseases. Similarly, the liver may be involved in certain of the primary etiologies of restrictive cardiomyopathy. Ascites is much more common in patients with restrictive or constrictive heart disease.

Extremities. Patients with pericardial, restrictive, and hypertrophic disease have less edema than patients with dilated cardiomyopathy, probably due to the lower cardiac output found in patients with dilated cardiomyopathy.

Subtle or Misleading Findings. Often the jugular venous pressure elevation is not appreciated. This is due to the dramatic distention in the veins when the patient is supine. The patient's head and upper body must be raised until a meniscus is evident in the vein to judge the height of the venous pressure. Even if the elevated venous pressure is appreciated, A and v waves are often not appreciated, nor are the x and y descents. Carotid pulsations may be mistaken for venous pulsations. The carotid pulse is medial to the venous pulse and protected by the two heads of the sternocleidomastoid muscle.

The point of maximal impulse is frequently missed due to the patient's habitus and should be felt for in the left lateral decubitus position if not apparent with the patient supine.

The differentiation of a pericardial knock from an S_3 gallop is difficult in timing but straightforward by the nature of the sound produced. The S_3 is a low-frequency sound, whereas the pericardial knock has a high frequency that is more like a typical first or second heart sound. Patients with midsystolic clicks are often misdiagnosed as having a pericardial knock or an S_3 gallop. Strict attention to the timing of the sound should differentiate systolic clicks from diastolic gallops. Rubs and murmurs may be misinterpreted.

DIAGNOSIS

Diagnostic Procedures

The transthoracic echocardiogram is the single most useful procedure to diagnose myocardial and pericardial disease. Patients with dilated cardiomyopathy characteristically have thin left ventricular walls, a dilated left ventricular internal diastolic dimension (greater than 2.7 cm/m^2 body area), and poor contractility (Table 68-1). Patients with hypertrophic cardiomyopathy have markedly thickened and often asymmetric left ventricular walls, small left ventricular cavities, and hyperdynamic contractility. Patients with restrictive cardiomyopathy have normal or slightly thickened walls, a normal ventricular cavity, and normal contractility until late in the disease when systolic dysfunction may occur. Patients with amyloidosis, hemochromatosis, or interstitial fibrosis may have a speckled pattern to the left ventricular myocardium, which is suggestive of an infiltrative process. Patients with pericardial effusions are easily diagnosed with echocardiography, which also determines diastolic compliance and assesses the presence or absence of valvular disease.

Etiology. A number of studies can be performed to determine the etiology of the identified abnormality. These include blood and urine studies as well as an array of noninvasive and invasive procedures.

Diagnostic Laboratory Studies

Dilated Cardiomyopathy. Routine screening for apathetic thyroid disease in elderly patients is recommended.[8] Otherwise, special studies, such as antinuclear antibody testing and iron studies, are reserved for those patients with findings on history or physical examination that are suggestive of a systemic disorder.

Hypertrophic Cardiomyopathy. Routine genetic screening to identify mutations is not yet available but probably will be shortly. Electrocardiography (ECG) and echocardiography remain the best screening tools for family members of those patients with hypertrophic cardiomyopathy.

Table 68-1. Echocardiographic Differentiation of Myocardial and Pericardial Disease

Disease	Contractility	Hypertrophy	Ventricular cavity
Cardiomyopathy			
Dilated	Decreased	Little	Large
Hypertrophic	Hyperdynamic	Massive (often asymmetric)	Small
Restrictive	Usually normal (speckled myocardium)	Little	Small
Pericardial			
Effusion	Normal (effusion)	None	Normal (compressed with tamponade)
Constriction	Normal	None	Compressed (thickened pericardium)

Restrictive Cardiomyopathy. Specific studies may be performed to identify the potential etiology of restrictive cardiomyopathy. Iron, ferritin, iron-binding capacity, and percent saturation studies are helpful in evaluating hemochromatosis. Patients with suspected amyloidosis, particularly those associated with multiple myeloma, should have serum and urinary protein electrophoresis performed. Some patients with hypereosinophilia may develop a restrictive-like cardiomyopathy due to endocardial fibrosis (Löffler's syndrome).

Pericardial Disease. Patients with constrictive pericarditis have no distinguishing blood laboratory studies. Patients with pericarditis or pericardial effusion may have laboratory values, such as an elevated sedimentation rate, that reflect the inflammatory nature of this process. Only with a suppurative infective pericarditis would blood cultures identify the etiology.

Electrocardiography. Patients with dilated cardiomyopathy may have atrial enlargement, low voltage, left bundle branch block, ventricular hypertrophy, and poor R wave progression, often in a pseudoinfarct pattern. Patients with a hypertrophic cardiomyopathy, on the other hand, have a dramatic increase in voltage and may display left ventricular hypertrophy with strain in addition to atrial enlargement. Restrictive cardiomyopathy patients display a dramatic decrease in voltage and are notorious for a pseudoinfarct pattern in the inferior or anterior leads. Patients with pericardial effusions similarly have low voltage but may also have electrical alternans due to swinging of the heart within the fluid-filled pericardium. Acute pericarditis is characterized by PR-segment depression and ST-segment elevation. The differentiation between pericardial inflammation and ischemia is often difficult in patients with ST-segment elevation. Patients with pericarditis always have a return of their ST-segments to baseline before inversion of their T waves, whereas patients with ischemia have persistent ST elevation while their T waves are inverted.

Chest Roentgenography. Patients with dilated cardiomyopathy have enlargement of their cardiac silhouette, usually with evidence of four-chamber involvement. Patients with hypertrophic cardiomyopathy have less enlargement of their ventricular silhouettes and tend to have less right ventricular prominence. Restrictive cardiomyopathy patients often have normal-appearing cardiac silhouettes despite an increase in pulmonary vascularity. Patients with constrictive pericarditis may have pericardial calcification. Significant pericardial effusion results in enlargement of the cardiac silhouette.

Chest Computed Tomography Scan or Magnetic Resonance Imaging. Constrictive pericarditis is diagnosed by the demonstration of pericardial thickening. Chest computed tomography (CT) and magnetic resonance imaging (MRI) are valuable tools in the evaluation of patients with putative constrictive pericarditis. MRI is probably the most sensitive imaging technique currently available for evaluating the thickness of the pericardium. In contrast, echocardiography is relatively insensitive.

Cardiac Catheterization. Coronary arteriography should be performed in patients over 35 years of age with dilated cardiomyopathy and standard risk factors for coronary disease. Often, however, the left ventricular dysfunction is in excess of that which could be attributed to the degree of coronary artery disease. For clinical purposes, the degree of aortic and mitral valve disease can usually be adequately judged by echocardiography using Doppler techniques.

Catheterization may be of benefit in patients with hypertrophic cardiomyopathy to rule out associated coronary artery disease and to assess the degree of outflow obstruction. The ventricular diastolic pressures in restrictive cardiomyopathy or constrictive pericarditis display a characteristic pattern of filling. Left and right ventricular end-diastolic pressures are elevated, and the early diastolic pressure has a square root configuration due to the rapid influx of blood and achievement of maximal cavity volumes early in diastole. Additionally, patients with significant constrictive and restrictive heart disease have equalization of the diastolic pressures. Patients with restrictive disease are more likely to have a higher left ventricular than right ventricular end-diastolic pressure and typically have higher systolic pulmonary artery pressures.

Endomyocardial Biopsy. Endomyocardial biopsy may be helpful in patients with dilated or restrictive cardiomyopathy. Table 68-2 lists the final diagnoses reached after performance of history, physical examination, routine blood work, endomyocardial biopsy, and coronary angiography, when necessary, in 673 patients referred to the Johns Hopkins Hospital for the evaluation of dilated cardiomyopathy.[7] Many of these diagnoses are made by histologic examination,

Table 68-2. Etiology of Dilated Cardiomyopathy

Diagnosis	Frequency	Percent (%)
Idiopathic	313	46.5
Myocarditis	81	12.0
Coronary artery disease	74	11.0
HIV	33	4.9
Peripartum	33	4.9
Chronic alcohol abuse	23	3.4
Drug-induced	21	3.1
Connective tissue diseases	15	2.2
Amyloidosis	14	2.1
Hypertension	14	2.1
Familial	12	1.8
Metabolic	10	1.5
Valvular myopathy	10	1.5
Congenital heart disease	4	0.6
Neuromuscular diseases	4	0.6
Postcoronary bypass surgery	4	0.6
Sarcoidosis	4	0.6
Atrial fibrillation	1	0.1
Endomyocardial fibroelastosis	1	0.1
Histiocytosis X	1	0.1
Thrombotic thrombocytopenic purpura	1	0.1
TOTAL	673	99.8

From Kasper EK, et al: The causes of dilated cardiomyopathy: a clinicopathologic review of 673 consecutive patients, *J Am Coll Cardiol* 23:586, 1994.

Box 68-3. Differential Diagnosis

Dilated Cardiomyopathy

Focal coronary disease
- Left ventricular aneurysm
- Left ventricular pseudoaneurysm

Valvular disease
- Aortic stenosis
- Aortic regurgitation
- Mitral stenosis
- Mitral regurgitation

Pericardial effusion

Hypertrophic Cardiomyopathy

Hypertensive hypertrophic cardiomyopathy
Aortic stenosis
Subaortic stenosis
Infiltrative cardiomyopathy

Restrictive Cardiomyopathy

Hypertrophic cardiomyopathy (any form)
Normal heart
Pericardial constriction
Liver disease

Pericardial Disease

Acute Pericarditis

Myocardial infarction
Pulmonary embolus
Aortic dissection

Constrictive Pericarditis

Restrictive cardiomyopathy
Liver disease

including myocarditis, amyloidosis, sarcoidosis, hemochromatosis, Adriamycin toxicity, histiocytosis X, scleroderma, and thrombotic thrombocytopenic purpura (TTP). Utilizing this approach, only 50% of the patients were considered idiopathic. Patients with new-onset dilated cardiomyopathy of less than 6-months' duration and those who are young or potential transplant candidates should undergo heart biopsy. Biopsy is of even greater benefit for patients with restrictive cardiomyopathy. The etiology can virtually always be established by endomyocardial biopsy in view of the common infiltrative causes of restrictive cardiomyopathy. The biopsy is particularly beneficial in patients with constrictive-restrictive hemodynamics, since it is less risky to perform an endomyocardial biopsy to rule out infiltrative disease than to submit the patient to an exploratory pericardiectomy to rule out constrictive pericarditis. Biopsy of patients with hypertrophic cardiomyopathy is rarely warranted.

Differential Diagnosis

See Box 68-3.

Dilated Cardiomyopathy

Focal Coronary Artery Disease

Left Ventricular Aneurysm. Patients with a proximal left anterior descending obstruction may develop massive degrees of dilation and dyskinesia of the anterior wall. This can produce a markedly enlarged cardiac silhouette and a falsely low ejection fraction by gated blood pool scanning. Echocardiography or ventriculography demonstrates active inferior and lateral walls, as well as the focal nature of the left ventricular aneurysm.

Left Ventricular Pseudoaneurysm. Patients may rarely suffer a rupture of the anterior wall that is confined to the pericardial space, which is adherent to the anterior wall due to focal pericardial inflammation. Such patients similarly show an enlargement of the left ventricular silhouette on noninvasive studies.

Primary Valvular Disease

Aortic Stenosis. Patients with end-stage aortic stenosis may develop significant ventricular dilation and contractile dysfunction. Due to the low cardiac output generated by the failing heart, the murmur of aortic stenosis may be markedly diminished in intensity or absent.

Aortic Regurgitation. Regurgitant lesions of the aortic and mitral valve result in a volume challenge to the left ventricle. This volume challenge is handled extraordinarily well until late in the course of decompensation. Because of the low aortic diastolic pressure and high left ventricular end-diastolic pressure, the diastolic pressure gradient is low and results in a barely audible murmur.

Mitral Regurgitation. Of all the valvular lesions, mitral regurgitation is the most difficult to distinguish, since patients with dilated cardiomyopathy develop this murmur due to annular dilation and papillary muscle malalignment. A prior history of mitral regurgitation and the finding of moderate to severe regurgitation by noninvasive or invasive studies, as well as a finding of primary valvular pathology by echocardiography, suggest that the mitral regurgitation caused the dilated cardiomyopathy.

Mitral Stenosis. Rarely, patients with severe mitral stenosis, pulmonary hypertension, and right heart failure develop massive enlargement of the right ventricle. This may result in a huge heart by chest x-ray and palpable as well as audible gallops.

Pericardial Disease. Pericardial effusions may produce marked cardiac silhouette enlargement and heart failure, while ventricular function remains entirely normal. This is the most important of the lesions in differential diagnosis in view of the treatability of the disorder.

Hypertrophic Cardiomyopathy

Hypertensive Hypertrophic Cardiomyopathy. Patients with longstanding hypertension may develop left ventricular hypertrophy and congestive heart failure.

Valvular Aortic Stenosis. Aortic stenosis results in a significant obstruction to flow through the aortic valve as the stenosis progresses. Patients develop progressive myocardial hypertrophy in response to this increased workload, resulting in myocardial thickness.

Subaortic Stenosis. Rarely, patients may present with discrete subaortic rings simulating hypertrophic subaortic stenosis and aortic stenosis.

Infiltrative Disorders. Patients with amyloidosis and other infiltrative disorders may appear to have significant ventricular hypertrophy with normal or enhanced contractility early in the natural history of the disease.

Restrictive Cardiomyopathy

Hypertrophic Cardiomyopathy. See above.

Hypertensive Hypertrophic Cardiomyopathy. See above.

Normal Heart Size and Function. Some patients with restrictive cardiomyopathy appear to have normal ventricular wall thickness and contractility early in their course, only to have wall thickness increase and contractility diminish over time.

Pericardial Disease

A pericardial effusion can be mistaken for any of the generalized causes of cardiomegaly noted above. Pericardial constriction may be mistaken for restrictive cardiomyopathy.

MANAGEMENT

The primary tenet is to treat the primary cause when it is identified and if treatment is appropriate. For example, patients with hypothyroidism should be treated with thyroid replacement. Patients with regurgitant or stenotic valvular lesions may be candidates for surgical correction. Similarly, patients with coronary artery disease may be appropriate for revascularization. Patients with pericardial effusions may benefit from pericardiocentesis while patients with constrictive pericarditis benefit from pericardiectomy. All of the cardiomyopathies as well as pericardial tamponade and constrictive pericarditis may present with signs and symptoms of the heart failure syndrome. It is necessary to define the cause of the heart failure syndrome to provide appropriate therapy.

Nonpharmacologic Therapy

Dilated Cardiomyopathy. Patients with dilated cardiomyopathy may benefit from dynamic cardiomyoplasty, left ventricular reduction surgery, or heart transplantation. Dynamic cardiomyoplasty is experimental and utilizes the latissimus dorsi wrapped around the heart muscle in a complicated surgical procedure. The latissimus is stimulated with a pacemaker to contract in conjunction with the left ventricle. This is thought to prevent further ventricular dilation and perhaps augment contractility. Left ventricular reduction surgery has been applied to patients with dilated cardiomyopathy. In this experimental operation, a significant amount of the left ventricular lateral wall is surgically removed. Results from this operation and cardiomyoplasty are mixed. Cardiac transplantation, on the other hand, is a well-established treatment for all forms of end-stage heart disease. It is, however, not available to all patients due to a lack of suitable donor organs. Significant limitations due to age, pulmonary vascular resistance, diabetes, excessive obesity, extracardiac vascular disease, other comorbidities, or psychosocial factors govern the utilization of this operation. Cardiac transplantation results in the replacement of an end-stage, life-threatening heart condition with a multitude of posttransplant medical problems associated with immunosuppressive drugs and their side effects.

Hypertrophic Cardiomyopathy. Patients with hypertrophic cardiomyopathy and an outflow gradient may benefit from atrioventricular (AV) sequential pacing, with improvement in symptoms and a decrease in the outflow gradient.[5] For those patients with hypertrophic cardiomyopathy and outflow tract obstruction that are not improved by medical or pacing therapy, septal myectomy may be indicated. This surgical procedure is characterized by the removal of a portion of the ventricular septum. Patients with hypertrophic cardiomyopathy may also undergo mitral valve replacement. This prevents mitral regurgitation and the anterior movement of the mitral leaflet that is associated with the left ventricular outflow tract obstruction.

Pericardial Disease. Pericardial effusions associated with tamponade may be drained, which results in immediate and dramatic improvement in the patient. The fluid removed must be carefully examined to determine the etiology of the effusion so that it may be appropriately treated to prevent recurrence. If no etiology is identified, antiinflammatory medications may be of benefit.

Surgery for pericardial constriction is virtually always of benefit. The degree of benefit depends on the magnitude of adherence of the pericardial surface to the epicardial surface. Some pericardial constrictions are as easy to remove as an orange peel, whereas others must be painstakingly chiseled from the heart. One must remember that a pericardiectomy is, in fact, only a release of the anterior pericardium between the vagus nerves, since the posterior pericardium cannot be reached.

Pharmacologic Therapy

The pharmacologic treatment for heart failure is covered in Chapter 65. There are several caveats to be observed. Diuretics may be harmful to individuals with small or fixed stroke volumes. This is the case for patients with hypertrophic cardiomyopathy, restrictive cardiomyopathy, pericardial effusion with tamponade, and constrictive pericarditis. Careful attention must be paid to excessive diuresis characterized by decreased cerebral or renal perfusion. Diuretics can be used in all forms of congestive heart failure in which the patient has peripheral, pulmonary, or hepatic venous congestion. The extent to which diuretics may be beneficial depends on the pathophysiology of the condition as noted in earlier sections of this chapter.

Vasodilators are potentially dangerous to patients with hypertrophic cardiomyopathy or pericardial disease. This is particularly the case with hypertrophic cardiomyopathy, in which afterload reduction may exacerbate the hyperdynamic contractility, outflow tract obstruction, and the associated predisposition toward syncope or presyncope.

β-Blockers may be useful for patients with hypertrophic or dilated cardiomyopathy. β-Blockers with intrinsic agonist activity should be avoided. Carvedilol, a nonspecific β-blocker with α-blocking properties, is now available for patients with dilated cardiomyopathy and stable, symptomatic heart failure.

Positive inotropic agents are of limited benefit to those with dilated cardiomyopathy, restrictive cardiomyopathy, or constrictive pericarditis. Positive inotropic agents are contraindicated for patients with hypertrophic cardiomyopathy where hypercontractility already characterizes the condition. The only exceptions are in patients with atrial fibrillation and hypertrophic cardiomyopathy, when digoxin may be utilized for rate control, and in advanced states of the condition, when patients develop systolic dysfunction and should be treated more like a dilated cardiomyopathy.

Patients with dilated cardiomyopathy are at risk for developing systemic and pulmonary emboli. Patients with any form of myocardial or pericardial disease may develop atrial fibrillation and may similarly be at risk for emboli, particularly if they have heart failure. Therefore patients with myocardial disease and atrial fibrillation or dilated cardiomyopathy with an ejection fraction below 30% should receive anticoagulants unless there is a contraindication.

Atrial fibrillation is commonly seen in patients with cardiomyopathy and pericardial disease. Patients with myocardial disease who develop atrial fibrillation have a significant decrease in their cardiac output due to the increased heart rate, decreased diastolic filling time, and lack of atrial systolic preloading of the ventricle before contraction. Control of rapid ventricular response in atrial fibrillation and conversion to sinus rhythm are important objectives for patients with myocardial or pericardial disease. Those with myocardial diseases, particularly dilated cardiomyopathy and hypertrophic cardiomyopathy, are markedly prone to ventricular dysrhythmias, including ventricular tachycardia, and are at risk for sudden death. There is as yet no convincing evidence to indicate that pharmacologic treatment of ventricular dysrhythmias prolongs survival in patients with dilated, hypertrophic, or restrictive cardiomyopathy. Nonetheless, for survivors of sudden death, an automatic implantable cardioverter defibrillator (AICD) is indicated. For patients with nonsustained ventricular tachycardia, serious consideration must be given to prophylactic treatment with drugs or devices. Electrophysiologic testing is of prognostic value in patients with ischemic cardiomyopathy. Patients who are inducible should undergo AICD placement.[12] For those patients who are noninducible yet symptomatic, β-blockers and amiodarone appear to be the most efficacious and least risky drugs. Antidysrhythmic drugs other than β-blockers and amiodarone in patients with ischemic cardiomyopathy are associated with increased mortality and should be avoided.[2,15]

Hypertrophic Cardiomyopathy. Negative inotropic agents, including β-blockers, calcium blockers, and disopyramide, improve symptoms in patients with hypertrophic cardiomyopathy. β-Blockers and calcium channel blockers, especially verapamil, decrease intrinsic heart rate, which allows greater ventricular filling and improved stroke volume. These agents also decrease the hypercontractility characteristic of this disorder, which may diminish the outflow tract gradient, angina, presyncope, syncope, and excessive fatigability.

Restrictive Cardiomyopathy. The symptoms caused by restrictive cardiomyopathy are difficult to treat. Careful use of low-dose diuretics and vasodilators may be of some benefit. Negative inotropic agents will be of no benefit to patients with restrictive cardiomyopathy. In fact, these agents may be harmful due to depression of the contractility necessary to maintain reasonable forward perfusion. Digoxin should be used with caution in patients with amyloid heart disease, since these patients appear to be particularly sensitive.

Specific treatment of the various causes of dilated and restrictive cardiomyopathy is beyond the scope of this chapter. Careful consideration must be given to the pros and cons of treatment of disorders such as myocarditis or ischemic cardiomyopathy. Consultation with a cardiologist is appropriate.

Pericardial Disease. The first step in the management of acute pericarditis is bed rest. The pain often responds to nonsteroidal antiinflammatory drugs (NSAID) such as ibuprofen. If the pain is severe and does not quickly respond to NSAID, corticosteroids may be efficacious. Large doses, such as 30 mg of prednisone twice daily, are typically used and tapered over 1 month. Colchicine, 1 mg per day, may be of benefit for those patients with recurrent episodes of acute pericarditis.[1]

Consultation

Consultation with a cardiologist should be sought for patients with newly diagnosed cardiomyopathies. Patients with New York Heart Association class III and IV symptoms of heart failure should be referred to a cardiologist with expertise in heart failure and a connection to a heart transplant program. Those patients with symptomatic dysrhythmias or sudden death should be seen and treated by an electrophysiologist. Recurrent pericarditis should be evaluated and treated by a cardiologist. Similarly, a cardiologist should help differentiate restrictive cardiomyopathy from constrictive pericarditis.

SPECIAL ISSUES

The management of patients with a cardiomyopathy is challenging. Patients must be seen frequently, especially when medications are changed or the patient has significant

... are symptomatic at rest, as well as ... with unstable angina, syncope, or symptomatic palpitations, should be hospitalized. Disease management using a team approach may be of benefit to those patients with New York Heart Association class III and IV symptoms.[13] Special emphasis must be placed on compliance, education, and the management of comorbidities such as hypertension, diabetes, and hyperlipidemia.

Patients with hypertrophic cardiomyopathy should refrain from competitive athletics.[11]

Patients with renal dysfunction represent a particular problem. Angiotensin-converting enzyme inhibitors may be difficult to use in these patients and require careful monitoring. A rising creatinine may indicate inadequate renal perfusion, due to poor stroke volume, or dehydration, due to excessive diuretic use. Evidence of congestion is usually seen in the former, whereas patients with the latter look dry. In ... right heart catheterization may be needed to ... volume from dehydration.

EBM EVIDENCE ...

The primary source for this chapter was MEDLINE. Electronic searches dating back to 1985 were conducted in November 1998. They focused on identifying reviews and large randomized trials.

REFERENCES

1. Adler Y, Finkelstein Y, Guindo J, et al: Colchicine treatment for recurrent pericarditis: a decade of experience, *Circulation* 97:2183-2185, 1998.
2. Cardiac Arrhythmia Suppression Trial (CAST) Investigators: Preliminary report: effect of encainide and flecainide on mortality in a randomized trial of arrhythmia suppression after myocardial infarction, *N Engl J Med* 321:406-412, 1989.
3. Codd MB, Sugrue DD, Gersh BJ, et al: Epidemiology of idiopathic dilated and hypertrophic cardiomyopathy: a population-based study in Olmsted County, Minnesota, 1975-1984, *Circulation* 80:564-572, 1989.
4. Dec GW, Fuster V: Idiopathic dilated cardiomyopathy, *N Engl J Med* 331:1564-1575, 1994.
5. Fananapazir L, Epstein ND, Curiel RV, et al: Long-term results of dual-chamber (DDD) pacing in obstructive hypertrophic cardiomyopathy, *Circulation* 90:2731-2742, 1994.
6. Fowler NO: Constrictive pericarditis: its history and current status, *Clin Cardiol* 18:341-350, 1995.
7. Kasper EK, Agema WRP, Hutchins GM, et al: The causes of dilated cardiomyopathy: a clinicopathologic review of 673 consecutive patients, *J Am Coll Cardiol* 23:590, 1994.
8. Konstam MA, Dracup K, Baker DW, et al: Heart failure: evaluation and care of patients with left-ventricular systolic dysfunction. *Clinical Practice Guideline number 11*. AHCPR Publication No. 94-0612 ed., Rockville, Md, 1994, Agency for Health Care Policy and Research, Public Health Service, U.S. Department of Health and Human Services.
9. Kushwaha SS, Fallon JT, Fuster V: Restrictive cardiomyopathy, *N Engl J Med* 336:267-276, 1997.
10. Malik MS, Watkins H: The molecular genetics of hypertrophic cardiomyopathy, *Curr Opin Cardiol* 12:295-302, 1997.
11. Maron BJ, Isner JM, McKenna WJ: 26th Bethesda conference: recommendations for determining eligibility for competition in athletes with cardiovascular abnormalities. Task Force 3: hypertrophic cardiomyopathy, myocarditis and other myopericardial diseases and mitral valve prolapse, *Med Sci Sports Exerc* 26:S261-S267, 1994.
12. Moss AJ, Hall WJ, Cannom DS, et al: Improved survival with an implanted defibrillator in patients with coronary disease at high risk for ventricular arrhythmia, *N Engl J Med* 335:1933-1940, 1996.
13. Rich MW, Beckham V, Wittenberg C, et al: A multidisciplinary intervention to prevent the readmission of elderly patients with congestive heart failure, *N Engl J Med* 333:1190-1195, 1995.
14. Richardson P, McKenna W, Bristow M, et al: Report of the 1995 World Health Organization/International Society and Federation of Cardiology Task Force on the definition and classification of cardiomyopathies, *Circulation* 93:841-842, 1996.
15. Singh SN, Fletcher RD, Fisher SG, et al: Amiodarone in patients with congestive heart failure and asymptomatic ventricular arrhythmia, *N Engl J Med* 333:77-82, 1995.
16. Wigle ED, Rakowski H, Kimball BP, et al: Hypertrophic cardiomyopathy: clinical spectrum and treatment, *Circulation* 92:1680-1692, 1995.

CHAPTER 69

Infective Endocarditis

Burke A. Cunha
Diane H. Johnson
Natalie C. Klein

EPIDEMIOLOGY AND ETIOLOGY

Infective endocarditis (IE) is defined as an infection of the valvular and nonvalvular endothelial surfaces of the heart. Although most frequently caused by bacteria, other microorganisms such as fungi, rickettsiae, mycoplasmas, or chlamydiae may also cause endocarditis.

Endocarditis is classified as acute or subacute depending on the clinical course of the untreated illness. Subacute bacterial endocarditis (SBE) usually occurs on previously damaged valves, and is due to relatively avirulent organisms (e.g., viridans streptococci). The course of illness is indolent and characterized by night sweats, fevers, and malaise. Acute bacterial endocarditis (ABE) occurs on normal and damaged heart valves and also in association with intravenous drug use or intravascular catheters or devices. ABE is caused by virulent microorganisms such as *Staphylococcus aureus, Streptococcus pneumoniae,* or *Pseudomonas aeruginosa*. The clinical course is fulminant with rapid valvular destruction and a high incidence of metastatic disease. IE should be viewed as subacute or acute. This clinical classification explains difference in signs, symptoms, laboratory abnormalities, and differing pathogens associated with SBE vs. ABE. Isolation of the organism in culture-positive endocarditis serves as a guide for antimicrobial therapy[2,7,13] (Box 69-1).

PATHOPHYSIOLOGY

The left side of the heart is more frequently involved in infection, with the mitral valve affected more frequently than the aortic valve. Rheumatic heart disease, congenital heart disease (e.g., bicuspid valves, ventricular septal defects, coarctation of the aorta), and degenerative disease such as calcific aortic stenosis all predispose a person to the development of IE.[10,12]

After the endothelial surface of the valve or cardiac structure is damaged by high velocity or turbulent blood flow, a sterile platelet or fibrin clot is formed that results in marantic or nonbacterial thrombotic endocarditis. When a transient bacteremia occurs, the platelet or fibrin thrombus may become colonized. As the bacteria multiply, there is

Box 69-1. Culture-positive and Culture-negative Endocarditis

Culture-positive

Acute

Normal Valve
- *Staphylococcus aureus**
- *Pseudomonas aeruginosa*†
- *Serratia marcescens*

Prosthetic Valve (Early)
- Staphylococcus aureus
- Streptococcus pneumoniae
- Pseudomonas aeruginosa

Subacute

Native Valve
- Viridans streptococci
- Enterococcal

Prosthetic Valve (Late)
- Staphylococcus epidermidis
- Viridans streptococci

Culture-negative‡

Apparently culture-negative endocarditis (fastidious organ with delayed growth)

Haemophilus species
Acinetobacter actinomycetemcomitans
Cardiobacterium hominis
Eikenella corrodens
Kingella kingae

True culture-negative endocarditis (serologic diagnosis)

Aspergillus
Legionella

*Normal hosts, procedure-related, IVDAs.
†IVDAs only.
‡Low-grade fevers, leukocytosis, with cardiac murmur/vegetations; should not be diagnosed as culture-negative endocarditis unless there are also signs of endocarditis present.

further disposition of fibrin and platelets that protect the pathogens from the host defenses. Portions of this vegetation may break off and embolize systemically. The valve may be damaged or destroyed, and the endocardium can be invaded by myocardial abscesses, resulting in the development of heart block or dysrhythmias.[10,14]

CLINICAL MANIFESTATIONS

The classic signs and symptoms of SBE are fever, anemia, splenomegaly, a cardiac murmur, and embolic phenomena. The clinical manifestations of IE depend on whether the patient has SBE or ABE.

The history of valvular disease, recent medical or dental procedures, infections, or intravenous drug abuse (IVDA) is important to obtain. The source of viridans streptococcal SBE is usually the mouth. The symptoms of SBE typically begin within 2 weeks of the initial bacteremia.[17] Nonspecific symptoms such as fever, weight loss, night sweats, low back pain, arthralgias, or malaise may be present in SBE due to relatively avirulent organisms (e.g., viridans streptococci).

Infection with more virulent pathogens such as *S. aureus* results in ABE.[10] Fever ≥102° F is the most common physical finding and is present in nearly all patients with ABE. Little or no fever may be due to recent antibiotic use. Fever may also be absent in elderly or debilitated patients, in patients with congestive heart failure or renal failure, or in IVDAs.[2,9] Heart murmurs are present in over 80% of patients, but may be absent in right-sided or mural endocarditis.[6] The physical examination may have findings of congestive heart failure in ABE. Splenomegaly is present in the minority of patients, but is most common in those with SBE.[15] Peripheral manifestations of endocarditis such as petechia or splinter hemorrhages are seen in about 15% of persons with IE. Osler's nodes (tender nodular lesions of the fingers and toes) and Janeway lesions (painless hemorrhagic macules [illegible] palms and soles) are uncommon. Clubbing may [illegible] secondary to *S. aureus*, and chronic [illegible] complicate SBE. Roth's spots [illegible] surrounded by hemorr[illegible] back pain, my[illegible] with IE [illegible] [illegible]mon in patients [illegible] low back pain suggests enterococcal [illegible]. Up to one third of patients may have a monoarticular or polyarticular septic arthritis with ABE. Focal neurologic deficits may occur as a result of systemic septic embolization in ABE or immunologic-mediated bland embolus (aseptic meningitis) in SBE.[8]

Laboratory abnormalities in patients with IE are nonspecific. The majority of patients have a normochromic, normocytic anemia; leukocytosis with a left shift is variably present. The erythrocyte sedimentation rate (ESR) is elevated, and positive Venereal Disease Research Laboratories (VDRL) and elevated rheumatoid factors are often present in SBE. Urinalysis findings in SBE consist of microscopic hematuria or proteinuria.[9,13] Blood cultures are positive in almost all patients with infectious endocarditis. Since the bacteremia is continuous, all cultures should be positive. Blood culture positivity is related to volume of blood cultured by one or more venipunctures from one or more sites. In SBE and ABE, blood cultures should be obtained prior to initiating therapy. The most common reason for negative blood cultures is prior antibiotic use. Infection with fastidious organisms such as the HACEK group (*Haemophilus, Actinobacillus, Cardiobacterium, Eikenella,* and *Kingella*) is rare. *Legionella* species and the nutritionally deficient streptococci may also result in negative cultures. The microbiologist should be alerted and specimens held for at least 3 weeks when a diagnosis of culture-negative IE is suspected.[9] Most patients with low-grade fevers, leukocytosis, and cardiac murmurs with or without vegetations by echocardiography do not have culture-negative endocarditis. Those who do will also have peripheral manifestations.

DIAGNOSIS

In addition to positive blood cultures with known endocarditis pathogens, echocardiography has been used to support the diagnosis of IE. Two-dimensional transthoracic echocardiography (TTE) has a sensitivity of approximately 50%, and is poor for detecting small vegetations and those on prosthetic valves. The larger the vegetation, the more likely the risk for systemic embolization. Transesophageal echocardiography (TEE) is more sensitive than TTE, but is invasive, not innocuous, and more expensive. TEE can detect small vegetations (<5 mm), perivalvular abscesses, and those on

Table 69-1. Clinical Differentiation of Acute vs. Subacute Endocarditis

	ABE	SBE
Symptoms		
Anorexia	−	+
Myalgias/arthralgias	+	±
Fatigue	−	+
Dyspnea/cough	+	−
Pleuritic chest pain/hemoptysis	+	−
Lumbar back pain	+	+
Weight loss	−	±
Headache	+	±
Mental status changes	+	±
Acute confusional states	+	−
Unexplained stroke	−	+
Sudden unilateral blindness	−	+
Left upper quadrant pain	Splenic abscess	Splenic infarct
CVA tenderness (renal abscess)	+	−
Signs		
Fever	>102° F	<102° F
New heart murmur	±	−
Splenomegaly	−	+
Petechiae	+	+
Osler's nodes	−	+
Janeway lesions	+	−
Splinter hemorrhages	±	+
Roth's spots	−	+
Congestive heart failure (LVF)	+	−
Laboratory Tests		
Anemia	−	+
Marked leukocytosis	+	−
Microscopic hematuria	±	+
Hematuria, proteinuria, RBC casts	−	+
Elevated ESR	≤50 mm/hr	≥50 mm/hr
Elevated RF titer	−	+
Elevated VDRL titer	−	+
Circulating immune complexes	−	+
Synovial fluid analysis	Septic arthritis	Aseptic arthritis
Cerebrospinal fluid (CSF)	Purulent meningitis profile	Aseptic meningitis profile
Heart block	+	−
Chest x-ray	Pneumonia (septic pulmonary emboli)	−
Brain CT/MRI	Positive if cerebritis, microabscesses or hemorrhage (pyogenic arteritis)	Negative unless mycotic aneurysms or embolic CVAs
Mycotic aneurysms (abdominal CT/MRI)	−	+

Modified from Cunha BA, Gill VM, Lazar JM: Acute infective endocarditis, *Infect Dis Clin North Am* 10:822, 1996.
+, Commonly present; ±, uncommonly present; −, rarely, if ever, present.

prosthetic valves.[2] Echocardiography of the heart should be obtained on all patients with suspected IE. However, vegetations without positive blood cultures do not signify IE, or even culture-negative IE.[5,11] Echocardiography should be obtained for baseline purposes in case of subsequent hemodynamic deterioration or congestive heart failure (CHF), or to rule out IE. The most common problem is that of interpreting the significance of viridans streptococci in blood cultures. High-grade bacteremia always represents SBE, but low culture positivity (e.g., one of three positive blood cultures for viridans streptococci) is never associated with SBE.

MANAGEMENT

Antibiotic Therapy

Empiric antimicrobial therapy is based on the presumptive organism causing infection.[18] Bacteriocidal antibiotics given in endocarditis doses for 4 to 6 weeks sterilize the vegetation. Current recommendations for treatment of IE in Table 69-2 are the consensus of the American Heart Association based on published studies and collective clinical experience of this group of experts.[18] The treatment of ABE is always urgent, but the start of SBE therapy is not time-critical. For native valve SBE, a β-lactam with or without gentamicin for viridans streptococci is appropriate empiric therapy. Nafcillin

Table 69-2. Suggested Empiric Therapy for Native Valve Endocarditis

Pathogen	Antibiotic*	Duration
Viridans streptococci and *Streptococcus bovis* (MIC ≤0.1 μg/ml)	Aqueous crystalline penicillin G sodium 18 MU/24h (IV) in 6 divided doses	4 weeks
	or	
	ceftriaxone sodium 2 gm (IV) q24h	4 weeks
	or	
	vancomycin† 1 gm (IV) q12h	4 weeks
Viridans streptococci and *Streptococcus bovis* (MIC >0.1 μg/ml and <0.5 μg/ml)	Aqueous crystalline penicillin G sodium 18 MU/24h (IV) in 6 divided doses	4 weeks
	with	
	gentamicin 1 mg/kg (IV) q24h	2 weeks
	or	
	vancomycin† 1 gm (IV) q12h	4 weeks
Enterococci	Aqueous crystalline penicillin G 18 MU/24h in 6 divided doses	4-6 weeks
	with	
	gentamicin 1 mg/kg (IV) q8h	4-6 weeks
	or	
	ampicillin sodium 2 gm (IV) q4h	4-6 weeks
	with	
	gentamicin 1 mg/kg (IV) q8h	
	or	
	vancomycin† 1 gm (IV) q12h	4-6 weeks
	with	
	gentamicin 1 mg/kg (IV) q24h	
Staphylococcus aureus	Nafcillin or oxacillin 2 gm (IV) q4h	4-6 weeks
	with	
	gentamicin 1 mg/kg (IV) q24h	3-5 days
	or	
	cefazolin 1 gm (IV) q8h	4-6 weeks
	with	
	gentamicin 1 mg/kg (IV) q24h	3-5 days
	or	
	vancomycin† 1 gm (IV) q12h	4-6 weeks
HACEK‡	Ceftriaxone 2 gm (IV) q24h	4 weeks
	or	
	ampicillin 2 gm (IV) q4h	4 weeks
	and	
	gentamicin 1 mg/kg (IV) q24h	4 weeks

*Dosage for normal renal function.
†For β-lactam allergic patient.
‡*Haemophilus parainfluenzae, Haemophilus aphrophilus, Actinobacillus actinomycetemcomitans, Cardiobacterium hominis, Eikenella corrodens,* and *Kingella kingae.*

or vancomycin combined with gentamicin, directed against *S. aureus,* is adequate empiric therapy for endocarditis in IVDAs.[18] For prosthetic valve endocarditis (PVE), a combination of vancomycin and gentamicin covering *Staphylococcus epidermidis* and *S. aureus* is adequate initial therapy. Once the organism is isolated, therapy may need to be changed based on organism or susceptibility testing[18] (Tables 69-1 and 69-2). After initiating appropriate therapy, fever should decrease within 72 hours and repeat blood cultures should be sterile.

Patients with continued fevers for more than 7 days on appropriate antibiotics, or who have persistently positive blood cultures, may have myocardial or metastatic abscesses. The most common sites for septic emboli are the spleen, liver, kidney, and lung, but emboli in the brain, bones or joints, or meninges may also occur. A computed tomography (CT) scan of the abdomen, pelvis and brain, or bone, or indium or gallium scan may be helpful in the diagnosis. Fever that abates after initiation of antibiotics but later recurs is usually due to recurrent septic emboli, noninfectious emboli phenomenon such as splenic infarct, or drug fever.

Surgical Indications

For most patients, medical therapy with 4 to 6 weeks of antibiotics is curative. However, valvular replacement may be necessary for certain complications: intractable heart failure, recurrent systemic emboli, inability to eradicate infection due to large vegetation or resistant organism, fungal endocarditis, myocardial abscess, or prosthetic valve dysfunction.

Prophylaxis

Although there are no randomized, controlled human studies to demonstrate that antibiotic prophylaxis prevents endocarditis, the use of prophylactic antibiotics in individuals with underlying cardiac abnormalities undergoing bacteremia-inducing procedures is common practice. Current guidelines from the American Heart Association are not universally agreed on.[3,4] Oral prophylaxis directed against viridans streptococci is now preferred to parenteral regimens (i.e., a single dose of amoxicillin, 2 gm (PO), given 1 hour before dental or upper respiratory tract surgical procedures is recommended for prophylaxis, with no further doses necessary). For the penicillin-allergic patient, a single dose of

Table 69-3. Prophylactic Antibiotic Regimens

Procedure	Antibiotic	Alternative
Dental, upper respiratory tract, or esophagus	Amoxicillin 2 gm	Clindamycin 600 mg or cephalexin 2 gm or azithromycin 500 mg
Gastrointestinal (GI) or genitourinary (GU)		
High risk*	Ampicillin 2 gm (IV/IM) plus gentamicin 1.5 mg/kg (IV) within 30 minutes prior to procedure and 6 hours later ampicillin 1 gm (IV) or amoxicillin 1 gm (PO)	Vancomycin 1 gm (IV) slowly over 1 hour and gentamicin 1.5 mg/kg (IM) or slowly (IV)
GI or GU		
Moderate risk†	Amoxicillin 2 gm (PO) 1 hr before procedure, or ampicillin 2 gm (IV/IM) within 30 minutes prior to procedure	Vancomycin 1 gm (IV) slowly over 1 hour

*Prosthetic valves, previous bacterial endocarditis, complex cyanotic congenital heart disease, surgically constructed systemic pulmonary shunts.
†Other congenital cardiac malformations, acquired valvular dysfunction, hypertrophic cardiomyopathy, mitral valve prolapse with murmur, and/or thickened leaflets.

clindamycin, cephalexin, or azithromycin is an alternative approach.

Prophylactic regimens for gastrointestinal or genitourinary procedures are IV/IM ampicillin and gentamicin for high-risk patients, or amoxicillin alone for moderate-risk patients. These are directed against enterococci, the sole cause of SBE acquired from a source below the waist (Table 69-3).

REFERENCES

1. Bush LM, Johnson CC: Clinical syndrome and diagnosis. Kaye D, editor: In *Infective endocarditis,* ed 2, New York, 1992, Raven, pp 99-113.
2. Cunha BA, Gill VM, Lazar JM: Acute infective endocarditis, *Infect Dis Clin North Am* 10:811-833, 1996.
3. Dajani AS, Taubert KA, Wilson W, et al: Prevention of bacterial endocarditis: recommendations by the American Heart Association, *JAMA* 277:1794-1801, 1997.
4. Durack DT: Antibiotics for prevention of endocarditis during dentistry: time to scale back? *Ann Intern Med* 129:829-831, 1998.
5. Durack DT, Lukes AS, Bright DR, et al: New criteria for the diagnosis of infective endocarditis, *Am J Med* 96:200-209, 1994.
6. Garvey GJ, Neu HC: Infective endocarditis—an evolving disease: a review of endocarditis at the Columbia-Presbyterian Medical Center 1968-1973, *Medicine* 57:105-127, 1978.
7. Harris SL: Definitions and demographic characteristics. In Kaye D, editor: *Infective endocarditis,* ed 2, New York, 1992, Raven, pp 1-18.
8. Hermans PE: The clinical manifestations of infective endocarditis, *Mayo Clin Proc* 57:15, 1982.
9. Kaye D, editor: *Infective endocarditis,* ed 2, New York, 1992, Raven.
10. Korzeniowski M, Kaye D: Endocarditis. In Gorbach SL, Bartlett JG, Blacklow NR, editors: *Infectious diseases,* ed 2, Philadelphia, 1998, WB Saunders, pp 663-674.
11. Lukes AS, Bright DR, Durack DT: Diagnosis of infective endocarditis, *Infect Dis Clin North Am* 7:1-9, 1993.
12. Pelletier LL, Petersdorf RG: Infective endocarditis: a review of 125 cases from the University of Washington Hospital 1963-1972, *Medicine* (Baltimore) 56:287, 1977.
13. Scheld WM, Vande MA: Endocarditis and intravascular infection. In Mandell GL, Bennett JE, Dolin R, editors: *Principles and practices of infectious diseases,* ed 4, New York, 1995, Churchill Livingstone, pp 740-783.
14. Sultan PM, Drake TA, Sande MA: Pathogenesis of endocarditis, *Am J Med* 78(Suppl B):110, 1995.
15. Terpenning MS, Buggy BP, Kaufman CA: Infective endocarditis: clinical features in young and elderly patients, *Am J Med* 83:626-634, 1987.
16. Weinstein L, Brusch J: Clinical manifestations of native valve endocarditis. In Weinstein L, Brusch J, editors: *Infective endocarditis,* New York, 1996, Oxford.
17. Weinstein L, Schlessinger JT: Pathoanatomic pathophysiologic and clinical correlations in endocarditis, *N Engl J Med* 291:832-836, 1974.
18. Wilson WR, Karchmer AW, Dajani AS, et al: Antibiotic treatment of adults with infective endocarditis due to streptococci, enterococci, staphylococci and HACEK microorganisms, *JAMA* 274:1706-1713, 1995.

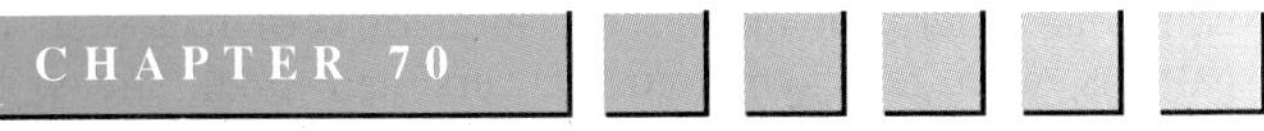

Peripheral Vascular Disease

Jay D. Coffman

OBSTRUCTIVE ARTERIAL DISEASE

Epidemiology and Etiology

Patients with obstructive arterial disease complain of pain, tightness of muscles, fatigue, or weakness of the legs on walking. Symptoms are relieved by rest within a few minutes. This symptom is termed *intermittent claudication,* which means to limp intermittently.[2] Most patients have arteriosclerotic obstructive arterial disease. About 2.1% of males and 1.6% of females have symptoms suggesting intermittent claudication. The prevalence is markedly increased in diabetic patients. The incidence is two times greater in smokers than in nonsmokers and increases with the intensity of the habit. The ratio of men to women is about 3 : 1. Females lag behind males by about 10 years in development of the disease.

Pathophysiology

The symptoms are usually caused by obstructive arterial disease due to arteriosclerosis. The obstructed or stenosed large or medium-sized artery limits blood flow to the active muscle. A decreased perfusion pressure distal to the lesion falls further with the vasodilation of exercise, and the muscle contraction may actually stop blood flow. Diabetic patients may have more severe and progressive arteriosclerosis obliterans than others. Other risk factors for arteriosclerotic occlusive disease are tobacco smoking, hypertension, and hyperlipoproteinemias.

History

The patient's muscle symptoms occur after walking a remarkably constant distance, except they are aggravated by walking on inclines or when heavy bundles are carried. The location of the discomfort sometimes helps define the vessel affected; however, calf claudication may occur with the disease at any vascular level, since these muscles are most involved in walking. Low back or buttock claudication suggests aortoiliac disease, thigh pain indicates iliac or common femoral artery disease, and foot symptoms point to diseased vessels at or below the popliteal artery. The most common lesion is an obstruction or stenosis of the superficial femoral artery in the adductor canal, and it causes calf claudication. The other symptoms of obstructive arterial disease of the limbs are rest pain, numbness, and paresthesia. When these occur, the circulation is severely compromised, since even the small nutritional requirements of the skin are not being met. These symptoms usually occur only in feet; rest symptoms in muscles are rare.

Physical Examination

Most patients with only intermittent claudication have normal appearing limbs. There may be global atrophy of the lower limbs in patients with aortoiliac disease. Hair may be sparse on the lower limbs and absent on the toes. Observation of the limbs in the dependent position may reveal dependent rubor, which is a purplish red discoloration of cool feet seen in patients with rest symptoms. Ulcers and small areas of gangrene may be present, usually on the toes.

All pulses are palpated, and auscultation for bruits over the femoral arteries and abdominal aorta is performed. A systolic bruit indicates an arterial lesion proximal to the point of auscultation, and if accompanied by a decreased pulse, it is a hemodynamically significant obstruction. A diastolic component to the bruit indicates poor collateral blood flow.

The collateral circulation to the affected limbs can be evaluated by a simple office test. With the patient supine, elevation of the limbs at a 45-degree angle should not produce pallor. If the feet become pale, the collateral circulation is not fully compensatory. The patient is then asked to assume a sitting position with the limbs dependent. The feet should flush immediately and the veins of the dorsal foot fill within 20 seconds. If the flushing and venous filling times exceed 30 seconds, the collateral circulation is borderline.

Laboratory Studies and Diagnostic Procedures

In the few patients in whom the diagnosis cannot be made by physical examination, the most valuable test is the measurement of ankle systolic blood pressure via Doppler methods. This pressure should be equal to or greater than the arm pressure. Arteriography or magnetic resonance arteriography defines the anatomy of the diseased vascular tree but yields little hemodynamic information. It is useful only if surgery is being considered and is rarely needed as a diagnostic test.

Differential Diagnosis

In over 90% of patients arteriosclerosis obliterans is the cause of intermittent claudication. There are other vascular and nonvascular etiologies (Table 70-1). Neurogenic claudication may be secondary to a prolapsed intervertebral disk, stenosis of the canal, or hypertrophic bony ridging in the intervertebral canal.

Thromboangiitis obliterans (Buerger's disease) is a rare cause of intermittent claudication.[4] The etiology is unknown. Small and medium-sized arteries and veins are affected by an inflammatory reaction; thrombosis in blood vessels may contain sterile microabscesses and multinucleated cells. There are characteristic areas of normal blood vessel between involved segments. The typical patient is a man 20 to 40 years of age, and almost all patients are smokers. Patients usually present with ischemic symptoms or signs in the feet or intermittent claudication. Vasospasm and migratory superficial thrombophlebitis may occur in up to 40% of patients.

Clinical Course

Several studies have shown that 60% to 90% of patients with intermittent claudication due to arteriosclerosis remain stable or improve over a 5- to 9-year period. Patients with diabetes

Table 70-1. Differential Diagnosis of Leg Pain with Exercise

	Sex	Age	Frequency	Cause	Pulses
Arteriosclerosis obliterans	M > F	Seventh decade	Very common	Occluded or stenosed large or medium-sized arteries; lower extremity involvement	Abnormal
Neurogenic	M = F	Sixth-seventh decade	Common	Spinal cord compression or ischemia	Normal
Thromboangiitis obliterans	M >> F	Third-fourth decade	Rare	Vasculitis of medium to small arteries; upper and lower extremity involvement	Abnormal; loss of ulnar pulse
Adventitial cysts	M > F	Fourth decade	Rare	Unknown	Usually normal
Popliteal artery entrapment syndrome	M > F	Third-fourth decade	Rare	Abnormal origin of muscles	Usually normal
Venous claudication	M = F	Any age	Rare	Iliofemoral thrombophlebitis	Normal
McArdle's disease	M = F	Any age	Rare	Deficient muscle phosphorylases	Normal
Shin splints	M = F	Any age	Common	Swollen anterior tibial muscle	Normal

mellitus usually have progressive disease; their amputation rate is four times greater than that in patients with obstructive arterial disease without diabetes. Acute ischemic events occur in 25% of patients over 4 to 7 years. The amputation rate is about 0.8% to 1% per year but is much higher in diabetics and smokers. Obstructive arterial disease is a marker for shortened survival. Most of these patients die a decade earlier of coronary artery disease and/or diabetes.

Management

Most patients with intermittent claudication should be treated conservatively. The immediate success rate of graft bypass surgery of the superficial femoral artery is 80% to 90%, and the 5-year graft patency rate is 70% in the best vascular centers. Balloon angioplasty of the iliac arteries can produce excellent results but not in more distal vessels. In Maryland it was found that the use of balloon angioplasty increased 24-fold and peripheral bypass surgery doubled, but the rate of lower extremity amputation did not change over 11 years.[11] Therefore patients should not be referred for surgery or balloon angioplasty unless the symptoms are interfering with their occupation or lifestyle or there are symptoms and signs of ischemia at rest.

General measures include advice to quit smoking and referral to a cessation program if needed. A graded exercise regimen improves walking distance in about 80% of patients. Patients are instructed to keep their feet warm, clean, and dry; toenails should always be cut straight across. Extremes of temperature should be avoided, since ischemic tissue burns at lower temperatures and is more susceptible to frostbite. Cuts or severe bruises on the limbs and feet should be reported to the physician immediately. Obesity and carrying bundles shorten the walking distance before symptoms, since the muscles receive only enough blood flow for a certain amount of work.

Most vascular specialists consider vasodilator drugs not to be of value. Pentoxifylline purportedly increases blood flow by a decrease in blood viscosity and has been reported to produce a small increase in walking distance. The recommended dosage is 400 mg three times a day with nausea and dyspepsia as side effects. Three meta-analyses have been done; two found pentoxifylline of questionable value, while the other reported it of benefit.[8] Cilostazol is a phosphodiesterase inhibitor that suppresses platelet aggregation and dilates arteries. It has been shown to significantly increase walking distance in patients with claudication at doses of 50 to 100 mg. Patients must be observed carefully for tachycardia; other frequent side effects are headache, diarrhea, dizziness, and nausea.[4a]

The treatment of thromboangiitis obliterans is similar to that for arteriosclerosis obliterans except sympathectomy may be helpful in cases with severe vasospasm and smoking must be stopped.

Vignette: An 85-year-old woman presents with limb-threatening ischemia[5] and a history of angina. The left leg is pale and cool, the toes are purplish. A vascular surgeon is consulted immediately and recommends an aortogram. An amputation in this patient is associated with a high mortality and, if successful, markedly decreases the quality of life. The aortogram shows a tight stenosis of the left external iliac artery and an occluded superficial femoral artery; the right iliac arteries are patent. Consultation with the interventional radiologist results in a successful balloon dilation and stenting of the iliac artery lesion. The left leg becomes warm and the toes pink. The patient is able to walk 100 yards without leg pain. Six months later, left foot pain recurs at rest. Consultation with the vascular surgeon results in an aortogram showing occlusion of the left common and external iliac arteries. The interventional radiologist explains that this lesion cannot be dilated. An anesthesiologist is consulted who recommends epidural anesthesia, which allows greater safety for surgery in the elderly. The vascular surgeon chooses to perform a femorofemoral bypass to supply the left leg, since the right iliac arteries are patent. He prefers this approach, although an axillofemoral bypass would be an alternative option. A cardiologist is consulted who recommends a dobutamine stress test and then clears the patient for surgery since it does not show reversible ischemia. Following surgery, the left leg again becomes warm and of good color. The patient's recovery is slow, and she finds it difficult to walk because of incisional discomfort. A physical therapist is consulted who recommends transfer to a rehabilitation unit where she works with the patient daily on walking and then stair climbing. In 10 days the patient is fully ambulatory and able to live independently because of the close collaboration of the primary care physician, vascular surgeon, anesthesiologist, cardiologist, and physical therapist.

ARTERIAL EMBOLI AND ACUTE THROMBOSIS

Epidemiology and Etiology

Typically in this disorder the patient calls the physician because of the sudden onset of severe leg pain that is secondary to abrupt interruption of the arterial supply by an embolus or acute thrombosis of a diseased blood vessel. In the differential diagnosis an embolus is unlikely if a source cannot be found (Box 70-1), and an acute thrombosis is likely if other evidence of chronic obstructive arterial disease is present. Paradoxical emboli originate from venous thromboses, travel to the right side of the heart, and reach the peripheral circulation through the foramen ovale. Emboli may also occur from thrombi in aneurysms or from atheromatous ulcers in any proximal vessel. Atheromatous emboli are often caused by catheterization procedures. Acute thrombosis of an artery usually occurs in a patient with stenosed blood vessels due to arteriosclerosis obliterans.

Pathophysiology

The clinical picture relates to the acute loss of blood supply to the distal extremity. The symptoms and signs are due to the lack of oxygen and the accumulation of toxic metabolites in

Box 70-1. Sources of Arterial Emboli

Myocardial infarction with mural thrombi
Atrial fibrillation
Cardiomyopathies
Prosthetic heart valves
Chronic congestive heart failure
Endocarditis
Left ventricular aneurysm
Left atrial myxoma
Sick sinus syndrome
Paradoxical embolus from venous thrombosis
Aneurysms of large blood vessels
Atheromatous ulcers of large blood vessels

the limb. In patients with atheromatous emboli, small vessels in skin and muscle are occluded by cholesterol crystals and atheromatous debris.

History

In 50% of patients, embolism or acute thrombosis of large or medium-sized arteries produces the sudden onset of severe pain in the extremity. The remaining patients complain of a more insidious onset of pain over several hours. Paresthesias and numbness are present in the majority of patients; muscular weakness or paralysis occurs in one of five cases. The pain is usually unrelenting. However, in patients with acute thrombosis of previously diseased arteries, collateral vessels may already be well developed and the symptoms may abate. Questions about the possible etiologies (e.g., heart disease, peripheral vascular disease, rhythm disturbances) are appropriate.

Physical Examination

Emboli usually lodge at bifurcations of arteries, and therefore the most common sites are the superficial femoral artery–deep femoral artery junction, the aorta at the origin of the iliac arteries, and the popliteal artery above the trifurcation of medium arteries to the calf. Distal to the embolus the extremity is cold, pale, and pulseless, and the veins are collapsed. The muscles may be tender. These manifestations are usually sharply demarcated at some distance distal to the embolus (e.g., the lower third of the thigh in femoral artery embolus).

Small atheromatous emboli produce a typical clinical picture. One or more digits may be cyanotic (blue toe syndrome), petechiae or ecchymoses may be apparent on the distal limb and foot, livedo reticularis is often present, and elevated reddened plaques may appear on the skin. The muscles are usually tender and the extremities cool, but pulses are often present and normal. If collateral circulation is inadequate, hemorrhagic blebs and gangrene may form.

In acute thrombosis of an artery, the clues to diagnosis are an absence of pulses in the unaffected extremity, a history of intermittent claudication, and the absence of a source of emboli.

Laboratory Studies and Diagnostic Procedures

The clinical picture of acute embolism or thrombosis is usually typical, and special tests are not needed. Devices that detect extremity pulsations show no pulsations. Ankle systolic pressure measured with a Doppler technique is absent (no arterial sounds detected) or very low. In microemboli a source may not be apparent. Atheromatous blood vessels may need to be sought by arteriography and aneurysms by ultrasound studies. In difficult diagnostic cases skin or muscle biopsy shows cholesterol crystals. In acute thrombosis arteriography shows the diseased blood vessels and the site of thrombosis.

Prognosis

The prognosis for patients with acute arterial embolism depends heavily on their underlying disease and the high incidence of recurrent emboli.[6] The mortality in most series is more than 20% because of these factors. The prognosis for a given limb depends on the vessel size, patient age, and ischemic time before operation. Larger vessel emboli (aortoiliac) require surgery or gangrene ensues. Smaller vessels may be managed with watchful waiting.

Management

A vascular surgeon should be consulted as soon as possible. Anticoagulation with heparin is started to prevent thrombus formation and recurrent embolization. Thrombolytic therapy may be used before anticoagulation and is successful in about one third of patients. The affected extremity is placed in the dependent position and the body and limb kept warm. Heat should not be applied directly to the extremity, since ischemic tissues burn at lower temperatures than normal tissue. Adequate analgesia must be given, since the pain is often intense. If conservative therapy does not improve the color and temperature of the extremity or the pain in 1 to 4 hours, and if the patient is stable, embolectomy is indicated. Following embolectomy, anticoagulation must be reinstituted.

Treatment of an acute occlusion of an artery narrowed by arteriosclerosis can be conservative with bed rest, anticoagulation, and analgesics. If the limb improves, no further therapy is necessary. If rest pain continues, vascular surgery may be necessary. If thrombolytic therapy is used and successfully dissolves the thrombus, the stenosed vessel must be dilated by angioplasty or bypassed to prevent recurrence.

The treatment of atheromatous emboli is often unsatisfactory. Anticoagulation with heparin or administration of antiplatelet agents has been advocated. Warfarin is usually avoided, since it has been implicated as a cause of the emboli.

ERYTHROMELALGIA

Patients with erythromelalgia complain of burning pain associated with a bright red color of the feet and, less commonly, the hands on exposure to warmth, on dependency of the limb, or during exercise.[10] It may occur idiopathically or be associated with hypertension, thrombocythemia, lupus erythematosus, or myeloproliferative diseases. There is no age or sex predilection. There is evidently a hypersensitivity of the skin to heat, but when a high platelet count is present, prostaglandins or thromboxane may be involved because aspirin relieves the pain. The attacks of burning pain may be mild to disabling, and often occur in bed at night. During an attack the affected areas are warm, red, very sensitive, and may sweat profusely. Arterial pulses are normal. Cyanosis and necrosis of the toes can occur in thrombocythemia. Attacks can be produced by exposure of the limb to 32° to 36° C water, dependency of the limb, or venous engorgement. Peripheral neuropathies should be ruled out; the dependent rubor of obstructive arterial disease is associated with a cold, pulseless foot. Attacks may be relieved by elevating the extremity and cooling. Treatment is generally unsatisfactory, requiring large doses of sedatives.

RAYNAUD'S PHENOMENON

Epidemiology and Etiology

Raynaud's phenomenon includes episodic, ischemic attacks of the digits induced by cold or emotional stimuli.[3] If no underlying cause can be found, the phenomenon is considered primary Raynaud's phenomenon. The primary syndrome occurs more frequently in females and is much more common than the secondary causes of the phenomenon. It may be present in as many as 16% of young women in cool climates. The onset of attacks is usually between puberty and 40 years of age. Raynaud's phenomenon may be secondary to a number of underlying causes, most of which involve ischemia or trauma to the digital tissue or its nerve or vascular supply (Box 70-2).

Pathophysiology

Evidence points to a local fault in the digital vessels, causing them to be abnormally reactive to cold; this local problem can be aggravated by a normal amount of reflex sympathetic nerve activity. The initial pallor of the attacks is due to digital artery vasoconstriction; this may be followed by cyanosis due to slow blood flow. When the vessels reopen, a reactive hyperemia occurs, imparting a bright red color to the digits. During the first phase numbness is usual; the patient often describes the part as dead. Pain is more common in the reactive hyperemic stage.

History

In Raynaud's phenomenon the patient may have only sharply demarcated blanching or cyanosis, or all three color changes, during attacks (Fig. 70-1). At first only one or two fingers may be affected, but later all fingers of both hands are involved. Episodes may last minutes to hours; they may terminate spontaneously or by warming the digits. The fingers are affected alone in the majority of cases, the fingers and toes next in frequency, and only the toes in few patients.

Box 70-2. Common Secondary Causes of Raynaud's Phenomenon

- Connective tissue diseases
  - Scleroderma
  - Lupus erythematosus
- Traumatic vasospastic disease
  - Chain saw workers
  - Pneumatic hammer workers
- Hammer hand syndrome
- Drugs
  - β-Receptor blockers
  - Ergot preparations
- Neurogenic causes
  - Thoracic outlet syndrome
  - Carpal tunnel syndrome
- Obstructive arterial disease

Physical Examination

Between attacks the digits appear normal in the primary form. Arterial pulses are normal. Trophic changes appear in progressive cases with the development of sclerodactyly. This is characterized by thin, tapering, contracted fingers with smooth, tight skin. Recurrent painful digital infections, blisters, and small areas of gangrene may occur. In patients showing these trophic changes, scleroderma may be present, although positive tests or other symptoms or signs may not appear until many years later. Patients with obstructive arterial diseases have an absence of pulses in the afflicted extremity. The attacks in patients with other secondary causes have no distinguishing features.

Laboratory Studies and Diagnostic Procedures

Important laboratory tests include the white blood cell count, hemoglobin, erythrocyte sedimentation rate, protein electrophoresis, urinalysis, complement levels, and tests for antinuclear antibodies and rheumatoid factor. In some cases cold agglutinins and cryoproteins are sought. The capillaries of the fingernail fold can be examined under a microscope. In scleroderma, mixed connective tissue disease, and dermatomyositis there are enlarged, deformed capillary loops surrounded by avascular areas, and hemorrhages may be present. The capillaries are normal in the primary syndrome.

Differential Diagnosis

Raynaud's phenomenon is often diagnosed from the history of well-demarcated color changes of the digits on exposure to cold, since attacks are difficult to induce in the physician's office. The diagnosis of primary Raynaud's phenomenon depends on exclusion of all secondary causes. A careful history and physical examination eliminates the drug- or work-related cases and elicits symptoms and signs of connective tissue diseases or occlusive arterial disease.

Patients who present with an unevenly blue-red discoloration of the digits that can extend to the wrists and ankles have acrocyanosis.[7] The etiology is unknown but is probably

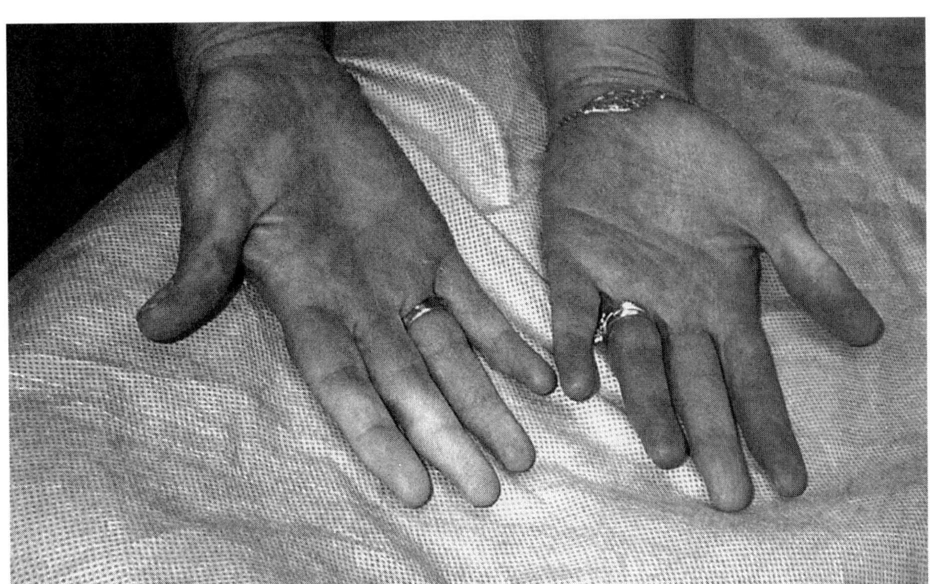

Fig. 70-1. Well-demarcated pallor of the fingers occurring during episodes of cold exposure in a young woman with Raynaud's phenomenon.

a vasospastic disturbance of the cutaneous arterioles due to cold hypersensitivity. Acrocyanosis has no special age or sex incidence; it may be associated with various endocrine diseases. The blue discoloration appears in cool environments; the hands usually sweat profusely and are persistently cool. The hands and/or feet are symmetrically involved. The digits may swell and mild hypesthesia may be present, but trophic changes do not occur. Acrocyanosis can be distinguished from Raynaud's phenomenon by the persistent nature of the discoloration in the former entity.

Prognosis

In primary Raynaud's phenomenon about one sixth of the patients improve or even recover, about one third progress, and the rest remain stable. The progressive form with sclerodactyly, recurring infection, or local gangrene can become a disabling, painful disease, but distal digital loss occurs in fewer than 1%. The prognosis for secondary Raynaud's phenomenon depends on the underlying cause.

Management

In most patients with primary Raynaud's phenomenon reassurance that the prognosis is benign and an explanation of the attacks is the only treatment necessary. The body and extremities must be kept warm to prevent reflex sympathetic vasoconstriction. Loose-fitting warm clothing should be worn. Tobacco smoking is discouraged because it causes cutaneous vasoconstriction, which aggravates the underlying disease. If these measures fail to allow the patient to engage in usual activities, drug therapy may be tried; it is palliative in approximately two thirds of patients. Nifedipine, a calcium channel blocker, decreases the frequency, severity, and duration of vasospastic attacks and is the most effective treatment. However, some patients cannot tolerate the side effects of headache, anxiety, nausea, edema, and reflex tachycardia. The extended action tablets (30 to 90 mg) given once daily have fewer side effects. Prazosin, an α-receptor blocker, 3 to 6 mg daily, may also be tried; side effects include dizziness, headaches, drowsiness, palpitations, and nausea. Although lumbar sympathectomy has successfully alleviated Raynaud's phenomenon involving the feet, cervicodorsal sympathectomy for the finger symptoms is not recommended. Symptoms usually return within 6 to 24 months after upper extremity sympathectomy.

LIVEDO RETICULARIS

In livedo reticularis the patient presents with a painless, reddish blue mottling of the skin of the extremities (reticular pattern, fishnet) or rarely on the trunk of the body on exposure to cold environments or during emotional upsets.[3] In the idiopathic type, there are no other physical findings or diagnostic tests. The blanched areas of skin are believed secondary to vasospasm of the perpendicular arterioles that perforate the skin from the subcutaneous tissue. The bluish periphery around the blanched area is caused by deoxygenated blood in the surrounding horizontally arranged venous plexuses. Besides the idiopathic type, livedo reticularis may accompany other vasospastic diseases or be a clue to systemic disease (Box 70-3). In the idiopathic type no treatment except reassurance is necessary. Rare patients develop cutaneous ulcerations in the winter, or even the summer. These patients actually have an underlying vasculitis for which no treatment has proved satisfactory.

Box 70-3. Secondary Causes of Livedo Reticularis

- Raynaud's phenomenon
- Acrocyanosis
- Obstructive arterial disease
- Connective tissue disease
- Hypertension
- Amantadine
- Hyperviscosity states
- Endocrine disorders
- Infections
- Neurogenic diseases
- Atheromatous embolism
- Sneddon's syndrome

POSTPHLEBITIC SYNDROME AND VARICOSE VEINS

Epidemiology and Etiology

The postphlebitic syndrome is a chronically swollen limb often with stasis dermatitis, subcutaneous tissue induration, and ulcerations.[1] It can appear soon after phlebitis or 10 to 20 years later and is due to incompetent superficial or deep veins.

Varicose veins are distended, tortuous veins with incompetent valves that may appear following phlebitis or pregnancy or with no apparent instigating cause.[7]

Pathophysiology

High venous pressure in the limb due to incompetent venous valves leads to capillary leakage of fluid and red blood cells. The tissue reacts to the hemoglobin from red blood cells with inflammation and fibrosis. A brown pigmentation occurs from the inflammatory reaction and deposition of hemoglobin. Ulceration is probably the result of stasis of blood with ensuing hypoxia of the tissue.

Varicosities are due to incompetent venous valves as a result of high venous pressure distending and stretching the veins or to destruction of the valves from thrombophlebitis. For the pathophysiology of ulcers see Chapter 93.

History

Patients with the postphlebitic syndrome have a chronically swollen extremity. Often medical care is not sought until very advanced disease with ulcers is present because of the absence of pain. Aching pain in the leg may occur after long periods of standing.

Most patients with varicose veins have no symptoms, whereas others complain of fatigue or aching in the lower part of the leg or swelling at the end of the day.

Physical Examination

In the postphlebitic syndrome varicose veins are usually present. The edema is pitting but later may become indurated. An itchy, inflamed, scaly rash above or below the medial malleolus is followed by brown pigmentation of the area and finally ulceration.

Varicose veins can be seen as dilated, tortuous, sacculated superficial veins.

Table 70-2. Differential Diagnosis of the Swollen Limb

	Pain	Inflammatory signs	Varicose veins	Noninvasive venous studies	Clues to diagnosis
Thrombophlebitis	+	+	±	+	Acute onset of swelling
Lymphedema	Usually absent	0	0	Negative	Gradual onset of swelling
Postphlebitic syndrome	+	±	+	Negative	Stasis pigmentation, subcutaneous tissue induration
Ruptured popliteal synovial membrane	+	+	0	Negative	Fluid in the knee joint, history of arthritis
Ruptured calf muscle	+	+	0	Negative	Ecchymoses around ankle, tender knot in muscle, sudden onset during exercise—may feel a pop
Myositis ossificans	+	+	0	Negative	Indurated area in thigh with localized swelling; positive bone scan

Laboratory Studies and Diagnostic Procedures

The clinical picture of the postphlebitic syndrome almost always is diagnostic. When the diagnosis is in doubt, a venogram shows the involved leg to contain an excessive number of veins often with valve destruction and a feathery appearance of the lining of some veins indicating previous phlebitis.

The incompetent valves of varicose veins can be demonstrated by applying a tourniquet on an elevated extremity so that the superficial veins are empty. The patient then stands; release of the tourniquet allows the vein distally to enlarge quickly if incompetent valves are present. If two tourniquets are applied, filling of the saphenous vein between the tourniquets delineates incompetent communicating (perforating) veins.

Differential Diagnosis (Table 70-2)

The postphlebitic syndrome should not be confused with lymphedema. Patients with lymphedema do not usually have varicose veins, stasis pigmentation, or ulcers. Venograms or lymphangiograms are rarely necessary in the differential diagnosis.

Management

Postphlebitic syndrome is difficult to treat and requires patient compliance. Heavy-gauge elastic support (30 mm Hg or greater) must be worn when the patient is ambulatory. Patients must usually sleep with the foot of the bed elevated above heart level to keep edema to a minimum. In elderly patients, especially with arthritis, some arrangement must be made to help them put on the stockings.

Uncomplicated varicose veins respond well to heavy-gauge elastic stockings. This prevents symptoms, edema, and further enlargement of the veins. Panty girdles or garters are never worn. Ligation and stripping of veins have decreased in popularity, since the veins may be needed in the future for arterial bypass.

LYMPHEDEMA

Epidemiology and Etiology

Lymphedema is a chronically swollen, painless limb[9] (see Box 70-4).

Box 70-4. Types of Lymphedema

- Primary lymphedema
  - Congenital (<2 yrs old)
  - Praecox (2-35 yrs)
  - Tarda (>35 yrs)
- Secondary lymphedema
  - Lymph node dissection
  - Neoplasms
  - Radiation
  - Lymphangitis/cellulitis
  - Filariasis

Pathophysiology

The chronic swelling of the limb is due to aplasia, hypoplasia, or varicosities of the lymphatic vessels that drain the tissue fluid. Subcutaneous fibrosis of the edematous tissue gradually occurs.

History

The swelling in lymphedema is usually gradual in onset and asymptomatic. Some patients do complain of a heaviness and pain. Patients should be questioned about a family history of leg swelling, episodes of cellulitis, radiation therapy, surgery, and travel to areas where filariasis is common. Recurrent lymphangitis can lead to lymphedema, and extremities inflicted with lymphedema are very susceptible to recurrent episodes of cellulitis.

Physical Examination

Lymphedema first involves the distal extremity or the entire limb and is soft, pitting, and reversible. Later the edema becomes indurated and nonpitting, the skin thickens and resists wrinkling, and hair follicles become prominent dimples. The skin finally becomes coarse, thick, folded, and hard; the extremely disfigured extremities have been aptly termed *elephantiasis*. The lower extremities are involved most often, and approximately 50% of patients have bilateral swelling. Secondary lymphedema usually involves only one extremity.

Laboratory Studies and Diagnostic Procedures

Lymphoscintigraphy may confirm the diagnosis but is usually not necessary.

Differential Diagnosis

Painless, chronic swelling of an extremity without varicosities, stasis dermatitis, and collateral veins are diagnostic of lymphedema. In lipodystrophy the subcutaneous tissue of the legs feels nodular; lymphoscintigraphy is necessary to demonstrate the normal lymphatics displaced by lipomatous masses.

Management

With lymphedema it is important to attempt to keep the involved extremities as free from edema as possible to prevent subcutaneous fibrosis and skin thickening as well as recurrent episodes of lymphangitis. Heavy surgical elastic support garments (30 to 50 mm Hg) covering the entire involved area with graded pressure from distal to proximal extremity must be worn whenever ambulatory. The patient should sleep with the involved extremity above heart level. In late, disfiguring cases surgical removal of the subcutaneous tissue has been performed, but it is itself a very disfiguring operation.

LYMPHANGITIS

Epidemiology and Etiology

In most cases of infection of the lymphatic vessels the agent is the hemolytic streptococcus or the coagulase-positive staphylococcus. Although a portal of entry for the bacteria is not always apparent, fungal infections of the toes are commonly present.

Pathophysiology

The bacterial infection spreads along lymphatics with an inflammatory response often spreading to surrounding tissues (cellulitis).

History

Patients often show systemic symptoms of infection: fever, shaking, chills, headache, general malaise, nausea, and vomiting.

Physical Examination

Red streaks appear, following the pathways of lymphatic vessels, and proximal lymph nodes are often enlarged and tender. The limb may be swollen, and there may be diffuse redness, increased temperature, and tenderness indicative of cellulitis.

Laboratory Studies and Diagnostic Procedures

The clinical picture is usually typical. Leukocytosis with a left shift in polymorphonuclear cells may be present. Culture of any open lesion may yield the inciting organism.

Management

Broad-spectrum antibiotics are administered in high doses intravenously until culture reports are obtained. Debridement or drainage of any focus of origin is also very important. Bed rest and extremity elevation may hasten healing by decreasing edema. In recurrent cases, especially with underlying lymphedema, a prophylactic antibiotic, usually penicillin, is administered on a long-term basis.

REFERENCES

1. Browse NL, Burnand KG, Lea Thomas M: *Diseases of the veins: pathology, diagnosis, and treatment,* London, 1988, Arnold.
2. Coffman JD: Intermittent claudication. In Tooke JE, Lowe GD, editors: *A textbook of vascular medicine,* London, 1996, Arnold, p 207.
3. Coffman JD: *Raynaud's phenomenon,* New York, 1989, Oxford University.
4. Cutler DA, Runge MS: 86 years of Buerger's disease: what have we learned? *Am J Med Sci* 309:74, 1995.

4a. Dawson DL, Cutler BS, Meissner MH, et al: Cilostazol has beneficial effects in the treatment of intermittent claudication, *Circulation* 98:678, 1998.

5. Dormandy JA, Loh A: Critical limb ischemia. In Tooke JE, Lowe GD, editors: *A textbook of vascular medicine,* London, 1996, Arnold, p 221.
6. Freund U, Romanoff H, Floman Y: Mortality rate following lower limb arterial embolectomy: causative factors, *Surgery* 77:201, 1975.
7. Goldman MP, Weiss RA, Bergman JJ: Diagnosis and treatment of varicose veins: a review, *J Am Acad Dermat* 31:393, 1994.
8. Hood SC, Moher D, Barber GG: Management of intermittent claudication with pentoxifylline: meta-analysis of randomized controlled trials, *Can Med Assoc J* 155:1053, 1996.
9. Kinmonth JB: *The lymphatics: diseases, lymphography, and surgery,* Baltimore, 1972, Williams & Wilkins.
10. Kurzrock R, Cohen PR: Erythromelalgia: review of clinical characteristics and pathophysiology, *Am J Med* 91:416, 1991.
11. Tunis SR, Bass EB, Steinberg EP: The use of angioplasty, bypass surgery, and amputation in the management of peripheral vascular disease, *N Engl J Med* 325:556, 1991.

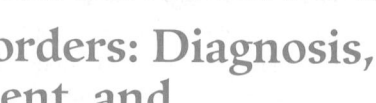

Lipid Disorders: Diagnosis, Management, and Controversy

David A. Halle
Joseph Loscalzo

Coronary heart disease (CHD) is the leading cause of death in the United States, with a prevalence that is equally distributed between men and women. Cholesterol is a well-known major modifiable risk factor for CHD, and several large prospective studies have convincingly demonstrated that lowering cholesterol improves CHD risk. This finding has broad-ranging implications for public health, as well as for the individual patient, that both society and the primary care physician need to address. Since there is not universal agreement among lipid experts, the primary care physician must make judicious decisions about whom to treat, with what therapies, and how to monitor the response to therapy. To understand the general principles of evaluation and management of lipid disorders, it is first necessary to review basic lipid metabolism.

LIPID METABOLISM

There are three major forms of lipid found in mammals: phospholipids, triglycerides, and cholesterol. Each has its own unique structure and purpose, with the liver playing a central role in the synthesis and metabolism of all classes.

Phospholipids

Phospholipids are synthesized in all cells, but most are produced in the liver and, to a lesser extent, the intestinal mucosa. These amphipathic molecules not only play vital roles in cellular membrane structure and in myelination of nerve fibers, but are also important in solubilizing more hydrophobic lipids, such as cholesterol and cholesteryl ester.

Triglycerides

Triglycerides are essentially the storage form of free fatty acids utilized as an energy source. They are retained primarily in the liver and in adipose tissue, where they are stored until needed and then released through the activity of lipases. Triglycerides consist of three fatty acid molecules esterified to one molecule of glycerol. Fatty acids differ in chain length and the number of double bonds between carbon atoms. The more double bonds there are, the more *unsaturated* the fat.

Hydrogenation is the process used in the food industry to convert the double bonds into single bonds with the addition of hydrogen atoms to the carbon atoms. This chemical process leads to *saturation* of fatty acids, and tends to solidify the fat at room temperature. The process of hydrogenation can also change the isomer configuration around a double bond from a *cis* to a *trans* configuration. The consumption of trans-unsaturated fatty acids, when compared to cis-unsaturated fatty acids, has been associated with a more atherogenic profile and increased CHD.[68]

Dietary triglycerides contain saturated, monounsaturated, and polyunsaturated fatty acids. Saturated fatty acids have the greatest impact on elevating low-density lipoprotein (LDL) cholesterol.[38] They are also the predominant fatty acid consumed in the American diet (15% of total calories) and are derived from meat products, dairy products (including eggs), and vegetable oils (Box 71-1).

Monounsaturated fatty acids are derived from vegetable and animal fats, and have a modest LDL cholesterol-lowering effect. Oleic acid is a monounsaturated fatty acid and a main component of olive oil. The low prevalence of CHD in Mediterranean populations, who consume large amounts of olive oil, has prompted its recommendation as a dietary replacement for saturated fatty acid.[91]

Polyunsaturated fatty acids (PUFAs) are the only essential fatty acids of the three groups because they are not synthesized by mammals de novo and need to be obtained from plants and cold-water fish. They are required for various metabolic activities, including the synthesis of arachidonic acid and prostaglandins. There are two principal groups of polyunsaturated fatty acids: the omega-6 fatty acids, and the omega-3 fatty acids.

Linoleic acid, the major omega-6 fatty acid, was considered to be the preferential fatty acid for replacement of saturated fatty acid consumption. However, this is now questioned because the long-term safety of a diet high in linoleic acid is not known. In contrast, the safety of oleic acid, a staple in the Mediterranean diet for a considerable amount of time, is not questioned. The consumption of linoleic acid should not exceed 7% of total calories. Omega-3 fatty acids, which are present in high concentrations in fish, can improve the lipid profile and inhibit platelet aggregation, which may reduce the risk of intravascular thrombosis. In one study, the consumption of omega-3 fatty acids decreased triglycerides by 30% compared with fasting levels in patients without CHD.[53] The benefits of lowering CHD risk are theoretic and have not been proven in large clinical trials.

Box 71-1. Sources of Dietary Fatty Acids

Cholesterol

Egg yolks
Organ meats: liver, sweetbreads, brain
Animal meats: beef, pork, lamb
Butter

Saturated Fatty Acids

Animal fat: beef, pork
Whole dairy products: milk, cream, ice cream, cheese
Palm oil
Coconut oil

Polyunsaturated Fatty Acids

Safflower oil
Sunflower oil
Soybean oil
Corn oil

Monounsaturated Fatty Acids

Olive oil
Canola oil

Cholesterol

Cholesterol is a critical lipid component of all cell membranes. In addition, it is a metabolic precursor for steroid hormones (adrenocortical hormones, estrogens, progesterone, and testosterone), and is used in the synthesis of cholic acid in bile. Cholesterol is obtained through dietary sources (exogenous pathway) or synthesized de novo (endogenous pathway). The exogenous pathway involves the absorption of dietary cholesterol through the gastrointestinal tract (250 to 500 mg per day). Endogenous synthesis, however, is the main source of cholesterol (600 to 1000 mg per day). Synthesis of cholesterol begins with the conversion of acetate into 3-hydroxy-3-methylglutaryl coenzyme A (HMG CoA), which is then converted to mevalonic acid by HMG CoA reductase. This is the rate-limiting step in the overall synthesis of cholesterol, and inhibition of this enzyme decreases cholesterol synthesis.

LIPID TRANSPORT

All lipids are transported in the circulation within large particles that also include a number of types of apoproteins. Together, these molecular assemblies form what are known as lipoproteins. Lipoproteins provide a means to solubilize their relatively hydrophobic components and, through specific apoproteins, engage in unique metabolic reactions. Clinically important lipoproteins are classified into six main categories: chylomicron, very low-density lipoprotein (VLDL), chylomicron remnant, intermediate-density lipoprotein (IDL), LDL,

Table 71-1. Lipoprotein Classes and Composition

Lipoprotein	Density (water = 1.000)	Composition (weight %)			Major apoprotein
		Cholesterol	Triglycerides	Protein	
Chylomicron	0.940	5	85-90	1-2	B-48, E, C-II
VLDL	0.940-1.006	20	60-70	5-10	B-100, E, C-II
Chylomicron remnant	1.006-1.019	30	30	15-20	B-48, E
VLDL remnant (IDL)	1.006-1.019	30	30	15-20	B-100, E
LDL	1.019-1.063	50-60	4-8	20	B-100
HDL	1.063-1.210	15-20	2-7	45-55	A-I, A-II

From Frishman WH, et al: Lipids and lipoproteins: atherosclerotic risk and management. In Frishman WH, editor: *Medical management of lipid disorders,* Mount Kisco, NY, 1992, Futura.

and high-density lipoprotein (HDL) (Table 71-1). They are named based on their relative protein content and its effect on particle density, with the least dense and most lipid-rich being chylomicrons and the most dense and least lipid-rich being HDL. Each lipoprotein has its own unique route of synthesis and functions.

Chylomicrons

On entering the gastrointestinal tract, phospholipids, triglycerides, and cholesterol are transported across the intestinal mucosa and assembled into chylomicrons (Fig. 71-1). Chylomicrons are triglyceride-rich particles that are absorbed in the intestinal lacteals where they enter the lymphatic system and, eventually, the bloodstream. Once in circulating blood, chylomicrons enter capillary beds in adipose tissue and liver where endothelial *lipoprotein lipase* acts to hydrolyze a majority of the triglycerides. Depending on the tissue, triglycerides may be stored for energy in adipocytes, undergo lipolysis so that free fatty acids can be used for immediate fuel in muscle, or undergo oxidation in the liver. The modified particle that remains, the so-called chylomicron remnant, is then removed from the circulation by the liver.

Very Low-density Lipoprotein

Lipids taken up as chylomicron remnants are reassembled with apoproteins synthesized by the liver and released in the form of VLDL. VLDL is also reasonably triglyceride-rich and is metabolized by capillary endothelial lipoprotein lipase to release free fatty acids for utilization or storage. The remaining VLDL remnants, which include small VLDL, β-VLDL, and IDL, are then either taken up by the liver or further metabolized to LDL.

Low-density Lipoprotein

LDL is the main cholesterol-containing lipoprotein and is the primary source of cholesterol delivery to peripheral tissues. LDL contains unique apoproteins (specifically apoproteins B and E) for which peripheral cells have specific receptors. The classic LDL receptor is responsible for the uptake of LDL by all nucleated cells. Approximately 75% of LDL receptors are found in the liver, and the expression of this receptor is feedback-regulated: increasing LDL concentration is associated with a reduction in LDL receptor density. A rising intracellular concentration of LDL also leads to negative feedback inhibition of HMG CoA reductase activity, thereby decreasing endogenous cholesterol production.

There are several consequences of increased LDL in the vasculature. First, when intravascular LDL increases, there is increased LDL entry into the intima of the artery wall. Second, LDL may be oxidized by smooth muscle cells and endothelial cells. Third, monocytes enter the vessel wall where they accumulate and take up the oxidized LDL via a unique class of unregulated receptors, the scavenger receptor class. This process leads to the formation of the lipid-laden macrophage or foam cell. Fourth, the lipid-laden macrophages accumulate to form the first visible sign of atherosclerosis—the fatty streak.

High-density Lipoprotein

HDL is the *reverse transport lipoprotein* and is responsible for taking cholesterol from the periphery back to the liver, where it may be used in the production of cholic acid and excreted in the form of bile salts. Increases in HDL are associated with a decreased risk of coronary heart disease.[10]

FACTORS INFLUENCING LIPID METABOLISM

Environmental

Dietary habits have some influence on serum cholesterol concentrations. A common misconception among patients, however, is that limiting dietary cholesterol intake will have a significant effect on lowering serum cholesterol levels. Reducing dietary cholesterol intake from standard Western dietary levels (approximately 300 mg daily) by as much as one third has only a modest effect, at best, on serum cholesterol concentrations. Exchanging polyunsaturated fats for saturated fats, in contrast, can have a marked effect on serum cholesterol levels. The Hegsted equation illustrates the relationship among the dietary consumption of cholesterol, saturated fats, and polyunsaturated fats on total serum cholesterol:

$$\text{Change in total serum cholesterol} = 2.10\,(\Delta S) - 1.16\,(\Delta P) + 0.0670\,(\Delta C)$$ [38]

ΔS and ΔP are the changes in the dietary content of saturated and polyunsaturated fatty acids in mg/dl, respectively. ΔC is the change in dietary cholesterol consumption expressed in mg/1000 kcal. As can be ascertained from this equation, a diet high in saturated fat contributes more of an effect than dietary cholesterol on the total serum cholesterol levels. This more profound effect of saturated fat has been attributed to its ability to alter (reduce) LDL receptor activity, thereby leading

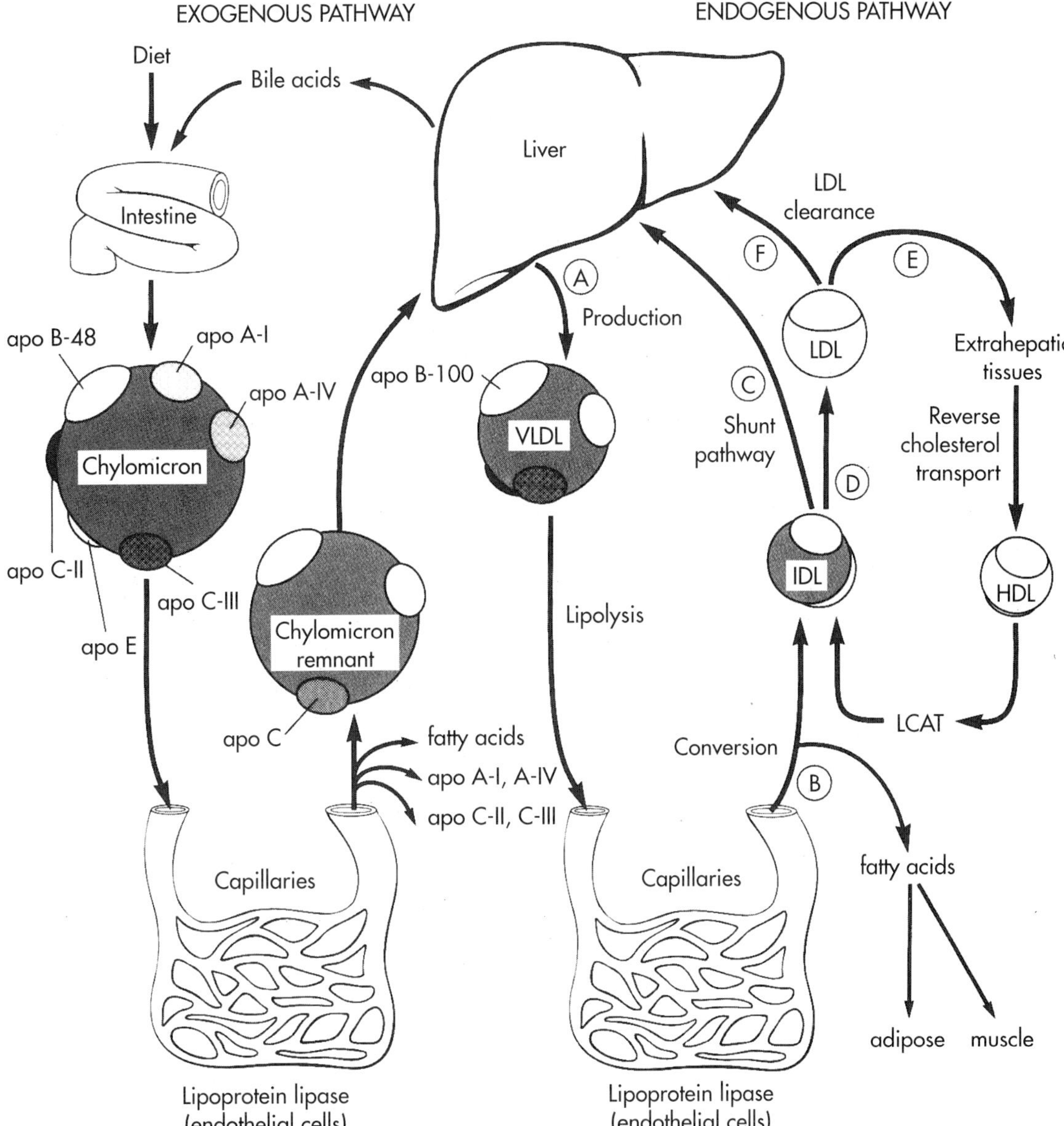

Fig. 71-1. Pathways of lipid metabolism. The exogenous pathway *(left)* describes the absorption of metabolism of fats ingested from dietary sources. Absorbed fats form chylomicrons, which move from lymph into the bloodstream where insulin activates lipoprotein lipase to release fatty acids for use by muscle or fat. The endogenous pathway *(right)* depicts formation of lipoproteins within the liver followed by metabolism in other parts of the body and return to the liver. After hepatic synthesis of VLDL with apo C, E, and B-100, lipoprotein lipase is stimulated in the same fashion as the exogenous pathway. The remnant IDL is either taken up by the liver through apo E receptors or further metabolized to LDL. LDL circulates through the periphery and is taken up at the liver by the LDL receptor. Although there is essentially no feedback mechanism within the exogenous pathway, the endogenous pathway can exert feedback inhibition through the receptors on the cell service. In the reverse transport pathway, free cholesterol is taken up by nascent HDL in peripheral tissues and transferred to apo E–containing lipoproteins which can then be taken up by apo I receptors in the liver. Direct hepatic uptake of HDL may also exist. (From Frishman WH, et al: *Medical management of lipid disorders*, Mount Kisco, NY, 1992, Futura.)

to elevated LDL cholesterol. With this knowledge and the fact that saturated fat is quite atherogenic, primary care physicians should counsel patients on modifying their dietary habits accordingly.

Lipid profiles, in general, are also negatively influenced by corticosteroids, anabolic steroids, cimetidine, thiazide diuretics, and β-blockers without intrinsic sympathomimetic activity. The importance of these factors in altering the course of CHD, however, has yet to be definitively proved.

Receptors, Enzymes, and Surface Proteins

Defects of certain receptors, enzymes, and apoproteins can lead to the elevation of lipids and lipoproteins. This more molecular understanding of dyslipidemias has led to a new empirical classification replacing the phenotypic classification of Fredrickson, Levy, and Lees (Types I-V) (Table 71-2).

Familial hypercholesterolemia (Type IIa) is the best studied molecular cause for hyperlipidemia, but it is not that common (minimal heterozygote frequency of 1:500). Many

Table 71-2. Primary Dyslipidemias and Their Treatment

Dyslipidemia	Defect	Lipoprotein	Lipid	Therapy: First-line	Therapy: Second-line	Therapy: Combination
Familial Hypercholesterolemia (IIa)	LDL receptor mutation	↑ LDL	↑ Cholesterol	Statin Bile acid sequestrant Nicotinic acid	Fibrate Probucol	Bile acid sequestrant + statin Bile acid sequestrant + nicotinic acid Bile acid sequestrant + fibrate
Familial Combined Hyperlipidemia (IIb)	↑ apo B-100 levels ↑ VLDL/LDL production ↓ VLDL/LDL clearance ↓ lipoprotein lipase activity	↑ LDL ↑ VLDL	↑ Cholesterol	Fibrate Nicotinic Acid	Statin	Bile acid sequestrant + fibrate Bile acid sequestrant + nicotinic acid Statin + fibrate
Familial Dysbetalipoproteinemia (III)	↓ apo E clearance	↑ VLDL remnants	↑ Cholesterol ↑ Triglyceride	Fibrate Nicotinic Acid	Statin	
Familial Hypertriglyceridemia (IV)	↓ insulin, apo C-II, or lipoprotein lipase activity	↑ VLDL	↑ Triglyceride	Fibrate Nicotinic acid		Fibrate + nicotinic acid
Primary Hyperchylomicronemia (I)	Inherited deficiency lipoprotein lipase	↑ Chylomicron	↑ Triglyceride	None	None	None
Secondary Hyperchylomicronemia (V)	Acquired deficiency lipoprotein lipase	↑ Chylomicron ↑ VLDL	↑ Triglyceride	Fibrate Probucol		Fibrate + nicotinic acid
Hypoalphalipoproteinemia	Primary: ↓ apo A-I, LCAT Secondary: obesity, tobacco, medications	↓ HDL	→↑ Triglyceride	Exercise + estrogen replacement + Rx of ↑ triglycerides (if present)		

Modified from Betteridge DJ: Combination drug therapy for dyslipidemia, *Curr Opin Lipodol* 4:49-55, 1993.

mutations in the LDL receptor gene can lead to this phenotype, but do so through different mechanisms. The basis for the resulting hyper-LDL-emia ranges from reduced affinity of the LDL-receptor for LDL to defective internalization of the LDL ~ LDL-receptor complex. Importantly, the atherogenic risk of hyper-LDL-emia is a consequence of enhanced LDL oxidation and uptake by the scavenger receptor in monocytes and vascular cells in a process that is not feedback inhibited.

Familial combined hyperlipidemia (Type IIb) occurs in approximately 1% of the U.S. population. Several abnormalities caused by genetic or secondary factors have been attributed to this phenotype. Increased accumulation of apo B-100 will increase the levels of apo B–containing lipoproteins (VLDL and LDL). Overproduction of VLDL and LDL, abnormal clearance of these lipoproteins, and decreased lipoprotein lipase activity can also contribute to this disorder.

Familial dysbetalipoproteinemia (Type III) is characterized by accumulation of β-VLDL (remnantlike lipoprotein) in the serum because an abnormal isoform of apo E slows hepatic clearance. The remnants circulate longer, accumulate cholesteryl esters, and are readily taken up by macrophage receptors to promote atherosclerosis. This is a rare disorder that may have important physical signs that suggest the diagnosis. These include yellow discoloration of palmar and digital creases by xanthomatous deposits (palmar xanthomas) and premature atherosclerosis.

A defect in lipoprotein lipase or one of its cofactors (insulin or apo C-II) will lead to hypertriglyceridemia. A defect in this enzyme is responsible for *familial hypertriglyceridemia* (Type IV), which is an autosomal dominant disorder found in 5% of all patients who sustain a myocardial infarction under the age of 60.

Chylomicronemia is diagnosed by the finding of chylomicrons in a fasting serum sample. Chylomicrons are not known to be atherogenic, but elevated levels are often seen in the setting of increased triglycerides, which have been linked to CHD risk (see Controversies and Future Considerations). Elevated triglyceride production has been associated with excessive alcohol consumption and obesity. Impaired activity of lipoprotein lipase can also cause elevated levels of triglycerides. This state can be acquired, as found in the endothelial dysfunction accompanying type II diabetes mellitus. Under these circumstances, *secondary hyperchylomicronemia* (Type V) occurs, which is manifest as greatly elevated serum triglycerides (>1000 mg/dl), and can be accompanied by lipemia retinalis and eruptive xanthomas. An absolute deficiency in lipoprotein lipase can also be inherited as an autosomal recessive trait, and is a cause of *primary hyperchylomicronemia* (Type I).

Low levels of HDL *(hypoalphalipoproteinemia)* can be primary or secondary in origin. Primary hypoalphalipoproteinemia is seen in the setting of normal cholesterol and triglyceride levels, and has been associated with genetic mutations in apoprotein A-I and lecithin:cholesterol acyltransferase (LCAT).[65a] Secondary hypoalphalipoproteinemia usually coexists with elevated triglyceride levels and is associated with obesity, tobacco use, reduced physical activity, and hypertriglyceridemia. HDL levels are also negatively influenced by progestins, corticosteroids, anabolic steroids, cimetidine, thiazide diuretics, and β-blockers without intrinsic sympathomimetic activity.

The mechanisms of HDL metabolism are not fully understood. Thus optimal drug therapy tailored to this condition is lacking. The approach to the patient with low HDL is to modify the risk factors that may be influencing it. Estrogen and exercise will increase HDL modestly. Hypertriglyceridemia is present in up to one half of individuals with low HDL, and therapy targeted at lowering triglycerides will be beneficial in this subset of patients.

Other Disease States

Various disease states are secondarily responsible for altered lipid metabolism, as well, including hypothyroidism, which leads to hypertriglyceridemia and hypercholesterolemia, and diabetes mellitus, which leads to hypertriglyceridemia. Obstructive liver disease causes increased serum cholesterol by blocking cholesterol excretion. The nephrotic syndrome may also increase LDL production by stimulating synthesis of lipoproteins and triglycerides as a partially compensatory mechanism by which to maintain plasma oncotic pressure in the face of hypoalbuminemia.

CHOLESTEROL AND THE RISK OF CHD

The risk of CHD directly correlates with total serum cholesterol concentration. Serum cholesterol levels beginning in the range of 150 to 180 mg/dl in men as young as 20 years old have been associated with a low subsequent CHD risk, but the risk increases in a curvilinear fashion (Fig. 71-2).[55] The steepest part of the curve, where CHD risk is compounded, occurs above total cholesterol levels of 240 mg/dl. In middle age, treatment trials have shown that for every 1% reduction in total cholesterol levels, the risk of CHD is lowered by 2% to 3%.[16] Women have half the risk of developing CHD compared with men at any given cholesterol level.

It is now recognized that the association between CHD risk and increasing total serum cholesterol levels is a direct consequence of the elevated LDL cholesterol component of the total cholesterol pool. HDL cholesterol is an independent risk factor for CHD, but is inversely related to CHD risk. When lipid profiles have been analyzed in men with CHD, 20% of them have a total cholesterol less than 200 mg/dl but

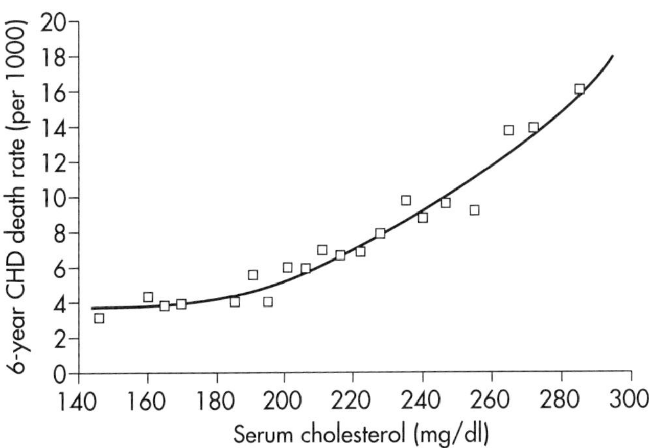

Fig. 71-2. Age-adjusted 6-year coronary heart disease (CHD) death rate (per 1000 men screened for Multiple Risk Factor Intervention Trial) according to serum cholesterol. (From Martin MJ, et al: Serum cholesterol, blood pressure, and mortality: implications from a cohort of 361,662 men, *Lancet* 11:933-936, 1986.)

a low HDL level of less than 35 mg/dl. From these observations, the National Cholesterol Education Program Adult Treatment Panel II (NCEP II) advocates that both total cholesterol and HDL cholesterol should be measured simultaneously for the screening and risk assessment of patients.[31]

Elevated levels of HDL cholesterol appear to offset risk attributed to elevated LDL cholesterol levels disproportionately. The precise mechanism by which HDL offers protection against atherosclerosis is not known. An inverse correlation exists between HDL levels and concentration of apo B–containing lipoproteins. Thus some of the increased risk attributed to low HDL levels may actually be a consequence of elevated levels of other lipoproteins. HDL, by serving as a reverse cholesterol transporter, may slow atherosclerotic progression by removing cholesterol from the arterial wall.[32] HDL may also prevent the oxidation and aggregation of LDL within the arterial wall.

Framingham Study data initially revealed the reduction in CHD risk attributed to HDL.[10] Individuals with high total cholesterol concentrations in association with HDL cholesterol levels greater than or equal to 60 mg/dl have no increased risk for CHD, a lipid profile common in postmenopausal women on estrogen therapy. Accordingly, the NCEP II supports subtracting one CHD risk factor when an individual's HDL cholesterol is greater than or equal to 60 mg/dl.

The accuracy of measuring serum cholesterol can be quite variable, with reported coefficients of variation as great as 14%. Levels depend on patient stress, collection technique, and variability in laboratory assay methods, among other factors. Cognizant of this variation, the Centers for Disease Control and Prevention has established a national standardization program to minimize variations both within and between laboratories, and many hospital laboratories participate in this program. Of the three lipids commonly measured, total cholesterol varies less than HDL cholesterol and triglycerides. When more precision is required, the average of two or more different measurements should be used.

THE EFFICACY OF PRIMARY PREVENTION

The importance of screening for dyslipidemias is supported by overwhelming evidence that cholesterol lowering in patients with high cholesterol reduces the risk of CHD and, in patients with documented CHD, improves morbidity and mortality. The benefit of identifying and treating patients for primary prevention of CHD stems from four large prospective trials, each using different agents: the World Health Organization Cooperative Trial (1978) with clofibrate, the Lipid Research Clinics Coronary Primary Prevention Trial (1984) with cholestyramine, the Helsinki Heart Study (1987) with gemfibrozil, and the West of Scotland Coronary Prevention Study (1995) with pravastatin.[23,67,76,85] These trials were similar in design, with the enrollment of middle-aged men who had elevated cholesterol levels (means ranging from 246 to 289 mg/dl) and no CHD. The incidence of cardiac events was reduced by 19% to 34% over a 5- to 7-year period. The West of Scotland Coronary Prevention Study was the only trial of the four to show a reduction in all-cause mortality (22%).

AFCAPS/TexCAPS (1998) is a more recent primary prevention study conducted on 6605 men and women with average total cholesterol levels (mean 228 mg/dl) and low HDL cholesterol (mean 40 mg/dl for women and 36 mg/dl for men).[19] Lovastatin of 20 or 40 mg daily was compared with placebo. After a mean follow-up of 5 years, cardiovascular events were significantly reduced (37%) in the lovastatin group. With the results of these latter two trials, lipid experts have attributed these benefits to the statin (HMG CoA inhibitor) class of lipid-lowering agents as a whole. They are more effective in lowering LDL cholesterol and their side effect profile makes them more tolerable for patients than the agents used in the earlier primary prevention trials.

THE EFFICACY OF SECONDARY PREVENTION

Improving dyslipidemia in patients with documented CHD also confers a marked benefit in preventing recurrent events (secondary prevention). One of the more notable trials to show the significant benefits for secondary prevention was the Scandinavian Simvastatin Survival Study (1994).[60] This prospective trial showed a decrease in cardiac mortality of 42% and in all-cause mortality of 30% over 5.4 years in 4444 patients with preexisting CHD. Importantly, patients treated with cholesterol-lowering therapy for secondary prevention derived much greater benefit than those treated for primary prevention after adjusting for the cholesterol level. This observation suggests that future approaches to identifying those individuals without clinical CHD and with hypercholesterolemia at greatest risk for a CHD event will be important for optimizing therapy among this broad population of individuals. A more recent notion is that the percent reduction of LDL may be more important than the absolute change in LDL concentration.[87]

The question of how much benefit, if any, accrues to CHD patients with average cholesterol levels was elucidated by the Cholesterol and Recurrent Events (CARE) trial (1996).[70] This trial enrolled over 4000 post–myocardial infarction patients with mean total serum cholesterol of 209 mg/dl and LDL cholesterol of 139 mg/dl, then subjected them to treatment with 40 mg of pravastatin daily or placebo. Five-year follow-up results showed a 24% reduction in coronary events, including death from CHD. A reduction was also noted in the need for percutaneous transluminal coronary angioplasty (PTCA) of 23% and coronary artery bypass graft (CABG) of 26%. Subgroup analysis showed that the magnitude of the benefit was proportional to the pretreatment LDL cholesterol level. Coronary events were reduced by 35% in patients who had pretreatment LDL cholesterol levels of 150 to 174 mg/dl, but patients with a pretreatment LDL cholesterol level of <125 mg/dl had no statistically significant reduction in cardiac events.

The AVERT trial (1999) compared the role of lipid-lowering drug therapy with PTCA in secondary prevention.[62a] Some 341 patients with stable CAD, LDL ≥115 mg/dl, and triglycerides ≤ 500 mg/dl were randomized to either aggressive lowering of LDL with atorvastatin (80 mg/d) or PTCA and usual care, which could include lipid-lowering therapy. High-risk patients were excluded if they had left main CAD, three-vessel CAD, ejection fraction < 40%, or recent MI or angina. Main outcome measures were ischemic events (including nonfatal MI, cardiac death, PTCA, CABG, or worsening angina requiring hospitalization), which were measured with intention-to-treat analysis at

18 months. The atorvastatin group had a reduced but not statistically significant rate of ischemic events (13.4% vs. 20.1%). This trial reassures that lipid-lowering therapy is safe and as good as PTCA for patients with stable CAD.

THE ROLE OF DIETARY INTERVENTION

The findings of the Oslo Study Group (1981) established the foundation for recommending dietary intervention and smoking cessation to improve lipid profiles.[40] This prospective, multifactorial intervention trial was conducted among middle-aged men who had very high cholesterol levels (320 mg/dl), had high saturated fat consumption (mean 44% of daily caloric intake), and smoked. Dietary advice with cessation of smoking lowered total cholesterol by 13% and reduced the incidence of CHD by 47%. Generalization of the impact of these two findings is limited by the extreme cholesterol and fat intake of the enrolled subjects prior to the intervention. Other similarly designed trials have only been able to show a reduction in total cholesterol of 0% to 5% in patients with low total cholesterol levels and without CHD, and were unable to demonstrate statistically significant effects on CHD incidence.

The impact of dietary fish consumption was examined in a cohort of 1822 men from the Chicago Western Electric Study.[17] The participants were 40 to 55 years old without known CHD; they were stratified into four groups based on fish consumption and followed prospectively for 30 years. Dietary consumption of fish (grams per day) was obtained from questionnaires at the onset of the study. Analysis of the data adjusted for demographics and other dietary factors revealed a significant inverse association between fish consumption and 30-year risk of death from all cardiovascular causes, especially non–sudden fatal myocardial infarction. The greatest protective effect was found in the participants who consumed 35 grams or more of fish per day. More recent evidence from the Physicians Health Study showed that men who ate fish (including shellfish) at least once a week had a 52% reduction of sudden cardiac death compared with those who consumed fish less than once per month.[1] In contrast, these data did not find an inverse association between fish consumption and the rate of myocardial infarction. The protective mechanism of fish consumption is not yet known, but may be related to the effects of omega-3 fatty acids on cardiomyocyte membrane stabilization (see Nutritional Supplements).

AGE GROUPS TO SCREEN

The strongest evidence for screening asymptomatic patients was shown for men between the ages of 35 to 65 years. The age at which to screen women is controversial because of the lack of trial data in which adequate numbers were enrolled. The onset of clinically apparent CHD is dependent on multiple factors, but the beneficial effects of estrogen delay the incidence in women by a decade, and the risk increases progressively after menopause. Most authorities agree that an effective screening program for asymptomatic women should begin at 45 years of age or later. However, the NCEP II expert panel holds a minority view and advocates screening all adults (men and women) 20 years of age or older (Box 71-2).[9,25,26,31,90]

Total cholesterol levels increase with age, most likely due to the proportional increase in the body mass index, and then plateau about age 65. Screening is less effective in patients after this age, especially if they have had a desirable lipid profile in their middle-aged years. Advocates of screening after this age point to the documented epidemiologic evidence that the risk of developing CHD is problematic until the age of 75. Most agree that elderly patients up to the age of 75 who have documented CHD will likely benefit from screening.

The appropriate interval for periodic screening has not been clearly defined. Five years is the standard presently proposed by the NCEP II for patients with desirable lipid profiles. Shorter intervals, in theory, would be more effective in perimenopausal women and in individuals with recent weight gain.

Box 71-2. Cholesterol Screening Criteria

National Cholesterol Education Program[31]

- Adults ≥20 yrs of age should have total and HDL cholesterol determined every 5 years
- Follow-up depends on risk factors and total and HDL cholesterol levels

U.S. Preventive Services Task Force[90]

- Screen men ages 35-65 years and women ages 45-65 years for total cholesterol every 5 years
- Follow-up depends on results

Canadian Task Force on the Periodic Health Examination

- Insufficient evidence to support routine screening; endorses case findings in men ages 30-59 years

American College of Physicians (ACP)[26]

- Appropriate but not mandatory in men ages 35-65 years and women ages 45-65 years
- Not recommended in younger individuals unless they have multiple cardiac risk factors or suspected familial lipoprotein disorders
- Insufficient evidence to recommend for or against screening asymptomatic individuals between 65-75 years, but recommend against screening after age 75

HDL, High-density lipoprotein.

SCREENING FOR DYSLIPIDEMIA

A HDL cholesterol of less than 35 mg/dl is classified as a major risk factor and a level of 60 mg/dl or greater is considered a negative risk factor by the NCEP II. Screening for dyslipidemia by measuring total and HDL cholesterol compared with total cholesterol alone has not been proven to have additional benefit in the general population.[9,26,90] However, it is helpful in identifying patients who will have the highest risk of developing CHD, especially when used to screen patients with other nonlipid risk factors for CHD.[31] At present, total serum cholesterol and HDL cholesterol levels are recommended by the NCEP II for screening selected patients for primary prevention.

The higher the ratio of total-to-HDL cholesterol, the higher the risk of CHD.[10] A ratio of five or greater is associated with increased CHD risk among men and women.

Nonfasting samples are acceptable because recent consumption of a high-fat meal will have minimal effects on these two levels, unless the individual has high triglyceride levels.

PRINCIPLES OF MANAGEMENT

The combined CHD risk of a patient should be used as the guide to therapy. In primary prevention, this assessment takes into account LDL cholesterol level, a low or high HDL cholesterol level, age, cigarette smoking, diabetes mellitus, family history of CHD, and hypertension (Box 71-3).[31] Those at higher risk of CHD should receive more aggressive intervention. Patients should be categorized into one of three groups according to risk: (1) highest risk—those with prior CHD or atherosclerotic disease, including peripheral arterial disease or symptomatic carotid disease; (2) high risk—those without CHD but multiple CHD risk factors; or (3) low risk—those with few CHD risk factors, especially men younger than 35 and premenopausal women.

The cornerstones of therapy for the patient with dyslipidemia include dietary counseling to reduce saturated and total fat consumption, weight loss, and drug therapy (if necessary). The possibility of adverse effects, as well as cost, warrants caution regarding the use of drug therapy in primary prevention for patients not at high risk. Cholesterol lowering through diet and physical activity is safer and should be the mainstay of therapy for primary prevention in most individuals.

Clinical trials have shown the strong benefit of lowering LDL cholesterol, but the evidence for raising HDL levels has only recently become elucidated. The VA-HIT study (1999) randomized 2531 men who were younger than 74 years old and had known CAD, low HDL levels (≤40 mg/dl), and moderate LDL (≤140 mg/dl) and triglyceride (≤300 mg/dl) levels.[67a] They were allocated to gemfibrozil (1200 mg/d) or placebo. The main outcome measures of nonfatal MI and death from CAD were significantly lower in the gemfibrozil-treated group (17.3% vs. 21.7%) over the median follow-up of 5.1 years. The evidence for using gemfibrozil over statins in men with CAD and low HDL levels has strengthened. However, the treatment of women with low HDL levels is likely to be similar, but has yet to be reported in a large clinical trial. Additionally low HDL levels should be treated with increased physical activity, smoking cessation, and weight loss. If a patient has concomitant high LDL and low HDL cholesterol levels, a drug that counteracts both should be prescribed.

Box 71-3. Risk Factors for Coronary Heart Disease (CHD)

Positive (↑ Risk)

- Elevated LDL cholesterol
- Age: men ≥45 years; women ≥55 years or premature menopause without estrogen replacement therapy
- Family history of premature CHD (definite MI or sudden death before age 55 in father or first-degree male relative or sudden death before age 65 in mother or first-degree female relative)
- Cigarette smoking
- Hypertension (≥140/90 mm Hg) or use of antihypertensive medications
- Diabetes mellitus
- HDL cholesterol ≤35 mg/dl

Negative (↓ Risk)

- High HDL cholesterol (≥60 mg/dl)

Modified from Grundy SM, et al: Summary of second report of the NCEP expert panel on detection, evaluation, and treatment of high blood cholesterol in adults, *JAMA* 269:3015-3023, 1993.
HDL, High-density lipoprotein; *LDL*, low-density lipoprotein; *MI*, myocardial infarction.

Table 71-3. National Cholesterol Education Program Categories for Cholesterol Levels

Lipid	Risk category (values in mg/dl)		
	Desirable	Borderline high	High
Total cholesterol	<200	200-239	≥240
HDL cholesterol	>60	—	<35
LDL cholesterol	<130	130-159	≥160
Triglycerides*	<200	200-400	400-1000 high >1000 very high

From Grundy SM, et al: Summary of the second report of the NCEP expert panel on detection, evaluation, and treatment of high blood cholesterol in adults, *JAMA* 269:3015-3023, 1993.
CHD, Coronary heart disease; *HDL*, high-density lipoprotein; *LDL*, low-density lipoprotein.
*Triglycerides in borderline high and very high categories may increase CHD risk. Levels greater than 1000 mg/dl are associated with increased risk of pancreatitis.

Primary Prevention

In patients without CHD, the first step is to measure the serum total and HDL cholesterol levels (Table 71-3).[31] Total cholesterol levels equal to or greater than 240 mg/dl are classified as *high blood cholesterol* and are the concentrations above which the risk for CHD is highest. A *borderline high blood cholesterol* concentration is a total cholesterol level between 200 and 239 mg/dl. Twenty percent and 31% of the U.S. adult population have levels within the high blood cholesterol and borderline high cholesterol categories, respectively.[75] A *desirable blood cholesterol* concentration is defined as a total cholesterol level below 200 mg/dl.

The second step, if required, is to perform a fasting lipoprotein analysis on all patients with a total cholesterol of 240 mg/dl or greater, or with a HDL cholesterol level lower than 35 mg/dl (Fig. 71-3). A lipoprotein profile includes measuring total cholesterol, HDL cholesterol, and triglycerides. The Friedewald formula is then used to calculate the LDL cholesterol:

$$\text{LDL cholesterol} = \text{total cholesterol} - \text{HDL cholesterol} + 0.16\ (\text{triglycerides})$$

This formula is valid for estimating LDL cholesterol if the triglyceride level is less than 400 mg/dl and if the individual does not have familial dysbetalipoproteinemia.

Further stratification is then based on LDL cholesterol levels. Three categories are used: *high LDL cholesterol* (levels equal to or greater than 160 mg/dl), *borderline-high*

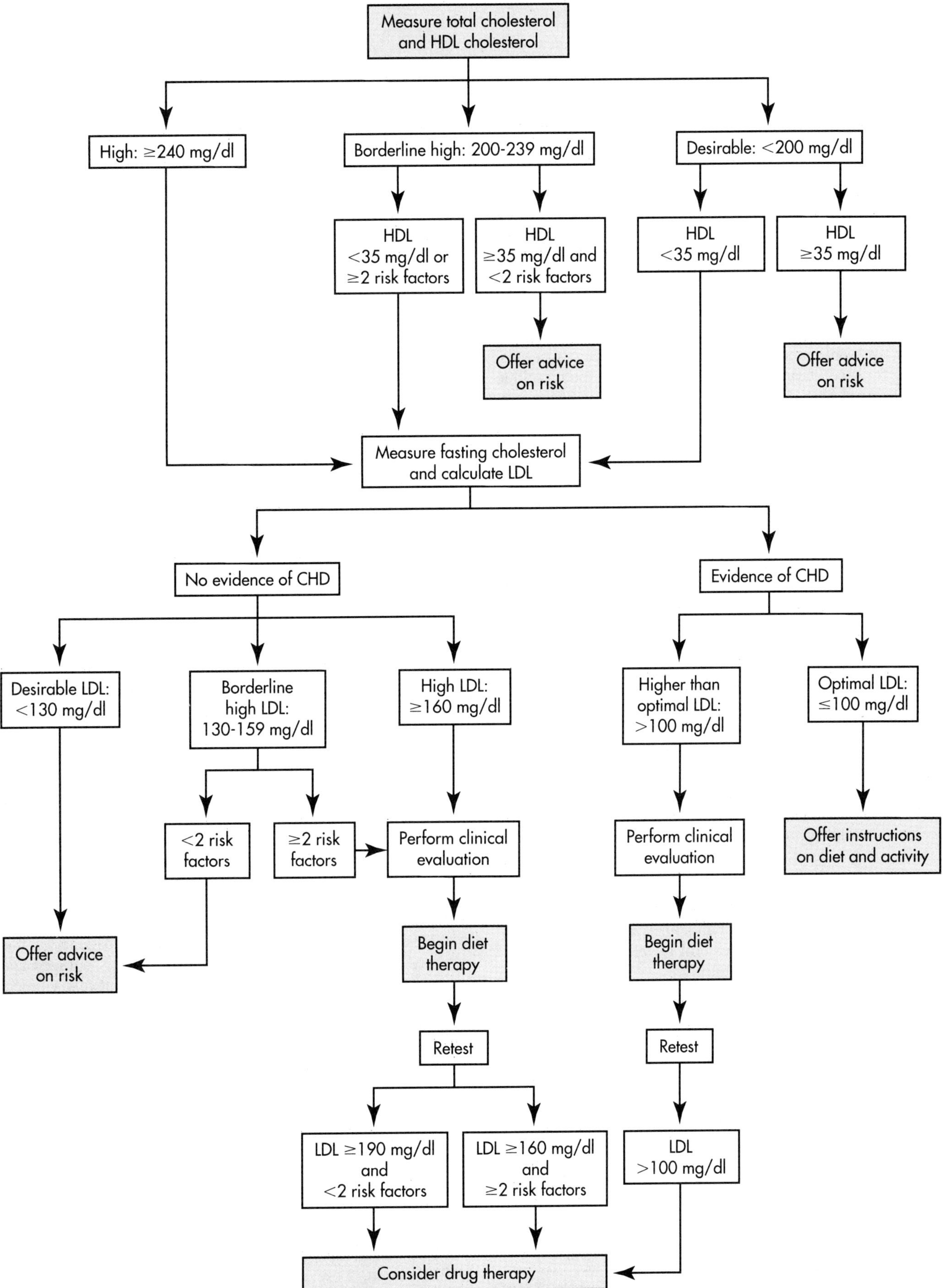

Fig. 71-3. Recommended advice and treatment for U.S. adults by cholesterol level. Shaded areas are the National Cholesterol Education Program's alternative recommendations for advice and treatment intensity. *CHD,* Coronary heart disease; *HDL,* high-density lipoprotein; *LDL,* low-density lipoprotein. (Redrawn from Grundy SM, et al: Summary of the second report of the NCEP expert panel on detection, evaluation, and treatment of high blood cholesterol in adults, *JAMA* 269:3015-3023, 1993.)

LDL cholesterol (levels 130 to 159 mg/dl), and *desirable LDL cholesterol* (levels below 130 mg/dl).

If a patient has a desirable LDL cholesterol, the physician should educate the patient on the on the use of a low-saturated-fat diet, physical activity, and risk factor reduction. The patient should have a repeat total cholesterol and HDL cholesterol measured at 5 years. If the patient has a borderline-high LDL cholesterol with one or no risk factors, the same advice should be given but the patient should be reevaluated in 1 year.

If a patient has a borderline-high cholesterol level with two or more risk factors or a high-risk LDL cholesterol level, a careful clinical evaluation should then be performed. The aim of the clinical evaluation is to identify any secondary causes of hyperlipidemia by reviewing pertinent family history, present medications, and concomitant diseases. Testing for secondary causes, when indicated, should include thyroid-stimulating hormone (TSH) for hypothyroidism, serum glucose for uncontrolled diabetes mellitus, urinalysis and creatinine for nephrotic syndrome, and hepatic enzymes for liver disease. Active cholesterol lowering with dietary intervention should be instituted in all these patients. In addition, if a patient has a high-risk LDL cholesterol with two or more risk factors or an absolute LDL cholesterol greater than or equal to 190 mg/dl regardless of the presence or absence of risk factors, drug therapy should be instituted. The cholesterol levels at which dietary or drug therapy should be instituted are shown in Table 71-4.

Secondary Prevention

Secondary prevention begins with the fasting lipid analysis to determine the LDL cholesterol.[31] The guidelines in these patients are much more stringent, and optimal LDL cholesterol levels are considered less than or equal to 100 mg/dl. Intervention for patients with LDL cholesterol levels above this value should begin with dietary modification. If the LDL cholesterol is greater than or equal to 130 mg/dl, drug therapy should not be delayed. With careful management, it is possible to achieve these goals within 3 to 6 months.

Table 71-4. Treatment Guidelines Based on LDL Cholesterol Level and Risk Factor Status

Status	Initiation level (mg/dl)	Goal level (mg/dl)
No CHD and <2 risk factors		
Diet	≥160	<160
Drugs	≥190	<160
No CHD and ≥2 risk factors		
Diet	≥130	<130
Drugs	≥160	<130
CHD		
Diet	>100	≤100
Drugs	≥130	≤100

Modified from Grundy SM, et al: Summary of the second report of the NCEP expert panel on detection, evaluation, and treatment of high blood cholesterol in adults, *JAMA* 269:3015-3023, 1993.

CHD, Coronary heart disease; *LDL*, low-density lipoprotein.

DIETARY THERAPY AND PHYSICAL ACTIVITY

The principal goal of dietary therapy is to lower an elevated serum cholesterol. The NCEP II expert panel has advocated dietary therapy that involves a two-step American Heart Association approach. The Step I diet consists of a daily cholesterol intake of less than 300 mg, as well as saturated and total fat consumption not to exceed 10% and 30% of total calories, respectively (Fig. 71-4). The Step II diet should be recommended to all patients with established CHD or patients who have not been able to achieve the targeted cholesterol level on a Step I diet. The goal of the Step II diet is to maintain saturated fat and cholesterol intake at a minimum by limiting daily intake of cholesterol to less than 200 mg and saturated fat to less than 7% of total calories.

A registered dietitian can be useful in helping patients with the difficult task of reducing their saturated fat and cholesterol intake, especially with the Step II diet. For the patient on the Step I diet, serum cholesterol levels should be monitored at 4 to 6 weeks and at 3 months following initiation of these changes. If the patient has achieved the targeted LDL cholesterol level, he or she can then be monitored with a total cholesterol measurement on a quarterly basis for the first year and biannually thereafter. At all visits, the primary care physician should reemphasize the adherence to diet and physical activity.

If the patient has not achieved the targeted cholesterol level on a Step I diet, the Step II diet should be prescribed. Total cholesterol levels should again be assessed at 4 to 6 weeks and at 3 months after instituting dietary therapy. If goals are achieved, monitoring as outlined above can begin. Otherwise drug therapy should be prescribed in addition to the Step II diet.

Aerobic exercise lowers total and LDL cholesterol and triglycerides, as well as increases HDL cholesterol. Exercise is also beneficial in decreasing a patient's weight toward ideal body weight. Weight reduction has been found to have benefits independent of exercise in improving dyslipidemia.

DRUG THERAPY

It is important to point out that even under the best of circumstances, rigorous nonpharmacologic therapy rarely yields more than a 10% to 15% reduction in total or LDL cholesterol. Physicians should apprise their patients of this likely outcome so that they do not become discouraged and choose to ignore the need to lower cholesterol levels. Clinical judgment is needed when patients have not met their target LDL cholesterol level by diet and physical activity, but do not meet the criteria for drug therapy. Patients with a low absolute risk of developing CHD but an abnormal cholesterol profile should be considered for delaying drug therapy. To illustrate this point, consider a 35-year-old premenopausal woman with a total cholesterol above 240 mg/dl, a LDL cholesterol greater than 160 mg/dl, and no family history of early CHD. Her CHD risk is higher than another 35-year-old woman with a normal cholesterol profile, but her *absolute risk* is still very small since she is unlikely to develop CHD for several decades. Nonpharmacologic interventions, including smoking cessation, diet, and physical activity, should be stressed to this patient. Low doses of bile acid sequestrants can be considered as an adjunctive therapy.

The major classes of drugs that reduce LDL cholesterol are HMG CoA reductase inhibitors, bile acid sequestrants, and nicotinic acid. Other classes of agents that have less of an effect on LDL cholesterol are fibric acid derivatives, probucol, and estrogen replacement therapy (Table 71-5). These will be discussed in turn.

HMG CoA Reductase Inhibitors (Statins)

As noted previously, large clinical trials have shown that lovastatin, pravastatin, and simvastatin reduce coronary events.[19,60,70,76] Other trials have shown modest regression of coronary lesions with lovastatin, fluvastatin, pravastatin, and simvastatin.[5,39,62,69] Lesion regression is likely less important than plaque stabilization. Recent data support this mechanism as a means to explain the reduction in acute clinical CHD events associated with the use of these drugs. These benefits are considered a class effect and are believed to carry over to the other statins.

As a group, the statins lower total cholesterol, LDL cholesterol, VLDL cholesterol, and triglycerides. They may also mildly increase HDL cholesterol. The efficiency of lowering LDL cholesterol, cost, and hepatic CYP3A4(P450)

Table 71-5. Lipid-modifying Drugs

Drug class	Initial dosage	Maximum dosage	Monthly cost* ($) (AWP)	Effect on lipoproteins: LDL	HDL	VLDL	Side effects
HMG CoA reductase inhibitors				↓↓↓↓	↑	↓	Elevated liver function tests Gastrointestinal symptoms Myalgia/myositis
Atorvastatin	10 mg qd	80 mg qd	56.36-209.88				
Cerivastatin	0.3 mg qd	0.3 mg qd	39.68				
Fluvastatin	20 mg qd	40 mg bid	37.70-75.27				
Lovastatin	20 mg qd	80 mg qd (40 mg bid)	69.85-251.48				
Pravastatin	20 mg qd	40 mg qd	64.95-106.77				
Simvastatin	10 mg qd	40 mg qd	59.13-196.39				
Bile acid sequestrants				↓↓↓↓	↑	→↓	Drug interactions Gastrointestinal symptoms Decreased absorption of vitamins A, D, E, and K
Cholestyramine	4 gm qd-bid	24 gm in divided doses	25.48-183.12				
Colestipol (granules & tablets)	5 gm qd	30 gm in divided doses	29.72-329.10				
Niacin	50-100 mg bid-tid	3 gm in divided doses	1.69-50.71	↓↓↓	↑↑↑↑	↓↓↓↓	Flushing/pruritus/rash Gastrointestinal symptoms Gout exacerbation Worsening of glycemic control Elevated liver function tests
Fibric acid derivatives				↓	↑↑	↓↓↓	Pruritus/rash Gastrointestinal symptoms Myositis Cholelithiasis
Gemfibrozil	600 mg bid	600 mg bid	10.80-81.75				
Fenofibrate (micronized)	67 mg qd	201 mg qd	20.62-61.88				

Modified from *Med Lett Drugs Ther* 40:117-122, 1998; and Betteridge DJ: Combination drug therapy for dyslipidemia, *Curr Opin Lipodol* 4:49-55, 1993.
AWP, Average wholesale price.
*Range provided is for minimum and maximum dosages.

Nutrient	Recommended intake: Step I diet	Step II diet
Total fat	← <30% of total calories →	
Saturated fat	8%-10% of total calories	<7% of total calories
Polyunsaturated fat	← Up to 10% of total calories →	
Monounsaturated fat	← Up to 15% of total calories →	
Cholesterol	<300 mg/d	<200 mg/d
Carbohydrates	← 50%-60% of total calories →	
Protein	← 10%-20% of total calories →	
Calories	← To achieve and maintain desired weight →	

Fig. 71-4. Comparison of the Step I and Step II diets for lowering serum cholesterol. (Modified from Grundy SM, et al: Summary of the second report of the NCEP expert panel on detection, evaluation, and treatment of high blood cholesterol in adults, *JAMA* 269:3015-3023, 1993.)

metabolism appear to be the basis for differences among the statins. Maximum daily doses of cerivastatin (0.3 mg), lovastatin (80 mg), pravastatin (40 mg), and simvastatin (40 mg) reduce LDL cholesterol by 30% to 40% when compared with the 25% reduction by fluvastatin (40 mg). Atorvastatin at maximum dosage (80 mg) has been reported to reduce LDL cholesterol by as much as 50% to 60%.[12]

The initial dose should be low and titrated every 4 to 6 weeks until the desired target LDL cholesterol is achieved. Typical dosing is once daily, and these agents are most efficacious when taken with the evening meal to reduce nocturnal hepatic synthesis of cholesterol.

The most common side effects include rash, headache, gastrointestinal distress, and myalgias. Patients with concomitant renal or hepatic dysfunction, hypothyroidism, advancing age, and bacteremia appear to have an increased risk of myalgias and myositis. If severe enough, myositis can lead to rhabdomyolysis, myoglobinemia, and acute renal failure. Myositis associated with an increase in serum creatine phosphokinase levels up to 10 times normal is reversible after discontinuation of the drug. Increases in hepatic transaminases may occur in 1% to 2% of patients taking higher doses of statins. Some lipid experts recommend obtaining hepatic transaminase measurements at 6-week intervals until a stable dose of the statin has been achieved. Thereafter, testing is recommended at 6-month intervals. A rare lupus-like syndrome and peripheral neuropathy have been reported with statin use.

Because statins are one of the newer classes of lipid-lowering drugs, their long-term sequelae are not known. At present, there are little data to suspect any long-term adverse outcomes. Despite higher cost, statins have proven effectiveness and good patient acceptability, making them the first choice for most patients with hypercholesterolemia.

Bile Acid Sequestrants

The bile acid sequestrants, cholestyramine and colestipol, bind bile acids and prevent their absorption in the ileum. The bile acids, including cholic and chenodeoxycholic acid, are derivatives of cholesterol. The depletion of the bile acid pool results in feedback to the hepatocytes to increase expression of LDL cholesterol receptors to enhance hepatic uptake of LDL. The net effect of bile acid sequestrants is to lower LDL cholesterol by increasing its catabolism.

Cholestyramine and colestipol lower LDL cholesterol by 15% to 30%, increase HDL cholesterol by 3% to 8%, but increase triglycerides by 10% to 50%. The effective dose is 2 to 6 packets or scoops per day (8 to 24 grams daily). Both drugs have nonlinear dose-response curves so that maximal doses of these agents have little additional benefit, but side effects increase proportionally. The main side effects are largely limited to gastrointestinal distress, including heartburn, bloating, constipation, and exacerbation of preexisting hemorrhoids or anal fissures. Adding fiber to the diet will improve constipation, and letting the resin stand in liquid before consumption will alleviate heartburn. Treatment should begin with two to four scoops per day as an initial dose, and the drug should be taken with meals to reduce side effects. Patients should be advised to take these resins separately from any other oral medications because they may bind to the resin and not be absorbed. The most important of these are digoxin, thyroxine, thiazide diuretics, β-blockers, and warfarin. A period of 1 hour before or 4 hours after taking oral medications should be allowed before a resin is consumed.

Because of their rather benign side effect profile, bile acid sequestrants are considered by the NCEP II expert panel to be a good choice for young patients who will be taking cholesterol-lowering therapy for decades. Similar recommendations apply to women of childbearing age.

Niacin

Nicotinic acid or niacin is a member of the B complex family of vitamins, but at higher doses also lowers cholesterol and is therefore classified as a drug. It is, however, available over-the-counter because the Food and Drug Administration (FDA) classifies it as a vitamin. Niacin lowers total and LDL cholesterol by 10% to 25% and triglycerides by 20% to 50%, and increases HDL cholesterol by 15% to 30%. Niacin is considered a very effective treatment for low HDL cholesterol and for the treatment of small, dense LDL (see Controversies and Future Considerations). The exact mechanism of action is not known, but it is thought to decrease the production of VLDL and LDL. The mechanism by which niacin increases HDL cholesterol is also not known.

Initiation of niacin therapy should begin with low doses of 50 to 100 mg BID to TID with meals. Niacin is available in regular-release and time-release capsules. The newer time-release agents have promoted increased patient acceptability. The dose is then increased over a period of 6 to 8 weeks to 1500 mg daily, and should be adjusted depending on the initial response of the cholesterol level. The usual effective dose is 1500 to 3000 mg daily in three divided doses.

The major side effect is flushing, and this unpleasant reaction often hampers patient compliance. Administration of 325 mg of aspirin 30 minutes before the administration of niacin and the avoidance of hot liquids and alcohol minimize or prevent most flushing episodes. Physiologic tolerance to this side effect eventually develops. Only after patients have developed tolerance at a specific dose should niacin therapy be increased.

Other side effects include pruritus, which may be ameliorated with antihistamines; rash; body odor; gastrointestinal distress; and exacerbations of gout. If the patient has concomitant diabetes mellitus, the physician should be aware of the possibility of worsening glycemic control. There is also dose-dependent hepatotoxicity, especially with the time-release capsules, termed *niacin hepatitis*.

Some key features of this uncommon disorder include a history of malaise, hepatomegaly, and elevated transaminases. Fortunately, the hepatitis begins to reverse within days of decreasing or stopping the drug, and this observation has led some lipid experts to recommend not exceeding 2000 mg daily.

Fibric Acid Derivatives

Fibric acid derivatives decrease hepatic VLDL synthesis and increase the effectiveness of VLDL and triglyceride removal from the circulation. Owing to the lower concentrations of circulating VLDL, there is less cholesterol to be transferred from HDL to VLDL. The net effect is that they are the most effective drugs for reducing triglyceride levels, with a subsequent HDL increase of approximately 10%. The effect on LDL cholesterol is variable and dependent on the initial level of triglycerides. In patients with very high triglyceride levels, the lowering of triglycerides may actually increase the LDL cholesterol level.

The fibric acid derivatives provide the most benefit in lowering CHD risk in patients with hypertriglyceridemia (including diabetics), combined hyperlipidemia, and familial dysbetalipoproteinemia. These agents are not effective in patients with isolated hypercholesterolemia.

Clofibrate was the first drug of this class to have been prescribed. A 1992 study that compared clofibrate with placebo found a higher incidence of cancer as well as other gastrointestinal diseases, including cholecystitis and gallstones requiring cholecystectomy, among patients treated with clofibrate.[36] This drug has since fallen out of favor and has been superseded by the use of gemfibrozil and the newest fibric acid derivative available in the United States, micronized fenofibrate.

Gemfibrozil is considered a safe drug on the basis of lengthy experience in the Helsinki Heart Study.[23] The recommended dose is 300 to 600 mg twice daily. Micronized fenofibrate (67 mg) is equivalent to the 100 mg of the nonmicronized form available in Europe and Canada. An equivalent dose of 200 to 400 mg daily is recommended. Micronized fenofibrate appears to be more effective in lowering triglycerides with a more favorable effect on LDL cholesterol levels than gemfibrozil.[22]

The main side effects of the fibrates include abdominal pain, nausea, diarrhea, rash, and pruritus. Transient elevations in hepatic transaminases have been noted. These drugs are conjugated in the liver and excreted in the urine, making them relatively contraindicated in hepatic or renal disease. As with clofibrate, the fibric acid derivatives as a class appear to increase the long-term risk of cholelithiasis.

Probucol

Probucol is a unique agent for the treatment of dyslipidemia whose mechanism of action is not fully understood. Proposed actions include removing LDL from the circulation by increased efficiency of LDL receptor binding and increased non–receptor-mediated catabolism of LDL. Probucol is also a highly effective antioxidant. While it lowers LDL by 10% to 20%, the drug also lowers HDL, leading to a neutral effect on the total-to-HDL cholesterol ratio. The usual dosage is 500 mg twice daily. Side effects are mostly limited to gastrointestinal distress. It is contraindicated in any patient with a prolonged QT interval or a history of ventricular dysrhythmias. Despite being on the market for over 2 decades, its role in lipid management is limited, largely owing to its adverse effects on HDL cholesterol. Its benefits as an antioxidant, however, may prove to modify and expand its use in the future.

Estrogen Replacement Therapy

A major question in the treatment of postmenopausal women with lipid disorders is the efficacy of estrogen replacement therapy, either alone or in combination with other lipid-lowering drugs. Clinical trials of large magnitude have yet to be performed, but a meta-analysis of some observational studies suggests a reduction of approximately 44% in the primary prevention of CHD risk by estrogen replacement therapy.[29] The NCEP II expert panel recommends estrogen replacement to all postmenopausal women with lipid disorders. This recommendation is controversial because there are incomplete data to support this stance.

Framingham Study data suggested a fourfold increase in CHD risk for women who experience menopause before 40 years of age.[49] They also noted that the risk of CHD increases twofold in women who underwent natural menopause in their sixth decade. There is agreement that CHD risk increases with age for both women and men, and that premature ovarian failure is associated with increased risk. The contribution of ovarian failure to CHD risk in women who undergo natural menopause is controversial. Benefit has yet to be proven in this population of women.

Estrogen replacement benefits the lipid profile by decreasing LDL and lipoprotein(a), and increasing HDL. However, triglycerides are also increased. The initial studies of estrogen replacement therapy used this therapy without progestins in women with an intact uterus. Current practice dictates prescribing progestins in women with an intact uterus because it is now known that estrogen therapy used in an unopposed manner increases the risk of endometrial cancer approximately sixfold. There is also an increase in the risk of deep vein thrombosis, pulmonary embolism, and possibly breast cancer with hormone replacement therapy (HRT).

The Postmenopausal Estrogen/Progestin Interventions (PEPI) Trial (1995) examined risk factor changes (HDL cholesterol, systolic blood pressure, serum insulin, and fibrinogen) as a surrogate marker for CHD events.[86] Combined estrogen/progestin therapy had a less desirable effect on HDL cholesterol than estrogen therapy alone. This has led some authorities to believe that combined therapy will not be as effective in lowering CHD risk. Proponents of estrogen replacement estimate that the effect of estrogen on lipids only accounts for about one third of its beneficial effect on CHD risk. Other cardiovascular benefits of estrogen include increased levels of nitric oxide, which allow less spasm of the coronary vasculature; increased insulin sensitivity; and its role as a possible antioxidant.[83]

The Heart and Estrogen/Progestin Replacement Study (HERS) (1998) randomized 2763 postmenopausal women with established CHD to either conjugated equine estrogen (0.625 mg/d) and medroxyprogesterone acetate (2.5 mg/d) or placebo.[42] After a mean follow-up of 4.1 years, the rate of nonfatal myocardial infarction and CHD mortality did not differ between the women who received HRT (12.5%) and those who received placebo (12.7%), despite significant improvements in LDL, HDL, and triglycerides in the HRT-treated group. From these results, some authorities are advocating the use of proven secondary prevention measures of lowering CHD risk (including other lipid-lowering agents) more strongly than HRT therapy.

The role of HRT in primary prevention will hopefully be evaluated by the ongoing Women's Health Initiative clinical trial. This study is attempting to recruit 27,500 women and to randomize them to either combined estrogen/progestin therapy or placebo if they have an intact uterus. If they had a hysterectomy, they will be treated with estrogen alone. The investigators plan to observe the response to treatment over 9 years, with results reported in the year 2005. Hopefully this trial and others to follow will elucidate the effect of progestin in combination with estrogen replacement therapy.

Other Drugs

Raloxifene is a nonsteroidal benzothiopene that inhibits the growth of estrogen receptor–dependent mammary tumors. It is classified as a selective estrogen-receptor modulator that has shown to be efficacious in preventing bone loss, having a less stimulatory effect on the endometrium compared with estrogen, and to lower serum total cholesterol and LDL cholesterol. Raloxifene has also been shown to decrease LDL oxidation, decrease vascular smooth muscle migration, and decrease restenosis in animal models. A recent study of 601 postmenopausal women who were randomized to receive 30, 60, or 150 mg of raloxifene daily or placebo daily were followed for 2 years.[18] Both groups also received 400 to 600 mg elemental calcium daily. In addition to improvements in bone mineral density, raloxifene was shown to have a dose-dependent reduction of serum concentrations of total cholesterol and LDL cholesterol of 9.7% and 14.1% respectively, in the group treated with raloxifene, 150 mg daily. Serum concentrations of HDL and triglycerides were not significantly different from placebo. Smaller studies have shown a trend for raloxifene decreasing lipoprotein(a) and apo B levels. Raloxifene may be found useful in the treatment of certain postmenopausal women with elevated levels of total cholesterol and LDL cholesterol with less risk of estrogen's stimulatory effect on mammary and endometrial tissue. Low HDL levels are, however, best improved with estrogen replacement in conjunction with exercise.

D-thyroxine lowers LDL cholesterol by 10% to 15% by enhancing its clearance from the circulation. This treatment makes the patient mildly hyperthyroid, and has been essentially abandoned because of the cardiac side effects. *Neomycin* decreases intestinal absorption of cholesterol when given in a dosage of 2 grams daily; it can lower LDL by 10% to 15%. Besides altering the native gut flora, neomycin has the potential to cause ototoxicity and renal insufficiency, and has not been approved by the FDA as a lipid-lowering agent. *Olestra* is a nonabsorbable sucrose polyester fat substitute that interferes with the absorption of cholesterol and fat-soluble vitamins by solubilizing cholesterol, making it unavailable for intestinal absorption. It is approved by the FDA for use in foods, but not as a drug.

Stanols and their saturated derivative *sterols* structurally resemble cholesterol except for the addition of a methyl or ethyl group. They are found exclusively in plants and are important for cellular membrane integrity. When dietary intake of plant sterols and stanols is higher than typical daily intake, they compete with cholesterol in the formation of mixed micelles and interfere with cholesterol absorption in the gastrointestinal tract. Evidence for this effect has been shown in several studies over the last 40 years.[11] Sitostanol-ester margarine is a pine tree–extract stanol that is esterified to allow solubilization in a low-saturated-fat vehicle (e.g., margarine). The RAISIO Group (1995) in Finland studied 153 nonobese subjects with mild dyslipidemia (total cholesterol levels greater than 216 mg/dl, triglycerides less than 265 mg/dl).[56] They were randomized to either sitostanol-ester margarine or placebo margarine. After 1 year, the sitostanol-ester group had a significant reduction of total cholesterol (10.2%) and LDL cholesterol (14.1%), and the agent was well tolerated. There was no significant difference in triglyceride or HDL cholesterol levels between the two groups. Sitostanol-ester margarine has recently been approved to be marketed in the United States, but its role has yet to be determined in the treatment of dyslipidemia.

Combination Therapy

The goal of combination therapy is to combine lipid-lowering drugs of different mechanisms of action in order to achieve an additive or synergistic therapeutic effect in patients with dyslipidemia.[48] In patients with severe dyslipidemia, such as familial hypercholesterolemia and familial combined hyperlipidemia, the use of combination therapy may be required to reach target LDL cholesterol levels (see Table 71-2).[4] Combination therapy has also proven useful in patients with less severe forms of dyslipidemia by using low doses of two agents rather than a high dose of a single agent. Not only may there be a potential decrease in clinical toxicity with combination therapy, but there also may be a cost advantage.

The bile acid sequestrants (cholestyramine and colestipol) are the most commonly used agents included in combination therapy. The benefits of these drugs are that they are not absorbed and have less drug interactions than their counterparts. Bile acid sequestrants have been shown to be efficacious in combination with nicotinic acid, the statins, the fibrates, and probucol. However, the most effective regimens have been bile acid sequestrants in combination with nicotinic acid or the statins. Nicotinic acid (4.5 to 5.5 grams/day) when combined with the full dose of a bile acid sequestrant can achieve a 32% to 55% reduction of LDL cholesterol, but it is poorly tolerated because of cutaneous flushing and gastrointestinal side effects. In addition to good tolerability, LDL cholesterol reductions of over 50% are commonly achieved with a bile acid sequestrant in combination with a statin, making them ideal drugs for combination therapy. Bile acid sequestrants should be taken at least 1 hour prior to the administration of a statin because of its ability to bind to a statin and make a statin less available for absorption. The combination of lovastatin, colestipol, and nicotinic acid has been shown in a limited number of studies of patients with severe dyslipidemia to lower LDL cholesterol by 60% to 70%.

Statins in combination with a fibric acid derivative have been reported to increase the risk of myositis more than that of statin therapy alone.[61] These two drugs should, in general, not be prescribed together. However, on occasion their combined use may be necessary for patients who are resistant to other forms of drug therapy.

PATIENT EDUCATION

The importance of the physician's role as patient educator cannot be overemphasized in the management of CHD risk. An interactive environment should be established, with the underlying theme being that the patient is an important participant in maintaining his or her wellness. Expecting patients to be compliant with a prescribed regimen without proper education will result in frustrations for both physician and patient. One study demonstrated that only approximately 50% of patients who were prescribed a lipid-lowering drug were taking it 1 year later.[78] In another study, 20% to 30% of women never filled their prescription for HRT, and only about 40% who did were still compliant with the regimen 1 year later.[66] One of the more commonly cited reasons for noncompliance was that the patients did not understand why they needed to be on the medication.

Compliance may be increased by reviewing the basics of dietary reduction of saturated fat and cholesterol and weight reduction at periodic visits. Since dietary therapy cannot be expected to reduce LDL by more than 10%, it is important to be nonjudgmental if a higher and unrealistic goal was initially established. Asking the patient his or her understanding about prescribed therapy may also curtail noncompliance and increase patient satisfaction.

CONTROVERSIES AND FUTURE CONSIDERATIONS

Hypertriglyceridemia

The role of elevated triglycerides in CHD risk has been more controversial than the association of high LDL cholesterol and low HDL cholesterol. Large studies initially linked elevated triglyceride levels with CHD. Subsequently, when HDL cholesterol levels were measured with triglyceride levels, elevated triglycerides were often found to coexist with low HDL cholesterol levels, and were not initially found to confer an independent CHD risk.[14] This observation led to the early conclusion that hypertriglyceridemia is not an independent risk factor for CHD, and that HDL cholesterol is the principal risk factor determinant. More recently, however, individuals with low HDL cholesterol and elevated triglyceride levels have been found to have a greater CHD risk than individuals with similarly low HDL cholesterol but normal triglyceride levels.[41,82] This type of observation gives some credibility to the independent association of elevated triglyceride levels and CHD risk, but that association appears to be less robust than that for low HDL cholesterol.

Nonpharmacologic therapy (weight reduction, increased physical activity, and alcohol restriction) is recommended for all patients with elevated triglycerides (200 mg/dl or greater).[31] There has yet to be conducted a clinical trial to establish a benefit, if any, of lowering triglyceride levels and improved CHD risk. Until intervention data are available, triglyceride-lowering agents should be reserved for patients with triglyceride levels of 400 mg/dl or greater and other cardiac risk factors.[47]

Small, Dense LDL and the Atherogenic Dyslipidemia Syndrome

LDL can be divided into four subclasses with differing density, size, and atherogenic risk. The largest, most buoyant subclass is LDL-I, followed in decreasing size and buoyancy by LDL-II, LDL-III, and LDL-IV. LDL-I and LDL-II subclasses are seen predominantly in patients with normolipidemic profiles and have been termed *pattern A*. LDL-III and LDL-IV as a group have been termed *pattern B,* also denoted as small, dense LDL particles.

The *atherogenic dyslipidemia syndrome* (ADS) includes the clustering of four different abnormalities: borderline high total cholesterol; high triglycerides; small, dense LDL particles (pattern B); and low levels of HDL cholesterol.[32,33] ADS is a dominant dyslipidemia and has been found in patients with CHD and familial combined hyperlipidemia. The lipid profile of ADS is similar to that of patients with type II diabetes mellitus, and it has been suggested that ADS is a risk factor for the development of type II diabetes mellitus. ADS in combination with type II diabetes mellitus, hypertension, central obesity, and a procoagulant state has been termed *syndrome X* or *the metabolic syndrome*. The morbidity associated with this metabolic derangement of proatherosclerotic risk factors is just beginning to become elucidated.

ADS is associated with at least a threefold increased risk of CHD.[8] The relative contribution of each of the four components to CHD risk is unclear because they usually coexist and separation of their individual risk has been unsuccessful.[32] In addition to what has been already suggested with hypertriglyceridemia, small, dense LDL may also be an independent CHD risk factor.* At present, the estimation of CHD risk is determined from the level of HDL and the ratio of total cholesterol-to-HDL cholesterol. In the future, triglycerides or small, dense LDL may be added to this analysis in order to increase the predictive power of the risk assessment.

Standard screening with total cholesterol and HDL cholesterol is not adequate for the identification of patients with ADS because the resulting "normal" lipid profile will overlook this atherogenic disorder.[32] The present challenge for primary care physicians in diagnosing ADS is to identify those patients at risk for premature CHD, or those with established CHD and seemingly "normal" lipid profiles. Future testing may include routine measurement of the various subclasses of lipoproteins including small, dense LDL. At present, this cannot be recommended until there is standardization of the laboratory measurement of lipoprotein subclasses.

Therapy is based on diet, exercise, and drug treatment. A subgroup of patients from the Helsinki Heart Study with ADS (pattern B), when compared with patients with pattern A, had a significant reduction of CHD events. Gemfibrozil-treated patients with ADS had increased levels of large LDL and decreased levels of small, dense LDL; gemfibrozil had no significant effect on pattern A subjects. The striking feature of this observation is that drug treatment improved the lipid profile of the pattern B patients, an effect that would not have been revealed by routine lipoprotein monitoring. Lipid experts believe there is no one ideal drug with which to treat this disorder; however, since ADS represents a combination of metabolic derangements, some combination of nicotinic acid, statins, and fibric acid derivatives may be effective.[32]

Hyperapobetalipoproteinemia (Hyperapo B)

Apolipoprotein B (apo B) is the component of LDL that serves as the ligand for its receptor. Apo B is also contained within VLDL, IDL, and chylomicrons. There is only one molecule of apo B in each of these lipoprotein particles. Therefore measuring fasting serum apo B should correlate on a 1:1 ratio with the total number of VLDL, LDL, IDL, and chylomicron particles.[65]

An increased apo B level in the absence of hyperlipidemia has been designated *hyperapo B,* which is found in hypertriglyceridemia.[6,77] Persistently elevated triglycerides replace the cholesteryl ester component of VLDL and LDL, while the apo B levels remain the same. When this occurs, the apo B level is a more accurate representation of the total number of VLDL and LDL particles as compared with the cholesterol measurement because the risk of CHD is greater than indicated by the measured cholesterol level.[6,79] Hyperapo B often accompanies ADS, but is not necessarily a component thereof.[32]

---

*References 2, 15, 27, 30, 32, 3345, 89.

Some recommendations for assessing CHD risk include the quantification of apo B in patients who have a family history of premature CHD, and patients with documented CHD who do not require lipid-lowering therapy based on the current NCEP II guidelines. Analysis of some clinical trials has recognized that apo B is a strong predictor of CHD risk, and that reduction of apo B lowers CHD.* Prospective studies are needed to determine if apo B is a better predictor of CHD risk than the current lipid measurements.

Lipoprotein(a)

Lipoprotein(a) or Lp(a), is a unique particle that contains a LDL component and a unique covalently linked protein component, apoprotein(a). Apo(a) is linked by a disulfide bridge to apo B-100 of the LDL component, and its structure is similar to that of plasminogen. The atherogenic potential of Lp(a) has been attributed to its competition with plasminogen for the plasminogen receptor on endothelial cells and for fibrin, thereby reducing fibrinolysis and promoting thrombosis.[57] Lp(a) is considered an independent risk factor for premature CHD, but its importance appears to lessen with advancing age.[51,64] Elevated Lp(a) levels are not always associated with increased CHD risk owing to variability within the apo(a) molecule allowing for some polymorphisms to have increased risk. The precise relationship between apo(a) structure and sequence and CHD risk is the subject of ongoing studies.

Levels of Lp(a) are genetically determined, but external factors may account for up to 10% of the variation in concentration. Renal impairment and nephrotic syndrome are among the best studied nongenetic factors. An inverse correlation exists between Lp(a) and creatinine clearance that may account for the greater prevalence of CHD in this population.[74] Genetic determinants of Lp(a) levels may cluster in certain ethnic groups. African-Americans have higher Lp(a) levels and Asians have lower Lp(a) levels when compared with the general U.S. population; yet, among the African-American population, the risk associated with any given level of Lp(a) is less clear than among Caucasians likely as a consequence of polymorphic differences in apo(a).[34,54,71-73,80]

Despite controversy, screening for Lp(a) has been recommended by some lipid experts to be measured in individuals with a family history of premature CHD, or in individuals with established premature CHD and a low risk factor profile with relatively normal lipid levels.[64] Treatment with niacin or neomycin has been shown to be effective in lowering Lp(a) levels. However, there have been no trials to support the view that lowering Lp(a) levels reduces CHD risk. In the future, Lp(a) may become an integral measurement of CHD risk, but not until we standardize its measurement, better define the isoforms and polymorphisms that confer the greatest risk, and more fully understand its impact on the development of atherosclerosis.[84]

Diabetes Mellitus

CHD is the principal cause of death in patients with diabetes mellitus. Subgroup analyses of secondary prevention trials of statin therapy indicate that lowering LDL levels in patients with diabetes mellitus is beneficial.[60,70] It is not clear if the target of therapy is the same as in the general population. Unanswered questions include whether the LDL goal of less than 100 mg/dl in diabetics with CHD should be further lowered. Also, we do not know how aggressively to treat patients with diabetes mellitus and no known CHD. There have as yet been no large clinical trials to answer these questions. At present, the NCEP II recommends a target LDL of 130 mg/dl for primary prevention, and less than 100 mg/dl for secondary prevention. Triglycerides are also an important risk factor in patients with diabetes, and it has been suggested that a level of less than 200 mg/dl be the goal. However, for those patients with established CHD or vascular disease, a triglyceride level of less than 150 mg/dl should be the goal.[58] Future trials will hopefully define the optimal approach to lipid-lowering therapy in patients with diabetes mellitus.

Cerebrovascular Disease

The role of dyslipidemia in cerebrovascular disease (stroke and transient ischemic attack [TIA]) is not well understood. CHD and stroke share many of the same risk factors including age, sex, blood pressure, preexisting vascular disease, diabetes mellitus, and smoking. A notable difference is dyslipidemia. Large population-based studies prior to the advent of computed tomography grouped cardioembolic, atherothrombotic, and hemorrhagic strokes together, which created conflicting data in the understanding of dyslipidemia and its association with stroke. Another difficulty has been the methodologic flaw in the design of studies, which predominantly looked at CHD as the endpoint. Cerebrovascular events only occurred in a small number of individuals in these studies because their incidence is delayed about 1 decade in respect to CHD.[63] There have been no large trials looking at all forms of cerebrovascular disease as an endpoint; however, secondary analysis of data from the CARE and the 4S trials has found a significant reduction in stroke among patients treated with statins. A systemic review of 16 trials using statin therapy found a 25% reduction in all forms of stroke when total cholesterol and LDL cholesterol were reduced 22% and 30% respectively.[37] In a case-controlled study of 90 patients with atherothrombotic stroke or TIA, subjects were found to have significantly higher levels of total cholesterol, LDL cholesterol, and triglycerides than a matched control group.[35]

These insights suggest that dyslipidemia is associated only with atheroembolic stroke. The attributable risk of dyslipidemia to stroke may be reduced after significant reductions of total cholesterol and LDL cholesterol with prolonged statin therapy. Clinical studies are needed that will improve our understanding of the interaction of dyslipidemia with this heterogeneous disorder.

Alcohol

Studies have shown that alcohol in moderation protects against CHD. A prospective study of 490,000 men and women found that participants who averaged one drink per day had a 21% decrease in all-cause mortality and a 30% to 40% decrease in mortality from CHD.[88] Another study found that men who drink moderate amounts of alcohol (two to six drinks per week) have a 28% reduction in all-cause mortality compared with light drinkers (one or fewer drinks per week).[7] The protective effect of moderate drinking was attributed to a 34% to 53% reduction in CHD mortality. However, when heavy drinkers (two drinks or greater per day) were compared

*References 3, 20, 21, 28, 44, 46, 50.

with the light drinkers, they were found to have a 51% increase in all-cause mortality.

Alcohol consumption is directly proportional to HDL and triglyceride levels. The greatest consumers of alcohol have both the highest levels of HDL and of triglycerides when compared with minimal consumers. However, a U-shaped association between alcohol consumption and CHD risk has been defined. Despite the elevated levels of HDL in the highest consumers of alcohol, the role of hypertriglyceridemia or some other unknown factor may have a greater adverse effect on CHD risk. Alcohol consumption appears to have no effect on LDL levels.

Recent data from the Helsinki Heart Study have shown that the beneficial effect of moderate alcohol consumption may be restricted to tobacco smokers only.[52] Future studies may clarify which subgroups of the population may benefit from moderate alcohol consumption. However, the current recommendation of the American Heart Association limits the health benefit of alcohol to one to two drinks per day.[59]

Nutritional Supplements

Epidemiologic data have suggested that there is a lowered prevalence of CHD in populations with a higher intake of fruits and vegetables. There is also a widespread belief that antioxidant vitamins (vitamins C and E) will reduce the risk of CHD. This premise is based on the belief that since LDL oxidation promotes atherogenesis, impairing oxidation should reduce CHD risk. However, the GISSI-Prevenzione trial (1999) showed vitamin E supplementation to have a neutral effect.[28a] This secondary prevention study randomized 11,324 patients who had suffered a recent myocardial infarction (within 3 months) to either dietary supplementation with omega-3 PUFAs (eicosapentaenoil acid, 850 mg, and decosahexaenoic acid, 1700 mg) or vitamin E (α-tocopherol, 300 mg), singly or in combination. Intention-to-treat analysis at 42 months revealed a significant reduction of nonfatal MI and cardiovascular death, in addition to all-cause death and stroke, in the omega-3 PUFA-treated group. Supplementation with vitamin E alone or in combination showed no effect. The more recent HOPE study (2000) did not find any discernible effect of vitamin E (400 IU/d) on cardiovascular events in subjects with CAD or diabetes mellitus over a duration of 4.5 years.[84a] These large clinical trials add to the strong but limited body of evidence of the beneficial effects of omega-3 PUFAs and the mixed results of vitamin E supplementation.[6a,65b,82a] Folic acid and vitamin B_6 are also thought to be beneficial in decreasing CHD risk by reducing elevated homocysteine levels, another known atherogenic factor. It is not clear whether folic acid and vitamin B_6 supplementation reduces the risk of CHD.[81]

Most of these current beliefs have yet to be proven by large clinical trials. In the future, nutritional prevention may expand to include these factors along with weight loss and reduced intake of saturated fat and cholesterol.

SUMMARY

The prevalence of CHD will continue to increase because more people will be living longer with CHD. A reduction in the prevalence of CHD in this new century will only come from prevention. Screening, diagnosing, and treating patients with abnormal lipid profiles will be major factors in this reduction. Great strides have been made in our understanding of the metabolism and complex interaction of the various lipoproteins and their components. Future research will help to enlighten the roles of apo B; Lp(a); small, dense LDL; triglycerides; and ADS. The effectiveness of lowering LDL beyond 100 mg/dl in certain subgroups of patients with CHD may also be elucidated. The expansion of pharmaceutical armamentarium, including gene therapy, will likely be more effective and possibly permanently cure atherogenic abnormalities. The screening guidelines that have been reviewed in this chapter will continue to evolve, and the challenge to the primary care physician will be to adapt them appropriately and effectively to clinical practice.

EBM EVIDENCE-BASED MEDICINE

Primary sources for this chapter were MEDLINE and the National Cholesterol Educational Program Adult Treatment Panel II (NCEP II) guidelines.[30] Electronic searches dating back to 1978 were conducted in April 2000. They focused on identifying systemic reviews, meta-analyses, and large randomized trials with clinical endpoints.

REFERENCES

1. Albert CD, et al: Fish consumption and risk of sudden cardiac death, *JAMA* 279:23-28, 1998.
2. Austin MA, et al: Low-density lipoprotein subclass patterns and risk of myocardial infarction, *JAMA* 260:1917-1921, 1988.
3. Barbir M, et al: High prevalence of hypertriglyceridaemia and apolipoprotein abnormalities in coronary heart disease, *Br Heart J* 60:397-403, 1988.
4. Betteridge DJ: Combination drug therapy for dyslipidemia, *Curr Opin Lipidol* 4:49-55, 1993.
5. Blankenhorn DH, et al: Coronary angiographic changes with lovastatin therapy: the Monitored Atherosclerosis Regression Study (MARS), *Ann Intern Med* 119:969-976, 1993.
6. Brunzell JD, et al: Apolipoproteins B and A-I and coronary artery disease in humans, *Arteriosclerosis* 4:79-83, 1984.

6a. Burr ML, et al: Effects of changes in fat, fish, and fibre intakes on death and myocardial reinfarction: diet and reinfarction trial (DART), *Lancet* 2:757-761, 1989.

7. Camargo CA, et al: Prospective study of moderate alcohol consumption and mortality in US male physicians, *Arch Intern Med* 156:79-85, 1997.
8. Campos H, et al: Low density lipoprotein particle size and coronary artery disease, *Arterioscler Thromb* 12:187-195, 1992.
9. Canadian Task Force on the Periodic Health Exam: Periodic health examination, 1993 update: 2. lowering the blood total cholesterol level to prevent heart disease, *Can Med Assoc J* 148:521-538, 1993.
10. Castelli WP, et al: Incidence of coronary heart disease and lipoprotein cholesterol levels: the Framingham Study, *JAMA* 256:2835-2838, 1986.
11. Cater NB, Grundy SM: Lowering serum cholesterol with plant sterols and stanols: historical perspectives, *Postgrad Med* Special Report s6, November 1998.
12. Choice of lipid-lowering drugs, *Med Lett Drugs Ther* 40:117-122, 1998.
13. Reference deleted in proofs.
14. Criqui M, et al: Plasma triglyceride level and mortality from coronary heart disease, *N Engl J Med* 328:1220-1225, 1993.
15. Crouse JR, et al: Studies of low density lipoprotein molecular weight in human beings with coronary artery disease, *J Lipid Res* 25:566-574, 1985.
16. Davis C, et al: A single cholesterol measurement underestimates the risk of CHD: an empirical example from the Lipid Research Clinics mortality follow-up study, *JAMA* 264:3044-3046, 1990.
17. Daviglus ML, et al: Fish consumption and the 30-year risk of fatal myocardial infarction, *N Engl J Med* 336:1046-1053, 1997.
18. Delmas PD, et al: Effects of raloxifene on bone mineral density, serum cholesterol concentrations, and uterine endometrium in postmenopausal women, *N Engl J Med* 337:1641-1647, 1997.

19. Downs JR, et al: Primary prevention of acute coronary events with lovastatin in men and women with average cholesterol levels: results of AFCAPS/TexCAPS. Air Force/Texas Coronary Atherosclerosis Prevention Study, *JAMA* 279:1615-1622, 1998.
20. Durrington PN, et al: Serum apolipoproteins AI and B and lipoproteins in middle-aged men with and without previous myocardial infarction, *Br Heart J* 56:206-212, 1986.
21. Durrington PN, et al: Apolipoproteins (a), AI, and B and parental history in men with early onset ischaemic heart disease, *Lancet* I:1070-1073, 1988.
22. Fenofibrate for hypertriglyceridemia, *Med Lett Drugs Ther* 40:68, 1998.
23. Frick MH, et al: The Helsinki Heart Study: primary-prevention trial with gemfibrozil in middle-aged men with dyslipidemia. Safety of treatment, changes in risk factors, and incidence of coronary heart disease, *N Engl J Med* 317:1237-1245, 1987.
24. Frishman WH, et al: Lipids and lipoproteins: atherosclerotic risk and management. In Frishman WH, editor: *Medical management of lipid disorders,* Mount Kisco, NY, 1992, Futura.
25. Garber AM, et al: Guidelines for using serum cholesterol, high-density lipoprotein cholesterol, and triglyceride levels as screening tests for preventing coronary heart disease in adults, *Ann Intern Med* 124:515-517, 1996.
26. Garber AM, Browner WS, Hulley SB: Cholesterol screening in asymptomatic adults, revisited, *Ann Intern Med* 124:518-531, 1996.
27. Gardner CD, Fortmann SP, Krauss RM: Association of small low-density lipoprotein particles with the incidence of coronary heart disease in men and women, *JAMA* 276:875-881, 1996.
28. Genest J Jr, et al: Lipoprotein cholesterol, apolipoprotein A-I and B and lipoprotein (a) abnormalities in men with premature coronary artery disease, *J Am Coll Cardiol* 19:792-802, 1992.
28a. GISSI-Prevenzione Investigators: Dietary supplementation with n-3 polyunsaturated fatty acids and vitamin E after myocardial infarction: results of the GISSI-Prevenzione trial, *Lancet* 354:447-455, 1999.
29. Grady D, et al: Hormone therapy to prevent disease and prolong life in postmenopausal women, *Ann Intern Med* 117:1016-1037, 1992.
30. Griffin BA, et al: Role of plasma triglyceride in the regulation of plasma low density lipoprotein (LDL) subfractions: relative contribution of small, dense LDL to coronary heart disease risk, *Atherosclerosis* 106:241-253, 1994.
31. Grundy SM, et al: Summary of the second report of the NCEP expert panel on detection, evaluation, and treatment of high blood cholesterol in adults, *JAMA* 269:3015-3023, 1993.
32. Grundy SM: Atherogenic dyslipidemia: lipoprotein abnormalities and implications for therapy, *Am J Cardiol* 75:45B-52B, 1995.
33. Grundy SM: Cholesterol and coronary heart disease: the 21st century, *Arch Intern Med* 157:1177-1184, 1997.
34. Guyton JR, et al: Relationship of plasma lipoprotein Lp(a) levels to race and to apolipoprotein B, *Arteriosclerosis* 5:265-272, 1985.
35. Hachinski V, et al: Lipids and stroke: a paradox resolved, *Arch Neurol* 53:303-308, 1996.
36. Heady JA, Morris JN, Oliver MF: WHO clofibrate/cholesterol trial: clarifications, *Lancet* 340:1405-1406, 1992.
37. Hebert PR, Gaziano JM, Hennekens CH: Cholesterol lowering with statin drugs, risk of stroke, and total mortality: an overview of randomized trials, *JAMA* 278:313-321, 1997.
38. Hegsted DM, et al: Dietary fat and serum lipids: an evaluation of the experimental data, *Am J Clin Nutr* 57:875-883, 1993.
39. Herd JA, et al: Effects of fluvastatin on coronary atherosclerosis in patients with mild to moderate cholesterol elevations: Lipoprotein and Coronary Atherosclerosis Study (LCAS), *Am J Cardiol* 80:278-286, 1997.
40. Hjermann I, et al: Effect of diet and smoking intervention on the incidence of coronary heart disease: report from the Oslo Study Group of a randomised trial in healthy men, *Lancet* 2:1303-1310, 1981.
41. Hokanson JE, Austin MA: Plasma triglyceride level is a risk factor for cardiovascular disease independent of high-density lipoprotein cholesterol level: a meta-analysis of population-based prospective studies, *J Cardiovasc Risk* 3:213-219, 1996.
42. Hulley S, et al: Randomized trial of estrogen plus progestin for secondary prevention of coronary heart disease in postmenopausal women: the Heart and Estrogen/Progestin Replacement Study (HERS), *JAMA* 280:605-613, 1998.
43. Reference deleted in proofs.
44. Kottke BA, et al: Apolipoproteins and coronary artery disease, *Mayo Clin Proc* 61:313-320, 1986.
45. Krauss RM: Dense low density lipoproteins and coronary artery disease, *Am J Cardiol* 75:53B-57B, 1995.
46. Kwiterovich, et al: Comparison of the plasma levels of apolipoproteins B and A-I, and other risk factors in men and women with premature coronary artery disease, *Am J Cardiol* 69:1015-1021, 1992.
47. LaRosa JC: Triglycerides and coronary risk in women and the elderly, *Arch Intern Med* 157:961-968, 1997.
48. Larsen ML, Illingworth DR: Drug treatment of dyslipoproteinemia, *Med Clin North Am* 78:225-245, 1994.
49. Lerner DJ, Kannel WB: Patterns of coronary heart disease morbidity and mortality in the sexes: a 26-year follow-up of the Framingham population, *Am Heart J* 113:383-390, 1986.
50. Levinson SS, Wagner SG: Measurement of apolipoprotein B–containing lipoproteins for routine clinical laboratory use in cardiovascular disease, *Arch Pathol Lab Med* 116:1350-1354, 1992.
51. Loscalzo J: Lipoprotein(a): a unique risk factor for atherothrombotic disease, *Arteriosclerosis* 10:672-679, 1990.
52. Manttari M, et al: Alcohol and coronary heart disease: the roles of HDL-cholesterol and smoking, *J Intern Med* 241:157-163, 1997.
53. Marckmann P, Bladbjerg EM, Jespersen J: Dietary fish oil (4g daily) and cardiovascular risk markers in healthy men, *Arterioscler Thromb* 17:3384-3391, 1997.
54. Marcovina SM, et al: Lipoprotein (a) concentrations and apolipoprotein(a) phenotypes in Caucasians and African Americans, *Arterioscler Thromb* 13:1037-1045, 1993.
55. Martin MJ, et al: Serum cholesterol, blood pressure, and mortality: implications from a cohort of 361,662 men, *Lancet* 11:933-936, 1986.
56. Miettinen TA, et al: Reduction of serum cholesterol with sitostanol-ester margarine in a mildly hypercholesterolemic population, *N Engl J Med* 333:1308-1312, 1995.
57. Miles LA, Plow EF: Lp(a): an interloper in the fibrinolytic system, *Thromb Haemost* 63:331-335, 1990.
58. O'Brien T, Nguyen TT, Zimmerman BR: Hyperlipidemia and diabetes mellitus, *Mayo Clin Proc* 73:969-976, 1998.
59. Pearson TA: Alcohol and heart disease: a statement from the Nutritional Committee, American Heart Association, *Am J Clin Nutr* 65:1567-1569, 1997.
60. Pederson TR, et al for the Scandinavian Simvastatin Survival Study Group: Randomized trial of cholesterol lowering in 4444 patients with coronary heart disease, *Lancet* 344:1383-1389, 1994.
61. Pierce LR, Wysowski DK, Gross TP: Myopathy and rhabdomyolysis associated with lovastatin-gemfibrozil combination therapy, *JAMA* 264:71-75, 1990.
62. Pitt B, et al, for the PLAC I Investigators: Pravastatin Limitation of Atherosclerosis in the Coronary Arteries (PLAC 1): reduction in atherosclerosis progression and clinical events, *J Am Coll Cardiol* 26:1133-1139, 1995.
62a. Pitt B, et al, for the Atorvastatin versus Revascularization Treatment Investigators: Aggressive lipid-lowering therapy compared with angioplasty in stable coronary artery disease, *N Engl J Med* 341:70-76, 1999.
63. Qizilbash N: Are risk factors for stroke and coronary disease the same? *Curr Opin Lipidol* 9:325 328, 1998.
64. Rader DJ, Brewer HB Jr: Lipoprotein (a): clinical approach to a unique atherogenic lipoprotein, *JAMA* 267:1109-1112, 1992.
65. Rader DJ, Hoeg JM, Brewer Jr HB: Quantitation of plasma apolipoproteins in the primary and secondary prevention of coronary artery disease, *Ann Intern Med* 120:1012-1025, 1994.
65a. Rader DJ, Ikewaki K: Unraveling high density lipoprotein-apolipoprotein metabolism in human mutants and animal models, *Curr Opin Lipidol* 7:117-123, 1996.
65b. Rapola JM, et al: Randomised trial of alpha-tocopherol and beta-carotene supplements on incidence of major coronary events in men with previous myocardial infarction, *Lancet* 349:1715-1720, 1997.
66. Ravnikar VA: Compliance with hormone therapy, *Am J Obstet Gynecol* 156:1332, 1987.
67. Report from the Committee of Principal Investigators: A cooperative trial in the primary prevention of ischaemic heart disease using clofibrate, *Br Heart J* 40:1069-1118, 1978.
67a. Rubins HB, et al, for the Veterans Affairs High-Density Lipoprotein Cholesterol Intervention Trial Study Group: Gemfibrozil for the secondary prevention of coronary heart disease in men with low levels of high-density lipoprotein cholesterol, *N Engl J Med* 341:410-418, 1999.

68. Sacks F: Dietary fats and coronary heart disease, *J Cardiovasc Risk* 1:3-8, 1994.
69. Sacks FM, et al, for the Harvard Atherosclerosis Reversibility Project (HARP) Group: Effect on coronary atherosclerosis of decrease in plasma cholesterol concentrations in normocholesterolemic patients, *Lancet* 344:1182-1186, 1994.
70. Sacks FM, et al, for the Cholesterol And Recurrent Events Trial investigators (CARE): The effect of pravastatin on coronary events after myocardial infarction in patients with average cholesterol levels, *N Engl J Med* 335:1001-1009, 1996.
71. Sandholzer C, et al: Effects of the apolipoprotein(a) size polymorphism on the lipoprotein(a) concentrations in 7 ethnic groups, *Hum Genet* 86:607-614, 1991.
72. Sandholzer C, et al: Apo(a) isoforms predict risk for coronary heart disease: a study in six populations, *Arterioscler Thromb* 12:1214-1226, 1992.
73. Sandholzer C, et al: Apolipoprotein(a) phenotypes, Lp(a) concentration and plasma lipid levels in relation to coronary heart disease in a Chinese population: evidence for the role of the apo(a) gene in coronary heart disease, *J Clin Invest* 89:1040-1046, 1992.
74. Sechi LA, et al: Increased serum lipoprotein(a) levels in patients with early renal failure, *Ann Intern Med* 129:457-461, 1998.
75. Sempos CT, et al: Prevalence of high blood cholesterol among US adults: an update based on guidelines from the Second Report of the National Cholesterol Education Program Adult Treatment Panel, *JAMA* 269:3009-3014, 1993.
76. Sheperd J, et al for The West of Scotland Coronary Prevention Study Group: Prevention of coronary heart disease with pravastatin in men with hypercholesterolemia, *N Engl J Med* 333:1301-1307, 1995.
77. Simons LA, Balasubramaniam S, Holland J: Low density lipoprotein metabolism in the normal to moderately elevated range of plasma cholesterol: comparisons with familial hypercholesterolemia, *J Lipid Research* 24:192-199, 1983.
78. Simons LA, Levis G, Simons J: Apparent discontinuation rates in patients prescribed lipid-lowering drugs, *Med J Aust* 164:208, 1996.
79. Sniderman AD, Silberberg J: Is it time to measure apolipoprotein B? *Arteriosclerosis* 10:665-667, 1990.
80. Srinivasan SR, et al: Racial (black-white) differences in serum lipoprotein(a) distribution and its relation to parental myocardial infarction in children: Bogalusa heart study, *Circulation* 84:160-167, 1991.
81. Stampfer MJ, Malinow MR: Can lowering homocysteine levels reduce cardiovascular risk? *N Engl J Med* 332:328-329, 1995.
82. Stampfer MJ, et al: A prospective study of triglyceride level, low density lipoprotein diameter, and risk of myocardial infarction, *JAMA* 276:882-888, 1996.
82a. Stephens NG, et al: Randomised controlled trial of vitamin E in patients with coronary disease: Cambridge Heart Antioxidant Study (CHAOS), *Lancet* 347:751-786, 1996.
83. Sullivan JM: Estrogen replacement, *Circulation* 94:2699-2702, 1996.
84. Superko HR: Beyond LDL cholesterol reduction, *Circulation* 94:2351-2354, 1996.
84a. The Heart Outcomes Prevention Evaluation Study Investigators: Vitamin E supplementation and cardiovascular events in high-risk patients, *N Engl J Med* 342:154-160, 2000.
85. The Lipid Research Clinics Coronary Primary Prevention Trial results: I. Reduction in incidence of coronary heart disease, *JAMA* 251:351-364, 1984.
86. The Writing Group for the PEPI Trial: Effects of estrogen or estrogen/progestin regimens on heart disease risk factors in postmenopausal women: The Postmenopausal Estrogen/Progestin Interventions (PEPI) Trial, *JAMA* 273:199-208, 1995.
87. Thompson GR, Hollyer J, Waters DD: Percentage change rather than plasma level of LDL-cholesterol determines therapeutic response in coronary heart disease, *Curr Opin Lipodol* 6:386-388, 1995.
88. Thun MJ: Alcohol consumption and mortality among middle-aged and elderly US adults, *N Engl J Med* 337:1705-1714, 1997.
89. Tornvall P, et al: Relationships of low density lipoprotein subfractions to angiographically defined coronary artery disease in young survivors of myocardial infarction, *Atherosclerosis* 90:67-80, 1991.
90. U.S. Preventive Services Task Force: Screening for high blood cholesterol and other lipid abnormalities, *Guide to clinical preventive services*, ed 2, Baltimore, 1996, Williams & Wilkins, pp 15-38.
91. Willett WC, et al: Mediterranean diet pyramid: a cultural model for healthy eating, *Am J Clin Nutr* 61(suppl):1402-1406, 1995.

PULMONARY DISEASE IV

CHAPTER 72

Asthma and Other Allergic Disorders

Richard M. Effros
Jack Kaufman

BRONCHIAL ASTHMA

Bronchial asthma is a clinical disorder in which the airways are hyperreactive to a variety of stimuli. After exposure to these stimuli, airway resistance increases because of smooth muscle contraction, increased secretions, and inflammation of the bronchial walls. In contrast to the relatively fixed airway obstruction encountered in emphysema, increased airway resistance in asthma is episodic and improves between attacks. During remissions the patient may be essentially asymptomatic, but in more severe forms of the disease, some bronchospasm may persist even between attacks. No evidence indicates that asthma shortens life span, although later onset and concomitant chronic obstructive pulmonary disease appear to shorten survival.[6,8]

Pathogenesis

Although asthma was once thought to result from an abnormal immune response of the lungs, multiple inflammatory factors are now known to play a role in its etiology[4] (Fig. 72-1). The primary immune mechanism of asthma involves the association of antigen with immunoglobulin E (IgE) bound to the cell surfaces, which triggers the release of histamine and a variety of other factors that promote both bronchospasm and local inflammation. Histamine increases leakage of protein and fluid from venules, increases airway secretions, and can stimulate irritant receptors in the airway walls. This in turn leads to reflex vagal release of acetylcholine near smooth muscles, promoting further bronchoconstriction. Although antihistamines are useful in the treatment of other allergic disorders such as allergic rhinitis, they are not helpful in asthma.

Many factors besides histamine participate in the pathogenesis of bronchial asthma, including the lipoxygenase products of arachidonate, the leukotrienes (formerly known as slow-reacting substance of anaphylaxis). Other mediators that may play a role in bronchospasm include platelet activating factor, bradykinin, substance P, oxidants, complement fragments, and a variety of other substances. Agents that inhibit the synthesis of leukotrienes or their receptors have proved helpful in some patients with asthma. The intensity of the eosinophilia observed in patients with asthma appears to be correlated with the severity of airflow obstruction, and eosinophil counts are increased in bronchoalveolar lavage fluid from asthmatic patients. Response to steroids is marked by a decrease in both airway resistance and eosinophil counts.

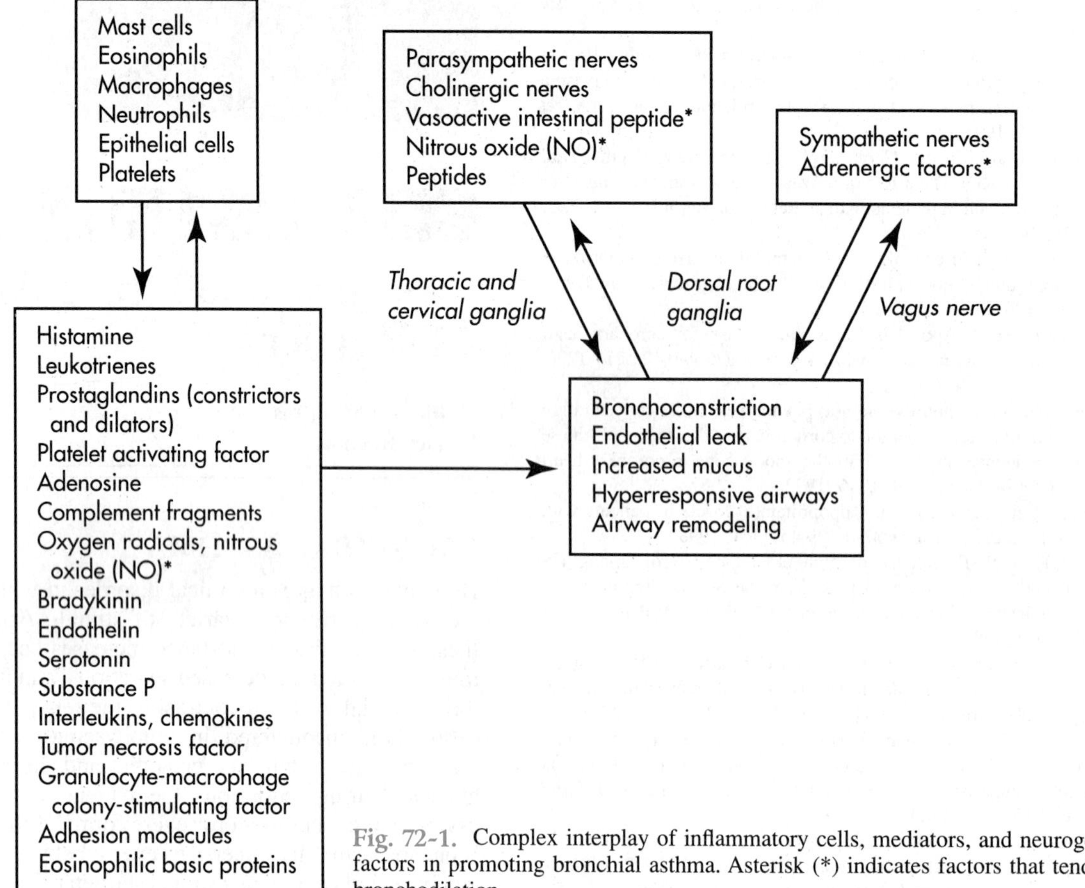

Fig. 72-1. Complex interplay of inflammatory cells, mediators, and neurogenic factors in promoting bronchial asthma. Asterisk (*) indicates factors that tend to cause bronchodilation.

Mast cells within the lung tissues of patients appear to be activated and probably play an important role in the early events preceding an asthmatic attack. Bronchospasm can be induced by cholinergic nerves that travel in the vagus nerve and may release acetylcholine reflexively when irritant receptors in the airways are stimulated. Stimulation of these same receptors is also responsible for cough. Although not as effective as β-adrenergic agents, anticholinergic drugs can relieve airway obstruction in some asthmatic patients.

Epidemiology

Bronchial asthma is a common clinical problem in the United States, affecting about 10 million people, or about 4% of the population. The economic cost of this disease in the United States was estimated at $6.2 billion in 1990,[10] and the incidence may be increasing in the general population.[3] Males predominate over females by a factor of 1.5 to 2.0 under age 10 years, but the incidence is approximately equal by age 30, after which incidence in women becomes greater. Black children have a higher incidence of asthma than other children. Airway hyperresponsiveness, as judged by methacholine challenges, is almost always present in asthmatic persons, but this observation is also seen in many asymptomatic subjects. Perhaps 20% of those with asymptomatic airway hyperreactivity eventually develop clinical asthma. Approximately half of those with asthma have a familial history of asthma, rhinitis, eczematous dermatitis, or urticaria. The onset of asthma is frequently associated with viral upper respiratory tract infections (e.g., respiratory syncytial virus disease in infancy, rhinovirus or influenza in older children and adults). Air pollutants such as ozone, nitrogen dioxide, and sulfur dioxide can initiate attacks in asthmatic persons and probably contribute to the incidence. Both active and passive smoking may predispose to the development of asthma.

About 50% of children with asthma improve or become symptom free on reaching early adulthood, but a very early onset of disease is associated with a less favorable prognosis. Mortality is uncommon in the United States, averaging 3000 per year. Despite the introduction of newer modes of therapy, the mortality rate for asthma has not declined, and some are concerned that mortality in the United States and elsewhere may be increasing.

Agents and Circumstances That Induce Asthma

Many patients with asthma tend to produce IgE to one or more antigens in the environment (designated as *allergens*) and are therefore referred to as *atopic*. Atopy may also be associated with eczema and hay fever. This form is sometimes referred to as *extrinsic asthma,* whereas the type unrelated to an atopic predisposition or to specific environmental antigens is designated as *intrinsic asthma*. Patients with extrinsic asthma generally contract their illness at a younger age. Pollens, molds, house dust, and animal dander are common antigens. Because the pollens are too large to reach the bronchi or reactive cells (mast cells), fragments of the pollens apparently are responsible for asthmatic attacks. Antigens associated with the skin mites *Dermatophagoides pteronyssinus,* especially the feces of these arthropods, are the principal allergenic factors in house dust. Cockroaches are a

... high-density ...gen associated with ...glands, and many patients

...cks related to foods are much less ...ose induced by inhaled antigens, but ...o specific foods and additives such as meta-...ites (sometimes used as a preservative for salads) can induce serious attacks. Reactions to foods are usually associated with either gastrointestinal symptoms or rashes. Gastroesophageal reflux is common in asthmatic patients, and treatment of this problem can relieve the asthma's severity.

A careful occupational history is essential in the evaluation of adults with bronchial asthma.[9] Substances that can cause asthma in the workplace can be divided into low-molecular-weight substances and proteins. Toluene diisocyanate (TDI), is an important ingredient of polyurethane foams that can foster asthma in workers who may have had no previous reaction to the substance over many months. Platinum salts and a variety of anhydrides may cause development of both IgE antibodies and asthma. Proteins that can cause asthma include enzymes used in detergents, which may result in hypersensitivity in approximately one fourth of workers exposed. A variety of wood dusts, particularly western red cedar, can also cause occupational asthma. Electricians may contract asthma from inhalation of fumes released during soldering. Exposure to cotton and other organic fibers can provoke bronchospasm by stimulating release of histamine, a condition referred to as *byssinosis* (see Chapter 76). Although formaldehyde appears to have been responsible for asthma in a few workers exposed to heavy concentrations, evidence regarding the small amounts released from fiberboard or foam in homes is not considered persuasive.

A single, direct exposure to high concentrations of toxic fumes (e.g., ammonia, bleach, TDI) can result in the onset of asthma in patients without previous airway disease.[2] This condition is referred to as *reactive airway dysfunction syndrome* (RADS). Patients with RADS characteristically become acutely ill and require medical attention during the first 24 hours after exposure. After recovery, airway hyperreactivity may be present, with asthmatic symptoms persisting indefinitely, or airway hyperreactivity may gradually decline over months. The hyperreactivity of the airways of asthmatic patients extends to a variety of nonspecific stimuli, including cold air, perfume, smoke, and sulfur dioxide. Vigorous exercise may be followed by bronchospasm, and hyperventilation (voluntary or associated with laughing and crying) can initiate an asthmatic attack. Exercise-induced asthma can be avoided by prior inhalation of cromolyn, nedocromil, or a β-adrenergic agent. Other nonspecific contributing factors are esophageal reflux and chronic sinus disease.

Drugs are responsible for approximately 10% of acute asthmatic attacks. Nonsteroidal antiinflammatory drugs (NSAIDs), particularly aspirin preparations, have been implicated in more than half these cases. Hypersensitivity to aspirin and other NSAIDs typically appears in the third and fourth decades of life and does not seem to be inherited. Intense vasomotor rhinitis frequently precedes asthmatic symptoms, and nasal polyps and sinusitis are common. Within several hours of ingesting aspirin, patients experience rhinitis and wheezing and may develop nausea, vomiting, facial edema, angioedema, and life-threatening anaphylaxis. The action of these drugs appears to be related to their ability to inhibit cyclooxygenase. Drugs that do not inhibit cyclooxygenase, such as salicylamide and sodium salicylate, are considered safe. Acetaminophen and dextropropoxyphene are also relatively safe in the great majority of these patients. Desensitization with daily administration of aspirin has been recommended but should be undertaken by an experienced allergist. Leukotriene receptor inhibitors may also be useful.

β-Adrenergic inhibitors, including those used in ophthalmic preparations and even those that enter the milk of nursing mothers, may induce asthmatic attacks. Because the lung, like the heart, contains some β_1-receptors as well as β_2-receptors, the physician must ensure that the action of these drugs is restricted to the heart. Many antibiotics and iodinated dyes may result in severe asthmatic responses, which can be ameliorated by prior treatment with antihistamines and steroids. Cocaine and a variety of anesthetic agents have also been associated with asthmatic attacks. Any of the angiotensin-converting enzyme inhibitors may cause a persistent cough that begins soon after administration or as late as 1 year after initiating therapy; however, these reactions are rarely associated with bronchospasm or changes in bronchial hyperreactivity and are relieved within weeks after the drug is discontinued. Rarely, they have been associated with acute angioedema, which may affect the mouth, tongue, and larynx, causing acute upper airway obstruction, which may require administration of epinephrine.

Patient Evaluation

History. More than in any other respiratory disease, the history plays a crucial diagnostic role in bronchial asthma. The patient usually gives a history of dyspnea with recurrences and remissions. Often the dyspnea worsens at night and may be initiated by viral infections or exposure to irritants or antigens, such as those already listed. Although intrathoracic obstruction leads to greater resistance during expiration, patients typically complain more of inspiratory distress. Fatigue of the inspiratory muscles probably occurs because they remain tonically contracted throughout the respiratory cycle and are disadvantaged by the high maintenance volumes in the lungs. Wheezing is apparent to both patient and physician but may disappear when tidal volumes become sufficiently compromised in severe asthma. Cough is a common manifestation of asthma and may be the only complaint; response to bronchodilators may reveal the cause. Frequently a cough productive of intrabronchial plugs may herald relief during an attack. Symptoms of asthma usually occur within 10 to 30 minutes of exposure to an irritant or antigen. Late responses are also common, however, occurring several hours after exposure. Usually an early response precedes the late response, but some patients with occupational asthma may have no early phase. Whereas the early response appears to be caused by bronchospasm, edema, and vascular congestion, the late response is associated with the appearance of inflammatory cells in the tissues.

Physical Examination. Wheezing is the most common physical finding in asthma and generally is audible during both inspiration and expiration rather than just expiration. If these sounds are audible only during inspiration, extrathoracic obstruction with stridor is probably present rather than intrathoracic obstruction from bronchial asthma. The time required for airway sounds to disappear over the trachea during expiration is characteristically increased to as long as 6 seconds in patients experiencing bronchospasm. In a severe attack the patient strains to inspire, often using both scalenus and sternocleidomastoid muscles, and then expires slowly, frequently against pursed lips, contracting abdominal muscles to force the diaphragm upward. Marked variation of intrathoracic pressures results in pulsus paradoxus, with systolic pressures falling by more than 15 mm Hg during inspiration. Pulsus paradoxus may become less prominent, however, if the patient tires; again, wheezing may disappear in severe attacks as tidal volume decreases.

Laboratory Studies and Diagnostic Procedures

Increases in airway resistance associated with bronchial asthma can be readily detected by spirometry. Forced vital capacity (FVC) maneuvers reveal decreased flow rates, forced expiratory volume in 1 second (FEV_1) and peak expiratory flow rate (PEFR) are most often used to assess alterations in airway obstruction. It is common practice to determine responsiveness to bronchodilators during the evaluation of pulmonary function. Failure to document a response is not particularly helpful, however, since patients who show no improvement in the laboratory may respond outside the laboratory; a clinical trial of bronchodilator therapy should generally be given regardless of the laboratory response. It is important to assess the FEV_1/FVC ratio, since a reduction of this ratio from expected values is specific for obstructive rather than restrictive disease. The severity of asthma can be judged on the basis of both pulmonary function studies and clinical presentation (Table 72-1).[5,7]

Differentiation between intrathoracic and extrathoracic obstruction is facilitated by obtaining a flow-volume loop. The total lung capacity and, during remission, the carbon monoxide diffusion test are frequently increased in asthmatic patients. Between bronchospastic episodes, pulmonary function may be completely normal; bronchoprovocation studies are then conducted, generally by having the patient inhale an aerosol containing methacholine. Patients with hyperreactive airways experience a decrease in airflow with very low methacholine concentrations. Documentation of a normal challenge test argues against bronchial asthma, but many normal subjects who have airway [illegible] bronchoprovocation tests may have no history of asth[illegible] these tests may become abnormal for several months after a viral infection in nonasthmatic individuals.

Arterial blood gases must be carefully followed in patients with severe asthma. Mild hypoxia and hypocapnia are usually observed in mild and moderate asthma. With more severe episodes, hypoxia worsens and carbon dioxide pressure (Pco_2) may rise to normal or greater levels, resulting in respiratory acidosis. If oxygen delivery to the tissues becomes inadequate, lactic acidosis ensues. If Pco_2 increases to normal or elevated levels in a patient in distress, respiratory failure may be present, and mechanical ventilation may become mandatory.

Eosinophilia is common in all forms of allergic diseases, including asthma, drug reactions, allergic rhinitis, angioedema, and eczema. As noted, the number of eosinophils tends to reflect the severity of asthma and may indicate whether steroid therapy is adequate.

The lungs are characteristically hyperinflated on radiographs. Chest films should be obtained in patients with severe asthma, since they may reveal unexpected findings (e.g., pneumothorax, atelectasis, pneumonia) that require immediate attention. The detection of central bronchiectasis with mucous plugs strongly suggests bronchopulmonary aspergillosis, which is usually accompanied by asthmatic symptoms.

Complications

Status asthmaticus, generally defined as life-threatening asthma that does not respond to standard medication, is one of the most serious complications in asthmatic patients. A patient who shows signs of respiratory failure with severe hypoxia and rising Pco_2 must be admitted to an intensive care unit, where mechanical ventilation can be properly managed (see Chapter 77). Other complications of acute asthma include pneumothorax, pneumomediastinum, and atelectasis from bronchial plugging.

Differential Diagnosis

Many clinical disorders can mimic bronchial asthma (Box 72-1). Manifestations of extrathoracic obstruction caused by lesions of the upper airways may be confused with those of

Table 72-1. Therapeutic Staging for Acute Bronchial Asthma Exacerbations in Adults

Stage	Symptoms	FEV_1 or PEFR*	Treatment
Mild	Mild wheeze, cough, dyspnea on exercise	>80%	Use metered-dose inhaler or nebulizer up to three times an hour; oral steroids if no response. Administer oxygen (O_2) to keep saturation at 90% or higher.
Moderate	Wheeze, cough, moderate dyspnea at rest	50%-80%	As above, with repeat bronchodilators every hour; if no response, call physician. In emergency room (ER), intravenous steroids and inhaled anticholinergic agent; admit to hospital if poor response.
Severe	Severe dyspnea at rest, accessory muscle use, retraction, difficulty talking, wheeze may disappear	<50%	As above, and go to ER; if no response, admit to hospital. If impending respiratory arrest, intubate and place on 100% O_2.

Modified from *Practical guide for diagnosis and management of asthma,* NIH Pub No 97-4053, Bethesda, Md, 1997, National Institutes of Health.
**PEFR,* Percentage of predicted peak expiratory flow rate; *FEV_1,* percentage of personal-best forced expiratory volume in 1 second.

intrathoracic obstruction caused by asthma. Because of injuries sustained to the larynx and trachea during intubation and tracheostomies, extrathoracic obstruction is increasingly common in general practice. Careful examination should allow detection of inspiratory stridor, which is loudest over the larynx and trachea. In some cases, laryngeal "dysfunction" may be a manifestation of psychiatric disorders. Patients with this disorder characteristically narrow their glottis during inspiration and expiration but do not have increases in alveolar-arterial oxygen differences. Wheezing is also often associated with early congestive heart failure (CHF) with edema of the airways, and CHF may cause a cough that worsens when the patient is recumbent. CHF patients have an increased incidence of bronchial hyperreactivity. Bronchial asthma must also be distinguished from *hypersensitivity pneumonitis,* which is related to inhalation of fungi or proteins. Unlike bronchial asthma, this condition is more often manifested by rales than wheezing, is frequently associated with pulmonary infiltrates and fever, and recurrent exposure may lead to chronic pulmonary fibrosis. Children who have had bronchopulmonary dysplasia or cystic fibrosis may develop airway obstruction that may be confused with bronchial asthma.

Bronchiolitis is a common disease in infants frequently associated with respiratory syncytial virus infections. It is also seen in adults after viral infections and may present with chronic cough and wheezing, which subside over weeks or months. *Bronchiolitis obliterans* is a more serious form of small-airway obstruction in which granulation tissue fills the smaller bronchioles. This disease may be idiopathic or may be caused by toxic fume exposure, connective tissue disorders (e.g., rheumatoid arthritis), and bone or organ transplantation (e.g., graft-vs.-host disease). Early inspiratory crackles are common, and chest radiographs may be normal or show patchy overinflation. *Bronchiolitis obliterans with organizing pneumonia* (BOOP) is characterized by small-airway obstruction with plugs of granulation tissue and accumulation of fibrinous exudates and foamy macrophages in inflamed alveoli. Patchy infiltrates are visible in chest radiographs, and BOOP frequently responds to steroid therapy.

Box 72-1. Disorders and Diseases Associated with or Mimicking Bronchial Asthma

Chronic obstructive pulmonary disease
Upper airway obstruction
Congestive heart failure
Bronchopulmonary aspergillosis
Pulmonary infiltration with eosinophilia
Churg-Strauss syndrome
Endobronchial sarcoid or tuberculosis
Angioedema
Carcinoid syndrome
Gastroesophageal reflux
Bronchiolitis
Cystic fibrosis
Factitious asthma
Pulmonary embolism

Management

Although considerable effort has been devoted to development of more effective treatment of asthma, progress has been slow, and many drugs represent variants of agents used for centuries. The complexity of the inflammatory events responsible for hyperreactive airways suggests that it is necessary to block multiple mediators and effectors to prevent and treat asthma more effectively. Many of the more effective drugs tend to have multiple biologic actions. Treatment should be graded in accordance with the severity and chronicity of the disorder (Table 72-2).[5,7] Asthma can be unpredictable, and the physician must use ingenuity in designing individualized regimens. Evidence indicates that frequency of hospitalization can be reduced if asthmatic patients are closely followed by their physicians, are instructed carefully in the use of their medications, and, in more labile patients, are taught to keep a record of their own pulmonary function with a peak flowmeter.

Sympathomimetic Agents. The recognition that different adrenergic receptors exist in different tissues has led to the development of β-adrenergic drugs that are more specific in their action to promote bronchodilation and less likely to be

Table 72-2. Stepwise Management of Chronic Bronchial Asthma in Adults and Children over 5 Years Old

	Frequency (day/night)		PEFR or FEV_1*		
Step	Day	Night	Value	Variability	Daily medications†
1: mild intermittent	≤2/week	≤2/month	≥80%	<20%	None
2: mild persistent	3-6/week	3-4/month	≥80%	20%-30%	Inhaled steroid: low dose; cromolyn, nedocromil, theophylline, or anti-leukotriene agent
3: moderate persistent	Daily	≥5/month	60%-80%	>30%	Inhaled steroid: medium dose plus step 2; sustained-release β_2-agonist
4: severe persistent	Continual	Frequent	≤60%	>30%	Inhaled steroid: high dose plus step 3; oral steroids with attempts to reduce

Modified from *Practical guide for diagonsis and management of asthma,* NIH Pub No 97-4053, Bethesda, Md, 1997, National Institutes of Health.
**PEFR,* Percentage of predicted peak expiratory flow rate; FEV_1, percentage of personal-best forced expiratory volume in 1 second.
†Short-acting β_2-agonist (2-4 puffs) is used for acute symptoms, regardless of step.

associated with side effects. α-Agonists cause vasoconstriction, whereas β_1-adrenergic agents increase cardiac contractility and heart rate, which is undesirable in patients undergoing therapy for asthma. In addition to promoting bronchodilation, β_2-adrenergic agents also increase secretion of electrolytes by the airways and enhance mucociliary activity. Protein kinase A levels increase within the smooth muscle cells, resulting in inhibition of myosin phosphorylation and smooth muscle cell relaxation. β_2-Agonists are not free from side effects, such as skeletal muscle tremor, hyperglycemia, and hypokalemia, as well as dilation of the vasculature of skeletal muscles. A transient decrease in oxygen saturation is sometimes observed after administration of these agents. This paradoxic effect is related to the effect of increased cardiac output, which can result in perfusion of underventilated regions of the lungs and is not a contraindication to continued use of these drugs.

Epinephrine was introduced in 1910 and continues to be administered subcutaneously, and less frequently by intravenous injections, in the treatment of severe asthmatic or anaphylactic attacks (see Anaphylaxis). Cardiac necrosis has been described after administration of parenteral epinephrine, and if at all possible, such injections should be avoided in older patients and those with history of coronary artery disease. Because epinephrine is the only aerosolized agent available without prescription, many patients continue to use it. However, epinephrine is associated with potent α-adrenergic and nonspecific β-adrenergic activity and has a very limited half-life; its use in aerosols has been largely replaced by newer, more specific agents. Ephedrine, an oral drug with weak properties similar to those of epinephrine, is of largely historic interest, since it was used for millennia in herbal form and was popular in various proprietary combinations for many years. Isoproterenol became popular after its introduction in the 1940s because it lacked α-adrenergic activity. Unfortunately, it is relatively nonspecific for β_1-adrenergic and β_2-adrenergic effects, and the former may have been responsible for an increased incidence of sudden death when it was widely used as a metered aerosol. Isoproterenol is still occasionally used intravenously in children with status asthmaticus to avoid the need for intubation and ventilation, but terbutaline is safer for this purpose.

Metered-dose inhalers (MDIs) containing β_2-agonists are widely available on the American market, including terbutaline (oral and subcutaneous forms), albuterol (aerosol and oral administration but not parenteral therapy), bitolterol, and pirbuterol. These drugs remain active for relatively longer periods than the earlier preparations and are less likely to cause unwanted cardiovascular effects. Salmeterol has a particularly long duration of action and is useful for preventing nocturnal bronchospasm. The onset of bronchodilation is also delayed, however, and salmeterol should not be used to treat acute bronchospasm. β_2-Adrenergic agents are best prescribed in aerosol form because much higher concentrations can be reached locally within the lungs than with oral and parenteral administration, and systemic effects can be minimized. The latter routes, however, may permit the drug to reach areas of the lung that are inaccessible to aerosols because of severe bronchoconstriction and mucous plugging, and oral and occasionally parenteral administration may be helpful. Studies suggest that MDIs are just as effective as aerosol generators, particularly if the patients are properly trained in inhaling during release of medication from the inhaler. For those who have difficulty with the MDI inspiratory maneuver, spacers can be used to permit administration of medication during tidal breathing. Considerably more medication is delivered with the aerosol generators, however, and they continue to be popular for patients with episodes of very severe asthma unresponsive to the MDIs.

Concern still exists that patients tend to develop tachyphylaxis to β-adrenergic therapy. Although laboratory models can show this phenomenon, the clinical significance of tachyphylaxis is not clear. Nevertheless, the physician must be alerted if the patient finds it necessary to use the medication more frequently, since this may signal worsening of the disease and mandate additional therapy. The usual recommendation has been that β-adrenergic aerosols should be used regularly (e.g., two breaths four times a day), but with concern about increased cardiac events or tachyphylaxis, the recommendation now is that patients with relatively mild asthma can use MDIs less frequently and as needed. Administration of aerosols is often increased to every 15 minutes for patients in the emergency room, but chronic administration of high doses should probably be avoided, since an increase in asthma mortality may be related to overuse of these agents.

Corticosteroids. The beneficial and deleterious effects of the glucocorticoids in asthma treatment are related in part to the specific cytoplasmic receptors for these agents in both inflammatory cells and many parenchymal cells, including those of the lungs. Subsequent activity requires interaction with regulatory elements of DNA, so the antiinflammatory actions of corticosteroids are not seen for 6 to 12 hours. Chronic administration can reduce nonspecific airway hyperresponsiveness, and single doses inhibit the late, inflammatory response to antigen exposure.

Parenteral administration is particularly valuable in patients with severe episodes of asthma (Table 72-3). Because the effects of these agents may not be clinically evident for as long as 12 hours and the course of the illness is so unpredictable, these drugs are administered as early as possible to patients who require hospitalization. High dosages of steroids may be continued in oral form until flow returns toward baseline levels, and then tapering may proceed over 1 or 2 weeks, with adjustment if peak flows begin to deteriorate (Table 72-4). Concomitant use of steroid aerosols is recommended both during and after tapering (see following discussion). Oral glucocorticoids can be used for recurrences in the home environment with appropriate tapering schedules. In a minority of patients, oral steroids must be used on a chronic basis with attempts at as slow a taper as possible. Longer exposure entails increased risk of side effects. Administration of more than the physiologic levels of glucocorticoids (7.5 to 10 mg/day of prednisone) leads to suppression of the hypothalamic-pituitary-adrenal (HPA) axis. This effect can be reduced by administering all the medication in the morning, when adrenocorticotropic hormone (ACTH) levels are maximal, rather than in multiple doses throughout the day. Alternate-day dosing is even more effective in preventing HPA axis suppression and, by allowing recovery of some inflammatory function, may reduce the incidence of infection; however, controlling asthmatic symptoms in many patients is difficult with this

Table 72-3. Parenteral Agents Used to Treat Asthma

Agent	Form/patient	Dose
β-Adrenergics		
Epinephrine	1:1000 solution	0.3-0.5 mg every 20 min × 3
Sus-Phrine	1:200 suspension	0.1-0.3 mg every 6 hr or more often
Terbutaline	1 mg/ml solution	0.25 mg every 20 min × 3
Theophylline		
Loading dose	Not receiving therapy	5 mg/kg IV in 20 min
	Receiving therapy	2.5 mg/kg IV in 20 min
Maintenance	Young smoker	0.7 mg/kg/hr
	Nonsmoking adult	0.43 mg/kg/hr
	Older adult, cor pulmonale	0.26 mg/kg/hr
Corticosteroids		
Methylprednisolone	Acute	40-120 mg q 4-6 hr
Prednisone	Exacerbation	100-400 mg q 4-6 hr

regimen. After prolonged glucocorticoid administration, weaning should be done slowly (e.g., by decreasing dosage by 1 mg/day for a month). Hypothalamic-pituitary function may remain suppressed for as long as a year, and the patient should keep steroids on hand for stressful circumstances and carry a card indicating possible need for steroid administration if stress or surgery occurs during the year after discontinuation of steroids.

Aerosolized steroids have gained considerable popularity in the treatment of asthma. These have been designed to exert maximal local activity while minimizing absorption and systemic effects. They can assist in withdrawal of chronic oral steroid therapy and may reduce dependence on β_2-adrenergic agents and the incidence of exercise dyspnea. Oropharyngeal candidiasis can be ameliorated or avoided by thoroughly rinsing the mouth after administration of aerosolized steroids. Dysphonia, manifested as hoarseness, is usually related to the effect of the drugs on the skeletal muscles of the larynx. It may respond to less frequent administration or use of spacers to improve more distal delivery of medication.

High dosages of inhaled steroids may have systemic effects, such as suppression of the HPA axis and bone formation, and the incidence of cataracts and glaucoma may be increased. Use of a spacer can decrease absorption through the membranes of the mouth and upper airways; patients should rinse their mouths after administration. It should be emphasized to patients that these aerosolized steroids do not provide immediate relief and must be taken on a regular basis for some weeks before improvement may occur and some months before maximal effect is observed (Table 72-5).

Methylxanthines. The popularity of methylxanthines for the treatment of asthma has waxed and waned dramatically. Although they cannot be considered primary drugs for asthma treatment because of a less favorable benefits/complications ratio than aerosolized β_2-adrenergic agents, they can be beneficial as ancillary therapy in many patients. Of the three most common derivatives of methylxanthine (theophylline, caffeine, theobromine), only theophylline is used to treat asthma. Theophylline is frequently formulated with ethylenediamine (aminophylline) to improve

Table 72-4. Oral Agents Used to Treat Asthma

Agent	Available tablets	Dose
β-Adrenergics		
Metaproterenol	10 and 20 mg	10-20 mg every 6 hr
Terbutaline	2.5 and 5 mg	2.5-5.0 mg every 6-8 hr
Albuterol	2 and 4 mg	2-4 mg every 6-8 hr
Leukotriene Modifiers		
Zafirlukast (Accolate)	20 mg	1 tab twice daily between meals
Montelukast (Singulair)	10 mg	1 tab each evening
Zileuton (Zyflo)	600 mg	1 tab four times daily
Theophylline		
Sustained release (once or twice daily forms)	100, 200, 300, 400 and 600 mg	Initial: 100-300 mg/day Maximum: 800 mg/day Routine serum levels: 5-15 μg/ml
Prednisone	1, 2.5, 5, 10, 20, 50 mg	1-2 mg/kg/day See text regarding taper
Methylprednisolone	2, 4, 8, 16, 24, 32 mg	0.8 mg/kg/day See text regarding taper

Table 72-5. Inhaled Steroids Used to Treat Asthma

Agent steroid	Daily dose (puffs) Low	Medium	High
Beclomethasone (Vanceril, Beclovent)			
42 μg/puff	4-12	12-20	>20
84 μg/puff	2-6	6-10	>10
Budenoside (Pulmicort Turbuhaler)	1-2*	2-3*	>3*
Flunisolide (AeroBid)	2-4	4-8	>8
Fluticasone (Flovent)			
44 μg/puff	2-6		
110 μg/puff		2-6	
220 μg/puff			>3
Triamcinolone (Azmacort)	4-8	8-12	>12

*Inhalations.

solubility by making the diluent solution more alkaline. Although the actions of methylxanthines were thought to be mediated by inhibition of phosphodiesterases, this requires concentrations much greater than those encountered clinically. In addition to bronchodilation, theophylline appears to increase diaphragmatic contractility, decrease pulmonary artery resistance, and act as a respiratory stimulant.

During acute attacks, aminophylline is often administered intravenously at a rate to maintain blood levels at 5 to 15 μg/ml. Lower blood levels are less effective but may help patients who cannot tolerate higher concentrations. Chronic therapy is generally administered with sustained-release oral medication. As blood concentrations increase, patients develop anorexia, nausea, and vomiting because of the central action of theophylline. The patient may also develop more serious symptoms, such as cardiovascular toxicity with tachycardia, tachyarrhythmias, and hypotension. Nervousness, insomnia, headache, and refractory seizures are central nervous system manifestations of toxicity. Drugs, illnesses, and smoking can have a profound effect on blood levels, complicating therapy. Dosage should be reduced by one third when a patient is given ciprofloxacin or erythromycin and by one half when fever develops or the patient is given cimetidine or oral contraceptives. Dosage should also be decreased in patients receiving zileuton or zafirlukast (see next section). Blood levels should be determined after the onset of therapy or a change in dosage and when bronchospasm worsens or symptoms are consistent with toxicity. Patients should be advised to refrain from taking their next dose and to contact their physicians when these symptoms appear. Theophylline is often recommended in patients with nocturnal asthma resistant to bedtime β-adrenergic agonists.

Leukotriene Inhibitors. Agents that inhibit the synthesis of leukotrienes (zileuton) or block leukotriene receptors (zafirlukast, montelukast) offer a new approach to treating mild or moderate bronchial asthma (see Table 72-4). Zileuton has been associated with elevations in liver enzymes, however, and patients should be monitored periodically for this complication. Also, zileuton should be avoided in patients with preexistent liver disease or alcoholism. Both zileuton and zafirlukast may elevate prothrombin times of patients receiving coumadin and may increase levels of theophylline if taken concomitantly. Churg-Strauss syndrome has occurred in patients taking zafirlukast who were withdrawn from steroids, but the drug has proved to be very safe. Current guidelines suggest that leukotriene inhibitors can replace inhaled steroids, nedocromil, or cromolyn in mild to moderate asthma, using inhaled β-agonists as needed.

Other Medications (Table 72-6). *Cromolyn* (disodium cromoglycate) helps prevent immediate and delayed bronchoconstriction after exposure to antigens. Although its exact mode of action is unclear, cromolyn inhibits release of mediators (e.g., histamine, leukotrienes) from mast cells and has other antiinflammatory properties. The liquid aerosol is less irritating than the powder formerly used. Cromolyn is particularly helpful in children and adults with asthma related to specific allergic responses. It is effective in airway challenges from exposure to animals and substances at work. Cromolyn is less effective than β_2-adrenergic agonists in preventing bronchospasm induced by exercise or exposure to cold. Response may take up to 2 months, and cromolyn provides no relief in an acute asthmatic attack. Cromolyn can prevent bronchospasm, however, if given just before exposure to exercise or a known offending agent. Side effects are rare but include local irritation, cough, hoarseness, and minor complications (dermatitis, myositis, gastroenteritis).

Table 72-6. Inhaled Drugs Other Than Steroids Used to Treat Asthma

Agent	Dose (puffs)
Short-acting β-agonists	
Albuterol	2 qid
Bitolterol (Tornalate)	1-3 qid*
Pirbuterol (Maxair)	2 qid
Terbutaline	2 qid*
Long-acting β-agonist	
Salmeterol (Serevent)	2 bid
Anticholinergic	
Ipratropium (Atrovent)	2 qid
Cromolyn and nedocromil	
Cromolyn (Intal)	2-4 qid
Nedocromil (Tilade)	2 qid
Combination	
Albuterol/ipratropium (Combivent)	2 qid

qid, Four times daily; *bid,* twice daily.
*Puffs separated by 1 to 3 minutes.

Nedocromil is an alternate agent that may have antiinflammatory effects in the airways and may also inhibit reflex reactions to exercise and cold. Although aerosolized anticholinergic drugs have been used primarily for chronic obstructive disease, some asthmatic patients respond to *ipratropium,* which has a slower onset of action than the β-agonists and requires 30 to 60 minutes before maximal effects are achieved. Antibiotics are indicated only if bacterial infection is associated with asthma. *Desensitization* may have a role in the treatment of asthma related to specific pollens and to mites if patients do not respond adequately to routine pharmacotherapy, but it is more effective in the treatment of allergic rhinitis. Magnesium, gold, methotrexate, and cyclosporin have been used to treat asthma but are potentially toxic and must be considered experimental at this time. Bronchoalveolar lavage for status asthmaticus can worsen bronchospasm and probably should be avoided.[1]

ANAPHYLAXIS

Pathophysiology

Anaphylaxis is the most dreaded complication of immediate hypersensitivity. As with other disorders of immediate hypersensitivity, anaphylaxis is initiated by binding of antigen to IgE attached to the surfaces of mast cells, with the subsequent release of agents that mediate vascular leak of protein, smooth muscle contraction, and mobilization of inflammatory cells. The relationship of anaphylaxis to prior atopy remains unclear; the incidence of anaphylactic reactions to both penicillin and bee stings is no more common in subjects with than without atopy. Antigenic substances include proteins and smaller solutes that combine with proteins. The offending agents range from foods, pollens, insect bites, and drugs to latex and ethylene oxide. Some drugs (e.g., NSAIDs) cause anaphylactic-like reactions that may result from direct effects on mast cells rather than from IgE-mediated events.

Etiology

Stings of bees, yellow jackets, wasps, and hornets (all of which are members of the order Hymenoptera) can induce reactions varying from local cutaneous symptoms to the characteristic manifestations of anaphylactic shock. Penicillin is the most common cause of drug-related anaphylaxis, and cross-reaction with cephalosporins is common. Other antibiotics, local anesthetics, and specific foods, such as eggs, seafood, nuts, beans, and chocolate, can also be associated with anaphylaxis. Blood products can cause anaphylactic reactions as well as more common complications such as hemolysis. Patients with an inherited absence of immunoglobulin A may develop severe anaphylaxis after administration of blood or plasma containing this protein.

Patient Evaluation

Within seconds to minutes after exposure (e.g., sting, ingestion, injection) the patient may experience symptoms related to both upper and lower airway obstruction, with hoarseness, stridor, chest tightness, wheezing, and shortness of breath. Pruritic, raised, and erythematous urticaria typically appears in a local or diffuse distribution over the skin. Angioneurotic edema is also common, with localized swelling that does not pit and may or may not be accompanied by local burning or stinging. Angioedema of the larynx and epiglottis may result in asphyxiation. Mucosal swelling, intense bronchospasm, and bronchial edema are found at autopsy with secondary emphysematous overdistention of the lungs. The patient may experience severe hypotension and syncope.

Laboratory Studies and Diagnostic Procedures

Skin tests and radioallergoabsorbent tests are available for both bee stings and penicillin allergies.

Management

Subcutaneous injection of epinephrine (0.2 to 0.5 ml of 1:1000 solution, repeated twice at 20- to 30-minute intervals if needed) remains the cornerstone for immediate treatment of anaphylaxis and should be given as early as possible. Antihistamines and steroids seem to have relatively little effect in the acute episode. Aerosolized bronchodilation and theophylline may be needed as well as oxygen if the patient is hypoxic. If the patient is in profound shock, 5 ml of 1:10,000 epinephrine should be administered intravenously every 5 minutes as needed; if no response is observed, 2 to 50 μg/kg of dopamine is indicated. Patients should wear bracelets indicating agents to which they are allergic; if drug therapy is essential, desensitization with increasing doses of medication administered intradermally, subcutaneously, and then intramuscularly can be tried with an allergist. Immunotherapy is particularly effective in preventing anaphylactic reactions to insect stings but may need to be continued indefinitely if the skin test remains positive. Allergic patients should carry kits for self-administration of epinephrine if they are not receiving immunotherapy.

ALLERGIC RHINITIS

Etiology and Epidemiology

IgE on mast cells and basophils in the nasal mucosa interacting with antigens causes allergic rhinitis, which affects at least 15 million Americans. Pollens are the most common antigens involved, and the disease is frequently seasonal. Many antigens causing asthma can also cause allergic rhinitis. However, many patients have perennial symptoms or vasomotor rhinitis unrelated to specific antigens but aggravated by changes in temperature, humidity, spicy foods, and inhaled irritants.

Patient Evaluation

The cardinal manifestations of allergic rhinitis are nasal obstruction and secretions, sneezing, and itching of the mucous membranes of the nose, eyes, posterior pharynx, and conjunctivae. When symptoms are severe, patients complain of fatigue, loss of appetite, and irritability. The nasal mucous membranes may appear blue with swollen turbinates, and the conjunctivae are injected. Nasal polyps are uncommon unless the patient has aspirin-type allergy, but serious otitis media is common and may lead to hearing defects, especially in young children. Chronic sinusitis may result in throbbing pain over the sinus areas.

Diagnostic Procedures

If negative, scratch, prick, and intradermal skin tests argue against allergic rhinitis. Radioallergoabsorbent and other in vitro tests also are available.

Management

Antigens (e.g., those associated with animals) can frequently be avoided, and levels of pollens can be decreased by remaining indoors and using electrostatic precipitators. The histamine (H_1) receptors can be blocked with a variety of antagonists. Many older agents crossed the blood-brain barrier and caused sleepiness. Loratidine, cetirizine, and fexofenadine are less likely to cause sedation and are not associated with the arrhythmias that were observed with terfenamide and astemizole (which are no longer available in the United States). Antihistamines should be given regularly because they are more effective if administered before than after exposure. Short-acting and long-acting α-adrenergic agents are effective when applied to the nasal mucosa. Continued use for more than a few days, however, results in rebound nasal congestion and reliance on the medication (rhinitis medicamentosa). Oral preparations are also effective but have systemic effects. Nasal steroid aerosols effectively treat allergic rhinitis, although they may not relieve ocular symptoms. Nasal cromolyn can be effective for both prevention and treatment, although a beneficial response may require weeks. Ipratropium nasal aerosol can effectively treat some patients with vasomotor rhinitis. Immunotherapy, using increasing doses of the offending antigen, can also help but requires prolonged therapy. Administration of antigen is believed to result in the development of IgG antibody, which binds to the antigen and limits access to IgE, but other mechanisms have also been proposed.

URTICARIA AND ANGIOEDEMA

Hives (urticaria) are often encountered in primary care practice and may or may not be a manifestation of an allergic reaction. These pruritic, raised lesions are caused by local vasodilation and accumulation of fluid in the superficial skin layers. Fluid entering the deeper tissues causes a nonpitting edema with erythema over a more diffuse area and is referred to as angioedema. Angioedema and urticaria may appear together or independently and more frequently affect young adults. Interaction of IgE on cutaneous mast cells with antigens causes the allergic forms of these disorders. Histamine is released from the mast cells and interacts with receptors in the venules, which dilate and leak fluid and inflammatory cells. If the symptoms persist for more than 6 weeks, the disorder is considered to be chronic. In the great majority of patients, no cause is ever found for chronic urticaria-angioedema. In addition to recurrent reactions to defined antigens, urticaria may be initiated by physical stimuli such as cold exposure or exercise (either of which can result in life-threatening anaphylaxis), heat, stroking (dermatographism), vibration, sun exposure, and pressure. Inherited and acquired deficiencies in the inhibitor (CINH) of the activated form of the first component of complement (C1) can result in angioedema not associated with urticaria. Urticaria can also be seen in some forms of vasculitis. Antihistamine therapy may be of some help in treating patients with these disorders, and steroids are also effective in some patients (see Chapter 95).

REFERENCES

1. Barnes PJ, Rodger IW, Thomson NC, editors: *Asthma: basic mechanisms and clinical management,* ed 3, Philadelphia, 1998, Academic Press.
2. Brookes SM, Weiss MA, Bernstein K: Reactive airways dysfunction syndrome (RADS): persistent asthma syndrome after high level irritant exposures, *Chest* 88:376, 1985.
3. Buist AS: Is asthma mortality increasing? *Chest* 93:449, 1988.
4. Djukanovic R, Roche WR, Wilson JW, et al: Mucosal inflammation in asthma, *Am Rev Respir Dis* 142:434, 1990.
5. *Guidelines for the diagnosis and management of asthma,* NIH Pub No 97-4051, Bethesda, Md, 1997, National Institutes of Health.
6. Lemanske RF Jr, Busse WW: Asthma, *JAMA* 278:1855, 1997.
7. *Practical guide for diagnosis and management of asthma,* NIH Pub No 97-4053, Bethesda, Md, 1997, National Institutes of Health.
8. Silverstein MD, Reed CE, O'Connell EJ, et al: Long-term survival of a cohort of community residents with asthma, *N Engl J Med* 331:1537, 1994.
9. Venables KM, Chan-Yeung M: Occupational asthma, *Lancet* 349:1465, 1997.
10. Weiss KB, Gergen PJ, Hodgson TA: An economic evaluation of asthma in the United States, *N Engl J Med* 326:862, 1992.

CHAPTER 73

Pneumonia

Randolph J. Lipchik

More than 2 million cases of community-acquired pneumonia (CAP) occur each year in the United States, resulting in approximately 10 million physician visits, more than 500,000 hospitalizations, and approximately 50,000 deaths. Over time the number of microorganisms identified as pathogens has increased, along with new broad-spectrum antibiotics available for treatment. At the same time, common pathogens have become increasingly resistant to frequently used antibiotics, complicating the management of CAP and prompting the development of management guidelines.

EPIDEMIOLOGY

The actual incidence of pneumonia in ambulatory patients is difficult to estimate because the etiologic agent is rarely identified except in clinical trials, and CAP is not currently considered a reportable disease. Each year in the United States there are 2 to 3 million cases of CAP. The incidence of hospitalization is estimated at 260 cases per 100,000 population but is about fourfold higher in those over age 65. CAP results in about 500,000 hospitalizations annually, with approximately 45,000 deaths; pneumonia is the sixth most common cause of death in the United States. Between 1979 and 1994, pneumonia and influenza–related death rates have increased because of the increasing number of patients over 65 and patients with underlying illnesses. Studies of patients with CAP report mortality rates of 5.1% to 36.5%, averaging about 14%.[4] An analysis of 1993 hospital discharge data from Washington, Illinois, and Florida revealed death rates of 7.0%, 8.1%, and 9.7%, respectively.[6] Risk factors for mortality include age, alcoholism, bacteremia, and multilobar involvement on radiographs. Contributing factors include underlying malignancy, immunosuppression, neurologic disease, congestive heart failure, and diabetes. Aspiration, postobstructive, gram-negative, and *Staphylococcus aureus* forms of pneumonia are also associated with higher mortality risk.

Pathophysiology

Traditionally thought to be responsible for 60% to 70% of pneumonias, the prevalence of *Streptococcus pneumoniae* has decreased with the identification of other agents (Table 73-1). The likelihood of each of these agents causing disease in a given patient is not certain, although certain host factors and geographic location may predispose to certain infections (Table 73-2). Travel to southwestern United States, including California and Texas, and contiguous areas of Mexico suggests *Coccidioides immitis. Histoplasma capsulatum* is endemic in states bordering the Mississippi and Ohio rivers. *Blastomyces dermatitidis* is endemic in southeastern United States but also in Wisconsin, Minnesota, and neighboring Canadian provinces. Exposure to birds necessitates the addition of psittacosis to the differential diagnosis, and exposure to parturient cats, cattle, or sheep suggests Q fever *(Coxiella burnetii).*

Table 73-1. Causes of Community-acquired Bacterial Pneumonia

Pathogen	Prevalence (%)
Streptococcus pneumoniae	30-75
Mycoplasma pneumoniae	5-35
Haemophilus influenzae	6-12
Staphylococcus aureus	3-10
Legionella pneumophila	3-30*
Gram-negative organisms	3-10
Chlamydia pneumoniae	5-12
Moraxella (Branhamella) catarrhalis	0.5-1
Viruses	2-10

*High prevalence in specific geographic locations.

Table 73-2. Association of Host Factors with Particular Pathogens

Condition	Pathogen(s)
Chronic obstructive pulmonary disease	*S. pneumoniae, H. influenzae, M. catarrhalis*
Alcoholism	*S. pneumoniae, Klebsiella pneumoniae, Staphylococcus aureus*
Diabetes	*S. aureus, S. pneumoniae*
Sickle cell anemia, asplenism	*S. pneumoniae, H. influenzae, S. aureus*
Postinfluenza status	*S. aureus, S. pneumoniae*
Neutropenia	*S. aureus, S. pneumoniae, enteric gram-negative bacteria*
Injection drug use	*S. aureus*
Human immunodeficiency virus (HIV) infection	*Pneumocystis carinii, S. pneumoniae*

The respiratory tract is a unique system in that it is open to the external environment and therefore continuously exposed to microorganisms, particulate matter, and fumes. In addition to all the organisms that are coughed or sneezed into the environment by others, humans regularly aspirate nasopharyngeal flora during sleep. Multiple defense mechanisms counteract these continuous exposures, including mechanical, anatomic, and immunologic barriers. The cough reflex, the mucociliary transport mechanism, and secretory immunoglobulins remove and neutralize microbes in the upper and central airways. In the alveoli the alveolar macrophages, immunoglobulins, and complement combine to clear organisms from the distal lung. Alterations in mental status may reduce the cough reflex; mucous production and ciliary function can be overcome by viral illness or tobacco smoke; and the immune response can be blunted by many illnesses or medications. Loss of these defenses in the setting of a large inoculum or particularly virulent organism can produce significant infection. Whether or not colonization of the upper airway is necessary before the development of pneumonia is unclear. In the outpatient population the carrier rate for *S. pneumoniae* is quite high but the incidence of pneumonia quite low. In hospitalized patients, however, colonization by gram-negative organisms probably occurs before development of pneumonia. In a few patients, pneumonia may result from hematogenously spread infection.

Annual vaccination against influenza should reduce its incidence and that of secondary bacterial pneumonias. Vaccination against pneumococcal infection is recommended for patients 65 years and older and for younger persons at increased risk, that is, with anatomic or functional asplenia (including sickle cell disease), cardiovascular disease, pulmonary disease, diabetes mellitus, alcoholism, cirrhosis, and cerebrospinal leaks. The current vaccine is a 23-valent preparation that provides coverage against approximately 90% of the most frequently reported capsular types. Routine revaccination of adults is not currently recommended unless the patient is at high risk for pneumococcal infection (asplenic) and originally received the 14-valent vaccine. Revaccination should also be considered for persons 65 or older who received the vaccine 5 or more years earlier and were under age 65 at the time of primary vaccination. Although evidence is lacking, single revaccination should also be considered in immunocompromised patients if 5 or more years have elapsed since initial vaccination.

PATIENT EVALUATION

History

Because of the multiple potential pathogens that cause pneumonia, the history becomes especially important in the evaluation of a patient with pneumonia. Presence or absence of fever, dry or productive cough, acute or gradual onset, and presence of chest pain and dyspnea may help distinguish upper from lower respiratory infection and a "typical" from an "atypical" pneumonia. In contrast to typical (pneumococcal) pneumonia, atypical pneumonia is characterized by lack of sputum production, lack of chest pain, and radiographic infiltrates that are not evident on physical examination. Agents causing atypical pneumonia are *Mycoplasma pneumoniae, Chlamydia pneumoniae,* viruses, and *Coxiella burnetii.* Concomitant medical conditions, recent travel, and animal exposure help to direct evaluation and therapy.

Physical Examination

Attention to all aspects of the physical examination is crucial to determining severity of illness, hospitalization, and possibly treatment. Fever is nonspecific, but a pulse-temperature disparity (normal pulse in the setting of high fever) suggests pneumonia from *Mycoplasma, Legionella, Chlamydia,* or virus. Tachypnea and cyanosis indicate significant respiratory compromise and thus careful consideration before choosing outpatient vs. inpatient therapy. Examination of the thorax may be unremarkable, reveal evidence of consolidation (dullness to percussion, increased tactile fremitus, egophony), suggest interstitial infiltrates (crackles), or present evidence of a pleural effusion (dullness to percussion, decreased tactile fremitus, decreased breath sounds). Extrapulmonary findings should not be overlooked and can offer clues to the underlying pathogen (Table 73-3). Neurologic disease, altered level of consciousness, and recent seizures suggest aspiration pneumonia. Periodontal disease makes an anaerobic infection more likely.

DIAGNOSIS

Diagnostic Procedures

The chest radiograph is the gold standard for determining the presence or absence of pneumonia. For many years, the radiographic pattern was thought to be useful in determining the etiology of the pneumonia, but with more pathogens and more elderly and immunocompromised patients, this has become less reliable. The presence of an abscess, central mass, or pleural effusion, however, is very helpful in management decision making. Because of the lack of specificity of the chest radiograph, supplemental studies are necessary to determine an etiology. Examination of a sputum sample provides data that are available at the presentation and may help guide therapy. Unfortunately, most patients cannot produce a sample, and if they do, it is often contaminated by oral flora. Nonetheless, a sputum smear with fewer than 10 squamous cells and greater than 25 neutrophils per high-power field should be representative of the secretions in the lung. Sputum culture requires 24 to 48 hours and may not provide diagnostic information. For example, the sensitivity for pneumococcus is only about 50%.

Several invasive methods can be employed when sputum is unobtainable, but the risks must be considered compared with the use of empiric antibiotics, a safe and usually successful treatment. Transtracheal aspiration consists of passing a catheter via a large-bore needle through the cricothyroid membrane to allow aspiration of material distal to the oropharynx, thus avoiding contamination by oral flora. Its sensitivity has been questioned, the potential for complications is real, and transtracheal aspiration is rarely employed. Bronchoscopy can be employed to obtain distal samples, but passage through the upper airway makes contamination difficult to avoid. Quantitative cultures obtained during bronchoscopy with a protected brush or by bronchoalveolar lavage may distinguish infection from colonization or contamination. If the patient has already received antibiotics, however, the results have poor predictive value. This approach does have a useful role in evaluating the immunocompromised patient and cases of nonresolving pneumonias, but routine use is not justified because standard antibiotics are effective and low risk.

In addition to sputum cultures, blood cultures should be obtained, although on average only 10% to 15% of patients hospitalized for pneumonia have bacteremia. If a pleural effusion is present, a thoracentesis is performed to obtain material for Gram's stain and culture. Infections with *Mycoplasma, Legionella, Chlamydia, Coxiella,* and some viruses can be proved with serologic assays, but because convalescent titers must be drawn at least 3 weeks after onset of illness, empiric therapy is still necessary. Cold agglutinins may rise after 7 to 14 days of infection in *Mycoplasma* infections but are nonspecific, and similar increases can also be seen with influenza. *Legionella* can be detected in sputum, pleural fluid, or tissue by direct immunofluorescent staining with a specificity of 90% to 100% but a sensitivity of only 25% to 50%. Detection of *Legionella* antigen in the urine

Table 73-3. Extrapulmonary Findings and Causes of Pneumonia

Finding	Organism(s)
Bullous myringitis	*Mycoplasma pneumoniae*
Erythema multiforme	*M. pneumoniae, Histoplasma capsulatum, Coccidioides immitis,* some viruses
Erythema nodosum	Tuberculosis, *Chlamydia* species, *H. capsulatum, C. immitis*
Absent gag reflex from seizure activity or central nervous system disease	*Bacteroides* species, aerobic and anaerobic streptococci; include *S. aureus* and gram-negative organisms for institutionalized patients
Periodontal disease	Anaerobes
Encephalitis	*Legionella pneumophila, M. pneumoniae, Coxiella burnetii*

Table 73-4. Differential Diagnosis of Pneumonia and Selected Noninfectious Pulmonary Diseases

Disease	Clinical features	Radiographic appearance
Pulmonary embolism	Sudden dyspnea, low-grade fever; cough not characteristic	Usually normal, but atelectasis or small pleural effusion may be seen; peripheral consolidation with infarct
Congestive heart failure	Increased jugular venous pressure, S_3 gallop, no fever or purulent sputum	Large cardiac shadow, bilateral infiltrates; may be asymmetric in chronic obstructive pulmonary disease
Lymphangitic carcinomatosis	Insidious, but progressive dyspnea	Resembles pulmonary edema
Alveolar hemorrhage		
Rapidly progressive glomerulonephritis	Abrupt dyspnea, falling hematocrit, hemoptysis (50%), abnormal urinalysis	Bilateral infiltrates
Systemic vasculitis: Wegener's granulomatosis, microscopic polyarteritis, systemic lupus erythematosus		
Hypersensitivity pneumonitis	Flulike illness, relevant exposure history	Diffuse bilateral reticulonodular infiltrates
Bronchiolitis obliterans with organizing pneumonia	Indistinguishable from pneumonia	Bilateral consolidation

is more useful, with sensitivity as high as 86%. Blood chemistries and leukocyte count with differential are quite nonspecific. An elevated leukocyte count with a left shift is common in any infection, and a low leukocyte count does not rule out a bacterial infection. Although hyponatremia, hypophosphatemia, and liver function abnormalities are associated with *Legionella* infection, these abnormalities can also be seen with other severe infections.

Differential Diagnosis

Radiographic pulmonary infiltrates, cough, dyspnea, and fever are the presenting features of not only pneumonia, but many noninfectious conditions as well, including pulmonary embolism, congestive heart failure (CHF), malignancy, vasculitis, collagen vascular disease, hypersensitivity, and idiopathic processes (Table 73-4). Often the presentation and clinical clues help distinguish these from a community-acquired infection, but failure to respond to standard empiric therapy or unexpected progression should alert the physician to reconsider the initial diagnosis. Pulmonary embolism usually presents with sudden onset of dyspnea and often in the setting of immobilization, the perioperative period, CHF, or malignancy. Chest pain and hemoptysis, which signify pulmonary infarction, occur in a minority of patients. The chest radiograph is usually normal in patients without infarction but may show evidence of atelectasis or a small pleural effusion. CHF is usually distinguishable from pneumonia because of elevated jugular venous pressure, no fever, and no productive cough. In patients with chronic obstructive pulmonary disease (COPD), pulmonary edema may produce infiltrates that are asymmetric or focal. Resolution within hours to a day with diuresis will confirm the presence of pulmonary edema.

Malignancy may present as a segmental consolidation, atelectasis, or diffuse interstitial pattern but presents clinically with a subacute development of cough or dyspnea. Fever, if present, is usually low grade, and the cough is frequently dry. Radiographic abnormalities are often present without significant symptoms. The abrupt onset of dyspnea, hypoxemia, radiographic infiltrates, variable degrees of hemoptysis, and a falling hematocrit are seen in alveolar hemorrhage. This can occur in the setting of rapidly progressive glomerulonephritis or systemic necrotizing vasculitis (e.g., Wegener's granulomatosis, microscopic polyarteritis, systemic lupus erythematosus). The rapid progression of renal abnormalities and extrapulmonary evidence of vasculitis should suggest a noninfectious process. The presentation of hypersensitivity pneumonitis (e.g., farmer's lung, humidifier lung) includes fever, dry cough, and pulmonary infiltrates within 4 to 6 hours of exposure to inhaled organic antigens (e.g., thermophilic actinomycetes). Eliciting the history of inhalational exposure is the only way to distinguish this illness from CAP.

Several medications have been associated with acute onset of a pneumonia-like illness. Nitrofurantoin can cause fever, dry cough, dyspnea, and infiltrates; a detailed history and peripheral blood eosinophilia are clues to the diagnosis. Amiodarone can also produce pulmonary infiltrates; the diagnosis is often one of exclusion because no distinguishing diagnostic features are specific for this process.

An idiopathic process such as bronchiolitis obliterans with organizing pneumonia (BOOP) may be initially confused with infectious pneumonia because of cough, dyspnea, alveolar infiltrates, and constitutional symptoms. Failure to respond to antibiotics may lead to open lung biopsy, the definitive way to confirm the diagnosis.

MANAGEMENT

Management of pneumonia must include both antibiotic therapy directed against the causative organism and supportive measures. The latter include rest, adequate hydration to correct for fever-induced fluid loss and poor intake, supplemental oxygen for saturation less than 90%, and analgesia for chest pain. Chest percussion and postural drainage may be useful in selected patients with bronchiectasis or those too weak to generate an adequate cough. Routine use of this time-consuming and labor-intensive modality, however, is not beneficial in uncomplicated pneumonias.

Antibiotic therapy should be administered as quickly as possible once the diagnosis has been confirmed radiographically. Ideally the choice of antibiotic should be guided by a

Table 73-5. Empiric Antibiotic Selection for Patients with Community-acquired Pneumonia

Group/factors	Antibiotic therapy
Outpatients	**Macrolides,* fluoroquinolones,† or doxycycline**
Modifying factors	
Suspected penicillin-resistant *Pneumococcus*	Fluoroquinolones
Aspiration	Amoxicillin/clavulanate
Young adults (ages 17-40 yr)	Doxycycline
Inpatients	
General medical ward	β-Lactam‡ with or without a macrolide, *or* a fluoroquinolone alone
	Cefuroxime with or without a macrolide, *or* azithromycin alone
Intensive care unit	Erthyromycin, azithromycin, or a fluoroquinolone *plus* cefotaxime, ceftriaxone, or a β-lactam/β-lactamase inhibitor§
Modifying factors	
Chronic obstructive pulmonary disease, bronchiectasis	Antipseudomonal penicillin, a carbapenem, or cefepime *plus* a macrolide or fluoroquinolone *plus* an aminoglycoside
Penicillin allergy	Fluoroquinolone with or without clindamycin
Suspected aspiration	Fluoroquinolone *plus* clindamycin or a β-lactam/β-lactamase inhibitor alone

Modified from Bartlett JG, Brieman RF, Mandell LA, File TM Jr: *Clin Infect Dis* 26:811, 1998.

*Azithromycin, clarithromycin, or erythromycin.

†Levofloxacin, sparfloxacin, grepafloxacin, trovafloxacin, or another fluoroquinolone with enhanced activity against *Pneumococcus*.

‡Cefotaxime, ceftriaxone, or a β-lactam/β-lactamase inhibitor.

§Ampicillin/sulbactam, ticarcillin/clavulanate, or piperacillin/tazobactam.

Table 73-6. Antibiotic Choices for Specific Pathogens

Pathogen	Antibiotic of choice	Alternative
Streptococcus pneumoniae		
Penicillin susceptible (MIC <0.1 μg/ml)	Penicillin, amoxicillin	Cephalosporins,* macrolides, clindamycin, FQ, doxycycline
Intermediate penicillin resistance (MIC 0.1-1 μg/ml)	Ceftriaxone, cefotaxime, FQ	Clindamycin, doxycycline, oral cephalosporins
Highly penicillin resistant† (MIC ≥2 μg/ml)	FQ, vancomycin, others based on in vitro testing	
Haemophilus influenzae	Second/third-generation cephalosporins, doxycycline, β-lactam/β-lactamase inhibitor, FQ	Azithromycin, TMP-SMX
Moraxella (Branhamella) catarrhalis	Second/third-generation cephalosporins, TMP-SMX amoxicillin/clavulanate	Macrolides, FQ, β-lactam/β-lactamase inhibitor
Anaerobes	Clindamycin, penicillin *plus* metronidazole, β-lactam/β-lactamase inhibitor	
Staphylococcus aureus†		
Methicillin susceptible	Nafcillin with or without gentamicin	Cefazolin, cefuroxime, vancomycin, clindamycin, TMP/SMX, FQ
Methicillin resistant	Vancomycin with or without gentamicin	Based on in vitro testing
Enterobacteriaceae		
Escherichia coli, Klebsiella, Proteus, Enterobacter†	Third-generation cephalosporin with or without an aminoglycoside, carbapenems	β-Lactam/β-lactamase inhibitor, FQ
Pseudomonas	Aminoglycoside *plus* antipseudomonal β-lactam‡	Aminoglycoside *plus* ciprofloxacin, ciprofloxacin *plus* antipseudomonal β-lactam‡
Legionella	Macrolides with or without rifampin, FQ	Doxycycline with or without rifampin
Mycoplasma	Doxycycline, macrolides, FQ	
Chlamydia pneumoniae	Doxycycline, macrolides, FQ	
Chlamydia psittaci	Doxycycline	Erythromycin, chloramphenicol
Coxiella	Tetracycline	Chloramphenicol

Modified from Bartlett JG, Brieman RF, Mandell LA, File TM Jr: *Clin Infect Dis* 26:811, 1998.

FQ, Fluoroquinolones: levofloxacin, sparfloxacin, grepafloxacin, trovafloxacin; ciprofloxacin is appropriate for *Legionella,* FQ-susceptible *S. aureus,* and most gram-negative bacilli; *MIC,* minimum inhibitory concentration; *TMP-SMX,* trimethoprim-sulfamethoxazole.

*Intravenous: cefazolin, cefuroxime, cefotaxime, ceftriaxone; oral: cefpodoxime, cefprozil, cefuroxime.

†In vitro susceptibility tests are required for optimal therapy; FQ and carbapenems are preferred for *Enterobacter*.

‡Piperacillin, ticarcillin, ceftazidime, cefepime, carbapenems.

Gram's stain of sputum. Many polymorphonuclear neutrophils (PMNs), no epithelial cells, and a predominant organism allow more specific therapy; most often, however, the choice is empiric, and all the clinical data must be considered before deciding on a regimen. In 1993 the American Thoracic Society published guidelines for the initial management of patients with CAP.[7] In 1998 the Infectious Diseases Society of America published their guidelines for CAP in immunocompetent adults, which is evidence based where possible.[2] Both these documents are guidelines and require prospective validation.

Unless the presentation or history suggests a particular pathogen, the macrolides, newer fluoroquinolones, and doxycycline are the drugs of first choice because they are effective for the agents causing the vast majority of CAPs (i.e., *S. pneumoniae, M. pneumoniae*). For sicker patients with comorbidities, initial therapy may need to be broader. Therapy can be altered or narrowed if sputum or blood cultures yield an organism (Tables 73-5 and 73-6).

Penicillin-resistant Pneumococci

The empiric use of penicillin for CAP is no longer acceptable given the rise of penicillin-resistant pneumococci. The incidence of penicillin resistance is approximately 23% in selected centers in western Europe and the United States[5] but as high as 50% to 60% in South Africa, Spain, eastern Europe, and Korea. The resistance is caused by alteration in penicillin-binding proteins, not the production of a β-lactamase. Of even more concern is the parallel resistance seen to other antibiotics, such as macrolides, trimethoprim-sulfamethoxazole (TMP-SMX), and tetracycline. About 30% of penicillin-resistant pneumococci are resistant to erythromycin, which predicts resistance to azithromycin and clarithromycin. Primary care physicians must be aware of the microbiology in their institutions and geographic locales to provide effective empiric antibiotic therapy.

Elderly Patients

The diagnosis of pneumonia and therapy in the geriatric population deserves special attention, particularly if the patient is a nursing home resident. Classic symptoms of cough, sputum production, chest pain, and fever occur much less often in weak, debilitated patients. Coughing requires adequate muscle strength, and pleuritic pain and fever result from a vigorous inflammatory response; these may be lacking in elderly patients with poor nutrition or poor general health.

Table 73-7. Pneumonia in Immunocompromised Patients

Condition/therapy	Pathogens
Leukemia/lymphoma, high-dose prolonged steroid therapy, organ transplants	CMV, PCP, *Cryptococcus, Nocardia, Legionella*
Neutropenia (<500 cells/mm^3)	Gram-negative bacteria, *Aspergillus, Mucor, Candida*
Immunosuppressive drug therapy (e.g., steroids, cyclophosphamide, methotrexate)	Gram-positive and gram-negative bacteria, PCP, CMV

CMV, Cytomegalovirus; *PCP, Pneumocystis carinii* pneumonia.

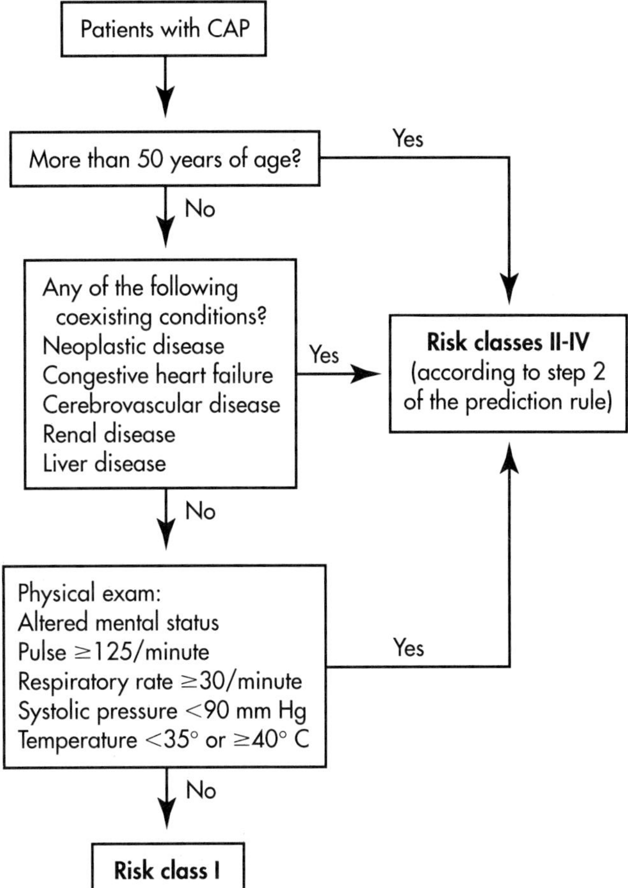

Fig. 73-1. Assessing risk in community-acquired pneumonia *(CAP)* and identifying patients in risk class I. (From Fine MJ, Auble TE, Yealy DM, et al: *N Engl J Med* 336:243, 1997.)

Box 73-1. Accepted Criteria for Hospital Admission in Treatment of Pneumonia

1. Inability to take oral medications
2. Multilobar involvement on chest radiograph
3. Severe vital sign abnormality (pulse >125/min, systolic blood pressure <90 mm Hg, respiratory rate >30/min
4. Acute mental status changes
5. Arterial hypoxemia (room air oxygen tension <60 mm Hg)
6. Secondary suppurative infection (e.g., empyema, meningitis, endocarditis)
7. Severe acute electrolyte, hematologic, or metabolic abnormality (serum sodium <130 mmol/L, hematocrit <30%, absolute neutrophil count <1000/mm^3, blood urea nitrogen >50 mg/dl, creatinine >2.5 mg/dl)
8. Acute coexistent medical conditions (e.g., suspected acute myocardial infarction, renal insufficiency, liver disease, malignancy)

Confusion and mental status changes may be the predominant clinical findings. Although *S. pneumoniae* is the most common pathogen, other agents such as *H. influenzae* (which produces β-lactamase in greater than 15% of cases) and *M. catarrhalis* must be considered, particularly in patients with COPD. Gram-negative bacilli are also more common, particularly in the chronically institutionalized patient. *M. pneumoniae* is an uncommon pathogen in the older patient. *Legionella* incidence is variable, being more prevalent in certain U.S. regions and during epidemic outbreaks.

Immunocompromised Patients

Altered immunity can result from HIV infection, leukemia or lymphoma, chemotherapy-induced granulocytopenia, or treatment for a variety of illnesses with long-term steroids and cytotoxic agents. The evaluation and treatment of a pneumonia in these patients should be in hospital. Because the morbidity and mortality of infections are much higher than in the general population, prompt empiric therapy and diagnostic procedures are essential. Initial empiric antibiotic therapy must cover multiple potential pathogens (Table 73-7). Because of the possibility of unusual and multiple pathogens, invasive diagnostic procedures such as bronchoscopy with bronchoalveolar lavage are considered in the first 24 to 48 hours in addition to cultures of sputum, blood, and other fluids. Although pulmonary infiltrates may also represent drug or radiation toxicity or an underlying leukemia or lymphoma, these can be considered only after an infectious etiology has been ruled out.

Once therapy has been initiated, fever, respiratory and cardiovascular status, and general features such as energy and appetite should be monitored. Most patients receiving appropriate antibiotics will improve within 48 to 72 hours. Fever that continues 24 hours into therapy is not necessarily a failure of antibiotics. A gradual decrease in the maximum daily temperature is the usual response to therapy. Persistent fever with worsening clinical status may indicate a suppurative complication (e.g., empyema), an inappropriate choice of antibiotics, the wrong diagnosis, or drug fever.

Few data address duration of therapy for pneumonia in general. *S. pneumoniae* should be treated until the patient has been afebrile for at least 72 hours. *Mycoplasma* and *Chlamydia* pneumonia should be treated for 14 days, and confirmed cases of *Legionella* require 14 to 21 days. For hospitalized patients, controversy surrounds when to switch from intravenous to oral antibiotics. In general, once a patient has become afebrile, is clinically improving, can tolerate oral intake, and has a functioning gastrointestinal tract, oral antibiotics can be considered. Radiographic infiltrates may completely clear only after many weeks, particularly with pneumococcal pneumonia. Slow radiographic resolution does not mean a failure of therapy in the face of clinical response, and frequent chest radiographs are not necessary. Consultation by a pulmonary or infectious diseases specialist should be considered for immunocompromised patients, those who fail to respond in a typical manner, and those with suppurative complications or respiratory compromise.

Table 73-8. Point Scoring System to Identify Risk in Patients with Pneumonia*

Characteristic	Points
Age	
Men	Age (years)
Women	Age (years) minus 10
Nursing home resident	+10
Coexisting illnesses	
Neoplasm	+30
Liver disease	+20
Congestive heart failure	+10
Cerebrovascular disease	+10
Renal disease	+10
Physical examination findings	
Acutely altered mental status	+20
Respiratory rate ≥30/min	+20
Systolic blood pressure <90 mm Hg	+20
Temperature <35° or ≥40° C	+15
Pulse ≥125/min	+10
Laboratory and radiographic findings	
Arterial pH <7.35	+30
Blood urea nitrogen ≥30 mg/dl	+20
Sodium <130 mmol/L	+20
Glucose ≥250 mg/dl	+10
Hematocrit <30%	+10
Partial pressure of arterial oxygen <60 mm Hg	+10
Pleural effusion	+10

From Fine MJ, Auble TE, Yealy DM, et al: *N Engl J Med* 336:243, 1997.
*Total score for a given patient is obtained by summing the patient's age in years and the points for each applicable characteristic. See Table 73-9.

Table 73-9. Hospitalization and Mortality According to Pneumonia Risk Class

Risk class (points)	Patients subsequently hospitalized	Mortality	
		Inpatients (%)	Outpatients (%)
I	587 (5.1)	185 (0.5)	587 (0.0)
II (≤70)	244 (8.2)	233 (0.9)	244 (0.4)
III (71-90)	72 (16.7)	254 (1.2)	72 (0.0)
IV (91-130)	40 (20.0)	446 (9.0)	40 (12.5)
V (>130)	1 (0.0)	225 (27.1)	1 (0.0)

Modified from Fine MJ, Auble TE, Yealy DM, et al: *N Engl J Med* 336:243, 1997.

Indications for Hospitalization

The need for hospitalization must be carefully considered because inadequate therapy can lead to increased morbidity and mortality (Box 73-1). Because rates of hospitalization vary greatly from region to region, data from more than 38,000 patients were used to develop a prediction rule to identify patients with CAP at low risk for mortality.[3] This was then validated prospectively on approximately 2200 patients in the pneumonia patient outcomes (PORT) cohort study. An algorithm stratifies patients into different risk groups (Fig. 73-1 and Tables 73-8 and 73-9). Outpatient therapy for patients in risk classes I and II, brief inpatient observation for risk class III, and standard inpatient care for risk classes IV and V would theoretically have reduced the number of patients receiving inpatient therapy by more than 30%. When this prediction rule was later used in an emergency department, the percentage of patients initially treated as outpatients increased from 42% to 57%, although this was offset somewhat by a 9% increase in the number of outpatients subsequently admitted to hospital.[1] Use of such a prediction rule requires further study. Clinical judgment must still ultimately guide such decisions in individual cases.

EBM EVIDENCE-BASED MEDICINE

The primary source for this chapter was MEDLINE. Electronic searches dating back to 1994 focused on systematic reviews, meta-analyses, and randomized trials.

REFERENCES

1. Atlas SJ, Benzer TI, Borowsky LH, et al: Safely increasing the proportion of patients with community-acquired pneumonia treated as outpatients, *Arch Intern Med* 158:1350, 1998.
2. Bartlett JG, Breiman RF, Mandell LA, File TM Jr: Community-acquired pneumonia in adults: guidelines for management, *Clin Infect Dis* 26:811, 1998.
3. Fine MJ, Auble TE, Yealy DM, et al: A prediction rule to identify low-risk patients with community-acquired pneumonia, *N Engl J Med* 336:243, 1997.
4. Fine MJ, Smith MA, Carson CA, et al: Prognosis and outcomes of patients with community-acquired pneumonia: a meta-analysis, *JAMA* 275:134, 1996.
5. Goldstein FW, Acar JF: Antimicrobial resistance among lower respiratory tract isolates of *Streptococcus pneumoniae:* results of a 1992-93 western Europe and USA collaborative surveillance study, *J Antimicrob Chemother* 38(suppl A):71, 1996.
6. Markowitz JS, Pashko S, Gutterman EM, et al: Death rates among patients hospitalized with community-acquired pneumonia: a reexamination with data from three states, *Am J Public Health* 86:1152, 1996.
7. Niederman MS, Bass Jr JB, Campbell GD, et al: Guidelines for the initial management of adults with community-acquired pneumonia: diagnosis, assessment of severity, and initial antimicrobial therapy, *Am Rev Respir Dis* 148:1418, 1993.

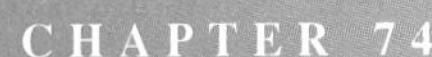

Tuberculosis and Nontuberculous Mycobacterial Diseases

David Rosenzweig

TUBERCULOSIS

Epidemiology

In the twentieth century the incidence of tuberculosis in the United States continuously declined until 1985. Between 1900 and 1985 annual tuberculosis mortality dropped from 200 to less than two per 100,000 population, more than a hundredfold decrease. From 1985 to 1993 the cases increased, but since then the decrease has resumed, and in 1997 the incidence was less than 20,000 new cases for the first time. Although declines have occurred worldwide, tuberculosis remains the most important fatal infection, accounting for 3 million deaths annually. Most deaths (2.5 million) occur in developing nations, where tuberculosis accounts for 6.7% of all deaths, 18.5% of deaths among persons 15 to 59 years of age, and 26% of all preventable deaths. Those who have been infected by *Mycobacterium tuberculosis* (i.e., tuberculin reactors) number almost 2 billion, more than one third of humankind.

Recently tuberculosis has been resurgent both in the United States and throughout the world, especially in Africa and Asia. Fueled by the acquired immunodeficiency syndrome (AIDS) epidemic and such factors as immigration, poverty, homelessness, and deterioration of public health programs, substantial increases in tuberculosis have occurred. In the United States these increases or outbreaks have been focused in larger cities and particularly in closed institutions (shelters, penal institutions, nursing homes, hospitals). Also, the age incidence of tuberculosis cases has shifted from elderly persons to younger adults, especially in minority populations, implying greater recent infection in these groups (Fig. 74-1). The problem has been compounded by an increase in drug-resistant cases. Drug resistance is especially prominent in Asia, Africa, Russia and other parts of eastern Europe, and Latin America, as well as the United States, but with modern travel, no part of the world is spared from drug resistance problems.

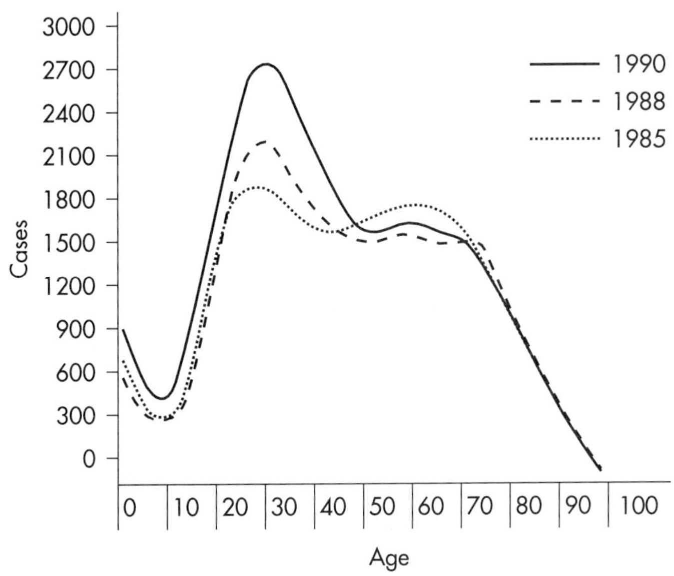

Fig. 74-1. Age distribution of reported tuberculosis cases by year of report, United States, 1985-1990. (From Jereb JA et al: *MMWR* 40:23, 1991.)

Etiology

In 1882 Robert Koch first demonstrated that tuberculosis is an infectious disease caused by *M. tuberculosis*. The bacillus is a rod 1 to 4 μm long with a waxy cell wall that accounts for its resistance to acid-stain decoloring, referred to as acid fastness. The organism is hardy, requiring minimal nutrients for culture and able to survive adverse conditions for long periods. A closely related organism, *M. bovis,* can cause bovine tuberculosis, a similar illness, but this infection has virtually disappeared from the United States due to elimination of its source in infected dairy herds and pasteurization of milk products.

Natural History

Airborne spread from an infected person, the usual mode of infection, is especially likely to occur during aerosolization of droplets in speaking, singing, coughing, or sneezing. Such droplets quickly evaporate to droplet nuclei, which are capable of penetrating deeply into the respiratory tract. Infected droplet nuclei of 1 to 5 μm can penetrate and be deposited at the alveolar level, where infection is likely to occur, especially with repeated exposure and close household contact.

Initially the host mounts no defense and the mycobacteria multiply, but within days, cellular and humoral defense mechanisms develop. At first, organisms are lysed within macrophages, and mycobacterial antigens become accessible to T and B lymphocytes. Sensitized T lymphocytes secrete lymphokines, which attract and enhance macrophage activity, making phagocytosis and bacterial killing much more effective. This process occurs over 4 to 6 weeks and parallels the development of tuberculin reactivity. This reaction, which depends on activated T lymphocytes, appears 3 to 12 weeks (mean 6 weeks) after inoculation.

The stage of primary tuberculosis also appears at about this time. It may be subclinical and is usually nonspecific with symptoms of fever and cough, which subside over 2 to 3 weeks. If tuberculosis is suspected and the patient is evaluated, the chest radiograph may show a middle or lower segmental infiltrate and enlarged hilar lymph nodes. Children may have atelectasis from lymph node compression. Mycobacterial stains and cultures of respiratory specimens, sputum, or bronchial lavage may be negative in more than half the cases because the organisms are still relatively few at this stage. Transient mycobacteremia occurs during primary tuberculosis, however, seeding distant sites for potential later reactivation of disease, most often the pulmonary apex, renal cortex, epiphyses of long bones, and meninges.

Primary tuberculosis can then spontaneously subside and lead to several outcomes: (1) no further disease and no residual lesions, or only a calcified parenchymal nodule and ipsilateral hilar lymph node calcification; this is called the *primary complex;* (2) manifestations of progressive primary infection with development of pleural effusion or mediastinal and cervical lymphadenitis (see Extrapulmonary Tuberculosis); (3) more serious life-threatening dissemination with development of miliary or meningeal tuberculosis; or (4) a dormant phase with development of reactivation disease years or decades later in distant sites, most frequently the lung apex. The immunocompromised host, especially with human immunodeficiency virus (HIV), is much more likely to develop progressive primary disease and extrapulmonary disseminated stages than the otherwise healthy host.

Conventional wisdom and historic data indicate that once infected an individual is relatively immune from subsequent new infection, and that later recurrences or relapses are caused by endogenous reactivation of the original strain. Recent data, however, show that this relative immunity can be overcome. In certain closed institutions (e.g., nursing homes, prisons) where exposure may be heavy, exogenous new infection with different strains may be identified. In AIDS patients during treatment for drug-susceptible tuberculous disease, new drug-resistant strains have emerged, reversing a favorable course.

Clinical Features

Tuberculosis disease is characteristically chronic or recurrent, but its manifestations range from an inapparent or subclinical infection in the majority of those affected to an acute and rapidly progressive illness, especially in immunocompromised hosts or small children.

Pulmonary Tuberculosis. Systemic manifestations are usually present. Fever occurs in 50% to 80% of patients, and malaise, weight loss, and night sweats also occur frequently. More than 85% of all forms of tuberculosis are pulmonary, so respiratory symptoms, especially cough, are common. The cough may be nonproductive in early stages, but patients may produce sputum later and less often, may experience hemoptysis. Pleuritic pain is occasionally seen even if overt pleural effusion is absent. Dyspnea, if present, is an ominous feature seen with widespread advanced disease. Crackles and bronchial breath sounds may be present, but more often there are no abnormal findings, even in well-developed pulmonary disease. Fatalities occur from wasting (consumption), hemorrhage, or respiratory failure.

Notable laboratory abnormalities include leukocytosis in 10% to 20% of patients, anemia in at least 10%, and hyponatremia in 10% to 15%. Anemia is more likely in more advanced disease and may be a sign of dissemination. Occasionally, anemia or pancytopenia may result from direct bone marrow involvement. Hyponatremia is usually of the normovolemic type and is a result of inappropriate antidiuretic hormone (ADH) secretion, marked by hyperosmolar urine in the presence of hyposmolar plasma. Hyponatremia is more often seen in advanced disease. Because these manifestations are nonspecific and often insensitive, a high index of suspicion may be needed for diagnosis. Screening and a careful diagnostic approach are justified in groups at high risk for tuberculosis (Box 74-1).

Extrapulmonary Tuberculosis. Tuberculosis can involve almost any organ, but only the more common types are discussed here. Extrapulmonary involvement is present in about 15% of all patients but is much more likely in immunocompromised hosts.

Pleuritis. Tuberculous pleural effusion results from a perforation of a subpleural focus of tuberculosis into the pleural space. The chest radiograph demonstrates an underlying parenchymal infiltrate, representing active pulmonary tuberculosis in only a minority of cases of tuberculous pleuritis. The purified protein derivative (PPD) skin test reaction may be temporarily suppressed, so when tuberculous pleuritis is suspected despite a negative PPD, the test should be repeated later. Evaluation of patients with suspected tuberculous pleural effusions includes sputum smear and culture, smear and culture of pleural fluid, and percutaneous pleural biopsy analyzed by smear, culture, and histopathology. The fluid features are characteristically a mononuclear cell and serous exudate. An elevated adenosine deaminase level may also be a helpful and specific marker. The analysis of the pleural fluid and pleural biopsy specimens diagnoses more than 90% of tuberculous pleural effusions, although the yield of pleural fluid culture alone is less than 25% (see Chapter 79). Diagnosis by thoracoscopic biopsy is occasionally needed. Untreated, most tuberculous pleural effusions spontaneously resolve in several weeks, although 65% of patients will develop active pulmonary tuberculosis within 5 years, underscoring the importance of diagnosis and treatment.

Box 74-1. High-risk Groups for Tuberculosis

Racial and ethnic minorities: 70% of all U.S. cases
Foreign-born persons: 37% of all U.S. cases
Substance abusers (drugs and alcohol): relative risk 5 to 20 times normal
HIV infection: relative risk 40 to 100 times normal
Predisposing medical condition (diabetes, immunosuppressive drugs, silicosis, cancer): relative risk 3 to 5 times normal
Residents of prisons, nursing homes, shelters: relative risk 2 to 10 times normal
Contacts of an active case: risk 3% within first year

Lymphadenitis. Hilar lymph node involvement with enlargement is a frequent sequela of primary tuberculosis. In children it can cause bronchial compression with atelectasis. Hilar and mediastinal lymphadenitis is also common in immunocompromised adults, especially HIV-infected patients.

Cervical lymphadenitis, formerly scrofula, presents as a firm group of supraclavicular or anterior nodes that are usually nontender and matted. Ulceration with sinus tracts is a later development. Diagnosis is usually made by aspiration or excision of the involved area. Granulomatous cervical lymphadenitis in younger children is rarely caused by tuberculosis in the United States. Most such cases now are caused by *Mycobacterium avium-intracellulare* complex (see later discussion).

Tuberculosis of Bone. This may involve the spine (Pott's disease) or the epiphyses of larger long bones, especially at the knees or hips, and occasionally the wrists or elbows. The lumbar spine is more frequently involved than the dorsal spine, and involvement of the cervical spine is rare. Manifestations include pain, compression fracture and deformity, and radiculopathy from compression. The gibbous deformity with sharp spinal angulation is characteristic. Diagnosis is usually suspected from the clinical and radiographic features. Early x-ray changes include soft tissue swelling, subchondral osteoporosis, cystic sclerosis, and later involvement of the synovial space. Diagnosis is best made by needle aspiration and occasionally by open biopsy.

Meningitis. Meningitis is the most common type of central nervous system tuberculosis. This dreaded disease was uniformly fatal before chemotherapy became available, and even with prompt and adequate treatment today, permanent sensory, motor, and cognitive impairment may be unavoidable; mortality may reach 40%. Usual features are basilar meningitis and cranial nerve involvement with headache, stiff neck, and obtundation. Lumbar puncture shows 100 to 1000 leukocytes, with lymphocytes predominant in two thirds of patients. Protein concentrations are high and glucose concentrations usually low. Acid-fast stains are positive in only 10% to 20% of patients, with culture confirmation later in 50% to 75%. Evidence indicating pulmonary or other forms of tuberculosis can assist diagnosis. If the diagnosis is suspected, early empiric therapy is prudent and may be lifesaving.

Disseminated or Miliary Tuberculosis. This may also carry a grave prognosis. Systemic manifestations are prominent, with fever, weakness, and malaise. Anemia or pancytopenia often occurs because of marrow involvement. The name *miliary* is derived from the characteristic innumerable fine nodules of uniform size (millet seeds) that appear on chest radiograph or on cut section of the lung at autopsy. In its earlier stages, however, the x-ray shadows may be inapparent. High-resolution computed tomography (CT) scanning can demonstrate such shadows more sensitively than plain films. Diagnosis can be made in half of cases by sputum examination, but invasive procedures, especially transbronchial lung biopsy and bone marrow biopsy, offer a much more reliable yield and should be considered early.

In addition to increased frequency of disseminated or extrapulmonary disease, the immunocompromised host, especially if HIV infected, exhibits many features of tuberculosis that differ from those in the immunocompetent host (Table 74-1).

Diagnostic Testing

Microbiology. The microbiology laboratory is essential for confirming the diagnosis by identification of *M. tuberculosis* as well as for following the course of disease by documenting the disappearance of organisms with successful therapy. In pulmonary disease the sputum first expectorated in the morning is the preferred specimen, usually on 3 successive days. If such sputum is unobtainable, sputum induction using hypertonic 3% saline aerosol is an alternative. If necessary, the next step is fiberoptic bronchoscopy with sampling by bronchoalveolar lavage, brushing, or biopsy of affected segments.

The initial examination is the acid-fast stain. Specimens generally give best results if they are examined after predigestion. Fluorescent stains using auramine-rhodamine improve the sensitivity and rapidity with which the slide can be screened, but false-positive results do occur, so a positive fluorescent specimen should be confirmed by the standard Ziehl-Neelsen or Kinyoun stain. A positive acid-fast stain does not identify *M. tuberculosis,* since all other mycobacteria as well as *Nocardia* species are acid fast. Acid-fast stains require a fairly heavy population of organisms for detection and thus may be falsely negative. Culture methods increase sensitivity, since 40% to 60% of eventual isolates may be negative on initial stains.

Classic culture methods require 3 to 8 weeks for identifiable growth. Because of this inordinate delay, other techniques, especially the Bactec methods, are being used to accelerate growth and provide identification in 10 to 14 days. These techniques are available in larger hospital and state reference laboratories. Genetic techniques (e.g., RNA sequencing, gas-liquid chromatography, high-performance

Table 74-1. Host Response Differences in Tuberculosis

Factor	Normal host	Immunocompromised host (especially HIV)
Pathologic response	Granuloma with caseation	Nonspecific inflammation or poorly organized granulomas
Tuberculin sensitivity	Usually reliable except in elderly patients or those with advanced disease	Unreliable
Chest radiograph	Nodular infiltrates, cavitations	Lymphadenopathy, diffuse infiltrates, sometimes no infiltrates
Chronicity	May appear after many years of dormancy	Frequently progressive within 3-12 months of infection
Extrapulmonary spread	15%	30%-50%

liquid chromatography) offer more precise and rapid identification in hours or days. The polymerase chain reaction technique offers promise as a rapid and sensitive test.

Drug susceptibility studies complement culture techniques. The proportion-plate method is being replaced by the more rapid and reliable broth (Bactec) technique. With recent increases in drug-resistant strains, susceptibility studies must be conducted on all initial isolates and must be repeated if organisms are still recovered after 2 to 3 months of treatment. The recent complete decoding of the tubercle bacillus genome holds great promises for advances in diagnostic methods as well as in drug and vaccine development.

Radiography. Routine chest radiography is highly sensitive for recognition of pulmonary tuberculosis. Supplementary x-ray techniques, especially CT scans, can give additional information in areas that are difficult to visualize with conventional films, such as the mediastinal, retrocardiac, or apical zones, which can be obscured by overlying structures. The characteristic features are nodular infiltrates and cavitation. Air-fluid levels are uncommon in cavities but suggest another problem (e.g., lung abscess). In later stages, when healing occurs, signs of fibrosis may include loss of volume, linear shadows, and traction deformities of the hilum and mediastinum. The most common areas of involvement are the apical and posterior segments of upper lobes and superior segments of lower lobes. Adjacent pleural thickening often occurs (Fig. 74-2, *A*). A normal chest radiograph may occur rarely in pulmonary tuberculosis, as in an isolated endobronchial lesion or a very early miliary stage.

In primary tuberculosis the radiographic picture is different and less specific. Infiltrates without nodularity, usually in the middle or lower zones, are seen. Hilar lymph node enlargement is a common feature. Lymphadenopathy is prominent in immunosuppressed patients, especially those with AIDS, and parenchymal infiltrates may be poorly defined, without nodularity or cavity formation (Fig. 74-2, *B* and *C*). Tuberculosis in AIDS can also have an interstitial pattern and be confused with *Pneumocystis carinii* pneumonia (Box 74-2).

Histology. The characteristic lesion of tuberculosis is the formation of granulomas, which represent aggregations of inflammatory cells, principally macrophages, many of which assume epithelioid forms and join to create giant cells. Caseation necrosis is a prominent feature. These features are not specific for tuberculosis and may be seen in infectious granulomas caused by fungi or other mycobacteria. Granulomas without caseation may be found in sarcoidosis and foreign bodies or as an adjacent reaction to neoplastic and inflammatory diseases. Specific recognition of the tuberculous granuloma depends on demonstration of the organism by stain or culture of this tissue, as well as on clinical circumstances. In the immunocompromised host, granulomas may not be seen or may be poorly formed, and the inflammatory response may be modest. In such cases the organisms may be abundant on tissue stains.

Tuberculin Test. The tuberculin reaction is the classic example of delayed hypersensitivity immune response. Tuberculin, an extract of killed tubercle bacilli, is now well standardized as PPD, and its activity is measured by bioassay. The standard test is the intradermal administration in the volar forearm of 5 units diluted to 0.1 ml (Mantoux test). The reaction is read at 48 to 72 hours as diameter of induration, not erythema. A positive reaction can be interpreted as infection with *M. tuberculosis.* The infection may be recent or remote, since persistence of reactivity is the rule. Up to 10% of reactors, however, may become negative on retesting a decade or more later.

The tuberculin test is plagued by uncertainties related to both sensitivity and specificity. In a diagnostic setting, sensitivity is as low as 70%, and false-negative results are likely when the diagnosis is most important: in overwhelming disease, in immunocompromised hosts, in elderly patients, and in sarcoidosis (Box 74-3). Cutaneous anergy may be present in such cases. Anergy is assessed by simultaneous intradermal testing with common antigens, such as mumps, tetanus toxoid, *Candida,* and *Trichophyton.* Unfortunately, anergic reactions offer little information. Specificity problems result from cross-reactivity with other mycobacterial infection (a common regional problem, especially in the southeastern United States) or with prior bacille Calmette-Guerin (BCG) vaccination. Such cross-reactivity usually gives weak reactions of 5 to 10 mm. In epidemiologic testing of healthy populations, tuberculin sensitivity is more reliable than for diagnostic use. In case contact surveys or employment screening programs the test is uniquely valuable.

Another difficulty is the *booster phenomenon.* A host who is weakly reactive may have an enhanced reaction on retesting a month or a year later. Since the implication is newly acquired vs. remote infection, interpretation can be confusing. This phenomenon is often seen in elderly patients and in annual nursing home surveys. One technique for clarifying the booster phenomenon is double testing, or repeating a negative test after 1 week. A positive reaction on second test represents a boost rather than a true conversion. This method is useful in screening persons over 60 years old.

Because of these difficulties, the American Thoracic Society has proposed a scaled interpretation of tuberculin tests based on clinical circumstances (Box 74-4). Although this interpretation formula is an improvement over the previous standard of 10-mm induration as the uniform positive threshold, the test still has intrinsic defects (e.g., 10% to 25% of AIDS patients have false-negative tests even at the 5-mm induration threshold).

Management

Comprehensive management of any contagious disease includes effective treatment of the source case as well as evaluation, prevention, and treatment of contacts. The cornerstone of effective treatment is multidrug chemotherapy, but the public health measures of contact surveys, isolation methods, and ensuring that the patient completes treatment are also important.

Tuberculosis is a reportable disease. Every case must be reported to the local health department when the diagnosis is made, but it is good policy to report cases even when tuberculosis is suspected but not proved. The public health officer should serve as a consultant to the primary care physician and is helpful in initiating the contact surveys of the patient's household and, if necessary, the patient's place of employment. Contact surveys begin as tuberculin testing followed by chest x-ray studies for reactors to evaluate them for active disease. A second round of tuberculin testing after 6 to 8 weeks is prudent for nonreactors to detect those who

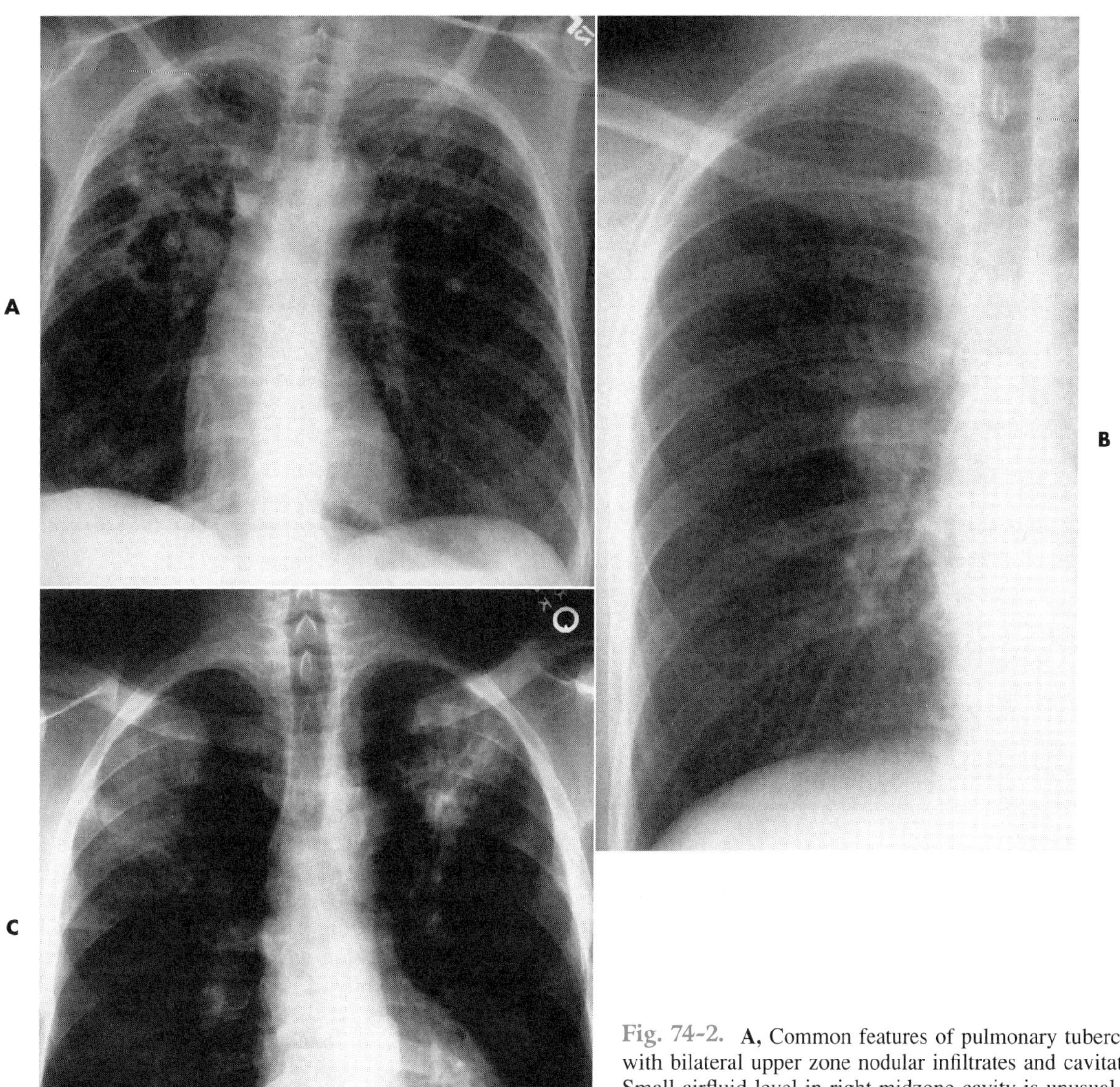

Fig. 74-2. **A,** Common features of pulmonary tuberculosis, with bilateral upper zone nodular infiltrates and cavitation. Small airfluid level in right midzone cavity is unusual. Target shadows are electrocardiographic lead artifacts. **B,** Tuberculosis in acquired immunodeficiency syndrome. Hilar and paratracheal lymph node enlargement is prominent, with faint infiltrate in lung apex. **C,** Tuberculosis in AIDS. Bilateral infiltrates resemble segmental pneumonitis, with moderate hilar node enlargement.

may have been very recently infected but who were not yet reactive on the initial survey. Preventive treatment is appropriately offered for contact reactors without evidence of clinical or radiographic disease. The health department also helps promote the successful completion of a prolonged course of patient treatment.

The decision for hospitalization is based on clinical circumstances. If the patient has pronounced symptoms and is seriously ill, if the patient requires extensive expedited diagnostic testing, or if drug resistance is suspected, hospitalization is indicated. On the other hand, many mildly ill patients can be managed at home. The hazard to household contacts is greatest before the diagnosis is made. Once effective treatment is begun, contagiousness rapidly decreases.

Chemotherapy. Successful chemotherapy is based on the prolonged use of multiple effective drugs. The earliest lesson in treatment of tuberculosis with streptomycin in 1946 was that early success but late relapse occurred because of the selective emergence of resistance of the organisms to a single drug. With the use of multiple drugs, and especially since the use of isoniazid-rifampin (INH-RIF) combinations, this risk of acquired drug resistance has been minimized. Prolonged uninterrupted treatment is needed because persistent, slowly growing or dormant bacilli can only be eliminated slowly, even though the main population of rapidly dividing organisms quickly responds to therapy.

Several large drug trials sponsored by the U.S. Public Health Service and the British Medical Research Council showed that the ideal course of therapy can be as short as

Box 74-2. Differential Diagnoses for Radiography of Tuberculosis

Multinodular Infiltrates

Other mycobacterial or fungal granulomatous infections
Hematogenous or lymphogenous metastases
Collagen vascular or vasculitic disease
Sarcoidosis

Cavitations

Lung abscess
Neoplasm
Septic infarction
Necrotizing pneumonia, especially staphylococcal or gram-negative organisms
Vasculitis

Lymphadenopathy

Neoplasm, especially lymphoma
Sarcoidosis

Pleural Effusion

Transudate
Malignant effusion
Parapneumonia effusion
Thromboembolism
Collagen vascular disease

Box 74-3. Conditions Predisposing to False-negative Tuberculin Reactions

Age: Newborns, elderly patients (>60 years)
Acute infection: Measles, mumps, chickenpox, typhoid fever, brucellosis, typhus, pertussis
Live virus vaccines: Measles, polio, mumps
Immunosuppressive states: HIV, chronic renal failure, drugs (e.g., corticosteroids, anticancer agents)
Overwhelming tuberculosis itself
Sarcoidosis
Neoplasm: Especially lymphomas and lymphoid leukemias
Errors in test administration or interpretation

6 months, if it has an intensive early three-drug phase followed by 4 months of INH-RIF. In the intensive phase, daily treatment is needed, but later the schedule may be daily or twice weekly. Demonstrated success in these drug trials included 95% or higher initial clearance of the disease, as well as freedom from relapse over 1 to several years after treatment. These trials established the standard of treatment as an initial 2 months of daily INH-RIF and pyrazinamide (PZA) followed by 4 months of INH and RIF either daily or two or three times weekly. If PZA cannot be tolerated, an alternative is INH-RIF for a 9-month course. Intolerance or drug resistance to either of the major drugs requires addition of two other drugs, usually ethambutol and streptomycin, and

Box 74-4. Thresholds for Positive Tuberculin Test Interpretation*

5 mm: Recent close contacts of infectious tuberculosis cases; patients with fibrotic or healed lesion on radiograph; HIV-infected patients
10 mm: Patients with special medical conditions (e.g., diabetes, silicosis, corticosteroid therapy); foreign-born persons from Asia, Africa, or Latin America; underserved or low-income groups or minorities, including African American, Hispanic, and Native American; injection drug users; residents of long-term care facilities
15 mm: All others

*Recommendations of American Thoracic Society and advisory committee of Centers for Disease Control and Prevention.

a more prolonged course of 12 to 18 months. These treatment programs need not be altered for extrapulmonary tuberculosis. In HIV-infected patients a minimum of 9 months is customary, although standard courses are likely to be effective (Table 74-2).

The recognition of drug-resistant strains affects the approach to therapy. In 1997 INH resistance occurred in 7.8% and INH-RIF resistance in 1.4% of cases in the United States. Substantially higher resistance rates were reported in California, Florida, New Jersey, and New York City, and 35 states reported INH resistance rates of 4% or higher. Thus an initial fourth drug, ethambutol or streptomycin, should be added in any region where INH resistance rates are greater than 4% or unknown. Treatment is then modified later based on susceptibility results, with reversion to standard regimens if resistance is not found and prolonged 18-month regimens if INH or RIF resistance is confirmed. Re-treatment of failed cases or treatment of multidrug-resistant cases is not the province of primary care, and cases should be referred. Treatment of diseases resistant to both INH and RIF is difficult, requiring less effective, more toxic drugs and prolonged administration.

Patient monitoring is necessary to ensure the safety and effectiveness of treatment. The patient should be seen at least monthly to discuss disease symptoms and side effects of therapy. For pulmonary tuberculosis, sputum studies should be done monthly for 3 months or until negative, at conclusion of treatment, and 3 to 6 months after treatment. Chest radiographs during therapy are desirable but not imperative because symptomatic and bacteriologic status indicators are more valuable; radiographic appearance should improve, but signs such as closure of cavities are not essential for success. Initial baseline complete blood count, blood urea nitrogen, liver enzymes, visual testing (for ethambutol), and uric acid (for PZA) are recommended. Since the three standard drugs are all potentially hepatotoxic, periodic monthly liver enzymes should be measured. Although modest elevations often subside with continued therapy, careful follow-up is necessary, but not discontinuance of treatment.

The most important and common reason for therapeutic failure is patient noncompliance. Education is helpful; the patient should understand the nature of the disease and the

Table 74-2. Recommended Drug for Treatment of Tuberculosis

Drug	Daily dosage		Twice-weekly dosage		Adverse reactions
	Children	Adults	Children	Adults	
Isoniazid	10-20 mg/kg PO or IM	5 mg/kg PO or IM, max 300 mg	20-40 mg/kg, max 900 mg	15 mg/kg, max 900 mg	Hepatic enzyme elevation, peripheral neuropathy, hepatitis hypersensitivity
Rifampin	10-20 mg/kg PO	10 mg/kg PO, max 600 mg	10-20 mg/kg, max 600 mg	10 mg/kg, max 600 mg	Orange discoloration or secretions and urine; nausea, vomiting, hepatitis, febrile reaction, purpura (rare)
Pyrazinamide	15-30 mg/kg PO	15-30 mg/kg PO, max 2 gm	50-70 mg/kg	50-70 mg/kg	Hepatotoxicity, hyperuricemia
Streptomycin	20-40 mg/kg IM	15 mg/kg* IM, max 1 gm*	25-30 mg/kg IM	25-30 mg/kg	Ototoxicity, nephrotoxicity
Ethambutol	15-25 mg/kg PO	15-25 mg/kg PO, max 2.5 gm	50 mg/kg	50 mg/kg	Optic neuritis (decreased red-green color discrimination, decreased visual acuity), skin rash

Data from *Core curriculum on tuberculosis: What the clinician should know,* ed 3, Washington, DC, 1994, US Department of Health and Human Services.
PO, Orally; *IM,* intramuscularly; *max,* maximum recommended dosage.
*In persons over age 60, daily dosage of streptomycin should be limited to 10 mg/kg with maximum of 750 mg.

need for adhering to prolonged treatment, long after feeling well. Another measure of proven effectiveness is supervised or directly observed therapy; a caregiver or dedicated family member dispenses each dose and observes the patient ingesting it. This method is most conveniently adapted for intermittent, thrice-weekly dosing. Directly observed therapy is appropriate for any patient who may be noncompliant. Although alcoholics and drug users might seem to be noncompliant groups, no basis exists for predicting compliance from any social, economic, or educational group. Given the gravity of the reemergence of tuberculosis, the recommendation is that all therapy should be directly observed. This advice applies to any setting where compliance is less than 90% or is unknown, or virtually everywhere. Involuntary confinement or other coercive measures are rarely used. Any measure that simplifies treatment (e.g., twice-weekly or thrice-weekly dosing) can improve compliance. Fixed-combination tablets containing INH-RIF or INH-RIF-PZA discourage taking only part of the regimen. Pyridoxine is often routinely given to prevent the rare INH-induced peripheral neuropathy; the patient may then take only the vitamins, however, so routine use of pyridoxine can be counterproductive. The best tactic is to "keep it simple."

Drug toxicity or intolerance accounts for much fewer treatment failures than patient compliance. Hepatotoxicity, even with three potentially toxic drugs (INH-RIF-PZA), occurs in less than 4% of cases but is seen more frequently in patients with preexisting liver disease. PZA usually produces hyperuricemia but rarely symptomatic gout. Optic neuritis caused by ethambutol is rare if the initial dosage of 25 mg/kg/day is reduced to 15 mg/kg/day after the first 6 weeks of use.

Adjunctive surgery has a minor role in tuberculosis treatment today. Occasional patients may require drainage of tuberculous empyema, decompression of constrictive pericarditis, or relief of neurocompression in spinal tuberculosis, but these are performed for specific reasons to improve organ function. Surgery could have a renewed role in multidrug-resistant disease, but this has yet to be demonstrated because successful surgery is not an alternative but an adjunct to effective chemotherapy.

Treatment of Children and Pregnant Women. Treatment of children is similar to that for adults in combinations and duration of treatment (see Table 74-2). Treatment of tuberculosis in pregnant women is essential and should not be deferred. The preferred initial treatment is INH-RIF and ethambutol. The teratogenicity of PZA is undetermined, so it should not be used unless resistance to other drugs is demonstrated or likely. Streptomycin is ototoxic to the fetus and should not be administered unless other options are lacking.

Preventive Treatment. Approximately 10% of persons who have been infected by the tubercle bacillus but have no disease (i.e., tuberculin reactors who have no active disease on radiographs) develop tuberculous disease at some point in their lifetime. This risk is greater within the year after infection and in immunosuppressed patients, such as those taking corticosteroids or chemotherapy, and patients with diabetes or cancer. The risk is extremely high in HIV-infected patients, 40 to 100 times that of the normal population. Several large field trials in the 1960s showed that INH given daily for 6 to 12 months provides effective protection in 80% to 90% of patients against this risk and that the protection endures in follow-up over at least a decade; subsequently, however, the hepatotoxic hazard of INH has curtailed its use in this setting. INH hepatotoxicity risk increases with patient age. The incidence is 2% to 3% in those over age 60, 1% in younger adults, and virtually nonexistent in children. INH is still recommended for most tuberculin reactors without disease, except those at lowest risk (Box 74-5). INH preventive treatment in the HIV-infected tuberculin reactor is strongly recommended. Other indications for such treatment in HIV patients include anergy and no apparent disease but

Box 74-5. Indications for Preventive Treatment of Tuberculosis

Skin test–positive persons in the following high-risk groups, *regardless of age:*

Persons with HIV infection
Close contacts of infectious tuberculosis cases
Recent tuberculin skin test converters
Previously untreated or inadequately treated persons with abnormal chest radiographs
Injection drug users
Persons with medical conditions that increase risk of tuberculosis

Skin test–positive persons in the following high-risk groups, *less than 35 years of age:*

Foreign-born persons from high-prevalence countries
Low-income populations, including high-risk minorities
Residents of long-term care facilities (including prisons)

From Core curriculum on tuberculosis: what the clinician should know, ed 3, Washington, DC, 1994, US Department of Health and Human Services.

Box 74-6. Managed Care Guide: Prevention of Tuberculosis

1. Identification and effective treatment of active tuberculosis cases. An undiagnosed, untreated active case will infect 10 to 14 other people in 1 year. Once a patient has been started on effective treatment, the risk of spread of disease diminishes rapidly, usually within the first 1 to 2 weeks.
2. *Reduction of infected aerosols.* Patients should be taught to cover their coughs. Effective masks capable of filtering particles as small as 0.1 μm are now available for patients and personnel.
3. *Ventilation.* Clearly beneficial, ventilation should be of negative pressure with exhaust to the outside and not recirculated. Air-change capacity of six times per hour is recommended.
4. *Ultraviolet air sterilizers.* These are inexpensive and relatively effective. They are mounted high in a room and directed upward to avoid possible visual damage.
5. *Tuberculin testing of personnel at risk of exposure.* This should be done at the start of employment and periodically every 6 to 12 months. Additional testing should follow known exposure to untreated active cases. Preventive treatment is recommended for all tuberculin converters.

high risk, as shown by a previous positive reaction, exposure to a patient with tuberculosis, a chest radiograph compatible with healed tuberculosis, or high likelihood of exposure (e.g., Haitian or Mexican immigrants, injection drug users).

Alternatives to INH have never been studied in a controlled way. If INH is indicated but cannot be given because of intolerance or suspected INH resistance, RIF would be the next drug of choice. Other inferior options include ofloxacin and ethambutol. BCG vaccine has uncertain and variable effectiveness. It is not used for tuberculin reactors and has no clear role for tuberculosis prevention in the United States. In addition, BCG is a live vaccine capable of causing progressive disease in immunocompromised patients, so it is clearly contraindicated in HIV disease.

Control Measures. With the reemergence of heightened risk of tuberculous infection, physicians in health care facilities and other close environments should know and help implement effective surveillance and preventive measures (Box 74-6).

NONTUBERCULOUS MYCOBACTERIAL DISEASES

Several dozen species of mycobacteria have been identified since the tubercle bacillus itself was discovered. Most are found in the environment. Many are saprophytes, and some are pathogenic for fish, amphibia, or birds; only a few species are important to humans. All are less virulent than *M. tuberculosis* and are most often seen as opportunistic infections. The most common and important group is *M. avium-intracellulare* complex (MAC); others include *M. kansasii, M. marinum,* and rapid growers such as *M. fortuitum-chelonae* complex. Laboratory differentiation is based on colonial morphology, growth rates, and a biochemical test battery, but genetic testing for rapid identification of MAC vs. *M. tuberculosis* is now replacing the cumbersome biochemical testing.

Diseases from *Mycobacterium Avium-intracellulare* Complex

Chronic Pulmonary Disease. MAC infection usually occurs in middle-aged men more often than women and may mimic pulmonary tuberculosis but has distinctive features. Respiratory symptoms often occur, but systemic symptoms are uncommon. Disease and progression are indolent, and radiographic features are usually limited to lung parenchyma, with thin-walled cavities and thickening of overlying pleura but rarely pleural effusion. Primary stages are rarely seen, and involvement usually occurs in a portion of the lung previously damaged by chronic bronchitis or bronchiectasis, emphysema, healed tuberculosis, or silicosis. Another distinct form of disease, with interstitial involvement and nodular bronchiectasis in the middle and lower zones, is seen in older women without preexisting lung disease. Extrapulmonary involvement is rare, but occasional cases of bone and joint disease occur. Because the MAC organisms may be casual isolates rather than disease producers, a firm diagnosis requires several criteria, including repeated isolates of the same organism over days or weeks in reasonable numbers, as well as a compatible radiographic and clinical picture.

Because of drug resistance, treatment is often of uncertain benefit. In mild disease, observation alone may be the best choice. In symptomatic cavitary disease, effective treatment often requires three or more drugs and a prolonged course of up to 2 years. If possible the choice of drugs should be guided by susceptibility studies. An initial recommended combination is clarithromycin or azithromycin, rifabutin or rifampin, and ethambutol, with an option of streptomycin initially. Adjunctive surgical resection can be beneficial if disease is well localized and the patient has acceptable surgical risks.

Cervical Lymphadenitis. This disease presents in children ages 1 to 5 as chronic nontender enlarged lymph nodes in the anterior or posterior chain. Cervical lymphadenitis is probably acquired by oral ingestion of contaminated materials from floors. It is a much more common cause of granulomatous lymphadenitis in children than is tuberculosis. Diagnosis is made by identification of the organisms from aspirated or resected material. The preferred treatment is complete surgical excision. Drugs are weakly effective, and untreated disease often progresses to draining fistulae or disfiguring scars.

Disseminated MAC Disease. This devastating disease occasionally occurs in immunosuppressed transplant or cancer patients, but its chief importance is in the late stages of AIDS. Disseminated MAC disease is marked by high fever, weakness, diarrhea, and pancytopenia that carries a poor prognosis. It is seen when marker CD4 T-lymphocyte counts are less than 50/mm^3 (often below 10) and may occur in 20% to 40% of late-stage AIDS patients. Diagnosis is most reliably made by blood or marrow culture. Stool cultures are usually positive as well but alone are inconclusive for diagnosis. If untreated, median life expectancy is 4 months. Survival can be doubled with multidrug treatment, similar to that used in chronic pulmonary disease. Drug toxicity often occurs, with special problems from antiviral/rifampin interactions. MAC prophylaxis using azithromycin is recommended in AIDS patients with CD4 counts less than 100/mm^3 (see Chapter 32).

Mycobacterium kansasii Infections

Although MAC can be widely found in the environment in soils and bodies of water, *M. kansasii* is rarely found in nature but can be found sporadically in tap water. The organism is beaded and larger than other mycobacteria, so an experienced microscopist can identify it from acid-fast stains alone. It shows the peculiar culture characteristic of pigmentation only if grown in light (photochromogen). *M. kansasii* shows limited virulence for humans. As with MAC, it can cause chronic pulmonary disease and disseminated disease in AIDS as well as the rare bone or joint disease. *M. kansasii* differs from MAC most importantly in its favorable response to therapy. Rifampin is highly effective in treatment, and the recommended current regimen is rifampin, isoniazid, and ethambutol for at least 9 months.

Mycobacterium marinum Cutaneous Infections

M. marinum infections occur as nodular ulcerations in swimmers (swimmers' itch), in fish processors, or from cleaning fish tanks (fish tank granuloma). Diagnosis is made by skin biopsy and identification of the organism. The disease may heal spontaneously, but deep infection should be treated for at least 3 months. The organism is usually susceptible to clarithromycin, sulfonamides, tetracycline, rifampin, and ethambutol, and monotherapy or a rifampin-ethambutol combination is appropriate.

Infections from Rapid-growing Mycobacteria

Rapid-growing mycobacteria, especially *M. fortuitum-chelonae* complex, are most important in wound infections and in contamination of implanted prosthetic materials, especially breast implants, long-term catheters, porcine heart valves, and bone wax. Occasional ocular or cutaneous infections are also seen, along with pulmonary disease resembling MAC. Diagnosis is usually evident; organisms are easy to grow, and cultures mature in 3 to 7 days. Successful treatment usually involves removal of prosthetics and wide excision of infected tissue. Chemotherapy is of variable effectiveness, but drugs, including amikacin, tobramycin, cefoxitin, sulfamethoxazole, imipenem, and ciprofloxacin, are likely to have some benefit.

ADDITIONAL READINGS

Bass JB Jr, American Thoracic Society: Treatment of tuberculosis and tuberculosis infection in adults and children, *Am J Respir Crit Care Med* 149:1359, 1994.

Core curriculum on tuberculosis: what the clinician should know, ed 3, Washington, DC, 1994, US Department of Health and Human Services.

Raviglione MC, Snider DE, Kochi A: Global epidemiology of tuberculosis: morbidity and mortality of a worldwide epidemic, *JAMA* 273:220, 1995.

Wallace RJ, American Thoracic Society: Diagnosis and treatment of disease caused by non-tuberculous mycobacteria, *Am J Respir Crit Care Med* 156:S1, 1997.

CHAPTER 75

Chronic Obstructive Pulmonary Disease

Ralph M. Schapira
Lynn F. Reinke

The term *chronic obstructive pulmonary disease* (COPD) refers to a spectrum of pulmonary disorders that have the common feature of impaired expiratory airflow, termed *airways obstruction.* COPD is diagnosed by a permanent reduction in the ratio of the forced expiratory volume in 1 second (FEV_1) to forced vital capacity (FVC). Clinically, the major disorders recognized as part of the spectrum of COPD are emphysema and chronic bronchitis. The many definitions of chronic bronchitis and emphysema have led to confusion among physicians. *Chronic bronchitis* is defined functionally as a disease characterized by cough and mucus hypersecretion (phlegm production) for at least 3 months of the year for 2 consecutive years, with airways obstruction defined by spirometry. Some authors use "simple chronic bronchitis" to differentiate those patients with mucus hypersecretion who do not have airways obstruction, so simple chronic bronchitis is not part of the spectrum of COPD. In contrast to chronic bronchitis, *emphysema* is an anatomic abnormality of the lung defined as abnormal permanent enlargement of the air spaces distal to the terminal bronchioles, with destruction of their walls but without obvious fibrosis. Although emphysema is an anatomic diagnosis, characteristic clinical features are associated with it. Chronic bronchitis and emphysema should not be considered isolated disorders, since most patients with COPD have clinical features of coexistent chronic bronchitis and emphysema. Clinical features of patients with predominant chronic bronchitis ("blue bloater") and predominant emphysema ("pink puffer") allow general qualitative differentiation between the two forms of COPD. Pure forms of chronic bronchitis and emphysema are exceptions. Cigarette smoking is the most important factor in the development of COPD.

Some patients with classic smoking-related COPD have clinically pronounced bronchial responsiveness manifested by episodes of wheezing and worsening of expiratory airflow superimposed on the permanent airways obstruction. This form of COPD must be differentiated from *asthma,* which is characterized by acute airways obstruction that remits between episodes (see Chapter 72). Thus, asthma is not part of the spectrum of COPD. However, some individuals with asthma develop irreversible obstruction to airflow even in the absence of smoking, a form of COPD termed *chronic asthmatic bronchitis.* Chronic asthmatic bronchitis can mimic the classic smoking-induced COPD with bronchial responsiveness, although clinical features can help differentiate these two entities.

EPIDEMIOLOGY AND ETIOLOGY

Approximately 15 million people in the United States are believed to have COPD. In 1994, COPD ranked fourth as the estimated cause of death in the United States, accounting for 4.5% of all deaths. COPD is a common disorder seen in outpatient settings, accounting for 17 million annual office visits in a recent survey. The prevalence of COPD and hospitalization for COPD are directly related to increasing age. Males are affected much more often than females, reflecting past gender-related patterns of smoking. With the gap narrowing, however, the number of women with COPD is increasing.

Cigarette smoking is the most important risk factor for the development of COPD. The risk of developing COPD is related to the number of cigarettes smoked and the duration of smoking. Cigar or pipe smoking also increases the risk of developing COPD, but to a much lesser extent than cigarette smoking. Individual host susceptibility to the effect of smoking is believed to be a key factor in the development of COPD, since only about 15% of smokers develop COPD. Smokers who develop COPD have a much greater annual decline in the FEV_1 than do nonsusceptible smokers or nonsmokers. This rate of decline can normalize to that of nonsmokers with smoking cessation. Recent evidence suggests that passive smoking may be a risk factor in the development of COPD in nonsmokers.

People with homozygous $alpha_1$-protease inhibitor (α_1-PI) deficiency (usually, PiZZ phenotype) are at risk for the development of emphysema, although this condition represents fewer than 2% of patients with emphysema. Certain chronic occupational exposures, particularly to inorganic dusts (coal, cement), grain dusts, or acid fumes (sulfuric acid), may result in chronic bronchitis. The role of indoor air pollution, ambient outdoor air pollution, and recurrent childhood respiratory infections in causing COPD in the absence of smoking has not been clearly established.

PATHOPHYSIOLOGY

Emphysema is an anatomic abnormality of the acinus, the portion of the lung parenchyma supplied by and distal to a terminal bronchiole (respiratory bronchiole, alveolar ducts, alveolar sacs). Emphysema is characterized by destructive changes of the acinus. In contrast, chronic bronchitis is a functional abnormality defined by clinical criteria and associated with pathologic changes in the airways.

The pathogenesis of emphysema is controversial, although emphysema probably is caused by an imbalance between proteinases and antiproteinases in the lung. Neutrophils are believed to be a major source of proteinases, such as elastase. Cigarette smoking causes a chronic inflammatory response in the lung characterized by a migration of neutrophils. The neutrophils in the lung release elastase, which overwhelms the local natural antiproteinase activity, resulting in the destruction of lung elastin. Cigarette smoke may inactivate α_1-PI, a major antiproteinase found in the epithelial lining fluid of the lung. In addition, some people with α_1-PI deficiency develop emphysema on the basis of inadequate antiproteinase protection. The resulting proteinase-antiproteinase imbalance in the lung leads to the destruction of elastin, an integral component of the structural framework of the lung parenchyma. Loss of elastin is associated with air space enlargement and reduction in the elastic recoil of the lung. Forms of emphysema include *centriacinar emphysema,* the type strongly associated with cigarette smoking. It predominantly involves the respiratory bronchiole, is irregular in severity, and most often involves the upper lobes. In contrast, *panacinar emphysema* is characteristic of α_1-PI deficiency but may be seen in patients who do not have this disorder. The entire acinus is uniformly enlarged and destroyed. Why some smokers develop emphysema and others do not is not known.

In contrast to emphysema, which involves the pulmonary parenchyma (acinus), the pathologic lesions of chronic bronchitis involve the airways. Morphologic changes in chronic bronchitis include hypertrophy of the submucosal glands and goblet cells of the large airways, clinically manifested as mucus hypersecretion and cough. In addition, infiltration of the submucosa by chronic inflammatory cells is common. Involvement of the small airways (bronchioles) is manifested by the abnormal presence of mucus-secreting cells, frequently accompanied by chronic inflammation. Smooth muscle hyperplasia and edema may also be present in the airways. The mucus hypersecretion seen in chronic bronchitis may be complicated by bacterial colonization and infection, potentially aggravating the underlying chronic inflammation.

Chronic bronchitis is believed to represent the airway epithelial response to chronic irritation by tobacco smoke or other agents. The pathogenesis of chronic bronchitis is less well understood than that of emphysema. In animal models the induction of airway injury by irritant gases, proteinases, and acids results in the pathologic changes in the airways seen in chronic bronchitis.

The final common pathway of the pathologic changes in COPD is chronic airflow obstruction. In emphysema the loss of radial support produced by a decrease in elastic recoil results in airflow obstruction. In chronic bronchitis, the obstruction to airflow is believed to result from chronic inflammatory changes and muscle hyperplasia of the airways. In addition to airway obstruction, major abnormalities of gas exchange can occur in COPD. Ventilation/perfusion ($\dot{V}/\dot{Q}$) relationships are altered by destruction of pulmonary parenchyma (emphysema) and airway abnormalities (chronic bronchitis). The changes in $\dot{V}/\dot{Q}$ relationships are highly complex but can result in hypoxemia and hypercapnia. It is speculated that the degree of hypoxemia and hypercapnia is related to such factors as severity and pattern of $\dot{V}/\dot{Q}$ mismatch, ventilatory drive response, and breathing pattern. The predominance of parenchymal abnormalities (emphysema) or airway inflammation (chronic bronchitis) as well as the level of alveolar ventilation help characterize a patient as having predominant emphysema or chronic bronchitis. In addition, patients with COPD who develop hyperinflation (predominant emphysema) have mechanically impaired muscles of respiration and respiratory muscle dysfunction. These changes increase the work of breathing, leading to respiratory muscle fatigue and potential respiratory failure. Hypoxemia results in pulmonary arterial hypertension and right ventricular failure.

PATIENT EVALUATION

History

COPD is typically a disease of older smoking or exsmoking adults (more than 20 pack-years), usually over age 50. The diagnosis of COPD is suggested by the history and confirmed by the criterion standard, spirometry. The cardinal symptom of COPD is progressive dyspnea, frequently accompanied by cough and phlegm production and episodes of wheezing. The cough usually precedes or accompanies the onset of dyspnea. Phlegm is whitish gray and expectorated in the morning but may continue intermittently during the day. A history of productive cough with relatively less prominent dyspnea suggests predominant chronic bronchitis.

In contrast, patients with predominant emphysema usually give a history of minimal productive cough but with marked dyspnea. Asthmatic bronchitis, a form of COPD, is suggested by a history of typical paroxysmal asthma, especially occurring at rest or during sleep, with no or minimal smoking history. Changes in the quality of expectorated sputum, from whitish gray and mucoid to purulent, suggest acute bacterial bronchitis. The wheezing in some patients with COPD may be from bronchospasm or from the flow of air through inflamed and narrowed airways. A history of wheezing predicts a beneficial response to inhaled bronchodilators. A family history of COPD suggests α_1-PI deficiency, particularly if the onset is during the fourth or fifth decade of life. Hemoptysis in patients with COPD usually results from acute bacterial bronchitis or pneumonia, but an underlying lung cancer must always be considered. A patient who presents with progressive dyspnea and a history of asthma, particularly a nonsmoker, may have asthmatic bronchitis. A detailed occupational history, including exposure to dusts and fumes, should be obtained.

Patients with predominant chronic bronchitis tend to remain relatively comfortable at rest but develop hypoxemia, which leads to pulmonary arterial hypertension and subsequent right ventricular failure (cor pulmonale). Their failure to complain about respiratory problems may be misleading. In contrast, patients with predominant emphysema tend to complain of dyspnea, even at rest. Patients with COPD may have complaints not directly related to the pulmonary system. The history, particularly in patients with severe COPD, may reveal easy fatigability, weight loss, and decreased appetite. Patients with COPD may have sleep disturbances and neuropsychiatric abnormalities such as depression, poor concentration, and memory impairment. A history of peripheral edema suggests cor pulmonale.

Physical Examination

Patients with predominant chronic bronchitis are usually of normal body weight or obese. The physical examination may reveal cyanosis and peripheral edema caused by right ventricular failure (blue bloater). The respiratory rate is usually normal, with no use of the accessory muscles of respiration. Chest percussion note is usually resonant, and auscultation may demonstrate wheezes and coarse rhonchi that may change in location and intensity after a cough. Physical findings compatible with allergic rhinitis or nasal polyps may be noted in patients with asthmatic bronchitis.

In contrast, patients with predominant emphysema are frequently asthenic with weight loss. Tachypnea, the use of accessory muscles of respiration, retraction of the lower intercostal spaces with inspiration, and the use of pursed lips during expiration are common. Cyanosis is uncommon until the disease becomes very advanced because the increased FEV_1 maintains a sufficient oxyhemoglobin saturation and prevents hypercapnia (pink puffer). The chest percussion note is usually resonant. Auscultation reveals diminished breath sounds.

A useful bedside diagnostic test for COPD is the forced expiratory time (FET), measured by timing a full exhalation of the vital capacity during chest auscultation. In a large clinical study[11] evaluating the FET, sensitivity and specificity of FET at a value of 6 or more seconds for the diagnosis of airways obstruction was 74% and 75%, respectively. The FET is most useful in patients older than 60.

DIAGNOSIS

Laboratory Studies and Diagnostic Procedures

Pulmonary function testing (spirometry) is the only criterion standard to demonstrate an obstructive ventilatory defect, the hallmark of COPD.[1] An obstructive defect is defined by a FEV_1/FVC ratio below the subject's predicted value. Alternatively, some pulmonary function laboratories use a percentage of FEV_1 or FVC (less than 70%) to define obstruction. Once airway obstruction has been documented from the FEV_1/FVC ratio, the severity of the obstructive abnormality can be graded by the patient's percentage of predicted FEV_1: down to 70%, mild; less than 70% to 60%, moderate; less than 60% to 50%, moderately severe; less than 50% to 34%, severe; and less than 34%, very severe. Patients with COPD have an irreversible obstructive impairment, as demonstrated by a persistently abnormal FEV_1/FVC ratio, although the FEV_1 and FVC may vary between bouts of wheezing or pulmonary infection and clinical stability during optimal therapy. Any changes in spirometry, either improvement or worsening, should be viewed cautiously unless serial tests show a consistent trend. In contrast, asthmatic patients have a reversible obstructive impairment, with normalization of the FEV_1/FVC ratio between clinical episodes of asthma. Spirometry can also be used to determine other parameters, such as the forced expiratory flow between the time 25% to 75% of the FVC is exhaled ($FEF_{25\text{-}75}$). A decrease in the $FEF_{25\text{-}75}$ is not used to diagnose an obstructive airways defect but does suggest obstruction of the small airways (less than 2 mm). Survival estimates of patients with COPD can be predicted based on the FEV_1. The 5-year survival begins to decrease at a FEV_1 of 1.15 to 1.5 L. At ranges of FEV_1 of 0.75 to 1.15 L, 5-year survival decreases to 66% and is even lower in this group if chronic hypercapnia is present.

The functional ability of a patient with COPD is more precisely defined by a formal pulmonary exercise evaluation than by the FEV_1 alone. Functional impairment of patients with COPD varies for any given FEV_1, although in general, functional ability decreases as the FEV_1 decreases. Exercise testing can also differentiate among limitations caused by gas exchange, ventilation, or cardiovascular abnormalities. Many patients with COPD are limited because of cardiovascular deconditioning and not by a gas exchange or ventilation impairment. An exercise test is not routinely recommended unless a major medical intervention is planned, for example, a lung resection in a patient when postoperative respiratory disability is a concern.

Spirometry in patients who demonstrate an obstructive defect typically includes measurement of the FEV_1 and FVC immediately after administration of an inhaled bronchodilator, the bronchodilator response. A widely used definition of a significant bronchodilator response is both a 12% increase *and* an absolute increase of 200 cc in the FEV_1 or FVC. Although not clinically proved, patients with a significant response are believed to derive the greatest benefit from inhaled bronchodilators and corticosteroids. The lack of a significant bronchodilator response, however, does not preclude clinical benefit, since the one-time administration of a bronchodilator during spirometry does not necessarily predict response with regular use. Therefore, inhaled bronchodilators should not be withheld from patients who do not exhibit a significant bronchodilator response. Some laboratories no longer perform a test of bronchodilator response in a patient with an established diagnosis of COPD, since the clinical practice is to prescribe a bronchodilator regardless of response. Finally, normalization of the FEV_1/FVC percentage after administration of a bronchodilator strongly suggests asthma.

Patients with predominant chronic bronchitis or asthmatic bronchitis tend to have a relatively mild reduction in diffusing lung capacity for carbon monoxide (DLco), since the principal abnormality is in the airways. In contrast, patients with predominant emphysema, a parenchymal abnormality, have a greater reduction in DLco, which tends to correlate with the anatomic extent of the emphysema. The lung volumes in predominant chronic bronchitis tend to show a normal or slightly increased total lung capacity (TLC). In predominant emphysema, however, the lung volumes often show hyperinflation, as manifested by a marked increase in TLC and residual volume (RV). The increase in RV may compromise the vital capacity. Arterial blood gas (ABG) results in patients with predominant bronchitis demonstrate marked hypoxemia and, in advanced cases or during exacerbations, hypercapnia. ABG abnormalities may be relatively modest in patients with predominant emphysema, however, demonstrating only mild hypoxemia without hypercapnia except in advanced cases. Significant ABG abnormalities in patients with COPD tend to be unusual until the FEV_1 drops below 1.25 to 1.5 L. Exercise may worsen hypoxemia in patients with COPD. Secondary erythrocytosis may ensue in severely hypoxemic patients.

Standard chest radiographs can suggest the diagnosis of emphysema. Marked overdistention of the lungs, as manifested by flattened diaphragms and an enlarged retrosternal air space, is highly suggestive of emphysema. A small and vertically oriented heart contour and hyperlucent lung fields due to oligemia are also suggestive of emphysema. Localized radiolucencies and upper lobe bullae may be visible on the chest radiograph. Lower lobe bullae are highly suggestive of emphysema associated with α_1-PI deficiency. Although the chest radiograph can provide only an approximation of the severity of emphysema, it is most useful in suggesting the presence of severe emphysema. Computed tomography (CT) and particularly high-resolution CT are much more sensitive than plain films in detecting emphysematous changes in the lung, such as small bullae. Neither the chest radiograph nor the CT scan replaces the criterion standard, spirometry.

Other helpful tests in the initial evaluation of a patient with COPD include Gram's stain of the sputum; a complete blood count and differential to identify eosinophilia, which may suggest asthmatic bronchitis; a baseline electrocardiogram to identify right atrial or ventricular abnormalities suggestive of cor pulmonale; and α_1-PI level if deficiency is suspected. Skin allergy tests and a serum IgE level should be considered in patients with suspected asthmatic bronchitis.

Differential Diagnosis

Chronic bronchitis and emphysema must be distinguished from other lung diseases that may cause obstructive ventilatory impairment on spirometry. Patients with an exacerbation of asthma may have impairment and radiographic abnormalities suggestive of emphysema. By definition, however, the airways obstruction in asthma is reversible between acute exacerbations. Patients with cystic fibrosis may have ventilatory impairment from airway inflammation and obstruction by secretions. Cystic fibrosis is differentiated from chronic bronchitis and emphysema by its numerous systemic nonpulmonary manifestations and early age of onset. Bronchiectasis, the persistent dilation and destruction of bronchi, represents the sequelae of other lung processes, such as granulomatous infections and an array of genetic defects. The spirometric results in patients with bronchiectasis vary, but those with diffuse bronchiectasis may have an obstructive ventilatory defect. The history, underlying disease process, and CT scan can help differentiate bronchiectasis from chronic bronchitis and emphysema.

MANAGEMENT

Nonpharmacologic Therapy

Lung Transplantation and Lung Volume Reduction Surgery. Lung transplantation has been used with success in patients with severe COPD, although clinical follow-up has been limited to a few years. Single-lung transplantation is usually preferred. In 1997, for example, more than 950 lung and heart-lung transplants were performed in the United States for COPD, including α_1-PI deficiency–related COPD. Patients being considered for lung transplantation should be referred to specialized centers. The resection of large bullae may improve gas exchange and improve symptoms in selected patients with bullae of sufficient size to compress normal lung parenchyma.

Lung volume reduction surgery (LVRS) is currently limited to certain designated, specialized centers participating in a National Institutes of Health–sponsored study. LVRS, the removal of emphysematous areas of lung, can improve some measures of pulmonary function and gas exchange, decrease dyspnea, and diminish or eliminate the need for supplemental oxygen. The criteria to select patients most likely to benefit from LVRS are uncertain, however, and await the results of the LVRS national multicenter study.

Smoking Cessation. Most patients (85%) with COPD are current or former cigarette smokers. Several investigations have clearly shown that smoking cessation will slow the annual decrement of FEV_1 to the level of a nonsmoker. In addition, the nonpulmonary benefits include improved cardiovascular status and a reduced risk of developing lung cancer. Comprehensive, multidisciplinary smoking cessation programs using nicotine replacement therapy, which includes nicotine chewing gum, nicotine transdermal patches, nasal spray, and an oral inhaler, have lead to long-term cessation rates as high as 50%. *Nicotine gum,* now available over the counter in 2-mg and 4-mg strengths, has been shown to improve smoking cessation rates when used in appropriate candidates. The gum helps to maintain a blood and tissue level at about that of a pack-a-day smoker and can be gradually decreased or stopped abruptly. Disadvantages include a bitter taste, which may lead to noncompliance, and improper chewing patterns, which result in poor absorption of the nicotine. Another method for nicotine replacement is the *transdermal patch.* The patch is available in three doses, which are tapered over 2 to 3 months during the smoking cessation program. Some physicians initiate therapy with a low-dose patch in patients with coronary artery disease. The patches' advantages over nicotine gum include (1) easy use and once-daily replacement and (2) a steady, unchanging dose of nicotine, unlike the boluses provided by gum. Studies have demonstrated that the nicotine patches double the quit rate achievable by various levels of behavioral modification used alone. *Nicotine nasal spray* delivers nicotine through the nasal mucosa. It is the fastest absorbed form of nicotine currently available and reduces cravings within minutes. The *nicotine oral inhaler* is the newest nicotine product on the market. It has a similar appearance to a cigarette but delivers nicotine into the mouth, not the lungs. It mimics the hand-to-mouth behavior of smoking and may be used as an adjunct tool along with other replacement therapies. The antidepressant *bupropion* (Zyban) is as effective as the nicotine patch in smoking cessation.[5] Patients who received 200 or 300 mg of bupropion per day had a quit rate at 1 year of 22.9% and 23.1%, respectively. The pill should be started at least 1 week before the target quit date and is contraindicated in patients with eating or seizure disorders.

Smoking results from many factors, such as learned behaviors, environmental influences, and chemical dependence. Therefore, in addition to temporary nicotine replacement, smoking cessation programs must address these various issues to achieve long-term success. Physician support and involvement are important in making smoking cessation efforts successful.

Preventive Measures. Exposure to occupational or environmental air pollutants may trigger an exacerbation of COPD, especially if the patient has asthmatic bronchitis. Assisting the patient to identify specific sensitivities and providing strategies to avoid these triggers may minimize exacerbations. Days with severe air pollution can exacerbate COPD.

Airway Clearance. The clearance of excessive secretions, particularly in patients with predominant chronic bronchitis, can result in significant subjective benefit.[6] Multiple approaches can be implemented to promote and maintain airways relatively free of excessive secretions. Most patients with COPD cough ineffectively, resulting in increased energy expenditure without adequate sputum expectoration to clear the airways. The simple combination of deep breathing and coughing is frequently overlooked as an effective method of airway clearance. One cough technique that may facilitate airway clearance is forced exhalation, which is especially valuable for patients with a weak or uncontrolled cough. This technique involves combining slow deep breaths, with 5 to 10 seconds of breath holding to increase intrathoracic pressure, then coughing on exhalation. Most patients find this cough technique easy to learn and effective for clearing secretions felt or heard in the large airways.

Another technique to aid in airway clearance is *chest physiotherapy* (CPT), which includes postural drainage and chest percussion and vibration either by hand or mechanical device. CPT allows gravity and applied external force to the chest wall to facilitate drainage of the dependent portions of the lung, thus improving airway clearance. Both postural drainage and CPT should always be followed with cough techniques to clear the airways. CPT can cause bronchospasm and worsening hypoxemia and should be performed by respiratory therapists or nurses who are well trained in its application.

Several new alternatives are available to percussion and postural drainage. The *flutter valve* is a hand-held mucus-clearing device that incorporates a steel ball resting in a hard plastic cone. As the patient exhales through the pipe, pressure builds in the airways and in the passage beneath the steel ball until the ball is forced to move and some gas escapes. This produces pressure oscillations that are transmitted throughout the tracheobronchial tree. In theory the oscillations dislodge mucus from the airway walls while back pressure supports smaller airways beyond the equal-pressure point; the expiratory flow helps to move the mucus toward the trachea, where it is coughed out. Although the flutter valve has been studied mainly in patients with cystic fibrosis, supporting evidence now indicates that flutter therapy is effective in patients producing more than 25 ml of sputum a day in other respiratory diseases. The main advantages of the flutter device are it is user friendly, does not require assistance from a caregiver, and is relatively inexpensive.

The ThAIRapy Vest is a high-frequency chest compression device that consists of a nonstretching inflatable vest attached by hoses to an air-pulse generator. Small volumes of gas are injected into and withdrawn from the vest at a rapid rate, pressurizing and releasing the chest with miniature hugs at frequencies from 5 to 25 Hz and generating pressures up to 53 cm H_2O. The minihugs from the vest create minicoughs in the patient, with increased mucus-airflow interaction and improved mucous rheology. Although the vest system was also developed for cystic fibrosis, any patients with excessive mucous production and difficulty clearing secretions would benefit from this therapy. An advantage of the vest is that it allows the patient to be passive, whereas the other clearance techniques require active participation. The major disadvantage is the expense of the vest system, which sells for approximately $16,000.

All these techniques can help to mobilize secretions, but deep breaths and gentle huff coughs are still required to move mucus into the central airways, where traditional cough or suction can remove it. Traditional CPT, once the predominant mucous clearance treatment, is now only one of a variety of modalities available.

Optimizing Functional Ability. Patients with COPD have many objective and subjective barriers to living an active and productive life. Comprehensive, multidisciplinary pulmonary rehabilitation programs offer patients education, exercise training and reconditioning, proper nutrition, and psychosocial interventions to decrease anxiety and other emotional disturbances related to the effects of COPD.[8] A recent literature review determined grades for each component of a rehabilitation program. Lower extremity and strength training was shown to improve exercise tolerance. Pulmonary rehabilitation improves dyspnea and health-related quality of life and reduces number and duration of hospitalizations. Expert opinion supports the inclusion of education and psychosocial interventions. Scientific evidence does not support the routine use of ventilatory muscle training in rehabilitation programs. Pulmonary rehabilitation may improve survival, but further research is needed, in addition to determining optimal methods for measuring outcomes and cost-effectiveness.

Pharmacologic Treatment

The aim of pharmacologic treatment of emphysema and chronic bronchitis is to improve symptoms and measurably improve lung function (Fig. 75-1). Inhaled medications (parasympatholytics, beta-adrenergic agonists (β-agonists, steroids) delivered by a metered-dose inhaler (MDI) are preferred in the pharmacotherapy of COPD, since inhalation

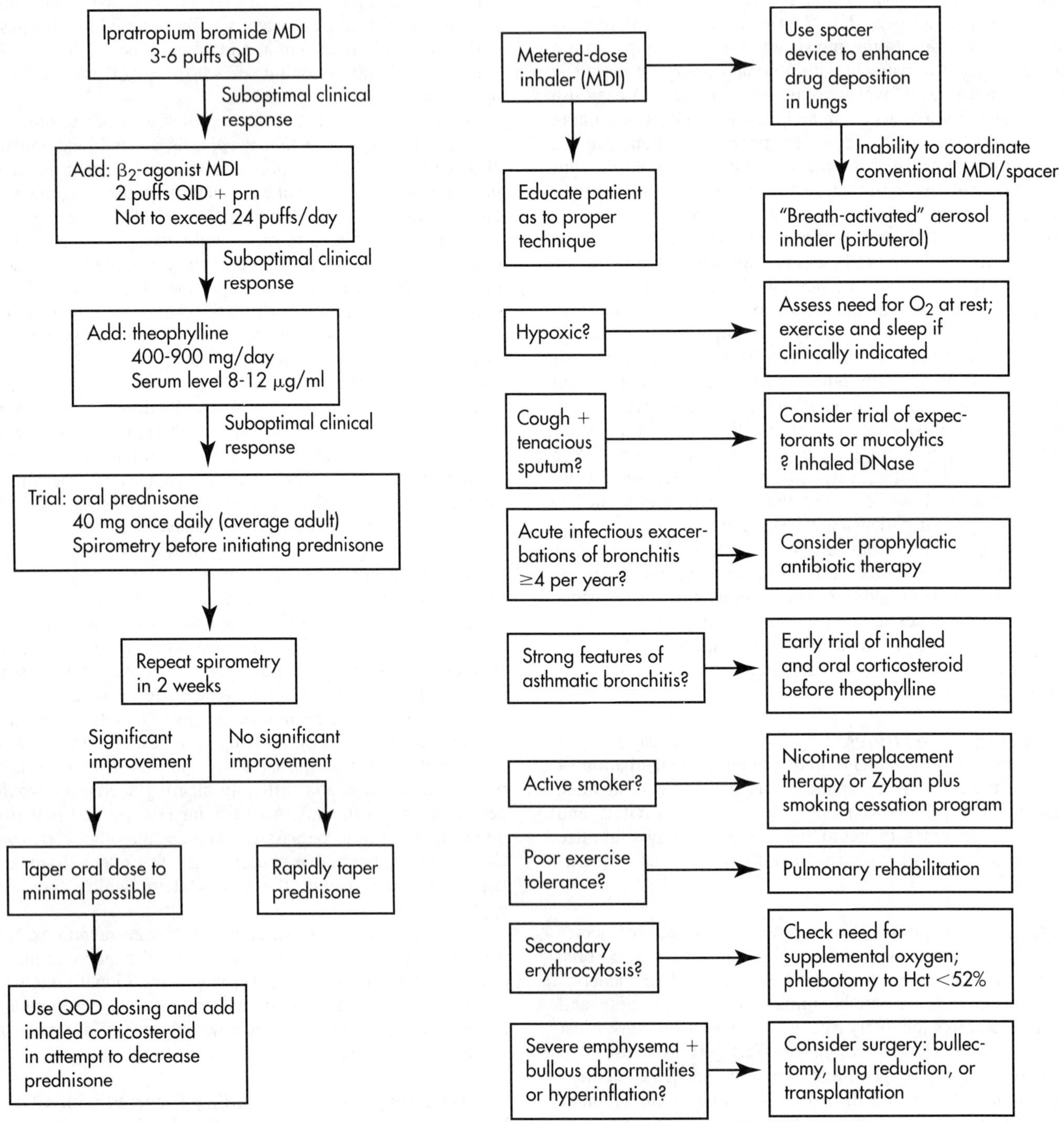

Fig. 75-1. Managed care guide: pharmacotherapy and general management approaches for chronic obstructive pulmonary disease (COPD). *QID*, Four times a day; *prn*, as needed; *QOD*, every other day; *DNase*, deoxyribonuclease; *Hct*, hematocrit.

allows direct deposition of medication in the airways and helps to minimize systemic side effects (Table 75-1). The delivery of all inhaled medications requires the use of a *spacer device,* which functions as a holding chamber reservoir that minimizes the need to coordinate simultaneous inhalation and depression of the MDI canister to deliver the dose. A spacer device used with an MDI provides greater drug deposition to the smaller airways, less accumulation in the oropharynx, and greater overall bronchodilator effect.

To ensure maximal drug deposition from the MDI, the patient must be given a spacer device and educated in inhalation technique. The patient should take a slow and complete inhalation from the end of a normal tidal breath (full exhalation to RV is not necessary) and hold inhalation for up to 10 seconds to allow for drug deposition (Box 75-1). Reevaluation and reinforcement of proper technique should occur regularly. The administration of nebulized medications by compressor-driven devices was once believed to be the optimal method of β-agonist delivery. Compared with the MDI, however, nebulization is no more effective, requires a larger dose of the drug, takes longer to administer, and is more costly. Some patients continue to report greater relief of dyspnea from a nebulized treatment than MDI delivery, possibly because nebulization provides more drug compared with an MDI. The use of a nebulizer should be reserved for patients with severe disease who are unable to hold their breath when using an MDI or who are unable, even with a spacer device, to coordinate MDI use.

Anticholinergics (Parasympatholytics). Anticholinergic drugs antagonize the effect of the parasympathetic system on the airways, which mediates bronchoconstriction. *Ipratropium,* a quaternary anticholinergic bronchodilator available by MDI, is more efficacious than inhaled β-agonist therapy and should supplant β-agonists as first-line therapy in COPD.

Table 75-1. Metered-dose Inhalers (MDIs) Used in Treatment of COPD

Agent	Action	Dose per inhalation (μg)
Albuterol (Proventil, Ventolin)	β_2-Agonist	90
Metaproterenol (Alupent)	β_2-Agonist	650
Pirbuterol (Maxair)	β_2-Agonist	200
Terbutaline (Brethine, Brethaire)	β_2-Agonist	200
Ipratroprium (Atrovent)	Anticholinergic (parasympatholytic)	18
Ipratropium and albuterol (Combivent)	β_2-Agonist and anticholinergic	103 and 18
Triamcinolone (Azmacort)	Antiinflammatory corticosteroid	100
Flunisolide (AeroBid)	Antiinflammatory corticosteroid	250
Beclomethasone (Beclovent, Vanceril)	Antiinflammatory corticosteroid	42
Fluticasone (Flovent)	Antiinflammatory corticosteroid	44 or 110 or 220

In clinical studies, ipratropium achieves greater bronchodilatory effect in COPD than β-agonists or theophylline when comparing FEV_1. In addition, ipratropium has a longer duration of action and wider margin of safety than β-agonists, making it a cornerstone of pharmacologic therapy for COPD. The traditional dosage of ipratropium (2 puffs, four times a day) may be suboptimal and can be safely increased to 3 to 6 puffs four times a day. Ipratropium is appropriate for maintenance treatment of COPD and is not indicated in the initial treatment of acute exacerbations because of its slow onset of action (about 20 minutes) compared with β-agonists. Ipratropium is poorly absorbed from the airways and thus has few systemic adverse effects, unlike with β-agonists. Potential side effects include dry mouth and cough. Ipratropium (available as MDI or for nebulization) is the only anticholinergic bronchodilator available in the United States.

Beta-adrenergic Agonists. Short-acting β-agonists have been the traditional cornerstone in the management of COPD. The role of β-agonists in COPD pharmacotherapy continues to evolve, however, particularly with the established efficacy and safety of the anticholinergic ipratropium. Most authorities recommend that short-acting β-agonists be used as second-line therapy, either to supplement or to replace ipratropium in patients who do not obtain satisfactory clinical benefit from ipratropium alone. Combivent combines a fixed dose of ipratropium and albuterol in a single MDI and may have an additive effect compared with using each agent alone for stable COPD.

The use of β-agonist bronchodilators can increase airflow, improve mucociliary clearance, and reduce dyspnea in patients with COPD. Administering higher doses of β-agonists (2 to 6 puffs four to six times a day) may result in greater achievement of airway bronchodilation without additional side effects than with the traditional dosage of 2 puffs four times a day. With concern over reported deaths associated with the overuse of β-agonists in patients with asthma, however, there is reluctance to recommend higher doses. In addition, tachyphylaxis, rebound bronchoconstriction, and bronchial hyperreactivity may occur with β-agonists.

The many short-acting β-agonist MDIs in clinical use are relatively selective for β_2-receptor sites that mediate

Box 75-1. Proper Use of a Metered-dose Inhaler (MDI)

1. Shake the inhaler.
2. Tilt the head back slightly and exhale normally. Forced exhalation to residual volume is not necessary.
3. Hold the mouthpiece 1 to 1½ inches away from open mouth. If using a spacer, however, seal lips around the mouthpiece.
4. Activate the MDI while simultaneously taking a slow, deep inhalation.
5. Hold breath at the end of inspiration for 5 to 10 seconds. Slowly exhale through mouth.
6. Wait 1 minute between puffs.
7. If using a steroid inhaler, rinse mouth after use to avoid thrush or dysphonia.

bronchial smooth muscle relaxation. Although the inhaled route helps to minimize systemic side effects, β-agonists can result in tachycardia, palpitations, tremor, and metabolic derangements such as hypokalemia. Patients should administer β-agonists prophylactically before engaging in physical activity known to provoke bronchospasm. A long-acting inhaled β-agonist, salmeterol, may improve lung function and symptoms in COPD, although it is formally approved only for asthma.[3] The use of oral β-agonists is strongly discouraged because they are no more effective than MDIs, absorption is unpredictable, and the incidence of systemic adverse effects is higher than from MDIs. However, patients with COPD who cannot use a MDI or who have nocturnal symptoms without relief from short-acting inhaled β-agonists may benefit from use of a sustained-release oral β-agonist. The latter group of patients may also benefit from salmeterol.

Theophylline. A methylxanthine derivative, theophylline, has been shown to act as a bronchodilator, improve gas exchange, decrease dyspnea, improve mucociliary clearance, enhance respiratory muscle performance, have a positive inotropic effect, and increase neuroinspiratory drive. The belief that theophylline relaxes bronchial smooth muscle by inhibiting phosphodiesterase has been supplanted by other proposed mechanisms, including antagonism of prostaglandins and adenosine, alteration of cellular calcium metabolism, and inhibition of phosphodiesterase isozymes. The precise role of theophylline in the management of COPD has been controversial, particularly with the availability of inhaled anticholinergics. Over the past few years, theophylline once again seems to have fallen out of favor.

The toxicity of theophylline and its interactions with other drugs make it a relatively complex drug to dose. Common side effects of theophylline include nausea, diarrhea, tremor, anxiety, and insomnia and even include life-threatening side effects such as seizures and cardiac dysrhythmias. A number of factors reduce the clearance of theophylline, which contributes to an increased risk for toxicity. These factors include antibiotics (e.g., erythromycin, quinolones), histamine blockers (e.g., cimetidine, calcium channel blockers), liver disease, cor pulmonale, and pregnancy. Although the therapeutic range for theophylline levels has been debated, the usual therapeutic serum level ranges from 10 to 20 μg/ml. However, most potential bronchodilation is believed to occur once levels of 10 to 15 μg/ml have been reached. Therefore a serum level of 8 to 12 μg/ml has been suggested as the therapeutic goal.

The decision to institute theophylline therapy must be individualized and should not be universally made in all patients with COPD. Theophylline may be added to the treatment plan in patients who have not achieved an optimal clinical response to β-agonist and ipratropium MDIs. Theophylline should be continued only if there is a clinical benefit to the patient, such as an objective improvement in spirometry or a decrease in dyspnea. The usual dose of theophylline is 400 to 900 mg/day of a long-acting preparation, but the precise dose depends on concurrent drug administration, the patient's medical problems, and the drug's metabolism. Serum theophylline levels must be checked in 1 to 2 weeks and dosages adjusted to achieve and maintain an adequate clinical response without side effects. Subsequent serum levels should be monitored twice annually and doses adjusted if levels are subtherapeutic or supratherapeutic, if drugs are prescribed that may alter the metabolism of theophylline, or if a change occurs in the patient's medical condition that might alter theophylline metabolism.

Systemic Corticosteroids. Unlike ipratropium, β-agonists, and oral theophylline, which are bronchodilators, corticosteroids are antiinflammatory agents. They objectively benefit about 10% of clinically stable outpatients with COPD and are thought to increase the clinical response to β-agonists, possibly by increasing β-adrenergic responsiveness of the airways. In addition, the antiinflammatory property of corticosteroids may decrease the airway inflammation seen in COPD. The onset of action of the antiinflammatory effect of corticosteroids is several hours.

The role of oral corticosteroids in COPD is not well defined, partly because of their serious adverse effects and lack of evidence in their favor. Oral corticosteroids should be considered in outpatients with stable COPD whose symptoms are not optimally controlled by a regimen of β-agonists, ipratropium, and possibly theophylline. Although it can be difficult to predict which patients with COPD will respond to corticosteroids, factors such as a significant response to bronchodilators during spirometry or clinical features of asthmatic bronchitis suggest that a trial of steroids is warranted. A therapeutic trial of corticosteroids must be preceded by spirometry to verify objective improvement in pulmonary function (FEV_1) after initiation of therapy. Prednisone (approximately 0.5 to 1 mg/kg once daily) is begun and spirometry repeated 2 weeks after start of therapy. Although no formal criteria exist, most providers continue prednisone only if significant improvement in FEV_1 (defined as greater than 20%) results. Subjective improvement in dyspnea alone without objective improvement in spirometry is not an indication for continuation of corticosteroids. It is not known whether oral corticosteroids ultimately affect the natural progression of COPD.

Oral corticosteroids are associated with significant toxicity when administered chronically. Potential adverse effects include adrenal suppression, osteoporosis, hypertension, cataracts, myopathy, diabetes mellitus, and rarely, opportunistic infections. Therefore, if a patient demonstrates a significant objective clinical response to oral corticosteroids, the dose should be promptly tapered to the lowest possible dose that continues to provide objective spirometric benefit. Subjective worsening, such as an increase in dyspnea during a corticosteroid taper, should not be equated with a worsening of the FEV_1. Spirometry should be repeated to determine whether a correlation exists between subjective worsening and a decrement in pulmonary function. Alternate-day oral therapy may minimize side effects, although this remains unproved. Patients taking corticosteroids should continue to receive maximal therapy with inhaled bronchodilators and theophylline in an effort to minimize the requirement of oral corticosteroids. Calcium, vitamin D, estrogen, or bisphosphonates should be considered, as applicable, to prevent glucocorticoid-induced osteoporosis.[9]

Inhaled Corticosteroids and Other Antiinflammatory Agents. Inhaled corticosteroids are an established part of asthma therapy. The role of inhaled steroids in the treatment of COPD is uncertain, however, leading some investigators to believe that the airway inflammation in COPD is fundamentally different from that of asthma. Despite the lack of evidence, many physicians prescribe inhaled corticosteroids to patients with COPD.[2,7] Inhaled corticosteroids cause less serious side effects than oral corticosteroids because lower doses are administered and minimal systemic absorption occurs, although with the availability of potent inhaled corticosteroids, side effects from these agents are being recognized. The main side effects at low doses include oropharyngeal candidiasis and dysphonia. Inhaled corticosteroids most likely benefit patients who have shown clinical benefit from oral corticosteroids or who have asthmatic bronchitis. Until additional clinical studies identify the subset of COPD patients who will benefit most from these inhaled agents, no firm recommendation can be made regarding their use in COPD.

Other antiinflammatory agents, such as cromolyn, nedocromil, or the leukotriene antagonists, have not been studied in COPD and cannot be recommended at this time. These agents have a clear role in some patients with asthma.

Mucolytics and Expectorants. The benefits of mucolytics and expectorants in the management of secretions are not well documented. Mucolytics, such as iodinated glycerol and acetylcysteine, are postulated to work by helping to liquefy tenacious mucus in the bronchial tree. The results from the National Mucolytic Study indicate that although patients with chronic bronchitis treated with iodinated glycerol reported subjective improvement in chest symptoms, pulmonary function was not affected. In contrast to mucolytics, oral expectorants such as guaifenesin may help to loosen bronchial secretions by stimulating the flow of respiratory tract fluid and facilitating the movement of secretions by ciliary motion and coughing. Patients with chronic bronchitis often subjectively report that these expectorants help them to raise their secretions more readily, but clinical efficacy of such products has not been demonstrated. No standard role exists for expectorants or mucolytics in symptomatic treatment of COPD.

Antibiotics. Antibiotics are frequently prescribed for patients with COPD to treat or prevent an acute infectious exacerbation of COPD. Three organisms, *Haemophilus influenzae, Streptococcus pneumoniae,* and *Moraxella (Branhamella) catarrhalis* have emerged as the major bacterial pathogens in infected patients with COPD. Acute infectious exacerbations, characterized by worsening dyspnea, increased cough, sputum production, and sputum purulence, may worsen pulmonary function during the infection, although controversy surrounds whether pulmonary function is permanently altered. Antibiotic prophylaxis with alternating agents administered 1 week a month may reduce the frequency of exacerbations in the subset of patients with COPD who have four or more exacerbations a year.

Although the role of antibiotics in managing exacerbations of COPD is controversial, it has become standard practice to prescribe a course of antimicrobial therapy when a patient presents with an acute exacerbation of COPD, particularly if the exacerbation appears infectious, as characterized by an increase in sputum volume and purulence. The most common antimicrobial agents used in the treatment of patients with acute infectious exacerbations of COPD include amoxicillin, amoxicillin/clavulanate, tetracycline, macrolides (e.g., erythromycin, clarithromycin, azithromycin), or trimethoprim-sulfamethoxazole. Gram's stain and culture of the sputum are important because *M. catarrhalis* and 15% to 25% of *H. influenzae* strains are typically resistant to amoxicillin.

α_1-Protease Inhibitor Replacement. Patients with COPD and a documented homozygous α_1-PI deficiency with serum levels less than 11 μM may potentially benefit from weekly intravenous α_1-PI replacement derived from human plasma. Although replacement therapy is safe and feasible and can increase levels of α_1-PI, the efficacy of replacement therapy in terms of preservation of pulmonary function is unknown. Patients with α_1-PI deficiency and COPD should be referred to specialty centers for evaluation for replacement therapy.

Relief of Dyspnea. The best way to relieve dyspnea in patients with COPD is through maximal use of bronchodilators, oral and inhaled corticosteroids, and theophylline. Benzodiazepines are generally of no clinical benefit, although opiates such as morphine may help relieve dyspnea. Opiates are associated with respiratory depression, however, and extreme caution is warranted when considering their use in disabling dyspnea.

Prevention of Influenza and Pneumococcal Pneumonia. Since pulmonary infection is a common complication in COPD that can lead to worsening pulmonary function and respiratory failure, an annual prophylactic vaccine against influenza is recommended in those individuals who are not sensitive to egg protein. This vaccine is associated with a 60% to 80% protection rate. Amantadine can be considered in patients with COPD who have not received the vaccination and who are at risk for influenza A or in patients with early influenza A. The polyvalent pneumococcal vaccination, administered one time, is also recommended for people with COPD over 50 years of age. Revaccination is currently advised only if the patient received the vaccine 5 or more years earlier and was under age 65 at the time of primary vaccination.[4] In immunocompromised persons an initial vaccine is recommended, and a single revaccination should be administered 5 years after the initial dose.

Supplemental Oxygen Therapy. Oxygen (O_2) is a component of the pharmacotherapy of COPD because it is a potent pulmonary arterial vasodilator.[10] Since hypoxemia can cause pulmonary arterial hypertension and right ventricular failure (cor pulmonale), supplemental O_2 would be expected to blunt pulmonary arterial hypertension and prevent cor pulmonale. The importance of supplemental O_2, termed *long-term oxygen therapy* (LTOT), in a subset of patients with COPD has been derived from two clinical trials conducted in the early 1980s. The trials demonstrated that supplemental O_2 therapy significantly decreased morbidity and mortality in COPD patients with chronic hypoxemia. Additional benefits included an improvement in neuropsychiatric functioning and an increase in exercise tolerance.

Box 75-2 lists the three criteria for the initiation of LTOT. ABGs should be obtained from an approved laboratory for the initial evaluation of the need for LTOT. Pulse oximetry is easily obtained, noninvasive, and less expensive but is less accurate and gives no information regarding arterial carbon dioxide pressure ($Paco_2$). The identification of patients with hypercapnia is extremely important, since hypercapnia may worsen with the institution of LTOT. A subset of patients with

Box 75-2. Indications for Long-term Supplemental Oxygen Therapy*

1. Resting state, room air Pa_{O_2} ≤55 mm Hg or Sa_{O_2} ≤88%.
2. Resting state, room air Pa_{O_2} of 56-59 mm Hg or Sa_{O_2} ≤89%, if patient has polycythemia (hematocrit ≤52%) or clinical or electrocardiographic evidence of cor pulmonale
3. Pa_{O_2} ≤55 mm Hg or Sa_{O_2} ≤88% during exercise (documented by 6- or 23-minute walk test) or sleep (documented by sleep study) regardless of Pa_{O_2} at resting state and room air.

Pa_{O_2}, Arterial oxygen partial pressure (tension); *Sa_{O_2}*, arterial oxygen saturation.

*All assessments must be done during a stable clinical state and not during an acute illness. When long-term O_2 therapy is initiated, arterial blood gases (room air, resting state) should be repeated within 3 months to confirm a continued need for oxygen.

COPD may be at risk for desaturation during exercise or sleep even if the patient does not meet the criteria for LTOT based on resting ABGs (criteria 1 and 2). Room air, resting arterial oxygen pressure (Pa_{O_2}) levels between 60 and 65 mm Hg, a reduced DLco, and complaints of dyspnea on exertion warrant consideration of a 6-minute standardized walk test with pulse oximetry to evaluate the need for supplemental O_2 during exercise (criterion 3). Some investigators also recommend a sleep study in this same group to evaluate for nocturnal desaturation that would warrant supplemental O_2 therapy during sleep, particularly in patients who are obese or hypercapnic or have erythrocytosis (hematocrit 52% or greater) or cor pulmonale. Most studies use resting oxyhemoglobin saturation criteria as the basis to prescribe LTOT. LTOT prescribed to patients who do not meet criteria at rest, however, but only with exercise or sleep, has been shown to improve exercise tolerance and quality of life and may improve survival.

The majority of patients who meet the indications for LTOT warrant the use of O_2 therapy on a continuous basis unless O_2 was prescribed based solely on exercise- or sleep-induced criteria. In these two instances, O_2 should be prescribed only during the times of desaturation. Dyspnea without evidence of significant hypoxemia at rest or exercise is not an indication for LTOT.

Components of Oxygen Prescription

Oxygen flow. The majority of patients with COPD can attain a Pa_{O_2} of 60 mm Hg or greater (corresponding to an oxyhemoglobin saturation of about 90%) on a flow of 1 to 2 L/min of supplemental O_2 while at rest. A small subset of patients with hypoxemic COPD develop hypercapnia with oxygen supplementation, and careful titration in these patients is essential. In addition to the flow prescribed at rest, some physicians prescribe a separate O_2 flow for exercise and sleep. This is usually accomplished by empirically increasing the resting O_2 flow by 1 L/min during exercise and sleep. A more precise method to evaluate the degree of desaturation with exercise and thus prescribe a more precise flow of O_2 is by conducting a 6- or 12-minute walk test. If sleep studies have been conducted, desaturation during the study will determine flow rates during sleep, although sleep studies should not be done unless clinically indicated.

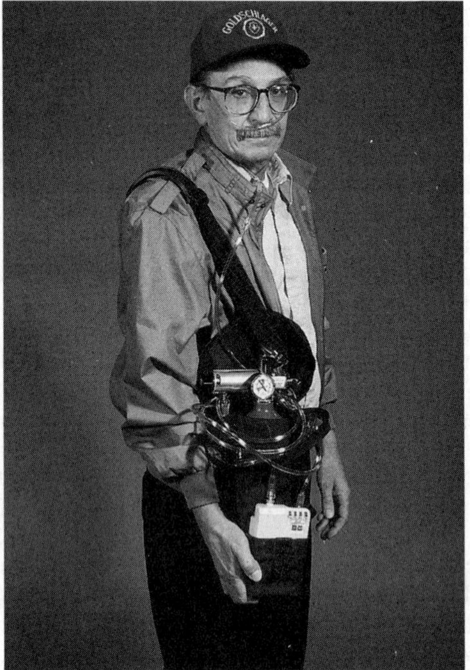

Fig. 75-2. Pulsed oxygen delivery device attached to ambulatory unit.

Routine delivery devices. The most often used O_2 delivery device for LTOT is the nasal cannula. It is easy for patients to use and has few side effects (dryness of the nasal membranes, facial irritation). A disadvantage of the nasal cannula is that the amount of O_2 inspired is variable because of variations in the breathing pattern, including breathing through the mouth. In addition, since O_2 flow is continuous, even during expiration, O_2 is wasted. LTOT can also be delivered through a tracheostomy mask in patients with a tracheostomy. Unlike delivery through a nasal cannula, humidification should be provided with a tracheostomy mask.

Oxygen-conserving delivery devices. Oxygen for LTOT is expensive. O_2-conserving devices decrease the waste of oxygen to cut costs and maximize the duration of use of portable systems. A conserving device should be considered for patients who require flow rates greater than 2 L/min, who use liquid O_2, or who are active and spend more than 6 hours a day away from the stationary O_2 delivery system. Examples of conserving devices include reservoir nasal cannulas, pulsed O_2 devices, and transtracheal (TT) O_2 therapy. The reservoir nasal cannula allows for O_2 conservation by storing O_2 delivered from the equipment system in a reservoir during exhalation, which can result in an O_2 savings of 50% or more during rest. The pulsed O_2 delivery device, which allows for O_2 flow only during inhalation, can be attached to an ambulatory O_2 unit (Fig. 75-2). The TT catheter delivers O_2 directly into the trachea through an 18-gauge catheter. This delivery method is very efficient, decreasing the amount of O_2 use by 33% to 50%. Oxygen delivered by TT catheter may increase exercise tolerance more than other methods of O_2 delivery by decreasing inspired minute ventilation. Since the TT catheter can be concealed under a scarf or necktie, the patient has no reason to remove the O_2 source, which can improve compliance. Insertion of a TT catheter is an invasive procedure, however, and catheters may become obstructed, and local infection may occur. Patients must take an active role in catheter care and must be able to problem solve to

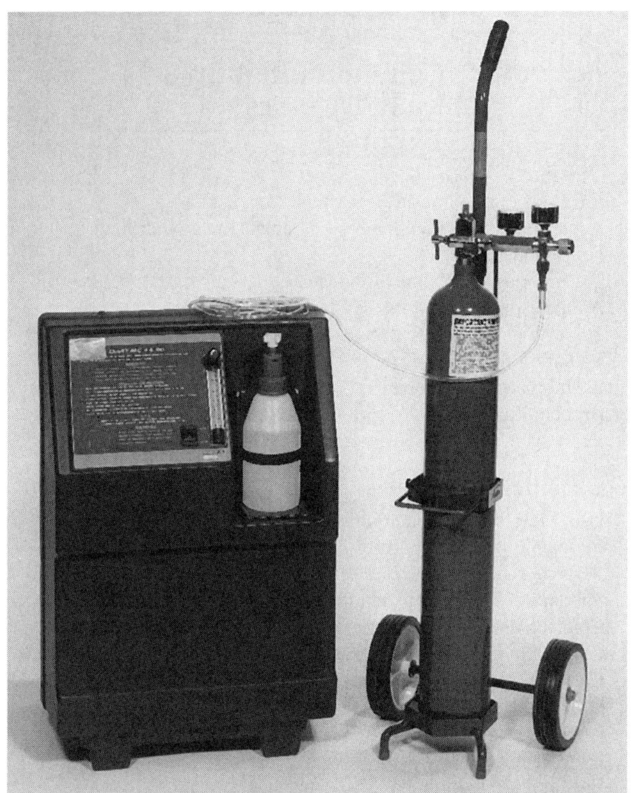

Fig. 75-3. Oxygen concentrator *(left)* with portable "E" tank cylinder *(right)*.

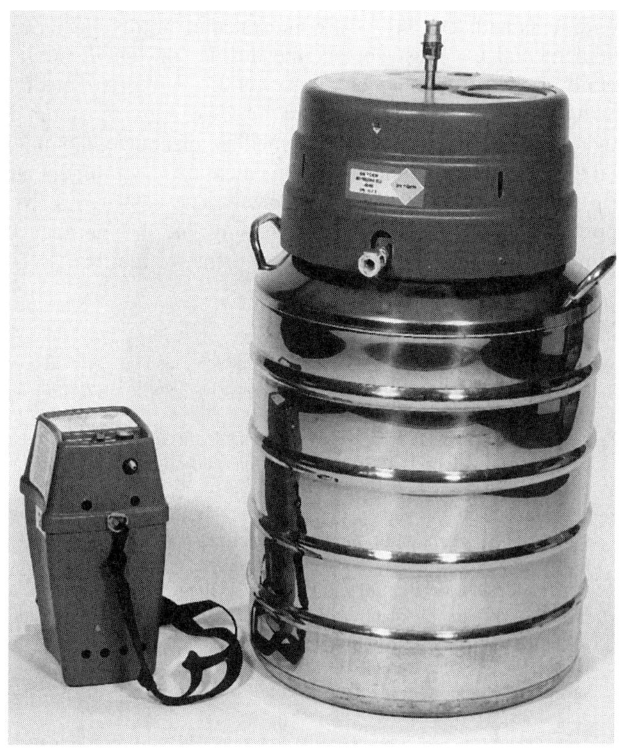

Fig. 75-4. Liquid oxygen stationary reservoir *(right)* with portable liquid system *(left)*.

achieve success. Interested patients should be referred to an established TT program for insertion and follow-up care.

Equipment systems. The three major types of O_2 systems for use in the home are the O_2 concentrator, compressed O_2, and liquid O_2. The O_2 concentrator separates atmospheric O_2 from nitrogen (N_2) and delivers O_2. This system operates by electrical power and is not portable; thus it is the most acceptable system for the homebound or less active patient. The concentrator is economical, is low maintenance, and refills are not needed. Compressed O_2 is usually prescribed in conjunction with the O_2 concentrator as a portable source of O_2 therapy for the patient when away from home (Fig. 75-3). Compressed O_2 tanks of various sizes are provided on a stroller. These compressed sources need to be exchanged for full tanks when empty. Delivery schedules are usually arranged between the O_2 vendor and the patient. A more recent advancement is a portable concentrator that weighs approximately 35 pounds. This concentrator is A/C battery driven and is rechargeable from a cigarette lighter in an automobile. This state-of-the-art technology permits patients to travel without the need for refilling O_2 tanks. This O_2 delivery system costs approximately $3000 and is not covered by medical insurance. Liquid O_2 is 100% pure and provided to the patient in cylinders filled with cryogenic O_2 (Fig. 75-4) When the system is turned on, the O_2 is warmed to room temperature before delivery to the patient. For portability the patient can fill a shoulder-bag tank by attaching the portable tank to the main liquid O_2 reservoir. This portable liquid system weighs approximately 8 to 10 pounds and allows about 6 hours of O_2 at 2 L/min. The liquid O_2 system requires frequent refills by the O_2 vendor depending on the prescribed liter flow; therefore this is the most expensive O_2 delivery system and should be reserved for patients who are active and mobile.

Follow-up Evaluations. LTOT is frequently initiated before discharge from an acute care facility before the patient's clinical pulmonary status has returned to baseline. Patients may no longer meet the criteria for LTOT after discharge. Therefore it is recommended that ABGs be repeated on room air, in a resting state, within 1 to 3 months after initiation of LTOT to reevaluate its need. If LTOT is continued, annual documentation of ABGs or oxyhemoglobin saturation by pulse oximetry is recommended to assess the patient's clinical and physiologic status. In contrast, if LTOT is discontinued, ABGs should be repeated 1 to 2 weeks after cessation to verify continued adequate oxygenation.

Air Travel

The pressure of inspired oxygen falls considerably with altitude because of a decrease in total barometric pressure. Commercial aircraft cruise between 22,000 and 44,000 feet above sea level. Hypoxemia can occur during air travel because the aircraft cabin is only pressurized to a median altitude of 6214 feet above sea level, which results in a significant decrease in inspired oxygen pressure. All travelers develop some degree of arterial oxygen desaturation during flight from the decrease in inspired oxygen, but patients with lung disease, including COPD, are particularly prone to develop significant hypoxemia. Patients at risk must be identified in advance. Those with ground-level, room air Pao_2 levels of less than 70 mm Hg should be referred to a pulmonary function laboratory for an evaluation that will determine the need for and amount of O_2 supplementation during flight. The most effective treatment of significant altitude hypoxemia is supplemental O_2 to attain a PaO_2 of at least 50 mm Hg during flight.

Patients with COPD who are interested in air travel and need supplemental O_2 must contact the airline for specific policy details and instructions for authorization. A written medical statement from a physician is required at least 48 hours in advance of a scheduled flight for medical clearance. Commercial airlines provide their own supplemental O_2 equipment and will not accept the patient's equipment. The cost varies from approximately $40 to $150, depending on the number of cylinders used and the number of segments of the trip.

REFERENCES

1. American Thoracic Society: Lung function testing: selection of reference values and interpretative strategies, *Am Rev Respir Dis* 144:1202, 1991.
2. Bourbeau J, Rouleau MY, Boucher S: Randomised controlled trial of inhaled corticosteroids in patients with chronic obstructive pulmonary disease, *Thorax* 53:477, 1998.
3. Cazzola M, Di Perna F, Noschese P, et al: Effects of formoterol, salmeterol or oxitropium bromide on airway responses to salbumatol in COPD, *Eur Respir J* 11:1337, 1998.
4. Centers for Disease Control and Prevention: Prevention of pneumococcal disease: recommendations of the Advisory Committee on Immunization Practices, *MMWR* 46:663, 685, 1997.
5. Hurt RD, Sachs DPL, Glover ED, et al: A comparison of sustained-release bupropion and placebo for smoking cessation, *N Engl J Med* 337:1195, 1997.
6. Langenderfer B: Alternatives to percussion and postural drainage, *J Cardiopulm Rehabil* 18:283, 1998.
7. Paggiaro PL, Ragnar D, Barkran I, et al: Multicentre randomised placebo-controlled trial of inhaled fluticasone propionate in patients with chronic obstructive pulmonary disease, *Lancet* 351:773, 1998.
8. Pulmonary rehabilitation: joint ACCP/AACVPR evidence-based guidelines, *Chest* 112:1363, 1997.
9. Saag KG, Emkey R, Schnitzer TJ, et al: Alendronate for the prevention and treatment of glucocorticoid-induced osteoporosis, *N Engl J Med* 339:292, 1998.
10. Schapira RM, Reinke LF: Long-term (home) oxygen therapy, *Clin Pulm Med* 7:69, 2000.
11. Schapira RM, Schapira MM, Funahashi A, et al: The value of the forced expiratory time in the physical diagnosis of obstructive airway disease, *JAMA* 270:731, 1993.

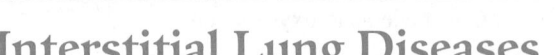

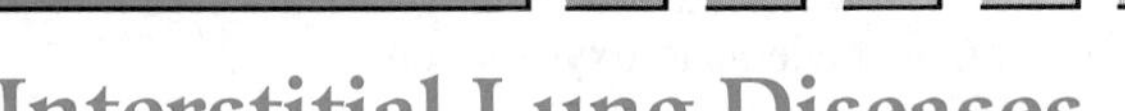

Interstitial Lung Diseases

Donald P. Schlueter

More than 130 acute and chronic diseases can involve the interstitium of the lung either as a primary disorder or as a secondary manifestation of a systemic disease (Box 76-1). They constitute a heterogenous group of disorders in which often no cause can be identified. The interstitium of the lung includes the connective tissue of the pleura, blood vessels and bronchi, and the alveolar walls. Interstitial lung disease has been defined as an inflammatory process involving all the components of the alveolar wall that may heal completely or may result in excess connective tissue with gross distortion of the lung architecture.[26] The initial event involves a focal or diffuse alveolitis caused by the accumulation in the alveolar walls of pulmonary macrophages, circulating lymphocytes, monocytes, and neutrophils that mediate acute and chronic inflammation. This inflammatory process results in the release of mediators that stimulate collagen production by fibroblasts and may eventually progress to *interstitial pulmonary fibrosis,* also known as *fibrosing alveolitis*. The clinical course depends on the pathologic diagnosis, and prognosis is quite variable. In some cases where a specific etiologic agent has been identified, simply removing the individual from exposure results in gradual recovery; others respond to steroid therapy, but in many patients the condition progresses despite treatment.

Box 76-1. Common Interstitial Lung Diseases

Acute

Infection (e.g., viral, mycoplasmal, fungal)
Acute interstitial pneumonitis (Hamman-Rich syndrome)
Drug-induced disease
Organic dust–or chemical-induced hypersensitivity pneumonitis
Adult respiratory distress syndrome (ARDS)
Toxic gas exposure (chlorine, nitrogen dioxide)
Radiation therapy
Eosinophilic pneumonia
Bronchiolitis obliterans with organizing pneumonia (BOOP)
Pulmonary vasculitis syndrome

Chronic

Usual interstitial pneumonitis (UIP)
Idiopathic pulmonary fibrosis (IPF)
Sarcoidosis
Pneumoconiosis due to inorganic dust
Connective tissue disorder
Chronic hypersensitivity pneumonitis due to organic dust
Carcinomatosis and alveolar cell carcinoma
Drug-induced disease
Goodpasture's syndrome
Lymphangioleiomyomatosis
Eosinophilic granuloma histiocytosis X

CLINICAL PRESENTATION

The most common presenting complaint of patients with interstitial lung disease is dyspnea.[26] Initially it may be present only with exertion, but as the disease process progresses, it may occur at rest. Since the loss of lung function may be gradual (because substantial functional reserve exists in the lung), the disease may progress significantly before the patient seeks medical attention. A nonproductive, irritating cough frequently aggravated by exertion and deep breathing and a feeling of chest tightness or heaviness may be present, especially as the fibrosis develops and progresses. Wheezing, sputum production, anorexia, and weight loss are not usually seen until the disease is more advanced. However, systemic symptoms may be present in patients whose interstitial lung disease is secondary to another condition, such as a connective tissue disorder.

PATIENT EVALUATION

History

A thorough and accurate history is extremely important in the evaluation of a patient with interstitial lung disease. This should involve potential environmental exposures at work.

The occupational history should include a detailed listing of all jobs held by the patient, the specific tasks performed, and materials used. Where potentially hazardous materials are used, the employer must provide the worker with the pertinent material safety data sheets (MSDS). This information should be helpful in considering the possible contribution of this source to the patient's problem. Since some exposures (e.g., asbestos) produce clinically apparent disease over a long latent period, usually 10 to 20 years, it may require considerable perseverance to obtain the appropriate information. The home environment should not be neglected, since contaminated humidifiers and air-conditioning systems can be a cause of interstitial lung disease in the form of hypersensitivity pneumonitis.[11] Prolonged low-level exposure, as may be encountered with exposure to an organic dust in the home environment, may not produce sufficient acute symptoms to cause the patient to seek medical attention and therefore results in a delay in diagnosis. With the acute form of hypersensitivity pneumonitis, symptoms of malaise, fever, dyspnea, and cough develop 4 to 8 hours after exposure to the offending agent. Because of this delay, the patient often does not recognize the causal relationship. Early recognition is essential, since avoidance of further exposure can result in resolution or at least stabilization of the interstitial process. A number of drugs, particularly cancer chemotherapeutic agents and illicit street drugs, have been implicated as causative agents in this disease, and their use should be carefully evaluated. A geographic history may be helpful in suggesting or excluding a chronic infectious process. Symptoms consistent with a connective tissue or vascular disorder should be sought.

Physical Examination

In the early stages of interstitial lung disease the physical examination, including auscultation of the chest, may be entirely normal. As the disease process progresses and dyspnea develops, basilar crackles (Velcro rales) signal the presence of interstitial pulmonary fibrosis. However, the absence of crackles does not exclude the diagnosis. Later, cyanosis and, in about 10% to 15% of patients, finger clubbing develop. The latter is more common in patients with idiopathic pulmonary fibrosis (IPF) and asbestosis. With advanced disease, cardiac involvement is common, with pulmonary hypertension and right-sided heart failure. With the exception of sarcoidosis and the collagen vascular diseases, the physical findings are generally limited to the chest.

LABORATORY STUDIES AND DIAGNOSTIC PROCEDURES

The chest radiograph is the most important piece of information in the initial evaluation of a patient with suspected interstitial lung disease and may be abnormal in the absence of significant respiratory symptoms. Some patients with dyspnea and interstitial lung disease, however, may have a normal chest film; in one series, 13% of patients with IPF, 37% with hypersensitivity pneumonitis, and 10% with sarcoidosis had normal chest radiographs.[4] The introduction of high-resolution computed tomography (HRCT) scanning of the lung has increased the sensitivity for detecting minimal interstitial disease not evident on conventional chest radiographs.[14] Early in the disease process, radiographic changes may be limited to an increase in interstitial markings, more prominent in the lower lung fields. Every effort should be made to obtain any existing chest radiographs, since subtle

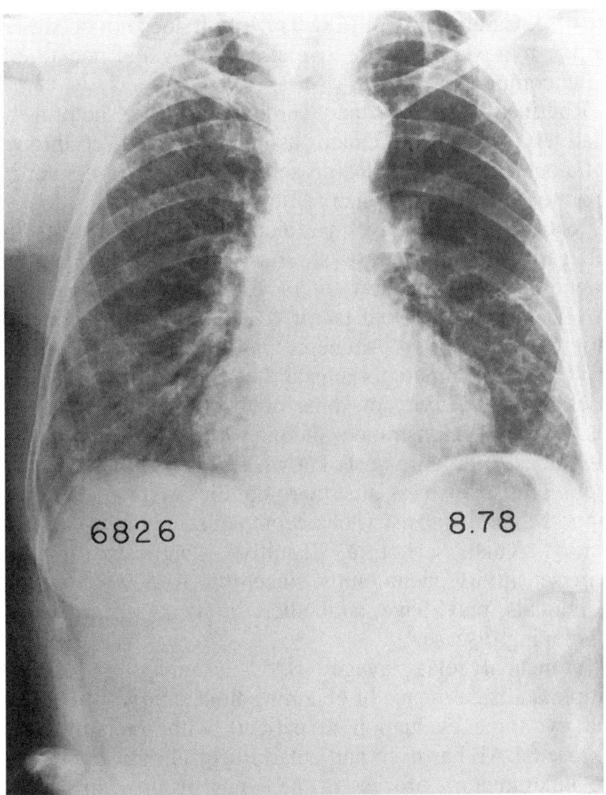

Fig. 76-1. Chest radiograph of 73-year-old woman showing diffuse linear opacities with honeycombing and early cor pulmonale. She had progressive dyspnea for 3 years, bilateral end-inspiratory crackles, and physiologic studies showing decreased vital capacity, very low single-breath diffusing capacity, and oxygen desaturation at rest that became more severe with exercise. Lung biopsy showed usual interstitial pneumonitis (UIP).

changes may become more obvious when previous chest films are available for comparison. They may also provide information on disease onset and progression. Hilar and mediastinal lymphadenopathy is usually associated with sarcoidosis, silicosis, and some lymphomas. Pleural disease is uncommon in interstitial lung disease. Pleural effusion and pleural thickening may occur with collagen vascular disease, lymphoma, asbestos-related disease, and a small percentage of patients with sarcoidosis. As the disease progresses, a more clearly defined reticulonodular pattern becomes evident with a decrease in lung volume, as indicated by elevation of the diaphragms (Fig. 76-1).

Pulmonary function studies reflect the structural changes that cause a stiff, noncompliant lung. All lung volumes are reduced, consistent with a restrictive ventilatory impairment. Spirometry shows a decrease in forced vital capacity (FVC) and forced expiratory volume in 1 second (FEV_1) but a normal FEV_1/FVC ratio. Usually, flow rates are not significantly decreased unless the restriction is severe, although evidence for small airways obstruction has been reported in interstitial lung disease.[7] Lung volume measurements show a decreased total lung capacity (TLC), functional residual capacity (FRC), and residual volume (RV), with a normal to low RV/TLC ratio. Most patients have a disturbance in gas exchange manifested by a significantly diminished single-breath diffusing lung capacity for carbon monoxide (DLco). Although arterial oxygenation may be normal at rest, arterial hypoxemia is usually present with exercise. Carbon dioxide (CO_2) retention does not occur, and despite hypoxemia, erythrocytosis and elevated hematocrits are uncommon.

Routine blood tests and serology may be helpful but relatively nonspecific, such as an increased erythrocyte sedimentation rate (ESR) or serum angiotensin-converting enzyme (ACE) level, which is elevated in about 29% to 93% of patients with active sarcoidosis. Serologic tests for collagen vascular disease are necessary to exclude these diagnoses, although low titers of antinuclear antibodies (ANAs) and rheumatoid factor (RF) have been reported in patients with IPF.[15] Antineutrophil cytoplasmic antibody (ANCA) determinations appear helpful in diagnosing and assessing the activity of some of the necrotizing vasculitides.[27] The demonstration of high titers of precipitating antibodies to organic dusts known to cause hypersensitivity pneumonitis, such as the thermophilic *Actinomyces,* may support this diagnosis when accompanied by an appropriate history. This is not a definitive diagnostic test for hypersensitivity pneumonitis, since 40% to 50% of exposed individuals may have antibodies in their serum without developing disease.[5]

Bronchoalveolar lavage (BAL) provides a relatively simple and safe means of obtaining fluid samples for culture and cytologic evaluation in patients with interstitial lung disease.[2] BAL has been particularly helpful in characterizing the inflammatory process in the lungs by providing viable cells for analysis of functional and secretory activity. Analysis of the cellular constituents has been suggested not only as a means for diagnosing the specific interstitial disease process, but also as guide for instituting and monitoring the effectiveness of therapy. A predominance of lymphocytes is found in sarcoidosis, hypersensitivity pneumonitis, and lymphoma, whereas polymorphonuclear neutrophils (PMNs) predominate in IPF, histiocytosis X, asbestosis, cigarette smokers, and infection. At present the use of BAL for diagnosing and staging of interstitial lung disease remains controversial, since the procedure is invasive, the technique is not standardized, and results show significant variability.

Radioactive gallium scanning has been used to evaluate patients with interstitial lung disease. Its role also remains somewhat controversial because of its nonspecificity; varied types of pulmonary inflammation as well as neoplasms can produce a positive result. Gallium is most likely taken up by activated alveolar macrophages or PMNs in the areas of inflammation, and the uptake may be a marker of alveolitis. This is supported by the finding of a better correlation of gallium uptake with the extent of inflammation on open lung biopsy compared with conventional chest radiographs. Gallium scanning has been used to follow the course of disease during treatment but has been disappointing in predicting responsiveness to corticosteroid or immunosuppressive therapy; only 10% to 30% of patients with increased uptake may respond to therapy.[9] Favorable responses to therapy have been noted even when the gallium scans are normal. Gallium scanning may be helpful in planning a biopsy procedure by identifying areas of active inflammation and thus increasing the probability of a positive result.

Despite the large number of causes, a definitive diagnosis of interstitial disease can often be made on the basis of the history, clinical findings, and laboratory data. Some examples include pneumoconiosis, hypersensitivity pneumonitis, and drug-induced lung diseases. Sarcoidosis could be included, particularly if organs other than the lung are involved. In most patients with interstitial lung disease, however, histologic examination of lung tissue is the most effective method of obtaining a definitive characterization of the extent and pattern of disease and determining the presence or absence of organisms that might be responsible. Fiberoptic bronchoscopy with transbronchial biopsy is the initial procedure of choice when the suspected diagnosis includes sarcoidosis, hypersensitivity pneumonitis, pulmonary alveolar proteinosis, eosinophilic granuloma or histiocytosis X, and malignancy.

Open lung biopsy remains the gold standard for a histologic diagnosis when the transbronchial biopsy is nondiagnostic or with a suspected disease process that is not likely to yield a definitive result by this procedure. In addition, it excludes other etiologies and directly assesses the inflammatory and fibrotic lesions. It also provides enough tissue to perform a variety of special tests, including electron microscopy, energy-dispersive x-ray analysis, and immunofluorescence.[8] Tissue can be obtained from several lobes and areas with different degrees of involvement. Video-assisted thoracoscopic lung biopsy can help in the diagnosis and staging of interstitial lung disease. This procedure involves two or three endoscopic trocars and instruments, with single-lung ventilation and collapse of the lung to be biopsied. Hospital stay and postoperative pain are reduced, and adequate tissue can be obtained in most patients.

ACUTE INTERSTITIAL PNEUMONIAS

Acute interstitial pneumonia, or *diffuse alveolar damage,* can result from a variety of insults to the lung. This response can be seen in viral pneumonias, adult respiratory distress syndrome (ARDS), toxic chemical exposures, antineoplastic drugs, active connective tissue diseases, radiation injury, and fat embolism syndrome. In most cases the pathologic changes of diffuse alveolar damage gradually resolve with minimal residual effect. In ARDS the chest radiograph shows a diffuse infiltrate consistent with pulmonary edema, whereas in the other conditions the infiltrates may be more patchy. The diagnosis usually can be suspected from the clinical setting; biopsy may be needed only when an infectious process is suspected. Treatment is supportive for most of these patients, but corticosteroids may accelerate recovery in those with acute interstitial pneumonia associated with connective tissue disorders or caused by chemical exposure, radiation therapy, or antineoplastic drugs.

CHRONIC INTERSTITIAL PNEUMONIAS

Idiopathic pulmonary fibrosis (IPF), or *cryptogenic fibrosing alveolitis* (a term preferred by the British), is one of the more common interstitial lung diseases of unknown etiology. IPF is a chronic progressive lung disorder associated with both inflammation and fibrosis of the lung parenchyma. Confusion has arisen concerning IPF and its relation to the morphologic classification of interstitial pneumonias, including desquamative interstitial pneumonitis (DIP) and usual interstitial pneumonitis (UIP).[13] Some recommend that this terminology not be applied to IPF, even though lung tissue from patients with IPF may show morphologic changes typical of DIP or UIP, since these changes are nonspecific and found in other interstitial lung diseases; however, this suggestion has not been generally accepted.[1] The distinction between DIP and UIP has some prognostic significance because patients with DIP are more likely to respond to corticosteroids. This has led to the conclusion that DIP is probably an early stage of UIP.

In addition, certain subgroups of interstitial pneumonias are based on the types of predominant inflammatory cells in the lung biopsy, including lymphocytic interstitial pneumonia (LIP), giant cell interstitial pneumonia (GIP), and plasma cell interstitial pneumonia (PIP).

IPF typically occurs in people 50 to 80 years old but may affect all age groups and is more common in men and in smokers. It occurs with a prevalence rate of three to five cases per 100,000 population. In 1935 Hamman and Rich first described five patients with rapidly progressive dyspnea, diffuse infiltrates in chest radiographs, and death occurring in 6 months of presentation. Recent studies suggest that this more fulminant type of pulmonary fibrosis occurs more often in connective tissue diseases, particularly rheumatoid arthritis. Although the course of IPF is variable, progressive deterioration in pulmonary function and exercise capacity, increasing hypoxemia, and radiographic evidence of extensive fibrosis and honeycombing over 2 to 8 years are typical features. Periods of stabilization may occur, but spontanenous improvement is rarely seen. Mean survival ranges from 3 to 5 years, with mortality exceeding 40% within 5 years of onset of symptoms.[17]

Patients with IPF typically present with a history of an insidious onset of progressive dyspnea on exertion and nonproductive cough. The cough often occurs with prolonged paroxysms and responds poorly to antitussives. Chest examination in most patients reveals bilateral late-inspiratory crackles (Velcro rales), predominantly over the lower lung fields. Wheezing is not a feature of IPF. Finger clubbing is relatively common, occurring in 40% to 75% of patients. Cardiac examination usually yields normal results, except in later stages of the disease, when signs of pulmonary hypertension and cor pulmonale may become evident. Cyanosis is also a late manifestation indicative of severe disease.

The chest radiograph is abnormal in the majority of patients with IPF, and these changes often alert the physician to the presence of interstitial lung disease. The most common abnormalities are a reticular or reticulonodular pattern diffusely involving the lower lung fields and volume loss. With advanced disease, multiple cystic or honeycombed areas may be seen. Although the correlation between the radiographic pattern and the stage of disease (clinical or histopathologic) is generally poor, chest radiographs and HRCT of the lungs are important in gauging progression or regression of disease in response to therapy. The HRCT may show the presence of interstitial fibrosis in a small percentage of patients with IPF who have a normal chest radiograph.

A variety of abnormal laboratory tests have been noted in IPF, including an elevated ESR, circulating immune complexes, RF, and ANAs. However, serologic parameters fail to correlate with activity of disease or predict responsiveness to therapy. Serum anticollagen antibodies may be a marker of IPF activity. The typical pulmonary function changes are consistent with a restrictive impairment, with reduction in all lung volumes, including FVC, FEV_1, TLC, FRC, and RV. Airways obstruction is not usually present unless there is complicating chronic obstructive lung disease. A major physiologic abnormality is a disturbance in gas exchange caused by ventilation/perfusion inequality and contraction of the pulmonary capillary volume. As a result the DLco is reduced, a change that may precede the reduction in lung volume. Although arterial oxygenation at rest may be normal, desaturation almost always can be demonstrated with exercise. Exercise testing is more sensitive in the detection of abnormalities in oxygen transfer and provides a more sensitive parameter for following the clinical course.

The clinical, physiologic, and radiographic manifestations of IPF are similar to those of other interstitial lung diseases; open lung biopsy is usually required to substantiate the diagnosis and exclude other etiologies. The lung biopsy in IPF shows a wide spectrum of histologic changes depending on the stage of the disease. The early stages involve an alveolitis characterized by an accumulation of mononuclear cells (lymphocytes, alveolar macrophages, and type II alveolar cells) in the alveolar spaces, with relative preservation of the alveolar walls (i.e., DIP). As the disease progresses, the alveolar walls are distorted with edema, mononuclear cell infiltration, and fibroblast proliferation (i.e., UIP). In advanced stages the alveolar walls are greatly thickened, and much of the alveolar architecture is destroyed and replaced by connective tissue and fibrosis.[25] Large cystic spaces forming the honeycomb lung and minimal inflammatory cells represent the end stage of this disease. Because of the small amount of tissue obtained by transbronchial biopsy (TBB), it is difficult to assess the degree of inflammation and fibrosis, and therefore TBB provides little prognostic information. Thoracoscopic lung biopsy may provide a compromise between TBB and open lung biopsy by minimizing operative risks yet providing adequate tissue for diagnosis. BAL is not specific enough to provide a definitive diagnosis of IPF but may predict therapeutic responsiveness, since the presence of BAL lymphocytosis has been associated with a greater responsiveness to corticosteroid therapy.[30]

The most effective treatment for IPF is corticosteroids, but response to therapy is inconsistent.[32] In general, patients with the shortest duration of symptoms, with BAL fluid showing greater than 5% lymphocytes and less than 10% neutrophils, and with a lung biopsy demonstrating more inflammation with less fibrosis will most likely respond to corticosteroids and have a more favorable prognosis.[31] Usually an initial dose of oral prednisone at 40 to 60 mg daily is given for several months, and if a favorable response is obtained, prednisone is tapered slowly to 15 to 20 mg daily or an equivalent alternate-day dosage. Corticosteroids should be continued for at least 1 year. If no response is observed in the initial therapeutic trial of corticosteroids, they should be rapidly tapered and discontinued. Cytotoxic agents, such as azathioprine and cyclophosphamide, are used as second-line drugs, usually in combination with oral corticosteroids; the efficacy of these treatments has not been definitively demonstrated, however, and they carry a considerably greater risk of adverse effects than corticosteroids alone. Colchicine has been suggested as a potentially useful agent in the treatment of IPF because of its antifibrotic properties.[18] No controlled prospective clinical studies are available to evaluate the efficacy of this therapy. Finally, single-lung transplantation is a consideration for patients with end-stage pulmonary fibrosis refractory to medical therapy.[10] Survival time has increased significantly since then, to more than 75% in some centers. Unfortunately, because of the shortage of donor organs, many patients with IPF die while awaiting transplantation.

HYPERSENSITIVITY PNEUMONITIS

Hypersensitivity pneumonitis, or *extrinsic allergic alveolitis*, is an immunologic-induced interstitial pneumonitis characterized by predominantly mononuclear cell inflammation of the

Table 76-1. Occupational Hypersensitivity Pneumonitides

Disease	Exposure	Specific inhalant
Farmer's lung	Moldy hay	*Thermoactinomyces vulgaris*
		T. candidus
		T. viridis
		Micromonospora faeni
Bagassosis	Moldy sugar cane	*T. vulgaris*
		T. sacchare
Maple bark–stripper's lung	Contaminated maple logs	*Cryptostroma corticale*
Bird-breeder's lung	Avian droppings	Serum protein
Air conditioner, humidifier lung	Contaminated water	*T. vulgaris*
		T. candidus
		Amoeba species
		Endotoxin
Mushroom-worker's lung	Mushroom compost	*T. vulgaris*
		M. faeni
Malt-worker's lung	Moldy barley	*Aspergillus clavatus*
		A. fumigatus
Bakers asthma	Flour dust	Wheat flour
Detergent-worker's lung	Detergent powder	*Bacillus subtilis*
Grain weevil (miller's) lung	Grain dust	*Sitophilus granarius*
	Flour	
Suberosis	Oak bark	*Penicillium frequentans*
	Cork dust	
Furrier's lung	Fox	Hair protein
Coffee-worker's lung	Coffee bean dust	Coffee bean protein
Vineyard-sprayer's lung	Spray solution	Copper sulfate
		T. viridis
Sequoiosis	Redwood sawdust	*Graphium* species
		Aureobasidium pullulans
Cheese-washer's lung	Cheese mold	*Penicillium caseii*
		P. roqueforti
Fish meal–handler's lung	Fish meal (pet food)	Fish proteins
Wood-dust disease	Mahogany and oak dust	Unknown
Wood pulp–worker's lung	Moldy logs	*Alternaria tenuis*
Paprika-slicer's lung	Moldy paprika pods	*Mucor stolonifer*
Fog fever	Cattle	*T. candidus*
Feather-plucker's lung	Chicken products	Chicken proteins
Tobacco-grower's lung	Tobacco plants	Unknown
Tea-grower's lung	Tea plants	Unknown
Bible-printer's disease	Moldy typesetting water	Unknown
Plastics and resin makers	Plastics industry	Toluene diisocyanate
	Polyurethane	Methylene diphenyldiisocyanate
	Paints	Hexamethylene diisocyanate
Painters and paint makers	Sand binders	Trimellitic anhydride

pulmonary parenchyma, terminal bronchioles, and alveoli. The antigenic agents include organic dusts derived from fungal, bacterial, or serum protein sources, as well as some reactive organic chemicals[20-22] (Table 76-1).

Because of the very small particle size, usually less than 5 μm, a large quantity of antigenic material can be delivered to the alveolar level. The clinical response to antigen exposure depends on the individual's immunologic reactivity, the nature of the dust or chemical, the size of the particles, and the intensity of the exposure, particularly whether it is regular or intermittent. The immunologic reactivity appears to be an important predisposing factor in the development of hypersensitivity pneumonitis, since large surveys of farmers and workers exposed to bagasse, the spent sugar cane after the sugar has been removed, and a number of organic chemicals reveal a high percentage with serum precipitating antibody against specific antigen, but a low incidence of lung disease. The immunologic hallmark of hypersensitivity pneumonitis is the presence of serum IgG and IgA precipitating antibody to the inhaled antigen, with precipitins present in more than 90% of patients.[5] This finding of precipitating antibody in studies of farmer's lung disease suggested a hypersensitivity reaction. Subsequent investigations have shown that multiple immunologic reactions are involved predominantly with cell-mediated delayed hypersensitivity, with or without amplification by immune complexes, lymphokines, and other biologic modifiers. The predominance of CD8% T lymphocytes in BAL fluid in farmer's lung disease shifts toward the CD4% predominance after removal from exposure.

Although exposure in the workplace has most often been the focus of reports of hypersensitivity lung disease, more recently the home environment and even the family automobile have been implicated as a source of respiratory problems. Air-conditioning systems, furnace and room humidifiers, cold steamers, saunas, and hot tubs can cultivate a variety of organisms identified as etiologic agents in hypersensitivity pneumonitis.[6] Alleviation of symptoms when away from home with recurrence on return, or changes in symptoms during the heating or cooling season, may also offer clues. Thus a patient's total environmental exposure must be considered when a hypersensitivity lung disease is suspected.

The clinical manifestations of hypersensitivity pneumonitis are similar, regardless of the organic dust or chemical inhaled; these diseases should be considered as a syndrome with a spectrum of clinical features. The patient with hypersensitivity pneumonitis may present with three different clinical pictures: acute, subacute, or chronic.

Acute Form

The classic and most readily recognized form of hypersensitivity pneumonitis results from intermittent exposure to antigen and resembles an acute viral or bacterial infection. Symptoms include chills, fever, malaise, headache, nonproductive cough, chest tightness, and dyspnea without wheezing. Symptoms develop 4 to 6 hours after exposure and resolve spontaneously in 12 to 24 hours but recur on reexposure. Fatigue and weight loss may follow frequent or severe episodes. Physical findings include fever, tachypnea, tachycardia, cyanosis, and bibasilar late-inspiratory crackles; wheezing is rarely heard. Laboratory studies reveal a leukocytosis without eosinophilia and elevated immunoglobulin levels. High titers of precipitating antibody against the offending antigen are characteristic. Because precipitins are also common in exposed individuals without disease, however, this finding is not sufficient to make a diagnosis of hypersensitivity pneumonitis.

The chest radiograph may be normal after a brief exposure. With an intense or more prolonged exposure, however, a diffuse pattern of small, somewhat discrete nodules or a diffuse, soft, stringy or patchy interstitial infiltrate may be seen. The typical physiologic change is restrictive, with a decrease in vital capacity and lung volumes without airways obstruction. Some patients, particularly with severe reactions, may demonstrate small airways obstruction. Bronchial hyperreactivity is found in a significant number of individuals, particularly after an acute attack. This enhanced responsiveness may be caused by mediators released in the inflammatory response. Hypoxia is usually present, and the DLCO is invariably reduced, particularly at the height of the reaction. This abnormality may persist for some time after other parameters have returned to normal. Long-term follow-up studies in patients who continue to have only brief and infrequent exposure to the antigens usually do not show a significant decrement in pulmonary function.

Subacute Form

Subacute hypersensitivity pneumonitis is much less common than the acute form and tends to develop with more chronic exposure. Symptoms develop insidiously, with features of progressive chronic bronchitis, including productive cough, dyspnea, easy fatigue, anorexia, and weight loss. Typical acute attacks, although infrequent, can be precipitated by heavy exposure. The chest radiograph may show diffuse nodulation or change consistent with interstitial fibrosis, but normal radiologic findings are not unusual. Both restrictive and obstructive defects in pulmonary function are seen, with the former predominating. DLCO is reduced, along with hypoxemia, at least with exercise if not at rest. Long-term avoidance of exposure and administration of corticosteroids usually result in reduced symptoms and physiologic abnormalities. This is the most difficult form of the disease to diagnose because of the insidious nature and nonspecific clinical findings.

Chronic Form

Recurrent intense exposure to antigen or prolonged low-level exposure can lead to the chronic form of hypersensitivity pneumonitis, with the gradual development of disabling respiratory symptoms and irreversible physiologic changes. Progressive dyspnea is the most common symptom, along with nonproductive cough and easy fatigue. Physical findings include tachypnea, bibasilar crackles (Velcro rales), and wheezing, which are heard in some patients with a predominantly obstructive profile. With advanced disease, signs of pulmonary hypertension and cor pulmonale may be present. The chest radiograph in this predominantly fibrotic phase shows contraction of the lungs, particularly in the upper lobes, more peripheral involvement, and development of a honeycomb appearance. Some nodulation may persist but probably does not represent active granulomatous disease. Avoidance of exposure for prolonged periods and administration of corticosteroids and bronchodilators afford only slight improvement.

Pathophysiology

The histologic pattern found in the lung in hypersensitivity pneumonitis depends at what stage of disease the biopsy is obtained. In the acute stage the primary process is an interstitial granulomatous pneumonitis with foreign body giant cells, large numbers of lymphocytes, and macrophages with abundant foamy cytoplasm. Eosinophilia may be seen in the perivascular areas; vasculitis is rare. In the subacute stage there is moderate interstitial thickening, with only slight fibrosis, along with changes consistent with chronic bronchitis. In the chronic stage, interstitial fibrosis is the predominant feature and may be focal or diffuse. Intraalveolar septa are infiltrated with lymphocytes, and collections of dust-laden macrophages may be seen in the alveolar spaces. Bronchiolitis obliterans, cystic changes, and honeycombing are found in association with densely fibrotic areas. Confluent fibrosis tends to occur predominantly in the upper lobes. Regardless of the disease stage, these changes are not specific for hypersensitivity pneumonitis and must be interpreted in the context of all the associated clinical information.

Diagnosis

The diagnosis of hypersensitivity pneumonitis requires a high index of suspicion, a thorough history focusing on potential exposures in both work and home environments, and the temporal relationship between development of symptoms and exposure. Familiarity with the variety of organic dusts and chemicals that can cause this disorder is helpful (see Table 76-1). Frequently a specific antigen is not readily identified, however, and environmental sampling and culturing are necessary to isolate the offending agent. This isolate can then be used to prepare an antigen to test the patient's serum for precipitating antibodies. The demonstration of precipitating antibody against a particular organic antigen reflects exposure and is not sufficient evidence alone to make a diagnosis of hypersensitivity pneumonitis. About 40% to 50% of exposed individuals may have antibodies present in their serum without developing disease. In addition, serum precipitins may disappear after exposure ceases. BAL studies show a predominance of lymphocytes, reflecting an active alveolitis, but this finding is not limited to hypersensitivity pneumonitis. The most specific diagnostic test at present, if the suspected antigen can be identified, is controlled inhalation challenge in the laboratory followed by serial pulmonary function tests and clinical response monitoring. In the sensitized patient the signs, symptoms, and physiologic changes are accurately reproduced.

Treatment

The major therapeutic approach to treatment is removal from exposure to the offending antigen. This could cause significant economic hardship, however, as in the case of an affected farmer. Efforts to reduce the intensity of antigen exposure by changes in work practices and use of personal protection with a respirator have been of some benefit. Cromolyn is capable of blocking the immediate and late reaction in some individuals, whereas corticosteroids block only the late reaction. It is not certain, however, that continued exposure to antigen and control of the symptoms with medication will prevent subsequent lung damage. In some patients, continued antigen exposure may not lead to clinical deterioration.[28]

INORGANIC DUST DISEASE: PNEUMOCONIOSIS

The word pneumoconiosis literally means dust in the lungs; however, not all dusts deposited in the lungs cause disease. A more widely accepted definition is from the International Labor Organization (ILO): "pneumoconiosis is the accumulation of dust in the lungs and the tissue reaction to its presence."[16] Inorganic dusts that do not disrupt the alveolar architecture or produce fibrosis when retained in the lung are classified as inert dusts or nuisance particulates, provided that they are free from toxic impurities and contain less than 1% quartz. These dusts ordinarily do not cause respiratory symptoms or functional abnormalities and may be cleared from the lung over time with avoidance of exposure; the term *benign pneumoconiosis* has been applied to this condition (Box 76-2). The most common example is *siderosis,* occurring primarily in welders and in workers mining and crushing iron ores. The inhalation of inorganic dusts that elicit a response in the lungs, eventually leading to irreversible fibrosis and structural and functional alterations, causes *fibrosing,* or collagenous, *pneumoconiosis*. The most important etiologic agents are silica and asbestos.[3]

Box 76-2. Inorganic Dusts Causing Pneumoconiosis

Benign Form

Iron oxide (siderosis)
Tin ore (stannosis)
Barium compounds (baritosis)
Antimony ore
Zirconium compounds
Chromite ore
Cerium dioxide
Titanium dioxide

Fibrosing (Collagenous) Form

Silica
- Quartz
- Cristobalite
- Tridymite

Diatomaceous (infusorial) earth
Beryllium
Asbestos
Coal dust
Graphite
Carbon black
Aluminum
Talc

Silicosis

Silicosis is a chronic fibrotic disease of the lungs resulting from prolonged and intense exposure to free crystalline silica. Industrial sources of free silica include mining, quarrying and tunneling, foundry work, sandblasting, stone cutting and polishing, glass manufacturing, ceramics, and vitreous enameling. Several different clinical forms of silicosis are seen. The most common type is *chronic classic silicosis,* which occurs with moderate exposure over 20 to 45 years, usually involving respirable dust with less than 30% quartz. The lesions are usually nodular with a predominance in the upper lobes, probably due to better clearance of dust from the lower lobes. This simple stage of silicosis is associated with nodules generally 5 mm or less and usually normal pulmonary function. However, silicosis may be complicated by coalescence of the nodular lesions into conglomerate or confluent lesions, called *massive fibrosis,* usually in the upper lobes (progressive massive fibrosis, PMF) (Fig. 76-2). High quartz content apparently is the primary factor in the pathogenesis of massive fibrosis in silicosis.

Accelerated silicosis occurs most frequently in sandblasters and silica flour workers. It results from moderately high exposure to dust containing 40% to 80% quartz and appears 5 to 15 years after the initial exposure. The nodular lesions tend to be smaller than in chronic silicosis, and the massive fibrosis favors the midzones of the lungs.

Acute silicosis (silicoproteinosis) is a rare form of silicosis occurring in workers with intense exposure to dust with very high concentrations of silica. It has been reported primarily in sandblasters. The disease develops over 1 to 3 years and progresses rapidly to death from respiratory failure. The characteristic histopathologic finding is a lipid-proteinaceous material filling the alveoli, which gives a strongly positive reaction to periodic acid–Schiff reagent, similar to that in idiopathic pulmonary alveolar proteinosis. Since acute silicosis is frequently associated with occupations in which freshly fractured crystalline silica of respirable size is generated, fracture-generated silicon-based radicals may play a significant role in the pathogenesis of this disease.

Pathogenesis. Inhalation of silica particles small enough to reach the alveolar level induces a series of events resulting in the activation and persistence of inflammatory cells, with the alveolar macrophage playing a central role in the development of pulmonary inflammation. Earlier studies in

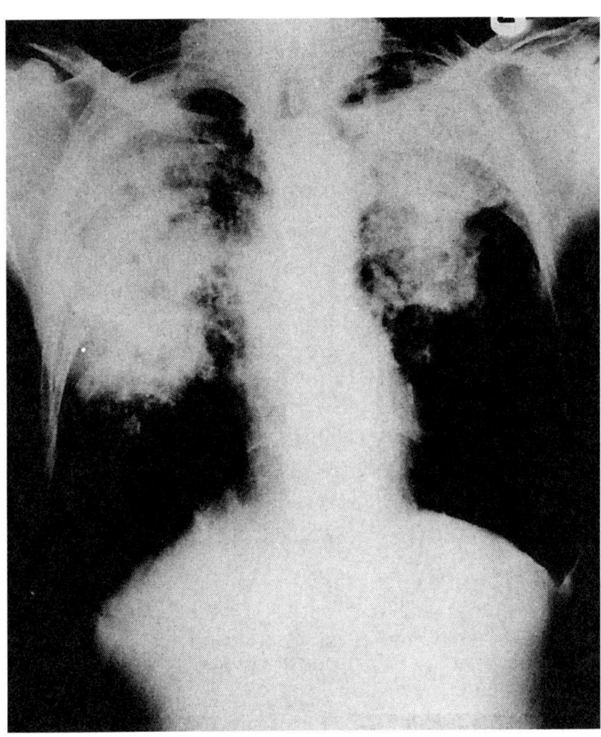

Fig. 76-2. Chest radiograph of coal worker 2 weeks before his death. Appearance is classic for progressive massive fibrosis (PMF), with larger conglomerate masses in both lung fields. (Courtesy JC Wagner.)

the pathogenesis of silicosis suggested that ingestion of silica particles by the macrophages resulted in an interaction of silica-containing phagosomes with lysozymes releasing enzymes, which caused rupture of the phagosome and freed the silica particles in the cell cytoplasm. This process eventually leads to death of the cell due to the release of lysosome enzymes. The cycle of cell destruction is perpetuated by ingestion of the silica particles by other macrophages. However, more recent studies have shown that silica-laden macrophages can maintain normal viability but may be activated to produce proinflammatory mediators such as cytokines, interleukin-1 (IL-1), and tumor necrosis factor alpha (TNF-α) that can participate in numerous inflammatory processes. Repeated inhalation of silica and slow clearance of silica-laden macrophages would keep the inflammatory mediators chronically activated and would perpetuate the inflammatory process, resulting in the development of granulomatous inflammation and fibrosis in the lung. Alveolar macrophages have also been shown to produce fibronectin and macrophage-derived growth factor (MDGF), which would also contribute to the subsequent progressive fibrosis.

The typical lesion of silicosis is the silicotic nodule. These well-circumscribed nodules consist of whorled zones of acellular hyalin surrounded by a moderately cellular collagenous capsule. The majority of the silica particles are found in the outer layers of the nodules. The silica can be demonstrated as birefringent particles when the tissue sections are viewed under polarized light. The nodules are usually associated with adjoining parenchymal fibrosis.

Clinical Features. Silicosis is a disease with a long latent period and usually requires 15 to 20 years of exposure before the chest film shows significant abnormality, except where very intense exposure has occurred. With simple silicosis, although a nodular infiltration may be seen on the chest radiograph, the worker is usually asymptomatic, and no functional impairment is evident. With progression of disease to a more advanced stage, shortness of breath with exertion is the major symptom. Often, poor correlation exists between the radiographic findings and the degree of functional impairment. Cough and sputum may develop, especially in smokers, as the disease progresses, but wheezing is not usually present. With development of PMF, normal lung structure is distorted from contraction of the upper lobes, and emphysematous changes occur in the lower lobes, resulting in airways obstruction. Silicosis is the only pneumoconiosis that predisposes to the development of tuberculosis and is most likely to occur after age 50 in association with moderate to severe silicosis. Incidence of atypical mycobacteriosis is also increased, primarily from *Mycobacterium avium-intracellulare* complex (MAC), which can be difficult to treat because of resistance to most antituberculosis drugs.

Physical findings in simple silicosis are nonspecific unless complicated by heart or other lung disease, such as congestive heart failure, chronic obstructive pulmonary disease, and tuberculosis. With complicated silicosis there are signs of fibrotic or obstructive lung disease. Finger clubbing is not a feature of this disease, even though significant hypoxemia may be present.

Lung Function. In simple nodular silicosis, lung function is usually normal. With progression of disease, a restrictive impairment gradually increases, with a reduced FVC, FEV_1, and TLC. DLco gradually decreases, and although hypoxemia may be absent at rest, it usually can be demonstrated during exercise. In the absence of PMF, hypoxemia at rest is rare. Associated airways obstruction may also be present, particularly in smokers with advanced disease. The latter suggests a synergistic effect between silica dust exposure and cigarette smoke.

Diagnosis. With an occupational history of significant silica exposure and a chest radiograph showing a discrete nodular infiltrate, a diagnosis of simple silicosis can be made with reasonable certainty. Obtaining previous chest films is helpful in establishing the stability and progression of the disease. Although a restrictive impairment and abnormal DLco may be demonstrated in some patients at this stage, pulmonary function studies are usually normal. A lung biopsy is rarely indicated to make a diagnosis. When the diagnosis is in question, a biopsy may be used to rule out a potentially treatable disease. If tissue is available, it can be examined under light and electron microscopy; examination under polarized light can identify birefringent foreign material. Spectroscopy and x-ray diffraction have been used for the qualitative and quantitative analysis of lung tissue, but these techniques require considerable lung tissue. Energy- dispersive x-ray analysis (EDXA) permits simultaneous multielemental analysis while examining the tissue in the scanning electron microscope (SEM) without destruction of the tissue sample.

Treatment. No specific treatment exists for silicosis. When a diagnosis has been made, the worker should be removed from further silica exposure. Although even simple silicosis may progress in the absence of further exposure, it is more likely to do so if exposure continues. Selected workers may continue working with the use of an external air–supplied airstream helmet, which does offer excellent dust protection. With advanced disease, treatment is supportive with oxygen, bronchodilators, cardiac medications, and antibiotics for infections.

Asbestos-related Disease

The term *asbestos* is given to a group of naturally occurring fibrous silicates with the unique property of great resistance to heat and chemical destruction. Asbestos was seldom used commercially until the Industrial Revolution, when the need arose to insulate the steam engine. Between 1877 and 1967 the world production of asbestos increased from 50 tons to 4 million tons per year. Of the various types of asbestos fibers, only chrysotile, crocidolite, and amosite are of economic importance. More than 90% of all asbestos used in the United States is chrysotile. With the wide use of asbestos, an estimated 2.5 million U.S. workers had potential exposure to asbestos by 1976.[33]

Asbestosis is a pneumoconiosis resulting from the inhalation of asbestos fibers and is characterized by diffuse interstitial fibrosis of the lung. These parenchymal changes may be associated with pleural fibrosis and parietal pleural plaques. The first detailed epidemiologic study of asbestos workers in the United States was undertaken by the Public Health Service in 1937. This study[33] demonstrated a relationship between the extent of exposure and clinical symptoms, prompting the recommendation of an exposure limit of 5 million particles per cubic foot of air. In 1965 Selikoff and colleagues[24] published a landmark survey of 1500 asbestos insulation workers. They found that nearly half of those examined had asbestosis and concluded that asbestosis and its complications were significant hazards among insulation workers. This was subsequently corroborated by other investigators.

Pathogenesis. Deposition of inhaled particles, in this case asbestos fibers, depends on the aerodynamic behavior of the fibers, the dimensions of the respiratory tract entered, and the pattern of breathing. Since the fibers tend to align with the airstream, large fibers (even greater than 50 μm) can reach peripheral locations. Longer fibers are retained and eventually gain access into the interstitium of the lung. Smaller fibers are cleared by the alveolar macrophages. Exposure to asbestos results in the accumulation of macrophages in the area of deposition, which may serve a protective role. Because alveolar macrophages can release mediators capable of injuring alveolar walls and stimulating fibroblast proliferation, however, the alveolar macrophage may play the central role in the production of fibrosis and asbestosis. Studies in animals and in humans exposed to asbestos using BAL have demonstrated an inflammatory process (alveolitis) preceding the development of pulmonary fibrosis. Alveolar macrophages contribute to the alveolitis and fibrosis by the direct release of tissue-destructive metabolites, release of growth factors (e.g., MDGF, fibronectin) that stimulate fibroblasts to replicate and synthesize collagen, and release of neutral proteases.[19] Active alveolitis appears predictive of disease progression and can be evaluated by BAL or gallium scan. Despite a clear understanding of the mechanisms involved in the development of lung fibrosis resulting from asbestos exposure, it is not clear why individuals with similar exposure may have very different responses in terms of the fibrotic process.

Pathophysiology. In the early stages of asbestosis, only microscopic changes are observed, manifested by fibrosis at the level of the respiratory bronchiole. As the disease evolves, the fibrosis extends peripherally, resulting in diffuse interstitial fibrosis most prominent in the lower lobes. Fibrous wall cysts may form, giving the lung a honeycomb appearance. Pleural fibrosis and circumscribed pleural plaques, involving the parietal pleura with or without calcification, may be present. *Asbestos bodies* are an indicator of asbestos exposure that differentiates it from other forms of lung fibrosis. They are considered an essential feature for the histologic diagnosis of asbestosis. Asbestos bodies tend to form a yellow-brown structure on the larger fibers that measures 20 to 150 μm in length. These bodies result from the deposition of an iron-protein complex on the core fiber by alveolar macrophages. Asbestos body content has been quantitated by counting asbestos bodies in tissue sections, by digesting lung tissue and extracting the bodies, and more recently by examination of BAL fluid. By employing a combination of ultrastructural morphology, electron microscopy, and EDXA, it is possible to identify almost every asbestos fiber found in the lung. From a medicolegal standpoint the number of fibers present would provide some estimate of the asbestos exposure, and data on the fiber type might allow identification of a source of exposure if the worker was thought to have been exposed to a specific type of asbestos.

Clinical Features. Asbestosis develops insidiously many years after the initial exposure, so the association may not be recognized. Symptoms and signs are not specific for asbestosis, since they do not differ from those found in diffuse interstitial fibrosis from a variety of other causes. The most common symptom is shortness of breath, particularly with exertion, which slowly progresses to breathlessness at rest. The dyspnea may be out of proportion to the radiographic abnormality, and cough is often present and may be productive, especially among smokers, due to coexisting chronic bronchitis. The most characteristic physical sign is bibasilar inspiratory crackles, which may be an early finding in asbestosis. Finger clubbing has been noted in 20% to 84% of patients. With advancing disease, cyanosis may become apparent, with signs of pulmonary hypertension and cor pulmonale.

Lung Function. A characteristic functional change in asbestosis is restrictive lung disease. All lung volumes are reduced, particularly the vital capacity, inspiratory capacity, and TLC. Lung compliance is reduced because of the pulmonary fibrosis. Airways obstruction is uncommon, except in cigarette smokers. However, varying degrees of small airways obstruction have been demonstrated in nonsmoking asbestos workers, attributable to distortion of the small airways with bronchiolar fibrosis.[12] The diffusing capacity is frequently reduced, and although hypoxemia may be absent at rest, it may first become evident only under the stress of exercise. In general the effects of asbestos on lung function are dose related, but functional abnormalities can be demonstrated in some asbestos-exposed individuals in the absence of definite radiologic change.

The radiographic appearance is characterized by linear and

irregular opacities predominant in the lower half of the lung fields, as opposed to the nodular changes seen in silicosis and coal worker's pneumoconiosis. The early changes of asbestosis consist of linear shadows of varying thickness, between 1 and 3 mm, most marked in the lower lung fields. As these lesions increase in profusion, the cardiac and diaphragmatic borders are gradually obscured. Irregular opacities may be seen, but discrete rounded opacities are not a feature of asbestosis. As the fibrotic process progresses, the linear and irregular opacities become thicker and spread into the middle zones but rarely reach the upper zones. Lung volume gradually decreases. The basilar fibrotic changes are bilateral, and although they tend to be more prominent in one side, they are never unilateral.

Diagnosis. A clinical diagnosis of asbestosis depends on a history of asbestos exposure and one or more of the following: radiographic changes of parenchymal/pleural fibrosis, basilar crackles, dyspnea on exertion, and abnormal pulmonary function that demonstrates restrictive impairment, low diffusing capacity, and hypoxemia at rest or with exercise. With all criteria present the diagnosis would be certain, but a history of exposure and a chest film consistent with asbestosis usually are sufficient. A lung biopsy is rarely indicated, but the pathologist cannot make a definite diagnosis of asbestosis in cases that show characteristic fibrosis in the absence of asbestos bodies or other evidence of asbestos fibers.

Treatment. Asbestosis has no specific treatment, although corticosteroids have been used with some symptomatic improvement but without evidence that they affect the course of disease. Removal from further exposure to asbestos is an accepted approach; eliminating further asbestos burden on the lungs at an early stage would favor arresting the disease. Despite removal from further exposure, however, disease can continue to progress slowly.

Pleural Disease. See Chapter 79.

Lung Cancer. The association between lung cancer and asbestos exposure was reported as early as 1935 and firmly established in 1964.[23] The effects of smoking and asbestos are multiplicative and result in a cancer risk over 50 times greater for a smoking asbestos worker compared with a nonsmoker with no asbestos exposure. The risk for nonsmokers exposed to asbestos is also slightly increased. Epidemiologic surveys indicate that the risk of lung cancer is dose related. Lung cancers tend to arise in relation to areas of fibrosis and therefore occur chiefly in the lower lobes and periphery. All major tumor cell types are seen, but adenocarcinoma is predominant. In the absence of asbestosis it is difficult to establish an asbestos etiology for the lung cancer, particularly in a smoker.

Clinical findings are those of the underlying asbestosis. A rapid increase in respiratory symptoms, appearance of hemoptysis, loss of appetite, and weight loss should alert the physician to the possibility of lung cancer. Chest radiographs should be taken and compared to previous radiographs. Since the changes of asbestosis progress slowly, any abrupt change should prompt further studies to include sputum cytology and a diagnostic bronchoscopy and biopsy. Once the cell type has been determined, appropriate therapy can be instituted. The most effective measure is to convince the worker to discontinue cigarette smoking.

Mesothelioma. The incidence of mesothelioma in the United States is estimated at 12 cases per 1 million population per year. The association of pleural mesothelioma and asbestos exposure was first demonstrated in 1960.[29] The latency period from first exposure to diagnosis is long, ranging from 20 to 40 years, with a mean of about 35 years. Although a dose-effect response has been shown in some groups, there is no threshold below which asbestos exposure is safe with regard to mesothelioma. In addition, mesothelioma may occur without radiologic evidence of asbestosis. In contrast to bronchogenic carcinoma, cigarette smoking does not play a synergistic role in the development of mesothelioma. Fiber type appears to be important, since a much higher mesothelioma death rate is seen in those individuals exposed to crocidolite.

A diagnosis of mesothelioma can be difficult for the pathologist, not only to recognize that the tumor is a mesothelioma, but also to distinguish it from metastatic adenocarcinoma or sarcoma. A thoracotomy and open biopsy are invariably required to obtain an adequate specimen for histologic evaluation.

The major presenting symptoms in patients with mesothelioma is chest pain of insidious onset. The pain is nonpleuritic, aching, and persistent and may be referred to the upper abdomen or shoulder. Progressive shortness of breath and cough may accompany the pain. The chest pain gradually becomes an incapacitating symptom, with dyspnea, anorexia, and weight loss. Physical findings vary with the stage of disease, but patients usually present with signs of fluid in the involved hemithorax; the fluid often is hemorrhagic. A chest film may show a pleural effusion and thickened pleura on the affected side. A CT scan may be helpful in determining the extent of the disease and separating fluid from tissue densities.

Most patients with mesothelioma die within 12 to 15 months from the onset of symptoms. Radical surgery, chemotherapy, and megavolt therapy have minimally improved survival and have not been curative.

REFERENCES

1. Crystal RG et al: Interstitial lung disease of unknown cause: disorders characterized by chronic inflammation of the lower respiratory tract, *N Engl J Med* 310:154, 1984.
2. Daniels RP et al: Bronchoalveolar lavage: role in the pathogenesis, diagnosis and management of interstitial lung disease, *Ann Intern Med* 102:93, 1985.
3. Dement JM, Merchant JA, Green FHY: In Merchant JH, editor: *Occupational respiratory diseases,* Washington, DC, 1986, US Department of Health and Human Services (NIOSH).
4. Epler GR, McLoud TC, Gaenslar EA: Normal chest roentgenogram in chronic diffuse infiltrating lung disease, *N Engl J Med* 298:934, 1978.
5. Fink JN, Deshazo R: Immunologic aspects of granulomatous and interstitial lung disease, *JAMA* 258:2938, 1987.
6. Fink JN, Banaszak EF, Barboriak JJ: Interstitial lung disease due to contamination of forced air systems, *Ann Intern Med* 84:406, 1976.
7. Fulmer JD, Roberts WC: Small airways and interstitial pulmonary disease, *Chest* 77:470, 1980.
8. Funahashi A et al: Value of in situ elemental microanalysis in the histologic diagnosis of silicosis, *Chest* 85:506, 1984.
9. Gelb AF et al: Immune complexes, gallium lung scan and bronchoalveolar lavage in idiopathic interstitial pneumonitis-fibrosis: a structure-function clinical study, *Chest* 84:148, 1983.
10. Grossman RF et al: Results of single-lung transplantation for bilateral pulmonary fibrosis, *N Engl J Med* 322:727, 1990.
11. Hodges GR, Fink JN, Schlueter DP: Hypersensitivity pneumonitis caused by contaminated cool mist vaporizer, *Ann Intern Med* 80:501, 1984.

12. Kilburn KH et al: Airway disease in non-smoking asbestos workers, *Arch Environ Health* 40:293, 1985.
13. Liebow AA, Carrington CB: The interstitial pneumonias. In Simon M, Potchen EJ, LeMay M, editors: *Frontiers of pulmonary radiology,* New York, 1969, Grune & Stratton.
14. Muller NL, Miller RR: State of the art: computed tomography of chronic diffuse infiltrative lung disease. Part 2, *Am Rev Respir Dis* 142:1440, 1990.
15. Nakos G, Adams A, Andriopoulos N: Antibodies to collagen in patients with idiopathic pulmonary fibrosis, *Chest* 103:1051, 1993.
16. Parkes WR: *Occupational lung disorders,* Boston, 1988, Butterworth.
17. Pratt DS et al: Rapidly fatal pulmonary fibrosis: the accelerated variant of interstitial pneumonitis, *Thorax* 34:587, 1979.
18. Rennard SI et al: Colchicine suppresses the release of fibroblast growth factors from alveolar macrophages in vitro: the basis of a possible therapeutic approach to the fibrotic disorders, *Am Rev Respir Dis* 137:181, 1988.
19. Rom WN, Travis WD, Brody AR: State of the art cellular and molecular basis of the asbestosis-related disease, *Am Rev Respir Dis* 143:408, 1991.
20. Rose C, King TE Jr: Controversies in hypersensitivity pneumonitis, *Am J Rev Respir Dis* 145:1, 1992 (editorial).
21. Schlueter DP: Infiltrative lung disease hypersensitivity pneumonitis, *J Allergy Clin Immunol* 70:50, 1982.
22. Schlueter DP: Response of the lung to inhaled antigens, *Am J Med* 57:476, 1974.
23. Selikoff IJ, Churg J, Hammond EC: Asbestos exposure and neoplasia, *JAMA* 188:22, 1964.
24. Selikoff IJ, Churg J, Hammond EC: The occurrence of asbestosis among insulation workers in the US, *Ann NY Acad Sci* 132:139, 1965.
25. Sheppard MN, Harrison NK: Lung injury, inflammatory mediators, and fibroblast activation in fibrosing alveolitis, *Thorax* 47:1064, 1992.
26. Snider GL: Interstitial lung disease: pathogenesis, pathophysiology, and clinical presentation. In Schevary MJ, King TE Jr, editors: *Interstitial lung disease,* Philadelphia, 1994, Decker.
27. Specks U et al: Anticytoplasmic autoantibodies in the diagnosis and follow-up of Wegener's granulomatosis, *Mayo Clin Proc* 64:28, 1989.
28. Trentin L et al: Longitudinal study of alveolitis in hypersensitivity pneumonitis patients: an immunologic evaluation, *J Allergy Clin Immunol* 82:577, 1988.
29. Wagner JC, Sleggs GA, Marchand P: Diffuse pleural mesothelioma and asbestos exposure in the Northwestern Cape Province, *Br J Ind Med* 17:260, 1960.
30. Wall GP et al: Comparison of transbronchial and open biopsies in chronic infiltrative lung diseases, *Am Rev Respir Dis* 123:280, 1981.
31. Walters LC et al: Idiopathic pulmonary fibrosis: pretreatment broncho-alveolar lavage cellular constituents and their relationships to lung histopathology and clinical response to therapy, *Am Rev Respir Dis* 135:696, 1987.
32. Winterbauer RH: The treatment of idiopathic pulmonary fibrosis, *Chest* 100:233, 1991.
33. Ziskind M, Jones RN, Weill H: State of the art silicosis, *Am Rev Respir Dis* 113:643, 1976.

CHAPTER 77

Respiratory Failure

Kenneth W. Presberg

Respiratory failure is defined as the failure of the respiratory system to provide for adequate gas exchange, that is, adequate oxygenation of the circulating blood for sufficient oxygen (O_2) delivery to tissues and adequate elimination of carbon dioxide (CO_2) produced by cellular metabolism. Arterial oxygen tensions (Pao_2) less than 50 mm Hg and arterial carbon dioxide tensions ($Paco_2$) greater than 50 mm Hg are generally accepted criteria for the presence of respiratory failure. However, severe abnormalities of the respiratory system's capacity may imminently lead to respiratory failure and may not be reflected in initial measurement of an arterial blood gas (ABG).

Patients may present with the signs and symptoms attributable to the primary process causing the gas exchange abnormality or may have manifestations secondary to the adverse end-organ effects of hypoxemia and hypercapnia. When confronted with a patient with evidence of respiratory failure, the physician must first ascertain whether the process is acute or chronic, then further delineate the cause and initiate treatment. The acute causes will require expeditious evaluation and treatment that is best handled in the inpatient setting. An acute process is often apparent early in the evaluation because of an obvious insult or symptoms that indicate a recent deterioration. Chronic respiratory failure is often suggested by an insidious progression of limitation along with evidence of a chronic thoracic or neuromuscular disorder. At times the patient may not mention any specific complaints, and respiratory failure is apparent after an ABG determination is performed for other reasons. Hypoxemia can be judged to be chronic if no history suggests a recent event, evaluation discloses signs and symptoms of a chronic cardiopulmonary disorder, and other findings of chronic hypoxemia are present (see later discussion). Chronic hypercapnia is easier to judge because it is accompanied by respiratory acidosis that is mild because of renal compensation. When chronic respiratory failure is discovered, evaluation and therapy can often proceed in the outpatient setting; however, daytime hypoxemia should be corrected early. *Acute on chronic* respiratory failure refers to the acute deterioration in the patient who previously had well-compensated chronic impairment. Severe, life-threatening hypoxemia and worsening hypercapnia with severe respiratory acidosis often occur in this setting.

Many of the chronic pulmonary and neuromuscular disorders are discussed in other chapters. Therefore more attention is given here to the causes of the acute decompensation in chronically impaired patients and the acute, fulminant processes leading to respiratory failure.

CHRONIC RESPIRATORY FAILURE

Pathophysiology: Overview of Gas Exchange Abnormalities

The lung can be considered conceptually as an alveolar-capillary gas exchange unit and the respiratory pump. The pump is driven by an integrated control center, the central nervous system (CNS). The pump (muscles of respiration) directs the bulk flow of gas through the airways to the gas exchange unit. Gas exchange failure caused by the respiratory system results from the malfunction of one or more of these many components. Disorders causing respiratory failure are often further categorized by the predominant gas exchange abnormality that is present. Mechanisms for these gas exchange abnormalities are discussed next.

Tissue Oxygenation Failure. Inadequate tissue oxygenation can result from other well-known mechanisms quite distinct from the respiratory system. These causes of tissue hypoxia need to be well understood for an expeditious and directed approach to the patient with oxygenation failure (Table 77-1). Failure to correct severe hypoxemia within minutes can result in irreversible organ damage. The CNS and cardiovascular system are particularly affected by hypoxemia. Treatment may require the rapid implementation of mechanical ventilatory and cardiac resuscitative support. Measurement of oxygenation is essential.

Table 77-2 summarizes and contrasts these various mechanisms of hypoxemia in terms of frequently measured and calculated variables. The degree of hypoxemia is often described by the ratio of Pao_2 to fractional inspired O_2 concentration (Fio_2). Values less than 200 are usually caused by significant degrees of physiologic shunting. Chronic lung disorders usually cause hypoxemia by ventilation/perfusion ($\dot{V}/\dot{Q}$) inequality. In contrast, acute lung injuries are associated with severe hypoxemia that is most often secondary to physiologic shunting or increased venous admixture. The hypoxemia in these latter cases often responds poorly to supplemental O_2. Patients with chronic hypoxemia may be relatively asymptomatic until pulmonary vascular, cardiac, and other end-organ sequelae ensue. These include cognitive impairment, weight loss, left-sided heart dysfunction, pulmonary hypertension with cor pulmonale, edema, cyanosis, and polycythemia. Hypoxemia should always be expeditiously corrected when found. If the pulmonary parenchyma appears normal and evaluation is also negative for the common cardiac abnormalities, the physician should consider the possibility of an intracardiac right-to-left shunt, pulmonary arteriovenous malformations, or the hepatopulmonary syndrome.

Table 77-1. Causes of Tissue Hypoxia

Condition	Measured abnormality
Hypoxemia caused by pulmonary disorders (see Table 77-2)	Decreased Pao_2
Decreased oxygen delivery	Low $Do_2 = Cao_2 \times$ cardiac output
Low cardiac output	Increased a-v O_2 content difference $= Cao_2 - Cvo_2$
Decreased Hgb-bound oxygen (e.g., anemia, carbon monoxide poisoning)	Low $Cao_2 = Sao_2 \times$ g% Hgb $\times$ 1.34
Increased oxygen consumption	High Vo_2 and high a-v O_2 content difference
Defects of oxygen extraction and utilization (e.g., cyanide poisoning, sepsis)	Low Vo_2 and low a-v O_2 content difference

Do_2, Oxygen delivery; Vo_2, oxygen consumption; Pao_2, arterial oxygen tension; Cao_2, arterial oxygen content; Cvo_2, mixed venous oxygen content; Sao_2, hemoglobin oxygen saturation of arterial blood; *a-v O_2 content difference*, arterial-to-mixed-venous oxygen content difference; *Hgb*, hemoglobin.

Mechanisms of Hypoventilatory Failure. The failure of ventilation to eliminate the CO_2 produced by cellular metabolism (Vco_2) can lead to hypercapnia and respiratory acidosis. Virtually all CO_2 is eliminated from the body through the lungs. $Paco_2$ is tightly controlled by the regulation of alveolar ventilation under the control of the central chemoreceptors. The failure of the combination of respiratory drive and the respiratory pump to meet the ventilatory requirement for adequate elimination of CO_2 results in hypoventilatory failure. Acute hypercapnia can lead to severe dyspnea, flushing of the skin, and vasodilation of the cerebral vessels, with an increase in intracranial pressure that may result in headache, papilledema, depressed consciousness, and frank coma. For every acute increase in $Paco_2$ of 10 mm Hg, there is a corresponding pH decrease of 0.08 pH units. Respiratory acidosis leading to a pH less than 7.20 or failure of ventilation to compensate for a metabolic acidosis to a pH greater than 7.20 can adversely affect myocardial function, predisposing the patient to hypotension and dysrhythmias (arrhythmias). The respiratory acidosis from chronic hypoventilatory respiratory failure associated with ongoing CO_2 retention is mild because of renal compensation. However, the renal compensation with the retention of bicarbonate does not totally correct the acidosis under these circumstances. No specific symptoms are related to chronic hypercapnia, and these patients can tolerate marked elevations in $Paco_2$ without experiencing adverse consequences. Many of the patients with chronic hypoventilation caused by central or extrapulmonary disorders, such as hypothyroidism or sleep apnea, have a blunted respiratory drive response to elevations in $Paco_2$. These patients also experience chronic hypoxia because of the alveolar gas relation described previously and $\dot{V}/\dot{Q}$ inequalities. Therefore patients with chronic hypoventilation often have the symptoms and signs related to coexistent hypoxemia described earlier.

Table 77-2. Mechanisms of Hypoxemia Caused by Pulmonary Disorders

Condition	Fio_2	PAo_2	Pao_2	Sao_2	$Paco_2$	A-a gradient
Normal	0.21 (room air)	100	90	95%	40	Normal
Hypoventilation	0.21	70	60	90%	70	Normal
Ambient hypoxia (low ambient Po_2)	0.21	75	60	90%	40	Normal
Shunt	0.21	100	45	75%	40	Increased
	1.00	650	50	80%	40	Increased
Ventilation/perfusion ($\dot{V}/\dot{Q}$) inequality	0.21	100	50	85%	40	Increased
	0.50	300	75	93%	40	Increased

Fio_2, Fractional inspired oxygen concentration; Po_2, oxygen tension; PAo_2, alveolar Po_2; Pao_2, arterial Po_2; Sao_2, hemoglobin oxygen saturation of arterial blood; $Paco_2$, arterial Pco_2; *A-a gradient* = ($PAo_2 - Pao_2$). All pressures in mm Hg. Note the different responses to supplemental oxygen between conditions with shunt and those with $\dot{V}/\dot{Q}$ inequality.

$Paco_2$ is determined by three key factors: CO_2 production (Vco_2), total minute ventilation (VE), and the physiologic dead space (Vd/Vt). Their relationship is described by the following equation, where k is a constant:

$$Paco_2 = k\ Vco_2\ [1/V_E\ (1 - Vd/Vt)]$$

Vco_2 can be increased in hypermetabolic states (e.g., acute illness), which also increase Vo_2. Therefore the acute increase in $Paco_2$ and decrease in Pao_2 in a patient with respiratory failure who develops a high fever are not necessarily caused by any change in pulmonary gas exchange efficiency or a new mechanical problem and may be secondary to changes in the patient's metabolic state. Dead space is increased in patients with underlying lung disease, particularly in those with chronic obstructive pulmonary disease (COPD). The increase in Vd/Vt increases the basal ventilatory requirement (VE) needed to maintain a normal $Paco_2$. Vd/Vt is also increased when positive-pressure ventilation is used and tends to increase as mean airway pressure increases. This increase in Vd/Vt can be mitigated if careful attention is paid to limiting mean airway pressure. Therefore the effect of ventilatory settings on Vd/Vt needs to be considered if the Pco_2 is not responding in the usual way to adjustments of VE. At times it is not possible to normalize the $Paco_2$ with mechanical ventilation without incurring prohibitive risks of complications. Certain strategies for mechanical ventilation of patients with severe adult respiratory distress syndrome (ARDS) and asthma have incorporated permissive hypercapnia to avoid barotrauma-related complications (see Acute Respiratory Failure). However, the safe threshold below which an elevation of $Paco_2$ does not lead to adverse CNS or other organ effects has not been determined.

Hypoventilatory respiratory failure occurs when the normal or increased ventilatory requirement of the patient cannot be met. It results from an imbalance between the work of breathing imposed by respiratory loads and the respiratory capacity, which is determined by the respiratory drive and the respiratory pump (Fig. 77-1). Normally the respiratory capacity reserve is sufficient to accommodate modest increases in respiratory loads (e.g., bronchospasm) without leading to hypoventilatory failure. Acute hypoventilatory failure with an underlying lung or muscular disease is usually caused by respiratory muscle fatigue, which reflects a reversible defect of strength. Treatment strategies for patients with respiratory failure critically depend on reversing respiratory muscle fatigue while reducing respiratory workloads.

Pathophysiology and Differential Diagnosis of Chronic Disorders

Box 77-1 lists the common causes of hypoventilatory respiratory failure. A further classification within this group distinguishes between disorders with normal and abnormal

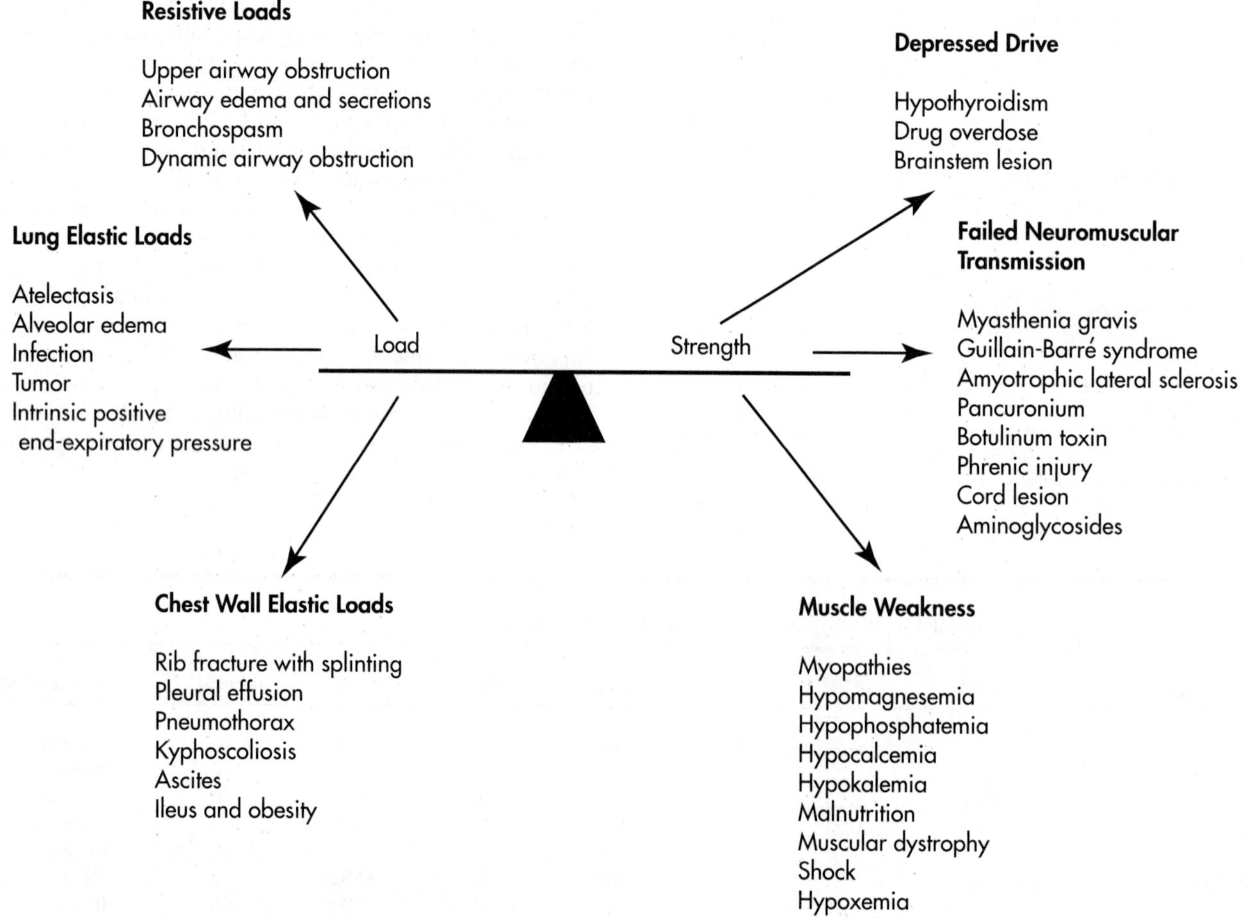

Fig. 77-1. Abnormalities that can increase the normal respiratory resistive and elastic workloads are listed on the left. Defects of the normal respiratory capacity are noted on the right. Unless respiratory capacity remains sufficient to counterbalance these workloads, respiratory failure will ensue. (From Schmidt GA, Hall JB: *JAMA* 261:3444, 1989.)

respiratory workloads. Those with normal respiratory workloads involve impaired respiratory capacity; these diseases include disorders of CNS control and intrinsic neuromuscular disorders. On the other hand, patients with abnormal respiratory workloads have pulmonary disorders or extrapulmonary thoracic disorders. Fig. 77-1 shows a classification of the abnormalities of respiratory loads and capacity. Table 77-3 further describes these abnormalities of respiratory mechanics, strength, and gas exchange for specific chronic disorders.

Central Hypoventilation Syndromes. Chronic central hypoventilation syndromes include acquired processes that result in an abnormal central respiratory drive to common stimuli, including hypoxemia and hypercapnia. This abnormal central regulation can result from specific vascular or anatomic insults, such as midbrain cerebrovascular accidents (CVAs, strokes) and multisystem atrophy syndrome (Shy-Drager syndrome). Metabolic abnormalities (hypothyroidism being the most common) can also lead to hypoventilation. Some patients with morbid obesity may also have chronic daytime hypoventilation, for which the exact cause is unknown, and severe obstructive sleep apnea syndrome. Daytime hypoventilation may improve with treatment of the sleep abnormalities alone. In patients with obesity-hypoventilation syndrome the P_{CO_2} can be voluntarily decreased with forced tachypnea. These patients may benefit from respiratory stimulants. In all these disorders, respiratory abnormalities and gas exchange may worsen during sleep. These aggravating sleep abnormalities may require specific evaluation and treatment (Box 77-2).

Box 77-1. Causes of Hypoventilatory Respiratory Failure

Abnormal Respiratory Capacity (Normal Respiratory Workloads)

- Acute depression of central nervous system
  - Various causes (see text)
- Chronic central hypoventilation syndromes
  - Obesity-hypoventilation syndrome
  - Sleep apnea syndrome
  - Hypothyroidism
  - Shy-Drager syndrome (multisystem atrophy syndrome)
- Acute toxic paralysis syndromes
  - Botulism
  - Tetanus
  - Toxic ingestion or bites
  - Organophosphate poisoning
- Neuromuscular disorders (acute and chronic)
  - Myasthenia gravis
  - Guillain-Barré syndrome
  - Drugs
  - Amyotrophic lateral sclerosis
  - Muscular dystrophies
  - Polymyositis
  - Spinal cord injury
  - Traumatic phrenic nerve paralysis

Abnormal Pulmonary Workloads

- Chronic obstructive pulmonary disease (COPD)
  - Chronic bronchitis
  - Asthmatic bronchitis
  - Emphysema
- Asthma and acute bronchial hyperreactivity syndromes
- Upper airway obstruction
- Interstitial lung diseases

Abnormal Extrapulmonary Workloads

- Chronic thoracic cage disorders
  - Severe kyphoscoliosis
  - After thoracoplasty
  - After thoracic cage injury
- Acute thoracic cage trauma and burns
- Pneumothorax
- Pleural fibrosis and effusions
- Abdominal processes

Neuromuscular Disorders. Neuromuscular disorders represent a heterogenous group of acute and chronic disorders (see Box 77-1). These diseases can affect the upper motor neurons, lower motor neurons, peripheral nerves, myoneuronal junction, or the muscle itself. Clinical signs and symptoms and patterns of weakness provide critical clues to the diagnosis. These disorders will lead to respiratory failure when muscles controlling the upper airway or the diaphragm or other respiratory muscles are involved. Chronic disorders include the muscular dystrophies, myopathies associated with polymyositis and the collagen vascular diseases, amyotrophic lateral sclerosis, myasthenia gravis, and those with persistent sequelae of the acute neuromuscular disorders. Some patients with chronic impairments do not experience respiratory symptoms with their everyday activities and only show evidence of mild respiratory muscle weakness on formal pulmonary function testing. However, these chronic, compensated patients are predisposed to early respiratory muscle fatigue with acute illnesses that may lead to acute respiratory failure. In contrast, others have significant exertional dyspnea, exercise intolerance, and symptoms attributable to sleep-disordered breathing. This latter group of patients would likely have chronic CO_2 retention, daytime hypoxemia, and little to no respiratory capacity reserve.

Obstructive and Restrictive Thoracic Disorders. These diseases are discussed in Chapters 72 to 76. Certain common diseases are readdressed here with regard to the specific mechanisms leading to their presentation with respiratory failure.

Chronic Obstructive Pulmonary Disease. It is estimated that more than 10 million Americans have COPD and that the majority of these patients will die of progressive respiratory failure. Patients with COPD can experience, on average, one to four exacerbations per year. An *exacerbation* is generally defined as an increase in dyspnea that is persistent for a few days and is not readily reversed with acute bronchodilator treatment. An exacerbation is usually accompanied by increased sputum production, sputum purulence, cough, and wheezing. In those with the most severe forms of disease, these episodes may lead to acute on chronic respiratory failure, which in turn requires hospital admission for treatment. Patients with COPD have a number of abnormalities that predispose them to respiratory pump failure (see Chapter 75 and Table 77-3). As a result, the patient with advanced COPD has a limited and often precarious reserve of respiratory capacity.

Box 77-3 lists common causes of a COPD exacerbation and other aggravating conditions that can lead to acute

Table 77-3. Basic Physiologic Abnormalities Associated with Hypoventilatory Respiratory Failure

Clinical disorder	Mechanical abnormality	Gas exchange
Central nervous system (CNS) insult	Depressed CNS drive	Secondary hypoventilation and hypoxemia
Neuromuscular disease	Respiratory muscle weakness	Same as above
Chronic obstructive pulmonary disease (COPD)	Increased inspiratory airway resistance Increased expiratory airway resistance Increased compliance Dynamic hyperinflation and intrinsic positive end-expiratory pressure Abnormal respiratory muscle length-tension relationship	Increased dead space (Vd/Vt) Hypoxemia from ventilation/perfusion ($\dot{V}/\dot{Q}$) inequality
Asthma	Increased large-airways resistance Dynamic hyperinflation Acute change in respiratory muscle configuration	Hypoxemia from $\dot{V}/\dot{Q}$ inequality Increased Vd/Vt
Interstitial lung disease	Increased elastic loads from parenchymal fibrosis	Increased Vd/Vt Hypoxemia from $\dot{V}/\dot{Q}$ inequality
Thoracic cage deformity	Increased elastic loads from atelectasis and chest wall malformations	Secondary hypoventilation Hypoxemia from $\dot{V}/\dot{Q}$ inequality and hypoventilation

Box 77-2. Managed Care Guide: Sleep Apnea

History and Physical Examination

History of snoring and excessive daytime somnolence

Obesity with body mass greater than 20% of normal, ear-nose-throat (ENT) examination, thyroxine (T_4) and thyroid- stimulating hormone (TSH) levels

Documentation

Syndrome confirmed by more than 15 apneic episodes per hour with desaturation of at least 4% by oximetry

Syndrome ruled out by normal overnight oximetry test or if arterial oxygen saturation (Sao_2) is less than 90%, less than 1% of total sleep time.

Treatment

Weight loss

Nighttime treatment with continuous positive airway pressure (CPAP) as necessary to overcome desaturation

Data from Matheson JK: Sleep and its disorders. In Stein JH: *Internal medicine*, St Louis, 1994, Mosby.

Box 77-3. Causes of Acute on Chronic Respiratory Failure in Patients with Chronic Obstructive Pulmonary Disease (COPD)

- Exacerbation of COPD (see text for definition)
  - Nonspecific bronchial irritants (e.g., dusts, air pollution, cigarette smoke)
  - Viral and bacterial respiratory infections
  - Gastroesophageal reflux disease
- Acute bronchospasm
  - Occupational exposures
  - Environmental exposures
  - Inhaled allergens (in "asthmatic bronchitis" patients)
  - Pharmacologic agents
- Pneumothorax: spontaneous or iatrogenic
- Pulmonary embolism
- Worsening coexistent cardiovascular disease
  - Decompensated cor pulmonale
  - Ischemic heart disease
  - Worsening left ventricular failure
  - Cardiac dysrhythmias
- Bronchogenic carcinoma
- Fungal or mycobacterial infections

respiratory failure. Overall, more than 50% of COPD patients over age 50 have a coexistent cardiovascular disease. Therefore early recognition of cardiac disease and cor pulmonale is important for directing other specific therapy. Signs of pulmonary hypertension are often difficult to discern in the patient with COPD. Edema is more readily apparent and suggests decompensated cor pulmonale in this patient population.

The severity of the patient's condition can be assessed by evaluating pulmonary function tests (PFTs), exercise capacity, and ABGs; examining for the presence of cor pulmonale; and documenting the frequency of exacerbations and hospital admissions. Recent reports indicate that the mortality rate for COPD patients requiring an intensive care unit (ICU) is only approximately 10%. Furthermore, mortality among patients with COPD who require ICU care for acute respiratory failure is no greater than that observed in patients matched for comparable degrees of respiratory impairment. Previous studies reported a 40% 2-year survival, however, after patients with COPD experienced their first episode requiring mechanical ventilation. Consequently, decisions about when to forego or limit mechanical ventilation remain difficult. A rational decision can often be made with patients using the previous information in conjunction with their beliefs and attitude toward their illness.

Interstitial Lung Disease. Patients with interstitial lung disease, especially idiopathic pulmonary fibrosis (IPF), often experience life-threatening respiratory complications, and many will unfortunately die of primary respiratory failure. Right ventricular failure due to pulmonary hypertension and cor pulmonale also contribute to the morbidity and mortality of these patients. Some patients with certain forms of interstitial lung disease, however, may exhibit mild to severe restrictive functional impairment and have a very stable respiratory status over a period of years. This latter course has been frequently described in patients with collagen vascular diseases. (see Chapter 76). The physiologic abnormalities include predominantly increased elastic loads that encroach on respiratory capacity, and these patients adopt breathing patterns that seek to decrease the work of breathing (see Table 77-3). Consequently, they function with little respiratory capacity reserve, and events that increase the work of breathing or compromise respiratory muscle strength can quickly lead to respiratory failure.

Common causes of deterioration in patients with interstitial lung disease include pulmonary infection, worsening pulmonary hypertension, decompensated cor pulmonale, and pneumothorax. This latter complication can be more recurrent and troublesome in these patients. Cardiovascular complications, bronchogenic carcinoma, and pulmonary embolism also need to be considered. Other specific causes of deterioration in these patients include adverse reactions to treatment with corticosteroids or cytotoxic agents and opportunistic infections. Fortunately, opportunistic infections still occur infrequently in this patient population despite the frequent use of corticosteroids and immunosuppressive agents. Many of these complications are associated with a more insidious disease process. Others, such as pulmonary embolism, pneumothorax, dysrhythmias, and infection, can be associated with abrupt clinical deterioration. Diagnostic evaluation and treatment need to be approached accordingly.

Thoracic Cage Abnormalities. Patients with severe kyphoscoliosis or thoracic cage deformities from trauma or surgery have decreased thoracic compliances primarily because of chest wall abnormalities and associated atelectasis. Given the abnormal configuration of the chest wall, cough and secretion clearance are also compromised. The high-energy cost of breathing from the increased elastic loads results in a pattern of rapid, shallow respirations. Chronic hypoventilation and secondary hypoxemia are common in these patients. Secondary cor pulmonale from hypoxemia and pulmonary vascular remodeling are frequently present. These disorders are also associated with many different respiratory abnormalities during sleep. These patients may have severe central apneas and hypopneas or obstructive events. These abnormalities are worse during rapid eye movement (REM) sleep and can be prolonged and associated with severe O_2 desaturation. These patients may be stable for years and then present with respiratory failure after minor insults such as a viral upper respiratory infection or illnesses that lead to mild decreases in muscle strength.

Diagnostic Evaluation

Arterial Blood Gases and Pulse Oximetry. Early evaluation of gas exchange by ABG analysis is important. The initial measurement of O_2 saturation by pulse oximetry is not sufficient in patients with a chronic respiratory disorder. Accuracy of these devices can vary by up to 5%, and falsely elevated arterial hemoglobin O_2 saturation (Sao_2) values obtained by pulse oximeters can be seen in smokers with elevated carboxyhemoglobin levels. Furthermore, Sao_2 tells the physician nothing about ventilation and the level of $Paco_2$. Attention to the pH associated with changes in $Paco_2$ is essential to make correct assessments of the acute gas exchange abnormalities. A pH that cannot be expeditiously corrected to above 7.20 with treatment often signals the need for mechanical ventilatory support. Hypoxemia in these chronic disorders is usually caused by $\dot{V}/\dot{Q}$ inequality and can be corrected with supplemental Fio_2 gas delivered at a sufficient flow. More severe hypoxemia heralds a complicating pneumonia or cardiac failure.

Radiologic Studies. A chest radiograph should be obtained early in all patients to rule out a pneumothorax, confirm the presence of a pneumonia, or detect signs of cardiogenic pulmonary edema. Additionally, the chest film can provide evidence of pulmonary hypertension if there is increased dilation of the pulmonary arterial tree. The value of chest radiograph, computed tomography (CT) scan, and high-resolution CT scan of the thorax in patients with interstitial lung disease is discussed in Chapter 76. In the patient with severe kyphoscoliosis the chest film can be difficult to interpret, and a chest CT scan may be necessary to evaluate the lung parenchyma adequately. Imaging studies should be considered for the evaluation of deep venous thrombosis and pulmonary embolism if no other apparent cause of respiratory failure is readily discernible (see Chapter 80). If necessary, lower extremity duplex Doppler ultrasound and lung perfusion scan can be done at the patient's bedside in most institutions.

Other Studies. An electrocardiogram (ECG) is necessary to rule out a dysrhythmia or cardiac ischemia early. Multifocal atrial tachycardia (MAT) is one of the dysrhythmias encountered in this patient group. Early recognition of MAT may lead to a reversal of its metabolic causes and may avoid potentially harmful and ineffective therapy typically used for other supraventricular dysrhythmias. Unfortunately, the ECG is not sensitive (approximately 33%) in detecting cor pulmonale in the COPD patient population. An echocardiogram is more accurate in this regard and is also sensitive for the detection of pulmonary hypertension and cor pulmonale in other chronic cardiopulmonary disorders. Measurements of respiratory muscle strength, spirometry, and lung volumes can be useful if the patient is able to cooperate and reproducible values can be obtained. Emergency clinical decisions are made without these measurements, however, and the physician must rely more on an assessment of the patient's clinical status and gas exchange. Evaluation for bronchitis and pneumonia should follow the guidelines in Chapter 73. Sputum Gram's stain and culture and blood cultures before antibiotic therapy are essential initial studies. Bronchoalveolar lavage (BAL) and perhaps transbronchial biopsy or open lung biopsy should be undertaken when opportunistic infection needs to be ruled out, most often in the immunocompromised patient. Indications for BAL, transbronchial biopsy, and open lung biopsy in the patient with interstitial lung disease are discussed in Chapter 76.

Nocturnal Oximetry and Sleep Studies. Nocturnal oximetry alone is most often used to detect significant nocturnal desaturation during sleep in patients with chronic pulmonary disorders. Patients with severe limitation or evidence of pulmonary hypertension or cor pulmonale are the best candidates for screening. Desaturation in these conditions usually occurs from worsening $\dot{V}/\dot{Q}$ inequality or hypoventilation during REM sleep and is readily treated with supplemental O_2. In patients with suspected primary or secondary severe respiratory abnormalities during sleep, however, a four-channel or full polysomnogram is indicated. These studies also include pulse oximetry.

Treatment

Oxygen Therapy. Acute O_2 therapy is often mismanaged in patients with chronic pulmonary disorders because of the concern about the known association between supplemental O_2 and further hypercapnia and respiratory acidosis. Ongoing hypoxemia, however, can result in severe end-organ damage and lead to rapidly progressive deterioration in respiratory muscle and cardiac function. Therefore O_2 should be provided in sufficient amounts to achieve an Sao_2 of at least 85% and preferably 90% saturation. Care must be taken not to decrease or to discontinue supplemental O_2 abruptly if Pco_2 is high, since this may result in a precipitous fall in Po_2. In most instances the Pco_2 will not rise more than 20 mm Hg, and therefore the pH will likely remain above the 7.20 to 7.25 range. If adequate Sao_2 cannot be met without resulting in severe hypercapnia and acidosis, the patient should be assessed for the need for assisted ventilation.

Long-term O_2 therapy (LTOT) has been well studied in the COPD patient population and increases quality of life and survival (see Chapter 75). Guidelines for COPD patients are also generally used for patients with other conditions causing chronic hypoxemia, although no similar multicenter trials have documented increased survival in these other groups. Intermittent O_2 therapy for desaturations that occur only at night or during exertion is less studied, and its benefits are not well documented. Nocturnal and exertional desaturation should be treated in patients with chronic pulmonary disorders, however, especially if the patient has any signs of pulmonary hypertension, cor pulmonale, or other coexistent cardiovascular disorder.

Pharmacologic Treatment. The standard accepted treatment approach for the patient with an exacerbation of COPD includes (1) maximal inhaled bronchodilator therapy with β_2-agonists and ipratropium bromide alone or in combination; (2) intravenous (IV) corticosteroids in initial doses equivalent to methylprednisolone, 0.5 mg/kg every 6 hours; (3) empiric antibiotics to cover common bacterial pathogens; (4) titrated O_2 therapy; and (5) electrolyte and nutritional supplementation. Theophylline is generally avoided acutely because of associated toxicities. The true efficacy of corticosteroids in this situation is debated, but little harm has been attributable to therapy with the above doses.

Specific pharmacologic treatment for progressive interstitial lung disease in the patient with acute on chronic respiratory failure has unpredictable effects, and unfortunately, benefit is often limited. Patients likely to respond to therapy are usually at a less precarious stage of their disease, and improvement is usually noticed after weeks of treatment. Corticosteroids and cyclophosphamide are typically prescribed for these patients. High-dose corticosteroids are indicated in the patient who experiences rapid deterioration soon after discontinuing or tapering corticosteroids. Other causes of respiratory failure that may mimic progressive interstitial lung disease need to be pursued and treated accordingly. These conditions most often include bacterial, viral, and opportunistic infections or left ventricular failure. Specific treatments for decompensated cor pulmonale may allow stabilization and significant improvement of the patient's condition (see Chapter 80).

Noninvasive Ventilation and Long-term Respiratory Aids. Noninvasive ventilation has been studied extensively over the last 10 years and has become an important advance in the treatment of patients with acute or chronic respiratory failure, acute pulmonary edema, and sleep-related breathing disorders. Box 77-4 lists the relative contraindications for noninvasive ventilation.

Respiratory assist devices and noninvasive ventilator strategies have been extensively used in patients with chronic neuromuscular impairments and are of proven benefit and generally well tolerated. These treatments can improve daytime $Paco_2$, decrease dyspnea, resolve symptoms attributed to sleep-disordered breathing, decrease hospitalizations, and improve survival in certain patient groups. Chronic support is frequently provided by positive-pressure assist devices, including intermittent ventilation, conventional ventilation by a tracheotomy or nasal mask, and bilevel positive-airway-pressure (BiPAP) device, also delivered by a nasal adapter. These machines are used intermittently throughout the day or just nocturnally. Other assist devices include rocker beds and externally applied negative-pressure respiratory devices, with the latter rarely used.

Patients with thoracic cage disorders can also benefit from noninvasive respiratory assistance with positive-pressure ventilation, typically delivered by nasal mask. Occasionally the patient must undergo a tracheotomy, and the intermittent ventilatory support must be delivered through the tracheotomy tube. Prolonged improvement in compliance and gas exchange has been reported after brief, intermittent pressure-assisted inflations, which appear to reverse underlying atelectasis. Daytime gas exchange and nocturnal desaturation improve with long-term use of nocturnal or intermittent ventilatory assistance. Noninvasive ventilation is less well

Box 77-4. Relative Contraindications to Noninvasive Ventilation

Hemodynamic instability or life-threatening dysrhythmias
High risk of aspiration
Impaired mental status
Life-threatening severe hypoxemia
Failed prior noninvasive ventilation
Intolerance to face mask, nasal mask, or nasal pillows

tolerated in patients with chronic respiratory failure from parenchymal lung diseases. However, noninvasive positive-pressure assistance can be provided intermittently and at night for select patients. The assist device is usually indicated for relief of symptoms caused by progressive hypercapnia.

Pulmonary Rehabilitation. A comprehensive discussion of the proven benefits and costs of pulmonary rehabilitation is beyond the scope of this chapter. Despite being considered essential and routine at some centers, this therapy has not been uniformly accepted by the medical community. However, these programs are integral to any lung transplantation or lung volume reduction surgery program. Pulmonary rehabilitation programs select for the most motivated patients, who in turn derive benefit in terms of increased exercise tolerance and physical conditioning, along with an improved quality of life and increased sense of well-being. Often, however, no other systematic improvements occur in pulmonary function, and no survival benefit has been shown. Variabilities in application and reimbursement and the failure of many patients to quit smoking are important obstacles that impede uniform successful utilization of pulmonary rehabilitation programs for the patient with a chronic pulmonary disorder.

Lung Transplantation. Heart-lung, double-lung, and single-lung transplantation are now options for patients with end-stage respiratory failure. Patients who are candidates are generally less than 65 years of age, are free of any significant systemic disorder, and have a poor prognosis related primarily to their underlying lung disease. Patients with COPD, end-stage emphysema from α_1-antitrypsin deficiency, cystic fibrosis, IPF, primary pulmonary hypertension, and pulmonary hypertension secondary to congenital heart defects have accounted for the vast majority of recipients to date. Detailed guidelines for recipient selection have been proposed. Patients with IPF, primary pulmonary hypertension, and cystic fibrosis have the highest mortality rates while awaiting transplantation; early referral of these patients is recommended. The time on the waiting list often exceeds 1 year. Therefore prolonged mechanical ventilatory support is not recommended for potential recipients, although some patients are now receiving transplants after being maintained on mechanical ventilation immediately before transplant.

The 1-year and 2-year posttransplant survival of these patients is about 80% and 70%, respectively. Early mortality is related to immediate postoperative complications and infections. Later mortality is seriously complicated by rejection and bronchiolitis obliterans. Recurrence of the underlying disease has been reported in sarcoidosis, lymphangioleiomyomatosis, giant cell interstitial pneumonitis, and eosinophilic granuloma. The number of lung transplants is increasing worldwide, but experience is more limited with lung transplantation relative to other common organ transplants due to (1) more limited donor acceptability because of pulmonary infection and other environmental exposures and (2) prior complications related to the bronchovascular blood supply and anastomotic healing. Long-term survival remains imperiled by chronic rejection, which manifests as bronchiolitis obliterans. Despite these limitations and the involved posttransplant medical regimen, lung transplantation has allowed for improved quality of life with prolonged survival for many recipients. It is hoped that experience, research, and technical advancements will make this a more successful and less costly option for patients in the future.

ACUTE RESPIRATORY FAILURE

Pathophysiology and Differential Diagnosis

Acute respiratory failure is often discussed in terms of the predominant gas exchange abnormality that occurs in the affected patient, that is, acute hypoventilatory failure and acute hypoxemic failure. The chronic lung disorders most often lead to *hypoventilatory* failure because of acute on chronic respiratory failure, as discussed earlier. In addition, diseases that acutely impair respiratory capacity (CNS drive, neuromuscular strength) also lead to hypoventilation and respiratory acidosis. In contrast, acute *hypoxemic* failure most often results from an acute parenchymal lung insult that may lead to life-threatening hypoxemia, even in the normal host.

Acute Hypoventilatory Respiratory Failure. A failure of ventilation with acute respiratory acidosis represents the predominant abnormality in a number of disorders. In patients with chronic restrictive or obstructive disorders, respiratory muscle fatigue ensues because of further increases in respiratory workloads or from causes that impair the respiratory muscles themselves. Acute asthma will also lead to respiratory muscle fatigue and hypoventilatory failure if the acute, severe bronchospasm cannot be expeditiously reversed. Neuromuscular disorders are not associated with any increased workloads but rather with a decreased capacity. Furthermore, diseased muscles are more prone to early failure leading to hypoventilation. In all these disorders, hypoxemia is often present as well but is caused by $\dot{V}/\dot{Q}$ inequalities and is often easily corrected with supplemental O_2 at low FIO_2 concentrations.

Acute on Chronic Respiratory Failure. The common causes of acute deteriorations in patients with chronic obstructive and restrictive thoracic disorders are discussed in the section on chronic failure. Most often, these patients present with hypoventilatory failure and hypoxemia. However, the hypoventilatory failure is usually the predominant abnormality and is the reason most require mechanical ventilatory support. If the hypoxemia is not readily reversible, causes of hypoxemic respiratory failure, such as pneumonia and cardiac failure, should be suspected.

Asthma. Fortunately, only a minority of patients with asthma will develop respiratory failure requiring mechanical ventilatory support. An estimated 4% of hospitalized asthmatic patients will require observation in the ICU, however, and the incidence of near-fatal and fatal asthma has increased in the United States and other countries. Patients with chronic severe disease, steroid dependency, undertreatment, and prior intubation are at particular risk for a severe exacerbation of their asthma. Underuse of corticosteroids and frequent daily treatment with inhaled β_2-agonists have also been associated with near-fatal and fatal presentations. Any asthmatic patient, however, can develop a severe, life-threatening episode of acute bronchospasm, at times linked to acute exposures to specific agents (see Chapter 72). Although significant morbidity and mortality are associated with positive-pressure ventilation, ventilator strategies designed to minimize barotrauma and adverse cardiopulmonary interactions have resulted in a very low mortality rate but significant remaining morbidity. Therefore prompt optimization of treatment during a severe exacerbation, careful monitoring for signs of compromise, and judicious use of assisted ventilation are important.

Asthmatic patients have certain physiologic abnormalities (Table 77-3), and common findings are associated with an asthma exacerbation (see Chapter 72). Diaphoresis, tachycardia greater than 120 beats/min, a pulsus paradoxus greater than 15 mm Hg, persistent dyspnea at rest, agitation and frequent repositioning, fragmented speech, and delirium are alarming signs of a severe exacerbation of asthma. Barotrauma is a serious complication and is indicated on physical examination by subcutaneous emphysema, tracheal deviation on palpation, and a mediastinal crunch or focal absence of breath sounds on auscultation. When signs and symptoms of a severe attack persist after early aggressive treatment, the condition is often referred to as *status asthmaticus*.

Upper Airways Obstruction. The primary physician may have difficulty distinguishing asthma from mechanical obstruction of the large airways, and the consequences of this missed diagnosis can be severe for the patient. *Stridor,* or a high-pitched inspiratory wheeze during inspiration, is a critical finding for the patient with a variable, extrathoracic lesion or a fixed trachea or major airways abnormality. If the large-airways obstruction is intrathoracic and is variable, or if it only occurs with expiration, it is often difficult to distinguish from common expiratory wheezing. Often these intrathoracic lesions are caused by bronchogenic carcinoma and occur in patients with underlying obstructive disease. Clues to a major airways obstruction in these patients include focal wheezes and wheezes that are heard best in the upper lung fields relative to the more peripheral areas. Gas exchange abnormalities usually only occur when these lesions are advanced and the narrowing is quite severe. Therefore early diagnosis based on clinical findings is required to avoid acute complications and the need for an emergency surgical airway.

Acute infectious processes leading to stridor from extrathoracic airway obstruction include epiglottitis, supraglottitis, and parapharyngeal abscesses. Symptoms and signs accompanying these acute processes help distinguish them from other causes of upper airway obstruction, which predominantly include tumors of the thyroid, trachea, and major bronchi. Vocal cord paresis, vocal cord dysfunction, and tracheal stenosis from prior intubation are other notable causes.

Depressed Central Nervous System Drive and Acute Neuromuscular Disorders. Acute insults to the CNS can impair the respiratory control and integrating center, resulting in ineffective transmission of efferent neurologic impulses to the muscles of respiration. Cranial nerve function and reflexes also may be impaired, leading to aspiration of oropharyngeal secretions. The result is acute hypoventilation, atelectasis, and aspiration pneumonia. Drug overdoses, metabolic encephalopathies, CVAs, and trauma are common causes of hypoventilatory failure. Seizures can also lead to respiratory insufficiency by central depression of the respiratory drive and by respiratory muscle dysfunction. Generalized or partial status epilepticus may also present with generalized, flaccid paralysis or a confusional state, respectively. Furthermore, the pharmacologic agents used to treat convulsions often suppress respiratory drive.

In disorders leading to acute neuromuscular failure (see Box 77-1), patients may have a history that indicates a definite process (e.g., bite, ingestion), or they may show a characteristic pattern of weakness that can help the physician to identify a specific disorder. Symptoms and signs of cholinergic excess can be seen with organophosphate poisoning and cholinergic crisis in patients with myasthenia gravis who are taking cholinesterase inhibitors. Signs include miosis, nausea and vomiting, excess salivation and diaphoresis, bronchorrhea, and bronchoconstriction. *Clostridium tetani* toxin causes local or generalized muscle rigidity and painful spasms. Sensory deficits should alert the physician to a spinal cord injury or compression or a generalized myelitis. An urgent workup should be undertaken to rule out these latter possibilities and circumvent further neurologic damage. Acute CVAs causing hemiparesis, including the muscles of respiration, do not usually lead to respiratory failure unless there is coexistent cardiopulmonary disease.

Acute Hypoxemic Respiratory Failure. In contrast to the causes of hypoventilatory failure, disorders associated with acute hypoxemic failure are often the result of an acute, severe, pulmonary insult (Box 77-5). These insults are sufficient to cause respiratory failure even in patients with previously normal pulmonary function, and life-threatening hypoxemia is often present. Hypoxemia may not be readily corrected with supplemental O_2 by face mask because it is often the result of "shunting." Therefore these patients may require prompt mechanical ventilation with settings that reduce the "shunt" and increase Pa_{O_2} to mitigate the adverse effects of tissue hypoxia. Because of the occasional prolonged need for high-Fi_{O_2} supplementation, the potential for oxygen toxicity arises. It is not a serious consideration, however, when Fi_{O_2} is less than 0.60 or if levels as high as 1.00 are given for less than 48 hours.

These disorders can be further divided into diffuse and focal processes. This distinction quickly directs the physician's attention to different sets of causes, diagnostic strategies, and treatment. *Diffuse* lung lesions are usually associated with more pronounced hypoxemia and mechanical abnormalities. Once cardiogenic pulmonary edema is ruled out, ARDS or diffuse lung infection must be considered.

Box 77-5. Causes of Acute Hypoxemic Respiratory Failure

Diffuse Pulmonary Abnormalities

Cardiogenic pulmonary edema
Adult respiratory distress syndrome (ARDS)
Diffuse infectious pneumonitis
Alveolar hemorrhage
Pulmonary alveolar proteinosis

Focal Pulmonary Lesions

Lobar pneumonia
Atelectasis
Pulmonary contusion
Alveolar and pulmonary hemorrhage
Reperfusion pulmonary edema
Reexpansion pulmonary edema

Diffuse alveolar hemorrhage is much less common but must not be overlooked. *Focal* lesions often result from obvious causes. Although hypoxemia is usually less severe than in the diffuse lesions, it may be disproportionate to the degree of lung involvement. Atelectasis is a common focal lesion that can complicate any of these respiratory disorders and should always be considered in any patient with a sudden decline in oxygenation (Fig. 77-2).

Diffuse Processes

Adult respiratory distress syndrome. ARDS has many different causes; an estimated 150,000 cases occur annually in the United States. Table 77-4 shows the variation in incidence and mortality among predisposing disorders. Twenty percent of patients with ARDS will experience a primary respiratory death. The mortality rate associated with ARDS has decreased, and younger patients (less than 60 years old) now do much better. Many patients who die from ARDS will succumb to infectious complications and multiorgan system dysfunction. The need for prolonged mechanical ventilation is a likely contributor to the increased incidence of infectious complications and death in these individuals.

ARDS is clinically defined by a limited number of diagnostic criteria that have been slightly modified since the early description of the syndrome. Current criteria for ARDS include (1) compatible clinical history and presentation of a severe lung injury, (2) signs of respiratory distress (tachypnea, dyspnea), (3) severe hypoxemia (Pa_{O_2} less than 50 mm Hg with Fi_{O_2} greater than 0.6, or Pa_{O_2}/Fi_{O_2} less than 200), (4) chest x-ray findings with bilateral infiltrates (Fig. 77-3), (5) exclusion of other causes (cardiogenic edema, progressive chronic respiratory failure), and (6) normal pulmonary capillary wedge pressure (PCWP) or no evidence for left atrial pressure elevation. Given the variability in presentation, severity, and course of ARDS, an expanded definition includes (1) a predisposing condition, (2) a lung injury score using physiologic parameters (chest film, Pa_{O_2}/Fi_{O_2}, PEEP, compliance), and (3) phase of the lung injury (acute or chronic). The criteria reflect a common injury response of the lung to a variety of insults. Box 77-6 lists these common pathophysiologic processes and the phases of ARDS. The key pathophysiologic abnormality is an *increase in alveolar-capillary permeability*. The Starling equation (see next) describes the forces governing capillary fluid filtration. Normally the hydrostatic forces favor fluid flux out of the capillary and into the perivascular tissues. This movement is usually counterbalanced by the oncotic forces that keep colloid in the vessels and favor fluid movement into the vascular space. The lung injury of ARDS results in an increase in the filtration coefficient, *Kf,* as follows:

$$\text{Capillary fluid flux (edema formation)} = Kf\,[(P_{\text{vascular}} - P_{\text{tissue}}) - (\pi_{\text{vascular}} - \pi_{\text{tissue}})\sigma]$$

where *Kf* is the filtration coefficient; σ is the reflection coefficient; *P* is the hydrostatic pressure; and π is the oncotic pressure. Increases in *Kf* encourage the flow of fluid into the interstitium and alveolar spaces. ARDS is also associated with a decrease in σ, from almost 1 to near 0. This parameter measures the efficiency of plasma proteins in returning fluid to the vasculature; σ decreases as the capillary membrane becomes more permeable to protein. These effects of ARDS result in the formation of exudative pulmonary edema at normal hydrostatic pressures.

In contrast, *cardiogenic edema* is caused by an increase in capillary hydrostatic pressure that results in the transudation of fluid into the tissues and air spaces of the lungs. *Kf* and σ remain normal under these conditions. The excess filtered fluid is initially located in the peribronchial tissue space and causes alveolar flooding only if this compartment is overwhelmed. This provides an additional safety factor with cardiogenic edema, unlike increased permeability states, since gas exchange and mechanical abnormalities are only appreciable when edema causes alveolar flooding. When cardiogenic edema results in respiratory failure, the gas exchange and mechanical abnormalities are similar to those seen in early ARDS.

A number of mediators have been implicated in the cellular injury, interstitial inflammation and fibrosis, and pulmonary and systemic hemodynamic changes seen in

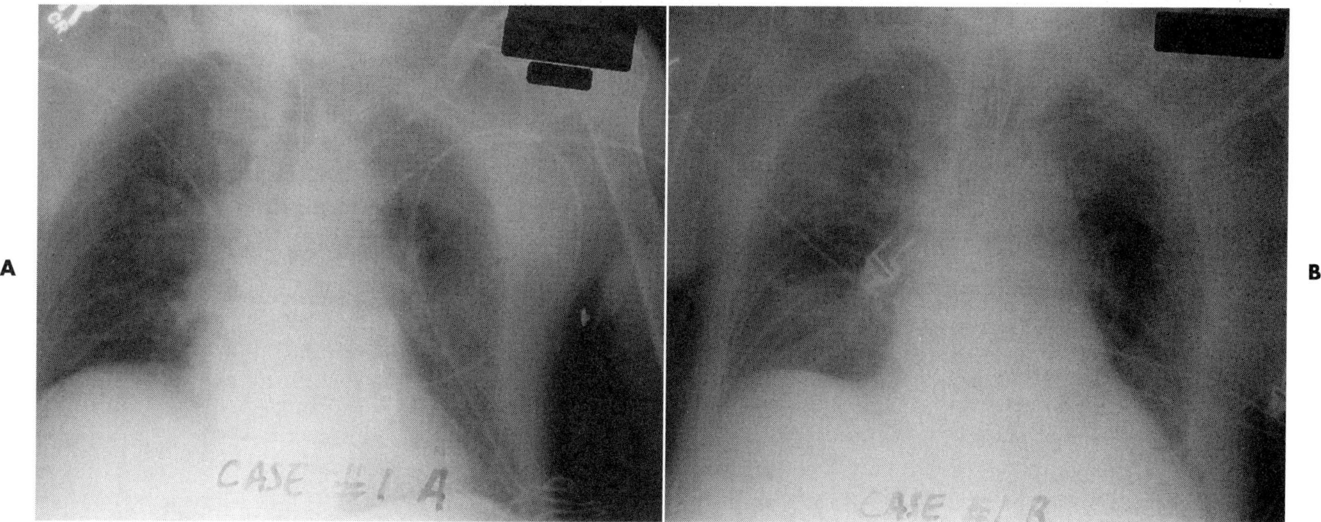

Fig. 77-2. **A,** Admission anteroposterior chest radiograph of man being monitored for exacerbation of COPD. He required intubation and later developed acute hopoxemia. **B,** Repeat chest film revealed silhouette sign of left hemidiaphragm consistent with left lower lobe atelectasis. Oxygenation improved quickly, with reversal of atelectasis.

Table 77-4. Selected Causes of Adult Respiratory Distress Syndrome (ARDS)

Cause	Incidence*	Mortality†
Infections		
Bacterial sepsis syndrome	High	High
Bacteremia	Low	High
Pneumonia treated in ICU	Moderate	High
Pneumocystis carinii pneumonia	High	High
Miliary tuberculosis and fungal disease	Low	High
Aspiration syndromes		
Acidic gastric aspiration	High	High
Near-drowning	High	Low
Coagulation and hematologic disorders		
Disseminated intravascular coagulation (various causes)	Moderate	High
Transfusion reactions	Low	Low
Thrombotic thrombocytopenic purpura	Low	N/A
Drugs		
Narcotics	Low	Low
Acetylsalicylic acid	Low	Low
Chemotherapy agents	Low	Low
Noninfectious embolic disorders		
Fat embolism	Low	Low
Amniotic fluid and venous air	Low	Low
Inflammatory and metabolic disorders		
Pancreatitis	Low	N/A
Acute fulminant liver failure	High	High
Vasculitis, collagen vascular disease‡	Low	N/A
Neurogenic pulmonary edema		
After grand mal seizure	Low	Low
After intracranial injury	Low	High
Toxic inhalational injuries	Low	N/A

*Rate among predisposed groups.
†N/A, Not available.
‡Only alveolar hemorrhage reported; see Box 77-5 and text.

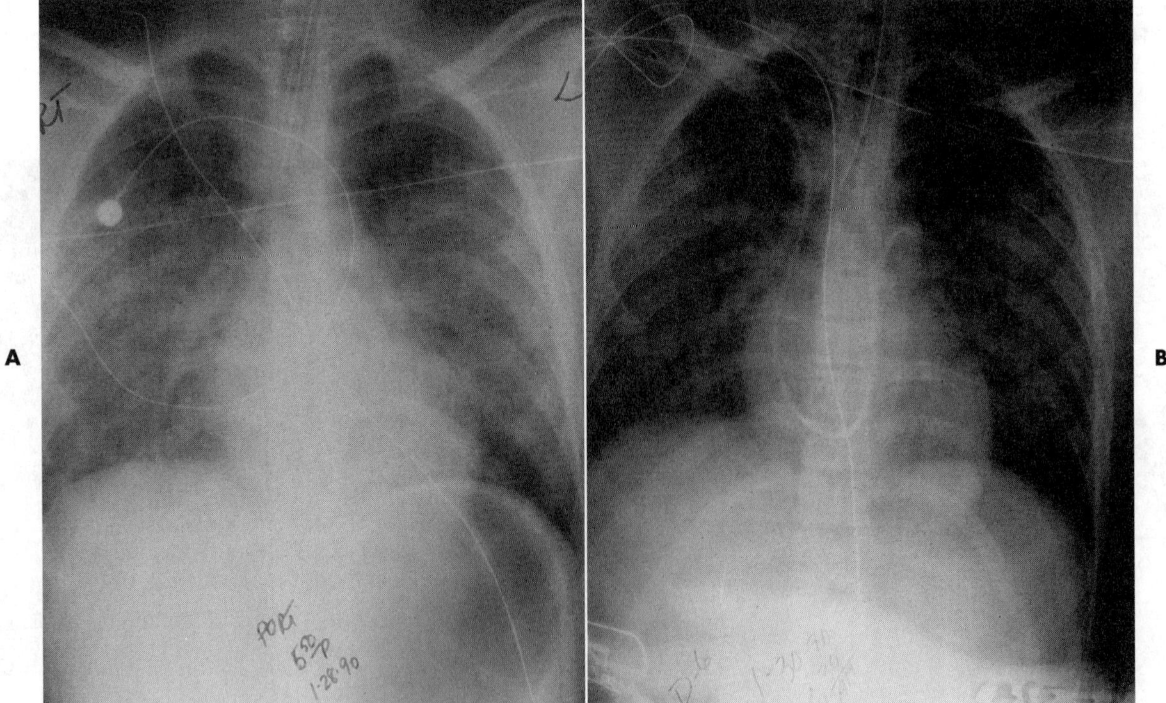

Fig. 77-3. **A,** Chest radiograph of 26-year-old male who developed confusion and ARDS 48 hours after intramedullary rodding procedure for femur fracture. **B,** Pulmonary artery catheter was placed to aid hemodynamic management. With diuresis the calculated shunt decreased from 35% to 20% over 48 hours, and patient was extubated shortly thereafter.

Box 77-6. Pathophysiologic Features and Phases of ARDS

Pathophysiologic Hallmarks

Increased alveolar-capillary permeability leading to edema formation at normal capillary hydrostatic pressures
Severe hypoxemia from shunt due to alveolar flooding
Decreased pulmonary compliance due to alveolar exudative edema and surfactant dysfunction
Increased pulmonary vascular resistance

Phases

Exudative and edemagenesis
Proliferative and reparative
Fibrotic and organizational

Box 77-7. Mediators of Acute Lung Injury

- Products of complement activation
  - C5a and related peptides
- Oxygen-reactive species
- Products of arachidonate-containing phospholipid metabolism
  - Cyclooxygenase products
  - Lipooxygenase products
  - Platelet-activating factor
- Proteolytic enzymes from neutrophils and macrophages
- Cytokines, including growth factors
  - Interleukins 1, 2, and 6
  - Tumor necrosis factor
  - Fibroblast growth factors
- Intravascular, extravascular, and intraalveolar coagulation abnormalities
- Endotoxin

ARDS (Box 77-7). Survivors of ARDS often recover remarkably. Some patients with the most severe lung injury can recover pulmonary function to within their normal predicted limits. Others may sustain a moderate decrease in function. Fortunately, the vast majority of survivors are not troubled by symptomatic respiratory insufficiency, although neuropsychiatric dysfunction and other limitations may impair their overall health after recovery.

Alveolar hemorrhage syndromes. Alveolar hemorrhage can lead to hypoxemia and can be associated with diffuse or focal hemorrhage (Fig. 77-4 and Box 77-8). Diffuse, fulminant alveolar hemorrhage can quickly lead to respiratory failure and death. The triad of hemoptysis, pulmonary infiltrates, and anemia is well described. Since the hemorrhage is distal to the ciliated central airways, however, hemoptysis may be scant or even absent. Patients also often have constitutional or other symptoms suggestive of a systemic disorder. Early recognition allows prompt treatment to prevent severe morbidity from fulminant alveolar hemorrhage, progressive renal failure, and severe anemia. Increasing infiltrates in the face of a rapidly declining hematocrit with no other source of

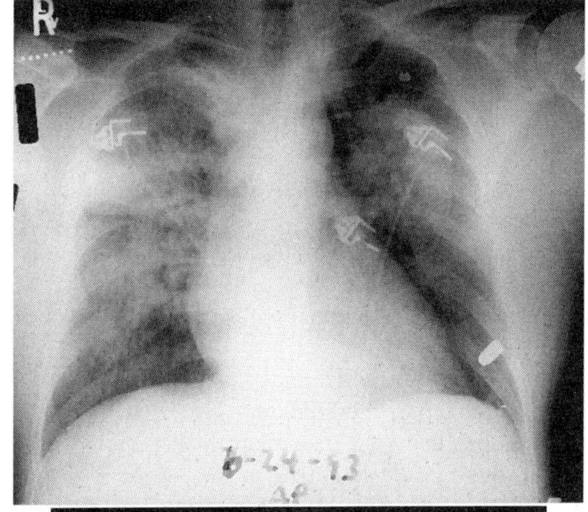

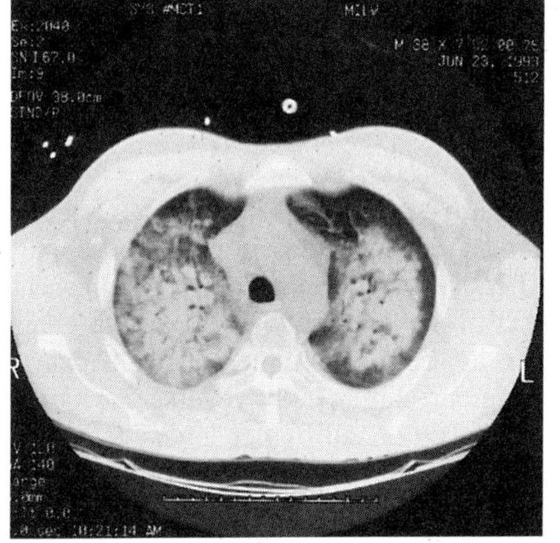

Fig. 77-4. Anteroposterior chest radiograph (**A**) and select view of CT scan of lung (**B**) of 37-year-old male with acute, severe alveolar hemorrhage from limited Wegener's vasculitis. Widespread dense consolidations with upper zone predominance were greatly increased from previous 36 hours, and hematocrit also decreased by 10%. Severe hypoxemia was corrected by using 60% Fi_{O_2} gas by face mask.

bleeding affords good presumptive evidence of pulmonary hemorrhage. Patients are often misdiagnosed as having an unresolving pneumonia with associated mild hemoptysis and are often treated with repeated antibiotic courses if their disease is mild at onset. Hypoxemia from shunt or increased venous admixture is quite common. If the process is diffuse, patients have the constellation of gas exchange and mechanical abnormalities that also affects patients with ARDS.

Focal Processes

Lobar pneumonia. Patients with lobar or multilobar pneumonia can have life-threatening hypoxemia without developing ARDS. Hypoxemia can be particularly pronounced when the pneumonia is most extensive in the well-perfused, gravity-dependent lung units. In addition, the venous admixture or shunt can be disproportionately elevated relative to the percentage of lung involved, if hypoxic pulmonary vasoconstriction is reversed by other vasoactive mediators of inflammation. Bacterial infection is by far the most likely cause of these consolidative processes (see Chapter 73).

Atelectasis. This occurs frequently in patients receiving mechanical ventilation with higher Fi_{O_2} gas. Problems with secretion clearance and prolonged supine positioning often lead to left and right lower lobe atelectasis. These changes can often be appreciated on routine daily chest films (see Fig. 77-2). Resorption atelectasis is promoted by high PA_{O_2} values

Box 77-8. Causes of Alveolar Hemorrhage

Anti–basement membrane antibody disease (Goodpasture's syndrome)
Immune complex–mediated vasculitides
Wegener's vasculitis
Other antineutrophil cytoplasmic antibody (ANCA)–associated vasculitides
Pauciimmune-associated vasculitides
Idiopathic pulmonary hemosiderosis
Hematologic disorders (e.g., coagulopathies, thrombocytopenia, bone marrow transplantation)
Other agents (e.g., penicillamine, trimellitic anhydride, lymph-angiogram contrast)

and low $\dot{V}/\dot{Q}$ ratios. At high levels of Fio_2, atelectasis of large lung unit areas can be radiographically apparent within minutes and cause hypoxemia from shunting. This needs to be considered in any patient with an abrupt change in Pao_2 without any other apparent clinical cause. Accurate recognition and treatment can quickly reverse the deterioration in Pao_2, can avoid prolonged higher levels of Fio_2 that further predispose to atelectasis, and can obviate the need for investigations into other potential causes of sudden O_2 desaturation, such as pulmonary embolus.

Diagnostic Evaluation

Arterial blood gases are necessary to determine the severity of hypoxemia and adequacy of ventilation. Once the patient is stable and has achieved an acceptable Sao_2, pulse oximetry can be used to assess the adequacy of oxygenation. The pulse oximeter needs to be intermittently correlated to ABGs. The $Paco_2$ needs to be measured independently according to the patient's clinical course. Serial ABGs are often necessary for the early evaluation of the patient with a severe asthma exacerbation or acute on chronic respiratory failure. Most patients initially have a respiratory alkalosis. A normal $Paco_2$ in a patient with persistent signs of respiratory distress indicates the potential for impending respiratory muscle fatigue and exhaustion. As the patient's clinical status improves, the $Paco_2$ will also naturally normalize. Therefore interpretation of laboratory data always requires close correlation with the patient's clinical condition. A progressively rising $Paco_2$ in the face of increasing respiratory efforts or signs of fatigue and exhaustion are common indications for assisted ventilation. No specific Pco_2 value, however, is sufficient to make a decision regarding mechanical ventilation without clinical correlation. The ABG may also show evidence of a metabolic acidosis, and the patient's ventilatory requirement may be increased accordingly.

An initial chest radiograph is warranted to delineate the pattern of abnormal pulmonary parenchymal processes, evaluate for pleural abnormalities, and provide information regarding any coexistent cardiac abnormality. Further thoracic imaging is usually not needed in the vast majority of cases. In addition to direct visualization, fluoroscopy and CT imaging of the thorax and neck are helpful in patients with upper airway lesions. Magnetic resonance imaging (MRI) or CT scans of the head are required for patients who have persistent, unexplained focal neurologic abnormalities and depressed CNS drive as the cause of their respiratory failure. Abdominal imaging may be necessary in the patient with ARDS and a likely undiagnosed infection. The lungs and abdomen are the most common sites of infection associated with ARDS.

For the acute neuromuscular disorders the history and clinical pattern of presentation are critical. In some conditions, such as tetanus, they may provide the sole means for diagnosis. *Early assessment of respiratory function is essential,* and respiratory failure represents the most life-threatening abnormality in these patients. Respiratory muscle weakness does *not* directly correlate with peripheral muscle strength and needs to be directly assessed (see following discussion). Some patients with Guillain-Barré syndrome may develop apnea at any time during their acute presentation. Therefore these patients require 24-hour monitoring until they start to improve. Early ICU care is justified in other conditions with signs of significant respiratory muscle involvement. ICU care has been clearly shown to decrease mortality in these patients, and a pulmonary or critical care consultant should be contacted early for assisting with respiratory care. Acute ABG abnormalities are a *late* sign of respiratory insufficiency in these patients. Therefore measurements of strength and mechanics should also be used to determine the need for ICU care. Acute hypercapnia and hypoxemia signal the need for ventilatory assistance.

Bedside measurements of respiratory muscle strength can be performed reproducibly by trained respiratory therapy personnel. Abnormalities of maximal inspiratory and expiratory pressures (MIP, MEP) are the most sensitive tests for respiratory muscle weakness. A MIP less than 15 to 20 cm H_2O is often incompatible with adequate ventilation. The MEP is generated by those muscles that can be recruited for active expiration and cough. A MEP less than 40 cm H_2O is associated with abnormal cough and clearance of respiratory secretions. Inability to clear respiratory secretions and an inadequate cough are common reasons for continued ventilation and reintubation in these patients. The forced vital capacity (FVC) determination is also useful. Values less than 30 ml/kg predispose to atelectasis; values less than 10 ml/kg, or approximately 1 L, are associated with inadequate ventilation. Bedside measurements of strength and volume should be done frequently throughout the day in the patient with an acute illness. Once the patient is at a stable, predictable level of function, treatments can be continued with less monitoring. The edrophonium test is recommended for the diagnosis of myasthenia gravis, but it can be positive in botulism as well.

Peak expiratory flow rates can be useful in the patient with acute asthma, but these data only complement careful clinical assessment (see Chapter 72). Values less than 100 L/min or decreased peak flow rates that increase by less than 10% after initial inhaled bronchodilator therapy indicate a severe attack. Patients who do not show significant improvement within the first 1 to 2 hours of treatment require close observation until consistent clinical improvement is noted on a stable treatment regimen. This observation may need to occur in the ICU setting. The flow-volume loop and airways resistance measurements can be helpful in identifying upper airway obstruction. Spirometry and ABGs alone will not identify lesions that cause variable obstruction only during inspiration.

In patients with pneumonia and risk factors or exposures that suggest an opportunistic infection or atypical pneumonia, more definitive diagnostic studies can be pursued. Broncho-alveolar lavage (BAL) can help to diagnose *Pneumocystis carinii* pneumonia and mycobacterial and fungal infections. Careful examination of the sputum and BAL results in a high yield for the diagnosis of blastomycosis when it leads to ARDS. The yield of sputum and BAL for other fungal infections and for miliary tuberculosis is less certain, and histologic tissue analysis may need to be pursued. Transbronchial biopsy carries a substantial risk of a complicated pneumothorax in a patient supported with mechanical ventilation and high cycling pressures. Open lung biopsy may need to be pursued to confirm or exclude these opportunistic and atypical pulmonary infections.

Fingerstick and serum glucose, basic chemistry and electrolyte panel, urine and blood toxicology screens, and specific serum drug levels are particularly valuable soon after the patient with depressed CNS drive arrives at the hospital. The ABG and electrolyte panel may provide early evidence of a severe underlying metabolic problem with life-threatening acid-base abnormalities. In patients with pulmonary or alveolar hemorrhage syndromes, serial blood counts, urinalysis, and biopsy of a suspicious skin lesion are studies that can be done promptly. Serologic tests should include the antinuclear antibody (ANA), anti–basement membrane antibody, and antineutrophil cytoplasmic antibody (ANCA). The ANCA can be very helpful in confirming a diagnosis of Wegener's vasculitis or an ANCA-associated vasculitis. Transbronchial biopsy is usually not helpful in making a specific histologic diagnosis with the immune alveolar hemorrhage disorders, but an open procedure can be considered for diagnosis.

Treatment: Pharmacologic and Supportive Care

Acute Hypoventilatory Respiratory Failure

Acute Central Nervous System and Neuromuscular Disorders. Treatment of ingestions may promptly restore consciousness and correct respiratory insufficiency. Rapid recovery may follow the administration of glucose, naloxone, and flumazenil for hypoglycemia, narcotic overdose, and benzodiazepine overdose, respectively. Flumazenil is useful for documenting benzodiazepine overdose but is not recommended in this general patient population because of its propensity to cause seizures. Other toxicology and critical care sources should be consulted for additional guidelines for treatment of these disorders.

The most immediate life-threatening abnormality in these conditions is respiratory insufficiency and hypoventilation. If patients have not responded promptly to a specific antidote or treatment, they should be expeditiously evaluated for airway protection and respiratory support (Box 77-9; see section on mechanical ventilation). Neurologic consultation is needed for all patients in whom a specific diagnosis is not readily apparent. Pulmonary or critical care consultation should be obtained for patients who require prolonged mechanical ventilation, have pulmonary complications, or have persistent problems requiring more expert management in the ICU.

Plasmapheresis for Guillain-Barré syndrome and other specific treatments for these disorders are covered elsewhere in this textbook. Adjunctive preventive therapies are very important for support of these patients. Deep venous thrombosis prophylaxis is essential (see Chapter 80). Combination therapy with sequential compression devices and subcutaneous heparin should be strongly considered in patients who cannot raise their legs against gravity. Additional treatments include stress ulcer prophylaxis, prevention of infectious complications, and management of autonomic dysfunction.

Box 77-9. Indications for Intubation and Mechanical Ventilation in Patients with CNS Abnormalities and Neuromuscular Insufficiency

Severely depressed or absent respiratory efforts
Aspiration or high risk for aspiration of oropharyngeal secretions or gastric contents
Persistent atelectasis with uncorrected gas exchange abnormalities
Acute decrease in maximal inspiratory pressure (MIP) to less than 20 cm H_2O
Acute decrease in forced vital capacity (FVC) to less than 10 ml/kg
Acute hypercapnia with or without hypoxemia (often a late finding)

Asthma. The patient's response to aggressive pharmacologic treatment must be carefully monitored. Specific therapies include aggressive treatment with inhaled bronchodilators and high doses of corticosteroids (see Chapter 72). IV aminophylline is generally avoided in the initial treatment of these patients, although ongoing debate surrounds this topic. IV magnesium sulfate, even with normal magnesium levels, may be helpful in improving the status of the patient with an acute exacerbation; however, this reported benefit has not been routinely reproduced. In refractory cases, inhaled general anesthetics and other agents have been employed.

Acute Hypoxemic Respiratory Failure

Adult Respiratory Distress Syndrome. The vast majority of patients with ARDS require mechanical ventilation because of the associated abnormalities (see Box 77-6). The intense supportive treatment needed by these patients requires expertise in mechanical ventilation, management of complications from barotrauma, hemodynamic management, and comprehensive care to avoid infection, gastrointestinal bleeding, and thromboembolic disorders. If these needs cannot be readily met at a certain medical center, it is strongly recommended that the patient be transferred to a center that is so equipped.

Appropriate hemodynamic and fluid management is crucial for the care of ARDS patients. Mechanical ventilation with the associated high levels of positive end-expiratory pressure (PEEP) and mean airway pressure can lead to impaired cardiac filling and a depressed cardiac output. O_2 delivery may fall and tissue hypoxia may ensue even if Sa_{O_2} has been normalized. Volume expansion could lessen the potential for this adverse consequence. Increases in fluid administration and PCWP, however, are associated with increases in edema formation and ventilatory requirements. Diuresis should be initiated and a negative fluid balance targeted if feasible. The physician should consider placement of a pulmonary artery catheter to guide fluid and hemodynamic management if high levels of PEEP are used (greater than 10 cm H_2O) and if hemodynamic instability is present. The goal for fluid management can be simply stated as to achieve the lowest pulmonary capillary filtration pressure associated with an adequate cardiac output and O_2 delivery. Output can be augmented by vasoactive agents to maintain an adequate O_2 delivery. Inotropic agents, such as dobutamine, should be the first-line agents. Increasing cardiac output may increase mixed-venous O_2 saturation and Sao_2 if shunt and O_2 consumption remain constant. This needs to be attempted on a trial-and-error basis, however, because increases in cardiac output may also increase shunt.

Pharmacologic treatments are being studied for ARDS and sepsis syndrome in general. Early administration of short-course, high-dose corticosteroids has been tested in various disorders leading to ARDS. The current consensus is *not* to give corticosteroids to patients early in their course. Nevertheless, case reports and a small, randomized study indicate that prolonged administration of lower doses of corticosteroids may have some benefit during the fibroproliferative phase of established ARDS in selected patients. Other pharmacologic treatments have failed to improve survival in ARDS and are not recommended. Inhaled nitric oxide given to patients with severe ARDS has decreased shunt, improved oxygenation, and decreased pulmonary artery pressure without systemic hemodynamic effects. No survival benefit has been demonstrated, and study results are pending. Nitric oxide is not approved by the U.S. Food and Drug Administration and is provided as an investigational drug at select medical centers. This therapy may save some patients with severe lung injury who cannot otherwise be oxygenated or who develop severe pulmonary hypertension in association with ARDS.

Alveolar Hemorrhage Syndromes. High-dose IV methylprednisolone can ameliorate the ongoing alveolar hemorrhage within 24 hours in most patients with these disorders. Correction of any coagulopathy and thrombocytopenia is an obvious priority. Cyclophosphamide and plasmapheresis can be added for other specific conditions. Prolonged supplemental O_2 may be required for the hypoxemia. If these patients require intubation and mechanical ventilation, they often have widespread hemorrhage, and their ventilator management can follow the guidelines given for the patient with ARDS. The patient must be assisted in the clearance of secretions; in particular, large blood clots may obstruct major airways and endotracheal tubes and may require emergency attention and therapy.

Atelectasis. Mechanical and pharmacologic strategies that promote lung inflation and secretion clearance should be vigorously pursued. Previous investigations showed no clear benefit to bronchoscopic treatment vs. these approaches. However, bronchoscopic clearance of tenacious mucus and other materials can be used early in patients with severe hypoxemia and those with unresolving large areas of atelectasis.

Focal Lesions. Prolonged administration of supplemental O_2 may be required in these patients. If the shunt is greater than 25%, mechanical ventilation may be necessary to provide adequate oxygenation. The patient can also be positioned more often with the most normal lung units in a gravity-dependent fashion in an attempt to improve $\dot{V}/\dot{Q}$ matching, but this may lead to atelectasis of these areas. Aggressive chest physiotherapy should be instituted to augment clearance of secretions and inflammatory debris.

Treatment: Mechanical Ventilation

Modes. Once the basic physiologic abnormalities of various disorders causing respiratory failure and the general features of the various modes of mechanical ventilation are understood, it becomes apparent that different modes of therapy may be suitable for the same patient (Tables 77-5 and 77-6). The first principle of using any mode of ventilation is that all operators should be familiar with it.

Noninvasive Ventilation. Noninvasive ventilatory strategies have been applied more extensively in patients with acute respiratory failure from various causes over the last 5 years. Recent prospective, randomized studies support the benefit of this strategy for selected patients with an acute exacerbation of COPD. These devices have also assisted select patients in other studied cohorts and have decreased complications relative to invasive ventilation. Assisted ventilation is delivered by nasal BiPAP system or face mask and a conventional mechanical ventilator. Necessary resources, essential monitoring, education, and guidelines for patient selection need to be clarified further before widespread application of this strategy. Randomized, controlled trials have shown noninvasive continuous positive airway pressure (CPAP) to be beneficial for patients with acute pulmonary edema from congestive heart failure (CHF). Most important, CPAP reduces the need for intubation and mechanical ventilatory support. Controlled trials of nasal BiPAP in patients with acute pulmonary edema from CHF showed improvement in respiratory parameters; however, more cardiovascular complications occurred with BiPAP compared with CPAP. Therefore, if used in this patient group, BiPAP should be titrated carefully; inspiratory and expiratory pressures should be initiated in the lower range and increased gradually.

Complications. Complications of mechanical ventilation are discussed throughout this chapter (Box 77-10). Appreciation of pressure-related and volume-related lung injury and occult intrinsic PEEP with its associated cardiac and respiratory complications have significantly impacted the approach to ventilation and monitoring in these patients. The risk of pneumothorax is not clearly defined, and certain conditions clearly predispose the patient to these complications. Peak airway pressures in excess of 45 cm H_2O have been associated with an increased incidence of pneumothorax in some retrospective reviews. Recent studies reported no increased mortality in ARDS patients who had a pneumothorax compared with other cohort patients. In certain conditions the plateau pressure and mean airway pressure are more indicative of the alveolar pressure. In general, plateau pressure should be maintained below 30 cm H_2O. PEEP can affect cardiovascular function by decreasing venous return (as occurs with other forms of positive intrathoracic pressure), decreasing right and left ventricular preload, increasing pulmonary vascular resistance, and altering venous admixture.

Table 77-5. Common Modes of Mechanical Ventilation

Ventilator mode	Breath initiated by	Set parameters	Monitored parameters
Volume controlled ("conventional")			
Controlled mandatory ventilation (CMV)	Ventilator	Vt, VE, peak flow and waveform	Airway pressures (peak, plateau, mean)
Assist-control ventilation (ACV)	Ventilator or patient	Vt, mininium VE, peak flow and waveform (spontaneous effort assisted by ventilator to set Vt)	Airway pressures, RR, total VE; flow limitation of patient effort with assisted breath
Synchronized intermittent mandatory ventilation (SIMV)	Ventilator or patient	Machine Vt, minimum VE, peak flow and waveform, synchronized spontaneous breath assisted to set Vt, (other spontaneous breaths not assisted)	Airway pressures, RR, total VE, spontaneous Vt (unassisted); flow limitation on assisted breaths
Pressure controlled			
Pressure-support ventilation (PSV)	Patient only	Inspiratory pressure (above set PEEP) during inspiratory flow only	Vt, VE, RR, mean airway pressure (no mandatory ventilation)
Continuous positive airway pressure (CPAP)	Patient only	Set positive pressure maintained during respiratory cycle	Vt, VE, RR (no mandatory ventilation)
Pressure-control ventilation (PCV)		Peak inspiratory pressure set; flow (pressure cycled) or inspiratory time (time cycled) set	Vt, VE, RR, mean airway pressure, inspiratory/expiratory ratio, intrinsic PEEP (at longer inspiratory times)
With CMV (PC-CMV)	Ventilator		As above
With ACV (PC-ACV)	Ventilator or patient	Spontaneous effort also assisted to set inspiratory pressure	As above
With SIMV (PC-SIMV)	Ventilator or patient	Synchronized spontaneous breath assisted	As above; also unassisted spontaneous Vt
Inverse-ratio ventilation			
Volume control (VC-IRV) or pressure control (PC-IRV)	Ventilator	See ARDS discussion	Also mean airway pressure and intrinsic PEEP

Vt, Tidal volume; *VE,* minute ventilation; *RR,* respiratory rate; *PEEP,* positive end-expiratory pressure.

Central Nervous System Disorders and Neuromuscular Insufficiency. Mechanical ventilation in these patients is straightforward, since they have only a deficiency in capacity and otherwise normal respiratory mechanics and gas exchange (see Box 77-9). A mandatory volume-controlled mode is necessary initially (see Table 77-6). These settings are intended to prevent atelectasis and barotrauma while providing for adequate gas exchange. An abnormal thoracic compliance and the need for an Fio_2 greater than 40% may signal an acquired pulmonary abnormality. Expeditious extubation of the patient once the condition has resolved will avoid complications of self-extubation and the paradoxic use of other sedative drugs. For patients with neuromuscular disorders who require more prolonged ventilatory support, daily measurements of respiratory muscle strength (MIP, MEP) and FVC are helpful. The patient can be evaluated for liberation from the ventilator once these parameters have sufficiently improved and the patient is able to clear secretions adequately and avoid significant problems with atelectasis.

Chronic Obstructive Pulmonary Disease. Box 77-11 lists indications for intubation and initiating mechanical ventilation in the patient with COPD (see Noninvasive Ventilation). Confused and agitated patients and those unable to clear secretions from the central airways because of weakness are most at risk for an imminent crisis; intubation and mechanical ventilation should be promptly initiated. These indications are not objective in all cases, and the decision to proceed with intubation and mechanical ventilation needs to be individualized (Box 77-12). Serious adverse consequences may occur with the initiation and subsequent titration of mechanical ventilation in patients with COPD. Therefore any clinician responsible for choosing ventilator settings for these patients should be familiar with these considerations (see Table 77-6).

Asthma. Indications for intubation and mechanical ventilation are again highly individualized; however, the indications in Box 77-11 are commonly accepted criteria. The reader is referred to other sources for consideration of noninvasive ventilation in this patient group. When the physician decides that intubation is necessary, it must proceed in a controlled, expert, and expeditious manner. The physician most experienced in airway management should oversee securing the airway. Because losing the airway after initial placement can be disastrous, heavy sedation and neuromuscular relaxants are often required initially. Patients

Table 77-6. Common Ventilator Machine Settings for Disorders Causing Respiratory Failure

Condition	Mode	Vt, VE	PEEP (cm H_2O)	Pressure targets (cm H_2O)	FiO_2
Depressed CNS drive	Mandatory ACV, SIMV	Vt = 10 ml/kg VE = 6-8 L/min	0-5	Peak usually <35	Minimum for SaO_2 >90%
Neuromuscular insufficiency	Acute: mandatory ACV, SIMV Mild, recovering: SIMV and PSV, PSV alone	Vt = 8-10 ml/kg VE = 6-8 L/min Guarantee Vt >350 ml with PSV breaths	0-5 0-5	Peak usually <35	As above
COPD	Early: ACV, SIMV Late: see text	Vt = 8 ml/kg VE: minimize, usually 8-10 L/min Peak flow ≥60 L/min	0*	Plateau <30; monitor for intrinsic PEEP (auto PEEP)	As above
Asthma	Early: ACV, SIMV	Vt = 8-10 ml/kg VE about 8 L/min Peak flows variable for sufficient expiratory time	0	Plateau <35; peak dependent on peak flow; monitor for intrinsic PEEP; neuromuscular blockade often needed early	As above
Interstitial lung disease	ACV, SIMV, PSV or PCV	Vt = 6-8 ml/kg VE = 8-10 L/min, peak flow ≥60 L/min	5	Plateau <35	As above
ARDS	ACV or PCV Severe, early: IRV (see text) Mild: consider PSV	Vt = 6-8 ml/kg VE > 10 L/min	7.5 (minimum), 20 (maximum)	Peak <45; plateau <30 Adjust to minimum mean airway pressure for adequate SaO_2	FiO_2 of 1.00 for 48 hours acceptable; attempt to decrease to ≤0.60

See Table 77-5 for abbreviations. *FiO_2*, Fractional inspired oxygen concentration; *CNS*, central nervous system; *COPD*, chronic obstructive pulmonary disease; *ARDS*, adult respiratory distress syndrome.
*PEEP added to obstructive disease only in special circumstances.

should continue receiving heavy sedation until signs of significant airways resistance abates. Once asthmatic patients are intubated and mechanically ventilated, they require frequent assessments and adjustments to machine settings to avoid complications from barotrauma. Further adjustments are best directed by a pulmonary or critical care specialist. The use of nondepolarizing neuromuscular relaxants in asthmatic patients has been associated with myopathy and prolonged muscular weakness on recovery. This may result from an adverse interaction between neuromuscular relaxants and high doses of corticosteroids. Therefore these drugs should be continued only when key therapeutic goals are not being met.

The physician should adhere to the recommended plateau pressure limits and be less scrupulous about the peak airway pressure for asthmatic patients (see Table 77-6). These patients also develop intrinsic PEEP, and settings should provide for prolonged expiration and a limited VE. This latter guideline often necessitates higher inspiratory flows and peak pressures, but plateau pressure can still be maintained. More conservative limits on peak pressure have been associated with hypotension and other adverse consequences consistent with increased intrinsic PEEP. If the patient does develop hypotension, the ventilator should be disconnected for a time (30 to 60 seconds) to release the trapped gas and relieve the intrinsic PEEP. A chest radiograph should be obtained to rule out a pneumothorax as well. Monitoring these airway pressures and the degree of intrinsic PEEP is essential for assessment of the patient's response to treatment while being supported on the ventilator. When ventilation to a normal $PaCO_2$ is not compatible with pressure targets, permissive hypercapnia has been used in an attempt to mitigate the risk of barotrauma and adverse cardiopulmonary interactions. This approach is controversial, and the reader is referred to other sources for further information. When the patient's clinical status improves, airway pressures fall toward normal, gas exchange normalizes, and the patient requires less sedation to coordinate with the ventilator. Since the patient may have labile airways resistance, the Vt may vary greatly on a pressure-controlled mode of ventilation (pressure support, pressure control), so Vt and VE must be monitored. Mechanical ventilation can be discontinued when the bronchospasm is well controlled and gas exchange, respiratory muscle strength, electrolyte balance, and nutritional status have returned to normal.

Restrictive Diseases (Interstitial Lung Diseases, Thoracic Cage Deformities). The causes of acute respiratory failure in these patients are generally not readily reversible. Therefore a decision to intubate does not have to

Box 77-10. Complications from Mechanical Ventilation

Alveolar injury from increased alveolar pressure and distention
Oxygen toxicity
Atelectasis
Barotrauma
- Pulmonary interstitial emphysema
- Pneumomediastinum and pneumopericardium
- Pneumothorax (often with tension)
- Systemic air embolism
- Gastric distention and pneumoperitoneum

Mechanical ventilator malfunctions
Endotracheal tube complications
- Mucus plugging
- Improper tube placement
- Tracheal injury and stenosis
- Laryngeal edema
- Bronchospasm and cough paroxysms

Adverse cardiopulmonary interactions
- Decreased venous return
- Impaired cardiac filling
- Increased pulmonary vascular resistance

Infections
- Nosocomial pneumonia
- Tracheotomy site infections
- Paranasal sinus infection

Prolonged diffuse muscular weakness
- Associated with neuromuscular blocking agents, especially with corticosteroids

Box 77-11. Indications for Intubation and Mechanical Ventilation in Patient with COPD

Hypoxemia that is unable to be corrected to an Sa_{O_2} of 85% or higher
Increasing Pa_{CO_2} despite therapy and with increased respiratory efforts
Persistent increase in respiratory rate to more than 40/min
Confusion, agitation, and altered sensorium
Increasing dyspnea with sense of exhaustion and fragmented speech
Inability to clear pooled secretions in central airways
Evidence of ongoing cardiac ischemia or failure
Need to pursue diagnostic or therapeutic procedures that place patient at risk for a respiratory crisis

await serial evaluations during acute therapy. However, patients with thoracic cage deformities may show a prompt, dramatic response to acute maneuvers that reverse atelectasis (see Table 77-6). Once reversible physiologic abnormalities are optimally treated and the patient has regained muscle strength, the patient's work of breathing can be increased while on the ventilator. This strategy can be continued until the patient's respiratory status is optimized and the patient is

Box 77-12. Managed Care Guide: Principles of Mechanical Ventilation in Patient with COPD

1. Provide *initial* total respiratory muscle rest.
2. Do not overventilate. Correct *acute* elevations in Pa_{CO_2} gradually (target patient's chronic compensated Pa_{CO_2} level).
3. Minimize ventilator requirement. Select ventilator settings with careful attention to intrinsic PEEP.
4. Provide minimal level of Fi_{O_2} to achieve Sa_{O_2} of 90% or higher.
5. Avoid deep sedation after 48 hours. Use paralysis only if essential.
6. Increase patient's work of breathing (weaning) as soon as tolerable.
7. Add PEEP *only* in specific circumstances to decrease patient work.
8. Provide periods for patient respiratory muscle rest until ready for focused trials of liberation from ventilator.
9. Attempt to treat true "panic" attacks while avoiding alteration of mechanical ventilation treatment plan.
10. Maintain nutrition and electrolyte balance.
11. Move to liberation from ventilation when:
    a. Reversible physiologic abnormalities are optimally treated.
    b. Patient has tolerated spontaneous or minimally assisted ventilation with signs of stable strength and gas exchange.

(See Table 77-6 for common ventilator machine settings.)

ready for focused attempts to be liberated from the ventilator. These patients normally breathe with a relatively rapid, shallow pattern, and a low Vt and FVC should be expected when weaning parameters are measured. A near-normal MIP (50 to 60 cm H_2O) suggests that the patient may be able to sustain ventilation in the face of the increased elastic loads when spontaneous breathing is resumed. Pressure support is a well-tolerated mode of ventilation for increasing these patients' work of breathing. Patients can be liberated from the ventilator once they have sustained prolonged assisted ventilation with a pressure-support level that is just sufficient to overcome the resistance of the endotracheal tube.

Adult Respiratory Distress Syndrome and Other Diffuse Lung Lesions. The general goals of mechanical ventilation are to reverse life-threatening hypoxemia quickly, limit the potential for oxygen toxicity, provide adequate ventilation to specific goals of Pa_{CO_2} and pH, limit barotrauma and alveolar damage by carefully monitoring airway pressure limits, and avoid adverse cardiopulmonary interactions. Important settings in these patients include lower physiologic tidal volumes with higher respiratory rates (see Table 77-6). A high V_E (greater than 10 L/min) almost always is required, and PEEP needs to be employed at a minimal level of 7 cm H_2O and adjusted judiciously according to important pressure targets. To avoid oxygen toxicity, the physician should attempt to reduce the Fi_{O_2} to less than 0.60 within 48 hours; first, however, an Sa_{O_2} greater than 90% and pressure targets must be met. Permissive hypercapnia may be allowed if an adequate ventilation cannot be achieved while meeting the key pressure targets with the desired lower physiologic Vt. The recommended limits of this approach are a $Paco_2$ less than 65 mm Hg and pH greater than 7.20. This alternative approach may improve survival compared with historic controls. The National Institutes of Health (NIH) ARDS Network recently released preliminary results from a randomized trial that separated patients into two groups based on selected Vt. The lower Vt group (6 ml/kg) had a significantly improved survival compared with the higher Vt group (12 ml/kg); the survival rates were 70% and 60%, respectively. These data strongly support the use of lower or physiologic tidal volumes in the ventilatory management of patients with ARDS.

The initial choice of mechanical ventilation mode should be well known to physicians and personnel (see Mechanical Ventilation). The minimum mean airway pressure needed to achieve adequate oxygenation is an important precept of ventilator management in these patients. These maneuvers may include inverse-ratio ventilation, which is usually most successful early in ARDS and should be abandoned if no benefit is seen within a few hours. Since pressure targets are prominent goals in the current ventilatory management of these patients, pressure-controlled modes are typically used, although conventional volume-controlled modes can achieve targets as well. When pressure targets are easier to achieve, the volume-controlled modes may be desirable to prevent hyperinflation and "volutrauma." Sedation and neuromuscular blockade should be used initially in almost all patients. Neuromuscular blockade should be prolonged only when the patient is not meeting other prominent therapeutic goals, including pressure targets. The patient's assistance with ventilation can be increased as physiologic abnormalities resolve. Once the Fio_2 is less than 0.4 with a PEEP of 5 cm H_2O or lower and a compliance greater than 25 ml/cm H_2O, patients can be evaluated for more specific trials to liberate them from the ventilator.

Focal Lesions and Hypoxemic Failure. Mechanical ventilation maneuvers used in the patient with ARDS and a more widespread pulmonary process may not be beneficial in patients with focal lesions. Therefore PEEP should be applied carefully and reversed if no benefit occurs. The physician may need to use high and potentially toxic Fio_2 levels of inspired gas until the process subsides. Cyclooxygenase inhibitors have been shown to improve shunt fraction and improve Pao_2 in animal models and during short administration periods in adults with pneumonia. The benefits and hazards of prolonged administration of these compounds are not known. Other causes of focal lesions, such as reperfusion edema and lung contusion, can be handled similarly.

Weaning and Liberation. Given the previously listed complications, some oppose use of the term *weaning* to refer to removing a therapy that poses such hazards to the patient. To emphasize that patients should be removed from mechanical ventilation as soon as feasible, they refer to the process as *liberation.* Predicting the success of liberation from mechanical ventilation has been extensively studied; however, the methods used rely on "static" indices regarding time to predict long-term patient endurance and have been less helpful for patients on prolonged mechanical ventilation (longer than 7 days). No substitute exists for ongoing assessment of the patient's respiratory loads and capacity and vigorous correction of reversible abnormalities before trials of liberation from ventilation. Of the indices studied, the simple parameters of respiratory rate, average Vt, and frequency (respiratory rate)/average Vt index have been most helpful. The frequency/Vt index during spontaneous or minimally assisted ventilation quantifies the well-known bedside observation for rapid, shallow breathing; an index less than 105 can predict a successful outcome from liberation in patients mechanically ventilated for less than 8 days. MIP, MEP, FVC, VE, and other indices are important for ongoing evaluation of the patient, with certain parameters more important for specific patient problems, but they have been less useful as an index to predict endurance once the patient is liberated from the ventilator.

In the patient who has a clear, acute process that is reversed, and when respiratory loads and capacity are normal, a very expeditious approach to liberation from mechanical ventilation is warranted. For other patients on mechanical ventilation, those ready for liberation can be most readily identified by a successful spontaneous breathing trial once other usual parameters for discontinuation have been satisfied, including a PEEP of 5 cm H_2O or less, Fio_2 of 0.40 or less, Pao_2/Fio_2 ratio less than 200, ability to clear secretions, and no hemodynamic instability. Some physicians only use this approach; others use a gradual approach to liberation in patients who cannot be weaned from the ventilator expeditiously. No mode has proved to be superior when a gradual increase in work of breathing is pursued before discontinuation of ventilation. PSV, SIMV with a decrease in rate, and CPAP are common modes employed for the patient who is weaned gradually (see Table 77-5).

ADDITIONAL READINGS

Ely EW et al: Effect on the duration of mechanical ventilation of identifying patients capable of breathing spontaneously, *N Engl J Med* 335:1864, 1996.

Green RJ et al: Pulmonary capillaritis and alveolar hemorrhage, *Chest* 110:1305, 1996.

Hillberg RE et al: Noninvasive ventilation, *N Engl J Med* 337:1746, 1997.

Kollef MH et al: The acute respiratory distress syndrome, *N Engl J Med* 332:27, 1995.

Marini JJ: Ventilatory management of COPD. In Cherniak NS, editor: *Chronic obstructive pulmonary disease,* New York, 1991, Saunders.

McKibben AW et al: Pressure-controlled and volume-cycled ventilation, *Clin Chest Med* 17:395, 1996.

Meduri GU et al: Effect of prolonged methylprednisolone therapy in unresolving acute respiratory distress syndrome: a randomized controlled trial, *JAMA* 280:159, 1998.

O'Connor MF et al: Acute hypoxemic respiratory failure. In Hall JB, Schmidt GA, Wood LDH, editors: *Principles of critical care,* New York, 1998, McGraw-Hill.

Pingleton SK: Complications of acute respiratory failure, *Am Rev Respir Dis* 137:1463, 1988.

Presberg KW et al: Pulmonary edema and other disorders in acute renal failure. In Ronco C, Bellomo R, editors: *Critical care nephrology,* Boston, 1998, Kluwer.

Yang KL, Tobin MJ: A prospective study of indexes predicting the outcome of trials of weaning from mechanical ventilation, *N Engl J Med* 324:1445, 1991.

CHAPTER 78

Sarcoidosis

Richard A. DeRemee

Sarcoidosis is a relatively common problem in a pulmonary disease practice. At the Mayo Clinic, approximately 100 new cases are evaluated each year. Among the diffuse interstitial pulmonary diseases, the two major entities are sarcoidosis and idiopathic pulmonary fibrosis (IPF).[4] Worldwide, the incidence of sarcoidosis ranges from 11 to 640 cases per 100,000 population. The mean age of affected patients is approximately 40 years, although the age range is broad and includes some patients in their 70s. Although many published series report a larger proportion of women than of men, data from the Mayo Clinic (unpublished) suggest that this seeming preponderance may be inaccurate because of a higher incidence of symptoms in women that probably leads to more frequent medical attention. Furthermore, sarcoidosis is often more symptomatic and aggressive in African-Americans than in Caucasians. Thus drawing firm conclusions from studies that combine data from African-American and Caucasian cohorts is unwise.

PATHOPHYSIOLOGY

Because the cause of sarcoidosis is unknown, a somewhat lengthy and descriptive definition is necessary. In a sense, sarcoidosis is a syndrome—a collection of signs, symptoms, and laboratory, radiologic, and pathologic data that presumably identify a group of patients for whom the prognosis and management are predictable. Authorities may offer various definitions, all of which should include four major points. First, a noncaseous or nonnecrotizing (the more modern parlance) granuloma is the characteristic pathologic finding. The granuloma is the result of a complex immunologic cascade probably driven by unspecified antigen(s).[1] The finding of nonnecrotizing granuloma is not specific for sarcoidosis but can be caused by specific agents or conditions, such as mycobacteria, fungi, beryllium, or syphilis. It may also be associated with Crohn's disease (regional enteritis). Thus the finding of noncaseous granuloma alone is nondiagnostic but must be assessed in the context of the total clinical framework, and reasonable efforts should be exerted to exclude these alternative causes. The second point is that, thus far, the cause of sarcoidosis is unknown. Continued investigations may eventually elucidate specific etiologic mechanisms. Third, sarcoidosis should be considered a systemic disease. For example, noncaseous granuloma isolated to skin in a foreign body reaction or in regional lymph nodes that drain areas of a malignant lesion represents a local "sarcoid reaction" and is not sarcoidosis. Fourth, sarcoidosis should have clinical consistency. This concept is the most difficult to convey but should be clarified by the subsequent discussion.

CLINICAL MANIFESTATIONS

In general, the initial manifestations and clinical picture are a function of the predominant organ involvement (Box 78-1). In more than 90% of patients the lungs or intrathoracic lymph nodes are affected. Paradoxically, few (if any) symptoms are attributable to lung involvement, at least in the early phase of the disease. In Caucasian cohorts, pulmonary symptoms such as dyspnea and cough may be absent, even with extensive lung disease manifested on a chest radiograph. Symptoms, particularly dyspnea, usually occur when the disease is in a late fibrotic phase associated with airways obstruction.[5] This characteristic contrasts with IPF, which has dyspnea as a cardinal, early symptom.

Box 78-1. Sites of Manifestation of Sarcoidosis

Lymph nodes (especially intrathoracic)
Lungs
Liver
Spleen
Eyes
Bones (especially small bones of hands and feet)
Salivary and lacrimal glands
Central nervous system
Skin
Heart (infrequently)

Sarcoidosis may be diagnosed because of involvement of the eyes with uveitis, iritis, conjunctivitis, or perhaps dry eyes from involvement of the lacrimal glands. Twenty-five percent of Mayo patients have such involvement. In approximately 20% of patients, characteristic skin involvement, such as erythema nodosum, lupus pernio, or salmon-colored to brown plaques, may be the first manifestation that leads to further investigations for sarcoidosis. In patients with a seventh cranial nerve palsy (Bell's palsy), an obscure peripheral neuropathy, or perhaps even a mass lesion in the central nervous system that proves to be noncaseous granuloma, sarcoidosis should be included in the differential diagnosis. Approximately 10% of patients with sarcoidosis have neurologic involvement. A physician may suspect sarcoidosis in patients with pituitary gland dysfunction or an increased serum calcium concentration. Other manifestations include hepatosplenomegaly, cystic or erosive lesions of bones (particularly in the hands), and symmetric ascending polyarthritis. Clinically significant heart involvement occurs infrequently, but sarcoidosis is a possible cause of conduction disturbances, dysrhythmias, and cardiomyopathies. Fever may be present in up to 10% of affected patients, particularly those with extensive involvement of retroperitoneal lymph nodes, as assessed by a computed tomography (CT) scan of the abdomen.

RADIOLOGIC STAGING SYSTEM

For more than 30 years a radiologic staging system has been used in the classification of sarcoidosis.[14] This system is based solely on the appearance of the plain chest radiograph and has no foundation in data from CT, gallium scanning, or other findings. Stage I consists of bilateral hilar adenopathy, often in conjunction with a right paratracheal node (Fig. 78-1). In stage II sarcoidosis, patients have bilateral hilar adenopathy and diffuse parenchymal infiltration, which

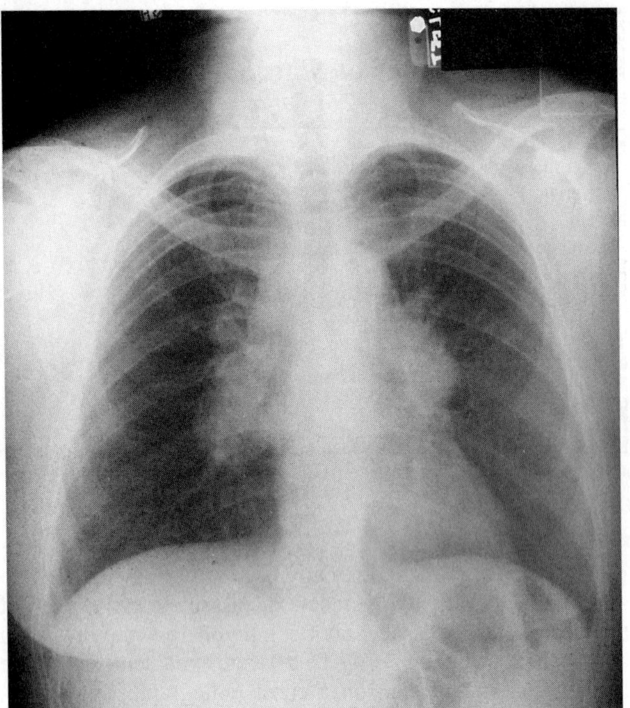

Fig. 78-1. Chest x-ray appearance of stage I sarcoidosis: bilateral hilar adenopathy without parenchymal infiltration.

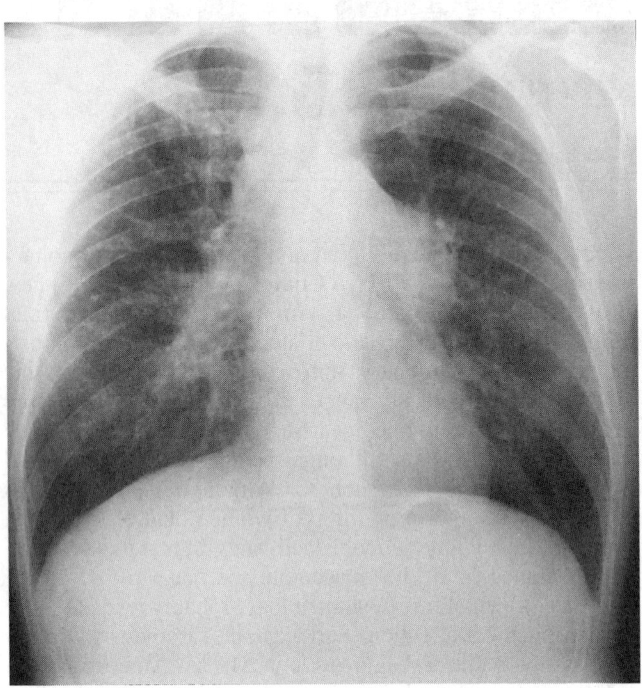

Fig. 78-2. Chest x-ray appearance of stage II sarcoidosis: bilateral hilar adenopathy with parenchymal infiltration.

usually is interstitial but occasionally is finely nodular or miliary (Fig. 78-2). Parenchymal infiltration without hilar adenopathy constitutes stage III (Fig. 78-3). Some authorities use a stage IV classification to indicate irreversible fibrosis, but this category must be based on information other than that available from the plain chest film and probably is not helpful.

More than simply transmitting radiologic visual information, the staging system also provides information on prognosis, frequency of symptoms, and degree of derangement of pulmonary function[5] (Table 78-1). Relative to prognosis, the probability of spontaneous remission is approximately 80% in patients with stage I sarcoidosis, 50% in those with stage II, and 30% in those with stage III. In a study of 256 Mayo patients (unpublished), only 1 of 125 with stage I sarcoidosis, 6 of 48 with stage II, and 30 of 83 with stage III complained of dyspnea. The complaint of dyspnea was correlated with the finding of airways obstruction.[6] In another study of pulmonary function, only 1 of 32 patients with stage I sarcoidosis had an abnormal finding, a mild obstructive change. Of 21 patients with stage II disease, seven had abnormalities (one obstructive and six restrictive patterns). Of 21 patients with stage III disease, 15 had abnormalities of pulmonary function, including 12 restrictive and three obstructive patterns (three had a combination of obstruction and impairment of diffusing capacity). Many patients with stage II or III sarcoidosis may have no symptoms and may have pulmonary function variables within normal limits at the initial assessment. Whereas CT has gained wide use in the evaluation of diffuse interstitial lung disease, its role in the overall diagnosis and management is currently controversial.

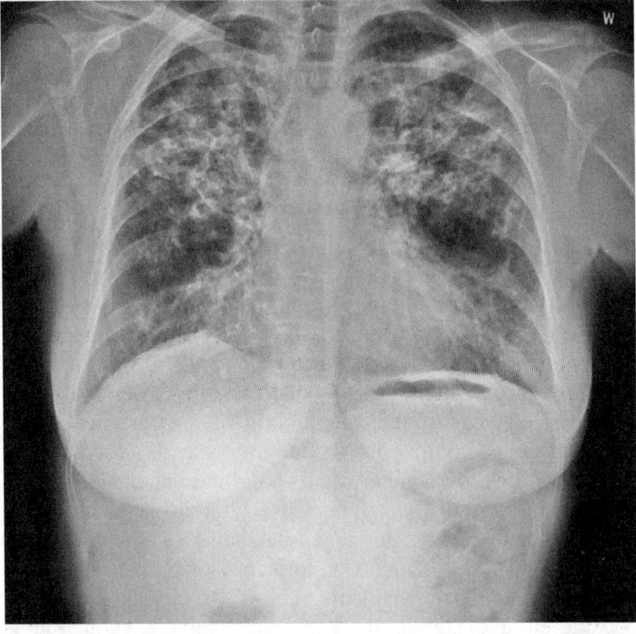

Fig. 78-3. Chest x-ray appearance of stage III sarcoidosis: parenchymal infiltration without hilar adenopathy. Note preponderant upper zone involvement.

LABORATORY STUDIES AND DIAGNOSTIC PROCEDURES

Because more than 90% of patients have intrathoracic disease often as the sole manifestation of sarcoidosis, many will likely be asymptomatic and are brought to medical attention

Table 78-1. Patient Variables in Radiologic Stages of Sarcoidosis

Stage	Remission	Symptoms (dyspnea)	Pulmonary function
I	>80%	<1%	Normal
II	50%	12%	Two-thirds normal
III	<30%	36%	One-third normal

only because of abnormal findings on a chest film. Chest radiographs may have been performed during a mass screening program (infrequent today), a routine physical examination, or an investigation of other problems or seemingly unrelated symptoms. As previously mentioned, other organ system involvement may have prompted clinical attention. Once the diagnosis of sarcoidosis is considered, tissue confirmation should be sought. In patients with stage I sarcoidosis, mediastinoscopy is recommended. Transbronchial biopsy is positive in about 50% of cases. Some clinicians might argue that an asymptomatic patient without physical findings but with stage I radiologic abnormalities needs no tissue confirmation. This may be a reasonable approach, but because the diagnosis necessitates tissue confirmation, the patient cannot be given a firm diagnosis or prognosis. If the patient is comfortable with this degree of uncertainty, tissue confirmation may be postponed, but careful follow-up is imperative, that is, chest films every 3 to 6 months until the course is clarified. For patients with stage II or stage III sarcoidosis, bronchoscopy in conjunction with bronchial and transbronchial lung biopsy is recommended. With experienced investigators, tissue confirmation should be achieved in more than 80% of cases.

If these measures fail, open lung biopsy can be considered. Before such a biopsy is done, however, a diligent search should be made for possible sarcoidal lesions in the skin or conjunctiva. A conjunctival biopsy is unlikely to reveal sarcoidosis if no gross abnormalities of the conjunctiva are evident on visual inspection. Open lung biopsy should be resorted to infrequently. In a series of 99 consecutive Mayo patients (unpublished), only five required open lung biopsy for final diagnosis. All biopsy material should be cultured for mycobacteria and fungi, and the diagnosis of sarcoidosis cannot be confirmed until a specific cause for the noncaseous granuloma has been excluded. The Kveim test is primarily of historic interest. Although it may still be used, the antigen is not commercially available, and few centers are actively engaged in its production and validation.

MANAGEMENT

The treatment of lung manifestations of sarcoidosis remains controversial more than 45 years after the introduction of glucocorticoids. On the basis of a large experience, use of glucocorticoids is advocated in all patients with stage II or III sarcoidosis if, after observation for 6 to 12 months, the disease either shows no evidence of spontaneous clearing or has worsened, as determined by serial radiographs and pulmonary function studies. Alternate-day regimens of prednisone, usually beginning at 40 mg, are usually

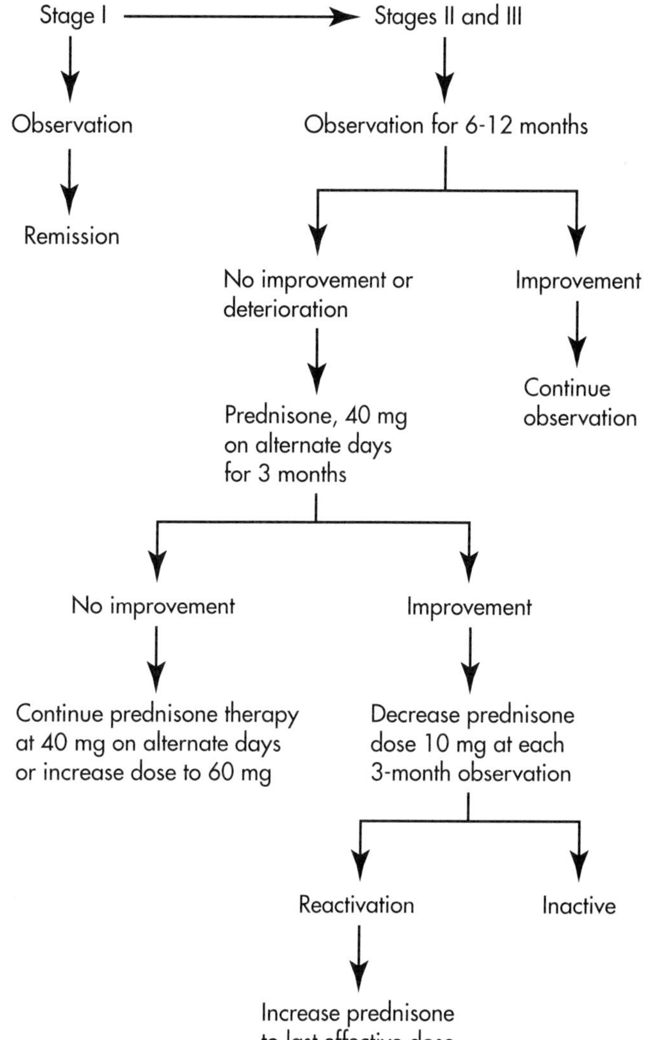

Fig. 78-4. Sarcoidosis treatment.

effective.[7] Fig. 78-4 outlines the recommended management approach. Stage I disease rarely is an indication for treatment unless symptoms of erythema nodosum and arthritis must be alleviated. If nonsteroidal agents such as indomethacin, 25 mg three times a day, are ineffective, a short course of alternate-day prednisone therapy beginning at 20 mg can be used. Although some authorities view pulmonary symptoms as an indication for treatment, research has found that dyspnea is a strong indicator of irreversible disease. Therefore glucocorticoid treatment is best administered in the presymptomatic phase of sarcoidosis to stave off irreversible changes. This approach has been supported by a recent prospective study done by the British Thoracic Society.[9]

Most authorities agree on the following indications for glucocorticoid treatment: (1) uveitis (local treatment may be attempted first), (2) hypercalcemia, (3) myocardial involvement (particularly cardiomyopathy), and (4) neurologic disease. If glucocorticoids cannot be used, other agents are available, but they are second-line drugs, seldom as effective as glucocorticoids, or have equally consequential side effects. These second-line agents include methotrexate, chloroquine, azathioprine, and oxyphenbutazone. Thalidomide and pentoxifylline may be effective in selected patients.[2,3]

Monitoring

Serial chest radiographs and pulmonary function studies are essential in the management of sarcoidosis. Their intervals are dictated by either the individual patient's course or the personal preferences of the managing physician. In addition, serum angiotensin-converting enzyme (SACE) determinations may be of value in monitoring the course. The level of SACE is thought to reflect the mass or "load" of granuloma in the individual patient.[10] Mayo studies have shown that the level of SACE is increased more than two standard deviations from the mean in 67% of patients with stage I sarcoidosis, in 87% with stage II, and in 95% with stage III.[13] A substantial number of patients deemed to have active sarcoidosis had SACE levels in the "normal" range.[8] Therefore the physician should not use an individual SACE determination in assessing a patient's clinical activity; the serial profile is indicative of activity. Patients with SACE levels in the normal range manifest appreciable decreases either in the course of spontaneous remission or under the influence of glucocorticoid treatment. Thus SACE levels can be used to detect the degree of granulomatous activity and, consequently, the adequacy of the glucocorticoid suppression. Increasing SACE levels should raise concern about an impending relapse or an inadequate glucocorticoid dose. The levels of SACE should never be used as the sole indication for treatment.

Involvement of additional sites necessitates assessment of changes pertinent to the organs affected. Relapse is common after effective treatment, occurring in as many as 25% of patients with stage II or III sarcoidosis. Thus physicians must be vigilant in maintaining periodic surveillance for years after treatment. If stability of the condition and signs of inactivity have been maintained for longer than 1 year after cessation of treatment, the possibility of relapse is considerably diminished.

Only a few laboratory studies other than those previously mentioned are helpful in the diagnosis and management of sarcoidosis. Some basic studies are reasonable, such as a complete blood cell count, serum creatinine and calcium concentrations, and urinalysis. A few patients with hypersplenism may have leukopenia and even mild anemia. Every patient should be tested for hypercalcemia, a prime indication for treatment. A urinalysis and serum creatinine determination can reveal the presence of hypercalcemic nephropathy and renal stones.[11,12] In the early 1980s, bronchoalveolar lavage (BAL) and gallium lung scanning were touted as important in determining the clinical course and need for treatment. Although BAL has led to important discoveries about the humoral and cellular mechanisms involved in the pathogenesis of sarcoidosis, neither of these procedures yields practical information for the day-to-day management of sarcoidosis.

REFERENCES

1. Agostini C, Costabel U, Semenzato G: Sarcoidosis news: immunologic frontiers for new immunosuppressive strategies, *Clin Immunol Immunopathol* 88:199, 1998.
2. American Thoracic Society: Statement on sarcoidosis, *Am J Respir Crit Care Med* 160:736, 1999.
3. Baughman RP, Lower EE: Steroid-sparing alternative treatments for sarcoidosis, *Clin Chest Med* 18:853, 1997.
4. DeRemee RA: *Clinical profiles of diffuse interstitial pulmonary disease,* Mount Kisco, NY, 1990, Futura.
5. DeRemee RA: The roentgenographic staging of sarcoidosis: historic and contemporary perspectives, *Chest* 83:128, 1983.
6. DeRemee RA, Andersen HA: Sarcoidosis, a correlation of dyspnea with roentgenographic stage and pulmonary function changes, *Mayo Clin Proc* 49:742, 1974.
7. DeRemee RA, Offord KP: The treatment of pulmonary sarcoidosis: the house revisited, *Sarcoidosis* 9(suppl 1):17, 1992.
8. DeRemee RA, Rohrbach MS: Normal serum angiotensin-converting enzyme activity in patients with newly diagnosed sarcoidosis, *Chest* 85:45, 1984.
9. Gibson GJ, Prescott RJ, Muers MF, et al: British Thoracic Society sarcoidosis study: effects of long term corticosteroid treatment, *Thorax* 51:238, 1996.
10. Gilbert S, Steinbrech DS, Landas SK, Hunninghake GW: Amounts of angiotensin-converting enzyme mRNA reflect the burden of granulomas in granulomatous lung disease, *Am Rev Respir Dis* 148:483, 1993.
11. Johns CJ, Michele TM: The clinical management of sarcoidosis: a 50-year experience at the Johns Hopkins Hospital, *Medicine* 78:65, 1999.
12. Newman LS, Rose CS, Maier LA, et al: Medical progress: sarcoidosis (review article), *N Engl J Med* 336:1224, 1997.
13. Rohrbach MS, DeRemee RA: Pulmonary sarcoidosis and serum angiotensin-converting enzyme, *Mayo Clin Proc* 57:64, 1982.
14. Wurm K, Reindell H, Heilmeyer L: *Der Lungenboeck im Roentgenbild,* Stuttgart, Germany, 1958, Thieme.

CHAPTER 79

Disorders of the Pleural Space

Basil Varkey
Ralph M. Schapira

Pleural effusion is an abnormal accumulation of fluid in the pleural space caused by either an intrinsic abnormality of the pleura (exudative effusion) or an imbalance in oncotic or hydrostatic pressures (transudative effusion) (Box 79-1). Other pleural disorders discussed in this chapter are fibrothorax, asbestos-related pleural disease, and pneumothorax.

PLEURAL EFFUSION

Pathophysiology

The pleura is a serous membrane made of a single layer of mesothelial cells. The *visceral pleura* covers the lung parenchyma, and the *parietal pleura* covers the remaining structures of the thoracic cavity. The airless space between the parietal and visceral pleurae is the *pleural space.* Because of a net gradient favoring movement of fluid through the parietal pleura into the pleural space, a nearly undetectable amount of clear, colorless pleural fluid with a low protein concentration (less than 1.5 gm/dl) is normally present, estimated at 10 ml in humans. The fluid in the pleural space is believed to be removed by the lymphatics of the parietal pleura, which normally maintain an equilibrium between the physiologic formation of pleural fluid and the removal of

Box 79-1. Causes of Pleural Effusions

Transudates
Common
Congestive heart failure
Cirrhosis

Less common
Nephrotic syndrome
Peritoneal dialysis
Urinothorax
Pulmonary embolism
Atelectasis
Superior venal caval obstruction

Exudates
Common
Parapneumonia
Malignancy
Pulmonary embolism

Less common
Tuberculosis
Nonbacterial infections: viral, fungal, parasitic
Pancreatitis, pseudocyst
Esophageal rupture
Endoscopic sclerotherapy
Subphrenic/liver abscess
Collagen vascular diseases
Dressler's syndrome
Drugs, including those causing drug-induced lupus
Benign asbestos effusion
Chylothorax
Uremia
Sarcoidosis
Meigs' syndrome
Yellow nail syndrome
Trauma
Amyloidosis
Vertebral osteomyelitis

Box 79-2. Clues to the Cause of Pleural Effusion

History
Smoking
Asbestos exposure
Trauma
Drugs
Tuberculosis exposure
Cough with purulent sputum
Hemoptysis
Chills, fever
Joint pains, swelling, stiffness
Urinary obstruction
Present or recent subclavian venous line insertion
Recent abdominal surgery, orthopedic surgery, parturition, vomiting, abdominal pain, upper gastrointestinal endoscopy, sclerotherapy
History of congestive heart failure, nephrotic syndrome, cirrhosis, deep venous thrombosis, any malignant disease, cardiac surgery

Physical Examination
Clubbing of fingers
Yellow nails
Superior vena cava syndrome
Horner's syndrome
Cervical/supraclavicular/other lymphadenopathy
Rheumatoid subcutaneous nodules, joint swelling, deformity
Sclerodactyly, malar rash, Raynaud's phenomenon
Putrid breath, purulent sputum
Herpes labialis, fever
Jugular vein distention, S_3, rales, leg edema
Ascites
Abdominal tenderness, mass

pleural fluid. (The visceral pleural lymphatics are poorly developed and do not contribute significantly to the removal of pleural fluid.) The parietal pleura receives its blood supply from systemic arteries of the adjacent chest wall, and the visceral pleura is supplied by the bronchial circulation. Much of the venous drainage of the visceral pleura is into the pulmonary veins; the parietal pleura drains into the bronchial veins and inferior vena cava.

Pleural effusions are caused by increased pleural fluid formation, decreased pleural fluid lymphatic drainage, or a combination of the two mechanisms. *Transudative pleural effusions* are caused by oncotic or hydrostatic factors that favor increased formation of pleural fluid, the most common cause being congestive heart failure. *Exudative pleural effusions* are caused by an increase in the permeability of the pleura; examples include malignant pleural effusions (usually caused by tumor invasion of the pleura) and bacterial pneumonia (parapneumonic effusion).

The presence of a pleural effusion limits expansion of the lung and may cause diaphragmatic dysfunction. Consequently, a restrictive ventilatory impairment can be noted on pulmonary function testing. The dyspnea associated with some pleural effusions, particularly those of large size, is believed to result from the mechanical disadvantage of the diaphragm. Hypoxemia associated with a pleural effusion results from intrapulmonary shunt caused by compression of the lung, ventilation/perfusion mismatch, and underlying lung disease. The drainage of a pleural effusion does not always improve gas exchange.[1]

Patient Evaluation

History. The three cardinal symptoms of a pleural effusion are dyspnea, chest pain (pleuritic or nonpleuritic), and a nonproductive cough. However, even large pleural effusions can be asymptomatic. The underlying disease producing the pleural effusion may play a role in the symptoms. For example, a patient with effusions from left ventricular failure may have symptoms from pulmonary edema rather than from the effusions. The history and physical examination can provide clues as to the cause of the effusion (Box 79-2).

Physical Examination. The findings on physical examination usually correlate with the size of the pleural effusion.

Inspection of the thorax in a patient with a large pleural effusion may reveal bulging intercostal spaces on the side of the effusion and a shift of the trachea away from the side of the effusion. Palpation reveals a decrease in tactile fremitus over the effusion. The percussion note is dull. Auscultation over the pleural effusion reveals decreased or absent breath sounds. Palpation, percussion, and auscultation are useful in delineating the superior border of the effusion, since the physical signs are normal above this level.

Diagnosis

Laboratory Studies and Diagnostic Procedures. The presence of an effusion is confirmed by chest radiographs. A small effusion (about 200 ml) obliterates the normally sharp costophrenic angle on a lateral view, and a decubitus film can detect as little as 100 ml of pleural fluid. A moderate effusion (about 500 ml) typically reveals a meniscus-shaped border laterally on a posteroanterior (PA) view. Subpulmonic effusions, loculated effusions, and underlying lung disease may alter the typical radiographic pattern. An ultrasonogram is more sensitive than chest radiographs in detecting pleural fluid and in differentiating a pleural effusion from pleural thickening.[6] When a pleural effusion is suggested on a radiograph, the physician must decide whether to obtain pleural fluid for analysis. If the cause of a pleural effusion is clearly evident, such as bilateral effusions in a patient with heart failure or asymptomatic effusions within 48 hours of parturition or abdominal surgery, the effusions may be observed and resolution documented on serial radiographs during treatment. If a pleural effusion is of unknown cause, however, an evaluation is mandatory. A diagnostic thoracentesis with removal of a small volume of pleural fluid (50 to 100 ml) is needed to define the effusion as a transudate or an exudate and for other tests.

To perform a thoracentesis safely, a lateral decubitus chest film with the effusion dependent should be taken to determine whether the suspected pleural fluid is free flowing. If the fluid layers along the inner chest wall, and if the distance between the inner chest wall and the superior surface of the effusion is at least 10 mm, a diagnostic thoracentesis can be performed on the location of the effusion as determined by physical examination. If the pleural effusion does not layer on the lateral decubitus film, however, or if the distance is less than 10 mm, three possibilities exist: (1) the effusion is small in volume, (2) the effusion is loculated, or (3) the radiographic abnormalities represent pleural thickening and not a pleural effusion. An ultrasound of the pleural space can differentiate among these possibilities and, if pleural fluid is present, can guide a diagnostic thoracentesis. A common error is for a patient's chest wall to be marked by the ultrasonographer for subsequent thoracentesis. Unless the patient is in precisely the same position as at the time of marking, the effusion may have shifted, making thoracentesis unsuccessful. Computed tomography (CT) scan of the chest is usually not necessary to identify a pleural effusion but does provide additional information on the underlying lung parenchyma and mediastinum, such as the presence of a mass or lymphadenopathy. Magnetic resonance imaging (MRI) of the chest has less utility than CT scan or ultrasound.

The major complications of thoracentesis are pneumothorax, pleural space infection, hemothorax, and reexpansion pulmonary edema. An end-expiratory PA chest radiograph should be performed after thoracentesis to check for a pneumothorax. Pleural fluid in patients with suspected or confirmed infections, such as human immunodeficiency virus (HIV) or hepatitis B, should be handled with special precautions to avoid transmission of these agents.

Invasive procedures are selectively employed to determine the cause of a pleural effusion if thoracentesis fails to provide a definitive answer. These invasive procedures include percutaneous parietal pleural biopsy (PPB), thoracoscopy (pleuroscopy), fiberoptic bronchoscopy (FOB), and thoracotomy with pleural biopsy.

Differential Diagnosis. To define an effusion as a transudate or an exudate, the total protein and lactate dehydrogenase (LDH) concentrations of the pleural fluid must be compared with those of simultaneously obtained serum. An exudative effusion has at least one of the following three criteria (Light's criteria): (1) a pleural fluid/serum protein ratio greater than 0.5, (2) a pleural fluid/serum LDH ratio greater than 0.6, or (3) an absolute LDH greater than two-thirds the upper limits of normal for the serum LDH. Transudative pleural effusions meet none of these three criteria. A study found that new criteria were not superior to Light's criteria in the differentiation of a transudative from an exudative effusion.[10] A meta-analysis determined that each of Light's three criteria had a similar diagnostic accuracy; paired or triplet combinations increased the diagnostic accuracy compared with any one of the criteria alone, but no combination of tests was found to be superior.[5]

Transudative Pleural Effusions. Congestive heart failure is the most common cause of pleural effusions. Typically the effusion is bilateral, the pleural fluid is serous in appearance, and chemical analysis reveals a transudate. Recent evidence suggests that biventricular failure is a requirement for the development of a pleural effusion and that right ventricular failure alone does not cause a pleural effusion. Diuresis usually does not convert a transudative pleural effusion from cardiac failure into an exudate. A patient who presents with typical clinical features of left-sided cardiac failure, a radiograph demonstrating cardiomegaly, and bilateral effusions usually does not require pleural effusion analysis. Patients with cardiac failure, however, may be at risk for pulmonary embolism; if a patient with cardiac failure presents with a unilateral pleural effusion or atypical features such as a fever or pleuritic chest pain, pulmonary embolism or pneumonia should be considered.

Another common cause of a transudative pleural effusion is hepatic cirrhosis. The pleural effusion of cirrhosis arises by movement of ascitic fluid from the peritoneal cavity through the diaphragm. The chemical characteristics of the pleural and ascitic fluid are usually similar. The chest radiograph typically shows a right-sided pleural effusion (70%) and a normal-sized heart. The patient usually has evidence of chronic liver disease and ascites, although if enough of the fluid in the peritoneum has traversed the diaphragm, clinical evidence of ascites may be lacking.

Although frequently associated with an exudative bloody pleural effusion, pulmonary thromboembolism can cause a typically unilateral pleural effusion, which can be a transudate in 20% of patients. Thus a transudative pleural effusion does not rule out a pulmonary embolism, and further diagnostic evaluation may be necessary.

Other less common causes of transudative effusions include the nephrotic syndrome (from decreased oncotic pressure), urinothorax (from retroperitoneal urinary leakage associated with urinary obstruction), and peritoneal dialysis (from movement of dialysate from the peritoneal to pleural space). Collapse of an entire lobe or lung by an endobronchial tumor or foreign body can cause a transudative pleural effusion because of a decrease in the negative pleural pressure, which favors an increase in pleural fluid formation. The cause of transudative effusions is usually apparent from the clinical history.

Exudative Pleural Effusions. A pleural effusion associated with bacterial pneumonia, termed a *parapneumonic effusion,* is the most common cause of an exudative pleural effusion. Parapneumonic effusions occur in about 40% of cases of bacterial pneumonia and are ipsilateral to the pneumonia; pleural fluids have leukocyte counts greater than 10,000 cells/mm^3, with a predominance of polymorphonuclear neutrophils (PMNs). A parapneumonic effusion is termed *uncomplicated* if it resolves with appropriate antibiotic therapy alone without sequelae and *complicated* if it requires chest tube drainage to avoid persistent pleural space infection, bronchopleural fistula, or pleural adhesions. A loculated parapneumonic effusion suggests a complicated form.

The differentiation between a complicated and an uncomplicated parapneumonic effusion is based on the gross characteristics of the pleural fluid, a Gram's stain and culture of the pleural fluid, and biochemical characteristics of the pleural fluid. Complicated parapneumonic effusions consist of empyemas (gross pus, Gram's stain demonstrating bacteria, or positive culture) or effusions with a pH less than 7.0 or glucose concentration less than 40 mg/dl. The pleural fluid LDH concentration alone does not define a parapneumonic effusion as complicated, although effusions with a pH value under 7.0 or glucose under 40 mg/dl are frequently associated with an LDH greater than 1000 IU/L. Bacteria vary greatly in their potential to cause complicated parapneumonic effusions. *Streptococcus pneumoniae,* although a common cause of pneumonia, seldom causes complicated parapneumonic effusion. In contrast, anaerobic bacteria, gram-negative bacteria, *Staphylococcus aureus,* and *Streptococcus pyogenes* are often associated with complicated parapneumonic effusions.

Malignant pleural effusions, usually caused by pleural invasion by malignant cells, are the second major cause of exudative pleural effusions. Carcinomas of the lung and breast are the leading causes of malignant effusions and, along with lymphomas, account for about 75% of cases. A malignant pleural effusion may be the presenting clinical evidence of cancer and implies an advanced stage and poor prognosis. Although most often caused by direct metastatic involvement of the pleura, pleural effusion may be caused by tumor invasion of mediastinal lymph nodes, atelectasis, or pneumonia rather than direct pleural involvement. These effusions are termed *paramalignant* by some authorities. Cytopathologic analysis of pleural fluid shows malignant cells in 60% to 80% of malignant effusions. The differentiation of a true malignant effusion (an effusion containing malignant cells) from a paramalignant effusion can be very important clinically. For example, lung cancer with a malignant effusion is surgically unresectable, whereas lung cancer with a paramalignant effusion (no malignant cells in the effusion) may be resectable.

The third most common type of pleural effusion is caused by *pulmonary* embolism (PE), which is an exudate about 80% of the time. Pleural effusions occur in up to 50% of patients with PE. The effusion usually is unilateral and may be bloody. An underlying pulmonary infiltrate may be present, but the history, physical examination, pleural fluid analysis, and chest radiographs are nonspecific in PE. Therefore the physician should always consider PE in the differential diagnosis of a patient who has a pleural effusion with symptoms or signs suggestive of a PE or risk factors for PE.

Disease caused by *Mycobacterium tuberculosis* can cause pleuritis with an associated unilateral exudative pleural effusion and should always be considered in the patient with a lymphocyte-predominant exudative pleural effusion (see Chapter 74). Glucose concentrations are frequently normal.

Upper abdominal disease (e.g., subphrenic abscess) resulting from perforation of an abdominal structure, a hepatic or splenic abscess, or viral hepatitis may cause upper abdominal or lower thoracic pain, fever, and a pleural effusion. Amebic abscess of the liver may cause right-sided pleural effusions as an inflammatory response to the abscess or, more often, as a result of rupture of the abscess through the diaphragm into the pleural cavity. These illnesses may mislead the physician into looking for pleuropulmonary disease, delaying early recognition of an intraabdominal problem. Acute and chronic pancreatitis may result in a high-amylase exudative pleural effusion, which is usually left sided. A pleural effusion with or without an associated pneumomediastinum or pneumothorax in a patient with a history of vomiting, chest pain, and dyspnea should lead the physician to consider esophageal rupture. The exudative effusion in esophageal rupture typically has a high salivary amylase level and a pH in the range of 6.0. In addition, the pleural space may be infected with oropharyngeal anaerobes. Early diagnosis and management are essential.

Collagen vascular diseases, particularly systemic lupus erythematosus (SLE) and rheumatoid arthritis (RA), may be complicated by effusions. Although pleural effusions usually complicate previously defined SLE and RA, an effusion may be the presenting clinical manifestation. Glucose levels in the pleural fluid are often greatly reduced in rheumatoid effusions, and physical examination almost invariably shows joint abnormalities. *Dressler's syndrome,* also known as *postcardiac injury syndrome* (PCIS), can occur after myocardial injury, such as infarction, trauma, or cardiac surgery. The syndrome includes pericarditis, pleural effusions, and pulmonary infiltrates associated with fever or chest pain, usually a few weeks to several months after myocardial injury. PCIS should be considered in any patient with a pleural effusion, unilateral or bilateral, after a myocardial infarction or cardiac surgery.

Exudative pleural effusions may result from medications, either directly or as a part of the drug-induced lupus syndrome (Box 79-3). Pleural effusion in a patient with a central venous catheter may result from erosion of the venous wall by the catheter tip. This complication most often occurs with left-sided venous catheters and is suggested by a hemothorax or an effusion with a composition similar to that of the infusate.

Utility of Diagnostic Tests. The key to ordering the appropriate tests is to form a pretest diagnosis based on integrated clinical information. Pleural fluid tests can be divided into four groups based on their relative usefulness

(Table 79-1). Observation of gross characteristics *(group A tests)* costs nothing but may provide a specific diagnosis or lead to individual tests that are diagnostic. Foul-smelling, yellow-green thick fluid is pus (empyema). Chocolate-colored (anchovy sauce) fluid strongly suggests a ruptured amebic liver abscess. White milky pleural fluid indicates a chylous or chyliform effusion and the need for triglyceride level and cytologic evaluation. A grossly bloody fluid suggests hemothorax, and the pleural fluid hematocrit must be checked. Protein and LDH along with serum protein and LDH separate transudates and exudates with a 95% accuracy. When a transudate is suspected, a two-step approach is appropriate, keeping some fluid in reserve pending protein and LDH determinations. If the effusion is confirmed as a transudate, no further analysis is necessary.

Group B tests have the potential to provide a definite diagnosis of empyema or malignant effusion. Although about 40% of bacterial pneumonias may be associated with a parapneumonic effusion, only a small percentage develop into an empyema. In contrast, cytologic examination proves malignancy in most cases of malignant effusions. In either case, negative studies do not exclude the diagnosis of a parapneumonic effusion or a malignancy.

Group C tests have a high specificity for diagnosing uncommon causes of pleural effusion. These tests should be selectively ordered based on clinical suspicion and gross appearance of the pleural fluid. Pleural fluid cultures for mycobacteria and fungi have a low sensitivity but should be obtained if these organisms may be the cause of the exudative effusion. Pleural effusions are present in 16% to 37% of patients with SLE. These patients are symptomatic with

Box 79-3. Drugs That Can Cause Pleural Effusion

Drugs that induce systemic lupus erythematosus (SLE): phenytoin, hydralazine, isoniazid, procainamide
Sclerosing agents for esophageal varices
Chemotherapeutic agents (e.g., procarbazine, methotrexate)
Tocolytics used for premature labor
Bromocriptine
Dantrolene
Methysergide
L-Tryptophan
Nitrofurantoin
Amiodarone

Table 79-1. Diagnostic Utility of Pleural Fluid Tests

Group	Tests	Utility
A (useful in all)	Observation of gross characteristics	May be diagnostic (e.g., empyema)
	Lactate dehydrogenase	Allows separation of transudates and exudates
	Protein	Allows separation of transudates and exudates
B (useful in exudates)	Stains, cultures for bacteria	Diagnostic if positive
	Cytology for malignant cells	Diagnostic if positive
C (selectively useful)	Stains, cultures for mycobacteria, fungi	Diagnostic if positive
	Antinuclear antibody and lupus erythematosus cells	Antinuclear antibody (ANA) titer ≥1:160 and pleural fluid/serum ANA ratio ≥1 are strongly suggestive of lupus pleuritis; LE cells in pleural fluid are diagnostic of lupus pleuritis.
	Amylase	Increased and above serum level in pancreatic effusion: amylase of salivary origin is elevated in esophageal rupture and may be increased in malignancies.
	Triglycerides, chylomicrons	>110 mg/ml indicates chylothorax. Presence of chylomicrons is diagnostic of chylothorax.
	Hematocrit	High hematocrit, approaching that of blood, indicates hemothorax. Hematocrit >1% suggests malignancy, trauma, or pulmonary embolism.
D (useful when combined with a strong prethoracentesis clinical diagnosis)	Red cell count	>100,000/mm^3 suggests same diagnosis as hematocrit >1%.
	White cell count, differential count	>10,000/mm^3 suggest parapneumonic effusions, pulmonary embolism, malignancy, tuberculosis, Dressler's syndrome, or lupus pleural effusion. Neutrophilic predominance indicates acute inflammation. Lymphocyte predominance suggests malignancy or tuberculosis.
	Glucose	<60 mg/ml suggests rheumatoid arthritis and parapneumonic and malignant effusions.
	pH	<7.2 results from various causes. <7.0 in parapneumonic effusion indicates chest tube drainage. <6.0 accompanied by elevated amylase indicates esophageal rupture.

pleuritic chest pain, and most have arthralgias or arthritis before the pleuritis. Measurement of the antinuclear antibody (ANA) level in pleural fluid and serum is helpful in diagnosing lupus pleuritis. Pleural fluid ANA titer is usually 1:160 or greater, and the pleural fluid ANA/serum ANA is 1 or greater. The finding of LE cells in pleural fluid is considered to be diagnostic of lupus pleuritis.

Pleural fluid amylase determination is indicated when pancreatitis or esophageal rupture is suspected. Pleural fluid amylase is above the upper limits of normal for serum and above the amylase level of a simultaneously sampled serum in pancreatitis. In chronic effusions caused by pancreatic pseudocyst, abdominal symptoms may be minimal and chest symptoms may predominate. In large left-sided effusions of unknown cause an effusion of pancreatic origin must be considered. Pleural fluid amylase is also elevated in esophageal rupture, but unlike with pancreatitis, the amylase is of salivary origin. Pleural fluid amylase may also be elevated in some malignant effusions, but the levels of amylase usually do not reach the levels seen in pancreatic disease and esophageal rupture, and the amylase is of salivary origin.

A triglyceride level greater than 110 mg/ml in the pleural fluid indicates *chylothorax*. If the level is indeterminate, 50 to 110, lipoprotein analysis is indicated. The detection of chylomicrons confirms the diagnosis of chylothorax. A chylothorax indicates disruption of the thorax duct, which allows chyle to enter the pleural space. The most common causes are malignancy, particularly lymphoma, and trauma.

The hematocrit of a bloody pleural effusion should be measured. A pleural fluid hematocrit approaching that of blood indicates a hemothorax and suggests trauma as the cause; chest tube drainage should be strongly considered. A hematocrit greater than 1% suggests malignancy, trauma, or pulmonary embolism. A hematocrit less than 1% is a relatively nonspecific finding.

Group D tests do not provide specific diagnoses, but integrated with clinical information, they often help the physician narrow the range of possible disorders. Red blood cell (RBC) count of pleural fluid should be interpreted with great caution, and RBC counts generated by an automated counter may not be reliable. RBC counts greater than $5000/mm^3$ may impart a bloodlike color (serosanguineous) to the fluid but are not very helpful, since 40% of exudative effusions and some transudates may be blood tinged. Effusions with RBC counts greater than $100,000$ cells/mm^3 suggest the same diagnostic possibilities as those with a hematocrit less than 1%.

A white blood cell (WBC) count greater than $10,000/mm^3$ is most often seen in parapneumonic effusions but also occurs in PE, malignancy, tuberculosis, pancreatitis, Dressler's syndrome, and SLE. Neutrophilic predominance indicates acute pleural inflammation. A predominance of small lymphocytes in an exudative effusion strongly suggests tuberculosis or malignancy. Eosinophilic effusions (more than 10% eosinophils) have a variety of causes. Malignant pleural effusions can be eosinophilic. Pleural effusions after trauma and thoracic surgery, as well as benign asbestos-related effusions, can show eosinophilia. Drug-induced pleural effusions are frequently eosinophilic, as are effusions caused by parasitic and some fungal diseases. Mesothelial cells are sparse (less than 5%) in tuberculous pleural effusions. This finding is not specific, however, since any extensive inflammatory process may diminish the number of mesothelial cells in the pleural fluid.

A low pleural fluid glucose level (less than 60 mg/ml) suggests a short list of possible causes of the effusion, primarily RA and parapneumonic and malignant effusions. Often the pleural fluid glucose in RA pleural effusions is strikingly low; in 80% of patients pleural fluid glucose levels are less than 30 mg/ml.[4a] In comparison, lupus pleuritis is less often associated with low glucose pleural effusions (in one study 21%[3a]), and the levels are not as low as in effusions associated with RA.

Pleural fluid acidosis (pH less than 7.2) can have a variety of causes, including infection, esophageal rupture, rheumatoid effusion, tuberculosis, malignancy, hemothorax, lupus pleuritis, and urinothorax. In combination with high pleural fluid amylase, a low pH (under 6.0) suggests esophageal rupture as a cause. At present the best use of pH testing is for parapneumonic effusions to decide if chest tube drainage is necessary, since effusions with pH under 7.0 generally require tube drainage to avoid serious pleural space complications (e.g., loculations, adhesions). Although helpful in this regard, pleural fluid pH is not foolproof in its predictive value.

Indications and Utility of Other Invasive Procedures. Consideration should be given to other invasive procedures when the cause of a pleural effusion remains unknown after thoracentesis and pleural fluid analysis.

Percutaneous pleural biopsy (PPB) is particularly useful in the diagnosis of tuberculous pleuritis or pleural malignancy (see Chapter 74). The predominance of lymphocytes in pleural effusion is predictive of a high diagnostic yield by PPB. The diagnostic yield of PPB in tuberculous pleuritis is 87% when two or more pleural samples are obtained and the tissue is analyzed by both histology and culture.[4] In malignant pleural effusions, the yield of pleural fluid cytopathologic analysis alone is 50% to 60%, and the gain from adding PPB to a negative cytologic study is only 7.1%.[2,9] The most common complication of PPB is pneumothorax, usually caused by entry of atmospheric air into the pleural space (3% to 15%). An end-expiratory PA chest radiograph should be performed after the procedure. PPB is most safely performed in a cooperative patient when a sufficient amount of pleural fluid is present in the biopsy area to minimize the chance of penetrating the underlying lung during the biopsy.

A PPB that yields a histologic diagnosis of nonspecific pleuritis is not helpful. The physician must then decide whether to observe the effusion without further diagnostic tests or proceed with thoracoscopy or fiberoptic bronchoscopy.

Thoracoscopy has replaced thoracotomy and open pleural biopsy as the preferred procedure in pleural diseases that are difficult to diagnose. In a study of thoracoscopy in 102 patients with undiagnosed pleural disease, a diagnosis of malignancy was established in 38 patients, yielding a sensitivity of 91% and a specificity of 100%. The four cases of malignancy that were missed by thoracoscopy were all malignant mesothelioma. Thoracoscopy is also useful in the diagnosis of tuberculous pleuritis. Some controversy remains on the role of thoracoscopy, however, since it may not add much to the diagnosis of metastatic pleural malignancy or tuberculous pleuritis compared with thoracentesis and PPB.

In addition, biopsies from other causes of exudative pleural effusions (e.g., rheumatologic disease or pulmonary embolism) may demonstrate a nonspecific pleuritis. Thus thoracoscopy should be considered when a diagnosis of tuberculous pleuritis has been missed despite negative cultures and nondiagnostic pleural histopathology or if the diagnosis of a malignant pleural effusion has not been established after cytopathologic analysis of at least three pleural fluid samples obtained by thoracentesis. Thoracoscopy is also useful in suspected malignant mesothelioma because of the relatively low yields of PPB and thoracentesis.

Fiberoptic bronchoscopy (FOB) after nondiagnostic thoracentesis and PPB is indicated only when the chest radiograph or CT scan demonstrates a lung parenchymal abnormality, such as a mass or collapse, or if the patient has a history of hemoptysis. In the absence of these features, FOB has a very low diagnostic yield.

Even after an evaluation that includes invasive procedures, the cause of a pleural effusion remains unknown in about 15% of patients, although the course and outcome are often favorable. In a study of 51 patients, 31 (60.8%) had spontaneous resolution of the effusion. In another study of 40 patients with an undiagnosed pleural effusion, 32 (80%) were not diagnosed even after prolonged follow-up. The remaining eight cases were eventually diagnosed as three asbestos-related effusions and one each of adenocarcinoma, mesothelioma, rheumatoid arthritis, cirrhosis, and heart failure.[3]

Management

The many causes of pleural effusions demand that treatment be directed at the specific etiology (see Box 79-1). In some patients, however, the pleural fluid must be drained for therapeutic or palliative reasons. Most transudative pleural effusions are treated by addressing the underlying cause of the effusion, such as heart failure. Video-assisted thoracoscopic surgery has been successfully used to localize and close diaphragmatic defects in select patients with recurrent effusions caused by cirrhosis and ascites.[7] Although critically ill medical patients frequently develop pleural effusions, 90% are small effusions and do not necessarily require evaluation by thoracentesis. Congestive heart failure, atelectasis, ascites, hypoalbuminemia, and atelectasis account for almost 75% of the effusions in these patients.[6] Other causes include uncomplicated parapneumonic effusion (11%); rare causes include malignancy, uremic pleurisy, pancreatitis, and empyema.

The appropriate initial method to drain an empyema is by tube thoracostomy using a closed system. Thoracoscopy (preferably with video assistance) is indicated with a loculated or poorly draining empyema to facilitate complete drainage, which may obviate the need for more invasive surgical procedures such as pleurectomy. A similar approach is needed in other types of complicated parapneumonic effusions that have a pH less than 7.0 or a glucose less than 40 mg/ml. Parapneumonic effusions with a pH greater than 7.2 usually respond to an appropriate antibiotic alone; a repeat thoracentesis in 5 to 7 days should be done only if fever or leukocytosis persists or the effusion is unchanged or enlarging. In parapneumonic effusions with pH of 7.0 to 7.2, thoracentesis should be repeated within 12 to 24 hours and chest tube drainage instituted if the pleural fluid pH has dropped further.

The palliation of dyspnea in patients with a recurrent malignant pleural effusion is an important goal. The instillation of agents such as talc, doxycycline, or bleomycin into the pleural space after chest tube drainage is an effective method to fuse the pleura *(pleurodesis)* and can prevent recurrence of the effusion. A success rate greater than 70% has been reported with talc or bleomycin instillation.[2] Ambulatory sclerotherapy is a possible alternative to inpatient treatment of malignant effusions.[8] The decision to perform these interventions depends on the patient's overall condition and life expectancy.

Certain caveats apply to the management of other conditions causing pleural effusions. In PE, neither the bloody character of the pleural fluid nor hemoptysis is a contraindication to anticoagulation treatment. A patient with an undiagnosed lymphocyte-predominant exudative effusion who has a positive intermediate-strength tuberculin skin test (PPD) should be considered for antituberculosis drug therapy. Pleural effusion and pleuritis caused by PCIS respond to nonsteroidal antiinflammatory agents; In severe cases of PCIS, glucocorticoids are also effective. In effusions caused by esophageal rupture or a pancreatic pseudocyst, thoracic surgical consultation should be promptly obtained.

FIBROTHORAX

Deposition of fibrous tissue results in a thick fibrotic visceral pleura that impairs the mobility of the pleura and the expansion of the underlying lung. This condition, fibrothorax, is often caused by pleural empyema, hemothorax, or tuberculous pleural disease. Other conditions that induce pleural inflammation, including uremia, collagen vascular disease, and pancreatitis, can also cause fibrothorax.

Dyspnea on exertion is a common symptom, and examination may reveal diminished expansion and narrowed intercostal spaces in the involved side. A tracheal shift toward the involved side may be noted on palpation of the suprasternal notch. Radiographic findings are an ipsilateral mediastinal shift and a dense pleural peel surrounding the lung. Calcification may be noted in the inner peel. Pulmonary function tests show restrictive ventilatory impairment. The only effective treatment is decortication with removal of the fibrous peel from the visceral pleura. The degree of impairment caused by the fibrothorax and the status of the underlying lung are the main factors in deciding whether decortication will be beneficial. In patients without significant lung disease, especially fibrosis, improvement after decortication can be expected.

ASBESTOS-RELATED PLEURAL DISEASE

Asbestos is a naturally occurring, fibrous silicate that causes a variety of pleural and pulmonary parenchymal diseases (see Chapter 76). Asbestos enters the respiratory tract through inhalation. Because of its size and shape, asbestos is only minimally cleared by the normal host defense system of the lungs. The retained fibers are found in both the lung parenchyma and the pleura, where they are believed to generate a chronic inflammatory response that causes tissue injury. Five pleural disorders are associated with asbestos exposure: benign pleural effusions, pleural plaques, pleural fibrosis, rounded atelectasis, and malignant mesothelioma.

Benign pleural effusion (BPE) is the most common asbestos-related disorder, occurring within 10 years of exposure. In some cases the latency period may be longer.

BPE may be incidentally discovered on a chest radiograph or may simulate a pneumonia with pleuritic pain and fever. The effusions more often are unilateral, and the natural history is spontaneous resolution with a tendency to recur. The pleural fluid may be blood tinged and often eosinophilic. The diagnosis of BPE is made by excluding other causes in a patient with a history of asbestos exposure.

Pleural plaques, the most common manifestation of asbestos exposure, are discrete areas of the parietal pleura that consist of an abnormal accumulation of mesenchymal cells and connective tissue matrix. They often become calcified. Asbestos can be found in plaques using electron microscopy. Pleural plaques are located on the parietal pleura, usually on the lateral and inferior aspects; frequently involve the diaphragmatic pleura; and may be bilateral. Plaques usually manifest at least 20 years after asbestos exposure, and pleural plaques usually do not cause pulmonary function abnormalities. CT scanning is much more sensitive in demonstrating pleural plaques than conventional chest radiography. No therapy is needed for pleural plaques, and they do not evolve into malignant mesothelioma. In contrast to pleural plaques, diffuse *pleural fibrosis* (which involves both the visceral and parietal pleura) is a rare manifestation of asbestos exposure than can cause a severe restrictive ventilatory impairment.

Rounded atelectasis is a pleuropulmonary process that usually occurs in patients with asbestos exposure. It is believed that an inflammatory process in the visceral pleura causes underlying lung parenchyma to collapse. On chest radiograph, rounded atelectasis can simulate a lung carcinoma, from which it must be differentiated. The CT scan is helpful in this situation, since the appearance can be diagnostic; a biopsy is necessary if doubt remains.

Patients with *malignant pleural mesothelioma* frequently complain of chest pain or dyspnea. About 80% of these patients have had asbestos exposure. The latency period from exposure to development of disease is usually 35 to 40 years. Chest radiographs demonstrate a unilateral pleural effusion and thickening. The diagnosis of malignant pleural mesothelioma usually requires thoracoscopy or thoracotomy, since PPB and cytologic specimens do not yield enough material for analysis, so confusion with other malignant or inflammatory processes is possible. Electron microscopy and advanced staining techniques have increased diagnostic accuracy. The prognosis of patients with malignant pleural mesothelioma is poor, although pleuropneumonectomy combined with chemotherapy shows some promise. In contrast to malignant pleural mesothelioma, fibrous mesothelioma is a benign disease unrelated to asbestos exposure.

PNEUMOTHORAX

A pneumothorax is an accumulation of air in the normally airless pleural space between the lung and chest wall. Pneumothorax can be divided into spontaneous or traumatic causes. Spontaneous pneumothoraces can be further subdivided into primary or secondary types. *Primary* spontaneous pneumothorax occurs in healthy persons without lung disease, whereas a *secondary* spontaneous pneumothorax occurs as a complication of underlying pulmonary disease. A primary spontaneous pneumothorax occurs more often in young, tall, asthenic men. A reasonable theory for this predisposition is that, because of the configuration of the thoracic cage, traction on the alveolar walls is increased, causing rupture of subpleural apical blebs. The most common underlying disease responsible for secondary pneumothorax is obstructive airways disease. Infections that cause necrosis (e.g., pulmonary tuberculosis, necrotizing pneumonias, lung abscess) can cause a pneumothorax. Other diseases that predispose to secondary pneumothorax include histiocytosis X, sarcoidosis, tuberous sclerosis, cystic fibrosis, pulmonary infarction, and primary lung carcinoma. *Catamenial pneumothorax* is an uncommon entity that recurs at menstrual periods. Although the exact pathogenesis of this disorder is unknown, it may be related to pleural and diaphragmatic endometriosis.

Traumatic (noniatrogenic) pneumothorax is caused by penetrating or nonpenetrating chest trauma. Iatrogenic pneumothorax, the most common type of pneumothorax diagnosed in the hospitalized patient, is a complication of procedures such as transthoracic needle aspiration, subclavian vein puncture, thoracentesis, pleural biopsy, and transbronchial lung biopsy. Another iatrogenic cause is positive-pressure mechanical ventilation, particularly with high airway pressures or airway obstruction.

Normally the pressure in the pleural space is negative with reference to atmospheric and alveolar pressures. Therefore, if a communication exists between the pleura and the atmosphere (e.g., after penetrating trauma) or between the pleura and the lung (e.g., after rupture of an emphysematous bulla), air continues to enter the pleural space until pleural pressure becomes atmospheric. This increased pleural pressure collapses the lung. In some cases a ball-valve communication is formed in which air can enter but cannot leave the pleural space. Intrapleural pressure may then exceed atmospheric pressure throughout expiration and often during inspiration. This *tension pneumothorax* is life threatening because it compromises ventilation by shifting mediastinal structures, impairing venous return, and diminishing cardiac output. Tension pneumothorax more often develops as a complication of mechanical ventilation or other secondary pneumothoraces rather than from primary spontaneous pneumothorax.

The main symptoms of pneumothorax are chest pain and dyspnea, which usually start abruptly. The severity of the symptoms depends on the volume of air in the pleural space and the degree of underlying disease. The physical signs are hyperresonance on percussion and diminished or absent tactile fremitus and breath sounds on the affected side. Patients with tension pneumothorax are in distress, with dyspnea, tachypnea, and tachycardia often accompanied by distended neck veins, thready pulse, and hypotension. Bulging of the ipsilateral intercostal spaces is sometimes observed, and mediastinal shift may be signaled by tracheal deviation to the contralateral side. The chest radiograph is diagnostic because the margin of the collapsed lung is separated from the parietal pleura by air.

The management options are observation only, small-catheter pleural aspiration or chest tube drainage to evacuate the air, and chemical pleurodesis or open thoracotomy or thoracoscopy with pleural abrasion to prevent a recurrence of pneumothorax. The choice depends on severity of the pneumothorax, predisposing state, and underlying disease.

Asymptomatic, unilateral, small (10% to 20% of the lung volume) primary spontaneous pneumothoraces can be observed, since most resolve within 10 days. A repeat chest radiograph in 6 to 12 hours should be done to check for progression of the pneumothorax. Supplemental oxygen is believed to hasten the resorption of air in the pleural space, since supplemental oxygen increases the gradient between nitrogen in the pleural space and nitrogen in the pleural capillary blood, favoring movement of nitrogen out of the pleural space. Progressively increasing spontaneous pneumothorax and large symptomatic pneumothoraces should be treated by evacuation of the pleural air. The preferred method is insertion of a small catheter (7 to 9 French) in the second anterior intercostal space in the midclavicular line using either a trocar or the Seldinger technique. Air is aspirated using a stopcock and a 60-ml syringe until a mild resistance is felt, and a Heimlich valve is attached to permit continued air evacuation. In large symptomatic pneumothoraces, suction can be added through the exhaust port of the Heimlich valve. After the pneumothorax is evacuated, with no evidence of reaccumulation of air on chest radiograph, the catheter can be removed. Chest tube insertion and drainage are indicated in a few cases of primary spontaneous pneumothorax when the initial volume of air evacuated is large (about 4 L) or when there is a persistent pneumothorax after catheter evacuation. Small-catheter pleural aspiration can also be used in iatrogenic pneumothoraces or selectively in patients with minor trauma.

Chest tube drainage is the preferred management in tension pneumothorax, hydropneumothorax, hemopneumothorax, and pneumothorax with underlying pulmonary disease. Tension pneumothorax is a medical emergency; if the diagnosis is suspected, a large-bore needle should be immediately inserted into the second anterior intercostal space to evacuate the air in the pleural space. A large amount of air coming through the needle confirms the diagnosis. The needle should be left in place until a chest tube is inserted and the air drained under water seal.

The recurrence rate of primary spontaneous pneumothorax is about 50% in 2 years. An ipsilateral recurrence should be treated with chest tube drainage and chemical pleurodesis. Open thoracotomy or thoracoscopy with pleural abrasion is indicated for subsequent recurrence.

REFERENCES

1. Agusti AG, Cardus J, Roca J, et al: Ventilation-perfusion mismatch in patients with pleural effusion, *Am J Respir Crit Care Med* 156:1205, 1997.
2. Belani CP, Pajeau TS, Bennett CL: Treating malignant pleural effusions cost consciously, *Chest* 113:78S, 1998.
3. Ferrer JS, Munoz XG, Orriols RM, et al: Evolution of idiopathic pleural effusion: prospective long-term follow-up study, *Chest* 109:1508, 1996.

3a. Good JT, King TE, Antony VB, et al: Lupus pleuritis: clinical features and pleural fluid characteristics with special reference to pleural fluid antinuclear antibodies, *Chest* 84:714, 1983.

4. Heffner JE, Brown LK, Barnieri CA: Diagnostic value of tests that discriminate between exudative and transudative pleural effusions, *Chest* 111:970, 1997.

4a. Joseph J, Sahn SA: Connective tissue diseases and the pleura, *Chest* 104:262, 1993.

5. Kirsch CM, Kroe DM, Azzi RL, et al: The optimal number of pleural biopsy specimens for a diagnosis of tuberculous pleurisy, *Chest* 112:702, 1997.
6. Mattison LE, Coppage L, Alderman DF, et al: Pleural effusions in the medical ICU, *Chest* 111:1018, 1997.
7. Mouroux J, Perrin C, Venissac N, et al: Management of pleural effusion of cirrhotic origin, *Chest* 109:1093, 1996.
8. Patz EF Jr: Malignant pleural effusions, *Chest* 113:74S, 1998.
9. Prakash UB, Reiman HM: Comparison of needle biopsy with cytologic analysis for the evaluation of pleural effusion: analysis of 414 cases, *Mayo Clin Proc* 60:158, 1985.
10. Vives M, Porcel JM, de Vera VM, et al: A study of Light's criteria and possible modifications for distinguishing exudative from transudative pleural effusions, *Chest* 109:1503, 1996.

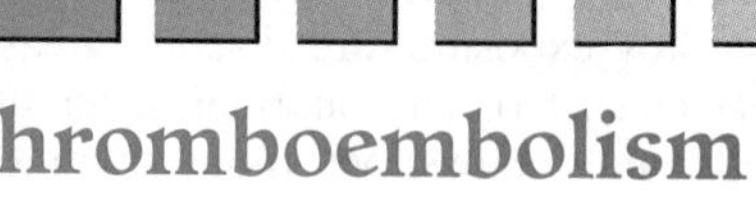

CHAPTER 80

Venous Thromboembolism and Pulmonary Hypertensive Diseases

Randolph J. Lipchik
Kenneth W. Presberg

VENOUS THROMBOEMBOLISM

Venous thromboembolism (VTE) remains a common and serious problem that can lead to premature mortality and long-term morbidity. Physicians in almost all areas of patient care will encounter patients at risk for this disease. VTE often occurs in patients with significant underlying medical problems.[8] In recent studies the overall 1-year mortality rate for patients who developed VTE was 20% to 40%. Cardiac disease, chronic lung disease, and malignancy accounted for the majority of the deaths.[4] The diagnosis of pulmonary embolism (PE) can be difficult because the signs and symptoms may be similar to the patient's chronic condition.

Epidemiology

More than 5 million cases of deep venous thrombosis (DVT) occur annually in the United States. Of these patients, approximately 500,000 will have a clinically apparent PE, about 10% of whom will die. The Prospective Investigation of Pulmonary Embolism Diagnosis (PIOPED) study found that 2.5% of patients who survive to hospitalization will die of PE and that 8% will experience a recurrence in the following months. A small percentage of survivors will fail to resolve the intravascular thrombi and will develop chronic pulmonary hypertension (Fig. 80-1). Current theory stipulates that PE is a complication of venous thrombosis, which is preventable and amenable to early diagnosis and treatment. Despite these advances, the overall incidence of VTE has not decreased, partly because of the increasing age of the U.S. population. Most patients enrolled in the PIOPED study were older than 60. The VTE incidence of 1 in 1000 at age 65 increases to approximately 3 in 1000 at age 85. Unfortunately, many cases still arise because of a failure to provide proven preventive therapy for patients at risk.

Approximately 90% of clinically significant PEs arise from the deep veins of the lower extremities; however, not all venous thrombi of the lower extremities or other venous systems pose such a serious risk. Thrombi that remain confined to the calf veins do not cause significant PE. Thrombi may also originate in the pelvic veins, but emboli are less hazardous from these smaller veins. Axillary and subclavian vein thrombosis is more often seen, with central venous catheterization a major risk factor. Axillary thrombus may also arise spontaneously in a young adult from exercise,

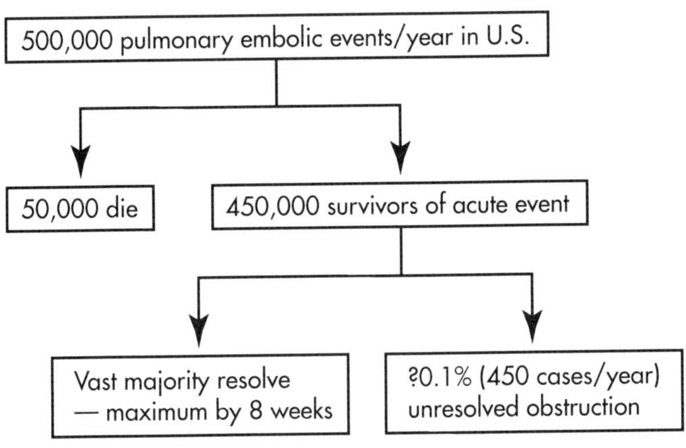

Fig. 80-1. Estimated incidence of venous thromboembolism and associated complications in the United States.

Box 80-1. Risk Groups for Venous Thromboembolism

Low: <40 years old, no other risk factors, general anesthesia <30 minutes
Medium: >40 years old, general anesthesia >30 minutes
High: Predisposing risk factors:
- Prolonged immobilization, intensive care
- Congestive heart failure, myocardial infarction
- Prior deep venous thrombosis or pulmonary embolism
- Inherited and acquired coagulation defects
- Malignancy
- Obesity
- Age >65 years
- Hip fracture/replacement, knee replacement
- Pelvic or lower extremity trauma or surgery

usually in the setting of thoracic outlet venous compression (Paget-Schroetter syndrome). Clinically significant PE occurs less often from thrombi involving these sites, but all DVT complications of the lower extremities have been described for thrombosis in these other locations.

Data from natural history studies of VTE indicate that the vast majority of patients who die from PE do so within the first few hours of the event, probably from recurrent embolism.[7] Almost all fatal recurrences are within the first week of presentation. Therefore overall morbidity and mortality can be significantly reduced only by prevention of DVT, and in-hospital mortality can be decreased by early initiation of effective therapy to treat VTE and prevent recurrent PE.

Pathophysiology

Risk Factors. Conditions that promote DVT were first described by Virchow and include vascular intimal injury, blood stasis, and hypercoagulability. Patients can be divided according to the degree of risk and their management directed accordingly (Box 80-1). In the low-risk group, DVT occurs in less than 0.5% of patients. Medium-risk patients are older, with a 2% to 10% incidence of DVT. DVT may occur in 20% of high-risk patients. In many patients, significant risks converge to promote DVT development.

A subset of patients may be predisposed to thrombotic events because of a primary or secondary imbalance in coagulation.[10] These conditions are generally referred to as *hypercoagulable states* (Box 80-2). These disorders are uncommon, and diagnostic screening is best directed toward those who are young, have a family history of thrombosis, had unexplained recurrent events, or had abnormal resolution despite adequate anticoagulation. Recently discovered genetic disorders associated with an increased risk of thrombosis include the factor V Leiden mutation, which imparts a resistance to activated protein C, and the prothrombin gene mutation (A^{20210} allele). Some of these genetic disorders are limited to certain ethnic groups, which may partly explain the variability in the incidence of VTE among different populations. Certain disorders, such as the antiphospholipid syndrome, may lead to recurrent devastating complications. Other individuals with inherited thrombophilias may not experience significant complications; a cohort of asymptomatic antithrombin III–deficient patients had a low prevalence of thrombotic events. Anticoagulation is not

Box 80-2. Hypercoagulable States

Primary Disorders
- Fibrinolytic defects
- Dysfibrinogenemia
- Factor XII deficiency
- Protein C deficiency
- Protein S deficiency
- Antithrombin III deficiency
- Antiphospholipid syndrome
- Homocysteinuria
- Factor V Leiden
- Prothrombin A^{20210} allele mutation

Secondary Disorders
- Nephrotic syndrome
- Vasculitides
- Liver disease
- Peripartum period
- Malignancy
- Estrogen therapy
- Acquired platelet disorders
- Hyperviscosity syndromes

necessary until patients are at risk or develop a complication. Long-term primary prophylactic anticoagulation has not been beneficial for any of these disorders.

Trousseau first described the well-known association of malignancy with VTE in 1865. A peculiar form of migrating superficial venous thrombosis may antedate the signs and symptoms of cancer by years. A new DVT in an otherwise healthy individual may also be an early clue to the presence of an occult malignancy; however, exhaustive diagnostic tests for an occult malignancy have no proven benefit. Directed examinations of the lung, gastrointestinal tract, breasts, and reproductive organs (the most common sites) are reasonable.

Complications. Death from this disease is the result of a PE arising from DVT. PE has multiple respiratory and hemodynamic consequences. Hyperventilation is almost universal and relatively proportional to the degree of vascular obstruction. The exact mechanisms are unknown, but lung mechanoreceptors may play an important role. The embolism leads to vascular obstruction and decreased perfusion, which increases alveolar dead space and ventilatory requirements. The obstruction may be relieved in hours by normal fibrinolysis, and dead space may return to normal shortly after the event. The many causes of hypoxemia include a decrease in mixed-venous oxygen pressure (Po_2) if cardiac output is decreased, ventilation/perfusion ($\dot{V}/\dot{Q}$) inequality, and occasionally an increase in right-to-left shunt through a patent foramen ovale. Hyperventilation tends to increase arterial Po_2 (Pao_2) toward normal, limiting the diagnostic utility of Pao_2 for PE. The alveolar-arterial (A-a) gradient, however, remains elevated in almost all patients. Severe hypoxemia in a patient without underlying lung disease signals a massive embolism.

Atelectasis appears after 24 hours of obstruction and partly results from depletion of surfactant secondary to an interruption of nutrient supply to the type II alveolar cells of the lung. Infarction is uncommon because of the dual arterial blood supply of the lung. Hemoptysis and other signs attributed to infarction occur 24 to 48 hours after the acute event but may be the first signs of PE. The hemodynamic consequences of PE may also be life threatening. If the embolism causes more than 50% of the vascular bed to be acutely obstructed, right ventricular afterload will increase precipitously, and right ventricular failure may ensue. The normal right ventricle can sustain adequate blood flow only up to a mean pulmonary artery pressure (PAP) of about 40 mm Hg or a systolic pressure of about 65 mm Hg. Compounds that lead to pulmonary vasoconstriction (e.g., serotonin, thromboxane A_2) are released by platelet aggregation and contribute to PAP elevation. The patient's ability to tolerate these insults largely depends on the underlying cardiopulmonary status, so the cardiopulmonary manifestations of PE can vary greatly among patients. Fortunately, the thrombus begins to resolve within hours after treatment, and restoration of 25% of the luminal diameter allows sufficient flow to normalize a perfusion scan. Much of the obstruction is relieved within days, and resolution is maximal at approximately 8 weeks.

Chronic thromboembolic pulmonary hypertension involving major vessels results from recurrent submassive or massive emboli that do not resolve.[6] Many of these patients do not have a documented history of PE and did not receive prior treatment. Most do not have recognized hypercoagulable states, but an intrinsic defect in fibrinolysis is strongly suspected; lupus anticoagulant has been found in 10% of these patients. When major vessel thromboemboli do not sufficiently resolve over weeks, the right ventricle adapts over time to the increased afterload, hypertrophies, and may sustain systemic or suprasystemic pressures. These chronic adaptations are usually documented by an electrocardiogram (ECG) or echocardiogram. Patient survival has been correlated to the mean PAP; 5-year survival is significantly decreased when the mean PAP is greater than 35 mm Hg. Patients with a mean PAP greater than 55 mm Hg have a very poor prognosis and are at risk of sudden death. Progressive right ventricular dysfunction is signaled by further increases in right atrial pressure and right-sided cardiac volumes. Hypoxemia in these patients does not correlate with the degree of pulmonary hypertension. Some may be candidates for surgical thromboendarterectomy, whereas others have very limited therapeutic options.

Patient Evaluation

History. The diagnosis of PE is one of the most difficult diagnoses to make on clinical grounds because the clinical signs, symptoms, and basic laboratory studies are neither sensitive nor specific, and the only definitive diagnostic test, pulmonary angiography, is invasive and expensive. The history may strengthen clinical suspicion of PE and with objective tests may allow the physician to rule in or rule out the diagnosis with reasonable certainty. Although PE can occur silently, the sudden onset of dyspnea is usually the most common symptom reported. The multicenter Urokinase Pulmonary Embolism Trial (UPET) identified the most common symptoms associated with angiographically proven PE (Table 80-1). Dyspnea, pleuritic chest pain, and cough were most often seen. The classic triad of dyspnea, pleuritic chest pain, and hemoptysis occurred in only 28% of cases, but two of the three symptoms were present in 65%. Dyspnea, chest pain of any quality, and a sense of apprehension were present in 44%; two of these three symptoms were reported in 81% of patients. Syncope, reflecting inadequate systemic perfusion from obstruction of the pulmonary vasculature, was seen in 13% of patients overall, usually with massive emboli.

In the more recent PIOPED study the subset of patients without prior cardiac or pulmonary disease was examined to identify symptoms that could be attributed solely to the pulmonary embolism (Table 80-1). Dyspnea was present in 73% of cases, pleuritic chest pain in 66%, and cough in 37%. Hemoptysis occurred in only 13% of patients. The lack of specificity of these symptoms was confirmed, since their prevalence was not significantly different in patients proven not to have PE. Since at least 90% of pulmonary emboli arise from the deep veins of the lower extremities, symptoms of DVT should also be elicited. With thrombosis of the iliac, femoral, or popliteal veins, unilateral leg swelling may be the only symptom. In calf vein thrombosis, pain is the most common symptom, but because of multiple veins and collaterals, an isolated clot may be asymptomatic. In UPET, symptoms of lower extremity DVT were present in only 21% of patients. In a small percentage, PE may arise from thrombosis of upper extremity veins, usually in association with a longstanding central line or in cases of trauma. Upper extremity thrombosis is often asymptomatic, but pain and swelling are the most common symptoms, when present. Although nonspecific, the symptoms discussed, in conjunction with the conditions associated with increased risk for venous thrombosis, are important diagnostic clues in the investigation of thromboembolic disease.

Physical Examination. In patients with PE the examination can be surprisingly unremarkable. Evidence of acute pulmonary hypertension (right ventricular heave, right-sided S_3, large jugular *a* wave, increased P_2) is seen infrequently and in the setting of massive embolism. Table 80-1 lists the most common signs of PE. In PIOPED, for patients with no prior cardiac or pulmonary disease, tachypnea was present in 70%, tachycardia in 30%, and rales in 51%. DVT was clinically evident in only 11%. In UPET these signs were present in 92%, 44%, and 58%, respectively. Phlebitis occurred in 32% of patients. The greater incidence of signs in UPET may have resulted from selection criteria. UPET

Table 80-1. Incidence of Symptoms and Signs Associated with Acute Pulmonary Embolism

	Percentage of patients	
	UPET*	PIOPED†
Symptoms		
Dyspnea	84	73
Pleuritic chest pain	74	66
Cough	53	37
Hemoptysis	30	13
Syncope	13	NR
Signs		
Tachypnea	92	70
Rales	58	51
Increased P_2	53	23
Tachycardia	44	30
Fever	43	7
Phlebitis	32	11
Leg edema	24	NR

NR, Not reported.

*Urokinase Pulmonary Embolism Trial, 327 patients. Modified from Bell WR, Simon TL, DeMets DL: The clinical features of submassive and massive pulmonary emboli, *Am J Med* 62:355, 1977.

†Prospective Investigation of Pulmonary Embolism Diagnosis, 117 patients. Modified from Stein PD et al: Clinical, laboratory, roentgenographic, and electrocardiographic findings in patients with acute pulmonary embolism and no preexisting cardiac or pulmonary disease, *Chest* 100:598, 1991.

patients were included only if the embolus involved at least one segmental artery, whereas PIOPED patients could have smaller emboli. All these findings are not very specific, however, since patients without PE have a similar incidence of the same signs. The physical findings for lower extremity DVT are also deceptive. Two thirds of DVTs are clinically silent, and in patients with leg swelling, tenderness, or a positive Homans' sign, only half will actually have DVT. Therefore the physical findings alone are not particularly helpful but can be additional diagnostic clues.

Laboratory Studies

General Tests. Again, routine laboratory studies are not particularly specific. Classically, arterial blood gases (ABGs) demonstrate hypoxemia and hypocapnia, the latter resulting from hyperventilation. These findings are supportive evidence but are also found in a variety of other settings. In patients without prior cardiac or pulmonary disease, Pao_2 was the same for patients with and without PE, and 26% of those with angiogram-proven PE had a normal Pao_2 (greater than 80 mm Hg). ECG abnormalities are common with PE and usually nonspecific. In UPET, ST-segment and T-wave abnormalities occurred in 64% of patients. Evidence of acute cor pulmonale ($S_1Q_3T_3$, right bundle branch block, p pulmonale, or right axis deviation) was less common, but one or more of these occurred in 25% of cases. Sinus tachycardia was present in 43%. Other rhythm disturbances (premature ventricular or atrial beats, atrial fibrillation) occurred in 11% of patients, with atrial fibrillation accounting for 3%. These abnormalities persisted for 5 to 6 days. The ECG was normal in only 13% of patients.

The chest radiograph most often demonstrates findings of atelectasis, small pleural effusion, infiltrates, or elevated hemidiaphragm but may be normal. Other features, such as a pleural-based density (Hampton's hump) and regional loss of vascularity with proximal vascular fullness or cutoff (Westermark's sign), have been associated with PE. Overall, however, the chest film has poor sensitivity and specificity for PE. Its main value is as an adjunct to the $\dot{V}/\dot{Q}$ scan and its ability to detect an alternate cause for the patient's symptoms.

Specific Tests. Pulmonary angiography is the definitive study for the diagnosis of PE. A catheter is introduced, most often through the femoral vein, and advanced to the main pulmonary artery of interest. PAP is measured and then contrast injected while films from multiple views are taken. Subselective injection of smaller arteries can be done if necessary. A thrombus must be clearly outlined to make the diagnosis of PE. Although definitive, angiography is not suitable as a routine test because it is invasive, expensive, not available at all centers, and has potential complications, such as anaphylactoid reactions to intravenous (IV) contrast and worsening of renal dysfunction, particularly in the diabetic patient. Pulmonary hypertension was once thought to be a contraindication to angiography, but in large centers with experience the procedure can be done safely. This modality is reserved for patients whose diagnosis of PE is uncertain after clinical evaluation and noninvasive imaging studies.

Perfusion lung scanning has been in use for 30 years and is a sensitive but nonspecific method for evaluating pulmonary perfusion. Macroaggregated albumin labeled with technetium 99m is injected intravenously, and anterior, posterior, lateral, and oblique views of the chest are taken. The distribution of particles in the lung reflects the distribution of blood flow. Localized defects can occur in areas of lung consolidation or collapse, with pulmonary vasoconstriction caused by local alveolar hypoxia and vascular obstruction. The chest radiograph is critical in evaluating lung scan perfusion defects. Abnormal perfusion without an abnormality on chest film is much more specific for pulmonary vascular obstruction (embolism) than abnormal perfusion that corresponds to an area of parenchymal consolidation. Ventilation scanning is often performed after the perfusion scan to increase its specificity. $Xenon^{133}$ is inhaled for several minutes to fill all areas of the lung. The patient then breathes ambient air, and the washout of the isotope is studied. With normal ventilation the lungs clear rapidly and symmetrically. Areas of retained radioactivity indicate abnormal ventilation. Areas of normal ventilation with abnormal perfusion (mismatch) are very suggestive of PE.

The PIOPED trial was unique in that it combined the clinical estimate of the likelihood of PE with the findings of $\dot{V}/\dot{Q}$ scanning in patients with angiographically proven PE, thus strengthening the diagnostic utility of lung scanning (Table 80-2).[11] With high clinical suspicion the probability of PE is as high as 40% when the $\dot{V}/\dot{Q}$ scan is read as low probability; however, when the scan is near normal or normal, the chance of PE is very low regardless of the level of clinical suspicion. However, the diagnosis of PE can still be difficult. Approximately 67% of PIOPED patients fell into nondiagnostic categories, and further testing was required. In patients with chronic obstructive pulmonary disease (COPD), up to 90% of scans are nondiagnostic.

Table 80-2. Likelihood of Pulmonary Embolism (PE) Based on Clinical Estimates and Ventilation/Perfusion Scans

	Clinical probability (% positive for PE)			
Scan category	**80%-100%**	**20%-79%**	**0-19%**	**All probabilities**
High probability	96	88	56	87
Intermediate probability	66	28	16	30
Low probability	40	16	4	14
Near normal/normal	0	6	2	4

Modified from Value of the ventilation/perfusion scan in acute pulmonary embolism: results of the Prospective Investigation of Pulmonary Embolism Diagnosis (PIOPED), *JAMA* 263:2753, 1990.

Because most pulmonary emboli arise from the lower extremity, techniques for the detection of DVT are important modalities to consider in a PE workup. Contrast venography is the definitive test for detection of DVT but is invasive and requires large amounts of IV contrast material. Noninvasive modalities include ^{125}I-fibrinogen scanning, impedance plethysmography (IPG), and venous compression ultrasound. ^{125}I-fibrinogen incorporated into freshly forming thrombus was a sensitive method for detecting thrombus formation in calf, popliteal, and distal thigh veins. This test required active thrombus formation so was of little value in the immediate diagnosis of DVT; because of the risk of transmissible infection, it is no longer available for clinical use. IPG assesses venous drainage from the thigh after partial release of an occlusive cuff. Using a mild electric current, the impedance of the thigh is measured after application of an occlusive cuff and should decrease as venous blood is allowed to drain proximally. Failure of impedance to fall suggests obstruction to venous outflow due to a thrombus. Calf thrombi do not usually affect venous outflow so are not detected reliably by IPG, and extrinsic compression of thigh vein(s) or elevated central venous pressure (congestive heart failure) may give false-positive results. Ultrasound examination of the proximal veins of the lower extremity is a sensitive and specific test for DVT. If the vessel is adequately visualized and cannot be compressed, the diagnosis of DVT is confirmed. Visualization of thrombus is unreliable, however, and ultrasound is somewhat operator dependent. The choice of IPG or ultrasound is usually based on local availability. More recent studies have shown that both IPG and ultrasound are much less sensitive than initially reported.

Helical (or spiral) computed tomography (CT) technology has greatly enhanced the diagnostic capability of CT scans. During continuous x-ray exposure the patient moves through the scanner without stopping, often during a single breath-hold. This results in a helix-shaped volume of data over a larger distance. Narrow slices and overlapping reconstruction result in vastly improved spatial resolution and imaging of small vessels. Therefore a relatively small bolus of IV contrast can opacify the pulmonary vasculature, allowing imaging of intravascular thrombi. Multiple studies have documented sensitivities and specificities for PE ranging from 79% to 95% and 93% to 97%, respectively. Helical CT often can provide an alternative cause for the patient's symptoms, which the $\dot{V}/\dot{Q}$ scan cannot. The major concern with helical CT is the small, peripheral emboli that are not easily seen. In recent studies, patients who received no anticoagulation after either a normal helical CT scan or a normal to low-probability $\dot{V}/\dot{Q}$ scan had similar risks of recurrent PE and mortality. This suggests a good outcome after a negative helical CT scan but requires further study. Whether the CT scan should replace the $\dot{V}/\dot{Q}$ scan or substitute for standard pulmonary angiography is the subject of ongoing debate. We favor the use of helical CT for chronically ill and hospitalized patients because they are more likely to have abnormal chest radiographs that result in nondiagnostic $\dot{V}/\dot{Q}$ scans. For most outpatients with normal chest films, the $\dot{V}/\dot{Q}$ scan should remain the initial imaging study.

The plasma concentration of D-dimer, a fibrin degradation product, is often elevated in patients with thrombosis, but a normal level may eliminate DVT and PE as diagnoses. Using a simple whole-blood D-dimer assay, available in Europe, Canada, and Australia, investigators have found that a normal test may help to exclude PE in patients with a low pretest probability of PE or a nondiagnostic $\dot{V}/\dot{Q}$ scan. This would obviate the need for further testing.

Diagnosis

A chest radiograph should be obtained, and if it does not reveal an alternate diagnosis or is normal, a $\dot{V}/\dot{Q}$ scan should follow. If the perfusion scan is normal, PE is essentially ruled out, and therapy or further workup is unnecessary. The lack of subsequent DVT or PE in this setting has been confirmed in several prospective studies. A high-probability $\dot{V}/\dot{Q}$ scan indicates an 85% to 90% probability of PE; if combined with a high clinical suspicion, however, the positive predictive value is as high as 96%. In this setting, treatment is initiated without further evaluation. Unfortunately, most patients do not have normal or high-probability scans and fall into more difficult categories. Of PIOPED patients, 73% had low-probability or intermediate-probability $\dot{V}/\dot{Q}$ scans, which, combined with different levels of clinical suspicion, indicate PE probabilities of 4% to 66% (see Table 80-2). This degree of uncertainty requires further diagnostic investigation. The first option is to perform pulmonary angiography, which is the definitive test but is invasive and not universally available. Helical CT scanning may be a more reasonable option. The alternative is to study the lower extremity for evidence of DVT. Contrast venography is an option, but for reasons previously mentioned, noninvasive studies have become more prevalent. Finding a proximal DVT with IPG or lower extremity ultrasound warrants therapy, making the diagnosis of PE unnecessary because the therapy is the same. With PE a proximal DVT is found in approximately half the cases.

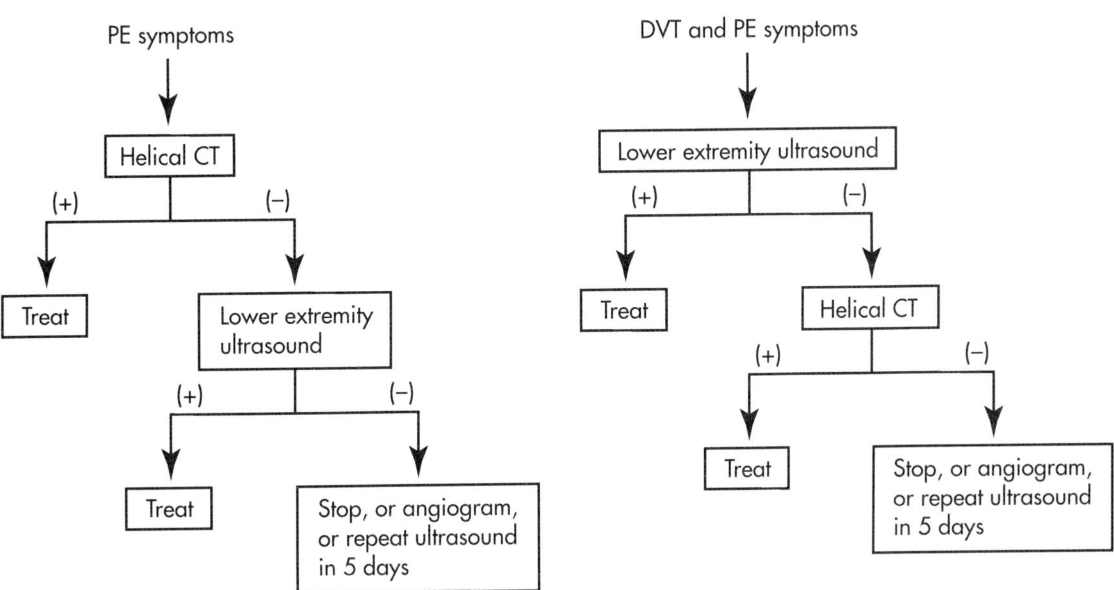

Fig. 80-2. Diagnostic algorithm for venous thromboembolic disease. *V̇/Q̇*, Ventilation/perfusion; *CT*, computed tomography; *PE*, pulmonary embolism; *DVT*, deep venous thrombosis. (From Lipchik RJ, Kuzo RS, Goodman LR: *Clin Pulm Med* 5:109, 1998.)

With a nondiagnostic V̇/Q̇ scan and a negative noninvasive leg study, probability of PE may still be as high as 30% to 50%, and pulmonary angiography or helical CT is indicated to clarify the diagnosis. Fig. 80-2 shows a diagnostic strategy for the diagnosis of PE that applies equally well for females as well as males. In a separate analysis of female PIOPED patients, signs, symptoms, and risk factors were essentially the same as in male patients, except that oral contraceptive use (not postmenopausal estrogen use) in the setting of surgery was associated with a more frequent diagnosis of PE. In addition, the sensitivity of a high-probability V̇/Q̇ scan was diminished in this group, and angiography was needed more frequently to confirm the diagnosis of PE.

Differential Diagnosis. Because the symptoms associated with pulmonary embolism are nonspecific, the initial evaluation of the patient with a chest radiograph and general laboratory studies usually identifies alternative diagnoses. For example, chest pain and dyspnea may indicate pneumococcal pneumonia, acute myocardial infarction, or pneumothorax. Fever, elevated white blood cell count, purulent sputum, and segmental infiltrate on the chest film occur with pneumonia. Signs of acute ischemia on the ECG with evidence of congestive heart failure should direct the focus toward ischemic heart disease. The chest radiograph alone should confirm the presence of a pneumothorax. Irritation of the diaphragm by abdominal processes such as pancreatitis or subdiaphragmatic abscess may also produce lower chest pain and a sense of dyspnea, but these can usually be distinguished from PE by physical examination. The failure to find a clear alternative diagnosis and the presence of predisposing factors for thromboembolic disease are the diagnostic clues that increase the suspicion for PE and lead to the next level of investigation.

Management

Prophylaxis for Deep Venous Thrombosis. Key principles for the administration of prophylactic regimens include (1) a well-defined risk group, (2) a simple and easily implemented modality, and (3) a modality that is safe for widespread use. The most frequently used modalities have varying efficacy among the different risk groups[5] (Table 80-3). Some, such as graded elastic stockings, should be limited to a few select patient groups and have little applicability to high-risk populations. The anticoagulant drugs, including heparin, warfarin, and low-molecular-weight heparin (LMWH), are effective in most high-risk groups. The LMWH enoxaparin is approved for DVT prophylaxis in patients undergoing hip or knee replacement surgery or general surgery. The different LMWHs have specific activities and safety profiles. They need to be individually studied in different clinical settings as they become available. They are not recommended for patients with lumbar puncture or spinal anesthesia and must be used with caution in patients with liver or kidney failure. For patients at high risk for VTE, a combination of intermittent compression devices and an anticoagulant should be strongly considered.

Treatment for Venous Thromboembolism. Heparin remains the initial treatment of choice for DVT and PE, unless specific contraindications exist, because it immediately inhibits thrombus formation. Heparin binds to antithrombin III, inducing a conformational change in its active center that allows antithrombin III to rapidly inactivate factors IIa (thrombin), Xa, and IXa so that the body's thrombolytic mechanisms can proceed unopposed. Although thrombus formation is arrested, heparin does not prevent embolization of established thrombus. The embolization risk decreases when the thrombus is either dissolved or organized; therefore thromboembolism within the first few days is not a failure of therapy. Heparin's efficacy increases with increasing doses, but at higher doses the risk of bleeding becomes significant. Therapy is usually adjusted to maintain the activated partial thromboplastin time (PTT) in a therapeutic range (1.5 to 2.5 times the control). A delay in achieving a therapeutic PTT or allowing the PTT to fall into a nontherapeutic range increases the risk of recurrent DVT from 7 to 15 times, whereas recurrent thrombus occurs in less than 5% of patients who are adequately anticoagulated. Heparin can be administered intravenously or by multiple daily subcutaneous injections. The IV route is most common and usually involves a bolus followed by a continuous infusion. The dose of heparin is adjusted according to the PTT drawn every 4 to 6 hours until a therapeutic range has been reached; thereafter the PTT is checked daily. Table 80-4 shows one nomogram for managing heparin therapy. Heparin is usually administered for 5 days, overlapping with oral anticoagulants.

Anticoagulation is continued for 3 to 6 months on an outpatient basis with coumadin, maintaining the prothrombin time (PT) at approximately 1.5 times control, or an international normalized ratio (INR) of 2.0 to 2.5. The INR, or ratio of patient PT/control PT^{ISI} (ISI, international sensitivity index for thromboplastin), allows the reporting of therapeutic range to be universally applicable. Coumadin can be started simultaneously with heparin so that after 5 days the INR should be in therapeutic range, allowing the discontinuation of heparin. Coumadin is usually initiated with daily 5-mg doses, with further adjustments made according to the INR. Coumadin should be continued for 3 to 6 months or indefinitely if a predisposing condition persists.

The use of oral anticoagulants alone for the initial treatment of proximal DVT results in three times the rates of thrombus extension and PE compared with IV heparin therapy. When properly diagnosed and treated, recurrence and mortality rates for PE are 8.3% and 2.5%, respectively. The major complications of these medications must also be considered. The major complication of heparin is hemor-

Table 80-3. Deep Venous Thrombosis (DVT) Prophylaxis

Condition	DVT incidence (%)	Prophylaxis	Risk reduction (%)
General surgery	25	ES	64
		ICD	60
		LDH	68
		LMWH	72
Hip replacement	50	LD warfarin	57
		Adjusted LDH	78
		LMWH	71
Spinal cord surgery	70-90	Adjusted LDH	>70
		LMWH	>70
Elective neurosurgery	25	ICD	74
Myocardial infarction	25	LDH	71
Ischemic stroke	47	LDH	63
		LMWH	75
Intensive care patients	50	LDH	50
Immobile patients		LDH	31*

ES, Graded elastic stockings; *ICD,* intermittent calf-thigh compression devices; *adjusted LDH,* low-dose heparin adjusted to high normal or PTT 1.5 × control; *LDH,* heparin 5000 units subcutaneously every 8-12 hours; *LMWH,* low-molecular-weight heparin (ardeparin, dalteparin, danaparoid, enoxaparin); *LD warfarin,* low-intensity warfarin.
*Reduction in hospital mortality.
Modified from Clagett GP et al: Prevention of venous thromboembolism, *Chest* 102:3915, 1992.

Table 80-4. Weight-based Heparin Therapy for Venous Thromboembolism

Unfractionated heparin: initial dose of 80 U/kg as IV bolus, then 18 U/kg/hr IV. Check activated partial thromboplastin time (PTT) in 6 hours, then:

PTT (sec)*	Dose (units)	Repeat PTT
<35 (<1.2 × control)	80 U/kg, +4 U/kg/hr	6 hours
35-45 (1.2-1.5 × control)	40 U/kg, +2 U/kg/hr	6 hours
46-70 (1.5-2.3 × control)	No change	Daily
71-90 (2.3-3 × control)	−2 U/kg/hr	6 hours
>90 (>3 × control)	Hold infusion 1 hour, then −3 U/kg/hr	6 hours
Low-molecular-weight heparin		
Enoxaparin	1 mg/kg subcutaneously every 12 hours	
	1.5 mg/kg subcutaneously every day	

*Check platelet count daily.
Modified from Raschke RA et al: The weight-based heparin dosing nomogram compared with a "standard care" nomogram, *Am Intern Med* 119:874, 1993.

rhage, which usually occurs with coexistent disease or coagulopathy (e.g., uremia, unsuspected peptic ulcer disease, thrombocytopenia, concomitant aspirin use) but can occur with a therapeutic PTT. Reversible *heparin-associated thrombocytopenia* (HAT), mediated by a heparin-IgG immune complex, has been noted more frequently with bovine-derived than porcine-derived heparin. With porcine heparin the incidence of HAT is 2.4% for therapeutic heparin and 0.3% for prophylactic heparin. The usual time of onset is between 3 and 15 days from the onset of therapy. The incidence of arterial or venous thrombosis after HAT is 0.4%. Other heparin complications include osteoporosis, alopecia, skin necrosis, and hypoaldosteronism.

As with heparin, warfarin's major complication is hemorrhage. The rare but serious complication of skin necrosis can occur with initiation of therapy and may be caused by a rapid fall in protein C, a vitamin K–dependent inhibitor of coagulation factors Va and VIIIa. A decrease in protein C before a reduction in the other factors results in a transient hypercoagulable state with thrombosis of subcutaneous vessels. Treatment requires discontinuation of warfarin and administration of vitamin K.

The LMWHs approved for use in orthopedic DVT prophylaxis offer an alternative to standard unfractionated heparin in the treatment of DVT and PE. Enoxaparin is approved by the U.S. Food and Drug Administration for DVT therapy. Subcutaneous LMWH in fixed body-weight-adjusted doses may be a better alternative than standard IV heparin in treating lower extremity DVT. No IV administration, no PTT monitoring, and the ease of outpatient therapy are major potential advantages. Considerable cross-reactivity occurs between heparin and LMWH in the setting of HAT, but danaparoid, a heparinoid, has been used successfully in such patients.

Because the greatest risk for PE occurs in patients with proximal DVT, some question whether venous thrombi in the calf need to be treated at all. Studies show good outcomes without anticoagulation in some patients. Using serial IPG of the lower extremities in patients with clinically suspected DVT, patients were not anticoagulated unless they had evidence of proximal extension of thrombus (confirmed venographically). When the IPG remained normal, there were no recurrences of DVT or episodes of symptomatic PE during follow-up. In a similar trial of patients with clinically suspected PE, anticoagulation was not initiated as long as serial IPG studies remained negative for proximal thrombus. At 3 months' follow-up the rate of PE was as low as for patients with normal perfusion scans, supporting the belief that thrombi from the proximal veins of the lower extremities are the usual cause of significant pulmonary emboli.[8a] Whether serial noninvasive studies are practical, cost-effective, and safe remains to be seen.

Thrombolysis. Tissue plasminogen activator, streptokinase, and urokinase are all approved for treatment of PE. The only consensus indication for thrombolytic therapy in acute PE is in the setting of submassive or massive embolism and hemodynamic compromise.[7] Many physicians would administer this therapy only after initial resuscitative efforts have failed to restore adequate hemodynamics. Thrombolysis accelerates clot lysis and improves hemodynamics within hours. Peripheral IV administration may be equivalent to intrapulmonary artery infusion, allowing for lesser delays until treatment. At day 7, however, the effects of thrombolysis plus heparin are equivalent to heparin alone. Furthermore, thrombolysis does not improve mortality in patients with PE.

The use of thrombolytic agents in patients with DVT without PE is more controversial. Many physicians will consider use of these drugs in a patient with acute iliofemoral thrombosis or with vascular compromise (phlegmasia) to improve symptoms and prevent long-term disability. Some studies have shown earlier and more complete recovery of venous flow, but long-term venous competence and decreased morbidity have yet to be demonstrated. The benefits of this treatment in patients with DVT alone need to be balanced with the small but serious risks of major hemorrhage, including intracranial bleeding. The standard of care for proximal DVT remains heparinization followed by warfarin therapy.

Inferior Vena Cava Filters. Inferior vena cava (IVC) ligation therapy has been used since the late 1800s. It caused severe venous stasis, however, and development of venous collateral flow may again lead to recurrent PE. Therefore alternative methods were needed to prevent PE when standard therapy had failed or was not feasible. For the last 25 years IVC filters have been in use, most widely the Greenfield filter, although newer designs have been implemented in the past 10 years. These filters can trap emboli as small as 2 mm in diameter and allow for a significant proportion of their volume to be obstructed while preserving a sufficient cross-sectional area for venous flow. Box 80-3 lists the recommended indications for and complications of IVC filters. None of the indications has been substantiated in controlled clinical trials, but the decreased rate of PE compared with untreated DVT supports their use when anticoagulation fails or cannot be administered. IVC filters have also been used successfully in trauma patients who cannot be anticoagulated. Complication rates of modern IVC filters are low.[3]

Thromboembolic Pulmonary Hypertension. Symptomatic patients with mean PAPs greater than 35 mm Hg should have a thorough evaluation to determine if they are candidates for surgical therapy.[6] The surgical options include pulmonary thromboendarterectomy or lung transplantation. Thromboendarterectomy has a 6% to 15% perioperative mortality risk, but survivors recover sufficiently to return to work or other usual activities. Candidates for this surgery need to have proximal organized vascular thrombosis, as determined by angiography or helical CT scan. Pulmonary angioscopy is available at select centers and allows for direct visualization of thrombus. $\dot{V}/\dot{Q}$ scanning invariably shows a segmental or larger defect but usually underestimates the degree of obstruction. Those who are not candidates for endarterectomy can be considered for vasodilator therapy or lung transplantation. All patients should have supplemental oxygen to keep their oxygen saturation above 90% at rest, during sleep, and with exertion. Most physicians recommend lifelong anticoagulation and an IVC filter. Thrombolytic therapy has no proven value once this condition is established.

Thromboembolic Disease in Pregnancy. Pregnancy presents unique problems in VTE and its management for a variety of reasons. During pregnancy, increases in clotting

Box 80-3. Inferior Vena Cava (IVC) Filters for Venous Thromboembolism

Recommended Indications

Prevention of PE in setting of documented DVT (standard practice)
- Treatment failure with anticoagulation
- Contraindication to anticoagulation

Prevention of death from recurrent PE in addition to anticoagulation (controversial)
- After acute, massive PE
- If IVC or large proximal thrombus visualized
- Chronic pulmonary hypertension caused by recurrent PE

Prevention of PE in patients at high risk for DVT (controversial)
- Trauma patients
- Other high-risk groups

Complications

- Incorrect placement
- Hematoma at insertion site
- Venous thrombosis at insertion site (2%-7%)
- Recurrent PE (2%)
- Worsened venous insufficiency (5%)
- Caval thrombosis (4%-19%)
- Migration of filter (rare)
- Fatal complications (<0.5%)

PE, Pulmonary embolism; *DVT*, deep venous thrombosis.

factors V, VII, VIII, IX, X, XII, and fibrinogen create a hypercoagulable state; however, this is usually balanced by an increase in baseline fibrinolytic activity. Other factors associated with an increased risk of PE are older maternal age, race (black vs. white), operative delivery, and prior thromboembolism. The diagnostic strategy is as discussed earlier. The total radiation dose to the fetus from a chest radiograph, $\dot{V}/\dot{Q}$ scan, and pulmonary angiogram (via the brachial vein) is approximately 0.05 rad, a low dose, particularly balanced against the potential mortality of a PE.

Heparin or an LMWH is the drug of choice during pregnancy for thromboembolic disease because their size precludes transit across the placenta. The daily requirement of IV heparin can be given subcutaneously in two or three daily doses, but monitoring is necessary to ensure that the PTT measured at the midpoint between doses is maintained at 1.5 to 2 times the control. The potential risk of osteoporosis with long-term heparin use becomes a problem in this setting; 20,000 U/day for more than 20 weeks is associated with an increased risk of bone demineralization, but even prophylactic heparin may result in vertebral compression fractions in up to 1.6% of pregnant women. The demineralization is reversible with discontinuation of heparin but may be a slow process. The incidence of osteopenia with LMWH appears to be less.

Warfarin is contraindicated during pregnancy because of well-known teratogenic effects. First-trimester exposure results in a characteristic set of findings, including nasal hypoplasia, depressed bridge of the nose, epiphyseal stippling, and a high rate of developmental impairment. Exposure in the second trimester is associated with central nervous system and ophthalmologic abnormalities. Overall, 13% of pregnancies exposed to warfarin result in abnormal infants. The use of thrombolytic agents is reserved for life-threatening situations and carries the risk of abruptio placentae and fetal death, although there are anecdotal reports of uncomplicated use of thrombolytic therapy during pregnancy.

PULMONARY HYPERTENSIVE DISEASES

Although flow through the pulmonary circulation usually equals that through the systemic circulation, PAPs are normally much lower than those in the systemic arteries. This difference in arterial pressure reflects the resistance of the pulmonary vessels being proportionately lower than that in their systemic counterparts. The pulmonary circulation has a high compliance because of nonmuscularized, distensible small vessels and capillaries. Therefore significant increases in pulmonary blood flow are accommodated with only slight increases in pressure. According to Poiseuille's equation (law) describing flow through a tube, resistance to flow is inversely proportional to the radius of the tube to the fourth power. Therefore, as vascular remodeling occurs and the pulmonary arterioles are narrowed, resistance may increase precipitously, leading to significant increases in PAP at normal blood flows. For obstructive vascular diseases such as PE, increases in PAP are usually not evident until more than 30% to 50% of the vascular bed has been lost. A diagnosis of pulmonary arterial hypertension is made when the mean PAP is greater than 18 mm Hg. Since extensive pulmonary vascular changes are often present before severe pulmonary hypertension results, many patients will develop symptoms and present at an advanced stage.

Pathophysiology

Box 80-4 lists disorders associated with pulmonary hypertension, presenting the chronic disorders according to the 1998 World Health Organization Classification of Pulmonary Hypertension. Although thromboembolic disease usually involves macroscopic clots that cause a heterogenous loss of vessels, resulting in abnormal perfusion scans or angiograms, multiple small emboli occasionally may result in a relatively uniform distribution of obstruction. In situ thrombosis is particularly common in patients with sickle cell disease and may also occur with the hypercoagulable states. The hypertensive effects of either the obstructive or restrictive lung diseases may be related to obliteration of pulmonary vessels along with the primary lung damage. Alternatively, hypoxia may contribute to the elevated PAP. Hypoxia is one of the most potent pulmonary vasoconstrictors, and administration of oxygen may acutely reverse some of the PAP elevation. Chronic hypoxemia, however, can lead to vascular remodeling, which may be only partially reversed with time. Chronic high blood flow through left-to-right shunts via atrial or ventricular septal defects may also result in irreversible pulmonary vascular remodeling. Similarly, chronically elevated left atrial pressure from mitral stenosis, atrial myxomas, or diseases that cause increased pulmonary venous resistance may also cause pulmonary hypertension. Collagen vascular disease may cause pulmonary hypertension secondary to interstitial lung disease or by primary vascular involvement. The prognosis is quite poor in patients who develop pulmonary vasculitis or other primary pulmonary vascular

Box 80-4. Pulmonary Hypertensive Disorders

Acute Disorders

Acute pulmonary embolism
Acute lung injury
Acute hypoxic vasoconstriction
Pulmonary hypertensive crisis with congenital heart or mitral valve disease

Chronic Disorders

- Pulmonary arterial hypertension
  - Primary pulmonary hypertension
  - Pulmonary hypertension caused by associated illness:
    - Collagen vascular disease
    - Congenital heart disease
    - Portal hypertension
    - Human immunodeficiency virus (HIV) infection
    - Drugs/toxins (anorexigens)
    - Persistent pulmonary hypertension of newborn
- Pulmonary venous hypertension
  - Left-sided heart disease
  - Compression of central pulmonary veins
  - Pulmonary venoocclusive disease
- Pulmonary hypertension associated with respiratory disorders and hypoxemia
  - Chronic obstructive pulmonary disease
  - Interstitial lung disease
  - Sleep-disordered breathing
  - Alveolar hypoventilation syndromes
  - Chronic exposure to high altitude
  - Neonatal lung disease
  - Alveolar-capillary dysplasia
- Pulmonary hypertension caused by chronic thrombotic and embolic disease
  - Thromboembolic obstruction of proximal pulmonary arteries
  - Obstruction of distal pulmonary arteries
- Pulmonary hypertension caused by disorders directly affecting pulmonary vasculature
  - Inflammatory disorders (e.g., sarcoidosis, schistosomiasis)
  - Pulmonary capillary hemangiomatosis

disease. Portal hypertension from hepatic or extrahepatic origin is associated with potentially severe pulmonary hypertension. These patients usually do not have hepatopulmonary syndrome, and therefore resting Pao_2 is usually normal.

Primary pulmonary hypertension (PPH) is a diagnosis of exclusion when no other cause can be found. PPH occurs more often among young adult women, but the pathogenesis remains obscure. A significant association exists between the use of fenfluramine-derived anorexic agents and PPH, and fenfluramine has been taken off the market in the United States.[1] More patients have been exposed to these drugs, and an increased number of PPH cases is expected.

Patient Evaluation

Unfortunately, most patients with pulmonary hypertension will develop symptoms late in the course. Dyspnea with effort and eventually at rest is the most common complaint of patients with severe pulmonary hypertension. Any persistent complaint of effort intolerance should be taken seriously. Pulmonary hypertension may be associated with substernal chest pain indistinguishable from angina but may result from pulmonary artery (PA) distention rather than from myocardial ischemia. As pulmonary vascular changes progress, resistance increases and cardiac output decreases, leading to further limitation and occasionally syncopal episodes. Hemoptysis is uncommon. As pulmonary vascular resistance becomes excessive, the right side of the heart dilates, and right atrial and ventricular end-diastolic pressure rises. Systemic venous hypertension is required for adequate venous return, and peripheral edema becomes apparent. Other signs of pulmonary hypertension include jugular venous distention and *v* waves, a palpable PA impulse, and a precordial lift from right ventricular hypertrophy and distention. A loud pulmonic component of the second heart sound and a right-sided S_3 or S_4 may be heard. Holosystolic and diastolic murmurs may be present when tricuspid or pulmonary valvular regurgitation are present, respectively. Flow murmurs over the lung fields have been described in patients with chronic pulmonary hypertension from PE. As cardiac function declines, peripheral edema, cyanosis, and other signs of hypoperfusion may be seen. Raynaud's phenomenon is often seen in patients with collagen vascular disease or PPH.

Diagnosis

The general diagnostic approach to the patient with suspected pulmonary hypertension is shown in Fig. 80-3. Chest radiographs can provide information regarding any lung disorder and secondary vascular changes. The central pulmonary vessels are often dilated, and a right descending PA greater than 19 mm in diameter suggests pulmonary hypertension. A main PA greater than 30 mm on CT scan is also suggestive. Oligemia can be present in the more peripheral regions of the lung. Disorders that raise pulmonary venous pressure, such as pulmonary venoocclusive disease, may lead to pulmonary edema. Pao_2 at rest may be normal but tends to fall with exercise, and as carbon dioxide pressure decreases, the A-a gradient increases. Hypoxemia stimulates ventilation, and a compensated respiratory alkalosis is a common finding. The alveolar dead space may be relatively high because some ventilated regions of the lungs are underperfused, and it may fail to decrease normally with exercise. Diffusing capacity usually decreases as pulmonary vasculature is lost; however, decreases in diffusing capacity can be mild in patients with PPH or other diseases that primarily affect the pulmonary blood vessels. ECGs are abnormal in most patients. Right axis deviation, right ventricular hypertrophy with strain, and right atrial enlargement are common. Echocardiography is useful because it permits evaluation of the right ventricle and estimation of systolic PAP. Studies with solutions that generate microbubbles, which serve as a contrast agent, help identify the presence of right-to-left shunts. Perfusion scans, helical CT scans, and pulmonary angiography are essential for detecting thromboembolic disease. Cardiac catheterization is frequently needed to rule out congenital heart defects, to obtain accurate hemodynamic measurements, and to evaluate the efficacy of therapy.

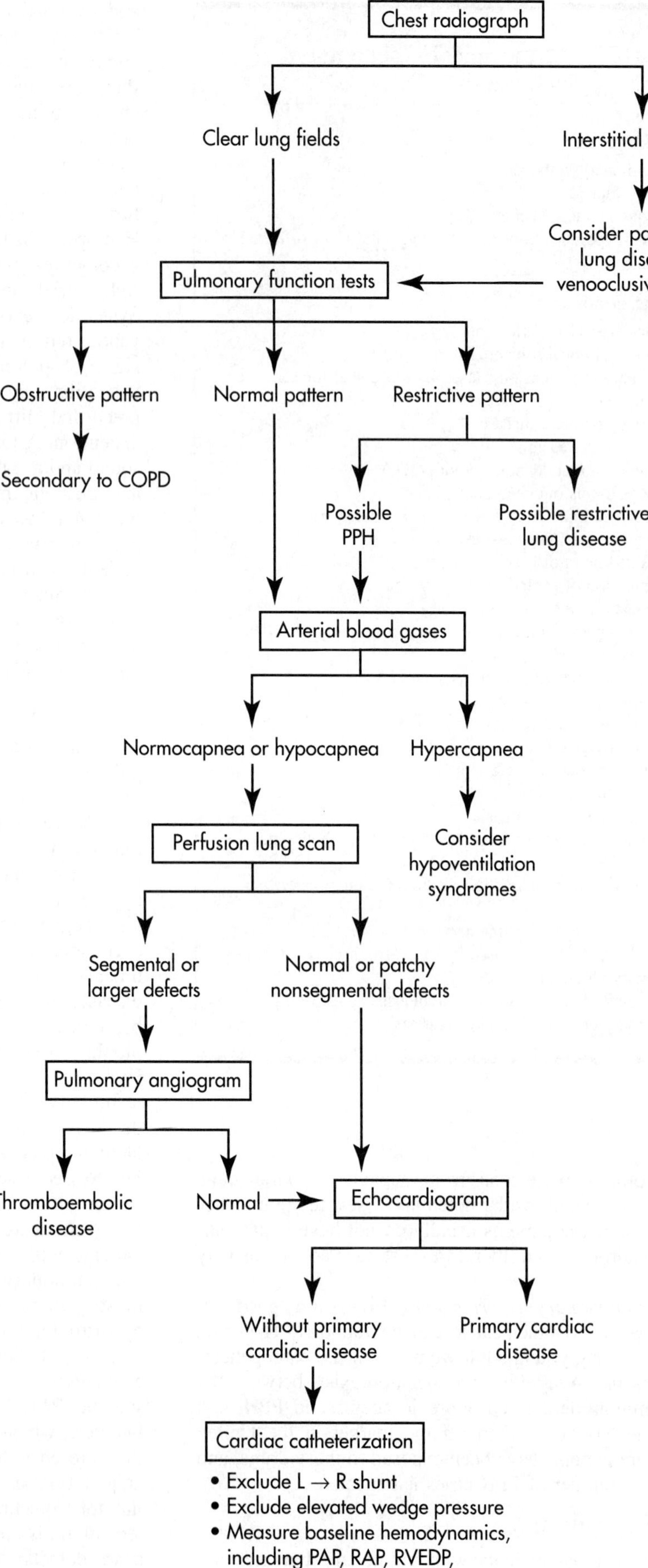

Fig. 80-3. Diagnostic algorithm for pulmonary hypertension. *COPD,* Chronic obstructive pulmonary disease; *PPH,* primary pulmonary hypertension; *L → R,* left to right; *PAP,* pulmonary artery pressure; *RAP,* right atrial pressure; *RVEDP,* right ventricular end-diastolic pressure. (From Rich S: *Prog Cardiovasc Dis* 31:205, 1988.)

Box 80-5. Treatment Options for Chronic Pulmonary Hypertensive Diseases

Medical Therapy

Treatment of underlying disorder
Supplemental oxygen to keep oxygen saturation >90%
Anticoagulation
Pulmonary vasodilator therapy (pulmonary arterial hypertension)
  Oral agents
  Continuous intravenous epoprostenol (prostacyclin)
Digoxin and diuretics

Surgical Therapy

Correction of specific cardiac lesion
Lung or heart-lung transplant
Blade septostomy for recurrent syncope
Thromboendarterectomy for chronic pulmonary embolism of major vessel

Treatment

General treatment options for pulmonary hypertension are summarized in Box 80-5. When pulmonary hypertension is secondary to an underlying disease, treatment of the primary disorder is the treatment of choice. For example, if pulmonary hypertension is caused by hypoxemia, supplemental oxygen may result in lower PAPs, improved right-sided heart function, and enhanced survival. On the other hand, many patients are quite ill at presentation, and treatment options may be limited. Patients with PA hypertension are candidates for vasodilator therapy. Oral and IV vasodilator agents can cause systemic hypotension, which limits their use and requires hemodynamic monitoring in an intensive care unit when they are initiated. Inhaled nitric oxide is used as a screening agent and is selective in that it does not cause systemic hypotension; it can predict acute responses to oral and IV vasodilators. Patients experience symptomatic benefit from vasodilator therapy if their pulmonary vascular resistance decreases by 30% or more.

Recent studies have shown improved survival with titrated high-dose calcium channel blockers or continuous IV epoprostenol (prostacylin) therapy in patients with PPH.[2] These patients uniformly have significant decreases in both PAP and pulmonary vascular resistance with therapy. Many of these patients who did not improve acutely with therapy did demonstrate improved hemodynamics with long-term IV epoprostenol. Similar benefits have been seen in some patients with scleroderma and other diseases.[9] Epoprostenol therapy is limited to patients with American Heart Association class III or IV symptoms; it is expensive and requires comprehensive patient training. Warfarin also improves survival in patients with PPH independent of their response to other therapy. Some patients with end-stage pulmonary hypertension are candidates for lung transplantation.

EBM EVIDENCE-BASED MEDICINE

The primary source for this chapter was MEDLINE. Electronic searches dating back to 1994 were conducted up to July 1999, focusing on systematic reviews and randomized trials.

REFERENCES

1. Abenhain L et al: Appetite-suppressant drugs and the risk of primary pulmonary hypertension, *N Engl J Med* 335:609, 1996.
2. Barst RJ et al: A comparison of continuous intravenous epoprostenol (prostacyclin) with conventional therapy for primary pulmonary hypertension, *N Engl J Med* 334:296, 1996.
3. Becker DM, Pholbrick JT, Selby JB: Inferior vena cava filters: indications, safety, effectiveness, *Arch Intern Med* 152:1985, 1992.
4. Carson JL et al: The clinical course of pulmonary embolism, *N Engl J Med* 326:1240, 1992.
5. Clagett GP et al: Prevention of venous thromboembolism, *Chest* 114:531S, 1998.
6. Fedullo PF et al: Chronic thromboembolic pulmonary hypertension, *Clin Chest Med* 16:353, 1995.
7. Goldhaber SZ: Pulmonary embolism, *N Engl J Med* 339:93, 1998.
8. Hyers TM: Venous thromboembolism, *Am J Respir Crit Care Med* 159:1, 1999.

8a. Kearon C et al: Noninvasive diagnosis of deep venous thrombosis, *Ann Intern Med* 128:663, 1998.

9. Sanchez O et al: Treatment of pulmonary hypertension secondary to connective tissue diseases, *Thorax* 54:273, 1999.
10. Thomas DP, Roberts HR: Hypercoagulability in venous and arterial thrombosis, *Ann Intern Med* 126:638, 1997.
11. Value of the ventilation/perfusion scan in acute pulmonary embolism: results of the Prospective Investigation of Pulmonary Embolism Diagnosis (PIOPED), *JAMA* 263:2753, 1990.

CHAPTER 81

Neoplasms of the Lung

Stephen Dolan
Akira Funahashi

BENIGN NEOPLASMS

Benign neoplasms of the lung account for about 5% of all lung neoplasms and include hamartoma, fibroma, leiomyoma, and lipoma. Of these, only hamartoma is clinically important.

Hamartoma

Hamartoma, the most common benign neoplasm of the lung, is believed to be congenital in origin. Histologically, hamartoma contains cartilage, smooth muscle, and mucus-secreting glands. The majority of hamartomas appear as a small, peripheral nodular density on the chest radiograph and may show a popcorn-type calcification. When no clear calcification is seen on the chest radiograph, a computed tomography (CT) scan may reveal a calcification or a characteristic fat density that allows the diagnosis of hamartoma. If no calcification indicates the benign nature of the lesion, a thoracotomy is often necessary for a definitive diagnosis, since commonly applied diagnostic procedures, such as fiberoptic bronchoscopy (FOB) and transthoracic needle aspiration (TNA), often do not yield a definitive diagnosis (see Solitary Pulmonary Nodule). Rarely a hamartoma presents as an endobronchial mass lesion with the clinical and radiographic signs of an obstructive endobronchial lesion, such as a cough, repeated episodes of pneumonia, and atelectasis.

If the radiographic or CT scan appearance confirms the diagnosis of hamartoma, no treatment is necessary. If the diagnosis is uncertain, however, the lesion should be excised. Generally, an endobronchial hamartoma also requires surgical resection because the diagnosis remains uncertain because of small biopsy samples obtained by FOB. If the diagnosis is certain, a local treatment with an yttrium-aluminum-garnet (YAG) laser can be considered.

Bronchial Adenoma

The term *bronchial adenoma* was once used to refer to bronchial carcinoid, bronchial cylindroma (adenoid cystic carcinoma), and mucoepidermoid carcinoma, accounting for approximately 90%, 8%, and 2% of cases, respectively. Because these tumors are histologically distinct, however, they are no longer categorized together under the heading of bronchial adenoma. All three are low-grade malignant tumors and should be separated from bronchial adenomas (bronchial cystadenoma and mucoepidermoid adenoma), which are rare, but truly benign, neoplasms.

Bronchial Carcinoid

The majority of bronchial carcinoids occur in the larger, centrally located bronchi, and only 20% or less originate in the peripheral airways. Bronchial carcinoids are believed to originate in the neurosecretory cells of the bronchial mucosa. Histologically they are composed of small polyhedral cells grouped in nests, trabeculae, or poorly developed tubercles.

The clinical presentation and radiographic findings of bronchial carcinoid differ greatly depending on the tumor's location and size. Centrally located bronchial carcinoids usually grow into the bronchial lumen; thus the patient typically presents with symptoms associated with airway involvement, such as cough and dyspnea. Because bronchial carcinoids are highly vascular, nearly 50% of the patients have hemoptysis. If a tumor obstructs the bronchus, the patient may present with symptoms of pneumonia distal to the obstructed bronchus. Unlike carcinoid tumor of the gastrointestinal (GI) tract, carcinoid syndrome with bronchial carcinoid is very rare. Radiographic findings of bronchial carcinoid also vary greatly. In patients with a centrally located bronchial carcinoid without bronchial obstruction, a chest radiograph often shows a centrally located mass lesion. If bronchial obstruction is present, the film usually shows atelectasis or pneumonic infiltrates distal to the obstruction. If tumor growth is limited within the bronchial lumen with no obstruction, the chest radiograph may be completely normal. When a relatively young individual, particularly a nonsmoker, presents with hemoptysis and a normal chest radiograph, the physician should suspect bronchial carcinoid and have an FOB performed. When bronchial carcinoid originates from a small peripheral airway, the patient is usually asymptomatic, and the lesion is discovered as an incidental finding on the chest radiograph. Establishing the diagnosis of a centrally located bronchial carcinoid is relatively easy once the diagnosis is suspected. In the past a forceps biopsy at bronchoscopy with a rigid bronchoscope was contraindicated because of the potential for massive bleeding. With the advent of FOB and the relatively smaller size of biopsy forceps, a forceps biopsy has been performed safely in some patients, although massive hemoptysis should be considered if a biopsy is performed. A thoracotomy is often required for the definitive diagnosis of a peripherally located carcinoid.

The treatment of bronchial carcinoid is a surgical resection. The prognosis after surgical resection is generally favorable (5-year survival is 90%). Bronchial carcinoids vary in their potential for malignancy, however, and metastases and death occur early in some patients.

Bronchial Cylindroma (Adenoid Cystic Carcinoma)

Unlike bronchial carcinoid, which arises from neurosecretory cells, bronchial cylindroma arises from the bronchial mucous gland. Microscopically it consists of interlacing cylinders of tumor cells, the centers of which are often canalized to form tubular spaces. Since this tumor grows into bronchial lumen, the clinical and radiographic presentations are those of endobronchial mass lesions that cause cough, dyspnea, and hemoptysis. Treatment is surgical excision, but local recurrence is possible.

BRONCHOGENIC CARCINOMA

Epidemiology and Etiology

An estimated 2 million people worldwide develop carcinoma of the lung annually. The highest incidence is found in the industrialized nations of England and Wales, the United States, and Japan. In the United States, although less common than breast and prostate cancer, carcinoma of the lung is the most frequently fatal cancer in men and women, accounting for 28% of all cancer deaths. It ranks second only to ischemic heart disease as the leading cause of death. In 1999 there were an estimated 171,600 new cases of lung cancer. In 1996, 158,900 died of this disease. Lung cancer occurs mainly in males between ages 50 and 80, although the incidence in U.S. women continues to rise, with 40% of all new lung cases involving women.

About 85% to 90% of all lung cancers are the result of cigarette smoking. A clear dose response rate accentuates a genetic predisposition. Male smokers have a 20-fold increased risk of developing lung cancer compared with nonsmokers. Those with chronic obstructive pulmonary disease (COPD) who smoke have an additional twofold to threefold increased risk. Pipe smoking does not carry the same risk as cigarette use, and chewing tobacco is not associated with lung carcinoma but rather malignancies of the upper aerodigestive tract. Passive smoking or environmental tobacco smoke has been demonstrated to be a risk factor for lung carcinoma in lifelong nonsmokers and accounts for an estimated 3000 cancer deaths annually. Other carcinogens linked to lung cancer include asbestos, radon products, polycyclic hydrocarbons, cadmium, chloromethyl ethers, chromium, nickel, and inorganic arsenic. The relative risk of asbestos exposure and tobacco use is multiplicative and estimated to be 100 times that of asbestos workers who do not smoke. Finally, a well-described association exists between bronchoalveolar cell carcinoma and scleroderma and that of adenocarcinoma with fibrocavitary lung disease following granulomatous infections.

Histopathology

Bronchogenic carcinoma can be classified according to four major cell types: squamous cell carcinoma, adenocarcinoma, large-cell carcinoma, and small-cell carcinoma. Because of the similarities in response to treatment and prognosis, the first three cell types are often grouped together as non–small-cell lung carcinomas (NSCLCs) to distinguish them from small-cell lung carcinomas (SCLCs), which are high-grade malignancies and carry an unfavorable prognosis. A significant number of tumors have more than one cell type in the same specimen and are classified as mixed NSCLCs. Squamous cell carcinoma and small-cell carcinoma are the cell types most closely associated with tobacco use. In recent years, adenocarcinoma has replaced squamous cell carcinoma as the most common presenting cell type.

Squamous Cell Carcinoma. Accounting for 30% to 35% of all lung carcinomas, squamous cell carcinomas originate from the respiratory epithelium of the proximal airway (trachea, mainstem bronchi, lobar and segmental bronchi). Typical radiographic features are those of centrally located mass with or without hilar adenopathy. Postobstructive atelectasis or pneumonitis is characteristic given the proximal endobronchial location; cavitation occurs in 5% of cases. Presentation as a small peripheral nodule is less common. Light microscopy features include a stratified layering of polygonal epithelial cells with prominent intercellular bridges and whorls of keratotic debris, the latter being responsible for the term *keratin pearls*. Doubling time is estimated at 3 months (longer for the more well-differentiated forms), and late distant metastases tend to occur. At presentation, therefore, patients are more often symptomatic from local disease spread than distant metastases.

Adenocarcinoma. Accounting for 35% to 40% of all lung carcinomas, adenocarcinomas probably arise from goblet cells in the major bronchi. Despite this, the typical presentation is that of a peripheral tumor in an asymptomatic patient. Adenocarcinoma is the cell type most often associated with lung cancer in nonsmokers or those with preexisting scars (scar carcinoma). Characteristic radiographic features are those of a peripheral mass or nodule in 65% of patients or hilar or mediastinal mass in approximately 40%. Malignant pleural effusion or chest wall involvement is seen in 15%.

Bronchoalveolar cell carcinoma, a subset of adenocarcinoma, presents as a single or multicentric infiltrate with air bronchograms and can mimic an infectious or inflammatory pneumonia. A presenting feature may be that of copious bronchorrhea. Characteristic light microscopy features of all adenocarcinomas include mucin production and gland formation. Bronchoalveolar carcinoma may present as tuftlike proliferation along the alveolar lining. Doubling time is estimated at 6 months, with a predilection to metastasize early to bone, brain, liver and adrenal glands.

Large-cell Carcinoma. Accounting for about 10% of all lung cancers, large-cell carcinomas are relatively undifferentiated; they are free of areas of squamous or small cells, gland formation, or carcinoid differentiation. Radiographically, large-cell carcinomas tend to appear as large peripheral mass lesions. Metastatic patterns are similar to adenocarcinoma, and 50% of patients develop brain metastases. Prognosis is poor, with median survival greatly below that of an equivalent stage of the other NSCLC cell types.

Giant-cell carcinoma, a subset of large-cell carcinoma, is an aggressive, highly malignant tumor composed of large, bizarre, multinucleated cells. Tumors are infiltrated with white cells, and peripheral white count can exceed 40,000. An advanced stage is often seen at presentation, and prognosis is very poor.

Small-cell Carcinoma. Accounting for 20% to 25% of all lung cancers, small-cell carcinomas are histologically subdivided into oat cell, intermediate, and combined cell types. They show finely distributed nuclear chromatin, inconspicuous nucleoli, and scant cytoplasm. The characteristic radiographic appearance is a rapidly enlarging hilar or perihilar mass with mediastinal adenopathy. A peripheral solitary mass is a rare presentation. Most tumors have extensive spread on presentation. Survival is influenced by stage, histology, and gender, with advanced stage (extensive), classic small-cell histology (absence of large polygonal cells), and male gender being poor prognostic features. Doubling time is estimated at 1 to 2 months, with a predilection for early metastasis to bone, liver, bone marrow, central nervous system (CNS), extrathoracic lymph nodes, and subcutaneous tissue. Median survival is much less than for NSCLC, with a 5-year survival of 27% for limited disease and 7 to 9 months for extensive disease.

Patient Evaluation

History. Most patients with bronchogenic carcinoma are symptomatic at presentation, although the symptomatology may not be specific to lung cancer. Signs and symptoms can be grouped according to those that result from local vs. distant manifestations of the disease.

Local Manifestations. Cough resulting from bronchial mucosal irritation is the most common presenting symptom (50% of patients). Airway obstruction presenting as focal wheezing, dyspnea, hoarseness, or even stridor is the result of endobronchial disease or mediastinal extension with involvement of phrenic or recurrent laryngeal nerves. Distal airway obstruction may present as postobstructive atelectasis or pneumonitis with or without cavitation. Hemoptysis, which is usually limited to blood-streaked sputum, suggests endobronchial pathology and warrants a chest radiograph and formal airway examination for smokers over age 40. Chest pain described as a dull ache may result from parietal pleural inflammation. *Superior vena cava syndrome* occurs in 5% of presenting patients and is caused by compression or invasion of the superior vena cava. Characteristic features include neck vein distention, facial and upper extremity edema, and engorgement of venous collaterals in the anterior chest wall. Patients complain of being unable to wear a necktie or having a tight collar. Tumors of the superior sulcus may involve the brachial plexus, resulting in arm and shoulder pain and weakness *(Pancoast's syndrome). Horner's syndrome* (ipsilateral miosis, ptosis, and anhydrosis) indicates involvement of the sympathetic stellate ganglia by this same tumor distribution.

Distant Manifestations. Extrathoracic manifestations of bronchogenic carcinoma primarily result from metastatic tumor spread or numerous paraneoplastic syndromes (Box 81-1). Bony pain and pathologic fractures associated with

Box 81-1. Paraneoplastic Syndromes Associated with Bronchogenic Carcinoma

Endocrine
Cachexia
Antidiuretic hormone secretion
Hypercalcemia
Ectopic adrenocorticotropic hormone secretion

Neuromuscular
Carcinomatous myopathy
Peripheral neuropathy
Eaton-Lambert syndrome
Cortical-cerebellar degeneration
Encephalomyelopathy

Skeletal
Clubbing
Pulmonary hypertrophic osteoarthropathy

Dermatologic
Dermatomyositis, polymyositis
Acanthosis nigricans

Cardiovascular
Migratory thrombophlebitis
Nonbacterial verrucous endocarditis

Hematologic
Anemia
Thrombocytosis
Leukocytosis

Renal
Proteinuria
Nephrotic syndrome

From Matthay RA: Lung neoplasms. In *Chest medicine*, Baltimore, 1990, Williams & Wilkins.

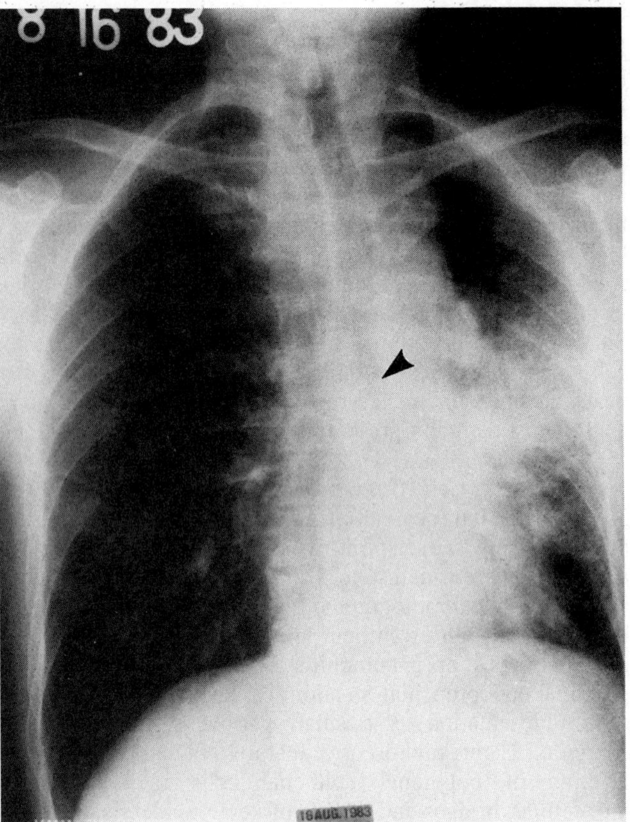

Fig. 81-1. Squamous cell carcinoma originating from distal left main stem bronchus *(arrow)*. Note shifting of mediastinum and trachea and elevation of left diaphragm.

bone metastases are the presenting symptoms in 1% of patients. Intracranial metastases occur in up to 6% of patients on presentation. Symptoms include confusion, lethargy, personality changes, a new-onset seizure disorder, or a speech defect. SCLC is the cell type most often associated with the paraneoplastic syndromes; the *syndrome of inappropriate antidiuretic hormone* (SIADH) is its most common manifestation (10% of patients). Hypercalcemia is primarily associated with squamous cell carcinoma and results from the release of a parathyroid hormone (PTH)–like peptide.

Physical Examination. Physical examination of patients with lung carcinoma is often unrevealing unless the carcinoma is sufficiently advanced to cause obstruction of major airways, a pleural effusion, or bone or brain metastases. Unilateral or localized wheezing suggests airway narrowing. Diminished breath sounds, egophony, and increased vocal fremitus suggest a postobstructive pneumonia, whereas contralateral tracheal deviation, diminished breath sounds, and diminished vocal fremitus without egophony suggest a massive malignant pleural effusion. Neck vein distention, upper extremity and facial edema, and engorged venous collaterals in the anterior chest wall suggest the superior vena cava syndrome, whereas anhydrosis, miosis, and ptosis suggest Horner's syndrome. A careful nodal examination emphasizing the supraclavicular, scalene, and axillary lymph nodes will identify these important sites of metastases in patients with advanced disease, obviating the need for further invasive evaluation. Digital clubbing of recent onset suggests bronchogenic carcinoma, not COPD. Weakness and fatigability of the proximal muscles, particularly in the legs, suggest Eaton-Lambert syndrome, which is associated with SCLC.

Diagnosis

Chest Radiograph. Because the history, physical examination, and laboratory findings are usually nonspecific, the chest radiograph becomes central to the diagnosis of bronchogenic carcinoma. Chest radiographs should be obtained for the evaluation of unexplained cough, hoarseness, dyspnea, or weight loss, as well as to investigate hemoptysis in a smoker. Typical radiographic features include a central or peripheral masslike lesion with or without hilar or mediastinal adenopathy. Central lesions with proximal endobronchial involvement may lead to lobar collapse as the result of resorptive atelectasis (Fig. 81-1). When this occurs, the chest radiograph reveals increased radiodensity of the collapsed lobe, ipsilateral tracheal and hilar deviation, elevation of the ipsilateral hemidiaphragm, and decreased size of the ipsilateral intercostal spaces. A pneumonia that recurs in the

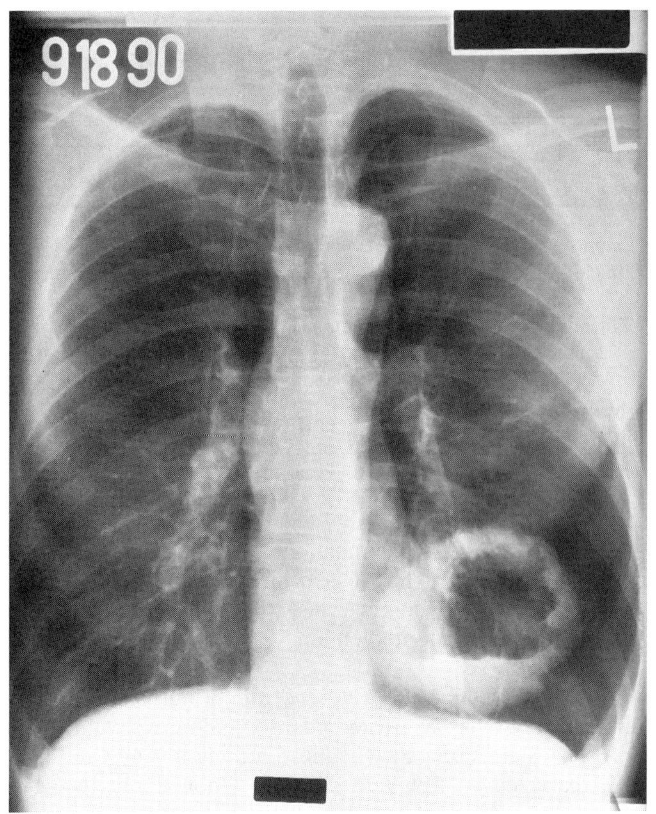

Fig. 81-2. Large peripheral squamous cell carcinoma. Fiberoptic bronchoscopy did not reveal endobronchial lesion. Note large cavity with air-fluid level.

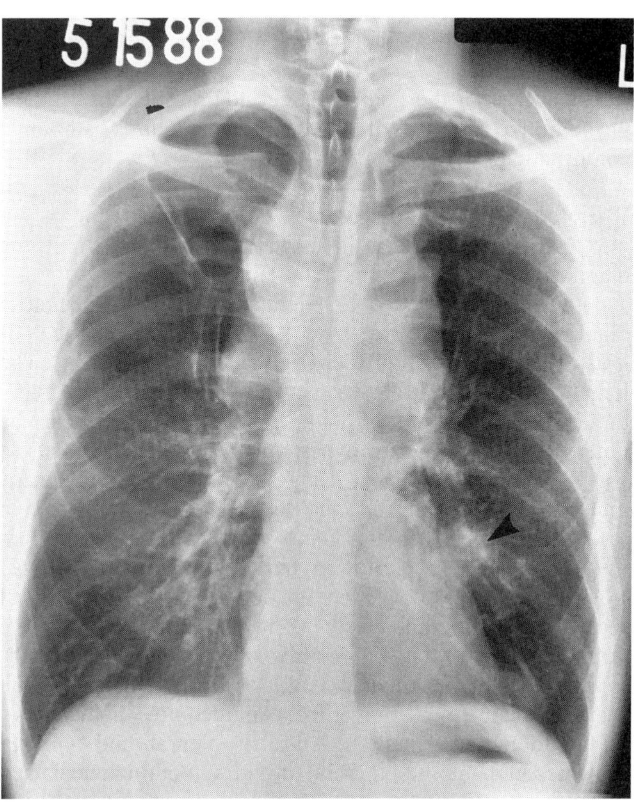

Fig. 81-3. Small-cell carcinoma. Note small parenchymal lesion *(arrow)* and massive mediastinal involvement.

same anatomic location or is slow to resolve radiographically (longer than 12 weeks) similarly suggests bronchial pathology, with either a partial intraluminal obstruction or an extrinsic compressing lesion. Thick-walled cavitary lesions with irregular intraluminal contours suggest squamous cell carcinoma (Fig. 81-2). Small-cell carcinomas tend to present as a rapidly progressing hilar or perihilar mass with mediastinal adenopathy (Fig. 81-3). Other unusual radiographic presentations of bronchogenic carcinoma include multicentric alveolar infiltrates that mimic an infectious or inflammatory process, as seen in bronchoalveolar cell carcinoma (Fig. 81-4).

Computed Tomography. A CT scan of the chest complements the radiographic information. For solitary pulmonary nodules, CT may clarify patterns of calcification and delineate border contours, which may assist in the assessment of benignancy. A chest CT scan offers superior visualization of the mediastinum, the site of early local metastases, and therefore can identify a more advanced stage than chest radiography. CT also clearly defines the anatomic location of the suspected lesion, characterizing its relationship to the pleura, chest wall, and mediastinum, which facilitates clinical staging and more invasive evaluation.

Magnetic Resonance Imaging. Compared with CT, MRI offers superior contrast resolution and excellent visualization of vascular structures without the need for intravenous contrast. Its major limitations are greater expense, limited availability, and inability to visualize

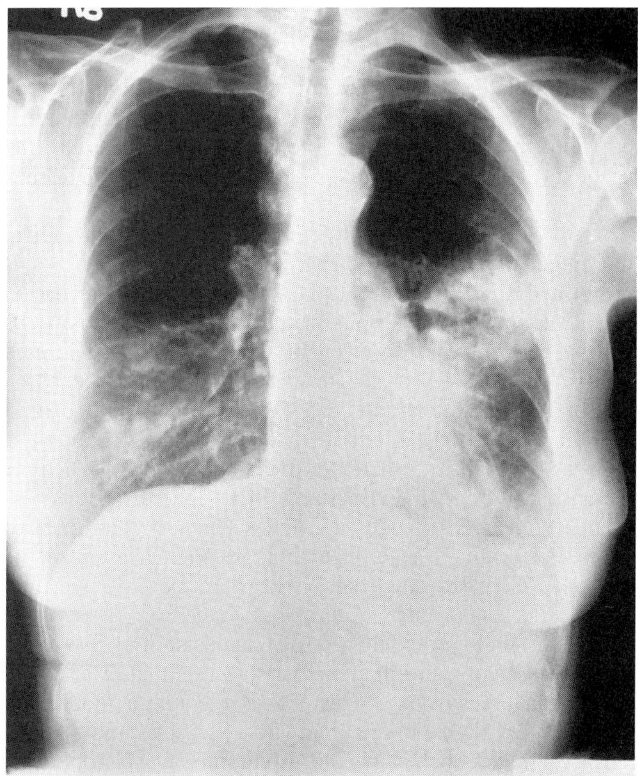

Fig. 81-4. Bronchoalveolar cell carcinoma, showing bilateral multiple pneumonic infiltrates.

calcium directly. The role of MRI is limited to assessment of vascular or chest wall invasion, as in tumors of the superior sulcus.

Regardless of the findings suggested on imaging studies, the definitive diagnosis of lung carcinoma requires pathologic confirmation.

Cytopathology. A sputum cytologic evaluation is an inexpensive and the least invasive means of confirming the diagnosis of lung carcinoma. The examination of five spontaneously collected or induced sputum specimens obtained on consecutive days offers a diagnostic yield of greater than 90% for squamous cell carcinoma histology. The larger and more centrally located the lesion, the more likely the cytology will be positive. Sputum induction can be obtained with aerosolized hypertonic 3% to 5% saline, sterile water, or propylene glycol using an ultrasonic nebulizer. Its major limitation is that it offers no insight into the anatomic location of the offending tumor; thus a positive sputum cytology should be followed by a bronchoscopic airway examination. This applies to all patients except when surgical resection is contraindicated, as in those with prohibitive pulmonary function or active coronary artery disease (CAD).

Pleural fluid in the presence of a suspected lung carcinoma may represent a malignant effusion and requires thoracentesis with cytologic examination. A positive pleural fluid cytology indicates inoperability, thereby providing both diagnosis and staging in a single minimally invasive procedure. Several hundred milliliters should be submitted for each examination. Blind closed-needle pleural biopsy adds little diagnostically to the cytologic evaluation, since pleural metastases are focal and begin near the mediastinum and diaphragm. Costal and cephalad spread occurs late with more advanced disease. Nonmalignant causes of a pleural effusion in the setting of lung carcinoma include parapneumonic effusion from postobstructive pneumonitis, pulmonary embolism from the hypercoagulable state, lymphatic or mediastinal lymph node obstruction from tumor involvement, and transudative effusion from low oncotic pressure associated with the cachexia and catabolic state associated with malignancies.

Fiberoptic Bronchoscopy. FOB is an important tool in the diagnosis and evaluation of carcinoma of the lung. It is performed under topical anesthesia with conscious sedation and does not require hospitalization. In skilled hands, FOB can be performed safely even in patients who have limited pulmonary reserve. The diagnostic yield of FOB depends on the tumor's location and size (Table 81-1). With central tumors greater than 2 cm in diameter, diagnosis by FOB approaches 60%. This increases to greater than 90% when the lesion can be directly visualized. In peripheral lesions less than 2 cm, FOB provides a diagnosis in less than 20% of cases. Performing transbronchial biopsies under fluoroscopic guidance increases diagnostic yield when the lesions cannot be directly visualized.

In addition to providing a tissue diagnosis, FOB also offers important staging information. Tumors less than 2 cm from the carina are labeled T_3 lesions by the tumor, node, and metastasis (TNM) classification (Box 81-2 and Table 81-2). Positive transbronchial needle aspiration of subcarinal and precarinal lymph nodes confirms N_2 nodal status. In 2% to 5% of patients with a unilateral lung mass, a synchronous endobronchial lesion in the contralateral lung is noted on a surveillance airway examination (M_1 lesion). All these findings suggest a higher stage with more advanced disease, limiting successful surgical resection and necessitating a different therapeutic intervention.

Table 81-1. Transthoracic Needle Aspiration (TNA) vs. Fiberoptic Bronchoscopy (FOB)

	TNA	FOB
Lesion size	≤2 cm	>2 cm
Clinical symptoms	None	Cough, blood-tinged sputum
Clinical diagnosis	Malignancy	Both malignant and benign processes
Airway examination (staging)	Not possible	Routine
Pneumothorax	25%-30%	<5%

Transthoracic Needle Aspiration. Fluoroscopic or CT-directed TNA has a greater positive predictive value than FOB in establishing the diagnosis of malignancy in small (less than 2 cm) peripheral lesions (see Table 81-1). Its major limitations are low negative predictive value (i.e., a negative TNA does not exclude the diagnosis of malignancy) and higher complication rate. The role of TNA in the diagnosis of lung cancer should be limited to (1) patients with multiple pulmonary nodules suggestive of metastatic disease and (2) when a definitive preoperative diagnosis of lung cancer is necessary to warrant the risks of general anesthesia and thoracotomy. An elderly patient with advanced COPD and active CAD is an ideal candidate for TNA. An otherwise healthy, middle-aged smoker with an enlarging peripheral, spiculated, noncalcified nodule should *not* be subjected to TNA but rather taken directly to surgical resection once the fiberoptic airway examination has excluded synchronous contralateral disease.

Mediastinoscopy and Thoracoscopy. Lymph nodes of the mediastinum are the usual sites of early metastases in NSCLC. These include the superior and inferior mediastinal, aortic, and hilar lymph nodes. In the patient with bronchogenic carcinoma, lymph nodes greater than 1 cm in their short axis (as visualized on chest CT scan) have an 80% probability of being malignant. Mediastinoscopy is a surgical technique that allows direct visualization of the superior mediastinum. Subcarinal, aortopulmonary window, and periaortic lymphadenopathy can be better assessed by an anterior mediastinotomy or Chamberlain procedure. Relative contraindications to mediastinoscopy include prior mediastinal radiation and previous tracheostomy. Similar to bronchoscopic attempts at transbronchial needle aspiration (TBNA) of pathologic lymph nodes, the role of mediastinoscopy is to detect advanced disease and therefore exclude patients from futile attempts at thoracotomy and lung resections. Perioperative identification of contralateral lymph node involvement (N_3) by mediastinoscopy or transbronchial aspiration is a contraindication to surgical resection (stage IIIb). Perioperative identification of N_2 lymph nodes by mediastinoscopy

Box 81-2. Tumor, Node, and Metastasis (TNM) Classification

Primary Tumor (T)

T_{is} Carcinoma in situ

T_1 Tumor 3 cm or less in greatest diameter, surrounded by lung or visceral pleura, without bronchoscopic evidence of invasion more proximal than lobar bronchus

T_2 Any of the following: tumor 3 cm or larger; tumor involving main bronchus 2 cm or more from carina; tumor invading visceral pleura; or atelectasis or obstructive pneumonitis extending to hilum but not involving entire lung

T_3 Tumor of any size that invades chest wall, diaphragm, or mediastinal, parietal, or pericardial pleura; tumor involving main bronchus 2 cm or less from but not involving carina; or atelectasis or postobstructive pneumonitis involving entire lung

T_4 Tumor of any size that invades mediastinum, heart, great vessels, trachea, esophagus, vertebral body, or carina; tumors that have malignant pleural or pericardial effusion; or satellite tumor nodules within ipsilateral primary tumor lobe of lung

Regional Lymph Node (N)

N_0 No regional lymph node metastasis

N_1 Metastasis to ipsilateral peribronchial or ipsilateral hilar lymph nodes and intrapulmonary lymph nodes

N_2 Metastasis to ipsilateral mediastinal or subcarinal lymph nodes

N_3 Metastasis to contralateral mediastinal, contralateral hilar, ipsilateral or contralateral scalene, and supraclavicular lymph nodes

Distant Metastasis (M)

M_0 No distant metastasis

M_1 Distant metastasis present

Modified from Mountain CF: Revisions in the international system for staging lung cancer, *Chest* 111:1718, 1997.

or TBNA (stage IIIa) carries a survival disadvantage (5-year survival of 9% vs. 24% if pathologically negative), and some thoracic surgeons believe this precludes candidacy for surgical resection.

Video-assisted thoracoscopy (VATS) or minimally invasive surgery results in less patient discomfort and shorter hospital stays compared with thoracotomy. The role of VATS in the surgical management of lung carcinoma has been questioned because incomplete visualization and inadequate mediastinal lymph node dissection make it inferior to standard thoracotomy. Staging is therefore inadequate using VATS, and candidates for combined-modality therapy for their advanced disease are missed. The ideal candidate for VATS has a small peripheral tumor and a normal mediastinum on chest CT or has marginal pulmonary function that allows only a wedge resection or segmentectomy. Alternatively, VATS-directed pleural biopsy is superior to pleural fluid cytologic examination obtained by thoracentesis and closed pleural biopsy in the diagnosis of malignant effusions.

Table 81-2. Stage Grouping of TNM Subsets in Lung Cancer

Stage	TNM subset(s)
Occult carcinoma	$T_{is}N_0M_0$
Ia	$T_1N_0M_0$
Ib	$T_2N_0M_0$
IIa	$T_1N_1M_0$
IIb	$T_2N_1M_0$, $T_3N_0M_0$
IIIa	$T_3N_1M_0$, $T_1N_2M_0$, $T_2N_2M_0$, $T_3N_2M_0$
IIIb	$T_4N_0M_0$, $T_4N_1M_0$, $T_4N_2M_0$, $T_1N_3M_0$, $T_2N_3M_0$, $T_3N_3M_0$, $T_4N_3M_0$
IV	Any T, any N, M_1

Modified from Mountain CF: Revisions in the international system for staging lung cancer, *Chest* 111:1718, 1997.

Staging

Once the diagnosis of lung carcinoma has been established, whether by sputum cytology, FOB, or TNA, staging is essential for the treatment planning and prognostication. A standardized staging system also allows comparison of results from multicenter treatment trials. The International Staging System was developed for staging of NSCLCs based on the TNM classification (see Table 81-2 and Box 81-2). Table 81-3 lists a recommended workup for staging both NSCLC and SCLC.

Clinical staging must be distinguished from pathologic or surgical staging. *Clinical staging* relies on the information obtained by noninvasive imaging and often underestimates the extent of disease and therefore survival. *Pathologic staging* is done at the time of mediastinal lymph node dissection and is more accurate. Table 81-4 shows the percentage of patients surviving 5 years after initial diagnosis and treatment. The cell type of NSCLC also adversely affects prognosis. For a similar stage, survival is least for giant cell and greatest for squamous cell, with large cell and adenocarcinoma interposed. Staging for small-cell carcinoma is much simpler because most patients with this type of carcinoma have distant metastases at diagnosis. Although the TNM staging system is appropriate, most oncologists use a modified staging system for SCLC (Table 81-5). The 5-year survival of patients with limited SCLC is 17% and for extensive disease is 3%.

Solitary Pulmonary Nodule

Solitary pulmonary nodule (SPN) is a fairly common radiographic entity. It is usually an incidental finding on a chest radiograph and is defined as a round or oval peripheral density surrounded by aerated lung tissue, with the largest diameter less than 4 cm and without associated hilar or mediastinal lymph node involvement or pleural effusion.

The etiology of an SPN differs greatly depending on geographic location. In developing countries, many SPNs represent infectious processes, particularly tuberculous granuloma. In the United States and other developed countries, approximately 40% of SPNs are the result of bronchogenic carcinoma. When a lung carcinoma presents as an SPN and is resected early, it is potentially curable, as evidenced by a 65% to 75% 5-year survival for $T_1N_0M_0$ lesions. Therefore the differentiation between a benign and malignant SPN is

Table 81-3. Recommended Staging Workup for NSCLC and SCLC

	NSCLC	SCLC
Initial diagnostic evaluation	H&P, CXR, chest CT, pulmonary function tests	H&P, CXR, chest CT, CBC with review smear, serum chemistry profile
Tissue confirmation	Sputum cytology, FOB vs. TNA, thoracentesis if pleural effusion	FOB, thoracentesis if pleural effusion, mediastinoscopy
Further studies	As indicated by initial evaluation	As indicated by initial evaluation
Neurologic symptoms	Brain MRI	Brain/spine MRI
Mediastinal adenopathy	Transbronchial needle aspiration, mediastinoscopy	Transbronchial needle aspiration, mediastinoscopy
Palpable lymph node	TNA	TNA
Elevated alkaline phosphatase or serum calcium	Bone scan with plain film correlation; biopsy if single lesion to confirm M_1 disease	Bone scan with plain film correlation; biopsy if single lesion to confirm extensive disease
Leukoerythroblastosis	—	Bone marrow biopsy
Elevated transaminases	Liver CT or ultrasound; biopsy if single lesion to confirm M_1 disease	Liver CT or ultrasound; biopsy if single lesion to confirm extensive disease

NSCLC, Non–small-cell lung carcinoma; *SCLC*, small-cell lung carcinoma; *H&P*, history and physical examination; *CXR*, chest radiograph; *CT*, computed tomography; *CBC*, complete blood count; *MRI*, magnetic resonance imaging; *FOB*, fiberoptic bronchoscopy; *TNA*, transthoracic needle aspiration.

Table 81-4. Five-year Survival According to Stage in NSCLC

Stage	TNM subset	5-year survival (%)
Ia	$T_1N_0M_0$	67
Ib	$T_2N_0M_0$	57
IIa	$T_1N_1M_0$	55
IIb	$T_2N_1M_0$ or $T_3N_0M_0$	39
IIIa	$T_{1-3}N_2M_0$	25
IIIb	T_4, any N M_0 or any T, N_3M_0	5
IV	Any T, any N, M_1	1

From Mountain CF: Revisions in the international system for staging lung cancer, *Chest* 111:1718, 1997.

Table 81-5. Modified Staging for SCLC

Stage	Description	Presenting stage (%)
Limited	Disease confined to one hemithorax with or without ipsilateral or contralateral mediastinal, supraclavicular lymph node, or ipsilateral pleural effusion	30-40
Extensive	Any disease at any site beyond limited definition	60-70

From Johnson BE: Management of small-cell lung cancer, *Clin Chest Med* 41:173, 1993.

crucial. The patient's age, smoking history, environmental tobacco exposure, occupational carcinogen exposure, and past residency are important clinical factors. Nonsmoking patients under age 35 have less than a 1% chance that their SPN is malignant. For smokers over 40 with more than 20 pack-years (pack/day) of smoking, the risk of malignancy equals their age.

The chest radiograph provides important findings to differentiate benign from malignant lesions. If the diameter of the lesion is smaller than 1 cm and borders are smooth and nonspiculated, it is most likely benign. If the SPN is larger than 3 cm, it has a 90% chance of being malignant. The presence and pattern of calcification are other important radiographic features. Benign patterns of calcification include central, lamellar, or popcorn calcification, with the latter suggesting a hamartoma, the most common benign neoplasm of the lung. Peripheral calcification suggests malignancy. Previous chest radiographs are essential. If the lesion is stable for more than 2 years, it is probably benign. Similarly, if the SPN doubles its volume in either less than every 20 days or more than 400 days, it is benign. Unfortunately, the smallest size at which a SPN can be reliably identified by chest radiography is a 1-cm nodule. At this size, it has already undergone 20 doubling times and consists of more than 1 million cells. When it has increased from 1 cm in diameter to 2 cm, 50% of patients already have evidence of metastases, increasing their concern when they are assigned to a watch-and-wait algorithm for management of their SPN.

When a standard chest radiograph does not show the characteristic calcifications and no previous chest radiographs are available, a chest CT scan should be obtained. If the CT scan does not demonstrate the benign nature of a lesion, a more invasive approach becomes necessary. FOB or TNA should be the next diagnostic procedure. FOB is useful for patients who have clinical complaints that suggest bronchial involvement, such as increased cough or blood-tinged sputum. TNA should be reserved for peripheral lesions and when a confirmed preoperative diagnosis of lung cancer is necessary to justify the perioperative risks of thoracotomy, as in patients with major surgical risk factors. All others should have thoracotomy. A watch-and-wait approach to an indeterminate SPN should be reserved for patients who have a low probability of cancer, have major surgical risk factors, or who refuse exploratory thoracotomy.

Management

Surgery. For NSCLC, surgery is the best method to achieve long-term survival or cure. All patients in clinical stages I and II should be offered surgery unless they have severely compromised pulmonary function or unstable CAD. Preoperative assessment should include spirometry, an electrocardiogram (ECG), and a thorough cardiac history. Cardiology consultation is necessary for patients with significant cardiac disease, since cardiac problems are the most common complications after lung cancer surgery. Surgical resection offers the best attempt at cure while preserving remaining lung function, thus ensuring a satisfactory quality of life. Determining postoperative pulmonary function is based on the extent of resection, preoperative spirometry, and the contribution of the diseased segment, lobe, or lung to total pulmonary function. An accepted approach is to retain at least 35% of normal pulmonary function values after a lobectomy and 40% after a pneumonectomy. In most patients this would result in a tolerable decrement in exercise tolerance, usually without the requirement of chronic ambulatory oxygen therapy. To determine the predicted postoperative forced expiratory volume in 1 second (FEV_1) and diffusing lung capacity for carbon monoxide (DLco), the following equation is used:

Predicted postoperative FEV_1 = Preoperative FEV_1 − [Preoperative FEV_1 × (Number of segments removed/Total number of segments) × Percent function of that lung]

Of the 19 total lung segments, three are in the right upper lobe, two in the right middle lobe, five in the right lower lobe, four in the left upper lobe, and five in the left lower lobe. A quantitative perfusion scan determines the percentage that the diseased lung contributes to the entire system, since substantial differences can occur in regional ventilation with bullous emphysema or a large mass. When the predicted postoperative FEV_1 is less than 40%, postoperative DLco and gas exchange at rest and with exercise are determined. If the predicted postoperative FEV_1 is less than 30%, the patient is not a candidate for a lobectomy. If it is greater than 40%, the patient is a candidate for a pneumonectomy. If the predicted postoperative FEV_1 is 30% to 40%, candidacy for a lobectomy depends on the predicted postoperative DLco being greater than 40% and a fall in Sao_2 being less than 2% at maximal exercise. For selected borderline patients, some centers advocate formal cardiopulmonary exercise testing, with a maximal oxygen consumption ($\dot{V}o_2$) greater than 20 ml/kg/min determining surgical candidacy.

Limited surgery that includes wedge resection and segmentectomy can be offered to patients with unsatisfactory pulmonary function. These surgical techniques, however, are associated with increased risk of local recurrence and decreased long-term survival, particularly with adenocarcinoma. A number of surgical techniques, such as sleeve resection and bilobectomy, have been developed to preserve nondiseased lung and thus postoperative pulmonary function. Tumor invasion of the intrapulmonary or hilar lymph nodes (N_1 disease, stage II NSCLC) decreases survival (67% vs. 55% 5-year survival for $T_1N_0M_0$ vs. $T_1N_1M_0$), and adjuvant therapy with radiation and chemotherapy is usually considered at this time. Many patients with clinical stage IIIa disease are potential surgical candidates, although long-term survival for this group is poor, with 5-year survival of 25%. Selected patients may qualify for neoadjuvant chemotherapy and radiation followed by surgical resection in a multicenter study using only the newer chemotherapeutic agents. Patients with stages IIIb and IV NSCLC are not considered surgical candidates. Management of small-cell carcinoma consists of chemotherapy and radiation. The value of surgery followed by chemotherapy in selected patients with limited SCLC has yet to be established.

Radiation Therapy. The efficacy of radiation therapy is limited in part by toxicity to the local tissues and adjacent organs. Lower, less toxic doses (and thus less effective therapy) are usually offered when the disease is deemed unresectable at thoracotomy or, regardless of stage, when the patient is deemed inoperable because of comorbid medical problems or when the patient refuses surgery. Postoperative or adjuvant radiation therapy does not increase survival in patients with stage I NSCLC who have complete surgical resection of their lesion. Because they are at risk for a second primary tumor involving their aerodigestive tract (3% to 5% per year), these patients should be followed closely for the first 5 years after resection. Patients with stage I NSCLC who are unwilling or unable to undergo resection should be offered radiation therapy with the intent to cure. A 5-year survival of up to 20% may be achieved for patients with small peripheral lesions. It is important to remember that lung function is lost through surgical resection and radiation-induced fibrotic changes. For patients with intrapulmonary and hilar lymph node metastasis (N_1 disease, stage II NSCLC), adjuvant radiation therapy offers improved control of local disease recurrence but has no effect on distant metastases or 5-year survival. Therefore the routine use of postoperative radiation therapy for completely resected stage II NSCLC is not supported.

Preoperative radiation therapy delivered outside a protocol is advocated only for superior sulcus tumors in patients with Pancoast's syndrome. In this setting, benefit is reported only from small, uncontrolled studies. Although patients with stage III disease often receive radiation treatment with a curative dose, long-term survival is seldom achieved. In stage IV disease, radiation therapy is used for palliative purposes, most often to control pain from bone metastases. Other indications include obstruction or narrowing of large airways that causes distal pneumonia or dyspnea and obstruction of a large vessel, as in superior vena cava syndrome. Radiation treatment often provides significant symptomatic relief in these patients. Brachytherapy is a form of local radiation in which a source of radioactivity is placed directly in the involved airway to minimize the effects on the surrounding normal lung tissue.

Chemotherapy. Chemotherapy is the preferred treatment in small-cell lung carcinoma. The use of traditional agents (etoposide and cisplatin or cyclophosphamide, doxorubicin and vincristine) has been disappointing, however, with only 17% and 3% 5-year survival for limited and extensive stages, respectively. A current approach uses etoposide and cisplatin with radiotherapy; however, the 5% increase in 2-year survival for those with limited disease is offset by increased pulmonary, bone marrow, and esophageal toxicity. Long-term survival can be achieved in a small percentage of patients with limited disease. Unfortunately, these long-term survivors have a 50% risk for cranial metastases and a 3% to 5% incidence per year of a second primary lung lesion.

The role of chemotherapy in NSCLC is undergoing intensive investigation. Studies have shown promising results for preoperative chemotherapy (neoadjuvant) in carefully selected stage II and IIIa NSCLC. Similarly, treatment of locally advanced or inoperable stage III and IV NSCLC with combined-modality therapy (radiation plus chemotherapy) that includes newer chemotherapeutic agents (e.g., paclitaxel) has shown promising results in patients with good performance status (e.g., Karnofksy, greater than 70%).

Other Treatment Modalities. Obstruction of the central airways is a common presenting feature of bronchogenic carcinoma, particularly among squamous cell and small-cell cancers. The proximal location of the lesion often leads to severe dyspnea or a postobstructive pneumonia with possible cavitation. Removal of the obstructing endobronchial component offers immediate palliative symptom control and may improve short-term survival. This can be achieved with a neodynium:YAG laser delivered either through a flexible fiberoptic or rigid bronchoscope under general anesthesia in the operating room by a bronchoscopist. The tissue effects of neodynium:YAG laser include photocoagulation and thermal necrosis, which can penetrate from several millimeters to several centimeters. Endobronchial radiation therapy (brachytherapy), another effective modality to treat centrally obstructing lesions, can be used either with laser bronchoscopy when the lesion has an endobronchial component or alone when there is extrinsic compression only. Bronchoscopically placed endobronchial catheters are afterloaded with radioactive seeds to deliver local radiation with controlled depth of penetration. The use of endobronchial stents to maintain airway patency is best suited for patients with extrinsic compression that is not controlled with brachytherapy.

Early Detection

Despite the observations that early-stage lung cancer is common, is usually asymptomatic, is amenable to surgical resection, and has the best 5-year survival rate, large-scale cooperative studies designed to detect early-stage lung cancer by chest radiograph and sputum cytology failed to show any benefit in overall mortality. Theories to account for this have included the heterogeneity of the disease itself, the limited sensitivity of radiography for all cell types and of sputum cytology for non–squamous cell carcinomas, and the ineffectiveness of current treatment strategies for advanced disease. Often-cited errors in the study design include biases of selection, lead time, length of time, overdiagnosis, and contamination by poor compliance to screening algorithm. Because of this the National Cancer Institute (NCI) has sponsored the Prostate, Lung, Colon, and Ovary Cancer Screening Trial. The lung cancer arm is designed to look at the usefulness of a yearly chest film in reducing cancer-specific mortality, but results will not be available for about 15 years. In the interim the American Cancer Society, American College of Radiology, NCI, and the U.S. Preventative Services Task Force do *not* advocate a routine chest radiograph for the mass screening of lung cancer in asymptomatic adults. We advocate annual screening chest radiography in high-risk patients, however, including those with a smoking history of greater than a 40 pack-years and any one or more of the following: COPD, family history of lung cancer, prior history of lung cancer, asbestos, radon or other occupational carcinogen exposure, and chronic fibrotic lung disease of any etiology.

Future developments in the field of lung cancer screening will include the use of serum biomarkers and diagnostic photodynamic therapy. The latter uses a photosensitizing agent and light source delivered through a fiberoptic bronchoscope to detect carcinoma in situ.

Prevention

Each day, 3000 U.S. teenagers take up the deadly, lifelong habit of cigarette smoking; 1 in 20 will develop lung cancer, and 90% will die from it. Less than 30% of individuals are successful in obtaining long-term smoking cessation, and the risk of developing lung cancer attributable to former cigarette smoking continues beyond 20 years after smoking cessation is complete. These facts emphasize the importance of primary prevention: discouraging those contemplating cigarette smoking from beginning. The physician's efforts at encouraging smoking cessation should not be discounted. The use of tobacco by white males has been declining for the past several decades as the result of intensive antismoking campaigns, and other demographic groups need to be targeted as well.

METASTATIC CARCINOMA OF THE LUNG

Because of their anatomic location, the lungs are common sites of metastases from malignant neoplasms outside the thorax. Patients with metastatic neoplasm of the lungs often have a known primary site or a recent history of malignancy, although occasionally the metastatic lesion is discovered without an identified site. Metastatic malignancy of the lung usually presents as multiple nodular lesions on the chest radiograph. When it appears as an SPN on the chest radiograph, a CT chest scan often reveals other lesions that are not apparent on the chest radiograph. Careful history, physical examination, and simple laboratory tests (e.g., urinalysis, stool guaiac test) usually suggest the primary site. Common primary sites are the genitourinary system in males (hypernephroma, transitional cell carcinoma of urinary bladder, germ cell tumor of testis) and the breasts and reproductive system in females (breast cancer, cervical cancer, choriocarcinoma). Gastrointestinal (gastric, pancreatic, and colorectal) carcinoma and head and neck carcinoma in smokers are frequent primary sites in both genders. In younger individuals the primary sites include muscle, bone, cartilage, and testes (e.g., leiomyosarcoma, osteosarcoma, synovial cell sarcoma). In some patients the metastasis occurs in the bronchial submucosa and causes an endobronchial lesion with associated symptoms and signs. In patients with endobronchial involvement the diagnosis can be made by FOB, whereas in those with single or multiple peripheral lesions the diagnosis is often made by TNA. Occasionally a thoracotomy is necessary to establish the diagnosis. The treatment of metastatic lesion(s) in the lung depends on the condition of the primary site. Surgery is usually not indicated after the lesions are diagnosed as metastatic neoplasms. Surgical resections have been performed occasionally, however, for select patients when primary tumors have been completely resected, there is no sign of local recurrence, and the lung lesion(s) can be completely resected without serious consequence to pulmonary function.

A less common but clinically important presentation is *lymphangitic metastasis*. This type of metastatic spread is usually seen in patients with carcinoma of the stomach, the pancreas, and the lung. The patient presents with rapidly progressive dyspnea, and the chest radiograph shows linear and coarse, irregular nodular infiltrates, often in the distribution of a segment or a lobe. Hilar and mediastinal lymph nodes are often enlarged. When a patient with carcinoma of the lung who underwent or is undergoing radiation treatment presents with lymphangitic metastasis, a differential diagnosis for radiation pneumonitis is important because this condition responds to treatment with steroids. Presumptive diagnosis of radiation pneumonitis can often be made on the basis of clinical and radiographic findings, and a trial of steroids may be given. Occasionally a lung biopsy is necessary to confirm the diagnosis.

LYMPHOMA

Lymphoma is a malignant disease of the lymphatic tissue and frequently involves the intrathoracic lymph node as well as the lung parenchyma. Lymphoma is usually divided into Hodgkin's disease and non-Hodgkin's lymphoma.

Hodgkin's Disease

Both Hodgkin's disease and non-Hodgkin's lymphoma occur in all age groups; however, Hodgkin's disease is more likely in younger persons. The peak incidence of Hodgkin's disease is the third decade, whereas non-Hodgkin's lymphoma is seen more often in patients over age 50. Involvement of the intrathoracic structures by Hodgkin's disease is usually a part of the generalized disease process, and primary pulmonary Hodgkin's disease is very rare. Patients with Hodgkin's disease usually have constitutional symptoms such as general malaise, easy fatigability, fever, and weight loss at presentation. Physical examination often reveals peripheral lymph node enlargement and anemia. When the disease involves the thorax, it usually presents as mediastinal and hilar lymph node enlargement on chest radiograph. The mediastinal and hilar lymph node enlargement is usually asymmetric but bilateral. The involvement of the lung parenchyma is uncommon and is almost always associated with a mediastinal mass. The lung parenchymal involvement is more often seen in patients with a nodular sclerosis type and is usually the result of direct extension of the mediastinal process. Occasionally it may cause a compression of the airway or actual invasion of the bronchus, resulting in atelectasis or distal pneumonia.

The major differential diagnosis of intrathoracic Hodgkin's disease is sarcoidosis (see Chapter 78). Patients with sarcoidosis who have bilateral hilar lymphadenopathy are usually asymptomatic unless there is a significant lung involvement. The diagnosis of sarcoidosis is usually made with FOB and transbronchoscopic lung biopsy, which has a very high diagnostic yield (80% to 85%), even for patients without appreciable lung parenchymal involvement on chest radiograph. The diagnosis of Hodgkin's disease confined in the mediastinum often requires mediastinoscopy.

Treatment of Hodgkin's disease is a combination of radiation and chemotherapy. The response to treatment and the prognosis for patients with Hodgkin's disease are generally better than for patients with non-Hodgkin's lymphoma.

Non-Hodgkin's Lymphoma

Non-Hodgkin's lymphoma is a heterogenous group of malignant diseases of lymphatic origin and frequently involves the mediastinum and the lungs. Non-Hodgkin's lymphoma is sometimes classified as primary and secondary lymphoma. In primary pulmonary lymphoma, only the lung is involved at diagnosis, with no evidence of extrathoracic dissemination for at least 3 months after the initial diagnosis. In secondary pulmonary lymphoma, patients are known to have disease outside the thorax before the pulmonary involvement. Pathologically the most common cell of primary pulmonary lymphoma is a small lymphocytic type. Radiographically, primary lymphoma manifests as reticulonodular, nodular, or parenchymal consolidation. Clinically, most patients with primary lymphoma are asymptomatic. The histologic diagnosis can be made by examination of FOB specimens but often requires thoracotomy. Secondary pulmonary lymphoma occurs much more frequently than primary pulmonary lymphoma. The most common radiographic manifestation of secondary pulmonary lymphoma is mediastinal and hilar lymph node enlargement. When the lungs are involved, the lesion may present as an SPN or as multiple nodules. Cavitation may occur, but less often than in Hodgkin's disease. The lesion may extend to the large airway and cause an atelectasis or a distal pneumonia. Clinical presentation depends on the extent of extrathoracic disease. Constitutional symptoms, such as fever, anorexia, and weight loss, typically occur.

Treatment of non-Hodgkin's lymphoma is a combination of chemotherapy and radiation. Response to treatment and prognosis are less favorable than for Hodgkin's disease.

ADDITIONAL READINGS

Bains MS: Surgical treatment of lung cancer, *Chest* 100:826, 1991.

Boring C, Squires TS, Tong T: Cancer statistics, *CA Cancer J Clin* 43:7, 1993.

Flehinger BJ, Kimmel M, Melmad MR: The effect of surgical treatment on survival from early lung cancer: implication for screening, *Chest* 101:1013, 1992.

Ihde DC: Chemotherapy of lung carcinoma, *N Engl J Med* 327:1434, 1992.

Jett J: Pretreatment evaluation of non-small-cell lung cancer, Am J Respir Crit Care Med 156:320-332, 1997.

Mountain CF, Greenberg SD, Fraire AE: Tumor stage in non–small-cell carcinoma of the lung, *Chest* 99:1258, 1991.

Murren JR, Buzaid AC: Chemotherapy and radiation for the treatment of non–small-cell lung cancer, *Clin Chest Med* 14:161, 1993.

V DERMATOLOGY

CHAPTER 82

Diagnosis and Examination Techniques

Frank Parker
James C. Shaw

AN APPROACH TO DIAGNOSING SKIN DISEASE

Dermatology is a visual specialty. The patient's skin condition is apparent and readily observed by the physician. Because there are hundreds of dermatoses, a logical process of elimination is needed to narrow the possibilities, first to a specific group of diseases and finally to one condition, when initially examining a patient with a skin disease. Such a diagnostic approach is based on specific morphologic description of the skin lesions along with an appropriate history and laboratory tests. This systems analysis approach to diagnosis involves three steps. First, the primary and secondary skin lesions are identified. Second the examiner places the patient in one of several major diagnostic groups of diseases. Many skin conditions are found in each of the groups, but all the diseases in a given group tend to manifest the same primary and secondary lesions. The third step involves selecting the one disease the patient has from the other conditions in the group. This step is accomplished by looking for specific features such as location and distribution of skin lesions, unusual shapes or arrangements of the lesions (annular, serpiginous, dermatomal), color, and surface characteristics (appearance of scales, verrucous or vegetative changes).

Step 1: Description of Primary and Secondary Skin Lesions

Primary skin lesions are uncomplicated lesions that represent the initial cutaneous pathologic changes uninfluenced by secondary alterations such as infection, trauma, or therapy. Secondary skin lesions are changes that occur as a result of progression of the disease, scratching, or infection of the primary lesion. At times primary changes also can occur as secondary manifestations (i.e., pustules may appear as primary lesions of folliculitis or as secondary lesions when pruritic primary lesions are scratched and infected). The challenge is to recognize a primary skin lesion as the initial change characteristic of a disease.

The terminology used to describe primary and secondary skin lesions is the basic language of dermatology, the means by which skin diseases are accurately described (Table 82-1). Each descriptive term is not only a short account of what is seen on the surface of the skin, but also implies specific information about pathologic processes within the skin.

Step 2: Assignment of Spectrum of Primary and Secondary Lesions to a Major Group of Skin Diseases

Each disease within a given group shares the same primary and secondary skin lesions. Because some diseases have overlapping traits, they may be assigned to more than one group. An arbitrary grouping of common skin diseases listed in Table 82-2 according to their dominant skin lesion is used in this section to facilitate discussion.

Step 3: Narrowing the Possibilities within a Given Group to the Exact Diagnosis

Several factors are important in identifying the specific skin condition within each group. The distribution of the skin lesions is important because many conditions have typical patterns or often affect specific regions. For example, psoriasis commonly affects extensor surfaces and atopic eczema involves flexor areas of extremities. Photoreactions are confined to the sun-exposed areas of the body. Involvement of the palms and soles is seen in erythema multiforme, secondary syphilis, psoriasis, and eczema. Contact dermatitis presents with unusual patterns corresponding to areas where the offending material contacts the skin.

A second important clue in differentiating diseases within a given group is the shape of individual lesions and the arrangement of lesions in relation to one another. For example the lesions of lichen planus characteristically are angular papules, whereas pityriasis rosea presents as oval, raised patches. A linear arrangement of lesions is typical of contact with an exogenous substance brushing across the skin or a cutaneous nevus. "Zosteriform" refers to lesions arranged along the cutaneous distribution of a spinal nerve in a bandlike, unilateral configuration (e.g., herpes zoster, dermatomal hemangiomas in Sturge-Weber syndrome) (Plate 16). Annular lesions are circular with normal skin in the center. Annular macules are observed in drug eruptions, secondary syphilis, and lupus erythematosus. Scaling annular lesions suggest dermatophytosis (Plate 17). Iris lesions are a special annular lesion in which a papule or vesicle evolves into the center-target or bullseye lesion typical of erythema multiforme (Plate 18). Urticaria polycyclic patterns evolve when numerous annular lesions enlarge and run together (hives). Serpiginous (snakelike patterns) are seen in creeping eruption (Plate 19). Herpetiform refers to the grouping of lesions seen in herpes simplex or dermatitis herpetiformis (Plate 5).

Other physical features are important in diagnosing skin diseases. Dry, lichenified lesions (Plate 10) suggest a chronic state of a disease, whereas wet, oozing, macerated lesions (Plate 15) suggest acute reactions. Nodular lesions that are soft, fluctuant, and tender suggest an abscess, whereas firm nodules are likely to be a benign or malignant tumor (Plate 1). Redness caused by dilation of superficial blood vessels blanches with pressure, whereas erythema caused by extravasated blood, as occurs in petechiae and purpura, does not blanch (Plate 20). Hues of blue and black indicate melanin pigment. The deeper the melanin pigmentation deposition in the skin, the bluer the color (Plate 21).

Table 82-1. Primary and Secondary Skin Lesions

Lesion	Description
Primary skin lesions	
Macule	Circumscribed change in skin color without elevation or depression of the surface, Example: erythema, purpura, café au lait, vitiligo (Plate 1).
Papule	A solid elevated area no more than 10 mm in diameter. Implies pathologic involvement of epidermis (especially if there is scaling or disturbance of the normal surface of the epidermis) or dermis (usually epidermal surface is normal but redness is present). Example: warts, molluscum contagiosum, lichen planus (Plate 2).
Nodule	Similar to a papule but larger (1 cm or larger in diameter) with visible elevation of the skin. It may represent a pathologic process in the epidermis, in which case it may be associated with scale, erosion, and loss of skin markings or dermis, where it may be fluctuant (if it is a cyst) or firm (if it is a skin cancer or granulomatous infiltrate). Example: cyst, basal cell carcinoma (Plate 21).
Plaque	Evolves from a confluence of papules leading to a flat-topped, circumscribed elevation. Example: psoriasis, urticaria, mycosis, fungoides (Plate 3).
Wheal	Special type of plaque. A slight elevation caused by movement of fluid out of blood vessels. Example: hives (Plate 4).
Vesicles and bullae	Circumscribed, elevated lesion with cavities containing free fluids that flow out if the lesion is pricked. Vesicles are less than 10 mm in diameter. Bullae are greater than 1 cm in diameter. Vesicles and bullae may evolve within the epidermis (Plates 5 and 6), in which case the fluid is usually clear serous. The lesions may be flaccid and easily break (i.e., very thin roof), or they may evolve at the DEJ, in which case the lesions are tense, may contain hemorrhagic fluid, and are less likely to rupture (thick roof). Umbilicated vesicles suggest viral-induced lesions (herpes simplex and zoster). Example: pemphigus, pemphigoid, porphyria cutanea tarda.
Pustule	A vesicle containing purulent exudate. Example: acne, folliculitis (Plate 7).
Scale	Desiccated thin plates of cornified epidermal cells that result from altered keratinization. Scale occurs when the epidermis is perturbed and involved scale assumes different appearances that can be useful in diagnosis, including, fine, thin squames seen in eczema or exfoliative dermatitis; thick, silvery scales typical of psoriasis (Plate 8).
Atrophy	Loss of tissue with depression of the surface of the skin. Atrophy may involve the epidermis with fine wrinkling and redness (stria) or the dermis with whitish depression (scleroderma) (Plate 9).
Telangiectasis	Persistent dilation of individual vessels in the skin, usually associated with alterations in the connective tissue of dermis. Example: connective tissue diseases, radiation skin damage (Plate 7).
Secondary skin lesions	
Lichenification	Dry, leathery thickening of the skin with exaggerated skin markings. Thickening of the epidermis resulting from repeated rubbing and scratching of the skin in chronic dermatitis. Example: atopic dermatitis, neurodermatitis (Plate 10).
Fissures	Erosion and breaks in the skin of varying depths and causes. Fissures are linear cracks in the skin, usually through the epidermis. Example: chronic eczema, perléche. Erosions are wide, shallow defects in the skin (Plate 11).
Ulcer	Deep loss of skin into the dermis and even into the subcutaneous tissue. Example: Venous and arterial ulcers (Plate 12).
Scar	An area of replacement fibrosis of the dermis or subcutaneous tissues. Scars vary in appearance and may be depressed or raised. Example: keloids may appear as nodules (Plate 13).
Crusts	Dried exudate of serum, blood, sebum, or purulent material on the skin surface after vesicles or bullae break down to release their contents (Plate 14).
Oozing	Loss of stratum corneum or breakdown of small vesicles with serum covering the skin surface. Example: acute dermatitis (Plate 15).

DEJ, Dermal-epidermal junction.

Dermatologic History

Although the clinical examination is vital in diagnosing skin disease, the history is also important and certain specific information should be determined if possible:

- *Onset:* Where precisely on the body did the condition begin? What did it look like? What are associated symptoms?
- *Course:* How did the disease progress and change? What has been done to treat the condition (by the patient or by physicians)? What is the relationship to vacations, seasons, the environment? Has the condition been continuous or intermittent?
- *Past Medical History:* Does the patient have other cutaneous diseases? Is there a history of atopy, endocrine conditions, skin, or other malignancies or autoimmune diseases?
- *Family History:* Is there a history of atopic diseases and allergies, psoriasis, or other inherited conditions in family members?
- *Work and Hobbies:* What work or hobbies of the patient may expose them to contactants?
- *Topical and Systemic Medications and Materials Used:* Because drug reactions are so common (both to topical and systemic medications—prescribed and over the counter), the physician should always be alert to this possibility. What medications does the patient apply,

Table 82-2. Major Groups of Skin Diseases

Skin disease	Dominant skin lesions
Dermatitis or eczemas	Erythema papules, vesicles, lichenification, oozing, crusts Example: contact dermatitis, atopic eczema, nummular eczema, stasis eczema
Papulosquamous skin diseases	Unique papules, plaques, and scales Example: psoriasis, pityriasis rosea, lichen planus
Pustular skin diseases	Papules and pustules Example: acne, rosacea, folliculitis
Nodular skin diseases	Epidermal and dermal nodules Example: benign skin tumors and malignant skin tumors
Vesiculobullous skin diseases	Vesicles and bullae Example: infectious—impetigo, herpes; immunologic—pemphigus and pemphigoid; mechanical—epidermolysis bullosa.
Pigmentary alterations of the skin	Hyperpigmented and hypopigmented macules Example: vitiligo, Addison's disease, albinism, melasma
Maculopapular eruptions	Macules and papules Example: childhood exanthems, drug eruptions, purpuric lesions
Special erythematous reactions of the skin	Macules and plaques Example: urticaria, dermatographism, insect bites
Ulcerative skin lesions	Example: pyoderma gangrenosum, ulcers due to vascular diseases, infectious ulcers

especially with rubber gloves? Does the patient use topical steroids? Are other cosmetics, anti-itch products, and other topical medications used? What medications are used in every orifice (i.e., eyedrops, eardrops, suppositories, oral). Even vitamins, cough medications, and birth control pills may cause skin reactions.

The chapters in this section deal with the major disease groups (e.g., dermatitis, papulosquamous, pustular). Not every skin group listed in Table 82-2 is identified as a separate chapter; some chapters are listed based on etiologic factors (e.g., infectious diseases of the skin, common reaction patterns [hives, erythema multiforme], and photoreaction). Nevertheless, it should be possible for the physician to "place" a patient presenting with a common skin condition into the appropriate chapter and further to arrive at a precise diagnosis if the steps in the preceding systematic clinical approach are followed.

In this section, skin conditions are discussed in association with internal diseases and in pediatric, geriatric, and black patients. Finally, a chapter on the general principles of dermatologic therapy is included to help the clinicians treat the common disorders.

EXAMINATION TECHNIQUES

The examination of the skin by inspection is the most valuable step in dermatologic diagnosis. The use of selected tests can be helpful in confirming or excluding suspected diagnoses. These include the potassium hydroxide (KOH) examination, Gram's stain, Tzanck smear, selected cultures, and skin biopsy for histologic examination. An understanding of when and how to perform these ancillary tests is essential in dermatologic diagnosis (Table 82-3).

Examination of the Skin

Morphology. Color, size, shape, texture, as well as the presence or absence of scale, serum crust, or pus, are a few important morphologic features of primary lesions that aid in making a correct diagnosis and communicating with dermatologists. Good lighting and magnification are important, and examination of the entire skin surface is frequently required.

Distribution. Certain diseases have characteristic distributions that are pathognomonic even if the primary lesions are not characteristic (i.e., herpes zoster in a dermatomal distribution and photo-related skin eruptions on sun-exposed areas: central face, extensor arms, and dorsal hands).

Palpation. While macules feel like normal skin, palpable lesions may reflect epidermal, dermal, or subcutaneous involvement. A rough surface or scaling suggests epidermal involvement; a smoother surface usually implies dermal or deeper involvement.

KOH Examination

KOH examination (Plates 22 and 23) of skin rapidly confirms or excludes tineas (dermatophyte fungi), candidiasis, scabies, or tinea versicolor (Fig. 82-1). The KOH examination helps dissolve keratin and allows for separation of aggregates of stratum corneum cells but does not disrupt the cell walls of fungi. All of the following steps must be optimal for a successful test:

1. Obtain copious scale with a no. 15 blade onto a glass slide. In annular lesions, scrape the peripheral scale. Center material on slide and place cover slip.
2. Apply KOH (10% to 20%). DMSO 5% helps with penetration of the KOH.*
3. Heat the slide, with gentle agitation. Blot excess fluid.
4. The microscope must have the appropriate optical settings. The ten power (10×) objective is the best to look for fungal hyphae. The four power (4×) is best for the larger scabies mites. In both cases, the visualization is optimal with a large depth of field made by closing down the iris or by

*Solution can be obtained from DELASCO, 800-831-6273.

Table 82-3. Ancillary Tests in Dermatology: When to Use Them

Test	Indications	Precautions
KOH (potassium hydroxide)	Fungal infections of skin or mucosa Tinea versicolor: short, plump hyphae and spores (see Fig. 82-1). Scabies: look for a linear burrow. Any red, scaly dermatosis where diagnosis uncertain	Large depth of field on microscope. Never need greater than 40× lens Debris can look like fungal hyphae Scabies: scan at low power (2× or 4×)
Gram's stain	Bacterial folliculitis (gram-positive cocci in clumps) Pustular eruption (sterile if psoriasis, drug reaction) Candida, when there are pustules (gram positive)	Federal regulations may not allow this test as an office procedure.
Tzanck smear	To confirm or rule out herpesvirus infection: HSV herpes zoster varicella Confirms molluscum bodies in material from molluscum lesions.	Frequently much cellular debris: PMNS, lymphocytes
Direct if for herpesvirus infection	Confirmation of herpesvirus Identifies HSV 1 and 2 and varicella-zoster virus	Requires special glass slides from laboratory.
Cultures	Bacterial infections Nasal staphylococcal carrier state Fungal disease: nail, scalp HSV: positive in 48-72 hours CMV infection	Negative result does not exclude infection. Positive bacterial culture may not be the primary cause of the disease (i.e., leg ulcers, mouth ulcers, crusted lesions)
Wood's light examination	Fungal infections (tinea capitis from *Microsporum* species fluoresces green) Inguinal dermatitis (erythrasma fluoresces coral red)	Not confirmatory Negative test does not rule out disease.
Skin biopsy	Any atypical dermatosis where a specific diagnosis will influence treatment. If malignancy is in the differential diagnosis If histologic confirmation is desirable by patient, epidemiologists, treating physicians Atypical presentations of common disorders Skin lesions in immunocompromised patients	Consultation by dermatologist may be more cost effective if no biopsy required. Many dermatoses do not have pathognomonic histologic findings. Sampling errors may hinder making a correct diagnosis. Pathology report without diagnostic possibilities (i.e., descriptive only) may not help in making the diagnosis.

HSV, Herpes simples virus; *PMNS*, polymorphonucleocytes; *CMV*, cytomegalovirus.

lowering the condenser lens. The forty power (40×) lens can be used to confirm findings but should not be used to search for fungi. The oil immersion (100×) lens is not necessary in the KOH examination and can actually hinder the chances of finding hyphae.

Gram's Stain

Once utilized and valued as a diagnostic test by physicians, recent federal regulations allow only certified laboratories to perform Gram's stains. Most specimens sent for culture will include a Gram's stain.

Tzanck Smear

The Tzanck smear is the most rapid way to identify herpesvirus infection, including herpes simplex virus (HSV), varicella, and herpes zoster. Any dark nuclear stain is acceptable. A 5% methylene blue solution is inexpensive and effective, but Wright's or Geimsa stain also work well.

Preparation. Open a vesicle and scrape the base or the under side of the blister roof. Smear onto a slide, air dry, and fix with absolute alcohol or gentle heating. Stain with Geimsa or Wright's for 1 minute or methylene blue for 15 seconds. Rinse, dry, and examine at 10× and 40× power. Immersion oil and a cover slip optimize the optics.

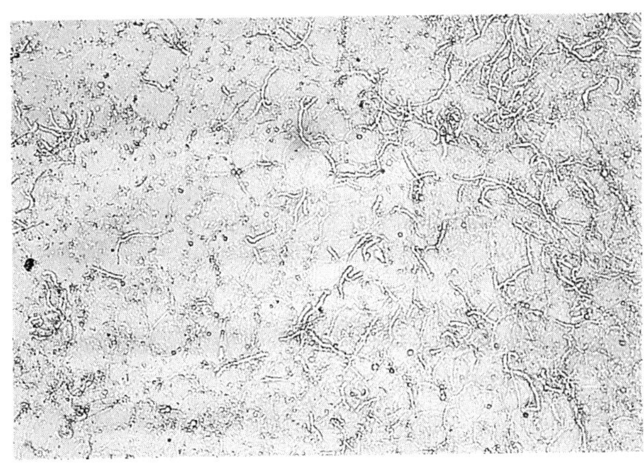

Fig. 82-1. KOH examination of tinea versicolor. Note shorter nonbranching hyphae.

Interpretation. Look for multinucleated keratinocytes (Plate 24). The keratinocytes become "fused" in herpesvirus infections and appear as large cells with multiple nuclei. Neutrophils and mononuclear cells frequently are also present on a Tzanck smear and are much smaller than the multinuclear keratinocytes.

Direct Immunofluorescence for Herpesvirus

Direct immunofluorescence (IF) is now available in most laboratories and is valuable in rapidly confirming the presence of HSV 1 or 2 or varicella-zoster virus. Obtain material as for a Tzanck smear and place in wells on special slides from the lab. Results are usually available within 2 hours.

Cultures

Fungal culture is most valuable in cases of tinea capitis and nail infections, both of which are difficult to diagnose by inspection and KOH examination. In tinea capitis, use either plucked hairs or swab/brush and place directly into media provided by the laboratory. Bacterial culture can be helpful in any atypical pustular eruption. Culture of the anterior nares is useful to diagnose a staphylococcal carrier state. HSV usually grows in 48 hours; varicella-zoster virus requires up to 4 weeks to grow and is frequently negative. Tissue cultures from biopsy specimens are indicated when deep fungi, atypical mycobacteria, or other deep bacterial involvement are suspected.

Wood's Light Examination

The use of a Wood's light (ultraviolet light, 360 nm) helps diagnose certain fungal and bacterial infections and helps delineate some disorders of pigmentation. Most tinea capitis does not fluoresce, since *Tinea tonsurans* became the predominant organism. Erythrasma, the intertriginous infection with *Corynebacterium minutissimum,* can fluoresce a coral-red color if the water soluble porphyrins have not been recently washed off.

Skin Biopsy

The punch biopsy is the most common form of skin biopsy, with punches ranging in size from 2 mm to 8 mm in diameter. Most skin diseases are best sampled by this method because the epidermis, dermis, and subcutaneous fat are present in one sample. If the skin lesion is raised above the skin surface, a shave biopsy of superficial skin can be used, and in cases where deep tissue or a larger sample are needed, an incisional or excisional biopsy is indicated.

Indications. There are no absolute indications for doing a skin biopsy. This is because there are frequently nonspecific histologic findings that do not allow confirmation of a particular diagnosis, and because management of the patient may not be affected by a histologic diagnosis. In cases where consultation by a dermatologist may obviate the need for biopsy, considerations pertaining to cost effectiveness may be important. In spite of these uncertainties, some general principles apply when considering performing a skin biopsy (see Table 82-3).

Procedure. In most cases the required materials include local anesthetic, a biopsy punch or scalpel, and means of achieving hemostasis. Healing is rapid after closure with sutures but usually is adequate when the wound is allowed to heal by granulation. Hemostatic products include aluminum chloride, silver nitrate, and Gelfoam packing.

Interpretation. Dermatopathology is a subspecialty of its own because of the complexity of skin pathology. A skin biopsy in the primary care setting may not always provide an answer to a dermatologic problem. The following factors determine the quality of the information from a biopsy:

1. Characteristic pathologic findings: Many skin diseases have nonspecific histologic changes, and skin biopsies may be noncontributory (e.g., atopic dermatitis, urticaria, drug eruptions, viral exanthems).
2. Sample location: A biopsy from the center of a lesion has the best chance of demonstrating pathology. Occasionally, a sample from the periphery of the lesion shows the characteristic changes (e.g., some bullous diseases).
3. Sample size or depth: A sample that is not large enough or deep enough may not demonstrate the pathologic changes.
4. The pathologist: The person who interprets the skin biopsy must be an expert in the histopathology of the skin. Dermatopathologists are the best trained in this field, although general pathologists and dermatologists receive training in skin pathology.

Ideally, a pathology report either confirms a specific diagnosis, or discusses differential diagnoses and suggests further diagnostic procedures if indicated.

ADDITIONAL READINGS

Habif TP: *Clinical dermatology,* ed 3, St Louis, 1996, Mosby.

Robinson JK, LeBoit PE: Biopsy techniques: description and proper use. In Arndt KA et al, eds: *Cutaneous medicine and surgery,* Philadelphia, 1996, Saunders.

CHAPTER 83

General Dermatologic Therapy

James C. Shaw

WOUND HEALING

The most important principle of wound healing is adequate hydration. Migration of keratinocytes and the making of collagen by fibroblasts are both dependent on a moist environment. Wet-to-dry dressings for wounds have been replaced by dressings that simulate a biologic environment. Biocclusive dressings can be designed at home or in the office with the use of antibacterial ointments covered with an occlusive film or gauze dressing (petrolatum-impregnated gauze), or they can be purchased as prepackaged dressings (e.g., DuoDerm, Vigilon, OpSite). Although these products are expensive, they can be helpful in the healing of large ulcers, abrasions, and burns.

TOPICAL CORTICOSTEROIDS

The Vehicle: Cream vs. Ointment

The vehicle containing a corticosteroid can be as important as the steroid itself. Creams and lotions are composed of a combination of oil and water. The higher the ratio of oil to water, the thicker the preparation. The presence of water in the vehicle may contribute to skin drying through evaporation. Vehicles containing water also must contain preservatives to prevent contamination with bacteria and fungi. Preservatives such as quaternium 15 and imidazolidinyl urea can occasionally cause allergic contact dermatitis. In general, patients tolerate creams and lotions better than ointments, but ointments have some inherent occlusive properties that enhance the penetration of steroids. Creams and lotions tend to be more effective in intertriginous or moist areas because of their drying properties. Ointments are used preferably on dry skin because their occlusive properties retard drying. Solutions usually contain alcohol and are best used on the scalp.

Side Effects

Corticosteroids are graded from class I (most potent) to class VII (least potent). Corticosteroids applied topically are generally safe when used for a short time. Chronic use can result in side effects if the steroid is stronger than class VII. The main side effect seen with chronic use of potent steroids is skin atrophy with thinned dermis with prevalent telangiectasis and increased friability. These changes can lead to the development of striae. When potent steroids are used on the face, a rosacea-like papular and pustular dermatitis, referred to as steroid-induced rosacea, can occur.

Use of Potent Steroids

In general, potency correlates with fluorinated or chlorinated steroids (Table 83-1). Class I (most potent) steroids should be considered in the most recalcitrant dermatoses as short-term treatment only. These steroids, in general, should never be used on the face. Class II through V levels of potency can be used on open areas of the skin for up to several months without concern but should be avoided in intertriginous areas. The weakest, Class VI and VII, are generally safe on the face and in intertriginous areas.

Occlusion

Steroids have increased effectiveness when they are occluded. The use of an ointment provides some natural occlusion, but additional occlusion can be provided with the use of a plastic or other synthetic dressing such as DuoDerm. Even simple tape increases the penetration of the steroid. Although occlusion increases effectiveness, it also increases the chances of side effects.

Intralesional Steroids

On occasion, when a recalcitrant dermatosis is of limited size, the use of intralesional steroids can be helpful. Either intralesional betamethasone valerate (Celestone) 6 mg/ml or triamcinolone acetonide (Kenalog) 5 mg/ml can be used judiciously in plaques of psoriasis, prurigo nodules, inflamed cysts, and in localized patches of alopecia areata. Skin atrophy is a risk whenever intralesional steroids are used.

COMPRESSES, SOAKS, AND WRAPS

Indications

Wet compresses are helpful in reducing itching and in drying areas of inflamed skin with serous oozing. The main goals of wet dressings are to cool the skin temperature, debride necrotic tissue, and dry out the skin through evaporation. Soaks are used to hydrate dry skin. A 10 to 15 minute soak in warm plain water hydrates dry skin before application of emollients.

Table 83-1. Selected Topical Corticosteroids

Strength	Class	Medication
Super potent	I	Diprolene, Temovate, Cormax, Psorcon
Potent	II	Fluocinonide 0.05%, betamethasone diproprionate 0.05%
Mid-potency	IV, V	Triamcinolone 0.1%, Elocon 0.1%
Low potency	VI, VII	Desonide 0.05%, hydrocortisone 1%

Table 83-2. Selected Emollients

Type	Brand
Ointments	Petrolatum, Vaseline, Aquaphor
Creams	Cetaphil, Eucerine
Lotions	Neutragena moisture SPF 15, Oil of Olay, Lubriderm, Eucerine, Eucerine for the face
With urea	Carmol 10, 20, 40; Aqua care, Eucerine plus
With α-hydroxy acids	Neutrogena healthy skin, Aqua glycolic, Lac-hydrin, Lacticare

Procedure

Generally, plain water can be used for wet dressings, but occasionally aluminum acetate (Burow's solution and others) aids in the drying of the skin. The compresses should not be occlusive and should allow for evaporation. A thin fabric is wetted and applied to the affected skin for 5 to 10 minutes and repeated for 30 minutes. This protocol can be followed two or three times a day until the skin has achieved the desired dryness.

Wraps can be beneficial, short-term treatment in any severe dermatitis. Petrolatum or a paste or ointment containing zinc oxide is applied to the skin and wrapped by a thin cotton or linen sheeting. Topical steroids may be added to the base ointment.

EMOLLIENTS

Emollients provide a barrier to evaporation and deliver some oil content to the skin. Emollients can be pure ointments (Vaseline), which deliver an oil product to the stratum corneum and which provide the greatest protection against evaporation (Table 83-2). Creams represent a combination of oil product plus water and are thinner and therefore easier to apply. Because of the water content, some evaporation takes place. In the most severe cases of dry skin, creams may not provide an adequate protective barrier. Lotions are the thinnest of the emollients because of a higher water content and a lower oil content. These preparations are effective in the mildest forms of dryness, but tend to be ineffective in severe xerosis.

Emollients contain petrolatum, mineral oil, or glycerin. The addition of urea or lactic acid promotes hydration and removal of excess keratin in the skin and can be helpful in the treatment of dry skin (see Table 83-2).

Emollients are best applied after the skin has been exposed to water through a shower, bath, or soak. Even dry skin absorbs some moisture through gentle bathing, especially if soap is avoided. Emollients can then be applied immediately after the bath or shower to protect the hydrated skin from evaporation.

ANTIHISTAMINES

Antihistamines are valuable in the treatment of numerous skin problems. The main use is for the treatment of histamine-mediated dermatosis, such as urticaria, as well as for the general treatment of pruritus (Table 83-3). For urticaria, any of the antihistamines can be used, and frequently a combination of antihistamines are effective, such as a nonsedating product during the day and a sedating one at night. For other pruritic dermatoses, only the sedating brands are beneficial.

ANTIBIOTICS

Topical Antibiotics

Numerous topical antibiotics are available for the treatment of acne and minor bacterial skin problems (Table 83-4).

Topical Antibiotic Ointments. Several topical antibiotic ointment preparations are available for use in minor wounds (see Table 83-4). Patients can develop allergic contact dermatitis to topical application of neomycin and bacitracin. A newer topical antibiotic, mupirocin (Bactroban ointment), is effective against infections with gram-positive cocci. This antibiotic is especially useful in patients who are carriers of *Staphylococcus aureus* in the nares. Topical clindamycin phosphate and metronidazole have become standards of care in the treatment of acne and rosacea, respectively.

Table 83-3. Selected Antihistamines Used in Dermatology

Type	Drug
Sedating	Diphenhydramine, hydroxyzine, doxepin
Less sedating	Ceterizine (Zyrtec)
Nonsedating	Loratadine (Claritin), astemizole (Hismanal)

Table 83-4. Topical Antibiotics*

Generic name	Brand name	Preparation
Bacitracin	Same	15, 30, 120 gm
Chloramphenicol	Chloromycetin cream	30 gm
Clioquinol (iodochlorhydroxyquin)	Vioform cream, lotion, ointment	15, 30 gm
	Vioform/hydrocort	15, 30 gm
Clindamycin phosphate (1%)†	Cleocin-T soln, gel	60 gm
Erythromycin 2%†	Ery-cette pledgets	box of 60
	Em-gel	30 gm
	Akne-Mycin ointment	25 gm
	A/T/S alcohol soln	60 ml
	Eryderm alcohol soln	60 ml
	Erymax alcohol soln	2 oz, 4 oz
	T-Stat alcohol soln	60 ml
	Staticin (1.5%) alcohol soln	60 ml
Erythromycin 3% and Benzoyl peroxide 5%	Benzamycin gel	23.3 gm
Gentamycin	Garamycin cream, ointment	15 gm
Gramicidin & hydrocortisone	Cortisporin ointment	15 gm
Iodoquinol & HC	Vytone	30 gm
Meclocycline†	Meclan cream	20, 45 gm
Mefenide acetate	Sulfamylon cream	60, 120, 480 gm
Metronidazole‡	Metrogel	30 gm
Mupirocin 2%	Bactroban ointment	15, 30 gm
Neomycin	multiple	7.5-60 gm
Nitrofurazone	Furacin cream	30 gm
Polymyxin/bacitracin	Polysporin (many)	15, 30 gm
Polymyxin/bacitracin/neomycin	Neosporin	15, 30 gm
	Mycitracin	15, 30 gm
Povidone-iodine	Betadine ointment	30 gm
Silver sulfadiazine	Silvadene cream	20-1000 gm
Sulfacetamide sodium‡	Sulfacet-R lotion	30 gm
	Novacet lotion	30 gm
	Sebizon lotion	85 gm
Tetracycline HCl†	Achromycin ointment	15, 30 gm
	Topicycline alcohol soln	70 ml

Modified from Habif TP: *Clinical dermatology*, ed 2, St Louis, 1990, Mosby.
*Application: Infections: multiple times daily. Acne: once or twice daily.
†Best for acne vulgaris.
‡Best for acne rosacea.

Antiseptic Cleansers. The main antiseptic cleansers include povidone iodine (Betadine), hexachlorophene (pHisoHex), and chlorhexadine gluconate (Hibiclens). These effective antibacterial cleaners are useful as adjunctive therapy in superficial skin infections.

Oral Antibiotics. Dermatologic uses of systemic antibiotics include bacterial infections, acne, rosacea, hidradenitis suppurativa, and folliculitis. The antiinflammatory effects of the tetracycline and erythromycin families of drugs may be of equal importance as the antibacterial effects in the treatment of inflammatory skin disorders.

ANTIFUNGAL THERAPY

Topical antifungal therapy is effective in tinea pedis (excluding onychomycosis), tinea crurus, tinea versicolor, and seborrheic dermatitis (Table 83-5).

SYSTEMIC ANTIFUNGAL THERAPY

Systemic use of antifungal drugs is indicated in the treatment of tinea corporis, tinea capitis, onychomycosis, all deep fungal infections, and most fungal infections that occur in the setting of human immunodeficiency virus (HIV) infection.

Griseofulvin, the first systemic antifungal for use in dermatology, is now limited in use. Its main use is in tinea capitis in children. Recent research, however, suggests that terbinafine and itraconazole may be as effective and will likely replace griseofulvin.

Ketoconazole, the first oral imidazole antifungal, is no longer used routinely because of potential liver toxicity and the advent of newer, less toxic, and more effective antifungals.

Fluconazole is effective against dermatophytes, *Candida* species, and *Malassezia furfur.* Its concentration in skin tissue lends to its use in skin infections. It is used commonly in the treatment of oral thrush (200 mg as the first dose, then 100 mg/day) and vaginal candidiasis (150 mg single dose). It has also been found to be effective as a single-dose therapy for tinea versicolor and as a weekly 200-mg dose for onychomycosis. Liver toxicity is a rare complication, and drug interactions can be significant.

Itraconazole, another imidazole antifungal, is approved for treating onychomycosis in a pulse regimen of 200 mg twice daily for 1 week per month, for a total of 3 months. Drug interactions and potential liver toxicity require monitoring.

Terbinafine is an allylamine derivative effective against most superficial skin fungal infections. Risks of liver toxicity and drug interactions are less than with imidazole antifungals. It is approved for the treatment of onychomycosis (250 mg/day for 3 months).

ANTIVIRAL THERAPY

Acyclovir is effective against herpesvirus infections, including herpes simplex virus (HSV) and herpes zoster. The antiviral activity of acyclovir requires activation by the viral enzyme thymidine kinase. Because of this requirement, acyclovir has little toxicity to human cells and therefore has relatively few systemic side effects. The specific treatment recommendations for HSV and herpes zoster are discussed in Chapter 91.

Table 83-5. Selected Topical Antifungal Agents

Generic name	Brand name	Activity	Packaging	Use
Ciclopirox	Loprox	Candida (C) Dermatophytes (D)	15, 30, 90 gm cream 30 ml lotion	Twice a day
Clotrimazole	Lotrimin AF (OTC) Mycelex	C, D	1, 2 oz 15, 30, 45, 90 gm cream 10, 30 ml lotion 10 mg troches	Twice a day Every 3-4 hr
Econazole	Spectazole	C, D	15, 30, 85 gm cream	Twice a day
Ketoconazole	Nizoral	C, D	15, 30, 60 gm cream	Twice a day
Miconazole	Monistat-Derm Micatin (OTC)	C, D	15, 30, 85 gm cream 30, 60 ml lotion 15 gm cream	Twice a day
Naftifine	Naftin	C, D	15, 30, 60 gm cream 20, 40 gm gel	Twice a day
Nystatin	Mycostatin	C only	15, 30 gm cream 15, 30 gm ointment 60 ml suspension	Twice a day 4 times a day (oral)
Oxiconazole	Oxistat	C, D	15, 30 gm cream	Twice a day
Sulconazole	Exelderm	C, D	15, 30, 60 gm cream 30 ml soln	Twice a day
Terbinafine	Lamisil	D only*	15, 30 gm cream	Twice a day
Tolnaftate	Tinactin (OTC)	D only	15 gm cream 10 ml soln	Twice a day
Undecylenic acid	Desenex (OTC)	D only	30 gm ointment 45 ml spray 42.5 gm foam	Once or twice a day

OTC, Over-the-counter.
*Terbinafine effective in candida skin infections in some studies.

Valacyclovir is used for the same indications as acyclovir. It achieves higher blood levels than acyclovir with oral dosing. After absorption, valacyclovir is metabolized to acyclovir.

Famciclovir is indicated for the treatment of acute herpes zoster and recurrent HSV. Its pharmacologic action is similar to acyclovir and valacyclovir.

Topical antivirals include penciclovir and acyclovir, both indicated in the treatment of recurrent HSV infections. Both drugs have demonstrated reduced healing time and viral shedding.

PROCEDURAL DERMATOLOGY

Skin Biopsy

Skin biopsy can be essential to making a correct dermatologic diagnosis, and all clinicians should know how to perform this procedure. See Chapter 82 for a detailed description of the skin biopsy.

Liquid Nitrogen Cryosurgery

Indications. The correct use of cryosurgery requires confidence in the diagnosis. This treatment should be avoided if the diagnosis is questionable. Liquid nitrogen is effective in treating small, superficial lesions of epidermal origin such as verruca, seborrheic keratoses, or actinic keratoses. Small lesions with a dermal component, such as acrochordons, also may respond to this treatment. Larger dermal lesions and skin malignancies can be treated with liquid nitrogen but require special temperature monitoring techniques to maximize the response and minimize complications. Liquid nitrogen should never be used to treat melanocytic nevi because of the possibility of misdiagnosing what is actually a malignant melanoma (Box 83-1).

Procedure. Liquid nitrogen (boiling point: 196° C) is commercially available and requires storage in an industrial container. It may be applied by cotton applicator or spray. Cotton applicators generally need to be tailored to a size slightly smaller than the lesion.

Warts. The amount of freezing required to adequately treat the lesion depends on the size and location. Flat warts and small warts on thin skin require the least amount of freezing. Large and deep warts, such as plantar/palmar warts, require a relatively more aggressive treatment. Repeated freezing-thawing produces more tissue damage. Although the treatment is painful, local anesthetic is usually not required except in large lesions on the palms, soles, and fingers.

Seborrheic Keratoses. Seborrheic keratoses, which are epidermal growths, tend to be more superficial than warts and therefore require less freeze time than large warts.

Actinic Keratoses. The time required to treat actinic keratoses with liquid nitrogen depends on the amount of keratinized surface and on the depth of involvement. These lesions generally require less freeze time than warts. If there is uncertainty about the diagnosis, cryosurgery should be avoided.

Box 83-1. Liquid Nitrogen Cryotherapy

The use of liquid nitrogen cryotherapy to treat melanocytic nevi is contraindicated.

Complications. Blister formation is common after cryosurgery. Pain may be severe in the 48 hours after treatment. The use of cryosurgery is limited in dark-skinned people because of the high frequency of healing with hypopigmentation. Infection rarely occurs after cryosurgery, and dressing changes are not required. In general, scarring is usually minimal but is more common on the face.

Cryotherapy in children and elderly patients should be performed with caution because of these patients' increased susceptibility to blister formation and scarring.

Skin Tag Removal

Acrochordons are treated by a variety of methods depending on the size of the lesions. The smallest lesions can be treated with liquid nitrogen. Larger lesions are best treated by removal with a scalpel or scissors. The need for local anesthesia depends on the size of the lesion, but most can be removed without anesthesia as long as the cutting of each lesion is swift.

Cyst Removal

Surgical excision of small cysts can be uncomplicated. Large lesions on the face or scalp require the same surgical precautions as larger excisions. In a noninflamed cyst, failure to remove the entire cyst wall can result in its recurrence. Small cysts are best excised after local anesthesia by means of an elliptical or punch incision to gain access to the cyst, and removal of the entire cyst wall is achieved with blunt and sharp dissection. Closure can require both dermal and surface suturing.

ADDITIONAL READINGS

Arndt KA: *Manual of dermatologic therapeutics,* ed 5, Boston, 1995, Little, Brown.

Habif TP: *Clinical dermatology,* ed 3, St Louis, 1996, Mosby.

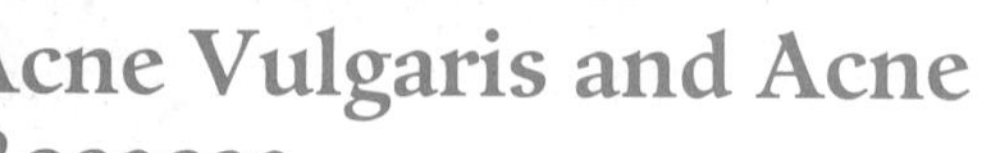

Acne Vulgaris and Acne Rosacea

Frank Parker
James C. Shaw

ACNE VULGARIS

Acne vulgaris, commonly referred to as "acne," is a multifactorial inflammatory disorder of the pilosebaceous units over the face, chest, and back areas where the greatest concentrations of these skin appendages are found. It is the most common cause of pustular reactions of the skin.

Epidemiology and Etiology

Acne occurs during the life of nearly every human being. Very mild cases go unnoticed, while severe cases result in significant physical and psychologic problems. Several factors play a role as individuals enter puberty: (1) androgenic stimulation of the sebaceous glands and increased serum production; (2) abnormal keratinization in the pilosebaceous canal with obstruction to sebum flow (comedones); and (3) proliferation of anaerobic bacteria, *Propionibacterium acnes,* which lead to rupture of the pilosebaceous unit, extravasation of sebum, and bacteria into the dermis, resulting in inflammatory papules, pustules, and cysts.

Pathophysiology

Weak and strong androgens stimulate the pilosebaceous units at the time of puberty to enlarge and produce large amounts of sebum (an oily substance composed in part of large quantities of triglycerides, diglycerides, and monoglycerides). The vast majority of patients secrete normal amounts of androgens from the ovaries, testes, and adrenal glands, but in occasional instances an underlying endocrine problem (polycystic ovarian syndrome, adrenal hyperplasia, adrenal or ovarian tumors) may cause acne. At the same time the increased sebum production is seen, the keratinization process in the pilosebaceous canal is disrupted with impaction and obstruction of the outflow of sebum (comedo formation—open blackheads and closed whiteheads). The wall of the closed comedo may rupture, spilling the follicular contents into the dermis. This leads to the development of inflammatory papules, pustules, and large cysts because under the influence of increased sebum production large numbers of *P. acnes* proliferate (sebum is the substrate for the *P. acnes*); these bacteria are chemotactic, bringing in neutrophils, which cause the inflammatory response. Stress may accentuate acne. Dietary factors seem to play little or no role in the pathogenesis.[2]

History

The comedones, papules, and pustules that evolve on the face, chest, and back early in puberty occur at the usual time of onset; but acne can occur in patients in their second and third decade. In women, cosmetics with oily bases may aggravate acne. A history of irregular menses or hirsutism should lead to an evaluation of possible endocrine disorder. Potent topical or large doses of corticosteroids can also induce an acneiform eruption.

Physical Examination and Clinical Features

In noninflammatory acne, comedones (plugged follicles—blackheads and whiteheads) are usually present in large numbers over the forehead, nose, cheeks, and occasionally in the ears and on the lower face, chest, and back. Inflammatory acne is classified as *papular* (mild, moderate, severe) or *nodular* (mild, moderate, severe) on the basis of size of lesions and degree of involvement[3] (Plate 25). Pustular components can be present in papular and nodular types. The term *cystic acne* has been recently discouraged because these lesions are not cysts but are large inflammatory nodules. True cysts can form in the wake of severe acne lesions, but this is uncommon. Acne scars can be discrete "ice-pick" scars or larger depressed areas. Some individuals develop hypertrophic scars or keloids in response to acne.

Several variants of acne vulgaris that are worth noting include the following:

- *Acne fulminans:* A rare, acute, severe variety of acne with widespread nodular lesions that contain large quantities of necrotic material that may break down, leaving eroded areas over the face and back accompanied by systemic findings of fever, leukocytosis, and arthralgias.
- *Acne due to drugs:* Several medications, including androgens, corticosteroids, and medications with halogens (iodides, bromides, anticonvulsants, and lithium), may lead to acne or exacerbate preexisting acne.
- *Gram-negative folliculitis:* A true bacterial infection that usually presents during the course of treatment with antibiotics or isotretinoin for acne. A sudden worsening of acne-like lesions is typical and requires culture for diagnosis and appropriate antibiotic coverage.

Differential Diagnosis

Rosacea may be confused with acne, but a history of flushing, the presence of telangiectases, and lack of comedones should help distinguish this condition. Flat warts on the face also should be in the differential diagnosis, but the lack of pustules and comedones help identify warts. Bacterial folliculitis can be diagnosed by Gram's stain and cultures of the pustules. Occasionally, acne is confused with adenoma sebaceum (angiofibroma), which consists of fleshy, red papules over the central face associated with tuberous sclerosis.

Management

The principles of therapy involve reversing the following etiologic factors that induce the acne lesions: decrease sebaceous activity, decrease *P. acnes* population, decrease follicular occlusion and inflammation, and decrease androgen stimulation of sebaceous glands.[1]

Topical Therapy

1. *Comedolytics:* Retinoic acid (tretinoin, Retin-A, Avita), adapalene (Differin), and azaleic acid (Azalex) are comedolytic agents available as gels, creams, or solutions in varying concentrations. They are applied to the affected areas once a day beginning with the weakest preparations to avoid its two major side effects, skin irritation and scaling. Although comedolytic agents are used mainly for comedonal acne, they are also beneficial in inflammatory acne.
2. *Antiseptics:* Benzoyl peroxide, an effective antibacterial agent, as well as a comedolytic agent, is most useful to treat inflammatory acne. It is available as an over-the-counter lotion base and in a gel base in 2.5%, 5%, and 10% concentrations as prescription items. Irritation may follow the use of benzoyl peroxide and allergic sensitization may occur. The preparation is usually applied once a day. At times it may be useful to use both comedolytics and benzoyl peroxide (inflammatory and comedonal acne).
3. *Antibiotics:* Topical antibiotics including erythromycin and clindamycin are effective in decreasing the *P. acnes* skin population. These preparations in solution, lotion, and gel are used twice a day, often in conjunction with comedolytics or benzoyl peroxide. Topical antibiotics are not quite as effective as systemic antibiotics, but they do alleviate the many side effects of oral antibiotics.

Systemic Therapy

1. *Antibiotics:* Tetracycline and erythromycin are effective in controlling mild to moderate papular or nodular inflammatory acne. Tetracycline 500 mg twice daily, or erythromycin 500 mg twice daily (or E.E.S. 400 mg three times daily) is commonly used. Gastrointestinal upset is common with both drugs, and tetracycline must be taken on an empty stomach. Alternatives include minocycline 100 mg/day and doxycycline 100 mg twice daily. Both of these drugs can cause photosensitivity. Sulfa drugs, although reportedly used in acne, have a high incidence of allergic reactions and should be avoided if possible. All of these drugs can cause candidal vaginosis. The length of treatment depends on the response but frequently requires up to 3 months before significant improvement is observed.
2. *Systemic retinoids:* Isotretinoin (Accutane) is a useful therapy in severe nodular acne that is unresponsive to other treatment regimens. The medication produces remarkable clearing in 95% of these patients, but it also provides persistent remissions in 85% of patients. The drug, usually given in doses of 0.5 to 1.0 mg/kg per day for 3 to 4 months, has many side effects characteristic of chronic hypervitaminosis A, including cheilitis, xerosis, epistaxis, eye irritation, myalgias, and bony hyperkeratosis. Accutane is a potent teratogen and is contraindicated during pregnancy. Dose-related elevations in serum triglycerides and night blindness also occur. Because of these potential problems, the medication should be given by those familiar with the use of this drug with frequent monitoring of complete blood count (CBC), serum chemistries (occasionally liver function test abnormalities are seen), and fasting blood lipids. Women of childbearing age must be on birth control measures (both birth control pills and barrier methods) and be monitored for pregnancy before and during treatment (usually at 2 and 4 weeks and then monthly).
3. *Hormonal therapies:* Adult women with acne or hirsutism present unique problems that go beyond the scope of this text. However, the selected use of hormonal treatments can be helpful in these women. Treatment options include ovarian androgen suppression with oral contraceptives, androgen receptor blockers (spironolactone, flutamide), and adrenal androgen suppression with corticosteroids.[4]

ROSACEA

Acne rosacea, commonly called *rosacea,* is a chronic inflammatory disorder of the blood vessels and pilosebaceous units of the face that occurs most often in middle-aged adults.

Pathophysiology

The cause of this condition is not completely understood.[5] Some studies suggested a role for the follicular mite Demodex. Other aggravating factors that have been incriminated but not well proved include ingestion of foods that cause flushing (hot liquids, caffeine-containing beverages, alcohol, spicy foods), stress, and sunlight.

History

Middle-aged adults are primarily affected. Erythema develops first, followed by telangiectasia, associated with increasing blushing and flushing over the central face and at times the neck and chest. Flushing is an important symptom, often precipitated by heat, hot foods, alcohol, and caffeine-containing beverages. Papules and pustules develop over the central face, nose, and chin. Eye symptoms of burning, itching, and irritation may also occur, as well as a history of chalazia.

Physical Examination

Typically papules and pustules are superimposed on a ruddy complexion and telangiectases most pronounced over the central face (see Plate 7). Sebaceous and fibrous enlargement of the nose (rhinophyma) may eventually ensue. Comedones are not present. In severe cases the pustular component may lead to cystic and granulomatous nodules. Ten percent of patients may have ocular complications, including blepharitis, conjunctivitis, chronic chalazia, and keratitis, that may impair vision. Some patients present with only ocular findings.

Laboratory Studies

The diagnosis is based on clinical findings. Laboratory findings are not helpful, and skin biopsy is seldom required.

Differential Diagnosis

Rosacea may be confused with acne vulgaris, but the former is found in older individuals, lacks comedones, and is accompanied by blushing and telangiectasis. Lupus erythematosus, photodermatitis, and seborrhea may be confused with the vascular element of rosacea, but none of these have pustules. The flushing component of rosacea might cause one to consider the carcinoid syndrome. Perioral dermatitis is considered a variant of rosacea seen in young women. It consists of papules and pustules around the mouth and nose. Steroid rosacea is a papulo-pustular eruption that mimics rosacea but is associated with the use of potent topical corticosteroids.

Management

Nonpharmacologic. Trigger factors in rosacea include sunlight, emotional stress, hot liquids, spicy foods, certain vasoactive foods (cheeses, chocolate, alcohol, especially red wine), and all of these should be avoided if possible. Daily use of sunscreens can help with the most common trigger factor: ultraviolet light.

Pharmacologic

Topical Therapy. Topical metronidazole (Metrogel, Metrocreme), 0.75% twice a day, often can control the condition without oral antibiotics. At times both tetracycline and topical metronidazole are needed. Topical sulfur-containing materials (Sulfacet-R) are also useful. Topical steroids should be avoided, especially fluorinated potent steroids, as they may exacerbate the problem and indeed can induce steroid rosacea.

Systemic Therapy. Low-dose tetracycline or erythromycin, 250 to 1000 mg/day, controls the papules and pustules, but the erythema and telangiectasis are resistant to therapy. The use of antibiotics must be continued lifelong, and some patients require tetracycline 250 mg two to three times a week to suppress the condition. Flushing can be treated with low doses of clonidine.[6]

Surgery. Severe telangiectasias can be treated with tunable dye laser. Rhinophyma can be treated with removal of the excess sebaceous and collagenous material with scalpel, electrosurgery, or laser technique.

Hidradenitis Suppurativa

Hidradenitis suppurativa is a chronic, suppurative, acne-like eruption occurring primarily in the axillae, inguinal and intergluteal folds, and inframammary areas. Frequently patients with hidradenitis suppurativa also suffer from severe acne (acne conglobata). The precise pathophysiology of this condition is not certain, but whereas early theories linked the apocrine glands to this disease, more recent evidence shows a histologic process identical to that seen in acne vulgaris. Mild cases exist, but the more familiar presentation is that of large draining nodules with sinus tract formation and fibrosis in the affected areas. The presence of double comedones is characteristic in early stages. Treatment is usually difficult. Standard therapy to control inflammation includes systemic antibiotics in maximal acne doses, occasional use of systemic corticosteroids, oral isotretinoin, and local care as needed with incision and drainage. Surgical excision of large areas of involvement is curative, and in severe cases, may be the only successful treatment approach.

REFERENCES

1. Leyden JJ: Therapy for acne vulgaris, *N Engl J Med* 336:1156-1162, 1997.
2. Leyden JJ: New understandings of the pathogenesis of acne, *J Am Acad Dermatol* 32(part 3):S15-25, 1995.
3. Pochi PE, Shalita AR, Strauss JS, et al: Report of the consensus conference on acne classification, *J Am Acad Dermatol* 24:495-500, 1991.
4. Shaw JC: Antiandrogen and hormonal treatment of acne, *Dermatol Clin* 14:803-811, 1996.
5. Wilkin JK: Rosacea: pathophysiology and treatment, *Arch Dermatol* 13:359-362, 1994.
6. Wilkin JK: The red face: flushing disorders, *Clin Dermatol* 11:211-223, 1993.

CHAPTER 85

Psoriasis and Other Papulosquamous Diseases

James C. Shaw
Frank Parker

The combination of papules and scales are the common features of papulosquamous skin diseases. The term *squamous* refers to scaling that represents thick stratum corneum and thus implies an abnormal keratinization process. In addition to unusual scales, lesions are characterized by sharply demarcated, red to violaceous papules and plaques that result from thickening of the epidermis or underlying dermal inflammation. The sharp delineation of the lesions in this group of diseases helps distinguish them from scaling lesions of eczematous diseases where the borders are usually indistinct (with two exceptions—nummular eczema and seborrheic dermatitis) (Box 85-1).

Box 85-1. Papulosquamous Diseases

- Psoriasis
- Pityriasis rosea
- Lichen planus
- Seborrheic dermatitis
- Pityriasis rubra pilaris
- Secondary syphilis
- Miscellaneous mycosis fungoides, discoid lupus erythematosus, ichthyoses

PSORIASIS

Epidemiology and Pathophysiology

The exact cause of psoriasis is unknown, but it appears to be a multifactorial disease with genetic influences and immune regulation.[1] The worldwide prevalence is 3%, with a 1% prevalence in North America. Onset can be at any age. Family history of psoriasis is found in about 40% of patients, and gene studies have shown linkage to several HLA loci.

The psoriasis phenotype is manifested by increased epidermal cell turnover (decreased turnover time), increased numbers of epidermal stem cells, and abnormal differentiation of keratin expression leading to thickened skin with copious scale. Immune regulation appears to be the largest influence of the abnormal phenotype, with numerous cytokines and growth factors required, and striking clinical improvement with immunomodulatory therapies (see Management section). Precipitating factors can trigger or worsen psoriasis. These include streptococcal infections, overuse of ethanol, psychologic stress, certain medications (beta blockers, lithium), and trauma to the skin (inducing the Koebner phenomenon, where new skin lesions evolve in areas of injury to the skin).

Patient Evaluation

History. The onset and course of the disease are highly variable. It usually begins gradually, confined to a few areas, but it can be explosive in onset. One cause of the latter presentation is a preceding streptococcal throat infection, which leads in 2 to 3 weeks to multiple, small guttate lesions generalized over the body. Once the disease appears, it follows an irregular, chronic, and unpredictable course. It may remain localized to a few areas or may cause intermittent or continuous generalized lesions.

Itching is usually not a problem in psoriasis but may be severe in individual patients.

Physical Examination. The lesions are erythematous papules and plaques surmounted by thick, silvery scales that resemble mica (micaceous) and that are not easily removed and often accumulate in the patient's clothing or bed (see Plate 3). When the scales are traumatically removed, multiple small bleeding sites appear (Auspitz's sign). In intertriginous areas, maceration and moisture prevent dry scales from accumulating, but the lesions remain red and sharply defined (inverse psoriasis) (Plate 26).

Lesions usually are distributed symmetrically over areas of body prominence such as elbows and knees. They also frequently occur on the trunk, penis (Plate 27), scalp, and intergluteal cleft and umbilicus. Nail involvement may include stippling or pitting of the nail plate or yellow or red-brown coloring ("oil-staining") of onycholytic patches with accumulation of yellow debris under nails (Plate 28). Psoriatic arthritis, occurring in less than one-third of patients with psoriasis, commonly presents with red, swollen distal interphalangeal joints and nail involvement.

Diagnosis

Laboratory Studies and Diagnostic Procedure. A skin biopsy can substantiate the diagnosis but is seldom necessary because the clinical features of psoriasis are so distinctive. No serologic or other diagnostic tests are available.

Differential Diagnosis. See Table 85-1.

Management

There are now numerous treatments available, both topical and systemic. Although there is no cure for the disease, considerable improvement can be achieved with well-selected treatments.

Nonpharmacologic Therapy. Avoidance of excessive alcohol consumption may benefit some patients. Many patients improve in the summer months on the basis of sun exposure, which can be recommended with caution. Soaking baths to remove scale, followed by liberal emollient use is also helpful. Stress reduction programs may help prevent exacerbations in some patients.

Topical Pharmacologic Therapy

Corticosteroids. Class I steroid ointments are a mainstay of psoriasis treatment and can be used as a short course therapy twice a day followed by a class III steroid for maintenance. On the face, only class VI or VII should be used. On the scalp, class I solutions are best, along with a medicated shampoo containing tar, selenium sulfide, or ketoconazole.

Tar. Coal tar is frequently added to a topical corticosteroid regimen. A 2% to 5% crude coal tar (CCT) compounded with the steroid, although messy, can be helpful.

Calcipotriol. Calcipotriol is a vitamin D derivative (calcipotriene, Dovonex) that affects keratinocyte differentiation. It has been successful when used twice a day on psoriasis plaques.[2] Recently, the combined use of calcipotriol and a class I corticosteroid has shown to be effective when used for a limited time to induce remission of plaques.

Topical Retinoids. The newest form of topical therapy in psoriasis is tazarotene, a topical retinoid that affects keratinocyte differentiation. Successful outcomes have been shown with once daily application. Tazarotene has been used in combination with ultraviolet light therapy.[3] Some irritation of the skin can be reduced with concomitant use of corticosteroids.

Ultraviolet Light Therapy. Treatment with ultraviolet B (UVB) and oral psoralen plus ultraviolet A (PUVA) are possibly the most successful of the nonsystemic therapies in psoriasis. Details of these treatments are beyond the scope of this text, but light therapy should be considered in any patient

Table 85-1. Differential Diagnosis of Psoriasis

Disease	Clinical features	Cause	Diagnosis
Tinea and onycholysis	Scaling annular to round patches and onycholysis and crumbling nails.	Dermatophyte infections	KOH
Seborrheic dermatitis	Diffuse lesions with greasy scales on scale behind ears, nasolabial folds and presternally.	Possibly overgrowth pityrosporum	Skin biopsy may help
Secondary syphilis	Guttate or small scaling plaques over trunk, like pityriasis rosea, but involves palms and soles.	Spirochete	Positive test for syphilis RPR
Cutaneous T-cell lymphoma	Flat to thick plaques with variable scaling, which may be identical to psoriasis anywhere on body. May be erythrodermic-Sézary syndrome.	T-cell lymphoma	Skin biopsy Sézary cells in circulation. T-cell gene rearrangement studies
Reiter's syndrome	Identical skin changes as psoriasis with pustular lesions on palms and soles (keratoderma blennorrhagicum), balanitis circinata; arthritis nail involvement. Mucous membrane changes not seen in psoriasis.	Unknown, but triggered by certain infectious agents	Clinical features, arthritis, conjunctivitis, urethritis
Pityriasis rubra pilaris	Diffuse salmon-colored papulosquamous lesion areas, normal skin in midst, involved skin—"island sparing," keratoderma palm. Keratotic papules on dorsum of fingers.	Unknown	Clinical features, skin biopsy
Pityriasis lichenoides et varioliformis acuta	Red, purpuric, vesicular lesions evolve into scaling macular and papular lesions that scar. Lesions occur over entire body.	Unknown	Clinical features, skin biopsy

KOH, Potassium hydroxide; *RPR,* rapid plasma reagin.

with widespread disease involving more than 20% of the skin surface.

Systemic Therapies

Methotrexate. Low doses of methotrexate given weekly have been used in widespread psoriasis or psoriatic arthritis for the last 25 years. The effect of methotrexate on T-lymphocytes appears to be responsible for the effect. Monitoring for side effects, including bone marrow suppression and liver disease, is essential when using this modality.

Systemic Retinoids. Acetretin (a metabolite of etretinate, its predecessor) is highly effective in selected patients with widespread disease, including those with severe pustular forms of psoriasis. Concerns about teratogenicity limit its use in women.

Cyclosporine. Another immune modulator with considerable success in psoriasis is cyclosporin A, which can be considered in severe disease. Monitoring of blood pressure, renal function, and blood levels is required.

Special Patients and Issues

Guttate psoriasis in the young patient should initiate a search for streptococcal pharyngitis.[5] The patient often is asymptomatic after a day or two of throat soreness. Antibiotic therapy and eradication of the streptococcus may induce a remission of the psoriasis.

Reiter's Syndrome

Reiter's syndrome (Plate 29) can be readily confused with psoriasis because the skin lesions of the two disorders are indistinguishable clinically and histologically. In Reiter's disease, pustular and keratotic papules and plaques commonly occur on the palms and soles (keratoderma blennorrhagicum) and scaling, red patches are found encircling the glans penis and within the groin (balanitis circinata). Other features of Reiter's syndrome may include a seronegative, asymmetric arthritis that may involve the sacroiliac joints, as well as uveitis, conjunctivitis, and mucous membrane lesions. The presence of asymptomatic erosions on the tongue and buccal mucosa, urethritis, and occasionally diarrhea distinguish Reiter's syndrome from psoriasis.

PITYRIASIS ROSEA

Epidemiology and Etiology

Pityriasis rosea is a self-limited papulosquamous eruption that occurs in young adults. A possible viral etiology has been suggested because of the increased incidence in the winter months and because patients report a history of a preceding upper respiratory infection.

Physical Examination

Oval or round, tan-, ink-, or salmon-colored, scaling papules and plaques appear rapidly over the trunk, neck, upper arms, and thighs (see Plate 8). Several features of this papulosquamous condition are unique. First, the generalized eruption is preceded by a single lesion, termed the *herald patch,* that is commonly misdiagnosed as tinea corporis. The herald patch can occur anywhere but often appears on the neck or lower trunk and precedes the general rash by several days to a week. Second, the oval patches have an unusual fine, white scale located near the border of the plaques, forming a collarette (Plate 30). Third, the lesions follow skin cleavage lines, with the long axis paralleling these lines in a Christmas tree pattern (see Plate 8).

Differential Diagnosis

Drug eruption and secondary syphilis must be considered in the differential diagnosis. If the rash persists beyond 3 months or generalizes to involve the extremities and face, a drug reaction should be considered (e.g., gold compounds, barbiturates, captopril, clonidine). Serologic tests for syphilis should be obtained if the rash involves the palms and soles and if fever, coryza, or mucous membrane erosions (mucous patches) are present.

Management

Treatment may not be necessary, although topical corticosteroids and antihistamines relieve itching and decrease erythema. Ultraviolet light (UVB) given as three to five treatments to give a mild erythema reaction often clears the rash.

LICHEN PLANUS

Epidemiology and Pathophysiology

Lichen planus is a chronic, pruritic, papulosquamous disease with a wide range of clinical manifestations. Lichen planus is considered an immune response to one or more antigenic stimuli. The association with infection with hepatitis C virus (HCV) has given increased importance to making the diagnosis of lichen planus.

Physical Examination

Lichen planus is included in the papulosquamous group of diseases because the primary lesion is a unique papule with an unusual surface configuration. The papules are flat topped (planus) and polygonal in configuration (i.e., the sides conform to normal fine skin folds and creases) and have a lilac or purple hue (Plate 31). They may have visible scales on their surface, but more characteristic are subtle, fine, white reticulated lines (Wickham's striae) surmounting the shiny flat tops of the papules (resembling lichen). Wickham's striae become more apparent under a hand lens after the application of a drop of mineral oil on the surface of the papules. Typical distribution is symmetric papules on the ankles, flexural wrists, mouth, and genitalia. Although the condition is extremely pruritic, one seldom sees excoriations or erosions induced by scratching. Mucous membranes are commonly involved, the lesions appearing most often as asymptomatic white streaks in a reticulate pattern on the buccal mucosa, tongue, gums, or lips (Plate 32). At times, blisters and erosions are superimposed on the mucous membrane areas (erosive lichen planus), causing severe discomfort.

Differential Diagnosis

See Table 85-2.

Management

Since up to 20% of patients with lichen planus have antibodies to HCV (compared to 2.4% of controls in a study from Spain), screening of all patients for HCV infection may be indicated.[4] Treatment is nonspecific and not always successful. For localized patches, topical steroids of the moderate to potent forms may be useful in suppressing the itching and inflammation. If the disease is widespread, a 4- to 6-week course of oral corticosteroids may reverse the course (40 to 60 mg/day) with tapering. Erosive oral lichen planus is particularly difficult to control, but at times intralesional steroid injections are helpful. Patients with widespread lichen planus or erosive painful oral lichen planus should be referred for dermatologic consultation.

Table 85-2. Differential Diagnoses of Lichen Planus-like Skin Conditions

Condition	Clinical feature	Etiology	Diagnosis
Discoid lupus erythematosus	Atrophic red patches with follicular plugging	Autoimmune	Skin biopsy for H&E DIF examination
Drug-induced lichen planus-like eruption	Skin biopsy same as lichen planus, except at times more eosinophiles in infiltrate	Medications: Thiazide, gold, Quinidine, antimalarials	History
Graft versus host	Identical clinical picture, but in patient in clinical situation where graft vs. host-reaction can occur	Immunologic reaction	Skin biopsy identical to lichen planus
Candidiasis and/or mouth cancer	Oral lichen planus can be white and eroded	Infection—*Candida,* r/o cancer	Swab and KOH of lesion to rule out cancer

H&E, Hematoxylin and eosin; *DIF,* direct immunofluorescence.

SEBORRHEIC DERMATITIS

Etiology

The cause of seborrheic dermatitis is not known; but overgrowth of a normally occurring yeast, *Pityrosporum ovale,* may play some role. The disorder is also possibly genetically determined, although its mode of inheritance is not clear.

Pathophysiology

Seborrheic dermatitis is an inflammatory scaling reaction that occurs in seborrheic areas of the skin (areas where large numbers of sebaceous glands are found, e.g., scalp, ears, head, and chest). Dandruff is merely a mild form of seborrheic dermatitis in the scalp.

History

In adults, the process can involve only the scalp or may also cause an erythematous, greasy, scaling rash in the nasolabial folds, eyebrows, beard area, external ears, and presternal areas. Blepharitis is also a manifestation. At times, stress may cause exacerbation of the condition. Seborrheic dermatitis is often one of the earliest cutaneous signs of human immunodeficiency virus (HIV) infection.

Physical Examination and Clinical Features

Ill-defined, erythematous patches with greasy yellow scales are typical of seborrheic dermatitis. They may or may not be pruritic. The location of the lesions is often the most important factor in diagnosing this condition; locations include scalp, retroauricular, external ears, eyebrows, nasolabial folds, presternal, and, at times, axillae, and groin (Plate 33).

Seborrheic dermatitis associated with HIV infection is often extensive and difficult to control. For reasons not clear, seborrheic dermatitis is common and often severe in patients with chronic neurologic conditions such as Parkinson's disease, cerebrovascular accident and spinal cord injuries. At times, it is difficult to distinguish seborrheic dermatitis from psoriasis; some patients appear to have both conditions.

Diagnosis

Differential Diagnosis. The differential diagnoses in adults include psoriasis, Reiter's disease, and atopic dermatitis.

Laboratory Evaluation. There are no specific diagnostic tests, although biopsy can distinguish between typical psoriasis and seborrheic dermatitis.

Management

Shampoos containing tar, sulfur, salicylic acid, ketoconazole, or selenium, if used daily on a prolonged basis, often control scalp and face lesions (when the shampoo is applied to these areas as well). Hydrocortisone cream 1% to 2.5% applied once or twice a day controls lesions on the ears and face. More potent topical steroids in solution form (flucinolone 0.01%) are useful in controlling scalp lesions when medicated shampoos do not provide complete clearing.

PITYRIASIS RUBRA PILARIS

Pityriasis rubra pilaris (PRP) is a rare papulosquamous disorder of keratinization. Its cause is unknown, although there are cases of familial PRP, as well as the more common sporadic cases. Clinical findings include widespread orange-red plaques that can involve the entire skin surface area, frequently with small islands of totally normal skin ("island sparing"), thickening of the palms and soles into a waxy keratotic shell, and in early stages, follicular accentuation. Treatment is with short courses of high-dose vitamin A (up to 300,000 IU/day), but frequently the disease is resistant to all therapies.

SYPHILIS

Secondary syphilis frequently presents with skin lesions that fit the category of papulosquamous diseases. Multiple, raised papules or small plaques with some scale are typical. The disease can resemble pityriasis rosea closely. Clues to suggest syphilis include involvement of palms and soles; lesions in inguinal, gluteal, axillary, or mucosal areas; scalp involvement with patchy alopecia; and a supportive sexual history. Serology and skin biopsy can help confirm the diagnosis. See Chapter 29 for management of syphilis.

REFERENCES

1. Gottlieb AB: Immunopathogenesis of psoriasis, *Arch Dermatol* 133:781, 1997.
2. Koo JY: Tazarotene in combination with phototherapy, *J Am Acad Dermatol* 39(part 2):S144-S148, 1998.

3. Lebwohl M, Yoles BS, Lombardi BS, et al: Calciptriene ointment and halobetasol ointment in the long-term treatment of psoriasis: effects on the duration of improvement, *J Am Acad Dermatol* 39:447-450, 1998.
4. Sanchez-Perez J, DeCastro M, Buezo GF, et al: Lichen planus and hepatitis C virus: prevalence and clinical presentation of patients with lichen planus and hepatitis C virus infection, *Br J Dermatol* 134:715-719, 1996.
5. Telfer NR, Chalmers RJ, Whale K, Coleman G: The role of streptococcal infection in the initiation of guttate psoriasis, *Arch Dermatol* 128:39, 1992.

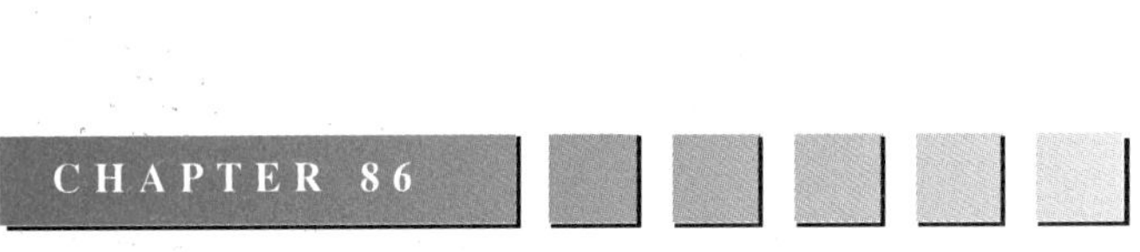

Dermatitis and Eczema

James C. Shaw

When the term *eczema* is used alone, it usually connotes atopic dermatitis. Dermatitis and eczema are frequently used interchangably for numerous disorders, each with qualifiers. Although these diseases have multiple etiologies, they have some clinical features in common and are therefore grouped. Symptoms of pruritus and morphologic features of erythema, papules, microvesicles, excoriation, and lichenification (in older lesions) are commonly found in all diseases within this category.

ATOPIC DERMATITIS

Atopic dermatitis is a chronic skin disease characterized by pruritus, erythema, skin inflammation, and lichenification typically distributed in flexural areas, plus a personal or family history of asthma, hay fever, or eczema. The term *atopy* refers to the triad of dermatitis, asthma, and hay fever.

Epidemiology

Atopy (atopic dermatitis, asthma, or hay fever) is present in 8% to 25% of populations. Atopic dermatitis is present in all races and geographic locations, but there appears to be a higher incidence in urban areas and developed countries. Although the trait runs in families, the precise genetics have not been fully elucidated. A family history of respiratory atopy can be obtained in almost 50% of patients with atopic dermatitis.[3] Mothers with respiratory atopy have atopic children more often (26%) than do fathers with respiratory atopy (13%),[5] and chromosome studies have suggested that the trait for atopy may be inherited on a maternal gene.[1]

Pathophysiology

Atopy is characterized immunologically by high concentrations of serum IgE, a high incidence of IgE-mediated response by skin test to common inhaled antigens, decreased numbers of immunoregulatory T cells, defective antibody–dependent cellular cytotoxicity, and reduced cell-mediated immunity.[3]

Criteria for making the diagnosis of atopic dermatitis have been proposed (Table 86-1). Three major criteria plus three minor criteria should be present to confirm the diagnosis.

Patient Evaluation

History. A suggestive history includes onset of a dermatitis at an early age (most patients have manifestations of atopic dermatitis by age 5), pruritus, the existence of exacerbating factors (Box 86-1), and a positive family history of atopy.

Examination. Papules, erythema, excoriations, and lichenification are the hallmarks of atopic dermatitis. In adults, flexural areas, such as the neck, antecubital fossae and popliteal fossae, are most commonly involved (Plate 34). The face, wrists, and forearms are also common sites of involvement. In severe cases, any area of the body can be involved. Infants usually present with pruritic patches of erythema and papules that can be present more centrally on the face, chest, and extensor extremities. Pustules suggest secondary infection with *Staphylococcus aureus.* Other physical findings that support the diagnosis include xerosis, the infraorbital skin fold (Dennie-Morgan line), periorbital darkening, hyperlinear palms, keratosis pilaris, and nipple dermatitis.

Diagnosis

Diagnosis is made on the basis of personal and family history and clinical features.[4] There are no definitive laboratory tests. The differential diagnosis includes the other diseases in this chapter (see Table 86-1).

Management

The treatment of atopic dermatitis centers around the following three principles:

1. Treatment of inflamed skin
2. Control of itching
3. Control of exacerbating factors

The first two usually require *pharmacologic* treatment, while control of exacerbating factors is usually *nonpharmacologic.*

To treat inflamed skin, topical corticosteroids are the primary modality. For mild disease, a low potency (class VI or VII) corticosteroid cream is effective. For more severe disease a medium potency (class IV or V) corticosteroid cream or ointment may be needed. Secondary infection requires oral antibiotics. Acute flares can sometimes be aborted by a short course of systemic corticosteroids (i.e., prednisone 40 to 60 mg/day for 3 to 4 days, then 20 to 30 mg/day for 3 to 4 days). The most severe cases require combinations of treatments that can include systemic corticosteroids, cyclosporin, FK-506, methotrexate, azothiaprine, and ultraviolet light therapy.

To control pruritus, antihistamines usually are helpful. Considerable trial and error may be required to identify the antihistamine best for the individual patient. Sedating H_1 blockers are best. Commonly used H_1 blockers include diphenhydramine, hydroxyzine, cetirizine, and doxepin. Tepid baths to hydrate and cool the skin can also relieve itching temporarily but must be followed immediately by emollients.

An important aspect of successful treatment of atopic dermatitis is the use of emollients. When used frequently and liberally, emollients can prevent drying of the skin, which is effective in the control of pruritus (see Chapter 83).

Controlling exacerbating factors can be helpful in the acute phase and in long-term management. There may be

Table 86-1. Differential Diagnosis of Dermatitis

Diagnosis	History	Physical examination	Laboratory	Management
Atopic dermatitis	Onset by age 5 Family history of atopy Pruritus Exacerbating factors Coexistent hay fever, asthma	Flexural distribution Lichenification Papules, erythema Pustules if secondary *Staphylococcus aureus*	Routine: none Consider: Culture/pustule IgE	Topical corticosteroids Control environment Antihistamines Emollients
Contact dermatitis				
Irritant type	Predisposing history of atopy Frequent water exposure Solvents Job description	Hands commonly Erythema, scale, fissuring	None	Topical steroid ointments Protect from wet exposures Gloves Emollients
Allergic type	Rapid onset Pruritus Exposures: Plants Cosmetics	Erythema, vesicles, oozing Location corresponds to exposure	None	Wet to dry dressings Topical or systemic corticosteroids Identify and avoid allergen
Stasis dermatitis	Gradual onset Distal legs Previous history of varicosities, leg trauma, etc	Erythema Pigmentation Edema Fibrosis	None	Acute: steroid ointments Long-term: compression, leg elevation, emollient ointments
Xerotic dermatitis	Winter Low humidity Frequent baths Soap use Pretibial common	Patchy erythema, scale on extensor areas Spares folds	None	Decrease soap and water exposure Liberal use of thick emollients, especially after bath Steroids: short-term prn
Dyshidrosis	Pruritic papules and vesicles on hands Recurrent	Papules and small vesicles on hands	None Exclude fungus with KOH Exclude allergen	Systemic or topical steroids Antibiotics
Nummular dermatitis	Gradual onset Pruritus Frequent history of exposure to drying (see Box 86-3)	Round patches Erythema Scaling Oozing	None KOH to exclude fungus	Steroid ointments Tar cream, gel Ultraviolet light

KOH, Potassium hydroxide.

multiple exacerbating factors that need to be controlled (see Box 86-1).

Allergy testing by prick test in atopic dermatitis is rarely beneficial. Atopic patients frequently have allergic responses to multiple allergens, and the elimination of these is usually not feasible. In individual cases, elimination of a particular food may help control exacerbations, but in the majority of cases, searching for foods to eliminate is without benefit.

CONTACT DERMATITIS

Contact dermatitis refers to any dermatitis caused by external substances that come in contact with the skin directly. Contactants can induce either allergic or irritant contact dermatitis, either of which can be acute, subacute, or chronic.[2]

Irritant Contact Dermatitis

Irritant contact dermatitis is more common than allergic contact dermatitis. It occurs when a chemical disrupts the normal epidermal barrier and causes an inflammatory response. Most irritants are those used on a daily basis and are found in most living and work environments. These generally are low-grade irritants that require repeated exposure to produce a dermatitis (soapy water, cleansers, rubbing alcohol). Some irritants are highly caustic, producing severe dermatitis after minimal exposure (bleach, strong acids, alkalis). Although anyone can develop irritant contact dermatitis, those with compromised skin (atopic dermatitis, dry skin) are at a higher risk.

Examination. Mild irritants produce erythema, chapped skin, dryness, and fissuring. Pruritus is usually mild to moderate. The hands are the usual site for irritant contact dermatitis (see Plate 11), but the face, especially the eyelids, may be affected. Severe cases can present with edema, serous oozing, and tenderness. Potent irritants cause painful bullae within hours of the exposure.

Management

The goals of treatment of irritant contact dermatitis are to restore a normal epidermal barrier and then protect it from the irritating substance. Reduced exposure to soap and water, use

Box 86-1. Controlling Atopic Dermatitis

Protect Skin From the Following Agents

Moisture
- Avoid frequent hand washing
- Avoid frequent bathing
- Avoid lengthy bathing
- Use tepid water for baths
- Avoid abrasive wash cloths

Foods
- Avoid prolonged contact (clean food around babies' mouth)

Rough clothing
- Avoid wool
- Use 100% cotton

Irritants and allergens
- Use soaps only in axilla, groin, feet
- Avoid perfumes or makeup that burns or itches
- Avoid fabric softeners

Scratching
- Do not scratch
- Pat, firmly press, or grasp the skin
- Apply soothing lubricants

Control Environment

Temperature
- Maintain cool, stable temperatures
- Do not overdress
- Limit number of bed blankets
- Avoid sweating

Humidity
- Humidify the house in winter

Airborne allergens and dust
- Do not have rugs in bedrooms
- Vacuum drapes and blankets
- Use plastic mattress covers
- Wet mop floors
- Avoid aerosols
- Ventilate cooking odors
- Avoid cigarettes
- Use artificial plants
- Avoid ragweed pollen contact
- Minimize animal dander–no cats, dogs, rodents, or birds

Change geographic location
- Sudden improvement may occur

Control Emotional Stress

Pleasant work environment

Learn relaxation techniques

Control Diet

Diet control is a controversial treatment method (see text for treatment)

From Habif TP: *Clinical dermatology: a color guide to diagnosis and therapy*, ed 2, St Louis, 1990, Mosby.

of emollient creams or ointments, and use of gloves in hand dermatitis may control a chronic irritant contact dermatitis. In more severe cases, corticosteroid ointments under occlusion may be necessary to treat the acute phase. Systemic corticosteroids, although potentially helpful in reducing acute inflammation, have no place in the treatment of chronic irritant contact dermatitis unless corrective measures are taken to avoid the offending contactants.

Allergic Contact Dermatitis

Allergic contact dermatitis occurs when a delayed (type IV) hypersensitivity to a substance develops. This hypersensitivity can occur after one exposure (poison ivy) or after years of repeated exposure to an antigen (fragrances, nickel).

Pathophysiology. The antigen, usually of low molecular weight, binds to epidermal proteins and is presented by Langerhans cells to T-lymphocytes in the dermis, as well as lymph nodes, where sensitized T-lymphocytes are expanded. The allergic dermatitis occurs when the sensitized lymphocytes encounter the antigen in the skin and release inflammatory mediators. The sensitization phase takes 10 to 14 days, but dermatitis may be seen in a sensitized individual within 12 to 48 hours after reexposure.

The most common sensitizer in the United States is the oleoresin of the Rhus family of plants (poison oak, poison ivy, poison sumac). Other common sensitizers include nickel in jewelry, fragrances, preservatives in topical preparations, components in rubber, and chemicals in shoes.

History. Intense itching in the area of exposure, followed by the development of a pruritic rash is typical of acute allergic contact dermatitis. The exposure can antedate the dermatitis by 2 weeks, if it is the result of a primary sensitization. Frequently an exact date of exposure is difficult to identify. In chronic cases, the dermatitis may have been present for months or years.

Examination. Clinical findings include erythema, edema, papules, vesicles, and serous oozing in the involved areas. In Rhus dermatitis there are frequently linear streaks of dermatitis corresponding to areas of contact with the plant resin (Plate 35). The extent of the dermatitis reflects the source of exposure, i.e., cosmetics on the face, nickel where jewelry is worn, rubber where elastic bands contact the skin, and points of shoe contact on the feet.

Management. Wet to dry compresses with water or aluminum acetate (Burow's solution) help dry the vesicular phase when indicated (see Chapter 83). Topical corticosteroids are helpful after the skin is dry enough to retain the topical preparation. In severe cases, systemic corticosteroids and antihistamines may be required. Usually, elimination of the offending antigen is curative, but in persistent cases, correct identification of the antigen may require patch testing. Referral to a dermatologist for possible patch testing is especially useful when multiple potential exposures exist such as in certain work environments.

Latex Dermatitis

Latex allergy has become an increasingly prevalent medical problem frequently presenting with hand dermatitis. Serious anaphylactic reactions, including several deaths, have been caused by latex allergy during procedures involving latex exposure, such as barium enemas, vaginal examinations, and dental procedures, all of which involve mucous membranes. In addition to type I hypersensitivity reactions, latex can cause allergic contact dermatitis (type IV) and irritant contact dermatitis.[6,7]

Epidemiology and Pathophysiology. The highest prevalence of latex sensitization (18% to 73%) occurs in individuals with spina bifida. Risk factors in this group include a history of more than five operations and atopy. Health care workers, especially those with atopy, have the second highest prevalence of latex sensitization (3% to 17%). Several foods cross react with latex; the most common of these are avocado, kiwi, banana, and chestnuts.

Clinical Manifestations and Diagnosis. Most cases of latex allergy present with a contact hand dermatitis, either irritant or allergic. Patients may present with rhinitis or asthma from inhalation of latex or anaphylactoid reactions from mucosal contact with latex during procedures.

Patient Evaluation. Avoidance of contact may serve as both diagnostic test and treatment in mild cases. In complicated cases, diagnostic evaluation requires patch testing with rubber additives, in vitro IgE antibody testing (radioallergosorbent test [RAST], enzyme-linked immunosorbent assay [ELISA], others), and direct skin testing with latex. Referral to an allergist or dermatologist is indicated in these instances.

Treatment. Avoidance of latex is the best treatment. Powder-free latex gloves can eliminate airborne latex exposure. Glove liners may prevent hand dermatitis. Latex sensitive individuals are at risk for anaphylaxis during procedures and should wear a *medical alert bracelet* to indicate their allergy and carry an anaphylaxis kit. Patients with spina bifida should be screened before surgical operations.

Stasis Dermatitis

Stasis dermatitis occurs on the legs as a result of chronic venous insufficiency. Incompetent venous valves, inadequate tissue support, and postural hydrostatic pressure contribute to the development of venous stasis. The dermatologic changes are secondary to the effects of extravasated blood, which induces a mild inflammatory response in the dermis and subcutaneous fat, plus the low grade tissue ischemia associated with stasis at the capillary level. Superimposed allergic contact dermatitis or recurrent infections are frequently the predominant finding in patients with stasis dermatitis.

History. Symptoms are mild in most cases of stasis dermatitis. There may be a sense of fullness or dull aching in the legs. The patient usually reports a gradual increase in pigmentation and redness.

Examination. In early stasis dermatitis there is mottled pigmentation and slight erythema. There may be evidence of varicosities, ankle edema, and mild tenderness to deep palpation. Pulses are usually normal. In chronic cases, fibrosis may be the predominant finding, resulting in a woody, hard sclerotic lower leg.

Differential Diagnosis. See Box 86-2.

Management

Nonpharmacologic. The main emphasis in the management of stasis dermatitis is to counteract the effects of gravity and posture on venous pressure. Leg elevation and compression with stockings are the most effective treatment. In mild cases, support hose alone may be sufficient. In more severe cases, daily leg elevation above the level of the head for varying amounts of time may be necessary. Exercise on a regular basis also helps to reduce venous pressure and edema.

Pharmacologic. The inflammatory component of stasis dermatitis is treated with low or medium potency topical corticosteroids. An ointment base avoids exposure to preservatives, which can cause allergic contact dermatitis.

Box 86-2. Differential Diagnosis of Stasis Dermatitis

Diabetic dermopathy
Allergic contact dermatitis
Cellulitis
Pigmented purpura (Schamberg's disease)

Box 86-3. Factors That Can Cause Xerosis

Excessive bathing
Long hot showers
Soap use
Swimming, hot tubs, jacuzzi
Electric blankets
Heated mattress or waterbed
Low humidity in home or office
Lotions (high water content)

Xerotic Dermatitis

Xerotic (asteatotic) dermatitis is a form of mild irritant dermatitis that occurs in areas of dry skin (Box 86-3). As the skin loses hydration the stratum corneum becomes scaly and develops small cracks that gradually enlarge to form patches of erythema with scaling (Plate 36). These areas are usually intensely pruritic and are worsened by low humidity and exposure to hot water, soap, or solvents. Pretibial areas are most common but the lower back, extensor arms, and thighs may be involved.

Management. Treatment of xerotic dermatitis consists of frequent use of emollients to the affected areas, especially after bathing or other water exposure. Topical medium strength corticosteroids help with the pruritus of the acute phase.

Dyshidrotic Dermatitis

Dyshidrotic dermatitis (pompholyx, dyshidrosis) is an intensely pruritic, chronic recurrent dermatitis that typically involves the palms and soles. The name is misleading, since the disorder has no relationship to eccrine sweating. The etiology of dyshidrosis is uncertain, although ingested allergens and emotional stress have been suggested Plate 37.

History. Intense pruritus on the palms or soles that progresses to multiple small vesicles is typical. The vesicles

Box 86-4. Differential Diagnosis of Dyshidrotic Dermatitis

Tinea (dermatophyte): Vesicles usually on feet only; KOH is positive.
Psoriasis: Pustules more common; less itching.
Id reaction: Can resemble dyshidrosis; look for fungal or bacterial antigen source.
Contact dermatitis: Can be superimposed on dyshidrotic dermatitis.

KOH, Potassium hydroxide.

gradually desquamate over 1 to 2 weeks. Recurrent episodes alternating with disease-free periods are common.

Examination. The presence of multiple small vesicles on the palmar or plantar skin, especially along the lateral aspects of the fingers, is suggestive. Desquamation, erythema, cracking, and fissuring may be seen in older lesions. The process is usually symmetric.

Differential Diagnosis. See Box 86-4.

Management. In mild cases, medium to potent topical corticosteroids can control outbreaks. Systemic corticosteroids are occasionally required in difficult cases.

Nummular Dermatitis

Nummular dermatitis is a chronic pruritic skin eruption consisting of circular raised patches of erythematous scaly skin. The etiology is not known, although xerosis and emotional stress have been implicated. Adults tend to be affected more than children.

History. Patients usually report patches of itchy skin that gradually enlarge in size and increase in number. Individual lesions tend to remain fixed for the duration of the disease process.

Examination. Round patches of erythema, scaling, and occasional crust or exudation are suggestive of nummular dermatitis (Plate 38). The term *nummular* translates literally to "coin shaped." The distribution is usually extensor areas of extremities, the back, and buttocks. The differential diagnosis includes psoriasis and tinea corporis. A potassium hydroxide (KOH) examination of any scaly lesions is indicated.

Management. To reduce acute inflammation, class I topical corticosteroids under occlusive dressings or intralesional corticosteroid injections (triamcinolone 5 mg/cc or betamethasone 6 mg/cc) may be necessary. Emollients throughout the day and especially after water exposure or bathing are essential. In severe cases systemic steroids, antihistamines, topical tar preparations (see Chapter 83) and ultraviolet light treatments can be used.

Lichen Simplex Chronicus and Prurigo Nodules

Lichen simplex chronicus is not a true dermatitis but the result of rubbing or scratching. Although lichen simplex chronicus is usually a patch or plaque of thickened skin, there is a nodular form (prurigo nodularis) that consists of raised thickened nodules with excoriations. A history of chronic persistent itching in the involved area is typical. Patients with renal or hepatic failure and late stage HIV infection commonly have this problem.

Examination. In lichen simplex chronicus there is thickened skin with erythema and accentuation of skin lines (lichenification). Usually there is only one area of involvement. Common sites include extremities, posterior neck, buttocks, vulva, scrotum, and anal area. In prurigo nodularis there are several to multiple nodules, 0.5 cm to 1.0 cm in size, scattered over the upper back, arms, and thighs. Areas that are not convenient to reach, such as the central back and posterior thighs, tend to be spared (Plate 39).

Management. The treatment of lichen simplex chronicus consists of breaking the itch-scratch cycle. Potent corticosteroids under occlusion may be successful. Intralesional corticosteroid injections and cryotherapy with liquid nitrogen may be required in nodular cases, although the treatment of prurigo nodularis is frequently unsuccessful. Topical capsaicin, ultraviolet light therapy, antihistamines, and antidepressants can be helpful, but persistence over years is common.

REFERENCES

1. Cookson WOCM, Young RP, Sanford AJ, et al: Maternal inheritance of atopic IgE responsiveness on chromosome 11q. *Lancet* 340:381-384, 1992.
2. Fisher AA: *Contact dermatitis*, ed 3, Philadelphia, 1986, Lea & Febiger.
3. Hanifin JM: Atopic dermatitis, *J Am Acad Dermatol* 6:1-13, 1982.
4. Hanifin JM, Rajka G: Diagnostic features of atopic dermatitis, *Acta Derm Venerol Suppl (Stockholm)* 92:44-47, 1980.
5. Kuster W, Peterson M, Christophers E, et al: A family study of atopic dermatitis: clinical and genetic characteristics of 188 patients and 2,151 family members, *Arch Dermatol Res* 282:98-102, 1990.
6. Michael T, Niggemann B, Moers A, et al: Risk factors for latex allergy in patients with spina bifida, *Clin Exp Allergy* 26:934, 1996.
7. Sussman G, Gold M: Guidelines for the management of latex allergies and safe latex use in health care facilities, *Am Coll Aller Asthma Immunol* August, 1996.

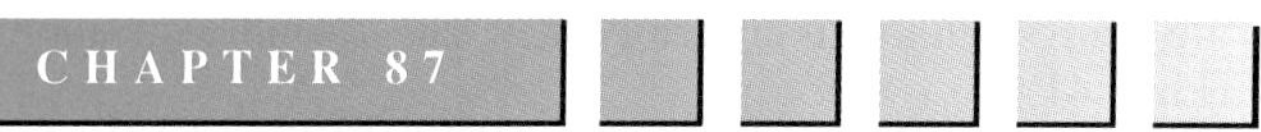

Neoplasms of the Skin

Bert G. Tavelli
James C. Shaw

BENIGN NEOPLASMS

There are easily dozens of benign proliferations of the skin and its appendages, each with numerous variations. Familiarization with the most common of these can help decide when it is best to treat or advise the patient and when it is best to refer.

Freckles and Lentigines

Freckles (ephelids) and *solar lentigines* (liver spots) are sun-induced, variably-pigmented macules that are characterized histologically by increased melanin along the basal layer of the epidermis. Solar lentigines are larger and more irregular in shape than freckles. *Simple lentigines* are similar in appearance to solar lentigines but appear in childhood, are symmetric, and are generally smaller. They are randomly distributed and not sun-sensitive. Histologically they have increased numbers of normal melanocytes, along with increased melanin pigmentation throughout the epidermis. No treatment is usually needed.

Melanocytic Nevi

Melanocytic nevi are a group of benign proliferations of nevus cells, forming symmetric, well-circumscribed, evenly pigmented lesions anywhere on the skin. Acquired melanocytic nevi vary considerably in clinical appearance. Typical benign nevi present as symmetric, round-to-oval lesions with distinct, rounded borders. They range in contour from flat (junctional) to slightly raised or papillated (compound) (Plate 40) to dome-shaped or pedunculated (intradermal); pigmentation may vary from tan to all shades of brown or black. Many intradermal nevi eventually become flesh colored or only slightly pigmented. They tend to enlarge in proportion to body growth and may do so more rapidly during pregnancy.

Although variations in size, shape, color, and growth characteristics occur within a given individual's nevi, the "ABCD's" provide a rationale for the clinical identification of lesions suggestive of melanoma. These ABCD's are the following:

Asymmetry (not round or oval)
Border irregularity (notching or poorly defined)
Color variegation (shades of brown, red, white, black, blue, or combinations of colors)
Diameter (greater than 6 mm)
Symptoms (persistent itch or other sensation)

In addition, an otherwise benign-appearing pigmented or nonpigmented nevus that changes rapidly in any way can also represent melanoma, which is presented later in this chapter.

Several clinical variants of melanocytic nevi deserve discussion. *Blue nevi* are acquired and are usually solitary dark blue or blue gray papules located anywhere on the skin or mucous membranes. They are thought to represent ectopic accumulations of melanocytes in the dermis that reflect light of a blue wavelength because of their density and depth. They are benign, although clinically they can resemble melanoma (Plate 41).

Atypical nevi are a more common but controversial variant that are difficult to classify and for which there are no strict diagnostic criteria. Previously referred to as "dysplastic nevi," they are generally larger than other acquired nevi, with somewhat indistinct or irregular borders (Plate 42). Pigmentation varies within lesions from dark brown to tan or flesh colored, often on a reddish background. They are usually flat but may have a centrally raised portion that can be darker than the surrounding macular area.

Clearly, an individual lesion that is large, has an asymmetric or irregular shape, and color variation might be suggestive of melanoma. However, when many such nevi occur on the same person, management becomes more difficult. Additionally, the histology of these lesions has been similarly difficult to define, with no clear-cut reproducible criteria with which to distinguish them from other pigmented lesions.

The main importance of atypical nevi lies in the possible increased risk of the development of melanoma, either in an individual lesion or in patients or families in whom these nevi are seen. These questions are highly controversial, and the field is constantly in flux, making clinical management difficult. A reasonable approach for the primary practitioner based in part on a recent National Institutes of Health consensus conference is summarized in Box 87-1.

Chondrodermatitis Nodularis

Chondrodermatitis nodularis (Plate 43) is a painful, pressure-induced papule or nodule occurring primarily along the helical rim of the ear. Lesions are precipitated by focal, often minor, trauma, and develop into inflamed, intensely painful papules with central necrosis or ulceration. They may resemble basal cell or squamous cell carcinoma. Treatment

Box 87-1. Managed Care Guide: Atypical Nevi

Terminology

The term *dysplastic nevi* is misleading and confusing and should be avoided. Nevi are presently classified clinically as "atypical nevi" or "nevi with atypical architecture," and histologically as "nevi with architectural disorder."

Frequency

Estimates vary by tenfold, but atypical nevi are common.

Familial Atypical Mole and Melanoma Syndrome

Familial atypical mole and melanoma (FAM-M) syndrome seems to be well-established and defines families with (1) occurrence of melanoma in one or more first or second degree relatives; (2) large numbers of nevi, some of which are atypical; and (3) nevi that show certain histologic features. Individuals with the FAM-M syndrome have a significantly high risk of developing melanoma. Referral to a dermatologist is required for intensive surveillance and to promote early diagnosis.

Nonfamilial Atypical Moles

The risk of development of melanoma in individuals with nonfamilial atypical nevi is unknown. The risk is certainly far less than with the familial type, but there may be an increased relative risk compared with the general population. These cases must be individualized and assessed by as many criteria as are available.

Management

Lesions that are clinically suggestive of malignant melanoma require biopsy. As with the clinical evaluation, where inspection of small portions of the lesion is inadequate for diagnosis, so it is with the histopathologic evaluation. When possible, total excisional biopsy is required. A large incisional-wedge biopsy is preferred for lesions that are too large or technically or cosmetically inappropriate for excision. Shave biopsies or punch biopsies are never acceptable. Because of the difficulty in diagnosing melanoma, both clinically and histopathologically, referral to a dermatologist should be strongly considered.

with intralesional corticosteroids may be useful, but surgical excision is often necessary.

Keloids

Keloids (Plate 44) are firm, smooth, often tender proliferations of scar tissue at sites of injury to the skin that occur mostly on the chest, shoulders, back, and earlobes. Treatment is problematic, since surgery usually results in a larger keloid. Early treatment is more successful, using a combination of silastic gel sheeting, intralesional corticosteroids, and specialized surgical techniques.

Seborrheic Keratoses

Seborrheic keratoses (Plate 45) are symmetric, keratotic papules or plaques that can arise anywhere on the skin and appear "stuck on." They range in color from light tan to dark brown or black and often have a waxy consistency. Seborrheic keratoses can be distinguished from melanoma, which at times they closely resemble, by the presence of multiple, dilated follicular ostia filled with keratin. Biopsy by excision is necessary when the diagnosis is uncertain. If needed, symptomatic lesions can be treated with a light liquid nitrogen spray.

Calluses and Corns

Both calluses and corns represent hyperkeratotic, thickened skin arising in response to chronic trauma from pressure or friction. A corn is generally smaller and more focal, occurring over bony pressure points on the sides of the toes or foot. Elimination of the abnormal pressure forces and manipulating or changing footwear is often successful.

Sebaceous Hyperplasia

Sebaceous hyperplasia is the term given to symmetric, raised, 2 to 4 mm papules that appear on the face in middle age. The distinctive yellow color and typical umbilication around a central pore (follicular ostium) help distinguish them from basal cell carcinoma and other epidermal neoplasms. No treatment is needed for these benign lesions.

Hemangiomas

Hemangiomas are benign proliferations of blood vessels forming variably sized, soft, red compressible papules that occur anywhere on skin. The most common is the "cherry hemangioma," which is small, usually less than 3 mm, and difficult to blanch. They are seen primarily on the chest and back and increase in number with age. No treatment is required, although laser removal for cosmesis has had some success.

Pyogenic Granuloma

Pyogenic granulomas (Plate 46) are reddish purple, friable, vascular tumors that range in size from several millimeters to greater than a centimeter. They can arise anywhere on the skin, usually as a response to local trauma. They bleed profusely when abraded and are often ulcerated or covered with scale crust. They usually require surgical excision, and recurrences are common. Occasionally, malignant melanoma can resemble a pyogenic granuloma and should be considered in the differential diagnosis.

Lipomas

Lipomas are subcutaneous tumors of adipose tissue, usually located on the trunk and proximal extremities. They are soft, symmetric, and easily movable over deeper structures and can be confused with various cystic lesions. They may be single or multiple and any size from 1 to many centimeters in diameter. The term *angiolipoma* is given to a variant that histologically contains multiple small blood vessels and clinically may be associated with pain. These symptomatic lesions may be surgically excised.

Follicular Cysts

Follicular cysts are dermal tumors containing sebum and keratin debris that are derived from the lining of the hair follicle. They appear as firm, raised, slowly enlarging nodules anywhere on the skin, predominantly the scalp, face, and trunk. They are also termed *wens* and erroneously referred to as epidermal, inclusion, or sebaceous cysts. Most lesions are left untreated, although surgical excision may be needed for larger cysts, those in sensitive anatomic sites, or those that have become recurrently infected.

Dermatofibromas

Dermatofibromas (Plate 47) are firm, scarlike, pigmented dermal nodules that occur most frequently on the extremities of women but can be found anywhere on the skin in either sex. Most present as slowly enlarging, reddish-brown, slightly elevated papules or nodules. Individual lesions can reach a centimeter or more in size and can be painful. They are not attached to fat or fascia but are affixed to overlying epidermis. Dermatofibromas should be referred for evaluation if they are large or rapidly enlarging, irregularly pigmented, bleeding, or painful, so that malignant melanoma, dermatofibrosarcoma protuberans, and other malignant processes can be excluded.

Fibrous Papule

Fibrous papules (adenoma sebaceum, angiofibroma) are smooth, 1 to 2 mm, grayish to flesh-colored papules that occur almost exclusively on the nose and central face. They are common in middle-aged individuals and usually solitary, although multiple lesions are sometimes seen and should alert the practitioner to the possibility of tuberous sclerosis. Biopsy is required at times to distinguish them from basal cell carcinoma.

Acrochordon

Acrochordons, which are also called skin tags, are extremely common. They most often involve the axillae, neckline, and groin, where they appear as pinpoint to 5 mm or larger flesh-colored papules. Acrochordons are most often confused with nevi or seborrheic keratoses. Surgical removal is used for those lesions that interfere with function or become persistently inflamed.

MALIGNANT NEOPLASMS

Nonmelanoma Skin Cancer

Epidemiology/Etiology. Basal cell carcinoma (BCC) and squamous cell carcinoma (SCC) represent the most common human malignancies. Nonmelanoma skin cancers account for greater than 1 million new cases of cancer annually in the United States and are responsible for 1200 to 1500 deaths per year. Costs of $500,000,000 have been estimated in the management of these malignancies. Fair-skinned caucasians have the highest risk for the development of nonmelanoma skin cancer. Ultraviolet (UV) light exposure has been implicated as the carcinogen most responsible for the development of these malignancies.[2] UV light has been shown to alter DNA, such as tumor suppressor genes (p 53), thymidine dimers, and ras oncogenes, all of which are thought to contribute to the development of skin cancer. UV light has also been shown to alter the immune system by damaging epidermal immune cells and modulating cytokine activity.

Basal Cell Carcinoma

Physical Examination. There are three main variants of BCC based on the clinical appearance.

Nodular BCC, the most common, usually develops as a papule and enlarges slowly into a nodule (Plate 48). The lesion is raised, pearly or translucent in color, with telangiectasias. Ulceration or surface crusting is common (Plate 49). The most common sites are the sun-exposed areas of the head and neck. Rarely, BCCs are pigmented and resemble malignant melanoma.

Sclerosing BCC (Plate 50) appears as a patch of indurated scarlike change, whitish in color, usually without telangiectasias or ulceration. This variant enlarges horizontally into plaques.

Superficial BCC (Plate 51) refers to a variant that resembles a dermatitis. In this variant, a patch of erythema with slight scale and friability gradually enlarges over years. A slightly raised, advancing border usually surrounds the lesion. The tumor process remains at the base of the epidermis for months to years before larger nodular growth develops.

Laboratory Evaluation. Histologic confirmation is important and helps direct treatment. The depth of involvement, histologic type, and whether there are aggressive features are important factors in designing therapy. A punch biopsy gives the best results. There are several histologic variants of BCC, as well as numerous benign skin tumors that resemble BCC histologically.

Management

Prevention. Sun protection beginning in childhood is the best preventive measure against BCC. This prevention includes educating adults and children about the damaging effects of excessive sun exposure, the early use of sun screens (minimum SPF 15), and protective clothing.

Treatment. Modalities for treating BCC include curettage surgery, excision, radiation, and Mohs' surgery. The choice of treatment depends on the location, size, histologic type, and history of previous treatment. For small lesions, simple excision is usually curative. Large tumors, recurrent tumors, and those on the central face and around the ears have a higher treatment failure rate.

For these types of BCC, the use of Mohs' surgery may be indicated. Mohs' surgery is a specialized procedure that utilizes excision with frozen-section control of all margins by means of quadrant mapping of the specimen (Fig. 87-1). Radiation may be indicated in patients who cannot tolerate excisional surgery or for lesions in difficult anatomic sites.

Squamous Cell Carcinoma

Physical Examination. There are several clinical presentations that are considered within the disease spectrum of SCC.

Actinic keratoses (solar keratoses) (Plate 52) are considered precursors to SCC. They begin as areas of rough or thickened skin, usually with some erythema, and slowly evolve into raised hyperkeratotic plaques or nodules. They are always found on sun-damaged skin. Histologically, actinic keratoses have atypical epidermal growth that is limited to the lower portion of the epidermis. The differential diagnosis of actinic keratosis are found in Box 87-2.

Bowen's disease (SCC in situ) (Plate 53) usually presents as a patch of erythematous or brown-red discoloration, slightly raised, with sharp borders. Sun-protected, as well as sun-damaged, skin can develop Bowen's disease, which demonstrates atypical epidermal growth throughout the entire thickness of the epidermis but no invasion into the dermis. Both actinic keratoses and SCC in situ have the potential to evolve into invasive SCC.

Keratoacanthoma (Plate 54) is a type of SCC that in the past has been called self-healing or benign. It develops rapidly as a dome-shaped nodule that can reach a size of 1 or 2 cm within 8 weeks. Histology can be indistinguishable from invasive SCC. Although past literature suggests that keratoacanthomas can resolve spontaneously, there have been reports of metastasis, and many authors now regard keratoacanthomas as a variant of well-differentiated SCC.

SCC arising de novo without a precursor lesion usually starts with a patch of hyperkeratosis with erythema, which grows slowly into a nodular tumor or a cutaneous horn (Plate 55).

Laboratory Evaluation. Skin biopsy is required to confirm the diagnosis. No other laboratory tests are useful.

Management. The treatment of choice for SCC is surgical excision. Actinic keratoses can be treated with cryotherapy using liquid nitrogen. Topical chemotherapy with 5-fluorouracil (5-Fu) is occasionally used when numerous actinic keratoses are present. Keratoacanthomas are treated with excision or intralesional injection with 5-FU or methotrexate. Systemic retinoids have been used in cases of multiple keratoacanthomas. SCCs in the setting of immunosuppression require aggressive treatment because of their rapid growth patterns.

Melanoma

Epidemiology/Etiology. The worldwide incidence of melanoma is increasing faster than any other malignancy. It is predicted that by the year 2000, 1 out of 75 persons will develop melanoma during their lifetime, compared with 1 out of 600 in 1960 and 1 out of 150 in 1985. While the incidence is increasing, the death rate from cutaneous melanoma can be reduced by early detection and treatment.[6]

Melanoma is a disease primarily of caucasians, although it does occur, although rarely, in darker-pigmented populations. Risk factors include multiple dysplastic nevi, family history of melanoma, multiple basal nevi, immunosuppression, fair skin, and a history of excessive childhood sun exposure.

Physical Examination. There are several characteristics of melanoma that are common and are the basis for the previously mentioned ABCD'S of melanoma recognition:

Asymmetry is a common feature of melanoma, whereas most benign tumors tend to be symmetric in shape.

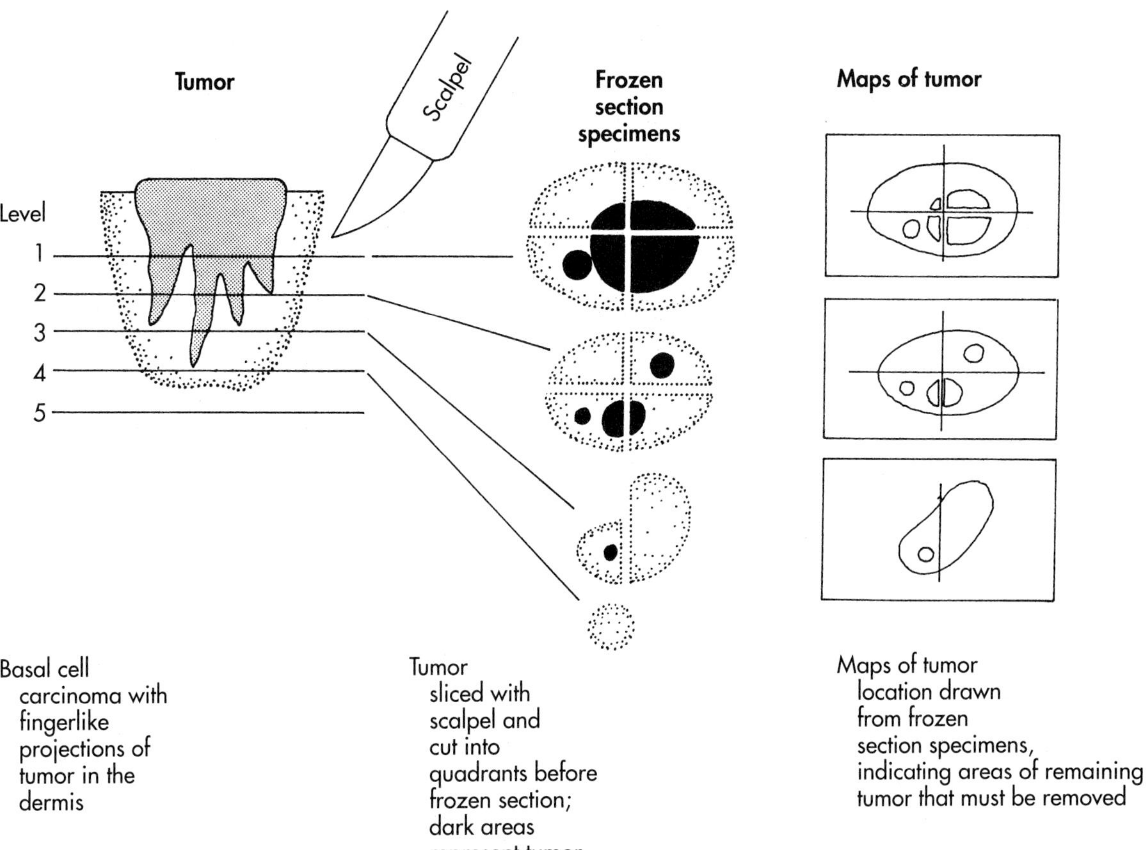

Fig. 87-1. Microscopically guided excision of cutaneous tumors—Mohs' micrographic surgery. (From Habif TP: *Clinical dermatology,* ed 3, St Louis, 1996, Mosby.)

Box 87-2. Differential Diagnosis of Actinic Keratosis

Superficial BCC
Verruca vulgaris
Seborrheic keratosis
SCC

Border irregularity, although not pathognomonic for melanoma, is a typical finding.

Color variegation is an important diagnostic feature. Black, blue, and red hues are commonly present. Colors of the brown spectrum (tan to dark brown) are characteristic of benign lesions (nevi, seborrheic keratoses) and are rarely part of a melanoma unless it arises from a preexisting nevus of that color.

Diameter of melanoma tends to enlarge with time, whereas benign lesions remain stable. Any lesion that enlarges significantly over a period of 1 to 3 months should be evaluated.

Symptoms, such as bleeding and ulceration, may be present in larger lesions.

When examining patients with melanoma, examination of the mucous membranes and lymph nodes should be included.

Clinical Variants. Historically, melanoma has been classified into variants based on appearance, histology, and biologic course. Although there is increasing evidence that the separations may not have prognostic significance, many authors continue to use the terms.

Superficial spreading melanoma (Plate 56) is the most common type of melanoma. It is found mostly on the upper back and on the legs in women. The horizontal growth pattern results in irregular shapes. Considerable color variation can be seen.

Nodular melanoma (see Plate 21) is a raised lesion found anywhere on the body. It can be black, reddish, or flesh colored. The early vertical growth pattern results in the clinical nodule.

Acral-lentiginous melanoma occurs on the palms, soles, finger tips, nails, and mucous membranes. It is most common in blacks and Asians. The lesions are usually flat but become nodular if left undiagnosed and untreated. Metastatic spread is common at the time of diagnosis.

Lentigo maligna refers to a melanoma in situ that develops on sun-damaged skin of elderly patients. An enlarging pigmented patch on the face is the most common presentation. The process can remain in situ for many years before evolving into melanoma.

Laboratory Evaluation. Expert pathologic interpretation is critical to the management of patients with melanoma. The implications of a missed diagnosis are obvious. The prognosis is based on the measured thickness of the tumor in

Table 87-1. 5-Year Survival Rates in Malignant Melanoma

Breslow tumor thickness (mm)	Survival (%)
<0.75	95-99
0.76-1.49	80-95
1.50-4.00	60-75
>4.00	<50

Modified from Johnson TM et al: *J Am Acad Dermatol* 32:689-707, 1995.

Box 87-3. Sun-avoidance Behavior

1. For type I or II skin (always burns or frequently burns), minimize exposure to the sun.
2. Avoid outdoor activities in mid-day sun.
3. Wear a broad-brimmed hat in the sun (7-inch brim ideally).
4. Wear long pants and long-sleeved shirts.
5. Sunscreens: SPF 15 minimum. Wear daily and reapply if planning sun exposure. Waterproof if swimming.

millimeters (Breslow level) more than any other histologic finding (Table 87-1). Ideally, the lesion should be excised entirely for diagnosis. Incisional biopsies may be performed for diagnosis when complete excision is not feasible. A shallow shave biopsy should be avoided, and freezing or burning of pigmented lesions is contraindicated with the sole exception of seborrheic keratoses. The use of the sentinel node biopsy has helped identify individuals with micrometastases who would benefit from lymph node dissection or adjuvant chemotherapy.[1] In this procedure, blue dye and radioisotope is injected into the melanoma site to identify the sentinal lymph node in the drainage site.

Management

Prevention. Sun-avoidance behavior (Box 87-3) is currently the main emphasis in melanoma prevention. Protecting young children from sun exposure may be the most important factor that can be monitored.

Early Detection. Early detection of melanoma can be lifesaving. The skin self-examination is now recommended to all patients with increased risk of melanoma.[4] This examination is analogous to the breast self-examination. Patients examine their entire skin surface (using mirrors and assistance when needed) on a monthly basis and seek medical advice for changing lesions or new suspicious lesions. Annual or semi-annual physician visits have also been recommended, but studies of cost effectiveness of this practice have not been done.

The management of a patient with stage I and II melanoma (local disease only) depends on the type of melanoma and the size and thickness of the lesion.[5] Recent studies have revised the concept of "deep and wide excisions for all melanomas." It is now felt that melanomas of a depth of less than 1-mm Breslow thickness can be excised with margins of 1 cm of normal skin. It is not clear what the optimal size of resection is for thicker melanomas, and wider resections continue to be done until this question is answered. The benefit of an elective lymph node dissection is also not established. For melanomas less than 1 mm thick, lymph node dissection is not needed, and for those greater than 4 mm thick, lymph node dissection does not prolong life. In lesions between 1 mm and 4 mm of thickness, there may be some value in performing a lymph node dissection, especially if a single drainage pathway can be identified. The sentinel node biopsy has been used in this group. Follow-up is every 6 to 12 months for thin melanomas (less than 1 mm thickness) and every 3 to 4 months for thicker lesions during the first 5 years, with gradual extension up to 10- to 12-month intervals. Patients need lifelong follow-up, since metastatic spread can become evident after 10 years. The management of stage III (lymph node involvement) and stage IV (systemic involvement) melanoma is beyond the scope of this section. Most treatments are designed for palliation or temporary remission.

Cutaneous T-Cell Lymphoma

Cutaneous T-cell lymphoma (CTCL) (mycosis fungoides) is a malignancy of CD4% T-lymphocytes with a predilection for involvement of the skin.[3] Men are affected twice as much as women and blacks twice as much as whites. The disease is usually diagnosed in the fifth and sixth decades, although a trend toward earlier diagnosis has been observed recently. The incidence in the United States is twice that observed in England, Wales, Norway, the Netherlands, and Western Australia. Although the etiology of CTCL is unknown, hypotheses concerning etiology include occupational exposure, chronic antigen stimulation, and retroviruses, although none have been proved.

Pathophysiology. The precise pathophysiology leading to the development of CTCL is uncertain. One theory is that CTCL begins as a malignancy of CD4% T-cells that is not easily detectable in early stages because of effective immune host response. The malignancy then becomes more aggressive as host response declines and the total number of malignant cells increases. An alternate theory is that CTCL is the result of chronic antigen stimulation (no antigen has yet been identified), which results in T-lymphocyte proliferation with the potential for transformation into malignant cell lines.

History. CTCL develops slowly in most cases. Patients usually seek medical attention because of asymptomatic or pruritic patches of abnormal-appearing skin. Patients commonly report a long history of a chronic dermatitis that is unresponsive to treatment. Rarely, CTCL presents with raised tumors noticed by patients. Constitutional symptoms are usually absent but may include fever, night sweats, and weight loss.

Physical Examination. There are three clinical stages in CTCL. The *patch stage* (Plate 57) consists of fixed erythematous patches with slight scaling and wrinkling of the epidermis. They range in size from a few millimeters to 10 to 20 cm in diameter and can be present anywhere on the body. The *plaque stage* evolves from the patch stage as the lymphocytic infiltrate in the dermis enlarges and the lesions develop a raised component. The plaques can be arcuate or irregular in shape and usually take on a red-brown color. The *tumor stage* (Plate 58) represents further evolution from the plaque stage, with raised red-brown to violaceous cutaneous tumors with central necrosis and ulceration. All three stages can be present simultaneously, and regional or generalized lymphadenopathy can be present during any of the stages. Occasionally, CTCL presents as a generalized exfoliative erythroderma. *Sezary syndrome* is a variant of CTCL presenting as a leukemic phase of the disease. Although this form can be present with any of the stages, it presents more frequently with erythroderma or an exfoliative dermatitis.

Diagnosis

Differential Diagnosis. The diagnosis of CTCL can be difficult to make on the basis of clinical appearance, especially in the early phases. Allergic contact dermatitis, other chronic dermatitis, pigmented purpura, psoriasis, and drug eruptions can be in the differential diagnosis of patch stage. Once raised lesions are present, the differential diagnosis includes other cutaneous malignancies, deep fungal infections, granulomatous disease, and deep forms of vasculitis. In all phases of CTCL, diagnosis is made by biopsy.

Diagnostic Procedures. Confirmation of the diagnosis requires histopathologic examination from lesional skin. The hallmark of CTCL is the presence of a dense accumulation of mature and atypical lymphocytes in the upper dermis. In most cases the lymphocytes are also present within the epidermis (epidermotropism), a feature that may be lost in late tumor stages. Multiple biopsies over time may be necessary to confirm the diagnosis. In addition to routine histopathologic examination, cell surface markers and gene rearrangement studies of the T-cell antigen receptors from sampled lymph node tissue can help make the diagnosis. Laboratory evaluation for evidence of systemic involvement includes routine hematology and chemistry, a Sezary cell count (greater than 5% Sezary cells is suggestive of Sezary syndrome), flow cytometry, molecular studies, and imaging studies of liver, spleen, and paraaortic lymph nodes. Staging is by the TNM classification (Table 87-2).

Table 87-2. Staging of Cutaneous T-Cell Lymphoma: TNM Classification

Classification	Description
T: Skin	
T_0	Lesions clinically and/or histopathologically suggestive of CTCL
T_1	Limited plaques, papules, or eczematous patches covering <10% of the skin surface
T_2	Generalized plaques, papules, or erythematous patches covering ≥10% of the skin surface
T_3	Tumors (>1)
T_4	Generalized erythroderma
N: Lymph nodes	
N_0	No palpable adenopathy, lymph node pathology negative for CTCL
N_1	Palpable adenopathy, lymph node pathology negative for CTCL
N_2	No palpable adenopathy, lymph node pathology positive for CTCL
N_3	Palpable adenopathy, lymph node pathology positive for CTCL
B: Peripheral blood	
B_0	Atypical circulating cells not present (<5%)
B_1	Atypical circulating cells not present (>5%); record total white blood cell count, total lymphocyte count, and number of atypical cells/100 lymphocytes
M: Visceral organs	
M_0	No visceral organ involvement
M_1	Visceral involvement (must have pathology confirmation and organ involved should be specified)

Management. The treatment of CTCL depends on the level of involvement and frequently requires a team approach utilizing the skills of dermatologists, oncologists, and radiation therapists. Because the therapies available for late stage disease are disappointing, early treatment of the patch and plaque stages of the disease yields the best responses. Topical nitrogen mustard has been used in early disease for many years and has been associated with remissions for up to 12 years in approximately 20% of those treated. UV light treatment (UVB or PUVA [psoralens plus UV light A]) is also effective in early disease, although recurrences usually develop if treatment is stopped. Total body electron beam therapy has been the most successful treatment, with total remissions achieved in 80% to 95% of patients with early disease and disease-free periods of up to 4 years. Other beneficial treatments include extracorporeal photopheresis (especially in erythodermic stages), single and multiple drug chemotherapy, and combinations of electron beam plus adjuvant chemotherapy. These treatments are palliative.

Lymphoma Cutis

All types of lymphoma can rarely involve the skin. The most common presentation is the development of asymptomatic erythematous to violaceous firm nodules that require biopsy for diagnosis. Treatment is systemic treatment of the underlying lymphoma.

Leukemia Cutis

Leukemia can rarely involve the skin with infiltrative nodules and plaques (Plate 59). Diagnosis is based on histopathologic examination, and treatment is directed toward the leukemic process.

Cutaneous Metastases

Cutaneous metastasis of an underlying malignancy is rare, occurring in approximately 1% or 2% of patients with malignancy. The incidence by tumor classification of cutaneous metastasis reflects the incidence of the underlying malignancy: lung cancer and colon cancer are most common in men, and breast cancer is most common in women. Any area of the body can be involved. Lesions usually develop rapidly and are usually asymptomatic. Cutaneous metastases usually consist of firm dermal nodules measuring 0.5 cm to 1.5 cm in diameter. The color is erythematous or red-brown with occasional violaceous hues (Plate 60). Diagnosis is made by biopsy, and treatment is directed toward the underlying malignancy.

REFERENCES

1. Brady MS, Coit DG: Sentinel lymph node evaluation in melanoma, *Arch Derm* 133:1014-1020, 1997.
2. Grossman D, Leffell DJ: The molecular basis of nonmelanoma skin cancer, *Arch Dermatol* 133:1263-1270, 1997.
3. Heald PW, Shapiro PE, Madison JF, et al: Cutaneous T-cell lymphoma. In Arndt KA et al, eds: *Cutaneous medicine and surgery,* Philadelphia, 1996, WB Saunders.
4. Howell JB: Skin self-examination for melanoma: another golden rule, *Semin Cutan Med Surg* 16:174-178, 1997.
5. Johnson TM, et al: Current therapy for cutaneous melanoma, *J Am Acad Dermatol* 32:689-707, 1995.
6. Rivers JK: Melanoma, *Lancet* 347:803-807, 1996.

ADDITIONAL READINGS

Elder D, editor: *Lever's histopathology of the skin,* ed 8, Philadelphia, 1991, Lippincott-Raven.

Maize JC, Ackerman AB, eds: *Pigmented lesions of the skin,* Philadelphia, 1987, Lea and Febiger.

National Institutes of Health (NIH): Diagnosis and treatment of early melanoma, *NIH Consensus Statement* 10(1):1992.

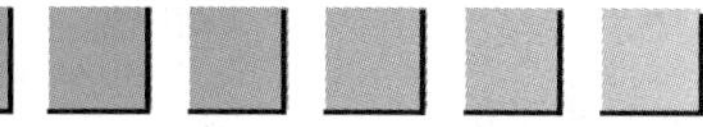

Cutaneous Manifestations of Systemic Disease

James C. Shaw

VASCULITIS, PURPURA, AND COAGULOPATHIES AFFECTING THE SKIN

Vasculitis represents a disease group that encompasses numerous disorders with varied etiologies (see Chapter 138). Vasculitis can affect large, medium, or small vessels, the latter two being most common in the skin. Purpuric lesions can be seen in the setting of vasculitis or can be a manifestation of hemorrhage into the skin. Hypercoagulable states frequently cause thromboses in the skin, with subsequent necrosis. The most common of these vasculopathies is discussed here.

Hypersensitivity Vasculitis

Hypersensitivity vasculitis, also known as leukocytoclastic vasculitis or cutaneous small vessel vasculitis,[4] is the most common of the cutaneous vasculitides and can be associated with numerous disorders and diseases (Box 88-1).

The clinical presentation of leukocytoclastic vasculitis is usually "palpable purpura," which translates to multiple nonblanchable hemorrhagic papules, usually on lower extremities and almost always bilateral (Plate 61). Symptoms are usually mild and can include pruritus, tenderness, and burning. Organ involvement other than skin is not common except in Henoch-Schönlein purpura and systemic lupus erythematosus (SLE) where renal, gastrointestinal, and occasionally other organ involvement can occur.

Skin biopsy is helpful in diagnosing leukocytoclastic vasculitis. Other directed tests, such as cryoglobulins, antinuclear antibodies, urinalysis, may be needed to confirm the etiology.

Treatment is frequently not required in leukocytoclastic vasculitis, which tends to be self-limited. In severe cases, systemic corticosteroids are helpful.

Box 88-1. Leukocytoclastic Vasculitis and Associated Disorders

Drug reactions
Infections (viral hepatitis, streptococcal)
Henoch-Schönlein purpura
Mixed cryoglobulinemia
Connective tissue disease (SLE, Behçet's disease, dermatomyositis)
Malignancy

SLE, Systemic lupus erythematosus.

Churg-Strauss Vasculitis

Churg-Strauss vasculitis is a small- to medium-sized vessel vasculitis with a characteristic clinical picture and cutaneous involvement in 40% of patients.[2] The vasculitis is preceded commonly by adult-onset asthma and allergic symptoms that can be present for several years. Since medium-sized vessels become involved, the clinical picture includes linear or livedo pattern inflammation, as well as small nodules (Plate 62). There is frequently a marked eosinophilia. Antineutrophil cytoplasmic antibody (ANCA) is usually negative, although a perinuclear pattern (P-ANCA) has been reported to be helpful in distinguishing Churg-Strauss syndrome from Wegener's granulomatosis. Most cases respond to treatment with systemic corticosteroids.

Wegener's Granulomatosis

Wegener's granulomatosis is a vasculitis involving arterioles that can affect the skin with palpable purpura and ulcerations. Noncutaneous involvement usually dominates the clinical picture.

Polyarteritis Nodosa

Polyarteritis nodosa (PAN), is a rare vasculitis involving medium-sized vessels. It can be localized to skin or be a systemic and life-threatening disease. In localized cutaneous PAN, a livedo pattern of vascular erythema, nodules, and painful ulceration is common. Biopsy is diagnostic if deep enough to visualize the larger vessels in the deep dermis and fascia. The systemic form can involve the kidneys, gastrointestinal tract, heart, and central nervous system (CNS). Immunosuppressive therapy with corticosteroids and cyclophosphamide are frequently helpful.

Disseminated Intravascular Coagulation

Rapidly evolving widespread purpura usually represents activation of the coagulation cascade as a result of severe multisystem disease. Coagulation factors are consumed, resulting eventually in hypocoagulability. A variant of disseminated intravascular coagulation (DIC), called purpura fulminans (see Plate 20), is seen in children after meningococcal, streptococcal, and sometimes viral infection.

Table 88-1. Xanthomas

Type	Clinical Features	Lipid Abnormality
Xanthelasma	Periocular, flat-topped, or papular	Apo E, hyperapo β-lipoproteinemia; occasionally, no abnormality found
Plane xanthoma	Palms, face, neck	Biliary cirrhosis: type III
Eruptive xanthoma	Eruptive crops of papular lesions on buttocks, extremities	Hypertriglyceridemia: primary types I, III, IV, V, or secondary (diabetes mellitus)
Tuberous	Large nodular lesions on elbows and knees	Hypertriglyceridemia: familial types II, III
Tendinous	Deep nodules over tendons: knees, elbows, hands, Achilles	Hypercholesterolemia: familial types II, III

Modified from Habif TP: *Clinical dermatology,* ed 3, St Louis, 1996, Mosby.

Antiphospholipid Antibody Syndrome

Antiphospholipid antibody syndrome[3] is a hypercoagulable state associated frequently with underlying collagen vascular diseases such as SLE and scleroderma. The syndrome can also be idiopathic. Clinical manifestations are those of thrombosis; cutaneous findings include a livedo reticularis pattern on lower extremities (Plate 63), with areas of necrosis if the disease progresses or is not treated. Laboratory evidence of the syndrome includes the presence of (1) lupus anticoagulant, (2) anticardiolipin antibody, and (3) β-2 glycoprotein 1. Treatment is anticoagulation with heparin initially, followed by warfarin for maintenance of an international normalized ratio (INR) of 3 or higher.

CUTANEOUS MANIFESTATIONS OF DIABETES MELLITUS

Diabetic dermopathy is a common cutaneous finding in patients with diabetes that consists of tan-brown macular areas on the pretibial areas. Whether these lesions represent a form of diabetic vasculopathy or are from minor trauma remains uncertain. There appear to be no potential complications from this disorder.

Necrobiosis lipoidica (NL) occurs only in approximately 1% of diabetics, but approximately two-thirds of patients who develop NL have overt diabetes. NL is a granulomatous skin disorder of uncertain etiology consisting of red-brown or red-orange plaques occurring mostly on the pretibial areas (Plate 64). Atrophy and telangiectasia are common features of NL plaques. Symptoms are mild, but disfigurement can be significant when lesions become large or ulceration occurs. Biopsy is diagnostic, showing pathognomonic granulomatous changes throughout the dermis. Treatment consists of potent topical or intralesional corticosteroids and standard ulcer care when ulcerated. Inhibition of platelet aggregation and pentoxyphylline have been helpful in isolated case reports. Treatment failures are common.

Eruptive xanthomas are described in the section on xanthomas (see below).

Pruritus without primary cutaneous lesions is a common complaint in patients with diabetes (see Chapter 96). Treatment consists of diabetic control, keeping the skin temperature cool, and judicious use of antihistamines.

Neurotrophic ulcers occur in patients with diabetes with peripheral neuropathy and loss of sensation. They are pressure-induced ischemic ulcers similar to those seen in patients with spinal cord injuries. Therapy, which requires avoidance of pressure, can be complicated by diabetic vasculopathy, which can compromise tissue perfusion.

Bullous disease of diabetes is an idiopathic disorder consisting of bullae on the distal extremities with little or no inflammation. The bullae can reach considerable size. The differential diagnosis can include bullous pemphigoid, burns, mechanical blisters, and porphyria cutanea tarda. Treatment is supportive, with attention to tight glucose regulation.

XANTHOMAS

Xanthomas are clinical lesions with a characteristic yellowish color resulting from lipid-filled histiocytes present in the dermis or deeper tissues. Several types of xanthomas have been described and are associated with different lipoprotein abnormalities, both familial and acquired (Table 88-1).

Eruptive xanthomas occur from acute elevations in triglycerides as a result of lipoprotein lipase deficiency or familial hypertriglyceridemia seen in types I, II, IV, and V dyslipidemias (see Table 71-2). Most cases are secondary to poorly controlled diabetes mellitus. A patient presenting with eruptive xanthomas requires evaluation of lipids, glucose, and thyroid function. Insulin and thyroid hormone stimulate lipoprotein lipase, the enzyme responsible for moving triglycerides from blood to tissues. Multiple yellow papules on the buttocks or extremities are typical (Plate 65). Diagnosis is made by clinical picture, history of rapid onset of lesions, and skin biopsy. When possible, correction of underlying disease and triglyceride levels result in gradual resolution of the lesions.

CUTANEOUS SARCOIDOSIS

Sarcoidosis is a granulomatous disease of uncertain etiology that can affect any organ (see Chapter 78). Cutaneous sarcoidosis is present in approximately 25% of patients with systemic sarcoidosis. Nonspecific cutaneous findings, such as erythema nodosum, can be associated with sarcoidosis but do not represent sarcoidal involvement of the skin.

The typical presentation of cutaneous sarcoidosis is papules or small plaques. These are common around the mouth, nose, and eyes (Plate 66). A red-brown color is common and is caused by the presence of histiocytes in the dermis. Larger plaques can be present elsewhere on the trunk and extremities (Plate 67). A less common presentation is a purple-red firm nodular plaque that commonly presents on the nose or ears (Plate 68). This lesion has been called "lupus pernio" from original descriptions but consists in fact of dermal infiltrates of sarcoidal granulomas.

Diagnosis is made by clinical presentation and biopsy confirmation. Treatment options for cutaneous sarcoidosis include potent topical or intralesional corticosteroids, systemic corticosteroids, antimalarial therapy, and immunosuppressive agents such as methotrexate and cyclosporin. Evaluation for systemic disease should be considered in all patients with cutaneous sarcoidosis.

PORPHYRIA CUTANEA TARDA

Porphyria cutanea tarda (PCT) is a cutaneous manifestation of a rare disorder of porphyrin and heme metabolism resulting in high levels of circulating porphyrins. There are several types of porphyria; PCT is the most common form. PCT requires a genetic defect in the hepatic enzyme porphyrinogen decarboxylase. In homozygous individuals, PCT occurs spontaneously in childhood and early adulthood. In heterozygotes, a second hepatic insult is usually required to produce the disease. Ethanol, other hepatotoxic drugs, and more recently, hepatitis B and C virus (HBV and HCV) infections have been associated with PCT.[1]

The skin findings in PCT are primarily from photodamage. Circulating porphyrins absorb ultraviolet (UV) light and cause cellular damage. Patients typically present with skin fragility and bullae on the dorsal hands (Plate 69). Facial hypertrichosis is a common finding of uncertain etiology.

Diagnosis is made by clinical presentation, skin biopsy, and serum and urine porphyrin studies. Serum studies show elevation in total body iron stores (ferritin >500µg/L), and urine porphyrin studies show a pattern characteristic of PCT.

Management. Patients with new onset of PCT need to be screened for underlying liver disease, including HBV and HCV infections. Sun protection is of utmost importance; complete avoidance of exposure to UV light can prevent blisters. Treatment of underlying liver disease is essential, as is avoidance of hepatotoxins. Specific treatment for PCT consists of removal of 500 ml of whole blood every 2 to 4 weeks until the serum ferritin and urine porphyrins return to normal levels and the clinical picture improves. An alternative therapy is the use of antimalarial drugs that facilitate renal excretion of porphyrins. This therapy can be associated with acute worsening of the disease before improvement is observed.

PYODERMA GANGRENOSUM

Pyoderma gangrenosum is an inflammatory, neutrophil-mediated skin disease of unknown etiology that can be associated with several internal diseases[6] (Box 88-2).

History and Physical Examination. The clinical presentation of pyoderma gangrenosum is usually a pustule that enlarges over days into a violaceous-erythematous plaque that frequently ulcerates (Plate 70). A typical appearance is a plaque with a reticulated (cribriform) ulceration pattern. Plaques can enlarge to greater than 10 cm within two to four weeks, and ulceration can progress in the same time period to depths that can expose subcutaneous fat and tendons. Pain is moderate to severe. Obtaining a complete history of underlying illness is important.

Diagnosis. The differential diagnosis of pyoderma gangrenosum includes numerous infectious diseases, including mycobacterial infection, deep fungal infection, and tertiary syphilis. It is common for pyoderma gangrenosum to be misdiagnosed and unsuccessfully treated multiple times with antibiotics before a correct diagnosis is made. Skin biopsy, while supportive, is not specific.

Box 88-2. Pyoderma Gangrenosum: Associated Diseases

Common

Inflammatory bowel disease: ulcerative colitis, Crohn's disease
Arthritis: rheumatoid, seronegative
Hematologic disorders: myelocytic leukemias, IgA gammopathy

Less common

Chronic active hepatitis
Polycythemia vera
SLE
Primary biliary cirrhosis
Malignancy

SLE, Systemic lupus erythematosus.

Management. Nonpharmacologic therapy consists of wound care (see Chapter 83). Pharmacologic therapy is essential and includes, as the mainstay of treatment, systemic corticosteroids in doses that range from 60 mg/day orally to intravenous methylprednisolone 1 gm daily. Cyclosporin A, 5 mg/kg/day, has been successful in steroid-resistant cases and has been recommended as first-line therapy by some authors.[5] Dapsone has been used for many years in acute disease and as maintenance therapy. Doses range from 50 to 200 mg per day orally.

ACANTHOSIS NIGRICANS

Acanthosis nigricans is associated with endocrine disorders that include obesity, with an underlying malignancy, or with a familial occurrence. Clinically, acanthosis nigricans consists of hyperpigmented areas of hyperkeratosis that result in plaques or patches of thickened skin with a velvety or slightly verrucous texture. Common sites of involvement are the skin fold areas of the neck, axillae, groin, and antecubital/popliteal fossae. In paraneoplastic acanthosis nigricans, involvement of the dorsal and palmar hands or other atypical sites are clues to the malignant association.

PRURITUS

Generalized pruritus (see Chapter 89) is associated with several systemic diseases, most notably obstructive liver disease, renal disease, diabetes mellitus, and iron deficiency. The most common malignancies associated with pruritus are lymphomas, polycythemia, and multiple myeloma.

SWEET'S SYNDROME

Sweet's syndrome (acute febrile neutrophilic dermatosis) may be associated with malignancy in approximately 10% of cases.[7] Hematologic malignancy is most common, usually acute myelogenous leukemia. Clinically, Sweet's syndrome consists of tender, erythematous dermal nodules anywhere on the body (Plate 71), with associated systemic findings of fever, malaise, arthralgias, and neutrophilia. Biopsy of skin lesions shows a neutrophilic dermal infiltrate. Response to treatment with systemic corticosteroids (i.e., prednisone 40 to 60 mg/day) is usually excellent regardless of whether or not there is an associated malignancy. Recurrences are common.

GLUCAGONOMA SYNDROME

There is a specific cutaneous finding associated with the α cell pancreatic malignancy, glucagonoma. The skin change, termed *necrolytic migratory erythema (NME),* consists of shallow erythematous erosions from superficial blisters, along with some scaling. The most common sites are the perineum and other periorificial areas, distal legs, and sites of trauma. Associated findings include stomatitis and glossitis, anemia, and hyperglycemia with glycosuria. Histopathology of the skin lesions can demonstrate pallor and necrotic cells in the epidermis that are characteristic of NME. The clinical and histologic differential diagnosis includes nutritional deficiencies (zinc, amino acid, thiamine), acrodermatitis enteropathica, and superficial blistering diseases such as bullous impetigo and pemphigus foliaceus. The definitive test is a serum glucagon level that is markedly elevated. The precise mechanism of the skin lesions is not clear, but rapid resolution occurs when the tumor is resected.

REFERENCES

1. Bonkovsky HL, Poh-Fitzpatrick M, Pimstone N, et al: Porphyria cutanea tarda, hepatitis C, and HFE gene mutations in North America, *Hepatology* 27:1661-1669, 1998.
2. Davis MDP, Daoud MS, McEvoy MT, et al: Cutaneous manifestations of Churg-Strauss syndrome: a clinicopathologic correlation, *J Am Acad Dermatol* 37:199-203, 1997.
3. Greaves M: Antiphospholipid antibodies and thrombosis, *Lancet* 353(9161):1348-1353, 1999.
4. Lotti T, Ghersetich I, Comacchi C, et al: Cutaneous small-vessel vasculitis, *J Am Acad Dermatol* 39:667-687, 1998.
5. Matis WL, Ellis CN, Griffiths CEM, et al: Treatment of pyoderma gangrenosum with cyclosporine, *Arch Dermatol* 128:1060-1064, 1992.
6. Seitzenger JW: Pyoderma gangrenosum, *N Engl J Med* 86:465-467, 1989.
7. Von den Driesch P: Sweet's syndrome (acute febrile neutrophilic dermatosis), *J Am Acad Dermatol* 31:535-556, 1994.

CHAPTER 89

Pruritus

Susan Tobey Denman

The skin is the largest organ in the human body, and the skin's most common symptom is itch. Thus pruritus presents a daily challenge to the clinician. Itch is defined as the unpleasant sensation that evokes the desire to scratch. Pruritus is present in every age group. It can be associated with many dermatologic, as well as systemic, diseases. Itch can also be generalized without an obvious etiology.

PATHOPHYSIOLOGY

Pruritus can be evoked by physical stimuli, such as a thin wire, electrical stimuli, and thermal heat, and chemical stimuli, such as histamine, serotonin, and substance P. Prostaglandins and dry skin, although not stimuli by themselves, both lower the threshold for evoking itch.

Itch receptors are free unmyelinated penicillate nociceptors in the epidermis.[4] Unmyelinated C fibers carry the sensation of itch along the afferent pathway. These enter the dorsal horn of the spinal cord, synapse, cross the midline, and ascend in the spinothalamic tracts closely associated with pain fibers to the thalamus. Tertiary neurons ascend from the thalamus to higher centers that regulate the conscious perception of itch.

Central nervous system (CNS) factors can modulate our perception of itch by either amplifying or inhibiting the sensation. An example of inhibition is the effect of scratching an itch. Scratching demonstrates the concept of gating of sensory afferent activity. In this system, simultaneous firing of large-diameter myelinated fibers can presynaptically inhibit firing of smaller afferent fibers so that the sensations they usually evoke would be diminished in intensity or not perceived. Scratching stimulates firing of large-diameter myelinated A fibers that can presynaptically inhibit the firing of smaller afferent C fibers carrying itch. Psychologic factors, such as emotion and past experience, may also act on the gate-control system and modify the perception of itch.

An additional central influence on itch involves the enkephalins and opioid receptors in the CNS. When enkephalins bind to opioid receptors, they relieve pain and may cause itch.[5] A pharmacologic example is the itching seen in more than 50% of patients who receive intraspinal or epidural morphine. When the opioid receptors are blocked by administration of a competitive antagonist, such as naloxone, itching is diminished or disappears. Parenteral naloxone has been used successfully in treating itching in cholestasis.[5]

Histamine is the classic mediator of pruritus. Derived from mast cells, histamine acts on H_1 receptors to cause itch.[1] But how histamine mediates itch in many dermatologic and general diseases is a paradox. Experimentally induced itching is always associated with wheal and flare, yet most clinical itch is not. Also, repeat injections of histamine at the same site results in tachyphylaxis. Antihistamines are often ineffective in relieving itch. An unknown cytokine has been proposed as mediator of itch in diseases such as atopic dermatitis.[5] Supporting this is the antipruritic effect of cyclosporin A (a cytokine inhibitor) in atopic dermatitis, lichen planus, and mycosis fungoides. Substance P and serotonin also mediate itch. Peptides, such as bradykinin, vasoactive intestinal polypeptide (VIP), neurotensin, secretin, and substance P, are potent histamine releasers rather than primary mediators of itch. Prostaglandins modulate rather than cause itch. Prostaglandin E lowers the threshold for histamine-induced itch.[5]

CLINICAL PRURITUS

Pruritus may be associated with numerous skin diseases (Box 89-1). Xerosis is the most common skin disease causing pruritus, particularly in the elderly. A careful history of bathing habits, use of emollients, whether patients experience concomitant burning and stinging, as well as physical examination showing increased skin markings with plates of scale and dryness, make this diagnosis.

Scabies can be difficult to find, especially in a fastidious patient. A single burrow on the heel of the foot is sometimes the only sign in these patients. If a patient has scabies, it should be possible to demonstrate a mite or eggs on skin scraping. Sometimes only part of a mite, such as a leg, will be found on skin scraping.

Atopic dermatitis is a very common, frustrating cause of severe itching. Often called the itch that rashes, patients report itching and scratching preceding the development of the rash characterized by eczematous dermatitis. Careful

Box 89-1. Skin Diseases Associated with Pruritus

Xerosis	Psoriasis
Scabies	Lichen planus
Dermatitis herpetiformis	Urticaria
Atopic dermatitis	Folliculitis
Pruritus vulvae	Lichen simplex chronicus
Pruritus ani	Sunburn
Miliaria	Bullous pemphigoid
Insect bites	Fiberglass dermatitis
Pediculosis	Trichinosis
Contact dermatitis	Onchocerciasis
Drugs	Echinococcosis
Pruritic urticarial papular eruption of pregnancy	

Box 89-2. Generalized Pruritus Associated With Systemic Disease

Uremia	Myeloproliferative disorders
Obstructive biliary disease	Hodgkin's disease
Primary biliary cirrhosis	Mycosis fungoides
Chlorpropamide	PCV
Contraceptive pills	Lymphoma
Extrahepatic biliary obstruction	Multiple myeloma
Intrahepatic cholestasis of pregnancy	Visceral malignancies
Endocrine disorders	Breast carcinoma
Thyrotoxicosis	Gastric carcinoma
Hypothyroidism	Lung carcinoma
Diabetes	Iron deficiency anemia
Carcinoid	Neurologic disorders
Psychiatric disorders	Multiple sclerosis
	Brain abscess
	CNS infarct

history usually elicits a personal or family atopic diathesis with allergies, hay fever, or asthma.

Contact dermatitis, either irritant or allergic, is a very common cause of itching. Irritant dermatitis is caused by a direct toxic effect of a substance on the skin, whereas allergic contact dermatitis is a type IV hypersensitivity reaction to substances such as fragrance, plants, preservatives, rubber products, dyes, and some topically applied medications (i.e., neomycin or diphenhydramine). Contact dermatitis begins as a local phenomenon, but when severe can become a generalized dermatitis, affecting areas of the skin that have never been in contact with the offending substance.

Dermatitis herpetiformis is a much rarer blistering disease, usually presenting with intense pruritus. Pruritus is usually the first symptom, and skin lesions include papules, wheals, and vesicles distributed symmetrically on the lumbosacral spine, elbows, and knees. The early vesicles are fragile and may be difficult to find intact.

Folliculitis often itches out of proportion to the clinically evident rash. The rash on the chest, back, or thighs consists of numerous small follicularly oriented pustules or papules.

Early bullous pemphigoid can present as pruritic urticarial patches that can be subtle and diagnosed on biopsy.

Lichen simplex chronicus is a secondary rather than primary skin lesion; it is thickened skin as a result of prolonged scratching or rubbing of an itchy area. The skin becomes thickened with exaggerated skin markings. This secondary finding can be present in patients with any of the listed dermatologic or systemic causes of itch.

SYSTEMIC DISEASES ASSOCIATED WITH PRURITUS

If no skin disease is evident, pruritus may be a symptom of one of the systemic diseases associated with pruritus (Box 89-2).

Uremic Pruritus

Itching in chronic renal failure is the most prevalent of all the systemic disorders listed in Table 89-2. A dramatic increase in the incidence of pruritus in chronic renal failure has occurred since the advent of hemodialysis: from 13% before the advent of dialysis in 1932 to 86% of dialysis patients at present. Currently, 25% of renal failure patients treated without dialysis complain of itching. The itch, often occurring in severe paroxysms, was generalized in 44% and localized in 56% of patients. Pruritus can be severe just before the patient's next dialysis, suggesting accumulation of pruritogenic metabolites; in other patients it is most severe during or immediately following dialysis and is often worse in summer.[3]

The pathophysiology of uremic pruritus is unclear. Many of the metabolic disturbances in uremia have been investigated. Secondary hyperparathyroidism with hypercalcemia, hyperphosphatemia, aluminum overload, mast cell proliferation in skin and elevated plasma histamine levels, atrophic sebaceous glands, atrophy of eccrine sweat glands, and microangiopathy are all present.[6] Unknown cytokines have been proposed as causative agents.[5]

Treatment with ultraviolet (UV) B or psoralen plus UVA (PUVA) has been successful with remissions of up to 18 months. The mechanism for UV effect on uremic pruritus is unknown but may be due to a systemic effect, since patients who receive this treatment to only half their body noticed a generalized improvement in their itch without localization to the treated side.

In addition to UV light, balneotherapy with polidocanol may be helpful if the patient is xerotic[6]; antihistamines are of little value unless used in large soporific doses. Activated charcoal, 6 gm/day, has been effective. Topical capsaicin cream 0.0255% was shown to be effective in moderate and severe uremic pruritus. Capsaicin acts by depleting substance P from type C sensory nerves (Table 89-1).

Cholestatic Liver Disease

Cholestatic liver disease is frequently associated with generalized pruritus. Pruritus can precede other signs and symptoms. It first appears in hands and feet and in areas of pressure and is worse at night. This itching can be very severe and is a serious clinical problem. Severe unrelieved itch in these patients can be an indication for liver transplantation.

Table 89-1. Management of Pruritus in Chronic Renal Failure

Treatment	Mechanism	Comments
Dialysis	? Removal of pruritogens	Not always effective
Phototherapy (UVB light)	Reduce dermal histamine	? Efficacy
TENS	? Lateral inhibition	Only temporary relief
Parathyroidectomy	Remove parathormone and Ca^{++}	
Antihistamines	H_1 blockade	Sedation; anticholinergic effects
Erythropoietin	Decrease plasma histamine	Expensive
Oral charcoal	Bind "toxins"	? Efficacy
Cholestyramine	Bind uric acid	? Efficacy

From Kam PCA, Tan KH: *Anaesthesia* 51:1133-1138, 1996.
TENS, Transcutaneous electrical nerve stimulation.

Accumulation of bile acids in skin and plasma has been implicated in the pathogenesis of this pruritus because patients have high levels of bile acids in their skin and serum. Application of pure bile acids to the skin causes pruritus. Patients experience relief of itch when serum bile concentration is lowered by oral cholestyramine or external biliary drainage. The relationship of itch to bile salts is unclear, however, because not all patients with elevated serum bile acid levels itch and itching can subside without any decrease in bile salt levels.

Although bile salts are not directly responsible for pruritus, treatment with cholestyramine that binds bile salts is effective in reducing itch in cholestatic disease. In addition to bile salts, cholestyramine binds other substances in the intestine that may be the basis for its effectiveness, since it has also been used successfully in uremic patients and in polycythemia vera. Patients who do not tolerate cholestyramine can be given colestipol hydrochloride (Colestid), another ion exchange resin that is less constipating.

Naloxone, an opiate receptor antagonist, given intravenously, improved pruritus in a double-blind, placebo-controlled trial of 20 patients with chronic cholestatic liver disease.[5] This suggests that central opiate receptors and enkephalins may mediate itch in cholestasis.

Odansetron, which blocks 5HT receptors, has also been shown to improve itching of cholestasis, suggesting that serotonin is involved in the itch (Table 89-2).

Hematologic Disorders Associated With Pruritus

An estimated 14% to 52% of patients with polycythemia vera (PCV) have pruritus. Pruritus triggered by a sudden decrease in temperature is considered a highly diagnostic symptom, especially when it occurs as a patient emerges from a warm bath and begins to cool off. The itch is pricking in quality and lasts for minutes or hours. In one study, two-thirds of patients with uncontrolled PCV had elevated plasma and urine histamine levels. Unfortunately, antihistamines are not usually successful. Two controlled studies suggest that antiserotonin agents relieve pruritus in PCV.[2]

Table 89-2 Pharmacologic Management of Pruritus in Cholestatic Jaundice

Agent	Mechanism	Disadvantage
First-line		
Cholestyramine	Bind bile salts in gut	Unpleasant taste; constipation; malabsoption
Ursodeoxycholic acid	Cholestasis Reduce salt pool	Diarrhea Paradoxic itch
Antihistamines	H_1 blockade	Sedation
Second line		
Rifampicin	Reduce bile salt uptake	Diarrhea; nausea; hepatitis
Phenobarbitone	Enzyme induction	Encephalopathy
Experimental		
Opiate antagonists	Block opiate receptors	Opiate withdrawal
Propofol (sub-hypnotic dose)	Inhibit spinal afferents	Requires administration intravenously
Ondansetron	Block $5HT_3$, receptors	Constipation; headache

From Kam PCA, Tan KH: *Anaesthesia* 51:1133-1138, 1996.

Iron deficiency can be associated with pruritus and may relate to underlying malignancy. Prolonged generalized pruritus is frequently experienced before the diagnosis of Hodgkin's disease is made.

Aquagenic pruritus is intense distressing itching after water contact without visible skin changes. There is an age range of 17 to 81 years, with a mean age of 40.5 years. It is more common in males and has a mean duration of 6.1 years.

A subset of aquagenic pruritus is aquagenic pruritus of the elderly, which happens after prolonged immersion in warm water when the patient dries off. This usually begins after age 60; 75% are women. Treatment of xerosis is key to management.

Patient Evaluation

To evaluate the itching patient, a careful history and physical examination of the entire body is important. In patients who have no visible rash, an unexplained adenopathy or organomegaly can indicate an occult malignancy.

If the physical examination is negative, symptomatic treatment for 2 weeks should be initiated. Patients will need specific instructions for bathing. They should bathe no more than once a day, use warm not hot water, and use of a mild soap, such as Dove unscented or Cetaphil, sparingly. They should pat their skin dry and use adequate amounts of emollients. A midpotency steroid cream can be applied to moist skin with emollient overlay twice daily.

If emollients alone are unsuccessful, antihistamines can be added to the regime. H_1 blockers, such as hydroxyzine, can be added. If patients do not respond to this empirical treatment, screening laboratory studies should be done to rule out systemic disease causing itch (see Box 89-2). If laboratory studies are negative and the patient has skin lesions, a skin biopsy should be done. If present, biopsy an early primary lesion. If no primary lesions are present, a biopsy of perilesional skin or skin near an area that has been scratched can be helpful in bullous pemphigoid or dermatitis herpetiformis.

If itch persists in spite of a thorough evaluation and conservative therapy, a multisystem therapeutic approach may be helpful. If patients have a localized area of itching or lichenification, a midstrength topical steroid applied with the Schotz regimen can be used. A nonsteroid alternative is tar emulsion; care should be taken to apply in the direction of hair growth (to prevent folliculitis). An unna boot can be used on localized area of itch to protect the area from scratching and reduce lichenification. Patients should be encouraged to continue emollients. Patients should avoid heat, dress coolly, and take warm not hot showers. Other antihistamines can be used. Doxepin has the advantage of a long-lasting therapeutic result. Because doxepin is variably absorbed, serum level, obtained 12 hours after the last dose, will help ensure that the patient has an adequate dose. Nonsedating antihistamines are not usually helpful. Pimozide may be used for opiate receptor antagonist effect. A transcutaneous electrical nerve stimulation (TENS) unit may help, via sensory gating mechanism, in some patients.

Patients who have persistent generalized pruritus should be regularly reevaluated with repeat screening laboratory tests, since itching can be the early presenting sign of occult malignancy.

REFERENCES

1. Davies MC, Greaves MW: The current status of histamine receptors in human skin: therapeutic implications, *Br J Dermatology* 104:601-606, 1981.
2. Fitzsimmons EJ, Pagg JH, McAllister EJ: Pruritus of polycythemia vera: a place for pizotifen? *Br Med J* 282:277, 1981.
3. Gilchrist BA, Stern R, Steinman TI, et al: Clinical features of pruritus among patients undergoing maintenance hemodialysis, *Arch Dermatol* 118:154-156, 1982.
4. Greaves MW: New pathological and clinical insights into pruritus, *J Dermatol* 20:735-740, 1993.
5. Hagermark O, Wahlgren CF: Some methods of evaluating clinical itch and their application for studying pathophysiological mechanisms, *J Dermatol Sci* 4:55-62, 1992.
6. Szepietowski JC, Schwartz RA: Uremic pruritus, *Intern J Dermatol* 247-253, 1998.

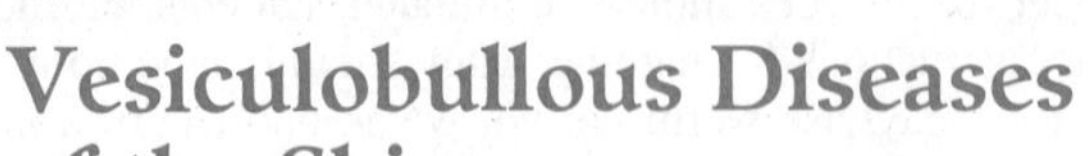

Vesiculobullous Diseases of the Skin

Lynne H. Morrison

The blistering diseases discussed in this chapter are immunologically mediated disorders that cause blisters, erosions, and erythema of both skin and mucous membranes. They are all uncommon. Although there are a variety of autoimmune bullous dermatoses, this chapter focuses on three major diseases—bullous pemphigoid, the major forms of pemphigus, and dermatitis herpetiformis. Patients with pemphigoid and pemphigus can be at risk for serious morbidity, especially if the disease becomes extensive; accurate diagnosis and early therapy are important issues in patient management. Bullous diseases can mimic one another not only clinically but also histologically. Therefore accurate diagnosis for all of these diseases requires a biospy for direct immunofluorescence (IF) studies to identify the presence of pathologic autoantibodies; biopsies for routine histology should be done.

BULLOUS PEMPHIGOID

Epidemiology

Bullous pemphigoid (BP) is an acquired bullous disease of the elderly. It is characterized histologically by subepidermal blisters and immunopathologically by deposition of autoantibodies and complement along the basement membrane zone (BMZ). Most patients also have circulating autoantibodies directed against the epithelial BMZ.[2,4] The true incidence of BP is unknown, but according to estimates there is one case per 100,000 annually. The vast majority of BP patients are over 60 years old at the time of presentation. In general, men and women are equally affected, there is no racial or geographic predilection, and there is no known HLA association.

Pathophysiology

BP is considered an autoimmune disease mediated by autoantibodies directed against two antigens (the bullous pemphigoid antigens) in the BMZ of stratified squamous epithelia. These antigens are proteins thought to be important mediators of dermal to epidermal adhesion.[2] Current evidence suggests the following hypothesis for subepidermal blister formation in BP:

1. *Initiating event:* immunologic recognition of the BP antigens causes production of IgG class anti-BMZ antibodies.
2. *Attachment:* autoantibodies attach to the pemphigoid antigen(s) in the BMZ.
3. *Complement activation:* complement is activated, which generates the anaphylatoxins C3a and C5a.
4. *Inflammatory response:* complement activation results in recruitment of eosinophils, mast cell degranulation, and release of multiple cytokines, histamine, and proteolytic enzymes. Injury to the BMZ is thought to be mediated by these enzymes and eventually produces dermal-epidermal separation.[1]

History and Physical Examination

Most patients with BP present with a pruritic eruption. The degree of pruritus varies from nearly nonexistent to intense. A few patients have prolonged pruritus that precedes the clinical appearance of bullous lesions. Most patients with BP are not systemically ill, although elderly patients with extensive blistering can become debilitated. Most large series concluded that there is no increased incidence of malignancy in patients with BP compared with age- and sex-matched controls. Several medications and therapies have been associated with the onset of BP, including furosemide, sulfasalazine, phenoxymethylpenicillin, topical 5-fluorouracil (5-FU), and both ultraviolet B (UVB) and psoralen plus UVA (PUVA) phototherapy.[1]

Frequently the earliest manifestation of BP includes

erythematous macules, papules, and urticarial plaques that may have a serpiginous configuration. Subsequently, tense bullae arise on these erythematous lesions, as well as on normal skin (see Plate 6). These tense bullae make up the most characteristic clinical feature of BP. The blisters may be filled with clear fluid or may be hemorrhagic; when they rupture, they leave denuded areas that become encrusted. The erosions tend to not spread peripherally and generally heal without scarring.[4,5]

Laboratory Studies/Diagnostic Procedures

Biopsies submitted for routine histology and for direct IF studies are essential in BP and other immunologically mediated blistering diseases. The most characteristic histologic finding is subepidermal separation with a mixed inflammatory infiltrate containing lymphocytes and eosinophils. Biopsies processed for IF studies show linear deposition of IgG and C3 along the BMZ. Biopsies taken for routine histology need to include part of the blister, whereas biopsies taken for IF studies should be from normal-appearing skin immediately adjacent to an urticarial lesion or a blister. Biopsies taken from blisters commonly give negative IF results. About 50% of patients show hypereosinophilia, and approximately 70% will have circulating anti-BMZ autoantibodies.

Differential Diagnosis

Differential diagnosis for BP can be found in Table 90-1.

Management

Determining the severity of the disease and identifying the patient's other medical problems are important in choosing a therapeutic agent. Systemic corticosteroids are still the mainstay of therapy in generalized BP. The majority of patients can be controlled with prednisone 40 to 80 mg/day. In general, mild disease usually responds to lower doses of prednisone than does moderate or severe disease. Once the disease is under control the goal of therapy is to taper the prednisone and eventually maintain the patient on alternate-day therapy to minimize long-term steroid side effects. In patients with mild to moderate disease or those who are not tolerating prednisone, dapsone or tetracycline would be reasonable alternative therapies. Most patients respond well to corticosteroids, but those who do not or those who require high doses may need the addition of azathioprine or methotrexate.[2,4,6]

PEMPHIGUS

The term *pemphigus* refers to a group of chronic blistering skin diseases (Tables 90-2 to 90-4) in which autoantibodies are directed against keratinocytes resulting in loss of epidermal cell-to-cell adhesion—a process termed *acantholysis*. This loss of epidermal cell cohesion causes intraepidermal blisters. In all types of pemphigus, IgG autoantibodies are bound in a characteristic pattern around the cell membrane of affected cells and are also found in patients' serum. The three major forms of pemphigus are pemphigus vulgaris (PV), with suprabasilar acantholysis (i.e., the split occurring above the basal or lowest layer of epidermal cells); pemphigus foliaceus (PF), with acantholysis in the superficial layers of the epidermis; and paraneoplastic pemphigus (PNP), which shows suprabasilar acantholysis and the histologic features of erythema multiforme and is seen in association with underlying malignant neoplasms.[4,5]

Both PV and PF have further variants that are not reviewed here. Each major form is associated with distinct autoantibodies that are directed against specific epithelial proteins that have been shown to be pathogenic.

Table 90-1. Differential Diagnosis of Bullous Pemphigoid

Disease	History	Physical	Laboratory	Management
BP	Elderly population: intense pruritus; tense bullae	Widespread bullae; urticarial lesions; distribution not diagnostic	Skin biopsy; direct IF; linear IgG along BMZ	Systemic oral corticosteroids occasionally azathioprine or cyclophosphamide
Cicatricial pemphigoid	Elderly; mucous membranes and conjunctivae	Erosive blisters on mucous membranes and conjunctivae; skin lesions in 20%	Skin biopsy; direct IF	Corticosteroids
Herpes gestationis	Pregnancy; intense pruritus	Vesicles and bullae; urticarial lesions	Skin biopsy, direct IF	Resolves after delivery; may require systemic corticosteroids
Epidermolysis bullosa acquisita	Adult onset; skin fragility and blisters, extensor areas, pruritus	Bullae and vesicles; erosions; healed areas with scars and milia	Skin biopsy, direct IF similar to BP; differentiation requires split skin direct IF	Corticosteroids; immunosuppressive agents; difficult to treat
DH	Intense pruritus; extensor areas; gastrointestinal symp. occasionally	Grouped (herpetiforme) vesicles; elbows, knees, back, buttocks	Skin biopsy: direct IF; gastrointestinal if diarrhea	Dapsone; gluten-free diet
Linear IgA bullous dermatosis	Pruritus; any age; vesicles and bullae	May be similar to DH or BP	Skin biopsy; direct IF	Dapsone

IF, Immunofluorescence.

Table 90-2. Differential Diagnosis of Pemphigus Vulgaris

Disease	History	Physical	Laboratory	Management
PV	Widespread erosions; oral lesions	Oral and cutaneous bullae and erosions	Skin biopsy; direct IF; indirect IF	Systemic corticosteroids; immunosuppressive agents; gold
BP	Elderly; intense pruritus; blisters	Bullae widespread; urticarial lesions common	Skin biopsy; direct IF	Corticosteroids
Cicatricial pemphigoid	Elderly; mucous membranes and conjunctivae	Bullae, erosions, and scarring on mucous membranes and conjunctivae	Skin biopsy; direct IF	Systemic corticosteroids
Erythema multiforme (oral)	Oral mucosal lesions; painful	Oral erosions; may have target lesions on skin	Skin biopsy; direct IF to exclude pemphigus	Supportive; eliminate or treat underlying cause
Erosive lichen planus	Oral mucosal and tongue lesions	Erosions; white lacy mucosal changes	Skin biopsy; direct IF to exclude pemphigus	Topical and systemic steroids; retinoids; cyclosporine topically

IF, Immunofluorescence.

Table 90-3. Differential Diagnosis of Pemphigus Foliaceus

Disease	History	Physical	Laboratory	Management
PF	Widespread crusted erosions; adult onset	Crusted, scaling plaques	Skin biopsy; direct IF	Systemic corticosceroids
Impetigo	Crusted lesions; face; children	Crusted plaques; honey crusts; serous oozing	Culture	Antibiotics

IF, Immunofluorescence.

Table 90-4. Differential Diagnosis of Paraneoplastic Pemphigus

Disease	History	Physical	Laboratory	Management
Paraneoplastic pemphigus	Erosions of skin and mucous membranes; associated malignancy	Oral and cutaneous erosions; polymorphous skin eruption	Skin biopsy; direct IF indirect IF	Treat malignancy; systemic corticosteroids; immunosuppressive agents
Erythema multiforme (major Stevens-Johnson syndrome)	Mouth, conjunctivae, ears, and widespread; history drug, viral infection	Erosions on mucous membranes; target lesions on skin	Skin biopsy	Supportive; treat or eliminate underlying cause

IF, Immunofluorescence.

Epidemiology

PV is the most common form of the disease and generally occurs during the fourth to sixth decades of life. It occurs worldwide with an annual incidence of about 0.1 to 0.5 per 100,000 population and is more common in the Jewish population. There is an increased incidence of HLA-DR4, HLA-DR6, and HLA-DR10 haplotypes. In the presteroid era, the disease had a nearly 100% mortality at 5 years. Currently, the mortality from PV is approximately 10% and often due to side effects of therapy. PF is generally less life-threatening than PV, which is likely due to the more superficial nature of the lesions.[2,5] Patients with PNP often have a high mortality rate with refractory cutaneous lesions.

Pathophysiology

Each major form of pemphigus is characterized by specific autoantibodies of the IgG class directed against epithelial desmosomal proteins. In PV and PF the antigens are found only in stratified squamous epithelia, whereas in PNP the antigens are found in all types of epithelia. The autoantibodies in each form of the disease are capable of reproducing the disease clinically and histologically, both in vivo and in vitro, indicating their pathogenicity.[2,3] Attachment of autoantibodies to desmosomal proteins is thought to be the first step in pathogenesis and is followed by acantholysis. The mechanism of acantholysis is not certain but some data suggest that binding of the autoantibody may induce release of proteolytic enzymes from epidermal cells. Antibodies alone in the absence of complement can induce acantholysis, although complement may augment the process. Other mechanisms, including the direct effect of the IgG autoantibodies on desmosomal integrity and cell adhesion, may also be important in the pathogenesis of this disease.

History and Physical Examination

PV is the most common form of pemphigus. Many patients present with painful oral erosions, which can precede the cutaneous lesions by weeks or months. Typically, oral lesions are painful and irregularly bordered erosions that extend peripherally, are persistent, and heal slowly. Other mucous membranes may be involved but less commonly than the oral mucosa. Patients who present with only cutaneous lesions eventually have mucous membrane involvement in almost all cases. Cutaneous lesions usually appear as flaccid bullae or erosions with a predilection for the scalp, face, upper trunk, axillae, and groin (Plate 72). The lesions may develop on normal skin or on erythematous base. They rupture easily to produce painful, red, weeping erosions that extend at the edges. It is not uncommon to see only erosions in these patients, as the fragile blisters break quite easily.[2-4] The ability to easily dislodge epidermis adjacent to an erosion with lateral pressure is referred to as a Nikolsky's sign and indicates active disease with potential to progress. When disease activity increases, large areas of a patient's skin can become denuded, resembling a burn patient, with marked susceptibility to secondary infection and fluid and electrolyte imbalance. Sepsis is a common cause of death in patients with widespread disease.

Patients with PF have a different clinical appearance than those with PV. PF usually presents with scaling, crusted lesions on the upper trunk and face, and patients rarely, if ever, have oral lesions. The primary lesions are flaccid, extremely fragile bullae that rupture to produce shallow erosions with subsequent scaling and crusting with relatively little weeping. They are not usually found intact. Mortality from this form of pemphigus is usually quite low.

PNP is a recently described variant in which the vast majority of patients have a recognized or occult malignant neoplasm, most often non-Hodgkin's lymphoma, thymomas, or hematologic malignancies.[1,2] Patients can have a polymorphous skin eruption that consists of large areas of erythema, bullae, and lesions resembling erythema multiforme. A consistent clinical finding is painful oral erosions often accompanied by an erosive conjunctivitis. Pulmonary and gastrointestinal tract involvement has been identified in some patients with PNP.

Laboratory Studies/Diagnostic Procedures

Skin biopsies for routine histopathology and IF are essential for accurate diagnosis.[5,6] PV histopathologically shows suprabasilar intraepidermal blister formation with acantholysis. In PF, the intraepidermal split is higher up on the plane of the epidermis, often within the granular layer just below the stratum corneum. The remainder of the epidermis stays attached to the BMZ. PNP characteristically shows a combination of suprabasilar acantholysis similar to PV, vacuolar interface change, and keratinocyte necrosis, which is similar to erythema multiforme.

Skin biopsies processed for direct IF in all three types of pemphigus show deposition of IgG autoantibodies and often, complement within the intercellular spaces of the epithelium. Biopsies from patients with PNP may also have linear or granular deposition of complement along the BMZ.

Obtaining indirect IF studies on a patient's serum and looking for the presence and titer of pemphigus autoantibodies are also useful for diagnosis management of pemphigus patients and can help differentiate PNP from other forms of pemphigus.[1]

Management

The mainstay of therapy for both PV and PF is corticosteroids, usually in the form of oral prednisone. The goal of therapy is to control the disease at the lowest possible dose of prednisone. When the disease is severe, achieving control in a hospital setting is appropriate. For severe disease, higher doses of prednisone, generally 80 mg a day or greater, is necessary to get the disease under control. Less severely affected patients can be started on lower doses. Once the disease is under control, the prednisone is tapered, if possible, to an alternate-day regimen. The goal is to control the disease at the lowest possible alternate-day dose of prednisone or discontinue prednisone if possible. This is a chronic disease, and although remission with therapy is possible, the disease generally recurs at some point after treatment has been discontinued. It is not unusual for PV patients to need immunosuppressive medications in addition to prednisone for control. Those most often used include azathioprine, cyclophosphamide, and gold and may be used in patients who are not responding well to higher doses of corticosteroids or not tolerating side effects of steroids. They can also be used as steroid-sparing agents.[2,4,5]

It is important early in the course of the disease to initiate osteoporosis evaluation and prevention therapies, since these patients are often subjected to long-term corticosteroid therapy.

DERMATITIS HERPETIFORMIS

Epidemiology

Dermatitis herpetiformis (DH) is a chronic, severely pruritic papulovesicular eruption distributed symmetrically over extensor areas, characterized by deposition of IgA in the upper dermis, and associated with a gluten sensitivity. DH usually has an onset between the second and fourth decades, with a male/female ratio of 3×2. The prevalence of DH in the United States is unknown; however, the prevalence in Utah has been estimated at 15×100,000. Scandanavian and Anglo-Saxon populations have a relatively high prevalence of DH, but it is uncommon in African-Americans and Asians. Patients with DH have an associated gluten-sensitive enteropathy that is present in the vast majority of patients but is most often asymptomatic. As in patients with isolated gluten-sensitive enteropathy, there is an increased frequency of the HLA-B8 antigen, which is noted in 80% to 90% of DH patients.[2,3] The frequency in the normal population is 20% to 30%. There is also an increased frequency of HLA-DR3 and HLA-DQW2 haplotypes.

Pathophysiology

The precise pathophysiology of DH is unknown. Features that suggest an immunologic basis include the presence of IgA in the upper dermis in essentially all patients, as well as marked HLA associations. The disease has not been clearly shown to be an immune complex–mediated process nor has pathogenicity of IgA autoantibodies been demonstrated. The association of a gluten-sensitive enteropathy and presence of granular IgA in the skin suggest that gluten may act as an antigen, inducing an abnormal mucosal permeability with subsequent production of IgA either locally in the gut mucosa or systemically. This IgA could then bind to the skin as either a cross-reacting antibody or possibly an immune complex. Gluten has been proposed as the dietary antigen important in producing the disease. A strict gluten-free diet controls both the cutaneous and gastrointestinal manifestations.[3,6] An alternative hypothesis is that a gluten-induced intestinal defect may allow passage of other dietary antigens that then could incite production of IgA that subsequently binds to the skin.

History and Physical Examination

Patients with DH typically have severe pruritus, often described as having a stinging or burning quality. The onset of pruritus commonly precedes the onset of new lesions by several hours. The typical primary lesion of DH is a erythematous papule or papulovesicle. Patients quite often excoriate the primary lesions quickly so that when they are examined only secondary changes of excoriations and crusts are apparent. The configuration of lesions is grouped or "herpetiform" with an erythematous base. Usually, the eruption of DH is very characteristic with symmetric involvement of extensor surfaces including elbows, knees, sacrum, upper back and shoulders, and posterior neck (Plate 73). Mucous membranes are characteristically spared. Oral involvement should raise suspicion of other immunobullous diseases. Because of the frequent lack of intact primary lesions, the diagnosis should be based on characteristic distribution. Although the activity of the disease may wax and wane, DH is generally a lifelong disease with spontaneous remissions considered rare.[2,3,5]

Patients frequently have a gluten-sensitive enteropathy, which is often clinically asymptomatic. Only 15% of DH patients have symptomatic malabsorption. Approximately 20% to 30% of patients show deficiencies of iron or folate, resulting in a mild anemia.[6] The enteropathy can be diagnosed by small intestinal biopsies showing varying degrees of villous atrophy and lymphocytic infiltrate, but this procedure is generally not warranted.

DH is associated with a variety of clinical diseases and serologic abnormalities, some of which are autoimmune in nature. Several investigators found an increased incidence of thyroid abnormalities in patients with DH, reporting an incidence of 5% to 34% of patients with thyroid disease and 20% to 48% with antithyroid antibodies.[2,5] Several studies found the presence of antigastric parietal cell antibodies in 10% to 25% of patients with DH, and a small number of these individuals will develop pernicious anemia.[5,6] Hypochlorhydria and atrophic gastritis has been identified in 50% to 70% of individuals with DH.

An important association with DH is the increased frequency of malignancy, particularly gastrointestinal lymphoma. Leonard and associates evaluated 109 patients with DH and found a 6.4% incidence of malignancy over 12 years, giving a relative risk of 2.38. Three of seven patients who developed malignancy had a lymphoma, giving a 3.00 relative risk for that specific malignancy.[2,5,6]

Laboratory Studies/Diagnostic Procedures

The diagnosis is most reliably established by direct IF biopsies taken from clinically normal-appearing skin immediately next to an area of inflammation or vesicle. These studies should be correlated with histologic findings and clinical picture. Histologically DH shows a subepidermal blister with infiltration of neutrophils in the papillary tips. Perilesional skin biopsies processed for direct IF studies show pathognomonic findings of granular deposition of IgA in papillary tips and along the dermal-epidermal junction.[4,5] Indirect IF studies typically are negative. Antiendomesial antibodies have been found in a number of these patients and tend to correlate with severity of underlying gastrointestinal abnormality. An iron deficiency anemia or folate deficiency anemia resulting from malabsorption may be noted in some patients, and appropriate laboratory testing should be done to evaluate these manifestations.

Differential Diagnosis

The diseases most likely to be confused with DH are linear IgA bullous dermatosis and BP. Linear IgA bullous dermatosis generally occurs after puberty and presents with heterogenous clinical features. Some cases are indistinguishable clinically from true DH. Unlike DH, however, mucous membranes are affected in up to 50% of patients with linear IgA bullous dermatosis. Pruritus is not as consistent a feature of linear IgA bullous dermatosis as in patients with DH. The disease tends to have exacerbations and remissions similar to DH; spontaneous resolution is noted in approximately one-third of the cases. There is no known association between linear IgA bullous dermatosis and gluten-sensitive enteropathy.

Management

There are two approaches to therapy for patients with DH. One is adherence to a strict gluten-free diet and the other is medical therapy, usually with dapsone.[2,5,6] Most patients can completely control their cutaneous disease with dapsone, 100 mg/day. Dapsone does not alter any morphologic changes noted in the intestine or change gastrointestinal symptoms, but it does control cutaneous manifestations of DH quite well. Patients who are glucose-6-phosphate dehydrogenase (G6PD)-deficient develop severe anemia on dapsone; screening for G6PD levels should be performed before initiating therapy with dapsone. Less common side effects of dapsone include toxic hepatitis, sensory and motor neuropathy, infectious mononucleosis–like syndrome, and agranulocytosis. Because of these potential side effects, complete blood counts and liver functions should be routinely monitored, more often early in therapy and less frequently later in the course of therapy.

Patients following a strict gluten-free diet may be able to significantly reduce the dose of dapsone needed to control the disease or control the eruption entirely by diet alone. This diet corrects the abnormality of the small bowel and results in a decrease or loss of cutaneous deposits of IgA. Adherence to this diet is difficult and requires support from a dietitian, as well as family members. The clinical benefits of a strict gluten-free diet may not be seen for up to 2 years.

REFERENCES

1. Anhalt GJ: *Paraneoplastic pemphigus, Adv Dermatol* 12:77-96, 1997.
2. Crosby DL, Diaz LA, editors: Bullous diseases. In *Dermatologic clinics,* Philadelphia, 1993, WB Saunders.
3. Fine JD, editor: Bullous diseases. In *Topics in clinical dermatology,* New York, 1993, Igaku-Shoin.
4. Fitzpatrick TB et al, editors: *Dermatology in general medicine,* New York, 1999, McGraw-Hill.
5. Sauder DN, editor: Immunodermatology. In *Dermatologic clinics,* Philadelphia, 1990, WB Saunders.
6. Wojnarowska F, Briggaman RA, editors: *Management of blistering diseases,* London, 1990, Chapman and Hall Medical.

CHAPTER 91

Infectious Diseases of the Skin

Bert G. Tavelli

BACTERIAL INFECTIONS

Impetigo

Impetigo is characterized by erythematous macules that evolve into vesicopustules, which quickly rupture to form the hallmark honey-colored crusts, usually on exposed skin of the face and extremities. Caused by *Staphylococcus aureus* or *Streptococcus pyogenes,* or both, it is typically seen in children, in whom it is highly contagious. Lesions may burn or itch, but constitutional symptoms are usually absent. Other forms of impetigo include a rare bullous type, mediated by toxins produced by group II *S. aureus* (which in its most severe form results in staphylococcal scalded skin syndrome), and impetiginized eczema, in which honey-colored crusts and pustules representing staphylococcal or streptococcal superinfection develop on dermatitic skin (see Plate 14).

Management. Small areas of superficial involvement respond to local cleansing with antibiotic soaps and topical treatment with mupirocin (Bactroban) ointment, applied three times daily until clear. Widespread and bullous lesions are best treated systemically with a penicillinase-resistant antibiotic. In penicillin-allergic patients, clindamycin or erythromycin may be substituted. In recurrent cases, positive nasal swab cultures indicate a carrier state, which responds to twice daily mupirocin ointment application.

Erysipelas and Cellulitis

Both erysipelas and cellulitis are caused by rapidly spreading infection with streptococcal or, less commonly, staphylococcal organisms. In erysipelas, more superficial skin and lymphatics are affected, resulting in raised, red, warm plaques with sharply demarcated borders and a brawny (orange-peel) appearance. The face is most commonly affected, and vesicles and bullae also may be seen (Plate 74). In cellulitis, deeper tissues and subcutaneous fat are involved, most often on the lower extremities (Plate 75), and the plaques are less well marginated or distinct. Local dermatitis, tinea pedis, trauma, surgical wounds, and stasis ulcers predispose to infection. Both erysipelas and cellulitis can be associated with fever, chills, local pain, lymphangitis, regional lymphadenopathy, and systemic toxicity with tachycardia and hypotension. Tissue culture is usually unnecessary and yields are low, but blood cultures should be obtained with extensive infection or marked toxicity.

Management. Treatment consists of systemic antibiotic therapy and support. Penicillin is usually adequate, but erythromycin, clindamycin, or cephalosporins may be used. Attention should be given to predisposing conditions to prevent recurrences, and prophylactic antibiotics (e.g., erythromycin 250 mg twice a day) in susceptible individuals help prevent chronic lymphedema, which is a condition causing progressive woody induration of the legs.

Necrotizing Fasciitis

In some cases, a combination of anaerobic and aerobic bacteria, including staphylococci and streptococci, causes an infection of the subcutaneous tissues called necrotizing fasciitis. Usually induced by trauma or extension of an antecedent infection, it rapidly spreads to cause bright red, edematous, tender plaques, associated with superficial gangrene, and marked systemic symptoms. This serious often fatal infection requires hospitalization, surgical exploration, and broad-spectrum antibiotics.

Ecthyma. Ecthyma is caused by streptococcal and staphylococcal infection, often in patients with poor hygiene or at sites of trauma, especially of the lower extremities. Multiple, discrete vesicopustules quickly enlarge and rupture to form purulent ulcers with overlying necrotic crust. Lesions often scar and spread if untreated but respond quickly to appropriate systemic antibiotics.

Erythrasma. Erythrasma is a superficial skin infection occurring in skin folds and toe webs, caused by the diphtheroid *Corynebacterium minutissimum.* Asymptomatic flat, dry, brown patches develop, which resemble tinea but can be distinguished by negative potassium hydroxide (KOH) examination and by their bright "coral" red fluorescence under Wood's light examination. Topical application of 2% erythromycin or 1% clindamycin for 5 to 7 days is rapidly effective.

Folliculitis, Furuncles, and Carbuncles. Folliculitis occurs around hair follicles, caused by occlusion of the ostium with accompanying superficial inflammation and infection. Precipitating factors include trauma, chronic friction, occlusive clothing and chemicals, and excessive sweating or exposure to water. With deeper involvement an inflammatory nodule, or furuncle, is formed, and multiple furuncles can coalesce to form a carbuncle, usually on the posterior neck. *S. aureus* is the cause in most cases. Simple folliculitis can be treated with chlorhexidine gluconate wash

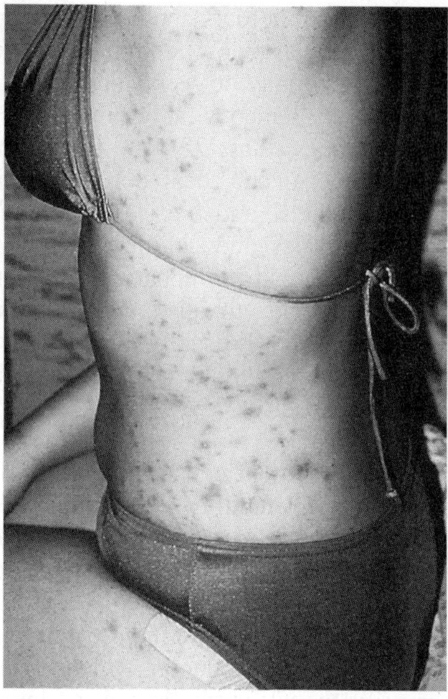

Fig. 91-1. Hot tub folliculitis. Note discrete pustules on an erythematous base distributed on the trunk.

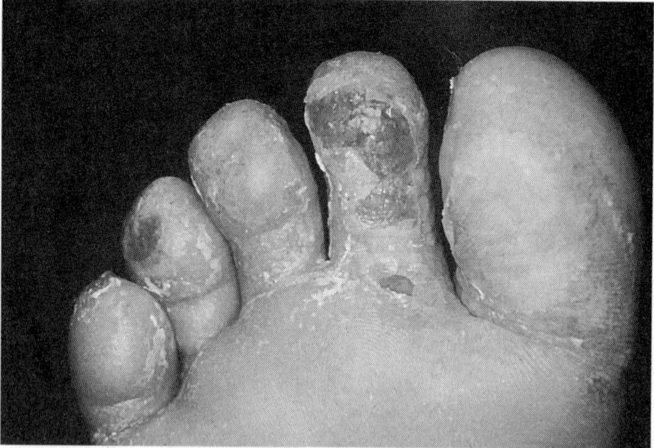

Fig. 91-2. Tinea pedis, vesicular inflammatory type. Note small vesicles and erosions.

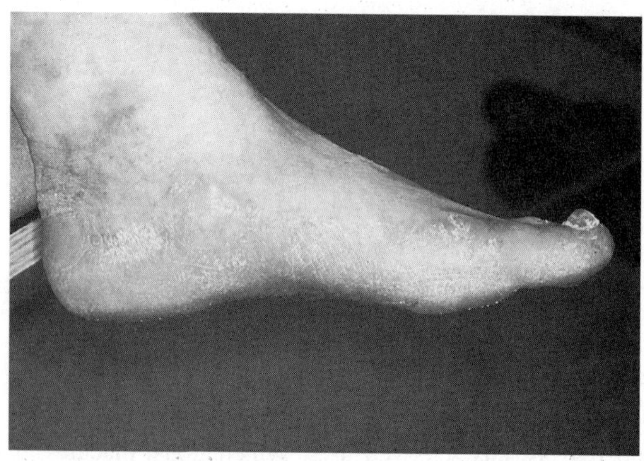

Fig. 91-3. Tinea pedis, chronic form. Note the moccasin distribution of scaling and slight erythema.

plus topical antibiotics. Recurrent folliculitis or furuncles respond to systemic antibiotics.

"Hot tub folliculitis" results from exposure to inadequately disinfected pools or spas contaminated by *Pseudomonas aeruginosa.* One to 2 days after exposure, pinpoint follicular pustules surrounded by large, bright red macules appear (Fig. 91-1), which resolve without treatment. Systemic infection is rare, but treatment with oral ciprofloxacin may be warranted in cases of widespread or highly symptomatic infection and in health care workers.

Tinea Pedis

Tinea pedis, or athlete's foot, is the most common dermatophytosis. It can present acutely as a blistering eruption with vesicles, pustules, fissures, and marked inflammation (Figs. 91-2 and 91-3). Lesions may burn or itch fiercely, and secondary bacterial infection is frequent. A more common chronic form presents either as maceration and fissuring in toe webs, or as dry, reddish scaly patches around the foot, often in a "moccasin" distribution. Topical treatment is usually sufficient for localized involvement, along with elimination of concominant hyperhidrosis and use of occlusive footwear. Highly inflamed, widespread, or resistant infection requires systemic treatment (see Management section).

Tinea Cruris

Raised, red, scaling, occasionally vesicular plaques, which can expand to involve the thigh, pubic, and perianal skin characterize tinea involvement of the groin area (jock itch). Candidiasis, psoriasis, and erythrasma must be considered in the differential diagnosis, although unlike candidiasis, the penis and scrotum are generally spared. Topical treatment for 3 to 4 weeks is effective for most cases, along with attempts to minimize the chafing and excess moisture that precipitate infection.

Tinea Corporis

Fungal involvement of the trunk and extremities most often begins as one or more slightly raised, reddish, scaly patches, which slowly enlarge while clearing centrally (see Plate 17). These annular lesions represent classic "ringworm," but tinea corporis also may be vesiculopustular, eczematous, or nodular. Furthermore, all annular lesions are not ringworm: sarcoidosis, granuloma annulare, urticaria, and gyrate erythema, to name a few, can present as annular lesions. Tinea faciale is a variant that is frequently difficult to recognize (Plate 76). Superficial, localized infection is usually cured with topical treatment applied twice a day for 2 to 4 weeks. Deeper or more inflamed areas require systemic treatment.

Tinea Capitis

Scalp ringworm occurs most often in urban children but is also seen in adults. It can present as one or more scaly plaques with short stalks of broken hair, resembling seborrheic dermatitis, or more commonly as smooth, alopecic plaques with pinpoint hair stubs, broken off at scalp level ("black dot" type), which can mimic alopecia areata. Occasionally, lesions are highly inflamed, resulting in an indurated, tender, boggy mass exuding pus called a kerion. Toxic symptoms and adenopathy may be present, and scarring alopecia can result

Table 91-1. A Comparison of New Medications for Dermatomycoses

	Itraconazole (Sporanox)	Fluconazole (Diflucan)	Terbinafine (Lamisil)
Drug class	Triazole	Triazole	Allylamine
Contraindications	Terfenadine (Seldane) Astemizole (Hismanal) Cisapride (Propulsid) Triazolam/alprazolam/midazolam Lovastatin/simvastatin	Terfenadine (Seldane) Astemizole (Hismanal) Cisapride (Propulsid) Triazolam/alprazolam/midazolam Lovastatin/simvastatin	None
Adverse reactions	Hematologic: none Hepatic: uncommon ↑ Liver function tests: rare Nausea/vomiting/abdominal pain: slight Rash: slight	Hematologic: none Hepatic: uncommon ↑ Liver function tests: Rare Nausea/vomiting/abdominal pain: slight Rash: slight	Hepatic: uncommon Neutropenia: uncommon Pancytopenia: uncommon Nausea/vomiting/abdominal pain: slight ↓ Taste: mild Rash: slight
Coverage	Dermatophytes *Candida* species Nondermatophyte molds	Dermatophytes *Candida* species ? Nondermatophyte molds	Dermatophytes
FDA approval			
Dermatomycoses	Yes	No	Yes
Candida	Yes	Yes	No
Antifungal action	Fungistatic	Fungistatic	Fungicidal
Dose schedule			
Fingernails	Two pulse packs*	200-300 mg/week × 4-6 months	250 mg/day × 6 weeks
Toenails	Three pulse packs*	200-300 mg/week × 9-12 months	250 mg/day × 12 week
Hands/feet	One pulse pack*	—	250 mg/day × 4-6 week
Trunk/groin	200 mg/day/1 week	—	250 mg/day × 2-4 week
Monitoring	Pulse mode: none Continuous mode: LFT's q 6 wks	Pulse mode: No recommendations Continuous mode: Liver function tests q 6 weeks	Liver function tests and CBC: q 4-6 weeks
Reservoir effect: nails	11-12 months	6 months	3+ months
Pregnancy/nursing	Not indicated	Not indicated	Not indicated

*Pulse packs are two 100 mg tablets twice a day for 7 days, then 21 days off.

if not treated. These lesions are often misdiagnosed as bacterial infections.

Treatment with systemic antifungals is required, along with aggressive local care and consideration of concomitant treatment with prednisone in the case of kerions.

Onychomycosis

See Chapter 92 for disorders of the nails.

Management. Numerous topical agents are available for treating superficial fungal infections.[5] The imidazoles, such as clotrimazole (Lotrimin AF), oxiconazole (Oxistat), and econazole (Spectazole) provide good broad-spectrum coverage against dermatophytes and *Candida*. They are used twice daily until infection is clear. Topical steroids, including those containing antifungals (Lotrisone), blunt local host defenses, may exacerbate infection, and lead to atrophy in occluded skin areas. They have no real place in the treatment of superficial fungal infections.

The emergence of three superior antifungal agents has recently supplanted griseofulvin and ketoconazole for systemic use[3] (Table 91-1). These agents provide better efficacy, shorter treatment times, and improved safety profiles. Itraconazole (Sporanox) provides the best broad-spectrum coverage; in the absence of several important drug interactions, itraconazole is safe and well tolerated. The pulse regimen improves compliance and is the preferred approach. A baseline liver profile should be considered. Terbinafine (Lamisil) has no significant drug interactions, but requires baseline and ongoing monitoring for possible hematologic effects and does not cover candida or most nondermatophyte molds. Fluconazole (Diflucan) is not approved for treatment of dermatomycoses. Its main use is for candidal skin infections.

Candidiasis

Cutaneous candidiasis is usually caused by *C. albicans* and may be associated with underlying conditions such as diabetes mellitus, immunosuppression, or use of systemic antibiotics. Moisture, heat, and maceration greatly predispose to infection, which preferentially involves skin folds of the axillae, groin, breasts, and corners of the mouth (perleche). Infection is characterized by burning, beefy red erythema with scale and adjacent ("satellite") pustules (Plate 77).

Candidal involvement of the nail unit presents most commonly with chronic redness, pain, and swelling of nail folds (paronychia). It greatly favors those exposed to constant wet work, including food industry and health care workers.

Management. KOH examination and cultures, including bacterial, are necessary for a rational approach to treatment. Most superficial infections respond to twice daily topical applications of nystatin or an imidazole cream, along with attention to any predisposing conditions. Severe, resistant, or paronychial infections require systemic treatment with one of the newer triazole agents (fluconazole or itraconazole).

VIRAL INFECTIONS

Human Papillomavirus Infection

Long considered benign and uninteresting, infection with human papillomavirus (HPV) has gained considerable importance, emerging as the second most common sexually transmitted disease in the United States and linked to development of genitourinary tract carcinomas. To date more than 60 specific subtypes of HPV have been identified. Although many of these subtypes have been loosely associated with a particular body region, for most purposes these associations are not clinically relevant.

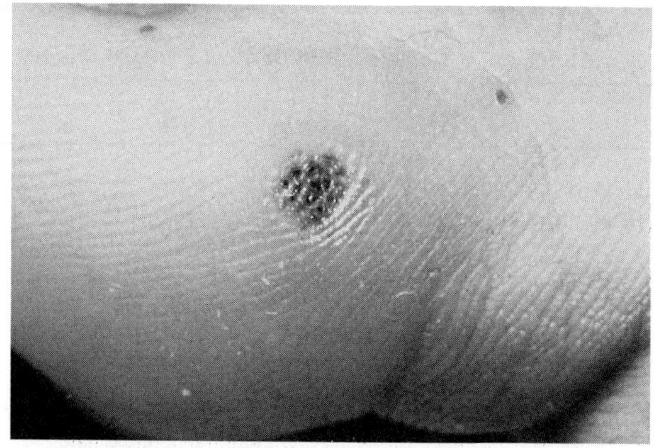

Fig. 91-4. Plantar wart (verruca). Note the pinpoint thromboses after the lesion is pared.

Common Warts. Common warts (verrucae vulgares) are quite polymorphous on skin. They begin tiny and smooth, but progress over weeks to months to become typical, raised, keratotic, and often cauliflower-like papules. Common warts occur most often on the extremities but can be found anywhere on the skin in persons of all ages (see Plate 2).

Planar, or flat warts, occur primarily on the face, hands, and pretibial surfaces as tiny, slightly raised, flesh-colored papules. They can be numerous and refractory to treatment.

Palmar and plantar warts present as thick, endophytic papules or plaques, often multiple, which may be exquisitely painful when located over pressure points. These warts may be distinguished from a callus, which they resemble, by the appearance of tiny black dots (sclerosed vessels), or by bleeding points after paring (Fig. 91-4).

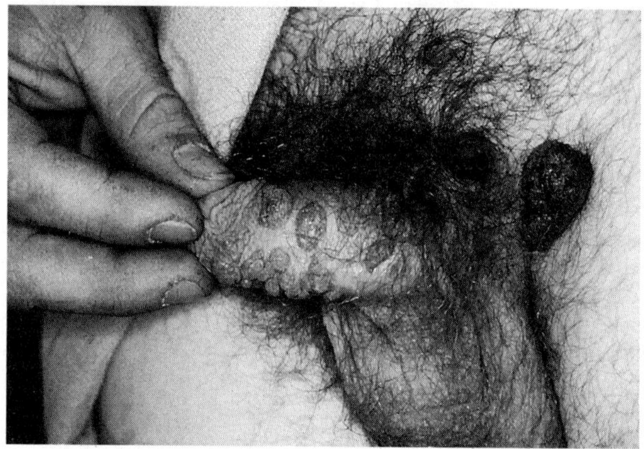

Fig. 91-5. Condylomata. Verrucoid pigmented lesions on the penis.

Genital Warts. An enlarging body of evidence documented the explosive rise in incidence of genital HPV infection and its recognition as a sexually transmitted disease (Fig. 91-5). Most important is the association of certain HPV types, including 16, 18, and 31, with the development of intraepithelial neoplasia of the uterine cervix. Recognition of genital HPV infection by the primary care practitioner is vital.

Genital warts, or condyloma accuminata, present as single or multiple papillary or fingerlike proliferations that may coalesce to form large, moist, cauliflower-like tumors on mucosal or nonmucosal skin. Presence on the vulva is an important indicator of vaginal or cervical involvement. Subclinical infection is common, and attempts at elucidation using acetic acid soaks are limited by frequent false positives.

Bowenoid papulosis is a clinicopathologic variant of HPV infection, in which multiple, smooth, slightly raised papules, ranging from flesh-colored to reddish-brown, develop on genital skin. These lesions show squamous cell carcinoma in situ on biopsy and are usually caused by HPV 16, one of the oncogenic subtypes. An affected female, or female sexual partner of an affected male, should be referred to a gynecologist.

Management. Because many warts regress spontaneously, some patients, especially children, may not require treatment. For common warts, topical application of keratolytics, such as salicylic acid (Occlusal), or salicylic and lactic acid in flexible collodion (Duofilm), is useful when applied directly to the wart at bedtime. Cryotherapy with liquid nitrogen for 10 to 20 seconds is also effective.

Flat warts often respond to cryotherapy, but subsequent pigment alteration occurs easily, especially on the face of darker-skinned individuals. Patients also should be advised to avoid shaving or scrubbing affected areas.

Palmar and plantar warts can be refractory, and aggressive treatment with keratolytics and liquid nitrogen is the usual initial approach. Surgical excision and laser ablation are treatments of last resort.

There are numerous approaches to treating genital warts[1]; none are superior and all have only modest efficacy and substantial rates of recurrence. Moist genital lesions respond to topical treatment with 25% to 40% podophyllin, applied weekly until lesions resolve. Treated areas are washed after 3 to 6 hours as tolerated. Podophyllin is toxic and can be a severe irritant and thus should not be dispensed. Podofilox 0.5% solution or gel (Condylox) is available by prescription for home use and is less irritating and more potent than podophyllin. It is applied twice daily for 3 consecutive days followed by 4 days off, repeating this cycle for up to 8 weeks. Imiquimod (Aldara) is a local immune-response modifier, applied at home 3 times a week for up to 16 weeks. Like Condylox, Aldara may be an effective, although expensive, alternative. Liquid nitrogen continues to be a reliable, efficacious, and cost-effective treatment.

Referral to a dermatologist should be considered for additional treatment modalities, and for evaluation of persistent lesions, especially of the mouth, genital and periungual areas, where occult squamous cell carcinoma is a concern.

Herpesvirus Infections

Herpes Simplex Virus. Herpes simplex virus (HSV) (see Plates) infection is an acute, self-limited eruption that is characterized by groups of small vesicles on an erythematous base. After infection by direct inoculation from another individual, the virus replicates within the skin where it involves the sensory nerves. The viral capsid is subsequently transported to the nerve root ganglion where it remains latent, with the potential for reactivation and reinfection at any time. Both the HSV-1 and HSV-2 subtypes can involve nearly any mucocutaneous site.

Oral-Facial Infection. Gingivostomatitis and pharyngitis are the most frequent primary HSV-1 infections, occurring primarily in children. Lesions develop anywhere in the mouth, on the lips, or on the face. Numerous rapidly evolving vesicles rupture to form painful, necrotic ulcers, associated with fever, malaise, anorexia, and cervical adenopathy. Infection lasts 1 to 3 weeks and heals without scarring. Recurrences present most frequently as herpes labialis (fever blisters, cold sores) where prodromal stinging or burning is quickly followed by one or more typical painful vesicles, usually located on the lips. Viral shedding lasts until the lesions have crusted over, approximately 5 to 7 days. Fever and ultraviolet (UV) light may precipitate the recurrences.

Genital Infection. Primary genital herpes, usually caused by HSV-2, is characterized by bilaterally distributed groups of vesicles. The infection may also involve the cervix and urethra, with accompanying fever, headache, and malaise. Local symptoms include pain, itching, dysuria, and tender inguinal adenopathy. Viral shedding may persist for 10 to 12 days or more, and the complete course lasts 3 to 4 weeks.

Recurrences vary considerably in severity and duration. Prodromal tingling or burning commonly precedes the eruption, which is unilateral, and usually without adenopathy. Lesions can be painful, but the course is milder than primary disease and lasts 7 to 10 days. Recurrence rates also vary greatly, averaging three to four recurrences per year, and patients should be reassured that these tend to become milder and less frequent over time. Unfortunately, asymptomatic shedding, also called subclinical reactivation, likely occurs in all persons infected with HSV, and results in transmission of infection despite the lack of physical evidence of active disease.

Herpetic Whitlow. HSV infection of the finger is characterized by redness, swelling, and painful vesicles or pustules resembling bacterial infection. Systemic symptoms and localized adenopathy accompany primary infection, but recurrences are infrequent.

Herpetic Eye Infection. See Chapter 108 for herpetic eye infection.

Eczema Herpeticum. Eczema herpeticum occurs in patients with an underlying skin problem, such as atopic dermatitis or Darier's disease, which causes altered skin integrity and thereby allows widespread superinfection with HSV. Diffuse vesiculopustular, eroded, and crusted lesions are accompanied by fever, pain, and adenopathy. Referral to a dermatologist should be considered.

Laboratory Evaluation. Most HSV infections can be diagnosed by the clinical presentation. When in doubt, the quickest and least expensive confirmatory test is the Tzanck smear (see Chapter 88), which like all tests for HSV should be taken from intact vesicles or fresh erosions.

Most laboratories now perform fluorescent antibody tests on specimens sent for culture, with initial results in 24 hours. These tests are highly specific but not very sensitive. Negative samples are then submitted for standard cultures, requiring 3 to 7 days. The polymerase chain reaction assay is rapid, highly sensitive and can distinguish HSV from varicella-zoster virus infection but is more costly and less readily available. It should be used when rapid diagnosis is required.

Serologic tests are unreliable in documenting acute HSV infection but can help demonstrate the presence of a previous infection and are useful in identifying asymptomatic infection in patients undergoing immunosuppressive regimens who should receive prophylactic treatment.

Management.[2] Most acute primary oral-facial or genital HSV infections can be safely treated with acyclovir, 400 mg orally 3 times a day for 7 to 14 days. Significant improvement in the rate of healing and the resolution of symptoms can be achieved, especially if initiated early (within 12 to 36 hours), but treatment has no effect on the development of recurrences.

The benefits of oral acyclovir for acute recurrent disease are less dramatic, but long-term daily therapy to suppress frequent recurrences is safe and effective. Initial doses of 400 mg twice a day can be tapered as tolerated, with periodic drug holidays to reassess the need to continue. Long-term suppressive therapy does not eliminate ganglionic latency, and reactivation occurs when treatment is stopped.

Two new oral antiviral agents have demonstrated superior pharmacokinetics vs. acyclovir, allowing less frequent dosing while achieving higher serum drug concentrations. Valacyclovir (Valtrex) is taken as 1 gm twice a day for 10 days with initial infection and 1 gram twice a day for 5 days with recurrences, or 500 mg each day for suppression. The dose for famciclovir (Famvir) is 125 mg twice daily for recurrences.

Topical acyclovir ointment has minimal effect on typical primary or recurrent HSV infection but has been used adjunctively for chronic disease. Intravenous acyclovir is generally reserved for immunocompromised patients and those with CNS involvement, but it can be used in severely ill patients with first-episode HSV infection. Other adjunctive therapies include analgesics, sitz baths, and topical xylocaine ointment or viscous xylocaine mouthwash.

Prevention. Because of frequent asymptomatic shedding, it is suggested that all patients with HSV-2, whether on oral antiviral therapy or not, should use condoms at all times, and abstain totally from sex during recurrences. Sunscreen agents to block UV-activated recurrent labial HSV are useful.

Herpes Zoster Virus. Herpes zoster (shingles) (Plate 78) is an acute vesicular eruption caused by reactivation of latent virus from a previous varicella infection. Reactivation can occur at any time and may be triggered by illness, immunosuppression, debilitation, and advancing age. The eruption is unilateral and follows the dermatome of the affected ganglion, although involvement of adjacent dermatomes is common.

History. A prodrome of 1 to 4 days or more is common, consisting of tingling, itch, or pain and tenderness, often accompanied by systemic symptoms. The pain can be severe, suggesting acute myocardial infarction or acute abdomen in thoracic or lumbar dermatomes. Following the prodrome, an eruption develops that consists of several or multiple groups of vesicles on an erythematous base. Vesicles umbilicate, become purulent, rupture and ulcerate, and over 10 to 14 days, progress to crusting and complete healing.

Infection may involve motor neurons as well, usually of the same dermatome, and can lead to nerve palsies, weakness, and urinary retention. Zoster in the ophthalmic distribution can lead to severe ocular complications. Dissemination of infection also can occur, primarily in immunocompromised individuals and those with certain underlying malignancies.

The most common sequela of zoster is postherpetic neuralgia, in which pain in the involved region may persist for months or rarely years. It occurs in 10% to 15% of patients and is more common in those over 60 years of age. Scarring may be seen, especially after severe infection.

Laboratory Evaluation. See diagnosis section for HSV.

Management. Pain control is the mainstay of treatment in zoster and should include narcotic analgesics when indicated. In younger and middle-aged patients, who tend to have milder disease courses, pain control and attention to possible secondary infection may be all that is necessary.

Acyclovir attenuates the course and symptoms of herpes zoster. For optimal effect, therapy must be initiated early at a usual adult dose of 800 mg taken orally five times a day. It is still considered safe at these doses, but gastrointestinal intolerance is greater; CNS effects, such as confusion and lethargy, can occur; and the patient should be well hydrated. In patients with reduced renal function, lower doses are required. The newer agents valacyclovir (Valtrex), at 1 gram three times a day or famciclovir (Famvir), at 500 mg three times a day, each for 7 days, are safe and excellent alternatives with more sane dosing schedules.

Unfortunately, antivirals have no effect on subsequent pain. Concurrent treatment with prednisone has traditionally been given to reduce the incidence of postherpetic neuralgia and is typically reserved for persons over age 55. The usual adult dose is 60 mg/day for 7 days tapered over 2 to 3 weeks. Its use is controversial, however, and must be weighed against known risks and side effects.

Molluscum Contagiosum. Molluscum contagiosum (Plate 79) is a benign papular eruption caused by a poxvirus. It is characterized by multiple, 2 to 5 mm, dome-shaped, flesh-colored papules with distinctive central umbilication from which caseous material can be expressed. After an average incubation period of 2 to 3 months, lesions develop primarily on the face, trunk, and extremities in children and on thighs, abdomen, buttocks, and genital areas in adults. The mode of transmission can be sexual, nonsexual, or by fomites. Autoinoculation is also possible, causing linear lesions and distant spread.

Diagnosis is usually clinical, but molluscum contagiosum can be mistaken for many lesions, including warts, nevi, adnexal tumors, and keratoacanthomas. Giant or widespread lesions should alert the practitioner to possible immunodeficiency.

Without treatment, the lesions can persist for months or years, but they respond to cryotherapy, light curettage, or any sufficiently destructive or irritating technique.

INFESTATIONS

Pediculosis

Three forms of lice infest humans: head lice (pediculosis capitis), body lice (pediculosis corporis) and pubic or "crab" lice *(Phthirus pubis)*. All are obligate blood-sucking ectoparasites, which produce eggs (nits) that attach firmly to the base of the human's hair shafts or to clothing. Adult lice appear as tiny rust-colored spots after feeding, but diagnosis is made more easily by finding nits, especially with the aid of a hand magnifier or microscope.

Head lice infestation occurs only on scalp hair, particularly the nape of the neck, where intense pruritus may lead to secondary excoriations and furunculosis.

Body lice are similar in appearance, but unlike head lice can be vectors for systemic diseases, such as typhus. Females lay eggs in clothing along seams, a good place to check in suspected individuals (Plate 80). Transmission occurs by contact with infested skin, clothing, or bedding. Widespread pruritic dermatitis can result, along with excoriations and secondary infection from scratching.

Pubic lice are usually contracted from sexual contact, but clothing or linen are possible sources. In addition to the genital area, skin, hair of the face, eyelashes, trunk, and axillae can be involved.

Management. Control of all types of louse infestation includes attention to affected clothing, bed sheets, towels, combs and brushes, and measures to limit spread to others. Hot water laundering, dry cleaning, and use of a disinfectant (e.g., Lysol) for combs and brushes are effective measures, as is isolation of fomites for 1 to 2 weeks.

Treatment of head lice in adults is best accomplished with 1% lindane shampoo (Kwell) applied to hair for 10 minutes and then thoroughly washed off, or 1% permethrin (Nix), applied as a cream rinse after shampooing, left on for 10 minutes, and then rinsed. Nonprescription products containing pyrethrins and piperonyl butoxide (Rid) are also quite effective. All of the treatments probably should be repeated in 1 week, and nits should be dislodged with tweezers or a fine-toothed comb.

Body and pubic lice are treated by application of 1% lindane (Kwell) lotion or shampoo for not more than 8 to 10 hours, then completely washed off. Over-the-counter regimens (Rid) are also effective.

Close contacts should be treated in all types of pediculosis. Lindane can be neurotoxic and should be avoided in patients with widespread dermatitis, pregnant or nursing women, and children less than 3 years of age.

Scabies

Scabies (Plate 81) is caused by infestation with the itch mite *Sarcoptes scabiei,* resulting in intensely pruritic vesicles,

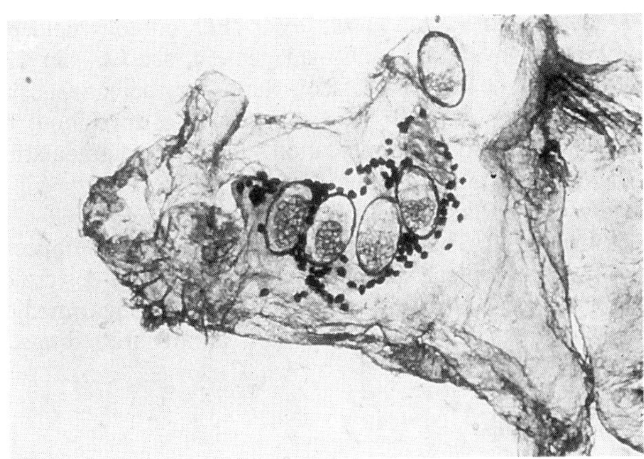

Fig. 91-6. Scabies. KOH preparation demonstrating scabetic mites and eggs.

faint red papules, or short linear burrows (Plate 82). Sites of predilection include finger webs, wrists, axillae, and elbows, with sparing above the neck except in infants. Typical red papules on the glans penis are nearly pathognomonic (Plate 83). Keratotic, crusted scabies (Norwegian scabies) is a variant seen mostly in institutionalized or immunosuppressed patients, in which widespread, crusted lesions teeming with mites are not accompanied by pruritus.

Because the differential diagnosis for scabies includes nearly all pruritic dermatoses, a slide prepared from scrapings of multiple suspected lesions should be prepared to demonstrate mites or ova (Fig. 91-6). Treatment of the nonpregnant adult is usually with 5% permethrin cream (Elimite), or 1% lindane, now somewhat less effective since resistance has emerged. Both are applied from the neck down (30 gm or 1 oz), washed off after 8 to 10 hours, then repeated once after 5 days. As described with pediculosis, infested clothing and bedding and close contacts should be treated simultaneously. Patients should be reminded that posttreatment hypersensitivity and pruritus can persist for several weeks.

REFERENCES

1. Beutner KR, Ferenczy A: Therapeutic approaches to genital warts, *Am J Med* 102(5a):28-37, 1997.
2. Erlich KS: Management of herpes simplex and varicella zoster virus infections, *West J Med* 166(3):211-215, 1997.
3. Katz HI: Systemic antifungal agents used to treat onychomycosis (review), *J Am Acad Dermatol* 38:S48-52, 1998.
4. Pereiva FA: Herpes simplex: evolving concepts (review), *J Am Acad Dermatol*, 35(4):503-20, 1996.
5. Smith EB: Topical antifungal drugs in the treatment of tinea pedis, tinea cruris, and tinea corporis, *J Am Acad Dermatol* 28:S24, 1993.

CHAPTER 92

Disorders of Hair, Nails, and Pigmentation

Janet Roberts
Phoebe Rich
Frank Parker

DISORDERS OF HAIR

Alopecia

The term *alopecia* means hair loss or baldness and requires an adjective to specify a given pathology. Hair loss is a common complaint, often confusing to both the patient and the treating physician. It can be emotionally devastating to some people.

Hair Physiology. Understanding hair growth cycles is essential to diagnosing hair disorders.[1] The hair shaft is keratin protein produced by hair matrix cells at the base of each follicle. These cells divide every 12 hours, which makes them vulnerable to physical insult. The active growth phase of hair follicles is the anagen phase and may last from several months to several years. The length of the growth phase is genetically determined, varies with different hair follicles in different parts of the body, and determines the length to which a person's hair will grow. At the end of the anagen phase, an unknown signal causes the hair follicle to undergo a brief transition or catagen phase, lasting only 2 to 3 weeks. After the catagen phase, the hair follicle enters a relatively long resting, or telogen, phase lasting 2 to 3 months. During this time a new anagen hair is forming beneath the resting hair. As it grows, the telogen hair is shed. Normally about 90% of scalp hair is in anagen phase. Approximately 100 scalp hairs are shed daily and are minimally observed by an individual.

History of Hair Loss (Box 92-1). The following points must be clarified: (1) whether the first observable change noticed by the patient is shedding (increased loss of hairs coming out by the roots), breakage (increased loss of hairs because of hair shaft fracture above the root level), or thinning (having less hair to cover the head); (2) duration, extent, and distribution of hair loss; (3) family history of hair loss; (4) associated abnormalities of nails and skin; (5) specifics of chronic or acute illnesses, surgeries, nutrition, and medications; (6) in females, hormonal status and hirsutism; and (7) cosmetic processing.

Physical Examination. The hair and scalp over the entire head must be examined carefully in a strong light. Check for excessive hair (hirsutism) or lack of hair in remote areas and note any associated lesions of skin, mucous membranes, and nails. Note the extent and pattern of hair growth on the scalp and body and any evidence of scalp disease, such as erythema, scaling, crusting, pustules, atrophy, telangiectasias, and presence or absence of follicular orifices. Note any discrete nodules or growths, either superficial or deep, which may suggest malignancy, either primary or metastatic, to the scalp. Short hairs, whether blunt

Box 92-1. History in Patients with Hair Loss

Type of hair loss:
- Shedding: Increased loss of hairs coming out by the roots
- Breakage: Increased loss because of hair shafts breaking above the root level
- Thinning: Having less hair to cover the head

Duration
Extent of hair loss
Distribution of hair loss
Family history of hair loss
Associated skin or nail abnormalities
Chronic illness
Surgical history
Nutritional history
Medication history
Women: hirsutism, hormonal status
Cosmetic processing

(broken off or cut) or tapered (regrowing or miniaturizing hairs) are more easily visualized when viewed against a card of a contrasting color—white for pigmented hairs and black for gray or white hairs.

Laboratory Findings Microscopic examination of the hair is indicated in patients with breakage problems such as tinea capitis, hair shaft abnormalities, or cosmetic breakage.

In preparing hairs to evaluate for fungus, pluck a few short or broken hairs and cover with potassium hydroxide (KOH) for 15 to 20 minutes. This procedure dissolves the hair keratin and allows for visualization of the fungal elements under high dry magnification. When preparing a hair mount to look for suspected hair shaft abnormalities, the goal is clear visualization of the hair shafts without optical distortion; so place segments of hairs on the slide and cover with a drop or two of Permount (available from most laboratory supply companies).

TYPES OF ALOPECIAS

Diseases resulting in alopecia are classified as scarring or nonscarring to facilitate making the correct diagnosis (Table 92-1). The nonscarring classification can be divided further into those conditions in which the hair is lost because of hair shaft breakage, hair shedding with the roots attached, and hair thinning with little-to-no discernible breakage or shedding.

Scarring Alopecias

Tinea Capitis.

Tinea Capitis. For etiology, epidemiology, and management, see Chapter 91.

History and Physical Examination. Tinea capitis may present either as hair breakage, accompanied by minor scaling, or as tender, boggy patches of alopecia (kerion). Symptoms range from none, to pruritus, pain, and tenderness.

Management. Usually systemic antifungal agents are required to treat tinea capitis. Combined use of systemic antifungal therapy and systemic corticosteroids are necessary to treat kerions (see Chapter 91).

Discoid Lupus Erythematosus. For etiology/epidemiology, pathophysiology, and management, see Chapter 135.

Physical Examination. Discoid lupus erythematosus presents as patches of hair loss with scarring throughout the affected area, hyperpigmentation and hypopigmentation, telangiectasias, and follicular hyperkeratosis.

Differential Diagnosis. See Table 92-1.

Management. Therapy of inflammatory scarring alopecias may include topical, intralesional or oral corticosteroids, topical or oral antibiotics, topical or oral antifungal medications, and in selected, severe cases, antimalarial drugs or dapsone (see Table 92-1).

Nonscarring Alopecias

Hair Shaft Disorders

Shedding Because of Breaking Hair Shafts. Structural hair shaft abnormalities can be acquired or congenital. Acquired forms are from breakage due to improper or too frequent use of chemicals for permanent waving, straightening, dying, or bleaching. Cessation of the offending cosmetic processing usually results in normal regrowth.

The major groups of congenital hair shaft abnormalities include fractures, irregularities, or twisting and coiling of the hair shafts. They may be seen as an isolated finding or be associated with abnormalities of nails, teeth, and sweat glands. A full discussion of these disorders is beyond the scope of this chapter. Microscopic examination of the hair under light magnification is usually sufficient for diagnosis by a sophisticated observer.

Trichotillomania. Trichotillomania is an abnormal compulsion to pull out one's own hair (Fig. 92-1).

Etiology/epidemiology. There are two types of trichotillomania. The first, which occurs in those less than 6 years, is usually self-limited, and is more common in boys. The second type begins in those over 6 years and females are affected ten times more often than males. This type has a chronic course. Scalp hair pulling predominates, but any site may be affected.

History. Although the cause is pulling of one's hair, frequently the patient does not admit to pulling and parents are not aware of the habit.

Physical examination. Clinically, trichotillomania presents as irregular, bizarre shapes of hair loss with stubble of different lengths, distorted hair tips from manipulation, and often retained bits of hair at scalp level, which appear as black dots.

Laboratory evaluation. In those patients who deny pulling their hair, a biopsy may be necessary. Pathognomonic histologic findings called trichomalacia (pigmented fragments of hair shafts within follicles) confirm the diagnosis.

Management. Treatment is difficult. Behavior modification training is sometimes helpful as may be newer medications used for treating obsessive-compulsive disorders such as clomipramine and fluoxetine.

Anagen Arrest. Anagen arrest refers to alopecia in patients receiving systemic chemotherapy or local irradiation. The insult to the matrix cells is severe enough to cause temporary cessation of mitosis of matrix cells in anagen phase, with a resultant breakage of the hair shafts below scalp level. Hairs are shed 2 to 3 weeks after treatment. Because about 90% of scalp hairs are in anagen phase at any given time, the resultant hair loss can be almost complete. Chemotherapy is

Table 92-1. Differential Diagnosis of Alopecias

Disease	History	Physical	Laboratory	Management
Scarring alopecias				
Congenital (aplasia cutis)	Present at birth	Alopecia Ulceration occasionally	None	Plastic surgery
Tinea capitis with inflammation (kerion)	Pruritic, scaly patches Pain and tenderness	Alopecia, scales Boggy patches Pustules	KOH positive Fungal culture	Oral antifungals
Bacterial folliculitis	Pruritic pustules	Pustules, papules Some alopecia	Gram's stain Bacterial culture	Antibiotics
Discoid lupus erythematosus	Pruritus occasionally Lesions other than scalp common	Erythema Scaly thick plaques Pigmentation	Skin biopsy Direct IF occasionally	Topical steroids Intralesional steroids Antimalarial agents
Lichen planopilaris	Pruritus occasionally	Alopecia Peripheral erythema Follicular accentuation	Skin biopsy	Topical steroids Intralesional steroids
Folliculitis decalvans	Rare Asymptomatic alopecia, inflammation	Patchy alopecia Follicular erythema at periphery	Skin biopsy	No effective Rx
Neoplasm	Asymptomatic alopecia	Evidence of tumor on the scalp	Skin biopsy	Treat tumor
Trauma	Hx of traction, excessive hair treatments	Distribution where traction is most severe	None	Eliminate trauma
Nonscarring alopecia				
Breakage of hairs				
Cosmetic treatment	Hx frequent or excessive hair Rx	Broken hairs	None	Eliminate trauma
Tinea capitis	Pruritic scaly patches	Erythema, scales	KOH positive Fungal culture	Oral antifungals
Structural hair shaft disease	Unmanageable hair Childhood onset usual	Kinky hair Broken hairs	Microscopic hair examination	No effective Rx
Trichotillomania (hair pulling)	Children Frequently no history	Hair loss in irregular, bizarre pattern	Skin biopsy in difficult to diagnose cases	Counseling Behavior modification Clomipramine
Anagen arrest	Hx chemotherapy Hx radiation Rx Rapid fallout	Widespread shedding	None	Self correcting
Shedding by roots				
Telogen effluvium (telogen arrest)	See Box 92-2 Occurs 3 months after physical insult	Diffuse alopecia or thinning	Hair pull >5-10 hairs Forced hair pull analysis for anagen: telogen ratio	Reassurance Correct any identified causes Eliminate offending drug
Alopecia areata	Asymptomatic patches of alopecia	Round patches Noninflammatory May be diffuse	Skin biopsy in difficult cases	Topical steroids Intralesional steroids Induce contact dermatitis (DNCB) UV therapy
Thinning without increased shedding				
Androgenetic alopecia (male pattern balding) (female diffuse thinning)	Gradual thinning	Men: temporal and vertex Women: thinning over crown area	None usually Skin biopsy occasionally Rule out other causes	Topical minoxidil Finasteride in men Hair transplant

IF, Immunofluorescence; *DNCB*, dinitrochlorobenzene.

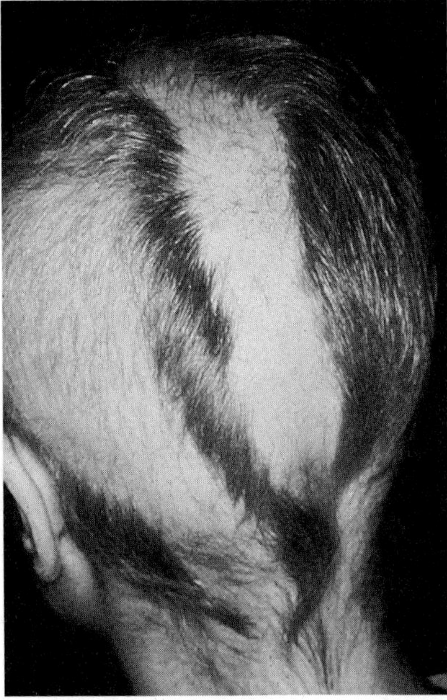

Fig. 92-1. Trichotillomania. Note large area of incomplete hair loss.

generally not scarring so that hair regrowth begins when treatments are stopped. Attempts at prevention include ice-filled "chemo-caps" to reduce circulation to the scalp during therapy.

Shedding with Roots Attached. See Table 92-1.

Telogen Arrest (Effluvium)

Pathophysiology. Telogen arrest is caused by insults to the growing hairs that are sufficient to cause a greater than usual number of anagen hairs to cycle prematurely into the resting or telogen phase. After 30 to 90 days in telogen phase, the hairs are shed. Daily hair counts exceed 100 a day. Acute and chronic causes exist (Box 92-2), and many drugs can cause this form of shedding (Box 92-3).

History. See Box 92-1.

Management. Treatment includes identification and elimination of any offending causes. It is usually self-limited and reversible.

Alopecia Areata. Translated literally, *alopecia areata* means patchy hair loss. However, the disease can be extensive resulting in loss of hair over the entire scalp (alopecia totalis) or over the entire body (alopecia universalis).

Etiology/epidemiology. Alopecia areata is a common cause of hair loss and can occur at any age. The peak incidence is between 20 and 50 years, and sex distribution is equal.

Pathophysiology. Alopecia areata is thought to be autoimmune in nature. The precise mechanism is not known.

History. The most common presentation is the sudden appearance of asymptomatic, round patches of complete hair loss, usually limited to the scalp, although any hair may be affected. In the most severe cases, rapid hair loss with extensive total scalp hair shedding can be seen.

Physical examination. Round patches of smooth alopecia with no inflammation are the usual finding (Plate 84). "Exclamation-point" hairs (short broken-off hairs) may be present around the perimeter of the patches. Loss may be either limited to an occasional inconspicuous spot or total or universal (Fig. 92-2).

Laboratory evaluation. Usually, laboratory evaluation is not required. In atypical cases, a skin biopsy can be helpful. In rare cases, there are coexistent autoimmune associations, including thyroid disease, vitiligo, diabetes mellitus, Addison's disease, pernicious anemia, and connective tissue disease. Laboratory evaluation to exclude these diseases should be based on suggestive history.

Differential diagnosis. Tinea capitis and scarring alopecias, such as folliculitis decalvans, should be considered.

Disease course. In general the disease is more extensive and chronic in childhood, with a poorer prognosis for spontaneous, permanent regrowth. The vast majority of adults with alopecia areata experience the intermittent occurrence of asymptomatic bare patches with spontaneous regrowth.

Management. No treatments are predictably effective, especially in extensive hair loss. Treatments include immune suppressants, such as UV light, potent topical corticosteroids, intralesional corticosteroids (betamethasone 6 mg/ml or triamcinolone 3 to 10 mg/ml given monthly), and rarely oral corticosteroids. Immune stimulation through irritant or allergenic compounds (squaric acid, anthralin) applied to the affected areas, and direct hair growth stimulation with topical minoxidil also can be effective. In cases of extensive hair loss, a well-styled wig is sometimes the best alternative. Oral

Box 92-2. Causes of Telogen Effluvium

Severe acute and chronic illnesses
Childbirth
Surgery with general anesthesia
High fevers
Rapid weight loss
Dietary: protein deficiency, iron deficiency, excessive vitamin A
Hypothyroid, hyperthyroid
Severe psychologic insult
Drugs (see Box 92-3)

Box 92-3. Drugs That May Cause Telogen Effluvium

Anticoagulants: coumarin, heparin
Nonsteroidal antiinflammatory drugs (including ASA)
Tricyclic antidepressants
Beta-adrenergic blockers (oral, ophthalmic): propranolol, metoprolol
H_2 antagonists: cimetidine, ranitidine, famotidine
Antikeratinizing: vitamin A toxicity, isotretinoin, etretinate
Heavy metals: lithium, arsenic, lead, gold
Gout medications: allopurinol, probenecid, colchicine
Hormones: oral contraceptives, progesterone, clomiphene, anabolic steroids
Antihyperlipemic drugs: clofibrate, lovastatin, niacin

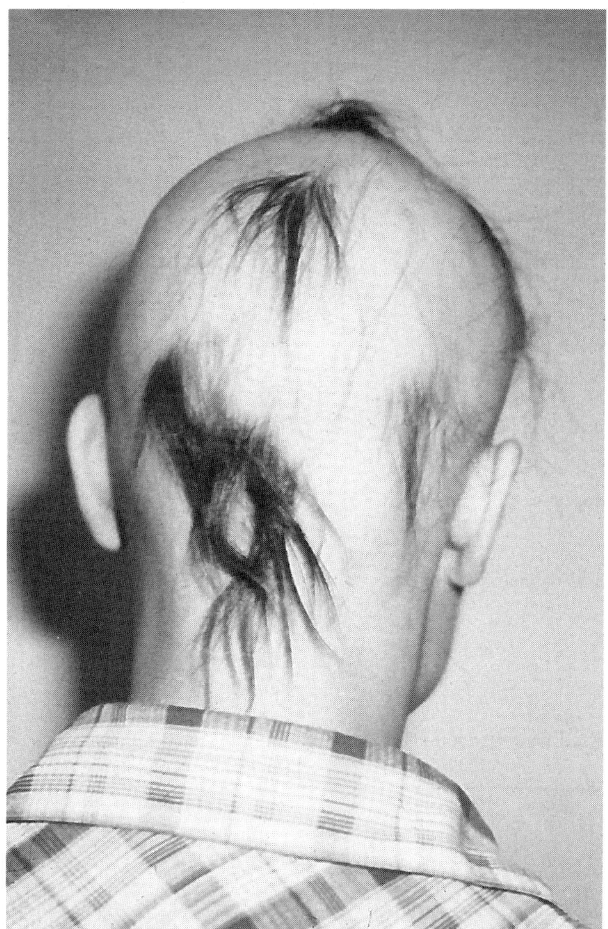

Fig. 92-2. Alopecia areata (alopecia totalis). Note completely smooth scalp where hair has fallen out.

corticosteroids should be used for limited periods of time, 3 to 6 months maximum. Intralesional corticosteroids are injected in small increments into the bare patches with a dosage totalling no more than 20 to 30 mg/month over the long term.

Androgenetic Alopecia

Etiology/epidemiology. Androgenetic alopecia, or male-pattern balding, affects up to about 50% of men.[3] Androgenetic alopecia can be present in as many as 37% of postmenopausal women. Asians appear to be less susceptible than whites or blacks. The genetic predisposition appears to be multifactorial rather than of a single maternal gene as was previously thought.

Pathophysiology. The metabolism of androgens within hair follicles and a genetic predisposition are the requirements for the development of androgenetic alopecia. The activity of the enzyme 5-α-reductase in the scalp, which converts testosterone to dihydrotestosterone (DHT), appears to play a role in the process of hair miniaturization. Serum levels of circulating androgens are not elevated in most cases. In both men and women there is a progressive shortening of the anagen phase, which leads to smaller, finer hairs with each succeeding cycle.

History. Gradual thinning of the scalp hair is typical. A history suggestive of masculinization requires evaluation for possible systemic androgen excess.

Physical examination. In men the usual pattern is temporal recession and thinning on the vertex with gradual progression to total balding of the frontal and vertex scalp. In women the thinning is more diffuse over the crown and usually spares the frontal scalp line and temporal areas. In both men and women, the parietal and occipital scalp are not involved.

Laboratory evaluation. In men the diagnosis is usually apparent. In women occasionally there can be uncertainty. In these cases, certain laboratory tests to exclude causes of telogen effluvium (see the box at top left) plus a scalp biopsy can be helpful.

Management. The only treatments currently available are the topical use of minoxidil (2% and 5%) in men and women and oral finasteride in men and surgical hair transplantation. Ongoing research in the use of androgen antagonists may possibly result in effective treatments.

NAIL DISEASES

Nail disorders (Table 92-2) are common complaints among patients. The physician treating nail disorders must have a thorough understanding of the anatomy of the nail and its growth pattern.[4-6]

Anatomy and Terminology

The *nail plate* is surrounded by folds on three sides: the two lateral *nail folds* and the proximal nail fold. The nail folds are collectively the *parionychium.* The area beneath the free edge of the nail, the *hyponychium,* is contiguous with the volar skin of the digit. The *nail bed* lies beneath the nail plate and contains the blood vessels and nerves. The *nail matrix* is the root of the nail, and its distal portion is visible on some nails as the half-moon shaped structure called the *lunula.*

Nail Growth and Kinetics

Nails grow at a rate of approximately 0.1 mm/day, which means it takes about 4 to 6 months to regenerate a fingernail and 8 to 12 months to replace a toenail. The nail matrix is the germinative portion of the nail and is responsible for the formation of the nail plate. Damage to the matrix usually results in an abnormal nail plate, which may result in a permanent nail dystrophy such as a split nail. Conversely, an injury to the nail plate or nail bed will usually allow for regrowth of a normal nail.

Infectious Nail Diseases

Onychomycosis (Fungal Nail Infection). Approximately 50% of all nail disorders are fungal in origin. Fungal infections of the nails are common worldwide without racial predilection. Some persons may have genetic predisposition to the development of chronic tinea unguium. Other factors that may increase the development of onychomycosis are humidity, heat, trauma, diabetes mellitus, and underlying tinea pedis.

Tinea Unguium. The most common type of onychomycosis, tinea unguium, is caused by a dermatophyte fungus. Nonfungal nail conditions, such as psoriasis, can be indistinguishable from onychomycosis; therefore it is important not to rely on clinical inspection alone to diagnose fungal infections of the nail. A potassium hydroxide (KOH) preparation or fungal culture should be performed to substantiate the diagnosis. An adequate culture requires

Table 92-2. Differential Diagnosis of Nail Disorders

Condition	PE/history	Laboratory	Management
Onychomycosis	Hyperkeratosis of nail bed, yellow-brown discoloration, onycholysis. Usually chronic.	KOH positive Culture positive	Systemic or topical antifungal therapy
Paronychia, acute	Red, warm, tender nail. Often follows injury to nail fold.	Positive bacterial culture, usually *Staphylococcus*	Systemic antibiotic
Paronychia, chronic	Boggy, swollen, red, inflamed nail folds. Usually occurs in people who have wet work jobs.	Pus is KOH positive and culture positive for *C. albicans*	Anticandida therapy, topical or systemic
Psoriasis	Usually associated with cutaneous psoriasis. Pitting, onycholysis, splinter hemorrhages, nail bed hyperkeratosis.	KOH negative	Topical or intralesional steroids
Lichen planus	Pitting and ridging early. Can eventuate in scarring and pterygium formation.	KOH negative	Systemic, topical, or intralesional steroids
Melanoma	Pigmented band in the nail that widens or darkens.	Biopsy nail bed or matrix depending on site of pigment	Wide excision
SCC	Hyperkeratosis, onycholysis.	Biopsy lesion	Excision, sometimes Mohs' surgery
Habit tic	Usually thumbs, horizontal parallel lines on nail plate. History of manipulating nail folds.	KOH negative	Explain cause to patient; occasionally wrapping nail
Mucous cyst	Occurs on proximal nail fold, and over DIP joint.	Mucin expressed from punctured lesion	Excision, repeated liquid N_2, intralesional cortisone

SCC, Squamous cell carcinoma.

obtaining subungual debris at least 1 or 2 mm under the nail.

Physical Examination. The various subtypes of tinea unguium are based on their pattern of involvement of the nail unit.

Superficial white onychomycosis (Fig. 92-3) is characterized by white discoloration on the surface of the patient's nail, which can be easily scraped away with a blade. It occurs only on the patient's toenails and is easily treated with any of the topical antifungal medications. The causative organism is *Trichophyton mentagrophytes* in most of the cases.

Distal subungual onychomycosis (DSO) (Fig. 92-4) is so named because the site of invasion is the distal nail bed and progression is distal to proximal. Nail bed hyperkeratosis and yellow brown discoloration is usually present, with eventual crumbling and disintegration of the nail plate. The most common dermatophytes are *T. rubrum* and *T. mentagrophytes,* although others also can be seen. DSO of the toenails is usually associated with tinea pedis. When it occurs in fingernails, it is often associated with scaling of the palm of the affected hand and both feet. The organism on the hands is usually *T. rubrum.*

Proximal subungual onychomycosis (PSO) occurs when the organisms invade the nail plate proximally from the proximal nail fold and involves the ventral nail plate. The clinical presentation is a white or yellow discoloration on the inferior surface of the nail plate extending out from the proximal nail fold. The causative organisms of this rare form are *T. rubrum, T. mentagrophytes, T. schoenleinii,* and *T. tonsurans.* In patients infected with human immunodeficiency virus, a variant called *proximal white subungual onychomycosis* (PWSO) is seen in which the nail is white proximally and with a superficial, as well as deep, involvement.

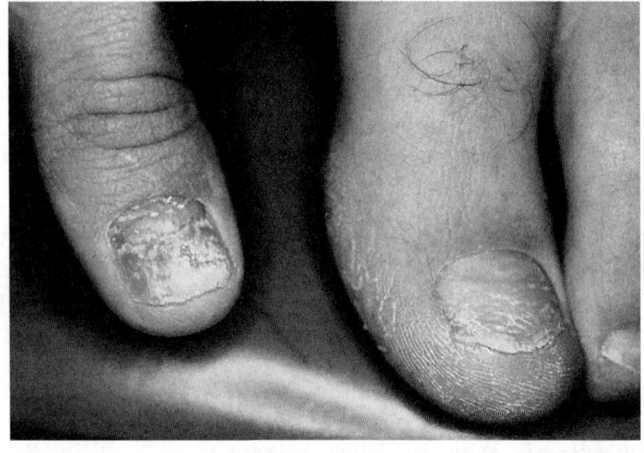

Fig. 92-3. Superficial white onychomycosis.

Differential Diagnosis. Psoriasis is the most common nail disorder that can be mistaken for tinea unguium. Usually other signs of psoriasis are present on the body. In certain cases, confirmation by KOH examination of nail debris and fungal culture for identification are required.

Management. Treatment of onychomycosis must be tailored to the type of infection and the individual patient's needs. Because onychomycosis is often overdiagnosed, it is important to demonstrate fungus by KOH or culture before initiating oral antifungal therapy. There are currently three medications approved for the indication of onychomycosis: griseofulvin, itraconazole, and terbinafine. The latter two drugs have become widely used for this condition because of shortened treatment times and increased efficacy. See Table 91-1 for a comparison of these antifungal drugs.

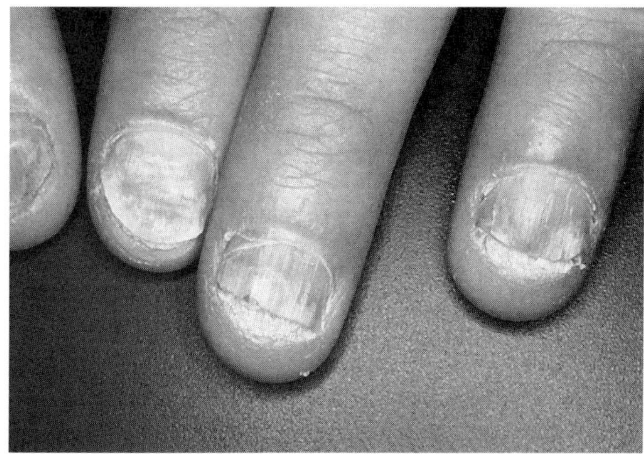

Fig. 92-4. Distal subungual onychomycosis.

Itraconazole (Sporanox) is a triazole antifungal that is fungistatic and has activity against dermatophytes, yeasts, and some molds. It is used continuously at a dose of 200 mg daily for 90 days or preferably in a pulse dose of 200 twice a day for 1 week per month for 2 months for fingernails and 3 months for toenails. When used in a pulse dose schedule, laboratory monitoring is optional.

Terbinafine (Lamisil) is an allylamine drug that is fungicidal. Its coverage is excellent for dermatophytes but is less active against yeasts and molds. The usual dose of terbinafine for toenail fungus is 250 mg daily for 90 days. Terbinafine remains in the nail plate for at least 3 months after discontinuing therapy. It has few drug-drug interactions and periodic laboratory monitoring is recommended.

Another newer oral antifungal drug with clinical usefulness in onychomycosis is fluconazole (Diflucan). This drug does not have FDA approval for the indication of onychomycosis; however, studies show that it has good efficacy and safety for nail fungus. It is given in a dose of 200 to 300 mg once weekly for the length of time it takes for the nail to become clinically normal (6 to 12 months). It is fungistatic and covers yeast, dermatophytes, and some molds.

Paronychia. Paronychia is defined by infection or inflammation of the nail folds. It can be acute or chronic based on the pathogenesis and organism.

Acute Paronychia. Acute paronychia results from a bacterial infection of the nail folds. It usually follows some kind of trauma to the nail folds such as overly aggressive manicuring or injury. The most common bacterial agents in acute paronychia are *Staphylococcus aureus* and *Pseudomonas* species. Treatment is similar to treatment of other bacterial infections of the skin and includes draining and administering culture-specific antibiotics.

Chronic Paronychia. Chronic paronychia causes swollen, red, tender, boggy nail folds. It occurs most frequently in people with wet work jobs or those whose hands are exposed to solvents and chemicals. The first occurrence is separation of the cuticle and nail folds from the nail plate, followed by the formation of a potential space for various microbes to invade, especially *C. albicans.*

Management. Treatment includes drying the area and applying anticandidal agents. In cases of severe paronychial inflammation, topical or intralesional steroids can be used. It is important to educate the patient about excessive water and chemical exposure.

DERMATOLOGIC DISEASES THAT AFFECT THE NAILS

Psoriasis

Psoriasis occurs in 2% to 3% of the population, and between 10% and 50% of psoriatics have nail involvement (see Chapter 85).

Physical Examination. Psoriasis of the nails can have a variety of clinical manifestations depending on the site of the involved nail unit. Nail pitting (in the nail plate) is due to involvement of the matrix; onycholysis, subungual hyperkeratosis, and yellow discoloration ("oil drop sign") are due to involvement of the nail bed. Psoriasis of the nail is often indistinguishable clinically from fungal infection of the nail (see Plate 28). Clinical inspection of other areas of the body that are prone to psoriasis (elbows, knees, scalp, gluteal cleft) and negative KOH examination and fungus culture can provide clues to the diagnosis of psoriasis of the nails. Approximately 5% of patients with psoriasis have psoriasis limited to the nails, a situation that poses a great diagnostic challenge.

Management. Treatment of psoriasis of the nails can be challenging. Often as cutaneous psoriasis clears, the nails clear as well. Topical steroids in a liquid or gel form may be helpful in some mild cases; however, results are usually disappointing in severe psoriatic involvement of the nails. Intralesional steroids (triamcinolone 3 mg/ml) injected into the nail fold overlying the matrix are generally more helpful, although not always welcomed by the patient. Psoralen plus UV A (PUVA) and grenz ray are sometimes beneficial in severe cases. A dermatologist should be consulted for these treatments.

Lichen Planus

Lichen planus is a relatively uncommon disorder that can affect the skin and/or nails (see Chapter 85). When it occurs in the nails, it can rapidly destroy the nail matrix, leading to onychorrhexis (longitudinal ridges) and occasionally eventual destruction of the nail plate. The end stage of lichen planus of the nails is destruction of the matrix so that portions of the nail fail to grow. The resultant defect is called a pterygium and is characterized by areas of the nail where the proximal nail fold adheres to the nail bed where the nail is absent.

Management. Potent topical corticosteroids can be tried, but systemic steroids are sometimes necessary for the treatment of rapidly destructive lichen planus of the nails.

Neoplastic Nail Conditions

Malignant Melanoma. Malignant melanoma of the nail unit is rare, accounting for only 1% to 4% of melanomas. Although 20% of these are amelanotic (containing little or no pigment), most start as a solitary longitudinal pigmented band in the nail. The band usually widens and darkens over time and frequently there is leaching of pigment into the proximal nail fold (Hutchinson's sign). The most commonly involved nails are the great toe and thumb. Over 25% of patients give a history of prior trauma to the digit, which in some cases causes delay in seeking medical attention. There are many benign causes of longitudinal pigmented bands in the nail ranging from hematoma and certain medications to a normal occurrence in blacks; but any solitary pigmented band that widens, darkens, or otherwise alters the nail plate needs further evaluation. The onus is on the physician to be certain that a pigmented band or spot on the nail is not a melanoma.

Management. Early detection and wide surgical excision are essential. When there is doubt about the diagnosis, referral to a dermatologist and biopsy of nail bed, nail matrix, or surrounding tissue are indicated. Once the diagnosis of malignant melanoma is confirmed, referral to an oncologic surgeon experienced in the management of malignant melanoma is mandatory (see Chapter 87).

Other cutaneous neoplasms occasionally are seen in the nail unit. Both basal cell carcinoma and squamous cell carcinoma occur rarely in the nail bed. A benign painful tumor that is often seen in a subungual location is a glomus tumor, an encapsulated tumor of the arteriovenous anastomosis in the nail bed. These tumors may be seen beneath the nail as a red or blue discoloration, but the main distinguishing feature is pain, which may be spontaneous or associated with cold. A benign bony growth called an exostosis can occur subungually, usually beneath the toenail, and often after trauma to the digit.

Other Common Nail Disorders

Habit Tic Disorder. Habit tic disorder (Plate 85) is a common disorder that is self-induced and characterized by horizontal parallel ridges in the nail plate. It results from frequent repetitive manipulation of the cuticle and nail fold overlying the matrix. The thumb is the most commonly involved digit. Once the cause of the problem is explained to the patient, the cure is simply a matter of leaving the nail alone.

Digital Mucous Cyst. Mucous cysts are the most common tumor of the digit and usually occur on the dorsal surface of the finger between the nail folds and the distal interphalangeal joint. They are not a true cyst because they lack a cystic lining but are more accurately called focal mucinosis.

Nail Changes in Systemic Disease. Some nail findings provide helpful clues for the diagnosis of systemic disorders. A few nail signs are specific for underlying medical problems. Nail fold telangiectases are associated with connective tissue disorders such as systemic lupus erythematosus and dermatomyositis. Clubbing is associated with pulmonary and gastrointestinal disorders. Other much less specific nail signs, such as splinter hemorrhages, may be seen in subacute bacterial endocarditis but are commonly seen in trauma (Table 92-3).

DISORDERS OF PIGMENTATION

Hyperpigmentation and hypopigmentation occur when a variety of things go wrong, including (1) changes in the number of melanocytes, (2) alterations in melanin synthesis, and (3) changes in hormonal balance. These alterations can be either congenital or genetic conditions or acquired diseases.

Hyperpigmentation

Generalized hyperpigmentation is usually caused by systemic conditions including endocrine, metabolic, and nutritional conditions. Addison's disease causes diffuse hyperpigmentation with accentuation in scars, palmar and plantar creases, and mucous membrane–pigmented patches. Secretion of cortisol from the adrenal glands suppresses melanocyte-stimulating hormone (MSH) and adrenocorticotrophic hormone (ACTH) release from the pituitary. Lack of cortisol with loss of adrenal gland function allows uninhibited release of MSH-stimulating melanocyte pigmentary synthesis. Glucocorticosteroid replacement slowly reverses the hyperpigmentation.

ACTH- and MSH-secreting tumors cause similar Addisonian pigmentation. Pregnancy and oral estrogen stimulate pigmentation of the nipples, areolae, and genitalia, as well as localized patches in the sun-exposed areas on the face (Plate 86). Several metabolic diseases (porphyria cutanea tarda, advanced liver disease, hemochromatosis, and chronic renal failure) and nutritional diseases (kwashiorkor, pellagra, inflammatory bowel disease, and malabsorption) cause hyperpigmentation. Hemochromatosis gives an unusual bronze hyperpigmentation. Certain drugs also cause hyper-

Table 92-3. Nail Signs of Systemic Disease

Nail sign	Nail appearance	Systemic disease
Clubbing	Increased unguophalangeal angle	Cardiopulmonary and gastrointestinal disorders
Half and half nail	Proximal half is brown, distal half is white	Renal failure
Nail fold telangiectases	Dilated vessels in proximal nail fold and cuticle	Dermatomyositis and systemic lupus erythematosus
Splinter hemorrhages	Longitudinal brown streaks under the nail	Trauma is the most common cause but also may be seen in subacute bacterial endocarditis
Mees' lines	Transverse white lines	Arsenic poisoning
Muehrcke's lines	Double white transverse lines	Chronic hypoalbuminemia
Koilonychia	Thin everted distal edge	Anemia, Plummer-Vinson syndrome
Azure lunula	Blue lunula	Hepatolenticular degeneration (Wilson's disease)
Terry's nails	Milky white nails with prominent onychodermal band	Cirrhosis, chronic congestive heart failure
Plummer's nails	Onycholysis	Thyrotoxicosis

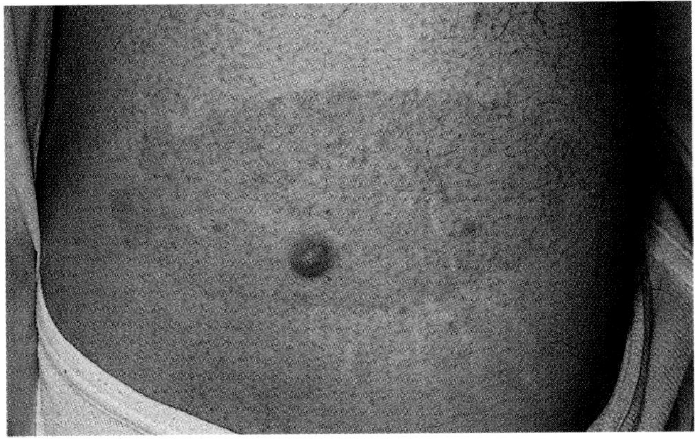

Plate 1. Macule (café au lait spot) plus a nodule (neurofibroma).

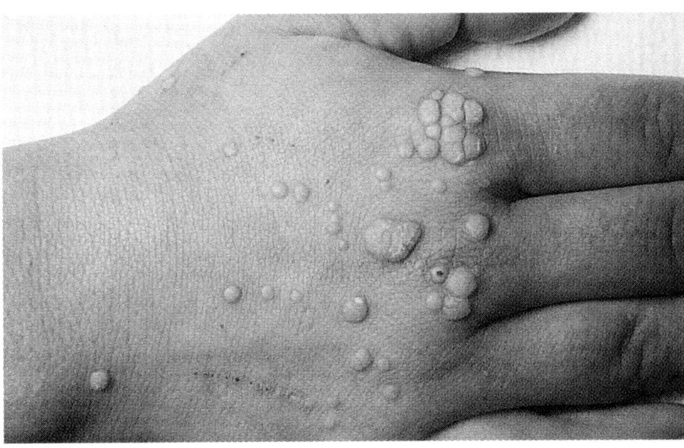

Plate 2. Common warts. Papules (verrucae). Note verrucous surface.

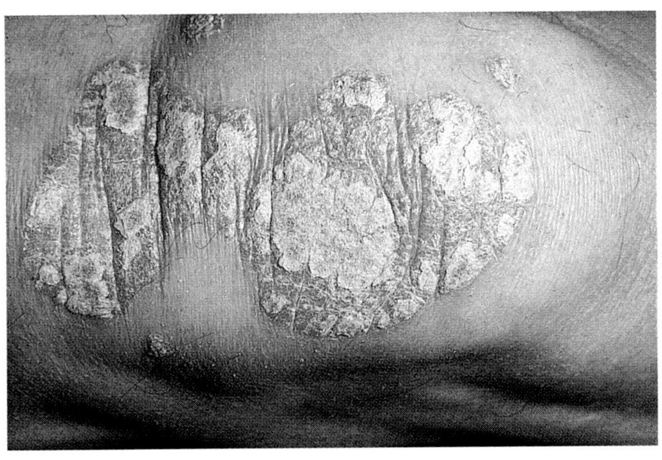

Plate 3. Plaques (psoriasis). Note special physical characteristic of scale (silvery, micaceous). Typical location: extensor surfaces (knee).

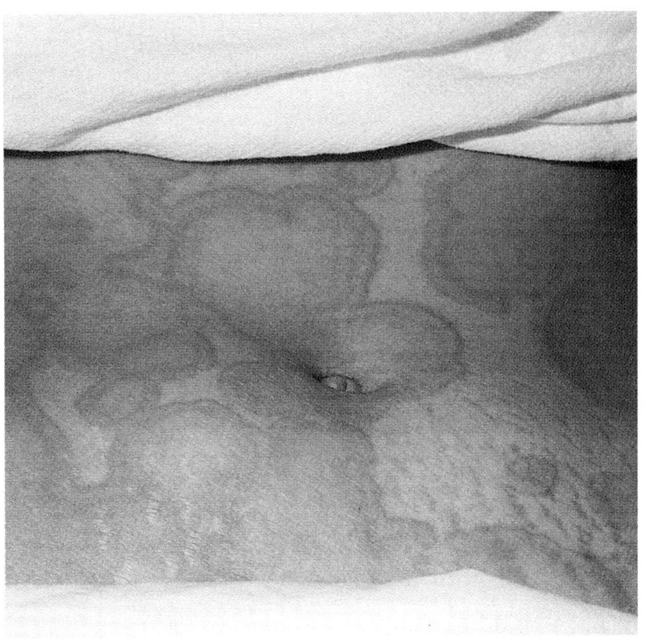

Plate 4. Wheal (urticaria). Note central cleaning, giving annular configuration.

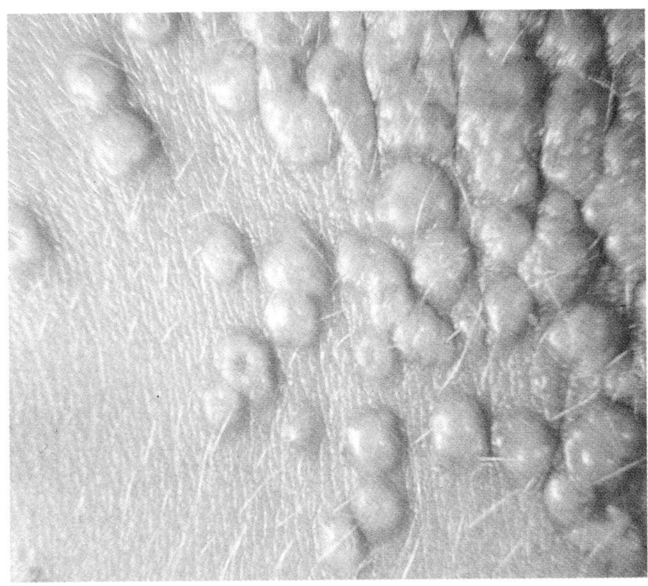

Plate 5. Vesicles (herpes simplex). Note umbilication characteristic of viral infection and herpetiform grouping.

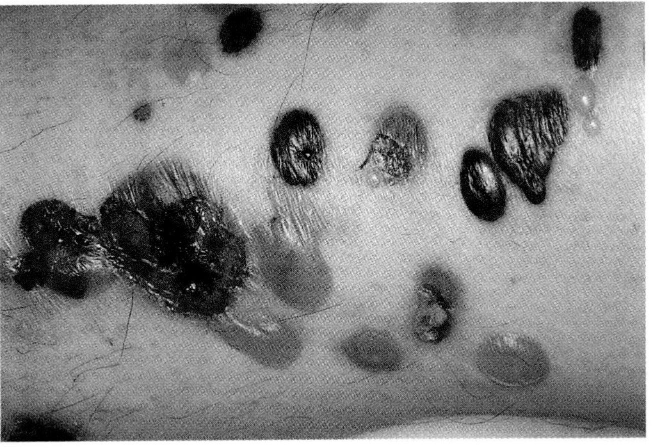

Plate 6. Bullae (bullous pemphigoid). Note hemorrhagic nature suggesting subepidermal process.

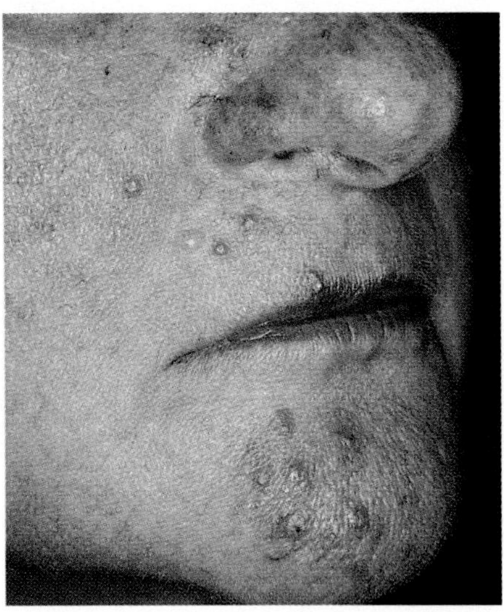

Plate 7. Pustules (rosacea). Note also the presence of telangiectasia.

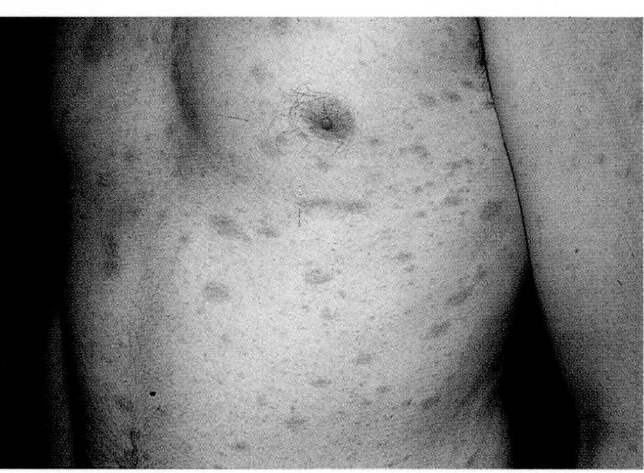

Plate 8. Scale (pityriasis rosea). Shows example of how unique scaling (collarette of fine scale within several lesions), distribution and shape of lesions (oval lesions with long axis paralleling natural skin cleavage lines), and color (salmon-pink) help in diagnosing skin disease.

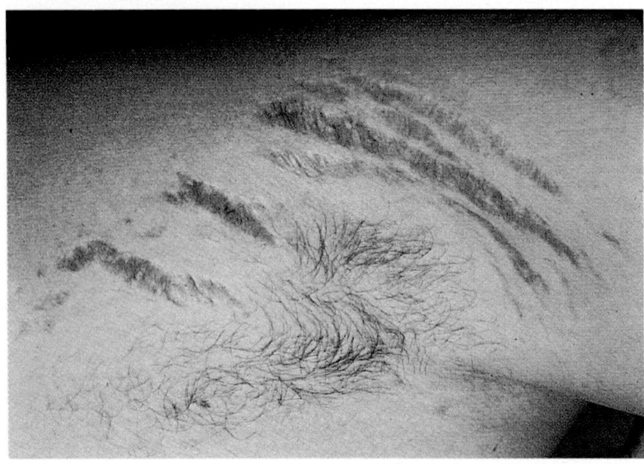

Plate 9. Atrophy (striae). Thinning of both the epidermis and dermis contributes to the development of striae.

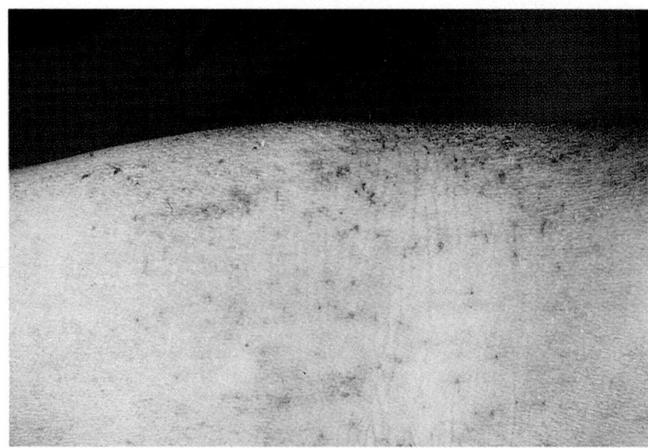

Plate 10. Lichenification (atopic dermatitis). Note erythema and pinpoint excoriations in antecubital fossa (typical location for atopic dermatitis—flexural).

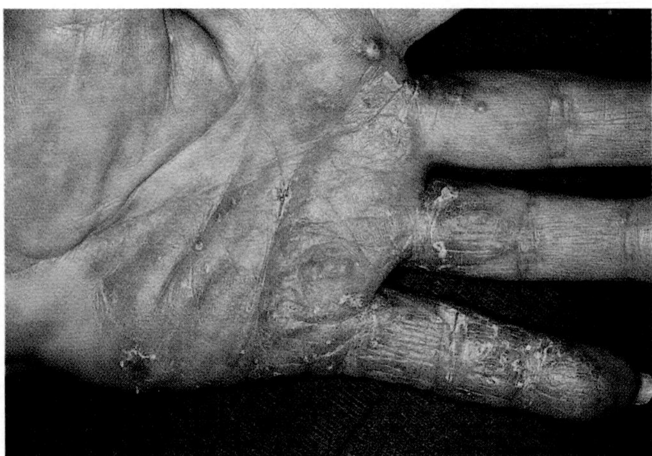

Plate 11. Fissures (chronic irritant hand dermatitis). Note superficial fissures in folds along with erythema, lichenification, scaling, and vesicles.

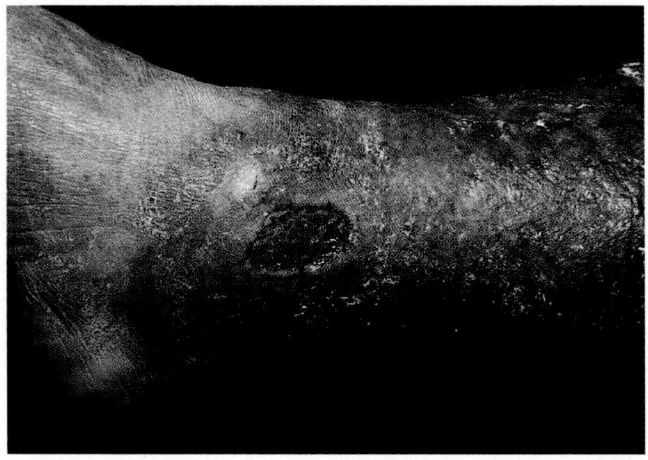

Plate 12. Ulcer (stasis dermatitis with ulcer). Note moist ulcer base and typical location near lateral malleolus plus associated dermatitis and stasis pigmentation.

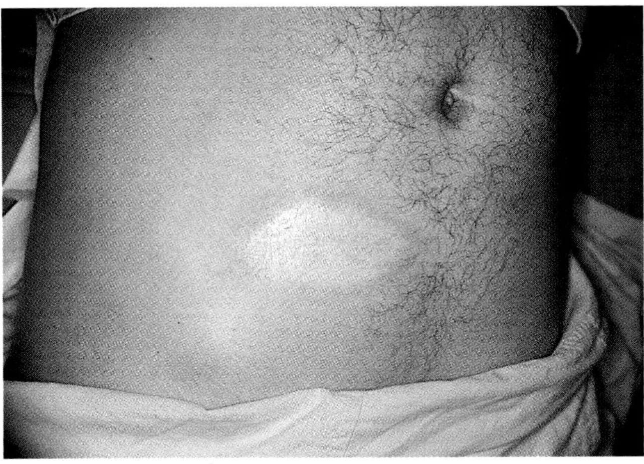

Plate 13. Scarring process (morphea). Note ivory white color due to deposition of collagen and loss of hair appendages.

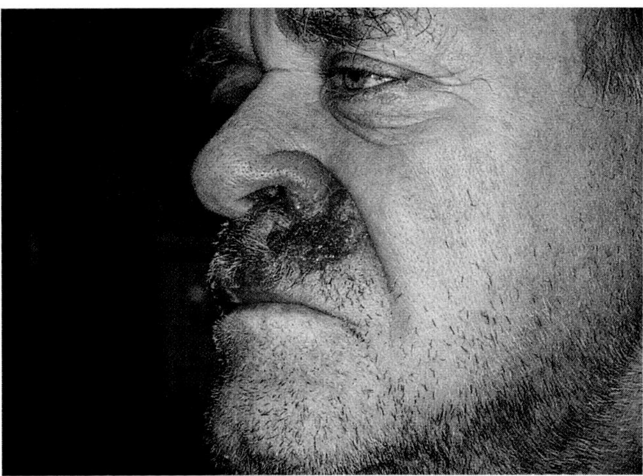

Plate 14. Crusts (impetigo). Note both hemorrhagic and honey-colored crust.

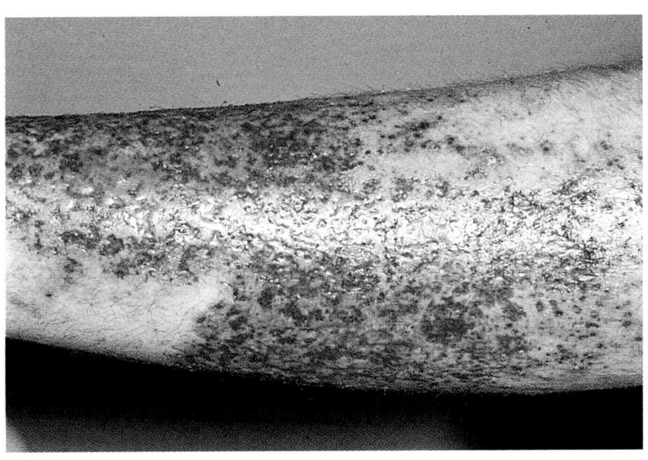

Plate 15. Oozing (acute dermatitis). Note multiple erosions with oozing wet glistening surface.

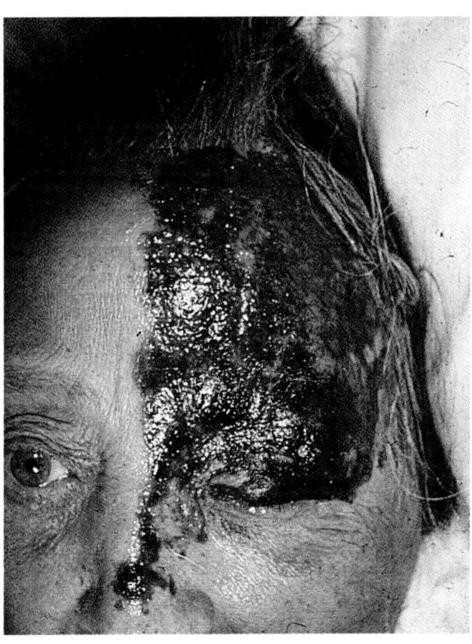

Plate 16. Zosteriform lesions (herpes zoster). Note hemorrhagic vesicular involvement of left VI cranial nerve.

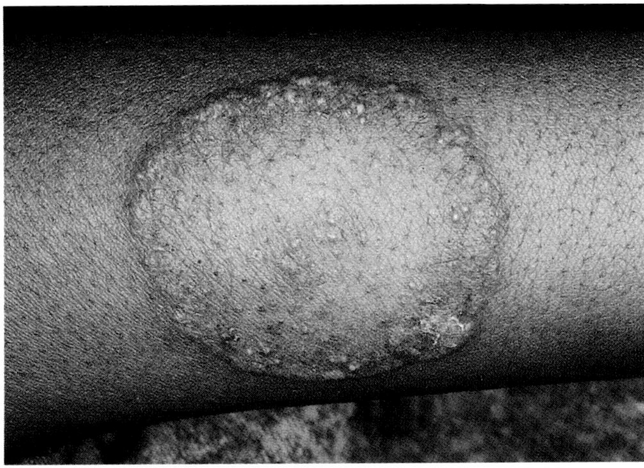

Plate 17. Annular lesion (tinea corporis). Note raised (expanding) erythematous scaling border and central clearing.

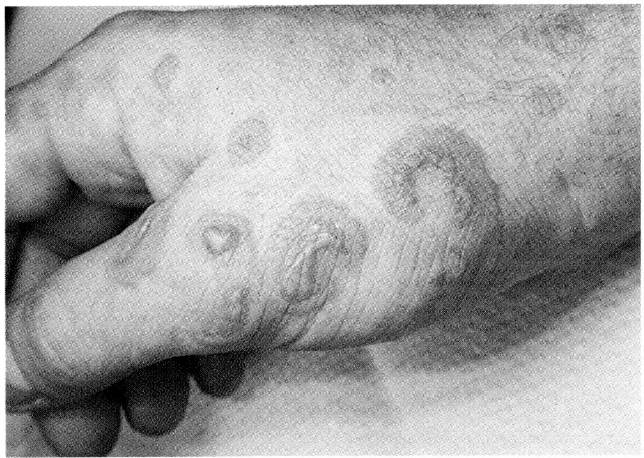

Plate 18. Iris and arcuate lesions (erythema multiforme). Note erythematous lesions with multiform configurations—target, arcuate, and vesicles.

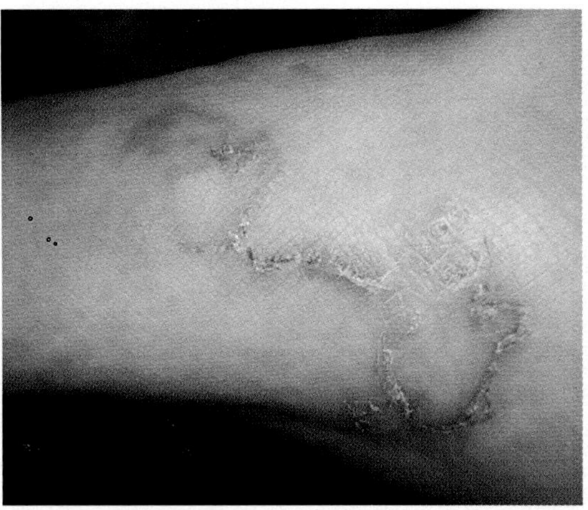

Plate 19. Serpiginous lesion (cutaneous larva migrans, creeping eruption). Note snakelike tract of ankylostoma or strongyloides larvae infection of the skin.

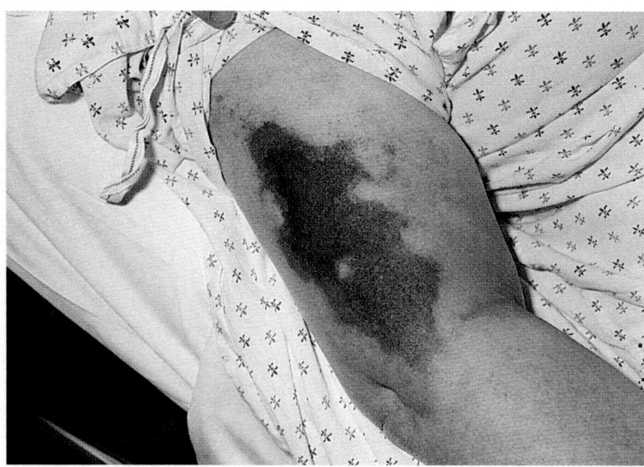

Plate 20. Purpuric lesion (purpura fulminans). Note stellate purpuric lesion with surrounding erythema characteristic of disseminated intravascular coagulation secondary to sepsis (e.g., meningococcemia).

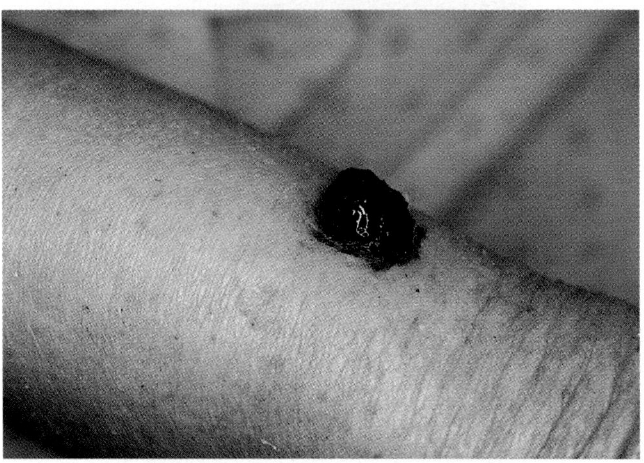

Plate 21. Melanin pigment (melanoma). Note variations of hues of color (black and blue) reflecting depth of melanin within the skin and pigment extending laterally at the base.

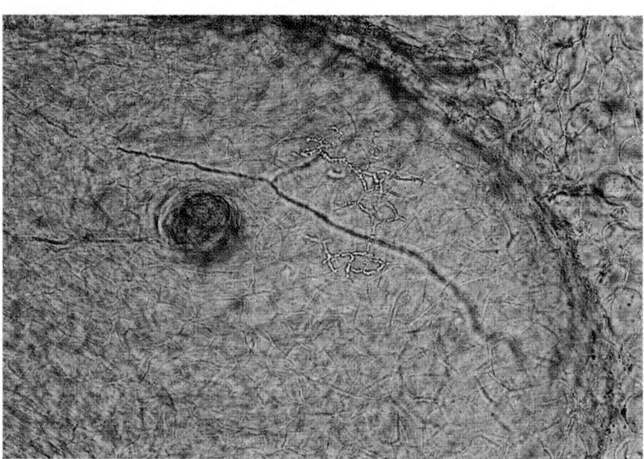

Plate 22. Linear hyphal element present within a clump of keratinocytes. (Courtesy James C. Shaw, MD.)

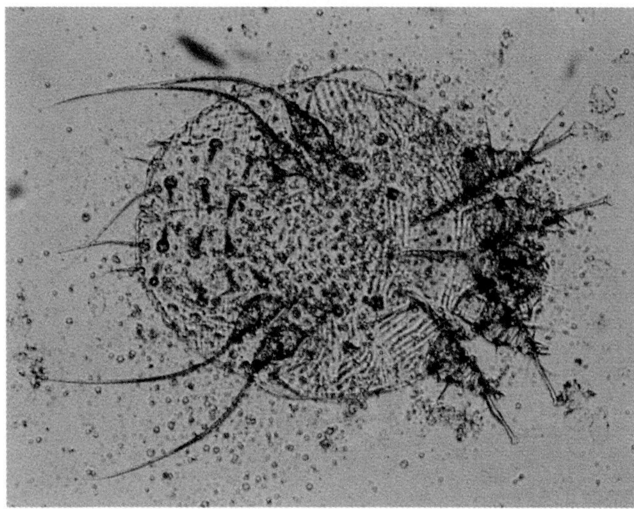

Plate 23. *Sarcoptes scabiei* in a potassium hydroxide wet mount (×40). (From Habif TP: *Clinical dermatology: a color guide to diagnosis and therapy,* ed 3, St Louis, 1996, Mosby.)

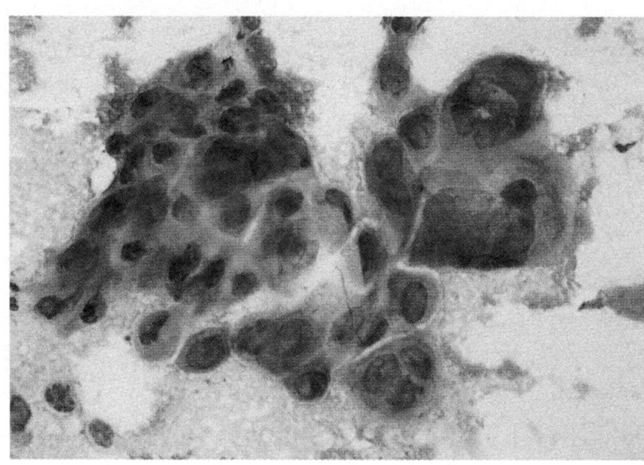

Plate 24. Multinucleated keratinocytes pathognomonic of herpes viral infections.

TYPES OF LESIONS

Noninflammatory lesions

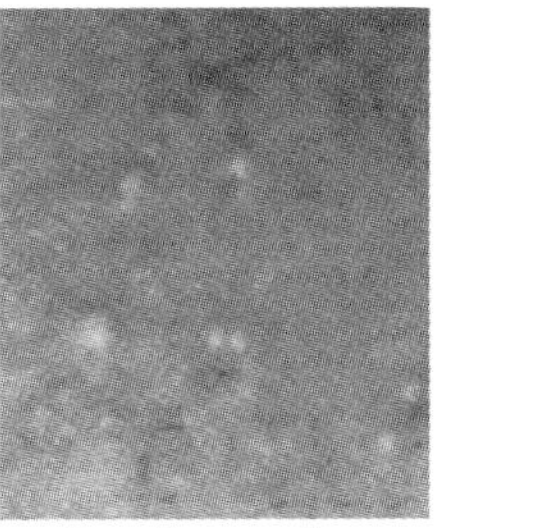
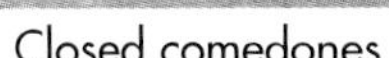

Closed comedones

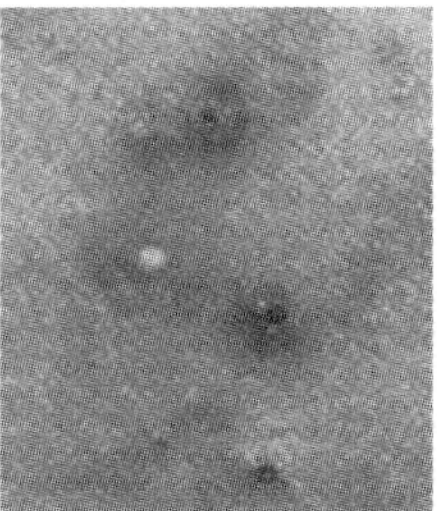

Open comedones

Inflammatory lesions

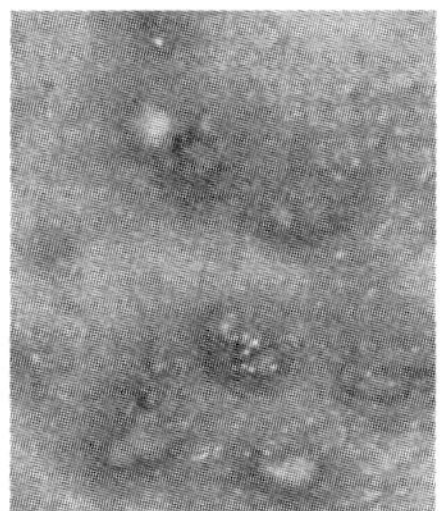

Papules/pustules

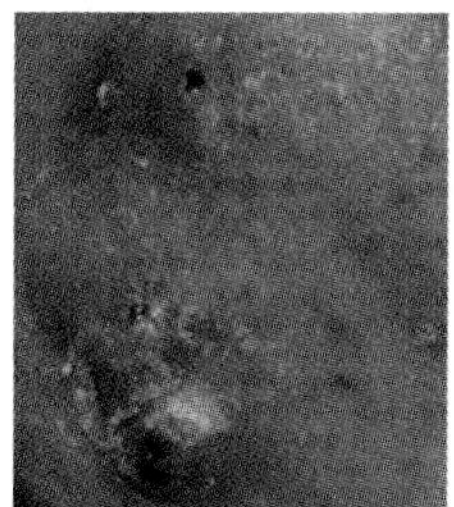

Nodules

ACNE CLASSIFICATION AND GRADING

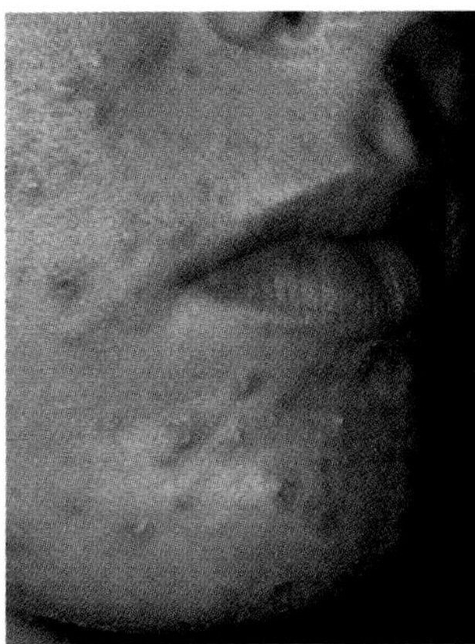

Mild
Papules/pustules +/++
Nodules 0

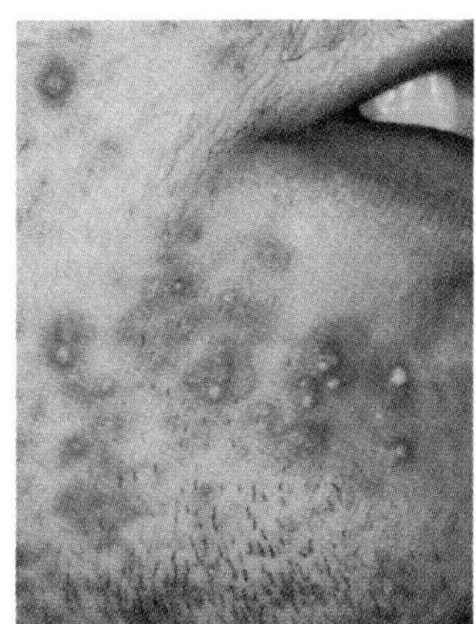

Moderate
Papules/pustules ++/+++
Nodules +/++

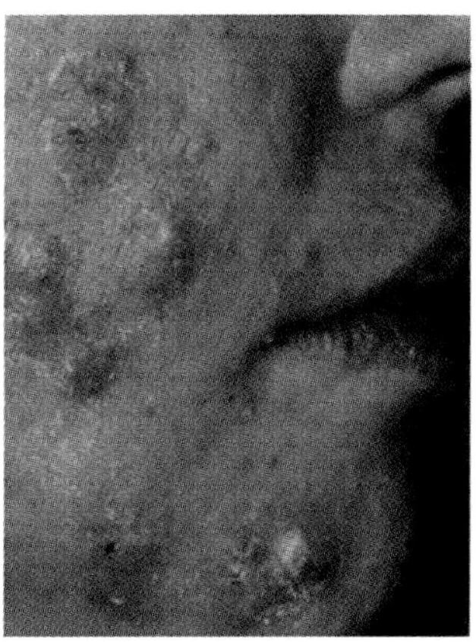

Severe
Papules/pustules +++/++++
Nodules +++

SEVERITY GRADING OF INFLAMMATORY LESION

Severity	Papules/pustules	Nodules	Additional factors that determine severity
Mild	Few to several	None	Psychosocial circumstances
Moderate	Several to many	Few to several	Occupational difficulties
Severe	Numerous and/or extensive	Many	Inadequate therapeutic responsiveness

Plate 25. Acne classification of lesions. (From Habif TP: *Clinical dermatology: a color guide to diagnosis and therapy,* ed 3, St Louis, 1996, Mosby.)

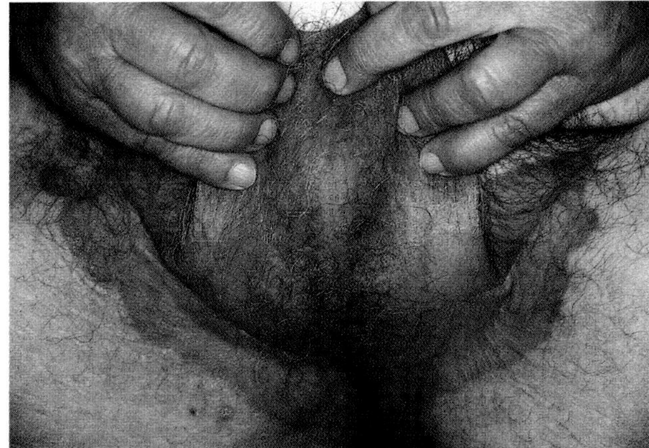

Plate 26. Inverse psoriasis. Sharp demarcation in the groin with scrotal involvement. (Courtesy James C. Shaw, MD.)

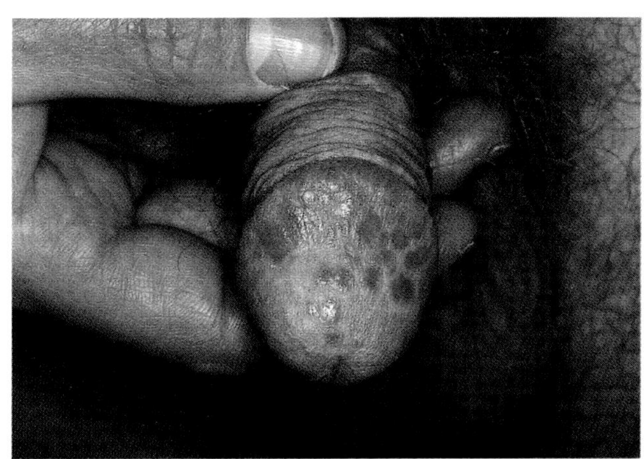

Plate 27. Plaques of psoriasis on the glans penis. (Courtesy James C. Shaw, MD.)

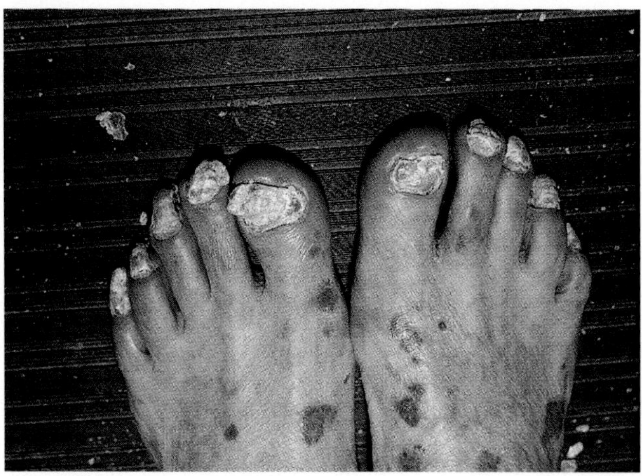

Plate 28. Psoriatic nail changes. Note nail dystrophy and accumulation of yellow subungual debris resembling onychomycosis, plus associated cutaneous psoriatic lesions.

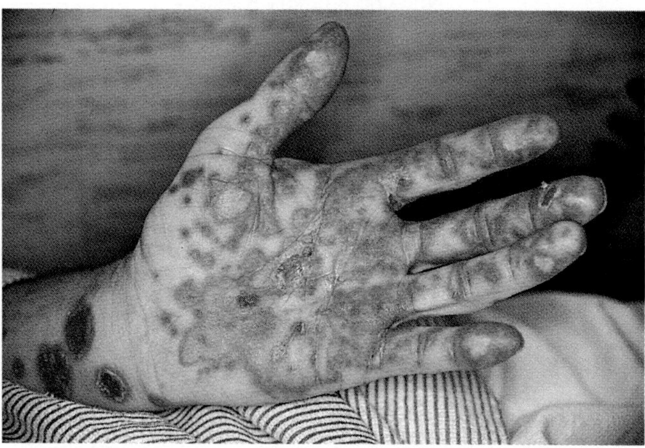

Plate 29. Reiter's syndrome (keratoderma blennorrhagicum). Note erythematous and pustular plaques on the palm.

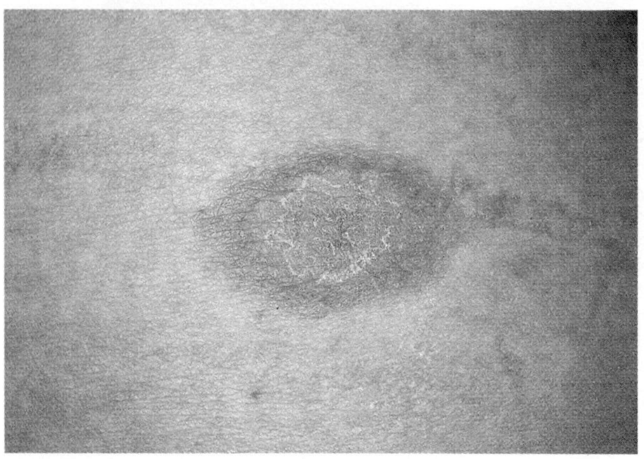

Plate 30. Pityriasis rosea. Herald patch. (Courtesy James C. Shaw, MD.)

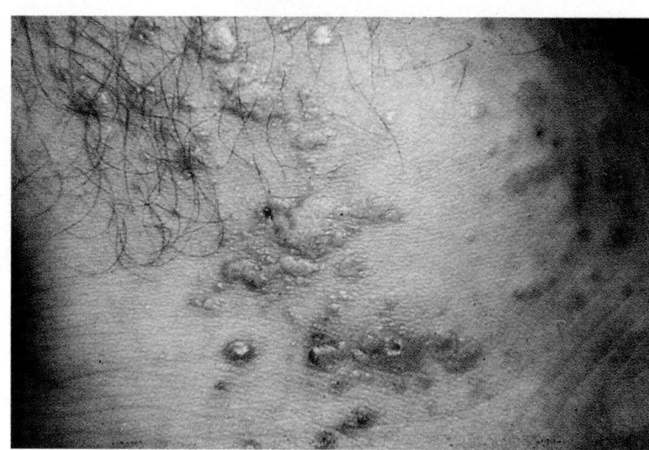

Plate 31. Lichen planus. Note polygonal purple, flat, shiny topped papules in typical area (ankles).

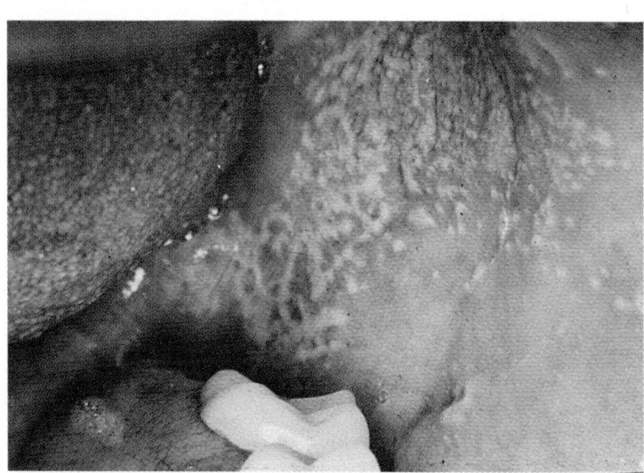

Plate 32. Oral lichen planus. Note lacy white streaks on buccal mucosa.

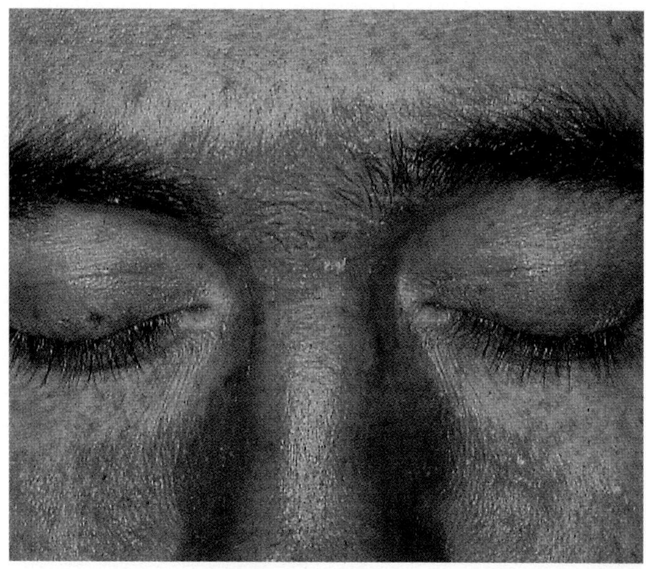

Plate 33. Seborrheic dermatitis. (From Habif TP: *Clinical dermatology,* ed 2, St Louis, 1990, Mosby.)

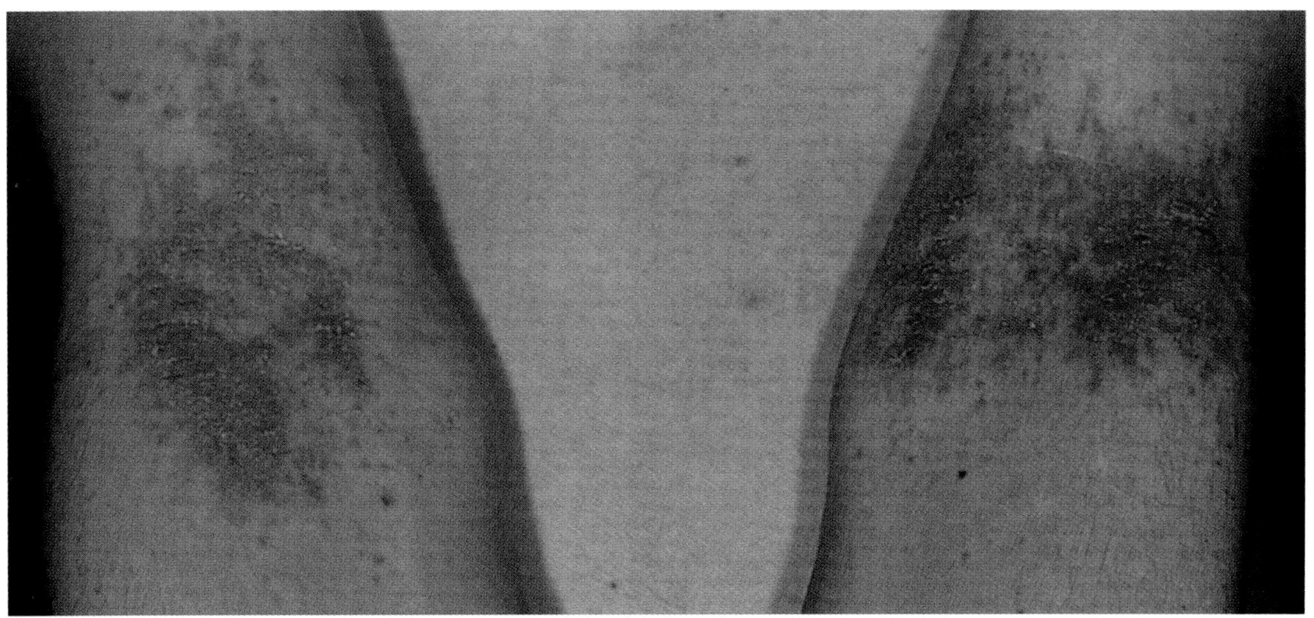

Plate 34. Atopic dermatitis. Classic appearance of confluent papules forming plaques in the antecubital fossa. (From Habif TP: *Clinical dermatology: a color guide to diagnosis and therapy,* ed 3, 1996, St Louis, Mosby.)

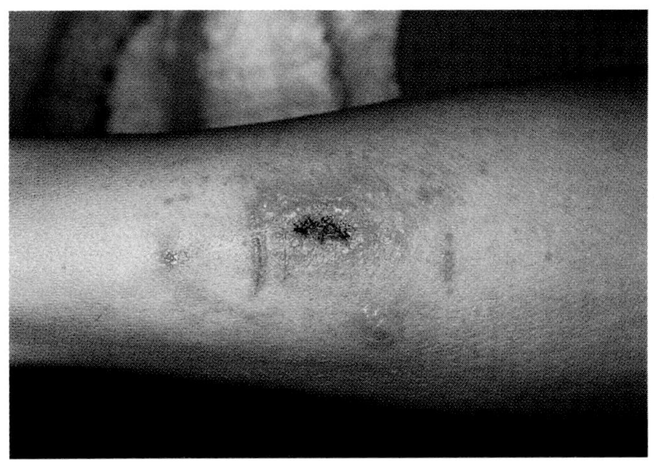

Plate 35. Allergic contact dermatitis (poison oak, acute vesicular reaction, and linear features). Dark central pigmentation is oxidized oleoresin.

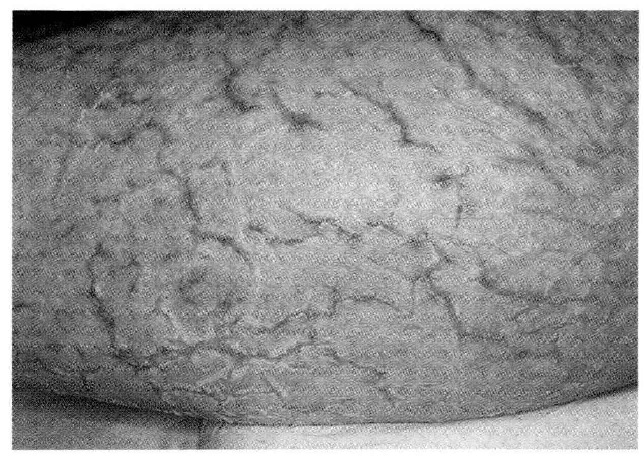

Plate 36. Xerotic dermatitis. (Courtesy James C. Shaw, MD.)

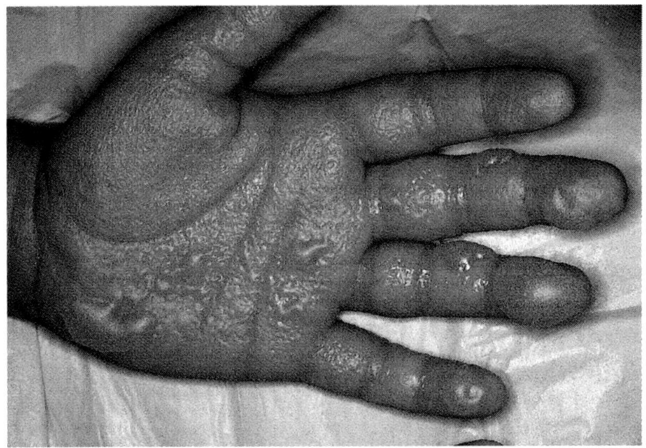

Plate 37. Dyshidrotic dermatitis. Severe vesicular hand eruption. (Courtesy James C. Shaw, MD.)

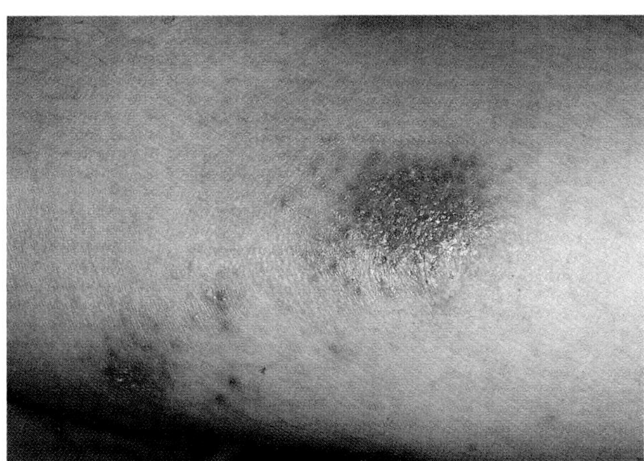

Plate 38. Nummular dermatitis. Typical localized patch of dermatitis. (Courtesy James C. Shaw, MD.)

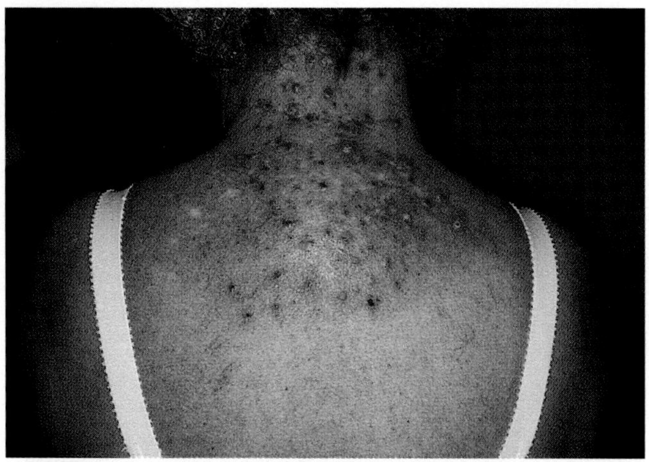

Plate 39. Lichen simplex chronicus and prurigo nodules. Note lichenification and excoriated papules that involve only an area on the back that can be reached.

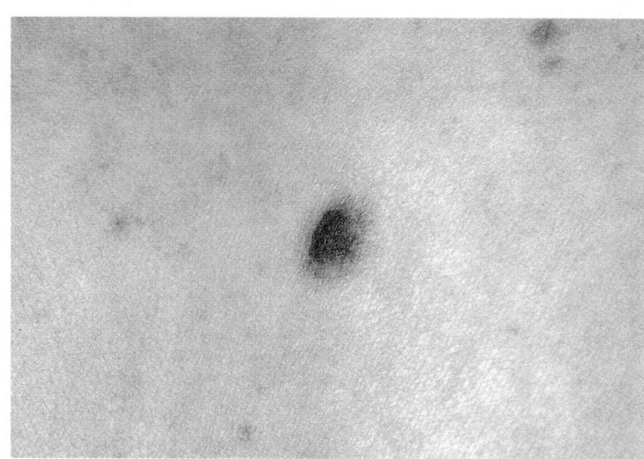

Plate 40. Melanocytic nevus. Note slightly raised tan brown papule. (Courtesy James C. Shaw, MD.)

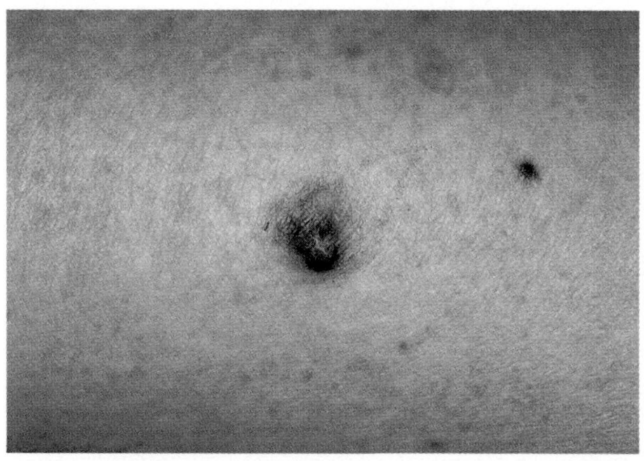

Plate 41. Blue nevus. Blue-gray color that can resemble melanoma. (Courtesy James C. Shaw, MD.)

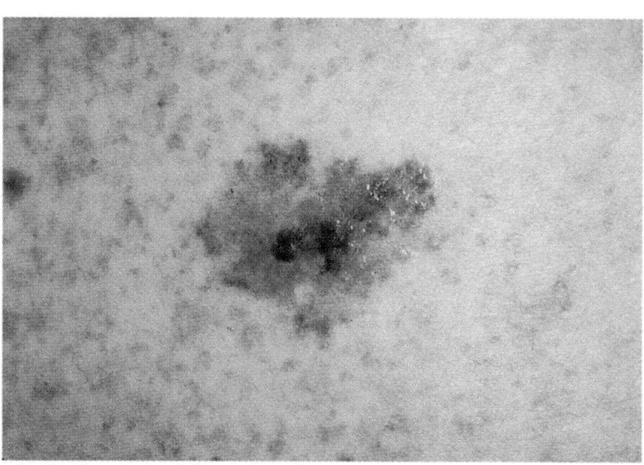

Plate 42. Atypical nevus. Note large irregular configuration with some red hue. (Courtesy James C. Shaw, MD.)

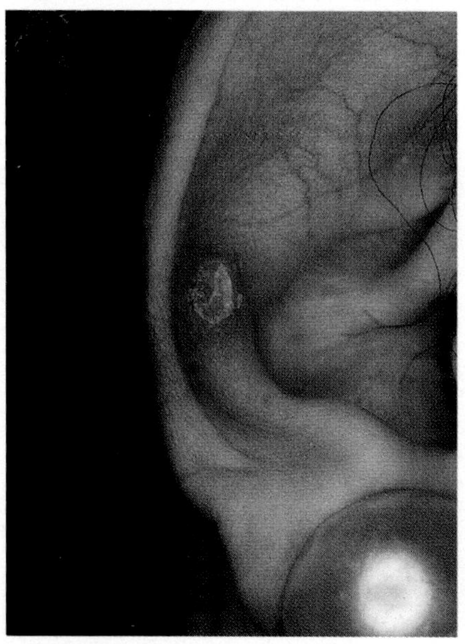

Plate 43. Chondrodermatitis nodularis. Note location on pressure point (antihelix). (Courtesy James C. Shaw, MD.)

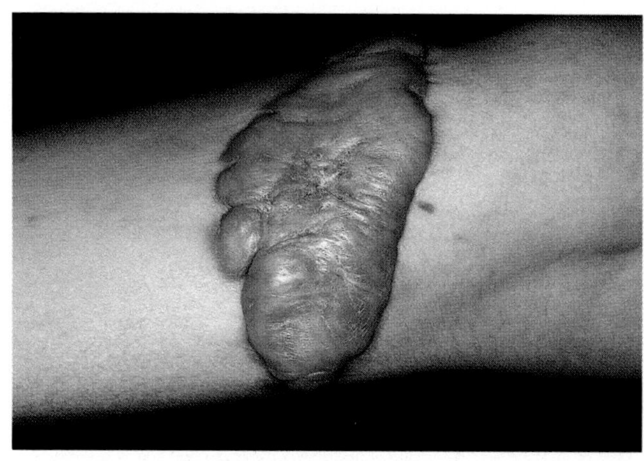

Plate 44. Keloid. Firm mass on extremity. (Courtesy James C. Shaw, MD.)

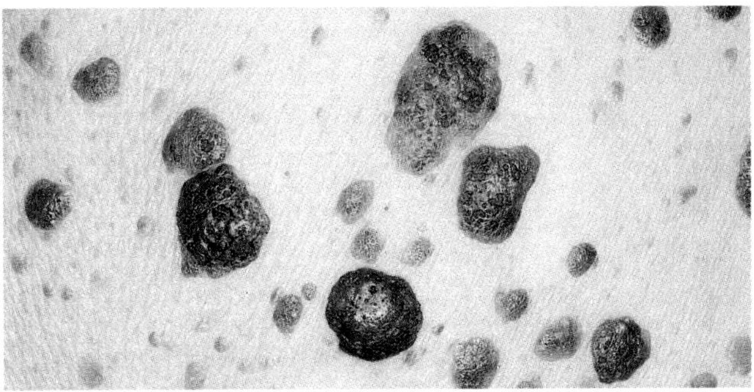

Plate 45. Seborrheic keratoses. Multiple dark epidermal lesions with obvious texture. (Courtesy James C. Shaw, MD.)

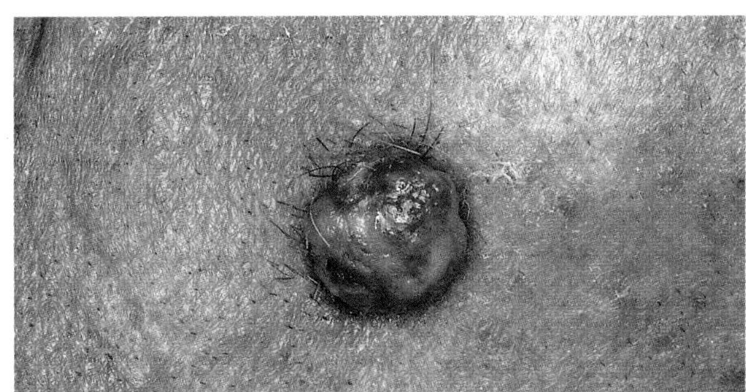

Plate 46. Pyogenic granuloma. Raised friable lesion resembling granulation tissue. (Courtesy James C. Shaw, MD.)

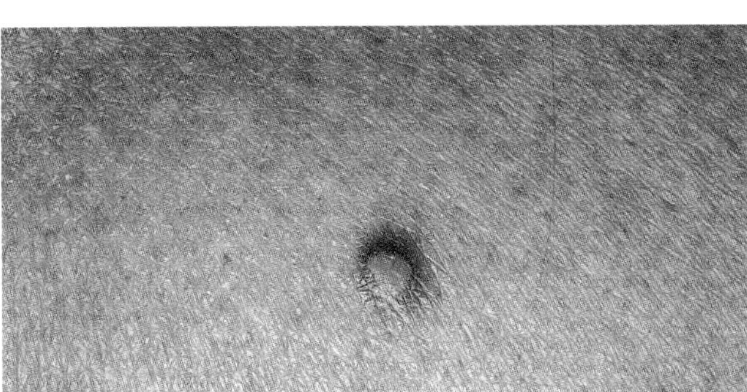

Plate 47. Dermatofibroma. Discrete firm nodule, frequently hyperpigmented. (Courtesy James C. Shaw, MD.)

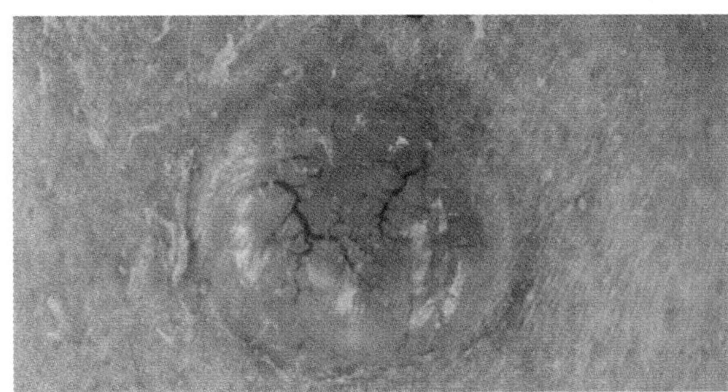

Plate 48. Basal cell carcinoma. The blood vessels are haphazardly distributed over the entire surface. (From Habif TP: *Clinical dermatology: a color guide to diagnosis and therapy,* ed 3, St Louis, 1996, Mosby.)

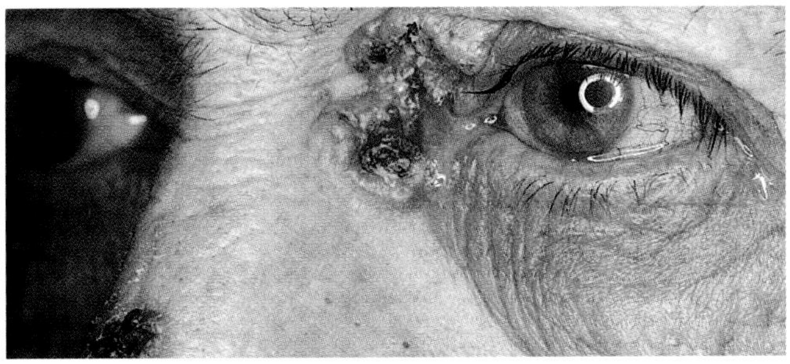

Plate 49. Basal cell carcinoma. Note rolled translucent border and central ulceration in typical facial location.

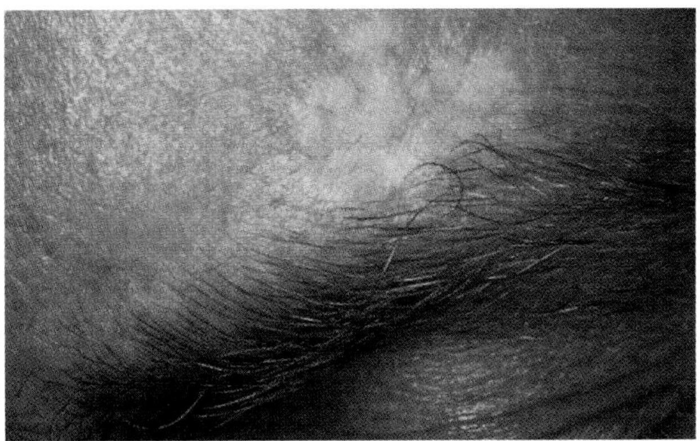

Plate 50. Sclerosing basal cell carcinoma. (From Habif TP: *Clinical dermatology: a color guide to diagnosis and therapy,* ed 3, St Louis, 1996, Mosby.)

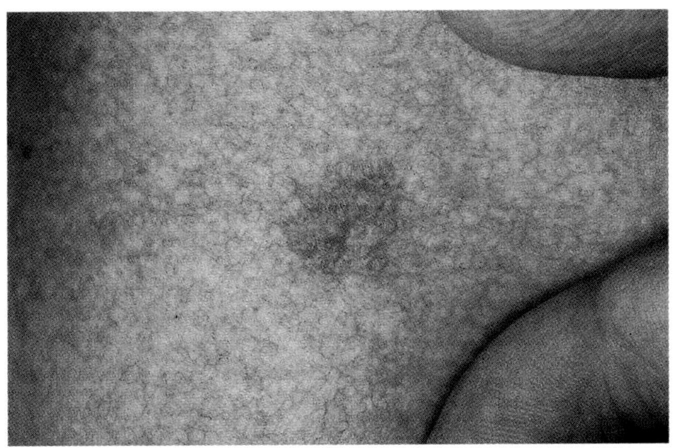

Plate 51. Superficial basal cell carcinoma. Subtle findings with slight raised pearly border. (Courtesy James C. Shaw, MD.)

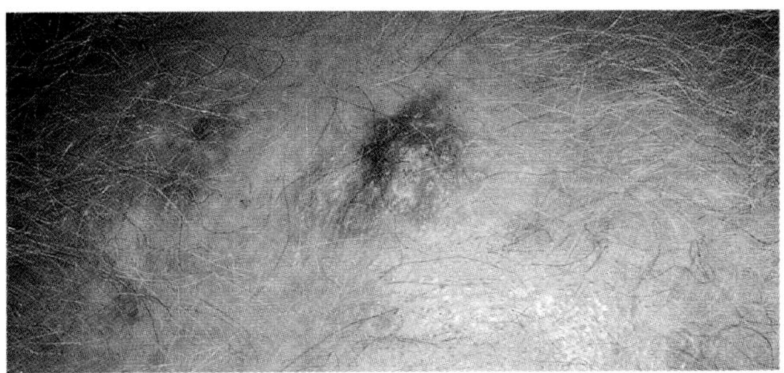

Plate 52. Actinic keratosis. Hyperkeratotic lesion on sun-exposed forehead. (Courtesy James C. Shaw, MD.)

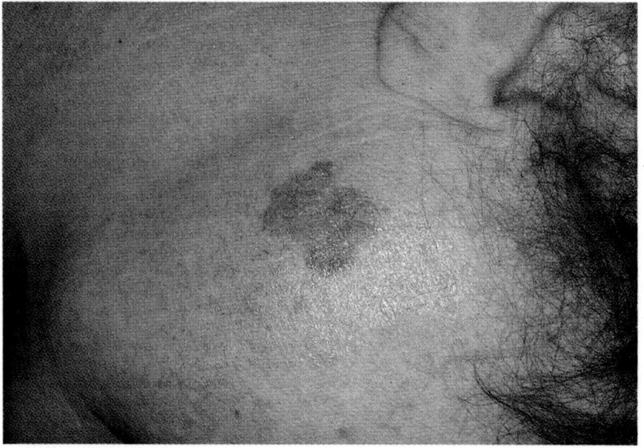

Plate 53. Bowen's disease (squamous cell carcinoma in situ). Thin erythematous-brown plaque. (Courtesy James C. Shaw, MD.)

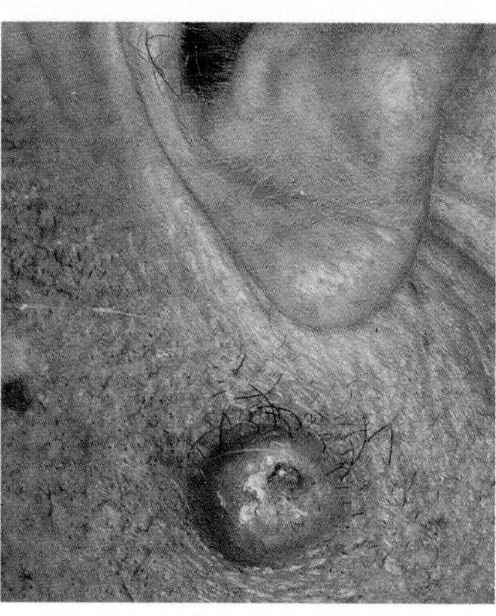

Plate 54. Keratoacanthoma. Typical dome-shaped nodule with central keratin plug. (Courtesy James C. Shaw, MD.)

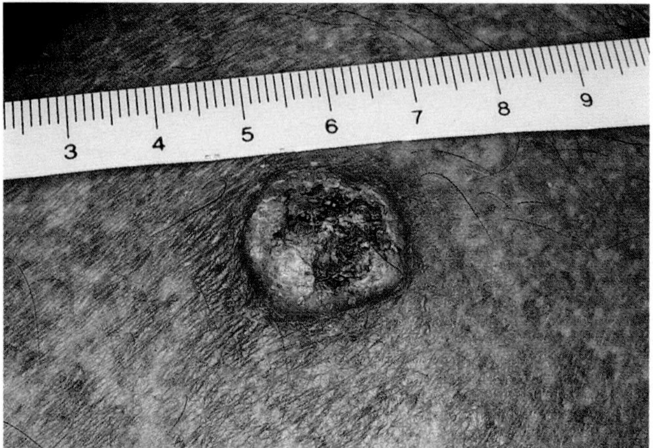

Plate 55. Squamous cell carcinoma. Nodular hyperkeratotic lesion with central erosion.

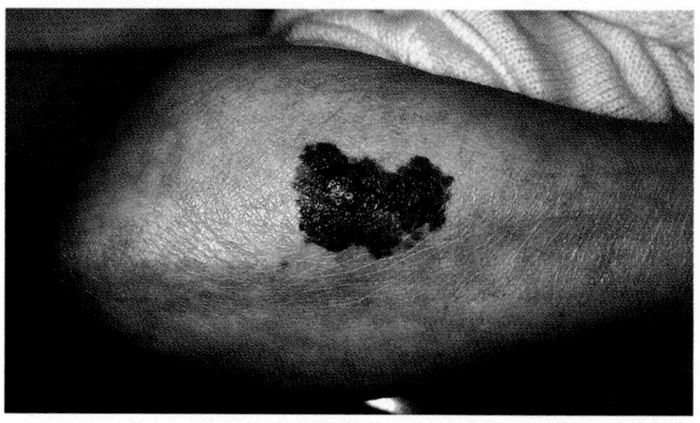

Plate 56. Melanoma—superficial spreading. Typical irregular border and variegate color. (Courtesy James C. Shaw, MD.)

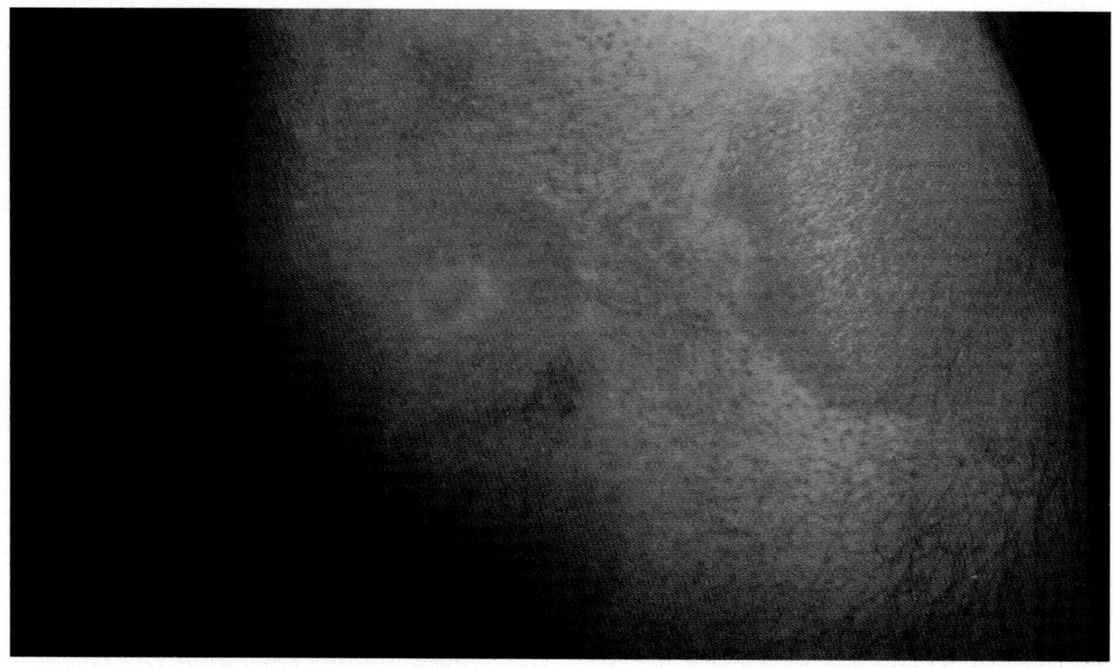

Plate 57. Mycosis fungoides. Lesions typical of the eczematous form or the patch stage. Persistent, flat, red, itchy, well-circumscribed patches can persist for months or years. (From Habif TP: *Clinical dermatology: a color guide to diagnosis and therapy,* ed 3, St Louis, 1996, Mosby.)

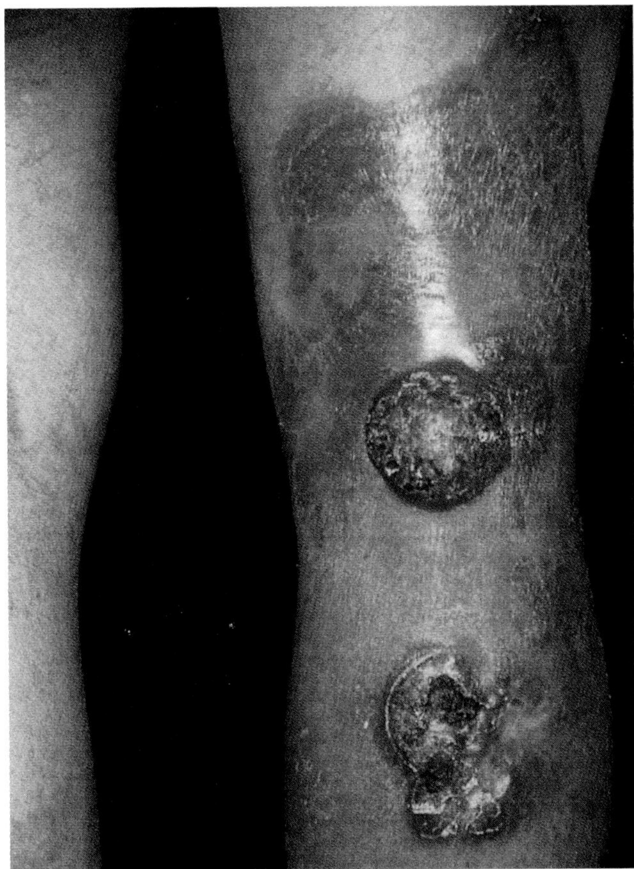

Plate 58. Mycosis fungoides. Plaque and tumor stages. (From Habif TP: *Clinical dermatology: a color guide to diagnosis and therapy,* ed 3, St Louis, 1996, Mosby.)

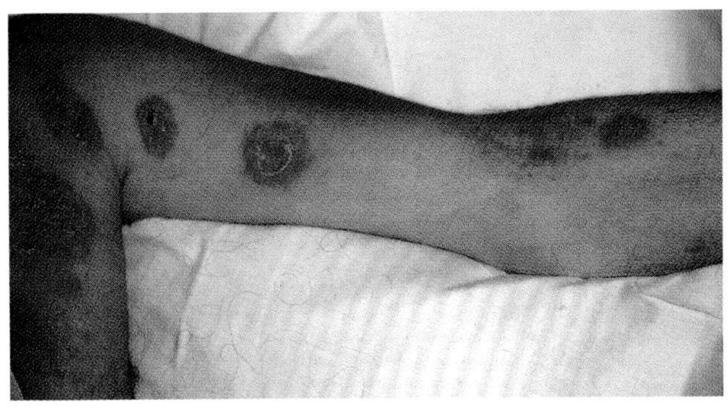

Plate 59. Leukemia cutis. Erythematous nodular tumors. (Courtesy James C. Shaw, MD.)

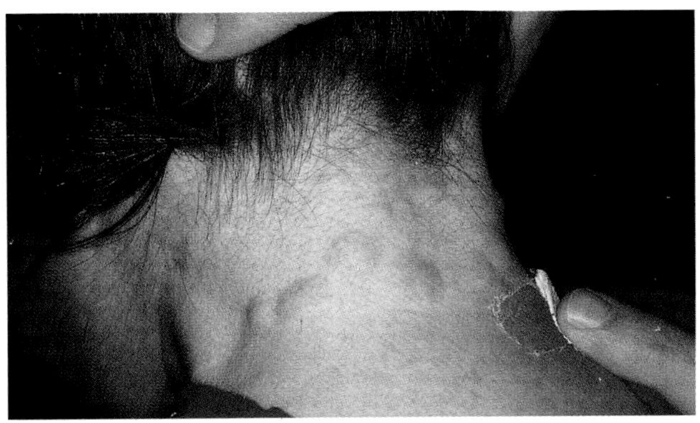

Plate 60. Firm red-brown dermal nodules in cutaneous metastatic breast carcinoma. (Courtesy James C. Shaw, MD.)

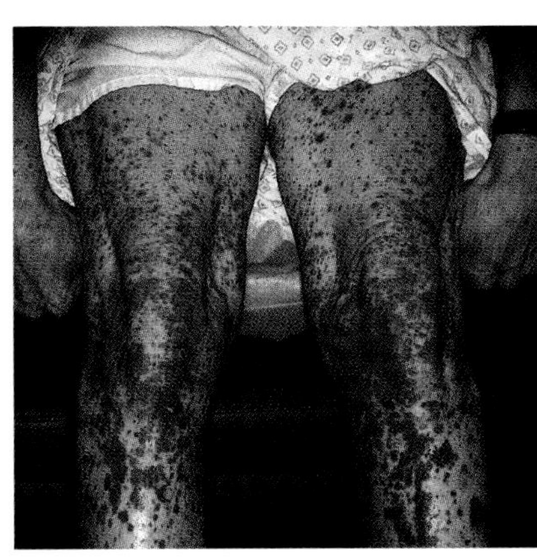

Plate 61. Leukocytoclastic vasculitis. Note bilateral purpuric lesions on distal lower extremity. (Courtesy James C. Shaw, MD.)

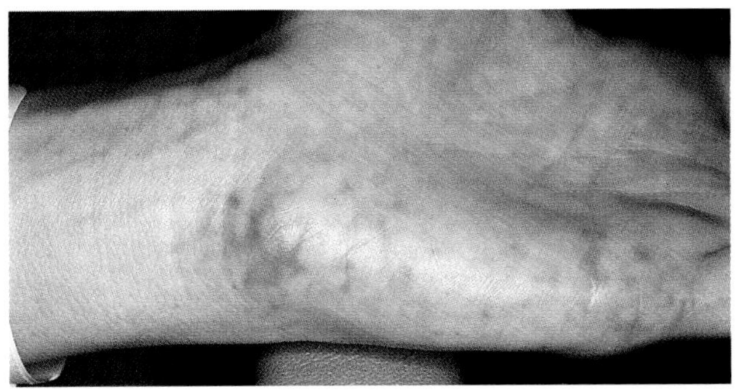

Plate 62. Churg-Strauss vasculitis. Erythematous nodules with vascular livedo pattern. (Courtesy James C. Shaw, MD.)

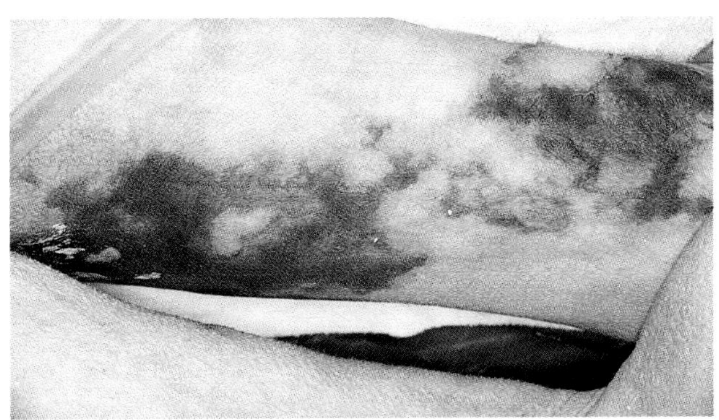

Plate 63. Antiphospholipid antibody syndrome. Livedo pattern of purpura. (Courtesy James C. Shaw, MD.)

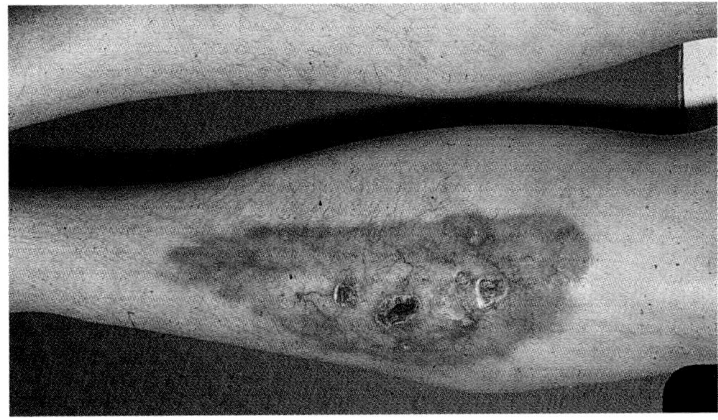

Plate 64. Necrobiosis lipoidica diabeticorum. Note red-brown atrophic plaque with telangiectasia.

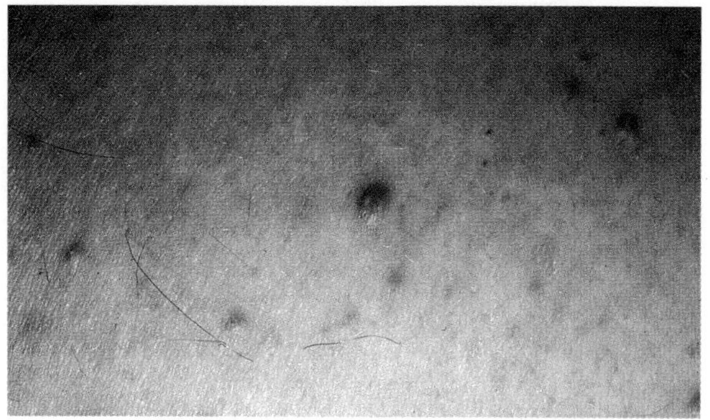

Plate 65. Eruptive xanthomas. Yellow to red papules. (Courtesy James C. Shaw, MD.)

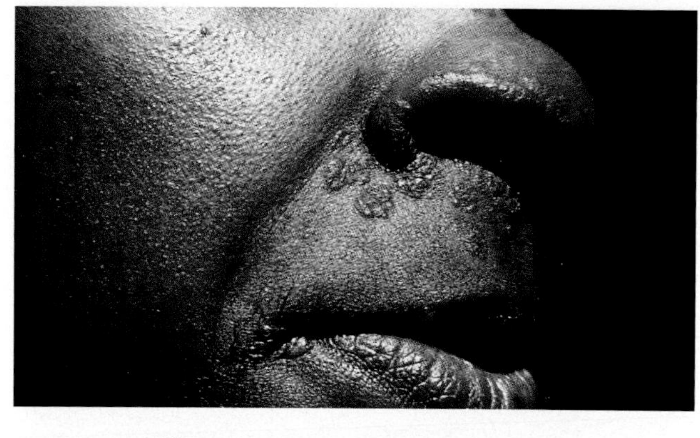

Plate 66. Sarcoidosis. Papular type.

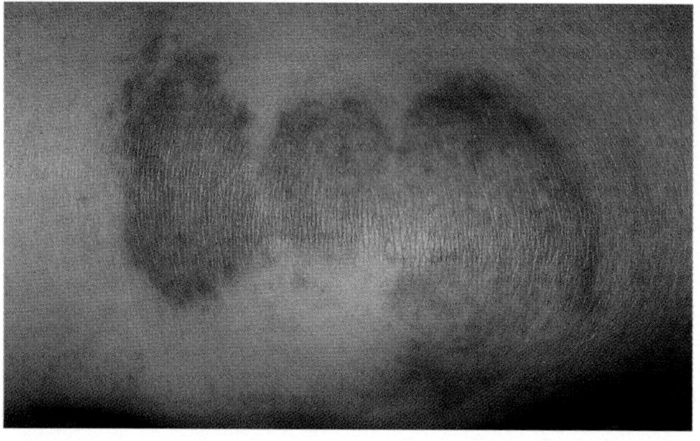

Plate 67. Sarcoidosis. Plaque type. (Courtesy James C. Shaw, MD.)

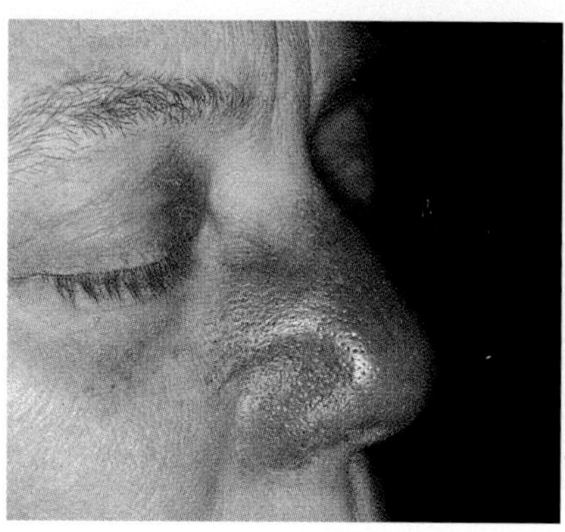

Plate 68. Sarcoidosis. Lupus pernio type. (Courtesy James C. Shaw, MD.)

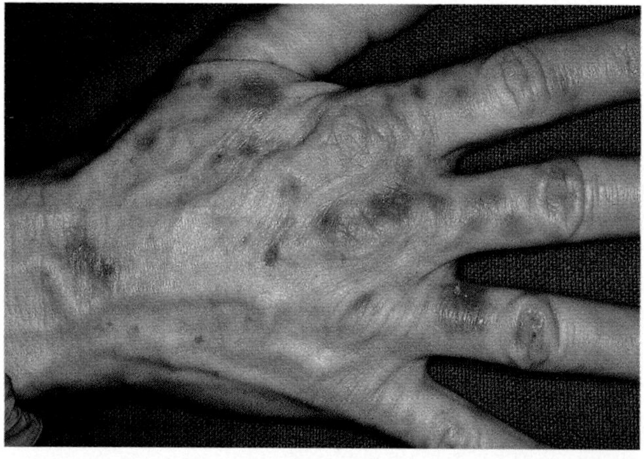

Plate 69. Porphyria cutanea tarda. Typical erosive changes on the sun-exposed hands. (Courtesy James C. Shaw, MD.)

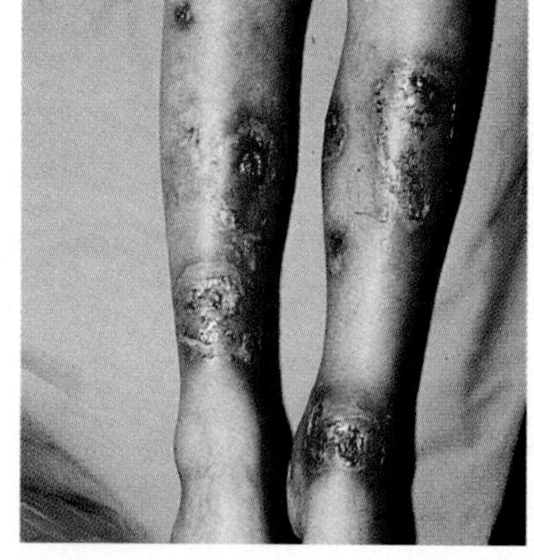

Plate 70. Pyoderma gangrenosum. Note ragged ulcerations with surrounding erythema.

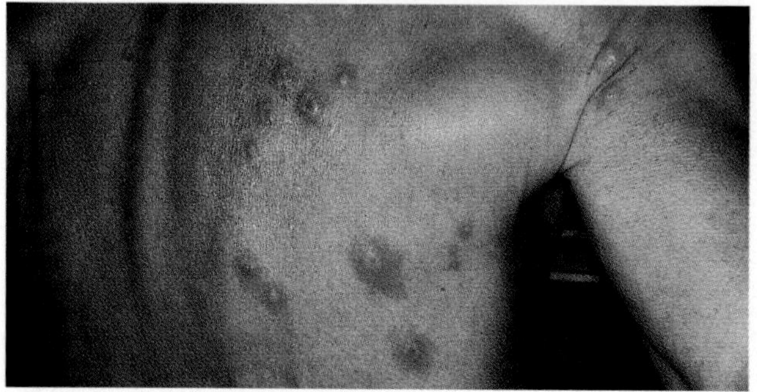

Plate 71. Sweet's syndrome. Typical erythematous nodules on the trunk. (Courtesy James C. Shaw, MD.)

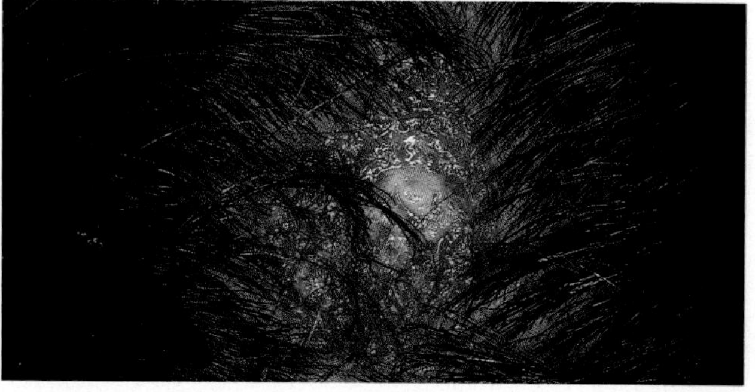

Plate 72. Pemphigus vulgaris. Large erosion on the scalp. (Courtesy James C. Shaw, MD.)

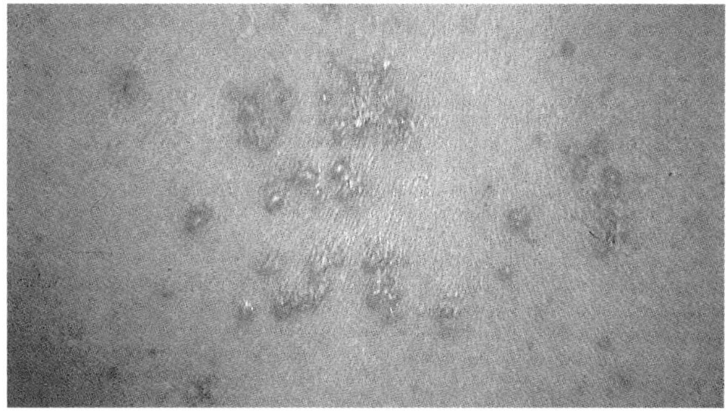

Plate 73. Dermatitis herpetiformis. Typical grouped papulovesicles. (Courtesy James C. Shaw, MD.)

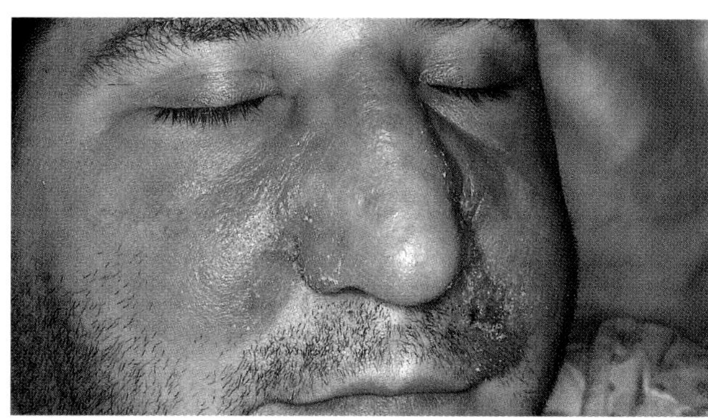

Plate 74. Erysipelas. Typical facial location with superficial cellulitis. (Courtesy James C. Shaw, MD.)

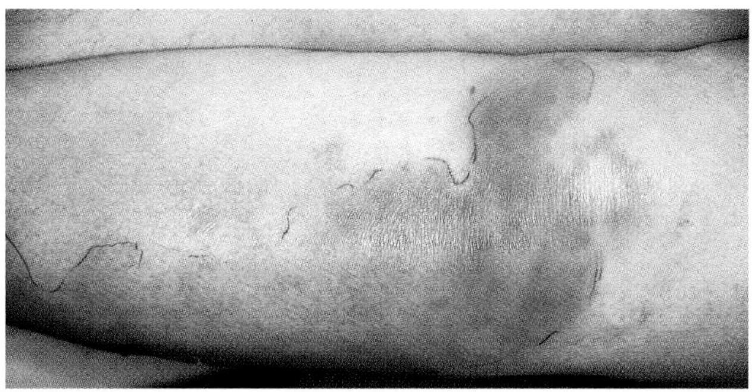

Plate 75. Cellulitis. Note advancing irregular border. (Courtesy James C. Shaw, MD.)

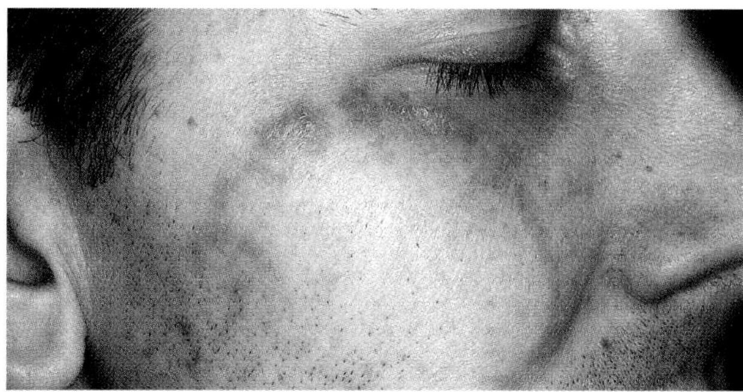

Plate 76. Tinea faciale. Annular scaling lesion. (Courtesy James C. Shaw, MD.)

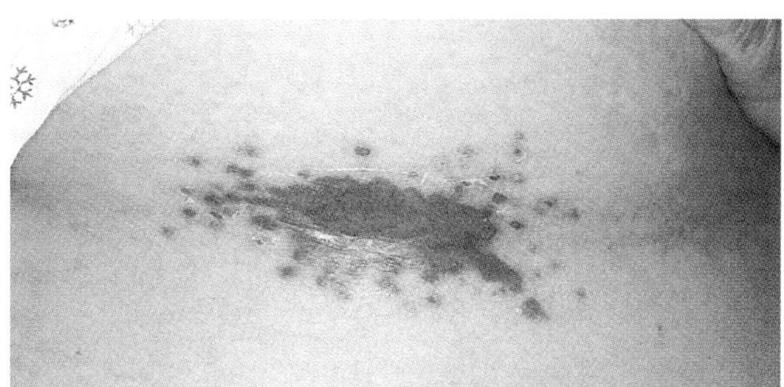

Plate 77. Candidiasis. Note erythematous erosive dermatitis with satellite pustules.

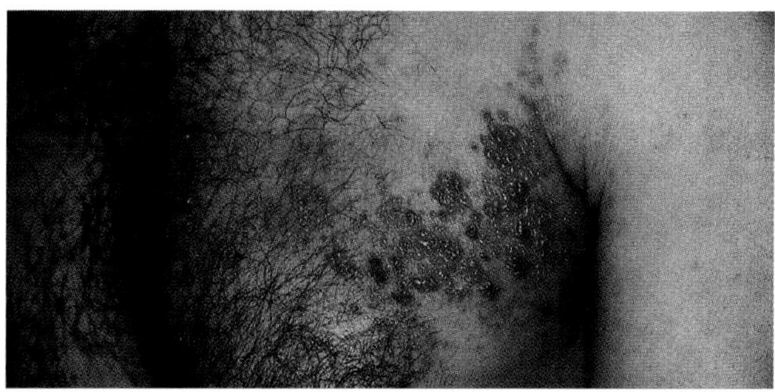

Plate 78. Herpes zoster. Typical dermatomal involvement. (Courtesy James C. Shaw, MD.)

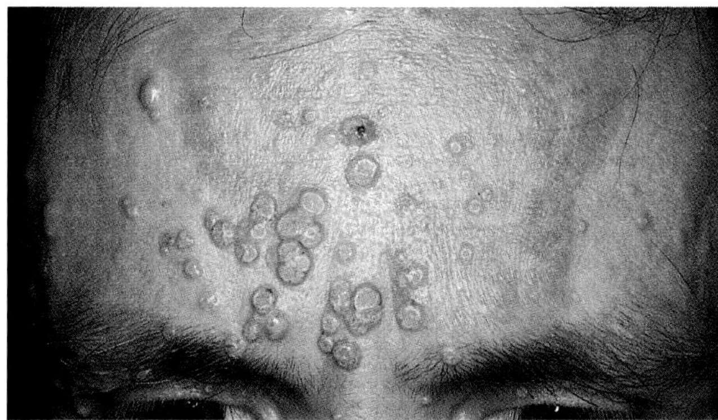

Plate 79. Molluscum contagiosum (may appear in atypical manner in HIV-positive patients). Note large-size varicoid appearance and central keratin plugging.

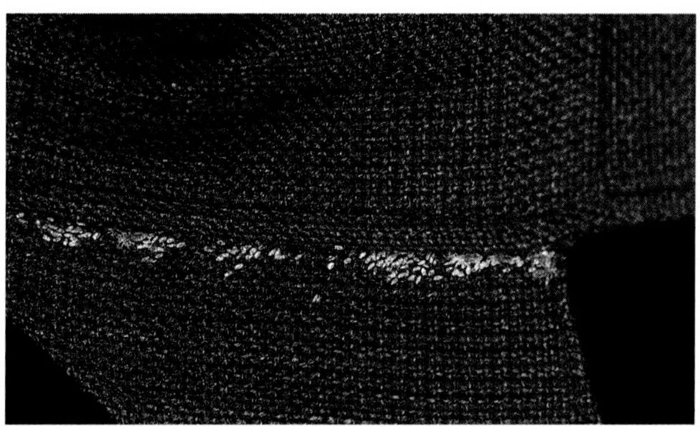

Plate 80. Body lice and nits on a patient's clothing. (Courtesy James C. Shaw, MD.)

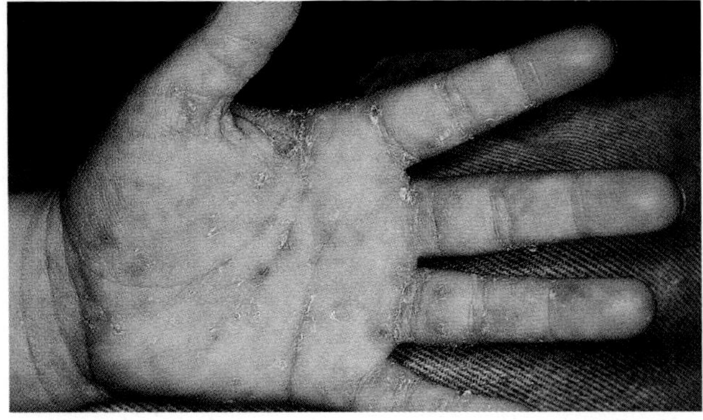

Plate 81. Scabies. Note involvement in web space and wrist. (Courtesy James C. Shaw, MD.)

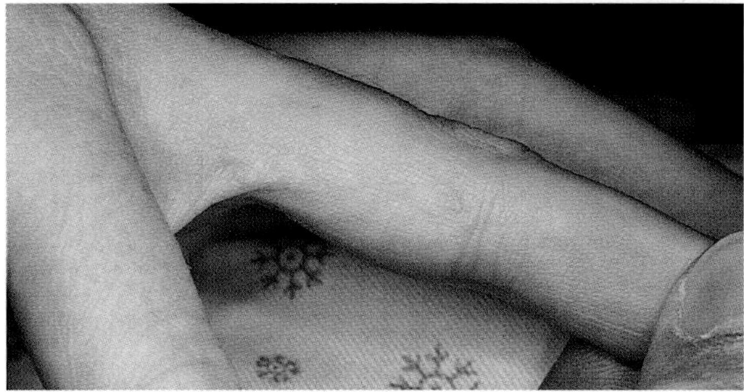

Plate 82. Scabies burrow. Note subtle raised linear lesion on the lateral aspect of the finger.

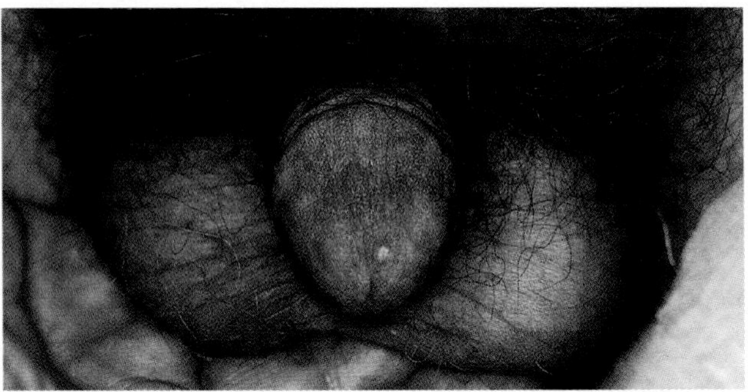

Plate 83. Scabies, penile involvement. (Courtesy James C. Shaw, MD.)

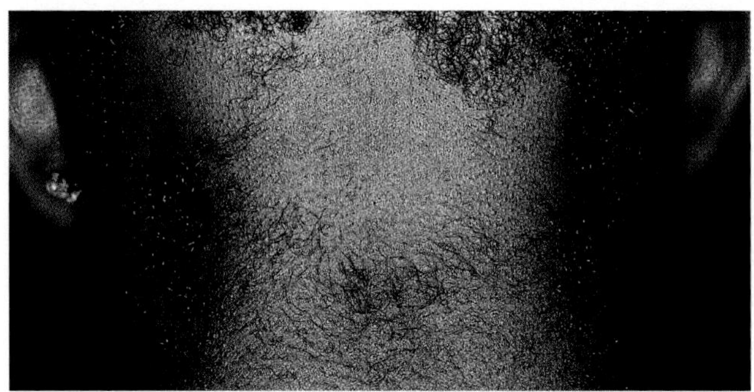

Plate 84. Alopecia areata. Circular patches of alopecia. (Courtesy James C. Shaw, MD.)

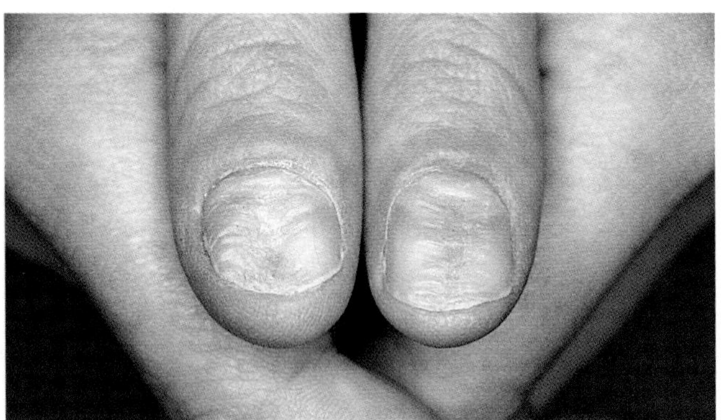

Plate 85. Habit tic deformity. Note the pathognomonic horizontal ridges.

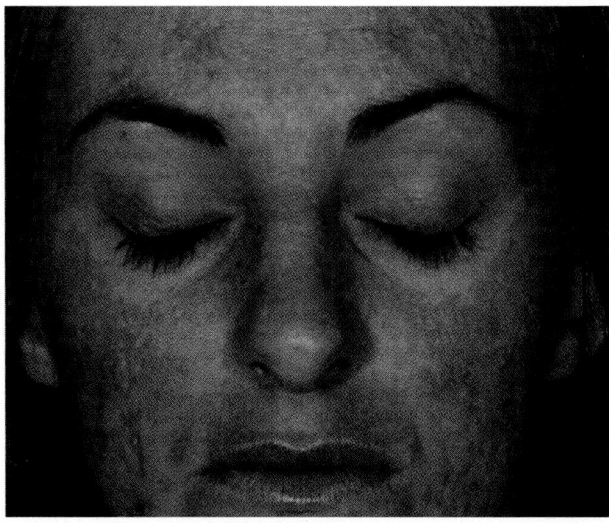

Plate 86. Melasma (mask of pregnancy). Diffuse brown hyperpigmentation may occur during pregnancy or while taking oral contraceptives. (From Habif TP: *Clinical dermatology: a color guide to diagnosis and therapy,* ed 3, St Louis, 1996, Mosby.)

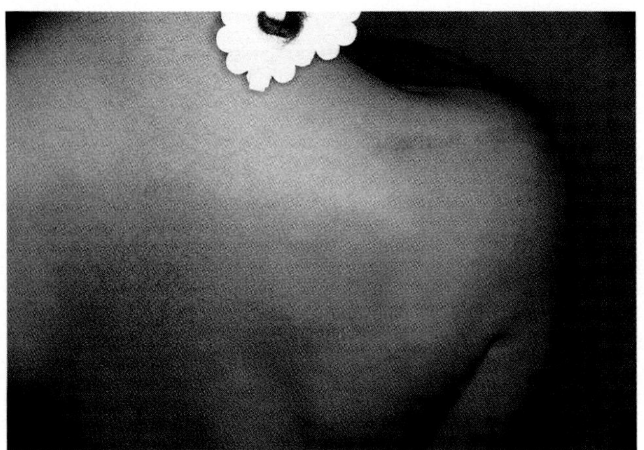

Plate 87. Mongolian spot. Bluish pigment reflects dermal melanin. (Courtesy James C. Shaw, MD.)

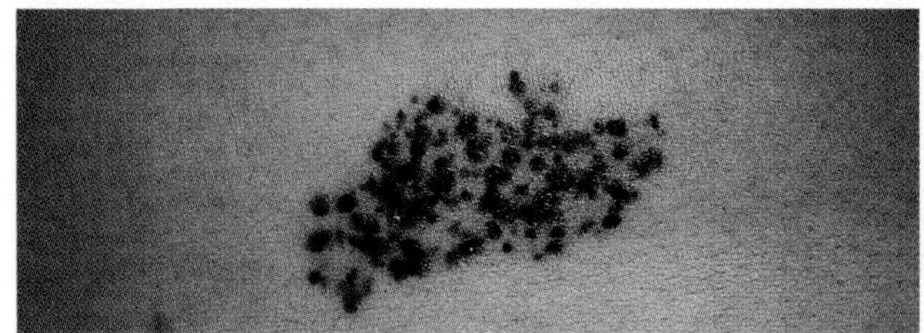

Plate 88. Nevus spilus. Typical speckled pigmentation. (Courtesy James C. Shaw, MD.)

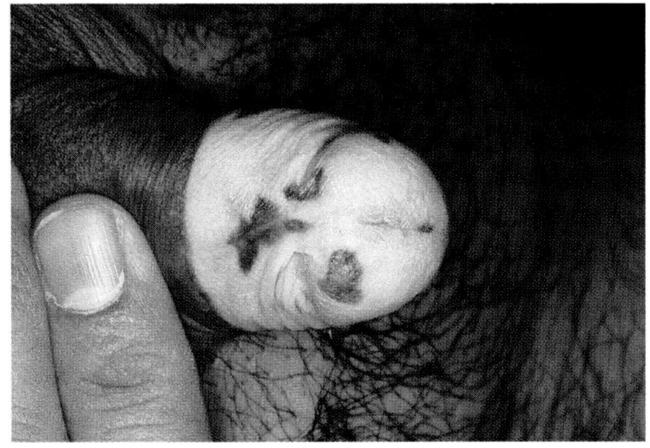

Plate 89. Vitiligo. Note complete absence of pigmentation in involved area. (Courtesy James C. Shaw, MD.)

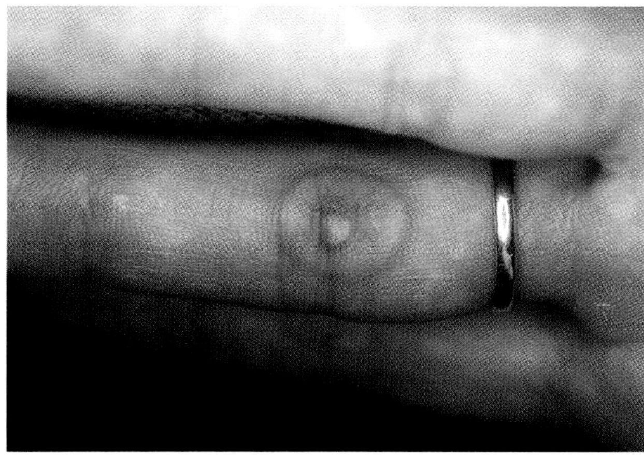

Plate 90. Erythema multiforme. Target lesion. (Courtesy James C. Shaw, MD.)

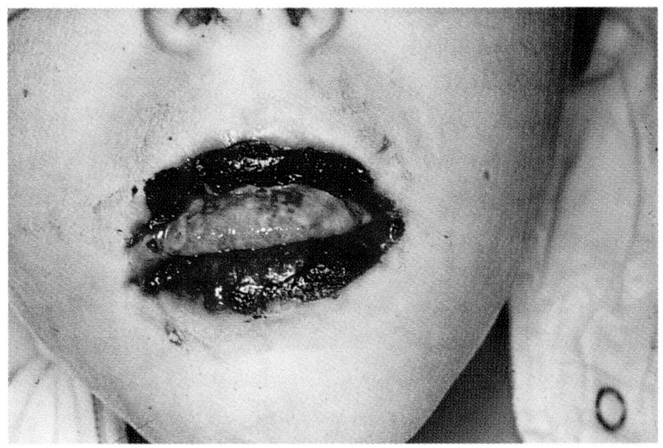

Plate 91. Stevens-Johnson syndrome (severe form of erythema multiforme with mucous membrane involvement). Note hemorrhagic erosive crusting of the lips and tongue.

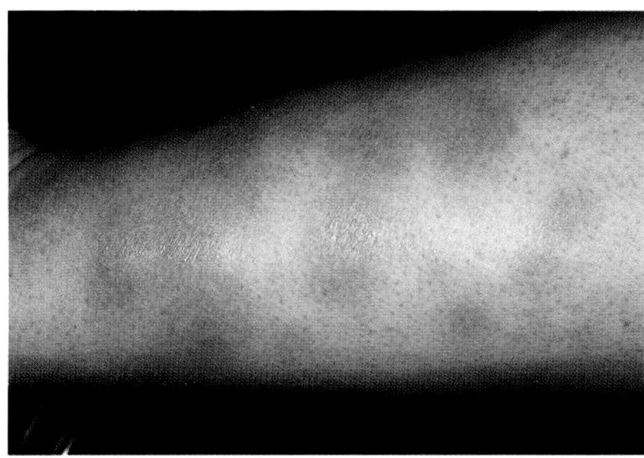

Plate 93. Erythema nodosum. Pretibial location typical. (Courtesy James C. Shaw, MD.)

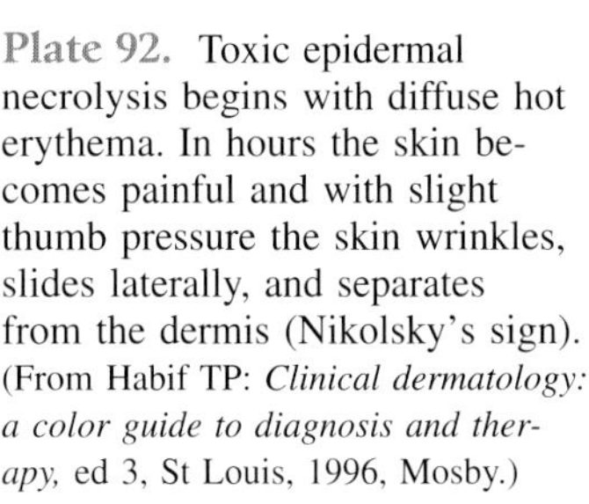

Plate 92. Toxic epidermal necrolysis begins with diffuse hot erythema. In hours the skin becomes painful and with slight thumb pressure the skin wrinkles, slides laterally, and separates from the dermis (Nikolsky's sign). (From Habif TP: *Clinical dermatology: a color guide to diagnosis and therapy,* ed 3, St Louis, 1996, Mosby.)

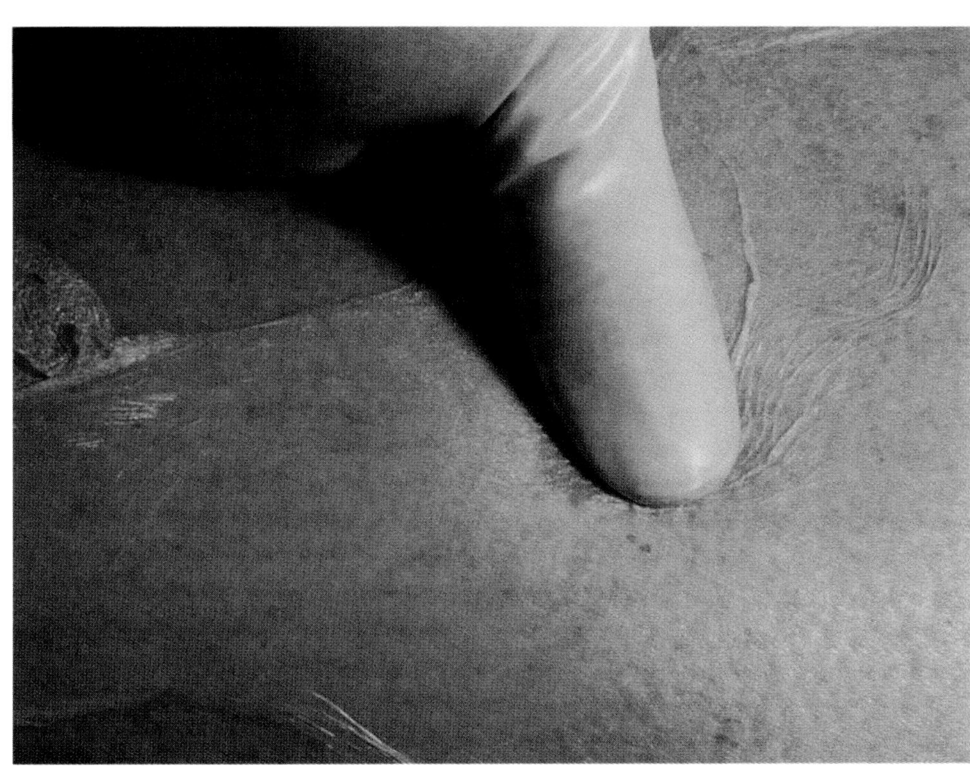

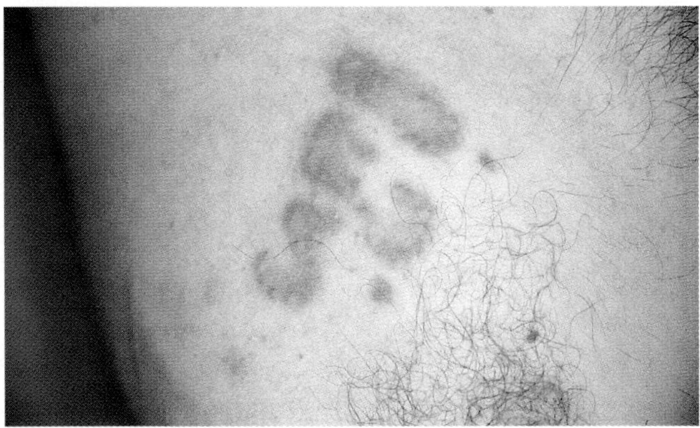

Plate 94. Granuloma annulare. Note erythematous plaques of confluent papules arranged in an annular shape.

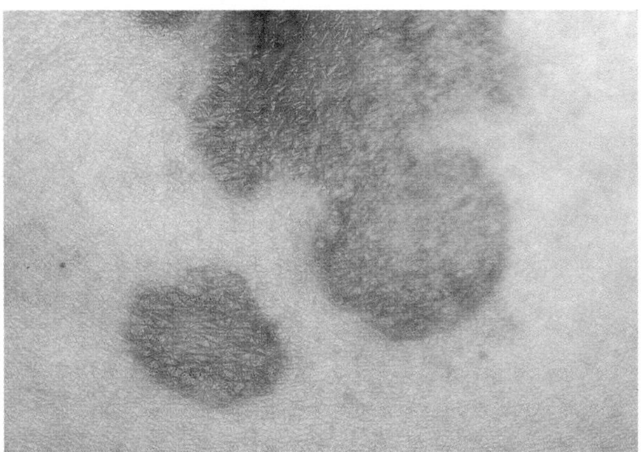

Plate 96. Minocycline pigmentation. Note typical blue-gray color. (Courtesy James C. Shaw, MD.)

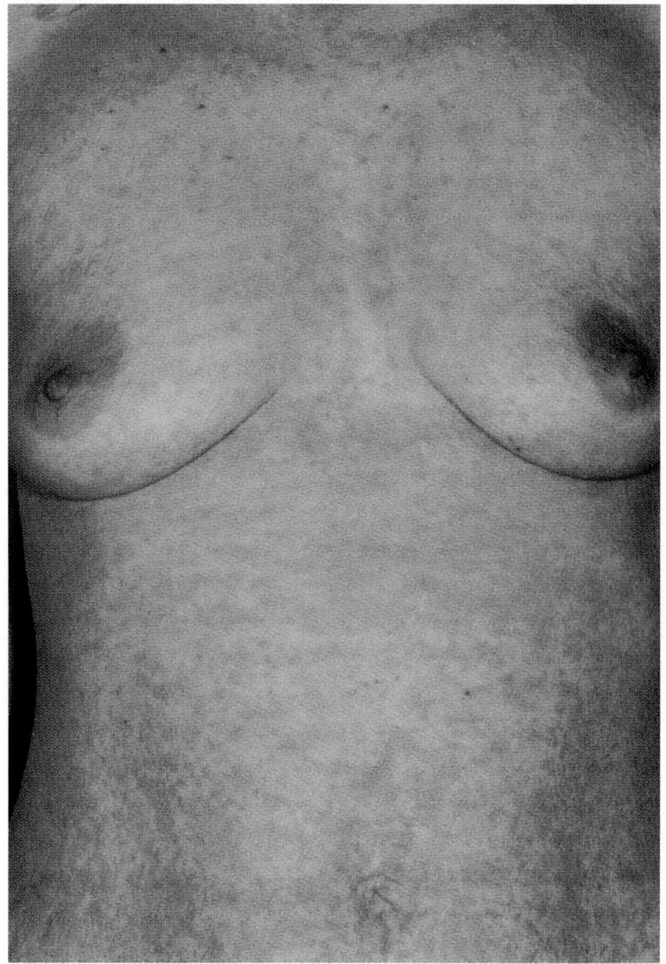

Plate 95. Morbilliform drug eruption. (From Habif TP: *Clinical dermatology: a color guide to diagnosis and therapy,* ed 3, St Louis, 1996, Mosby.)

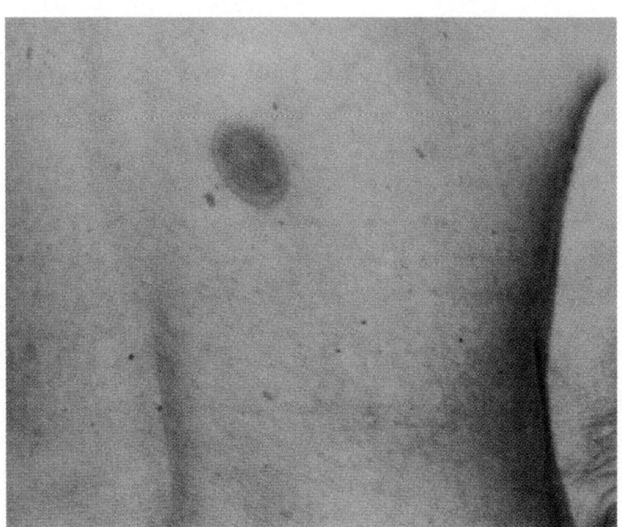

Plate 97. Fixed drug eruption. A single sharply demarcated, round plaque appeared shortly after trimethoprim was taken. (From Habif TP: *Clinical dermatology: a color guide to diagnosis and therapy,* ed 3, St Louis, 1996, Mosby.)

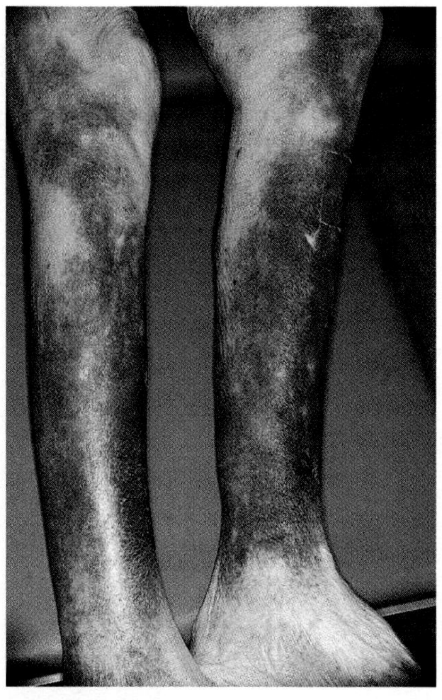

Plate 98. Lichenoid drug eruption from penicillamine. (Courtesy James C. Shaw, MD.)

pigmentation, including bleomycin, fluorouracil, and busulfan (see Chapter 99).

Several genetic and acquired conditions cause the following pigmented lesions:

Simple lentigo: Flat brown to black spots, 2 to 3 mm in diameter on the trunk and proximal extremities, due to an increase in melanocytes at the dermal-epidermal junction; they do not hyperpigment with UV light exposure.

Freckles (ephelides): Tan macules in sun-exposed areas that darken with sun exposure; they are the result of increased melanin synthesis within a normal number of melanocytes.

Solar lentigo: Brown flat lesions on sun-exposed areas due to increased numbers of melanocytes; these lesions increase in numbers in individuals over 40.

Various nevi: Including mongolian spots (Plate 87)—blue-black pigmentation in sacrogluteal region present at birth; nevus spilus—light brown patch with speckled dark, brown macules within (Plate 88).

Miscellaneous localized pigmented lesions in inherited conditions: Café au lait macules in neurofibromatosis. *Brown to black macules* on the lips and buccal mucosa in Peutz-Jeghers syndrome. Associated polyposis of the large and small intestine are a prominent part of this condition. *Incontinentia pigmenti* in an X-linked dominant disease with streaks and whorls of hyperpigmentation following the lines of Blaschko[2] that is seen in females and associated with ophthalmologic, bony, and CNS abnormalities.

Postinflammatory hyperpigmentation: Common in dark-skinned individuals; occurs after any inflammatory process including acne, folliculitis, minor injuries, and numerous other skin disorders.

Management. Replacing cortisone in Addison's disease will result in slow resolution of the hyperpigmentation. Hyperpigmentation of a variety of types can be improved using creams containing hydroquinone (3% to 4%) applied twice a day in conjunction with avoidance of sun and the use of sunscreen. Hydroquinone suppresses pigmentation by interfering with tyrosinase activity.

Hypopigmentation

Generalized loss of pigment is usually the result of oculocutaneous albinism, a group of genetic diseases that are associated with light hair color, nystagmus, and poor visual acuity.

Localized Hypopigmentation. Vitiligo (Plate 89) is a condition in which melanocytes are destroyed, possibly on an immunologic basis, resulting in symmetric or segmental white macules. Common areas of involvement include perioral, periocular, genital areas, and hands. Spontaneous repigmentation occurs in some patients. Vitiligo may be seen in association with the autoimmune conditions, including Hashimoto's thyroiditis, diabetes mellitus, pernicious anemia, and Addison's disease.

Piebaldism or white forelock consists of depigmentation due to an absence of melanocytes over the forehead and frontal scalp, chest, mid arms, and thighs.

Waardenburg's syndrome is an inherited defect of neural crest–derived elements consisting of poliosis (white forelock), deafness, broad nasal root, epicanthic eyefolds, and heterochromia of the irides.

Tuberous sclerosis is a phakomatosis and one of the earliest signs is hypopigmented macules present at birth. Typically, these macules are "ash leaf" in shape but may be polygonal. Wood's lamp examination of skin accentuates these areas of depigmentation.

Chemically induced depigmentation is caused by exposure to rubber products, germicidal agents, and industrial cleaning solutions. This exposure can cause irregular depigmented areas simulating vitiligo. These chemicals contain phenols and hydroquinones that destroy melanocytes.

Treatment of Hypopigmentation Conditions. Vitiligo is difficult to treat. Sunscreens are necessary to prevent burning. PUVA therapy has had limited success. Patients should be referred to a dermatologist for PUVA therapy. Chemically induced depigmentation also may benefit from PUVA therapy. If the vitiligo is extensive, depigmentation of the remaining normally pigmented skin may be a reasonable option. This procedure should also be supervised by a dermatologist.

REFERENCES

1. Baden HP: *Diseases of the hair and nails,* ed 1, Chicago, 1987, Mosby.
2. Bolognia JL, Orlow SJ, Glick SA: Lines of Blaschko, *J Am Acad Dermatol* 31:157-90, 1994.
3. Roberts JL: Androgenetic alopecia: treatment results with topical minoxidil, *J Am Acad Dermatol* 16:705, 1987.
4. Samman PD, Fenton DA, editors: *The nails in disease,* ed 4, Chicago, 1986, Year Book.
5. Scher RK, Daniel CR: *Nails: therapy, diagnosis, surgery,* Philadelphia, 1990, WB Saunders.
6. Zaias N: *The nail in health and disease,* ed 2, Norwalk, Ct, 1990, Appleton and Lange.

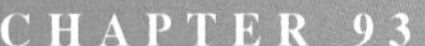

CHAPTER 93

Leg Ulcers

Carolyn I. Hale

EPIDEMIOLOGY/ETIOLOGY

There are many causes of leg ulcers (Box 93-1). Venous insufficiency accounts for 80% to 90%, arterial insufficiency for 5%, and a mixture of arterial and venous accounts for another 5%. Approximately 2% of ulcers are caused by diabetes and only 1% of ulcers will be caused by one of the many diseases listed in Box 93-1. Ulcers are costly to treat, cause loss of work time, and tend to be chronic and recurrent. Median duration of ulceration was 9 months, and 20% had not healed in over 2 years. The great majority of patients have recurrence.

Box 93-1. Differential Diagnosis of Leg Ulcers

Vascular

Arterial
- Arteriosclerosis
- Thromboangiitis obliterans
- Cholesterol emboli
- Hypertension
- Arteriovenous malformation

Venous
- Superficial varicosities
- Deep venous thrombosis
- Incompetent perforators

Lymphatics—elephantiasis

Vasculitis

Small vessel
- Hypersensitivity vasculitis (leukocytoclastic vasculitis)
- Lupus erythematosus
- Rheumatoid arthritis
- Scleroderma
- Livedo vasculitis (atrophic blanche)
- Pyoderma gangrenosa
- Antiphospholipid antibodies (anticardiolipin or lupus anticoagulant)

Medium and large vessel
- Polyarteritis nodosa
- Nodular vasculitis

Hematologic
- Sickle cell anemia
- Spherocytosis
- Thalassemia
- Polycythemia rubra vera
- Leukemia
- Dysproteinemias
  - Cryoglobulinemia
  - Cold agglutinin disease
  - Macroglobulinemia
- Deficiencies of coagulation inhibitors
  - Protein C and S deficiency

Infectious

Fungus
- Blastomycosis
- Coccidioidomycosis
- Histoplasmosis
- Sporotrichosis

Bacterial
- Furuncle
- Ecthyma
- Ecthyma gangrenosum
- Septic emboli
- Pseudomonas
- Mycobacterial (typical and atypical)

Protozoal
- Leishmaniasis

Metabolic

Diabetes
- Necrobiosis lipoidica diabeticorum

Gout
Gaucher's disease
Prolidase deficiency
Calcinosis cutis
Localized bullous pemphigoid

Tumors

Basal cell carcinoma
Squamous cell carcinoma
Melanoma
Kaposi's sarcoma
Metastatic tumors
Lymphoproliferative
Cutaneous T cell lymphoma (mycosis fungoides)

Trauma

Insect bites
Pressure
Cold injury (frostbite, pernio)
Radiation dermatitis
Burns
Factitial

Neuropathic

Diabetic trophic ulcers
Tabes dorsalis
Syringomyelia

Drug

Halogens
Methotrexate
Coumarin necrosis
Ergotism
Hydroxyurea

Panniculitis

Weber-Christian disease
Pancreatic fat necrosis
Alpha 1 antitrypsinase deficiency

PATHOPHYSIOLOGY

Venous ulcers, also known as varicose ulcers, venous hypertension ulcers, venous stasis ulcers, or postphlebitic ulcers are caused by the common mechanism of too much hydrostatic pressure in the superficial venous system of the leg. At least 80% of the time this is caused by incompetent valves in deep veins. In the leg, venous blood is returned to the heart via the deep venous system and the superficial venous system. The superficial system, consisting of the short and greater saphenous veins and their tributaries, is emptied into the deep system via perforating veins. Directional flow is maintained by a series of one-way valves. Flow is maintained by the pump action of the calf muscle or elevation of the leg above the level of the heart. Alteration in this system by a previous deep venous thrombosis is the most common predecessor of leg ulcers, although frequently there is no clinical history of thrombosis. Incompetent superficial veins leading to varicose veins account for less than 20% of leg ulcers. This group can be surgically cured and should be identified. Trauma to the leg and rare congenital fistulas can

Table 93-1. Physical Examination

	Venous	Arterial	Diabetic	Vasculitic
Location	Medial malleolus, gaitor area.	Toes, heels, bony prominences of foot, lateral malleolus, rarely over medial malleolus.	Same as arterial trophic ulcers on pressure points on the plantar foot, especially metatarsal heads.	Pretibial and dorsum of foot but may be anywhere and frequently is also on other areas.
Appearance	Irregularly shaped, surrounded by brown pigmentation with edema or sometimes fibrotic, hard skin (lipodermatosclerosis). Ulcer base has granulation tissue and exudate, and the borders may be hyperkeratotic.	Punched out ulcer with round well-demarcated borders and pale or white ulcer bed. Sometimes covered with dry eschar. Surrounding skin cool atrophic and hairless.	Punched out, often surrounded by hyperkeratotic borders; purulent drainage may indicate osteomyelitis.	Palpable purpura, hemorrhagic vesicle, typically small and multiple, with black, gray, or yellow base and minimal or no granulation tissue; may have thin undermined border; surrounding skin shows reticulated vascular pattern.
Pain	Increases with leg dependency, decreases with elevation.	Frequently very painful. Decreases with leg dependency, increases with exercise and leg elevation.	Painless but associated with paresthesia, anesthesia, inconstant, mostly at night.	Extremely painful.
Vascular examination	Ankle/brachial index greater than 0.9. Pulses present. Plethysmography or Doppler studies show abnormal venous system.	Ankle/brachial index less than 0.9. Pulses decreased. Abnormal pallor of leg with elevation, and subsequent rubor with dependency. Delayed venous filling.	Mixed, usually associated with arterial disease.	Normal.
History	Edema, trauma, rapid onset. Thrombophlebitis 20% varicosities.	Arteriosclerosis, claudication. Usually >45 yr. Slow progression.	Diabetes mellitus; peripheral neuropathy.	Association with other systemic disease; rapid onset.
Treatment	Leg elevation, compression by elastic bandages or stockings, 30 mm Hg, moist wound dressings. Grafts.	Vascular surgical consultation. No compression. Moist wound dressings. Pentoxyphylline?	Control diabetes; careful wound care, early intervention for infections; vascular surgical consult.	Control underlying disease; nonadherent dressings; oral steroids, ASA, bed rest.

cause arteriovenous fistulas, which also result in venous hypertension.

Basically, an increased venous pressure results in increased pressure in the capillary bed, transudation of fluid and protein into the interstitial space, and altered delivery of oxygen and nutrients to the skin and subcutaneous tissues resulting in ulceration of the overlying tissue. Current theories of the pathophysiology are more complex than this. In 1982, Browse and Burnand suggested that increased back pressure into the capillaries distended endothelial gaps, allowing for leaky capillaries. Fibrin then forms around the capillaries and impedes oxygen diffusion. These findings of pericapillary fibrin cuffs have been confirmed with immunologic staining. It is also known that fibrinolysis is abnormal in this group of patients, but the clinical importance of this is unknown. More recent evidence supports a trapped leukocyte theory. With decreased perfusion pressure, white cells become trapped in the capillaries and release proteolytic enzymes and superoxide radicals that cause endothelial damage. This damage may result in leaky capillaries and fibrin deposition, as well as blockage of local capillary filling and resultant ischemia.

Arterial ulcers are primarily a result of arteriosclerosis obliterans of the lower extremity as previously described. Although this accounts for only 5% to 10% of all leg ulcers, by the age of 80, over 90% of patients have an arterial component. In other words, a venous ulcer at age 50 will become a mixed venous and arterial ulcer by the time the patient reaches 80 and treatment will need to be changed to address the arterial component. Risk factors are diabetes mellitus, smoking, hyperlipidemia, hypertension, and early menopause in women.

Diabetes mellitus results in ulceration from atherosclerosis, peripheral neuropathy, and less commonly necrobiosis lipoidica, diabetic dermopathy, and bacterial and fungal infections. Hyperemia and capillary hypertension, loss of

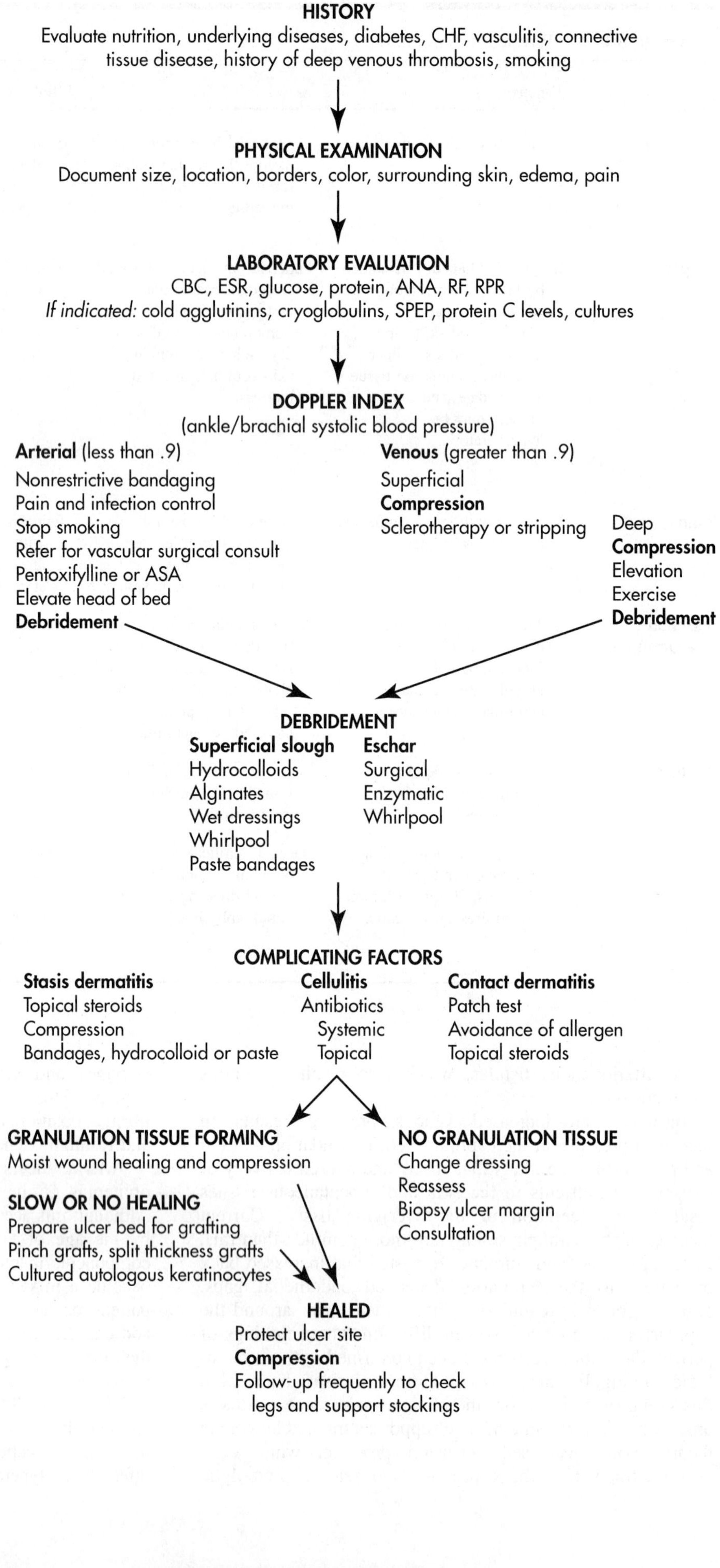

HISTORY
Evaluate nutrition, underlying diseases, diabetes, CHF, vasculitis, connective tissue disease, history of deep venous thrombosis, smoking

↓

PHYSICAL EXAMINATION
Document size, location, borders, color, surrounding skin, edema, pain

↓

LABORATORY EVALUATION
CBC, ESR, glucose, protein, ANA, RF, RPR
If indicated: cold agglutinins, cryoglobulins, SPEP, protein C levels, cultures

↓

DOPPLER INDEX
(ankle/brachial systolic blood pressure)

Arterial (less than .9)
Nonrestrictive bandaging
Pain and infection control
Stop smoking
Refer for vascular surgical consult
Pentoxifylline or ASA
Elevate head of bed
Debridement

Venous (greater than .9)
Superficial
Compression
Sclerotherapy or stripping

Deep
Compression
Elevation
Exercise
Debridement

DEBRIDEMENT

Superficial slough
Hydrocolloids
Alginates
Wet dressings
Whirlpool
Paste bandages

Eschar
Surgical
Enzymatic
Whirlpool

↓

COMPLICATING FACTORS

Stasis dermatitis
Topical steroids
Compression
Bandages, hydrocolloid or paste

Cellulitis
Antibiotics
Systemic
Topical

Contact dermatitis
Patch test
Avoidance of allergen
Topical steroids

GRANULATION TISSUE FORMING
Moist wound healing and compression

SLOW OR NO HEALING
Prepare ulcer bed for grafting
Pinch grafts, split thickness grafts
Cultured autologous keratinocytes

NO GRANULATION TISSUE
Change dressing
Reassess
Biopsy ulcer margin
Consultation

HEALED
Protect ulcer site
Compression
Follow-up frequently to check legs and support stockings

Fig. 93-1. Flowchart for the management of leg ulcers. (Modified from Ryan TJ: Current management of leg ulcers, *Drugs* 30:461, 1985.)

autoregulation and neurogenic regulation, disturbed endothelial function, and abnormal rheology also play a part in the abnormal microcirculation of diabetic patients.

The pathophysiology of other leg ulcers varies with the disease. A few of these are mentioned briefly. Rheumatoid arthritis is associated with ulcers both from vasculitis and from immobility of the leg with resultant inadequate venous return. In sickle cell anemia there is an incidence of ulcers of 25% to 75%, probably from the abnormal rheologic properties of the red blood cells resulting in an ulcer that resembles venous ulcers. Recurrent hemorrhages and infections also play a role. Other hematologic diseases also share common factors with venous ulcers. Polycythemia vera results in increased viscosity, as do various dysproteinemias.

Pyoderma gangrenosum most likely represents a small vessel vasculitis, although not all cases show vasculitis. It may be associated with ulcerative colitis, rheumatoid arthritis, leukemias, regional enteritis, or may occur without any underlying disease.

Drugs may cause ulcers by a number of mechanisms. Hydroxyurea may cause ulcerative lichen planus or a livedo vasculitis-like picture. Some drugs, such as corticosteroids, alter wound healing, although low antiinflammatory products (e.g., cortisone acetate and prednisone in oral doses under 10 mg daily) have no appreciable effect on wound healing. Coumarin necrosis is a rare disease caused by an imbalance in the anticoagulant and procoagulant factors. Inhibition of production of protein C and protein S in hereditary deficiency states or rarely acquired deficiencies associated with disseminated intravascular coagulation, multiple myeloma, and the lupus anticoagulant may disproportionately balance the coagulation system toward thrombosis in early coumarin treatment (see Chapter 115).

Antibodies to phospholipids cause recurrent thrombosis with a vasculitic-appearing ulcer. These antibodies are manifested by false positive VDRL, a lupus anticoagulant, or anticardiolipin antibodies, and may be associated with lupus and lupus-like diseases and livedo vasculitis and may cause their effects through interactions with protein C or protein S. It has been proposed that they may promote thrombosis by binding to endothelial cells and impairing prostacyclin release or damaging platelet adhesiveness.

The clinical features of leg ulcers are frequently nonspecific, although several characteristics can help identify the most common types of ulcers (Table 93-1).

Extensive laboratory testing is not necessary except in unusual ulcers. Generally a complete blood count, glucose, sedimentation rate, albumin, protein, and thyroid screen are sufficient. If a vasculitis is suspected an antinuclear antibody, rheumatoid factor, syphilis serology, cold agglutinins, cryoglobulins, serum protein electrophoresis, protein C and S levels, and anticardiolipin antibodies may be evaluated.

Bacteriologic cultures of the wound are not necessary and are frequently misleading as most wounds are colonized. If there is clinical evidence of cellulitis, a culture should be taken to direct antibiotic therapy. A tissue biopsy is the most accurate method and is necessary if deep fungal or acid-fast organisms are suspected by the clinician.

Biopsies of a leg ulcer should be undertaken with caution. Frequently the biopsy site will not heal, and the patient is left with another ulcer. However, if an ulcer does not heal for 4 months on adequate therapy, a biopsy from the ulcer edge should be taken.

Vascular studies are needed when pulses are nonpalpable. An ankle/brachial pressure index should be measured in all patients. Venous studies are indicated if needed to confirm the diagnosis of venous ulcers or in the case that superficial varicose veins are the cause. In this case, surgical intervention can prevent recurrent disease and compression stockings will not be needed.

MANAGEMENT

Although there are a number of causes of leg ulcers, the most common cause is venous insufficiency. Compression therapy is the most important treatment for these ulcers. Moist wound dressings, growth factors, and grafting, although beneficial in treatment of venous ulcers, pale in comparison to the use of adequate compression of the leg. Arterial ulcers, however, should *not* be compressed for fear of further arterial compromise. Treatment of this condition is discussed in Chapter 70. Once an ulcer is healed continued care will be needed to prevent recurrences (Fig. 93-1).

ADDITIONAL READINGS

Burnand KG et al: Pericapillary fibrin deposition in the ulcer bearing skin of the lower limb, the cause of lipodermatosclerosis and venous ulceration, *Br Med J* 285:1071, 1982.

Callam MJ, Harper DR, Dale JJ et al: Chronic ulcer of the leg: clinical history, *Br Med J* 294:1389, 1987.

Coleridge-Smith PD et al: Causes of venous ulceration: a new hypothesis, *Br Med J* 296:1726, 1988.

Flynn MD, Tooke JE: Aetiology of diabetic foot ulceration: a role for the microcirculation? *Diabet Med* 8:320, 1992.

Harahap M et al: Leg ulcers, *Clin Dermatol* 8:3-4, 1990.

Phillips TJ et al: Leg ulcers, *J Am Acad Dermatol* 25:965, 1991.

Renfro L, Moy J, Sanchez M: Cutaneous ulcers caused by drugs, *Wound* 2(6):236-246, 1990.

Ryan TJ: Current management of leg ulcers, *Drugs* 30:461, 1985.

Young JR: Differential diagnosis of leg ulcers, *Cardiovascular Clin* 13:171, 1983.

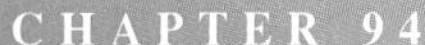

CHAPTER 94

Bites and Toxic Envenomation

Ann Gateley

Patrick McKinney

Human encounters with the animal world, both in the domestic setting and in the wild, provide ample opportunities for bites and envenomations. The primary care physician is often called on to treat or triage these wounds.

ANIMAL AND HUMAN BITES

Dog Bites

Dog bites are the most frequently reported bite, averaging over 500,000 reported per year in the United States. The human victim is usually a 7- to 9-year-old boy, who is often teasing or playing with a dog. The dog is most often a working dog, such as a boxer, collie, German shepherd, Great Dane, or a sporting dog, such as a pointer, setter, or retriever.

Occasionally, dogs inflict extensive wounds resulting in death by trauma.

Cat Bites

Cat bites are less frequently reported. Because of their size and the sharpness of their teeth, domestic cats deliver puncture wounds, mainly in the hand. It is estimated that over 50% of cat bites become infected. Serious complications include infectious tenosynovitis, closed space infection of the hand, and inoculation of the periosteum, leading to osteomyelitis.

Management of Dog and Cat Bites. Evaluation and treatment of bite wounds depends on the immune status of the victim, site of the bite, and extent of the wound. Most wounds should be irrigated and left open. Deep wounds can be closed by delayed primary closure after 3 days if there is no apparent infection. Facial wounds are usually referred to a surgeon and can be closed after careful irrigation, exploration, and cautious debridement. Hand wounds should be followed closely for closed space infection. Splenectomized patients or other immunocompromised patients should be treated with prophylactic antibiotics. Tetanus immune status should be evaluated, and rabies immunization considered in certain cases.

A prospective study of infected wounds from dog and cat bites found that infection was due to aerobes and anaerobes together or singly in over 90% of the cases. *Pasteurella* species were the most common isolates in both cat bites (75%) and dog bites (50%). Other common aerobic isolates included streptococci, staphylococci, *Moraxella,* and *Neisseria* organisms. Therefore, if wounds become infected or prophylaxis is indicated, a β-lactam and β-lactamase inhibitor (e.g., amoxicillin/clavulanic acid) would be appropriate. Treatment recommendations are summarized in Box 94-1.

Box 94-1. Recommendations for Treatment of Dog and Cat Bites

1. Explore the wound for injuries involving joints, tendons, and periosteum.
2. Irrigate the wound copiously.
3. Leave wound open if it is superficial, punctate, greater than 6 to 8 hours old and on the extremities, and greater than 12 to 24 hours old and on the face.
4. Reserve antibiotics for high risk wounds, i.e., a deep puncture wound by a cat, immunocompromised patients, wounds involving a fracture, or wounds requiring surgical repair.
5. Empirical therapy should be directed against *Pasteurella,* streptococci, staphylococci, *Moraxella,* and *Neisseria* organisms and anaerobes (e.g., a β-lactam/β-lactamase inhibitor).
6. Tetanus hyperimmune globulin should be given to patients with two or less of the primary immunization series, and a toxoid booster should be given if the last booster was more than 5 years before.

Special Issues with Dog and Cat Encounters

Cat-scratch Disease. Cat-scratch disease (CSD) is a worldwide bacterial infection of the *Bartonella* species. In the United States, CSD typically occurs in children or adolescents most often in the fall or winter. Over 95% have had a history of contact with cats, usually kittens. Cats act only as vectors; they do not become ill themselves. Fleas appear to transmit the bacteria among cats, but data do not support flea-to-human transmission.

The typical history includes a scratch, perhaps a bite as well, 3 to 10 days before developing a round, reddish, nontender papule at the site (Fig. 94-1). Proximal lymphadenopathy develops, often the epitrochlear, axillary, or cervical nodes, within a week to 2 months after appearance of the papule. These nodes may be tender or nontender and may suppurate and drain late in the course. Systemic symptoms may include fever, headache, or malaise. Rare complications include encephalopathy, endocarditis, stellate retinitis, or oculoglandular disease (Parinaud's syndrome, which is preauricular lymphadenopathy with conjunctival granulomas), and systemic dissemination with hepatosplenomegaly. The diagnosis is suggested by a history of regional lymphadenopathy developing slowly over weeks after a cat scratch. The history of a prior papule is highly supportive of the diagnosis. Rarely, bacteria can be recovered from blood or lymph nodes. Positive serology for *Bartonella henselae* is confirmatory.

In the immunocompetent host, the disease is granulomatous, suppurative, and usually self-limited. In the immunocompromised patient, the disease is vasculoproliferative and can be progressive and fatal if untreated. Antibiotics that appear to be the most effective include macrolides, tetracyclines, aminoglycosides, and quinolones.

Rabies. Humans are at risk for acquiring various zoonoses from domestic and wild animal bites. However, in the case of the viral infection of rabies, no effective treatment exists for the full-blown clinical syndrome of encephalomyelitis. Therefore, preexposure and postexposure prophylaxis are critical considerations.

The virus of rabies is introduced into the body through the bite of an infected animal. The virus travels centrally along

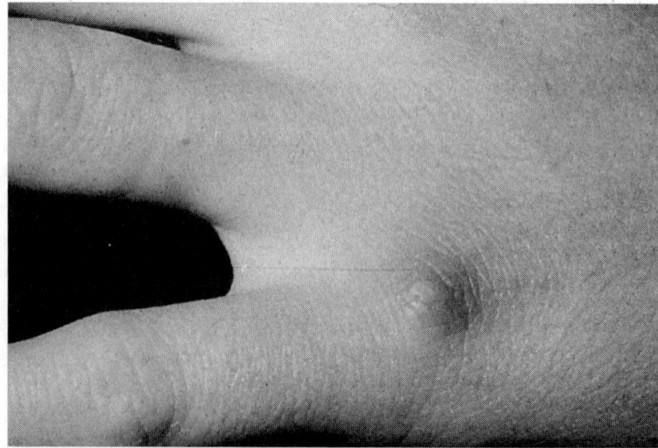

Fig. 94-1. Primary lesion of cat-scratch disease is a tender papule occurring 3 to 10 days after a scratch.

peripheral nerves, producing a focal encephalitis that mainly involves the cervical cord, the brainstem, and the temporal lobes (Fig. 94-2). The latent period between the bite and the clinical features of the disease may be as long as a year.

Clinically, early irritability and agitated delirium lead on to muscle hypertonia especially affecting the pharyngeal muscles, which go into spasm—thus the term *hydrophobia*. Convulsions and death usually occur within 10 days of the onset.

Fortunately, because of effective vaccination of domestic animals, the human disease is rare in the United States with fewer than five cases reported per year. Although dogs account for most cases of rabies worldwide, the sylvatic reservoir of skunks, raccoons, wolves, bats, woodchucks, and foxes account for 90% of rabid bites in North America. The infected animal has the rabies virus proliferating in the salivary glands (see Fig. 94-2). Any introduction of this saliva into skin or mucous membranes constitutes an exposure.

The decision to prophylactically treat for rabies is based on the history (species of animal, apparent state of health of the animal, and circumstances of the attack) and local public health data on the prevalence of rabies and examination of the wound. Significant risk of exposure is based on the extent and depth of the wound. If the decision to offer postexposure prophylaxis is made, the wound should be cleaned thoroughly and a virucidal agent used if available (e.g., povidine iodine). Both passive and active immune products should be used. The passive agent (rabies immune globulin) should be infiltrated around the wound at 20 IU/kg body weight. The active immune–response producing product should be given in the deltoid area on days 0, 3, 7, 14, and 28.

Preexposure prophylaxis is offered to individuals, such as veterinary personnel, laboratory workers, and spelunkers, who may be members of high-risk groups. The recommendations for preexposure prophylaxis are summarized in Box 94-2.

Human Bites

Human bites deserve special attention because a large percentage of them become infected with aerobic and

Box 94-2. Recommendations for Preexposure Rabies Prophylaxis

High Risk Group

- Rabies research workers
- Rabies biologic production workers

Offer primary course (3 vaccinations/1 month) with serologic testing every 6 months

Moderate Risk Group

- Animal workers in endemic areas
- People living in hyperendemic areas for more than 1 month
- Spelunkers
- Rabies diagnostic laboratory workers

Offer primary course (3 vaccinations/1 month) and serologic testing every 2 years

Lower Risk (Higher Than the General Population) Group

- Animal workers in low endemic areas

Offer primary course without serologic follow-up

Modified from Advisory Committee on Immunization Practice (ACIP): CDC 1999.

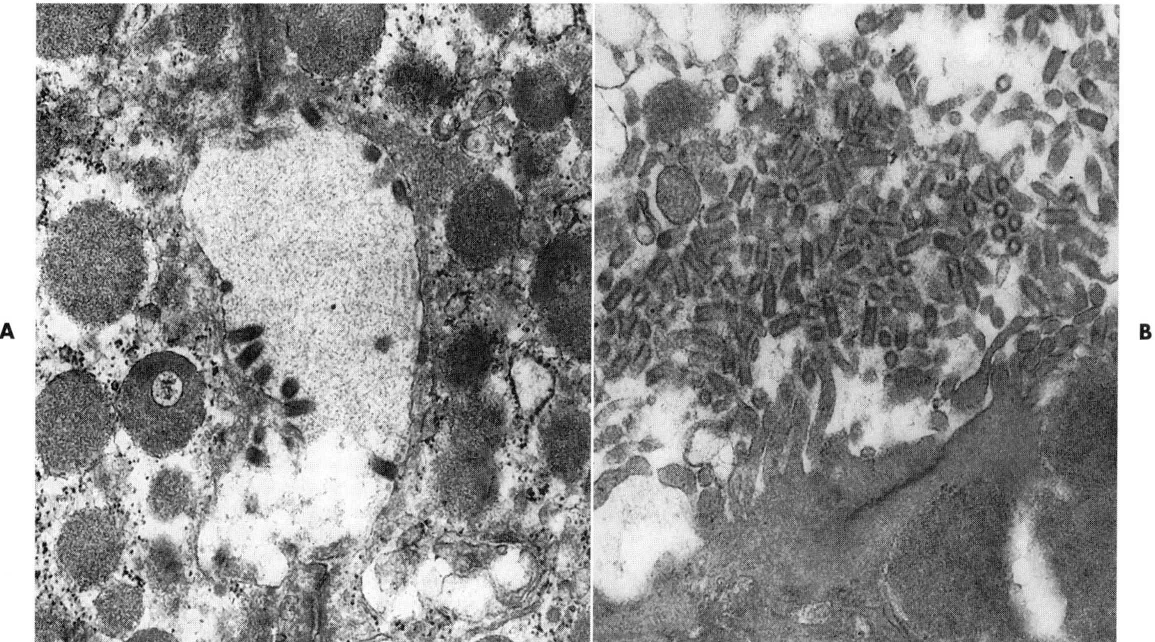

Fig. 94-2. Rabies virus proliferates abundantly in the salivary glands of infected animals. Bullet-shaped rabies virions can be seen budding through the plasma membrane **(A)** and extracellular to the acinar cells **(B)**. (Courtesy Frederick A. Murphy and Alyne K. Harrison, Viral Pathology Branch, Centers for Disease Control and Prevention.)

Box 94-3. Recommendations for the Treatment of Human Bites

1. Explore for wounds that may involve joints and concomitant fractures.
2. Irrigate.
3. Prescribe antibiotic prophylaxis to cover mouth flora (e.g., amoxicillin/clavulanic acid).
4. Refer the following to hand surgeon: wounds acquired by punch injury, wounds with a question of deep space infection, and wounds with possible joint or bone contamination.
5. Consider HIV and HBV prophylaxis, if bites are obtained from high-risk individuals.

anaerobic mouth organisms. A bite to the hand is at risk for a serious closed-space infection. The physical examination should be thorough with special attention to those wounds over a joint or deeply penetrating with possible periosteal contamination. The wound should be irrigated copiously and left open. The patient should be started on oral antibiotics and referred to a hand surgeon if there is a question of deep space or joint and bone infection. Additionally, referral should be made if a hand wound is sustained at high velocity (e.g., a punch to the mouth) since these wounds are deep and at high risk for infection.

Special Issues with Human Bites. Human bites now include concern for inoculation of the human immunodeficiency virus (HIV) and hepatitis B virus (HBV). If the bite is from a high-risk individual, prophylaxis with antiviral agents or immunoglobulin may be indicated. Management recommendations for human bites are summarized in Box 94-3.

ARTHROPOD ENVENOMATION

Spiders and Scorpions (Arachnida)

Over 20,000 species of spiders are found in the United States and almost all produce venom. About 50 of these species have fangs large enough to penetrate human skin. Bites from the majority of these 50 species produce only minor local pain or mild cutaneous reactions. Two spiders with medical significance to humans account for the two main envenomation syndromes, the black widow syndrome or Latrodectism, and a dermonecrotic syndrome, which may be produced by brown spider members of the genus Loxosceles, as well as several others.

Black Widow (Latrodectus). Members of the Latrodectus genus are found throughout the continental United States. Typically, only the female is large enough to envenomate humans. The spider is easily recognizable with a shiny, round abdomen, small cephalothorax, and long, spindly legs. Although known as the "black" widow, the spider may be black, brown, tan, or even variegated, and the classic red hourglass on the ventral abdomen may be an indistinct yellow or orange spot. The web is coarse and irregular and is often found in brush piles, around stacks of firewood, and in garages and basements. The venom contains multiple fractions that activate cation channels, resulting in sympathetic and parasympathetic activation and muscular spasm.

Most bites occur on the lower extremity and may occur when the spider has crawled into clothing or bedsheets. The initial black widow bite is sharp and mildly painful. The bite site is often not remarkable. One or two small punctures may be seen 1 or 2 mm apart with a zone of erythema or a target lesion. Thirty minutes to 12 hours after the bite, muscular cramping begins, usually in the large muscle groups of the back, thighs, and stomach. Hypertension and diaphoresis may occur. Severe envenomations may cause a maculopapular rash and periorbital edema, salivation, lacrimation, tachypnea, tachycardia, convulsions, and respiratory failure. Deaths are extremely rare. Untreated, the symptom complex may last several days, although weakness and spasm may recur for weeks to months.

Therapy is directed primarily toward relieving muscle pain and spasm. A combination of an opioid and a benzodiazepine is often successful. Parenteral administration of these drugs is often necessary. Calcium gluconate intravenous injection may be used; however, relief is inconsistent and often transient. Hypertension usually resolves when adequate analgesia is administered; however, calcium channel blockers and β-adrenergic blocking agents are two reasonable choices if therapy were needed. An equine-derived antivenin is available, but its use should be limited to severe envenomations because of the risk of anaphylaxis and serum sickness. Antivenin may be indicated for severe symptoms that are not responsive to conservative therapy and for higher risk patients including children, pregnant women, geriatric patients, and those with preexisting hypertension or vascular disease. Symptoms typically resolve almost immediately with 1 to 2 vials of antivenin. Most patients treated with antivenin improve within 24 to 48 hours.

Brown Spiders (Loxosceles). The brown recluse spider, *Loxosceles reclusa,* is found primarily in the Midwestern United States, but other members of the genus Loxosceles are distributed across the United States. Loxosceles spiders are less distinct than black widows and can easily be mistaken for a variety of other spiders. They are brown-to-tan in color, with a hair-covered abdomen and a cephalothorax marked by a darker inverted violin or "fiddle" on the dorsal side. Loxosceles spiders are often found indoors, hiding in clothes and bedsheets. The spider is usually not seen at the time of the bite, making definitive diagnosis problematic. The venom contains various proteases, peptides, and sphingomyelinase D that result in local inflammation, polymorphonuclear cell attraction, local small vessel thrombosis, and tissue necrosis. The venom has hemotoxic constituents as well.

The initial Loxosceles bite is mildly painful and may not be noticed at all. An area of redness develops surrounded by pallor then ecchymosis within hours. Vesicle formation may occur within the first 2 hours. Mild systemic symptoms, such as malaise, chills, sweats, dizziness, gastrointestinal upset, and headache may occur. Within 24 to 48 hours, an area of central necrosis may be seen that may continue to enlarge for several days. In a minority of cases, large slow-healing ulcers are formed.

A systemic syndrome of toxicity may occur marked by fever, myalgias, chills, hemolysis, disseminated intravascular coagulation (DIC), and, rarely, renal dysfunction and death. The development of the systemic syndrome does not appear to be correlated to the appearance of the necrotic lesion.

Initial treatment should be directed toward local wound

Box 94-4. Spiders That May Produce a Dermonecrotic Lesion

Brown spiders
Hobo spiders
Wolf spiders
Orb weavers
Jumping spiders
Crab spiders

care. In the case of suspected infection, an antibiotic with coverage of skin flora, such as cephalexin or erythromycin, is indicated. Early excision is to be avoided because appropriate wound margins are difficult to identify, and a large surgical wound with necrotic margins may result. Other therapies, such as dapsone, hyperbaric oxygen, and corticosteroids, are controversial and should not be routinely recommended pending more favorable data.

Hobo Spider (Tegenaria). The hobo spider, *Tegenaria agrestis,* is found in the Pacific Northwest and is a common cause of necrotic bites in this area. Local necrosis resembling a brown spider bite may occur and similar systemic syndromes have been reported.

The great majority of patients who present with a presumed necrotic bite did not see the spider or insect and often were not aware of the bite at the time. Because of this, diagnosis must be presumptive and the differential diagnosis of cutaneous necrosis (diabetic ulcers, herpes simplex, pyoderma gangrenosum, Lyme disease, purpura fulminans, foreign body, factitious ulcer, fat necrosis, vasculitis, or heparin or warfarin necrosis) should be kept in mind. It is important not to diagnose beyond the limits of the history and examination to avoid undue patient anxiety and potential adverse effects of unnecessary therapy. In many cases, the diagnosis of "necrotic skin lesion" or "necrotic insect bite" may be as specific as the history and examination allow. Box 94-4 lists spiders that may produce a dermonecrotic lesion.

Scorpions (Centruroides). Scorpions are large arachnids (2 to 8 cm) with pincers, a segmented body, and a tail equipped with a stinging apparatus (Fig. 94-3). Scorpion envenomation is a common occurrence in the southwestern United States, but the majority of bites produce only local pain. The only indigenous scorpion with a medically significant envenomation syndrome is *Centruroides exilicauda,* which is found in Arizona, Texas, Nevada, New Mexico, California, and Mexico. This scorpion is slender yellow or brown and is also known as the bark scorpion.

Severe local pain and hyperesthesias, restlessness, hypertension, and autonomic dysfunction mark Centruroides syndrome. Roving eye movements, dysphagia, respiratory distress, salivation, slurred speech, and rarely, pancreatitis, rhabdomyolysis, metabolic acidosis, and pulmonary edema can be seen. The majority of severe envenomations occur in young children. Diagnosis is usually made in conjunction with the observations of a scorpion bite, but in cases where the bite was not witnessed, appropriate signs and symptoms may strongly suggest the diagnosis. Treatment is primarily supportive.

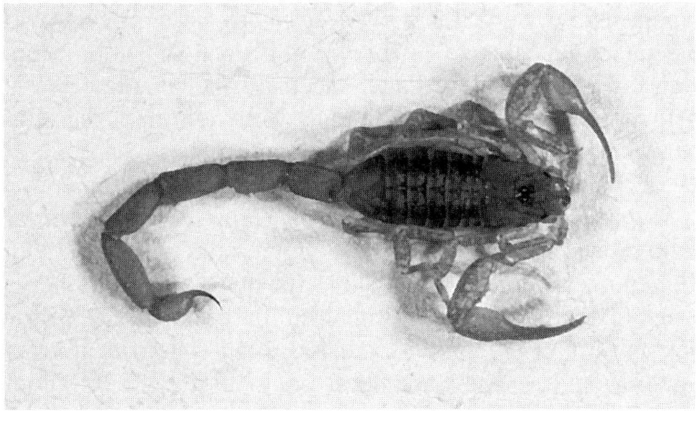

Fig. 94-3. Scorpion.

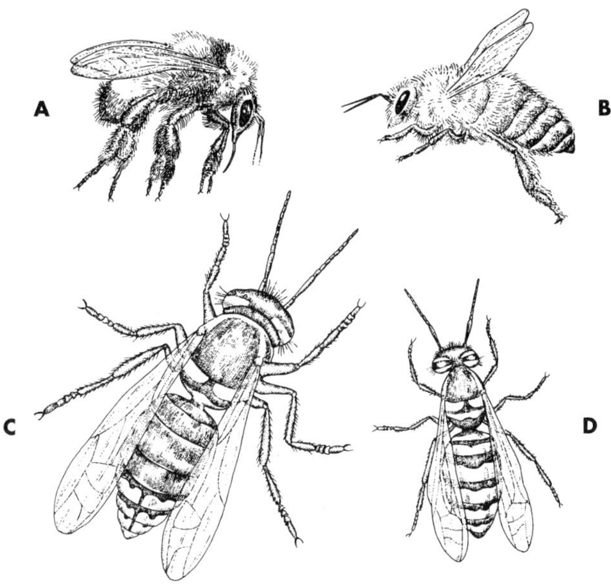

Fig. 94-4. Vespidae and Apidae insects. (**A**) Boribus sonorus, the bumblebee. (**B**) Apix mellifera, the honeybee. (**C**) Vespula maculata, the white-faced wasp. (**D**) Vespula maculifrous, the yellow jacket. (From Lichenstein LM: *Hosp Pract* 10:3, 1975. Drawing by Nancy Lou Makris.)

Wasps, Bees, and Ants

The order, Hymentoptera (Insecta), includes three families of medical importance: Vespidae (wasps, yellow jackets, hornets), Apidae (bees) (Fig. 94-4), and Formicidae (ants). Hymenoptera stings are responsible for more deaths than rattle snake bites every year in the United States. Most of these deaths are due to anaphylaxis, although massive envenomations may result in serious toxicity and even death. It is speculated that up to 50% of sudden deaths occurring outdoors may be due to Hymenoptera-induced anaphylaxis. Groups at risk include the elderly, those with preexisting cardiac disease, and those with multiple previous stings. Hymenoptera sting anaphylaxis is probably an IgE-mediated hypersensitivity reaction. However, many cases of Hymenoptera anaphylaxis have no previous history of sting, which suggests a non-IgE-mediated mechanism may play a role. Hymenoptera venoms are antigenically similar, therefore there may be some cross reactivity among families.

Wasps, Yellow Jackets, and Hornets (Vespidae). Yellow jackets are the most aggressive of the flying Hymenoptera and are responsible for the greatest number of stings (excluding bee stings incurred by beekeepers). Yellow jackets nest in the ground and are often found in areas of human activity. They are attracted to bright colors, floral patterns, sweet floral scents, and carrion. Hornets and wasps typically nest off the ground and are less likely to be found in areas where human contact is likely. The vespidae stinging apparatus is located at the distal end of the abdomen, and they may sting more than once. In contrast, honeybee stingers are barbed, and the stinger usually remains embedded in the victim, mortally wounding the bee. Potential venom allergens and toxins include phospholipase A, hyaluronidase, acid phosphatase, mellitin, kinins, serotonin, dopamine, apamin, and other polypeptides.

Africanized Honeybees (Apidae). Most North American honeybees are descendants of European strains and are generally docile unless provoked. In the 1950s, African honeybees were imported to Brazil in hopes of producing a hybrid better suited to tropical climates. The resulting "Africanized honeybees" (sometimes referred to as "killer bees") are much more aggressive than their European cousins and more cold tolerant than pure African strains. Thus hives composed of very aggressive bees have been migrating northward. The northernmost limit of their range is not known. Africanized honeybees swarm frequently and will attack at seemingly minimal provocation. They are capable of stinging in massive numbers and will recruit other hive members through pheromone signaling. Once agitated, the hive will remain active for many hours, endangering other people or animals that wander into its range. The primary danger of the Africanized bee is the potential for massive numbers of stings, numbering in the hundreds or even thousands. It is estimated that 2000 stings may be fatal to a healthy adult, although far fewer may be dangerous to children or older patients with cardiopulmonary disease. Massive stings may cause acute renal failure, rhabdomyolysis, and hemolysis independent of any immune mechanism.

If attacked by a swarm of bees, the most effective strategy is to run from the scene. Africanized bees reportedly will not pursue aggressors more than ¼ to ½ mile. Avoid smashing the bees as pheromones will be released that may agitate and recruit other hive members.

Fire Ants: Solenopsis (Formicidae). Imported fire ants can be found across the southeastern United States. Fire ants are small black or red ants and appear similar to other native ant species. Their mounds are composed of loose dirt and may house hundreds of thousands of individuals. Mounds extend far underground, making eradication very difficult. Stings occur when the mound is disturbed; agitated ants stream out and hundreds of bites can occur in seconds. The ant grabs the skin with large mandibles and envenomates with the distal stinger (which it may swivel around its head), producing a circular series of stings. The venom has necrotic and hemolytic effects and produces painful, edematous lesions, which usually form pustules. Scarring can occur. Extensive local reaction with persistent pain and swelling may be seen. Although the pustules are sterile, cellulitis and superinfection can occur. Systemic symptoms including DIC, seizures, rhabdomyolysis, and mononeuritis may be seen in 1% to 2% of cases. In the Southeast, fire ant stings are now the leading cause of insect sting hypersensitivity.

Management of Hymenoptera Stings. Local sting reactions begin with immediate pain and swelling. Symptoms typically resolve within 24 to 48 hours. Cold packs and antihistamines are occasionally required. Severe local reactions, such as massive swelling of the stung extremity, may occur. Corticosteroids and H_1 and H_2 blockers may provide benefit. Stings in proximity to the airway may compromise respiratory status. Most serious envenomations are due to anaphylaxis. Following the sting, symptoms reflecting mast cell degranulation occur in sensitized individuals. Hoarseness, wheezing, and laryngotracheal swelling may occur, along with pruritus and urticaria. Anxiety and gastrointestinal symptoms, such as nausea and vomiting, may be seen. In more severe reactions, cardiovascular toxicity including hypotension and myocardial ischemia may develop. Deaths due to Hymenoptera stings that do not show evidence of airway obstruction may be due to direct cardiovascular causes.

Symptoms of anaphylaxis including hypotension, hoarseness, or other evidence of airway compromise should be treated aggressively. An IV line should be established, and the patient should be placed on a cardiac monitor. Epinephrine 0.3 to 0.5 mL 1:1000 should be given subcutaneously, if there are no contraindications. Antihistamines should be given (H_1 and H_2 blockers); diphenhydramine 25 to 50 mg IV and cimetidine 300 mg IV are reasonable choices. For cases with severe airway compromise or hypotension, epinephrine 1 mL 1:10,000 can be given intravenously. Orotracheal intubation or cricothyrotomy may be necessary.

Patients with moderate to severe allergic reactions to Hymenoptera stings should be monitored for a minimum of 8 to 12 hours to watch for recurrence or delayed manifestations of anaphylaxis. All patients with allergic reactions should be counseled about insect stings and be provided with an autoinjectable epinephrine device and oral antihistamines and instructed about their use. They should be told to seek emergency health care immediately if they are stung again. The purchase of a medical alert bracelet should be considered. These patients, like any with anaphylaxis, should also be referred to an allergist for consideration of immunotherapy. Venom immunotherapy has been associated with an overall desensitization rate of 98%.

If one is stung by a bee, the stingers should be promptly removed because the venom sac remains attached and may contract, injecting more venom. It is generally recommended to scrape the stingers out rather than grasping them with fingers or tweezers to avoid squeezing the venom sac. Box 94-5 summarizes the management of Hymenoptera stings.

REPTILIAN ENVENOMATION

About 8000 poisonous reptile bites (mostly snake bites) are reported each year. Usually less than three deaths per year result from these bites. The vast majority of envenomations occur in intoxicated young men and in children. Regionally, the largest number of reported bites are from the Southwest and the Gulf Coast area. Ninety percent of these reported bites occur from April through October. The majority of the bites are on extremities.

To avoid bites, it is important to understand reptiles. Because reptiles cannot regulate their body temperature, they are most active in the evening of hot summer days. They will inevitably seek relief from heat on hot days and seek warmth on cool days. Careful foot placement in wooded areas and the avoidance of casual hand placement in concealed areas are important. Wearing long loose pants with high top boots are helpful strategies to help prevent bites.

The two major families of poisonous snakes in North America are the Crotalidae (pit vipers) and Elapidae (coral snakes). One family of poisonous lizards, Heloderma (Gila monsters), is found in southern Arizona, New Mexico, and Nevada.

Box 94-5. Recommendations for the Treatment of Hymenoptera Stings

1. Control local symptoms with cold applications and oral antihistamines.
2. Treat severe local reactions with the addition of H_1 blockers and glucocorticoids.
3. Observe patient for 8 to 12 hours if progressive local symptoms and for delayed manifestations of anaphylaxis.
4. Treat anaphylaxis with the following:
   A. Epinephrine 0.3 to 0.5 ml of 1/1000 subcutaneously.
   B. Give H_1 and H_2 blockers IV.
   C. For hypotension or airway obstruction, consider epinephrine 1 mL 1/10,000 IV.

Pit Vipers (Crotalidae)

Crotalidae are represented by rattlesnakes, copperheads, and water moccasins (cottonmouths). These snakes have a triangular head and a heat-sensing maxillary pit located between each nostril and eye. They have vertical pupils and an obvious neck between the head and body (Fig. 94-5). Most of this country's venomous bites are from rattlers, which usually strike after a warning rattle. These snakes' venom is complex with variable enzymes and toxic proteins that serve to decrease the escape of the prey and to increase digestion. Crotalid proteolytic enzymes result in significant local necrosis, as well as increased capillary permeability leading to hypotension. The venom is delivered via dual fang hypodermic injection.

Clinical Syndrome and Management. The degree of toxicity of envenomation depends on the type and size of pit viper. Copperhead venom and water moccasin venom, although similar to rattlesnake venom, are less potent. The larger the snake, the more potentially serious the envenomation. Up to 30% of pit viper bites deliver little or no venom.

Most envenomations are marked by instant pain, followed by swelling and ecchymosis within the first 15 minutes. Usually one or two puncture sites or a scratch can be located. Initial first aid includes calming the victim, immobilizing the limb below the level of the heart and rapidly transporting the patient to a health care facility. There is no clear documented benefit of electric shock administration, cryotherapy, or tourniquet placement. Only the Sawyer Extractor, a powerful suction device applied within 3 minutes and left on for 30 minutes has been demonstrated in animal studies to be helpful in extracting venom.

After transportation to the emergency room, priorities include establishing a physiologic baseline and IV access. The next step is to assess the degree of envenomation and the need for antivenin by noting the advancing borders and the increasing circumferential swelling, as well as laboratory

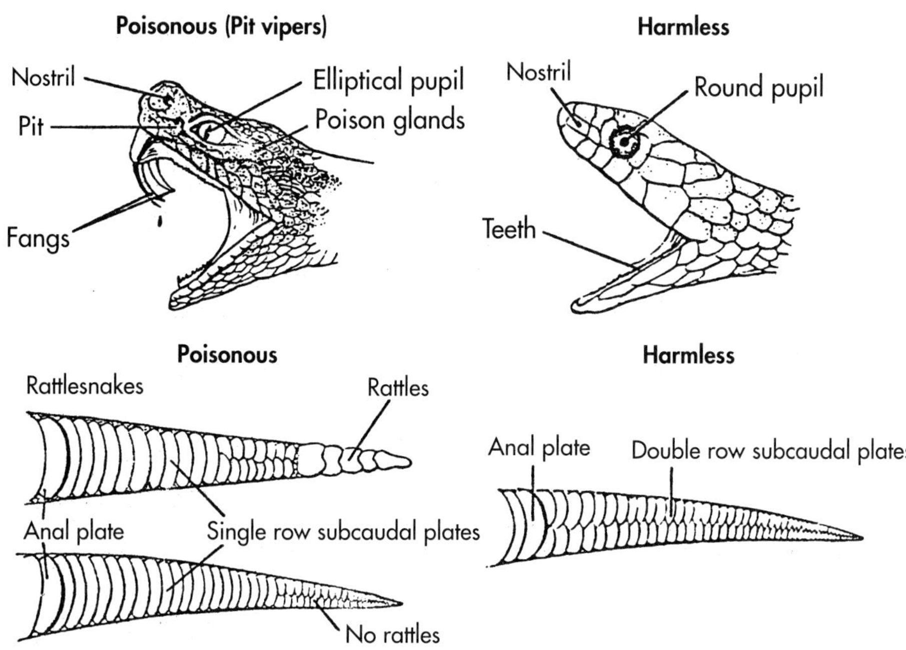

Fig. 94-5. The differentiation of crotalids from harmless snakes. (From Wingert WA, Wainschel J: *Resident and Staff Physician* 23:56, 1977.)

abnormalities. The examination and laboratory studies should be repeated every 6 hours until the patient is stable. Before administration of antivenin, the patient should be skin tested for hypersensitivity. Commercial antivenin is a pooled hyperimmune serum from a equine source and is suitable for all Crotalid envenomations but is highly allergenic. Table 94-1 summarizes IgG antivenin administration.

A new product of sheep-derived, highly-purified polyspecific crotalid antivenin consisting of Fab fragments is now available at several locations in areas where snake bites are highly prevalent. The Fab fragment binds with the toxins as does the older IgG antivenin. However, the Fab toxin is smaller than the IgG toxin, has a larger volume of distribution, and can be more rapidly eliminated by renal clearance. Case studies have suggested immediate reversal of clinical deterioration, including neurotoxicity, with Fab-antivenin administration in mild-to-moderate cases of envenomation. Repeat doses over 36 hours may be necessary for local control of symptoms. This newer antivenin appears to have less allergic complications.

Coral Snakes (Elapidae)

Coral snakes are found primarily in the Southeastern United States (Eastern coral snake) and in the Western United States (Western or Sonoran coral snake). These snakes are typically small and colorful with black noses and round pupils. Because of their short, fixed fangs and small mouths, they rarely cause significant envenomation. Elapidid venom has significant neurotoxicity. The clinical envenomation syndrome may initially cause few local symptoms but may be followed after 15 minutes to an hour with extremity weakness, paresthesias, and fasciculations. Several hours later, systemic toxicity may become manifest. These symptoms may include tremors and paresthesias. Late (5 to 10 hours) symptoms may include cranial nerve palsies. Death is rare. Therapy includes antivenin for the Eastern coral snake envenomation and supportive care.

Gila Monster and Mexican Beaded Lizard (Helioderma)

The only species of venomous helioderma lizards found in the United States are found in southern Arizona, New Mexico, and Nevada. The Gila monster and the Mexican beaded lizard are large with flat heads and bulging mandibular areas. The envenomation occurs through capillary action after the lizard has grasped the victim and punctured the skin. Not all bites result in envenomation but both lizards, particularly the Gila monster, may hang on and require assistance in dislodging. The clinical syndrome usually involves intense, severe pain at the wound site, edema, and systemic symptoms of mild hypotension. Severe local or systemic complications are rare. Treatment involves cleaning the wound and providing analgesia.

Table 94-1. Guide for IgG Crotalid Antivenin Administration

Level of envenomation	Administration
No envenomation	No antivenin
Mild envenomation	5-10 vials
Moderate envenomation	10-20 vials
Severe envenomation	>20 vials

MARINE TOXIC ENVENOMATION

Many sea creatures are capable of inflicting serious injury and toxic envenomation. Two common sources of marine envenomation in the United States are jellyfish and stingrays.

Jellyfish (Cnidaria)

The Cnidaria are represented along all three coasts in the United States. Toxic jellyfish possess venom discharging cells called *nematocysts* that are found in their tentacles. The sea nettle *(Chyrsaora quinqecirrha)* is one of the most common of the jellyfish found along the Atlantic and Gulf coasts (Fig. 94-6). Its close relative, the lined sea nettle, is commonly encountered along the Alaska and California coasts. Contact with a sea nettle usually produces a mild pruritic rash. Extensive contact may produce a systemic reaction, including severe cramps and respiratory difficulty.

Highly toxic reactions may result from contact with two common, large jellyfish. The first, the Portuguese man-of-war *(Physalia physalis),* is a jellyfish that floats on the surface by means of a gas-filled float that changes shape to catch the prevailing wind. Its tentacles contain an extremely toxic

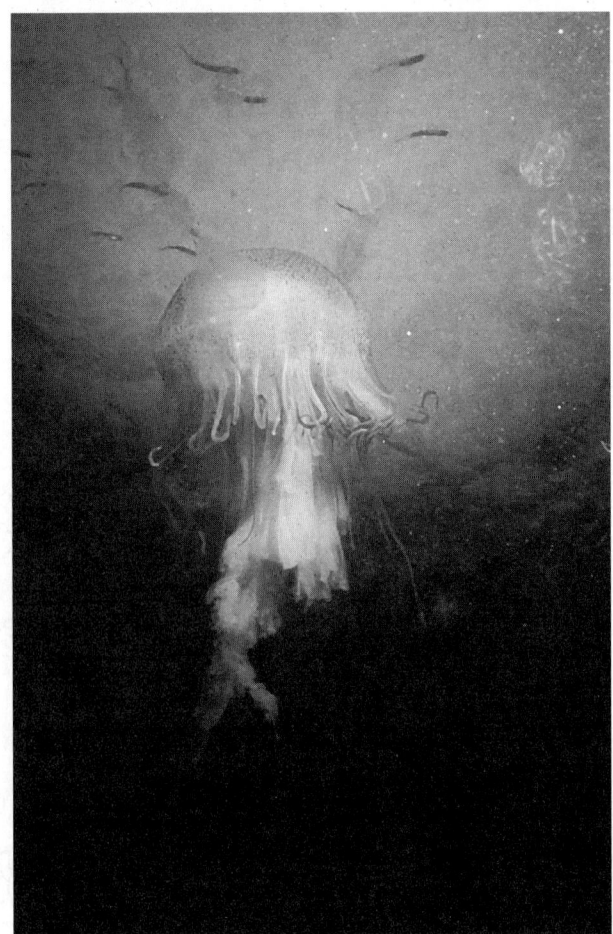

Fig. 94-6. Sea nettle, a common toxic jellyfish along the Atlantic and Gulf coasts. This specimen was photographed in Block Island Sound, Rhode Island. (Courtesy Harold Wes Pratt.)

poison that can produce severe burns and blisters even when the jellyfish is dead and has washed up on the beach.

The lion's mane *(Cyanea capillata)* is the other highly toxic jellyfish. It is prevalent along the Pacific, Atlantic, and Gulf coasts. This jellyfish has a bell-like saucer shape and develops a reddish-brown color as it grows larger. It has 16 marginal lobes and shaggy clusters of more than 150 tentacles below. Lion's mane is the largest jellyfish in the world, sometimes attaining a diameter of 8 feet. Its tentacles produce severe burning and blistering, and exposure may cause muscle cramps and respiratory difficulty.

Management. A swimmer who sustains major contact with any poisonous jellyfish should be brought aboard a boat or assisted to the beach because swimmers can panic and drown when stung. Ocean water should be poured over the wound; sand should not be rubbed on the wound because this will fire the nematocysts that have not discharged. Alcohol or acetic acid (vinegar) inactivates the penetrating nematocysts. An attempt should be made to remove the tentacles with protective gloves. A paste of talc or shaving cream may be used with subsequent skin scraping. A traditional but unproved treatment is to cover affected areas of skin with meat tenderizer. The papain present in most of the preparations supposedly digests the nematocysts and tentacles and alleviates the discomfort. Hot water should not be used on coelenterate stings; it may also cause firing of the nematocysts. No systemic drugs have shown to be helpful except for analgesia.

Stingray (Rajiformes)

On the North American coasts, several spiny groups of fish contain poison. This group includes the stingray, which is responsible for most human envenomations by fish.

Stingrays abound off the coast of southern California, the south Atlantic states, and the Gulf coast. The stingray body is flattened, and the pectoral fins broadened laterally so that they present a flat disk. The tail is long and equipped with barbs (Fig. 94-7). The barb often penetrates a foot of a wader, releases venom, and lacerates tissue on coming out. The pain is sharp and immediate. The jagged wound bleeds and may contain torn integumentary sheath. The leg becomes edematous, and if a large amount of venom is inoculated, systemic symptoms may also occur.

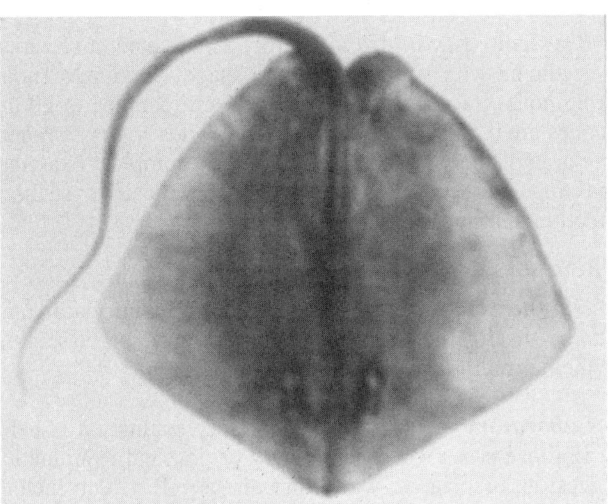

Fig. 94-7. Stingray, commonly found along the southern California and south Atlantic coasts.

Management. Treatment starts with immediate and thorough irrigation of the wound with a cold diluent (e.g., salt water) to remove the venom and act as a vasoconstrictor. The wound is then immersed in hot water to tolerance for at least ½ to 1 hour. The heat will neutralize the toxin. Finally, remaining pieces of sheath should be searched for. In general, wounds are to be left open. Tetanus toxoid should be given if the last booster was more than 5 years before, and antibiotics should be prescribed to cover marine organisms such as the vibrio species.

ADDITIONAL READINGS

Bass JW, Vincent JM, Person DA: The expanding spectrum of Bartonella infections. II. Cat-scratch disease, *Pediatr Infect Dis J* 16:163-79, 1997.

Berg RA et al: Envenomation by the scorpion *Centruroides exilicauda (C. sculpturatus)*: severe and unusual manifestations, *Pediatrics* 87:930-933, 1991.

Dart RC et al: Affinity-purified, mixed monospecific crotalid antivenom ovine Fab for the treatment of crotalid venom poisoning, *Ann Emerg Med* 30(1):33-39, 1997.

Davidson TM et al: North American pit vipers, *J Wildern Med* 3:397-421, 1992.

DeShazo R, Butcher BR, Banks WA: Reactions to the stings of the imported fire ant, *N Engl J Med* 303:462-465, 1990.

Human Rabies Prevention: Recommendations of the advisory committee on immunization practice (ACIP), *MMWR* 48:RR-1, 1999.

Jerrard DA: ED management of insect stings, *AJEM* 14(4):429-433, 1996.

Stewart C: Emergency management of arachnid envenomations: spider bites and scorpion stings, *Emerg Med Rep* 14:75-82, 1993.

Talan D et al: Bacteriologic analysis of infected dog and cat bites, *N Engl J Med* 340:85-92, 1999.

Wilson DC, King L Jr: Spiders and spider bites, *Dermatol Clinics* 8:277-286, 1990.

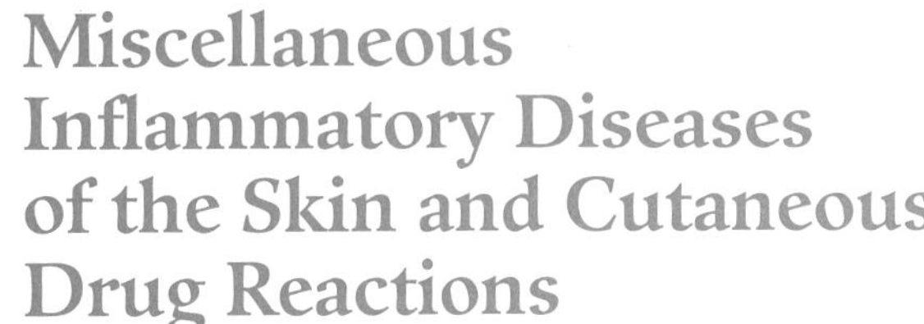

CHAPTER 95

Miscellaneous Inflammatory Diseases of the Skin and Cutaneous Drug Reactions

James C. Shaw

URTICARIA

Epidemiology

Urticaria (hives) occurs at any age without preference to genetic population, age, or sex. Up to 20% of the population is affected at some time with urticaria. The majority of cases are acute and self-limited. A small number persist beyond 6 weeks and are termed *chronic urticaria*. Multiple causative factors exist (Box 95-1).

Box 95-1. Common Causes of Urticaria

Foods
Nuts, strawberries, fish, shellfish, eggs, chocolate, tomatoes

Food Additives
Benzoates, dyes (Tartrazine), sweeteners (Aspartame), salicylates

Drugs*
Penicillin, sulfonamides, aspirin, morphine and other opiates, polymyxin, dextran, quinine

Infections
Hepatitis A, B, and C, mononucleosis, Coxsackie virus, dental abscesses, sinusitis, fungal infections (dermatophytes or candida species), intestinal parasites (helminths or protozoa)

Inhaled Allergens
Pollens, mold spores

Internal Disease
Collagen vascular disease (systemic lupus erythematosus, Sjögren's syndrome), autoimmune thyroid disease, malignancies

Physical Urticarias
Dermographism, cold, heat, water (aquagenic urticaria), vibration, pressure, exercise, ultraviolet light

Miscellaneous
Pregnancy, hormones, mastocytosis, contact urticaria, hereditary angioedema

*Any drug should be considered a possible cause.

Autoantibodies. Recently, autoantibodies to IgE receptors on mast cells have been demonstrated in patients with chronic idiopathic urticaria. Up to one-third to one-half of patients with chronic urticaria have demonstrated such autoantibodies.[7] This information may help to explain the large group of patients with no known trigger factor identified.

Pathophysiology

Urticaria occurs when cutaneous mast cells release histamine and other inflammatory mediators into the dermis, causing capillary fluid leakage, inflammatory cell infiltrate, and stimulation of sensory nerves. The results are pruritic raised lesions observed clinically.

Immunologically induced urticaria is most commonly a type 1 IgE-mediated process in which circulating antigens bind with IgE receptors at the cell membrane and trigger the enzyme-activated degranulation. In up to half of patients with chronic idiopathic urticaria, there are circulating autoantibodies against the high affinity IgE receptor, or IgE, or both. Less commonly, immune complexes cause urticaria through the activation of complement. In nonimmunologically induced urticaria, the same enzymatic cellular response is induced by certain pharmacologic or physical stimuli such as morphine, strawberries, or vibration.

Box 95-2. History in Patients with Urticaria

Pattern of Development
Time of day
Acute or chronic pattern
Associated activities (physical urticaria)

Food History
Processed foods (food additives)
Other prepared foods (restaurants)
Snacks, candies, diet drinks

Medications
Aspirin
Over-the-counter products
Medications taken occasionally

Environment
Home (improvement when away from home?)
Work (improvement when away from work?)

General Health
Underlying chronic illness
Autoimmune diseases
Malignancy
Occult infection (dental, sinus, genitourinary)

Patient Evaluation

History. The diagnosis of urticaria is usually evident after a brief history and examination. The history of pruritic wheals lasting up to several hours is typical. The pruritus can be intense. A history of a swollen tongue or lips and epigastric discomfort can imply gastrointestinal involvement, and the presence of wheezing or pharyngeal swelling suggests an anaphylactic reaction. Obtaining a detailed history is an essential part of determining the cause of the urticaria. Box 95-2 lists some important points to consider when taking a history.

Physical Examination. Sharply demarcated raised areas of erythema with variable size and shape (circular, annular, serpiginous), ranging in size from 0.5 cm papules to 20 cm plaques are typical (see Plate 4). Central clearing is common. Any area of the body can be involved. A complete examination may be needed to identify possible causes such as infection and internal disease.

Diagnosis

Diagnostic Procedures. Biopsy can be confirmatory and can be useful in excluding the presence of vasculitis, erythema multiforme, or drug reactions.

Laboratory Evaluation. Laboratory evaluation is helpful in those cases where the history or physical examination suggest an association with other disease. Tests can include complete blood count, serum chemistries, urinalysis, and antinuclear antibodies.

Management. If a cause can be identified and eliminated, pharmacologic treatment of the urticaria may not be required. Frequently the cause cannot be identified and management consists of controlling the development of new lesions and reducing symptoms. Antihistamines control the majority of patients with acute and chronic urticaria. Antihistamines competitively block histamine receptors, but do not prevent mast cell release of inflammatory mediators. They are therefore most effective when administered continuously as a preventive therapy. Combinations of antihistamines may be necessary to suppress the development of urticaria. The H_1 blockers diphenhydramine and hydroxyzine are commonly used in doses ranging from 25 mg to 100 mg every 8 hours as tolerated by sedation. The nonsedating H_1 blockers (cetirizine, loratidine, fexofenadine) can be useful during the day in patients who are intolerant of the sedation. The tricyclic antidepressant doxepin is a potent H_1 blocker that can be used in difficult cases. Because of sedation, doxepin is best administered at night. Evidence for the addition of H_2 blockers (cimetidine, ranitidine) is lacking, and these drugs should not be considered unless maximal use of H_1 blockers has failed.

Systemic corticosteroids can be tried in recalcitrant cases to suppress autoantibody formation. Although many cases ultimately resolve spontaneously without a proved cause, a systematic elimination of some ingested substances can be helpful (Box 95-3).

Box 95-3. Urticaria Elimination List

Dietary

Beer, alcohol
Chocolate
Eggs
Fish, shellfish
Milk
Nuts (including peanuts)
Citrus fruits
Strawberries
Cinnamon
Peas, beans
Pork
Cola
Diet drinks
Artificial sweeteners
Tonic water (quinine)

Medications

Aspirin
Vitamins
Laxatives
Lozenges
Mouthwashes
Eyedrops

Miscellaneous

Candies
Cigarettes
Toothpaste
Perfume and perfumed soaps
Cosmetics
Chewing gum

ERYTHEMA MULTIFORME

Erythema multiforme is an acute self-limited disease of skin and mucous membranes that consists of characteristic clinical lesions and histopathology. The severity of erythema multiforme is variable, ranging from mild cases with few lesions to a widespread vesiculobullous form (Stevens-Johnson syndrome), which is discussed later in this chapter.

Epidemiology

The true incidence of erythema multiforme is not known. Estimates range from 1 in 1000 to 1 in 10,000 persons. It is generally a disease of children, adolescents, and young adults.

Etiology

Infections and medications are the most common causes of erythema multiforme. The most common association is with either recurrent Herpes Simplex virus (HSV) infection[1] or mycoplasmal pneumonia. Boxes 95-4 and 95-5 list the infections and drugs that can cause erythema multiforme.

Box 95-4. Etiology of Erythema Multiforme

- Infections
  - Herpes simplex
  - Epstein-Barr virus
  - Streptococcal
  - Mycoplasmal pneumonia
  - Syphilis
- Immunizations
  - Hepatitis B vaccine
  - Immunotherapy (allergy shots)
- Drugs (see Box 95-5)
- Malignancy
- Radiation therapy
- Connective tissue disease
- Hormonal
  - Pregnancy
  - Menstruation

Pathophysiology

An immunologic mechanism of disease has been postulated as the cause of erythema multiforme. This is supported by the frequent association with the administration of medications and with some infections plus the finding of immune complexes containing herpesvirus DNA around the microvasculature of involved skin.

Patient Evaluation

History. Patients usually report a rapid onset of lesions that may follow a short prodrome of malaise. The hands and feet are commonly involved in early stages. Mouth tenderness is common if there is mucosal involvement.

Box 95-5. Drugs Commonly Associated with Erythema Multiforme, Stevens-Johnson Syndrome, and Toxic Epidermal Necrolysis

Sulfonamides
Trimethoprim/sulfamethoxazole
Dapsone

Anticonvulsants
Diphenylhydantoin (Dilantin)
Carbamazepine (Tegretol)

Nonsteroidal Antiinflammatory Drugs
Oxyphenbutazone
Phenylbutazone
Piroxicam (Feldene)

Barbiturates

Allopurinol

Other Antibiotics
Penicillins
Tetracyclines
Erythromycin
Cephalosporins

Salicylates

Furosemide

A detailed history of recent illnesses, medications, and infections, including a past history of herpetic infection, is essential to identifying the cause.

Physical Examination. The classic lesions of erythema multiforme are raised circular erythematous lesions, 0.5 cm to 3 cm in diameter. Central epidermal pallor with surrounding erythema produces the "target" or "iris" lesions that are described (Plate 90). The central dusky gray pallor is caused by epidermal necrosis and can be mistaken for pustule formation. Mucosal lesions erode easily, presenting as shallow ulcerations. Although the distribution of erythema of erythema multiforme can be widespread, the distal extremities, including palms and plantar surfaces, are most commonly involved.

Diagnosis

Diagnostic Procedures. Biopsy shows a lymphocytic infiltrate at the dermal-epidermal junction with a characteristic vacuolization of epidermal cells and necrotic keratinocytes within the epidermis. Blood studies may show a slight leukocytosis and elevation of the erythrocyte sedimentation rate. However, no consistent laboratory abnormalities are associated with erythema multiforme. The differential diagnosis of erythema multiforme can include other annular eruptions, such as urticaria and other figurate erythemas, and in the mouth, herpesvirus infection and blistering diseases in the pemphigus group.

Management. Erythema multiforme is usually self-limited without treatment. Identification and treatment of any underlying illness may prevent recurrent episodes. In cases without an obvious trigger, the use of empiric treatment to suppress HSV infection has been shown to be effective in a majority of patients.[8] Analgesics may be necessary in some cases. The use of systemic corticosteroids is controversial but may be helpful early in the disease.

STEVENS-JOHNSON SYNDROME

A widespread vesiculobullous form of erythema multiforme with involvement of mucosal surfaces is called *Stevens-Johnson syndrome*. The two diseases have been thought to represent variations of the same pathophysiologic mechanism. A recent review suggests that on the basis of different trigger factors Stevens-Johnson syndrome may be a different disease process than erythema multiforme.[5]

Etiology

The causes of both erythema multiforme and Stevens-Johnson syndrome are similar (see Box 95-5). Radiation therapy and particularly cranial x-ray therapy, in association with the administration of antiseizure medications, appears to be associated with an increased incidence of erythema multiforme and Stevens-Johnson syndrome.

Patient Evaluation

History. A rapid onset of skin and mucosal lesions associated with variable symptoms of malaise and fever are typical in Stevens-Johnson syndrome. Pain or burning in the conjunctivae and mouth are common early symptoms that may at first suggest an infectious etiology until more skin involvement is apparent. A detailed history of underlying diseases and exposure to medications is essential.

Physical Examination. The extensive distribution and severity of the lesions are what distinguish Stevens-Johnson syndrome from erythema multiforme. Erosive changes on the lips, mouth, conjunctivae, anogenital area, and ears are typical (Plate 91). Intact vesicles and bullae are uncommon in these areas. Cutaneous lesions may involve the entire skin surface. Individual lesions may be characteristic circular lesions of erythema multiforme, but it is more common to find large confluent areas of dusky erythematous skin, with occasional flaccid vesicles, bullae, and erosions. The lesions are usually tender to touch.

Diagnosis

Diagnostic Procedures. Biopsy is frequently helpful in confirming the diagnosis. Histologic features are those of erythema multiforme. Viral cultures of intact vesicular lesions or mucosal erosions may be indicated to exclude herpesvirus infection.

Differential Diagnosis. Stevens-Johnson syndrome should be differentiated from staphylococcal scalded skin syndrome, vesicular viral exanthems, Kawasaki's disease, toxic shock syndrome, and paraneoplastic pemphigus. The presence of the classic circular "target" or "iris" lesions plus the erosive changes on the mucous membranes should allow for making the correct diagnosis.

Management. While supportive treatment is essential, recent evidence supports the early use of high doses of corticosteroids. Control of pain and treatment of secondary infection may require narcotic analgesics and antibiotics. Patients with large areas of denuded skin need fluid and electrolyte management. Liquid diet or intravenous nutrition may be required when mouth lesions prevent intake by mouth. Eroded areas of skin should be cleansed gently and kept covered with occlusive compresses to prevent drying. Mucosal lesions should be kept moist by frequent application of antibacterial ointments or other protective agents.

The use of systemic corticosteroids has been controversial. Early studies demonstrated delayed healing and higher incidence of complications when steroids are used. More recent studies have demonstrated clear benefit when high doses of corticosteroids are used early in the disease course.[2]

TOXIC EPIDERMAL NECROLYSIS

The widespread blistering disease called toxic epidermal necrolysis (TEN), or Lyell's syndrome, has many similarities to Stevens-Johnson syndrome and many consider the two to be variations of the same disease. Most authors agree that TEN and Stevens-Johnson syndrome are differentiated on the basis of the percentage of total body surface area involved, with TEN having greater than 30% to 40% involvement. Histologic differences between the two diseases suggest different mechanisms of disease.

Etiology

Clinical evidence points to drugs as the main cause of TEN. The list of drugs associated with TEN is similar to that associated with Stevens-Johnson syndrome, with anticonvulsants, nonsteroidal antiinflammatory agents and antibiotics being most commonly involved (see Box 95-5). Immunizations, some viral infections, and graft-vs.-host disease have also been implicated.

Pathophysiology

The pathophysiology of TEN is not known but most evidence supports an immune-mediated process. A genetic predisposition is suggested by the increased incidence of HLA B12 in patients with TEN. An interaction between the normally expressed Fas receptor and Fas ligand on keratinocytes has been recently demonstrated in TEN, with blockade of this interaction resulting in disease improvement.[9]

Patient Evaluation

History. The prodrome in TEN is similar to that of Stevens-Johnson syndrome, with two or three days of fever and malaise. The history of a new drug taken within one to three weeks before the onset of the illness is strong evidence of a causal relationship.

Physical Examination. Extensive epidermal sloughing along with severe mucosal changes are characteristic of TEN (Plate 92). The mucosal changes, which are present in over 90% of cases, frequently precede the skin involvement. The percentage of skin surface involvement can range from 40% up to 100%. The full-thickness epidermal detachment leaves painful areas of denuded dermis. Primary target lesions can also be seen occasionally.

Complications. Complications contribute to the mortality rate in TEN that ranges between 25% and 70%. Sepsis is the main cause of death. Gastrointestinal hemorrhage, hypovolemia, and pulmonary edema have also contributed to mortality. Ocular complications include conjunctival scarring, corneal ulceration, and photophobia. Cutaneous complications include alopecia, loss of nails, pigmentary changes, and hypertrophic scarring with contractures.[9]

Diagnosis

Diagnostic Procedures. Biopsy can be helpful in differentiating between TEN and a less severe form of drug eruption. Epidermal separation with scant dermal infiltrate and characteristic necrotic keratinocytes is suggestive of TEN.

Differential Diagnosis. Staphylococcal scalded skin syndrome in children is the main differential diagnosis to consider. Bullous graft vs. host disease can mimic TEN.

Management

Nonpharmacologic Therapy. A burn center provides the best environment for the treatment of TEN. The skills and materials needed to treat TEN are similar to those used in burn care, including xenografts, temperature control, and nutritional management. Treatment consists of supportive measures designed to prevent complications and allow healing of all affected tissue. A successful approach requires the help of the surgical team, intensivist or internist, ophthalmologist, physical therapist, and expert nursing staff.

Pharmacologic Treatment. Although there are no established treatments of TEN, recent work with intravenous immune globulin (IVIG) is promising. IVIG is thought to block the interaction between Fas receptor and Fas ligand to prevent keratinocyte death and was successfully used in a pilot study of 10 patients with TEN, in whom the disease reversed rapidly and all patients recovered.[9]

ERYTHEMA NODOSUM

Erythema nodosum (EN) is the most common of a group of diseases under the heading of 'panniculitis'.

Epidemiology

EN occurs mostly in young adults, with women affected more than men in a ratio of approximately 3-6:1. Since EN is considered an immunologic response to a variety of antigenic stimuli, prevalence rates vary on the basis of regional antigen exposures. Overall prevalence rates are in the range of 1:1000/year.

Pathophysiology

EN is thought to be a hypersensitivity reaction, but the exact type has not been determined. The immunologic reaction is centered in the subcutaneous fat. Numerous causes of EN have been reported including infections with bacteria, viruses, fungi, and parasites, medications (especially oral contraceptives), sarcoidosis, inflammatory bowel disease, malignancies, and collagen vascular diseases. A recent study from France demonstrated predominance of streptococcal infections and sarcoidosis in patients with EN.[3]

Patient Evaluation

History. A prodrome that can include malaise, low grade fever, or arthralgias can be reported in the majority of patients with EN. This is followed in several days by characteristic tender lesions usually on extensor legs. A complete history looking for underlying disease, medications, and infections is essential.

Physical Examination. Tender erythematous, smooth-topped, subcutaneous nodules present on extensor surfaces are characteristic (Plate 93). Pretibial location is most common, but lesions may be present on upper extremities and trunk.

Diagnosis

Diagnostic Procedures. A biopsy that includes involved subcutaneous fat is usually helpful, although the histologic findings are not pathognomonic. Other diagnostic evaluation is based on evidence from the history and physical examination and may include blood studies, chest x-ray, and cultures for bacterial or viral infection.

Differential Diagnosis. The main differential diagnosis in EN is nodular vasculitis, sometimes called erythema induratum, which is associated with prior infection with *Mycobacterium tuberculosis.* Occasionally, it is difficult to differentiate between these two.

Management

Nonpharmacologic Therapy. The disease is usually self-limited; thus identification and treatment of underlying disease or offending medication is most important. Bed rest with leg elevation is a time-honored treatment usually combined with pharmacologic treatment.

Pharmacologic Treatment. Nonsteroidal antiinflammatory drugs (NSAIDs) are the treatment of choice, in conjunction with bed rest. In some cases, systemic corticosteroids (approximately 40 mg/day) for 1 or 2 weeks may be needed.

GRANULOMA ANNULARE

Granuloma annulare (GA) is an uncommon inflammatory skin disease that has a characteristic clinical presentation. The cause of GA is not known.

Epidemiology

Two forms of GA are seen most often. The localized form is most common and is a disease of men and women usually under age 50. A generalized form is seen between the ages of 40 and 70. Some studies have suggested an association between GA, especially the generalized form, and diabetes mellitus.

Pathophysiology

The pathophysiology of GA is not well understood. The presence of histiocytes and mucin in the dermis suggests an interaction between immune mediators and dermal fibroblasts.

Patient Evaluation

History. A rapid onset of one or more areas of pruritus, commonly on the hands, feet, or elbows, is typical. Usually there are no identifiable trigger factors.

Physical Examination. GA has a characteristic color and shape (Plate 94). The color is a red-brown, reflecting histiocytes in the dermis. This color is similar to other granulomatous (histiocytic) diseases including sarcoidosis and leprosy. The shape is usually one or more annular ring of confluent papules. Individual papules may or may not be evident. The size of the annular ring can vary from 1 to 10 cm diameter. The center of the rings is usually clear, and there are usually no epidermal changes such as scaling or crust.

Diagnosis

Diagnostic Procedures. A biopsy is usually diagnostic. The presence of histiocytes in a palisaded array surrounding dermis with increased mucin is typical.

Differential Diagnosis. Other granulomatous diseases should be considered, such as sarcoidosis, leprosy, and other mycobacterial diseases, and necrobiosis lipoidica.

Management. Although not life-threatening, this disease causes pruritus that can be severe, especially in the generalized form. Topical, intralesional, and systemic corticosteroids are the usual treatments. Dapsone and niacinamide have been used in the generalized form.

DRUG REACTIONS

Cutaneous reactions to drugs are common, can mimic virtually all forms of skin conditions, and should be in the differential diagnosis in all patients presenting with skin complaints.

Epidemiology

Drug rashes account for 2% of skin reactions in the hospital setting. They can affect all ages. Those most commonly associated with adverse reactions are antibiotics and nonsteroidal anti-inflammatory agents.[6]

Pathophysiology

The cellular mechanisms of cutaneous drug reactions are largely unknown. Only about 25% of drug reactions have a clearly identified immunologic cause, i.e., one of the four types of hypersensitivity reactions. The mechanisms of nonimmunologic-mediated drug reactions include toxic overdose, idiosyncratic, drug interactions, and pharmacologic side effects. The mechanisms involved are urticaria, Stevens-Johnson syndrome, and EN, all of which are commonly drug induced and discussed earlier in this chapter.

Patient Evaluation

History. The onset of a drug eruption is usually 5 to 10 days after the initiation of the drug or 2 days after reexposure in a sensitized patient. Drugs that are chemically related can cross-react (thiazides and sulfonylureas). All ingested chemicals are suspected, including vitamins, herbs, other over-the-counter preparations, recreational drugs, and food additives. When multiple drugs are being used, carefully noting the dates of administration and doses of each drug may be useful.

Box 95-6. Drug Reactions and the Drugs that Cause Them

Maculopapular (Exanthematous) Eruptions

Ampicillin
Barbiturates
Diflunisal (Dolobid)
Gentamicin
Gold salts
Isoniazid
Meclofenamate (Meclomen)
Phenothiazines
Phenylbutazone
Phenytoin
(5% of children: dose dependent)
Quinidine
Sulfonamides
Thiazides
Thiouracil
Trimethoprim/sulfamethoxazole
(in patients with AIDS)

Anaphylactic Reactions

Aspirin	Sera (animal derived)
Penicillin	Tolmetin (Tolectin)
Radiographic dye	

Serum Sickness

Aspirin	Sulfonamides
Penicillin	Thiouracils
Streptomycin	

Acneiform (Pustular) Eruptions

Bromides	Iodides
Hormones	Isoniazid
ACTH	Lithium
Androgens	Phenobarbital (aggravates acne)
Corticosteroids	Phenytoin
Oral contraceptives	

Alopecia

Allopurinol
Anticoagulants
Antithyroid drugs
Chemotherapeutic agents
Alkylating agents
Antimetabolites
Cytotoxic agents
Colchicine
Hypocholesteremic drugs
Indomethacin
Levodopa
Oral contraceptives
Propranolol
Quinacrine
Retinoids
Thallium
Vitamin A

Erythema Nodosum

Iodides
Oral contraceptives
Sulfonamides

Exfoliative Erythroderma

Allopurinol	Hydantoins
Arsenicals	Isoniazid
Barbiturates	Lithium
Captopril	Mercurial diuretics
Cefoxitin	Paraaminosalicyclic acid
Chloroquine	Phenylbutazone
Cimetidine	Sulfonamides
Gold salts	Sulfonylureas

Fixed Drug Eruptions

Aspirin	Phenylbutazone
Barbiturates	Sulfonamides
Methaqualone	Tetracyclines
Phenazones	Trimethoprim/sulfamethoxazole
Phenolphthalein	Many others reported

Lichen Planus-like Eruptions

Antimalarials	Methyldopa
Arsenicals	Penicillamine
Beta-blockers	Quinidine
Captopril	Sulfonylureas
Furosemide	Thiazides
Gold salts	

Erythema Multiforme-like Eruptions

Allopurinol	Penicillin
Barbiturates	Phenolphthalein
Carbamazepine	Phenothiazines
Hydantoins	Rifampin
Minoxidil	Sulfonamides
Nitrofurantoin	Sulfonylureas
NSAIDs	Sulindac

Lupus-like Eruptions

Common	*Uncommon*	*Probable*
Hydralazine	Chlorpromazine	Acebutolol
Procainamide	Hydrochlorothiazide	Carbamazepine
	Isoniazid	Ethosuximide
	Methyldopa	Lithium carbonate
	Quinidine	Penicillamine
		Phenytoin
		Propylthiouracil
		Sulfasalazine

Photosensitivity

Amiodarone
Carbamazepine
Chlorpropamide
Furosemide
Griseofulvin
Lomefloxacin
Methotrexate (sunburn reactivation)
Nalidixic acid
Naproxen
Phenothiazines
Piroxicam (Feldene)
Psoralens
Quinine
Sulfonamides

Continued

Box 95-6. Drug Reactions and the Drugs that Cause Them—cont'd

Photosensitivity—cont'd

Tetracyclines
- Demeclocycline
- Doxycycline (less frequently with tetracycline and minocycline)

Thiazides
Tolbutamide

Skin Pigmentation

ACTH (brown as in Addison's disease)
Amiodarone (slate-gray)
- Anticancer drugs
- Bleomycin (30%—brown, patchy, linear)
- Busulfan (diffuse as in Addison's disease)
- Cyclophosphamide (nails)
- Doxorubicin (nails)

Antimalarials (blue-gray or yellow)
Arsenic (diffuse, brown, macular)
Chlorpromazine (slate-gray in sun-exposed areas)
Clofazimine (red)
Heavy metals (silver, gold, bismuth, mercury)
Methysergide maleate (red)
Minocycline (patchy or diffuse blue-black)
Oral contraceptives (chloasma-brown)
Psoralens
Rifampin—very high dose (red man syndrome)

Pityriasis Rosea-like Eruptions

Arsenicals
Barbiturates
Bismuth compounds
Captopril
Clonidine
Gold compounds
Methoxypromazine
Metronidazole
Pyribenzamine

Toxic Epidermal Necrolysis

Large areas of skin become bright red, then slough at the dermoepidermal border. This is a life-threatening reaction.
Allopurinol
Phenylbutazone
Phenytoin
Sulfonamides
Sulindac

Small-vessel Cutaneous Vasculitis

Allopurinol
Diphenylhydantoin
Hydralazine
Penicillin
Piroxicam (Feldene) (Henoch-Schönlein purpura)
Propylthiouracil
Quinidine
Sulfonamides
Thiazides

Vesicles and Blisters

Barbiturates (pressure areas—comatose patients)
Bromides
Captopril (pemphigus-like)
Cephalosporins (pemphigus-like)
Clonidine (cicatricial pemphigoid-like)
Furosemide (phototoxic)
Iodides
Nalidixic acid (phototoxic)
Naproxen (like porphyria cutanea tarda)
Penicillamine (pemphigus foliaceus-like)
Phenazones
Piroxicam (Feldene)
Sulfonamides

Ocular Pemphigoid

Demecarium bromide
Echothiophate iodide
Epinephrine
Idoxuridine
Pilocarpine
Timolol

Chemotherapy-induced Acral Erythema

Cyclophosphamide
Cytosine arabinoside
Doxorubicin
Fluorouracil
Hydroxyurea
Mercaptopurine
Methotrexate
Mitotane

From Habif TP: *Clinical dermatology,* ed 3, St Louis, 1996, Mosby.

Knowledge of which drugs are most likely to cause a rash is also crucial[4] (Box 95-6).

Physical Examination

Common Types of Drug Reactions. Morbilliform (exanthematous, toxic erythema, maculopapular) eruptions are the most common of all drug rashes (Plate 95). These eruptions often begin on the trunk and evolve onto the extremities. Pruritus is common, and mild fever can occur. Both usually begin within the first 2 weeks after a variety of drugs are taken and clear within 2 to 3 weeks after the drug is withdrawn. Fortunately, these are not associated with organ damage.

Lichen planus-like drug eruptions (lichenoid drug reaction) resemble lichen planus, with pruritic violaceous papules and plaques (Plate 96). Gold and antimalarials are the most common culprit drugs (see Box 95-6).

Fixed drug eruptions (Plate 97) are frequently misdiagnosed because of their unique presentation. One or several circular areas of violaceous erythema that may become bullous, followed by healing that leaves postinflammatory hyperpigmentation is the usual presentation. The same presentation recurs every time the offending drug is ingested. A common site of involvement is the penis. In addition to common offenders, such as tetracycline and sulfa drugs, over-the-counter drugs such as pseudoephedrine and phenolphthalein found in some wines may cause this reaction.

Photosensitivity induced by drugs occurs by two main mechanisms: phototoxicity and photoallergic reactions. Phototoxicity can occur after the first exposure to the drug and results in cellular damage resembling a sunburn. Tetracyclines, thiazides, sulfonylureas, and NSAIDs are the usual causes of phototoxic reactions. Photoallergic drug reactions require sensitization and repeated exposure and are usually manifested by an eczematous pruritic eruption. Common causes of photoallergic reactions include chlorpromazine, promethazine, and topical sunscreen agents PABA, benzophenone, and cinnamates.

Drug-induced pigmentation can be caused by several drugs, either as a chemical pigment deposition or by stimulation of melanogenesis. Minocycline pigmentation is a blue-gray-black pigment deposit, commonly in scars but can be widespread (Plate 98). Antimalarial pigmentation is also from a deposit of chemical pigment. Bleomycin causes an unusual streaked pigmentation that suggests prior scratching on the skin. Nail pigmentation can be seen with nucleoside antiretroviral drugs.

Diagnosis

Laboratory Studies/Diagnostic Procedures. No laboratory tests can diagnose a drug eruption or identify a specific drug. Skin biopsy can help to identify the specific clinical form of the skin rash, but not whether a drug is the etiology. Skin tests for penicillin are only of use for predicting immediate hypersensitivity reactions such as hives and anaphylaxis. Rechallenging with the suspected agent is potentially dangerous.

Differential Diagnosis. Viral exanthems, scarlet fever, Kawasaki disease, and exfoliative erythroderma can resemble drug eruptions. Viral exanthems are associated with enanthems, fever, and other viral symptoms. Exfoliative erythroderma also can be due to drugs, psoriasis, eczema, or cutaneous T-cell lymphoma.

Management

Nonpharmacologic Therapy. Ideally, a nonpharmacologic approach, discontinuing the offending drug, clears the skin rash. When the patient is on multiple drugs, a drug should be withdrawn or switched when possible. Most cutaneous drug reactions remit within 2 to 3 weeks after the drug is stopped. Some drug reactions are serious, such as TEN, vasculitis, erythema multiforme, and exfoliative erythroderma and take a longer period to resolve.

Pharmacologic Treatment. Judicious use of antipruritics, antihistamines, and occasionally systemic corticosteroids is helpful. Treatment of life-threatening drug eruptions is discussed in Chapter 86.

REFERENCES

1. Aslanzadeh J, Helm KF, Espy MJ, et al: Detection of HSV-specific DNA in biopsy tissue of patients with erythema multiforme by polymerase chain reaction, *Br J Dermatol* 126:19-23, 1992.
2. Cheriyan S, Patterson R, Greenberger PA, et al: The outcome of Stevens-Johnson syndrome treated with corticosteroids, *Allerg Proc* 16:151-155, 1995.
3. Cribier B, Caille A, Heid E, et al: Erythema nodosum and associated diseases. A study of 129 cases, *Int J Dermatol* 37:667-672, 1998.
4. Habif TP: Exanthems and drug eruptions. In *Clinical dermatology,* ed 3, St Louis, Mosby, 1996.
5. Roujeau JC: Stevens-Johnson syndrome and toxic epidermal necrolysis are severity variants of the same disease which differs from erythema multiforme, *J Dermatol* 24:726-729, 1997.
6. Roujeau JC, Stern RS: Severe adverse cutaneous reactions to drugs, *N Engl J Med* 331:1272-1285, 1994.
7. Sabroe RA, Greaves MW: The pathogenesis of chronic idiopathic urticaria, *Arch Dermatol* 133:1003-1008, 1997.
8. Tatnall FM, Schofield JK, Leigh IM: A double-blind, placebo-controlled trial of continuous acyclovir therapy in recurrent erythema multiforme, *Br J Dermatol* 132:267-270, 1995.
9. Viard I, Wehrli P, Bullani R, et al: Inhibition of toxic epidermal necrolysis by blockade of CD95 with human intravenous immunoglobulin, *Science* 282(5388):490-493, 1998.

ENDOCRINE, DIABETES, AND METABOLISM VI

CHAPTER 96

Diabetes Mellitus

Jay S. Skyler
Irl B. Hirsch

Diabetes mellitus is a group of metabolic diseases characterized by hyperglycemia resulting from defects in insulin secretion, insulin action, or both. As a function of time, the chronic hyperglycemia of diabetes is associated with long-term damage, dysfunction, and failure of various organs, especially the eyes, kidneys, nerves, heart, and blood vessels.

The vast majority of cases of diabetes fall into two broad categories. In one category (type 1 diabetes), the cause is an absolute deficiency of insulin secretion, a result of autoimmune destruction of the pancreatic islet β-cells. In the other, much more prevalent category (type 2 diabetes), the cause is a combination of resistance to insulin action and an inadequate compensatory insulin secretory response.

EPIDEMIOLOGY AND PUBLIC HEALTH ASPECTS

In the United States today, diabetes mellitus is a public health nightmare.[8] Consider the following:

- Of the estimated 15.6 million people nationwide who have diabetes (approximately 1 in 16 people), a projected 5.4 million people are unaware of it.
- Nearly 800,000 Americans develop diabetes every year, or approximately 2,200 every day, but individuals may have diabetes and remain undiagnosed for an average of 5 to 10 years.

- Each year 182,000 deaths are linked to diabetes, making it the third largest killer in the country, with 57,000 of those deaths directly attributable to diabetes.
- Diabetes has the highest direct costs for health care of any disease category (estimated by the National Institutes of Health [NIH] to be $91.1 billion in 1995), and is responsible for one in every seven health care dollars spent in the country.
- Total medical costs for diabetic patients are staggering, per capita almost fourfold that of people without diabetes.
- Diabetic retinopathy is the leading cause of blindness in working age adults—24,000 cases of legal blindness every year—but an estimated 90% of lost vision is preventable.
- Diabetic nephropathy is the leading cause of end-stage renal disease (ESRD)—42% of all cases—but an estimated 90% of future ESRD is preventable.
- Diabetes is the leading cause of nontraumatic amputations—67,000 limbs lost per year, a rate of amputation fifteenfold to fortyfold greater than that in the nondiabetic population—but an estimated 85% of limb loss is preventable.
- Diabetes results in a twofold to sixfold increased risk of heart disease and a twofold to fourfold increased risk of stroke.
- Risk can be dramatically reduced by careful glucose control, aiming for near-normal levels of hemoglobin A_{1c} (HbA_{1c}), but national surveys demonstrate that only 12% of patients achieve that, with the average HbA_{1c} among diabetic patients 9.1% (normal 3.9% to 6%); even worse, the majority of patients do not have HbA_{1c} measurements performed at all.

PATHOPHYSIOLOGY

The brain and nervous system are obligate users of glucose for fuel metabolism (Fig. 96-1). They do so independent of insulin. In contrast, insulin-stimulated glucose uptake occurs in most peripheral tissues (e.g., muscle, adipose), with muscle consuming the largest portion of postprandial glucose (see Fig. 96-1). Glucose entry into the circulation is from the gastrointestinal system as a consequence of food consumption and metabolism of carbohydrates to monosaccharides. In nondiabetic individuals, hepatic glucose production (HGP) matches brain and nervous system glucose utilization in the basal state, almost on a precise quantitative basis. Basal insulin secretion modulates HGP, thus regulating glycemia (see Fig. 96-1).

Hyperglycemia emerges when there is relative deficiency of insulin action at target tissues—muscle and peripheral tissues in the postprandial state, liver in the basal state. Thus hyperglycemia occurs either when circulating levels of insulin are low or when cellular sensitivity to insulin is impaired. Without insulin to stimulate glucose transport into cells, blood glucose concentrations increase and symptoms of diabetes, including polyuria, polydipsia, polyphagia, and fatigue, develop. With milder degrees of insulin deficiency, the abnormalities may be manifest only during the fed state when plasma insulin levels are normally high. With more severe degrees of insulin deficiency, the effects that insulin normally has in the fasted state (i.e., modulation of hepatic glucose production and inhibition of catabolism) are also impaired, and thus the metabolic derangement is more severe (e.g., proteolysis, lipolysis, weight loss). The most extreme degree of impairment results in ketogenesis and ketoacidosis.

Diabetic ketoacidosis (DKA) develops when excess free fatty acids taken up by the liver are preferentially shunted toward the formation of acetoacetate and β-hydroxybutyrate. As the concentration of ketone bodies increases, serum buffering capacity is exceeded and metabolic acidosis occurs. Hyperglycemia induces an osmotic diuresis that eventually leads to dehydration and volume depletion.

Type 1 Diabetes

Type 1 diabetes mellitus arises as a consequence of selective destruction of the insulin-producing β-cells in the pancreatic islets of Langerhans.[7] Thus there is absolute insulinopenia, and the dependence on exogenous insulin therapy for survival. Because of the absolute insulinopenia, patients with type 1 diabetes are prone to ketosis (and possible ketoacidosis) even under basal conditions. Type 1 diabetes generally has its onset in the first 2 decades of life (thus the previous name *juvenile-onset diabetes*), but may occur at any age. In the United States, among Caucasians, the

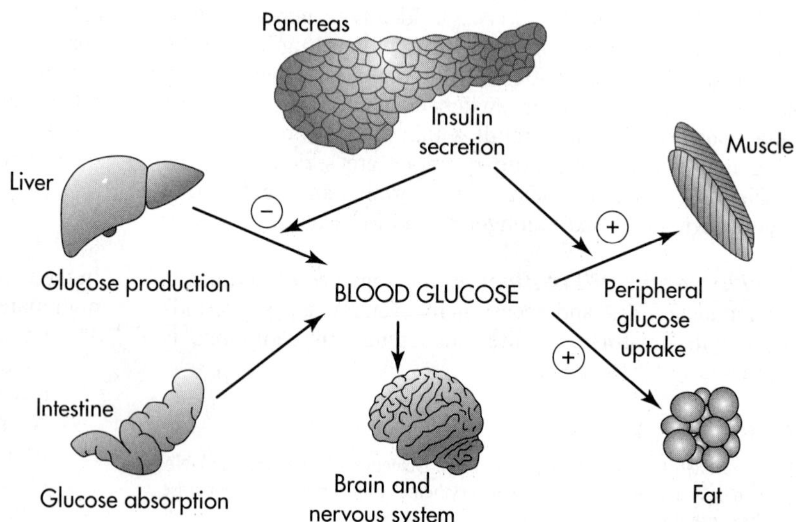

Fig. 96-1. Scheme of regulation of blood glucose. Glucose input is from food intake via the gastrointestinal system, or during the basal state from hepatic glucose production, which is modulated by basal insulin secretion. The brain and nervous tissue use glucose independent of insulin, while insulin stimulates glucose uptake and utilization by peripheral tissues (here represented by muscle and adipose tissue).

disease typically affects 1 in 300 persons in the population. Relatives of type 1 patients have a higher risk (approximately 3% to 6%), the highest risk being in monozygotic twins (30% to 50%).

Multiple loci have demonstrated associations or linkages to type 1 diabetes. Both human leukocyte antigen (HLA) and non-HLA genes contribute to diabetes susceptibility. The best characterized susceptibility loci are *IDDM1* (HLA) and *IDDM2* (*INS*-VNTR), while several other loci linked to diabetes await further characterization. *IDDM1* appears to confer ~50% of the genetic susceptibility to type 1 diabetes. Interestingly, genetic protection from type 1 diabetes is associated with specific alleles at the *IDDM1* (DQB1*0602) and *IDDM2* (*INS*-VNTR class III) loci.

The current concept is that islet β-cells in genetically susceptible individuals are destroyed by an autoimmune response mediated by T lymphocytes (T cells) that react specifically to one or more β-cell proteins (autoantigens). The disease process is insidious, evolving over a period of years. During this time, a number of immune markers appear that indicate the presence of ongoing β-cell damage (e.g., immunofluorescent islet cell autoantibodies [ICA], insulin autoantibodies [IAA], and autoantibodies to glutamic acid decarboxylase [GAD65] and to a transmembrane tyrosine phosphatase [ICA512]). This is accompanied by a progressive decline of β-cell function (loss of first-phase insulin response (FPIR) during an intravenous glucose tolerance test (IVGTT). Ultimately, the clinical syndrome of type 1 diabetes becomes evident when a majority of β-cells have been destroyed and hyperglycemia supervenes.

The generally accepted sequence, genetic susceptibility → environmental trigger → immunologically mediated pancreatic islet β-cell destruction, however, is not straightforward. Rather, the pathogenesis of type 1 diabetes appears to involve a disruption of balance between forces propelling the progression of disease and forces retarding or preventing that progression. Diabetes appearance is influenced by the net effects of genetic and environmental factors on immunoregulatory responses. Thus there are susceptibility genes and protective genes; environmental triggers and environmental factors associated with protection; and autoreactive immune/inflammatory processes leading to insulitis and immunoregulatory mechanisms restraining the destructive processes. The predominant regulatory cells appear to be various subsets of helper T cells, acting via the cytokines they produce. Thus β-cell destruction is enhanced by the T-helper-1 (Th1) subset of $CD4^+$ T cells and the *type 1* cytokines (interleukin-2 [IL-2] interferon-γ [IFN-γ], tumor necrosis factor-β [TNF-β]) they produce. In contrast, there is inhibition of β-cell destruction by the T-helper-2 (Th2) and T-helper-3 (Th3) subsets of $CD4^+$ T cells and the *type 2* cytokines (IL-4, IL-5, IL-10) and *type 3* cytokines (transforming growth factor-β [TGF-β]) they respectively produce. The cytokines produced by Th1-cell activation activate lymphocytes and macrophages to kill islet β-cells by a variety of mechanisms. Nonspecific immune/inflammatory killing mechanisms involved in islet β-cell destruction are mediated by molecules released from activated T cells (both $CD4^+$ and $CD8^+$ T cells) and macrophages. These include destructive cytokines (IL-1, TNF-α, TNF-β, IFN-γ), oxygen free radicals ($O_2^{\bullet -}$, H_2O_2, $OH^{\bullet}$), nitric oxide ($NO^{\bullet}$), and peroxynitrite ($ONOO^-$). These reactions may be counterbalanced by endogenous or exogenous protective mechanisms (e.g., antioxidants, nicotinamide, or superoxide dismutase activity). Antigen-specific $CD8^+$ cytotoxic-T cells (that interact with a β-cell autoantigen-MHC class I complex) may kill β-cells by receptor (Fas/FasL)-mediated mechanisms and/or by secretion of cytotoxic molecules (granzymes and perforin). Once the initial immune destruction commences, secondary and tertiary immune responses also are activated, with virtually the whole immunologic army attacking β-cells.

Enhancement of protective forces has been demonstrated in animal models of diabetes. For example, diabetes development can be prevented by administering β-cell autoantigens—insulin or GAD—by the parenteral, oral, intranasal, or aerosol inhalation routes. The protective effects of these treatments have been attributed to activation of T cells that produced one or more suppressor cytokines (IL-4, IL-10, and TGF-β). Based on this, plus pilot studies in high-risk relatives of type 1 diabetic patients, a full-scale randomized, controlled clinical trial, the Diabetes Prevention Trial of Type 1 Diabetes (DPT-1), is being conducted to determine whether intervention with insulin (parenteral or oral) can delay the appearance of overt clinical diabetes. Also underway is another randomized, prospective, controlled clinical trial, the European Nicotinamide Diabetes Intervention Trial (ENDIT), to evaluate the effects of nicotinamide in high-risk relatives of individuals with type 1 diabetes. The concept is that nicotinamide may work by restoring β-cell content of nicotinamide adenine dinucleotide (NAD) toward normal (via inhibition of poly-ADP-ribose polymerase), by scavenging free radicals, or by inhibiting cytokine-induced islet nitric oxide production.

Type 2 Diabetes

Type 2 diabetes mellitus is a heterogeneous disorder characterized by impaired β-cell function (defective insulin secretion) and by diminished tissue (liver, muscle, adipose) sensitivity to insulin (insulin resistance).[9] Insulin secretion is not absent, so that these individuals are not dependent on exogenous insulin for survival, and are not prone to ketosis. It is the more common form of the disease, accounting for over 90% of all cases. There is a higher risk among relatives of type 2 patients, with the highest risk being in monozygotic twins (80% to 90%). Thus there appears to be an important genetic predisposition. However, central obesity, a sedentary lifestyle, and the sarcopenia of aging are all contributing factors. Type 2 diabetes generally has its onset after age 40 (thus the previous name *adult-onset diabetes*), but may occur at any age. Indeed, there is a growing epidemic of type 2 diabetes in adolescents, perhaps related to the epidemic of obesity in that age group, accelerated by a progressively sedentary lifestyle.

Multiple genetic loci have demonstrated associations or linkages to type 2 diabetes. These associations and linkages are not observed in all populations studied. The most important locus found thus far is on chromosome 2 *(NIDDM1)*. In the study group of Mexican-American sibling pairs with type 2 diabetes from Starr County, Texas, *NIDDM1* accounted for ~30% of genetic susceptibility to type 2 diabetes.

There has been considerable debate as to which of the two defects, impaired insulin secretion or insulin resistance, is the initial lesion in the pathogenesis of type 2 diabetes. For individuals with significant fasting hyperglycemia (plasma glucose > 180 to 200 mg/dl [>10 to 11.1 mmol/L]), it is clear that both defects are present. Furthermore, defects in insulin secretion can lead to insulin resistance and vice versa. Thus, in a given individual it is impossible to determine if the initial defect was the impairment of insulin secretion or the impairment of insulin action.

Most individuals with genetic defects in insulin secretion do not develop hyperglycemia (glucose intolerance or diabetes) unless there is superimposed insulin resistance (e.g., pregnancy, weight gain, physical inactivity) or the simultaneous presence of diabetogenic genes predisposing to insulin resistance. Likewise, insulin resistance alone does not result in hyperglycemia unless there is an impairment in the ability of the β-cell to compensate for the insulin resistance. Although patients with type 2 diabetes may have insulin levels that seem normal or elevated, the higher blood glucose levels in these diabetic patients would be expected to result in even higher insulin values had their β-cell function been normal. Thus insulin secretion is defective in these patients and insufficient to compensate for the insulin resistance.

The impairment in β-cell function is manifest in several ways. There is an attenuated sensitivity of insulin response to glucose, or "blindness" to hyperglycemia. This blindness is selective for glucose, and the insulin response to other stimuli is not impaired. In addition, there is blunted or absent first-phase insulin response to glucose, so that insulin secretion is delayed and fails to restore prandial glycemic excursions in a timely manner. Insulin response is normally biphasic. The first phase is the critical determinant of the magnitude of hyperglycemia following carbohydrate intake. Its decrease results in an overall delayed insulin secretory response. Although variable, in mild and moderate type 2 diabetes, second-phase insulin response is sufficient to restore prandial plasma glucose excursions to basal levels. With more significant hyperglycemia, both the first phase and second phase of insulin release are impaired, and there is decreased overall insulin secretory capacity.

Decreased insulin action (insulin resistance) has been demonstrated in type 2 diabetes, in impaired glucose tolerance (IGT), and in first-degree relatives of individuals with type 2 diabetes despite having normal glucose tolerance. It is also seen in obesity, essential hypertension, and acromegaly, or with use of glucocorticoids or estrogens.

Insulin resistance occurs at several sites. Normally, insulin binds to its receptor on a target cell, initiating a signaling cascade that eventually results in the effects of insulin, including glucose entry into the cell. Abnormalities before insulin's interaction with the cell are termed *prereceptor* defects. These include binding of insulin by antibodies, increased degradation of insulin, and molecular abnormalities in the structure of the insulin molecule that make it difficult to bind to its receptor. These causes of insulin resistance are rare. At the *receptor* level, insulin resistance may be caused by decreased binding of insulin to the insulin receptor due to decreased number or affinity of receptors for insulin, or by decreased ability of the receptor to generate a transmembrane signal for example, by decreased receptor tyrosine kinase activity for both autophosphorylation and phosphorylation of substrates (e.g., insulin receptor substrate-1 [IRS-1]). Beyond the level of insulin interaction with its receptor, *postreceptor* defects may occur. There may be an impairment in any number of the biologic effects of insulin (e.g., translocation of the glucose transporter [GLUT4] to the cell membrane).

Hyperglycemia itself may aggravate the impairments both in insulin secretion and in insulin action. The components of defective insulin secretion and action that are reversible by lessening of hyperglycemia are known as *glucose toxicity*.

There is a progressive loss of β-cell function during the course of type 2 diabetes. This may be related to amyloid deposits that are seen in the islets of most people with type 2 diabetes. The material consists of fibrils formed by a 37–amino acid peptide called islet amyloid polypeptide (IAPP) or amylin. Within the β-cell, a precursor is cleaved to form IAPP, which is contained within secretory granules and cosecreted with insulin. IAPP accumulation within the β-cells may contribute to their destruction via some form of direct cytotoxicity.

Other Types

There are a number of other specific types of diabetes.[2] One is a group of disorders associated with monogenetic defects in β-cell function. These are frequently characterized by onset of mild hyperglycemia at an early age (generally before age 25 years) and were formerly referred to as maturity-onset diabetes of youth (MODY). They are characterized by impaired insulin secretion with minimal or no defects in insulin action. They are inherited in an autosomal dominant pattern. Abnormalities at three genetic loci on different chromosomes have been identified to date: MODY1, mutations on chromosome 20q in a hepatic transcription factor (HNF-4α) gene region; MODY2, mutations in the glucokinase gene on chromosome 7p; and MODY3, mutations on chromosome 12 in a hepatic transcription factor (HNF-1α) gene region. Point mutations in mitochondrial DNA are associated with diabetes mellitus and deafness. Genetic abnormalities that result in the inability to convert proinsulin to insulin have been described. There are rare genetic defects in insulin action, previously termed *type A insulin resistance*. Leprechaunism and the Rabson-Mendenhall syndrome are two syndromes that have mutations in the insulin receptor gene. In addition, there are a number of genetic syndromes sometimes associated with diabetes.

Secondary diabetes can occur as a consequence of diseases of the exocrine pancreas or endocrinopathies. The pancreatic diseases may include pancreatitis, trauma, infection, pancreatectomy, pancreatic carcinoma, cystic fibrosis and hemochromatosis. Fibrocalculous pancreatopathy may be accompanied by abdominal pain radiating to the back and pancreatic calcifications on x-ray. Pancreatic fibrosis and calcium stones in the exocrine ducts have been found at autopsy. Endocrinopathies that may cause diabetes include acromegaly, Cushing's syndrome, glucagonoma, and pheochromocytoma, particularly in individuals with preexisting defects in insulin secretion. Somatostatinoma- and aldosteronoma-induced hypokalemia can cause diabetes by inhibiting insulin secretion.

Many drugs can impair insulin secretion (e.g., thiazide diuretics, β-blockers), and thereby precipitate diabetes in individuals with insulin resistance. There are also many drugs and hormones that can impair insulin action (e.g., nicotinic acid and glucocorticoids).

Atypical diabetes mellitus (ADM) is a form of diabetes that may be seen in African-Americans. In ADM, there is acute onset of hyperglycemia, with ketosis or ketoacidosis as a common feature, followed by a clinical course more characteristic of type 2 diabetes. It appears to be inherited as an autosomal dominant disorder, often being seen in two to three consecutive generations. In one of 10 families with ADM, a unique glucokinase mutation was identified.

Gestational diabetes mellitus (GDM) is defined as any degree of glucose intolerance with onset or first recognition during pregnancy. The definition applies regardless of whether insulin or only diet modification is used for treatment or whether the condition persists after pregnancy. In the majority of cases of GDM, glucose regulation will return to normal after delivery.

DIAGNOSIS

The diagnosis of diabetes mellitus is established by the demonstration of hyperglycemia (Table 96-1). The diagnostic criteria for diabetes mellitus were changed in 1997.[2] The previous criteria were based mainly on the use of the oral glucose tolerance test (OGTT), which was sufficiently inconvenient not to be used in clinical practice. As a consequence, the default criterion for diagnosis became the fasting glucose alone, which was pegged at a plasma glucose level of 140 mg/dl (7.8 mmol/L). There were at least two problems with this cut point. One, it simply was too high, based on retinopathy risk. Two, it did not correspond to the OGTT level. This left undiagnosed patients with disease sufficient to lead to complications. Consequently, the American Diabetes Association (ADA) commissioned an expert committee to examine the available data and make recommendations that might allow individuals with diabetes to be more easily diagnosed in clinical practice. The expert committee analysis found that by lowering the fasting plasma glucose (FPG) cut point to ≥126 mg/dl (7 mmol/L), most people with undiagnosed diabetes would become recognized, without very much risk of false-positive diagnosis. Moreover, those at risk of retinopathy would be detected earlier. Thus 126 mg/dl (7 mmol/L) is a surrogate for an OGTT 2-hour value of 200 mg/dl (11.1 mmol/L). This change does not increase the number of people *with* diabetes. Rather, it increases the number of people with *known* diabetes.

The revised criteria include three ways to diagnose diabetes, each of which must be confirmed on a subsequent day by any one of the three methods. The criteria are (1) unequivocal symptoms (polyuria, polydipsia, unexplained weight loss) and casual (any time of day regardless of time since last meal) plasma glucose ≥200 mg/dl (11.1 mmol/L); (2) fasting (no caloric intake for at least 8 hours) plasma glucose ≥126 mg/dl (7 mmol/L); and (3) 2-hour plasma glucose ≥200 mg/dl (11.1 mmol/L) during an OGTT using a 75-gram oral glucose load.

The old criteria used a FPG of <115 mg/dl (6.4 mmol/L) for normal. In contrast, the new criteria use a FPG of <110 mg/dl (6.1 mmol/L) for normal. Individuals having FPG levels 110 to 125 mg/dl (6.1 to 6.9 mmol/L) are now defined as having *impaired fasting glucose* (IFG) (Table 97-1), and are at increased risk of diabetes, similar to those with IGT, who have OGTT 2-hour values of 140 to 199 mg/dl (7.8 to 11 mmol/L).

HbA_{1c} measurement is not currently recommended for diagnosis of diabetes, although some studies have shown that the frequency distributions for HbA_{1c} have characteristics similar to those of the FPG and the 2-hour PG. However, both HbA_{1c} and FPG (in type 2 diabetes) have become the measurements of choice in monitoring the treatment of diabetes, and decisions on when and how to implement therapy are often made on the basis of HbA_{1c}. The revised criteria are for diagnosis and are not treatment criteria or goals of therapy.

Screening is important because meticulous glycemic control slows the course of development of diabetic complications. Thus prolongation of normoglycemia should reduce risk of complications. Studies suggest that in the earlier stages (IFG and IGT) interventions, such as diet and exercise, may forestall the evolution of type 2 diabetes. Screening for type 2 diabetes is simple, only a FPG is needed. The OGTT is no longer the primary screening tool. Screening and early diagnosis of type 2 diabetes should be highly cost-effective. All adults over age 45 should be screened every 3 years. All individuals at higher risk (based on obesity, ethnicity, family history, previous gestational diabetes) should be screened annually, starting at an earlier age.

Table 96-1. Categories of Glycemia

	Fasting		2-Hour
Normal	<110		<140
Impaired fasting glucose	110-125		NA
Impaired glucose tolerance	NA		140-199
Diabetes mellitus	≥126	or	≥200

NA, Not applicable.

PATIENT EVALUATION

A comprehensive medical history can uncover symptoms that may help establish the diagnosis in a patient with previously unrecognized diabetes. It provides information essential for providing high-quality care. The hallmark symptoms of diabetes mellitus are polyuria, polydipsia, and polyphagia. However, many individuals with type 2 diabetes present only with fatigue, which may be dismissed as related to aging. Patients with type 2 diabetes may have only a gradual onset of frequent urination that prevents recognition of symptoms. Many attribute their polyuria to their polydipsia and do not seek medical attention. Nocturia is a particularly helpful indicator of polyuria and the onset of significant hyperglycemia; most patients remember how many times they get up during the night. The association of thirst or dry mouth with frequent nocturia is more consistent with elevated nighttime blood glucose than with benign prostatic hyperplasia or other urogenital conditions. Visual changes such as transient blurriness are very suggestive of fluctuating hyperglycemia.

In patients with known diabetes, the history should review previous treatment, evaluate glycemic control, seek evidence of complications, assist in formulating a management plan, and provide a basis for continuing care. It should focus on the following 15 elements:

- Details of previous treatment programs, including nutrition and diabetes self-management education
- Current treatment program, including medications, meal plan, and results of glucose monitoring and patients' use of the data
- Prior HbA_{1c} records
- Nutritional status, weight history, and eating patterns
- Physical activity and exercise pattern

- Lifestyle, cultural, and psychosocial factors that might influence diabetes management
- Growth and development in children and adolescents
- History of acute complications (e.g., ketoacidosis and hypoglycemia)
- Prior or current infections
- Symptoms and treatment of chronic complications (eye; kidney; nerve; genitourinary, including sexual; bladder; gastrointestinal; cardiovascular; cerebrovascular; peripheral vascular; foot)
- Other medications
- Risk factors for atherosclerosis (smoking, hypertension, obesity, dyslipidemia, family history)
- History and treatment of other conditions
- Family history of diabetes
- Gestational history (hyperglycemia, delivery of an infant weighing >9 lb, toxemia, stillbirth, polyhydramnios, or other complications of pregnancy)

The physical examination in people with diabetes should note the following:

- Height and weight measurement (and comparison with norms in children and adolescents)
- Blood pressure determination (with orthostatic measurements when indicated)
- Ophthalmoscopic examination (preferably with dilation)
- Cardiac examination
- Abdominal examination (for hepatomegaly)
- Evaluation of pulses
- Foot examination
- Skin examination (including insulin-injection sites)
- Neurologic examination

Laboratory evaluation focuses on determination of the degree of glycemic control and the identification of complications and risk factors. These include FPG; HbA_{1c}; fasting lipid profile (total cholesterol, high-density lipoprotein [HDL] cholesterol, triglycerides, and low-density lipoprotein [LDL] cholesterol); serum creatinine; urinalysis (glucose, ketones, protein, and sediment) test for microalbuminuria (e.g., timed specimen or the albumin-to-creatinine ratio) in pubertal and postpubertal type 1 patients who have had diabetes for at least 5 years and in all patients with type 2 diabetes); urine culture if sediment is abnormal or symptoms are present; thyroid function tests when indicated; and electrocardiogram.

Comprehensive dilated eye and visual examinations should be performed annually by an ophthalmologist or optometrist who is knowledgeable and experienced in the management of diabetic retinopathy for all postpubertal patients who have had diabetes for 3 to 5 years, all patients diagnosed after age 30, and any patient with visual symptoms and/or abnormalities.

All individuals with diabetes should receive a thorough foot examination at least once a year to identify high-risk foot conditions. This examination should include an assessment of protective sensation, foot structure and biomechanics, vascular status, and skin integrity.

MANAGEMENT

Type 1 Diabetes

Goals of Therapy. The importance of glycemic control in diminishing risk of complications in type 1 diabetes was unambiguously demonstrated by the Diabetes Control and Complications Trial (DCCT).[10] The DCCT showed that intensive treatment with a goal of meticulous control decreased the frequency and severity of retinopathy, nephropathy, and neuropathy, by 50% to 70% (Fig. 96-2). The intervention group in DCCT achieved a HbA_{1c} of 7.2%. However, there was a continuous relationship between glycemic exposure and risk of complications, without a "glycemic threshold." Similar findings were also obtained in the Stockholm Diabetes Intervention Study (SDIS).[24] The beneficial effects and impact of effective glycemic control in type 1 diabetes also have been seen in a number of other smaller intervention studies, which collectively were subjected to a meta-analysis[31] that produced findings consistent with the DCCT. Thus there are a number of randomized controlled clinical trials that support the ADA Standards of Medical Care for Patients With Diabetes Mellitus,[4] which recommend the treatment targets shown in Table 96-2.

Medical Nutritional Therapy. Contemporary dietary practice allows flexibility in when and what individuals eat. A meal plan based on the individual patient's lifestyle, food preferences, and eating habits should be determined and used as a basis for integrating insulin therapy into lifestyle. Insulin regimens are integrated with lifestyle and adjusted for deviations from usual eating and exercise habits. Patients monitor blood glucose levels and adjust insulin doses for the amount of food usually eaten. To accomplish this, patients and their families learn a system that incorporates calorie and nutrient content of foods (e.g., exchanges, carbohydrate counting). They also should learn general principles of the influence of various foods and of activity on glycemia, and the balancing of these to achieve glycemic control.

Diabetic patients should follow sound general nutritional practices. This particularly means avoiding excess intake of saturated fats and cholesterol, which influence serum lipids, which also may be elevated if there is suboptimal diabetic control. It also means limiting salt consumption, which may aggravate the risk of blood pressure elevation and may alter vascular reactivity.

Dietary protein should be ~10% to 20% of total caloric content, with the other 80% to 90% of calories distributed between dietary fat and carbohydrate. In general, 30% or less of the calories should be from total fat, with less than 10% of calories from saturated fats and up to 10% calories from polyunsaturated fats. This leaves 60% to 70% of total calories from monounsaturated fats and carbohydrates. Dietary cholesterol is limited to 300 mg or less daily. Sucrose and sucrose-containing foods must be substituted for other carbohydrates and not simply added to the meal plan. In making such substitutions, nutrient content of concentrated sweets and sucrose-containing foods, as well as the presence of other nutrients frequently ingested with sucrose such as fat, must be considered. Saccharin, aspartame, and acesulfame-K may be used as nonnutritive sweeteners.

Exercise. Regular physical activity contributes to the determination of dietary calorie content and insulin dose and regimen. Sporadic physical activity, which departs from daily routine, requires compensatory action to avert hypoglycemia (e.g., 10 to 15 grams of carbohydrates every 30 to 45 minutes during the activity). Blood glucose monitored before, during, and after the activity determines effectiveness of the extra carbohydrate. Insulin dose reductions may be used in addition to or instead of extra carbohydrate. Quick-acting, rapidly

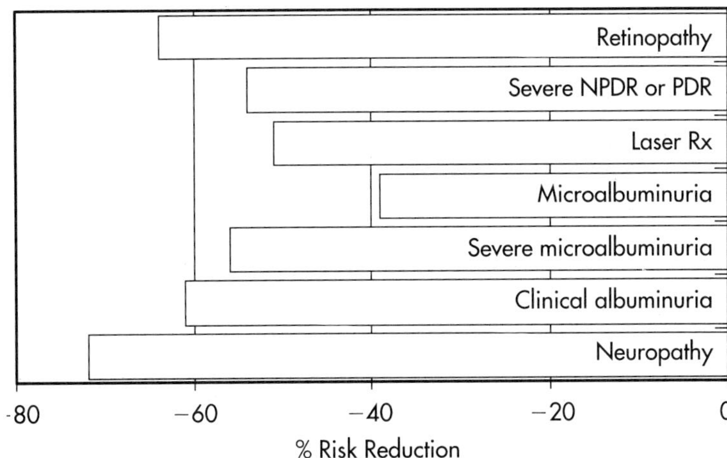

Fig. 96-2. Relative risk reductions for microvascular complications, seen with intensive glycemic control, as demonstrated in the DCCT.

Table 96-2. American Diabetes Association Glycemic Targets

Parameter	Normal	Goal	Additional action suggested
Fasting (or preprandial) glucose	<110	80-120	<80 or >140
Bedtime glucose	<120	100-140	<100 or >160
HbA_{1c} (DCCT method)	<6%	<7%	>8%

absorbed carbohydrate should be available during activity in case of hypoglycemia.

Moderately intensive exercise may deplete glycogen stores, resulting in sustained food requirement to replace the glycogen. Thus may occur well after exercise (e.g., 12 hours later). Therefore patients should be cautious when planning evening physical activity.

Insulin. Although any discussion on the treatment of type 1 diabetes focuses on insulin therapy, successful treatment cannot be accomplished without sufficient understanding about how physical activity and diet affect blood glucose levels. Furthermore, it is critical to appreciate that a team of individuals expert in diabetes therapy is required to achieve optimal goals. This team does not need to be located in the same clinic or office as the physician supervising the care, but all team members need to be aware of everyone else's responsibilities. At the least, a diabetes nurse educator and a nutritionist need to be available for routine treatment. Furthermore, these other team members should be *certified diabetes educators* (CDEs), which guarantees they have the fundamental skills required to teach and manage many aspects of diabetes therapy.

Modern management of type 1 diabetes focuses on replication of normal insulin secretion.[13,25] Also called *flexible diabetes therapy,* this strategy calls for insulin delivery that comprises a basal and prandial component, frequent home self-monitoring of blood glucose, and less restrictive dietary plans (compared with previous recommendations), yet with specific guidelines on how to alter therapy based on carbohydrate intake. Most important, patients require the self-management skills to correct alterations in metabolic control at the time such occur. This could include a change in insulin dose for premeal hyperglycemia, treatment of hypoglycemia, or addition of carbohydrate at bedtime to compensate for exercise earlier in the day. In addition, patients should understand basic principles of diabetes management during illness—*sick day guidelines.* All too often, patients with type 1 diabetes either fail to administer enough insulin during a viral gastroenteritis or they fail to measure urinary ketones during illness. As a consequence, life-threatening ketoacidosis may develop.

Available insulins are noted in Table 96-3. Although insulins have traditionally been categorized as being long-acting, intermediate-acting, and short-acting, it would be more relevant to consider them as being used as a basal or prandial insulin component. The former is that part of the regimen responsible for suppression of hepatic glucose (and ketone) production, and the latter is the insulin available for mealtime caloric ingestion. There are several options patients may choose, and each one has advantages and disadvantages.

A diabetes *algorithm* is the term used to describe actions patients take to prevent or correct any alteration in diabetes management. These include insulin *supplements* (additional insulin used to correct hyperglycemia) and *adjustments* (a change in the usual or prevailing dose of insulin). Supplements usually are with rapid-onset insulin (regular insulin, insulin lispro, or insulin aspart), whereas adjustments may be made to any insulin component. An adjustment is made when a pattern of blood glucose levels outside the target range is noted. For example, for an individual who takes bedtime NPH insulin and fasting blood glucose levels are consistently above target, an adjustment—in this case an increase—in the bedtime dose of NPH would be suggested. Another important part of a diabetes algorithm is altering the *lag time* for the onset of a dose of prandial insulin. Premeal hyperglycemia, for example, in a patient using a rapid-onset insulin analog (lispro or aspart) may be effectively treated by increasing the lag time between the dose and eating from 5 minutes to 15 or 20 minutes.

The traditional *split-mix* regimen (Fig. 96-3) may seem to be less complex than others, but it limits flexibility, especially with timing of lunch. Even if lunch is not delayed, many patients find it necessary to consume a midmorning snack to prevent hypoglycemia. Because both regular and NPH insulin have actions around lunchtime, many patients find it difficult

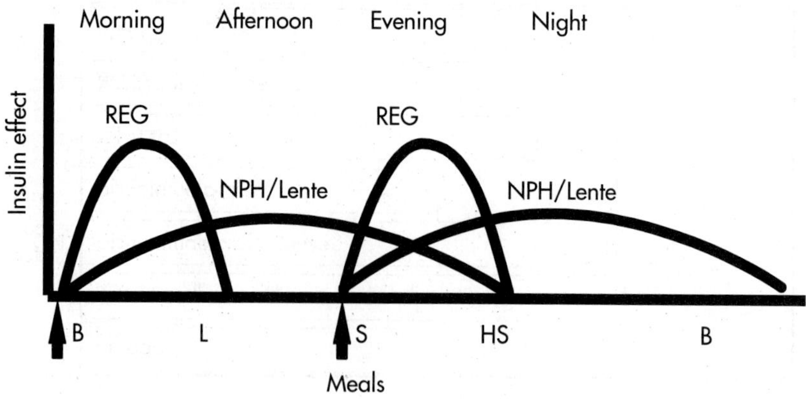

Fig. 96-3. Schematic representation of idealized insulin effect provided by insulin regimen consisting of two daily injections of regular (REG) insulin and intermediate-acting insulin (NPH or lente). *Arrows* indicate time of insulin injection, 30 minutes before meals. *B*, Breakfast; *L*, lunch; *S*, supper; *HS*, bedtime snack.

Table 96-3. Time Course of Action of Human Insulin Preparations

Insulin Preparation	Onset of action (hours)	Peak action (hours)	Effective duration of action (hours)	Maximum duration of action (hours)
Rapid-acting				
Insulin lispro (analog)	¼-½	½-1½	3-4	4-6
Rapid-acting				
Insulin aspart (analog)	¼-½	½-1½	3-4	4-6
Short-acting				
Regular (soluble)	½-1	2-3	3-6	6-8
Intermediate-acting				
NPH (isophane)	2-4	6-10	10-16	14-18
Intermediate-acting				
Lente (insulin zinc suspension)	3-4	6-12	12-18	16-20
Long-Acting				
Ultralente (extended insulin zinc suspension)	6-10	10-16	18-20	20-24
Long-acting				
Insulin glargine (analog)	3-4	8-16	18-20	20-24
Combinations				
70/30—70% NPH, 30% regular	½-1	Dual	10-16	14-18
Combinations				
50/50—50% NPH, 50% regular	½-1	Dual	10-16	14-18

to avoid midday hypoglycemia. Furthermore, many (if not most) patients are above their blood glucose target by dinner, due to dissipation of NPH insulin effect. An increase of the morning NPH dose creates more problems with midday hypoglycemia and assists little with late afternoon hyperglycemia. In addition, NPH insulin dissipation from the presupper injection results in similar problems in the morning with fasting hyperglycemia. Nocturnal hypoglycemia also is more problematic with presupper NPH insulin. One solution to these problems is adding a prandial injection of regular insulin at lunchtime and moving the NPH injection to bedtime (Fig. 96-4). The morning NPH insulin now does not have to act as a prandial insulin component for lunch and thus can better function as a basal component. Nocturnal control, often considered the Achilles' heel of type 1 diabetes therapy, should provide less of a risk of hypoglycemia and provide higher levels of insulin when they are often required (i.e., around the time of awakening, to counteract the *dawn phenomenon*).

For an improved flexible regimen, prandial insulin may be administered with each meal. Patients learn to estimate the appropriate dose based on anticipated carbohydrate intake and the prevailing blood glucose at the time of the meal. Often, individual patient experience becomes an important part of daily management. What becomes clear is that frequent home blood glucose monitoring is required, and patients need to be able to review the large amount of information they may generate. Written glucose log books allow patients to think about each glucose level at the time it is tested. Among other things, insulin doses may be written down, and comments for changes in daily schedule may be noted. Many blood glucose meters now have memories that can be downloaded to a computer. A vast array of statistical information, graphs, and charts can be generated. These may suggest trends in glucose that are not obvious with the log book. Therefore many patients and physicians prefer using both of these techniques for reviewing blood glucose data.

For the basal insulin component, one may use bedtime NPH or lente insulin, with or without a morning injection of the same insulin (Fig. 96-4). Alternatively, ultralente insulin or the new basal insulin analog, insulin glargine, may be used. These have less of a peak than NPH or lente. If ultralente or

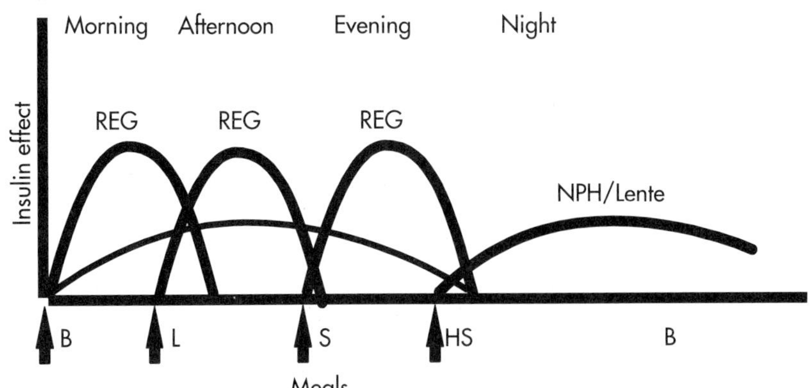

Fig. 96-4. Schematic representation of idealized insulin effect provided by multiple-dose regimen providing preprandial injections of regular (REG) insulin before meals, and basal regimen consisting of two daily injections of intermediate-acting insulin (NPH or lente). *Arrows* indicate time of insulin injection, 30 minutes before meals. *B,* Breakfast; *L,* lunch; *S,* supper; *HS,* bedtime snack.

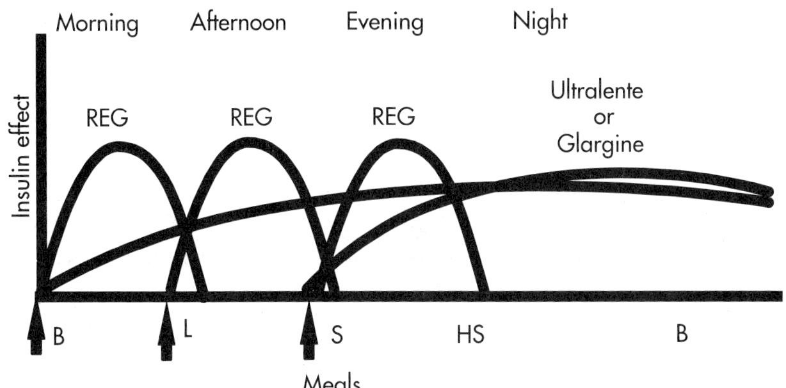

Fig. 96-5. Schematic representation of idealized insulin effect provided by multiple-dose regimen providing preprandial injections of regular (REG) insulin before meals, and basal long-acting insulin (ultralente or insulin glargine). *Arrows* indicate time of insulin injection, 30 minutes before meals. *B,* Breakfast; *L,* lunch; *S,* supper; *HS,* bedtime snack.

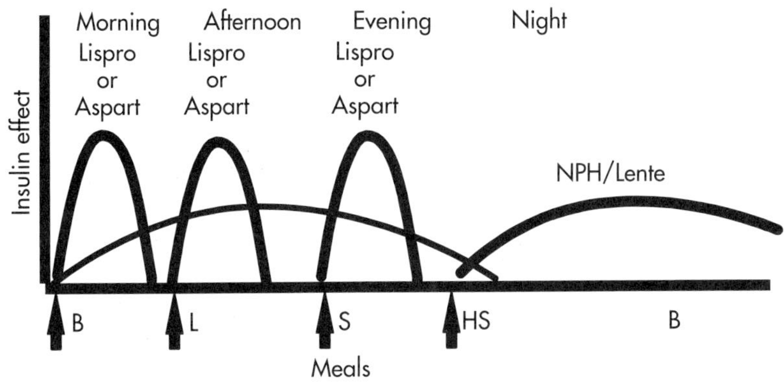

Fig. 96-6. Schematic representation of idealized insulin effect provided by multiple-dose regimen providing preprandial injections of rapid-acting insulin (insulin lispro or insulin aspart) before meals, and basal regimen consisting of two daily injections of intermediate- acting insulin (NPH or lente). *Arrows* indicate time of insulin injection, 30 minutes before meals. *B,* Breakfast; *L,* lunch; *S,* supper; *HS,* bedtime snack.

glargine is used as the basal component, it still may be desirable to use two daily doses (before breakfast and dinner [Fig. 96-5]). Another option is to give ultralente or insulin glargine before breakfast, together with bedtime NPH as the overnight basal component, the latter to target the severe insulin resistance some patients experience in the mornings, and thus overcome the dawn phenomenon.

There are also several options for the prandial insulin component. Regular insulin has the advantage of being better suited for meals high in fat and protein. However, postprandial hyperglycemia occurs with higher carbohydrate meals. Furthermore, to be most efficacious, regular insulin should be administered 20 to 30 minutes prior to eating, unless there is premeal hyperglycemia in which case one should wait longer. The rapid-onset insulin analogs, insulin lispro and insulin aspart, are better suited for higher carbohydrate-containing meals. Slower absorbed meals that are high in fat and protein content may result in greater problems with postprandial hyperglycemia after the analog (lispro or aspart) has dissipated. These analogs can be used as prandial insulin together with basal insulin provided either by intermediate-acting insulin, NPH or lente (Fig. 96-6), or by long-acting insulin, ultralente or insulin glargine (Fig. 96-7). Compared with regular insulin, hypoglycemia is decreased with insulin lispro and insulin aspart, since there is less interaction with basal insulin, especially NPH. Hypoglycemia related to exercise also tends to be less problematic when the activity occurs greater than 2 hours after the last injection of lispro or aspart.

Many patients have learned that for certain situations they do better by mixing regular insulin and a rapid-onset analog. For example, if insulin lispro or aspart is usually used but a

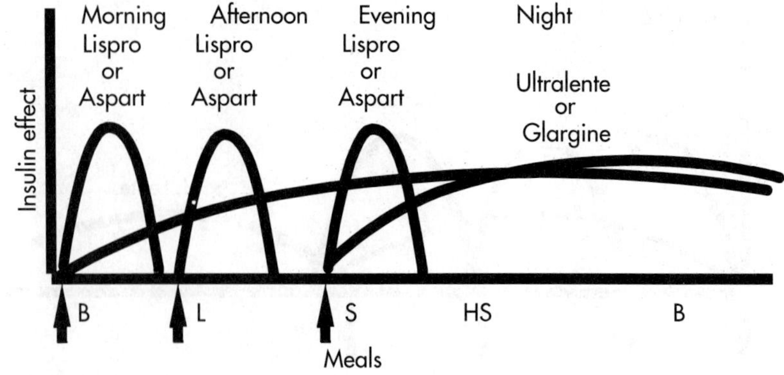

Fig. 96-7. Schematic representation of idealized insulin effect provided by multiple-dose regimen providing preprandial injections of rapid-acting insulin (insulin lispro or insulin aspart) before meals, and basal long-acting insulin (ultralente or insulin glargine). *Arrows* indicate time of insulin injection, 30 minutes before meals. *B*, Breakfast; *L*, lunch; *S*, supper; *HS*, bedtime snack.

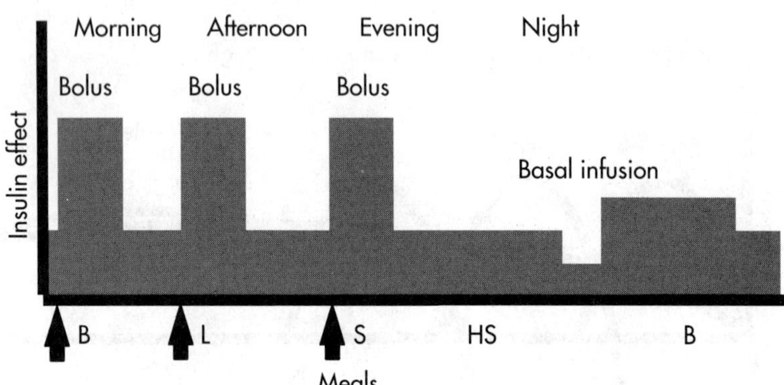

Fig. 96-8. Schematic representation of idealized insulin effect provided by continuous subcutaneous insulin infusion using insulin lispro or insulin aspart. *B*, Breakfast; *L*, lunch; *S*, supper; *HS*, bedtime snack.

particular meal will have more fat than usual, it might be wise to mix half the dose as regular insulin. Alternatively, for individuals who are doing well on regular insulin, insulin lispro or insulin aspart may be used as supplemental insulin for premeal hyperglycemia.

The most precise way to replicate normal insulin secretion is to use an insulin pump in a program of continuous subcutaneous insulin infusion (CSII) (Fig. 96-8). By delivering microliter amounts of insulin on a continual basis, basal insulin secretion is replicated. Programming a variable basal rate counteracts the dawn phenomenon and other variations in insulin sensitivity that otherwise result in disruption of glycemic control. The pump is activated before meals to provide prandial insulin increments as meal *boluses,* allowing total flexibility in meal timing and replicating physiologic prandial insulin availability. If a meal is skipped, the prandial bolus is omitted. If a meal is larger or smaller than usual, a larger or smaller bolus is used.

Typical insulin dose in type 1 diabetes is 0.5 to 1 unit per kg body weight per day, less during the "honeymoon" period of relative remission early in the disease, more during the adolescent growth spurt or intercurrent illness. Basal insulin is about 40% to 60% of the total daily insulin dose, with the rest divided among the meals.

Self-monitoring of Blood Glucose (SMBG). SMBG is essential for guiding the therapeutic plan. At a minimum, SMBG should be done four times daily—before meals and at bedtime. Nocturnal measurements and occasional postprandial values also are helpful. It is important that the patient understands his or her individualized target blood glucose levels (Table 96-4).

Table 96-4. Representative Target Blood Glucose Levels Suitable for a Young Otherwise Healthy Patient With Type I Diabetes Mellitus

	mg/dl	mmol/L
Preprandial	70-130	3.9-7.2
1-hour postprandial	100-180	5.6-10.0
2-hour postprandial	80-150	4.4-8.3
2 to 4 AM	100-140	5.6-7.8

Type 2 Diabetes

Goals of Therapy. The importance of glycemic control in diminishing risk of complications in type 2 diabetes was demonstrated by the large United Kingdom Prospective Diabetes Study (UKPDS)[28,29] and a small study from Kumamoto University in Japan.[19] In both of these studies, meticulous glycemic control decreased the frequency and severity of microvascular complications (Fig. 96-9). The intervention group in UKPDS achieved a HbA_{1c} of 7%. Moreover, a linear relationship between glycemic exposure and risk of complications was found across the spectrum of HbA_{1c}, without a *glycemic threshold.* The consistent and substantial beneficial effects of improved glycemic control in both type 1 and type 2 diabetes suggest that the impact of glycemic control on complications may be generalized to all categories of patients. This supports the ADA standards and treatment targets shown in Table 96-2.

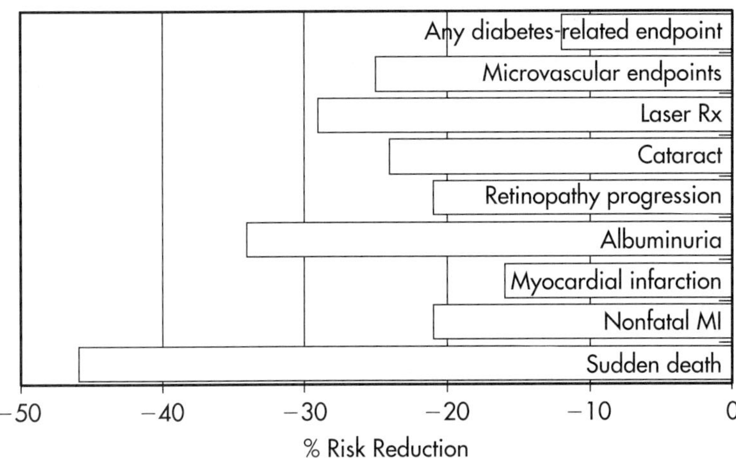

Fig. 96-9. Relative risk reductions for major endpoints, seen with intensive treatment policy, as demonstrated in the UKPDS.

Medical Nutrition Therapy. Medical nutrition therapy is an essential component of successful diabetes management. The emphasis in the plan in type 2 diabetes should be placed on achieving glucose, lipid, and blood pressure goals.

In obese patients with type 2 diabetes a major focus is weight reduction and restriction of total calorie intake. Even mild to moderate weight loss (10 to 20 pounds [5 to 10 kg]) improves short-term glycemic control. Weight loss is best approached by a moderate decrease in calorie intake, coupled with an increase in caloric expenditure.

Additional principles that facilitate glycemic control are a balanced nutrient intake; emphasis on appropriate alterations for achieving lipid and blood pressure goals; adequate spacing between meals (i.e., 4 to 5 hours apart); consumption of dietary fiber; and avoidance of excessive intake of rapidly absorbed, simple sugars (i.e., sucrose, glucose, maltose), confining their use to substitution for other carbohydrates and not as simply added to the meal plan. Coexisting conditions—dyslipidemia, renal disease, hypertension—may require alteration in nutrient content.

Exercise. Exercise improves insulin sensitivity and facilitates insulin action; increases energy expenditure; improves cardiovascular conditioning; facilitates control of hypertension; and improves dyslipidemia. A formal exercise training program is not necessary. Patients should increase physical activity to a tolerable level. Evaluation should include an exercise-stress electrocardiogram in all individuals >35 years old to detect silent ischemic heart disease. Patients should self-monitor their glycemic response to exercise.

Pharmacologic Therapy. One of the greatest changes in the past several years in clinical medicine is the increase in treatment options for management of type 2 diabetes (Table 96-5). With all these options, it is tempting to disregard the dramatic effects of exercise and diet on glycemic control. Nonpharmacologic treatments need to be emphasized indefinitely because none of the drug therapies will have their maximum impact otherwise. Despite all of the medications, there appear to be "secondary failures" after initial response. These are recognized by deterioration of glycemic control. Such deterioration in control may occur because of disease progression, lack of dietary adherence, intercurrent illness, or loss of pharmacologic effect (drug failure). Usually, however, these are not true drug failures, but masking of pharmacologic effect by disease progression. The fact that the underlying pharmacologic effect remains intact can be demonstrated by adding another agent with a different mode of action. In clinical trials with that design, marked improvement of glycemic control is seen when a second agent is added, whereas little change in glycemia is seen by switching to the new agent. Nevertheless, in view of possible loss of effect of any pharmacologic agent, glycemia should be regularly monitored to regulate dosage and verify that beneficial effects are sustained.

Including insulin, there are currently six classes of drugs available for the treatment of type 2 diabetes. There is no consensus as to which drug should be used first, although the UKPDS suggested that metformin may be preferable as first-line therapy in obese patients with diabetes.[29]

Insulin Secretagogues. Two categories of drugs, sulfonylureas and meglitinides, act to stimulate insulin secretion. Secretagogues improve β-cell function, thus correcting one of the two fundamental defects that characterize type 2 diabetes. They act by binding to a receptor unit on the β-cell, which results in closure of an ATP-dependent potassium ion channel. This causes depolarization of the plasma membrane, resulting in intracellular calcium accumulation, that in turn causes migration of insulin secretory granules to the membrane surface, there poised for insulin release on signaling in response to hyperglycemia. Excess hepatic glucose production is suppressed by secretagogues, presumably as a result of secretion of insulin into the portal circulation. Some studies suggest chronic improvement in insulin sensitivity, presumably secondary to correcting glucose toxicity.

The newest sulfonylurea formulations, glipizide-GITS and glimepiride, are long-acting sulfonylureas taken once daily, with sufficient duration to both control fasting glycemia and improve meal-related insulin secretion. Traditional formulations of second-generation drugs—glipizide and glyburide—must be taken two to four times daily, and less adequately control fasting glycemia, while increasing the risk for hypoglycemia due to large sustained postprandial peaks of drug. First-generation sulfonylureas have a greater likelihood of side effects and of interactions with other drugs, and are only rarely used.

On the other hand, the meglitinides such as repaglinide and nateglinide are ultrashort in duration of action, stimulating insulin to coincide with meals, and thus are taken

Table 96-5. Characteristics of Oral Antidiabetic Agents Available in the United States

Generic name	Brand name	Dosage range (mg/day)	Duration of action (h)	Dosing frequency (per day)
Sulfonylureas				
Tolbutamide	Orinase	500-3000	6-12	2-3 times
Chlorpropamide	Diabinese	100-500	60	Once
Tolazamide	Tolinase	100-1000	12-24	Twice
Acetohexamide	Dymelor	250-1500	12-18	Twice
Glipizide	Glucotrol	2.5-40	12-24	Twice
Glipizide-GITS	Glucotrol-XL	5-20	24	Once
Glyburide	DiaBeta, Micronase	1.25-20	16-24	Twice
Glyburide (micronized)	Glynase	0.75-12	12-24	Twice
Glimepiride	Amaryl	1-8	24	Once
Meglitidinides				
Repaglinide	Prandin	1.5-16	½-2	3 times
Nateglinide	Starlix	120-180	½-2	3 times
Biguanide				
Metformin	Glucophage	1000-2550	5-6	2-4 times
α-Glucosidase Inhibitors				
Acarbose	Precose	150-300	6	3 times
Miglitol	Glyset	75-300	6	3 times
Thiazolidinediones				
Rosiglitazone	Avandia	2-8	24+	1-2 times
Pioglitazone	Actos	15-45	24+	Once

together with any meal consumed. This offers flexibility in dosing, which some patients may find advantageous.

There is a high initial response rate to secretagogues, with 80% to 90% of subjects showing a response (defined as a decrement in plasma glucose of at least 30 mg/dl). Moreover, the response time is rapid, with improvements in glycemia seen within 24 to 48 hours. As monotherapy, these agents result in a HbA_{1c} decrease of ~1.5% to 2%. Although very effective, they may lose their effectiveness over time. One clue that a secretagogue is still effective during a period of otherwise high blood glucose levels is when hypoglycemia occurs, perhaps after exercise or a missed meal. The presence of hypoglycemia proves that the secretagogues are still effective.

Disadvantages of secretagogues include the major side effects of hypoglycemia (which in some instances may be prolonged or severe); weight gain; drug interactions (especially with the first-generation compounds); and hyponatremia with chlorpropamide.

Advantages of secretagogues include improvement in a primary pathophysiologic impairment, that of insulin secretion; a physiologic route of insulin delivery (from the pancreas into the hepatic portal circulation); a high initial response rate; and no lag period before response. Additional advantages of repaglinide are that it may be used in renal insufficiency and that there is flexible dosing in relationship to meals.

Biguanides. The glucose-lowering effects of the biguanides were first shown in the nineteenth century, although this class was not introduced clinically until the 1950s. One biguanide, phenformin, was withdrawn by the Food and Drug Administration (FDA) in 1977 because of propensity to lactic acidosis, sometimes fatal. Another biguanide, metformin, which had been available for 4 decades, was released in the United States in 1995. Biguanides have a complex and poorly understood mechanism of action, but appear to directly effect glucose metabolism, thus improving insulin sensitivity, particularly at the liver, where they decrease hepatic glucose output, while also increasing peripheral (muscle) glucose uptake and utilization.

Metformin may be used as initial monotherapy in type 2 diabetes, particularly in obese patients because, unlike secretagogues, it is not associated with weight gain on improvement in glycemia, and in fact a modest weight loss may be seen. Metformin enjoys particular success in combination with secretagogues, since biguanides and secretagogues have complementary mechanisms of action. Indeed, most patients require this combination to achieve glycemic targets. On the other hand, in the setting of inadequate glycemic regulation, switching from a secretagogue to metformin, or vice versa, does not result in improvement of glycemic control.

As monotherapy, metformin results in a HbA_{1c} decrease of ~1.5% to 2%. There is a high initial response rate, with 80% to 90% of subjects showing a response (defined as a decrement in plasma glucose of at least 30 mg/dl). Because of the need for slow dose titration in order to minimize the gastrointestinal side effects (nausea, abdominal discomfort, and less frequently, diarrhea) that are seen on initiation of therapy, the full effectiveness of metformin may not be seen for 4 to 6 weeks.

It is important to be sure that patients receive adequate

doses of metformin. A dose-response study demonstrated that maximum glucose lowering was achieved with a dose of 1000 mg twice daily, which is substantially higher than that prescribed by most physicians.

Unlike phenformin, metformin is rarely associated with lactic acidosis, provided its use is avoided in patients with elevated serum creatinine, hepatic disease, congestive heart failure, or cardiovascular compromise. Following radiographic procedures involving contrast dyes, metformin should be withheld until it is ensured that acute renal insufficiency has not been induced by the contrast media.

Disadvantages of metformin include gastrointestinal side effects on initiation of metformin (forcing gradual dose increments) and the risk of lactic acidosis in the circumstances noted above.

Advantages of metformin include improvement in a primary pathophysiologic impairment, that of insulin resistance; a high initial response rate; a long record (40 years) of relative safety; and the fact that it is associated with absence of weight gain and may result in modest weight loss.

α-Glucosidase Inhibitors. The α-glucosidase inhibitors competitively bind to the carbohydrate-binding region of α-glucosidase gastrointestinal enzymes (sucrase, maltase, isomaltase, amylase, glucoamylase), thus slowing digestion of complex carbohydrates, oligosaccharides, and disaccharides. These actions result in retardation of gut glucose absorption. In the United States, acarbose became available in 1996, miglitol in 1999, and voglibose is in clinical trials. These agents inhibit intestinal brush border enzymes and reduce postprandial hyperglycemic excursions. This results in a modest improvement in HbA_{1c}, which on average is about 0.5% to 1%. Although occasionally used alone, their primary role is in combination with other agents when glycemic targets are not met.

Because carbohydrates remain in the gut, these drugs frequently produce gastrointestinal side effects, particularly high frequency of flatulence, which is often severe. Other gastrointestinal side effects include nausea, abdominal discomfort, borborygmi, and diarrhea. To some extent, these can be reduced by very slow dose titration to therapeutic levels, but continuing flatulence is bothersome to many patients.

Caution must be exerted in treatment of hypoglycemia by patients using α-glucosidase inhibitors. Because these enzymes are inhibited, hypoglycemia cannot be treated with sucrose, maltose, or starch, since glucose is not readily available for gut absorption. On the other hand, lactose (e.g., milk) may be used to treat hypoglycemia, since lactase is a β-glucosidase and not inhibited. Monosaccharides, including glucose itself and fructose, may be used to correct hypoglycemia.

Disadvantages of α-glucosidase inhibitors include the fact that a high carbohydrate diet is required for efficacy, since it is a competitive enzyme inhibitor; the flatulence and other gastrointestinal side effects; its limited effect on fasting plasma glucose; and the need to alert patients about the ineffectiveness of many usual treatments of hypoglycemia.

Advantages of α-glucosidase inhibitors include a good safety profile; lack of weight gain with improved glycemic control; and a unique mechanism of action that allows these drugs to be combined with any other class of glucose-lowering agent.

Thiazolidinediones. The most recent class of oral agents for the treatment of diabetes is the thiazolidinediones (glitazones). These agents act by binding to nuclear receptors called peroxisome proliferator-activated receptors (PPARs). These receptors are important regulators of lipid homeostasis, adipocyte differentiation, and insulin action. The thiazolidinediones act by binding to the PPAR gamma subtype (PPARγ), resulting in the expression of a number of gene-encoding proteins that enhance cellular insulin action on glucose and lipid metabolism. As a consequence, there is improvement in insulin sensitivity, particularly resulting in increased peripheral (muscle and adipose) glucose uptake and utilization, with only a modest effect at the liver. The effect of thiazolidinediones on improving target cell insulin action has been demonstrated in type 2 diabetes, in IGT, and in obese individuals with normal glucose tolerance.

In the United States, troglitazone became available in 1997 and rosiglitazone and pioglitazone in 1999, and several other thiazolidinediones are in various stages of development.

Thiazolidinediones are most effective when given in conjunction with insulin in patients with type 2 diabetes, in which circumstance insulin doses can be lowered and improvement in glycemic control achieved, including attaining control in some individuals who previously were refractory to glucose lowering in spite of large doses of insulin. Effectiveness is also seen in combination with secretagogues, metformin, or both (so-called *triple therapy*). When used in monotherapy, the response rate is variable, and there is no easy way to anticipate who will be "responders." Rosiglitazone and pioglitazone appear to have a higher response rate than troglitazone, although this point is moot, since troglitazone is no longer on the market.

The major problem with troglitazone was that of idiosyncratic liver disease, which in some cases was associated with acute hepatic necrosis, resulting either in death or need for liver transplantation. It was recommended that liver enzyme levels be measured at the start of therapy and monthly thereafter. In spite of monitoring, cases of severe liver dysfunction were missed. Although this was a rare problem, it is unfortunately unpredictable. Therefore troglitazone was withdrawn from the market. Fortunately, the clinical trial experience with rosiglitazone and pioglitazone suggests that these agents appear devoid of this risk of liver disease. If that proves to be the case, this class of agents will enjoy widespread usage.

Other disadvantages of thiazolidinediones include the fact that there is a delayed onset of action (up to 3 weeks) and a prolonged time to see the full effect (10 to 12 weeks); weight gain; a relatively high nonresponse rate in monotherapy; increased levels of LDL cholesterol; and unknown long-term side effects since this is a relatively new class of drug.

Advantages of thiazolidinediones include improvement in a primary pathophysiologic impairment, that of insulin resistance; a unique mechanism of action that allows it to be combined with any other class of glucose-lowering agent; once-daily dosing; lowering of serum triglycerides and increase in HDL cholesterol; and that some agents may be used in renal insufficiency.

Insulin Therapy in Type 2 Diabetes. Because of the progressive nature of β-cell dysfunction in type 2 diabetes, insulin therapy often becomes necessary. It should also be appreciated that enough insulin will almost always overcome insulin resistance and improve glucose metabolism. In addition, insulin therapy can be used to overcome glucose toxicity and correct the reversible components of the defects in insulin secretion and insulin action.

Disadvantages of insulin therapy in type 2 diabetes include induction of hypoglycemia, weight gain, the need for injections and nonacceptance of that by patients or physicians, and the fact that subcutaneous injections represent a nonphysiologic route of administration (i.e., the peripheral circulation rather than the hepatic portal circulation).

Advantages of insulin therapy in type 2 diabetes include flexibility in dosing and lifestyle by virtue of the multiple preparations with different action profiles, the ability to control all patients (although this may require very high doses), and that it can be used to overcome glucose toxicity.

It should be noted that temporary insulin therapy may be used to attain glycemic control, to overcome glucose toxicity, or to re-regulate decompensated patients. Insulin often is used in combination with various oral medications. All classes of oral medications can be used with insulin. In combination therapy, bedtime NPH insulin has been shown to be an effective strategy of initiating insulin therapy in patients with type 2 diabetes already on an oral agent. It targets the fasting glucose, and thus lowers the level of glycemia above which daytime glucose excursions occur. Alternatively, such basal insulin may be given as ultralente insulin or insulin glargine, both long-acting insulins, or by continuous insulin infusion. However, over time, insulin deficiency becomes more pronounced and a more physiologic regimen will be required, similar to what is used in individuals with type 1 diabetes (see above).

Insulin therapy is often used in the elderly as a last resort, after failure of dietary management and maximum doses of oral hypoglycemic agents. The aim of therapy in the elderly is to relieve symptoms and prevent both hypoglycemia and acute complications of uncontrolled diabetes (e.g., hyperosmolar states). Schedules for the injection of insulin should be kept as simple as possible, since self-administration may be difficult and dosage errors are not uncommon. Premixed insulins may be particularly desirable due to their simplicity of use.

Insulin therapy in type 2 diabetes need not be permanent. With correction of glucose toxicity, there is improvement in both endogenous insulin secretion and insulin sensitivity. As a consequence, it may be possible to discontinue exogenous insulin therapy.

A Therapeutic Strategy. Although there is controversy about which drug to use initially, it is clear that many agents work well in combination. It also is clear that most patients need more than one drug. It would seem logical to favor combinations of drugs that work by complementary mechanisms of action, such as a secretagogue with either metformin or a thiazolidinedione. Although both are insulin sensitizers, metformin and a thiazolidinedione may be used together, since the former has its greatest effect on the liver, and the latter has its greatest effect on peripheral glucose utilization. Adding oral agents, especially metformin or a thiazolidinedione to insulin may be very effective, or initiating insulin therapy to a patient not reaching targets on sulfonylureas, metformin, or a thiazolidinedione may be very effective.

It is important to emphasize that frequent SMBG levels at home and regular HbA_{1c} measurements are required to assist in deciding how to optimally use the diabetes drugs. SMBG in particular has become a critical tool because it allows patients to see how different foods and exercise change blood glucose, but it also assists patients to make changes in insulin at the time the test is performed. Furthermore, one should not assume that a deterioration of glycemic control is from the failure of the agent, although that may be the case. If diabetes control is achieved initially but is not maintained (secondary failure), other possibilities should be entertained before taking further action. For example, life stresses, illness, travel, or a change in activity may all cause a deterioration of glycemic control and should not necessitate the addition of a new agent. Temporary insulin therapy may be considered in such circumstances, even if it is just an injection or two of rapid-acting insulin (e.g., insulin lispro or insulin aspart) to correct prevailing hyperglycemia.

ACUTE COMPLICATIONS

Diabetic Ketoacidosis

DKA occurs in 2% to 5% of patients with type 1 diabetes each year. Depending on the age group and population, death still occurs in 1% to 10% of patients. The metabolic derangements in DKA result from absolute or relative insulin deficiency and elevated counterregulatory hormones, resulting in severe hyperglycemia, ketonemia and acidemia, and volume depletion.

Laboratory values for DKA include an arterial pH < 7.3, plasma bicarbonate ≤ 15 meq/L, blood glucose usually >250 mg/dl, and ketonuria with ketonemia. Although the clinical diagnosis is usually apparent in an individual with known type 1 diabetes, it also needs to be considered in a comatose elderly patient with type 2 diabetes or a child with rapid breathing perceived as having a respiratory tract infection. The clinical signs and symptoms of DKA are noted in Box 96-1. Abdominal pain in association with a leukocytosis and high amylase level is not uncommon, but if it persists with therapy, consideration should be given to appendicitis or bowel perforation.

Any intercurrent illness or stress may precipitate DKA, including myocardial infarction, stroke, trauma, and particularly infection. Some patients may mistakenly withhold their insulin during an acute illness due to decreased appetite. This is particularly common during a bout of gastroenteritis, during which patients may be prone to ketosis anyway. Alternatively, some patients (especially adolescent girls) intentionally withhold insulin as a strategy for weight loss.

The most important component for the treatment of DKA is close monitoring. For this reason, many believe that it is best to treat these individuals in an intensive care unit. There should be frequent assessment of fluid intake and output, vital signs, and pertinent laboratory values (glucose, bicarbonate, potassium, sodium, urea nitrogen, and creatinine). Although some authors recommend the measurement of a routine arterial blood gas, especially on admission, this is probably not necessary. Indeed, if a simple metabolic acidosis is discovered, there is no need for subsequent blood gas measurements. A flow sheet with all of the pertinent clinical and laboratory information is invaluable. The essential elements of treatment are listed in Box 96-2.

Volume depletion is present in all patients. It is reasonable to assume a weight loss of 5% to 10% of total body weight,

Box 96-1. Symptoms and Signs in Diabetic Ketoacidosis

Symptoms

Nausea and vomiting
Thirst and polyuria
Anorexia
Abdominal pain
Visual disturbances
Somnolence

Signs

Tachycardia
Hypotension
Dehydration
Hyperpnea or Kussmaul's breathing
Impaired consciousness and/or coma
Weight loss
Fruity odor of ketones

or 3.5 to 7 L of fluid in a 70-kg patient. Isotonic solutions are the fluids of choice; hypotonic solutions run the risk of rapid reduction of plasma osmolality, with large fluid shifts precipitating cerebral edema and hypovolemia. Appropriate solutions are either 0.9% saline or, alternatively, a solution of one ampoule (~50 mEq) of sodium bicarbonate (plus appropriate potassium supplements) added to each liter of 0.45% saline.

Insulin replacement should be accomplished by an intravenous infusion of regular insulin. Insulin should be delayed if the patient is hypokalemic. A bolus of 0.1 units/kg may be administered, and then infused at 0.1 units/kg/hr. Only in unusual situations (e.g., myocardial infarction or sepsis) will this amount of insulin not result in an improvement in the acidemia and the anion gap. For this situation, the rate of insulin infusion should be doubled and consultation with a diabetologist should be considered.

Glucose is always normalized more quickly than the acidosis is corrected, but the *insulin infusion needs to be continued until both are corrected.* Five percent dextrose is added to the infusion when the blood glucose reaches 250 mg/dl. When plasma bicarbonate level reaches 18 meq/L and the anion gap has decreased to 15 meq/L, the insulin infusion may be reduced (by about 50%).

All patients with DKA are total body potassium depleted, even if they present with normokalemia or hyperkalemia. Prior to initiating potassium replacement, it is necessary to establish urine output and obtain an electrocardiogram to quickly estimate hyperkalemia or hypokalemia. If low T waves with U waves are noted (indicative of severe hypokalemia), potassium should be initiated even if the serum potassium level is not available from the laboratory. For most situations, potassium replacement should be initiated no later than 1 to 2 hours after starting the insulin infusion.

The use of bicarbonate in the treatment of DKA is controversial. Although bicarbonate may be used as part of the intravenous solution, routine bolus bicarbonate infusion is not recommended. Some authorities recommend bicarbonate only for severe acidemia (i.e., pH < 7), particularly when associated with hypotension, shock, and arrhythmias. When needed, bicarbonate may be given as an infusion of 1 to 2 meq/kg over 2 hours, and then the plasma bicarbonate level should be remeasured.

Phosphate replacement in the treatment of DKA also is controversial. Routine phosphate replacement has not been shown to be of significant benefit. However, with low initial phosphate levels, it is reasonable to replace phosphate as potassium phosphate.

Other considerations in the treatment of DKA are the following. Low-dose subcutaneous heparin is recommended in the elderly. Cerebral edema has been described in children, most likely due to correction of the hyperglycemia too quickly and using excessive amounts of hypotonic saline. Therefore, in children blood glucose should be maintained at 250 mg/dl for the first 12 to 24 hours. Overaggressive fluid replacement may induce congestive heart failure. Frequent auscultation of the lungs is recommended.

Box 96-2. Essential Elements in the Treatment of DKA

Fluid Replacement

- 2-3 L isotonic solution over the first 3 hours
- Subsequent fluid at 150-300 ml/hr
- More cautious replacement in the elderly or if heart disease is present
- Add 5% glucose when blood glucose reaches 250 mg/dl
- Continue intravenous fluids (including insulin) until acidemia is corrected and food is tolerated

Insulin Administration

- Bolus 0.1 unit/kg
- Continuous infusion of 0.1 units/kg/hr
- Before connecting tubing to patient, run 30 ml of insulin solution through tubing to saturate tubing absorption sites
- If no biochemical response in 2-4 hours, double infusion rate (ensure patency of infusion lines, and that insulin was actually added to the infusion)
- When plasma bicarbonate has increased to 18-20 meq/L and the anion gap has decreased to 15 meq/L the insulin dose may be reduced
- Most patients may be maintained on ~2 units/hour with
- 5-7.5 grams glucose/hour to clear any residual ketosis
- Discontinue intravenous insulin and resume subcutaneous insulin when oral intake is resumed

Potassium Replacement

- Initially, if urine output adequate, ECG (lead 2) may be used as a guide for potassium replacement
- Replacement rate based on plasma potassium levels
  If serum potassium <3 meq/L, infuse at ≥ 0.6 meq/kg/hr
  If serum potassium 3-4 meq/L, infuse at 0.6 meq/kg/hr
  If serum potassium 4-5 meq/L, infuse at 0.2-0.4 meq/kg/hr
  If serum potassium 5-6 meq/L, infuse at 0.1-0.2 meq/kg/hr
  If serum potassium ≥ 6 meq/L, withhold infusion until serum potassium is <6 meq/L
- Remeasure potassium every 2 hours if plasma concentration is <4 or >6 meq/L

Hyperosmolar Hyperglycemic Nonketotic Syndrome (HHNS)

If DKA is at one end of the spectrum of severe metabolic decompensation, HHNS is at the other end. With HHNS there is a lack of significant ketosis and higher average glucose levels than noted with DKA. By definition, plasma glucose is above 600 mg/dl and plasma osmolality is greater than 320 mOsm/L. Many cases of HHNS are associated with acidemia, often related to lactic acid accumulation or uremia. Average initial laboratory values include a plasma glucose of 1000 mg/dl, serum osmolality of 360 mOsm/L, and a blood urea nitrogen (BUN) and creatinine of 65 mg/dl and 3 mg/dl, respectively. Precipitating factors are similar to those seen in DKA.

The cornerstone of HHNS therapy is fluid replacement. These patients are both volume contracted (loss of isotonic saline), resulting in tachycardia and hypotension, and dehydrated (pure water loss), reflected by hypertonicity. Since the tonicity of isotonic saline (308 mOsm/L) is always hypotonic to the patient's tonicity, most authors suggest initially infusing isotonic saline (usually at 1 L/hr) until blood pressure and heart rate are normalized. With more severe dehydration and hypernatremia, some combination of isotonic saline (to correct volume deficits) and hypotonic saline (to correct hypertonicity and water deficits) will be required. Most patients respond well to receiving the first liter of fluid in the first hour, and then the next liter over the next 2 hours. Thereafter, the rate and tonicity of the fluid must depend on the clinical status of the patient. Elderly patients need to be managed more cautiously.

Rehydration itself will dramatically lower blood glucose levels. However, all patients require insulin therapy, although they are less resistant than those in DKA. Most authors recommend 3 to 4 units/hour initially, although many do well with 1 to 2 units/hour, especially once plasma glucose levels reach 250 mg/dl. At this stage, 5% dextrose should be added to the intravenous solutions, as in the treatment of DKA.

Hypokalemic emergencies are less of a concern in HHNS compared with DKA, most likely because these patients usually have less vomiting before admission. Therefore the rates of potassium replacement should be more cautious, based on renal function and serum potassium level.

MICROVASCULAR COMPLICATIONS

Retinopathy

Diabetic retinopathy is the leading cause of blindness in the United States.[1] Approximately 5% of patients with diabetes progress to severe visual loss of 5/200 or less. Several risk factors exist for the development of diabetic retinopathy. The first is duration of disease. The risk of having any diabetic retinopathy after 15 years duration is 98% for individuals with type 1 diabetes and 78% for those with type 2 diabetes. The second risk factor, now definitively proven, is glycemic control, which should be conceptualized as *glycemic exposure*. This is considered the amount of time exposed to a given level of hyperglycemia. For example, in the DCCT it was shown that 9-years' exposure to a HbA_{1c} level of 8% yields approximately the same risk of retinopathy as 2.5 years at a HbA_{1c} level of 11%. The final important risk is hypertension. In the UKPDS, an average blood pressure of 144/82 compared with 154/87 resulted in a 47% decreased risk in the deterioration of visual acuity from diabetic retinopathy.[30]

Diabetic retinopathy may be classified as nonproliferative (background) or proliferative retinopathy. Nonproliferative diabetic retinopathy (NPDR) is characterized by structural abnormalities of the retinal vessels, varying degrees of retinal hypoperfusion, retinal edema, lipid exudates, and intraretinal hemorrhages. Neovascularization is the hallmark of proliferative diabetic retinopathy (PDR), and may occur on the optic disc, elsewhere in the retina, or on the iris (rubeosis iridis). Neovascular tissue contains both a vascular and fibrous component. The former may cause preretinal or vitreous hemorrhage, and the latter may interact with the vitreous to produce traction on the retina and subsequent retinal detachment. It needs to be appreciated that both PDR and NPDR may result in visual loss. For example, macular edema is a serious form of NPDR that may only be diagnosed by viewing the macula stereoscopically.

For the primary care physician caring for the patient with diabetes, management of diabetic retinopathy can be divided into prevention, screening, and treatment. For prevention, it is clear that both blood glucose control and blood pressure control can decrease the risk for the development and progression of diabetic retinopathy.

Because treatments for diabetic maculopathy and proliferative retinopathy are most effective when initiated early, it is incumbent on the physician to obtain ophthalmic consultation on patients with diabetes who complain of decreasing vision and/or demonstrate any retinal vascular abnormalities. Screening recommendations include a yearly dilated retinal examination for individuals with type 2 diabetes. For those with type 1 diabetes, yearly screening examinations should begin after 5 years of disease but not before puberty. Women with diabetes who become pregnant should have a dilated eye examination in the first trimester of pregnancy and close follow-up throughout the pregnancy. Screening examinations should be performed by a trained eye care professional and should include a stereoscopic examination.

The Diabetic Retinopathy Study proved that argon laser panretinal photocoagulation significantly decreases the likelihood that eyes with proliferative retinopathy will progress to severe visual loss.[11] Other controlled studies proved the effectiveness of focal argon laser photocoagulation in decreasing or stabilizing diabetic macular edema and the value of vitrectomy in managing the severe complications of diabetic retinopathy.

It needs to be appreciated that numerous studies have shown that rapid improvement of glycemic control may actually result in a worsening of preexisting retinopathy. Patients at highest risk of this are those with longstanding poor control and a moderate stage of NPDR. Although there was no serious visual loss noted in subjects participating in the DCCT, other reports have noted a decrease in visual acuity. Patients at high risk of early worsening should have more frequent ophthalmologic evaluations. Although not yet formally studied, many recommend a slower improvement of glycemic control in these patients. For those individuals who already have advanced retinopathy, it would be prudent to delay improvement of glycemic control until after photocoagulation treatment is completed.

Although not considered microvascular disease, there are other ocular complications that occur more frequently in people with diabetes. The first is cataract formation, which is present in 22% of adults with diabetes compared with 3% of those without. For those diagnosed with diabetes after reaching the age of 30 years, cataract formation is responsible for more decrease in vision than diabetic retinopathy. Similarly, glaucoma is more common, being present in 7% of individuals with diabetes compared with 1% in the general population. Glycemic control may be important for these complications as well. For example, in the UKPDS the intensive group had a 24% reduction in need for cataract extraction.[28]

Nephropathy

Diabetic nephropathy occurs with an overall prevalence of approximately 20% to 30%. Although it is often noted that nephropathy is more common in type 1 than in type 2 diabetes, this point is now under some debate. Younger patients with type 1 diabetes frequently develop ESRD without significant cardiac disease. On the other hand, older individuals with type 2 diabetes may have significant nephropathy (manifested by heavy proteinuria) with normal renal function when they succumb to coronary artery disease. Proteinuria is an independent risk factor of cardiac death, and these older patients have other risks such as dyslipidemia and hypertension. Furthermore, diabetic nephropathy is more common in certain ethnic populations (African-Americans, Native Americans, Mexican-Americans) for which the prevalence of type 2 diabetes is increasing. Individuals with type 2 diabetes are the largest group entering treatment programs for ESRD in the United States. The mean 5-year life expectancy for patients with diabetes-related ESRD is less than 20% in the absence of transplantation.

The major risk factors for the development or progression of diabetic nephropathy are poor glycemic control and the presence of hypertension. Both of these risk factors are well supported by both observational and prospective studies. Other reported risk factors include duration of diabetes, family history of diabetic nephropathy, male gender, cigarette smoking, and ethnicity (as noted above). There is increasing support that one or several genes may predispose to nephropathy. Hypercholesterolemia may be an independent risk factor for the development and progression of diabetic nephropathy. Indeed, it has been reported that treating patients with nephropathy with a 3-hydroxy-3-methylglutaryl coenzyme A (HMG CoA) reductase inhibitor may slow the progression of established renal disease.

Although the natural history of diabetic nephropathy has been described for type 1 diabetes, it appears to be similar in type 2 diabetes. The hallmark of diabetic nephropathy is albuminuria, which reflects both histologic and functional abnormalities of the kidney. Microalbuminuria is the earliest laboratory finding in nephropathy, and occurs 5 to 8 years before the onset of overt proteinuria. Normoalbuminuria is present with albumin excretion rates below 30 mg/day, whereas microalbuminuria is defined by an albumin excretion rate of 30 to 300 mg/day. An albumin excretion rate greater than 300 mg/day defines clinical nephropathy, also known as overt proteinuria, dipstick positive proteinuria, or macroalbuminuria. At this stage, the usual commercial dipstick for proteinuria is positive.

Without intervention, there is relentless progression from microalbuminuria to clinical nephropathy. Intervention in the microalbuminuria stage (at which time renal function is normal) can reverse the albuminuria and halt or slow the progression of the nephropathy. If intervention does not occur until clinical nephropathy is present (when renal function is normal or slightly decreased), the progression of the nephropathy can be slowed considerably, but it is rare to have it stabilize and at this point it will not reverse. Without any intervention at this stage, the average rate of decline in glomerular filtration rate (GFR) is about 1 ml/min/month, but there is wide variation in this. Without intervention, most patients with type 1 diabetes develop ESRD within 18 years after the diagnosis of their diabetes. With improved screening and intervention, this dismal figure hopefully will improve.

There are four interventions to consider once albuminuria is discovered. The first is meticulous glycemic control. Numerous studies have shown that near-normal glucose control can reduce the albumin excretion rate and prevent the progression to overt proteinuria. There are less data about the impact of glycemic control with more advanced nephropathy, but available evidence suggests the more advanced the renal disease the less impact glycemic control will have on slowing its progression.

The second intervention is scrupulous blood pressure control. Studies from the early 1980s clearly showed that controlling systemic blood pressure slows the rate of decline of renal function and improves survival.[20] In these studies, the primary drugs used were cardioselective β-blockers and loop diuretics.

Later, it was shown that angiotensin-converting enzyme (ACE) inhibitors have an incremental beneficial effect, by virtue of selective efferent arteriolar dilation.[18] Indeed, ACE inhibitors offer beneficial effects on microalbuminuria even in the absence of systemic hypertension.[23] ACE inhibitors also have proven to be of benefit in patients with established nephropathy and mild renal insufficiency.[17]

The fourth intervention for diabetic nephropathy is dietary protein restriction.[21] It is thought that this strategy is useful in reducing renal plasma flow, thus improving glomerular hemodynamics in diabetic renal disease. The ADA currently recommends 0.8 grams of protein/kg/day (or about 10% of daily total calories) in patients with clinical nephropathy.

With the identification of these intervention strategies, screening for diabetic nephropathy needs to be a routine aspect of diabetes care. The ADA recommends yearly screening for individuals with type 2 diabetes, and yearly screening for those with type 1 diabetes after 5-years' duration of disease (but not before puberty).[4] Several screening techniques are available; a random albumin-to-creatinine ratio from a spot collection and a timed (e.g., overnight) or 24-hour urine collection for albuminuria and creatinine are all acceptable. Positive results need to be confirmed with a second measurement due to the high variability in albumin excretion in people with diabetes. Box 96-3 lists substances and circumstances that may result in false-positive screening. Urine dipsticks for microalbuminuria are reasonable for an initial screen but are "semiquantitative," and long-term data on their use are not available.

With our increasingly effective interventions for diabetic nephropathy, one of the most debilitating of diabetic complications, it is imperative that screening becomes routine. Due to the great expense of dialysis and renal transplantation, it is not surprising that screening has been shown to be extremely cost-effective.

Neuropathy

There are several classifications of the various diabetic neuropathies. One such clinical classification is noted in Box 96-4.

Box 96-3. Etiologies of False-positive Measurements for Albuminuria

- Uncontrolled hyperglycemia
- Uncontrolled hypertension
- Menstrual bleeding
- Urinary tract infection
- Exercise just prior to or during collection
- Thyrotoxicosis

Box 96-4. Clinical Classification of Diabetic Neuropathies

Peripheral Neuropathies
Polyneuropathies

Distal symmetric neuropathy
Sensory loss with numbness
Dysesthesias
Paresthesias
Chronic sensorimotor
Acute sensory
Muscle pain
Neuropathic foot ulceration
Neuroarthropathy (Charcot's joint)

Mononeuropathies

Mononeuropathy
  Cranial neuropathies
  Compression or entrapment neuropathies
Isolated peripheral
Proximal motor
Mononeuropathy multiplex
Plexopathy
Diabetic truncal neuropathy or radiculopathy

Autonomic Neuropathies
Cardiovascular autonomic neuropathy

Cardiac denervation syndrome
Postural hypotension

Gastrointestinal neuropathy

Gastroparesis diabeticorum
Diabetic diarrhea
Fecal incontinence
Constipation

Genitourinary neuropathy

Diabetic cystopathy
Impotence
Female sexual dysfunction

Sudomotor dysfunction

Pupillary abnormalities

Painful chronic sensorimotor neuropathy (symmetric polyneuropathy) is one of the most common complaints of individuals with diabetes. Estimates vary, but two large studies noted that symptomatic neuropathy had a prevalence of almost 30% in people with diabetes. Another report noted that only 13% of the diabetic population had symptomatic neuropathy, yet more than half of the study sample had clinical evidence of neuropathy on examination. Thus careful clinical examination is important to identify which patients are affected, since an insensate foot is a strong predictor of neuropathic ulcer and lower extremity amputation. Although decreased vibratory sensation and absent ankle reflexes are the hallmarks of this complication, the inability to appreciate the 10-gram (5.07) Semmes-Weinstein monofilament is the simplest and cheapest way to determine if plantar sensation is sufficient to protect from future ulceration. The inability to detect this pressure necessitates further education regarding frequent foot inspection, proper foot care, and the need for extra-depth shoes.

The exact pathogenesis of diabetic symmetric polyneuropathy is not entirely clear. It is likely that the pathogenesis is multifactorial, with both hyperglycemia and other factors playing a role. Therefore it is not surprising that there is not a single, definitive treatment to relieve the pain, although improved glycemic control is effective in some patients. Certainly, improving glycemic control can delay progression of neuropathy. There is some suggestion that in addition to improvement of HbA_{1c}, glycemic stability is also important. Rapid swings from hypoglycemia to hyperglycemia may aggravate neuropathic pain and may actually be more detrimental than continued hyperglycemia.

Tricyclic antidepressants have been the first-line drug for the treatment of painful symmetric polyneuropathy. They are not efficacious, however, in everyone and there is no way to predict whom they will benefit. Some prefer to use amitriptyline for those patients who have difficulty falling asleep. A number of other drugs have been reported to be useful. These include phenytoin, carbamazepine, mexiletine, lidocaine, and topical capsaicin. There has recently been great enthusiasm for the use of gabapentin, and one large clinical trial reported this agent to be beneficial. Unfortunately, there is no mechanism to predict which drug will benefit which patient.

Autonomic neuropathy is common but its clinical presentation is quite variable. Parasympathetic dysfunction, which may only be manifested by an increase in heart rate, has been shown to be present in 65% of patients with type 2 diabetes 10 years after diagnosis. Gastroparesis is one of the most frustrating of the autonomic neuropathies. Mild cases can often be treated by the avoidance of high-fat foods in conjunction with either metoclopramide or cisapride. Cases presenting with refractory nausea and vomiting often require hospitalization with intravenous metoclopramide. Some patients respond to prochlorperazine, and there are data to suggest that erythromycin, especially if given intravenously, may be effective. Abnormal sweating is another common type of autonomic neuropathy. Gustatory sweating is particularly troublesome, with profuse sweating of the face, trunk, and upper neck associated with eating. More common is reduced sweating of the feet, a form of sympathetic dysfunction. This is potentially a risk factor for plantar fissures, and in combination with sensory polyneuropathy adds to the risk of a neuropathic ulcer. Moisturizing creams should be used daily in these individuals.

MACROVASCULAR COMPLICATIONS

Cardiovascular (CV) disease is the major cause of death in patients with diabetes. Individuals with diabetes have a twofold to sixfold increased risk of having a CV event compared with age-matched controls. Heart failure is the most common cause of hospitalization for patients with diabetes, increased by sixfold in men and ninefold in women.

Although patients with diabetes have a higher prevalence of the traditional risk factors for coronary artery disease (CAD), these risk factors account for less than half of the excess mortality seen in this population. Thus diabetes per se is an independent risk factor for the development of CAD.

The mechanisms by which diabetes increases CV risk are complex. Nonenzymatic glycation of proteins appears to promote atherosclerosis. The resultant insoluble proteins, called advanced glycation end products (AGEs), are increased in diabetes. AGEs accelerate atherosclerosis in a variety of ways. In addition, glycation of lipoproteins enhances their atherogenic potential. Both the degradation and release of LDL cholesterol are impaired by glycation, while glycated HDL results in increasing HDL clearance.

A clustering of risk factors for CV disease is termed the *insulin metabolic syndrome* (IMS), also known as the *syndrome of insulin resistance* or *syndrome X*. The components of this syndrome are noted in Box 96-5. Any individual may have various components of this syndrome present at any one time. It is thought that insulin resistance is the key underlying factor in this syndrome. Compensatory hyperinsulinemia develops, and is a marker of the insulin-resistant state. Unfortunately, much confusion exists about this, principally because hyperinsulinemia is easily measured, whereas direct measurement of insulin resistance is complex. Thus, in many epidemiologic studies, insulin was measured as a surrogate for insulin resistance. These studies have often found a correlation between hyperinsulinemia and CV outcome. Yet, hyperinsulinemia is not an independent risk factor for CV disease, although insulin resistance may be a risk factor. Most important, the circulating insulin levels that are a consequence of exogenous insulin therapy do not increase risk. This was shown in the UKPDS, where there was no added risk in subjects randomized to insulin therapy. Indeed, there tended to be an improvement of risk for CV events when insulin was used.

In view of the increased CV risk in patients with diabetes, current recommendations are for aggressive control of all CV risk factors, as well as increased screening for heart disease, even in asymptomatic individuals. Box 96-6 presents the best evidence and summarizes indications for CAD testing.[3]

Box 96-5. Components of the Insulin Metabolic Syndrome

- Insulin resistance
- Hyperinsulinemia
- Glucose intolerance or type 2 diabetes
- Hypertension
- Dyslipidemia—hypertriglyceridemia and decreased HDL cholesterol
- Small, dense LDL cholesterol particles
- Increased uric acid
- Increased plasminogen activator inhibitor
- Coronary artery disease

Box 96-6. Indications for Cardiac Testing in Diabetic Patients

Testing for CAD is Warranted in Patients with the Following:

Typical or atypical cardiac symptoms

Resting electrocardiograph suggestive of ischemia or infarction

Peripheral or carotid occlusive arterial disease

Sedentary lifestyle, age ≥35 years, and plans to begin a vigorous exercise program

Two or more of the following risk factors in addition to diabetes:

- Total cholesterol ≥240 mg/dl, LDL cholesterol ≥160 mg/dl, or HDL cholesterol <35 mg/dl
- Blood pressure > 140/90 mm Hg
- Smoking
- Family history of premature CAD
- Positive microalbuminuria/macroalbuminuria

From Consensus Development Conference on the Diagnosis of Coronary Heart Disease in People With Diabetes, *Diabetes Care* 21:1551-1559, 1998.

Lipids

The most characteristic pattern of dyslipidemia in type 2 diabetic patients is elevated triglyceride levels and decreased HDL cholesterol levels. Yet, LDL cholesterol levels likely are more important in conferring risk. Although the concentration of LDL cholesterol in type 2 diabetic patients (without nephropathy) is usually not significantly different from nondiabetic individuals, LDL cholesterol elevations are common in both diabetic patients and the general population. Moreover, type 2 diabetic patients typically have a preponderance of small, dense LDL particles, which are more atherogenic than typical big, fluffy LDL particles.

There are new recommendations for treatment of dyslipidemia for adults with diabetes. These recommendations are based on recent prospective randomized intervention studies that included subjects with diabetes. The most important of these are the Scandinavian Simvastatin Survival Study (4S)[22] and the Cholesterol and Recurrent Events (CARE) trial.[14] 4S was a trial in patients, including 202 with diabetes, with known coronary heart disease (CHD) manifested by angina pectoris or previous myocardial infarction, who had serum cholesterol levels of 213 to 310 mg/dl (5.5 to 8 mmol/L) while on a lipid-lowering diet. Among the diabetic patients, active treatment with simvastatin reduced total mortality by 43%, major CV events by 55%, and any atherosclerotic event by 37%. CARE was a trial in patients, including 586 with diabetes, with myocardial infarction who had LDL cholesterol levels of 115 to 174 mg/dl (3 to 4.5 mmol/L). Among the diabetic patients, active treatment with pravastatin reduced the absolute risk of

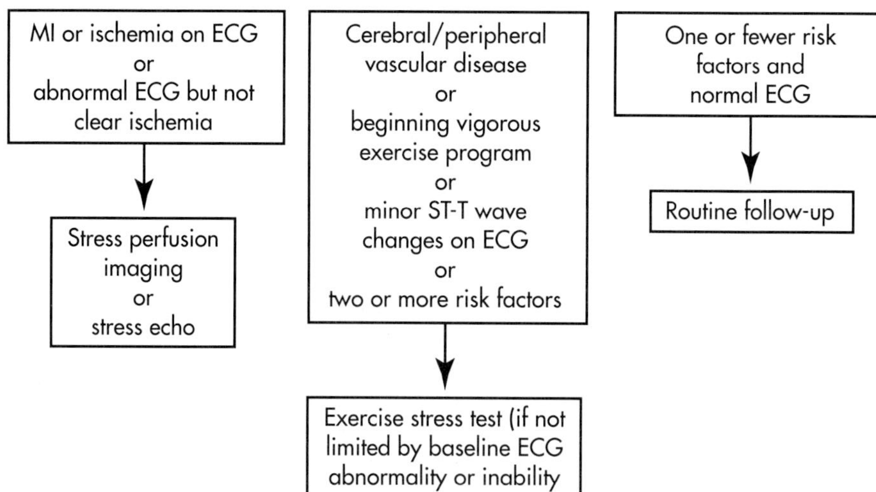

Fig. 96-10. Cardiac testing of the asymptomatic diabetic patient. (From Consensus Development Conference on the Diagnosis of Coronary Heart Disease in People With Diabetes, *Diabetes Care* 21:1551-1559, 1998.)

coronary events for the diabetic patients by 8.1% and the relative risk by 25%, and reduced the relative risk for revascularization procedures by 32%.

These and other studies have resulted in a revised set of recommendations from the ADA for lipoprotein goals for individuals with diabetes.[5] The goal is to achieve LDL cholesterol level of ≤100 mg/dl (2.60 mmol/L). Medical nutrition therapy should be instituted in all patients with values above this level. Pharmacologic agents should be added if this level is not reached, unless there is no history of CHD and no other risk factors are present, in which case pharmacologic agents are used only if LDL cholesterol level is above 130 mg/dl (3.35 mmol/L). Since a large proportion of diabetic patients die before they reach the hospital, a preventive strategy based solely on secondary intervention would not be able to "save" large numbers of these diabetic patients. Furthermore, the ADA has developed an algorithm for the screening of CAD (Fig. 96-10).[3]

Blood Pressure

Several randomized controlled clinical trials have addressed the influence of blood pressure control in diabetes. The Hypertension in Diabetes Study (HDS) was embedded in the UKPDS by using a factorial design, and included 1148 patients with type 2 diabetes with coexisting hypertension.[30] Risk reductions among patients assigned "tight" control were substantial: 24% for "any diabetes-related endpoint," 32% for diabetes-related deaths, 56% for heart failure, 44% for stroke, and 37% for microvascular disease. The Hypertension Optimal Treatment (HOT) Study included 1501 patients with diabetes.[15] They were randomly assigned to different target diastolic blood pressure groups: ≤90 mm Hg, ≤85 mm Hg, and ≤80 mm Hg. In patients with the lowest target blood pressure (≤80 mm Hg), there was a decline in the rate of major CV events, CV mortality, and total mortality. The Systolic Hypertension in Europe (Syst-Eur) Trial included 492 patients with diabetes.[27] Active treatment to reduce systolic blood pressure by at least 20 mm Hg and to less than 150 mm Hg among the diabetic patients reduced overall mortality by 55%, mortality from CV disease by 76%, all CV events combined by 69%, fatal and nonfatal strokes by 73%, and all cardiac events combined by 63%.

The primary goal of therapy for (nonpregnant) adults (>18 years of age) with diabetes is to decrease blood pressure to and maintain it at <130 mm Hg systolic and <85 mm Hg diastolic. It should be noted, however, that the risks for end-organ damage appear to be lowest when the systolic blood pressure is <120 mm Hg and the diastolic blood pressure is <80 mm Hg.

Aspirin

A number of studies have established the beneficial effect of aspirin therapy on CV risk. In the Physicians' Health Study diabetic physicians had risk reductions for myocardial infarction of 61% and for peripheral artery surgery of 46%.[26] In the Early Treatment Diabetic Retinopathy Study (ETDRS), risk reduction for myocardial infarction in those randomized to aspirin was 28%.[12] In the HOT Study, aspirin reduced major CV events by 15% and myocardial infarction by 36%.[15] Risk reduction was also seen among diabetic patients in a meta-analysis of antiplatelet therapy involving ~100,000 patients.[6]

Thus there are beneficial effects of antiplatelet therapy, particularly with aspirin, in diabetic patients, impacting on various diabetic complications. The ADA advocates use of aspirin therapy as a secondary prevention strategy in diabetic men and women who have evidence of large vessel disease, including a history of myocardial infarction, vascular bypass procedure, stroke or transient ischemic attack, peripheral vascular disease, claudication, and/or angina. ADA also recommends considering aspirin therapy as a primary prevention strategy in high-risk men and women with type 1 or type 2 diabetes.

PREGNANCY AND DIABETES

Pregnancy in Women With Diabetes

During the past 2 decades, perinatal outcome has improved remarkably in this high-risk group.[16] Excellent control of maternal diabetes will reduce the risks of fetal demise, excessive fetal growth, and delayed pulmonary maturation. Except for deaths due to major fetal malformations, the perinatal mortality rate for women with diabetes who receive optimal care now approaches that of the general obstetric population.

Table 96-6. Representative Target Glucose Levels for a Pregnant Woman with Type 1 Diabetes

	mg/dl	mmol/L
Fasting	60-90	3.3-5.0
Preprandial	60-105	3.3-5.8
1-hour postprandial	70-140	3.9-7.8
2-hour postprandial	60-120	3.3-6.7
Bedtime	60-120	3.3-6.7
2 to 4 AM	60-100	3.3-5.5

To prevent early pregnancy loss and to reduce the risk of fetal malformations and maternal and fetal complications, pregnant women and women planning pregnancy require excellent blood glucose control. Therefore optimal medical care and patient education and training must begin before conception. Because of the need for prepregnancy planning and excellent glucose control, pregnancy in women with diabetes should be planned in advance. Therefore women not attempting to conceive should use effective methods of contraception.

Glycemic targets during pregnancy are more stringent than otherwise, because of the profound potential adverse impact of even modest hyperglycemia on the fetus (Table 96-6). Treatment should include more frequent SMBG, extra snacks to avert hypoglycemia, and expectation of progressive increase of insulin requirement during the course of gestation, as a consequence of insulin resistance induced by placental hormones.

Maintaining maternal glucose levels in the desired range throughout gestation is difficult. During the first trimester, morning sickness may be troublesome and the risk of hypoglycemia increased; hypoglycemia is most likely during the night, when the mother is fasting but the fetus and placenta continue to consume glucose. In contrast, during the early third trimester, when the diabetogenic stress of pregnancy is greatest, insulin needs may rise 50% to 100% over 4 to 6 weeks, heightening the risk for ketoacidosis. The total insulin dose may double, or even treble, compared with the prepregnancy dose.

The outcome for both mother and baby is generally more favorable when an experienced team is responsible for management during pregnancy, delivery, and the perinatal period. The team ideally includes an experienced medical management team, including internist or endocrinologist, obstetrician or maternal-fetal specialist, pediatrician or neonatologist, teaching nurse, dietitian, and the patient and her partner. Pregnant women are usually highly motivated; therefore this time is ideal for teaching self-care skills they can use for the rest of their lives.

Delivery can be safely delayed until term in most pregnancies complicated by type 1 diabetes. Labor may then be induced when the cervix is favorable, or the onset of spontaneous labor may be awaited. Patients must continue excellent glycemic control, and all parameters of antepartum fetal surveillance should remain normal. The timing and site of delivery must be discussed and coordinated with the neonatologists who are to be present.

Box 96-7. Diagnostic Criteria: Gestational Diabetes Mellitus

Procedure

Oral glucose is administered in a dose of 100 grams (in adults). A fasting baseline sample is obtained (at 0 minutes) before glucose is consumed. Blood samples are obtained at 60, 120, and 180 minutes after glucose consumption is complete for the determination of plasma glucose.

Interpretation

Gestational diabetes mellitus (GDM) is diagnosed if two or more values equal or exceed those listed.

	mg/dl	mmol/L
Fasting	105	10.5
1 hour	190	10.6
2 hour	165	9.2
3 hour	145	8.1

Gestational Diabetes Mellitus

Gestational diabetes mellitus (GDM) has its onset during pregnancy, with virtually all women returning to normal glucose tolerance after parturition. A history of GDM, however, heralds a marked increased risk of future diabetes.

As a consequence of the potential dangers to the fetus of GDM, it is recommended that all pregnant women be screened for abnormal glucose levels at approximately 26 to 28 weeks gestation. The recommended screening test is measurement of plasma glucose 1 hour after consumption of 50 gm of glucose. Values $140 mg/dl warrant a full OGTT (performed according to pregnancy protocol [Box 96-7]).

SUMMARY

The impact of diabetes is staggering. In the future, this need not be. Future development of blindness, kidney failure, amputation, and heart disease can be markedly lessened by scrupulous attention to therapies and preventive approaches demonstrated to be effective.

Since the discovery of insulin in the 1920s, the seminal question for physicians caring for diabetic patients, and for the patients themselves, has been whether the risk of diabetic complications can be altered by careful control of glycemia. For decades, this crucial question vexed all concerned. Finally, the question has been answered in the affirmative as a consequence of carefully conducted, prospective, randomized controlled clinical trials. The landmark DCCT, first reported in 1993, established this relationship for type 1 diabetes. The DCCT convincingly and unequivocally verified the then-growing database derived from smaller randomized (mostly European) prospective intervention trials of meticulous control in type 1 diabetes. Subsequently, again with prospective, randomized trials, the importance of glycemic control was demonstrated in type 2 diabetes, first in the relatively small Kumamoto Study using insulin therapy, and then in the monumental UKPDS.[19,28,29]

UKPDS demonstrated risk reductions in spite of the fact that the degree of glycemic separation was less than 1% for HbA_{1c}. The mean HbA_{1c} in the conventional group was less than 8%, with risk reductions clearly seen when HbA_{1c} was 7%. Given the relatively low glycemic exposure and the small differences between groups, an important conclusion is that appropriate treatment targets should be HbA_{1c} of ~7%, as recommended by ADA. The 8% ADA "action suggested" threshold is simply not good enough. More intensive glycemic control leads to reduced risk of diabetic complications.

In addition to attainment of meticulous glycemic control, randomized controlled clinical trials, completed over the last several years, have clearly demonstrated the benefits in diabetic patients of aggressive blood pressure control, lowering of LDL cholesterol, and use of aspirin therapy. There can no longer be any excuse to ignore these important risk factors. To reduce the burden of diabetes also requires the appropriate use of proven therapies and technologies (e.g., laser photocoagulation, early introduction of ACE inhibitors or angiotensin receptor blockers, and routine foot care.

EBM EVIDENCE-BASED MEDICINE

Primary sources for this chapter were MEDLINE and American Diabetes Association Clinical Practice Recommendations (Diabetes Care 1999; 22:Supplement 1). Electronic searches, conducted between January and April 1999, focused on randomized controlled clinical trials and meta-analyses.

REFERENCES

1. Aiello LP, Gardner TW, King GL, et al: Technical review: diabetic retinopathy, *Diabetes Care* 21:143-156, 1998.
2. American Diabetes Association: Report of the Expert Committee on the Diagnosis and Classification of Diabetes Mellitus, *Diabetes Care* 20:1183-1197, 1997.
3. American Diabetes Association: Consensus statement: diagnosis of coronary heart disease in people with diabetes, *Diabetes Care* 21:1551-1559, 1998.
4. American Diabetes Association: Standards of medical care for patients with diabetes mellitus, *Diabetes Care* 23: (Suppl 1):S32-S42, 2000.
5. American Diabetes Association: Position statement: management of dyslipidemia in adults with diabetes, *Diabetes Care* 23: (Suppl 1):S57-S61, 2000.
6. Antiplatelet Trialists' Collaboration: Collaborative overview of randomised trials of antiplatelet therapy. I: Prevention of death, myocardial infarction, and stroke by prolonged antiplatelet therapy in various categories of patients, *BMJ* 308:81-106, 1994.
7. Bach JF: Insulin-dependent diabetes mellitus as an autoimmune disease, *Endocrine Reviews* 15:516-542, 1994.
8. Centers for Disease Control and Prevention: *The public health of diabetes mellitus in the United States,* Atlanta, 1997, US Department of Health and Human Services.
9. DeFronzo RA, Bonadonna RC, Ferrannini E: Pathogenesis of NIDDM: a balanced overview, *Diabetes Care* 15:318-368, 1992.
10. Diabetes Control and Complications Trial Research Group: The effect of intensive treatment of diabetes on the development and progression of long-term complications in insulin-dependent diabetes mellitus, *New Engl J Med* 329:683-689, 1993.
11. Diabetic Retinopathy Study Research Group: Photocoagulation treatment of diabetic retinopathy: clinical application of Diabetic Retinopathy Study (DRS) findings: DRS report number 8, *Ophthalmology* 88:583-600, 1981.
12. ETDRS Investigators: Aspirin effects on mortality and morbidity in patients with diabetes mellitus. Early Treatment Diabetic Retinopathy Study Report 14, *JAMA* 268:1292-1300, 1992.
13. Farkas-Hirsch RM, editor: *Intensive diabetes management,* ed 2, Alexandria, Va, 1998, American Diabetes Association.
14. Goldberg RB, Mellies MJ, Sacks FM, et al: Cardiovascular events and their reduction with pravastatin in diabetic and glucose-intolerant myocardial infarction survivors with average cholesterol levels: subgroup analyses in the Cholesterol and Recurrent Events (CARE) trial, *Circulation* 23:2513-2519, 1998.
15. Hansson L, Zanchetti A, Carruthers SG, et al: Effects of intensive blood-pressure lowering and low-dose aspirin in patients with hypertension: principal results of the Hypertension Optimal Treatment (HOT) randomised trial, *Lancet* 351:1755-1762, 1998.
16. Jovanovic L, editor: *Medical management of pregnancy complicated by diabetes,* ed 2, Alexandria, Va, 1998, American Diabetes Association.
17. Lewis EJ, Hunsicker LG, Bain RP, et al for the Collaborative Study Group: The effect of angiotensin-converting-enzyme inhibition on diabetic nephropathy, *New Engl J Med* 329:1456-1462, 1993.
18. Microalbuminuria Captopril Study Group: Captopril reduces the risk of nephropathy in IDDM patients with microalbuminuria, *Diabetologia* 39:587-593, 1996.
19. Ohkubo Y, Kishikawa H, Araki E, et al: Intensive insulin therapy prevents the progression of diabetic microvascular complications in Japanese patients with non–insulin-dependent diabetes mellitus: a randomized prospective 6-year study, *Diabetes Res Clin Pract* 28:103-117, 1995.
20. Parving H-H, Andersen AR, Smidt UM, et al: Early aggressive antihypertensive treatment reduced rate of decline in kidney function in diabetic nephropathy, *Lancet* i:1175-1179, 1983.
21. Pedrini MT, Levey AS, Lau J, et al: Dietary protein restriction on the progression of diabetic and nondiabetic renal diseases: a meta-analysis, *Ann Intern Med* 124:627-632, 1996.
22. Pyrälä K, Pedersen TR, Kjekshus J, et al: Cholesterol lowering with simvastatin improves prognosis of diabetic patients with coronary heart disease: a subgroup analysis of the Scandinavian Simvastatin Survival Study (4S), *Diabetes Care* 20:614-620, 1997.
23. Ravid M, Lang R, Rachmani R, et al: Long-term renoprotective effect of angiotensin-converting enzyme inhibition in non–insulin-dependent diabetes mellitus: a 7-year follow-up study, *Arch Intern Med* 156:286-289, 1996.
24. Reichard P, Nilsson BY, Rosenqvist U: The effect of long-term intensified insulin treatment on the development of microvascular complications of diabetes mellitus, *New Engl J Med* 329:304-309, 1993.
25. Skyler J, editor: *Medical management of type 1 diabetes mellitus,* ed 3, Alexandria, Va, 1998, American Diabetes Association.
26. Steering Committee of the Physicians' Health Study Research Group: Final report on the aspirin component of the ongoing Physicians' Health Study, *New Engl J Med* 321:129-135, 1989.
27. Tuomilehto J, Rastenyte D, Birkenhager WH, et al, for the Systolic Hypertension in Europe Trial Investigators: Effects of calcium-channel blockade in older patients with diabetes and systolic hypertension, *New Engl J Med* 340:677-684, 1999.
28. UK Prospective Diabetes Study Group: Intensive blood-glucose control with sulphonylureas or insulin compared with conventional treatment and risk of complications in patients with type 2 diabetes (UKPDS 33), *Lancet* 352:837-853, 1998.
29. UK Prospective Diabetes Study Group: Effect of intensive blood-glucose control with metformin on complications in overweight patients with type 2 diabetes (UKPDS 34), *Lancet* 352:854-865, 1998.
30. UK Prospective Diabetes Study Group: Tight blood pressure control and risk of macrovascular and microvascular complications in type 2 diabetes (UKPDS 38), *BMJ* 317:703-713, 1998.
31. Wang PH, Lau J, Chalmers TC: Meta-analysis of effects of intensive blood glucose control on late complications on type I diabetes, *Lancet* 341:1306-1309, 1993.

CHAPTER 97

Thyroid Gland Disorders

Alan P. Farwell
Susana A. Ebner

Clinical disorders of the thyroid gland are the most common endocrinopathies. As such, it is essential for the primary care physician to recognize the clinical features of the various forms of thyroid dysfunction. In addition, subclinical thyroid disease, a disorder in which mild abnormalities in circulating thyroid hormones are present in the absence of overt symptomatology, is present in up to 17% of patients based on population screening studies. The diagnosis of subclinical thyroid disease allows the identification of clinically euthyroid patients at risk to develop overt thyroid dysfunction. To appropriately identify and manage patients with clinical and subclinical thyroid dysfunction, the physician must first possess an understanding of the fundamentals of thyroid hormone economy, the laboratory evaluation of thyroid function, and the availability of thyroid imaging techniques.

NORMAL THYROID HORMONE ECONOMY

Regulation of the Thyroid-Pituitary Axis

Synthesis and secretion of thyroid hormone is under the control of the anterior pituitary hormone, thyrotropin (thyroid-stimulating hormone [TSH]). TSH secretion increases when serum thyroid hormone concentrations fall, and decreases when they rise, in a classic negative feedback system. TSH is also under the regulation of the hypothalamic hormone, thyrotropin-releasing hormone (TRH). The negative feedback of thyroid hormone is targeted mainly at the pituitary level but probably affects TRH release from the hypothalamus as well. In addition, input from higher cortical centers affects TRH secretion.

Under the influence of TSH, the thyroid gland synthesizes and releases thyroid hormone. Thyroxine (T_4) is the principal secretory product of the thyroid gland, constituting about 90% of the secreted hormone under normal conditions. T_4 is also the most abundant thyroid hormone in serum. Although some effects of thyroid hormone are attributed specifically to T_4, for the most part T_4 functions as a hormone precursor that is metabolized in peripheral tissues to a more active form.

Metabolic Pathways

The major pathway of metabolism of T_4 is by sequential monodeiodination. Removal of the 5′-, or outer ring, iodine is the activating metabolic pathway, leading to the formation of the metabolically active form of thyroid hormone, L-3,5,3′-triiodothyronine (T_3). Removal of the inner ring, or 5-, iodine is an inactivating pathway, producing the metabolically inactive hormone, L-3,3′,5′-triiodothyronine (reverse T_3 [rT_3]). Under normal conditions about 41% of T_4 is converted to T_3, about 38% is converted to rT_3, and about 21% is metabolized via other pathways, such as conjugation in the liver and excretion in the bile.

T_3 is the metabolically active thyroid hormone and exerts its actions via binding to chromatin-bound nuclear receptors and regulating gene transcription in responsive tissues. Only about 10% of circulating T_3 is secreted directly by the thyroid gland, whereas more than 80% is derived from conversion of T_4 in peripheral tissues, primarily in the liver. Thus factors that affect peripheral T_4 to T_3 conversion have significant effects on circulating T_3 levels. Peripheral T_4 to T_3 conversion is catalyzed by type I 5′-deiodinase, which is found primarily in the liver. Serum levels of T_3 are about 100-fold less than those of T_4 and, like T_4, T_3 is metabolized by deiodination, forming diiodothyronine, and by conjugation in the liver.

Serum-binding Proteins

Both T_4 and T_3 circulate in the serum bound to several proteins that are synthesized in the liver. Thyronine-binding globulin (TBG) is the major serum-binding protein and binds about 80% of the serum thyroid hormones. The affinity of T_4 for TBG is about tenfold greater than that of T_3 and is part of the reason that circulating T_4 levels are higher than T_3 levels. Other serum-binding proteins include transthyretin, which binds about 15% of T_4 but little if any T_3, and albumin, which has a low affinity but a very large capacity for binding T_4 and T_3. Overall, 99.97% of circulating T_4 and 99.7% of circulating T_3 are bound to plasma proteins.

Thyroid Function Tests

The development of immunoassays has allowed the easy and reliable measurement of circulating T_4 and T_3 concentrations (Table 97-1). The most widely available assays measure total hormone levels, consisting of both bound and free hormone. Essential to the understanding of the regulation of thyroid function is the *free hormone concept* (i.e., only the unbound hormone has any metabolic activity). Because of the high degree of binding of T_4 and T_3 to the serum-binding proteins, changes in either the concentrations of these proteins or the binding affinity of thyroid hormone to the serum-binding proteins would have major effects on the total serum hormone levels. However, since the pituitary responds to and regulates the circulating free hormone levels, minimal changes in the free hormone concentrations and thus overall thyroid function are seen.

The gold standard for the direct measurement of free T_4 concentrations is equilibrium dialysis. However, this technique requires expertise and is time-consuming. The free T_4 index (FTI) is the most widely available test of free T_4 concentrations and is determined by multiplying the total T_4 concentration by a factor that corrects for changes in serum-binding proteins. This factor is often the T_3 resin uptake, which is an inverse estimate of serum TBG concentrations and is expressed as a percent. The T_3 resin uptake is reduced if the capacity of serum-binding proteins is high and is increased when serum-binding proteins have diminished ability to bind hormone. An attempt to improve on the accuracy of the FTI multiplies the total T_4 by the thyroid hormone binding ratio (THBR), which is determined by dividing the T_3 resin uptake by a standardized "normal" T_3 resin uptake. Other methods to directly measure free thyroid hormone levels besides equilibrium dialysis are also available but are more expensive than the FTI and may be no more accurate. Direct measurements of free T_3 concentrations are also available, but are of limited utility. Serum T_3 concentrations are only useful in the evaluation of thyrotox-

Table 97-1. Tests of Thyroid Function

Test	Typical normal range	Use
TSH	0.4-5.0 mU/L	Best initial test to determine biochemical thyroid status in healthy patients
Total T_4	4-12 μg/dl	Measures bound and free hormone in serum
T_4 or T_3-resin uptake	25-35%	Estimate of the serum-protein binding sites
Thyroid hormone binding ratio (THBR)	0.8-1.15	Estimate of the serum-protein binding sites
Free T_4 Index (FTI)	1-4—if use resin uptake 4-12—if use THBR	Estimate of free T_4 concentrations
Free T_4, equilibrium dialysis method	0.7-2.1 ng/dl	Gold standard for measurement of free T_4 concentrations, expensive, time-consuming to measure
Free T_4, analog method	0.7-1.85 ng/dl	Direct measurement of free T_4 concentrations, may not be more reliable than FTI
Total T_3	75-180 ng/dl	Second-line test, measures bound and free hormone in serum
Free T_3, analog method	200-400 pg/dl	No advantage over total T_3
Reverse T_3	95-350 pg/ml	Inactive T_4 metabolite, rarely clinically indicated
Thyroid antibodies (anti-Tg, anti-TPO)	Negative	Second-line test, determines presence of autoimmune thyroid disease
Thyroglobulin	0-55 ng/ml	Second-line test, intrinsic thyroid protein, useful as a marker for differentiated thyroid cancer

icosis and, for the most part, measurements of total T_3 are sufficient. Assays that measure serum levels of rT_3 are also available but are of little use clinically.

Sensitive TSH Assays. Serum determination of TSH by a sensitive TSH assay is currently the best first test of thyroid status in ambulatory patients. Although TSH assays have been available since 1965, the first-generation assays were useful only for diagnosing primary hypothyroidism, since a lower limit to the normal range could not be reliably measured. The first sensitive TSH assay was developed in 1985, resulting in the expansion of the assay detection limit below the normal range. The main utility of the sensitive TSH assay is to differentiate between normal and thyrotoxic patients, who should exhibit suppressed TSH values. Currently, commercially available TSH assays have a limit of detection of 0.05 mU/L or lower.

With the advent of the sensitive TSH assay came the realization that abnormal TSH values, especially subnormal values, were very common. Abnormal TSH values have been reported in over 15% of hospitalized patients, with more than two thirds of these patients having no intrinsic thyroid dysfunction on follow-up testing after recovery from illness. In addition, 20% to 30% of patients over the age of 60 have abnormal TSH values. The vast majority of these abnormal TSH values are associated with normal FTI determinations, giving rise to the syndromes of subclinical thyroid disease (discussed below). Despite these pitfalls, the following conclusions can be made regarding sensitive TSH assays: (1) normal TSH values are both sensitive and specific to identify normal patients; (2) subnormal and suppressed TSH values are sensitive but not specific to identify thyrotoxic patients; (3) abnormal TSH values require additional biochemical and clinical evaluation before a diagnosis of thyroid dysfunction can be made.

Thyroid Antibodies. Antibodies directed against the thyroid proteins thyroglobulin (Tg) and thyroid peroxidase (TPO, formerly microsomal protein) are markers of autoimmune thyroid disease and are often helpful in determining the etiology of thyroid dysfunction. Of the two, anti-TPO antibodies are most closely associated with autoimmune thyroid disease. Measurement of these antibodies is always a secondary test and may be useful to predict the development of overt thyroid dysfunction. Thyroid-stimulating immunoglobulins (TSI) are the cause of Graves' disease, the most common form of thyrotoxicosis. However, the routine measurement of TSI is not indicated in most patients with Graves' disease. Determination of TSI titers is best reserved for special circumstances, such as in the pregnant patient with Graves' disease (see below).

Thyroid Imaging Studies. Thyroid imaging studies can be divided into those that provide an assessment of gland function vs. those that provide imaging alone. Radioisotope imaging with radioiodine (^{123}I) is commonly utilized to determine the overall activity of the gland in patients with thyrotoxicosis (24-hour radioactive iodine uptake [RAIU]) as well as to provide information regarding the function of parts of the gland, such as nodules. Nodules that take up radioiodine are considered to be functioning, or *warm*. If all of the radioiodine is concentrated within a solitary nodule and serum TSH values are suppressed, the nodule is considered to be toxic, or *hot*. Nodules that fail to concentrate radioiodine are considered to be hypofunctioning (*cool* or *cold*), increasing the chances that those nodules harbor a malignancy. Radioisotope imaging with technetium (^{99m}Tc pertechnetate) provides information on the regional function within the gland but is less informative regarding the overall function of the gland. In addition, an occasional nodule that is functioning with technetium will be cold on imaging with radioiodine. Thus most physicians prefer radioiodine imaging.

Ultrasound provides only structural information and is helpful in identifying cysts and in following the size of nodules, and occasionally is necessary to guide the fine-needle aspiration biopsy of a nodule. Other anatomic imaging modalities include magnetic resonance imaging (MRI) and computed tomography (CT). These latter two studies should never be first-line tests and should be reserved for specialized indications.

HYPOTHYROIDISM

Hypothyroidism is the most common disorder of thyroid function. Worldwide, hypothyroidism is most often the result of iodine deficiency. In the United States, where iodine is sufficient, autoimmune processes account for the majority of cases. The prevalence of newly diagnosed overt hypothyroidism in the United States ranges from two to six cases per 1000 women, and the prevalence of established cases is in the range of 20 to 40 per 1000 women. The prevalence of overt hypothyroidism worldwide is ~5%.

Failure of the thyroid to produce sufficient thyroid hormone is the most common cause of hypothyroidism and is referred to as primary hypothyroidism (Box 97-1). Central hypothyroidism occurs much less often and results from diminished thyroidal stimulation by TSH due to pituitary failure (secondary hypothyroidism) or hypothalamic failure (tertiary hypothyroidism). Chronic autoimmune thyroiditis accounts for about 60% of the cases of hypothyroidism in the United States and is further subdivided into goitrous (Hashimoto's thyroiditis) and atrophic forms. As with other autoimmune diseases, females are affected much more frequently than males (~8:1). Chronic autoimmune thyroiditis is characterized by the presence of thyroid antibodies, which are present in about 7% of the population.

Hypothyroidism resulting from the treatment for hyperthyroidism is the second most common cause and accounts for about 30% of cases. Secondary and tertiary hypothyroidism constitute less than 5% of cases. Congenital hypothyroidism occurs in about 1 in 4000 live births and is the major preventable cause of mental retardation in the world today. Untreated congenital hypothyroidism results in multiple developmental abnormalities known as cretinism. Diagnosis is made primarily through newborn thyroid function screening. Early institution of thyroid hormone replacement therapy results in normal IQ values in treated infants. A rare but increasingly recognized cause of hypothyroidism is generalized thyroid hormone resistance. Serum thyroid hormone concentrations are elevated but unable to exert any action due to genetic defects in the nuclear receptors for thyroid hormone.

Transient hypothyroidism is, by definition, the only reversible form of hypothyroidism. Postpartum thyroiditis, occurring 1 to 6 months after delivery, approaches an incidence of 20% in some series. A hypothyroid phase occurs in more than 60% of individuals and may last up to 1 year. Permanent hypothyroidism occurs in 20% to 30% of those affected. Subacute thyroiditis is also associated with a hypothyroid phase in over two thirds of patients; however, the incidence of permanent hypothyroidism is ~5%.

Box 97-1. Causes of Hypothyroidism

Primary Hypothyroidism

Chronic autoimmune thyroiditis

Goitrous (Hashimoto's)
Atrophic

Therapy for hyperthyroidism

^{131}I therapy
Thyroidectomy
Use of antithyroid drugs

Congenital abnormalities

Thyroid agenesis or dysgenesis
Biosynthetic defects in hormone synthesis

Other

Iodine deficiency
Thyroidectomy for benign or malignant conditions
Head/neck irradiation

Secondary Hypothyroidism

Hypopituitarism
Isolated TSH deficiency

Tertiary Hypothyroidism

Hypothalamic dysfunction
Isolated TRH deficiency

Generalized Thyroid Hormone Resistance

Transient Hypothyroidism

Postpartum thyroiditis
Silent (painless) thyroiditis
Subacute thyroiditis

Patient Evaluation

Regardless of the etiology, the clinical features of hypothyroidism are similar (Box 97-2). The onset of symptoms is usually insidious; thus hypothyroidism may be present for years before it is diagnosed. Despite the fact that every organ system can be involved, most of the symptoms and signs of hypothyroidism are nonspecific. Indeed, in one series a diagnosis of hypothyroidism was established in less than 4% of ambulatory patients with symptoms potentially attributable to the disease. In addition, symptoms do not always correlate with the severity of the hypothyroidism and may be lacking altogether in individuals with overt biochemical evidence of the disease. Weakness, lethargy, constipation, dry skin, and hair loss are common nonspecific symptoms. Characteristic clinical features of hypothyroidism include cold intolerance, facial puffiness, deepening of the voice, and carpal tunnel syndrome (Fig. 97-1).

Some presentations are age specific, such as delayed growth in the child, menorrhagia in premenopausal women, and dementia in the elderly. The clinical picture of florid myxedema includes dull, expressionless facies; slow movements; periorbital puffiness; sparse, coarse hair; macroglossia; and cool, pale, coarse skin (Table 97-2) (Figs. 97-2 and 97-3). The most characteristic clinical finding in hypothyroidism is the delayed relaxation phase of deep tendon reflexes. This is most commonly seen with the Achilles reflex. Small pericardial and pleural effusions are common and occasionally may be massive. Hypothyroid-related pericardial effusions typically do not cause tamponade and nearly always resolve with T_4 therapy.

Sinus bradycardia and flattened T waves are characteristic electrocardiographic (ECG) findings in hypothyroidism.

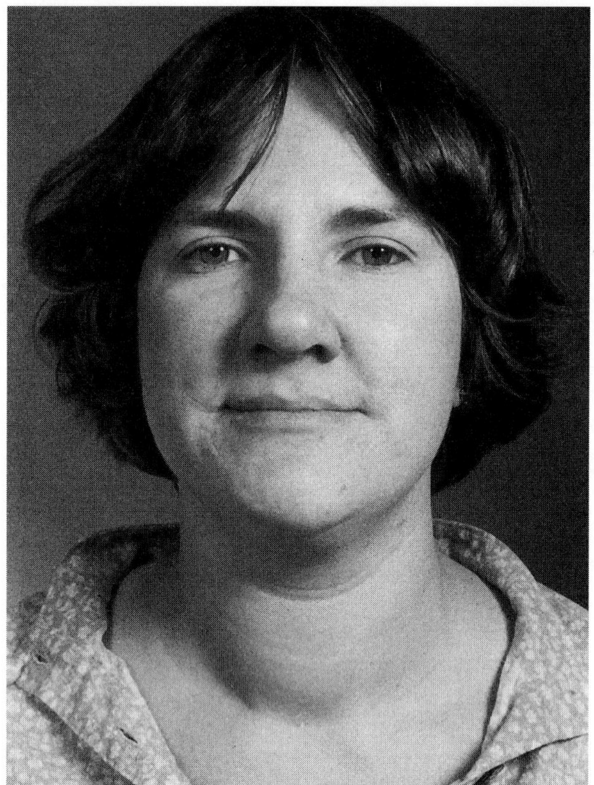

Fig. 97-1. Thirty-year-old patient with Hashimoto's thyroiditis and hypothyroidism. Presenting complaint was thyroid enlargement. T_4 = 4.5 µg/dl, TSH = 84 µU/ml. Note puffiness of face and visible goiter.

Table 97-2. Signs of Hypothyroidism

Sign	Physical examination	Laboratory values
Common (seen in >50% of patients)	Coarse skin Cold skin Pallor of skin Coarse hair Periorbital edema Hoarse voice Goiter Nonpitting edema (myxedema) Delayed relaxation of reflexes	Pericardial effusion Pleural effusion Hyponatremia Hypercholesterolemia Normochromic, normocytic anemia Elevated CPK (MM variant) Decreased basal metabolic rate
Less common (seen in <50% of patients)	Slow speech Sleep apnea Joint effusions Hypothermia Hypertension Hypoventilation Macroglossia Myopathy Cardiomegaly	Sinus bradycardia Flattened T waves Prolonged QT interval Low amplitude QRS complexes Coagulopathy Elevated lactic dehydrogenase Elevated transaminases Hyperprolactinemia

Box 97-2. Symptoms of Hypothyroidism

Common (Seen in >50% of Patients)	Less Common (Seen in <50% of Patients)
Weakness	Depression
Fatigue	Anorexia
Lethargy	Muscle cramps
Decreased energy	Musculoskeletal pain
Cold intolerance	Arthralgias
Dry skin	Infertility
Decreased sweating	Menorrhagia and anovulation
Hair loss	Carpal tunnel syndrome
Inability to concentrate	Decreased hearing
Memory loss	
Constipation	
Weight gain	
Dyspnea	
Peripheral paresthesias	

Hypercholesterolemia occurs in 95% of patients due to impaired clearance of low-density lipoprotein (LDL) and very low-density lipoprotein (VLDL) particles. Dilutional hyponatremia is common due to impaired water excretion. Increased free water retention also produces increased diastolic blood pressure. Elevated creatine phosphokinase (CPK) concentrations (MM variant), occasionally over 1000 U/L, are often seen due to impaired clearance and may raise the possibility of a myocardial infarction until fractionation is performed. A normochromic, normocytic anemia is frequently found.

Diagnosis

The best initial test in the evaluation of hypothyroidism is a sensitive TSH, since 95% of hypothyroid patients have primary thyroid failure. Indeed, increased serum TSH concentrations are the most sensitive indicator of the failing thyroid. However, modest elevations of TSH (usually under 15 mU/L) are often associated with normal T_4 values, identifying those individuals with subclinical hypothyroidism. At present there is no consensus on the indications for treatment in healthy individuals with subclinical hypothyroidism (see further).

Since the hallmark of hypothyroidism is the presence of decreased serum concentrations of thyroid hormones, the measurement of T_4 should be considered in most individuals (see Table 97-1). Since alterations in serum hormone binding capacity can alter total T_4 concentrations and obscure the diagnosis of hypothyroidism (Box 97-3), an estimation of free T_4 concentrations by the FTI method is often valuable. The measurement of serum T_3 concentrations has a low sensitivity in the laboratory evaluation of hypothyroidism and is almost never indicated. T_3 values can be normal in up to one third of patients with overt hypothyroidism and are commonly depressed in euthyroid patients with nonthyroidal illness (see further).

The vast majority of cases of hypothyroidism can be diagnosed based on clinical findings and the serum FTI and TSH concentrations. Thyroid antibodies (see Table 97-1) are

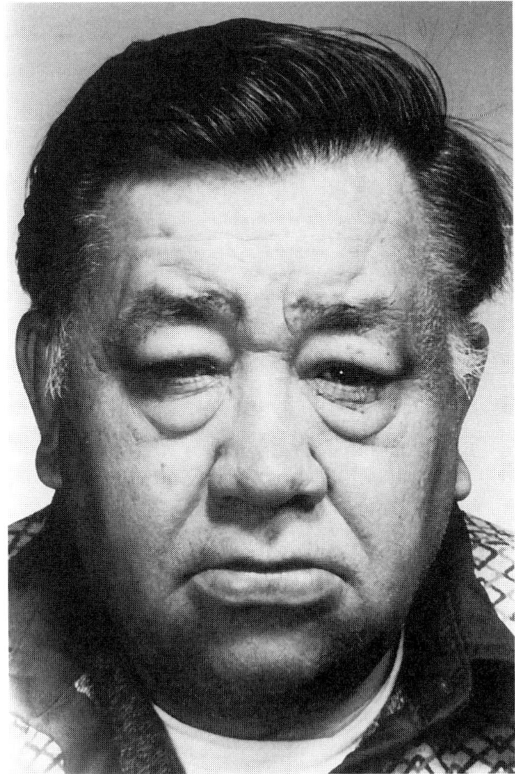

Fig. 97-2. Advanced hypothyroidism. Note dulled expression, facial puffiness, and periorbital edema.

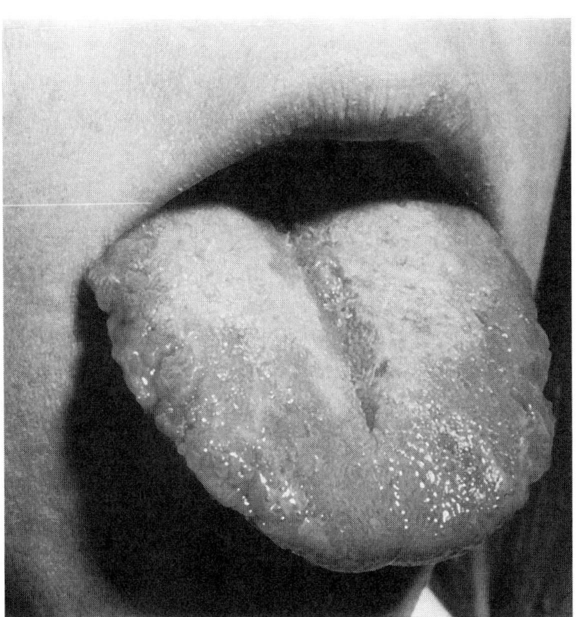

Fig. 97-3. Macroglossia of hypothyroidism.

helpful in providing an etiology for the hypothyroidism and to identify a population with subclinical hypothyroidism that has a high risk of progression to overt disease. Radioisotope scanning is almost never indicated unless used either to document congenital thyroid abnormalities or to evaluate a nodular goiter (see further).

Box 97-3. Factors That May Obscure the Diagnosis of Thyroid Dysfunction

Mask Hypothyroidism/ Mimic Thyrotoxicosis (Increased TBG Binding)	Mimic Hypothyroidism/ Mask Thyrotoxicosis (Decreased TBG Binding)
Drugs	
Estrogens	Glucocorticoids
Methadone	Androgens
Clofibrate	L-asparaginase
5-fluorouracil	Salicylates
Heroin	Mefenamic acid
Tamoxifen	Antiseizure medications (phenytoin, Tegretol)
	Furosemide
Systemic factors	
Pregnancy	Inherited
Neonatal period	Acute illness
Liver disease	
Familial dysalbuminemic hyperthyroxinemia	
Porphyria	
HIV infection	

Differential Diagnosis

Changes in serum TBG concentrations can have marked effects on serum T_4 values and may obscure the diagnosis of hypothyroidism (see Box 97-3). Factors that either decrease TBG concentrations or interfere with binding to TBG can result in low T_4 values in the hypothyroid range. Drugs such as dilantin and salicylates are the most common cause of low serum T_4 levels in euthyroid ambulatory individuals. FTI values are often low as well, but a normal serum TSH value in the absence of signs or symptoms of pituitary or hypothalamic failure confirms the diagnosis of drug effect in most cases. Conversely, factors that increase TBG concentrations can result in T_4 values in the normal range in the hypothyroid patient.

Abnormal thyroid function tests are often seen in patients with nonthyroidal illness (see further). In one large series fewer than 10% of hospitalized patients with elevated serum TSH values less than 20 mU/L and only 50% of those with serum TSH values over 20 mU/L were subsequently diagnosed with hypothyroidism. Retesting thyroid functions 2 to 3 months after complete recovery from an acute illness usually distinguishes nonthyroid illness from hypothyroidism.

Management

The synthetic preparation of levothyroxine sodium (L-T_4) is the drug of choice for thyroid hormone replacement therapy. T_4 is converted to T_3 in peripheral tissues such as the liver, which produces >80% of the circulating T_3 in both euthyroid and T_4-treated hypothyroid individuals. The hormonal content of the various brands of synthetic L-T_4 is reliably standardized; however, clinical experience suggests that it is best to stay with a single brand for an individual patient due to potential small deviations of a specific dose between manufacturers.

The use of liothyronine (L-T_3) alone should be discouraged, due to the need for multiple daily doses and peak-and-valley serum concentrations, as well as the need for target tissues such as the brain to locally convert T_4 to T_3. Similarly, synthetic fixed combinations of L-T_4 and L-T_3 are expensive relative to L-T_4 alone and are unnecessary except in a few highly unusual circumstances. Desiccated thyroid preparations, derived from bovine thyroid, contain T_4 and T_3 and have drawn some interest as a "natural" thyroid hormone replacement. However, desiccated thyroid also contains thyroidal proteins and hormone precursors and metabolites that do not usually find their way into the circulation. In addition, these preparations have a highly variable biologic activity. Since the synthetic T_4 is identical to the T_4 produced by the thyroid, there is no indication for the use of desiccated thyroid in the management of hypothyroidism.

The average replacement dosage of L-T_4 in the United States is 0.112 mg (112 μg) per day. Institution of therapy in healthy individuals under the age of 60 can begin at dosages of 0.05 to 0.1 mg (50 to 100 μg) per day (Table 97-3). Adequacy of the replacement dose can best be determined by serum TSH measurements. Because of the prolonged half-life of T_4 (7 days), new steady-state concentrations of T_4 are not achieved until 4 to 6 weeks after a change in dosage. Thus measurement of serum TSH values should not be performed any earlier than this time frame. The goal of L-T_4 replacement therapy is to achieve a TSH value in the normal range, since overreplacement of L-T_4 suppressing TSH values to the subnormal range has been shown to have a deleterious effect on bone density (see further). Once a normal serum TSH value is achieved, monitoring replacement therapy by determining serum TSH concentrations at 6- to 12-month intervals is appropriate.

Certain drugs can interfere with the absorption of L-T_4 in the gut. Iron and calcium supplements are the most common interfering agents; others include sucralfate, cholestyramine, and certain antacids. L-T_4 administration should be spaced as far apart as possible from these medications. Higher L-T_4 doses may be necessary in patients who are taking drugs that accelerate the metabolism of T_4, such as anticonvulsants and rifampin.

In individuals over the age of 60, institution of therapy at a lower daily dosage (0.025 mg) of L-T_4 is indicated to avoid exacerbation of cardiac disease. The dosage can be increased at a rate of 0.025 mg per day every 4 to 6 weeks, with reevaluation after a total daily dose of 0.075 mg is achieved. For individuals with preexisting cardiac disease an initial dosage of 0.0125 mg with increases of 0.0125 to 0.025 mg per day every 6 to 8 weeks is indicated.

Table 97-3. T_4 Replacement Therapy in Hypothyroidism

	Initial dose	Incremental period
Patient <60 years	0.05-0.1 mg/d	Every 4-6 weeks
Patient >60 years	0.025-0.05 mg/d	Every 4-6 weeks
Preexisting cardiac disease	0.0125-0.025 mg/d	Every 6-8 weeks

Daily doses of L-T_4 may be interrupted periodically because of intercurrent medical or surgical illnesses that prohibit taking anything by mouth. A lapse of several days of hormone replacement usually has no metabolic consequences. However, if more prolonged interruption is necessary, L-T_4 may be given parenterally at a dosage 25% to 50% less than the daily oral requirements.

Special Considerations

Myxedema Coma. Myxedema coma is a rare syndrome that represents the extreme expression of severe, longstanding hypothyroidism. It is a medical emergency, and even with early diagnosis and treatment the mortality can be as high as 60%. Myxedema coma occurs most often in the elderly during the winter months. Common precipitating factors include pulmonary infections, cerebrovascular accidents, and congestive heart failure. The clinical course of lethargy proceeding to stupor and then coma is often hastened by drugs, especially sedatives, narcotics, antidepressants, and tranquilizers. Indeed, many cases of myxedema coma have occurred in the undiagnosed hypothyroid patient who has been hospitalized for other medical problems.

Cardinal features of myxedema coma are (1) hypothermia, which can be profound, (2) respiratory depression, and (3) unconsciousness. Other clinical features include bradycardia, macroglossia, delayed reflexes, and dry, rough skin. Dilutional hyponatremia is common and may be severe. Elevated CPK and lactate dehydrogenase (LDH) concentrations, acidosis, and anemia are common findings. Lumbar puncture reveals increased opening pressure and high protein content. Hypothyroidism is confirmed by measuring serum FTI and TSH values. Ultimately, however, myxedema coma is a clinical diagnosis.

The mainstay of therapy is supportive care, with ventilatory support, rewarming, correction of hyponatremia, and treatment of the precipitating incident. Because of a 5% to 10% incidence of coexisting adrenal insufficiency in patients with myxedema coma, intravenous steroids are indicated before initiating T_4 therapy. Parenteral administration of thyroid hormone is necessary due to uncertain absorption through the gut. A reasonable approach is an initial intravenous loading dose of 200 to 300 μg L-T_4, with a second dose of 100 μg given 24 hours later. Simultaneously, with the initial dose of L-T_4, some physicians recommend adding L-T_3 at a dosage of 10 μg intravenously every 8 hours until the patient is stable and conscious. The dose of thyroid hormone should be adjusted on the basis of hemodynamic stability, the presence of coexisting cardiac disease, and the degree of electrolyte imbalance.

Subclinical Hypothyroidism. Subclinical hypothyroidism is defined as mild elevations of serum TSH in conjunction with normal serum thyroid hormone concentrations and lack of any overt clinical manifestations of hypothyroidism. The prevalence of subclinical hypothyroidism ranges from 10% to 20%, depending on the population, and is frequently observed in the elderly. The presence of thyroid antibodies in these patients clearly identifies a subset of patients who are at high risk of progressing to overt hypothyroidism. Potential benefits of instituting L-T_4 therapy in patients with subclinical hypothyroidism include prevention of overt hypothyroidism, improvement in mild metabolic and physiologic abnormalities, and improvement in symptoms not originally attributed to thyroid dysfunction. Several small studies have demonstrated that treatment of subclinical hypothyroidism with L-T_4 improved serum lipid profiles in patients with hypercholesterolemia, improved cognitive function in the elderly, and relieved hypothyroid-related symptoms in patients who initially characterized themselves as asymptomatic.

Although there is currently no consensus for the management of patients with subclinical hypothyroidism, an approach to the management, based on the published literature, is shown in Table 97-4. In addition, a therapeutic trial of L-T_4 is reasonable in individuals with symptoms that are out of proportion to the TSH elevations and that do not fit any of the criteria listed. In these individuals, and in those with hypercholesterolemia or cognitive dysfunction, reassessment after 6 months of L-T_4 therapy that normalizes the serum TSH is reasonable to determine if therapy should be continued. All individuals with subclinical hypothyroidism who are not treated should be followed with periodic determination of serum TSH concentrations (i.e., semiannually or annually).

Thyroid Hormone Replacement and Osteoporosis. Thyroid hormone has a direct effect on bone resorption and has been shown in several studies to decrease bone density in women taking thyroid hormone in suppressive doses for many years. When analyzed carefully, a significant decrease in bone density has been demonstrated in women taking doses of L-T_4 that result in undetectable TSH values, with the hip affected to a greater degree than the spine. This is mainly seen in those individuals requiring suppressive therapy after surgery for thyroid cancer, in whom TSH suppression is the goal of therapy. However, increased fracture rates have not been demonstrated in patients taking L-T_4. Women on replacement therapy with normal serum TSH concentrations show no changes in bone mineral density compared with age-matched women not on L-T_4 therapy. Thus, as stated above, the goal of replacement therapy in patients with hypothyroidism should be to achieve a serum TSH in the normal range.

Table 97-4. Management of Subclinical Hypothyroidism

Therapeutic indication	Reason
Therapy probably indicated	
Presence of thyroid antibodies	High risk for progressing to overt hypothyroidism
Presence of goiter	Decrease size or prevent further growth of goiter
Prior therapy for hyperthyroidism	High risk for progressing to overt hypothyroidism
Pregnancy	Optimize maternal thyroid status to preserve maternal contribution to fetal thyroid economy
Hypercholesterolemia	Correct mild thyroid-related abnormalities in lipid metabolism
Cognitive dysfunction	Improve memory and mood
Therapy probably not indicated	
Absence of thyroid antibodies	Low risk for progression to overt hypothyroidism
Lack of goiter	Low risk for progression to overt hypothyroidism
Recovery from nonthyroidal illness	Low risk for progression to overt hypothyroidism

Thyroid Hormone Replacement in Pregnancy. In general, L-T_4 replacement requirements increase during pregnancy. This is primarily due to an estrogen-dependent increase in serum TBG concentrations that occurs during the first trimester. In addition, gastrointestinal absorption of L-T_4 may be decreased during pregnancy. Approximately 80% of hypothyroid patients need an increase in their replacement dosage during pregnancy, with an average increase equivalent to about 45% of the basal dosage. In addition, pregnancy may unmask hypothyroidism in patients with decreased thyroid reserve, such as those residing in areas of iodine deficiency or those with euthyroid chronic autoimmune thyroiditis. Thus all patients receiving thyroid hormone replacement who become pregnant should have a serum TSH determination at or near the end of their first trimester. Similarly, evaluation of thyroid function during pregnancy in normal patients is indicated in those patients at high risk for hypothyroidism, such as those residing in areas of iodine deficiency or with a family history of thyroid or other autoimmune disease.

THYROTOXICOSIS

Thyrotoxicosis is a condition caused by elevated concentrations of the circulating free thyroid hormones T_4 and T_3. Various disorders of different etiologies can result in this syndrome. The term hyperthyroidism should be restricted to those conditions in which thyroid hormones are overproduced due to hyperfunction, rather than thyroid inflammation or destruction or thyroid hormone administration.

Etiology

For practical purposes hyperthyroidism can be classified according to the 24-hour radioactive iodine uptake (RAIU) (Box 97-4). An elevated RAIU indicates that the etiology of the elevated serum thyroid hormones is a hyperfunctioning thyroid gland. Graves' disease is the most common cause of high RAIU thyrotoxicosis. It accounts for 60% to 90% of the cases, depending on age and geographic region. Toxic nodular and multinodular goiter follows in frequency, accounting for 10% to 40% of the cases, and is more common in older patients. A low RAIU is seen in destructive thyroiditides and in thyrotoxicosis resulting from exogenous thyroid hormone. Low RAIU thyrotoxicosis caused by subacute and painless thyroiditis represents about 5% to 20% of all cases. Other causes of thyrotoxicosis are much less common.

Patient Evaluation

Thyroid hormone excess affects multiple organ systems. Although the resulting signs or symptoms in thyrotoxicosis can be nonspecific, their combination usually creates a characteristic clinical picture. Age, presence of other underlying disturbances, and rapidity of onset of the disease can modify both the type and severity of the clinical presentation. Symptoms of thyrotoxicosis may start slowly or precipitously and may range from subtle to florid.

Box 97-4. Use of the RAIU in the Diagnosis of Thyrotoxicosis

Causes of High RAIU Thyrotoxicosis (Hyperthyroidism)

Graves' Disease
Toxic multinodular goiter
Solitary hot nodule
TSH secreting pituitary tumor
Molar pregnancy
Choriocarcinoma

Causes of Low RAIU Thyrotoxicosis

Subacute thyroiditis thyroditis
Sporadic silent thyroiditis
Postpartum lymphocytic thyroiditis
Radiation-induced thyroiditis
Iodine-induced thyroiditis
Thyrotoxicosis factitia
Metastatic follicular thyroid cancer
Struma ovarii

Box 97-5. Symptoms of Hyperthyroidism

Common (Seen in >50% of Patients)	Less Common (Seen in <50% of Patients)
Nervousness	Nausea and vomiting
Irritability	Dysphagia
Hyperactivity	Decreased libido
Insomnia	Impotence
Hand tremor	Dyspnea on exertion
Excessive sweating	Periodic paralysis
Palpitations	Exacerbation of angina
Weight loss	
Increased appetite	
Heat intolerance	
Pruritus	
Hyperdefecation	
Oligomenorrhea	

Typical patient complaints include nervousness, irritability, hyperactivity, insomnia, hand tremor, excessive sweating, and palpitations (Box 97-5). Most of these symptoms are due to increased sympathetic tone. Weight loss, despite an increased appetite, and heat intolerance are common due to increased energy production and utilization. Pruritus, when present, results from increased blood flow to the skin. Proximal muscle weakness is often manifested as difficulty climbing stairs or standing up. Increased gut motility may result in hyperdefecation and occasionally in malabsorption or diarrhea. Hyperthyroidism may exacerbate angina pectoris. Oligomenorrhea in women and decreased libido and impotence in men are described.

Less often patients develop nausea, vomiting, and dysphagia. Dyspnea on exertion, due to increased oxygen consumption and respiratory muscle weakness, can be seen. Rarely tracheal compression from a large goiter can cause dyspnea. Periodic paralysis is rare and is seen usually in Asian males usually in association with low serum potassium levels.

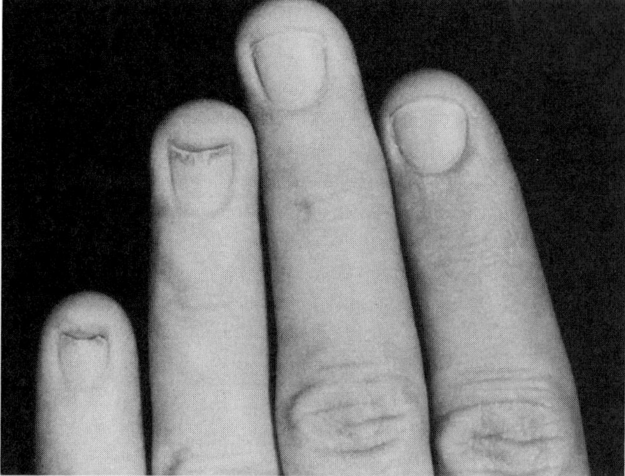

Fig. 97-4. Onycholysis involving the ring finger in a patient with Graves' disease.

The thyroid gland is diffusely enlarged in most patients with Graves' disease. Typically both thyroid lobes are symmetrically enlarged, firm, and nontender. The gland may be particularly firm in those thyroids with coexistent Hashimoto's thyroiditis. In patients with a multinodular goiter the thyroid gland is often asymmetric, irregular, and bumpy. A unilateral nodule, usually larger than 3 cm, is found in a solitary toxic adenoma. A tender thyroid raises the possibility of subacute thyroiditis. A normal or nonpalpable thyroid gland points toward a diagnosis of thyrotoxicosis factitia (see further) or painless thyroiditis, although goiter may rarely be absent in Graves' disease. Hyperthyroidism without goiter is more common in the elderly. Because of increased blood supply to the thyroid, a systolic bruit and a thrill may be present in Graves' disease.

Cardiac findings are the result of both direct thyroid hormone effects on the cardiovascular system and indirect effects through the increased metabolism and oxygen consumption. Sinus tachycardia, elevated systolic blood pressure, and widened pulse pressure are common. A systolic ejection flow murmur may be present. Although sinus tachycardia is the most common rhythm in thyrotoxicosis, other arrhythmias, especially atrial fibrillation, occur in 10% to 25% of patients. Atrial fibrillation is more common in older patients and may be the presenting feature of thyrotoxicosis. In these patients the presence of left atrial enlargement is the rule. Arterial embolism occurs in about 10% of patients with atrial fibrillation.

The skin is often warm, moist, and smooth. Onycholysis, or separation of the nail from the nailbed, is often seen in thyrotoxicosis (Fig. 97-4). Acropachy and clubbing are associated with Graves' disease. Hair texture is fine and alopecia may occur. Hyperpigmentation of the skin may be observed. Vitiligo is associated with Graves' disease. Distal fine tremor, brisk deep tendon reflexes, and proximal muscle weakness are common neurologic findings. Ophthalmopathy associated with thyrotoxicosis is classified as noninfiltrative

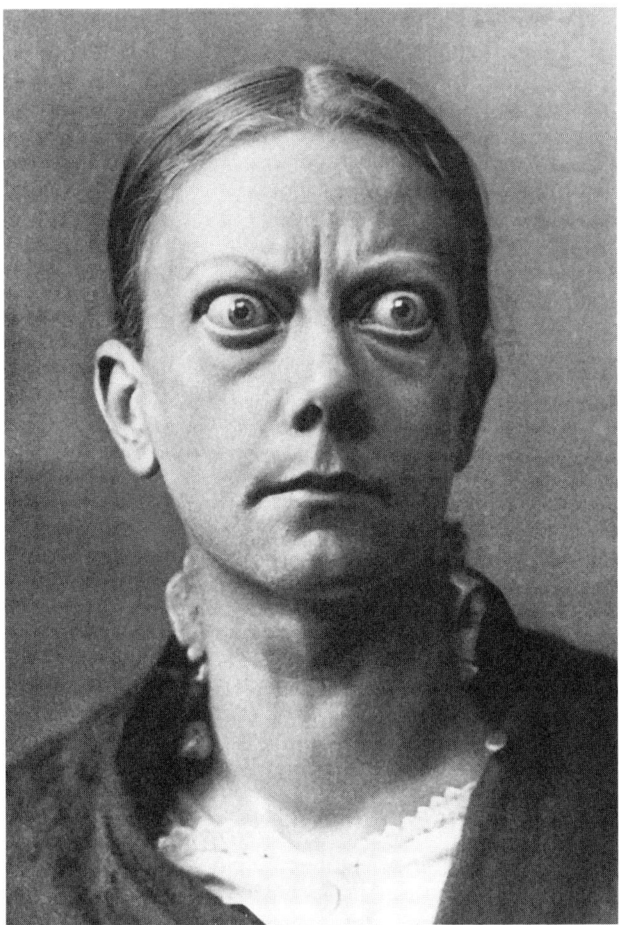

Fig. 97-5. Classic appearance of Graves' disease with advanced hyperthyroidism. (From Bramwell B: *Atlas of clinical medicine*, Edinburgh, 1892, University Press.)

or infiltrative. Noninfiltrative ophthalmopathy is associated with thyrotoxicosis of any origin. It is characterized by upper lid retraction, which results in lid lag and stare (Fig. 97-5). Infiltrative ophthalmopathy is specifically associated with Graves' disease and is discussed later.

Diagnosis

Elevated serum concentrations of thyroid hormones and suppressed serum TSH concentrations are the hallmarks of thyrotoxicosis. Both total and free thyroid hormone concentrations are elevated, although isolated increases of either T_4 or T_3 may also occur. An increase in serum T_4 binding protein concentrations or capacity, as seen during pregnancy and estrogen replacement therapy, can result in an increase of total T_4 concentrations into the thyrotoxic range. Therefore estimation of free T_4 concentrations by the FTI is helpful to clarify the diagnosis in these situations. Disorders that are associated with elevated total T_4 concentrations, but normal free T_4 concentrations (see Box 97-3), may mimic the diagnosis of thyrotoxicosis and are collectively known as the *euthyroid hyperthyroxinemia syndrome*. In these patients serum T_3 and TSH concentrations are normal.

T_4-toxicosis is described in thyrotoxic patients with concomitant diseases, such as hospitalized patients, in whom T_4 to T_3 conversion in peripheral tissues is inhibited because of nonthyroidal illness or drugs. On the patient's recovery from the acute illness, serum T_3 levels may rise up to the hyperthyroid range. Similarly, hyperthyroid patients who received iodinated preparations, for example, those used for radiologic studies, may also develop T_4-toxicosis. Occasionally patients may have increased serum T_3 levels and normal T_4 levels. Hyperthyroidism due to T_3 alone is referred to as T_3-toxicosis. This disorder is more frequent in areas of iodine deficiency, in patients with solitary nodules, and in early or relapsing Graves' disease.

Serum TSH determination by a sensitive TSH radioimmunoassay (limit of detection <0.05 mU/L) is a very accurate indicator of thyrotoxicosis. Serum TSH levels should be low or undetectable. Indeed, with the rare exception of a TSH-secreting pituitary tumor, a serum TSH concentration in the normal range rules out the diagnosis of hyperthyroidism. The new sensitive TSH assays have replaced the thyrotropin-releasing hormone stimulation test as a tool in the diagnosis of hyperthyroidism.

Thyroid autoantibody titers (antithyroglobulin and anti-TPO) are elevated in up to 70% of patients with Graves' disease. Their measurement is not routinely necessary but many times is helpful in establishing the diagnosis, especially in the absence of ophthalmopathy. TSH receptor antibodies can be commercially measured as thyroid-stimulating (TSI) or thyroid-binding inhibitor (TBII) immunoglobulins. TSI is more sensitive than TBII, but both are very specific. Nevertheless, their measurement is costly and is not routinely recommended. Measurement of TSH receptor antibodies in pregnant women is helpful in predicting the risk of developing neonatal Graves' disease (see below). TSI measurements can occasionally be useful in the diagnosis of euthyroid Graves' disease and in the differential diagnosis of Graves' disease from other hyperthyroid disorders.

Normochromic normocytic anemia and mild neutropenia with lymphocytosis are sometimes found in Graves disease. Liver enzymes (alanine aminotransferase, aspartate aminotransferase) may be minimally increased. Mild elevations of serum calcium levels are seen in up to 20% of thyrotoxic patients. This is due to increased bone resorption by thyroid hormones, and resolves with the treatment of hyperthyroidism. Bone and liver alkaline phosphatase fractions may also be elevated. Serum cholesterol levels may be decreased.

As mentioned previously, the 24-hour RAIU separates thyrotoxicosis into two categories. When the diagnosis of Graves' disease is clinically obvious, especially in the presence of coexisting Graves' ophthalmopathy, RAIU determination is unnecessary. However, RAIU is a useful tool in the differential diagnosis of thyrotoxicosis in unclear cases. Whereas RAIU distinguishes etiology based on iodine uptake, thyroid radionuclide imaging can distinguish different forms of goiter. A thyroid scan should be requested when the thyroid gland appears to be nodular on physical examination to establish the diagnosis of toxic nodular or multinodular goiter. In addition, a thyroid scan may be ordered in a patient with Graves' disease when a thyroid nodule is palpated so as to rule out a coexistent cold nodule.

Differential Diagnosis

When the clinical picture is classic with a diffuse goiter and ophthalmopathy, the diagnosis of Graves' disease is straightforward. The absence of ophthalmopathy or the presence of subtle hyperthyroid symptoms may obscure the diagnosis. This is particularly true in the elderly (Fig. 97-6). Certain

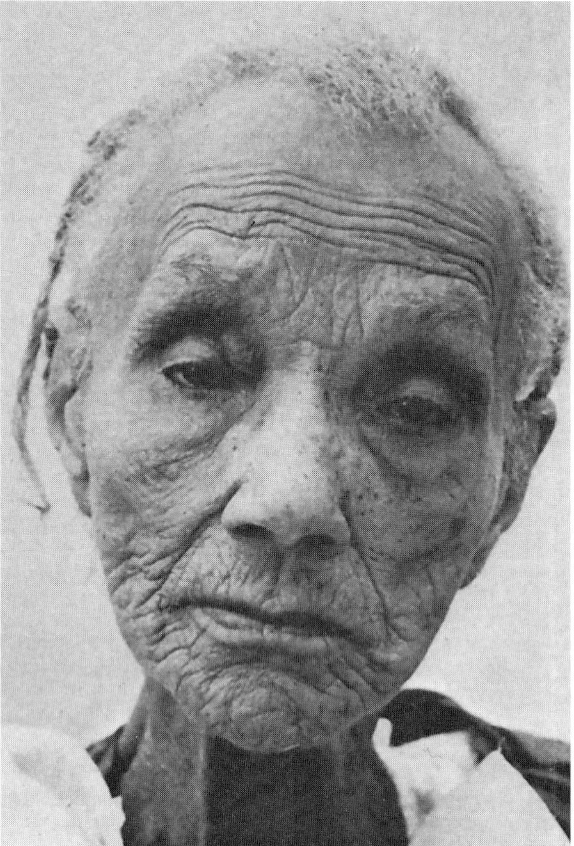

Fig. 97-6. Apathetic hyperthyroidism in an older patient. (From Thomas FB, et al: *Ann Intern Med* 72;679, 1970.)

psychiatric diseases, such as anxiety and bipolar disorder, can mimic thyrotoxicosis. Conversely, thyrotoxicosis can be manifest as a psychiatric disorder or can expose a previously unrecognized one.

History, physical examination, and determination of serum FTI, T_3, and TSH concentrations usually provide enough information to make the diagnosis. RAIU is helpful in borderline patients or in those with atypical or few clinical manifestations. High T_3/T_4 ratios (greater than 20) are suggestive of Graves' disease. In contrast, inflammatory thyroiditis or exogenous L-T_4 administration is characterized by a low T_3/T_4 ratio, usually less than 15. TSH receptor antibody determinations and radionuclide imaging studies can be helpful but should be reserved for unusual cases (see above). An elevated sedimentation rate is essential for a diagnosis of subacute thyroiditis (see below). Serum thyroglobulin concentration, which is elevated in most forms of thyrotoxicosis, is low or suppressed in thyrotoxicosis factitia.

Graves' Disease. Graves' disease, or toxic diffuse goiter, is an autoimmune disorder characterized by thyrotoxicosis, diffuse goiter, and antibodies directed against the TSH receptor. This is a relatively common disorder, with an incidence of 0.02% to 0.4% in the United States. Endemic areas of iodine deficiency have a lower incidence of autoimmune thyroid disease. As with most types of thyroid dysfunction, women are affected more than men, with a ratio of 5 to 7:1. Graves' disease is more common between the ages of 20 and 50 but can occur at any age. HLA B8 and DR3 haplotypes are associated with Graves' disease in the white population. The disease is commonly associated with other autoimmune disorders (Box 97-6).

Box 97-6. Autoimmune Diseases Associated with Graves' Disease

Hashimoto's thyroiditis
Vitiligo
Pernicious anemia
Insulin-dependent diabetes mellitus
Adrenal insufficiency
Myasthenia gravis
Idiopathic thrombocytopenic purpura
Sjögren's syndrome
Systemic lupus erythematosus

Pathogenesis. Hyperthyroidism results from the stimulation of TSH receptors on thyroid cells by TSH receptor antibodies. The TSH receptor antibody is believed to stimulate the generation of cyclic adenosine monophosphate in the thyroid, resulting in the increased synthesis and release of the thyroid hormones. Proposed hypotheses regarding the abnormal generation of thyroid-stimulating antibody include (1) a primary defect on antigen-specific suppressor T cells that results in unregulated helper T cell function and therefore abnormal antibody synthesis, (2) direct helper T cell activation by thyroid follicular cells expressing HLA class II antigens, and (3) cross-reactivity between bacterial or parasitic antigens and the TSH receptor, provoking the generation of autoantibodies.

The abnormal function of the immune system found in patients with this disease is strongly linked to a genetic predisposition. However, the specific genes involved have not been identified. Concurrence rates for Graves' disease are approximately 50% for monozygotic twins and 5% for dizygotic twins. This lack of complete concordance suggests that environmental factors, including infectious agents such as *Yersinia enterocolitica* or retrovirus, and stressful events, either physical or psychologic, may be involved.

Specific Clinical Manifestations. The general manifestations of thyrotoxicosis have already been described. Specific findings in Graves' disease include infiltrative ophthalmopathy, pretibial myxedema, and acropachy.

Graves' ophthalmopathy. The infiltrative ophthalmopathy associated with Graves' disease is considered an autoimmune-mediated inflammation of the periorbital connective tissue and extraocular muscle. This disorder is clinically evident with various degrees of severity in about 50% of patients with Graves' disease but is present on radiologic studies, such as ultrasound and CT scan, in almost all patients. The majority of patients have mild or moderate disease. Euthyroid Graves' disease refers to patients with ophthalmopathy who have not developed hyperthyroidism; only 5% of these patients remain euthyroid indefinitely. Overall, ophthalmopathy precedes the diagnosis of hyperthyroidism in 15% of patients, coincides with the diagnosis of hyperthyroidism in about 40% of patients, and develops after the diagnosis and treatment of hyperthyroidism in the remaining patients.

Although there is good evidence that this disorder is autoimmune in origin, the target antigen in the orbital tissue has not yet been identified. Thyroid and orbital tissue, such as the eye muscle, may share antigens toward which autoantibodies react. Smoking appears to be a risk factor for the development or worsening of Graves' ophthalmopathy. Graves' ophthalmopathy may also be exacerbated after radioactive iodine therapy, and this exacerbation can be prevented by the use of high-dose corticosteroids.

Patients with Graves' ophthalmopathy may complain of retroocular pressure, photophobia, lacrimation, and blurred vision. Muscle inflammation and fibrosis can result in ophthalmoplegia and diplopia. Optic nerve damage due to increased intraocular pressure can lead to decreased vision and blindness, although this is quite rare. On physical examination the most obvious sign is proptosis. Although usually bilateral, only one eye may be involved. Conjunctival injection, chemosis, and periorbital and eyelid edema may also be present. The combination of proptosis and lid retraction may lead to corneal exposure and ulceration.

The diagnosis of ophthalmopathy is based on the findings just described. Proptosis is measured with a Hertel exophthalmometer, with a reading of 20 to 22 mm suggestive and more than 24 mm diagnostic of exophthalmos. Similarly, an asymmetric reading of more than 2 mm is abnormal. Orbital ultrasound, CT, or MRI will show the thickened eye muscle and increased orbital content. These radiologic studies are not routinely ordered to assess the ophthalmopathy, but they may be occasionally useful in the differential diagnosis of exophthalmos, especially if the patient is euthyroid. Unilateral exophthalmos should be evaluated by imaging studies even in patients with documented Graves' disease so as to exclude other causes of orbital pathology (Fig. 97-7).

Treatment of Graves' ophthalmopathy should be performed in conjunction with an ophthalmologist. Conversion to euthyroidism, preferably with antithyroid drugs, is first required. Radioactive iodine treatment should be avoided in patients with clinically significant ophthalmopathy due to potential worsening of the eye disease after treatment, although the frequency with which this occurs is controversial. If the eye disease is mild, local, nonspecific measures should be prescribed for symptom relief and to protect the eye from corneal exposure, including lubricants, dark-colored glasses, and adhesive taping of eyelids during sleep.

Systemic treatments with immunosuppressive drugs (high-dose steroids or cytotoxic agents) are reserved for severe cases with active and progressive inflammation. Orbital radiation is also used in severe disease. Similar results are obtained with both treatments. When systemic treatment is ineffective or contraindicated, surgical orbital decompression may be beneficial. In patients with severe diplopia, surgical release of the fibrosed extraocular muscle is indicated. Lid retraction that persists after the patient is rendered euthyroid can be corrected with Müller myotomy.

Pretibial myxedema. Pretibial myxedema is an uncommon autoimmune disorder associated with Graves' disease that is present in fewer than 5% of patients. It is characterized by localized dermal accumulation of mucopolysaccharides, most commonly over the tibial surface. It may present as a diffuse nonpitting lesion of the anterior lower leg or as a sharply circumscribed lesion (Fig. 97-8). An elephantiasis form is rare. The lesions are usually asymptomatic. Rarely, they may cause pain or ulcerate. Topical occlusive treatment with potent fluorinated steroids has been reported to be successful.

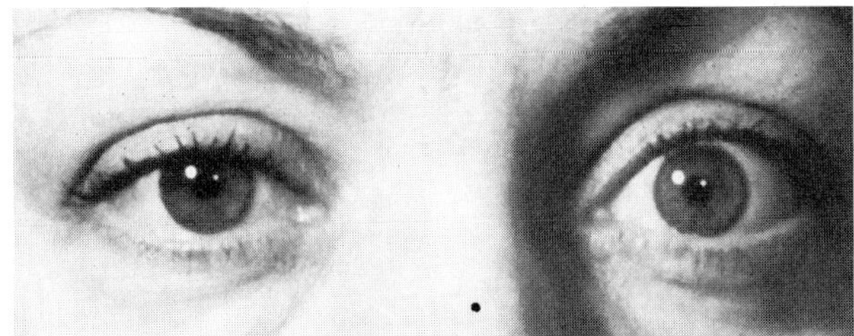

Fig. 97-7. Unilateral *(left)* lid retraction in a patient with hyperthyroidism.

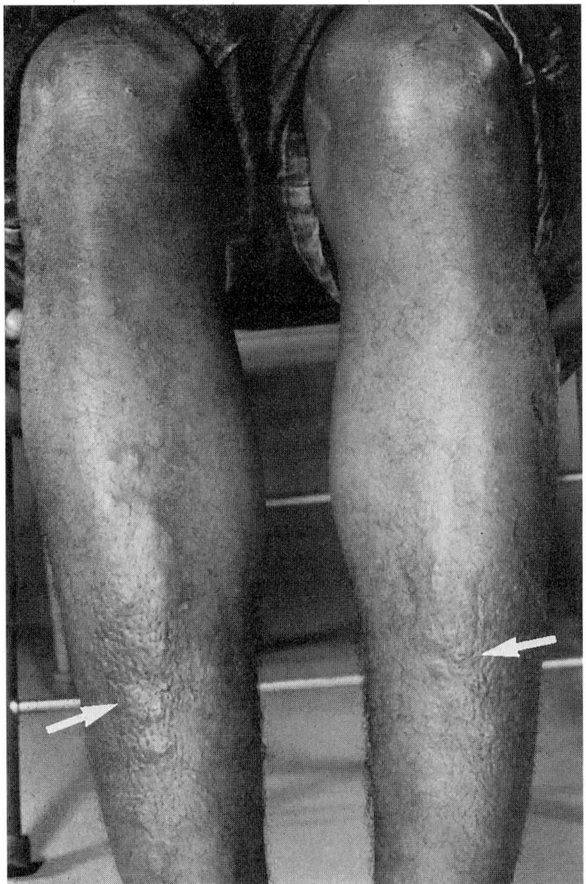

Fig. 97-8. Pretibial myxedema *(arrows)* in a patient with Graves' disease.

Thyroid acropachy. Thyroid acropachy is the rarest manifestation of Graves' disease. It is characterized by subperiosteal new bone formation, predominately of the digits, associated with clubbing of the fingers and localized soft tissue swelling. There is no effective treatment for acropachy.

Management. The course of hyperthyroidism in Graves' disease is characterized by cycles of relapse and remission of variable duration, although an unremitting course or a single episode of the disease is also possible. There is no available treatment aimed at the cause of Graves' disease, namely antibodies to the TSH receptor, thus there is no true cure for this disorder. Instead, treatment is aimed at decreasing circulating thyroid hormone levels either by inhibiting thyroid hormone production or by destroying thyroid tissue. There are three major ways of achieving these goals: (1) antithyroid drugs, (2) radioactive iodine, and (3) surgery. The goal of treatment with antithyroid drugs is to alter the natural history of the disease and to induce a remission of the hyperthyroidism. Radioactive iodine and surgery seek to alter the natural history of the disease by decreasing the amount of thyroid tissue available to respond to stimulation by TSH receptor antibodies. The choice of therapy should be individualized based on the patient's interest and the availability of experienced thyroid surgeons.

Antithyroid drugs. Antithyroid drugs (ATDs) belong to a group of compounds known as thionamides. They act by inhibiting thyroid peroxidase and therefore block iodine organification and thyroid hormone synthesis. In addition, they exhibit extrathyroidal actions that may be beneficial (Table 97-5). The two available antithyroid drugs in the United States are propylthiouracil (PTU) and methimazole (Tapazole). Both are effective in controlling hyperthyroidism. In most cases the choice between the two drugs is up to the physician's individual experience and preference. PTU is recommended for use during pregnancy because its transplacental passage is much less than that of methimazole (see further). PTU is also transmitted into breast milk to a lesser degree than is methimazole and has the additional benefit of inhibiting T_4 to T_3 conversion, allowing for a more rapid fall in serum T_3 concentrations and thus a more rapid improvement in symptoms than methimazole. However, in practice this effect of PTU is important only in the most severely toxic individuals.

The usual starting dosage of methimazole is 20 to 40 mg daily as a single dose; for PTU it is 100 to 150 mg two to three times daily. Higher dosages may be required for the severely toxic patient, as well as those with very large goiters. After treatment is initiated, patients should be examined and thyroid function tests (FTI and serum T_3 levels) monitored every 4 to 6 weeks. Once euthyroidism is achieved, usually within 12 weeks, the dosage of the antithyroid drug can be decreased. Maintenance dosages are usually 5 to 10 mg daily for methimazole and 50 to 200 mg daily for PTU. Thereafter, follow-up visits every 3 months are reasonable.

Remission rates after a treatment course with ATDs vary from 10% to 90% 1 year after stopping the drug, with a mean remission rate of about 50%. Longer durations of therapy have been associated with higher remission rates. We recommend that therapy be administered for 1 to 2 years. Remission rates have been lower in recent years compared with those initially described in the 1950s and 1960s. Increased dietary iodine has been implicated in the latter, less favorable, rates. Although it is difficult, if not impossible, to predict which individual patient will go into remission with ATDs, factors associated with higher chances of remission after discontinuation of ATD treatment include negative TPO antibody titers, HLA DR3 negative haplotype, milder thyrotoxicosis at presentation, and reduction in goiter size with ATD therapy. Conversely, patients with large goiters and a long duration of symptoms are less likely to go into remission with ATDs. Among those patients who experience remission, about 25% ultimately become hypothyroid, probably due to concurrent Hashimoto's thyroiditis.

Concomitant use of L-T_4 therapy along with ATDs, primarily methimazole, has been reported to increase rates of remission in Japan. However, similar studies carried out in Europe and in the United States, as well as a subsequent study in Japan, have shown no advantage to concomitant use of L-T_4 and ATDs. Thus the use of combination L-T_4 and ATD therapy is not recommended.

Relapse of Graves' disease after discontinuation of ATDs usually occurs within the first few months. In that case a repeat course of ATDs may be indicated; however, ablation therapy should be considered. In any event, long-term (years) use of ATDs appears to be safe in the patient who is unable to achieve a drug-free remission and is not interested in radioactive iodine or surgery. Patients who remain in remission should be reevaluated for a relapse every 3 to 6 months or with the recurrence of symptoms.

The most serious side effect of ATDs is agranulocytosis, which usually, but not always, occurs within the first 3 months of treatment. The incidence of agranulocytosis is the same for both PTU and methimazole (0.1% to 0.5%). There is some evidence that methimazole-induced agranulocytosis is dose-related and is rarely seen at dosages under 30 mg daily, whereas there is no relationship between dose and agranulocytosis with PTU. Patients should be instructed to discontinue the medication and to contact the physician in case of fever or sore throat. Any patient taking ATDs who develops a fever or a sore throat should have an urgent white blood cell (WBC) count and differential performed, and the ATD should not be resumed until the results of the WBC count are obtained. Since ATD-related agranulocytosis occurs rapidly, routine monitoring of complete blood counts (CBCs)

Table 97-5. Characteristics of Antithyroid Drugs

	PTU	Methimazole
Intrathyroidal Effects	Inhibition of iodination and iodotyrosine coupling	
Extrathyroidal Effects	Possible immunomodulation	
	Inhibition of T_4 to T_3 conversion	No effect on T_4 to T_3 conversion
Serum half-life	75 min	4-6 h
Transplacental passage	Low	High
Breast milk levels	Low	High
Usual daily dose	100-300 mg	10-30 mg
Dose frequency	BID-TID	QD
Agranulocytosis	Not dose-related	Dose-related

is not recommended. It is useful to check a pretreatment CBC, since WBCs are often depressed by Graves' disease itself. If agranulocytosis occurs, preparations for definitive therapy with radioactive iodine or surgery should be made because it is not recommended to rechallenge the patient with the other ATD due to cross-reactivity between drugs. Minor side effects, such as rash and urticaria, are relatively more common (1% to 5%). If acceptable to the patient, the medication can be safely continued and an antihistaminic may be added. Otherwise, one can replace one ATD for the other, realizing that cross-reactivity for minor side effects has also been reported.

Radioactive iodine treatment. Radioactive iodine (RAI) in the form of ^{131}I is taken up by the thyroid gland and produces destruction of thyroid follicular cells. Use of RAI is recommended by many physicians, especially in the elderly. RAI is generally avoided in children and is contraindicated during pregnancy and breastfeeding. The dosage of ^{131}I to be administered is usually in the range of 5 to 10 mCi, with the dosage calculation based on thyroid size (80 to 120 μCi/gm tissue) and 24-hour RAIU. Administration of ATDs before radioiodine treatment is recommended to decrease thyroid hormone storage and prevent transient worsening of symptoms of hyperthyroidism or development of thyrotoxic storm. The ATDs should be stopped at least 3 to 5 days prior to the RAI treatment. About 75% of patients are rendered euthyroid after one dose of radioiodine. The rest of the patients require a second and rarely a third dose. RAI treatment often produces mild thyroidal pain, which may be managed by nonsteroidal antiinflammatory medications. In addition, the radiation thyroiditis that is produced after RAI therapy may result in transient worsening of the thyrotoxic state 7 to 14 days after treatment, especially if the patient has not been pretreated with ATDs. Supportive treatment with β-blockers is occasionally necessary for a short (2 to 3 weeks) period of time.

Normalization of thyroid function, including normalization of serum TSH, usually takes 1 to 2 months but may be delayed for up to a year. Retreatment should not be considered for at least 3 to 6 months after the initial treatment in order to document a treatment failure, except in extenuating circumstances. Permanent hypothyroidism is the major complication of radioactive iodine treatment. Hypothyroidism eventually develops in about 80% of the patients; therefore lifelong follow-up is warranted. Extensive studies involving over 5000 patients for up to 40 years have revealed no increase in the incidence of any malignancy after the RAI treatment for hypothyroidism. Radioiodine may cause exacerbation in Graves' ophthalmopathy, the risk of which may be reduced with the concomitant use of corticosteroids.

Surgery. Subtotal thyroidectomy is reserved for the following conditions: (1) patients with large goiters, (2) children who are allergic to ATDs, (3) pregnant women (usually in the second trimester) who are allergic to ATDs, and (4) patients who prefer surgery over ATDs or RAI. Preparation of the patient before undergoing surgery involves depletion of the gland of thyroid hormone with ATDs and decreasing the vascularity of the gland with iodide administration (1 to 3 drops of super-saturated potassium iodide (SSKI) or Lugol's solution daily for 10 days). β-Adrenergic blockers alone have been used in some cases to prepare toxic patients for thyroidectomy.

The two most common complications from subtotal thyroidectomy are hoarseness due to recurrent laryngeal nerve damage and hypoparathyroidism. Complication rates in the hands of an experienced thyroid surgeon are low (less than 1%). Hyperthyroidism recurs in about 5% of patients and hypothyroidism develops in up to 60% of patients. RAI should be considered for surgically treated patients who relapse.

Adjuvant therapy. Iodide inhibits synthesis and release of thyroid hormones, but its effect is transient and may result in eventual exacerbation of the hyperthyroid state if not administered concomitantly with ATDs. Iodide, in the form of Lugol's solution or SSKI (8 drops every 6 hours), is used in the treatment of thyroid storm and for preparation of patients for surgery. Iodinated contrast agents (e.g., iopanoic acid [Telepaque], 1 gm/day) have the additional advantage of inhibiting peripheral T_4 to T_3 conversion and may be used in the management of thyrotoxic crisis.

β-Adrenergic blockers and calcium channel blockers are useful drugs in the symptomatic treatment of hyperthyroidism and are quite effective in decreasing heart rate. Propranolol, 20 to 40 mg four times daily, or atenolol, 100 to 200 mg daily, is the usual starting dosage. Propranolol and esmolol can be given intravenously if needed. Diltiazem can be used for heart rate control if β-blockers are contraindicated. These drugs should be discontinued once the patient is euthyroid.

Toxic Multinodular Goiter. Typically, toxic multinodular goiter presents in older patients who have longstanding asymptomatic nodular goiters. Administration of iodine-containing preparations, such as radiographic contrast media, amiodarone, or cough medicines, can precipitate hyperthyroidism in these patients. The onset of hyperthyroidism is more gradual and symptoms are usually milder than those of Graves' disease. Weight loss, atrial fibrillation, and depression are common presentations.

Physical examination usually reveals a large and firm goiter. Discrete nodules may be palpable. Lid lag can be observed, but infiltrative ophthalmopathy is absent. Borderline serum T_4 and T_3 levels and suppressed serum TSH concentrations are frequent. Radionuclide thyroid imaging is characterized by multiple functioning areas with suppression of other portions of the gland. Substernal thyroid extension may be detected. RAIU is usually elevated but may be normal.

Once hyperthyroidism occurs, it follows an unremitting course; therefore definitive treatment by ablation therapy is recommended. RAI is the treatment of choice in the elderly and large doses of ^{131}I are usually required. Surgical removal of the thyroid is advised in patients with large, compressive goiters. Subtotal thyroidectomy is commonly performed in these cases. ATDs are given to render the patient euthyroid before radioiodine treatment or surgery to avoid the precipitation of cardiac arrhythmias or thyrotoxic crisis in an unprepared patient. In contrast to Graves' disease, ATD treatment of the toxic multinodular goiter does not result in remission of the hyperthyroidism, and discontinuation of ATDs without ablative therapy will result in the return of the thyrotoxic state.

Autonomously Functioning Thyroid Nodules (AFTNs). In this condition, hyperthyroidism is associated with a single thyroid nodule that functions independently of the normal thyroid regulatory axis. About 75% of patients with functioning nodules are euthyroid at diagnosis, 20% are overtly hyperthyroid, and 5% are borderline thyrotoxic. AFTNs are more frequent in areas of iodine deficiency, such as Europe, than in the United States and account for 5% of all solitary nodules. In patients with euthyroid AFTNs, factors that increase the likelihood of developing thyrotoxicosis include (1) nodule size 3 cm or larger, (2) older age, and (3) serum T_3 levels in the upper normal range. Overall, about 20% to 25% of functioning nodules eventually become thyrotoxic.

A laboratory picture of T_3 toxicosis can be observed, since nodules secrete relatively more T_3 than T_4. Radionuclide thyroid imaging with either ^{123}I or ^{99m}Tc shows a concentration of radioisotope in a single area corresponding to the nodule. There is partial or complete suppression of the rest of the thyroid gland.

In thyrotoxic patients treatment options and considerations are similar to those discussed for a toxic multinodular goiter. For those patients who are asymptomatic, observation and periodic thyroid function monitoring are reasonable, especially if the patient is young and healthy. In older patients and in those with preexisting medical conditions, such as cardiovascular disease, ablation treatment may be indicated.

Thyroiditis

Subacute Thyroiditis. Subacute thyroiditis, the most common cause of the painful thyroid, is a self-limited inflammation of the thyroid, probably due to a viral infection of the gland. Transient thyrotoxicosis results from leakage of large quantities of stored thyroid hormones from the inflamed gland. The thyrotoxic phase lasts weeks to months and is followed by a euthyroid then a hypothyroid phase as the gland is depleted of hormone. Normal thyroid function recovers in 95% of patients within 6 to 12 months.

A prodromal upper respiratory tract illness is common. Typical symptoms include pain in the thyroid area with radiation to the ears or jaw, malaise, and low-grade fever. Thyrotoxicosis is present in ~50% of patients. On physical examination a tender, mildly enlarged thyroid is characteristic. Acute hemorrhage into a thyroid nodule and suppurative thyroiditis can also cause a painful thyroid, but are less common. In addition to elevated serum thyroid hormone concentrations and suppressed serum TSH values in the toxic phase, an elevated erythrocyte sedimentation rate and a low RAIU are essential to confirm the diagnosis. Thyroid antibodies (antithyroglobulin and anti-TPO) are usually absent or only weakly positive. Although most patients are only mildly to moderately ill, subacute thyroiditis may have a dramatic presentation, with marked fever and severe thyrotoxicosis.

Treatment is aimed at the relief of symptoms. Aspirin or other nonsteroidal antiinflammatory agents are very effective for mild to moderate thyroid pain. Steroid administration (prednisone 20 to 40 mg/d) may be necessary for treatment of severe thyroid pain. Up to 20% of patients will have recurrence of pain on discontinuation of the steroids, which responds to the reinstitution of the drug. In general, steroids should be tapered over a 2 to 4 week period. Subacute thyroiditis rarely recurs. Control of the thyrotoxic symptoms can be achieved with β-adrenergic blockers, while L-T_4 replacement may be indicated for relief of symptoms in the hypothyroid phase.

Postpartum and Painless Thyroiditis. Postpartum and painless thyroiditis are also inflammatory thyroid disorders; in contrast to subacute thyroiditis, the thyroidal injury is immune-mediated. Postpartum thyroiditis is very common, affecting up to 20% of women in the postpartum period, usually within the first 4 months. Painless thyroiditis is much less common and can occur in both men and women.

Similar to subacute thyroiditis, inflammation and destruction of thyroid tissue results in the release of thyroid hormone, resulting in a thyrotoxic phase. As the gland becomes depleted, the thyrotoxicosis abates and a hypothyroid phase ensues, followed by restoration of normal thyroid function within 1 year. In general, one third of patients will demonstrate the classic biphasic pattern, one third will have only the thyrotoxic phase, and one third will present with only the hypothyroid phase. In contrast to subacute thyroiditis, the hypothyroid phase is permanent in up to 20% of patients and relapse of postpartum thyroiditis after subsequent pregnancies is common.

As in subacute thyroiditis, elevated serum thyroid hormone concentrations, suppressed serum TSH values, and a low RAIU are observed in the toxic phase. In contrast to subacute thyroiditis, thyroid antibodies (antithyroglobulin and anti-TPO) are usually present in high titer. Measurement of the serum thyroglobulin concentration is helpful to differentiate thyroiditis (high serum thyroglobulin concentrations) from surreptitious thyroid hormone administration (low serum thyroglobulin concentrations). Control of the thyrotoxic symptoms can be achieved with β-adrenergic blockers, while L-T_4 replacement may be indicated for relief of symptoms in the hypothyroid phase in these self-limited disorders. L-T_4 replacement, if begun, should be discontinued after 6 to 9 months to determine if there has been recovery of thyroid function.

Rare Causes of Thyrotoxicosis (Box 97-7). TSH-induced hyperthyroidism results from both tumoral and nontumoral TSH hypersecretion from the pituitary. In a hyperthyroid patient the finding of normal or high serum TSH concentrations in conjunction with elevated serum T_4 levels is the most distinctive feature of this disorder. Pituitary TSH-secreting tumors are usually macroadenomas and identifiable on MRI scan of the sellar region and require surgical excision. Although medical therapy is limited, octreotide, a long-acting somatostatin analog, has been successfully used as adjunctive therapy in these patients. Nontumoral pituitary TSH hypersecretion may be due to the

Box 97-7. Rare Causes of Thyrotoxicosis

TSH-secreting pituitary adenoma
Selective pituitary thyroid hormone resistance
Trophoblastic tumors: choriocarcinoma and hydatidiform mole
Differentiated follicular thyroid carcinoma
Struma ovarii
Thyrotoxicosis factitia
Autosomal dominant nonautoimmune hyperthyroidism

rare syndrome of thyroid hormone resistance. Thyrotoxicosis is seen in a subset of these patients with selective pituitary thyroid hormone resistance.

Trophoblastic tumors, either hydatidiform moles or choriocarcinomas, secrete human chorionic gonadotropin (hCG), which has weak TSH-like biologic activity. Very high concentrations of serum hCG, such as those detected in patients with these tumors, can result in hyperthyroidism. Therapy is aimed at either surgical removal of the tumor or appropriate chemotherapy. Differentiated follicular thyroid carcinoma, particularly if metastatic, is a rare cause of thyrotoxicosis. A whole-body ^{131}I scan shows increased uptake in thyroidal and extrathyroidal areas. High-dose radioiodine ablation treatment is warranted in these situations. Struma ovarii is a benign ovarian tumor that contains ectopic thyroid tissue. Very rarely this tumor produces enough thyroid hormone to cause thyrotoxicosis. Surgical removal of the tumor treats the thyrotoxicosis. Autosomal dominant nonautoimmune hyperthyroidism has been described in children, including newborns. It is caused by constitutively activating germline mutations in the TSH-receptor gene.

Thyrotoxicosis factitia results from the ingestion of large doses of thyroid hormone. The self-administration of thyroid hormones is often surreptitious. Occasionally accidental ingestions can occur, especially in children. Thyrotoxicosis may be clinically evident, but the thyroid gland is not enlarged. A low RAIU and a low serum thyroglobulin concentration are characteristic findings. Depending on the thyroid preparation ingested, either or both serum T_4 and T_3 concentrations are elevated.

Special Considerations

Hyperthyroidism in Pregnancy. Thyrotoxicosis occurs in about 0.2% of pregnancies and is most frequently caused by Graves' disease. Physiologic changes that occur in pregnancy result in clinical features that resemble those of hyperthyroidism (i.e., increased heart rate, palpitations, heat intolerance, diaphoresis). Signs that are more specific to thyrotoxicosis include lid lag, tremor, and diffuse goiter. Weight gain during pregnancy may be inappropriately low.

High serum total T_4 and T_3 concentrations and low serum THBR values are characteristic findings in normal pregnancy and may obscure the diagnosis of thyrotoxicosis (see Box 97-3). As in the nonpregnant patient, thyrotoxicosis is confirmed biochemically with an elevated FTI, an elevated total T_3, and a suppressed TSH. Mild hyperthyroidism may be seen in association with hyperemesis gravidarum during or at the end of the first trimester. This is due to thyroidal stimulation from elevated serum hCG concentrations and rarely requires the institution of antithyroid therapy. The hyperthyroidism resolves as serum hCG concentrations fall.

RAIU and radioisotope imaging studies are contraindicated in the pregnant patient. ATDs are the treatment of choice. PTU is preferred over methimazole because of lower transplacental passage and extensive clinical experience with PTU in pregnancy. PTU dosage should be minimized to keep serum FTI in the upper half of the normal range. As pregnancy progresses, Graves' disease often improves. Indeed, it is not uncommon for patients to require daily PTU dosages of less than 100 mg or to be off all ATDs by the end of pregnancy. Therefore PTU dosage should be reduced and maternal thyroid function should be frequently monitored to decrease chances of fetal hypothyroidism. Relapse or worsening of Graves' disease is common after delivery, and patients should be monitored closely in the postpartum period.

If the pregnant woman is allergic to thionamides, subtotal thyroidectomy in the second trimester is recommended. As indicated above, RAI therapy is contraindicated because it can cause fetal hypothyroidism. Similarly, iodide administration is associated with fetal goiter and hypothyroidism and should be avoided. Since ATDs are transferred in small amounts to breast milk, the infant's thyroid function should be frequently monitored if nursing is desired.

Transplacental passage of maternal thyroid-stimulating immunoglobulins may result in fetal or neonatal hyperthyroidism. In the fetus, the diagnosis is based on increased fetal heart rate and hyperactivity. In this situation increased doses of ATDs may be advised and methimazole, with its higher degree of transplacental passage, may be preferable. Therapy is titrated based on the fetal heart rate. Neonatal Graves' disease occurs in 2% of the infants born to mothers with Graves' disease. Very high values of TSI (over 500% of controls) measured in the mother during the third trimester of pregnancy should alert the physician to the possibility of fetal and neonatal hyperthyroidism. ATDs and iopanoic acid (Telepaque) have been used to manage this disorder. Therapy is rarely required longer than 6 to 8 weeks.

Thyroid Storm. Thyroid storm is an uncommon but life-threatening complication of thyrotoxicosis in which a severe form of the disease is usually precipitated by an intercurrent medical problem. It occurs in untreated or partially treated thyrotoxic patients. Precipitating factors associated with thyroid storm include infections, stress, trauma, thyroidal or nonthyroidal surgery, diabetic ketoacidosis, labor, heart disease, and RAI treatment (especially if there was no pretreatment with ATDs).

Clinical features are similar to those of thyrotoxicosis, but more exaggerated. Cardinal features include fever (temperature usually over 38.5°C) and tachycardia out of proportion to the fever. Nausea, vomiting, diarrhea, agitation, and confusion are frequent presentations. Coma and death may ensue in up to 20% of patients. Thyroid function abnormalities are similar to those found in uncomplicated hyperthyroidism. Therefore thyroid storm is primarily a clinical diagnosis.

Treatment includes supportive measures such as intravenous fluids, antipyretics, cooling blankets, and sedation. ATDs are given in large doses. PTU is preferred over methimazole due to its additional advantage of impairing peripheral conversion of T_4 to T_3. Recommended initial dose for PTU is 200 to 300 mg every 6 hours. PTU and methimazole can be administered by nasogastric tube or rectally if necessary. Neither of these preparations is available for parenteral administration.

Iodides, orally or intravenously, may be used only after ATDs have been administered. The radiographic contrast dye iopanoic acid (Telepaque), 1 gm daily, is used to block thyroid hormone release and to inhibit T_4 to T_3 conversion. β-Adrenergic blockers, such as propranolol (oral or IV) and esmolol (IV), are given for heart rate control. Calcium channel blockers may also be used to control tachyarrhythmias. High-dose dexamethasone (0.5 to 1 mg every 6 hours IV) is recommended both as supportive therapy and as an inhibitor of T_4 and T_3 conversion. Plasmapheresis has also been used in severe cases. Finally, treatment of the underlying precipitating illness is essential to survival in thyroid storm.

Subclinical Hyperthyroidism. Subclinical hyperthyroidism is defined as TSH values in the subnormal or suppressed range, normal circulating thyroid hormone levels, and no specific signs of thyrotoxicosis. The prevalence of subnormal TSH concentrations varies depending on the patient population sample, ranging from 4% in an ambulatory setting to 30% in a hospitalized setting. The majority of the patients with subclinical hyperthyroidism are receiving exogenous thyroid hormone therapy. Endogenous subclinical hyperthyroidism is commonly associated with an autonomous nodular or multinodular goiter and, to a lesser degree, with early Graves' disease, thyroiditis, or an iodine load. Other causes of subnormal and suppressed TSH values that must be differentiated from subclinical hyperthyroidism include hypopituitarism and nonthyroidal illness (see below).

The slight increases in thyroid hormone production or intake that translate in the low serum TSH values seen in subclinical hyperthyroidism have been reported to have adverse effects on both the skeletal and the cardiovascular systems. As noted above, a significant reduction in bone mineral density, especially among postmenopausal women, has been reported in several studies in patients taking suppressive doses of L-T_4. Adverse cardiac effects include arrhythmias, such as atrial fibrillation, and worsening of angina. Up to 10% of patients presenting with atrial fibrillation have suppressed serum TSH values, with up to 40% of these patients fitting the definition of subclinical hyperthyroidism.

Management of subclinical hyperthyroidism in patients receiving L-T_4 replacement therapy is straightforward. The dosage should be titrated to maintain a serum TSH value within the normal range. In patients taking suppressive doses of L-T_4 for goiter reduction or thyroid cancer, in whom a low TSH is the goal of therapy, the administered dosage should be the lowest necessary to keep serum TSH concentrations in the target level.

Treatment of endogenous subclinical hyperthyroidism should be considered based on the individual situation. Factors such as age, preexisting medical conditions (i.e., coronary artery disease, osteoporosis, hypertension, arrhythmias), and the likelihood of becoming overtly hyperthyroid should be taken into account. A trial of ATDs to normalize the TSH is reasonable to determine if symptoms possibly related to subclinical hyperthyroidism may improve. RAI therapy may be the best option in patients with a multinodular goiter.

THYROID NODULES

Nodular thyroid disease is the most common endocrinopathy. The prevalence of clinically apparent nodules is 4% to 7% in the United States, with the frequency increasing throughout adult life. When ultrasound and autopsy data are included, the prevalence of thyroid nodules approaches 50% by age 60. As with other forms of thyroid disease, nodules are more frequent in women. Nodules have been estimated to develop at a rate of 0.1% per year. In individuals exposed to ionizing radiation, the rate of nodule development is twentyfold higher. Although the presence of a nodule raises the question of a malignancy, only 8% to 10% of patients with thyroid nodules have thyroid cancer. There are about 14,000 new cases of thyroid cancer diagnosed annually, with about 1000 deaths from the disease per year. However, many more people have clinically silent thyroid cancer: up to 35% of thyroids removed at autopsy or at surgery harbor a small (under 1 cm), clinically silent papillary cancer.

Table 97-6. Differential Diagnosis of Thyroid Nodules

Type	Incidence (%)
Benign nodules	**83-92**
Colloid (adenomatous)	42-77
Follicular adenomas	15-40
Thyroiditis	<5
Nonthyroid	<5
Congenital abnormalities	<1
Other	<1
Malignant nodules	**8-17**
Papillary	50-70
Follicular	10-15
Anaplastic	5-10
Medullary	5-10
Lymphoma	1-5
Metastatic	<5
Thyroid cysts	**15-25**
Benign	85
Malignant	15

The mechanism underlying nodule growth and development in most cases remains unknown. Thyroid cancer is more frequent in patients exposed to ionizing radiation, such as radiation treatments for acne, tonsillitis, enlarged thymus, or cheloid scars or exposure to nuclear fallout (i.e., Chernobyl, Three Mile Island, Nevada atomic bomb tests). In the latter situation, the risk is highest in children exposed to nuclear fallout, with little increased risk observed in adults who were exposed. Nodules in general are more frequent in patients exposed to ionizing radiation, as are multiple nodules in a single exposed patient. In addition, nodules are more frequent in individuals residing in regions of endemic iodine deficiency.

The vast majority (over 90%) of thyroid nodules are benign lesions (Table 97-6). The most common benign nodule is the colloid, or adenomatous, nodule, followed by follicular adenomas. Thyroiditis is unusual in a solitary nodule but common in a multinodular gland. Of the malignant nodules, papillary cancer is most common, followed by follicular and then anaplastic carcinoma. Medullary carcinoma occurs most often over the age of 40, with about 20% of cases being associated with the familial multiple endocrine neoplasia type IIA (MEN IIA) and mutations in the RET proto-oncogene. Cysts make up 15% to 25% of all nodules and include simple cysts, hemorrhagic adenomas, parathyroid cysts, and necrotic papillary cancers. Rare causes of a solitary thyroid nodule include metastatic carcinoma and fungal or parasitic infection in the immunocompromised patient.

Patient Evaluation

Nodules that occur at the extremes of age are more likely to be malignant. Rapid growth and symptoms of local invasion (i.e., vocal cord paralysis, dysphagia) are poor prognostic signs, but few patients present with these symptoms. The most common presentation is that of a nodule discovered incidentally during a physical examination performed for other reasons. Once the nodule is discovered, the patient should be asked about symptoms of hyperthyroidism, exposure to radiation, and family history of medullary or papillary thyroid cancer or familial polyposis (Gardner's syndrome).

Physical examination should reveal nodules larger than 1 cm unless they lie deep in the neck. The physical characteristics may give clues as to the malignant potential of the nodule. However, a hard, firm nodule can be seen in Hashimoto's thyroiditis and a cystic papillary carcinoma may be soft and mobile. Cancers are more often found in patients with solitary nodules, although when examined by ultrasound or at surgery multiple nodules are found in up to two thirds of thyroid cancer patients. Most thyroid cancers metastasize locally, so the presence of suspicious lymph nodes in the cervical and supraclavicular regions should be noted.

Diagnosis

In the absence of signs of hyperthyroidism, thyroid function tests are usually normal. Serum TSH measurement is often the only test needed. Management principles are outlined in Box 97-8. If medullary carcinoma is suspected, serum calcitonin should be measured. Once a diagnosis of medullary carcinoma is confirmed, testing for mutations in the RET proto-oncogene should be performed to identify hereditary disease. Mutations in the RET proto-oncogene are present in 90% to 95% of hereditary disease and 25% of sporadic disease.

Box 97-8. Evaluation of Thyroid Nodules

1. Evaluation of thyroid nodules with a full array of diagnostic techniques is costly.
2. If the diagnosis of a nodule or diffuse goiter is uncertain, the most cost-effective approach is to have another physician assess the findings.
3. A discrete, firm, irregular mass associated with suspicious lymphadenopathy is strongly suggestive of malignancy.
4. Thyroid dysfunction implies a background of diffuse and almost always benign disease.
5. Approximately 90% of uninodular thyroid disease proves to be cold on isotopic screening. The 10% of nodules that are hot do not usually require evaluation for malignancy. Clinical follow-up is indicated to detect the rare malignant hot nodule.
6. Isotopic scanning may be 3 to 5 times as expensive as fine-needle aspiration biopsy (FNAB). By performing FNAB first, isotopic scans may be reduced by 50%, saving both time and money.
7. Thyroid ultrasounds are not employed in early diagnostic assessment of thyroid nodules because of poor diagnostic discrimination between benign and malignant processes. They may be utilized, however, to accurately guide FNA and to delineate small or posterior masses.
8. Controversy currently exists over whether to perform isotopic scans on all patients before biopsy to identify cold nodules at greater cost and inconvenience or whether to perform FNAB first and run the risk of indeterminate or false-negative biopsy results. Community standards and consultation with an endocrinologist provide the best guide at this time.

Modified from Clinical Guidelines and Algorithms, Harvard Community Health Plan.

Fine-needle Aspiration Biopsy. The most cost-effective initial test in the nontoxic patient with a thyroid nodule is fine-needle aspiration biopsy (FNAB), which is a safe and accurate method to diagnose the presence of a thyroid malignancy. Essential to the accuracy of the FNAB is the presence of a cytopathologist skilled in the interpretation of the results. Four cytologic results are possible: (1) benign (negative), (2) malignant (positive), (3) suspicious (possible follicular or Hürthle cell tumor), and (4) nondiagnostic (inadequate) (Table 97-7). Benign conditions identified by FNAB include colloid goiter, cysts, and thyroiditis. Benign FNAB smears are obtained in the vast majority of patients. Positive FNAB smears include papillary, medullary, and anaplastic primary thyroid cancer; metastatic cancer; and lymphoma. Since the diagnosis of follicular carcinoma requires the documentation of vascular or capsular invasion, the finding of follicular cells on FNAB may indicate either a benign or malignant neoplasm and thus falls into the suspicious category. Nondiagnostic FNAB smears often occur in the setting of vascular or cystic lesions or when performed by less experienced physicians. Repeat FNAB yields a satisfactory smear in up to 50% of cases that were initially nondiagnostic. FNAB is very accurate, with a false-positive rate of 2.9% and a false-negative rate of 5.2%, representing the average in seven published series.

Table 97-7. Cytologic Categories in Fine-needle Aspiration Biopsy of the Thyroid

Cytologic diagnosis	Frequency (%)*
Benign	70.3
Malignant	3.6
Suspicious	10.1
Nondiagnostic	16.3

*Average of eight published series.

Imaging Studies. The function of the thyroid nodule can be addressed through the use of radionuclide imaging with either iodine or technetium isotopes. If the FNAB is performed as the initial test, all patients with suspicious biopsy results should undergo a radionuclide scan to determine whether or not the nodule is functioning, since the incidence of malignancy in a functioning adenoma is under 1%. Although radioisotope scanning is unnecessary preoperatively in patients with thyroid malignancies, patients whose benign nodules are most likely to decrease in size with thyroid hormone suppression therapy may be identified with

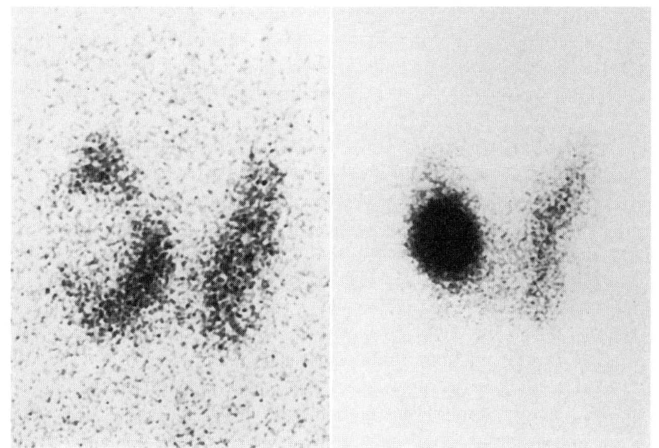

Fig. 97-9. Radioiodine imaging in the evaluation of the solitary thyroid nodule. Two patients presented with a solitary 2.5-cm nodule in the right lobe of the thyroid. Thyroid imaging with ^{123}I was obtained. **A,** This scan represents a hypofunctioning, or cold, nodule, with decreased uptake in the region of the palpable nodule. Uptake in the rest of the gland is homogeneous. This patient was referred for FNAB of the nodule. **B,** This scan represents a functioning nodule, with partial suppression of the remaining thyroid tissue. This patient was placed on L-T_4 suppression and a suppression scan was obtained.

radioisotope imaging (see further). When used as the initial test, radioiodine scans will identify those patients who will benefit the most by a biopsy of the nodule (i.e., those with a hypofunctioning, or cold, nodule). Shown in Fig. 97-9 are radioiodine scans of two asymptomatic patients presenting with a 2.5-cm solitary nodule in the right lobe of the thyroid. The patient in Fig. 97-9, *A,* has a hypofunctioning (cold) nodule, as shown by the absence of radionuclide uptake in the region of the nodule. This patient was referred for biopsy of the nodule. The patient in Fig. 97-9, *B,* has a functioning nodule that is concentrating almost all of the radionuclide; this patient was placed on thyroid hormone in an attempt to suppress and shrink the nodule.

Ultrasound rarely adds more to the evaluation of the thyroid nodule over and above the physical examination and a radioisotope scan and cannot discriminate between a benign and malignant nodule. Ultrasound can readily diagnose a cyst; however, cysts show up as cold nodules on scans and thus are referred for biopsy, where the diagnosis is made. Ultrasound is most useful in documenting the size of the nodule, identifying the presence of nonpalpable nodules, and assessing the effect of thyroid hormone on shrinking benign nodules. Ultrasound is also useful in guiding FNAB of nodules that are difficult to palpate, such as those deep in the neck, or those with significant substernal extension. However, physical examination by an experienced physician is adequate in most cases.

Nonpalpable Nodules. Occasionally, thyroid nodules will be identified during an imaging study performed for another reason, such as carotid ultrasound or chest CT. The evaluation of these thyroid "incidentalomas" should include a physical examination and TSH testing and, if the nodule is palpable, the approach indicated above should be followed. If the nodule is nonpalpable and less than 1 cm on the initial imaging study, follow-up thyroid palpations every 6 months to a year are reasonable. If the nonpalpable nodule is 1 cm or greater, ultrasound-guided biopsy is a reasonable approach.

Management

Surgery is indicated for patients with FNAB smears in the malignant category. The management of those patients with suspicious FNAB results depends on the sequence of procedures performed. If radioisotope imaging is performed first, only those patients with a hypofunctioning nodule will be referred for FNAB; thus all suspicious FNAB results would be referred for surgery. If FNAB is the initial procedure, patients with suspicious FNAB smears are referred for radioisotope scanning, after which those with hypofunctioning nodules are referred for surgery (see Box 97-8). Surgery is indicated for large benign nodules and any nodule that continues to increase in size, especially if the patient is placed on L-T_4 suppression (see below).

Thyroid Cancer. The extent of surgery for thyroid cancer is controversial and recommendations vary significantly. Factors affecting surgery include the size of the lesion, pathology, and experience of the surgeon. Lobectomies are performed less frequently since the publication of data demonstrating cancer foci in the opposite lobe in up to 35% of patients. A near-total thyroidectomy is thought by many to be appropriate for most lesions and affords less risk of either vocal cord paralysis or hypoparathyroidism compared with total thyroidectomy.

In patients with differentiated thyroid cancer, total body scanning with ^{131}I should be performed 6 to 8 weeks after near-total thyroidectomy surgery to identify metastatic disease. Radioiodine scanning is of no value in the patient with medullary thyroid cancer, since this tumor does not take up iodine. Postoperative radioiodine scanning is done when the patient is hypothyroid (TSH over 50 mU/L) in order to maximally stimulate any remaining thyroid remnants with endogenous TSH; thus the patient should not be started on L-T_4 therapy postoperatively. To minimize the time the patient is hypothyroid, L-T_3 (Cytomel, 50 to 75 μg per day) may be administered for 3 to 4 weeks after surgery, then discontinued for 2 weeks. Depending on the residual uptake or the presence of metastatic disease, an ablative dose of ^{131}I ranging from 30 to 150 mCi is administered and a repeat total body scan is obtained 1 week later. The precise amount of ^{131}I needed to treat residual tissue and metastases is also controversial. Foci of metastatic disease outside the neck should be imaged by CT or MRI to follow the progression or regression of the disease.

Suppressive therapy with L-T_4 is indicated in all patients after treatment for thyroid cancer. The goal of therapy is to keep serum TSH levels in the subnormal range. Serum thyroglobulin, which is only produced by differentiated thyroid tissue, is a valuable tumor marker after treatment for thyroid cancer, since the goal of surgery and radioiodine ablation is the elimination of all thyroid tissue, both malignant and normal. Follow-up evaluation every 6 months with a physical examination and measurement of serum TSH and thyroglobulin concentrations is reasonable. A rise in serum thyroglobulin concentration is often the first indication of recurrent disease.

Repeat total body radioiodine scanning should be performed 1 year after the initial surgery and patients retreated if residual uptake is found. This usually means withdrawing the patient from L-T_4 to increase endogenous TSH and obtaining a radioiodine scan, resulting in the patient becoming symptomatically hypothyroid. Recently, recombinant human TSH (rhTSH [Thyrogen]) has become available and has been shown to stimulate radioiodine uptake in, and release of thyroglobulin from, thyroid remnants that persist in patients with metastatic differentiated thyroid cancer. The use of Thyrogen allows the patient to remain on L-T_4 suppression and precludes the morbidity of severe hypothyroidism associated with withdrawal of radioiodine scanning. Thyrogen scanning should be limited to those patients with previously negative (outside of the neck) postablative radioiodine scans or those with low (<2 ng/ml) thyroglobulin concentrations while on L-T_4 suppression therapy. At present, Thyrogen is approved only for radioiodine scanning and not for primary radioiodine therapy. Thus individuals with rising thyroglobulin concentrations on L-T_4 suppression or significant uptake on a Thyrogen scan will have to be withdrawn from L-T_4 to undergo repeat radioiodine therapy. If no uptake is seen on the 1-year scan, follow-up scans can be obtained every 3 to 5 years as long as serum thyroglobulin measurements while on L-T_4 suppression therapy remain stable.

Prognosis in patients with thyroid cancer depends on the pathology and size of the tumor and is generally worse in the elderly. Overall, the vast majority of patients with thyroid cancer will not die of their disease. Papillary cancer is the least aggressive tumor, metastasizes locally, and has a 10-year survival rate greater than 90%. Lymph node metastasis at the time of diagnosis does little to alter the prognosis. Follicular cancer is more aggressive and can metastasize via the bloodstream. Still, prognosis is fair and long-term survival is common. Anaplastic cancer is the exception, since it is highly malignant with survival usually less than 6 months.

Benign Nodules. Two options are available for the patient diagnosed with a benign nodule: observation or suppressive L-T_4 therapy. The rationale behind suppressive L-T_4 therapy is that the benign nodule will either stop growing or decrease in size after TSH stimulation to the thyroid gland is turned off. The success rate of such therapy ranges from 0% to 68% in different studies.

Identification of those patients who are most likely to benefit from thyroid hormone therapy can be achieved through measurement of the serum TSH concentration and radioisotope scanning. Suppression therapy has no value if thyroid nodule autonomy exists, as evidenced by a subnormal TSH value. Functioning nodules are the most likely to respond to suppression therapy. However, once TSH concentrations are suppressed, a repeat radioisotope scan (suppression scan) should be obtained. If significant uptake persists on a suppression scan, the nodule is autonomous and L-T_4 therapy should be discontinued. Suppression therapy needs to be considered carefully in older patients or those with coronary artery disease. Hypofunctioning nodules are much less likely to respond to suppression therapy. However, a 6-month trial of L-T_4 suppression is reasonable and L-T_4 therapy should be continued for as long as the nodule is decreasing in size. Once the size of a nodule remains stable for 6 to 12 months, therapy should be discontinued and the nodule observed for recurrent growth. Any nodule that grows during suppression therapy requires repeat biopsy and/or surgical excision.

Box 97-9. Changes in Thyroid Hormone Economy Due to Nonthyroidal Factors

Inhibition of $T_4 \rightarrow T_3$ Conversion	Decrease in TSH Secretion
Acute illness	Acute illness
Chronic illness	Chronic illness
Caloric restriction	Caloric restriction
Glucocorticoids	Glucocorticoids
β-Blockers	Dopamine agonists
Amiodarone	Adrenergic agonists
	Acute psychosis
	Surgical stress

SICK EUTHYROID SYNDROME

Widespread changes in thyroid hormone economy occur in all critically ill patients and in many others with less severe illnesses, leading to alterations in thyroid function tests that may lead to the mistaken determination of thyroid dysfunction in euthyroid patients. The sick euthyroid syndrome is one of the most common disorders in hospitalized patients and results in frequent consultation to the endocrine service. The changes in thyroid hormone economy in ill patients occur as a result of alterations in: (1) the peripheral metabolism of the thyroid hormones, (2) TSH regulation, and (3) the binding of thyroid hormone to TBG (Boxes 97-3 and 97-9).

The changes in serum concentrations of thyroid hormone that are observed in ill patients represent a continuum of changes that depends on the severity of the illness (Fig. 97-10). Thus the wide spectrum of thyroid function tests observed often results from the differing points in the course of the illness that the thyroid function tests were obtained. Over half of the patients admitted to the medical service will demonstrate depressed serum T_3 concentrations due to inhibition of T_4 deiodination, which can occur within 24 hours after the onset of illness *(low T_3 state)*. This can lead to elevated serum T_4 levels *(high T_4 state)* early on in an acute illness, but soon T_4 levels return to the normal range. Since the most common finding in hospitalized patients is a low serum T_3, the only time a serum T_3 should be measured is if there is a high clinical suspicion of thyrotoxicosis. Clinically, hospitalized patients with low T_3 concentrations appear euthyroid, although mild prolongation in Achilles reflex time is found in some patients.

As the severity and the duration of the illness increase, serum total T_4 levels decrease into the subnormal range *(low T_4 state)*. Contributing to this decrease in serum T_4 levels are: (1) a decrease in the binding of T_4 to serum carrier proteins, (2) a decrease in serum TSH levels leading to decreased thyroidal production of T_4, and (3) an increase in nondeiodinative pathways of T_4 metabolism. The decline in serum T_4 levels correlates with prognosis in the critically ill medical patient, with mortality increasing as serum T_4 levels drop below 4 μg/dl and approaching 80% in patients with serum T_4 levels < 2 μg/dl. Treatment of these patients with T_4 or T_3 fails to alter this grave prognosis, and is not indicated, suggesting that the low T_4 state is probably more of a marker of multisystem failure in these critically ill patients.

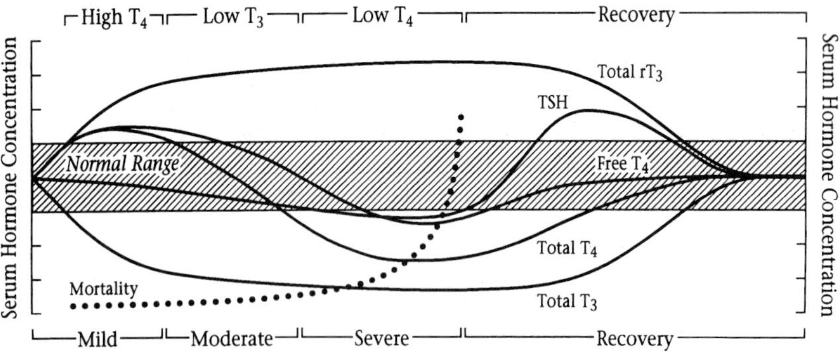

Fig. 97-10. Alterations in thyroid hormone concentrations with critical illness. Schematic representation of the continuum of changes in serum thyroid hormone levels in patients with nonthyroidal illness. These alterations become more pronounced with increasing severity of the illness and return to the normal range as the illness subsides and the patient recovers. A rapidly rising mortality accompanies the fall in total and free T_4 levels. (From Farwell AF: Sick euthyroid syndrome in the intensive care unit. In Irwin RS, Cerra FB, Rippe JM, editors: *Intensive care medicine,* ed 4, Philadelphia, 1999, Lippincott-William & Wilkins.)

As acute illness resolves, so do the alterations in thyroid hormone concentrations *(recovery state).* This stage may be prolonged and is characterized by modest increases in serum TSH levels. Mild to moderate elevations of serum TSH concentrations have been reported in up to 20% of hospitalized patients. Full recovery, with restoration of thyroid hormone levels to the normal range, is observed in ~90% of individuals with mildly elevated TSH values within several months after they are discharged from the hospital.

The spectrum of alterations in thyroid function tests seen in patients with nonthyroidal illness is the result of a coordinated systemic reaction to illness and most likely represents an adaptive response of the endocrine system to the acute illness. The interpretation of thyroid function tests in the ill patient and the identification of those patients with intrinsic thyroid dysfunction are often difficult and must take into consideration both the clinical assessment of the patient and the duration and severity of the illness. Thyroid hormone replacement therapy is not indicated in the vast majority of patients. Whenever possible, it is best to defer the evaluation of thyroid function until the patient has recovered from the critical illness.

SCREENING FOR THYROID DISEASE

Screening for thyroid disease would appear to be beneficial due to the subtle and nonspecific nature of the symptoms of thyroid dysfunction and the fact that thyroid disorders are eminently treatable. In a large study in Wickham, England, about 7.5% of women and 2.8% of men were found to have TSH levels > 6 mU/l. Review of several studies indicates that the worldwide prevalence of thyroid gland failure is ~5%. The Framingham Study revealed that 10.3% of women over the age of 60 had a TSH > 5 mU/l. Subsequent studies in Michigan and Colorado have demonstrated a prevalence of elevated TSH values of 7.5% and 9.5%, respectively, and a prevalence of low TSH values of 2.5% and 2.2%, respectively. In all studies, the prevalence of abnormal TSH values increases with age and is far more common in women than men.

Case-finding, or identifying disease in patients who seek medical attention for unrelated reasons, is a reasonable screening approach to detect thyroid disease. Although most medical societies now agree that screening women older than 50 years of age for thyroid dysfunction is reasonable, a case can be made that screening patients beginning at age 35 has equal or better cost-effectiveness than other widely accepted preventative medical interventions. In addition, patient subpopulations that do have a higher incidence of thyroid dysfunction can be identified, including elderly individuals of both sexes and patients with preexisting autoimmune diseases, diabetes, hypercholesterolemia, atrial fibrillation, or carpal tunnel syndrome. Case-finding for thyroid disease is not helpful in patients admitted to an acute care medical or psychiatric ward. Abnormal test results are common and rarely indicate previously unrecognized thyroid dysfunction. In these patients, thyroid function testing should be reserved for those individuals in whom the clinical suspicion of thyroid disease is high.

The best single screening test is a TSH determination by a sensitive TSH assay, since the specificity of a normal TSH value in ruling out thyroid disease is close to 100%. In all cases when an abnormal result is obtained, the diagnosis should be confirmed with other tests of thyroid function as well as a directed clinical evaluation. Therapy should not be instituted on the basis of a single abnormal thyroid function test.

EBM EVIDENCE-BASED MEDICINE

The primary sources for this chapter were evaluated MEDLINE, PUBMED, and the previous edition of this textbook. Electronic searches dating back to 1990 were conducted, identifying systemic reviews, meta-analyses, large clinical trials, and medical society guidelines.

ADDITIONAL READINGS

Arem R, Escalante D: Subclinical hypothyroidism: epidemiology, diagnosis and significance, *Adv Intern Med* 41:213-250, 1996.

Astakhova LN, et al: Chernobyl-related thyroid cancer in children of Belarus: a case-control study, *Radiation Research* 150:349-356, 1998.

Braverman LE, Utiger RD, editors: *The thyroid,* ed 8, Philadelphia, 2000, Lippincott Williams & Wilkins.

Bartalena L, Marcocci C, Bogazzi F, et al: Use of corticosteroids to prevent progression of Graves' ophthalmopathy after radioiodine therapy for hyperthyroidism, *N Engl J Med* 321:1349-1352, 1989.

Bartalena L, et al: Relation between therapy for hyperthyroidism and the course of Graves' ophthalmopathy, *N Engl J Med* 338:73-78, 1998.

Bartalena L, et al: Cigarette smoking and treatment outcomes in Graves' ophthalmopathy, *Ann Intern Med* 129:632-635, 1998.

Brucker-Davis F, Skarulis MC, Grace MB, et al: Genetic and clinical features of 42 kindreds with resistance to thyroid hormone: the National Institutes of Health Prospective Study, *Ann Intern Med* 123:572-583, 1995.

Cooper DS: Subclinical thyroid disease: a clinician's perspective, *Ann Intern Med* 129:135-138, 1998.

Cooper DS: Antithyroid drugs for the treatment of hyperthyroidism caused by Graves' disease, *Endocrinol Met Clin North Am* 27:225-247, 1998.

Cooper DS, et al: Thyrotropin suppression and disease progression in patients with differentiated thyroid cancer: results from the National Thyroid Cancer Treatment Cooperative Registry, *Thyroid* 8:737-744, 1998.

Delange F: Neonatal screening for congenital hypothyroidism: results and perspectives, *Hormone Res* 48:51-61, 1997.

Danese MD, Powe NR, Sawin CT, et al: Screening for mild thyroid failure at the periodic health examination: a decision and cost-effective analysis, *JAMA* 276:285-292, 1996.

Farwell AP, Braverman LE: Thyroid and antithyroid drugs. In Hardman, JG, Limbird, LE, editors: *Goodman and Gilman's the pharmacological basis of therapeutics,* New York, 1996, McGraw-Hill, pp 1383-1410.

Farwell AP, Braverman LE: Inflammatory thyroid disorders, *Otolaryngol Clin North Am* 29:541-556, 1996.

Farwell AP: Sick euthyroid syndrome, *J Intensive Care Med* 12:249-260, 1997.

Gharib H, Mazzaferri EL: Thyroxine suppressive therapy in patients with nodular thyroid disease, *Ann Intern Med* 128:386-394, 1998.

Gharib H: Changing concepts in the diagnosis and management of thyroid nodules, *Endocrinol Met Clin North Am* 26:777-800, 1997.

Helfand M, Redfern CC: Screening for thyroid disease: an update. American College of Physicians, *Ann Intern Med* 129:144-158, 1998.

Kaplan MM: Assessment of thyroid function during pregnancy, *Thyroid* 2:57-61, 1992.

Ladenson PW, et al: Comparison of administration of recombinant human thyrotropin with withdrawal of thyroid hormone for radioactive iodine scanning in patients with thyroid carcinoma, *N Engl J Med* 337:888-896, 1997.

Laurberg P, Nygaard B, Glinoer D, et al: Guidelines for TSH-receptor antibody measurements in pregnancy: results of an evidence-based symposium organized by the European Thyroid Association, *Eur J Endocrinol* 139:584-586, 1998.

Lazarus JH, et al: The clinical spectrum of postpartum thyroid disease, *Quart J Med* 89:429-435, 1996.

Leenhardt L, et al: Indications and limits of ultrasound-guided cytology in the management of nonpalpable thyroid nodules, *J Clin Endocrinol Metab* 84:24-28, 1999.

Nicoloff JT, Spencer CA: The use and misuse of the sensitive thyrotropin assays, *J Clin Endocrinol Metab* 71:553-558, 1990.

Ron E, et al: Cancer mortality following treatment for adult hyperthyroidism. Cooperative Thyrotoxicosis Therapy Follow-up Study Group, *JAMA* 280:347-355, 1998.

Reference deleted in proofs.

Singer PA, et al: Treatment guidelines for patients with hyperthyroidism and hypothyroidism, *JAMA* 273:808-812, 1995.

Singer PA, et al: Treatment guidelines for patients with thyroid nodules and well-differentiated thyroid cancer, *Arch Intern Med* 156:2165-2172, 1996.

Tan GH, Gharib H: Thyroid incidentalomas: management approaches to nonpalpable nodules discovered incidentally on thyroid imaging, *Ann Intern Med* 126:226-231, 1997.

Tunbridge WMG, et al: The spectrum of thyroid disease in a community: the Wickham survey, *Clin Endocrinol* 7:481-493, 1977.

Vanderpump MPJ, Tunbridge WMG: The epidemiology of thyroid disease. In Braverman LE, Utiger RD, editors: *The thyroid,* ed 8, Philadelphia, 2000, Lippincott Williams & Wilkins, pp 467-473.

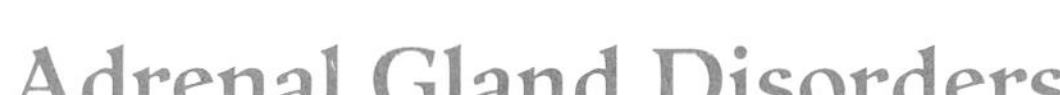

Adrenal Gland Disorders

Melanie J. Brunt
James C. Melby

ADRENAL ANATOMY AND PHYSIOLOGY

In the adrenal cortex, which constitutes 80% of the total adrenal weight, three zones are responsible for corticosteroid synthesis. The outermost layer, the zona glomerulosa, synthesizes aldosterone, which is the predominant mineralocorticoid responsible for sodium retention and potassium excretion. The middle and inner layers, the zona fasciculata and the zona reticularis, produce glucocorticoids (principally cortisol) and the sex steroids and their precursor, dehydroepiandrosterone (DHEA). Cortisol functions to promote protein and lipid catabolism and gluconeogenesis. Catecholamines are synthesized in the adrenal medulla, and they are regulated via the autonomic nervous system.

All corticosteroids are derived from cholesterol, which is found in abundance in the adrenal cortex. Regulatory systems for cortisol and aldosterone are outlined in Fig. 98-1. Cortisol is subject to negative feedback regulation via the hypothalamic-pituitary axis (HPA). The majority of the daily cortisol production of 15 to 25 mg is produced between 5 and 9 AM. Metabolic stress such as sepsis or myocardial infarction can raise production levels to 250 mg per day. Aldosterone is regulated via the renin-angiotensin feedback loop, through which low renal perfusion pressure stimulates increased aldosterone production. Extracellular potassium concentration also affects aldosterone secretion, and the HPA plays a small role as well, regulating about 15% of aldosterone production via adrenocorticotropic hormone (ACTH) stimulation.

ADRENOCORTICAL HYPOFUNCTION

Pathophysiology

Adrenocortical hypofunction can result from primary destruction of the adrenal cortex, with consequent loss of all corticosteroid hormone production. It may also be secondary, due to diminished ACTH production by the pituitary. In the latter disorder only glucocorticoid and androgen production are affected. Mineralocorticoid production remains largely intact because ACTH plays only a small role in aldosterone regulation. Angiotensin II and potassium are the principal factors affecting aldosterone production, and the renin-angiotensin II-aldosterone regulatory axis is independent of regulation by the pituitary. In both disorders the clinical consequences related to loss of cortisol, a hormone essential for survival, are paramount. Cortisol is essential for the maintenance of vascular tone and cardiovascular output due to its positive inotropic effects; thus hypotension may be present in either disorder. Hypoglycemia also occurs due to the loss of the permissive effects of cortisol on glycogenolysis and gluconeogenesis. Hypercalcemia may be present due to the loss of cortisol inhibition of intestinal absorption and renal reabsorption of calcium. Hyponatremia can also occur. In primary adrenal insufficiency this is due to loss of the

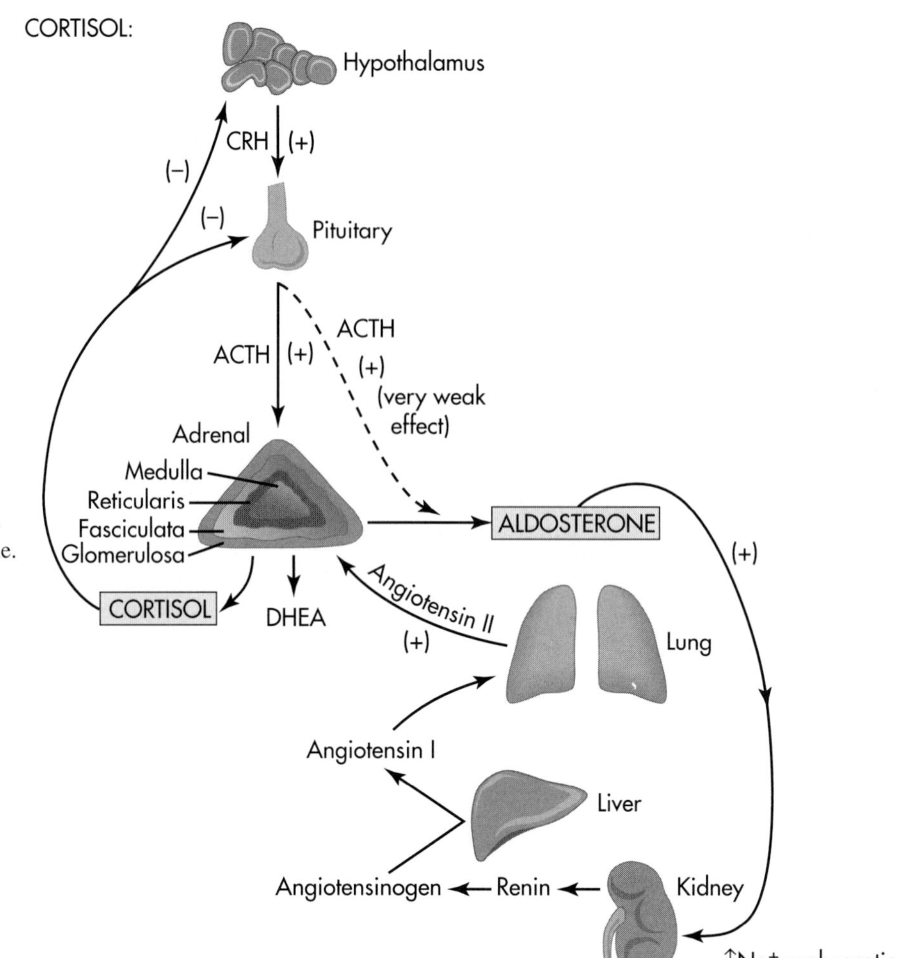

Fig. 98-1. Regulatory systems for cortisol and aldosterone. *CRH,* Corticotropin-releasing hormone; *ACTH,* adrenocorticotropic hormone; *DHEA,* dehydroepiandrosterone.

sodium-retentive properties of aldosterone. In secondary insufficiency it can occur despite normal aldosterone levels due to (1) decreased cortisol-mediated renal free water clearance and (2) compensatory elevations of antidiuretic hormone (ADH).

Hyperpigmentation is seen only in primary adrenal insufficiency and is due to increased secretion of β-lipotropin, a component of the precursor peptide that also contains ACTH. Also in primary insufficiency, the loss of aldosterone, the principal regulator of potassium excretion in the body, can result in potentially life-threatening hyperkalemia. Increased sodium excretion in the absence of aldosterone can result in profound volume depletion.

History and Physical Findings

Adrenal insufficiency often fails to be diagnosed because the clinical presentation can be quite nonspecific. Key clinical features include weakness, fatigue, anorexia, nausea/vomiting, weight loss, and symptoms of volume depletion. Box 98-1 lists the predominant clinical features of primary adrenal insufficiency, or Addison's disease, which is the most common type. Skin changes in this disease include diffuse hyperpigmentation with accentuation in palmar folds, scars, and oral mucosa (Fig. 98-2); longitudinal pigmented bands under nails; vitiligo in up to 15% of patients; and decreased pubic and axillary hair in females. Associated problems include weakness, fatigue, nausea and vomiting, and a craving for salt. It may be associated with other endocrine insufficiencies, such as hypothyroidism and hypoparathyroidism, pernicious anemia, thyroiditis, and alopecia areata. Treatment is to replace adrenal hormones. Secondary adrenal insufficiency most commonly occurs in the setting of panhypopituitarism; thus most patients have clinical signs and symptoms suggestive of secondary hypothyroidism and hypogonadism in addition to evidence of cortisol deficiency (see Chapter 99). Rarely secondary adrenal insufficiency is due to isolated ACTH deficiency. In this disorder symptoms and signs of cortisol deficiency such as hypotension, hyponatremia, malaise, and fatigue are present without concomitant evidence of secondary thyroid and gonadal failure.

The following cases illustrate the difficulty in making a diagnosis of adrenal insufficiency:

Case 1 A 50-year-old U.S. citizen living overseas in a tropical climate developed malaise, weakness, intermittent abdominal pain, and diarrhea a few months after a brief febrile illness. Physicians prescribed antibiotics without effect. During a visit to the United States he saw his internist, who referred him to a gastroenterologist. Several radiographic studies were performed, no diagnosis was found, and he was treated symptomatically. The patient continued to experience the same symptoms and became depressed, for which he pursued counseling. Upon his permanent return to the United States over a year later, he sought further

Box 98-1. Frequency of Clinical Features of Primary Adrenal Insufficiency

Symptoms

Weakness and fatigue (100%)
Anorexia (100%)
Nausea and diarrhea (56%)

Signs

Weight loss (100%)
Hyperpigmentation (97%)
Hypotension (91%)
Vitiligo (rare)

Laboratory Findings

Hyponatremia (90%)
Hyperkalemia (66%)
Hypoglycemia (40%)
Hypercalcemia (6%)

counseling and was started on a tricyclic antidepressant. A few weeks thereafter he experienced two falls, the second of which was associated with a loss of consciousness. He was brought to an emergency ward, where laboratory data revealed a sodium level of 110 mEq/L. Hyperpigmentation in sun-exposed areas was noted; the patient attributed this to frequent sun exposure. A workup revealed low cortisol levels with absent response to synthetic ACTH (cosyntropin) injection. A purified protein derivative (PPD) test was positive, and calcification was noted in the area of the right adrenal gland on computed tomographic (CT) scan of the abdomen. All symptoms resolved promptly with glucocorticoid replacement.

Case 2 A 35-year-old non–English-speaking immigrant from the Caribbean had a medical history remarkable only for a motor vehicle accident involving a brief loss of consciousness 5 years previously. He was brought to an emergency ward on many occasions over a 3-year period by family members due to confusional episodes associated with violent behavior, recurrent fevers, weight loss, and malaise. The patient was admitted to the hospital from the emergency ward on several occasions. On some of these admissions infections were documented, including streptococcal pharyngitis, pneumococcal pneumonia, and urinary tract infection; on other occasions extensive sepsis evaluations were unrevealing. His mental status remained abnormal but no explanation was found. Electrolytes were consistently within normal limits, although potassium was usually ≥4.5 mEq/L, sodium ≤140 mEq/L, and blood glucose 60 to 70 mg/dl. A blood glucose level of 29 mg/dl finally prompted evaluation of the adrenal axis, and poor response to synthetic ACTH injection was documented.

In both cases primary adrenal insufficiency was finally diagnosed, but the delay led to significant morbidity.

Etiology and Differential Diagnosis

Primary Adrenal Insufficiency. Idiopathic Addison's disease is the predominant cause of primary adrenal insufficiency (Box 98-2). This is thought in most cases to be an autoimmune disorder of the adrenal cortex characterized by lymphocytic infiltration on histologic examination. The prevalence of antiadrenal antibodies in patients with idiopathic Addison's disease is 70%; therefore the absence of antibodies does not rule out the diagnosis. Nearly half of Addison's disease patients develop associated endocrine disorders with organ-specific antibodies, such as pernicious anemia, gonadal failure, insulin-dependent diabetes mellitus, hypoparathyroidism, vitiligo, or thyroid disorders.

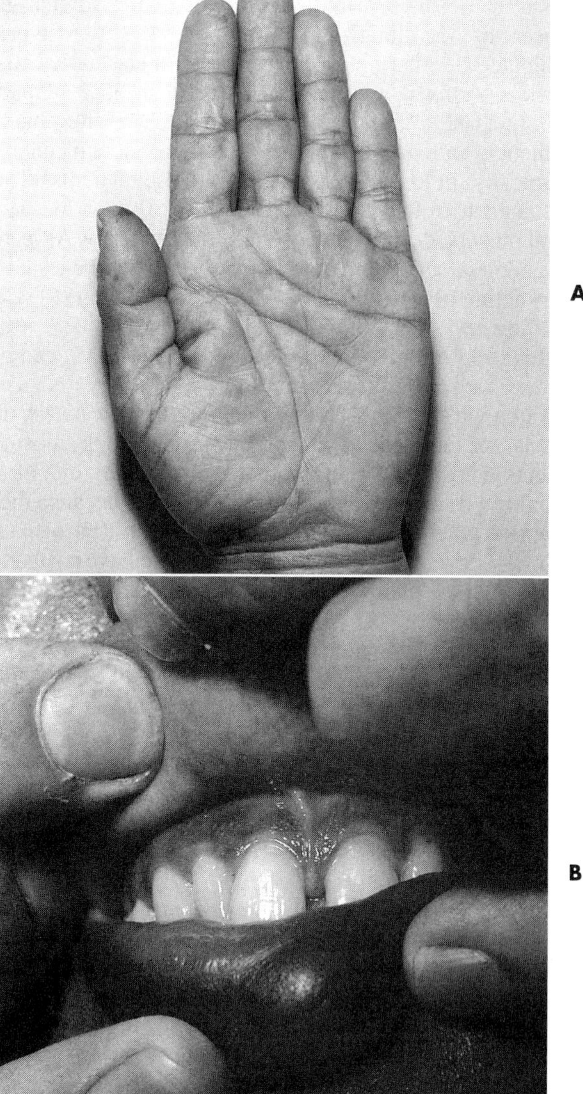

Fig. 98-2. Hyperpigmentation of almar folds **(A)** and gums in Addison's disease **(B).**

Tuberculosis once accounted for over 75% of all cases of Addison's disease. Although it is now less common, the emergence of resistant strains of tuberculosis among human immunodeficiency virus (HIV)-infected persons and increased immigration from countries with a high prevalence of tuberculosis may lead to a resurgence of this type of Addison's disease. Features of tuberculous adrenal insufficiency include adrenal enlargement in the early stages (within the first 5 years) followed by adrenal atrophy with calcification. Absence of these features does not rule out tuberculosis as a cause; thus skin testing for tuberculosis should be a standard part of the evaluation of patients with Addison's disease.

Metastatic disease frequently involves the adrenal gland. Cancer of the lung and breast are the two types of malignancies that most commonly metastasize to the adrenals. Adrenal metastases are found in 35% of patients with metastatic lung or breast cancer. Despite this high frequency, adrenal insufficiency can be documented biochemically in only about 20% of these patients. This is presumed to reflect the fact that over 90% of the adrenal gland must be destroyed to produce insufficiency. All patients with bilateral adrenal metastatic disease should be tested with short-acting synthetic α-1,24 ACTH (cosyntropin) to rule out insufficiency.

Acquired immunodeficiency syndrome (AIDS) can cause primary adrenal insufficiency. The etiology is usually infection with cytomegalovirus (CMV), *Cryptococcus*, tuberculosis, or atypical *Mycobacterium*. Although most HIV patients with evidence of adrenal infiltration by one of these organisms do not have adrenal insufficiency because there is sufficient adrenal function preserved, about 20% of patients with HIV have been found in some series to have a subnormal response to injected synthetic ACTH consistent with adrenal insufficiency.[4] Also, medications such as ketoconazole, rifampin, and megestrol, which are commonly used in patients with HIV disease, can cause adrenal insufficiency. Ketoconazole inhibits adrenal steroidogenesis by blocking cholesterol desmolase, 11β-hydroxylase, and aldosterone synthase, which can result in primary insufficiency. Megestrol has glucocorticoid receptor agonist activity, which has resulted in both Cushing's syndrome and secondary adrenal insufficiency. Rifampin induces cortisol-metabolizing enzymes.

Box 98-2. Causes of Adrenal Insufficiency

Primary

Autoimmune/idiopathic (70%)
Tuberculosis (20%)
Other (10%)
Fungal infections
Adrenal hemorrhage
Congenital adrenal hyperplasia
Sarcoidosis
Amyloidosis
HIV/AIDS
Adrenoleukodystrophy
Metastatic disease

Secondary

Iatrogenic (following exogenous glucocorticoids) (common)
Isolated ACTH deficiency (uncommon)
Hypothalamic/pituitary lesions (uncommon)

Secondary Adrenal Insufficiency. Secondary adrenal insufficiency can be related to panhypopituitarism, isolated ACTH loss, or exogenous glucocorticoid suppression of the HPA (see Box 98-2). Panhypopituitarism is discussed in detail in Chapter 99. Pituitary tumor, infiltration, and infarction are common etiologies. Cases have been reported in the literature of isolated ACTH loss due to selective failure of pituitary ACTH-producing cells. The etiology is unknown in most cases, but an association with other autoimmune endocrinopathies, the postpartum occurrence in some patients, and the measurement of serum antipituitary antibodies have suggested an autoimmune etiology. Exogenous suppression of the HPA during glucocorticoid therapy for nonendocrine disorders is common. This can occur up to 12 months after treatment of at least 3 weeks' duration with pharmacologic dosages of these medications. A pharmacologic dosage is defined as any dosage exceeding the 24-hour adrenal replacement dosage (Table 98-1). Although most cases of adrenal suppression follow prolonged use of oral or parenteral glucocorticoids, cases of adrenal suppression following the use of high dosages of inhaled or topical glucocorticoids have been reported as well. In general, the likelihood of suppression increases with dosage and duration of therapy and with use of longer acting agents. However, it is impossible to predict the exact dosage or duration of glucocorticoid use that will produce HPA suppression in an individual patient. Clinically some patients undergoing a taper from prolonged use of glucocorticoids can experience the glucocorticoid withdrawal syndrome, which includes fatigue, weakness, arthralgias, anorexia, nausea, abdominal pain, skin desquamation, and dizziness. This clinical syndrome may or may not be associated with evidence of endogenous adrenal suppression upon testing. In some cases testing is completely normal, suggesting that this syndrome

Table 98-1. Glucocorticoid Characteristics

Medication	$t_{1/2}$	Dosages		Potencies	
		Replacement*	Stress†	GC‡	MC§
Hydrocortisone (cortisol) (Cortef, Solu-Cortef)	8-12 hr	20 mg	200 mg	1	1
Prednisone	12-36 hr	5 mg	50 mg	4	0.25
Methylprednisolone (Solu-Medrol)	12-36 hr	4 mg	40 mg	5	0.25
Dexamethasone (Decadron)	36-72 hr	0.75 mg	7.5 mg	25	0
Fludrocortisone (Florinef)	12-20 hr	0.05-2 mg	Increase dietary sodium	10	125

*Refers to the dosage required to replace the 24-hour cortisol production of nonstressed adrenal glands.
†Refers to the dosage required to replace the 24-hour cortisol production of the adrenals in situations of severe metabolic stress.
‡Refers to the glucocorticoid potency of the medication as compared with cortisol (note the 1,4,5,25 rule may be a helpful way to recall relative potencies).
§Refers to the mineralocorticoid potency of the medication as compared with cortisol.

may reflect physiologic and/or psychologic dependence on high doses of glucocorticoids.

Laboratory Studies and Diagnostic Procedures

As shown in Box 98-1, hyperkalemia occurs in 66%, hyponatremia in 90%, and hypoglycemia in 40% of cases. However, as illustrated by Case 2, they can be mild and easily missed. Dynamic endocrine testing is necessary to establish a diagnosis, since random cortisol levels are usually not helpful. Indications for such testing, in addition to electrolyte abnormalities, may include repeated episodes of syncope or hypotension, significant weight loss, unexplained fevers, or fever disproportionate to the type of infection. Fig. 98-3 is an algorithm of the diagnostic evaluation.

Plasma ACTH Level. A plasma ACTH assay differentiates between primary adrenal insufficiency and insufficiency at a higher level when the rapid ACTH stimulation test yields abnormal results. Patients with primary failure have elevated ACTH levels, whereas patients with secondary failure have normal or low levels. A normal plasma ACTH level is 20 to 80 pg/ml. Careful attention must be paid to specimen collection, since falsely low results can occur.

Rapid ACTH Test. The rapid ACTH stimulation test is highly accurate in establishing or excluding adrenal insufficiency. The test measures only adrenal response to injected synthetic ACTH and does not test for endogenous ACTH or corticotropin-releasing hormone (CRH) deficiency. However, the adrenal atrophy that occurs with chronic endogenous ACTH or CRH deficiency often results in poor adrenal response to injected ACTH. Correlation has been demonstrated between rapid ACTH testing results and results of direct testing at higher levels, so the test can be used to assess all levels of adrenal dysfunction. A bolus intravenous injection of 0.25 mg of synthetic α-1,24 ACTH (cosyntropin) is administered. Plasma cortisol levels are measured at 0 and 30 to 60 minutes. A 30- to 60-minute plasma cortisol level of greater than 18 to 20 μg/dl excludes the diagnosis of primary adrenal insufficiency and usually excludes chronic

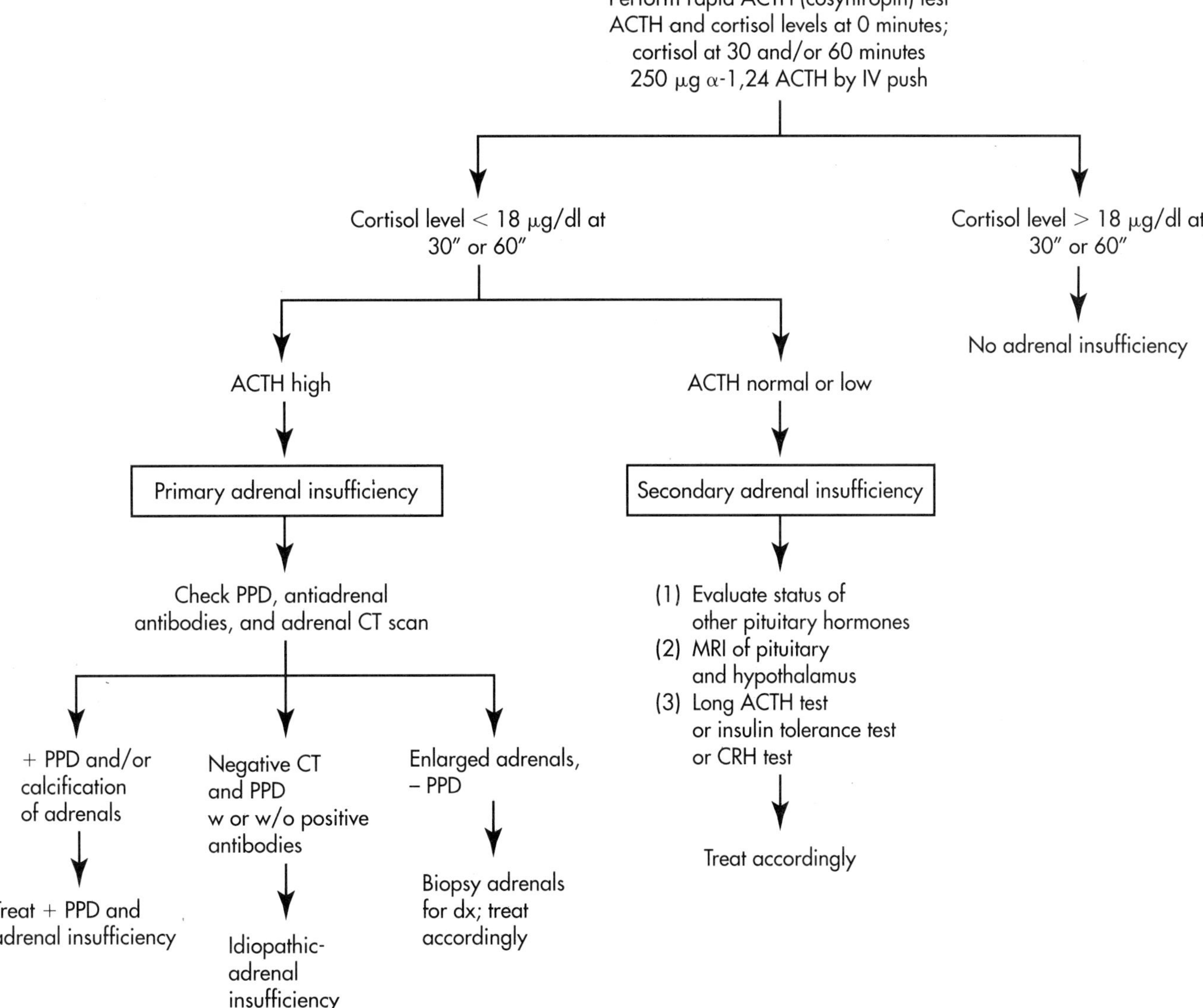

Fig. 98-3. Algorithm for adrenal insufficiency.

secondary adrenal insufficiency as well. However, in acute secondary adrenal insufficiency, cortisol response to cosyntropin may be normal.

Other Tests. These tests are usually reserved for endocrine/metabolic units and are not essential for diagnosis if the combined cortisol and ACTH test results establish the level of dysfunction. A long ACTH test involves the administration of 500 μg/dl cosyntropin as a continuous infusion over 48 hours, with measurement of urinary free cortisol and serum cortisol levels. An insulin tolerance test involves the administration of insulin to invoke hypoglycemia, which is a stimulus to pituitary ACTH secretion. Endogenous ACTH levels are measured as hypoglycemia occurs. This test requires close supervision by experienced personnel. The metyrapone test uses the drug metyrapone to block the final step in cortisol synthesis, thus stimulating an ACTH response to a temporary decrease in cortisol production. Those who are confirmed to have secondary adrenal insufficiency may require additional testing to rule out secondary thyroid or gonadal failure.

Radiologic Imaging. If a biochemical diagnosis of primary adrenal insufficiency is established, imaging of the adrenal glands may be helpful in distinguishing etiology. CT scan may be preferable to magnetic resonance imaging (MRI) in this setting, because detection of calcification in the area of the adrenals by CT scan is suggestive of prior adrenal tuberculosis. Infiltrative disorders such as metastatic disease, sarcoidosis, and tuberculosis may cause adrenal enlargement detectable by CT or MRI in the early stages of disease. If antiadrenal antibodies are negative and calcification is present in the area of the adrenal glands, the presumed etiology is tuberculosis. Patients who have neither adrenal calcification nor positive tuberculin skin testing must be presumed to have idiopathic Addison's disease regardless of antibody status. There is no role for adrenal imaging in patients who have biochemical evidence of secondary adrenal insufficiency.

For patients who appear to have secondary adrenal insufficiency on biochemical testing, MRI of the brain with views of the pituitary is necessary to rule out a midline central nervous system (CNS) lesion.

Management

The emergency treatment of acute adrenal crisis is outlined in Box 98-3. Empiric treatment for adrenal crisis should be considered in all severely ill patients with shock refractory to volume expansion or pressor agents. Factors that would argue strongly for such treatment include risk factors for adrenal insufficiency such as anticoagulant therapy, bleeding diathesis, disseminated intravascular coagulation, disseminated tuberculosis, AIDS, sepsis, or a history of glucocorticoid therapy within the previous 12 months. Treatment is not likely to benefit patients whose refractory hypotension is clearly related to cardiogenic shock. Treatment should be continued until results of the diagnostic evaluation are available. The dosage of glucocorticoid can be tapered at a rate appropriate to the clinical condition of the patient. In patients who are clearly improving clinically, the dosage can be tapered by 50% daily, with a change to oral maintenance therapy within several days.

Maintenance therapy for adrenal insufficiency consists of daily oral glucocorticoid, most commonly hydrocortisone or prednisone, plus the mineralocorticoid fludrocortisone in primary adrenal insufficiency (see Table 98-1). For primary adrenal insufficiency, hydrocortisone may be a better choice than prednisone because of its higher mineralocorticoid activity. Thus, for some patients taking hydrocortisone, mineralocorticoid replacement with fludrocortisone may not be necessary. Prednisone is less expensive than hydrocortisone but often requires the concurrent use of fludrocortisone for mineralocorticoid replacement. The need for mineralocorticoid therapy can be monitored via electrolytes and postural blood pressure measurements. Plasma renin activity levels can also be used, since they are elevated if mineralocorticoid replacement is insufficient. Patients should be given the minimum amount of glucocorticoid and mineralocorticoid required to prevent symptoms and maintain normal electrolyte and blood pressure status.[9] Care must be taken to ensure that the patient is indeed on the minimum required dosage, since even small excesses of glucocorticoid therapy can cause osteoporosis and metabolic complications such as hyperglycemia (see the discussion on iatrogenic Cushing's syndrome in this chapter). Excess mineralocorticoid therapy can cause hypertension and hypokalemia.

In secondary or tertiary adrenal insufficiency, only glucocorticoid replacement is required, unless any concurrent deficiencies of the other pituitary hormones are present.

Patients with adrenal insufficiency should wear some form of easily visible identification stating their diagnosis and therapy. They also must be instructed to increase their medication dosage if any significant illness occurs. Medication should be doubled for illnesses associated with vomiting and/or diarrhea. For milder febrile illnesses dosages should be increased somewhat less. Major medical stresses such as trauma or a surgical procedure require parenteral therapy. For surgery 100 mg of hydrocortisone should be given 8 hours preoperatively and repeated at 1 hour preoperatively. Hydrocortisone should also be added as a continuous infusion to the intravenous fluids at 5 mg/hour during the surgical procedure. A total of 150 to 200 mg should be given in the first 24 hours, with tapering of dosage by 50% per day assuming continued uneventful recovery.

Box 98-3. Management of Acute Adrenal Insufficiency

Draw blood for measurement of cortisol and ACTH.
Infuse sufficient normal saline with 5% dextrose to restore normotension.
Administer 2 mg dexamethasone IV immediately (which will not interfere with further testing)
Give 250 μg Cortrosyn (ACTH) IV and measure 30-minute cortisol level.
Begin IV hydrocortisone as a continuous infusion to total 200 mg in 24 hours; or doses can be given in bolus form, 50 mg every 6 hours.
Investigate underlying etiology of adrenal insufficiency with plain film of abdomen to rule out adrenal calcification, tuberculosis testing, and evaluation of thyroid and gonadal status.
Chronic oral replacement therapy can begin as soon as the patient is medically stable and able to take medication orally.

Box 98-4. Principles of Glucocorticoid Use and Withdrawal

Use the smallest dosage of glucocorticoid for the shortest time possible.
Use shorter-acting agents (prednisone, cortisol) given as early in the day as possible and avoid twice daily administration.
Use alternate day therapy when possible (if underlying condition is responsive to this regimen).
Give all patients supplemental calcium and vitamin D; consider pharmacologic prophylaxis of osteoporosis.
Educate the patient as to the appropriate response to major medical stress for 1 year following exogenous glucocorticoid replacement.
To begin to taper, change to the shortest acting agent administered once daily early in the day.
Taper dosage further and switch to alternate day therapy as tolerated by the underlying disease.

Management of Glucocorticoid Withdrawal

Sudden cessation of therapy following at least 3 weeks of supraphysiologic doses of glucocorticoids can precipitate acute adrenal insufficiency (see Table 98-1). Guidelines to prevent adrenal crisis during withdrawal from therapy are outlined in Box 98-4. Changing therapy to shorter acting agents and using alternate day therapy are features that allow HPA axis recovery. The rate of taper of a pharmacologic glucocorticoid dosage depends primarily on the underlying nonendocrine disorder for which the medication is being used. As noted, there may be significant adrenal suppression for up to 1 year after discontinuation of steroids. Major stresses, including surgery, require stress dose steroid therapy (see Box 98-4 and Chapter 13). If patients have symptoms of adrenal insufficiency on withdrawal of steroids, it may be reasonable to perform a cosyntropin stimulation test to assess adrenal responsiveness.

ADRENOCORTICAL HYPERFUNCTION (CUSHING'S SYNDROME)

Pathophysiology

Cushing's syndrome is a constellation of symptoms, signs, and biochemical abnormalities that result from prolonged exposure to excess levels of glucocorticoids. The principal glucocorticoid, cortisol, has primarily catabolic effects in most tissues. Collagen production is impaired, which reduces the tensile strength of dermal structures, including blood vessels, resulting in spontaneous ecchymoses, purple striae, and poor wound healing. Cortisol excess can also result in diffuse fine body hair growth, known as lanugo hair. Muscle wasting and weakness occur due to generalized protein catabolism. Catabolic effects on bone are also seen, since cortisol decreases intestinal calcium absorption, which in turn results in increased bone reabsorption and hypercalciuria, progressing to osteoporosis. Hyperglycemia results from the direct anti-insulin effect of cortisol and a cortisol-mediated increase in hepatic gluconeogenesis and glycogenolysis. Impaired immune and inflammatory response is seen due to a variety of immunologic effects, including impairment of polymorphonuclear cell phagocytosis; depletion of T lymphocytes, monocytes, and eosinophils; and decreased antibody formation. Cell-mediated immune response, vascular permeability, and histamine release are also impaired. The clinical result is an increased susceptibility to bacterial and fungal infections, most commonly with opportunistic organisms such as *Pneumocystis carinii, Aspergillus, Nocardia,* and *Cryptococcus.* Hypertension is also seen due to the permissive effect of cortisol on catecholamine activity and its positive inotropic effects on the heart. The increased catecholamine also has lipolytic effects, as does excess cortisol. This appears to affect adipocytes differentially. In the extremities fat wasting occurs, while fat deposition is increased centrally in the face, neck, and trunk, resulting in the typical Cushing's features of centripetal obesity, moon facies, and buffalo hump.

Clinical manifestations of androgen or mineralocorticoid excess may also be present, depending on the etiology of the syndrome. In the ACTH-dependent forms of Cushing's syndrome, in which excess pituitary or ectopic ACTH production is the primary pathologic feature, signs of androgen excess occur due to stimulation of adrenal androgen production by the excess ACTH. Androgen excess is clinically apparent only in women, resulting in coarse terminal hair growth in androgen-sensitive areas, such as the face, chest, and upper back. Acne, oligomenorrhea, temporal balding, and deepening of the voice may also occur. In the ACTH-independent forms of Cushing's syndrome primary overproduction of cortisol results in suppression of ACTH production, which in turn reduces adrenal androgen production, so that features of androgen excess do not occur.

Cushing's syndrome is also associated with accelerated atherosclerosis. In the years before effective treatment evolved, patients with Cushing's syndrome commonly experienced early death from myocardial infarction or stroke. Vascular endothelial cell damage and elevated serum lipid levels due to cortisol excess are thought to be the pathogenic factors.

Endogenous (noniatrogenic) Cushing's syndrome is a serious disorder with a 5-year mortality of 50% if left untreated. The majority of deaths are due to infection, cardiovascular disease, and suicide. Treatment confers a dramatically improved prognosis.

History and Physical Findings

Many of the features of Cushing's syndrome are seen with high frequency in the general population, as shown in Box 98-5. In particular, the triad of obesity, hypertension, and glucose intolerance or diabetes is commonly encountered in an outpatient general medical practice. Alternately, among patients with documented Cushing's syndrome, the presentation is often nonspecific, and typical clinical features may be absent. For example, among patients with pituitary Cushing's syndrome the prevalence of symptoms is obesity 79%, hypertension 77%, easy bruisability 77%, hirsutism 64%, proximal muscle weakness 48%, psychiatric disturbances 48%, abnormal glucose tolerance 39%, clinical diabetes 13%, and hypokalemia 24%. Psychiatric symptoms most frequently include affective changes (mania, depression) but may also present as toxic psychoses, often with paranoia. Symptoms are typically dose-related, although they occasionally follow use of low-dose steroids. Onset is usually within 5 days of starting glucocorticoid therapy, often in the setting of prior psychiatric problems. Resolution is typically within 1 week of discontinuation of glucocorticoids.

Rapid or subacute onset of obesity, hypertension, or other features of Cushing's syndrome is one clue that there is an underlying pathologic process that merits investigation.

Etiology and Differential Diagnosis

The differential diagnosis for Cushing's syndrome and the features unique to each type of the syndrome are outlined in Table 98-2.

Box 98-5. Clinical Features of Cushing's Syndrome

Nonspecific Features

Generalized obesity
Hypertension
Abnormal glucose tolerance
Amenorrhea or impotence
Hirsutism

Specific Features

Central obesity
Ecchymoses
Pigmented striae (>1 cm)
Osteopenia
Muscle weakness
Spontaneous hypokalemia
Erythrocytosis

Features Unique to Iatrogenic Cushing's Syndrome

Aseptic necrosis of femoral and humeral heads
Glaucoma
Cataracts
Benign intracranial hypertension
Pancreatitis

Iatrogenic Cushing's Syndrome. Iatrogenic Cushing's syndrome is the most common type seen clinically. Any prolonged use of glucocorticoid at dosages above replacement (see Table 98-1) can result in the adverse metabolic effects and/or clinical features of Cushing's syndrome. Osteoporosis can be a serious problem, with an incidence of 30% to 50% among those treated chronically with glucocorticoids. Reductions in trabecular bone density have been measured after as little as 8 mg of prednisone daily for 4 months. At prednisone dosages of over 10 mg daily for at least 2 months, an increased prevalence of infection is seen. Atherosclerotic disease may also be increased and steroid myopathy may be very disabling (see Chapter 175). Several pathologic features of iatrogenic Cushing's syndrome are unique to exogenous glucocorticoid use and are not seen in other types of the syndrome. These include aseptic necrosis of the femoral or humeral heads (which can occasionally occur even with short-term steroid therapy), glaucoma, cataracts, benign intracranial hypertension, and pancreatitis. Signs of androgen excess are not a feature, since exogenous glucocorticoids cause HPA suppression, resulting in decreased ACTH-mediated adrenal androgen production.

Pituitary Cushing's Syndrome (Cushing's Disease). Pituitary Cushing's syndrome accounts for approximately 60% of cases of endogenous hypercortisolism. This is due to an ACTH-secreting pituitary adenoma. These adenomas are often small, resulting in sella turcica enlargement in only 10% of cases. Signs of androgen excess are often present in this disorder due to ACTH-mediated adrenal overproduction of androgen precursors. The HPA appears to be intact but has an abnormally high set point of ACTH feedback regulation. Thus circulating cortisol production can be suppressed with high-dose dexamethasone testing but not with low-dose or overnight testing.

Ectopic ACTH Syndrome. Ectopic ACTH syndrome accounts for about 10% of endogenous hypercortisolism. The

Table 98-2. Cushing's Syndrome: Etiology and Differential Diagnosis

Type	Frequency	Unique features
Iatrogenic	Common	Absence of signs of androgen excess due to suppression of adrenal androgen production
Pituitary (Cushing's disease)	60%	Signs of androgen excess present; pituitary tumor; suppresses with high-dose dexamethasone testing
Adrenal neoplasms	30%	
Adenoma	~30%	Absence of signs of androgen excess; no suppression with high-dose dexamethasone testing
Carcinoma	Rare	May or may not have features of androgen excess; 50% metastatic at diagnosis; no suppression on testing
Bilateral nodular hyperplasia	Uncommon	Features of androgen excess present; suppression with high-dose dexamethasone testing; may be Cushing's disease without visible pituitary lesion
Ectopic ACTH syndrome	10%	Most common tumors associated with this are small cell carcinoma of lung, pancreatic carcinoma, bronchial adenoma, thymoma; features of androgen excess may be present; lack of suppression to high-dose dexamethasone
Alcoholic pseudo-Cushing's syndrome	Common	Endogenous cortisol overproduction; hypogonadism also present due to direct gonadotoxic effects of alcohol

source of ectopic ACTH production is a thoracic tumor in 79% of patients. The most common thoracic tumors are small-cell carcinoma of the lung, bronchial carcinoid, and thymoma. Extrathoracic tumors such as pancreatic carcinoma can also produce ACTH. Both bronchial carcinoid and thymoma are usually benign tumors with a clinical course typical of Cushing's syndrome. The malignant tumors resulting in this syndrome often have a poor prognosis, and patients seldom live long enough to manifest the typical Cushing's stigmata. Metabolic features, such as severe hypokalemia, may predominate. Hyperpigmentation, leg edema, and weight loss may also be predominant features. These tumors are autonomously functioning; thus cortisol and ACTH production are not suppressed following the administration of high doses of the glucocorticoid dexamethasone. Symptomatic treatment may improve quality of life or prolong life and should be pursued.

Adrenal Neoplasms. Adrenal tumors account for about 30% of cases of endogenous Cushing's syndrome. The majority of these are benign adenomas, which are autonomously functioning and secrete primarily cortisol. Excess cortisol suppresses pituitary production of ACTH; thus, clinically, signs of cortisol excess without androgen excess predominate. These tumors are autonomous and do not decrease cortisol production in response to dexamethasone.

Bilateral nodular adrenal hyperplasia is a poorly understood entity. It is characterized by autonomous cortisol overproduction, but production can be suppressed with high doses of dexamethasone. This may represent a variant of Cushing's disease in which a pituitary adenoma is not visible, since ACTH levels are often elevated.

Adrenal carcinomas are rare, accounting for only 0.2% of cancer deaths in the United States per year. The mean age of presentation is 46 years, with a female/male ratio of 2.5 : 1. In those cases with hormonal overproduction the majority present with clinical features of Cushing's syndrome. In one series 30% presented with pure glucocorticoid excess, 27% had combined glucocorticoid and androgen excess, 8% had androgen excess alone, 2% had mineralocorticoid excess, 1% had estrogen excess, and the remainder (32%) had no hormone overproduction. At diagnosis 50% had regional or distant metastases. Median survival was 21 months, with only 10% surviving for 5 years.

Alcoholic Pseudo-Cushing's Syndrome. Chronic alcoholism may have many of the stigmata of Cushing's syndrome. Cortisol dynamics are abnormal and cortisol overproduction can be documented. Following abstinence the cortisol dynamics usually return to normal within 3 to 7 days.[6]

Diagnostic Tests

An algorithm that outlines a diagnostic approach to Cushing's syndrome is outlined in Fig. 98-4. The initial step is to perform a screening test to confirm the presence of Cushing's syndrome.

Hormonal Tests. The overnight dexamethasone suppression test (ONDST) is the most widely used screen for this disorder. It involves the oral administration of 1 mg of dexamethasone at 11 PM, with measurement of plasma cortisol at 8 AM the following day. The normal cortisol response is suppression to less than 5 mg/dl. This test has an extremely low false-negative rate of <2%, but a high false-positive rate. Obesity, stress, psychiatric disease (especially depression), and medications that increase hepatic metabolism of cortisol and dexamethasone, such as antiseizure medications, estrogen, and rifampin, can falsely elevate the results of this test. If any of these conditions are present, the ONDST should not be performed, and either of the following two tests should be used as the initial screening maneuver (these tests are also used to confirm the diagnosis when the ONDST is positive): (1) the 24-hour urinary free cortisol test is a measurement of unbound, biologically available cortisol; (2) the low-dose dexamethasone suppression test (LDDST) is done by administering 0.5 mg of dexamethasone orally every 6 hours for 2 days. A serum cortisol measured at 8 AM after 48 hours of dexamethasone administration should be suppressed to less than 5 mg/dl. However the diagnostic accuracy of the LDDST is only 71%.[10] A recent modification, which has been shown to increase diagnostic accuracy to 100%, is the LDDST-CRH, in which the dexamethasone is initiated at noon, so that the eighth dose is taken at 6 AM 2 days later. CRH (corticotropin-releasing hormone) as a 1 μg/kg IV bolus is injected at 8 AM after the last dose of dexamethasone, and a 15-minute serum cortisol is drawn. A cortisol result of >1.4 μg/dl is diagnostic of Cushing's syndrome.[13] This modification of the LDDST can be performed in patients with positive ONDST results, whose LDDST is negative but in whom clinical suspicion is extremely high for Cushing's syndrome.

If Cushing's syndrome is confirmed, further testing is pursued to differentiate among the types of the syndrome. The high-dose dexamethasone suppression test in conjunction with an ACTH level is the first step. ACTH measured by immunoradiometric assay rather than by radioimmunoassay (RIA) more accurately identifies ACTH-independent forms of Cushing's syndrome. A single 8-mg dose of dexamethasone is given at 11 PM following a baseline 8 AM cortisol measurement. The cortisol is then repeated the following morning. This test has a higher sensitivity of 70% to 90% compared with the traditional test in which dexamethasone is given every 6 hours for 2 days and urine and serum cortisols are monitored (60% to 70% sensitivity).[10] Lack of suppression of the cortisol level, in conjunction with an undetectable to low ACTH level, is diagnostic of adrenal Cushing's syndrome. Suppression to 50% or less of the baseline cortisol level with normal to elevated ACTH is diagnostic of pituitary Cushing's syndrome. Lack of suppression of cortisol in conjunction with a normal to elevated ACTH suggests the ectopic ACTH syndrome.

If results do not localize the source of the excess cortisol production, further testing must be performed via inferior petrosal sinus sampling. This consists of measuring ACTH levels in blood drawn directly from the petrosal sinuses, which receive the venous drainage from the pituitary. A central/peripheral ACTH ratio of 2 : 1 or greater indicates a pituitary source of ACTH hypersecretion. A ratio of 1.5 : 1 or less supports an ectopic cause. If a pituitary source is evident from petrosal sinus sampling, levels may also help to indicate whether it is located on the right or left side of the pituitary.

Radiologic Studies. Radiologic studies are performed after localization of the site of excess cortisol production. It is

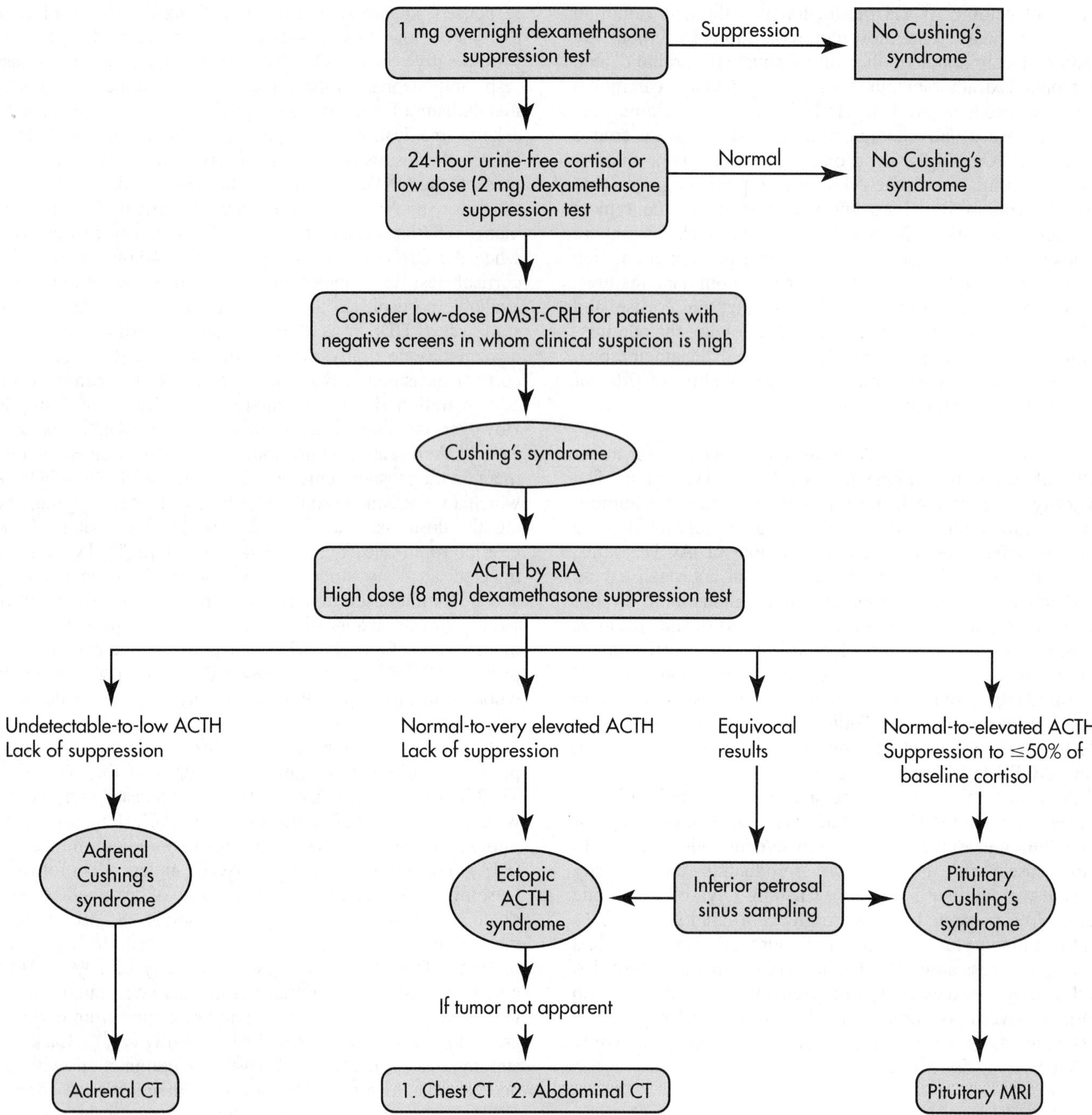

Fig. 98-4. Diagnostic algorithm for Cushing's syndrome. (Modified from Kaye TB, Crapo L: *Ann Intern Med* 112:434, 1990.)

critical that imaging studies be deferred until hormonal studies have been completed, since incidental adrenal or pituitary adenomas are common, occurring in 1% to 8% of normal individuals. If hormonal studies indicate an adrenal source of cortisol overproduction, adrenal imaging is performed. CT scanning of the adrenal has a sensitivity of almost 100% and is generally the preferred initial imaging modality.[10] MRI or adrenal scintigraphy with ^{131}I-iodomethylnorcholesterol (NP-59) may be helpful in localizing adenomas not seen by CT scan.

If hormonal studies indicate that cortisol overproduction is localized to the pituitary, MRI has higher sensitivity for pituitary imaging than CT scan and should be the diagnostic study of choice. When gadolinium contrast is used, pituitary MRI has approximately 80% sensitivity.[10]

Management

The treatment of iatrogenic Cushing's syndrome once it has occurred is to taper the dosage of glucocorticoid as tolerated by the underlying disease. Some of the metabolic effects of excess glucocorticoid use, such as the loss of bone mass, are not reversible. Thus prevention by minimizing dosage and duration of glucocorticoid therapy is critical. Principles of glucocorticoid use and withdrawal are outlined in Box 98-4. Use of the shortest acting preparation for the shortest time possible is a key feature. Additionally, to minimize bone loss, calcium and vitamin D supplementation should be given to those in whom glucocorticoid use is expected to exceed 1 month. Calcium intake from all sources should total at least 1000 mg per day, and vitamin D, 400 IU per day, should also be administered. Also, pharmacologic prevention of glucocorticoid-induced osteoporosis should be strongly considered; regimens demonstrated to be effective include alendronate 5 mg qd, etidronate 400 mg/day for 14 days every 3 months, and risedronate 5 mg/day.[1] For women who are estrogen deficient due to menopause, other disorders, or the effects of the glucocorticoid therapy, estrogen therapy should be strongly considered.

The treatment of choice for pituitary Cushing's syndrome is surgery. A transsphenoidal microsurgical approach is used. The surgery is safe and effective, with tumor localization and removal occurring in approximately 90% of patients without subsequent pituitary hypofunction in most. If no adenoma is visible at operation, total or partial hypophysectomy is sometimes recommended, because very small tumors can be found on careful sectioning of the pituitary. Tumor lateralization with inferior petrosal sinus sampling can be used to guide hemihypophysectomy if no tumor is seen on MRI. Surgical cure rates are high, and surgical morbidity and mortality are low. For pituitary microadenomas (under 10 mm), the 10-year cure rate is over 90%, while for macroadenomas, 10-year cure rates are lower at 55%, but survival rates remain high due to a variety of adjunctive therapies to control hypercortisolism, including medications, irradiation, and bilateral adrenalectomy.[5,12]

For Cushing's syndrome due to adrenal adenoma, surgical resection is the treatment of choice and is usually curative. Surgery may have to be delayed for a few months while medical adrenolytic agents (see below) are administered to avoid problems with poor wound healing or with metabolic derangement. Surgical resection after medical preparation is also used for adrenal carcinoma, even if metastases are documented preoperatively. If metastatic disease is present, postoperative medical therapy is usually necessary on an indefinite basis to control symptoms and metabolic manifestations. Similarly, the hypercortisolism of ectopic ACTH syndrome is usually controlled with medical therapy, even if the ACTH-secreting malignancy confers a poor prognosis. Medical therapy can substantially improve the quality of life in terminally ill patients by ameliorating the myopathy, hypokalemia, and catabolism of Cushing's syndrome.

Options for medical therapy of Cushing's syndrome include ketoconazole, the most commonly used medication, which reduces or normalizes cortisol levels in about 40% of patients. Other drugs that may be effective in lowering cortisol overproduction include mitotane, an adrenolytic agent, and aminoglutethimide, a more rapidly acting adrenolytic agent that blocks the conversion of cholesterol to pregnenolone, a cortisol precursor. This is extremely effective for the rapid reduction of cortisol overproduction. Metyrapone, another effective drug sometimes used in conjunction with aminoglutethimide, is an inhibitor of the adrenocortical enzyme 11β-hydroxylase. Physiologic doses of hydrocortisone must usually be administered with these drugs to avoid adrenal insufficiency. In Cushing's syndrome caused by ectopic ACTH production or adrenal carcinoma, mifepristone (RU 486) is effective. In Cushing's disease cyproheptadine, an antiseratoninergic agent, has been shown to induce clinical and biochemical remission in a small number of patients. Bromocriptine, a dopaminergic agonist, has also produced temporary remission in Cushing's disease.

Finally, alcoholic pseudo-Cushing's syndrome is best treated by detoxification from alcohol. Calcium and vitamin D supplementation should also be considered as osteoporosis prophylaxis in all alcoholics, and estrogen replacement should be considered in amenorrheic alcoholic women.

MINERALOCORTICOIDS

Aldosterone is the major mineralocorticoid produced by the adrenal gland. Its production is affected primarily by angiotensin II and extracellular potassium, with ACTH playing a small role as well (see Fig. 98-1). Angiotensin II, the predominant factor controlling aldosterone secretion, is in turn responsive to renin, which is secreted by the renal juxtaglomerular apparatus in response to low renal perfusion pressure and low extracellular sodium concentration. Renin stimulates hepatic conversion of angiotensinogen to angiotensin I, which is in turn converted in the lungs to angiotensin II. Stimulation of this axis results in increased aldosterone production, resulting in distal tubular sodium retention and in renal potassium excretion. Disorders of aldosterone may result from excess production, as in primary hyperaldosteronism, or inadequate production, as in hypoaldosteronism.

Primary Hyperaldosteronism

Pathophysiology. Estimates of the incidence of primary hyperaldosteronism in the hypertensive population of the United States vary from 0.05% to 2%. Excess mineralocorticoid results in hypokalemia, metabolic alkalosis, and sodium retention. Sodium retention in turn leads to volume expansion and hypertension. Hypokalemia and sodium retention occur because aldosterone acts on the cortical collecting tubules within the kidney to retain sodium and increase potassium excretion. The mechanism is increased aldosterone-mediated synthesis of sodium-potassium-ATPase, which in turn increases the activity of the sodium-potassium pump that draws sodium into the tubular cells and secretes potassium into the lumen. Excess secretion of hydrogen ion into the tubular lumen, resulting in metabolic alkalosis, occurs in the renal medullary collecting tubules under aldosterone's influence as well. Renin and angiotensin II levels are both suppressed due to primary overproduction of aldosterone.

History and Physical Findings. This disorder presents between the third and fifth decades and is more common in women. The hypertension is clinically indistinguishable from essential hypertension in most cases, since most patients with this disorder are asymptomatic. When symptoms occur, the most commonly reported are headache, easy fatigability, and weakness. The most consistent and overt biochemical manifestation is hypokalemia, which results from renal potassium wastage. More than 50% of hypertensive patients with spontaneous hypokalemia are found to have primary aldosteronism; thus hypokalemia in the absence of diuretic therapy should prompt testing for aldosterone excess, even if the hypokalemia is mild (3.4 to 3.5 mEq/L). It should also be suspected in patients who become severely hypokalemic with the administration of diuretics and who remain so after diuretics are stopped. The hypokalemia causes no symptoms in a substantial proportion of patients. In others, nocturnal polyuria and polydipsia and neuromuscular manifestations

Box 98-6. Frequency of Primary Aldosteronism

APA (65%)
IHA (34%)
Aldosterone-producing carcinoma (<1%)
Glucocorticoid-suppressible hyperaldosteronism (<1%)

APA, Aldosterone-producing adenoma; *IHA*, idiopathic hyperaldosteronism.
Modified from Melby JC: Clinical review 1: Endocrine hypertension, *J Clin Endo Metab* 69:697, 1989.

such as weakness, paresthesias, intermittent paralysis, and frank tetany can occur. The degree of hypokalemia is related in part to sodium intake. Sodium restriction leads to potassium retention, whereas sodium excess promotes further renal potassium wastage.

Etiology and Differential Diagnosis. The causes of primary hyperaldosteronism and their frequencies are illustrated in Box 98-6. An aldosterone-producing adenoma (APA) of the adrenal, also known as Conn's syndrome, is the most common cause. These adenomas are usually unilateral, more commonly on the left, and less than 2 cm in size. Aldosterone excess is more pronounced than in other forms of primary hyperaldosteronism. Although plasma renin is completely suppressed by the excess aldosterone, synthesis of aldosterone is only partly autonomous. In about 80% of patients, plasma levels still exhibit a circadian rhythm that parallels the plasma cortisol and ACTH levels (corticotropin-responsive). About 20% maintain some response to angiotensin II and postural changes (renin-responsive). The latter is also true of idiopathic hyperaldosteronism (IHA), which is due to bilateral nodular hyperplasia of the adrenal cortex. The histologically normal but hypertrophic adrenal glands found in this condition are thought to result from stimulation by an abnormal secretagogue or an amplifier of angiotensin II that has yet to be identified. There is partial suppression of plasma renin, and there is no parallel between cortisol and aldosterone levels. Rarely, primary hyperaldosteronism is due to production of aldosterone by an adrenal carcinoma. Another unusual etiology is glucocorticoid-suppressible hyperaldosteronism, a rare hereditary autosomal dominant trait in which there is ACTH-mediated hypersecretion of aldosterone and little or no regulation of aldosterone by angiotensin II.[3] This disorder often presents in children or young adults as hypertension, with or without a family history. Typically, hypokalemia is mild or absent. APA is more common in young adult to middle-aged females, and IHA more typically occurs in middle-aged males.

Diagnostic Tests. Screening for primary hyperaldosteronism can be performed in the outpatient setting. Currently, the most widely recommended screening test is the ratio of the plasma aldosterone level to plasma renin activity.[3a] Patients should be off all antihypertensive medications for at least 2 weeks (calcium channel blockers can be continued until 3 days prior to testing). Hypertension can be controlled with prazosin, doxazosin, or clonidine during this time if diastolic blood pressures exceed 110 mm. The blood should be drawn in the morning, with the patient in the upright position, preferably after 2 hours of ambulation. An aldosterone : renin ratio of >30 is an indication for further evaluation. Definitive diagnosis is best established by the saline infusion test, in which 1.25 L over 2 hours, or 2 L of normal saline over 4 hours, is infused and plasma aldosterone is measured. An aldosterone level of <8.5 ng/dl (240 pmol/L) rules out all types of primary aldosteronism.

Once a diagnosis of primary hyperaldosteronism is established, the cause must be determined (Fig. 98-5). The renin-aldosterone stimulation test (posture test) results can be helpful in differentiating IHA from APA in 90% of cases of confirmed primary hyperaldosteronism. Starting at 7:30 AM the patient remains recumbent for 30 minutes. Plasma renin and aldosterone levels are drawn at 8 AM. The patient then remains upright for 4 hours, and the levels are repeated. Whereas most patients with APA have a decline in aldosterone levels at 4 hours, patients with IHA experience a normal rise in levels. Additional testing may be necessary to identify those patients who have corticotropin-responsive APA or glucocorticoid-remediable hyperaldosteronism.

Bilateral adrenal venous sampling continues to be the most accurate test. Normal adrenal venous aldosterone concentration is from 100 to 400 ng/dl. In APA the ipsilateral adrenal venous aldosterone concentration is usually 1000 to 10,000 ng/dl, and the ratio of ipsilateral to contralateral aldosterone levels is usually greater than 10 : 1. Correct placement of the catheter in the adrenal vein is essential and can be verified by administration of synthetic ACTH with subsequent bilateral cortisol measurements. An aldosterone ratio greater than 10 : 1 in the presence of a symmetric ACTH-induced cortisol response is diagnostic of APA.

Radiologic Studies. CT scanning can detect most aldosterone-producing adenomas. Another promising radiologic maneuver in those unable to undergo adrenal venous sampling is adrenal scanning with ^{131}I-iodomethylnorcholesterol (NP-59). Patients are pretreated with dexamethasone to suppress normal adrenal functioning, and radioisotope is administered. Imaging is deferred for 5 days, since adrenal uptake and concentration of the isotope are maximal at that time. APA is manifested as lateralization of isotope to one adrenal gland. Accuracy may be as high as 90%, but false-negative results have been reported, so this test has not supplanted adrenal venous sampling.

Management. Surgery is the treatment of choice once APA is identified. Hypokalemia resolves permanently following surgery in all patients, but hypertension may persist. One year after surgery over 70% of patients are normotensive, whereas only 50% remain so at 5 years. With IHA fewer than 30% of patients are cured by surgery, so this approach, which invariably results in permanent adrenal insufficiency, is not indicated. Potassium-sparing diuretics are quite effective in IHA. Normokalemia is restored with spironolactone, amiloride, or triamterene/hydrochlorothiazide, although additional antihypertensives may be required to control blood pressure.

Secondary Hyperaldosteronism

Secondary hyperaldosteronism describes renin-mediated aldosterone excess, which is characterized by high renin and aldosterone levels. This can occur in edematous states

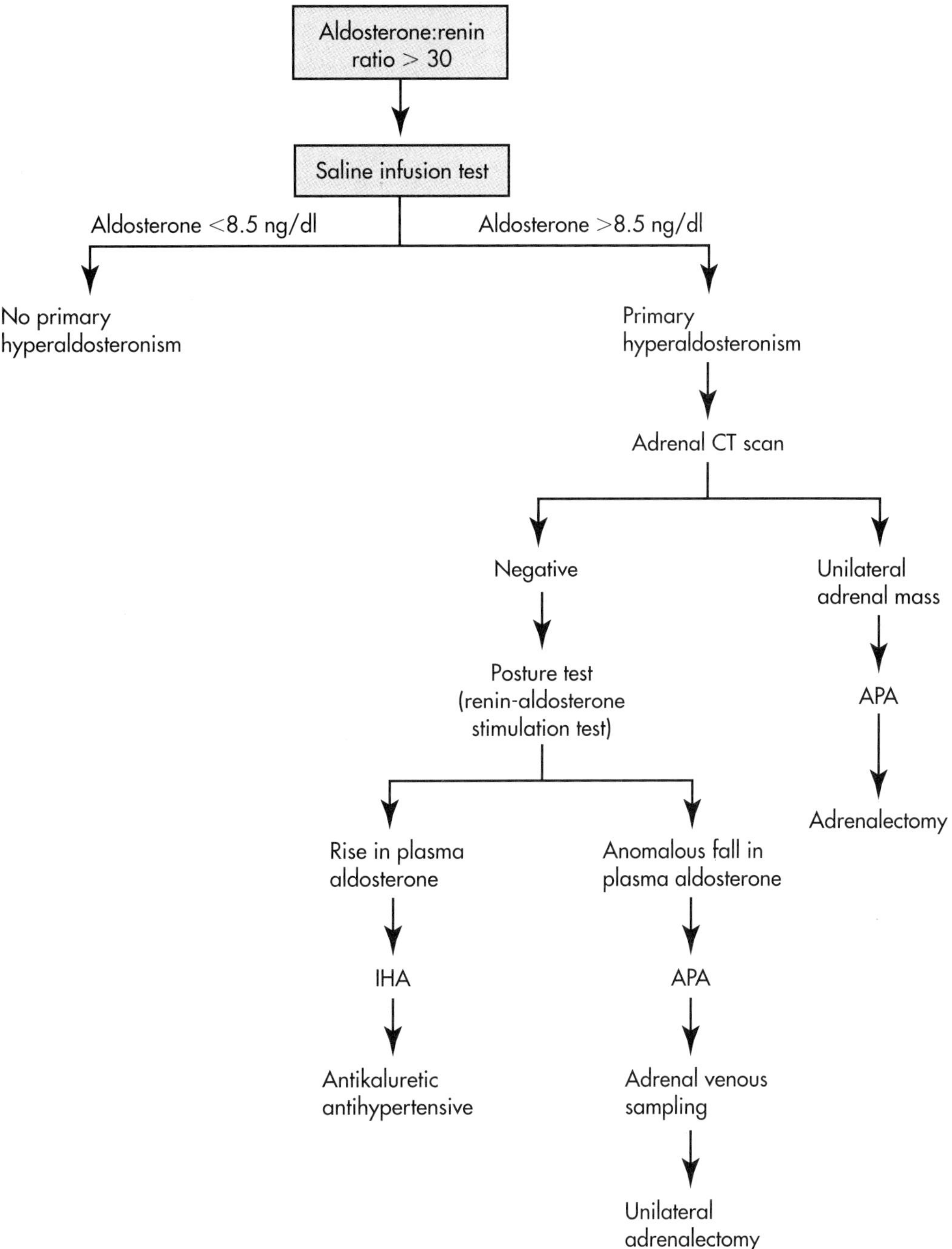

Fig. 98-5. Diagnostic approach to primary hyperaldosteronism. (Modified from Melby JC: *J Clin Endocrinol Metab* 69:697, 1989.)

such as congestive heart failure (CHF) or cirrhosis, in which intravascular volume depletion stimulates the renin-angiotensin axis. It also can occur in association with hypertension, in disorders such as renal artery stenosis, malignant hypertension, and juxtaglomerular cell tumor. Box 98-7 outlines the causes of secondary hyperaldosteronism. Hypokalemia may not be a prominent feature. Other unusual causes of secondary hyperaldosteronism include Bartter's syndrome. In this disorder chloride absorption is impaired in the ascending limb of the loop of Henle. Impaired chloride reabsorption in turn increases distal tubular delivery of sodium, resulting in increased sodium exchange for potassium in the distal tubule, with loss of potassium. This disorder can be mimicked by diuretic abuse or by chronic self-induced vomiting. Surreptitious vomiting can be recognized from a low urinary chloride level, and diuretics can be detected by a urine screen. Excess ingestion of true licorice, which contains substances that have mineralocorticoid-like effects, can also cause a metabolic picture that mimics endogenous aldosterone excess.

Disorders of Mineralocorticoid Deficiency

Pathophysiology. In hypoaldosteronism there is a decrease in aldosterone-mediated synthesis of sodium- potassium ATPase in renal tubular cells; thus the activity of the renal tubular sodium-potassium pump is diminished.

Box 98-7. Causes of Secondary Hyperaldosteronism

Secondary Hyperaldosteronism with Edema
Nephrotic syndrome
Hepatic cirrhosis
Congestive heart failure
Severe malabsorption

Secondary Hyperaldosteronism with Hypertension
Renovascular hypertension
Malignant hypertension
Primary hyperreninism (juxtaglomerular cell tumor)

Secondary Hyperaldosteronism Without Hypertension or Edema
Bartter's syndrome

Secondary Hyperaldosteronism (Miscellaneous)
Diuretics
Vasodilators (except prazosin)
Chronic self-induced vomiting
Excess licorice ingestion

Box 98-8. Causes of Hypoaldosteronism

Hyporeninemic Hypoaldosteronism
Diabetes mellitus
Hypertensive nephrosclerosis
β-Adrenergic blocking agents
Chronic volume expansion

Hyperreninemic Hypoaldosteronism
Aldosterone enzyme defect
Heparin
Lead poisoning
ACE inhibitor
Severe illness

Pseudohypoaldosteronism
Chronic interstitial nephritis
Systemic lupus erythematosus
Amyloidosis
Type 2 pseudohypoaldosteronism
Spironolactone

Hyperkalemia and sodium wasting are the result. The hyperkalemia can be severe, causing arrhythmias and even sudden death. The sodium wasting is more modest. Although decreased effective blood volume, mild hyponatremia, and postural hypotension may be present, there is often no clinical evidence of volume depletion. Metabolic acidosis may also be present due to decreased aldosterone-mediated renal tubular secretion of hydrogen ion.

Etiology and Clinical Findings. Box 98-8 outlines the etiologies of this syndrome, which can occur at several levels of the renin-angiotensin axis. Hyporeninemic hypoaldosteronism, previously known as type IV renal tubular acidosis, is the most common of these disorders, usually presenting as unexplained hyperkalemia in a patient with diabetes, hypertension, and mild renal insufficiency, occurring spontaneously or with use of ACE inhibitors or administration of a potassium load. Hypochloremic acidosis may also be present. The production of renin by the renal juxtaglomerular apparatus is permanently diminished or absent, presumably due to local tissue damage.

Hyperreninemic hypoaldosteronism is seen when renin production by the kidney is intact and the defect is either in the biosynthesis or action of angiotensin II or in aldosterone biosynthesis. This may be due to a genetic disorder of aldosterone production. It is also the mechanism of action of ACE inhibitors, which interfere with angiotensin II synthesis. Heparin and lead induce hypoaldosteronism as well by interfering with aldosterone synthesis at the level of the adrenal gland. This pattern of elevated renin and low aldosterone is also sometimes seen in critically ill patients with hypotension.

Pseudohypoaldosteronism is characterized by renal resistance to aldosterone, despite high aldosterone and renin levels. The pharmacologic antagonist spironolactone has this effect by interfering with the effect of aldosterone at the receptor level. Less commonly it is caused by a renal resistance to aldosterone seen in association with interstitial nephritis, systemic lupus erythematosus, or amyloidosis. Type 2 pseudohypoaldosteronism is a rare syndrome characterized by the features of hyporeninemic hypoaldosteronism, including low renin and aldosterone levels, but with a normal glomerular filtration rate. A distal tubule defect in chloride reabsorption that increases distal sodium chloride reabsorption and a collecting tubule defect in potassium secretion have both been postulated.

Diagnosis and Management. In most cases the clinical setting points to the diagnosis. The level of the defect can be confirmed, however, with the previously described renin-aldosterone stimulation test. Low stimulated renin and aldosterone levels point to a diagnosis of hyporeninemic hypoaldosteronism. Treatment consists of avoidance of potassium loads or inciting pharmacologic agents such as ACE inhibitors or potassium-sparing diuretics. A low-potassium diet with liberalization of sodium intake, potassium-wasting diuretics, or fludrocortisone 100 to 500 μg (0.01 to 0.05 mg) per day may be necessary in some patients. High stimulated renin and low aldosterone levels point to a defect at the level of the adrenal, and high stimulated renin and aldosterone levels point to end-organ refractoriness to aldosterone's effects. Treatment options are the same for these disorders as for hyporeninemic hypoaldosteronism, although treatment of pseudohypoaldosteronism may not be as effective due to renal insensitivity.

ADRENAL MEDULLA

The adrenal medulla has a different embryologic origin from the adrenal cortex, being composed of chromaffin tissue derived from neural crest ectoderm. Its location next to the adrenal cortex appears to be critical to the synthesis of its major catecholamine, epinephrine. The enzyme critical to epinephrine formation is inducible by high levels of glucocorticoids, delivered from the cortex to the medulla by a rich blood supply. The adrenal medulla is the source of all epinephrine, whereas norepinephrine is produced by extra-adrenal chromaffin cells.

Pheochromocytoma

Pheochromocytoma is the most important disease of the adrenal medulla. It is a tumor of the chromaffin cells that is an uncommon but serious cause of hypertension, with an incidence of 0.1% to 0.4% among hypertensive patients. Autopsy series indicate that it may be substantially underdiagnosed, since about 40% of all pheochromocytomas detected at autopsy in patients with a history of hypertension are not identified during life. About 90% of pheochromocytomas are found in the adrenal medulla, and 10% are extraadrenal. In general, once spread occurs to outside the chromaffin tissue, the tumor is considered malignant. This occurs in fewer than 10% of the cases. Intraadrenal tumors are usually unilateral. In the 10% of the cases in which adrenal pheochromocytoma is bilateral, patients often are found to have polyglandular multiple endocrine neoplasia (MEN) type II. Most extraadrenal pheochromocytomas are intraabdominal and can be found anywhere along the sympathetic ganglion chain, which is also composed of chromaffin tissue.

Pathophysiology. Excess production of catecholamines has a variety of physiologic effects. Catecholamines stimulate renal sodium retention by a direct tubular effect, by increased renin secretion, and by reduced intrarenal hydrostatic pressure. Shunting of blood toward the heart, increased cardiac inotropy, and increased peripheral resistance due to vasoconstriction are also consequences of catecholamine excess. Metabolic effects include hyperglycemia, hyperlipidemia, hypokalemia, and increased tissue oxygen consumption. Most of these effects occur due to increased β-receptor–mediated stimulation of adenyl cyclase in cell membranes, which results in increased conversion of ATP to cAMP. Hyperglycemia occurs due to catecholamine-mediated increases in glycogenolysis and gluconeogenesis. Catecholamines also diffusely inhibit gut motility.

History and Physical Findings. Most patients have persistently elevated blood pressure with superimposed paroxysms of severe hypertension. Despite the hypertension, patients are usually orthostatic due to volume contraction. A minority of patients are normotensive between paroxysmal hypertensive episodes. Episodes are accompanied by headache, sweating, palpitations, anxiety, tremulousness, and nervousness lasting from 15 to 30 minutes. The symptom triad of headache, palpitations, and diaphoresis in association with hypertension has been found to have a high specificity (93.8%) and sensitivity (90.9%) for the diagnosis in hypertensive patients. Other symptoms of pheochromocytoma may include dizziness, constipation, weight loss, flushing, and psychiatric symptoms. Laboratory findings may include hyperglycemia, hyperlipidemia, and hypokalemia. The presentation may be less typical among the elderly, since cardiomegaly and left ventricular hypertrophy (LVH) were the only features recognized retrospectively among elderly hypertensives found at autopsy to have pheochromocytoma in one series.[7]

Table 98-3. Normal Catecholamine Values

	Range
Urine	
Metanephrine	<1.3 mg/24 hr
VMA	2-7 mg/24 hr
Epinephrine	0-34 μg/24 hr
Norepinephrine	550 μg/24 hr
Plasma	
Norepinephrine	60-400 pg/ml
Epinephrine	10-55 pg/ml
Dopamine	<100 pg/ml

From Melby JC: Clinical review 1: Endocrine hypertension, *J Clin Endo Metab* 69:697, 1989.

Diagnosis. Excess production of epinephrine and/or norepinephrine is best determined by measurement of their excreted metabolites. Normal urinary values for catecholamines are listed in Table 98-3. Care must be taken in determining who to screen for this disorder. Because of its low prevalence among hypertensives, even a highly specific screening test results in a significant number of false-positives. Therefore screening should be performed only in those in whom clinical suspicion is truly high. In particular, it should be reserved for those with uncontrollable hypertension; for those with hypertension and the above-mentioned symptom triad of headache, palpitations, and sweating; or for those with a personal or family history of disorders suggestive of the MEN syndromes.

The 24-hour urine collection must be performed carefully. Chlorpromazine, the benzodiazepines, α-methyldopa, and the β-blockers should be eliminated 2 weeks before testing. Ethanol, amphetamines, quinidine, theophylline, tetracycline, reserpine, clofibrate, and disulfiram can also interfere with the test results by raising or lowering catecholamine levels. If antihypertensive agents must be continued, diuretics or vasodilators such as hydralazine and minoxidil cause minimal interference. Levels of metanephrines, vanillylmandelic acid (VMA), and catecholamines can be measured. Total or fractionated urinary catecholamines using the high-performance liquid chromatography (HPLC) method may be the most sensitive and specific urinary test, with twofold elevations in over 95% of patients with pheochromocytoma. Urinary free norepinephrine was 100% sensitive and 98% specific for pheochromocytoma in one series. Mildly elevated values of all the catecholamine metabolites are common among hypertensives; only very high values are consistent with a diagnosis of pheochromocytoma. Plasma catecholamine measurements can also be used and may be as reliable as urinary measurements, but can be artificially elevated by stress, volume depletion, activity, anoxia, smoking, and medications; thus they must be performed under idealized conditions at complete bed rest. A clonidine suppression test can also be used when the diagnosis is uncertain and plasma norepinephrine levels are only modestly elevated (500 to 1000 pg/ml). Clonidine, 0.3 mg, is given and plasma norepinephrine levels are measured 3 hours later. Virtually all patients with essential hypertension suppress norepinephrine levels to below 500 pg/ml, whereas patients with pheochromocytoma do not.

Localization of pheochromocytoma after biochemical confirmation may be performed with adrenal CT scan or MRI. CT scan is the most cost-effective initial study, and has >98% sensitivity for detection of adrenal tumors, but a specificity of only 70%.[7] MRI has comparable sensitivity, but has higher specificity in distinguishing medullary pheochromocytoma from adrenal cortical tumors. The latter may be superior in the detection of small tumors. Extraadrenal pheochromocytomas or very small adrenal tumors are harder to localize and may require ^{131}I metaiodobenzylguanidine (MIBG) scanning. This isotope, although expensive, is specific for catecholamine-producing tissue and has 80% sensitivity and over 95% specificity for localization of malignant pheochromocytomas. Another effective isotope used for imaging, which is reported to be of similar sensitivity, is ^{111}In-pentetreotide (Octreoscan). Those who are found to have bilateral adrenal tumors should be screened for other manifestations of the MEN syndromes.

Management. Surgical removal is the treatment of choice in most cases of benign and malignant pheochromocytoma. Medical treatment must begin at least 2 weeks before surgery to avoid intraoperative hypertensive crisis or hypotension after resection. This includes restoration of plasma volume, which is usually profoundly depleted by catecholamine-induced vasoconstriction, and α- and β-blockade. Phenoxybenzamine is the α-blocker of choice, starting at 10 mg twice daily and increasing as tolerated to 0.5 to 1 mg/kg/day until near normotension and control of symptoms are achieved. Prazosin may also be effective preoperatively; however, it does not control intraoperative hypertension well, so phenoxybenzamine must be used intraoperatively. Prazosin is started slowly at 1 mg three times a day to avoid postural hypotension and increased to 2 to 5 mg three times a day. After α-blockade has been achieved, β-blockers can be added if needed to control tachycardia, arrhythmias, or angina. β-Blockers should never be administered before α-blockade because they can precipitate hypertensive crisis due to unopposed α-receptor stimulation. Calcium channel blockers have also been used successfully preoperatively and intraoperatively. During surgery volume expansion with blood or plasma is advocated to keep blood pressure normal.

The same medications are used to manage the symptoms of malignant pheochromocytoma when complete surgical resection is not possible. An additional agent, α-methylparatyrosine, a catecholamine synthesis inhibitor, actually lowers serum catecholamine levels and can also be effective for these patients. ^{131}I-MIBG also shows promise in the treatment of unresectable pheochromocytoma.

INCIDENTAL ADRENAL MASS

The ability of abdominal CT scan or MRI performed for unrelated reasons to detect adrenal masses of 0.5 cm or smaller has resulted in a diagnostic dilemma. The prevalence of such incidentally discovered masses is 1% to 4% depending on the series. These small adrenal tumors are not new, having been previously reported at autopsy in up to 30% of patients without known endocrinopathy; what is new is our ability to detect them during life.

Evaluation Criteria

Once these lesions are detected, a limited hormonal evaluation is considered appropriate to rule out occult hypersecretory states. Although most (up to 94%) are nonsecretory, clinically silent hypersecretory pheochromocytomas, aldosteronomas, and cortisol-secreting tumors have been extensively reported, and between 50% to 70% of adrenal carcinomas are secretory; thus, a hormonal evaluation should be performed for all patients.[8] Table 98-4 indicates the frequency of the various diagnoses to be excluded and the appropriate hormonal evaluations necessary. Identification of hormonal activity indicates the need for surgical removal.

Adrenal masses found to be nonhypersecretory require an investigation to rule out malignancy. Prior treatment algorithms based on the presumption that malignancies are usually over 3 cm in size have low sensitivity and specificity. In one series of 86 adrenal masses, all eight lesions found to be primary carcinomas of the adrenal were 3 cm or larger, but over 60% of lesions found to be metastatic to the adrenal from other primary sites were 3 cm or smaller.[8] Those with known primary malignancies and extensive metastatic disease elsewhere do not need further investigation. Those with primary malignancies in other sites without known metastases require biopsy of the adrenal lesion for appropriate staging of their primary tumor. In those patients who have nonhypersecretory lesions without known primary malignancies elsewhere, CT and MRI imaging features may be more accurate than size criteria in distinguishing benign vs. malignant adrenal lesions. Non-contrast CT attenuation characteristics may be helpful, as an attenuation coefficient of <10 Hounsfield units (HU) has been shown to be highly specific (92%) for benign adenomas. However, sensitivity is low (58%), as many benign adenomas have higher values.[11] MRI T1- and T2-weighted imaging may have similar utility, but at least one study found CT attenuation coefficients to be better discriminators. If contrast CT is performed, delayed images at 1 hour may distinguish between benign lesions (<30 HU) and malignant ones (>30 HU). Chemical shift MRI for lesions with >10 HU on non-contrast CT or >30 HU on contrast CT shows promise in distinguishing those lesions with high fat content (adenomas, myelolipomas) from those with low fat content (hemorrhages, pheochromocytomas, metastases, cysts). Loss of signal with MRI chemical shift imaging indicates high fat content, while no signal loss is seen in lesions with low fat content, indicating the need for biopsy. An algorithm using these imaging criteria to determine the need for biopsy is outlined in Fig. 98-6. This strategy has been shown to correctly characterize over 90% of incidental adrenal masses. Biopsy is recommended for all lesions >3 cm and those <3 cm with suspicious radiologic characteristics. An alternate approach recommended by some experts is performance of ^{131}I-iodomethylnorcholesterol (NP-59) imaging in all patients with nonhypersecretory lesions, regardless of size, with biopsy of those with imaging patterns more characteristic of malignancy (decreased, absent, or distorted radioisotope distribution).[8] In all cases, hormonal studies must be completed before needle biopsy, since manipulation of an unsuspected pheochromocytoma is quite dangerous.

Monitoring

Those who do not meet the criteria for further investigation should be followed clinically, with yearly history and physical examination. Some experts recommend repeat CT scan or MRI in 3 months, with removal of tumors evidencing growth to >3 cm at 3 months. Small lesions of less than 3 cm that are stable in size for 1 year in asymptomatic patients can be monitored infrequently.

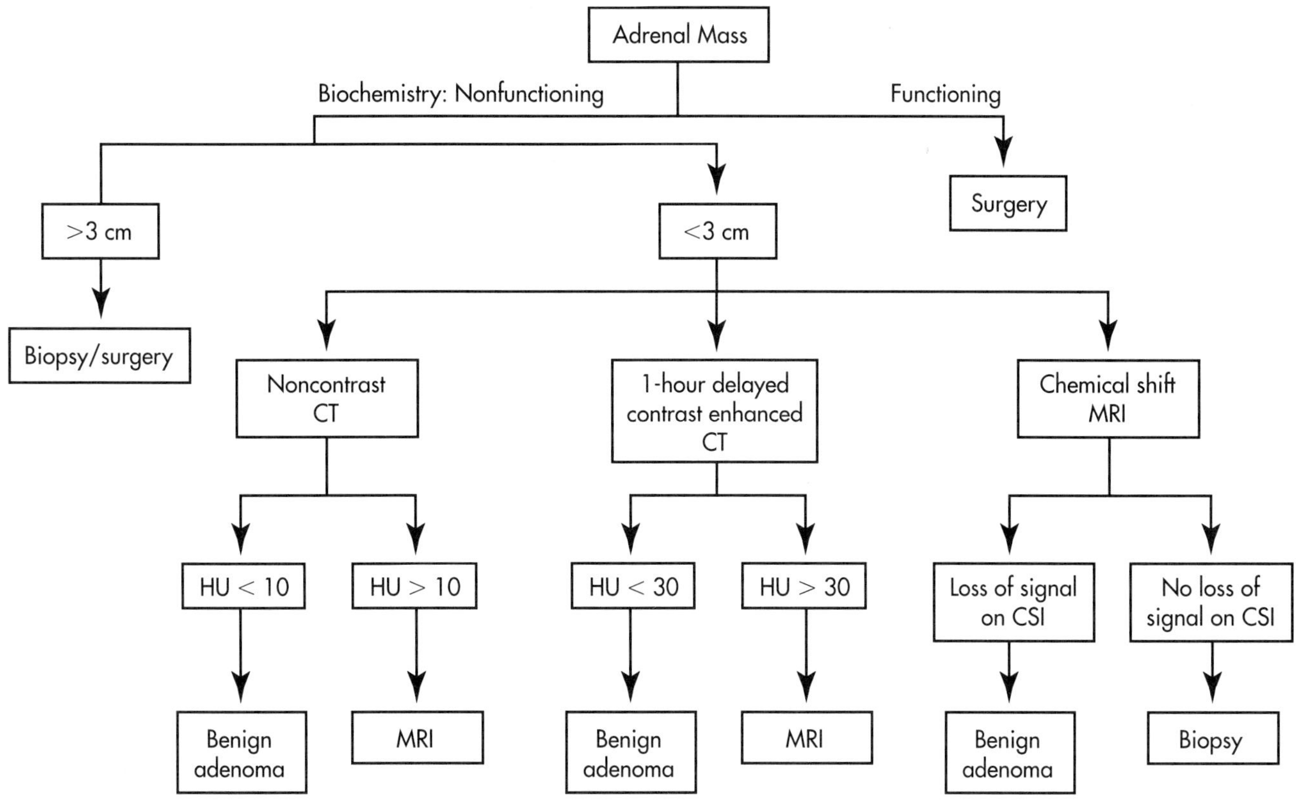

Fig. 98-6. Diagnostic approach to incidental adrenal mass. (From Peppercorn PD, Grossman AB, Reznek RH: *Clin Endocrinol* 48:379-388, 1998.)

Table 98-4. Recommended Biochemical Screening Tests for All Incidental Adrenal Masses

Hypersecretory state	Frequency among incidentalomas	Screening test
Pheochromocytoma	0-11%	24-hr urine catecholamines
Cushing's syndrome	0-12%	Overnight dexamethasone suppression test
Aldosterone-producing adenoma	0-7%	Blood pressure and serum K^+; if HTN, do renin/aldosterone ratio
Masculinizing tumor	0-11%	Serum dehydroepiandrosterone sulfate
Feminizing tumor	Rare	Serum estradiol in feminized men

Modified from Kloos RT, Gross MD, Francis IR, et al: *Endocrine Reviews* 16:460-484, 1995.

REFERENCES

1. Amin S, LaValley MP, Simms RW, et al: A meta-analysis ranking efficacy of treatments for corticosteroid-induced osteoporosis, *Arthritis Rheum* 41:S137, 1998.
2. Dluhy R: Uncommon forms of secondary hypertension in older patients, *Am J Hypertension* 11(3, Part 2):52S-56S, 1998.
3. Dluhy R, Williams G: Glucocorticoid-remediable aldosteronism, *Cardiovascular Research* 31:870-872, 1996.

3a. Ganguly A: Current concepts: primary aldosteronism, *New Engl J Med* 339:1828-1834, 1998.

4. Hofbauer LC, Heufelder AE: Endocrine implications of human immunodeficiency virus infection, *Medicine* 75(5):262-278, 1996.
5. Invitti C, Giraldi FP, De Martin M, et al: Diagnosis and management of Cushing's syndrome: results of an Italian multicenter study, *J Clin Endocrinol Metab* 84:440-448, 1999.
6. Jeffcoate W: Alcohol-induced pseudo Cushing's syndrome, *Lancet* 341(8846):676, 1993.
7. Kenady DE, McGrath PC, Sloan DA, et al: Diagnosis and management of pheochromocytoma, *Curr Opin Oncol* 9:61-67, 1997.
8. Kloos RT, Gross MD, Francis IR, et al: Incidentally discovered adrenal masses, *Endocrine Reviews* 16(4):460-484, 1995.
9. Oelkers W, Diederich S, Bahr V: Diagnosis and therapy surveillance in Addison's disease, *J Clin Endocrinol Metab* 75:259, 1992.
10. Orth DN: Medical progress: Cushing's syndrome, *New Engl J Med* 332:791-803, 1995.
11. Peppercorn PD, Grossman AB, Reznek RH: Imaging of incidentally discovered adrenal masses (Review), *Clinical Endocrinology* 48:379-388, 1998.
12. Swearingen B, Biller BM, Barker FG, et al: Long-term mortality after transsphenoidal surgery for Cushing's disease, *Ann Intern Med* 130:821-824, 1999.
13. Yanovski JA, Cutler GB, Chrousos GP, et al: Corticotrophin-releasing hormone stimulation following low-dose dexamethasone administration: a test to distinguish Cushing's syndrome from pseudo-Cushing's states, *JAMA* 269:2232-2238, 1993.

CHAPTER 99

Disorders of the Hypothalamus and Pituitary Gland

Janet Schlechte

Hyperprolactinemia, acromegaly, and hypopituitarism are common neuroendocrine disorders that are likely to be encountered in the primary care setting. Although all will be managed in conjunction with an endocrinologist, the primary care physician needs to be familiar with the clinical presentation, appropriate screening tests, and treatment options for these disorders.

HYPERPROLACTINEMIA

Although most anterior pituitary hormones, including growth hormone (GH), adrenocorticotropic hormone (ACTH), luteinizing hormone (LH), and thyroid stimulating hormone (TSH), are stimulated by hypothalamic releasing factors, the secretion of prolactin (PRL) is under inhibitory hypothalamic control. Dopamine is the predominant PRL inhibitory factor and disruption of hypothalamic dopaminergic pathways or alteration of dopamine synthesis leads to hypersecretion of PRL. The primary action of PRL is to stimulate lactation and growth of mammary tissue. PRL levels gradually increase throughout pregnancy, with a tenfold elevation at term. Four to 12 weeks after delivery PRL levels return to normal unless breastfeeding occurs. Serum levels of PRL are usually under 20 ng/ml in females and under 10 ng/ml in males.

Clinical Presentation

The major consequence of hyperprolactinemia is reproductive dysfunction. High levels of PRL suppress the pulsatile secretion of gonadotropin releasing hormone, leading to low LH and follicle stimulating hormone (FSH) secretion and impaired production of estradiol and testosterone. In women the classic symptoms of hyperprolactinemia are amenorrhea, galactorrhea, and infertility. However, amenorrhea may occur without galactorrhea, galactorrhea may occur alone, and some women with hyperprolactinemia have regular menses. The hypogonadism induced by PRL excess also leads to dyspareunia or hot flashes. Hyperprolactinemia in males causes impotence, decreased libido, infertility, and gynecomastia. Galactorrhea is present in only 10% to 20% of men with hyperprolactinemia.

Causes

Although PRL-secreting pituitary tumors are the most common cause of hyperprolactinemia, the first step in evaluating a patient is to rule out causes unrelated to the pituitary or hypothalamus (Box 99-1). A variety of medications cause hyperprolactinemia by altering hypothalamic dopamine levels. Dopamine receptor antagonists such as neuroleptic agents and metoclopramide may be associated with PRL levels that exceed 200 ng/ml. Histamine type 2 receptor blockers cause hyperprolactinemia through centrally mediated mechanisms, and peripheral decarboxylase inhibitors like carbidopa interfere with dopamine biosynthesis. Verapamil may raise PRL levels in about 10% of patients taking the drug. PRL levels usually return to normal 48 to 96 hours after the medication is discontinued.

Box 99-1. Causes of Hyperprolactinemia

Prolactinoma
Hypothalamic disease
GH-secreting pituitary tumors
Drugs
- H_2-blockers
- Metoclopramide
- Estrogen
- Phenothiazines
- Verapamil

Primary hypothyroidism
Nipple stimulation
Chest trauma
Renal insufficiency

PRL levels rise during the menstrual cycle, and oral contraceptives cause a mild elevation of PRL. In patients with renal insufficiency the clearance of PRL is decreased. Chronic nipple stimulation and chest trauma increase PRL secretion and psychic stress has a variable effect. Primary hypothyroidism may be associated with an elevated PRL, and the pituitary enlargement that may accompany longstanding primary hypothyroidism mimics the presentation of a prolactinoma. A careful history and physical examination, measurement of thyroid function, and a pregnancy test will rule out most causes of hyperprolactinemia. Stimulation or suppression tests of PRL secretion using thyrotropin releasing hormone, L-dopa, or insulin-induced hypoglycemia are not valuable in the differential diagnosis of hyperprolactinemia.

Prolactinomas

Prolactinomas account for over 80% of all functioning pituitary tumors. In women prolactinomas are usually microadenomas (less than 10 mm) and are rarely associated with visual loss or hypopituitarism (Fig. 99-1). Fewer than 30% of women with hyperprolactinemia will have a macroadenoma (greater than 10 mm), but the majority of prolactinomas in men are large tumors (Fig. 99-2). PRL-secreting macroadenomas are more likely to be associated with visual loss, neurologic deficits, and loss of anterior pituitary hormones. Although males with prolactinomas develop impotence and decreased libido due to hyperprolactinemia, they usually seek medical attention because of headaches or visual loss.

Diagnosis. The diagnosis of a prolactinoma is confirmed by demonstration of sustained hyperprolactinemia and radiographic evidence of a pituitary tumor. Because PRL secretion is episodic and PRL levels can be increased with stress, minimally elevated levels (20 to 30 ng/ml) should be confirmed by obtaining several samples.

When no obvious cause of an elevated PRL is apparent the hypothalamus and pituitary should be imaged. Magnetic

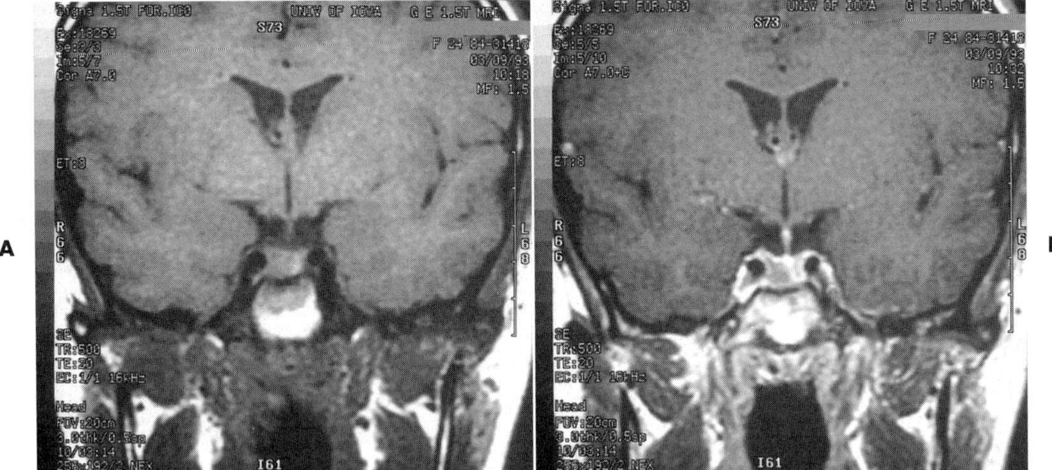

Fig. 99-1. Coronal T_1-weighted images before *(left)* and after *(right)* administration of gadolinium. After administration of contrast the pituitary microadenoma is hypodense compared with surrounding pituitary tissue.

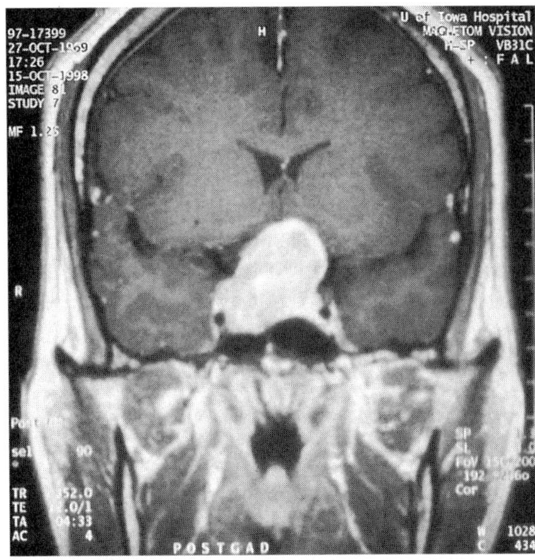

Fig. 99-2. Coronal T_1-weighted image of a pituitary macroadenoma extending into the cavernous sinus and displacing the optic chiasm.

resonance imaging (MRI) is superior to computed tomography (CT) in delineating tumor size and evaluating suprasellar or lateral tumor extension. PRL-secreting macroadenomas are virtually always accompanied by marked elevations of PRL (over 1000 ng/ml). In fact, a large pituitary tumor that is associated with a PRL of less than 200 ng/ml is unlikely to be a prolactinoma. Formal testing of visual fields and assessment of anterior pituitary function should always be undertaken when a macroadenoma is detected. Small prolactinomas are so rarely associated with hypopituitarism or visual loss that formal visual field testing and tests of anterior pituitary function are not necessary.

Management. The two established indications for treatment of a prolactinoma are infertility and the presence of a macroadenoma. The goals of therapy are to normalize PRL, restore menses or erectile function, and decrease tumor size. The treatment of choice, regardless of tumor size, is a dopamine agonist. Pituitary surgery is not generally recommended because it is associated with a high rate of recurrence of hyperprolactinemia. Radiation is not used as primary therapy because of the time required to normalize PRL and gonadal function and because it may lead to hypopituitarism.

In the majority of cases treatment should be initiated with bromocriptine. This dopamine agonist causes rapid normalization of PRL and restoration of menses in 80% to 90% of patients. Treatment is usually started with a bedtime dose of 1.25 mg, which is slowly increased to 5 mg daily. A PRL level should be checked 3 to 4 weeks after reaching the target dose. If the PRL has not normalized, the dose should be increased slowly and the level should be repeated. Most women with a microadenoma will require 5 to 7.5 mg of bromocriptine daily. Gonadal function usually normalizes within 3 months, and after 4 to 6 weeks of therapy there will be a reduction in tumor size. Women with macroadenomas and men may require higher doses of bromocriptine to normalize PRL and cause tumor shrinkage.

Bromocriptine may be associated with nausea, nasal stuffiness, and orthostatic hypotension. All of these symptoms can be reduced if the drug is started at a low dose and increased slowly. If bromocriptine is not effective or is not well tolerated, another dopamine agonist such as pergolide (Permax) or cabergoline (Dostinex) may be substituted. Cabergoline has a high specificity for the dopamine D2 receptor and a long half-life and can be given twice weekly. Doses of cabergoline ranging from 0.5 to 2 mg weekly are as efficacious as 5 to 7.5 mg of bromocriptine and may be associated with fewer side effects. However, cabergoline is expensive and should be reserved for patients with resistant tumors or for those who cannot take bromocriptine. All dopamine agonists must be taken regularly to be effective. Discontinuation leads to a rapid return to pretreatment PRL levels and tumor regrowth (Box 99-2).

When treatment with bromocriptine is initiated, mechanical contraception should be used until two to three menstrual cycles have occurred. When pregnancy is documented, the dopamine agonist should be discontinued. Although dopamine agonists are not associated with an increased rate of

Box 99-2. Dopamine Agonist Therapy

Start with bromocriptine
5-7.5 mg is the usual dose required to restore menses
Needs to be taken continually to be effective
Use pergolide or cabergoline if bromocriptine is poorly tolerated or in resistant cases

spontaneous abortion or congenital defects, fetal exposure should be limited. PRL normally rises after conception, and it is not necessary or cost-effective to monitor levels throughout pregnancy. The pituitary gland will increase in size during pregnancy and the high estrogen levels achieved during pregnancy will stimulate lactotroph hyperplasia, but pregnant women with PRL microadenomas rarely develop symptomatic tumor enlargement. A pregnant woman with a macroadenoma, however, should have a formal visual field examination each trimester and MRI scanning if symptoms of tumor expansion occur. The primary care physician may institute and manage dopamine agonist therapy for a microadenoma but treatment of a PRL-secreting macroadenoma will require a multidisciplinary approach involving an endocrinologist, neuro-ophthalmologist, and neurosurgeon.

Management of Prolactinomas When Pregnancy Is Not an Issue. When a prolactinoma is small and fertility is not an issue, there is no clear consensus on whether to treat the hyperprolactinemia or to monitor the patient without therapy. PRL-secreting microadenomas have a benign natural history and do not progressively increase in size over time. Elevated PRL levels do, however, suppress production of estradiol and testosterone and may place these patients at risk for premature bone loss. Women with hyperprolactinemic amenorrhea have been shown to have 25% lower spinal bone mass than women with regular menses but do not have an increased fracture rate. The use of dual-energy x-ray absorptiometry to quantitate bone mass in hyperprolactinemic women may help with treatment decisions in individual patients. An amenorrheic woman with elevated PRL who is not desirous of pregnancy or a postmenopausal woman with hyperprolactinemia may be treated with estrogen. Since estrogen may induce pituitary enlargement, these women should be monitored closely for clinical signs of tumor growth. Alternatively, they can be treated with a combination of estrogen and bromocriptine.

Idiopathic Hyperprolactinemia. Some women with amenorrhea, galactorrhea, and hyperprolactinemia have no evidence of a tumor on MRI, and this condition is termed *idiopathic hyperprolactinemia.* A tumor may actually be present but is too small to be detected radiographically. In most of these patients PRL levels remain stable and progression toward a macroadenoma or microadenoma is uncommon.

ACROMEGALY

Secretion of GH is regulated by two hypothalamic peptides, GH releasing factor and somatostatin. The releasing factor stimulates synthesis and release of GH, while somatostatin is inhibitory and maintains low levels of GH secretion. Insulin-like growth factor (IGF-1) is the peripheral target for GH and the anabolic effects of GH are mediated through IGF-1, which is produced in the liver. GH secretion is pulsatile and is stimulated by exercise, stress, and estrogen.

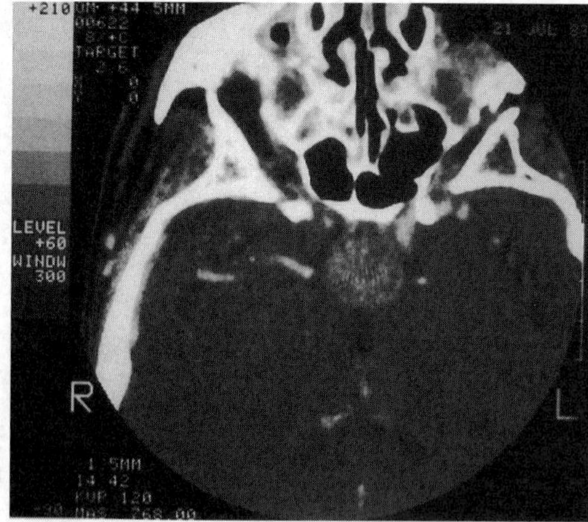

Fig. 99-3. Computed tomography (CT) scan of large pituitary tumor in a patient with acromegaly.

GH secreting tumors account for 10% to 15% of pituitary adenomas and are usually discovered in the third to fifth decade. GH secreting tumors grow slowly, and about 80% of patients have tumors larger than 10 mm on presentation (Fig. 99-3). Headache is present in about 50% of patients at diagnosis, and a patient with a rapidly enlarging tumor may present with a visual field defect or cranial nerve palsy. Primary care physicians need to be aware of the clinical presentation of acromegaly and how to screen for GH hypersecretion.

Clinical Presentation

Typical findings of GH excess include coarsening of facial features, increasing hand and foot size, frontal bossing, oily skin, and hyperhidrosis (Fig. 99-4). With enlargement of the mandible, malocclusion of the jaw may occur, and the diagnosis of acromegaly may first be considered during a dental evaluation. Sleep apnea occurs in 50% of patients with acromegaly and degenerative arthritis is common. Diabetes mellitus occurs in 10% to 25%. Cardiovascular disease is prevalent and is the most common cause of death in patients with acromegaly. Acromegaly is associated with an increased frequency of colonic polyps, uterine leiomyomata, and gastrointestinal malignancies. Early recognition of GH excess is important since patients with acromegaly have two to three times the expected mortality rate, which decreases after GH levels return to normal.

Diagnosis

GH secretion is pulsatile with undetectable levels between pulses. Because of this pulsatility random measurement of GH will not suffice to make the diagnosis of acromegaly. The diagnosis of GH excess can be confirmed by measurement of IGF-1 or by measurement of GH during a glucose tolerance test. After the oral administration of 75 or 100 grams of glucose, GH levels in healthy individuals will fall to less than 2 ng/ml, whereas patients with acromegaly will show no suppression or may show a paradoxical increase in GH (Fig. 99-5). The best single test for diagnosis of acromegaly

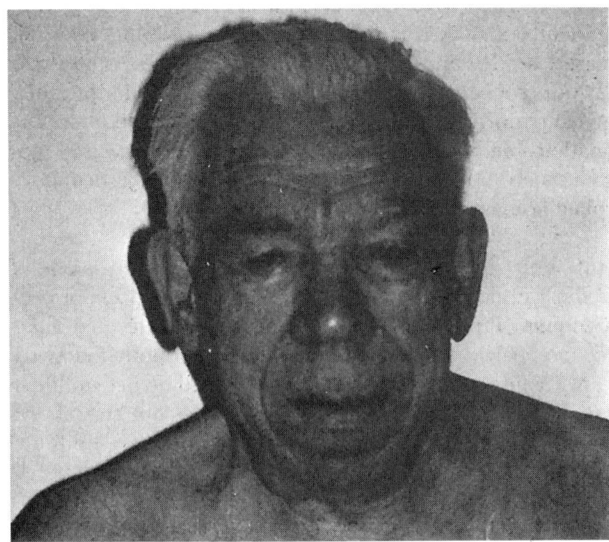

Fig. 99-4. Typical facial features of acromegaly.

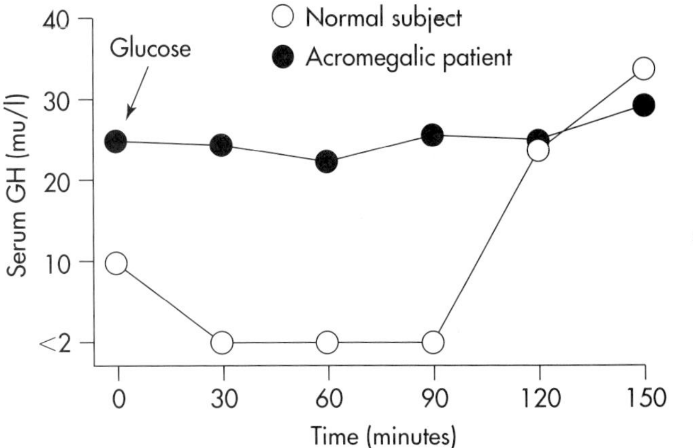

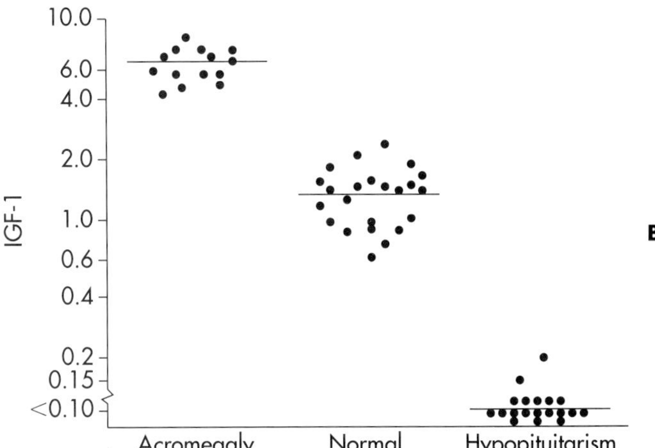

Fig. 99-5. **A,** Lack of suppression of GH after oral administration of glucose in patient with acromegaly. Levels less than 2 ng/ml are normal. **B,** IGF-1 levels in normal subjects and patients with acromegaly.

is measurement of IGF-1. IGF-1 values are not affected by exercise and reflect integrated GH secretion over the previous 24 hours (see Fig. 99-5). Other laboratory abnormalities in patients with acromegaly include elevated triglycerides, hyperglycemia, and hyperphosphatemia. The elevated phosphate may be due to direct stimulation of renal tubular phosphate reabsorption by IGF-1. One third of individuals with GH excess will have hyperprolactinemia due to co-secretion of GH and PRL by the tumor. When GH excess is confirmed, a MRI of the pituitary should be done and the patient should be referred to an endocrinologist for treatment.

Management

The treatment of choice for a GH-secreting tumor is transsphenoidal surgery. This procedure should be performed by an experienced neurosurgeon, and preoperative and postoperative care should be coordinated by the primary care physician, endocrinologist, and neurosurgeon. Surgical success rates range from 78% to 90% for small GH-secreting tumors and from 33% to 80% for macroadenomas. Unsuccessful surgery may necessitate treatment with a dopamine agonist, a long-acting analog of somatostatin, or radiation therapy.

HYPOPITUITARISM

Hypopituitarism results from failure of all or portions of the anterior pituitary. The clinical manifestations of pituitary insufficiency depend on the process responsible for the hormone loss and the type and number of hormones that are absent. Hormone loss may be total (panhypopituitarism) or partial, and in some cases hormone deficiency is due to loss of a single hypothalamic releasing hormone. In a patient with a large pituitary mass, visual loss or headache may bring the patient to medical attention before the hormone loss becomes clinically apparent. In contrast, a patient with a slow-growing pituitary tumor may present with nonspecific symptoms such as fatigue.

Causes

The most common cause of hypopituitarism is a hypothalamic or pituitary tumor. Infiltrative processes such as sarcoidosis account for only 1% of cases of pituitary dysfunction, and postpartum hemorrhage (Sheehan's syndrome) leading to hypopituitarism is rare. Hormone loss can occur from a few months to years after radiation therapy. Sudden hemorrhage into a large pituitary tumor may lead to headache, diplopia, and acute pituitary failure (pituitary apoplexy). Head trauma may lead to direct fracture of the sella turcica, causing hemorrhage within the gland or rupture of the pituitary stalk. In older subjects a rare cause of hypopituitarism is vascular insufficiency sustained during coronary artery bypass surgery (Box 99-3).

Clinical Presentation

The endocrine symptoms that accompany pituitary failure mimic the symptoms that develop with the loss of the target organs (thyroid, ovary, testes, adrenal). Although there is no fixed order in which anterior pituitary hormones are lost, GH, LH, and FSH usually disappear before ACTH or TSH. The clinical manifestations that accompany loss of the anterior pituitary hormones are discussed below. When hormone deficiency is due to failure of the target organ the disorder is termed *primary* hormone insufficiency. When the hormone deficiency is due to loss of a hypothalamic or pituitary hormone it is termed *secondary* hormone insufficiency.

LH and FSH. Loss of gonadal function is perhaps the most common presentation of hypopituitarism in adults.

Box 99-3. Causes of Hypopituitarism

Pituitary and hypothalamic tumors
Pituitary radiation or surgery
Infiltrative processes
- Hemochromatosis
- Sarcoidosis

Pituitary infarction
Pituitary apoplexy
Head trauma

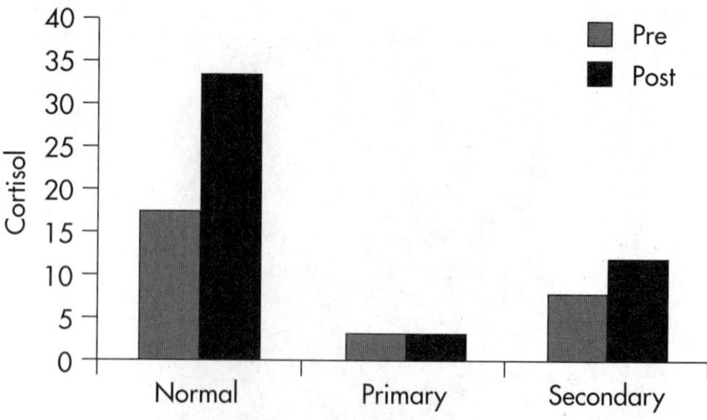

Fig. 99-6. Cortisol response to ACTH in healthy subjects and patients with primary and secondary adrenal insufficiency. The flat response in primary adrenal insufficiency is due to adrenal failure. The blunted response in secondary adrenal insufficiency is due to insufficient stimulation of the adrenals by ACTH.

Attention to clinical symptoms is important, since normal semen analysis in a male and regular menstrual function in a female make hypogonadotropic hypogonadism extremely unlikely. In premenopausal women loss of LH and FSH leads to oligomenorrhea, amenorrhea, infertility, dyspareunia, and decreased libido. In males, decreased testicular function is manifested by decreased libido, decrease in ejaculate volume, infertility, and change in beard and body hair growth.

Evaluation of the pituitary-gonadal axis involves measurement of LH, FSH, and testosterone or estradiol. Patients with ovarian or testicular failure will have low testosterone and estradiol levels with an elevated FSH and LH, whereas those with hypogonadotropic hypogonadism will have low LH and FSH levels and low sex steroid levels.

TSH. Secondary hypothyroidism that develops due to loss of TSH is less common than thyroid failure and accounts for less than 5% of all cases of hypothyroidism. It is not possible to distinguish primary and secondary hypothyroidism on clinical symptomatology alone, and common findings include cold intolerance, constipation, dry skin, myalgias, delayed deep tendon reflexes, and bradycardia.

The most reliable test to document secondary hypothyroidism is measurement of free thyroxine, and a normal serum thyroxine indicates that the pituitary-thyroid axis is intact. A TSH alone should not be used as a screening test in patients with pituitary disease because most patients with secondary hypothyroidism will have a TSH within the normal range. With symptoms of hypothyroidism a subnormal serum thyroxine and a low or normal TSH should suggest pituitary insufficiency.

ACTH. ACTH deficiency is potentially the most serious outcome of pituitary hormone loss. The symptoms associated with loss of ACTH usually occur gradually, and patients who develop secondary adrenal insufficiency usually present with fatigue, weight loss, and lassitude. Patients with secondary adrenal insufficiency do not develop hyperpigmentation and rarely have the salt wasting, volume contraction, or hypokalemia that is seen in patients with primary adrenal failure. Hypotension and electrolyte abnormalities are absent in secondary adrenal insufficiency because the renin-angiotensin-aldosterone system in the adrenal glands remains intact. Patients with ACTH deficiency do not develop hyperpigmentation because the pituitary cannot produce ACTH or other components of the proopiomelanocortin molecule, which is responsible for skin darkening in primary adrenal insufficiency. Patients with severe ACTH deficiency may develop hypoglycemia after a prolonged fast and some patients may present with abdominal pain, arthralgias, and myalgias. Patients with ACTH deficiency occasionally develop hyponatremia as a consequence of inappropriately elevated levels of antidiuretic hormone (ADH). Since ACTH stimulates production of adrenal androgens, ACTH deficiency may also lead to loss of axillary and pubic hair. This is more likely to occur in women where it may also contribute to decreased libido. In some cases impairment of ACTH secretion is only partial and patients may be asymptomatic unless they become severely ill or have surgery. Long-term administration of glucocorticoids is a common cause of secondary adrenal insufficiency. Any glucocorticoid given in supraphysiologic doses or over a prolonged period of time will suppress hypothalamic production of corticotropin releasing factor and lead to decreased ACTH secretion.

When ACTH deficiency is suspected it is important to determine whether the hypothalamic-pituitary-adrenal axis is intact *and* whether it can respond to stress. A plasma cortisol greater than 18 mg/dl excludes adrenal insufficiency but a normal cortisol does not exclude partial ACTH deficiency. Provocative testing may be needed to document adrenal cortical reserve. A normal cortisol response to the administration of Cortrosyn indicates that the adrenal cortex can respond and excludes primary adrenal insufficiency but does not exclude partial ACTH deficiency (Fig. 99-6). A patient with low serum cortisol or an inadequate response to Cortrosyn should be referred to an endocrinologist for provocative testing of the pituitary-adrenal axis.

Growth Hormone Deficiency. For many years GH deficiency was not thought to have any adverse effects in adults. Recent studies suggest that lack of GH may lead to decreased muscle mass, increased fat mass, decreased muscle strength, reduced aerobic exercise capacity, low bone density, and increased low-density lipoprotein (LDL) cholesterol. Patients with GH deficiency have also been shown to have a higher mortality rate than age- and sex-matched subjects.

Measurement of IGF-1 and random GH cannot be used to diagnose GH deficiency. The diagnosis can only be made when a patient has a subnormal response to a test of GH reserve. Provocative tests to assess GH reserve include

Box 99-4. Hormone Replacement Therapy for Hypopituitarism

Pituitary-gonadal axis
- Estrogen/progesterone
- Testosterone

Pituitary-adrenal axis
- Prednisone
- Cortisone acetate
- Hydrocortisone

Pituitary-thyroid axis
- Levothyroxine

Growth hormone deficiency
- ?Recombinant GH

insulin-induced hypoglycemia, L-dopa, clonidine, or arginine, and all should be performed in consultation with an endocrinologist.

Management of Hypopituitarism

Hypogonadism. The treatment of hypopituitarism requires replacement of hormones normally produced by the target organs (Box 99-4). Treatment of gonadotropin deficiency is accomplished by replacing gonadal steroids except when fertility is an issue. Estrogen is indicated for maintenance of secondary sex characteristics and prevention of osteoporosis. A variety of estrogen preparations are available. Postmenopausal women can be adequately treated with estrogen and progesterone, but it may be more convenient to treat a premenopausal woman with an oral contraceptive. In women with an intact uterus estrogen should be used in conjunction with a progestational agent like medroxyprogesterone acetate to avoid the development of endometrial hyperplasia. In women with gonadal dysfunction due to loss of gonadotropins the response to therapy cannot be monitored by changes in LH and FSH.

Parenteral testosterone preparations are the agents of choice for androgen replacement therapy and can be administered intramuscularly every 2 to 4 weeks. The consequences of androgen therapy include salt and fluid retention, edema, gynecomastia, and occasional aggressive behavior. Worsening of benign prostatic hypertrophy in middle-aged and elderly men may also occur. Oral testosterone preparations are not recommended because of low potency and an association with peliosis hepatitis and hepatoma.

Hypoadrenalism. The cortisol deficiency induced by loss of ACTH can be effectively treated with hydrocortisone, cortisone acetate, or prednisone. Since the renin-angiotensin-aldosterone system is intact in patients with secondary adrenal insufficiency, mineralocorticoid replacement is usually not required. Serum and urine cortisol and ACTH levels cannot be used to monitor the efficacy of replacement, and assessment of electrolytes and clinical symptoms will be used to guide therapy. In patients with partial ACTH deficiency enough cortisol may be secreted to take care of daily needs but secretion may be inadequate in times of stress. Patients must be alert to the requirement for additional glucocorticoids during periods of illness. Occasionally administration of glucocorticoid replacement will unmask central diabetes insipidus leading to polyuria (see Diabetes Insipidus). In patients with pituitary disease it is important to establish that ACTH secretion is normal prior to initiating thyroid hormone therapy. Treatment with thyroid hormone accelerates cortisol metabolism and could precipitate an adrenal crisis.

Hypothyroidism. The goal of therapy in patients with TSH deficiency is to restore the euthyroid state. Synthetic levothyroxine preparations should be used because of their uniform potency, and the usual replacement dose is 0.1 to 0.15 mg daily. Elderly patients and those with cardiovascular diseases should be started on lower doses (0.025 to 0.05 mg daily) and the dose should be increased slowly. Measurement of TSH cannot be used to confirm the euthyroid state, and free T4 levels should be used to monitor therapy.

Growth Hormone Deficiency. Recombinant GH therapy is only indicated for select patients with GH deficiency. In order to qualify for GH therapy an adult must have a subnormal GH response to a standard stimulation test (see above) and evidence of hypopituitarism secondary to pituitary or hypothalamic disease. The optimal dose of recombinant GH for adults has not been determined and the drug should be administered by an endocrinologist. Side effects include edema, arthralgias, carpal tunnel syndrome, and glucose intolerance.

Disorders of the Posterior Pituitary

Diabetes Insipidus. Diabetes insipidus develops when the posterior pituitary cannot produce adequate amounts of ADH. The principal manifestation of diabetes insipidus is polyuria and some patients may excrete more than 15 liters of urine daily. Central diabetes insipidus is caused by any process that damages the hypothalamic nuclei that synthesize ADH or the axons extending into the pituitary, and about one third of cases of central diabetes insipidus are idiopathic. Other patients develop diabetes insipidus because the kidneys are incapable of responding to ADH (nephrogenic diabetes insipidus). Common causes of nephrogenic diabetes insipidus include hypokalemia, hypercalcemia, and the use of lithium and demeclocycline.

The diagnosis of diabetes insipidus requires the demonstration of an inability to concentrate the urine. The second step in the evaluation is to determine whether the inability to concentrate the urine is due to deficient production of ADH from the pituitary or hypothalamus or is due to insensitivity of the kidney to the hormone. A formal water deprivation test measuring pituitary and kidney responses to exogenous ADH is usually required to make the diagnosis. A water deprivation test should be done under close medical supervision and in consultation with an endocrinologist.

Desmopressin is an analog of ADH with a prolonged half-life and is the primary therapy for central diabetes insipidus. Two daily doses are usually efficacious. Patients who require long-term use of ADH should be cautioned about the potential for water intoxication and hyponatremia.

EMPTY SELLA

During radiographic evaluation of the central nervous system it is not uncommon to discover an enlarged sella that is not completely filled with pituitary tissue. An empty sella may result from herniation of the suprasellar cistern through an incompetent diaphragm sella, and the pituitary gland may be flattened on the floor of the sella. A partial empty sella occurs in obese and multiparous middle-aged women who are often hypertensive. An empty sella alone is not an indication for therapy and clinical symptoms should determine the need for tests of hormone function. In general pituitary function remains normal in patients with the empty sella syndrome.

PITUITARY INCIDENTALOMA

With the widespread use of MRI to evaluate central nervous system disorders it is not unusual to detect unsuspected abnormalities in the pituitary glands of patients who have no symptoms of pituitary disease (pituitary incidentaloma). Asymptomatic patients with an incidentally diagnosed pituitary adenoma that is less than 10 mm will not require extensive tests of hormone function if there is no clinical evidence of hormone hypersecretion. In the absence of clinical signs of hormone excess a single measurement of serum PRL is a cost-effective approach. An MRI can be repeated in 1 to 2 years. If the adenoma has not changed in size, no further testing is required. Patients with an incidentaloma larger than 10 mm should be evaluated for hormone excess and should have formal visual field testing. In general, incidentally discovered pituitary adenomas do not progressively increase in size or become hormonally active over time.

ADDITIONAL READINGS

Hall WA, et al: Pituitary magnetic resonance imaging in normal human volunteers: occult adenomas in the general population, *Ann Intern Med* 120:817-820, 1994.

Melmed S: Acromegaly, *New Engl J Med* 966-977, 1990.

Molitch ME, Thorner MO, Wilson C: Therapeutic controversy: management of prolactinomas, *J Clin Endocrinol Metab* 82:996-1000, 1997.

Schlechte J, et al: The natural history of untreated hyperprolactinemia: a prospective analysis, *J Clin Endocrinol Metab* 68:412-418, 1989.

Shimon I, Melmed S: Management of pituitary tumors, *Ann Intern Med* 129:472-483, 1998.

Vance ME: Hypopituitarism, *New Engl J Med* 330:1651-1662, 1994.

CHAPTER 100

Evaluation and Treatment of Disorders in Calcium, Phosphorus, and Magnesium Metabolism

Michael F. Holick

CALCIUM METABOLISM

Calcium is an important mediator of cell signaling, neurotransmission, and a variety of intracellular biochemical activities. In addition, calcium is the major building block that provides structural integrity to the skeleton. Therefore it is no wonder that the body requires that the circulating concentrations of calcium be tightly regulated. The three hormones responsible for maintaining the blood calcium in the normal range are vitamin D (1,25-dihydroxyvitamin D [$1,25(OH)_2D$]), parathyroid hormone (PTH), and calcitonin. A variety of factors and disease states can alter calcium metabolism, leading to either hypocalcemic or hypercalcemic disorders.

There are approximately 1000 gm of calcium in the adult human body. About 99% of the calcium is found in the skeleton and approximately 1% is freely disassociable from the skeleton. The three major sources of calcium that contribute to the blood calcium are the intestine, bone, and kidney (Fig. 100-1). The normal blood calcium range is 8.4 to 10.4 mg/dl. Approximately 40% of the blood calcium is protein bound, 50% is in the ionized form, and an additional 10% is complexed to citrate and phosphate ions. At a

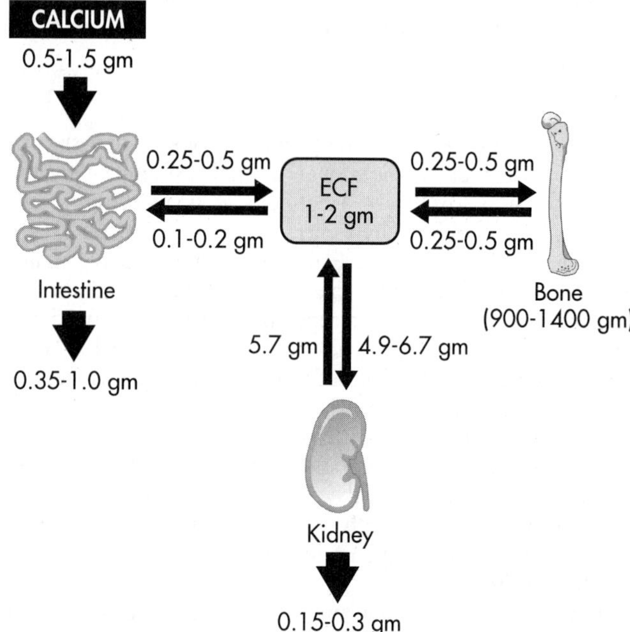

Fig. 100-1. Calcium homeostasis. Schematic illustration of calcium content of extracellular fluid (ECF) and bone as well as of diet and feces; magnitude of calcium flux per day as calculated by various methods is shown at sites of transport in intestine, kidney, and bone. Ranges of values shown are approximate and chosen to illustrate certain points discussed in text. In intestine, absorption efficiency varies inversely with dietary calcium (chronic adaptation). This is reflected in typical quantities absorbed and excreted in feces; with 0.5 gm intake, 50% absorption is depicted to occur (0.25 gm), but at 1.5 gm, only 30% (0.5 gm). Endogenous fecal calcium, the 0.1 to 0.2 gm secreted into the intestinal lumen daily, is constant and does not vary with calcium intake or absorption. Quantities of calcium depicted as filtered, reabsorbed, and excreted at the kidney are chosen arbitrarily to indicate that at lower rates of filtration of calcium (expected at lower glomerular filtration rates), most is reabsorbed (e.g., 5.85 of 6 gm), leading to urinary excretion of 150 mg; at higher rates of filtration (at high dietary calcium intake), slightly less is reabsorbed (e.g., 9.7 of 10 gm), leading to a higher urinary excretion, 300 mg. In all situations, renal calcium reabsorption exceeds 95% of filtered load. Urinary calcium excretion is seen, therefore, to increase by only 150 mg despite a 1 gm increase in dietary intake. In conditions of calcium balance, rates of calcium release from and uptake into bone are equal.

physiologic pH of 7.4, 1 gm of albumin binds 0.8 mg/dl of calcium; therefore the total serum calcium concentrations need to be corrected when circulating albumin levels are abnormal. For example, at pH 7.4 if the total calcium is 7 mg/dl with an albumin of 2 gm/dl, then the corrected calcium is $(4\ \text{gm/dl} - 2\ \text{gm/dl}) \times 0.8\ \text{mg/dl} \times 7\ \text{mg/dl} = 8.6\ \text{mg/dl}$. When the pH is below 7.4, less calcium is bound to albumin; thus a higher fraction is in the ionized form. When pH is above 7.4, the reverse is true. Calcium concentrations are usually reported in mg/dl and can be converted to molar units by dividing the calcium concentrations in mg/dl by 4.

Magnesium is the most abundant intracellular divalent cation and plays an important role in a number of enzymatic reactions and neuromuscular excitability. Since 1% of the total body magnesium is contained in the extracellular compartment, its concentration in the plasma does not provide a reliable index of either total body or soft tissue magnesium content. There is an integral relationship between magnesium and calcium in the body (see magnesium section later).

There is an abundance of phosphorus in the diet, mostly as phosphoproteins. Approximately 85% of the body's phosphorus is present in the skeleton and the other 15% resides in the extracellular fluids and soft tissues. Because our diet has a high phosphorus content, including meats and soft drinks, hypophosphatemia becomes a medical concern only when there is either a phosphate leak in the kidney, malnutrition, or secondary hyperparathyroidism (see phosphate section later).

The three principal hormones that regulate calcium and phosphorus metabolism are PTH, calcitonin, and vitamin D. PTH is a polypeptide that is secreted from the parathyroid glands in response to a decrease in serum ionized calcium concentrations. It acts on calcium and phosphorus metabolism by (1) increasing tubular reabsorption of calcium in the proximal and distal convoluted tubules in the kidney, (2) decreasing tubular reabsorption of phosphate, thereby causing increased loss of phosphate into the urine, (3) mobilizing stem cells to become osteoclasts to liberate calcium and phosphate from the bone, and (4) stimulating the production of $1,25(OH)_2D$ in the kidney, which in turn increases the efficiency of intestinal calcium and phosphate absorption. The precise physiologic function of calcitonin is unknown. Calcitonin interacts with its receptors on mature osteoclasts and decreases osteoclastic function, thereby decreasing mobilization of calcium and phosphate from bone.

Vitamin D can be obtained either from exposure to sunlight (vitamin D_3) or from dietary sources (vitamin D_2 or vitamin D_3), including fortified foods such as milk, some cereals, some breads, fatty fish such as salmon and mackerel, and cod liver oil. Vitamin D is biologically inactive and requires successive hydroxylations first in the liver to 25-hydroxyvitamin D (25[OH]D) and then in the kidney to $1,25(OH)_2D$ (Fig. 100-2). 25(OH)D is the major circulating form of vitamin D, and its measurement in the blood is useful to the physician as an indicator of the vitamin D status of a patient. $1,25(OH)_2D$ is the biologically active form of vitamin D that is responsible for increasing the efficiency of intestinal absorption of calcium. In addition, $1,25(OH)_2D$ mobilizes stem cells to become osteoclasts, which in turn mobilize calcium and phosphorus stores from the bone. Measurement of $1,25(OH)_2D$ has value in patients with hypocalcemia and hypercalcemia disorders when there is suspicion that there is an acquired or inherited disorder in the metabolism of 25(OH)D to $1,25(OH)_2D_3$ or that there is an abnormal or deficient response to $1,25(OH)_2D$.

PTH and calcitriol ($1,25(OH)_2D_3$), when produced in excess, cause hypercalcemia by either directly or indirectly increasing the efficiency of intestinal calcium absorption and by mobilizing calcium stores from bone. Excess production of PTH causes hypercalcemia and hypophosphatemia, whereas excess vitamin D or $1,25(OH)_2$ D can cause hypercalcemia and hyperphosphatemia (although most often the serum phosphate is in the high normal range). A deficiency or defect in the recognition of PTH or vitamin D or an abnormality in the synthesis of $1,25(OH)_2$ D can result in hypocalcemia. A PTH deficiency leads to hypocalcemia and hyperphosphatemia, whereas vitamin D deficiency causes hypocalcemia and hypophosphatemia. Although calcitonin is not absolutely necessary for maintaining calcium homeostasis, when provided in pharmacologic concentrations from an exogenous or endogenous source it transiently lowers blood calcium levels.

Hypercalcemia

Epidemiology and Etiology. Most often hypercalcemia is picked up on a routine blood laboratory evaluation. Although there are a large number of possible causes for hypercalcemia (Table 100-1), approximately 90% of hypercalcemic patients suffer from either a malignancy or primary hyperparathyroidism. Primary hyperparathyroidism is a relatively common endocrine disorder with estimates of incidence as high as 1 in 500. Primary hyperparathyroidism occurs at all ages but is most frequent in the sixth decade of life, affecting women more often than men by a ratio of 3 to 2. The hallmark of primary hyperparathyroidism is hypercalcemia associated with inappropriately normal or overtly elevated levels of PTH. The disease is most often benign, and 85% of cases are caused by a solitary adenoma. Approximately 15% of patients have a pathologic process characterized by hyperplasia of all four parathyroid glands. Hyperplasia may occur sporadically, but more likely the multiglandular disease is associated with multiple endocrine neoplasia (MEN) type I or II. Very rarely primary hyperparathyroidism is caused by parathyroid carcinoma, occurring in fewer than 1% of patients. With the exception of the presentation of a kidney stone in about 20% of patients with hypercalcemia, there are very few symptoms associated with primary hyperparathyroidism, especially when it is detected early. The hypercalcemia is often mild, no more than 1.5 mg/dl above the upper limit of normal (less than 12 mg/dl). Patients who suffer with malignancy are often more ill and manifest the classic signs and symptoms of hypercalcemia. Usually the malignancy is easily detected; however, sometimes an occult malignancy can be the cause.

Pathophysiology. There are three principal causes for hypercalcemia (i.e., PTH, vitamin D, and malignancy related) and several other less common causes (see Table 100-1). PTH and $1,25(OH)_2$ D are the major regulators of calcium metabolism; excess production of these hormones can lead to hypercalcemia. A third hormone that affects calcium metabolism only during malignancy is parathyroid hormone related peptide (PTHrP). As the name implies, the first part of the structure of PTHrP is very similar to PTH (nine of the first 20 amino acids in the N-terminal part of PTHrP are identical to those in PTH). When produced in large amounts by the

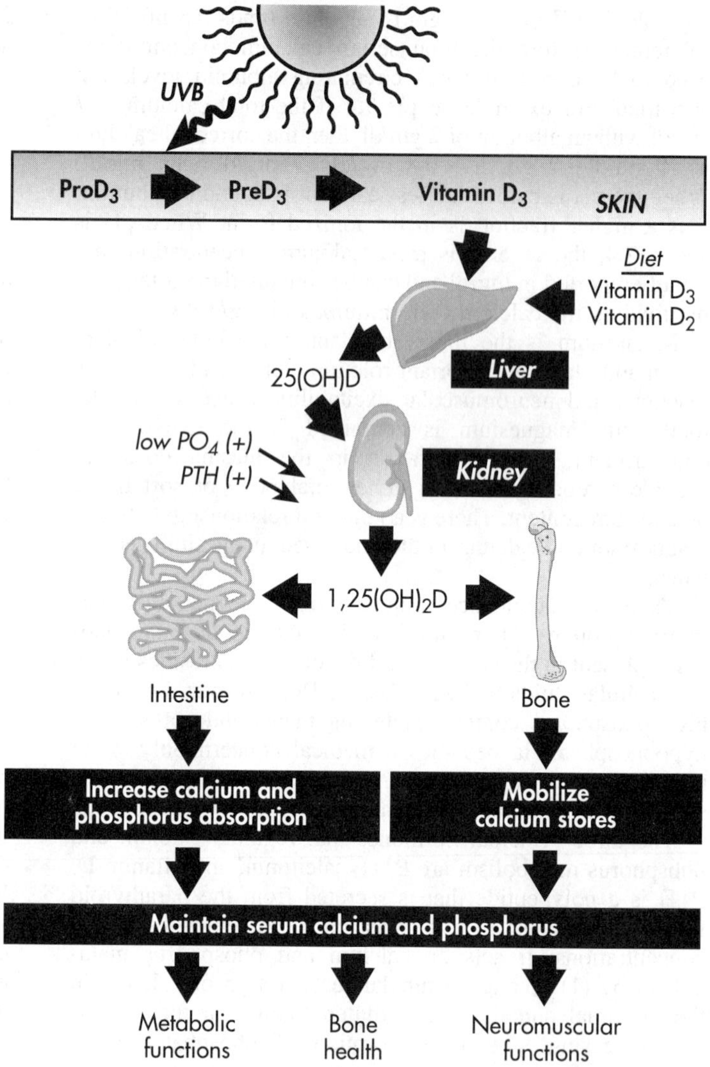

Fig. 100-2. Photosynthesis of vitamin D_3 and the metabolism of vitamin D_3 to $25(OH)D_3$ and $1,25(OH)_2D_3$. Once formed, $1,25(OH)_2D_3$ carries out the biologic functions of vitamin D_3 on the intestine and bone. Parathyroid hormone (PTH) promotes the synthesis of $1,25(OH)_2D_3$, which in turn stimulates intestinal calcium transport and bone calcium mobilization and regulates the synthesis of PTH by generative feedback. Calcium and phosphorus homeostasis promotes normal neuromuscular function and bone health.

tumor during malignancy, it can act like PTH on bone to mobilize calcium stores. It is estimated that greater than 50% of all hypercalcemia associated with malignancy is due to the abnormal production of PTHrP (especially carcinomas of the head, neck, breast, kidney, lung, ovary, and bladder). The other 50% of tumors that cause humoral hypercalcemia produce other osteoclast activating factors (OAFs) such as interleukin-1, prostaglandins, and other cytokines. Activated macrophages in chronic granulomatous diseases and activated lymphocytes in some lymphomas can produce hypercalcemia by an unregulated extrarenal metabolism of 25(OH)D to $1,25(OH)_2D$.

The availability of highly sensitive and specific assays for these calciotropic hormones allows ready identification of the underlying etiology of most hypercalcemic disorders. The etiology of hypercalcemia does affect prognosis. The interval between detection of hypercalcemia associated with malignancy and death is often less than 6 months. As shown in Table 100-1, although several cancers are associated with hypercalcemia, the majority are squamous cell carcinomas of the lung and kidney.

Patients with chronic granulomatous disorders often have hypercalciuria and may have hypercalcemia. For example, in sarcoidosis approximately 50% of patients are hypercalciuric and about 10% are hypercalcemic. The cause for the abnormality in calcium metabolism is due to the unregulated synthesis of $1,25(OH)_2D$ by the granulomatous tissue. Besides treating the underlying disorder, control of the hypercalcemia can often be achieved by inhibiting the extrarenal metabolism of 25(OH)D to $1,25(OH)_2$ D by either high-dose glucocorticoids or the cytochrome P-450 inhibitor ketoconazole. In addition, limiting vitamin D intake and decreasing exposure to sunlight decreases the amount of substrate, thus limiting the extrarenal production of $1,25(OH)_2D$. However, the patient should not be made intentionally vitamin D deficient, since that would cause osteomalacia.

The rare inherited disorder familial hypocalciuric hypercalcemia (FHH) is due to a defect in the calcium sensor in the parathyroid glands, which causes a set point defect and an inappropriate secretion of PTH, resulting in hypercalcemia and hypocalciuria due to increased tubular reabsorption of calcium by PTH. Hypercalcemia may be detected in the first decade of life, whereas hypercalcemia due to primary

Table 100-1. Causes of Hypercalcemia

	PTH	PTHrP	25(OH)D	$1,25(OH)_2D$
Parathyroid gland related				
Primary hyperparathyroidism	↑	nl or ↓	nl	nl or ↑
Adenoma (~85%)	↑	nl or ↓	nl	nl or ↑
Hyperplasia (~15%)	↑	nl or ↓	nl	nl or ↑
Carcinoma (<1%)	↑	nl or ↓	nl	nl or ↑
Multiple endocrine neoplasia (hyperplasia)	↑	nl or ↓	nl	nl or ↑
Familial hypocalciuric hypercalcemia	↑	nl or ↓	nl	—
Tertiary hyperparathyroidism	↑	nl or ↓	nl	nl or ↓
Severe secondary hyperparathyroidism	↑↑	nl or ↓	nl	↓
Malignancy related				
Bone involvement (breast, multiple myeloma, lymphoma)	↓	nl or ↓	nl	↓
Humoral hypercalcemia (lung, esophagus, cervix, vulva, head, neck, skin, renal, breast, and ovarian carcinomas)	↓	↑↑	nl	↓
Vitamin D related				
Vitamin D intoxication	↓	nl	↑↑↑	nl, ↓ or ↑
Granulomatous disorders (e.g., sarcoidosis, tuberculosis)	↓	nl	nl or ↓	↑↑
Williams syndrome	—	—	nl	↑
Drug related				
Lithium	↑	—	nl	—
Thiazides	nl or ↓	—	nl or ↑	nl
$1,25(OH)_2D_3$, 1α-OH-D_3, calcipotriene, dihydrotachysterol	↓	—	nl or ↑ for DHT	↑ Calcipotriene, nl
Androgens (breast cancer therapy)	↓	—	nl	—
Estrogens and antiestrogens	↓	—	nl	—
Vitamin A	↓	—	nl	—
Aluminum intoxication	↓ or ↑	—	nl	nl
Aminophylline	↓	—	nl	—
Miscellaneous				
Immobilization	↓	—	nl	↓
Milk-alkali syndrome	↓	—	nl	↓
Hypophosphatasia	↓	—	nl	—
Acute and chronic renal failure	↑	—	nl	↓
Hyperthyroidism	↓	—	nl	↓

PTH, Parathyroid hormone; *PTHrP*, parathyroid hormone related peptide; *nl*, normal; ↑, elevated; ↓, decreased; *DHT*, dihydrotachysterol.

hyperparathyroidism and MEN syndromes is usually not observed then. The serum PTH values may be elevated in FHH, but they are usually normal or lower for the same degree of calcium elevation when compared with patients with primary hyperparathyroidism. It is difficult to make the diagnosis based on 24-hour urinary calcium excretion because the excretion depends on the glomerular filtration rate (GFR). However, the ratio of calcium clearance to creatinine clearance is helpful. The clearance ratio for FHH is usually one third of that in a hyperparathyroid patient and is less than 0.01. These patients are usually identified because of asymptomatic hypercalcemia. The parathyroid glands demonstrate mild hyperplasia. Partial parathyroidectomy is not recommended because the remaining parathyroid tissue continues to secrete excessive amounts of PTH.

Vitamin D intoxication is a rare cause of hypercalcemia. The most likely settings are ingestion of foods inadvertently overfortified with vitamin D or incorrect prescribing or ingestion by patients (often elderly) who may take 50,000 IU of vitamin D daily instead of biweekly or monthly. Excessive exposure to sunlight does not produce vitamin D intoxication. However, the use of active vitamin D compounds for treating illnesses such as renal osteodystrophy and osteoporosis with oral calcitriol ($1,25[OH]_2D_3$) or dihydrotachysterol, and psoriasis with topical calcipotriene (Dovonex), can cause hypercalcemia.

It is estimated that about 1% of the calcium stores in bone can be mobilized during each month of strict bed rest. Immobilization of adults often causes hypercalciuria. Hypercalcemia is seen only when there is an underlying cause for a high bone turnover such as Paget disease, early or subclinical malignancy-associated hypercalcemia, hyperthyroidism, hyperparathyroidism, secondary hyperparathyroidism associated with renal failure, and in patients with spinal cord injury and paraplegia or quadriplegia; patients can mobilize up to 50% of the calcium from their skeleton within 6 months.

Thiazide diuretics, in combination with hyperparathyroidism, can exacerbate hypercalcemia due to the increased tubular reabsorption of calcium. Vitamin A intoxication is a rare cause of hypercalcemia, as is the hypercalcemia associated with renal failure that is often considered to be due to aluminum intoxication. Lithium carbonate in dosages of 900 to 1500 mg/day causes hypercalcemia in about 5% of patients taking this drug and may be associated with increased PTH levels.

Milk-alkali syndrome, which was much more common several decades ago, is caused by excessive ingestion of calcium and absorbable antacids. It causes hypercalcemia in conjunction with some degree of renal failure.

History. It is often difficult to make the diagnosis of hypercalcemia simply based on symptoms unless the patient has a history of kidney stones. The symptoms are often very subtle and limited to the patient or family member reporting increased fatigability, increased sleep requirement, and a change in the ability to concentrate. In more severe cases of hypercalcemia, symptoms may gradually progress to depression, confusion, and even coma. A history of kidney stones (either calcium oxalate or calcium phosphate) or a reduction in height due to spinal compression fractures may be the first presenting symptom. Gastrointestinal symptoms are often prominent with constipation, anorexia, nausea, and vomiting. Pancreatitis and peptic ulcer disease are unusual but have been associated with hypercalcemia. Polyuria and polydipsia are often present but subtle. Chondrocalcinosis and pseudogout may be the first symptoms of hyperparathyroidism. Hypercalcemia increases the rate of cardiac repolarization, thus shortening the QT interval on the electrocardiogram (ECG). Bradycardia and first-degree atrioventricular (AV) block as well as arrhythmias may occur. Hypercalcemic patients who take digitalis may have an increased sensitivity to the drug. Patients should be asked if they take lithium, thiazide diuretics, excessive quantities of either vitamin A or vitamin D, aminophylline, aluminum-containing antacids, androgens, estrogens, or antiestrogens, since all have been associated with hypercalcemia.

Because of the non–life-threatening and often subtle symptoms associated with mild hypercalcemia, it is not unusual to see an elderly patient complaining of mild confusion, constipation, and fatigue. Thus it is only after a routine blood laboratory evaluation that hypercalcemia is identified.

Physical Examination. The physical examination is not particularly helpful in the diagnosis of hypercalcemia. Clinical signs are not usually seen until the corrected total calcium is above 12 mg/dl and are more prominent when the total calcium is above 14 mg/dl. Muscle atrophy and proximal muscle weakness may be associated with symptoms of increased fatigue. However, patients with longstanding hyperparathyroidism can have a substantial reduction in their height due to multiple spinal compression fractures. Generalized or local bone pain due to osteitis fibrosa cystica may also be present. Muscle weakness, fatigue, depression, and mental status change in the setting of malignancy or other chronic illnesses could be caused by hypercalcemia. Calcifications in the cornea (band keratopathy) can sometimes be seen in severe chronic hypercalcemia. About 15% to 20% of patients with hyperparathyroidism may suffer from a kidney stone. Soft tissue calcifications are rarely observed in primary hyperparathyroidism because the elevated serum calcium is associated with a low or normal serum phosphorus; thus the Ca × phosphate product is not elevated. However, in situations where there are chronically elevated levels of both calcium and phosphorus (e.g., severe renal failure with secondary hyperparathyroidism and hyperphosphatemia), soft tissue calcifications especially along the tendons and ligaments and ends of digits can be found.

Laboratory Studies and Diagnostic Procedures. The most cost-effective way of determining the etiology of hypercalcemia is to obtain at least two fasting serum calcium, phosphorus, and albumin determinations. The reason for a second analysis is that there may be a laboratory error or inadvertent hemoconcentration during blood collection or elevation in serum proteins, particularly albumin. Although fasting does not significantly affect serum calcium or albumin, it is more difficult to evaluate the serum phosphorus level in a nonfasting state. Dietary sources of phosphorus will transiently increase phosphorus levels and a glucose load will decrease serum phosphorus. There is little advantage to obtaining an ionized calcium because of its cost.

Differential Diagnosis. If hypercalcemia is confirmed with two calcium and albumin levels (preferably in a fasting state), then a determination of intact PTH will differentiate between primary hyperparathyroidism and other causes. Other clinical cues, such as a low or low normal fasting phosphorus level in a patient in the fifth or sixth decade of life, suggest hyperparathyroidism. Because the PTH immunoradiometric assay (IRMA) is so specific (the C-terminal, N-terminal, and midmolecule PTH assays are used less frequently because they often give false-positive results in hypercalcemia of malignancy caused by PTHrP), an elevation in the circulating PTH levels in association with hypercalcemia essentially makes the diagnosis of some abnormality in the parathyroid glands. There is no need to do an extensive evaluation for other etiologies. All other hypercalcemic disorders, with the exception of FHH and chronic renal failure, will have either suppressed or undetectable levels of intact PTH when the serum calcium is elevated. If a malignancy is found associated with hypercalcemia, it is likely that the two are related and that there is no particular need to measure a PTHrP, which just adds cost to the evaluation. In addition, PTHrP is of no prognostic value. Thus the PTHrP assay is not routinely used for known malignancies. If there is a concern about an occult malignancy, it may be reasonable to measure IRMA PTHrP blood levels, since 50% of occult malignancies in hypercalcemic patients are associated with increased circulating levels of

PTHrP. Disorders in extrarenal synthesis of $1,25(OH)_2D$ can be detected by measuring circulating levels of $1,25(OH)_2D$ in conjunction with hypercalcemia. Chronic granulomatous disorders (e.g., sarcoidosis) or lymphoma should be suspected in hypercalcemic patients with low or undetectable PTH levels and high normal or elevated $1,25(OH)_2D$. Since the extrarenal 1α-hydroxylase is sensitive to prednisone, a course of prednisone (40 mg/day) with an associated drop in serum calcium often makes the diagnosis of a chronic granulomatous disease. To rule out vitamin D intoxication, a markedly elevated 25(OH)D that is at least two times above the upper limit of normal (over 100 ng/ml) is usually necessary.

Management. Hypercalcemia is caused by an increase in (1) the mobilization of calcium from the bone, (2) intestinal calcium absorption, and (3) tubular reabsorption of calcium. Thus when the cause is in part due to an increase in intestinal calcium absorption such as patients with hyperparathyroidism, vitamin D intoxication, chronic granulomatous disorders, or lymphoma, patients can benefit by decreasing their dietary calcium intake to 600 to 800 mg a day and increasing their hydration. For patients with mild hypercalcemia (under 12 mg/dl) and no clinical manifestations, this often suffices until a cause is determined. Patients with a moderate elevation (12 to 14 mg/dl), with or without symptoms, usually benefit from treatment because the patients are often dehydrated, leading to a decrease in the GFR and the renal clearance of sodium and calcium. Patients with severe hypercalcemia (over 14 mg/dl) usually require immediate therapeutic intervention (Table 100-2).

Hydration with isotonic saline is an important first step in correcting the extracellular fluid deficit. Hydration can usually be achieved by continuous infusion of 3 to 4 L of 0.9% sodium chloride over 24 to 48 hours. This usually results in increased urinary excretion of calcium (100 to 300 mg/dl) and a lowering of the serum calcium by about 1.5 to 2 mg/day. Hydration alone will not return the serum calcium to normal in moderate or severe hypercalcemia. When treating elderly patients with compromised cardiac or renal function in the hospital, fluid inputs and outputs need to be documented. A loop diuretic can help prevent fluid overload.

After hydration has been achieved, a loop diuretic can be used to inhibit tubular reabsorption of sodium and calcium. Usually small doses of furosemide (10 to 20 mg) or ethacrynic acid (50 to 100 mg) will be of benefit. Excessive use of loop diuretics causes dehydration and electrolyte abnormalities, including hypokalemia and hypomagnesemia. Only in life-threatening situations is aggressive hydration with up to 6 L of isotonic saline along with a loop diuretic such as furosemide, 50 to 100 mg every 1 to 2 hours, warranted. Urinary excretion of calcium of up to 1000 mg/day and a decrease of about 3 to 4 mg/dl of serum calcium can be achieved.

Bisphosphonates, in particular intravenous pamidronate or etidronate, have been of great value in inhibiting bone calcium mobilization due to hypercalcemia of malignancy. Daily infusion of 30 to 90 mg of pamidronate for 3 days or 7.5 mg/kg of etidronate over 2 to 4 hours for 3 days causes the calcium to decrease within 2 days and reach a nadir after 7 days. Intravenous etidronate is as well tolerated and safe as pamidronate. Some patients (about 20%) receiving pamidronate develop a transient fever that is usually controlled with acetaminophen. Mild, usually asymptomatic, hypercalcemia

Table 100-2. Management of Hypercalcemia

Therapy	Dosage	Onset	Side effects
Hydration and diuresis			
Hydration	3-4 L saline/24 hr	Rapid	Congestive heart failure
Furosemide	10-40 mg IV	Rapid	Hypokalemia
Ethacrynic acid	50-100 mg IV	Rapid	
Inhibition of calcium mobilization from skeleton			
Calcitonin	4-8 U/kg SQ, IM, or IV 6-12 hr	2-6 hr	Nausea, rapid tolerance (1-2 weeks)
Etidronate	7.5 mg/kg IV 2-4 hr	1-2 days	
Pamidronate	30-90 mg IV 2-4 hr	1-2 days	Transient fever
Plicamycin (Mithracin)	15-25 μg/kg IV 4-6 hr	12-24 hr	Thrombocytopenia, neutropenia, nausea, nephrotoxicity, hepatic toxicity
Gallium nitrate	200 mg/m^2 IV 24 hr	3-5 days	Nephrotoxicity, hypophosphatemia
Phosphate	250-350 mg PO qid; 1-1.5 g IV 6-8 hr	Rapid	Soft tissue calcification can cause rapid decline in serum calcium
Decreased intestinal calcium absorption			
Hydrocortisone	100-200 mg/day	2-3 days	Cushing's syndrome
Prednisone	40-80 mg/day	2-3 days	Cushing's syndrome
Decrease dietary calcium intake to 600-800 mg/day			
Miscellaneous			
Dialysis			
Mobilization			

lasting for several days to several weeks may develop when using a bisphosphonate. Oral etidronate therapy has not been found to be useful for treating hypercalcemia of malignancy.

Calcitonin is very effective in rapidly lowering hypercalcemia associated with increased bone calcium mobilization. The dosage of calcitonin is 4 to 8 U/kg, given either intravenously, subcutaneously, or intramuscularly every 6 to 8 hours. The serum calcium will begin to decrease within 2 hours. However, tachyphylaxis often occurs, and therefore this drug is only of value for a few days to a few weeks. This drug is especially useful in life-threatening hypercalcemia while waiting for the more sustained effects from intravenous etidronate or pamidronate or other calcium-lowering drugs such as plicamycin and gallium nitrate. Calcitonin therapy may be associated with transient nausea, cramping, abdominal pain, and flushing.

Plicamycin (Mithracin) is a cytotoxic drug that inhibits bone resorption. It has lost favor with the advent of intravenous bisphosphonate therapy because of associated toxicities. The usual dosage of 15 to 25 μg/kg intravenously over 4 to 6 hours causes the serum calcium to decrease within 12 to 24 hours. The serum calcium usually reaches a nadir by 48 to 72 hours. If hypercalcemia recurs, treatment with 10 to 15 μg/kg twice a week often returns the serum calcium to normal. Toxicity is usually associated with the frequency of treatment and total dosage; side effects include thrombocytopenia, hepatocellular necrosis leading to transient increases in transaminases, decreased levels of clotting factors resulting in bleeding, azotemia, proteinuria, and hypocalcemia. Because of the toxicities, plicamycin is of limited value in treating chronic hypercalcemia. Its major benefit is in the rapid control of severe symptomatic hypercalcemia.

Gallium nitrate also inhibits bone resorption. A 5-day infusion of 200 mg/m^2/day normalizes calcium in about 75% of patients. However, because of its relatively slow onset and associated nephrotoxicity and severe hypophosphatemia, this therapy has been of limited value.

Other therapies include glucocorticoids, which increase urinary calcium excretion and decrease intestinal calcium absorption when given in a dosage of 40 to 200 mg of prednisone daily in divided doses, or 200 to 300 mg of hydrocortisone or its equivalent intravenously for 3 to 5 days. Glucocorticoids are very effective in treating hypercalcemia from vitamin D intoxication as well as hypercalcemia from extrarenal production of $1,25(OH)_2D$ associated with chronic granulomatous disorders and some lymphomas. They have been less effective in patients with hypercalcemia of malignancy and primary hyperparathyroidism.

Phosphate therapy is effective for treating chronic hypercalcemia and acute hypercalcemia. However, it is important not to increase the blood levels of phosphate so as to cause a high calcium/phosphate product that will increase risk of nephrocalcinosis and soft tissue calcification. The usual treatment is 1 to 1.5 gm of phosphate daily for several days, given in four divided doses to minimize chances of developing hyperphosphatemia. Intravenous phosphate is one of the most effective treatments for treating severe hypercalcemia; however, because of its associated toxicity (nephrocalcinosis and hypocalcemia), it is rarely used except in the most severe hypercalcemic patients with cardiac or renal failure. A dosage of 1500 mg of phosphate intravenously over 6 to 8 hours leads to a prompt and precipitous decrease in serum calcium by as much as 3 to 6 mg/dl in patients with initially normal serum inorganic phosphate concentrations. Since the serum calcium concentrations can rapidly drop, it is important to monitor the serum calcium frequently to prevent potentially fatal hypocalcemia.

Thus there are several therapies for treating hypercalcemia. Mild hypercalcemia can usually be treated by decreasing dietary intake of calcium and by hydration. In a hospital setting intravenous isotonic saline with a loop diuretic is reasonable. However, more severe hypercalcemia (over 14 mg/dl) often requires rapid correction. Calcitonin acts rapidly (within hours) and is usually very effective with minimal side effects. At the same time aggressive hydration and sodium and calcium diuresis should be instituted. The bisphosphonates have become the standard treatment for chronic management of hypercalcemia. Because of the associated side effects with phosphate, gallium nitrate, and plicamycin, these agents are less often used.

Patients over the age of 50 with mild hypercalcemia and documented hyperparathyroidism who do not have a history of radiopaque kidney stones, nephrocalcinosis, generalized bone pain, or multiple nontraumatic fractures and have normal renal function and bone mass can be followed with careful monitoring. Patients under age 50 should have surgery, given the high likelihood of osteoporosis and the long surveillance that would be required. Guidelines recommended for surgery in patients with asymptomatic hyperparathyroidism include (1) elevated serum calcium of more than 1 to 1.6 mg/dl above the upper limit of normal of the laboratory, (2) history of a life-threatening hypercalcemia, such as an episode induced by dehydration and recurring illness, (3) the presence of kidney stones, (4) a recent reduction in creatinine clearance by greater than 30% compared with aged-matched controls, (5) elevation of 24-hour urine calcium excretion above 400 mg or a urinary Ca/Cr of over 0.35, and (6) reduction in bone mass more than 2 S.D. below the normal by one of several noninvasive methods for measuring bone mass. In patients who do not want immediate surgery, it is advisable to follow bone density measurements regularly. If documented demineralization is found, the potential positive impact of surgery can be stressed more. Also, some postmenopausal women who decline surgery may benefit from estrogen therapy, which may decrease bone turnover.

Hypocalcemia

Epidemiology and Etiology. Hypocalcemia is not often encountered in an outpatient setting because it is corrected physiologically by an increase in the secretion of PTH and the production of $1,25(OH)_2D$, which mobilize calcium stores from bone and increase the efficiency of intestinal calcium absorption. However, a defect in the production or recognition of PTH or $1,25(OH)_2D_3$ or a chronic deficiency of vitamin D can precipitate hypocalcemia. Chronic hypocalcemia is caused by vitamin D deficiency, chronic renal failure, hereditary and acquired hypoparathyroidism, pseudohypoparathyroidism, hereditary disorders in vitamin D metabolism and vitamin D resistance, and hypomagnesemia (Table 100-3).

There are occasions when total serum concentrations of calcium do not reflect the free ionized calcium available to cells. Up to 50% of patients in an intensive care setting are reported to have calcium concentrations below 8.5 mg/dl; however, fewer than 10% have a reduction in ionized

Table 100-3. Causes of Hypocalcemia

Disorder	PTH	25(OH)D	$1,25(OH)_2D$
PTH deficiency			
Hereditary (idiopathic)	↓	nl	nl or ↓
Postsurgical	↓	nl	nl or ↓
Hypomagnesemia	↓	nl	nl or ↓
DiGeorge syndrome	↓	nl	—
Neonatal hypocalcemia	↓	nl or ↓	—
Vitamin D deficiency			
Malabsorption syndromes	↑	↓↓	↓, nl, or ↑
Liver disease	↑	↓↓	↓, nl, or ↑
Lack in diet	↑	↓↓	↓, nl, or ↑
Sunscreen use	↑	↓↓	↓, nl, or ↑
Lack of exposure to sunlight	↑	↓↓	↓, nl, or ↑
Antiseizure medications	↑	↓↓	↓, nl, or ↑
PTH resistance			
Pseudohypoparathyroidism	↑	nl	nl or ↓
Hypomagnesemia	↓	nl	—
$1,25(OH)_2D$ insufficiency			
Chronic renal failure	↑	nl	↓
Hyperphosphatemia	↑	nl	↓
Vitamin D–dependent rickets type I	↑	nl	↓
Oncogenic osteomalacia	↑	nl	↓
X-linked hypophosphatemic rickets	↑	nl	nl or ↓
$1,25(OH)_2D$ resistance			
Vitamin D–dependent rickets type II	↑	↓ or nl	↑↑
Miscellaneous			
Acute pancreatitis	↑	nl	—
Citrated blood transfusion	↑	nl	—
Osteoblastic metastases	↑	nl	—
Acute rhabdomyolysis	↑	nl	—
Acute renal failure	↑	nl	—
Hungry bone syndrome after parathyroidectomy	nl or ↓	nl	—
Foscarnet	↑	nl	—
Radiographic dyes containing EDTA	—	nl	—

nl, Normal; ↓, decreased; ↑, increased; *EDTA*, ethylenediaminetetraacetic acid.

calcium. Patients who are critically ill may have transient hypocalcemia in association with burns, severe sepsis, acute renal failure, and extensive transfusions with citrated blood. Acidosis will increase ionized calcium concentrations, whereas alkalosis will decrease ionized calcium concentrations due to decreases and increases in the binding of calcium to albumin, respectively. In many chronic illnesses substantial reductions in serum albumin concentrations are often seen, and this may lower total serum calcium concentrations while the ionized calcium concentration remains normal. At pH 7.4, hypoalbuminemia can be corrected by adding 0.8 mg/dl to the total serum calcium for every 1 gm/dl by which serum albumin is lower than 4 gm/dl (see previous discussion). Medications such as heparin, glucagon, and protamine may cause transient hypocalcemia. Also, patients with acute pancreatitis have varying degrees of hypocalcemia that usually resolves with the resolution of the acute inflammatory process.

Pathophysiology. The calcium sensor in the parathyroid glands is exquisitely sensitive to small changes in serum ionized calcium concentrations. A small decrease in Ca^{++} results in an increase in the synthesis and secretion of PTH. If a defect in either the synthesis or recognition of PTH is present, hypocalcemia can occur. Idiopathic hypoparathyroidism is manifested by hypocalcemia with a low or absent PTH level. It most often occurs as part of an autoimmune syndrome. Congenital aplasia of the parathyroid glands is rare and usually is in conjunction with a defective development of the thymus (DiGeorge syndrome). Surgical hypoparathyroidism can be transient or permanent following neck surgery for thyroid disease due to inadvertent removal of or damage to the parathyroid glands or their vascular supply. The most common form of transient or permanent hypoparathyroidism occurs after surgical correction for primary hyperparathyroidism. Calcium levels decrease for several reasons. In patients with an autonomous parathyroid adenoma the chronic hypercalcemia suppresses the normal parathyroid tissue. Chronic hyperparathyroidism also results in osteitis fibrosa cystica, which causes a calcium deficit in the skeleton. Immediately after removal of the adenoma, PTH levels precipitously drop, resulting in hypocalcemia. The remaining suppressed parathyroid glands usually begin secreting PTH, and correction of the hypocalcemia is seen within days. However, hypocalcemia can persist for days to several weeks as the calcium-deficient "hungry bones" begin to remineralize.

Hypomagnesemia below 1 mg/dl is often associated with hypocalcemia. Low magnesium impairs both the release and responsiveness of PTH. Correcting the hypomagnesemia results in an increase in PTH levels and a normalization of serum calcium. Other syndromes associated with a defective production of PTH are listed in Table 100-3.

Hypocalcemia, in association with elevated PTH levels, is most commonly seen in patients with chronic renal failure, vitamin D deficiency, abnormalities in the recognition or metabolism of vitamin D, PTH-resistant syndromes, and other miscellaneous causes (see Table 100-3).

In chronic renal failure there is a decrease in the clearance of phosphate, causing hyperphosphatemia, which leads to a decreased production of $1,25(OH)_2D$ and a decrease in the efficiency of intestinal calcium absorption. This results in increased PTH levels, which mobilizes calcium stores from the bone to satisfy the body's calcium requirement. Thus maintaining normal serum phosphate concentrations in the early stages of chronic renal failure ameliorates the secondary hyperparathyroidism that results from mild to moderate renal failure. When the GFR is below about 30% normal, the reserved capacity to produce $1,25(OH)_2D$ is so compromised that, even with a normal serum phosphate, PTH levels rise because of hypocalcemia. Thus, initially, careful management of patients before dialysis with restriction of dietary phosphate and the use of phosphate-binding antacids is of great value (see hyperphosphatemia section). Later calcium supplementation (800 to 1000 mg/day) along with calcitriol (0.25 to 0.5 μg once or twice a day) will maintain serum calcium in the normal range and prevent secondary hyperparathyroidism. Secondary hyperparathyroidism should be avoided because of its devastating consequences to the skeleton causing renal osteodystrophy.

Since it is often assumed that vitamin D deficiency causes hypocalcemia, when the routine blood workup reveals a normal calcium, the diagnosis of vitamin D deficiency is dismissed. However, in the early stages of vitamin D insufficiency the transient hypocalcemia is quickly corrected by secondary hyperparathyroidism. Thus patients with vitamin D insufficiency and early vitamin D deficiency initially have low normal serum calciums with low normal fasting serum phosphorus, an elevated PTH level, and a normal or even elevated $1,25(OH)_2D$ level. If vitamin D deficiency persists, hypocalcemia and hypophosphatemia with low 25(OH)D (under 10 ng/ml) and elevated PTH levels are often seen. Any reduction in the production of $1,25(OH)_2D$ by the kidney can lead to hypocalcemia and secondary hyperparathyroidism. Vitamin D–dependent rickets type I is an inherited disorder of the renal 25(OH)D-1α-hydroxylase leading to low or undetectable levels of $1,25(OH)_2D$. In oncogenic osteomalacia usually a benign tumor secretes a substance that inhibits 1α-hydroxylation of 25(OH)D and causes phosphaturia, resulting in low blood levels of $1,25(OH)_2D$ and phosphorus and painful bones. Patients with vitamin D–dependent rickets type II have markedly elevated levels of $1,25(OH)_2D$ because of a vitamin D receptor defect. This rare disorder is often associated with alopecia totalis.

Vitamin D deficiency is being recognized as a common problem for the elderly, who are less likely to be outdoors where sunlight can stimulate vitamin D_3 production in the skin. In addition, aging and sunscreen use substantially diminish the synthesis of vitamin D_3 in the skin. Although aging does not decrease the intestinal absorption of vitamin D, intestinal malabsorption syndromes that affect the small intestine (especially the duodenum and jejunum) can markedly reduce the absorption of vitamin D. Similarly, patients with chronic severe parenchymal and cholestatic liver disease often have vitamin D deficiency due to the associated malabsorption syndrome as well as a decreased hepatic capacity to convert vitamin D to 25(OH)D. Patients with seizure disorders who are institutionalized and are not obtaining an adequate source of vitamin D either from the diet or exposure to sunlight are more prone to developing vitamin D deficiency (25[OH]D under 10 ng/ml) and the associated bone disease (rickets or osteomalacia). This is most often seen when patients take more than one antiseizure medication (e.g., phenytoin and phenobarbital). This deficiency state is usually easily corrected by increasing the vitamin D intake to 800 to 1000 IU daily or increasing exposure to sunlight.

Pseudohypoparathyroidism is a hereditary disorder that is associated with elevated PTH levels, hypocalcemia, and hyperphosphatemia. Features such as short stature, round face, skeletal abnormalities (brachydactyly), and heterotrophic calcifications are associated with Albright's hereditary osteodystrophy. A defective renal response to PTH can be demonstrated by measuring the urinary output of cyclic adenosine monophosphate (AMP) in response to PTH administration. Other causes of hypocalcemia include acute pancreatitis, multiple citrated blood transfusions, osteoblastic metastases, and hyperphosphatemia associated with extensive tissue or cell damage such as acute rhabdomyolysis. Usually in these acute and chronic situations the secondary hyperparathyroidism is unable to compensate for the hypocalcemic stimulus, and hypocalcemia ensues.

History. A gradual lowering of the serum calcium or a corrected calcium of more than 8 mg/dl often will not cause any symptoms. However, precipitous drops in the serum calcium by 2 to 3 mg/dl observed after surgery for a parathyroid adenoma or after aggressive therapy to treat hypercalcemia can cause neuromuscular irritability, sensations of numbness, and tingling involving fingertips, toes, and the circumoral region (Box 100-1). When the corrected calcium is below about 7 mg/dl, patients often complain of carpopedal spasms.

Physical Examination. Increased neuromuscular irritability can be demonstrated by eliciting a positive Chvostek's sign by gently tapping the facial nerve just anterior to the ear, resulting in the twitching of the circumoral muscles. Trousseau's sign is a carpal spasm elicited by inflation of a blood pressure cuff to 20 mm Hg above the patient's systolic blood pressure for 3 to 5 minutes. Flexion of the wrist and metacarpophalangeal joints, extension of the interphalangeal

Box 100-1. Signs and Symptoms Associated with Hypocalcemia

Chvostek's sign	Tetany
Trousseau's sign	Laryngospasm
Neuromuscular irritability	Bronchospasm
Paresthesias	Seizures

joints, and adduction of the digits reflect the heightened irritability of the nerves to ischemia in the region below the cuff. Whereas approximately 10% of normal individuals demonstrate a slight positive Chvostek's sign, a positive Trousseau's sign is rarely seen in the absence of significant hypocalcemia. In more severe hypocalcemia muscle cramps of the legs and feet progress to spontaneous carpopedal spasm (tetany), laryngeal spasm or bronchospasm, seizures of all types, and respiratory arrest. Mental changes include irritability, psychosis, and depression. The QT interval on the ECG is prolonged, and arrhythmias can occur.

Patients with longstanding hypocalcemia due to idiopathic hypoparathyroidism or pseudohypoparathyroidism may have calcification of the basal ganglia and extrapyramidal neurologic symptoms. Subcapsular cataracts and abnormal dentition are also common in these patients.

Laboratory Studies and Diagnostic Procedures. The diagnosis of hypocalcemia is most easily made when the serum calcium is below the normal range (usually 8.4 mg/dl) with a normal serum albumin. When hypoalbuminemia exists and the correction for the hypoalbuminemia does not correct the serum calcium, then hypocalcemia is also diagnosed. A low serum PTH associated with hypocalcemia is most likely caused by either idiopathic hypoparathyroidism, surgically induced hypoparathyroidism, or hypomagnesemia (see Table 101-3). An elevated PTH associated with hypocalcemia is due either to a primary defect in the recognition of PTH or secondary hyperparathyroidism. The most common cause of hypocalcemia associated with elevated PTH is secondary hyperparathyroidism due to vitamin D deficiency. A low serum 25(OH)D (usually less than 10 mg/ml) with or without hypophosphatemia and secondary hyperparathyroidism is diagnostic. Measurement of $1,25(OH)_2D$ is of little value in evaluating vitamin D deficiency because it can be low, normal, or elevated depending on the degree and duration of the deficiency except in acquired and inherited disorders of vitamin D metabolism such as chronic renal failure, vitamin D–dependent rickets type I, and oncogenic osteomalacia, where low circulating levels of $1,25(OH)_2D$ with secondary hyperparathyroidism and hypocalcemia are usually seen.

Differential Diagnosis. Care must be taken to ensure true hypocalcemia is present. Chronic hypocalcemia can usually be associated with the absence of PTH or its ineffectiveness, the absence of vitamin D, or a defect in vitamin D metabolism or in the recognition of $1,25(OH)_2D$ by its target tissues. Since hypoparathyroidism, pseudohypoparathyroidism, and vitamin D–dependent rickets types I and II are typically lifelong illnesses, the recent onset of hypocalcemia in an adult is usually due to renal failure, small intestinal malabsorption disorders, vitamin D deficiency, magnesium deficiency, or an acquired defect in the metabolism of vitamin D.

Hypomagnesemia can cause neuromuscular irritability and paresthesias similar to hypocalcemia, and this should be ruled out whether hypocalcemia is present or not. Hypocalcemia can also be precipitated by the aggressive treatment of medications intended to reverse hypercalcemia such as plicamycin, bisphosphonates, calcitonin, and oral or parenteral phosphate. Radiographic dyes that contain the calcium chelater ethylenediaminetetraacetic acid (EDTA), citrated blood, and the phosphorus-containing drug foscarnet (trisodium phosphonoformate) that is used to treat opportunistic infections in acquired immunodeficiency syndrome (AIDS) patients can cause reductions in total and ionized serum calcium concentrations.

Management. Management approaches for hypocalcemia depend in part on the severity of the hypocalcemia, the acuteness of onset, and the symptoms. For acute symptomatic hypocalcemia the intravenous administration of calcium salts such as calcium gluconate (90 mg elemental calcium/10 ml ampule) is recommended. Calcium chloride (272 mg elemental calcium/10 ml ampule) should be used with caution because it causes irritation of the veins. Initially 1 or 2 ampules of calcium gluconate diluted in 50 to 100 ml of 5% dextrose (180 mg elemental calcium) should be infused over 5 to 10 minutes. This procedure should be repeated as necessary to control symptomatic and potentially life-threatening hypocalcemia. Persistent or less severe hypocalcemia can be managed by administration of more dilute calcium solutions over a longer period. Infusion of 15 mg/kg of elemental calcium over 4 to 6 hours will raise the serum calcium by 2 to 3 mg/dl (0.5 to 0.75 mmol/L). For example, to initiate therapy in a 60-kg patient with a calcium level of 4.5 mg/dl, 10 ampules of calcium gluconate (900 mg Ca^{++}) in 1 L of 5% dextrose infused at a rate of 50 ml/hour will provide approximately 45 mg of elemental calcium per hour. The rate of infusion can be regulated based on the serum calcium and symptoms. Hypomagnesemic patients who have concomitant hypocalcemia require magnesium supplementation before the hypocalcemia can resolve (see hypomagnesemia section).

Patients with vitamin D deficiency and no associated intestinal malabsorption syndrome can be given 50,000 IU of vitamin D_2 once a week for 2 months. Once the 25(OH)D levels have returned to normal (optimally 25 to 45 ng/ml), the patient usually remains vitamin D sufficient if provided a multivitamin containing 400 IU of vitamin D. There is no need for concern about potential vitamin D intoxication for a patient who may drink a quart of milk containing 400 IU of vitamin D, take a multivitamin containing 400 IU of vitamin D, and be exposed to sunlight. Vitamin D intoxication is usually seen when patients ingest over 5000 IU of vitamin D daily. Patients with small intestinal malabsorption syndromes can obtain their vitamin D from exposure to sunlight (suberythemal doses on hands, arms, and face two or three times a week; in northern latitudes little vitamin D is produced in the skin in the winter), artificial ultraviolet B radiation, or intramuscular injections of 50,000 to 100,000 IU of vitamin D_2. Patients on total parenteral nutrition (TPN) usually get their vitamin D from the multivitamin preparation that is added to their TPN solution. Patients with a partial malabsorption syndrome may benefit from increased doses of vitamin D either with 50,000 units of vitamin D or using the liquid vitamin D (8000 IU/ml) and titrating their dose to maintain their serum 25(OH)D level in the midnormal range (about 25 to 45 ng/ml).

Patients with severe liver disease and malabsorption may benefit from calcidiol (25[OH]D_3) therapy. One capsule (20 or 50 µg of 25[OH]D_3 [Calderol]) per day is helpful in treating vitamin D deficiency associated with severe hepatic dysfunction.

Hypocalcemia associated with hypoparathyroidism, pseudohypoparathyroidism, renal failure, and acquired and inherited disorders of vitamin D metabolism and recognition have benefited greatly with the oral or intravenous use of calcitriol (1,25[OH]$_2D_3$). Calcium supplementation of 800 to 1000 mg along with calcitriol of 0.25 µg twice a day is often adequate to increase the efficiency of intestinal calcium absorption to restore serum calcium into the normal range. However, sometimes a dosage as high as 0.5 to 1 µg twice a day is required. Intravenous calcitriol after dialysis has gained favor because of the drug's effect on reversing hypocalcemia and possibly having a direct inhibitory effect on the parathyroid glands. Caution should be exercised when using calcium in combination with calcitriol because hypercalcemia can occur. Therefore this therapy requires frequent serum calcium determinations until a stable dosage of calcium and calcitriol is established. This problem is especially important in treating surgically induced hypoparathyroidism, since the hypocalcemia is transient. Initially, more calcium and calcitriol are needed to satisfy the hungry bone syndrome. However, once normal parathyroid function is restored and the hungry bone is satisfied, calcitriol therapy can often be stopped. Dihydrotachysterol, which is a pseudo–1α-hydroxy analog that mimics the actions of 1,25$(OH)_2D$, has lost favor because of its long half-life in the circulation and potential toxicity.

PHOSPHORUS METABOLISM

An adult body contains approximately 600 gm of phosphorus; 85% is present in the crystalline structure of the skeleton, and the other 15% is found in extracellular fluids. Most of the phosphorus in the circulation is in the form of inorganic phosphate ions $(PO_4)^{-3}$, and in soft tissues the phosphorus is found as phosphate esters such as adenosine triphosphate (ATP). Only about 10% of the inorganic phosphorus is bound to protein. In addition to age, sex, and pH, the serum phosphorus concentration is affected by diet, thus making a nonfasting level difficult to interpret. For example, after a meal, the increase in insulin enhances cellular phosphorus uptake, thereby decreasing serum phosphorus levels. Serum phosphorus levels are higher in children and in women after the menopause. There is a circadian variation in phosphorus concentration even during a 24-hour fast; the nadir occurs between 9 AM and noon followed by an increase to a plateau in the afternoon and another small peak after midnight. Alkalosis and acidosis cause a decrease and increase in serum phosphorus, respectively.

Phosphorus is efficiently absorbed by the small intestine (Fig. 100-3). Although most phosphorus absorption is passive, 1,25$(OH)_2D$ increases phosphorus absorption in the duodenum, jejunum, and ileum. A low phosphorus intake increases the efficiency of intestinal absorption to 80% to 90%. Up to 70% of phosphorus in foods with a high phosphorus content, such as dairy products, meats, and eggs, can be absorbed. Thus hypophosphatemia due to deficient intestinal absorption is unusual except when nonabsorbable antacids like aluminum hydroxide are consumed.

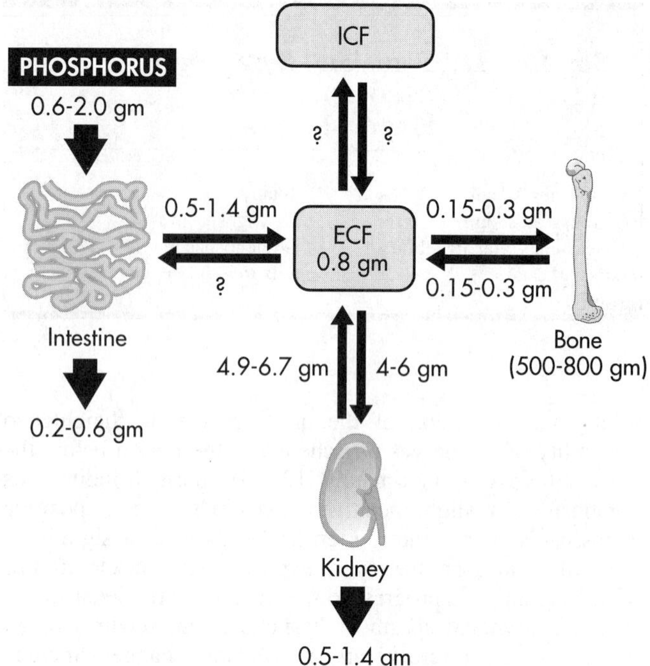

Fig. 100-3. Phosphate homeostasis. Schematic illustration of inorganic phosphorus content (termed here phosphate) in extracellular fluid (ECF) and bone as well as diet and feces; magnitude of phosphorus flux per day as estimated by various methods is shown at transport sites in intestine, kidney, and bone. Range of values shown illustrates special features of phosphorus metabolism discussed in text. Intestinal phosphorus absorption is highly efficient, 85% at lower intake (0.5 gm of a 0.6 gm intake) and 70% at a higher intake (1.4 gm of a 2.0 gm intake). Estimates of magnitude of endogenous fecal phosphate are less well established than for calcium. Contribution of at least 0.15 gm is estimated to be added to the nonabsorbed phosphorus to provide a total of 0.2 gm fecal phosphorus at the low intake level. At high phosphorus dietary intakes, no correction for endogenous fecal phosphate is calculated. Higher quantities of phosphorus are excreted in urine at all levels of dietary intake than for corresponding intakes of calcium; quantities excreted match closely the quantities absorbed, thereby maintaining phosphorus balance (no correction in this illustration is made for endogenous fecal phosphorus). Note that renal phosphorus reabsorption, in contrast to high and relatively invariant renal calcium reabsorption, varies from a low of 75% of filtered load to greater than 85%. The compartment labeled ICF refers to intracellular phosphorus, both organic and inorganic; rapid shifts of phosphorus into cells (and corresponding, possibly slower, efflux of phosphorus from cells) contribute to changes in ECF phosphorus. These shifts between ECF and ICF and phosphorus release from and uptake by bone are equal in conditions of phosphorus balance.

The major control of phosphorus balance is exerted by the kidney (see Fig. 100-3). About 90% of the phosphorus in the circulation is filtered through the glomerulus and is largely absorbed in the proximal tubule, so only 10% to 15% of the filtered load is normally excreted. Urinary excretion of phosphorus reflects dietary intake. Although proximal reabsorption of phosphorus depends on parallel sodium reabsorption in the proximal tubule, sodium reabsorption in the distal convoluted tubule is independent of phosphorus. Therefore volume expansion and decreased sodium reabsorption increase phosphorus clearance.

Hypophosphatemia

Pathophysiology. Hypophosphatemia can be caused by decreased intestinal absorption of phosphorus, increased losses of phosphate in the urine, and a shift of phosphorus from extracellular to intracellular compartments (Box 100-2). Increased renal secretion of phosphorus occurs in states of excess PTH such as primary hyperparathyroidism, vitamin D deficiency, vitamin D–resistant and vitamin D–dependent rickets, as well as hyperglycemic states and oncogenic osteomalacia. Serum phosphorus is low in vitamin D deficiency, due not only to the secondary hyperparathyroidism but also to a decrease in efficiency of intestinal phosphorus absorption. In X-linked hypophosphatemic rickets and oncogenic osteomalacia there is a severe renal leak of phosphorus into the urine. In hyperglycemic states associated with polyuria and acidosis, inorganic phosphorus is lost in the urine in excessive amounts. Ketoacidosis enhances intracellular organic phosphorus degradation, thereby releasing large amounts of inorganic phosphorus into the plasma that is cleared into the urine. In a ketotic patient the serum phosphorus is often normal because of the continuous shift of phosphorus from intracellular to extracellular pools. However, when the ketoacidosis is corrected, hypophosphatemia often becomes manifest because of the return of phosphorus into the intracellular compartment. Rarely, hypophosphatemia is a paraneoplastic syndrome, most often associated with benign bone tumors but occasionally with small cell lung or prostate cancers.

Alcohol abuse is the most common cause of severe hypophosphatemia. Alcoholics usually have a low dietary phosphorus intake, and the use of calcium- or aluminum-containing antacids and vomiting contribute further. Ethanol also enhances urinary inorganic phosphorus excretion, and marked phosphaturia often occurs during episodes of alcoholic ketoacidosis. Intense hyperventilation for prolonged periods may depress serum phosphorus levels due to the associated alkalosis. Advanced leukemia with blast crisis (leukocyte counts usually above 100,000) has been associated with severe hypophosphatemia; the likely cause is rapid uptake of phosphate into rapidly dividing cells.

Box 100-2. Causes for Hypophosphatemia

Decreased Intestinal Phosphate Absorption

Vitamin D deficiency
Vitamin D–dependent rickets types I and II
Malabsorption
Antacid abuse
Alcohol abuse
Intracellular shift of phosphorus to extracellular compartment
Ketoacidosis

Increased Renal Phosphate Excretion

Hyperparathyroidism
Vitamin D deficiency
Vitamin D–dependent rickets types I and II
X-linked hypophosphatemic rickets
Oncogenic osteomalacia
Hyperglycemic states
Alcohol abuse

Other

Respiratory alkalosis
Blast crisis in leukemia
Starvation

Box 100-3. Clinical Signs and Symptoms of Severe Hypophosphatemia

Encephalopathy	Bone pain
Seizures	Rickets/osteomalacia
Muscle weakness	Cardiomyopathy
Rhabdomyolysis	Red cell dysfunction

History and Physical Examination. Mild hypophosphatemia is usually not associated with any clinical symptoms. However, severe hypophosphatemia can cause a variety of clinical symptoms compatible with metabolic encephalopathy, as outlined in Box 100-3. Patients may appear irritable and apprehensive and complain of muscle weakness, numbness, and paresthesias. In the most severe form they appear severely confused or are obtunded and suffer from seizures and coma. Diffuse slowing of the EEG can be observed.

Since phosphorus is essential for muscle action through the high-energy bonds (ATP and creatine phosphate), patients with severe hypophosphatemia may suffer from muscle weaknesses, myalgia, and myopathy. Patients with preexisting phosphate deficiency who develop acute hypophosphatemia may develop rhabdomyolysis. Chronic hypophosphatemia causes rickets in children and osteomalacia in adults. Patients with oncogenic osteomalacia with chronic low phosphorus levels often complain of severe bone pain, especially of their long bones. Severe hypophosphatemia has also been associated with cardiomyopathy characterized by a low cardiac output.

Management. Mild hypophosphatemia usually corrects when the underlying cause is addressed. Oral phosphate replacement is sufficient if serum phosphorus is greater than 1 mg/dl and the patient is without symptoms. Milk is an excellent source of phosphorus, containing 1 gm of inorganic phosphorus per quart. Neutra-Phos-K or K-Phos tablets, which contain 250 mg of inorganic phosphate per tablet as a sodium and potassium, or potassium salt, respectively, can provide up to 3 gm a day (3 tablets every 6 hours). The serum phosphorus level rises by as much as 1.5 mg/dl within 1 to 2 hours after ingestion of 1000 mg of phosphorus.

Severe hypophosphatemia with serum levels lower than 0.5 mg/dl may require as much as 3 gm of phosphorus per day over several days to replete the body stores. In patients with severe symptomatic hypophosphatemia who are unable to eat, intravenous phosphorus can be given—up to 1 gm in 1 L of fluid over 8 to 12 hours. Some caution is necessary because of the potential for developing associated hypocalcemia and soft tissue calcification. A 15- to 30-ml phosphosoda enema solution composed of buffered sodium phosphate three to four times a day is also useful in correcting severe hypophosphatemia in patients who are unable to take oral phosphorus.

Hyperphosphatemia

Pathophysiology. Hyperphosphatemia of clinical significance occurs in renal failure and hypoparathyroid states (Box 100-4). In renal failure the loss of glomerular and tubular function results in impaired phosphorus excretion. Increasing the serum phosphorus level causes a decreased renal production of $1,25(OH)_2D_3$, often producing hypocalcemia. In the absence of renal failure a defect in the renal excretion of phosphorus may be found in pseudohypoparathyroidism and tumor calcinosis. The bisphosphonate etidronate increases renal phosphorus reabsorption and can cause hyperphosphatemia. Vitamin D intoxication due to excessive ingestion of vitamin D or one of its metabolites or analogs can cause hyperphosphatemia along with hypercalcemia. Severe hyperthermia, crush injuries, nontraumatic rhabdomyolysis, and cytotoxic therapy of hematologic malignancy such as acute lymphoblastic leukemia are also associated with hyperphosphatemia.

History and Physical Examination. When there is a rapid elevation in serum phosphorus levels, the associated hypocalcemia can cause symptoms such as neuromuscular irritability and tetany (see the hypocalcemia section). Chronic hyperphosphatemia in association with a normal calcium can cause nephrocalcinosis and soft tissue calcifications.

Management. The goal is to treat the underlying disorder and return the serum phosphorus to the normal range.

Box 100-4. Causes of Hyperphosphatemia

Decreased Renal Phosphate Excretion

Acute renal failure
Chronic renal failure
Hypoparathyroidism
Tumor calcinosis
Bisphosphonates
Hypoparathyroid states
Idiopathic hypoparathyroidism
Pseudohypoparathyroidism

Other

Vitamin D intoxication
Metabolic and respiratory acidosis
Crush injuries
Rhabdomyolysis
Cytotoxic therapy

Because most foods have a high phosphorus content, it is often very difficult to limit dietary phosphorus intake. However, the goal is to decrease dietary phosphorus to approximately 600 to 1000 mg per day with modest protein restriction. Aluminum hydroxide and aluminum carbonate bind phosphorus in the intestine; therefore 30 to 60 ml of gel or 1 to 4 tablets with each meal help decrease phosphorus absorption. This has been of particular value to patients with renal failure. However, concern about aluminum toxicity causing encephalopathy, osteomalacia, proximal myopathy, and anemia are of concern. Therefore it is now recommended that calcium salts be used in place of aluminum salts as the first line of phosphate binders. Initially 1 gm of calcium carbonate with each meal can be gradually increased to 8 to 12 gm of calcium carbonate a day; this can be associated with constipation. If the hyperphosphatemia is due to vitamin D intoxication, calcium salts are contraindicated because they will induce severe hypercalcemia.

MAGNESIUM METABOLISM

Magnesium is the most abundant intracellular divalent cation. It is an essential cofactor for a variety of enzymatic reactions related to the transfer of high-energy phosphate groups from ATP. The maintenance of serum magnesium results from the intestinal absorption of magnesium and the conservation magnesium in the kidney. Approximately 30% of dietary magnesium is absorbed in the small intestine. However, when dietary magnesium is very low or in excess, there is an increase and decrease in the efficiency of magnesium absorption, respectively. It does not appear that either $1,25(OH)_2D$ or PTH regulates magnesium absorption in any significant manner. Approximately 96% of magnesium is absorbed along the nephron and about 4% is excreted into the urine.

Approximately 30% of magnesium in the serum is protein bound and 55% is ionized; the remaining 15% is complexed. Similar to calcium, magnesium is bound principally to albumin. Ionized magnesium is the fraction that is important for physiologic processes, including neuromuscular transmission and cardiovascular tone. The serum concentration of magnesium is closely maintained within a narrow range of approximately 1.7 to 2.6 mg/dl. There are no significant differences in magnesium concentration between men and women or with respect to age. Prolonged standing or hemolysis of a blood specimen can lead to a spurious increase in serum magnesium concentrations.

Hypomagnesemia

Pathophysiology. Magnesium deficiency is a common problem in clinical medicine. It has been estimated that 10% of patients admitted to city hospitals are hypomagnesemic and as many as 65% of the patients in an intensive care unit may be hypomagnesemic. The principal causes of hypomagnesemia are renal or gastrointestinal losses and a decrease in intestinal magnesium absorption. Reduced renal tubular reabsorption of magnesium is the most common cause of hypomagnesemia. Renal magnesium reabsorption is proportional to tubular fluid flow as well as to sodium and calcium excretion. Thus chronic parenteral fluid therapy, especially with saline, and volume expansion states such as primary hyperaldosteronism may result in hypomagnesemia. Hypercalcemia and hypercalciuria decrease renal magnesium reabsorption and contribute to the hypomagnesemia observed in hypercalcemic states. Osmotic diuresis in diabetes mellitus is one of the more common causes of hypomagnesemia.

The magnesium content of upper intestinal tract fluids is about 1 mEq/L; thus vomiting and nasal gastric suctioning can contribute to magnesium depletion. Similarly, magnesium content in diarrheal fluids can be as high as 15 mEq/L; therefore magnesium depletion is common in acute and chronic diarrhea, Crohn's disease, ileitis, ulcerative colitis, and intestinal and biliary fistulas. Malabsorption syndromes may also be a contributing factor for magnesium depletion. Hypomagnesemia occurs in 30% of severe alcoholics and 80% of those with delirium tremens. The fall in magnesium levels within the first 24 to 48 hours of alcohol cessation is presumably due to intracellular shifts of magnesium following hydration. Drugs associated with renal wasting of magnesium include diuretics (especially loop diuretics, although renal magnesium loss occurs with thiazides), aminoglycosides, cisplatin, cyclosporin A, and amphotericin B (Box 100-5).

History and Physical Examination. Neuromuscular hyperexcitability similar to that caused by hypocalcemia is often the presenting complaint in hypomagnesemia. Many of the signs and symptoms of hypomagnesemia are similar to those of hypocalcemia, including muscle weakness, prolonged PR and QT intervals, and cardiac arrhythmias. Chvostek's and Trousseau's signs may be present and the patient may complain of spontaneous carpopedal spasm.

Since magnesium is required for the secretion of parathyroid hormone and the function of parathyroid hormone in the bone, hypomagnesemia can cause hypocalcemia, with its associated symptoms and signs.

Laboratory Studies and Management. Serum magnesium levels less than 1.5 mEq/L usually indicate magnesium deficiency. Treatment of hypomagnesemia should first be directed at the underlying cause. For a mild deficiency oral magnesium replacement is satisfactory. Diarrhea is the most common side effect. When a patient's magnesium level is less than 1.0 mEq/L, this suggests that there is a significant depletion of total body magnesium stores. The total body magnesium deficit can be as high as 400 mEq. Under these circumstances parenteral magnesium administration is usually indicated. Administration of 2 gm magnesium sulfate (16.2 mEq magnesium) can be given intravenously up to 48 mEq over 24 hours. Alternatively, a 50% solution can be given every 8 hours intramuscularly; but these injections can be painful. Patients with severe hypomagnesemia with seizures or acute arrhythmias may be given 8 to 16 mEq magnesium as an intravenous injection over 5 to 10 minutes, followed by 48 mEq per day.

It should be noted that the restoration of a normal serum magnesium concentration does not indicate repletion of magnesium stores. Therapy should be continued for 3 to 7 days. Once magnesium replacement has been achieved, dietary magnesium is adequate to satisfy the body's requirement. However, patients who have magnesium loss from the intestine or kidney may require continued oral magnesium supplementation of a daily dosage of 300 mg of elemental magnesium given in divided doses. The major side effect is diarrhea. Patients who suffer from renal failure should be monitored carefully to prevent hypermagnesemia.

Box 100-5. Causes of Hypomagnesemia

Increased Renal Excretion

Volume expansion
Hypercalcemia
Osmotic diuresis

Increased Intestinal Losses

Vomiting
Nasogastric suctioning
Malabsorption syndromes
Ileitis
Colitis
Intestinal and biliary fistula
Ketoacidosis with treatment
Acute and chronic diarrhea

Drugs

Diuretics
Aminoglycosides
Cisplatin
Cyclosporin A
Amphotericin B
Ethanol

Hypermagnesemia

Pathophysiology and Laboratory Studies. Hypermagnesemia is most often caused by renal failure and can be worsened by the use of magnesium-containing antacids. Elevated magnesium levels encountered in patients with ketoacidosis are often a reflection of dehydration. These patients frequently have a magnesium-deficiency. Modest elevations in serum magnesium may be seen in familial hypocalciuric hypercalcemia, with lithium ingestion, and during volume depletion (Box 100-6).

History and Physical Examination. Neuromuscular symptoms are the most common complaint in patients with magnesium intoxication. Deep tendon reflexes are often absent when magnesium concentrations reach 4 to 7 mEq/L. Depressed respiration and apnea due to paralysis of voluntary musculature may be seen in severe magnesium intoxication. Magnesium concentration greater than 5 mEq/L causes a prolonged PR interval as well as increased QRS duration and QT interval. Complete heart block and cardiac arrest may occur at concentrations greater than 15 mEq/L. Hypermagnesemia causes a suppression of PTH secretion and therefore can be associated with hypocalcemia.

Box 100-6. Causes of Hypermagnesemia

Renal failure with magnesium-containing antacid
Ketoacidosis without treatment
Familial hypocalciuric hypercalcemia
Volume depletion
Lithium

Management. Patients with renal failure who are taking magnesium antacids should be carefully monitored. If hypermagnesemia is present and the patient's antacid contains magnesium, a different antacid such as calcium carbonate should be used. Patients with severe magnesium intoxication require intravenous calcium. Calcium will antagonize the toxic effects of magnesium. The usual dosage is infusion of 100 to 200 mg of elemental calcium over 5 to 10 minutes. The antagonistic effect of calcium is short lived. Patients whose severe magnesium intoxication causes cardiovascular, neuromuscular, and CNS symptoms may require peritoneal dialysis or hemodialysis against a low-dialysis magnesium bath.

ADDITIONAL READINGS

Attie MF: Treatment of hypercalcemia, *Endocrinol Metab Clin North Am* 18:807, 1990.

Burtis WJ, et al: Immunochemical characterization of circulating parathyroid hormone–related protein in patients with humoral hypercalcemia, *N Engl J Med* 322:1106, 1990.

Desai TK, Carlson RW, Geheb MA: Prevalence and clinical implications of hypocalcemia in acutely ill patients in a medical intensive care setting, *Am J Med* 84:209, 1988.

Dunlay R, et al: Calcitriol in prolonged hypocalcemia due to tumor lysis syndrome, *Ann Intern Med* 110:162, 1989.

Favus MJ, editor: *Primer on the metabolic bone diseases and disorders of mineral metabolism,* ed 3, New York, 1996, Lippincott-Raven.

Holick MF, Krane S, Potts JR, Jr: Calcium, phosphorus, and bone metabolism: calcium-regulating hormones. In Isselbacher KJ, et al, editor: *Harrison's principles of internal medicine,* ed 14, New York, 1998, McGraw-Hill, pp 2214-2226.

Jacobus CH, et al: Hypovitaminosis D associated with drinking milk, *N Engl J Med* 326:1173, 1992.

Malabanan A, Veronikis IE, Holick MF: Redefining vitamin D insufficiency, *Lancet* 351:805-806, 1998.

Pollak MR, et al: Mutations in the human $Ca^{2\%}$-sensing receptor gene cause familial hypocalciuric hypercalcemia and neonatal severe hyperparathyroidism, *Cell* 75:1297, 1993.

Potts JT, Jr: Diseases of the parathyroid gland and other hyper- and hypocalcemic disorders. In Isselbacher KJ, et al, editors: *Harrison's principles of internal medicine,* ed 14, New York, 1998, McGraw-Hill, pp 2227-2246.

Ryzen E, et al: Parenteral magnesium tolerance testing in the evaluation of magnesium deficiency, *Magnesium* 4:137, 1985.

Shane E: Medical management of asymptomatic primary hyperparathyroidism, *J Bone Miner Res* 6(suppl 2):S131, 1991.

GASTROINTESTINAL DISEASE VII

CHAPTER 101

Esophageal Disease

Robert Burakoff
Scott David Lippe

REFLUX ESOPHAGITIS

Reflux esophagitis refers to pathology resulting from frequent contact between the esophageal mucosa and gastric acid. This is the most common disease affecting the esophagus. The resting lower esophageal sphincter (LES) pressure is mainly responsible for preventing reflux of the gastric acid and esophageal mucosal contact. When resting LES pressure decreases, reflux of acid occurs. Whether the decrease of LES pressure precedes or results from reflux is still unknown. Factors contributing to reflux include transient LES relaxations, low or hypotensive LES, and anatomic disruption of the sphincter associated with hiatus (hiatal) hernia. All three mechanisms do not occur in all patients. Also, patients with reflux clear acid more slowly than normal individuals.

Clinical Presentation

The most common reflux symptom is *heartburn,* a burning sensation in the chest usually after meals, when lying down, or bending over. Specific foods can provoke heartburn, and certain foods (e.g., chocolate, caffeine) can decrease LES pressure, promoting reflux (Box 101-1). When heartburn is severe, the patient may experience a bitter or sour taste in the mouth or a mouthful of fluid *(water brash).* Relief with antacids helps confirm the presence of heartburn.

Odynophagia, or chest pain on swallowing, is usually seen only in severe and usually longstanding reflux, particularly in patients with severe esophagitis or ulceration of the esophagus. *Dysphagia* is a transient sensation of food sticking in the esophagus and may result from esophagitis. Organic strictures produce a persistent dysphagia despite repeated swallowing. *Night sweats* have been associated with esophageal reflux in many patients. The sweating is usually mild, and patients usually do not mention it spontaneously. A history of night sweats suggests gastroesophageal reflux, which may also be causing chest pain, asthma, or chronic cough while not necessarily causing heartburn.

Diagnosis

Although the symptoms of gastroesophageal reflux disease (GERD) can be characteristic, patients with features of angina pectoris should undergo an electrocardiogram (ECG) and exercise stress testing before evaluation for GERD. No single test provides the diagnosis of GERD in all patients. If a patient presents with isolated heartburn without dysphagia, the best approach is to avoid testing and start a therapeutic

Box 101-1. Substances that Affect Lower Esophageal Sphincter (LES) Pressure

Increase

Protein meal
Coffee*
Bethanechol (Urecholine)
Metoclopramide (Reglan)
Antacids
α-Adrenergic agents
β-Adrenergic agents

Decrease

Alcohol
Chocolate
Essence of peppermint
Smoking
Fatty foods
β-Adrenergic agents
Estrogen and progesterone
Caffeine*
Calcium channel blockers
Diazepam
Barbiturates

*Coffee contains a protein that increases LES pressure, whereas caffeine decreases LES pressure.

trial (Fig. 101-1). If symptoms do not improve with acid-suppressing medication and dietary changes, testing is appropriate.[1]

If reflux is present, the simplest, least sensitive, and most common test is a barium swallow. This test can determine if a stricture is present but only demonstrates reflux in 25% of patients and usually the most severe cases. The most sensitive test for reflux is the use of a pH probe during esophageal manometry. Reflux can be determined by a decrease in pH, as seen in 85% of GERD patients. Concurrently, resting LES pressure can be determined with an esophageal manometry catheter; it is usually at least 10 mm Hg greater than gastric pressure in normal controls. About 85% of reflux patients also have decreased LES pressure.

Once reflux has been demonstrated, it is necessary to determine the condition of the esophageal mucosa, ideally using endoscopy and biopsy. The physician then determines whether the patient's symptoms are caused by the acid reflux. A positive esophageal acid infusion (Bernstein) test confirms the diagnosis of reflux. If this test is negative and biopsies are inconclusive, a 24-hour ambulatory pH recording is indicated to determine whether the patient has prolonged acid reflux or if the symptoms are temporally related to acid reflux (Fig. 101-2).

Complications

Esophageal stricture occurs with severe reflux esophagitis and results from an extension of the inflammatory process into the submucosa. The stricture usually occurs at the distal esophagus and is smooth, contrasting with the irregular stricture of carcinoma. The presenting symptom of dysphagia is most often progressive. Patients initially complain of dysphagia with solids, not liquids, but with an increasingly tight stricture, dysphagia for liquids can develop. A barium swallow with a bread bolus or barium tablet can determine the stricture's diameter (Fig. 101-3). When a stricture is demonstrated, endoscopy and biopsy are mandatory to help rule out esophageal carcinoma.[6] The medical treatment of esophageal strictures, in addition to an antireflux regimen (see next section), involves dilation with mercury-filled rubber bougies or dilators to a diameter of 15 mm. This allows patients to swallow a typical well-chewed meal. Esophageal dilation is successful in most patients and therefore avoids the need for surgery. Patients whose strictures are long or tortuous usually require esophageal stent placement or surgery.

Esophageal ulceration and hemorrhage from esophagitis are uncommon, but if they do not respond promptly to medical therapy, surgery is indicated. An esophageal ulcer is usually diagnosed with a barium swallow and often presents with worsening of reflux symptoms, from episodic heartburn to a more continuous pain pattern. The diagnosis of hemorrhage from esophagitis can be confirmed only by endoscopy.[5] Another uncommon but significant complication of chronic reflux esophagitis is *Barrett's esophagus,* or columnar dysplasia of the esophagus. A portion of the squamous epithelium is replaced with columnar epithelium. Esophageal adenocarcinoma may develop in up to 10% of patients with Barrett's esophagus. Patients should have endoscopy with biopsy every 2 years or yearly if low-grade dysplasia is present.[2] GERD also should be considered in the differential diagnosis of adult-onset asthma. Some patients show improvement in pulmonary function tests and symptoms after treatment of GERD.

Treatment

The primary goal of medical therapy is to keep gastric acid from contacting the squamous epithelium of the esophagus (Box 101-2 and Table 101-1). Treatment involves three goals. First, to prevent reflux, the head of the bed is elevated at bedtime, and lying down after meals is avoided. Eating is also avoided for 3 hours before sleep to prevent the acid load produced by a meal. Second, an attempt is made to neutralize gastric acidity with antacids, histamine receptor antagonists (H_2 blockers), or proton pump inhibitors (PPIs). Patients should avoid calcium-containing antacids because calcium stimulates acid production through gastrin; they should take other antacids whenever symptoms occur. If antacids are ingested several times each day or diarrhea results, an H_2 blocker is taken twice daily to reduce gastric acid secretion for more than 6 hours. For patients who do not experience relief with H_2 blockers or who have moderate to severe esophagitis on endoscopy, the use of PPIs is indicated. Omeprazole (Prilosec) or lansoprazole (Prevacid) provides much greater acid suppression than H_2 blockers. Omeprazole is superior to H_2 blockers in treating severe esophagitis and heals almost 90% of patients over 12 weeks. PPIs have now been approved for long-term use.

The third goal in treating reflux is to increase the LES pressure when the patient still has nocturnal reflux while taking an H_2 blocker or a PPI. Metoclopramide, approved in the United States for diabetic gastroparesis, is a potent dopamine inhibitor that increases LES pressure for 2 hours and increases gastric emptying. Metoclopramide, 10 mg

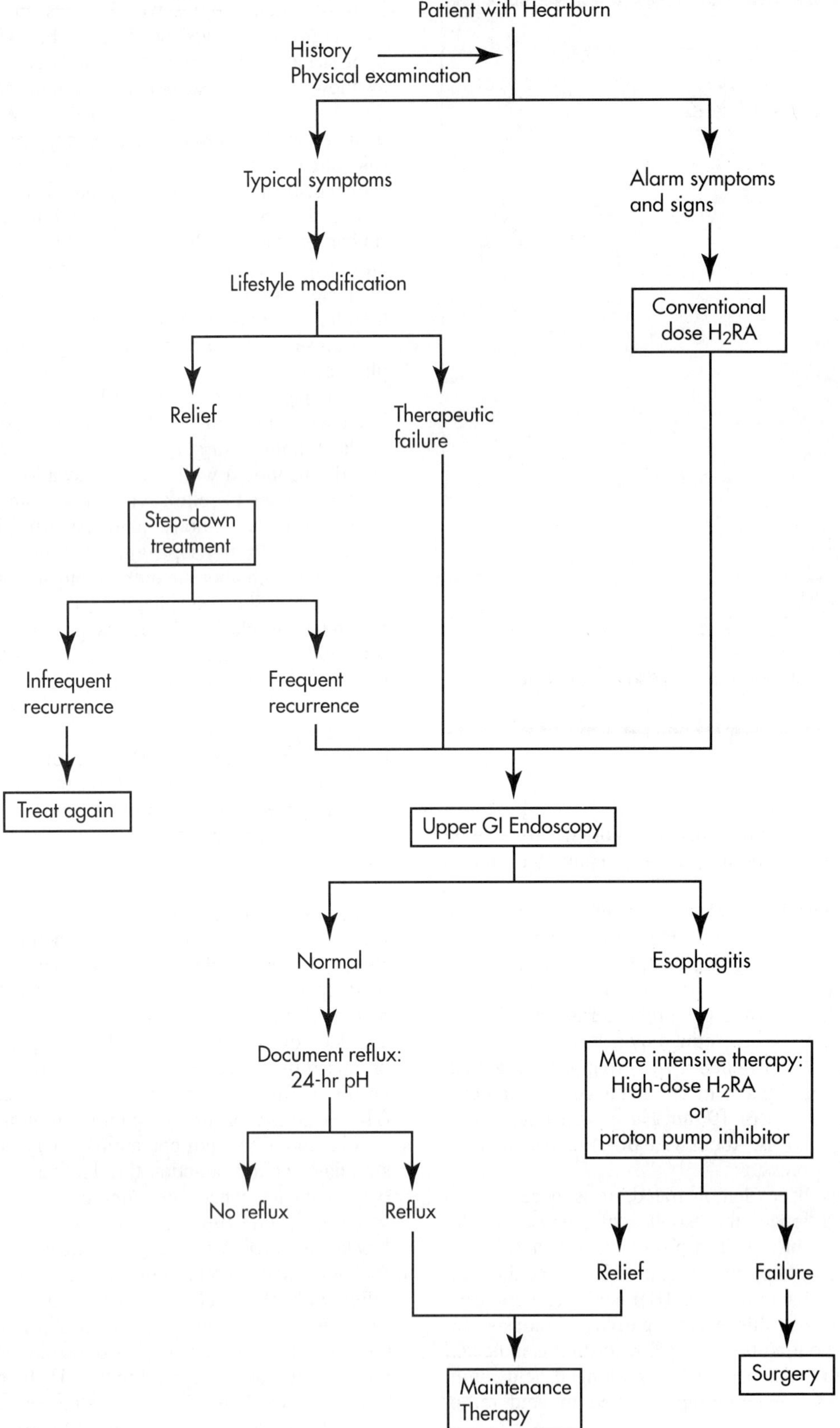

Fig. 101-1. Algorithm for treatment of patient with heartburn and possible gastroesophageal reflux disease (GERD). *H_2RA*, H_2 receptor antagonist. (Modified from Sampliner RE: Heartburn. In Greene HL, Johnston WP, Maricic MJ, editors: *Decision making in medicine,* St Louis, 1992, Mosby.)

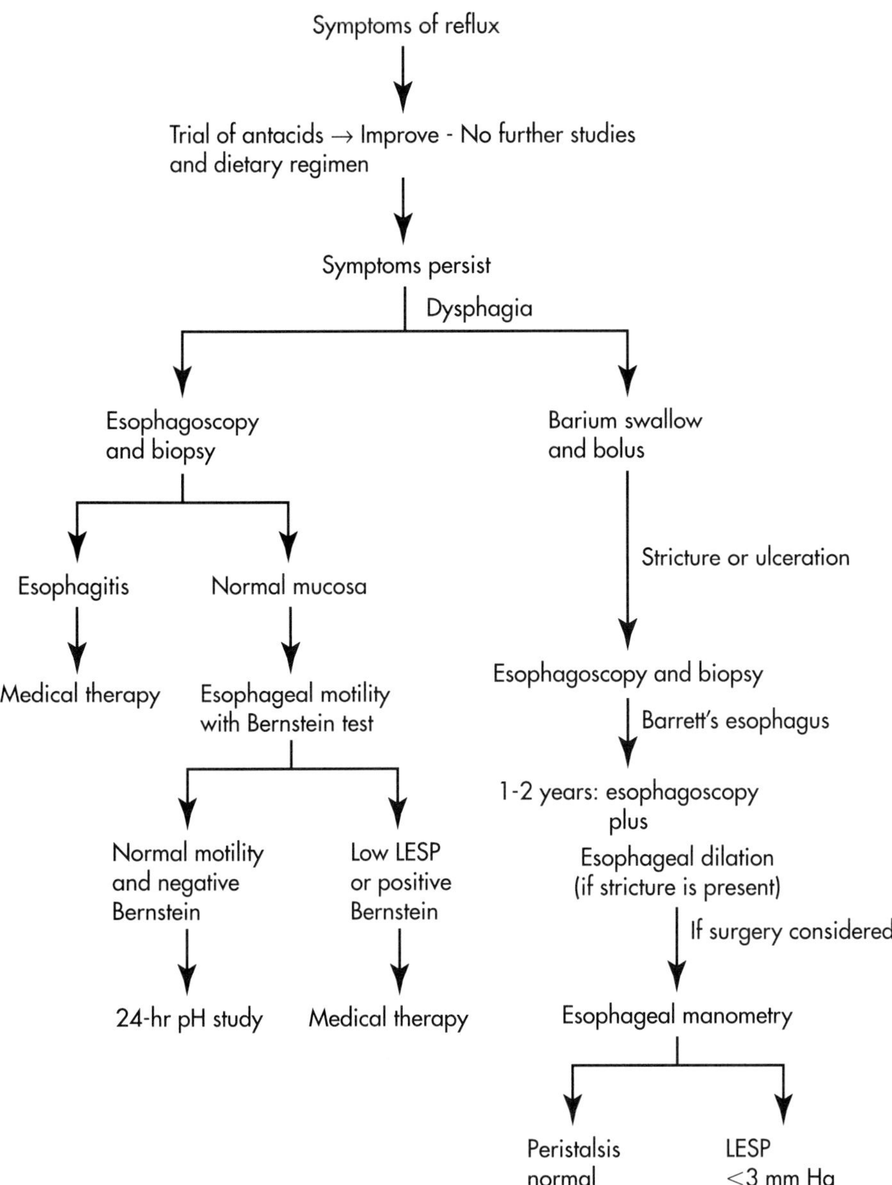

Fig. 101-2. Approach to patient with reflux esophagitis. *LESP,* Lower esophageal sphincter pressure.

before meals and at bedtime, is usually given as adjunctive therapy with H_2 blockers or PPIs, although 25% to 50% of patients experience restlessness, tremors, parkinsonism, and tardive dyskinesia. The typical patient should avoid foods and drinks that affect LES pressure (see Box 101-1). Most patients respond to the simple three-pronged regimen of elevating the head of the bed, controlled diet, and postprandial antacids.[9]

ACHALASIA

Achalasia is a diffuse motor disorder of the esophagus characterized by incomplete relaxation of the LES and loss of peristaltic activity in the esophageal body. These abnormalities result in a functional obstruction of the lower esophagus. The etiology is unknown, but a consistent pathologic finding is a significant decrease in or absence of ganglion cells in Auerbach's plexus of the esophagus.

Clinical Presentation

This relatively rare disease has a prevalence of approximately 1 in 100,000 per year. Achalasia rarely appears in members of the same family, and onset of symptoms often occurs between ages 20 and 40, although the disease can affect any age group, including infants. The typical patient presents with dysphagia for solids and liquids, which is often of several years' duration. The patient often regurgitates retained material from the esophagus after lying down or with exercise. Heartburn is rarely a complaint. Further questioning may reveal that the dysphagia worsens with stress or rapid eating. Some patients learn to avoid these symptoms by regurgitating before meals to empty the esophagus. As the disease progresses and the esophagus dilates further, episodes of aspiration pneumonia occur. Odynophagia is seen at the beginning of the illness but abates as the esophagus dilates. Persistent chest pain may indicate a variant called *vigorous achalasia*.

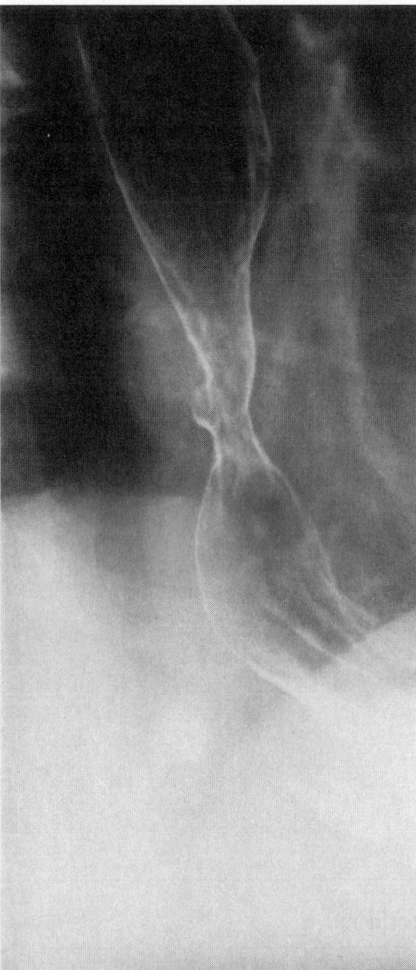

Fig. 101-3. Barium swallow demonstrating esophagitis with hiatal hernia, stricture, and ulceration.

Box 101-2. Medical Therapy for Gastroesophageal Reflux

Mild: Normal Esophageal Mucosa

1. Antireflux regimen: avoid substances that decrease pressure of lower esophageal sphincter (see Box 101-1)
2. Aluminum hydroxide/magnesium hydroxide antacids: 30 ml after each meal and at bedtime; avoid in renal failure: use aluminum hydroxide only

Moderate: Erosive Esophagitis

1. Antireflux regimen
2. Elevate head of bed
3. H_2 receptor antagonist twice daily for 12 weeks: cimetidine (Tagamet), 400 mg; ranitidine (Zantac), 150 mg; famotidine (Pepcid), 20 mg; or nizatidine (Axid), 150 mg
4. Proton pump inhibitors (PPIs) bid for 8 weeks

Severe

1. Antireflux regimen
2. Elevate head of bed
3. PPIs bid for 8 weeks

Table 101-1. Medical Therapy for Gastroesophageal Reflux Disease*

Drug	Dosage	Healed (8 weeks)
Cimetidine (Tagamet)	400 mg bid	30%-50%
Ranitidine (Zantac)	150 mg bid 150 mg qid†	30%-50%
Famotidine (Pepcid)	20 mg bid 40 mg bid†	30%-50%
Nizatidine (Axid)	150 mg bid	30%-50%
Omeprazole (Prilosec)	20 mg qd	75%-85% (4 weeks)
Lansoprazole (Prevacid)	30 mg qd	75%-85% (4 weeks)

bid, Twice daily; *qid,* four times daily; *qd,* every day.
*Patients with erosive esophagitis may require up to 12 weeks of treatment.
†Patient with erosive esophagitis may require higher doses.

Diagnosis

The physical examination is rarely helpful in diagnosing achalasia, except for the findings of halitosis and weight loss. In longstanding achalasia a presumptive diagnosis can be made from a chest radiograph showing retained material in the esophagus (sometimes misdiagnosed as a mediastinal mass on the right side) and absence of air in the stomach. The simplest method for diagnosis is a barium swallow (Fig. 101-4). This test is performed in the supine position to demonstrate loss of peristalsis, which always involves the lower two thirds of the esophagus. The esophagus is usually quite dilated, and an air-fluid level may be secondary to retained secretions. The classic finding is a gradual tapering at the end of the esophagus, similar to a bird's beak, a result of the incomplete relaxation of the often hypertonic sphincter. The differential diagnosis of these radiologic findings includes a stricture from reflux esophagitis and secondary achalasia from carcinoma involving the fundus of the stomach or distal esophagus. Possible tumors include adenocarcinomas of the stomach, pancreas, and lung. Secondary achalasia typically occurs in patients over age 60 with symptoms for less than 1 year.

A radiologic clue in the diagnosis of secondary achalasia is asymmetric narrowing in the distal esophagus. Endoscopy can rule out a stricture or tumor, since the endoscope can be passed into the stomach in the presence of achalasia but not with a peptic stricture or cancer. Also, in reflux esophagitis the esophagus appears erythematous and friable. Biopsies of the stomach fundus are done to rule out adenocarcinoma. Confirmation of the presumptive diagnosis of primary achalasia requires esophageal manometry, which characteristically shows an elevated LES pressure. The barium swallow shows that the sphincter pressure does not relax to gastric baseline. Esophageal body contractions are usually simultaneous or nonperistaltic. Secondary achalasia, however, can give the same manometric tracings.

Treatment

No medical or surgical therapy for achalasia can restore normal esophageal function. Therefore the goal of therapy is to weaken the LES to allow solids and liquids to empty by gravity. Medical therapy involves pneumatic (balloon) dilation of the LES. Under fluoroscopic guidance a firm balloon is inflated to a predetermined diameter, thus tearing

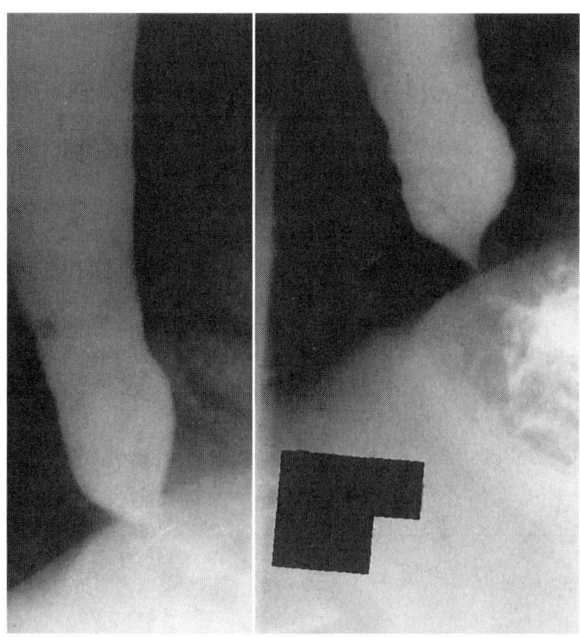

Fig. 101-4. Barium swallow demonstrating classic findings in achalasia, with dilated esophagus *(left)* terminating at gastroesophageal junction in beaklike narrowing *(right)*.

some of the muscle fibers in the LES. Success is obtained in approximately 75% of patients in one or two sessions and is determined by more rapid emptying of barium on radiography and cessation of dysphagia. The major complication of balloon dilation is a mediastinal tear. This occurs in less than 5% of patients and can usually be treated nonsurgically with nasogastric suction and antibiotics.

Calcium channel blockers are potent smooth muscle relaxants and may help in treatment of achalasia. Botulinum toxin is a new therapeutic modality in which the toxin is injected endoscopically into the LES muscle fibers to paralyze the muscle. This therapy seems more effective in elderly patients, in whom effects can last longer than 6 months. Unfortunately, many patients develop antibodies to this treatment, and the efficacy decreases with repeated treatments.[8] Balloon dilation therapy is still the definitive medical therapy, but botulinum toxin should be considered in all patients.

If medical therapy is unsuccessful, a myotomy (Heller's procedure) can be performed, which involves an incision through the circular muscle down to the mucosa over the entire length of the LES. At least 80% of patients have acceptable results. The major problem after myotomy is severe reflux esophagitis, which occurs in 5% to 25% of patients, depending on the surgeon's experience.

SMOOTH MUSCLE SPASTIC DISORDERS

Diffuse Esophageal Spasm

Although diffuse esophageal spasm has never been clearly defined, these criteria provide a working definition: (1) chest pain and dysphagia, (2) spontaneous *nonperistaltic* contractions ("tertiary contractions") on barium swallow, and (3) repetitive simultaneous contractions on manometry in 50% or more of the esophagus. With these strict criteria, esophageal spasm is much less prevalent than achalasia. The etiology is unknown, and consistent pathologic findings have not been documented. The diagnosis is usually considered after a complete cardiac evaluation, often including coronary angiography. Diffuse esophageal spasm should be considered before cardiac disease if the patient complains of sharp retrosternal chest pain when eating solids or liquids. This pain can awaken the patient from sleep. Patients may complain of dysphagia for solids and liquids, but unlike achalasia, the symptoms are intermittent and not progressive. The barium swallow may show spontaneous random contractions, also called "corkscrew esophagus," most often in the lower two thirds of the esophagus. Normal individuals also may show spontaneous or tertiary contractions on barium swallow. Esophageal manometry reveals an LES with normal relaxation after a swallow, although resting pressure may be higher than normal, with spontaneous, high-amplitude, and often repetitive contractions.

Nutcracker Esophagus

Another motor abnormality of the smooth muscle, nutcracker esophagus, is characterized by chest pain and dysphagia and occurs more often in women (mean age, 40). This disorder is more common than diffuse esophageal spasm and involves high-amplitude *peristaltic* contractions in the lower two thirds of the esophagus.

Diagnosis

Since some patients with noncardiac chest pain secondary to an esophageal smooth muscle spastic disorder have normal asymptomatic resting manometry, provocative testing is recommended to increase diagnostic yield. Intravenous edrophonium (Tensilon) can provoke the patient's typical chest pain but does not affect the coronary arteries. Esophageal balloon distention can also provoke a positive response. For those patients with continued noncardiac chest pain with normal manometry and negative provocative testing, 24-hour ambulatory motility manometry is available.

Treatment

No definitive medical therapy exists for diffuse esophageal spasm or nutcracker esophagus. The goal of therapy is to relieve pain and dysphagia, especially during meals. Nitrates (e.g., sublingual nitroglycerin) or longer-acting preparations (e.g., isosorbide dinitrate) are variable and unpredictable. Calcium channel blockers (e.g., nifedipine, diltiazem) have yielded symptomatic improvement and a decrease in amplitude contractions. Antidepressant therapy (e.g., trazodone) has been used successfully in these conditions, with the rationale of treating an "irritable esophagus" syndrome.

NONCARDIAC CHEST PAIN

More than 50,000 new cases of noncardiac chest pain occur annually, based on the percentage of normal coronary angiographies done in the United States. In patients with atypical chest pain and normal cardiac evaluation, an esophageal cause for the pain must be considered. The typical patients with noncardiac chest pain are females between ages 30 and 60. The etiology of the pain is most often acid reflux or less often an esophageal motility disorder (Fig. 101-5). Acid reflux should prompt an aggressive antireflux regimen using PPIs (e.g., omeprazole) once or twice daily. If a motility disorder is revealed, other agents are considered (Table 101-2).

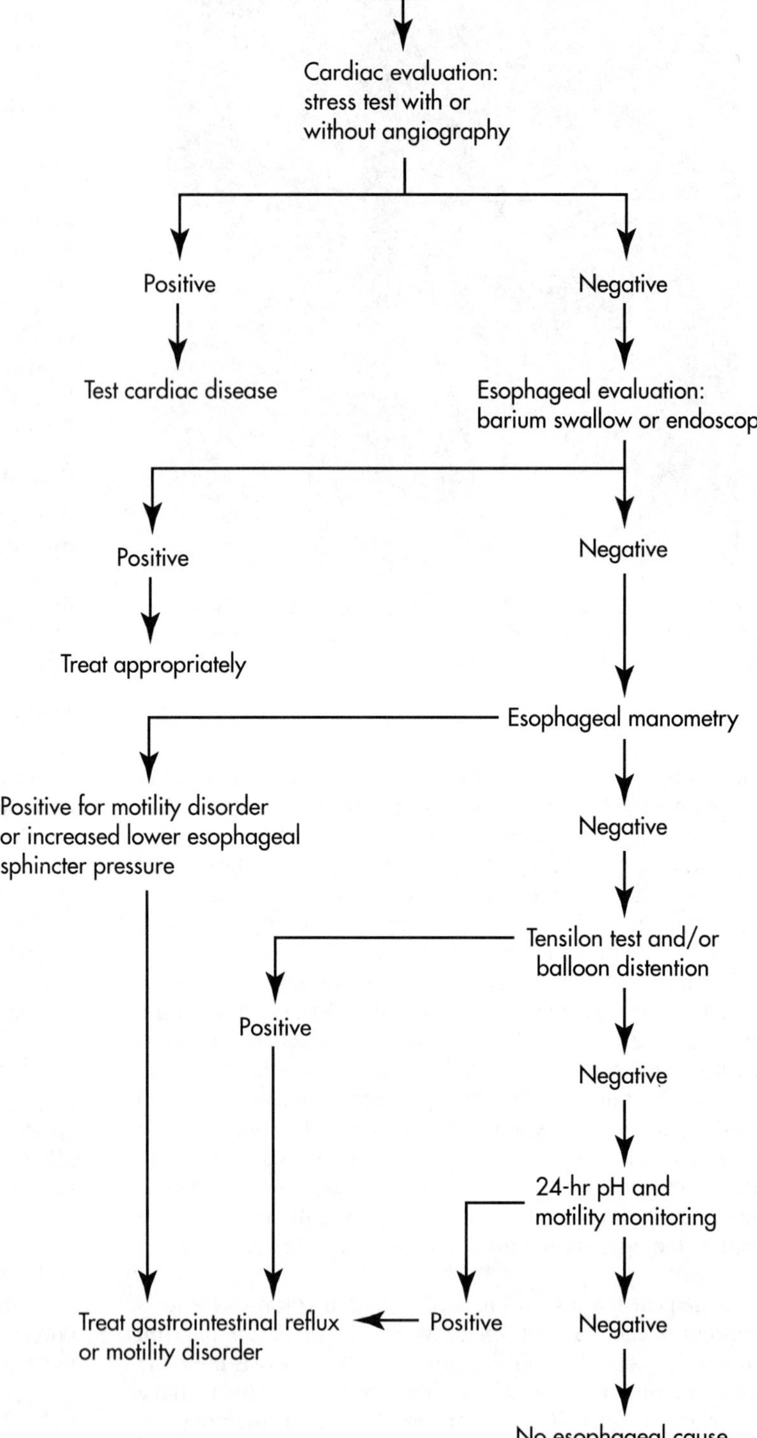

Fig. 101-5. Diagnosis of noncardiac chest pain.

ESOPHAGEAL CANCER

The most common tumors of the esophagus are malignant. Squamous cell carcinoma is decreasing in frequency, whereas adenocarcinoma is becoming more common. Adenocarcinoma usually arises from an extension of the stomach mucosa or can result from malignant degeneration of Barrett's esophagus. Benign tumors are usually an incidental finding without clinical importance.

Squamous Cell Carcinoma

Squamous cell carcinoma is relatively rare, occurring in two to four white individuals per 100,000 and as many as 15 black males per 100,000. The highest incidence is found in northern China, with 130 cases per 100,000. Certain etiologic factors have been associated with squamous cell esophageal cancer, such as tobacco and alcohol use, as well as long-term stasis, as occurs in achalasia. Lye ingestion and radiation exposure

Table 101-2. Treatment for Noncardiac Chest Pain

Drug	Dosage
Nitrates	
Nitroglycerin	0.4 mg sublingually as needed 30 min before meals
Isosorbide dinitrate	10-20 mg orally 30 min before meals
Calcium channel blockers	
Nifedipine	10-20 mg sublingually or orally 30 min before meals *or* 10-20 mg orally 30 min before meals and at bedtime
Diltiazem	90-120 mg orally 30 min before meals and at bedtime
Verapamil	80-160 mg orally 30 min before meals and at bedtime
Sedatives/tranquilizers	
Trazodone (for example)	100-150 mg orally daily

also increase the risk. Patients present with progressive dysphagia for solids, then liquids. Most have unresectable disease by the time of presentation. As such, any patient over age 40 who has progressive dysphagia of less than 6 months' duration is presumed to have esophageal cancer until proved otherwise. Many patients also have anorexia and weight loss by the time they see their physician. The physical examination is not usually helpful unless supraclavicular lymph node enlargement or hepatomegaly is found, indicating metastatic disease. Less common presenting symptoms include hoarseness secondary to involvement of the recurrent laryngeal nerve; coughing secondary to aspiration or a tracheoesophageal fistula; and rarely hematemesis.

The presumptive diagnosis can be made by a barium swallow showing mucosal irregularity and tumor encroaching on the lumen (Fig. 101-6). Difficulty in diagnosis arises when the tumor causes a smooth narrowing, mimicking a benign stricture. Definitive diagnosis is made by esophagoscopy with biopsy and brush cytology in 95% of patients. Endoscopic ultrasound is the most reliable diagnostic technique in staging local cancer. Computed tomography (CT) scan of the chest continues to be useful for determining metastatic disease.

Regardless of the type of therapy, the 5-year survival of all patients with esophageal cancer is approximately 5% to 15%. Surgery is the treatment of choice for cancer of the lower third of the esophagus, whereas irradiation is used for involvement of the upper two thirds. The extent of the disease should be determined before surgery. In patients with metastatic disease, surgery is reserved for palliation. Endoscopic techniques for palliation include esophageal dilation or the placement of stents.[7]

Adenocarcinoma

Adenocarcinoma arising from the mucous glands of the esophagus is extremely rare, but adenocarcinoma arising in columnar epithelium (Barrett's esophagus) is becoming more common. Barrett's esophagus, as noted earlier, results from reflux esophagitis. Approximately 10% of patients with

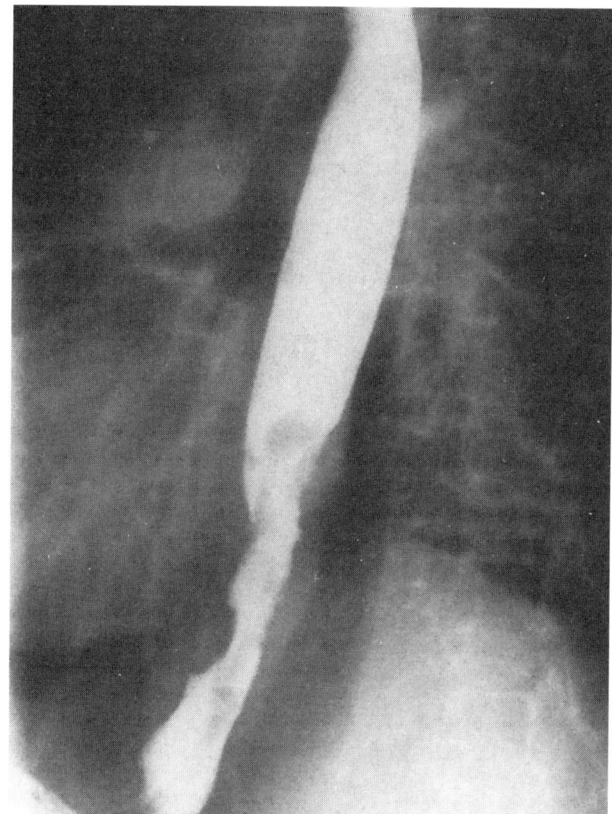

Fig. 101-6. Barium swallow demonstrating classic findings in cancer of distal third of esophagus.

biopsy-proven Barrett's esophagus develop adenocarcinoma. Patients give a history of heartburn progressing to dysphagia. Diagnosis is made by endoscopic biopsy and brush cytology. Surgery is the treatment of choice, but 5-year survival is only about 5%. As a result, surveillance of Barrett's esophagus with endoscopy is recommended.

ESOPHAGEAL RINGS

The lower esophageal ring, also called Schatzki's ring or the B ring, marks the junction of the esophageal and gastric mucosa (Fig. 101-7). It is composed of squamous epithelium superiorly and gastric epithelium inferiorly and is frequently associated with hiatal hernias. It is the most common clinical entity among esophageal rings and webs, often resulting in clinical symptoms. A patient without heartburn who reports that solid food, invariably meat or bread, intermittently becomes lodged in the lower end of the chest probably has a lower esophageal ring. It is not known whether lower esophageal rings are congenital or acquired. Patients may develop the condition in their 20s or present initially in the fifth to seventh decades.

The diagnosis is made by barium swallow if care is taken to distend and adequately fill the lower end of the esophagus (Fig. 101-8). A bolus is also swallowed during this test, which demonstrates a holdup at the gastroesophageal junction. The ring appears as a symmetric indentation at the junction and is usually less than 5 mm thick. If the ring is thicker, an esophageal stricture must be considered. Endoscopy is done to rule out carcinoma or stricture. For treatment, passage of mercury-filled bougies relieves symptoms.[4]

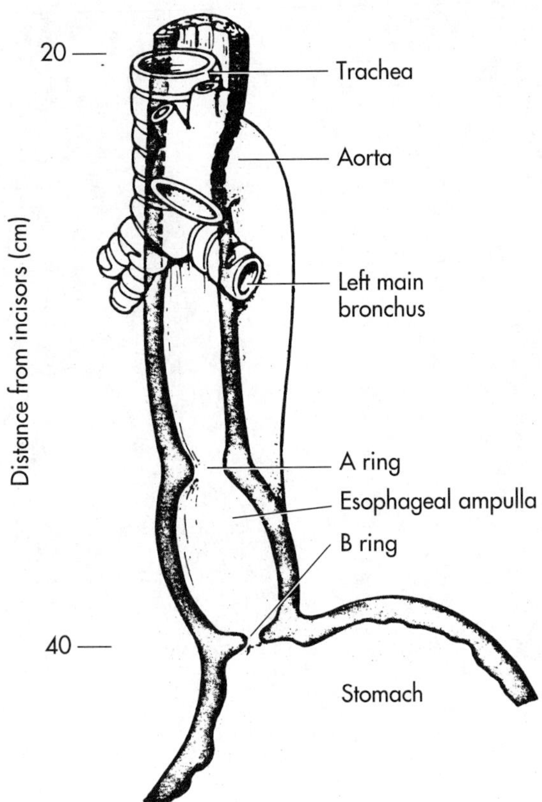

Fig. 101-7. The esophagus in relation to the trachea and aorta. (From Spechler S, Burakoff R: The esophagus. In Wilkins R, Levinsky N, editors: *Medicine: essentials of clinical practice,* ed 3, Boston, 1983, Little, Brown.)

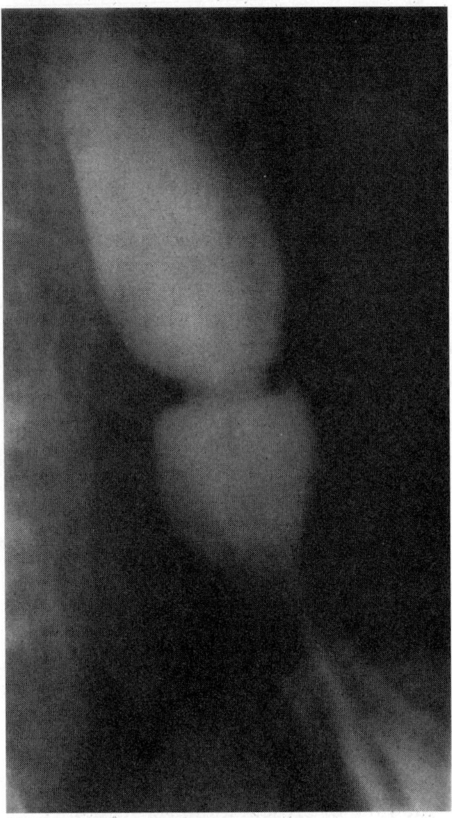

Fig. 101-8. Barium swallow demonstrating lower esophageal ring (B ring) at gastroesophageal junction.

ESOPHAGEAL DIVERTICULA

Esophageal diverticula represent outpouchings of one or more layers of the esophagus. *Zenker's diverticulum* occurs above the upper esophageal sphincter (cricopharyngeus) and may be associated with incoordination of the pharynx and cricopharyngeus during swallowing (Fig. 101-9, *A*). The patient presents with intermittent dysphagia. As the pouch enlarges, symptoms progress to aspiration of liquids and regurgitation of food into the mouth. Diagnosis is by barium swallow. Zenker's diverticulum usually requires no therapy, but surgery is available for problematic cases.

Epiphrenic diverticulum occurs just above the LES and is associated with failure of the LES to relax and with increased amplitude of esophageal contractions. Patients present with dysphagia and may regurgitate large amounts of accumulated fluid when recumbent. Diagnosis is by barium swallow (Fig. 101-9, *B*). Esophageal manometry is then performed to rule out an associated motility disorder. Surgery is indicated only if clinical symptoms are significant.

SYSTEMIC DISEASE WITH ESOPHAGEAL INVOLVEMENT

Several diseases can secondarily involve the esophagus (e.g., diabetes, alcoholism with neuropathy, amyloidosis), but none demonstrates a consistent characteristic abnormality. Collagen vascular disease can also involve the esophagus, resulting in varying degrees of aperistalsis. Invariably, these abnormalities are associated with *Raynaud's phenomenon,* which is seen with esophageal aperistalsis. Except for scleroderma, these diseases rarely result in significant functional impairment.

Scleroderma causes clinical problems resulting from aperistalsis of the lower two thirds of the esophagus and incompetence of the LES. The combination of these defects produces severe reflux esophagitis. The abnormalities result from atrophy of the smooth esophageal muscle and an abnormality of LES innervation. Patients have symptoms of heartburn and dysphagia for solids. Physical examination reveals evidence of Raynaud's phenomenon. Over time, heartburn may lessen while the dysphagia worsens from stricture development. A presumptive diagnosis is made based on the history and examination. A barium swallow demonstrates aperistalsis from the aortic arch to the LES and barium reflux. A stricture may be seen with longstanding disease. The diagnosis is confirmed with esophageal manometry, demonstrating aperistalsis of the distal two thirds of the esophagus and decreased LES pressure. All patients should undergo esophagoscopy at some point in their illness to evaluate the severity of the esophagitis and to determine if Barrett's esophagus is present.

No specific treatment exists for scleroderma involving the esophagus except aggressive reflux control. This includes the lifestyle modifications noted earlier and either H_2 blockers or PPIs, which decrease the reflux symptoms and the severity of esophagitis seen endoscopically. If a stricture develops, dilation with bougies is usually successful. Surgery is avoided because of the poor peristalsis in the distal esophagus. If the

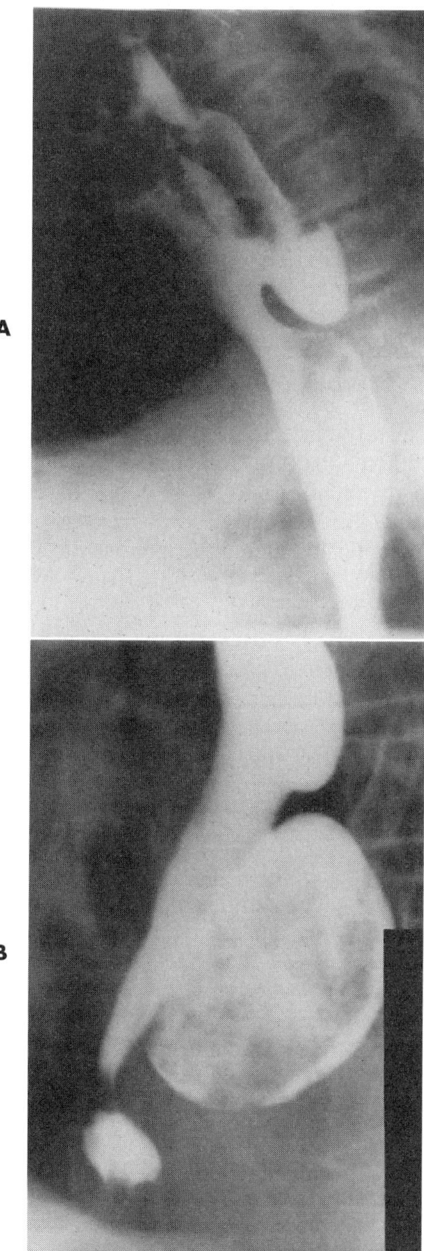

Fig. 101-9. Barium swallow demonstrating Zenker's diverticulum (**A**) and large epiphrenic diverticulum of distal esophagus (**B**).

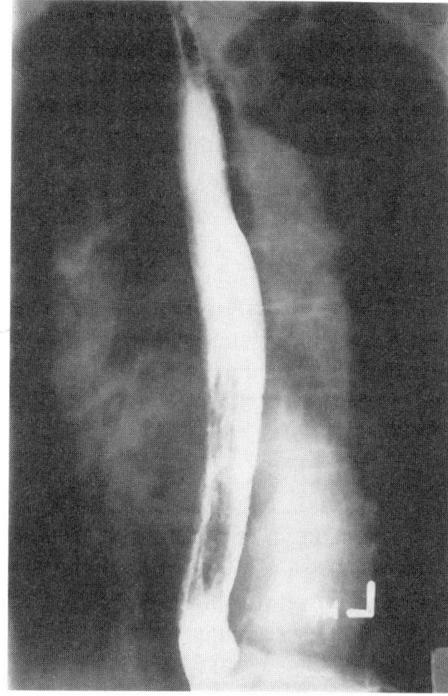

Fig. 101-10. Barium swallow demonstrating mucosal ulcerations of candidal esophagitis.

reflux esophagitis cannot be treated medically, surgical fundoplications may be of some benefit.

DISEASES OF THE HYPOPHARYNX AND PROXIMAL ESOPHAGUS

Systemic diseases can involve the smooth portion of the esophagus. Several diseases, primarily neurologic, can affect the hypopharynx, upper esophageal sphincter, and striated portions of the esophagus. Diseases involving the upper esophagus in patients with dysphagia for solids and liquids include amyloidosis, dermatomyositis, polymyositis, myasthenia gravis, myotonic dystrophy, myxedema, oculopharyngeal muscular dystrophy, and thyrotoxicosis. Patients with difficulty initiating swallowing may have had cerebrovascular accidents (CVAs), strokes, amyotrophic lateral sclerosis, multiple sclerosis, poliomyelitis, or tetanus. Those recovering from CVAs may benefit from speech therapy, with swallowing exercises to improve deglutition. Involvement of the striated muscle is diagnosed by barium swallow and cineradiology and confirmed by demonstrating aperistalsis in the upper third of the esophagus by manometry. The dysphagia may be alleviated by treating the systemic disorder.

ESOPHAGEAL INFECTIONS

The incidence of infectious diseases of the esophagus has increased primarily because of acquired immunodeficiency syndrome (AIDS). These patients may have candidiasis, herpes simplex virus type 1 (HSV-1), and cytomegalovirus (CMV). *Candidiasis* is seen with increased frequency in patients with neoplastic diseases, diabetes mellitus, chronic renal failure, and other conditions with immune incompetence. Patients develop severe odynophagia, dysphagia, and if severe, hematemesis. Oral candidiasis *(thrush)* may be present on physical examination. Barium swallow may reveal ulceration of the esophageal mucosa, but the diagnosis is best confirmed by endoscopy (Fig. 101-10). Brushings show yeast forms, and biopsy of the ulcerations demonstrates the fungus. Treatment of the immunocompetent patient is usually successful with nystatin oral suspension, 250,000 U every 2 hours for 1 week. A total dose of up to 12 million U a day may be required. In the immunocompromised patient, excellent results have been achieved with fluconazole (Diflucan), 50 to 200 mg once daily.[3]

Patients with HSV-1 and CMV usually complain of odynophagia. Diagnosis is by endoscopy and biopsy of the esophageal mucosal lesion with staining and cultures. Successful treatment includes acyclovir (Zovirax) for HSV-1 and ganciclovir (Cytovene) for CMV.

MISCELLANEOUS DISORDERS

Mallory-Weiss Syndrome

Mallory-Weiss syndrome consists of a mucosal tear at the gastroesophageal junction as a result of retching or emesis. It is found in 15% of patients with hematemesis. The classic description is forceful retching followed by hematemesis. As many as 25% of patients vomit blood with the initial emesis. Diagnosis is made by endoscopy, and the tear is usually evident on the gastric side of the gastroesophageal junction. Treatment consists of observation, since nearly all episodes stop spontaneously. Somatostatin can be used if bleeding continues, as can electrocautery. Surgery is rarely required.

Foreign Bodies

Most often, foreign bodies are the result of poorly chewed, hastily swallowed food, especially bread or meats. Food impaction usually occurs in edentulous elderly or very young patients. Animal bones and other objects, including pins or coins, pass through the gastrointestinal tract more than 90% of the time. Patients describe ingestion of the food or object followed by acute chest pain and salivation. A plain radiograph of the chest or neck frequently visualizes the object. A patient who cannot swallow secretions should undergo prompt endoscopic removal of the object. A nonobstructing foreign body that has not caused a perforation within 24 hours usually passes into the stomach. If the object is impacted or fails to pass, it is removed with a snare by flexible upper endoscopy. Often a lower esophageal ring is found when food impaction occurs. After removal of the object, the ring can be dilated with a bougie.

REFERENCES

1. Burakoff R: Noncardiac chest pain, *Emerg Med* 22:49, 1990.
2. Cameron AJ: Management of Barrett's esophagus, *Mayo Clin Proc* 73:457, 1998.
3. Darouiche RO: Oropharyngeal and esophageal candidiasis in the immunocompromised patients: treatment issues, *Clin Infect Dis* 26:259, 1998.
4. DeVault KR: Lower esophageal (Schatzki's) ring: pathogenesis, diagnosis and therapy, *Dig Dis* 14:323, 1996.
5. Hirschowitz BI: Management of refractory and complicated reflux esophagitis, *Yale J Biol Med* 69:271, 1996.
6. Kahrilas PJ: Gastroesophageal reflux disease, *JAMA* 276:983, 1996.
7. Lambert R: An overview of the management of cancer of the esophagus, *Gastrointest Endosc Clin N Am* 8:415, 1998.
8. Pasricha PJ, Ravich WJ, Hendrix TR, et al: Intrasphincteric botulinum toxin for the treatment of achalasia, *N Engl J Med* 322:774, 1995.
9. Walker SJ: What's new in pathology, pathophysiology and management of benign esophageal disorders? *Dis Esophagus* 10:282, 1997.

CHAPTER 102

Acid-Peptic Disorders, Gastritis, and *Helicobacter pylori*

Robert C. Lowe
M. Michael Wolfe

The incidence of peptic ulcer disease (PUD) has been decreasing steadily since the 1950s, but PUD continues to affect 200,000 to 400,000 people each year, with estimated annual costs of $3 billion to $4 billion. The discovery of *Helicobacter pylori* in the early 1980s and its association with PUD have dramatically altered the approach to management of this condition. Despite the importance of *H. pylori* infection, however, gastric acid continues to play a critical role in the pathogenesis of ulcers, and "no acid, no ulcer" remains a valid principle.

EPIDEMIOLOGY

PUD affects 1.8% of the U.S. population and, despite previous studies suggesting male predominance, appears to affect males and females equally. A study of male physicians reported a 10% lifetime risk of developing a duodenal ulcer (DU). The most common risk factors for ulcer development are use of nonsteroidal antiinflammatory drugs (NSAIDs), infection with *H. pylori*, and cigarette smoking. The common belief that alcohol, stress, and spicy food are important in ulcerogenesis has not been borne out in clinical studies. A family history of DU is reported in 20% to 50% of DU patients in published series, compared with 10% of patients without ulcer disease. These epidemiologic studies, however, antedate the discovery of *H. pylori*, and fecal-oral transmission of *H. pylori* or a genetic predisposition to *H. pylori* infection may be responsible for this apparent familial clustering. Previous studies showing an association of DU with blood type O may also reflect a predisposition to *H. pylori* infection in persons with this blood type. Some patients, however, may have a genetic predisposition to gastric acid hypersecretion that contributes to DU pathogenesis. The incidence of PUD is also increased in patients with underlying illnesses (e.g., cirrhosis, chronic obstructive pulmonary disease, renal failure) and after renal transplantation.

ANATOMY AND PHYSIOLOGY

The proximal stomach (i.e., cardia, fundus, body) is compliant and, besides secreting acid and pepsin, functions as a reservoir for the mixing of food and gastric secretions. The distal stomach (antrum and pylorus) is more muscular, provides the force to mix food and gastric juice, and propels chyme into the small intestine for further digestion and subsequent absorption. The stomach possesses an extensive blood supply that forms two vascular arcades along the greater curvature (left and right gastroepiploic arteries) and lesser curvature (left and right gastric arteries). Lymphatic drainage parallels this vascular supply. The vagus nerve provides parasympathetic input to the stomach that modulates both motor function and acid secretion.

Functionally the stomach can be divided into two areas: the oxyntic gland and pyloric gland regions. Oxyntic glands are located in the gastric fundus and body and are composed of several cell types, including parietal cells (which secrete hydrochloric acid [HCl] and intrinsic factor), chief cells (which secrete pepsinogen), mast and enterochromaffin-like (ECL) cells (which generate histamine), D cells (which produce somatostatin), and mucus-secreting cells. The pyloric glands are located in the antrum and contain mucus- secreting cells, D cells, and G cells, which synthesize and secrete gastrin. Parietal cells generate hydrogen ions (H^+), which are secreted into the lumen by a cellular H^+/K^+ (potassium ion) adenosinetriphosphatase (ATPase) that constitutes the final common pathway of H^+ secretion.

The generation of H^+ is mediated by three pathways: neurocrine, paracrine, and endocrine (Fig. 102-1). The principal neurocrine transmitter is *acetylcholine,* which is released by vagal postganglionic neurons and causes parietal cells to increase gastric acid secretion both directly and indirectly by stimulating histamine release from ECL cells. *Histamine* (H_2) is the primary paracrine transmitter that binds to H_2-specific receptors on parietal cells; adenylate cyclase is then activated, leading to an increase in cyclic adenosine monophosphate (cAMP) levels and subsequent generation of H^+. Histamine receptors can be selectively and competitively blocked by H_2 receptor antagonists (H_2RAs, H_2 blockers), agents that constituted the mainstay of ulcer therapy during the 1980s and early 1990s. The secretion of *gastrin* from antral G cells constitutes the endocrine pathway and stimulates gastric acid secretion predominantly by stimulating histamine secretion from ECL cells. Gastrin represents the principal pathway by which acid secretion is stimulated during the gastric phase of a meal. Antral distention provides the initial stimulus for gastrin release through a β-adrenergic pathway in humans. The effect of antral distention is transient, however, and the maintenance of gastrin release is mediated by two principal components of the ingested meal: protein content and pH. Gastrin is secreted when the luminal pH increases above 3.5, whereas gastrin release is abolished at a pH of less than 1.5.

These neurocrine, paracrine, and endocrine pathways are not independent; interactions among them are coordinated to promote or inhibit the secretion of gastric acid. Histamine appears to represent the dominant route because gastrin and (to some extent) acetylcholine stimulate H^+ secretion principally by promoting histamine release from ECL cells. Thus ECL cells are often referred to as *controller cells* in the process of gastric acid secretion.

Acid secretion in response to a meal can be divided into three phases: cephalic, gastric, and intestinal. The *cephalic phase* is mediated by the vagus nerve in response to the sight, smell, or thought of food and accounts for 30% to 35% of the total acid output in response to a meal. Basal and nocturnal acid secretion is also mediated by the vagus nerve; thus both the cephalic phase of a meal and the basal circadian rhythm of acid secretion can be abolished by vagotomy. The *gastric phase* of acid secretion accounts for 50% to 60% of total meal-stimulated acid release, and more than 90% of this phase is mediated by gastrin release from antral G cells. The *intestinal phase* of acid secretion plays only a minor role, accounting for less than 5% of the acid response to a meal, and appears to result from the effects of absorbed amino acids.

A negative feedback loop governs the means by which both gastrin release and acid secretion return to basal levels. This process represents a vital autoregulatory mechanism for preventing postprandial acid hypersecretion. After ingestion of a meal, gastrin release stimulates the secretion of gastric acid. The intraluminal pH begins to decrease as the buffering capacity of the meal is overwhelmed by continued acid secretion. The increasing acidity appears to stimulate the release of somatostatin from antral D cells. Somatostatin in turn acts through a paracrine mechanism to inhibit the further release of gastrin from G cells, and acid secretion is subsequently diminished. D cells may also directly inhibit acid secretion from parietal cells or may suppress histamine release from ECL cells.

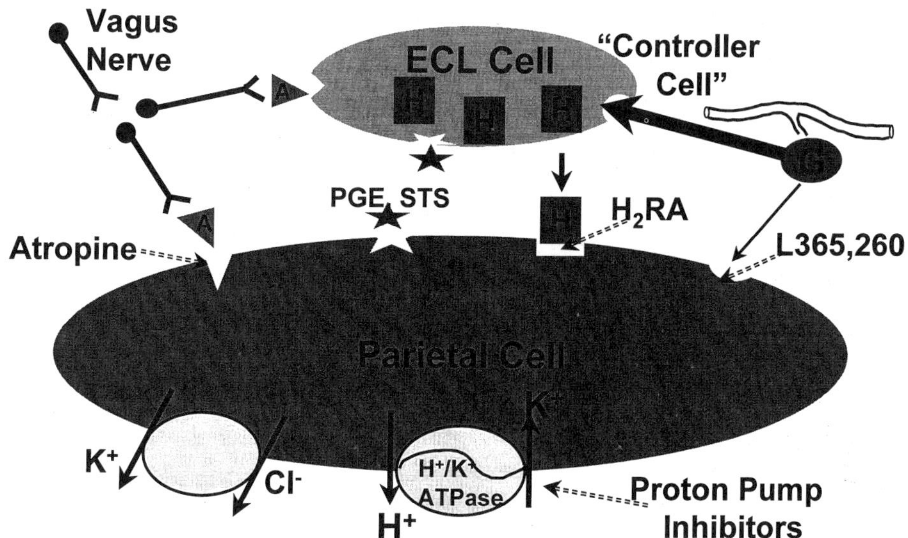

Fig. 102-1. Gastric acid secretion by parietal cell, as influenced by neurocrine (acetylcholine [*A*] from vagal efferent neurons), paracrine (histamine [*H*] release from gastric enterochromaffin-like [*ECL*] cells), and endocrine (circulating gastrin [*G*]) factors. Dashed arrows indicate potential sites of pharmacologic inhibition of acid secretion, either through receptor antagonism or inhibition of H^+/K^+ ATPase, the common pathway for gastric acid secretion. *H_2RA,* Histamine receptor antagonists; *L365,260,* synthetic gastric receptor antagonist; *PGE,* prostaglandin E.

PATHOPHYSIOLOGY

Historically, acid and pepsin have been considered the sole determinants of ulcer pathogenesis. Although patients with gastric ulcers tend to have normal or reduced levels of acid secretion, DU patients on average are hypersecretors of acid. When compared with age-matched controls, DU patients secrete approximately 70% more acid during the day (meal stimulated) and about 150% more acid at night (basal secretion). As noted, gastric acid secretion during the day is regulated primarily by postprandial gastrin release and subsequent inhibition of the hormone's secretion after acidification of the gastric lumen. Individuals infected with *H. pylori* have diminished antral D cells, which decreases the magnitude of the somatostatin response during acidification of the gastric lumen. Thus, in patients with infection limited to the antrum, the negative feedback inhibition of gastrin release is attenuated, resulting in higher postprandial gastrin levels and hypersecretion of acid.

Despite the enhanced daytime rate of acid secretion in DU patients, the presence of food in the stomach has a buffering effect that helps protect the mucosa from acid-induced injury. At night, however, acid bathes the bare mucosa, and in DU patients the increase in nocturnal acid secretion magnifies this effect. Also, duodenal bicarbonate secretion is impaired in patients with DU, as well as in those infected with *H. pylori*, making the mucosal exposure to acid even greater. These observations, as discussed later, form the rationale for single nocturnal dosing of H_2RAs in the treatment of DU, which is at least as effective as multiple dosing regimens. Vagotomy also provides an effective means of healing DUs because nocturnal acid secretion is mediated primarily by vagal activity and appears to be predominantly *H. pylori* independent.

Factors other than acid and pepsin are involved in the pathogenesis of PUD, since only 30% of patients with DUs and very few patients with gastric ulcers are acid hypersecretors. Another important element is the balance between aggressive factors that act to injure the gastroduodenal mucosa and defensive factors that normally protect against noxious agents; when this balance is disrupted for any reason, an ulcer may develop (Fig. 102-2). The aggressive factors include acid (dominant role), pepsin, and bile salts. The mucosal defensive factors include (1) mucus secretion, which traps H^+ and permits bicarbonate secreted by surface epithelial cells to titrate acid effectively; (2) mucosal blood flow, which delivers oxygen, nutrients, and bicarbonate and removes metabolites ("alkaline tide"); (3) intercellular tight junctions that prevent transepithelial penetration of H^+; and (4) cell restitution and epithelial renewal, which enable the mucosa to repair itself after injury. These defensive properties appear to be mediated largely by endogenous prostaglandins. When prostaglandin synthesis is diminished by the use of NSAIDs, the ability of the gastroduodenal mucosa to resist injury is decreased. Thus even normal rates of acid secretion may be sufficient to injure the mucosa and produce gastroduodenal ulcers.

ETIOLOGY

H. pylori infection, NSAID use, and hypersecretory states (e.g., Zollinger-Ellison syndrome) appear to account for the vast majority of gastric and duodenal ulcers.

Helicobacter pylori

Chronic antral infection with *H. pylori* results in increased postprandial acid secretion through increased and prolonged gastrin release. This abnormality occurs as a result of a

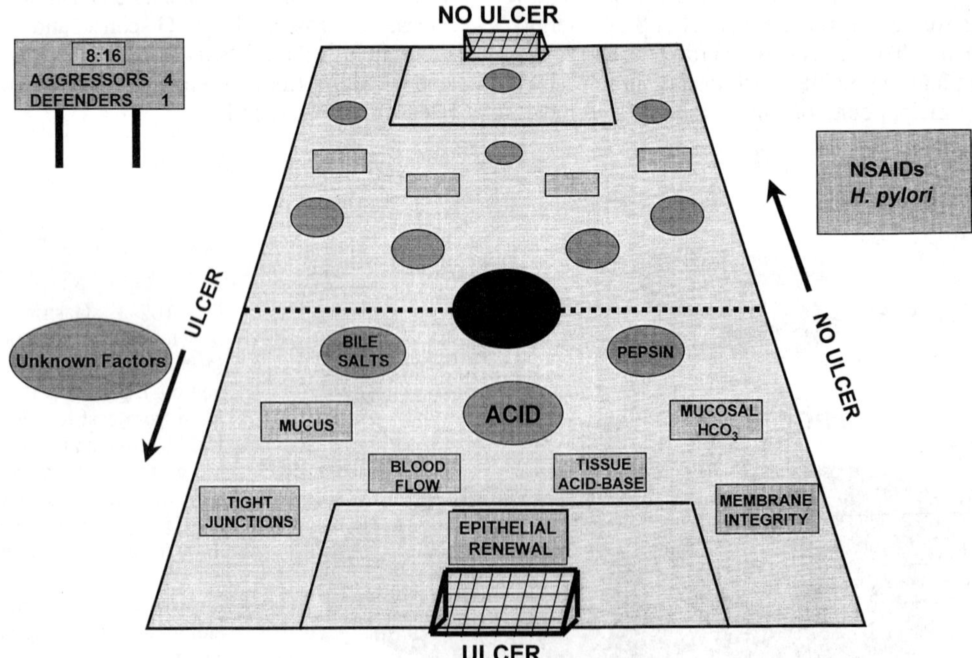

Fig. 102-2. Pathogenesis of peptic ulcer modeled as an imbalance between aggressive and defensive factors within gastroduodenal mucosa. Ulcers form when aggressive factors (e.g., acid, pepsin) overwhelm defensive mechanisms normally present within mucosa. In most instances, acid and pepsin secretion is not increased; rather, mucosal resistance is diminished by factors such as ingestion of nonsteroidal antiinflammatory drugs *(NSAIDs)* or infection with *Helicobacter pylori*.

marked decrease in the number of D cells in the antrum, which decreases somatostatin activity and consequently diminishes inhibitory signaling to antral G cells and possibly ECL and parietal cells. DU patients infected with *H. pylori* have an increased acid secretory response to gastrin compared with volunteers who are *H. pylori* negative and who do not have ulcers. Thus *H. pylori*–infected DU patients not only secrete more gastrin but also are more responsive to the hormone. These abnormalities are largely reversible after successful eradication of the organism.

H. pylori and pH are closely related etiologic factors in PUD (Fig. 102-3). Unknown genetic factors lead to gastric acid hypersecretion, which can produce gastric metaplasia of the duodenum. Because of a predilection for infection of gastric-type mucosa, secondary colonization of the duodenum with *H. pylori* may occur, which may in turn incite an immune response, leading to duodenitis and DU. Despite the clear epidemiologic association between *H. pylori* and PUD, however, the percentage of ulcers associated with *H. pylori* may not be 90% to 95% but as low as 32% in nonreferral-based populations. Thus peptic ulceration is not caused solely by *H. pylori*, but rather involves several factors, most notably the erosive properties of acid and pepsin.

Nonsteroidal Antiinflammatory Drugs

Approximately 15% to 20% of chronic NSAID users develop gastroduodenal ulcers. Although NSAIDs damage the gastric mucosa more frequently than the duodenal mucosa, the mechanisms of injury are the same: the disruption of mucosal defenses by both topical and systemic effects. The topical effects of NSAIDs, seen primarily in the stomach, result from a direct toxic insult by these agents or their metabolites on the gastric mucosal surface. The systemic effects are mediated through inhibition of cyclooxygenase in the gastric epithelium and consequently a decrease in the production of mucosal prostaglandins. The diminished prostaglandin levels alter gastric mucus secretion, mucosal blood flow, ion transport, and other defensive properties of the gastroduodenal mucosa, allowing acid and pepsin to induce mucosal damage, which results in formation of peptic ulcers. Even enteric-coated or intravenous NSAID formulations can induce gastroduodenal ulcers because of their systemic effects.

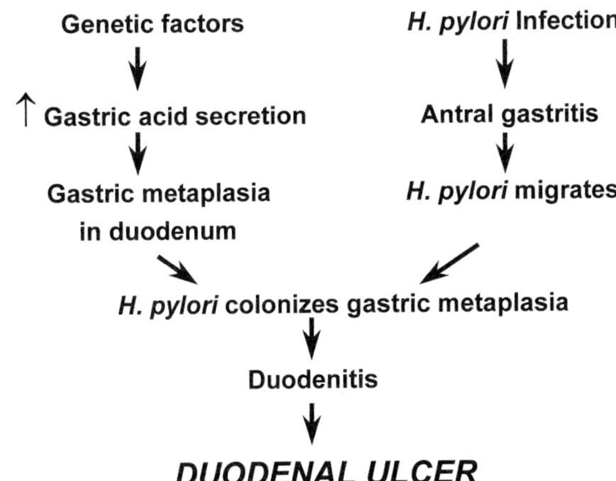

Fig. 102-3. Pathways depicting postulated pathogenesis of *Helicobacter pylori*–associated duodenal ulcer. Gastric metaplasia in duodenum provides environment that enhances colonization by *H. pylori*, with subsequent duodenal inflammation and possible progression to peptic ulcer.

Risk factors for PUD and its complications include age over 65 years, prior history of PUD, use of high doses of NSAIDs, and concurrent steroid use. Patients with these risk factors or those who would poorly tolerate any complications of PUD may benefit from ulcer prophylaxis. Both proton pump inhibitors (PPIs) and misoprostol (a prostaglandin E_1 analog) provide effective ulcer prophylaxis in users of NSAIDs. Misoprostol is clearly superior to H_2RAs in the prevention of gastric ulcers, whereas both are equally effective in preventing DUs. Famotidine in high doses (40 mg twice daily) may also offer some protection against gastric ulcers, although not as effectively as misoprostol or PPIs. PPIs may be as effective as misoprostol in the prevention of gastroduodenal ulcers caused by NSAIDs. In addition to the use of prophylactic agents, new NSAIDs have been developed that may lack the ulcerogenic properties of earlier preparations. Agents such as meloxicam, celecoxib, and rofecoxib preferentially or selectively inhibit inducible cyclooxygenase II (COX-II), which is responsible for inflammation, while having a minimal effect on constitutively expressed cyclooxygenase I (COX-I), the enzyme that plays a key role in preserving mucosal integrity.

Hypersecretory States

Hypersecretory states such as Zollinger-Ellison syndrome (ZES), antral G-cell hyperplasia, and systemic mastocytosis are also associated with PUD. A reported 0.1% of all DUs are caused by ZES. Classically, hypersecretory states are associated with multiple DUs, ulcers in unusual locations (beyond the first portion of the duodenum), or ulcers that fail to respond to standard therapy. More often, however, they behave as ulcers associated with *H. pylori*, often with additional symptoms, such as pyrosis, diarrhea, or cutaneous flushing.

A significant number of patients with PUD are *H. pylori* negative, and the appropriate evaluation of such patients is presently unclear. A number of these patients are taking NSAIDs (57% to 75% in studies), whereas others have an underlying hypersecretory state or another illness associated with gastroduodenal ulceration (e.g., Crohn's disease). The remaining patients with truly "idiopathic" ulcers may have a disturbance of gastric motility; delayed gastric emptying may predispose to gastric ulceration by increasing the contact time between acid and the mucosa, and rapid gastric emptying may have similar consequences for the duodenal mucosa. Most authorities recommend that patients with PUD who are *H. pylori* negative and who deny NSAID use should be evaluated with a fasting serum gastrin level (to identify a hypergastrinemic syndrome) and a biopsy of the ulcer to look for granulomatous infiltration or evidence of neoplasia (adenocarcinoma or lymphoma).

CLINICAL PRESENTATION

The most common symptom of PUD is nonradiating epigastric pain. The pain of DU is classically described as occurring 2 to 3 hours after a meal, improving with food or antacids, and awakening patients at night several hours after retiring (2 to 4 AM). Gastric ulcer pain is said to worsen with food, although the response to a meal cannot reliably distinguish gastric ulcers from DUs. Other symptoms of PUD include nausea and vomiting, which may occur in up to 60% of patients, especially those with prepyloric or pyloric channel ulcers. Unfortunately, the classic symptom complex occurs only in a minority of patients with PUD, and it is difficult even to determine the percentage of patients who experience pain, since a significant number of patients with PUD lack any symptoms. In one study, 10% of patients presenting with a complication of ulcer disease (perforation or hemorrhage) reported no prior symptoms. In studies of patients with hemorrhage from NSAID-induced gastroduodenal ulcers, as many as 50% to 60% had no antecedent symptoms. Another confounding factor is that the relief of pain has not proved to be a reliable indicator of a successful response to therapy, since some patients will have continued pain despite ulcer healing, whereas others will report relief of their symptoms in the presence of a persistent ulcer.

The physical examination in patients with uncomplicated PUD is largely unrevealing, with most patients having little more than epigastric tenderness. When complications supervene, however, the range of clinical presentations includes an acute abdomen after perforation, hematemesis and melena after hemorrhage, and early satiety, nausea, and vomiting from gastric outlet obstruction.

DIAGNOSIS

Although some authors report accurately predicting endoscopic findings in 66% of patients with PUD, establishing the diagnosis solely on the basis of history and examination is usually difficult and uncertain. Given the nonspecific symptoms and signs of PUD, the differential diagnosis is broad and includes gastroesophageal reflux disease (GERD), gastric cancer, gastroduodenitis, cholecystitis, biliary tract disease, pancreatic cancer, pancreatitis (acute or chronic), intestinal ischemia, pain associated with ischemic heart disease, and nonulcer dyspepsia. The diagnosis of PUD is most often made by esophagogastroduodenoscopy (EGD) or upper gastrointestinal (UGI) series. The two modalities tend to correlate well, although reported sensitivities and specificities may not be applicable to all centers because they depend largely on examiners' expertise in radiology and gastroenterology. In the *best* hands, using double-contrast fluoroscopic technique, EGD and UGI series correlate 80% to 90% of the time in diagnosing duodenal ulcers. The UGI series is not as effective in detecting small ulcers (less than 0.5 cm) and does not allow for biopsy. Therefore, if available, endoscopic evaluation is clearly preferred for patients with suspected PUD.

Laboratory tests are generally of little help in evaluating patients with uncomplicated PUD. A fasting serum gastrin level for the presence of ZES may be useful in DU patients with a reasonable index of suspicion. Measurement of gastric acid secretion is generally helpful only in patients with elevated serum gastrin levels. In these patients a gastric pH measurement at endoscopy is useful in distinguishing atrophic gastritis or other causes of decreased acid secretion from ZES. A pH greater than 2.5 in the absence of antisecretory medication (not taking H_2RAs for 24 hours or PPIs for 5 days) virtually excludes the diagnosis of ZES.

Laboratory tests do play an important role in the diagnosis of *H. pylori* infection, most often through serologic determination of immunoglobulin G (IgG) antibodies in peripheral blood, which is greater than 90% sensitive and 90% specific for *H. pylori* infection. ^{13}C-urea and ^{14}C-urea breath tests also can establish *H. pylori* infection and are the most sensitive methods (invasive or noninvasive) for determining successful eradication of the organism. The patient ingests urea labeled with carbon-13 or carbon-14. If *H. pylori* is present on the gastric mucosa, bacterial urease metabolizes the urea into ammonia and labeled carbon dioxide, which is absorbed into the bloodstream and excreted through the lungs. Breath samples are collected at intervals after urea ingestion and are analyzed using either mass spectrometry (^{13}C) or a scintillation counter (^{14}C). Urea breath testing is 95% sensitive and 98% specific for the diagnosis of *H. pylori* infection. The high diagnostic accuracy and noninvasive nature make the test a superior means of documenting *H. pylori* and confirming eradication of the organism at 4 to 6 weeks after cessation of treatment.

For patients undergoing upper endoscopy, several tests for *H. pylori* can be performed on biopsy specimens of the gastric mucosa. Culture of *H. pylori* is difficult and at present is rarely used to diagnose infection in clinical practice. Direct histologic examination of biopsy specimens is a sensitive and specific means of diagnosing *H. pylori* infection and remains the gold standard. The rapid urease test provides a faster and less expensive way of establishing *H. pylori* infection from a biopsy specimen. These tests use a gel matrix impregnated with both urea and a pH-sensitive color indicator. Gastric biopsies are placed into the gel, and in the presence of *H. pylori*–associated urease, ammonia is generated from urea, and the gel turns red as the pH becomes increasingly alkaline. Rapid urease testing is 92% sensitive when read at 3 hours and 98% sensitive at 24 hours, with 100% specificity.

TREATMENT

The treatment of PUD has changed dramatically since the discovery that ulcer recurrence rates decrease dramatically after eradication of *H. pylori* infection, compared with annual recurrence rates of 50% to 80% when antisecretory therapy alone is used (Table 102-1). Determining whether a patient with PUD is infected with *H. pylori* is critical to appropriate

Table 102-1. Healing Rates with Pharmacologic Treatments of Peptic Ulcer

Medication	Dose	Healing rate
Antacids	>200 mEq of neutralizing capacity	70%-80% at 4 weeks
Sucralfate	1 g qid	70%-80% at 4 weeks
H_2 receptor antagonists	Famotidine, 40 mg qhs	
	Ranitidine, 300 mg qhs	70%-80% at 4 weeks
	Nizatidine, 300 mg qhs	87%-94% at 8 weeks
	Cimetidine, 800-1200 mg qhs	
Proton pump inhibitors	Omeprazole, 20 mg QAM	80%-100% at 4 weeks
	Lansoprazole, 30 mg QAM	
	Rabeprazole, 20 mg QAM	
	Pantoprazole, 40 mg QAM	

qid, Four times daily; *qhs,* every evening before bedtime; *QAM,* every morning (before breakfast).

management. If a patient is not infected with *H. pylori*, an alternative etiology must be sought, such as NSAID use, hypersecretory states, or less common causes.

Nonpharmacologic Therapy

Historically, bed rest and dietary modification were the mainstays of treatment for PUD. Bland diets rich in milk were advocated with recommendations to eat smaller, more frequent meals to decrease gastric distention and subsequent acid secretion. These treatments were never evaluated in controlled clinical trials, and it was later discovered that milk itself was a potent stimulus of gastric acid secretion. Dietary modification is thus no longer advised, besides counseling patients to avoid any specific foods that precipitate dyspepsia. General measures recommended in the treatment of ulcer disease include cessation of smoking and alcohol and, if possible, discontinuation of NSAID use.

Pharmacologic Therapy

Antacids. Antacids are effective in relieving the symptoms of PUD, and a double-blind study demonstrated that antacids are superior to placebo in healing DUs (although no difference in symptom relief was noted in that trial). Later studies evaluated the dose and dose intervals of antacids and found that as little as a single antacid tablet before meals or at bedtime was effective in healing ulcers with minimal side effects. The toxicity of antacids is generally low, with the predominant side effects of diarrhea with magnesium hydroxide–containing preparations and constipation with aluminum hydroxide–based formulations.

H_2 Receptor Antagonists. The discovery of the role of selective histamine receptors in regulating gastric acid secretion generated a search for a receptor antagonist, culminating in the introduction of cimetidine in the mid-1970s. As with antacids, cimetidine (0.8 to 1.2 gm/day) promotes healing of duodenal ulcers in 70% to 80% of patients after 4 to 6 weeks, compared with placebo healing rates of 20% to 45%. Later formulations (ranitidine, famotidine, nizatidine) retained the basic structure of cimetidine, with minor modifications affecting potency, bioavailability, and side effect profile. Overall, H_2RAs are among the safest classes of drugs available. They may cause mild central nervous system (CNS) effects, including drowsiness, agitation, and headache, because of their ability to cross the blood-brain barrier and cross-react with CNS histamine receptors. Cimetidine and ranitidine both interact with the hepatic cytochrome P-450 system (ranitidine having fivefold to tenfold less avidity than cimetidine) and may affect the metabolism of various drugs. However, only patients receiving warfarin sodium, theophylline, or phenytoin are at small risk of developing a clinically significant alteration in drug levels; since monitoring of drug levels and coagulation parameters is routine in these patients, an adverse outcome rarely results from this interaction. Other reported side effects of H_2 blockers include gynecomastia (cimetidine only) and rarely thrombocytopenia. In general, a 50% dose reduction is recommended in patients with a glomerular filtration rate of 30 ml/minute or less. All the H_2RAs are equally effective in healing duodenal ulcers, with 90% to 95% healing rates achieved after 8 weeks of therapy. Twice-daily dosing regimens have been replaced by a single evening-dose regimen (with an equivalent total daily dose), since ulcer healing is proportional to the effectiveness of *nocturnal* acid secretion. Although both modes of therapy are equally effective, patient compliance improves with the single-dose regimen, which is thus preferred for treatment of PUD with H_2RAs.

Sucralfate. Sucralfate (an aluminum salt of sucrose octasulfate) has been used for the past two decades in the treatment of PUD and possesses healing rates similar to antacids and H_2RAs. Although sucralfate has no effect on gastric acid secretion, it is thought to protect the gastroduodenal mucosa through adhesion to the ulcer base, adsorption of bile acids, inactivation of pepsin, and stimulation of bicarbonate and mucus secretion. In addition to its use as primary therapy for PUD (1 gm orally four times daily), sucralfate is also effective in preventing DU relapse (1 gm twice daily). Sucralfate is generally well tolerated and has an excellent safety profile because only 3% to 5% of a single dose is absorbed into the circulation. In patients with renal disease, however, sucralfate must be used cautiously, since even this small systemic dose may lead infrequently to aluminum toxicity.

Prostaglandin Analogs. The prostaglandin analogs misoprostol, arbaprostil, and enprostil have been used in the treatment of PUD; only misoprostol is available in the United States. These agents protect the gastroduodenal mucosa by stimulating the secretion of bicarbonate and mucus and by enhancing mucosal blood flow and mucosal cell restitution. When given at higher doses, these drugs also exhibit an antisecretory effect. These agents are effective in healing peptic ulcers and in preventing ulcer recurrence, but only when given in antisecretory doses. Thus the relative contributions of mucosal protection and inhibition of gastric acid secretion are difficult to distinguish clinically. Because prostaglandin analogs require frequent dosing (for misoprostol, 200 μg two to four times daily) and are associated with significantly more side effects than H_2RAs, they are generally not used in the treatment of PUD. Currently, these agents are primarily used to prevent NSAID-induced gastroduodenal ulceration. Diarrhea is the most frequently reported side effect of these agents, occurring in up to 20% to 30% of patients. The diarrhea is dose dependent and is related to the drug's ability to increase cAMP levels in intestinal mucosal cells, thereby inducing a secretory diarrhea. Prostaglandin analogs also possess abortifacient properties and should not be used during pregnancy or in women of childbearing age.

Proton Pump Inhibitors. The PPIs, which include omeprazole, lansoprazole, rabeprazole, and pantoprazole, are the most powerful inhibitors of gastric acid secretion available. These agents are substituted benzimidazoles that irreversibly inhibit the activity of H^+/K^+ ATPase. Administered as prodrugs with a pK_a of approximately 4.0 (5.0 for rabeprazole), they become concentrated in the secretory canaliculus of the activated parietal cell, where the local pH is less than 1.0. In this acidic environment these agents are protonated to form sulfonamides, which then irreversibly bind H^+/K^+ ATPase. PPIs are most effective when the parietal cell is stimulated to secrete acid in response to a meal; thus these drugs should *only* be taken before a meal and should *not* be used in conjunction with H_2RAs or other antisecretory agents, including prostaglandins. PPIs are extremely potent inhibitors of acid secretion and are also the agents of choice for treatment of ZES.

The safety profile of PPIs is similar to that of H_2 blockers. Although high doses of PPIs precipitated ECL cell hyperplasia and subsequent gastric carcinoid tumors in rats, these drugs have been used for more than 15 years in Europe and 10 years in the United States with no increased tumor incidence. This interspecies difference may be related to a lower mucosal ECL density and a less pronounced increase in circulating gastrin in humans vs. rodents in response to antisecretory medications. PPIs heal peptic ulcers more rapidly than H_2RAs; lansoprazole (30 mg daily) healed 74% of duodenal ulcers after 2 weeks vs. 51% with ranitidine, although at 4 weeks, healing rates were comparable, 95% and 89%, respectively. PPIs are best administered when parietal cells are stimulated (i.e., with meals, optimally before breakfast). Although these agents are less effective in patients not receiving enteral nutrition, evidence suggests that they can be given in suspension through a nasogastric tube in critically ill patients and still induce a significant but inconsistent decrease in acid secretion.

Summary. All peptic ulcers eventually heal, as evidenced by placebo responses. Antisecretory therapy accelerates healing and allows more rapid relief of symptoms. Antacids, sucralfate, H_2RAs, prostaglandin analogs, and PPIs have similar healing rates when given for at least 4 weeks, although PPIs appear to heal ulcers more rapidly than the others. Moreover, because they are often used in *H. pylori* eradication regimens and because they heal gastroduodenal ulcers in patients continuing NSAIDs, PPIs have become the mainstay of therapy for healing peptic ulcers.

Maintenance Therapy

The practice of continuing antisecretory therapy after ulcer healing evolved from observations regarding the natural history of PUD. In both preendoscopy and postendoscopy studies, up to 82% of DU patients had persistent symptoms after the initial diagnosis, with some lasting up to 30 years. Only 26% of patients with an untreated DU were free of symptoms 1 year after diagnosis. After a median follow-up of 38 weeks, only 12% of patients who underwent *H. pylori* eradication relapsed, compared with 95% of patients who received H_2RAs alone. Other studies report similar relapse rates after *H. pylori* therapy, so the maxim "once an ulcer, always an ulcer" no longer holds true.

The role of maintenance antisecretory therapy has changed in recent years. Before embarking on long-term therapy, the most important risk factors for ulcer recurrence, *H. pylori* infection and NSAID use, must be eliminated. Several studies have demonstrated the cost-effectiveness of *H. pylori* eradication compared with maintenance antisecretory therapy, which may cost more than $1200 per year. The American College of Gastroenterology currently recommends that only high-risk ulcer patients receive maintenance antisecretory therapy. This group includes patients with a history of ulcer complications, those with frequent recurrences, those who are *H. pylori* negative, and those who fail to clear *H. pylori* infection despite appropriate therapy. Some experts, however, state that even patients with a complication of PUD do not require maintenance therapy provided *H. pylori* infection is cured. Thus, although maintenance therapy plays a role in select situations, the most important principles in treating PUD are to identify and treat *H. pylori* infection and to discontinue or minimize the use of NSAIDs.

Box 102-1. Treatment Recommendations for *Helicobacter pylori* Infection

Proven Effective

Active duodenal ulcer with proven *H. pylori* infection
All patients on maintenance therapy for past ulcer with proven *H. pylori* infection
Active gastric ulcer
- Only if *H. pylori* positive
- History of NSAID ingestion should not alter treatment of *H. pylori*

Mucosa-associated lymphoid tissue (MALT) lymphoma

Controversial

Gastric cancer relatives: no proven benefit in preventing development of cancer
Antral (type B) gastritis
- Will cure gastritis, but no known clinical benefit
- Best done under protocol

Nonulcer dyspepsia: data equivocal

Helicobacter Pylori Infection

Optimal treatment of *H.* pylori infection continues to be an area of active research, with a plethora of therapeutic regimens currently available and many others being studied in clinical trials. The two important issues are (1) the determination of which patients should be treated for *H. pylori* infection and (2) the choice of one effective therapeutic regimen from the many available to the practicing physician (Box 102-1). Recurrence rates of DU in *H. pylori*–infected patients decrease significantly after eradication of infection, both in patients with active ulcers and those with a past history of DU disease who are *H. pylori* positive. Patients with gastric ulcer and *H. pylori* infection should also be treated, even if NSAID use is the etiologic factor in the ulcer's pathogenesis. The diagnosis of a gastric mucosa-associated lymphoid tissue (MALT) lymphoma in an *H. pylori*–infected patient is also an indication for treatment, since eradication of infection may induce regression of the malignant lesion. See Chapter 105 for the relationship between *H. pylori* and MALT and gastric carcinoma.

Although *H. pylori* has been associated with an increased incidence of gastric adenocarcinoma, mass screening and eradication of infection as a chemopreventive strategy is not currently recommended. Eradication of infection in patients with a strong family history of gastric cancer, however, can be considered a reasonable strategy. Similarly, patients with type B antral gastritis and *H. pylori* infection may benefit from treatment, but this issue is still unresolved; optimally, patients should be treated in the context of a clinical trial. The treatment of *H. pylori* infection in patients with nonulcer dyspepsia is controversial (see later discussion).

Once the decision to treat *H. pylori* infection is made, a regimen should be chosen that meets two important criteria: (1) it must be effective against the organism, and (2) it must be simple and inexpensive enough to ensure patient

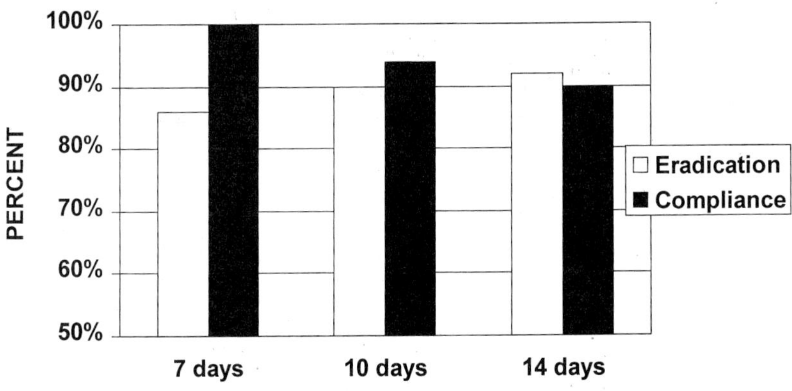

Fig. 102-4. Effect of duration of therapy on compliance and rate of eradication of *Helicobacter pylori*. Oral twice-daily regimen consisted of omeprazole (20 mg), clarithromycin (500 mg), and amoxicillin (1 gm) for 7, 10, or 14 days.

compliance. The first effective therapies against *H. pylori* combined bismuth subsalicylate with two antimicrobial agents, tetracycline and metronidazole. In clinical trials, eradication rates of 77% to 89% were obtained. Although inexpensive, however, this therapy has a complex dosing regimen that decreases compliance outside clinical studies. In addition, the rising rate of metronidazole resistance among strains of *H. pylori* further decreases the efficacy of this regimen, and the need for concurrent antisecretory therapy during treatment of active PUD further increases its cost and complexity.

Dual therapies consisting of a PPI and an oral antibiotic have the advantages of easy use and high compliance. Unfortunately, the combination of amoxicillin and omeprazole has an eradication rate of only 30% to 50% and clarithromycin with omeprazole only 70% to 74%. These low rates of clearance of *H. pylori* make these regimens suboptimal for the treatment of *H. pylori*–associated PUD.

At present, three-drug regimens consisting of clarithromycin, a PPI, and either metronidazole or amoxicillin are the most frequently used therapies for *H. pylori* in the United States. The three agents are given twice daily, which improves compliance, and eradication rates are high (Fig. 102-4). Duration of treatment has an important effect on eradication rates. Although European studies reported clearance rates of 90% to 95% using 7-day regimens, U.S. clinical trials have shown rates less than 90% for 7-day regimens; eradication in 14-day regimens has been as high as 92%, however, even though compliance decreases as duration of therapy increases.[4] The Food and Drug Administration (FDA) has approved the following twice-daily oral regimen for treatment of *H. pylori:* clarithromycin, 500 mg; amoxicillin, 1 gm; and lansoprazole, 30 mg. In practice, any PPI may be used (e.g., omeprazole, 20 mg), and metronidazole (500 mg) may replace amoxicillin, with eradication rates possibly lower in areas where metronidazole-resistant *H. pylori* is prevalent.

COMPLICATIONS OF PEPTIC ULCER DISEASE

Despite a decreasing incidence of PUD, the incidence of the major complications of ulcer disease—hemorrhage (see Chapter 109), ulcer perforation, and gastric outlet obstruction—has not diminished, and the rate of hospitalization for complications of gastric ulcer disease is increasing.

Ulcer Perforation

Perforation of a gastric or duodenal ulcer occurs most often in the fifth or sixth decade of life, with an approximate incidence of 7 to 10 cases/100,000 persons/year. The risk factors for ulcer perforation are similar to those for PUD in general: *H. pylori* infection, NSAID use, and smoking. The use of NSAIDs in particular is associated with a high risk of complications from PUD (hemorrhage and perforation), and although the use of steroids alone is not considered a risk factor for peptic ulcer, the combined use of systemic steroids and NSAIDs carries a significant risk of ulcer complications. The most common presenting symptom of gastric or duodenal ulcer perforation is severe abdominal pain. The pain is sudden in onset and most severe in the epigastrium, but with time the pain may become more diffuse and radiate to the lower quadrants or be referred to the shoulders due to diaphragmatic irritation. Nausea and vomiting may occur, and 10% to 15% of patients present with concomitant gastrointestinal (GI) hemorrhage. A history of prior PUD can be elicited in 60% to 75% of patients.

On examination, patients may have a low-grade fever but are often afebrile. Tachycardia and tachypnea are common, and the abdomen is usually diffusely tender, with signs of peritonitis (guarding, rebound tenderness, or rigidity). Laboratory examination often reveals a mild leukocytosis. Serum amylase is generally normal but may be elevated above 200 Somogyi units in up to 15% of patients. Plain films of the chest and abdomen reveal free air under the diaphragm or on decubitus films in 70% of cases; patients should remain upright or in the decubitus position for 10 to 15 minutes before obtaining these films so that intraperitoneal air can percolate to the highest point. Contrast radiographs are usually unnecessary, but when the diagnosis is unclear, an upper GI series using water-soluble contrast may be helpful.

The treatment of a perforated peptic ulcer is surgical in approximately 95% of patients, and consultation with an experienced surgeon is essential, even if medical management is contemplated. Medical therapy may be considered in patients who meet these criteria: longstanding perforation (more than 24 hours), evidence of a contained perforation on contrast upper GI study, absence of peritoneal signs, and presence of a comorbid illness that significantly increases the risk of operative repair. These criteria apply only to perforated DUs; gastric ulcer perforation should always be managed surgically. Medical management consists of nasogastric suction, intravenous (IV) hydration, and the continuous IV infusion of an H_2RA or pantoprazole.

Gastric Outlet Obstruction

Gastric outlet obstruction is a common complication of PUD, with an incidence ranging from 6% to 21.5%. Effective antisecretory therapy for PUD has decreased the incidence of ulcer-induced obstruction. Case series before 1975 reported PUD as the most common cause of gastric outlet obstruction, whereas more recent studies demonstrate that gastric carcinoma has surpassed PUD as the leading cause of this syndrome. Patients with gastric outlet obstruction generally have a long history of peptic ulcer pain. The obstruction is marked by the onset of nausea and vomiting in about 90% of patients. Additional symptoms include early satiety, bloating, and a sense of fullness in the epigastrium. Patients report progressive weight loss if the obstruction develops slowly, but an acute presentation with dehydration and electrolyte disturbances can occur. Physical examination is remarkable for signs of weight loss and a succussion splash over the epigastrium while the abdomen is shaken from side to side. This sign is present in 25% to 49% of patients with outlet obstruction from any cause. The diagnosis can be confirmed with barium contrast radiography, which reveals a greatly dilated stomach and delayed emptying of contrast from the stomach. Endoscopy is recommended to visualize the gastric outlet and biopsy the obstructed region to look for malignancy.

Initial treatment of gastric outlet obstruction consists of nasogastric suction, IV hydration, antisecretory therapy, and depending on the patient's nutritional status, hyperalimentation. Once a diagnosis of an ulcer-induced benign obstruction is established, a treatment plan is made in consultation with both a gastroenterologist and a GI surgeon. Medical therapy alone may often relieve edema-related obstruction in the short term, although recurrence is common. More definitive therapy can be performed using endoscopic dilation of the stenotic region or a surgical drainage procedure.

GASTRITIS

Gastritis refers to inflammation of the gastric mucosa; it is a nonspecific lesion observed in a number of unrelated disorders. *H. pylori* is responsible for most episodes of gastritis. Acute inflammation with *H. pylori* causes gastric mucosal inflammation that is often asymptomatic but may be associated with mild epigastric discomfort. Persistent infection results in a chronic inflammatory state known as type B gastritis. Usually confined to the antrum, this inflammatory process may extend proximally with time to involve the body and fundus of the stomach as well. *H. pylori* gastritis may also progress to atrophic gastritis, which is associated with transformation into gastric adenocarcinoma in a minority of patients. The natural history of *H. pylori* also includes the development of lymphoproliferative diseases, such as T-cell-derived lymphoma and the rare low-grade, B-cell-derived MALT lymphoma (Fig. 102-5).

Other infectious agents may also cause acute gastritis, and most infections occur in immunocompromised hosts. Among patients with human immunodeficiency (HIV) disease, gastritis caused by herpes simplex virus (HSV) or cytomegalovirus (CMV) infection has been recognized, as has gastritis caused by mycobacterial infections and syphilis. In immunocompetent hosts, bacterial gastritis is uncommon but is often life threatening and associated with systemic sepsis; predominant organisms in these cases include *Streptococcus, Staphylococcus,* and enteric gram-negative rods. In all such patients, treatment consists of appropriate IV antimicrobial therapy, with gastric resection reserved for the most severe cases of bacterial gastritis.

Noninfectious gastritis accounts for most cases of chronic gastritis not attributable to *H. pylori*. The classic type A gastritis is characterized by involvement of the fundus and body, in contrast to the antral predominance of the type B lesion. Type A gastritis is considered autoimmune in origin because it is often associated with circulating antibodies to parietal cells or intrinsic factor and, in many cases, with frank pernicious anemia. This form of gastritis usually progresses to mucosal atrophy, resulting in decreased acid secretion and subsequent hypergastrinemia. Atrophic changes predispose to gastric carcinoma, whereas persistent high gastrin levels are associated with the development of carcinoid tumors.

Other types of chronic gastritis include the eosinophilic and lymphocytic gastritidies, as well as granulomatous gastritis from fungal, mycobacterial, or treponemal infection and rarely from gastric Crohn's disease or sarcoidosis.

NONULCER DYSPEPSIA

The term *dyspepsia* refers to a constellation of symptoms, including upper abdominal pain or discomfort, often accompanied by bloating, abdominal distention, nausea, or early satiety. Despite this vague definition, dyspepsia is a common problem, with a 14% to 26% prevalence. Up to 5% of office visits in general medical practice are for dyspeptic symptoms. The differential diagnosis of dyspepsia is similar

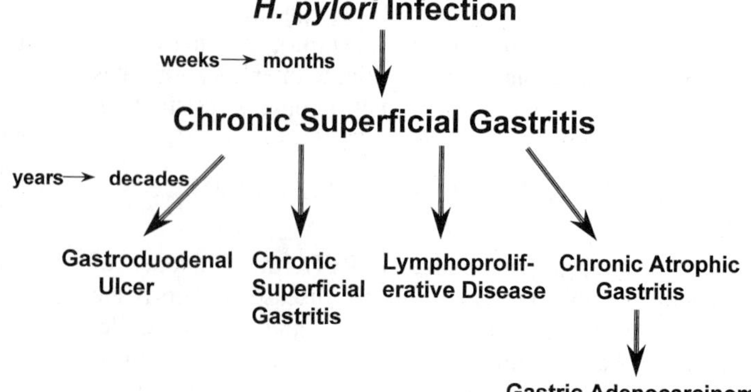

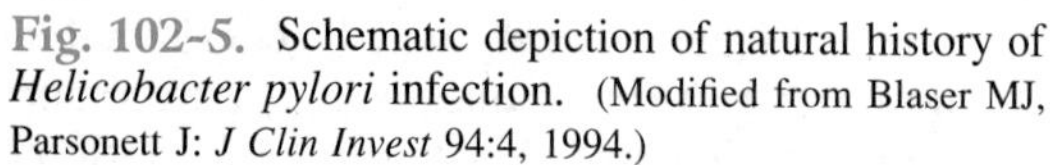
Fig. 102-5. Schematic depiction of natural history of *Helicobacter pylori* infection. (Modified from Blaser MJ, Parsonett J: *J Clin Invest* 94:4, 1994.)

to that of PUD, as detailed earlier. In addition, numerous medications cause dyspepsia, including NSAIDs, antibiotics (most often macrolides and metronidazole), estrogens, narcotics, and digitalis preparations. Certain systemic illnesses may also present with dyspepsia, including hyperthyroidism, hyperparathyroidism, and rheumatologic disorders.

In 40% to 60% of patients with dyspepsia, no organic cause is discovered, a condition known as *functional* (nonulcer) *dyspepsia*. The pathogenesis of this disorder is not well understood and may involve heightened visceral sensitivity to painful stimuli, abnormal gastric and duodenal motility, and psychologic factors. The role of *H. pylori* infection in nonulcer dyspepsia is controversial, but studies show no clear-cut relationship between *H. pylori* status and presence of dyspeptic symptoms (Fig. 102-6).[2,3]

The diagnostic evaluation of dyspepsia begins with a thorough history and physical examination, with particular attention to alarm symptoms and signs that necessitate prompt endoscopic examination. These include *age over 45 years,* weight loss, dysphagia, significant vomiting, a palpable epigastric mass, or guaiac-positive stools. The presence of any of these or the finding of iron deficiency anemia on laboratory examination is associated with a greater prevalence of structural disease (malignancy, PUD) and warrants early endoscopy.

Several strategies have been proposed for the evaluation of dyspepsia in patients younger than 45 without alarm symptoms. The American Gastroenterological Association[1] proposes that dyspeptic patients first undergo serologic testing for *H. pylori* infection. Patients with documented infection are treated empirically; if symptoms fail to resolve within 4 to 8 weeks, endoscopy should be performed. In patients who are *H. pylori* negative, an empiric trial of an H_2RA or PPI or a prokinetic agent for 4 to 8 weeks is recommended, with endoscopy reserved for patients who fail to improve or who relapse after cessation of therapy. This strategy attempts to treat PUD (the cause of dyspepsia in 15% to 20% of patients) without invasive testing. However, the widespread use of antibiotics in dyspeptic patients infected with *H. pylori,* although often advocated, will likely hasten the development of antibiotic-resistant strains of *H. pylori*. In addition, *H. pylori* may be responsible for a smaller proportion of peptic ulcers than originally postulated, further decreasing the effectiveness of empiric treatment. Finally, as noted, the eradication of *H. pylori* improves dyspeptic symptoms in a minority of individuals, if at all (see Fig. 102-6). Thus alternative approaches have been recommended (Fig. 102-7).

Pharmacologic treatment of nonulcer dyspepsia is not well established, and clinical studies have been hampered by differing definitions of symptoms, small patient numbers, and high placebo response rates. Antisecretory agents (H_2RAs, PPIs) may improve dyspeptic symptoms in patients with

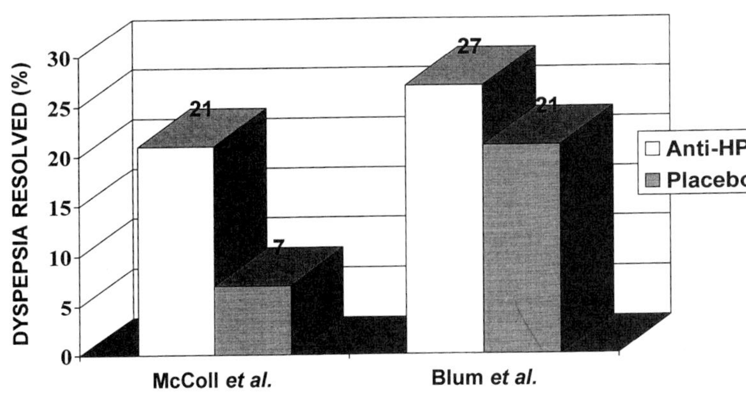

Fig. 102-6. Results of two randomized, controlled trials for treatment of *Helicobacter pylori* (HP) infection in patients with nonulcer dyspepsia. (Data from Blum AL, Tallet NJ, O'Marain C, et al: *N Engl J Med* 339:1875, 1998; and McColl K, Murray L, El-Omar E, et al: *N Engl J Med* 339: 1869, 1998.)

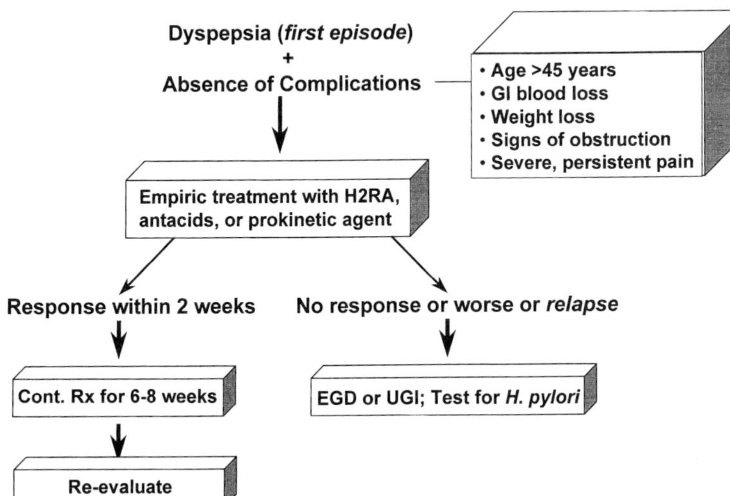

Fig. 102-7. Algorithm for evaluation and treatment of dyspepsia. *H_2RA,* Histamine receptor antagonist (H_2 blocker); *EGD,* esophagogastroduodenoscopy; *UGI,* upper gastrointestinal series.

refluxlike symptoms but not necessarily in those with other symptom complexes. Prokinetic agents, if available, may confer a benefit in dyspeptic patients, with response rates of 65% to 90% vs. 13% to 42% for placebo. Tricyclic antidepressants, effective in several pain syndromes, have not been adequately studied in dyspepsia. In Europe the opioid agonist fedotozine has been shown to be superior to placebo in treating dyspepsia, presumably by decreasing visceral sensitivity to painful stimuli; this agent is not currently available in the United States.

Since drug therapy is not reliably effective in treating nonulcer dyspepsia, the focus of treatment is a supportive physician-patient relationship. After ruling out structural disease and symptoms caused by medications or exogenous agents, the physician should explain to the patient that nonulcer dyspepsia is not psychosomatic but a real disorder likely related to abnormal pain sensitivity of the GI tract. Patients should be reassured that their illness is not life threatening, and the physician and patient should work together to develop a plan for symptomatic relief without multiple diagnostic tests. Stress management, tailoring of diet to avoid symptom-inducing foods, and attention to psychologic factors that may contribute to dyspepsia are important components of therapy. Pharmacologic agents are used with caution because placebo response rates are high and symptoms may recur over time; if a medication proves ineffective, the patient should switch to another agent, since "stacking" of medications is ineffective and costly.

REFERENCES

1. American Gastroenterological Association: Medical position statement: evaluation of dyspepsia, *Gastroenterology* 114:579, 1998.
2. Blum AL, Tallet NJ, O'Marain C, et al: Lack of effect of treating *Helicobacter pylori* infection in patients with nonulcer dyspepsia, *N Engl J Med* 339:1875, 1998.
3. McColl K, Murray L, El-Omar E, et al: Symptomatic benefit from eradicating *Helicobacter pylori* infection in patients with nonulcer dyspepsia, *N Engl J Med* 339:1869, 1998.
4. Walsh JH, Peterson WL: The treatment of *Helicobacter pylori* infection in the management of peptic ulcer disease, *N Engl J Med* 333:984, 1995.

ADDITIONAL READINGS

Blaser MJ, Parsonnet J: Parasitism by the "slow" bacterium *Helicobacter pylori* leads to altered gastric homeostasis and neoplasia, *J Clin Invest* 94:4, 1994.

DeBoer W, Driessen W, Jansz A, Tytgat G: Effect of acid suppression on efficacy of treatment for *Helicobacter pylori* infection, *Lancet* 345:817, 1995.

Feldman M, Burton ME: Histamine$_2$-receptor antagonists: standard therapy for acid-peptic diseases, *N Engl J Med* 323:1672, 1990.

Hansson L-E, Nyren O, Hsing AW, et al: The risk of stomach cancer in patients with gastric or duodenal ulcer disease, *N Engl J Med* 335:242, 1996.

Hawkey CJ, Karrasch JA, Szczepanski L, et al: Omeprazole compared with misoprostol for ulcers associated with nonsteroidal antiinflammatory drugs, *N Engl J Med* 338:727, 1998.

Jaspersen D, Koerner T, Schorr W, et al: *Helicobacter pylori* eradication reduces the rate of rebleeding in ulcer hemorrhage, *Gastrointest Endosc* 41:5, 1995.

Lichtenstein DR, Syngal S, Wolfe MM: Nonsteroidal anti-inflammatory drugs and the gastrointestinal tract: the double-edged sword, *Arthritis Rheum* 38:5, 1995.

NIH Consensus Conference: *Helicobacter pylori* in peptic ulcer disease, *JAMA* 272:65, 1994.

Ofman JJ, Etchason J, Fullerton S, et al: Management strategies for *Helicobacter pylori*–seropositive patients with dyspepsia: clinical and economic consequences, *Ann Intern Med* 126:280, 1997.

Parsonnet J: *Helicobacter pylori* in the stomach: a paradox unmasked, *N Engl J Med* 335:278, 1996.

Raskin JB, White RH, Jackson JE, et al: Misoprostol dosage in the prevention of nonsteroidal anti-inflammatory drug–induced gastric and duodenal ulcers: a comparison of three regimens, *Ann Intern Med* 123:344, 1995.

Rokkas T, Karameris A, Mavrogeorgis A, et al: Eradication of *Helicobacter pylori* reduces the possibility of rebleeding in peptic ulcer disease, *Gastrointest Endosc* 41:1, 1995.

Silverstein FE, Graham DY, Senior JR, et al: Misoprostol reduces serious gastrointestinal complications in patients with rheumatoid arthritis receiving nonsteroidal anti-inflammatory drugs: a randomized, double-blind, placebo-controlled trial, *Ann Intern Med* 123:241, 1995.

Talley NJ, Silverstein MD, Agreus L, et al: AGA technical review: evaluation of dyspepsia, *Gastroenterology* 114:582, 1998.

Vicari JJ, Peek RM, Falk GW, et al: The seroprevalence of *cagA*-positive *Helicobacter pylori* strains in the spectrum of gastroesophageal reflux disease, *Gastroenterology* 115:50, 1998.

Wallace JL: Nonsteroidal anti-inflammatory drugs and gastroenteropathy: the second hundred years, *Gastroenterology* 112:1000, 1997.

Wolfe MM, editor: *Therapy of digestive disorders: a companion to Sleisenger and Fordtran's Gastrointestinal diseases,* Philadelphia, 2000, Saunders.

Wolfe MM, editor: *Gastrointestinal pharmacotherapy,* Philadelphia, 1993, Saunders.

Wolfe MM, Soll AH: The physiology of gastric acid secretion, *N Engl J Med* 319:1707, 1988.

Wolfe MM, Lichtenstein DR, Singh G: Gastrointestinal toxicity of nonsteroidal antiinflammatory drugs, *N Engl J Med* 340:1888, 1999.

Yeomans ND, Tulassay Z, Juhasz L, et al: A comparison of omeprazole with ranitidine for ulcers associated with nonsteroidal antiinflammatory drugs, *N Engl J Med* 338:719, 1998.

CHAPTER 103

Biliary Tract Disease

Nezam H. Afdhal

The major function of the gallbladder is the interprandial storage and concentration of hepatic bile, which consists of cholesterol, bile salts, and phospholipids. Bile is also the major excretory route for excess cholesterol and organic compounds metabolized in the liver. Postprandially, fat in the duodenum results in the release of the hormone cholecystokinin, which in turn triggers contraction of the gallbladder with ejection of concentrated gallbladder bile through the cystic duct and then the ampulla of Vater into the duodenum. The gallbladder is lined by simple absorptive columnar mucosa whose major functions are the absorption of water and the secretion of mucin glycoprotein and hydrogen ions. The majority of disorders of the gallbladder relate to an inability to maintain cholesterol solubility, resulting in gallstones and their complications.

CHOLELITHIASIS

Epidemiology

Because the greatest risk factor for the development of gallstones is increasing age, the incidence of gallstones is on the rise. In the United States, approximately 30 million people have gallstones, and approximately 1 million new cases are diagnosed annually. According to the National

Table 103-1. Pathophysiology of Cholesterol Gallstone Formation in High-risk Patients

High-risk groups	Cholesterol supersaturation of bile	Nucleation	Gallbladder stasis
Female	+	+	+
Pregnancy	++	+	++
Ileal disease (e.g., Crohn's disease)	+++	?	?
Obesity	+++	+	+
Rapid weight loss	++	++	++
Spinal cord injury	+	+	+++
New World Indians (e.g., Pima)	+++	+	+
Diabetes mellitus	+	+	+++
Cholesterol-lowering fibric acid agents (e.g., clofibrate, gemfibrozil, bezafibrate)	++	+	?
Somatostatin analogs (e.g., octreotide)	++	+	+++

Institutes of Health, nearly 900,000 cholecystectomies were performed in 1996, with an estimated health care cost of over $5 billion. Although gallstones can be classified into cholesterol stones and pigmented stones, each with distinct mechanisms of pathogenesis, the vast majority (more than 75%) of gallstones in Western countries are primarily composed of cholesterol.[3]

Pathophysiology

Cholesterol Gallstones. Three simultaneous defects are necessary for cholesterol gallstone formation: (1) secretion of a cholesterol-supersaturated bile by the liver; (2) nucleation of cholesterol monohydrate crystals from gallbladder bile; and (3) gallbladder stasis with an adequate residence time of crystals within the gallbladder so that they can grow to a size that prevents them from being expelled from the biliary tract.[1,2] The majority of patients have all three defects, but in certain clinical situations one particular factor may predominate[3,9] (Table 103-1). Recognition of the pathophysiologic mechanism of gallstone formation in high-risk groups has led to attempts at prophylaxis. Ursodeoxycholic acid, an orally administered, naturally occurring, hydrophilic bile acid, completely prevented gallstone formation in a group of obese patients rapidly undergoing weight loss (more than 20 kg/16 weeks), whereas the incidence was 25% in similar patients receiving placebo. The use of cholecystokinin (CCK) and CCK analogs in long-term total parenteral nutrition (TPN) has been associated with a reduction in gallstone formation secondary to TPN-induced biliary stasis.

Pigmented Stones. Pigmented stones make up approximately 20% to 25% of cases of cholelithiasis in Western industrialized nations. Pigmented stones are more common in elderly patients, in patients after cholecystectomy, and in those who reside in the Orient. Although the two types of pigment stones, brown and black, are primarily composed of calcium bilirubinate, they occur in very different clinical settings. *Black stones* are formed in the gallbladder and are more common in patients with chronic hemolysis, cirrhosis, or alcoholism and in those receiving TPN. Black stones have an irregular surface, are usually small and hard, and consist of fully cross-linked calcium bilirubinate. *Brown stones* are usually formed within the bile ducts, consist of calcium bilirubinate, mucin, and cholesterol, and are often soft and friable. Brown stones are more common in the Orient, particularly in patients with cholangiohepatitis, a condition associated with infection by *Opisthorchis sinensis,* a liver fluke (Fig. 103-1). In the United States, brown stones usually occur in patients after cholecystectomy in which bile may be chronically infected with microorganisms that are able to deconjugate bilirubin, such as *Escherichia coli.*

Biliary Sludge. Biliary sludge is most often identified by ultrasound examination of the gallbladder as echogenic material that layers out in the dependent portion of the gallbladder and is composed of a mixture of mucin, cholesterol crystals, and calcium bilirubinate granules (Fig. 103-2). Previously assumed to be a completely benign, incidental finding usually associated with conditions of impaired gallbladder emptying (e.g., TPN, pregnancy), it is now recognized that 30% of patients with sludge develop gallstones and that biliary sludge can result in complications of gallstone disease (e.g., pancreatitis, cholangitis). In a study of 23 patients on TPN, sludge developed in 30% by 3 weeks, in 50% by 4 weeks, and in 100% after more than 6 weeks. Stones formed in almost half (43%) of patients who developed sludge. Half these patients developed complications necessitating cholecystectomy after a mean of 43 days.[7,8]

Although biliary sludge formed during pregnancy disappears in the majority (60%) of patients after delivery, postpartum ultrasound examinations have demonstrated the persistence of sludge in 20% of patients and the formation of gallstones in the remaining 20%. Therefore biliary sludge should be considered part of the clinically relevant spectrum of gallstone disease. On occasion, especially in patients with idiopathic pancreatitis, sludge may not be visible by imaging tests, and examination of gallbladder bile during endoscopic retrograde cholangiopancreatography (ERCP) for small cholesterol crystals (microlithiasis) is required to make the diagnosis. These patients with recurrent pancreatitis respond well to cholecystectomy.

Clinical Presentation

Gallstones are usually asymptomatic within the gallbladder. They may transiently obstruct the cystic duct, however, producing biliary colic or, with more significant obstruction, cholecystitis and its complications. Stones small enough to pass into the common bile duct may obstruct there; the most

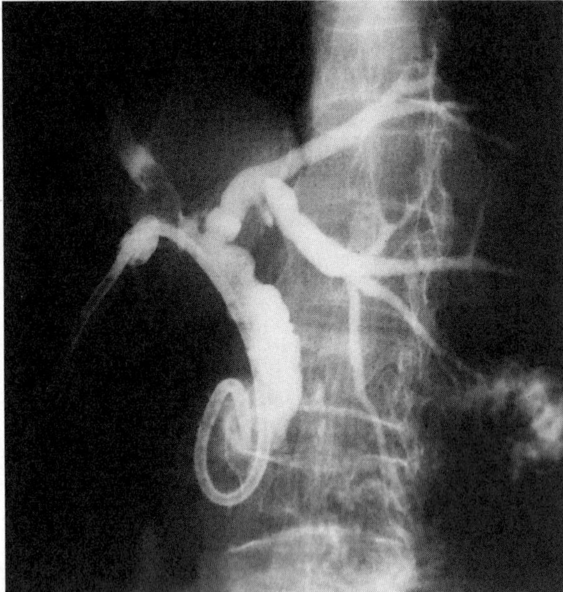

Fig. 103-1. Percutaneous transhepatic cholangiogram after placement of stent across large stone in right hepatic duct, obstructing entire right hepatic system in Chinese immigrant with Oriental cholangiohepatitis.

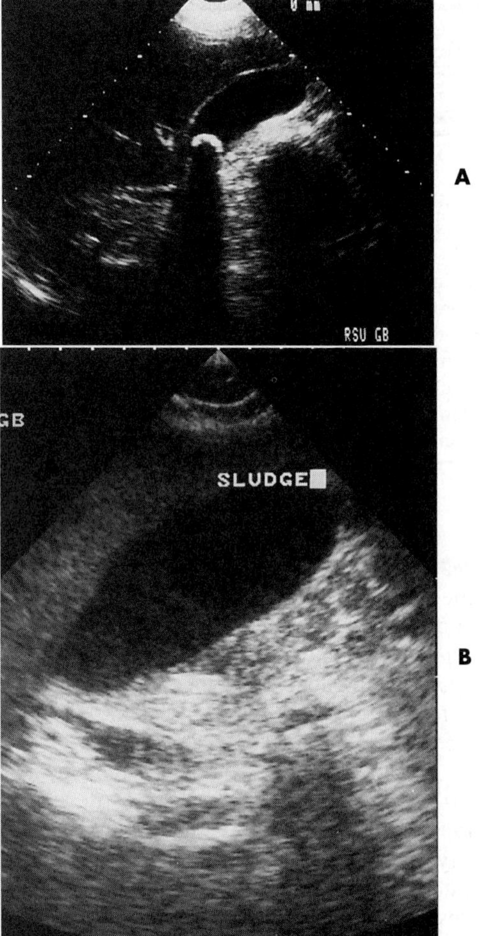

Fig. 103-2. **A,** Longitudinal ultrasound scan of gallbladder demonstrating gallstone. Characteristic shadowing occurs from base of stone. **B,** Longitudinal ultrasound scan demonstrating sludge within gallbladder. Unlike stones, sludge casts no acoustic shadow.

common site is at the ampulla, where obstruction may be associated with the development of cholangitis or gallstone pancreatitis. Since none of the treatments for any of these conditions is without risk, a knowledge of their natural history and the treatment options is essential (Fig. 103-3).[10] The assessment of patients with gallstones is based on whether they are symptomatic.

Asymptomatic Gallstones. Many medical centers once performed a cholecystectomy when gallstones were found, regardless of whether the patient had symptomatic cholelithiasis. This was especially true for patients with diabetes, a condition thought to increase the risk of complications of cholecystitis and cholangitis. In the past 5 years, however, a thorough evaluation of the natural history of asymptomatic gallstones has altered this approach. With rare exceptions, cholecystectomy is not required for most patients with asymptomatic cholelithiasis. Patients with asymptomatic gallbladder stones have a 2% to 3% risk of developing biliary pain each year for the first 10 years after the diagnosis of stones. After 10 years the risk decreases to less than 1% annually. Postmortem studies have demonstrated that of known gallstone patients, the cause of death is related to gallstone disease in fewer than 3%. In general, therefore, surgical treatment for gallstones is recommended only for patients with symptomatic disease.

Symptomatic Gallstones. In patients whose conditions become symptomatic, the most common presentation is *biliary colic.* Biliary colic is not colicky in nature. It is usually steady, intense, and located in the right upper quadrant, although the pain may be referred to the right shoulder or scapular region, the midepigastrium, or elsewhere in the chest or abdomen. Peptic symptoms, belching, bloating, fatty food intolerance, and chronic pain should not be confused with biliary colic. The patient has no associated laboratory abnormalities. In 60% of cases the acute attack resolves spontaneously. Recurrent attacks of pain may occur in up to 70% of patients weeks to years after the initial episode. Biliary complications, such as acute cholecystitis, cholangitis, and gallstone pancreatitis, occur in 10% to 20% of patients with symptomatic gallstones. For these reasons, treatment, usually cholecystectomy, is often advised for patients with symptomatic gallstones.

Diagnosis

Although pain in the right upper quadrant should always raise suspicion for gallstone-related disease, it is not pathognomonic for these conditions (Box 103-1). Acute hepatitis is often associated with pain in this location, which results from acute hepatic inflammation stretching the liver capsule. The liver edge is often tender. Characteristically, transaminase levels in viral or toxin-mediated hepatitis are elevated at least 5 to 10 times normal, compared with less than twice normal in cholecystitis and with normal values in biliary colic. Using the symptom and laboratory complex to differentiate between alcoholic hepatitis and acute cholecystitis, however, can be more difficult. Although alcoholic hepatitis is usually

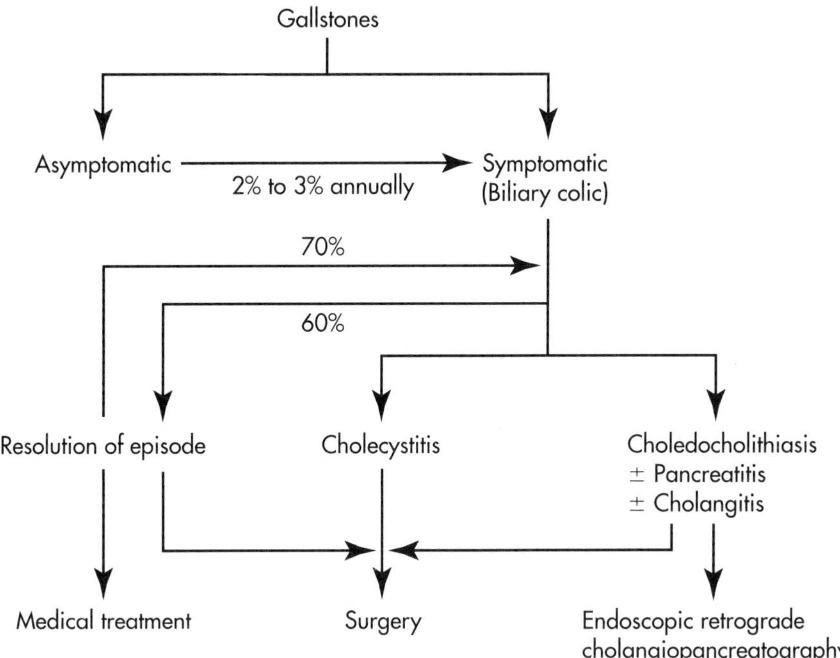

Fig. 103-3. Natural history and management of gallstones.

Box 103-1. Differential Diagnosis of Biliary Pain

Peptic ulcer disease
Acute hepatitis
Renal colic
Appendicitis
Ileitis
Colitis

associated with characteristic hepatic enzyme elevations, both conditions generally produce low levels of transaminases, and both may be associated with fever and leukocytosis. Taking a thorough history is essential. Although classically producing midepigastric pain, peptic ulcer disease may also present with pain in the right upper quadrant. Unlike pain of biliary origin, however, peptic symptoms often improve or resolve with antacid therapy. Rarely, appendicitis, colitis, or terminal ileitis may also present with right upper quadrant pain.

Atypical presentations of biliary tract disease may occur as well. Pain may rarely occur in the right lower quadrant, left upper quadrant, or even the chest, where it may occasionally be confused with angina pectoris.

Management

In general, treatment of gallstone disease is directed at alleviating symptoms and preventing complications. Medical and surgical options for symptomatic gallstone disease have expanded in the last 15 years. Whereas surgery can permanently resolve disease associated with gallbladder stones of any size, number, and makeup, medical therapy can be used only in specific situations, with significant risk of recurrence after discontinuation of therapy. Medical therapy still is occasionally recommended in certain patients, particularly those with extremely high surgical risk.

Surgery. Surgery has historically been the mainstay of treatment for symptomatic gallstone disease. *Cholecystectomy* is generally a very safe procedure with an overall mortality rate of 0.1% to 0.3%. It relieves the characteristic biliary type of pain in approximately 90% of patients and prevents future recurrences. In addition, cholecystectomy is also responsible for the incidental discovery and removal of early gallbladder cancers. Before 1987, cholecystectomy was performed only as an open procedure through one of several possible laparotomy incisions. The operative mortality rates for elective open cholecystectomy in men are estimated at 0.11% for those under age 30, 0.24% for those 31 to 40, 0.54% for those 41 to 50, 1.22% for those 51 to 60, 2.73% for those 61 to 70, 6.15% for those 71 to 80, and 13.84% for those aged 81 to 90.[10] Women are apparently more tolerant of this procedure, since their mortality rates are approximately half those in men at all age groups. Elective ("late") surgery, performed 6 to 8 weeks after an episode of biliary colic or uncomplicated acute cholecystitis, had formerly been preferred over earlier surgery because actively inflamed tissues were believed to complicate surgery and increase the risk of secondary complications. Prospective randomized controlled trials, however, have demonstrated that early surgery is associated with lower morbidity and mortality rates.

Although open cholecystectomy is relatively safe and simple, *laparoscopic cholecystectomy,* first performed in 1987, now accounts for 90% of all cholecystectomies performed in the United States.[11] Laparoscopic surgery reduces patient hospitalization, time away from work, and postoperative pain and complications. Bile duct injuries are no more common with laparoscopic than with open surgery. Conversion from a laparoscopic to an open approach is necessary in approximately 5% of patients because of difficulty in identifying anatomy, excessive bleeding, or intraoperative complications. Open cholecystectomy is still the preferred route in patients with peritonitis, sepsis, severe acute pancreatitis, and end-stage cirrhosis. Initially it was thought that laparoscopic cholecystectomy would reduce the cost of gallstone disease to both the patient and society. Although each patient's unit cost has decreased, however, annual total cholecystectomy costs are rising because of an increase in laparoscopic procedures.

Cholecystectomy should only be performed in symptomatic patients. Large clinical series have confirmed that laparoscopic cholecystectomy is as safe and effective as open cholecystectomy for gallstone disease.[11]

Postcholecystectomy Syndrome. After cholecystectomy, fewer than 5% of patients have recurrent or persistent abdominal pain months to years later. Persistence or early recurrence of pain may imply, however, that the initial diagnosis of gallbladder-related pathology causing the pain was incorrect. Biliary sources of postcholecystectomy pain include retained common bile duct stones, postsurgical bile duct strictures, and sphincter of Oddi dysfunction. Although controversial, sphincter of Oddi dysfunction after cholecystectomy appears to be more common in women and may result in typical biliary pain months to years after surgery. Elevated pressures (greater than 40 mm Hg) within the sphincter of Oddi result in intermittent biliary obstruction at the sphincter's level. In addition to their pain, affected patients may demonstrate: (1) a dilated common bile duct, (2) delayed emptying (more than 45 minutes) of contrast material from the duct after ERCP, and (3) hepatic enzyme elevations (usually low grade), especially during episodes of pain. Approximately 95% of patients with two of the three findings appear to respond to biliary sphincterotomy, with resolution of biliary-type pain.

Medical Therapy. The nonsurgical approaches to gallstone disease include bile acid dissolution therapy and fragmentation of stones with extracorporeal shock wave lithotripsy (ESWL). These approaches offer the benefit of potentially avoiding surgery in patients at high risk of significant morbidity and mortality from cholecystectomy. Nonsurgical measures have important disadvantages, however, especially high recurrence rates after discontinuation of therapy. At present, fewer than 10% of patients with symptomatic gallstones are suitable candidates for nonsurgical therapy.

Bile Acid Dissolution Therapy. Oral dissolution therapy should be considered for patients with suspected cholesterol gallstones and high surgical risk. Oral dissolution agents include ursodeoxycholic acid (UDCA) and chenodeoxycholic acid (CDCA). Although both work by reducing cholesterol secretion into bile and enhancing cholesterol solubilization, UDCA also inhibits cholesterol crystal nucleation. Because these agents have no effect on calcium bilirubinate stones, candidates for therapy should have noncalcified (cholesterol) gallstones. In addition, an oral cholecystogram should reveal a functioning gallbladder and thus these agents' ability to reach the gallbladder lumen. UDCA is more expensive than CDCA, but CDCA may be associated with diarrhea and hepatotoxicity in a significant number of patients. Combination therapy with both agents reduces the cost and diminishes side effects without substantially affecting dissolution rates. The ideal patient for oral dissolution is not obese and has small (less than 1 cm), floating stones. Success rates in such patients are as high as 70% total dissolution at 1 year. Biliary colic is alleviated in the majority of patients, even those who do not have complete dissolution. Gallstone recurrence is about 10% per year over the first 5 years, and the role of maintenance therapy is unclear. Gallstones, when they recur, are often small and again symptomatic.

Contact Dissolution Therapy. Direct instillation into the gallbladder of powerful cholesterol-solubilizing solvents, such as methyltertbutyl ether (MTBE) and ethyl propionate (EP), has been associated with almost 100% dissolution of cholesterol gallstones. A major drawback of this therapy is the need to catheterize the gallbladder directly by a radiologically placed percutaneous catheter. MTBE is more toxic and volatile than EP and can cause damage to the duodenal mucosa, with drowsiness and hemolysis when systemically absorbed. Automated pump systems can decrease operator and patient contact with the solvents, reduce spillage of solvent from the gallbladder, and result in complete dissolution of large stones in hours. If delivery systems can be further perfected, this therapy may benefit critically ill patients unable to withstand surgery.

Extracorporeal Shock Wave Lithotripsy and Oral Bile Acid Therapy. ESWL is similar to that used for fragmentation of renal calculi. Shock waves are produced by lithotriptors and delivered to the gallbladder using ultrasonic guidance. Oral bile acid therapy is begun simultaneously because the resulting stone fragments are more amenable to dissolution therapy and because such therapy promotes bile acid flow for enhanced clearance of stone fragments. ESWL has had variable success; experience in the United States has demonstrated 50% stone clearance, compared with greater than 90% in West Germany.[4] Successful lithotripsy is more likely to occur when stones are radiolucent, solitary, and less than 2 cm in size. Normal gallbladder motility is required for fragment passage. Although the addition of ESWL to dissolution therapy for large stones is theoretically better than either alone, ESWL has risks. Through the process of fragmentation, larger stones become smaller and may more easily pass into the cystic and common bile ducts, where they may cause acute obstruction. In the 6 months after ESWL, severe biliary pain was noted in 1.5%, acute cholecystitis in 1.0%, and acute pancreatitis in 1.5% of patients. Also, the high costs of lithotriptors have made access prohibitive for many centers. Because of these factors, ESWL has not gained its initially expected acceptance.

Complications

Acute Cholecystitis. Acute inflammation of the gallbladder and adjacent peritoneum usually occurs as a result of a stone impaction within the cystic duct. Affected individuals have a history of biliary colic. The pain associated with cholecystitis is similar in location to colic but is usually more severe and persistent, lasting at least 6 hours. In the absence of complications such as gangrene or perforation, fevers are usually low grade and rigors uncommon. The right upper quadrant is very tender, and localized rebound may be present. On examination the patient cannot take a deep breath while the physician's hand is palpating the right upper quadrant because of increased pain as the gallbladder descends to touch the hand (Murphy's sign). Bilirubin levels may be elevated, but jaundice is rare. Transaminase levels are rarely greater than three times normal. Leukocytosis with band forms is common. Radiologic imaging is recommended to confirm the diagnosis and to rule out complications such as gallbladder perforation or gangrenous cholecystitis. Ultrasound usually demonstrates stones, gallbladder distention, wall thickening, and localized edema but is often nondiagnostic. Cholescintigraphy, using ^{99m}Tc-hepatic iminodiacetic acid (HIDA) analogs, is more sensitive than ultrasound for uncomplicated cholecystitis, characteristically demonstrating nonvisualization of the gallbladder in patients with acute cholecystitis. In most cases, however, ultrasound is usually recommended before HIDA scanning because of its added sensitivity in evaluating the anatomy adjacent to the gallbladder. Although most patients with acute cholecystitis respond to conservative management, surgery is recommended because of the high recurrence rate and significant incidence of complications. In patients with a prohibitively high acute surgical risk, a drainage tube can be placed by radiologic guidance into the gallbladder (percutaneous cholecystostomy) during the acute period.

Complications of acute cholecystitis include gangrenous cholecystitis, emphysematous cholecystitis, and gallbladder perforation. Although their presentation is usually associated with a higher incidence of fevers, rigors, and peritoneal signs, these problems may not appear different from those in uncomplicated cholecystitis and thus may not be suspected before surgery. These complications have a significantly increased incidence of morbidity and mortality that necessitates emergency surgery. Gangrenous cholecystitis implies necrosis of the gallbladder wall. The diagnosis is suggested during cholescintigraphy by visualization of a rim of increased radioactivity around the gallbladder and within the adjacent hepatic parenchyma. Diabetic and elderly patients appear to be at increased risk of developing emphysematous cholecystitis, a severe form of acute cholecystitis associated with gas-forming organisms, particularly *Clostridium perfringens*. Emphysematous cholecystitis is suggested by the findings of gas bubbles within the gallbladder wall or lumen on plain radiographs and by irregular, indistinct shadowing from the gallbladder on ultrasound (Fig. 103-4). All diabetic persons with symptoms of acute cholecystitis should have a plain film of the abdomen to search for emphysema. Gangrenous and emphysematous forms of cholecystitis greatly increase the risk of gallbladder perforation.

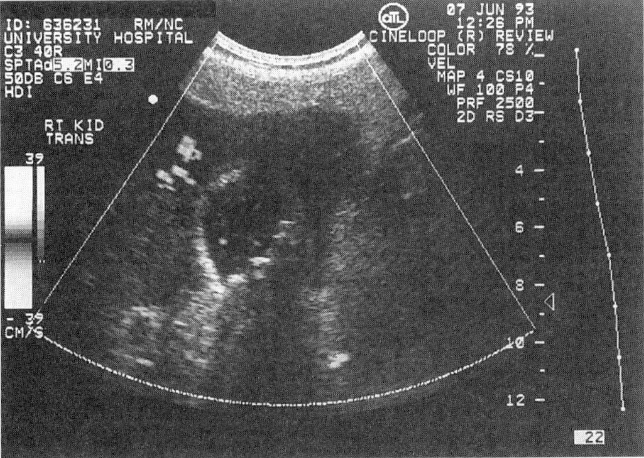

Fig. 103-4. Ultrasound demonstration of air within lumen of gallbladder and adjacent hepatic parenchyma in diabetic patient with emphysematous cholecystitis.

Other complications of calculous cholecystitis include gallstone ileus, a gallstone obstruction of the distal small bowel that usually results from erosion of a gallstone through the gallbladder wall into the duodenal bulb. The most common site of bowel obstruction is the ileocecal valve. Bouveret's syndrome occurs when the stone obstructs the duodenal bulb, producing gastric outlet obstruction. Another rare complication of cholecystitis is Mirizzi's syndrome, in which bile duct obstruction occurs secondary to stone impaction within the cystic duct when the impacted stone and its secondary inflammatory mass impinge on the lumen of the adjacent bile duct.

Choledocholithiasis. Stones within the bile duct usually originate in the gallbladder but may arise de novo (see earlier discussion on brown pigment stones). Up to 15% of patients with cholelithiasis develop choledocholithiasis. Although it is occasionally asymptomatic, the characteristic presentation is jaundice and cholestatic biochemical serum studies. Bilirubin levels rise in proportion to the degree of obstruction, are primarily the direct (conjugated) form, and may be elevated 20 to 30 times normal values. Alkaline phosphatase levels are usually three to six times normal but may be only mildly elevated. In contrast to the generally benign course in most patients with incidentally found gallbladder stones, 25% to 50% of patients with bile duct stones may develop serious complications of obstruction (i.e., cholangitis, gallstone pancreatitis); therefore bile duct stones should always be removed.

Radiologic identification of biliary tract stones is not as sensitive as for gallstones. Ultrasound examinations demonstrate stones within the bile duct in 20% to 50% of cases but have an 80% sensitivity for demonstrating bile duct dilation, a marker for extrahepatic obstruction. Magnetic resonance cholangiography (MRCP) is a novel technique with an ability to detect small stones in the gallbladder comparable to more invasive tests such as ERCP. In experienced centers, MRCP can detect more than 90% of common bile duct stones greater than 5 mm in size. Bile duct dilation occurs in virtually all cases of chronic obstruction (i.e., malignancy) but may take up to 2 weeks to develop in some patients with acute obstruction from stones. Thus a patient with acute obstruction who initially had nondilated ducts on ultrasound may benefit from repeating the examination 2 weeks later. Cholangiography is the most sensitive test for identification of dilation, stones, and other causes of obstruction. Cholangiography can be performed by the gastroenterologist (ERCP), the radiologist (percutaneous transhepatic cholangiography [PTC]), or the surgeon during surgery. ERCP and PTC have very high success rates, can be performed in elective and emergency situations, and can obviate the need for surgery. ERCP is successful in obtaining a cholangiogram in more than 90% of cases and is generally preferred by most patients and physicians because it is more comfortable for the patient and allows for therapeutic intervention during the same session.

Endoscopic stone removal is performed by making a small cut in the ampulla, a sphincterotomy, to enlarge this opening to the bile duct. A basket or balloon can then be introduced into the bile duct through the ERCP scope to clear the duct of stones. In the hands of an experienced endoscopist, this procedure has an 85% to 90% success rate, with complications such as pancreatitis, perforation, and bleeding occurring in 2% to 5% of cases. The most common complication, pancreatitis, occurs in approximately 2% and is usually mild.

PTC is successful in demonstrating the bile ducts in more than 95% of cases when the intrahepatic ducts are dilated but significantly less when they are not. Stones can be removed by choledocholithotomy, but several weeks are required to form a dilated tract across the liver and into the bile duct, through which the stone can be removed or manipulated.

Cholangitis. The biliary tree is normally an open, sterile system that behaves as a closed system when obstructed. Regardless of the cause of obstruction, impaired biliary excretion into the intestine results in jaundice and the spilling of conjugated bilirubin into the urine. When bacteria are introduced into the system, as occurs often with stones and occasionally with malignancy, the resulting closed system behaves as an abscess. In addition to jaundice, the patient develops significant inflammation of the bile duct, often with abdominal pain, intermittent fevers and rigors, and jaundice. These three form the classic symptom triad of cholangitis, referred to as *Charcot's triad.* Although obstructive cholangitis is frequently referred to as pus under pressure, frank pus (suppuration) is not usually seen within the bile duct. The term *suppurative cholangitis,* however, is used to refer to severe cholangitis, regardless of the presence or absence of pus. This condition is an emergency, requiring emergency ductal decompression. *Reynold's pentad,* which adds hypotension and altered mental status to the signs of Charcot's triad, is considered pathognomonic for suppurative cholangitis. Clinical findings suspicious for suppurative cholangitis include fever above 104° F, hypotension, abdominal rebound, leukocytosis greater than 20,000/mm^3, and bilirubin over 9 mg/dl. A mortality rate of 40% has been associated with suppurative cholangitis, compared with 10% in the less toxic cases.

The intermittent fevers and rigors seen with cholangitis are presumed to result from bacteremia. Although the bile in 90% of affected individuals contains many different microbes, blood cultures are positive in 40% of patients and usually for only one strain of organism. The most common organisms are *Escherichia coli* (60%), *Klebsiella pneumoniae* (30% to 40%), *Bacteroides fragilis* (5% to 10%), and *Enterococcus faecalis* (5% to 10%). Initial antibiotic therapy is usually broad based and empiric to cover these organisms. Antibiotic coverage should also be widened to include *Pseudomonas aeruginosa,* if the patient has recently had an ERCP, since scope contamination by *P. aeruginosa* has been reported. Although all patients should receive antibiotic and intravenous fluids, the mainstay of treatment is biliary decompression. This can be achieved by ERCP with sphincterotomy or stone extraction, by stenting (placing a drainage tube across the site of obstruction via the endoscope), by PTC, or by surgery. ERCP or PTC should be used initially. Even when the condition cannot be cured (i.e., by removal of stones), these treatments may allow for long-term palliation of an otherwise moribund patient.

Gallstone Pancreatitis. Overall, approximately 40% of cases of acute pancreatitis are related to choledocholithiasis. Surgical series have demonstrated stones within the biliary tree in up to 75% of patients during the initial presentation of presumed gallstone pancreatitis but in as few as a third of such patients if evaluated after their pancreatitis has improved. The mechanism of pancreatic injury may be that of elevated pressure within the pancreatic duct as a result of more distal obstruction from stones and secondary inflammation.

The physician should suspect "gallstone" pancreatitis when a patient with acute, often recurrent pancreatitis has a present or past history of gallstones or common bile duct stones, especially when there are no other known risk factors for pancreatitis. Although patients classically complain of epigastric pain radiating to the back with nausea, vomiting, and anorexia, the symptoms and physical findings may be difficult to differentiate from those of acute cholecystitis. Acute cholecystitis occurs concomitantly with gallstone pancreatitis 5% of the time, so serum amylase levels should be measured in all patients with presumed cholecystitis. Elevation of alkaline phosphatase or bilirubin levels at the onset of an attack of pancreatitis often suggests gallstone pancreatitis but may also occur secondary to compression of the intrapancreatic portion of the common bile duct as it passes through an inflamed pancreas.

The diagnosis of gallstone pancreatitis is confirmed by cholangiography, usually by ERCP. Since the optimal timing for ERCP and possible sphincterotomy was controversial, however, studies compared early (within 24 to 72 hours of admission) vs. late ERCP with or without papillotomy for pancreatitis presumed secondary to choledocholithiasis. Complications, including biliary sepsis and death, were reduced when ERCP was performed early in patients with moderate to severe pancreatitis. A similar effect was shown for mild pancreatitis as well. When performed within 72 hours of admission in patients with severe pancreatitis, early intervention with ERCP also significantly reduced the length of hospitalization.[6]

Based on these results, the present recommendation is ERCP with possible sphincterotomy performed within 48 hours of the onset of moderate to severe pancreatitis presumed secondary to choledocholithiasis. The treatment of mild pancreatitis is primarily supportive care. Affected patients require aggressive fluid resuscitation because of sequestration of fluids into the inflamed retroperitoneum and their inability to eat. Conservative management alone in patients with mild pancreatitis is associated with a success rate of approximately 80%.

ACALCULOUS DISEASES OF THE GALLBLADDER

Acute Acalculous Cholecystitis

Overall, approximately 5% to 15% of patients with acute cholecystitis have acalculous disease, but estimates are as high as 87% and 50%, respectively, in patients with acute cholecystitis postoperatively and in children. Most patients are older (over 55), and gender does not affect the incidence. Acalculous cholecystitis is most often seen in the intensive care unit in patients with multiorgan system failure, trauma (especially after major surgery), burns, and sepsis. Although in most patients the pathogenesis is unclear and is likely multifactorial in origin, the process is believed to be one of secondary infection in a functionally obstructed gallbladder. Rarely, primary infections of the gallbladder with *Salmonella* and *Candida* organisms and cytomegalovirus may cause this condition in patients with severe immunosuppression.

Regardless of the etiology, however, the clinical scenario is similar to that of acute calculous cholecystitis. Patients may become bacteremic and septic if the condition is not treated promptly. Delays in diagnosis or treatment have led to a high incidence of complications (e.g., gangrene, empyema, perforation) before surgery. The mortality rate may be at least twice as high in acalculous cholecystitis as in calculous disease because of the high incidence of comorbid conditions and the delay in diagnosis. The timely diagnosis of acute acalculous cholecystitis requires awareness of this entity and suspicion. Laboratory findings are similar to those seen in acute calculous cholecystitis; most patients demonstrate leukocytosis and mild elevations in the alkaline phosphatase, bilirubin, and transaminase levels. HIDA scanning confirms the diagnosis, and ultrasound may detect complications. Optimal treatment is emergency cholecystectomy, but a percutaneous cholecystectomy is alternative therapy in patients with extremely high surgical risk.

Hyperplastic Cholecytoses

Hyperplastic cholecytoses represent abnormalities of the gallbladder wall with an unclear etiology. They are usually clinically silent but may be associated with symptoms of cholelithiasis that respond to cholecystectomy. These conditions may be associated with the formation of nodules. When large in size, they may present as a fundal "polyp" on gallbladder ultrasound or oral cholecystogram. The most common forms of hyperplastic cholecytoses are cholesterolosis and adenomyomatosis. *Gallbladder cholesterolosis,* or *cholesterosis,* involves deposition of triglycerides and cholesterol within the gallbladder wall. These yellowish deposits lying within a mildly inflamed, reddened background have given rise to the term *strawberry gallbladder.* The deposits may form small polypoid projections that can break off and serve as seeds for gallstone formation. Gallstones are seen in 10% to 15% of patients with cholesterolosis, but this condition is present in a minority of all patients with gallstones. *Adenomyomatosis,* or *adenomyosis,* implies hyperplasia of the gallbladder mucosa and muscular coat. Gallbladder wall thickening can increase three to five times that of normal gallbladders. Intramural diverticula, crypts, or sinus tracts (Rokitansky-Aschoff sinuses) may be seen on ultrasound of the gallbladder, and adenomyosis may present as localized, segmental, or diffuse disease. The localized disease may produce a nodule that is sometimes referred to as an *adenomyoma,* a pseudotumor with no potential for neoplasia. The segmental form produces a constricting ring or septum in the fundus or body, and the diffuse form produces generalized thickening of the gallbladder wall. *Hyalocalcinosis,* also referred to as the *porcelain gallbladder* because of its eggshell appearance on plain film, ultrasound, or computed tomography (CT) scan, has been associated with a 22% chance of developing gallbladder cancer. Prophylactic cholecystectomy is generally recommended in these patients.

GALLBLADDER NEOPLASIA

Gallbladder cancer is the fifth most frequent digestive tract cancer. Epidemiologic studies have demonstrated an association between gallbladder cancer and gallstones. The risk associated with stones larger than 3 cm is estimated to be nine times that of 1-cm stones. Certain ethnic groups, in particular Native Americans and Mexicans, have increased risk over the general population. The risk is also increased in patients with the porcelain gallbladder and with anomalous connections between biliary and pancreatic ducts.

Primary gallbladder cancers are usually adenocarcinomas and are thought to arise in adenomatous polyps. Polyp size appears to be an important risk factor for the presence of carcinoma. In one study, all benign adenomas were less than 12 mm in diameter, whereas those with carcinomatous foci were greater than 12 mm. Most invasive carcinomas were more than 30 mm in diameter. The prognosis associated with gallbladder cancer is uniformly poor when the process has extended beyond the gallbladder wall, with 5-year survival rates of less than 5%. Although distant metastasis of the tumors occurs late, aggressive local extension of the disease along the biliary tract and into the liver is seen very early. This, in combination with late diagnosis, accounts for the poor survival. In general, surgery is curative only when a carcinoma is found incidentally during routine cholecystectomy for other indications. Curative surgery often involves not only cholecystectomy but also segmental or local liver resection. Because of the aggressive nature of this disease, its poor outcome, and the inability radiologically to differentiate early gallbladder cancers arising in a polyp from benign polyps or pseudotumors (as may occur in the hypertrophic cholecystoses), cholecystectomy should be performed when ultrasound or CT scanning demonstrates a focal, irregular thickening of the gallbladder wall or a polyp. Prophylactic cholecystectomy should be considered in patients with porcelain gallbladders and perhaps in young Native Americans with very large gallstones. Chemotherapeutic trials for gallbladder cancer have demonstrated no benefit. The use of external beam radiation therapy and local radiotherapy using implantable iridium (^{192}Ir) wires for patients with localized disease and pain or jaundice is being evaluated.

REFERENCES

1. Afdhal NH, Smith BF: Pathogenesis of cholesterol gallstones, *View Dig Dis* 22:13, 1990.
2. Apstein MD, Carey MC: Pathogenesis of cholesterol gallstones: a parsimonious hypothesis, *Eur J Clin Invest* 26:343, 1996.
3. Attili AF, Capocaccia R, et al: Factors associated with gallstone disease in the MICOL experience: Multicenter Italian Study on Epidemiology of Cholelithiasis, *Hepatology* 26:809, 1997.
4. Barkun ANG, Ponchon T: Extracorporeal biliary lithotripsy, *Ann Intern Med* 112:126, 1990.
5. Donohue JH, Stewart AK, et al: "The National Cancer Data Base Report on carcinoma of the gallbladder, 1989-1995, *Cancer* 83:2618, 1998.
6. Fan S-T et al: Early treatment of acute biliary pancreatitis by endoscopic papillotomy, *N Engl J Med* 328:228, 1993.
7. Ko CW, Sekijima JH, et al: Biliary sludge, *Ann Intern Med* 130:301, 1999.
8. Lee SP, Nicholls JF, Park HZ: Biliary sludge as a cause of acute pancreatitis, *N Engl J Med* 326:589, 1992.
9. Misciagna G, Centonze S, et al: Diet, physical activity, and gallstones: a population-based, case-control study in southern Italy, *Am J Clin Nutr* 69:120, 1999.
10. Ransahoff DF, Gracie WA: Treatment of gallstones, *Ann Intern Med* 119:606, 1993.
11. Steiner CA, Bass EB, Talamini MA, et al: Surgical rates and operative mortality from open and laparoscopic cholecystectomy in Maryland, *N Engl J Med* 330:403, 1994.

CHAPTER 104

Liver Disease

Raymond S. Koff

GENERAL DIAGNOSIS

Accurate diagnosis and optimal management of patients with liver disease are common concerns of primary care physicians. Since liver diseases are prevalent and screening tests for liver disease are widely available, both symptomatic and asymptomatic patients often seek assistance. Effective approaches are essential to avoid diagnostic or management errors. Clinical assessment has been enhanced by the development of serologic tests for viral hepatitis, noninvasive hepatobiliary imaging, and increased sophistication in the use of invasive procedures.

Unconjugated Hyperbilirubinemias

Hyperbilirubinemias result from overproduction of bilirubin, impaired hepatic uptake, and impaired conjugation of bilirubin in the absence of intrinsic liver disease. They are suspected in the jaundiced patient whose urine is normal in color and lacking in detectable bilirubin. Causes of bilirubin overproduction include hemolysis, ineffective erythropoiesis, and breakdown of large hematomas. When evidence of these is absent and the patient seems generally healthy, impaired bilirubin uptake and conjugation resulting from *Gilbert syndrome* are suspected. In Gilbert syndrome, other liver tests are usually normal, a family history of unconjugated hyperbilirubinemia may be present, and fasting for 2 or more days may raise the serum bilirubin to levels that trigger recognition of jaundice. Patients should be reassured that they do not have a serious disorder. Affected patients should carry identification indicating that they have Gilbert syndrome.

Cholestatic Syndromes

Decreased flow of hepatic bile is known as *cholestasis* (Box 104-1). The associated pruritus, presumably related to serum retention and sequestration in the skin of poorly defined pruritogenic bile salts, may be extremely distressing. Intrahepatic cholestasis results from parenchymal liver disease or disorders affecting the small intrahepatic bile ducts. Extrahepatic biliary obstruction leading to cholestasis may result from stones, strictures, or cancer in larger bile ducts. Cholestasis is accompanied by elevation of serum bilirubin, bile acids, cholesterol, and alkaline phosphatase. Serum aminotransferase levels are usually only slightly elevated, and serum albumin is at near-normal levels. Malabsorption of fat-soluble vitamins may result from inadequate bile salt micelle formation, leading to hypoprothrombinemia that is responsive to parenteral administration of vitamin K. If cholestasis is prolonged, vitamin D deficiency may result in osteomalacia.

Drug-induced liver injury, alcoholic hepatitis, and acute viral hepatitis top the list of likely causes of intrahepatic cholestasis. Primary biliary cirrhosis, postoperative intrahepatic cholestasis, and gram-negative or gram-positive septicemia should also be considered. *It is critical to distinguish patients with intrahepatic cholestasis from those with extrahepatic bile duct obstruction, who may require surgery.* In addition to the clinical and laboratory manifestations of cholestasis, patients with extrahepatic cholestasis are at risk for ascending cholangitis, with fever, chills, and right upper quadrant pain. After many months or years of unrelieved extrahepatic obstruction, secondary biliary cirrhosis may develop.

In all patients with jaundice, ultrasonographic examination of the biliary tree to detect dilation of ducts, presence of gallstones, and level of anatomic obstruction is the first step. Ductal dilation may be found in as many as 90% of patients with extrahepatic obstruction of 2 or more weeks' duration. In patients with obstruction of shorter duration, dilation of the ducts may not be detected. If evidence of obstruction is present on ultrasonography or if obstruction is still suspected despite absence of ductal dilation, endoscopic retrograde cannulation of the common bile duct and pancreatic ducts is undertaken for diagnosis and possible endoscopic intervention (i.e., removal of impacted stones). If ultrasonography and cholangiographic techniques indicate the absence of extrahepatic cholestasis, needle biopsy of the liver may provide a specific diagnosis of intrinsic liver disease.

ACUTE HEPATITIS

Viral hepatitis is encountered often in the office and clinic; more than 250,000 new infections occur annually in the United States. The major objectives of management are supportive care of the symptomatic patient and interruption of hepatitis transmission by patient education and, where available, by immunoprophylaxis.

Etiology and Epidemiology

Most cases of acute viral hepatitis seen in clinical practice in the United States result from hepatitis A virus (HAV), hepatitis B virus (HBV), and hepatitis C virus (HCV) (Fig. 104-1). A very small proportion of reported HBV infections actually may be coinfections with the hepatitis D virus (HDV), a defective virus requiring the simultaneous presence of HBV for its expression. Although rare in the United States,

Box 104-1. Clinical and Laboratory Features of Cholestasis

Clinical Features

Jaundice
Dark urine
Light-colored stools
Pruritus

Laboratory Features

Increased serum bilirubin
Increased serum bile acids
Increased serum cholesterol
Increased serum alkaline phosphatase
Slight increase in serum alanine (ALT) and aspartate (AST) transaminases
Prolonged prothrombin time (PT)
Normal serum albumin

infections resulting from hepatitis E virus (HEV) are common in developing nations.

In addition to acute infection, HBV, HDV, and HCV may result in persistent infection associated with chronic hepatitis, cirrhosis, and an increased risk of hepatocellular carcinoma, one of the most prevalent nondermatologic malignancies in the world. In contrast, HAV and HEV infections do not lead to persistent infection.

Hepatitis A Virus. Infection by HAV, a 27-nm picornavirus containing ribonucleic acid (RNA), leads to the formation of a specific antibody: anti-HAV. In acute-phase sera, anti-HAV belongs to the immunoglobulin M (IgM) class, whereas in convalescent sera, immunoglobulin G (IgG) anti-HAV predominates. Anti-HAV confers prolonged, probably lifelong immunity to reinfection. The incubation period of HAV infection is about 30 days; viremia is short-lived and occurs during the late incubation period and early acute phase. Fecal shedding of HAV is more prolonged, beginning during the second half of the incubation period and persisting for several days and rarely for weeks after the onset of symptoms or jaundice. Peak fecal HAV shedding and maximal communicability occur at the onset of illness in most patients. Fecal-oral spread is the predominant mode of HAV transmission and is responsible for community-wide outbreaks[4] (Table 104-1). HAV outbreaks have occurred in day-care centers, neonatal intensive care units, and institutions, as well as among injection drug users (IDUs), homosexual and bisexual men, and recipients of certain clotting factor concentrates. Contaminated water and foods, such as raw or inadequately cooked clams, oysters, and mussels, have been implicated in common-source epidemics. Parenteral transmission of HAV appears to be rare because of the brief period of viremia, although outbreaks among IDUs are well known. Maternal-neonatal HAV transmission is not an established epidemiologic entity.

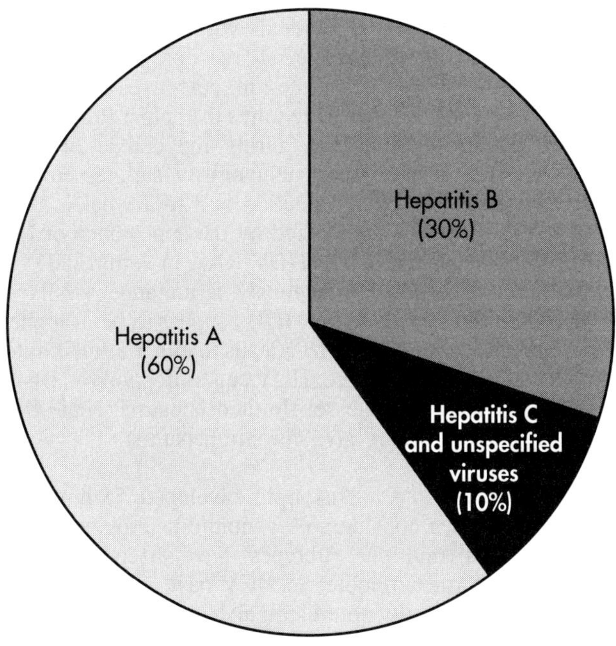

Fig. 104-1. Acute viral hepatitis in United States. Hepatitis A is now the predominant etiologic form.

Hepatitis E Virus. HEV, a 32-nm agent believed to belong to the alpha-like supergroup of RNA viruses, is responsible for large waterborne outbreaks of hepatitis in developing nations; it is the most common cause of sporadic hepatitis in young adults in the third world. Pregnant women who acquire HEV infection appear to be at very high risk for acute liver failure. Cases in the United States are seen in travelers or visitors from endemic regions. The incubation period is about 6 weeks, with a range of 2 to 9 weeks. Assays for serologic identification of anti-HEV are available.

Hepatitis B Virus. Although this 42-nm virus has not been efficiently propagated in cell culture, cloning of HBV deoxyribonucleic acid (DNA) in bacteria and yeast has permitted expression of HBV antigens. The surface of HBV contains a specific antigenic material, the hepatitis B surface antigen (HBsAg), which is also found in excess of the intact virus in the form of smaller 22-nm spheres and tubular particles in the circulation of HBV-infected patients (Fig. 104-2). HBV DNA and the hepatitis B core antigen (HBcAg) have been identified in the core of the virus. The HBeAg, derived from HBcAg, is found in the serum of most individuals with active HBV replication. HBsAg is the first serologic marker of HBV to appear and precedes elevation of the serum alanine aminotransferase (ALT). HBeAg appears a few days to a week or so later but disappears well before HBsAg (Fig. 104-3). HBeAg is detected only in HBsAg-positive sera and is a marker of infectivity. In one HBV variant, however, HBeAg is not expressed but viral replication still occurs. Antibody to HBeAg (anti-HBe) becomes detectable as HBeAg declines in titer.

Table 104-1. Routes of Hepatitis Virus Transmission

Mode of spread	HAV	HEV	HBV	HDV	HCV
Percutaneous					
Inoculation	Injection drug users	No	Yes	Yes	Yes
Transfusion	Very rare	No	Uncommon		Rare since 1992
Permucosal					
Fecal-oral	Community-wide outbreaks	Waterborne outbreaks	No	No	No
Sexual	Homosexual and bisexual men	No	Yes	Yes	Low frequency
Maternal-neonatal	No	Rare	Yes	Yes	Low frequency

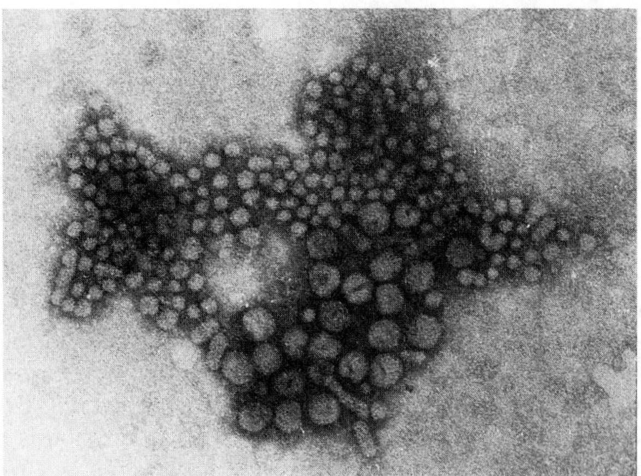

Fig. 104-2. Hepatitis B virus. Small particles are composed of hepatitis B surface antigen. Large particles are intact viruses. (Original magnification × 130,000.)

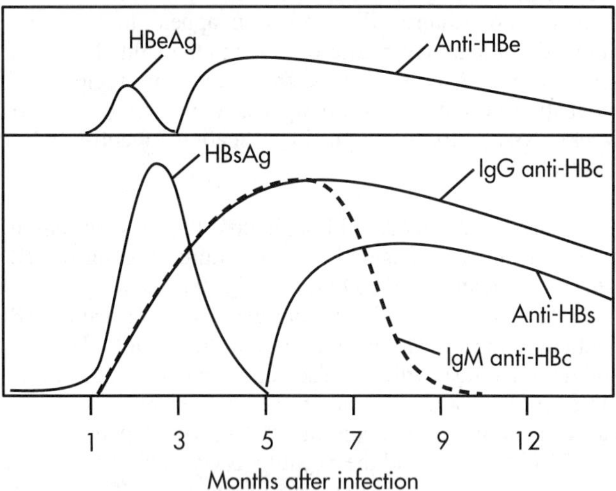

Fig. 104-3. Sequential appearance of serologic markers in acute hepatitis B infection. See text for abbreviations.

IgM antibody to HBcAg (IgM anti-HBc) appears in sera after HBsAg and HBeAg become detectable and persists for several months. It is replaced by an IgG anti-HBc, which persists for decades. In some patients, HBsAg may no longer be detectable during the acute phase of infection. In this circumstance, IgM anti-HBc is invariably present. Antibody to HBsAg (anti-HBs) is the last serologic marker of HBV to appear, usually in the late convalescent phase. This antibody is neutralizing, persists for decades, and is highly correlated with immunity to reinfection. HBV infection is self-limited in 95% to 98% of adults, and persistent infection occurs more often in neonates, infants, and young children.[6] Persistent infection is characterized by the prolonged presence of HBsAg and anti-HBc with little or no detectable anti-HBs. Some carriers are asymptomatic; others have chronic hepatitis. The prevalence of the carrier state varies widely, but 0.2% to 0.5% of the U.S. population are HBsAg positive. Among Asian-Americans, Pacific islanders, Native Alaskans, IDUs, homosexual men, and immunosuppressed populations, the carrier rate may exceed 5%.

The long incubation period of HBV infection, averaging from 60 to 90 days, is responsible for the efficiency of blood-borne spread. Viremia begins late in the incubation and persists for several weeks to months or, in the case of individuals destined to become carriers, years. Although screening of blood donors for HBsAg has dramatically reduced the frequency of transfusion-associated HBV infection, transfusion of blood products that cannot be sterilized, injection drug use, and accidental needle sticks or splashing accidents in unvaccinated health care workers remain sources of HBV transmission. Permucosal transfer of HBV plays an even more important role. HBV has been identified in semen, menstrual blood, and saliva, and transmission from acutely infected patients and HBsAg carriers has been established by follow-up study of their sexual contacts. Permucosal transfer during parturition is responsible for maternal-neonatal spread. Women who are HBsAg carriers, particularly those who are HBeAg positive, and women with acute disease in the third trimester may infect their infants. Since infection early in life often results in persistent infection, maternal-neonatal spread serves to perpetuate HBV infection in successive generations. Neither food nor water has been implicated in the spread of HBV.

Hepatitis D Virus. Individuals with acute or persistent HBV infection appear to be at risk of coinfection or superinfection with HDV, a 36-nm defective agent. This HBsAg-enveloped RNA virus requires the helper functions of HBV for its expression, and during the course of HDV infection, HBV replication is temporarily suppressed. The incubation period of HDV infection is 3 to 7 weeks. Acute HDV infection can be recognized by the appearance of IgM anti-HDV, HDV antigen, and HDV RNA in serum. HDV is believed to be spread percutaneously, in a manner similar to HBV, and in the United States, IDUs appear to be at highest risk. HDV coinfection with HBV leads to either a self-limited hepatitis or acute liver failure. HDV superinfection of HBsAg carriers may lead to acute self-limited hepatitis, acute liver failure, or rapidly progressive chronic hepatitis.

Hepatitis C Virus. This lipid-enveloped 55-nm RNA virus demonstrates considerable genomic heterogeneity. Six genotypes and multiple subtypes have been identified. Current assays for antibodies to HCV have 95% sensitivity and specificity but do not distinguish between active and resolved infections. Polymerase chain reaction (PCR) amplification to detect HCV RNA in serum permits the identification of viremia. Viremic patients may be acutely infected or may have chronic infection. Although HCV usually has an incubation period of about 7 to 10 weeks, the range is extremely wide. HCV has been identified in serum during the late incubation period, the acute phase of illness, and for prolonged periods after convalescence in those with persistent infection. HCV RNA has been identified in hepatocytes and lymphocytes; HCV may be present in low concentrations in some body fluids.

HCV is a blood-borne pathogen spread predominantly by percutaneous transmission. Injection drug use, cocaine snorting, maintenance hemodialysis, and transfusion before 1992 are known risk factors. However, the introduction of anti-HCV screening of blood donors has dramatically reduced the frequency of transfusion-associated HCV infection. Sexual transmission occurs but is less common than with HBV. Maternal-neonatal spread occurs infrequently unless the mother is also HIV positive or has high titers of HCV RNA. Tattooing and body piercing may also be risk factors.

Clinical Presentation and Natural History

The spectrum of illness in acute viral hepatitis is broad. Many patients have no recognized clinical illness and do not seek care. In others the presence of viral hepatitis may be signaled by recognition of biochemical abnormalities or serologic markers of recent infection. Patients with anicteric illness may have transient gastrointestinal (GI) or upper respiratory symptoms suggestive of a nonspecific viral infection, short-lived anorexia and fatigue, and a day or two of fever. The decision to seek medical aid is often delayed and then canceled as the illness wanes. In contrast, viral hepatitis with jaundice has a longer, more striking clinical presentation, although it is usually self-limited as well. The illness may begin with a prodrome of malaise, anorexia, nausea and vomiting, fatigue, influenza-like symptoms, diarrhea, arthralgias, right upper quadrant abdominal discomfort, low-grade fever, and distaste for or actual aversion to cigarettes and their smoke. This may last a few days to a few weeks. A transient syndrome resembling serum sickness with polyarthritis, urticaria or maculopapular rashes, angioneurotic edema, and hematuria may be the earliest manifestation of hepatitis B but is unusual in the other infections. Deposition of immune complexes in the joints, skin, small blood vessels, and kidneys appears to be responsible.

Prodromal symptoms resolve with the development of jaundice, which is usually preceded by the appearance of dark-brown urine. Mild hepatic enlargement with mild tenderness is typical, and the spleen is enlarged in about 20%. Jaundice typically is maximal during the second week after onset and then disappears during the next 2 to 8 weeks, marking clinical recovery in most patients. Symptomatic improvement occurs concomitantly with the resolution of the biochemical abnormalities.

The natural history of acute viral hepatitis remains incompletely defined (Table 104-2). HAV infection, whether silent or symptomatic with or without jaundice, is rarely fatal (fatalities from acute liver failure are seen in about 2% of patients over 40 years old). In symptomatic HBV infection with jaundice the case fatality rate approaches 1% and is adversely influenced by increasing age, debility, the coexistence of malignancy, and coinfection or superinfection with HDV. HCV is rarely associated with acute liver failure. Persistent infection, chronic hepatitis, cirrhosis, and hepatocellular carcinoma are sequelae of HBV, HDV, and HCV infections.

Table 104-2. Natural History of Viral Hepatitis

Outcome or sequela	Estimated frequency (%)				
	HAV	HEV	HBV	HDV	HCV
Complete recovery	>99	>90-99*	95-97	95	15
Acute liver failure	<0.1-2	<1-10	1	1-2	<0.1
Persistent viremia	0	0	2-5†	1-5	85
Chronic hepatitis	0	0	1-3	1-5	75
Progression to cirrhosis	0	0	33	33-50	2-20
Progression from cirrhosis to hepatocellular carcinoma	0	0	5-40	5-40‡	15-40

*Among pregnant women, case fatality rates may exceed 10% in acute HEV infection.
†Carrier rates of 50%-80% may follow HBV infection in neonates and infants.
‡HDV infection may promote the development of hepatocellular carcinoma in HBV-infected chronic hepatitis/cirrhosis patients.

Laboratory Studies

During the prodrome and early acute phase of the illness, leukocyte counts may be normal or low normal. Atypical lymphocytes may be seen. Serum aminotransferase elevations are detected during the prodrome and rise progressively. ALT levels are usually higher than those of aspartate aminotransferase (AST). In icteric patients, serum bilirubin levels usually peak in the second week of the acute illness and vary between 5 and 20 mg/dl. Serum alkaline phosphatase levels are either normal or mildly increased. Serum albumin is usually normal or slightly decreased, whereas serum globulins may be mildly elevated. The prothrombin time (PT) is normal or minimally prolonged, usually to within a few seconds over the control values. Serologic studies defining the responsible virus are undertaken during the acute phase of illness and, if necessary, during convalescence (Table 104-3).

The presence of anti-HAV of the IgM class in acute-phase sera is diagnostic for acute HAV infection. Anti-HAV of the IgG class is a marker of prior HAV infection. The presence of HBsAg or, if HBsAg is absent, IgM anti-HBc in acute-phase sera is indicative of HBV infection. The development of anti-HBs in late convalescent-phase sera is also indicative of HBV infection or immunization to HBsAg (see Prevention). The diagnosis of HDV infection is only considered in HBsAg-positive individuals. Diagnosis of acute HCV infection requires detection of anti-HCV or HCV RNA.

Clinical Variants

Acute Liver Failure. The most dreaded variant of viral hepatitis, acute liver failure, is seen almost exclusively in patients with symptomatic hepatitis with jaundice and is characterized histopathologically by massive hepatic necrosis. Acute liver failure is manifested by signs of hepatic encephalopathy accompanied by profound PT prolongation. Decreased liver size is a characteristic feature, and GI bleeding and ascites are common complications. The course in 65% to 95% of patients is rapidly downhill, with death occurring in 1 to 4 weeks of onset. Early referral for liver transplant is mandatory. Sepsis, cerebral edema, respiratory and renal failure, and refractory hypotension punctuate the course and contribute to the mortality. Hypoglycemia is observed in about 5% of patients. Survivors have no evidence of chronic liver disease.

Cholestatic Hepatitis. This uncommon variant is usually caused by HAV infection. Serum bilirubin levels as high as 30 mg/dl and severe pruritus may persist for many weeks, although other symptoms of hepatitis are less prominent. Serum ALT levels are elevated early in the course but may decline with time, whereas serum alkaline phosphatase levels

Table 104-3. Serologic Diagnosis of Viral Hepatitis

Agent	Acute phase	Convalescence
HAV	Presence of IgM anti-HAV	Development of IgG anti-HAV
HEV	Presence of IgM anti-HEV and/or HEV RNA	Loss of HEV RNA; development of IgG anti-HEV
HBV	Presence of HBsAg and/or IgM anti-HBc	Loss of HBsAg: development of anti-HBs and IgG anti-HBc
HDV	Presence of HDV RNA or HDV antigen or IgM anti-HDV in HBsAg-positive patient	Loss of HDV RNA or antigen; development of IgG anti-HDV or loss of anti-HDV
HCV	Presence or development of anti-HCV, presence of HCV RNA	Loss of HCV RNA

may remain elevated by twofold to sixfold. Although the course is prolonged, the prognosis is excellent, with full recovery anticipated. If the diagnosis of viral hepatitis cannot be confirmed by serologic studies, further studies are necessary to exclude other causes of cholestasis.

Relapsing Hepatitis. Several weeks to a few months after clinical recovery from acute hepatitis, recurrent symptoms and liver test abnormalities may be detected. HAV appears to be the most common virus associated with relapsing disease. During the relapse, IgM anti-HAV remains positive, and fecal shedding of HAV may recur. Despite the prolonged course and multiple relapses in some patients, full recovery is invariable, and chronic hepatitis is not seen. Cutaneous vasculitis and arthralgias may occur in some patients.

Consultation and Hospitalization

Most patients with uncomplicated viral hepatitis are managed at home. Consultation with a specialist is necessary for patients with severe clinical variants (e.g., acute liver failure) for whom a gastroenterologist-hepatologist may expedite management. Referral is also reasonable when the diagnosis remains uncertain after initial evaluation and observation. Hospitalization is restricted to those few patients with dehydration as a result of persistent vomiting in whom parenteral fluids are given until adequate oral intake can be resumed. Hospitalization is also indicated for patients with acute liver failure.

Management

Typical Viral Hepatitis. Treatment is largely supportive. The goals are to provide adequate nutrition, reduce discomfort and distressing symptoms, avoid exposure to known or suspected hepatotoxic drugs, and interrupt transmission of infection when possible (see Prevention). Limited experience with HCV suggests that treatment with α-interferon during the acute phase may reduce the risk of chronic infection. Interferon treatment of other forms of acute viral hepatitis is not recommended. Monitoring is necessary to identify clinical variants and to intervene as needed. A clear discussion of the illness, its typical course, and reassurance about the generally self-limited nature of the disorder may reduce anxiety and prevent psychogenic disability.

Adequate caloric intake of a balanced diet may require multiple small meals. Because anorexia and nausea usually worsen during the day, breakfasts are often best tolerated, and the bulk of calories may be consumed in the morning. Self-selection of foods is usually highly satisfactory, and no foods need to be restricted on medical grounds. High-protein diets have no important influence on recovery rates. Enforced bed rest has no value, but if fatigue is extreme, bed rest for a few days may be beneficial. Mild physical exercise is generally well tolerated. Restrictions in physical activity are progressively lifted as symptoms diminish, the sense of well-being returns, and biochemical studies reflect waning of the hepatitis. Complete resumption of normal activities should not be hampered by the persistence of minor ALT or AST elevations during convalescence.

All nonessential medications are discontinued. Oral contraceptives may be continued during the illness, however, and do not adversely influence the course. Alcohol ingestion is prohibited until the convalescent phase, when social use may be resumed without harm. Corticosteroid therapy has no benefit. Drug treatment of severe nausea and vomiting remains unsatisfactory. For patients who cannot retain oral fluids or food, home health care or brief hospitalization is required. Intravenous glucose with supplemental potassium, sodium, thiamine, and vitamin B complex is used to restore body water, provide calories, and maintain electrolyte balance.

Monitoring the course of hepatitis requires semiweekly or weekly visits to the physician's office or clinic, supplemented by telephone contact. At each visit, symptoms and physical findings are reviewed and serum bilirubin, ALT, and PT measured. Progressive PT prolongation necessitates further evaluation for severe disease. When the clinical illness is over, further monitoring is done at 3 months to determine, in the case of HBV, that HBsAg has cleared and ALT levels are once again normal. Persistent abnormalities after HBV or HCV infection may be rechecked at 6 months and, if present, require further evaluation for chronic hepatitis.

Clinical Variants

Acute Liver Failure. Patients with liver failure should be hospitalized in centers with liver transplantation programs as soon as their illness is identified. Previous survival rates of 10% to 35% are now 65% to 70% if liver transplantation is promptly performed before the development of irreversible brain injury.

Cholestatic Hepatitis. No specific therapy is available. Pruritus may respond to oral administration of the anion-exchange resin cholestyramine or to treatment with ursodeoxycholic acid. A brief course of corticosteroids may accelerate recovery.

Box 104-2. High-risk Groups Recommended for Hepatitis A Immunoprophylaxis

Travelers to endemic regions
Military and peace-keeping personnel
Sewage and waste water plant workers
Caregivers of children
Injection drug users
Men who have sex with men
Food handlers in endemic areas
Patients with chronic liver diseases
Patients with clotting disorders

Prevention

HAV Infection. Immunoglobulin may be given as postexposure immunoprophylaxis (0.02 ml/kg) to household and intimate contacts of an index case within 2 weeks of exposure. Protective efficacy approaches 90%, and the duration of protection is about 2 to 3 months. Casual contact is not an indication for prophylaxis. Preexposure immunoprophylaxis with inactivated HAV vaccine is recommended for high-risk populations (Box 104-2). Protective efficacy for HAV vaccines in the preexposure setting should approach 100%, and protection may last 10 to 20 or more years. HAV vaccines may also be effective in the control of community-wide, common-source, and institutional outbreaks. Transient pain at the injection site is the major adverse effect of HAV vaccine.

HEV Infection. Passive immunoprophylaxis is not available. A recombinant vaccine is under study.

HBV Infection. Universal preexposure immunization with recombinant HBV vaccine (HBsAg subunit vaccine) of neonates, infants, children, and adolescents through 18 years of age may eventually result in HBV eradication in the United States.[6,7] Until that time, postexposure prevention will continue to require use of hepatitis B immunoglobulin (HBIG), containing large amounts of anti-HBs, together with HBV vaccine. This is indicated in three major settings: (1) after accidental inoculation, ingestion, or splashing of HBV-positive blood or secretions onto mucous membranes or conjunctivae in nonvaccinated individuals; (2) for the susceptible sexual contacts of the acutely infected patient; and (3) for the neonate of HBsAg-positive mothers. In the first two settings, intramuscular HBIG (0.04 to 0.07 ml/kg) is given as early as possible and may be repeated 1 month later. For the neonate at risk, HBIG (0.5 ml) is given shortly after birth (within hours) and HBV vaccine administered in a three-or four-dose schedule beginning early within the first week of life. Combined immunization can prevent 95% of neonatal infections.

Preexposure immunoprophylaxis with HBV vaccine is recommended for certain patient groups and high-risk populations (Box 104-3). Preexposure HBV vaccine protective efficacy rates are about 90% to 95%. They are administered intramuscularly, into the deltoid or, in infants, the anterolateral thigh muscle. In the three-dose schedule, after the initial injection a second injection is given at 1 month and a third 6 to 12 months after the first. In the four-dose schedule the third dose is given 2 months after the first, and the fourth is given 12 months after the first. The recombinant vaccines induce seroprotective levels of anti-HBs in more than 95% of recipients. Booster doses are recommended only in immunosuppressed patients whose antibody levels fall below the seroprotective threshold. Except for transient soreness at the injection site in 10% to 15% and fever of less than 24-hours' duration in fewer than 3%, no important adverse reactions have been attributed to the vaccine.

Box 104-3. Patient and High-risk Groups Recommended For Preexposure Hepatitis B Immunoprophylaxis

Patient Groups

Neonates/infants of HBsAg-negative women

Catch-Up Vaccination of Adolescents (Through 18 Years of Age)

High-risk Populations

Family/household contacts of HBsAg carriers
Health care workers
Homosexual and bisexual men
Individuals with multiple sexual partners or sexually transmitted diseases
Injection drug users
Patients with non-HBV chronic liver disease
Patients with hemophilia or thalassemia
Hemodialysis patients
Prisoners
Pacific islanders and Native Alaskans

HDV Infection. Active immunization against HBV is the only current method of preventing HDV infection.

HCV Infection. Conventional immunoglobulin preparations are ineffective. A hyperimmune globulin and a prototype recombinant vaccine are currently in early trials.

Drug-induced Hepatitis

Drug-associated liver disease may simulate acute viral hepatitis and its variants or extrahepatic bile duct obstruction. It may also induce chronic liver disease, including chronic hepatitis, cirrhosis, granulomatous disease, and even malignant disorders of the liver.

Because drug hepatotoxicity is often severe and rarely anticipated, the physician should document all drug exposures in any patient with abnormal liver tests or jaundice. All prescribed and over-the-counter medications, including herbal remedies, vitamins, and food supplements, regardless of where purchased, are enumerated. Consumption of medications prescribed for other household members should be questioned. Although most drug-induced hepatotoxicity occurs within the first few months after the drug is taken, hepatic injury may not become manifest until after several months of drug use. Rarely, drug-induced injury is seen after a year or more of drug use.

Liver disease induced by drugs is occasionally accompanied by extrahepatic clinical manifestations that can cause confusion with other forms of liver disease. For example, the presence of rash, arthralgias, and fever may be seen in liver injury resulting from sensitizing drugs as well as in viral hepatitis. The absence of extrahepatic features, however, does not exclude drug-induced hepatotoxicity. Similarly, although the presence of eosinophilia suggests drug sensitivity, it is not an invariable finding.

Practitioners must become familiar with the hepatotoxicity of commonly prescribed drugs and maintain a high index of suspicion when dealing with less well-known and newer agents. If liver injury is recognized, all nonessential drugs are discontinued. Although consistent with drug-induced disease, improvement is not necessarily diagnostic, and further evaluation for other causes of liver disease is necessary. Drug rechallenge is potentially dangerous, requires informed consent, and should not be undertaken unless the drug is essential and cannot be substituted. Drug rechallenge is rarely required for the patient's care. Suspected drug-induced liver injury should be reported to the pharmaceutical manufacturer and to the Food and Drug Administration (FDA) on their adverse-reaction forms.

After discontinuation of the suspected drug, liver tests should be sequentially measured to ascertain that improvement in laboratory studies occurs concomitantly with clinical improvement. Many patients show clinical and biochemical improvement within a few days of drug discontinuation. For some drugs, however, liver injury progresses and peaks at variable times thereafter; acute liver failure occasionally ensues. Progression of disease for more than a few days after drug discontinuation requires reassessment to ensure that other hepatic disorders have not been missed. Referral to a gastroenterologist-hepatologist is appropriate.

Clinically important drug-induced liver disease should be distinguished from transient minor aminotransferase elevations in the asymptomatic patient. A number of drugs, in many different therapeutic classes, may produce minor increases in serum enzyme levels in as many as 15% of patients during the first several weeks of treatment. This adaptive phenomenon, in which enzyme levels may be as high as two or three times the upper limits of normal, is not a precursor of symptomatic drug hepatotoxicity. If the patient is asymptomatic when the abnormality is found, the drug may be continued if (1) it is still needed, (2) enzyme levels are sequentially measured and do not exceed three times the upper limit of normal, and (3) the patient fails to develop symptoms suggestive of hepatotoxicity. The drug must be immediately discontinued if these conditions cannot be met.

Alcoholic Hepatitis

Although a form of drug-induced liver disease, the contribution of alcoholic hepatitis to the development, morbidity, and mortality of cirrhosis mandate that it receive special attention. Management of the patient with alcoholic hepatitis presents issues that are distinctly different from those concerned with viral or drug-induced hepatitis.

Epidemiology and Pathophysiology. Alcoholic liver disease is one of the most common causes of liver disease in the United States, and alcoholic hepatitis, both as a precursor and a part of alcoholic cirrhosis, is responsible for a large proportion of hospital admissions for alcohol-related liver disease, including many of those directly related to cirrhosis and its complications. In contrast to alcoholic fatty liver, which is a universal feature of excessive alcohol consumption, alcoholic hepatitis is seen in only about 10% to 20% of heavy imbibers. The bulk of men with recognized alcoholic hepatitis have consumed more than 70 gm of alcohol daily for more than 10 years.[2] In women the threshold appears to be as low as 20 to 40 gm for the same period. The role of malnutrition or nutrient deficiency in the pathophysiology remains to be established. Direct ethanol toxicity, mediated by acetaldehyde and acetaldehyde adducts, may play a role in the initiation of liver injury, but perpetuation of injury may be linked to cell-mediated immune mechanisms.

Clinical Presentation and Natural History. Early in alcoholic hepatitis, most patients are asymptomatic. Denial of excessive alcohol ingestion is common, and family members may be unaware of the patient's alcohol abuse. Minor abnormalities of liver chemistries (e.g., AST elevations with normal ALT levels) may provide the sole clue to the presence of liver disease. In some patients a workup for pancreatitis or erosive gastritis may reveal incidental evidence of alcoholic hepatitis. In other patients the diagnosis of alcoholic liver disease is preceded by hepatitis-like complaints, such as anorexia, nausea, vomiting, abdominal pain, malaise, fever, and weight loss. Jaundice may be striking, particularly in patients who have had repeated bouts of alcoholic hepatitis superimposed on alcoholic cirrhosis. The clinical picture occasionally resembles that of extrahepatic bile duct obstruction. There is a broad spectrum of severity, and case fatality rates of 2% to 10% are reported. Hepatomegaly with or without mild tenderness is a characteristic feature of alcoholic hepatitis. Spider angiomas are common, and ascites may be present in as many as 25% of patients without cirrhosis. When cirrhosis is present, the frequency of ascites in alcoholic hepatitis may exceed 80%.

With discontinuation of alcohol, most patients recover over weeks to months. If cirrhosis is absent and abstinence is maintained, the lesion is reversible. In some patients, particularly those with underlying alcoholic cirrhosis, the disease is rapidly progressive over weeks and ultimately leads to death from hepatic failure despite alcohol withdrawal. In as many as one quarter to one third of patients with alcoholic hepatitis, markers of active HCV infection may be present. The degree to which chronic HCV infection contributes to the morbidity and mortality of alcoholic liver disease remains to be determined.

Complications and Clinical Variants. The major complication of alcoholic hepatitis is the development of alcoholic cirrhosis. Even in the absence of cirrhosis, evidence of portal hypertension may be recognized. Ascites, splenomegaly, and esophagogastric varices may reflect elevation of portal venous pressure because of the combined effects of perivenular fibrosis, venoocclusive disease, hepatic inflammation, hepatic triglyceride accumulation, and increased hepatocyte water content. The management of portal hypertension and its manifestations in alcoholic hepatitis is identical to that for portal hypertension in the cirrhotic patient. However, to the extent that the underlying lesions of alcoholic hepatitis are reversible with abstinence, portal pressure falls and clinical manifestations of portal hypertension abate.

Alcoholic hepatitis may simulate extrahepatic biliary tract obstruction. The presence of jaundice, fever, leukocytosis, and liver tests compatible with cholestasis suggests ascending cholangitis. Painless, unrecognized pancreatitis leading to compression of the common bile duct may be responsible for a few such cases. In a smaller number of patients, choledocholithiasis resulting from gallstones may be responsible. In most patients with alcoholic hepatitis, evaluation with ultrasonography fails to disclose bile duct dilation, and cholangiography confirms the absence of an obstructing anatomic lesion. Evidence of cholestasis subsides with resolution of alcoholic hepatitis. The precise mechanism responsible for cholestasis in these patients remains to be established.

Laboratory Studies. Anemia is present in about two thirds of patients and reflects folate deficiency, alcohol-induced marrow depression, iron deficiency secondary to GI bleeding as a result of alcoholic gastritis, or hemolysis. Even without folate deficiency or reticulocytosis the mean corpuscular volume of the red cell may be strikingly increased. Leukopenia may occur (10% to 20%), and leukocytosis is seen in about 40% of patients. A leukemoid reaction is seen in fewer than 5%. Thrombocytopenia may be present in about 10% to 15%. Serum bilirubin is elevated, but the range of values may be extreme, and levels exceeding 30 mg/dl are found in about 10% of patients. In about 80% to 90% the serum AST level is at least twice as high as the ALT, which is often normal or only slightly elevated. Peak levels of AST exceed 300 IU in fewer than 10% of patients. The serum alkaline phosphatase is usually elevated, often to levels two or three times the upper limit of normal. Serum albumin levels may be depressed, and globulins are elevated because of increases in IgG and IgA levels. PT is prolonged in severe disease.

Consultation and Hospitalization. Liver biopsy is useful in confirming the diagnosis and in determining the reversibility of the liver lesion. Consultation is also necessary when the clinical picture suggests extrahepatic bile duct obstruction. Hospitalization is necessary for symptomatic patients who have fever, persistent vomiting, or signs of hepatic failure (e.g., hepatic encephalopathy). Home management is particularly difficult because cessation of alcohol ingestion can rarely be ensured, and failure to improve may indicate continuing alcohol consumption. Consultation with an alcoholism treatment program may be initiated during hospitalization or on an ambulatory basis.

Management. Specific drug therapy is not available. Mortality of severe alcoholic hepatitis is manifested by spontaneous hepatic encephalopathy and a calculated discriminant function greater than 32 based on the serum bilirubin and prothrombin time (PT), as follows:

Discriminant function =
4.6 × (Patient's PT in seconds − Control PT in seconds) +
Serum bilirubin (mg/dl)

Discriminant function of 32 or greater is associated with a 50% case fatality rate in alcoholic hepatitis. This value can be reduced with corticosteroids. The efficacy of corticosteroid treatment is reduced in patients with acute GI bleeding. The major objectives of management are to ensure alcohol withdrawal, provide supportive care during the symptomatic illness, and offer extended counseling and intensive medical supervision supporting continued abstinence.

CHRONIC LIVER DISEASE

Chronic Viral Hepatitis

Chronic viral hepatitis refers to a virus-induced necroinflammatory disorder persisting for more than 6 months. It is characterized histopathologically by the presence of hepatocyte necrosis, a dense mononuclear and plasma cell infiltration of the portal triads variably spilling into the adjacent parenchyma, with or without fibrosis. Progression of fibrosis, with distortion of the normal hepatic architecture and development of cirrhosis, is seen in some patients. Patients with chronic viral hepatitis, particularly those with cirrhosis, also are at risk for the development of hepatocellular carcinoma.

Epidemiology and Etiology. Chronic viral hepatitis attributed to persistent HBV, HBV/HDV, and HCV infections is the major cause of nonalcoholic chronic hepatitis in the United States. No more than 5% of adult patients with acute HBV infection will develop chronic hepatitis B. As many as 85% of patients with HCV infection, however, develop chronic hepatitis C. Approximately 40% of the chronic viral hepatitis cases in the United States are attributable to HCV infection, about 25% to HBV infection, and about 5% to HBV and HDV infection. The remainder are attributed to currently unknown agents.

Clinical Presentation and Natural History. Many patients with chronic viral hepatitis are asymptomatic or have nonspecific symptoms such as fatigue. In a small percentage, end-stage liver disease, with the complications of cirrhosis, may be the earliest clinical manifestation of the disease. Some patients may be identified on follow-up after acute viral hepatitis, and their serum ALT levels remain elevated or fluctuate in and out of the normal range for prolonged periods. Multiphasic health screening tests demonstrating elevation of serum ALT or positive tests for HBsAg or anti-HCV may be the sole abnormalities pointing to the presence of chronic viral hepatitis. Other patients are identified through blood donor screening programs. Recently, public education programs designed to identify and test individuals with a history of risk factors for the acquisition of HCV or HBV have been endorsed by government agencies.

Although chronic viral hepatitis can remain clinically and biochemically unchanged over many years, the disease may progress silently to cirrhosis after decades. In a very small proportion of patients the disease is rapidly progressive, and evidence of hepatic failure or cirrhosis manifests within 5 years. As many as 50% of patients with chronic hepatitis B may develop cirrhosis; 10% to 20% of those with chronic hepatitis C develop cirrhosis. A large number of HBV-infected individuals with detectable HBsAg have repeatedly normal biochemical tests and little evidence of disease on liver biopsy. These "healthy" HBsAg carriers represent the largest reservoir of HBV-infected and infectious individuals. Although patients are at risk for important sequelae, the natural history of the HBsAg carrier state remains incompletely defined.

Laboratory Studies. Serum aminotransferase levels are variably elevated and occasionally may be normal, even on sequential studies. Peak serum ALT levels are usually increased less than tenfold. Serum AST levels are equal to or lower than the ALT levels. Hyperbilirubinemia is variable, and many patients have normal levels. If present, increases in serum alkaline phosphatase levels are usually mild. Hypoalbuminemia and PT prolongation are found in severe disease.

Diagnosis. Criteria for the diagnosis of chronic viral hepatitis include laboratory documentation of liver disease for 6 or more months. Persistently elevated or fluctuating serum ALT levels may be sufficient to raise suspicion of chronic viral hepatitis. In patients with chronic hepatitis B, tests for HBsAg are positive, and in those with biochemically active disease, HBeAg and HBV DNA are usually detected. In a small proportion of patients with HBsAg-positive chronic hepatitis, positive tests for HDV infection indicate superinfection by this agent. HBsAg-positive, HBV DNA–positive, chronic hepatitis B patients without HBeAg are infected by a HBV variant (the precore mutation). Positive tests for anti-HCV and the presence of HCV RNA are characteristically found in chronic hepatitis C. Liver biopsy may be undertaken to confirm the diagnosis and to assess the severity of the lesion but is not a requirement for the initiation of therapy.

Management. Consultation is necessary for liver biopsy, for patients with clinical or biochemical evidence of incipient hepatic failure, and for initiation of antiviral therapy.

HBV Infection. Treatment with injections of 5 million units (daily) or 10 million units (three times weekly) of interferon alfa-2b for 4 to 6 months is indicated for patients with compensated chronic hepatitis B, who have HBeAg and HBV DNA and elevated serum aminotransferase levels.[3] Treatment has resulted in HBV clearance, biochemical resolution, and histologic improvement in 30% to 40% of patients. These responses are maintained for at least a decade and probably longer. During treatment, adverse reactions are common and include a flulike syndrome, bone marrow suppression, and depression. Patients must be monitored frequently, and dose reductions may be necessary in as many as 25% of treated patients. Unfortunately, interferon treatment of patients with HBV and HDV chronic hepatitis has produced few sustained responses. Patients with decompensated disease, signs of liver failure, GI bleeding, ascites, or encephalopathy should not be treated except by experienced investigators following a defined protocol.

Treatment with other antiviral drugs (e.g., lamivudine) is well tolerated and apparently as effective as interferon-α in chronic hepatitis B. Long-term maintenance therapy may be required and drug resistance frequently develops.

HBsAg Carriers. Counseling of the carrier and the family is necessary to avoid maladaptive anxiety reactions, depression, and the social isolation responses associated with stigmatization of the carrier as someone with inordinately high personal health risks and high risks of infectivity. The HBsAg carrier state is not invariably lifelong, however, and HBsAg may be cleared with time. Effective antiviral or immunologic measures to accelerate clearance of HBV in carriers without active liver disease are not yet available. Susceptible household and family members living with carriers and neonates of carrier women should receive the HBV vaccine.

HCV Infection. Treatment of patients with compensated chronic hepatitis C with interferon-α, 3 million units or 9 μg per injection (depending on the preparation) three times weekly for 12 months, produces a sustained biochemical and virologic response in about 10% to 20% 6 months after treatment. Higher doses, daily therapy, pegylated interferons (interferon attached to polyethylene glycol [PEG] for slow, sustained release), and combination therapy with the guanosine analog ribavirin may increase the sustained response rate to 40% or even higher in some patient groups. Retreatment of relapsed patients may result in a sustained response in about 50%. In contrast, retreatment of nonresponders to an initial course of interferon has been disappointing.

Liver Transplantation. In patients with life-threatening, end-stage chronic hepatitis B in whom HBV replication is active, liver transplantation is not curative, and the newly grafted liver is likely to be infected. An accelerated course of HBV infection may lead to liver failure and the need for recurrent transplantation. Immunotherapy with hepatitis B immune globulin and antiviral treatment with interferon or lamivudine may reduce or postpone the risk of graft infection. In contrast, although HCV infection may recur when transplantation is undertaken in the patient with end-stage chronic hepatitis C, clinically important injury of the graft is uncommon. Treatment to reduce the risk of posttransplant chronic hepatitis C in the new liver is under study.

Autoimmune Hepatitis

Autoimmune hepatitis is a chronic, progressive, inflammatory disease of the liver of unknown etiology, predominantly affecting young women and frequently associated with hypergammaglobulinemia.[5] Several markers of autoimmunity and extrahepatic autoimmune manifestations may be present, suggesting an immunologically mediated disorder; a response to immunosuppressive therapy also is characteristic.

Etiology and Classification. Autoimmune hepatitis may take a variety of serologic forms, based on the presence of different autoantibodies. The best known is *classic* autoimmune hepatitis, also known as *type I* autoimmune hepatitis, a disease found predominantly in women and associated with antinuclear and anti–smooth muscle (antiactin) antibodies. Evidence of genetic susceptibility and an association with HLA-A1-B8-DR3 haplotypes has been found.

Clinical Presentation and Natural History. Jaundice and fatigue accompanied by extrahepatic manifestations of systemic disease may be presenting features. Abdominal pain, severe acne, arthralgias or polyarthritis, amenorrhea, pleuritic pain, diarrhea, and fever may be prominent. In the absence of jaundice these features may fail to raise the suspicion of underlying liver disease unless hepatomegaly or splenomegaly is detected. In the fully expressed disorder, jaundice is present in as many as 80% of patients, hepatomegaly is found in a similar percentage, and the spleen is enlarged in about 50%. Spider angiomas may be present, and signs of portal hypertension (e.g., ascites) may develop. Complications of cirrhosis may be presenting features or sequelae.

The course of the disease is variable. Inactive phases may occur in as many as 20% of untreated patients, and the lesion may resolve before the development of cirrhosis. However, severe disease, if untreated, is associated with high morbidity and mortality, particularly within the first few years after diagnosis. Approximately one third of patients succumb to hepatic failure within 5 years, and about three-fourths have died at the end of 10 years, if untreated.

Laboratory Studies and Diagnosis. Anemia, leukopenia, and thrombocytopenia may be present and may reflect hypersplenism. Elevations of gamma globulin and IgG levels are typically found. High titers of antinuclear and anti–smooth muscle antibodies are typical. Liver biopsy reveals the lesions of chronic hepatitis with or without cirrhosis.

Differential Diagnosis. Drug-induced chronic hepatitis may closely simulate autoimmune hepatitis. In general, implicated drugs cause an acute hepatitis–like illness; women are at highest risk, and regression usually occurs after cessation of the offending drug. Drugs associated with chronic hepatitis include isoniazid, nitrofurantoin, and phenytoin. Chronic viral hepatitis must be considered, as well as other disorders that may masquerade as autoimmune hepatitis, such as Wilson's disease and α_1-antitrypsin deficiency. Iron overload may be considered, although the serum aminotransferase levels tend to be lower than in autoimmune hepatitis.

Management. Corticosteroids with or without azathioprine are the mainstays of treatment. In severe disease, corticosteroid treatment prolongs life but may not reduce the risk of progression to cirrhosis. Side effects temper enthusiasm for corticosteroid therapy, and prednisone-azathioprine regimens require frequent white cell and platelet counts to monitor for azathioprine toxicity.

Therapy may be initiated with high-dose prednisone (60 mg) daily, moderate-dose prednisone (30 mg), or even a maintenance dose of 10 to 20 mg. Azathioprine may be added from the beginning or shortly thereafter. The high-dose and moderate-dose prednisone regimens are tapered to maintenance levels (10 to 20 mg) over 4 to 8 weeks. Symptomatic improvement on these regimens is expected within 3 months and biochemical remission within 6 months. Histologic remission may be delayed for 1 to 2 years. Treatment should be continued for 1 to 2 years before an attempt is made to discontinue therapy. Relapse is common, and repeated courses or maintenance regimens may be needed. After induction of remission with prednisone and azathioprine, prednisone may be discontinued, and azathioprine alone may maintain remission in some patients. Liver transplantation has been successful for patients with end-stage liver disease. Recurrence is uncommon.

Cirrhosis

Cirrhosis is one of the 10 leading causes of death for both sexes in the United States. Cirrhosis implies irreversible hepatic injury in which diffuse disorganization of the lobular architecture results from the combined effects of connective tissue proliferation and nodular regeneration of surviving hepatocytes. Hepatic necrosis and inflammation appear to be responsible for collapse and collagenization (fibrosis) of the reticulin framework of hepatocyte cords. Total liver cell mass is reduced. Distortion of the microcirculation of the liver and collagen deposition lead to impaired sinusoidal transport and reduced extraction of protein-bound substrates, as well as increased resistance to blood flow. Portal venous hypertension, intrahepatic anastomotic channels between inflow and outflow veins, and extrahepatic collaterals between the portal and systemic veins are sequelae.

Alcoholic Cirrhosis. After chronic HCV infection, alcoholic cirrhosis is the second major cause of cirrhosis and end-stage liver disease in the United States.

Clinical Presentation and Natural History. Alcoholic cirrhosis may be clinically latent and discovered incidentally, during evaluation of unrelated illness, or as a consequence of complications, such as portal hypertension. Cirrhosis may be detected during the workup of impotence, infertility, hepatosplenomegaly, or minimal abnormalities of liver biochemical tests. Evaluation of alcoholic hepatitis may lead to identification of underlying cirrhosis. Since alcoholic cirrhosis is usually not detected until after 10 or more years of excessive alcohol ingestion, children and adolescents are unaffected. The incidence of the disease peaks in midlife, and affected men exceed affected women by about 2:1. Presenting features may include jaundice, particularly in patients with alcoholic hepatitis or those with far-advanced disease. Associated complaints include nausea, vomiting, anorexia, fatigue, weight loss, low-grade fever, and decreased libido. Evidence of portal hypertension, hepatic encephalopathy, or abnormalities of hemostasis may be presenting features.

The liver may be enlarged, with a rounded edge and a firm consistency. In advanced disease, however, the liver may be smaller than normal, and the liver edge may be grossly irregular because of macroscopic nodular regeneration. Splenomegaly is common, and venous collaterals in the abdominal walls may be striking. Spider angiomas, palmar erythema, evidence of muscle wasting, and an emaciated appearance accompanied by parotid gland enlargement are typically found. Gynecomastia and testicular atrophy are frequent findings.

The course of alcoholic cirrhosis depends on the stage and activity of the disease at diagnosis, subsequent alcohol consumption, and the occurrence of complications, which in themselves are life-threatening. Variceal bleeding because of portal hypertension, progressive hepatic encephalopathy, intercurrent bacterial infections, and hepatocellular carcinoma are the major causes of death. Life expectancy is reduced in alcoholic cirrhotic patients. Five-year survival rates vary between 25% and 60%.

Laboratory Studies and Diagnosis. Hematologic abnormalities are similar to those found in alcoholic hepatitis, and liver chemistries may reflect the presence of alcoholic hepatitis superimposed on alcoholic cirrhosis. Patients without evidence of acute alcoholic hepatitis have a wide spectrum of biochemical abnormalities. In patients who have abstained for prolonged periods, results of liver tests may be completely normal despite established cirrhosis. In most patients, particularly those who continue to imbibe, mild elevations of serum bilirubin, serum AST, and serum alkaline phosphatase are found. Patients with progressive disease may have PT prolongation resulting from reduced synthesis of prothrombin precursor proteins, impaired conversion of the inactive protein to the active molecule, and consumption coagulopathy. Hypoalbuminemia is common in severe cases and malnourished patients. Serum globulins and the gamma globulin fraction may be mildly to moderately elevated. Hyponatremia, hypokalemia, and low blood urea nitrogen levels are characteristic. However, cirrhosis may be complicated by the development of progressive azotemia, the hepatorenal syndrome (see Ascites).

The clinical diagnosis of alcoholic cirrhosis is based on recognition of the characteristic clinical features, physical findings, and laboratory studies in the alcoholic patient. Since alcoholic hepatitis, a reversible disorder, may simulate alcoholic cirrhosis, an irreversible one, and because both may be present, liver biopsy is a useful confirmatory procedure. Histologic examination helps define the stage of the disease and exclude other disorders that may affect the alcoholic patient (e.g., iron overload disease).

Complications, Consultation, and Hospitalization. Complications of alcoholic cirrhosis, such as variceal bleeding, infection, nonresponsive ascites, and progressive hepatic failure, are indications for consultation and should prompt hospitalization. Surgery in a patient with alcoholic cirrhosis often is associated with excessive operative morbidity-mortality and should be avoided or delayed unless failure to intervene is life-threatening.

Management. No specific therapy is known to reverse cirrhosis or to halt disease progression in the patient who continues to consume alcohol. Complete abstinence is the major goal of management, since compliance with such a regimen may lead to clinical and biochemical improvement and slow the rate of loss of hepatic mass. Although a balanced and nutritious diet containing more than 2000 kcal and 1 gm of protein per kilogram of body weight is prescribed, except for patients with hepatic encephalopathy, dietary treatment has limited value in the patient who continues to drink. Thiamine and multivitamins may be given, as well as supplemental folic acid, magnesium, and pyridoxine or pyridoxal phosphate.

Because occult sepsis is common, careful evaluation for bacterial infection is warranted even in the absence of high fever or shaking chills. Patients with cirrhosis, including those with nonalcoholic disease, should be cautioned about the high risk of *Vibrio* septicemia resulting from ingestion of raw or undercooked mollusks. The primary care physician should seek evidence of encephalopathy, fluid retention, and GI bleeding at each visit. Successful long-term management requires that the physician be sympathetic and supportive but also firm in stressing a program of abstinence. Referral to a formal alcohol withdrawal program may be useful. Counseling of the patient's family and employer may facilitate adherence to such a program. Psychotropic drugs (e.g., hypnotics, sedatives, tranquilizers) are best avoided, since their administration is potentially hazardous in this setting. Disulfiram has induced acute liver failure in a number of patients and should not be used.

Primary Biliary Cirrhosis. This chronic, progressive inflammatory disease of the liver is characterized by destruction of the intrahepatic bile ducts and eventual development of cirrhosis. In contrast to secondary biliary cirrhosis, a complication of prolonged anatomic obstruction of the extrahepatic biliary tree, the extrahepatic biliary tree is normal in patients with primary biliary cirrhosis.

Etiology and Epidemiology. Although the cause is unknown, an autoimmune mechanism may be involved; cytotoxic T lymphocytes infiltrate and attack the bile duct epithelium, granulomas surround injured bile ducts, circulating antibodies against mitochondria are present in nearly all patients, immune complexes may be found in the circulation, and other autoimmune disorders are seen in 10% to 15% of patients. A disorder resembling primary biliary cirrhosis has been described in a few patients after exposure to chlorpromazine, tolbutamide, methyltestosterone, and oral contraceptives.

The disease primarily affects women between ages 35 and 65; the range is wide, however, and onset in the third and eighth decades of life has been described. Fewer than 15% of patients are men. Familial cases of primary biliary cirrhosis are documented, and some family members may have the antimitochondrial antibody characteristic of the disease, but no association with HLA types has been recognized.

Clinical Presentation and Natural History. As many as 50% of affected patients are asymptomatic at diagnosis. These patients are usually identified through evaluation of unexplained hepatomegaly or by elevated serum alkaline phosphatase or, more rarely, serum aminotransferase levels during routine evaluation. Many patients remain asymptomatic for decades, although the liver lesion may progress silently. Pruritus with or without fatigue is usually the earliest symptom, followed months to years later by jaundice, xanthomas, and the clinical picture of prolonged and slowly progressive intrahepatic cholestasis. Weight loss, right upper quadrant abdominal pain, anorexia, nausea and vomiting, and increased skin pigmentation are described in 5% to 15% of patients. The CREST syndrome (calcinosis, Raynaud's phenomenon, esophageal hypomotility, sclerodactyly, telangiectasia), Sjögren's syndrome, or renal tubular acidosis may be present. Although variceal bleeding, ascites, and hepatic failure are terminal features of disease progression, these are presenting features in a few patients. Bone thinning secondary to osteomalacia and osteoporosis may lead to vertebral collapse.

Hepatomegaly is present in 50% to 75% of patients at diagnosis and splenomegaly in 10% to 50%. Hyperpigmentation and xanthomas are present in 10% to 30% at diagnosis, but the frequency of physical abnormalities increases with time. The rate of progression of the disease is highly variable. In asymptomatic patients, life expectancy may be minimally reduced. In symptomatic cases, average survival appears to vary between 6 and 12 years, but the range is wide. Jaundice, weight loss, ascites, bridging fibrosis, and cirrhosis on presentation are correlated with a poor prognosis.

Laboratory Studies and Diagnosis. Isolated elevation of serum alkaline phosphatase of liver origin, exceeding twice the upper limits of normal with or without mild increases in serum aminotransferase levels, is an early feature. Mild elevations of serum bilirubin and hypercholesterolemia are present in about half of asymptomatic patients and may become more prominent with time. Elevated serum IgM levels may be found in about 50% of patients. In patients with cholestasis, malabsorption of vitamin K, secondary to impaired bile salt excretion, leads to PT prolongation. Antimitochondrial antibodies are found in 95% of patients, and the titer exceeds 1:500 in about half. Antimitochrondrial antibodies also are found in some patients with autoimmune chronic hepatitis, but low titers are characteristic.

The diagnosis can be confirmed by liver biopsy, which demonstrates destruction of portal triad bile ducts; these ducts are surrounded by mononuclear and plasma cells resembling lymphoid follicles, with or without granulomas and piecemeal necrosis. Portal fibrosis, bridging fibrosis, and cirrhosis may be present. Cholestasis is prominent in most specimens and may be accompanied by increased hepatic copper concentrations. Patients with a suggestive liver biopsy but absent anti–mitochondrial antibodies may require endoscopic retrograde cholangiography to exclude secondary biliary cirrhosis.

Consultation and Hospitalization. Consultation is necessary for liver biopsy and for patients with progressive disease manifested by hepatic failure or complications of cirrhosis. In the latter circumstances, referral to a liver transplantation center is appropriate.

Management. Ursodeoxycholic acid (UDCA), in a dosage of 13 to 15 mg/kg, has improved biochemical tests and pruritus and is generally well tolerated. UDCA has not had a major effect on the histologic lesion but appears to delay the development of hepatic failure and improve survival.[8] UDCA is the current treatment of choice. Corticosteroids, azathioprine, and D-penicillamine have been studied but cannot be recommended. Colchicine has been used, but evidence of efficacy is minimal. Methotrexate also has been used, but efficacy is uncertain and pulmonary fibrosis may complicate treatment. The efficacy and safety of the combination of UDCA plus methotrexate is under study.

Supportive, symptomatic therapy includes oral administration of vitamins D, A, and K and oral vitamin E and calcium supplements. Pruritus nonresponsive to UDCA may be controlled by administration of cholestyramine with each meal. Rifampin, naltrexone, plasmapheresis, or ultraviolet light may lessen pruritus for those who cannot obtain relief with UDCA or cholestyramine.

Liver transplantation should be considered for patients with intractable pruritus, bilirubin levels of 10 mg/dl or greater, or evidence of hepatic failure. Posttransplantation recurrence of disease has been reported but is rare.

Wilson's Disease. This rare, autosomal recessive disorder of copper metabolism affects children and young adults and leads to chronic hepatitis and cirrhosis. If untreated, Wilson's disease inevitably leads to progressive and fatal liver and central nervous system (CNS) damage.

The gene for Wilson's disease has been localized to the long arm of chromosome 13 at the ATP7B site. More than 40 mutations have been identified in this gene, which controls the expression of a liver-specific copper transporter protein. About 1 in 30,000 individuals are homozygous for two copies of the abnormal gene. Production of the defective protein results in impaired biliary excretion of copper from the hepatocyte and the accumulation of toxic amounts of copper in the liver and subsequently in the brain, cornea, lens, and kidney.

Liver involvement, resembling acute viral hepatitis or acute liver failure often complicated by hemolytic anemia and chronic hepatitis with or without cirrhosis (or cryptogenic cirrhosis), is the usual presenting manifestation of affected children and young adolescents. In adults, neurologic or psychiatric features may be more prominent, and liver disease may be inapparent, although it is invariably present. Parkinson-like tremors, dysphagia, dysarthria, and dystonia are typically seen. Emotional lability, adolescent adjustment problems, depression, and psychosis are well-known findings. Golden-brown Kayser-Fleischer rings, a result of the deposition of copper in Descemet's membrane of the cornea, are usually demonstrable by slit-lamp examination in patients with CNS involvement.

Liver chemistries are usually abnormal but nonspecific, reflecting variable degrees of hepatocyte necrosis, fatty infiltration, and inflammation. Reduced serum levels of ceruloplasmin, the copper-binding serum glycoprotein, are found in 95% of patients, but only 85% of children with symptomatic liver disease have low levels. Hypouricemia, hypophosphatemia, uricosuria, aminoaciduria, and phosphaturia may be present. Diagnosis requires a high index of suspicion as well as documentation of low serum ceruloplasmin levels, increased urine copper, and increased hepatic copper concentrations in specimens obtained by biopsy.[10]

Management. Testing for mutations in the Wilson's disease gene is not yet practical. If Wilson's disease is suspected, the patient should be referred to a specialist familiar with the disease. Screening of family members may permit detection of asymptomatic Wilson's disease. Both the propositus and identified asymptomatic individuals require lifelong treatment with the copper-chelating agents D-penicillamine or triethylene tetramine to reduce copper stores. Oral zinc salts and avoidance of high-copper foods may be useful adjunctive maneuvers. Successful decoppering prevents disease when begun early, improves liver and neurologic symptoms, and prolongs survival. Liver transplantation is indicated for those with acute liver failure and patients with decompensated cirrhosis who are unresponsive to decoppering.

Iron Overload Disease. The accumulation of excessive amounts of iron in the liver and extrahepatic tissues may result from a genetic disorder or a complication of chronic hemolysis, transfusion therapy, porphyria cutanea tarda, alcoholic cirrhosis, portacaval anastomosis, or dietary iron overload. Hepatic fibrosis, cirrhosis, complications of portal hypertension, and an increased risk of hepatocellular carcinoma are sequelae of the progressive liver disease in untreated patients and may be accompanied by diabetes, dilated cardiomyopathy, hypogonadism, hyperpigmentation, and arthropathy. This section discusses the genetic disorder.

Genetic iron overload, the most common inherited liver disease, is transmitted as an autosomal recessive disease. The responsible gene, the HFE gene, has been localized to the short arm of chromosome 6. The most common mutation of this gene, the C282Y mutation, is found in both copies of the gene in homozygous patients and in one copy among heterozygotes. Other mutations also have been reported, but their role is less clear. Precisely how the C282Y mutation in the HFE gene results in enhanced intestinal iron absorption and altered iron metabolism is unknown.

Although iron accumulation begins early in life, clinical manifestations may not be seen until the fifth decade or later. Iron overload is about 10 times more common in men than women and usually begins earlier. Most patients identified by laboratory studies are asymptomatic. Those with early symptoms most frequently have weakness, lethargy, arthralgias, loss of libido, and weight loss. Hepatomegaly, splenomegaly, and signs of cirrhosis and portal hypertension may be found. The development of hepatocellular carcinoma is the most devastating complication of liver involvement. Diabetes is present in a minority of patients at diagnosis but diabetic retinopathy, renal involvement, and neuropathy may complicate the course. Impotence and testicular atrophy in men and secondary amenorrhea and early menopause in women may be seen. Patients with iron overload disease appear to be at increased risk of *Listeria, Yersinia,* and pathogenic *Vibrio* infections.

Serum aminotransferase levels may be slightly elevated but usually do not exceed three times the upper limits of normal. Diagnosis requires demonstration of increased serum iron levels and decreased transferrin levels, yielding a

Table 104-4. Results of Effective Iron Depletion in Patients with Hemochromatosis

Complication	Expected result of treatment
None present	Normal life expectancy
Hyperpigmentation	Usually resolves
Hepatomegaly	Often improves
Cardiac dysfunction	Improvement may occur
Glucose intolerance	May improve but rarely disappears
Arthropathy	Minimal improvement
Cirrhosis	No change
Progression of cirrhosis to hepatocellular carcinoma	No change
Hypogonadism	No change

Table 104-5. Risks and Survival with Bleeding Esophagogastric Varices

Risk/survival	Mortality (%)
Development of varices	25-35
Mortality for hemorrhage	30-50
Recurrent hemorrhage in survivors	30-70
5-year survival after hemorrhage	5-20

transferrin saturation usually in excess of 60%, elevated serum ferritin levels (often above 1000 ng/ml), and quantitative evidence of increased hepatic iron concentration, permitting estimation of the hepatic iron index. The latter is defined as the hepatic iron concentration (in micromoles of iron per gram dry liver) divided by the age of the patient (in years). A hepatic iron index greater than 1.9 is generally considered diagnostic, but exceptions exist.[9]

Management. Patients with suspected iron overload disease should be referred to a specialist for definitive diagnosis (liver biopsy with quantitative hepatic iron determinations) and initiation of iron depletion by phlebotomy. Subsequent management can be undertaken by the primary care physician. Phlebotomies are undertaken weekly or biweekly and continued at that rate until the hemoglobin falls because of mild iron deficiency anemia. Transferrin saturation may decline precipitously just before the decrease in hemoglobin levels. Maintenance of iron balance thereafter may require occasional phlebotomy. Siblings and other first-degree relatives of the propositus may be tested for HFE mutations and iron parameters. If they are homozygous for the C282Y mutation or have evidence of iron overload, phlebotomy therapy must be initiated, since effective iron depletion prevents all clinical manifestations and results in normal life expectancy. Treatment of patients with clinical complications of iron overload disease may reverse some but not all manifestations (Table 104-4).

COMPLICATIONS OF CIRRHOSIS

Regardless of the etiology of cirrhosis, the complications are often life-threatening in themselves and may contribute to reduced life expectancy. The primary care physician must be familiar with these complications, recognize them early, and plan a course of appropriate management. Early consultation with an experienced gastroenterologist-hepatologist may be helpful, since management of the major complications of cirrhosis is difficult and the efficacy and safety of many therapeutic measures remain controversial. Furthermore, early referral for consideration for hepatic transplantation is recommended for most patients with cirrhosis, except those with alcoholic cirrhosis who have continued to drink.

Esophagogastric Varices

Portal hypertension secondary to cirrhosis leads to the development of extensive collateral channels between the left gastric and azygos veins in 30% to 75% of patients. These esophagogastric varices are most prominent in the lower third of the esophagus and fundus of the stomach. They may be asymptomatic for prolonged periods, but when varices are large and associated with marked elevations of portal pressure, the risk of hemorrhage is 25% to 35%. No specific precipitants of bleeding from esophagogastric varices are recognized. Impaired hemostasis may contribute to the initiation or perpetuation of variceal bleeding in some patients. Thrombocytopenia in cirrhosis may reflect hypersplenism secondary to congestive splenomegaly resulting from portal hypertension, disseminated intravascular consumptive coagulation, or alcohol-induced bone marrow depression. Prolongation of the PT in cirrhosis may be multifactorial (see Alcoholic Cirrhosis) and may also contribute to bleeding.

Hematemesis and melena are the cardinal manifestations of bleeding esophagogastric varices. Because patients with cirrhosis may bleed from other lesions, such as erosive gastritis, peptic ulcer disease, and Mallory-Weiss tears, endoscopic visualization of the bleeding site is essential as soon as hemodynamic stabilization is achieved after emergency hospital admission. Hemorrhage from esophagogastric varices is associated with reduced survival (Table 104-5).

Management. Consultation with a gastroenterologist is appropriate for patients with cirrhosis. In those with large varices, treatment with nonselective β-adrenergic blockers reduces the risk of the first variceal bleed by about 40%. In patients without contraindications to β-blockers and who can tolerate therapy, it should be continued indefinitely. For the patient with acute variceal hemorrhage, resuscitation in the intensive care unit is essential to establish airway protection and hemodynamic stability. Transfusion of whole blood and, if necessary, fresh-frozen plasma and platelet concentrates may improve circulating blood volume and improve clotting. Endoscopy is mandatory for both diagnosis and endoscopic treatment (injection of varices by sclerotherapy or variceal ligation by banding). Pharmacologic therapy with vasopressin and nitroglycerin or octreotide through a peripheral vein may provide temporary control of hemorrhage. The combination of endoscopic and pharmacologic therapy may be superior to either alone, but improved survival rates have yet to be shown. Prevention of recurrent bleeding may be achieved by endoscopic variceal ligation, which appears superior to sclerotherapy, or by use of nonselective β-blockers.

For patients with variceal bleeding that fails to respond to conventional treatment, the construction of a transjugular intrahepatic portal-systemic shunt (TIPS) by an interventional radiologist or a surgically constructed distal splenorenal shunt may be effective. This approach may be most appropriate for the liver transplantation candidate in whom bleeding cannot be controlled by other techniques and immediate transplantation is not possible.

Hepatic Encephalopathy

This neuropsychiatric syndrome is a complication of cirrhosis, portal-systemic shunting, or acute liver failure. Hepatic encephalopathy may develop insidiously or abruptly and may be transient, recurrent, or chronic. The pathogenesis remains uncertain; both hepatic detoxification of intestine-derived neuroactive compounds and hepatic production of substances essential for normal CNS function may be impaired. Elevated CNS and peripheral blood levels of ammonia, methanethiol, false neurotransmitter amines, aromatic amino acids, short-chain fatty acids, γ-aminobutyric acid, and benzodiazepine ligands have been reported. With the exception of the encephalopathy seen in acute liver failure, which is often associated with cerebral edema and responds poorly to treatment, most episodes of hepatic encephalopathy are precipitated by exogenous factors (Table 104-6). Correction of these factors leads to reversal of the encephalopathy.

The earliest phases of hepatic encephalopathy may be subclinical or subtle and difficult to recognize unless formal neuropsychologic (trail-making) testing is undertaken. Electroencephalography and study of sensory-evoked potentials have been used to assess subclinical encephalopathy but have little value in diagnosis of the overt syndrome. Episodic slowing of speech and alertness and reversal of sleep patterns may be followed by confusion, slurred speech, and movement disturbances. Asterixis, the flapping tremor, is usually present, as is constructional apraxia. Muscle rigidity, pyramidal tract signs, and seizures are prominent features in some patients. Those with longstanding hepatic encephalopathy may have psychosis, choreoathetosis, dementia, or myelopathy. The diagnosis of hepatic encephalopathy is clinical based on the characteristic clinical picture in advanced liver disease. An elevated arterial ammonia level may be found but is not diagnostic; normal levels do not exclude hepatic encephalopathy. Because other disorders may resemble hepatic encephalopathy, further evaluation may be necessary (Box 104-4). The clinical importance of abnormalities on cerebral imaging in hepatic encephalopathy remains uncertain.

In its early phases and in acute episodes with an identifiable precipitant, the syndrome is completely reversible and the brain histologically normal. In some forms of chronic hepatic encephalopathy and myelopathy, however, reversibility is less likely, and structural changes may be found.

Table 104-6. Precipitants of Hepatic Encephalopathy in Cirrhosis

Precipitating factor	Examples
Drug administration	Antianxiety agents (particularly benzodiazepines), sedative-hypnotics, analgesics
Electrolyte and acid-base abnormalities	Hypokalemia, metabolic alkalosis, severe hyponatremia, azotemia
Hypovolemia	Overzealous diuresis, dehydration
Increased gastrointestinal intraluminal nitrogenous materials	Gastrointestinal bleeding, excessive dietary protein, azotemia, constipation
Miscellaneous catabolic states	Infection; surgical anesthesia; portacaval, splenorenal, or other portal-systemic shunting; superimposed acute hepatic injury; hypoxemia

Box 104-4. Disorders Simulating Hepatic Encephalopathy

Subdural hematoma, brain tumor, brain abscess
Meningitis
Sepsis
Alcohol intoxication or withdrawal
Drug overdose
Uremia
Respiratory failure
Hyperosmolar states
Hypoglycemia

Management. Hospitalization is usually required if encephalopathy is more than mild. In addition to initiating supportive therapy to maintain vital functions, identification of other causes of encephalopathy and possible precipitating factors and their elimination or correction are the first steps of treatment. Concurrently, encephalopathy is controlled by intestine-cleansing enemas, restriction of dietary protein to near-zero levels, and oral or nasogastric tube administration of lactulose, a synthetic nonabsorbable disaccharide that acts as a cathartic, lowers the pH in the lumen of the colon, traps ammonia as ammonium ions, favors the bacterial assimilation of ammonia, and reduces the concentration of short-chain fatty acids in the colon. Overdoses of lactulose may induce severe diarrhea with crampy abdominal distress, bloating, and electrolyte disturbances. If lactulose fails, neomycin may be used (0.5 gm every 6 hours) with or without continued lactulose. Metronidazole and vancomycin may be effective, but experience with these agents is limited. For patients with intractable or recurrent encephalopathy or those only responsive to low protein intake, liver transplantation should be considered.

Ascites

The accumulation of fluid in the peritoneal cavity is a cardinal feature of advanced liver disease (cirrhosis and alcoholic hepatitis are the major causes) but may also be seen in peritoneal tuberculosis, nephrotic syndrome, congestive heart failure, and neoplastic diseases. In patients with advanced liver disease, retention of sodium and water leading to ascites formation is caused by the combined effects of portal hypertension, increased hepatic lymph production, hypoalbuminemia, splanchnic venous pooling, and peripheral arterial vasodilation resulting from release of vasodilator factors and

Box 104-5. Mechanisms of Ascites Formation

Initiating Factors

Portal hypertension and splanchnic venous pooling
Increased hepatic lymph flow with accumulation in peritoneal space
Hypoalbuminemia and decreased colloid osmotic pressure
Peripheral arteriolar dilation resulting from vasodilator factors and arteriovenous shunting

Secondary Factors

Enhanced sympathetic efferent discharge
Nonosmotic release of arginine vasopressin
Activation of renin-angiotensin-aldosterone system
Resistance to atrial natriuretic factor
Impaired escape from aldosterone-induced sodium retention

Consequences

Avid distal renal tubular sodium reabsorption
Increased proximal renal sodium reabsorption
Impaired free water clearance

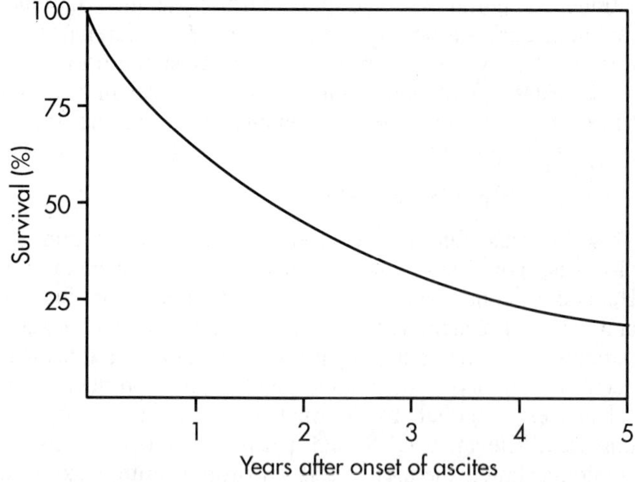

Fig. 104-4. Reduced survival rate after onset of ascites in patient with cirrhosis.

arteriovenous shunting (Box 104-5). The precise mechanisms and the sequence in which they occur remain controversial. Systemic vasodilation with arterial underfilling, enhanced sympathetic efferent discharge, release of arginine vasopressin through nonosmotic baroreceptor mechanisms, and activation of the renin-angiotensin-aldosterone system may result in decreased renal perfusion pressure and increased proximal sodium and water reabsorption. Distal renal tubular sodium reabsorption is also increased, and free water clearance is impaired.

Although ascites may be insidious and unrecognized by the patient, its development portends premature death (Fig. 104-4). When extensive, ascites may lead to abdominal discomfort, respiratory compromise, umbilical hernia, impaired sense of well-being, and early satiety. Spontaneous bacterial peritonitis is rarely seen in the cirrhotic patient without ascites; it should be considered in every cirrhotic patient with ascites. When clinical examination at the bedside is equivocal, abdominal ultrasonography may confirm the presence of fluid. Diagnostic paracentesis with removal of 50 to 100 ml of fluid is necessary in all patients with new-onset ascites and in those with longstanding ascites in whom fever, abdominal pain, leukocytosis, azotemia, or hepatic encephalopathy may indicate a complicating disorder. In uncomplicated ascites secondary to cirrhosis, the serum-ascitic albumin gradient is typically 1.1 gm/dl or more. The ascitic fluid total protein is usually less than 2.5 gm/dl in the ascites of cirrhosis but may exceed this level in cardiac ascites. Cell counts in uncomplicated ascites are usually less than 400 leukocytes/mm^3, with fewer than 25% polymorphonuclear neutrophils (PMNs). The presence of more than 250 PMNs strongly suggests bacterial infection. In spontaneous bacterial peritonitis the serum-ascitic albumin gradient is unchanged, the cell count is elevated, PMNs predominate, and lactic acid dehydrogenase of ascitic fluid may be increased. Bacterial culture of the fluid is mandatory.

Management. In the stable cirrhotic patient with uncomplicated ascites, management is initiated in the office. Dietary sodium is restricted to 0.5 to 2.0 gm daily, and nonsteroidal antiinflammatory drugs (NSAIDs) are avoided. Consultation with a dietitian is often necessary. In patients with severe dilutional hyponatremia (serum sodium less than 125 mEq/L), fluid intake should be limited to 1500 ml daily. If weight reduction, diminution in abdominal girth, and diuresis are not achieved within a few days after dietary sodium restriction, spironolactone, in a single oral dose of 100 mg daily, is the initial drug of choice for single-agent therapy. However, a combination regimen of spironolactone (100 mg) and furosemide (40 mg) once daily may be more effective. The goal of diuretic treatment in the patient with ascites without peripheral edema is a loss of no more than 0.4 kg of body weight daily. In patients with extensive edema, the latter serving as a reserve for plasma volume, no limit on daily weight loss is needed until edema disappears. Throughout treatment, serum electrolytes and renal function must be monitored regularly. Diuretic-induced hypovolemia, hypokalemia or hyperkalemia, hyponatremia, hyperchloremic metabolic acidosis, azotemia, or encephalopathy may require temporary cessation of therapy and, if severe, corrective measures.

Large-volume paracentesis with removal of 4 to 6 L of fluid appears to be as safe and effective as diuretic therapy and considerably more rapid in achieving a therapeutic effect. For patients with tense ascites and respiratory embarrassment or imminent rupture of an umbilical hernia and for those who are refractory to diuretic therapy, paracentesis is the treatment of choice.[1] Some centers where ascites is treated by multiple large-volume paracenteses use intravenous colloid infusion with albumin or dextran to prevent volume depletion.

In patients with intractable ascites, prophylactic antibiotics (e.g., fluoroquinolones) may reduce the risk of spontaneous bacterial peritonitis, which may also be responsible for failure to respond to diuretics. If spontaneous bacterial peritonitis is suspected, parenteral broad-spectrum antibiotics are begun while cultures of ascitic fluid are pending. Use of a third-generation broad-spectrum cephalosporin is a reasonable approach until sensitivity tests dictate the need for altered therapy. For the patient who has recovered from spontaneous bacterial peritonitis, a high recurrence rate can be anticipated; recurrences are reduced by prophylactic antibiotic treatment with norfloxacin or triple oral nonabsorbable antibiotic regimens.

Another contributor to treatment failure is the *hepatorenal syndrome,* characterized by oliguria and progressive azotemia, with a low urinary sodium concentration. This almost invariably fatal syndrome, linked to intense renal vasoconstriction-induced hypoperfusion with renal cortical ischemia, is characterized by a marked diminution in glomerular filtration rate in the absence of structural renal disease.[1] Management for this form of oliguric renal failure should be undertaken in consultation with the nephrologist. Liver transplantation can reverse the renal failure and should be considered in suitable patients. A transplant also may be required for patients with refractory ascites.

REFERENCES

1. Arroyo V, Gines P, Gerbes AL, et al: Definition and diagnostic criteria of refractory ascites and hepatorenal syndrome in cirrhosis, *Hepatology* 23:164, 1996.
2. Bellentani S, Saccoccio G, Costa G, et al: Drinking habits as cofactors of risk for alcohol-induced liver damage, *Gut* 41:845, 1997.
3. Hoofnagle JH, Di Bisceglie AM: Treatment of chronic viral hepatitis, *N Engl J Med* 336:347, 1997.
4. Koff RS: Hepatitis A, *Lancet* 341:1643, 1998.
5. Krawitt EL: Autoimmune hepatitis, *N Engl J Med* 334:897, 1996.
6. Lee WM: Hepatitis B virus infection, *N Engl J Med* 337:1733, 1997.
7. Lemon SM: Vaccines to prevent viral hepatitis, *N Engl J Med* 163:196, 1997.
8. Poupon RE, Lindor KD, Cauch-Dudek K, et al: Combined analysis of randomized controlled trials of ursodeoxycholic acid in primary biliary cirrhosis, *Gastroenterology* 113:884, 1997.
9. Powell LW, George DK, McDonnell SM, Kowdley KV: Diagnosis of hemochromatosis, *Ann Intern Med* 129:925, 1998.
10. Schilsky ML, Sternlieb I: Overcoming obstacles to the diagnosis of Wilson's disease, *Gastroenterology* 113:350, 1997.

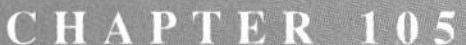
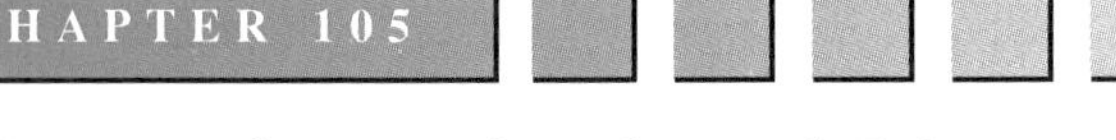

CHAPTER 105

Gastrointestinal and Liver Tumors

Paul C. Schroy, III

TUMORS OF THE STOMACH

A variety of benign and malignant tumors can arise in the stomach (Table 105-1). Adenocarcinomas are the most common malignant neoplasms, followed by lymphomas and leiomyosarcomas. Leiomyomas are the most common benign neoplasms but are rarely clinically significant. Benign gastric polyps tend to be more relevant clinically but are relatively uncommon. Carcinoid tumors may also arise in the stomach. In general these tumors are detected during radiographic or endoscopic evaluation of patients with nonspecific gastrointestinal (GI) complaints such as epigastric pain, nausea, vomiting, and bleeding. Progressive weight loss and the presence of a palpable mass are more ominous signs suggestive of advanced malignancy. Because these tumors share similar radiographic appearances with each other as well as with benign diseases, particularly gastric ulcer, endoscopy with biopsy and brush cytology is the diagnostic modality of choice. Management varies considerably depending on tumor type and, in the case of malignancy, tumor stage.

Table 105-1. Most Common Gastrointestinal and Liver Tumors

Site	Benign	Malignant
Stomach	Leiomyoma Hyperplastic polyp Adenomatous polyp Hamartomatous polyp	Adenocarcinoma Primary lymphoma Leiomyosarcoma Carcinoid
Small bowel	Adenomatous polyp Leiomyoma Lipoma	Adenocarcinoma Primary lymphoma Carcinoid Leiomyosarcoma
Large bowel	Adenomatous polyp Hyperplastic polyp Juvenile polyp Pseudopolyp Lipoma	Adenocarcinoma
Liver	Hemangioma Adenomanoma Focal nodular hyperplasia	Hepatocellular carcinoma Cholangiocarcinoma

Gastric Cancer

Gastric cancer is one of the most common cancers worldwide, even though both incidence and mortality have declined dramatically worldwide over the past 50 years. Recent advances in understanding the epidemiology and pathogenesis have helped identify etiologic factors. Recent interest has focused on substantiating the causal role of these factors to develop rational preventive strategies. Meanwhile, early diagnosis remains the key to prolonged survival and reduced mortality.

Epidemiology. The incidence of gastric cancer varies worldwide. In general the disease is more common in developing countries than industrialized nations and has a predilection for urban and lower socioeconomic groups. Japan, China, South America, and Eastern Europe have the highest rates, whereas the United States, Canada, parts of Africa (e.g., Uganda), and Southeast Asia have the lowest rates. Migrants typically acquire the risk of their host countries, suggesting an important role for environmental factors. Gastric cancer rarely occurs before age 40, after which the incidence rises steadily, peaking in the seventh decade. Men are affected almost twice as often as females.

Curiously, incidence rates have declined steadily in both high-risk and low-risk countries, except in Poland and Portugal. In the United States the annual incidence of gastric cancer declined from more than 30 cases per 100,000 population in the 1930s to less than 10 cases per 100,000 in the 1990s. Nevertheless, gastric cancer remains an important public health concern, with estimates of more than 22,000 new cases and 14,000 deaths for 1999. African, Hispanic, and Native Americans are 1.5 to 2.5 times more likely to develop gastric cancer than whites.

The global decline of gastric cancer incidence rates reflects a decrease in the incidence of cancers arising in the distal stomach (body and antrum); in contrast, the incidence of cancers in the proximal stomach (cardia) and gastroesophageal (GE) junction has steadily increased at a rate exceeding that of any other cancer, except melanoma or lung cancer. Unlike cancers of the distal stomach, cancers of the proximal stomach and GE junction are more common among higher socioeconomic groups.

Etiology. The etiology of gastric cancer is obscure. Epidemiologic data provide strong evidence that environmental factors, particularly diet, play a dominant role. Diets rich in complex carbohydrates (e.g., fava beans), salt, pickled or smoked foods, dried fish, and poorly preserved foods have all been linked with an increased risk of gastric cancer. Conversely, diets rich in fresh fruits and vegetables have a negative association. Dietary nitrates have also been implicated on the basis of both epidemiologic evidence and rodent models of gastric carcinogenesis. Dietary nitrates may be reduced by bacteria into nitrites, which then combine with secondary amines in food, drugs, or pesticides to form carcinogenic nitrosamines.

Chronic *Helicobacter pylori* infection, a causative agent of chronic antral gastritis and peptic ulcer disease (PUD), has also been implicated in the etiology of gastric cancer (see Chapter 102). Both descriptive and observational epidemiologic studies have consistently demonstrated a strong association between *H. pylori* infection and gastric cancer. By 1994 the World Health Organization (WHO) concluded that sufficient evidence had accumulated to classify *H. pylori* as a group 1 human carcinogen.[11] More recently, a meta-analysis of existing cohort and case-control studies found that *H. pylori*–infected individuals were nearly twice as likely to develop gastric cancer as uninfected controls (summary odds ratio, 1.9; confidence interval, 1.3 to 2.8).[5] The relative risk was found to be greatest for younger individuals (9.3 for under age 29), in whom the absolute risk is quite low. The relative risk was also greater for cancers in the distal stomach than for those located in the cardia but was comparable for intestinal and diffuse cancers.

Genetic factors also play a role in etiology. Gastric cancer is one of the extracolonic malignancies associated with *hereditary nonpolyposis colorectal cancer* (HNPCC), or *Lynch syndrome,* a genetic disease caused by germ-line mutations of repair genes with mismatched deoxyribonucleic acid (DNA). Gastric cancer has also been reported in patients with *familial polyposis* (polyposis coli), a distinct genetic syndrome caused by mutations of the *APC* gene. As with colorectal cancer, familial clustering has also been observed in the absence of these well-defined genetic syndromes. First-degree relatives (e.g., parent, sibling) of patients with gastric cancer have a twofold to threefold increased risk of developing the disease. Familial risk is more strongly associated with the diffuse histopathologic type of gastric cancer than the intestinal type. Risk of gastric cancer is also increased among persons with blood group A.

Predisposing Conditions. A variety of conditions have been associated with an increased risk of gastric cancer. Chronic atrophic gastritis with intestinal metaplasia and achlorhydria is found in the majority of patients with gastric cancer, but its etiologic role is unclear, since fewer than 10% of patients with this condition ultimately develop gastric cancer. Chronic *H. pylori* infection and pernicious anemia, both also associated with chronic atrophic gastritis, reduced gastric acidity, and intestinal metaplasia, are well-recognized predisposing conditions. Prior gastric surgery for PUD, particularly partial gastrectomy with Billroth II anastomosis, is associated with an increased risk of cancer in the gastric remnant 15 to 20 years after the initial surgery. Other premalignant conditions include gastric adenomatous polyps and Ménétrier's disease (giant hypertrophic gastritis). Although each of these conditions is associated with cancers of the distal stomach, Barrett's esophagus is the only recognized premalignant condition linked with cancers of the cardia and GE junction. Periodic endoscopic surveillance is currently recommended only for patients with adenomatous polyps and Barrett's esophagus. A baseline screening endoscopy has also been recommended for patients with newly diagnosed pernicious anemia, but data are insufficient to warrant long-term surveillance for this condition.

The relationship between chronic gastric ulcer and gastric cancer is controversial. Most authorities currently agree that gastric ulcer does not predispose to gastric cancer, but recent evidence suggests an association with benign duodenal ulcer disease. Because gastric cancers may present as an ulcer, however, histologic and cytologic assessment is recommended for all gastric ulcers, regardless of their radiographic or endoscopic appearance. Follow-up endoscopy after 8 to 12 weeks of appropriate medical therapy is also indicated, since a small but significant number of malignant ulcers can demonstrate healing by radiographic criteria alone.

Histopathology. Gastric cancers can arise in any region of the stomach and can assume a myriad of gross morphologic configurations. *Early gastric cancers* (i.e., tumors confined to the mucosa or submucosa regardless of lymph node status) may appear as a subtle polypoid protrusion, superficial plaque, mucosal discoloration, depression, or ulceration. More advanced cancers typically present as polypoid or fungating masses with ulceration (Fig. 105-1*A*); superficial spreading or infiltrating (linitis plastica) forms are encountered less often. Histologically the vast majority of malignant neoplasms of the stomach are adenocarcinomas. These can be subdivided into diffuse and intestinal types (Lauren's classification) or infiltrative and expanding types (Ming's classification). The intestinal or expanding type tends to predominate in high-risk populations, is more common in men and older patients, is associated with a relatively better prognosis, and is preceded by a prolonged precancerous state. In contrast, the diffuse or infiltrative type predominates in women and younger patients, carries a poorer prognosis, and is not preceded by a known precancerous lesion.

Clinical Presentation. Although routine endoscopy and biopsy may diagnose early gastric cancers, 90% of patients with gastric cancer seek medical help only when the cancer has progressed to a more advanced stage. Persistent abdominal pain and weight loss are the most common presenting symptoms. Weight loss may be caused by anorexia, nausea and vomiting, or early satiety. Although

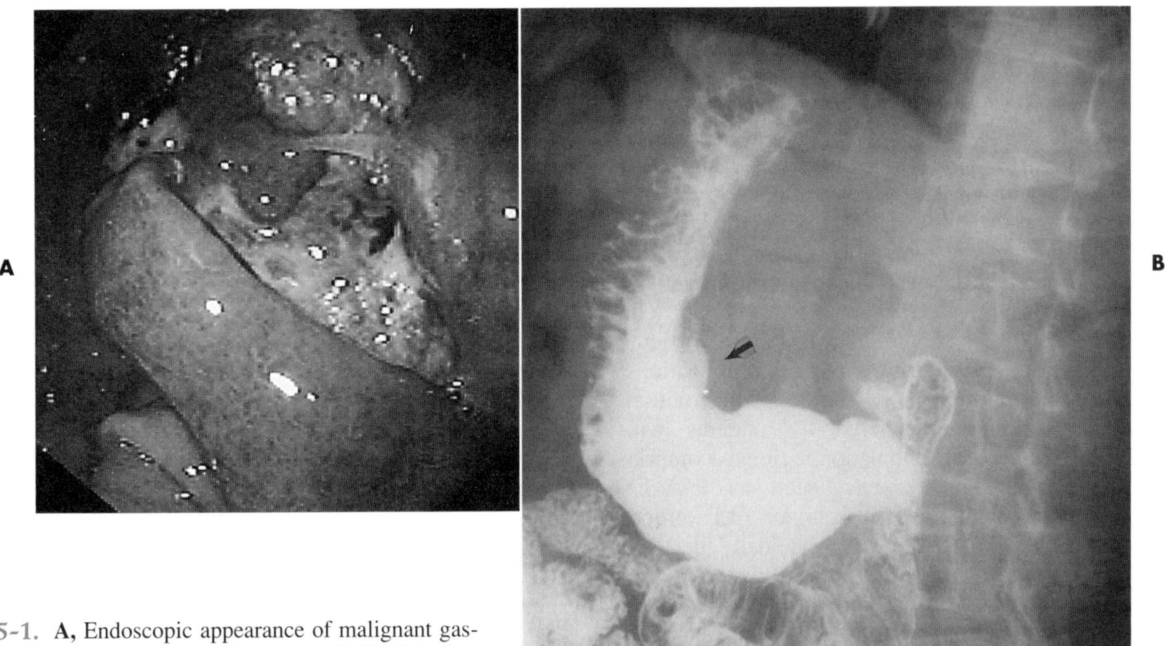

Fig. 105-1. **A,** Endoscopic appearance of malignant gastric ulcer arising in the fundus of stomach. **B,** Radiologic appearance of malignant gastric ulcer on upper gastrointestinal series. Note that ulcer *(arrow)* is within a mass.

occult GI blood loss with or without iron deficiency anemia is common, gross hematemesis is rare. Dysphagia and weight loss are typical presenting symptoms in patients with tumors of the gastric cardia or GE junction. A palpable mass may be detected in up to 50% of patients and indicates longstanding advanced disease. Jaundice, ascites, a periumbilical metastatic nodule (Sister Mary Joseph node), left supraclavicular adenopathy (Virchow's or signal node), a palpable enlarged ovary (Krukenberg's tumor), or a firm mass palpable on rectal examination in the anterior cul-de-sac (Blumer's shelf) all suggest widespread metastases and a poor prognosis. Gastric cancer is also associated with a variety of paraneoplastic phenomena, including the sudden appearance of diffuse seborrheic keratoses (Leser-Trélat sign), pigmented dermal lesions (acanthosis nigricans), microangiopathic hemolytic anemia, membranous nephropathy, hypercoagulability with thrombosis (Trousseau's syndrome), and dermatomyositis.

Diagnosis. In high-risk countries such as Japan, mass screening of asymptomatic individuals with endoscopy, double-contrast radiography, and cytology has been successful in detecting a high percentage of early gastric cancers. Unfortunately, mass screening cannot be justified in the United States because of the relatively low incidence. Physicians must therefore rely on a high degree of suspicion when evaluating patients with vague nonspecific GI complaints, particularly older patients with new dyspeptic symptoms or high-risk patients. Upper gastrointestinal (UGI) endoscopy, or esophagogastroduodenoscopy (EGD), is widely accepted as the diagnostic procedure of choice because of its superior accuracy. Referral for early endoscopy is indicated for patients over age 45 with new-onset dyspepsia, patients of any age with alarm symptoms (e.g., weight loss, recurrent vomiting, dysphagia, evidence of bleeding, or anemia), or younger patients who fail empiric antisecretory or prokinetic therapy.[1] At endoscopy a minimum of six biopsies and brush cytology should be obtained of any mass lesion, ulceration, area of discoloration, unexplained mucosal depression, or prominent fold(s). Repeat endoscopy with tissue sampling may be necessary if histologic or cytologic assessment is nondiagnostic.

UGI radiography is an alternative diagnostic strategy if upper endoscopy is not readily available. Double-contrast studies afford greater accuracy, particularly for early mucosal abnormalities. Abnormal findings such as a mass with or without ulceration (Fig. 105-1, *B*), enlarged gastric folds, and lack of distensibility (leather bottle appearance) require endoscopic follow-up and tissue confirmation. Endoscopy is also warranted for patients with equivocal radiographic findings and those with suspicious clinical presentations but negative x-ray results.

Once the diagnosis is established, evaluation for the extent of disease is warranted to optimize treatment planning and determine prognosis. Endoscopic ultrasound provides an accurate assessment of depth of tumor invasion into the bowel wall and may give useful information regarding perigastric lymph nodes. Computed tomography (CT) provides an accurate assessment of regional and retroperitoneal lymph node involvement, direct extension into contiguous organs, liver metastases, and ascites. Paracentesis with cytologic examination should be performed if ascites is present. Laparoscopy may also be useful in the evaluation of patients with unexplained ascites and negative or equivocal CT scans. Enlarged peripheral lymph nodes (e.g., Virchow's node) require biopsy. Additional studies, such as abdominal ultrasound, radionuclide scanning, magnetic resonance imaging (MRI), and angiography, may be useful in select cases.

Treatment. Surgical or endoscopic resection is the only potentially curative treatment for gastric cancer. Tumors amenable to endoscopic removal should be confined to the mucosal layer of the stomach, as determined by endoscopic ultrasound and confirmed histologically. All other patients should be considered for surgery unless (1) there is evidence of widespread metastatic disease, (2) the patient is a poor surgical candidate, (3) the primary tumor is clearly unresectable, or (4) total gastrectomy is required with only palliative intent. Curative resection requires wide excision of the primary tumor and en bloc removal of regional lymph nodes and contiguous structures. The actual extent of resection is determined at surgery and depends on several factors, most notably tumor size, location, and lymph node status. A palliative resection should be considered in patients with incurable disease to diminish the risk of complications, such as bleeding, perforation, or gastric outlet obstruction. Chemotherapy should be considered for patients with surgically incurable disease. Combination regimens comprising the most active single agents, such as FAMTX (5-fluorouracil, doxorubicin, methotrexate) or ELF (etoposide, leucovorin, 5-fluorouracil) have yielded the best response rates but have had little impact on long-term survival. Radiotherapy has been used primarily as a palliative approach to specific tumor-related problems, such as bleeding, obstruction with pain from local extension, liver infiltration, and bone metastases.

Palliation is an important aspect of gastric cancer treatment. With any palliative therapy the physician must consider the patient's overall prognosis to avoid excessive morbidity and mortality or lengthy hospital stays for patients with a limited life span. Although surgical resection and intestinal bypass may be therapeutic options for some patients with obstruction, nonsurgical candidates may benefit from endoscopic approaches (e.g., laser ablation, stent placement) and radiation therapy, which are also preferred for the management of acute or chronic tumor-related bleeding in nonsurgical patients. Decisions regarding nutritional support need to be individualized, but in general, enteral feeding via endoscopically placed gastrostomy (PEG) or jejunostomy (PEJ) tubes is preferred over parenteral feeding.

Follow-up. Postoperative management of patients with gastric cancer depends on disease status after resection. Patients with residual or inoperable disease should be considered for radiation or chemotherapy. Those without evidence of disease should be closely monitored for signs or symptoms of recurrence. Since 85% occur within the first 2 years, patients should be evaluated frequently during this period. Follow-up should include a careful history, physical examination, and routine laboratory tests (complete blood count, liver profile) every 3 to 6 months for the first 2 years and every 6 to 12 months thereafter. In addition, a CT scan of the abdomen, chest radiograph, and UGI endoscopy with biopsy of the anastomosis should be obtained 6 to 12 months after surgery, then yearly. Suspicious findings warrant aggressive diagnostic evaluation and tissue confirmation.

Prognosis. Prognosis depends on tumor stage at diagnosis. The tumor, node, and metastasis (TNM) classification system is currently the most widely used staging system (Table 105-2). Based on this system, 5-year survival rates range from 85% to 90% for stage I disease to 3% for stage IV. Unfortunately, overall survival is only 18% to 20%, indicating that most patients present with advanced, incurable disease.

Gastric Polyps

Gastric polyps are uncommon, occurring in less than 2% of autopsy surveys, so epidemiologic and etiologic data are scant. *Hyperplastic* polyps are most common (75% to 90%) and occur frequently in association with *H. pylori*–associated chronic gastritis; malignant transformation is rare. *Adenomatous* polyps are much less common (10% to 20%), but unlike hyperplastic polyps, adenomatous polyps are true neoplastic lesions that carry a significant risk of malignant transformation, particularly if greater than 2 cm in size. Although most occur sporadically, adenomatous polyps have been described in patients with pernicious anemia and familial adenomatous polyposis or Gardner's syndrome. *Hamartomatous* polyps, also referred to *fundic gland* polyps because of their predilection for the proximal stomach, are the rarest type of gastric polyp and have no malignant potential. These lesions may occur sporadically or in association with a variety of inherited polyposis syndromes, including familial adenomatous polyposis and Gardner's syndrome, Peutz-Jeghers syndrome, Cronkhite-Canada syndrome, and Cowden disease.

Gastric polyps are almost always asymptomatic and usually discovered incidentally at endoscopic or radiologic examination. Patients may complain of vague epigastric pain unrelated to eating, bloating, belching, or nausea. Occult GI bleeding and iron deficiency anemia may also occur, but hematemesis is rare. Patients with pedunculated polyps near

Table 105-2. Gastric Cancer: 5-year Survival by Disease Stage at Diagnosis

Stage	TNM		Description	5-year survival (%)
I	$T_1N_0M_0$	T1	Tumor limited to mucosa or submucosa	85-90
		N0	No lymph node metastases	
		M0	No distant metastases	
II	$T_{2\text{-}3}N_0M_0$	T2	Tumor involves muscularis, does not penetrate serosa	52-55
		T3	Tumor penetrates serosa, does not involve contiguous structures	45-47
III	$T_{1\text{-}3}N_{1\text{-}3}M_0$	N1	Involvement of perigastric nodes within 3 cm of tumor	17-20
		N2	Involvement of regional nodes more than 3 cm from tumor, resectable	5-10
		N3	Other intraabdominal and nonremovable nodes involved by tumor	
IV	$T_4N_{1\text{-}3}M_0$	T4	Tumor invades contiguous structures (includes unresectable tumors)	3
	$T_{1\text{-}4}N_{0\text{-}3}M_1$	M1	Distant metastases present	

the pylorus may present with symptoms of intermittent gastric outlet obstruction caused by prolapse.

Management of gastric polyps depends on clinicopathologic considerations. All polypoid gastric lesions require biopsy to establish a histologic diagnosis. All symptomatic polyps should be removed either endoscopically or surgically. Asymptomatic hyperplastic or hamartomatous polyps, if small and adequately biopsied, do not need to be removed. Eradication of *H. pylori* has been reported to induce regression of hyperplastic polyps and should be considered if coinfection is present. Adenomatous polyps should be completely excised because of their premalignant nature. Surgical resection is indicated for any polyp containing malignant tissue, adenomatous polyps not amenable to complete endoscopic removal, and polyps with nondiagnostic histology. Patients with adenomatous gastric polyps require annual endoscopic surveillance because of the risk of developing new polyps or cancer. Surveillance is not recommended for patients with only hyperplastic or hamartomatous polyps.

Gastric Lymphoma

Primary gastric lymphoma accounts for 1% to 5% of all gastric malignancies and is anatomically the most common extranodal type of non-Hodgkin's lymphoma. The stomach is also often involved in patients with disseminated disease arising elsewhere. Most primary gastric lymphomas arise from preexisting mucosa-associated lymphoid tissue (MALT) lymphomas. Recent epidemiologic studies support a strong association between MALT lymphomas and chronic *H. pylori* infection.[11] MALT lymphomas can also occur in association with various autoimmune and immunodeficiency syndromes. Most develop in individuals over age 50, and there is a slight male predominance. Symptoms are nonspecific and include abdominal pain, nausea, vomiting, anorexia, weight loss, and bleeding.

Grossly, MALT lymphomas are often indistinguishable from gastric adenocarcinomas and may present as unifocal ulcerated, polypoid, or infiltrating mass lesions involving the antrum and prepyloric region or body of the stomach (Fig. 105-2, *A*). Multifocal or diffuse involvement is uncommon. Histologically, MALT lymphomas are of B-cell origin and classified as low grade or high grade. *Low-grade* MALT lymphomas are characterized by the presence of nonneoplastic reactive lymphoid follicles surrounded by small to medium-sized centrocyte-like (CCL) tumor cells that extend into the surrounding tissue and invade individual gastric glands to form lymphoepithelial complexes (Fig. 105-2, *B*). *High-grade* MALT lymphomas are characterized by confluent sheets or clusters of centroblastic (large, noncleaved) or plasmablastic tumor cells outside of colonized follicles. Reactive lymphoid follicles and lymphoepithelial lesions may or may not be present; if absent, high-grade MALT lymphomas may be histologically and cytologically indistinguishable from other high-grade B-cell lymphomas.

The diagnosis of gastric lymphoma should be considered in any person found to have diffuse mucosal hypertrophy with irregular thickening of the rugal folds or an ulcerated or polypoid mass at endoscopy or on UGI series. Endoscopic biopsies and brush cytology or fine-needle aspiration should be obtained to establish the diagnosis. Endoscopic ultrasound, CT of the abdomen and chest, and bone marrow aspiration with biopsy provide additional staging information.

Histologic grade and stage of disease dictate the treatment of gastric lymphomas (Table 105-3). Eradication of *H. pylori* is the treatment of choice for stage IE low-grade lymphomas, with complete regression rates in the range of 70%. Coincident high-grade disease missed on biopsy is the most common reason for resistance. Because of the potential for sampling error and relapse, close follow-up with periodic UGI endoscopy and biopsy is indicated every 4 weeks until resolution, then every 3 to 6 months. Patients who do not respond or relapse still have a high rate of cure. Five-year survival for such patients is as high as 80% to 90% after single-agent chemotherapy (e.g., cyclophosphamide or chlorambucil) or radiation therapy. Multiagent chemotherapy, such as CHOP (cyclophosphamide, doxorubicin, vincristine, prednisone), is reserved for the small percentage of patients who fail to respond or who relapse after other, less aggressive

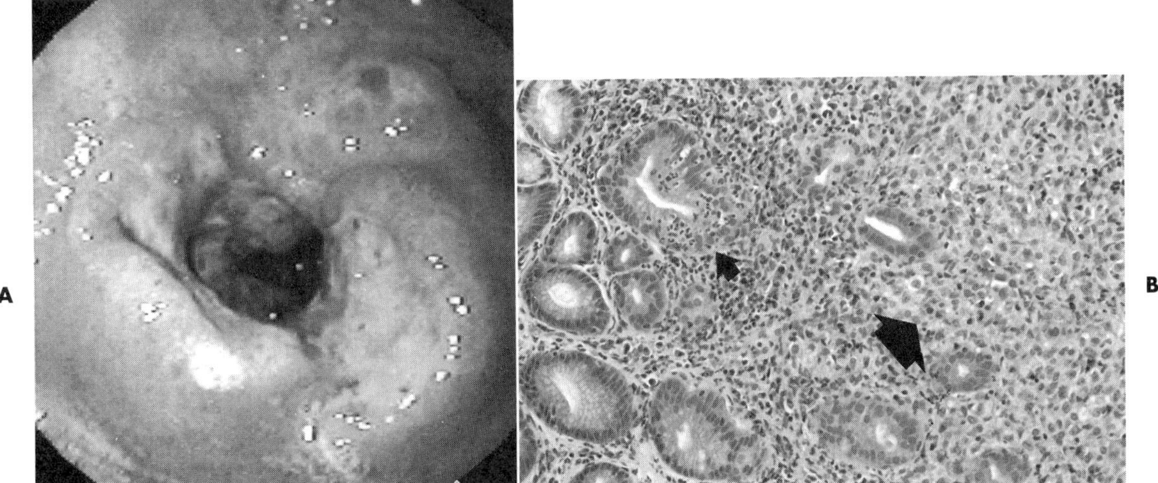

Fig. 105-2. **A,** Endoscopic appearance of large, ulcerated gastric MALT lymphoma. **B,** Histologic appearance of low-grade gastric MALT lymphoma with characteristic lymphoepithelial complex *(small arrow)* on left, and coincident high-grade MALT lymphoma on right *(wide arrow)*.

Table 105-3. Ann Arbor Classification of Gastric Lymphomas

Stage	Extent of disease
IE	Disease limited to stomach
IIE	Extention to abdominal nodes
IIIE	Involvement of stomach, abdominal nodes, and nodes above diaphragm
IV	Disseminated

E, Extranodal site.

therapies. CHOP chemotherapy is also the treatment of choice for patients with extensive mucosal involvement or advanced (stage IIIE or IV) disease.

Optimal treatment for early-stage high-grade lymphomas remains controversial. Historically, surgery, alone or in combination with radiation therapy or chemotherapy, was the mainstay of therapy for stages IE and IIE disease. Although surgery remains an option, particularly for patients with bulky disease, recent studies suggest that systemic chemotherapy with multiagent regimens (e.g., CHOP) alone may be superior. CHOP chemotherapy remains the treatment of choice for stages IIIE and IV disease. Overall survival for high-grade gastric lymphomas is about 45%.

Stromal Tumors

Leiomyomas are the most common benign stromal tumor of the stomach, occurring in up to 50% of persons over age 50. The vast majority are small (less than 2 cm) and clinically silent. Larger lesions may ulcerate and produce bleeding or abdominal pain. These tumors arise from the smooth muscle layer of the stomach and therefore appear as intramural filling defects with or without superficial ulceration on UGI series or as submucosal masses endoscopically. Endoscopic biopsies are frequently nondiagnostic, unless the lesion is ulcerated. Local surgical excision is the treatment of choice for symptomatic lesions.

Leiomyosarcomas account for approximately 1% of gastric malignancies. These tumors are sometimes difficult to distinguish from benign leiomyomas unless evidence suggests local extension or distant metastasis. As with leiomyomas, GI bleeding and abdominal pain are the most common presenting symptoms. A palpable abdominal mass and weight loss are highly suggestive of malignancy. Surgical resection is the treatment of choice, but unfortunately, two thirds of patients have extragastric spread at initial laparotomy. Neither radiotherapy nor chemotherapy has demonstrated significant efficacy. Five-year survival rates are 25% to 50%.

Gastric Carcinoids

Carcinoid tumors of the stomach are rare. They can be separated into three distinct groups: those associated with chronic atrophic gastritis type A, those associated with Zollinger-Ellison syndrome, and so-called sporadic carcinoids. Carcinoids associated with chronic atrophic gastritis (75%) may be unifocal or multifocal and typically present in the sixth or seventh decade of life; most are small (less than 1 cm) and rarely metastasize. Carcinoids associated with Zollinger-Ellison syndrome (5% to 10%) occur almost exclusively in patients with multiple endocrine neoplasia (MEN) type 1 and behave similar to those associated with chronic atrophic gastritis. Sporadic gastric carcinoids (15% to 25%) are much more aggressive and often fatal. Most present with metastatic disease, which may be accompanied by an atypical carcinoid syndrome manifested primarily by flushing.

Most gastric carcinoids, except for the sporadic type, are small and asymptomatic. Grossly they may resemble an ordinary ulcer, polyp, or tumor mass; occasionally, multiple lesions are present. Histologically it is often difficult to distinguish between benign and malignant tumors unless metastases are present. Gastric carcinoids arise in the foregut and may secrete a variety of hormones, including 5-hydroxytryptophan, adrenocorticotropic hormone (ACTH), or 5-hydroxytryptamine (serotonin). Thus patients may present with clinical manifestations of the carcinoid syndrome or Cushing's syndrome, but both are rare in the absence of liver metastases. An elevation in 24-hour urinary levels of 5-hydroxyindoleacetic acid (5-HIAA) confirms the diagnosis in such patients. Decisions regarding management depend on tumor size and histology. Complete endoscopic or surgical excision is the treatment of choice for small (less than 1 cm), incidentally discovered lesions. Larger lesions tend to exhibit more aggressive biologic behavior and warrant wide surgical resection with lymph node dissection. Management of metastatic disease and the carcinoid syndrome is discussed in the next section.

TUMORS OF THE SMALL BOWEL

Primary tumors of the small bowel are uncommon compared with other sites in the GI tract. The relative paucity of small bowel tumors is intriguing particularly because the small bowel accounts for 75% of the length of the GI tract and more than 90% of its mucosal surface area. Neutral or alkaline luminal pH, rapid transit, the liquid nature of the luminal contents, few anaerobic bacteria, and the presence of detoxifying enzymes (e.g., benzopyrene hydroxylase) capable of nullifying the effects of carcinogens have all been implicated as causing this phenomenon. Despite their rarity, small bowel tumors should be considered in the differential diagnosis of patients with symptoms suggestive of intermittent partial small bowel obstruction or unexplained occult GI blood loss (see Table 105-1).

Epidemiology

The epidemiology of benign small bowel tumors is not well defined because most are asymptomatic and not evident clinically. Conversely, accurate epidemiologic data for malignant small bowel tumors are available because of their progressive and ultimately symptomatic nature. Overall, tumors of the small bowel account for approximately 1% of all GI malignancies. In 1998, approximately 4500 new cases and 1200 deaths from malignant small bowel tumors occurred in the United States. Adenocarcinomas, carcinoid tumors, and primary lymphomas are the most common small bowel malignancies. Incidence figures suggest a slight male predominance for all three types of malignancies, with an overall incidence of less than one case per 100,000 population. Malignant small bowel tumors tend to be more common in developed countries, with the exception of *immunoproliferative small intestinal disease* (IPSID), also known as α-chain disease, Mediterranean lymphoma, or diffuse primary small intestinal lymphoma, which predominates in impoverished geographic regions.

Etiology

The etiology of most small bowel tumors is poorly understood. Although causative factors undoubtedly vary with histologic type, common factors must exist because patients with celiac sprue are predisposed to both adenocarcinoma and lymphoma of the small bowel. As in the colon, small bowel adenocarcinomas probably arise from preexisting benign adenomas, but the molecular mechanisms responsible for malignant transformation are unknown. Microbial colonization appears to be an important etiologic factor in the IPSID form of primary small bowel lymphoma based on its epidemiology and the observation that the disease is reversible if treated with tetracycline at the early prelymphomatous stage. Infectious etiologies have also been linked to other forms of small bowel lymphoma, most notably Epstein-Barr virus and both Burkitt's and Burkitt's-like (sporadic Burkitt's) small bowel lymphomas. Impairment of the normal mechanical or immunologic barriers, resulting in increased mucosal penetration of deleterious pathogens and antigens, has also been implicated in the etiology of small bowel tumors in patients with Crohn's disease and celiac sprue.

Predisposing Conditions

A number of mostly rare conditions appear to be associated with an increased risk of malignant small bowel tumors. Celiac sprue, Crohn's disease, familial adenomatous polyposis or Gardner's syndrome, neurofibromatosis, and various reconstructive procedures involving the ileum (e.g., ileal conduit, ileocystoplasty, ileostomy) have all been associated with an increased risk of small bowel adenocarcinomas. Celiac sprue, Crohn's disease, nodular lymphoid hyperplasia, autoimmune diseases, and immunodeficiency syndromes, including acquired immunodeficiency syndrome (AIDS), predispose to small bowel lymphomas. With the exception of familial adenomatous polyposis, periodic surveillance is generally not recommended for these conditions.

Histopathology and Differential Diagnosis

Benign Tumors. Adenomas, leiomyomas, and lipomas are the most common benign tumors of the small bowel. *Adenomas* arise from the epithelial elements and can display tubular, tubulovillous, or villous growth patterns. Although the natural history of small bowel adenomas is not well defined, they probably have a similar malignant potential to colorectal adenomas. Most are small and may be sessile or pedunculated. Both sporadic adenomas and those associated with familial polyposis syndromes have a predilection for the proximal small intestine, particularly in the periampullary region of the duodenum. Periampullary adenomas, particularly of the villous type, are associated with a high risk of invasive adenocarcinoma.

Leiomyomas and *lipomas* arise from smooth muscle and fatty tissue, respectively. It is unknown if they can degenerate into malignant forms, but if this occurs, it must be very rare. Other benign tumors are curiosities.

Malignant Tumors. Adenocarcinomas are the most common malignant tumors of the small bowel. Most originate in the proximal small bowel, from the second part of the duodenum to about 20 to 30 cm distant to the ligament of Treitz. Structurally they may be flat, stenosing, infiltrating, ulcerating, or polypoid lesions. Histologic appearance is similar to that of colorectal adenocarcinomas.

Primary small bowel *lymphomas* are a heterogenous group of unique B-cell and T-cell lymphoid malignancies with distinctive epidemiologic and clinicopathologic features (Table 105-4). The most common are B-cell lymphomas of the MALT type. IPSID is a specialized type of MALT lymphoma that occurs almost exclusively in the Middle East and is characterized by the synthesis of α-heavy chain paraprotein.

As with benign leiomyomas, *Leiomyosarcomas* arise from smooth muscle cells. Early-stage tumors may be difficult to distinguish from leiomyomas. More advanced tumors tend to be less differentiated and easier to diagnose histologically.

Small bowel *carcinoid tumors* (carcinoids) are thought to arise from serotonin-producing intraepithelial neuroendocrine cells. The ileum is the most common site of malignant tumors. Besides serotonin, these tumors may secrete a variety of biologically active substances, including gastrin, histamine, somatostatin, pituitary hormones, catecholamines, kinins, and prostaglandins. In general, localized tumors are rarely associated with the carcinoid syndrome because they secrete only small amounts of hormone(s), which are rapidly inactivated by the liver. The carcinoid syndrome is much more frequently associated with bulky metastatic disease involving the liver.

Histologically, it is often difficult to distinguish benign from malignant tumors. Localized tumors less than 1 cm are generally regarded as benign and those greater than 2 cm as malignant.

Clinical Presentation

Benign tumors are often asymptomatic and clinically insignificant. Fluctuating abdominal pain from intermittent partial small bowel obstruction is the most frequent presenting manifestation of symptomatic lesions. Obstruction is often caused by intussusception; benign small bowel tumors, particularly lipomas, are the most common cause of intussusception in adults. Occult GI bleeding may also be seen, but frank hematemesis or rectal bleeding is rare.

Because of their progressive nature, malignant tumors eventually become symptomatic and ultimately fatal unless detected early. Abdominal pain is the most common presenting symptom and may be colicky or more constant. Occult GI blood loss and iron deficiency anemia are also common, but frank bleeding is rare except with leiomyosarcomas. Weight loss occurs in up to 50% of patients and may be secondary to malabsorption, particularly with IPSID. Perforation is rare but may be seen with lymphomas or leiomyosarcomas. Jaundice is a common presenting feature of malignant periampullary tumors. Flushing, diarrhea, abdominal pain, and valvular heart disease typify the carcinoid syndrome, but other manifestations may also be present (Table 105-5). Foregut carcinoids may also cause symptoms of hypoglycemia, gastric hypersecretion, or Cushing's syndrome.

Diagnosis

Barium contrast radiography has been the principal modality for the preoperative detection of small bowel tumors. The

Table 105-4. Clinicopathologic Features of Primary Gastrointestinal Non-Hodgkin's Lymphomas

Type of lymphoma	Clinical features	Site(s) of involvement	Pathologic features	Associated conditions
B cell				
Mucosa-associated lymphoid tissue (MALT) Western type	Adults: fifth to sixth decade Males > females Abdominal pain, nausea/vomiting, occult bleeding, weight loss, diarrhea	Stomach > terminal ileum > jejunum > duodenum > colon > esophagus ± Mesenteric nodes (late) ± direct extension to adjacent organs (late)	Ulcerated, exophytic, or infiltrating mass (unifocal > diffuse) Low grade Reactive lymphoid follicles Parafollicular small to medium-sized centrocyte-like (CCL) tumor cells Lymphoepithelial complexes High grade Sheets/clusters of centroblastic (large, noncleaved) or plasmablastic tumor cells ± Reactive lymphoid follicles ± Lymphoepithelial complexes	*Helicobacter pylori* infection Autoimmune disease Immunodeficiency syndromes Inflammatory bowel disease Nodular lymphoid hyperplasia
Immunoproliferative small intestinal disease (IPSID) (α-chain disease, Mediterranean, diffuse small intestinal lymphoma)	Young adults: second to third decade Males ≥ females Mediterranean, Middle East regions Low socioeconomic status Poor sanitation, low hygiene Abdominal pain, malabsorption, diarrhea, weight loss, clubbing, edema α-Chain paraproteinemia	Small intestine (proximal >> distal) ± Mesenteric nodes (late) ± Direct extension to adjacent organs (late)	Diffuse, infiltrating tumor Prelymphomatous stage: mature plasma cell infiltrate in mucosa and mesenteric lymph nodes Lymphomatous stage Low grade: extension of plasma cell infiltrate into submucosa and features of low-grade Western-type MALT High-grade: resemble high-grade Western-type MALT	Small intestine bacterial overgrowth and parasitosis

Mantle cell	Sixth to seventh decade Males > females Abdominal pain, diarrhea, weight loss, hematochezia, fatigue	Colon, small bowel > stomach Mesenteric nodes Early spread to liver, spleen, peripheral nodes, and bone marrow	Multiple nodules or polypoid lesions Resemble peripheral nodal-type lymphomas Dense, monotonous infiltrate of small intermediate-sized cleaved cells Nodular or mixed nodular/diffuse pattern	?
Burkitts/Burkitt-like	Adults, children (50%) Industrialized societies Abdominal pain, obstruction, diarrhea, bleeding	Children: ileocecal region Adults: small bowel, rectum	Bulky mass ± ulceration Small noncleaved tumor cells "Tingible body" macrophages leading to "starry sky" appearance	? Epstein-Barr virus infection Immunodeficiency syndromes (e.g., AIDS) Immunosuppression (e.g., posttransplantation)
T cell				
Enteropathy associated	Adults (mean age, 60 years) Abdominal pain, diarrhea, weight loss, bleeding, perforation, obstruction	Jejunum > duodenum > ileum Mesenteric nodes	Large circumferential ulcer > bulky mass Variable histology Medium to large blast cells *or* Pleomorphic cell infiltrate with multinucleated cells *or* Tumor cells resembling small lymphocytes ± Intense inflammatory infiltrate	Longstanding celiac sprue ± Dermatitis herpetiformis

Table 105-5. Clinical Manifestations of Carcinoid Syndrome

Organ	Manifestation
Skin	Flushing
	Telangiectasia
	Cyanosis
	Pellagra
Gastrointestinal tract	Diarrhea
	Cramping
Heart	Valvular lesions
Respiratory tract	Wheezing
Kidney	Peripheral edema
Joints	Arthritis

routine small bowel follow-through after oral ingestion of barium is useful in assessing the terminal ileum but less sensitive than enteroclysis (small bowel enema) in assessing other parts of the small bowel. Since enteroclysis requires duodenal intubation, it is reasonable to obtain a routine small bowel study, with compression views of the terminal ileum as the initial diagnostic study, in patients with suspected small bowel tumors. If this examination is negative or inconclusive, enteroclysis should be performed.

Endoscopic approaches are also useful in the diagnosis of small bowel tumors. In addition to direct visualization, endoscopy provides a means of obtaining tissue for histologic evaluation. Endoscopy is the procedure of choice for patients with occult GI blood loss. Otherwise asymptomatic patients, however, should first undergo colonoscopy to exclude the presence of a colonic neoplasm. Evaluation of the UGI tract is indicated if the colonoscopy is negative or if the condition suggests UGI disease. UGI endoscopy is done to further evaluate abnormal radiographic findings. Other diagnostic modalities, particularly for preoperative staging of malignant tumors, include CT scan, MRI, and in select cases arteriography.

Urinary 5-HIAA, a metabolite of serotonin, should be measured in patients with clinical features suggestive of carcinoid syndrome. Serotonin-containing foods and drugs (e.g., phenothiazines) that elevate serotonin levels can give false-positive results and should be withheld during testing. Malabsorption and chronic intestinal obstruction can also cause modest elevations in urinary 5-HIAA levels. Plasma or platelet serotonin levels can also be measured, but these tests are not widely available. Scintigraphy with radiolabeled octreotide, a long-acting somatostatin analog, is useful in localizing both primary and metastatic carcinoid tumors, with a sensitivity of about 90%.

Treatment and Prognosis

Benign Tumors. Adenomas of the small bowel should be treated because of their premalignant status. Appropriate therapy depends on several factors, including location, size, shape (sessile or pedunculated), and histologic type (tubular or villous). Duodenal adenomas, with the exception of periampullary lesions, are usually amenable to endoscopic removal or ablation. Although some periampullary adenomas can also be treated endoscopically, surgical resection is preferred for most because of their sessile shape, villous histology, and propensity for malignant transformation. Local resection is considered adequate for completely benign tumors; more radical resection (i.e., pancreaticoduodenectomy [Whipple procedure]) is indicated for adenomas containing carcinoma. Unlike with colonic adenomas, long-term surveillance is not indicated for sporadic small bowel adenomas unless incomplete removal is a concern. Surveillance is recommended for patients with familial polyposis or Gardner's syndrome. Although strict guidelines have not been adopted, before prophylactic colectomy it is reasonable to perform a UGI endoscopy in these patients at age 30, then every 3 years.

Limited resection is adequate treatment for other benign tumors of the small bowel. Observation alone may be sufficient for asymptomatic tumors discovered incidentally at endoscopy, assuming biopsies confirm benign histology.

Malignant Tumors. Surgical resection is the only potentially curative treatment for adenocarcinomas of the small bowel. Palliative resection or bypass should be considered if curative resection is not feasible. Palliative procedures should also be considered to control bleeding or relieve obstruction. Unfortunately, neither chemotherapy nor radiation therapy is effective in the treatment of advanced disease. Overall 5-year survival is only 10% to 20% even after "curative" resection.

Optimal treatment of primary small bowel lymphomas depends on extent of involvement, stage, and to a lesser degree, type. Broad-spectrum antibiotics (e.g., tetracycline) alone or in combination with corticosteroids are recommended for the treatment of early-stage (prelymphomatous) IPSID, with response rates of 33% to 71%. Regardless of type, surgical resection is indicated for localized lymphomas confined to the bowel wall (stage IE) or involving contiguous nodes only (stage IIE). The role of adjuvant radiation therapy or chemotherapy after curative resection is controversial. Resection should also be considered for more advanced segmental disease to reduce tumor burden, relieve symptoms (e.g., obstruction), and obviate the risk of bleeding or perforation induced by radiation therapy or chemotherapy. Radiation therapy, alone or in combination with chemotherapy is the treatment of choice for patients with diffuse, unresectable small bowel disease. Disseminated disease is usually treated with radiation therapy plus combination chemotherapy. Overall 5-year survival rates vary but are about 50% for Western-type MALT lymphomas, 67% for IPSID, 60% for mantle cell lymphomas, and less than 10% for enteropathy-associated T-cell lymphoma. Prognosis for Burkitt's-like lymphomas is very good for children, with 5-year survival rates of 75%, but poor for adults, particularly in association with human immunodeficiency virus (HIV) infection.

Carcinoid tumors of the small bowel should be resected because of their potential to invade and metastasize. Tumors less than 1 cm are usually benign and can be cured with a limited surgical resection. Larger tumors, particularly those greater than 2 cm, require more radical surgical resection. Surgical resection of liver metastases should be considered for patients with limited hepatic disease, since it offers the most effective long-term palliation of symptoms and may prolong survival. Hepatic artery occlusion or embolization are alternatives for patients who are not candidates for resection, but responses tend to be of short duration. Cytotoxic chemotherapy is rarely of benefit and should be reserved for patients with significant symptoms or those who exhibit poor prognostic signs, such as impaired liver function, clinically evident carcinoid heart disease, or very high levels of urinary 5-HIAA. Synthetic analogs of somatostatin (e.g., octreotide) are highly effective in relieving the symptoms of carcinoid syndrome and have emerged as the treatment of choice for symptomatic disease. Although overall 5-year survival is only about 54%, prolonged survival does occur, even in the patient with metastatic disease.

Surgical resection is the treatment of choice for leiomyosarcomas. Chemotherapy with doxorubicin-containing regimens and radiation therapy both have a role in the management of unresectable disease. Surgery has also been advocated in the treatment of solitary liver or lung metastases. Overall 5-year survival rates of 20% to 50% have been reported.

TUMORS OF THE LARGE BOWEL

Colorectal tumors are often encountered in the evaluation of both symptomatic and asymptomatic patients. Polyps are the most common benign tumors and may be classified as neoplastic (adenomatous polyps), nonneoplastic (e.g., hyperplastic polyps), or submucosal (e.g., lipomas). Adenomatous polyps (adenomas) are premalignant precursors of most colorectal cancers; in contrast, nonneoplastic polyps have little or no malignant potential. Adenocarcinomas are by far the most common malignant tumors. Lymphomas, carcinoids, sarcomas, and a variety of extremely rare malignant tumors may also occur in the large bowel. This discussion focuses primarily on adenocarcinoma of the large bowel, commonly referred to as colorectal cancer, and its precursor, the adenomatous polyp.

Epidemiology

Worldwide incidence and mortality of colorectal cancer vary considerably. With the notable exception of Japan, industrialized countries are at greatest risk. High rates are found in North America, Western Europe, and New Zealand, whereas lower rates are found in Eastern Europe, most South American countries, Asia, and Africa. In the United States, both incidence and mortality rates have declined in recent years. Nevertheless, colorectal cancer remains the third most common form of cancer, with a standardized age-adjusted incidence of approximately 31 cases per 100,000 population, and the second leading cause of cancer-related death. In 1999 approximately 129,000 new cases were diagnosed and 56,600 persons died from their disease. Americans of average risk have approximately a 6% chance of developing colorectal cancer during their lifetime. Age is an important determinant of risk. Although extremely uncommon in persons under age 35 (except with rare predisposing genetic syndromes), the incidence of colorectal cancer increases steadily with age, particularly after age 50. Cancers of the colon affect men and women at similar rates, whereas cancers of the rectum are more common in men. Overall 5-year survival rates have improved significantly in recent years, presumably because of improved therapy and early detection, and are currently about 60%. Low-income minority groups, particularly black males, tend to have lower survival rates even after adjustment for tumor stage.

The epidemiology of colorectal adenomas is similar to that of colorectal cancer. In general the prevalence of colorectal adenomas in a given country parallels the prevalence of colorectal cancer. Age is an important determinant of prevalence in high-risk countries. U.S. autopsy studies suggest an overall prevalence of 50%, from about 30% at age 50 to 55% at age 80. Unlike colorectal cancer, adenomas are more common in men.

Etiology

The etiology of colorectal adenomas and subsequent colorectal cancer is unknown but seems related to both environmental and genetic factors. The importance of environmental factors is supported by the wide geographic variation in incidence rates and studies of migrant populations. Diet is probably the major environmental factor that explains these epidemiologic associations. In general, populations with a relatively high prevalence of colorectal adenomas and cancer consume high-calorie, high-fat diets. Conversely, populations at low risk consume diets rich in fruits, vegetables, and crude fiber. Observational studies have suggested that red meat rather than total fat may be responsible for the increased risk. Such studies have also challenged the protective effect of fiber.

Environmental factors other than diet have been linked with colorectal cancer risk. Lack of physical activity, obesity, daily alcohol consumption, and long-term exposure to cigarette smoke all appear to increase risk, whereas high levels of physical activity, multivitamins containing folic acid, regular use of aspirin, and for women, use of postmenopausal hormones and possibly oral contraceptives may reduce risk. More than 50% of colorectal cancers could be prevented if these lifestyle modifications were adopted at an early enough age to reverse risk.

Genetic factors are also important in the etiology of colorectal adenomas and cancers. It is now well established that germ-line mutations of the *APC* (adenomatous polyposis coli) tumor suppressor gene are responsible for familial adenomatous polyposis (FAP) and its variants. Germ-line mutations of at least five DNA-mismatch repair genes (*hMLH1, hMSH2, hMSH3, hPMS1,* and *hPMS2*) have also been identified as the causal events in HNPCC. Somatic mutations of *APC* and the DNA-mismatch repair genes, particularly *hMLH1,* and alterations in a number of other genes, including the *K-ras* protooncogene, p53 tumor suppressor gene, and *DCC* (deleted in colon cancer) gene, have also been identified in a variable percentage of familial and sporadic colorectal cancers and adenomas.

Predisposing Conditions

A number of conditions have been associated with an increased risk of colorectal cancer (Box 105-1). Recognition of these high-risk groups has important implications for screening.

Personal History. With rare exception, virtually all colorectal cancers arise from adenomas. Metachronous adenomas can be identified in 12% to 60% of patients at follow-up colonoscopy, depending on the surveillance interval employed, with a 5% to 8% risk of developing a cancer within 15 years of follow-up. Patients with a history of colorectal cancer have a 5% to 10% risk of developing a metachronous cancer with 15 years and a 30% risk of developing metachronous adenomas.

Box 105-1. Risk Factors for Colorectal Cancer

Average Risk

Age 50 or older, asymptomatic

Increased Risk

Past history
- Colorectal cancer
- Colorectal adenoma
- Breast, ovarian, and uterine cancer

Family history
- Colorectal cancer
- Colorectal adenomas before age 60

Inflammatory bowel disease
- Chronic ulcerative colitis
- Crohn's colitis

Hereditary nonpolyposis colorectal cancer (HNPCC, Lynch syndrome)

Adenomatous polyposis
- Familial polyposis (polyposis coli)
- Gardner's syndrome
- Turcot's syndrome

Nonadenomatous polyposis
- Peutz-Jeghers syndrome
- Juvenile polyposis

Familial Adenomatous Polyposis. The inherited polyposis syndromes, including FAP, Gardner's syndrome, and Turcot's syndrome, account for about 1% of colorectal cancer cases. FAP is a rare autosomal dominant condition characterized by the presence of 100 or more colorectal adenomas. The disease is caused by mutations of the *APC* gene on chromosome 5. The polyps are not present at birth but appear during the second or third decade of life. If left untreated, the risk of colorectal cancer is 100% by age 40. The incidence of gastric and small bowel polyps is also increased. The duodenal papilla and periampullary region have a particular propensity for adenomatous and occasionally carcinomatous change. *Gardner's syndrome* is a variant of FAP and can be distinguished from FAP by extraintestinal manifestations, including desmoids, osteomas, benign soft tissue tumors (e.g., lipomas), and dental abnormalities. Congenital hypertrophy of the retinal pigment epithelium is an early manifestation of both FAP and Gardner's syndrome. *Turcot's syndrome* is another rare genetic condition sometimes associated with *APC* mutations and characterized by colorectal adenomatous polyposis and brain tumors.

Two other conditions have been linked to mutations of the *APC* gene and are believed to be FAP variants: an attenuated form typically presenting later in life, with far fewer, predominantly right-sided adenomas, and the so-called flat adenoma syndrome, which is phenotypically similar to the attenuated form except that the adenomas are flat rather than polypoid.

Hereditary Nonpolyposis Colorectal Cancer. HNPCC is an autosomal dominant condition caused by mutations of at least five different DNA-mismatch repair genes with high penetrance. The syndrome accounts for 5% to 10% of colorectal cancer cases and is characterized by early-onset colorectal cancer (average age, 44 years) in the absence of polyposis, a predominance of tumors proximal to the splenic flexure (approximately 70%), and an excess of both synchronous and metachronous colorectal cancers. Patients are also at increased risk of cancers at other sites, including the endometrium, ovaries, stomach, small intestine, upper urinary tract, biliary tract, and brain (Turcot's syndrome). *Torre's syndrome* (Muir-Torre syndrome), a rare familial condition characterized by multiple sebaceous gland tumors and colorectal cancer, is a subtype of HNPCC. The estimated lifetime risk of developing colorectal cancer in any of the HNPCC syndromes is 80% to 90%, with approximately 50% of cases occurring before age 50. Patients tend to develop multiple, predominantly right-sided, flat adenomas at a higher frequency and younger age than sporadic cases. These adenomas typically exhibit an aggressive histology and diminished dwell time, even though HNPCC-associated cancers have a better prognosis stage for stage than those arising in the general population. Revised criteria have been adopted by which to identify HNPCC families (Box 105-2).

Box 105-2. Revised Amsterdam Criteria for Hereditary Nonpolyposis Colorectal Cancer (HNPCC)

Three or more relatives should have HNPCC-associated cancer (colorectal, endometrial, small bowel, ureter, or renal pelvis).
One relative should be a first-degree relative of the other two.
At least two successive generations should be affected.
At least one relative should be diagnosed before age 50.
Familial adenomatous polyposis (FAP) should be excluded in colorectal cancer cases, if any.
Tumors should be verified by pathologic examination.

Family History. It has long been recognized that a family history of colorectal cancer increases an individual's risk of colorectal cancer. Results of several epidemiologic surveys indicate that individuals with a single first-degree affected relative have a twofold to threefold increased lifetime risk of developing colorectal cancer compared with the average person in the general population. Individuals with two first-degree affected relatives are at even greater risk. The same is true for persons with a first-degree affected relative diagnosed with a colorectal adenoma before age 60.

Inflammatory Bowel Disease. Patients with both chronic idiopathic ulcerative colitis and Crohn's disease have an increased risk of colorectal cancer. The actual degree of risk, however, is debatable. For ulcerative colitis the duration of disease and extent of involvement are important determinants of risk. Patients with pancolitis of greater than 7 years' duration or left-sided colitis of 15 years' duration are at increased risk. Duration of disease also appears to be a factor for patients with Crohn's disease. Unlike most colorectal cancers that arise from adenomas, cancers associated with inflammatory bowel disease tend to arise in flat mucosa and therefore are more difficult to detect at an early stage. Dysplasia, the presence of DNA aneuploidy, and mutations of the p53 tumor suppressor gene are early markers of neoplastic transformation.

Inherited Nonadenomatous Polyposis Syndromes. Generalized juvenile polyposis and Peutz-Jeghers syndrome are both associated with an increased risk of colorectal cancer. *Generalized juvenile polyposis* is an autosomal dominant condition characterized by numerous juvenile polyps of the colon. Juvenile polyps are nonneoplastic hamartomas composed of a fibrovascular stroma, cystic epithelial glandular structures, and a conspicuous inflammatory component. The increased risk of colorectal cancer, although small, is related to the presence of adenomatous epithelium in some juvenile polyps. Single juvenile polyps are not associated with an increased risk of colorectal cancer. *Peutz-Jeghers syndrome* is another autosomal dominant hereditary disease characterized by hamartomatous polyposis of the small and large bowels and by mucocutaneous pigmentation. A small percentage of patients develop colorectal cancer at a young age, presumably related to the occasional presence of adenomatous epithelium within the hamartomas.

Miscellaneous Conditions. Women with a history of breast, ovarian, or endometrial cancer are at increased risk of colorectal cancer, as are patients with a history of abdominal or pelvic irradiation. Additional risk factors include the presence of a ureterosigmoidostomy, *Streptococcus bovis* bacteremia and endocarditis, *Schistosoma japonicum* infections of the colon, and Bloom syndrome. The association between cholecystectomy and colorectal neoplasia appears to be relatively weak.

Histopathology and Differential Diagnosis

Adenomatous Polyps. Adenomatous polyps are benign glandular neoplasms. They are classified as tubular, villous, or tubulovillous. Clinicopathologic studies suggest a strong correlation between extent of the villous component and adenoma size. Based on endoscopic surveys, approximately 80% of adenomas are tubular, 5% to 15% tubulovillous, and 3% to 5% villous. The distribution of adenomas is similar to that of colorectal cancers.

All adenomas display some degree of *dysplasia,* which is defined on the basis of cytologic atypia and architectural abnormality. According to the WHO classification system, *low-grade* dysplasia incorporates the categories of mild and moderate dysplasia, whereas *high-grade* dysplasia incorporates the categories of severe dysplasia and carcinoma in situ. Adenomas with mild dysplasia exhibit few of the pathologic criteria of malignancy; those with severe dysplasia have most of the cytologic and structural characteristics of cancer, but the glands themselves are not invasive. Adenomas containing invasive cancer are referred to as *malignant polyps.* It is estimated that fewer than 5% of adenomas undergo malignant transformation. The likelihood of finding invasive cancer in an adenoma increases with size (larger than 2 cm), villous component, and presence of high-grade dysplasia. Multiplicity and age may also be determinants.

Nonadenomatous Polyps. In addition to adenomas, other types of benign polyps arise in the colon and rectum. The most common of these is the *hyperplastic polyp.* Hyperplastic polyps tend to be small (under 5 mm) and have a predilection for the rectum and sigmoid colon. Depending on the method of study, hyperplastic polyps may be found in up to 80% of individuals. As with adenomas, their frequency increases with age. Hyperplastic polyps are nonneoplastic and have no malignant potential. Although subtle differences have been described in terms of gross appearance, it is nearly impossible to distinguish these lesions from small adenomas endoscopically.

Juvenile polyps are nonneoplastic hamartomas with a characteristic histology. They are the most common polyps of childhood. Bleeding and rectal prolapse are the most common clinical manifestations. Many will infarct and pass spontaneously. Unlike generalized juvenile polyposis, isolated juvenile polyps have no malignant potential. *Pseudopolyps* are nonneoplastic polypoid remnants seen in longstanding inflammatory bowel disease. Multiple lesions are usually found throughout the involved area of colon and frequently have a friable, inflamed appearance. Although these pseudopolyps are not themselves neoplastic, the entire colon of a patient with inflammatory bowel disease is at risk of developing a malignancy.

Lipomas originate within the wall of the colon, but as they enlarge, they frequently become polypoid. They may be found anywhere in the colon but are usually seen near the ileocecal valve. The surface is smooth and red and may have a yellow tinge reflecting the fat content. Usually these tumors are asymptomatic and do not require removal. *Leiomyomas* and *lymphoid polyps* are very unusual. When seen, they are smooth, sessile, and firmly attached to the wall. They rarely cause symptoms. *Carcinoid tumors* of the colon are almost always benign. They are usually seen as small yellow nodules in the rectum. No treatment is needed unless they enlarge.

Cancers. Colorectal cancers may present as exophytic, ulcerative, infiltrating, or annular lesions. With the exception of the cecum, where exophytic, polypoid lesions predominate, no correlation exists between site and configuration. The anatomic distribution of colorectal cancers has shifted proximally in recent decades. Currently, approximately 30% of cancers arise in the rectum, 25% in the sigmoid, 6% in the descending colon, 11% in the transverse colon, 9% in the ascending colon, and 13% in the cecum. Histologic grades for colorectal adenocarcinomas include well differentiated, moderately differentiated, poorly differentiated, and undifferentiated or anaplastic, depending on the degree of cytologic atypia and glandularity. Mucinous or signet cell carcinomas are variants of undifferentiated tumors.

Metastatic pathways usually involve lymphatic invasion with spread to mesenteric lymph nodes or hematogenous spread through the portal system to the liver. Ultimately, spread occurs through the systemic circulation to the lungs and other parts of the body. Rarely, tumors in the rectal region metastasize directly to the lungs, presumably by hemorrhoidal veins that connect directly to the systemic circulation.

Occasionally, other types of colorectal tumors are encountered. Malignant tumors of the anorectal junction are squamous cell or cloacogenic carcinomas. These metastasize through lymphatics to groin nodes before spreading systemically. These tumors are rare, comprising only about 1% of colorectal tumors. Lymphomas, leiomyosarcomas, and liposarcomas may also occur but are even rarer. Direct invasion of the colon from adjacent malignancy (ovary or prostate) or metastasis to the colon from distant sites (breast, lung, stomach, and melanoma) may occur late in the disease course but rarely presents a diagnostic problem.

Staging and Prognosis

Since Dukes' original staging system for rectal cancers in 1932, several modifications have been made in an attempt to incorporate additional prognostic information. The Astler-Coller system and the TNM system (proposed by the American Joint Committee on Cancer and International Union Against Cancer) are currently the most widely used and are applicable to both colon and rectal cancers (Table 105-6). Both are defined on the basis of depth of mural invasion and lymph node status. Prognosis, as defined by a 5-year survival rates, is closely correlated with tumor stage at diagnosis and ranges from 97% for stage I tumors to only 4% for stage IV tumors.

Poorly differentiated histology, mucin production, abnormal DNA content (aneuploidy), perforation, tumor invasion of adjacent organs, venous involvement, and a preoperative elevation in the plasma carcinoembryonic antigen (CEA) titer are also correlated with a poor prognosis. Loss of the *DCC* tumor suppressor gene has been identified as a poor prognostic factor in patients with stage II (Dukes' B) tumors but not stage III (Dukes' C) tumors. Loss of the p53 tumor suppressor gene has also been identified as a poor prognostic factor independent of stage. Unlike most other carcinomas or sarcomas, prognosis is not influenced by tumor size.

Clinical Presentation

Adenomas. Adenomatous polyps usually are asymptomatic. Intermittent bleeding, which is usually occult, is the most common manifestation. Visible but scant bleeding occasionally occurs, either mixed in the stool or on its surface; massive bleeding is rare. Patients may complain of a change in bowel habits, but this is unusual. Rarely, profuse watery diarrhea, resulting in dehydration and electrolyte abnormalities, is associated with large villous adenomas of the distal colon and rectum. Patients may also complain of vague discomfort; more severe pain is very uncommon and may be attributable to intussusception. Rectal prolapse of polyps has also been described.

Cancers. The clinical manifestations of colorectal cancers tend to vary with anatomic location. Cancers of the right colon most often present with occult bleeding and iron deficiency anemia. Obstruction is unusual because of the voluminous and distensible nature of the cecum. Occasionally a mass may be palpated in the right lower quadrant. Since stool becomes more concentrated as it passes through the transverse and descending colon, cancers of these sites cause crampy abdominal pain, obstruction, or less often, perforation. Cancers of the transverse colon may also present with occult bleeding but more often with obstruction. Cancers of the left colon and sigmoid typically produce rectal bleeding or symptoms related to partial bowel obstruction, such as crampy abdominal pain, change in bowel habits, and changes in stool size and consistency. Cancers of the rectum characteristically produce increased stool frequency, changes in stool caliber or consistency, small amounts of bright-red bleeding, rectal urgency, tenesmus, and incontinence. Advanced tumors may also produce perianal pain, hematuria, urinary frequency, or vaginal fistula caused by local invasion. Cancers of any site may perforate, resulting in signs and symptoms of a localized abscess or peritonitis.

Anorexia and weight loss are common systemic symptoms, although their presence is not specific for colorectal cancers; patients may have far-advanced colon cancers without these findings. When they are present, however, especially in the older age group, colon cancer must be a prime diagnostic possibility. Signs and symptoms of metastatic disease vary according to the site of involvement.

Evaluation of Symptomatic Patients: Diagnosis

Colonoscopy is the most widely used diagnostic modality for symptomatic patients, since it permits direct visualization of the entire large bowel in 90% to 95% of patients, as well as a means of obtaining tissue for histologic evaluation of suspicious lesions or removal of polyps. Depending on the nature of the symptoms or other mitigating circumstances, a sigmoidoscopy and barium enema may also be obtained. If a lesion is found by sigmoidoscopy or barium enema, a colonoscopy should be performed to ascertain the nature of the lesion, obtain tissue for histologic evaluation, and

Table 105-6. Staging Classifications and Prognosis of Colorectal Cancer

Dukes'	Astler-Coller	AJCC/UICC	Description	5-year survival (%)
A			Penetration into bowel wall	Stage I: 90-97
	A	T1 } Stage 1	Submucosa	
	B1	T2 } Stage 1	Muscularis	
B	B2	T3 } Stage II T4 } Stage II	Penetration through bowel wall ± involvement of adjacent organs	Stage II: 63-78
C			Lymph node involvement	Stage III: 37-66
	C1		Without penetration of bowel wall	
	C2	Stage III	With penetration of bowel wall	
		N1	1-3 nodes	
		N2	>4 nodes	
		N3	Any node along a major vascular trunk	
D	D	Stage IV M1	Any T, any N, distant metastases present	Stage IV: 4

AJCC, American Joint Committee on Cancer; *UICC*, International Union Against Cancer.

determine whether synchronous lesions are present elsewhere in the bowel. A colonoscopy should also be performed in patients with persistent symptoms and negative sigmoidoscopy or barium studies. If the entire bowel is not well visualized because of an obstructing lesion, technical difficulties, or poor patient tolerance, a double-contrast barium enema should be obtained. Once the diagnosis is established, preoperative staging is pursued with a CT scan of the abdomen, chest radiograph, and for patients with rectal cancer, endoscopic ultrasound. MRI, scintigraphy with radiolabeled anti-CEA monoclonal antibodies, and intraoperative ultrasound may also be of value in select patients.

Evaluation of Asymptomatic Patients: Screening and Surveillance

Although the survival rates from colorectal cancer have improved significantly in recent years, more than 40% of patients still die from their disease. As with many other cancers, prognosis is closely correlated with stage of disease at diagnosis. Despite improvements in diagnostic capability, almost 40% of patients have locoregional spread of their tumors, and another 20% have metastatic disease. This is largely because most patients remain entirely asymptomatic until their tumors reach an advanced stage. Sufficient evidence has accumulated to suggest that colorectal cancer screening is effective in reducing not only colorectal cancer mortality but also its incidence through the identification and removal of adenomatous polyps.

Proponents of colorectal cancer screening agree that case finding rather than mass screening is the most appropriate approach for early detection. *Case finding* refers to the performance of screening individuals at increased risk for the disease of interest. High-risk groups have been identified for colorectal cancer. Patients in whom age (50 or older) is the only risk factor are considered to be of average risk (Table 105-7). Fecal occult blood testing (FOBT), sigmoidoscopy, double-contrast barium enema, and colonoscopy have all been advocated as appropriate screening tests for average-risk individuals, beginning at age 50. The digital rectal examination (DRE) has not been shown to be effective and thus is no longer recommended as a screening test for colorectal cancer, although it should still be performed as part of a routine physical examination in persons over age 40. The common practice of using DRE to obtain a stool sample for fecal occult blood testing should be discouraged, except perhaps in noncompliant patients, since it compromises both the sensitivity and the specificity of FOBT.

It has long been recognized that occult bleeding is an early sign of colorectal cancer. The tests used most often to detect occult bleeding are based on hemoglobin's peroxidase activity, which can be easily detected at the bedside by the addition of a hydrogen peroxide reagent to a guaiac-impregnated slide (e.g., Hemoccult II, Hemoccult II Sensa). These guaiac-based tests are not specific for blood; foods containing peroxidase and pseudoperoxidase, such as red meat and certain vegetables, will also produce a positive test. Immunologic assays for hemoglobin (e.g., HemeSelect) or its porphyrin derivatives (e.g., Hemoquant) are more costly and less amenable to widespread clinical use. Three separate randomized controlled trials demonstrated that FOBT followed by diagnostic colonoscopy significantly reduces colorectal cancer mortality by 15% to 18% if performed biannually and 33% if performed annually.[4,6,7] The major limitations of FOBT relate to test sensitivity and specificity. Although the trials reported sensitivities of 72% to 78% for nonhydrated slides and 88% to 92% after hydration, other studies have observed false-negative rates as high as 75% for cancers and greater than 90% for adenomas. False-negative tests result primarily because not all neoplasms bleed and those that do may bleed only intermittently.

Table 105-7. Colorectal Cancer Screening and Surveillance Strategies

Risk group	Strategy
Average risk	
Age 50 or older	Beginning at age 50, *one* of the following: Annual fecal occult blood testing (FOBT)* Flexible sigmoidoscopy every 5 years Annual FOBT plus flexible sigmoidoscopy every 5 years Double-contrast barium enema every 5-10 years Colonoscopy every 10 years
Increased risk	
Family history†	Same as average risk, except beginning at age 40
Familial adenomatous polyposis (FAP) and variants	Genetic counseling/screening at age 10; if positive, flexible sigmoidoscopy yearly beginning at puberty
Hereditary nonpolyposis colorectal cancer (HNPCC, Lynch syndrome)	Genetic testing/counseling at about age 25; if positive, colonoscopy every 2 years until age 40, then yearly
Inflammatory bowel disease	Colonoscopy every 1-2 years beginning after 8 years of pancolitis or after 15 years of distal colitis
Prior colorectal cancer	Colonoscopy at 1 year, then every 3-5 years
Prior colorectal adenoma	Colonoscopy at 3 years, then every 3-5 years

*Two samples should be taken from each of three consecutive bowel movements. Restricted diet is recommended before test. Test is positive if one or more of the six samples are positive.

†Family history of one or more affected first-degree relatives with colorectal cancer or adenoma before age 60.

Another typical screening test for average-risk individuals is sigmoidoscopy. The rationale for sigmoidoscopy is that it permits direct visualization of the distal large bowel and biopsy of any abnormal lesions. Several types of sigmoidoscopes are available, including the 25-cm rigid scope, the 60-cm flexible fiberoptic scope, and the 60-cm flexible videoscopes. Flexible instruments afford a significantly higher diagnostic yield than the rigid scopes and have demonstrated much better patient tolerance and acceptance. Case-control studies suggest that periodic sigmoidoscopy, even every 5 to 10 years, can reduce mortality from colorectal cancers arising in the distal large bowel as much by 70% to 80%.[9,13] Since both studies used rigid instruments, they provide only indirect evidence of the effectiveness of flexible sigmoidoscopy. Additional studies suggest that sigmoidoscopy may also reduce the incidence of colorectal cancer through the identification and removal of adenomas. The major disadvantage of sigmoidoscopy is that only the distal half of the large bowel can be visualized, and thus only about half of all colorectal cancers and adenomas can be detected by this technique alone.

Colonoscopy is the only screening strategy that allows direct visualization of the entire large bowel, biopsy of suspicious lesions not amenable to endoscopic removal, and polypectomy. Overall sensitivity for polyps and cancer is about 90%, ranging from 75% to 85% for polyps less than 1 cm in diameter to 95% for larger polyps and cancers, whereas specificity approaches 100% for all lesions. Failure to reach the cecum and suboptimal bowel preparation account for the majority of missed lesions. No direct evidence proves that colonoscopy is an effective screening test, but extrapolation of data from the FOBT trials, screening sigmoidoscopy studies, and the National Polyp Study indicates that screening colonoscopy can reduce both the incidence of and the mortality from colorectal cancer. The major disadvantages of colonoscopy relate to higher procedural costs and risk of complications.

Double-contrast barium enema (DCBE) offers a less expensive, less invasive, and safer alternative to colonoscopy for evaluating the entire colon. As with colonoscopy, however, no direct evidence shows that DCBE is an effective screening test for colorectal cancer. The sensitivity of DCBE ranges from 50% to 80% for polyps less than 1 cm, 70% to 90% for polyps 1 cm or greater, and 55% to 85% for Dukes' A and B cancers. Specificity also varies according to polyp size, ranging from about 50% for small polyps to 90% to 95% for large polyps and more than 95% for cancers. Sensitivity increases slightly when sigmoidoscopy is combined with DCBE. Besides sensitivity and specificity concerns, the major limitation of DCBE is the need for follow-up colonoscopy to evaluate abnormal findings.

The optimal strategy for colorectal cancer screening remains controversial (see Table 105-7). Although widely endorsed by authoritative groups, guidelines vary and might include any of the following options: annual FOBT, sigmoidoscopy every 5 years, the combination of annual FOBT and flexible sigmoidoscopy every 5 years, DCBE every 5 to 10 years, *or* colonoscopy every 10 years.[2,12,15] One analysis suggested that these strategies have comparable and favorable cost-effectiveness ratios (less than $20,000 per year of life saved) and should be offered to all average-risk individuals beginning at age 50.[15] Selection of a given strategy needs to be individualized on the basis of potential risks and benefits, compliance issues, availability, insurance coverage, and local expertise. Decisions about when to stop screening also needs to be individualized, but in general, screening should be discontinued in patients with significant comorbidity or when the lead time between screening and its benefits (about 10 years) is longer than the patient's life expectancy.

Individuals at risk of FAP or HNPCC should be offered genetic counseling and testing. Because of the potential for false-negative results, affected relatives should be screened first. Those who test positive for *APC* mutations should undergo flexible sigmoidoscopy every 6 to 12 months beginning at puberty (age 10 to 12 years). Those who test positive for one of the DNA-mismatch gene mutations associated with HNPCC should undergo colonoscopy every 2 years beginning at age 25 and then yearly after age 35. When affected relatives test negative or refuse testing, individuals should be offered similar screening as those who test positive. Individuals with a positive family history of colorectal cancer or adenomas before age 60 should be offered the same options as for average-risk individuals but beginning at age 40. Patients with longstanding ulcerative colitis should undergo colonoscopy with biopsy for dysplasia beginning 8 years after age of onset for pancolitis and at 15 years for distal disease. Recommendations for surveillance of patients with a history of colorectal cancer or adenoma(s) are discussed under Treatment.

Evaluation of Patients with Positive Screening Tests. Colonoscopy is the diagnostic procedure of choice for patients with positive FOBT. The likelihood of finding a neoplastic lesion in these patients increases with age. Approximately 50% of positive-FOBT patients have either an adenoma (38%) or cancer (12%). Colonoscopy is also indicated for patients with distal adenomas detected at sigmoidoscopy, particularly those with advanced histology (i.e., 1-cm or larger lesion, villous growth, or high-grade dysplasia). Up to 50% of patients with adenomas detected by sigmoidoscopy have a proximal adenoma, and a small percentage have a proximal cancer. Colonoscopy is not recommended for patients with only a hyperplastic polyp found by sigmoidoscopy.

Treatment

Adenomas. Endoscopic polypectomy is the treatment of choice for all colorectal adenomas, regardless of whether they are symptomatic or discovered incidentally. Since histologic evaluation is the only reliable means of distinguishing adenomas from nonneoplastic polyps, particularly for diminutive lesions (5 mm or smaller), endoscopic removal or ablation is recommended for all colorectal polyps. The major risks of endoscopic polypectomy are bleeding and perforation. If a polyp cannot be removed endoscopically, surgical resection should be considered after careful assessment of the patient's operative risk vs. the risk of malignancy. Periodic endoscopic assessment and piecemeal removal every 6 months to 1 year is a reasonable alternative in poor surgical candidates. Laser ablation is also an option in such patients.

The treatment of malignant polyps (i.e., adenomas containing invasive cancer) depends on polyp morphology and histology. Endoscopic polypectomy is considered curative for pedunculated polyps if (1) there is a "clean" margin (1 mm or more) of resection, (2) there is no lymphatic or vascular invasion, (3) the cancer is well or moderately differentiated, and (4) there is no residual or recurrent tumor at the polypectomy site on follow-up examination. If all these criteria are not met, surgical resection is warranted. Surgical resection is recommended for all patients with malignant sessile polyps if they have acceptable surgical risks.

Cancer. Surgical resection is the only potentially curative treatment for colorectal cancer. Curative resection requires wide excision of the primary tumor and en bloc removal of draining lymph nodes, lymphatics, and contiguous structures. The actual extent of resection varies according to anatomic location. The introduction of stapling devices has been an important advance in that it has shortened operative time, reduced the incidence of anastomotic leaks and infection, and reduced the need for colostomy in patients with low-lying rectal cancers. Although an abdominoperineal resection with colostomy is often recommended for rectal tumors not amenable to low anterior resection with primary anastomosis, alternate sphincter-sparing approaches, including coloanal anastomosis and local excision, may be curative in select patients. Tumors amenable to local excision should be less than 4 cm in size, mobile, and confined to the mucosa (T1) or submucosa (T2) and limited to one quadrant of the rectal circumference. Endoscopic ultrasound is particularly valuable in identifying lesions amenable to local excision. A more limited palliative resection is recommended for patients with metastatic disease at diagnosis.

Evidence supports the use of adjuvant therapy after curative resection.[10] Combined-modality treatment with chemotherapy (5-fluorouracil alone or in combination with levamisole or leucovorin) and postoperative radiation has been shown to reduce local recurrence rates and improve disease-free survival and overall survival in patients with Astler-Coller (modified Dukes classification) B2 and C rectal cancers (see Table 105-6). Combination chemotherapy with 5-fluorouracil and levamisole or leucovorin has also been shown to improve disease-free survival and overall survival in patients with C cancers arising above the pelvic-peritoneal reflection; its efficacy in the treatment of B2 tumors remains unproven.

Chemotherapy is the treatment of choice for patients with metastatic disease. Since this approach is rarely curative, efficacy is generally defined in terms of initial response rates (i.e., tumor shrinkage) and improved 5-year survival. 5-Fluorouracil is the most active single agent, with response rates of about 20%. Combination chemotherapy with 5-fluorouracil plus leucovorin has replaced single-agent therapy as the standard for patients with advanced, unresectable colorectal cancer. Intraarterial hepatic infusion of 5-fluorouracil or floxuridine has demonstrated superior efficacy in the treatment of hepatic disease but has had little impact on survival and is associated with significant toxicity.

Aggressive surgical intervention may be warranted with isolated hepatic or pulmonary metastases in an otherwise healthy patient. Although the cure rate is not high, many case reports document the value of attempting tumor removal in this otherwise 100% fatal situation.

Palliation is the goal of treatment for patients with advanced, incurable disease. Segmental resection of the primary tumor is generally recommended to reduce the morbidity associated with recurrent bleeding and obstruction. Diverting colostomy should be considered for unresectable tumors, particularly low-lying rectal cancers. Radiation therapy is often effective in the management of advanced or recurrent pelvic disease, particularly in patients with pain unresponsive to chemotherapy. Endoscopic approaches, such as laser ablation or stent placement, may also be of value in the management of tumor bleeding or obstruction in select patients.

Follow-up

Adenomas. Periodic surveillance colonoscopy is warranted in patients with a history of colorectal adenomas because of the risk of metachronous adenomas and cancer. An interval of at least 3 years has been recommended for repeat colonoscopy after removal of all adenomas.[16] If the initial follow-up examination is negative for adenomas, subsequent examination can be deferred for at least 5 years. Patients with malignant polyps or large sessile adenomas, multiple adenomas, and identified polyps that have not been removed may require more frequent examinations.

Cancer. Close surveillance is also indicated for patients with colorectal cancer after curative resection. A reasonable follow-up program includes office visits every 3 months for the first 3 years and then every 6 months, with CEA determination every visit and complete blood count (CBC) and liver profile every 6 months. An annual CT scan of the abdomen and pelvis and a chest radiograph should also be obtained for the first 5 years. Colonoscopy should also be performed at 1 year to detect anastomotic recurrences, then every 3 years to detect metachronous adenomas or cancer. Patients in whom a complete preoperative colonoscopy or DCBE could not be performed because of obstructing tumors should undergo a postoperative examination at 3 to 6 months.

The detection of a rising CEA level after stable low levels necessitates thorough evaluation. Scintigraphy with radiolabeled anti-CEA antibodies may be of value in localizing recurrences; if negative, some oncologists and surgeons suggest exploratory second-look laparotomy in hope of finding resectable disease.

TUMORS OF THE LIVER

Tumors of the liver are frequently encountered in clinical practice. Depending on geographic location, the majority of such tumors may be either primary liver tumors or metastatic tumors. Primary liver tumors may be benign or malignant and may arise from hepatic parenchymal tissue, the biliary tree, or vascular structures (see Table 105-1). *Hepatocellular carcinomas (hepatomas)* and *cholangiocarcinomas* are the most common malignant tumors; *hemangiomas* are the most common benign tumors. All other types of benign or malignant primary tumors are rare.

Epidemiology

The global distribution of hepatocellular carcinoma correlates with the geographic prevalence of chronic hepatitis B virus (HBV) carriers. Incidence rates range from less than 2% of malignant tumors found at autopsy in North and South America and Europe to 20% to 30% in parts of Africa and Asia. Although still a rare disease (2.4 cases per 100,000 population) in the United States, incidence rates have nearly doubled over the past two decades and will continue to rise because of the large pool of persons infected with hepatitis C virus (HCV).[3] Hepatocellular carcinoma is up to four times more common in men than women. The peak incidence occurs in the fifth or sixth decades of life in low-risk countries but one to two decades earlier in high-risk areas.

Unlike hepatocellular carcinoma, the incidence of cholangiocarcinoma is dispersed more evenly throughout the world. Peak incidence is in the sixth decade of life, and there is no male predominance.

Hemangiomas occur in approximately 5% of the population, based on all autopsies. The epidemiology of other types of benign tumors is essentially unknown.

Etiology

Between 30% and 70% of patients with hepatocellular carcinoma have underlying cirrhosis. The risk of hepatocellular carcinoma varies with the type of cirrhosis. Cirrhosis from hemochromatosis has the highest risk; up to 22% of such patients develop hepatocellular carcinoma even if treated with phlebotomy. Hepatocellular carcinoma also occurs in approximately 2% to 3% of patients with alcoholic cirrhosis and up to 10% of patients with postnecrotic cirrhosis associated with chronic HBV or HCV infection. Other forms of chronic liver disease, such as chronic HCV infection, α_1-antitrypsin deficiency, and tyrosinemia, are also predisposing conditions. In parts of Asia, chronic parasitic infection with *Opisthorchis sinensis* is associated with the development of cholangiocarcinoma.

Epidemiologic studies have established a close association between hepatocellular carcinoma and chronic HBV infection. In high-risk areas, 90% to 95% of patients with hepatocellular carcinoma have serologic evidence of active or remote infection. Approximately 60% to 70% have evidence of chronic hepatitis or cirrhosis at presentation. Integration of HBV DNA into the host genome appears to be an inciting event. Chronicity of infection and vertical transmission predispose to HBV DNA integration and thus hepatocellular carcinoma.

Chronic HCV infection has also emerged as an important risk factor, particularly in developed countries (e.g., United States, Japan). Once cirrhosis is established, hepatocellular carcinoma develops at a rate of 1% to 4% per year. Alcohol, iron overload, and coincident chronic HBV infection potentiate risk. Controlled trials in Japan and France suggest that antiviral therapy with interferon may reduce risk, even in the absence of a complete virologic response.

Environmental carcinogens have also been implicated in the etiology of hepatocellular carcinoma. Mycotoxins derived from saprophytic fungi (e.g., *Aspergillus flavus*), particularly aflatoxin B1, are potent hepatocarcinogens and are believed to contribute to the increased incidence of hepatocellular carcinoma in high-risk areas such as Africa and China. Vinyl chloride and the contrast agent Thorotrast are associated with angiosarcomas of the liver. Oral contraceptives (OCs) and pregnancy have both been associated with liver cell adenomas and focal nodular hyperplasia. Rare cases have involved malignant transformation of liver cell adenomas into hepatocellular carcinomas.

Long-term use of androgenic steroids is also associated with an increased risk of hepatocellular carcinoma.

Histopathology and Differential Diagnosis

Benign Tumors. Hemangiomas are typically solitary and small but may be multiple or large. Most are subcapsular and have a predilection for the right lobe of the liver. Two forms typically occur in the liver: (1) the cavernous hemangioma, the more common and caused by dilation of existing blood vessels, and (2) the true hemangioma, which results from a proliferation of embryonic vascular tissue.

Liver cell adenomas are rare benign tumors associated with OCs and pregnancy. They are usually large with a smooth appearance and soft consistency. They occur with equal frequency throughout the liver and are usually visible at the surface. The histologic differentiation of a liver cell adenoma from a well-differentiated liver cell carcinoma can be quite difficult.

Focal nodular hyperplasias are also rare benign tumors associated with OCs and pregnancy. They are usually solitary, often less than 5 cm in diameter, and occur in either lobe of the liver. Like adenomas, these lesions occur with equal frequency throughout the liver and are usually located peripherally. Unlike adenomas, they are nonneoplastic hamartomas. Focal nodular hyperplasias are often pedunculated and highly vascular.

MRI with contrast enhancement can differentiate adenomas from hepatomas, hemangiomas, focal nodular hyperplasias, and metastatic disease.

Malignant Tumors. Hepatocellular carcinomas account for 80% to 90% of primary liver cancers. Grossly, they may present as a focal mass or exhibit a nodular pattern characterized by multiple small nodules throughout the liver. A diffuse fibrolamellar type occurs primarily in younger, noncirrhotic patients and carries a better prognosis. Histologically, it is sometimes difficult to distinguish benign lesions from malignant tumors and even from normal parenchymal cells in the case of well-differentiated tumors.

Cholangiocarcinomas are glandular malignancies that arise from bile duct epithelium. Although these tumors may be found coincidentally within hepatocellular carcinomas, cholangiocarcinomas are generally not associated with underlying cirrhosis. *Angiosarcomas* are rare hepatic malignancies that arise from vascular elements. Hepatoblastomas are rare tumors seen primarily in infants and young children. Unlike other types of liver cancer, these tumors tend to be unifocal, resectable, and highly curable.

In the United States the incidence of clinically significant metastatic disease is at least 20 times greater than that of primary hepatic malignancies. The liver is the most frequent site of blood-borne metastases, which occur in about 30% of all cancers, including half of those from stomach, breast, and lung, and tumors arising in the portal venous drainage system.

Clinical Presentation

Benign Tumors. Most benign tumors of the liver are asymptomatic. Vague right upper quadrant pain or discomfort is often the major complaint in symptomatic patients. Severe right upper quadrant pain with hypotension suggests spontaneous rupture, which can be fatal. Physical examination is often normal but may reveal a palpable mass, hepatomegaly, or in the case of large hemangiomas, a vascular hum. Thrombocytopenia from platelet adherence has been reported in patients with large hemangiomas.

Malignant Tumors. The onset of symptoms in patients with hepatocellular carcinoma may be insidious or sudden. In general, symptomatic patients have advanced, incurable tumors. Abdominal pain is the most common presenting feature. The pain may be characterized as a dull, localized ache resulting from stretching of the liver capsule or sudden and severe from spontaneous rupture. Patients may also complain of diffuse pain caused by rapidly accumulating ascites. Weakness, anorexia, and weight loss also frequently occur. Early satiety may result from liver enlargement or ascites. Occasionally, patients present with manifestations of Budd-Chiari syndrome from hepatic venous thrombosis or variceal hemorrhage from portal venous thrombosis. Tender hepatomegaly (often with a palpable mass), ascites, and in some cases a bruit are the most common physical findings. Overt jaundice is often a late finding, except in patients with cholangiocarcinomas.

A variety of paraneoplastic syndromes have been described in patients with hepatocellular carcinoma. Hypercalcemia, erythrocytosis, hypoglycemia, hyperlipidemia, sexual precocity or feminization, coagulopathy from dysfibrogenemia, hyperthyroidism, and pseudoporphyria have all been reported.

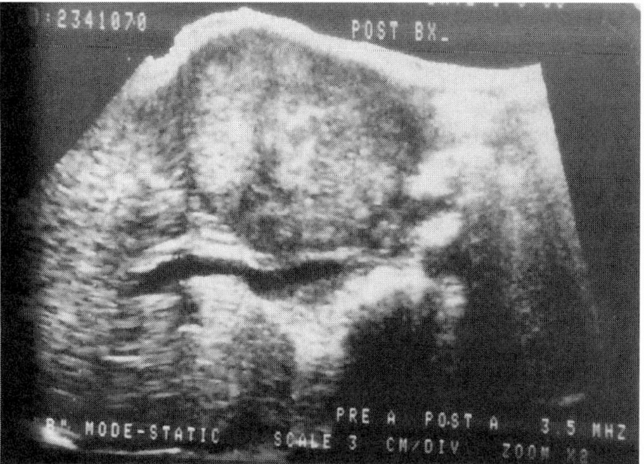

Fig. 105-3. Ultrasound of liver demonstrating solid mass of left lobe with areas of central necrosis. Mass proved to be a hepatocellular carcinoma.

Diagnosis

Accurate diagnosis of hepatic tumors relies on clinical suspicion, radiologic imaging, serologic testing for tumor markers, and tissue confirmation. The vast majority of benign or malignant tumors present as space-occupying lesions easily detectable by a variety of imaging modalities (Figs. 105-3 and 105-4). Ultrasonography is most widely employed because it is readily available, reliable, inexpensive, and noninvasive and avoids the potential risks of radiation. CT scan and MRI are useful for confirming the findings at ultrasound, distinguishing benign from malignant tumors, and assessing extent of disease. Dynamic CT scanning (CT angiography) and MRI may be particularly useful in detecting small tumors and in evaluating invasion of vascular structures. Hepatic arteriography is also useful for characterizing vascular status of small lesions, determining operability, and defining anatomy in potentially resectable tumors.

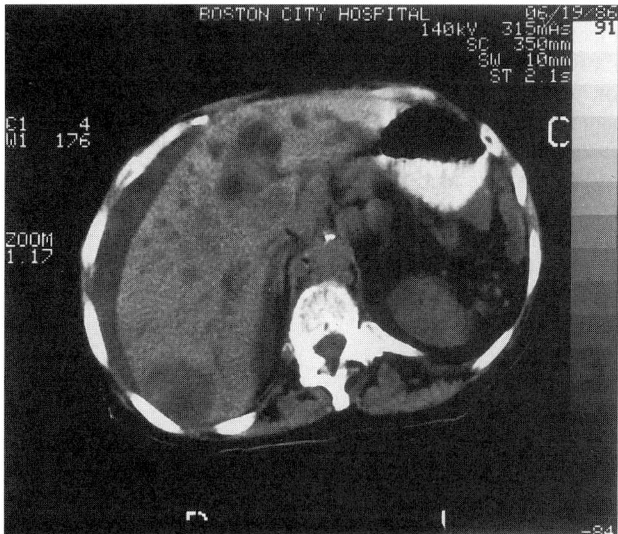

Fig. 105-4. CT scan of metastatic carcinoma of liver with ascites. Note multiple filling defects.

Hepatic isotope scans have limited utility in the detection of many primary tumors. Technetium-labeled red blood scans are most useful in the diagnosis of hemangiomas but otherwise lack both sensitivity and specificity, particularly in the setting of cirrhosis. Dynamic CT scanning using a bolus injection is helpful in distinguishing hemangiomas from other hepatic tumors. Gallium scans may be useful because this tracer preferentially accumulates in some hepatocellular carcinomas but not in normal liver or cirrhosis. Gallium does accumulate, however, in liver abscesses and granulomas.

Most patients with hepatocellular carcinoma at some time have elevated serum levels of α-fetoprotein; levels greater than 500 ng/ml are diagnostic. Lower levels are less specific because they may also be seen in the setting of hepatitis or active cirrhosis. High-risk patients, particularly those with cirrhosis associated with chronic HBV infection, chronic HCV infection, or hemochromatosis, should have annual α-fetoprotein determinations and ultrasound studies in hope of detecting early, potentially curable tumors. Measurement of serum CEA levels is another useful tumor marker in the diagnosis of metastatic disease, particularly for primary cancers of the GI tract, breast, or lung.

Liver biopsy is often necessary to confirm the diagnosis of most liver tumors. Although a blind percutaneous biopsy may suffice for patients with large tumor masses, ultrasound or CT-guided biopsies have a much higher yield. Laparoscopy with directed liver biopsy is an even more accurate method for establishing the diagnosis. Caution is warranted for patients with localized tumors, since skin metastases at the biopsy site have been reported.

Treatment

Benign Tumors. Most benign tumors are asymptomatic and do not require treatment. Both adenomas and focal nodular hyperplasias are known to regress in patients taking OCs once the drugs are discontinued. Surgical resection may be indicated in rare patients with intractable pain or with a strong possibility of rupture. Corticosteroids are effective in the treatment of thrombocytopenia associated with large hemangiomas.

Malignant Tumors. Surgical resection is the only proven effective treatment for hepatocellular carcinoma or cholangiocarcinoma.[8] Unfortunately, few patients have localized, potentially curable disease. Even if an early, resectable lesion is detected, which rarely occurs, the presence of cirrhosis often precludes aggressive surgical intervention. Careful preoperative assessment is essential, including evaluation for the extent of the disease and workup of hepatic functional reserve in patients with known or suspected cirrhosis. Because of advances in surgical technique and perioperative care, resections as extensive as a trisegmentectomy have an acceptable operative mortality in carefully selected patients. Palliative surgery is generally not recommended except for patients with obstructive jaundice.

The treatment of advanced primary malignancies of the liver is often disappointing. The role of liver transplantation for patients with unresectable disease confined to the liver is still under investigation, but results have been unimpressive, except for young patients with the fibrolamellar variant of hepatocellular carcinoma. Chemotherapy delivered either systemically or by hepatic artery infusion is often used but rarely effective. Of the many agents studied, 5-flourouracil and doxorubicin (Adriamycin) have been the most active agents currently available. Radiation therapy has no role because of its lack of efficacy and risk of radiation hepatitis. Minimally invasive methods, such as percutaneous ethanol injection and transarterial chemoembolization, are effective in providing temporary local control and palliating symptoms for patients with small, unresectable tumors and in select patients with advanced tumors but have little impact on survival.[8]

The management of patients with metastatic liver disease varies according to the site of origin. In general, chemotherapy is most often used. Embolization and hepatic artery ligation have been used for palliation in select patients. Surgical resection has been advocated for patients with very limited involvement.

Prognosis

The overall prognosis for patients with malignant tumors of the liver is poor. Although cure rates as high as 30% have been reported after surgical resection, the median survival without resection is 4 to 6 months.

EBM EVIDENCE-BASED MEDICINE

Electronic searches dating back to 1985 were conducted using MEDLINE. The searches focused on systematic reviews, meta-analyses, large randomized trials with clinical end points, and position statements by authoritative groups.

REFERENCES

1. American Gastroenterological Association: Medical position statement: evaluation of dyspepsia, *Gastroenterology* 114:579, 1998.
2. Byers T, Levin B, Rothenberger D, et al: American Cancer Society guidelines for screening and surveillance for early detection of colorectal polyps and cancer: update 1997, *CA Cancer J Clin* 47:154, 1997.
3. El-Serag HB, Mason AC: Rising incidence of hepatocellular carcinoma in the United States, *N Engl J Med* 340:745, 1999.
4. Hardcastle O, Chamberlain JO, Robinson MHE, et al: Randomized controlled trial of faecal occult blood screening for colorectal cancer, *Lancet* 348:1472, 1996.
5. Huang J-Q, Subbaramiah S, Chen Y, Hunt R: Meta-analysis of the relationship between *Helicobacter pylori* seropositivity and gastric cancer, *Gastroenterology* 114:1169, 1998.
6. Kronberg O, Fenger C, Olsen J, et al: Randomized study of screening for colorectal cancer with fecal occult blood test at Funen in Denmark, *Lancet* 348:1467, 1996.
7. Mandel JS, Bond JH, Church TR, et al: Reducing mortality from colorectal cancer by screening for fecal occult blood: Minnesota Colon Cancer Control Study, *N Engl J Med* 328:1365, 329:672 (erratum), 1993.
8. Mor E, Kaspa RT, Sheiner P, Schwartz M: Treatment of hepatocellular carcinoma associated with cirrhosis in the era of liver transplantation, *Ann Intern Med* 129:643, 1998.
9. Newcomb PA, Norfleet RG, Storer BE, et al: Screening sigmoidoscopy and colorectal cancer mortality, *J Natl Cancer Inst* 84:1572, 1992.
10. NIH Consensus Conference: Adjuvant therapy for patients with colon and rectal cancer, *JAMA* 264:1444, 1990.
11. Parsonnet J, Jansen S, Rodriguez L, et al: *Helicobacter pylori* infection and gastric lymphoma, *N Engl J Med* 330:1267, 1994.
12. Preventive Services Task Force: *Guide to clinical preventive services*, ed 2, Baltimore, 1996, Williams & Wilkins.
13. Selby JV, Friedman GD, Quesenberry CP, Weiss NS: A case-control study of screening sigmoidoscopy and mortality from colorectal cancer, *N Engl J Med* 326:653, 1993.
14. Vasen HFA, Watson P, Mecklin J-K, et al: New clinical criteria for hereditary nonpolyposis colorectal cancer (HNPCC, Lynch syndrome) proposed by the International Collaborative Group on HNPCC, *Gastroenterology* 116:1453, 1999.
15. Winawer SJ, Fletcher RH, Miller L, et al: Colorectal cancer screening: clinical guidelines and rationale, *Gastroenterology* 112:594, 1997.
16. Winawer SJ, Zauber A, O'Brien MJ, et al: Randomized comparison of surveillance intervals after colonoscopic removal of newly diagnosed adenomatous polyps, *N Engl J Med* 328:901, 1993.

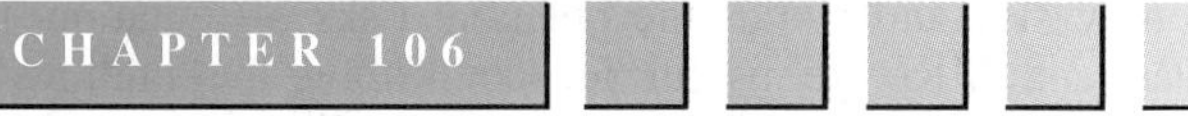

Pancreatic Disease

Norton J. Greenberger

ACUTE PANCREATITIS

Epidemiology and Etiology

The incidence of pancreatitis varies in different countries and depends on etiologic factors (e.g., alcohol, gallstones), metabolic factors, and drugs (Box 106-1). In the United States, acute pancreatitis is related to alcohol ingestion more often than to gallstones, whereas in England the opposite is true. Pancreatitis is classified as acute or chronic. An attack is defined as acute if the patient becomes asymptomatic after recovery, whereas with chronic pancreatitis the patient has persistent pain or insufficient exocrine or endocrine pancreatic function. Autopsy surveys in the United States indicate that the overall prevalence of acute pancreatitis is approximately 0.5%; the annual death rate is an estimated 1.5 per 100,000, or approximately 4000 cases per year.

Pathophysiology

Many causative factors exist in the pathogenesis of acute pancreatitis, but the mechanism by which the conditions trigger pancreatic inflammation have not been clearly elucidated. The final common pathway is thought to be autodigestion by activated enzymes. The autodigestion theory postulates that proteolytic enzymes (e.g., trypsinogen, chymotrypsinogen, proelastase, phospholipase) are activated within the pancreas rather than the intestinal lumen. A variety of factors (e.g., endotoxins, exotoxins, viral infections,

Box 106-1. Causes of Acute Pancreatitis

Common

Alcoholism
Gallstones
Postoperative complications (abdominal, coronary bypass)
Drugs
Post-ERCP
Abdominal trauma
Hypercalcemia (drugs, TPN)
Hypertriglyceridemia

Less Common

Vasculitis (SLE)
Thrombotic thrombocytopenic purpura
Refeeding after fasting (anorexia nervosa)
Periampullary duodenal diverticulum
Pancreas divisum
Cancer of the pancreas
End-stage renal disease

ERCP, Endoscopic retrograde cholangiopancreatography; *TPN,* total parenteral nutrition; *SLE,* systemic lupus erythematosus.

Box 106-2. Drugs Causing Acute Pancreatitis

Definite

Thiazides
Furosemides
Sulfonamides
Estrogens
Azathioprine/6-mercaptopurine (6-MP)
Angiotensin-converting enzyme (ACE) inhibitors
Didanosine (ddI)
Valproic acid
Pentamidine
L-Asparaginase

Probable

Ethacrynic acid
Acetaminophen
5-Aminosalicylic analogs
Codeine

ischemia, noxae, direct trauma) activate these proenzymes. Activated enzymes then digest cellular membranes and cause proteolysis, edema, interstitial hemorrhage, vascular damage, coagulation necrosis, fat necrosis, and parenchymal cell necrosis. In addition, activation of bradykinin peptides and vasoactive substances (e.g., histamine) produces vasodilation, increased vascular permeability, and edema. Thus a cascade of events culminates in the development of acute necrotizing pancreatitis. A second theory postulates that inappropriate release of pancreatic lysosomal hydrolases activates zymogens and autodigestion. Several factors normally protect the pancreatic acinar cell: (1) zymogens and lysosomal hydrolases are packaged in intracellular organelles; (2) pancreatic tissue and juice contain inhibitors of pancreatic trypsin; and (3) plasma contains antiproteases (e.g., α_1-antitrypsin, α_2-macroglobulin).

The two most common causes of acute pancreatitis are alcohol ingestion and gallstones. Alcoholic pancreatitis develops in susceptible persons after heavy ethanol ingestion for many years. Chronic alcoholism may produce proteinaceous plugs in the small pancreatic ducts, causing atrophy of pancreatic parenchyma drained by the obstructed duct. Thus in first episodes of alcohol-associated acute pancreatitis, approximately 50% of patients already have evidence of chronic pancreatic disease. Patients with gallstone pancreatitis frequently have occult gallstones in their feces. Certain clinical features suggest the diagnosis of gallstone-associated pancreatitis. Drugs have also been implicated as a cause of acute pancreatitis (Box 106-2).

Patient Evaluation

History. Abdominal pain is the cardinal symptom of acute pancreatitis. This pain may vary from a mild and tolerable discomfort to severe, constant, and incapacitating distress. Characteristically the pain, which is steady and boring, is in the epigastrium and periumbilical region and often radiates to the back as well as to the chest, flanks, and lower abdomen. Pancreatic pain frequently is more intense when the patient is supine, and patients often obtain relief by sitting with the trunk flexed and knees drawn up. Nausea, vomiting, and abdominal distention from gastric and intestinal hypomotility and chemical peritonitis are frequent complaints.

Physical Examination. The patient is typically distressed and anxious. Low-grade fever, tachycardia, and hypotension are common. Shock may result from (1) hypovolemia secondary to exudation of blood and plasma proteins in the retroperitoneal space (i.e., a retroperitoneal burn); (2) increased formation and release of kinin peptides, which cause vasodilation and increased vascular permeability; (3) impairment of myocardial contractility by kinins and other poorly characterized peptides; and (4) systemic effects of proteolytic and lipolytic enzymes released into the circulation. Jaundice occurs in approximately 10% of patients and usually is caused by edema of the pancreatic head with compression of the intrapancreatic portion of the common bile duct. Abdominal tenderness and muscle rigidity are present to a variable degree, but when compared with the intense pain, these signs may be unimpressive. Bowel sounds usually are diminished or absent. A pancreatic pseudocyst may be palpable in the upper abdomen. A faint blue discoloration around the umbilicus (Cullen's sign) may result from hemoperitoneum. A blue, red, purple, or green-blue discoloration of the flanks (Turner's sign) reflects tissue catabolism of hemoglobin. The last two findings are uncommon but indicate severe necrotizing pancreatitis. Approximately 10% to 20% of patients develop pulmonary findings, which include atelectasis, basilar rales, mediastinal abscesses, and pleural effusion, most often left sided. Erythematous skin nodules that mimic erythema nodosum may result from subcutaneous fat necrosis.

Findings that indicate severe disease include hypotension, tachycardia greater than 130 beats/min, altered sensorium, abnormal physical examination of the lungs, and Cullen's and Turner's signs.

Laboratory Studies and Diagnostic Procedures

The diagnosis of acute pancreatitis usually is established by an increased serum amylase level exceeding two times the upper limit of normal values. No definite correlation exists between the severity of pancreatitis and the degree of serum amylase elevation. In acute pancreatitis the serum amylase usually is elevated within 24 hours and remains so for 1 to 3 days. Levels return to normal values within 3 to 5 days unless there is extensive pancreatic necrosis, incomplete ductal obstruction, or pseudocyst formation. Approximately 75% of patients with acute pancreatitis have an elevated serum amylase. Normal values, however, may occur if (1) there is a delay of 2 to 5 days in obtaining appropriate blood samples; (2) the underlying disorder is chronic pancreatitis with an acute exacerbation rather than acute pancreatitis; and (3) hypertriglyceridemia is present. Serum lipase levels are increased in approximately 70% to 85% of patients, and lipase may be the best enzyme to measure for the diagnosis of acute pancreatitis. If both serum amylase and serum lipase levels are determined, one test is abnormal in approximately 80% to 85% of patients with acute pancreatitis.

Serum amylase is often elevated in other conditions (Box 106-3). The enzyme is found in many organs besides the pancreas (salivary glands, liver, small intestine, kidney, fallopian tubes) and can be produced by various tumors (carcinoma of lung, esophagus, breast, and ovary). No blood test is reliable for the diagnosis of acute pancreatitis in patients with renal failure. The serum amylase can become elevated when the creatinine clearance is less than 50 ml/min. In such patients the serum amylase is usually less than 500 IU/L in the absence of other objective evidence of pancreatitis. A serum amylase may be spuriously normal in certain conditions (e.g., hypertriglyceridemia). In this setting, values for urine amylase and serum lipase are often abnormal, thus supporting the diagnosis of acute pancreatitis. Imaging procedures such as ultrasound and computed tomography (CT) scan are helpful in further confirming the diagnosis (Fig. 106-1). Imaging techniques show a diffusely enlarged pancreas in 70% to 90% of patients during an acute attack. In patients with clinical findings suggesting a *severe* attack (Box 106-4), a contrast-enhanced CT scan provides the best means to visualize the pancreas and is very accurate in diagnosing pancreatitis and detecting its local complications. More than 90% of CT scans performed within 72 hours of admission are abnormal in patients with acute pancreatitis. Identification of pancreatic and peripancreatic necrosis by dynamic CT scanning is useful in distinguishing between mild and severe pancreatitis. Areas of the pancreas not enhanced by contrast are thought to be necrotic, and the extent of pancreatic necrosis does correlate with severity of disease. The vast majority of patients with acute pancreatitis do not require a CT scan, which should be reserved for patients with more than three prognostic signs, one or more major factors, or evidence of one or more systems undergoing organ failure.[3,13]

Other routine studies in patients with acute pancreatitis include chest radiograph, electrocardiogram (ECG), arterial blood gases, and routine serum chemistries. Careful attention is given to the white blood cell count, blood glucose, liver tests, blood urea nitrogen (BUN), serum calcium, serum albumin, and arterial oxygen pressure, which are also of prognostic value (see Box 106-4).

Box 106-3. Causes of Hyperamylasemia

Pancreatic Disease

Acute pancreatitis
Pancreatic pseudocyst
Pancreatic trauma
Pancreatic carcinoma

Nonpancreatic Disease

Renal insufficiency
Salivary gland lesions*
Tumor (lung, esophagus,* ovary, breast)
Diabetic ketoacidosis*
Burns
Pregnancy
Renal transplantation
Drugs (morphine, codeine)
Macroamylasemia

Other Abdominal Disorders

Biliary tract disease (cholecystitis, choledocholithiasis)
Perforated peptic ulcer
Intestinal obstruction or infarction
Postoperative hyperamylasemia
Peritonitis
Ruptured ectopic pregnancy

*Salivary isoamylase elevated and not pancreatic isoamylase.

Differential Diagnosis

Any severe acute pain in the abdomen or back should suggest acute pancreatitis. The diagnosis usually is considered when a patient has severe and constant abdominal pain, nausea, emesis, fever, tachycardia, and abnormal findings on abdominal examination. Laboratory studies frequently reveal leukocytosis, abnormal radiographs of the abdomen, hyperglycemia, hypocalcemia, increased BUN levels, and decreased serum albumin values. The diagnosis usually is confirmed by finding an elevated serum amylase or serum lipase. The diagnosis should be considered in terms of definite, probable, and possible pancreatitis (Table 106-1). Acute appendicitis must be considered in all patients with acute abdominal pain (Box 106-5). Localization of pain to the right lower quadrant, low-grade fever, and moderate leukocytosis point to the diagnosis of acute appendicitis. It may be quite difficult to distinguish between acute cholecystitis and acute pancreatitis, since an increased serum amylase may be found in both disorders. The pain of biliary tract origin is more right sided and gradual in onset, and ileus usually is absent; these clues suggest acute cholecystitis. A perforated duodenal ulcer is usually diagnosed by free intraperitoneal air, which is present in more than 75% of patients. Alcoholic hepatitis should be considered in patients with a history of excessive alcohol ingestion, hepatomegaly, and elevated values for mean corpuscular volume (MCV), γ-glutamyltransferase (GGT), and serum aspartate transaminase (AST) and an AST/ALT (alanine) ratio greater than 3:1. The diagnosis of intestinal obstruction caused by mechanical

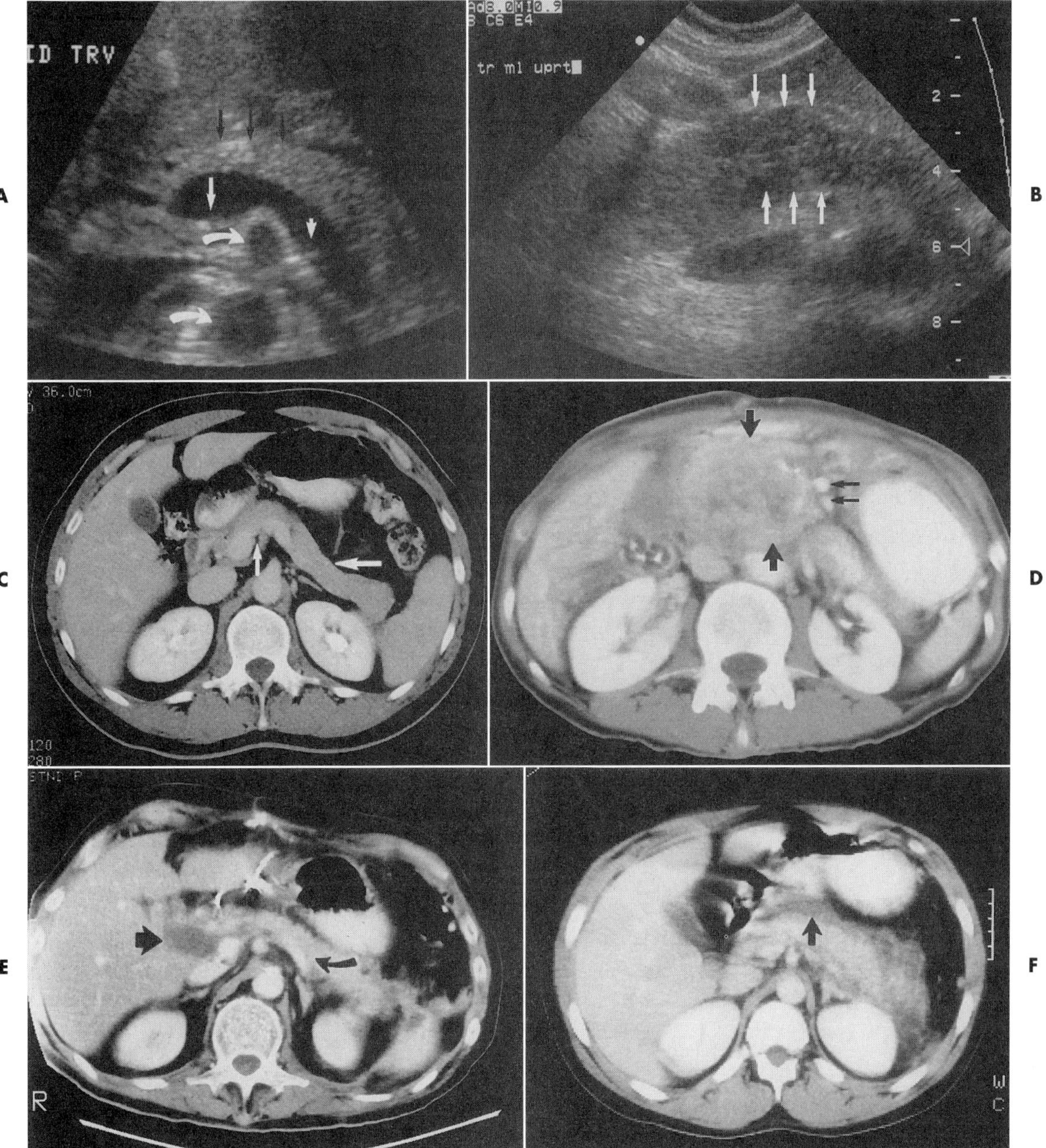

Fig. 106-1. Normal pancreas and pancreatitis. **A,** Normal pancreas *(black arrows)* and normal landmarks. Portal vein *(large white arrow),* splenic vein *(white arrowhead),* superior mesenteric artery *(top curved arrow),* and aorta *(lower curved arrow).* **B,** Ultrasound demonstrating enlarged pancreas outlined by arrows in acute pancreatitis. **C,** Dynamic (contrast-enhanced) CT scan showing normal pancreas *(arrows).* **D,** CT scan showing a necrotic pancreas *(thick arrows)* impinging on the superior mesenteric artery and vein *(thin arrows).* **E,** Dynamic CT in acute pancreatitis showing viable pancreas *(curved arrow)* and necrotic pancreas *(broad arrow).* **F,** CT scan in acute pancreatitis showing enlarged pancreas and peripancreatic fluid collection *(arrow).*

factors is suggested by a history of colicky abdominal pain, compatible findings on physical examination of the abdomen, and radiographs of the abdomen showing characteristic changes of mechanical obstruction. Acute mesenteric vascular occlusion should be considered in elderly debilitated patients with a history of weight loss, postprandial abdominal pain, and an abdominal bruit who present with brisk leukocytosis, abdominal distention, and bloody diarrhea. Arteriography in such patients frequently shows evidence of vascular occlusion in two or more major arteries. Serum amylase levels are increased in approximately 25% of patients. In patients with systemic lupus erythematosus (SLE) or polyarteritis nodosa, it may be difficult to differentiate abdominal pain caused by vasculitis and gut ischemia (with or without infarction) from pain caused by pancreatitis.

Diabetic ketoacidosis often is accompanied by abdominal pain, leukocytosis, and elevated serum amylase levels, thus simulating acute pancreatitis. However, the serum amylase frequently is of salivary and not of pancreatic origin.[9] Metabolic acidosis can result in elevated serum amylase levels (especially salivary isoamylase). The serum lipase level is not elevated in diabetic ketoacidosis, however, and

Box 106-4. Assessing the Severity of Acute Pancreatitis

Prognostic Signs (Modified Ranson)
At admission or diagnosis

Age > 55 years
WBC > 16,000
Blood glucose > 200 mg/dl
Serum LDH > 350 IU/L
AST > 250 IU/L

During initial 48 hours

↓ Hct > 10% with hydration or Hct ≤ 30%
↑ BUN > 5 mg/dl
Serum calcium < 8 mg/dl
Pao_2 < 60 mm Hg
Fluid sequestration > 5000 ml
Interpretation: Mortality increases with three or more signs.

Major Factors Adversely Influencing Survival

Hypotension
Need for massive fluid and colloid replacement
Respiratory failure
Hypocalcemia
Chocolate brown (hemorrhagic) peritoneal fluid
Interpretation: If three or more factors present, mortality can be as high as 50%.

Banks' Clinical Criteria for Grading Severity

Cardiac: Shock, tachycardia > 130 beats/min
Pulmonary: Pao_2 < 60 mm Hg; acute respiratory distress syndrome
Renal: Azotemia, urine output < 50 ml/hr with hydration
Metabolic: ↓ Serum albumin, ↓ serum calcium
Hematologic: ↓ Hct > 10% with hydration
Neurologic: Confusion, obtundation
Abdominal: Hemorrhagic peritoneal fluid, tense ascites
Interpretation: One or more signs indicate severe disease.

WBC, White blood cell count; *LDH*, lactate dehydrogenase; *AST*, aspartate aminotransaminase; *Hct*, hematocrit; *BUN*, blood urea nitrogen; Pao_2, arterial oxygen pressure.

with an imaging procedure is useful in excluding a diagnosis of acute pancreatitis. Renal colic usually is associated with an abnormal urinalysis and sonogram and often with an abnormal intravenous pyelogram. All patients with acute abdominal pain must have a chest film examination to exclude acute pneumonia, which can mimic a surgical abdomen. A constellation of the following clinical features should suggest the diagnosis of gallstone-associated acute pancreatitis: (1) age over 50 years; (2) female; (3) serum amylase over 1000 U; (4) serum AST over 100 U; and (5) serum bilirubin over 2 mg/dl. If all five features are present, there is an 85% probability the diagnosis is gallstone pancreatitis.

Although the vast majority of patients with acute pancreatitis recover without major complication, 5% to 10% develop severe pancreatitis. Accordingly, it is important to identify factors that increase the likelihood of a fatal outcome in patients with acute pancreatitis (see Box 106-4). Patients with severe acute pancreatitis need to be hospitalized in the intensive care unit (ICU), and consultation with a surgeon and gastroenterologist is indicated.

Management and Complications

In most patients with acute pancreatitis (85% to 90%) the disease is self-limited and subsides spontaneously, usually within 3 to 5 days after treatment is initiated. Medical treatment is aimed at reducing pancreatic secretion and, in essence, putting the pancreas at rest. Conventional measures include (1) analgesics for pain; (2) intravenous (IV) fluids and colloids to maintain normal intravascular volume and correct electrolyte abnormalities; (3) no oral alimentation; and (4) nasogastric suction. Since nasogastric suction offers no clear-cut advantages in the treatment of mild to moderately severe acute pancreatitis, however, its use should be considered elective rather than mandatory. The patient with mild to moderate pancreatitis usually requires treatment with IV fluids, no oral intake, and possibly nasogastric suction for 3 to 5 days. A clear-liquid diet frequently is started on the fifth day and a regular diet by the seventh day.

No drugs have been demonstrated to improve the course of mild, moderate, or severe pancreatitis. The list includes

Table 106-1. Diagnosis of Acute Pancreatitis

Criterion	Definite	Probable	Possible
1. Causal factor identified	X	X	X
2. Compatible physical examination	X	X	X
3. Nonspecific indications of an inflammatory response: Fever, tachycardia, increased WBC	X	X	±*
4. Biochemical confirmatory tests: Serum amylase three times normal or higher; Serum lipase twice normal or higher; Urine amylase increased; Other reasons for elevated serum amylase excluded	X†	—	—
5. Imaging procedures: ultrasound, CT scan	X†	—	—

*All three are not present.
†If 1 to 3 and either 4 or 5 are positive, a definite diagnosis of acute pancreatitis is established.

anticholinergic drugs (which are contraindicated), antibiotics (except for infected pancreatic necrosis and other infections), somatostatin analogs (e.g., octreotide), H_2 receptor antagonists (H_2RAs, H_2 blockers), calcitonin, and lexiplafant, an inhibitor of platelet-activating factor.

The patient with fulminant pancreatitis requires intensive therapy. This usually includes large amounts of IV fluids, treatment of cardiovascular collapse and respiratory insufficiency, and management of hypocalcemia. Removal of toxic pancreatic exudate from the peritoneal cavity may alter the course of the disease, although controlled trials of peritoneal lavage have not established that this procedure is effective. In patients with failure in one or more organ systems (Box 106-6), intensive supportive therapy, preferably in an ICU, is indicated. Such patients with severe acute pancreatitis usually require parenteral nutrition. Consultation with a surgeon or gastroenterologist should be obtained.

In patients acutely ill with severe pancreatitis and major risk factors, pancreatic abscess or infected pancreatic necrosis needs to be excluded, usually by CT-guided biopsy, aspiration of pancreatic tissue, and preparation of appropriate cultures.[10] Infected pancreatic necrosis should be removed by debridement; this is done surgically because it is difficult to evacuate solid infected material by percutaneous catheter drainage. Current evidence favors the use of prophylactic antibiotics in severe acute pancreatitis. Results of four randomized trials[4,5] restricted to patients with prognostically severe acute pancreatitis demonstrated improved outcome (i.e., decreased rate of infection, reduced mortality) with antibiotic treatment. The carbapenem group of antibiotics, including imipenem, has a very broad spectrum, including activity against *Pseudomonas, Staphylococcus,* and *Enterococcus,* and achieves good penetration into pancreatic tissue. Secondary infection of necrotic pancreatic tissue (abscess, pseudocyst, obstructed biliary passages with ascending cholangitis complicating choledocholithiasis) contributes to much of the late mortality

Box 106-5. Differential Diagnosis of Acute Pancreatitis

- Acute appendicitis
- Acute cholecystitis
- Perforated viscus, especially peptic ulcer
- Alcohol hepatitis
- Mesenteric vascular occlusion
- Connective tissue disorders with vasculitis (SLE, polyarteritis nodosa) and related disorders (TTP, Henoch's purpura, Schönlein purpura)
- Renal colic
- Dissecting aortic aneurysm
- Gynecologic problems (pelvic inflammatory disease, ectopic pregnancy, mittelschmerz, ruptured ovarian cyst)
- Medical problems that can cause acute abdominal pain (pneumonia, myocardial infarction, diabetic ketoacidosis, sickle cell anemia, porphyria)

SLE, Systemic lupus erythematosus; *TTP,* thrombotic thrombocytopenic purpura.

Box 106-6. Complications of Acute Pancreatitis

Local

- Pancreatic necrosis
- Pancreatic pseudocyst
  - Pain
  - Rupture with/without hemorrhage
  - Hemorrhage
  - Infection
- Pancreatic ascites
  - Disruption of main pancreatic duct
  - Leaking pseudocyst
- Pancreatic abscess
- Involvement of contiguous organs by necrotizing pancreatitis
  - Massive intraperitoneal hemorrhage
  - Thrombosis of blood vessels
  - Bowel infarction
- Obstructive jaundice

Systemic

- Pulmonary
  - Atelectasis
  - Pneumonitis
  - Pleural effusion
  - Mediastinal abscess
  - Adult respiratory distress syndrome
- Cardiovascular
  - Hypotension
    - Hypovolemia
    - Sepsis
  - Sudden death
  - Nonspecific ST-T changes in ECG simulating myocardial infarction
  - Pericardial effusion
- Hematologic
  - Disseminated intravascular coagulation (DIC)
- Gastrointestinal hemorrhage
  - Peptic ulcer disease
  - Erosive gastritis
  - Hemorrhagic pancreatic necrosis with erosion into major blood vessels
  - Portal vein thrombosis; variceal hemorrhage
- Renal
  - Oliguria } usually caused by hypovolemia
  - Azotemia }
  - Renal artery/vein thrombosis
- Metabolic
  - Hyperglycemia
  - Hypertriglyceridemia
  - Hypocalcemia
- Central nervous system
  - Psychosis
  - Fat emboli
  - Encephalopathy
- Fat necrosis
  - Subcutaneous tissues; erythematous nodules
  - Bone
  - Other organs (mediastinum, pleura, nervous system)
- Miscellaneous
  - Sudden blindness (Purtscher's retinopathy)

Modified from Greenberger NJ et al: *The medical book of lists: a primer of differential diagnosis in internal medicine,* ed 5, St Louis, 1998, Mosby.

from pancreatitis, so appropriate antibiotic therapy of established infections is especially important. The optimum treatment of patients with severe pancreatitis and *sterile* pancreatic necrosis is controversial. If such patients develop organ failure or have acute physiologic and chronic health evaluation scores (APACHE II, a scale used to assess severity of illness) greater than 13, surgical debridement is reasonable because the mortality in this setting can be as high as 40%.

PSEUDOCYST

Pseudocysts of the pancreas are collections of tissue, fluid, debris, pancreatic enzymes, and blood that develop over 1 to 4 weeks after the onset of acute pancreatitis. In contrast to true cysts, pseudocysts do not have an epithelial lining, and the walls consist of necrotic, granulation, and fibrous tissue. Disruption of the pancreatic ductal system is common. Transient edema and fluid collections within the pancreas may give rise to epigastric pain, a palpable abdominal mass, and distortion or displacement of the upper gastrointestinal (UGI) tract on barium study, thus mimicking a pancreatic pseudocyst. The use of ultrasonography and CT scanning should permit differentiation between an edematous and inflamed pancreas and an actual pseudocyst.

Etiology

Pseudocysts are preceded by pancreatitis in approximately 90% of cases. In several reports the incidence of acute and chronic alcoholism in patients with pseudocysts has ranged from 88% to 93%. Gallbladder disease was identified in approximately 5% and trauma in approximately 10% of cases; other etiologic factors rarely exist.

Clinical Presentation

Pseudocysts develop in 10% to 15% of patients with acute pancreatitis. Pseudocysts are solitary lesions in more than 90% of patients and multiple in less than 10%. Approximately 90% of pseudocysts are located in the body or tail of the pancreas and 10% in the head.[12] Abdominal pain is a cardinal symptom and is present in more than 90% of patients. Nausea and vomiting, anorexia, and weight loss are common symptoms, whereas diarrhea and fever occur infrequently. A palpable mass, often tender and usually in the midabdomen or left upper quadrant, is present in approximately 50% of patients. On the basis of physical examination alone, however, it is difficult to differentiate between an edematous, inflamed pancreas (which can give rise to a palpable mass) and a pseudocyst. Ascites is present in approximately 20% and jaundice in 10% of patients.

Several laboratory tests are important in the evaluation of patients with pseudocysts. Serum amylase is elevated in approximately 75% of patients. The WBC is 12,000/mm^3 or higher in approximately half of patients, the blood sugar is elevated in one third, and the hemoglobin level is less than 10 gm/dl in approximately one fourth of patients. Chest x-ray evidence of pulmonary and pleural disease is found in approximately 25% of such patients. The serum bilirubin is elevated to values greater than 2 mg/dl in approximately 10% of patients, usually from compression of the intrapancreatic portion of the common bile duct. Ultrasound, CT scan, and endoscopic retrograde cholangiopancreatography (ERCP) help identify pancreatic pseudocyst (Fig. 106-2).

Differential Diagnosis

The diagnosis of pseudocyst often is difficult, however, because the clinical features, physical examination, and conventional radiologic evaluations are both insensitive and nonspecific. An ultrasound or CT scan should be obtained to confirm the diagnosis. The differential diagnosis of pancreatic cysts includes (1) pseudocysts, (2) retention cysts, (3) neoplasms (e.g., cystadenoma, cystadenocarcinoma), (4) congenital causes, and (5) desmoids.

In studies using serial ultrasound or CT scan, pseudocysts resolved in 25% to 40% of patients. However, pseudocysts greater than 5 cm and present for longer than 6 weeks infrequently disappear. Persistent pseudocysts can be treated by CT-guided percutaneous drainage (if the location is favorable) or by surgical or endoscopic cystogastrostomy or cystoenterostomy.

Natural History and Complications

The major complications of pseudocyst include pain, rupture with and without bleeding, gastrointestinal bleeding, abscess, and pancreatic ascites. Rupture with hemorrhage is the most serious, with mortality rates of 50% to 60%. Pancreatic abscess can occur (1) because of communication of the pseudocyst with the colon; (2) after inadequate surgical drainage of a pseudocyst; (3) after needling a pseudocyst; and (4) with infected severe pancreatic necrosis. In addition, pancreatic abscess is much more common in patients with severe pancreatitis. In a representative series, pancreatic abscess occurred in 28 of 330 patients with pancreatitis. The cause of pancreatitis in patients with pancreatic abscess most often was surgery; alcoholism and biliary tract disease caused only 6.6% and 3.0%, respectively. In patients with lethal pancreatitis, evidence of pancreatic abscess is found at autopsy in more than 90%. The incidence of pancreatic abscess rises appreciably with an increasing number of risk factors present in a given case, being less than 3% with fewer than three risk factors and greater than 50% with five or more risk factors. Characteristic signs of pancreatic abscess are the development of fever, tachycardia, leukocytosis, toxicity, and rapid deterioration after initial stabilization. Serial CT scans may provide additional evidence to support a diagnosis of infected pseudocyst and pancreatic abscess, but the absence of telltale gas on a CT scan does not exclude a diagnosis of pancreatic abscess.

Pancreatic ascites occurs because of one of two factors: (1) disruption of the main pancreatic duct or (2) a leaking pseudocyst. The diagnosis is established by the triad of findings of (1) persistently increased serum amylase; (2) elevated ascitic fluid amylase; and (3) increased ascitic fluid protein concentration (more than 3 gm/dl). Patients frequently require surgery.

Management

If the patient is stable and serial ultrasound examinations show that the pseudocyst is decreasing in size, observation only is indicated. However, patients with an expanding pseudocyst or those complicated by rupture, hemorrhage, or abscess should undergo surgery. Elective cyst drainage usually is indicated if pseudocysts persist for longer than 6 weeks. ERCP may be important in this setting because a leaking pancreatic duct can be identified and treated by stenting (see Fig. 106-2, *C*). The long-acting somatostatin

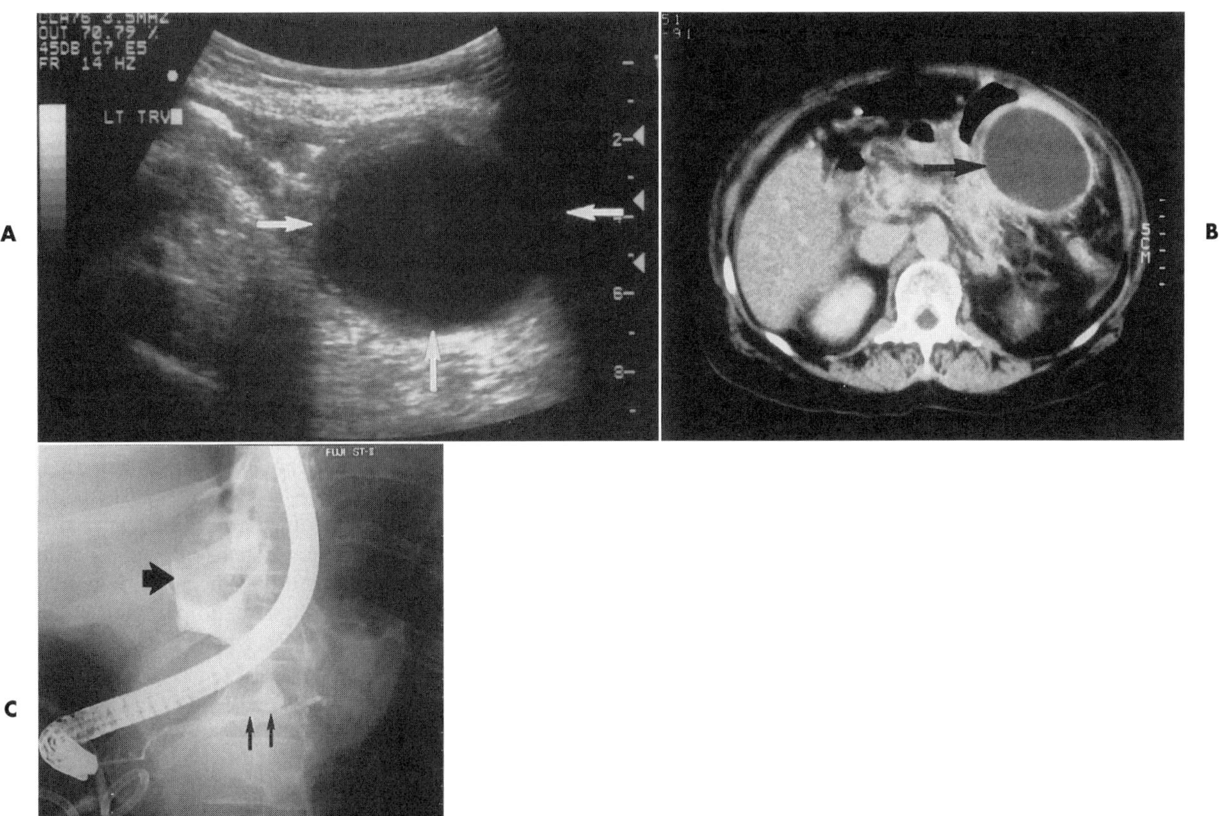

Fig. 106-2. Pseudocyst of pancreas. **A,** Ultrasound showing large pancreatic pseudocyst *(arrows).* **B,** CT scan showing well-encapsulated pseudocyst *(arrow).* **C,** ERCP showing a disrupted pancreatic duct *(thin arrows)* communicating directly with pancreatic pseudocyst *(broad arrow).*

analog octreotide, which inhibits pancreatic secretion, is also useful in these patients.

CHRONIC PANCREATITIS

Epidemiology and Etiology

Chronic pancreatitis is usually characterized by recurring or persistent abdominal pain with or without steatorrhea or diabetes. Morphologically, chronic pancreatitis is characterized by irregular sclerosis with destruction and permanent loss of pancreatic parenchyma that may be focal, segmental, or diffuse and with variable dilation of the pancreatic ducts.

Chronic pancreatitis may present as episodes of acute inflammation superimposed on a previously injured pancreas or as chronic damage with persistent pain or malabsorption. Box 106-7 lists the causes of both chronic pancreatitis and pancreatic exocrine insufficiency. Patients with chronic pancreatic damage of mild to moderate severity usually come to medical attention because of chronic abdominal pain. Often the only abnormal laboratory test at this stage of the disease is a test of pancreatic exocrine function such as the secretin test. Patients with extensive chronic pancreatic damage frequently present with diarrhea, steatorrhea, and weight loss; these patients have pancreatic exocrine insufficiency. Because of the enormous reserve capacity of the pancreas, malabsorption is a late manifestation of chronic pancreatitis resulting only when more than 90% of the exocrine pancreas is destroyed.

In several patients with hereditary chronic pancreatitis, researchers were able to identify a genetic defect that affects the gene and coding for trypsinogen. The defect seems to allow trypsinogen to resist the effect of trypsin inhibitor and thus become spontaneously activated and remain activated. This continual activation of digestive enzymes within the gland is believed to lead to continued injury and ultimately chronic pancreatitis.[14]

In the United States, alcohol is by far the most common cause of clinically apparent pancreatic exocrine insufficiency, whereas cystic fibrosis (CF) accounts for the majority of cases in children. Approximately 85% of CF patients have impaired pancreatic exocrine function. With improved treatment of their pulmonary problems, an increasing number of CF patients are reaching adulthood, when their pancreatic exocrine insufficiency can become clinically relevant. In adult patients 20 to 40 years of age with exocrine pancreatic insufficiency without obvious cause, the diagnosis of CF should be excluded. In recent studies of patients with idiopathic chronic pancreatitis, an appreciable number of patients had gene mutations of CF, and classic stigmata of CF, such as abnormal spirometry or respiratory tract disease, were usually absent.[7] In adult patients over age 40 with pancreatic insufficiency without obvious cause, pancreatic cancer needs to be excluded (Box 106-8). In up to 25% of U.S. adults with chronic pancreatitis, the disorder is idiopathic.

Box 106-7. Causes of Chronic Pancreatitis and Pancreatic Exocrine Insufficiency

Chronic Pancreatitis

Chronic alcoholism*
Etiologic factor unknown (idiopathic)*
Hereditary pancreatitis
Hemochromatosis
Radiation injury
Trauma
Sicca syndrome

Cystic Fibrosis*

Postoperative

Gastric surgery (e.g., subtotal gastrectomy, antrectomy, vagotomy, pyloroplasty)
Whipple's procedure
95% or greater pancreatic resection for chronic pancreatitis

Neoplasms

Adenocarcinoma of pancreas*
Islet cell tumors (e.g., gastrinoma, VIPoma)
Duodenal adenocarcinoma obstruction of pancreatic duct

Severe Protein-Calorie Malnutrition

VIP, Vasoactive intestinal polypeptide.
*Most common.

Box 106-8. Recurrent Bouts of Acute Pancreatitis Without Obvious Cause

Biliary microlithiasis (most common; 60%-75% of cases)
Occult disease of biliary tree, pancreatic duct system, ampulla of Vater
Hypertriglyceridemia
Pancreas divisum
Hereditary pancreatitis
Drugs

Pathophysiology

The pancreas has an enormous reserve capacity for the digestion of nutrients. An inverse relationship exists between intraduodenal and intrajejunal levels of lipase and development of steatorrhea, as well as between intraluminal trypsin and chymotrypsin levels and the development of azotorrhea (increased nitrogen in the stool) and creatorrhea (undigested muscle fibers in the stool).[8] Steatorrhea, azotorrhea, and creatorrhea are late manifestations of pancreatic exocrine insufficiency and develop when the capacity of the exocrine pancreas to secrete these enzymes is less than 10% of normal values. Thus patients may have evidence of exocrine dysfunction, that is, an impaired response to intravenously injected secretin or secretin plus cholecystokinin or an abnormal pancreatic ductal system demonstrated by ERCP but without any obvious impairment in digestive function.

Many patients with chronic pancreatitis have persistent abdominal pain as the major manifestation of their disease. Pain in chronic pancreatitis may be caused by (1) persistence of pseudocysts with perifocal inflammation, (2) dilation of the pancreatic duct from elevated ductal pressures, (3) continued pancreatic parenchymal inflammatory processes, (4) pressure of an enlarged or inflamed gland on retroperitoneal structures, and (5) infiltration or entrapment of sensory nerves.[6] Pseudocysts can be important in the pathogenesis of pancreatic pain, as evidenced by the repeated observation that up to 50% of patients with chronic pancreatitis have obtained pain relief by simple drainage of pseudocysts. Therefore, in all patients with chronic pancreatic pain, imaging studies (preferably a CT scan) are performed to rule out an underlying pseudocyst. An abnormal pancreatic ductal system is frequently documented in patients with chronic pancreatitis, although no consistent relationship exists between severity of pain and presence of strictured or dilated ducts. Some patients with pancreatic pain and stenotic ducts may obtain relief, however, when the pancreatic ductal system is stented.

Studies support the concept of an enteropancreatic axis. After initiation of intraluminal digestions by pancreatic enzymes, increased levels of proteases in the duodenal and jejunal lumen act in a feedback manner to decrease release of cholecystokinin from the small bowel mucosa, which in turn results in decreased stimulation of the pancreas. This concept has led to the use of pharmacologic doses of pancreatic enzymes, rich in protease content, in the treatment of persistent pain in patients with chronic pancreatitis.

Patient Evaluation

History. Although patients with chronic pancreatitis may have symptoms identical to those found in patients with acute pancreatitis, patients with chronic pancreatitis often complain of persistent or recurring pain. Although many patients may have severe epigastric pain that radiates through to the back, the pain pattern often is atypical. The pain may be maximal in the right upper or left upper quadrant, in the back, or diffuse throughout the abdomen; it may even be referred to the anterior chest or flank. Characteristically the pain is severe, persistent, deep seated, unresponsive to antacids or food ingestion, and increased by alcohol ingestion or heavy meals (especially foods rich in fat). Often the pain is so severe as to require the frequent use of narcotics. Nausea, vomiting, and abdominal distention are seen less frequently and usually are secondary to the pain and use of medications (especially narcotics), which decrease gastric and intestinal motility.

Weight loss, diarrhea, and steatorrhea frequently are present. However, clinically apparent deficiencies of fat-soluble vitamins are noted less frequently than in patients with steatorrhea secondary to small bowel disease. The stool characteristically has an oily appearance and may cling to the sides of the toilet bowl.

Physical Examination. The physical findings in patients with chronic pancreatitis or pancreatic exocrine insufficiency usually are not impressive. Indeed, the disparity between the severity of the abdominal pain and the paucity of physical findings is remarkable. Abdominal tenderness and mild fever may be seen, especially in those with episodes of acute superimposed on chronic pancreatitis. Weight loss may be profound. Jaundice may be noted in 10% to 20% of patients from obstruction of the common bile duct secondary to edema or fibrosis of the duct above or in the head of the pancreas. Ascites and a palpable abdominal mass (pseudocyst) may be noted in 2% to 5% of patients. Patients with severe malabsorption often show evidence of malnutrition with cachexia, muscle wasting, edema, and stigmata of vitamin deficiencies.

Laboratory Studies and Diagnostic Procedures

Several studies can be used to evaluate pancreatic exocrine function, but many of these are not widely available. Direct tests of pancreatic secretory capacity include the secretin test or the secretin plus cholecystokinin test. These tests are usually available only in academic health centers. A reliable test to document evidence of intraluminal maldigestion is to examine stools for evidence of fatty acid globules and for crystals and undigested muscle fibers (creatorrhea). The finding of more than five muscle fibers in the stool provides strong evidence of impaired intraluminal digestion. Although a very specific test, this test is rather insensitive in that positivity requires that more than 95% of the exocrine pancreas has been destroyed.

Several diagnostic procedures are available to image the pancreas. The simplest test is the plain film of the abdomen; if this shows evidence of pancreatic calcification, it establishes the diagnosis of chronic pancreatitis (Fig. 106-3). Ultrasound studies may reveal evidence of pancreatic calcification (before it is evident on the plain film), enlargement of the pancreas, or irregularities in the pancreas. The CT scan is the diagnostic procedure of choice to evaluate the pancreas in patients with suspected chronic pancreatitis. In addition to showing evidence of calcification, it may show evidence of duct dilation, focal enlargement, fluid collections, biliary ductal dilation, alterations of peripancreatic fat, or fascia. A normal-appearing pancreas appears in only 10% of the patients with chronic pancreatitis. ERCP often shows varying degrees of ductular dilation and may show marked dilation of areas of stenosis as well.

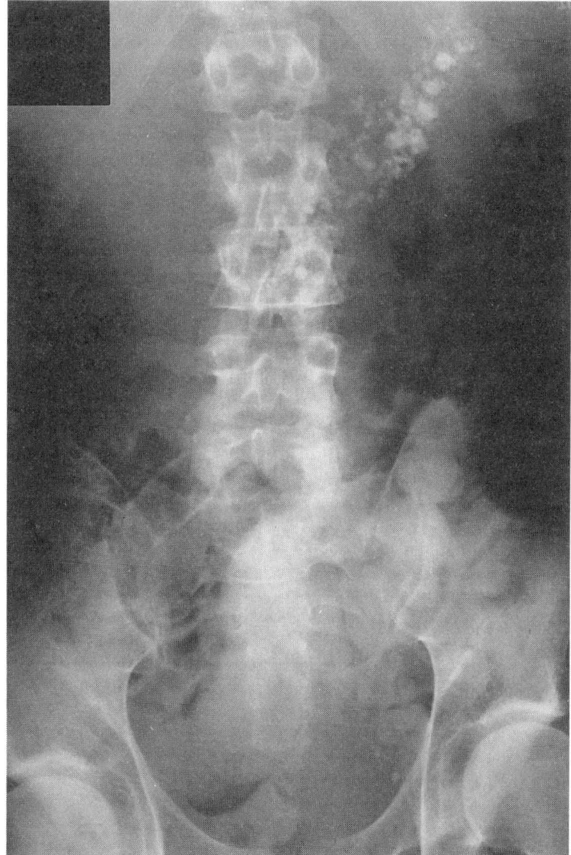

Fig. 106-3. Calcification in pancreas.

Differential Diagnosis

First, the etiology of pancreatic insufficiency must be identified (see Box 106-7). In adults past age 40 and especially past age 60 who present with evidence of pancreatic malabsorption (steatorrhea, creatorrhea) the diagnosis of pancreatic cancer must be excluded. If the classic diagnostic triad for pancreatic exocrine insufficiency (steatorrhea, pancreatic calcification, diabetes mellitus) is present, no need exists for additional tests of pancreatic secretory capacity. Unfortunately, only one fourth of the patients with pancreatic exocrine insufficiency manifest the diagnostic triad, so other tests are often needed (e.g., qualitative examination of stool). The criteria for diagnosis of chronic pancreatitis are shown in Box 106-9. Absorption of vitamin B_{12} (Schilling test) is often done, since over 40% of patients with pancreatic exocrine insufficiency have impaired absorption of vitamin B_{12}. In patients with malabsorption, as evidenced by the presence of steatorrhea, tests must confirm that mucosal function is normal. These include a normal D-xylose test, normal small bowel radiographs, and a normal small bowel biopsy. An important parameter that confirms the presence of malabsorption due to pancreatic exocrine insufficiency is a positive response to pancreatic enzyme replacement therapy. Such a positive response is characterized by gain in weight and amelioration of diarrhea, steatorrhea, and creatorrhea.

Box 106-9. Diagnosis of Pancreatic Exocrine Insufficiency

Identify etiology of pancreatic insufficiency (e.g., alcoholism, pancreatic cancer)

Steatorrhea
Pancreatic calcification
Diabetes mellitus
} Classic diagnostic triad

Undigested muscle fibers in stool (creatorrhea)

Secretin/cholecystokinin test of pancreatic exocrine function; frequently necessary since diagnostic triad found in approximately 20% of patients

Decreased absorption of vitamin B_{12} (Schilling test)

Normal tests of mucosal function (D-xylose, small bowel biopsy)

Response to pancreatic enzyme replacement therapy
- Gain in weight
- Amelioration of diarrhea/steatorrhea

Pancreatic function tests may correlate poorly with ERCP findings

In patients with chronic pancreatitis manifested only by chronic abdominal pain, it is important to exclude other painful conditions and to confirm that patients are not surreptitiously using alcohol. If available, the secretin test is useful in establishing the diagnosis of chronic pancreatitis, since patients with pain from chronic pancreatitis almost invariably have a peak bicarbonate concentration less than 80 mEq/L.

The differential diagnosis of pain in chronic pancreatitis should include (1) pseudocysts, (2) peptic ulcer disease, (3) cholelithiasis, (4) pancreatic cancer, (5) biliary tract obstruction, (6) pancreatic stones, and (7) narcotic addiction. The latter is an important issue and can usually be diagnosed by taking a careful history and trying to wean the patient off narcotics under clonidine cover. This usually requires hospitalization and administration of clonidine (usually as a patch, but at least in a dosage of 5 μg/kg). Because the drug may cause hypotension, it should be done in a hospital setting, where the narcotic dosage can be reduced by 20% to 25% each day.

Management and Complications

Management of patients with pancreatogenous steatorrhea usually starts with pancreatic enzymes that have both potent lipase and protease content, with 6 to 18 capsules per day depending on the lipase and protease content of the enzyme preparation (Fig. 106-4). If diarrhea or steatorrhea persists, the fat content in the diet should be reduced. If problems persist with steatorrhea or diarrhea, either bicarbonate or an H_2 RA can be added. The evidence that H_2 RAs bring about additional improvement in this setting is still somewhat controversial.

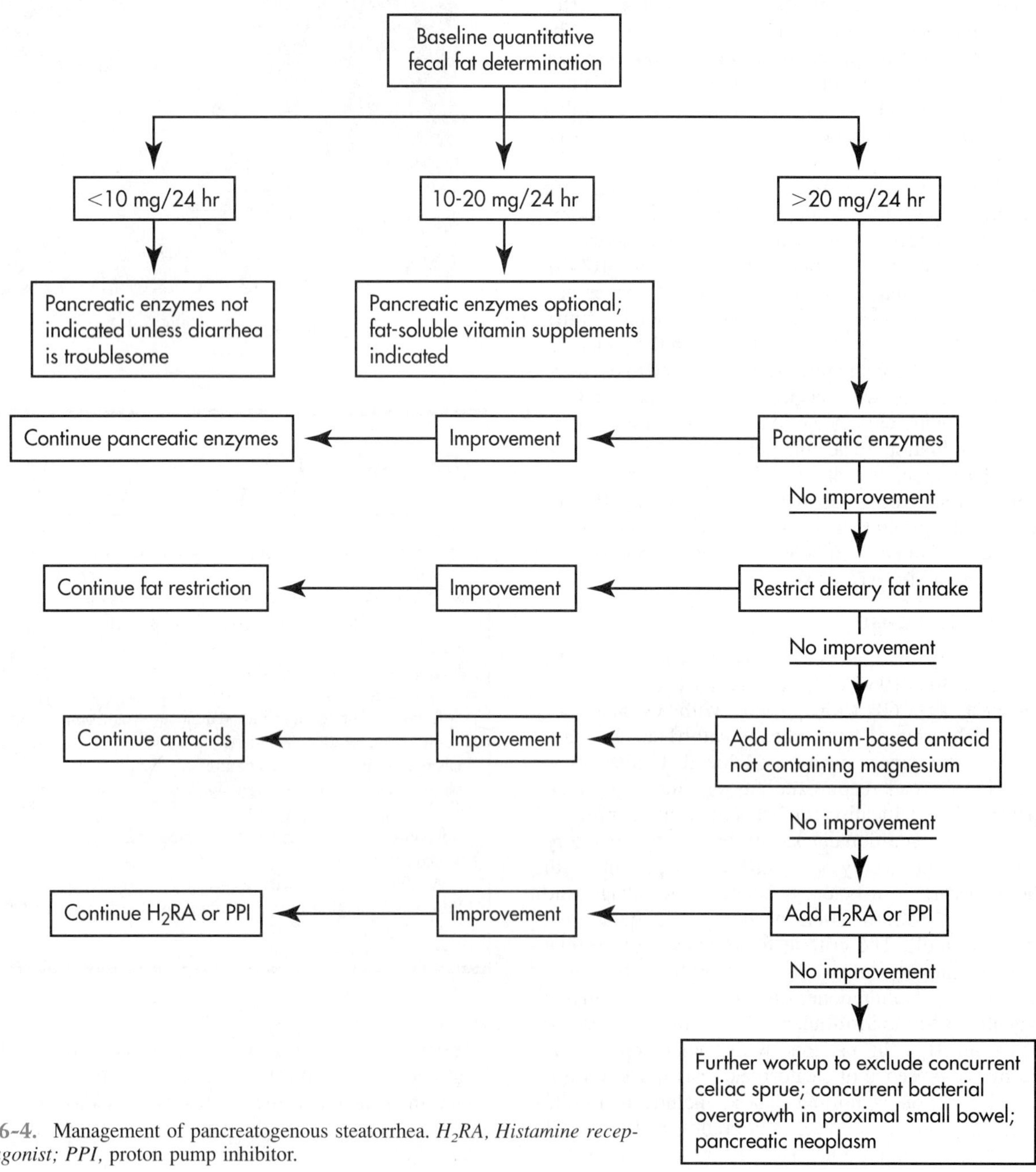

Fig. 106-4. Management of pancreatogenous steatorrhea. *H_2RA, Histamine receptor antagonist; PPI,* proton pump inhibitor.

The management of pain in chronic pancreatitis requires an understanding of the natural history of this problem. A classic study evaluated 245 patients with chronic pancreatitis and persistent pain for an average of 10 years.[1] Alcohol was the etiologic factor in 173 patients, 58 had idiopathic chronic pancreatitis, and 14 had various rare disorders. Regardless of medical or surgical therapy, 85% of the patients obtained lasting pain relief within 4½ years. In many patients, pain relief was accompanied by further pancreatic dysfunction and the development of malabsorption. The physician must ensure that the use of alcohol is discontinued in all patients with chronic pancreatitis, especially those with persistent pain. This simple expedient will result in pain relief in approximately 50% of patients with chronic pancreatitis.

Because evidence supports an enteropancreatic axis, a trial of high-dose pancreatic enzyme therapy rich in pancreatic proteases should be considered in all patients who have pain from chronic pancreatitis (Fig. 106-5).[2,4,5] This should include pancreatic enzyme therapy (18 to 24 capsules per day), and the capsules should not be enteric coated or slow release. The patients most likely to respond to pancreatic enzyme replacement therapy are females with idiopathic pancreatitis, in whom a response rate of about 75% may be seen. By contrast, the response rate is much less in males (20% to 25%), male alcoholics (12% to 15%), and males and females with severe chronic pancreatitis (25%). In all patients with chronic pancreatitis and persistent pain, it is important to exclude the presence of the pseudocyst, since drainage of the pseudocyst often results in amelioration of pain. Risk of narcotic addiction is high, and the pain in such patients should be controlled by using nonnarcotic analgesics. Drugs such as Darvon plus Tylenol combinations or nonsteroidals such as ketorolac, taken orally, are often effective. A regular schedule of Extra Strength Tylenol (1 gm every 8 hours) is also effective. Patients who have been alcoholic should be cautioned about using even small doses of alcohol if they are taking 3 gm of Tylenol per day.

Serious complications of chronic pancreatitis include pancreatogenous ascites, which can result from a leaking pseudocyst or a disrupted pancreatic duct (Box 106-10). Common bile duct obstruction is associated with abnormal liver function tests and development of secondary biliary cirrhosis. Accordingly, in all patients with chronic pancreatitis who have persistent and sustained elevation of the serum alkaline phosphatase to values greater than twice normal for more than 2 months, studies should be undertaken to evaluate for extrahepatic biliary tract obstruction, usually with ERCP. If this shows evidence of a stricture, a liver biopsy should be performed. If this suggests secondary biliary cirrhosis, the biliary tract obstruction should be decompressed.

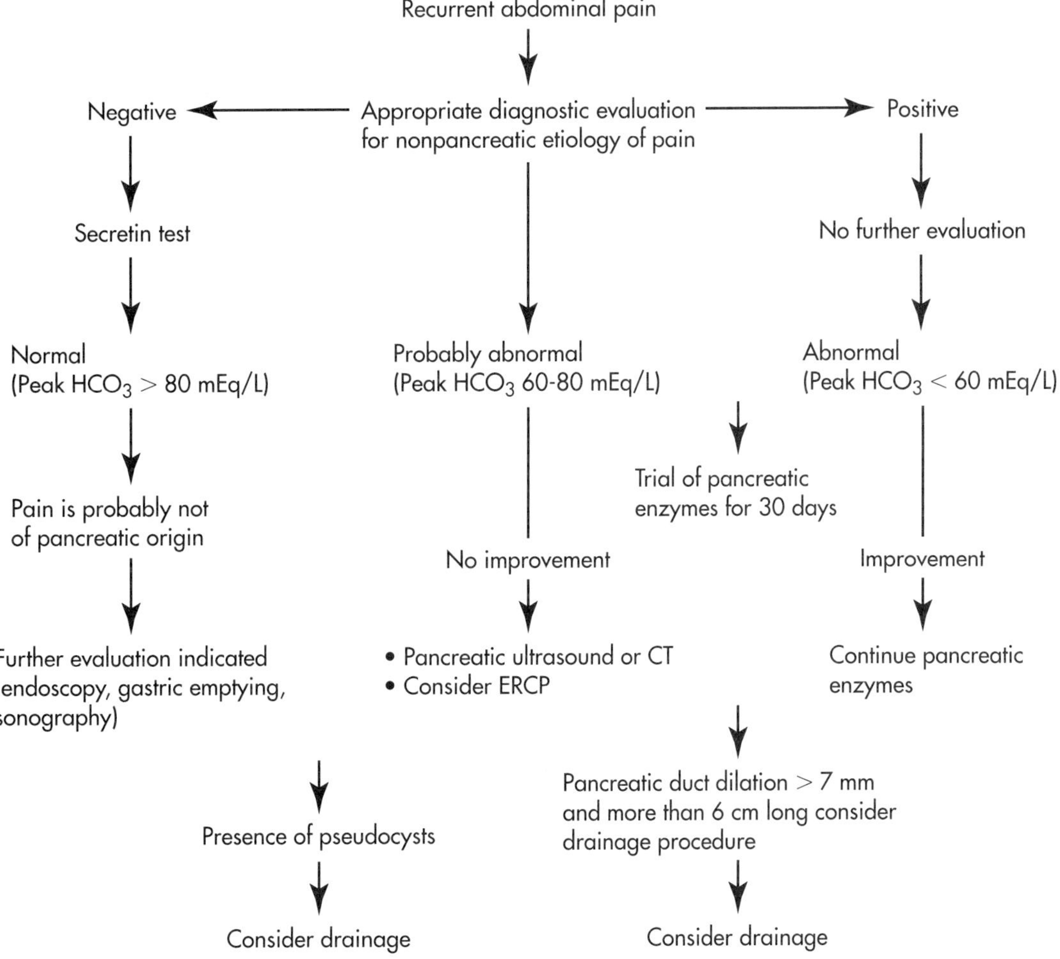

Fig. 106-5. Management of chronic pancreatic pain. HCO_3, Bicarbonate.

Box 106-10. Complications of Chronic Pancreatitis and Pancreatic Exocrine Insufficiency

Pancreatic ascites
Chronic pain
Narcotic addiction
Steatorrhea and diarrhea
Diabetes mellitus
Cobalamin malabsorption
Ascites
Common bile duct obstruction
Biliary cirrhosis
Splenic vein thrombosis
Portal hypertension
Nondiabetic retinopathy
Pancreatic cancer

Box 106-11. Clinical Presentations of Pancreatic Carcinoma

New onset of persistent abdominal pain without an obvious cause
Onset of diarrhea (irritable bowel–type symptoms) without obvious cause in adult over age 50
Unexplained weight loss
Onset of diabetes without obvious risk factors
Onset of obstructive-type jaundice in adults over age 50
Onset of depression without obvious cause
Onset of malabsorption with stigmata of pancreatic exocrine insufficiency in adults over age 50
Metastatic adenocarcinoma with primary lesion of unknown origin
Malignant ascites
Recurrent thrombophlebitis
Onset of symptoms of gastric outlet obstruction (nausea, post-prandial distention)

PANCREATIC CANCER

Epidemiology

Carcinoma of the pancreas, one of the most dreaded of all tumors, strikes adults in all age groups; the peak age of risk is about 60 years. The overall incidence has risen 300% over the past 30 years, and pancreatic cancer now ranks as the fourth most common tumor behind lung, colorectal, and breast cancer. The disease attacks men twice as frequently as women.

Only a few risk factors have been clearly identified as predisposing to the development of pancreatic cancer. These include cigarette smoking, diabetes, and chronic pancreatitis.[11] However, the vast majority of patients with this tumor have none of these risk factors. This inability to identify subgroups at risk for the disease is one of the major problems limiting the development of screening techniques for early detection.

Pathophysiology

The clinical presentation of pancreatic carcinoma, at least initially, can be quite variable (Box 106-11). The most common presentation (new onset, obscure and unrelenting abdominal pain) results from an enlarging mass in the pancreas causing pressure on retroperitoneal structures and the stomach and duodenum. Presentation with diarrhea and malabsorption can be caused by a localized obstruction of the main pancreatic duct and head of the pancreas, resulting in pancreatic exocrine insufficiency and steatorrhea with diarrhea. New onset of an irritable bowel–type syndrome in any patient past 50 with no prior history of such a disorder should always suggest pancreatic cancer. Pancreatic cancers located at the head of the pancreas often cause obstruction of the common bile duct, resulting in new onset of jaundice with obstructive features. Approximately 40% of patients with pancreatic carcinoma have an abnormal blood glucose level detected within 2 years before diagnosis. Therefore, in any patient past age 50 who develops signs of unexplained carbohydrate intolerance, especially if this is accompanied by abdominal pain or weight loss, the diagnosis of pancreatic carcinoma should be excluded.

Patient Evaluation

History. Persistent abdominal pain, weight loss, and unremitting jaundice are the outstanding symptoms of pancreatic carcinoma. The site of the lesion, however, greatly influences the character and time of onset of symptoms. Obscure abdominal pain is one of the most difficult of all symptoms to evaluate. Clues to a pancreatic origin include a persistent gnawing, boring upper abdominal discomfort referred through to the back. This upper abdominal pain may have no particular exacerbating or relieving factors. If there is already some mechanical compromise to gastric emptying, the patient may complain of vague abdominal distress and fullness made worse by eating. Cancer in the body or tail of the pancreas frequently produces more severe pain, and its unrelenting nature should suggest pancreatic cancer, especially if the pain is worse when lying supine and relieved by sitting forward. Although painless jaundice is touted as a presentation of pancreatic cancer, more often the patient complains of vague abdominal distress that may be difficult to characterize. In adults over age 50 presenting with irritable bowel–type symptoms without any prior such history, and especially if this is accompanied by weight loss, the diagnosis of pancreatic cancer should be considered. Similarly, new onset of malabsorption with stigmata of pancreatic exocrine insufficiency in adults past age 50 without an obvious reason for pancreatic insufficiency should also suggest pancreatic cancer. Patients with anaplastic carcinoma of the pancreas have a lesion that grows rapidly and spreads quickly to distant locations, and this can result in evidence of malignant ascites or metastatic carcinoma at presentation. Finally, patients with obstructive type jaundice often complain of intense and persistent pruritus.

Physical Examination. Pertinent physical findings in the patient with suspected pancreatic cancer include (1) jaundice; (2) excoriations or scratching that may reflect pruritus; (3) evidence of recent weight loss; (4) Virchow supraclavicular adenopathy; (5) hepatomegaly, especially with the palpable left lobe of the liver; (6) a palpable gallbladder (Courvoisier's sign), which occurs in one fourth

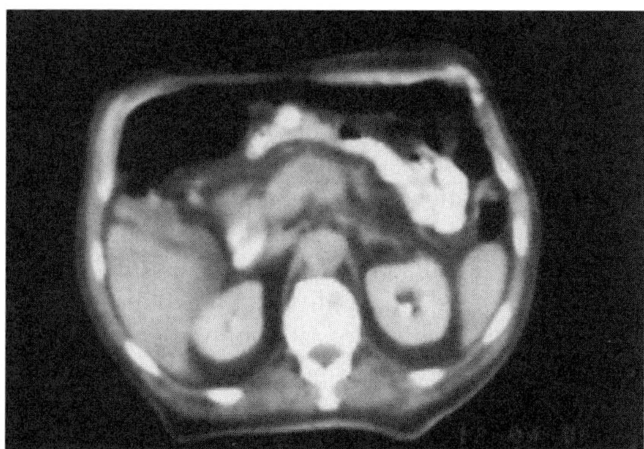

Fig. 106-6. CT scan demonstrating mass in pancreas.

to one third of patients; (7) palpable periumbilical (Sister Mary Joseph) lymph nodes; (8) splenomegaly, which may be caused by splenic vein thrombosis because of invasion of the splenic artery and vein by the tumor; and (9) new detection of a left upper quadrant bruit, again due to invasion of the splenic artery or vein (this occurs in approximately 25% of patients with carcinoma of pancreatic body and tail).

Laboratory Studies and Diagnostic Procedures

Routine studies to obtain in patients suspected of harboring a pancreatic cancer include CBC, chemistry profile, and chest film. A disproportionately elevated serum alkaline phosphatase may provide an initial clue to the presence of metastatic disease. In patients with classic obstructive jaundice the serum transaminases, are less than 400 IU, if elevated. The serum alkaline phosphatase may be 2 to 10 times normal, and markers for viral hepatitis should be negative. Key tests to confirm suspected pancreatic cancer include ultrasound, CT scan, ERCP, CT-guided biopsy of a pancreatic mass lesion, and arteriography if surgery is contemplated (Fig. 106-6).

For a patient with obstructive-type jaundice the ultrasound study is an important initial consideration. The presence of dilated intrahepatic ducts suggests a mechanical, obstructive process, whereas the absence of dilated ducts indicates intrahepatic cholestasis. CT scan, especially contrast-enhanced (dynamic) scan, is abnormal in approximately 90% of the patients with carcinoma of the pancreas, especially if the lesion is more than 2 cm in diameter. When an obvious lesion is detected by CT scanning, a CT-guided percutaneous biopsy may establish the diagnosis. ERCP may also provide important diagnostic information as well as affording an opportunity to decompress the obstructed bile duct. If CT scanning shows evidence of potentially resectable disease, an arteriogram can assist the surgeon and exclude sheathing of the pancreaticoduodenal artery and splenic vein thrombosis, which preclude a curative resection if present.

Differential Diagnosis

For any patient presenting with new onset of persistent abdominal pain, jaundice with obstructive-type liver tests, new onset of diarrhea, and malabsorption, the diagnosis of pancreatic carcinoma must be considered. In patients past age 60 with jaundice and obstructive-type liver tests, the differential diagnosis in 80% of cases lies between pancreatic cancer and choledocholithiasis, with viral hepatitis, posttransfusion hepatitis, drug-induced jaundice, and alcoholic liver disease in the other 20%. Therefore, if the history suggests none of the latter four disorders, an imaging procedure can determine whether the biliary ducts are dilated and, if so, further studies are indicated. Choledocholithiasis is rarely painless. Carcinoma of the ampulla of Vater can mimic many of the features of carcinoma of the pancreas but has a much better prognosis. This condition is diagnosed by ERCP, which reveals a tumor protruding into the duodenal lumen. CT-guided percutaneous biopsy of the pancreas is an effective means of establishing the diagnosis and provides positive results in approximately 85% of patients. For pancreatic duct adenocarcinomas, ERCP has a sensitivity of approximately 90% and a similar specificity. Arteriography has a sensitivity of approximately 65%, with a specificity of 90% for vessel sheathing and splenic vein thrombosis.

Management

For patients with a lesion demonstrable by CT scan that measures less than 3 cm and in whom arteriography shows no evidence of vessel involvement or metastases, exploration with planning for Whipple's procedure is recommended. If the operative findings confirm a lesion that is 3 cm or less in size with no adenopathy and no extension, Whipple's procedure results in a 2-year survival of up to 40%. The resectability rate in patients with pancreatic carcinoma is only about 20% because of the presence of small metastases at presentation not detectable by CT scan. The 5-year survival rate is still only 5% or less in patients with nonresectable lesions. For patients with obstructive jaundice and evidence of metastases or nonresectability, it is reasonable to attempt stenting of the common bile duct to relieve symptoms and sequelae of high-grade extrahepatic obstruction. If a carcinoma of the pancreatic head is causing gastric outlet obstruction, exploration and a gastric bypass procedure as well as cholecystojejunostomy are reasonable. These procedures are palliative and will not affect the patient's long-term survival. Only 10% of patients with pancreatic cancer survive 1 year. No effective chemotherapy or radiation therapy exists for carcinoma of the pancreas. Approximately 15% of patients will respond briefly to chemotherapy. The addition of radiotherapy to chemotherapy results in an increased survival of only 1 to 2 months.

Glucagonoma Syndrome

Tumors of the pancreatic alpha cells result in high levels of circulating glucagon. This syndrome is associated with angular cheilitis, glossitis, and necrolytic migratory erythema—intertriginous, red, scaling, arcuate, erosive lesions in the body folds. The lesions are often confused with candidiasis. Skin biopsy is often diagnostic of glucagonoma syndrome. Diabetes, anemia, and weight loss are commonly seen. Removal of the tumor results in healing of the cutaneous lesions.

REFERENCES

1. Ammann RW et al: Course and outcome of chronic pancreatitis: longitudinal study of mixed medical-surgical series of 245 patients, *Gastroenterology* 86:820, 1984.
2. Balthazar EJ et al: Acute pancreatitis: value of CT in establishing prognosis, *Radiology* 174:331, 1990.
3. Banks PB: Acute pancreatitis: identification of high risk patients and aggressive treatment, *Gastrointest Dis Today* 2:2, 1993.
4. Baron TH et al: Acute necrotizing pancreatitis, *N Engl J Med* 340:1412, 1999.

5. Bassi C et al: Controlled trial of perfloxacin versus imipenem and severe acute pancreatitis, *Gastroenterology* 115:1513, 1998.
6. Campbell DR, Greenberger NJ: Management of pain in chronic pancreatitis. In Burn GR, Bank S, editors: *Disorders of the pancreas,* New York, 1992, McGraw-Hill.
7. Cohn JA et al: Relations between mutations of cystic fibrosis gene in idiopathic pancreatitis, *N Engl J Med* 339:653, 1998.
8. DiMagno EP, Go VLW, Summerskill WH: Relations between pancreatic enzyme outputs and malabsorption in severe pancreatic insufficiency, *N Engl J Med* 288:813, 1973.
9. Eckfeldt JH, Lentherman JH, Levitt MD: High prevalence of hyperamylasemia in patients with acidosis, *Ann Intern Med* 104:362, 1986.
10. Karimgani I, et al: Prognostic factors in sterile pancreatic necrosis, *Gastroenterology* 103:1636, 1992.
11. Lowenfels AB et al: Pancreatitis and the risk of pancreatic cancer, *N Engl J Med* 328:1433, 1993.
12. O'Malley VP et al: Pancreatic pseudocysts: cause, therapy, and results, *Am J Surg* 150:680, 1985.
13. Ranson JHC: Risk factors in acute pancreatitis, *Hosp Pract* 20:69, 1985.
14. Whitcomb DC et al: Hereditary pancreatitis is caused by a mutation in the cationic atrypsinogen gene, *Nature Genet* 13:141, 1991.

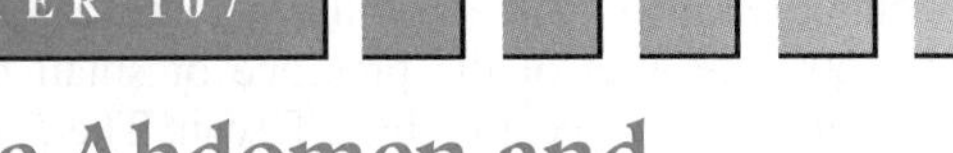

Acute Abdomen and Common Surgical Abdominal Problems

Eric S. Lambright
Noel N. Williams

The patient with acute abdominal pain offers a diagnostic challenge to the physician because of the wide spectrum of disease processes that present with this symptom. Abdominal pain can represent processes as varied as a benign, self-limited viral gastroenteritis to a perforated hollow viscus that is uniformly fatal without intervention. As with all other acute disease processes, accurate diagnostic evaluation and prompt implementation of definitive therapy are essential. The diagnostic evaluation of acute abdominal pain requires a focused and precise history, complete physical examination, and appropriate complementary radiographic and laboratory studies.

PATIENT EVALUATION

History

The diagnosis of processes causing acute abdominal pain can often be made by the history alone. The symptom of pain must be precisely defined. Other symptoms helpful in the evaluation of acute abdominal pain include vomiting, anorexia, changes in bowel habit, and in females the time in the menstrual cycle.

Pain. Knowledge of physiology and anatomy should be applied to mediators of visceral pain and location of intraperitoneal organs. Abdominal pain is mediated by the autonomic nervous system and the intercostal nerves from the fifth to eleventh spinal cord segments. The autonomic response to pain is poorly localized, reported as "deep," and associated with systemic responses such as diaphoresis, nausea, tachycardia, and decrease in blood pressure. Chemical irritation, mechanical stimulation, contraction against resistance, or sudden distention will stimulate afferent visceral nerve fibers and cause pain. In contrast to viscerally mediated symptoms, irritation of the parietal peritoneum causes a more localized sharp pain, and the resultant abdominal tenderness and rigidity can be elicited on physical examination. This duality of abdominal pain is exemplified by the pain of acute appendicitis, which classically begins as a viscerally mediated, periumbilical dull ache that "migrates" to the right lower quadrant as the parietal peritoneum becomes progressively inflamed. Pain from intraperitoneal viscera may occur at sites distant from the abdomen. This referred pain has significant clinical implications, as exemplified by the pain felt at the tip of the scapulae from acute cholecystitis or the shoulder pain experienced with diaphragm irritation.

The symptom of pain must be precisely characterized as to onset, duration, character, and radiation. Pain that begins suddenly in a previously well patient suggests a perforated hollow viscus, a vascular catastrophe, or acute pancreatitis. Pain of severe intensity that began acutely and lasts longer than 6 hours is often associated with a surgical disease process. In contrast, progressive pain may reflect a worsening intraperitoneal inflammatory process (e.g., diverticulitis, cholecystitis, appendicitis) or may indicate intestinal obstruction. The character of the pain is helpful in the diagnostic evaluation: the "burning" of a perforated ulcer, the "tearing" of an aortic dissection, or the "crampy" pain of intestinal obstruction. The radiation of pain can also be helpful. Classically, in biliary system processes, pain will radiate to the scapulae; in ureteral processes, to the groin; inflammation of the pancreas, to the back; and diaphragm irritation, to the shoulder.

Emesis. The patient with an acute abdomen often complains of vomiting. In acute abdominal processes, vomiting is caused by acute gastric irritation, severe visceral afferent nerve irritation, or obstruction of an involuntary muscular tube (e.g., bowel, biliary duct, ureter, appendix). The frequency and the character of the vomitus should be characterized. Frequent, scanty emesis is associated with pancreatitis, in contrast to the intermittent, voluminous emesis seen in a distal small bowel obstruction. The absence of vomiting, however, does not rule out an intraabdominal catastrophe.

Bowels. A change in a patient's bowel habits is often associated with an acute intraabdominal process. Obstipation (an absence of the passage of gas or stool) is often indicative of intestinal obstruction. Melena or occult blood in the stool may reflect underlying ulcer disease or malignancy. Diarrhea is sufficiently common that it provides little specific information in the diagnostic workup. Tenesmus often reflects pelvic inflammatory disease, pelvic appendicitis, or ectopic pregnancy with hemorrhage and may indicate inflammatory bowel disease.

A review of systems must also be included in a thorough history. The physician should obtain a surgical history and determine if the patient ever had the symptoms. Extraabdominal disease processes also may be present with abdominal pain, such as atypical angina, diabetic ketoacidosis, sickle cell crisis, or pyelonephritis. The patient's physiologic reserve is assessed for any underlying cardiac, pulmonary, endocrine, or renal disease that may complicate medical or surgical management.

Physical Examination

Examination of the patient provides further data to support the preliminary diagnosis established by a thorough history. During the abdominal examination the physician should "think anatomically" and apply relationships between intraabdominal structures. For example, pain localizing to the right upper quadrant may be caused by the liver, biliary system including gallbladder, duodenum, hepatic flexure, or right kidney (Box 107-1).

The examination begins with the patient's general appearance. A patient with an acute inflammatory process in the abdomen causing peritonitis remains still and shows obvious pain with any movement. In contrast, the patient with intestinal obstruction or ureteral stone is restless and has intermittent episodes of agony. A patient's vital signs are nonspecific but helpful in defining physiologic stability.

Vital Signs. The patient with acute abdominal disease may be febrile, normothermic, or hypothermic. High fever (greater than 104° F [40° C]) is suggestive of renal, biliary, or pulmonary sepsis. A low-grade fever (100° to 101.5° F [37.7° to 38.5° C]) is consistent with most abdominal inflammatory processes, such as appendicitis, diverticulitis, cholecystitis, or pancreatitis. A normal temperature does not rule out intraabdominal disease and is often seen in the early stages of ulcer perforation. Hypothermia suggests severe sepsis and is a poor prognostic indicator. The pulse rate, blood pressure, and respiratory rate are nonspecific indicators as well. Tachycardia may reflect hemorrhage or hypovolemia related to "third space" fluid accumulation or vomiting. Cardiovascular collapse associated with acute abdominal pain indicates intraabdominal hemorrhage and requires aggressive surgical therapy. Tachypnea may reflect a primary intrathoracic process or may be a physiologic response to a metabolic acidosis secondary to an abdominal process.

Abdominal Examination. A general inspection of the abdomen can identify areas of abnormal distention or surgical scars, with specific attention to areas of potential hernia formation. Findings on abdominal auscultation are nonspecific. Any inflammatory process within the abdomen may cause a paralytic ileus, and examination reveals a "quiet" abdomen. Hyperactive bowel sounds can be found in intestinal obstruction but are also heard in viral gastroenteritis. It is dangerous to dismiss the presence of an acute abdominal process because "the patient had normal bowel sounds."

Palpation and percussion of the patient with abdominal pain require gentleness and should proceed from areas of least to most pain. Percussion may demonstrate abnormal areas of dullness consistent with fluid or areas of increased tympany, which reflects an air-filled viscus or, when demonstrated over the liver, often signifies pneumoperitoneum. Gentle percussion also may demonstrate areas of "rebound" tenderness and more accurately localize an area of peritoneal inflammation. Palpation of the abdomen can localize tenderness, identify any unique masses within the abdomen, or determine the presence of swelling from a hernia and the extent of muscle rigidity. Deep palpation over the abdomen with sudden release can produce "rebound" tenderness in almost all patients, and gentle palpation or percussion of the abdomen can elicit more useful diagnostic information.

In addition to examination of the main abdominal cavity, digital rectal examination is important and informative. Rectal masses such as tumors, stool, or strictures can be identified. The pelvic peritoneum can be examined for areas of local tenderness or masses. Tenderness laterally to the right is consistent with acute appendicitis and intussusception, whereas tenderness laterally to the left may reflect diverticulitis and possible abscess. In females a bimanual examination can identify an adnexal mass that may reflect an abscess, ovarian mass, or ectopic pregnancy. The stool is examined for gross blood or melena and tested for occult blood.

Box 107-1. Differential Diagnosis of Abdominal Pain by Anatomic Location

Right Upper
- Hepatitis
- Cholecystitis
- Choledocholithiasis
- Peptic ulcer
- Appendicitis
- Pancreatitis
- Hepatic abscess
- Hepatomegaly
- Hepatic metastasis
- Subphrenic abscess
- Choledochocyst
- Pneumonia
- Pulmonary infarct

Right Lower
- Appendicitis
- Crohn's disease
- Ulcerative colitis
- Ectopic pregnancy
- Pelvic inflammatory disease
- Gastroenteritis
- Ruptured peptic ulcer
- Endometriosis
- Ovarian cyst
- Diverticulitis
- Cholecystitis
- Renal calculi

Left Upper
- Splenomegaly
- Pancreatitis
- Splenic infarct
- Gastritis
- Pneumonia
- Myocardial infarct
- Splenic artery aneurysm
- Empyema
- Pulmonary infarct

Left Lower
- Diverticulitis
- Colon cancer
- Intestinal obstruction
- Endometriosis
- Ovarian cyst
- Ectopic pregnancy
- Pelvic inflammatory disease
- Ulcerative colitis
- Renal calculi

Epigastrium
- Peptic ulcer
- Pancreatitis
- Cholecystitis
- Reflux esophagitis
- Myocardial ischemia

Diffuse
- Appendicitis
- Spontaneous bacterial peritonitis
- Abdominal aortic aneurysm
- Intestinal obstruction
- Intestinal ischemia
- Gastroenteritis
- Colitis
- Inflammatory bowel disease
- Pancreatitis
- Sickle cell crisis
- Toxic/metabolic etiology

LABORATORY STUDIES AND DIAGNOSTIC PROCEDURES

A thorough history and physical examination can provide an accurate diagnosis in two thirds of patients with acute abdominal pain. Laboratory and radiographic evaluation can supplement the clinical examination and assist in preoperative preparation. Tests should only be performed, however, if the results would alter patient management.

Blood should be drawn for laboratory analysis and cross-matching performed in most patients with acute abdominal pain. A complete blood cell count (CBC) with differential is useful but never diagnostic. A rising or significant leukocytosis supports the diagnosis of an acute infectious or inflammatory process. Anemia may reflect acute or chronic blood loss and often requires correction before surgical intervention. An electrolyte panel is important, especially in the patient who requires hydration or who has had significant fluid shifts. Arterial blood gases should be obtained in critically ill patients or those with significant underlying cardiopulmonary disease. A metabolic acidosis often reflects a serious intraabdominal process. Liver function tests and pancreatic enzymes should be obtained when hepatobiliary disease is suspected. Prothrombin time (PT) and partial thromboplastin time (PTT) are necessary when surgery is planned. Urinalysis may reveal hematuria or pyuria consistent with a urologic process, and specific gravity measurement reflects hydration status. Stool studies should be performed in patients with a suspected infectious process (e.g., *Clostridium difficile* colitis) but are rarely helpful in the acute setting.

Radiographic Evaluation

An upright chest film is essential in evaluating the patient with acute abdominal pain. It may reveal thoracic pathology that has presented with intraabdominal symptoms or free intraperitoneal air under the diaphragm. A film is also vital to the preoperative assessment. Plain radiographs of the abdomen (flat plate and upright views) are useful in the patient with suspected intestinal obstruction but are often not helpful and should be used selectively. An abdominal series may reveal an abnormal bowel gas pattern, free air, pneumatosis (air in the bowel wall), or pneumobilia (air in the biliary system); suggest an intraabdominal mass lesion; or define radiopaque densities such as renal or biliary calculi.

In patients with acute abdominal pain a computed tomography (CT) scan of the abdomen is most useful in evaluating the organs of the retroperitoneum or assessing localized infections. CT is helpful in the management of patients with pancreatitis and diverticulitis and may be useful in the evaluation of appendicitis when the diagnosis is unclear. An abdominal CT scan should be used selectively in patients with acute abdominal pain and may provide confusing information if an adequate history and physical examination were not performed.

Ultrasonography is useful in evaluating the hepatobiliary tree and gallbladder, assessing intraabdominal masses, and studying the adnexal structures. Ultrasound can identify gallstones, pericholecystic fluid, and common bile duct dilation. Ultrasound also should be used selectively.

Angiography is indicated in the patient with acute abdominal pain if intestinal ischemia is suspected. Mesenteric infarction may be revealed by visceral arteriography. Angiography has no role in the patient with suspected ruptured abdominal aortic aneurysm except at centers where endovascular aortic tube grafts are a possible therapeutic option.

Gastrointestinal contrast studies should not be used as initial tests in the evaluation of acute abdominal pain. A water-soluble contrast study may be useful in the patient with suspected ulcer perforation without free air on plain films. A limited barium enema can identify the lesion causing large bowel obstruction. A radionuclide excretion study using technetium-labeled derivatives of iminodiacetic acid (HIDA) to image the biliary ductal system and gallbladder may be used to complement ultrasound in the evaluation of acute cholecystitis. Gallium scans are useful to identify abscesses. These studies have little utility, however, in the initial evaluation of acute abdominal pain.

SPECIFIC DISEASE PROCESSES

Peptic Ulcer Disease

Free perforation of a peptic ulcer is always fatal if untreated, emphasizing the need for early diagnosis and treatment. Perforation and the resultant spillage of acidic secretions cause sudden epigastric burning pain. Early symptoms are marked by generalized pain that often radiates to the shoulders, with associated nausea. Initially the patient is diaphoretic and tachycardic and appears unwell. After the initial perforation the patient may show clinical improvement over several hours; the pain may subside, vomiting may cease, and general appearance may improve. However, the physical examination confirms abdominal tenderness with abdominal wall rigidity but without significant distention, decreased liver dullness, and severe pain with any movement. Subsequently, within 12 to 24 hours the patient shows signs of severe peritonitis with abdominal distention and hypotension and tachycardia from hypovolemic shock. At this point the pathologic process is probably irreversible, and death is imminent.

The diagnosis of ulcer perforation is relatively easy based on a thorough history and physical examination. A history of chronic indigestion or known ulcer disease may be obtained. A sudden onset of burning epigastric pain with evidence of peritonitis on physical examination is most consistent with ulcer perforation. An upright plain radiograph of the chest may often be diagnostic of pneumoperitoneum (Fig. 107-1); however, free air is not seen on plain radiographs in approximately 30% of patients with ulcer perforation.[3] An abdominal CT scan may be helpful when plain radiographs are nondiagnostic but the history and physical examination are consistent with the diagnosis. Treatment requires restoration of intravascular volume, antibiotics, nasogastric decompression, and surgical exploration with definitive treatment of the perforation.

Hepatobiliary Tract

Acute Cholecystitis. Inflammation of the gallbladder is a common cause of acute abdominal pain. Acute cholecystitis is linked to the presence of gallstones and is a result of cystic duct occlusion by a stone impacted in Hartmann's pouch. Classically, this disease process affects middle-age women who are overweight. Typically, pain in the right upper quadrant is associated with nausea and emesis, often with a history of intermittent, vague, postprandial abdominal discomfort. Physical examination reveals fever (usually low grade) and tenderness in the right upper quadrant, scleral

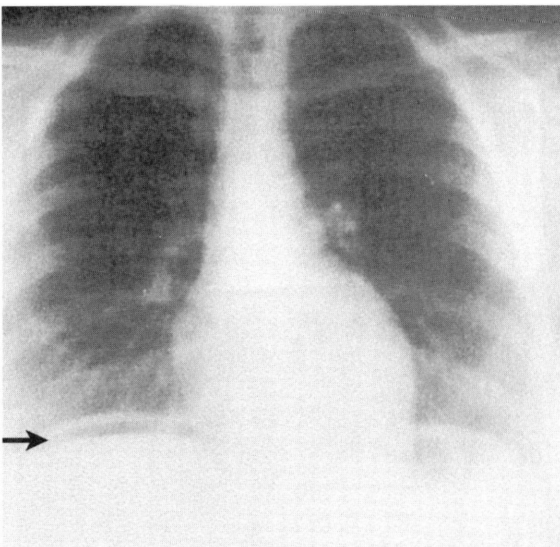

Fig. 107-1. Upright chest radiograph reveals free intraperitoneal air under right hemidiaphragm in patient with perforated duodenal ulcer.

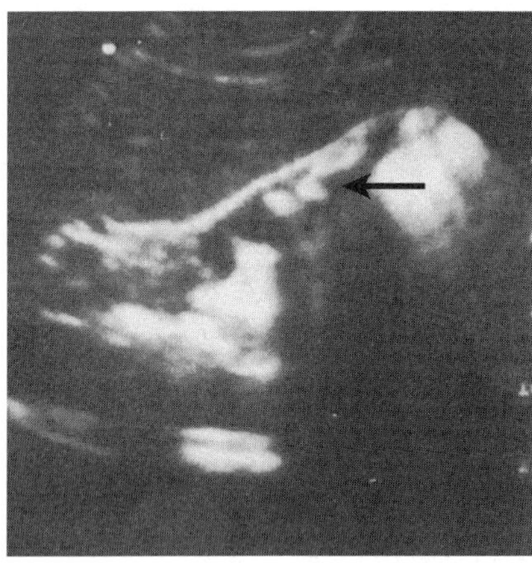

Fig. 107-2. Right upper quadrant ultrasound reveals gallstones in patient with symptoms of biliary colic.

icterus may be present, and a palpable inflammatory mass is occasionally appreciated. Leukocytosis and hyperbilirubinemia are often present, although a greatly elevated bilirubin level is more suggestive of choledocholithiasis. Ultrasonography can confirm the diagnosis and determine the presence of gallstones, evaluate for thickening of the gallbladder wall or pericholecystic fluid, and measure the size of the common bile duct (Fig. 107-2). If the diagnosis is still unclear, a nuclear medicine study with cholescintigraphy (HIDA scan) can confirm acute cholecystitis if gallbladder filling is absent. Therapy for uncomplicated acute cholecystitis is hydration, bowel rest, antibiotics, analgesia, and after stabilization, cholecystectomy.

Cholangitis. Cholangitis is an imminently life-threatening disease process characterized by the classic symptoms of fever, jaundice, and right upper quadrant abdominal pain (Charcot's triad). Cholangitis results from obstruction of the biliary system from choledocholithiasis or from a bile duct stricture secondary to malignancy or previous surgery. This results in a buildup of purulence within the biliary ductal system and ascending infection of the liver. The patient with cholangitis is acutely ill, jaundiced, pyrexic, and hypotensive and has significant right upper abdominal tenderness, often with a history of gallstones or previous biliary surgery. Laboratory evaluation reveals leukocytosis, hyperbilirubinemia, and electrolyte abnormalities consistent with hypovolemia. Therapy requires aggressive resuscitation, antibiotics, and surgical decompression of the biliary system. Decompression can be achieved by endoscopic methods to retrieve obstructing gallstones. A sphincteroplasty can also be performed endoscopically to improve drainage through the sphincter of Oddi. Decompression may be performed by percutaneously draining a dilated biliary system retrograde through the liver under ultrasound guidance. Open surgical drainage is required if these interventions are not successful.

Acute Pancreatitis. An extremely painful and potentially life-threatening disease process, acute pancreatitis is diagnosed by the history and physical examination. A history of untreated cholelithiasis or a recent alcohol binge is often elicited. The clinical presentation of pancreatitis is variable and may be confused with other upper abdominal processes, such as peptic ulcer disease, acute biliary disease, or intestinal obstruction. Pain in the upper abdomen in the midline with radiation to the back associated with nausea and vomiting is typical of acute pancreatitis. Physical examination reveals tachycardia and mild hypotension secondary to fluid shifts. Tenderness is found in the epigastrium, often with evidence of peritoneal irritation. Leukocytosis, elevated serum amylase, and mild liver function test abnormalities are seen on laboratory evaluation. Ultrasound may reveal offending gallstones. CT scan of the retroperitoneum can evaluate the extent of pancreatic inflammation and exclude other etiologies for the abdominal pain. Treatment of uncomplicated pancreatitis is supportive, with volume expansion, analgesia, nasogastric decompression, and ventilatory support, if needed.

Small Intestine

Acute Mechanical Small Bowel Obstruction. A relatively common cause of intestinal pain and a life-threatening process, small bowel obstruction has widely variable symptoms based on the site and underlying cause. Management requires prompt diagnosis and treatment to prevent intestinal strangulation and its associated high mortality. The most common causes are adhesions, hernia, and malignancy.

The patient with small bowel obstruction presents with often severe pain that is referred to the umbilical or epigastric areas. The pain is often spasmodic, which reflects bowel peristalsis attempting to alleviate the obstruction. Vomiting is almost always present; the frequency of emesis corresponds to the anatomic location of the obstruction. Patients with proximal obstruction have frequent, scant bilious vomiting, whereas those with distal obstruction tend to have infrequent, feculent emesis. The patient's initial vital signs are often normal. Tachycardia suggests dehydration and relative hypovolemia but also may reflect bowel ischemia. The temperature and blood pressure are usually normal. Physical examination shows evidence of dehydration with dry mucous

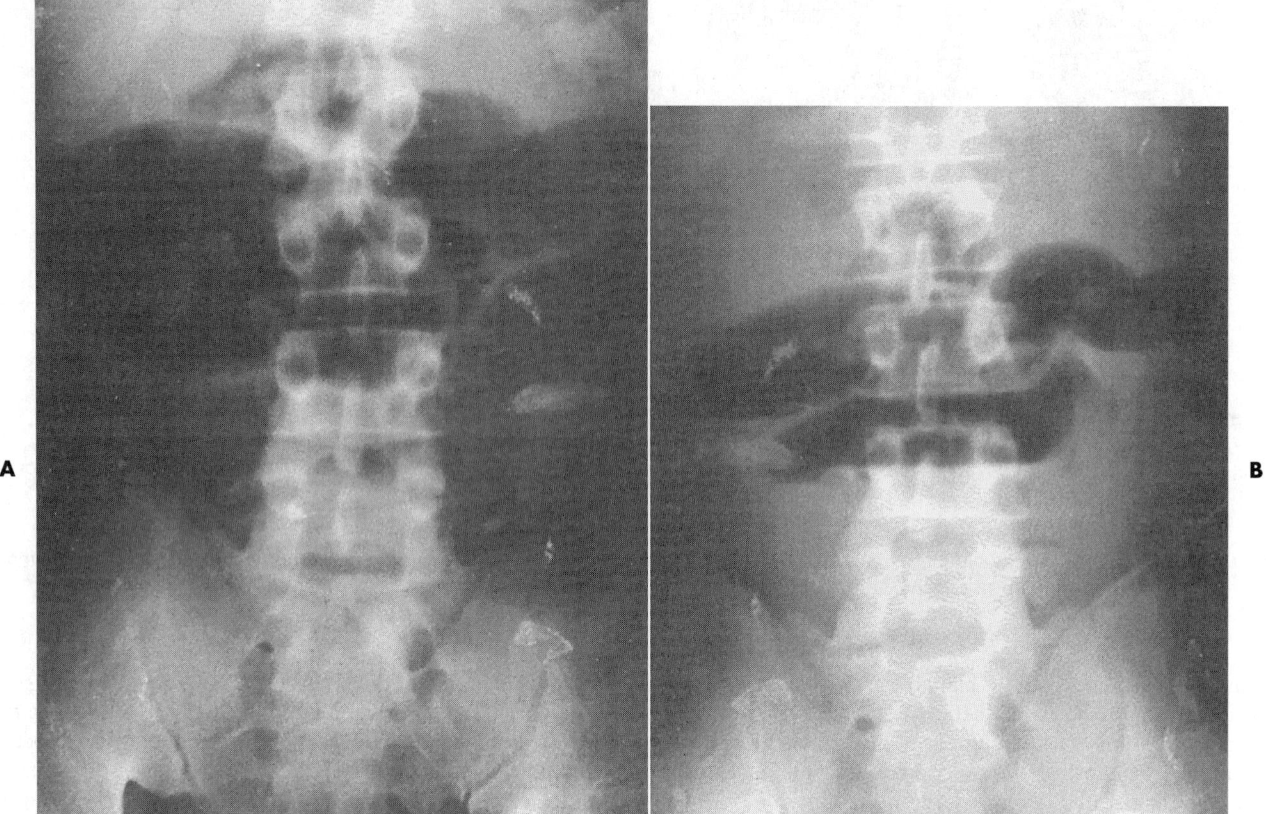

Fig. 107-3. Upright (**A**) and supine (**B**) abdominal films reveal multiple loops of distended small bowel with air-fluid levels in patient with abdominal pain, nausea, and vomiting. Radiographic findings are diagnostic of small bowel obstruction.

membranes and wasted facies. Examination of the abdomen may reveal scars from previous abdominal surgery and varying degrees of abdominal distention. Distention is minimal or absent in patients with proximal obstruction and is often pronounced in those with distal obstruction. Bowel sounds may still be active in patients with early small bowel obstruction, intussusception, or ischemia. Mild abdominal tenderness is present. Evidence of localized peritonitis is an ominous finding and often reflects ischemic or strangulated bowel. All possible hernial orifices must be thoroughly examined. Laboratory data are often nondiagnostic. Elevated blood urea nitrogen and creatinine levels often reflect the degree of dehydration. Leukocytosis may indicate bowel ischemia in the patient with bowel obstruction. The diagnosis of obstruction is confirmed by supine and upright plain films of the abdomen, which reveal a ladderlike pattern of bowel loops with air-fluid levels (Fig. 107-3).

The initial management of the patient with small bowel obstruction is nasogastric decompression and volume resuscitation. After correction of volume status, laparotomy is often required to alleviate the obstruction.

Meckel's Diverticulum. The most common developmental abnormality of the small bowel is a Meckel's diverticulum, which is present in approximately 2% of the population. The omphalomesenteric duct fails to disappear completely, resulting in several possible anomalies, most often a diverticulum of the distal ileum. Patients may develop complications of ulceration, obstruction, bleeding, and acute inflammation. Symptoms may mimic appendicitis if acute inflammation is present, or the patient may present with obstructive symptoms. The diagnosis is often difficult to make preoperatively; however, a small bowel contrast study may demonstrate the offending diverticulum. Treatment is diverticulectomy when complications occur.

Colon

Acute Appendicitis. Approximately 7% of individuals in Western countries develop appendicitis during their lifetime.[1] Appendicitis should be included in the differential diagnosis of patients with abdominal pain because the physician rarely sees a patient with "classic" signs and symptoms of appendicitis. Prompt diagnosis is essential, since delay often will result in appendiceal rupture with increased morbidity and mortality. The peak age of acute appendicitis is approximately 20 years, although 10% of patients are younger than 10 or older than 50.[1] These two populations are at highest risk of perforation because of atypical presenting symptoms and delay in diagnosis. Acute appendicitis must be included in the differential diagnosis of *all* patients presenting with acute abdominal pain.

The patient with appendicitis frequently has a history of "indigestion" and vague periumbilical discomfort. This is associated with vomiting and anorexia and alterations in bowel habit, with resulting diarrhea or increased flatulence. These early symptoms reflect the visceral response to the inflamed appendix. After these initial symptoms, the patient often describes movement of the pain from the periumbilical area to the right lower quadrant, with increased intensity. Vital signs may be within normal limits but usually reveal low-grade fever, typically 2° or 3° F above normal, and tachycardia. Abdominal examination shows tenderness in the right lower quadrant with evidence of local peritonitis. Tenderness at McBurney's point is not required for the diagnosis of appendicitis. Rectal examination reveals tenderness in the right hemipelvis, and at times an inflammatory mass can be palpated. Laboratory data may reveal a leukocytosis with a left shift, although the white blood cell count is normal in 20% of patients.[2] In the female patient a pelvic ultrasound may be helpful to rule out a gynecologic process. Abdominal CT scan can be helpful when the diagnosis is unclear.

The history and physical examination are often sufficient to diagnose appendicitis. If the physician waits until diffuse peritonitis and abdominal rigidity are present, the diagnosis of appendicitis has been made too late and perforation has probably occurred. Treatment of appendicitis requires intravenous (IV) antibiotics and appendectomy.

Acute Diverticulitis. *Diverticulosis,* the presence of multiple false diverticula of the colon, is a common disease in modernized countries and is found in approximately 50% of individuals over age 50 and almost 75% over 80.[1] Diverticulosis remains asymptomatic in most patients, but about 20% develop the complications of bleeding or inflammation, leading to diverticulitis. Acute diverticulitis, which most often occurs in the sigmoid colon, is similar to appendicitis because both result from obstruction of a colonic diverticulum. The resulting increased intraluminal pressure subsequently causes the diverticulum to perforate. The paracolic tissues may locally contain this perforation, with a focal inflammatory process, or more extensive bacterial spillage may occur, with abscess formation or frank fecal peritonitis. Thus this disease process may have a varied clinical presentation.

An acute attack closely resembles the symptom complex of appendicitis except that the pain is in the left side of the abdomen. The pain often starts as vague discomfort in the midabdomen and then migrates to the left lower quadrant or suprapubic area. Anorexia, changes in bowel habit with either increased defecation or constipation, and dysuria secondary to bladder inflammation are also common symptoms. Physical findings include fever, left lower quadrant tenderness with evidence of local peritonitis, and abdominal distention; often a mass is palpated on abdominal examination and leukocytosis is found on laboratory evaluation. Rarely, there is free perforation of an inflamed diverticulum into the peritoneal cavity. The patient may present with systemic evidence of sepsis, including hemodynamic compromise and mental status deterioration. The abdomen is tender with evidence of diffuse tenderness.

Radiographic studies complement the clinical evaluation of diverticulitis. A plain film of the abdomen may reveal pneumoperitoneum if there is free perforation, or evidence of ileus may be seen. CT scan of the abdomen with oral and IV contrast shows effacement of the pericolic fat and may identify an abscess that could be drained under radiographic guidance. CT scan also helps identify other complications, such as fistulization.

Management of acute diverticulitis requires close observation; approximately 25% of hospitalized patients require surgical therapy. Initial treatment should include hospitalization for bowel rest, hydration, and appropriate IV antibiotics. Urgent surgery is required for patients with general or progressing peritonitis or evidence of systemic sepsis. Most patients improve in 2 to 3 days. If the patient has persistent pain, fever, leukocytosis, or peritonitis after 3 to 4 days of medical therapy, however, surgery is necessary. Diverticulitis recurs in approximately one third of medically treated patients, usually within the first 5 years. Indications for elective resection include recurrent diverticulitis, persistent symptoms, and the inability to rule out malignancy.

Inflammatory Bowel Disease. See Chapter 108.

Obstruction of the Large Intestine. Unlike obstruction of the small bowel, colonic obstruction often presents with more subacute symptoms because of the large reservoir capacity of the colon and the slower peristaltic transit time. Colon cancer causes approximately 75% of colonic obstructions. Diverticular disease and acute volvulus are the other main causes.[4]

The acute symptoms of colonic obstruction include colicky pain, increasing abdominal distention, and obstipation. Obstruction secondary to cancer or diverticular disease is precipitated by firm stool occluding a narrowed colonic lumen and occurs much more frequently in the left and sigmoid colon than the right colon. In contrast, a volvulus is caused by a twisting of the intestine on its mesentery, resulting in a closed-loop obstruction and subsequent vascular compromise of the gut; this usually occurs in the cecum or sigmoid colon. A thorough history often reveals previous symptoms, such as changes in stool caliber, episodes of hematochezia, and gradually increasing constipation that alternates with diarrhea. Vomiting is present if the ileocecal valve is incompetent. Physical examination is most remarkable for abdominal distention. Vital signs are usually within normal limits. A rectal examination may reveal an obstructing mass or demonstrate Hemoccult-positive stool. Laboratory data are usually unrevealing but may demonstrate iron deficiency anemia. An obstruction series shows a dilated colon with a lack of air in the rectum. If the ileocecal valve is incompetent, air is also seen in the small bowel, and this may resemble a partial small bowel obstruction. The plain radiograph of patients with volvulus reveals an extremely distended colonic coil with proximal dilated loops. If the diameter of the cecum is greater than 12 to 14 cm on radiographs, cecal ischemia and perforation are imminent. Barium enema may be helpful in diagnosing some obstructions and may be therapeutic in patients with sigmoid volvulus, but an enema should be reserved for select patients and only after discussion with a surgeon. Patients with suspected sigmoid volvulus may be treated with rigid sigmoidoscopy to untwist the loop of colon. Colonic obstruction requires urgent surgical intervention. Treatment includes IV hydration, appropriate preoperative antibiotics, gastric decompression, and urgent laparotomy.

Vascular Lesions

Aneurysmal disease of the abdominal aorta and intestinal ischemia can present as acute abdominal catastrophes.

Abdominal Aortic Aneurysm. Abdominal pain associated with an aortic aneurysm is a symptom of present or impending rupture. The pain is throbbing in character and localizes to the back or loins. Cardiovascular collapse in the patient with a known aneurysm indicates rupture. Abdominal examination often reveals a pulsatile mass. The diagnosis of a leaking abdominal aortic aneurysm must be considered in the patient with acute abdominal and back pain. If the diagnosis is suspected, prompt surgical evaluation must be obtained before further workup. A history and physical examination consistent with a rupturing aneurysm are sufficient to implement surgical exploration.

Intestinal Ischemia. Intestinal ischemia results in severe abdominal pain. Occlusive lesions secondary to mesenteric arterial thrombosis or embolism and low-flow states with resultant hypoperfusion of the gut can cause intestinal ischemia. The patient with occlusive vascular disease of the abdomen complains of cramping periumbilical pain and often has a history of postprandial abdominal angina or other clinical manifestations of atherosclerotic disease. A history of atrial dysrhythmias should increase suspicion of an embolic event. Nausea and diarrhea are often present. Abdominal examination may be unrevealing, but rectal examination is positive for gross or occult blood. Classically, pain out of proportion to physical findings is intestinal ischemia until proved otherwise. Radiographic evaluation may demonstrate ileus but is often nonspecific. The findings of fever, shock, and abdominal distention occur late in the disease process and often indicate a fatal outcome. Therefore close monitoring of all patients presenting with abdominal pain out of proportion to physical signs is essential. Premature discharge home may be followed by extensive bowel infarction.

Intestinal ischemia may involve the large or small bowel and can occur without any vascular occlusive lesion. Arteriography is indicated to evaluate the vascular anatomy and to rule out a correctable occlusive lesion. Treatment includes optimization of hemodynamic parameters with volume resuscitation and inotropic support as appropriate. Laparotomy with embolectomy or mesenteric revascularization is often required for definitive therapy. Bowel resection may be required if nonviable intestine is present. Surgery, however, is rarely beneficial. The prognosis for patients with nonocclusive ischemia is poor, with a mortality rate greater than 50%.

Urogenital Disease

Patients with processes involving the urinary or genital system may present with abdominal pain, although characteristically the pain is located in the groin or flank. Renal colic results from obstruction of a ureter secondary to a kidney stone, blood clot, or pus. The prominent symptom is sudden severe pain in the flank, often radiating to the groin, and is associated with emesis and dysuria. Abdominal examination demonstrates no tenderness. A urinalysis may reveal hematuria and pyuria. A plain film may demonstrate the offending calculus, but an IV pyelogram may be necessary to provide a definitive diagnosis.

Acute infection of the kidney may also present with abdominal pain, but pain is typically described in the flank. High fever (greater than 103° F [39.4° C]) and shaking chills with dysuria are typical symptoms. Examination may reveal abdominal tenderness, although costovertebral angle tenderness is more common. Laboratory evaluation reveals leukocytosis and pyuria. Treatment is with hydration and IV antibiotics.

In the female patient, gynecologic causes for acute abdominal pain must also be included in the differential diagnosis. Ectopic pregnancy, pelvic inflammatory disease, ovarian torsion, and ovarian cystic disease can mimic gastrointestinal disease. A thorough history, physical examination, and appropriate laboratory evaluation, including a pregnancy test, are required for accurate diagnosis. A transvaginal ultrasound of the pelvic organs supplements the history and examination. These gynecologic disease processes are discussed under Women's Health (see especially Chapters 44 and 46).

MEDICAL DIAGNOSES THAT SIMULATE ACUTE SURGICAL PROCESS

Several medical causes of the acute abdomen should be included in the differential diagnosis of the patient with acute abdominal pain. A thorough history, with attention to past medical problems, and physical examination can usually identify these conditions. Abdominal pain must not be attributed to a medical etiology, however, until acute surgical disease processes are ruled out conclusively, which may require laparotomy (Box 107-2).

Box 107-2. Nonsurgical Causes of Acute Abdominal Pain

Infectious and Inflammatory

Tabes dorsalis
Henoch-Schönlein purpura
Lupus
Acute rheumatic fever
"Food poisoning"
Polyarteritis nodosa

Toxic

Lead
Narcotic withdrawal
Venoms (snake, spider)

Hemotologic

Sickle cell crisis
Acute leukemia

Metabolic

Uremia
Porphyria
Diabetic ketoacidosis
Addisonian crisis

Cardiopulmonary

Pericarditis
Myocardial infarct
Pneumonia
Empyema

Neurogenic

Vertebral osteomyelitis
Herpes zoster
Spinal cord tumor

REFERENCES

1. Boey JH: Acute abdomen. In *Current surgical diagnosis and treatment,* Norwalk, Conn, 1994, Lange.
2. Liu CD, McFadden DW: Acute abdomen and appendix. In *Surgery: scientific principles and practice,* Philadelphia, 1997, Lippincott-Raven.
3. Morris JA, Sawyers JL: The acute abdomen. In *Sabiston's Essentials of surgery,* Philadelphia, 1987, Saunders.
4. Silen W: *Cope's Early diagnosis of the acute abdomen,* New York, 1991, Oxford University Press.

CHAPTER 108

Inflammatory Bowel Disease

Ciarán P. Kelly
Pierre F. Michetti

Inflammatory bowel disease (IBD) is characterized by idiopathic, chronic, or recurrent intestinal inflammation. Based on clinical, endoscopic, and histologic patterns, IBD is divided into two categories: ulcerative colitis and Crohn's disease.[1] In ulcerative colitis, inflammation is confined to the mucosa and submucosa of the large intestine. In Crohn's disease, inflammation can affect any part of the intestinal tract and all layers of the intestinal wall, from mucosa to serosa.[2-5]

IBD is more prevalent in North America and Northern Europe, where Caucasians have the highest incidence, estimated at 35 to 100 cases per 100,000 population for ulcerative colitis and 10 to 50 for Crohn's disease.[1] IBD is reportedly fourfold higher among the Ashkenazi Jewish population of Europe and America. The prevalence of IBD among family members of IBD patients is 50 times higher than in the general population. Family members tend to be affected by the same form of IBD (ulcerative colitis or Crohn's disease), although not always. A study of monozygotic twins showed 6% concordance for ulcerative colitis and 44% concordance for Crohn's disease.[1] These observations suggest a genetic predisposition to IBD, particularly Crohn's disease, and a requirement for unidentified environmental agents (e.g., bacterial, dietary) for disease expression.

Despite numerous studies, no specific dietary factor has been linked reproducibly with Crohn's disease or ulcerative colitis.[8] The search for an infectious cause has also been unrewarding. Both mycobacterial and measles infection have been studied, but a firm causative link has not been established for either agent. In genetically modified mice, disruption of various immune response genes (e.g., interleukins 2 and 10) leads to intestinal inflammation that is similar to human IBD, and animals raised in a germ-free environment do not develop intestinal disease.[1a] Thus IBD may develop in genetically susceptible individuals because of a heightened or inappropriate immune response to commensal or pathogenic intestinal flora.[9]

The peak age of onset of IBD is in early adult life (15 to 25 years). Symptoms may develop in childhood or in later life, however, and in some series a second peak of onset in men aged 55 to 65 years is reported. Cigarette smoking has a protective effect in ulcerative colitis but not in Crohn's disease. Prior appendectomy is also associated with a significant reduction in the risk of developing ulcerative colitis.

ULCERATIVE COLITIS

Clinical Presentation

The two main symptoms of ulcerative colitis are diarrhea and the passage of blood in the stool. Other common symptoms include cramping lower abdominal pain, abdominal tenderness, fever, and rectal symptoms. Patients with severe disease may develop weight loss and symptomatic anemia. Ulcerative colitis usually follows a chronic, intermittent course, with periods of disease activity interspersed with periods of spontaneous remission. However, as many as 18% of patients have only one episode of colitis, whereas 7% show chronic unremitting disease activity. For patients under age 50 the median time to relapse after a first episode is 2 years, with lower relapse rates in older patients.

Key elements in the evaluation of patients with ulcerative colitis are a determination of disease severity and disease extent, since these two factors will influence clinical presentation, management, and prognosis. Disease severity is determined mainly by clinical evaluation of the frequency of diarrhea, the amount of blood visible in the stool, abdominal tenderness or distention, and the presence or absence of systemic manifestations of disease (fever, tachycardia, postural hypotension, fatigue, anemia, hypoalbuminemia, electrolyte disorders, particularly hypokalemia) (Table 108-1).

Ulcerative colitis always involves the lower rectum; colonic mucosal inflammation extends proximally in a contiguous manner to a varying extent (Fig. 108-1). The extent of disease involvement is often described by the terms *ulcerative proctitis* (rectum only), *distal* or *left-sided colitis* (disease distal to the splenic flexure), and extensive colitis or *pancolitis* (disease proximal to the splenic flexure). In ulcerative proctitis, rectal symptoms predominate (fecal urgency, tenesmus, rectal pain, passage of bright-red blood

Table 108-1. Severity of Ulcerative Colitis Based on Disease Manifestations

Manifestation	Mild	Moderate	Severe
Bowel frequency (daily)	<4	4-9	>9*
Blood in stool	+/–	+	++
Fever	–	+	+
Tachycardia	–	+/–	+†
Abdominal tenderness	–	+/–	+
Anemia	–	+/–	+‡
Erythrocyte sedimentation rate	Normal	Elevated	Elevated
Electrolyte disturbances	–	+/–	+
Hypoalbuminemia	–	+/–§	+

*Passage of diarrhea may decrease in toxic megacolon.
†Heart rate may drop in fulminant colitis.
‡May require blood transfusion.
§May develop in prolonged, moderately active, extensive colitis.

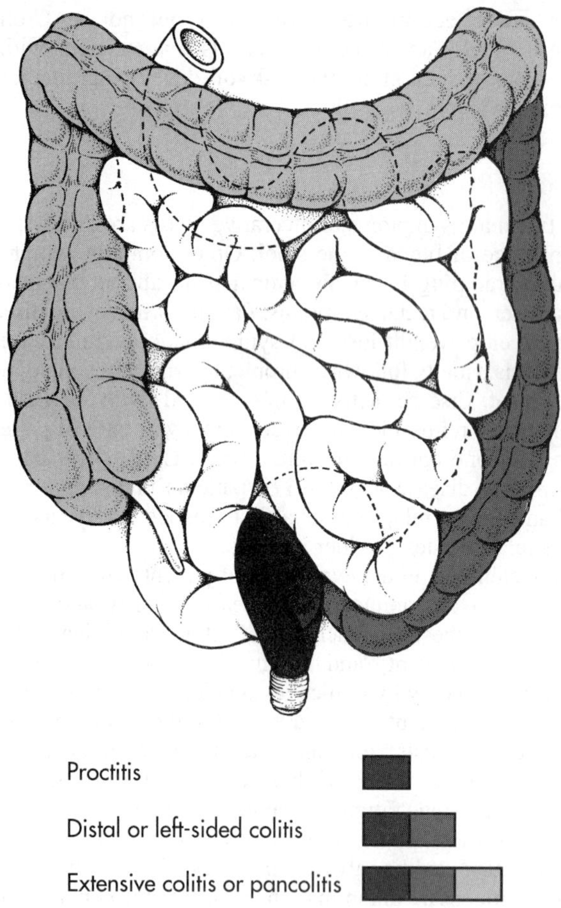

Fig. 108-1. Extent of disease involvement in ulcerative colitis.

coating the stool). With more extensive disease, diarrhea tends to increase, and blood becomes mixed into the stool. Only one quarter of patients with ulcerative colitis have extensive disease; this subgroup is at greater risk for severe disease requiring colectomy. The extent of disease involvement in individual patients usually remains constant, but about 10% of those who present initially with proctitis or distal colitis later develop more extensive disease. Neither disease severity nor disease extent influence the risk of relapse.

Diagnosis

Colonoscopy with biopsy is the best diagnostic study for ulcerative colitis. At colonoscopy the severity of colonic inflammation and ulceration and the proximal extent of disease involvement can be evaluated by endoscopic appearance and by histologic examination of mucosal biopsies. In active disease, histologic examination reveals an acute colitis with neutrophil infiltration of the colonic glands, crypt abscess formation, and surface erosions. Architectural changes in the colonic glands reflect a chronic colitis and may be helpful in differentiating between an acute, self-limited infectious colitis and chronic IBD. Radiographic studies are useful in the diagnosis and management of Crohn's disease but play a lesser role in ulcerative colitis.

The most common diagnostic difficulty in ulcerative colitis is excluding infectious colitis (Box 108-1). This is particularly relevant in patients who present after a short duration of symptoms (less than 4 to 6 weeks) and in patients with risk factors for enteric infectious disease, such as recent travel to endemic areas, contact with cases, antibiotic use, receptive anal intercourse, and immunosuppression, including human immunodeficiency virus (HIV) infection. An infectious agent should be excluded by testing stool samples for relevant enteric pathogens, including *Shigella, Yersinia, Campylobacter, Clostridium difficile,* and *Amoeba.* In patients with a previous diagnosis of ulcerative colitis, enteric infection should also be considered as a possible cause of relapsing colitis.

Radiation colitis is suggested by the patient's history. Ischemic colitis should be considered in elderly patients and in those with risk factors for atherosclerotic, thromboembolic, or inflammatory vascular disease.

Clinical, endoscopic, radiographic, and histologic criteria are used to differentiate between ulcerative colitis and Crohn's disease of the colon (Box 108-2). In approximately 10% of patients it is not possible to differentiate with certainty between Crohn's disease and ulcerative colitis, and the term *indeterminate colitis* is used. Differentiation between ulcerative colitis and Crohn's disease becomes most important if surgery is being considered, since the surgical treatment of ulcerative colitis differs substantially from that of colonic Crohn's disease.

Box 108-1. Differential Diagnosis of Proctocolitis

Ulcerative colitis
Infectious colitis
Crohn's disease of the colon
Ischemic colitis
Radiation proctitis or colitis

Box 108-2. Findings Indicative of Colonic Crohn's Disease Used to Differentiate from Ulcerative Colitis

Small bowel involvement
Rectal sparing
Less bleeding
Perianal disease
Focal colonic involvement
Fistulas
Granulomas

Treatment

Medical Therapy. For many years, sulfasalazine (Azulfidine) was the mainstay of therapy for mild or moderately severe ulcerative colitis. It is inexpensive and effective in controlling active disease. Its efficacy is dose dependent, however, and side effects such as nausea and headache are

Table 108-2. Sulfasalazine and 5-Aminosalicylic Acid (5-ASA) Preparations*

Agent	Composition	Sites of activity	Treatment dose†	Maintenance dose
Sulfasalazine‡	Sulfapyrine and 5-ASA	Colon	2-6 gm/day	2-4 gm/day
Pentasa (mesalamine)	5-ASA (sustained release)	Pylorus to rectum	1.5-4.8 gm/day	1.5-4 gm/day
Asacol (mesalamine)	5-ASA (pH-dependent release)	Distal small intestine and colon	1.6-4.8 gm/day	1.6-4 gm/day
Dipentum (olsalazine)	5-ASA dimer	Colon	1.5-3 gm/day	0.75-3 gm/day
Rowasa (mesalamine)	5-ASA (enema or suppository§)	Rectum and distal colon	One or two daily	One daily

*Only those currently approved for use in the United States are listed.
†Administered in two to four divided doses.
‡1 gm of sulfasalazine contains approximately 500 mg of 5-ASA.
§Each enema contains 4 gm of 5-ASA and each suppository 500 mg of 5-ASA.

frequent at higher doses. These effects may be reduced by taking the medication with food, using gradual dose escalations, or using an enteric-coated preparation. Other side effects include allergic reactions, hemolysis, folate deficiency, male infertility, and occasionally, life-threatening agranulocytosis or other severe drug reactions. Thus patients are monitored by periodic blood counts, including reticulocyte counts, and folic acid supplements are given to prevent folate deficiency.

Sulfasalazine comprises 5-aminosalicylic acid (5-ASA) linked by an azo bond to sulfapyridine. The sulfapyridine prevents 5-ASA absorption and degradation in the upper intestinal tract. The azo bond is cleaved by the action of colonic bacteria releasing the active 5-ASA moiety in the colon, where it is poorly absorbed. Most of the sulfasalazine's toxicity is attributed to the sulfapyridine moiety, which is well absorbed from the colon. A variety of 5-ASA preparations use different release systems to deliver 5-ASA to the inflamed intestinal mucosa while avoiding sulfa-related side effects (Table 108-2). These 5-ASA preparations are more expensive than sulfasalazine but have fewer side effects and avoid the need for routine hematologic monitoring and folate supplementation. As with sulfasalazine, they are effective in controlling active disease and in maintaining remission. Their efficacy is dose dependent, and high doses are usually well tolerated. Many patients with newly diagnosed ulcerative colitis are treated using a 5-ASA preparation. Patients who previously tolerated sulfasalazine well can continue to take it.

Ulcerative proctitis and left-sided colitis can be treated effectively using enemas containing either 5-ASA or hydrocortisone. Enemas are usually administered once or twice daily for 7 to 14 days to control active disease. An hydrocortisone foam enema is available for patients who have difficulty retaining the liquid enema preparation. Some patients prefer 5-ASA suppositories.

Systemic corticosteroid therapy is used for patients with severe ulcerative colitis and extensive disease involvement and for patients with moderately severe disease who fail to respond to high-dose 5-ASA treatment. Depending on the severity of disease and the patient's response to previous steroid therapy, daily doses of 15 to 60 mg of prednisone are used. Therapy is tapered over 2 to 8 weeks as disease activity decreases. Since corticosteroid side effects are common and can be severe, the lowest effective dose should be used. Relapse may occur as the dose of prednisone is decreased, however, necessitating further dose escalation.

Severe Disease. Severe ulcerative colitis, particularly if extensive, may be incapacitating and may require hospital admission for intravenous (IV) fluid and electrolyte repletion and high-dose IV corticosteroid therapy (hydrocortisone, 300 mg/day, or methylprednisone, 48 to 60 mg/day). Since diarrhea is exacerbated by oral intake, patients should fast until the colitis is under control. A nasogastric tube may be required for decompression if an ileus exists. Blood transfusion may also be needed for marked anemia or acute severe bleeding. If fasting is prolonged for more than 4 to 5 days, if the patient is already malnourished from the disease, or if urgent colectomy may be required, parenteral nutrition should be administered. Abdominal symptoms and signs should be monitored frequently for evidence of colonic distention or peritoneal inflammation indicating toxic megacolon or risk of perforation. If patients have not responded after 7 to 10 days of IV corticosteroid treatment, colectomy must be considered. IV cyclosporine has been used in these circumstances and may be effective in averting urgent colectomy in more than 50% of patients. Many subsequently relapse, however, and potential adverse effects of cyclosporine are a concern.

Refractory Disease. Refractory disease occurs with incomplete response to systemic corticosteroid therapy or with relapse of symptoms as the steroid dose is reduced despite concurrent treatment with high-dose sulfasalazine or 5-ASA. Chronic treatment with corticosteroids should be avoided when possible, since these agents do not alter disease progression or relapse and are frequently associated with substantial drug-induced side effects. Alternatives include colectomy or immunosuppressive agents. Azathioprine or the closely related 6-mercaptopurine (6-MP) is effective in approximately two thirds of patients and allow reduced dosage or complete discontinuation of steroid therapy. Their onset of action is slow (3 to 6 months for maximal effect), and frequent monitoring is needed for neutropenia and other adverse effects. In patients who respond, maintenance treatment with azathioprine or 6-MP is usually given because discontinuation of therapy is often followed by disease relapse.

Surgical Treatment. Fewer than 10% of patients undergo surgical treatment for ulcerative colitis. Surgery is required most often in patients with extensive colitis, for whom the colectomy rate is 20% to 25%. The most common indication for surgery is persistently active disease with an inadequate response to medical therapy or unacceptable medication-induced side effects. Colonic dysplasia or carcinoma is another common indication for elective colectomy. Urgent colectomy is occasionally required for fulminant colitis, toxic megacolon, or persistent severe colonic hemorrhage. Colonic perforation is an absolute indication for surgery in ulcerative colitis and is associated with a reported mortality rate of 40%.

Surgical treatment of ulcerative colitis consists of proctocolectomy. Partial or subtotal colectomy is not recommended because colitis frequently recurs in the remaining colon. The simplest procedure combines proctocolectomy with the formation of a Brooke's end ileostomy. This is associated with the lowest risk for perioperative complications and subsequent stoma dysfunction. Ileoanal anastomosis, with the formation of a pelvic pouch of small intestine, is technically more difficult and often requires more than one procedure. Fecal urgency, frequency, and incontinence are common after ileoanal anastomosis. Severe inflammation of the pouch (pouchitis), intractable diarrhea, or pelvic sepsis may require removal of the pouch and conversion to an end ileostomy. Despite these limitations, most patients undergoing colectomy for ulcerative colitis choose ileoanal anastomosis over a permanent end ileostomy. Surgical outcomes are excellent, with fewer than 5% of patients requiring conversion to an end ileostomy. Patients with Crohn's disease are poor candidates for an ileoanal anastomosis, which is an important consideration when patients with indeterminate colitis are evaluated for surgery.

Maintenance Therapy. Strong evidence supports the use of oral sulfasalazine or 5-ASA as maintenance therapy in ulcerative colitis. In one study, 73% of patients with ulcerative colitis in remission treated by placebo relapsed within 1 year, whereas only 21% of patients treated with sulfasalazine (2 gm/day) had a relapse.[3a] Similar results have been obtained using 5-ASA preparations. The duration of maintenance therapy varies depending on disease severity. A patient with a single episode of mild colitis may discontinue therapy after 1 year, whereas a patient with previous repeated episodes of severe colitis may choose to continue therapy indefinitely. The efficacy of sulfasalazine or 5-ASA in preventing disease relapse is dose dependent.

5-ASA enemas, used daily or every second day, help to maintain remission in patients with proctitis or limited colitis. 6-MP prevents relapse in patients whose active colitis responded to this agent. Corticosteroids have no role in maintenance therapy because they do not prevent disease relapse.

CROHN'S DISEASE

Crohn's disease is manifest by chronic or recurrent transmural inflammation that may involve any part of the digestive tract, from mouth to anus. Its distribution is characteristically focal or segmental rather than uniform and diffuse. The most frequent symptoms are abdominal pain and diarrhea. Intestinal fistula formation and bowel obstruction are common complications. Disease recurrence is highly likely, even after surgical resection. The term *Crohn's disease* has replaced other designations, such as granulomatous enteritis and regional or terminal ileitis, because granulomas are not always present and ileal involvement is common but not universal (Table 108-3). The three main patterns of involvement are isolated small bowel disease, ileocolitis, and isolated Crohn's colitis. In all locations, transmural inflammation results in thickening of the bowel secondary to edema and inflammatory cell infiltration, as well as narrowing of the lumen secondary to fibrosis.

Table 108-3. Sites of Involvement in Crohn's Disease

Site	Prevalence (%)
Mouth	8-9
Esophagus	<1
Stomach or duodenum	0.5-5
Small bowel alone	30-40*
Small and large intestine	40-55*
Large intestine alone	15-25
Perianal	3-36

*The terminal ileum is involved in 80% of patients.

Early lesions consist of hyperemia, edema, and discrete superficial ulceration, or aphthous ulcers. As the disease progresses, these mucosal lesions coalesce into deep transverse and longitudinal serpiginous ulcers accompanied by swelling of the intervening mucosa, providing the characteristic "cobblestone" appearance of the mucosa. Over time the bowel wall thickens and becomes fibrotic and stenotic, setting the stage for chronic, recurrent bowel obstruction. The mesentery participates in the chronic inflammatory process and is greatly thickened and edematous, generating fingerlike projections encasing the bowel called "creeping fat." Microscopically the inflammatory infiltrate is composed of neutrophils, plasma cells, lymphocytes, and macrophages; crypt abscesses are evident. Macrophages aggregate in noncaseating granulomas that may be recognized in all layers of the bowel wall. Microscopic focality is also a characteristic feature of Crohn's disease.

Clinical Presentation

Signs and symptoms of Crohn's disease are secondary to chronic transmural inflammation of the bowel. The onset of symptoms is usually insidious but occasionally is abrupt. In active ileal disease, pain is usually colicky and located in the right lower quadrant or suprapubic region. Because it is often associated with the passage of intestinal contents through the congested and narrowed segments of inflamed bowel, pain precedes evacuation of liquid stools. When cramping pain follows food intake along with nausea and abdominal distention, more proximal disease (gastroduodenitis or jejunitis) or chronic partial obstruction caused by fibrotic cicatrization must be suspected.

Intestinal inflammation is associated with increased fluid secretion and impaired absorption, resulting in diarrhea. Distal colitis and proctitis are associated with fecal urgency, tenesmus, and passage of mucus, pus, and blood. Bacterial overgrowth, fistula formation, impaired bile acid absorption, and generalized malabsorption can contribute to diarrhea in Crohn's disease. Low-grade fever, chills, and nocturnal sweats can result from chronic inflammation. High-grade fever suggests a suppurative complication. In contrast, fibrostenotic disease and remission are marked by a normal temperature. A 10% to 20% loss of body weight often results from anorexia and diarrhea. In the absence of intestinal resection, enterocolonic fistula formation, or bacterial overgrowth, malabsorption rarely plays a major role. In longstanding disease without signs of activity, weight loss should suggest a small bowel or colonic adenocarcinoma.

Visible blood is evident in the stool in about 50% of patients with Crohn's colitis and in less than 25% of those with ileal disease. Bleeding occurs less often in Crohn's disease than in ulcerative colitis (see Box 108-2). Massive bleeding is a rare but dangerous and sometimes recurrent complication of Crohn's disease. Perianal disease is present in 30% of patients. Fissures, fistulas, and abscesses can be a presenting or predominant feature of Crohn's disease. These lesions develop after occlusion of circumanal glands, creating abscesses that dissect into the intersphincteric plane.

Intestinal Complications. The inflammatory process of Crohn's disease tends to evolve into two distinct patterns, fibrostenotic obstructing or penetrating fistulous, with different implications for therapy and prognosis. Chronic partial intestinal obstruction with episodes of acute complete obstruction is common in Crohn's disease (Figure 108-2). In the early stages, obstruction results from edema and spasm. Diarrhea and inflammatory signs are present, and medical therapy is usually effective. Later, obstructive symptoms result from fibrosis, and constipation typically replaces diarrhea. Surgery is often required at this stage because the obstruction will not be reversed by antiinflammatory agents.

Transmural inflammation results in the formation of sinus tracts that may either end blindly, creating abscesses, or break into adjacent organs, creating fistulas. Mesenteric abscesses are most common, but retroperitoneal and psoas abscesses also occur, usually on the right side. Symptoms include abdominal pain, spiking fevers, and pain referred to the hip, thigh, or knee. A palpable tender mass and psoas sign may be evident on examination.

Enteroenteric fistulas, usually ileoileal, ileocecal, or ileosigmoid, are the most common fistulas. They are often relatively asymptomatic and found during barium studies or surgery. In contrast, the rare cologastric or coloduodenal fistulas, always originating from Crohn's colitis, result in foul-smelling eructation, feculent vomiting, and malabsorption from a combination of "short circuiting" and small intestinal bacterial overgrowth. Enterovesical fistulas typically present with dysuria and recurrent bladder infections and less often with pneumaturia and fecaluria. An intraabdominal abscess is present in about 50% of cases. Enterovaginal fistulas present with dyspareunia or feculent, foul-smelling vaginal discharge. They can arise from the ileum in women with prior hysterectomy but are much more frequently rectovaginal, secondary to extension of penetrating perianal and rectal disease. Enterocutaneous fistulas follow the planes of least resistance, typically through prior surgical scars, to the periumbilical area along a persistent urachal segment or along the psoas muscle to the groin. These fistulas may also develop after drainage of an intraabdominal abscess, indicating persistent underlying disease. Periileostomy fistulas complicate 2% of ileostomies and manifest recurrent proximal disease. Enterocutaneous fistulas rarely heal spontaneously.

Free perforation is uncommon (1% to 2% of patients) because transmural inflammation promotes extensive adhesions that generate pathways for abscess or fistula formation rather than free perforation. Perforations arise from the ileum or jejunum or secondary to toxic megacolon. Generalized peritonitis may also result from rupture of an intraabdominal abscess.

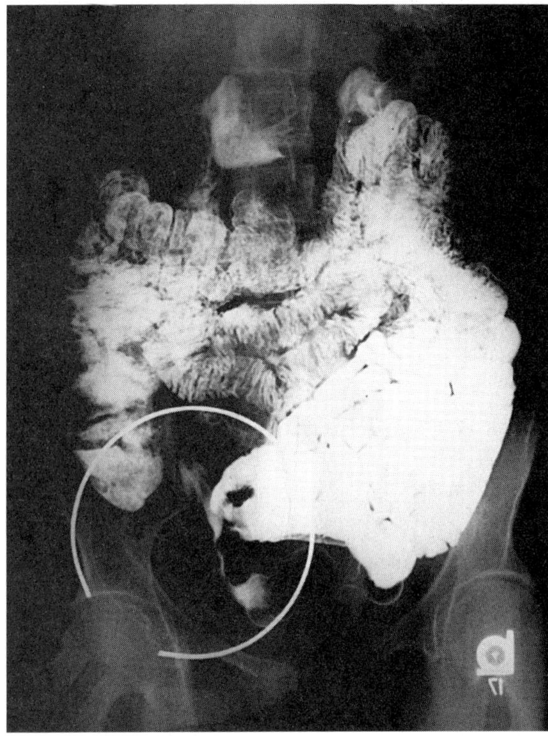

Fig. 108-2. Terminal ileal stricture in 39-year-old woman with 8-year history of Crohn's disease who reported postprandial cramping abdominal pain and distention. Small bowel follow-through demonstrated fixed narrowing of terminal ileum with some dilation of ileum proximal to stricture. No other areas of intestinal disease were identified.

Diagnosis

In patients with a brief history of right lower quadrant pain, the first step in the differential diagnosis of Crohn's disease is to exclude acute appendicitis (Box 108-3). A history of diarrhea or the presence of palpable mass should prompt evaluation by abdominal computed tomography (CT) scan. Stool cultures and examination for ova and parasites are done to rule out infection. Because enteric infection may trigger a recurrence, these stool studies should also be considered in patients with established Crohn's disease. The presence of peritoneal signs should trigger the search for extramural complications.

A small bowel follow-through study is used for diagnosis and to delineate the extent of disease (see Figure 108-2). Because the anatomic location of Crohn's disease rarely changes (except after surgery), repeat examinations are performed only if symptoms change or a major change in medical therapy or surgery is contemplated. Barium enema is complementary to colonoscopy and is especially useful before surgery and in evaluating fistulas and narrow strictures. Colonoscopy is the examination of choice to evaluate possible segmental colonic involvement and allows biopsy of inflamed and adjacent normal mucosa, strictures, and mass lesions. Routine colonoscopy, however, is not used to follow response to therapy. Histology may be useful in

Box 108-3. Differential Diagnosis of Crohn's Disease

Inflammatory Disorders of Appendix and Cecum
Appendicitis
Cecal diverticulitis

Tuboovarian Pathologies
Pelvic inflammatory disease
Ectopic pregnancy
Ovarian cysts and tumors
Endometriosis

Neoplastic Disorders of Intestine
Carcinoma
Carcinoid tumor
Lymphoma

Vascular Diseases
Ischemic colitis or ileitis
Systemic vasculitides: polyarteritis nodosa, systemic lupus erythematosus, rheumatoid arthritis, necrotizing angiitis, dermatomyositis, Behçet's disease
Radiation enteritis

Infectious Diseases
Ileocecal tuberculosis
Amebiasis
Yersinia, Salmonella, Shigella, Campylobacter, Chlamydia, or Clostridium difficile infection
Mycobacterium avium complex (AIDS patients)
Anisakiasis

Other Intestinal Inflammatory Disorders
Ulcerative jejunoileitis
Eosinophilic gastroenteritis

differentiating Crohn's colitis from ulcerative colitis. Intubation of the ileocecal valve allows examination and biopsy of the terminal ileum. Upper intestinal endoscopy with biopsy is more sensitive than barium studies for diagnosis of gastroduodenal Crohn's disease. The presence of noncaseating granulomas is considered almost pathognomonic of Crohn's disease, but granulomas are found only in 30% of biopsies and 50% of surgical specimens. Multiple biopsies can confirm the focality of disease involvement.

CT plays an important role in patient evaluation. It can demonstrate transmural intestinal thickening and is the modality of choice to evaluate extramural complications (e.g., fistulas, phlegmons, abscesses). Magnetic resonance imaging (MRI) is inferior to CT in demonstrating intraperitoneal lesions but is useful to evaluate pelvic lesions (e.g., ischiorectal abscesses, perirectal fistulas). Ultrasonography is useful in the initial evaluation of right lower quadrant pain to rule out tuboovarian pathology and extrauterine pregnancy.

Treatment

Medical Therapy

Gastroduodenal Crohn's Disease. Omeprazole, sucralfate, or histamine receptor antagonists (H_2RAs) may induce partial or even complete remission of symptoms. Slow-release mesalamine in methylcellulose granules (Pentasa) is partly released in the proximal small intestine and may be useful in duodenal Crohn's disease, but its benefit has not been tested in clinical trials. Patients who do not respond to these therapies are treated with prednisone. Azathioprine or 6-MP is indicated for patients who remain symptomatic despite steroid therapy or who are steroid dependent. Duodenal strictures associated with Crohn's disease have been treated by balloon dilation with good long-term results.

Ileitis, Ileocolitis, and Colitis. When systemic symptoms are absent or minimal, treatment can be initiated with an oral 5-ASA agent. Sulfasalazine has limited efficacy in ileitis, probably related to its need for bacterial degradation for activation. Mesalamine (Pentasa, 4 gm/day) has some efficacy in ileitis. 5-ASA therapy is started at a low dose to evaluate the patient's tolerance, then increased to a higher dosage (see Table 108-2). Both sulfasalazine and mesalamine can induce remission in ileocolitis or colitis. Improvement should be noted in 2 to 4 weeks. Treatment with antibiotics can be tried in patients with ileitis who do not respond to 5-ASA. Metronidazole is the preferred antibiotic in Crohn's ileocolitis or colitis, starting at 10 mg and increasing to 20 mg/kg/day if tolerated. A clinical response is expected within 3 to 4 weeks; prolonged treatment with metronidazole can cause peripheral neuropathy. Ciprofloxacin and clarithromycin can be used as alternatives.

Corticosteroid therapy should be considered for patients with marked systemic symptoms and those who fail to respond to 5-ASA compounds and antibiotics. Prednisone, 30 to 60 mg daily by mouth, is the usual starting dose depending on the patient's clinical state. An aggressive approach is favored, using 60 mg for 10 days before initiating a slowly tapering schedule. Steroids with reduced systemic penetration have a role in these patients. In two well-controlled and randomized studies a controlled-release form of budesonide induced remission in about 50% of patients. This steroid is more potent than prednisone and is largely degraded during first hepatic passage, leading to minimal systemic delivery of the drug. The overall efficacy of budesonide in Crohn's disease may be reduced compared with systemic steroids, however, and this agent is not yet approved for this use in the United States.

Severely ill patients with ileocolitis or colitis may require immediate hospitalization for bowel rest, rehydration, parenteral steroids, and possibly antibiotic therapy. These patients should be monitored for anemia, severe intestinal bleeding, or toxic megacolon.

Localized Peritonitis. Patients with localized peritoneal signs should be evaluated for extramural complications, and treatment with broad-spectrum antibiotics should be started. The combination of metronidazole with a broad-spectrum cephalosporin or with ampicillin plus gentamicin provides appropriate coverage. The use of steroids is controversial because they may mask and facilitate progressive sepsis and peritonitis.

Chronic Small Bowel Obstruction. Obstruction can result from a stricture, intestinal adhesion, or rarely an enterolith. Obstructive episodes are often precipitated by inflammation or spasm of the narrowed segment, and patients usually respond to medical therapy. Nasogastric suction, IV fluids, and steroids often lead to prompt improvement. Patients who fail to improve or who depend on high-dose steroids should undergo surgery.

Refractory and Steroid-dependent Disease. Controlled trials and a meta-analysis indicate that azathioprine and 6-MP are effective in both refractory and steroid-dependent Crohn's disease.[7] Treatment is initiated at 50 mg/day with either of these purine analogs. If no improvement is obtained after 4 weeks, the dose is increased by 25-mg increments every month, to a maximum of 2.5 mg/kg/day of azathioprine or 1.5 mg/kg/day of 6-MP. The prolonged time to peak response (3 to 6 months) suggests that a reduction in steroid dosage should be delayed. Clinical remission occurs in 60% to 70% of patients with resistant small or large bowel Crohn's disease. Intramuscular or oral methotrexate is effective in patients who do not respond or are intolerant to purine analogs. A liver biopsy is recommended for patients who receive a cumulative dose of 1 to 1.5 gm of methotrexate. Folic acid supplements are given to patients taking methotrexate to decrease side effects.

Parenteral infusion of monoclonal chimeric anti–tumor necrosis factor (TNF)-α antibodies is now approved for severe Crohn's disease. In one study, 65% of patients with moderate to severe Crohn's disease showed improvement and 33% entered remission, compared with 17% and 4% in the placebo group, respectively.[6] Caution should be used in administering this new drug until its safety profile is better defined.[10] The development of anti-DNA antibodies and some cases of lymphoma have been reported in patients receiving this compound. Other agents currently under evaluation for use in Crohn's disease include anti-CD4 antibodies, recombinant interleukin-10, and intercellular adhesion molecule 1 (ICAM-1) antisense oligonucleotides.

Perianal Disease. Metronidazole, 10 to 20 mg/kg/day, is the drug of choice for perianal disease. Because high dosages may need to be maintained for a prolonged period, patients should be made aware of potential side effects, particularly the occurrence of paresthesias, that may persist for long periods after discontinuation of the drug. A 50% relapse rate follows cessation of metronidazole. Abscesses require surgical drainage. Patients who do not improve with metronidazole and local surgical management are candidates for 6-MP therapy.

Fistulas. Attempts should be made to manage fistulas medically because of the high rate of recurrence after surgery. Metronidazole is initiated at 10 mg/kg/day and increased to 20 mg/kg/day if needed and tolerated. 6-MP is the second-line agent. Patients with jejunocolic fistulas may have bacterial overgrowth responsive to antibiotics. In one study, anti-TNF-α antibodies induced closure of 46% of fistula vs. 13% in the placebo group.[6] Treatment of enterovesical fistulas should include antibiotics to control the urinary tract infection as well as therapy for the underlying active Crohn's disease. 6-MP is the agent of choice for enterovesical fistulas, but most patients will require surgery because of progression of the underlying bowel disease.

Dietary Management. No compelling evidence exists to recommend a specific diet for all patients with Crohn's disease. Those with active disease or chronic strictures often benefit from a low-residue diet. Severely ill patients should be treated by bowel rest. Enteral feeding with an elemental diet or total parenteral nutrition may be used in patients with steroid-refractory or steroid-resistant Crohn's disease. Both these nutritional approaches seem to be equally effective in inducing remission.

Maintenance of Remission. Although less successful in Crohn's disease than in ulcerative colitis, 5-ASA agents are indicated for maintaining remission (see Table 108-2). The role of steroids as maintenance agents in Crohn's disease is still unclear, but their systemic toxicity make them less than ideal. Both azathioprine and 6-MP are used to maintain remission, especially for patients who entered remission while taking these agents.

Surgical Treatment. Approximately 70% of patients with Crohn's disease require surgery at some point in their disease course. Because recurrence after surgery is the rule rather than the exception, surgery should always be as conservative as possible. Abscesses should be drained under CT guidance when feasible, but the frequent occurrence of secondary enterocutaneous fistulas is an indication for surgical resection. Symptomatic ileal strictures may require surgical correction by stricturoplasty or resection. Gastroduodenal strictures are managed by gastrojejunal anastomosis. If proctocolectomy is indicated, a permanent ileostomy is necessary because patients with Crohn's disease are not good candidates for an ileoanal anastomosis with pouch. A surgeon should be involved in the management of patients with perianal Crohn's disease.

Slow-release mesalamine (Pentasa), metronidazole, and 6-MP have shown efficacy in preventing postoperative relapse after ileal resection and anastomosis. The effect of metronidazole does not appear to exceed 1 year, and its toxicity may not be compatible with long-term use.

COLON CANCER SURVEILLANCE

Patients with ulcerative colitis are at increased risk for colon cancer. Cancer risk increases with duration of disease and disease extent. Disease activity is not closely associated with cancer risk. Patients with extensive colitis have a 5% risk of colon cancer after 20 years of colitis, 12% after 25 years, and 25% after 35 years. Colon cancer surveillance is usually recommended for patients with extensive colitis for 8 to 10 years or left-sided colitis for 12 to 15 years. Colonoscopy is performed initially every 2 years and annually after 15 years of colitis. Serial biopsies are done to look for histologic evidence of dysplasia. Colon cancer in ulcerative colitis is frequently a flat, broad-based lesion rather than an exophytic mass, so even small, sessile, mucosal lesions should be biopsied. Indications for colectomy include carcinoma, confirmed high-grade dysplasia, or dysplasia in a mucosal plaque or nodule (dysplasia-associated lesion or mass). Patients with low-grade dysplasia should undergo repeat surveillance within 6 months. Recommendations for colon cancer screening in ulcerative colitis have not been tested by controlled clinical trials, and the cost-effectiveness is questionable.

Patients with Crohn's disease are at increased risk for small bowel adenocarcinoma and probably also for colon cancer. Colonoscopic screening may be appropriate for patients with longstanding, extensive Crohn's colitis, but no established screening protocols exist for intestinal carcinoma in Crohn's disease.

EXTRAINTESTINAL MANIFESTATIONS

The most common symptomatic extraintestinal manifestation of IBD is an asymmetric, nondeforming, pauciarticular, migratory arthralgia affecting the knees, hips, ankles, or

Box 108-4. Extraintestinal Manifestations of Inflammatory Bowel Disease

Joints
Polyarthralgia
Sacroileitis
Sacroileitis with ankylosing spondylitis*

Skin
Erythema nodosum
Pyoderma gangrenosum
Cutaneous fistula

Eyes
Uveitis
Episcleritis

Urinary Tract
Calcium oxalate stones†
Ureteric obstruction
Enterovesical or colovesical fistula

Hepatobiliary Tract
Cholesterol gallstones†
Sclerosing cholangitis*
Pericholangitis
Chronic active hepatitis

Other
Amyloidosis
Thromboembolic events

*Severity and progression do not correlate with severity or extent of intestinal disease.
†Complicates ileal disease or resection.

elbows (Box 108-4). It is most common in Crohn's colitis, less common in ulcerative colitis, and rarely complicates Crohn's disease isolated to the small intestine. This arthritis follows the activity of the colitis and responds to effective treatment of the colonic disease. Arthralgia may occur in combination with other extraintestinal manifestations of IBD that mirror disease activity, such as erythema nodosum and uveitis. Erythema nodosum is more common in Crohn's disease, usually occurs during a disease flare, and seldom recurs. Pyoderma gangrenosum is characterized by large skin ulcers, typically on the lower limbs. It usually develops in patients with extensive and active ulcerative colitis and usually resolves when the colitis remits.

Patients with ulcerative colitis have a 30-fold increased risk for developing the rare condition of sacroileitis with ankylosing spondylitis. The majority of affected IBD patients are HLA-B27 positive. The progress of ankylosing spondylitis does not reflect the severity of intestinal disease and is not altered by medical management of IBD or by colectomy. Sacroileitis alone is more common than sacroileitis with ankylosing spondylitis and is often asymptomatic and nonprogressive.

Sclerosing cholangitis is characterized by inflammation and fibrosis of the intrahepatic and extrahepatic biliary-tree leading to cholestasis. Most patients with sclerosing cholangitis have ulcerative colitis. Their colitis is frequently mild or even asymptomatic, however, and the course of the liver disease does not parallel that of their colonic disease. Sclerosing cholangitis frequently progresses to severe cholestatic liver disease and liver failure requiring transplantation. Cholangiocarcinoma develops in approximately 15% of patients with chronic sclerosing cholangitis and ulcerative colitis.

Patients with Crohn's disease of the terminal ileum and ileal resection are at increased risk for developing cholesterol gallstones due to interruption of the enterohepatic circulation of bile salts. Calcium oxalate renal stones are also more common in Crohn's disease as a result of fatty acid malabsorption. The fatty acids sequester calcium, thereby reducing the luminal formation of poorly absorbed calcium oxalate. Instead, sodium oxalate forms and is readily absorbed in the colon, leading to increased urinary oxalate secretion. Urinary tract complications may also occur in Crohn's disease when intestinal inflammation involves the ureter or fistula formation involves the urinary bladder.

SPECIALIST REFERRAL

The majority of patients with IBD are managed in consultation with a gastroenterologist. After initial diagnosis, patients with mild, limited ulcerative colitis that responds well to 5-ASA or sulfasalazine therapy may not require regular specialist consultation and management. Patients with severe, extensive ulcerative colitis and most patients with Crohn's disease should have regular consultation with a physician experienced in the treatment of IBD.

REFERENCES

1. Allan RN, Rhodes JM, Hanauer SB, et al: *Inflammatory bowel diseases,* ed 3, New York, 1997, Churchill Livingstone.
1a. Elson CO, Sartor RB, Tennyson GS, et al: Experimental models of inflammatory bowel disease, *Gastroenterology* 109:1344-1367, 1995.
2. Kornbluth A, Sachar DB, Salomon P: Crohn's disease. In Feldman M, Scharschmidt BF, Sleisenger MH, editors: *Sleisenger & Fordtran's Gastrointestinal and liver diseases,* vol 2, ed 6, Philadelphia, 1998, Saunders.
3. Michetti P, Peppercorn MA: Medical therapy of specific clinical presentations, *Gastroenterol Clin North Am* 28:353-370, 1999.
3a. Misiewicz JJ, Lennard-Jones JE, Connell AM, et al: Controlled trial of sulfasalazine in maintenance therapy for ulcerative colitis, *Lancet* 1:185-188, 1965.
4. Podolsky DK: Inflammatory bowel disease. Part 1, *N Engl J Med* 325:928, 1991.
5. Podolsky DK: Inflammatory bowel disease. Part 2, *N Engl J Med* 325:1008, 1991.
6. Present DH, Mayer L, van Deventer SJ, et al: Anti-TNF-alpha chimeric antibody (cA2) is effective in the treatment of the fistulae of Crohn's disease: a multicenter, randomized, double-blind, placebo-controlled study, *Am J Gastroenterol* 92:A648, 1997.
7. Sachar DB: Maintenance therapy in ulcerative colitis and Crohn's disease, *J Clin Gastroenterol* 20:117, 1995.
8. Stenson WF: Inflammatory bowel diseases. In Yamada T, Alpers DH, Owyang C, et al, editors: *Textbook of gastroenterology,* volume 2, ed 2, Philadelphia, 1995, Lippincott.
9. Targan SR, Shanahan F: *Inflammatory bowel disease, from bench to bedside,* Baltimore, 1994, Williams & Wilkins.
10. Targan SR, Hanauer SB, van Deventer SJ, et al: A short-term study of chimeric monoclonal antibody cA2 to tumor necrosis factor alpha for Crohn's disease, Crohn's Disease cA2 Study Group, *N Engl J Med* 337:1029, 1997.

CHAPTER 109

Gastrointestinal Hemorrhage

David Lichtenstein
Umar Beejay

The management of patients with gastrointestinal (GI) hemorrhage constitutes a major problem that mandates close cooperation among primary care providers, gastroenterologists, surgeons, and interventional radiologists. Pragmatically, GI bleeding is divided into upper and lower GI hemorrhage, with the ligament of Treitz being the anatomic dividing line. Bleeding can be *acute,* with hematemesis, melena, and hematochezia, or *chronic,* presenting as iron deficiency anemia or guaiac-positive stool. The clinical approach depends not only on the acuity and localization of the bleeding, but also on patient characteristics and the medical skills and resources available. A consistent, planned approach to GI hemorrhage optimizes patient management, reduces hospital length of stay and expenditures, and improves patient survival.

INITIAL MANAGEMENT

The initial approach to the patient with acute GI hemorrhage includes assessing the severity of hemorrhage, initiating resuscitative efforts, and performing a brief history and limited physical examination (Fig. 109-1). The key to the successful management is the rapid institution of fluid resuscitation to maintain organ perfusion and tissue oxygenation. Depending on the acuity of illness, patients can be triaged to the intensive care unit (ICU) or a less intensively monitored setting. In those with severe bleeding, a multidisciplinary approach should be instituted early.

Clinical Assessment

The primary initial objective of the clinical evaluation is to assess the patient's severity of hemorrhage by determining hemodynamic status. This assessment takes precedence over measures aimed at localizing and directing treatment of the bleeding site. Vital signs are monitored frequently, including blood pressure, pulse, and postural changes. The patient's ability to manifest compensatory hemodynamics is often influenced by other factors, such as medication intake (e.g., β-adrenergic blocker), age, vascular integrity, and the intactness of the autonomic nervous system. Initial hematocrit (Hct) determination can be misleading at presentation because vascular fluid redistribution requires 24 to 72 hours to equilibrate (Fig. 109-2). The patient's general appearance is also important; skin turgor and jugular venous pressure supplement vital signs in determining the level of volume depletion. Whether the patient is pale or jaundiced should also be noted. Cachexia, lymphadenopathy, and abdominal masses suggest malignancy. The abdominal examination should evaluate for tenderness, masses, hepatosplenomegaly, ascites, and bowel sounds. A rectal examination provides valuable information on the color and consistency of the stool (e.g., maroon vs. bright red, melena vs. occult blood). Cutaneous stigmata may suggest the etiology of GI

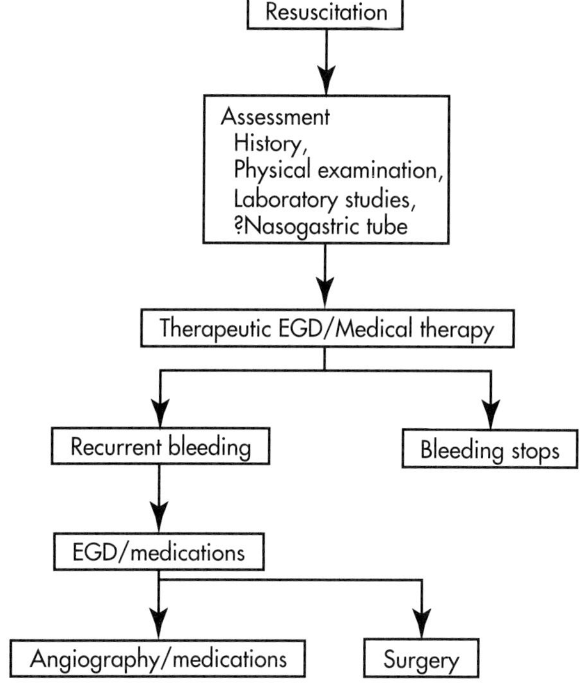

Fig. 109-1. Approach to patient with acute gastrointestinal hemorrhage. *EGD,* Esophagogastroduodenoscopy.

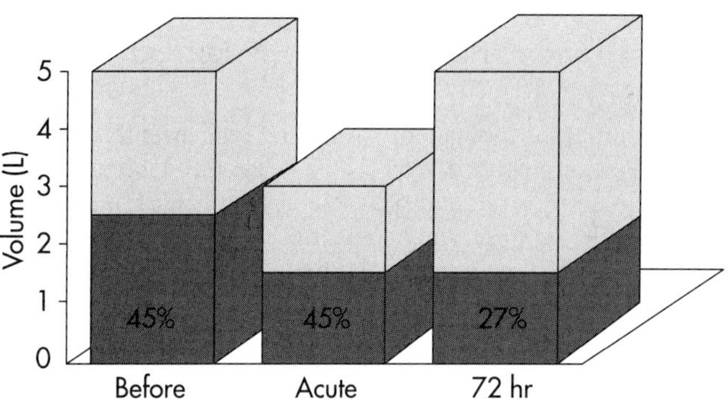

Fig. 109-2. Reliability of hematocrit (Hct) as indicator of severity of gastrointestinal bleeding. In acute period after hemorrhage, plasma volume and red blood cell volume have decreased in parallel so that Hct remains essentially unchanged. Over the ensuing 72 hours, however, equilibration of extravascular and intravascular fluid spaces results in Hct that accurately reflects total blood losses.

hemorrhage. Jaundice, spider nevi, palmar erythema, and ecchymoses suggest liver disease, whereas orofacial telangiectasias suggest Osler-Weber-Rendu syndrome (hereditary hemorrhagic telangiectasia). Café au lait spots suggest neurofibromatosis, and eythema nodosum is associated with inflammatory bowel disease (IBD).

Clinical assessment is poor at predicting the source of bleeding, but the history helps direct therapy because the distribution of etiologies varies with patient age, particularly in lower GI bleeding. Thus in young patients the diagnosis frequently includes IBD, Meckel's diverticulum, and juvenile polyps; in middle-aged patients, polyps, hemorrhoids, and diverticula; and in elderly patients, angiodysplasia, malignancy, ischemia, diverticulosis, and polyps. With lower GI hemorrhage the presence or absence of abdominal pain is also important (see Chapter 107). Diffuse abdominal pain can suggest inflammatory bowel disease or ischemic bowel, whereas painless bleeding is common with diverticula, angiodysplasia, malignancy, polyps, and Meckel's diverticulum. Bloody diarrhea may indicate infectious (e.g., *Clostridium difficile*) colitis or IBD, or recent antibiotic use. Recent constipation suggests anorectal sources, such as hemorrhoidal bleeding, anal fissure, or solitary rectal ulcer syndrome. The physician should inquire about symptoms of extraintestinal manifestations of IBD (see Chapter 108). The history should include prior episodes of bleeding, family history of GI diseases (e.g., hereditary hemorrhagic telangiectasia), known illnesses (e.g., ulcers, cirrhosis, cancer, bleeding diathesis), and previous abdominal surgery. A prior aortic aneurysm repair suggests aortoenteric fistula; undiagnosed bleeding from an aortoenteric fistula is ultimately fatal. The medication profile is important, especially use of nonsteroidal antiinflammatory drugs (NSAIDs) and anticoagulants. Within the spectrum of upper GI hemorrhage, classic features of epigastric pain relieved by food suggests peptic ulcer disease, whereas chronic renal failure should suggest arteriovenous malformations. Similarly, a classic history of retching followed by hematemesis should suggest a Mallory-Weiss tear, although this classic history, which was initially considered to be a prerequisite for the syndrome, is now known to occur in only 30% to 50% of patients. Many patients experience hematemesis without previous retching or present infrequently with melena alone.

Resuscitation and Transfusion of Blood Products

Resuscitation of the patient is initiated concurrently with the clinical assessment. Blood is sent to the laboratory for determination of the complete blood count (CBC), coagulation profile, and serum chemistries, including blood urea nitrogen (BUN), creatinine, and liver function tests. Blood is also sent to the blood bank for typing and crossmatching. While obtaining blood specimens, at least two large-bore (14- to 18-gauge) intravenous (IV) catheters should be placed for the administration of fluids and blood products. More aggressive invasive monitoring may be needed in those with significant cardiorespiratory disease. Strict charting of fluid intake and output is helpful to assess tissue perfusion. Patients in shock unresponsive to fluid resuscitation require IV pressors. The type and quantity of fluid replacement must be tailored to the patient's specific needs.

The use of rigid transfusion guidelines, such as maintaining Hct above 30%, should be avoided. A hemoglobin (Hb) level greater than 7 to 8 g/dl is generally acceptable if the patient is young and not actively bleeding and if fluid resuscitation has achieved a near steady-state value. In elderly patients or those with known cardiovascular disease, an Hb level of approximately 10 g/dl should be maintained. Empiric transfusion of fresh-frozen plasma (FFP) or platelets after packed red blood cells (PRBCs) is unnecessary provided rapid access to the coagulation profile and platelet count is available. FFP may be used to reverse the effect of warfarin; correct deficiencies of coagulation factors (II, V, VII, VIII, IX, X, XI, XIII), antithrombin III, heparin cofactor II, protein C, and protein S; and correct deficiencies of multiple factors, as in severe liver disease and vitamin K depletion. Early factor replacement should be considered in patients with known cirrhosis, with an average requirement of 1 unit of FFP for every 4 units of PRBCs. Factor VII biologic half-life is only 6 hours, and additional infusions may need to be repeated every 6 to 12 hours. The usual adult dosage of FFP is 3 to 5 units (12 to 15 ml/kg) given over 1 hour to several hours, depending on the patient's cardiac status. Platelet counts less than 80,000/dl are associated with increased bleeding and, in the setting of active GI bleeding, should be corrected with transfused platelets. If existing platelets are dysfunctional, as with recent aspirin or NSAID use, platelet replacement should be considered for the actively bleeding patient even when platelets are quantitatively normal.

The majority of patients who develop GI bleeding while taking anticoagulants have underlying mucosal pathology. When bleeding occurs in the setting of anticoagulation, the degree of bleeding and the reason for anticoagulation need to be reassessed for possible reversal of therapy. Patients with GI bleeding who are taking warfarin may require only discontinuation of their anticoagulation therapy if bleeding is not severe and if the coagulation profile is within the therapeutic range. When warfarin is discontinued, the international normalized ratio (INR) does not normalize for 3 to 4 days. Alternatively, a low dose of vitamin K (1 mg) or FFP may be given intravenously. Heparin therapy can simply be stopped, unless bleeding is severe, in which case the anticoagulant effects of heparin should be reversed with protamine sulfate.

Patients with renal failure often have an underlying bleeding diathesis reflected in a prolonged bleeding time. The hemostatic defects in patients with chronic renal failure are caused by abnormalities in platelet function, vessel wall–coagulation interaction, and plasma coagulation factor deficiencies. Desmopressin (DDAVP) is a synthetic analog of arginine vasopressin that possesses hemostatic properties because of the release from vascular endothelium of preformed high-molecular-weight multimers of von Willebrand's factor and factor VIII:C. DDAVP has a rapid onset of effect but is limited by its short duration of action of 6 hours. The IV dose is 0.3 μg/kg diluted in 50 ml of normal saline given over 15 to 30 minutes. Repeat dosing in 12 to 24 hours reproduces an increase in coagulant factors, although a decreased physiologic response is then seen because of depletion of preformed factors from vascular endothelium. Although DDAVP is frequently used to correct the bleeding diathesis in uremic patients with acute bleeding, improved survival has not been shown. Uncontrolled trials also report improved bleeding times and reduced rebleeding rates and transfusion requirements after administration of cryoprecipitate, conjugated estrogens, or combined estrogen and progesterone.

Localization of Gastrointestinal Hemorrhage

The initial challenge after stabilization of the patient is to determine whether the hemorrhage is emanating from above (upper intestinal) or below (lower intestinal) the ligament of Treitz. The presence of hematemesis is virtually always indicative of an upper gastrointestinal (UGI) hemorrhage; however, epistaxis or oropharyngeal bleeding may infrequently simulate a UGI bleed. Melena usually indicates UGI bleeding and occurs as a result of bacterial degradation of Hb to hematin and other hemochromes as blood traverses the small bowel and colon. Melena can result from as little as 50 to 100 ml of blood introduced into the UGI tract. Rarely, melena will occur during a lower GI bleed, but only when bleeding is slow and is localized to the right colon or small bowel. Other clinical findings suggestive of UGI hemorrhage include hyperactive bowel sounds and elevated BUN out of proportion to serum creatinine.

The passage of red blood from the rectum usually indicates a lower GI bleed. A brisk upper GI bleed can present similarly, however, and therefore nasogastric (NG) tube aspiration should be performed in all patients with suspected lower GI bleeding. Patients with hematochezia from UGI bleeding usually have evidence of volume depletion from the history and physical examination. NG tube placement and lavage are not recommended for suspected UGI hemorrhage (provided endoscopy is planned within several hours) because of (1) delays in definitive therapy caused by prolonged efforts to clear the stomach of its contents; (2) risks of pulmonary aspiration, intestinal perforation, incorrect tube placement into the respiratory tree, and mucosal suction artifacts, which can be indistinguishable from true mucosal vascular lesions; and (3) lack of evidence that gastric lavage is capable of stopping active bleeding or preventing recurrence. NG aspiration should be considered in patients with suspected UGI hemorrhage when esophagogastroduodenoscopy (EGD) will be delayed in order to (1) confirm the upper tract nature of bleeding when melena or hematochezia is present rather than hematemesis, (2) provide prognostic information, and (3) cleanse the stomach to facilitate endoscopic examination. The presence of gross blood or "coffee grounds" on gastric aspirate confirms an UGI source. A clear aspirate does not exclude an upper bleed, however, since bleeding may be episodic or the lesion may be distal to the stomach, with a competent pylorus preventing duodenogastric reflux of blood. Bile in a nonbloody aspirate makes an upper source less likely, although this can be misleading because the visual appearance of the aspirate does not reliably discriminate between the presence and absence of bile. When NG aspiration is performed, the use of chemical tests (e.g., guaiac reaction) are of little clinical value and should be avoided.

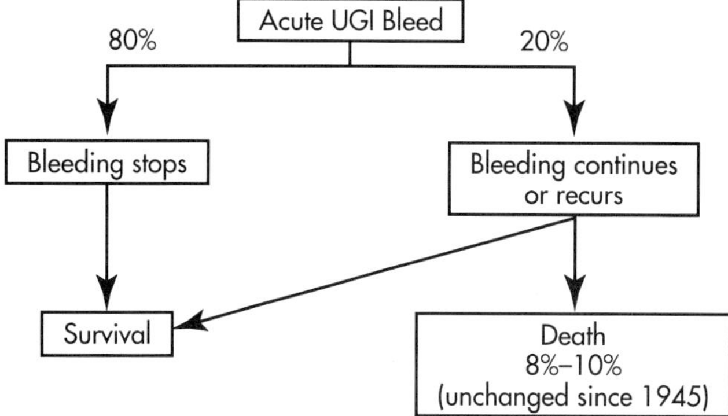

Fig. 109-3. Outcome of acute upper gastrointestinal (UGI) bleeding.

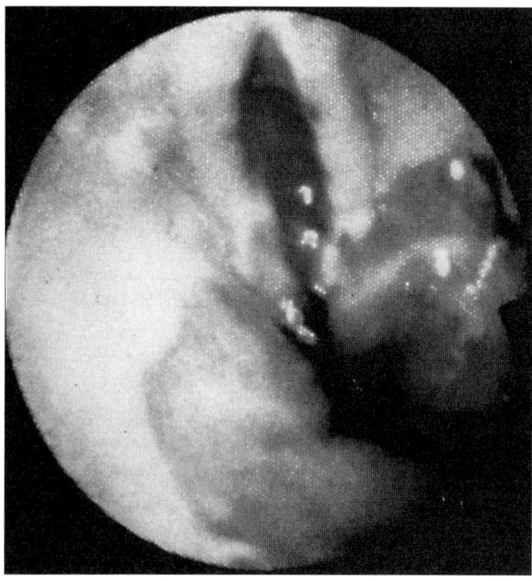

Fig. 109-4. Endoscopic view of Mallory-Weiss tear, with linear mucosal laceration at gastroesophageal junction.

NONVARICEAL UPPER GASTROINTESTINAL HEMORRHAGE

Nonvariceal UGI bleeding continues to rank among the most common emergencies encountered by physicians, with more than 300,000 hospital admissions annually in the United States. With only supportive therapy, approximately 80% to 85% of patients with UGI hemorrhage will stop bleeding (Fig. 109-3). The remaining 15% to 20% who continue to bleed or have recurrent hemorrhage account for the majority of complications and deaths. It is these high-risk patients who require early identification and in whom endoscopic, surgical, and angiographic therapies have improved patient outcome. Severe UGI hemorrhage is most often caused by peptic ulcer disease, Mallory-Weiss tears (Fig. 109-4), esophageal varices, vascular malformations, and erosive gastroduodenal lesions (Table 109-1).

Prognostic Factors

Clinical factors that predict a poor outcome include advanced patient age, comorbid medical illnesses, onset of bleeding while already hospitalized, recurrent hemorrhage, and specific etiology and severity of the bleeding episode (Box 109-1). Clinical indicators of severe bleeding include hemodynamic instability on presentation, persistent hypotension, transfusion requirements in excess of 4 to 6 units within 24 hours of hospital admission, or bleeding manifested as hematemesis, hematochezia, or a bloody gastric aspirate that does not clear with lavage.[4]

Although clinical criteria are useful predictors for determining outcome, the endoscopic information indicating the cause of bleeding (and in the case of ulcers the appearance of the ulcer base) provides equally important prognostic information (Fig. 109-5). The bleeding ulcer may have no stigmata of recent hemorrhage (SRH), that is, a clean base. Major SRH include active bleeding (oozing or spurting) or visible vessel, and minor SRH include an adherent clot or flat pigmented spots (red, black, purple, or brown) (Table 109-2).[4] An actively bleeding ulcer predicts continued or recurrent bleeding in more than 85% of cases (Fig. 109-6). The term *nonbleeding visible vessel* describes a 2-mm to 3-mm protuberance in the floor of an ulcer crater that is typically the vessel itself or more often represents an adherent clot plugging the eroded artery (Fig. 109-7). The visible vessel is found in 17% of bleeding ulcers; 43% of patients

Table 109-1. Common Causes of Upper Gastrointestinal (UGI) Hemorrhage

Lesion	Prevalence (%)	Comments
Peptic ulcer disease (PUD)	21 (gastric ulcer) 24 (duodenal ulcer) 2 (anastomotic ulcer)	Account for up to 50% of all UGI bleeds. Up to 40% may lack dyspeptic symptoms before bleed. Any age, but more common in elderly persons. Mortality rate of 5%.
Erosive gastritis	5-25	Bleeding usually self-limited and treated similar to PUD. Multiple etiologies: stress, drugs (NSAIDs, alcohol, iron, potassium chloride), corrosives, ischemia, vasculitis, radiation, mechanical causes, portal hypertension.
Esophageal varices	9-21	Responsible for a high proportion of severe hemorrhage.
Mallory-Weiss tear	11-14	Arterial bleeding from longitudinal mucosal lacerations. Retching and vomiting preceding vomiting occurs in only 50%, but 90% experience hematemesis. Bleeding stops spontaneously in up to 90%.
Erosive duodenitis	5-9	Most cases are a primary nonspecific form, but some result from stress, alcohol, NSAIDs, ischemia, infection, inflammatory bowel disease, or renal failure.
Malignancy	~3	Clinically significant bleeding in UGI neoplasms is uncommon. If bleeding occurs, endoscopic therapy is usually temporizing measure before definitive surgery.
Esophagitis	2-8	Occult more common than overt blood loss. Most respond to conservative medical therapy. Multiple etiologies: gastroesophageal reflux, infection, pills, corrosives, radiotherapy, nasogastric trauma.

Modified from Gilbert DA, Silverstein FE, Tedesco FJ, et al: The national ASGE survey on upper gastrointestinal hemorrhage. Part III. Endoscopy in upper gastrointestinal bleeding, *Gastrointest Endosc* 27:94, 1981.
NSAIDs, Nonsteroidal antiinflammatory drugs.

Box 109-1. Adverse Prognostic Factors for Upper Gastrointestinal (UGI) Hemorrhage

- Age > 60
- Continued or recurrent bleeding
- Comorbid illness
- Onset of UGI hemorrhage in hospital
- Severity of hemorrhage
  - Red nasogastric aspirate
  - Hematemesis/hematochezia
  - Multiple transfusions
  - Hemodynamic instability
- Type of lesion
- Need for emergency surgical intervention
- Endoscopic criteria
  - Stigmata of recent hemorrhage (SRH)
  - Ulcer location (posterior duodenal bulb, higher lesser gastric curvature)
  - Ulcer size

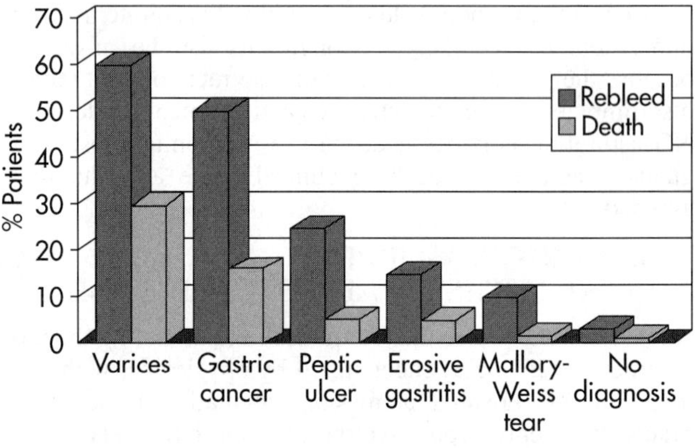

Fig. 109-5. Influence of diagnosis on outcome of UGI hemorrhage.

have rebleeding, 34% require emergency surgery, and 11% die when endoscopic therapy is withheld. A clean ulcer base (i.e., without endoscopic SRH) is found in 20% to 50% of bleeding ulcer patients and reliably predicts a benign course with a negligible risk for rebleeding (0% to 5%) and virtually no mortality. Ulcers with minor SRH of flat spots or adherent clots account for approximately one third of the ulcers found at endoscopy (Fig. 109-8). These patients have a slightly increased incidence of rebleeding, surgery, and mortality, with mean rates of 10% to 20%, 5% to 10%, and 3% to 7%, respectively. Other endoscopic prognostic factors shown to influence outcome include ulcer location and size. Ulcers greater than 1 to 2 cm diameter more often have SRH and indicate an increased likelihood of rebleeding and death. Ulcers located in the posteroinferior duodenal bulb and to a lesser extent the high lesser gastric curve may adversely influence outcome because of their proximity to large vessels, the gastroduodenal artery and left gastric artery, respectively.

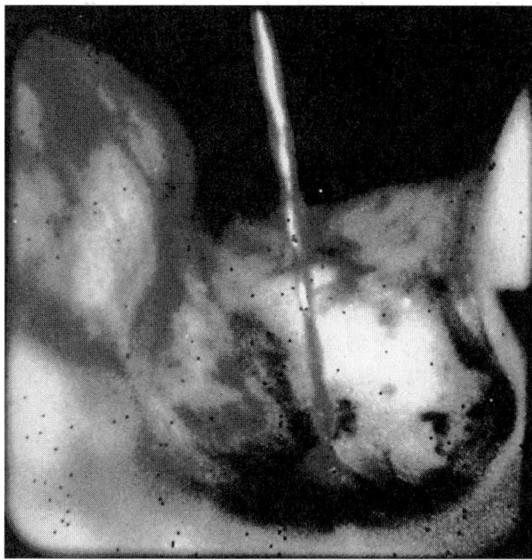

Fig. 109-6. Endoscopic view of a spurting ulcer.

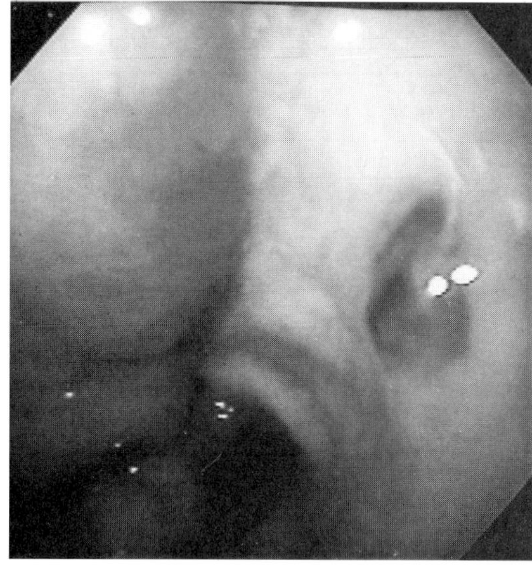

Fig. 109-7. Gastric ulcer containing nonbleeding visible vessel, manifested by raised red spot within ulcer crater.

Table 109-2. Endoscopic Stigmata of Recent Hemorrhage (SRH) in Peptic Ulcer Bleeding

	Mean of range (%)			
Characteristic	Prevalence	Rebleeding	Surgery	Mortality
Clean base	42	5*	0.5	2
Flat spot	20	10	6	3
Adherent clot	17	22	10	7
Visible vessel	17	43	34	11
Active bleeding†	18	55	35	11

Modified from Laine L, Peterson WL: Bleeding peptic ulcer, *N Engl J Med* 331:717, 1994.
*0% to 2% in most studies.
†Usually includes oozing and spurting.

Patient Triage

A treatment and triage algorithm incorporates clinical criteria with endoscopic findings (Fig. 109-9). Patients can be divided on clinical grounds into two groups: those with hemodynamically significant bleeding at high risk for rebleeding and death and those at low risk with limited blood loss. The high-risk group requires admission to a monitored unit or ICU. The low-risk group can be triaged in the emergency room with diagnostic endoscopy or admitted to the ward before EGD. Endoscopy in both groups can predict the likelihood of further bleeding and guides further decisions regarding therapy, feeding, and length of hospitalization.

Patients with major SRH of active bleeding or nonbleeding visible vessels are treated endoscopically and observed for 24 hours in an ICU and then transferred to the ward if there are no signs of rebleeding. The patients with an uncomplicated hospital course can safely be discharged after 3 to 4 days of observation, since the vast majority of ulcer rebleeding occurs within 72 hours of bleeding onset. Patients with endoscopic SRH predicting a high likelihood of rebleeding should receive nothing by mouth or a clear-liquid diet for 24 hours after endoscopic therapy so that food in the

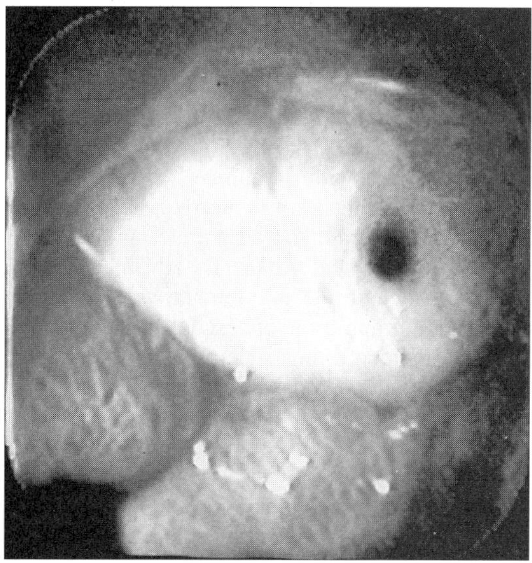

Fig. 109-8. Duodenal ulcer with minor stigmata of recent hemorrhage (SRH), manifested by nonraised black spot within ulcer crater.

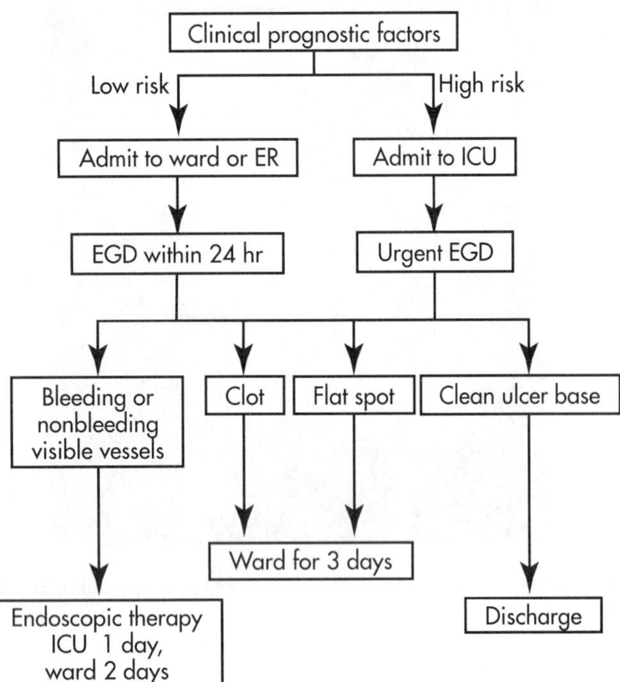

Fig. 109-9. Proposed algorithm to triage and manage patients with UGI hemorrhage from peptic ulcer disease. *EGD,* Esophagogastroduodenoscopy; *ER,* emergency room; *ICU,* intensive care unit.

stomach does not interfere with an urgent endoscopic or surgical procedure, which may be necessary if rebleeding occurs. Patients with clean ulcer bases can be fed and discharged on the first day of admission immediately after volume resuscitation and stabilization. Factors favoring outpatient care include absence of severe anemia, serious comorbid medical illness, or liver disease; lack of concomitant anticoagulation therapy or coagulopathy; no signs of active bleeding; and adequate volume resuscitation and home support.[3,7] Patients with intermediate risk of rebleeding, characterized by minor SRH, should be refed early and observed on a medical ward for up to 3 days before discharge.

Diagnostic Studies

EGD is the most useful study for determining the location and type of lesion responsible for UGI hemorrhage. The skilled endoscopist can identify the bleeding source in more than 95% of cases and can offer a number of therapeutic options for the endoscopic control of hemorrhage and prevention of rebleeding. Radiographic contrast studies should be avoided in the setting of acute hemorrhage. Disadvantages of the early use of barium include (1) interference with diagnostic and therapeutic angiographic and endoscopic procedures; (2) lack of sensitivity in identifying superficial mucosal sources of bleeding (e.g., Mallory-Weiss tear, gastritis, vascular malformation); and (3) inability to distinguish the source of hemorrhage in patients with more than one mucosal lesion.

EGD should be performed urgently for the high-risk bleeder and within 12 to 24 hours for all others with an acute, self-limited episode of UGI bleeding. Included in the high-risk category are patients with chronic liver disease, suspected aortoenteric fistula, large-volume blood loss, and active hemorrhage, as well as patients experiencing or unlikely to tolerate a recurrent episode of hemorrhage, including those who have comorbid illness or who object to blood transfusions on religious grounds. Uncorrectable coagulopathy is a relative contraindication to endoscopic hemostasis in the patient who is not actively bleeding; this should not preclude attempts to control active bleeding, however, despite that effective hemostasis may be only temporary. Airway protection with endotracheal intubation is recommended in the pediatric, obtunded, or massively bleeding patient. EGD in the bleeding patient is technically more demanding than an elective endoscopic procedure. Although complications occur slightly more often in the actively bleeding patient, the procedure is usually well tolerated and safe, with a reported rate of major complications (e.g., perforation, pulmonary aspiration, induced bleeding) of only 0.5% and a mortality of less than 0.1%. Recent myocardial infarction is not an absolute contraindication to EGD, and a risk-benefit assessment needs to be individualized for each patient.

Management

Management of UGI hemorrhage may be divided into acute treatment of the bleeding lesion and strategies for prevention of rebleeding. It is important to develop both a short-term and a long-term strategy for preventing recurrent ulceration and rebleeding, since recurrent hemorrhage may develop acutely during the initial hospitalization (typically within 24 to 48 hours) or may be delayed for months to years after peptic ulcer bleeding.

Acute Treatment

Medical Therapy. Theoretically, by slowing or halting bleeding, pharmacologic agents may be useful in the resuscitative phase of management and in enhancing the visualization of lesions during endoscopy. Iced saline gastric lavage has been a time-honored treatment considered essential for controlling UGI hemorrhage; however, the therapeutic value of lavage has since been refuted. Pharmacologic agents that act as antifibrinolytics (e.g., tranexamic acid), reduce gastric acid (e.g., histamine receptor antagonists [H_2RAs], proton pump inhibitor [PPIs], and prostaglandin analogs), act as mesenteric vasoconstrictors (e.g., vasopressin), or both reduce acid and act as vasoconstrictors (e.g., somatostatin) have been studied in an attempt to control actively bleeding ulcers. Although a few studies have reported benefit, most have found these agents to be ineffective, and at present, no medical therapy can be strongly recommended for the acute treatment of nonvariceal UGI bleeding. Data from in vitro studies suggest that clotting occurs more effectively and that lysis of clots by proteolytic enzymes occurs more slowly at high intraluminal pH levels.[8a] This forms the basis for regimens designed to reduce gastric acidity in patients with intestinal bleeding. No single trial has convincingly demonstrated an overall benefit of H_2RAs in stopping active bleeding or preventing rebleeding. The availability of the more potent PPIs to control peptic ulcer bleeding has renewed interest in antisecretory therapy. The available information is promising but inconclusive.[2,6] Therefore it is reasonable to initiate treatment with a PPI for the potential benefit and as an alternative therapy when endoscopy is unsuccessful, contraindicated, or unavailable. PPIs also may be used once the diagnosis of an acid-peptic disorder is confirmed, acutely to promote healing of the lesion and as maintenance therapy to prevent recurrence.

Endoscopic Therapy. A National Institutes of Health (NIH) Consensus Conference[8] on therapeutic endoscopy and bleeding ulcers concluded that endoscopic therapy should be limited to patients at high risk for persistent or recurrent bleeding and death. This group includes those with clinical evidence of significant blood loss and endoscopic evidence of active bleeding or a nonbleeding visible vessel. Meta-analysis of studies evaluating endoscopic hemostasis for nonvariceal UGI bleeding found a significant reduction in mortality (relative risk reduction of 30%) and a decrease in both continued or rebleeding rates (69%) and need for emergency surgery (62%).[1] Ulcers with minor SRH or a clean base have a much lower rate of rebleeding and do not benefit from endoscopic therapy. Other nonulcer lesions amenable to endoscopic therapy include select vascular malformations, Dieulafoy's lesion, and Mallory-Weiss tears. The two major complications of endoscopic therapy are the induction of bleeding (0.5%) and intestinal perforation (0.3%).

Prevention of Ulcer Rebleeding. Effective endoscopic hemostasis decreases the risk of acute rebleeding to approximately 10% to 20% in patients presenting with peptic ulcer hemorrhage. Repeat upper endoscopy and retreatment are reserved for patients with recurrent bleeding; permanent hemostasis is achieved in about 50% of these patients, for an overall endoscopic success rate of approximately 90%. Although no known pharmacologic intervention has been shown to reduce reliably the incidence of acute rebleeding in patients with peptic ulcer hemorrhage after endoscopic hemostasis, acid-suppressive medication, eradication of *Helicobacter pylori,*[10] and cessation of NSAIDs greatly reduce delayed rebleeding. The presence of *H. pylori* is determined at the initial EGD, with gastric biopsy for rapid urease testing or histologic examination, or subsequently with noninvasive breath testing or serology. Follow-up endoscopy is recommended to document healing, exclude malignancy, and assess for *H. pylori* eradication in patients with bleeding from a gastric ulcer. The less expensive and noninvasive breath testing alone is recommended 4 to 6 weeks after completion of antimicrobial therapy for bleeding duodenal ulcer disease. Antisecretory therapy is continued until *H. pylori* eradication is documented. Although previously recommended for all peptic ulcer–related bleeds, maintenance antisecretory therapy should be restricted to select patients, including ulcer patients not infected with *H. pylori,* those with failed *H. pylori* eradication, and successfully treated patients who are likely to tolerate poorly recurrent hemorrhage because of concurrent illness. Patients with *H. pylori* infection and a history of NSAID use should have both problems corrected; when therapy is successful, maintenance ulcer therapy generally is not recommended. Although eradication of *H. pylori* infection would also seem to decrease the risk of delayed recurrent hemorrhage in patients continuing to use NSAIDs, the extent of this reduction has not been evaluated. Patients still requiring NSAIDs should receive long-term prophylactic therapy with misoprostol or preferably a PPI and then a selective cyclooxygenase II (COX-II) inhibitor.

Angiographic Intervention. Angiographic therapy is used infrequently to treat patients with UGI bleeding and should be considered only for severe, persistent bleeding if surgery confers a high risk and endoscopic therapy is not available or has been unsuccessful. Uncontrolled studies suggest that arterial embolization with absorbable gelatin sponge (Gelfoam) and autologous clot or with nonabsorbable polyvinyl alcohol and sponge-wire coils may control bleeding identified angiographically in 75% to 80% of patients, although recurrent bleeding may occur in more than half. Alternatively, selective intraarterial vasopressin infusion may temporarily stop bleeding in up to 50% of patients. Complications of angiographic therapy include allergic reactions, renal insufficiency, ischemia, and perforation in target and nontarget organs.

Emergency Surgery. All patients with UGI bleeding severe enough to cause significant hemodynamic instability that requires ICU admission warrant evaluation by a surgeon. Criteria for emergency surgery include (1) failure to control bleeding with nonoperative means; (2) severe rebleeding despite two attempts at endoscopic hemostasis; (3) a lesion inaccessible to endoscopy because of prior surgery, anatomic anomaly, or pyloric stenosis; (4) severe shock when emergent surgery may prevent exsanguination; and (5) a severe complication of endoscopic therapy (e.g., perforation, worsening bleeding lesion).

ACUTE LOWER GI BLEEDING[12]

It is helpful to divide the common causes of lower GI bleeding by age and clinical presentation, since knowledge of the etiology helps plan optimal management (Tables 109-3 and 109-4). After initial evaluation and volume resuscitation, further management depends on the results of an NG tube aspirate. About 1000 ml or more of blood is required to cause hematochezia from an upper source, and hemodynamic compromise is typically an accompanying feature. If copious nonbloody bile is seen on NG aspiration, the physician should proceed directly to a colonoscopy. In all other cases, however, the colonoscopy should be preceded by an EGD because as many as 10% to 15% of patients with suspected lower GI bleeding have a UGI source. The diagnostic yield from colonoscopy ranges from 60% to 80%. Timing of endoscopy has not been systematically studied but should be performed as soon as possible in patients with continuous hematochezia. Patients who have stopped bleeding can undergo examination on a semielective basis.

The three outcomes to colonoscopy are source identification, negative examination, or incomplete colonoscopy secondary to severe bleeding. If identified, the source of bleeding should be treated appropriately. If the examination is unsuccessful in identifying the source because the bleeding is sudden and intermittent or is severe, arteriography is indicated. In some patients a bleeding scan is an appropriate initial step before arteriography. Abdominal scintigraphy plays a limited diagnostic role, however, because it requires active bleeding, is often obscured by liver and spleen tracer uptake, and does not provide information on the nature of the bleeding site. Angiography may be helpful when bleeding is active and has not been localized endoscopically. The bleeding must be arterial and at least 0.5 ml per minute. A negative colonoscopy and arteriographic study may require further evaluation with a Meckel's scan, small bowel enteroscopy, or a repeat colonoscopy if bleeding recurs. A Meckel's scan with technetium-99m pertechnetate should be considered in young patients to exclude Meckel's diverticulum. If bleeding has ceased, contrast radiography to evaluate

Table 109-3. Age and Clinical Presentation of Lower Gastrointestinal Bleeding

Clinical presentation	Child	Young adult	Middle-age adult	Elderly
Abdominal pain	IBD, intussusception	IBD	IBD	Ischemia
Painless bleeding	Meckel's juvenile polyp	Meckel's diverticulum	Diverticulosis, polyp, malignancy	Angiodysplasia, diverticulosis, polyp, malignancy
Diarrhea	IBD, infection	IBD, infection	IBD, infection	Ischemia, infection
Constipation/dyschezia	Fissures	Hemorrhoids, fissures, rectal ulcers	Hemorrhoids, fissures	Malignancy, hemorrhoids, fissures

IBD, Inflammatory bowel disease.

Table 109-4. Common Causes of Lower Gastrointestinal Bleeding

Lesion	Prevalence (%)	Comments
Diverticular disease	17-40	80% are self-limited.
Colonic vascular ectasia	2-30	Frequency varies widely in clinical series. Source tends to be proximal colon in acute bleeding.
Colitis (ischemic, infectious), IBD, radiation proctopathy	9-21	Ischemic colitis often presents with pain and limited hematochezia. Bloody diarrhea is most common symptom of infectious colitis and IBD.
Colonic neoplasia, postpolypectomy bleed	11-14	Postpolypectomy bleeds are usually self-limited and tend to occur 7-14 days after polypectomy.
Anorectal causes	4-10	Proctoscopy can be helpful in initial evaluation.
UGI source	0-11	Although bilious nasogastric aspirate makes UGI source unlikely, it cannot totally eliminate UGI tract as source.
Small bowel source (Crohn's ileitis, Meckel's diverticulum, vascular ectasia, tumors)	2-9	Diagnosis is often made by radiologic studies and enteroscopy after acute bleed has resolved.

IBD, Inflammatory bowel disease; *UGI*, upper gastrointestinal.

for small bowel pathology with enteroclysis is preferred to standard barium small bowel series because of greater sensitivity. The technique requires intubation of the small bowel to the duodenojejunal junction, with controlled infusion of barium, methylcellulose, and water to achieve a double-contrast effect. If the results of small bowel studies are negative and the blood loss is self-limited or maintained by oral iron supplementation, further evaluation may not be necessary. Surgery is reserved for treatment of a defined site of hemorrhage or for diagnostic purposes when combined with intraoperative endoscopy.

CHRONIC GASTROINTESTINAL HEMORRHAGE

Occult Bleeding[9]

The most common presentation of occult GI bleeding includes a positive fecal occult blood test with or without concomitant iron deficiency anemia. Although fecal occult blood tests were designed as a screening test for colorectal carcinoma, they are used to obtain evidence of blood loss in any acute or chronic bleeding lesion. The standard workup for occult GI blood loss in the adult population is to perform a colonoscopy. In the presence of UGI symptoms or iron deficiency anemia, a negative colonoscopy should be followed by an EGD.

Obscure Bleeding

Obscure bleeding is defined as active or recurrent hemorrhage that evades diagnosis on routine endoscopic and radiologic evaluation. It has an estimated prevalence of 5% to 10% in patients with GI bleeding. A wide range of diagnostic studies are available for evaluating bleeding of obscure origin, and the choice depends on severity of bleeding and availability of endoscopic, radiologic, and surgical expertise. Initially, standard UGI endoscopy should be repeated, particularly if blood prevented adequate mucosal inspection, since missed lesions account for a significant proportion of identified lesions on subsequent enteroscopy evaluation. Patients with massive or acute recurrent bleeding require a more invasive approach, including small bowel enteroscopy and angiography. Small bowel enteroscopy can be accomplished with push, sonde, or intraoperative techniques.[5,11] *Push enteroscopy* permits inspection of the entire duodenum and proximal jejunum to a level 40 to 50 cm beyond the ligament of Treitz. *Sonde enteroscopy* or intraoperative techniques examine the length of small intestine to the level of the terminal ileum. An etiology of bleeding can be determined in up to 35% of cases evaluated. Most patients with a small bowel source have bleeding from vascular malformations, but other lesions occasionally can be identified, including celiac disease, tumor, and occult IBD.

REFERENCES

1. Cook DJ, Giuatt GH, Salena BJ, Laine LA: Endoscopic therapy for acute nonvariceal upper gastrointestinal hemorrhage: a meta-analysis, *Gastroenterology* 102:139, 1992.
2. Khuroo MS, Yattoo GN, Javid G, et al: A comparison of omeprazole and placebo for bleeding peptic ulcer, *N Engl J Med* 336:1054, 1997.
3. Lai KC, Hui WM, Wong BCU, et al: A retrospective and prospective study on the safety of discharging selected patients with duodenal ulcer bleeding on the same day as endoscopy, *Gastrointest Endosc* 45:26, 1997.
4. Laine L, Peterson WL: Bleeding peptic ulcer, *N Engl J Med* 331:717, 1994.
5. Lewis BS: Small intestinal bleeding, *Gastroenterol Clin North Am* 23:67, 1994.
6. Lin H-J, Low W-C, Lee F-Y, et al: A prospective randomized comparative trial showing that omeprazole prevents rebleeding in patients with bleeding peptic ulcer after successful endoscopic therapy, *Arch Intern Med* 158:54, 1998.
7. Longstreth GF, Feitelberg SP: Successful outpatient management of acute upper gastrointestinal hemorrhage: use of practice guidelines in a large patient series, *Gastrointest Endosc* 47:219, 1998.
8. NIH Consensus Conference: Therapeutic endoscopy and bleeding ulcers, *JAMA* 262:1369, 1989.

8a. Patchett SE, Enright H, Afdhal N, et al: Clot lysis by gastric juice: an in vitro study, *Gut* 30:1704, 1989.

9. Rockey DC: Occult gastrointestinal bleeding, *N Engl J Med* 341:38, 1999.
10. Rokkas T, Karameris A, Mavrogeorgis A, et al: Eradication of *Helicobacter pylori* reduces the possibility of rebleeding in peptic ulcer disease, *Gastrointest Endosc* 41:1, 1995.
11. Waye JD: Enteroscopy, *Gastrointest Endosc* 46:247, 1997.
12. Zuccaro G Jr: Management of the adult patient with acute lower gastrointestinal bleeding, *Am J Gastroenterol* 93:1202, 1998.

CHAPTER 110

Functional Gastrointestinal Disease

Richard I. Rothstein

Functional gastrointestinal diseases consist of varying combinations of chronic or recurrent symptoms with no identifiable physiologic, biochemical, infectious, anatomic, or structural cause. These disorders comprise a large percentage of primary care patient visits and account for about 40% of visits to gastroenterologists. A random survey of the U.S. population revealed that 69% reported having at least one of 20 defined functional gastrointestinal (GI) symptoms during the previous 3 months. With significant overlap, symptoms were attributed to four major regions: esophagus (42%), gastroduodenum (26%), bowel (44%), and anorectum (26%). In general, symptom reporting declined with increasing age, and low socioeconomic status was associated with increased symptom reporting. The rate of physician visits and work or school absenteeism was increased for those having a functional GI disorder.

The functional GI disorders encompass those related to the esophagus (globus, rumination, atypical chest pain), gastroduodenum (nonulcer dyspepsia, aerophagia), bowel (irritable bowel syndrome, chronic constipation, painless diarrhea, bloating/excessive gas, chronic abdominal pain), pancreaticobiliary tree (pancreaticobiliary dyskinesia, pancreatitis), and anorectum (proctalgia fugax, levator syndrome). The unifying pathophysiology for functional GI disorders is probably a primary disorder of gut motility. With no specific gold standard to assist in identification, these disorders require comprehensive histories, physical examinations, and laboratory studies. Diagnostic criteria for functional disorders based on epidemiologic and clinical research have enhanced diagnostic certainty and the ability to make a positive diagnosis rather than a diagnosis of exclusion.

The functional GI diseases share similar biopsychosocial models and a close relationship of psychophysiologic effect. Stress, anxiety, depression, and heightened emotional states affect symptom production and response (Fig. 110-1). The seeking of medical attention for functional symptoms may be prompted by increased frequency or severity of symptoms, reduced coping mechanisms or concomitant illness, or fear of serious illness. Individuals with functional complaints who seek medical attention have significant psychiatric disorders more frequently diagnosed than those who do not seek care. Psychologic factors influence the decision to seek health care, and examining the motivation for an office visit is a key step in evaluation and management.

IRRITABLE BOWEL SYNDROME

Some physicians use the term *irritable bowel syndrome* (IBS) to connote all the functional GI disorders, from globus to proctalgia fugax. IBS has provided a general diagnosis for complaints not attributable to organic disease. The shared

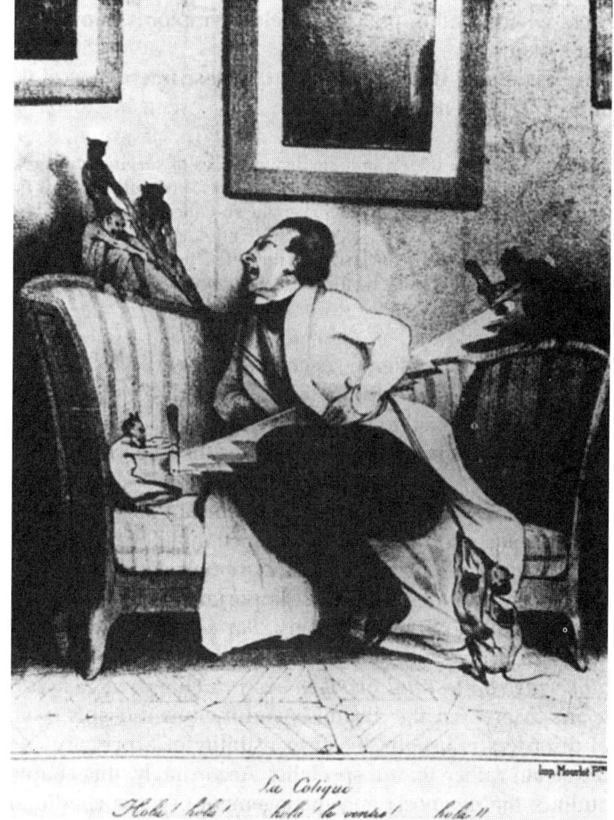

Fig. 110-1. *La colique*. Honoré Daumier, Paris, 1848.

Box 110-1. Rome Diagnostic Criteria for Irritable Bowel Syndrome (IBS)

Continuous or recurrent symptoms for at least 3 months
Abdominal pain, relieved by defecation or associated with changes of frequency or consistency of stool
An irregular pattern of defecation at least 25% of the time, with two or more of the following:
- Altered stool frequency
- Altered stool form (scybala or loose and watery)
- Altered stool passage (straining, urgency, feeling of incomplete evacuation)
- Passage of mucus, usually with bloating or feeling of abdominal distention

From Drossman DA et al: *Gastroenterol Int* 3:159, 1990.

similarities of the various functional syndromes in pathophysiology and presentation have suggested the concept of the irritable gut or irritable person syndrome, with symptoms arising principally from global physiologic changes that accompany emotional tension. IBS is defined as a functional GI disorder attributed to the intestine and includes chronic or recurrent abdominal pain, altered bowel habit (consistency, frequency, feeling of incomplete evacuation), abdominal bloating with feelings of excessive intestinal gas, and mucus in the stools. These symptoms are continuous or intermittent and should be present for at least 3 months (Box 110-1).

Epidemiology and Etiology

The syndrome of IBS occurs in 15% to 20% of adults, with a predominance among women in the United States (nearly 2:1) but a reported predominance among men in other parts of the world (e.g., India). In the United States, no difference exists among racial subgroups. Symptoms usually begin in young adulthood and persist throughout life, although intermittently. The childhood GI disorder of recurrent abdominal pain may be equivalent in symptoms and pathophysiology to IBS, and about one third of affected children have IBS in adulthood. Less than half the people with irritable bowel symptoms seek medical attention and become *patients* with IBS. The overall prevalence of IBS in a population remains stable, although dynamic shifting occurs, with some individuals becoming asymptomatic and others developing symptoms or having a recurrence.

Pathophysiology

Pain in the lower abdomen, relief of pain on defecation, and passage of scybala (pelletlike stools) implicate irritability of the distal colon as a principal mechanism of IBS. Sigmoid contractions are paradoxically increased in patients with symptoms of constipation, causing increased segmentation and decreased propulsive movement, with resultant scybala and distention. Segmental contractions may be decreased in diarrhea-prone patients, with more rapid intestinal transit time. Abdominal pain in IBS most likely arises from areas of intestinal distention occurring proximal to areas of spasm.

Altered myoelectric activity of the colon, with a higher proportion of slow waves in the frequency range of 2 to 4 cycles per minute, has been reported for patients with IBS. The specificity of this marker has been questioned, however, since it also occurs in psychoneurotic patients who have no bowel symptoms. Small intestinal transit is more rapid in diarrhea-prone IBS patients, whereas it is prolonged in those with constipation and abdominal pain or distention.

An altered sensation of visceral pain may occur in IBS, with a lowered threshold for gut distention. Balloon distention of the lower bowel provokes pain in patients with IBS at volumes that do not usually cause symptoms in controls. Patients with IBS frequently complain of bloating and increased gas; however, studies have shown that IBS patients have abdominal symptoms with the same or lower colonic gas volumes as nonsymptomatic controls. Balloon distention at various sites along the large or small bowel during colonoscopy or during the passage of a small bowel tube resulted in the exact reproduction of right upper quadrant pain in a group of patients initially thought to have gallbladder symptoms. All patients had negative screening tests for gallbladder disease. This possibly explains the return or persistence of symptoms in patients who undergo cholecystectomy for right upper quadrant pain suspected to be biliary in origin, who may have had a silent gallstone but noisy gut.

The pathophysiology of IBS involves the enteric nervous system, visceral smooth muscle, and neurohumoral control of gut function. Symptoms arise as the lower gut participates in the total-body response to emotional arousal, as part of the fight-or-flight emergency reactions. Release of neurotransmitters and interchange of information from the central nervous system to the enteric nervous system modulate the activity of the bowel and its irritability. Measured alterations in bowel motility occur in response to such stimuli as eating, stressful interviews, and acute psychologic or physical stress. Measurement of sigmoid motility during hypnosis, using an indwelling transrectal manometric catheter, has provided information about brain-gut emotional relationships, with the ability to isolate an emotion (e.g., hostility, anger, sadness) and its related manometric pattern. The prevalence of psychologic symptoms and psychoneurotic personality traits in patients with IBS is higher than in non-IBS controls and, importantly, higher than in those with IBS who do not seek medical care. Depression, somatization, and frequency of consulting a physician for minor complaints (learned illness behavior) are found more frequently in patients than nonpatients with IBS. These psychologic factors relate to the health care–seeking behavior in patients with IBS and not to the illness itself. Patients presenting to primary care practices may demonstrate less somatization than those referred to gastroenterologists, although mood disturbances are often present in IBS patients visiting primary care settings.

The patient's total dependency needs must be recognized, including attitude toward illness and the sick role. Surveys of IBS patients and matched controls have shown that childhood physical, emotional, and sexual abuse occurred more often in IBS patients and that abuse was not confined to women. Childhood sexual abuse was associated with findings of depression, increased medical visits, and multiple somatic complaints in IBS patients.

Clinical Presentation and Patient Evaluation

A wide range of symptoms prompts the division of IBS into symptom-predominant subtypes, although it may be best considered as a single entity with variable manifestations. Patients who offer one of the predominant IBS symptoms (pain, constipation, diarrhea) as their chief complaint usually have all three symptoms after rigorous history taking and stool inspection. Dyspepsia, without organic explanation, affects most patients with IBS, and symptoms of esophageal dysfunction occur in 50%. The noncolonic GI symptoms of nausea, vomiting, dysphagia, and early satiety were found more often in IBS patients than in matched controls. In two studies of IBS patients and age-matched controls who were 90% to 100% female and middle aged, anxiety, fatigability, hostile feelings, sadness, and sleep disturbances were reported more often in the IBS group, as were palpitations, hand tremor, and fear of serious disease. Bladder dysfunction symptoms (nocturia, frequency and urgency of micturition, feeling of incomplete bladder emptying) were present more often in the IBS patients, as were the symptoms of back pain, unpleasant taste in the mouth, constant feelings of tiredness, and dyspareunia. This range of symptom reporting represents global physiologic responses and heightened emotional arousal.

The usual patient with IBS has had at least months of symptoms, and many relate a lifelong history of altered bowel habits and abdominal distress. New onset of IBS symptoms in an elderly patient should prompt a thorough examination for organic etiology, although prevalence of functional symptoms may be level throughout all age groups. Patients may describe the initial passage of a formed bowel movement, possibly after straining, with a sense of incomplete evacuation. Subsequent need to defecate results in several looser bowel movements, which may be described as diarrhea. Other patients may relate the passage of pelletlike stools and a changing frequency of bowel habits. IBS patients may report alterations in stool consistency, color, and shape. Patients may have long periods of normal stool habits and no abdominal symptoms, only to develop sudden recurrence of symptoms. Crampy lower abdominal pain, usually on the left, may be worsened or precipitated by eating (gastrocolic reflex); it is relieved, perhaps only transiently, by passage of flatus or stool. Some patients complain of bloating and being full of gas with variable increases in eructation or passage of flatus, although most do not have demonstrable changes in abdominal girth. Occasional patients have abdominal protrusion caused by contraction of the diaphragm and lumbar muscles.

Female patients may relate exacerbations of symptoms to phases of their menstrual cycle, with exacerbation of diarrhea often occurring during menstrual or premenstrual phases. About half of IBS patients may describe episodes of fecal or mucous incontinence, and many complain of stool urgency. Sleep disturbances may relate to exacerbation of symptoms. A history of rectal bleeding, weight loss, fever, and nocturnal diarrhea or pain awakening the patient from sleep is not part of IBS and should prompt investigation for other causes. Although bleeding may result from hemorrhoids or an anal fissure caused by straining from constipation, bleeding is not part of IBS and should always be fully investigated.

The physical examination in patients with IBS is usually normal, although fullness and tenderness may be found during palpation of the left lower quadrant, associated with sigmoid colon spasm and distention. This finding is not specific for IBS and may occur in diverticular disease. The digital rectal examination can help determine stool character.

Box 110-2. Manifestations and Associated Features of IBS

Key Features

Abdominal pain; relief with defecation
Irregular bowel habits with alternating diarrhea and constipation
Feeling of incomplete bowel evacuation
Passage of mucus
Bloating with abdominal distention
Absence of weight loss
Absence of rectal bleeding
Left lower abdominal tenderness to palpation

Common Associated Features

Dyspepsia, nausea, heartburn, dysphagia
Fatigability, sleep disturbances, sadness, anxiety
Fear of serious disease
Bladder dysfunction symptoms, back pain
Multiple abdominal surgical procedures

Patients with a chief complaint of diarrhea may have formed, hard scybalous stool in the rectal vault; an empty rectum can be found in constipated patients. A careful bimanual pelvic examination should be done for female patients with lower abdominopelvic pain to check for a possible gynecologic cause of symptoms (Box 110-2).

Laboratory Studies and Diagnostic Procedures

The range of symptoms of IBS encompasses those found in the organic diseases that form its differential diagnosis. Abdominal pain and altered bowel habit are common symptoms in a variety of GI illnesses, and a review of the disorders that produce symptoms of IBS should always be undertaken. When diarrhea is a predominant symptom, stool samples should be analyzed for fecal leukocytes and ova and parasites to check for infectious or inflammatory colitis. Depending on the specific clinical situation, a stool culture for enteric pathogens and assay for *Clostridium difficile* toxin may be sent. The stool *Giardia* antigen immunoassay requires only one sample and has excellent sensitivity and specificity.

In most patients, flexible sigmoidoscopy and stool analysis for occult blood are necessary diagnostic tests. Biopsy of the bowel mucosa to check for microscopic or collagenous colitis or possible mast cell disease may be considered. Young patients with infrequent symptoms and good response to initial treatments do not require endoscopic examination of the lower bowel. Those with diarrhea or who do not improve with initial treatment should undergo this procedure. Reproduction of the patient's usual abdominal pain during air insufflation of the sigmoid and its reduction with removal of the air and endoscope are typically elicited in IBS patients undergoing sigmoidoscopy. Any patient with rectal bleeding requires lower GI endoscopy because hematochezia is not part of IBS, and its source must be determined.

Lactose intolerance should be considered, since it may result in altered bowel habit, bloating, and excess intestinal gas and can be easily identified by the lactose hydrogen breath test or lactose tolerance test. An inexpensive lactose tolerance test involves asking the patient to drink a quart of milk at one sitting and record the ensuing gut symptoms, if any. This usually works better to identify lactose-related symptoms than the dairy-free diets sometimes recommended.

A complete blood cell count (CBC) is recommended to check for anemia or inflammation. Tests for thyroid disease, carcinoid, or other systemic disease are usually not done unless specific clinical indicators are present in the history or physical examination. Depending on the situation, barium enema studies or colonoscopy may be done to examine the proximal colon and ileocecal region. Localized pain and other features may dictate an ultrasound study of the gallbladder, liver, and pancreas; computed tomography (CT) scan of these organs; or imaging studies of the colon, as in suspected diverticulitis. Small bowel radiography may be done in patients with periumbilical pain and other symptoms possibly related to Crohn's disease. Some patients with constipation, especially those with laxative abuse or dependency, benefit from study of colonic transit, and those who complain of fecal incontinence may be studied with anorectal manometry. Dyspeptic patients may require upper GI radiography or endoscopy. Patients with unexplained diarrhea should have a stool sample alkalinized to check for phenolphthalein from surreptitious laxative abuse; a few drops of sodium hydroxide on a small stool smear results in a red color change if the laxative is present. Laxative abuse was the cause in about one third of patients who came to a tertiary medical center because of chronic diarrhea.

At present the minimal workup for IBS should include the history and physical examination of the stools, CBC, and in most patients, flexible sigmoidoscopy. Tests for lactose intolerance should be considered. Other possible tests should be reserved for specific clinical indicators based on patient age or should be done later if subsequent clinical information suggests alternative etiologies (Box 110-3).

Box 110-3. Laboratory and Diagnostic Tests for IBS

Initial

History: check for positive IBS features
Physical examination: include digital rectal examination
Complete blood count, stool guaiac test
Flexible sigmoidoscopy for most patients
Rule out lactose malabsorption

Subsequent or Symptom Directed

Stool analysis for leukocytes, ova and parasites
Stool for *Giardia* antigen, *C. difficile* toxin
Gastrointestinal radiography or ultrasound
Upper and lower gastrointestinal endoscopy
Blood studies for thyroid disease, other metabolic disorders
Colonic transit marker study, anorectal manometry
Alkalinization of the stool: check for laxative abuse

Differential Diagnosis

The symptoms of IBS are not specific for it. Abdominal distress with altered bowel habit may result from many conditions affecting the GI tract. Complaints of diarrhea should prompt a search for lactose intolerance, an extremely common condition that can result in loosening of bowels, increased bowel frequency, increased intestinal gas and passage of flatus, and feelings of bloating. The amount of lactose load determines symptoms, and patients should look for a relationship between dietary intake and gut symptoms. Prevalence of lactose intolerance ranges from about 6% in white Americans to 75% to 90% in groups of Native Americans, African-Americans, and Asian-Americans. No relationship exists between lactose intolerance and IBS, and since both occur with relative frequency, they will affect some individuals concomitantly. Tests for lactase deficiency should be done, and if confirmed, most patients are easily managed with lactase supplements without altering dairy intake. Other patients may need to reduce the total intake of lactose-containing foods.

Giardiasis, sprue, Crohn's disease, bacterial overgrowth, and other small bowel disorders should be considered. Food intolerance, different from true food allergy, can cause abdominal pain and diarrhea in patients who are often atopic. Food diaries to record intake and symptoms may assist in discovering food relationships. The history taking should include possible sorbitol ingestion from sugarless gums, candies, or soft drinks, since many adults have sorbitol intolerance because of excessive intake and may experience abdominal pain, cramping, bloating, and altered bowel habit.

Abdominal symptoms arising from peptic ulcer disease or gallbladder disease are not generally accompanied by altered bowel habit and should not usually be confused with IBS. Upper GI radiography or abdominal ultrasound should be reserved for patients with an unclear clinical picture. Inflammatory bowel disease, and less often, infectious colitis, may give rise to symptoms simulating IBS. The common feature of hematochezia in ulcerative colitis separates it from IBS, which lacks rectal bleeding. Collagenous colitis, microscopic colitis, and eosinophilic gastroenteritis are unusual disorders with features overlapping those of IBS, with chronic diarrhea and abdominal discomfort predominating. Symptoms of diarrhea, abdominal pain, urinary frequency, headache, flushing, hives, and dermatographia are seen in some patients with mast cell–mediated disease, and increased numbers of mast cells may be found in colonic or terminal ileal mucosal biopsies. Lower abdominal pain may arise from pelvic processes (e.g., ovarian cysts, pelvic inflammatory disease, endometriosis) and can be investigated with pelvic examination, ultrasound, or CT scan.

Constipation may result from anatomic obstruction (e.g., bowel malignancy), a medication side effect, or sigmoid spasm in diverticulosis. It may be part of idiopathic pseudoobstruction, Hirschsprung's disease, or a sequela of laxative abuse. Sigmoidoscopy allows screening for luminally obstructing processes, the presence of diverticulosis, or melanosis coli (resulting from laxative abuse). Since the pathophysiology of colonic diverticulosis involves sigmoid spasm and segmentation, some patients with diverticulosis have symptoms similar to those of IBS patients, and the two disorders may coexist. The majority of patients with diverticulosis are asymptomatic. Patients with constipation and abdominal symptoms since infancy should be considered for anorectal manometry to determine the presence of reflex internal sphincter relaxation, which is absent in Hirschsprung's disease.

The physician must avoid extensive, expensive, repetitive, or hazardous workups in approaching an IBS diagnosis as a

Table 110-1. Differential Diagnosis of IBS

Condition	Evaluation
Lactose intolerance	Tests of lactase deficiency
Giardiasis	Stool O&P, *Giardia* antigen
Sprue, other mucosal diseases	Malabsorptive tests, small bowel biopsy
Crohn's disease	Small bowel radiography
Bacterial overgrowth	Lactulose hydrogen breath test
Food intolerance	Food diaries and avoidance
Sorbitol intolerance	Dietary elimination
Hyperthyroidism	Thyroid function tests
Peptic ulcer disease	Upper GI radiography/ endoscopy
Gallbladder disease	Abdominal ultrasound, ERCP
Inflammatory bowel disease	Endoscopy, mucosal biopsy, barium enema
Infectious colitis	Stool O&P, culture, *Clostridium difficile* toxin
Mast cell disease	Rectal biopsy
Painful diverticulosis	Flexible sigmoidoscopy
Diverticulitis	Abdominal CT scan
Laxative abuse	Alkalinization of stool for phenolphthalein
Abdominal angina	Doppler ultrasound to check vascular flow
Gynecologic disorders	Pelvic examination, ultrasound, CT scan
Bowel neoplasia	Flexible endoscopy, barium radiography
Hirschsprung's disease	Anorectal manometry, rectal biopsy
Intestinal pseudoobstruction	Colonic transit marker studies

O&P, Ova and parasites; *CT,* computed tomography; *ERCP,* endoscopic retrograde cholangiopancreatography.

diagnosis of exclusion. Using a strict definition for IBS and following a limited workup, investigators have shown that a positive diagnosis can be made with excellent reliability. Positive historic features favoring the functional diagnosis of IBS include (1) pain eased by a bowel movement, (2) looser stools and more frequent bowel movements at onset of pain and abdominal distention, (3) scybala, (4) diarrhea alternating with constipation, (5) passage of mucus, and (6) absence of weight loss. A normal screening CBC and flexible sigmoidoscopy confirm the diagnosis. Rectal bleeding, fever, anemia, evidence of malnutrition, and other atypical features in presentation or laboratory findings are not part of the IBS and should prompt investigation into the differential diagnosis (Table 110-1).

Management

The physician-patient relationship is important in caring for patients with IBS. A willingness to provide ongoing care, with appropriate consultation as indicated, is prerequisite for successful management. Many patients search for an explanation of their symptoms and might be shunted around a primary care physician as multiple specialists do extensive medical investigations or invasive surgery.

The initial encounters should provide adequate time for exploration of symptoms and explanation of GI function and dysfunction. Some patients are able to correlate the onset or recurrence of symptoms with critical or stressful life events. Many IBS patients demonstrate excessive somatic focusing and more health-related fears, a common feature of patients in referral practices. They complain of more nongastrointestinal symptoms and more frequently utilize health care services than their IBS counterparts who tolerate their symptoms without consulting a physician. This illness behavior may be based on familial factors, such as learning a sick role, being reinforced for symptoms, or even undergoing physical or sexual abuse. A significant minority of patients meet the criteria for a psychiatric illness (e.g., depression, anxiety, somatoform disorder, posttraumatic stress disorder), which should be recognized and managed. IBS patients in primary care practices may demonstrate less chronic somatization than those in referral gastroenterology practices, although mood disorders are common in IBS patients at primary care sites.

A positive diagnosis of IBS must be established beginning with the first encounter if it appears to be the reason for the patient's symptoms. Confidence minimizes the desire for more testing "to be sure no other hidden disease exists" to explain the symptoms. Scheduling return visits demonstrates an ongoing interest, and follow-up encounters enable the assessment of changes in clinical features and response to treatment. As the clinical course progresses, less frequent and shorter appointments are needed as the patient responds to treatment and gains an understanding of the disease.

The impact of irritable bowel symptoms on the quality of a patient's life is often underrecognized or insufficiently explored. In a group of patients, two thirds of whom were female with a mean age of 45 and mean duration of symptoms of 7 years, the reported areas impacting quality of life were activities and schedules, diet and nutrition, lack of social support and interpersonal relationships, and mood changes. Patients were concerned about not being taken seriously, being told "it's in your head," undergoing many tests without adequate explanation, and a perceived lack of physician concern for their symptoms. Many of these issues are easily avoided through adequate patient education and empathic listening. Failure to attend to these issues contributes to "doctor shopping" and alternative health care venues.

Management of IBS may involve dietary, pharmacologic, and psychologic intervention (Box 110-4). The intermittent nature of IBS directs intervention to symptomatic relapses and to strategies for management of its chronic forms. Patients with IBS have a marked placebo response rate, and many interventions appear successful, at least initially. Patients need to be reassured that the disorder is benign, waxes and wanes, has an excellent prognosis, and is not related to colon cancer. Although most patients respond to reassurance and supportive therapy, along with symptom-specific medical treatment, some require frequent telephone or office contact. The dependency issues in these patients are related to their more common psychopathology, especially neuroticism and hypochondriasis. When psychiatric disease is identified in IBS patients, appropriate referral is indicated.

Specific dietary recommendations involve lactose avoidance for IBS patients who also have lactase deficiency, or they may use lactase supplements when eating foods containing dairy products. Yogurt and aged cheeses may be better tolerated because lactose is diminished by the

Box 110-4. Management of IBS

Key is ongoing supportive physician-patient relationship. Therapy is directed to initial predominant symptom.

Abdominal Pain

Anticholinergics: hyoscyamine, 0.125-mg tablets 20 minutes ac and hs; dicyclomine, 20 mg qid
Anticholinergics/anxiolytics: clidinium, 2.5 mg, with chlordiazepoxide, 5 mg 20 minutes ac and hs; hyoscyamine, atropine, scopolamine with phenobarbital, 16.2 mg tid to qid
Tricyclic antidepressants: amitriptyline, 50-100 mg hs
Behavioral therapy, psychotherapy, hypnotherapy

Diarrhea

Antidiarrheals: loperamide, 2 mg bid to qid prn; diphenoxylate, 2.5 mg, with atropine, 0.025 mg qid prn
Fiber: bran, psyllium seed husk, methylcellulose daily to tid
Calcium, cholestyramine, cholestipol
Tricyclic antidepressants
Psychotherapy, hypnotherapy, behavioral therapy
Alosetron, 1 mg bid

Constipation

Fiber, fluids, exercise
Occasional stool softeners
Lactulose, colonoscopy prep solution (rarely)

Gaseousness and Bloating

Lactase supplement/lactose reduction in lactose intolerance
Food diaries to correlate symptoms and dietary intake
Avoidance of specific offending dietary components
Trial of activated charcoal with meals

ac, Before meals; *hs*, at bedtime; *qid*, four times daily; *tid*, three times daily; *prn*, as needed; *bid*, twice a day.

microbial action in those products. Specific foods that trigger symptoms should be avoided. For some patients with either constipation or diarrhea, bulking the stools with fiber may be helpful through increased bran in the diet. A significant number of patients are intolerant of excessive bran, however, and develop bloating and increased intestinal gas. The fiber supplements of hydrophilic colloid (psyllium, methylcellulose) may be better tolerated and can be ingested as liquids, tablets, or even cookies. Patients with constipation and those taking fiber supplements should be encouraged to drink at least 2 quarts of fluid each day. Bland or restrictive diets do not generally benefit the IBS patient and may be harmful over time.

Although patients with an initial complaint of constipation, diarrhea, or abdominal pain have all three identified after careful questioning and physical examination, medication therapy should focus on the chief complaint. Patients with abdominal cramps or spastic abdominal pain may obtain benefit from anticholinergic agents, which function to diminish sigmoid contractility and decrease intestinal distention occurring proximally. Hyoscyamine and dicyclomine are frequently prescribed for this effect, and patients need to be aware of the side effects of dry mouth, dizziness, and possible blurred vision. Anticholinergics coupled with minor tranquilizers (e.g., phenobarbital, chlordiazepoxide) may be of benefit for patients with anxiety, although controlled trials demonstrating clinical efficacy are lacking. The natural antispasmodic peppermint oil may be of benefit; its encapsulation allows dissolution distal to the stomach to avoid the possible side effect of pyrosis, caused by lowering of esophageal sphincter tone if the oil is released at a higher level. Tricyclic antidepressants can help manage symptoms of abdominal pain, perhaps because of their anticholinergic effect and central effects.

Diarrhea may be controlled with diphenoxylate or loperamide; the latter is particularly useful with concomitant fecal incontinence. Some patients benefit from stool bulking to solidify their looser stools; calcium supplements are potentially useful, as are cholestyramine and cholestipol. Although diarrhea may not be fully controlled with these measures, urgency and frequency may be reduced. Some patients with diarrhea may also benefit from treatment with the tricyclic antidepressants. Long-term use of paregoric or codeine is not recommended. The new $5HT_3$ antagonist, Alosetron, has been shown to be of benefit in diarrhea-predominant women with IBS.

Constipation in IBS usually responds to bulking agents, increased fluids, and exercise. Stool softeners (dioctyl sodium sulfosuccinate) are of occasional benefit, but patients should be counseled to avoid long-term use of laxatives. Infrequently a patient may require treatment with lactulose or polyethylene glycol and electrolytes (colonoscopy prep solution) to enhance colonic transit. Initial use of enemas may help wean a patient from laxative use.

For patients with intestinal gas or bloating, specific food avoidance (e.g., leguminous vegetables, beans) may be of benefit. The yeast-derived enzyme food supplement Beano, marketed to diminish intestinal gas production, is not likely to offer benefit, nor will simethicone products, whose target is gas bubble dissolution in the upper GI tract. Activated charcoal capsules taken with meals can reduce intestinal fermentation and gas production, although patients should be advised that charcoal will darken their stools.

Psychotherapy, behavioral therapy, and hypnotherapy offer alternative approaches or can assist in management of the IBS patient. Compared with continued medical therapy, dynamically oriented short-term psychotherapy is more likely to reduce abdominal pain and bowel dysfunction. Patients refractory to at least six different therapeutic regimens over a year or more had significantly improved symptoms of abdominal pain and bowel irregularity after hypnosis compared with medically treated controls. The improvement persisted in long-term follow-up and in patients who underwent group hypnotherapy. Behavioral therapies such as biofeedback have met with mixed success and may be considered.

The future management of IBS may include therapies directed at neuroendocrine manipulation (e.g., leuprolide, 5HT-receptor antagonists) or prokinetic motility stimulation, but further clinical evaluation is needed. No one management strategy works for all patients. Directing therapy at the initial or chief complaint should effect symptom relief and may permit identification and modification of stressful situations. Patients need to be educated about the relationship of IBS symptoms to diet and stress. Although most patients with IBS can be managed completely in a primary care practice, referral to a gastroenterologist should occur when endoscopic examination is anticipated, when the patient fails to respond to initial therapies, for second opinions, and for periodic follow-up assessments. The primary care physician serves a critical role as health adviser and counselor for the patient with IBS, and the most important tool of management is the ongoing, supportive physician-patient relationship.

GLOBUS

The sensation of a lump or ball in the throat that occurs independently of the act of swallowing is called globus. Typically this sensation is present all the time and seems to interfere with swallowing and breathing. Often the onset may follow a swallowing event in which the patient believes a food item may have gotten stuck or caused irritation, such as a fishbone or seed. Many individuals with globus sensation relate significant stress or anxiety as a precipitant to symptom onset. Globus can be a common complaint; it was experienced by about one third of patients with IBS, was present in 18% of a control group of women in a gynecology clinic, and accounted for 4% of new otolaryngologic clinic appointments. In younger patients, globus was three times more prevalent in women than men, but after age 50 the prevalence is equal.

Although its pathophysiology is not understood, globus sensation is presumably caused by cricopharyngeal spasm, which may occur during heightened emotional arousal. A tense individual may become aware of the previously subconscious act of swallowing; coupled with anxiety-related reduction of saliva, this may result in further tension and spasm. Manometric studies to document increased cricopharyngeal tone have been contradictory. In about one fourth of globus patients, abnormal gastroesophageal reflux may be present, although the nature of its association or its relationship to symptoms is not clear.

Globus should be differentiated from true dysphagia, which may be high, with difficulties in initiating a swallow, or may be low, with the typical symptom of food or pills lodging substernally in the esophagus. A careful history allows separation of globus from dysphagia, the latter occurring only with swallow attempts (Table 110-2). If high or low dysphagia is suspected, investigation should identify an anatomic obstruction or motility disorder. Barium radiography, laryngoscopy, upper GI endoscopy, esophageal manometry, and other specialized tests may identify oropharyngeal or cricopharyngeal disorders, esophageal stenosis from ring or stricture, or possible motility disorder. The workup for globus may involve cineradiography to evaluate the swallowing function and to provide reassurance. Globus sensation may occur in some patients with reflux esophagitis.

Management of the globus sensation requires adequate explanation of the mechanism of symptom production and reassurance. Some patients with gastroesophageal reflux disease (GERD) may benefit from acid suppression or prokinetic agents. Treatment of globus sensation is often difficult, and recurrence is common. Determining stressful trigger events and providing supportive therapy may be helpful. Some patients benefit from treatment with antidepressants, behavioral therapy, or psychotherapy.

RUMINATION

Rumination, also called *merycism,* involves painless regurgitation of swallowed food into the mouth. The regurgitated food is rechewed and reswallowed; this behavior does not upset the individual, who considers the regurgitated material pleasant tasting. The process is involuntary, usually begins shortly after meals, lasts about a half hour, and decreases as the regurgitant material changes its taste from increased acidity. In contrast to vomiting, rumination is not associated with nausea. In contrast to GERD, patients have no pain. The motility of the esophagus and stomach is normal in ruminators. The habit begins in childhood, sometimes persisting into adulthood. Although this behavior is unusual, within certain families it may be fully acceptable, with familial ruminators developing in several generations. Rumination appears to be a learned behavior and is upsetting to the patient only when it results in social embarrassment. It is important to distinguish rumination from vomiting or GERD to avoid unnecessary treatments. Some ruminant patients respond to behavioral therapies.

Table 110-2. Comparison of Globus and Dysphagia

Findings	Globus sensation	Dysphagia
Timing	Not related to swallow	With swallowing
Location	Upper chest, throat	Neck, esophagus
Associated symptoms	Difficulty breathing, anxiety	Regurgitation, weight loss
Psychologic stress	Common	Uncommon
Barium x-ray endoscopy	Normal	Usually abnormal

ATYPICAL CHEST PAIN

Patients with chest pain are regularly evaluated in primary care practices and emergency departments. Diagnosing possible coronary artery disease is the first step in the evaluation of chest pain, resulting in about 600,000 coronary arteriograms annually in the United States. With up to one third of these examinations having normal results, about 200,000 new cases of noncardiac chest pain are diagnosed each year. The number is actually higher, since younger patients or those without classic anginal symptoms do not undergo catheterization. Within this group of noncardiac chest pain patients, about one third have an esophageal cause of the pain after investigation, with GERD a more common finding than esophageal dysmotility or spasm. Noncardiac chest pain assumes the exclusion of valvular heart disease and pericarditis; disorders of the lung or pleura (tumor, pleurisy) and chest wall conditions of musculoskeletal origin (costochondritis) are part of the differential diagnosis.

The term *chest pain of unknown origin* (CPUO) is used to describe a chest pain syndrome without a discernible cause. The pain is often atypical for classic angina. Patients with CPUO have a high prevalence of anxiety disorders, depression, somatization, and perceived vulnerability to serious heart disease. High levels of neuroticism and poor coping strategies are found in some CPUO patients, with less symptom improvement, more frequent pain episodes, and greater social maladjustment. Patients with CPUO may have a lower threshold to visceral sensation and may interpret normal physiologic events as uncomfortable. Studies incorporating balloon inflation in the esophagus show that CPUO patients experience chest discomfort at significantly smaller balloon volumes than do asymptomatic volunteers. The pathophysiology of CPUO may parallel that for IBS, with a lowered threshold to visceral stimulation (sensing distention above an area of spasm), induction of abnormal motility during acutely stressful stimulation, a close relationship with emotional arousal, and similar psychometric profiles for personality characteristics. About one third of CPUO patients have panic disorder, with features of tachycardia, sweating, dyspnea, dizziness, hot flashes, nausea, choking, trembling, depersonalization, paresthesias, fear of dying, or fear of "going crazy."

The diagnostic investigation for a patient with chest pain involves a careful history and physical examination (checking for chest wall tenderness), an electrocardiogram (ECG), and a chest radiograph. Echocardiography may be indicated, and treadmill exercise tolerance testing evaluates for a possible cardiac origin of symptoms. Some patients need referral to cardiologists for assessment and coronary catheterization. Microvascular angina (syndrome X) may be diagnosed during atrially paced coronary catheterization, as may coronary spasm during ergonovine stimulation. When coronary disease is ruled out as the cause of chest pain, or if the pain is accompanied by esophageal symptoms initially (e.g., dysphagia, reflux), esophageal investigation should be performed. Upper GI radiography or endoscopy provides information on possible GERD. Endoscopy allows acquisition of esophageal biopsies for histologic evidence of reflux esophagitis, even when the endoscopic view is normal. Referral to a GI motility laboratory for ambulatory 24-hour pH probe testing allows quantification of esophageal acid exposure and correlation of reflux events to symptoms. Stationary or ambulatory esophageal motility testing may reveal a baseline dysmotility associated with the chest pain (e.g., achalasia, diffuse spasm, nutcracker esophagus), and provocative testing with edrophonium or balloon inflation may implicate a probable esophageal cause for symptoms.

The differential diagnosis for CPUO includes the disorders just reviewed with consideration of peptic ulcer disease, biliopancreatic disease, IBS, upper GI malignancy, and panic disorder.

Management of patients with CPUO begins with the reassurance that none of the determinable disorders that cause its symptoms has been found. Patients should be educated about the possible mechanisms of pain production and assessed for psychologic disease. They should know that the prognosis in CPUO is excellent, with no increased risk of mortality. Patients with reflux-type symptoms or evidence of increased esophageal acid exposure may benefit from acid suppression or prokinetic medications. If esophageal motility changes are evident on manometric studies or by clinical suspicion, nitrates, calcium channel blockers, or anticholinergics should be tried. Some patients may respond to low-dose anxiolytics or to antidepressant therapies. Behavioral therapies may also be of benefit for some patients with CPUO.

AEROPHAGIA

Aerophagia means excessive air swallowing followed by belching. Normal individuals swallow approximately 2 to 3 ml of air with each swallow, accumulate air in the gastric fundus as a bubble, and intermittently eructate (burp). After a meal or the ingestion of carbonated beverages, large amounts of gas may be belched from the stomach, and depending on the norms of a society, burping may be socially appropriate and expected or inappropriate and discouraged.

Patients with aerophagia complain of excessive stomach gas and feel bloated after meals. They may have abdominal pain or dyspepsia in addition to distention. Eructating seems to offer relief of symptoms, and the patient complains of constant need to belch, which can be accompanied by some regurgitation. Individuals with aerophagia may believe that their gas results from poor digestion or fermentation. Although these two mechanisms account for production of gas in the colon, gas in the stomach is primarily derived from swallowed air and has a composition similar to that of room air. Anxiety increases the frequency of swallowing and may contribute to the excess ingestion of air.

Patients with aerophagia should be observed during the initial visit for repetitive air swallowing, which usually precedes a belch. The mechanism of air intake into the esophagus and stomach, with forced expulsion, can be easily explained by making the person aware of the activity. Attention during eating often reveals excessive air intake, with slurping of some foods or high intake of carbonated drinks.

The symptoms of bloating, abdominal distention, pain, and eructation may be found in other GI conditions, such as peptic ulcer disease, giardiasis, and IBS. Some of these symptoms may be seen in patients with GERD, gallbladder disease, and gastroparesis. Bloating, distention, and abdominal pain with increased flatus but not excessive eructation are characteristic of lactose intolerance and some malabsorptive diseases. In select patients, barium radiography, abdominal ultrasound, upper GI endoscopy, and tests of lactase deficiency may be indicated. Most patients require minimal workup, especially if active air swallowing is witnessed during the initial encounter.

Patients with aerophagia should be educated about the origin of their symptoms. Pointing out each air-swallowing event, as observed during the office visit, can demonstrate the mechanism and frequency of aerophagia to the patient. An explanation of the mechanism of esophageal speech taught to patients with laryngectomies is often helpful in understanding air intake and belching. The physician's demonstration of air swallowing and belching can be effective. Patients must be more aware of the frequency of their maladaptive behavior, and this awareness often reduces the frequency of air swallowing. Simethicone, with an ability to coalesce smaller air bubbles into larger ones, does not reduce total ingested air but does offer significant placebo effect. Again, reassurance and education provide impressive benefit in managing patients with aerophagia.

PANCREATICOBILIARY DYSKINESIA

Dysfunction of the sphincter of Oddi can result in biliary and pancreatic disorders. Biliary dyskinesia results in elevated common duct pressure because of increased sphincteric resistance to bile flow, either from sphincter stenosis, hypertonicity (spasm), or dyssynergic motility. Sphincter stenosis may occur from passage of a stone, with resultant papillitis and fibrosis. Dysfunction of the sphincter from spasm or abnormal contractile activity has been variously termed *tachyoddia, sphincterismus,* and *dyssynergia.* Abdominal pain is presumed to develop when elevated bile duct pressure is transmitted to liver ductules. Cholecystectomy removes the capacitor for bile storage, with more direct pressure changes exerted on the proximal biliary tract, and biliary dyskinesia should be considered in the evaluation of the postcholecystectomy syndrome. Sphincter of Oddi dysfunction has also been implicated in the pathophysiology of pancreatitis and pancreatic pain.

Pancreaticobiliary dyskinesia most often affects women and is usually seen after cholecystectomy. Other functional GI disorders are frequently found in patients with biliary dyskinetic syndromes, including IBS, esophageal dysmotility, and gastroparesis. Dyskinetic patients have more neuropsychiatric complaints and increased somatization scoring on psychometric testing than controls, as well as increased incidence of temporomandibular joint syndrome and hysterectomy.

Most patients with biliary dyskinesia report a recurrence of the same pain that led to gallbladder removal. The pain is usually episodic, located in the epigastrium or right upper abdominal quadrant, and may radiate to the back or flank. The pain in some patients is more chronic, with variations in intensity. Pancreatic dyskinesia may produce chronic or intermittent pancreatic-type pain, epigastric in location with radiation to the back. Initial diagnostic studies to define pancreaticobiliary dyskinesia include screening for elevations in liver function tests or in amylase and lipase during or after pain episodes and ultrasound for a dilated common bile duct or pancreatic duct. Referral for endoscopic retrograde cholangiopancreatography (ERCP) allows definition of ductal anatomy and bile duct drainage time, and some specialists can perform sphincter of Oddi manometry along with ERCP to determine ductal pressures and sphincteric function. Diagnosis of pancreaticobiliary dyskinesia is based on the history of classic symptoms, with elevated liver or pancreatic enzymes, dilated biliary or pancreatic ducts, and often delayed ductal drainage at ERCP. Sphincter of Oddi manometry has become a gold standard to demonstrate elevated ductal pressures and dysfunction of sphincter motility. The differential diagnosis includes other disorders of the biliopancreatic ducts (e.g., stones, strictures, tumors). Patients with postcholecystectomy pain should be reevaluated for possible IBS or peptic diathesis.

Management of pancreaticobiliary dyskinesia includes pharmacologic agents that lower sphincteric tone (calcium channel blockers, nitrates, anticholinergics). Pancreatic enzyme supplementation may lessen pancreatic pain by suppressing pancreatic exocrine secretion and decreasing ductal pressure. Endoscopic sphincterotomy and surgical sphincteroplasty are effective in reducing or alleviating symptoms in selected patients with elevated sphincter of Oddi pressures determined by manometry. Patients with pancreaticobiliary dyskinesia should benefit from the behavioral and supportive therapies found useful in the other functional disorders.

CHRONIC ABDOMINAL PAIN

Chronic functional abdominal pain is defined as pain persisting at least 6 months for which no defined cause is discernible after extensive review of the history, physical examination, and laboratory testing. The majority of patients with this syndrome are women, and many had chronic abdominal pain as children. The true prevalence is not known, but patients with this disorder are frequent users of the health care system, often for multiple chronic pain syndromes (see Chapters 14 and 107).

Pain is usually reported to be present constantly and not related to positional changes, diet, eating, or defecation. The patient may have fixed beliefs about the cause of the pain that do not correlate with anatomic or physiologic processes. Increased symptom reporting is usually associated with heightened stress and emotional arousal. Many patients with chronic pain have experienced sexual or physical abuse in childhood. Some individuals manifest depression, and somatoform disorders are often present.

The physical examination usually elicits pain with palpation of the abdomen but without focality. Patients asked to demonstrate the area of pain with one finger often rub the entire abdomen with the whole hand. Multiple surgical scars are often present. The laboratory evaluation should be directed at symptoms suggestive of particular organ systems, and often patients are extensively studied. It is important to review prior studies and avoid unnecessary repetition.

The differential diagnosis is extensive; however, features of the history and laboratory should guide the appropriate workup (Table 110-3).

Management of patients with chronic pain is best accomplished with a multidisciplinary team approach including the primary care physician and referral specialists. Some institutions have a pain clinic with a coordinated program of analgesic, behavioral, psychologic, and medical management. The physician should establish an ongoing relationship with the patient and provide reassurance. Goals should focus on minimizing the impact of the illness on the patient and family and not on curing the illness. The patient must be an active participant in the treatment process. Various pharmacologic agents have been used in managing chronic abdominal pain, including opiate analgesics, tricyclic antidepressants, and anxiolytics. Psychologic treatments have encompassed behavioral therapy, psychotherapy, and hypnotherapy. Chemical or surgical nerve destruction has been successful in some patients with intractable chronic abdom-

Table 110-3. Differential Diagnosis of Chronic Abdominal Pain

Condition	Evaluation
Intestinal angina	Doppler ultrasound
Crohn's disease	GI radiography/endoscopy
Pancreatic disease	ERCP, CT scan
Slipping rib syndrome	Trial of nerve block, rib resection
Gynecologic disorders	Pelvic examination, ultrasound, CT scan
Metabolic disorders	Porphyrin screen, check for diabetes, uremia, and Addison's disease
Poisoning	Lead and arsenic levels
Adhesions	Laparoscopy
Muscular hematoma	Ultrasound
Superior mesenteric artery syndrome	Upper GI radiography, check for impingement
Miscellaneous	Rule out familial Mediterranean fever, sickle cell disease, paroxysmal nocturnal hemoglobinuria, and tabes dorsalis

inal pain, and transcutaneous electrical nerve stimulation (TENS) and acupuncture have helped others. Relaxation training and biofeedback techniques are useful adjuncts in comprehensive multidisciplinary treatment.

CHRONIC CONSTIPATION AND LAXATIVE ABUSE

Chronic constipation is a common disorder that can lead to chronic laxative abuse and resultant colonic dysmotility. Constipation in IBS often alternates with diarrhea and is associated with abdominal pain, whereas chronic functional constipation may be painless and constant. Some patients with lifelong symptoms may defecate once weekly or even less frequently. Individuals with chronic constipation often begin their symptoms in childhood, related to improper toilet training, lack of bathroom privacy, or embarrassment. With suppression of the normal urge to defecate the rectum fills with stool and becomes capacious. Subsequent stool passage may be painful due to hardness or volume of the feces or because of an associated anal fissure or inflamed hemorrhoid. This prompts further stool holding and leads to reduced rectal sensation of the urge to defecate. The capacious rectum affects normal anorectal reflex relaxation of the internal sphincter, requiring ever-increasing volumes of rectal contents to trigger this initial defecatory event. Some children and elderly patients may develop *encopresis,* described as involuntary fecal incontinence resulting from overflow of looser stool past a full rectum. Encopresis in childhood is usually accompanied by behavioral or personality changes and may be secondary to significant family psychopathology. Occasionally, elderly patients have an associated stercoral ulcer of the rectum.

Constipation in adult patients is usually related to dysfunction of the colon in one of three patterns: pancolonic inertia, sigmoid spasm, or anorectal dysmotility. *Pancolonic inertia* may result from neuropathic illnesses, medication side effects, or laxative abuse. *Sigmoid spasm* is a mechanism for diminished bowel transit in IBS or diverticulosis, resulting from paradoxic hypermotility of the left colon and excessive segmental contractions. *Anorectal dysmotility* may result from rectal distention and diminished rectal sensitivity or from failed relaxation of the internal sphincter with megacolon in Hirschsprung's disease. *Hirschsprung's disease* involves congenital absence of ganglion cells in a segment of bowel wall, with resultant chronic segmental contraction and failure of relaxation of the anal sphincter. The colon dilates above the hypertonic segment with ensuing megacolon. The affected segment varies in length and usually produces symptoms in childhood or adolescence, although some individuals with short-segment involvement might not show symptoms until adulthood. Treatment involves surgical resection of the aganglionic segment.

The diagnostic evaluation in chronic constipation involves a complete history and physical examination, with attention to signs of possible metabolic or neurologic illness. The digital rectal examination may reveal a fecal impaction in the rectum and defines the anal sphincter. Patients with Hirschsprung's disease have large amounts of stool in the colon but none palpable with the examining finger, whereas patients with functional constipation but not IBS usually have abundant stool felt in the rectum by digital examination. Anoscopy is important to search for an anal fissure if painful defecation is present. Flexible sigmoidoscopy permits screening for left-sided colonic lesions associated with obstruction (e.g., neoplasia, stricture, myochosis [spastic, thickened bowel wall] with diverticulosis). Endoscopy can reveal *melanosis coli,* a brown pigment found in the colonic wall in patients who chronically ingest anthroquinone laxatives (e.g., senna, cascara, aloe). Barium enema examination depicts form and function of the colon, and plain radiographs are helpful to quantify stool content and distention of bowel loops.

The most important examination in chronically constipated patients may be the marker study of colonic transit. Patients ingest a gelatin capsule containing 20 plastic opaque 1-mm rings, and the progress of these markers is documented with plain abdominal films over the next 5 days. Patients must not take laxatives and should supplement their diets with 30 g of fiber daily, beginning 3 days before swallowing the marker capsule and throughout the radiographic study. The location of the markers at the end of 5 days directs further investigation and management: for pancolonic inertia if the markers are scattered throughout the colon, for sigmoid spasm or obstruction if markers pile up at the left colon, and for possible Hirschsprung's disease if markers make it to the rectum but do not exit by the end of the study. If Hirschsprung's disease is suspected, anorectal manometry is done to investigate sphincter function. Often, all markers are gone from the intestine by day 5, indicating normal colonic function, and patients attribute an improvement in their symptoms to fiber supplements. Fiber then becomes a basis for treatment.

The differential diagnosis for constipation is broad, but the usual chronic nature of functional constipation allows it to be distinguished from metabolic, neurologic, or anatomic causes. Appropriate evaluation screens for these other etiologies.

The management of chronic constipation begins with educating the patient about the physiology of defecation and the pathophysiology of constipation. Bowel retraining should be instituted, with encouragement to visit the toilet after a meal, taking advantage of the gastrocolic reflex, and regular exercise to help stimulate colonic transit. Judicious use of laxatives initially may assist in regularizing the bowel habit, but long-term use is prohibited. High intake of supplemental fiber (e.g., bran, hydrophylic colloid) is safe and effective and should be accompanied by generous intake of fluids. Dried fruits and fiber-rich fruit juices are excellent adjuncts. Stool softeners or glycerin suppositories are of occasional benefit. Some patients require initial and periodic enemas to help empty the lower bowel, but chronic enema therapy should not be necessary. Long-term management may include daily lactulose, a nonabsorbed carbohydrate fermented by colonic bacteria that results in increased stool fluidity and colonic output. A rare patient may require intermittent use of colonoscopic prep solutions (polyethylene glycol with electrolytes), with small daily amounts effecting increased stool output. All treatment regimens need to be individualized, and response depends on duration of symptoms, antecedent laxative abuse, and general activity status.

LEVATOR SYNDROME

The levator syndrome is characterized by a dull ache or firm pressure felt higher in the rectum than the anal location of proctalgia. More women than men experience this discomfort, usually in middle age. Unlike the fleeting pain in *proctalgia fugax,* patients with levator syndrome, also called *coccygodynia,* experience pain for hours to days. The pain is most often constant or rhythmic and may be likened to sitting on a ball or feeling like a ball (or corncob) was inside the rectum. Precipitants include defecation, sexual intercourse, sitting for long periods, and stress or anxiety. The pathophysiology probably involves spasm of the pelvic floor muscles.

Digital rectal examination in levator syndrome demonstrates tender rectal muscles. Palpation of the coccyx may reveal tenderness or excessive mobility from traumatic injury, suggesting an alternative diagnosis. As with proctalgia, patients with levator syndrome should undergo flexible sigmoidoscopy to screen for other anorectal diseases. Careful pelvic and prostate examinations need to be conducted, and ultrasound or CT scan of the pelvis may be warranted.

Management of levator syndrome and proctalgia fugax has included digital puborectal muscle massage, sitz baths, electrogalvanic stimulation, and biofeedback training utilizing electromyography. Medications that may help control symptoms include muscle relaxants, nonsteroidal antiinflammatory drugs, and calcium channel blockers.

ADDITIONAL READINGS

Almy TP, Rothstein RI: Irritable bowel syndrome: classification and pathogenesis, *Annu Rev Med* 38:257, 1987.

Camilleri M, Prather CM: The irritable bowel syndrome: mechanisms and a practical approach to management, *Ann Intern Med* 116:1001, 1992.

Drossman DA, Thompson WG: The irritable bowel syndrome: review and a graduated multicomponent treatment approach, *Ann Intern Med* 116:1009, 1992.

Drossman DA et al: Identification of subgroups of functional gastrointestinal disorders, *Gastroenterol Int* 3:159, 1990.

Lynn RB, Frieman LS: Current concepts: irritable bowel syndrome, *N Engl J Med* 329:1940, 1993.

Talley NJ, Philips SF: Non-ulcer dyspepsia: potential causes and pathophysiology, *Ann Intern Med* 108:865, 1988.

Thompson WG, Pigeon-Reesor H: The irritable bowel syndrome, *Semin Gastrointest Dis* 1:57, 1990.

Whitehead WE, Crowell MD, Schuster MM: Functional disorders of the anus and rectum, *Semin Gastrointest Dis* 1:74, 1990.

Zighelboim J, Talley NJ: What are functional bowel disorders? *Gastroenterology* 104:1196, 1993.

CHAPTER 111

Gastrointestinal Infections

Subhas Banerjee
J. Thomas Lamont

Infections of the gastrointestinal tract are seen in about 10% of patients examined in medical practice. Worldwide, infectious diarrheas are second only to cardiovascular disease as a cause of death. The primary care physician can evaluate and treat these common disorders in the office; only a minority require specialist consultation.

OFFICE DIAGNOSIS OF INFECTIOUS DIARRHEA

The cornerstone in diagnosing intestinal infection is a meticulous history of the present illness, especially duration of the illness and exposure to possible sources of infective pathogens (Table 111-1). Viral gastroenteritis and toxin-mediated food poisoning are brief illnesses with short incubation periods, as is traveler's diarrhea. Bacterial dysenteries are generally longer in duration, more severe, and accompanied by more serious signs and symptoms of colitis, including bloody diarrhea, fever, prostration, and weight loss. Familiarity with the basic patterns of these dysenteries allows a tentative diagnosis to be made at the initial visit.

A simple algorithm can be used to categorize the usual infectious diarrheas encountered in office practice (Fig. 111-1). Acute diarrhea lasting less than 1 week indicates infectious diarrhea. The physician should ask about antibiotic exposure, recent travel, exposure to infected persons, and homosexual contacts. Patients with bloody diarrhea, fever, chills, and dehydration are likely to have bacterial or amebic dysentery, whereas watery diarrhea with only mild cramps suggests viral infection.

Infectious diarrhea can be categorized according to the agent involved (viral, bacterial, parasitic), the mode of acquisition (food poisoning, traveler's diarrhea), and the pathophysiologic mechanism (ingestion of preformed toxin, epithelial invasion) (Table 111-2). A brief physical examination of the abdomen may provide additional diagnostic information. Tenderness in both lower quadrants suggests infectious colitis (*Shigella, Campylobacter, Entamoeba histolytica*), whereas middle or upper abdominal tenderness suggests *Salmonella* or *Campylobacter* infection or viral gastroenteritis. In some elderly patients, *Clostridium difficile* infection may cause an ileus with only minimal diarrhea, abdominal distention, and reduced bowel sounds. Rectal examination provides the opportunity to examine the stool for blood or mucus and to test for occult blood. Significant abdominal tenderness, rebound, and rigidity indicate severe disease and the need for hospital admission and prompt surgical consultation.

After a careful history the physician should obtain a fresh stool specimen for bacterial culture, parasite examination, and testing for leukocytes (Box 111-1). Invasive pathogens such as *Shigella, Campylobacter,* and enteropathogenic or enteroinvasive strains of *Escherichia coli* produce a leukocyte-containing diarrhea, whereas viral gastroenteritis and some toxin-mediated diarrheas are rarely accompanied by fecal leukocytes. However, stool leukocytes are absent in 40% to 50% of stool specimens from patients with proven bacterial enteritis. Stool leukocytes are also present in idiopathic inflammatory bowel disease and ischemic colitis, but these conditions can generally be excluded by a careful history. Flexible sigmoidoscopy or colonoscopy can provide useful diagnostic information in selected patients with acute infectious diarrhea, particularly those with pseudomembranous colitis, amebic dysentery, or sexually transmitted anorectal disease. However, these invasive tests are generally reserved for evaluation of severe or chronic diarrhea that has not been diagnosed by simpler tests.

In office practice, a specific etiologic agent is not identified for most patients. Even in prospective studies using a sophisticated battery of stool culture techniques, more than half of outpatient acute diarrheas cannot be ascribed to a

Table 111-1. Clinical Features of Common Infectious Diarrheas

Class	Typical agent	Incubation period	Duration of illness	Epidemiology
Viral gastroenteritis	Norwalk agent	1-2 days	1-2 days	Family and school outbreaks, usually in winter and summer
Food poisoning	*Staphylococcus aureus*	4-8 hours	12-24 hours	Point source outbreaks common
Bacterial dysentery	*Shigella sonnei*	1-2 days	3-7 days	Contaminated food and water
Enteric fever	*Salmonella typhi*	3-10 days	3-6 weeks	Contaminated food and water, often via asymptomatic carrier
Traveler's diarrhea	*Escherichia coli*	4-6 days	2-4 days	Common in Mexico, Latin America, and Far East; usually transmitted via uncooked foods, salads, and tap water
Antibiotic-associated pseudomembranous colitis	*Clostridium difficile*	1-3 days	3-10 days	Usually acquired in hospital during or after antibiotic therapy

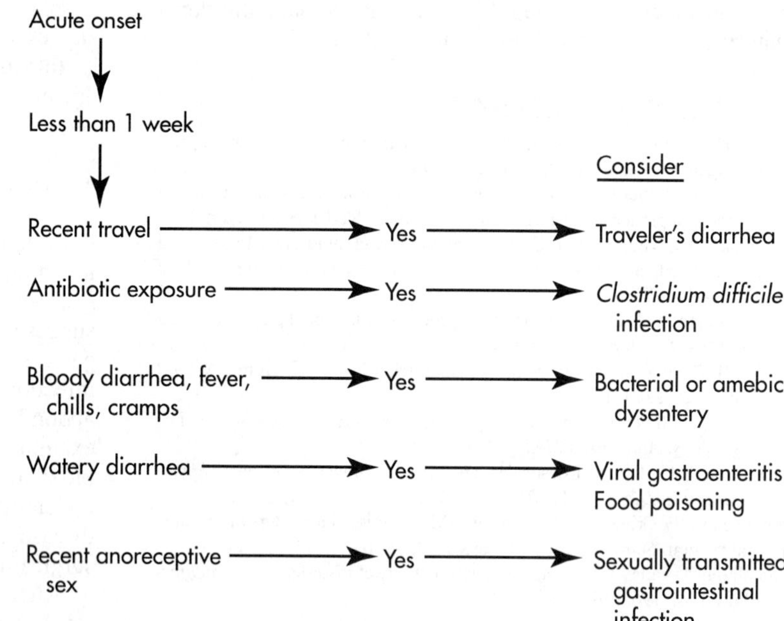

Fig. 111-1. Diagnostic algorithm for infectious diarrhea.

Table 111-2. Classification of Infectious Diarrheas

Mechanism	Bacterial pathogen	Source of pathogen
Ingestion of preformed exotoxin	*Staphylococcus aureus*	Custard, pudding, potato salad, mayonnaise
	Bacillus cereus	Rice
Colonization of bowel together with enterotoxin production	*Vibrio cholerae*	Contaminated food or water
	Enterotoxigenic *Escherichia coli*	Contaminated food or water
	Clostridium difficile	Hospital environment
Epithelial invasion	*Salmonella* spp.	Eggs and poultry
	Shigella spp.	Various
	Campylobacter spp.	Various
	Yersinia enterocolitica	Milk, meat
	Vibrio parahaemolyticus	Fresh or cooked seafood
	Enteroinvasive *E. coli*	Various

Box 111-1. Incidence of Leukocytes in Infectious Diarrheas

Usually (≥50%)
Shigella dysentery
Campylobacter dysentery
Amebic colitis
Enterohemorrhagic or enteroinvasive *Escherichia coli*

Sometimes (30%-50%)
Yersinia enterocolitica
Clostridium difficile
Salmonella gastroenteritis
Giardia duodenalis

Rarely (<5%)
Viral gastroenteritis
Acute food poisoning
Enterotoxigenic *E. coli*, enteric or typhoid fever

specific pathogen. In a typical office setting, 25% or fewer patients with acute, presumably infectious diarrhea will have a positive stool culture. Patients with negative tests may be infected with fastidious organisms or may have noninfectious causes of acute diarrhea (e.g., food intolerance, stress).

VIRAL GASTROENTERITIS

The major viral agents causing gastroenteritis are *Rotavirus* and Norwalk virus, which account for approximately 30% to 40% of gastrointestinal infections worldwide.

Rotavirus

Rotavirus is the most important etiologic agent in severe dehydrating diarrheal illness of children aged 6 to 24 months.[12] Older family members may develop a mild or asymptomatic infection. The annual epidemic starts in southwestern states in the late fall and spreads across the United States during winter, reaching the northeastern states by spring. Transmission is fecal-oral, and asymptomatic shedding of the virus before and after clinical diarrhea aids its spread, particularly in day-care centers. After an incubation period of 1 to 2 days, the child develops a 5- to 6-day illness, with vomiting followed by watery diarrhea. Fecal leukocytes are absent, and the stool may be acidic and test positive for reducing substances, indicating carbohydrate malabsorption from lactase and sucrase deficiency as a result of villous damage from the infection. The diagnosis can be confirmed by detection of rotavirus antigen in stool. Treatment is supportive, with fluid and electrolyte replacement using oral rehydration or intravenous (IV) solutions in severe cases. Infection is followed by antibody-mediated protection from reinfection in more than 90% of patients. *Rotavirus* vaccines tested in field trials provide 50% overall protection against all rotavirus diarrheas and 70% protection against severe diarrhea.

Norwalk Virus

Norwalk virus predominantly affects older children and adults, and the resulting gastroenteritis is one of the most common causes of work absenteeism in U.S. society.[5] Transmission is fecal-oral with a high attack rate, and outbreaks have occurred in hospitals, in nursing homes, and on cruise ships resulting from food handlers contaminating food and drink; family outbreaks are also common. Oysters and shellfish have been responsible for several outbreaks. The incubation period is approximately 1 to 2 days. Symptoms of gastroenteritis are mild and brief, usually lasting 24 to 48 hours. The disease tends to be self-limited in most patients and rarely requires special treatment. Occasionally it can be quite debilitating with vomiting, frequent loose watery stools, diffuse myalgias, chills, and fever. As with other viral gastroenteritides, fecal leukocytes are absent. Specific culture or serologic tests are not currently available. The diagnosis can be established by viral antigen detection in the stool, but given the mild nature of the illness, this is rarely necessary except for epidemiologic studies. Transient disaccharidase deficiency due to small bowel villous damage may result in diarrhea persisting for 1 to 2 weeks after the initial attack. The antibody response does not appear to protect against reinfection.

BACTERIAL DIARRHEAS

Bacterial enteropathogens can cause diarrhea by several well-defined mechanisms: (1) secretion of a preformed exotoxin during storage of food, (2) colonization of the intestinal tract without mucosal invasion but with release of enterotoxin, and (3) invasion of the intestinal epithelium with or without enterotoxin production (see Table 111-2). "Food poisoning" refers to infectious diarrhea of various etiologies acquired by eating contaminated food.[17] Outbreaks of food poisoning are typically more common in warm weather, when food is stored at higher room temperatures, which allows bacterial multiplication and release of protein exotoxins. These organisms or their toxins are then ingested and cause an acute illness within a few hours.

Staphylococcus aureus

Food poisoning caused by *Staphylococcus aureus* is now the second most common cause of reported outbreaks of food-borne illness, after *Salmonella*. The illness is caused by ingestion of one of five preformed enterotoxins (A through E, most often A) produced by certain strains of *Staphylococcus*.[18] Skin lesions on the hands of food handlers are typically responsible for introducing the bacteria into food. Improper food handling practices, including slow cooling of food and reheating before serving, allow for proliferation of the bacteria and toxin production. Previously cooked proteinaceous foods that have been reheated are most often implicated. Because the illness results from a preformed enterotoxin, its onset is swift and abrupt, occurring 4 to 8 hours after ingestion of the contaminated food. The cardinal manifestations of nausea and vomiting, followed by abdominal colic, profuse watery diarrhea, and prostration, rarely last more than 24 hours. Fever is usually absent. Most sufferers do not seek medical attention, but occasional patients may become dehydrated and require IV fluid replacement. The diagnosis of *S. aureus* food poisoning is suggested when several people who share the same contaminated food develop the clinical picture just described, with the characteristically short incubation period. A definitive diagnosis can be made only if the contaminated food is shown to contain large numbers of enterotoxin producing staphylococci or by enterotoxin detection in the implicated food; however, this is impractical in office or hospital practice. Antibiotic treatment is not indicated for this short-term disease, since bacterial proliferation in the host does not occur.

Clostridium perfringens

Clostridium perfringens type A is primarily responsible for food poisoning in humans.[10] *C. perfringens* type C produces a severe necrotizing enteritis rarely if ever seen in the United States. *C. perfringens* is ubiquitous in the environment and can be routinely isolated from human and animal feces, air, water, and soil. Fortunately, only small numbers of naturally isolated *C. perfringens* strains carry the gene for the enterotoxin (CPE gene) responsible for the food poisoning syndrome. The usual vectors are meat and poultry, which are often contaminated with heat-resistant *C. perfringens* spores. The spores are able to germinate if the food is stored after cooking with slow or inadequate cooling. Reheating to an inadequate temperature then allows further bacterial proliferation, producing an inoculum capable of causing disease. Symptoms may occur simultaneously in several individuals who ate the same meal 6 to 24 hours previously. Diarrhea and cramping abdominal pain lasting 12 to 24 hours are the typical symptoms. Nausea may be present, but vomiting is distinctly rare, as is fever. Stool cultures are not helpful because *C. perfringens* is part of the normal fecal flora. If necessary for epidemiologic investigation of an outbreak, the diagnosis can be established by polymerase chain reaction (PCR) of the CPE gene from stool specimens or by an enzyme-linked immunosorbent assay (ELISA) for enterotoxin in stool. Antibiotic treatment is not indicated.

Bacillus cereus

Bacillus cereus, an organism increasingly implicated as a cause of food poisoning, is ubiquitous in soil and frequently present in raw, dried, and processed foods.[3] The organism is able to produce two distinct enterotoxins, one similar to the heat-labile *E. coli* enterotoxin that causes watery diarrhea and one similar to the enterotoxin of *S. aureus* that produces emesis. *B. cereus* food poisoning is usually associated with rice dishes that have initially been boiled, which *B. cereus* spores can withstand, and then left to simmer or kept warm in steam heaters for prolonged periods, during which the pathogen multiplies and produces toxins. Outbreaks are therefore more common in countries where rice is a staple; for example, *B. cereus* accounts for up to 28% of food poisoning in Taiwan. Diarrhea and abdominal cramping are the most common symptoms, followed by nausea and less often vomiting. The illness is short-lived, and recovery usually occurs within 48 hours. Two cases of fulminant hepatic failure have been reported in association with*B. cereus* food poisoning in youngsters.[9]

Shigella Species

Shigellosis, an acute self-limited enteric infection, is a common cause of bacillary dysentery[16] and accounts for up to 20% of all cases of infectious diarrhea worldwide, particularly in areas of poor hygiene and overcrowding. The four major groups are *S. dysenteriae, S. flexneri, S. boydii,* and *S. sonnei.* The most important isolates in the United States are *S. sonnei,* which accounts for three fourths of isolates, and *S. flexneri,* which accounts for most of the remaining cases. U.S. outbreaks tend to be sporadic, but minor epidemics from a single food source or in custodial institutions or day-care centers have been described. The mode of spread is predominantly fecal-oral, with infected food handlers posing the major health hazard. A distinguishing feature of this pathogen is the small number of organisms required for an infective dose, thus explaining its rapid spread within closed groups.

Shigella causes disease primarily by invasion of and multiplication within the colonic epithelium, which induces an acute colitis. Certain strains release an enterotoxin that causes a profuse watery diarrhea in early stages, before colonic inflammation and dysentery. After an incubation period of 24 to 48 hours, the onset of diarrhea is heralded by abdominal pain, tenderness, and cramping. Fever may occur, but bacteremia is rare. The diarrhea is liquid and greenish with strands of mucus, blood, and leukocytes. The entire colon may be involved, and 20% to 30% of patients may pass gross blood (hematochezia). In general, *Shigella* dysentery is a self-limited disease; fever abates within approximately 4 days, and diarrhea and abdominal cramping subside in a week. Bacteremia, leukemoid reactions, thrombocytopenia, seizures, colonic perforation, and the hemolytic uremic syndrome have been reported in severe childhood shigellosis. Reactive arthritis may subsequently occur in patients with the histocompatibility antigen HLA-B27.

Sigmoidoscopic appearances in severe cases may mimic ulcerative colitis, with mucosal hyperemia, friability, and ulceration. The diagnosis is made by isolation of the organism from stool cultures or rectal swabs. Stool cultures typically remain positive for several days or weeks after clinical illness has subsided. Antibiotic therapy is indicated (see Treatment).

Salmonella Species

Salmonella is one of the major diarrheal pathogens of the world, with more than 40,000 cases reported annually in the United States. Since most diarrheal infectious diseases are underreported, the actual figure is likely much higher. *Salmonella* is divided into three species: *S. typhi,* the causative agent of classic typhoid fever; *S. choleraesuis;* and *S. enteritidis,* which is divided into many serotypes. *Salmonella* species, particularly *S. enteritidis* and *S. choleraesuis,* can be cultured from a variety of nonhuman hosts, including poultry, rats, reptiles, wild birds, and flies. The main animal reservoirs for human disease are poultry and livestock. Supermarket chicken and eggs are often contaminated with *Salmonella* species, which are present in the intestinal tracts of commercially raised poultry and animals. An estimated 85% of community-acquired salmonellosis in the United States is related to ingestion of contaminated food, whereas 15% arises from person-to-person spread. In contrast to *Shigella* species, where small inocula can cause disease, infection with *Salmonella* requires ingestion of 10,000 to 100 million organisms, although smaller numbers will cause infection in patients with hypochlorhydria. *Salmonella* infection produces two forms of illness. The gastroenteritis is similar to other bacterial diarrheas, and typhoid (enteric) fever comprises a profound systemic illness lasting 4 to 6 weeks if left untreated. Diarrhea does not usually occur until the later weeks of the illness.

Salmonella *Gastroenteritis.* Caused primarily by serotypes of S. enteritidis, including *S. typhimurium, S. heidelberg, S. newport,* and *S. agona,* this disease shows seasonal variation, with the highest incidence reported during July through November. It is usually associated with infection from poultry products and eggs.[2] Poultry from avian carriers becomes contaminated during evisceration and packing. Thus adequate cooking of poultry and poultry products is important in disease prevention. The high incidence of *Salmonella* in raw poultry and eggs makes food handlers particularly susceptible to infection. Onset of clinical symptoms occurs 8 to 48 hours after ingestion of organisms, reflecting the time required for multiplication and invasion of the small bowel epithelium. Nausea and vomiting are prominent initially, followed by colicky abdominal pain and diarrhea, which is frequently mixed with mucus and blood. Fever and bacteremia may occur. The course of the disease is 2 to 5 days, followed by a gradual reduction of symptoms. Reactive arthritis or Reiter's syndrome may develop in patients with HLA-B27. The carrier state occurs much less often after gastroenteritis than enteric fever. In previously healthy hosts the illness is usually mild, and antimicrobial therapy may not improve the course of gastroenteritis and prolongs the carrier state (Fig. 111-2). Patients with immunosuppression, diabetes, hypochlorhydria or achlorhydria, sickle cell disease, and other chronic debilitating conditions may develop bacteremia and sepsis with osteomyelitis and metastatic abscess formation after a bout of *Salmonella* gastroenteritis. These patients require antibiotic therapy.

Typhoid (Enteric) Fever. Classic enteric fever is caused by *S. typhi,* although other species of *Salmonella*, including *S. paratyphi,* produce a similar illness with a shorter and milder course. About 70% of U.S. cases occur in patients with a history of recent travel abroad, with the highest risk in Mexico, the Indian subcontinent, and the Phillipines.[11] In this form of salmonellosis the organism multiplies in the small intestine and invades the epithelium but produces minimal inflammation and cell destruction. *S. typhi* appears to use the cystic fibrosis transmembrane regulator (CFTR) for entry into intestinal epithelial cells. The organisms then gain access to the bloodstream through intestinal lymphatics, and a short-lived primary bacteremia ensues 24 to 72 hours after inoculation. This primary bacteremia is transient and terminated by phagocytosis of the organisms by the cells of the reticuloendothelial system. The organisms survive intracellularly and continue to multiply, giving rise to a second, more prolonged bacteremia accompanied by high fever with a relative bradycardia, headaches, abdominal pain in right lower quadrant, and myalgias that can last days to weeks. During this phase of continuous bacteremia, all organs are exposed to viable organisms, and metastatic infection may lead to complications (e.g., pneumonia, meningitis, myocarditis, septic arthritis, osteomyelitis). Delirium, diarrhea, and small bowel ulceration with perforation or bleeding may occur later. Patients with sickle cell disease, aortic aneurysms, cancer, hemolytic anemia, and valvular heart disease are more prone to developing prolonged bacteremia and tissue abscesses. For unknown reasons the gallbladder is almost universally infected during this period, and organisms multiply to a higher titer in bile, usually without the production of cholecystitis.

Diagnosis is made by blood cultures early in the disease. Stool cultures become positive secondary to the shedding of a large number of organisms into the bile during the third to fourth week of disease. At this time the serologic test (Widal's test) also becomes positive. Antibiotic therapy considerably shortens the course of this otherwise prolonged illness (see Treatment). Chronic carriage of *Salmonella*, resulting from chronic infection of the gallbladder after enteric fever, provides a human reservoir for this organism. Approximately 50% of patients continue to shed organisms in the stool at 6 weeks, and 5% to 10% continue to excrete up to the third month. The chronic carrier state occurs in 1% or fewer patients and is defined as positive stool cultures 1 year after initial infection.

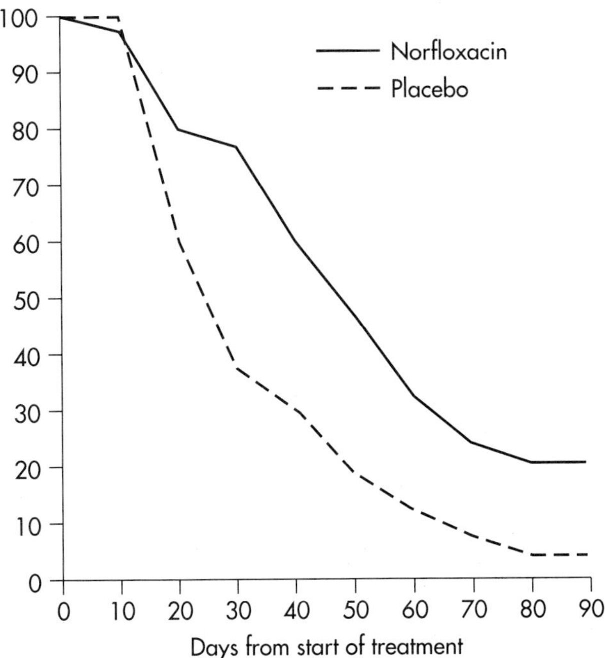

Fig. 111-2. Effect of antibiotic therapy in prolonging carrier state in acute *Salmonella* gastroenteritis. (From Wistrom J et al: *Ann Intern Med* 17:207, 1992.)

Escherichia coli

Diarrhea-producing strains of *E. coli* can be classified into five groups based on the mechanisms of diarrhea: enterotoxigenic, enteropathogenic, enteroadherent, enteroinvasive, and enterohemorrhagic. These groups produce different clinical syndromes that vary in clinical features, geographic incidence, and host susceptibility (Table 111-3). Specific strains are diagnosed by serotyping the flagellar and somatic antigens, which is useful in the study of *E. coli* epidemics. In clinical practice the results of specific typing on stool samples are not available for at least several days, by which time patients have often recovered.

Enterotoxigenic *E. coli* (ETEC) organisms adhere to the small bowel mucosa and produce diarrhea by release of several toxins. LT, or heat-labile toxin, resembles cholera toxin and produces a watery diarrhea by triggering fluid secretion in the intestine. ST, or heat-stable toxin, is a peptide that stimulates intestinal guanylate cyclase, causing fluid secretion. ETEC is a major cause of diarrhea in travelers from industrialized societies who are visiting developing or third-world countries (traveler's diarrhea) and in infants and children in these countries. The usual mode of transmission is contaminated food or water. ETEC produces a mild illness

Table 111-3. Mechanisms of Diarrhea in *Escherichia coli* Infection

E. coli strains	Typical illness	Epidemiology
Enterotoxigenic (ETEC)	Watery diarrhea for 2-4 days	Travelers to and infants in developing countries
Enteropathogenic (EPEC)	Mild watery diarrhea	Rare cause of sporadic diarrhea in United States
Enteroadherent (EAEC)	Mild diarrhea without blood or leukocytes	May cause outbreaks of food poisoning
Enteroinvasive (EIEC)	Dysentery as in *Shigella* infections but milder	Food poisoning outbreaks in developing countries; rare in United States
Enterohemorrhagic (EHEC)	Hemorrhagic colitis occasionally with hemolytic uremic syndrome	Epidemics related to ingestion of meat and dairy products; infants and elderly most severely affected

Box 111-2. Effectiveness of Antibiotic Therapy for Bacterial Diarrheas

Effective
Salmonella enteric fever
Shigella dysentery
Clostridium difficile
Yersinia septicemia
Traveler's diarrhea, severe or with bloody stools
Campylobacter dysentery or sepsis

Possibly Effective
Enteroinvasive *E. coli*
Enteropathogenic *E. coli*
Campylobacter enteritis

Probably Not Effective
Enterohemorrhagic *E. coli*
Salmonella gastroenteritis
Yersinia enteritis without septicemia
Acute food poisoning (*S. aureus, B. cereus*)

lasting 2 to 4 days and characterized by abdominal cramps, low-grade fever, and diarrhea with the passage of watery stools. Anorexia and vomiting may occur early in the illness.

Enteropathogenic *E. coli* (EPEC) organisms are an occasional cause of profuse watery diarrhea in infants in the United States and Europe. These strains possess a virulence factor, with the ability to adhere to intestinal epithelial cells, a property lacking in nonpathogenic *E. coli*. As with ETEC, diarrhea associated with EPEC is usually self-limited, except in infants, in whom massive dehydration may occur.

Enteroadherent strains of *E. coli* (EAEC) are seldom encountered in clinical practice, and the mechanism for diarrhea is still not clear. These strains adhere to liver cells in culture, a feature that distinguishes them from other pathogenic strains. Infected individuals develop a mild, nonbloody diarrhea.

The enteroinvasive and enterohemorrhagic forms of *E. coli* involve the colon primarily and produce a clinical picture of acute dysentery. Enteroinvasive *E. coli* (EIEC) may cause traveler's diarrhea or rarely food-borne outbreaks of dysentery with bloody diarrhea, especially in children in developing countries. The main pathogenic feature is invasion of and proliferation within enterocytes, a feature that also characterizes *Shigella* species. Patients infected with EIEC complain of fever, malaise, anorexia, cramps, watery diarrhea, or the passage of mucus or blood. The diarrhea is short-lived, with spontaneous recovery within 2 to 4 days of onset, and complications are rare except in malnourished infants. Although not well studied, antibiotics may reduce the duration of illness, as in shigellosis (Box 111-2).

The most serious form of *E. coli* diarrhea is caused by infection with enterohemorrhagic *E. coli* (EHEC). EHEC accounts for up to a third of all cases of hemorrhagic colitis in the United States. The 0157:H7 strain of *E. coli* was first identified as the cause of hemorrhagic colitis after the ingestion of contaminated hamburger. Outbreaks are now reported with increasing frequency, particularly from the Pacific Northwest region of the United States, but sporadic cases are diagnosed in all areas. Although undercooked ground beef remains the major source of infection, outbreaks have also been reported after consumption of unpasteurized milk and apple juice and after swimming in contaminated lakes. *E. coli* 0157:H7 produces two *Shigella*-like toxins that inhibit protein synthesis within intestinal cells, but their role in hemorrhagic colitis is obscure. As with all types of dysentery, a wide range of symptoms follows infection with EHEC.[6] In a typical case 12 to 24 hours of abdominal cramps and watery diarrhea are followed by fever and bloody stools. Severe cases of EHEC infection are often accompanied by white blood cell counts in excess of 20,000/mm^3, dehydration, and azotemia. Severe infection, particularly in children and the elderly, may be complicated by the hemolytic uremic syndrome (HUS), which carries a fatality rate of 25%. *E. coli* 0157:H7 may be the major etiologic factor in HUS in children, with 77% of patients of HUS showing recent infection with the organism.[15] Antibiotic treatment does not decrease the duration of symptoms or the risk of progressing to HUS. Preventive measures include adequate cooking of ground beef, pasteurization of milk and cider, and strict hygienic measures at food-processing centers and by food handlers.

Campylobacter Species

Campylobacter jejuni, C. coli, and C. fetus are the most common causes of bacterial diarrheal illness in the United States, with isolation rates exceeding those of *Salmonella* and *Shigella*. *Campylobacter* species are also a major cause of traveler's diarrhea in winter months in subtropical areas.

Campylobacter resembles *Salmonella* in its mode of transmission to humans from eggs and poultry. In addition, sick pets and other domestic animals may harbor *Campylobacter* as a pathogen and may serve as reservoirs of human disease. The pathogenesis of *Campylobacter* colitis involves invasion of the mucosa and toxin production, as in *Shigellosis*.

Typically, *C. jejuni* and *C. coli* produce moderate to severe diarrhea that may be watery or bloody, fever, constitutional symptoms, and abdominal pain. Pain may be so severe that it mimics an acute surgical condition (e.g., appendicitis, diverticulitis). Rarely, toxic megacolon with perforation can occur. The illness usually lasts less than a week. One study showed that 26% of patients with Guillain-Barré syndrome had *Campylobacter* infection in the preceding month, compared with only 1% to 2% of controls.[13] Cross-reacting serum antibodies to *C. jejuni* antigens and brain gangliosides have been implicated in this association. HUS has also been associated with *Campylobacter* infections, and reactive arthritis may develop in patients with HLA-B27. Fecal leukocytes are usually present, and the diagnosis can be established by stool cultures and occasionally by blood cultures in febrile patients. Sigmoidoscopy may reveal evidence of an acute proctocolitis resembling inflammatory bowel disease. Antibiotic treatment is indicated if the clinical presentation suggests bacteremia or if severe acute dysentery is present.

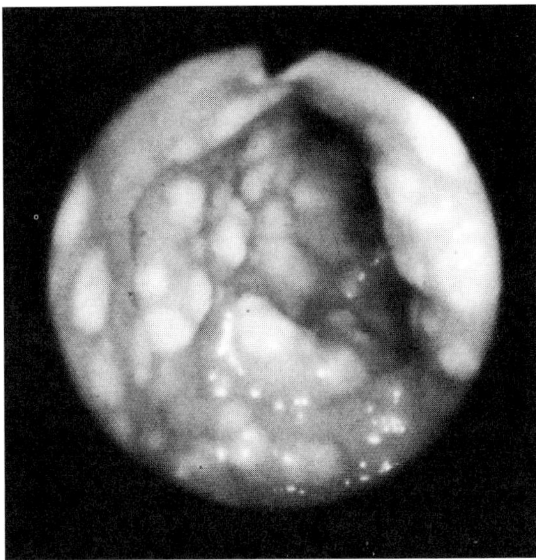

Fig. 111-3. Proctoscopic appearance of pseudomembranes in rectum. White raised plaques scattered over mucosa are typical of acute pseudomembranous colitis secondary to *C. difficile* infection. (From Triadafilopoulos G, LaMont JT: In Walker WA et al, editors: *Pediatric gastrointestinal disease*, vol 1, Philadelphia, 1991, Decker.)

Clostridium difficile

Clostridium difficile, the pathogen responsible for antibiotic-associated colitis and diarrhea, is a common cause of nosocomial infections.[7] The organism is a gram-positive anaerobe whose spores are widely distributed in hospital rooms and soil. Colonization of the large bowel occurs only when the normal colonic microflora is altered by antibiotics or cancer chemotherapy drugs. Once it has colonized, *C. difficile* releases two potent toxins, A and B, which are implicated in pathogenesis.

Diarrhea occurs in up to 25% of patients receiving antibiotics. In most patients this is not related to *C. difficile* infection, particularly in outpatients, in whom this infection is uncommon. The cause of noninfectious antibiotic diarrhea is related to antibiotics interfering with the ability of the colonic microflora to metabolize dietary carbohydrates to short-chain fatty acids and other end products. During antibiotic therapy the bowel flora cannot digest this carbohydrate, allowing it to remain in the lumen, where it attracts water and causes diarrhea.

C. difficile infections primarily are hospital acquired; outpatient cases account for less than 1% of total cases. Patients in the hospital are often exposed to the two conditions necessary to develop disease: antibiotic therapy and *C. difficile* spores. These spores persist for months or even years on commodes, toilets, soiled bed linen, bed rails, call buttons, and floors. Hospital personnel, although not infected or colonized, often carry *C. difficile* on their hands, rings, or stethoscopes and thus can spread the infection within the hospital. Risk factors associated with *C. difficile* infection include recent exposure to antibiotics in the hospital, occupying a hospital room with an infected roommate, exposure to rectal thermometers, sigmoidoscopy or enema, and treatment in an intensive care unit. Approximately one patient in five acquires *C. difficile* infection after admission, and a third of these develop clinical illness with diarrhea or colitis. Most culture-positive patients remain asymptomatic and probably serve as a reservoir for infection of other patients. At discharge, some patients are still culture positive for *C. difficile* and presumably carry the organism home or to long-term care facilities.

C. difficile causes a wide spectrum of disease, ranging from the asymptomatic carrier state to life-threatening colitis with toxic megacolon and perforation. In a typical case, diarrhea starts during the administration of antibiotics or within a few days of stopping antibiotics. The most frequently implicated antibiotics are ampicillin, amoxicillin, cephalosporins, and clindamycin, but almost all antibiotics (including metronidazole) have been implicated. Diarrhea is usually watery or mushy and may be blood tinged, but frank rectal bleeding is rare and should suggest another diagnosis. Lower abdominal cramps, distention, and low-grade fever may occur. Persistent or worsening fever, abdominal pain, and distention may indicate severe disease with impending megacolon or perforation. Elevation of the white blood cell count above 20,000/mm^3, hypoalbuminemia, ascites, and metabolic acidosis indicate severe colitis.

Diagnosis of *C. difficile* infection is based on demonstration of the cytotoxin in stools with either the cytotoxin assay or an immunoassay for toxins A and B. Culture of the organism is considered too sensitive for routine clinical use, since up to 20% of inpatients treated with antibiotics become transient carriers without diarrhea or other symptoms and do not require treatment. Diagnosis can be easily confirmed by bedside sigmoidoscopy without bowel preparation; pseudomembranes are visible as yellow or white raised plaques studding the rectal mucosa (Fig. 111-3).

Treatment

Oral rehydration with clear liquids or Gatorade is the mainstay of therapy for patients with mild viral or bacterial diarrhea. IV hydration may be required in the patient with severe diarrhea or abdominal pain. Most authorities caution

Table 111-4. Treatment of Viral and Bacterial Diarrheas

Infection	Treatment	Comment
Viral gastroenteritis	Rehydration for infants, loperamide	Transient lactose intolerance is common in children.
S. aureus, C. perfringens, or *B. cereus* food poisoning	None required	Illness lasts less than 24 hours.
Shigella dysentery	Quinolone antibiotic	Antibiotic resistance is common in strains acquired in subtropical areas.
Salmonella enteric fever	Antibiotic selected on basis of drug sensitivity, usually ciprofloxacin, third-generation cephalosporin, or chloramphenicol	Chronic carriers may require prolonged therapy, especially *S. typhi.*
Traveler's diarrhea	Quinolone antibiotic or TMP-SMX	Mild diarrhea may be treated with antidiarrheals without antibiotics.
Hemorrhagic colitis (EHEC)	Antibiotics not effective	Observe for hemolytic-uremic syndrome.
Campylobacter colitis	Antibiotics indicated for septicemia; quinolones may reduce duration of diarrhea if started early.	Quinolone resistance is increasing rapidly.
Clostridium difficile colitis	Metronidazole or vancomycin	20% relapse rate; patient may be treated with further courses of same drug.

against the use of antidiarrheal agents (e.g., diphenoxylate, codeine, paregoric) because these drugs interfere with the flushing effect of diarrhea that eliminates organisms and their toxins. However, bismuth subsalicylate suspensions (Pepto-Bismol), 2 tablespoons four times daily, or kaopectate in the same dose is useful in controlling diarrhea, nausea, and other symptoms in mild infectious enteritis.

The effectiveness of antibiotics for bacterial dysentery is controversial. Confusion arises because some bacterial infections of the bowel respond to antibiotic therapy. Also, the specific diagnosis of the offending organism is usually not available for 3 or 4 days or longer after stool samples are submitted to the laboratory, by which time the patient is usually better. Antibiotic therapy clearly benefits patients with *Salmonella* enteric fever, shigellosis, *C. difficile* infection, and traveler's diarrhea (Table 111-4). *Campylobacter* septicemia responds to antibiotics, but their benefit in uncomplicated *Campylobacter* enteritis is unproved. Antibiotic treatment is not indicated for most patients with uncomplicated *Salmonella* gastroenteritis and may even increase the incidence and fecal shedding of the organism (see Fig. 111-2).

Another problem in the antibiotic treatment of enteric infections is the rapid acquisition of antibiotic resistance by *Shigella, Salmonella,* and *Campylobacter* species. Recent studies indicate that many strains of *Shigella* isolates in developing countries are resistant to ampicillin (28% to 90%), tetracycline (56% to 100%), and trimethoprim- sulfamethoxazole (TMP-SMX, 56% to 92%).[16] Fortunately, the quinolone antibiotics are still effective against most strains of *Shigella.* The quinolone antibiotics also remain effective against *Salmonella typhi* and nontyphoid *Salmonella,* although resistance is starting to emerge, with 4% to 7% low-level resistance and less than 1% high-level resistance. Up to 6% of *E. coli* isolates in the United Kingdom are now resistant to ciprofloxacin, as are a startling 41% to 88% of *Campylobacter* strains in Europe and Asia.

A practical approach is to avoid antibiotics in patients with mild gastroenteritis or acute food poisoning (predominantly vomiting). For patients with moderate or severe diarrhea with fever, tachycardia, chills, rectal bleeding, or abdominal pain, empiric broad-spectrum antibiotic coverage can be instituted with ciprofloxacin (500 mg) or norfloxacin (300 mg) twice daily. Antibiotics can be stopped or changed once stool culture and antibiotic sensitivity results are available. The duration of treatment is 3 to 5 days for traveler's diarrhea and 5 days for most other uncomplicated bacterial dysenteries other than *Salmonella typhi,* which is usually treated for 2 weeks. The asymptomatic carrier state, with fecal shedding of enteric pathogens, often occurs after clinical recovery from most forms of bacterial dysentery, but this does not necessarily indicate relapse and usually does not require therapy.

C. difficile can be treated with metronidazole (250 mg four times a day for 10 days) or vancomycin (125 mg). The response to therapy is rapid, with symptoms often disappearing in 3 to 5 days; 125 mg of vancomycin is just as effective as 500 mg (Fig. 111-4). Because of its lower cost, metronidazole is the drug of choice. Relapse of *C. difficile* colitis occurs in 15% to 20% of patients after successful initial therapy and should be treated with a second course of metronidazole or vancomycin. Multiple relapses occur in some patients and may respond to tapering doses of either agent for 1 to 2 months.

TRAVELER'S DIARRHEA

Epidemiology

Traveler's diarrhea disrupts the vacations of millions of travelers, primarily those visiting developing countries, where sewage disposal systems tend to be inadequate. The incidence of traveler's diarrhea varies considerably with the destination, and attack rates in developing countries approach 50% (Box 111-3). Longer journeys are associated with an increased risk of developing a diarrheal illness. Younger tourists are more likely than older adults to develop diarrhea because they may eat in lower quality restaurants or from street vendors. Patients with immunodeficiency, hypochlorhydric patients, and those with a history of prior gastrointes-

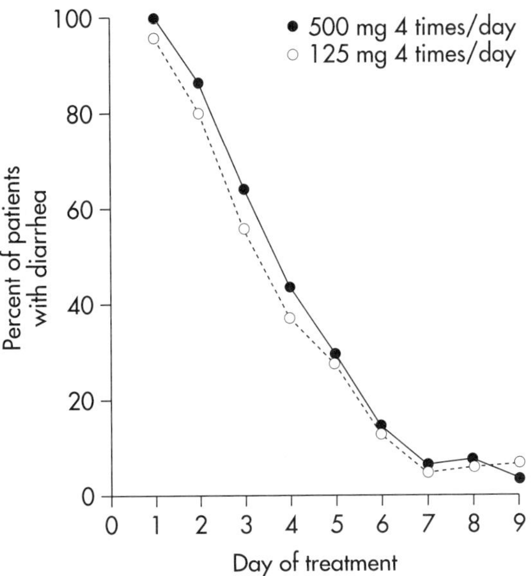

Fig. 111-4. Response to treatment of pseudomembranous colitis with 125 vs. 500 mg of vancomycin. (From Fekety R et al: *Am J Med* 86:15, 1989.)

Box 111-3. Geographic Incidence of Traveler's Diarrhea

High Risk (20%-50%)

Indian subcontinent
Southeast Asia
Africa
Mexico
Developing countries in Latin America and Middle East

Intermediate Risk (10%-20%)

Eastern Europe
Former Soviet Republics
Caribbean countries
China
Mediterranean European countries

Low Risk (<10%)

Canada, United States
Northern Europe
Japan
Australia, New Zealand
Developed areas of Latin America and the Caribbean

tinal disease (e.g., inflammatory bowel disease) are at increased risk for acquiring traveler's diarrhea. Older travelers, those with extensive travel experience, and those undertaking organized travel through a tour company are at a lower risk.

Traveler's diarrhea is acquired through consumption of contaminated food and drink. Even intelligent travelers fail to heed common sense dietary advice; traveler's diarrhea was reported in 50% of gastroenterologists attending a conference in Mexico City. Common sources of acquisition include tap water, ice cubes, unpasteurized milk products, uncooked vegetables and salads, unpeeled fruit, and raw or undercooked shellfish, seafood, and meat.

Microbiology

The pathogens isolated from patients with traveler's diarrhea vary with the country visited and the timing and techniques of stool culture.[1] Most pathogens are bacterial, and *E. coli* species account for the majority of infections, especially ETEC (up to 70%) and EAEC (up to 15%). *Campylobacter* and *Shigella* species are the other two important bacterial offenders, each accounting for approximately 10% to 15% of infections. Other rare bacterial pathogens include *Salmonella, Aeromonas,* and *Vibrio.* In high-risk areas such as Thailand, up to one third of diarrheal illnesses may be caused by polymicrobial infection, with two to four pathogens isolated on stool culture. Such parasites as *Entamoeba, Giardia, Cryptosporidium,* and *Cyclospora* are isolated rarely (1% to 2%). Viral infections are found in less than 1% of returning travelers with diarrhea. No pathogen has been isolated in up to 40% of cases in series worldwide.

Clinical Presentation

The clinical features of traveler's diarrhea depend on the pathogen involved, but the vast majority of cases are relatively mild. ETEC accounts for most cases and produces a mild 2- to 4-day illness with acute watery diarrhea (usually less than five bowel movements a day), abdominal cramps, and mild nausea without vomiting. Usually the patient is confined to bed for a day or two, but a change in itinerary is not required. Up to 10% of patients traveling to high-risk areas may develop a more serious illness with fever and bloody stools, often related to infection with *Shigella* or *Campylobacter* species. Less than 1% of patients require hospital admission with fever, severe dysentery, and dehydration. Dehydration often occurs in patients with associated vomiting, which limits maintenance of oral hydration. Importantly, no deaths have been reported from traveler's diarrhea.

About 2% of patients may experience protracted diarrhea after returning home, and parasitic infection should be considered, particularly *Cryptosporidium* and *Cyclospora* species. Protracted diarrhea may also result from secondary disaccharidase deficiency; this usually resolves in 6 to 8 weeks. Postinfectious irritable bowel syndrome occurs in 1% to 4% of patients after acute infectious gastroenteritis and may persist for months or years. This condition is indistinguishable from idiopathic irritable bowel syndrome (see Chapter 110).

Prevention and Prophylaxis

Avoidance of tap water, raw foods, and foods from street vendors decreases the risk of traveler's diarrhea. Washed citrus fruits, carbonated drinks, and dried foods are usually safe. Pretravel consultation and education allow travelers to cope better with their illness; despite a higher attack rate with travel to high-risk areas, they are less likely to require medical help or seek posttravel consultation. Routine antibiotic prophylaxis should be discouraged because of the risks of side effects and possible development of resistant strains of bacterial pathogens in the community. Prophylaxis is appropriate for high-risk patients, however, including those with other significant illness (e.g., diabetes mellitus, severe heart disease), for whom diarrhea would be especially deleterious. Prophylaxis can also be considered for some business travelers. In most travelers, however, short-term treatment of illness once it develops is preferable to antibiotic prophylaxis.

Bismuth subsalicylate has the advantages of protection, no effect on bacterial resistance, and low cost; the protection rate is about 66%. Two tablespoons (15 ml each) or two well-chewed tablets (262 mg each) should be taken four times a day with meals. The dosing frequency often makes compliance difficult. TMP-SMX offers satisfactory prophylaxis for travelers to Mexico, with protection rates up to 95%. It is taken in a dose of one tablet (160 mg TMP, 800 mg SMX) once a day. It is less useful in Africa, Asia, and South America, where resistance to TMP-SMX is high. The major adverse reaction is photodermatitis, a particularly undesirable risk for vacationers to beach resorts. Ciprofloxacin or norfloxacin provides protection rates of up to 95% in most parts of the world. A once-daily dose is taken for prophylaxis, 500 mg for ciprofloxacin or 300 mg for norfloxacin. These drugs are safer than TMP-SMX, with fewer reported adverse effects. Their use in children is not recommended because of possible effects on joint cartilage.

Treatment

Travelers should be advised about oral rehydration with mineral water, bottled drinks, and high-salt foods (e.g., crackers, chips, soup).[1] Healthy travelers should be given two medicines to carry on their journey: loperamide or a similar antidiarrheal agent, and a broad-spectrum antibiotic effective against enteric organisms (e.g., quinolone, TMP-SMX). The patient with mild diarrhea should avoid milk, alcohol, and spicy food; take loperamide only; and increase intake of fluids and salt. Moderate diarrhea (more than 10 watery stools a day, abdominal cramps) can be treated with loperamide with the addition of ciprofloxacin (500 mg) or norfloxacin (200 mg) twice daily for 3 to 5 days. In severe diarrhea with fever greater than 100.4° F (38° C) or bloody stools, loperamide should not be used, and the patient should be treated only with antibiotics. If dysentery symptoms persist for more than 3 to 4 days, medical consultation is recommended to exclude parasites or other conditions and to ensure adequate rehydration.

PARASITIC INFESTATIONS CAUSING DIARRHEA

The diagnosis of parasitic infestation requires proper stool examination by an experienced parasitologist. In this age of international travel, many parasitic infections are acquired abroad and become symptomatic after the patient returns home. A careful travel history and a high index of suspicion are critical to the diagnosis of parasitic disease.

Giardia duodenalis

The organism is distributed worldwide, with the vast majority of infestations being asymptomatic.[4] *Giardia* is a common cause of diarrhea among travelers, with certain areas posing exceptionally high risks, such as St. Petersburg, Russia, where attack rates of up to 30% have been reported in travelers. In the United States, *Giardia* infestations are acquired mainly from contaminated water supplies, many of which are located in frequently visited, remote wilderness settings. Patients with hypogammaglobulinemia, particularly selective immunoglobulin A deficiency, are at highest risk. Hypochlorhydric or achlorhydric patients, including those with a prior gastrectomy, are also more susceptible.

The major symptom of giardiasis is diarrhea, which may be acute, intermittent, or chronic and is often accompanied by dull cramping pain above the umbilicus, anorexia, nausea, bloating, and flatulence. A less common but important presentation is steatorrhea and progressive weight loss. Diagnosis of giardiasis can be made in 50% of patients by stool examination, but the remainder require examination of a duodenal aspirate for the characteristic organisms. The duodenal aspirate is best obtained at endoscopy, which also allows duodenal mucosal biopsies to be examined for the organisms. Patients with giardiasis and underlying immunoglobulin deficiency syndromes frequently have flat or club-like villi on duodenal biopsy as well as diminished plasma cells in the lamina propria, in contrast to celiac disease, where villous flattening is accompanied by an intense plasma cell infiltrate.

Metronidazole, 250 mg three times a day for 7 days, is highly effective therapy. For patients with immunoglobulin deficiency, long-term metronidazole can restore the normal villous architecture and reverse the malabsorption syndrome.

Entamoeba histolytica

Of the seven species of amebae known to parasitize the human intestinal tract, only *Entamoeba histolytica* is pathogenic.[8] Infection with this organism occurs worldwide but is much higher in tropical areas where poor sanitary conditions prevail. Clinical symptoms of amebiasis occur more often in endemic areas, in military personnel returning from the Far East, and in migrant laborers from Mexico, but the disease also occurs in individuals who have not traveled outside the United States. Humans are the principal host and reservoir for *E. histolytica,* and infection occurs through ingestion of cysts from contaminated water or food sources. Spread is predominantly fecal-oral, although venereal transmission is a significant hazard among homosexuals.

Most isolates of *E. histolytica* are nonvirulent, and the trophozoites lack the ability to invade tissue. Thus the most frequently encountered clinical variant of this disease is the asymptomatic cyst passer. In these asymptomatic patients, *E. histolytica* exists as a commensal in the large intestine. Once the ameba is encysted and passed into the environment, it is relatively resistant and can survive up to 10 days. The invasive motile trophozoite of *E. histolytica* cannot survive in the environment and plays no role in fecal-oral spread of the disease. Occasionally an asymptomatic cyst passer develops acute invasive amebiasis, and current recommendations are that all symptomatic cyst passers (except in highly endemic areas) be treated, since they are the reservoir of disease and pose an infective risk to others.

Symptomatic disease produces a variety of presentations. Some patients have chronic disease characterized by bouts of diarrhea, abdominal pain, and weight loss. The diarrhea usually contains blood and mucus, and tender hepatomegaly and pain over the cecum and ascending colon may be present. Occasionally a mass lesion called an *ameboma,* comprising a fibrous and granulomatous reaction to the infection, may develop in the large bowel, causing confusion with colon carcinoma. Other individuals have an acute dysenteric illness with fever, abdominal pain, tenesmus, and bloody diarrhea. Massive colonic bleeding, toxic megacolon, and perforation are potential complications. Extraintestinal invasion most

Table 111-5. Sexually Transmitted Anorectal Infections

Disease	Signs and symptoms	Diagnosis	Treatment
Anorectal gonorrhea	Often asymptomatic; creamy rectal discharge, constipation, and pain may occur; erythema and purulent exudate on sigmoidoscopy	Culture of *Neisseria* on selective media	Ceftriaxone, 250 mg IM, then doxycycline, 100 mg bid for 7 days *or* spectinomycin, 2 gm IM, if allergies to prior drugs
Herpes simplex	Extreme rectal pain and tenderness, bloody discharge, constipation, perianal vesicles; ulcers on sigmoidoscopy	Viral isolation from stool, discharge, or acute and convalescent sera	Acyclovir, 5 mg/kg IV every 8 hours for 7 days
Anorectal syphilis	Mild or no symptoms, with anorectal ulcers and tender inguinal nodes	Dark-field examination of ulcer, serologic testing	Benzathine penicillin, 2.4 million units IM (single dose), *or* doxycycline, 100 mg bid for 15 days
Amebiasis	Diarrhea with mucus and blood, diffuse proctitis with scattered ulcers at sigmoidoscopy	Motile trophozoites or cysts in stool, serologic studies	Metronidazole, 750 mg qid for 10 days
Lymphogranuloma venereum (LGV) (*Chlamydia trachomatis*)	Bloody diarrhea, rectal pain, discharge; diffuse proctitis at sigmoidoscopy; rectal strictures in chronic cases	Granulomas in rectal biopsy, serology	Doxycycline, 100 mg orally bid for 1 week (acute proctitis) or 3 weeks (LGV)

IM, Intramuscularly; *IV*, intravenously; *bid*, twice daily; *qid*, four times daily.

often affects the liver, where hepatic abscesses form. A critical concern is to distinguish amebiasis from ulcerative or Crohn's colitis, since mistaken treatment with corticosteroids can accelerate amebic colitis and foster systemic invasion.

Diagnosis can be established by examining fresh stool specimens, which may show cysts in asymptomatic carriers and characteristic trophozoites containing ingested red blood cells in patients with dysentery. Sigmoidoscopy may reveal discrete yellow-based rectosigmoid ulcers with undermined edges and characteristically normal intervening mucosa. The disease may be predominantly right sided, however, resulting in a normal sigmoidoscopic appearance. Serologic tests are sensitive in detecting invasive amebic disease, including hepatic abscess and colonic mucosal invasion, but remain positive for an extended period after treatment of the disease. Metronidazole, 750 mg three times a day for 10 days (active against trophozoites), followed by diloxanide furoate, 500 mg three times a day for 10 days (to eliminate cysts), is effective therapy for active intestinal infection with *E. histolytica.*

SEXUALLY TRANSMITTED GASTROINTESTINAL INFECTIONS

Two forms of sexually transmitted gastrointestinal infections are described: a diarrheal syndrome and acute proctitis.[14] Venereal transmission of enteric pathogens such as *Shigella, Salmonella, E. histolytica, G. duodenalis,* and *C. jejuni* occurs through oral-anal contact and may produce a picture of acute diarrhea or dysentery.

Acute proctitis occurs in men who have sex with men and in women who participate in anoreceptive sexual intercourse. The classic sexually transmitted pathogens, such as *Neisseria gonorrhoeae, Treponema pallidum, Chlamydia trachomatis, Haemophilus ducreyi,* herpes simplex virus, and human papillomavirus, have all been identified in anorectal lesions in acute proctitis (Table 111-5). The clinical features of acute proctitis are nonspecific and mimic idiopathic inflammatory bowel disease. The most common presenting symptoms include discharge, rectal pain, tenesmus, hematochezia, and diarrhea. Likewise, the sigmoidoscopic appearance of the rectal mucosa is nonspecific and includes mucosal erythema, granularity, friability, and ulceration. A specific infectious agent usually cannot be identified on the basis of clinical symptoms or sigmoidoscopic appearance. Before the institution of therapy, cultures must be obtained for the variety of organisms expected in this setting. Rectal swabs should be cultured for *N. gonorrhoeae* and *C. trachomatis*, and viral cultures should be sent to a reference laboratory for herpes simplex isolation. Routine bacterial stool cultures and stool examination for *E. histolytica* are also obtained. After identification of specific pathogens, therapy is directed toward each of the organisms identified; broad-spectrum empiric therapy is avoided.

EBM EVIDENCE-BASED MEDICINE

The primary source for this chapter was MEDLINE. Electronic searches dating back to 1994 were conducted in April 1999.

REFERENCES

1. Caeiro JP, DuPont HL: Management of traveler's diarrhoea, *Drugs* 56:73, 1998.
2. Centers for Disease Control and Prevention: Outbreaks of *Salmonella* serotype *enteritidis* infection associated with consumption of raw shell eggs—United States, 1994-1995, *JAMA* 276:1017, 1996.
3. Drobniewski FA: *Bacillus cereus* and related species, *Clin Microbiol Rev* 6:324, 1993.
4. Farthing MJ: Giardiasis, *Gastroenterol Clin North Am* 25:493, 1996.
5. Green KY: The role of caliciviruses in epidemic gastroenteritis, *Arch Virol Suppl* 13:152, 1997.

6. Griffin PM, Ostroff SM, Tauxe RV, et al: Illnesses associated with *Escherichia coli* 0157:H7 infections: a broad clinical spectrum, *Ann Intern Med* 109:705, 1988.
7. Kelly CP, LaMont JT: *Clostridium difficile* infection, *Annu Rev Med* 49:375, 1998.
8. Li E, Stanley SL Jr: Protozoa: amebiasis, *Gastroenterol Clin North Am* 25:471, 1996.
9. Mahler H, Pasi A, Kramer JM, et al: Fulminant liver failure in association with the emetic toxin of *Bacillus cereus, N Engl J Med* 336:1142, 1997.
10. Meer RR, Songer JG, Park DL: Human disease associated with *Clostridium perfringens* enterotoxin, *Rev Environ Contam Toxicol* 150:75, 1997.
11. Mermin JH, Townes JM, Gerber GE, et al: Typhoid fever in the United States, 1985-1994: changing risks of international travel and increasing antimicrobial resistance, *Arch Intern Med* 158:633, 1998.
12. Parashar VD, Bresee JS, Gentsch JR, Glass RI: Rotavirus, *Emerg Infect Dis* 4:561, 1998.
13. Rees JH, Soudain SE, Gregson NA, et al: *Campylobacter jejuni* infection and Guillain-Barré syndrome, *N Engl J Med* 333:1374, 1995.
14. Rompalo AM: Diagnosis and treatment of sexually acquired proctitis and proctocolitis: an update, *Clin Infect Dis* 28:S84, 1999.
15. Rowe PC, Orrbine E, Lior H, et al: Risk of hemolytic uremic syndrome after sporadic *Escherichia coli* 0157:H7 infection: results of a Canadian collaborative study, *J Pediatr* 132:777, 1998.
16. Shears P: *Shigella* infections, *Ann Trop Med Parasitol* 90:105, 1996.
17. Shewmake RA, Dillon B: Food poisoning: causes, remedies, and prevention, *Postgrad Med* 103:125, 1998.
18. Wieneke AA, Roberts D, Gilbert RJ: Staphylococcal food poisoning in the United Kingdom, 1969-90, *Epidemiol Infect* 110:519, 1993.

CHAPTER 112

Anorectal Disorders

David McAneny

Anorectal disorders are common and often readily managed in a primary care setting. Nevertheless, some physicians regard the anorectal canal with trepidation. This may be the result of medical education and a reluctance to examine this part of the body, as evidenced by the written response "deferred" on this portion of many physical examinations. This chapter clarifies anatomy and evaluation of the anorectum to help physicians more confidently diagnose and treat anorectal disorders.

ANATOMY

The anatomy of the anorectal canal is somewhat confusing because of the various descriptions and terms applied to this region. The levator ani and coccygeus muscles form the floor of the pelvis. The puborectalis muscle is a component of the levator and contributes to the anorectal sling that maintains rectal continence (Fig. 112-1). During a digital examination the anorectal sling is especially appreciated along the lateral walls of the anorectal canal, where the digit extends over the floor of the pelvis. This identifies the superior portion of the sphincter mechanism and is an important consideration in the management of rectal tumors.

Conceptually, the anus is comprised of two concentric muscular cylinders. The voluntary external sphincter and puborectalis form the outer muscle layer and are confluent with the levator ani. The inner cylinder is a continuation of

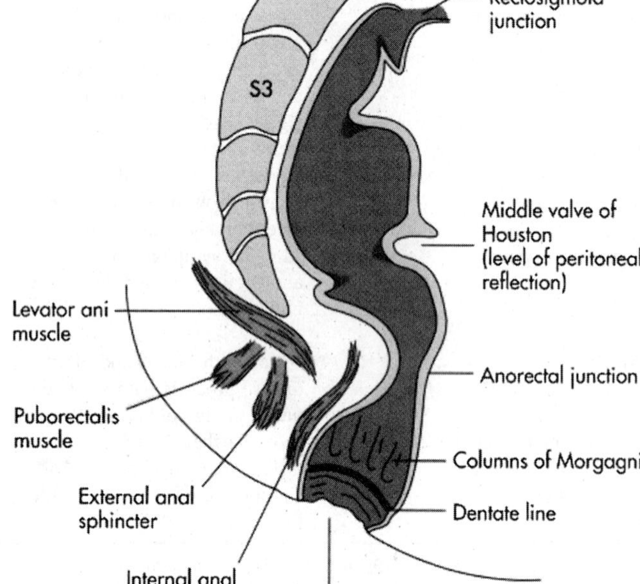

Fig. 112-1. Anorectal anatomy. (From Coates W: Disorders of the anorectum. In Rosen P et al: *Emergency medicine: concepts and clinical practice,* ed 4, St Louis, 1998, Mosby.)

the mucosa, submucosa, and circular and longitudinal muscle layers of the distal gut. The latter muscle bundle is the involuntary component of the sphincter mechanism. Everting the buttocks, the examiner can palpate the intersphincteric groove between these two cylinders.

The *anal verge* refers to the junction between pigmented cutaneous tissue and the sensate stratified squamous lining distal to the dentate (or pectinate) line. This area is of ectodermal origin, drains into the systemic veins and inguinal nodes, and harbors the external hemorrhoids. On the other hand, the mucosa of the true anal canal extends from the dentate line to the anorectal sling. This portion of the anus contains the endodermal, simple columnar mucosa that drains into the portal vein and the pelvic and lumbar nodes. Internal hemorrhoids arise at this level and are relatively insensate. Glands are concentrated at the dentate line and are the source of anal suppurative diseases.

PATIENT EVALUATION

History

Both the lay public and physicians use "hemorrhoid" to describe a myriad of anorectal complaints, just as "stomach" is applied to the abdomen. Patients should be queried about what hemorrhoid means to them. The history should ascertain whether the patient has felt and reduced any protrusions, whether symptoms occur during or after defecation or at night, bleeding frequency and volume, if mucus is expressed with stools or between bowel movements, and whether anal or pelvic pain is associated with passage of stool. If the anal area is pruritic, the patient may frequently rub or scratch thc surrounding area to obtain relief. Previous anorectal conditions and treatments, local operations, and obstetric trauma are critical. Determining the patient's daily diet is helpful, including the amounts of high-fiber foods and non-diuretic fluids. Bowel habits must be established, particularly the frequency, bulk, and firmness. Precise definitions of constipation or diarrhea should be elicited, and continence of solid stool, liquid feces, and flatus is relevant.

Patients should be questioned about nonprescription creams, ointments, and suppositories and whether any objects have been inserted into the rectum. A history of anoreceptive sex and sexually transmitted diseases can be elicited. Additional aspects include systemic illnesses, medications, a family history of gastrointestinal pathology (e.g., inflammatory bowel disease or tumors), and constitutional symptoms (e.g., fever, weight loss). Genitourinary symptoms are also associated with anorectal disorders.

Physical Examination

In conjunction with a thorough history, a proper examination should provide the diagnosis of most anorectal conditions. Besides the patient's general health, the physician should first assess the abdomen, genitalia, surrounding skin, and regional lymph nodes. This also creates a level of trust and comfort before probing the anorectum.

Patients may be examined in the prone or lateral decubitus positions. Although the latter is usually preferable for an examination, the jackknife prone position is valuable for rigid sigmoidoscopy. The left-side-down lateral decubitus position best serves the right-handed examiner. Certain conditions (e.g., rectal prolapse) warrant special positions and activities, such as performing Valsalva's maneuver while standing or squatting. The patient in the lateral decubitus position should move the buttocks to the examiner's side of the table and draw the knees to the chest. The examiner should first inspect the perianal region and evaluate the local skin for excoriations, external fistula orifices, protruding or thrombosed hemorrhoids, signs of infection, and skin lesions (e.g., tumors, condylomata, hidradenitis suppurativa). Pilonidal disease is located farther superiorly in the gluteal cleft and is often misinterpreted by patients as an anal problem. The buttocks are carefully retracted, everting the anus, and fissures are observed. When patients have severe anal pain, the examination may be limited to inspection alone. When reassured that a digital examination or an endoscopic procedure is not planned, patients often relax enough to permit identification of an anal fissure. An examination under anesthesia is an option for patients with severe discomfort or great anxiety.

The gloved digit should be well lubricated in preparation for a gentle insertion into the anorectal canal. The prostate gland or cervix is palpated through the anterior rectal wall, and tenderness can be elicited. A boggy, tender fullness in the intersphincteric, ischiorectal, or supralevator spaces typically connotes an abscess. Masses are sought, with particular attention to the relationship to the anorectal sling. The examiner should discern a tumor's morphology, extent of penetration into the rectal wall, and any suggestion of fixation to the surrounding pelvic tissues. Sphincter tone is noted and stool examined as to characteristics and presence of occult blood. The rectum also provides a "window" for the recognition of extrarectal pelvic pathology, such as tumors and abscesses.

Endoscopic Techniques

Primary care physicians should perform anoscopy with ease. When an endoscopic evaluation of the anorectum is anticipated, a mechanical preparation (e.g., Fleet's enema) is advised. Disposable anoscopes are readily available and permit visualization of the anal canal, including mucosal lesions, the dentate line, fissures, hemorrhoids, and purulence. Tumors, proctocolitis, ulcers, and extrinsic compression are apparent with a sigmoidoscope. The rigid sigmoidoscope should be another familiar instrument in the primary care setting. Air is insufflated through the sigmoidoscope to inflate and expose the rectal lumen and permit safe passage up to 20 cm from the anal verge. Suction equipment and cotton swabs might be necessary to eliminate residual stool. This device allows visualization of the entire rectum and a portion of the distal colon. The flexible sigmoidoscope can be passed as proximal as the hepatic flexure and is more comfortable than its rigid counterpart. Furthermore, the televised digital images enhance recognition of pathology. Biopsies and cultures can be obtained during sigmoidoscopy.

Anal manometry, defecography, electromyography, and endorectal ultrasonography are useful adjuncts in the evaluation of some anorectal disorders, although they are not usually available or indicated in primary care practice.

ANAL PAIN

Anal pain is usually diagnosed and treated with simple measures. The three most common causes are fissures, thrombosed external hemorrhoids, and abscesses (see later discussions). Each of these conditions is usually identified on careful inspection and palpation of the perianal tissues and does not require endoscopy or advanced diagnostic procedures. In fact, patients with severe anal pain typically do not tolerate digital examinations or anoscopy. Less frequent causes of anal pain include sexually transmitted infections (e.g., lymphogranuloma venereum, herpes simplex, condyloma acuminatum [see Chapter 29]), tumors, proctitis, coccygodynia, and proctalgia fugax.

PRURITUS ANI

Pruritus ani is especially common among men and is caused by a variety of local and systemic disorders, although it is frequently a primary condition. Pruritus ani is a *symptom,* not necessarily a diagnosis, and an underlying source should be sought. A prospective study evaluated 109 patients with pruritus ani as the only presenting symptom.[2] More than half the patients had an underlying benign anorectal condition, such as hemorrhoids, fissures, idiopathic or ulcerative proctitis, condylomata, fistulas, and abscesses. More importantly, 23% of the patients had occult neoplasms, including rectal cancer, epidermoid anal cancer, adenomatous polyps, colon cancer, and a premalignant anal lesion. Only one quarter were diagnosed with primary, or idiopathic, pruritus ani. Whereas most studies suggest that only 5% to 25% of patients with this symptom have an inciting source, selection criteria and referral practices could have biased this series. The report clearly affirms, however, that patients with pruritus ani should be thoroughly evaluated to diagnose underlying and correctable pathology. Appropriate studies include a careful inspection, digital rectal examination, anoscopy, rigid sigmoidoscopy, and perhaps colonoscopy.

The most common precipitants of secondary pruritus ani are the benign and malignant conditions already cited. Other causes include Crohn's disease, hidradenitis, pilonidal disease, uncommon tumors (e.g., melanoma, Bowen's disease, Paget's disease), rectal prolapse, dermatologic conditions (e.g., psoriasis, lichen sclerosus, various dermatitides), infections (fungal, parasitic, bacterial), sexually transmitted diseases (e.g., gonococcus, herpes, syphilis), systemic diseases (e.g., jaundice, lupus, diabetes), and psychologic disorders. These problems are identified with proper evaluation.

Primary pruritus ani is a cyclic, self-propagating phenomenon. An itching or burning sensation prompts the patient to scratch or rub the perianal area. The resultant abrasion of the tissues causes further itching and thus more scratching and local trauma. The leakage of anal mucus or stool permits fecal bacterial neuraminidases to irritate any excoriations of the thin and well-innervated perianal skin, resulting in pruritus. If the initial evaluation fails to reveal a precipitant, efforts should focus on local hygiene and bowel habits. Patients are specifically advised not to scratch the itchy area. The anus must be kept clean and dry and should be gently blotted with nonscented toilet paper after bowel movements rather than vigorously rubbed. Patients should cleanse especially after activities that promote heavy sweating. Powders, creams, and soaps are avoided, and white cotton underwear is encouraged. A bowel regimen is prescribed to provide stool bulk, promote complete fecal evacuation, and diminish perianal soiling (Box 112-1). Diet is modified to contain fiber foods and to exclude spices, tomatoes, coffee and tea, carbonated beverages, cheese, nuts, citrus, and chocolate. A particularly effective maneuver is the application of a wisp (not a ball) of cotton to the perianal area. The cotton wisp absorbs anal mucus discharge and is exchanged after bowel movements and baths. A short course of a topical steroid (1% hydrocortisone cream) is occasionally administered to disrupt the itch-scratch cycle.

Box 112-1. Recommended Bowel Regimen*for Patients with Anorectal Disorders or Discomfort

1. Increase the amount of fluid in the diet. Drink at least 6 to 8 large glasses of fluid every day. The fluid should be water, juices, or sport drinks; do not include coffee, tea, or soft drinks in this total.
2. Eat at least 4 or 5 servings of fruits and vegetables every day.
3. Take a fiber supplement (e.g., Metamucil, Citrucel): 1 tablespoon in 8 ounces of water once or twice every day. Take docusate sodium (e.g., Colace): one tablet once or twice a day. These products are available over the counter.†
4. Take a Sitz bath or tub bath of warm water twice daily. Avoid applying soap to the anal area because it can be irritating. A Sitz bath can be purchased at the pharmacy.
5. After each bowel movement, pat the anal area with toilet tissue, but do not rub or scratch the area. (After Sitz baths or bowel movements, place a wisp of cotton over the anus. Replace the wisp of cotton after baths and bowel movements.‡)
6. Do not sit on the toilet for prolonged periods; do not read in the bathroom.
7. Avoid or at least minimize taking narcotic analgesics (e.g., codeine, Percocet), since these medications can be constipating.
8. Do not spend prolonged periods sitting. Frequently assume a prone position with pillows beneath the hips to elevate the anal area.§

*This is a practical guide for the management of a variety of anorectal conditions, including hemorrhoids, fissures, pruritus ani, and postoperative care. Portions are modified to address the particular clinical situation.
†Apply step 3 if steps 1 and 2 do not result in soft, bulky stools.
‡Recommended for pruritus ani.
§Valuable advice after anal surgery, especially for hemorrhoids.

ANAL BLEEDING

Although lower gastrointestinal (GI) tract bleeding is distressing to patients, it is usually from a benign cause and not a harbinger of malignancy. Bright-red blood coating the stool or on the toilet paper generally implies an anorectal source, whereas darker hemorrhage indicates a more proximal lesion. Drops of blood associated with pain on defecation suggest a fissure. A thrombosed external hemorrhoid often presents with the passage of some blood from an acutely painful perianal lump. Bloody diarrhea occurs with proctocolitis, including infectious, ischemic, and inflammatory variants. The major sources of significant lower GI bleeding are diverticular disease and vascular ectasias, primarily involving the colon. Anorectal lesions rarely cause massive hemorrhage.

In the evaluation of lower GI bleeding, a thorough examination with anoscopy and sigmoidoscopy is valuable, especially if the characteristics of the bleeding and local symptoms suggest an anorectal source (see Chapter 109). The physician should exercise caution about casually ascribing hemorrhage to hemorrhoids, particularly in light of their prevalence. If hemorrhoids appear quiescent or if bleeding persists, neoplasms and other colorectal pathology must be considered and identified.

HEMORRHOIDS

Even when another clinician has assigned a patient a diagnosis of hemorrhoids, the physician should still obtain a precise description of what this term means to the patient. Hemorrhoids affect most people over age 50. Three dominant groups of vascular cushions normally reside in the left lateral, right anterolateral, and right posterolateral portions of the anal submucosa. These cushions may become engorged with blood during defecation to protect the anal canal. With age and various stresses, the buttressing muscularis submucosa deteriorates, resulting in venous distention. The cushions are then disposed to thrombosis and ulceration. The upright position and a low-fiber, constipating Western diet promote straining with defecation, making the hemorrhoid cushions more prominent. The numerous theories of the pathogenesis of hemorrhoids suggest a multifactorial process.

External and internal hemorrhoids are differentiated by their location relative to the dentate line, although the external and internal components can also create a confluent complex. Hemorrhoids are graded by size. *First-degree* hemorrhoids protrude into the anal lumen but do not prolapse. *Second-degree* hemorrhoids prolapse through the anal canal but spontaneously return to their original position. *Third-degree* hemorrhoids also prolapse but require manual reduction. *Fourth-degree* hemorrhoids remain prolapsed and are not reducible. This grading system is valuable in the selection of therapy.

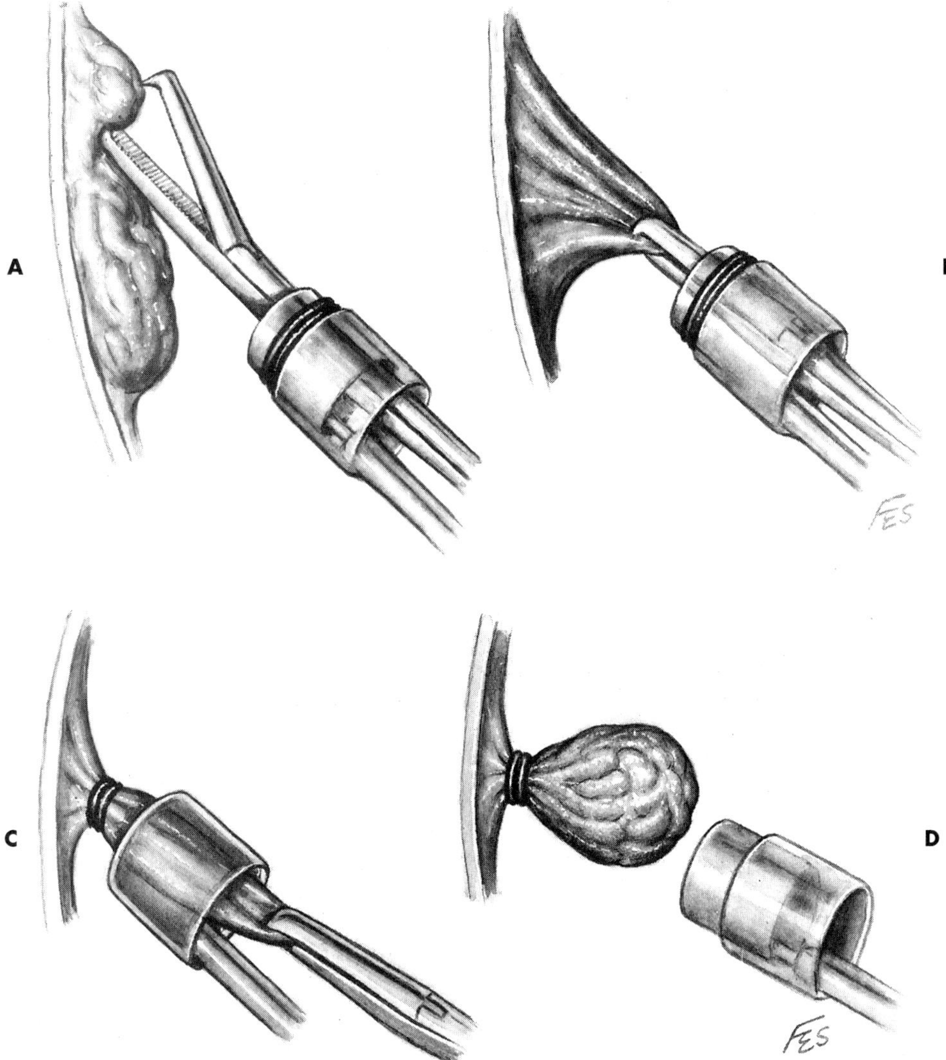

Fig. 112-2. Rubber band ligation of hemorrhoids. **A,** Redundant mucosa grasped at base of hemorrhoid within lower rectum. **B,** Excess tissue drawn into ligator, if not painful for patient. **C,** Band attached; hemorrhoid ligated. **D,** Instrument fired.

External Hemorrhoids

External hemorrhoids manifest with discharge, modest bleeding, and thrombosis. Mucous discharge occurs when the hemorrhoid no longer apposes the adjacent anal mucosa, which can also precipitate pruritus ani. Of greater concern, external hemorrhoids are prone to thrombosis, a particularly painful condition as a result of the sensate, overlying modified squamous epithelium. A thrombosis often develops after an episode of constipation.

External hemorrhoids generally respond to a bowel regimen that improves stool bulk and texture (see Box 112-1). Local anal hygiene measures are also instituted, including Sitz baths and the avoidance of prolonged sitting and straining to defecate. Explaining the rationale of this bowel regimen fosters compliance. Acutely thrombosed hemorrhoids can be excised under local anesthesia, if performed within 2 to 3 days after onset of symptoms.

Internal Hemorrhoids

Internal hemorrhoids are relatively insensate, so pain is not a common feature. Associated with bleeding and prolapse, internal hemorrhoids are identified by anoscopy and are elusive to detection by digital examination. Again, proper diet and bowel habits, along with local care, suffice for many first-degree and second-degree hemorrhoids. When these measures fail, more sophisticated options are available.

Less than 10% of patients with symptomatic hemorrhoids require surgery. First-, second-, and some third-degree internal hemorrhoids have been obliterated with cryotherapy, bipolar diathermy, laser, infrared photocoagulation, injection sclerotherapy, and rubber band ligation; none has proved to be clearly advantageous. A meta-analysis of five trials using infrared photocoagulation, sclerotherapy, and rubber band ligation found that ligation provides the most effective long-term outcome and is inexpensive[3] (Fig. 112-2). Rubber band ligation causes more discomfort, however, and is associated with rare episodes of serious complications (e.g., tetanus, perineal soft tissue sepsis). Therefore infrared photocoagulation may be the best nonsurgical approach. Proper training and recognition of complications are essential for any treatment.

Hemorrhoidectomy is reserved for third-degree and fourth-degree lesions, smaller hemorrhoids that do not respond to nonsurgical techniques, and complexes of internal and external components. Costly lasers have been employed for hemorrhoidectomy but have not demonstrated greater efficacy or less pain than standard surgery. Although outpatient procedures can be performed, the physician must be judicious about patient selection. An overnight observation or short hospital stay for intensive analgesia can be beneficial. Age, debilities, social situation, travel distance, and pain threshold are factors to consider.

ANAL SUPPURATIVE DISEASES

About 6 to 10 anal gland orifices reside along the dentate line. These glands extend through the submucosa, pierce the underlying muscularis, and often track to the intersphincteric groove. Fecal bacteria are exposed to these glands, and an acute perirectal abscess develops when the orifice is occluded. A fistula in ano represents the chronic version of this infection.

Abscess

An infected anal gland tracks along various planes and results in a focal abscess (Fig. 112-3). A submucosal tract leads to a perianal abscess. If the infected gland traverses the adjacent musculature, the abscess cavity can rest in the intersphincteric space or in the ischiorectal fossa. Conversely, a proximal dissection within the intersphincteric groove creates a supralevator abscess. Abscesses present with pain and possibly discharge. A digital examination can be superfluous and painful if fluctuance is readily apparent, as usually occurs with perianal and ischiorectal infections. Intersphincteric abscesses are less visible but cause much pain and throbbing with defecation because of their tight confines. A digital examination should identify this source. Supralevator abscesses are uncommon and may manifest as occult sepsis. Digital examination or cross-sectional imaging can be diagnostic.

A pervasive misconception is that perirectal abscesses should be managed with antibiotics to "bring them to a head." In the immunocompetent patient, pus is present within the indurated phlegmon, even when fluctuance is not yet evident. Therefore these abscesses warrant incision and drainage. Antibiotics are an adjunct among patients with cardiac valve considerations or with significant cellulitis. An exception is the human immunodeficiency virus (HIV) or otherwise immunocompromised host with marked granulocytopenia and perianal sepsis; this patient is best treated with antibiotics alone. This situation is a rare and challenging problem requiring teamwork among surgeons, hematologists, oncologists, and infectious disease experts.

Perianal and ischiorectal abscesses are evacuated by placing a curvilinear incision through the overlying skin. The incision should be parallel to the underlying musculature to minimize the likelihood of sphincter disruption. In addition, the incision should be as close as possible to the anal verge so that, if a fistula develops, its tract will be limited and a fistulotomy will disturb less tissue. The abscess cavity is thoroughly laid open, and loculations are digitally disrupted to release all the pus. The anorectal canal is also evaluated to exclude underlying disease, and the wound is packed open. Because one third to one half of patients with acute abscesses eventually develop fistulas, some surgeons advocate a search for the gland's internal orifice during the incision and drainage, and they perform an empiric fistulotomy. A prospective trial demonstrated that this approach resulted in a

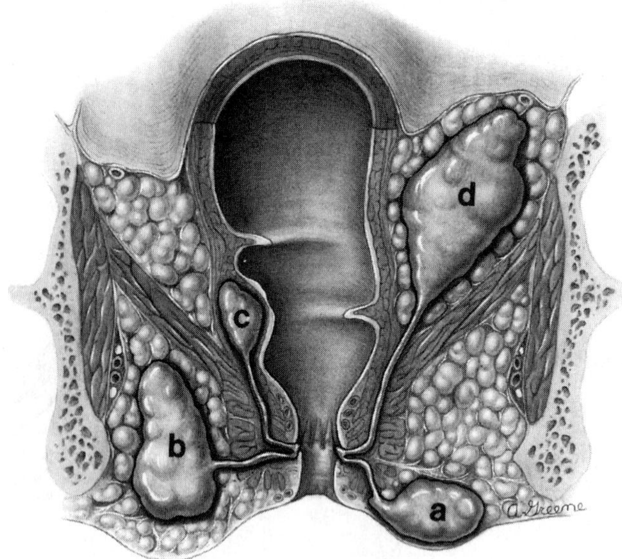

Fig. 112-3. Common sites of anorectal abscesses: perianal *(a)*, anorectal *(b)*, intersphincteric *(c)*, and supralevator *(d)*.

reduced risk of recurrent abscess and fistula compared with incision and drainage alone (3% vs. 41%).[8] However, an immediate fistulotomy was also associated with an increased risk of impaired anal function. Most surgeons treat the active infection and deal with a fistula later, when the tissues are not acutely inflamed.

Intersphincteric and supralevator abscesses are special problems that demand surgical expertise.

Fistula

A fistula is defined as a communication between epithelialized viscera. A few patients with an acute anorectal abscess develop a fistula in ano. These fistulas extend from the anorectal mucosa to the skin, although the tracts can be circuitous and envelop the entire sphincter mechanism. The tract is a function of the plane of dissection of the original septic focus in conjunction with the site of drainage. Fistulas in ano have been classified as intersphincteric, transsphincteric, suprasphincteric, and extrasphincteric[6] (see Fig. 112-3).

Patients with anal fistulas describe sporadic discharge that is occasionally stained with blood. New abscesses periodically form and spontaneously drain. The examiner recognizes the characteristic external orifice with surrounding heaped-up granulation tissue, suggesting chronic inflammation. In accordance with the cryptoglandular genesis of anorectal sepsis, the internal orifice is located along the dentate line. The course of the tract is predicted by Goodsall's rule (Fig. 112-4). If an imaginary line bisects the anus in the coronal plane, external orifices anterior to the line communicate with the internal orifice via the most direct radial tract. On the other hand, posterior external orifices correspond to an internal orifice in the posterior midline.

Once a fistula has formed, it does not spontaneously close because the sphincter mechanism acts as a distal obstruction to the flow of gas and liquid stool through the anorectal lumen. Therefore the tract must be laid open by an experienced surgeon. Although most fistulas are intersphincteric or low transsphincteric and traverse minimal muscula-

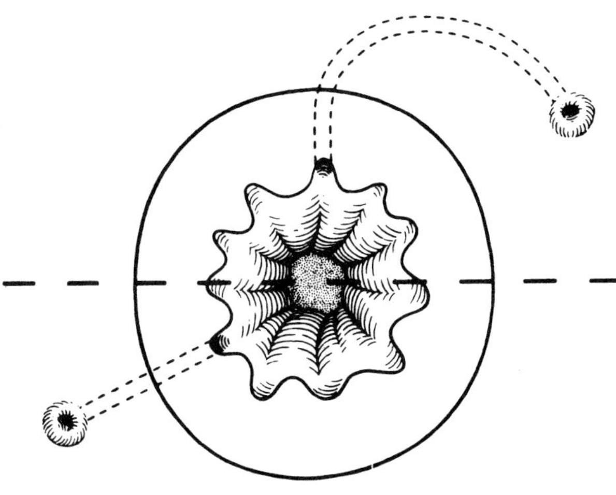

Fig. 112-4. Graphic representation of Goodsall's rule.

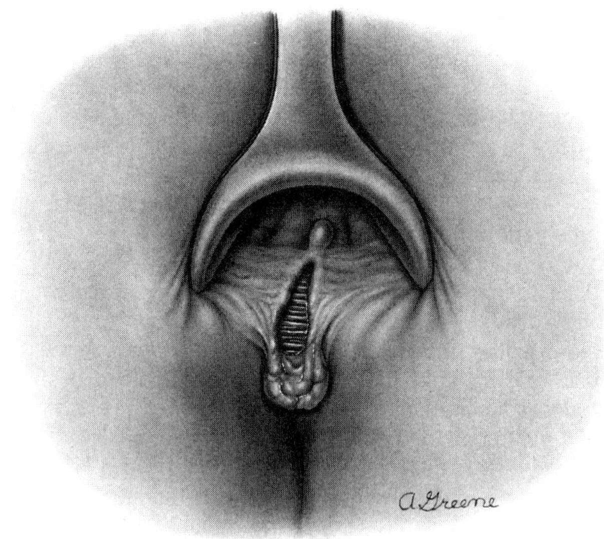

Fig. 112-5. Chronic anal fissure. Note sentinel pile, indurated ulcer, and hypertrophied papilla.

ture, the sphincter is at risk if the tract is not fully appreciated. Extrasphincteric and suprasphincteric fistulas are challenging and suggest inflammatory bowel disease.

Pilonidal Disease

Although pilonidal disease is not an anal suppurative problem, the sacrococcygeal pilonidal sinus resides in the superior pole of the gluteal cleft, and infections are often confused with perirectal sepsis. Congenital theories for the etiology of pilonidal disease were once favored, but now this is believed to be an acquired condition. Pilonidal disease begins with hair follicles burrowing into the underlying subcutaneous fat. Other hairs and debris are propelled into this sinus over time, creating a foreign body reaction and a soft tissue infection.

Long-term hygiene is emphasized, with initially weekly shavings to prevent additional hairs from being drawn into the pilonidal cavity.[1] Once the inciting foreign bodies have been eradicated, the inflammation should subside and the sinus will obliterate. An acute pilonidal abscess is incised and drained, preferably with a lateral vertical incision parallel to the midline cleft. Hairs are removed to the extent possible during the original drainage and in subsequent visits while the wound heals. Extensive and recurrent pilonidal disease may demand more aggressive surgical debridement and wound closure. However, it is critical to confine the dissection to the chronic fibrous tracts that contain the foreign debris and to spare the normal surrounding subcutaneous fat.

ANAL FISSURE

An anal fissure results from a disruption of the mucosal integrity of the anal canal. This usually follows a traumatic hard stool, although instrumentation or other local insults can also be the cause. Acute fissures are common and ordinarily heal spontaneously in a few days. The intense pain of a fissure engenders a reluctance to defecate, however, compounding the constipation and the aggravating effects of subsequent bowel movements. This cycle can produce a chronic fissure (Fig. 112-5). Anal manometry has demonstrated that some patients have a propensity to develop fissures as a result of increased anal sphincter resting pressures. Local ischemia is likely responsible as well.[5]

Anal fissures present with dramatic pain that is exacerbated by defecation. Bleeding and pruritus may also occur. Inspection and light palpation suffice to diagnose most fissures, although an examination under anesthesia may be necessary when pain is severe. A sentinel skin tag at the external portion of the fissure implies chronicity, as does a hypertrophied papilla at the proximal pole. Fissures are predominantly located in the posterior midline, but about 10% of fissures in women are in the anterior midline. Lateral or multiple fissures should arouse suspicions of underlying conditions, such as Crohn's disease, tuberculosis, HIV, chronic ulcerative colitis, leukemia, and sexually transmitted diseases (e.g., lymphogranuloma venereum).

The institution of a bowel regimen to create soft, bulky, atraumatic stools disrupts the provocative cycle and allows the fissure to heal in about half of patients (see Box 112-1). Surgery is necessary for chronic or refractory acute fissures to provide a wider aperture for stool to pass and to interrupt the internal sphincter spasm. Anal dilation accomplishes these goals, although the extent of sphincter disruption is unpredictable, causing undesirable rates of recurrence and of anal incontinence. Lateral internal sphincterotomy involves a more precise division of the distal portion of the internal sphincter muscle; success rates are greater than 90%, and incontinence is uncommon. The anorectum is also evaluated during surgery to identify underlying causes, such as inflammatory bowel disease.

PERIANAL CROHN'S DISEASE

Crohn's disease often involves the anus, and surgeons must be particularly circumspect about performing anal procedures on these patients, limiting the surgery to the minimal trauma necessary to relieve symptoms. When possible, it is prudent to defer surgery until the active Crohn's disease has subsided with medical management. Perianal Crohn's disease is associated with edematous discolored skin tags that can be mistaken for hemorrhoids, which are uncommon among Crohn's patients. When they do occur, hemorrhoids are best managed nonsurgically because of wound healing concerns and because proctectomy has been necessary for postoperative complications. However, surgery can be safely performed on select patients with quiescent Crohn's disease and symptomatic hemorrhoids that have failed to respond to nonsurgical measures.[9]

Anal suppurative disease is common among patients with Crohn's disease. This diagnosis should be strongly suspected in those with multiple, recurrent, or complex anal abscesses or fistulas. Suppurative disease often heals spontaneously or with local supportive care and medical management. The most common procedure for septic complications is a simple incision and drainage. A limited fistulotomy can often be done safely without disturbing anorectal function once the acute inflammation has resolved. Although a proctectomy may eventually be necessary for some patients with perianal Crohn's disease, it is generally conducted for the complications of the disease rather than for nonhealing surgical wounds.[7,9]

Most anal fissures associated with Crohn's disease are painless. However, a judicious internal sphincterotomy is successful in the minority of patients who require surgery.[7]

HUMAN IMMUNODEFICIENCY VIRUS

Up to one third of homosexual men with HIV experience anorectal problems. In fact, these conditions constitute the most common indications for surgery in this population. Condylomata may be the most common anal disorder among HIV-positive patients (see Chapter 29), although suppurative diseases, fissures, ulcers, hemorrhoids, and various malignancies occur as well. Interestingly, anal fissures are typically situated in the posterior midline, as they are in the general population. Anal ulcers are a peculiar phenomenon and are likely associated with chronic fissures. These patients present challenging clinical dilemmas because of their immunocompromised states and impaired wound healing.

A series of 1502 patients with HIV, predominantly homosexual men, revealed that 101 of them had undergone 161 anorectal procedures.[4] Pain was the most common symptom, followed by purulent discharge and bleeding. The indications for surgery, in decreasing order, were anorectal sepsis, fissures, condylomata, tumors, and hemorrhoids. Bacterial and viral cultures revealed fecal organisms, staphylococci, herpes simplex, cytomegalovirus, human papillomavirus, *Neisseria gonorrhoeae*, and cryptosporidia. Malignancies were identified in one quarter of the patients who underwent biopsies (10% of overall series). Lesions were often occult and included Kaposi's sarcoma, non-Hodgkin's lymphoma, anaplastic lymphoma, leukemia, and squamous cell carcinoma. Because only 40% of anorectal surgical wounds had healed by 3 months, a multivariate logistic analysis was done to identify critical factors.[4] Independent predictors of poor healing included a CD4 count less than 50 cells/μl and surgery within the first year of the diagnosis of acquired immunodeficiency syndrome (AIDS). Conversely, the Centers for Disease Control and Prevention stages of HIV and AIDS were not significant determinants of wound healing. Chronic fissures were the least likely lesions to heal (16% at 3 months).

The ideal treatments for the numerous anorectal conditions of HIV patients have not been clearly established. The physician must cautiously select appropriate candidates for surgery, although cultures and biopsies should be liberally performed (see Chapter 32).

ANAL TUMORS

Anal tumors are relatively uncommon, accounting for only 4% of anorectal malignancies (see Chapter 105). Although these tumors occur infrequently, the primary care physician plays an important role in detection because the lesions typically present with bleeding, pain, pruritus, or a mass. Appropriate evaluation of these symptoms should result in the recognition of tumors. Squamous cell carcinomas constitute about two thirds of malignancies of the anal canal and anal margin. Other cell types include cloacogenic, mucoepidermoid, small cell, adenocarcinoma, basal cell, Bowen's disease (squamous cell carcinoma in situ), Paget's disease (adenocarcinoma in situ), melanoma, lymphoma, and leukemia. Over the last two decades the philosophy of care for anal epidermoid tumors has dramatically shifted from radical, ablative surgery to combined regimens of radiation and chemotherapy. This has resulted in improved local control and survival as well as sphincter preservation.

REFERENCES

1. Armstrong JH, Barcia PJ: Pilonidal sinus disease: the conservative approach, *Arch Surg* 129:914, 1994.
2. Daniel GL, Longo WE, Vernava AM: Pruritus ani: causes and concerns, *Dis Colon Rectum* 37:670, 1994.
3. Johanson JF, Rimm A: Optimal nonsurgical treatment of hemorrhoids: a comparative analysis of infrared coagulation, rubber band ligation, and injection sclerotherapy, *Am J Gastroenterol* 87:1601, 1992.
4. Lord RVN: Anorectal surgery in patients infected with human immunodeficiency virus: factors associated with delayed wound healing, *Ann Surg* 226:92, 1997.
5. Neufeld DM et al: Outpatient surgical treatment of anal fissure, *Eur J Surg* 161:435, 1995.
6. Parks AG, Gordon PH, Hardcastle JD: A classification of fistula-in-ano, *Br J Surg* 63:1, 1976.
7. Sangwan YP et al: Perianal Crohn's disease: results of local surgical treatment, *Dis Colon Rectum* 39:529, 1996.
8. Schouten WR, van Vroonhoven TJMV: Treatment of anorectal abscess with or without primary fistulectomy: results of a prospective randomized trial, *Dis Colon Rectum* 34:60, 1991.
9. Wolkomir AF, Luchtefeld MA: Surgery for symptomatic hemorrhoids and anal fissures in Crohn's disease, *Dis Colon Rectum* 36:545, 1993.

VIII HEMATOLOGY/ONCOLOGY

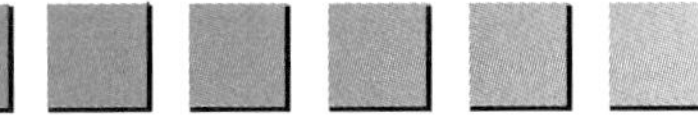

Cardinal Manifestations of Hematologic Disease, Anemias, and Related Conditions

Jack E. Ansell

A wide range of hematologic disorders can be diagnosed and treated by the primary care physician, although many complex or life-threatening conditions, sometimes presenting very subtly, require referral for more specialized care. Given the vast knowledge encompassed by the field of hematology, what is a primary care physician expected to know, and when is referral to a hematologic subspecialist appropriate? A primary care physician must be familiar with the basic physiology of red blood cells (RBCs), white blood cells (WBCs), platelets, coagulation, and elements of the lymphoreticular system. This knowledge provides a background for understanding the relevant pathophysiology, developing a diagnostic approach, acquiring diagnostic acumen, and selecting therapeutic interventions.

GENERAL APPROACH TO HEMATOLOGIC DISORDERS

The diagnostic and therapeutic approach to hematologic disorders is quite simple. Symptoms and signs of disease are based on a derangement in the normal function of one of the cellular elements of the blood or of the hemostatic system. Hallmark findings include fatigue, fever, bleeding, or thrombosis. Similarly, the pathophysiology of blood disorders can be viewed in the context of abnormal production (too much or too little) or excessive destruction or loss of a cellular element. Although this is an oversimplified approach, it does set the framework for understanding hematologic disease.

When interviewing the patient and establishing the history of an illness, genetic and inheritable factors tend to play an important role in hematologic disease, and thus one must pay attention to ethnic background and family history. The cellular elements of the blood are also exquisitely sensitive to environmental toxins, medications, and illicit drugs. Thus work experience and social history must not be neglected. Finally, the interpretation of hematologic parameters must be done with the understanding that (1) each cell line has specific cellular pools, (2) the distribution that one measures in the circulating blood can be dramatically affected by hydration or fluid shifts, and (3) the peripheral blood does not always reflect what is happening in the bone marrow or peripheral tissues.

Red Blood Cell Disorders: Anemia

Anemia is best defined as a reduction in hemoglobin that leads to a reduction in oxygen supply to peripheral tissues. Anemia may be clinically difficult to identify, and a routine blood count is usually required. It is important to remember that anemia is not a disease, but a manifestation of an underlying illness, and its presence should lead to a search for its etiology.

Classification. A common classification scheme of anemia is based on its pathophysiologic mechanism and the morphologic appearance of the red cells. Such an approach leads to an understanding of the etiology, as demonstrated in the algorithm presented in Fig. 113-1. According to this approach, anemia is due either to failure of the bone marrow to produce enough RBCs (hypoproliferative anemia) or excessive and premature destruction of RBCs in the circulation (hemolytic anemia). The former category also includes anemias due to red cell maturation abnormalities, and the latter includes anemias due to excessive loss of RBCs (i.e., bleeding). Morphologically, anemias can be characterized by RBCs that are large, normal, or small (macrocytic, normocytic, or microcytic) and normal colored or pale (normochromic, hypochromic). Densely colored cells are referred to as spherocytes. Table 113-1 categorizes a number of RBC shape abnormalities that might be seen on the peripheral blood smear.

Symptoms. The symptoms of anemia depend on the duration of onset, the pathophysiologic mechanism, and the specific etiology. Anemias that develop over hours or a few days are usually due to blood loss. They produce symptoms of intravascular volume depletion (hypotension, cardiac strain, shock). Such rapidly developing anemias can also be the result of fulminant hemolysis, but in the latter, symptoms are primarily attributable to the deleterious effects of hemoglobin metabolites. Anemias that develop slowly are more likely to be better tolerated at lower levels of hematocrit than those that develop rapidly because of a compensatory plasma volume increase. Symptoms are primarily related to tissue hypoxia and cardiac strain (fatigue, irritability, headache, dyspnea, orthopnea, palpitations, and angina).

Diagnostic Approach. The diagnostic approach to evaluating anemia starts with its signs and symptoms, but final conclusions regarding the etiology cannot be made until specific laboratory tests are performed. Most blood counts today are performed by electronic particle counters and are exceedingly accurate. A complete blood count (CBC) includes a WBC count, RBC count, hemoglobin, hematocrit (Hct), red cell indices, and differential count of the WBCs. RBCs can be morphologically categorized by examining the peripheral blood smear under a microscope, as well as by calculating the red cell indices, which denote average cell size, hemoglobin content, hemoglobin concentration, and distribution of RBC width (RDW) (Table 113-2). Microscopic examination of the peripheral blood smear may provide additional information about the potential etiology of anemia.

A reticulocyte count should always be considered when anemia is present. The reticulocyte percentage gives an indication of the bone marrow's capacity to respond to

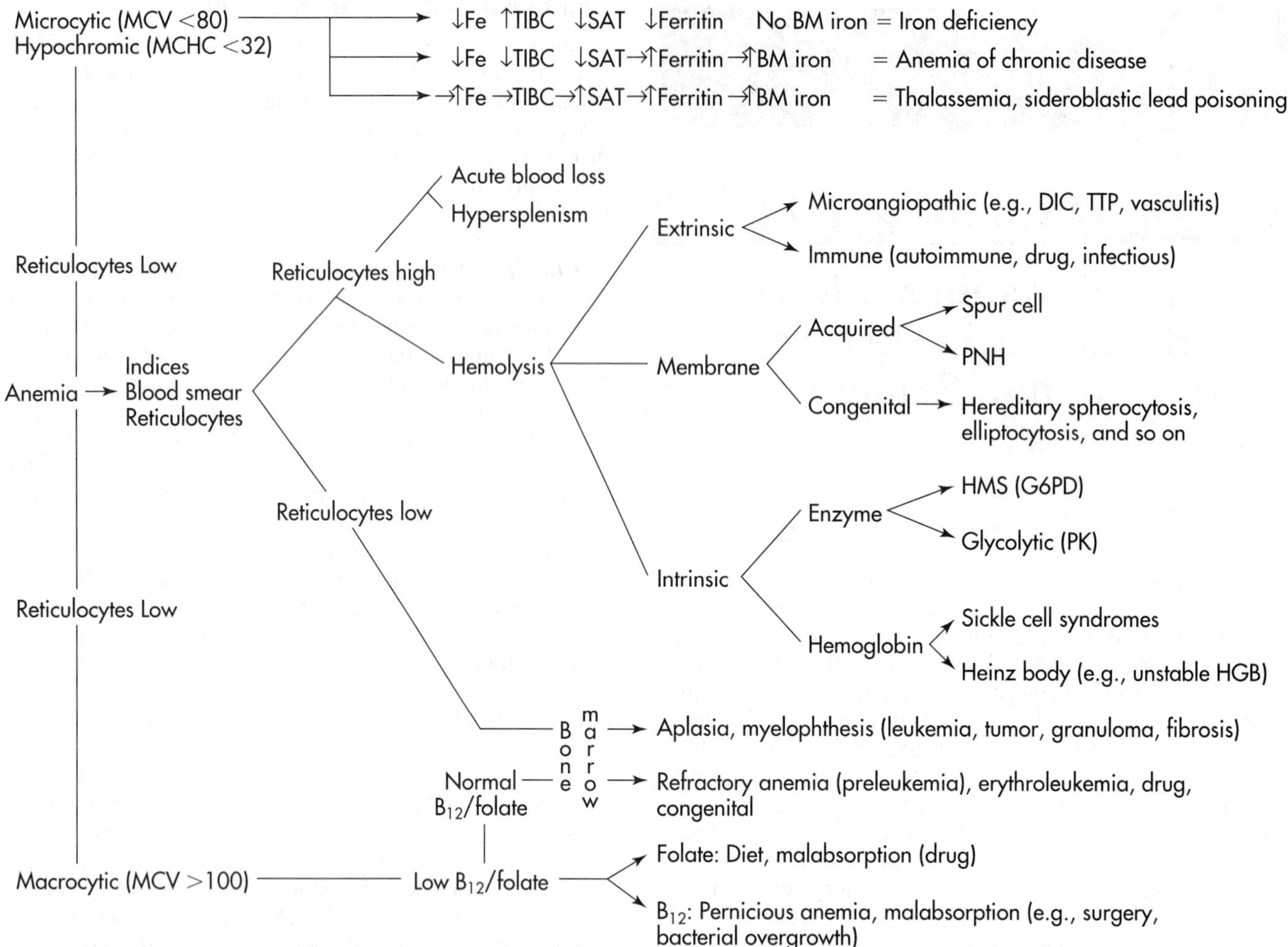

Fig. 113-1. Systematic laboratory approach to the patient with anemia is based on pathophysiologic and morphologic criteria and takes into consideration cost-effectiveness. Results of a CBC, red cell indices, reticulocyte count, and blood smear should indicate which pathway of analysis to pursue. Patients may have combined defects, thus disease processes do not always adhere to a textbook description. A disheartening observation is the all-too-frequent request for a CBC, serum iron, TIBC, serum ferritin, B_{12}, and folate level. This "shotgun" approach to the initial evaluation of anemia must be avoided. Consider the potential mechanism of the anemia and the RBC morphology and then order appropriate and specific diagnostic tests. *MCV,* Mean corpuscular volume; *MCHC,* mean corpuscular hemoglobin concentration; *Fe,* iron; *BM,* bone marrow; *TIBC,* total iron binding capacity; *SAT,* saturation; *DIC,* disseminated intravascular coagulation; *TTP,* thrombotic thrombocytopenic purpura; *PNH,* paroxysmal nocturnal hemoglobinuria; *PK,* pyruvate kinase; *HGB,* hemoglobin; *HMS,* hexose monophosphate shunt.

anemia by increased production. Reticulocytes show up as bluish-colored cells (polychromatophilia) on a standard peripheral smear, and this can provide a rough estimate of an elevated count. Otherwise, a specific stain must be made to determine the reticulocyte percentage. A reticulocyte count is a relative number and should be corrected by multiplying it by the patient's Hct divided by the normal Hct (corrected reticulocyte count) or by determining the absolute number of reticulocytes per microliter of blood by multiplying the reticulocyte count by the RBC count (absolute reticulocyte count). Examples are illustrated in Fig. 113-2. In general, corrections are not necessary when the reticulocyte count is markedly elevated or low in the setting of significant anemia.

Examination of the peripheral blood smear to assess morphologic abnormalities of RBCs is imperative in the evaluation of anemias. Simple observation of the blood smear may lead directly to the diagnosis, avoiding the cost and time of various diagnostic rests. Table 113-1 lists the commonly seen abnormalities in RBC shape and their pathophysiologic significance. Included in this table are various red cell inclusions and their clinical significance.

White Blood Cell Disorders

Alterations in the WBC count occur frequently in response to other disorders, such as inflammation or infection, but few if any symptoms are directly produced by such changes. When confronted with an abnormal WBC count, the physician should obtain a differential count and determine the absolute number of specific cell types. Percentages are relative and may be abnormal when the absolute number of a cell type is normal. Granulocytes predominate in most inflammatory states and counts as high as 20,000/μl are not uncommon and rarely may be as high as 40,000 to 50,000/μl. Such a reaction is called a *leukemoid response,* and there may be a number of less mature forms present. A leukocyte alkaline phosphatase (LAP), which usually increases with increasing WBC, helps

Table 113-1. Common Abnormalities in RBC Shape or Inclusions Seen in the Wright's Stain Blood Smear

Shape/inclusion abnormality	Description	Associated disease
Target cell	Circular midzone of pallor, with peripheral and central color	Liver disease, hemoglobinopathy, thalassemia, after splenectomy
Spherocyte	Round, frequently small, with no central pallor	Hereditary spherocytosis, acquired autoimmune hemolytic anemia
Schistocyte	Helmet- or triangular-shaped cell; fragmented RBC	Microangiopathic hemolytic anemias (e.g., DIC)
Burr cell	Scalloped perimeter, ecchinocyte, crenated	Uremia
Spur cell	Acanthocyte, spiculated	Advanced liver disease, abetalipoproteinemia
Teardrop cell	Pear- or teardrop-shaped	Myelofibrosis and other myeloproliferative diseases, thalassemia major, severe iron deficiency
Macroovalocyte	Large, egg-shaped	B_{12} or folate deficiency
Howell-Jolly body	Dark purple, dotlike inclusions, often at the periphery of cell; represents nuclear remnant	After splenectomy or splenic dysfunction, severe megaloblastic anemia
Heinz body	Dark purple, irregularly shaped by supravital stain (crystal violet); represents denatured hemoglobin	G6PD deficiency, unstable hemoglobins, thalassemia
Basophilic stippling	Dark purple, pinpoint stippling in RBC on Wright's stain; represents polyribosomes	β-Thalassemia, lead poisoning, and many toxic states
Siderocyte	Dark cluster of three to four granules in RBC; represents iron granules	After splenectomy
Normoblast	Nucleated RBC	After splenectomy, leukoerythroblastic anemia (myelophthisis), tumor, and other infiltrative disease in bone marrow

DIC, Disseminated intravascular coagulation; *G6PD,* glucose-6-phosphate dehydrogenase.

Table 113-2. Formulas Used to Determine MCV, MCH, MCHC, and RDW*

Formula	Normal range
$MCV = \frac{Hct(L/L)}{RBC\ count\ (\times 10^{12}/L)} \times 1{,}000$	80-100 fl (10^{-15} L)
$MCH = \frac{Hemoglobin\ (g/dl)}{RBC\ count\ (\times 10^{12}/L)}$	27-32 pg (10^{-12} g)
$MCHC = \frac{Hemoglobin\ (g/dl)}{Hct\ (L/L)}$	32-36 g/dl
$RDW = \frac{(SD\ of\ red\ cell\ volume)}{MCV} \times 100$	11%-15%

*Normal ranges may vary from laboratory.

MCV, Mean corpuscular volume; *MCH,* mean corpuscular hemoglobin; *MCHC,* mean corpuscular hemoglobin concentration; *RDW,* distribution of RBC width.

differentiate a leukemoid response from some myeloproliferative diseases such as chronic myelocytic leukemia (LAP high in the former, very low in the latter). In polycythemia vera, agnogenic myeloid metaplasia, and essential thrombocythemia, which are the other myeloproliferative disorders, the LAP is inappropriately elevated in comparison to the mild elevation of the WBC count.

Extremely high WBC counts (~100,000/µl or more), especially with immature cells as in acute leukemia, can produce leukostasis with signs of headache, dizziness, confusion, pulmonary congestion and hypoxia, retinal hemorrhages and papilledema, and digital ischemia.

A blood smear with granulocyte precursors and nucleated RBCs is characterized as a *leukoerythroblastic* blood smear. In agnogenic myeloid metaplasia, teardrop-shaped RBCs are also noted. Such findings also occur with other invasive diseases of the bone marrow, such as cancer or granulomas. This process is called *myelophthisis* and creates a myelophthisic anemia.

As with most cases of leukocytosis, leukopenia yields few symptoms unless the absolute granulocyte or lymphocyte count reaches significantly low levels. Infection is the major symptom of neutropenia. Its risk increases significantly when the absolute neutrophil count falls below 1000/µl. Patients with severe neutropenia may not be able to mount the same degree of inflammatory response normally seen (e.g., collections of pus), and thus infections may be difficult to diagnose. Drug reactions are often implicated as a cause of neutropenia and must be considered. Drug-induced agranulocytosis is a life-threatening emergency requiring cessation of all suspected medicines and close monitoring of the patient for infection.

Changes in the lymphocyte count present a different spectrum of possibilities. Lymphocytosis is typically seen in acute viral infections such as mononucleosis due to Epstein-Barr virus. Atypical appearing lymphocytes are also present (large cells with abundant cytoplasm, an immature nuclear chromatin pattern with or without nucleoli, and indentation or scalloped cytoplasmic membrane) and usually represent stimulated T cells. Stimulated B cells have a plasma cell–like appearance (smaller, dark blue cytoplasm, displaced nucleus, and clumped chromatin). Lymphopenia can occur in some inherited immunodeficiency disorders but is most often seen today in the setting of human immunodeficiency virus (HIV) infection and acquired immunodeficiency syndrome (AIDS).

Patient A: Hct, 20%; RBC count, $1.5 \times 10^6/\mu l$; reticulocyte count, 4%

Corrected reticulocyte count

$$4 \times \frac{20}{45} = 1.8\%$$

Absolute reticulocyte count

$$(0.04) \times (1.5 \times 10^6) = 60{,}000 \text{ reticulocytes}/\mu l$$

Patient B: Hct, 20%; RBC count, $1.5 \times 10^6/\mu l$; reticulocyte count, 15%

Corrected reticulocyte count

$$15 \times \frac{20}{45} = 6.6\%$$

Absolute reticulocyte count

$$(0.15) \times (1.5 \times 10^6) = 225{,}000 \text{ reticulocytes}/\mu l$$

Fig. 113-2. Even though the reticulocyte count is elevated in both patients, patient A clearly has an inadequate response, with a corrected reticulocyte count of 1.8%, suggesting that the bone marrow is not responding to the anemia and that deficient or defective RBC production may be the cause or is contributing to the anemia. *Patient B* has a good response to the anemia, suggesting that the bone marrow is normal and that the cause may be hemolysis or blood loss. A normal bone marrow is able to increase erythroid production sixfold to eightfold. If the average absolute reticulocyte count is 50,000/µl (1% of 5 million RBCs), the maximum increase in reticulocyte count in response to hemolysis or blood loss should range between 250,000 and 400,000 reticulocytes/µl.

Disorders of leukocyte function are even more difficult to detect than quantitative disorders of leukocytes. They usually represent congenital disorders and may require the services of an experienced laboratory for detection. Qualitative disorders produce symptoms according to the cell line affected (see Chapter 114).

Platelet and Coagulation Disorders

Platelet and coagulation disorders are manifest by either bleeding or thrombosis. Hypercoagulability (thrombophilia) is more likely to predispose to thrombosis than is a platelet abnormality.

Thrombocytopenia as a risk for bleeding is usually not a problem until the count falls below 50,000/µl, and especially below 10,000/µl. If the cause of the low platelet count is failure of production, then the risk of bleeding may be greater at low counts than if the cause is peripheral destruction as in immune thrombocytopenia because of the presence of younger more hemostatically effective platelets in the latter. Platelet-related bleeding can also occur even with normal counts if the platelets are qualitatively defective.

The cardinal sign of a platelet defect is the presence of *petechiae,* which are pinpoint hemorrhages in the skin that often appear on the lower extremities where hydrostatic pressure is greatest. Coalesced petechiae are referred to as *purpura. Ecchymoses,* however, are deep-seated hemorrhages in the subcutaneous tissue, usually indicative of a coagulation disorder. Platelet-related bleeding also tends to occur in the oral mucosa or gastrointestinal tract (GI), and bleeding tends to be immediate in onset since platelets are responsible for the primary hemostatic plug. Coagulation disorders may predispose to more delayed-onset bleeding, and bleeding may occur in intramuscular tissues and joints, as well as the skin and GI tract.

Coagulation disorders may be inherited, in which case they are usually single factor deficiencies (e.g., factor VIII), or acquired, in which case multiple factors are affected (e.g., vitamin K deficiency, liver disease). Recently, a number of new inherited coagulation disorders have been uncovered, accounting for a propensity for thrombosis.

In the final analysis, the diagnosis of a hemostatic disorder of platelets or coagulation depends greatly on the laboratory, and the clinical history simply provides the clues as to where to focus the initial evaluation. Given the complexity of hemostatic disorders, it is helpful to have the assistance of a specialist in the field of coagulation (see Chapter 115).

ANEMIAS AND RBC DISORDERS

Microcytic Anemias

Microcytic anemias are characterized by RBCs with a mean corpuscular volume (MCV) that is usually less than 80 fl. Microcytosis is often but not always associated with hypochromia (mean corpuscular hemoglobin concentration [MCHC] < 32 g/dl). Iron deficiency produces microcytic, hypochromic RBCs, but other causes of small cells can be anemia of chronic disease, thalassemia, and lead poisoning.

Iron Deficiency

The most common cause of anemia in the United States is iron deficiency. It results in a maturation abnormality with decreased hemoglobin and red cell production, and it represents one-quarter of anemias seen in a population of hospitalized patients. Typical patients include infants on a prolonged milk diet with no other nutrients, multiparous women, and patients with bleeding from a GI or gynecologic neoplasm. When iron deficiency is diagnosed, the etiology must be ascertained because of the potential for serious underlying pathology.

Iron homeostasis is finely regulated by absorption, rather than excretion, to meet metabolic needs. Iron is absorbed most effectively in the duodenum and upper jejunum. Absorption is mainly responsive to changes in total RBC mass and tissue hypoxia and not simply to total body iron stores. Iron loss in the GI tract and elsewhere approximates 1 mg daily, the amount absorbed per day. In the menstruating woman, approximately 2 mg daily are lost when averaged over the month, and during pregnancy, the need for absorbed iron reaches 2.5 to 3 mg per day to meet the demands of the fetus.

Etiology. Iron deficiency is almost exclusively caused by excessive blood loss in adults except in pregnancy where fetal needs can outstrip average daily intake. In the United States, dietary deficiency of iron is most often found in infants on a prolonged milk diet or in elderly people with inadequate diets. The daily recommended iron intake for infants is 1 mg/kg/day beginning at approximately 3 to 4 months of age. The infant consuming 1 quart of human milk per day receives only 0.4 mg of iron; those consuming cow's milk receive less than 0.1 mg. Female adolescents may develop

Table 113-3. Results of Laboratory Tests in Iron Deficiency, Anemia of Chronic Disease, or Both

Laboratory test	Normal	Iron deficiency	Anemia of chronic disease	Both
RBC indices	Normal	Microcytic hypochromic	Normal to hypochromic, microcytic	Microcytic, hypochromic
Serum iron	Normal	Low	Low	Low
TIBC	Normal	High	Low	Low
% Saturation	Normal	Low	Low	Low
Serum ferritin	Normal	Low	High	Low
BM iron stores	Normal	Absent	High	Absent

BM, Bone marrow.

NOTE: In the presence of combined iron deficiency and anemia of chronic disease, the serum iron, TIBC, and % saturation often reflect the anemia of chronic disease, while the serum ferritin reflects the iron deficiency. In general, the serum ferritin is a much more interpretable measure of iron stores, even though it is an acute phase reactant and might be raised to the normal range in the setting of combined iron deficiency and anemia of chronic disease. As such, it is the preferred diagnostic assay to assess iron stores in patients with suspected iron deficiency with or without anemia of chronic disease.

iron deficiency due to heavy menstrual bleeding as in adult women. Iron deficiency can also occur as a result of surgical resection of the proximal intestine, inflammatory bowel disease, and sprue. Chronic intravascular hemolysis as may be seen in a malfunctioning prosthetic cardiac valve can also result in iron deficiency due to loss of iron in the urine (hemosiderinuria).

Clinical Findings and Diagnosis. The clinical manifestations of iron deficiency include fatigue, weakness, and headache as in many anemias. Iron deficiency may produce specific signs and symptoms including chelitis, stomatitis, a spoonlike deformity of the finger nails (koilonychia), dysphagia (esophageal webs), and pica (especially pagophagia or ice craving). Occasionally, iron deficiency can cause splenomegaly. The laboratory diagnosis is based on the presence of anemia with microcytic, hypochromic RBCs with varying RBC size and shape leading to an elevated RDW. The diagnosis is confirmed by the findings of a low serum iron, elevated total iron binding capacity (TIBC), and very low TIBC saturation or a low serum ferritin (Table 113-3). The serum ferritin is the preferred measure of iron stores since the serum iron and TIBC are more readily influenced by associated inflammatory conditions making them more difficult to interpret.

Therapy. Iron therapy can start, even while the underlying cause is pursued. Ferrous sulfate, containing 60 mg of elemental iron, is the least expensive form of iron supplement. To avoid GI irritation, it may be advisable to start with one tablet daily and slowly increase to two or three per day depending on the severity of the iron deficiency. A response should be noted in 1 week with a mild increase in the reticulocyte count. Iron therapy should be continued for several months after correction of the Hct to replenish iron stores.

Anemia of Chronic Disease

Anemia of chronic disease denotes a chronic, mild-to-moderate normochromic normocytic or mildly hypochromic microcytic anemia that occurs in the setting of chronic inflammation from a variety of causes including autoimmune disorders, infections, cancer, and so on. In the presence of inflammatory mediators, but based on poorly explained mechanisms, the anemia is caused by a block in iron utilization by RBC precursors. Thus storage iron tends to increase, which results in an elevated ferritin, but circulating iron is low, which is reflected by a low serum iron. Transferrin production is also depressed, leading to a reduced TIBC. The RBC count settles in the range of a Hct of 30% and rarely goes below 28%. An anemia with a Hct below 28% may in part be due to chronic inflammation, but other factors should be considered as well. Anemia of chronic disease requires no specific treatment other than treatment of the underlying inflammatory process. Anemia of chronic disease and iron deficiency anemia often occur together or the potential for each may commonly be present. Since iron studies may be confusing, differentiating one from the other is not always easy. Table 113-3 summarizes the findings in each condition alone and when combined and recommends the most useful screening tests.

Macrocytic Anemia

Macrocytic anemia is characterized by large red cells in the peripheral blood smear and is defined by an elevated MCV. Many factors can lead to macrocytosis besides a deficiency of vitamin B_{12} or folic acid. These include an elevation in the reticulocyte count (reticulocytes are younger and larger cells), the presence of target cells typically seen in liver disease or post splenectomy (large cells with excess membrane), hypothyroidism, the myelodysplastic syndromes and in response to a number of cancer chemotherapeutic drugs.

Vitamin B_{12} and Folic Acid Deficiency

In vitamin B_{12} and folic acid deficiency, RBC maturation is characterized as megaloblastic, which refers to a specific maturation abnormality and morphologic appearance of RBC precursors. RBCs show a delay in nuclear maturation (immature nuclear appearance) while cytoplasmic maturation proceeds. The pathophysiology can be traced to the folic acid cycle and impaired production of purine nucleotides (Fig. 113-3). This is certain for folic acid, but it is not entirely clear whether the B_{12} defect is mediated through its relationship to the folic acid cycle or through some other mechanism.

Etiology. In theory, deficiencies of vitamin B_{12} or folic acid can occur as a result of inadequate intake, absorption, or excessive demand. In some cases there may be interference with folate metabolism. In practice, however, vitamin B_{12} deficiency is virtually always due to a problem with

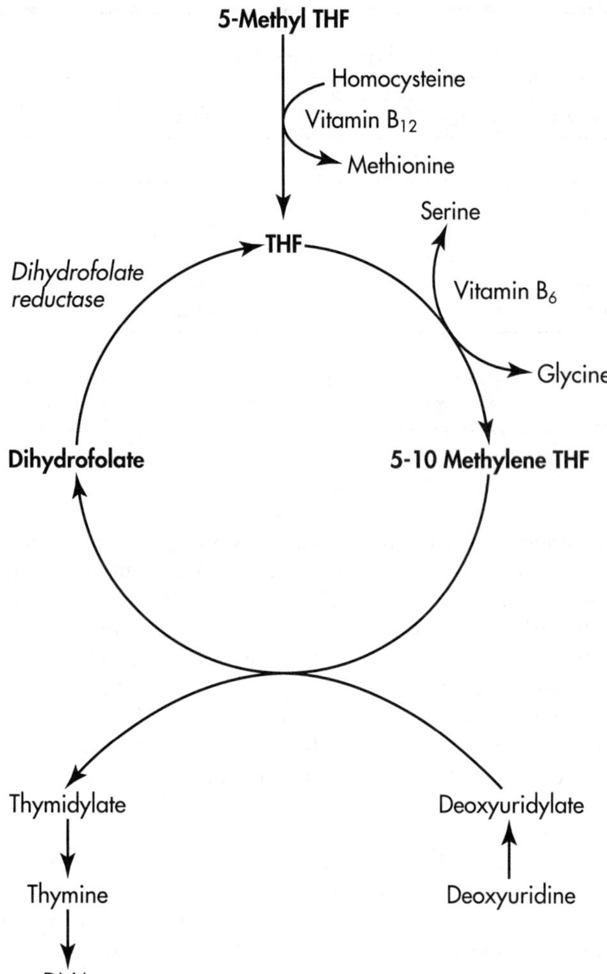

Fig. 113-3. Folic acid metabolism and interaction with vitamin B_{12}. Dietary folates enter the cycle as formyl, methyl, and methylene THF. Vitamin B_{12} serves as a cofactor in the conversion of 5-methylene THF to THF and homocysteine to methionine. Nucleic acid synthesis is integrated at the 5,10-methylene THF to dihydrofolate (DHF) step. *THF,* Tetrahydrofolate.

absorption, while folate deficiency spans the whole spectrum of possibilities. Box 113-1 summarizes the potential causes of deficiency of each vitamin. Pernicious anemia is a special case of vitamin B_{12} deficiency. Pernicious anemia may be an autoimmune disorder resulting in a deficiency of intrinsic factor, a protein secreted by parietal cells of the stomach that facilitates vitamin B_{12} absorption in the terminal ileum.

Clinical Findings and Diagnosis. Anemia develops insidiously and symptoms may not appear until the Hct is severely reduced. Folic acid stores are limited and a deficiency can develop over a 3 month period with inadequate intake. Vitamin B_{12} stores are enough to sustain an individual for up to 3 or more years. Since vitamin B_{12} is required for normal neurologic function, a disorder of impaired vibratory and position sense and ataxia or spastic gait can develop called *subacute combined systems disease* (affects lateral and dorsal columns of spinal cord). Mental status changes may also develop with B_{12} deficiency. If left untreated, these findings may become irreversible. It has recently become clear that these problems can develop in the setting of vitamin B_{12} deficiency without significant anemia.

Box 113-1. Causes of Vitamin B_{12} and Folic Acid Deficiency

Vitamin B_{12} Deficiency

Inadequate intake (rare)
Malabsorption (usual cause)
- Pernicious anemia (lack of intrinsic factor)
- Intestinal disease or surgical absence of terminal ileum
- Competition from bacterial overgrowth (blind loop) or fish tapeworm
- Transcobalamin II transport protein deficiency (rare)

Folic Acid Deficiency

Inadequate intake/availability
- Poor diet
- Long-term oral antibiotics

Malabsorption
- Sprue, celiac disease in children

Increased demand
- Pregnancy
- Chronic hemolysis
- Exfoliative dermatitis

Interference with metabolism
- Alcohol abuse
- Anticonvulsants
- Oral contraceptives
- Antimetabolites

The peripheral blood shows macrocytic RBCs (typically, oval macrocytes) and hypersegmented neutrophils. A diagnosis is established by measuring a low B_{12} or folate level. Sometimes, the RBC folate level can be helpful since it remains low for some time even after correction of the plasma level. A bone marrow, if necessary, if usually hypercellular and shows megaloblastic maturation in all three cell lines. In vitamin B_{12} deficiency, the presumed site of malabsorption can be determined by performing a Schilling test, which involves administering oral radioactively-labeled vitamin B_{12} with or without intrinsic factor attached, followed by an intramuscular injection of vitamin B_{12} to saturate binding sites, and then measuring urinary excretion of absorbed, labeled B_{12}.

Therapy. Therapy consists of administering folic acid daily, 1 mg per day, in the case of folate deficiency or vitamin B_{12}, 100 μg intramuscularly once monthly. Vitamin B_{12} deficiency is initially treated with higher doses (1000 μg) weekly for the first 4 weeks. It is imperative to make a correct diagnosis of the cause of a megaloblastic anemia because the administration of folic acid can improve the anemia of vitamin B_{12} deficiency, but it has no effect on the neurologic impairment that can become irreversible if untreated.

Hemolytic Anemias

The pathophysiologic abnormality in hemolysis is a shortening of the red cell survival, which is normally 100 to 120 days. Regardless of the primary cause, the final hemolytic event is a result of injury to the RBC membrane. Any disorder that affects the membrane may result in a shortened red cell survival. The hemolytic anemias are broadly categorized as those resulting from an intrinsic defect

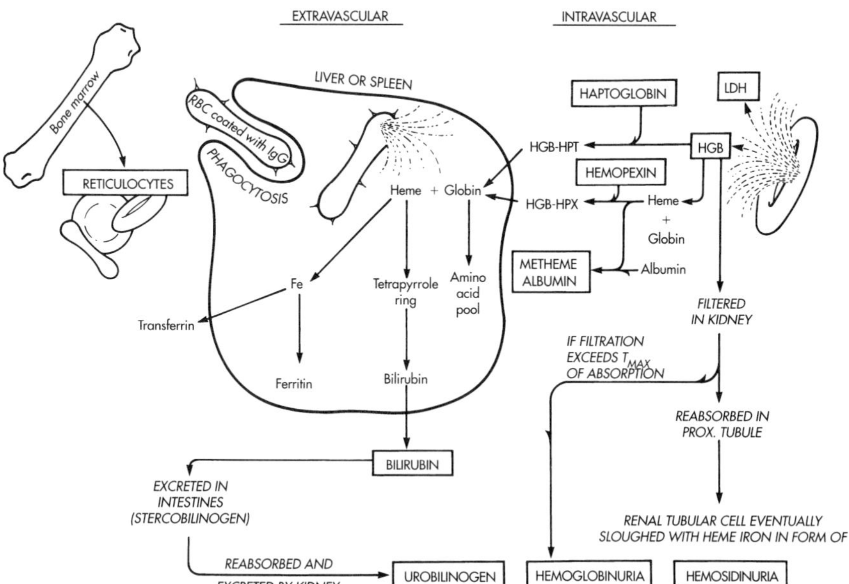

Fig. 113-4. Pathways of hemoglobin metabolism in extravascular or intravascular hemolysis. Items enclosed in rectangles indicate assays routinely obtained that reflect hemolysis. These tests are more likely to be positive with intravascular hemolysis than with extravascular hemolysis. Note that certain tests are not included here, e.g., a Coombs test. A Coombs test is a diagnostic test looking at a specific etiology for hemolysis, whereas these tests are more generic in that they simply reflect the presence of hemolysis and not necessarily its etiology. Once the presence of hemolysis is determined, tests are ordered that look for specific etiologies. *HGB,* Hemoglobin; *HPT,* haptoglobin; *HPX,* hemopexin; *LDH,* lactic dehydrogenase.

of red cells, usually congenital, and those related to an extrinsic defect, usually acquired. They can also be categorized by the site of RBC destruction: in some situations the major site is in the circulation (intravascular), whereas in others it is extravascular, primarily by macrophages in the spleen. The usual response of the bone marrow to hemolysis is an increase in erythropoiesis, reflected by an elevated reticulocyte count.

Symptoms due to hemolysis depend on its severity and the rapidity with which anemia develops. Jaundice is a common underlying finding. A history of cholelithiasis and splenomegaly may be found in association with congenital or long-standing hemolysis. Similar hereditary forms may exist in the family, and a study of parents or siblings may reveal reticulocytosis, splenomegaly, or both in otherwise compensated, silent cases. In chronic hemolytic syndromes, exacerbation of hemolysis may produce a hemolytic crisis with a severe worsening of anemia. Hemolysis should be suspected whenever the reticulocyte count is increased without evidence of blood loss. Depending on the cause of the hemolysis, spherocytes or other abnormalities in red cell shape may be present on the peripheral blood smear. In fulminant cases of hemolysis, the diagnosis is often not difficult. In more subtle cases, the physician may be confronted with the question of whether or not hemolysis is present. In this case, one needs to look for the breakdown products of hemoglobin. Fig. 113-4 is an illustration of the pathways of hemoglobin metabolism in the setting of either intravascular or extravascular hemolysis.

Hemolysis Due to Extrinsic RBC Defects

Immune Hemolysis. Immune hemolysis resulting from antibody damage to the RBC membrane may be a result of an autoimmune, alloimmune, or drug-induced process. Autoimmune hemolytic anemias (AIHA) can occur in the setting of a well-characterized autoimmune disease, or more commonly may be idiopathic. IgG-mediated AIHAs are more common and primarily produce extravascular breakdown of RBCs (Box 113-2). IgM-mediated AIHAs, also called cold AIHA or cold agglutinin disease because the antibodies are most reactive at low temperatures, produce complement activation and intravascular hemolysis. The Coombs test or direct antiglobulin test is positive in the vast majority of cases of AIHA. The reticulocyte count is typically elevated, and breakdown products of hemoglobin may be present in variable amounts depending on the intensity of hemolysis and whether it is predominantly intravascular or extravascular. Treatment for AIHAs always involves looking for an underlying cause such as lupus, lymphoma, or infection. A

> **Box 113-2. Disorders Associated with Warm (IgG) Autoimmune Hemolytic Anemia***
>
> **Reticuloendothelial Disease**
> Chronic lymphocytic leukemia
> Hodgkin's disease
> Non-Hodgkin's lymphomas
> Thymoma
> Multiple myeloma
> Waldenström macroglobulinemia
>
> **Collagen Disease**
> Systemic lupus erythematosus
> Scleroderma
> Rheumatoid arthritis
>
> **Infectious Diseases, Especially Childhood Viral Syndromes**
>
> **Immunologic Diseases**
> Hypogammaglobulinemia
> Dysglobulinemias
> Other immune deficiency syndromes
>
> **GI Disease**
> Ulcerative colitis
>
> **Benign Tumors**
> Ovarian dermoid cyst
>
> *Does not include drugs that cause AIHA.

drug-induced cause must also be considered, and if found, removal of the drug resolves the process in most cases. Steroids are the mainstay of treatment for IgG-mediated AIHA, and splenectomy may be necessary in some cases. Intravenous IgG may also be beneficial. Steroids are not as beneficial in IgM-mediated cold agglutinin AIHA, and various chemotherapeutic agents may be tried.

Mechanical Hemolysis. Mechanical or physical injury to RBCs is characterized by a microangiopathic hemolytic anemia and the finding on blood smear of RBC fragments called *schistocytes* and *helmet cells.* These nonpliable cells circulate poorly and are rapidly removed from the circulation. This problem may be seen in such conditions as disseminated intravascular coagulation (DIC), thrombotic thrombocytopenic purpura (TTP), and damaged prosthetic cardiac valves. Specific treatment involves removing the offending underlying problem or process.

Hemolysis Due to Intrinsic RBC Defects. Intrinsic defects include direct abnormalities of the RBC membrane (e.g., hereditary spherocytosis) or abnormalities of hemoglobin or enzymes of the Embden-Meyerhof pathway.

Hereditary Spherocytosis. Hereditary spherocytosis (HS) is typically an autosomal dominant disorder characterized by anemia, jaundice, splenomegaly, and spherocytes. There is usually a positive family history of anemia. The RBC membrane abnormality most often involves a deficiency of spectrin, one of the major supporting elements of the membrane, although HS can result from defects of other structural elements. Patients are often symptomatic in childhood. Cholelithiasis is common. Aplastic crises can develop (temporary decrease in bone marrow RBC production). The spherocytic cells typically show greater fragility in the osmotic fragility test. Treatment in patients with recurrent problems usually involves splenectomy.

Hemoglobinopathies. More than 300 types of hemoglobinopathies have been described, most being characterized by single or rarely multiple amino acid substitutions in the globin chains, which reduce the solubility of hemoglobin leading to increased RBC intracytoplasmic viscosity, decreased membrane pliability, and shortened RBC survival. Two major hemoglobinopathies are considered here: the sickle cell syndromes and the thalassemias. A hematologist should be involved in managing patients who are severely affected (usually homozygotes). The thalassemias are characterized by reduced synthesis of either α-chains (α-thalassemia) or β-chains (β-thalassemia), which results in precipitation of the normal (but excess) β- or α-chains, respectively, and causes membrane rigidity and shortened RBC survival. In both situations the final hemolytic event is precipitated by a change in the properties of the cell membrane. The electrophoretic mobility of hemoglobins with amino acid substitutions is usually abnormal and can be identified by hemoglobin electrophoresis.

Sickle Cell Disease

Etiology. Homozygous sickle cell anemia is an inherited disease found primarily in people of African ancestry, the gene having originated in two regions of West Africa and providing a possible survival advantage to individuals infected with the malarial parasite. The basic defect in sickle cell disease is replacement of glutamic acid by valine at position 6 of the β-chain, leading to hemoglobin S (two normal α and two β_s chains). Polymerization of deoxyhemoglobin is the ultimate cause of the sickling phenomenon. The end result of sickling is occlusion of precapillary arterioles and infarction of surrounding tissues. Hemolysis occurs because of increased membrane rigidity of the deformed cells.

Patients with sickle cell trait or the heterozygous condition have erythrocytes that contain 20% to 40% hemoglobin S, with most of the remainder being normal adult hemoglobin (hemoglobin A_1). Sickle cell trait may be associated with a mild renal tubular defect that results in an inability to concentrate urine, but generally the condition is completely asymptomatic. Rarely, on exposure to severe hypoxia, the sickling phenomenon can be induced and can lead to symptoms. Sickle cell trait is present in approximately 8% to 10% of African-Americans. Hemoglobin S also occurs in association with other abnormal hemoglobins, such as hemoglobin C and hemoglobin D, or with thalassemia trait. These are called sickle cell variants and produce symptoms of varying severity.

Clinical Findings and Diagnosis. Sickle cell anemia is a severe, constant, hemolytic anemia interrupted by vasoocclusive (painful) or aplastic crises. Symptoms first occur during the second half of the first year of life when most fetal hemoglobin has been replaced by hemoglobin S. Patients become progressively more anemic and develop splenomegaly. Eventually splenic function is lost from repeated thromboses (autosplenectomy), which can lead to an increased risk of infections during childhood.

Pain crises (vasoocclusive episodes) are caused by infarctions that lead to recurrent attacks of pain involving the chest, abdomen, and skeleton. Aplastic crises resulting in acute exacerbation of anemia develop as a result of infections when compensatory RBC production is impaired. Bone disease develops because of multiple infarctions and expansion of the bone marrow cavity. Vascular occlusions may cause avascular necrosis of the hip or shoulder. Osteomyelitis caused by *Salmonella* organisms is not an uncommon sequela. The sequence of marrow infarction, necrosis, and the healing process results in new bone formation, which produces characteristic radiographic changes. Cardiomegaly and pulmonary disease develop secondary to anemia and repeated infections and infarctions. The acute chest syndrome is a complication characterized by fever, pleuritic pain, lung infiltrates, and hypoxemia. It is fatal in 2% to 14% of cases due to infection, infarction, or both.

Stroke may be another catastrophic complication of sickle cell anemia. If CT scan or MRI examination is considered, one must be careful with the use of contrast dyes, even the nonionic contrast agents, unless the hemoglobin is at least 5 g/dl. Hyposthenuria, hematuria, priapism, and the nephrotic syndrome are occasionally encountered. Retinal detachment, blindness, and vitreous hemorrhages are common ocular complications. As a result of complications and repeated crises, patients often do not survive beyond the third decade.

Hemoglobin electrophoresis demonstrates only a hemoglobin S band in sickle cell anemia, and both hemoglobin A_1 and hemoglobin S in sickle cell trait. Hemoglobin F may be slightly elevated. Screening tests are based on rapid sickling of red cells under hypoxic conditions on peripheral smears or on solubility properties that allow distinction between Hb AS, SS, and A. In sickle cell anemia the presence of numerous sickled cells on Wright-stained blood smears is easily seen. Technical advances in amniocentesis have enabled the diagnosis of sickle cell anemia as early as the sixteenth week of gestation. When this is not feasible, fetoscopy and fetal blood sampling are required, although these procedures are associated with an increased risk of fetal loss and occasional false-positive or false-negative results. Because one out of four offspring has the homozygous disease if both parents have sickle cell trait, genetic counseling of young couples carrying the sickle cell gene can prevent the trauma of caring for a child afflicted with sickle cell anemia.

Treatment of sickle cell anemia is aimed at relieving the painful vasoocclusive crises, treating the secondary effects of the chronic anemia, and if possible correcting the anemia. Treatment also requires supplementation with folic acid (1 mg daily) and prevention of infections with prompt antibiotic treatment or by vaccination (pneumococcal vaccine). The treatment of vasoocclusive crises relies on supporting measures: analgesics, intravenous fluids, and oxygen. With severe and prolonged pain, narcotic analgesics are often necessary. Oxygen is commonly used to diminish hypoxia, but its benefits have not been substantiated. If acidosis is present, sodium bicarbonate is added, usually one ampule (44 mEq) to each liter of 0.45% saline in 5% glucose, but as with oxygen therapy its benefits have not been proved. Partial exchange transfusions may be indicated in situations of prolonged vasoocclusive crises, before elective surgery, for priapism, or during pregnancy. It is advisable to maintain the hematocrit at 25% throughout pregnancy, since sickle cell blood is closest to normal viscosity at this level. At delivery, regional or spinal anesthesia should be used and proper oxygenation ensured. Recently efforts to optimize erythropoiesis by administering erythropoietin and to increase fetal hemoglobin with hydroxyurea or butyrate have undergone initially promising trials.

Hemoglobin C Disease. Hemoglobin C disease is found in approximately 3% of heterozygotes in the United States. The interaction between hemoglobin S trait and hemoglobin C trait is quite common, occurring once in every 833 births to African-Americans. Individuals with hemoglobin SC disease tend to have a variable course, with complications occurring less frequently than with sickle cell anemia but with more symptoms than either trait alone. These patients have been reported to develop thromboembolic complications, retinopathy, and renal papillary necrosis more frequently than patients with sickle cell anemia.

Thalassemias. The thalassemia syndromes are a heterogenous group of inherited disorders resulting from suboptimal synthesis of either the α- or β-globin chains, called, respectively, α- and β-thalassemia. They result from genetic defects at any one of a number of sites in the production of globin. The clinical expression of the thalassemic defect depends on the globin chain involved, the extent of the defect, and the adequacy of compensatory adjustments in the production of other globin chains. The normal globin chains become unbalanced because of a decrease in the affected chains, forming intraerythrocytic inclusions that damage the RBC membrane and lead to hemolysis. For instance, in homozygous β-thalassemia, excess α-chains precipitate on the red cell membrane, forming inclusions called *Heinz bodies*. These inclusions in turn cause increased red cell rigidity, membrane damage, and subsequent hemolysis. The homozygous thalassemias should be treated in specialized centers.

β-Thalassemia. β-Thalassemia major (Cooley's anemia, Mediterranean anemia) is a severe, transfusion-dependent anemia that can be fatal by late childhood or early adolescence. It is found in persons homozygous or doubly heterozygous for a mutation that affects the capacity for synthesis of β-globin subunits of hemoglobin. In the full-blown case a severe anemia with drastically reduced MCV and MCHC is always found. In β-thalassemia trait (heterozygous β-thalassemia) normal α-chains are synthesized in parallel with decreased (but not absent) β-chains. Patients develop hypochromic, microcytic indices, mild poikilocytosis, and anisocytosis and are often misdiagnosed as having iron-deficiency anemia. In β-thalassemia trait, however, the RBC count is normal or even elevated in relation to the hematocrit, whereas it is decreased in iron-deficiency anemia. The two conditions must be distinguished and a firm diagnosis of β-thalassemia trait established for purposes of genetic counseling and to avoid iron therapy. With β-thalassemia trait, hemoglobin A_2 levels average 5.1% (normal upper limit is 3.7%), and in 50% of cases the hemoglobin F levels are mildly elevated to 2% to 5% (the upper normal limit being 2%).

The major problem in β-thalassemia major is the severity of the anemia. Compensatory mechanisms result in extramedullary hematopoiesis with hepatosplenomegaly. Expansion of the bone marrow leads to skeletal abnormalities, secondary thinning of cortices of long bones, and pathologic fractures. Patients require frequent transfusions, which result in hemosiderosis. Elimination of excess iron may be achieved with iron chelators (e.g., deferoxamine B) administered intramuscularly or via continuous intravenous infusion. Such treatment may result in a significant decrease in iron accumulation in tissues and hopefully longer and healthier survival. Bone marrow transplantation or molecular manipulations that would allow insertion of messenger RNA containing normal genetic information for the synthesis of β-chains are in preliminary stages of research.

α-Thalassemia. The α-thalassemia syndromes are a group of inherited disorders with decreased synthesis of α-chains. They are especially common in Chinese and southeast Asians but may also be encountered in people originating from Africa, the Middle East, and the Mediterranean area. In contrast to β-thalassemia, hemoglobins A_2 and F are decreased because of decreased α-chains, which are constituents of both A_2 and F hemoglobins. α-Thalassemia trait should be suspected in a patient belonging to the appropriate ethnic group who presents with microcytic, hypochromic anemia, normal or decreased hemoglobins A_2 and F, and in whom iron-deficiency anemia has been ruled out. A definitive diagnosis is made by proving defective synthesis of α-chains. This can be done only in specialized laboratories, since it will not show on routine hemoglobin electrophoreses.

Enzymopathies. Hemolytic anemias due to hereditary red cell enzyme deficiencies are exceedingly rare except for the deficiency of glucose-6-phosphate dehydrogenase (G6PD). G6PD is an enzyme vital to the RBC integrity, since it catalyzes the first step in the hexose monophosphate shunt, counteracting oxidative processes (Fig. 113-5). The gene for its synthesis is carried on the X chromosome. G6PD deficiency is fully expressed in heterozygous men and homozygous women and only partially expressed in heterozygous women. The enzyme deficiency appears to offer a selective advantage against the malarial parasite. There are two normal variants of the enzyme differing by one amino acid and designated A+ and B+ (+ denotes the presence of

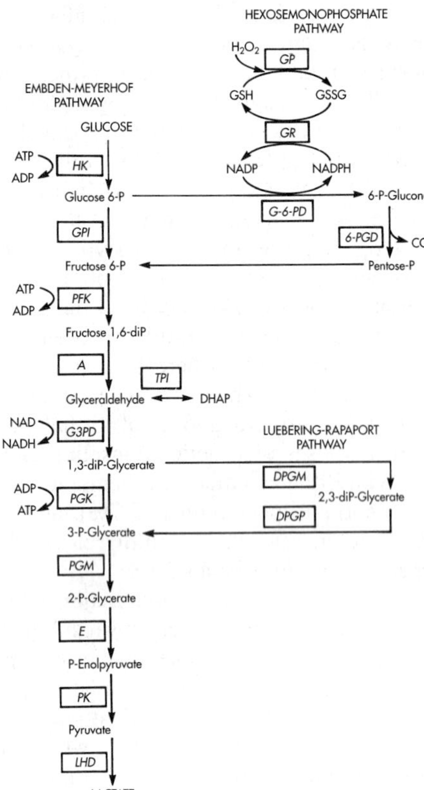

Fig. 113-5. Embden-Meyerhof pathway and hexose monophosphate shunt in RBCs.

the enzyme and – denotes its absence), the former of which is prevalent in people of African ancestry. In the United States the most common deficiency is the A– type: approximately 12% of African-Americans are affected, and 20% of African-American women are heterozygous. Among Mediterranean persons a more severe type of G6PD deficiency is common, designated G6PD Mediterranean or B–. The mechanism of hemolysis in G6PD deficiency is related to the inability of RBCs to regenerate reduced glutathione (GSH) when it has been oxidized. Individuals with the A– variant are usually not anemic unless exposed to an oxidant drug (Box 113-3), whereas in the Mediterranean variant hemolysis is chronically present and exacerbated by exposure to oxidants. In the A– variety the clinical manifestations are episodic, with complete recovery between hemolytic episodes. This can occur even if the chemical exposure is continued because the new, younger RBCs contain greater amounts of the G6PD.

POLYCYTHEMIAS

The term *polycythemia* refers to an absolute increase in the red cell mass as reflected by the hematocrit. However, if there is a significant reduction in plasma volume, a false or spurious polycythemia exists, such as in stress erythrocytosis and excessive use of diuretics. A true increase in red cell mass is either primary or secondary, the former being known as polycythemia vera. Determination of the red cell mass is often not needed if the hemoglobin and hematocrit are extremely elevated but may be of help with moderate elevations. Table 113-4 describes criteria for distinguishing these three entities. The various conditions resulting in

Box 113-3. Drugs That Can Produce Hemolysis of G6PD-Deficient RBCs

Sulfonamides
Antimalarials
Nitrofurans (nitrofurantoin)
Analgesics (aspirin, phenacetin)
Diuretics (thiazides, acetazolamide)
Hypoglycemic agents (tolbutamide, chlorpropamide)
Sulfones
Miscellaneous (naphthalene, vitamin K, quinidine, probenicid, isoniazid)

secondary polycythemia are listed in Box 113-4. In these cases, erythropoietin is increased and the primary stimulus for its secretion must be found.

Polycythemia Vera

Polycythemia vera is a chronic myeloproliferative disease. It occurs mostly after the fifth decade and is characterized by an increased production of RBCs with variable increases in granuloycytes and platelets. The red cells are responsive to but not dependent on erythropoietin for their maturation. The disease starts insidiously with fatigue and weakness. When hyperviscosity develops, the patients present with dizziness, headaches, and visual problems. Occasionally the disease is discovered after an episode of acute thrombosis or during investigation of a bleeding tendency. Some patients complain of itching, particularly after a warm bath. The typical patient is plethoric with congestion of the oral mucosa and a ruddy complexion. Splenomegaly is present in more than two-thirds of patients.

To establish the diagnosis of polycythemia vera, two groups of criteria have been established (Box 113-5). The diagnosis is considered firmly established if the three major criteria are present or if the first two major criteria plus two minor criteria are documented.

Polycythemia vera is a chronic disorder with a median survival of 9 years. The disease transforms into acute nonlymphocytic leukemia in some patients. Most patients become progressively anemic with increasing bone marrow fibrosis and reduction of hematopoietic tissue (i.e., spent polycythemia). Extramedullary hematopoiesis may develop, and the spleen may become enormous. Complete bone marrow failure with severe pancytopenia develops in the final phase of such cases.

Once the diagnosis of polycythemia vera has been established, the red cell mass should be reduced to normal levels. This is best managed in collaboration with a hematologist. Therapy must be individualized for the stage of disease and for symptoms. Therapeutic approaches include phlebotomy, myelosuppressive agents, interferon-α, and radioactive phosphorus (^{32}P), although the latter is used less in recent years. Phlebotomy and hydroxyurea tend to be the mainstay of therapy. Recent studies indicate that Interferon-a is a promising agent. Elective surgery should not be performed until polycythemia vera has been well controlled because of the high incidence of postoperative thrombotic and hemorrhagic complications.

Table 113-4. Differential Diagnosis of Relative Erythrocytosis, Secondary Erythrocytosis, and Polycythemia Vera

Examination	Relative erythrocytosis	Secondary erythrocytosis	Polycythemia vera
RBC mass	N	I	I
Plasma volume	D	N or I	N or I
Granulocytes	N	N	N or I
Platelets	N	N	N or I
Serum vitamin B_{12}	N	N	I
Transcobalamin 1	N	N	I
Serum iron	N	N	Usually D
Leukocyte alkaline phosphatase	N	N	N or I
Arterial oxygen saturation	N	N or D	N
Bone marrow	N	Erythroid hyperplasia	Panhyperplasia
Erythropoietin	N	I	N or D
Splenomegaly	Absent	Absent	Usually present

N, Normal; *D*, decreased; *I*, increased.

Box 113-4. Causes of Secondary Polycythemias

Appropriate Increase in Erythropoietin Production

High altitude
Chronic lung disease
Right-to-left cardiovascular shunt
High oxygen affinity hemoglobinopathy
Massive obesity with chronic hypoxia
High concentration of carboxyhemoglobin

Inappropriate Increase in Erythropoietin Production

Tumor
Renal carcinoma
Hepatoma
Cerebellar hemangioblastoma
Pheochromocytoma
Carcinomas of the ovary, prostate, lung, breast, adrenal cortex
Uterine fibroid

Renal Abnormalities

Hydronephrosis
Nephrotic syndrome
Renal cysts
Kidney transplantation

Benign Familial Erythrocytosis

Box 113-5. Criteria for the Diagnosis of Polycythemia Vera

Major Criteria

RBC mass: Male > 36 ml/kg
Female > 32 ml/kg
Arterial O_2 saturation > 92%
Splenomegaly

Minor Criteria

Thrombocytosis > 400,000/µl
Leukocytosis > 12,000/µl
Leukocyte alkaline phosphatase activity > 100 (no fever or infection)
Serum vitamin B_{12} > 900 pg/ml or unbound vitamin B_{12} binding capacity > 2200 pg/ml

Polycythemia vera is considered present if the patient has all three major criteria or the first two major criteria plus any two minor criteria.

Modified from Wasserman IR: The management of polycythemia vera, *Br J Haematol* 21:371, 1971.

ADDITIONAL READINGS

Berlin NI: Polycythemia vera, *Semin Hematol* 34:1-80, 1997.

Bini EJ, Micale PL, Weinshel EH: Evaluation of the gastrointestinal tract in premenopausal women with iron deficiency, *Am J Med* 105:281-286, 1998.

Bunn HF: Pathogenesis and treatment of sickle cell disease, *N Engl J Med* 337:762-769, 1997.

Carmel R: Prevalence of undiagnosed pernicious anemia in the elderly, *Arch Intern Med* 156:1097-1100, 1996.

Gladwin MT, Schecter AN, Shelhamer JH, et al: The acute chest syndrome in sickle cell disease. Possible role of nitric oxide in its pathophysiology and treatment, *Am J Respir Crit Care Med* 159:1368-1376, 1999.

Izaks GJ, Westendorp RGJ, Knook DL: The definition of anemia in older persons, *JAMA* 281:1714-1717, 1999.

Looker AC, Dallman PR, Carroll MD, et al: Prevalence of iron deficiency in the United States, *JAMA* 277:973-976, 1997.

Massey AC: Microcytic anemia: Differential diagnosis and management of iron deficiency anemia, *Med Clin N Am* 76:549-566, 1992.

Moore DF, Sears DA: Pica, iron deficiency, and the medical history, *Am J Med* 97:390-393, 1994.

Olivieri NF: The β-thalassemias, *N Engl J Med* 341:99-109, 1999.

Sears DA: Anemia of chronic disease, *Med Clin N Amer* 76:567-579, 1992.

Snow CF: Laboratory diagnosis of vitamin B_{12} and folate deficiency: A guide for the primary care physician, *Arch Intern Med* 159:1289-1298, 1999.

Wilcox CM, Alexander LN, Clark S: Prospective evaluation of the gastrointestinal tract in patients with iron deficiency and no systemic or gastrointestinal symptoms or signs, *Am J Med* 103:405-409, 1997.

CHAPTER 114

Nonmalignant White Blood Cell Disorders

Philip A. Lowry

The primary nonmalignant disorders of white blood cells encountered in adult practice represent abnormalities of number, although repetitive or unusual infections in face of normal leukocyte counts may suggest a functional abnormality. This chapter initially recounts the normal mechanisms of hematopoiesis, then reviews the various nonmalignant abnormalities of leukocyte subclasses. It concludes with a brief discussion of the role of hematopoietic growth factors in the treatment of these disorders.

NORMAL HEMATOPOIESIS

An understanding of the basic concepts of normal hematopoiesis forms the foundation for approaching the diagnosis and therapy of both malignant and nonmalignant blood disorders. Normal hematopoiesis proceeds from a pluripotent hematopoietic stem cell in the bone marrow that is theoretically capable of both self-renewal and proliferation and differentiation into all the mature hematologic lineages. This process is under the control of the various hematopoietic cytokines. Fig. 114-1 summarizes this scheme. Leukocytes derived from this process can be divided into two general classes: the myelomonocytic and lymphocytic. All leukocytes function to monitor for and react to infection, inflammation, and endogenous tissue damage or degeneration.

Myelomonocytic cells (neutrophils, eosinophils, basophils, and monocyte/macrophages) are capable of phagocytosis of infecting agents or cellular debris and release of inflammatory or chemotactic mediators. These cells have no inherent specificity but react to foreign antigens that have been *opsonized* by antibody or complement. Mature segmented neutrophils are released from the marrow and circulate for 6 to 8 hours before migrating to extravascular tissues, where they perform their bactericidal function and persist for only a few days. Less is known about the kinetics of basophils and eosinophils though they are probably similar. They participate in allergic reactions and in the response to parasitic and fungal infections.

Monocytes have a similarly short half-life in circulation but are longer lived in extravascular tissues. Monocytes that have developed specialized phagocytic function are recognized as macrophages. In addition to phagocytic functions, monocyte/macrophages play a key role in antigen presentation.

Lymphocytes synthesize specialized reactive molecules that interact with foreign antigens, forming the specific arm of the immune response. Differentiated B cells are responsible for *humoral* immunity through production of immunoglobulins, which circulate and initiate complement

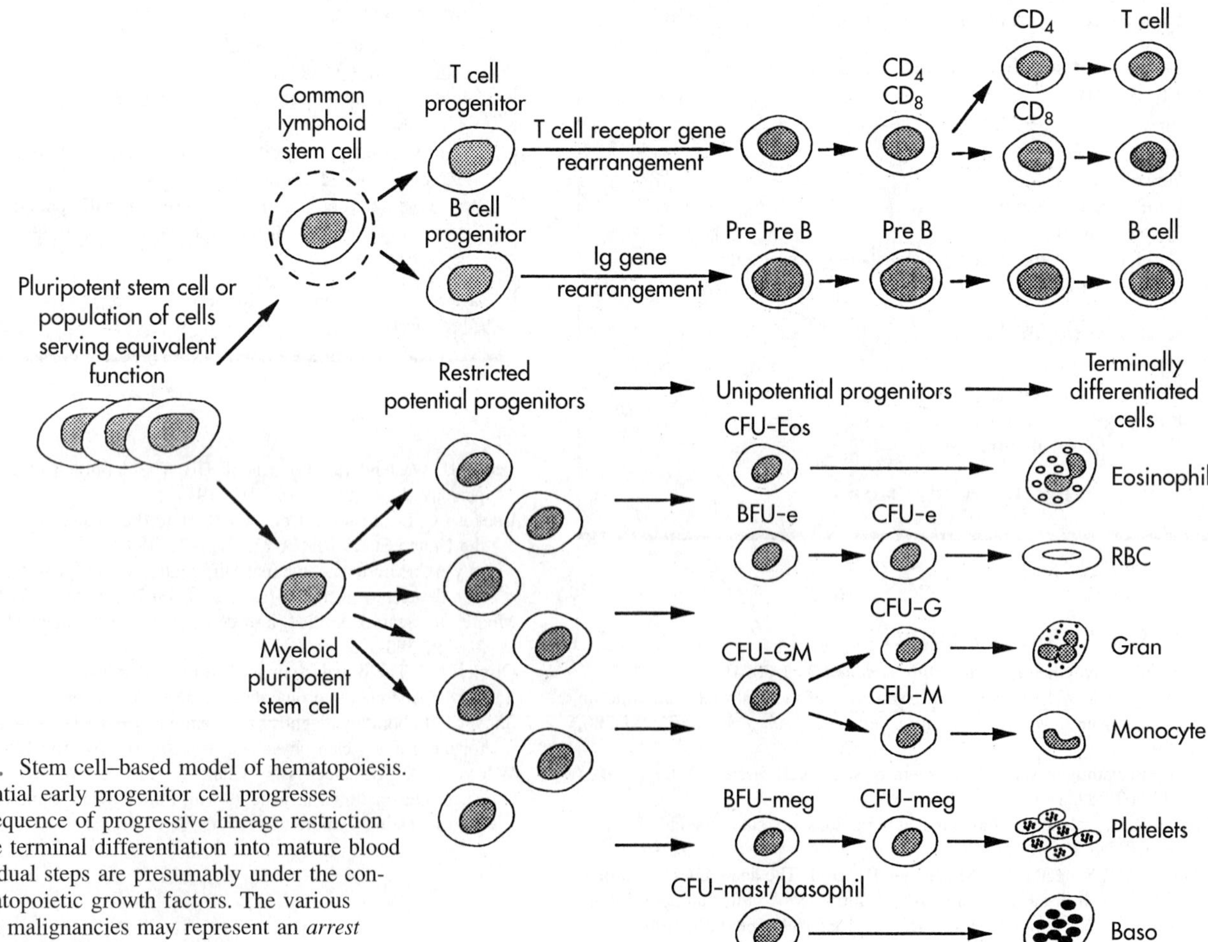

Fig. 114-1. Stem cell–based model of hematopoiesis. A pluripotential early progenitor cell progresses through a sequence of progressive lineage restriction and ultimate terminal differentiation into mature blood cells. Individual steps are presumably under the control of hematopoietic growth factors. The various hematologic malignancies may represent an *arrest* at one of these developmental stages.

mediated lysis or opsonized phagocytosis, particularly of bacterial pathogens. Differentiated T cells have a surface-bound T cell receptor that is similar to immunoglobulin in its unique structure and specificity for a limited antigen repertoire. T cells control cell-mediated immunity and, in addition to specific recognition and destruction of endogenous tissues altered by viral infection or neoplastic degeneration, modulate the overall immune response through direct cell-cell interaction with B cells and monocytes and the release of lymphokines and inflammatory modulators.

Development of these specialized reactive molecules starts with apparently random rearrangements of multiple genetic loci, which are ultimately combined to produce mature immunoglobulin and T cell receptor molecules. After initial development in the marrow, final lymphocyte proliferation and differentiation proceed in specialized tissues capable of antigen presentation, with selection of appropriate clones and elimination of pathologically autoreactive cells. This final lymphocyte development is summarized in Fig. 114-2.

GENERAL FEATURES OF NONMALIGNANT LEUKOCYTE DISORDERS

Abnormalities of leukocytes most often present as susceptibility to infections or inflammation. Inherent qualitative abnormalities are rare, and most are typically congenital and manifest in childhood, with the notable exception of the acquired immunodeficiency syndrome (AIDS). Table 114-1 presents a general approach to the evaluation of a patient with suspected immunodeficiency.[2]

Adult practitioners will more often encounter problems related to quantitative leukocyte disorders. Depression of leukocyte counts results from either an abnormality of production or an increased rate of loss or destruction. Production problems typically reflect abnormalities of the marrow due to inherent abnormalities of the hematopoietic stem cell, to acute toxic insults such as the cytopenias following chemotherapy or irradiation, to a metabolic abnormality such as vitamin deficiency, or to malignant or storage disorders that invade or replace the marrow cavity. These mechanisms affect all of hematopoiesis and therefore rarely manifest as a single lineage deficit and more often as pancytopenia.

Unusual disorders may be due to specific growth factor abnormalities. These disorders are rare, but those such as cyclic neutropenia and Kostmann's syndrome are now recognized to be the result of specific deficiencies of granulocyte colony-stimulating factor, a cytokine involved in the direction of terminal granulocyte differentiation and ultimate function. Increased loss or destruction may relate to severe infections, extensive tissue necrosis, splenic hyperfunction, or autoimmune mechanisms.

Syndromes of cellular excess are most typically due to malignant transformation with autonomous proliferation or

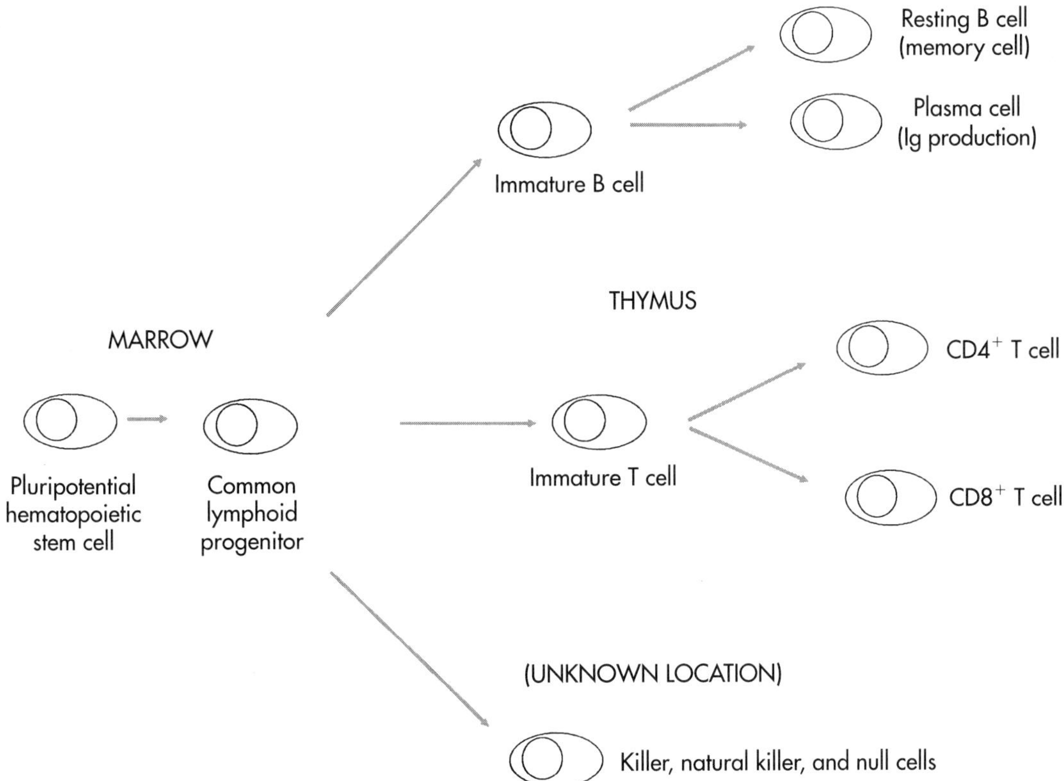

Fig. 114-2. Lymphopoiesis begins with the formation of a common lymphoid progenitor in the marrow derived from the pluripotential hematopoietic stem cell. After initial commitment to B or T cell lineage and initial random rearrangement of loci for immunoglobulin or T cell receptor molecules, final proliferation and differentiation proceed in specialized tissues and are subject to antigen presentation and the control of modulating cells and lymphokines. Killer, natural killer, and null cell subsets are rare, are poorly characterized, and apparently do not undergo antigen-dependent and restricted proliferation and differentiation.

Table 114-1. Approach to the Patient With Suspected Immunodeficiency

Step	Comment
History and physical examination	Establish frequency and type of infections, signs or symptoms of other congenital problems, signs or symptoms of autoimmune or lymphoproliferative disorder, medications, family history, risk factors for HIV infection
Complete blood count and differential	Screen for quantitative leukocyte abnormalities
HIV serology	Screen for acquired immunodeficiency syndrome
Nitroblue tetrazolium test	Screen for phagocytic defect (recurrent pyogenic infections)
Quantitative immunoglobulins	Screen for B cell defect
Candida skin test	Screen for T cell defect
CH_{50}	Screen for complement deficiency
Flow cytometric analysis of peripheral blood	Evaluate for the presence of a clonal lymphoproliferative disorder; screen for CD11b deficiency on granulocytes as indicator of Chédiak-Higashi syndrome

Data from Buckley RH: Immunodeficiency diseases, *J Am Med Assoc* 268:2797, 1992.

are *reactive* to a specific pathologic state. Table 114-2 lists normal ranges of leukocyte numbers and related evaluations, and Box 114-1 summarizes the quantitative leukocyte disorders.

GRANULOCYTE DISORDERS

Qualitative granulocyte defects are rarely encountered de novo in adult practice. They are marked by recurrent suppurative bacterial infections, but can sometimes be successfully managed with antibiotics. The nitroblue tetrazolium test is a rapid screen for neutrophil dysfunction. One specific defect, the Chédiak-Higashi syndrome, can be diagnosed by flow cytometric demonstration of altered CD11b expression on the neutrophil cell surface.

Neutropenia is probably seen most often in the context of previous treatment with cytotoxic therapy and in such a situation is usually anticipated and recognized prior to the onset of major secondary problems. Acute neutropenia may be due to acute destruction complicating certain severe infections, particularly bacterial sepsis; due to vitamin B_{12} or folate deficiency resulting from abnormal maturation (usually in combination with macrocytic anemia); or seen as the first manifestation of an acquired marrow disorder such as myelodysplasia, aplastic anemia, or leukemia or other malignancy involving the marrow leading to decreased production of normal elements. More chronic forms of neutropenia may be seen as an expression of a congenital disorder such as cyclic neutropenia; maybe seen in the context of autoimmune disease, particularly with systemic lupus erythematosus or Felty's syndrome; or may be a manifestation of hypersplenism.

Neutropenia, particularly when the absolute count is less than 500 neutrophils per mcl, constitutes a potential medical emergency requiring prompt evaluation and, in the context of manifestations of infection, immediate intervention to forestall life-threatening complications. A complete history and physical examination should focus on antecedent treatments or conditions. Review of peripheral blood and marrow smears may identify potential malignant forms or signs of vitamin deficiency. Additional tests that may be helpful include antinuclear antibody, rheumatoid factor, serum immune electrophoresis, and determination of folic and vitamin B_{12} levels. Antineutrophil antibodies are available on an investigational basis, but are rarely returned in time to help with acute decision making and may not be sufficiently reliable to determine treatment.

Although definitive therapy for neutropenia and its underlying causes may require the intervention of a hematologist, several immediate measures may be required and often should be instituted by the initial identifying physician, even in advance of hematologic consultation. Potential toxic drugs should be eliminated and other contributing causes immediately obvious at the time of diagnosis should be appropriately addressed. Any signs of infection including fever, even without other localizing signs, require prompt initiation of broad-spectrum antibiotics. This issue has been nicely reviewed in the classic monograph by Pizzo.[6]

Neutrophilia, in contrast, is rarely a medical emergency in and of itself except as a marker of a more serious underlying disorder. Neutrophilia is seen acutely most often as a manifestation of underlying infections, particularly those caused by bacterial organisms. It may also be seen in response to acute stress related to burns, major trauma, or organ infarction. In all these cases, the primary disorder is usually manifestly evident from the history and physical examination. Treatment with drugs such as epinephrine, corticosteroids, or the more recently available recombinant growth factors may also induce neutrophilia. A mild neutrophilia may be seen occasionally as a response to extreme heat or cold exposure, or with exercise, convulsions, or severe pain.

Chronic neutrophilia may be seen in the context of persistent infections or inflammatory conditions or occasionally as a chronic response to untreated malignancies of another organ system. Chronic neutrophilia may complicate chronic therapy with steroids or lithium or may be a manifestation of certain endocrinologic disorders such as adrerocorticotropic hormone (ACTH)- or glutocorticoid-producing tumors or occasionally thyroid storm. Chronic neutrophilia is rare as a congenital abnormality, although it may be seen particularly in association with Down's syndrome. In all these forms, the neutrophilia represents a reactive process, and its treatment is simply the treatment of the primary disorder.

The primary differential concern in neutrophilia is to detect a primary myeloproliferative disorder. Although a definitive evaluation may require bone marrow aspiration and biopsy with performance of cytogenetics to search for the characteristic Philadelphia chromosome (t9:22 translocation), a screen of leukocyte alkaline phosphatase levels may provide initial clues as to which of these two diagnoses is operative. Whereas leukemoid reactions or other reactive causes of neutrophilia are usually associated with an elevated leukocyte alkaline phosphatase level, chronic myelocytic

Table 114-2. Summary of Normal Values

Cell Type	Normal total and differential white blood cell counts	
	Absolute number (× 10^9/L)	Differential percentage
Total leukocytes	4.5-11.0	100
Neutrophils (total)	1.8-7.7	59
Lymphocytes	1.5-4.8	34
Monocytes	0-0.8	4
Eosinophils	0-0.45	2.6
Basophils	0-0.2	0.4

Normal values for selected additional laboratory determinations	
Test	Normal values
Serum vitamin B_{12}	160-1000 pg/ml
Serum folate	6-21 ng/ml
Leukocyte alkaline phosphatase	13-130 (rating score)
Serum IgG	8-16 mg/ml
Serum IgM	0.5-2 mg/ml
Serum IgA	1.4-4 mg/ml

Modified from Williams W, et al, editors: *Hematology,* ed 5, New York, 1995, McGraw-Hill.

leukemia is typically associated with the depression of its value.

EOSINOPHIL DISORDERS

Worldwide, the most common cause of eosinophilia is infection with helminthic parasites, particularly schistosomiasis but also ascariasis, *Toxocara* infection, filariasis, strongyloidiasis, trichomoniasis, and *Echinococcus* infection. In industrialized countries, allergic conditions, underlying malignancy, allergic bronchopulmonary aspergillosis, and primary eosinophil proliferations figure more prominently in the differential diagnosis.

Polyarteritis nodosa and Churg-Strauss syndrome may be accompanied by eosinophilia, but have a clinical presentation dominated more by the clinical consequences of systemic vasculitis. Of historic significance are the toxin-induced eosinophilic syndromes eosinophilic myalgia due to contaminated tryptophan ingestion and the toxic oil syndrome in Spain in 1981 due to substitution of rapeseed oil for olive oil.

Patients presenting with excess numbers of eosinophils require evaluation of stool for ova and parasites; cultures and evaluation for fungal, mycobacterial, or other chronic bacterial diseases; and evaluation for autoimmune or chronic allergic disorders, all of which may be associated with a reactive eosinophilia. Extreme hypereosinophilia or eosinophilia that persists for more than 6 months where reactive forms of eosinophilia have been excluded suggests a primary hypereosinophilic syndrome.

Hypereosinophilic syndrome most often afflicts caucasian males. Total white blood cell counts may be elevated to the range of 10 to 50 × 10^9 per liter, with differential showing that 30% to 70% of cells are mature-appearing eosinophils. Hypereosinophilic syndrome is an idiopathic syndrome that may range from totally mature-appearing eosinophils to a very immature eosinophilic leukemic-like picture.

Chronic eosinophilia from any cause may result in severe cardiac toxicity with restrictive congestive heart failure and

Box 114-1. Myeloid Cytokines

Current Uses

Definite utility: G-CSF for congenital neutropenia; myeloid cytokines for facilitation of prior stem cell collection and subsequent recovery from both autologous and allogeneic stem cell transplant

Probable utility: To facilitate more rapid recovery in patients with febrile neutropenia complicated by pneumonia, hypotension, multiorgan dysfunction, or fungal infection; to speed recovery postinduction for acute leukemia in patients over 55 years of age; periodically in cytopenic infections complicating myelodysplastic syndromes

Possible utility: To support dose-intensive chemotherapy; to maintain dose intensity or schedule in patients with delayed recovery from a previous chemotherapy although in neither situation has a clear benefit over traditional dose reduction been established

No data: Use in established, uncomplicated neutropenia after chemotherapy

Adverse effects: Possible acceleration of leukemic transformation in myelodysplastic syndromes and stimulation of solid tumor growth

Toxicities

GM-CSF: Fever, bone pain, myalgias, edema/pericarditis, first-dose reaction

G-CSF: Bone pain, splenomegaly (with prolonged use), neutrophilic dermatitis (rare)

GM-CSF, Granulocyte-macrophage colony-stimulating factor; *G-CSF,* granulocyte colony-stimulating factor.

From Anonymous: Update of recommendations for the use of hematopoietic colony-stimulating factors: evidence-based clinical practice guidelines, *J Clin Oncol* 14:1957, 1996; and Demetri GD: Hematopoietic growth factors: current knowledge, future prospects, *Curr Prob Cancer* 16, Number 4, 1992.

mitral valve regurgitation and also may be associated with chronic pulmonary infiltrates or effusions. Primary hypereosinophilic syndrome was uniformly fatal historically when severe and prolonged. More recently the prognosis has dramatically improved with treatment including steroids, hydroxyurea and leukapheresis.

BASOPHILIA

Basophilia may be seen in association with allergic or inflammatory conditions or with certain infectious conditions such as viral or tuberculosis infection. The underlying cause is usually obvious in these conditions and the treatment is directed toward it. Basophilia may also be a marker, particularly for the myeloproliferative diseases or for occult carcinoma, and a search for these disorders should be undertaken when no other cause for the abnormality is manifest.

MONOCYTE DISORDERS

Monocytosis is most often the result of underlying malignant disease such as myelodysplastic or myeloproliferative disorders or occasionally is a marker of underlying lymphoma or carcinoma. Monocytosis may also be noted with chronic inflammatory and immune disorders and may be particularly seen in the context of mononucleosis syndromes, collagen vascular disease, inflammatory bowel disease, sarcoidosis, or chronic infectious states, particularly tuberculosis, subacute bacterial endocarditis, and, historically, syphilis. Monocytopenia may nonspecifically result from marrow aplasia or may accompany human immunodeficiency virus (HIV) infection, hairy-cell leukemia, or treatment with radiotherapy, steroids, or interferon.

Although the role of monocytes and monocyte-derived tissue-based cells in antigen presentation has long been recognized conceptually, the specific mechanisms of that process are just now being characterized. That characterization will probably shed light on previously unrecognized subtle or perhaps not-so-subtle functional defects.

LYMPHOCYTE DISORDERS

Lymphocytopenia or qualitative lymphocyte disorders may be due to a variety of causes and, although perhaps not associated with the immediately explosive infectious susceptibility of severe neutropenia, may nevertheless be a marker of severe immune compromise, with significant consequences for the patient. Congenital lymphocyte disorders typically present in childhood with variable infectious complications; they may be fatal at an early age, particularly in the case of the *combined* disorders.

B cell disorders such as X-linked agammaglobulinemia are associated with recurrent pyogenic infections due to loss of opsonization, but can also be associated with autoimmune disorders. Common variable immunodeficiency is an acquired condition with similar clinical characteristics and a particular predilection toward the development of a sprue-like syndrome. Both disorders can be reasonably managed with regular immunoglobulin replacement and prompt antibiotic therapy for infections. More focused IgG subclass deficiencies have also been described with variable infectious risk.

IgA deficiency is the most common congenital *immunodeficiency* disorder affecting 1 in 700 people. About 80% of affected patients do not show a clinically significant increased risk of infection, but 20% have simultaneous deficiencies of IgG_2 and IgG_4 subclasses and show a pattern of infections similar to other hypoglobulinemic syndromes, with a similar response to immunoglobulin maintenance and antibiotics. All patients with IgA deficiency are at risk for developing an IgE directed against IgA, with the clinical consequence of anaphylactic reactions to the infusion of IgA-containing blood products. IgA deficiency should be suspected as the cause of any severe, unexplained reaction to transfusion.[8]

Qualitative T cell disorders produce a more severe, so-called *combined* immune compromise, both directly from impaired T cell immune function and the indirect compromise of B cell function due to loss of T cell modulation. Severe combined immunodeficiency, ataxia telangiectasia, and the Wiskott-Aldrich syndrome are congenital conditions that have unique individual features but share a susceptibility to severe and often fatal infection early in life. Homologous stem cell transplantation offers the possibility for cure. The DiGeorge syndrome is a noninherited developmental disorder resulting in congenital thymic aplasia and a pattern of infectious risk similar to the above conditions. Transplantation of fetal thymic tissue may help correct the deficiency.

Lymphopenias or abnormalities of lymphocyte function also are often a secondary manifestation of a variety of other autoimmune states and of malignancies such as lymphoma and Hodgkin's disease. Chronic therapy with glucocorticoids or antineoplastic agents may induce functional or numerical abnormalities of lymphocytes as well. With the recent emergence of AIDS, an entirely new category of lymphopenia and lymphocyte functional abnormalities has emerged (see Chapter 32). Screening for HIV infection should be a standard part of the evaluation of a patient presenting with lymphopenia.

Lymphocytosis, as with the other disorders of white cell excess, can be divided into two broad categories: a manifestation of a primary hematologic malignancy is a reactive process. Lymphocytosis may be particularly seen with the various mononucleosis syndromes due to Epstein-Barr virus, cytomegalovirus, or toxoplasma infection, and may also be paradoxically seen in early presentation of HIV-1 infection. Acute lymphocytosis may be seen with a number of other viral infections and may also be manifest in the context of noninfectious inflammatory processes particularly associated with autoimmune disease or hypersensitivity reactions.

With the increasing use of screening laboratories, patients with chronic lymphocytic leukemia (CLL) are frequently diagnosed in an asymptomatic and early stage on the basis of an elevated lymphocyte count noted on a "routine" complete blood count determination. CLL is discussed more completely in Chapter 119. Lymphocytosis is best evaluated initially by a complete history and physical examination, light microscopic inspection of the peripheral blood smear, and flow cytometric analysis of the peripheral blood.

HEMATOPOIETIC GROWTH FACTORS

A major addition to the therapeutic armamentarium in the treatment of hematologic disorders has been the identification, production, and clinical administration of the hematopoietic growth factors. Particularly notable in this regard are the dramatic increase and use of agents such as erythropoietin, granulocyte-macrophage colony-stimulating factor (GM-CSF), and granulocyte colony-stimulating factor (G-CSF).

Erythropoietin first saw use in the clear deficiency state associated with renal failure, with dramatic reduction in transfusion requirements and improvements in quality of life. Its use has now been extended to patients with chronic

Table 114-3. Quantitative Leukocyte Disorders

Cell type	Differential diagnosis of excess cell numbers	Differential diagnosis of deficiency of cell type	Comments
Neutrophils	Pyogenic infection Noninfectious tissue damage Malignant disorder, especially CML	Marrow production defect (e.g., aplastic anemia, leukemia) Drug-induced Folate or B_{12} deficiency Rickettsial or viral infections Alcoholism Chemotherapy or radiation therapy	Need to rapidly institute antibiotic therapy for infection in neutropenia particularly if ANC <500/mcl.
Eosinophils	Parasitic infection Allergy or hypersensitivity Malignant disorder Primary proliferation	Glucocorticoids Certain infections Hyperadrenalism	Eosinophilia of any etiology causes cardiac and neurologic damage and may require therapy; eosinopenia has no apparent functional consequence.
Basophils	Ulcerative colitis or other autoimmune disorders Chronic myelogenous leukemia Acute nonlymphocytic leukemia Urticaria pigmentosa	Glucocorticoids Depletion postallergic reactions	Unexplained basophilia should prompt an evaluation for an underlying leukemic process, particularly CML.
Monocytes	Hematologic disorders such as lymphoma, leukemia, ITP CMML Recovery from agranulocytosis Collagen vascular disease Viral and atypical infections, SBE Malignancy, especially ANLL	Aplastic anemia Hairy-cell leukemia HIV infection Glucocorticoids Interferon administration Radiotherapy	Monocyte-derived cells serve critical antigen-presenting roles in the response to infection and malignancy. As these mechanisms are better characterized, the significance of qualitative and quantitative defects will be better understood.
Lymphocytes	Mononucleosis syndromes and other infections Syphilis Lymphoma or lymphocytic leukemia Thyrotoxicosis	AIDS and other immunodeficiency disorders Glucocorticoids Hodgkin's disease Infectious hepatitis, TB, typhoid	Flow cytometry will frequently distinguish reactive from malignant lymphocyte abnormalities.

CML, Chronic myelogenous leukemia; *ANC*, absolute neutrophil count; *ITP*, idiopathic thrombocytopenic purpura; *CMML*, chronic nyelomonocytic leukemia; *SBE*, subacute bacterial endocarditis; *ANLL*, acute nonlymphoblastic leukemia; *HIV*, human immunodeficiency virus; *AIDS*, acquired immunodeficiency virus; *TB*, tuberculosis.

anemias complicating HIV infection, malignancy, and their treatment. The evolution of more practical weekly administration schedules has particularly fueled a modest but nevertheless improved quality of life for these patients as well. Attempted facilitation of autologous blood donation and better tolerance of surgery through preoperative or perioperative erythropoietin administration have not borne fruit, and alternate strategies such as acute hemodilution will probably better serve this purpose.

Myeloid cytokines arrived with even greater expectations. However, other than in the treatment of usual congenital neutropenic disorders or in the context of stem cell transplant, myeloid cytokines have not yet shown clear improvement in patient outcomes as measured by survival. The greatest temptation has been to apply G-CSF in the context of acute febrile neutropenia with the hopes of reducing the duration and severity of that illness. Although its application in this context seems logical, there is as yet no definitive scientific data as to the efficacy in this regard, with the possible exception of cases complicated by particularly resistant infections or signs of high patient threat such as hypotension or multi-organ failure. Particularly in the context of the need to control health care costs, it is essential that the medical community continue to critically evaluate the efficacy of these new agents and rigorously establish the appropriate contexts for their use.[1] Table 114-3 summarizes current uses of the myeloid growth factors.

REFERENCES

1. Anonymous: Update of recommendations for the use of hematopoietic colony-stimulating factors: evidence-based clinical practice guidelines, *J Clin Oncol* 14:1957, 1996.
2. Buckley RH: Immunodeficiency diseases, *J Am Med Assoc* 268:2787, 1992.
3. Cazzola M, et al: Use of recombinant human erythropoietin outside the setting of uremia, *Blood* 89:4248, 1997.
4. Demetri GD: Hematopoietic growth factors: current knowledge, future prospects, *Curr Prob Cancer* 16, Number 4, 1992.
5. Mazza JJ, editor: *Manual of clinical hematology*, ed 2, Boston, 1995, Little, Brown.
6. Pizzo PA: Management of fever in patients with cancer and treatment-induced neutropenia, *N Engl J Med* 328:1323, 1993.
7. Rothenberg ME: Eosinophilia, *N Engl J Med* 338:1590, 1998.
8. Williams WJ, Beutler E, Erslev AJ, et al, editors: *Hematology*, ed 5. New York, 1998, McGraw-Hill.
9. Yang KD, HR Hill. Neutrophil function disorders: pathophysiology, prevention, and therapy, *J Pediatr* 119:343, 1991.

CHAPTER 115

Hemorrhagic and Thrombotic Disorders

Jack E. Ansell

Primary care physicians often encounter clinical problems of bleeding or thrombosis. Easy bruising is a common complaint in the office setting. Posttraumatic or postsurgical bleeding in a hospitalized patient may first be seen by the family physician for management. Physicians are commonly faced with an unexpected or unexplained prolonged partial thromboplastin time or bleeding time. Deep venous thrombosis of a lower extremity, although a common medical condition, is notoriously tricky to diagnose, and its treatment may be fraught with complications. Accordingly, primary care physicians must have a working knowledge of the rudiments of hemostatic and thrombotic reactions, associated pathologic conditions, and especially appropriate treatment of disorders that can evolve into life-threatening emergencies. This discussion touches on a wide range of hemorrhagic and thrombotic disorders and their treatment, beginning with a brief overview of coagulation and platelet physiology.

NORMAL HEMOSTASIS

Normal hemostasis depends on the close interaction of platelets and the coagulation proteins in a normally functioning vascular system. As a consequence of vascular injury, platelets exposed to subendothelial collagen are stimulated to undergo a sequence of reactions leading to primary platelet plug formation. This plug is then reinforced by the activation of coagulation and fibrin formation to form a stable hemostatic plug.

Platelet reactions can be divided into three physiologic processes: adhesion to subendothelial collagen; activation, shape change, and secretion of a number of substances; and aggregation between adjacent activated platelets. Adhesion depends on specific platelet membrane receptors (glycoprotein Ib) and on von Willebrand's factor, a plasma factor that serves as a bridge between platelets and collagen. Deficiencies of either can lead to platelet dysfunction and bleeding. Platelet secretion depends on a sequence of reactions in the platelet membrane, which leads to calcium mobilization in the platelet cytosol, release of arachidonic acid, and the formation of thromboxane A_2. As a result, platelets secrete a number of endogenous proteins, platelet agonists, and vasoactive factors. This process also exposes the glycoprotein IIb-IIIa complex on the platelet membrane, which binds fibrinogen and serves as a linking site to bind other platelets and thus complete the process of platelet aggregation.

As platelets are activated, the coagulation cascade is also initiated, leading to fibrin formation and stabilization of the primary platelet plug (Fig. 115-1). A number of proenzymes require activation, while cofactors accelerate the enzymatic reactions, and inhibitors limit the reactions. Factors XII and XI in the intrinsic system are activated by contact with damaged endothelial cells. Kallikrein accelerates the reaction and high-molecular-weight kininogen serves as a cofactor. Factor IX in turn is activated by XIa but can also be activated through the extrinsic system by factor VII–tissue factor. Factor VIII is a cofactor accelerating the activation of factor X by IXa. Factor X can also be activated through the extrinsic system by factor VII and tissue factor. Factor VII is activated by the release or exposure of tissue factor from injured endothelial cells. The common pathway proceeds with activation of factor II (prothrombin), with factor V serving as a cofactor. Factor IIa, or thrombin, then cleaves two small peptides from fibrinogen (peptides A and B), and the remaining fibrin monomers polymerize to form long fibrin strands and ultimately a fibrin clot. Factor XIII stabilizes the association of fibrin monomers by introducing covalent disulfide bonds between strands.

There are a number of natural inhibitors in this process serving to limit fibrin formation. These include antithrombin, heparin cofactor II, protein C, protein S, and tissue factor pathway inhibitor (Fig. 115-2). Deficiencies of any of these proteins can lead to hypercoagulable or prethrombotic conditions.

Last, fibrin formation is limited by the fibrinolytic system, the principal factor being plasminogen (see Figs. 115-1 and 115-2). The primary activator of plasminogen is tissue plasminogen activator (t-PA) released from damaged endothelial cells. t-PA has its own natural inhibitor, plasminogen activator inhibitor, which can be altered in disease states.

DIAGNOSIS

There are a large number of assays of the functional status of the coagulation and platelet mechanisms, but many are relevant only to the coagulation specialist consulting in the evaluation of complex hemorrhagic or thrombotic disorders. The primary care physician, however, should be familiar with the usual screening tests and the conceptual approach to evaluating hemostatic disorders.

History and Physical Examination

The evaluation begins with the clinical history to determine whether a patient truly has a bleeding tendency based on history (if acute bleeding is not currently present), and whether it is congenital or acquired based on data such as family history, male or female occurrence, and childhood bleeding. Clues to a coagulation vs. platelet defect can also be discerned by noting the history of petechiae (platelet defects) or ecchymoses (coagulation defects). None of these historical elements is definitive, but they do help in the overall evaluation. A detailed medication history is imperative, particularly noting aspirin or nonsteroidal antiinflammatory agent use. Physical examination provides limited clues in this evaluation but may help support a platelet or coagulation defect by the presence of petechiae or ecchymoses. Furthermore, the presence of other abnormalities may indicate an underlying systemic illness associated with specific hemorrhagic or thrombotic disorders.

Laboratory Evaluation

The laboratory evaluation can be extensive, but the initial tests almost always include a prothrombin time (PT) and activated partial thromboplastin time (aPTT) for screening of the entire coagulation cascade, and a platelet count and bleeding time to screen for quantitatively and qualitatively normal platelets. The bleeding time has been shown not to be a good preoperative screening test to predict bleeding potential, but it is useful for evaluating suspected qualitative

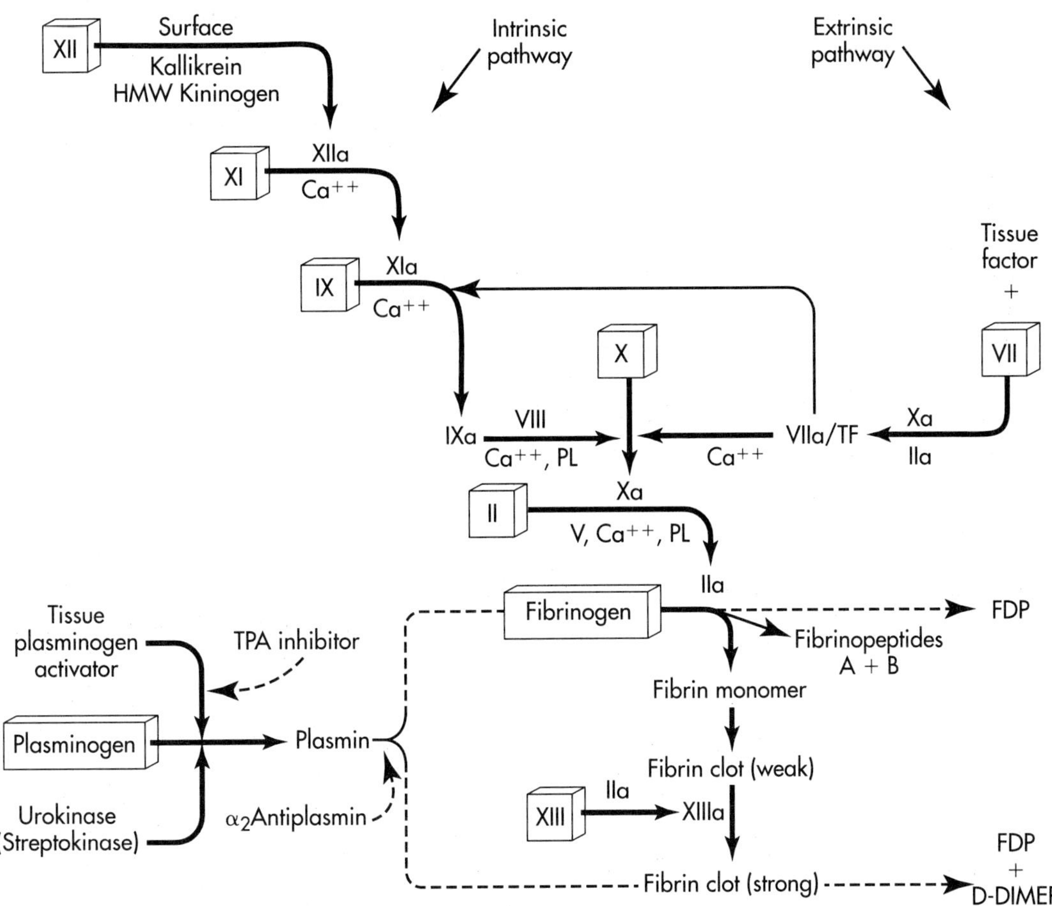

Fig. 115-1. Coagulation cascade. Fibrin clot formation results from the generation of thrombin, which is dependent on the sequential interaction of proenzymes and activated coagulation factors in the intrinsic, extrinsic, and common pathways of coagulation. *HMW,* High molecular weight; *PL,* phospholipid.

platelet defects. The platelet count is obviously useful to detect reduced or increased platelet numbers. Fig. 115-3 highlights the approach to evaluating an abnormal PT or aPTT and the diagnostic possibilities. A prolongation of either test can be the result of a coagulation factor deficiency or circulating inhibitor (antibody). The distinction between these two possibilities is made by performing a mixing assay with patient and normal plasma and repeating the abnormal test. A correction in the result suggests a factor deficiency, whereas no correction suggests an inhibitor. Factor assays or other tests can then be performed to further distinguish the abnormalities.

Additional assays with which physicians should be familiar include a thrombin time (an indirect measure of fibrinogen) and assays of fibrin(ogen) degradation products (FDP) or D-dimers. A positive FDP assay can result from plasmin lysis of fibrinogen or fibrin, whereas a positive D-dimer indicates plasmin lysis of fibrin, an indicator that thrombin has been generated and has converted fibrinogen to fibrin (i.e., intravascular coagulation).

Clinicians should not feel reticent about seeking consultative help from a coagulation specialist when confronted with a hemorrhagic or thrombotic disorder. Given their usual complexity, these disorders may require extensive laboratory evaluation. Table 115-1 illustrates some of the more common disorders and how they would alter the usual screening tests just discussed.

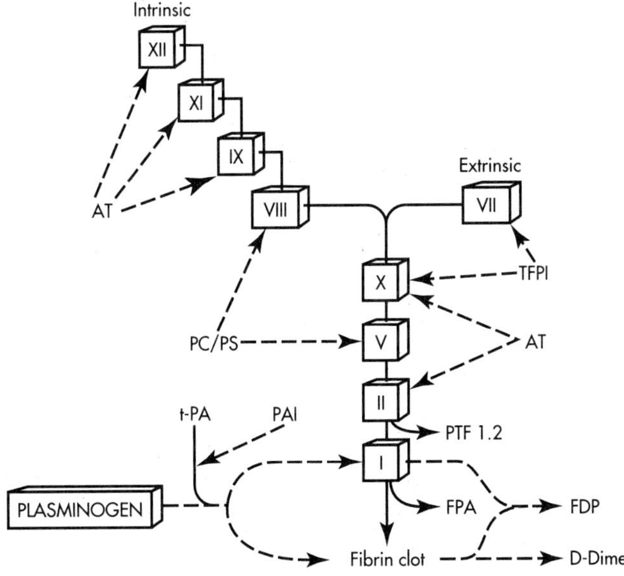

Fig. 115-2. Coagulation cascade illustrating the site of action of coagulation inhibitors and the fibrinolytic system. *AT,* Antithrombin; *PC/PS,* protein C/protein S; *t-PA,* tissue plasminogen activator; *PAI,* plasminogen activator inhibitor; *TFPI,* tissue factor pathway inhibitor; *PTF 1,2,* prothrombin fragment 1,2; *FDP,* fibrin(ogen) degradation products.

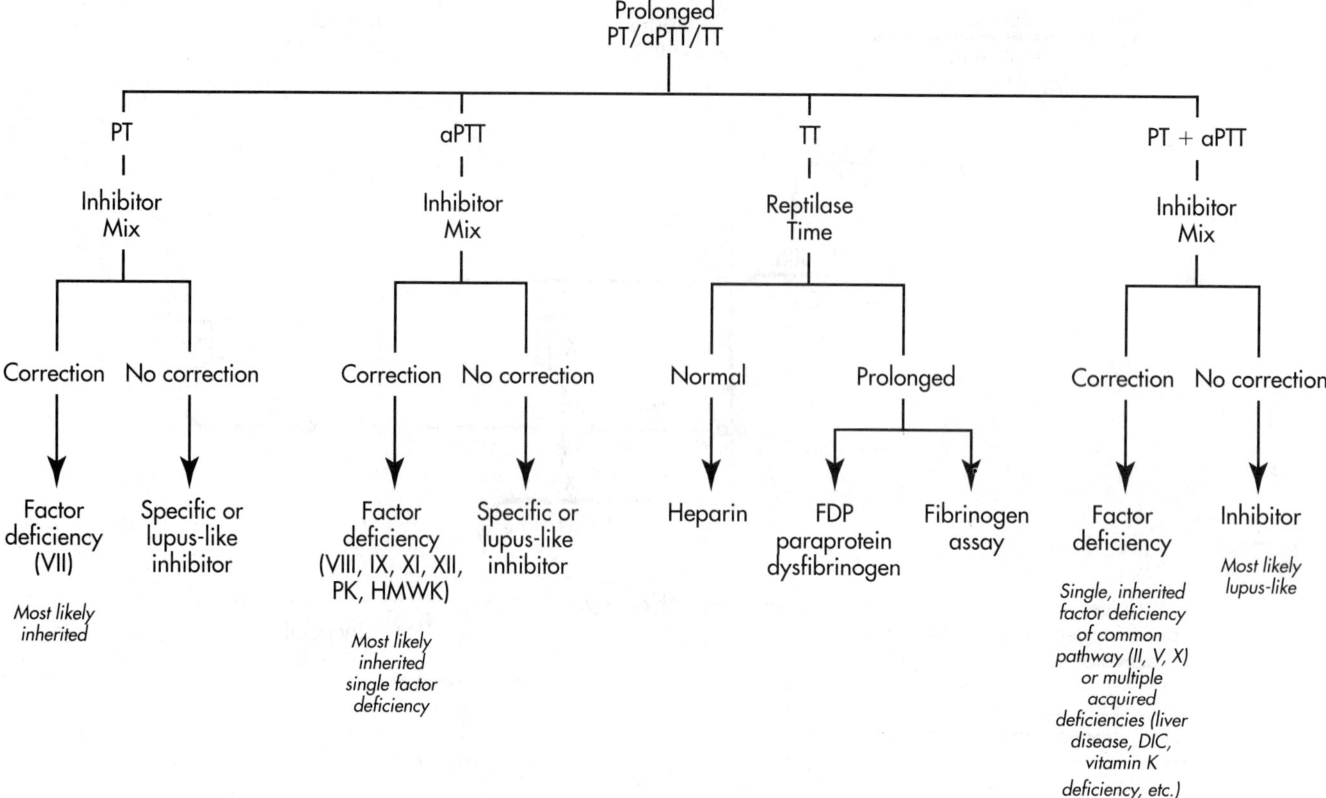

Fig. 115-3. Approach to the evaluation of a prolonged prothrombin time (PT), activated partial thromboplastin time (aPTT), or thrombin time (TT).

Table 115-1. Presumptive Diagnosis of Common Bleeding Disorders Based on Routine Screening Tests

Platelet count	Bleeding time	PT	PTT	TT	Miscellaneous	Presumptive problem
↓	N-↑	N	N	N		Thrombocytopenia
N	↑	N	N	N		Platelet function defect or vascular defect
N	↑	N	↑	N	↓ VIII_c, ↓ VIII_{ag}, ↓ VIII_{vWF}	von Willebrand's disease
N	N	↑	N	N		Extrinsic pathway defect (VII)
N	N	N	↑	N		Intrinsic pathway defect (VIII, IX, XI, XII, prekallikrein, high-molecular-weight kininogen, inhibitor)
N	N	↑	↑	N		Common pathway or multiple pathway defects excluding fibrinogen
N	N	↑	↑	↑	High levels of FDP	Fibrinogen deficiency or dysfunction, vitamin K deficiency, liver disease, primary fibrinolysis
↓	N-↑	↑	↑	↑	High levels of FDP/D-dimer	DIC
N	N	N	N	N	Positive clot solubility	XIII deficiency

N, Normal; ↓, decreased; ↑, increased; *FDP*, fibrin(ogen) degradation products; *DIC*, disseminated intravascular coagulation.

HEMORRHAGIC DISORDERS AND THEIR TREATMENT

Thrombocytopenia

A prolonged bleeding time as a result of thrombocytopenia does not develop until the platelet count reaches the 50,000 to 75,000/µl range (normal 150,000 to 350,000/µl). The risk of significant spontaneous bleeding, however, is not present until the count reaches the 10,000 to 20,000/µl level. Furthermore, the risk of bleeding is somewhat less for the same level of platelet count when the thrombocytopenia is due to peripheral destruction vs. inadequate production of platelets as determined by bone marrow biopsy.

Inadequate production of platelets may result from a stem cell defect and usually affects all three cell lines, as in the myeloproliferative and myelodysplastic syndromes. Invasion of the marrow by carcinoma, granuloma, or fibrosis also interferes with thrombopoiesis. Cancer chemotherapy is probably the most common cause today for a drug-induced reduction in platelet production, although some other drugs can also interfere, usually in an idiosyncratic fashion. Vitamin B_{12} and folic acid deficiencies are well-known causes of ineffective thrombopoiesis. Platelet transfusions are indicated to treat bleeding in these situations, but prophylactic platelets are not generally recommended unless the platelet count is reduced to the 5,000 to 10,000/µl range. When platelets are transfused, the quantity obtained from a single apheresis donor is used, which is equivalent to the platelets obtained from approximately 6 to 8 random donor units. Alternatively, random donor platelets can be used.

Thrombocytopenia in the setting of a normal bone marrow can be attributed to either immune or nonimmune peripheral destruction, and rarely to excessive dilution. Nonimmune thrombocytopenia is most often encountered with disseminated intravascular coagulation (DIC), where platelets are activated and destroyed when they come in contact with intravascular fibrin or are exposed to thrombin (see Disseminated Intravascular Coagulation). Severe thrombocytopenia can also occur in the rare disorder of thrombotic thrombocytopenic purpura (TTP), a primary disorder of platelet consumption. The TTP syndrome consists of thrombocytopenia, microangiopathic hemolytic anemia, often transient neurologic deficits, renal impairment, and fever. TTP, once a highly fatal disorder, is responsive to the simultaneous administration of fresh frozen plasma (FFP) and plasmapheresis. High-dose adrenal corticosteroids may provide some benefit, and in some cases splenectomy may also be of benefit. With these treatments mortality has been reduced considerably, but TTP and DIC are still life-threatening emergencies that require hematologic consultation.

Immunologic thrombocytopenia may be mediated by drug-induced antibodies, isoantibodies, or autoantibodies. Drug-induced antibodies may attach to platelet membranes by an innocent bystander mechanism (immune complex deposition), in response to neoantigen formation by a drug and platelet membrane complex, or by specific membrane receptor targeting induced by a drug. Heparin is the most common cause of drug-induced thrombocytopenia. Heparin-induced thrombocytopenia (HIT) usually occurs after 6 to 8 days of intravenous heparin therapy, although it can occur sooner, especially in patients recently exposed to heparin, and it may develop after exposure to subcutaneous therapy or even heparin flushes used to maintain catheter patency. It is an immune-mediated thrombocytopenia. The diagnosis is based on the clinical presentation with other causes being excluded. Heparin-induced platelet aggregation or serotonin release assays may help confirm a diagnosis, but are rarely useful in managing the acute situation because of limited availability or prolonged turnaround.

Although platelet counts may be low, bleeding is unusual. Rather, paradoxical thromboembolism is the most worrisome complication and may be attributable to in vivo heparin-induced platelet aggregation. HIT occurs in about 1% to 5% of patients taking heparin for 5 to 10 days, and heparin-induced thrombosis occurs in one third to one half of these patients. Cessation of heparin is mandatory, and alternative anticoagulation is initiated with either a low-molecular-weight heparinoid called danaparoid (Orgaran) or a recently approved hirudin derivative called lepirudin (Refludan). Substitution with one of the low-molecular-weight heparin products is contraindicated because of the high cross reactivity of the heparin-induced platelet antibody.

Idiopathic (immune) thrombocytopenic purpura (ITP) is the most common form of immunologic thrombocytopenia. It occurs in acute (often in children) and chronic (in adults) forms. In children 90% or more of cases have an acute onset, often preceded by a viral illness, and resolve on their own over the course of 1 to 3 months. Physical findings are limited to the skin, where petechiae may be seen, especially in the dependent extremities. Splenomegaly is not seen. Specific treatment is often unnecessary, although corticosteroids may be given to boost the count from very low levels until spontaneous recovery occurs. ITP in the adult is most often chronic with an insidious onset of easy bruising or minor bleeding noted over the preceding months. Women are more commonly affected. Bleeding manifestations include petechiae, ecchymoses, menorrhagia, hematuria, melena, epistaxis, and gingival bleeding. The onset is not associated with an antecedent infection. The physical examination is unremarkable. The diagnosis is traditionally based on clinical grounds (i.e., the exclusion of other causes of thrombocytopenia in the setting of peripheral destruction of platelets as determined by a bone marrow biopsy). A platelet antibody assay may be helpful but should not be used as a definitive test. Treatment is more complex than for childhood ITP. Corticosteroids are indicated initially, but definitive responses are uncommon. Splenectomy is generally indicated next in low-surgical-risk candidates. Other treatment modalities include intravenous γ-globulin, attenuated androgens, immunosuppressive agents, staphylococcal protein A columns, and plasmapheresis. After all therapeutic modalities are exhausted, about 10% of patients continue to have serious thrombocytopenia for which no therapy is effective. Table 115-2 highlights the differences between the acute and chronic forms of ITP.

Thrombocytopenia resulting from isoantibodies occurs after multiple platelet transfusions, or in a syndrome called posttransfusion purpura caused by transfusion of mismatched platelets. Thrombocytopenia can also occur on a dilutional basis in individuals transfused large volumes of blood over a short interval (e.g., 10 to 20 units of blood over a 24-hour period). Finally, thrombocytopenia can occur as a result of a hyperfunctioning spleen (hypersplenism) in individuals with splenomegaly for a variety of reasons.

Qualitative Platelet Disorders

Functional platelet defects produce a long bleeding time in the presence of a normal platelet count and may predispose to bleeding. Inherited disorders are uncommon, the most likely one being von Willebrand's disease, which is a defect or deficiency in von Willebrand's factor, a component of the factor VIII complex that is important for normal platelet adhesion. Acquired defects are much more common and are usually the result of drugs, aspirin being the major offender. Aspirin and other nonsteroidal antiinflammatory drugs (NSAIDs) impair platelet prostaglandin production and induce a release defect; aspirin-induced impairment is irreversible, whereas NSAID effect is not. Rarely platelet transfusions are needed to correct an aspirin defect in the face of serious bleeding. Uremia also produces a qualitative defect that can sometimes be improved by dialysis or by the infusion of cryoprecipitate or the use of deamino-8-D-arginine vasopressin (DDAVP). Last, myeloproliferative disorders can be associated with a platelet defect resulting from an abnormal stem cell.

Table 115-2. Clinical Features of the Acute and Chronic Forms of Idiopathic Thrombocytopenic Purpura

	Acute (predominating in children)	Chronic (predominating in adults)
Age of onset	2-6 yr	20-40 yr
Sex predilection	None	3 females : 1 male
Presentation	Sudden	Insidious
Preceding illness	Common	Unusual
Onset of bleeding	Abrupt	Insidious
Serious bleeding	Uncommon	Uncommon
Palpable spleen	Rare	Rare
Platelet count	<20,000/μl	20,000-80,000/μl
Clinical course	2-6 wk	Months to years

Acquired Coagulation Disorders

A discussion of the inherited coagulation disorders is a pediatric topic, but the more common acquired disorders are important to review, since the primary care physician will be called upon to diagnose and treat these problems. The reader is referred to other texts listed at the end of the chapter for a more detailed discussion of the congenital factor deficiencies.

Vitamin K Deficiency. Vitamin K deficiency is most often seen in seriously ill patients, especially in the postoperative state when patients are poorly nourished and receiving antibiotics. Poor nutrition removes vitamin K from the diet, and antibiotics suppress gut bacteria that produce vitamin K. Vitamin K deficiency produces an initial rise in the prothrombin time because of the rapid decline of factor VII activity, the vitamin K–dependent factor with the shortest metabolic half-life. An elevation of the activated partial thromboplastin time follows as other vitamin K–dependent factors decline (factors IX, X, and II). This condition, which often leads to serious bleeding, is easily reversed by parenteral vitamin K_1 therapy (5 to 10 mg subcutaneous).

Liver Disease. Impairment of the synthetic capacity of the liver is one of the most common causes for an acquired hemostatic defect. Hemostatic failure usually reflects the degree of liver failure and is usually subtle in acute liver failure unless the destruction of parenchymal tissue is fulminant. The PT, dependent on the short 6-hour half-life of factor VII, is prognostically helpful. Patients with biliary tract disease and obstructive jaundice may also develop a coagulopathy, but the mechanism in this situation is closely linked to levels of the vitamin K–dependent coagulation factors resulting from impaired absorption of vitamin K.

Hemostatic failure in liver disease involves both the platelet and coagulation phases of clotting. Mild thrombocytopenia is frequently encountered because of hypersplenism that accompanies portal hypertension. Qualitative defects in platelet function are probably not a major factor.

Coagulation is impaired primarily because of decreased factor synthesis, but abnormal factors may be produced, excessive consumption can occur, and fibrinolysis may be enhanced as contributing causes of hemostatic failure. A low fibrinogen, one of the last factors to be reduced, is a poor prognostic sign.

Treatment depends on the severity of the coagulopathy and the presence of bleeding and usually includes FFP. Treatment simply for the purpose of correcting an abnormal PT and aPTT, however, is not recommended, since it takes a large volume of plasma to correct the abnormality, the correction is short lived, and the protein load contained in the plasma may be enough to induce hepatic encephalopathy in a patient who is so predisposed. Platelet transfusions can be given in the face of clinically important bleeding with a very low platelet count, but generally they are not indicated in hypersplenism.

Disseminated Intravascular Coagulation. DIC often occurs in critically ill patients and is common in the intensive care setting. However, DIC can also occur in relatively well patients, a result of certain underlying diseases such as malignancy. Its onset can be fulminant and rapidly fatal or can be more subtle and gradual. Although its name implies a disorder of intravascular clotting, its clinical expression is often one of a diffuse hemorrhagic disorder.

DIC involves the pathologic activation of coagulation by an underlying disease process that leads to fibrin clot formation and secondary fibrinolysis, which then cause further consumption of coagulation factors, platelets, and red cells. In the fulminant syndrome bleeding results from factor deficiency (primarily factors I, II, V, VIII, and XIII), thrombocytopenia, excessive fibrinolysis, and high levels of FDP superimposed on a vascular system already damaged by diffuse microvascular thrombi. Bleeding is typically manifested by diffuse superficial hemorrhage in the form of ecchymoses and petechiae as well as oozing from the gingiva, the oral mucosa, or the gastrointestinal and urinary tracts. Most hemorrhage tends to be from the microvasculature, although major vascular hemorrhage and central nervous system bleeding can occur.

The pathophysiology of the consumption process depends on the underlying disease process or initiating event. The common mechanism is activation of a pathway of coagulation, usually the tissue factor pathway. Box 115-1 summarizes those conditions likely to cause a DIC syndrome.

The diagnosis of DIC is complicated by the fact that the clinical manifestations range from no findings to those of an extensive thrombotic or hemorrhagic disease. Bleeding is usually generalized and from the microvasculature. Table 115-3 highlights those tests commonly used to diagnose DIC. The most important component in the treatment of DIC is correction of the underlying disease. Supportive measures include FFP and platelet transfusions. Recent studies suggest a benefit to infusions of antithrombin concentrates, but it is too premature to recommend their use. In rare cases low doses of intravenous or subcutaneous heparin may be useful to interrupt the process of consumption by neutralizing activated coagulation factors. This may be most helpful in well-characterized conditions such as acute promyelocytic leukemia associated with a high incidence of DIC. Efficacy of therapy can be monitored by looking for a decrease in FDP, or D-dimer, an increase in fibrinogen, or the normalization of the PT and aPTT.

THROMBOTIC DISORDERS AND THEIR TREATMENT

The evaluation of an individual with thrombosis or suspected of having an increased risk of thrombosis should focus on abnormalities of one of the three elements of Virchow's triad—blood vessels, blood flow, or blood constituents. In the

Box 115-1. Causes of Disseminated Intravascular Coagulation

- Infection
  - Gram-negative endotoxemia with hypotension or shock
  - Severe gram-positive septicemia
  - Rocky Mountain spotted fever
  - Viral infections (herpes)
  - Malaria *(Plasmodium falciparum)*
  - HIV-1 infection
- Complications of pregnancy and delivery
  - Gram-negative sepsis
  - Abruptio placentae
  - Amniotic fluid embolism
  - Retained dead fetus
  - Toxemia
- Pediatric disorders—especially in newborns
- Malignant disease
  - Metastatic carcinoma (prostate, pancreas, lung, stomach, colon, breast)
  - Leukemia, especially APL
- Liver disease (cirrhosis)
- Complications of surgery
  - Extracorporeal circulation
- Critical tissue damage
  - Brain tissue destruction
  - Massive trauma
  - Heat stroke
  - Extensive burns
- Miscellaneous
  - Hemolytic transfusion reactions
  - Vasculitis
  - Aneurysms
  - Giant hemangioma
  - Snakebite

search for the etiology of a thrombotic event it is essential to take into account factors known to enhance the risk of thrombosis (Box 115-2). When a primary disorder of coagulation is the suspected cause, one begins by measuring the activities of the principal inhibitors of coagulation, including antithrombin, protein C, and protein S. Recently described genetic abnormalities of Factor V (Factor V_{Leiden}), leading to resistance to protein C inactivation, and prothrombin^{20210}, leading to increased circulating prothrombin, are relatively common causes of hypercoagulability and are found in as many as 6% or 3%, respectively, of the white population in the United States. Fibrinolytic system disorders can also be investigated. Analysis is best done when the acute thrombotic episode has stabilized and ideally when the patient is not receiving anticoagulants.

Antithrombotic Therapy

The following discussion focuses on the major antithrombotic agents in clinical use. Discussion of the various thromboembolic syndromes can be found elsewhere in this text.

Anticoagulants

Heparin. Heparin is a glycosaminoglycan of heterogeneous molecular weight derived from porcine intestinal mucosa or bovine lung. Heparin causes its anticoagulant effect through high-affinity binding with circulating antithrombin (AT). Binding with heparin produces a conformational change of AT, which greatly accelerates its inactivation of coagulation factors Xa, IXa, and thrombin, thereby causing a rapid anticoagulant effect.

Heparin is given parenterally as a constant intravenous infusion. Heparin dosing nomograms have recently been shown to provide for a more rapid achievement of therapeutic

Table 115-3. Laboratory Findings in Disseminated Intravascular Coagulation

Test	Low-grade DIC	Fulminant DIC
Blood smear (microangiopathic)	±	+
Platelets	Low normal to low	Very low
PT	Normal; short	Long
PTT	Normal; short	Long
TT	Normal; short; long	Long
Fibrinogen	Elevated; normal; low normal	Low
Fibrin monomers (protamine sulfate, ethanol gelation)	±	+
Fibrin(ogen) degradation products or D-dimer	Mildly elevated	High

All tests are easily obtainable within a short period of time (e.g., 1 to 2 hours) and constitute a DIC screen.

Box 115-2. Factors That Enhance the Risk of Thromboembolism

- Acquired risk factors
  - Age > 40 years
  - Prior major surgical procedures
  - Prior thromboembolism
  - Immobilization
  - Stasis (e.g., congestive heart failure, edema)
  - Malignancy
  - Sepsis
  - Stroke
  - Obesity
  - Inflammatory bowel disease
  - Pregnancy
  - Estrogen therapy
  - Nephrotic syndrome
  - Polycythemia rubra vera
  - Lupus anticoagulant
  - Paroxysmal nocturnal hemoglobinuria
- Inherited
  - Antithrombin deficiency
  - Protein C deficiency
  - Protein S deficiency
  - Factor V_{Leiden}
  - Prothrombin^{20210}
  - Dysfibrinogenemia
  - Disorders of plasminogen and plasminogen activator

anticoagulation, and their use is recommended (Table 115-4). Heparin may also be given by intermittent intravenous bolus at 4-hour intervals, but such therapy has been shown to be less effective than continuous infusions.

When heparin is given intravenously, the intensity of anticoagulation is monitored using the aPTT. The heparin infusion is adjusted to prolong the aPTT to the recommended therapeutic range depending on the aPTT reagent. Reagent differences can be overcome by performing in vitro heparin titration curves to determine the correlation of the aPTT with therapeutic heparin concentrations in the range of 0.2 to 0.4 U/ml. The overall variability of response to heparin demands frequent monitoring of the aPTT while treatment with heparin proceeds. Physicians encounter considerable variability in patients' heparin requirements not only because of differences in aPTT reagent sensitivity to heparin, but also because of differences in heparin clearance and neutralization by heparin-binding proteins.

Bleeding is the most common adverse effect of heparin therapy and is influenced by anticoagulation intensity, duration of heparin therapy, concomitant use of other drugs, and severity of illness. Heparin anticoagulation may be rapidly reversed with protamine sulfate, given at a ratio of 1 mg per 100 U of estimated heparin reserve (the amount of heparin thought to remain in the body). Heparin-associated thrombocytopenia occurs in approximately 1% to 5% of patients receiving heparin and is occasionally associated with venous and arterial thrombosis and bleeding (see discussion of heparin-induced thrombocytopenia earlier in this chapter). Chronic subcutaneous heparin therapy may cause osteoporosis in a minority of patients, leading to spontaneous fractures. Heparin does not cross the placenta and may be used for thromboembolic treatment during pregnancy.

Table 115-4. Guidelines for Dosing Heparin According to a Weight-based Nomogram

aPTT response*	Heparin dosage
Initial dose	80 U/kg bolus, then 18 U/kg/hr
aPTT <35 sec* (<1.2 × control)	80 U/kg bolus, then ↑ by 4 U/kg/hr
aPTT, 35-45 sec* (1.2-1.5 × control)	40 U/kg bolus, then ↑ by 2 U/kg/hr
aPTT, 46-70 sec* (1.5-2.3 × control)	No change
aPTT, 71-90 sec* (2.3-3.0 × control)	↓ infusion rate by 2 U/kg/hr
aPTT >90 sec* (>3 × control)	Hold × 1 hr, then ↓ rate by 3 U/kg/hr

From Raschke RA et al: The weight-based heparin dosing nomogram compared with a "standard care" nomogram, *Ann Intern Med* 119:874, 1993.

*The therapeutic range will vary depending on the aPTT reagent in use. Each laboratory must perform its own in vitro heparin titration curve to establish the therapeutic range for the specific aPTT reagent in use that is equivalent to a heparin concentration of 0.2-0.4 U/ml.

Low-molecular-weight Heparin. Low-molecular-weight heparins (LMWHs) are obtained by enzymatic or chemical depolymerization of unfractionated heparin. They have a more uniform distribution by molecular weight and shorter chain length of polysaccharides, with an average molecular weight of 4500 to 6000. LMWHs are advantageous compared with standard heparin in their greater ability to neutralize factor Xa compared with thrombin. They have less binding to heparin-binding proteins and platelets, have a longer half-life, are more uniformly absorbed from subcutaneous depots, and cause less heparin-induced thrombocytopenia. They can be given subcutaneously once or twice daily depending on the indication and the preparation. Dosages are determined on a fixed or weight basis and do not require monitoring, at least when used for primary prophylaxis. Several LMWH preparations are FDA approved in the United States for different prophylactic indications and for treatment of venous thromboembolism. One must become familiar with the different preparations and use them by name since dosage and indications vary. The differences between LMWH and regular heparin and the advantages of LMWH are illustrated in Table 115-5.

Oral Anticoagulants (Warfarin). Patients requiring intermediate-term or chronic anticoagulation are treated with warfarin, the most widely used oral anticoagulant.

Warfarin exerts its anticoagulant effect through competitive interference with vitamin K, which is essential for the normal synthesis of factors II, VII, IX, and X, and the antithrombotic factors protein S and protein C. Vitamin K serves as a cofactor that catalyzes the γ-carboxylation of

Table 115-5. Advantages of Low-molecular-weight Heparin

	Unfractionated heparin	Low-molecular-weight heparin	Observed advantage
Administration	IV/continuous infusion	Subcutaneous	Simpler administration
Half-life	Short	Longer	Less frequent dosing; once or twice daily
Subcutaneous absorption	Poor; erratic	Predictable, complete	Can be given subcutaneously
Protein binding	Increased, variable	Decreased, insignificant	Predictable dose response; less heparin resistance; fixed or weight-based dosing possible
Monitoring assay	Inadequate	None needed	Monitoring not required
Resistance	Frequent	Not apparent	Therapeutic efficacy
Side effects	Bleeding; thrombocytopenia; thrombosis	Bleeding; less thrombocytopenia; less thrombosis	Appears to be safer

certain glutamic acid residues on the vitamin K–dependent coagulation factors; the reaction provides critical calcium binding sites essential for full function. By competitive inhibition of microsomal reductases warfarin interferes with the conversion of oxidized vitamin K to its active reduced form, causing an acquired vitamin K deficiency and hepatic production of functionally inactive coagulation factors. Because the half-lives of the vitamin K–dependent factors vary, the full effect of a given dose of warfarin on the PT is not seen for several days after initiation of therapy. Early prolongation of the PT is due to depletion of factor VII, which has an estimated half-life of 6 to 8 hours.

Conversely, treatment with intravenous vitamin K reverses warfarin-induced anticoagulation via synthesis of new vitamin K–dependent factors within 24 to 48 hours. When necessary, treatment with intravenous FFP gives a rapid (although temporary) reversal of warfarin effect by direct replacement of active vitamin K–dependent factors.

Warfarin therapy is usually initiated with a dosage of 5 to 10 mg, with subsequent doses based on the response of the international normalized ratio (INR). When heparin anticoagulation precedes warfarin therapy, treatment with warfarin should begin 3 to 5 days before termination of heparin to permit full depletion of vitamin K–dependent factors and achieve a therapeutic PT. Usually both heparin and warfarin can be started at the same time when a patient enters the hospital with a deep venous thrombosis or pulmonary embolism.

The INR is the standard reporting methodology for monitoring warfarin anticoagulation; earlier monitoring methods using the PT fail to correct for differences in reagent sensitivity, and thus PTs from different laboratories are not comparable. The INR provides a method to compare different PTs based on an international standard. It is calculated by raising the laboratories' PT ratio (PT) mean normal range) to the power expressed by the international sensitivity index, a measure of thromboplastin reagent sensitivity. Two intensity levels of warfarin anticoagulation are currently recommended: less intense warfarin therapy (INR of 2 to 3) is sufficient for most thromboembolic indications, and more intense warfarin therapy (INR of 2.5 to 3.5) is reserved for mechanical heart valves and failure of less-intensive treatment with warfarin (Table 115-6). During warfarin treatment the patient's INR must be monitored regularly to ensure the desired intensity of anticoagulation. After initiating therapy the INR is checked at least weekly, adjusting the warfarin dose when necessary. When stable anticoagulation is attained, the frequency of INR testing may be reduced, based on the patient's compliance with medication and follow-up. Compliance can be improved significantly with regular education about warfarin dosing, drug interactions, and potential side effects of warfarin therapy.

Table 115-6. Therapeutic Range for Oral Anticoagulant Therapy Based on the International Normalized Ratio

Indication	Recommended INR
Prophylaxis of venous thrombosis Treatment of venous thrombosis Treatment of pulmonary embolism Prevention of systemic embolism Tissue heart valves Valvular heart disease Atrial fibrillation	2.0-3.0
Acute myocardial infarction Mechanical prosthetic valves Recurrent systemic embolism	2.5-3.5

Variations in dietary vitamin K, drug interactions with warfarin, and patient compliance all may cause rapid fluctuations in response to a given warfarin dose. Physicians must be aware of the many potential drug interactions with warfarin and should avoid those medications known to alter warfarin's anticoagulant effect. As a precaution, anticoagulated patients starting a new medication should be monitored with more frequent INR testing to detect any changes in anticoagulant effect induced by the drug.

Bleeding is the most frequent side effect of warfarin therapy. The risk increases with greater intensity of anticoagulation, history of previous bleeding, concurrent use of antiplatelet agents, severe intercurrent illness, and old age. Bleeding during warfarin anticoagulation may unmask occult pathology, such as lung, colon, uterine, or bladder neoplasia. Physicians must consider obtaining appropriate diagnostic studies if anticoagulated patients develop hemoptysis, rectal or vaginal bleeding, or hematuria. Warfarin-induced skin necrosis is a rare complication caused by thrombosis of small vessels supplying subcutaneous fat, often associated with occult protein C or protein S deficiency. Warfarin is contraindicated during pregnancy because of fetal bleeding and multiple teratogenic effects. Women of childbearing age who require warfarin therapy should be counseled in effective methods of birth control, and a pregnancy test is a prudent precaution for such patients before beginning treatment with warfarin.

Antiplatelet Agents

Aspirin. Aspirin and most other NSAIDs inhibit platelet aggregation by interfering with cyclooxygenase, an enzyme important in the generation of prostaglandins. Aspirin irreversibly inhibits this enzyme, whereas NSAIDs usually cause reversible inhibition of cyclooxygenase. Only small doses of aspirin are needed (less than one 5-grain tablet) to affect most of the platelets in the circulation. This effect persists for the lifetime of those platelets affected (about 10 days). Nonacetylated forms of salicylate (e.g., choline, sodium salicylate) do not have this inhibitory effect. Dipyridamole and sulfinpyrazone, agents used in the past for their supposed antiplatelet effect, have been shown not to have any beneficial effect mediated by antiplatelet activity.

Ticlopidine and Clopidogrel. Ticlopidine and clopidogrel are similarly acting antiplatelet agents that mediate their effect by inhibiting the adenosine diphosphate pathway for platelet activation. Their onset of action is slow, with a cumulative effect over 8 to 10 days and a similar time for recovery of platelet function once discontinued. Ticlopidine was the first of these two agents that was shown to be an effective platelet inhibitor in a number of conditions, but its use has been limited because of potentially serious side effects, including neutropenia and a syndrome of thrombotic thrombocytopenic purpura. More recently clopidogrel has

Table 115-7. Approved Indications and Suggested Dosages for Thrombolytic Agents

Thrombolytic agent	Deep venous thrombosis	Pulmonary embolism	Acute myocardial infarction	Occluded catheters/ arteries/veins
Streptokinase	250,000 IU × 30 min, then 100,000 IU/hr × 24 hr	250,000 IU × 30 min, then 100,000 IU/hr × 24 hr	1.5×10^6 IU × 20 min	250,000 IU × 60-120 min
Urokinase	4400 IU/kg × 10 min, then 4400 IU/hr × 24 hr	4400 IU/kg × 10 min, then 4400 IU/hr × 24 hr	2×10^6 IU bolus or 3×10^6 IU over 90 min	5000 IU
Alteplase (t-PA)	—	100 mg over 2 hr	60 mg × 1 hr (6-10 mg as bolus), 20 mg over second hr, 20 mg over third hr	—
Anistreplase	—	—	30 U (1.25×10^6 IU streptokinase) bolus	—

been available as an agent with effective antiplatelet properties and a reasonable substitute for individuals unable to take aspirin.

Thrombolytic Agents. The major fibrinolytic or thrombolytic agents currently in use include streptokinase, urokinase, t-PA, and anisoylated plasminogen-streptokinase activator complex (APSAC or anistreplase). These agents are most often used in ischemic cardiovascular disease (see Chapter 63). They are also recommended in fulminant pulmonary embolism and some cases of deep venous thrombosis, but because of a high-risk profile they should be used with great care and in those with no risk factors for bleeding. At a minimum, these agents are contraindicated in the setting of active internal bleeding, recent (within 2 months) cerebral vascular event or intracranial/intraspinal surgery, intracranial neoplasm, arteriovenous malformation or aneurysm, severe uncontrolled hypertension, or a known bleeding diathesis. Thrombolytic agents are used for the clearance of thrombi that obstruct indwelling catheters such as those used in cancer patients.

Streptokinase, the least expensive agent, binds to plasminogen, and the streptokinase-plasminogen complex activates other plasminogen molecules to the active enzyme plasmin. Urokinase directly activates plasminogen. t-PA, which also activates plasminogen directly, has a greater affinity for clot-bound plasminogen than circulating plasminogen and thus is less likely to activate plasminogen in a systemic fashion, leading to hypofibrinogenemia. However, in the dosages needed to be effective, some of this specificity is lost. Through molecular manipulation anistreplase has greater affinity for fibrin than circulating fibrinogen and thus on a theoretic basis is less likely to produce systemic hypofibrinogenemia. It also has a longer half-life than the three other agents.

Thrombolytic therapy does not require close monitoring of coagulation parameters, since a fixed dosage is given in most situations. The major reason to monitor therapy in some cases is to ensure that a lytic state has been achieved; this can easily be determined by a thrombin time that should be at least 3 seconds above baseline value or a fibrinogen level that should be reduced to the 1.5 gm/L level. Streptokinase has the problem of being susceptible to neutralization by existing antistreptococcal antibodies as well as producing allergic reactions resulting from these antibodies. It is recommended to coadminister corticosteroids with streptokinase to prevent such reactions, and if a lytic state cannot be achieved, another thrombolytic agent should be used. Table 115-7 summarizes the recommended dosages of these agents for their currently approved indications.

ADDITIONAL READINGS

American Society of Hematology ITP Practice Guideline Panel: Diagnosis and treatment of idiopathic thrombocytopenic purpura: recommendations of the American Society of Hematology, *Ann Intern Med* 126:319-326, 1997.

Ansell J: Oral anticoagulant therapy: fifty years later, *Arch Intern Med* 153:586, 1993.

Bick RL: Platelet function defects: a clinical review, *Semin Thromb Hemost* 18:167, 1992.

Broze GJ: The role of tissue factor pathway inhibitor in a revised coagulation cascade, *Semin Hematol* 29:159, 1992.

Clouse LH, Comp PC: The regulation of hemostasis: the protein C system, *N Engl J Med* 314:1298, 1986.

Hirsh J: Heparin, *N Engl J Med* 324:1565, 1991.

Landefeld SC, Beyth RJ: Anticoagulant-related bleeding: clinical epidemiology, prediction, and prevention, *Am J Med* 95:315, 1993.

Lane DA, Mannucci PM, Bauer KA, et al: Inherited thrombophilia: Part I, *Throm Hemostas* 76:651-662, 1996; Part II 76:824-834, 1996.

Raschke RA et al: The weight-based heparin dosing nomogram compared with a "standard care" nomogram, *Ann Intern Med* 119:874, 1993.

Redei I, Rubin RN: Recognizing the most common causes of bleeding in the ICU: how to diagnose and treat platelet and coagulation disorders, *J Crit Illness* 10:121-132 and 133-137, 1995.

Schmaier AH: Disseminated intravascular coagulation: pathogenesis and management, *J Intens Care Med* 6:209, 1991.

Stein JH, McBride PE: Hyperhomocysteinemia and atherosclerotic vascular disease, *Arch Intern Med* 158:1301-1306, 1998.

Weitz JI: Low molecular weight heparins, *N Engl J Med* 337:688-698, 1997.

CHAPTER 116

Transfusion Therapy in General Practice

Irma O. Szymanski

Blood transfusion is an intrinsic part of both medical and surgical practice. To meet the nation's blood needs, about 12 million volunteer blood donations are given annually in the United States. Modern transfusion practice utilizes *blood component therapy* instead of whole blood transfusions to provide specific therapy. The method of preparation of blood components is discussed briefly so that the reader can appreciate the relationship between the content and function of blood components. Despite our ability to prepare sophisticated blood components, both infectious and immunologic adverse effects still occur.

The *risk* of transmitting infectious diseases by blood components has decreased greatly in recent years, mainly because powerful methods are used to detect infectious disease markers in donor blood. The risk of transfusion-associated (TA) infection is now so small that it is immeasurable, and the degree of risk is calculated on the basis of mathematic models, taking into account the length of the seronegative window period of various viral infections. Current estimates of the risks of TA infection are given in Table 116-1. In the near future, blood safety will increase even further since nucleic acid amplification technology (NAT) will be adapted for detection of the RNA of the human immunodeficiency virus (HIV) and hepatitis C virus (HCV) in donor blood. Furthermore, methods to inactivate all pathogens in blood components have been introduced so that in the future the blood components will be practically sterile.

The *appropriate* use of blood components has been debated greatly in the last few years. Current understanding of the use of blood components is discussed in the next section.

BLOOD COMPONENTS

Preparation

During a blood donation a donor gives about 450 ml of whole blood, which is anticoagulated with 63 ml of citrate-phosphate-dextrose anticoagulant. The whole blood is centrifugally separated within 8 hours of collection into packed red cell concentrate, random platelet concentrate, and plasma. The red cells are stored in a preservative solution (Adsol or Nutricel) for up to 42 days at 4° C. Platelet concentrates are stored at 22° C in special gas-permeable plastic bags for 5 days while being agitated. Plasma is frozen and stored at −18° C for up to 1 year.

Random platelet concentrates separated from whole blood are transfused as pools of 5 or 6 units, but a therapeutic dose of platelets (total of about 3×10^{11} platelets) is obtained from a single donor using *apheresis* technique.

White Blood Cells in Blood Components

Centrifugally separated cellular blood components contain between 10^8 to 10^9 white blood cells (WBC)/unit. These "passenger" leukocytes may carry such infectious agents as cytomegalovirus (CMV), human T-cell leukemia/lymphoma virus (HTLV) I/II, and possibly the prion causing new variant Creutzfeld-Jakob disease (nvCJD). These leukocytes may also sensitize recipients to human leukocyte antigens (HLA), subsequently preventing a good response to platelet transfusions, cause graft vs. host disease (GvHD), as well as cause subtle changes in a patient's immune response (immune modulation). These complications can be avoided or minimized by using leukocyte-reduced red cells and platelets (containing less than 5×10^6 WBC/unit) that are prepared by high-efficiency filtration, preferably in the laboratory under standardized conditions, either before or during the early period of storage of the blood component (Table 116-2). The effectiveness of bedside filtration is variable.

Certain plateletpheresis techniques are designed to remove leukocytes from the product during collection (COBE Spectra LRS platelets) so that platelets prepared by this method need not be filtered.

Presently about 20% of red cell and platelet transfusions are leukocyte reduced. A change to universal leukocyte reduction of cellular blood components may occur since several European countries have recently switched to transfusing only leukocyte-reduced cellular blood components to all patients. Such a recommendation was also issued by the Blood Products Advisory Committee of the Food and

Table 116-1. Estimated Risks of TA Infections

Infection	Risk per unit
HIV	1/200,000-1/2,000,000
HBV	1/30,000-1/150,000
HCV	1/30,000-1/150,000
HTLV I/II	1/250,000-1/2,000,000
Parvovirus B19	1/10,000
CMV	Unknown
Bacterial contamination of red cells	1/500,000
Bacterial contamination of platelets	1/12,000
Malaria, Chagas' disease	Rare in United States
Babesiosis	Rare

Data from Goodnough LT et al: *N Engl J Med* 340:438, 1999.
HIV, Human immunodeficiency virus; *HBV,* hepatitis B virus; *HCV,* hepatitis C virus; *HTLV,* human T-cell leukemia/lymphoma virus; *CMV,* cytomegalovirus.

Table 116-2. "Regular" and Leukocyte-reduced (Containing $<5 \times 10^6$ WBC/Unit) Red Cell and Platelet Products

Regular blood products	Leukocyte-reduced blood products
Packed red cells	*Filtered packed red cells
Random platelet concentrates ($>5 \times 10^{10}$ platelets/unit)	*Filtered random platelet pools ($>3 \times 10^{11}$ platelets/pool)
Apheresis platelets	LRS apheresis platelets ($>3 \times 10^{11}$ platelets/concentrate) and *filtered apheresis platelets

*High-efficiency filtered.

Drug Administration (FDA) in September 1998, presaging the change to leukocyte-reduced blood product transfusion in the United States.

Washing, Irradiation, and Freezing of Cellular Blood Components

To prevent both allergic and anaphylactic transfusion reactions as well as TA-GvHD, cellular blood products can be further "customized" as follows:

- *Washing* cellular blood components prevents allergic and anaphylactic reactions caused by plasma present in components.
- *Irradiation* of blood components (about 3000 rads/unit) will prevent TA-GvHD, which may occur in susceptible patients even if they receive leukocyte-reduced blood components.
- *Frozen red cell programs* permit availability of fully typed, rare red cells and autologous red cells. Red cells can be stored at −80° C for up to 10 years.

Patient populations benefiting from the transfusion of customized products are listed in Table 116-3.

Table 116-3. Benefits of Customized Cellular Products (RBCs or Platelets)

Procedure	Usage	Recommended patient populations
Leukocyte reduction by high-efficiency filtration	Prevent disease transmission and immunization to HLA	Patients with leukemia and lymphoma, AIDS, long-term transfusion therapy
Washing	Prevent allergic or anaphylactic reactions	Previous reactions, patient is IgA negative, with anti-IgA
Irradiation	Prevent TA-GvHD	Patients with leukemia, lymphoma, premature babies, some malignancies, family donors
Freezing	Prolonged storage of red cells for up to 10 years (platelet freezing not routinely available)	Storage of rare cells, autologous blood

INFECTIOUS DISEASE TRANSMISSION

As shown in Table 116-1, the risks of transmitting infectious diseases by blood transfusion are currently quite low because of careful donor-screening techniques. These risks can be further decreased by using autologous blood, blood substitutes, and inactivating pathogens in blood components.

Autologous donations currently constitute a little more than 3% of total units, but they are feasible only before surgical procedures. Patients with bacteremia, severe aortic stenosis, and significant left coronary artery disease do not qualify. Since it is difficult to predict accurately the need of blood transfusion during surgery, only about 50% of the autologous blood is transfused. For safety reasons it is recommended that autologous blood not be "crossed over" to other patients. Thus autologous blood tends to be more expensive than homologous blood.

Various hemoglobin preparations have been tested in laboratory and in clinical settings. Due to their relatively short half-life and vasotoxicity, they have not yet been accepted in routine use. Perfluorocarbons are still being perfected, but the current preparations function only when recipients breathe 100% oxygen.

The desire to further reduce the risks of allogeneic blood transfusions has produced the following FDA-approved approaches:

- *Solvent/detergent (S/D) treatment* of *pooled fresh frozen plasma (FFP)* (pool size about 2500 units). The S/D process destroys lipid envelope viruses including HIV, HCV, and HBV, but not hepatitis A virus (HAV), or human parvovirus B19. The final product is expensive, and questions remain about the use of pooled product. Therefore many transfusion services have not adopted the routine use of S/D FFP.
- In the "delayed release" method, each individual unit of FFP is released for use only after a second donation from the same individual (given a minimum of 112 days after the first) tests negative for infectious disease markers.

Several methods of inactivation have shown promise but are not used routinely in clinical setting. Baxter/Fenwal introduced the use of methylene blue for destruction of viral RNA or DNA in FFP. This approach avoids using pools of plasma because the dye is added to individual units of FFP.

A photochemical treatment (PCT) using Psoralen S-59 with activation by long–wavelength ultraviolet A light (UVA) is a promising nucleic acid–targeted approach to inactivate pathogens in platelet concentrates. PCT requires 3 minutes of UVA exposure, is compatible with single-donor and pooled platelet concentrates, and inactivates high titers of enveloped and nonenveloped viruses, bacteria, and protozoa. In addition, leukocytes, including T cells, are inactivated in the process, with inhibition of proliferation and cytokine synthesis. A passive adsorption process of the S-59 is needed before transfusion. Clinical trials are currently ongoing.

Frangible anchor linker effectors (FRALEs) are being developed to inactivate pathogens in red cell concentrates. These agents cross-link nucleic acids without the need for light inactivation. A compound, *S-303*, is being evaluated for clinical use.

TRANSFUSION THERAPY

Acute Blood Loss

After acute blood loss the most important, immediate therapeutic goal is to restore the blood volume (Table 116-4). This can be accomplished with crystalloid or colloid infusion. However, recent studies have indicated that albumin use in critically ill patients is associated with higher mortality than is the case in patients who did not receive albumin. Patients who are treated in intensive care units tend to get red cells, FFP, and platelets. All of these products are probably over-used. A recent published study showed that liberal use of RBCs to maintain hemoglobin concentration between 10 and 12 gm/dl by transfusion was associated with higher in-hospital mortality than was the case when a patient's hemoglobin was kept between 7 and 9 gm/dl. The reason for this adverse effect was not clear, but it could be related to the poorly understood adverse effects of red cell transfusions

Table 116-4. Blood Component Transfusion During Acute Blood Loss

Blood component	Indications	Endpoint of therapy
Crystalloids	First-line therapy, blood loss >10% blood volume	Vital signs normalized
Red cells	Crystalloid therapy not effective, blood loss >15%	Surgical treatment effective, Hct stable
FFP	Initially abnormal coagulation tests	PT <15 s., PTT within normal range
Platelets	Microvascular bleeding while Hct within normal range, platelet count <50,000/μl	No microvascular bleeding, platelet count >50,000/μl

PT, Prothrombin time; *PTT,* partial thromboplastin time.

such as passenger leukocytes or the large number of nonviable red cells in the stored red cell product, compromising the function of the reticuloendothelial system of these patients. Some of the principles of blood component transfusion after acute blood loss are as follows.

Crystalloid infusions should be given as first-line therapy when acute blood loss exceeds 10% of blood volume. The treatment can be considered effective when vital signs have normalized. Red cell transfusions are helpful if blood loss exceeds 15% of the blood volume. In addition to increasing red cell mass and oxygen delivery capacity, red cell transfusions also increase plasma volume, by recruiting plasma proteins and extracellular fluid into the vascular compartment.

In most cases crystalloids and red cell transfusions are sufficient to correct all adverse effect of the blood loss. FFP transfusion might be useful if coagulation abnormalities exist (international normalized ratio [INR] >1.5 and PTT >60 sec).

Chronic Anemia

Long-term red cell transfusions are required for patients with bone marrow failure or when the purpose of the transfusions is to suppress bone marrow (as is in the case of thalassemia), or if patient's chronic hemolytic anemia does not respond to other therapy. Some principles of transfusion therapy in these cases include: leukocyte-reduced red cells should be given to chronically transfused patients, and, if possible, it would be helpful to limit the number of donors (using the same, dedicated donors repeatedly). Complete blood typing (for the minor antigens) may be helpful to avoid immunization to them.

At what level of hemoglobin should the patients be kept? In thalassemia, hypertransfusion requires that the hemoglobin is maintained above 10 gm/dl (hematocrit[Hct] >30%). In other conditions, patients might remain asymptomatic when hemoglobin concentration is at least 8 g/dl (Hct 24%). Erythropoietin has replaced transfusion therapy in patients suffering from chronic renal disease. Iron overload is a severe complication of chronic red cell transfusion therapy. It should be treated with iron chelators.

Table 116-5. Indications for Prophylactic Platelet Transfusions

Platelet count/μl	Associated conditions
<5000	None
5000-10,000	Fever or minor hemorrhage
10,000-20,000	Heparin therapy, coagulation disorder
<50,000	Surgery contemplated
>100,000	Bleeding time >15 min and surgery contemplated

Table 116-6. Reasons for Accelerated Platelet Destruction

Pathophysiology	Confirmatory tests, if available	Specific therapy
Medication (quinidine, quinine, heparin)	Drug-induced antibody tests	Discontinue the offending medication
DIC, fever, sepsis	PT/PTT, D-dimer, AT III, clinical evaluation	Treatment of the basic disease
Autoimmunization (ITP, antiphospholipid antibodies)	Antibodies to platelets antiphospholipids	IVIG, corticosteroids
Posttransfusion purpura	Anti-Pl^{A1} or other platelet-specific antibodies	IVIG or plasma exchange
Immunization to HLA	Anti-HLA	HLA matched platelet transfusions
Thrombotic thrombocytopenic purpura	Clinical diagnosis	FFP or plasma exchange; platelet transfusions contraindicated

Platelet Transfusions

Guidelines for platelet transfusion are given in Table 116-5. Although the transfusion trigger is based on platelet count, a low platelet count by itself is not an indication for platelet transfusion. Before initiation of platelet transfusions the etiology of thrombocytopenia must be established. The best results are obtained in patients whose platelet production is impaired. If it is likely that the reason for thrombocytopenia is accelerated peripheral destruction of platelets, the cause should be elucidated (Table 116-6). Useful principles of platelet transfusion are as follows:

1. The response to platelet transfusion should be evaluated by measuring the change in platelet count 1 hour and 24 hours after completion of the transfusion. Corrected count increment (CCI) is a measure of the effectiveness of the platelet transfusion.

$$CCI = (\Delta Pl) \times BSA/(\#Pl)$$

Table 116-7. Use and Properties of Plasma Products and Derivatives

Product	(Volume), content	Indications
FFP	(200-300 ml) All plasma constituents	Bleeding or surgery with coagulation factor deficiencies other than FVIII or FIX, when PT>16s. or PTT>16s. TTP*
S/D treated FFP, aliquots of pooled plasma	(200 ml) Low in vWF multimers Normal coagulation factor levels	Same as for FFP, may be useful in TTP
Cryoprecipitate	(10-20 ml) About 50% of FI, FVIII, FXIII, vWF, & fibronectin present in a unit of FFP	DIC, bleeding in uremia, vWF deficiency
FFP, cryoprecipitate removed	(150-250) Low levels of coagulation factors FI, FVIII, FXIII, vWF, fibronectin	TTP, coagulation factor deficiency in liver disease
Albumin, 5% Albumin, 25%	(Variable volumes) 96% albumin, 4% globulin	Hypovolemia
Intravenous IgG IVIG	Prepared as 6%, mostly IgG, minimal IgA and IgM	ITP, Kawasaki disease, agammaglobulinemia
Antithrombin III	AT III	To prevent thrombosis in congenital AT III deficiency, ?DIC
Coagulation Factor VIII	Factor VIII, some contain vWF (Humate P, Alphanate)	Hemophilia A and vWD
Factor IX complex	Factors IX, II, VII, X	Hemophilia B

TTP, Thrombotic thrombocytopenic purpura.

where ΔPl = change in platelet count (#/μl), BSA = body surface area (m^2), and #Pl = total number of platelets transfused.

2. CCI of 7500 or higher is considered a good response.
3. Since there is a negative correlation between anemia and platelet function, as measured by bleeding time, patients with low platelet counts should be kept at higher Hct values (about 30%) to improve the functional status of platelets and minimize the need to transfuse platelets.

Transfusion of Plasma and Plasma Products

The use and properties of plasma products and derivatives are presented in Table 116-7. FFP transfusions should not be given for plasma volume expansion, but to correct coagulation factor deficiencies. Patients with abnormal liver function should be transfused with FFP if INR > 1.5, when surgery or an invasive procedure is planned. Plasma exchange, in which a volume of the patient's plasma is removed and replaced with an equal volume of donor FFP, is used to correct coagulation factor deficiencies in patients who cannot tolerate increases in plasma volume. An overdose of Coumadin can be corrected by transfusion of FFP (10 to 20 ml/kg).

Patients with thrombotic thrombocytopenic purpura are treated either with FFP infusions or with plasma exchange using FFP as a replacement fluid. FFP from which cryoprecipitate has been removed, is also an acceptable, and maybe even a superior, replacement fluid for this purpose. Patients with disseminated intravascular coagulation (DIC) will benefit from infusions of cryoprecipitate, FFP, and additionally, if platelet counts are low, from platelet transfusions. It might be beneficial to give AT III infusions when the levels are very low (below 25%). Patients with hemophilia A are treated with purified coagulation factors. The current preparations are safe because they are either prepared with recombinant methods or treated with solvent/detergent. Patients with von Willebrands disease may be treated with cryoprecipitate or with purified coagulation factors containing vWF (Humate P or Alphanate). Purified AT III is now available to treat patients with congenital deficiency of AT III who undergo surgery. Albumin transfusions are much overused. A recent meta-analysis showed that critically ill patients who received albumin infusions had 6% higher mortality rate than similar patients who received crystalloid infusions.

TRANSFUSION REACTIONS

The incidence of noninfectious transfusion reactions is shown in Table 116-8. A brief description of various types of transfusion reactions follows.

Hemolytic Transfusion Reactions

Acute reactions occur during transfusion or within a few hours afterward. Delayed reactions occur within days to weeks after transfusion, and often go unnoticed. Donor red cells hemolyze intravascularly or extravascularly when patient's serum contains antibodies that combine with antigens on donor red cells. Complement binding antibodies (e.g., anti-A/B, anti-Kell, or anti-Jk^a) produce the most severe reactions. A common cause of a hemolytic transfusion reaction is an inability of the health care personnel to identify correctly the patient or the blood component. Transfusion reactions may be unavoidable when the antibody titer is too low to be detectable at the time of cross-match, or when the antibody is nonreactive by the normally used screening techniques. The symptoms of hemolytic transfusion reaction

Table 116-8. Etiology and Frequency of Immunologic Complications of Transfusion

Complication	Etiology	Frequency
Immediate hemolytic reactions	Antibody-induced destruction of donor red cells	1/250,000-1/1,000,000
Delayed hemolytic reactions	Destruction of donor red cells appearing after transfusion	1/1000
Febrile nonhemolytic transfusion reactions (FNHTR)	Reaction of antibodies to donor WBC or development of bioreactive substances during storage	1/200
Transfusion-related acute lung injury (TRALI)	WBC antibodies in donor plasma or reactive lipid products that may arise during storage	1/5000
Allergic reactions (mild)	Allergens in donor plasma	1/100
Allergic reactions with bronchospasm or laryngeal edema	Allergens in donor plasma	1/1000
Anaphylactic reactions	Immunizations of IgA-deficient recipients to IgA	1/150,000
Transfusion-associated graft vs. host disease (TA-GvHD)	Inability of the recipient to reject donor lymphocytes	Not defined

may include shock, DIC, and kidney failure. The principles of treatment of the patient who has hemolytic transfusion reaction are as follows:

- Monitor the vital signs frequently.
- Administer IV fluid to normalize vital signs.
- Do not give the patient epinephrine because it can increase the chance of kidney damage. Dopamine is acceptable.
- Monitor the patient for the laboratory signs of DIC.
- Treat the DIC, if necessary, with component therapy (cryoprecipitate, FFP, possibly platelet transfusions).
- If the patient becomes anemic, do not hesitate to give compatible red cell transfusions.
- Heparin therapy is rarely indicated, particularly in a postoperative patient. In order to prevent kidney damage, give the patient IV furosemide as soon as the transfusion reaction is identified. Monitor the urine output.

Patients in whose serum blood group antibodies are once detected must always receive red cell transfusions that are negative for the corresponding antigens.

Allergic Reactions

Allergic reactions occur in patients who receive donor plasma. The reactions can manifest themselves as local urticaria or as severe geographic urticaria, with joint involvement, laryngeal edema, pulmonary signs reminiscent of asthma, abdominal pains, and headaches. Depending on the severity of symptoms, the treatment may require antihistamines, corticosteroids, or epinephrine. In mild cases the transfusion can be started again after administering antihistamines.

Anaphylactic Reactions

Anaphylactic reactions occur within minutes of initiating a transfusion containing plasma or immunoglobulins. The symptoms include severe flushing of the skin, severe anxiety, laryngospasm, and shock. These types of reactions occur in IgA-deficient patients (frequency about 1/500) who have developed anti-IgA. The treatment may include intravenous fluids, epinephrine, and corticosteroids.

Febrile Nonhemolytic Transfusion Reactions

FNHTR occur after red cell and platelet transfusions. The risk is highest after platelet transfusions. FNHTR usually manifest themselves as fever above the baseline value (increase of at least 2° F), chills, and slight elevation of blood pressure. Occasionally, respiratory symptoms may occur.

Although most FNHTR are mild, some are life-threatening. The symptoms occur during or within 2 hours of transfusion. Treatment includes administration of a fever-lowering drug such as acetaminophen. It was previously assumed that FNHTR are caused by interactions between alloantibodies in the recipient's plasma and donor WBC, but now it appears more likely that they are mediated by bioreactive substances produced by WBC during blood component storage. Progressive increases in IL-1β, IL-6, IL-8, and TNF-α have been documented in platelet concentrates during storage. These increases are prevented by removal of leukocytes from platelet concentrates prior to storage.

Transfusion-related Acute Lung Injury (TRALI)

TRALI, a respiratory distress syndrome, occurs in patients within 4 hours after receiving plasma products, often derived from the blood of multiparous women. It is characterized by development of acute respiratory distress, severe hypoxemia, acute bilateral pulmonary edema, hypotension, and fever. There is no evidence of heart failure. In many cases of TRALI, HLA or granulocyte antibodies can be demonstrated in donor plasma, with specificity to antigenic determinants on patients' WBC. Recently, reactive lipid products that arise during storage of blood products have been implicated in the pathophysiology of TRALI. The complement reacting nature of these HLA or WBC antibodies results in generation of complement component C5a, which causes WBC clumping in pulmonary vasculature and increase in vascular permeability. TRALI is potentially life-threatening, but with prompt and vigorous respiratory support, at least 90% of patients recover.

Transfusion-associated Graft vs. Host Disease

Patients with impaired cellular immunity, and healthy patients who receive blood from relatives or from donors whose HLA type is homozygous and identical to one of the haplotypes of the patient, are at risk for developing TA-GvHD. Normally after transfusion the patient's immune system destroys donor lymphocytes. If, for reasons mentioned above, this does not occur, the donor lymphocytes may mount an immune attack against the patient's tissues. Within 5 to 30 days after transfusion the patient develops intractable skin rash, diarrhea, liver involvement, bone marrow failure, and eventually multiorgan failure. TA-GvHD is uniformly fatal. However, it can be prevented by irradiating blood products given to patients who are susceptible to this complication.

ADDITIONAL READINGS

American College of Physicians: Practice strategies for elective red blood cell transfusion, *Ann Intern Med* 116:403-406, 1992.

Goodnough LT, Brecher ME, Kanter MH, et al: Medical progress in transfusion medicine—blood transfusion, *N Engl J Med* 340:438-447, 1999.

Hebert PC, Wells G, Blajchman MA, et al: A multicenter, randomized, controlled clinical trial of transfusion requirement in critical care, *N Engl J Med* 340:409-417, 1999.

Horowitz B, Prince AM, Hamman J, et al: Viral safety of solvent/detergent-treated blood products, *Blood Coag Fibrin* 5:521-528, 1994.

Schierrhout G, Roberts I: Fluid resuscitation with colloid or crystalloid solutions in critically ill patients, *Br Med J* 316:961-964, 1998.

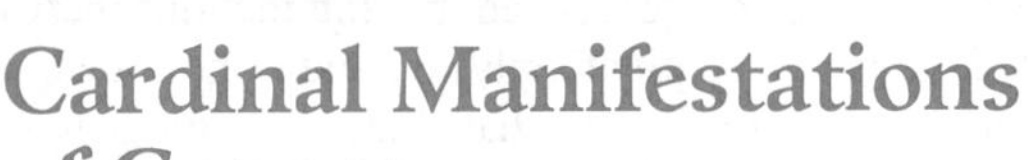

Cardinal Manifestations of Cancer

Kathryn L. Edmiston

Cancer is the second leading cause of death in the United States and as such is a concern for most patients seeing their primary care physicians (Table 117-1). The magnitude of the cancer problem is likely to increase in the coming decades as the U.S. population ages. At the beginning of the twentieth century fewer than 10% of Americans were over the age of 55. By 1989 this figure had doubled, and it is expected to increase through the year 2030. The risk of developing cancer increases dramatically with age. The age distribution of cancer deaths is shown in Fig. 117-1.[5a] Because patients frequently visit their primary care physician for routine health maintenance or the evaluation of new symptoms, primary care physicians need to have a thorough knowledge of the clinical signs and symptoms associated with cancer and the initial evaluation of the patient who is suspected of having cancer.

Table 117-1. Estimated Incidence and Mortality of Common Cancers in the United States in 2000

Primary cancer	Incidence	Deaths
Bronchogenic	164,100	156,900
Breast	184,200	41,200
Colorectal	130,200	56,300
Prostate	180,400	31,900
Head and neck	40,300	11,700

ASYMPTOMATIC PATIENTS

Patients may be diagnosed with cancer before symptoms occur or may come to medical attention because of symptoms resulting from their cancer. For most types of cancer, diagnosis in the early stages of disease before symptoms have occurred is critical. Treatment of early stage lung cancer may be cured, whereas advanced lung cancer is never curable even with aggressive treatment. This creates a particular dilemma for the primary care physician. How can cancer be diagnosed in its earliest and potentially curable stages before the patient has developed any symptoms? A thorough risk assessment during a routine visit and the appropriate use of cancer screening tests may lead to the diagnosis of cancer in the asymptomatic patient.

A thorough risk assessment can easily be accomplished during the medical interview. Risk assessment should include a history of habits such as smoking and alcohol use, occupational and other environmental exposures, diet, and family history. Cancers associated with specific risks are shown in Table 117-2. Once a patient is found to be at risk, what interventions are necessary? First, and most important, the patient should be counseled regarding the elimination of cancer-causing behaviors. Patients who smoke should be advised of the increased frequency of lung cancer and other cancers of the aerodigestive tract, as well as the risk of cardiovascular and peripheral vascular disease. It is estimated that 90% of all lung cancers are directly caused by tobacco use. Patients who wish to discontinue smoking should be provided with smoking cessation tools (see Chapter 57).

Early intervention to prevent the development of cancer may be warranted for patients with certain types of risk. For example, patients with familial adenomatous polyposis are almost certain to develop colon cancer by age 50 if left untreated. Prophylactic colectomy is recommended for prevention. Similarly, patients at high risk for breast cancer may wish to consider tamoxifen for chemoprevention,[5] genetic screening, or even prophylactic bilateral mastectomy in selected cases.

Finally, careful evaluation of organ systems at risk should be performed during the routine physical examination. Patients with heavy sun exposure or a family history of melanoma should have a thorough skin examination. A thorough inspection and manual examination of the oral cavity in patients with a history of tobacco and alcohol use may detect premalignant lesions or potentially curable invasive carcinomas of the oral cavity. The breasts should be carefully examined, particularly in women over the age of 50 or any woman with a family history of breast cancer.

Cancers that are frequently detected by screening are listed in Table 117-3. A number of cancer screening tools such as mammography,[8] prostate specific antigen,[11] and sigmoidoscopy[2] are recommended by the American Cancer Society for the early detection of cancer.

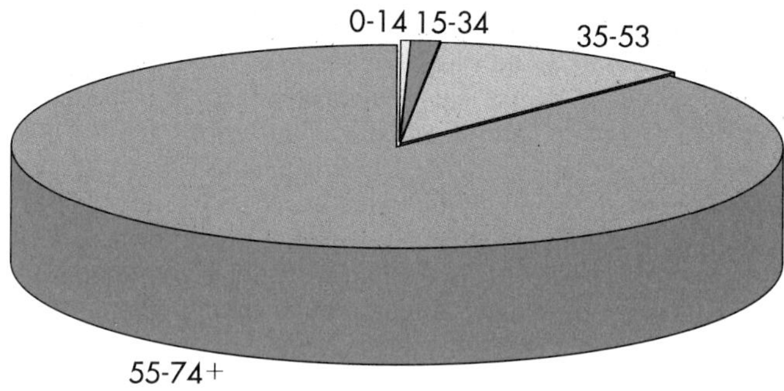

Fig. 117-1. Distribution of cancer deaths in the United States by age.

Table 117-2. Risk Factors Associated With Common Primary Cancers

Primary cancer	Risk factors
Bronchogenic carcinoma	Tobacco Asbestos Radiation exposure
Breast carcinoma	First-degree relative with breast cancer Prior personal history of breast cancer Nulliparity Early menarche Late menopause
Colon carcinoma	High-fat, low-fiber diet Personal history of colonic adenomatous polyps or previously resected colon cancer Inflammatory bowel disease
Cervical carcinoma	Multiparity Infection with human papillomavirus
Esophageal cancer and head and neck cancer	Tobacco and alcohol use

Table 117-3. Cancers Frequently Detected by Screening Tests

Primary cancer	Screening test
Breast cancer	Mammography
Colon cancer	Stool guaiac, sigmoidoscopy
Cervical cancer	Papanicolaou test
Prostate cancer	Prostate specific antigen

SYMPTOMATIC PATIENTS

Symptoms of cancer may be vague and nonspecific, such as weight loss, fatigue, and malaise. Specific symptoms may occur because of physiologic or mechanical effects of the primary tumor or metastases at distant sites.

Weight loss occurs commonly at the time of diagnosis in many patients with advanced cancer. Although a wide constellation of gastrointestinal symptoms are common in patients with cancer, decreased caloric intake may not be sufficient to explain weight loss. An aggressive search for an undiagnosed cancer is probably not warranted in most patients with unexplained weight loss as their only symptom until changes in dietary intake, depression, and stresses at work or in family have been assessed. Patients at high risk for cancer, such as smokers or those with additional symptoms, should undergo further evaluation without delay.

Table 117-4. Characteristics of Cancer Pain

Site	Characteristics of pain
Long bones	Localized, increased with weight bearing
Vertebrae	Localized or radicular, increased in supine position
Bowel	Intermittent, crampy
Liver	Sharp, throbbing, radiates to right shoulder
Lung/pleura	Sharp, increased with deep breathing
Neuropathic	Burning, tingling

Pain is the most feared symptom resulting from cancer. Pain occurs at some time during the clinical course of most cancer patients and may be a result of the treatment or the underlying malignancy. The characteristics of cancer pain originating from different sites are listed in Table 117-4. Although chronic pain affects nearly all patients with advanced cancer it usually can be adequately controlled as described in Box 117-1.

Trousseau first described superficial migratory thrombophlebitis associated with gastrointestinal malignancies in 1865. Since that time it has been noted that a hypercoagulable state is frequently associated with a diagnosis of cancer. Patients with advanced cancer are clearly at increased risk for the development of deep venous thrombosis (DVT). In 1951 Ackerman suggested that DVT may be the presenting problem of patients with undiagnosed cancer. This continues to be debated. About 70% of patients with DVT have an identifiable risk factor for thrombosis such as bed rest, recent surgery, or varicosities. The risk of occult malignancy in this group is less than 5%. In patients with idiopathic DVT the incidence of undiagnosed cancer is 30% to 35%. Many

Box 117-1. Principles of Pain Control in Cancer Patients[6,9]

Treat the underlying malignancy with surgery, radiation, or chemotherapy as appropriate for the primary tumor

Mild pain
- Acetaminophen
- Nonsteroidal antiinflammatory agents

Moderate to severe pain
- Opioid analgesics via oral, topical, parenteral, or epidural routes
- Local nerve blocks

patients with idiopathic DVT who are concurrently diagnosed with cancer after an extensive screening evaluation (abdominal ultrasonography, abdominal computed tomography [CT], and upper gastrointestinal endoscopy) are found to actually have symptoms of the primary cancer. The appropriate evaluation for patients with idiopathic DVT should be a complete history and physical examination, complete blood count and differential, serum lactic dehydrogenase (LDH), chest x-ray, and evaluation of any additional signs or symptoms consistent with a diagnosis of malignancy.[3]

PHYSICAL EXAMINATION

Skin

A thorough inspection of the skin is useful for detecting skin cancer. The incidence of malignant melanoma has increased dramatically over the last 6 decades. The principal risk factor is sun exposure. The prognosis for patients with deeply invasive primary lesions or regional or distant metastases is grim, so early detection is paramount. Pigmented skin lesions should be examined for size, color, shape, and symmetry. Guidelines for assessing hyperpigmented skin lesions (the ABCD acronym) and the characteristics of suspicious lesions are described in Chapter 87. Patients with suspicious lesions should be promptly referred to a dermatologist or plastic surgeon for excisional biopsy (see Chapter 87).

Oral Cavity

A careful inspection and manual examination of the oral cavity should be a routine part of the physical examination, particularly in patients over the age of 40 who use tobacco and alcohol. Tobacco and alcohol are the principal etiologic factors in these cancers. About 90% of oral cancers occur in regions easily visualized during the routine physical examination. Premalignant lesions such as leukoplakia and erythroplakia may also be detected and treated early. Leukoplakia appears as thick, white hyperkeratotic plaque most commonly on the buccal mucosa, dorsal tongue, and alveolar ridge. Although considered a premalignant lesion, there is a low frequency of transformation to invasive cancer. Erythroplakia appears as an erythematous granular lesion most commonly on the floor of the mouth, ventral tongue, and soft palate. About 60% to 85% of patients with erythroplakia have early invasive squamous cell cancer at biopsy. Patients with the above diagnoses should be advised to stop smoking and drinking alcohol and should continue under routine surveillance. Vitamin A derivatives may help prevent the subsequent development of second primary tumors of the head and neck in patients previously treated for squamous carcinoma of the oral cavity. See Chapter 183 for further information.

Lymphadenopathy

Inflammatory adenopathy, congenital abnormalities, and neoplasia are all broad categories that need to be considered when evaluating cervical adenopathy. In the pediatric population, inflammatory and congenital lesions are the most common cause of neck masses. In young adults the frequency of neoplasia, especially lymphoma, increases but it is still less common than inflammatory adenopathy. In contrast, 50% of patients over the age of 40 with an enlarged asymmetric neck mass are diagnosed with carcinoma or lymphoma (see Chapter 183). If a careful head and neck examination fails to reveal any abnormalities, a fine-needle aspiration biopsy can usually be performed as an outpatient procedure. Special stains may be necessary to determine the precise nature of the abnormality. If the cytology is consistent with a diagnosis of lymphoma, an excisional biopsy may be required for more precise diagnosis.

Axillary adenopathy is a frequently encountered abnormality in clinical practice and most often is due to benign processes. Large, multiple, matted or enlarging lymph nodes should be biopsied. Supraclavicular adenopathy is almost always of pathologic significance and requires further evaluation. Lung cancer is the most common cancer to metastasize to supraclavicular lymph nodes, and a chest x-ray should be obtained promptly. A Virchow's node in the left supraclavicular fossa may represent involvement from a gastrointestinal cancer.

Breast Mass

The breast examination is a complex and difficult part of the routine physical examination because of the wide variability in normal anatomy. The breast is a composite of fat and glandular tissue that changes throughout the menstrual cycle. These changes are typically referred to as fibrocystic change and should not be considered abnormal. However, any discrete palpable mass in the breast requires further evaluation. Although mammography is a useful screening test for breast cancer, it should not be used alone in the diagnosis of a palpable breast mass. A normal mammogram particularly in a young, premenopausal woman does not definitively exclude the diagnosis of cancer.

The differential diagnosis of a palpable breast mass includes fibroadenoma, benign cyst, and carcinoma. See Chapter 43 for a detailed presentation of breast diseases.

Signs on physical examination that require urgent evaluation are redness, warmth, and tenderness of the breast. There may or may not be a palpable mass in the breast. Although a biopsy is required to confirm the diagnosis, these may be signs of inflammatory breast cancer and prompt staging and treatment are indicated.

Chest

A chest x-ray is the most important diagnostic test in a patient with pulmonary complaints. Pleural effusions may result from inflammatory, cardiovascular, and neoplastic disorders. Thoracentesis obtains fluid that may yield a precise diagnosis. Fluid should be analyzed for LDH and protein content, cell count and differential, culture, pH, and cytology. The characteristics of a malignant pleural effusion are listed in

Box 117-2. Characteristics of Malignant Pleural Effusions

Appearance
- Bloody or serous

Biochemistry
- LDH_{pl}/LDH_{ser}>0.6
- TP_{pl}/TP_{ser} > 0.5
- pH may be <7.10

Cytology
- Malignant celis-identified

LDH_{pl}/LDH_{ser}. Ratio of lactic acid dehydrogenase in pleural fluid to LDH in serum: TP_{pl}/TP_{ser} ratio of total protein in pleural fluid to total protein in serum.

Box 117-2. Malignant pleural effusions occur most commonly in patients with lung and breast cancer. A chylous effusion with high lipid content occurs most commonly from lymphomatous involvement of lymph nodes in the retroperitoneum and mediastinum.

A solitary pulmonary nodule (SPN) is an opacity seen on chest x-ray measuring less than 4 cm and completely surrounded by lung parenchyma. It is a common incidental finding that requires further evaluation. The purpose of further diagnostic evaluation is to distinguish malignant neoplasms that are potentially curable with surgery from benign lesions and incurable malignant lesions. If the patient has had prior chest x-rays, these should be obtained for comparison with the most recent examination. If the SPN has been present and unchanged over 2 years, it is probably benign and a subsequent chest x-ray should be obtained to ensure stability. If previous chest x-rays are not available, further study is warranted. Fluoroscopy may be useful for clarifying subtle or questionable abnormalities on chest x-ray. For larger lesions or when the fluoroscopy is equivocal, CT scanning is the most useful diagnostic test. Lesions with benign appearing calcifications or CT-detectable fat in a well-circumscribed pulmonary nodule are probably benign and do not require further evaluation. The presence of enlarged mediastinal or hilar lymph nodes or multiple nodules is more likely to occur with malignant disease. See Chapter 81 for a presentation of neoplasms of the lung.

Abdomen

Unexplained ascites, hepatomegaly, or a palpable abdominal mass may all suggest the presence of an intraabdominal malignancy. Ascites in a middle-aged woman is a common presentation for ovarian cancer. The first step in evaluating such a patient is a pelvic examination to assess the presence of an adnexal mass. Additional studies should include transvaginal ultrasound or an abdominal CT scan to assess the extent of disease and a blood test for CA 125. CA 125 is a marker for ovarian cancer and is elevated in 80% of patients with ovarian cancer.

When the pelvic examination is normal, and for men with unexplained ascites, paracentesis should be performed. Malignant ascites typically is bloody, with malignant cells seen on cytologic analysis.

Hepatomegaly can occur as a result of benign infiltrative disease of the liver or involvement of the liver by tumor. Involvement of the liver by metastasis is far more common than the occurrence of primary hepatocellular carcinoma. Lung, colon, and breast cancer frequently metastasize to the liver, and a prior history of these cancers should raise the clinical suspicion of metastatic liver disease in a patient with hepatomegaly. A CT scan provides the most diagnostic information in evaluating hepatomegaly. If lesions consistent with metastatic or primary liver cancer are seen, a biopsy may be required to establish the precise diagnosis (see Chapter 105).

A palpable abdominal mass should be evaluated by a CT scan to determine its origin and relation to normal intraabdominal organs. A tumor mass in the abdomen may be a primary or metastatic focus of disease. Further evaluation and biopsy depend on the location and radiographic appearance of the mass. A mass arising from the large bowel may be further evaluated with colonoscopy (see Chapter 105). Upper gastrointestinal endoscopy may be indicated for upper abdominal masses or those that may be of pancreatic origin. A percutaneous fine-needle aspiration biopsy under CT or ultrasound guidance is the procedure of choice for diagnosing a renal mass.

Testing for fecal occult blood is recommended as part of the routine physical examination for patients over the age of 40. Those patients who are found to have occult blood in the stool or iron-deficiency anemia may have an occult gastrointestinal malignancy. Further evaluation should be guided by the presence of any associated symptoms (see Chapter 105 for a detailed presentation of GI neoplasms).

Prostate

Prostate cancer is the most common cancer affecting men in the United States. The American Cancer Society estimated that there would be 180,400 new cases of prostate cancer diagnosed in the United States in 2000. Enlargement of the prostate is part of the normal aging process and often results in symptoms of frequency, urgency, and hesitancy. It is often very difficult to distinguish on clinical criteria alone whether symptoms are due to benign prostatic hypertrophy or cancer. Patients who are symptomatic, even if the digital rectal examination (DRE) is normal, should probably be evaluated with the following tests.

Patients with prostate cancer may be asymptomatic or have symptoms similar to those in patients with benign disease. Asymptomatic patients may come to attention because of palpable findings on DRE such as diffuse enlargement or focal, well-localized nodules. Any hard area or discrete nodule detected on routine DRE should arouse suspicion for carcinoma. Transrectal ultrasound (TRUS) and determination of the prostate specific antigen (PSA) add significantly to the information obtained during the DRE. The diagnostic workup for prostate cancer is presented in detail in Chapter 152.

Testis

Testicular cancer is the most common malignancy occurring in young men between ages 20 and 35. The only identifiable risk factor for testicular cancer is cryptorchid testis. There is an eleven-fold to fifty-fold increased risk in the undescended testis compared with the frequency in normally located organs. Orchiopexy does not decrease this risk but may allow for earlier diagnosis.

Table 117-5. Differential Diagnosis of a Testicular Mass

Diagnosis	Age	Symptoms	Location	Ultrasound
Tumor	20-45	Painless swelling	Attached to testis	Solid
Epididymitis	Any	Acute painful swelling with or without fever	Around testis	—
Hydrocele	Any	None	In vaginal sac around testis	Cystic
Spermatocele	Middle	Painless swelling	On top of testis	Cystic
Varicocele	Young	None; bag of worms	Left > right	Cystic

Since the diagnosis of testicular cancer is frequently delayed and often misdiagnosed, young men are now being instructed in testicular self-examination as a means of improving early diagnosis of testicular cancer. The differential diagnosis of a testicular mass is shown in Table 117-5 and includes acute and chronic epididymitis, varicocele, hydrocele, and inguinal hernia.

Transscrotal ultrasound is a useful diagnostic tool in the evaluation of a testicular mass. Patients who are found to have a solid mass should be referred for inguinal orchiectomy (see Chapter 155).

DIAGNOSIS

Symptomatic or asymptomatic patients may have a variety of findings consistent with a diagnosis of cancer. Although patients may be suspected of having cancer based on abnormal physical findings or radiographic studies, a diagnosis of cancer always requires a biopsy. A biopsy may confirm the diagnosis of malignancy and may provide important prognostic information. Biopsy material may be obtained in a variety of ways depending on the site.

A fine-needle aspiration biopsy can be accomplished with a minimum of morbidity in the outpatient department. Material is sent to the pathology lab for cytologic evaluation. This is a particularly useful procedure for evaluating palpable masses in the breast and enlarged palpable lymph nodes. Needle aspiration biopsy guided by ultrasound or CT can be used to biopsy abnormalities in a variety of sites including breast, thyroid, and essentially all abdominal and pelvic organs except bowel and bladder. Incisional or excisional biopsy or a more extensive procedure may be necessary to obtain tissue for diagnosis if the fine-needle aspiration biopsy is nondiagnostic or if additional material is thought to be necessary for a complete histologic evaluation.

The pathologist plays an essential role in evaluating the patient with a suspected diagnosis of cancer. The patient's age, symptoms, physical findings, suspected diagnosis, and the site of the biopsy should all be communicated to the pathologist before the procedure to be certain that an optimal specimen is obtained, handled, and fixed in a manner that maximizes diagnostic accuracy. The pathologist has a variety of tools that are used to establish a precise diagnosis of cancer. Immunohistochemical markers may help to distinguish a carcinoma from a sarcoma or a lymphoma. Additional special stains may be necessary to reach a precise diagnosis or to identify a primary site when it is not clinically evident.

Once a diagnosis of cancer has been established, further studies may be needed to determine the extent of the disease and the precise stage of the cancer even if the patient is otherwise healthy. All patients should have a complete history and physical examination. Laboratory evaluation should include a complete blood count and differential and blood tests to screen for kidney, liver, and bone disease. Any abnormalities in the history, physical examination, or laboratory studies that may be due to cancer require further diagnostic evaluation. Even if all of the above studies are normal, selected radiographic studies may be required based on the natural history and usual pattern of metastases from the specific primary site. For example, all patients with cancer do not require a head CT unless there are symptoms, abnormalities in the neurologic examination, or if cancer from the patient's primary site frequently involves the brain.

Complete staging evaluation is essential for further management. Most solid tumors are staged by the TNM classification and grouped in stages 1 to 4 as described in Box 117-3. Unique TNM classifications exist for each primary site.[1] The stage at diagnosis often determines the appropriate treatment modality. Patients with localized disease may require only local therapy such as radiation or surgery, whereas patients with disseminated disease may be considered for systemic therapy. Second, the stage at diagnosis has a major impact on prognosis. Patients with localized disease may be curable, in contrast to most patients with disseminated cancer in whom the disease may be treatable but not curable. Finally, it is essential that patients enrolled in clinical trials be uniformly staged so that the results are generally valid.

Carcinoma of Unknown Primary Site

Most patients with metastatic cancer have a clinically obvious primary site where the tumor began. However, approximately 5% of patients with metastatic cancer have a clinically occult primary site despite a complete history, physical examination, routine laboratory studies, and a chest x-ray. Myriad extensive diagnostic testing can be undertaken in an attempt to identify the primary site, but this is generally futile because a primary site is not identified.[10] Moreover, specific identification of the primary site usually does not have a major impact on the subsequent outcome. Efforts should be directed at identifying treatable tumors such as the lymphomas, hormonally responsive malignancies such as breast and prostate carcinomas, germ cell tumors, and small cell carcinoma of the lung.

Some situations need special consideration.[4] Poorly differentiated carcinoma or poorly differentiated adenocarcinoma of unknown primary site describes a subset of patients who may have a favorable response rate to cisplatin-based combination chemotherapy. The most favorable responses occur in young patients with a limited number of metastases located in the retroperitoneum or peripheral lymph nodes.

Box 117-3. TNM Staging

T: Size and extent of the primary tumor
N: Involvement of *regional lymph nodes*
M: Absence or presence of distant metastases

About 30% of these patients are disease-free after treatment, and prolonged complete remissions may be achieved.

Adenocarcinoma in an axillary node in an otherwise asymptomatic woman should be treated as an occult breast primary. Immunohistochemical stains for estrogen and progesterone on the biopsy specimen may provide corroborative evidence of a breast primary. Mammography may be useful in identifying an occult breast cancer, but a normal mammogram does not rule out the possibility of a breast primary. Women who have adenocarcinoma of unknown primary only in an axillary lymph node should undergo breast surgery and axillary dissection and receive adjuvant therapy similar to that for patients with stage 2 breast cancer. In contrast to other patients with adenocarcinoma of unknown primary, the prognosis is good with approximately 65% 5-year disease-free survival.

Patients with upper or midcervical lymphadenopathy secondary to squamous cell carcinoma should be evaluated for a head and neck primary. This should include a chest x-ray and endoscopic evaluation of the whole upper aerodigestive tract. If no primary is identified, aggressive combined modality therapy with radiation therapy and neck dissection should be prescribed in the same dosage and fields as in patients with a known head and neck primary. With this approach the 5-year survival is 30% to 50%.

Occult prostate cancer should be searched for in men with osteoblastic metastases involving the axial and appendicular skeleton, since patients with diffuse metastatic prostate cancer are likely to benefit from hormonal therapy. In a male patient with diffuse osteoblastic metastases and adenocarcinoma on biopsy, an elevated serum PSA or immunohistochemical staining of the biopsy specimen for PSA is sufficient to initiate treatment for metastatic prostate carcinoma.

The Multidisciplinary Approach

Once the diagnosis of cancer is established, it should be communicated and explained to the patient. It is always helpful to have a family member or significant other present during this discussion. A thorough explanation of the treatment plan, potential complications, and expected outcome is essential.

Although many specialists are frequently involved in caring for the patient with cancer, the primary care physician is a vital part of the multidisciplinary team. Patients often look to their primary provider to help them understand the complicated aspects of their cancer management. Subspecialists also appreciate the unique perspective of the primary care physician for assessing the impact of other chronic diseases on future care. The primary care physician should continue to counsel the patient and family even after the diagnosis of cancer is established.

When the diagnosis of cancer is made, referral to the appropriate subspecialist is often necessary. This may include a medical oncologist, radiation oncologist, and surgical oncologist. Nurses, social workers, physical therapists, enterostomal therapists, occupational therapists, and clergy are also important members of the health care team.

FUTURE DIRECTIONS

Clinical research is being done to improve the care of patients with most solid tumors. Patients who are referred to tertiary care cancer centers are often candidates for participation in clinical research trials either through cooperative groups or pharmaceutical companies. Patients should be encouraged to participate in clinical trials to obtain the best possible care for their cancer and to help develop new and innovative cancer treatments for the future.

REFERENCES

1. American Joint Committee on Cancer: In Fleming ID, Editor: *AJCC cancer staging handbook,* Philadelphia, 1998, Lippincott-Raven.
2. Byers T, Levin B, Rothenberger D, et al: American Cancer Society Guidelines for screening and early detection of colorectal polyps and cancr: update 1997, *Ca Cancer J Clin* 47:154, 1997.
3. Cornuz J, Pearson SD, Creager MA, et al: Importance of findings on the initial evaluation for cancer in patients with symptomatic idiopathic deep venous thrombosis, *Ann Intern Med* 125:785, 1996.
4. Ettinger DS, Abbruzzese JL, Gams RA, et al: NCCN practice guidelines for occult primary tumors, *Oncology* 12:226, 1998.
5. Fisher B, Costantino JP, Wickerham L, et al: Tamoxifen for the prevention of breast cancer: report of the National Surgical Adjuvant Breast and Bowel Project P-1 Study, *J Natl Cancer Inst* 90:1371, 1998.

5a. Greenlee RT, Murray T, Bolden S, et al: Cancer statistics 2000, *CA Cancer J Clin* 50:7-33, 2000.

6. Jacox A, Carr DB, Payne R, et al: *Management of cancer pain: adults quick reference guide no. 9.* AHCPR Publication No 94-0593. Rockville, MD. Agency for HealthCare Policy and Research, U.S. Department of Health and Human Services, Public Health Service, 1994.
7. Reference deleted in pages.
8. Leitch AM, Dodd G, Costanza ME, et al: American Cancer Society screening guidelines for the early detection of breast cancer: Update 1997, *Ca Cancer J Clin* 47:150, 1997.
9. Levy MH: Pharmacologic treatment of cancer pain, *N Engl J Med* 335:1124, 1996.
10. Schapira DV, Jarrett AR: The need to consider survival, outcome and expense when evaluating and treating patients with unknown primary carcinoma, *Arch Intern Med* 155:2050, 1995.
11. von Eschenbach A, Ho R, Murphy GP, et al: American Cancer Society guideline for the early detection of prostate cancer: Update 1997, *Ca Cancer J Clin* 47:261, 1997.

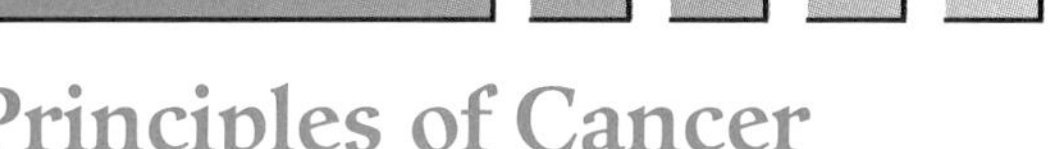

Principles of Cancer Therapy

Diane Savarese

Despite recent advances, cancer remains the second leading cause of death in the United States. Historically, resection offered the only possibility of cure, however small. This changed with the introduction of radiation therapy and combination chemotherapy in the mid-twentieth century. The modern approach to cancer therapy usually involves an integrated approach by medical, surgical, and radiation oncologists; nursing; nutrition; social work; and physical therapy.

SURGICAL MANAGEMENT

Surgery may play a role in the diagnosis, staging, primary therapy, and palliation of malignant disease. The suitability of primary surgical therapy for the treatment of a malignancy depends on the patient, the tumor type, and the extent of disease (stage). Most physicians use the American Joint Committee on Cancer (AJCC) staging system to classify tumor extent.[1] In general, primary surgical treatment is most appropriate for early stage tumors, whereas more advanced disease implies spread beyond locoregional areas and the inability of even aggressive surgery to cure the patient. For some tumors, chemotherapy or radiation therapy is preferable for primary treatment (e.g., lymphomas, small cell lung carcinoma). In other malignancies patients who have even disseminated (stage IV) disease may be amenable to surgical intervention for cure (e.g., osteogenic sarcoma, Wilms' tumor). Surgical debulking of large tumor masses may enhance the effectiveness of subsequent radiation or chemotherapy (e.g., advanced epithelial ovarian cancer). Palliation of specific complications from local tumor growth may also require surgical intervention (e.g., diverting colostomy for bowel obstruction in advanced colorectal cancer).

RADIATION THERAPY

Irradiation destroys cancer cells because, unlike normal cells, they cannot repair the cumulative cellular deoxyribonucleic acid (DNA) damage induced by x-rays administered in multiple doses over several days (fractionated radiation therapy). There are two types of radiation therapy in clinical use: external beam and interstitial radiotherapy (brachytherapy). External beam radiation is delivered by a source outside of the patient such as an x-ray generator, cobalt unit, or linear accelerator. Interstitial therapy entails placing the radiation source within an adjacent cavity or directly into the tumor itself. Radiation therapy may be delivered with curative intent, resulting in total and permanent eradication of tumor (e.g., early laryngeal or prostate cancer, Hodgkin's disease), or palliatively to relieve symptoms or reduce tumor bulk (e.g., brain metastases, epidural spinal cord compression, pain from bone metastases) (Table 118-1).

There is a direct relationship between the radiation dose administered, tumor cell kill, and the likelihood of complications (Fig. 118-1). In general, the larger the tumor, the higher the dose needed to sterilize the area. Preoperative radiotherapy may be used to reduce tumor volume, making a locally advanced tumor more amenable to surgical removal (e.g., rectal cancer). More commonly, postoperative radiotherapy is used to eradicate gross or microscopic disease left behind at the time of surgery. One example is the use of breast conservation therapy for early stage breast cancers. Treatment with lumpectomy followed by radiation therapy has shown equivalent long-term results when compared with modified radical mastectomy.[3] Postoperative radiotherapy is most useful in decreasing locoregional recurrences, but it usually has little effect on overall survival from cancer. Radiation may also be used with chemotherapy to maximize both systemic and locoregional control (e.g., Hodgkin's disease with bulky mediastinal masses and limited stage small cell lung cancer). Low-dose chemotherapy has also been used to sensitize cells to radiation therapy. This approach has been most useful for tumors of the cervix, rectum, pancreas, and head and neck.

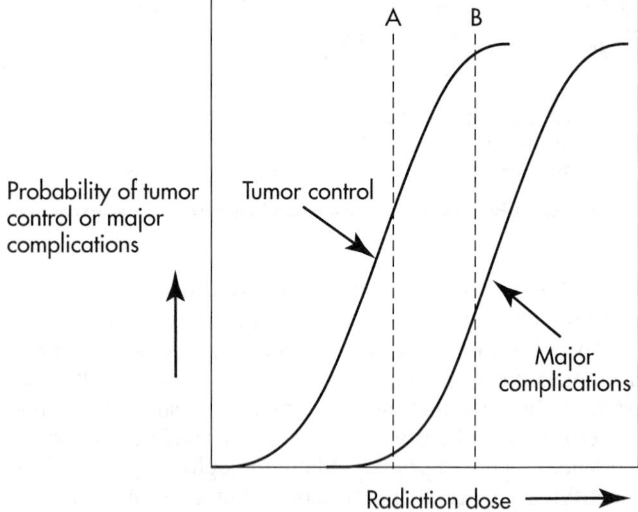

Fig. 118-1. Therapeutic index of radiation portrayed as two parallel sigmoid curves indicating the likelihood of tumor control and the likelihood of significant toxicity. *A*, Dose required for tumor control with minimum complications; *B*, dose resulting in maximum tumor control. (Adapted from DeVita FT Jr, et al, editors: *Cancer: principles and practice of oncology,* ed 2, Philadelphia, 1993, JB Lippincott.)

Table 118-1. Results from Palliative Radiotherapy

Reason for irradiation	Likelihood of response/relief of symptoms
Brain metastases	80%
Bone metastases	80%-90% (50% complete)
Spinal cord compression	
Ambulatory patient	70%-85%
Nonambulatory patient	16%
SVC obstruction	50%-70%
Bronchial obstruction	25%-60%

SVC, Superior vena cava.

DRUG TREATMENT OF CANCER

Useful chemotherapy agents include not only classic cytotoxic drugs but also hormones, biologic response modifiers, therapeutic immunoconjugates, and other drugs that by themselves have no or limited antitumor activity but instead act to modify the activity or toxicity of other drugs.

Cytotoxic Chemotherapy Agents

Cytotoxic chemotherapy agents directly kill tumor cells by interfering with cellular mechanisms such as DNA, ribonucleic acid (RNA), and protein synthesis. The mechanism of action is generally different for different classes of antineoplastic agents (Box 118-1). Although some drugs are designed to be selectively more toxic to malignant cells (e.g., 5-fluorouracil [5-FU], methotrexate), all agents are somewhat toxic to normal cells, resulting in side effects.

Box 118-1. Classes of Cytotoxic Chemotherapy Drugs

Antimetabolites
Methotrexate
5-Fluorouracil (5-FU)
6-Mercaptopurine
6-Thioguanine (6-TG)
Deoxycoformycin
Cytarabine (Ara-C)
Gemcitabine
Cladribine
Fludarabine

Alkylating Agents
Nitrogen mustard
Melphalan
Cyclophosphamide
Ifosfamide
Chlorambucil
Busulfan
Thiotepa

Nitrosoureas
Carmustine (BCNU)
Lomustine (CCNU)
Semustine (methyl-CCNU)
Streptozocin

Antitumor Antibiotics
Doxorubicin
Daunorubicin
Mitoxantrone
Mitomycin
Bleomycin
Actinomycin D
Mithramycin

Vinca Alkaloids
Vincristine
Vinblastine
Vindesine
Vinorelbine

Epidophyllotoxins
Etoposide (VP-16)
Teniposide (VM-26)

Miscellaneous
Cisplatin
Carboplatin
Hexamethylmelamine
Dacarbazine
Hydroxyurea
L-Asparaginase
Procarbazine
Amsacrine (m-AMSA)
Paclitaxel
Docetaxel
Irinotecan

The normal tissues most commonly affected by toxicity are those with the highest intrinsic turnover rate: bone marrow, hair follicles, gastrointestinal tract, and skin. Most cytotoxic drugs exhibit a dose-response relationship, a characteristic that is exploited in high-dose chemotherapy regimens that require bone marrow rescue because of limiting bone marrow toxicity (see below). In general, cytotoxic drugs are administered in combination rather than as single agents because simultaneous interference with multiple biochemical pathways may result in more tumor cell kill with a delay in the appearance of drug resistance. To diminish the likelihood of additive toxicity, drugs with non-overlapping side effects are combined. Commonly prescribed combination therapy regimens for several solid tumors are presented in Table 118-2.

Hormonal Therapy

Steroid hormones are useful for the therapy of tumors whose growth is hormone-dependent (Table 118-3). These agents are usually minimally toxic and are used most often for palliation of advanced disease, except for glucocorticoids, which may be useful for the primary treatment of hematologic malignancies.

Table 118-2. Commonly Used Combination Chemotherapy Regimens

Disease	Regimen
Breast cancer	Cyclophosphamide, methotrexate, 5-FU (CMF)
	Cyclophosphamide, doxorubicin (Adriamycin), 5-FU (CAF)
Lung cancer	Cisplatin, etoposide
Colorectal cancer	5-FU, leucovorin
Lymphoma	
Non-Hodgkin's	Cyclophosphamide, doxorubicin, vincristine, prednisone (CHOP)
Hodgkin's	Nitrogen mustard, vincristine, procarbazine, prednisone (MOPP)
	Doxorubicin, bleomycin, vinblastine, dacarbazine (ABVD)
Bladder cancer	Methotrexate, vinblastine, doxorubicin, cisplatin (MVAC)
Testicular cancer	Cisplatin, etoposide, bleomycin (PEB)

Table 118-3. Hormone Therapy of Malignant Disease

Disease	Hormone agent	Mechanism of action
Breast cancer	Tamoxifen	Antiestrogen
	Aminoglutethimide	Steroidogenesis inhibitor
Prostate cancer	Leuprolide	LHRH agonist
	Flutamide	Antiandrogen
Endometrial cancer	Medroxyprogesterone	Progestin
Lymphomas	Glucocorticoid	Lymphocytolytic

LHRH, Luteinizing hormone-releasing hormone.

Biologic Response Modifiers

Biologic response modifiers include an ever-expanding array of molecules that augment the natural immune-mediated host response to malignant cells. The interferons are molecules that are normally produced in vivo in response to viral infection and other antigenic stimuli but are synthesized for clinical use by recombinant DNA techniques. Interferons have shown activity in hairy-cell leukemia, Kaposi's sarcoma, chronic myelogenous leukemia (CML), and non-Hodgkin's lymphoma.[4] Interleukins, especially IL-2, have demonstrated activity against melanoma and renal cell cancer. Multiple ongoing trials are examining the role of these and other cytokines either alone or in combination with cytotoxic chemotherapy drugs in the management of malignant disease. A new class of agents, the therapeutic immunoconjugates, has become available with the recent introduction of Rituxan, a humanized anti-CD20 monoclonal antibody directed against antigenic molecules on the surface of non-Hodgkin's lymphoma tumor cells.[7]

Table 118-4. Results of Combination Chemotherapy for Initial Treatment of Stage IV Disease

Tumor type	Overall response rate (%)	Complete response rate (%)	Response duration (mo)	Median survival (mo)
Breast	60-70	<20	12	24
Colorectal	25-35	<10	12-18	12-24
NSCLC	20-40	<5	2-4	5-6
Bladder	30-50	10-20		9-18
Head and neck	50-70	15-30	3-5	5-8

NSCLC, Non-small cell lung cancer.

Adjuncts to Therapy

Some drugs used to treat cancer do not kill tumor cells directly but instead act to enhance the activity of other drugs (e.g., levamisole and leucovorin used with 5-FU in the treatment of colorectal cancer) or to ameliorate chemotherapy-associated toxicity (e.g., leucovorin rescue after high-dose methotrexate). Cytokines, including granulocyte colony-stimulating factor (G-CSF) and granulocyte-macrophage colony-stimulating factor (GM-CSF), have also been used to mitigate neutropenia after cytotoxic chemotherapy. Erythropoietin has become a valuable adjunct to chemotherapy, resulting in a decrease in the need for red blood cell transfusions, and improving fatigue and overall quality of life.

Indications for Systemic Chemotherapy

Primary Systemic Therapy. Chemotherapy alone as the primary treatment modality with curative intent may be useful for lymphomas, advanced testicular cancer, and small cell lung cancer.

Palliation of Advanced Disease. Palliation represents the use of chemotherapy to achieve objective tumor shrinkage, subjective improvement in symptoms, and prolongation of life. Unfortunately, improved survival is difficult to demonstrate for most patients with solid tumors. Response rates of selected metastatic cancers to typical chemotherapy regimens are presented in Table 118-4.

Combined-modality Therapy. Combined-modality therapy refers to regimens that incorporate chemotherapy and/or radiotherapy with or without surgery to achieve maximal tumor cell kill. Some tumors that are apparently localized at presentation have a high likelihood of systemic relapse despite optimal initial surgery or radiotherapy. Occult micrometastases left behind may provide a nidus for regrowth of tumor at a later time, resulting in clinically evident metastatic disease. Adjuvant therapy is systemic chemotherapy administered after primary curative therapy by other means (usually surgery) in an attempt to eradicate these micrometastases. For women with resectable breast cancer, a highly significant decrease in the rate of breast cancer recurrence and death follows the use of adjuvant chemotherapy or tamoxifen.[2] Adjuvant treatment with 5-FU–based regimens reduces recurrence rates and mortality in patients with lymph node–positive (stage III) colon cancer. For rectal cancers, adjuvant treatment with both 5-FU and radiation therapy can decrease recurrence and mortality in patients with either stage II or III disease.

Neoadjuvant therapy refers to the use of chemotherapy with or without radiotherapy before definitive local therapy (usually surgery). This approach is used most often for head and neck cancer and esophageal or rectal tumors in an attempt to increase surgical resectability or preserve organ function (e.g., anal sphincter, larynx). Although this approach may enhance local control and preserve organ function, many controlled trials have failed to show a significant survival advantage compared with that of conventional treatment.

Experimental vs. Standard Therapy. Some patients with cancer may be asked to participate in a clinical trial. Cancer clinical trials are no longer restricted to specialized large cancer centers; community physicians are increasingly being asked to participate. Clinical trials fall into phase I, II, and III categories. The goal of phase I studies is to determine the relationship between toxicity and dose. Phase II studies attempt to identify specific tumor types for which a new treatment may be promising. In general, patients who have failed standard therapy or for whom no standard therapy exists are appropriate for these types of studies. Phase III trials are randomized trials designed to compare standard treatment for a specific tumor or tumor-related condition with a newer treatment to determine whether the new treatment may be more efficacious and/or less toxic. These trials are usually offered to previously untreated patients. Randomized trials with concurrent control groups are necessary to definitively demonstrate the superiority of one treatment over another. The randomization procedure, which may be difficult to understand from the viewpoint of the patient, is necessary in trials of this design to prevent bias.

Evaluation of the Benefit of Chemotherapy

Risk/Benefit Ratio. Choosing optimal cancer therapy is not always easy. Guidelines for new regimens are frequently published, and it may be difficult to recommend a potentially beneficial new program of treatment without much knowledge of the results. Usually a rough estimate of the relative benefit from chemotherapy (likelihood, quality, and duration of response) may be compared with an estimate of the likelihood and severity of the side effects involved in the therapy (risk/benefit ratio). To accurately determine the value of a given response and what constitutes acceptable risk (toxicity), each patient's values and preferences, the impact of the therapy on lifestyle, and the repercussions of therapy on the patient's family must be considered.

Definition of Response Status. Objective response refers to measurable shrinkage of tumor masses as assessed by physical examination or radiologic studies. A complete response (CR) implies eradication of all clinically apparent tumor. CR is not necessarily synonymous with cure. Patients who have a CR may harbor residual tumor cells, and the rapidity of recurrence depends on the number of cells and how quickly they grow. Cure implies the persistent eradication of tumor for a proscribed period, the duration of which depends on differences in growth rate and biologic behavior. For example, of the patients destined to relapse after potentially curative treatment of early stage breast cancer, 65% to 85% do so within 2 years; however, the risk of relapse persists for 10 to 20 years. By contrast, over 95% of expected relapses from testicular cancer occur within 2 years of the original treatment, and late relapses are rare. In general, a CR is a necessary prerequisite for cure. Chemotherapy regimens expected to result in CR and cure should be administered aggressively, with a fair amount of toxicity accepted.

Many tumors fail to be completely eradicated with chemotherapy, representing a partial response (PR) to therapy. Treatments that result in a PR may lead to clinical improvement but may not have any meaningful impact on survival. Subjective response is a patient-reported sense of improved well-being after treatment; most subjective responses occur in the setting of objective response. Attempts to quantify this measure of improvement have included the use of quality of life scales, which assess functional status by using indirect measures such as performance status (Box 118-2), weight, and amount of analgesics or other supportive measures used by the patient.

Prognostic Factors. In general, good performance status and low tumor burden correlate most closely with better survival and higher response rates. More specific prognostic factors, such as the panel presented for early stage breast cancer (Table 118-5), may be helpful in identifying patients with a higher risk of relapse who may benefit from further systemic chemotherapy after definitive local therapy.

High-dose Therapy. Most cytotoxic drugs display a dose-response relationship with higher doses resulting in greater tumor cell kill and, theoretically, better cure rates. The limiting factor in increasing drug dose is toxicity, usually bone marrow toxicity. Hematopoietic support with bone marrow and/or peripheral blood stem cell transplantation has been used in an attempt to improve cure rates by allowing administration of higher-dose chemotherapy. Unfortunately, for most solid tumors, this approach has not yet been shown to result in greater survival compared with standard-dose chemotherapy and remains experimental.[8] It is most widely accepted for hematologic malignancies such as relapsed lymphoma and multiple myeloma.

Risks and Side Effects of Chemotherapy

All organ systems may be adversely affected by chemotherapy, with a wide variation in severity. In addition to anticipated tissue toxicity to bone marrow, hair, GI tract, and skin, other less common toxicities may be characteristic of particular drugs (Table 118-6). Chemotherapy-related toxicity, especially myelosuppression, may result in dose reduction to more tolerable levels but efficacy may be adversely affected.

Many patients are fearful of chemotherapy. The primary physician may be able to reduce anxiety by realistically defining and quantifying the specific risks involved. Not all potential side effects occur in all patients. When toxicity does occur, it is often of limited duration and reversible.

Box 118-2. Eastern Cooperative Oncology Group (ECOG) Performance Status Scale

0 Normal activity
1 Symptoms of disease, but ambulatory and able to carry out activities of daily living
2 Out of bed more than 50% of the time; occasionally needs assistance
3 In bed more than 50% of the time; needs nursing care
4 Bedridden; may need hospitalization

Table 118-5. Prognostic Factors for Axillary Node Negative Breast Cancer

Prognostic factor	Risk of relapse: Lower	Risk of relapse: Higher
Tumor size	Small	Large
Hormone receptors	Present	Absent
Nuclear grade	Low	High
Proliferative rate/S phase	Low	High
DNA-ploidy	Diploid	Aneuploid
HER-2/*neu* oncogene amplification	Absent	Present
Cathepsin D overexpression	Absent	Present

Occurrence and Management of Chemotherapy Toxicity by Organ Site

Postchemotherapy side effects may be acute or short term and generally reversible, or they may be long-term chronic toxicities, which may be irreversible. A brief synopsis of selected adverse effects by organ system follows. An extensive discussion of the adverse effects associated with biologic response modifiers is beyond the scope of this text.[4]

Bone Marrow

Leukocytes. Myelotoxicity may range from clinically insignificant decreases in the formed elements of the blood to life-threatening cytopenias. The nadir count refers to the lowest absolute value of the circulating blood cells after chemotherapy. Different chemotherapy drugs result in variable degrees of myelosuppression (see Table 118-6), but it may vary depending on the dose (methotrexate) or schedule of administration (5-FU). The time to the nadir averages 9 to 12 days after chemotherapy. Some agents cause prolonged or delayed granulocyte nadirs (nitrosoureas, chlorambucil, mitomycin C, busulfan, procarbazine). Patients whose neutrophil nadir is under 1000/μl have severe myelotoxicity; fever in the presence of neutropenia (less than 500/μl) is a medical emergency, and should be managed with prompt institution of broad-spectrum antibiotics.

Prophylactic antibiotics are usually not indicated for patients who are neutropenic from standard-dose chemother-

Table 118-6. Hematologic and Nonhematologic Toxicity

Drug	Bone marrow toxicity	Skin*			GI Tract		
		Necrosis	Rashes	Hair	Mucositis	Nausea and vomiting	Hepatic
Actinomycin D	3	3	3	3	3	3	0
Amsacrine (AMSA)	2	3	0	3	1	1	1
Ara-C (cytarabine)	3	0	0	0	2	2	3
L-Asparaginase	0	0	0	0	0	2	3
Azathioprine	—						3
Bleomycin	0	0	3	2	3	1	0
Busulfan	—	0	2	0	0	1	1
Carboplatin	3	0	1	1	0	1	0
Carmustine (BCNU)	3	2	2	1	0	3	3
Chlorambucil	2	0	1	0	0	1	1
Cisplatin	1	0**	0	0	0	3	0
Cladribine	3	0	2	0	0	2	0
Cyclophosphamide	3	0	1	3	1	2	1
Dacarbazine (DTIC)	1	2	0	0	0	3	2
Deoxycoformycin	1	0	1	0	0	1	2
Daunorubicin/ doxorubicin	3	3	3	3	3	3	0
Docetaxel	2	0	2	2	0	1	2
Etoposide/teniposide	2	2	0	1	1	1	2
Fludarabine	2	0	2	0	1	2	1
Fluorouracil	1-2	1	2	2	3	1	2
Gemcitabine	2	0	1	1	1	1	1
Hexamethylmelamine	1	0	0	0	0	1	0
Hydroxyurea	3	0	1	1	0	1	0
Ifosfamide	2		0	3	1	2	1
Irinotecan	2	0	1	2	0	2	0
Lomustine (CCNU)	3	0	0	0	0	3	3
Melphalan	3	0	0	0	0	1	1
Mercaptopurine	2	0	1	0	2	1	3
Methotrexate	1-2	0	1	1	3	1	3
Mithramycin	1	2	2	0	2	3	3
Mitomycin C	1	3	1	0	0	1	0
Mitotane	—	0	1	0	0	2	0
Mitoxantrone	2	3	0	1	2	2	1
Nitrogen mustard	3	3	2	1	1	3	0
Procarbazine	2	0	1	0	0	2	0
Streptozocin	1	2	0	0	0	3	3
Taxol (paclitaxel)	3		1	3	2	2	2
Thioguanine (6-TG)	2	0	1	0	2	1	2
Thiotepa		0	0	1	0	0	0
Vincristine	1	3	0	2	1	1	2
Vinblastine	3	3	0	2	2	1	0
Vindesine	2	3	0	2	1	1	0
Vinorelbine	3	2	1	1	0	2	1

0, Very mild or very rare; *1*, occasional, usually not severe; *2*, moderately severe; *3*, frequent or severe; *SIADH*, syndrome of inappropriate antidiuretic hormone; *MAO*, monoamine oxidase; *RTA*, renal tubular acidosis; *XRT*, radiation therapy.

*Necrosis if extravasted, or phlebitis; rashes, pruritus, changes in pigmentation; alopecia.

‡Arrhythmias or congestive heart failure.

§Hypersensitivity reactions.

||CNS toxicity.

¶Peripheral neuropathy.

#Toxicity unique to agent.

**High drug concentration infusion.

Cardiac‡	Allergic§	Pulmonary fibrosis	Nephrotic	Neurologic		Other#
				Central‖	Peripheral¶	
1	0	0	0	0	0	Fever, radiation recall
3	0	0	0	1	0	Cardiac arrhythmias
0	1	2	0	2	2	Fever, conjunctivitis
0	2	0	0	2	0	Fever, coagulopathy, pancreatitis
2		1	0	0	0	—
1	1	3	0	1	0	Pericarditis, fever
0	0	2	0	0	0	Addisonian syndrome, cataracts
0	2	0	0	1	1	Cumulative myelosuppression
0	0	2	2	2	0	Prolonged nausea and vomiting
0	1	1	0	1	0	
1	3	0	3	2	3	Vascular toxicity, prolonged nausea and vomiting
0	0	0	0	1	1	Fever, infection, decreased CD4 count, cough
0	1	2	0	0	0	Fever, SIADH, cystitis
0	0	0	0	1	0	Flulike syndrome
0	1	—	2	1	0	
3	1	0	0	0	0	Radiation recall
1	2	0	0	0	1	Fluid retention (pretreat with steroid)
0	2	0	0	1	2	
0	1	1	1	3	1	
1	1	0	0	2	1	Conjunctivitis
0	0	0	1	0	1	Fever, dyspnea, edema
0	0	0	0	2	2	
0	1	0	0	1	0	
1	1	0	2	2	1	Prolonged nausea and vomiting, cystitis, fever
0	0	0	0	0	0	Diarrhea: (early [cholinergic], late)
0	0	1	2	0	0	Prolonged nausea and vomiting
0	1	1	0	0	0	
0	0	0	0	0	0	
0	1	2	2	2	0	Fever, conjunctivitis
0	0	0	3	0	0	Coagulopathy, fever
1	0	2	2	0	0	Hemolytic-uremic syndrome
0	1	0	0	2	0	Adrenal insufficiency
1	0	0	0	0	0	
0	0	0	0	1	0	
0	2	2	0	2	2	MAO inhibitor
0	0	0	3	0	0	Prolonged nausea and vomiting; proximal RTA
3	3	0	—	0	0	Cardiac arrhythmias, fever
0	0	0	0	0	0	
0	0	0	0	0	0	
1	0	0	0	2	3	Hepatotoxic with XRT, SIADH
0	0	1	0	0	1	
0	0	1	0	2	3	
0	0	0	0	0	2	Shortness of breath

apy. While neutropenic, patients should avoid persons who are ill and should report fever immediately. When fever does occur, patients must receive parenteral broad-spectrum antibiotics until the neutropenia resolves. Visitors and medical personnel should observe strict handwashing techniques. Unnecessary instrumentation and invasive procedures should be avoided. Granulocyte transfusions are not generally used because of the high risk of complications. Recombinant colony-stimulating factors such as G-CSF and GM-CSF decrease the duration of the neutrophil nadir and the duration of empiric antibiotic use and hospitalization when administered prophylactically during the chemotherapy cycle. They have not been shown to alter the course of febrile neutropenia once it develops. Nevertheless, despite their expense, they are frequently prescribed in this scenario.

Platelets. Some agents are relatively less toxic to platelets than to other bone marrow cells (cyclophosphamide, etoposide, vinca alkaloids, mitoxantrone). A platelet decrease to under 50,000/μl represents severe thrombocytopenia, but in general, spontaneous bleeding rarely occurs unless platelet counts fall below 5000/μl.

It is important to avoid intramuscular injections, unnecessary instrumentation, and the use of medications (such as aspirin or nonsteroidal antiinflammatory drugs) that could exacerbate a bleeding tendency. Platelet transfusions should be reserved for patients with platelet counts under 5000/μl, patients with significant bleeding, and patients in whom invasive procedures become unavoidable.

Erythrocytes. Hypoproliferative anemia secondary to chemotherapy is less common than thrombocytopenia and leukopenia, although cisplatin and the nitrosoureas can cause refractory anemia. Cisplatin may also cause hemolytic anemia. In addition, a syndrome of microangiopathic hemolytic anemia, renal insufficiency, and thrombocytopenia has been described with mitomycin.

In the differential diagnosis for all of these myelotoxicities, one must consider tumor replacement of the marrow, autoimmune destruction, sepsis, and myelosuppression from other drugs. If cytopenias do not resolve within the expected time, it may be appropriate to perform a diagnostic aspiration and/or biopsy of the bone marrow.

Hair. Alopecia usually begins 2 to 3 weeks after the institution of cytotoxic chemotherapy. Not all cytotoxic agents produce the same degree of hair loss (see Table 118-6). Hair usually regrows after chemotherapy discontinuation. Although hair loss from the scalp is most noticeable, it may occur from all areas of the body, including eyebrows, axillary, and pubic areas.

Patients should be forewarned of this complication; a wig may be purchased if desired. Scalp hypothermia reportedly decreases the amount of hair loss, but protection depends on the type and dosage of drug. These devices should not be used during leukemia treatment, since circulation of the drug to the scalp may be impaired.

Gastrointestinal Tract

Mucositis. Mucositis usually presents as a burning or tingling sensation, especially in response to acid foods, and may be followed by erythema, superficial erosions, ulcerations, and sloughing of the mucosa. The oral mucosa is most commonly symptomatic. However, any mucosal area may be involved. Symptoms usually last 3 to 7 days. The worst drugs are bleomycin, doxorubicin, 5-FU, and methotrexate (see Table 118-6).

In the differential diagnosis, herpesvirus and *Candida albicans* mucosal infections should be considered. The patient should avoid dentures and irritating foods and rinse the mouth frequently with a salt or baking soda solution. Oratect gel, "miracle mouthwash" (mixture of viscous lidocaine, diphenhydramine elixir, and/or nystatin), and systemic pain medication may help a great deal. In severe cases the patient may require hospitalization for nutrition and fluid support.

Nausea and Vomiting. Symptoms may range from mild nausea to intractable vomiting. Symptoms usually begin 1 to 6 hours after chemotherapy and last less than 24 hours. Cisplatin, ifosfamide, and nitrosoureas may result in protracted nausea and vomiting up to 72 hours. Psychologic factors can influence vomiting, and anticipatory nausea and vomiting may occur when patients anticipate receiving treatment.

The differential diagnosis includes tumor obstruction, ileus, metabolic abnormalities (especially hypercalcemia), and brain metastases. Prophylaxis is important in management. Mildly emetogenic drugs (see Table 118-6) may be accompanied by oral phenothiazines. Moderately emetogenic drugs may require a combination of agents, including lorazepam, phenothiazines, metoclopramide, and serotonin antagonists with steroids. More severely emetogenic drugs such as cisplatin are usually managed with a serotonin antagonist like ondansetron and granisetron plus steroids. Other effective agents include haloperidol and droperidol. Patients with anticipatory nausea and vomiting may benefit from behavioral techniques, hypnosis, or the use of lorazepam.

Heart and Lungs. Transient dysrhythmias may occur during or shortly after the administration of amsacrine, paclitaxel, or doxorubicin. Anthracyclines and amsacrine may lead to a characteristic dose-dependent cardiomyopathy. The differential diagnosis should consider volume overload, intrinsic cardiac disease, cor pulmonale, and malignant pericardial effusion. To avoid cardiomyopathy, the total doxorubicin dosage should be limited to less than 450 mg/m^2. If this is exceeded or if patients have a higher than usual risk of developing cardiomyopathy, serial radionuclide ventriculograms should be followed. If congestive heart failure occurs, it is frequently irreversible but can be managed with diuretics, inotropic agents, and afterload reduction.

Pneumonitis and/or pulmonary fibrosis may be caused by bleomycin, Ara-C, paclitaxel, mitomycin C, nitrosoureas, alkylating agents, procarbazine, and methotrexate. Patients usually present with insidious onset of fever, dyspnea, and nonproductive cough. Pulmonary lymphangitic spread of tumor, adult respiratory distress syndrome (ARDS), infection, and other toxins should be considered in the differential diagnosis. Discontinuation of the offending agent and treatment with corticosteroids may help, although pulmonary fibrosis is frequently irreversible. Chest x-ray studies and single breath diffusing capacity of the lungs for carbon monoxide (DLCO) are not perfect screening tests for early bleomycin pulmonary toxicity, but they should be done periodically during therapy. Patients should inform anesthesiologists about prior bleomycin exposure, and inspired oxygen concentration should always be less than 30% (lifelong).

Kidneys. Renal insufficiency may be the result of direct tubular damage (cisplatin, streptozocin), glomerular injury (nitrosoureas), acute tubular necrosis from drug precipitation (high-dose methotrexate), or drug-induced vasculitis (mitomycin C). Differential diagnosis includes prerenal azotemia, diabetic nephropathy, paraprotein-induced renal insufficiency, other drugs, ureteral obstruction or direct kidney invasion by cancer or amyloid, infection, tumor lysis syndrome, and paraneoplastic syndromes.

For cisplatin use prevention is best accomplished by aggressive prechemotherapy hydration with 1 to 2 L of saline over several hours. Alkaline hydration should be used for high-dose methotrexate. The use of concomitant nephrotoxins such as radiographic contrast media or aminoglycosides should be avoided if possible. If renal insufficiency develops, potentially reversible causes should be ruled out and all drugs discontinued if possible. Patients with renal insufficiency may require dose reduction of chemotherapeutic agents whose excretion is predominantly renal. Chemotherapy agents excreted by the hepatic route may need dose adjustments in the presence of hepatic insufficiency also.

Genitals. Azoospermia and anovulation develop in the majority of patients treated with alkylating agents. Cisplatin causes temporary infertility in most patients. Reversibility depends on drug dosage, concomitant radiotherapy, and age.[6] Children treated before puberty are most likely to recover normal sexual development and fertility. Adult women older than 25 years are least likely to recover normal fertility after treatment. Many drugs are teratogenic, especially in the first trimester, but pregnancies have been successfully completed in the second or third trimester despite treatment with chemotherapy. There appears to be little if any increase in birth defects in children born of parents who have received prior chemotherapy.

Pretreatment factors may cause anovulation (stress, weight loss, heavy exercise) or azoospermia (Hodgkin's disease). Hypothyroidism, sometimes treatment related, may be a potentially reversible cause of infertility.

Patients should be counseled before therapy. The opportunity for sperm banking should be explored if pretreatment sperm counts are adequate. Unfortunately, oocyte cryopreservation is not routinely available in this country.

Second malignancies, both hematologic and solid tumors, may occur after chemotherapy, particularly when long-term treatment with alkylating agents is combined with radiation therapy. The risk for acute leukemia peaks at about 5 years, whereas that of secondary solid tumors may peak later, at 10 years.

Other side effects may also occur with various chemotherapy drugs. A full enumeration is beyond the scope of this text. They are summarized in Table 118-6.

APPROACH TO CANCER PAIN

Pain is one of the most frequent and least well-managed aspects of cancer care. Undertreatment of pain is a common problem despite the widespread availability of effective pharmacologic agents and other nonpharmacologic means of pain control. Barriers to effective pain management are summarized in Box 118-3. An excellent recent review of cancer-related pain is available.[5]

Box 118-3. Barriers to Effective Pain Management

Problems Related to Health Care Professionals

Inadequate knowledge of pain management
Poor assessment of pain
Concern about regulation of controlled substances
Fear of patient addiction
Concern about side effects of analgesics
Concern about patients becoming tolerant to analgesics

Problems Related to Patients

Reluctance to report pain
- Concern about distracting physicians from treatment of underlying disease
- Fear that pain means disease is worse
- Concern about not being a "good" patient

Reluctance to take pain medications
- Fear of addiction or of being thought of as an addict
- Worries about unmanageable side effects
- Concern about becoming tolerant to pain medications

Problems Related to the Health Care System

Low priority given to cancer pain treatment
- Inadequate reimbursement
- The most appropriate treatment may not be reimbursed or may be too costly for patients and families

Restrictive regulation of controlled substances
Problems of availability of treatment or access to it

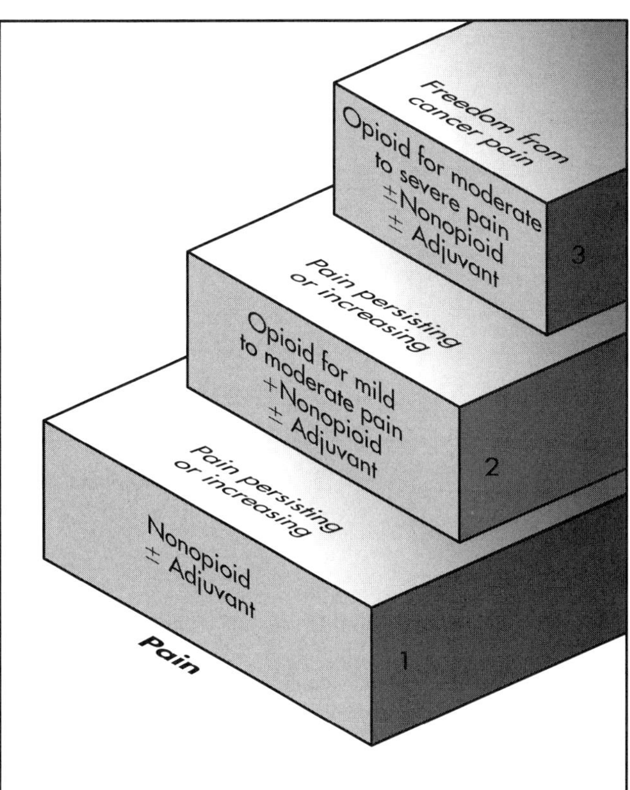

Fig. 118-2. The World Health Organization (WHO) three-step analgesic ladder. (Adapted from the World Health Organization.)

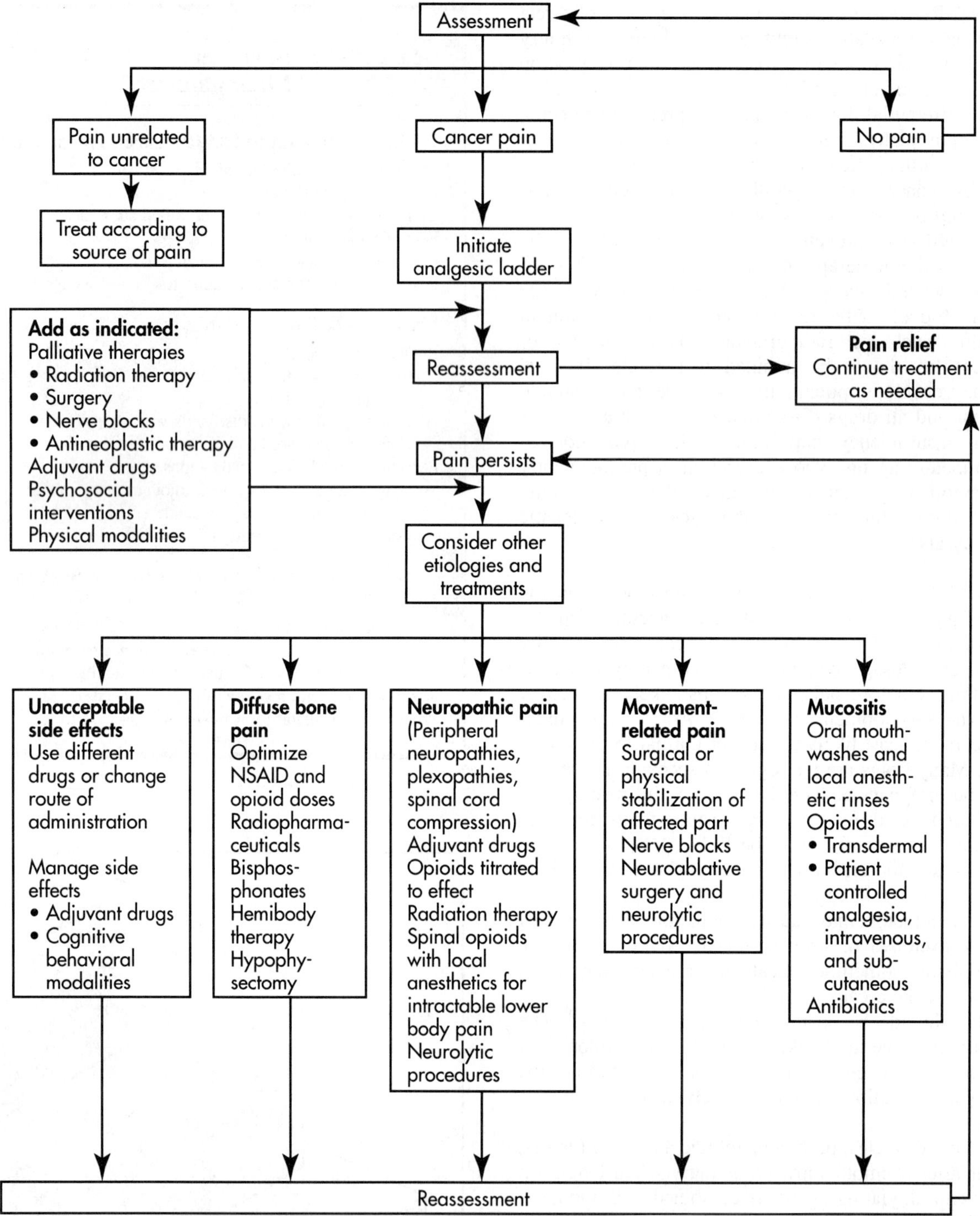

Fig. 118-3. Algorithm for pain management in patients with cancer.

Assessment of Pain

The initial assessment should focus on identifying the cause of the pain, and should include a detailed history of pain intensity, character, and location. Physical examination should place emphasis on the area affected by pain and, in particular, the neurologic examination.

Management of Cancer-related Pain

Specific antineoplastic therapy should be considered to control cancer-related pain. Surgery for curative excision or palliative debulking has the potential to reduce pain; however, many painful oncologic problems are not amenable to surgery. Radiotherapy may be particularly helpful in alleviating the pain of tumor invasion or compression. Alternatively, pharmacologic or neurosurgical/anesthetic approaches may be used to control pain. The World Health Organization (WHO) pain ladder (Fig. 118-2) portrays a rational progression in the doses and types of analgesic drugs for effective pain management. Fig. 118-3 is a flow chart depicting an algorithm for cancer pain management from initial assessment of pain to the various treatment modalities, including the WHO analgesic ladder and other pharmacologic and nonpharmacologic methods.

Pharmacologic Management of Cancer Pain. Nonsteroidal antiinflammatory drugs (NSAIDs) are especially useful in patients with bone pain or inflammatory lesions. They may also provide additive analgesia when combined with opioids. Their usefulness is limited to mild to moderate pain, and there is a ceiling dose above which no further analgesia occurs despite increasing doses. Adverse effects include gastritis, impaired platelet function, and renal insufficiency.

Opioids are the analgesics most used in managing moderate to severe pain. Opioids are classified as full agonists, partial agonists, or mixed agonist/antagonists. Commonly used narcotic agonists include morphine, codeine, hydromorphone, oxycodone, methadone, and fentanyl. These opioids are classified as full agonists because they do not reverse or antagonize the effects of other opioids within this class; they do not have a ceiling to their analgesic effect. Mixed agonist/antagonists and partial agonists are rarely used in chronic management of cancer pain, since they may reverse opioid effects and can precipitate abstinence syndrome in patients who are opioid-dependent.

Adjuvant medications, or co-analgesics, are used to enhance the analgesic efficacy of opioids. Corticosteroids, anticonvulsants such as phenytoin and carbamazepine, antidepressants, bisphosphonates, and antihistamines may all be useful in various settings.

Side effects of opioids are numerous and may result in a failure of opioid treatment, even when managed judiciously. Opioids decrease peristalsis and GI secretions, leading to increased transit time and desiccated, difficult to pass feces. A prophylactic bowel regimen should be prescribed to elderly patients, nonambulatory patients, those with intrinsic bowel disease, and patients receiving concurrent constipating drugs. Unfortunately, tolerance usually does not occur to this side effect. Management may include stool softeners, bulk agents such as psyllium, or mild stimulant laxatives.

Over 50% of patients receiving opioids experience nausea; it is usually multifactorial in etiology; constipation, CNS effects, delayed gastric emptying, and increased vestibular sensitivity may all contribute. Treatment with phenothiazine antiemetics or prokinetic agents (e.g., metoclopramide) may help.

Sedation is a property of all opioids. Fortunately, tolerance usually develops within several days. Excess sedation may be managed by administering smaller, more frequent doses of narcotic. Mental status changes including euphoria, dysphoria, and confusion may occur, especially with the initiation of narcotic therapy. Patients receiving long-term opioid therapy usually develop tolerance to the respiratory depression effects of these agents. Occasionally, respiratory depression may occur when sedative effects of opioids are no longer opposed by the stimulatory effects of pain. If rapid reversal of opioid effect resulting from excessive respiratory depression is necessary, repetitive doses of a dilute solution of naloxone should be used.

Tolerance refers to the need to increase doses over time to maintain pain relief. Increasing dose requirements are most consistently correlated with progressive disease. Opioid tolerance and physical dependency are expected with long-term opioid treatment and should not be confused with psychologic dependency (addiction). Patients should be warned not to abruptly discontinue narcotics; when a decrease is warranted, they should be tapered gradually.

Box 118-4. Managed Care Guide: General Principles of Narcotic Analgesic Management

1. Start with the lowest doses possible (equivalent to 5 to 10 mg IM morphine)
2. Titrate dose to desired effect OR to intolerable side effects
3. Use the appropriate route of administration
4. Anticipate pain; most patients require around-the-clock dosing plus additional "as needed" rescue doses
5. Know equianalgesic doses; knowledge of relative potency important
6. Use a combination of drugs: addition of co-analgesics (NSAID or adjuvant)
7. Manage side effects judiciously
8. Understand physical dependence and tolerance

NSAID, Nonsteroidal antiinflammatory drugs.

Nonpharmacologic Management of Cancer Pain. Nonpharmacologic management may include psychosocial interventions such as relaxation and imagery and anesthetic/ neurosurgical approaches. A full discussion of anesthetic techniques such as nerve blocks, intraspinal or epidural administration of narcotics or local anesthetics, and neurosurgical approaches such as rhizotomy, cordotomy, commissural myelotomy, or hypophysectomy is beyond the scope of this text.

Practice Guidelines and Recommendations. It is common clinical practice to initiate opioid therapy with a "weak" opioid such as codeine, oxycodone, or hydrocodone. These agents are most commonly available in fixed combination with acetaminophen or aspirin. In many cases the limiting factor to obtaining adequate analgesia with these agents is ingestion of maximal doses of the co- analgesic. If pain relief is inadequate with these agents, then it is appropriate to switch to a stronger opioid. Some general principles of narcotic management are listed in Box 118-4. The oral route is safe, acceptable to patients, economical, and effective. Morphine is the drug of choice in most patients requiring long-term analgesia for severe pain. Immediate- release oral morphine has a short half-life and must be dosed every 3 to 4 hours (Table 118-7). It is especially useful for "rescue" doses, when breakthrough pain necessitates the use of an opioid with a rapid onset of action. Sustained-release oral morphine eliminates the need for frequent dosing of oral morphine. Because many patients have persistent or daily pain, it is important to use opioids on a regular schedule rather than as needed.

A transdermal preparation of fentanyl, a potent narcotic absorbed through skin, is available. Advantages include convenience of dosing every 3 days and the avoidance of peaks and troughs during continuous dosing. Disadvantages include expense, poor adhesion to hairy or sweaty skin, and

Table 118-7. Equianalgesic Doses of Narcotic Agonists

Opiate	Equianalgesic dose (mg)	Usual dosing interval (hr)	Plasma half-life (hr)	Comment
Morphine	10 IM	3-4	2-3	Standard comparison for opioids
	5 IV	2-4		
	30-60* po			
Controlled-release morphine	30-60 po	8-12	—	Cannot be crushed
Codeine	200 po	3-4	2-3	Combination product with acetaminophen or aspirin
Oxycodone	30 po	3-4	2-3	Combination product with acetaminophen or aspirin
Hydromorphone	7.5 po	3-4	2-3	
Meperidine	75 IM	3-4	2-3	Toxic metabolite leads to CNS excitation
	300 po	4-6		
Methadone	20 po	4-6	15-30	Delayed toxicity due to accumulation with chronic dosing causing excessive sedation
Fentanyl	25 μg/hr	48-72	—	Patches should be initiated at lowest dose and titrated every 3d as needed

*1:6 relative potency po: IM changes to 1:3 during chronic dosing.

the long elimination half-life that results in a slow titration of effect.

Cross tolerance is not universal among the various members of the class of narcotic agonists. If one agent is not effective, another may be tried. It is important to be aware of equianalgesic doses (Table 118-7).

REFERENCES

1. American Joint Committee on Cancer: *Manual for staging of cancer,* ed 5, Philadelphia, 1997, JB Lippincott.
2. Early Breast Cancer Trialists' Collaborative Group: Systemic treatment of early breast cancer by hormonal, cytotoxic, or immune therapy, *Lancet* 339:1,71, 1992.
3. Fisher B, et al: Eight-year results of a randomized clinical trial comparing total mastectomy and lumpectomy with or without irradiation in the treatment of breast cancer, *N Engl J Med* 320:822, 1989.
4. Hansen RM, Borden EC: Current status of interferons in the treatment of cancer, *Oncology* 6:19, 1992.
5. Levy MH: Pharmacologic treatment of cancer pain, *New Engl J Med* 335:1124-1132, 1996.
6. Myers SE, Schilsky RL: Prospects for fertility after cancer chemotherapy, *J Clin Oncol* 19:5597, 1992.
7. Press OW: Prospects for the management of non-Hodgkin's lymphomas with monoclonal antibodies and immunoconjugates, *Cancer J Sci Amer* 4:S19-S26, 1998.
8. Savarese DM, Hsieh C-c, Stewart FM: Clinical impact of chemotherapy dose escalation in patients with hematologic malignancies and solid tumors, *J Clin Oncol* 15:2981-2995, 1997.

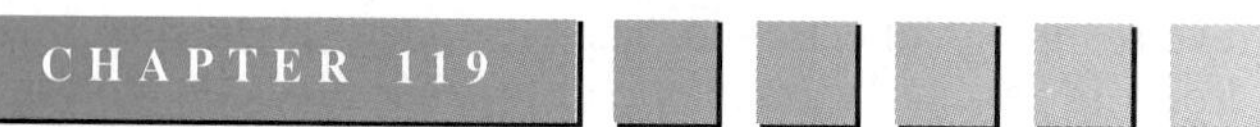

Hematologic Malignancies

Philip A. Lowry

Hematologic malignancies range in their presentation from the indolent disorders whose course is insidious and prolonged to the highly aggressive leukemias and lymphomas whose explosive onset and rapid progression are among the most dramatic in all of medicine. A thorough history and physical examination, complete blood count (CBC), basic chemistry determination, and evaluation of the peripheral blood smear remain the central pillars of the initial diagnosis of all hematologic disorders. A well-focused differential diagnosis and initial management plan can frequently be constructed from these alone.

The primary care physician must be more concerned to appropriately raise the general suspicion of hematologic malignancy than to make the final specific diagnosis. Particularly with the resurgence of primary care–centered medical practice, the physician will need to efficiently distinguish benign, self-limited conditions needing no further attention from the sometimes subtle signs and symptoms of the earliest and most treatable stages of hematologic malignancy. This chapter will focus on those initial signs of hematologic malignancy and the basics of their diagnosis and initial therapy.

SYSTEMIC SYMPTOMS

Involuntary weight loss, fevers, or night sweats may indicate an underlying malignancy, particularly the lymphoproliferative disorders; pruritus specifically suggests a diagnosis of Hodgkin's disease or polycythemia vera. Splenomegaly associated with hematologic malignancy may cause abdominal distention and discomfort, and back pain may reflect retroperitoneal adenopathy, direct spinal involvement with lymphoma, or compression fractures due to myeloma. Myeloma can additionally produce punched-out skeletal lesions, pathologic fractures elsewhere, or premature osteoporosis.

Hematologic malignancies frequently suppress normal bone marrow function, resulting in fatigue secondary to anemia, recurrent or serious infections due to neutrophil or lymphocyte defects, or petechiae or bleeding due to platelet deficiencies. Acute nonlymphocytic leukemia may induce frank disseminated intravascular coagulation (DIC). Myeloproliferative disorders may present with thrombosis because of quantitative and qualitative platelet abnormalities.

LYMPHADENOPATHY AND SPLENOMEGALY

Lymphadenopathy should particularly focus the attention of the primary care physician on the possibility of an underlying hematologic malignancy. Causes of lymphadenopathy are summarized in Box 119-1 and a general scheme for its evaluation presented in Fig. 119-1.

Lymphadenopathy most frequently reflects a benign, localized infectious process and usually resolves spontaneously with simple therapy. Persistent lymphadenopathy of greater than 2 weeks duration or lymphadenopathy with pathologic characteristics such as firm to hard or very large and/or unusually placed lymph nodes unassociated with obvious localized infection requires prompt diagnostic consideration. It is not acceptable to pursue multiple empiric antibiotic courses in the vain hope that adenopathy will resolve.

Early diagnosis should be the rule. A complete history and physical examination may suggest other less invasive diagnostic evaluations prior to definitive biopsy. Young patients or others with potential exposure should be screened for human immunodeficiency virus (HIV) infection. Severe or persistent pharyngitis should suggest the possibility of infectious mononucleosis with the diagnosis confirmed serologically.

Accompanying symptoms of fever, weight loss, or night sweats particularly suggest lymphoma. Chest x-ray and computed tomography (CT) scans of the chest and abdomen screen for occult mediastinal and retroperitoneal adenopathy. Chest tightness, progressive dysphagia or dyspnea, or facial plethora is often the result of a primary lung or esophageal process. Changes in bowel habits or abdominal discomfort points to an occult gastrointestinal malignancy. Cervical adenopathy in an older man who smokes suggests a primary head and neck cancer and should prompt full ear, nose, and throat evaluation prior to lymph node biopsy, since that biopsy may compromise subsequent lymph node dissection.

Supraclavicular adenopathy is frequently an indicator of more distant disease in the lung, breast, or abdomen. Axillary adenopathy suggests lymphoma or carcinoma of the breast, lung, skin, or even occasionally prostate. Workup of axillary or supraclavicular adenopathy should include a chest x-ray, mammography, a careful physical examination, and frequently body CT scans to look for a primary lesion elsewhere.

Many individuals may have longstanding, rubbery inguinal nodes that are non-pathologic. Small nodes that are by history unchanged over a long period of time and unassociated with focal signs of pelvic disorder may not require further evaluation. Adenopathy of more suspicious nature should prompt a thorough evaluation of the rectal and perineal regions, as well as specific genital examination.

Box 119-1. Common Causes of Lymphadenopathy

- Infections
  - Acute suppurative lymphadenitis
    - *Staphylococcus aureus*
    - *Streptococcus pyogenes*
    - Tuberculosis
  - Viral infections: rubella, rubeola, mumps, roseola (predominantly in children), infectious mononucleosis (EBV-positive, EBV-negative), toxoplasmosis
- Immune disorders
  - Systemic lupus erythematosus
  - Rheumatoid arthritis
  - Sjögren's syndrome
    - Benign adenopathy
    - Malignant adenopathy
  - Dermatomyositis
  - Sarcoidosis
  - Serum sickness
  - Hypersensitivity reaction
- Endocrine disorders
  - Hyperthyroidism
  - Adrenocortical insufficiency
- Dermatopathic diseases
- Drug-induced disorders
  - Benign
  - Malignant
- Neoplastic disorders
  - Leukemia
  - Lymphoma
  - Myeloproliferative syndromes
  - Metastatic
- Miscellaneous disorders
  - Angioimmunoblastic lymphadenopathy
  - Lipid-storage disorders
    - Gaucher's disease
    - Niemann-Pick disease
  - Other disorders

EBV, Epstein-Barr virus.

If a diagnosis is not clear from other evaluation, fine-needle aspiration of a pathologic lymph node may initially suggest a diagnosis but definitive excisional biopsy is often required to give more complete structural information as to the pathologic process. In all cases, the least invasive procedure to make a diagnosis should be selected first.

Other than the occasional young, aesthenic individual whose normal-sized spleen is palpable solely due to body habitus, palpable splenomegaly also suggests an underlying hematologic malignancy. Mild splenomegaly may be noted in the context of congestive heart failure, chronic inflammatory conditions, or autoimmune disease. It may be appropriate to cautiously follow splenomegaly in these circumstances without further diagnostic procedures, though indirect evaluation with flow cytometric analysis of blood and marrow is relatively simple to obtain and can more completely evaluate for the possibility of an underlying hematologic malignancy without abdominal surgery.

Moderate splenomegaly may be associated with chronic hemolytic anemias, cirrhosis with portal hypertension,

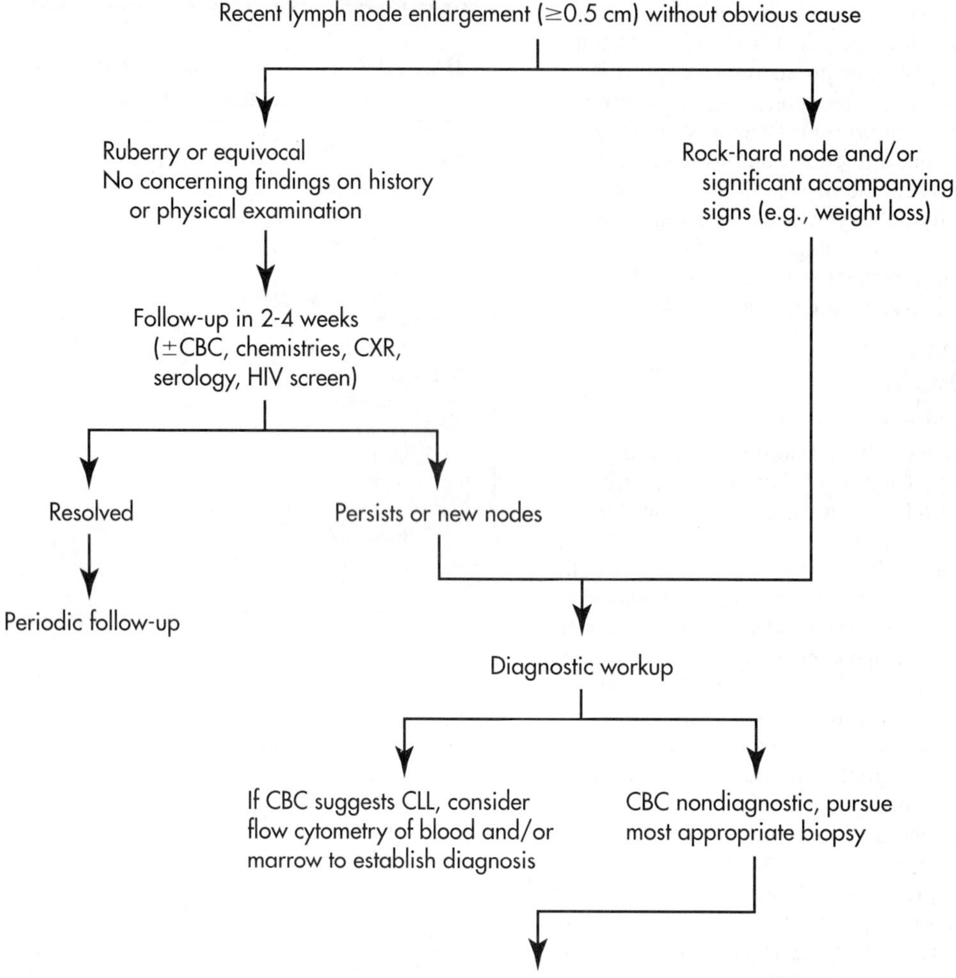

Prebiopsy workup: Consider CT scans to indicate other occult disease or potential sites for biopsy as well as to begin staging and focused studies (PSA, mammogram, etc.) suggested by initial H & P and lab screens; ENT evaluation should precede cervical node biopsy, especially in individuals with significant alcohol and tobacco use or upper respiratory symptoms; marrow aspiration and biopsy may be done first if abnormal but nondiagnostic CBC and may give a diagnosis obviating need for node biopsy.

Biopsy most accessible node or abnormal area. Alert pathology department in advance so that appropriate samples for flow cytometry, genetic studies, etc. may be preserved before tissue is fixed. Needle aspiration may give an initial indication, and be particularly useful if a nonhematologic malignancy is suspected, but excisional biopsy will be required for full diagnosis of lymphoma.

Institute appropriate subspecialty consultation and therapy.

Fig. 119-1. The workup of lymphadenopathy.

infectious mononucleosis, amyloidosis, or subacute bacterial endocarditis.[3] Primary hematologic disorders should be suspected and a vigorous search undertaken for associated adenopathy or hematologic abnormalities.

Massive splenomegaly presenting in the adult population is usually indicative of an underlying malignant disorder. Myeloproliferative diseases, particularly chronic myelocytic leukemia and myelofibrosis (agnogenic myeloid metaplasia), may present with massive splenomegaly. Hairy-cell leukemia may present in similar fashion.[3] Bone marrow biopsy and aspiration are usually diagnostic of these conditions. Inherited storage diseases may also result in massive splenomegaly but are usually diagnosed at an earlier age and rarely present de novo to the adult primary care physician.

Diagnostic splenectomy is rarely required, and a definitive diagnosis can frequently be obtained from careful examination of the peripheral blood or from node or marrow biopsy. Splenectomy for the staging of Hodgkin's disease has

Box 119-2. Causes of Splenomegaly

- Infections
  - Subacute bacterial endocarditis
  - Brucellosis
  - Infectious mononucleosis, cytomegalovirus infection
  - Tuberculosis
  - Parasites
    - Malaria
    - Schistosomiasis
    - Kala-azar
    - Other
  - Sepsis
- Immune disorders
  - Systemic lupus erythematosus
  - Sarcoidosis
  - Rheumatoid arthritis (Felty's syndrome)
- Hematologic disorders
  - Hemolytic anemias, acute and chronic
  - Lymphomas
  - Leukemias
  - Myeloproliferative diseases
- Metastatic diseases
- Infiltrative splenomegaly
  - Lipid storage disease
  - Amyloidosis
  - Diabetic lipemia
  - True cysts
    - Epithelial
    - Endothelial
    - Dermoids, lymphangiomyomatosis, hydatid
- Vascular Congestion
  - Congestive heart failure
  - Portal hypertension secondary to cirrhosis
  - Splenic vein obstruction
  - Budd-Chiari syndrome

essentially disappeared. Immune cytopenias complicating lymphoproliferative disorders, cytopenias resulting from splenic sequestration, and intractable symptoms from massive splenomegaly may require therapeutic splenectomy. Causes of splenomegaly are summarized in Box 119-2.

LABORATORY ABNORMALITIES

Basic laboratory evaluation can focus the differential diagnosis of hematologic malignancy and will occasionally be the first clue as to its presence. Anemia or other cytopenias due to marrow replacement or immune destruction frequently accompany an underlying hematologic malignancy. A monotonous, sustained increase in a single cell population without an obvious inciting event suggests a myeloproliferative or leukemic process; basophilia may be a specific marker of myeloproliferative disorder. An abnormal machine-generated CBC should prompt inspection of the peripheral smear, with a particular evaluation for abnormal morphology and the presence of blasts. Bone marrow evaluation may be necessary to establish a final diagnosis.

Elevated serum protein levels may indicate the presence of an underlying monoclonal protein associated with myeloma or another lymphoproliferative process. Aggressive hematologic disorders may produce elevations of calcium, uric acid, or lactic dehydrogenase. Flow cytometric analysis of blood and marrow is increasingly used in conjunction with traditional light microscopy in the characterization of hematologic malignancies.

SPECIFIC DISEASES

Myeloproliferative Disorders

The myeloproliferative disorders represent an abnormal proliferation of relatively mature-appearing cells of the erythrocyte, megakaryocytic, and/or myeloid lineage, although the abnormality resides in the earliest stem cell. Although the cells in excess may appear at least superficially normal on morphologic examination, they may be functionally abnormal. The myeloproliferative disorders are usually classified based on the primary cell in excess, although all lineages are affected.[13] Clinical features of these disorders are summarized in Table 119-1.

An excessive proliferation of myeloid cells and granulocytes characterizes chronic myelocytic leukemia (CML). The primary differential diagnosis of mature granulocytosis is between CML and a benign *leukemoid* reaction. Patients with a leukemoid reaction will frequently have a history of infection or other inciting process, will lack splenomegaly, and will have an elevated leukocyte alkaline phosphatase (LAP) score. Patients with CML, in contrast, have low LAP scores and lack signs or symptoms of a clear inciting event. CML is confirmed by bone marrow examination, with identification of a characteristic reciprocal genetic translocation involving the *bcr* locus on chromosome 22 and c-*abl* locus on chromosome 9 that frequently produces the abnormal *Philadelphia chromosome*.

CML typically presents as an indolent disorder, with patients remaining in the *chronic* phase for several years before it transforms in time to acute leukemia. Marrow or stem cell transplantation is the treatment of choice in younger patients, with well-matched donors inducing "cures" in 60% to 80%. Interferon treatment is an important alternative, with frequent responses and some long-term remissions. Prior interferon therapy may compromise the success of transplantation, especially from unrelated donors, so should be used judiciously in potential transplant candidates. Hydroxyurea can temporarily control cell counts and symptoms, and may be a less toxic approach for older patients.[13]

Polycythemia vera is a disorder manifested primarily as a proliferation of red blood cells. Patients may be diagnosed on the basis of an abnormal CBC or present with thrombosis due either to vascular sludging associated with the polycythemia or related to associated quantitative or qualitative platelet defects; gastrointestinal hemorrhage from qualitative platelet defects; or pruritus.

The specific diagnosis of polycythemia vera is historically based on the determination of an elevated red blood cell mass and evaluation for other indicators including splenomegaly and associated leukocytosis or thrombocytosis. The history and physical examination, measurement of arterial oxygen saturation, and determination of carboxyhemoglobin can exclude *reactive* polycythemias caused by chronic obstructive pulmonary disease, congenital or other cardiopulmonary disease, inheritance of a hemoglobin with abnormal oxygen affinity, or elevated carboxyhemoglobin levels due to smoking. Direct assay of circulating erythropoietin levels is becoming a useful adjunctive procedure as erythropoietin levels are elevated in reactive polycythemias but depressed in

Table 119-1. Clinical Features of Myeloproliferative Disorders

	Essential thrombocytosis	Chronic myeloid leukemia	Polycythemia vera	Myelofibrosis with myeloid metaplasia
Symptoms And Signs	Hemorrhage, thrombosis, increased platelets	Bone pain, fever/ sweats, pruritus	Hemorrhage, thrombosis, portal HTN	Hemorrhage, thrombosis, massive spleen
Splenomegaly, megaly	30%-40%	95%	90%	100%
White blood cell count	10,000-20,000	20,000-600,000	10,000-20,000	10,000-25,000
Differential	Rare basophil	Immature myeloid cells, basophilia	Usually normal	Immature myeloid cells, basophilia
Red cell	Normal	Normal	Normal*	Teardrops, nucleated RBCs, polychromatophilia
Hematocrit	Normal	Normal or decreased	Increased*	Decreased
LAP	→↑↓	↓	↑	↑
Cytogenetics, genetics	Normal	Ph[1] chromosome†	Normal	Normal
Marrow	↑ Megakaryocytes	↑ All lines	↑ All lines	↑ All lines, fibrosis
Progression to leukemia	Rare	Most	1%-2% (13% if treated with radioactive phosphorus)	6%

*Platelet defects may induce occult gastrointestinal blood loss, producing an artifactually normal or decreased hematocrit and morphologic changes consistent with iron deficiency.
†Gross chromosomal translocation may occasionally be absent, but genetic rearrangements involving the *bcr* locus on chromosome 22 and *c-abl* locus on chromosome 9 should be detectable on Southern Blot analysis.

polycythemia vera. Neoplasms of the kidneys or liver may occasionally produce erythropoietin autonomously, inducing a secondary polycythemia, and should be sought in patients with unexplained elevations of erythropoietin.

Unlike chronic myelogenous leukemia, polycythemia vera has a very low tendency toward transformation into acute leukemia and many patients enjoy relatively long survival. Treatment goals are directed at reduction of the effects of hyperviscosity with improved vascular flow as well as reductions in the risk of hemorrhage and thrombosis. Simple phlebotomy is the mainstay of therapy, but may be paradoxically associated with an increased thrombotic risk during the initial months of treatment. Elderly patients who cannot tolerate phlebotomy may be treated pharmacologically or with radioactive phosphorus to suppress red cell production, although such treatment raises the risk of leukemic transformation.[13]

Essential thrombocytosis is a less frequent syndrome associated with a predominant proliferation of platelets. Patients may present with either hemorrhage or thrombosis due to quantitative and qualitative platelet abnormalities, or may be diagnosed incidentally on *routine* CBC. Essential thrombocytosis must be differentiated from reactive thrombocytosis due to inflammation, iron deficiency anemia, or thrombocytosis postsplenectomy. Reactive thrombocytoses rarely achieve levels greater then 10^9 platelets per mcl.

The approach to patients with thrombocytosis is largely empiric. Any patient with an unexplained, persistent platelet count elevation above 600,000 per mcl and hemorrhage or thrombosis should be considered for therapy. Platelet apheresis is acutely effective and may immediately alleviate the symptoms of essential thrombocytosis. Aspirin has historically been avoided in the treatment of thrombocytosis associated with myeloproliferative disorders, but low-dose therapy may be useful, particularly in occasional patients who have severe or recurrent thromboses. Survival with essential thrombocytosis is variable: some patients are highly resistant to therapy, suffering multiple and severe thrombotic or bleeding complications that lead to their premature death, whereas others enjoy long, symptom-free survival. Anagrelide, hydroxyurea, or interferon therapy may be used to suppress excessive platelet production.

Myelofibrosis with myeloid metaplasia may present primarily or as an end stage of other myeloproliferative disorders. Patients present with marked splenomegaly and hepatomegaly and have variable, but often decreased, circulating cell counts and a leukoerythroblastic peripheral smear with teardrop red blood cells, nucleated red blood cells, and immature myeloid cells. Myelofibrosis with myeloid metaplasia probably represents a proliferation of megakaryocytes with a secondary release of a factor or factors that stimulate fibroblast proliferation within the marrow, which "displaces" hematopoiesis to extramedullary sites producing both the characteristic organomegaly and the changes seen on peripheral smear. Treatment of myelofibrosis is disappointing, with only occasional, transient responses, and short survival. Patients with massive splenic enlargement may benefit from splenectomy or splenic irradiation.[13]

Myelodysplastic Syndromes

The terms *myelodysplastic* and *myeloproliferative* are often confused. Whereas myeloproliferative disorders demonstrate

Box 119-3. Myelodysplastic Syndromes

General Features

Myelodysplastic syndromes show abnormal (dysplastic) hematopoietic maturation. Marrow cellularity is *increased,* reflecting "ineffective" hematopoiesis, but inadequate maturation results in peripheral *cytopenias.*

Syndromes

Refractory anemias: Refractory anemias typically present in older patients, with anemia the most prominent feature, although it is accompanied by mild to moderate pancytopenia. These syndromes include

	% Blasts in Marrow	*Survival*
Refractory anemia	<5%	2-4 years
Refractory anemia with ringed sideroblasts	<5%	3-5 years
Refractory anemia with excess blasts	5%-20%	1-2 years
Refractory anemia in transformation	20%-30%	<1 year

Chronic myelomonocytic leukemia (CMML): CMML presents with splenomegaly, monocytosis, and mild leukocytosis, which may be confused with chronic myelocytic leukemia. In contrast to CML, marrow maturation is dysplastic and the Philadelphia chromosome is absent. The clinical course is more similar to the refractory anemias.

Miscellaneous primary myelodysplasia: Patients may present with dysplastic marrow maturation but not the specific features of the above syndromes. Cytogenetic abnormalities involving chromosomes 5 or 7 are frequent. Those with a deletion of 5q may show a more indolent course and prolonged survival.

Secondary myelodysplasia: Previous exposure to benzene or other toxins, or treatment with chemotherapy, may induce myelodysplasia.

Treatment

Myelodysplastic syndromes and their resulting leukemias tend to be highly resistant to chemotherapy and are best treated with supportive measures employing antibiotics and transfusion. Occasional young patients may be considered for allogeneic bone marrow transplantation. The role of myeloid growth factors (G-CSF and GM-CSF) is undefined with possible stimulation of leukemic progression in others. Recent protocols using amifostine or Topotecan have generated initial cautious enthusiasm for new approaches, but require further testing.

proliferation of morphologically relatively normal-appearing cells, the myelodysplastic syndromes present an inherently different problem of abnormal maturation with typical cytopenias rather than cellular excess in the peripheral blood. As with the myeloproliferative disorders, the myelodysplastic syndromes originate in the transformation of a very early hematopoietic stem cell and typically have effects in multiple cell lineages. Because of the high frequency of acute leukemic evolution, these disorders are often referred to as *preleukemic.*

The median age of patients affected with myelodysplastic syndromes is 60 to 70 years old, although younger patients may occasionally present with similar abnormalities, particularly 5 to 10 years after intensive chemotherapy or radiotherapy for other malignant disorders. Presenting signs may be fatigue or weakness related to anemias, bleeding related to thrombocytopenia, and more infectious complications related to leukopenia. CBC and differential will frequently reveal cytopenias, and morphologic changes may include poorly granulated or hyposegmented neutrophils and hypochromic red cells, frequently with moderate to marked anisocytosis and poikilocytosis. Because of the marked maturation abnormalities, developing hematologic cells are incapable of normally completing their maturation sequence and thus accumulate in increased numbers within the marrow. Reflecting the preleukemic nature of this disorder, myeloblasts are often increased in number. Chromosome abnormalities are frequent with these syndromes, particularly those involving chromosomes 5, 7, 8, 17, and 21, and chromosomal analysis of marrow samples has become a mainstay of diagnosis.[7] Box 119-3 summarizes the myelodysplastic syndromes.

Chronic Lymphocytic Leukemia

The proliferating cell of chronic lymphocytic leukemia (CLL) is a mature-appearing lymphocyte that is morphologically indistinguishable from its normal counterpart. The morbidity of CLL is rarely attributable directly to the malignant cell. Patients with CLL can tolerate white blood cell counts exceeding 1 million per mcl without leukostasis or other major direct sequelae. Rather, patients ultimately die either from cytopenias resulting from marrow replacement or, more frequently, from infectious complications resulting from disordered lymphocyte development or function. In contrast to the acute leukemias and to chronic myelocytic leukemia, survival in patients with CLL is frequently prolonged and may not be dramatically different from that age-matched controls in patients presenting at a relatively low stage.

Patients are typically over 60 years of age and are frequently discovered incidentally based on the differential obtained with a routine CBC. They may occasionally present with mild symptoms of peripheral lymphadenopathy, splenomegaly, fatigue related to anemia, or infectious complications. Demonstration of a monoclonal circulating B cell clone in excess of 5×10^9 cells/L expressing the CD5 antigen makes a diagnosis of CLL. Although marrow evaluation is no longer required for diagnosis, establishment of the pattern of marrow involvement as nodular or diffuse provides important prognostic information.[6] Additionally, where cytopenias are present, marrow evaluation may help distinguish their etiology as due to loss of marrow production vs. immune destruction.

In the absence of marked cytopenias, excessive adenopathy or organomegaly, or major symptoms of fatigue or infection, a simple policy of "watchful waiting" may be the most effective initial therapy. Once specific therapy is required, the traditional approach has been to combine an oral alkylator with prednisone in pulse or continuous therapy. More recently, fludarabine has been found to produce dramatic responses and is favored by some as initial therapy, particularly for patients with good performance status. The vast majority of patients with CLL are elderly and not good candidates for allogeneic bone marrow transplantation. The occasional younger patient presenting with this disease should be considered for such therapy because it offers the potential for a permanent cure, although the complication rate is high; investigational autologous stem cell transplantation approaches are currently in development.[6]

Acute Leukemias

Acute leukemia can be considered a *maturation arrest* of an immature hematopoietic progenitor that rapidly proliferates and displaces normal elements within the marrow and peripheral blood. Classification schemes were historically based on morphologic and immunohistochemical criteria and divided the acute leukemias into lymphoblastic and nonlymphoblastic categories, depending on the presumed cell of origin. Monoclonal antibodies detecting specific cell surface markers have provided a more rapid and precise means of separating the various types of acute leukemia. Where possible, leukemias are increasingly classified on the basis of specific chromosomal or oncogene rearrangements.[4,7,9] Classification schemes and treatment outlines for acute lymphoblastic and nonlymphocytic leukemia are summarized in Boxes 119-4 and 119-5.

Acute leukemias are rapidly fatal if not successfully treated, most often due to infections related to granulocytopenia or bleeding related to thrombocytopenia. Occasional individuals presenting with hyperleukocytosis, particularly of immature blasts, may develop leukostasis reactions in the pulmonary or cerebral circulations and require immediate leukapheresis. Patients with acute promyelocytic leukemia or the monocytic variants may present with DIC, necessitating factor transfusion and platelet support in the face of active bleeding. Immediate all trans retinoic acid (ATRA) therapy for acute promyelocytic leukemia has substantially reduced the risk and morbidity of DIC, and significantly improved the prognosis of that disorder.[9]

Patients with acute leukemias have high levels of spontaneous cell turnover, which increases after the institution of therapy. The sudden transfer of the intracellular contents and cellular breakdown products to the extravascular space can cause life-threatening elevations of uric acid, potassium, and phosphate in the so-called *tumor lysis syndrome*. Thus patients presenting with acute leukemia should be routinely initiated on fluid support and allopurinol therapy in anticipation of rapid application of definitive chemotherapy. Many patients may already be cytopenic, and aggressive antibiotic and transfusion support may need to be initiated even before a final diagnosis has been made.

Definitive treatment of acute leukemia requires aggressive chemotherapy, usually in a tertiary care center. Consolidating allogeneic bone marrow transplantation in first complete remission may be associated with long-term disease-free survival rates approaching 50% among appropriately selected patients, although newer protocols with autologous transplant or even high-dose ara-C without stem cell support as consolidation produce increasingly similar results, particularly in individuals with "good risk" cytogenetics.[4,7]

Box 119-4. Acute Lymphoblastic Leukemia

Classification Schemes

Morphologic classification

L1: Small, regular blasts
L2: Larger blasts, irregular nuclei
L3: Burkitt's leukemia/lymphoma

Immunologic classification

"Null" cell (pre-B cell, CALLA$^+$) vs. T cell vs. B cell (Burkitt's)

Genetic classification

Karyotypic abnormalities in up to 50%
t12:21 (TEL-AML1 gene) good prognosis
t8:2, t8:14, t8:22 (involving c-*myc* on chromosome 8): Burkitt's
t9:22; t4:11; t1:19 poor risk
Altered ploidy

Prognostic Features

Poor-risk features

Age < 2 or > 9
White blood cell count at presentation >30-50 × 10^9/L
T cell phenotype with mediastinal mass
CNS involvement
Chromosome changes including t9:22, t4:11, t1:19, hypodiploidy

Treatment Considerations

Induction with vincristine and prednisone
Add anthracycline, intensive postinduction therapy for poor risk
CNS directed therapy
Prolonged maintenance therapy
B cell (Burkitt's) subtype—focused short-course regimens
Bone marrow transplantation in first remission for poor risk; second remission for others

Hodgkin's Disease

Hodgkin's disease probably represents a more diverse group of disorders than previously recognized. The Reed-Sternberg cell is the putative malignant cell without whose presence it

Box 119-5. Acute Nonlymphocytic Leukemia

Classification Schemes

Morphologic classification

M0: Primitive stem cell–like leukemia
M1: Undifferentiated myelogenous leukemia
M2: Acute myelogenous leukemia
M3: Acute promyelocytic leukemia
M4: Acute myelomonocytic leukemia
M5: Acute monocytic leukemia
M6: Acute erythroleukemia
M7: Megakaryoblastic leukemia

Immunologic classification

Morphologic classification schemes are supplemented by determination of leukemia cell expression of surface antigens including CD34 (expressed on stem cell–like leukemias), HLA-DR, CD11 (myelomonocytic cells), CD14 (monocytic cells), glycophorin A (erythroleukemia), and glycoprotein Ia/IIb (megakaryoblastic leukemia)

Genetic classification

t8:21—M2 (good prognosis)
t15:17—M3 (rearrangement of the retinoic acid receptor, good prognosis)
inv16—M4 with eosinophilia (good prognosis)
t9:22—ANLL complicating previous CML (poor prognosis)
del 5, del 7, $5q^-$, $7q^-$, tri 8, tri 13—(poor prognosis)
t1:3, t3:3—increased platelets (poor prognosis)
t4:11—biphenotypic (features of both ALL and ANLL, poor prognosis)

Prognostic Features

Poor prognostic features include infection at diagnosis; ANLL arising from previous chemotherapy, radiation therapy, or myelodysplasia; older age; cytogenetics (see above); hyperleukocytosis

Treatment Considerations

Induction with cytosine arabinoside (ara-C) and anthracycline followed by intensive consolidation
Inclusion of high dose ara-C with initial induction and/or consolidation may prolong survival
Treatment with all trans retinoic acid (ATRA) has dramatically improved APML (M3) prognosis but still requires subsequent chemotherapy
Allogeneic stem cell transplant for CR2 or CR1 with poor prognosis
Use of autologous transplant or "mini" allogeneic transplant a consideration for patients not considered candidates for traditional allogeneic transplant
Most patients with ANLL are older (>65 years of age): reduced-dose treatment is ineffective; either treat with full-dose therapy or a supportive approach; growth factors may reduce toxicity

Box 119-6. The REAL Classification Scheme of Lymphomas

B Cell Neoplasms

I. Precursor B cell neoplasm
II. Precursor B-ALL
III. Peripheral B cell neoplasms
Common disorders
B cell CLL, plasmacytoma/myeloma, diffuse large B cell lymphoma, Burkitt's and Burkitt's-like lymphoma
Additional entities
Immunocytoma, mantle cell lymphoma, marginal zone B cell lymphoma (nodal and MALT types), hairy-cell leukemia

T cell Neoplasms

I. Precursor T cell neoplasm
T lymphoblastic lymphoma/leukemia
II. Peripheral T and NK cell neoplasms
T cell CLL, large granular lymphocyte leukemia (LGL), mycosis fungoides/Sézary syndrome, peripheral T cell lymphoma, angioimmunoblastic T cell lymphoma, angiocentric lymphoma, adult T cell lymphoma/leukemia (ATL/L), anaplastic large cell lymphoma
Provisional: anaplastic large cell lymphoma (Hodgkin's-like)

Hodgkin's Disease

I. Lymphocyte predominance
II. Nodular sclerosis
III. Mixed cellularity
IV. Lymphocyte depletion
V. Provisional: lymphocyte-rich classical Hodgkin's disease

Harris NL, et al: A revised European-American classification of lymphoid neoplasms: a proposal from the International Lymphoma Study Group, *Blood* 84:1361, 1994.

is difficult or impossible to establish a diagnosis of Hodgkin's disease. The precise origin of this cell remains a subject of debate, and indeed it is possible that it may have different lineage derivations in the different subtypes of Hodgkin's disease.

Hodgkin's disease has a bimodal age distribution, with peaks in the second and third decades and then again in the sixth and seventh decades of life. Typical presentation is with cervical or axillary adenopathy or the detection of a medial mediastinal mass on chest x-ray. Patients may also frequently present with associated symptoms of fevers, night sweats, weight loss, or pruritus. The diagnosis is established by characteristic lymph node histology. Based on that histology, patients may be subcategorized as having lymphocyte-predominant, mixed cellularity, or lymphocyte-depleted disease. A separate category of Hodgkin's disease is the so-called nodular-sclerosing Hodgkin's in which bands of sclerosis are noted dividing the affected node into lobules; this has a somewhat better prognosis. The histologic classification is summarized in Box 119-6.

Spread is usually by lymphatic or hematogenous routes to contiguous lymphoid groups. Staging is largely based on physical examination; CT scans of the chest, abdomen, and pelvis; and bone marrow examination (Table 119-2). Lymphangiograms are used less often, while gallium scans are a newer and increasingly useful adjunct. Splenectomy is rarely performed now for staging.

The more economic staging approaches, and in particular elimination of splenectomy, represent both an improvement

Table 119-2. Staging Classification of Hodgkin's Disease (Modified Ann Arbor)

Stage	Definition
I	Single lymph node region (I) or a single extralymphatic site (I_E).
II	Two or more lymph node regions on the same side of the diaphragm (II) or a localized site of extralymphatic involvement plus one or more node regions on the same side of the diaphragm (II_E).
III	Lymph node regions on both sides of the diaphragm (III), which may include the spleen (III_S), a single extralymphatic site (III_E), or both (III_{SE}).
IV	Diffuse or disseminated involvement of one or more extralymphatic organs: Marrow = M+ Lung = L+ Liver = H+ Pleura = P+ Bone = O+ Skin = D+

The suffix "A" (e.g., Stage IIA) is added if there are no "B symptoms"; if the patient has one of the three B symptoms (fever, night sweats, or unexplained loss of 10% or more of the body weight), staging includes the suffix "B."

in noninvasive diagnostic modalities and a shift in the basic paradigm of treatment for Hodgkin's disease. Although limited stage disease, especially IA and IIA, has been a traditional target for radiotherapy alone, there is increasing sentiment for the use of chemotherapy in essentially all patients with Hodgkin's disease. With newer combination chemotherapy regimens such as ABVD associated with better tolerance and less long-term side effects, most oncologists now advocate that limited stage disease be treated either with a truncated chemotherapy regimen combined with involved field radiation, or even with chemotherapy alone.

Advanced stage disease is still treated with full course chemotherapy, with adjunctive radiotherapy included for patients with bulky mediastinal disease or poorly resolving disease elsewhere. Long-term disease-free survival rates appear to be improved both for advanced and limited stage Hodgkin's disease with the more universal application of chemotherapy. Bone marrow transplantation may be useful in the treatment of relapsed disease.[11]

There is an unfortunate increase in late secondary leukemias or solid malignancies complicating treatment for Hodgkin's disease, especially with older nitrogen mustard–based regimens and extensive irradiation ports. Secondary malignancies are also seen after stem cell transplantation. Patients must be closely counseled that even successful therapy will carry this risk, and appropriate screening measures should be instituted after successful primary therapy. This especially focuses on breast cancer screening for young women treated for Hodgkin's disease. Cardiovascular disease is also significantly increased after mediastinal irradiation for Hodgkin's disease.

Non-Hodgkin's Lymphoma

Non-Hodgkin's lymphomas are predominantly of B cell origin and typically present as adenopathy or an abdominal mass. Non-Hodgkin's lymphomas are classified based on morphology, immunophenotype, genetic features, and clinical characteristics. A recent revision of the classification system is summarized in Box 119-6 and anticipates the ultimate dissemination of a World Health Organization classification system to be published in the near future. Lymphomas were previously grouped into three broad clinical categories: *indolent, intermediate,* and *highly aggressive.* Better characterization of the clinical features of individual diagnostic categories shows a more heterogeneous outcome, and suggests that prognosis and treatment should be more individualized.

Approximately 20% of lymphomas are B cell follicular lymphomas constituting the bulk of the category previously referred to as indolent lymphomas, and typically present in older patients. Affected nodes are composed of relatively small, well-differentiated cells organized in a nodular pattern. Genetic analysis usually demonstrates the t(14:18) translocation with overexpression of *bcl-2*. Although slow growing, this group of lymphomas often present at an advanced stage because of the insidious symptoms associated with them. The indolent nature of these neoplasms usually results in relatively prolonged survival that may approach that of age-matched controls in selected patients.

Diffuse large B cell lymphoma constitutes 30% of Non-Hodgkin's lymphoma. Left untreated, the natural history of this aggressive subtype is more rapid, resulting in death within a short period of time, although a significant proportion of patients can be cured with chemotherapy. Lymphoblastic lymphoma, a T cell disorder, and the B cell–derived Burkitt's lymphoma are acute leukemia-like disorders whose onset tends to be explosive, with a high predilection toward involvement of the central nervous system (CNS) or other "sanctuary sites." Their course rapidly progresses to death unless successfully treated.

Several new diagnostic categories have been developed to account for entities with unique genetic or clinical characteristics. Mucosal-associated lymphoid tumors (MALT) are frequently present in extranodal tissues and pursue a typically indolent course. Gastrointestinal presentations may be associated with *Helicobacter pylori* infection and remit with antibiotic therapy directed against that organism. Mantle cell lymphomas are B cell neoplasms previously grouped with the indolent lymphomas. They are typically associated with the t(11:14) translocation and overexpression of cyclin D1. Mantle cell lymphoma has an aggressive and relatively inexorable clinical course that is resistant to standard-dose chemotherapy. Anaplastic large cell lymphoma is a histologically aggressive–appearing T cell malignancy that overexpresses CD30 (Ki-1) but seems to respond quite well to standard lymphoma chemotherapy, particularly the variant associated with the t(2:5) translocation.[11,12]

Non-Hodgkin's lymphomas have historically been staged in a manner analogous to that of Hodgkin's disease, although the lack of orderly spread and more unitary treatment approaches make that form of staging less useful in this context. The *International Prognostic Index* classification system, based on age, a more general distinction of localized vs. advanced disease, extent of extranodal involvement, performance status, and a biologic assessment of disease as reflected by serum LDH, has emerged as a more useful predictor of prognosis and guide to therapy,[14] superseding the previous histologic distinction of indolent, intermediate, and aggressive.

Treatment is most dependent on histologic subtype, stage, and status of the patient. Patients who present with apparently localized follicular lymphoma after full staging may enjoy prolonged disease-free survival after regional irradiation. For the advanced stage follicular lymphomas, therapy is historically minimalistic and often delayed until necessary to treat symptoms.

Monoclonal antibody–based therapies targeted against the CD20 molecule expressed on the surface of many of these lymphomas have provided an interesting new treatment option. Monoclonal antibody treatment combined with aggressive chemotherapy produces very high response rates, although the effect on long-term survival has yet to be fully determined. The occasional low grade–lymphoma patient who presents at a young age or with very good performance status may benefit from autologous or allogeneic bone marrow transplantation, although the toxicities are potentially significant and cure rates disappointing.

In the treatment of the large B cell lymphomas, a recently completed large cooperative group trial indicated no difference between more involved, and toxic, regimens and the standard combination of Cytoxan, Adriamycin, vincristine, and prednisone (CHOP), which has re-emerged as primary therapy. Patients with limited stage disease are often treated with three cycles of CHOP followed by involved field irradiation; more advanced disease is treated with six to eight cycles of chemotherapy. Monoclonal antibody therapy and stem cell transplantation may be useful to treat relapse.

Although Burkitt's and lymphoblastic lymphomas may be very chemotherapy responsive, their aggressive growth and extensive nature make them more challenging to treat than the aggressive lymphomas. A fulminant treatment-related tumor lysis syndrome may precipitate renal failure, cardiac arrhythmias, or other serious sequelae. Younger patients with good initial organ function and performance status may enjoy good survival after treatment with intensive but relatively short course therapy with aggressive CNS prophylaxis patterned after successful pediatric protocols.[11,12]

Myeloma and Related Plasma Cell Disorders

Myeloma is a disease of plasma cells, the terminally differentiated, immunoglobulin-secreting B cell. The classic presentation of myeloma is that of "punched-out" lytic lesions of the major marrow-containing bones, including the skull, proximal long bones, and axial skeleton, along with a monoclonal immunoglobulin spike detectable in the peripheral blood or urine. Plasmacytoma is a histologically similar plasma cell lesion presenting as a soft tissue mass.

Myeloma should be suspected in cases of pathologic fracture, unexplained anemia, unexplained renal failure, unexplained hypercalcemia, or unexpectedly severe osteoporosis, or with the detection of a monoclonal protein. Diagnosis is made by serum protein electrophoresis combined with marrow evaluation. Treatment includes chemotherapy and radiotherapy to skeletal lesions. Long-term survival is achievable with marrow transplantation in selected individuals.

Patients with low levels of monoclonal protein, less than 10% plasma cells in the marrow, and no other stigmata of myeloma such as lytic lesions or renal failure are labeled as having a "monoclonal gammopathy of unknown significance." Most such patients are elderly at diagnosis and more often die of unrelated causes, although long-term survivors may evolve frank myeloma. Watchful waiting may be the most appropriate initial intervention.

Box 119-7. General Concepts of Stem Cell Transplantation

Types of Bone Marrow Transplantation

Syngeneic: Donor is an identical twin.

Allogeneic: Donor is typically a sibling matched at the A, B, DR loci of the major histocompatibility (HLA) complex.

Unrelated: HLA-matched volunteer (unrelated) donor; results comparable to standard transplant when done with careful matching in experienced center.

Autologous: Use of marrow previously harvested from patient and cryopreserved until time of use.

Peripheral stem cell: Use of cells derived from blood rather than marrow, typically autologous.

Cord blood: Use of cells derived from the umbilical vein shortly after delivery.

Phases of Transplantation

Initial evaluation: Evaluation for ability to tolerate and benefit from transplant.

Marrow harvest: Autologous transplant patients have stem cells harvested in advance and cryopreserved.

Preparative phase: Patients receive high-dose chemotherapy/radiotherapy to suppress or eradicate malignant cells and, in heterologous transplantation, to suppress recipient immunity sufficiently to "receive" the donor marrow.

Transplant: Previously harvested autologous marrow is thawed or heterologous marrow harvested and infused into the patient via a central vein. Cells then "home" to marrow cavities.

Immediate recovery: Immediate recovery period is similar in all patients: with the possibility of acute pulmonary, hepatic, or cardiac toxicity from the preparative regimen and a period of absolute cytopenias resulting in bleeding or infectious risk.

Long-term recovery: Although patients undergoing autologous transplantation typically return to relatively normal status with hematologic recovery, heterologous transplant recipients may have additional complications related to graft-versus-host disease and related immune deficiencies.

STEM CELL TRANSPLANTATION

Bone marrow and stem cell transplantation are increasingly important therapies used in the treatment of hematologic malignancies. The general features of stem cell transplantation are summarized in Box 119-7.

Autologous transplant approaches are primarily a mechanism for chemotherapy dose escalation. The established role for autologous transplant is in the treatment of relapsed lymphoma, where a significant proportion of patients enjoy long-term disease-free survival. Selected patients with myeloma and acute nonlymphoblastic leukemia may also benefit from an autologous approach. The most common application of autologous transplant is in breast cancer, but its efficacy remains controversial. Ongoing clinical trials will hopefully better define the role of transplant there, although initial review suggests no dramatic improvement in survival.

Allogeneic transplant is an important option in the treatment of advanced malignant and nonmalignant bone marrow disorders. Chemotherapy and radiation dose escalation explain only a portion of the effects of allogeneic transplant; more important may be the replacement of marrow function from a new source, particularly the introduction of the donor immune system. Although this new immune functionality produces the primary danger of allogeneic transplant, graft-versus-host disease, the altered immune reactivity against residual malignant clones may explain their ultimate disappearance. Indeed, several centers are actively investigating the ability to introduce allogeneic transplants after much more modest preparative regimens, with interesting preliminary results. For patients who do not have appropriate sibling donors, unrelated donors or, especially for the pediatric population, cord blood transplantation may be an important alternative.[15]

A final word regarding cord blood banking is in order. The rapid evolution and increasing application of stem cell transplantation has spawned a number of proprietary enterprises that will indefinitely bank cord blood collected at birth for possible autologous or other family use at a later date. Potential parents find themselves in an emotional dilemma when promotional materials from these companies suggest that they may harm the prospects for their child if they do not bank the cord blood.

Although many individuals are indeed destined to contract a malignancy at some point in their lives, the subset who would actually benefit from autologous transplant is only a small fraction of those who have cancer. The expense of banking, the small likelihood of the later use of the cells, the increasing availability of alternate-treatment means, and the unknown durability of the technologies of storage make a recommendation of cord blood banking seem ill-advised in all but the very affluent for whom the investment in this procedure will not divert much-needed funds from more fruitful uses.

REFERENCES

General

1. DeVita VT, Jr, Hellman S, SA Rosenberg: *Cancer: principles and practice of oncology,* ed 5, Philadelphia, 1997, JB Lippincott.
2. Hillman RS, Ault KA: *Hematology in clinical practice,* ed 2, New York, 1998, McGraw-Hill.
3. Williams WJ, Beutler E, Lichtman MA, et al, editors: *Hematology,* ed 5, New York, 1998, McGraw-Hill.

Focused

4. Bloomfield CD, Herzig GP, editors: *Advances in the management of adult acute leukemia, Hematol Oncol Clin North Am* 7:1, 1993.
5. Boccadoro M, Pileri A: Diagnosis, prognosis, and treatment of multiple myeloma, *Hematol Oncol Clin North Am* 11:111, 1997.
6. Cheson BD, et al: National Cancer Institute-sponsored Working Group Guidelines for Chronic Lymphocytic Leukemia: revised guidelines for diagnosis and treatment, *Blood* 12:4990, 1996.
7. Cripe LD: Adult acute leukemia, *Current Probl Cancer* 21:1, 1997.
8. Forman SJ, editor: Bone marrow transplantation, *Hematol Oncol Clin North Am* 4:3, 1990.
9. Grignani F, et al: Acute promyelocytic leukemia: from genetics to treatment, *Blood* 83:10, 1994.
10. Harris NL, et al: A revised European-American classification of lymphoid neoplasms: a proposal from the International Lymphoma Study Group, *Blood* 84:1361, 1994.
11. Reference deleted in proofs.
12. Liebowitz DA, Williams SM, Golomb HN: Lymphomas, *Semin Oncol* 25:419, 1998.
13. Rosenthal DS: Clinical aspects of chronic myeloproliferative diseases, *Am J Med Sci* 304:109, 1992.
14. Shipp MA, et al: A predictive model for aggressive non-Hodgkin's lymphoma, *New Engl J Med* 329:987, 1993.
15. Thomas ED, Blume KG, Forman SJ, editors: *Hematopoietic cell transplantation,* ed 2, Malden MA, 1999, Blackwell Science.

CHAPTER 120

Management of Oncologic Emergencies

Ana Maria Lopez

Although patients with cancer often have chronic medical problems, oncologic emergencies arise as predictable complications of malignant primaries, metastases, or their treatments. The generalist is responsible for pursuing the signs and symptoms of these emergent problems, which if unrecognized, could result in patient morbidity and mortality.

METABOLIC EMERGENCIES

Hypercalcemia

Etiology. Malignant hypercalcemia is the leading cause of hypercalcemia in hospital practice. The most common cause of hypercalcemia in the outpatient setting is hyperparathyroidism. Malignant hypercalcemia may be associated with solid tumors or hematologic diseases. The solid tumors most often associated with hypercalcemia are of squamous cell origin. Elevation in the calcium level is the most common life-threatening metabolic disorder associated with cancer, affecting 10% to 20% of all patients. Approximately 150 new cases per million people are diagnosed each year (Box 120-1).

Pathophysiology. Malignant hypercalcemia may result from bone resorption secondary to skeletal invasion or from production of humoral factors, specifically parathyroid-like hormone. Elevated calcium levels impair the kidneys' ability to concentrate urine, resulting in further volume depletion.

Box 120-1. Malignant Etiologies of Hypercalcemia

Solid Tumor	Hematologic
Lung (squamous cell)	Multiple myeloma
Other squamous cell cancer	Leukemia
Head	Lymphoma
Neck	
Female genital tract	
Breast	
Renal cell	

Signs and Symptoms. Clinical suspicion in recognizing the symptom complex is the first step in making the diagnosis of malignant hypercalcemia. The clinical findings in hypercalcemia have been well documented and range from constipation to obtundation and death. Rapid recognition of this symptom complex may be lifesaving (Box 120-2). Symptoms may occur at calcium levels lower than those noted with benign hypercalcemia, perhaps because of the more rapid rate of calcium elevation in malignant hypercalcemia.

Diagnosis. Hypercalcemia is an elevation in unbound, ionized serum calcium concentration. Serum calcium levels measure total calcium values. Calcium is normally bound to albumin in the serum. Since many patients with underlying malignancies have low albumin levels because of poor nutrition and depletion of protein stores, a normal calcium level may actually represent hypercalcemia. The unbound calcium level may be calculated based on the albumin concentration as follows:

Corrected calcium (mg/dl) = Measured calcium (mg/dl) + 0.8 mg/dl for each gram of measured albumin less than 4.5 gm/dl.

Treatment. The goal of treatment is to improve the patient's quality of life. Hypercalcemia may be reversed by reducing or eliminating tumor burden, increasing renal clearance of calcium, and inhibiting osteoclastic bone resorption (Fig.120-1). Since most cases of malignant hypercalcemia occur late in the course of the disease, curative options are usually limited. The cornerstone of therapy is volume replacement with isotonic fluid. Rehydration alone is effective in 30% of cases. Furosemide may be added to promote calciuria but may increase dehydration. The response to fluids is usually not long lasting, since the underlying process has not been affected. Drug therapy is usually required to provide longer control.

Bisphosphonates inhibit osteoclastic function directly. Pamidronate is used in malignant hypercalcemia: 60 mg over 2 to 3 hours for calcium levels less than 13.5 mg/dl and 90 mg over 2 to 3 hours for calcium levels greater than 13.5 mg/dl. Patients may experience a febrile reaction. Phlebitis at the intravenous site is not uncommon. New agents in this class are being investigated and appear promising.

Other drugs that have been effective in hypercalcemia are calcitonin and mithramycin. Calcitonin is a potent inhibitor of bone resorption that acts within 12 to 24 hours. Although drug effects last approximately 72 hours, patients may quickly become refractory to the drug. Mithramycin is an antineoplastic antibiotic that possesses direct osteoclast inhibitory effects. The standard dose of mithramycin (25 μg/kg IV) usually leads to a decline in serum calcium levels in 6 to 48 hours. If no response is evident in 48 hours, the dose may

Box 120-2. Symptoms of Hypercalcemia

Nervous System
- Lethargy
- Weakness
- Decreased deep tendon reflexes
- Confusion
- Apathy
- Agitation
- Psychosis
- Stupor
- Obtundation
- Coma
- Death

Gastrointestinal
- Constipation
- Obstipation
- Ileus
- Anorexia
- Nausea
- Vomiting

Renal
- Diabetes insipidus-like syndrome
- Nocturia

Cardiac
- Short QT complex
- Broad T wave

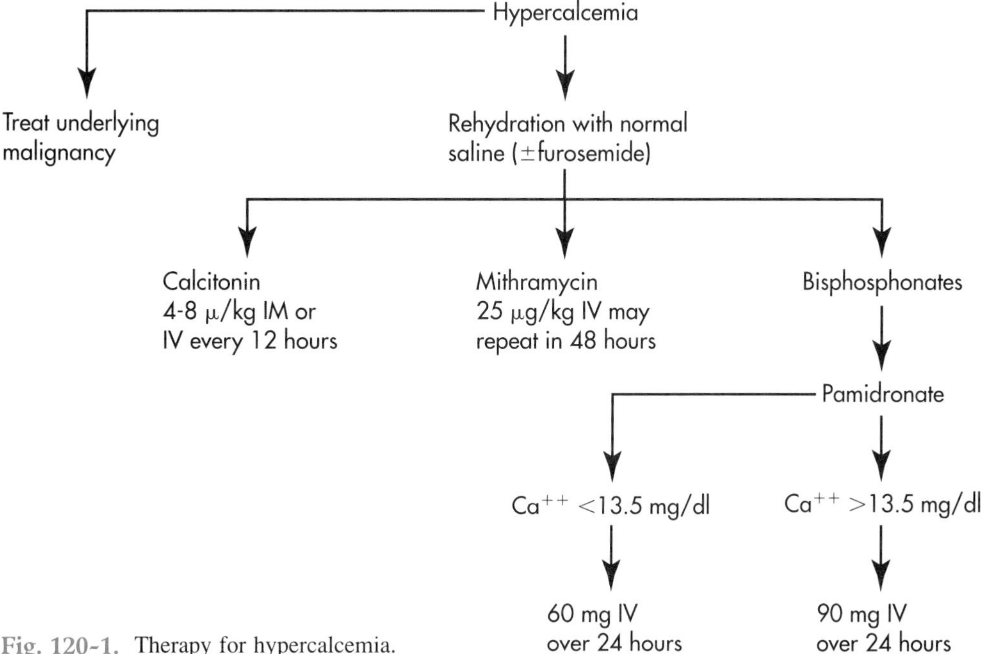

Fig. 120-1. Therapy for hypercalcemia.

be repeated. Mithramycin has renal, hepatic, and bone marrow toxicities.

Syndrome of Inappropriate Antidiuretic Hormone

Etiology. Syndrome of inappropriate antidiuretic hormone (SIADH) is a common cause of hyponatremia and is associated with a plethora of benign causes that must be considered before deciding that cancer is responsible. Pulmonary infections such as pneumonia, tuberculosis, and lung abscesses may produce SIADH. Abnormalities in the central nervous system may also result in SIADH. Medications such as opiates, thiazides, chlorpropamide, and the chemotherapeutic agents cyclophosphamide and vincristine may also contribute to SIADH.

Pathophysiology. Malignancy-related SIADH is thought to result from tumor secretion of humoral factors with ADH-like activity. Vasopressin acts on the renal tubule to conserve water, resulting in dilutional hyponatremia. In a typical patient, water retention results in a weight gain of approximately 3 kg or roughly 10% of body water. Increased volume status promotes water and sodium losses despite a low serum sodium level. Natriuresis produces the characteristically elevated urinary sodium concentration coupled with serum hyponatremia.

Signs and Symptoms. Clinical findings in SIADH are related to water intoxication. Initial drops in the serum sodium level cause the patient to complain of nausea, anorexia, fatigue, headache, and myalgia. When the serum sodium level drops below 120 mEq/L, increases in the total body water level result in brain swelling. At this level of hyponatremia an extensive range of neurologic symptoms are evident. Hyponatremia is a medical emergency that, if progressive and untreated, is uniformly fatal (Box 120-3).

Diagnosis. Diagnostic evaluation of hyponatremia may be prompted by a sudden change in mental status or by the incidental finding of a low serum sodium level (less than 130 mEq/L). A careful physical examination and history, laboratory evaluation of renal function, and measurement of urinary and serum osmolality and sodium concentration allow the physician to determine the physiologic appropriateness of the patient's hyponatremia. An elevated urine osmolality (>120 mOsm/kg) associated with a decreased serum osmolality (<280 mOsm/kg) is consistent with a diagnosis of SIADH (Table 120-1).

Treatment. The goal of therapy is to restore serum osmolality to normal. If efforts to control the tumor with chemotherapy are instituted, care must be taken not to promote hyponatremia with the pretreatment hydration required by some chemotherapeutic regimens. In mild cases of hyponatremia, fluid restriction to 1000 ml per day may be sufficient to produce volume contraction with an approximate 2- to 3-kg weight loss, reverse sodium wasting, and correction of serum sodium.

If the patient is unable to comply with fluid restriction, demeclocycline may be used. Demeclocycline restores sodium homeostasis by interfering with the renal tubular effects of vasopressin. Demeclocycline's main side effect is azotemia. Hypersensitivity to the sun and decreased gastrointestinal absorption with antacids, milk, and vitamins may also occur. Demeclocycline at a daily dose of 600 mg may be used in two or four divided doses. Dosages should be reduced for patients with renal insufficiency. To correct severe hyponatremia (less than 120 mEq/L), serum sodium levels may be corrected slowly with normal or hypertonic saline. The latter may be necessary in life-threatening hyponatremia. Sodium replacement needs may be calculated as follows:

Box 120-3. Symptoms of SIADH

Early	Late
Nausea	Mental status changes
Anorexia	Confusion
Fatigue	Lethargy
Headache	Pathologic reflexes
Myalgia	Papilledema
	Seizures
	Focal deficits
	Coma
	Death

Table 120-1. Diagnostic Criteria of SIADH

	Serum	Urine
Osmolality	Low (<280 mOsm/kg)	High (>120 mOsm/kg)
Sodium level	Low (<130 mmol/L)	High (>20 mEq/L)

Sodium deficit (mEq/L) = 125 mEq/L − (Measured serum sodium [mEq/L] × 0.6 × body weight in kg)

The goal is to correct the serum sodium level to 125 mEq/L at a rate of 0.5 mEq/L per hour or 14 mEq per day to minimize the risk of central nervous system damage in the form of central pontine myelinolysis (CPM). CPM is characterized clinically by dysphagia, facial weakness, flaccid quadriplegia or paraplegia, and eventually coma resulting from demyelination in the pons (Fig. 120-2).

Tumor Lysis Syndrome

Etiology. Tumor lysis syndrome occurs due to the effects of chemotherapy or rapid tumor growth, either of which may result in the rapid release of the products of cytolysis into the systemic circulation. This syndrome may lead to irreversible renal compromise and death.

Pathophysiology. Patients with both solid tumors and hematopoietic malignancies are at risk for tumor lysis syndrome, particularly if the tumor burden is high or the tumor is in a stage of rapid cell division, in which sensitivity to chemotherapy is increased. The rapid release of the products of cytolysis into the systemic circulation leads to elevations in the levels of uric acid, potassium, and phosphate, all of which may contribute to renal failure.

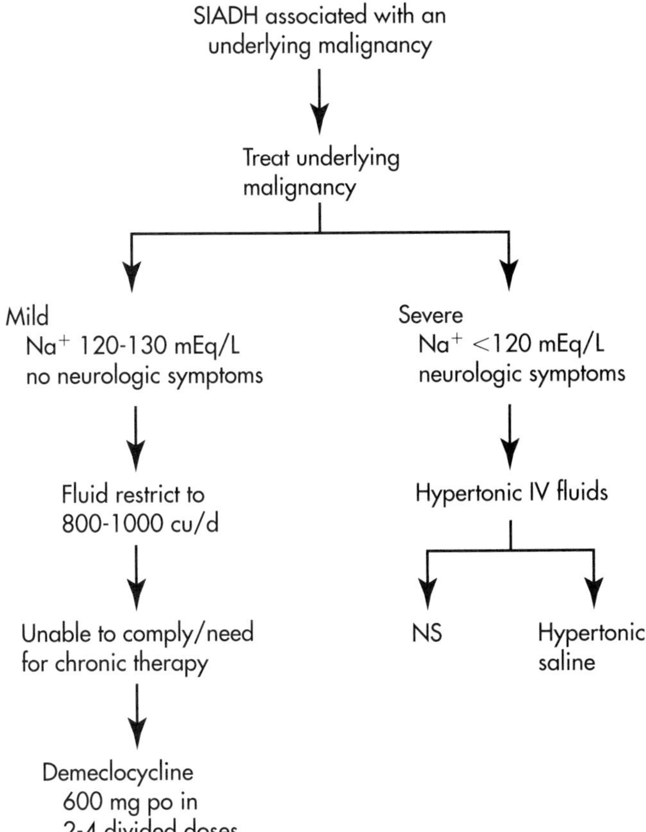

Fig. 120-2. Treatment for SIADH associated with malignancy.

Hyperphosphatemia promotes hypocalcemia. The release of these intracellular metabolites occurs at a rate that exceeds the excretory capacity of the kidneys. Uric acid and phosphorus may precipitate in the renal tubules, impairing renal excretory function and causing further elevations in these metabolites. At particular risk is the patient who is dehydrated or who has baseline renal insufficiency.

Signs and Symptoms. One of the earliest clinical signs of nephropathy related to uric acid elevation is oliguria. Signs and symptoms of uremia (nausea, vomiting, mental status depression, fluid overload), edema, and congestive heart failure may follow. High phosphate levels contribute to the nephropathy, and acidosis and anuria may develop.

Hyperkalemia and hypocalcemia primarily affect cardiac function. Dysrhythmias may be asymptomatic and seen only on the electrocardiogram (ECG). Hypocalcemia may result in complaints of muscle cramps, tetany, and seizures (Box 120-4).

Diagnosis. In the oliguric cancer patient, tumor lysis syndrome should be considered when ultrasound evaluation of the kidneys rules out obstruction. Elevated uric acid levels and electrolyte abnormalities may be noted. Microscopic examination of the urine may reveal the precipitated uric acid crystals confirming the diagnosis of tumor lysis syndrome; however, their absence does not exclude the diagnosis.

Treatment. Since tumor lysis syndrome is a common and predictable complication of certain malignancies, therapeutic intervention is primarily focused on prevention with hydration and the prophylactic use of allopurinol to impair the production of uric acid (Fig. 120-3). Normal saline rates, 100 to 150 ml per hour, are usually sufficient to produce a dilute urine. Allopurinol at oral dosages of 300 mg per day should be initiated 48 hours before the onset of chemotherapy, and continuation is advised until tumor lysis risk has passed. The dose of allopurinol should be adjusted for renal function. Electrolytes, renal function, and uric acid levels should be monitored daily to detect metabolic aberrations early. Furosemide may be used cautiously to aid with diuresis.

Hemodialysis is considered when potassium levels are greater than 6 mEq/L, uric acid levels are greater than 10 mg/dl, or phosphate levels are greater than 10 mg/dl. These interventions have resulted in a significant decline in mortality resulting from tumor lysis.

Box 120-4. Signs and Symptoms of Tumor Lysis Syndrome

- Oliguria
- Uremia
  - Nausea
  - Vomiting
  - Mental status depression
- Hypervolemia
  - Congestive heart failure
  - Edema
- Hyperkalemia
  - Ventricular tachycardia
- Hypocalcemia
  - Muscle cramps
  - Tetany
  - Seizures
- Hyperphosphatemia
  - Worsened nephropathy
- Acidosis
- Anuria

CARDIAC EMERGENCIES

Superior Vena Cava Syndrome

Etiology. The etiology of superior vena cava syndrome (SVCS) has changed since Ehrlich's review in 1934 (Table 120-2). At that time, 46% of the cases were associated with malignancies, 36% were due to aortic aneurysms, and 18% were due to infectious or other benign etiologies. Recent reviews have demonstrated that malignant causes account for 97% of the cases of SVCS, with most attributed to lung cancer or lymphoma.

Pathophysiology. The mass effect of a tumor or other space-occupying lesion may be a partial or complete obstruction of blood flow through the SVC to the right atrium, producing SVCS. The SVC is sensitive to mass effect because of its thin walls and low pressure.

Signs and Symptoms. The most dramatic presentation of SVCS is a rapid progressive development of facial and upper body edema. Alternatively, clinical symptoms may develop slowly over the course of several weeks. The patient may complain of headache, nausea, dizziness, vision changes, hoarseness, cough, dysphagia, and syncope. Stridor and dyspnea, especially when the patient is supine, are associated with airway obstruction. Increased intracranial pressure and consequent cerebral edema result in nightmares, stupor, and seizures, but death is rarely attributed to SVCS.

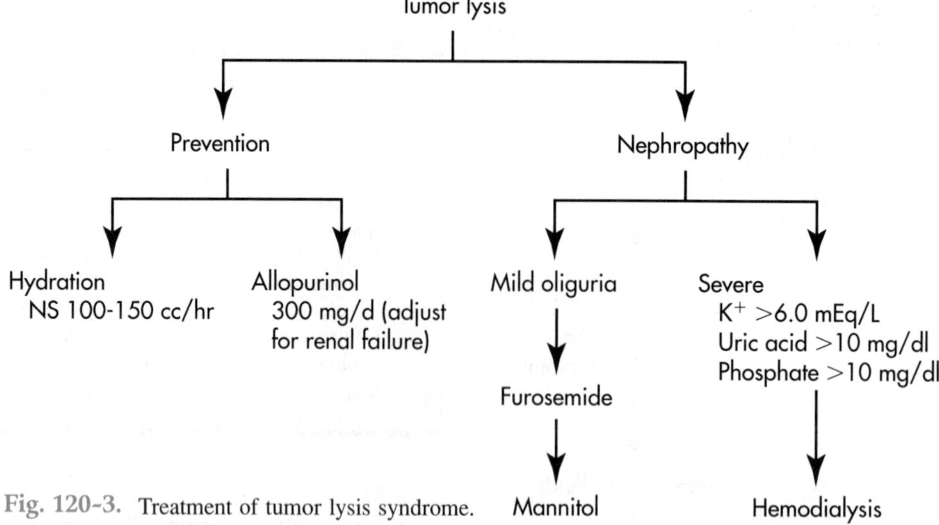

Fig. 120-3. Treatment of tumor lysis syndrome.

Table 120-2. Etiology of SVCS

	1934	1990
Cancer	46%	97%
Benign causes	54%	3%

Physical examination is often remarkable for neck vein distention, facial edema, and trunk and upper extremity swelling. Enlarged, dilated, cutaneous vessels in the anterior chest and upper abdomen provide evidence for collateral blood flow. Plethora and tachypnea may also be noted. In later stages, papilledema, lethargy, mental status changes, seizures, and coma may develop (Box 120-5).

Box 120-5. Signs and Symptoms of SVCS

Nervous System
Headaches
Nightmares
Nausea
Dizziness
Vision changes
Papilledema
Lethargy
Mental status changes
Syncope
Seizures
Stupor
Coma
Death

Respiratory
Hoarseness
Cough
Dyspnea
Tachypnea
Stridor

Vascular
Collateral flow
- Plethora
- Dilated cutaneous vessels

Obstruction
- Neck vein distention
- Facial edema
- Upper extremity and trunk swelling

Diagnosis. The diagnosis of SVCS is based primarily on the patient's symptoms and the physical examination findings. Chest radiographs may reveal a superior mediastinal mass or hilar adenopathy. Computed tomography (CT) scan allows for visualization of the obstruction and evaluation of the extent of the disease.

SVCS usually arises as a subacute oncologic problem and not as a true emergency, since unrelieved obstruction is not life threatening except when tracheal obstruction is also present. In most previously undiagnosed cases, measures to determine the etiology of the mass lesion may be performed and serve as essential guides to therapy. Radiation therapy induces necrosis; therefore, when initiated before the diagnosis, it may impair diagnostic efforts.

Treatment. Interim therapeutic measures such as elevation of the head, diuretics, and supplemental oxygen may be instituted for symptomatic relief. Dexamethasone may be used in patients with evidence of intracerebral edema. In patients with highly chemosensitive tumors, lymphoma, germ cell carcinoma, and small cell carcinoma of the lung, chemotherapy plays a significant role in treatment; however, in most patients, radiotherapy is the cornerstone of therapy. Balloon angioplasty and stent placement have been used to relieve the obstruction, but experience is limited (Fig. 120-4).

Cardiac Tamponade

Etiology. Cardiac tamponade is a life-threatening condition that, when recognized early, is treatable and often reversible. Tamponade occurs when fluid accumulates in the pericardial space and impairs adequate filling of the atria and ventricles. When caused by a malignant condition, this fluid contains malignant cells.

Pathophysiology. The pericardial space normally contains approximately 20 ml of fluid maintained at a very low pressure. Malignant cells bring about changes in oncotic pressures that cause fluid to accumulate. Increased pericardial fluid increases the intrapericardial pressure, which may lead to hemodynamic compromise and collapse. The amount of pericardial fluid does not directly correlate with the

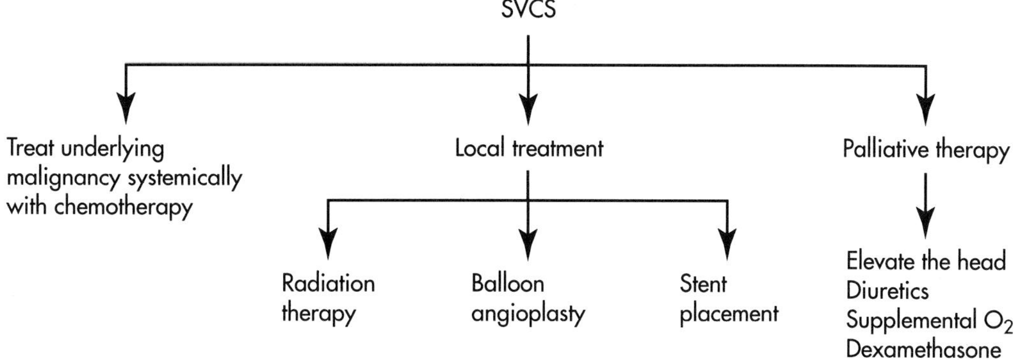

Fig. 120-4. Treatment of superior vena cava syndrome.

Box 120-6. Symptoms of Cardiac Tamponade

Symptoms	**Signs**
	Early
Nausea	High jugular venous pressure
Hiccups	Tachycardia
Cough	Pulsus paradoxus
Hoarseness	***Late***
Chest pressure	Bradycardia
Dyspnea	Low-output heart failure
	Shock
	Death

Box 120-7. Diagnostic Findings of Cardiac Tamponade

Chest radiograph: Globular cardiac shadow
ECG: Electrical alternans
Echocardiogram: Intrapericardial fluid and collapse of atrial and/or ventricular walls from increased pressure
Swan-Ganz measurement: Equalization of pressures

intrapericardial pressure. Fluid that accumulates quickly may reach a hemodynamically significant pressure earlier than fluid that accumulates slowly and provides time for the heart to adapt to the hemodynamic changes.

Signs and Symptoms. The patient's symptom complex is variable and may range from mild nausea and hiccups to cough, hoarseness, chest pressure, and dyspnea. Physical examination is often notable for tachycardia and high jugular venous pressures. Pulsus paradoxus is pathognomonic for tamponade. With frank tamponade bradycardia, low-output failure, shock, and death may occur (Box 120-6).

Diagnosis. Once the diagnosis of cardiac tamponade is suspected clinically, a definitive evaluation must be pursued. The chest radiograph is often remarkable for a large, globular heart shadow. ECG may reveal sinus tachycardia, low voltage, and electrical alternans. Echocardiogram allows for the visualization of the pericardial fluid and the collapse of the atrial and ventricular walls caused by high intrapericardial pressure. Swan-Ganz pressure measurements characteristically reveal equalization of the right atrial, right ventricular, pulmonary artery, and pulmonary capillary wedge pressures (Box 120-7).

Treatment. The goal of intervention is to decompress the heart with pericardiocentesis. The pericardial fluid may be serous, serosanguineous, or hemorrhagic. It may be distinguished from cardiac chamber blood because of its absence of clot formation and because its hematocrit is lower than that of venous blood. Once it is identified as pericardial fluid, a sample should be sent for culture, sensitivity, and cytologic testing. Potential complications of pericardiocentesis are laceration of the myocardium or coronary artery, hemorrhage, arrhythmia, and cardiac arrest.

If due to a malignant etiology, the fluid will reaccumulate without a more definitive intervention. An intrapericardial catheter may be placed in the pericardial space and left to drain. Sclerosis of the pericardial space may be successful. The significant chest discomfort often requires narcotic analgesia. Creation of a pericardial window is reserved for cases that are difficult to control. Whenever possible, treatment options should address the underlying malignancy (Fig. 120-5).

HEMATOLOGIC EMERGENCIES

Disseminated Intravascular Coagulopathy

Etiology. After infection and trauma, cancer is the third most common cause of disseminated intravascular coagulopathy (DIC). DIC is the principal coagulopathy encountered in cancer patients (Box 120-8). The most common malignant associations are melanoma; acute myelogenous leukemia (AML), especially the M3 promyelocytic subtype (APL); and mucin-producing adenocarcinomas such as those from the gastrointestinal tract, prostate, lung, and breast.

Pathophysiology. DIC results from general activation of the coagulation system. The formation of small thrombi throughout the microvasculature results in the consumption of platelets and coagulation factors associated with the

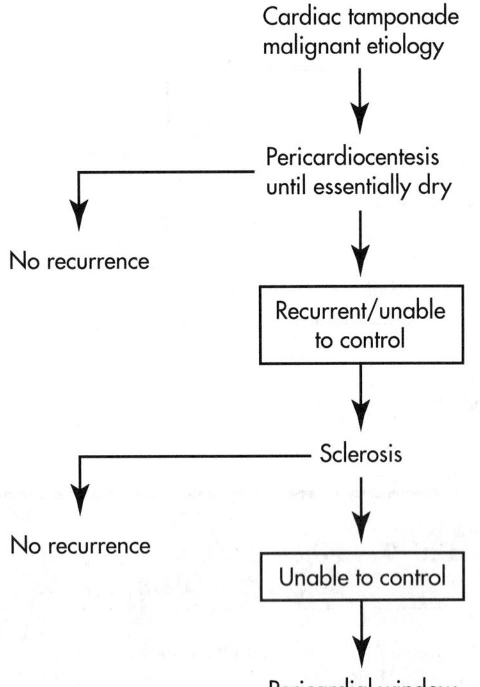

Fig. 120-5. Management of malignant pericardial effusion producing cardiac tamponade.

Box 120-8. Malignant Etiologies of DIC

AML (especially M3)
Adenocarcinoma
- Gastrointestinal
- Prostate
- Lung
- Breast

hemorrhagic phase of DIC. Procoagulants induce the thrombotic phase of DIC. Thrombotic events may produce ischemia and subsequent tissue damage.

Signs and Symptoms. Patients may have hemorrhagic or thrombotic events. Any site of trauma such as a venipuncture site or surgical incision may demonstrate poor hemostasis associated with the depletion of coagulation factors and thrombocytopenia. Thrombotic complications are less common than hemorrhagic ones but may be seen if significant blood flow obstruction takes place. Cancer patients may be asymptomatic.

Diagnosis. DIC is characterized by specific laboratory findings, including a prolonged prothrombin time (PT), partial thromboplastin time (PTT), and thrombin time (TT) accompanied by evidence of clotting factor consumption with low fibrinogen levels, elevated fibrin split products, and thrombocytopenia. Examination of the peripheral smear may reveal schistocytes. In chronic DIC, laboratory abnormalities may be only minimally out of range (Box 120-9).

Box 120-9. Diagnostic Characteristics of DIC

Increased PT
Increased PTT
Increased TT
Decreased fibrinogen level
Increased fibrin split products
Decreased platelets

Treatment. Once it is recognized, DIC should be urgently addressed to prevent potentially fatal complications (Fig. 120-6). When feasible, control of the underlying malignancy is essential; however, symptom control and subsequent prevention of recurrence often constitute the sole therapeutic option. Blood product support with platelets, packed red cells, cryoprecipitate, and fresh frozen plasma is frequently necessary. The use of heparin is controversial but is generally favored in conditions in which the thrombotic component predominates.

Migratory Thrombophlebitis: Trousseau's Syndrome

Etiology. Various malignant conditions are thought to be associated with hypercoagulability and thrombosis and are clinically characterized primarily as a migratory superficial thrombophlebitis, although larger vessels also may be affected. Clinical thromboembolic disease has been estimated to occur in 10% of patients, although postmortem studies often reveal a higher incidence. On occasion a thrombotic event may be the harbinger of an underlying malignancy. The most common malignancies associated with increased thrombotic events are melanoma, lymphoma, leukemia, and carcinoma of the lung or gastrointestinal tract, etiologies similar to those that result in DIC. As in all patients, hypercoagulability is heightened in the postoperative period and with bed rest.

Pathophysiology. The mechanism of migratory thrombophlebitis is not clearly understood and may precede detection of the underlying malignancy by several months. Normal hemostasis may be disrupted mechanically or biochemically by the presence of the tumor. Disseminated clotting may be triggered by the release of procoagulant substances from mucin-producing carcinomas. The role of other hypercoagulability risk factors such as advanced age and sedentary lifestyle also needs to be considered.

Signs and Symptoms. The patient typically comes to the primary care physician with complaints of a swollen, erythematous, and tender extremity consistent with deep venous thrombosis or with evidence of superficial thrombophlebitis. Less commonly, symptoms of pulmonary embolus with dyspnea and acute-onset pleuritic chest pain occur and require urgent attention. The hallmark of this syndrome is its recurrent nature.

Diagnosis. The usual diagnostic approach to superficial thrombophlebitis, deep venous thrombosis, and pulmonary

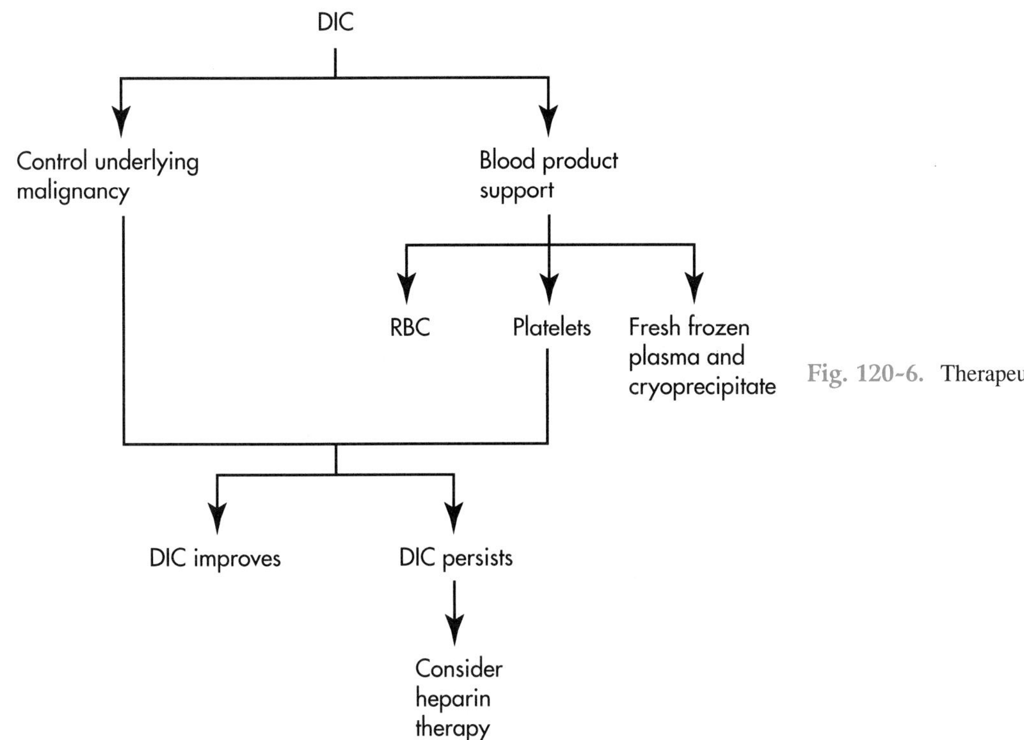

Fig. 120-6. Therapeutic approach to DIC.

embolus should be pursued and is not reviewed here. Although the presence of a malignancy may predispose to hypercoagulability, a single thrombotic event does not mandate an extensive search for a malignancy. Recent investigation, however, reveals a higher incidence of subsequent carcinoma in patients who have idiopathic deep venous thrombosis or pulmonary embolism.

Treatment. The therapeutic approach is not particular to cancer patients. The use of heparin quickly followed by oral anticoagulants is standard. Hypercoagulable cancer patients require anticoagulation for as long as the malignancy is active, which for many patients is the remainder of their life. For patients who are refractory to anticoagulation or in whom anticoagulation is contraindicated, a Greenfield filter may be surgically placed in the inferior vena cava (see Chapter 4).

NEUROLOGIC EMERGENCIES

Cord Compression

Etiology. Since new onset back pain in a patient with a known malignancy may be secondary to cord compressions, prompt diagnosis and urgent intervention may prevent serious and permanent neurologic impairments and result in a marked improvement in the patient's quality of life. Nearly 20% of patients develop neurologic complications related to their underlying cancer. Spinal cord or cauda equina compression occurs in 5% to 10% of patients with cancer, affecting approximately 20,000 persons annually. An increased incidence of this oncologic complication appears to be related to the increased survival of patients with cancer (Box 120-10).

Box 120-10. Malignant Etiologies of Cord Compression

Primary Malignancy	Metastatic Malignancy
Lymphoma	Lung
Melanoma	Breast
Sarcoma	Prostate
Multiple myeloma	
Renal cell carcinoma	

Pathophysiology. The most common scenario for cord compression is the direct extension of a metastatic lesion from the vertebrae into the epidural space. Although metastatic lesions are more common, cord compression may be the initial presentation of the tumor. Half of the metastatic lesions are due to lung, breast, or prostate cancer. The most common site of compression is the thoracic spine (70%). The lumbar spine is affected 20% of the time, with the cervical spine affected in 10% of cases.

Signs and Symptoms. About 95% of patients have new onset back pain, which is worse with movement and is accompanied by motor and sensory deficits that progressively move upward. In time, autonomic dysfunction may take place, with bladder and bowel incontinence. In contrast, back pain caused by degenerative joint disease is often improved with recumbency. It is not associated with progressive neurologic impairment and is most frequent in the cervical or lumbar spine.

Physical examination is remarkable for tenderness to percussion of the involved vertebrae, brisk deep tendon reflexes, and motor and sensory deficits. Sequential neurologic examinations may be used to clinically document the progression of the cord compression.

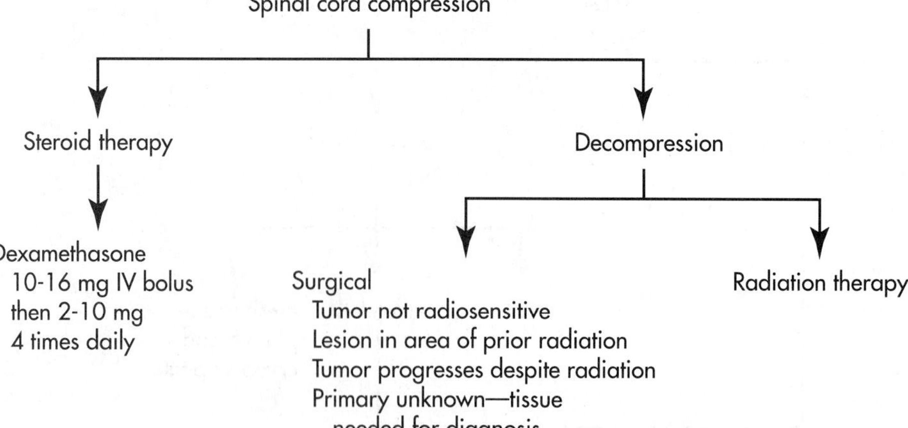

Fig. 120-7. Management of spinal cord compression.

Diagnosis. Clinical suspicion of cord compression is based on a thorough history and physical examination. In over half of cases the malignant lesion may be visualized on plain radiographs of the spine. Although better visualized on either a spinal myelogram or magnetic resonance imaging (MRI), MRI is noninvasive, has no radiation exposure, and carries no risk of allergic reaction to dye. Intramedullary disease may be visually enhanced with the use of gadolinium.

Treatment. Untreated sensory loss produces progressive anesthesia; motor deficits result in paralysis and loss of sphincter control. The best prognostic markers regarding the potential effectiveness of treatment are the patient's physical findings and functional status at the time that therapy is instituted. The majority of patients who are ambulatory at the time of diagnosis are ambulatory at the completion of treatment. Approximately 20% of patients who are paraplegic at the onset of treatment are able to ambulate after treatment, but fewer than 10% of patients who begin treatment with paralysis are ambulatory at the end of treatment.

The goal of therapy is to decompress the spinal cord (Fig. 120-7). Traditionally, a bolus of 10 to 20 mg of dexamethasone given intravenously is followed by oral doses of 2 to 10 mg four times daily. Decompression with radiotherapy can then be pursued. Surgical decompression is considered if the lesion is not radiosensitive, progresses despite appropriate radiation doses, occurs in an area of prior radiation, or is the only site of disease and a tissue diagnosis has not been made. Definitive decompression efforts should be instituted as soon as possible after the diagnosis is made.

Intracerebral Metastases

Etiology. Metastases to the brain are a frequent complication of bronchogenic carcinoma, lymphoma, melanoma, as well as other adenocarcinomas.

Pathophysiology. As with any other mass lesion within the skull, the mass may produce edema and elevated intracranial pressure. Metastatic lesions are often multiple and less amenable to resection.

Signs and Symptoms. Patients frequently visit the physician at the urging of family members who express concern regarding changes in mental status or personality. Focal neurologic deficits and new-onset seizures may also be noted. The clinical spectrum of increased intracranial pressure can range from headache and papilledema to loss of consciousness associated with frank herniation.

Diagnosis. The neurologic symptoms described should lead the physician to obtain a thorough history and to perform a complete physical examination. The diagnosis of intracerebral metastases relies on a thorough evaluation of the symptoms, a thoughtful consideration of the differential diagnoses, and an imaging study to visualize the lesion. The greatest risk of a mass-producing lesion is increased intracranial pressure with potential uncal herniation, which carries a grave prognosis.

Treatment. The initial treatment goal is to decrease the edema caused by the mass. This is accomplished with steroids as described in the management of spinal cord compression. Radiotherapy is the key therapeutic intervention for radiosensitive metastases. Because of their multiple nature, surgical resection of intracerebral metastases is usually not a therapeutic option.

End of life care and resources for supporting patients in the terminal phase of illness are presented in Chapters 9 and 164.

ADDITIONAL READINGS

Bryne TN: Spinal cord compression from epidural mets, *N Engl J Med* 327:614, 1992.

Helms SR, Carlson, MD: Cardiovascular emergencies, *Semin Oncol* 6:463, 1989.

Kamholtz R, Sze G: Current imaging in spinal metastatic disease, *Semin Oncol* 18:158, 1991.

Paterson AHG, et al: Double-blind controlled trial of oral clodronate in patients with bone metastases from breast cancer, *J Clin Oncol* 11:59, 1993.

Prandoni P, et al: Deep venous thrombosis and the incidence of subsequent symptomatic cancer, *N Engl J Med* 327:1128, 1992.

Ratnoff OD: Hemostatic emergencies in malignancy, *Semin Oncol* 16:561, 1989.

Silverman P, Distelhorst CW: Metabolic emergencies in clinical oncology, *Semin Oncol* 16:504, 1989.

Singer FR: Treatment of hypercalcemia of malignancy with intravenous etidronate, *Arch Intern Med* 151:471, 1991.

Sundersan N, et al: Treatment of neoplastic spinal cord compression: results of a prospective study, *Neurosurgery* 29:645, 1991.

Theriault RL: Hypercalcemia of malignancy: pathophysiology and implications for treatment, *Oncology* 7:47, 1993.

Walpole HT, et al: Superior vena cava syndrome treated by percutaneous transluminal balloon angioplasty, *Am Heart J* 115:1303, 1988.

Willson JKV, Masaryk TJ: Neurologic emergencies in the cancer patient, *Semin Oncol* 16:490, 1989.

CHAPTER 121

Living With Cancer: Psychosocial Implications

Debra M. Lundquist

Coping with cancer means more than coping with a chronic disease. It is coping with the human predicament. Cancer can be an exhausting, relentless, and resourceful foe.[16]

The very thought of cancer is frightening to most people. The diagnosis of cancer is devastating and affects every aspect of the person's life. It is often the first time one confronts mortality, questioning life and its meaning. To many, cancer implies a death sentence; to others it implies suffering and pain. Despite advances in diagnosis and treatment, cancer remains a fatal disease for a significant number of patients.

Cancer is a heterogeneous group of diseases characterized by uncontrolled growth and spread of abnormal cells. Many cancers can be cured if detected and treated promptly. However, if the spread of disease is not controlled or checked, it results in death.

In the United States, cancer is the second leading cause of death and accounts for 23% of all deaths. There were approximately 1.23 million new cases diagnosed in 1998 with 565,000 deaths in the United States. For women ages 35 to 74, cancer is the leading cause of death. Cancer is the second leading cause of death for men in the United States.[7]

In the early 1900s few cancer patients survived. By the 1940s only one patient in four was alive 5 years after diagnosis, and in the 1960s, it was one cancer patient in three. Today, there are more than 10 million living Americans who have a history of cancer. More than seven million persons were diagnosed 5 or more years ago. The 5-year survival rate is projected to reach 67% by the early twenty-first century.[5,11]

TRANSITION POINTS ALONG THE CANCER TRAJECTORY (BOX 121-1)

Meaning of a Cancer Diagnosis

The diagnosis of cancer elicits a wide range of emotions, including shock, disbelief, denial, anger, sadness, and depression. One may also experience feelings of powerlessness and vulnerability. It is a time of shock and disbelief for the individual as well as for that person's loved ones. Concerns about death and the feeling that time is running out are common. Many persons also experience a period of isolation and intense aloneness, but fear of dying creates an urgency to seek out information about treatment options and support from others. For most people, the reality of the situation is accepted, followed by feelings of anxiety, anorexia, irritability, and difficulty concentrating. It is common for patients to ask "Why me?" The person who is diagnosed with cancer finds the diagnosis is only the beginning of many life changes.[3,4]

Cancer is regarded as a chronic illness that affects every aspect of a person's life. It is no longer regarded as an immediate death sentence, although there are many concerns about death. As with most chronic illnesses, periods of stress and feelings of uncertainty characterize cancer, whether it involves unpredictable disease trajectories, uncertain remissions, or recurrence of disease. According to Weisman, like cancer's ability to spread through the body, it also is able to spread into the emotional and social domains of an individual, causing disruptions in families and causing one to question the meaning of life.[15] Weisman also identified uncertainty as a major coping problem.[16]

Box 121-1. Transition Points Along the Cancer Trajectory

1. Cancer diagnosis
2. Treatment-related concerns
3. Cancer recurrence
4. Palliative care
5. Survivorship

A diagnosis of cancer is considered a catastrophic event that causes physical and psychologic changes to the individual and family. Weisman identified seven major areas of concern for these individuals: health, self-appraisal, work and finances, family and significant relationships, religion, friends and associates, and existential issues. Weisman identified coping with the problems associated with a cancer diagnosis as a major task of the individual and family. He described good coping as an action that consists of the principal parts of hope, trust, quality of survival, and reasonable control of symptoms.[15,16]

Researchers have identified three general theoretic coping methods: active behavioral coping, which refers to behaviors directed toward the problem and its effects, including reliance on others for informational and emotional support; active cognitive coping, which involves one's thoughts, attitudes, and beliefs about the illness; and avoidance coping, which refers to attempts at actively avoiding the problem.[4]

These behaviors can be further categorized into eight strategies that provide a framework for classifying coping reactions. The strategies can be identified as those that are effective in most situations and those that are less effective. The effective strategies include: active positive involvement (increasing involvement, living one day at a time); active expressive/information-seeking (talking with others to gain information or offer support); active reliance on others; cognitive positive understanding/create meaning; and distraction (doing something nice for oneself). The less effective strategies are: cognitive passive/ruminative (daydreaming); passive resignation (fearing the worst, not sharing feelings); and avoidance solitary/passive behavior (avoiding others, using drugs).[4]

In general, those patients who demonstrate effective coping strategies report more positive affective states, higher levels of self-esteem, and fewer physical symptoms.[4]

In a study done by Weisman and Worden, 120 newly diagnosed cancer patients were interviewed in 4- to 6-week intervals, beginning 10 days after diagnosis. The purpose of the study was to further explore the impact of a cancer diagnosis. This study examined how newly diagnosed cancer patients coped with the existential plight of being diagnosed with a life-threatening illness. Existential plight was defined as "a luckless predicament in which one's very existence seems endangered." This study confirmed that newly diagnosed cancer patients are most concerned about dying regardless of their prognosis. These concerns occur most intensely during the first 100 days, the time known as *existential plight*.[16]

This finding was supported by a study done by McCorkle and Quint-Benoliel. Their study revealed that newly diagnosed lung cancer patients experienced more health and existential concerns than those newly diagnosed with myocardial infarction. The cancer patients also experienced more mood disturbances than the myocardial infarction group. An interesting finding was that, although symptom distress remained the same for both groups at interviews done at 1 and 2 months after diagnosis, both groups of patients reported being less worried as well as in better spirits than at the first interview. This led to the inference that as patients understand more about their illness, they may conclude that their situation is not as life threatening as previously thought.[12] Mood disturbances are not uncommon in the newly diagnosed cancer patient. Northouse interviewed women with breast cancer and found the level of mood changes improved over time, although the subjects' levels of distress did not.[14]

Treatment-related Concerns

The initiation of treatment for cancer is a time characterized by fear, uncertainty, and feelings of loss of control. Patients realize that treatment is essential to combat the disease. However, fears related to the physical and psychologic aspects of the treatment as well as the impact on the family and financial ramifications can be overwhelming. Concerns about the physical aspects of treatment include potential side effects, changes in body image, and changes in functional status. Psychologic concerns include the fears related to the outcome of treatment, the uncertain future, and the ability of the individual to cope with the treatment. Feelings of uncertainty are paramount. Common questions asked by newly diagnosed patients with cancer include: How will I be affected by the treatment? Will the treatment help me? Will I be cured? and Is it really worth it? Many patients fear being a burden to their family and have concerns about their ability to maintain employment. Concerns about employment and the financial implications predominate, particularly if the individual with cancer is the provider for the family.

The treatment itself is a source of anxiety. Many individuals have misconceptions based on the public perception of cancer and its treatment. It is important to clarify misconceptions before initiating treatment. This knowledge helps the person regain a sense of control in a situation that causes many to feel out of control.

Patients also experience difficulties at the completion of treatment.[3] For many, there is often a sense of ambivalence. Patients are happy at the thought of completing treatment but fear distancing themselves from the health care team. There is also a sense that they are no longer actively fighting the cancer. It is not unusual for some patients to develop behaviors such as hypochondriasis as a means of coping with anxiety about completing treatment. Reassurance about the availability of the health care team is encouraged, as is education about symptoms that would need to be reported. Routine checkups and yearly comprehensive examinations help alleviate anxiety. As the duration of time from the completion of treatment increases, patients become more comfortable with the distance that has developed from the health care team.

Cancer Recurrence

Cancer recurrence poses as great a threat as, if not greater than, the initial diagnosis of cancer. Many persons with cancer will experience one or more episodes of recurrence. Little is known about the psychosocial implications of recurrence. Mahon et al found the time of recurrence of cancer was more upsetting than the initial diagnosis and that people were less hopeful than at the time of initial diagnosis.[9] Fear of recurrence is almost always present whether the prognosis is excellent or poor. A number of psychosocial stressors are experienced at the time of recurrence. For most patients the realization that the focus of treatment shifts from cure to control of disease is extremely stressful and frightening. Many patients perceive that, once treated, cancer is cured and will not recur. Therefore when the recurrence is confirmed, feelings of disbelief, uncertainty, anger, and fear are experienced. Many patients experience feelings of hopelessness and depression and question the benefit of additional treatment if cure is no longer the goal.

Mahon et al interviewed 20 subjects at the time of first recurrence to understand the meaning of recurrence and to explore the differences between the initial diagnosis of cancer and the diagnosis of recurrence. Five themes emerged concerning the interpretation of recurrence: issues before recurrence; the diagnosis of recurrence; prior experience with cancer; death and death-related issues; and positive aspects of recurrence. In regards to the differences between initial diagnosis and the diagnosis of recurrence, subjects identified that recurrence makes one more aware of the cancer diagnosis; treatment and extent of disease created feelings of fear because they had already been through treatment once and worried about side effects as well as effectiveness; and lastly, in patients where the extent of disease was unclear there was more anxiety and they felt more threatened.[8,9]

In addition, Mahon et al identified health and health-related concerns, work and financial issues, and self-appraisal issues. It is important to assess patients and families who are most vulnerable to the stressors that result from recurrence and provide support and guidance to facilitate adjustment.[9] For many patients and families the opportunity to verbalize feelings of grief, anger, and fear enables them to move forward and make decisions regarding treatment and the future. Chekryn identified several stressors experienced at the time of recurrence by both patients and spouses (Box 121-2).[2]

Box 121-2. Chekryn's Stressors at Time of Cancer Recurrence

Difficulty with closure related to the expectation of cure or remission
Pervasive feelings of uncertainty
Grief about present and potential losses
Feelings of injustice, anger, and fear
Existential concerns
Concerns related to ability to cope with recurrence
Impact on the marital relationship

From Chekryn J: *Cancer Nurs* 7(6):491, 1984.

Palliative Care

The transition from active treatment to supportive care of the dying patient is important in the cancer continuum. Palliative care is the shift in treatment goals from a curative intent to providing relief from suffering. Relief from suffering for the dying patient goes beyond the management of physical symptoms. The emotional, spiritual, and existential concerns must all be addressed.

Martinez and Wagner identified the principles of palliative care, as shown in Box 121-3.[10]

When the decision is made to shift the focus to palliative care, persons experience many responses, often in a cyclic process. Initially, one may experience shock and denial at the realization that no further treatment will stop the cancer's spread. This is followed by varying degrees of denial, bargaining, sadness, anger, and acceptance.[10] Coping patterns in the terminal phase can be predicted by the patient's history of coping with past events.

Many patients choose to die at home with hospice services (if available). Hospice care and death at home give the patient and family a sense of control over their environment at a time when they feel out of control. Remaining at home in familiar surroundings is also comforting for many people. However, this option is not feasible for all dying persons. Some patients may be too acutely ill to be managed at home. Lack of resources to provide adequate care in the home is another barrier.

For patients who choose to die at home, an individualized plan of care must be developed with the involvement of the patient and family. Information regarding the dying process, including anticipated signs and symptoms of approaching death, is important to best prepare the family to care for the dying patient. Anticipation of predictable changes in the patient who is dying can help the patient and family effectively cope. The major processes underlying cancer death include infection, organ failure, extensive carcinomatosis, pulmonary problems, myocardial infarction, and hemorrhage. Common symptoms include dyspnea, pain, altered elimination, and seizures.[10] Assessment and care of the dying patient need to focus on the physical, psychosocial, and spiritual aspects of the individual. The focus shifts to maintaining comfort and managing symptoms to promote a peaceful death with dignity. See Chapters 9 and 164 for further discussion of death and dying.

Box 121-3. Managed Care Guide: Principles of Palliative Care

The goal of treatment is to optimize quality of life.

Death is regarded as a natural process, to be neither hastened nor prolonged.

Diagnostic tests and other invasive procedures are minimized unless the intervention will result in the alleviation of symptoms.

Use of heroic treatment measures is discouraged.

When using narcotic analgesics, the right dosage is the one that provides pain relief without unacceptable side effects.

The patient is the expert on whether pain and symptoms have been adequately relieved.

Patients eat if they are hungry and drink if thirsty; fluids and feeding are not forced.

Care is individualized and based on the goals of the patient and family, as the unit of care.

From Martinez J, Wagner S: Hospice care. In Groenwald S, et al, editors: *Cancer nursing: principles and practice,* ed 3, Boston, 1993, Jones & Bartlett.

Survivorship Issues

Early detection and intervention using a multimodality treatment approach have significantly increased the number of cancer survivors. Cancer is now considered a chronic, life-threatening illness rather than a terminal illness.

Cancer survivorship can be described as the experience of living through or beyond illness. It is a process that encompasses all phases of survival but is best defined as long-term survival.[5] Historically, cancer survivors were considered cured of their disease 5 years after the completion of treatment. When thinking of cancer survivorship, the term cure is not accurate because some persons have cancers that may be controlled for several years. Although these individuals are not cured, they are indeed survivors with a chronic disease. Long-term survivors may experience a variety of problems ranging from minor, short-term difficulties to major psychosocial crises.

Mullan describes the three seasons of survival: diagnosis of cancer, a time dominated by treatment; extended survival, a period of waiting during which the patient fears recurrence; and permanent survival, in which the likelihood of recurrence is quite small and the disease appears cured.[5]

The major psychosocial themes identified for cancer survivors include interrelationships between long-term physical effects and psychosocial outcomes, fears of relapse and death, dependence on health care providers, survivor guilt, uncertain sense of longevity, social adaptation dilemmas, and the effects on the family. The ability of a person to cope as a survivor of cancer is influenced by the degree of physical changes experienced relating to treatment. Certainly, fear of recurrence and death is present to some degree regardless of the time since initial diagnosis.[5,18] This is probably the most common concern for cancer survivors. Dependence on health care providers is often the result of ambivalence that develops as the patient completes treatment. There is a sense of euphoria about completing treatment, which is in conflict with fears experienced relating to the change in intensity and frequency of interactions with health care providers.

Feelings of survivor guilt are common for cancer survivors. These feelings may be experienced on routine follow-up visits when there is interaction between the survivor and others in the waiting room.

Many cancer survivors experience a sense of uncertainty regarding the future. Concerns focus on the potential long-term implications after having survived a chronic illness. Many persons identify a greater appreciation of life and the desire to live life in a more meaningful way as positive approaches to this uncertainty.

An additional area of difficulty is the transition from the sick role to the healthy role. This is not always easy for cancer survivors. Welch-McCaffrey and co-workers identified the presence of physical disability, negative expectations from the support network, personal concerns about the ability to readjust, and social stigma as social dilemmas encountered by the cancer survivor.[18] These are areas that require exploration and discussion. The ability of a member of the health care team to discuss these concerns may help the individual to look at them in a more objective manner.

Finally, the effects on the family of the survivor need to be considered. There is limited information regarding the effects of long-term psychologic stress on the family. However, this is an area of assessment that must not be minimized. The diagnosis of cancer affects not only the individual but also those around him or her. Throughout the diagnostic and treatment phases the family often struggles to respond and support the loved one with cancer. Health care professionals must be sensitive to the needs of families of survivors.

Additional areas of concern for the cancer survivor include financial, employment, and insurance issues. Access to insurance is usually through employment. Unfortunately, some cancer survivors experience discrimination in the workplace. Welch-McCaffrey and co-workers identified three categories of employment-related concerns: dismissal, demotion, and reduction or elimination of work-related benefits; problems resulting from co-workers' attitudes about cancer; and problems arising from attitudes of the survivor regarding how he or she should be perceived in the workplace.[18] Federal and state laws were developed to prohibit discrimination against qualified individuals with a history of cancer. Both the Federal Rehabilitation Act of 1973 and the more recent Americans with Disabilities Act prohibit discrimination against cancer survivors in the workplace.

Access to comprehensive insurance continues to be problematic. The availability of adequate insurance is not a guarantee for many people. Unfortunately, there is no state or federally mandated legal right to health insurance, although this may change in the future. Barriers to obtaining insurance include refusal of new applications, waived or excluded preconditions, policy cancellations or reductions, higher premiums, and extended waiting periods. These barriers may also affect the spouse or family member who carries the insurance. Studies have found that 25% to 30% of cancer survivors experience some form of insurance discrimination.[18]

In an effort to protect survivors of cancer, the American Cancer Society published the Cancer Survivor's Bill of Rights. The goal of this document was to call public attention to the needs of the cancer survivor, to enhance cancer care, and to bring greater satisfaction to cancer survivors. Resources are becoming increasingly available to better support cancer survivors, on both the local and national levels. The National Coalition for Cancer Survivorship (NCCS) serves as a resource for those interested in issues of survivorship. The continued development of programs, support networks, and resources is essential to ensure that cancer survivors are treated fairly and maintain their quality of life.

COMPLEMENTARY AND ALTERNATIVE THERAPIES

The use of complementary and alternative therapies has been gaining more attention from patients over the last several years. Many patients choose to use these therapies in addition to conventional treatment; however, there is a growing number of patients who choose to discontinue conventional therapy and pursue complementary and alternative therapies. Cassileth reviewed 26 surveys of cancer patients from 13 countries, including five studies from the United States, and found the utilization of complementary and alternative therapy was 31%. The following therapies were used: herbs, homeopathy, hypnotherapy, imagery/visualization, meditation, megavitamins, relaxation, and spiritual healing. Across samples, the prevalence in the United States ranged from 7% to 16%, with the exception of one study that revealed a rate of 54%.[1]

Patients who choose complementary therapies in addition to conventional treatment often do so due to some dissatisfaction with their treatment. The discomfort related to treatment is tolerated, but at the same time the patient may be drawn to the benefits of complementary therapies and feel more in control of their situation by taking a more active role. These therapies are usually self-managed, thus giving the person real control. Complementary therapies are used to reduce pain, stress, and anxiety, not to cure disease. The use of complementary therapies can enhance quality of life and feelings of well being.[1] For additional information refer to Chapter 12.

IMPACT OF CANCER ON THE FAMILY

Cancer is a disease that affects not only the patient, but also the entire family. One in four Americans will be diagnosed with cancer in his or her lifetime and two of every three families will have at least one member diagnosed with cancer. Some families may have multiple members of more than one generation being treated for cancer at the same time. It is essential that the health care team assesses the ability of the family to mobilize itself and its resources in response to the needs of the person with cancer. Acknowledgment of the importance of the family enhances the care of the person experiencing the disease.[6,20]

Worry about the impact of the illness on loved ones is very real. The diagnosis of cancer places a strain on the entire family, and often the person experiencing the disease expresses feelings of guilt or worry because of what "I'm putting my family through." This concern reinforces the need to include the family in the plan of care.

The major issues affecting the family and its ability to cope with a cancer diagnosis were identified by Woods, Lewis, and Ellison (Box 121-4). Whether the family can respond to these issues is related to disease characteristics such as the patient's age at diagnosis, prognosis, disease severity and progression, the duration of illness, and associated disabilities.[19]

Box 121-4. Issues Affecting the Family and Its Coping Ability

Emotional strain
Physical demands of care
Uncertainty
Fear
Altered roles and lifestyles
Financial considerations
Comforting the patient
Perceived inadequacy of services
Philosophic and spiritual concerns
Sexuality
Incongruent needs and perceptions

From Woods NF, Lewis FM, Ellison ES: *Cancer Nurs* 12(1):28, 1989.

The location of the person in the cancer trajectory is an important point to consider. Morse and Fife studied the impact of cancer on the lives of partners of people with cancer at four different points in the cancer trajectory: diagnosis, first remission, first recurrence, and metastatic disease. They noted three significant findings: psychologic distress increases and adjustment becomes more difficult as patients progress through the disease trajectory. Other researchers who have found that adjustment to recurrence is more difficult than at the time of diagnosis also support this finding. The second finding is that female partners experienced more psychologic distress than male partners. This was believed to be related to financial concerns as well as women's dependence on their husbands. And lastly, social support correlated with the adjustment of partners, with family support most significant.[13]

Families may remain at a transition point for an extended time or may progress quickly from one point to the next. The movement through these transition points serves as a reminder of the many changes experienced by the family that drain family strength and resources. Compounding this are the uncertainty and fear experienced at each transition point by the person with cancer and the family.

Family members may assume many different roles throughout the cancer experience. They may function in the role of partner, actively participating in decision making with the person with cancer and providing care to the ill family member. A family member fulfills the participant role by taking an active role in care and being included in decisions. However, the ill patient remains responsible for decision making. As an observer the family member does not participate in the care or decision making. It is important to identify who is functioning in the different roles to better care for the patient and family.[6,19]

In a study of 41 family members of adult cancer patients, Welch identified five specific family needs when a family member has cancer. These are: knowing the patient is receiving excellent care, being informed about cancer and treatment, participating in patient care, communicating with the health care team, and participating in a support group.[17]

Similar concerns of the family were identified by Wright and Dyck. The primary concerns of the family include dealing with symptoms, waiting, fear of the future, and obtaining information. Families of patients who had a recurrence had significantly higher needs. The highest priority of all families regardless of phase of illness was the need to be kept informed about the patient's condition and to be assured that the patient was comfortable.[20]

Research in this field has identified three consistent findings: the family affects the patient's adjustment to cancer, family members do not necessarily share the same concerns about cancer, and family members cope with cancer in individual ways. Regardless of the person's phase of illness, care of the family is critical in caring for the person with cancer. In caring for the family, the needs of the individual with cancer are best met.

HEALTH CARE TEAM

Use of a multidisciplinary team is essential in helping the patient adapt to the many changes encountered as the result of a cancer diagnosis. Involvement of the team in planning care for the individual facilitates the restoration of physical and emotional well being as the members focus on the goal of promoting quality of life. In addition to the patient and family, members of the team include physicians, nurses, social workers, clergy, nutritionists, and physical therapists. When appropriate, other members are psychologists, occupational therapists, and other health care providers. Regular team meetings are essential to maximize care and identify potential obstacles of goal attainment.

The goals are individualized to the patient. To formulate realistic goals, a thorough discussion of the treatment plan, potential complications, and expected results is essential. For some the goal is curative, whereas for others it may be palliative. Regardless of the goal, maintaining quality of life underlies all interventions.

In addition to the resources available by the members of the team, knowledge of additional resources available is important in providing care. Community-based resources include support groups, educational groups, and organizations such as the American Cancer Society and the Leukemia Society of America, both of which offer programs and services to persons with cancer. Most major cities and towns have local chapters. Written publications are available. These materials are written for medical professionals and laypersons; they are free of charge and informative.

REFERENCES

1. Cassileth BR: Complementary and alternative therapies, *Oncol Nurs Updates* 5(4):1-11, 1998.
2. Chekryn J: Cancer recurrence: personal meaning, communication, and marital adjustment, *Cancer Nurs* 7(6):491, 1984.
3. Coward DD: Constructing meaning from the cancer experience, *Semin Oncol Nurs* 13(4):248-251, 1997.
4. Fawzy NW: A psychoeducational nursing intervention to enhance coping and affective state in newly diagnosed malignant melanoma patients, *Cancer Nurs* 18(6):35-46, 1995.
5. Fredette SL: Breast cancer survivors: concerns and coping, *Cancer Nurs* 18(1):35-46, 1995.
6. Jassak P: Families: an essential element in the care of the patient with cancer, *Oncol Nurs Forum* 19(6):871, 1992.
7. Landis SH, Murray T, Bolden S, et al: Cancer statistics, *CA Cancer J Clin* 48(1):6-29, 1998.
8. Mahon SM, Casperon DM: Exploring the psychosocial meaning of recurrent cancer: a descriptive study, *Cancer Nurs* 20(3):178-186, 1997.
9. Mahon SM, Cella DF, Donovan MI: Psychosocial adjustment to recurrent cancer, *Oncol Nurs Forum* 17(3)(suppl):47, 1990.
10. Martinez J, Wagner S: Hospice care. In Groenwald S, et al, editors: *Cancer nursing: principles and practice,* ed 3, Boston, 1993, Jones & Bartlett.
11. Mayer D: The healthcare implications of cancer rehabilitation in the twenty-first century, *Oncol Nurs Forum* 19:23-27, 1992.
12. McCorkle R, Quint-Benoliel J: Symptom distress, current concerns and mood disturbance after diagnosis with a life-threatening disease, *Soc Sci Med* 17:431-438, 1983.
13. Morse SR, Fife B: Coping with a partner's cancer: adjustment at four stages of the illness trajectory, *Oncol Nurs Forum* 25(4):751-760, 1998.
14. Northouse L: A longitudinal study of the adjustment of patients and husbands to breast cancer, *Oncol Nurs Forum* 16(4):511-516, 1989.
15. Weisman AD: *Coping with cancer,* New York, 1979, McGraw-Hill.
16. Weisman AD, Worden JW: The existential plight in cancer: significance of the first 100 days, *Int J Psychiatry Med* 7:1, 1976-77.
17. Welch D: Planning nursing interventions for family members of adult cancer patients, *Cancer Nurs* 4:365, 1981.
18. Welch-McCaffrey D, et al: Psychosocial dimensions: issues in survivorship. In Groenwald S, et al, editors: *Cancer nursing: principles and practice,* ed 2, Boston, 1990, Jones & Bartlett.
19. Woods NF, Lewis FM, Ellison ES: Living with cancer: family experiences, *Cancer Nurs* 12(1):28, 1989.
20. Wright K, Dyck S: Expressed concerns of adult cancer patients' family members, *Cancer Nurs* 7:371-374, 1984.

CHAPTER 122

Cancer Prevention, Screening, and Follow-up

Linda M. Sutton

As a result of decades of research in the laboratory and in clinical practice, optimism in cancer care is now well founded. Although nearly 1.25 million Americans will be diagnosed with cancer in 1999, the incidence of cancer overall has declined 0.7% from 1990 to 1995 in contrast to increasing trends in earlier years. The downward trend in incidence has also been seen for the individual leading cancer types. There have been similar improvements in cancer-related mortality. Since the 1950s cancer has been the second leading cause of death in the United States, and an estimated 538,000 deaths in 1999 will be attributed to cancer.[8] Box 122-1 details the five primary sites of invasive malignancy, which account for nearly 60% of the estimated annual cancer incidence and mortality. However, when compared with the early 1960s, the rate of survival at 5 years after diagnosis has increased for a majority of cancer types. The last half of the 1990s has witnessed the fruition of several approaches to the prevention of cancer mortality. Improvements in cancer treatments, improved supportive care of those with cancer, and better detection of early-stage disease have contributed to decreased mortality. Perhaps more exciting are recent results suggesting that, at least for some individuals, the development of cancer may be prevented through interruption of the progression of neoplastic growth toward invasive malignancy.

Box 122-1. Leading Sites of Estimated Cancer Incidence and Mortality for 1999

Incidence	Mortality
Prostate	Lung
Breast	Colorectal
Lung	Breast
Colorectal	Prostate
Bladder	Pancreas

From Landix SH, Murray T, Bolden S, et al: Cancer statistics, 1999, *CA Cancer J Clin* 49:8-31, 1999.

PREVENTION

Prevention of cancer-related mortality has been a health care priority for the United States for a majority of the twentieth century. The deceptive simplicity of neoplastic growth clouded initial progress. Early tools in the preventive armamentarium consisted largely of antineoplastic therapies. Unfortunately, this tertiary prevention led to declines in cancer-related morbidity and mortality for only a minority of malignancies. Lack of curative therapies for the majority of cancers and a limited knowledge base precluded effective use of other preventive approaches.

We now understand that cancer is not a single target at which preventive strategies can be aimed. Rather, cancer is the collective term for many distinct neoplasms with different etiologies, risk factors, and behavioral characteristics. Carcinogenesis is a multistep process with long periods of latency for individual steps. This complicates but does not preclude effective preventive programs. There are several levels in the ontogeny of an invasive neoplasm at which specific interventions may prevent subsequent morbidity and mortality. An improved understanding of the process of carcinogenesis has allowed better identification of high-risk groups and has led to enthusiasm for primary and secondary preventive strategies.

Primary preventive strategies seek to interrupt neoplastic development before a malignant growth is established. This can be accomplished through modification of patient characteristics or environmental factors that have been identified through epidemiologic studies as being associated with increased cancer risk. Although risk factors such as age and gender are not amenable to modification, other risk factors such as tobacco use are believed to play a causative role in the transformation of a normal host cell to a neoplastic clone. Elimination of such causative factors can have a major impact on cancer incidence and mortality. Alternatively, neoplastic development could be reversed or inhibited through chemoprevention. A number of chemical agents, both naturally occurring and pharmaceutically engineered, have been shown to inhibit carcinogenesis in experimental systems. Recent clinical trials, such as the Tamoxifen Prevention Trial conducted by the National Surgical Breast and Bowel Project (NSABP), have documented reduction in short-term breast cancer incidence through chemoprevention. Whether the improvement in incidence rates, seen in the time interval over which the chemoprevention trials have been conducted, will translate into improved cancer-related mortality in the long term is unclear.

High-risk Groups

Successful preventive interventions require that factors associated with an increased risk of developing cancer can be defined and individuals or groups who possess these high-risk characteristics and behaviors can be identified prior to the diagnosis of cancer. Furthermore, the identified risk factors must be amenable to modification such that for individual patients the development of a particular cancer is delayed or prevented. It has been estimated that between 75% and 80% of cancers in the United States could be avoided through alterations in behavior.[2] Box 122-2 summarizes the categories of factors that are associated with enhanced cancer risk.

Tobacco. Tobacco is responsible for more cancer-related deaths than any other single risk factor and accounts for nearly one third of all cancer deaths. Box 122-3 underscores the impact of tobacco use on cancer incidence. Clearly, tobacco use is a high-risk behavior and its elimination would have a profound impact on cancer-related mortality in the United States. For example, the incidence of lung cancer would decline by approximately 90%, with an estimated 25% reduction in overall cancer mortality if smoking alone were completely eradicated. Elimination of other forms of tobacco use would further decrease cancer incidence and mortality.

Box 122-2. Risk Factors Associated With Cancer Mortality

Tobacco
Diet
Alcohol
Radiation exposure
  Ultraviolet
  Ionizing
Chemical exposure
  Drugs
  Pollution
  Occupational
Reproductive factors
Infections
Genetic predisposition

Box 122-3. Tobacco-related Cancers

Lung
Oral cavity
Larynx
Esophagus
Pancreas
Kidney
Bladder
Uterine cervix

Box 122-4. Tobacco Cessation Recommendations

1. Physicians should provide cessation advice to all smokers during each encounter.
2. Additional supportive interventions (e.g., follow-up telephone calls, self-educational materials) add to effectiveness but are less cost-effective.
3. The efficacy of intervention is high in high-risk situations such as pregnancy and ischemic heart disease.
4. Nicotine-replacement products add to effectiveness, particularly in those with higher levels of nicotine dependence.
5. Behavioral modification techniques such as aversion therapy and sensory deprivation are not supported by the data.
6. Adjunctive pharmacologic measures might include bupropion initiated prior to planned smoking cessation.
7. Recommendations on non–smoking tobacco cessation is limited by scant data.

There would be additional health benefits in the form of decreased incidence of cardiovascular and respiratory disease.

Numerous clinical trials have demonstrated that physicians are a powerful force in shaping the behavior of individual patients. Physician-based smoking cessation trials have repeatedly demonstrated that *any* intervention can effectively reduce tobacco use by smoking patients. A systematic review of 188 randomized controlled trials by Law and Tang demonstrated a modest but highly cost-effective benefit of a single episode of advice and encouragement on smoking cessation from a physician.[9] Brief advice by a physician to quit smoking can lead to sustained abstinence (at 1 year) for an estimated 2% of patients. Although this degree of efficacy may not seem worth the bother to individual physicians, the time involved is usually less than 5 minutes and the public health impact is significant. Additional supportive measures such as follow-up letters or visits increase efficacy to a variable extent. However, when these simple interventions are offered to populations with enhanced risk, such as pregnant women or patients with ischemic heart disease, there is a dramatic impact on efficacy. While the efficacy of smoking cessation advice increases an impressive fourfold for pregnant women, following a myocardial infarction (MI) efficacy can be as high as 35%. It is unclear whether efficacy is maintained when advice and encouragement are provided by health care providers other than the physician. Nurses in health promotion clinics have variable results, but advice, counseling, and follow-up provided by dental hygienists to those using chewing tobacco were significantly more effective than routine care.[14] Behavior modification therapy, such as relaxation or visualization techniques or avoidance of stimuli that trigger the urge to smoke, was no more effective than simple advice. Nicotine replacement can be an important adjunct for nicotine-dependent smokers who seek help in stopping. Nicotine replacement products are available as nasal spray, transdermal patch, and gum. These pharmacologic aids may enhance sustained abstinence for 13% of smokers. Finally, a recently reported randomized placebo controlled trial of sustained-release bupropion demonstrated improved 1-year abstinence rates over control, documented with carbon monoxide measurements.[6] The effect was dose responsive and statistically significant at the higher doses used (300 mg and 150 mg daily). At 1-year following intervention, approximately one fifth of the bupropion-treated groups maintained abstinence, whereas only 12.4% in the placebo group were able to remain smoke-free. Side effects of the bupropion were minimal. One interesting side effect was reduced weight gain, particularly at higher doses, with those in the 300-mg group gaining an average of 1.5 kg.

Recommendations for tobacco cessation are listed in Box 122-4.

Diet. There is a substantial body of evidence supporting the role of diet in both the development and inhibition of neoplastic growth. The evidence linking factors in the human diet to neoplastic growth is largely derived from epidemiologic studies conducted either at the population level or through specific cohort or case-control studies. The interpretation of such epidemiologic data is complicated by numerous factors. Retrospective epidemiologic studies attempting to link nutrient intake to risk of subsequent cancer suffer from recall bias, inaccurate knowledge of the composition of prepared foods, and confounding variables such as physical activity. In addition, the culprit in carcinogenesis may well be the intake of foodstuffs many years prior to a particular study. Finally, the role of genetic polymorphisms that may moderate the effects of particular risk factors for individuals is only beginning to be understood. Inherited changes in enzymes known to detoxify carcinogenic metabolites may enhance cancer risk when individuals are exposed to a carcinogen in the presence or absence of another factor. For example, smokers for whom the carcinogen detoxifying enzyme GSTM1 is genetically deleted appear to have an increased

Box 122-5. Nutrient Categories

Macronutrients	Micronutrients
Carbohydrates	Vitamins
Proteins	Minerals
Fiber	Trace elements
Fat	

risk of developing cancer only when low plasma concentrations of micronutrients such as α-tocopherol and specific carotenoids are also present.

The human diet is composed of macronutrients and micronutrients, as defined in Box 122-5. Both deficiencies and excesses of these elements within the diet appear to contribute to the development of specific malignancies. Epidemiologic studies have identified populations with high calorie and fat intake and low consumption of fiber, fruit, and vegetables, as well as certain micronutrients, in which there is an increased risk of developing a number of malignancies. How this risk should be interpreted for individual patients is unclear. Whether dietary modification for individual patients will alter neoplastic development is controversial. Kritchevsky, in a review of cancer and diet, emphasizes that a high-fiber diet may not be equivalent to a low-fiber diet supplement with fiber.[7] Vitamin and mineral supplementation may be complicated by unexpected toxicities and may not decrease cancer risk as well as adoption of a diet containing foods rich in these same vitamins and minerals. The increased incidence of lung cancer and lung and cardiovascular deaths among the 18,314 smokers and asbestos-exposed workers in the CARET study of β-carotene and vitamin A supplementation highlights the need for caution regarding dietary supplementation.[16]

A number of dietary intervention trials designed to address the impact of dietary modifications on neoplastic development and growth are currently underway. The number of these trials is limited by the large number of patients required to achieve statistically reliable results and the long duration between neoplastic incitement and clinically detectable cancer. Several studies have used intermediate markers of neoplastic transformation, such as colonic polyp formation or indicators of proliferative activity within target tissues, as a means of restricting study length. Although colonic polyps are established neoplastic precursors, the import of increased proliferative activity for malignant transformation in other tissues is not clearly established. There is currently a large research effort aimed at the identification and validation of intermediate markers of cancerous growth. An alternative approach is to modify the diet of patients diagnosed with cancer who are at high risk of recurrence or a second primary cancer. The ongoing Women's Intervention Nutrition Study (WINS), which addresses the impact of low-fat diet as an adjuvant to hormonal or chemotherapy for women with early-stage breast cancer, is one example.

Fat. The role of fat and fiber intake in carcinogenesis has been widely studied. Clinical studies have demonstrated an association between excessive consumption of fat and calories and cancers of the breast, colon, prostate, ovary, endometrium, kidney, and pancreas. International epidemiologic studies have identified strong associations between per capita fat intake and age-adjusted rates for specific cancers. The prevalence of breast, colon, and prostate cancers is much higher in the Western world than in countries such as Japan. The Western world derives approximately 35% to 40% of its calories from fat, whereas the amount of fat consumed in the Japanese diet is more limited. Interestingly, the incidence of breast cancer has risen in Japan as fat consumption has risen from about 10% of the caloric intake in the 1950s to the current 25%.

The increased risk of these cancers may not be uniform for all types and amounts of fat consumed. The components of a high-fat diet that is causally related to increased cancer risk clearly remain to be identified. It is known that the incidence of colorectal, breast, prostate, pancreatic, and possibly lung cancers increases directly in proportion to the amount of meat, particularly red and processed meat, consumed. Esophageal cancer is increased by ingestion of barbecued meat. Whereas diets rich in omega-3 fatty acids have been shown to retard tumor development in animal models, those relatively rich in omega-6 fatty acids enhance tumor development.

The mechanism by which dietary fat effects carcinogenesis is unclear. The heterocyclic amines present in cooked meat may be partially responsible for the carcinogenic effect. Omega-3 fatty acids, abundant in fish products, interfere with the inflammatory response through competitive inhibition of the cyclooxygenase pathway in prostaglandin formation. Overexpression of the gene for inducible cyclooxygenase was identified as an early critical step in colon carcinogenesis.[5] In addition, dietary fat may enhance the development of colon cancer by increasing the concentration of bile salts within the colon. Bile acids alter the metabolic activity of microbial flora within the colon such that the colonic mucosa is increasingly exposed to weakly carcinogenic bile acid metabolites. Mechanisms of mutagenesis in other malignancies are less well defined.

Whether dietary alteration has the potential to abrogate malignant growth remains controversial. The prospective Nurses' Health Study failed to document a decline in breast cancer risk for 88,795 women when the lowest quintile was compared with highest quintile for intake of total, polyunsaturated, or monounsaturated fat. More optimistically, the Lyon Diet Heart Study of 605 patients with coronary heart disease, who were randomized to a Mediterranean-type diet or a control diet (approximating a Step 1 American Heart Association prudent diet), demonstrated a statistically significant 65% reduction in cancer incidence for those on the Mediterranean-type diet during 4 years of follow-up.[3] The diet consisted of higher levels of bread, cereals, fresh fruit and vegetables, legumes, and fish. The diet prescribed fewer delicatessen foods, less meat, and no butter and cream, which were to be replaced with an experimental canola oil–based margarine rich in oleic and α-linolenic acids. Compliance with this α-linolenic acid–rich diet was excellent.

Fiber. Numerous case-control and retrospective studies have suggested a link between a low-fiber diet and subsequent development of colorectal cancers. It is hypothesized that a high-fiber diet may lower the risk of colon cancer by increasing fecal bulk and diluting the concentration of carcinogens within the colon, thereby limiting the exposure of colonic mucosa to potential mutagens. However, prospective trials have failed to demonstrate a protective effect of dietary fiber against the development of colorectal cancer or adenomas. The largest prospective trial to address this, the Nurses' Health Study, showed no association between dietary fiber intake and colorectal risk in 88,757 women, in the context of a Western diet.

Fruits and Vegetables. Fruits and vegetables are almost invariably protective for the major cancers. Conjecture regarding the micronutrients responsible for this beneficial effect has been extensive. The antioxidant vitamins (vitamin A and related compounds such as β-carotene, as well as vitamins C and E) are prominent components of many fruits and vegetables. The antioxidant vitamins function as scavengers for DNA-damaging, mutagenic oxygen free radicals. Epidemiologic studies suggest that diets deficient in vitamins A, C, and D have been associated with increased cancer risk, whereas those diets composed of foods rich in vitamin A, C, and E are associated with decreased cancer incidence.

Vitamin A is essential for the normal growth and development of epithelial tissue. A deficiency of this important vitamin can increase the susceptibility of normal tissues to mutagens. Dietary deficiency of vitamin A has been implicated in the development of cancers of the lung, breast, oropharynx, stomach, bladder, prostate, and colon. Squamous tissues deficient in vitamin A exhibit metaplastic differentiation that can be reversed by administration of vitamin A and related compounds. There is evidence to suggest that diets rich in vitamin A and related compounds not only diminish the risk but are also protective against the development of certain cancers. While vitamin C appears to inhibit the formation of carcinogenic nitrosamines that have been associated with the development of gastric cancer, vitamin E inhibits mutagenesis and cell transformation mainly through its antioxidant function. Nonetheless, the role of vitamins C and E in neoplastic development remains particularly unclear. Although vitamins C and E function as antioxidants, there is little evidence to support any direct role for these vitamins in the inhibition or reversal of neoplastic growth and development.

Among the many minerals required for normal tissue development, calcium and selenium have received the most attention with regard to carcinogenesis. There are laboratory as well as preliminary clinical data to support a role for calcium deficiency in the development of colon cancer. Results of the numerous studies focusing on the role of dietary selenium are contradictory and inconclusive, but consensus on its beneficial effects is building. Data on other micronutrients, such as molybdenum and zinc, are scant, and further investigations are necessary.

Several recent studies of dietary supplementation highlight the importance of clinical trials in defining benefit.[11] Both the CARET (β-carotene and retinol) and the α-tocopheral, β-carotene trials suggest that pharmacologic doses of β-carotene *increase* the risk of lung cancer among smokers or those with asbestos exposure. β-Carotene, vitamin C, and vitamin E were also unable to prevent the development of colorectal adenomas in a placebo-controlled trial of 864 patients. A large, four-arm clinical trial of multiple dietary supplements in 30,000 subjects in Linxian, China, demonstrated no significant effect on cancer incidence. However, those subjects who received treatment with a combination of selenium, β-carotene, and α-tocopherol enjoyed statistically significantly lower total and gastric cancer-specific mortality rates. A notable study of selenium supplementation in 1312 patients was clearly unable to protect against the recurrent development of basal and squamous cell carcinomas in the skin. Nonetheless, secondary end point analyses reveal a statistically compelling reduction in prostate, lung, and colon cancers, as well as significant reductions in total cancer mortality. On the other hand, a nonsignificant increase was noted in leukemias/lymphomas as well as breast and bladder cancers.

Alcohol. The chronic consumption of alcohol is strongly associated with cancers of the oropharynx, larynx, and esophagus. The risk of these cancers is greatly magnified by concomitant use of both alcohol and tobacco. Nonetheless, there is a dose-response relationship between alcohol consumption and the development of oral and esophageal cancers that is independent of concomitant tobacco use. In addition, there is some evidence—although not conclusive—that cancers of the liver, stomach, pancreas, colon, and breast are also associated with increased alcohol consumption. The risk of moderate or occasional alcoholic intake for cancer development is not well established. The mechanism through which alcohol influences carcinogenesis is currently under investigation. Animal studies have failed to identify pure ethanol as a carcinogen. Alcohol may exert its influence through alterations in cellular metabolism and permeability that permit carcinogenic disruption of normal cellular behavior by other chemical substances. Alternatively, alcohol consumption may contribute to malnutrition and increase consumption of other substances associated with enhanced cancer risk.

Dietary Recommendations. Many authorities believe that the complexity of the human diet with too many undefined interactions with other factors such as physical activity precludes firm dietary recommendations for individual patients. Other authorities such as the American Cancer Society (ACS), the National Research Council, and the National Cancer Institute (NCI) recommend general dietary guidelines for dietary components with sufficient data. The NCI recommends a diet that includes five or more servings of fruits and vegetables per day. Specific dietary instructions must be individualized, with consideration to comorbid illnesses and conditions. Notably most authorities that offer dietary guidelines include limitation of alcohol intake.

Radiation Exposure. Radiation comes in a variety of forms and energies. Nearly all tissues within the body are susceptible to its carcinogenic effects. It is an omnipresent risk factor within the environment. Background radiation provides the largest source of exposure for the general population. Light emitted from the sun contains a broad spectrum of radiation energies. The ultraviolet portion of these energies is a major risk factor for the development of basal and squamous cell carcinomas of the skin, as well as melanoma. Ultraviolet radiation is thought to be directly carcinogenic, and risk of subsequent malignancy is directly proportional to received dose. The risk of developing a skin cancer, particularly melanoma, is highest in populations who have the highest exposure by virtue of geographic latitude and skin type. The worldwide incidence of melanoma increases with increasing proximity to the equator. Skin cancers occur most frequently on those areas of the body with the greatest exposure to sunlight. In addition, there are genetically determined differences in susceptibility in ultraviolet radiation. Patients with conditions such as xeroderma pigmentosum are exquisitely sensitive to sunlight-induced skin damage, and are at very high risk of developing skin cancer.

Ionizing radiation is also thought to be directly mutagenic. Much of the data regarding the role of ionizing radiation in neoplastic development is derived from studies of individuals exposed to the radiation fallout of the atomic bomb and those receiving medical x-rays for either diagnostic or therapeutic purposes. These populations generally have exposure in excess of 50 Gy and clearly have an increased risk of leukemias and lung and breast cancers. There is also an increased incidence of thyroid and bone cancers within the field of radiation in some studies. Age at the time of exposure appears to be an important ameliorating factor, since the latency period for radiation-induced cancers is often years to decades.

Although exposure to ultraviolet radiation and the consequent risk of skin cancers can be minimized through the use of protective clothing and sunscreens, the largest source of radiation exposure is from the general background. This exposure is not only difficult to quantify and almost impossible to limit, it is likely to increase with progressive deterioration of the atmospheric ozone layer. However, exposure to medical and dental radiation, the second largest source of radiation exposure, can be limited. Physicians should demonstrate restraint in the use of diagnostic and therapeutic radiation, particularly in patients who are young, who are pregnant, or who have benign medical conditions. The cumulative exposure to medical radiation can be monitored by carefully recording within a patient's medical record all diagnostic radiographic studies as well as the total dose and target of any therapeutic radiation administered. The careful recording of radiation exposure as routinely practiced by radiation oncologists might serve as a paradigm for primary care physicians as a mechanism for monitoring individual patient exposures.

Chemical Exposure. The number of chemicals with carcinogenic potential seems to be endless. The daily exposure of individual patients to carcinogenic chemicals is difficult to accurately assess given the number and variety of chemicals present in the air, water, and food. Exposures occur within the home as well as through recreational and occupational activities. Certain chemicals have well-documented associations with human neoplasms (Table 122-1). In addition, some medical therapies are also closely linked with increased risk of subsequent cancer. Alkylating agents, such as chlorambucil, cyclophosphamide, and melphalan, were originally developed for use in antineoplastic regimens. These agents are associated with increased risk of subsequent malignancies when used to treat patients with collagen vascular diseases such as rheumatoid arthritis as well as those with cancers.

Hormonal therapy with estrogens or androgens has also led to increases in the incidence of particular malignancies. The use of androgens in male athletes has been associated with increased risk of liver cancers. In women the use of exogenous estrogens has been associated with an increased risk of endometrial and breast cancers. Use of diethylstilbestrol (DES) in pregnant women is associated with the development of vaginal clear cell adenocarcinoma in female offspring. Tamoxifen, a selective estrogen receptor modifier used in the treatment—and, most recently, prevention—of breast cancer, stimulates endometrial proliferation that contributes to an increased risk of endometrial cancer.

Table 122-1. Chemically Induced Tumors

Chemical	Tumor site
Arsenic	Lung, skin
Asbestos	Lung
Bis (chloromethyl) ether	Lung
Chromium	Lung
Nickel	Lung, nasopharynx
Betel nut	Oropharynx
Isopropyl alcohol	Nasopharynx
Cutting oils	Skin
Soot, coal, tar	Skin
Nitrosamines	Stomach
Aflatoxin B_1	Liver
Vinyl chloride	Liver, bladder
Aromatic amines	Bladder
Benzene	Leukemia
Radiopharmaceuticals	Liver, bone

The use of immunosuppressive therapy following organ transplantation is also associated with a dramatic increase in the incidence of lymphoma.

The potential neoplastic risk of any proposed medical therapy must be clearly understood and weighted carefully against the expected benefit. In a fashion similar to documentation for radiation exposures, patients who receive treatment with medications, such as alkylating agents and hormones, that carry an increase risk of subsequent malignancy should have the dose and duration of treatment carefully monitored in the medical record. Prominent labeling of individual patient charts can facilitate a monitoring program. The risks and benefits of these potentially carcinogenic therapies should be reviewed periodically in any patient who receives treatment for prolonged periods.

Exposure to occupational and industrial carcinogens can be minimized by the use of equipment such as gloves, protective clothing, and masks in appropriate situations. Physicians should encourage the use of such protective gear. However, often the hazards of chemical substances are unknown or patients are unaware of the specific exposures they have experienced. Recent legislation requiring employers to inform workers of potentially hazardous substances in the workplace may improve patient's cognizance of exposures. This in turn might lead to a better understanding of the role some chemical substances play in carcinogenesis in humans. Discussion of the occupational environment of individual patients and documentation of reported exposures within the medical record may serve several purposes. The patient may not be aware of the risk inherent in agents that are currently known to have carcinogenic potential and therefore may not adequately employ protective equipment. Secondly, documentation of exposures may allow associations to be identified at a future date.

Infectious agents play an important role in neoplastic development worldwide. There are well-documented associations between a number of agents and specific cancers (Table 122-2). The contribution of infectious agents to cancer

Table 122-2. Cancers Associated With Infectious Agents

Infectious agent	Neoplasm
Human immunodeficiency virus	Lymphoma, Kaposi's sarcoma
Human T-cell lymphotrophic virus	T-cell lymphoma/leukemia
Human papillomaviruses	Anogenital carcinoma
Herpes simplex virus VIII	Kaposi's sarcoma
Herpes simplex virus II	Cervical cancer
Epstein-Barr virus	Nasopharyngeal cancer, African Burkitt's lymphoma
Hepatitis B	Hepatocellular cancer
H. pylori	Gastric cancer, MALT lymphoma

morbidity and mortality within the United States is more limited. Nonetheless, the prevalence of certain infectious agents, particularly herpes simplex II (HSV II), hepatitis B virus, and the human immunodeficiency virus (HIV), mandates heightened public awareness of the role of these agents in neoplastic development. In addition, the recent association of *Helicobacter pylori* infection and subsequent gastric cancer may allow significant reduction in gastric cancer incidence through aggressive antibiotic therapy. *H. pylori* gastric infection has been strongly linked to mucosa-associated lymphoid tissue (MALT) neoplasms. Eradication of *H. pylori* leads to histologic regression of early MALT lymphoma. Attempts to eradicate *H. pylori* are underway in China, where gastric cancer is the second most common malignancy.

Alterations in sexual behavior might well lead to diminished risk for those cancers that are associated with sexually transmitted infectious agents such as HSV II and HIV. Patients who engage in unprotected sexual activities with multiple partners are at particularly high risk of becoming infected. Physicians should ask about sexual practices and advise patients of the associated risks of infection and subsequent malignancy. This is particularly important in those patients who have no current evidence of infection with these agents. Patients who do manifest evidence of infection should receive regular follow-up, with attention to evaluating the presence of neoplastic processes.

Patients with exposure to blood-borne agents should be encouraged to take appropriate precautions. Those individuals with occupational exposures to blood and body fluids should be advised to routinely employ protective gear. Intravenous drug users should be discouraged from sharing hypodermic needles. Finally, the hepatitis B vaccine should be offered to all individuals at high risk of exposure to this infectious agent.

SCREENING

Early detection of cancers through screening provides secondary prevention of cancer-related mortality. It is estimated that successful implementation of screening programs could reduce the mortality of specific cancers by 3% to 60%.[15] Screening for breast and cervical cancers alone could reduce overall cancer mortality by 3%, for an equivalent of nearly 15,000 lives saved per year. The potential public health impact of early diagnosis and detection of malignancy is clear. Yet, not all malignancies are amenable to screening programs. Although lung cancer is the leading cause of cancer-related mortality in the United States, no screening program has proven to be effective for reduction of lung cancer mortality. Indeed, for many cancers, the utility of secondary prevention is hampered by the lack of adequately sensitive and specific screening tests as well as the low prevalence of cancers at individual primary sites. Even for those malignancies that yield to screening programs, the divergent guidelines and recommendations of professional bodies such as the ACS and the NCI can be confusing. Finally, noncompliance by both patients and physicians further compromises the efficacy of available screening tests.

Box 122-6. Requirements for Effective Cancer Screening Programs

1. Screening test/procedure with adequate sensitivity, specificity, and positive predictive value to detect early disease
2. Effective therapy for early-stage disease
3. High degree of patient acceptability
4. Reasonable cost
5. Continued efficacy over time

Screening Program Development

The impetus for the development of cancer screening programs and early detection efforts is the direct correlation between the extent of disease (or stage) at diagnosis and cancer-related mortality. Patients diagnosed with early stages of cancer have improved survival and decreased mortality over those patients diagnosed with more advanced stages of disease. Thus the fundamental goal of screening is to reduce cancer-related mortality through early detection and diagnosis. However, for a screening program to successfully reduce mortality, several prerequisites must be fulfilled (Box 122-6). Mammography and cervical cytologic sampling are examples of moderately priced screening tests with high patient acceptability that can identify asymptomatic individuals within a population who have a higher probability of having a particular cancer than the population as a whole. Unfortunately, there are many common malignancies such as ovarian cancer for which screening tests are overly sensitive and inadequately specific, with a positive predictive value too low for use in the general public. Other cancers, such as leukemia with no identifiable localized phase, elude early detection.

The cancer screening protocols advocated by professional agencies are based on demonstration of improved outcomes over what would be expected without screening. It is important to note that the definition of a *better outcome* underlies the divergence in cancer screening recommendations and guidelines by these well-respected agencies. A reduction in mortality in a screened population over that of an unscreened population, as demonstrated in a randomized clinical trial, provides the strongest evidence of improved outcome and establishes the efficacy of a screening technique. Currently, evidence of this strength only exists for breast and colon cancer. Other measures of improved

Table 122-3. Evidence of Benefit for Cancer Screening Strategies

Measures of improved outcome	Advantages	Disadvantages
Decreased mortality	The academic standard, when demonstrated in randomized trials	Requires long follow-up; costly
Stage shift	Stage closely correlates with mortality	Length bias (may be detecting disease with no clinical consequence)
Increased survival	Shortens duration of study necessary	Length bias: Lead-time bias (earlier detection allows survival to appear longer even if therapy is ineffective)
Increased detection	Often the first evidence of efficacy of a screening tool	Length bias

outcome, such as a shift to earlier stage at diagnosis, an increase in survival, and an increase in detection rates, serve only as flawed substitutes for the gold standard of mortality reduction. These alternative measures suffer from inherent biases (Table 122-3), minimized by randomized clinical trials using mortality reduction as a primary end point. However, randomized clinical screening trials are not feasible for every malignancy and screening procedure. The number of patients required to perform randomized studies that will generate statistically and clinically significant results is prohibitive except for the three or four most common malignancies. For example, a screening study designed to detect a 25% reduction in mortality from prostate cancer would require >100,000 participants. A screening study of the same statistical design in testicular cancer would require over 6.5 million participants.[17] Furthermore, a screening study designed to detect mortality differences often requires many years of follow-up with the inherent complexity and expense of long-term follow-up.

Consequently, cancer screening recommendations based only on those screening protocols that manifest mortality reduction in randomized trials would abrogate all efforts at early detection through public education and all physical examinations on asymptomatic individuals. Self-examinations of the skin, testes, and breasts also would be eliminated by this strict approach. However, many authorities agree that this strict approach is not warranted for all screening techniques, in view of the fact that randomized clinical trials are not feasible for every malignancy. Although invasive or expensive screening strategies should be supported by the strongest possible evidence, the evidence required to document the efficacy of public education or self-examinations need not be as stringent.

Screening Methods

There is a broad array of methods that can be employed to enhance early detection of cancers. The spectrum includes public education to heighten awareness of malignancies and increase familiarity with early warning signs (Box 122-7), as well as risk assessment, health surveys, instruction in self-examination, physician examination, and mass screening. The vast majority of these methods are directly within the purview of the primary care physician. However, the extent of screening activity varies widely among physicians' practices. Those with a systematic approach to the preventive services are often the most successful at achieving and maintaining high levels of screening. Box 122-8 outlines the components of a successful practice-based implementation of cancer screening.

Box 122-7. CAUTION: Cancer's Warning Signals

Change in bowel or bladder habit
A sore that does not heal
Unusual bleeding or discharge
Thickening or lump in breast or elsewhere
Indigestion or difficulty in swallowing
Obvious change in wart or mole
Nagging cough or hoarseness

Box 122-8. Implementation of Office-based Cancer Screening Program

1. Determine level of current practice screening activity
2. Set measurable screening goals
3. Develop a comprehensive plan to achieve and maintain goals
4. Encourage staff training and active participation in screening activities
5. Ensure that office systems, design, and organization facilitate screening
6. Develop state-of-the-art skills in early detection and screening techniques
7. Develop state-of-the-art counseling and communication skills
8. Use reminder systems to ensure that patients at risk are identified, screened, and followed
9. Exploit every opportunity to perform screening and prevention
10. Minimize cost barriers for patients whenever possible

Early Detection Guidelines

The ACS was among the first professional medical organizations to advocate screening protocols. Numerous other groups such as the American Medical Association, the

Table 122-4. Cancer Screening Recommendations/Guidelines of the American Cancer Society and the National Cancer Institute

Cancer site	Gender and age	ACS recommendations	NCI guidelines
Breast	Women 20-39	Clinical breast examination every 3 years and monthly breast self-examination	
	Women 40+	Screening mammography yearly with clinical breast examination and monthly breast self-examination	Screening mammography on a regular basis every 1-2 years; a clinical breast examination should be included as part of routine health care
Colorectal	50+	FOBT annually with a flexible sigmoidoscopy and DRE every 5 yrs OR Colonoscopy with DRE every 10 years OR Double contrast BE with DRE every 5-10 years	FOBT annually or biennially up to age 80; sigmoidoscopy may decrease colorectal mortality; data are insufficient to recommend an interval
Prostate	Men 50+	DRE and PSA annually; information should be provided to patients regarding risks/benefits of intervention	
Uterine cervix	Women 18+ or sexually active	Pap test and pelvic examination every 1 year; after ≥3 consecutive, satisfactory normal annual examinations, the Pap can be performed less frequently at the discretion of the physician	Regular screening with Pap tests
Skin	Adults	Practice skin self-examination regularly; periodic total skin examination	
Oropharynx	Adults		
Testicle	Males 18+	Periodic self-examination; clinical testicular examination as part of periodic health examination	

ACS, American Cancer Society; *NCI*, National Cancer Institute; *FOBT*, fecal occult blood testing; *DRE*, digital rectal examination; *BE*, barium enema; *PSA*, prostate-specific antigen.

American College of Obstetricians and Gynecologists, and the American College of Radiology have promulgated recommendations or guidelines for screening of one or more malignancies. In 1987, the NCI convened representatives from many of these and similar organizations with the goal of establishing working guidelines for early cancer detection based on the best available statistical and clinical evidence. The NCI sought to establish working guidelines rather than firm recommendations in recognition of the fact that much of the available data was imperfect, with guidelines subject to change as new evidence develops. In addition, physicians might well adjust screening programs appropriately for individual patient circumstances that would include family and personal history as well as concomitant medical illnesses.

The NCI effort led to working guidelines for the early detection of cancers of the skin, oropharynx, breast, colon, rectum, cervix, prostate, and testes. Data for early detection of other malignancies were insufficient to support guidelines. These guidelines, compared with those of the ACS, are presented in Table 122-4. The individual organ sites are discussed below.

Breast Cancer. The landmark study opened in 1963 by the Health Insurance Plan of New York (HIP) demonstrated a statistically significant mortality reduction following annual screening mammography and clinical breast examination for women ages 40 to 64. In the years since the inception of the HIP trial, numerous controlled trials have confirmed the benefit of screening mammography for women older than 50 years of age.[2] Until recently, only the HIP study has provided direct evidence of benefit (mortality reduction) for screening mammography in women 40 to 49 years of age. This paucity of evidence supporting a direct benefit for younger women persisted despite population surveillance data (SEER) demonstrating a decline in breast cancer mortality in the face of rising incidence for women under age 50. Consequently there has been persistent controversy over screening mammography guidelines. The controversy was fueled in late 1993 when the NCI dropped its guideline for screening mammography in women ages 40 to 49 after several published trials failed to demonstrate benefit for women of this age group. However, evidence of benefit from screening mammography for women in their forties has emerged with longer follow-up of previously completed trials. The current NCI guidelines reflect the updated trial results.

Women at increased risk for breast cancer through an inherited predisposition as a result of one or more germline mutations in BRCA1 or BRCA2 deserve special consideration with regard to cancer screening. The Cancer Genetics Studies Consortium points out that the benefit of cancer surveillance and other measures to reduce inherent risk in individuals who possess cancer-predisposing mutations is presumptive at best.[1] Nonetheless, monthly self-examination beginning in early adulthood and annual or semiannual physician examinations in conjunction with annual mammography beginning at age 25 to 35 are suggested recommendations for this population whose lifetime risk of breast cancer may exceed 85%.

Colorectal Cancer. Colorectal cancer affecting both men and women is the second leading cause of cancer-related deaths in the United States. Both incidence and mortality are decreasing. Although the recommendations of the ACS are in concert with the guidelines of the NCI, several agencies, such as the U.S. Preventive Services Task Force, have found insufficient evidence to support firm recommendations. Virtually all screening studies using any of these modalities, either singly or in combination, have demonstrated a shift to earlier stage at diagnosis as well as an increase in survival. Yet, despite a wealth of indirect evidence supporting screening for colon cancer, direct evidence of benefit in the form of a mortality reduction was lacking until the Minnesota Colon Cancer Control Study demonstrated a 33% decrease in mortality following annual fecal occult blood testing (FOBT) in a randomized study in over 46,000 volunteers.[13] The paucity of direct evidence has prompted alternative approaches to the formulation of screening recommendations for colon cancer. Based on a mathematical model of 11 possible colon cancer screening strategies that incorporates the natural history of the disease, individual screening test performance, and costs associated with the individual strategies, Eddy suggests that annual FOBT and flexible sigmoidoscopy every 5 years might reduce mortality by 40% in individuals of average risk.[4] Notably, the estimated reduction in mortality is even greater when colonoscopy or barium enemas are substituted for flexible sigmoidoscopy in the screening strategy but are more costly and less well tolerated by patients. Other investigators confirm that the benefits of colonoscopy in detecting treatable neoplasms are compromised by the costs of the procedure. A cost-effectiveness model for colon cancer screening created by Lieberman illustrates the compromises required during selection of appropriate screening strategies for individual patients. In his model, FOBT alone was clearly the most cost-effective, but with fewer cancer deaths prevented than other strategies. Flexible sigmoidoscopy in conjunction with FOBT increases the rate of cancer prevention, but one-time colonoscopy (e.g., age 60) had the greatest impact on colorectal cancer mortality.[10]

Individuals with cancer-predisposing germline mutations, such as with hereditary nonpolyposis colorectal cancer, should undergo colonoscopy every 1 to 3 years beginning at age 25 years. In addition, endometrial cancer screening is also recommended. Although individuals who possess BRCA1 mutations are possibly at increased risk of colorectal cancer, no special screening strategies are recommended at this time.

Prostate Cancer. Screening and early detection of prostate cancer remain very controversial. To date, no randomized controlled studies have demonstrated prostate cancer mortality reduction for any test or procedure, including digital rectal examination (DRE). Consequently, many organizations decline to recommend any specific prostate screening strategies. The NCI makes no recommendations for screening based on the profound lack of evidence to establish prostate cancer–specific mortality reduction with DRE, transrectal ultrasound (TRUS), or serum markers (i.e., prostate-specific antigen [PSA]). However, several, although not all, studies have suggested improved survival and a shift to earlier stage at diagnosis for men diagnosed with prostate cancer following annual DRE. Nonetheless, some experts feel that the DRE alone is too insensitive to significantly alter prostate cancer mortality. The ACS has included PSA screening in its recommendations for early cancer detection. Results from the National Prostate Cancer Detection Project, conducted by the ACS on over 2400 men undergoing DRE, PSA, and TRUS screening, have suggested that DRE used in combination with PSA screening may be more cost-effective than DRE alone. The cost of DRE as the only screening technique rose significantly when DRE was not performed by a highly skilled examiner such as a urologist.[12] Interestingly, the ACS recommends that prostate cancer screening only be performed on men who have at least a 10-year life-expectancy. The ACS further recommends that younger African-American men and those at increased risk with two or more affected first-degree relatives also undergo regular screening.

Cancer of the Cervix. The guidelines and recommendations for early detection of cervical cancer of the various professional organizations are generally concordant. The NCI notes that strong evidence from case-controlled and cohort studies suggests a decline in mortality following regular screening with Pap tests. However, the ACS suggests that the recommendation for pelvic examination be similar to the recommendation for Pap testing (i.e., a pelvic examination should be performed with Pap testing every 1 to 3 years for women between the ages of 18 and 40). In addition, the ACS recommends that yearly pelvic examinations be performed on women over the age of 40. The U.S. Preventive Services Task Force has suggested that Pap testing may be discontinued at 65 if previous examinations have been consistently normal.

Although direct evidence of mortality reduction is lacking, several large studies in Sweden, Finland, the United States, and Canada have demonstrated reductions in cervical cancer incidence and mortality rates following initiation of screening programs.[1a,7a,15a,16a] In Canada, the reduction in mortality correlated with the intensity of screening. Cost-sensitive scrutiny of the available data has led several independent investigators to conclude that healthy women, with prior normal examinations, can be screened every 3 years, with the optimal screening interval potentially even less frequent. The wealth of indirect evidence of benefit and the widespread acceptance of regular Pap testing in conjunction with pelvic examination in screening for cervical cancer make a randomized controlled trial of the efficacy of this screening strategy improbable.

Skin Cancer. Skin cancers, melanoma in particular, are ideal candidates for early detection. Not only can physical examination detect over 90% of melanomas arising in the skin, but the vast majority of melanomas have a prolonged horizontal growth phase prior to the vertical invasion that correlates with prognosis. This prolonged period of horizontal growth provides lead time in which locally confined lesions can be detected. Aggressive public and professional education in Australia has led to an increase in the proportion of patients diagnosed with early-stage melanoma, as well as

Table 122-5. Possible Strategies for Follow-up of Selected Cancers

Cancer site	Follow-up frequency	Regimen for each follow-up visit	Additional follow-up
Prostate	Every 3-4 mo × 3 yr; then every 6 mo × 2 yr; then annually	Complete history Physical examination Complete blood count Hepatic transaminases Alkaline phosphatase PSA	
Breast	Every 3 mo × 3 yr; then every 6 mo × 2 yr; then annually	Complete history Physical examination Complete blood count Hepatic transaminases Alkaline phosphatase Calcium	Mammography every 12 mo; CXR every 6-12 mo
Lung	Every 3 mo × 3 yr; then every 6 mo × 3 yr; then annually	Complete history Physical examination Complete blood count Hepatic transaminases Alkaline phosphatase BUN/creatinine Calcium phosphate CXR	Chest CT with cuts through the liver and adrenals every 6-12 mo
Colorectal	Every 3 mo × 2 yr; then every 6 mo × 3 yr; then annually	Complete history Physical examination Complete blood count Hepatic transaminases Alkaline phosphatase CEA (if elevated before surgery) Sigmoidoscopy (if S/P anterior resection of rectal lesion)	CXR annually Colonoscopy (every 3-6 mo after surgery in patients with obstructing lesion) *or* Colonoscopy (at 1 yr after surgery; if negative then every 2-3 yr in patients without an obstructing lesion)
Bladder	Every 3 mo × 2 yr; then every 6 mo × 3 yr; then annually	Complete history Physical examination Complete blood count Hepatic transaminases Alkaline phosphatase BUN/creatinine Urinalysis, urine cytology	Cystoscopy and urethral washings with each visit (when organ has been preserved)
Uterine cervix	Every 3 mo × 1 yr; then every 4 mo × 1 yr; then every 6 mo × 3 yr; then annually	Complete history Physical examination Complete blood count Hepatic transaminases Alkaline phosphatase BUN/creatinine Urinalysis CXR Colposcopy	Abdominal/pelvic CT every 6-12 mo × 3-5 yr
Testicular	Every 1 mo × 1 yr; then every 2 mo × 1 yr; then every 3-6 mo thereafter	Complete history Physical examination Complete blood count Hepatic transaminases Alkaline phosphatase CXR Serum tumor markers (α-fetoprotein, β-subunit of human chorionic gonadotropin)	Abdominal/pelvic CT every 2-3 mo × 1 yr; then every 6 mo
Oropharyngeal	Every 1 mo × 1 yr; then every 2-3 mo × 2 yr; then every 6 mo × 2 yr; then annually	Complete history Physical examination	CXR Indirect laryngoscopy Sputum cytology
Skin (melanoma)	Every 3 mo × 2 yr; then every 6 mo × 4 yr; then annually	Complete history Physical examination Complete blood count Hepatic transaminases Alkaline phosphatase	

BUN, Blood urea nitrogen; *CXR*, chest x-ray; *CT*, computed tomography; *CEA*, carcinoembryonic antigen.

improvement in survival. Similar trends have been noted in Scotland and the United States. Although studies designed to document mortality reduction following screening are lacking, the indirect evidence of benefit, in conjunction with the low cost, absence of morbidity, ease of performance, and patient acceptability, provides ample justification for this guideline. Individuals with pigmented nevi or personal or family history of skin cancer or dysplastic nevi should be targeted for special surveillance.

Oral Cancer. Routine annual oral examination can lead to a shift in the proportion of patients diagnosed with early-stage disease. Physicians should pay special attention to those at high risk due to socioeconomic status and tobacco and alcohol use. More than 90% of oral cancers occur in patients over the age of 45. The oral cavity is unique in that careful physical examination can detect premalignant lesions such as leukoplakia and erythroplasia that are asymptomatic. The white patches that constitute leukoplakia occur most commonly on the lower lip, floor of the mouth, buccal mucosa, lateral tongue back, and retromolar region. Erythroplasia occurs as velvety patches on the floor of the mouth, lateral tongue, and soft palate. Over 90% of these lesions are found to harbor severe epithelial dysplasia, carcinoma in situ, or frankly invasive carcinoma. Identification of these early lesions is an important means of distinguishing high-risk patients who can be targeted for intensive counseling (tobacco and alcohol cessation) and close follow-up. Unfortunately, there is only scant evidence supporting a role for screening. In the future, patients with premalignant lesions may benefit from chemopreventative strategies.

Testicular Cancer. The most common malignancy in men aged 20 to 34, testicular cancer is most often discovered by patients themselves. Localized and regional testicular cancer is highly curable. The accessibility of the testicles allows for earlier detection of testicular masses than might otherwise be possible. The benefit of testicular examination is unlikely to be conclusively demonstrated in clinical trials given the low prevalence of this disease. Nonetheless, the low cost and morbidity of self-examination and physician examination support incorporation of these techniques into an early detection program.

Finally, many sites of potentially malignant growth are within reach of a skilled examiner's eyes and hands. Sarcomas, lymphoid malignancies, and thyroid cancers initially may be palpable or even visible as subtle alterations in body contours. Every opportunity should be exploited to detect and diagnose abnormalities that might otherwise go unnoticed until more advanced disease creates symptoms that demand medical attention.

FOLLOW-UP

Cancer is increasingly curable. Approximately 40% to 50% of those diagnosed with cancer will survive the disease. Countless others will live for extended periods of time with treatment-responsive disease. These numbers are likely to increase in the future as the anti cancer armamentarium expands with new strategies and methodologies. All of these patients require follow-up to monitor for distant effects of cancer therapy, recurrence of disease, or development of additional primary tumors.

Table 122-6. Tumor-associated Antigens With Efficacy in Follow-up

Serum tumor marker	Useful in following
Prostate-specific antigen	Prostate cancer
Carcinoembryonic antigen	Colon cancer
CA 125	Ovarian cancer
α-Fetoprotein	Testicular, liver cancer
β-Subunit of human chorionic gonadotropin	Testicular cancer

A reasonable follow-up strategy for the most common and/or most treatable malignancies is suggested in Table 122-5. The natural history of the primary cancer determines the frequency and procedures of follow-up. In addition, cancer survivors may be at increased risk for primary cancers in second or third sites and should continue to undergo routine cancer screening. It is important to note that few follow-up strategies have been subjected to the same rigorous analyses that have been required for screening strategies. Nonetheless, early detection of recurrent tumors may allow some patients to be salvaged with additional treatment. For example, a rising carcinoembryonic antigen (CEA) following resection of a colon cancer might detect isolated hepatic or pulmonary metastases. Some patients with hepatic metastases confined to one lobe or region of the liver can be cured by hepatic resection. Whereas the mean survival for patients with metastatic disease is 24 months, the 5-year survival for patients with isolated hepatic or pulmonary metastases is approximately 30%.

Some investigators question the benefit of periodic follow-up, suggesting that the improved survival associated with detection of occult recurrences may result from lead time and length bias. The increasing use of tumor markers for periodic follow-up has fueled the controversy over what constitutes appropriate follow-up. Many tumor markers are nonspecific and can be elevated by nonmalignant as well as malignant processes. An elevated CEA following breast cancer can lead to an extensive, costly search for a pathologic etiology. The sensitivity of the CEA assay may exceed the ability to detect recurrent lesions. The resultant fruitless search may leave the alarmed patient and physician unsatisfied and frustrated. Some tumor markers have well-defined roles in cancer follow-up, as outlined in Table 122-6. Although controversy over appropriate follow-up regimens persists, detection of abnormalities in any follow-up study should prompt a complete diagnostic evaluation and referral when appropriate.

REFERENCES

1. Burke W, Daly M, Garber J, et al: Recommendations for follow-up care of individuals with an inherited predisposition to cancer: II. BRCA1 and BRCA2, *J Am Med Assoc* 277(12):997-1003, 1997.

1a. Christopherson WM, Lundin FE, Mendez WM, et al: Cervical cancer control: a study of morbidity and mortality trends over twenty-one year period, *Cancer* 38(3):1357-1366, 1976.

2. Cullen JW, Greenwald P: Prevention of cancer. In Edelstein GA, Michelson L, editors: *Handbook of prevention,* New York, 1986, Plenum, pp 307-341.

3. De Lorgeril M, Salen P, Martin JL, et al: Mediterranean dietary pattern in a randomized trial: prolonged survival and possible reduced cancer rate, *Arch Intern Med* 158(11):1181-1187, 1998.

4. Eddy DM: Screening for colorectal cancer, *Ann Intern Med* 113(5):373-384, 1990.
5. Hong WK, Sporn MB: Recent advances in chemoprevention of cancer, *Science* 278(5340):1073-1077, 1997.
6. Hurt RD, Sachs DP, Glover ED, et al: A comparison of sustained-release bupropion and placebo for smoking cessation, *New Engl J Med* 337(17):1195-1202, 1997.
7. Kritchevsky D: Diet and cancer, *CA Cancer J Clin* 41(6):328-333, 1991.
7a. Laara E, Day NE, Hakama M: Trends in mortality from cervical cancer in the Nordic countries: association with organised screening programmes, *Lancet* 1(8544):1247-1249, 1987.
8. Landis SH, Murray T, Bolden S, et al: Cancer statistics, 1999, *CA Cancer J Clin* 49:8-31, 1999.
9. Law M, Tang JL: An analysis of the effectiveness of interventions intended to help people stop smoking, *Arch Intern Med* 155(18):1933-1941, 1995.
10. Lieberman DA: Cost-effectiveness model for colon cancer screening, *Gastroenterology* 109(6):1781-1790, 1995.
11. Lippman SM, Lee JJ, Sabichi AI: Cancer chemoprevention: progress and promise, *J Natl Cancer Inst* 90(20):1514-1528, 1998.
12. Littrup PF, Goodman AC, Mettlin CJ: The benefit and cost of prostate cancer early detection, *CA Cancer J Clin* 43(3):134-149, 1993.
13. Mandel JS, Bond JH, Church TR, et al: Reducing mortality from colorectal cancer by screening for fecal occult blood, *New Engl J Med* 328(19):1365-1376, 1993.
14. Masouredis CM, Hilton JF, Grady D, et al: A spit tobacco cessation intervention for college athletes: three-month results, *Adv Dent Res* 11(3):354-359, 1997.
15. Miller AB: Screening for cancer: state of the art and prospects for the future, *World J Surg* 13(1):79-83, 1989.
15a. Miller AB, Lindsay J, Hill GB: Mortality from cancer of the uterus in Canada and its relationship to screening for cancer of the cervix, *Int J Cancer* 17(5):602-612, 1976.
16. Omenn GS, Goodman GE, Thornquist MD, et al: Effects of a combination of beta carotene and vitamin A on lung cancer and cardiovascular disease, *N Engl J Med* 334(18):1150-1155, 1996.
16a. Sigurdsson K: Effect of organized screening on the risk of cervical cancer: evaluation of screening activity in Iceland, 1964-1991, *Int J Cancer* 54(4):563-570, 1993.
17. Smart CR: Screening and early cancer detection, *Semin Oncol* 17(4):456-462, 1990.

IX MUSCULOSKELETAL DISEASE

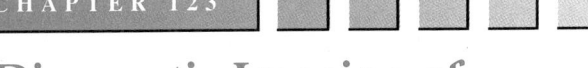

Diagnostic Imaging of Rheumatologic Disorders

James M. Coumas
Brian A. Howard
Eric W. Jacobson

The final diagnosis of immune-mediated rheumatologic disease is based on integration of clinical features with laboratory and imaging results. Rheumatologic screening tests should be ordered selectively based on the patient's clinical presentation. Such tests are frequently nonspecific, however, and results must be interpreted in the context of the particular clinical situation. Joint aspiration (arthrocentesis) is performed for both diagnostic and therapeutic purposes. Synovial fluid analysis is important in the evaluation of acute or chronic arthropathy of unknown cause. In general, patients with acute monoarthritis require joint aspiration to exclude joint infection (septic arthritis) or to confirm the presence of a crystal-induced arthropathy. Long-acting corticosteroid preparations can be injected directly into a noninfected joint to relieve the inflammatory arthritic symptoms. Selective imaging studies are important in the evaluation of the articular components of rheumatologic disorders. Conventional radiographs help distinguish inflammatory from noninflammatory arthropathies. Certain observed radiographic features help differentiate various arthritides.[2,4,5]

LABORATORY TESTS

Acute-phase Response

The acute-phase response refers to the change in systemic and metabolic factors that occurs in response to inflammatory stimuli such as infection or tissue injury. The most dramatic aspect of the acute-phase response is a rapid change in the concentration of certain plasma proteins produced primarily in the liver, including increased production of fibrinogen, haptoglobin, C-reactive protein, and serum amyloid A. The erythrocyte sedimentation rate (ESR) and C-reactive protein (CRP) are used most often to assess for an acute-phase response.

Erythrocyte Sedimentation Rate. Erythrocyte sedimentation depends on the ability of red blood cells (RBC) to aggregate and form linear clumps (rouleaux). When large amounts of acute-phase proteins (e.g., fibrinogen) are produced, binding of these proteins to erythrocytes neutralizes the negatively charged, repulsive electrostatic forces and allows the erythrocytes to aggregate and thus sediment more quickly. This forms the basis of the ESR. The more rapidly the RBCs sediment, the higher the ESR. The normal range for the Westergren method is usually less than 20 mm/hour. This range may vary among laboratories.

The ESR tends to be higher in women than in men, probably because androgens in men may lower the ESR. ESRs increase steadily with age, presumably due to increased levels of fibrinogen. They also can increase in the presence of certain medications (e.g., oral contraceptives, heparin).

The ESR may be falsely lowered by any condition that interferes with the ability of RBCs to aggregate (Box 123-1), including diseases in which (1) erythrocyte shape is abnormal, thus interfering with rouleaux formation (e.g., sickle cell disease, hereditary spherocytosis, anisocytosis); (2) hepatic dysfunction is present, which impairs production of acute-phase proteins; and (3) fibrinogen is consumed (such as disseminated intravascular coagulation). Corticosteroid preparations and high-dose antiinflammatory agents may lower the ESR. Congestive heart failure and diseases associated with an extreme elevation of the white blood cell (WBC) count (e.g., chronic lymphocytic leukemia) also may be associated with low ESRs.

The ESR is a nonspecific test; it can be elevated in many conditions associated with inflammation and tissue necrosis. The disease states most often associated with dramatically elevated (more than 100 mm/hour by Westergren technique) ESRs are malignancy (10%), collagen vascular disease (25%), and infection (50% to 60%). A thorough history,

Box 123-1. Conditions that Falsely Lower Erythrocyte Sedimentation Rate (ESR)

- Abnormal red blood cell shape
  - Sickle cell disease
  - Hereditary spherocytosis
  - Anisocytosis
- Hepatic dysfunction
- Hypofibrinogenemia
  - Hereditary
  - Fibrinogen consumption: disseminated intravascular coagulation
- Medications
  - Corticosteroids
  - High-dose antiinflammatory agents
- Congestive heart failure
- Extreme elevations of white blood cells: chronic lymphocytic leukemia

Box 123-2. Diseases that Typically Manifest Rheumatoid Factor (RF)

Rheumatic

Rheumatoid arthritis
Sjögren's syndrome
Systemic lupus erythematosus
Polymyositis, dermatomyositis
Mixed connective tissue disease
Scleroderma

Infectious

Subacute bacterial endocarditis
Tuberculosis
Infectious mononucleosis
Hepatitis
Syphilis
Leprosy
Influenza

Malignant

Lymphoma
Multiple myeloma
Waldenström's macroglobulinemia
Postradiation, postchemotherapy

Miscellaneous

Normal adults, especially elderly
Sarcoidosis
Chronic pulmonary disease (e.g., interstitial fibrosis)
Chronic liver disease (e.g., chronic active hepatitis, cirrhosis)
Mixed essential cryoglobulinemia
Hypergammaglobulinemic purpura

physical examination, and routine laboratory screens usually suggest the correct diagnosis.

C-Reactive Protein. CRP is one of the acute-phase proteins. The properties of CRP include the ability to bind to phosphocholine, to activate the complement cascade, and to interact with polymorphonuclear neutrophil leukocytes (PMNs). It tends to rise and fall quickly in response to acute-phase stimulation.

The CRP and ESR do not always correlate. CRP is a direct measure of one acute-phase protein, whereas the ESR reflects multiple processes. The CRP concentration rises and falls rapidly in response to inflammation or necrosis. Therefore it accurately reflects *acute* changes in clinical status. The ESR tends to rise more slowly and remain elevated for prolonged periods in response to acute-phase stimulation. Thus CRP level may be more indicative of a patient's clinical status at any point in time.

As with ESR, CRP can be used to assess for underlying inflammation or necrosis. It can also be used to follow the course of a disease and response to treatment. In chronic inflammatory states, CRP levels rarely exceed 6 to 8 mg/dl. Levels greater than this should suggest superimposed infection. Interestingly, CRP levels are frequently normal in active systemic lupus erythematosus (SLE). Therefore, when CRP levels are elevated, infection should be considered.

Rheumatoid Factor

Rheumatoid factor (RF) is an antibody directed against the Fc portion of human immunoglobulin G (IgG). The classic RF is an IgM antibody; however, all immunoglobulin classes of RF have been described. Only IgM RF is assayed routinely.

Several methods can be used to detect IgM RF. The most common are the latex fixation agglutination assay (LF) and the sensitized sheep RBC agglutination assay (SSCA). The LF and SSCA are considered to be positive at a dilution of 1:20 or greater. The importance of RF lies in its incidence and distribution in disease, its association with the course and severity of rheumatoid arthritis (RA), and its possible pathogenic role in RA. RF is positive in approximately 80% of patients with RA; however, it is nonspecific and is also present in many other diseases (connective tissue diseases, chronic inflammatory diseases, certain malignancies) as well as in up to 5% of the normal population, especially the elderly (Box 123-2). It is often present in high titers in mixed essential cryoglobulinemia.

The probability that a patient has RA increases in direct proportion to the titer of RF. In patients with RA, high titers of RF correlate with more severe and active joint disease, as well as rheumatoid nodules, systemic complications, and a poorer prognosis. Titers are not typically helpful in following the course of the disease over time. RF's role in the pathogenesis of RA is unclear. Possible pathophysiologic roles include (1) enhanced clearance of immune complexes, (2) increased complement fixation, (3) enhanced inflammatory response, and (4) antiviral properties. The physician should order RF test when considering a diagnosis of RA. A positive result supports the diagnosis of RA if the clinical features are consistent.

Antinuclear Antibodies

Antibodies to various nuclear (or cytoplasmic) antigens are found in the serum of many patients with systemic rheumatic diseases. A search for antinuclear antibodies (ANAs) may be

Table 123-1. Agents Associated With Antinuclear Antibodies (ANAs)

Category	Drug
Cardiovascular/antihypertensives	Procainamide
	Quinidine
	β-blockers
	Hydralazine
	Methyldopa
	Captopril
Antimicrobial	Isoniazid
	Sulfonamides
	Nitrofurantoin
Anticonvulsants	Phenytoin
	Ethosuximide
	Trimethadione
Psychotropics	Chlorpromazine
	Lithium carbonate
Antithyroid	Propylthiouracil
	Methylthiouracil
Miscellaneous	D-penicillamine
	Oral contraceptives
	Sulfasalazine

appropriate as a screen for autoimmune disease if the clinical situation suggests an autoimmune illness. Beside supporting a diagnosis of autoimmune disease, ANAs may define a specific subset of disease based on staining patterns and further identification of the specific target antigen.

ANAs are detected by an indirect immunofluorescent assay (IFA). Many different tissues or cell lines may be used as a substrate for this assay. If ANAs are present, the pattern and intensity of nuclear staining are documented. ANAs of all immunoglobulin classes will be detected, but IgM and IgA antibodies are detected with less sensitivity than IgG. False-positive tests are common with serum dilutions of less than 1:20; positivity at lower titers is considered a negative result.

ANAs are positive in more than 95% of patients with SLE and thus are an excellent screening test but are nonspecific for SLE. ANAs are present in other autoimmune diseases, chronic infections, certain neoplasms, chronic liver disease, pulmonary fibrosis, hypergammaglobulinemia, multiple sclerosis, and after other illnesses. ANAs can be produced transiently after viral illnesses or burns and can be induced by certain drugs, with or without associated clinical symptoms (Table 123-1). Procainamide is the medication most often associated with ANAs; up to 80% of patients taking this medication exhibit ANA. Only about 20% of these patients, however, experience a lupuslike illness. ANAs also are seen in normal people; the incidence increases steadily with age.

Four main staining patterns are observed with ANAs and suggest the etiology of the ANA. One pattern is homogeneous (or diffuse), in which the entire nucleus is fluorescent. It is produced by antibodies to deoxyribonucleoprotein (or the DNA-histone complex) and is nonspecific. In the speckled pattern the nucleus appears spotted. The speckled pattern occurs with antibodies directed against the extractable nuclear antigens (ENAs), which include Smith (Sm), ribonucleoprotein (RNP), Ro (formerly SS-A), and La

Table 123-2. Common Staining Patterns of ANAs

Pattern	Antigen	Disease association
Homogeneous (diffuse)	Deoxyribonucleoprotein	Nonspecific
Speckled	Extractable nuclear antigens (e.g., Smith, RNP, Ro, La)	Nonspecific
Rim (peripheral)	Double-stranded (native) DNA	SLE
Nucleolar	Nucleoli	Scleroderma

(formerly SS-B). Sm is highly specific for SLE but found in only 20% to 30% of cases. RNP is nonspecific but found in high titer in mixed connective tissue disease. Ro and La are strongly associated with Sjögren's syndrome but also are nonspecific. A third pattern is rim or peripheral, a pattern produced by antibodies directed against double-stranded (native) DNA, which is specific for SLE. The outer rim of the nucleus is stained. In the last pattern, nucleolar, the nucleoli are stained. This pattern is most often seen in scleroderma (Table 123-2).

The physician should order an ANA when considering a connective tissue disease. As with other rheumatologic tests, the result must be interpreted in the context of the particular clinical situation. Typically, the higher the titer, the more significant is the finding of a positive ANA. Rim or nucleolar patterns are more specific, and their presence indicates SLE or scleroderma, respectively. Speckled and homogeneous patterns are less specific. A positive speckled result can be further evaluated by ordering an ENA panel. Anti–double-stranded deoxyribonucleic acid (aDNA) and complement levels can provide additional important information when pursuing a workup of a positive ANA.

Anti–double-stranded DNA

aDNA is found almost exclusively in non–drug-induced SLE. Antibody titers often correlate with clinical disease activity, although changes may precede relapse or remission by several months. aDNA also correlates with development of lupus nephritis, in which it probably plays a direct pathogenic role.

Complement

The complement system comprises a group of distinct glycoproteins involved in clearance of immune complexes and microorganisms from the circulation and promotion of the inflammatory response. The measurement of complement factors and function identifies complement-consuming diseases and hereditary complement deficiencies. A screening test for complement levels is the quantitative CH_{50} photometric assay. The dilution of the patient's serum that will induce 50% lysis of antibody-coated sheep RBCs is measured. For suspected complement deficiency, CH_{50} will be low. C_3 and C_4 may be measured directly if specific quantitation is desired.

Complement glycoproteins are acute-phase reactants; *elevated* levels may be present in several conditions, including many inflammatory diseases. Elevations also occur in noninflammatory diseases (e.g., diabetes mellitus), obstructive jaundice, and acute myocardial infarction.

Decreased levels of complement factors can result from (1) decreased production, (2) in vivo activation and consumption of complement factors, or (3) in vitro consumption (e.g., postphlebotomy). The first mechanism is seen in hereditary factor deficiencies and severe liver disease. The second mechanism occurs with classic immune complex deposition and other infectious and inflammatory conditions. In vitro activation can be the result of poor specimen handling or the presence of complement activators in the serum. Inflammatory diseases result in normal complement levels when increased production equals in vivo consumption.

Complement levels are measured to assess for immune complex–mediated diseases such as active SLE and vasculitis. When immune complexes are produced, the classic pathway is activated. As complement is consumed, levels decline. Other disease states in which complement levels may be reduced by consumption include serum sickness, chronic active hepatitis, subacute bacterial endocarditis, glomerulonephritis, malaria, and mixed essential cryoglobulinemia. In SLE and vasculitis, complement levels may correlate with disease activity. Patients with inherited complement deficiencies also have low levels of complement. Some complement deficiencies (e.g., C_4) have been associated with autoimmune diseases, possibly from the inability to clear immune complexes from the circulation. Deficiencies of factors C_5 through C_9 predispose to recurrent infections with encapsulated microorganisms (e.g., *Neisseria* species), presumably because of reduced ability to lyse these organisms.

Antiphospholipid Antibodies

Antibodies to phospholipids are a heterogeneous group of "autoantibodies" that have been associated with thrombotic events. Some of the more common antigens to which these antibodies are produced include cardiolipin, phosphatidylserine, and phosphatidic acid. They are uniformly present in the primary antiphospholipid syndrome, which is characterized by venous and arterial thrombosis, recurrent fetal loss (typically in the second or third trimester), thrombocytopenia, and Coombs-positive hemolytic anemia. These antibodies are seen frequently in SLE (20% to 30%) and may be associated with certain drugs and other chronic inflammatory and infectious diseases.

Multiple laboratory assays may detect antiphospholipid antibodies. Their presence may be indicated by a false-positive Venereal Disease Research Laboratories test (VDRL) or prolongation of clotting time, as measured by the partial thromboplastin time (PTT) or Russell's viper venom time (RVVT). Antiphospholipid antibodies bind to the prothrombin activation complex (which consists of activated factor X [Xa], factor V, factor II [prothrombin], ionized calcium, and a phospholipid template) and delay the conversion of prothrombin to thrombin. Prolongation of in vitro clotting times is a paradox because these antibodies predispose to thrombosis in vivo. Antiphospholipid antibodies also may be detected by an enzyme-linked immunosorbent assay (ELISA), which identifies the specific subclass of immunoglobulin present (IgG, IgA, or IgM). Most pathogenic antiphospholipid antibodies are of the IgG variety.

The physician should consider screening for antiphospholipid antibodies when a patient presents with recurrent arterial or venous thrombi, emboli, and recurrent second- or third-trimester miscarriages. Screening may be especially important in younger patients with myocardial infarction or cerebrovascular accident in the absence of classic risk factors.

Antineutrophil Cytoplasmic Antibodies

Antineutrophil cytoplasmic antibodies (ANCAs) are directed against cytoplasmic antigens (lysosomal enzymes) of neutrophils. ANCAs may be detected using IFAs similar to those used to detect ANAs. Two different granular immunofluorescent patterns are typically described: (1) staining in granules in the *peri*nuclear region of the neutrophil (P-ANCA) and (2) granular staining more diffusely throughout the *cyto*plasm (C-ANCA). ANCAs are used to screen for the presence of vasculitis. C-ANCAs are strongly associated with Wegener's granulomatosis. P-ANCAs are less specific but have been described in patients with systemic necrotizing vasculitis associated with glomerulonephritis (e.g., polyarteritis nodosa) and idiopathic crescentic glomerulonephritis.

Lyme Antibodies

See Chapter 141.

HLA-B27

See Chapters 133 and 137.

ARTHROCENTESIS

Arthrocentesis is a safe and relatively simple procedure in which a needle is introduced into the joint space to remove synovial fluid. It is an essential part of the evaluation of any arthritis of unknown cause and is required to diagnose an infection in the joint. Arthrocentesis also can be used therapeutically, either to drain an inflamed joint or to introduce long-acting corticosteroids into the joint.

Joint aspiration requires sound knowledge of the joint anatomy, including the bony and soft tissue landmarks used for joint entry. Strict aseptic technique is crucial to minimize the risk of infection. The physician must practice universal precautions. The procedure is accomplished more easily when the patient is able to relax the muscles surrounding the joint.

Absolute contraindications to performing arthrocentesis include local infection of the overlying skin and severe coagulopathy. If coagulopathy is present and if septic arthritis is suspected, every effort should be made to correct the coagulopathy (with fresh-frozen plasma or alternate factors) before joint aspiration. Therapeutic anticoagulation is not an absolute contraindication, although every effort should be made to avoid excessive trauma during the aspiration.

The major complications of arthrocentesis include iatrogenically induced infection and bleeding. Both are extremely rare. The risk of infection after arthrocentesis is less than 1 in 10,000.[2] Correction of prominent coagulopathy before arthrocentesis reduces the risk of excessive hemorrhage.

The knee is one of the most accessible joints for aspiration. The physician should describe the procedure to the patient, including risks of complications. The entry site should be cleaned with an iodine-based antiseptic solution. After the area dries, it should be wiped once with alcohol. Local anesthesia (subcutaneous lidocaine or topical ethyl chloride) may be applied. With the patient supine and the knee fully extended, the knee joint is entered medially, under the patella (Fig. 123-1). The joint should be fully drained if possible. The needle is then removed, and pressure is applied to the

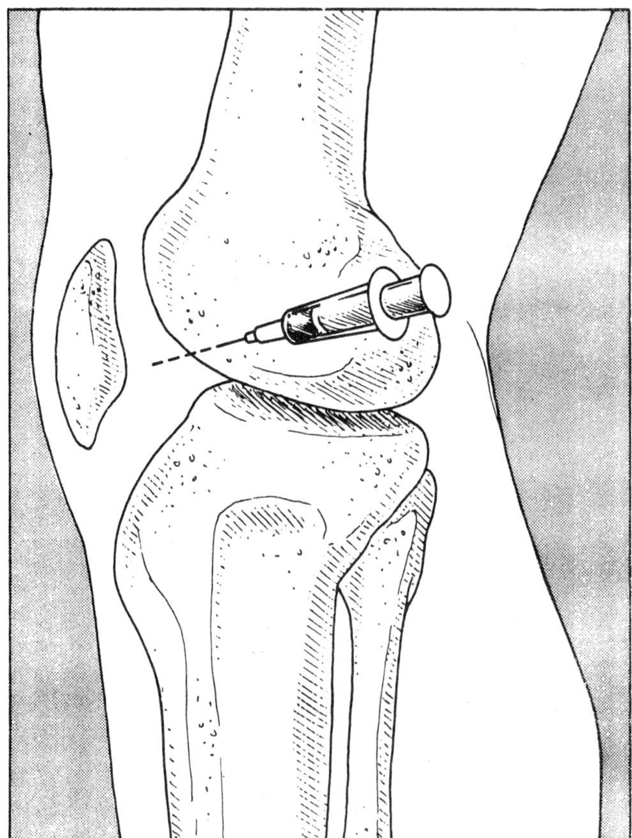

Fig. 123-1. Technique for arthrocentesis of the knee: medial approach.

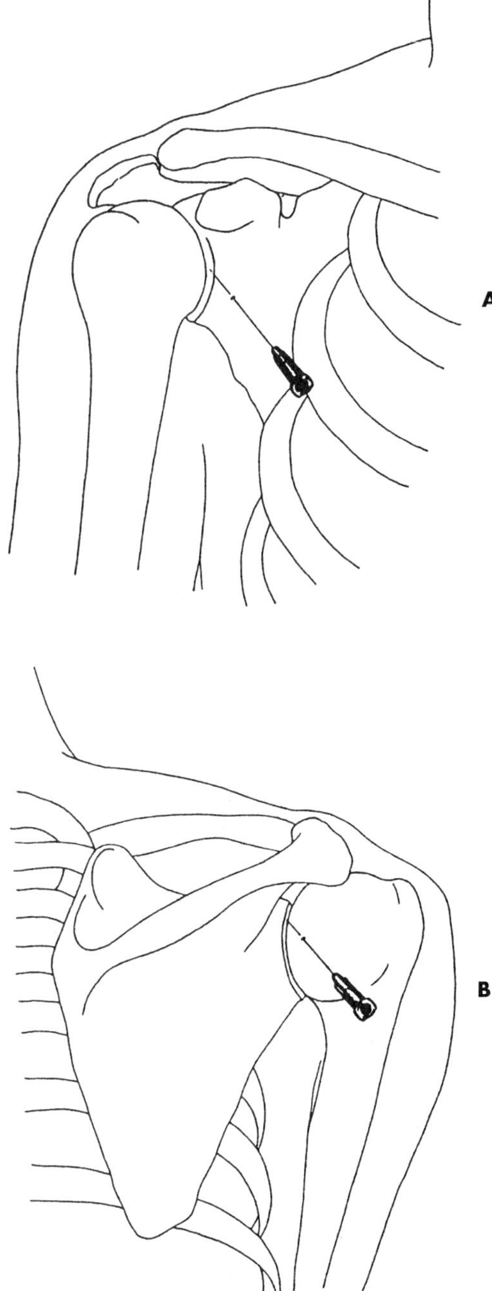

Fig. 123-2. Technique for arthrocentesis of the shoulder: anterior (**A**) and posterior (**B**) approach.

site until bleeding has stopped. The area is cleaned with alcohol and a bandage applied. Other joints that may be aspirated include shoulder, elbow, and ankle (Figs. 123-2 through 123-4).

Once fluid is obtained, synovial fluid analysis is performed to distinguish noninflammatory from inflammatory fluid. Less than 2000 WBCs/mm^3 is consistent with noninflammatory fluid, as in osteoarthritis. Greater than 2000 WBCs/mm^3 indicates inflammatory fluid (Box 123-3). In addition to absolute nucleated cell count, synovial fluid is divided into various categories based on the gross appearance, viscosity, WBC differential, and culture results (Table 123-3).

Synovial fluid analysis begins with bedside observation of the fluid. Normal synovial fluid is colorless. Both noninflammatory fluid and mildly inflammatory fluid appear yellow or straw colored. Septic effusions frequently appear purulent and whitish. Hemorrhagic effusions appear red or brown. The clarity of synovial fluids depends on the number and types of cells or particles present. To test clarity, a glass tube filled with synovial fluid is placed in front of black print on a white background. If the print is easily read, the fluid is transparent, indicating normal and noninflammatory fluid. If the print is distinguishable from the background but is not clear, the fluid is translucent, indicating inflammatory effusions. Grossly inflammatory, septic, and hemorrhagic fluids are opaque, preventing any visualization through the tube.

Synovial fluid viscosity, the result of hyaluronic acid content, also can be assessed at the bedside. Degradative enzymes (e.g., hyaluronidase) released from inflammatory cells produce a thinner, less viscous fluid. Viscosity can be assessed using the *string sign* while adhering to universal precautions. A drop of fluid is allowed to fall from the end of the needle or syringe, and an estimate is made of the length of the continuous "string" that forms. Normal fluid forms at least a 6-cm continuous string. Inflammatory fluid will not form a string; it drops like water dripping from a faucet.

After bedside assessment, the synovial fluid is sent to the laboratory for a cell count and differential, crystal analysis, Gram's stain, and culture. Cell counts approaching 100,000 WBCs/mm^3 suggest septic arthritis or a crystal-induced arthritis. Normally, synovial fluid has a predominance of

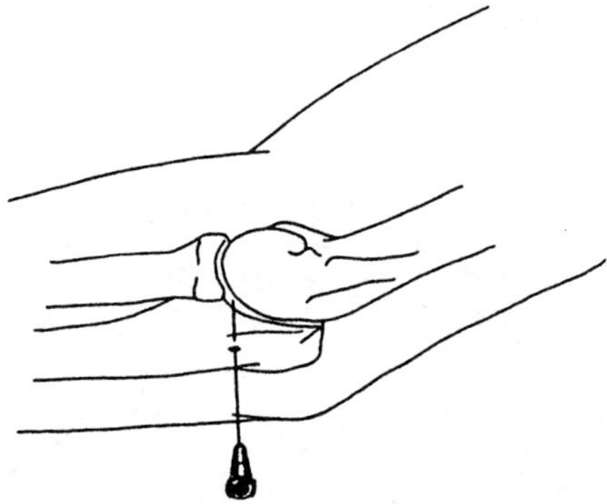

Fig. 123-3. Technique for arthrocentesis of the elbow.

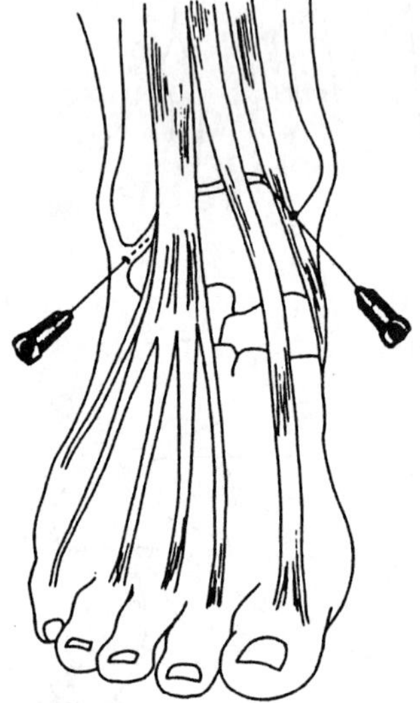

Fig. 123-4. Technique for arthrocentesis of the ankle: medial and lateral approach.

lymphocytes. The percentage of PMNs increases with inflammatory conditions. In most circumstances an infected joint has synovial fluid with more than 75% PMNs (see Table 123-3).

All fluid should be assessed for the presence of crystals, specifically monosodium urate and calcium pyrophosphate dihydrate, using a compensated polarized light microscope (see Chapter 136). If the fluid cannot be examined immediately, refrigeration of the fluid helps preserve the crystals.

Gram's stain and culture should be performed on most synovial fluid specimens. Cultures for aerobic and anaerobic bacterial organisms are performed routinely. In certain patients (e.g., with chronic monoarticular arthritis), fluid may be cultured for mycobacteria and fungi. If disseminated gonorrhea is suspected, fluid should be plated directly onto chocolate agar or Thayer-Martin media. A positive culture confirms septic arthritis. Other studies on synovial fluid (glucose, protein, complement) usually are not helpful.

Arthrocentesis also is used therapeutically. In septic arthritis, serial joint aspirations are required to remove accumulated inflammatory or purulent fluid. This allows serial monitoring of the total WBC count, Gram's stain, and culture to assess response to treatment and provides complete

Box 123-3. Common Causes of Inflammatory Arthritis

Rheumatoid arthritis
Spondyloarthropathies
- Psoriatic arthritis
- Reiter's syndrome/reactive arthritis
- Ankylosing spondylitis
- Ulcerative colitis/regional enteritis (Crohn's disease)

Crystal-induced arthritis
- Monosodium urate (gout)
- Calcium pyrophosphate dihydrate (CPPD, pseudogout)
- Hydroxyapatite

Infectious arthritis
- Bacterial
- Mycobacterial
- Fungal

Connective tissue diseases
- SLE
- Vasculitis
- Scleroderma
- Polymyositis

Hypersensitivity: serum sickness

drainage of a "closed space." Inflammatory fluid contains many destructive enzymes that contribute to cartilage and bony degradation. Removal of the fluid may slow this destructive process.

Arthrocentesis is necessary for intraarticular injection of long-acting corticosteroid preparations. Corticosteroids also are frequently injected into soft tissue sites such as bursae, tendon sheaths, and myofascial trigger points (Figs. 123-5 to 123-7). The dose of corticosteroid used depends on the size of the particular joint or soft tissue site being injected (Table 123-4). Three common corticosteroid preparations are triamcinolone diacetate (e.g., Aristocort Forte, Amcort), methylprednisolone acetate (e.g., Depo-Medrol, Medralone), and triamcinolone hexacetonide (e.g., Aristospan). Triamcinolone hexacetonide has a longer duration of action than the other two preparations. It is more likely to produce tissue atrophy or tendon injury and thus is mainly used for intraarticular injections. A local anesthetic such as lidocaine is frequently mixed with the corticosteroid before injection.

In addition to infection and bleeding, other complications must be considered with injection of a corticosteroid. Lipoatrophy and skin discoloration can occur with any of the steroid preparations, especially when injecting superficial soft tissue areas. Tendon rupture also can occur when injecting tendon sheaths, possibly from a weakening effect caused by the corticosteroid. A brief postinjection "flare" has been described in up to 1% to 2% of intraarticular injections. This complication generally occurs within the first few hours after the injection. If marked inflammatory symptoms persist for more than 24 hours, the joint or soft tissue region requires reaspiration to rule out infection. Finally, systemic absorption of the corticosteroid may be associated with a transient increase in blood glucose in patients with diabetes.

Repeated injections with corticosteroid preparations into the same joint (or soft tissue region) may accelerate connective tissue degradation. Generally, at least 3 to 4

Table 123-3. Joint Fluid Characteristics

	Normal	Group I (noninflammatory)	Group II (inflammatory)	Group III (septic)
Color	Clear	Yellow	Yellow or opalescent	Variable, may be purulent
Clarity	Transparent	Transparent	Translucent	Opaque
Viscosity	Very high	High	Low	Typically low
WBCs/mm^3	200	200-2000	2000-100,000	>50,000, usually >100,000
PMNs (%)	<25	<25	>50	>75
Culture	Negative	Negative	Negative	Usually positive

PMNs, Polymorphonuclear neutrophil leukocytes.

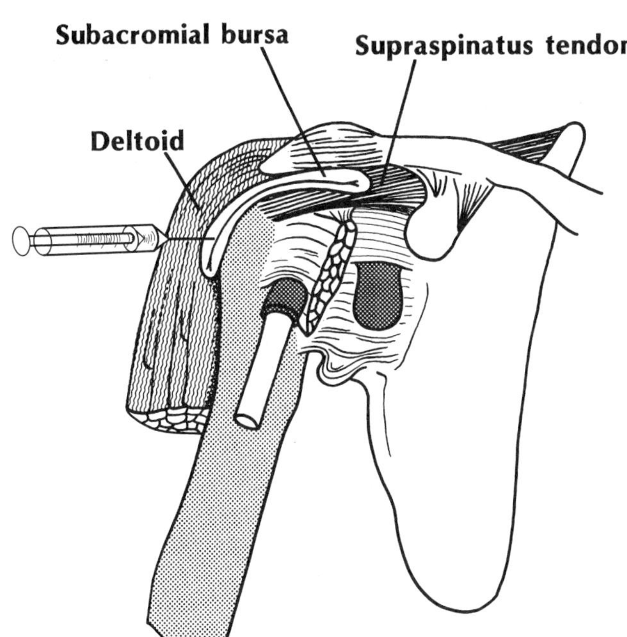

Fig. 123-5. Technique for injection of the subacromial bursa.

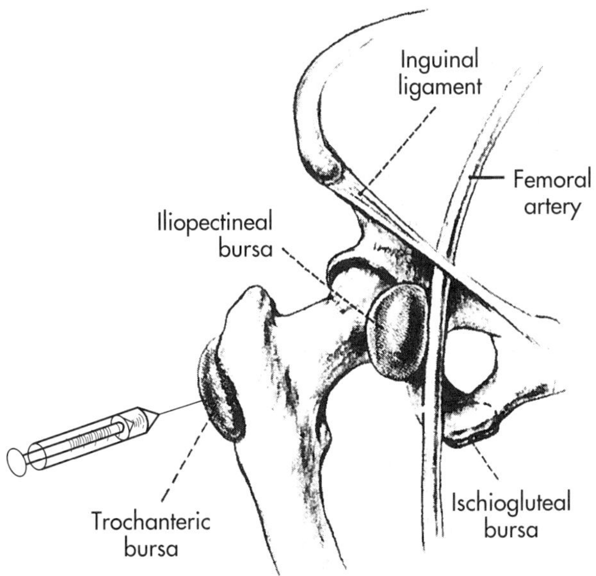

Fig. 123-6. Technique for injection of the trochanteric bursa.

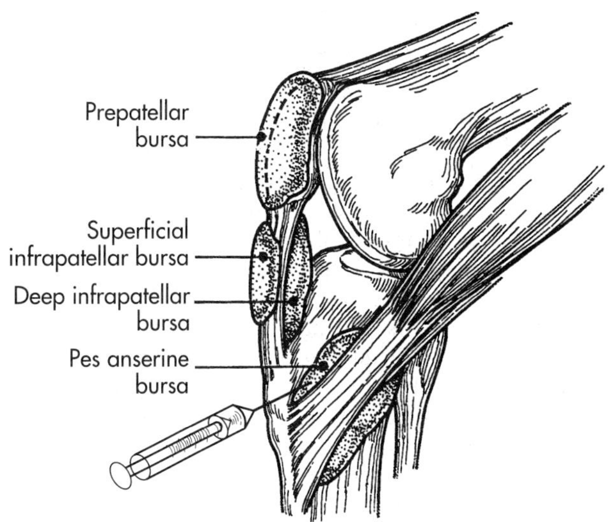

Fig. 123-7. Technique for injection of the anserine bursa.

Table 123-4. Dose of Corticosteroid Preparation Used in Injections

	Triamcinolone diacetate (Aristocort Forte, Amcort)	Methylprednisolone acetate (Depo-Medrol, Medralone)	Triamcinolone hexacetonide (Aristospan)
Joint			
Small joint of hand/foot		2.5-10 mg	2-5 mg
Wrist/elbow		10-30 mg	10 mg
Knee/ankle/shoulder		20-40 mg	20-40 mg
Bursae	20-40 mg	20-60 mg	
Trigger points	5-10 mg		
Epicondyles	5-10 mg		

months should pass before reinjecting a site. If a single site is injected regularly for more than 1 year, an alternate approach should be considered.

RADIOLOGIC EVALUATION

The common rheumatologic joint disorders (arthropathies) have a characteristic radiologic appearance. Diagnostic imaging technologies, in order of accessibility, include conventional radiography, ultrasound, nuclear scintigraphy, conventional or computed tomography (CT), and magnetic resonance imaging (MRI). Each modality has strengths and limitations. Conventional radiographic imaging (plain film) remains the most cost-effective approach to the diagnosis, evaluation, and assessment of disease progression. The history, physical examination, radiographic assessment, and laboratory results play synergistic roles in the diagnosis of joint disease.[2] Conventional radiographs should provide standardized views of the symptomatic joint of interest and the immediate regional articulations. A structured approach to plain film analysis and interpretation provides valuable information. A typical approach involves evaluation of anatomic *a*lignment, *b*ony mineralization, joint space or *c*artilage thickness, and adjacent *s*oft tissues changes, the ABCs of radiographic evaluation.[4,5,9]

Rheumatoid Arthritis

RA is a common rheumatologic disorder that affects synovial-lined joints, bursae, tendon sheaths, and ligamentous and tendinous bony attachments (entheses). Abnormalities of the adjacent soft tissues, bone, and cartilaginous joints may also be seen (see Chapter 133). In general, a symmetric polyarticular disorder principally involving the small and large joints of the appendicular skeleton is seen. Radiographic views of the hands and wrists are obtained in posteroanterior (PA) and semisupinated oblique (Norgaard) positions. Early observable findings include the following:

1. Soft tissue swelling caused by periarticular inflammation.
2. Juxtaarticular osteopenia, diminished bony trabecular pattern, and indistinct joint margin cortex.
3. Uniform cartilage thinning resulting in symmetric joint space narrowing, with a predilection for the metacarpophalangeal (MCP), proximal interphalangeal (IP), radiocarpal, and midcarpal joint spaces.
4. Early focal bony erosions at the peripheral margin of the joint adjacent to the capsular insertion, often referred to as the *bare area*. These erosions may appear as subtle craters or cystlike changes. In the wrist, erosions of the ulnar styloid process, radial styloid process, and middle scaphoid body are common.

Late observable changes include the following:

1. Subluxation or dislocation of the MCP and IP joints caused by loss of ligamentous restraints. Classic swan-neck and boutonniére deformities and ulna deviation of the digits may be seen. At the wrist, radiocarpal and intercarpal subluxations result in various malalignment patterns.
2. Generalized or diffuse osteopenia.
3. Progressive articular surface erosion and destruction.
4. Ankylosis of the carpal bones.
5. Synovial cyst formation with dissection into the soft tissues.
6. Soft tissue rheumatoid nodules.
7. Superimposed degenerative arthritis.

Changes similar to those in the hand (Figs. 123-8 and 123-9) occur in the feet in approximately 80% of patients. The knee, hip, elbow, and shoulder are the next most frequently involved joints. Approximately 60% to 70% of patients with RA develop neck symptoms (Fig. 123-10). Erosions and symmetric narrowing of the posterior apophyseal joints of the cervical spine with accelerated diskal resorption lead to vertebral body subluxation at multiple levels ("staircasing") below C2. Craniocervical involvement may result in anterior or lateral atlantoaxial instability (transverse ligament insufficiency), which can be associated with cervical myelopathy. More ominously, cranial settling caused by occipitocervical joint destruction can predispose to medullary brainstem compression.[2,8]

Men with a high level of physical activity have a specific radiographic appearance termed *robust rheumatoid arthritis,* with prominent subchondral cyst formation produced by high intraarticular pressure and intravasation of synovial fluid or granulation tissue through fissures in the articular cartilage. Nuclear scintigraphy has been used to evaluate the "activity" of the inflammatory process and assess therapeutic management. More recently, MRI is used to evaluate the extent of synovial hypertrophy and pannus formation at specific targeted joints. Ultrasound is helpful in the differentiation of solid vs. fluid-filled juxtaarticular soft tissue masses. Common clinical indications for MRI include neurologic deficits, suggestive of compressive myelopathy or basilar invagination; suspicion of subarticular ischemic necrosis; and soft tissue abscess formation with or without associated osteomyelitis.

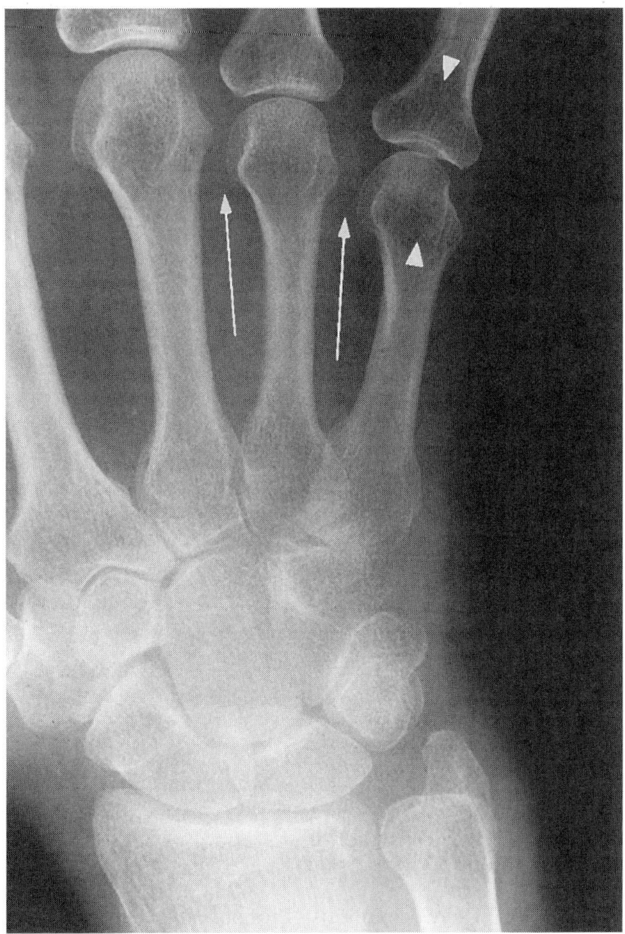

Fig. 123-8. Rheumatoid arthritis. Early changes may be confined to juxtaarticular osteopenia *(arrowheads)*, periarticular soft tissue swelling *(arrows)*, and loss of normal fat fascial planes (i.e., navicular fat stripe) and superficial fat fascial border along ulna styloid.

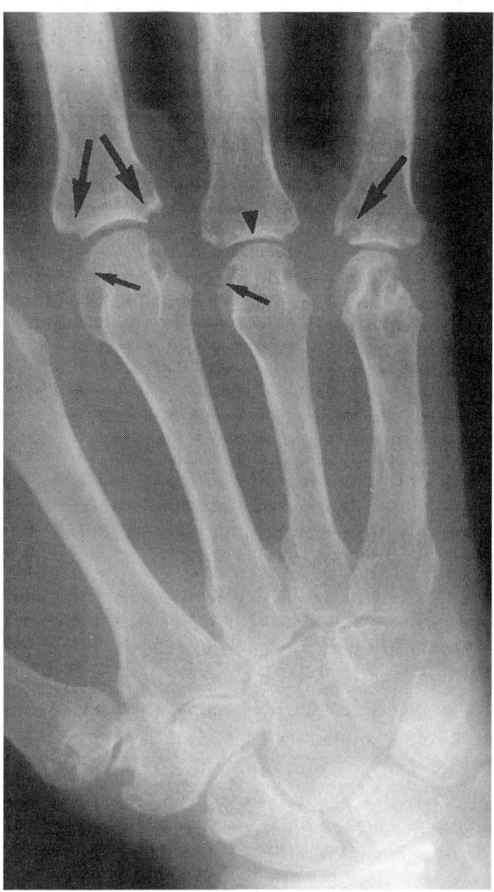

Fig. 123-9. Rheumatoid arthritis. Later changes include symmetric joint space narrowing *(arrowhead)*, loss of subchondral cortical margin *(small arrows)*, and marginal erosions *(large arrows)*.

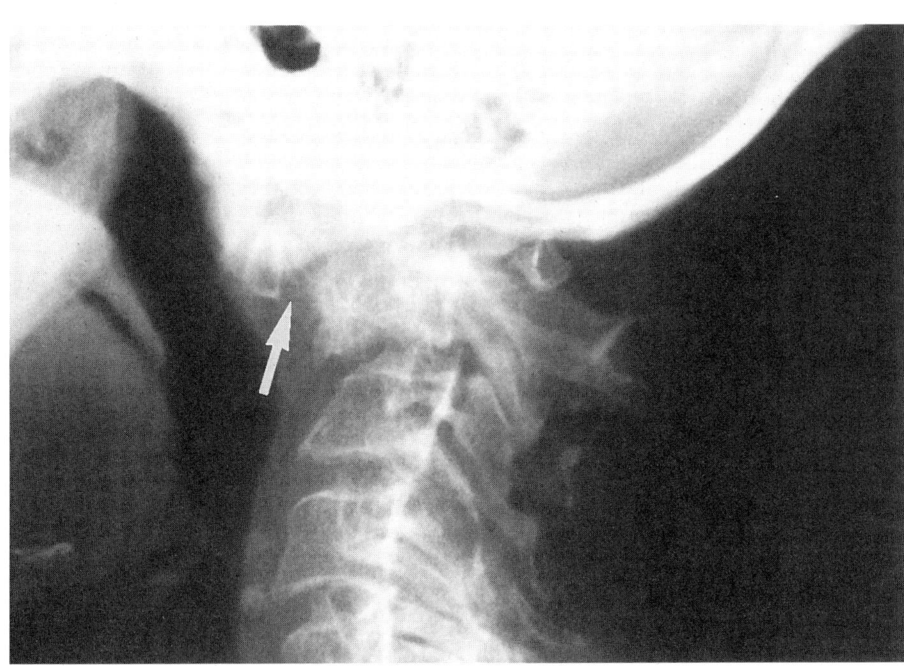

Fig. 123-10. Rheumatoid arthritis of the axial skeleton. Osteopenia, "staircasing" (multilevel subluxation), and erosion/subluxation at atlantoaxial articulation are common, with widening of atlanto-dens interval *(white arrow)*.

Seronegative Spondyloarthropathies

Psoriatic Arthritis. This common skin disease may present as a monoarticular or distal interphalangeal (DIP) polyarticular disorder or spondylitis (see Chapter 137). Psoriatic arthritis involves the synovial-lined joints, tendon sheath, and periarticular soft tissues, with specific entheseal involvement of ligamentous and tendinous attachments to bone. Radiographic articular changes may precede the appearance of any skin disease. However, the frequency of joint disease increases with chronicity and severity of the psoriatic skin manifestations. Plain film radiographs of the hand and wrist or feet may show classic radiographic features.[2] The distribution of joint involvement is distinct from RA. Early findings may include the following:

1. Normal plain radiographs.
2. Fusiform periarticular soft tissue swelling typically confined to a single IP joint without associated bony changes. Diffuse involvement of digits, joints, tendon sheath, and soft tissues is referred to as a *sausage digit*.
3. Maintenance of normal bone mineralization.
4. Asymmetric or unilateral joint involvement.
5. Distal phalangeal tuftal erosions.

Later radiographic changes include the following:

1. Joint space narrowing involving the DIP and proximal interphalangeal (PIP) joints.
2. Bone proliferation, typically adjacent to sites of articular erosion. An irregular, poorly defined marginal surface bony accretion, proliferative *enthesitis* indicates reactive change at the insertion of the capsule, ligament, and tendon.
3. Periosteal reaction along the diaphyseal shaft *(periostitis)*.
4. Erosions are marginal but may extend subchondrally to produce central erosions with apparent "widening of the joint."
5. Progressive joint surface destruction. Proximal articular surface tapering results from marginal erosions. Distal articular surface central erosions and enthesitic proliferation lead to the classic pencil-in-cup radiographic deformity.
6. Subluxation with distal-proximal telescoping of digit.
7. Bony ankylosis of the digits.

Although the pattern of distribution of joint disease is variable, characteristic areas of involvement include the DIP and PIP joints (Figs. 123-11 and 123-12). A high incidence of the first MCP joint involvement is noted. Wrist involvement usually follows that of the hand. Forefoot changes parallel those of the hand, with bilateral and asymmetric disease of the IP joints but a predilection for the IP joint of the great toe. In the hindfoot, characteristic erosive changes of the calcaneus are seen around the retrocalcaneal bursa. Proliferative *enthesopathy,* or poorly defined bony calcaneal spurs, is seen at the insertion of the plantar aponeurosis to the calcaneus[2,9] (Fig. 123-13).

Classic involvement of the axial skeleton occurs principally in the thoracolumbar spine, with paravertebral ossification that is bulky and asymmetric. Vertically oriented, lateral paravertebral spondylophytes are different from the osteophytes of degenerative disk disease and the syndesmophyte of ankylosing spondylitis. In the cervical spine, posterior apophyseal joints narrow, erode, and ankylose. Anteriorly, however, erosive diskovertebral changes may be combined with osseous bridging, which is more typical of syndesmophytic ossification similar to other seronegative spondyloarthropathies. At the atlantoaxial articulation, erosive changes and anterolateral instability mimic RA.

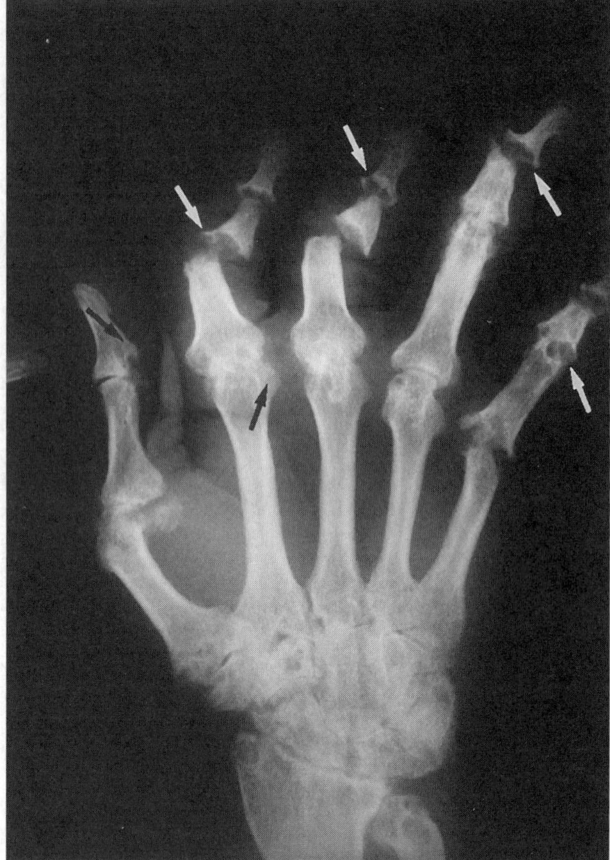

Fig. 123-11. Psoriatic arthritis. Erosions involving distal and proximal interphalangeal joints *(white arrows)* with associated periosteal reaction and proliferative change *(black arrows)*. Note pencil-in-cup configuration.

Up to 50% of patients with psoriatic arthritis develop bilateral asymmetric radiographic changes at the sacroiliac (SI) joints. Superficial and deep erosions of the iliac more than the sacral joint surfaces are associated with reactive subchondral sclerosis. Erosive changes are typically confined to the synovial-lined aspect of the SI joint. SI and other pelvic ligaments may ossify from underlying enthesopathy. Psoriatic arthritis usually can be differentiated from RA on plain radiographs by the presence of periosteal and entheseal new bone formation, IP joint predilection, distal tuftal resorption, bony ankylosis, and lack of juxtaarticular demineralization. Differentiating psoriatic arthritis from other seronegative spondyloarthropathies, however, may prove difficult. As in RA, further imaging modalities may be indicated as follows:

1. Total-body bone scan to screen for other sites of activity.
2. Spinal MRI to assess neuroaxis compromise.
3. Joint MRI to exclude complications (e.g., osteonecrosis, osteomyelitis, deep abscess, occult trauma).
4. CT scan to assess bony destruction or confirm SI joint disease.
5. Ultrasound to assess Baker's cyst–like masses vs. deep venous thrombosis.

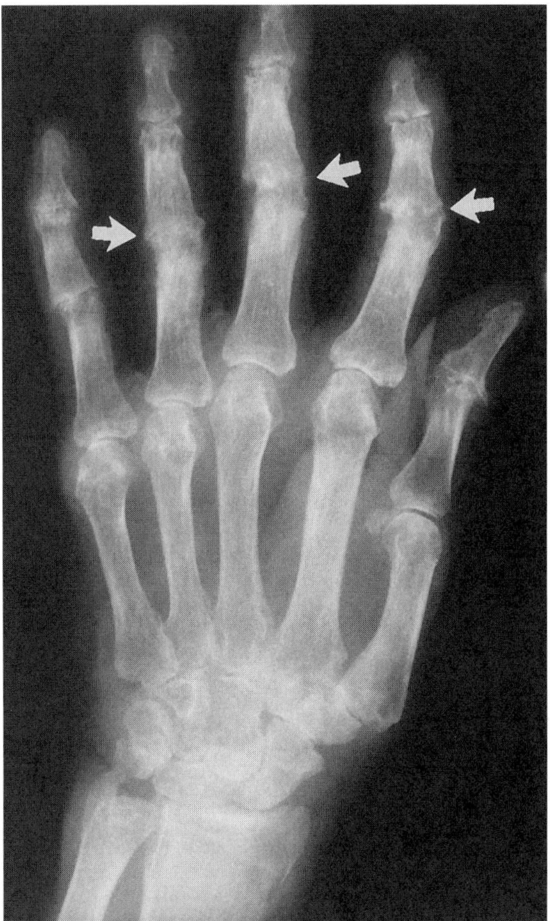

Fig. 123-12. Psoriatic arthritis. Bony ankylosis *(white arrows)*, maintenance of bone mineralization, and localization to target sites (interphalangeal involvement) help differentiate this arthritis from rheumatoid arthritis.

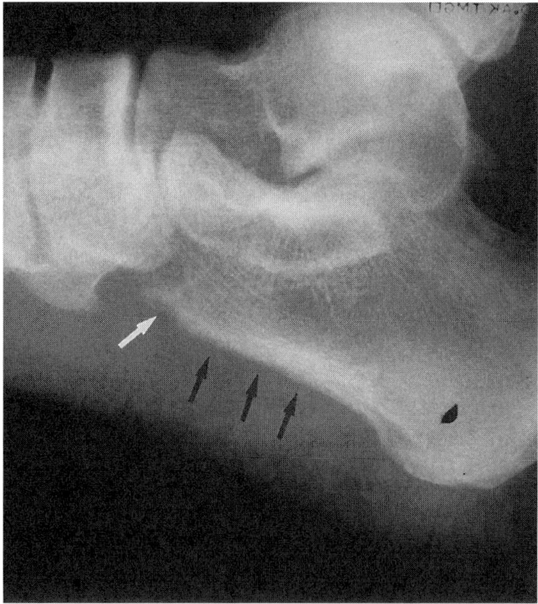

Fig. 123-13. Psoriatic arthritis. Periostitis along plantar calcaneus *(black arrows)* and poorly delineated erosion *(white arrow)* support the diagnosis.

Reiter's Syndrome. Reiter's disease is a reactive arthritis with a typical clinical syndrome consisting of the triad of urethritis, conjunctivitis, and inflammatory arthritis. The arthritic component of this seronegative spondyloarthropathy can be identified on plain films (see Chapter 137). The joint disease is an asymmetric, unilateral or bilateral polyarticular disorder of synovial-lined joints, with entheses and a predilection for involvement of the feet (lower extremities). Early radiographic changes seen in the metatarsophalangeal (MTP) and IP joints of the forefoot include the following:

1. Periarticular soft tissue swelling with early demineralization. Normal-appearing plain radiographs may be seen with resolution of the acute inflammatory phase.
2. Symmetric joint space narrowing.
3. Periostitis is often poorly defined or "fluffy" in appearance at joint margins or along the shaft.
4. Proliferative enthesopathy at the Achilles tendon and plantar aponeurosis attachments to the calcaneus, resulting in erosions and spurs.
5. Bursal and tendon sheath inflammation, with a predilection for the retrocalcaneal bursa.
6. Erosions are marginal early in the disease process. Narrowing may appear asymmetric but ultimately leads to uniform joint space narrowing.

Late radiologic findings include the following:

1. Uniform joint space loss at multiple articulations.
2. Bulky, well-defined enthesophytes.
3. Subluxation about the MTP joints, referred to as a *Launois deformity.*

Reiter's syndrome may involve the larger joints of the lower extremities (e.g., knee, ankle) but tends to spare the hip. Upper extremity involvement is less common and shows a predilection for the PIP joints of the hand. The SI joints show a bilateral asymmetric involvement confined to the true synovial-lined portion of the joint, which parallels the findings of psoriatic arthritis. Changes in the axial skeleton also parallel those of psoriatic arthritis.

Differentiating Reiter's syndrome from the other seronegative spondyloarthropathies can be difficult. Reiter's arthritis typically shows less upper extremity involvement, axial skeleton involvement, and ankylosis than psoriatic arthritis or ankylosing spondylitis. Intraarticular bone production, adjacent sites of bone erosion, and poorly defined, fluffy periostitis also are hallmarks of Reiter's arthritis[9] (Figs. 123-14 and 123-15). The plantar and retrocalcaneal changes are highly characteristic of Reiter's syndrome. Minimal axial skeleton involvement is helpful in differentiating Reiter's disease from peripheral ankylosing spondylitis. Nuclear scintigraphy may help detect subtle proliferative and inflammatory changes not apparent on plain radiographs. Early asymmetric, bilateral polyarticular involvement with changes involving both the hindfoot and the forefoot are helpful in establishing the early diagnosis of Reiter's syndrome.

Ankylosing Spondylitis. Ankylosing spondylitis is a chronic inflammatory disorder that predominantly affects the spine but may also involve appendicular joints (see Chapter 137). With the onset of spinal symptoms, earlier radiographic changes may start and progress in the SI joints with

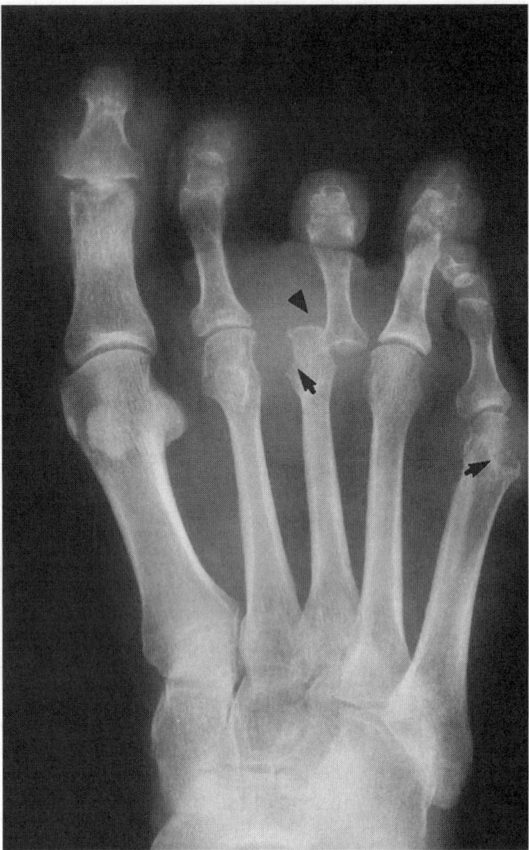

Fig. 123-14. Reiter's arthritis. Joint space narrowing, erosions *(black arrows)*, and subluxation *(arrowhead)* make it difficult to differentiate Reiter's syndrome from other seronegative spondyloarthropathies.

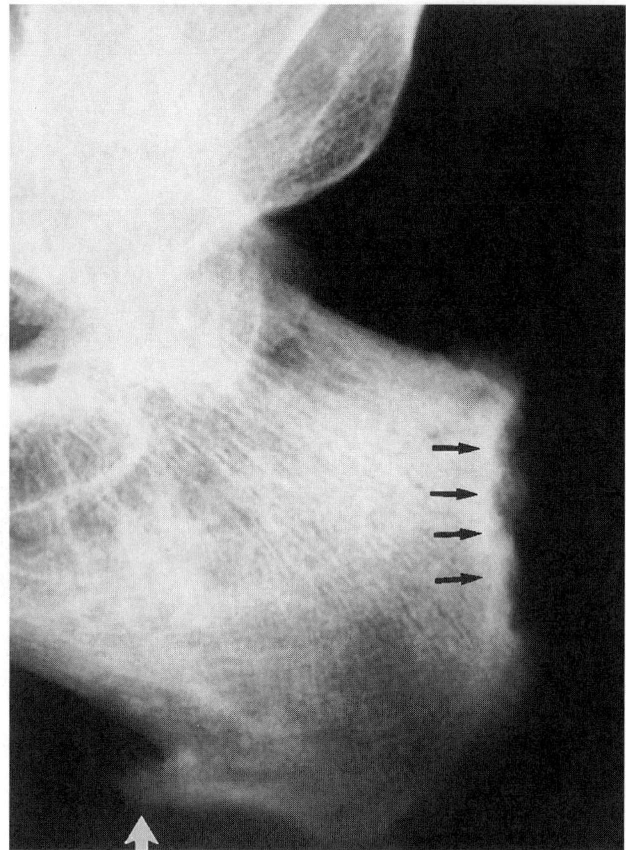

Fig. 123-15. Reiter's arthritis. Retrocalcaneal bursitis with associated erosions *(black arrows)* and prominent plantar calcaneal spur *(white arrow)* with poor cortical delineation.

symmetric erosions, reactive sclerosis, and subsequent fusion (Fig. 123-16). Early spinal involvement may occur at the thoracolumbar junction, with squaring of the vertebral body contours, corner erosions, and sclerosis, followed by formation of symmetric syndesmophytes bridging the vertebral bodies. Posterior apophyseal joint ankylosis and ligamentous ossification follow (Fig. 123-17). Contiguous progression of this reactive process up and down the spine results in the end-stage ankylosed spinal changes with a bamboo appearance. Radiographic findings include the following:

1. Bilateral, symmetric, apparent SI widening with loss of cortical definition of the iliac articular margin.
2. Erosions and reactive sclerosis of the articular surfaces, especially the lower third of the SI joint.
3. Subsequent narrowing and obliteration of the SI joint, with similar changes at the symphysis pubis.
4. Inflammatory resorption of the anulus fibrosus insertion at the corners of the vertebral end plates resulting in squaring of the vertebral body contours, marginal erosions, and reactive sclerosis.
5. Bony proliferation at the vertebral corners, which forms delicate vertical bridges of bone that create marginal syndesmophytes best appreciated on oblique views. Occasionally, destruction of the diskovertebral joint simulates septic diskitis.
6. Apophyseal and costovertebral joint ankylosis.
7. Craniocervical junction disease may be associated with transverse ligament insufficiency and resultant anterolateral instability.
8. Hips, heels, and shoulders may be affected with diffuse inflammatory narrowing, erosive destruction, and proliferative "whiskering" periostitis, respectively.
9. The ankylosed spine is rigid and osteoporotic. Minimal trauma may produce unstable, life-threatening spinal fracture, especially at the cervicodorsal junction.
10. The peripheral joints may undergo ankylosis.

Initial radiographic evaluation to help confirm the diagnosis of ankylosing spondylitis includes AP and lateral views of the lumbar spine and AP craniad angled view of sacroiliac joint (Hibbs-Ferguson view). A CT scan performed preferentially in the coronal plane of the SI joint may demonstrate erosive disease before findings are evident on plain films.[6] MRI has been used to assess associated spinal cord arachnoiditis, spinal canal stenosis, and posttraumatic cord changes.

Osteoarthritis

The term *osteoarthritis* is typically used interchangeably with *degenerative joint disease* (DJD). Osteoarthritis is characterized by asymmetric joint space narrowing secondary to articular cartilage thinning, subchondral eburnation or sclerosis, subchondral cystic changes, and marginal osteophyte formation (Fig. 123-18). Osteoarthritis may occur as a primary process or secondary to another joint insult or destructive joint process. Radiographic features may help in differentiating a primary from secondary process. In the appendicular skeleton, osteoarthritis is characterized as a

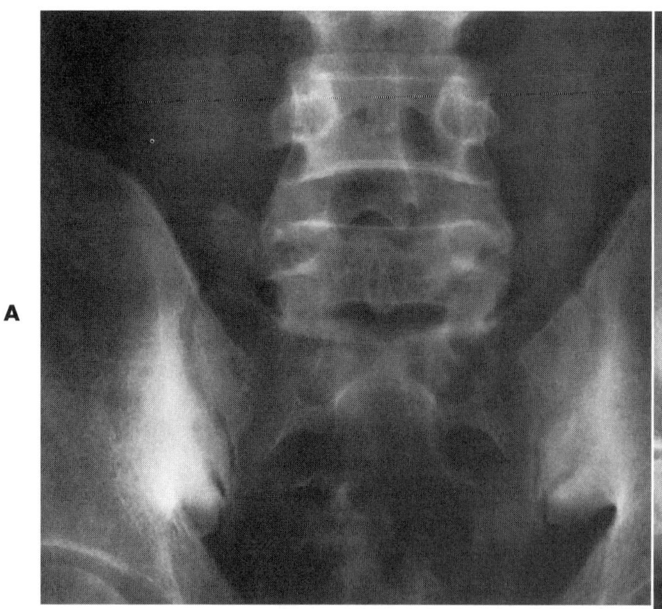

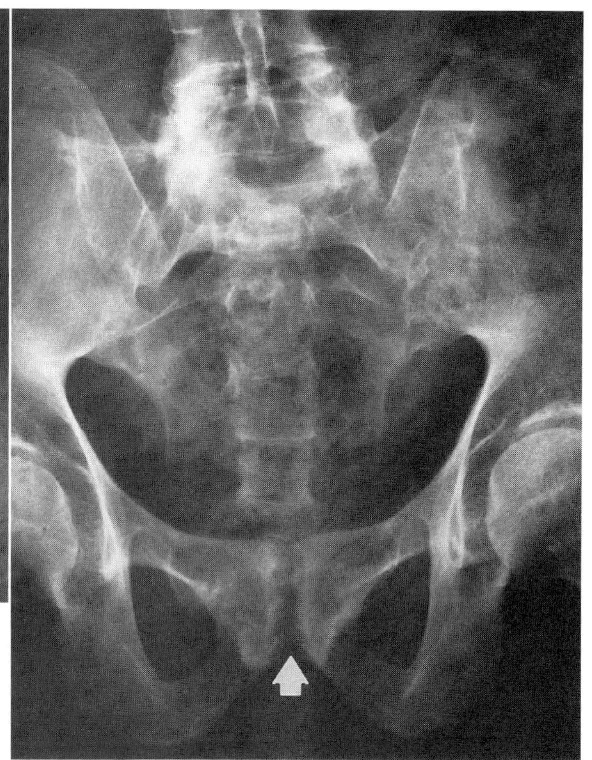

Fig. 123-16. Ankylosing spondylitis. **A,** Bilateral symmetric reactive sclerosis and erosions predominantly involving iliac wing aspect of sacroiliac joint. **B,** Late changes include bony ankylosis and obliteration of sacroiliac joint. Note symphysis pubis erosions *(white arow)*.

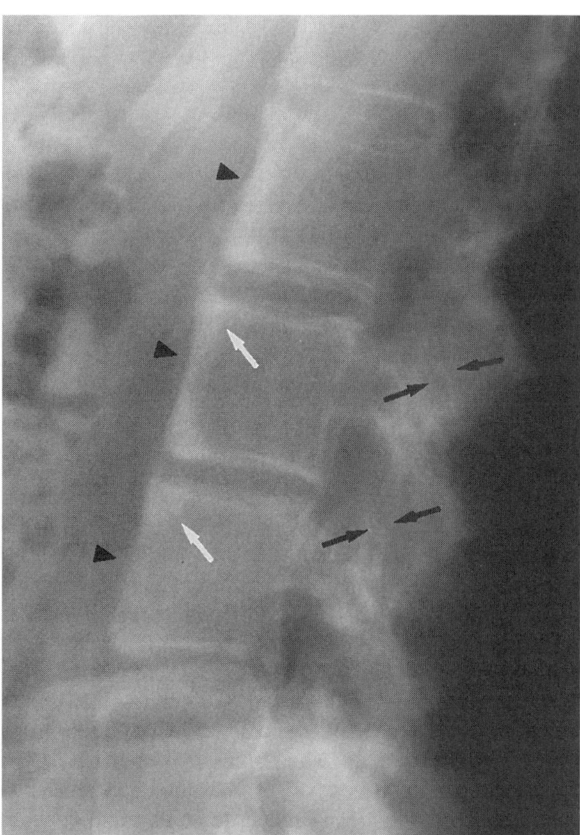

Fig. 123-17. Ankylosing spondylitis. Axial skeleton shows squaring of vertebral bodies *(arrowheads)*, classic "shiny corners" *(white arrows)*, and ankylosis of interarticular facet joints *(black arrows)*.

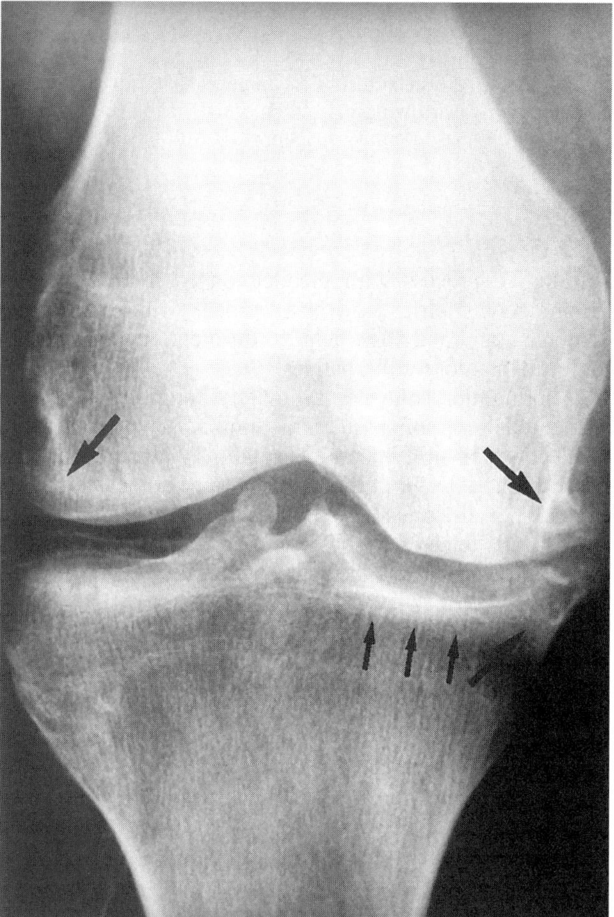

Fig. 123-18. Osteoarthritis. Proliferative marginal osteophytes *(larger arrows)*, narrowing of medial weight-bearing joint space, and subchondral eburnative changes *(smaller arrows)*.

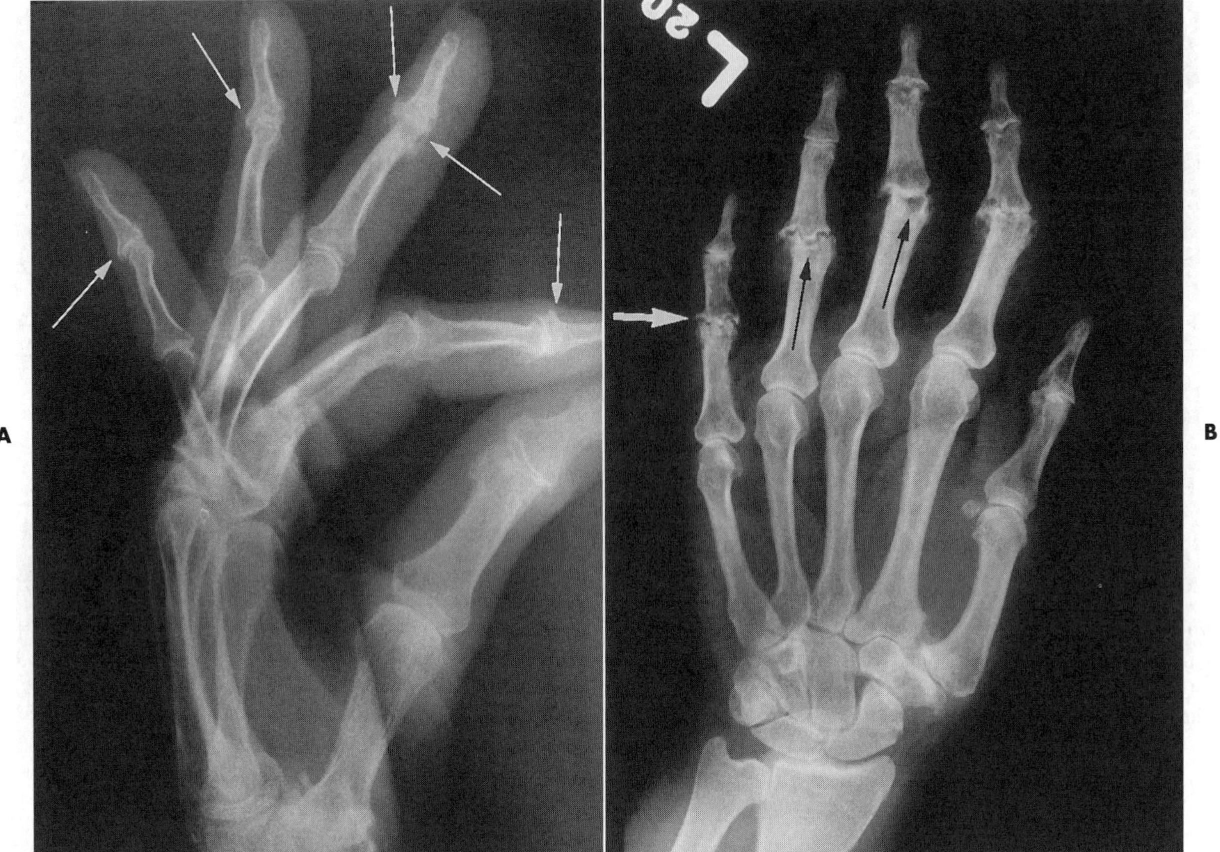

Fig. 123-19. A, Osteoarthritis. Asymmetric extensor and volar proliferative spurs *(arrows)* with associated subchondral eburnative reaction and asymmetric narrowing of joint space. **B,** Erosive osteoarthritis. Prominent central erosions of proximal interphalangeal joints *(black arrows);* gull-wing deformity, bet shown at fifth posterior interphalangeal joint *(white arrow);* and subluxation.

proliferative process with predilection for osteophyte formation. Asymmetric joint involvement without erosions, osteopenia, and ankylosis helps to differentiate osteoarthritis from inflammatory arthropathies.

Abnormalities of the synovial lining and adjacent ligamentous and soft tissue structures occur secondarily. A predilection for hips, knees, and small DIP joints of the hand is seen (Fig. 123-19). In the wrist the trapeziometacarpal and scaphotrapezial joints are typically involved. Secondary osteoarthritis tends to involve the elbow and shoulder. Early radiographic changes in the appendicular skeleton include the following:

1. Asymmetric joint space narrowing accentuated with weight-bearing or stress films.
2. Subchondral reactive sclerosis frequently seen in the large weight-bearing joints.
3. Subchondral changes seen on both sides of the joint space.
4. Effusions that are activity related.
5. No juxtaarticular osteopenia.

Late radiographic findings in the appendicular skeleton include the following:

1. Prominent marginal osteophyte formation.
2. Subchondral cyst formation with a corticated margin.
3. Malalignment or angular deformity, especially in weight-bearing joints.
4. Loose intraarticular bodies (cartilaginous or osseous).
5. Altered mechanical stress bearing, resulting in cortical and trabecular remodeling and buttressing.
6. Chronic effusions.

In the axial skeleton, osteoarthritis specifically refers to changes at the apophyseal joints. Disk space narrowing or changes of the end plates resulting from diskal resorption are more properly termed *intervertebral osteochondrosis.* The changes of osteoarthritis at the apophyseal joints parallel those in the appendicular skeleton. In addition to the classic radiographic findings of cartilaginous thinning, marginal proliferation, subchondral eburnation, and cystic changes, capsular and ligamentous laxity foster segmental anterior, posterior, and lateral subluxation.

Erosive or inflammatory osteoarthritis refers to a specific clinical arthritic pattern seen principally in women and characterized by central erosions of the IP joints.[1] A predilection for the PIP and DIP joints is noted. Monoarticular erosive osteoarthritis can be confused with septic arthritis. Marginal proliferative changes characteristic of osteoarthritis in the appendicular skeleton also are present. The central erosion and marginal proliferative changes with joint space narrowing are termed *gull-wing deformity.* Late radiographic changes may include angulation around the joint and ankylosis.

Calcium Pyrophosphate Dihydrate Arthropathy

Calcium pyrophosphate dihydrate (CPPD) crystals are deposited in articular cartilage and fibrocartilage, ligament,

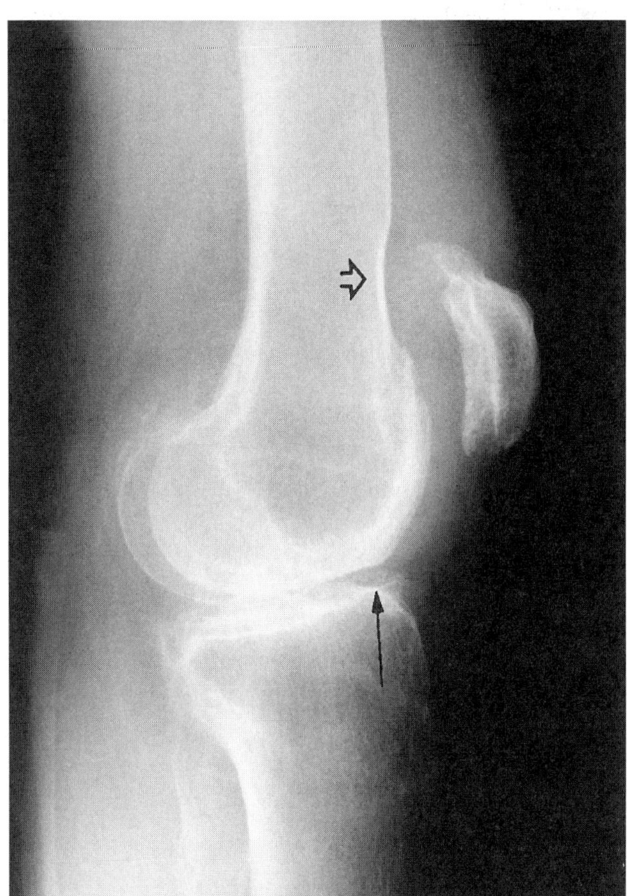

Fig. 123-20. Calcium pyrophosphate deposition disease (CPDD). Chondrocalcinosis of menisci, best shown anteriorly *(black arrow)*, and characteristic distal femoral cortical notching *(open arrow)*.

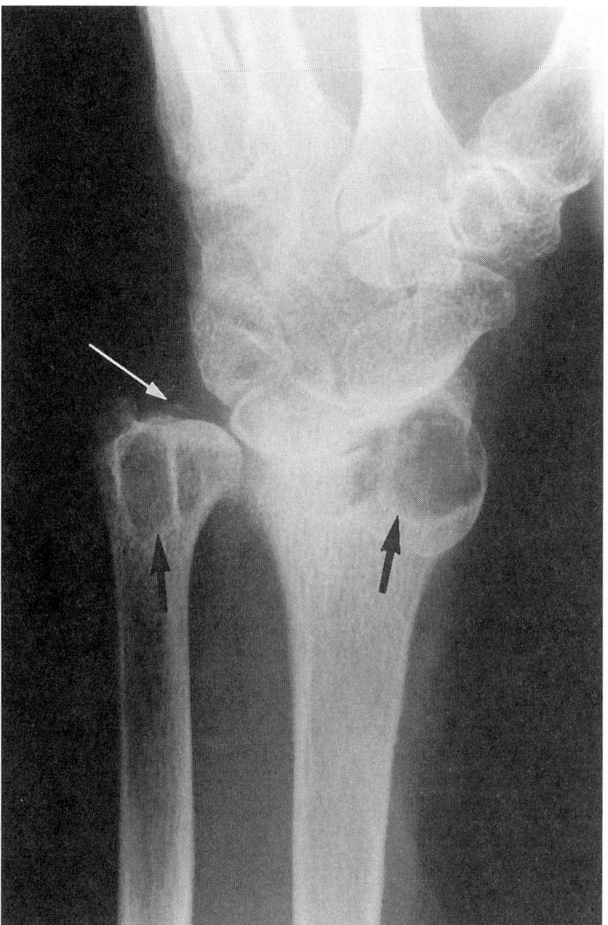

Fig. 123-21. Calcium pyrophosphate dihydrate arthropathy, or CPDD. Chondrocalcinosis of triangular fibrocartilage *(white arrow)* and large subchondral cyst formation *(black arrows)*.

tendon, capsule, synovium, and synovial fluid (see Chapter 134). Radiologic hallmarks of chondrocalcinosis or abnormal mineralization of hyaline and fibrocartilage are seen. Target areas for chondrocalcinosis include the menisci of the knee, triangular fibrocartilage complex of the wrist, articular cartilage of the hips, and fibrocartilage of the symphysis pubis.[6] Plain films of the knee (AP view), wrist (posteroanterior view), and pelvis (AP view) are the standard radiographs initially ordered to evaluate calcium pyrophosphate deposition disease (CPDD).

Although the radiologic findings simulate those of a degenerative process, an atypical pattern of distribution is noted. Chondrocalcinosis of the large weight-bearing joints and smaller non-weight-bearing joints with associated capsular and soft tissue mineralization indicates a systemic process of calcium crystal deposition arthropathy. Unicompartmental or bicompartmental involvement of the knee with isolated or severe patellofemoral disease is a common radiologic presentation. A characteristic notching (erosion) of the anterior distal femur also is seen frequently (Fig. 123-20). Subtle articular mineralization involving the small joints of the wrist and hand and mineralization of the triangular fibrocartilage complex suggest the diagnosis (Fig. 123-21). Early radiographic changes include the following:

1. Normal plain radiograph.
2. Subtle chondrocalcinosis in one or more target areas (knee, wrist, pelvis).
3. Mild symmetric joint space narrowing.
4. Subtle subchondral cyst formation.
5. Effusion.

Later radiographic findings include the following:

1. Prominent chondrocalcinosis.
2. Mineralization of ligaments, tendons, capsule, synovium, and periarticular soft tissues.
3. Prominent symmetric joint space narrowing.
4. Prominent subchondral cyst formation with disproportionately large cysts.
5. Subchondral eburnation.
6. Disproportionately small amount of osteophyte formation for the degree of joint space narrowing and subchondral change.
7. Bilateral weight-bearing and non-weight-bearing joint involvement, suggesting a systemic disorder.

The AP view of the pelvis is radiologically helpful because early or subtle chondrocalcinosis may be seen in the superolateral articular cartilage of the hips, in the synovial-lined SI joints, or at the level of the symphysis pubis.

In the axial skeleton, multilevel peripheral anular and central nuclear diskal calcification are clues. The radiographic features mimic those of a degenerative arthritic process, except for more florid and widespread involvement. Calcification of associated paraspinal ligaments is characteristic. Currently, nuclear scintigraphy and MRI are not helpful in the evaluation of this disorder. CT scan characterizes the

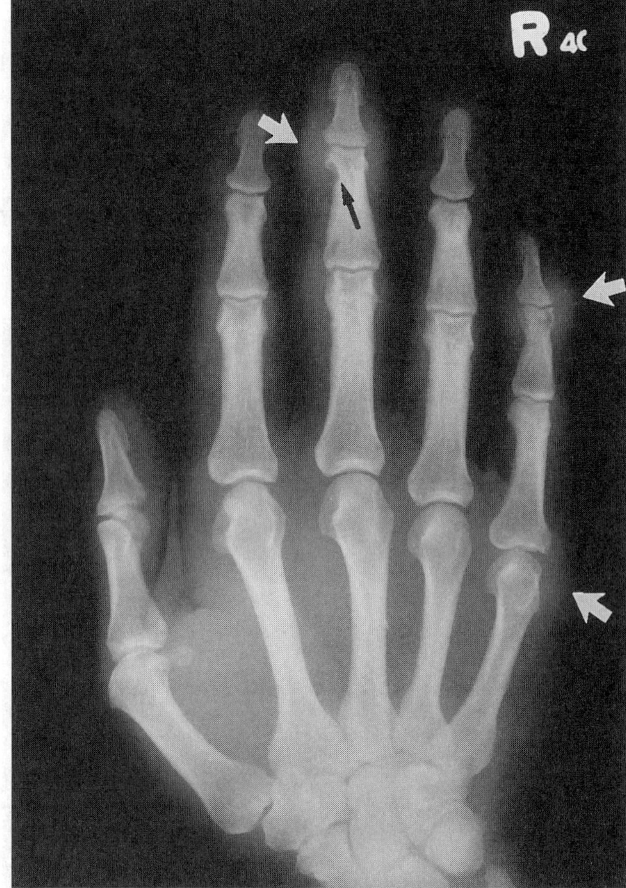

Fig. 123-22. Gouty arthritis. Prominent soft tissue tophi *(white arrows)* and associated bony erosion with geographic sclerotic margination *(black arrow)*.

diskal calcification of paravertebral calcific deposits. The diagnosis is most frequently suggested by plain films and corroborated through crystal isolation from joint aspirate.

Gout

Gout is a crystal deposition arthropathy secondary to deposition of monosodium urate crystals in soft tissues, synovium, cartilage, and joint capsule (see Chapter 136). Soft tissue changes and subsequent osseous remodeling characterize the radiologic findings of primary gouty arthritis (Fig. 123-22). Radiographs of initial episodes of gouty arthritis do not show articular abnormality. Juxtaarticular soft tissue swelling is the typical presenting finding. Bony demineralization is not noted. Less than 50% of patients with documented gouty arthritis show osseous change. Radiologic findings of bony change, which typically requires more than 5 years, document the chronicity of the disease process. The first MTP joint is the articulation most often involved (Fig. 123-23). Besides the feet, the ankle, knees, hands, and elbows can be affected. Bilateral olecranon bursitis is a clinical and radiologic clue to the diagnosis of gouty arthritis. Tophaceous deposits may occur juxtaarticularly, causing pressure erosion to the underlying bone. Deposits are seen in tendons, ligaments, capsule, and bursa. Extraarticular deposits are seen in the helix of the ear, palm of the hand, sole of the foot, and fingertip. Deposits may simulate the amyloid arthropathy seen in chronic renal failure patients, especially those on long-term hemodialysis.[8] Involvement of the axial skeleton is uncommon. In rare cases of SI joint involvement, changes are similar to those in other articulations, including large cystic or erosive changes of the true synovial-lined joint in an asymmetric unilateral or bilateral pattern of involvement.

Early radiologic findings of gouty arthritis include the following:

1. Normal mineralization.
2. Soft tissue swelling without articular abnormality.
3. Asymmetric monoarticular or polyarticular involvement.

Late radiologic findings include the following:

1. Soft tissue tophi with or without mineralization.
2. Chondrocalcinosis.
3. Osseous erosions with a characteristic overhanging bony margin.
4. Geographic sclerotic margination to bony erosion.
5. Intraosseous mineralization.

Gouty arthritis is differentiated from RA by the absence of juxtaarticular osteopenia, symmetric joint space loss, and symmetric polyarticular involvement. The peripheral distribution of joint involvement is also different in these two joint diseases. Differentiating a seronegative spondyloarthropathy such as psoriatic arthritis from gout may be more difficult due to the overlap of target sites (e.g., first MTP joint). Periosteal reaction, progressive bony erosive destruction without an associated soft tissue mass or tophus, and ankylosis of an articulation make gouty arthritis less likely. The high incidence of axial skeleton involvement in ankylosing spondylitis and its low occurrence in gouty arthritis help distinguish these two disorders. Differentiating gout from

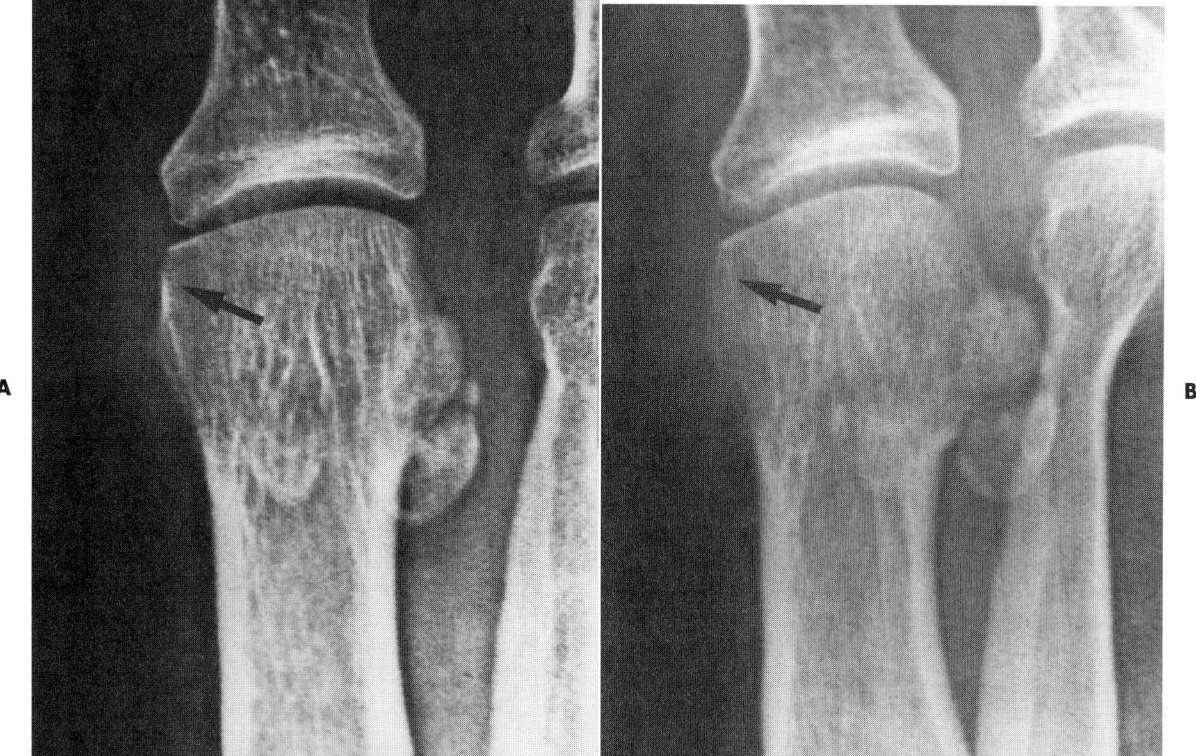

Fig. 123-23. **A,** Gouty arthritis. **B,** Progressive erosion of first metatarsal head with loss of subchondral cortical delineation over 8 months *(black arrows).*

other crystal deposition arthropathies (e.g., CPDD) can be challenging, especially early in the disease process. Joint fluid aspiration and crystal evaluation are most helpful. Radiologic findings of extensive chondrocalcinosis, joint space narrowing, and large subchondral cyst formation without associated soft tissue tophi are helpful in excluding gouty arthritis.

Alternate radiologic imaging modalities do not provide diagnostic or therapeutic advantage in the evaluation of gouty arthritis. The diagnosis is most often suggested by plain radiographs and corroborated by crystal isolation from joint and periarticular sites.

REFERENCES

1. Belhorn LR et al: Erosive osteoarthritis, *Semin Arthritis Rheum* 22:298, 1993.
2. Brower AC: *Arthritis in black and white,* ed 2, Philadelphia, 1997, Saunders.
3. Doherty M et al: *Rheumatology examination and injection techniques,* Philadelphia, 1992, Saunders.
4. Dussault RG, Samson L, Fortin MT: Plain film diagnosis of joint disease, *Can Assoc Radiol J* 42:87, 1991.
5. Forrester DM, Brown JC: *The radiology of joint disease,* Philadelphia, 1987, Saunders.
6. Freidman L et al: Limited low-dose computed tomography protocol to examine the sacroiliac joints, *Can Assoc Radiol J* 44:267, 1993.
7. Hayes CM, Conway WF: Calcium hydroxyapatite deposition disease, *Radiographics* 10:1031, 1990.
8. Loevner LA et al: Dialysis-related arthropathy in patients on long-term hemodialysis: radiographic features, *J Clin Rheum* 1:81, 1995.
9. Resnick D, Niwayama G: *Diagnosis of bone and joint disorders,* Philadelphia, 1988, Saunders.

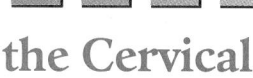

CHAPTER 124

Disorders of the Cervical Spine

John H. Bland

The extremely flexible cervical spine is the body's most complicated and mobile articular system; it is designed for mobility at the expense of stability. The seven small, comparatively fragile cervical vertebrae (C1 to C7) with their extensive ligaments, capsules, tendons, and muscle attachments are poorly designed to protect their contents compared with the skull above and the thorax below. The cervical spine balances a 10- to 15-pound ball, the head, on the lateral masses of the atlas.

Many clinically reported and distinct syndromes arise from abnormalities of the tissues of the cervical spine alone. Even more syndromes arise from distant structures, but they are associated with signs and symptoms referable to the cervical spine, head, shoulders, and upper extremities. These disorders constitute a considerable portion of any physician's practice.

EPIDEMIOLOGY

More than 10% of the Swedish population recalled having at least three episodes of pain in the neck in a 1984 study. Up to 12% of women and 9% of men experienced neck pain with or without associated arm pain. Seventy percent of adults who visited their physicians for neck pain were well or were improving within 1 month. Neck pain is a recurring clinical event and for most patients a mild to modest, transitory nuisance.

ANATOMY

The nucleus pulposus, present at birth, gradually disappears between ages 12 to 14 years and 35 to 40 years. Little if any nucleus pulposus remains in any of the disks in the cervical spine. Thus persons over age 40 cannot herniate the nucleus pulposus. The uncinate process, a bony development laterally and posterolaterally, enlarges with increasing age and presents a bulwark that prevents herniation of the intervertebral disks posterolaterally.[1]

From the level of C3-4, the posterior nerve root exits are below the level of the vertebral disk. Thus the nerve roots are found regularly with increasing obliqueness from above downward. Clinically, it is impossible for the disk to compress nerve roots within the spinal canal, because the root exit zone is below the level of the disk. After age 40 to 45, all dural root sleeves (exit sites) become fibrotic and stiff. All zygapophyseal joints (posterior joints) have menisci capable of proliferation into a pannuslike structure over the cartilage surface, which is clinically significant.[5] The anterior nerve root is low in the intervertebral foramen and thus is unlikely to be compressed. The posterior root is well protected from the point of view of any disk herniation; however, the zygapophyseal joints can become enlarged, osteoarthritic, and osteophytic and compress the posterior nerve roots. Any radiculopathy (although radiculopathy itself is rare) is a consequence of the zygapophyseal joint abnormality, not of the uncinate process or the alleged joints of Luschka.

Considerable disparity exists between the anteroposterior diameter and the transverse measurement of the spinal cord as it relates to the internal diameter and transverse diameter of the spinal canal. "Fat" cords and "thin" cords are seemingly a genetic endowment; the ideal is a thin cord and a capacious spinal canal, a constitutional characteristic.

Preganglionic sympathetic fibers are not present in the cervical spine because they originate from thoracic (T1, T2, and T3) levels and have their first synapse in one or more of the three cervical sympathetic ganglia. The postganglionic fibers travel in three directions: (1) distributing into the upper extremity, providing all autonomic function to the arm and hand; (2) reentering the intervertebral foramina and the spinal cord, with connections in the vestibular apparatus, cerebellum, hypothalamus, and thalamus as well as to the spinal nerves; and (3) accompanying vertebral and carotid arteries, following their distribution in the brain with multiple connections.[4]

The anterior portion of the spinal canal is characterized universally by bars of osteophytes at the level of the intervertebral disks, sometimes compressing the cord to varying degrees. The ligamentum flavum is usually hypertrophic and hyperplastic, projecting into the posterior spinal canal. A 30-degree turn of the head normally kinks the ipsilateral vertebral artery. A 45-degree turn kinks both vertebral arteries. In the presence of osteoarthritis, disk disorders, and facet disease, vertebral artery compression is not rare and can become symptomatic.

Physiologically, the cervical spine is characterized by a high degree of motion. When any part of the musculoskeletal system is put to complete rest, series of events will culminate in total destruction of a joint in approximately 4 to 6 months. Wherever there is the least motion, there will be the greatest degree of pathophysiologic change in the involved tissues. Because the cervical spine is virtually never completely still, it is especially vulnerable to partial immobilization and at considerable risk by total immobilization. Prolonged immobilization in a cervical collar may result in stiffness, pain, and limited motion. Immobilization, partial or total, should be avoided as much as possible.[2]

PATIENT EVALUATION

History

Knowing the patient's age and occupation is extremely important. Cervical osteoarthritis with myriad syndromes is a disease of later life. Trauma and "crick" (spasmodic torticollis) occur in younger people. Occupations requiring continued or intermittent hyperflexion, hyperextension, or overrotation of the cervical spine may produce and prolong symptoms. Details about previous injury are important. Whether the patient wears bifocal glasses may be pertinent because bifocals usually require the patient to extend the occiput, atlas, and axis complex and to flex the lower cervical spine. Inquiry about the type of pillow the patient uses, if any, frequently reveals useful information.

Physical Characteristics. Physical characteristics such as neck length, receding mandible, high arched palate, crooked teeth, and asymmetry of facial bones and muscles should be noted. Information about temporomandibular joint (TMJ) function is important. Investigation of a painful bite, limited jaw opening, or swelling of the TMJ area may lead to a proper diagnosis.

Pain Characteristics. Three phases or periods of the patient's pain history should be investigated during the interview: onset, course, and present status. The location, size, distribution, quality, intensity, severity, and duration of the first pain should be noted. Fig. 124-1 illustrates patterns of reflexly referred pain from visceral and somatic structures. Box 124-1 lists for common disorders causing cervical and shoulder pain. Head pain is common in and characteristic of cervical syndromes. A lesion at the C6-7 level may cause neurologic or myalgic pain and muscular tenderness in the precordial or scapular region and may suggest angina pectoris.

Paresthesia and Weakness. Numbness and tingling occur in the segmental distribution of the nerve roots, often with no demonstrable objective sensory change. Weakness is uncommon but requires inquiry. Patients who have trouble balancing their heads because of muscle weakness have clearly lost power.

Symptoms. Eye symptoms and signs associated with cervical syndromes include blurring of vision, frequent change of glasses without improvement, relief of pain by changing neck position, increased tearing, retroorbital pain, and strange description of eyes "being pulled backward or pushed forward." These signs and symptoms likely result from irritation of the cervical sympathetic nerve supply to eye structures. Change in equilibrium occurs because of irritation of sympathetic plexuses surrounding the vertebral arteries or

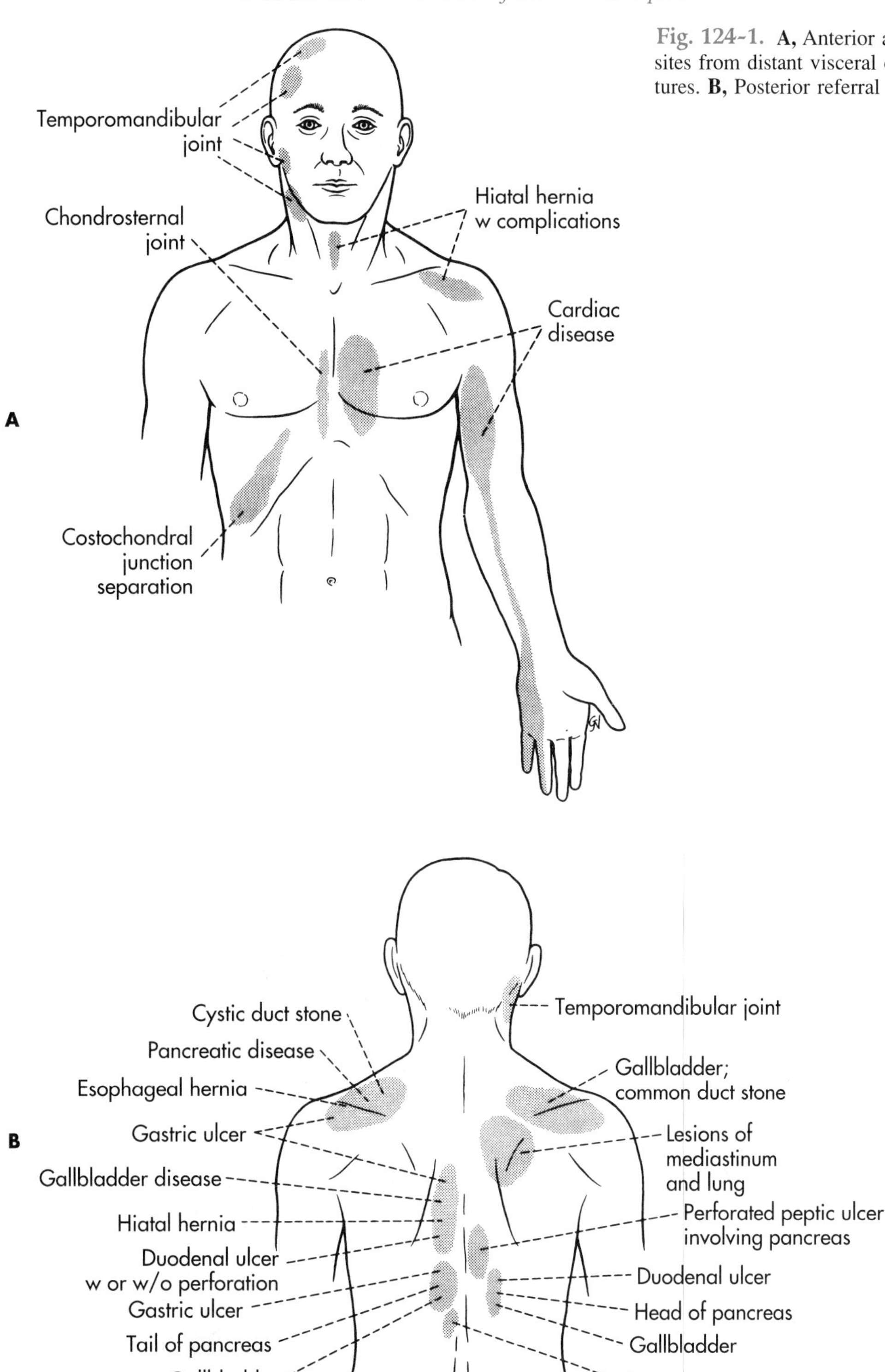

Fig. 124-1. A, Anterior and posterior referral sites from distant visceral or somatic structures. **B,** Posterior referral sites.

Continued

from vascular insufficiency. Dysphagia can be caused by muscle spasm and anterior osteophyte compression of the pharynx and esophagus (Fig. 124-2).

Multivalent pathogenetic mechanisms explain many bizarre symptoms, some of which are unrelated. A patient comment such as "I can't get a deep breath" may be caused by C3 to C5 lesions whose roots innervate the diaphragm and other respiratory muscles. Cardiac palpitation and tachycardia may result from unusual positions or hyperextension of the neck caused by irritation of the C4 nerve root supplying the diaphragm and pericardium or by irritation of the cardiac sympathetic nerve supply. Nausea and vomiting, poorly defined pain, and paresthesia may be caused by cord compression. Drop attacks may result from abrupt loss of proprioception; the patient may collapse without loss of consciousness, often with the ability to rise and continue with previous activity. Differentiating psychoneurosis from cervical syndromes is a common problem, usually reflecting the

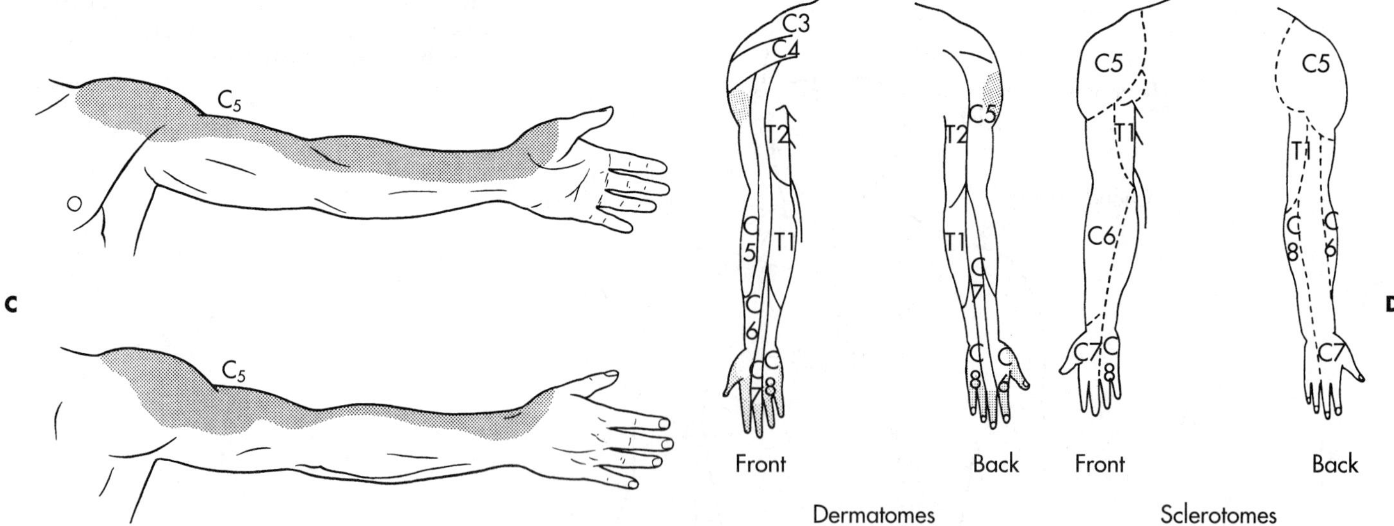

Fig. 124-1, cont'd. **C,** Distribution of all shoulder structures derived from fifth cervical (C5) dermatome-myotome-sclerotome. **D,** Distribution of dermatomes and sclerotomes of upper extremities. (**D** from Lance JW, McLeod JG: *A physiological approach to clinical neurology,* ed 2, Reading, Mass, 1975, Butterworth.)

Box 124-1. Cervical Disorders that Cause Neck and Shoulder Pain

Spasmodic torticollis
Intervertebral disk protrusion
Osteoarthritis
Fibromyalgia syndrome
Trauma, fracture
Injuries from hyperflexion or hyperextension (whiplash)
Rheumatoid arthritis
Ankylosing spondylitis
Infection
Thoracic outlet syndromes
Metastatic malignant disease
Carotid and vertebral artery atherosclerosis

examiner's inexperience with nerve root compression, sympathetic nervous system involvement, cervical cord compression, vascular insufficiency, and diseases and trauma of cervical bone, muscle, and joint.

Physical Examination

Most patients with cervical spine syndromes require a complete physical examination in addition to a thorough musculoskeletal examination with appropriate regional focus.

Posture and Movement. The patient should be gowned and sitting upright to determine the range of motion of the cervical spine. The patient's posture should be observed from the front, back, and side while the patient is sitting, standing, and walking. Anatomic details such as scapular height, spinal curves, head tilt, and head position should be noted. The cervicothoracic and thoracolumbar junctions and the sacral area should be examined. The presence of cervical lordosis, kyphosis, and lumbar lordosis should be specifically investigated. Gait analysis may help in making a diagnosis such as scoliosis, congenital lesions, or even a lumbar spondylolisthesis, which is reflected clinically in the cervical spine. The patient's ability and willingness to move should be

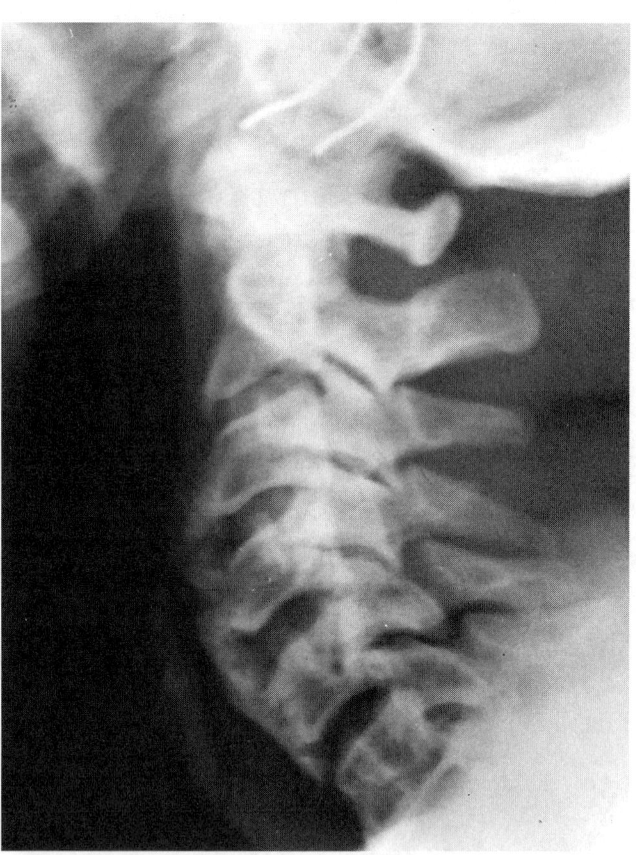

Fig. 124-2. Diffuse idiopathic skeletal hyperostosis. Laminar bone at C3-4 level has pushed esophagus forward, stretching tissues and causing dysphagia.

Table 124-1. Neurologic Screening Tests

Action/tendon/site	Nerve(s)
Motor function (active and against resistance)	
Rotation of ceivical spine	C1,2,3
Shrug	C2,3,4,5
Arm abduction	C5
Forearm flexion, supination	C5,6
Forearm extension	C7
Wrist extension (with elbows extended)	C6
Wrist flexion	C7
Thumb extension	C8
Fifth finger abduction	C8
Interosseal and lumbrical muscle function	T1
Deep tendon reflexes	
Pectoral	C5-T1
Deltoid	C5-6
Biceps	C5-6
Triceps	C7
Brachioradial	C5-6
Somite areas (light touch, pinprick, and vibration)	
Acromioclavicular joint	C4
Deltoid; lateral arm	C5
Thumb	C6
Middle finger	C7
Fifth finger	C8
Forearm, medial border	T1
Arm, medial border	T2

observed, looking particularly for head or neck guarding. The acuteness of the problem should be assessed.

Physical Abnormalities. The patient should be observed for any abnormal appearance such as extreme height or shortness, an unusually long or short neck, retracted mandible, crooked teeth, or high palate. These abnormalities, as well as facial asymmetry, abnormal facial development, and asymmetric bone and muscle development, suggest congenital anomalies of the cervical spine, particularly the upper third.

Neurologic Examination. Table 124-1 lists screening tests.

Spinal Movement. With the patient standing, movement of the entire spine in flexion, extension, lateral flexion, and rotation should be observed. Passive ranges of motion should be determined, then actively increased. All four motions should be tested against resistance to observe the patient's motor power and to determine whether muscle contraction against resistance produces pain. The goal is to produce signs and symptoms that will identify the pain-sensitive structure for a precise diagnosis.

Shoulder Examination. The examiner should determine whether the shoulder or any structures within it are contributing to pain in the neck (see Chapter 125).

Testing for Nerve Root Compression. The quadrant position is used to alter the size of the intervertebral foramina and determine whether the nerve root can be compressed. Head extension is tested first, so that the inferior facet of the vertebra above glides posteriorly on the facet of the vertebra below, thereby narrowing the foramina. If this maneuver produces shoulder pain, paresthesia, or numbness, the nerve root is compressed in the foramina. Other maneuvers should not be attempted. If the patient does not experience these symptoms, lateral flexion should be attempted, which closes the foramina toward the side of the flexion and opens it on the opposite side. If this maneuver produces the syndrome, other maneuvers should not be made. If it does not produce the pain or dysesthesia syndrome, full rotation should be added, which maximally closes the foramina on one side and opens it on the opposite side. If active range of motion produces the syndrome, the examiner need not use the quadrant position.

Head Compression Test (Spurling Test). Compression of the head, causing force transmission to the cervical spine, may induce pain by narrowing the intervertebral foramina. Upper extremity radicular pain or paresthesia produced or intensified by this maneuver is indicative of nerve root irritation. Localized, nonradicular pain suggests that soft tissue or joints are the pain-sensitive structures. The test is performed with the patient sitting. The physician places one hand across the other on the top of the patient's head and gradually increases downward pressure. The patient is instructed to report pain or paresthesia and its distribution. Repeating the test with the patient's head tilted to either side, backward, and then forward increases the test's sensitivity.

Distraction Test. This test predicts the effect of cervical spine traction in relieving pain or paresthesia. Nerve root compression may be relieved, with disappearance of the symptoms and signs, if the intervertebral foramina are opened or the disk spaces extended. Pressure on joint capsules of apophyseal joints is also decreased by distraction. Muscle spasms of any cause may be relieved. The test is performed with the patient sitting. The physician places the palm of one hand under the patient's chin and the other under the occiput and gradually increases the force of lifting, removing the weight of the skull and distracting the foramina, disks, and joints. This test is continued for 30 to 60 seconds.

Palpation. The examiner palpates the anterior and posterior cervical triangles for the brachial plexus and examines the site of the subclavian artery. Deep palpation also allows examination of the transverse processes of the atlas and axis and sometimes the third vertebra. Identification of landmarks in the anterior triangle assists in clinical orientation, such as in the identification of a fractured cervical vertebra. The hyoid bone is at the C3 level. If signs and symptoms are associated with C3, tenderness may be present at this level. The thyroid cartilage is at the upper level of C4, the thyroid gland at the lower level of C5, and the first ring of cricoid cartilage at the C6 level.

Appearance of the Back. The levator muscle of the scapula, the trapezius, rhomboid and scalene muscles, and superior angle of the scapula should be observed for atrophy, weakness, and neurologic signs. The deltoid, supraspinatus, and infraspinatus muscles should be observed for atrophy. The skin should be examined for thickness, color, scars, temperature, past incisions, and ecchymoses. The carotid arteries are palpated for tenderness. The sternocleidomastoid

Table 124-2. Cervical Spine Diseases With Uunusual Pathogenesis

Condition	Pathogenic process
Ankylosing spondylitis	Inflammation
Osteomyelitis	Infection
Bursitis in cervical spine	Inflammation
Neoplastic lesion (Horner's syndrome)	Neoplastic disease
Hyoid bone syndrome	Tendinitis
Neck-tongue syndrome	Nerve entrapment
Calcific retropharyngeal tendinitis	Tendinitis
Ligamentum flavum calcification	Calcific deposits
Occipital neuralgia	Neuritis of second cervical nerve
Simple long neck	Normal anatomic variant, extracervical vertebra
Syndrome of third neuron of cervical sympathetic system	Neoplastic or vascular disease, trauma
Neck sprain	Trauma (whiplash injury), psychologic mechanisms
Fibrous dysplasia of bone progress	Genetic
Atlantooccipital and atlantoaxial dislocation	Trauma, infection, inflammation
Bilateral facet dislocation below C3 level	Trauma
Tennis elbow, carpal tunnel syndrome, rotator cuff lesion	Secondary to cervical osteoarthritis
Posterior cervical sympathetic syndrome, Barré-Lieou syndrome	Inflammation, sepsis, neoplasm, psychologic/psychiatric mechanisms
Psychiatric syndrome of cervical spine	Mental mechanism (e.g., hysteria)
Paget's disease	Unknown, possibly viral origin
Vertebral artery syndromes	Osteoarthritis, trauma, atherosclerosis, rheumatoid arthritis
Esophageal syndromes	Osteoarthritis, hyperostosis
Axial osteomalacia	Metabolic bone disease
Osteoporosis	Metabolic bone disease (idiopathic)
Radiculopathy	Osteoarthritis, various root entrapment diseases
Peripheral neuropathy of C1-T1 peripheral nerves	Neuritis (multiple causes)
Myelopathy	Osteoarthritis intervertebral disks, trauma, others
Vertebrobasilar insufficiency syndromes	Vascular; osteoarthritis, atherosclerosis
Thoracic outlet syndrome	Vascular/neuropathic
Subclavian steal syndrome	Variety of causes
Gout	Monosodium urate crystal deposition
Double-crush syndrome	Nerve entrapments
Postural cervical syndromes	Abnormal posture
Levator scapulae muscle syndrome	Specific muscle strain, trauma, postural defects

muscle and its function are examined. Sites of tenderness are marked with a felt-tipped pen and correlated, if possible, with the local structures. Table 124-2 lists cervical spine diseases with unusual pathogenesis. Fig. 124-3 outlines the pathophysiologic mechanisms of common soft tissue cervical spine syndromes.

RADIOLOGIC EVALUATION

Technologic advances have greatly improved imaging of the cervical spine. Arthrography and diskography are rarely used. Development of low-toxicity, water-soluble myelographic contrast has ushered in the era of computed tomography (CT) myelography. Magnetic resonance imaging (MRI), with continuing refinements in software technology and surface coils, has added a new dimension of noninvasive evaluation of the cervical spine and spinal cord.

Conventional radiography of the cervical spine includes anteroposterior (AP), AP odontoid, lateral, and right and left oblique views. Two AP views are needed. The AP odontoid through the open mouth demonstrates the entire odontoid process and may also show atlantooccipital or atlantoaxial joints. The second AP view includes the lower cervical spine from C3 to T1. A lateral cervical spine radiograph should show the base of the skull, seven cervical vertebrae, and the end plate of the first thoracic vertebrae. If shoulders prevent clear imaging of the lower vertebral bodies, a coned-down, or "swimmer's view," of the cervicothoracic junction is obtained. Oblique views illustrate the neural foramina, pedicles, and the superior and inferior articulating facet joints.

The radiographic evaluation of trauma patients must be carefully tailored to prevent further neurologic injury. In a cooperative, neurologically intact patient, AP, AP odontoid, lateral, and right and left oblique views are obtained. Only if these radiographs are normal is it safe to proceed to flexion-extension views. In severely traumatized patients or those with neurologic deficits, only AP and lateral survey films are obtained without moving the patient. Further cervical spine evaluation of trauma patients is accomplished by CT scan. CT scanning accurately demonstrates fractures and displaced bone fragments that could cause serious neurologic injury by compromising either the spinal canal or neural foramina.

In radiologic evaluation of the cervical spine, MRI has several advantages over CT scanning. In contrast to CT, no ionizing radiation is involved. MRI has a higher contrast resolution, allowing it to differentiate between soft tissues, both normal and pathologic, with great sensitivity. Unlike CT

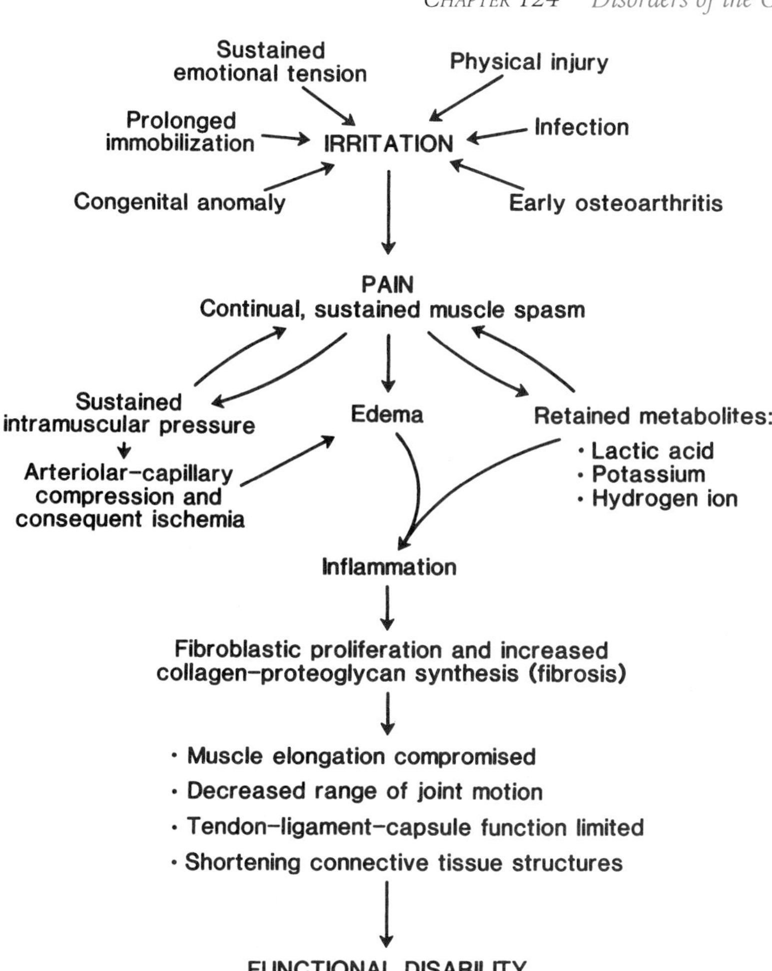

Fig. 124-3. Pathophysiologic mechanisms of soft tissue cervical spine syndromes.

scans, bone artifact does not degrade MR images. Multiple imaging planes (e.g., sagittal, axial, coronal, oblique) are available without repositioning the patient or significantly prolonging the length of the examination, an important advantage in the injured patient. The entire cervical spine is studied in sagittal and coronal images.

MRI study requires a cooperative patient. Disadvantages include extreme motion sensitivity. In addition, dense cortical or compact bone has few hydrogen protons and therefore is seen as a signal void on MR images with limited spatial resolution. Thus MRI may fail to delineate fractures and poorly defines bone spurs and calcification. MRI is more expensive than CT scanning, and patients occasionally are too claustrophobic to endure the study.

LABORATORY STUDIES AND DIAGNOSTIC PROCEDURES

Few laboratory studies are guided by results of the history and physical examination (e.g., occasional spinal tap, HLA typing, immunoglobulins, rheumatoid factor, antinuclear antibody). Diagnostic procedures include radiologic evaluation, occasional biopsy or electrodiagnostic studies, and less often CT scans, MRI, angiogram, or radionuclide studies. These diagnostic studies, as well as chest radiographs and electrocardiograms (ECGs), also help to exclude neck pain from metastatic disease and referred pain from chest pathology (e.g., Pancoast tumor, pneumonia, heart disease).

GENERAL MANAGEMENT

Maintaining optimum overall fitness contributes significantly to the success of management of cervical spine disorders and disease. Management and active treatment of disease, as well as rehabilitation of cervical spine disorders, are strongly linked to the rest of the spine and to the body as a whole.[6,7] Patient education contributes greatly to success. Classes about arthritis are available through the Arthritis Foundation. Patient handbooks and educational materials may be helpful. Physical therapy modalities can be categorized as *cryotherapy,* the use of physical cold; *thermotherapy,* both superficial and deep, the use of heat by any method that provides heat; *mechanical therapy,* the use of massage, whirlpool, and methods that move the tissues about in various ways; and *electrotherapy,* stimulation of nerve and muscle by electric current. Cervical collars play a relatively small role in stabilizing the spine but remind the patient to minimize neck motion. The cervical spine is particularly vulnerable to loss of function when immobilized. The collar may provide comfort and warmth, psychologic benefit, and marginal control of movement.[6-8]

Cervical Spine Pillows. The use of pillows specifically designed for cervical spine disorders is an important part of management. They usually provide comfort and relief of pain and allow for normal sleep. A frequent complaint in cervical spine patients is night pain. Correction of poor sleeping posture is often successful in alleviating discomfort. Most people sleep on one or more pillows, promoting long flexion of the neck, with subsequent aggravation of or increase in pain due to muscle spasm. Sleeping with no pillow almost always makes symptoms worse. To sleep prone is to keep the neck rotated, strained, and laterally flexed for long periods. When poor sleeping posture results in head and neck pain, the use of a pillow may be helpful.

Cervical pillows vary in size and types, from air pillows blown up to the thickness that raises the head to the most comfortable level, to a tubular-shaped pillow (Cervipillow), to a multipurpose pillow (Wal-Pil-O). Wal-Pil-O provides four combinations of head and neck support, one of which is proper for almost all cervical spine problems. The Wal-Pil-O cradles the head and supports the neck in both side-lying and back-lying postures. It comprises four pillows in all, with soft and medium centers for head and narrow and wide, firmer borders for the neck. The Shape of Sleep pillow features a neck support ridge that fits under the neck and is a physiologic, biomechanically sound model. Bolster-type pillows in different diameters and pillows with a contour cutout for the head are also available.[9]

Cervical Spine Traction

The usefulness and effectiveness of cervical spine traction are well established; it does cause vertebral distraction. This separation allows alteration of the pathologic relationship between the nerve root and compressing disk or between the nerve root and zygapophyseal joints. About 75% to 80% of patients with radicular symptoms receive clear benefit, usually lasting months to years, from optimally applied traction.

Intermittent traction is the best initial application. The clinical problem may be solved that simply. The weight applied ranges from a minimum of 10 pounds to a maximum of 50 pounds (rarely) over 15 to 20 minutes. If significant improvement does not occur over 8 to 10 sessions of optimally administered traction, it should be discontinued. If symptoms have worsened, the physician should identify precisely why the therapy was not successful. The amount of weight used in traction is a function of the patient's size, the presence of neurologic symptoms or signs, the specific lesion for which traction is prescribed, and the patient's general sense of comfort and improvement. The physician is guided by the results of each traction session. With secure improvement, patients may purchase home equipment and continue traction until all symptoms resolve, maintaining close contact with a medical authority.

Continual traction does not permit as much weight as intermittent traction. Increments of weight are added with each session, usually beginning with about 10 pounds, depending on the degree or lack of progress. Trial and error is used to determine distance from the traction pulley, direction of traction, and position. An average level of traction is 15 to 20 pounds for 20 minutes. The patient sits in slight cervical spine flexion facing the door or apparatus, and the angle of the rope is 20 to 30 degrees from vertical; this is a physiologic position (Fig. 124-4, *A*). In general, pain relief occurs sooner and more completely in patients with radicular symptoms than in those with symptoms arising from the connective tissue structures of the neck (ligaments, tendons, muscles, joints). Symptoms related to the upper extremities are much more likely to be relieved by traction, whereas symptoms related to connective tissue structures are more likely to respond to other measures. Traction is manipulative therapy, but it is vastly different from adjustments involving rotational and lateral stretches, which pose a greater risk of root irritation.

Cervical traction may be achieved manually. Some authors prefer manual traction because of the immediate sensory feedback and the specificity of treatment (Fig. 124-4, *B*). In manual traction, one hand is placed under the chin with the other under the occiput, or both hands are placed under the occiput. A longitudinal force is exerted at varying angles of cervical flexion, extension, lateral flexion, and rotation. Degree, direction, and duration of the tractive force are guided by the patient's response, the clinical disorder, and the goal of treatment. Relaxation is urged before initiating traction. The degree to which a patient relaxes can be used as a method of assessing potential response to mechanical traction.

Self-administered or home traction should always be undertaken initially in a teaching session so that the patient completely understands the procedures and probable perceptions in the process. Self-traction can be performed with the patient in a supine or sitting position (Fig. 124-4, *C*). The supine position combines the advantages of increased stability and the possibility of relaxation of muscles.

The angle of traction is between 15 and 35 degrees, depending on the clinical response and the patient's interpretation of its efficacy. The type of head halter used affects the angle of traction provided. The perception of force should be about equal under the occiput and the chin. In most patients, slight cervical flexion is preferred because in this position the posterior zygapophyseal joints are separated, the intervertebral foramina are enlarged, and the lateral nerve root canals are released. The application of moist heat before traction is recommended.

The decision for traction is based on the patient's history and physical examination. Two mechanisms by which cervical spine soft tissues can be damaged and fail are short-duration, high-amplitude loading and long-duration, low-amplitude loading. The first represents an obvious acute trauma—the classic automobile collision from the rear with whiplash injury. The second is a chronic sprain of soft tissues that occurs inconspicuously and gradually, usually with some final event that precipitates a more acute syndrome superimposed on a chronic condition.

Pharmacologic Treatment

Drugs have a relatively small role in the management of cervical spine syndromes unless specifically indicated.

Rest and Exercise

Stretching exercises for the cervical spine are used for the same reasons they are used elsewhere in the body: to prevent contracture, to increase range of motion if contracture has occurred, and to maintain biomechanical function of the supporting structures in the cervical spine. Range of motion exercises maintain or increase a limited range. Strengthening exercises are especially important because the cervical spine is extremely mobile compared with other areas of the body.

INDICATIONS FOR CONSULTATION

Neurologic consultation is indicated if the patient has rheumatoid arthritis (RA) of the cervical spine and sublux-

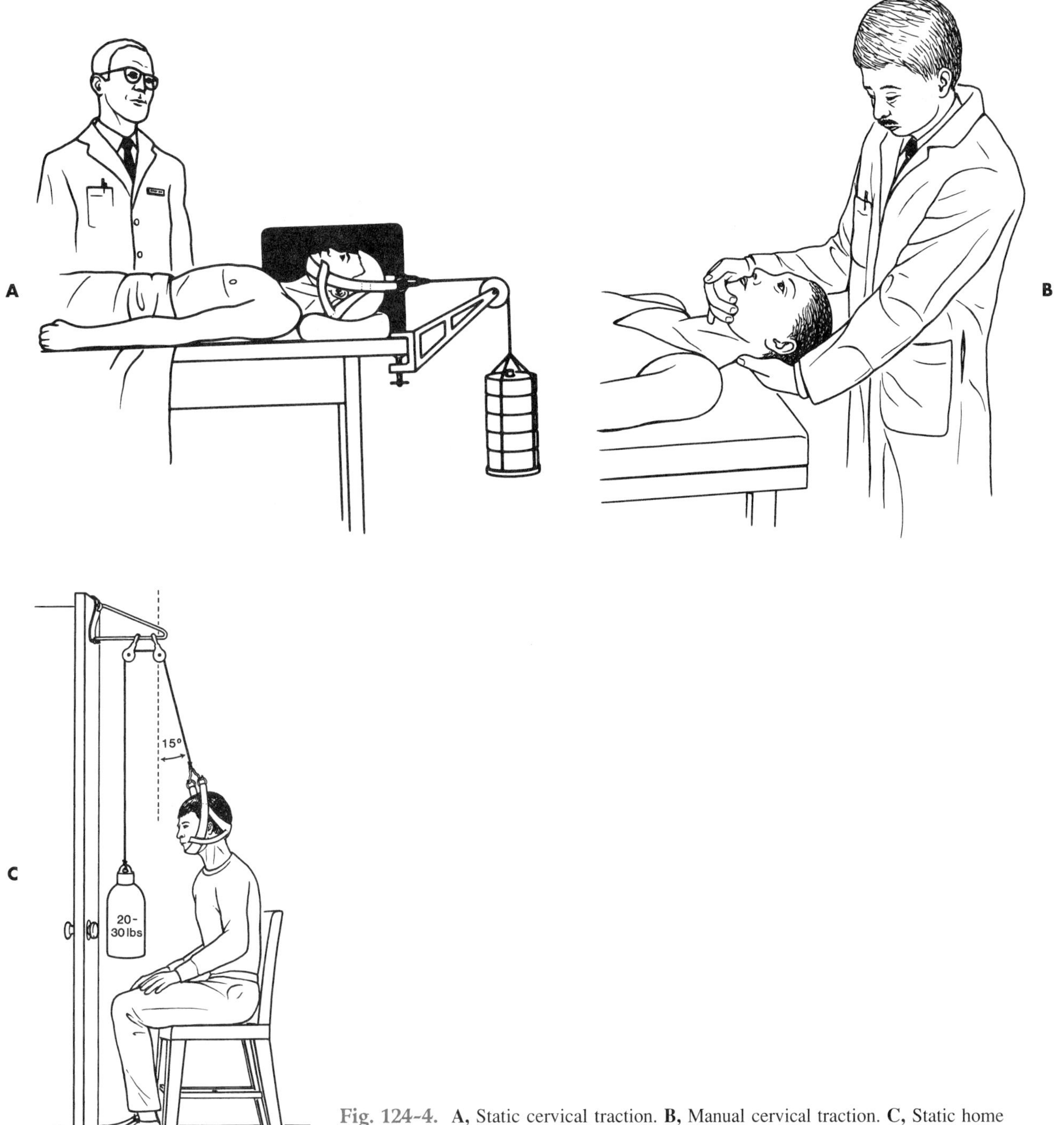

Fig. 124-4. **A,** Static cervical traction. **B,** Manual cervical traction. **C,** Static home cervical traction.

ations associated with neurologic symptoms and signs. If these signs are progressive, the indication becomes urgent. Unidentified peripheral neuropathy or entrapment neuropathy at the thoracic outlet, at the elbow, and associated with carpal tunnel syndrome at the wrist may indicate cervical myelopathy. Neurologic consultation also may be necessary when neurosurgical or orthopedic surgery (e.g., facetectomy, laminectomy, chondroosteophyte removal) is being contemplated for a patient with cervical osteoarthritis and when progressive inflammatory muscle disease (e.g., polymyositis, dermatomyositis) is present.

Neurosurgical consultation may be needed in RA patients with cervical spine subluxations who require surgical stabilization of the spine or have RA signs and symptoms of myelopathy, radiculopathy, and peripheral neuropathy. Other indications for neurosurgical consultation include osteoarthritis of zygapophyseal joints, overproduction of osteophytes in the uncinate processes, or vertebral chondral osteophytes with progressive symptoms; cervical spine fractures, particularly in ankylosing spondylitis, RA with subluxations, or juvenile polyarthritis with soft tissue injury; and any trauma with fracture, dislocation, or both.

Consultative services provided by the orthopedic surgeon and the neurosurgeon overlap. In general, orthopedic consultation is indicated when reconstructive surgery is being considered, as in ankylosing spondylitis; in the hip, lumbar spine, and cervical spine; and with surgical subluxations in RA, with fusions and wiring techniques to stabilize the cervical spine.[3]

CERVICAL SPONDYLOSIS (OSTEOARTHRITIS OF CERVICAL SPINE)

Osteoarthritis describes all joint involvement in the cervical spine, including all secondary manifestations in vertebrae, tendons, ligaments, capsules, muscles, and hyaline cartilage.[2,10] Primary generalized osteoarthritis has strong genetic implications. This disorder is dominant in women and recessive in men. Further hereditary factors occur in ochronosis, calcium pyrophosphate dihydrate (CPPD) crystal disease, gout, and RA, all of which may play a role in secondary osteoarthritis. Cervical spine osteoarthritis affects virtually all persons age 50 and older. Clinical syndromes, symptoms, and signs in osteoarthritis of the cervical spine are divided into five general categories, with considerable overlapping: (1) involvement of the joints, or intraarticular and extraarticular structures, with clinical reflections; (2) involvement of nerve rootlets, or anterior and principally posterior nerve roots; (3) compression of the spinal cord, or cervical myelopathy; (4) involvement of the vertebral artery by the osteoarthritic process, notably at the atlas-axis-occipital level; and (5) esophageal involvement.

Attacks occur approximately once a year. The patient awakes with severe unilateral pain in the neck; the neck is sometimes fixed by definite deformity; acute torticollis with constant severe pain may last 2 to 3 days, with recovery in 7 to 10 days. Pain caused by joint involvement is more likely to arise from the upper cervical spine, whereas pain caused by intervertebral disk osteoarthritis is more likely to arise from the lower cervical spine. These attacks occur from about ages 35 and 40 to 55 and 60 and gradually become more frequent, depending on the progression of the pathologic events. Pain may be variably severe and referred to the occipital, retroorbital, and forehead areas. Pain is usually worse in the morning and associated with stiffness, making neck rotation difficult. Moderate to severe unilateral cervical posterior root pain may occur after age 35; it is worse at night, with paresthesias in the hands. Arm pain is maximal for 2 to 3 weeks, lasts for 1 to 2 months, and subsides gradually. A pain episode may last about 3 months. When bilateral disk protrusion occurs, pain is present in both upper limbs, and paresthesia occurs in the digits of both hands. Central protrusion may press on the posterior longitudinal ligament and dura mater, becoming adherent, fibrotic, and adhesive and resulting in constant bilateral aching from occiput to scapula. Bilateral disk protrusion occurs primarily in patients age 60 and older. Motion is usually in only one to three of the six classic movements of the cervical spine; flexion is usually preserved, with limited lateral flexion, extension, and rotation. Painless restriction (painless stiffness) is interpreted as resulting from osteoarthritis. Manual compression of the zygapophyseal joints elicits tenderness. Osteoarthritis of zygapophyseal, atlantoaxial, and atlantooccipital joints causes ligamentous contracture.

Radiologic characteristics of cervical spondylosis include zygapophyseal and uncinate processes, with increased density of bone, varying degrees of chondroosteophytosis, irregular narrowing of joint spaces, and sometimes pseudocysts. There are no specific laboratory findings. Occasionally, routine radiologic studies are supplemented by CT or MRI.

Management

The patient is taught the natural history of osteoarthritis of the cervical spine. The majority of patients continue to be functional and effective. Daily stretching and range of motion exercises are emphasized, including cervical, thoracic, and lumbar portions. Physical therapy involves heat, ultrasound, diathermy, heating pads, infrared lamps, hot wet packs (hydrocollator), hot tub baths, Hubbard tank, and special pillows. Analgesic, antiinflammatory, and muscle relaxant drugs may be helpful. Special attention is needed for patients with complications of cervical spine osteoarthritis: radiculopathy, peripheral neuropathy, myelopathy, esophageal involvement by osteophytes, and vertebral artery compressive syndromes, with appropriate neurologic, neurosurgical, or orthopedic consultation. Other strategies include traction in select patients; relaxation techniques two or three times a day, particularly at night; and cervical massage. The prognosis is generally good.[11]

NEUROLOGIC DISORDERS

The clinical manifestations of nerve root involvement include compression of the posterior root and dorsal root ganglia infection by viruses such as herpes zoster. The anterior or motor root is well protected and anatomically low in the intervertebral foramen and thus rarely involved. Most of these syndromes are sensory, involving the posterior nerve root and the dorsal root ganglia. Sensory changes include functional disturbances, pain, paresthesia, anesthesia, hypesthesia, and hyperesthesia, which are confined to the dermatomes (skin areas supplied by specific cord segments, dorsal roots, or ganglia). Symptoms of nerve root irritation, termed *radicular,* are increase exacerbated by motion, coughs, sneezes, strain, nerve root stretching, and increased intraspinal pressure. The pain is lancinating in character, intermittent, and rarely constant. Etiologies for nerve root involvement are osteoarthritis, pachymeningitis, extramedullary tumors, protruded intervertebral disks, extradural abscesses, and a variety of viral disorders and active inflammation (e.g., nonspecific, noninfectious granuloma of RA). Muscle spasm alone can cause nerve root compression.

Cervical Radiculopathy

Cervical radiculopathy of osteoarthritis may be single or multiple, bilateral, symmetric, or asymmetric, with varying degrees of involvement of each separate root, and is often associated with myelopathy. Clinical syndromes are divided into acute, subacute, and chronic radiculopathies.

Acute Type. Acute radiculopathy is characterized by an abrupt onset of severe pain and aching in the dermatomal distribution of the cervical root involved. Pain perception affects bone, joints, muscles, blood vessels, and skin, with wide radiation involving the neck, shoulder, down the arm and forearm, and to the digits. Pain may extend into the chest anteriorly and posteriorly, especially with C5 to C7 nerve root involvement. Pain is altered by head or neck position. Scalp, retroorbital, and cervical pain worsens with both active and passive rotation; lateral flexion, extension, and rotation are most painful. Pain is not exacerbated by coughing unless there is acute intervertebral disk protrusion. In a few patients, muscular weakness or decreased to absent reflexes are seen, reflecting involvement of the motor and sensory root.

Atrophy may occur rapidly with fasciculations. Tendon reflexes are diminished or lost.

Subacute Type. With subacute radiculopathy, or typical "brachial neuritis," usually more than one root is involved. It is characterized by pain in the neck with associated paresthesias and severe muscle spasm. Mild muscle atrophy, hypotonia, and muscle weakness are uncommon. Frozen shoulder is a frequent complication, as are tennis elbow and carpal tunnel syndrome.

Chronic Type. Chronic radiculopathy usually follows unaccustomed exercise or work in an awkward position. Symptoms and signs develop insidiously, only partially clearing after an acute attack with lingering pain. Radiologic characteristics include narrowing of intervertebral disk spaces and zygapophyseal joints, along with chondroosteophytes of the uncinate processes. Special studies include electromyography and special radiologic views to identify narrowed intervertebral foramina. Occasionally, MRI is required.

Management. Patient education focuses on outcome, usually a good prognosis with optimum management. Physical therapy includes heat, cold therapy occasionally, and both alternating at times; gentle stretching and strengthening exercises; range of motion exercises; and intermittent use of a soft or hard plastic collar. Antiinflammatory drugs and occasional analgesics are helpful, but with little or no role for narcotic or potentially addictive drugs. Traction is judiciously applied with close follow-up and monitored according to specific results. Other therapies include a cervical spine pillow, massage, occasional lidocaine and corticosteroid injection in areas of pain and spasm, and hydrotherapy.

Cervical Myelopathy. Symptoms of cervical myelopathy are related to ischemia and compression of the spinal cord by osteoarthritic bars, hypertrophied ligamenta flava (posteriorly), cervical disk material anteriorly, and surrounding structures. Clinical symptoms vary greatly. Disability increases subtly, often preceded by a history of radicular symptoms and recurrent attacks of brachial neuritis. The patient also may experience paresthesias and dysesthesia of the hands, weak and clumsy hand functioning, weakness in the lower limbs, and vague deep pain in the lower extremities. Numbness and tingling occur in the finger tips. The pain is often radicular. Touch perception is usually not compromised, but the patient may have vague impairment of light touch and tactile discrimination, with pinprick sensation diminished to absent. Sensory loss may be one or two dermatomes above the upper segmental level of spinal compression. Vibration sense is impaired or lost below the iliac crest or costal margin; some loss may occur over the digits of the hands. Perception of passive movement in fingers and toes is slightly impaired. Acute cervical disk protrusion may involve sudden spinal cord compression, severe disabling neck pain and weakness, and paresthesias of the upper or all four extremities. Paresthesias in the soles of the feet are increased by neck flexion.

Onset of myelopathy may be painless and slow, with difficulty in gait and upper motor neuron signs affecting both legs. Both hands and feet are paresthetic, and the patient experiences the sensation of pins and needles from the anterior knees to all toes. Myelography shows often multiple protrusions, with several sites of spinal cord compression, and both chondroosteophyte formation and disk herniation, distinguishable only at laminectomy. The posterior longitudinal ligament has adhesions to the dura mater resulting from proliferative, thick fibroses. Neck flexion causes overstretching and further damage to the spinal cord. Pressure on the anterior spinal artery may cause widespread ischemia and cord infarction with paraplegia.

Atrophy of the upper limbs is variable. If upper cervical enlargement is compromised, the supraspinatus and infraspinatus muscles and the deltoid-triceps-biceps–greater pectoral muscles may be involved, as well as the dorsiflexors of the wrists and fingers. If the lower part of the cervical enlargement is involved, most wasting is in the flexors of the wrist and fingers and intrinsic muscles of the hands; wasting is variable. Corticospinal tract involvement is below the level of other involvement if motor radiculopathy coexists. If only the corticospinal tract is involved, symptoms are limited to the lower limbs, with spastic paraplegia and no upper limb symptoms. Rarely, symptoms are motor only, with muscular wasting of the upper limbs and spastic weakness of the lower limbs simulating motor neuron disease. Severe paraplegia or quadriplegia and loss of sphincter control also occur rarely. Muscular wasting and pain may be associated with concomitant osteoarthritis of the lumbar spine.

Tendon reflexes have diagnostic importance. A normal jaw jerk with exaggerated tendon reflexes of the upper extremity suggests that the lesion is below the level of the foramen magnum. An exaggerated, diminished, or absent jaw jerk suggests a lesion above the level of the pons. Tendon reflexes in myelopathy are a function of both upper and lower motor neuron lesions. Compression of the anterior horn cells causes lower motor nerve dysfunction, whereas compression of the corticospinal tract causes upper motor neuron dysfunction. Ultimately, reflexes disappear, but this is preceded by an exaggeration of reflexes, inverted radial reflex, extreme flexor finger jerks, and positive Hoffmann's and Babinski's reflexes. Abdominal reflexes diminish but are rarely lost; clonus, bowel, and bladder symptoms and signs rarely if ever disappear.

Cerebrospinal fluid often shows increased protein content (18 to 125 mg/dl). Pressure may be elevated, and Queckenstedt's test may be positive. Passive extension of the neck may raise the pressure, indicating partial but not complete block. Laboratory data are not usually helpful. Radiologic studies reveal the usual changes of osteoarthritis. Special studies show narrowing of the sagittal diameter of the spinal canal, as measured on standard radiographic films. MRI may be required for precise diagnosis.

Management

Special adaptations are provided for patients with problems of cervical cord compression. Surgical therapy is indicated only in unusual circumstances. Extensive laminectomy, foraminotomy, and excision of osteophytes are often unsuccessful. The natural history of cervical osteoarthritic myelopathy is one of mild disability. After initial deterioration, a static period may last for several years.

FRACTURES

As a rule of thumb, any patient with a severe head injury should also be evaluated for possible neck injuries. Cervical spine fractures must be ruled out in any patient who has multiple trauma or is unconscious. Every patient holding the head and complaining of neck pain should also be treated for a fracture until proved otherwise. The head and neck are stabilized first to prevent further spinal cord damage. Patients with head injuries, in shock, or with multiple trauma are frequently combative, requiring restraints. Every emergency room (ER) should be equipped with rigid and adjustable cervical collars to stabilize the spine until radiographs are obtained.

Fractures of the cervical spine are usually the result of severe trauma to the head or head and neck, usually from an axial load or flexion and rarely from an extension force on the head and neck. These forces may have a rotatory component that adds to the displacement. The neurologic examination should be properly documented as soon as the patient arrives at the ER. Radiographs should include an AP or swimmer's view of all the vertebrae, including C7. In a swimmer's view, while one arm is abducted 180 degrees, the other arm is pulled down and a radiograph taken at T1. Oblique views, tomograms, or CT scan may also be necessary.

C1 trauma may result in fracture of the posterior arch and anterior tuberosity that constitute the C1 vertebral body. If no subluxation or dislocation occurs, C1 fracture does not involve spinal cord damage. The diagnosis can be overlooked if the posterior arch of C1 is not properly visualized. CT scans or tomograms are helpful, and immediate treatment is immobilization of the spine (Fig. 124-5). Cranial-skeletal traction is preferable until swelling and muscle spasm subside. The neck can then be immobilized in a cervical brace until bony union occurs.

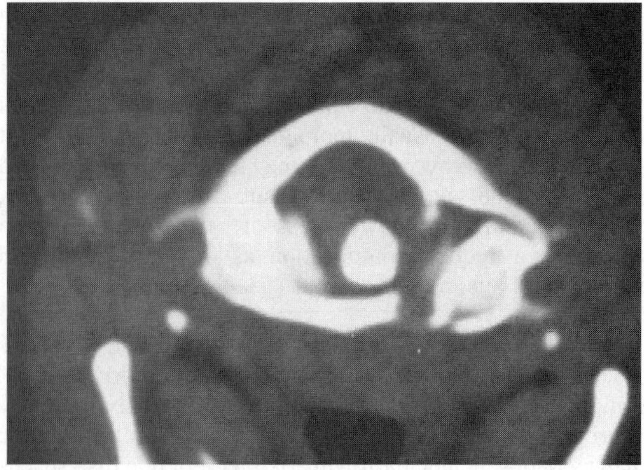

Fig. 124-5. CT scan of first cervical (C1) vertebra, or atlas, showing fracture of ring structure without compression of internal neural structures.

Odontoid Fractures

Fractures of the odontoid are increasingly recognized, usually associated with motor vehicle accidents. Different classifications exist for this fracture, which can be high or low on the odontoid process. Lower fractures, where the odontoid is essentially part of the C2 vertebral body, have a greater incidence of bony union. Fractures at or above the "waistline" of the odontoid have a high incidence of nonunion. These fractures should be differentiated from a congenital os odontoideum, a failed union between separate ossification centers.

With the exception of the lower type, the preferred treatment for odontoid fractures is fusion of C1 and C2. Immediate treatment consists of rigid immobilization with a cervical brace, cranial-skeletal traction, or a halo vest, depending on the associated soft tissue injuries. This helps protect against further spinal cord injury.

Hangman's Fracture

Hangman's fracture occurs through the pedicles of C2 and is associated with capital punishment. To eliminate the slow deaths from asphyxiation, the long drop was employed at hangings in London first in 1784. This resulted in a C2 fracture. The submental knot, applied in judicial hangings, causes a traumatic spondylolisthesis of the axis (C2). This injury can also occur in head-on automobile collisions with the victim's head hitting the windshield, causing extension with fractures of the pars of C2. When these fractures are associated with severe displacement, the spinal cord is damaged and the patient cannot survive (Fig. 124-6). Undisplaced fractures, however, frequently cause no neurologic symptoms. Occasionally, pain occurs along the greater occipital nerve, but more often, neck pain and muscle spasm are the presenting symptoms.

Treatment should be cranial-skeletal traction and then rigid immobilization, usually in a halo vest. The traction may need to realign minor displacement of the fragments. Surgery is rarely if ever indicated.

Fractures and Dislocation of C3 to C7

Injuries to the area of C3 to C7 can be devastating and are frequently associated with spinal cord injuries. Depending on the level of paralysis, the extent of the neurologic loss can vary from complete quadriplegia involving paralysis of the upper and lower extremities to high paraplegia with sparing of the upper extremities. The neurologic deficit results from ischemia, bleeding, decreased blood supply, or contusion of the cord, followed by swelling and oligemia, which result in cord necrosis with complete paralysis below the level of injury. The diagnosis is established after careful neurologic evaluation confirmed by radiologic findings.

The first treatment for fractures of the lower cervical spine is immediate immobilization with cranial-skeletal traction to provide temporary stabilization and alignment of the fracture. Patients may require surgical stabilization of the fracture and rarely a decompression laminectomy later, when their condition has improved. Spinal stabilization permits earlier rehabilitation and less time on bed rest or in a surgical orthosis. Surgery does not alter or lessen the neurologic deficit.

Minor, less devastating injuries to the cervical spine include stable fractures without neurologic deficit. The clay shoveler's fracture, for example, is an avulsion injury of the posterior spinous process.

ESOPHAGEAL COMPRESSION IN OSTEOARTHRITIS

Osteoarthritis can cause esophageal compression by osteoarthritic chondroosteophytes or by subluxated cervical vertebrae (atlantoaxial subluxation or subaxial subluxation in RA). Dysphagia may manifest as difficulty swallowing (atlantoaxial subluxation), discomfort or pain during swallowing, and pain from the esophagus or gastroesophageal junction referred to the chest. Evidence of radiologic esophageal compression by anterior chondroosteophytes in osteoarthritis

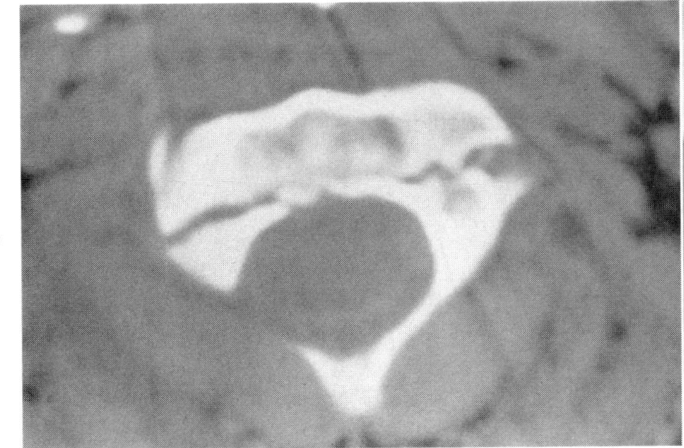

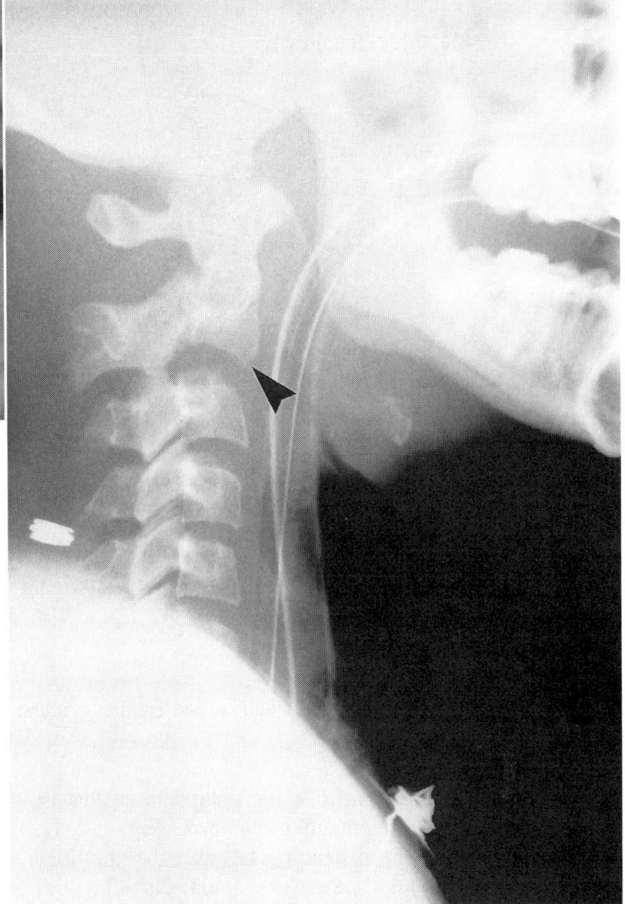

Fig. 124-6. **A,** CT scan of second cervical (C2) vertebra, or axis, showing fracture and discontinuity of ring structure. **B,** Lateral view showing C2 fracture (*arrow*) complicated by almost total ligamentous disruption between C2 and C3.

is noted on lateral cervical spine films. Some lesions may be asymptomatic even though they appear grossly compressive. Esophageal compression also can be demonstrated by barium swallow, lateral views of the cervical spine (neutral, flexion, extension), and esophagoscopy or gastroscopy if ulceration is suggested at sites of pressure by chondroosteophytes.

No treatment is indicated unless the patient has symptoms (see therapeutic maneuvers listed earlier). Surgical removal of anterior osteophytes may be necessary.

REFERENCES

1. Akeson WH et al: The chemical basis of tissue repair. In Hunter LY, Fink FJ, editors: *Rehabilitation of the injured knee,* St Louis, 1984, Mosby.
2. Bland JH: *Disorders of the cervical spine: diagnosis and medical management,* ed 2, Philadelphia, 1994, Saunders.
3. Bland JH: Rheumatoid arthritis of the cervical spine, *J Rheumatol* 1:3, 1974.
4. Bland JH, Boushey DR: Anatomy and physiology of the cervical spine, *Semin Arthritis Rheum* 20:1, 1990.
5. Brain WR, Wilkinson M: *Cervical spondylosis,* Philadelphia, 1967, Saunders.
6. British Association of Physical Medicine: Pain in the arm and neck: a multicenter trial of the effects of physical therapy, *Br J Med* 1:253, 1966.
7. Cailliet R: *Neck and arm pain,* ed 3, Philadelphia, 1991, Davis.
8. Hult L: The Munkfors investigation, *Acta Orthop Scand Suppl* 16:1, 1954.
9. McKenzie R: *Treat your own neck,* Lower Hutt, New Zealand, 1983.
10. Shernk HH, Cervical Spine Research Society: *The cervical spine,* ed 2, Philadelphia, 1989, Lippincott.
11. Wilkinson M: *Cervical spondylosis: its early diagnosis and treatment,* Philadelphia, 1971, Saunders.

CHAPTER 125

Disorders of the Shoulder

John H. Bland

In a general medical practice, shoulder pain is a common complaint in the outpatient setting. As the link between arm and thorax, the shoulder is susceptible to injury that can masquerade as a nonarticular disorder. With the exception of dislocation, shoulder syndromes are more common after age 40. Shoulder lesions occur more often in men than in women. Lesions of the cervical spine, nerves, and blood vessels entering the upper extremity and even functional abnormalities of remote structures, diaphragm, and thoracoabdominal viscera may be perceived symptomatically in the shoulder.

On assumption of erect posture in evolutionary development, primates freed the upper extremity for prehension, sacrificing shoulder joint stability for remarkably increased mobility. No other joint has such extensive, free-ranging mobility. The shoulder joint is strikingly unstable, highly mobile, and continually subject to injury, strain, sprain, and a variety of diseases.[2]

ANATOMY

Medically, the word *shoulder* means much more than the glenohumeral joint; it includes the complex mechanism of the

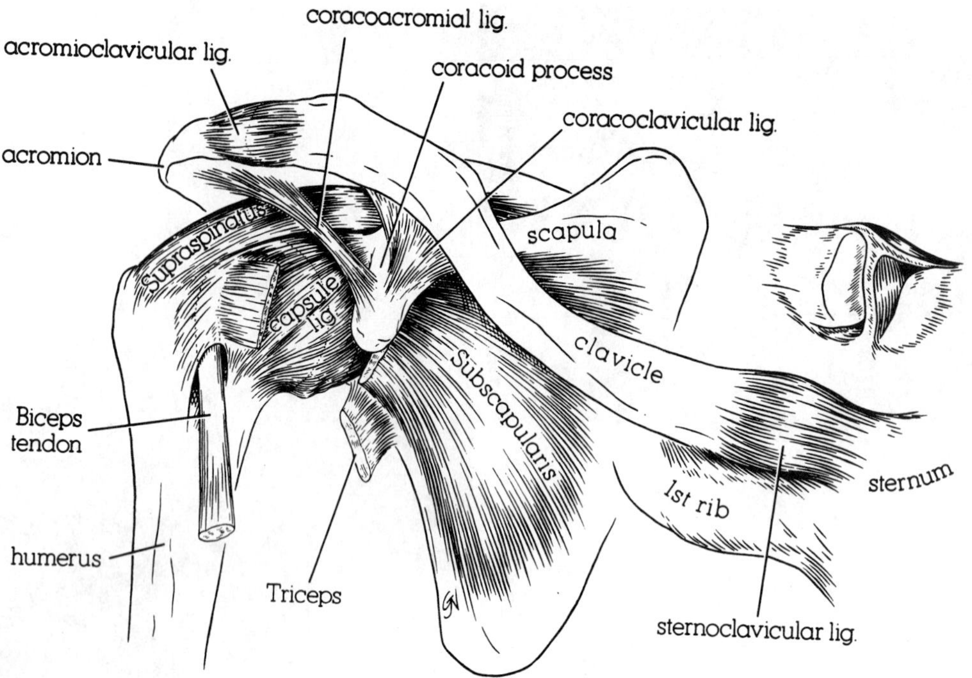

Fig. 125-1. Glenohumeral, acromioclavicular, and sternoclavicular joints. Thoracoscapular joint is between anterior scapular surface and chest wall.

entire shoulder girdle, each part of which plays an important role in the coordinated movements of the arm (Fig. 125-1). The term *shoulder joint* is misleading because the shoulder includes three large bones (humerus, scapula, clavicle) and four joints (sternoclavicular, acromioclavicular, scapulothoracic, glenohumeral). Shoulder motion is a summation of movement resulting from synchronous movement of all these joints; no unit moves without the others. The scapula is free floating and suspended by its muscles; the only connection to the axial skeleton is the sternoclavicular joint. When shoulder movement is started, rhythm and coordinated motion occur as the muscles attached to clavicle, humerus, and scapula increase or decrease in contraction while the scapula seeks its position of greatest stability, the *scapular setting phase*.

The term *scapulohumeral rhythm* describes events noted on inspection of the normally moving scapula and humerus (Fig. 125-2). This broad concept allows greater comprehension and interpretation in examination of the shoulder.

The acromion is large and powerful to stabilize the joint as a non-weight-bearing, hypermobile, prehensile structure. The acromion functions like the mast of a derrick, providing attachment to the large deltoid muscle. The supraspinatus muscle, relatively small, is used to hold the boom, the humerus, on the fulcrum, the glenoid. The clavicle is also like a boom that holds the entire shoulder out away from the body, allowing extensive hypermobility, adduction, and abduction (Fig. 125-3).

Muscles

Three topographic groups of muscles act on the shoulder: from scapula to humerus (scapulohumeral group), from trunk to humerus (axiohumeral group), and from trunk to scapula.

The *scapulohumeral group* is the supraspinatus, infraspinatus, teres minor, subscapularis, deltoid, and teres major. The first four are commonly called the *rotator cuff,* or the short rotators; the first three insert on the greater tuberosity; and the subscapularis tendon inserts on the lesser tuberosity. The tendons are broad and flat, and about 1 inch (2.5 cm) in length. It is impossible to dissect the tendons from the capsule; it is useful to think of the capsule of the glenohumeral joint as a conjoined tendon containing insertions of the powerful capsular muscles. The subscapularis and teres major are medial rotators; the supraspinatus, infraspinatus, and teres minor are lateral rotators. The subscapularis, teres minor, and infraspinatus functional groups depress and rotate the head of the humerus (Fig. 125-1 and 125-4).

The *axioscapular group* consists of the trapezius, rhomboids, serratus anterior, and levator scapulae. The trapezius rotates the scapula, raising the point of the shoulder and holding the scapula at a certain distance from the vertebral border, important to the setting phase of scapular fixation. The serratus anterior and levator scapulae originate on the transverse processes of the cervical vertebrae and upper eight or ten ribs, inserting on the vertebral border of the scapula. These muscles are also important for scapular fixation. The rhomboids, antagonists to the trapezius, pull the shoulders backward; they arise from the ligamentum nuchae and the spine of the seventh cervical (C7) and first to fifth thoracic (T1 to T5) vertebrae and insert on the medial border of the scapula. The trapezius overlies the rhomboids (see Fig. 125-4).

The *axiohumeral group* consists of the pectoralis major, pectoralis minor, and latissimus dorsi, the muscles connecting the humerus to the trunk. The pectoralis major arises from the manubrium and body of the sternum and medial clavicle and inserts into the lateral lip of the bicipital groove of the humerus. The pectoralis minor arises from the third, fourth, and fifth ribs under the pectoralis major and inserts into the coracoid process. The latissimus dorsi forms the posterior axillary fold and arises from the lower six thoracic vertebrae and the heavy lumbar fascia, inserting into the floor of the bicipital groove of the humerus (Fig. 125-5).

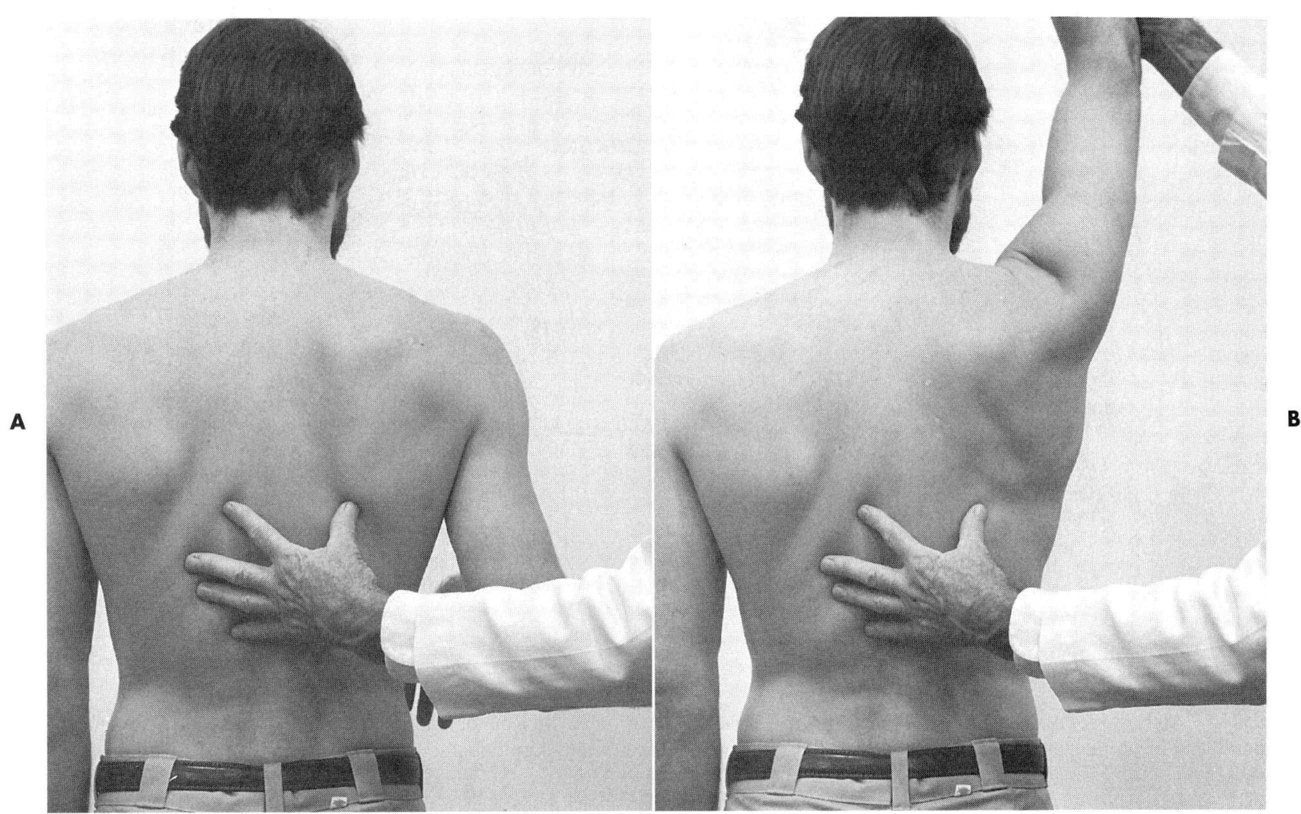

Fig. 125-2. **A,** Examiner's thumb is at inferior angle of scapula, with bone prominent and in slight shrug and elbow in flexion. **B,** Scapula has moved anteriorly, upward, and laterally on passive abduction, elevation, and hyperabduction. Normal passive scapulohumeral rhythm.

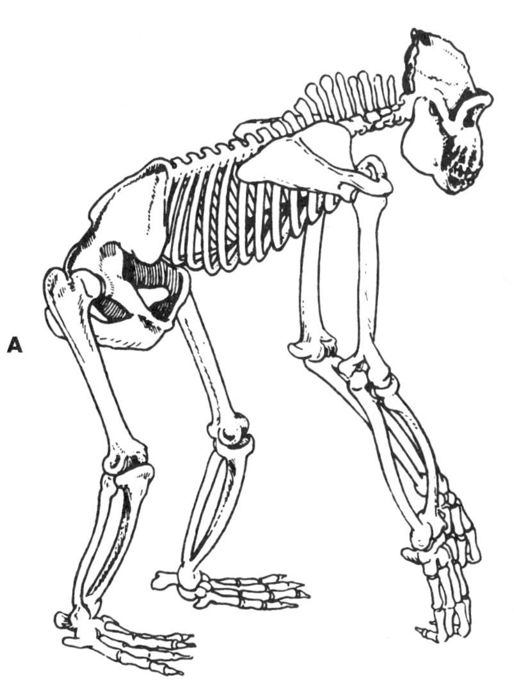

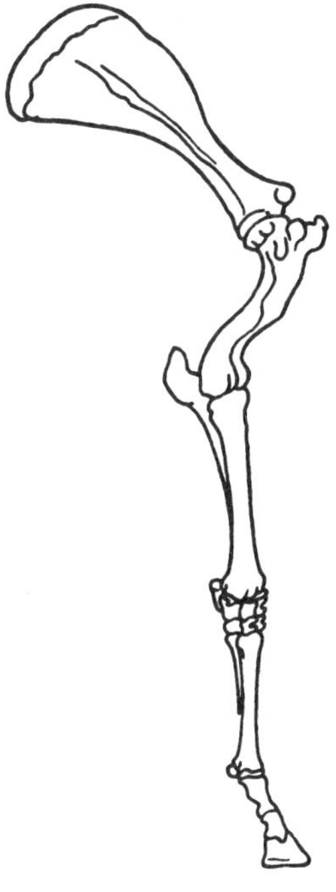

Fig. 125-3. **A,** Gorilla shoulder has massive acromion, broad scapula, very large clavicle, relatively large deltoid muscle, and small supraspinatus muscle. **B,** Horse shoulder with long thin scapula positioned on side of thorax (rather than posteriorly as in humans), no clavicle, tiny acromion, and very large supraspinatus muscle that efficiently accelerates pendulum action of foreleg. Deltoid is absent. (From Codman EA: *The shoulder: rupture of the supraspinatus tendon and other lesions in or about the subacromial bursa,* Boston, 1934, Thomas Todd.)

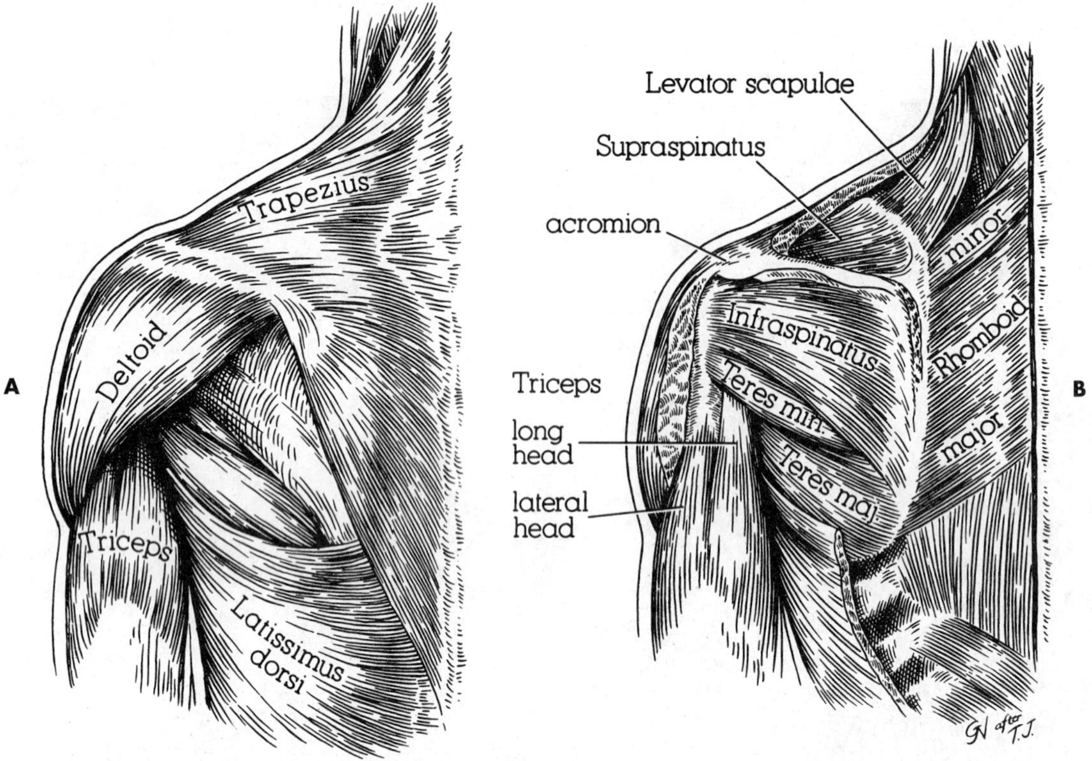

Fig. 125-4. **A,** Posterior view of the shoulder: surface muscles, all groups. **B,** Rotator cuff; subscapularis not shown (medial rotator). Rhomboids and levator scapula displace scapula medially toward midline, while scapulohumeral group rotates humerus laterally.

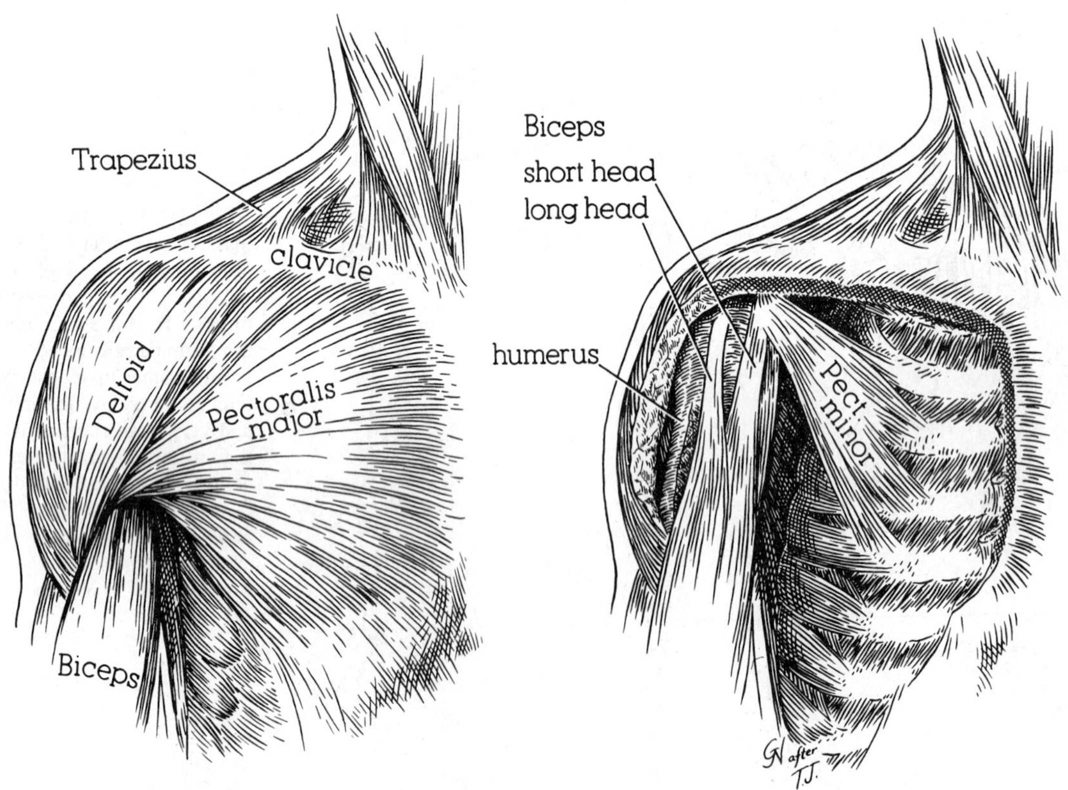

Fig. 125-5. Interior view of the shoulder: surface muscles and deep layer of muscles.

The biceps and triceps are a special category, connecting the scapula and the bones of the forearm. If the arm is externally rotated, the bicipital tendon is restored to its original position and can abduct the shoulder. The triceps arises by three heads, with lateral and medial heads from the humerus and a long head from the intraglenoid tubercle of the scapula, inserting into the posterior proximal humeral olecranon and the deep fascia on either side of it.

Bursae

Bursae provide easy gliding movement in areas with extensive movement but no need for a complete diarthrodial joint, such as where two muscles cross each other in opposite directions or where tendon or muscle must move on one another without real articular contact. Synovial sacs are formed, allowing smooth gliding movement. The only significant bursa around the shoulder is the *subacromial bursa;* such designations as subdeltoid, subcoracoid, and supraspinatus bursae describe extensions of the subacromial bursa or the glenohumeral capsule. Some of the subacromial bursal base covers the bicipital grooves; the roof is attached to the underside of the acromion and the coracoacromial ligament. The roof and base are in intimate contact. This bursa is an essential component of the shoulder mechanism. The subacromial bursa normally provides a smooth gliding mechanism between the coracoacromial arch above and the rotator cuff tendons below. When bursal surfaces are inflamed, the friction is so painful as to preclude arm abduction or rotation. Adhesive bursitis grossly limits serviceable motion (Fig. 125-6).

Coracoacromial Arch

The coracoacromial ligament is a tough, triangular structure joining the coracoid and the acromion, overhanging the humeral head anteriorly (Fig. 125-7). The combination of the bony acromial roof and this ligamentous arch protects both the rotator cuff tendons and the humeral head from direct trauma. However, the close relationship of the humeral head in abduction reduces the space available for rotator cuff tendons to glide beneath. Chronic impingement and tendon attrition with or without calcific tendinitis may result in a painful arc on abduction. The subacromial bursa may be secondarily inflamed by calcific deposits in the tendon, ultimately rupturing into the bursal sac or rotator cuff. Tendon tears may result in spread of inflammation to the bursa (see Fig. 125-6, *A*).

Articular Capsule

The capsule of the glenohumeral joint has a demonstrated volume twice as large as that of the humeral head, allowing unusual mobility and some obvious instability. The capsule arises from the glenoid labrum and surrounding bone and inserts into the upper anatomic neck and the periosteum of the humeral shaft. It is lined with synovium around the periphery of the articular cartilage. Synovial membrane extends into the lining of the biceps tendon sheath, an extension of the joint cavity.

Some areas of the fibrous capsule are thickened to ligamentous proportions. The coracohumeral ligament arises from the lateral edge of the coracoid process and extends over the top of the humerus to insert on the greater tuberosity. The

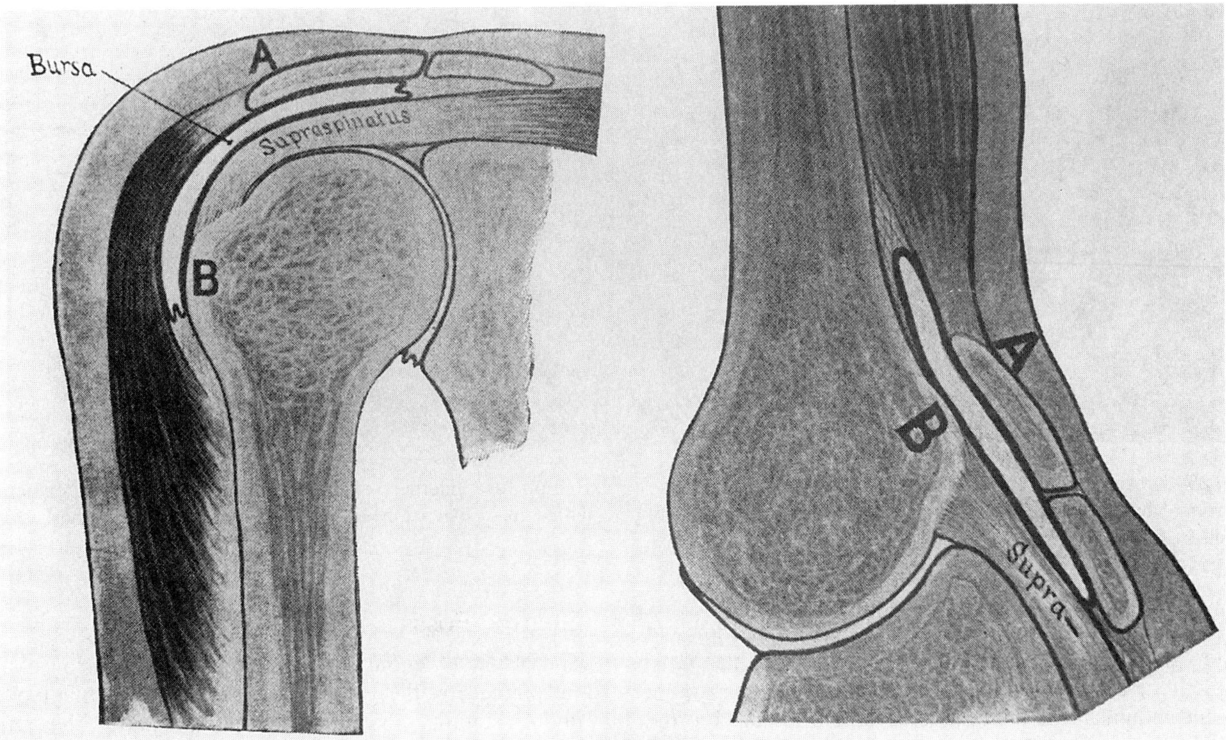

Fig. 125-6. *Left,* Subacromial bursa in normal anatomic position: supraspinatus insertion. After normal anatomic position: acromion *(A)* and greater tuberosity/supraspinatus insertion *(B)*. *Right,* Position of bursa in extreme abduction; deltoid muscle *(A)* and greater tuberosity of humerus *(B)*.

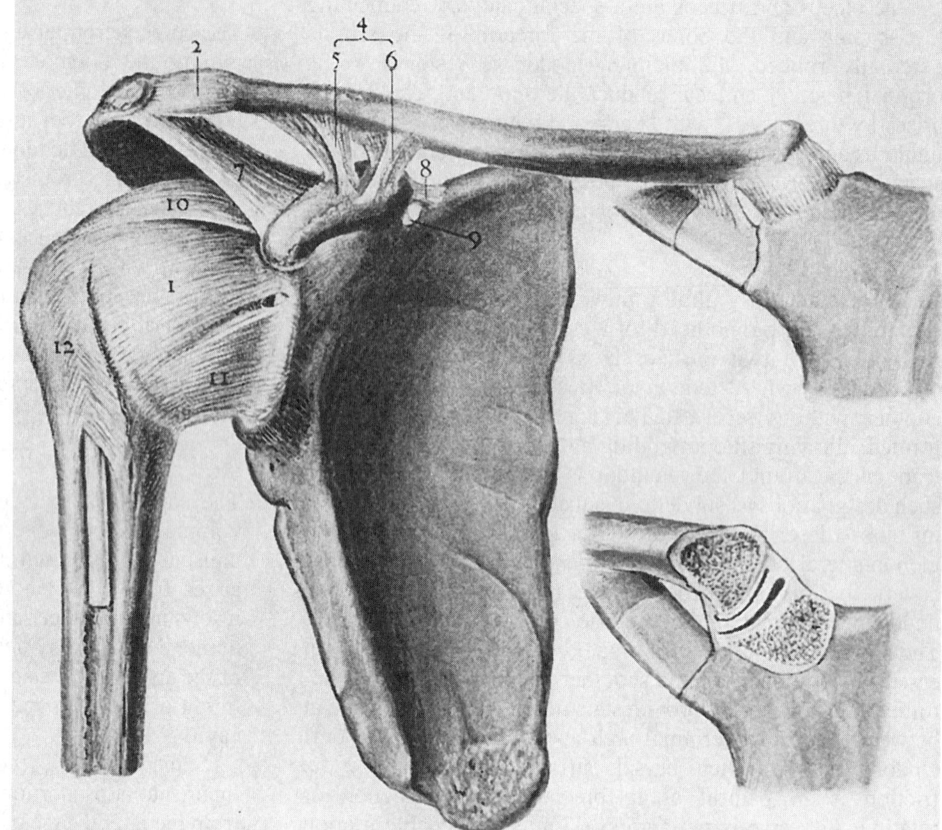

Fig. 125-7. Ligaments of the shoulder joint. *1*, Capsule blends with rotator cuff tendon; *2*, acromioclavicular ligament; *4*, coracoclavicular ligament; *5*, trapezoid ligament; *6*, conoid ligament; *7*, coracoacromial ligament or arch; *8*, *9*, superior and inferior transverse ligament; *10*, coracohumeral ligament; *11*, glenohumeral ligament; *12*, transverse humeral ligament.

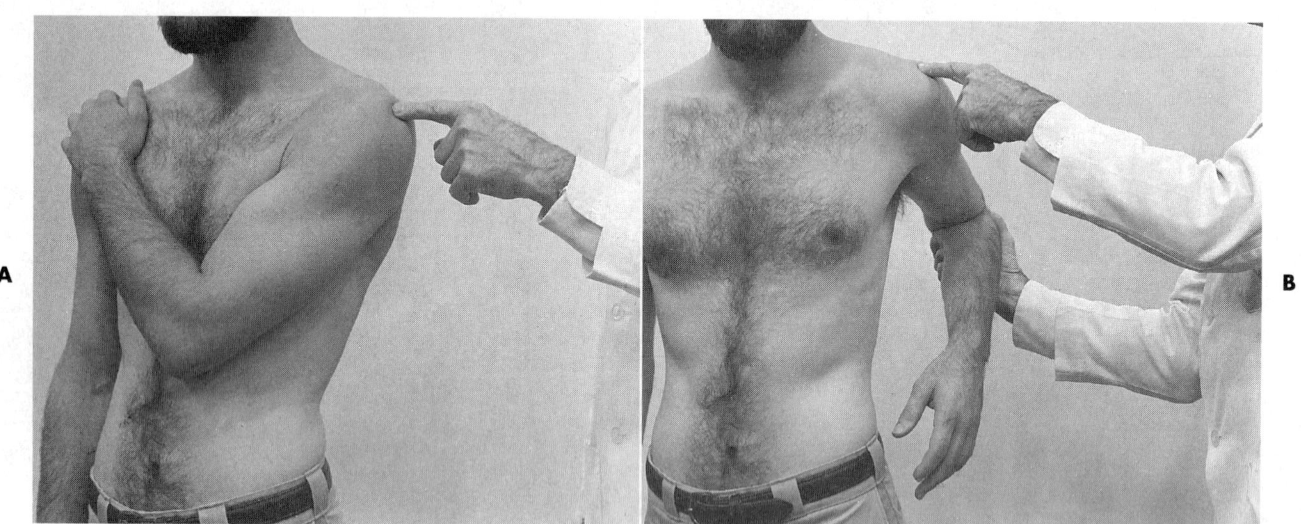

Fig. 125-8. **A,** Examiner palpates under shelving edge of posterior acromion for tenderness of rotator cuff or swelling and tenderness of subacromial bursa. **B,** Anterior aspect is exposed to examining fingers with arm in extension or with hand behind back in marked medial rotation.

capsule thickens anteriorly, forming the superior, inferior, and middle glenohumeral ligaments. These ligaments have variable recesses formed between them, sometimes quite large and redundant. If the fibrous capsule is attached to the neck of the scapula rather than the glenoid, a large anterior pouch appears. The middle glenohumeral ligament is absent or too thin; anterior dislocations may occur (Fig. 125-8).

Glenoid Fossa

The scapular glenoid fossa, broad below and narrow above, is surrounded by the glenoid labrum, a fibrocartilaginous rim giving stability to the glenohumeral joint. The articular surface of the humeral head is oriented posteriorly, medially, and upward; only a fraction of the surface is in contact with the glenoid surface at any time. The greater tuberosity directed laterally forms the outer wall of the bicipital groove, and the lesser tuberosity forms the inner wall. New bone formation in and around the bicipital groove may result in damage, fraying, and even rupture of the long head of the biceps tendon.

Blood Supply

Six major arteries supply the shoulder: the suprascapular, anterior circumflex humeral, and posterior circumflex humeral are always present; the thoracoacromial, suprahumeral, and subscapular arteries are present less often. An area of severe undervascularization exists in the distal part of the supraspinatus tendon proximal to its insertion in the greater tuberosity. The infraspinatus and subscapularis tendons may also show hypovascularization but less frequently. This is the critical zone, and the pathogenetic assumption is that the ischemic area is subject to cellular hypoxia, fiber tears, release of lysozymes with further destruction of tendons, and spread of traumatic inflammation. Such areas have limited repair potential for attritional tears. A further contributing force to tendon damage is the sharp angulation of the rotator cuff tendons over the humeral head, with vessel compression in the tissue of the tendon.

Nerve Supply

Only two sensory nerves supply the shoulder region: the axillary, or circumflex, and the suprascapular. The *axillary nerve* courses to the anterior surface of the capsule, sending branches into the joint from below. The *suprascapular nerve* separates from the superior division of the brachial plexus, courses laterally and downward under the trapezius muscle to the upper border of the suprascapular notch, passes under the supraspinatus muscle, and penetrates the infraspinatus fossa, where it divides into terminal branches. The suprascapular nerve supplies the superior and posterior portions of the joint capsule, most of the tendon sheath, and the acromioclavicular joint. Both nerves supply the coracoclavicular, coracoacromial, coracohumeral, and glenohumeral ligaments. The long thoracic nerve sends a branch to the coracoid process and the acromioclavicular joint. Cartilage and bone are not very pain sensitive. The tissues of the shoulder can be listed in decreasing degree of pain sensitivity: tendons, bursae, ligaments, synovial tissue, joints, their capsular reinforcements, and muscles.

PATIENT EVALUATION

History

Details of the patient's history should include type of pain of onset, location of initial pain, pain behavior from onset, history and nature of injury, type and degree of pain, rapidity of onset, magnitude of disability, spread of symptoms and their precise timing, true appearance of reproducible signs, relieving or aggravating factors, effect of position, relationship to time of day or night, effect of passive or active movements, and presence or absence of neurologic symptoms or signs. The patient's age, habitus, occupation, body type, posture, mental state, and intellectual status are important. Emotional tension, complaint threshold, anxiety states, and hysteria affect shoulder complaints.

Pain is most often in the lower part of the deltoid area, the referral area for the supraspinatus tendon. Although the lesion may be only millimeters in size, the pain can be great, often involving most of the deltoid area and the proximal arm. Pain at the acromioclavicular joint area indicates a problem in and around that joint. Pain in any other part of the arm, shoulder, or neck or in the C5 sclerotome is common to all other possible shoulder lesions (Fig. 125-9).

Initial symptoms in supraspinatus tendinitis are pain in the deltoid insertion area initiated by abduction, especially active but also on passive abduction. Spread of inflammation to the subacromial bursa is characterized by extension of the pain to the distal arm and into the forearm. Pain involving the forearm as far as the wrist indicates that the process has spread to the capsule and has been present for 3 to 6 months. If the entire arm is painful with severe limitation of motion, the inflammation has spread to involve the capsule and synovium, and a frozen shoulder is developing or already present.

Other joint involvement suggests rheumatoid arthritis, gout, or some systemic rheumatic disease. Osteoarthritis rarely involves the shoulder primarily. If preceding injury has occurred, osteoarthritis may gradually develop. Tears in the supraspinatus tendon or capsule and other injuries to the shoulder may appear later, long after the primary injury. The more the arm is involved by pain, the more extensive is the lesion. Tendinitis evolves into subacromial bursitis, which becomes capsulitis and then synovitis. Pain when lying on the side of the affected shoulder suggests supraspinatus tendinitis. Spontaneous pain indicates an extensive spread, from tendinitis to bursitis and later capsulitis. Head, neck, chest, or upper abdominal pain suggests a lesion separate from the shoulder, such as diaphragmatic hernia, cervical spondylosis, or cardiac involvement.

Physical Examination

Inspection should include the head, cervical spine, shoulder, arm, forearm, wrist, and hand, including the area the patient designates as the painful site. The effect of gravity is an important consideration (Fig. 125-10).

Cervical Spine. The cervical spine is examined by active flexion, extension, lateral flexion, and rotation to determine if any of these movements causes pain. Passive flexion, extension, lateral flexion, and rotation of the cervical spine are then demonstrated to determine if these movements produce the characteristic pain. The aim is to determine whether mobile structures (muscles and tendons) are pain sensitive or whether capsules, ligamentous structures, joints, osteophytes, and anterior and posterior longitudinal ligaments are the source of pain. To identify pain-sensitive structures by selective tension, the patient flexes, extends, laterally flexes, and rotates the cervical spine against resistance. These maneuvers also identify lesions at the origin and insertion of muscle.

Shoulder. The examiner inspects the painful shoulder anteriorly, laterally, and posteriorly, comparing it to the unaffected side. Observations of scapulohumeral, claviculohumeral, and arm trunk rhythm may be revealing and often diagnostic. Key characteristics are atrophy, loss of muscle tone, fasciculations, reflex changes, and sensory alterations. The entire upper limb should be inspected for color change, swelling, skin changes, and abnormal posturing.

Full range of active motion is then inspected. Shoulder flexion, extension, adduction, abduction, and medial and lateral rotation are observed anteriorly, posteriorly, and

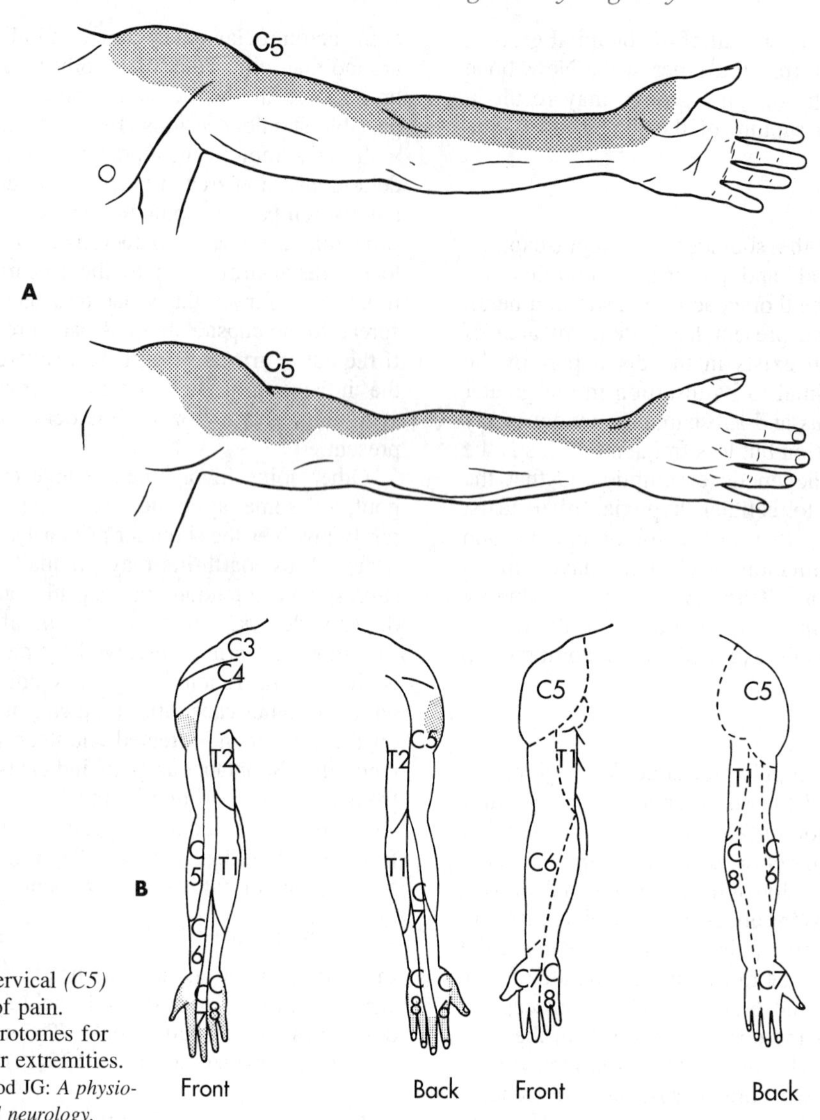

Fig. 125-9. **A,** Fifth cervical *(C5)* sclerotome distribution of pain. **B,** Dermatomes and sclerotomes for pain distribution in upper extremities. (**B,** From Lance JW, McLeod JG: *A physiological approach to clinical neurology,* ed 2, Reading, Mass, 1975, Butterworth.)

laterally. The examiner notes whether abduction is accomplished by shrugging and observes the clavicular movements. Posterior inspection centers on the scapular motion, the scapulohumeral rhythm, and the lower angle of the bone moving out or in as it seeks stability. At about 45 degrees the outward movement accelerates laterally, forward, and upward as the serratus anterior muscle moves (Fig. 125-11).

If the glenohumeral or acromioclavicular joint is fixed, the humerus and scapula move as one, and abduction to as much as 60 degrees occurs by the shrugging mechanism. The lateral view focuses on the deltoid muscle. A look from above with the patient seated is helpful, with occasional inspection in supine and prone positions to see the relaxed musculature and conformation of the shoulders.

The full range of these motions is noted passively, with the examiner lifting the shoulder and arm through its motions. Full passive motion, gently and slowly done, is common in shoulder problems, even with marked limitation of various active ranges of motion in the presence of muscle and tendon lesions. In tears or ruptures of the rotator cuff, active abduction may be impossible or grossly limited, whereas with assisted complete passive motion, abduction to 90 degrees can be shown. When the support is removed, however, marked weakness in holding the abduction is noted, the *drop-arm sign.* Rotation of the humeral head in the glenoid should be shown in both adduction and abduction (to 90 degrees). Humeral rotation must be distinguished from pronation and supination of the hand. To study lesions at the origin and insertion of tendons and ligaments, the patient demonstrates the ranges of motion against resistance.

Palpation. All landmarks are palpated: sternoclavicular and acromioclavicular joints, coracoid process, spine of scapula and clavicle, acromion around its periphery, rotator cuff, and muscles of the shoulder joint (adductors, latissimus dorsi, teres major, pectoralis major and minor, deltoid). The posterior aspect of the rotator cuff is readily palpable with the arm adducted across the chest.

Acromioclavicular lesions are detected by pain in the superior aspect of the shoulder, referral to the neck and jaw, and local joint tenderness exaggerated by adduction of the arm across the chest. *Crepitus* is elicited by placing the palm

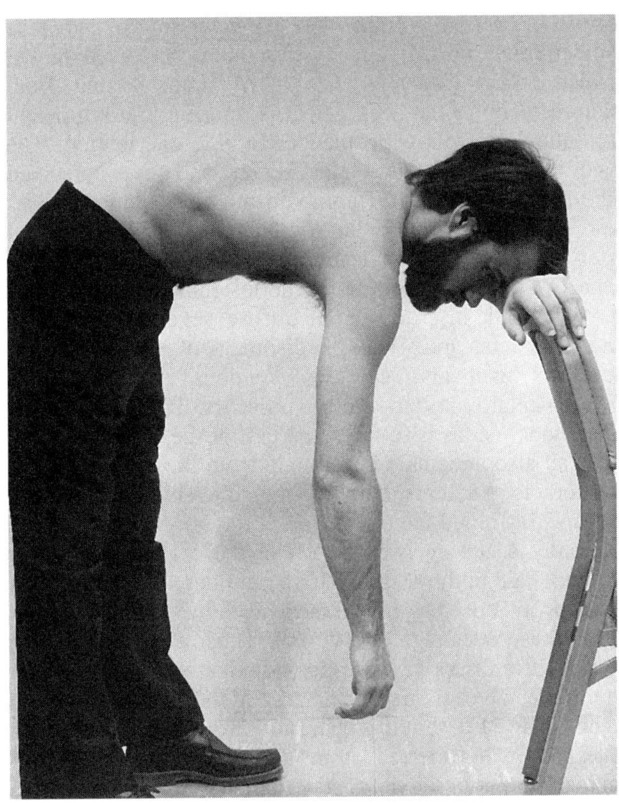

Fig. 125-10. Effect of gravity on shoulder (full trunk and hip flexion) separates pain-sensitive structures, relieving pain.

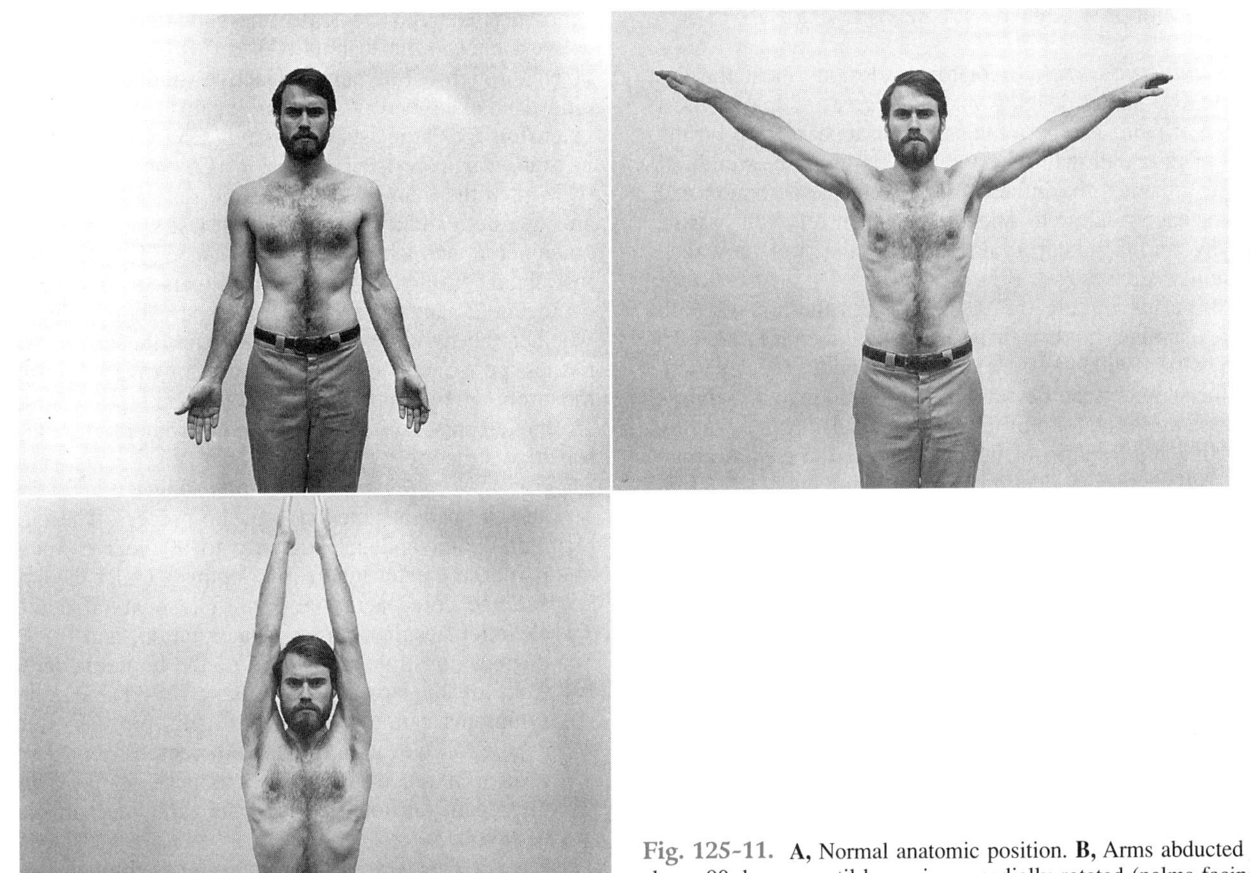

Fig. 125-11. **A,** Normal anatomic position. **B,** Arms abducted just above 90 degrees until humeri are medially rotated (palms facing down). Next 60 degrees of abduction cannot occur. **C,** With palms facing, scapulae have rotated, allowing 60 degrees more; last 30 degrees, with distal arm touching head, are achieved by abduction of humerus across front of scapula, coracoid, and acromion.

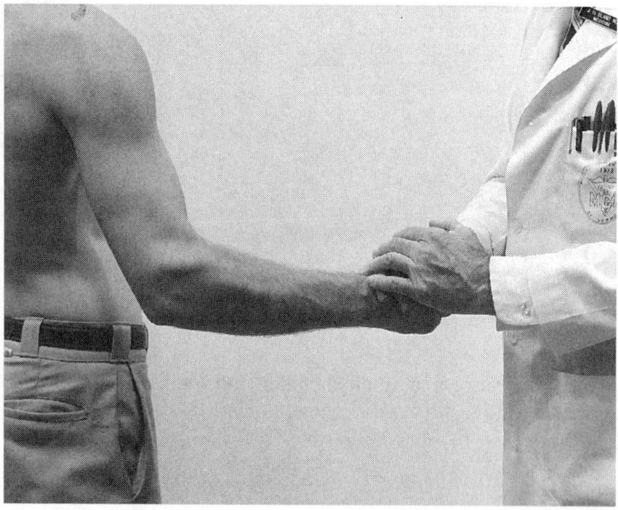

Fig. 125-12. Right arm abduction to just 30 degrees when pain is felt.

of the examiner's hand over the top of the patient's shoulder while the other hand rotates the humerus at various angles of adduction, abduction, and rotation. Crepitus is indicative of severe rotator cuff disease with secondary osteoarthritis of the glenohumeral joint. The *painful arc* is pain production at about 60 degrees of abduction, with freedom from pain before and after this level. This indicates impingement of the greater tuberosity under the acromion, a supraspinatus tendinitis with or without calcific deposits (Fig. 125-12).

Special Procedures. In rotator cuff lesions, most muscles around the shoulder develop varying degrees of spasm, itself a source of pain. The pain frequently disappears in full trunk and hip flexion, allowing the arm to hang limp; the weight of the arm separates the inflamed area from the acromion and the coracoacromial arch. The muscles then relax on passive swinging and pendular movements of the arm, so-called pendulum exercises (see Fig. 125-10).

With partial rupture the patient swings the arm forward and the examiner holds it there; the patient then returns to an erect position with the arm in full abduction, or elevation. Thus the shoulder can be put through a full range of painless motion. Pain in rotator cuff tendinitis may also be relieved by supporting the forearm in flexion, putting the arm at about 30 to 40 degrees abduction, and exerting gentle traction downward.

Lidocaine (Xylocaine) infiltration in the tissues of suspected involvement is often helpful, diagnostically and therapeutically. In rotator cuff tears, with the pain gone, painless movements allow determination of loss of power. With normal movement and power after lidocaine infiltration, nonsurgical therapy is promising.

Systematic Clinical Plan

A systematic clinical approach to identification of the pain-sensitive structure leads to a precise diagnosis and successful management in the vast majority of patients. With the exception of the acromioclavicular joint (derived from the C4 sclerotome embryologically), all structures of the shoulder, which include subacromial bursa, capsule, synovium, glenohumeral joint, periosteum, biceps tendon (long head), and rotator cuff muscles and tendons, are derived entirely or partially from the C5 sclerotome, and thus shoulder pain originating in any structure is perceived only in its distribution (see Fig. 125-9, *A*). Pain arising from structures deep to the deep fascia is referred in a segmental distribution not following the dermatome distribution. The area of pain is always very large, severe, and never perceived at the site of the lesion. Rhomboid muscle irritation causes severe transient pain over the shoulder region anteriorly and posteriorly, following the deep segmental sensory distribution of the C5 root. Irritation of the periosteum of the humerus near the capsule insertion causes diffuse, severe pain over the same segmental area. Thus in disorders of deep structures (muscles, ligaments, capsules, tendons, fascia), broad intrasegmental distribution of pain occurs. Thus pain caused by shoulder lesions is felt in some part of the C5 sclerotome. Pain may also arise as referred pain from the cervical spine, intrathoracic structures, diaphragm, and even intraabdominal structures, as noted later.

Initially a survey is made of all the segments possibly involved. Pain in the scapular area, shoulder, or arm indicates a lesion in one of the tissues forming the C5 to T2 sclerotomes (see Fig. 125-9, *B*). Thus a survey of the segments from neck to fingertips tells the examiner whether there is a lesion of tissues in and around the shoulder, a lesion perceived in the shoulder but not arising from shoulder tissues, or pain referred from a distant site, visceral or somatic; hysteria, anxiety state, and psychoneurosis are detectable through clinical inconsistencies. The patient is first asked to actively flex, extend, laterally flex, and rotate the cervical spine; next to shrug the shoulders maximally and actively elevate the scapula (C3 to C4); next the shoulder is taken through a full range of active motion (C5); then the elbow is examined in flexion, against resistance and in extension against resistance to study C5 to C7; next the wrist is examined in resisted extension (C6) and resisted flexion (C7); then the thumb is examined in resisted extension (C8) and resisted adduction (C8); and last the fifth finger is examined in adduction against resistance (T1). The patient is instructed during all these maneuvers to describe pain occurring at any point. The examiner should then know whether the tissues of the shoulder are the cause, whether tissues peripheral to that area are involved, or whether the problem is nonorganic or psychogenic. The following 12 movements, systematically done, determine the pain-sensitive structure:

1. *Elevation of the arm.* The arm is abducted to 90 degrees, and the patient notes pain in the process. The glenohumeral joint abducts normally to 90 degrees, at which point the greater tuberosity impinges under the coracoid and the coracoacromial arch. The next 60 degrees of elevation result from scapular rotation, and the last 30 degrees constitute adduction of the humerus across the front of the scapula (see Fig. 125-11). Psychogenic symptoms can be identified in this process, since the degree of elevation minus 60 degrees represents the abduction range at the glenohumeral joint. If marked discrepancy is noted later, psychogenic mechanisms may be invoked.
2. *Passive elevation.* The examiner goes through the same motions as in step 1. Pain is noted, and the "end feel" is observed (i.e., whether the movement comes to an abrupt or gradual stop at the extreme of the range, a perception that comes with experience).

3. *Painful arc.* The patient abducts the shoulders. Pain between 60 and 120 degrees indicates impingement between the acromion, the greater tuberosity, and the supraspinatus tendon (Fig. 125-12).
4. *Passive scapulohumeral abduction.* The thumb is placed at the lower angle of the scapula to determine whether it moves. The other hand elevates the arm until the examiner feels the scapula begin to rotate. This occurs normally at 90 degrees (see Fig. 125-2).
5. *Passive lateral rotation.* The patient's elbow is bent at a right angle, and the forearm (as a lever) rotates it outward in the sagittal plane. Normal range is 90 degrees; range, end feel, and pain are noted.
6. *Passive medial rotation.* The examiner rotates the humerus medially, noting how far behind the patient's back the forearm can be placed. Normal range is 90 degrees; restriction and pain are noted.
7. *Resisted abduction.* With the elbow tight against the body, the patient is asked to abduct against resistance by the examiner, who prevents the joint from moving. Resisted abduction examines the deltoid and supraspinatus. Since the deltoid muscle rarely if ever has painful lesions, pain with abduction generally indicates supraspinatus tendinitis (Fig. 125-13, *A*).
8. *Resisted medial rotation.* With the elbow fixed against the body, the patient is asked to rotate medially against resistance, testing pectoralis major, teres major, latissimus dorsi, and subscapular muscles (Fig. 125-13, *B*).
9. *Resisted lateral rotation.* This rotation tests the infraspinatus and teres minor muscles; if lateral rotation results in pain, only the infraspinatus tendon is at fault (Fig. 125-13, *C*).
10. *Resisted adduction.* This adduction tests the thoracohumeral group of muscles (Fig. 125-13, *D*).
11. *Resisted flexion at the elbow.* Resisted flexion tests biceps and brachialis function, but if supination against resistance is painful, the lesion is bicipital.
12. *Resisted extension at the elbow.* This extension tests triceps function (Fig. 125-13, *E*).

Shoulder Range of Motion. The shoulder lends itself well to measurements of range of motion: extension, 35 degrees from neutral; flexion, 95 to 100 degrees from neutral; adduction, 25 to 30 degrees; abduction, 90 degrees before gross scapular movement; and medial and lateral rotation, either from neutral or 90 degrees of abduction and 90 degrees both ways. In the superior plane the hands are placed behind the head and the elbow braced backward as far as possible; with palms facing and extending maximally vertically over the head, arms touch the sides of the head. In the inferior plane the dorsum of the hand is noted reaching variably up the back, the buttock, the small of the back, or up between the shoulder blades, all reflecting varying degrees of shoulder mobility (Fig. 125-14).

Muscle Power. Each muscle or muscle group can be tested for power by having the patient make the appropriate effort against resistance. Weakness may result from loss or impairment of nerve supply, rupture of tendons, or pain too severe to allow movement.

Laboratory Studies. Few laboratory studies are needed in studying the painful shoulder. Erythrocyte sedimentation rate (Westergren), latex fixation, antinuclear antibody, serum calcium, phosphorus, alkaline phosphatase, quantitative immunoglobulins, culture of joint fluids, synovial fluid analysis, and various metabolic and endocrine studies may be helpful in the diagnosis of rheumatoid arthritis, thyroid and parathyroid disease, septic arthritis, and neoplasms involving the shoulder.

Radiologic Studies. Most shoulder problems are diagnosed and treated using the history and physical examination. For more difficult presentations or cases of tendinitis with persistent disability, radiographs are useful. The standard views are anteroposterior (AP); the beam is centered on the coracoid process, with both medial and lateral rotation views of the humerus. These views document and locate a calcific deposit in the cuff or in the bursa (Fig. 125-15). Plain films may suggest a full-thickness rotator cuff tear. Subluxation of the acromioclavicular joint occurs as the patient laterally rotates the arm (Fig. 125-16, *A*). The freed humeral head drives the acromion upward. Full-thickness tears may appear simply as a narrowing of the acromiohumeral gap. Superior migration of the humeral head is a direct consequence of the loss of supraspinatus function (Fig. 125-16, *B*). The acromioclavicular joint is best studied with the beam passing anteroposteriorly, with 30 to 35 degrees angulation upward.

A chest film offers diagnostic clues to the origin of shoulder pain. It may reveal a cervical rib, a past clavicular fracture with malalignment, or an apical lung tumor (Pancoast's tumor).

Shoulder arthrography demonstrates the shape and capacity of the glenohumeral joint space (Fig. 125-17). A contrast study is the only way to distinguish between complete and incomplete tears of the rotator cuff. Complete ruptures can be surgically repaired. Arthrography may be helpful in adhesive capsulitis and recurrent shoulder dislocations. It is not helpful in bicipital rupture.

THE PAINFUL SHOULDER

Pain syndromes arising from structures in and around the shoulder joint have a surfeit of names in textbooks and the published literature, with subsequent confusion of terminology, diagnosis, and treatment. The following syndromes refer to the same basic process: supraspinatus tendinitis, rotator cuff tendinitis, subacromial bursitis, subdeltoid bursitis, painful arc syndrome, calcific tendinitis, calcific bursitis, and impingement syndrome. Overlapping and usually following these are a group of names also referring to the same process: periarthritis, adhesive capsulitis, frozen shoulder, adhesive bursitis, periarticular adhesions, and check rein shoulder.

The great majority of painful nontraumatic lesions and syndromes around the shoulder are caused by *tendinitis of the rotator cuff.* There are four rotator cuff tendons inserting into the greater and lesser tuberosities. The long head of the biceps tendon passes through the intertubercular groove to insert on the superior rim of the glenoid. The supraspinatus tendon is usually the first and ultimately the most involved of the cuff tears. The initial lesion is almost always a localized supraspinatus tendinitis with subsequent extension to other members of the rotator cuff and the subacromial bursa, later extending to the joint capsule and intraarticular and extraarticular structures and leading to frozen shoulder. The pathologic process of rotator cuff tendinitis may be a continuum of inflammation, degeneration, and attrition of

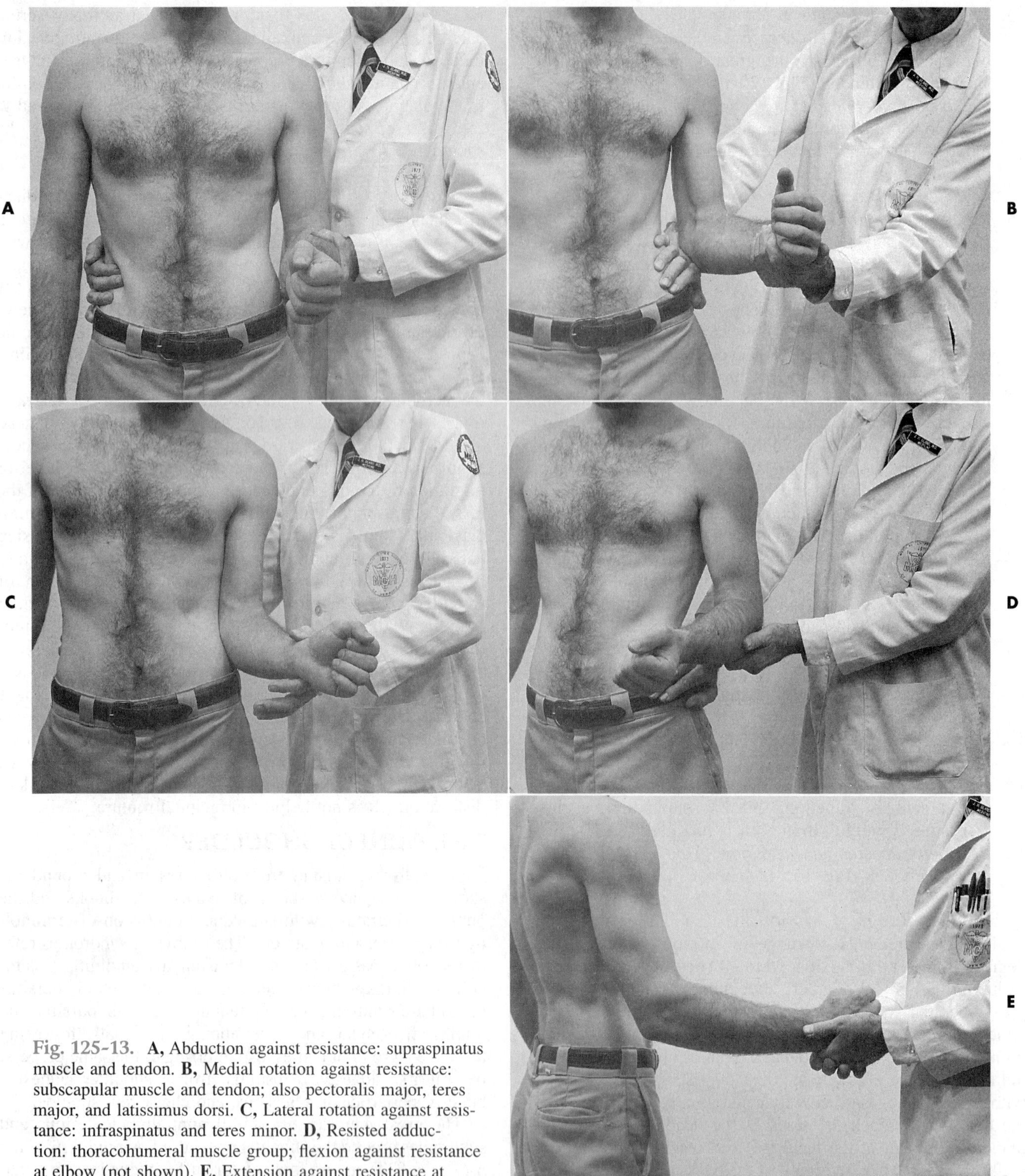

Fig. 125-13. **A,** Abduction against resistance: supraspinatus muscle and tendon. **B,** Medial rotation against resistance: subscapular muscle and tendon; also pectoralis major, teres major, and latissimus dorsi. **C,** Lateral rotation against resistance: infraspinatus and teres minor. **D,** Resisted adduction: thoracohumeral muscle group; flexion against resistance at elbow (not shown). **E,** Extension against resistance at elbow: triceps.

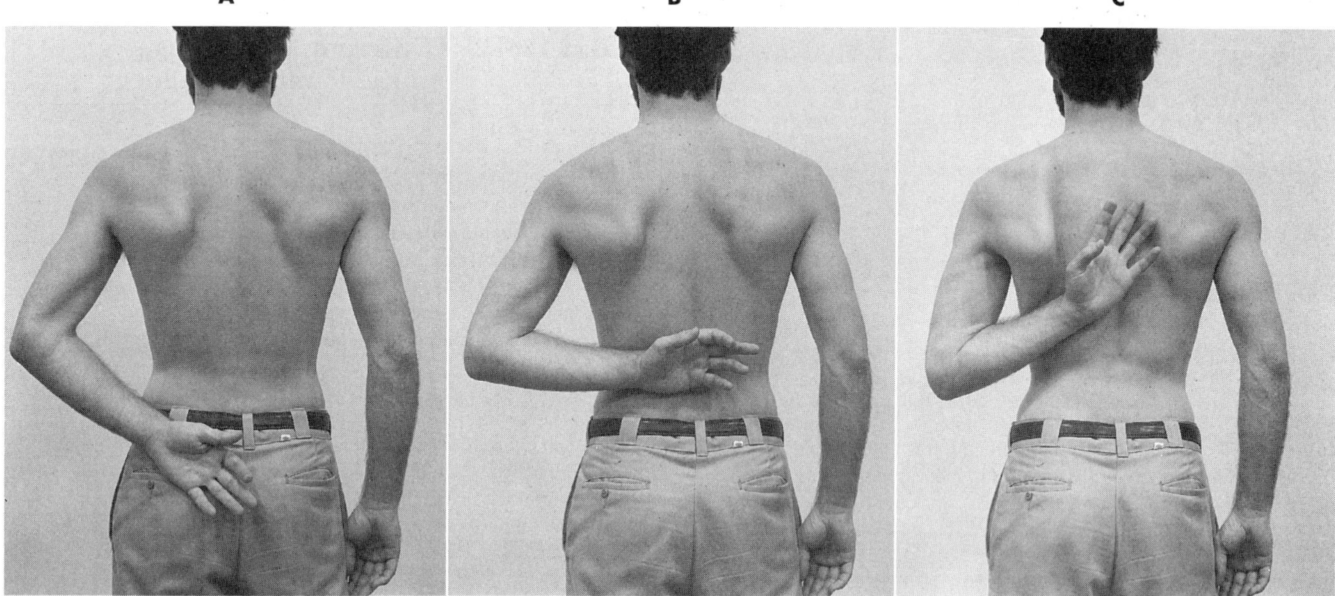

Fig. 125-14. Parameters of progress. **A,** Hand at buttock only. **B,** Hand can reach to flank. **C,** Hand can reach to interscapular area.

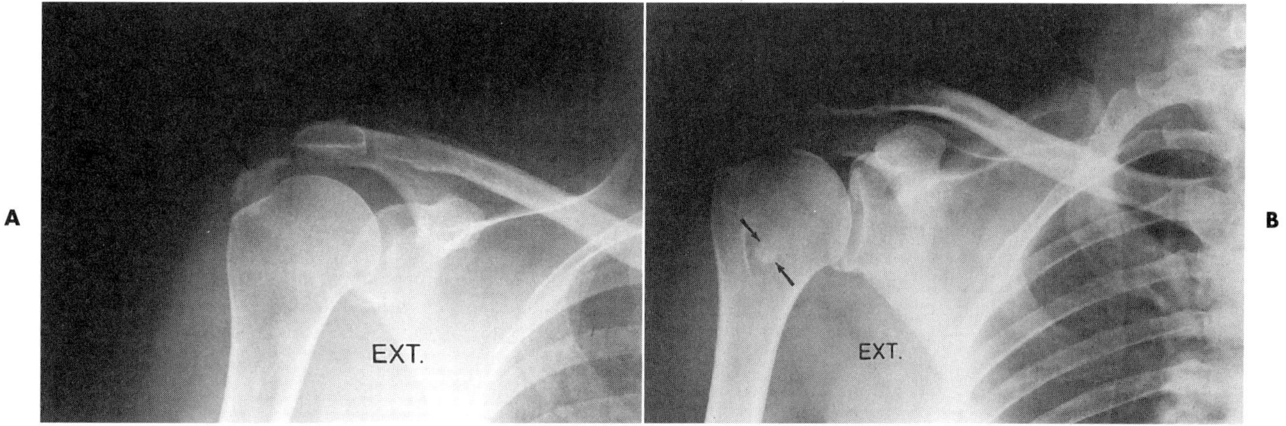

Fig. 125-15. **A,** Calcific tendinitis localized by AP radiographs. Supraspinatus tendon with extensive calcific deposit. **B,** Subscapularus tendon with calcific deposits; deposit moves across front of humeral head on medial rotation.

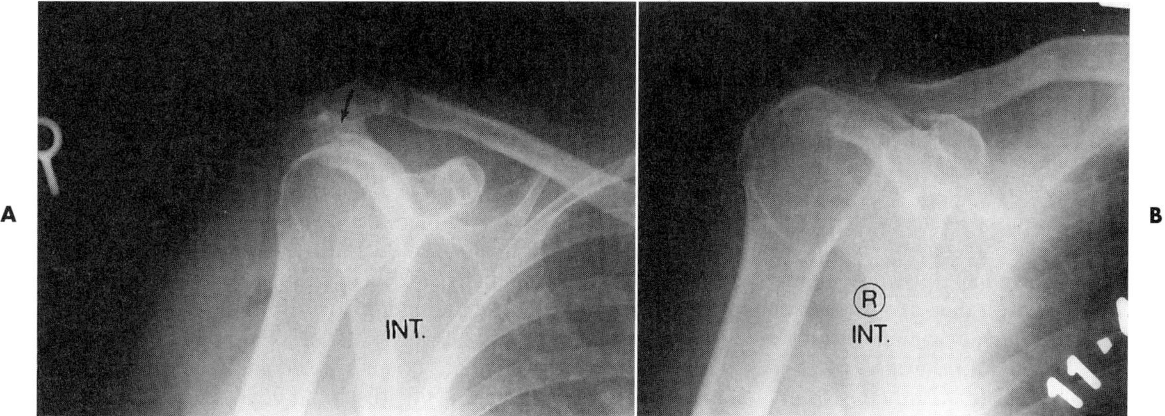

Fig. 125-16. **A,** Normal film in lateral rotation. **B,** Humeral head is elevated 2 years later; patient had full-thickness tear.

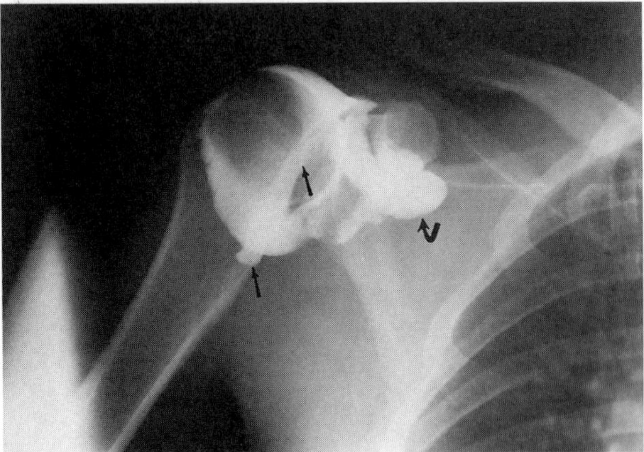

Fig. 125-17. Normal radiographic contrast study, with dye in biceps sheath *(straight arrows)* and subscapular recess *(curved arrow)*.

Box 125-1. Impingement Syndrome in Rotator Cuff Tendinitis

Clinical Characteristics

Sudden incapacitating or dull ache; painful arc as arm is abducted and elevated forward
Tenderness in anterior edge of acromion and bicipital groove
Symptoms relieved with instillation of short-acting local anesthetic in subacromial space, confirming diagnosis

Radiologic Findings

Normal in stage I
Sclerosis, periostitis, and cyst formation in stage II; traction osteophyte under surface acromion
Narrowing of acromiohumeral gap, superior subluxation of humeral head in relation to glenoid, and erosions of anterior acromion in stage III; arthrography shows full-thickness tear and communication between joint space and subacromial bursa

Treatment

Stage I: rest, graduated exercise; strictly avoid immobilization (risk of adhesive capsulitis); stretching and strengthening exercises; aspirin or other nonsteroidal antiinflammatory agents
Stage II: as for stage I; local injection of anesthetic and corticosteroid; recommended combination of 3 ml 1% lidocaine, 3 ml 0.5% bupivacaine, and 20 mg triamcinolone; i.e., short-acting anesthetic for diagnosis, long-acting anesthetic for analgesia, and steroid preparation in depot form
Stage III: as for stages I and II; anterior acromioplasty

the rotator cuff by impingement on the anterior edge of the acromial process, the coracoacromial ligament, and sometimes the acromioclavicular joint. The wear and attritional tears of the cuff occur on the supraspinatus tendon and may extend into the infraspinatus tendon and the long head of the biceps tendon (Box 125-1). Most cases of rotator cuff tendinitis improve with time, and conservative management is usually advised.

Some experts conclude that stiff and painful shoulders all improve regardless of treatment, whereas others strongly advocate localized steroid injections in all cases of both intracapsular and extracapsular lesions affecting tendons, their sheaths, and bursae.

Box 125-2. Differential Diagnosis of the Painful Shoulder

Musculoskeletal Syndromes

Supraspinatus and rotator cuff tendinitis and tenosynovitis
Calcific tendinitis of rotator cuff and biceps tendon
Calcific periarthritis involving multiple sites
Rotator cuff rupture, partial or complete (full thickness)
Bicipital tendinitis and tenosynovitis
Bicipital rupture, long head, partial and complete
Subacromial bursitis (almost always secondary to tendinitis and tenosynovitis)
Capsulitis, adhesive, secondary to tendinitis and bursitis
Frozen shoulder
Myositis, fasciitis, muscle contracture, and adhesions in and around the shoulder
Osteoarthritis, usually secondary, acromioclavicular, glenohumeral, osteophytic overgrowth in bicipital groove and sternoclavicular joints
Primary septic arthritis (rare)
Scapulothoracic syndromes
- Coracoclavicular disruption
- Fibrositis (fibromyalgia)
- Scapulothoracic grating
- Scraping scapula

Trauma

Acromioclavicular separation, partial or complete
Direct capsular injury
Dislocation with secondary trauma to soft bursa
Fractures of scapula, clavicle, and proximal humerus
Nerve injuries
Various injuries: automobile, athletic, vocational

Systemic Disease

Rheumatoid arthritis or other nonspecific inflammatory arthritis
Septic joint superimposed on rheumatic disease
Metabolic and endocrine disease
- Hyperthyroidism
- Myxedema
- Acromegaly
- Hyperparathyroidism
- Chondroclavicular disease and pseudogout
- Gout

Reflex Sympathetic Dystrophy (Shoulder-hand Syndrome)

The term *periarthritis* has become an umbrella term to describe inflammatory syndromes involving all structures about the shoulder. It describes a continuum of pathology with many subsets of sufficient clinical distinction to separate them, culminating in the frozen shoulder. Most physicians specializing in shoulder syndromes believe that the continuum should be interrupted and reversed before it reaches the extreme of this disabling condition.

Inflammation of the supraspinatus or bicipital tendon may spread by contiguity to the tendon sheaths, other tendons and

Box 125-3. Calcific Tendinitis

Pathophysiology

Most common cause of shoulder pain in young patients
Calcific mass 1 to 1.5 cm in diameter
- Always symptomatic
- Involves overlying subacromial bursa distended with fluid
- Tendinitis and bursitis coexistent

Rotator cuff calcification in 8% of asymptomatic population over age 30; one third of calcific deposits cause symptoms; 75% with multiple or bilateral deposits
Hydroxyapatite crystals identified

Clinical Characteristics

Young patient
Severe aching pain 1-4 days
All positions painful, unable to sleep
All movement painful
Pain relief if and when deposit inspissates from toothpaste consistency to powder or ruptures along fascial planes into bursa

Physical Examination

Allows no movement
Palpation in rotator cuff, point of maximum tenderness, fullness and swelling
Marked spasm in all shoulder muscles

Radiologic Findings

Round or oval deposit between acromion and humeral head, possibly several centimeters in length

Management

Nonsteroidal antiinflammatory drugs
Temporary rest in sling
Local heat or cold, or both serially
Injection of deposit with local anesthetic and steroid, needling the area at same time
With relief of pain, physical therapy and range of motion exercises
If calcific boil does not rupture, surgery may be necessary; over 90% of patients recover completely, most of calcification disappears

Box 125-4. Rupture of Rotator Cuff

Pathophysiology

Supraspinatus component most frequently torn, varies from few fibers to massive tears, full thickness of the cuff, even the capsule and floor of overlying bursa, resulting in communication between shoulder joint and subacromial bursa
Rare before age 50, common after age 60 (nearly impossible to rupture tendons in a healthy, young adult)
Occurs at insertion of cuff into bone
Supraspinatus and infraspinatus atrophy in 3 weeks
Shoulder muscles in severe spasm

Etiology

Degenerative changes
Fraying
Attritional wear
Minor recurrent trauma culminating in loss of collagen fibrillar structure

Clinical Characteristics

Over age 50, often a laborer; abrupt pain in deltoid area; snap after strain or fall
Pain very severe for 6 to 12 hours; cannot continue working if rupture extensive
Abduction mainly affected; patient shrugs to move arm; scapulohumeral rhythm lost; arm can be lifted passively in abduction; power to maintain arm gone (drop-arm sign)
Lidocaine infiltration relieves pain; range of motion serviceable if tear incomplete

Radiologic Findings

Humeral head high on the glenoid on adduction
Shoulder held in adduction

Physical Examination

Pain relieved by pendulum exercise position (see Fig. 125-10) or downward traction on arm (depression of head test)
Extreme tenderness over greater tuberosity

Management

Complete ruptures recognized early, surgically repaired
Partial ruptures heal surprisingly well, good return of function with conservative management

their sheaths (tenosynovitis), the bursa, capsule, synovium, cartilage, bone, and surrounding muscles.

Box 125-2 lists the differential diagnosis of shoulder pain. Uncomplicated supraspinatus tendinitis and tenosynovitis (with or without extension to other members of the rotator cuff) and bicipital tendinitis and tenosynovitis are associated with the normal range of passive motion. Involvement of the capsule (adhesive capsulitis), the bursa, muscles, and synovium is associated with limited range of motion.[4]

SUPRASPINATUS TENDINITIS, TENOSYNOVITIS, AND ROTATOR CUFF LESIONS

The first pathologic event occurs in the supraspinatus tendon. After the fifth decade of life, thinning, fraying, fissuring, and fibrillation of the distal tendon in the critical zone of hypovascularity result from the mechanical disadvantage and the constant stress on the tissue by humeral impingement against the coracoacromial arch. Traumatic inflammation occurs, possibly with an autoimmune mechanism producing antibody against denatured collagen and other structural proteins, and spreads to the contiguous tendon sheath, subacromial bursa, and other joint structures.

The patient is usually over 45 years of age with an occupation or leisure activity that entails unusual shoulder stress. The pain is a dull ache in the deltoid insertion area, often over a wider area, even the entire C5 sclerotome, with acute and severe pain on certain movements (abduction to 60 degrees or more, reaching over the head, putting on a coat). There is usually no arm or neck radiation. Night pain is characteristic, and the patient cannot lie on the affected side in bed because of increased pain. The patient often grabs the

Box 125-5. Bicipital Syndromes

Anatomy

Intraarticular: bicipital groove between greater and lesser tuberosities

Extraarticular: lies between subscapularis and supraspinatus tendons in synovial sheath, an extension from the shoulder joint proper

Tendinitis and Tenosynovitis

History

Chronic pain in anterolateral shoulder

Pain in trapezius, scalene, and deltoid, sometimes extending into arm and forearm

No history of acute trauma

Pain on repetitive activity over head

Physical examination

Shoulder stiffness, limited movement

Extreme tenderness in bicipital groove

Audible click when fully abducted and laterally rotated arm slowly brought to side (from tendon being dislocated)

Pain caused on resistance against flexed elbow and supinated hand (Yergason sign)

Management

Rest, heat, gentle exercise, nonsteroidal antiinflammatory drugs

Physical therapy

Avoidance of excessive tendon use

Local steroid/lidocaine injection

Elongation of Bicipital Tendon

Pathophysiology

Related to dislocation from groove

Part of attrition wear and tear

History

Shoulder pain and stiffness

Usually in older patient

Physical examination

Tenderness in bicipital groove

Crepitus on marked rotary movements

Laxity in long belly of biceps

Laxity with elbow flexed 90 degrees and forearm supinated against resistance

Audible click, as with tendinitis

Management

Conservative

Occasionally surgery

Tendon Dislocation

History

Painful audible click in external rotation of shoulder

Arm locking in painful condition, relieved by reversing movement, i.e., medial rotation

Physical examination

Manual pressure over groove with humerus rotated prevents tendon from dislocating

Management

Surgery if disability severe

Rupture of Long Head of Biceps

History

Chronic stiffness, shoulder pain

May or may not be history of a snap

Lump appears with elbow flexion

Acute traumatic rupture

Abrupt sharp pain, loss of power

Examination

Lump appears

Management

Young patient: surgical repair

Older patient: usually conservative

Box 125-6. Frozen Shoulder

Etiology and Pathogenesis

Most likely a reflex sympathetic dystrophy (shoulder-hand syndrome, Sudeck's atrophy)

Onset follows prolonged, sustained immobilization of arm (shoulder sling for trauma, rotator cuff or bicipital tendon lesions, myocardial infarction); immobilization may promote autonomic circulatory impairment, muscle contracture, fibrosis, and osteoporosis

History and Clinical Characteristics

Middle-aged people, more common in women than men

Associated with diabetes mellitus

Appears at varying rates and intensity; limitation of motion in one plane to complete fibrous ankylosis with glenohumeral motion compromise, development of pain and restricted motion and duration a few months to several years

Pain severe, worse at night, radiates into neck and down arms to fingers

Physical Examination

Tender anterior capsule, rotator cuff, and bicipital tendon

Disrupted scapulohumeral rhythm

Extremely restricted passive and active shoulder motion in all planes

Patient may appear systemically ill

Radiologic and Pathologic Findings

Osteopenia of humeral head with cystic changes

Narrowing of space between acromion and humeral head

Periarticular soft tissue calcifications on occasion

Great thickened, contracted fibrotic capsule, adherent to humeral head with adhesion of long head of biceps tendon in its sheath

Glenohumeral joint space contraction to 0.5-3 ml vs. normal volume of 30-40 ml

Management

Rest

Physical therapy with graded passive and active exercise program

Nonsteroidal antiinflammatory drugs

Systemic corticosteroids in tapering schedule (i.e., 15 mg prednisone twice a day for 5 days, then taper by 5 mg every 5 days for 4 to 5 weeks, then discontinue)

Injection of periarticular and intraarticular structures with depot corticosteroids and local anesthetic

Manipulation of shoulder under anesthesia

Prevention

Avoid immobilization

Exercise shoulder to pain limit

Box 125-7. Acromioclavicular Syndromes

Lesions in Differential Diagnosis of Shoulder Pain

Acromioclavicular joint contains meniscus.

Minor injuries (without clavicle dislocation) and negative radiograph may be symptomatic due to internal derangement of meniscus.

Osteoarthritis, rheumatoid arthritis, and direct or indirect trauma may cause pain.

Subacromial bursa just below acromioclavicular joint and critical zone of supraspinatus tendon and biceps tendon are in close relationship.

Acromioclavicular joint osteoarthritis is associated with osteophytes and joint space narrowing on radiographs.

Spread of inflammation from acromioclavicular to contiguous structures accounts for cases of periarthritis.

Clinical Characteristics

Pain is in superior aspect of shoulder.

Sharply localized tenderness is at joint.

Pain radiates toward perceived base of neck and in jaw on side of lesion.

Motion of throwing a ball overhand produces or exaggerates characteristic pain.

Adduction of arm across chest in horizontal plane causes severe pain.

Management

Nonsteroidal antiinflammatory drugs

Physical therapy

Surgical repair or resection of outer ½ inch of clavicle rarely necessary (joint is never fused)

affected shoulder with the opposite hand, complaining of a "catch," or a severe twinge in the shoulder. The shoulder is diffusely tender, especially over the humeral head lateral and posterior to the acromion and over the supraspinatus insertion. More posterior tenderness suggests teres minor and infraspinatus involvement. Pain in resisted medial rotation suggests subscapularis involvement. The anterior and superior aspects of the rotator cuff can be examined by having the patient reach behind the low back.

The posterior aspect of the rotator cuff can be best examined by adducting the arm across the chest. Downward pull on the relaxed arm is painful because of tension in the rotator cuff. Adduction and forward-backward swing cause no pain. Scapulohumeral rhythm is reversed, with the patient shrugging to rotate the scapula with the least glenohumeral adduction. The pain is greatly increased by forced abduction against resistance, and there is a painful arc of 10 to 15 degrees just beyond 60 degrees' abduction (as the tendons and cuff impinge over the coracoacromial arch). Passive range of motion is normal.

Radiographs are usually not helpful, although calcific densities may be seen later; bony flakes, spicules, sclerosis, and osteophytosis of the tuberosities occur, followed by eburnation and cystic changes. Infiltration of the cuff with 1% lidocaine with relief of pain, especially the arc of pain, is both diagnostic and therapeutic (see Figs. 125-15 and 125-16).

Management of rotator cuff tendinitis includes (1) extensive patient education with definition of the problem, prognosis, and reassurance regarding recovery; (2) heat as well as cold intermittently; (3) pendulum exercises (see Fig. 125-10); (4) range of motion exercises; (5) nonsteroidal antiinflammatory drugs; (6) injection of steroid and local anesthetic agents;

Box 125-8. Reflex Sympathetic Dystrophy Syndrome

Synonyms

Causalgia, Sudeck's atrophy, traumatic angiospasm, reflex dystrophy of extremities, postinfarction sclerodactyly, shoulder-hand syndrome, reflex neurovascular dystrophy, reflex sympathetic dystrophy

Pathophysiology

Arterial blood: vessels mainly on volar side of arm; lymphatics on dorsal side; venous return aided by pumping through muscle contractions in hand, forearm, and arm

Derangement of pumping mechanism
- Swelling and limitation of shoulder and hand motion
- Shoulder contraction
- Limitation of wrist movement

History

May involve wrist, elbow, and other arm tissue, other extremities; most striking usually in hand and shoulder

Painful, stiff shoulder; pain in arm and hand

Hyperesthesia

Physical Examination

Limitation of shoulder motion (may reach magnitude of frozen shoulder)

Swelling, edema, diffuse tenderness

Painful dystrophy in hand and fingers

Often bilateral; one side can be subtly affected, often later

Incomplete and painful digital flexion

Vasospasm, vasodilation, vasomotor instability

Trophic skin and nail changes
- Swelling, cyanosis, shiny skin
- Hypertrichosis and hyperhidrosis
- Hypertrophic nails

Radiologic Findings

Early: subchondral bone erosion (as early as a few days after onset)

Late: diffuse extensive osteoporosis

Precipitating Events

Myocardial infarction

Painful trauma

Cerebrovascular accident, epilepsy, other central nervous system disease

Cervical spine disk disease

Painful intrathoracic or upper intraabdominal disorder, Pancoast's tumor

Herpes zoster

Calcific tendinitis of shoulder

Clinical Course: Three Stages

Rapid or gradual onset of painful shoulder; periarthritis of shoulder, arm, hand, and fingers with redness, duskiness, and edema; progressive limitation of movement

Duration: weeks to 6 months

Decreased pain; increased shoulder mobility; decreased hand edema; skin, subcutaneous, and muscle tissue atrophy; palmar fascia contractures (simulates Dupuytren's contracture); months in duration

Dystrophic changes; inelastic skin; cold, cyanotic hands; nail changes; frozen shoulder in adduction; hand and fingers in stiff flexion deformity; muscle atrophy

Management

Early mobilization; maximal movement, active and passive

Avoidance of immobilization

Physical therapy: active and passive exercises

Corticosteroids: prednisone, 30 mg/day in divided doses, reducing dose by 5 mg each 5 days, for 5 to 6 weeks

Nonsteroidal antiinflammatory drugs

Analgesics

(7) pain medication; and (8) occasionally, a short course of steroids (e.g., prednisone, 15 mg in the morning and at supper for 5 days, reduced by 5 mg every 5 days until cessation). About 90% of patients recover with this therapy.

Boxes 125-3 to 125-10 summarize calcific tendinitis,[8] rupture of the rotator cuff, bicipital syndromes (Fig. 125-18), frozen shoulder[1,3,10] (Fig. 125-19), acromioclavicular syndromes, reflex sympathetic dystrophy syndrome,[7] neurovascular syndromes, and visceral and somatic lesions.[6]

SHOULDER ARTHROCENTESIS AND INTRAARTICULAR INJECTION

Shoulder arthrocentesis is best accomplished with the patient seated and the shoulder internally rotated. The skin is marked just medial to the head of the humerus and slightly inferior and just lateral to the coracoid process; both structures are readily palpable with practice. Using strict sterile skin preparation, a wheal is raised in the skin using a syringe with lidocaine and a 26-gauge needle at the marked spot. A 20- to 22-gauge needle is then directed posteriorly, slightly superiorly, and laterally. Ideally , the physician should feel the needle enter the joint space. If bone is hit, the physician should pull back and redirect the needle at a slightly different angle[9] (see Fig. 125-1).

For injection into the subacromial bursa the physician follows the clavicle laterally to palpate the shelving edge of the acromion process, which is usually readily identified; the needle is directed under the edge. Entry into the bursa can usually be perceived. A lateral approach to both the shoulder joint and the subacromial bursa can also be used, inserting the needle between the acromion process of the scapula and the head of the humerus.

Corticosteroids are often mixed with a local anesthetic, typically procaine or lidocaine. Package inserts from the major pharmaceutical manufacturers advise against this practice. Most local anesthetics contain preservatives that

Box 125-9. Thoracic Outlet Syndrome

Anatomy

Upper extremity neurovascular supply exits arm at root of neck.
Clinical syndromes result from compression of brachial plexus and subclavian vein or artery.
Medial cord (C8-T1) ulnar distribution (most inferior portion of brachial plexus) is often involved.
Sites of compression on neurovascular structures:
- Cervical ribs and fascial connections
- Thoracic rib anomalies
- Between scalene muscles
- Rib-clavicle
- During hyperabduction or other unusual positions with normal anatomy

Clinical Characteristics

Rare causes of shoulder pain; diagnosis best made on basis of history and examination

History

Paresthesias (numbness, tingling)
Pain
Weakness in shoulder, arm, forearm, and hand
Swelling, coldness of extremity
Pain on arising from sleep, related to sleep position

Physical Examination

Sensory loss
Muscle atrophy (especially hand) (late finding)
- Hypothenar, interosseus with ulnar involvement
- Abductor pollicis brevis, opponens pollicis with medial nerve involvement
- Fasciculations

Pallor, edema, cyanosis, coldness of involved extremity
Blood pressure discrepancies between arms
Provocative maneuvers (may produce abnormal responses in normal patient)
- Adson: neck extension, chin rotated toward affected side, deep inspiration, pulse obliterates or decreases in intensity, symptoms reproduced (tenses anterior and middle scalene muscles, decreasing interscalene space)
- Costoclavicular: exaggerated military posture (bracing shoulders back and down); pulse intensity decreases
- Pain exacerbation by downward traction on shoulder

Management

Conservative measures effective in 80% of patients
- Reassurance
- Education
- Exercise and physical therapy to correct faulty posture and strengthen shoulder girdle musculature
- Situational change (e.g., occupation, redesign of kitchen or work area)
- Treatment of muscle spasm

Surgery considered only after conservative treatment has failed

Box 125-10. Visceral and Somatic Lesions (Diaphragmatic Disorders) and Diseases Characterized by Referred Pain to the Shoulder

Pain referred via phrenic nerve (C3-4 and C4-5) to supraclavicular region, trapezius, and superior angle of scapula
Gallbladder and hepatic parenchymal disease: scapular and shoulder top pain associated with epigastric tenderness
Gastric and pancreatic disease: interscapular pain
Perforated hollow viscus via phrenic nerve distribution
Pulmonary infarction: diaphragmatic irritation
Pancoast's or apical lung tumor, may have coincident Horner's syndrome
Myocardial ischemia: pain infraclavicular, ulnar, and at base of neck
Transverse and descending aortic arch disease: pain in left side of neck and shoulder
Cervical osteoarthritis with neural, muscle, joint, and ligamentous (deep pain) referral pattern at C5-T1 levels
Pleural disease: diaphragmatic irritation
Peritoneal disease: diaphragmatic irritation
Neoplasms of cervical cord and nerve roots
Neurovascular syndromes (see text)
Objective clinical findings in shoulder joint usually absent in referred visceral or somatic disease; active and passive shoulder motion not limited, and pain or other symptoms not caused by movement; inclusive differential diagnosis imperative due to complexity and diversity of shoulder disorders

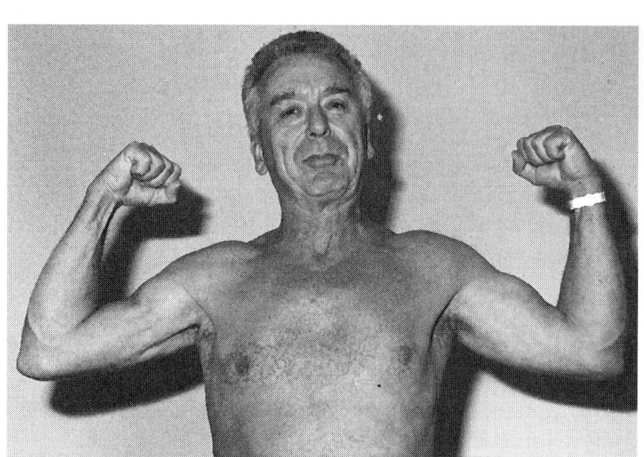

Fig. 125-18. Note "lump" in right biceps *(left side of photograph)* compared with left biceps. Long head of biceps tendon is completely ruptured.

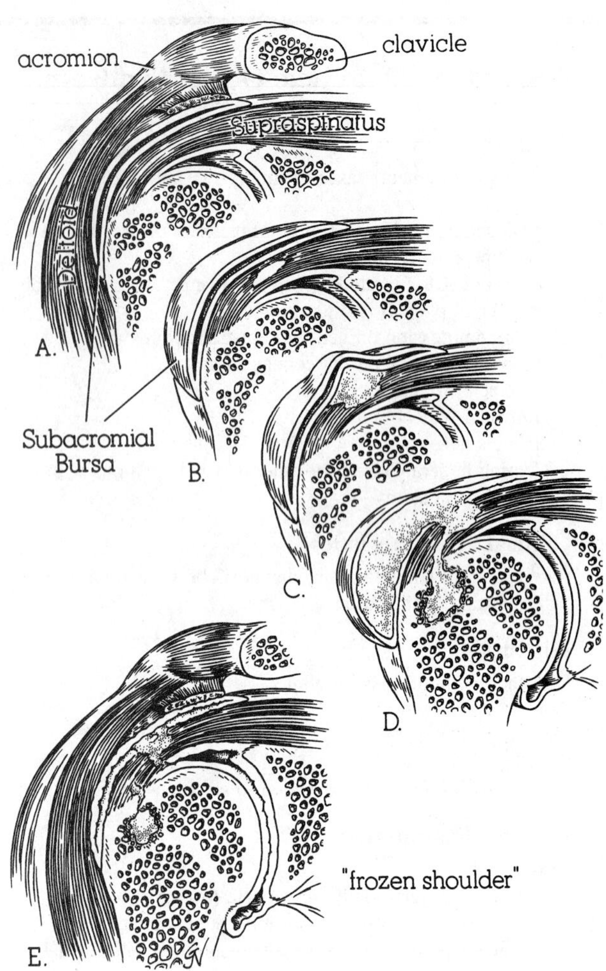

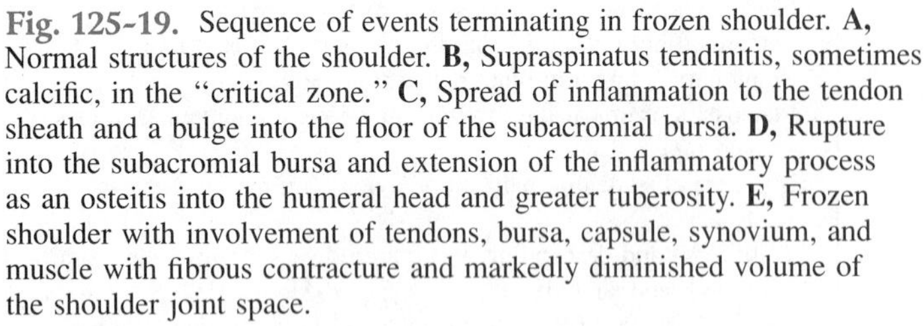
Fig. 125-19. Sequence of events terminating in frozen shoulder. **A,** Normal structures of the shoulder. **B,** Supraspinatus tendinitis, sometimes calcific, in the "critical zone." **C,** Spread of inflammation to the tendon sheath and a bulge into the floor of the subacromial bursa. **D,** Rupture into the subacromial bursa and extension of the inflammatory process as an osteitis into the humeral head and greater tuberosity. **E,** Frozen shoulder with involvement of tendons, bursa, capsule, synovium, and muscle with fibrous contracture and markedly diminished volume of the shoulder joint space.

Box 125-11. Corticosteroid Injections and Possible Sequelae

Corticosteroid Preparations

Methylprednisolone acetate (Depo-Medrol), 20, 40, and 80 mg/ml
Triamcinolone hexacetonide (Aristospan), 20 mg/ml
Betamethasone sodium phosphate and a citrate suspension (Celestone Soluspan), 6 mg/ml
Dexamethasone acetate (Decadron LA), 8 mg/ml
Hydrocortisone acetate (Hydrocortone), 25 mg/ml
Prednisolone tebutate (Hydeltra-T.B.A.), 20 mg/ml

Sequelae to Intraarticular and Soft Tissue Injections

Tendon rupture
Iatrogenic infection (rare)
Deterioration of joints, evidenced radiologically: steroid arthropathy, Charcot-like arthropathy, osteonecrosis
Nerve damage
Postinjection flare
Tissue atrophy, fat necrosis
Pancreatitis (rare side effect from systemic absorption)

may result in flocculation of the corticosteroid. Lidocaine for intravenous use does not contain a preservative. A conservative approach is advised. A short- or intermediate-acting steroid preparation such as triamcinolone diacetate or methylprednisolone acetate is recommended for periarticular injections. A long-acting preparation such as triamcinolone hexacetonide may be used for intraarticular injection (see Chapter 123). No consensus exists on the ideal volume and dose of corticosteroid for injection into joints. The shoulder is a large joint with considerable intrasynovial volume; 2 to 3 ml is advised (Box 125-11).[9]

REFERENCES

1. Binder AL et al: Frozen shoulder: a long-term prospective study, *Ann Rheum Dis* 43:361, 1984.
2. Bland JH, Merrit JA, Boushey DR: The painful shoulder, *Semin Arthritis Rheum* 7:21, 1977.
3. Bulgen DY et al: Frozen shoulder: prospective clinical study with an evaluation of three treatment regimens, *Ann Rheum Dis* 43:353, 1984.
4. Chard MD, Hazleman BL: Shoulder disorders in the elderly (a hospital study), *Ann Rheum Dis* 46:684, 1987.
5. Dacre JE, Beeney N, Scott DL: Injections and physiotherapy for the painful stiff shoulder, *Ann Rheum Dis* 48:322, 1989.
6. Halverson PB et al: Milwaukee shoulder. II. Synovial fluid studies, *Arthritis Rheum* 24:474, 1981.

7. Kozin F et al: The reflex sympathetic dystrophy syndrome. I. Clinical and histologic studies: response to corticosteroids and articular involvement, *Am J Med* 60:321, 1976.
8. Mavrikakis ME et al: Calcific shoulder periarthritis (tendinitis) in adult onset diabetes mellitus: a controlled study, *Ann Rheum Dis* 48:211, 1989.
9. McCarty DJ et al: Milwaukee shoulder—association of microspheroids containing hydroxyapatite crystals, active collagenase, neutral protease with rotator cuff defects. I. Clinical aspects, *Arthritis Rheum* 24:464, 1981.
10. Parker RD et al: Frozen shoulder, *Orthopedics* 12:869, 1989.

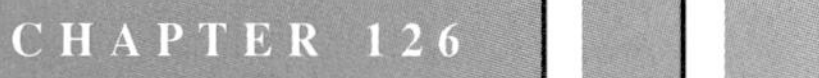

Disorders of the Hand

Joseph M. Lenehan

Approximately one third of all injuries involve the upper extremities. The National Safety Council estimated that 1.8 million disabling work injuries occurred in 1990, with 60,000 resulting in some permanent impairment. Upper extremity injuries accounted for 31% and hand injuries 24% of the cases. Thus these injuries represent a significant percentage of injuries seen by primary care physicians. Hand injuries cause not only significant physical disability but also deformities that are often a source of major psychologic trauma.

PATIENT EVALUATION

History

In addition to information regarding the patient's age, occupation, dominant hand, previous injury, and general health, a detailed history of the injury is needed. This should include the position of the fingers and hand at the time of injury, the degree of contamination, the initial treatment, and the interval between the injury and initial care.

Physical Examination

An understanding of functional anatomy is important in assessing the injured hand. Physical examination should be performed systematically to assess the skin, musculotendinous units, nerve and vascular supply, and bone and joint function. This is best accomplished by obtaining as much information by inspection as possible before asking the patient to actively move the hand, which may cause discomfort. Any gross positional deformity indicative of tendon or bone injury should be noted. The skin should be inspected for penetrating wounds or gross lacerations. An examination of the sensation in all digits, using the Weber two-point discrimination test, is important in determining median, ulnar, and radial nerve function (Fig. 126-1). The vascular supply should be assessed by inspecting color and capillary filling. Once this information has been obtained, the musculotendinous units and motor function can be assessed.

Extrinsic Muscles. The extrinsic muscles of the hand consist of the digital flexors and extensors; they should be tested individually. The flexor digitorum profundus tendons of the fingers are tested by stabilizing the proximal interphalangeal (PIP) joint of the fingers and asking the patient to flex the distal interphalangeal (DIP) joint actively (Fig. 126-2). The flexor digitorum superficialis tendons of the fingers are tested by holding the adjacent fingers in full extension and asking the patient to flex the PIP joint of the involved digit (Fig. 126-3). This effectively prevents the profundus tendon from acting on the digit being tested. The flexor pollicis longus tendon is tested by stabilizing the metacarpophalangeal (MCP) joint of the thumb and asking the patient to flex the interphalangeal (IP) joint (Fig. 126-4). The extrinsic extensor muscles are first tested by passive motion at the level of the wrist to check for any gross positional deformities. Each extensor tendon is then tested individually for active function with the wrist held in the

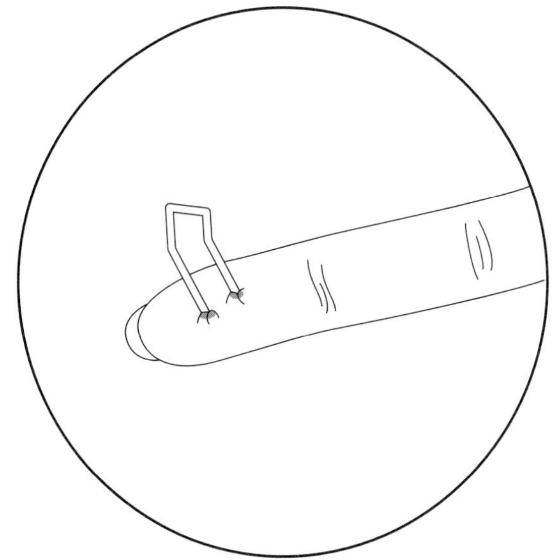

Fig. 126-1. Weber two-point discrimination is most sensitive test to detect intact sensation. Normally, two points can be distinguished when 6 mm apart. Testing should be longitudinally oriented along the radial and ulnar borders of the pulp to test individual proper digital nerve sensation.

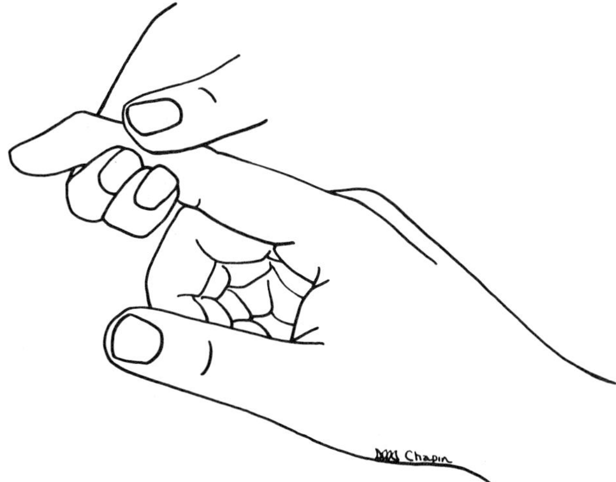

Fig. 126-2. Testing of flexor digitorum profundus tendon.

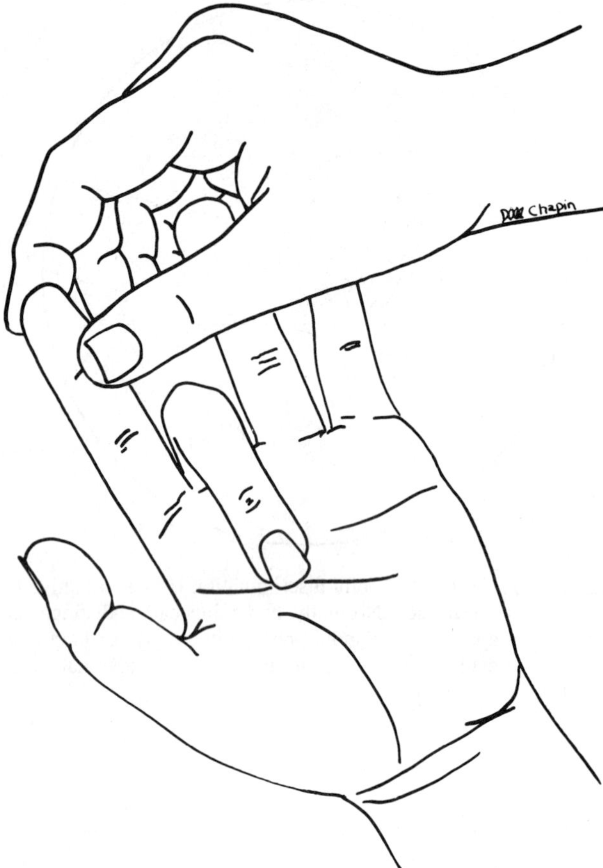

Fig. 126-3. Testing of flexor superficialis tendon.

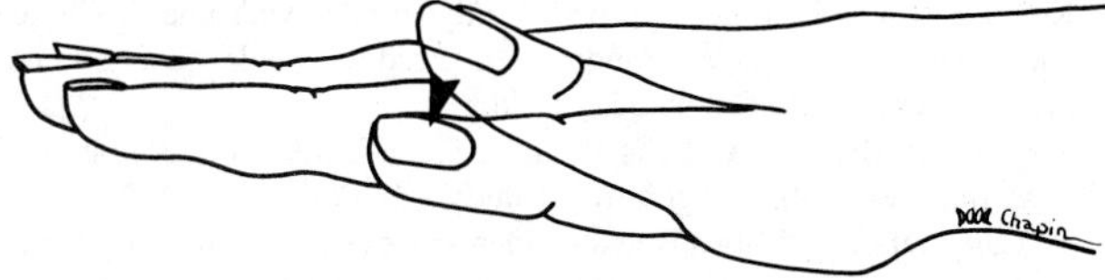

Fig. 126-5. Testing of extensor pollicis longus tendon.

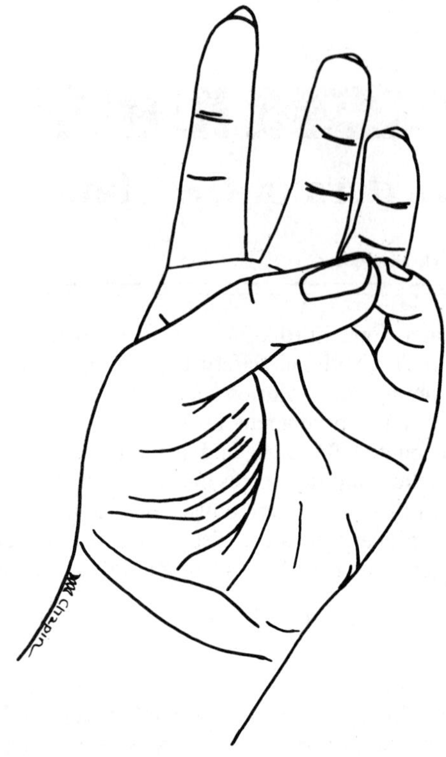

Fig. 126-6. Motor supply from median nerve to abductor pollicis brevis, opponens pollicis, and superficial head of flexor pollicis brevis muscle.

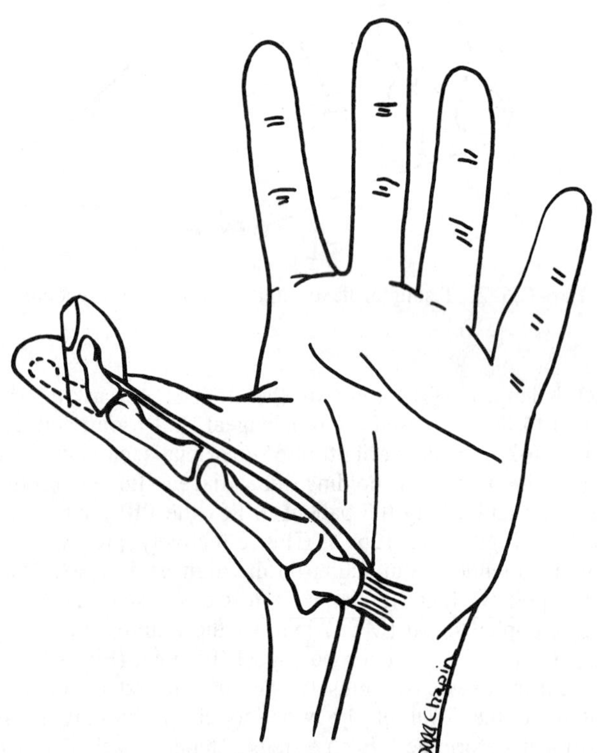

Fig. 126-4. Testing of flexor pollicis longus tendon.

slightly extended position. The index and the little fingers have an additional tendon, the extensor indicis proprius and the extensor digiti minimi tendons, respectively. These can be tested by asking the patient to extend one digit alone while holding the others flexed. The extensor pollicis longus tendon is best tested by asking the patient to hold the hand flat on the table and then extend the thumb (Fig. 126-5). The wrist extensors are tested by active extension against gravity with the fingers fully flexed in a fist with simultaneous palpation of the distal tendons.

Intrinsic Muscles. Testing the intrinsic muscles requires a clear understanding of the motor supply from the median and ulnar nerves. The median nerve supplies the abductor pollicis brevis, opponens pollicis, and the superficial head of the flexor pollicis brevis muscles, which contribute to opposition of the thumb (Fig. 126-6). The ulnar nerve supplies the interosseous muscles, the deep head of the flexor pollicis brevis muscle, the adductor pollicis muscle, and the hypothenar musculature. The lumbrical muscles to the index and long fingers are supplied by the median nerve and those

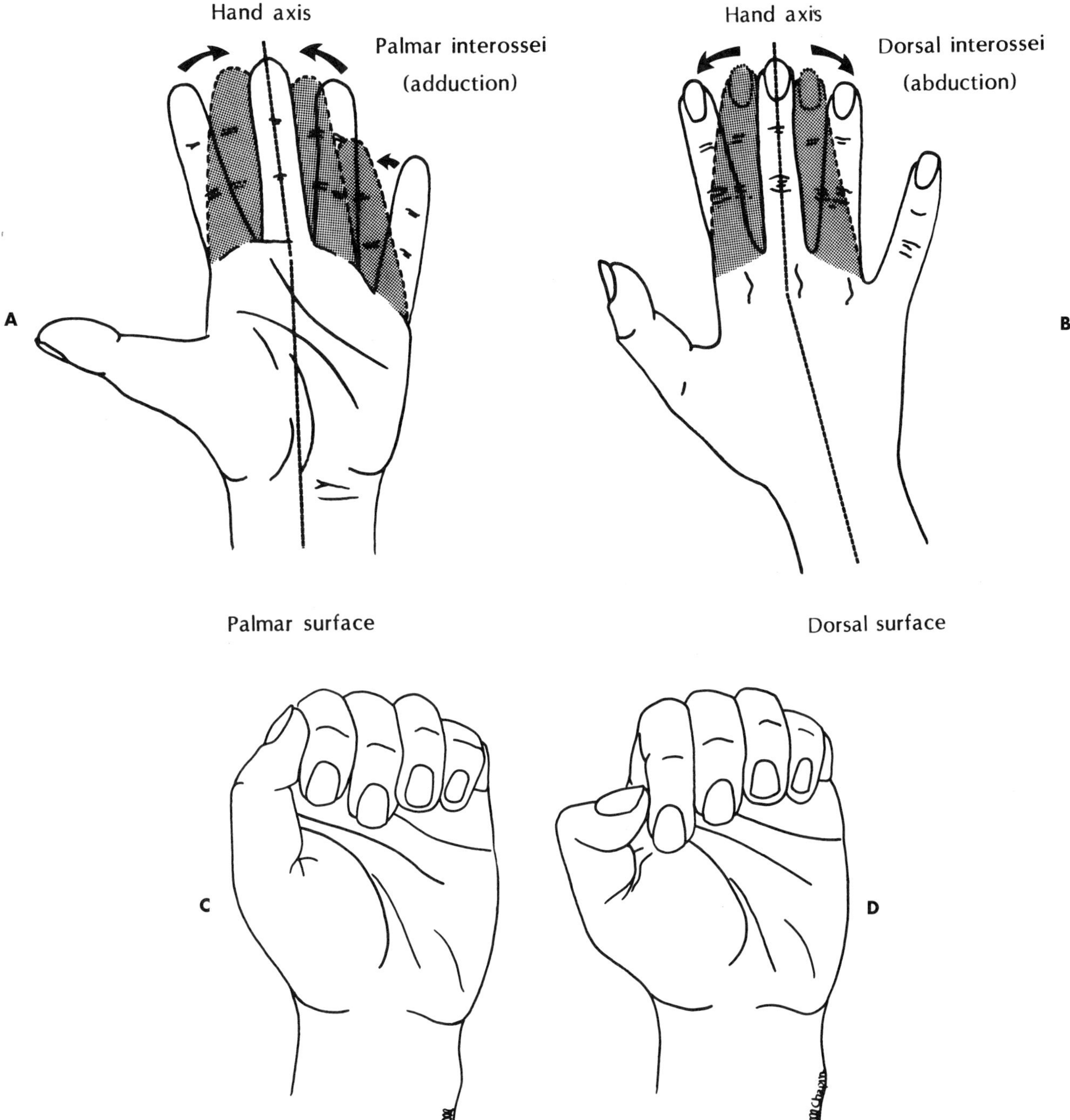

Fig. 126-7. Ulnar nerve testing. Weakness of intrinsic muscle is revealed by adduction (**A**) and abduction (**B**) when there is ulnar nerve injury. When ulnar innervation to adductor pollicis (**C**) is intact, Froment's test reveals a normal pinch. Injury to ulnar nerves results in an abnormal pinch (**D**), which can only be performed by using flexor pollicis longus, innervated by median nerve.

to the ring and little fingers by the ulnar nerve. To test for thenar muscle function supplied by the motor branch of the median nerve, the patient must demonstrate opposition of the thumb, with the examiner palpating the thenar muscle group. Ulnar nerve motor function is tested (1) by observing the patient's ability to abduct and adduct the fingers and to flex the MCP joints with the IP joints in the extended position and (2) by checking the adequacy of the adductor pollicis muscle by assessing the power of a key pinch (Fig. 126-7).

Sensory Testing. A sensory examination should include mapping of the areas of diminished sensation that are revealed by light touch and use of the Weber two-point discrimination test (see Fig. 126-1). Normal subjects can distinguish two points 6 mm apart. Besides assessing pallor and capillary filling, vascular examination should include palpation of pulses and an Allen's test at wrist and, if indicated, digital levels. This may be accompanied by a Doppler examination.

INJURIES

The patient with an acutely traumatized upper extremity should have a routine examination of all potentially involved structures. A sterile saline gauze dressing should be applied to the wound and the patient placed in the supine position with the hand elevated. Bleeding in the hand should be controlled by direct pressure alone; clamping a bleeding vessel is avoided because of its proximity to vital structures (e.g., nerves, tendons). The sterile saline gauze dressing should be left in place and the extremity assessed distal to the site of injury. A systematic examination can determine whether tendon, vascular, or nerve injuries exist. This is especially true for children, who often become uncooperative once the physician causes pain when examining the injury or exploring the wound.

Tendons

Tendon injuries can occur with small, superficial-appearing wounds if the tendon is under tension at the time of injury. This is most evident with superficial lacerations over the flexor creases of the fingers or wrist, which often result in significant nerve and tendon injuries.

Flexor Tendons. The flexor creases have no subcutaneous fat at the IP joint level, and a small puncture wound to that area often results in an injury to the flexor sheath. The patient with a partial tendon injury may not have a gross positional deformity but may complain of pain when flexing the finger actively. Testing finger flexion against resistance may elicit pain if there is a partial tendon injury; such testing must be done with caution, however, because it may cause a partial tendon transection to rupture. Critical areas include the flexor digitorum profundus tendon distal to the superficialis tendon insertion and distal to the flexor crease at the PIP joint. The transection of the flexor pollicis longus tendon at the level of the flexor crease at the MCP joint is also a common injury. In examining for flexor tendon injuries, the flexor digitorum superficialis and profundus tendons should be tested independently (see Figs. 126-2 and 126-3). Examination of the flexor pollicis longus tendon requires demonstration of active flexion at the IP joint (see Fig. 126-4). Many patients do not have significant independent flexion at the PIP joint of the little finger. The superficial tendon of the opposite little finger should be tested (Fig. 126-8). A closed rupture of the flexor digitorum profundus tendon can occur. Usually it involves the ring finger in a sports-related grasping injury. If this injury is recognized early, the tendon can be reinserted on the distal phalanx.

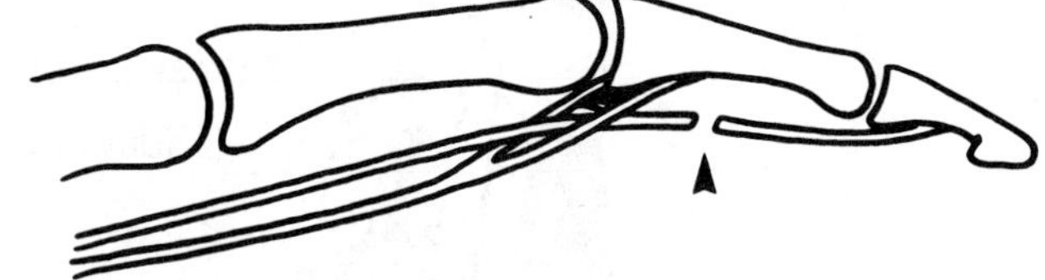

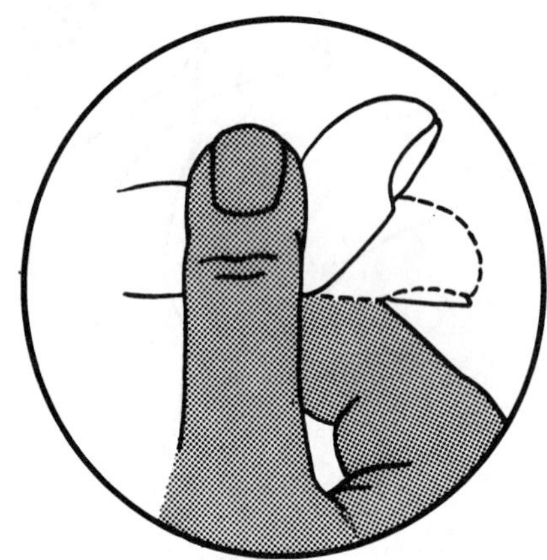

Fig. 126-8. Transection of flexor digitorum profundus tendon distal to superficialis insertion.

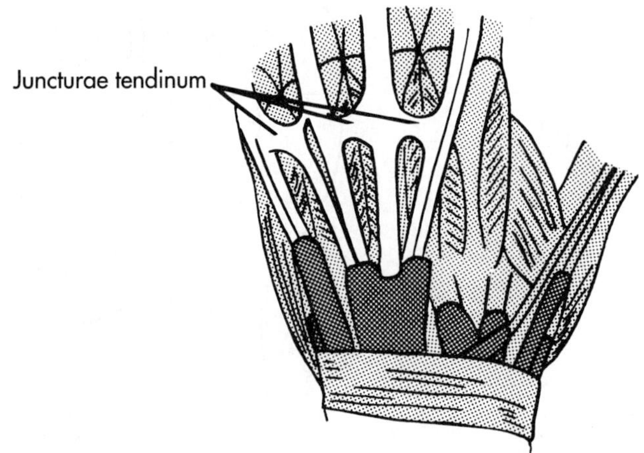

Fig. 126-9. Role of juncturae tendinum.

Extensor Tendons. Extensor tendon injuries occur with the fingers fully flexed or extended. Thus all dorsal wounds should be explored for tendon injuries. The fingers should be flexed and then extended so that the tendon can be examined through the full range of its excursion. The two tendons to the index and little fingers, which allow for independent extension of these digits, must be identified. When examining dorsal wounds for possible extensor tendon injuries, the physician must recognize the role of the *juncturae tendinum,* which are communications between the common digital extensor tendons on the dorsum of the hand (Fig. 126-9). Lacerations over the dorsum of the MCP joint area usually result in a lack of MCP extension, provided the transection is distal to the juncturae tendinum. IP joint extension results from intrinsic muscle function and MCP joint extension from extrinsic tendon function. In the absence of the extrinsic tendons the IP joints can be completely extended. Any laceration over the MCP joint should suggest a human bite wound.

Nerves

When assessing lacerations of the hand, the physician should understand the anatomic characteristics of the nerves potentially involved (Fig. 126-10). The proper digital nerves on the volar aspect of the thumb are immediately adjacent to the flexor pollicis longus tendon sheath near the MCP joint

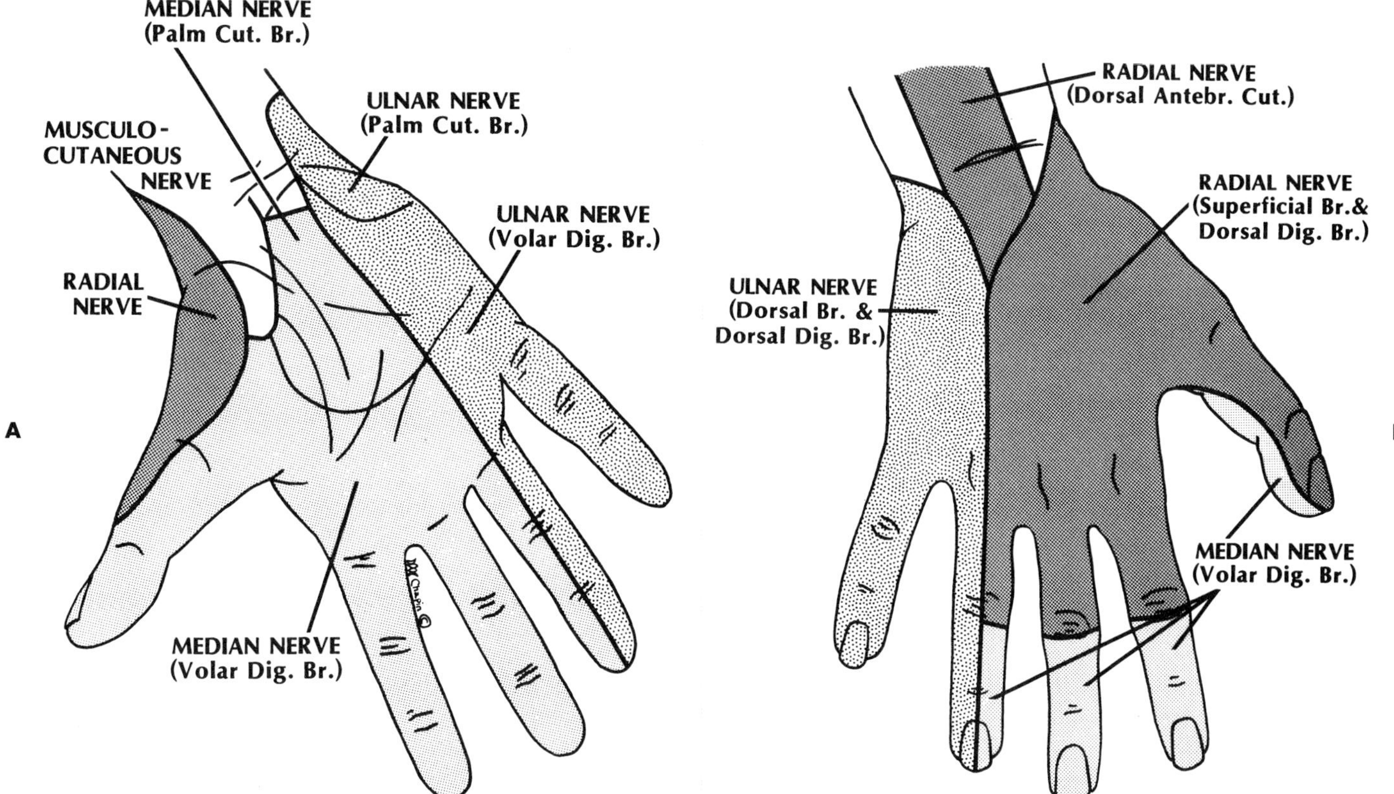

Fig. 126-10. Nerves of the hand. **A,** Volar aspect. **B,** Dorsal aspect. *Cut. br.,* Cutaneous branch; *dig. br.,* digital branch; *antebr.,* antebrachial.

and are susceptible to injury. The radial and ulnar proper digital nerves at this point are approximately 1 to 1.5 cm apart. The dorsal sensory branch of the ulnar nerve and the superficial radial nerve with its multiple branches pass in the subcutaneous tissue over the dorsal ulnar and dorsal radial aspect of the wrists, respectively. They are easily palpated and susceptible to injury by relatively superficial lacerations. On the volar aspect of the fingers the proper digital nerves are volar to the digital arteries. A patient presenting with a volar finger laceration and arterial bleeding most likely has a transected digital nerve in addition to the transected artery. A digital sensory examination using a paper clip should be performed to determine two-point discrimination before any anesthesia is instilled. In addition, if regional block anesthesia is performed, motor muscle testing of the intrinsic musculature should be done first. Regional nerve blocks include the intermetacarpal block and, at the wrist, the superficial radial nerve, dorsal sensory branch of the ulnar nerve, the median nerve, and the ulnar nerve blocks. With the widely used techniques of magnification for nerve repairs, a proper digital nerve can be repaired at the level of the DIP joint. The timing of nerve repair is controversial, but for sharp, clean wounds with nerve injury, primary repair is usually indicated.

Radiographic Examination

X-ray examination of the hand or finger is needed for most hand injuries and for lacerations resulting from glass; however, wood and nonopaque glass often are not demonstrated radiographically. In addition to searching for foreign bodies, a radiograph should be obtained to assess the hand for fractures, puncture wounds of the bone, dislocations, and ligamentous injuries with small avulsion fragments. Additional x-ray studies can provide true lateral views of the PIP joint for assessment of intraarticular fractures or dislocations and oblique views of the ring and little metacarpals for assessment of fractures or dislocations of the carpometacarpal joints. Once a nerve, tendon, joint, or open fracture is confirmed, further exploration of the wound is not indicated. The injury requires surgical exploration and repair in the operating room. Local exploration of the wound only increases the risk of contamination and may cause a blood clot to be dislodged, resulting in bleeding and requiring emergency interventions.

Diagnostic Considerations

In the hand, vital structures lie immediately beneath a thin covering of skin, especially over the joint surfaces on the dorsum and over the flexor creases on the volar aspect. In open injuries it is important to recognize a partial flexor or extensor tendon laceration, a transection of the flexor digitorum profundus tendon distal to the superficialis insertion (see Fig. 126-8), a transection of the common digital extensor tendon without extension lag because of the junctura tendons (see Fig. 126-9), digital nerve injuries, and crush injuries to the fingertip with subungual hematoma and nail bed injuries.

In closed injuries, long-term morbidity can result from mallet deformity at the DIP joint, boutonnière deformity at the PIP joint, collateral ligament injuries at the MCP joint of the fingers and thumb and PIP joint of the fingers, and rupture of the flexor digitorum profundus tendon from its insertion. Minor hand injuries must be properly splinted to allow uncomplicated wound healing in areas over mobile joint surfaces.

SPECIFIC DISORDERS AND TREATMENTS

Fractures

Basic orthopedic principles for the treatment of fractures apply to the hand, with the understanding that accurate reduction is required to restore maximum function to small hand bones and joints. Stable fractures usually can be treated by closed reduction and splinting. Unstable and displaced intraarticular fractures often need open reduction with internal fixation. Fractures are classified as either open or closed; an *open fracture* communicates with the wound.

Rotational Deformities. Gross angular or rotational deformity may allow easy recognition of a bone or joint injury. Palpation for tenderness at the injury site can be performed before x-ray examination. Motion or stress examination is usually reserved until after adequate radiographic assessment, which often includes anterior and true lateral views. Careful examination is required to evaluate for rotational deformities. Flexed fingertips normally point toward the scaphoid (Fig. 126-11). Overlapping or malpositioning of the fingertips should be observed in both flexed and extended positions. In the extended position, rotation is assessed by noting the relationships of the curve of the fingernails with the adjacent fingers and comparing this with the opposite hand.

Radiographic Examination. X-ray films may be misleading because overlapping structures can obscure a small fragment of bone. In hand injuries, small fragments of bone are often attached to a collateral ligament, a volar plate, or a displaced tendon (Fig. 126-12). The fragment may signify a potentially unstable condition that must be treated to avoid deformity. Particular attention should be directed to intraarticular fractures. In the case of specific ligamentous injuries, x-rays should be obtained before testing for instability (e.g., MCP joint of thumb). Stress testing may displace a previously undisplaced intraarticular fracture that could have been treated by immobilization alone.

Terminal Phalanx. Fractures of the terminal phalanx are usually the result of crush injuries and are associated with subungual hematomas and nail bed injuries. In most cases the subungual hematoma should be evacuated; if nail bed injuries exist, the nail should be removed and the laceration of the nail bed repaired with fine absorbable sutures. Adequate repair of the nail bed in soft tissue injuries usually results in a satisfactory reduction of the fracture fragments. Occasionally, with more proximal terminal phalanx fractures, open reduction and internal fixation are indicated. If there is a concomitant flexion deformity at the DIP joint, a tendon injury may exist in addition to the fracture.

Middle and Proximal Phalanx. Fractures of the middle and proximal phalanx can be displaced by a number of forces. Because of the extrinsic flexor and extensor tendons' longitudinal pull and the potential for rotational deformities, these fractures must be assessed for both rotational and angulation deformities (see Fig. 126-11). Furthermore, intraarticular fractures at the PIP and DIP joints may produce unstable fragments involving the articular surface (see Fig. 126-12). These fractures may be complicated by subluxation or fracture dislocation, requiring open reduction and internal fixation. Small fractures involving one fourth of the articular surface on the volar lip of the middle phalanx may be associated with late dorsal dislocation. Intraarticular injuries with small fragments, even if not displaced, have a potential for significant morbidity.

Metacarpal. Fractures of the metacarpal are usually treated by closed reduction. These fractures must be assessed for overriding with shortening and angulation. Rotational alignment is critical in metacarpal fractures and is checked by observing position of the fingernails and alignment of the

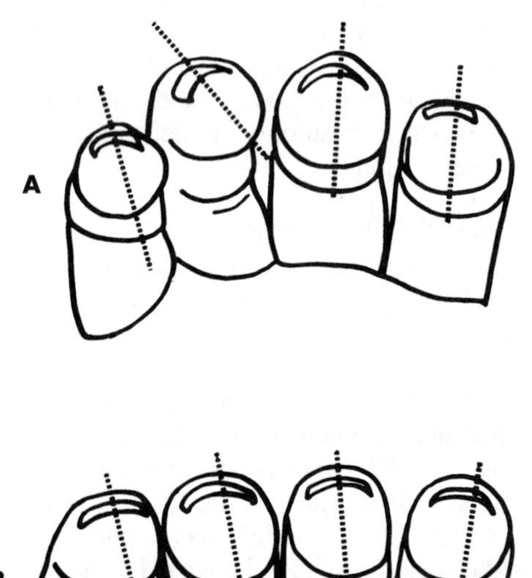

Fig. 126-11. Flexed fingertips should be checked for rotational alignment. **A,** Rotational malalignment of fourth finger caused by metacarpal or phalangeal fracture. **B,** Normal alignment.

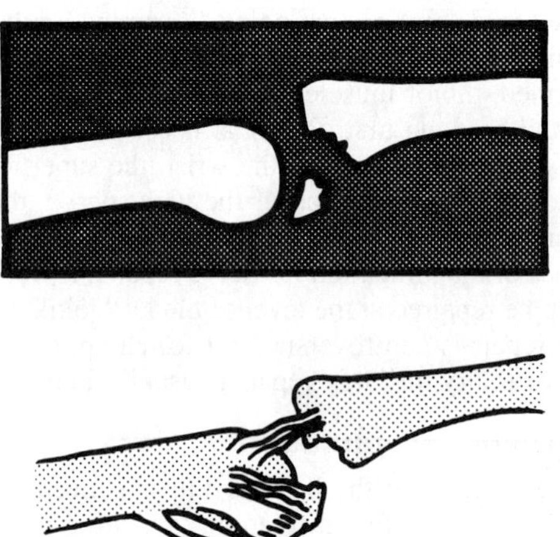

Fig. 126-12. Unstable fracture of proximal interphalangeal joint.

fingertips (see Fig. 126-11). Postreduction rotation should be checked clinically and radiographically. With open injuries and multiple displaced fractures, internal fixation is often recommended.

Bennett's fracture is an oblique intraarticular fracture through the base of the thumb (Fig. 126-13). The metacarpal shaft, the larger segment, is displaced proximally by the pull of the thumb's long abductor tendon. The volar ulnar fragment of the metacarpal usually remains in its normal position because of ligamentous attachments; it requires reduction and often internal fixation. A similar intraarticular fracture or fracture dislocation can occur at the base of the fifth metacarpal, involving the carpometacarpal joint. This fracture also requires reduction and frequently internal fixation.

Scaphoid. Fracture of the scaphoid usually results from a fall on an outstretched hand. The patient presents with

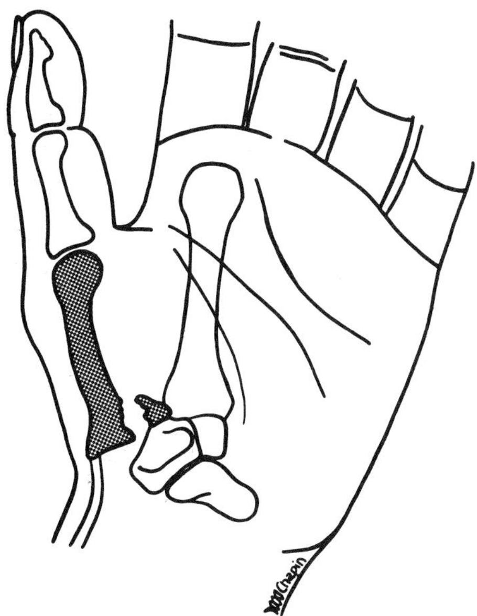

Fig. 126-13. Bennett's fracture.

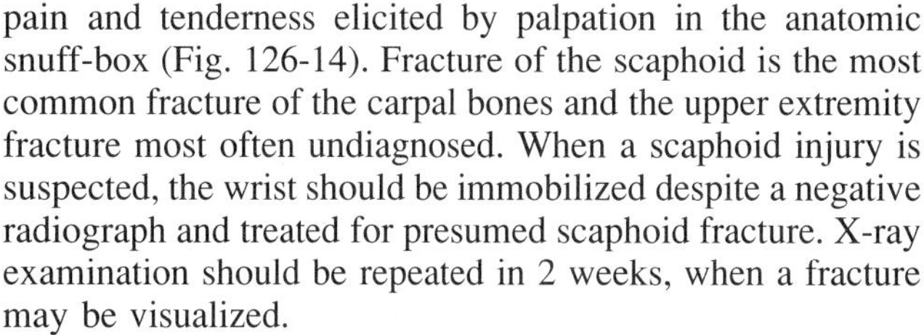

pain and tenderness elicited by palpation in the anatomic snuff-box (Fig. 126-14). Fracture of the scaphoid is the most common fracture of the carpal bones and the upper extremity fracture most often undiagnosed. When a scaphoid injury is suspected, the wrist should be immobilized despite a negative radiograph and treated for presumed scaphoid fracture. X-ray examination should be repeated in 2 weeks, when a fracture may be visualized.

Dislocations

Dislocations in the hand occur primarily at the IP and MCP joint levels. At the IP level, fractures result from hyperextension force or direct trauma on the fingertip and may produce a burst wound along the flexor crease at the DIP or PIP joint. Closed injuries often can be reduced without difficulty and splinted in slight flexion at the IP joint level. MCP joint dislocation usually results from a hyperextension injury. The volar plate is usually disrupted proximally at its metacarpal attachment, and the joint is dislocated so that the proximal phalanx lies dorsal to the metacarpal head. The metacarpal head can become trapped through a buttonhole of tissue and usually cannot be reduced by closed technique. The thumb MCP joint often can be reduced closed, but it occasionally requires open reduction. The most common dislocation of the carpals is a volar dislocation of the lunate, which may be associated with acute median nerve compression, requiring immediate reduction. If the physician is not familiar with techniques of reduction, the patient should be referred.

Ligamentous Injury

Injury to the ulnar collateral ligament at the MCP joint of the thumb usually results from acute radial deviation of the thumb at the MCP joint (Fig. 126-15). This injury usually is caused by a skiing fall and results in a complete or incomplete tear of the ulnar collateral ligament. The patient presents with swelling, pain, and tenderness on the ulnar side of the thumb's MCP joint. The area should be examined radiographically, and if no fracture is found, stress testing is recommended. With an incomplete lesion and minimal deviation on stress testing, immobilization with a thumb spica cast may be satisfactory. Significant laxity associated with complete

A

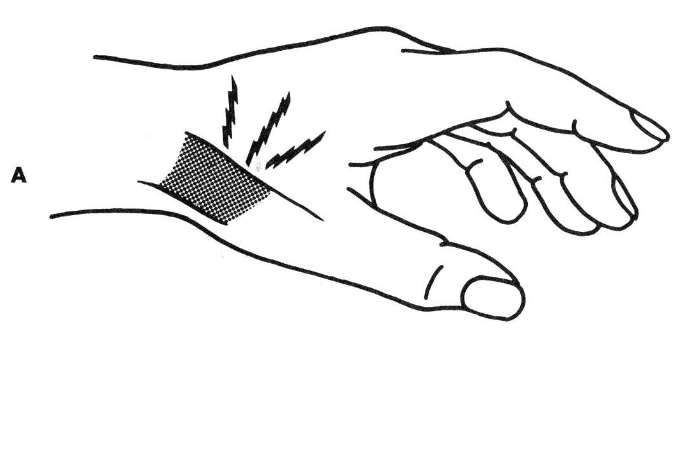

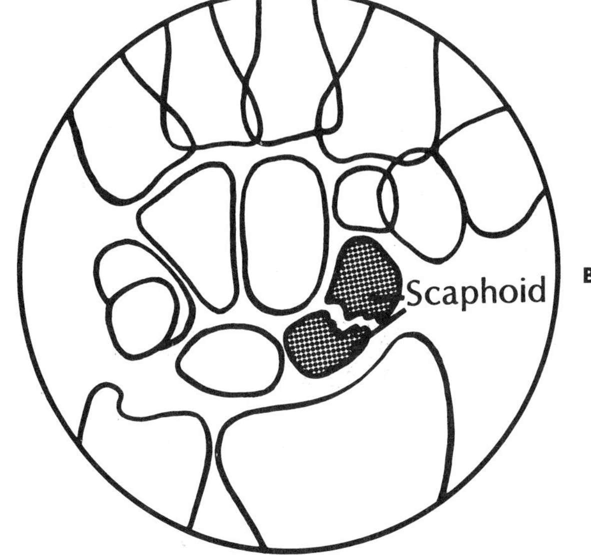

B

Fig. 126-14. **A,** Pain in anatomic snuff-box. **B,** Fracture of scaphoid.

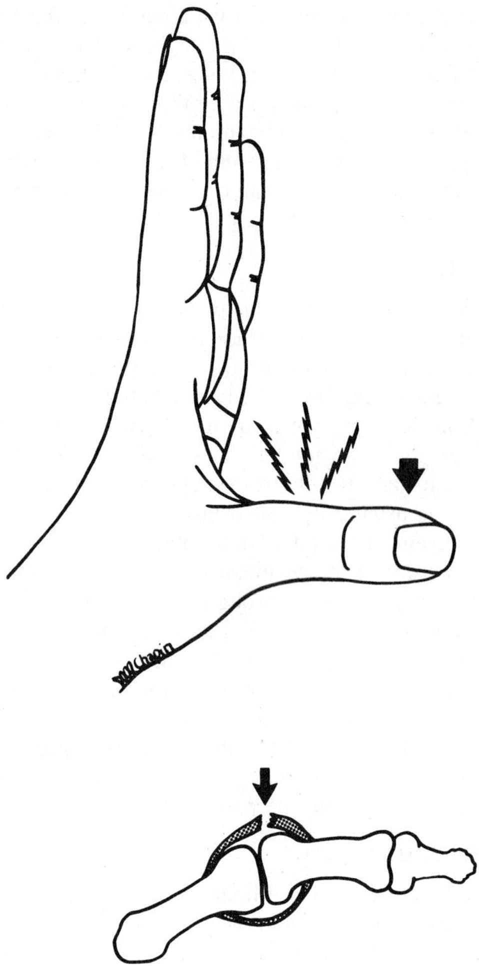

Fig. 126-15. Injury to ulnar collateral ligament at metacarpophalangeal joint of thumb.

disruption of the ulnar collateral ligament requires surgical repair of the ligament.

Mallet Finger

Mallet finger is a flexion deformity of the fingertip at the DIP joint secondary to avulsion of the extensor tendon from its insertion on the dorsal surface of the distal phalanx (Fig. 126-16). The patient presents with absent or incomplete active extension at the DIP joint. The mechanism of injury is often direct trauma to the fingertip, resulting in an avulsion of the extensor tendon. Treatment of a closed injury with a tendon avulsion or a tendon avulsion with a small fragment consists of splinting the DIP joint in the neutral position for 6 weeks and night splinting for an additional 2 or more weeks. When a larger fragment representing one third or more of the articular surface is present, or when a fragment is associated with volar subluxation of the terminal phalanx, open reduction and internal fixation are indicated. Radiographic assessment requires a true lateral view of the DIP joint.

Boutonnière Deformity

Boutonnière deformity is a flexion deformity of the finger at the PIP joint with hyperextension of the DIP joint (Fig. 126-17). This injury results from a rupture or laceration

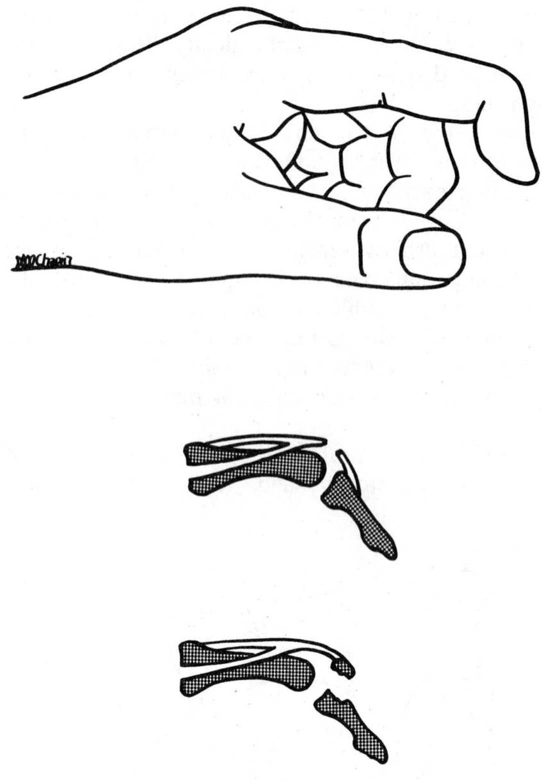

Fig. 126-16. Mallet finger.

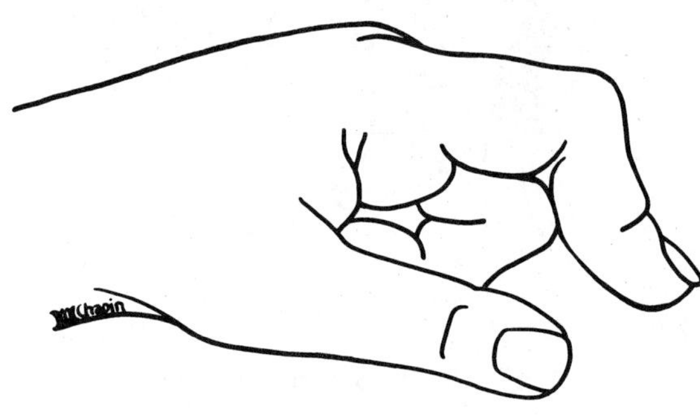

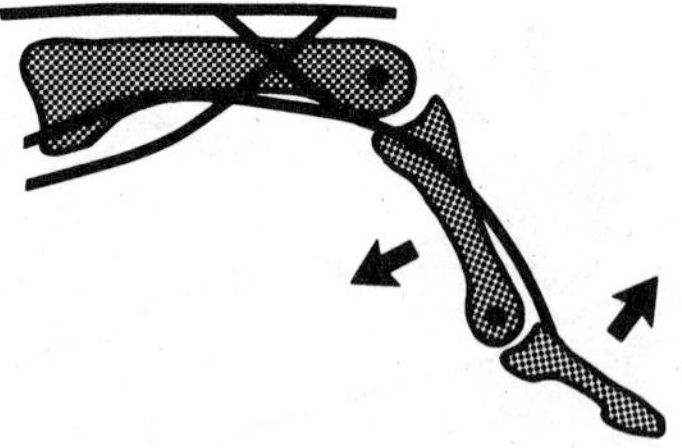

Fig. 126-17. Boutonnière deformity.

of the central slip of the extensor mechanism at or near its insertion into the base of the middle phalanx. The lateral bands of the extensor mechanism progressively dislocate in a volar direction from tearing or stretching of the transverse retinacular ligament, which normally maintains the position of the lateral bands dorsal to the axis of the PIP joint. As the

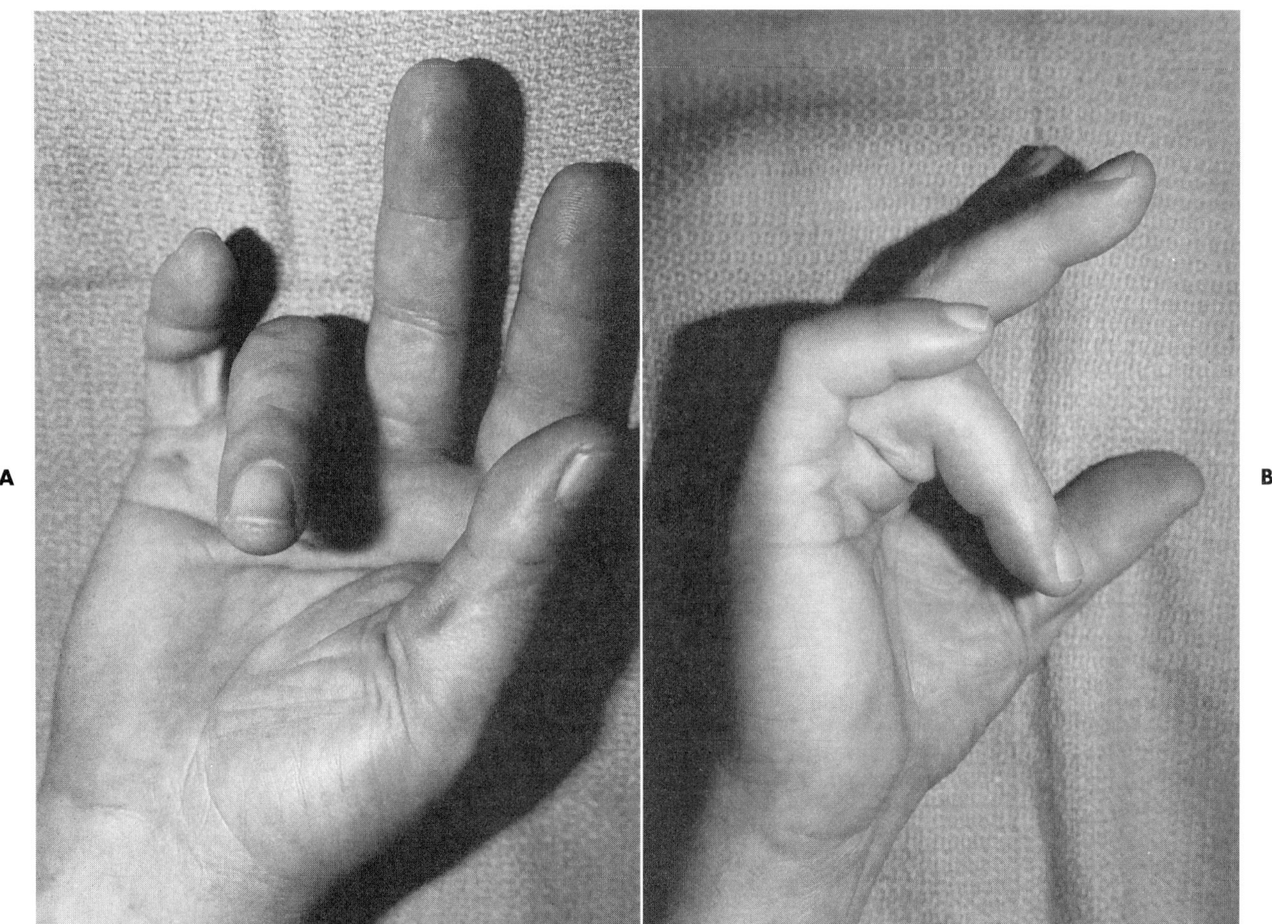

Fig. 126-18. Dupuytren's contracture, anteroposterior (**A**) and lateral (**B**) views.

lateral bands slip volar to the axis of the PIP joint, a flexion deformity of the PIP joint is created; shortening of the lateral bands results in a hyperextension deformity at the DIP joint. This deformity often is not present at the time of injury but develops slowly over weeks as the lateral bands drift progressively in a volar direction. If the injury is caused by an open wound, the central slip should be surgically repaired. The deformity is often seen late, and late closed injuries should be treated by splinting the PIP joint in extension and allowing active flexion at the DIP joint to stretch the shortened lateral bands. This injury requires a prolonged period of carefully supervised splinting.

Swan-neck Deformity

In a swan-neck deformity of the finger the PIP joint is in hyperextension and the DIP joint is in flexion. This condition can be caused by traumatic injury to the volar plate, a previous mallet finger deformity, rheumatoid arthritis, or intrinsic contraction.

Dupuytren's Contracture

Dupuytren's contracture results from a proliferative fibroplasia of the longitudinal band of the palmar aponeurosis that forms in nodules and cords (Fig. 126-18). The area involved is between the skin and the flexor tendon in the distal palm and fingers and can produce contractures at the metacarpal and PIP joints. The flexor tendons are not involved. The cause of this disorder is unknown, although heredity is a factor. The most common areas affected are the ring and little fingers, with occasional involvement of the thumb and long fingers. The condition may be associated with thickened knuckle pads over the PIP joint of the fingers and involvement of the plantar fascia. Surgical intervention is not recommended until definite flexion contracture develops at the metacarpal or PIP joints.

Trigger Finger and Thumb

Trigger finger and thumb may be congenital, occurring in infancy, but usually develops in adulthood from a nonspecific tenosynovitis of the flexor tendon sheath. The inflammation at the level of the proximal pulley of the flexor sheath produces a stenosis of the sheath, termed *stenosing tenosynovitis.* This causes telescoping of the fibers of the flexor tendon and results in a discrepancy between the size of the tendon and the opening at the level of the proximal pulley. The patient presents with a locking or snapping of the finger or thumb, with point tenderness and a nodule over the base of the flexor sheath near the MCP joint. The finger may be locked in the flexed or extended position. If the condition is chronic, referral for steroid injection or surgical treatment is often required.

Bowler's Thumb

Bowler's thumb is an injury to the ulnar proper digital nerve of the thumb at the level of the MCP joint secondary to repetitive trauma while grasping a bowling ball or heavy tools. Repetitive trauma can lead to perineural fibrosis. The patient presents with a tender mass on the ulnar aspect of the thumb just distal to the metacarpal joint, which usually represents a swelling of the nerve, with decreased sensation on the ulnar tip of the thumb. With early presentation, avoidance of the repetitive trauma usually allows the condition to resolve.

De Quervain's Stenosing Tenosynovitis

De Quervain's stenosing tenosynovitis is a nonspecific inflammatory condition involving the abductor and extensor pollicis tendons at the level of the first dorsal compartment. The condition usually affects women 30 to 50 years of age, who present with pain and tenderness, with palpable thickening in the first dorsal area. Finkelstein's test may be positive (Fig. 126-19). De Quervain's tenosynovitis must be differentiated from a bony pathologic condition of the distal radius or carpus and from carpal metacarpal joint degenerative arthritis. Recommended early treatment consists of splint immobilization and antiinflammatory medications. Chronic conditions may require referral for steroid injection or surgical intervention.

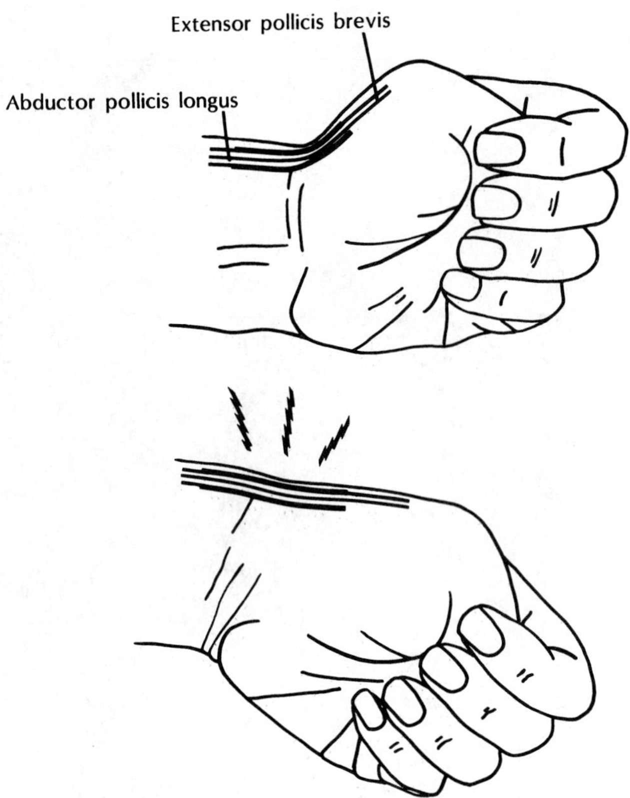

Fig. 126-19. Positive Finkelstein's test in de Quervain's stenosing synovitis. Ulnar flexion of wrist produces pain over dorsal compartment containing extensor pollicis brevis and abductor pollicis longus tendons.

Carpal Tunnel Syndrome

Carpal tunnel syndrome is a median nerve compressive neuropathy that occurs at the level of the wrist where the median nerve passes deep to the transverse carpal ligament. The condition usually affects women 30 to 60 years of age. The patient complains of numbness in the median nerve distribution, which may be exacerbated at night and is associated with some pain on the volar aspect of the forearm. The patient also may note tingling in the thumb, index, and long fingers and may tend to drop small objects. The condition usually involves the dominant hand but can be bilateral. Carpal tunnel syndrome may be associated with trauma (e.g., Colles' fracture), repetitive activity, edema secondary to trauma or infection, space-occupying lesions (e.g., lymphoma, ganglion), or systemic medical conditions (e.g., diabetes mellitus, thyroid dysfunction, amyloidosis, pregnancy). Often the cause is nonspecific but accompanies inflammatory conditions and rheumatoid tenosynovitis.

On examination the patient may have slight atrophic changes of the fingertips in the median distribution and atrophy of the thenar muscles, particularly the abductor pollicis brevis. Sensory testing may indicate abnormal two-point discrimination. Tinel's sign, the production of paresthesias in the hand by tapping over the median nerve at the level of the wrist or carpal tunnel, is often present with carpal tunnel syndrome (Fig. 126-20). When a degree of compressive neuropathy exists, Phalen's test, flexing of the wrist for 1 minute, causes increased paresthesias in the median nerve distribution resulting from increased pressure within the carpal tunnel. Symptoms may improve with a volar carpal splint and antiinflammatory medications. Otherwise the patient should be referred for consideration of steroid injection of the carpal tunnel or surgical release.

Arthritis

The major forms of arthritis that affect the hand are osteoarthritis and rheumatoid arthritis (see Chapters 132 to 134). Osteoarthritis involves the IP joints and the carpometacarpal joint of the thumb and often presents with swelling, stiffness, pain, and deformity. At the DIP joints, osteophytes may be associated with mucous cyst formation dorsally over the joint or in the eponychium. Rheumatoid arthritis affects the MCP and PIP joints and presents with pain, swelling, and stiffness. The condition may progress to deformity.

Tumors

Ganglions. Ganglions are the most common soft tissue tumor of the hand. These cystic masses arise from the tendon sheath or joint and may be related to acute trauma or recurrent chronic injury. The most common location is on the dorsum of the wrist over the radiocarpal joint in the area of the scapholunate ligament. Other locations include the volar surface of the wrist near the flexor carpi radialis tendon and the flexor sheaths of the fingers. Ganglions may present as an asymptomatic mass or may be associated with aching, pain, and weakness. They may disappear spontaneously. Persistent symptomatic ganglions may be referred for aspiration or removed completely through surgical intervention.

Lipomas. Unusual soft tissue tumors of the hand, lipomas present as a soft, asymptomatic mass. They may be deceptively large, extending deep beneath the fascia of the hand.

Giant Cell Tumors of Tendon Sheath. The second most common tumor in the hand, giant cell tumors of tendon sheath can occur at any age and are more common in women. They usually present as a painless, slow-growing mass on the volar or dorsal aspect of the finger. Giant cell tumors have

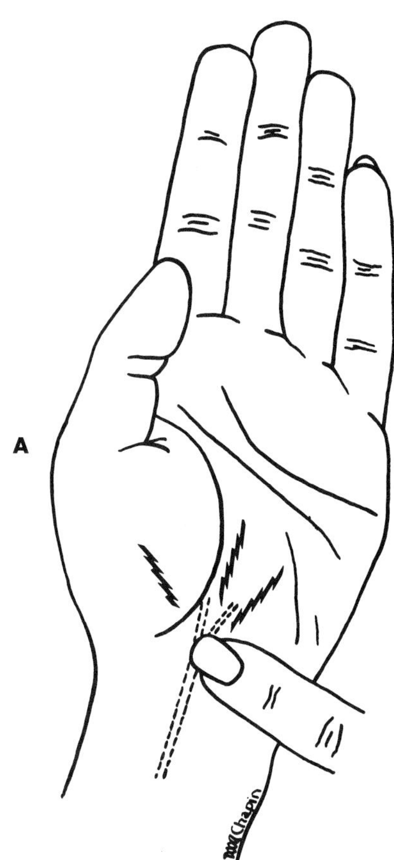

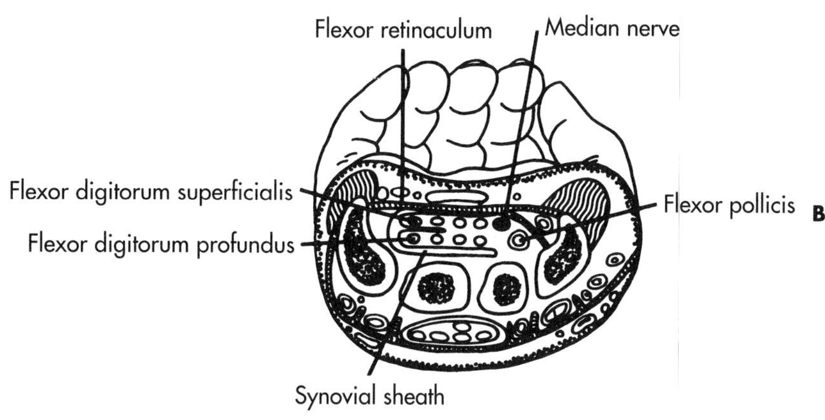

Fig. 126-20. **A,** Tinel's sign in carpal tunnel syndrome. **B,** Cross-sectional anatomy of wrist. Tendons and median nerve may be compressed by inflammation or infection because they are encompassed by synovial sheath and flexor retinaculum.

been associated with repetitive trauma. These benign lesions may enter joint spaces and create extrinsic pressure defects on the bone. They should be distinguished from giant cell tumors of the bone, which are malignant lesions.

Inclusion Cysts. Inclusion cysts of the digits result from penetrating trauma with implantation of epidermal elements beneath the skin. These painless cystic masses usually occur in the palm or on the volar aspect of the finger.

Glomus Tumor. An abnormal growth from an arteriovenous anastomosis normally present in the digits, glomus tumor usually occurs in the nail beds and fingertips. Patients often complain of severe pain exacerbated by exposure to cold. Alteration in color of the nail bed may be associated with point tenderness over the area of the lesion. The lesion is often less than 1 cm in diameter. If large enough, glomus tumor may erode the bone of the terminal phalanx, as demonstrated radiographically.

Bone Tumors. Usually benign, bone tumors are most often an *enchondroma,* or cartilaginous growth. They may present with posttraumatic pain and a pathologic fracture or may be discovered as an incidental finding on x-ray examination.

Infections

Infections can result in significant morbidity and functional loss; they are usually caused by a minor injury such as an abrasion. A significant infection can result in edema, tissue necrosis, and fibrosis and contracture. Antibiotics have significantly decreased the rate of mortality from hand infections but have not eliminated the need for incision and drainage. The timing and technique of surgical drainage are important in minimizing the degree of morbidity with infections.

The majority of hand infections are caused by coagulase-positive *Staphylococcus aureus* and *Streptococcus.* Infections caused by staphylococci often require incision and drainage. Streptococcal infections usually present as cellulitis with lymphangitis and lymphadenopathy. Human bite infections, common in the hand, often present with an injury over the MCP joint and sometimes with septic arthritis. The onset of symptoms resulting from the injury is rapid; classic signs of joint involvement include pain on passive range of motion at the MCP joint and point tenderness over the joint's volar aspect. The pathogenic organisms include anaerobic mouth organisms in addition to *S. aureus* and *Streptococcus.* An injury suggestive of a human bite infection with involvement of the MCP joint requires surgical exploration. In certain anatomic spaces the organisms may develop a localized abscess, requiring surgical incision and drainage.

Paronychia. An infection of the soft tissue around the fingernail, paronychia usually begins as a hangnail (Fig. 126-21). The most common organism is *S. aureus,* with the portal of entry being the eponychium. Paronychia may involve one corner of the nail or extend to the opposite side under the eponychium or fingernail. The patient presents with pain, erythema, and tenderness in the area of the eponychium or paronychium. Incision and drainage are indicated when a localized purulent collection is present. This may require

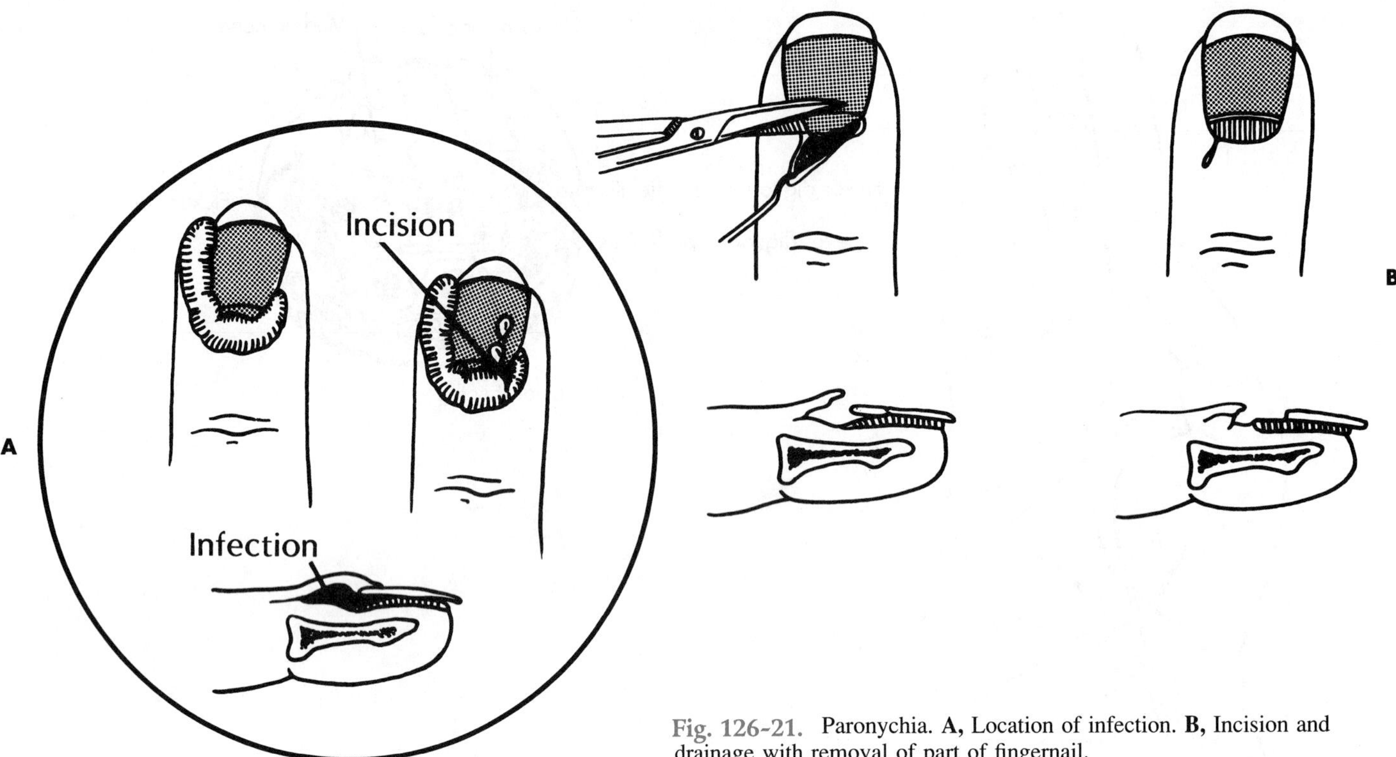

Fig. 126-21. Paronychia. **A,** Location of infection. **B,** Incision and drainage with removal of part of fingernail.

removing a portion of the nail to obtain adequate drainage. Chronic recurrent paronychia should suggest a fungal infection.

Herpetic Whitlow. Herpes infection can involve the fingertip (herpetic whitlow) and may resemble a bacterial paronychia. The distinction is important because incision does not help and may delay healing. Herpetic whitlow is a viral infection, and medical and dental personnel are at particular risk. Usual symptoms include pain or pruritus followed by the formation of vesicles, which may coalesce. The pain may become intense and is occasionally accompanied by bacterial infection. Healing usually takes 2 to 3 weeks. Therapy includes analgesia, saline soaks, and local wound care.

Felon. A felon is a digital pulp space abscess (Fig. 126-22). It usually causes significant throbbing pain, which develops over 48 to 72 hours. The fingertip is extensively involved and may become necrotic from ischemia. Interference with the blood supply to the diaphysis of the terminal phalanx may also result in aseptic necrosis. The bone can become secondarily infected, and osteomyelitis may develop. Treatment consists of incision and drainage after adequate anesthesia. In making the incision, the physician must avoid the digital nerves and not create painful scars on the contact points of the digit's volar pad.

Deep Space Infections. The deep palmar space lies between the fascia covering the metacarpals and the fascia below the flexor tendon sheaths on the volar aspect of the palm (Fig. 126-23). This space is divided into the thenar and midpalmar spaces by a septum that passes from the fascia beneath the index flexor sheath dorsally to the third metacarpal shaft. The adductor muscle of the thumb rises from the entire length of the third metacarpal bone and inserts in the thumb in the area of the MCP joint. This muscle divides the thenar space into anterior and posterior divisions. Both deep space infections cause systemic signs as well as local pain, tenderness, and decreased active range of motion of the fingers. A thenar space abscess causes tenderness over the thenar half of the palm and marked swelling of the thumb-index web space, which requires drainage. A midpalmar space abscess causes tenderness and swelling over the palm on the ulnar aspect with decreased range of motion of the middle, ring, and little fingers (Fig. 126-24). This space is drained through a transverse incision at the level of the distal palmar crease.

Tenosynovitis. Acute or purulent tenosynovitis is an infection of the flexor sheath that usually results from a penetrating wound over a flexor crease of the finger or palm. The patient usually presents with rapidly developing signs of infection (Fig. 126-25). The four signs of flexor sheath infection are uniform swelling of the digit, slight flexion of the involved finger, tenderness over the length of the involved flexor tendon sheath, and increased pain on passive extension of the finger. The patient cannot actively flex the finger and experiences pain in the attempt.

Acute purulent tenosynovitis is a closed-space infection and often requires incision and drainage. The flexor sheath of the thumb extends from the tip of the thumb proximally through the carpal canal into the radial bursa on the distal forearm. The flexor sheath of the little finger extends from the tip of the little finger throughout the carpal canal into the ulnar bursa on the distal forearm. The flexor sheaths on the index, long, and ring fingers extend to the level of the proximal palmar crease (see Fig. 126-23). Surgical drainage

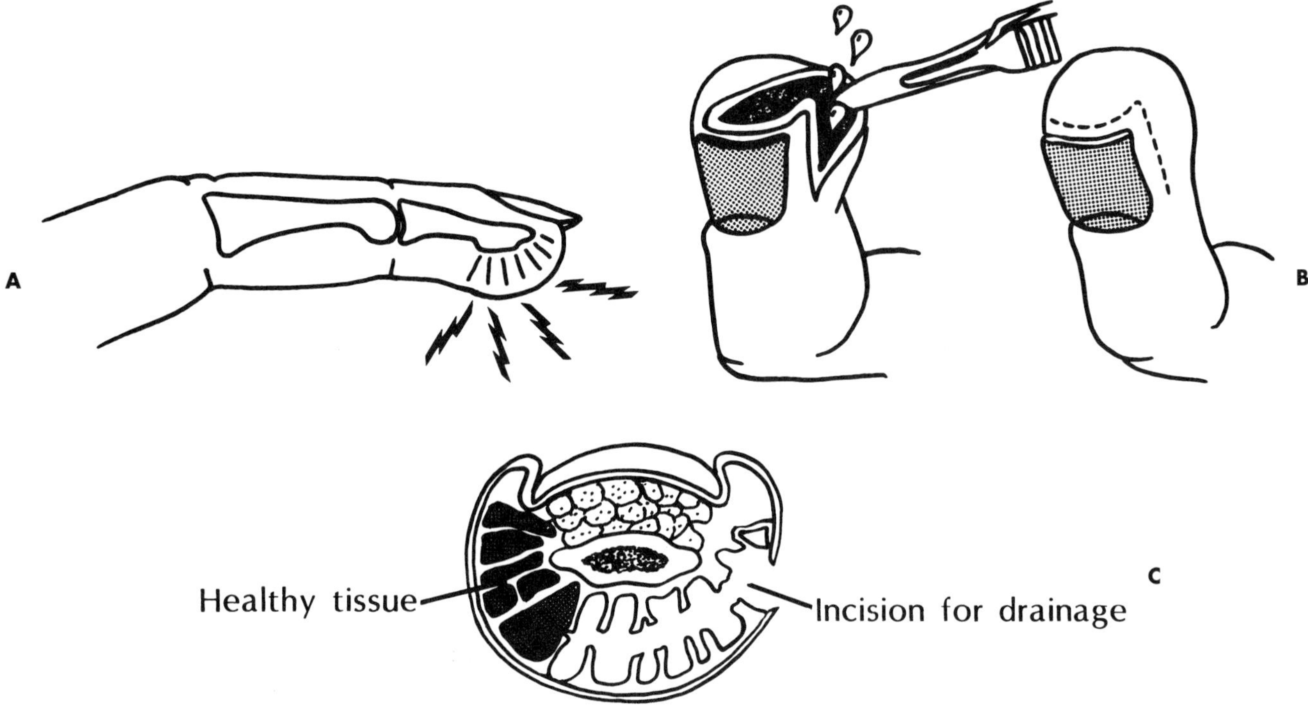

Fig. 126-22. **A,** Felon. **B,** Complete drainage of infected tissue. **C,** Incision must be made into each infected portion of the pulp space.

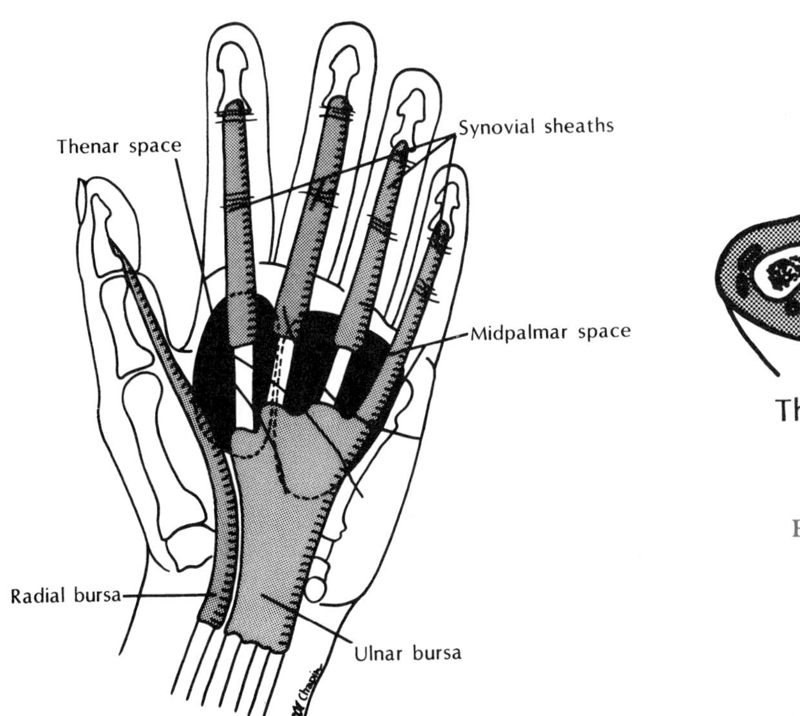

Fig. 126-23. Normal bursal anatomy.

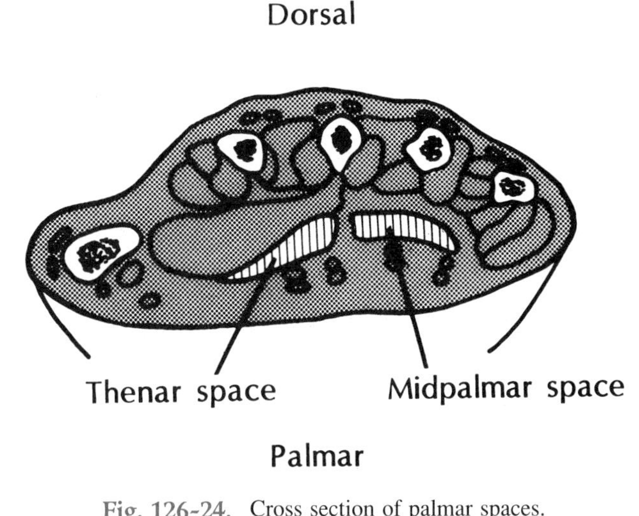

Fig. 126-24. Cross section of palmar spaces.

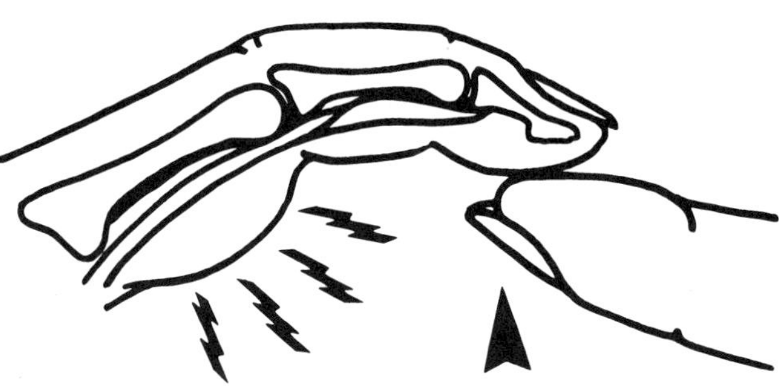

Fig. 126-25. Cardinal points of tenosynovitis as emphasized by Kanavel.

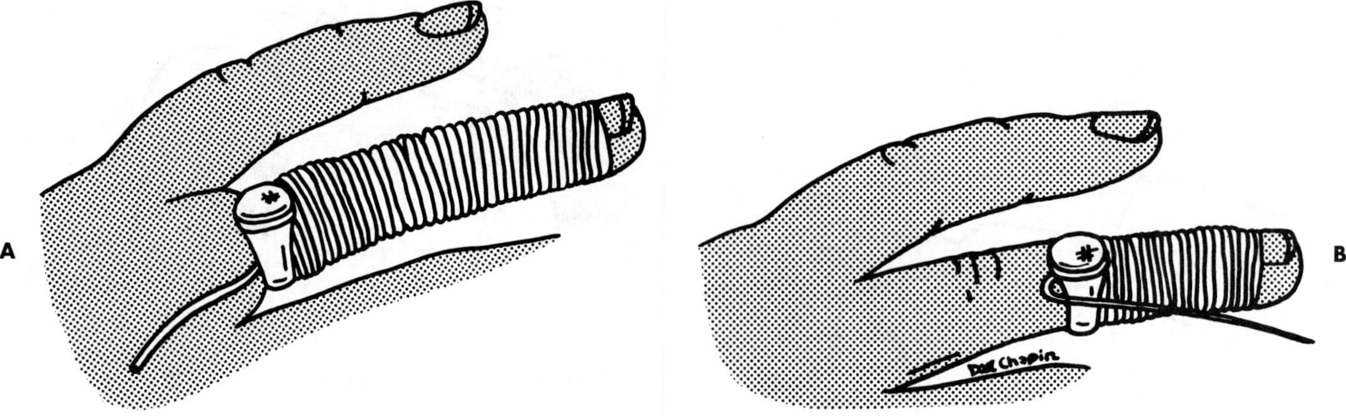

Fig. 126-26. Technique for removing ring from swollen finger. **A,** Wrap string snugly about finger and insert proximal end under ring. **B,** Unwind string slowly from proximal end.

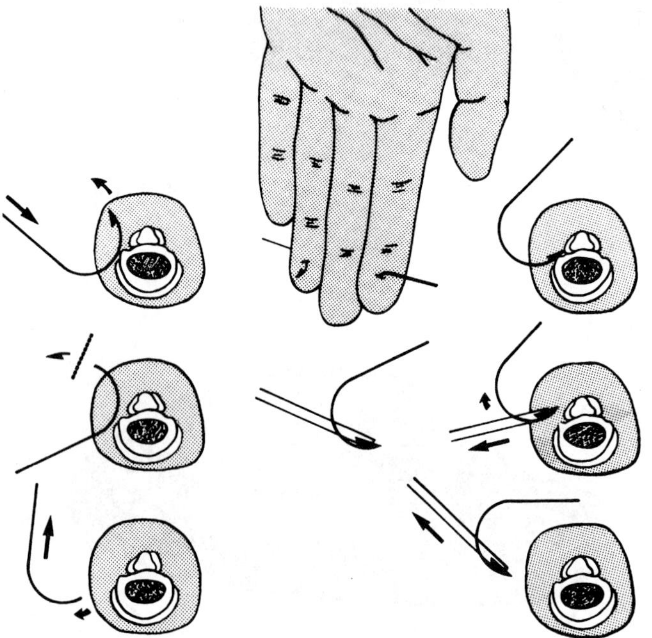

Fig. 126-27. Technique for removing fishhooks embedded in tissue by either snapping off barb or using bevel of a needle to minimize further injury.

usually requires an incision in the palm and in the affected digit and, in the case of the thumb and little finger, possibly at the level of the distal forearm.

Interventions. The general principles for treatment of hand infections are immobilization; incision and drainage when indicated; elevation of the infected part; systemic antibiotics; placement of the wrist, hand, and fingers in the position of function; and treatment of systemic diseases that can be exacerbated by the infection. Surgical intervention for closed-space infections of the hand should be carried out in a bloodless field under adequate anesthesia. Significant infection with associated edema may result in fibrosis and contracture of the affected area despite long-term therapy.

The removal of rings from a swollen finger is important. Rings usually can be removed with a soapy solution. Other techniques include using a ring cutter or the spiral string technique (Fig. 126-26).

Removing fishhooks can be accomplished after adequate anesthesia by either pushing the tip through and cutting it off or trying to pass the bevel of a needle over the barb and removing the needle in a retrograde manner (Fig. 126-27).

ADDITIONAL READINGS

American Society for Surgery of the Hand: *The hand: examination and diagnosis,* New York, 1990, Churchill Livingstone.

American Society for Surgery of the Hand: *The hand: primary care of common problems,* New York, 1990, Churchill Livingstone.

American Society for Surgery of the Hand: *Hand surgery update,* Rosemont, Ill, 1996, American Academy of Orthopaedic Surgeons.

Green DP: *Green's operative hand surgery,* ed 4, New York, 1999, Churchill Livingstone.

Jupiter JB: *Flynn's hand surgery,* Baltimore, 1991, Williams & Wilkins.

Lucas GL: *Examination of the hand,* Springfield, Ill, 1972, Thomas.

Milford L: *The hand,* St Louis, 1982, Mosby.

Zenz C: *Occupational medicine,* St Louis, 1994, Mosby.

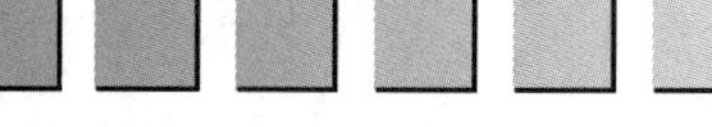

CHAPTER 127

Low Back Pain

James J. Heffernan

Low back pain is the most common musculoskeletal complaint among adult patients seen in primary care practice and second only to limb pain (generally related to injury) among patients seen in urgent care settings. Potential causes of low back pain are legion, but a specific pathoanatomic diagnosis is established in fewer than 20% of patients.

The back is a complex mechanical structure, a composite of vertebrae, intervertebral disks, and apophyseal joints stabilized by ligaments and the paraspinal and abdominal musculature. It supports the trunk and transmits, through the sacroiliac joints, upper body loads to the pelvis and lower extremities. The posterior vertebral elements encase and protect the spinal cord and cauda equina. Connections to the bulk of the body's peripheral nervous system run through the vertebral neural foramina. The spine and its supporting structures have extensive innervation. The posterior rami of the lumbosacral spinal nerves supply the apophyseal joints, the interspinous ligament, the paravertebral muscles, and associated cutaneous areas; at each vertebral level, the sinuvertebral nerve, joined by a sympathetic branch, innervates the anterior dura mater and dural sleeve, the posterior vertebral periosteum, the posterior longitudinal ligament, epidural blood vessels, and the anulus fibrosus.

Most episodes of low back pain arise from regional (i.e., nonsystemic) processes, a result of mechanical derangements to the complex anatomic relationships within and around the spine. Approximately 1% of patients with acute low back pain have *sciatica,* defined as pain in the distribution of a lumbar or sacral nerve root, with or without associated neurosensory and motor deficits. The presence of sciatica increases the likelihood that a herniated intervertebral disk is the cause of back pain. Systemic causes and the more serious local pathologic processes generally present with specific clinical features.

EPIDEMIOLOGY

Low back pain is extremely common, producing at least short-term impairment in 70% to 80% of a general population. The point prevalence of low back pain is 5% to 7% among adults. Nearly 2% of adults lose time from work annually as a result of low back pain, and 2% to 5% consult a physician for treatment. This ailment takes its toll in the productive years, with most patients between ages 30 and 60. Although most cases resolve in a relatively short period, 14% of adults report at least one episode lasting longer than 2 weeks, and 1.6% have features of sciatica.

Among chronic conditions, back and spine impairment is the leading cause of disability in persons under age 45 and ranks third behind heart disease and arthritis in the 45 to 64 age range.[5] It is the second most common complaint of pain for which treatment by a physician is sought. The annual cost of direct medical care for low back pain has been estimated at $13 to $16 billion, and the total annual societal costs in the United States are estimated at $20 to $50 billion.[12]

Men and women are comparably affected, but the incidence is somewhat higher for women in occupations requiring heavy exertion. Women also report low back symptoms more often after age 60, whereas men more frequently present with low back pain in their younger adult years. Most studies have demonstrated a precipitating event in a minority of cases (6% to 28%). The natural history of low back problems is one of recurrence, reported variably in 33% to 60% of patients with occupational low back pain during the ensuing 1 to 3 years. Symptoms tend to be mild and transient in young workers but more persistent and severe with increased age. Incidence rates are similar among heavy, light, and sedentary workers, although a higher proportion of heavy workers are incapacitated with low back pain. Those bored or dissatisfied with their occupations are more likely to report low back problems. In a given work setting, low back pain appears more frequently in those who consider their work to be physically demanding. Specific risk factors include occupations that require repetitive lifting in a forward bent-and-twisted position, exposure to vibrations caused by vehicles or heavy machinery, and cigarette smoking. Low back pain is common in persons who either sit or stand for prolonged periods; however, jobs requiring sudden maximal efforts are also associated with higher incidence rates.

No convincing evidence shows that patients with moderate kyphosis, scoliosis, or lordosis are more at risk for low back pain than those with normal spine curvature. Likewise, moderate differences in body habitus do not predict differences in incidence rates, although massive obesity and major skeletal abnormalities are associated with increased rates of low back pain. Isthmic spondylolisthesis, spinal osteochondrosis, and the spinal stenosis associated with achondroplasia appear to predispose affected patients to low back problems. Recreational activities have not been associated convincingly with low back pain syndromes, although isthmic spondylolisthesis is reportedly increased fourfold among gymnasts and interior linemen on football teams.

Attempts to characterize the low back pain patient psychologically have produced a variety of profiles. Although most studies have been performed retrospectively on patients in treatment programs, patients with low back pain have demonstrated greater levels of psychopathology than extremity-injured peers or noninjured industrial workers. A tendency toward neurotic depression rather than hysteria has been described, although other data support increased rates of hysteria and hypochondriasis along with anxiety and depression. Increased rates of alcoholism and divorce have also been noted among individuals disabled by low back pain.

PATHOPHYSIOLOGY

The potential causes of low back pain are myriad (Box 127-1). Systemic illness, regional cancer, and local infection account for only a trivial percentage of total cases. Most low back pain arises from uncharacterized regional processes. Although many putative causes have been identified by invasive studies and postmortem examinations, the specific anatomic cause of backache in a given patient most often goes unidentified (Figs. 127-1 and 127-2).

The herniated vertebral disk is probably the best known cause of low back pain (Fig. 127-3). Disk herniations tend to occur in a lateral or central posterior direction. Posterior prolapse of a herniated vertebral disk accounts for only a small subset of cases, however, and generally manifests through the classic neural impingement syndrome of sciatica. Herniation of the nucleus pulposus occurs in 95% to 98% of cases at the disk between the fourth and fifth lumbar vertebrae (L4-5) or between the fifth lumbar vertebra and sacrum (L5-S1), with herniation at two levels in 10% of cases. Older individuals have an increased risk of disk herniation at higher lumbar disk levels. Other causes of sciatica include spinal stenosis, synovial cysts, congenital anomalies of lumbar nerve roots, primary neural and osseous tumors, metastatic cancer, and epidural abscesses. Retroperitoneal neoplastic processes and endometriosis may cause sciatica by involvement of the lumbosacral plexus. Sciatica from local pressure to the sciatic nerve may result from toilet seats, especially in thin individuals, or from habitual placement of a wallet in a back pocket.

With aging the intervertebral disk degenerates, and much low back pain is probably related to small tears in the anulus fibrosus, compression of end plate cartilage, and microfractures of subchondral bone in the end plates; these processes cannot be demonstrated acutely. As these processes continue

Box 127-1. Causes of Low Back Pain

Primary Mechanical Derangements (Generally Putative)

Ligamentous strain
Muscle strain/spasm
Facet joint disruption/degeneration
Intervertebral disk degeneration/herniation
Vertebral compression fracture
Vertebral end plate microfractures
Spondylolisthesis
Spinal stenosis
Diffuse idiopathic skeletal hyperostosis
Severe scoliosis or kyphoscoliosis
Scheuermann's disease (vertebral epiphyseal aseptic necrosis)

Infection

Epidural abscess
Vertebral osteomyelitis
Septic diskitis
Pott's disease (tuberculosis)
Nonspecific manifestation of systemic illness
  Bacterial endocarditis
  Influenza

Neoplasia

Epidural/vertebral carcinomatous metastases
Multiple myeloma, lymphoma
Primary epidural or intradural tumors

Metabolic Disease

Osteoporosis
Osteomalacia
Hemochromatosis
Ochronosis

Inflammatory Rheumatologic Disorders

Ankylosing spondylitis
Reactive spondyloarthropathies (including Reiter's syndrome)
Psoriatic arthropathy
Polymyalgia rheumatica

Referred Pain

Abdominal or retroperitoneal visceral process
Retroperitoneal vascular process
Retroperitoneal malignancy
Herpes zoster

Other Causes

Paget's disease of bone
Primary fibromyalgia
Psychogenic pain
Malingering

over time, however, subtle anatomic derangements are integrated, and spondylosis develops, manifested radiographically in thinning of the intervertebral disk with narrowing of neural foramina and bony spurring and lipping, especially at the disk margins. *Spondylolisthesis* refers to slippage of one vertebra over another, usually at the L5-S1 level. Studies using fluoroscopically directed injections of hypertonic saline and anesthetic agents with or without corticosteroids have reproduced and relieved low back pain, respectively, in a variety of patients. Injection sites have included the facet joints, ligamentum flavum, interspinous and supraspinous ligaments, intradiskal space, and epidural space. Derangement of posterior structures may therefore cause or contribute to low back pain in a given patient.

Spinal stenosis resulting from bony encroachment by osteoarthritis, generally superimposed on congenital narrowing of the lumbar spinal canal, can result in lumbosacral radiculopathy and neural claudication (or pseudoclaudication) with pain on ambulation or standing, relieved by sitting. The pain of spinal stenosis probably represents reversible cord or root ischemia.

Muscle pain and spasm are common features in low back pain, but a primary role for muscle strain remains uncertain. Axial myalgias associated with polymyalgia rheumatica and the low back pain and tender points associated with idiopathic fibromyalgia (fibrositis) are relatively common syndromes that cause low back pain nonskeletally. An inflammatory spondyloarthropathy may affect up to 2% of the population and most often presents as low back pain and stiffness, especially in the morning after sleep. Diffuse idiopathic skeletal hyperostosis, noted predominantly in middle-aged and elderly men, may be dominated by complaints of low back pain and stiffness.

The systemic process of osteoporosis is a major public health problem (see Chapter 45). This condition can produce back pain by the mechanism of vertebral collapse, though more often in the thoracic spine. Chronic, poorly localized back pain associated with osteoporosis in the absence of overt vertebral collapse probably results from multiple microfractures near vertebral end plates and can be a debilitating condition among the elderly population.

The spectrum of causes of back pain differs above and below the lumbosacral area. The thoracic spine is the region most often affected by vertebral compression fractures resulting from osteoporosis; the lower thoracic and upper lumbar vertebrae are the most common sites of bony metastatic disease. Middle and upper back pain may result from axial loading of the spine, as in football or jumping injuries, or after strenuous upper extremity trauma, as in the vertebral spinous process avulsion fractures or "clay shoveler's back," a condition noted among manual laborers in whom shear forces are transmitted to the spine from abrupt unloading of upper extremity loads. Sacral fractures, a form of traumatic spondylolisthesis, may result from direct trauma to a flexed hip and extended leg. Coccygeal fracture may likewise result from direct trauma, usually a fall, and rarely from difficult childbirth. Pelvic malignancies may involve coccyx or sacrum by direct extension and lymphatic or hematogenous spread.

The clinical course of low back pain associated with systemic illness is that of the underlying disease. Excluding such patients from consideration, as well as those few with local infections and neoplastic processes whose prognosis depends on the specific cause and available treatment, the physician is left with the core of typical patients with low back pain. Among this group the natural course is remission and recurrence. Acute low back pain is generally a self-limited disease, with remission rates of 40% after 1 week, 50% to 85% in 3 weeks, and 90% in 2 months. Even

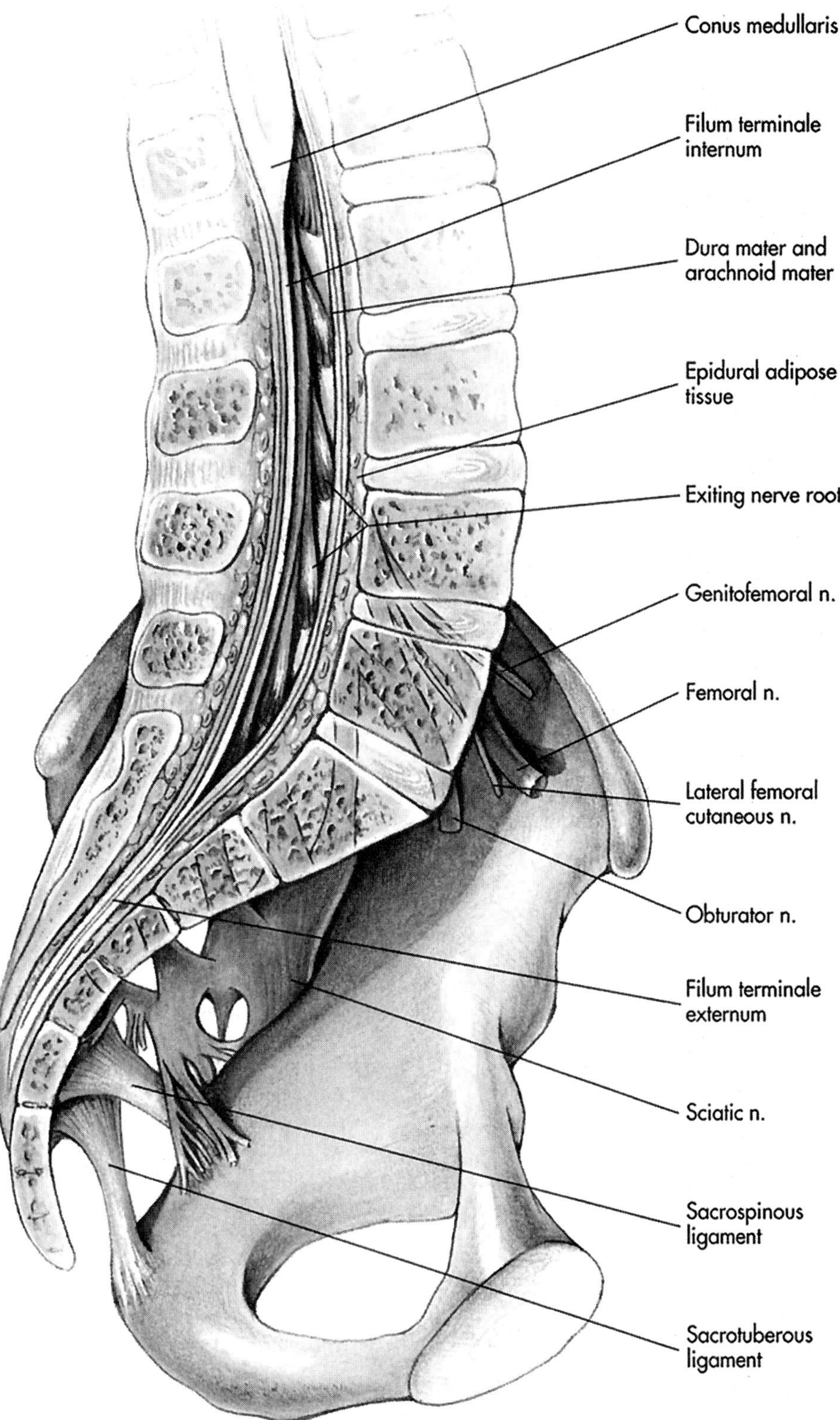

Fig. 127-1. Anatomy of the lumbosacral spine, lateral view. *n.*, Nerve. (From Cramer GD, Darby SA, editors: *Basic and clinical anatomy of the spine, spinal cord, and ANS,* St Louis, 1995, Mosby.)

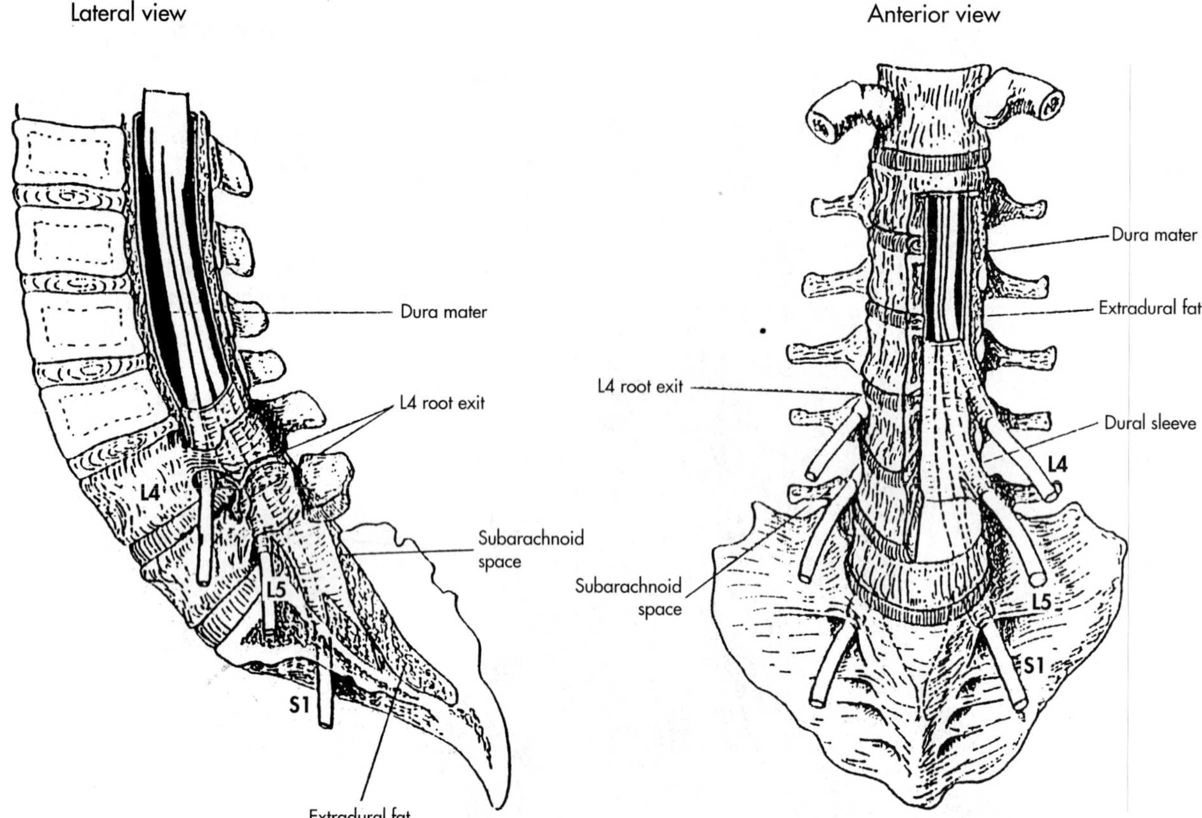

Fig. 127-2. Relationships of lumbar nerve roots to vertebrae and disk.

when low back pain is considered a work-related compensable injury, 85% to 90% of patients return to work within 12 weeks. Among patients who have sought medical attention for low back pain, recurrences are noted in 90% and are generally longer lasting than the initial attack.

PATIENT EVALUATION

Although a firm anatomic diagnosis is seldom made, the history and physical examination are generally discriminating enough to focus attention on the more serious causes of low back pain.

History

Severe backache after serious trauma suggests a fracture or acute disk herniation. Pain after a pure flexion injury suggests a pathologic condition of the disk or end plate, whereas pain after a torsional injury is more often associated with disruption of posterior structures (e.g., facet joint) and ligamentous injury. With either injury, pain may radiate to the buttocks or upper thigh. The pain associated with an acutely herniated intervertebral disk is often sharp or lancinating with radiation down the back of a leg, often to the ankle or foot. The patient resists movement and generally finds relief in a fixed, somewhat awkward supine posture or in the lateral decubitus position with the leg of the affected side in partial flexion. Bilateral sciatica associated with bowel or bladder dysfunction (incontinence or retention) and weakness suggests a massive central disk herniation or another epidural (and rarely intradural) mass lesion, especially hemorrhage, abscess, or metastasis. A patient writhing in pain suggests a visceral or vascular source (e.g., rupturing abdominal aortic aneurysm, ureteral colic). Backache, associated with fever, especially when unremitting or progressive, may represent vertebral osteomyelitis, septic diskitis, epidural abscess, or Pott's disease. Other febrile processes associated with back pain include early herpes zoster, influenza, or the nonseptic musculoskeletal manifestations of bacterial endocarditis.

Morning back pain and stiffness persisting several months after an insidious onset in a younger man who derives relief from exercise indicate ankylosing spondylitis. Similar symptoms coupled with conjunctivitis, urethritis, skin rash, balanitis, and diarrheal illness suggest a reactive inflammatory arthropathy (e.g., Reiter's syndrome; see Chapter 137). Most patients with typical mechanical low back pain present with pain, often severe, and muscle stiffness involving the back, buttocks, and often the thigh. Pain typically arises hours or days after a new or unusual exertion and is generally relieved by assumption of the supine position. In the patient with chronic sciatica, pain is often confined to the buttocks and leg and is usually described as dull or aching and exacerbated by sitting. Low or middle back pain in an elderly patient may result from osteoporosis with or without overt compression fractures, from polymyalgia rheumatica, or from neoplasia. Dull, progressively worsening bone pain in an elderly patient, especially pain that worsens with recumbency, suggests metastatic carcinoma or multiple myeloma. Spinal stenosis may also present as pain in a recumbent or standing position, relieved by sitting. Diffuse, poorly

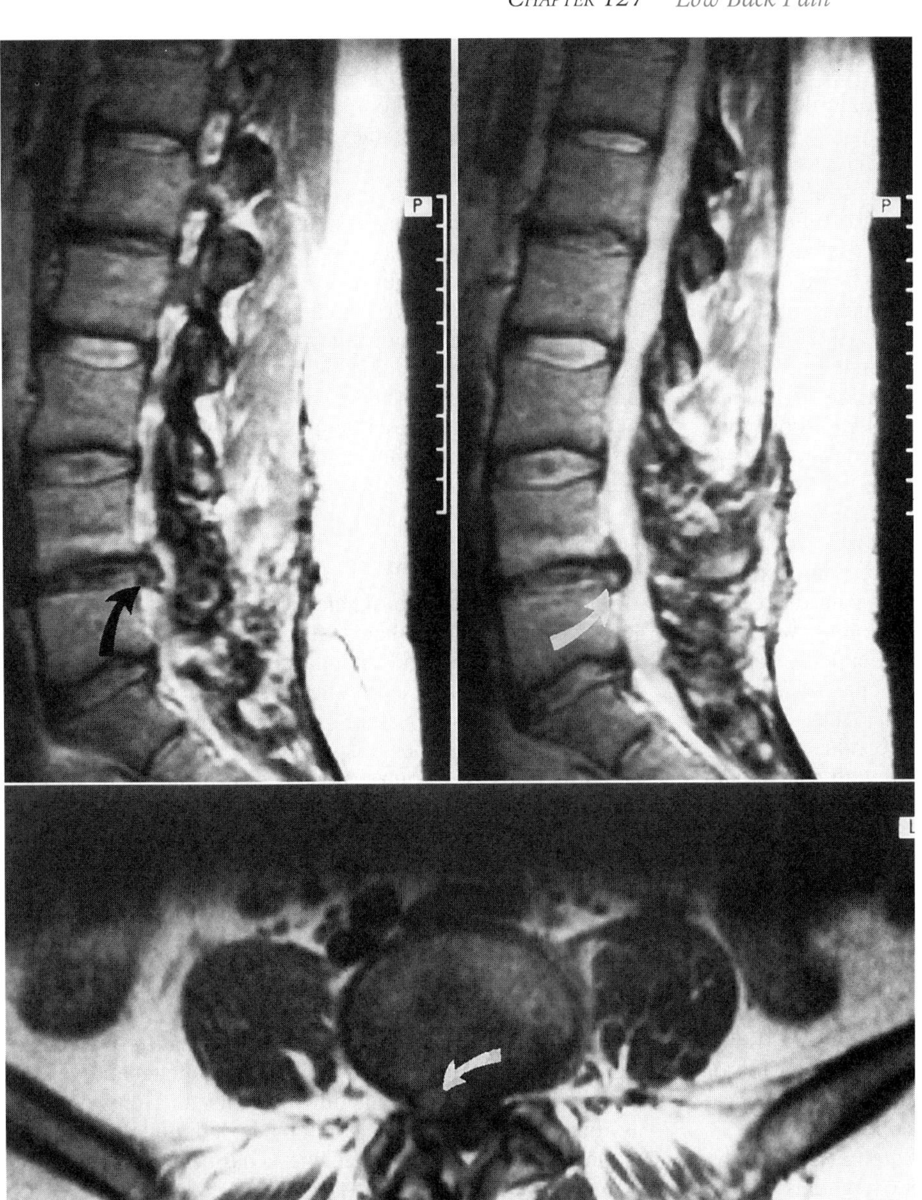

Fig. 127-3. Magnetic resonance images demonstrating right posterior herniated L4-5 disk.

localized back pain may be a manifestation of Paget's or Cushing's disease. Associated pelvic or abdominal disease may refer pain to the low or middle back.

Physical Examination

A systematic approach to examination of the back complements the history in focusing attention on the identifiable causes of low back pain. Inspection and palpation yield important initial clues. Severe idiopathic kyphoscoliosis is associated with degenerative arthritis; mild scoliosis or loss of lumbar lordosis is a common finding in the acute setting, the result of paravertebral spasm. Prominent dorsal kyphosis in an elderly patient suggests vertebral collapse as a result of osteoporosis or malignancy. Most patients with acute low back pain have restricted vertebral mobility. However, diminished chest expansion (less than 3 cm) in association with decreased mobility of the spine, especially when sacroiliac joint tenderness coexists, strongly suggests ankylosing spondylitis (see Chapter 137). Tenderness of the sciatic nerve in the sciatic notch suggests a component of radiculopathy or neuropathy.

A tender spinous process in the setting of fever and backache suggests vertebral osteomyelitis, septic diskitis, or an epidural abscess; a tender spinous process in the setting of malignancy and backache suggests vertebral or epidural metastatic disease. In both cases, aggressive emergency evaluation is indicated, especially if neurologic deficits are noted.

Simple maneuvers can provide further diagnostic clues. Induction of pain on torsion or hyperextension of the spine suggests ligamentous or facet joint injury, most often at the L4-5 level. Increased discomfort with spinal extension also suggests spinal stenosis. Reduction of lateral flexion is more suggestive of spondyloarthropathy than a herniated disk or other cause of mechanical low back pain.

The most useful simple maneuver in assessing nerve root impingement is the straight leg raising (SLR) test, which places the lower lumbosacral nerve roots under tension. With the patient supine the examiner slowly raises the straightened leg of the affected side through the arc of hip flexion. If pain occurs in a radicular distribution with straight leg elevation through an arc of 60 degrees or less, the test is positive. The probability that herniation is the cause of back pain increases as the angle necessary to produce radicular pain decreases, although there is little or no traction on nerve roots with arcs of less than 20 to 30 degrees. This test is moderately sensitive (80%) for herniated lumbosacral disks, but not specific (40%).[8] To exclude false-positive results, the examiner should attempt repeated trials, some conducted while distracting the patient. The angle associated with pain should be reproducible when the examiner passively flexes the patient's hip with the knee in flexion, then slowly extends the foreleg. An important supplement to the direct SLR is the crossed SLR, which entails elevation of the unaffected leg in the patient with sciatica. A positive test results when radicular pain is produced in the unraised leg. The crossed SLR is substantially less sensitive (25%) but strikingly more specific (90%) than the direct SLR.[8] A similar but less well-quantified provocative test for eliciting pain in the setting of L3-4 disk herniation involves forcing full or exaggerated extension of the hip of the affected side while the knee is flexed and the patient is prone or in the lateral decubitus position.

In most patients, deep tendon reflexes are not affected by mechanical low back pain. The ankle jerk (Achilles tendon reflex), however, is subserved by the S1 root and is often diminished or absent in the compression radiculopathy produced by L5-S1 disk herniation. The Achilles tendon reflex is frequently absent in normal, elderly individuals. No reflex deficits occur with L4-5 disk herniations. The infrequent occurrence of L3-4 disk herniation with L4 root compression is manifested as a diminished knee jerk (patella tendon reflex).

Motor deficits are often subtle but can usually be demonstrated in the setting of true sciatica. Compression radiculopathy of the S1 root by L5-S1 disk herniation is associated with weakness of plantar flexion, best demonstrated by having the patient walk on the toes. Dorsiflexion weakness is associated with L5 radiculopathy from L4-5 disk herniation, as demonstrated by the patient walking on the heels or dorsiflexing the great toe against resistance. Quadriceps weakness results from L4 radiculopathy associated with L3-4 disk herniation.

Sensory deficits with sciatica are also often subtle but demonstrable. Compression of the S1 root by L5-S1 disk herniation may result in sensory deficits of the posterior calf and lateral aspect of the foot. Compression of the L5 root by disk herniation at L4-5 manifests as hypesthesia on the dorsum of the foot and great toe, especially in the first web space. Hypesthesia over the lateral aspect of the thigh is consistent with L4 root compression from L4-5 disk herniation. Saddle anesthesia in the patient with bilateral sciatica and loss of anal sphincter tone suggests the cauda equina syndrome from massive central disk herniation or another space-occupying lesion and warrants further emergency evaluation.

Hallmarks of malingering or of a psychiatric origin for low back pain include overreaction; reproduction of back pain by "tests" that should not elicit such pain on physiologic grounds (e.g., axial loading by the application of downward pressure on the head of the standing patient); variable results of true provocative tests (e.g., SLR) when the patient is distracted; superficial, nonanatomic tenderness; and motor or sensory disturbances with nonphysiologic components.

DIAGNOSIS

Diagnostic Procedures

Blood tests are of little diagnostic use in most patients with low back pain. Leukocytosis, an elevated erythrocyte sedimentation rate, and anemia are nonspecific markers of possible infection, neoplastic disease, or inflammatory spondyloarthropathy. Serum or urine immunoelectrophoresis may corroborate the suspicion of multiple myeloma. Abnormalities of serum calcium, phosphate, and alkaline phosphatase are crude indices of metabolic bone disease. The diagnosis of spondyloarthropathy usually rests firmly on the history, physical examination, and radiographs of the spine and sacroiliac joints; HLA-B27 determination is corroborative.

Lumbosacral spine radiographs are abnormal in most persons over age 50 and often in younger persons. Radiographs are neither sufficiently sensitive nor sufficiently specific to justify routine use in evaluating backache, especially in the acute setting. Findings of degenerative disk disease, osteoarthritis, spina bifida occulta, and transitional or asymmetric vertebrae are common in individuals with and without back pain. Spondylolisthesis has been noted in 5% to 20% of spinal radiographs (Fig. 127-4).

Radiographs may be extremely helpful, however, if an inflammatory spondyloarthropathy or a destructive lesion associated with either malignancy or an infectious process is suspected. Anteroposterior and lateral views may also provide an overall view of the degree of osteoporosis and associated vertebral collapse. In major trauma, radiographic studies may demonstrate fractures and dislocations. Oblique views may better visualize the facet joint but rarely add to the evaluation process. Selective use of spinal radiographs based on specific criteria may increase the diagnostic yield threefold. Indications for spinal radiography in the patient with acute low back pain may include (1) age over 50, (2) history of serious trauma, (3) known cancer, (4) pain at rest, (5) unexplained weight loss, (6) drug or alcohol abuse, (7) treatment with corticosteroids, (8) temperature above 38° C, (9) suspicion of ankylosing spondylitis, and (10) demonstrable neuromotor deficit.[6] Spinal radiographs may also be appropriate for a patient with pain that persists beyond 3 to 4 weeks, even without neurologic findings.

Until the 1980s, contrast myelography was the procedure of choice when epidural compression by a tumor or infectious process was suspected or when neurologic deficits suggested intervertebral disk herniation, especially when a surgical

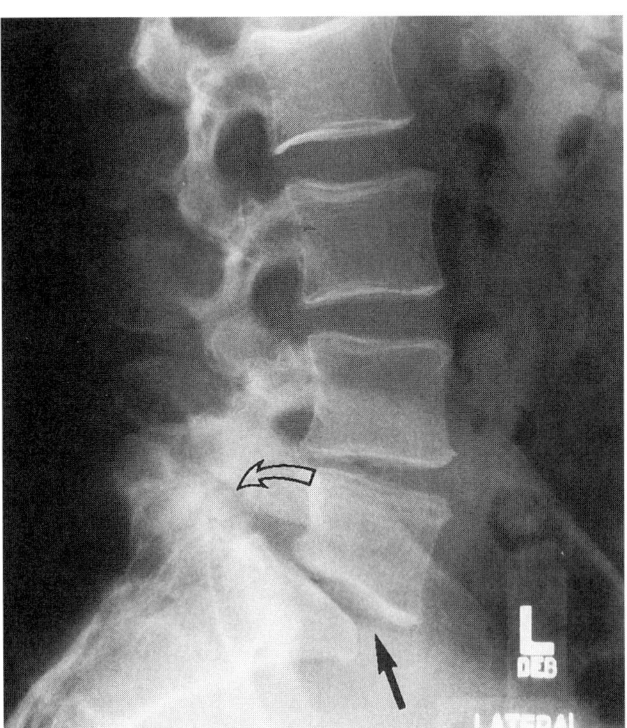

Fig. 127-4. Spondylolisthesis.

procedure was contemplated. The sensitivity of contrast myelography for herniated lumbar disk is 90% and the specificity 70% to 90%. Diskography demonstrates disk herniation reliably at a given level only, is somewhat less sensitive and specific than myelography, and is seldom necessary.

Computed tomography (CT) scans of the lumbosacral spine have better sensitivity and specificity than myelography for herniated intervertebral disks and may also reveal bony abnormalities, tumors, and vascular lesions. Unfortunately, CT scans of the lumbosacral spine demonstrate significant abnormalities in more than one quarter of asymptomatic persons. CT has often been employed in place of or in addition to myelography when evaluating patients with low back pain.

In studies comparing different diagnostic modalities, CT, magnetic resonance imaging (MRI), and CT with myelography have demonstrated comparable true-positive and true-negative rates for diagnosing lumbar disk herniation, and all are more accurate than traditional myelography.[3] MRI best differentiates between recurrent disk herniation and scar tissue and is recommended when imaging is indicated in the patient who has undergone previous surgery. As with CT, MRI identifies substantial abnormalities (e.g., disk herniation, spinal stenosis) in up to one third of patients with no prior low back pain[4]; disk bulging or degeneration at least one lumbar level is found in nearly all individuals over age 60 (see Fig. 127-3). Where available, MRI has generally become a standard in evaluating patients with suspected epidural abscess or malignancy.

Radionuclide bone scans are more sensitive than standard radiographs in identifying metastatic lesions (other than the plasmacytomas of multiple myeloma) and are also useful in characterizing the spondylolysis associated with isthmic spondylolisthesis. Nuclear medicine studies are sometimes helpful in identifying abscesses and osteomyelitis. When nerve root compression is suspected, electromyography may be confirmatory. "Therapeutic" facet joint injections are not beneficial, and injection studies to localize the source of low back pain are generally not indicated.

Differential Diagnosis

See Tables 127-1 and 127-2.

MANAGEMENT

An exhaustive evidence-based review of the management of acute low back pain culminating in a detailed clinical practice guideline was published by the Agency for Health Care Policy and Research (AHCPR) of the U.S. Public Health Service in December 1994.[3] Algorithms incorporating elements of assessment and treatment were promulgated, keying on the presence or absence of clinical "red flags" (Figs. 127-5 to 127-9 and Table 127-3).

Nonpharmacologic Therapy

The favorable short-term prognosis of most variants of low back pain supports a standard approach of conservative management for 4 weeks, even with suspected intervertebral disk herniation. The generally self-limited course of low back pain has made it difficult to interpret the success of interventions other than in prospective clinical trials. Invasive studies have shown reductions of intradiskal pressure with subjects in the supine position. Previous management recommendations, based to some extent on a study of military recruits, included substantial periods of bed rest. Subsequent data demonstrated that 2 days of bed rest is as effective as 7 days and results in 45% less time lost from work.[7] In ambulatory patients with acute low back pain, continuation of ordinary activities, as permitted by the pain, may lead to more rapid recovery than either bed rest or back-mobilizing exercises.[11] While on bed rest, partial flexion of the hips and knees while in the supine or lateral decubitus position further reduces symptoms. Sitting in bed to read or watch television should be prohibited when disk herniation is suspected, because sitting increases intradiskal pressure. Intradiskal pressures are only minimally higher in the standing position than they are lying on the side, and it is reasonable to allow ambulation to the bathroom and brief periods of walking to prevent deconditioning.

In the experimental setting, traction has been shown to reduce intradiskal pressure; however, the weight required to overcome lower segment resistance and produce dimensional changes in the intervertebral disk space approximates 60% of total body weight. Clinical trials of "therapeutic" vs. "sham" traction have demonstrated no convincing benefit from the former.[2] No trials have studied inversion devices or other gravity traction methods.

No well-designed studies have demonstrated benefit from physical measures.[3] Ice massage or local heat, however, may reduce pain from muscle spasm in select patients; heat may be more effective when muscle stiffness is prominent. No data support the use of transcutaneous electrical nerve stimulation (TENS) in acute back pain, with only weak support in chronic back pain. Studies of acupuncture in the treatment of low back pain are generally of poor quality and do not support a recommendation.[3] Spinal manipulation has some benefit, particularly among patients with uncomplicated

Table 127-1. Differential Diagnosis of Common Low Back Pain Syndromes

Clinical entity	History	Physical examination	Supporting studies
Mechanical low back pain	Pain in back, buttocks, possibly thigh; may be severe Onset after new or unusual exertion No history of major trauma, systemic infection, or malignancy Relief of pain in supine position	Paravertebral tenderness/spasm Scoliosis or loss of lumbar lordosis common No neurologic signs (see Table 127-2)	None necessary
Herniated intervertebral disk	Acutely, pain in back severe and lancinating Antecedent flexion strain injury or trauma Sciatica Relief of pain supine with hip flexed Bilateral weakness, possible bowel/bladder dysfunction with massive central disk prolapse With chronic disk herniation, pain usually dull and possibly confined to leg	Striking paravertebral tenderness/spasm with splinting in awkward postures Signs of radicular irritation/injury usually present in acute setting	MRI, CT, or myelogram Electromyography may provide supporting documentation of level of denervation
Referred visceral or vascular pain	Patient writhes in discomfort, with no relief in any position Pain may occur in waves	Abdominal findings usually predominate Fever or incipient shock often present	Imaging studies directed at abdomen and retroperitoneum may visualize aortic aneurysm or abnormality of viscera (e.g., ureteral calculus, pancreatitis)
Metastatic malignancy (or multiple myeloma)	Unremitting or progressive pain at rest Known or suspected malignancy Weight loss, fever, other systemic symptoms History of weakness, possible bowel/bladder dysfunction	Tender spinous process at level of involvement Variable neurologic findings, up to full paraplegia	Standard radiographs may reveal destructive bony lesions Radionuclide bone scan sensitive for metastatic carcinoma but not for myeloma Epidural impingement of spinal cord or roots best delineated by MRI, myelography, or CT ESR elevated

[illegible] vertebral osteomyelitis, or septic diskitis	Unremitting or progressive pain at rest Fever Drug abuse, diabetes mellitus, immunosuppression Suspected or known systemic infection Previous spinal or genitourinary surgery History of weakness, possible bowel/bladder dysfunction	Tender spinous process at level of involvement Variable neurologic findings, up to full paraplegia Stigmata of systemic infection	Standard radiographs may reveal destructive bony lesions Radionuclide scans may suggest abscess Blood cultures often positive MRI probably best imaging modality to delineate extent of lesion and neural impingement ESR elevated
Ankylosing spondylitis	Insidious onset Progressive morning back pain and stiffness over several months Relief with exercise Age at onset: 40 years or younger	Painful or ankylosed sacroiliac joints Reduced mobility of spine Reduced chest wall expansion Possible associated uveitis	Sacroiliac joints and lumbosacral spine ankylosed on standard radiographs ESR elevated HLA-B27 confirmatory Uveitis may be confirmed on ophthalmologic examination
Reactive spondyloarthropathies	As with ankylosing spondylitis Antecedent urethritis, rash, or colitis	As with ankylosing spondylitis Conjunctivitis, balanitis, urethritis, keratoderma blennorrhagicum Psoriasis	As with ankylosing spondylitis Bowel studies may reveal infectious or idiopathic inflammatory bowel disease Infectious urethritis may be confirmed
Spinal stenosis	Back pain may vary from severe to absent Pseudoclaudication often prominent, often involving L4 root (anterior thigh) Pain worsens during the day, aggravated by standing and relieved by rest Weakness, possible bladder/bowel dysfunction	Neurologic findings vary: often evidence of impairment at multiple spinal levels Findings of osteoarthritis may be prominent	Standard radiographs generally show extensive vertebral osteophytes and degenerative disk disease Imaging with MRI or CT/myelography supports diagnosis if neurologic and imaging findings are concordant

CT, Computed tomography; *MRI,* magnetic resonance imaging; *ESR,* erythrocyte sedimentation rate.

Table 127-2. Radiculopathies Associated With Intervertebral Disk Herniations

Disk syndrome	Root	Rate (%)*	Pain radiation	Sensory deficit	Motor deficit	Reflex deficit
L5-S1	S1	45-55	Posterior thigh Posterior and lateral calf Heel	Posterior calf Lateral foot	Plantar flexors	Ankle
L4-5	L5	30-40	Lateral thigh Anterior calf and dorsum of foot ± Great toe	Anterior calf Medial foot First web space ± Great toe	Dorsiflexors	None
L3-4	L4	2-12	Lateral and anterior thigh Medial calf and foot ± Great toe	Medial calf and foot ± Great toe	Quadriceps	Knee
Cauda equina (massive central anterior prolapse)	Multiple	<1	Bilateral, including any or all of the above	Saddle anesthesia Any or all of the above, usually bilaterally	Multiple, including any or all of the above Bladder/bowel dysfunction	Any or all of the above Anal wink Cremasteric

*More than one level of involvement in up to 10% of cases. *L*, Lumbar; *S*, sacral.

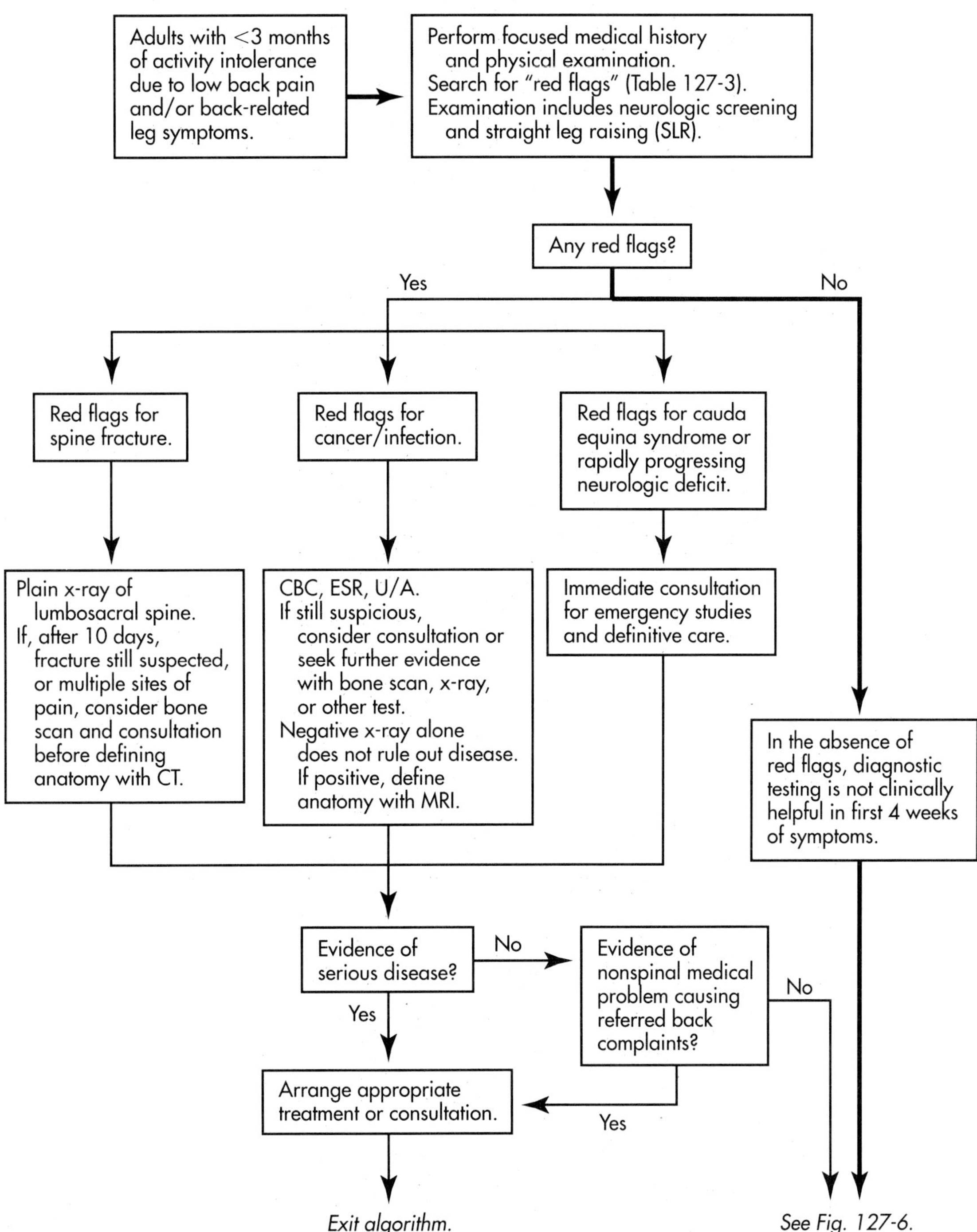

Fig. 127-5. Initial assessment of acute symptoms of low back pain. *CBC,* Complete blood count; *ESR,* erythrocyte sedimentation rate; *U/A,* urinalysis; *CT,* computed tomography; *MRI,* magnetic resonance imaging. (From Bigos S, Bowyer O, Braen G, et al: *Acute low back problems in adults,* Clinical practice guideline no 14, AHCPR pub no 95-0642, Rockville, Md, 1994, Agency for Health Care Policy and Research, Public Health Service, US Department of Health and Human Services.)

acute low back pain,[13] whose probability of recovery at 3 to 4 weeks is slightly increased. Manipulation is not recommended for patients with radiculopathy.[3]

In experimental situations, corsets and braces can reduce intradiskal pressure, the load on the lumbar spine, and the arc of motion in flexion; however, no convincing clinical data from controlled trials demonstrate their effectiveness for acute low back pain. Their use in the chronic setting also carries the risk of muscular disuse atrophy. Nonetheless, patients sometimes derive relief from low back pain with binders or braces. Lumbar corsets, used preventively, may reduce time lost from work due to low back problems in workers who do frequent lifting.[3] Flexion braces are generally most effective for patients with lumbar spinal stenosis or when examination suggests predominantly facet joint injury (with pain on spine extension and torsion). Other patients with less well-defined sources of low back pain may obtain relief with the hydraulic splinting of abdominal

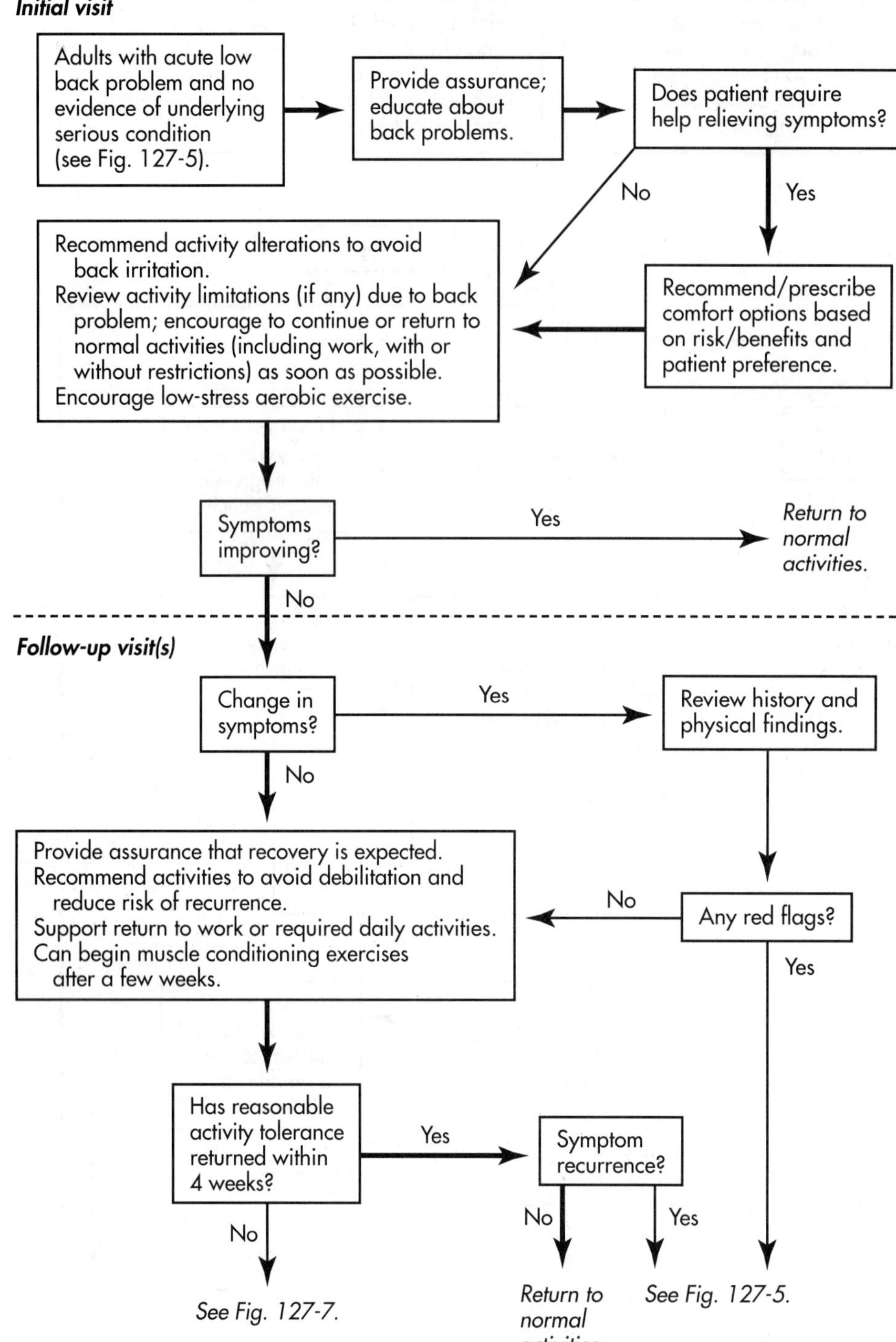

Fig. 127-6. Treatment of acute low back problems on initial and follow-up visits. (From Bigos S, Bowyer O, Braen G, et al: *Acute low back problems in adults,* Clinical practice guideline no 14, AHCPR pub no 95-0642. Rockville, Md, 1994, Agency for Health Care Policy and Research, Public Health Service, US Department of Health and Human Services.)

binders. The choice of device and restriction of a specific range of motion are best established after assessment by a physical therapist. Serious injury from use of back braces has been associated primarily with rigid devices in patients with scoliosis.

Low-stress aerobic exercise can prevent debilitation caused by inactivity during the first month of acute low back pain.[3] In general, patients can safely begin a slowly graduated endurance training program when they can sit comfortably. Advocated back exercise regimens include (1) spinal mobilization exercises emphasizing flexion, (2) paravertebral strengthening exercises stressing extension, and (3) modified isometric exercises directed at strengthening abdominal muscles and hip extensors. The few randomized controlled trials evaluating specific exercises for acute low back pain are limited in scope and size. The general consensus is that a

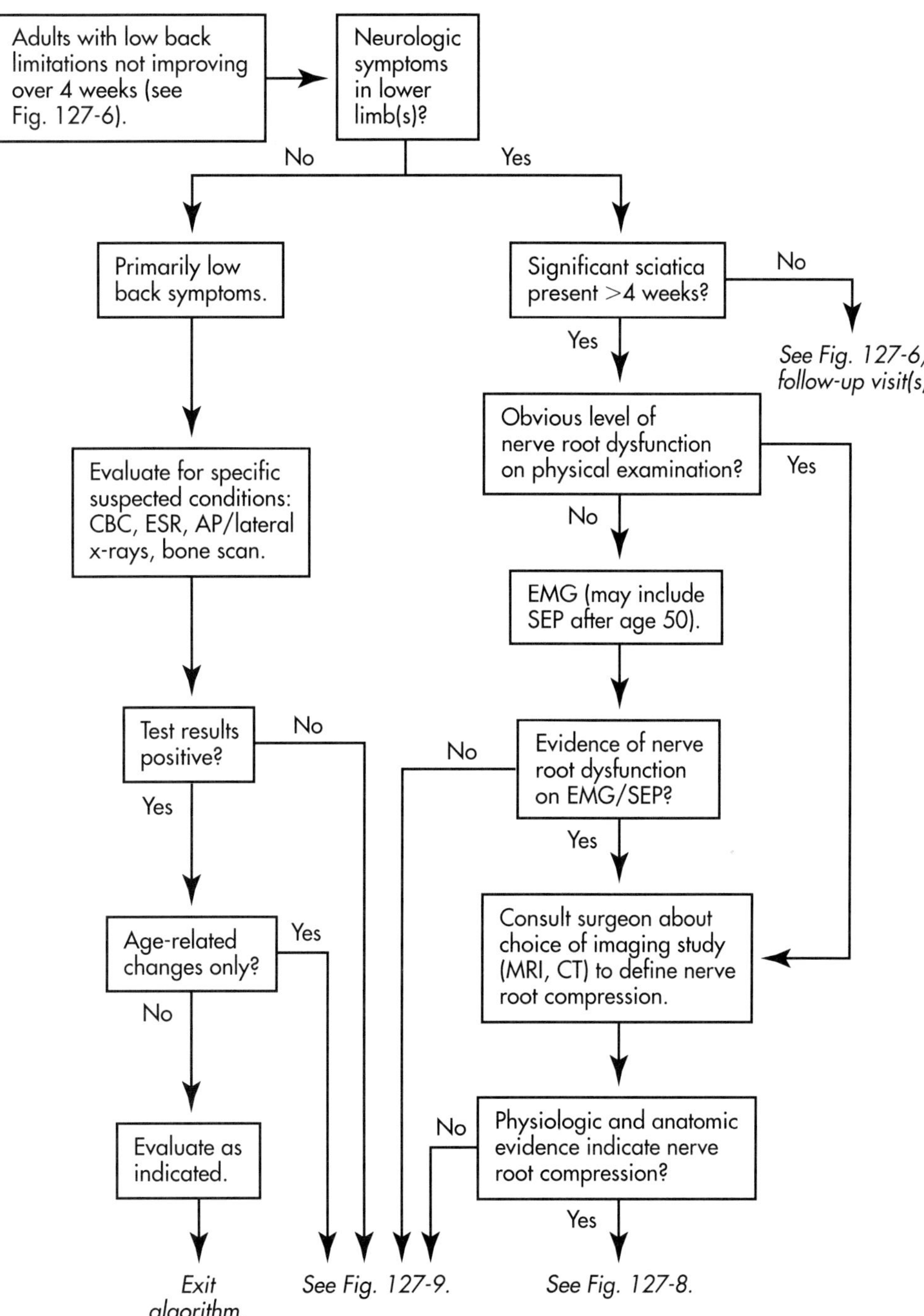

Fig. 127-7. Evaluation of low back symptoms in patient with slow recovery and limitations beyond 4 weeks. *AP,* Anteroposterior; *EMG,* electromyography; *SEP,* serum electrophoresis. (From Bigos S, Bowyer O, Braen G, et al: *Acute low back problems in adults,* Clinical practice guideline no 14, AHCPR pub no 95-0642, Rockville, Md, 1994, Agency for Health Care Policy and Research, Public Health Service, US Department of Health and Human Services.)

program of gradually increased aerobic activity and back-strengthening exercises is superior to no exercise.

In occupational settings an effective low-technology intervention for backache is low back school, a multifaceted educational course on body mechanics and back care. Although results have been variable, low back schools appear to help injured workers return to their jobs more quickly than manipulation or detuned diathermy and may reduce the incidence of injuries.

Pharmacologic Therapy

Analgesics and muscle relaxants are often prescribed to treat low back pain. Several randomized, double-blind studies demonstrated that nonsteroidal antiinflammatory drugs (NSAIDs) are superior to placebo for short-term relief from low back pain.[3] A recent meta-analysis reported a pooled odds ratio for pain relief after 1 week of 0.53 (95% confidence interval, 0.32 to 0.89) in four evaluable trials comparing NSAIDs with placebo in low back pain.[10] A

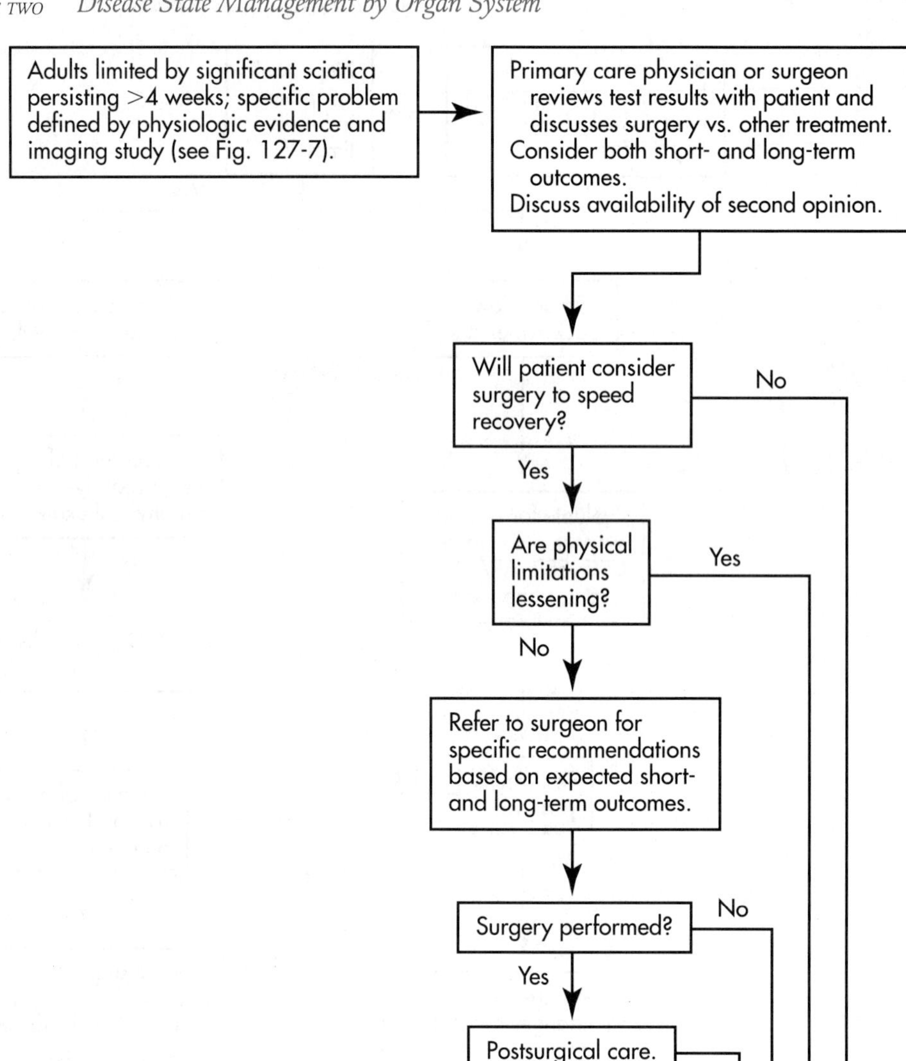

Fig. 127-8. Surgical considerations for patients with persistent sciatica. (From Bigos S, Bowyer O, Braen G, et al: *Acute low back problems in adults,* Clinical practice guideline no 14, AHCPR pub no 95-0642, Rockville, Md, 1994, Agency for Health Care Policy and Research, Public Health Service, US Department of Health and Human Services.)

number of NSAIDs have demonstrated efficacy. Some patients with mild low back pain respond adequately to therapeutic doses of acetaminophen, 1 gm every 4 to 6 hours, although no placebo-controlled studies have been reported. Since no data support one NSAID over any other in treating low back pain, choice of therapy may be based on cost and side effects. Patients with moderate or severe low back pain who are either intolerant of or allergic to NSAIDs may take a narcotic such as codeine or oxycodone with acetaminophen, but for no more than 7 days, given the natural history of most low back pain and the potential for abuse of these agents. No clinical trials have studied the cyclooxygenase-2 inhibitors in the management of low back pain, but in prerelease studies they were no more effective than NSAIDs in treating osteoarthritis and rheumatoid arthritis.

The putative muscle relaxants carisoprodol, diazepam, and cyclobenzaprine have also proved beneficial in controlled studies of patients with low back pain, although their efficacy is partly related to central nervous system effects. No data support improved efficacy over NSAIDs, although use of one of these agents in conjunction with an NSAID may have additive benefit. Cyclobenzaprine, carisoprodol, and diazepam are all sedating. Carisoprodol and diazepam possess significant addiction potential; cyclobenzaprine, which is similar in structure to the tricyclic antidepressants, has a striking atropine-like effect. As with narcotics, these agents generally should be taken by patients with acute low back pain for no more than 7 days.

More limited clinical data exist for orphenadrine and chlorzoxazone. These agents demonstrate muscle relaxant capabilities in animals and have reduced discomfort in humans, but the mechanism is more likely related to central analgesia and mild sedation than to muscle relaxation.

In patients with chronic low back pain, tricyclic antidepressant agents have demonstrated efficacy.[1] Response to a tricyclic antidepressant may reflect a combination of mood elevation with improvement in pain threshold, improved sleep pattern with reduction in symptoms of associated fibromyalgia, and a direct effect on neuropathic pain pathways by norepinephrine reuptake blockade. Pain

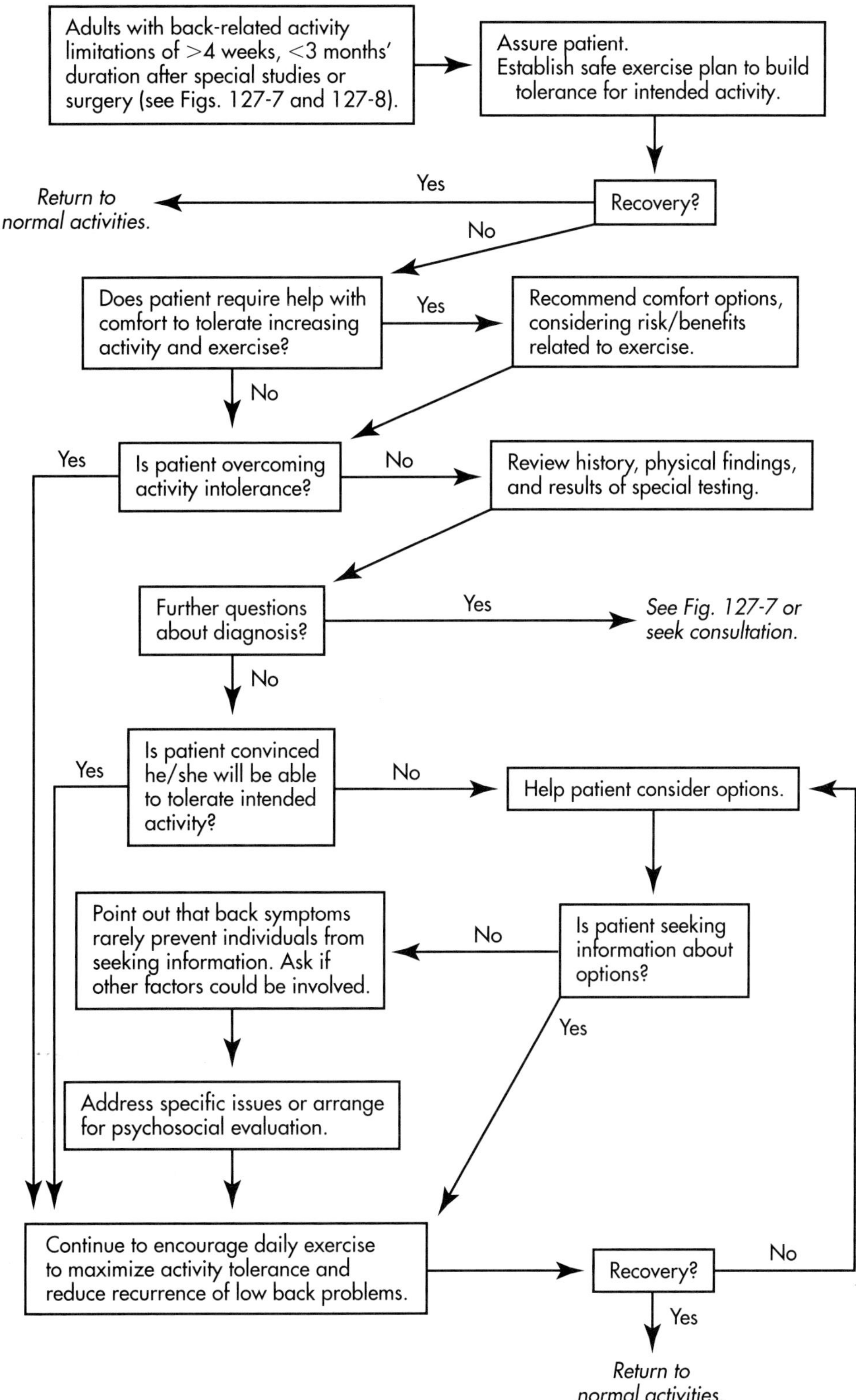

Fig. 127-9. Further care of acute low back problems. (From Bigos S, Bowyer O, Braen G, et al: *Acute low back problems in adults,* Clinical practice guideline no 14, AHCPR pub no 95-0642, Rockville, Md, 1994, Agency for Health Care Policy and Research, Public Health Service, US Department of Health and Human Services.)

Table 127-3. Clinical "Red Flags" for Use With Management Algorithms

Suspected clinical condition	"Red flag"
Cancer or infection	History of cancer Unexplained weight loss Duration of pain longer than 1 month Immunosuppression (e.g., corticosteroids, transplant, HIV infection) Fever Urinary infection Intravenous drug use Back pain not improved with rest, or worse supine Age >50
Spinal fracture	History of "significant" trauma Major trauma at any age Minor trauma if potentially osteoporotic Prolonged use of corticosteroids Age >70
Cauda equina syndrome (severe compromise)	Acute onset urinary retention/ overflow incontinence Loss of anal sphincter tone or fecal incontinence Saddle anesthesia Global or progressive lower extremity weakness

Modified from Bigos S, Bowyer O, Braen G, et al: *Acute low back problems in adults*, Clinical practice guideline no 14, AHCPR pub no 95-0642, Rockville, Md, 1994, Agency for Health Care Policy and Research, Public Health Service, US Department of Health and Human Services.

reduction may be noted at doses less than those effective in treating depression.

No data support the use of oral corticosteroids in the management of either acute or chronic low back pain.

Injection of long-acting anesthetic agents and corticosteroids into facet joints, ligamentous structures, or the epidural space has often been used to treat low back pain. Because corticosteroid injection into facet joints is no better than saline injection, however, and because 80% of low back pain patients have no definitive anatomic diagnosis and thus no specific target for injection, this therapy should not be considered part of the standard of care for low back pain.

Chemonucleolysis involves the injection of a chymopapain to dissolve herniated disk material. It was developed as a less invasive and potentially safer intervention than disk surgery in the treatment of sciatica. Although chemonucleolysis proved effective in relieving sciatica in a prospective clinical trial—77% of those treated with chymopapain responded 6 weeks after injection, compared with 47% of controls—both anaphylaxis and severe neurologic complications (e.g., transverse myelitis) have been reported. Morbidity is comparable to or worse than that associated with disk surgery, and surgery yields more predictable early relief from sciatica.

Emotional and Behavioral Therapy

Because conservative therapy is usually effective, the initial management of most patients with acute or recurrent low back pain should be at home; this avoids reinforcing illness behavior through hospitalization and reduces health care costs and inconvenience. A major source of patient dissatisfaction is the failure of health care providers to adequately describe the problem. Because the natural history of low back pain and sciatica is generally favorable, reassurance and education are important. Prescriptions for bed rest and graded activity should be explicit, with the anticipated course of improvement. Medications should be presented as temporary adjuncts to rest and graded exercise. The physician should also discuss recurrence and encourage lifestyle changes, including weight reduction, cessation of tobacco use, and regular exercise, to minimize long-term risk. Ergonomic changes at work (e.g., work position, lifting posture) and at home (e.g., firm mattress, chairs with firm lumbar support, elevated toilet seat) reduce ongoing discomfort and lower the risk of recurrence.

The patient impaired by chronic low back pain poses a special challenge. Attention must be directed at disruptions in family dynamics caused by this chronic condition, which may have no physical findings. Substance abuse is common among patients with chronic pain and includes alcohol, prescription medications, and illegal substances. Headache, fibromyalgia, and other somatic complaints may be a proxy for depression; the patient may benefit from counseling and pharmacologic intervention. Exercise and retraining programs with psychologic support may result in a return to work.

Surgery

Emergency surgical referral is clearly indicated when epidural abscess, malignancy, or hematoma is suspected; when neurologic deficits are severe or progressive (e.g., cauda equina syndrome); or when the pattern suggests referred pain from an impending intraabdominal or retroperitoneal catastrophe (e.g., leaking abdominal aortic aneurysm). Elective surgical referral is also appropriate when severe pain and neuromotor deficits from sciatica persist despite 4 to 8 weeks of appropriate conservative therapy and are associated with clinical evidence of root compression. Surgery is also considered for persistent pain or neurologic deficits from spondylolisthesis or spinal stenosis, but generally not until at least 3 months of conservative management have been completed.

During the past decade, nearly 200,000 diskectomies were performed annually in the United States, most electively to relieve sciatica. An estimated 5% to 15% of these procedures resulted in poor outcomes and reoperation, largely because of inappropriate patient selection.[9] Serious complications occur in less than 1% of patients. The results of standard diskectomy are excellent for short-term relief from sciatica in appropriate patients. Three quarters of such patients are sciatica-free 1 year after surgery, compared with one third of patients treated conservatively. Approximately one half of patients are completely pain-free (i.e., without sciatica or back pain) 1 year after surgery. However, long-term outcomes of diskectomy and conservative care are comparable after 4 to 10 years.[3] Standard diskectomy entails a posterior longitudinal incision, removal of laminar bone, incision of the ligamentum flavum, exploration for other abnormalities, and removal of herniated disk material. Complications include dural tears, diskitis, nerve root damage, and spinal instability. Recuperation is often lengthy.

Microdiskectomy employs a magnifying scope, allowing smaller incisions with fewer anatomic disruptions. Disk fragments are more likely to be missed than with standard diskectomy, and occasionally the wrong level is entered. However, microdiskectomy and standard diskectomy have similar efficacy.

Percutaneous diskectomy uses an automated percutaneous cutting and suction probe to aspirate the nucleus pulposus of the herniated disk, with minimal risk to the spinal cord or posterior elements. Few patients are candidates for this procedure, and recurrent herniation from the same disk is common. Percutaneous diskectomy is less efficacious than chymopapain injection therapy, and neither is as effective as standard diskectomy or microdiskectomy.

Overall, only a small percentage of patients with back pain and sciatica should require surgery. Those who meet criteria for surgery generally do well, with 90% achieving at least partial relief from sciatica and back pain. Preoperative markers of a poor outcome include physical findings suggesting a behavioral disturbance; distribution and quality of pain that deviate from expected anatomic pain radiation; pending workers' compensation claims; and psychologic tests showing hysteria, hypochondriasis, and somatization. A delay in surgery beyond 12 weeks may compromise the ultimate result, especially in patients with demonstrable weakness.

EBM EVIDENCE-BASED MEDICINE

Primary sources for this chapter include MEDLINE, searched through PUBMED, and the clinical practice guideline *Acute Low Back Problems in Adults* of the Agency for Health Care Policy and Research of the U.S. Public Health Service, published in December 1994. Electronic searches dating back to 1994 were conducted through May 1999, with a focus on systematic reviews, meta-analyses, and large randomized clinical trials.

REFERENCES

1. Atkinson JH, Slater MA, Williams RA, et al: A placebo-controlled randomized clinical trial of nortriptyline for chronic low back pain, *Pain* 76:287, 1998.
2. Beurskens AJ, de Vet HC, Koke AJ, et al: Efficacy of traction for nonspecific low back pain: 12-week and 6-month results of a randomized clinical trial, *Spine* 22:2756, 1997.
3. Bigos S, Bowyer O, Braen G, et al: *Acute low back problems in adults*, Clinical practice guideline no 14, AHCPR pub no 95-0642, Rockville, Md, 1994, Agency for Health Care Policy and Research, Public Health Service, US Department of Health and Human Services.
4. Boden SD, Davis DO, Dina TS, et al: Abnormal magnetic-resonance scans of the lumbar spine in asymptomatic subjects, *J Bone Joint Surg* 72A:403, 1990.
5. Cunningham LS, Kelsey JL: Epidemiology of musculoskeletal impairments and associated disability, *Am J Public Health* 74:574, 1984.
6. Deyo RA, Diehl AK: Lumbar spine films in primary care: current use and effects of selective ordering criteria, *J Gen Intern Med* 1:20, 1986.
7. Deyo RA, Diehl AK, Rosenthal M: How many days of bed rest for acute low back pain? A randomized clinical trial, *N Engl J Med* 315:1064, 1986.
8. Deyo RA, Rainville J, Kent DL: What can the history and physical examination tell us about low back pain? *JAMA* 268:760, 1992.
9. Hoffman RM, Wheeler KJ, Deyo RA: Surgery for herniated lumbar discs: a literature synthesis, *J Gen Intern Med* 8:487, 1993.
10. Koes BW, Scholten RJ, Mens JM, Bouter LM: Efficacy of non-steroidal anti-inflammatory drugs for low back pain: a systematic review of randomised clinical trials, *Ann Rheum Dis* 56:214, 1997.
11. Malmivaara A, Hakkinen U, Aro T, et al: The treatment of acute low back pain: bed rest, exercises, or ordinary activity? *N Engl J Med* 332:351, 1995.
12. Nachemson AL: Newest knowledge of low back pain: a critical look, *Clin Orthop* 279:8, 1992.
13. Shekelle PG, Adams AH, Chassin MR, et al: Spinal manipulation for low-back pain, *Ann Intern Med* 117:590, 1992.

CHAPTER 128

Disorders of the Hip

Jerry M. Greene
Elinor A. Mody

PATIENT EVALUATION

Pain in the hip is a frequent complaint of patients seen by primary care physicians (Fig. 128-1). A mnemonic device for recalling the many causes of pain in or around a joint is PODAGRA HOT JOINT (Box 128-1).[3]

History

The most important elements of the history include the precise location of the pain, its character, areas to which pain radiates, its severity, activities or other factors that aggravate or alleviate the pain, and any functional impairment (Box 128-2).

Location of Pain. Patients use the term *hip* to refer to areas from the lower back to midthigh, and many complaints of hip pain do not arise from the hip joint itself. The patient should localize the painful area early in the interview, preferably by pointing to it. Pain in certain areas suggests particular anatomic structures as the possible sites of the problem (Box 128-2).

Anterior hip, inguinal, proximal thigh, medial thigh, and occasionally knee pain may be caused by an intraarticular process. Pain in these areas may also originate in the iliopectineal bursa; quadriceps, iliopsoas, or adductor muscles; femoral artery, nerve, or vein; inguinal lymph nodes; superior and inferior pubic rami; obturator nerve; or structures within the bony pelvis, especially the adnexa, appendix, and small and large intestines. Inguinal pain may also be referred from the kidney or ureter, may be caused by upper lumbar radiculopathy, or may arise from spinal facet joints, intervertebral disk, or vertebral bodies of the lumbar spine.

Lateral hip pain may arise from the greater trochanter of the femur, trochanteric bursa, lateral femoral cutaneous nerve, or iliotibial band. Lateral hip pain may be caused by a back problem, such as fourth lumbar vertebra (L4) root irritation or L4-5 or L5-S1 (first sacral vertebra) facet joint arthritis; intervertebral disk degeneration or infection; vertebral fracture, infection, or neoplasm; or myofascial pain with trigger points.

Posterior hip or buttock pain may also arise from the hip joint. Other structures associated with posterior hip pain

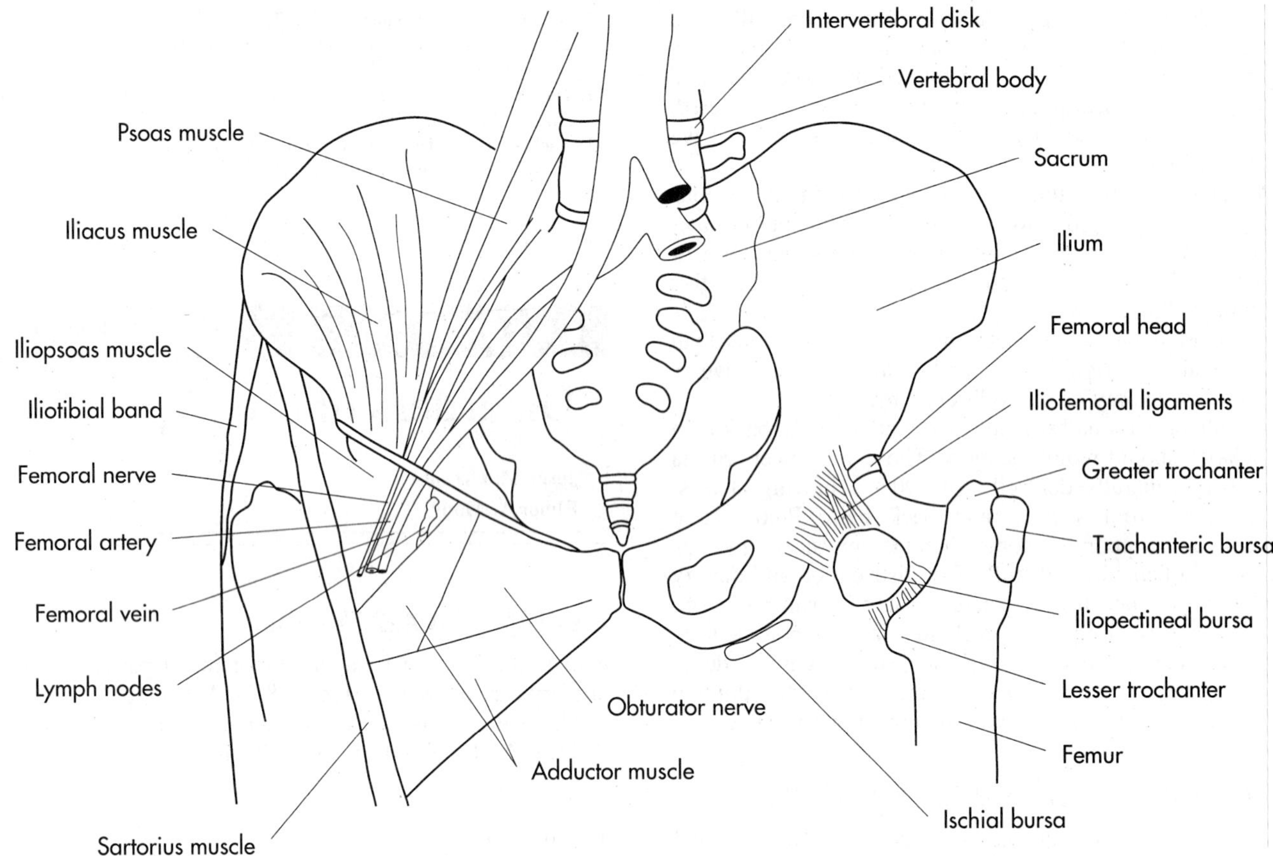

Fig. 128-1. Regional anatomy of the hip and lower back.

Box 128-1. Mnemonic for Pain in Area of Joint: PODAGRA HOT JOINT

*P*olyarthritis: rheumatoid arthritis, rheumatic fever, systemic lupus erythematosus
*O*steoarthritis: primary, posttraumatic, postinflammatory
*D*erangements: loose bodies, ligamentous tears, dislocation
*A*vascular necrosis: hemoglobinopathies, decompression
*G*out: pseudogout, apatite crystal–associated arthritis
*R*eactive arthritis: Reiter's syndrome, inflammatory bowel disease, psoriatic arthritis
*A*myloid: and other accumulations (e.g., Gaucher's disease)

*H*emorrhage: hemophilia, anticoagulation, posttraumatic, tumor
*O*steochondromatosis: also synovial chondromatosis
*T*umors: benign and malignant

*J*uxtaarticular: especially bursitis, tendinitis
*O*steitis deformans: Paget's disease
*I*nfection: including gonococcal and nongonococcal bacterial
*N*europathic: Charcot's disease, referred, radicular
*T*rauma: including fractures, foreign bodies, contusions

From Gravallese EM et al: Synovitis of the knee in a 42-year-old man: clinicopathologic conference, *Arthritis Rheum* 36:860, 1993.

include the ischial bursa, sciatic nerve, gluteal muscles, sacroiliac joints, the ischium, and the sacrum. Processes within the pelvis may also cause pain that is experienced in the posterior hip region. Neoplasms or abscesses arising from the rectum, prostate, adnexa, uterus, bladder, and bowel may involve the lumbosacral plexus or cause referred pain. Vascular insufficiency, especially of the external iliac arteries, may cause gluteal claudication. Lumbar spinal stenosis may cause pseudoclaudication (neurogenic) in the buttocks.

Character of Pain. Descriptions of the pain may be helpful in determining the underlying pathophysiology. Dysesthesia, paresthesia, and numbness suggests a neuropathic process. Constant pain, including pain at rest and especially pain that interferes with sleep, is most often seen with neurologic, inflammatory, and neoplastic processes. Pain with use and decreased pain with rest suggests a mechanical process and is classic for osteoarthritis of the hip. After characterizing the hip pain, the examiner should determine if

Box 128-2. Causes of Pain in Area of Joint

Anterior Hip, Medial Thigh, Knee

Acute

Acute rheumatic fever
Adductor muscle strain
Avascular necrosis
Crystal arthritis
Femoral artery (pseudo) aneurysm
Fracture (femoral neck or intertrochanteric)
Hemarthrosis
Hernia
Herpes zoster
Iliopectineal bursitis
Iliopsoas tendinitis
Inguinal lymphadenitis
Osteomalacia
Painful transient osteoporosis of hip
Septic arthritis

Subacute and chronic

Adductory muscle strain
Amyloidosis
Acute rheumatic fever
Femoral artery aneurysm
Hernia (inguinal or femoral)
Iliopectineal bursitis
Iliopsoas tendinitis
Inguinal lymphadenopathy
Osteochondromatosis
Osteomyelitis
Osteitis deformans (Paget's disease)
Osteomalacia (pseudofracture)
Postherpetic neuralgia
Sterile synovitis (e.g., rheumatoid arthritis, psoriatic, systemic lupus erythematosus)

Lateral Hip, Lateral Thigh

Acute

Herpes zoster
Iliotibial tendinitis
Impacted fracture of femoral neck
Lateral femoral cutaneous neuropathy (meralgia paresthetica)
Radiculopathy: L4-5
Trochanteric avulsion fracture (greater trochanter)
Trochanteric bursitis
Trochanteric fracture

Subacute and chronic

Lateral femoral cutaneous neuropathy (meralgia paresthetica)
Osteomyelitis
Postherpetic neuralgia
Radiculopathy: L4-5
Tumors

Posterior Hip, Thigh, Buttock

Acute

Gluteal muscle strain
Herpes zoster
Ischial bursitis
Ischial or sacral fracture
Osteomalacia (pseudofracture)
Sciatic neuropathy
Radiculopathy: L5-S1

Subacute and chronic

Gluteal muscle strain
Ischial bursitis
Lumbar spinal stenosis
Osteoarthritis of hip
Osteitis deformans (Paget's disease)
Osteomyelitis
Osteochondromatosis
Osteomalacia (pseudofracture)
Postherpetic neuralgia
Radiculopathy: L5-S1
Tumors

any trauma, recent or remote, has occurred to the hip, pelvis, or lower back. The remaining elements of a general history include medication use, habits, occupation, concomitant medical illnesses, prior surgery, any prior episodes of joint pain, sexual history, history of illicit drug use, and episodes of chills, fevers, and rigors (Table 128-1).

Physical Examination

The physical examination should be tailored to the acuteness, severity, and complexity of the complaints. The goal is to reproduce the pain through palpation or maneuvers.[4] The essential elements of an examination for hip pain include observing for deformities in patients who cannot walk. A flexed, externally rotated, shortened leg is seen with hip fracture, whereas an internally rotated shortened leg suggests posterior dislocation. Patients with either of these deformities should not undergo hip maneuvers until fracture or dislocation has been ruled out by radiographic studies.

The gait of patients who can walk may demonstrate a limp. The patient with an *antalgic gait* bears weight only briefly on the affected side. The patient with an *adductor lurch* shifts upper body weight to the side of the painful hip. Having the patient attempt to stand on one leg at a time (Trendelenburg's test) may demonstrate an inability to bear weight on the affected side or an inability to keep the pelvis level while doing so. The examiner should assess whether the patient rising from sitting to standing exacerbates the pain. The painful hip is inspected for swelling, erythema, and rash. Active range of motion of the hip, knee, and lower back is then assessed. Palpation helps identify masses and tenderness of the vertebral spines; paravertebral muscles; bursae, especially greater trochanteric, ischial, and iliopectineal; inguinal lymph nodes; femoral artery and vein; quadriceps, adductor, and gluteal muscles; superior pubic ramus; symphysis pubis; and sciatic notch.

Table 128-1. Selected Causes of Hip Pain

Disorder	Epidemiology	History	Physical examination	Diagnostic tests	Differential diagnosis	Management
Acute rheumatic fever	Children and young adults; poverty and overcrowding, epidemics of arthritogenic strains of streptococci	Preceding pharyngitis (may be asymptomatic), arthralgia, rash, involuntary movements, migratory oligoarthritis	Fever, evanescent salmon-colored rash, synovitis, heart murmur, CHF, chorea, subcutaneous nodules	ASLO titer increased, ESR increased, ECG PR interval prolonged, echocardiogram may demonstrate regurgitation, pericardial effusion	As for rheumatoid arthritis (see also Chapter 133)	Salicylates in anti-inflammatory dosages, steroids for resistant cases at dosages of 1 mg/kg/day, long-term prophylactic use of penicillin
Amyloidosis	Hip involvement unusual but may occur with chronic renal dialysis due to β_2-microglobulin–related amyloid deposition, amyloidosis with chronic infections, chronic inflammatory diseases, and with paraproteinemias	Gradual onset of hip pain, symptoms of carpal tunnel syndrome (numbness, paresthesia, pain in thumb, index, and middle fingers), shoulder pain due to rotator cuff infiltration, easy bruising	Skin: waxy appearance, bruises and echymoses; abdomen: hepatosplenomegaly; musculoskeletal: pseudohypertrophy of deltoid muscles (shoulder pad sign) due to amyloid infiltration, limited shoulder motion; neurologic: peripheral neuropathy and Tinel's sign at wrist common	Plain radiographs demonstrate cysts or erosions in femoral head or neck; needle biopsy of lytic lesions; serum and urine immunoelectrophoresis; abdominal fat pad aspiration with Congo red staining is least invasive biopsy method	In chronic renal failure with patient on dialysis, hyperparathyroidism with brown tumors, other neoplasms (see tumors)	Control of underlying disease may prevent progression; for amyloid associated with myeloma or paraproteinemia: chemotherapy may be indicated; for dialysis-related amyloid: renal transplantation if possible
Avascular necrosis[1]	Predisposing condition; alcohol, glucocorticosteroids, sickle cell disease, decompression, pancreatitis, trauma, SLE, hyperlipoproteinemias, radiation therapy	Sudden onset of pain, moderate to severe, limits weight bearing, predisposing factors may be present	Despite pain, passive ROM is normal in early disease; motion may be limited once collapse of cartilage and subchondral bone occurs	MRI most sensitive for early disease, demonstrates decreased T1 and increased T2 signal; plain films insensitive until late in course, may show subchondral collapse	Painful transient osteoporosis of hip, bone bruise, pelvic or sacral insufficiency fractures, osteomyelitis, neoplasm	Core decompression with or without vascularized bone or soft tissue grafting; rotational osteotomy; total replacement for hips with collapse and secondary osteoarthritis
Fracture of femoral neck	Increased risk with age; osteoporosis due to postmenopausal status; corticosteroid use; alcoholism; anticonvulsant drugs	Severe hip pain and inability to bear weight after fall	Deformity of hip with external rotation, slight flexion; assess neurovascular integrity; monitor vital signs carefully	Plain radiographs of hip and pelvis with minimal movement of affected leg	Pathologic fracture due to tumor or infection of femur; osteomalacia with Looser's line; impacted fracture; SI or pubic ramus fracture	Motion of affected hip should be minimized while assessment proceeds; if fracture documented: provide analgesia, monitor vital signs, obtain orthopedic consultation

[illegible]	Men twice as often as women, predominantly after adolescence; drugs may elevate uric acid level, especially hydrochlorothiazide, pyrazinamide, cyclosporine	Prior episodes of self-limited arthritis, severe pain, sudden onset, fever may be noted by patient	Fever may be present, usually <39° C; tophi; extremely limited ROM in all directions	Plain film may suggest effusion; aspiration positive for needle-shaped, brightly birefringent crystals on compensated, polarized microscopy; synovial WBC 10-100,000/mm^3; Gram's stain negative	Septic arthritis, pseudogout, apatite arthritis, RA, ARF, SLE, Reiter's syndrome, reactive arthritis	See Chapter 136
Hemorrhage	Children with hemophilia, adolescents with trauma, adults with trauma or anticoagulation	Sudden onset of pain after minor trauma, or no history of trauma; pain at rest and with use, usually severe with antalgic gait or inability to walk, history of prior bleeding diathesis or anticoagulant drug use	Signs of intraarticular process, evidence of bleeding diathesis (bruising, mucosal bleeding)	Plain radiograph to exclude fracture; CBC, PT/PTT, platelet count; aspiration yields blood; fat droplets on surface of aspirate (after specimen stands) suggest intraarticular fracture; hematocrit on synovial fluid <5% suggests hemorrhagic effusion, not hemorrhage	Hemorrhage: trauma, excessive anticoagulation, bleeding diathesis; bloody effusion: CPDD, pseudogout, apatite arthritis, neuropathic joint, pigmented villonodular synovitis, other joint tumors	Replacement of deficient clotting factors; partial correction to therapeutic range for excessive anticoagulation and clear indication (e.g., prosthetic valve); aspiration of as much fluid as possible; rest; analgesics; ROM exercises after 48 hours
Hernias	Associated with strenuous lifting, coughing, or Valsalva's maneuver	Anterior hip pain; patients sometimes note bulge	Hip motion normal; inguinal or femoral hernia palpated with Valsalva's maneuver or cough	If definite hernia, no further tests necessary	Inguinal mass may be tumor, lymphadenopathy, phlebothrombosis, arterial aneurysm, necessitating abscess from pelvis, abdomen, or psoas muscle, or synovial cyst from hip joint	Emergency repair for incarcerated hernia; elective repair for reducible hernia

See end of table for abbreviations.

Continued

Table 128-1. Selected Causes of Hip Pain—cont'd

Disorder	Epidemiology	History	Physical examination	Diagnostic tests	Differential diagnosis	Management
Iliopectineal bursitis	Most frequent in athletic males and dancers	Anterior hip pain; limited to hip extension, so running or brisk walking is painful; standing or slow walking does not increase pain	Affected hip may be flexed slightly; extension of hip aggravates pain; possible tenderness in anterior hip and inguinal region; palpate inguinal area for inguinal or femoral hernia, mass, aneurysm, lymph-adenopathy; examine abdomen to exclude sigmoid colonic or appendiceal disease; pelvic exam for women	Plain films usually negative, rarely demonstrate calcific periarthritis or intra-bursal calcifications; CBC, ESR, U/A to exclude infection and ureteral stone	If severe with limited hip ROM: infectious and other hip synovitis; if local anterior pain: iliopsoas tendinitis, psoas abscess, inguinal or femoral hernia, radicular pain, referred pain from kidney, ureter, obturator nerve irritation from pelvic mass or infection, femoral artery aneurysm	Analgesics, rest, local heat, NSAIDs, therapeutic ultrasound; for refractory cases: local corticosteroid injection (referral if necessary); refractory pain warrants bone scan, CT scan
Iliopsoas tendinitis	Athletes or coexisting osteoarthritis of hip	Anterior hip pain, active hip flexion may be most painful; stair climbing and putting on shoes and stockings may be difficult	Affected hip may be slightly flexed; possible anterior hip tenderness; pain reproduced by attempted hip flexion against resistance	Plain films negative; CBC, ESR normal	As for iliopectineal bursitis	As for iliopectineal bursitis
Iliotibial tendinitis	Athletes, overuse with repeated sitting and standing, leg length discrepancy	Lateral hip pain, aggravated by standing, walking, arising from chair	Tenderness along lateral thigh; pain with forced adduction or resisted abduction of hip	History and physical findings; diagnostic injection with local anesthetic of trochanteric bursa to distinguish trochanteric bursitis	As for trochanteric bursitis	Physical therapy with ultrasound, local heat, stretching of iliotibial band; analgesics, NSAIDs
Insufficiency (stress) fractures	Young people after repeated vigorous exercise; anyone after prolonged immobility or limited weight bearing, e.g., after total joint replacement in RA	Onset of pain with activity, aggravated with weight bearing, some relief with rest; may be severe and prevent weight bearing; pain may radiate widely to thigh or buttock	Passive hip motion usually preserved and does not aggravate pain; active motion may be limited by pain; pelvic compression (anteroposterior or lateral) or rocking may reproduce pain	Plain films of hip and pelvis relatively insensitive for insufficiency fracture of sacrum and ilium, better for pubic rami; bone scan sensitive; CT scan helps confirm fracture as cause	Metastatic and primary bone lesions, (see tumors), osteomyelitis, lumbar disk disease, referred pain	Analgesics and rehabilitation with partial weight bearing using walker; avoid prolonged bed rest; assess for osteoporosis or osteomalacia if indicated

Ischial bursitis (ischiogluteal bursitis)	Activities that cause repeated trauma to gluteal region predispose to condition, e.g., horseback riding, weaving, skating	Posterior hip pain, increased with forward bending, sitting on hard surface	Tenderness over ischial tuberosity, preserved hip ROM, no sciatic notch tenderness, normal neurologic exam	Plain radiographs usually normal	Pelvic fracture (traumatic, stress related), sciatic nerve compression, pyriformis syndrome, radicular pain, referred pain from within pelvis, bone lesions in ischium	Avoid further repetitive trauma to ischial area; analgesics, NSAIDs, local heat, therapeutic ultrasound, local injection with corticosteroids
Lateral femoral cutaneous neuropathy	Recent weight loss or weight gain predisposes to pressure on lateral femoral cutaneous nerve as it passes over pelvic brim	Sudden or gradual onset of pain confined to lateral hip and thigh, accompanied by numbness and paresthesia, in absence of back pain or sensory changes below knee	Decreased sensation over lateral hip and thigh; preserved DTRs; no tenderness over trochanteric bursa	Plain films of pelvis to exclude lytic or blastic lesion of iliac crest	Lumbar radiculopathies should produce neurologic symptoms extending below knee; iliotibial tendinitis or trochanteric bursitis should have local tenderness	Avoid tight-waisted clothing; use suspenders rather than belts; analgesic medications may be necessary; low-dose amitriptyline, imipramine, or desipramine at bedtime; gabapentin
Lumbar radiculopathies	May occur in young adults from herniated disks and in older persons from lumbar spondylosis (degenerative disk and facet joint disease) with compression of spinal canal (spinal stenosis) or impingement on exiting nerve roots (lateral recess stenosis)	Posterior, lateral, or anterior pain, extending from back beyond hip, usually below knee; change in sensation; pain aggravated by walking; patient sitting to obtain relief suggests lumbar spinal stenosis	Tenderness of lumbar spine, paraspinal muscle spasm, positive straight leg raising, diminished sensation in dermatomal distribution, loss of DTRs, muscle weakness, no exacerbation of pain with hip motion	LS spine and pelvic radiographs; if cancer diagnosis and radicular pain without weakness: bone scan and follow-up CT scan of involved area; if weakness, bowel/bladder incontinence: MRI or CT scan of LS spine	See Chapter 127	See Chapter 127
Lyme disease	Children and adults with exposure to ticks in areas with endemic *Borrelia burgdorferi*	Travel or residence in endemic area, tick bite or removing ticks, slowly enlarging circular or oval erythematous rash, history of painful radiculopathy or cranial nerve palsy, especially Bell's palsy	Fever, usually low grade if present; possible skin rash, usually polycyclic erythematous eruption; hip motion diminished in all directions; cranial nerve VII weakness or other cranial neuropathy or radiculopathy	Aspiration of hip reveals inflammatory fluid with lymphocytic predominance; plain films: swelling or normal; CBC normal; ESR: elevated moderately; Lyme titer usually elevated	Other chronic synovitis: as for rheumatoid arthritis (see also Chapter 133)	For proven Lyme arthritis: ceftriaxone 1 gm IV every 12 hr for 2 wk

See end of table for abbreviations.

Continued

Table 128-1. Selected Causes of Hip Pain—cont'd

Disorder	Epidemiology	History	Physical examination	Diagnostic tests	Differential diagnosis	Management
Osteitis deformans (Paget's disease of bone)	Middle-aged to older adults	Pain anywhere in hip; may occur with activity and weight bearing, especially with osteoarthritic change of involved hip joint; rest and night pain with bony involvement alone or advanced osteoarthritis	Preserved ROM without exacerbating pain suggests pain from bony involvement; pain with motion suggests concomitant osteoarthritis of hip	Plain films demonstrate coarse trabeculi; increased size of bone, thickening of cortex, areas of lucency; possible osteoarthritis of hip; alkaline phosphatase elevated; prostate-specific antigen in men	Prostate cancer, sclerosing osteomyelitis, other blastic metastatic disease (e.g., thyroid, breast), transformation of Paget's disease to osteogenic sarcoma (suggested by marked change, rise or fall, in alkaline phosphatase unrelated to therapy)	Alendronate, etidronate, or calcitonin; if severe associated osteoarthritis: total hip replacement, treatment with etidronate or calcitonin for 6 wk to 3 mo before surgery
Osteoarthritis	Older more than younger persons; some heritable forms with epiphyseal dysplasias and defined collagen mutations	Pain with use, better with rest, gel phenomenon common; with advanced disease: continuous pain, difficulty sleeping	Antalgic gait or adductor lurch, positive Trendelenburg's sign, limited ROM, pain reproduced by motion, no tenderness, leg lengths may differ slightly	Plain radiographs show joint space narrowing, osteophyte formation, sclerotic bone, subchondral cysts	Secondary osteoarthritis, septic arthritis complicating osteoarthritis, crystal disease	Weight loss, moderate low-impact exercise, cane, acetaminophen, NSAIDs, hip replacement for severe symptomatic disease or rotational osteotomy for younger patients
Osteochondromatosis[2]	Rare cause of large joint pain and chronic synovitis	Slowly developing pain, restricted motion in hip	Swelling may be apparent in anterior hip, joint motion restricted	Plain radiographs may demonstrate multiple osteochondral bodies within joint capsule or may suggest joint swelling or effusion; MRI can distinguish multiple cartilaginous bodies from joint fluid when calcification is absent	Chronic inflammatory synovitis (see rheumatoid arthritis), especially with rice bodies, pigmented villonodular synovitis	Synovectomy is curative, secondary osteoarthritis may progress following synovectomy
Pseudogout	Older persons; men same as women; some predisposing conditions, including hyperparathyroidism, hypothyroidism, hemochromatosis	Sudden onset of pain; history may suggest disorder associated with pseudogout	Fever possible; pain and limited ROM consistent with intraarticular process; features may suggest underlying disease	Plain radiographs may be normal, suggest effusion, or demonstrate chondrocalcinosis; WBC normal to mildly elevated; aspiration: weakly birefringent, stubby rhomboidal crystals; elevated synovial WBC 10-100,000/mm^3	As for gout; if aspiration proven or chondrocalcinosis extensive, consider hyperparathyroidism, hypothyroidism, hemochromatosis, hypomagnesemia, ochronosis, Wilson's disease, acromegaly	As for gout (see also Chapter 136)

Reactive arthritis	Sexually active patients at risk for postgonococcal arthritis; HLA-B27 often present, especially with sacroiliac or spinal involvement and in Reiter's syndrome; may follow dysentery	Antecedent urethritis, dysentery, inflammatory bowel disease, psoriasis, known HIV infection, previous or current eye pain, photophobia, conjunctivitis, iritis, back pain, back stiffness, skin rash, especially on palms or soles or genitalia	Psoriasis or psoriasiform lesions on glans penis, vesiculopustular hyperkeratotic lesions on palms or soles, nail pitting or onycholysis, painless oral ulcers, conjunctivitis, irregular pupils, limited back motion, tenderness over sacroiliac region, tenosynovitis, peripheral arthritis	If acute gonococcal dermatitis/arthritis suspected, appropriate cultures should be obtained (see septic arthritis); if risk factors for HIV, counseling and testing; SI joint plain films may demonstrate sacroiliitis; ANA and RF are negative; consider small bowel series for occult Crohn's disease	With evidence of synovitis of hip: gonococcal arthritis, other septic arthritis; if posterior hip pain and evidence of Reiter's syndrome: sacroiliitis	Indomethacin and naproxen may be more effective than other NSAIDs for Reiter's and spondylitis; phenylbutazone effective but risk of marrow aplasia; sulfasalazine or methotrexate for resistant disease; corticosteroids for severe disease; local injection of involved joint
Referred pain		Pain may be referred from many structures; pelvic and retroperitoneal inflammation or tumors; ureteral stones; osteoarthritis of facet joint, intervertebral disks of spine, pelvic bones	Hip motion usually preserved and does not exacerbate pain; palpable mass may be present in pelvis on abdominal, pelvic, or rectal examination	Plain films of hip and pelvis help to exclude bony pathology; U/A to assess for ureteral stone; consider pregnancy; ultrasound or CT scan of pelvis for pain that remains obscure	Other causes of pain discussed above and below	For pain referred from back; see Chapter 127; pain due to tumors or infections should be treated while underlying problem addressed
Rheumatoid arthritis	1% of population, any age, females more than males	Morning stiffness, symmetric pain in hands and feet, fatigue	Limited hip ROM in all directions, nodules, tenderness of small joints of hands and feet	ESR elevated, RF elevated in 80%, joint fluid WBC elevated	Septic arthritis, gout, pseudogout, apatite arthritis, psoriatic and other seronegative arthritis, rheumatic fever, SLE, viral arthritis (parvovirus B19), Lyme disease, sarcoidosis	Rule out septic arthritis with cultures if monoarthritis; NSAIDs, disease-modifying drugs, oral or injected corticosteroids (see Chapter 133)

See end of table for abbreviations.

Continued

Table 128-1. Selected Causes of Hip Pain—cont'd

Disorder	Epidemiology	History	Physical examination	Diagnostic tests	Differential diagnosis	Management
Septic arthritis	Children: *Haemophilus influenzae,* staphylococcal, streptococcal infection; adolescents and young adults: often gonococcal; older adults: impaired hosts (alcoholic, renal disease, immunosuppressed); staphylococcal, streptococcal, gram-negative bacteria; prior joint damage or chronic inflammation predisposes to infection	Anterior hip pain, usually sudden to subacute onset, generally severe; fever and rigors may occur; skin rash may have been noted; source of sepsis should be sought, e.g., cough, dysuria	Fever in 50%; maculopapular, vesicular, or vesiculopustular rash suggests gonococcal dermatitis arthritis; hip motion reduced in all directions; leathery crepitance may be felt	Blood cultures positive in 50% of nongonococcal bacterial arthritides; synovial WBC usually >50,000/mm^3, often >100,000/mm^3; peripheral WBC elevated in 50%; synovial Gram's stain positive in 50%; plain radiographs may demonstrate effusion or adjacent osteomyelitis; urethral, pharyngeal, rectal, or cervical cultures if appropriate	Purulent fluid aspirated; gonococcal and nongonococcal bacterial arthritis, fungal, mycobacterial infectious arthritis, Lyme disease, Whipple's disease, gout, pseudogout, apatite arthritis, rheumatoid psoriatic arthritis, Reiter's syndrome and reactive arthritis, ankylosing spondylitis, septic iliopectineal bursitis, psoas abscess	Drainage: requires arthrotomy or percutaneous placement of drain under CT guidance; antibiotics: ceftriaxone 1 gm IV every 12 hr for gonococcal arthritis: penicillinase-resistant penicillin (e.g., nafcillin) IV; add aminoglycoside if documented or strongly suspected gram-negative infection, e.g., neutropenic or immunosuppressed patients; analgesics; passive ROM after about 48 hr of treatment
Systemic lupus erythematosus	Young women: women more than men; African-American and Hispanic more than white, complement deficiencies, especially C2; drugs, especially INH, hydralazine, procainamide	Arthralgia, arthritis, malar skin rash, pleurisy, pericarditis, nephritis, seizures, psychosis, fever, malaise, fatigue	Oral ulcers, fundal hemorrhages or exudates; skin rash, especially malar or photosensitive; pleural or pericardial rubs; lymphadenopathy; arthritis of small joints of hands, wrists, feet (symmetric)	ANA present in 90%; anti-SM more specific, as are anti-dsDNA antibodies; anti-ssDNA and antihistone antibodies in drug-induced SLE; Coombs' test, VDRL	Pain may result from avascular necrosis of hip, septic arthritis, synovitis due to SLE, bursitis; most other causes of hip pain may occur in patients with SLE	For arthritis due to SLE, NSAIDs are mainstay; antimalarials (e.g., hydroxychloroquine) for arthritis; corticosteroids generally reserved for treatment of life-threatening disease

bursitis	Bursitis and tendinitis may result from overuse and may be seen in athletic adolescents; post-traumatic trochanteric bursitis may occur at any age: bursitis and tendinitis may be more common in diabetics and those with chronic inflammatory disorders, especially RA, SLE	Lateral hip pain, often aggravated by weight bearing, rising from chair, climbing or descending stairs; patients may note increased pain lying on affected side at night; night pain may be prominent; some patients unable to walk due to severe pain	Tenderness over greater trochanter of femur, reproduces pain; hip motion may be decreased by pain but internal and external rotation relatively preserved; forced adduction may aggravate pain	Plain radiographs show calcific deposits superior and lateral to greater trochanter, irregularity of trochanter, normal hip joint or early osteo-arthritic changes; for severe pain: CBC, ESR may exclude very uncommon septic trochanteric bursitis	Trochanteric fracture or bone bruise due to trauma; impacted fracture of femoral neck; avulsion fracture of greater trochanter (in athletic adoles-cents); meralgia paresthetica (lateral femoral cutaneous neuropathy); radicu-lopathy should not produce local tenderness; herpes zoster before appearance of rash	Conservative: local heat, analgesics or NSAIDs, rest, ultrasound with or without 10% hydrocortisone cream (phonopheresis) for 4-6 wk; local injection: 20-40 mg depomethyl-prednisolone and 2 ml 1% or 2% lidocaine, injected deeply with 1.5-inch 25-gauge or 3.5-inch 22-gauge spinal needle into area of maximal tenderness
Tumors	In childhood: leukemia, neuroblastoma most common solid tumor; in adults: metastatic cancer, lymphoma, soft tissue sarcomas	In children: limp may be noted by parents; in adults: hip pain may be aggravated by weight bearing but often prominent at night, gradual worsen-ing, may be severe, other constitutional symptoms, especially weight loss; review of systems important if no cancer history	If bone lesion: joint motion may be unrestricted and does not reproduce pain; if intrasynovial tumor: restricted joint motion, palpation may detect mass or tenderness of bones or soft tissues; thyroid, chest, breast, rectal, prostate, pelvic exam for suspected primary	Plain films may demonstrate lytic or blastic lesions or erosion of bone; bone scans sensitive for metastatic deposits; CT helpful to define bone lesions and guide biopsy if necessary; MRI useful for soft tissue tumors; CBC, ESR, SPEP, CXR, U/A, VDRL, liver enzymes (chest CT if sarcoma)	Infection, especially osteomyelitis, gummatous syphilis, histiocytosis, amyloidosis, tophaceous gout, hyperparathyroidism, Paget's disease	Analgesia including narcotics if necessary; tricyclics in low dose may be helpful; local or regional nerve blocks for proven malignant neoplasms; radiation therapy; consider prophylactic pinning if lesion is large and involves femoral neck or shaft

ROM, Range of motion; *ESR*, erythrocyte sedimentation rate; *RF*, rheumatoid factor; *WBC*, white blood cell count; *SLE*, systemic lupus erythematosus; *NSAIDs*, nonsteroidal antiinflammatory drugs; *CHF*, congestive heart failure; *RA*, rheumatoid arthritis; *ARF*, acute rheumatic fever; *TSH*, thyroid-stimulating hormone; *DIP*, distal interphalangeal; *SI*, sacroiliac; *ANA*, antinuclear antibodies; *PT*, prothrombin time; *PTT*, partial thromboplastin time; *CPDD*, calcium pyrophosphate deposition disease; *CBC*, complete blood count; *SPEP*, serum protein electrophoresis; *CXR*, chest x-ray; *CT*, computed tomography; *MRI*, magnetic resonance imaging; *HIV*, human immunodeficiency virus; *U/A*, urinalysis; *DTRs*, deep tendon reflexes; *LS*, lumbosacral; *ASLO*, antistreptolysin O; *ECG*, electrocardiogram; *VDRL*, Venereal Disease Research Laboratories; *IV*, intravenously.

Limitation of movement can be assessed by passively taking the hip through its range of motion, which normally consists of 90 to 100 degrees of flexion, 30 degrees of extension, and 30 to 45 degrees of rotation, abduction, and adduction. Palpation and passive motion may reproduce the patient's usual hip pain. A regional neurologic examination should be performed if the history or examination suggests a neuropathic process. Provocative testing, including straight leg raising (SLR) and Lasègue's sign (tensing the sciatic nerve by SLR, then dorsiflexing the foot) for nerve root irritation, are also useful (see Chapter 127). If the history and examination have not led to a definite working diagnosis, a complete physical examination may be necessary, including abdominal, rectal, and pelvic examinations.

LABORATORY TESTS AND DIAGNOSTIC PROCEDURES

Laboratory testing is guided by the findings on the history and physical examination. No standard panel of tests is appropriate for all cases of hip pain. (See Table 128-1.)

Depending on the history and physical findings, radiographs may be unnecessary, especially if (1) symptoms are mild; (2) symptoms result from muscular strain, bursitis, or tendinitis, for which conservative therapy is indicated; or (3) the patient can be relied on to return if symptoms persist or worsen. For more severe pain, when conservative therapy has failed, or when local injection of corticosteroids (e.g., trochanteric bursal injection) is anticipated, plain radiographs of the hip and pelvis are indicated to assess for fractures, neoplasm, or infection. (See Table 128-1.)

Aspiration of fluid from the hip is more difficult than from other, more superficial joints. Failure to obtain fluid with blind aspiration is not adequate to rule out an effusion. In patients with suspected septic arthritis or more chronic undiagnosed arthritis of the hip, arthrocentesis should be performed with fluoroscopic guidance and with instillation of contrast medium to confirm the intraarticular location of the needle tip. This procedure is most often performed by interventional or musculoskeletal radiologists or orthopedic surgeons. Any synovial fluid obtained should be analyzed for glucose, cell count and differential, Gram's stain, and crystals by compensated polarized microscopy. Joint fluid should be cultured routinely for aerobic and facultative anaerobic bacteria. If tuberculosis or opportunistic fungal infection is suspected, additional stains and cultures for mycobacteria and fungi should be obtained.

If the history, physical examination, routine laboratory tests, plain radiographs, and aspiration (if appropriate) do not provide a diagnosis, other tests may be helpful. Technetium pyrophosphate bone scans may demonstrate increased tracer uptake in neoplastic and infectious foci before they are apparent on plain radiographs. Bone scans can also identify stress fractures that may be difficult or impossible to detect on plain films. Gallium scans may detect infectious foci or tumors around the hip or within the pelvis. Computed tomography (CT) scans are useful for providing more detailed bone and soft tissue images and are particularly useful for evaluating pelvic structures, spinal elements, and the sacroiliac joints. CT scans are also moderately sensitive for avascular necrosis of the femoral head. Magnetic resonance imaging (MRI) is currently the most sensitive tool for early detection of avascular necrosis and is also very useful for evaluating the spinal canal, neural foramina, intervertebral disks, muscles, and bursae. With gadolinium enhancement, MRI is very useful in delineating septic diskitis. (See Table 128-1.)

DIFFERENTIAL DIAGNOSIS

See Boxes 128-1 and 128-2 and Table 128-1 for possible causes of pain in the area of the hip.

MANAGEMENT

See Table 128-1 for treatments appropriate in specific diseases. See chapters on specific diseases for additional information on management.

REFERENCES

1. Coombs RR, Thomas RW: Avascular necrosis of the hip, *Br J Hosp Med* 51:275, 1994.
2. Gilbert SR, Lachiewicz PF: Primary synovial osteochondromatosis of the hip: report of two cases with long term follow up after synovectomy and a review of the literature, *Am J Orthop* 26:555, 1997.
3. Gravallese EM et al: Synovitis of the knee in a 42-year-old man: clinicopathologic conference, *Arthritis Rheum* 36:860, 1993.
4. Roberts WN, Williams RB: Hip pain, *Prim Care* 15:783, 1988.

CHAPTER 129

Disorders of the Knee

Elinor A. Mody
Jerry M. Greene

The knee is one of the most frequently injured joints and the joint most often affected by systemic inflammatory and neoplastic disease. The physician must be familiar with the regional anatomy, especially the bony structures, ligaments, tendons, bursae, and cartilage, to perform a focused physical examination of the knee, to order the appropriate diagnostic tests, and to determine the differential diagnosis of the painful knee.

ANATOMY

The knee, one of the largest joints in the body, is formed from the femur, tibia, fibula, and patella. The femoral condyles and tibial plateaus create a hinge, capped by the patella within its tendinous mechanism. The cartilaginous medial and lateral menisci cushion the tibial plateaus and femoral condyles and distribute the forces across these areas. The medial and lateral collateral ligaments and the anterior and posterior cruciate ligaments provide stability to the knee. Several bursae are located external to the synovial membrane and capsule of the knee joint (Figure 129-1).

PATIENT EVALUATION

History

Important historic features include the temporal course of the knee pain and the nature of onset. Pain tends to be acute in cases of trauma, crystal diseases, sepsis, and hemorrhage. A

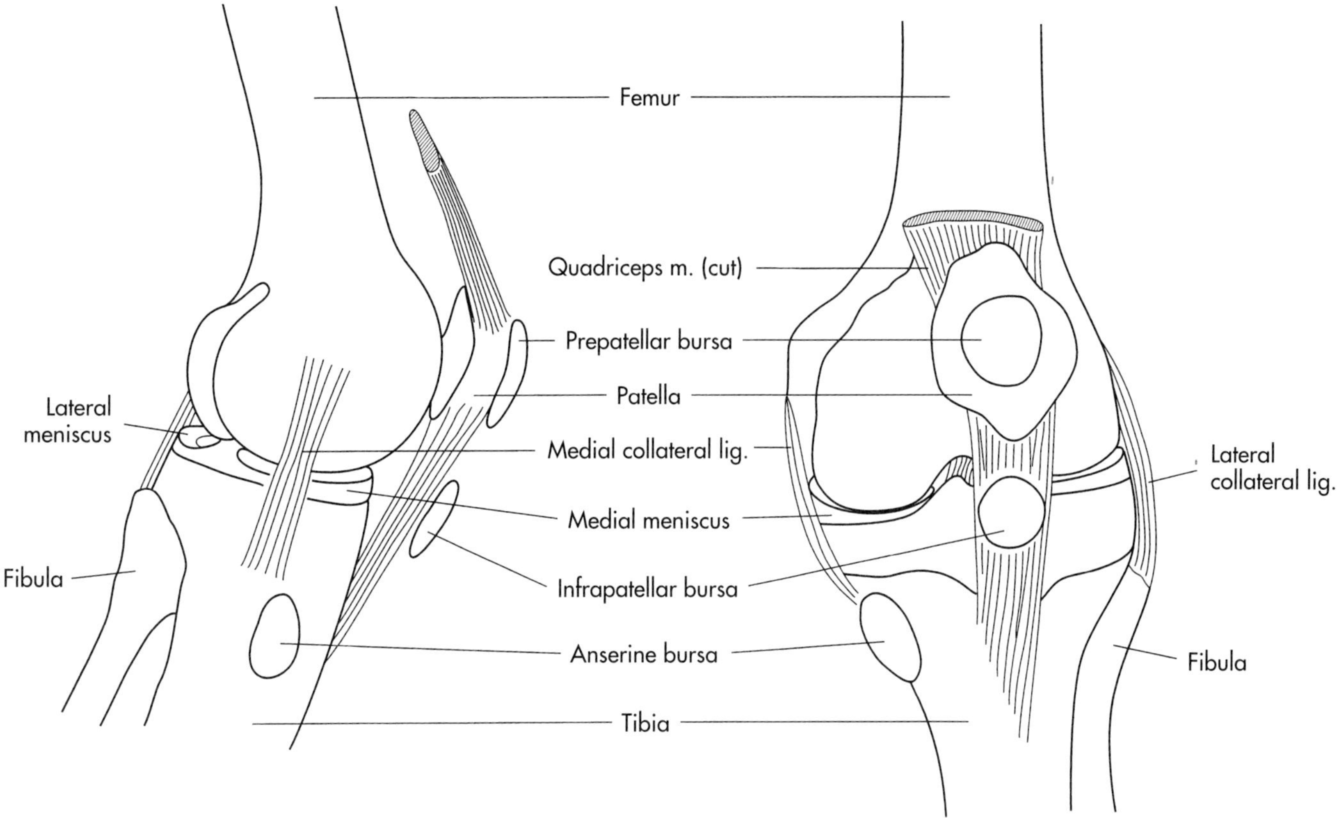

Fig. 129-1. Anatomic landmarks of the knee.

subacute or insidious onset is more consistent with a systemic inflammatory disease, tumor, or osteonecrosis. The location, character, radiation, aggravating and relieving factors, severity of the pain, and associated local symptoms (e.g., swelling, stiffness, redness, limitation of motion) are important historic features to elicit. Systemic symptoms (e.g., weight loss, fever, chills, malaise) are also significant.

The hallmarks of inflammatory synovitis are morning stiffness and pain at rest. Pain only during certain activities suggests a mechanical or traumatic disorder. Involvement of other joints should be assessed. In particular, polyarticular involvement of the joints of the wrists, hands, and feet suggests an inflammatory synovitis such as rheumatoid arthritis. Back pain with morning stiffness suggests spondylitis. A review of systems for rash, myalgias, pleuritic chest pain, mucosal lesions, fever, diarrhea, weight loss, neurologic symptoms, and malaise may suggest other etiologies, such as Lyme disease, inflammatory bowel disease, or systemic lupus erythematosus (SLE).

Hyperparathyroidism, hypothyroidism, hemochromatosis, and aging predispose to calcium pyrophosphate arthropathies, and alcohol abuse predisposes to gout. Unprotected sexual activity and intravenous drug use predispose to gonococcal and nongonococcal bacterial arthritis. Medication history is important. For example, diuretic use may contribute to gouty arthritis, and anticoagulation may increase the risk for hemarthrosis. Review of medical problems is important to assess for contraindications to drug therapy, such as peptic ulcer disease or renal disease when considering nonsteroidal antiinflammatory drug (NSAID) therapy. Family history is always important, since several types of arthritis have a heritable component.

Physical Examination

Inspection of the affected knee should include observation for erythema, ecchymosis, swelling, abrasions, puncture wounds, and active range of motion. The examiner should palpate the joint line, bursae, muscle, tendons, ligaments, and bones in an attempt to localize tenderness. Joint line tenderness may suggest meniscal or ligamentous injury. An effusion may be demonstrated by eliciting a *bulge sign* (Fig. 129-2). As the patient lies supine with knees fully extended and the quadriceps muscle relaxed, the medial aspect of the knee is massaged in a cephalad direction. The lateral aspect of the knee is then stroked inferiorly. An effusion is detected by the resultant bulge sign. Another maneuver to elicit excessive synovial fluid in the knee is to apply rapid, downward pressure on the patella; if a click is felt as the patella touches the femoral condyle, an effusion is probably present. This is also referred to as *patellar ballottement*. Occasionally, obesity or synovial bogginess (as often present in rheumatoid arthritis) may result in a false-positive ballottement sign. The examiner should also palpate the popliteal space for swelling that may occur with popliteal artery aneurysm, Baker's cysts, and tumors. Passive range of motion of the knee should also be performed.

Several maneuvers may help elicit mechanical disorders. *McMurray's test* is useful for diagnosing meniscal injury. This is performed by passive flexion of the knee with the patient lying supine. The lower leg is externally rotated at full

A

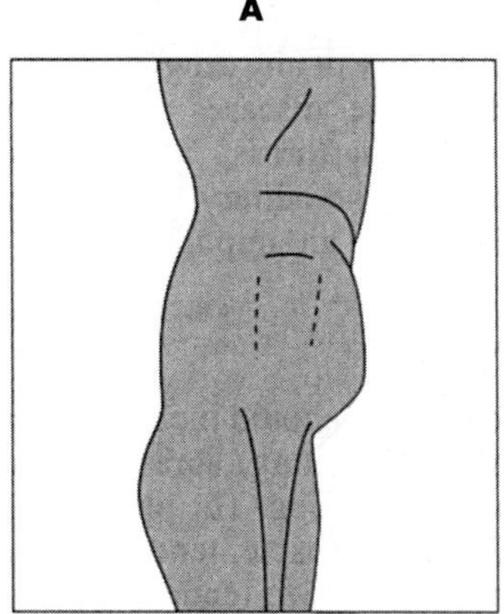

B

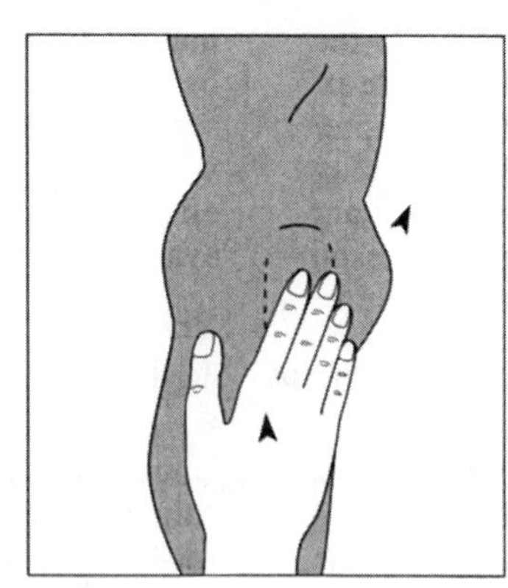

C

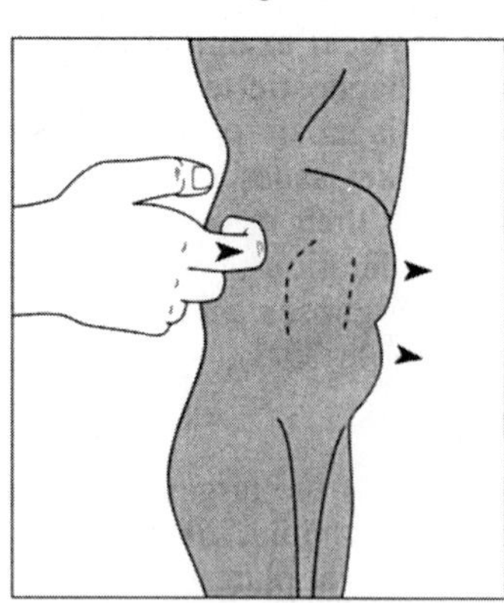

Fig. 129-2. **A,** Bulge sign for knee effusion. **B,** Fluid is palpated into suprapatellar bursa. **C,** Downward pressure exerted along the lateral aspect of the knee produces a bulge down the medial aspect.

flexion, then held in external rotation, and the knee is passively extended. A painful click near the top of the extension arc is a positive finding. The maneuver is then repeated with the lower leg in internal rotation. This tests for both medial and lateral meniscal tears or injury. Simply taking the knee through flexion and extension while feeling and listening for crepitus is also helpful in assessing such mechanical problems as a loose body in the knee joint. In the absence of signs of inflammation, crepitus suggests osteoarthritis.

A general examination may reveal evidence of a systemic disease associated with knee pathology. The nervous system, back, and hip merit particular attention because of possible referred pain to the knee. Cutaneous clues to the cause of arthritis include psoriasis, erythema chronicum migrans, rheumatoid nodules, and tophi.

LABORATORY TESTS AND DIAGNOSTIC PROCEDURES

Often the first diagnostic test sought after a thorough physical examination is a radiograph, particularly if there is a history of trauma or if a mechanical disorder is suspected. The most useful view is an anteroposterior (AP) film, which allows visualization of the medial and lateral femorotibial compartments of the knee. If fracture is not suspected, weight-bearing AP radiographs most accurately assess narrowing of the cartilage of the femorotibial joint. The skyline, or sunrise, view allows the physician to visualize the patella and the patellar surfaces that contact the femoral condyles. Tunnel views may also help, particularly in assessing ligamentous injuries, osteoarthritis, intraarticular loose bodies, and osteonecrosis. The lateral view is particularly helpful in assessing for effusion in the suprapatellar recess.

Synovial fluid analysis is important in distinguishing noninflammatory conditions from inflammatory joint disease. Arthrocentesis should always be performed under aseptic conditions to prevent infection and to obtain a sterile specimen for bacterial cultures. In immunocompromised patients, fungal and mycobacterial cultures should be sent as well. Another specimen should be sent for white blood cell count (WBC) and differential. If WBC reveals more than $1000/mm^3$, the fluid is inflammatory. WBC may also reveal evidence of intraarticular bleeding. If the synovial fluid is inflammatory, Gram's stain and culture should be performed to evaluate for joint sepsis. The fluid is examined with polarizing microscopy for birefringent crystals, specifically sodium urate and calcium pyrophosphate. With alizarin red staining of joint fluid smears, hydroxyapatite crystals may be visualized. The presence of fat droplets in synovial fluid suggests fracture of the bone into the marrow space.

Several blood tests may help in evaluation of knee pain. Erythrocyte sedimentation rate is a general screen for inflammatory disorders, as is a complete blood count, particularly WBC and differential. A routine chemistry panel is useful to assess for renal disease because renal insufficiency may affect therapeutic options. Depending on the clinical setting, serum urate level, rheumatoid factor, or antinuclear antibody level may also be helpful. Serum calcium, phosphate, magnesium, alkaline phosphatase, thyroid function, and iron studies should be considered in patients with pseudogout or chondrocalcinosis.

Magnetic resonance imaging (MRI) allows visualization of joint fluid, synovial swelling, ligaments, menisci, cartilage, and bone (including marrow). If infection is suspected and cannot be completely characterized by the routine methods, arthroscopy with synovial biopsy may be considered; this is particularly helpful if fungal or mycobacterial arthritis is suspected. Arthroscopy may also assist in the evaluation and treatment of internal derangements of the knee, such as meniscal tears.

SELECTED CAUSES OF KNEE PAIN

Inflammatory Arthritis

Any arthritis causing a purulent effusion is regarded as inflammatory. Although this category includes many different diseases, some general patterns occur; frequently more than one joint is affected, and the conditions tend to be chronic or recurrent. Knee arthritis may be a prominent manifestation of the disease. Inflammatory joint diseases that frequently involve the knee include gout, calcium pyrophosphate arthropathy (pseudogout), rheumatoid arthritis, the spondyloarthropathies (e.g., ankylosing spondylitis, Reiter's syndrome), septic arthritis, Lyme disease, mechanical disorders, and tumors (Table 129-1).

Mechanical Disorders

Mechanical disorders of the knee may involve bone, cartilage, and periarticular structures such as bursae, tendons, and ligaments.

Fracture. Most fractures within the knee involve the tibial plateaus or patella. A history of trauma followed by acute onset of pain and swelling suggests intraarticular fracture, and physical examination should be limited to assessing neurovascular integrity of the leg. Swelling and limited range of motion are usually present. The thigh, knee, and lower leg should be immobilized and radiographs obtained (AP, lateral, sunrise views). If a fracture is documented, aspiration may be deferred unless septic arthritis is strongly suspected as well. Occasionally the diagnosis of fracture is not definite even with radiographs. Aspirated synovial fluid may reveal a bloody effusion or frank blood, and Sudan red stain to detect fat droplets from the marrow should be performed. Computed tomography (CT) or MRI may help detect fractures not evident on plain films. The differential diagnosis includes other traumatic injuries (e.g., meniscal tear, ligamentous injury), other causes of hemarthrosis (e.g., pigmented villonodular synovitis), and bleeding disorders (e.g., hemophilia, anticoagulant therapy). Management of an intraarticular fracture includes immobilization and prompt orthopedic consultation.

Ligamentous Injury. Ligamentous injuries often result from athletic injuries and frequently involve the knee. The history usually reveals pivoting on the knee after a jump, excessive extension, or medial or lateral stress. Often the patient describes the feeling of something "giving" within the joint, followed by acute onset of pain and swelling.[5] Joint laxity may be apparent if the ligament tear is complete. Physical examination may reveal swelling and, depending on the ligament involved, point tenderness over the medial joint line (medial collateral ligament) or lateral joint line (lateral collateral ligament). To test for a cruciate ligamentous tear, instability of the joint may be assessed with the *anteroposterior drawer test.* With the knee flexed 90 degrees, the examiner attempts to pull the tibia forward, away from the femur. If laxity is detected, an anterior cruciate ligament tear is likely. By reversing the force, the posterior cruciate ligament is tested. Medial and lateral collateral ligaments are tested by applying pressure on the lateral aspect of the knee, stressing the medial collateral ligament. These forces are reversed to test the lateral collateral ligament while the patient lies supine with the knee extended. Laxity indicates a collateral ligament injury. As with fractures, neurovascular examination is important. Although plain radiographs help rule out fracture, the imaging study of choice to diagnose ligamentous tears is MRI. Joint aspiration generally reveals either serosanguineous, noninflammatory fluid or a bloody effusion. Differential diagnosis includes meniscal tear, fracture, or sprain. Management for complete tear in active patients is usually surgical repair.

Meniscal Tear. The two groups of patients likely to have meniscal tears are young adults with a history of trauma and middle-aged or elderly patients with osteoarthritis. Medial are more common than lateral meniscal tears. A meniscal tear presents with acute or subacute pain. Patients may experience the knee "giving way" or have painful popping or locking. On examination, swelling is common, with warmth and point tenderness over either the medial or the lateral joint line. Physical examination includes the McMurray's test, although a negative test does not exclude meniscal pathology. Diagnostic tests include radiographs to evaluate for fractures, osteoarthritis, and intraarticular loose bodies. Aspiration generally yields noninflammatory fluid that may be bloody, depending on the extent of the tear. The best imag ing study to diagnose a meniscal tear is MRI, generally done only if the diagnosis is in doubt or surgical intervention is anticipated. Initial management is conservative: rest, crutches, and analgesics. If symptoms do not resolve within several weeks, orthopedic referral is appropriate. The dif ferential diagnosis includes fracture, avascular necrosis, intraarticular loose bodies, and ligamentous injury.

Osteonecrosis. Sickle cell anemia, corticosteroid therapy, decompression illness, alcoholism, trauma, SLE, and dyslipoproteinemias predipose to osteonecrosis, also known as *avascular necrosis.* Osteonecrosis presents as acute pain, sometimes accompanied by swelling. Physical examination may reveal an effusion and tenderness over the lateral or medial joint line.[4] Range of motion may vary. If the process has been limited and painful, an AP radiograph may reveal an area of sclerosis and collapse of the affected femoral condyle or tibial plateau. Patients who are examined earlier may have normal radiographs. At this stage, MRI is the diagnostic study of choice. A bone scan may also reveal changes before a plain radiograph does. The differential diagnosis includes fracture, meniscal tear, neoplasm, osteomyelitis, and osteoarthritis. Initial management is conservative, with rest, NSAIDs, and muscle strengthening. If this is not effective, orthopedic consultation is recommended for possible tibial osteotomy or, in the case of established secondary osteoarthritis, hemiarthroplasty or total knee replacement.[2,3,6]

Osgood-Schlatter Syndrome. Osgood-Schlatter syndrome is a benign condition seen in adolescents. The patient complains of pain inferior to the patella. On physical examination, pain is elicited by palpation of the patellar tendon's attachment to the tibial tuberosity. The condition is typically self-limited and requires no therapy other than avoiding stress to the quadriceps tendon mechanism.

Chondromalacia. Also known as the *patellofemoral syndrome,* chondromalacia is also a disease of predominantly young, active individuals, particularly women. This overuse syndrome often affects the weekend athlete. The onset of knee pain is often subacute and is worse with use, particularly on climbing stairs and standing up after sitting. At rest, pain is generally minimal. Physical examination may reveal an effusion and warmth. Pain may be reproduced by direct downward pressure of the patella against the femoral condyles while the patient lies supine. Routine radiographs may reveal irregularity of the patella's undersurface. Synovial fluid is characteristically noninflammatory. The differential diagnosis includes tendinitis, bursitis, meniscal tear, and

Table 129-1. Selected Causes of Knee Pain

Disorder	Epidemiology	History	Physical examination	Diagnostic tests	Differential diagnosis	Management
Gout	Middle age, elderly, overproducers of urate, transplant patients	Acute onset of pain, often with previous attack in first MTP	Warmth, erythema, effusion, exquisite tenderness	High synovial WBC, urate crystals seen under polarizing microscope, "rat bite" erosions on radiograph	RA, spondylitis, other crystal-induced arthropathy, infection	NSAIDs, colchicine, local corticosteroid injection (acute), allopurinol or uricosuric (chronic)
Pseudogout	Elderly, patients with metabolic disorders, e.g., hypothyroidism, hypomagnesemia, ochronosis, hemochromatosis, Wilson's disease, hyperparathyroidism	Acute onset of pain; if metabolic disease, systemic complaints	Similar to gout	High synovial WBC, calcium pyrophosphate crystals seen under polarizing microscope, chondrocalcinosis on radiograph	Gout, RA, spondylitis, infection	NSAIDs, colchicine, local corticosteroid injection (acute), daily colchicine as prophylaxis against further attacks[1]
Rheumatoid arthritis	Age varies, usually female	Morning stiffness, involvement of joints of hand, multiple joint involvement, fatigue, multiple attacks	Warmth, erythema with effusion, "boggy" synovium with longstanding disease, symmetric involvement of joints, decreased ROM	High synovial WBC, RF often positive, elevated ESR, anemia, consistent with chronic disease, bone erosions on radiographs	Crystal-induced arthropathy, spondylitis, infection	NSAIDs, local corticosteroid injection, second-line agents (e.g., methotrexate, gold)
Spondyloarthropathy (reactive arthritis, Reiter's syndrome)	Young adults, male predominance; patients with associated disorders, e.g., IBD; psoriasis; *Chlamydia*, *Yersinia*, or *Shigella* infection; ankylosing spondylitis	Acute or subacute onset of pain, often with low back pain; pain in other joints; component of morning stiffness; possible systemic complaints related to underlying condition	Warmth, erythema, with effusion; "boggy" synovium with longstanding disease; evidence of underlying disease (e.g., oral ulcers, rash, nail changes); decreased ROM of spine	High synovial WBC, erosions on radiograph, sacroiliitis on radiograph, squaring of vertebral bodies, syndesmophytes	RA, crystal-induced arthritis, infection	NSAIDs, local corticosteroid injection, sulfasalazine, methotrexate
Gonococcal infection	Young adults predominantly, but any age if sexually active	Acute onset of symptoms, may complain of GU symptoms, recent menses, general malaise	Warmth, erythema, with very large tense effusion, decreased ROM, maculopapular rash over trunk, fever, urethral or cervical discharge, arthritis of other joints, tenosynovitis	High synovial WBC, positive culture for gonococci from genitourinary tract, blood, or synovial fluid	RA, spondylitis, crystal-induced arthropathy, nongonococcal infection, Lyme disease	Ceftriaxone, penicillin G for sensitive strains

Nongonococcal infection	IV drug abusers, severely debilitated, patients prone to fulminant sepsis or endocarditis	Acute onset of severe pain, swelling, redness, decreased ROM, possible associated systemic symptoms, and arthritis in other joints	Warmth, erythema, effusion, decreased ROM, signs of source for bacteremia (e.g., pneumonia, UTI)	Very high synovial WBC, positive synovial or blood culture or Gram's stain, high ESR, elevated peripheral WBC, periosteal elevation on radiograph suggests concomitant osteomyelitis	RA, spondylitis, crystal-induced arthritis, gonococcal infection	IV antibiotic therapy guided by Gram's stain, culture results, sensitivities; drain with needle aspiration or arthroscopically; ROM exercises; analgesics
Lyme disease	Travelers to or residents of endemic areas	Subacute onset of symptoms, swelling, warmth, decreased ROM, pain, history of ECM skin lesion(s), Bell's palsy, other painful joints	Warmth, erythema, effusion, "boggy" synovium with longstanding disease	Lyme titers, synovial fluid culture rarely positive, radiographs may eventually show erosions	RA, spondylitis, gonococcal and other nongonococcal infection, crystal-induced arthropathy	IV penicillin G, ceftriaxone
Fracture	Any age, risk factors include steroid use, osteoporosis, metastatic malignancy	History of trauma, sudden onset of pain, swelling, warmth	Swelling, tenderness over affected area, pain on weight bearing, decreased ROM	Bloody synovial fluid, may show fat droplets under polarizing microscopy, fracture seen on radiograph, bone scan may detect stress fractures inapparent on radiograph	Meniscal tear, ligamentous tear, hemophilia, PVNS, anticoagulant therapy	Splinting to protect against additional neurovascular injury, reduction, casting
Ligamentous injury	Young adults, athletes	Trauma with pivoting or hyperextension, feeling of "giving way," acute pain and swelling	Swelling, point tenderness medial or lateral joint line, positive anterior/posterior drawer sign, medial or lateral laxity depending on ligament disrupted	Bloody or serosanguineous noninflammatory synovial fluid, radiographs to rule out fracture, MRI reveals high T2 signal in area of ligamentous tear	Meniscal tear, fracture, hemophilia, PVNS, anticoagulant therapy	Analgesics, knee immobilizer, orthopedic consultation for surgical repair of complete tears in active patients
Meniscal tear	Two groups: elderly with OA and young adults, athletes	Acute or subacute onset of pain, locking, painful popping	Swelling, tenderness over the lateral or medial joint line, positive McMurray's test	Bloody or serosanguineous synovial fluid, radiograph to rule out fracture; MRI, arthrography, or arthroscopy diagnostic	Fracture, ligamentous tear, hemophilia, PVNS, anticoagulant therapy, worsening OA	Initial conservative (rest, NSAIDs), if unsuccessful, orthopedic referral for arthroscopic debridement, or total knee replacement if concomitant severe OA

See end of table for abbreviations.

Continued

Table 129-1. Selected Causes of Knee Pain—cont'd

Disorder	Epidemiology	History	Physical examination	Diagnostic tests	Differential diagnosis	Management
Osteonecrosis (AVN)	Any age, patients with sickle cell anemia, chronic steroid use, alcoholism, decompression illness, trauma, SLE, dyslipoproteinemia	Acute onset of pain, swelling, rest pain, increased pain with weight bearing	Swelling, tenderness, decreased ROM	Area of subchondral collapse appears after weeks on plain radiograph, MRI most sensitive for AVN before subchondral collapse	Tumor, fracture osteomyelitis, OA, meniscal tear	Conservative initial (no weight bearing, NSAIDs, analgesics); if unsuccessful, tibial osteotomy, hemiarthroplasty, or total knee replacement
Osgood-Schlatter syndrome	Young adolescents	Pain at the inferior aspect of the patella, subacute to chronic onset	Tenderness to palpation, occasionally swelling in region of tibial tubercle	None	Fracture, tendinitis of patellar tendon, tumor, osteomyelitis	Reassurance, analgesics
Chondromalacia	Young active persons, either gender	Subacute onset of patellar pain, worse walking stairs, little pain at rest	Reproduction of pain on pressing patella against femoral condyles	Synovial fluid noninflammatory, sunrise radiograph may reveal irregularity of articulating surface of patella	Tendinitis, bursitis, meniscal injury	Isometric quadriceps-strengthening exercises, NSAIDs, pure analgesics
Anserine bursitis	Middle age, elderly with OA, young active patients	Subacute onset of pain localized to the posteromedial aspect of knee	Point tenderness over anserine bursa, rarely palpable swelling	None	OA, medial meniscal injury	NSAIDs, local heat, local corticosteroid injection
Prepatellar bursitis	Those who kneel on hard surfaces, especially carpenters, plumbers, roofers, carpet layers	Subacute onset of pain in prepatellar area; swelling, erythema, desquamation, or purulent discharge suggests septic bursitis	Tenderness, erythema, fluctuant swelling of bursa anterior to patella, knee flexion may be limited but full extension possible without increased pain	Bursal aspirate, culture, Gram's stain, crystal search	Cellulitis, gouty bursitis, hemobursa, septic bursitis, patellar fracture, fat necrosis, erythema nodosum	If septic: antibiotics, repeated needle aspiration for drainage; if nonseptic: NSAIDs, local heat, activity modification

	Middle aged, elderly, athletes, obese, those with prior knee trauma	Progressive, pain, stiffness, decreased ROM over years, "cracking" of joint, no rest pain unless very advanced arthritis, short-lived morning stiffness (minutes)	Decreased ROM, swelling, crepitation, bony prominence	Synovial fluid noninflammatory, osteophyte formation, subchondral cysts, sclerosis, joint space narrowing seen on radiograph	Inflammatory arthritis, meniscal tear, anserine bursitis, secondary forms of OA: hemochromatosis, Wilson's disease, ochronosis, gout, acromegaly, hypothyroidism, hyperparathyroidism	Analgesics or NSAIDs, quadriceps-strengthening exercises, weight loss if appropriate, use of cane Consider surgical intervention (tibial osteotomy or total knee replacement) for unremitting pain
Malignancy	Metastatic cancer most common; primary bone and soft tissue sarcomas less likely; leukemia; lymphoma; myeloma	Slowly worsening pain, swelling, stiffness, prominent night pain is suggestive	Decreased ROM, diffuse tenderness, effusion	Synovial fluid with lymphocytic predominance, tumor cells sometimes seen, periosteal disruption or lytic bone lesions on plain radiograph; MRI defines bone and soft tissue involvement; biopsy if no known primary	Inflammatory arthritis, benign tumors, osteomyelitis	Primary tumors: surgical excision or amputation, adjuvant chemotherapy or radiation therapy Metastatic tumors: radiation therapy for pain control, other treatment based on type of malignancy

MTP, Metatarsophalangeal joint; *WBC*, white blood cell count; *RA*, rheumatoid arthritis; *NSAIDs*, nonsteroidal antiinflammatory drugs; *ROM*, range of motion; *RF*, rheumatoid factor; *ESR*, erythrocyte sedimentation rate; *IBD*, inflammatory bowel disease; *IV*, intravenous; *UTI*, urinary tract infection; *ECM*, erythema chronicum migrans; *PVNS*, pigmented villonodular synovitis; *OA*, osteoarthritis; *SLE*, systemic lupus erythematosus; *AVN*, avascular necrosis; *MRI*, magnetic resonance imaging.

osteoarthritis. Management is conservative, with quadriceps-strengthening exercises and NSAIDs.

Anserine Bursitis. Anserine bursitis generally affects middle-aged and elderly individuals with osteoarthritis of the knee, although it can occur in young, active individuals. Pain is subacute at onset and localized to the inferomedial aspect of the knee. Physical examination reveals point tenderness on palpation of the anserine bursa (see Fig. 129-1). Signs of osteoarthritis of the knee may be found. The differential diagnosis includes osteoarthritis and medial meniscal injury. Management includes local corticosteroid injection, NSAIDs, heat, and ultrasound, which may be combined with topical 10% hydrocortisone cream.

Prepatellar Bursitis. Also called *housemaid's knee,* prepatellar bursitis often results from prolonged kneeling on a hard surface and tends to be an occupational injury. Inflammation occurs in the prepatellar bursa (see Fig. 129-1). Pain, swelling, and erythema over the patella are often present. Knee extension is generally full, but flexion is limited because of traction on the inflamed soft tissues. Relatively painless motion from full extension to about 90 degrees of flexion helps distinguish prepatellar bursitis from inflammation of the true knee joint. If a bursal effusion is present, aspiration of the bursa should be attempted. If fluid is obtained, WBC should be obtained. If the fluid is inflammatory, septic bursitis must be considered. Since fever, peripheral leukocytosis, and positive bursal fluid Gram's stain for bacteria may be present, aspirated fluid should be cultured. The differential diagnosis includes septic bursitis, patellar fracture, arthritis of the knee, and cellulitis. Management is conservative and includes NSAIDs, rest, protective knee pads, and avoidance of further trauma. If septic bursitis is likely, empiric antibiotics to cover staphylococcal and streptococcal species should be given after bursal fluid aspiration, Gram's stain, and culture.

Synovial Tumors

In general, tumors of the synovium and bone are rare causes of knee pain. The diverse malignancies that involve the knee include chondrosarcoma, synovial sarcoma, lymphoma, osteosarcoma, neuroblastoma, and metastatic carcinomas of many origins. Marrow involvement with leukemia may also produce knee pain, especially in children. Pain from knee involvement is similar, regardless of the underlying neoplasm, being subacute to chronic and becoming constant with progression. Swelling of the joint and decreased range of motion are variable. Physical examination may reveal knee warmth, swelling, restricted motion, effusion, and tenderness over the affected area. Routine radiographs may reveal disruption of the periosteum and trabeculae and a soft tissue mass. If plain films do not reveal changes, CT or MRI scans may suggest the disease. Biopsy is necessary for diagnosis and should be performed carefully to avoid seeding uninvolved tissues. Synovial fluid is usually inflammatory with a lymphocytic predominance. Tumor cells are sometimes seen in synovial fluid. Differential diagnosis includes inflammatory arthritis and infection with concomitant osteomyelitis, particularly if the leukocyte count is greater than 10,000. Local management includes radiation and surgical debridement. Fixation with intramedullary rods may be needed for large lytic lesions, which predispose to pathologic fracture. Systemic management is determined by the nature of the malignancy.

REFERENCES

1. Alvarellos A, Spilberg I: Colchicine prophylaxis in pseudogout, *J Rheumatol* 13:804, 1986.
2. Case report, *N Engl J Med* 316:736, 1987.
3. Lotke P et al: Osteonecrosis of the knee, *Orthop Clin North Am* 16:593, 1985.
4. Mankin H: Nontraumatic necrosis of bone (osteonecrosis), *N Engl J Med* 326:1473, 1992.
5. McCune J et al: Evaluation of knee pain, *Prim Care* 15:795, 1988.
6. Spiera H: Osteoarthritis as a misdiagnosis in elderly patients, *Geriatrics* 42:37, 1987.

CHAPTER 130

Disorders of the Foot and Ankle

Robert G. Frykberg

Foot problems, although usually not serious, can be a significant source of discomfort or morbidity. A simple ingrown toenail may first be only an annoyance that limits one's ability to walk comfortably and that is easily treated. When left unattended or improperly treated, however, this common malady can progress to cellulitis or osteomyelitis. In the patient with diabetes mellitus or significant peripheral vascular disease, an infected ingrown toenail can lead to gangrene and subsequent amputation. Once a lower extremity amputation has been performed in these high-risk patients, their 5-year survival rates approach only 50%. Although this is a rather dramatic scenario not common to most foot disorders, it illustrates the significance of failing to manage properly an easily treatable condition at an early stage. As with any medical problem, most foot and ankle disorders can be effectively resolved with early diagnosis and appropriate intervention.

In an attempt to quantify the incidence and prevalence of foot disorders in the civilian noninstitutionalized U.S. population, the National Center for Health Statistics designed and conducted the 1990 National Health Interview Survey (NHIS) with a special supplement dealing exclusively with the foot.[5] From the 120,000 responses to the podiatry supplement, data were available for the first time on the magnitude and range of specific problems afflicting the general U.S. population. *Incidence* was defined by the number of respondents or family members who had foot trouble within the previous 12 months, and *prevalence* was defined by those who currently had the problem at the time of interview. The results represent age-adjusted values, using the age distribution of the U.S. population as the standard (Table 130-1). Of the estimated 43.1 million people with foot problems in the 12-month period (175 per 1000 population), toenail problems (ingrown or other), foot infections (including athlete's foot and warts), and corns or calluses each affected more than 11 million. Corns and calluses have the

Table 130-1. Incidence and Prevalence of Foot Problems in the United States, 1990

Problem	People who reported having had this problem in the past 12 months: Number (in millions)	People who reported having had this problem in the past 12 months: Rate per 1000 population	People who reported having this condition now: Number (in millions)	People who reported having this condition now: Rate per 1000 population
Ingrown toenails or other toenail problems	11.3	46	7.3	30
Foot infection, including athlete's foot, other fungal infections, and warts	11.3	46	6.2	25
Corns and calluses	11.2	45	9.2	38
Foot injury (sprain, strain, fracture, or dislocation)	5.6	23	1.8	7
Flatfeet or fallen arches	4.6	19	4.4	18
Bunions	4.4	18	3.8	16
Arthritis of toes	3.9	16	3.5	14
Toe and joint deformities (hammer toe, claw toe, missing toes)	2.5	10	2.2	9
Bone spurs	0.95	4	0.67	3
Nerve damage to foot	0.23	0.9	0.17	0.7
Clubfoot	0.16	0.6	0.13	0.5
Others	2.7	11	2.2	9
Total number of conditions reported	58.8	239	41.6	170
Unduplicated number of persons involved	43.1	175	31.7	129

From Greenberg L, Davis H: Foot problems in the US: the 1990 National Health Interview Survey, *J Am Podiatr Med Assoc* 83:475, 1993.

Table 130-2. Number of People per 1000 Who Reported Having Specific Foot Problems in the Past 12 Months, by Gender and Race, 1990

Problem	Total US	By gender: Men	By gender: Women	By race: White	By race: Black
Toenail problems	46	42	49	48	33
Foot infections	46	61	31	49	28
Corns and calluses	45	30	60	45	56
Foot injuries	23	23	22	24	15
Flatfeet	19	19	18	18	25
Bunions	18	6	29	18	17
Arthritis of toes	16	10	22	17	13
Toe and joint deformities	10	6	14	11	5
All foot problems combined	175	163	186	182	144

From Greenberg L, Davis H: Foot problems in the US: the 1990 National Health Interview Survey, *J Am Podiatr Med Assoc* 83:475, 1993.

greatest prevalence of all disorders, with 9.2 million people affected and a prevalence rate of 38 per 1000. The second most prevalent condition is toenail problems, which chronically affect more than 7 million people at a rate of 30 per 1000. A common and often neglected deformity, hallux valgus (bunion), affects 3.8 million people, or 16 per 1000, ranking second only to flatfeet as one of the most prevalent recognized foot deformities in the U.S. population. Table 130-2 presents the incidence of specific foot problems stratified by gender and race. Females report foot problems much more frequently than males, especially bunions, which are five times more common in women than in men. Whites report foot problems more often than blacks, although blacks report corns and calluses 30% more often than whites. Incidence of all disorders rises significantly with age (Table 130-3). In the age group under 5 years, the incidence of all foot problems combined is only 26 per 1000 but dramatically rises to 336 per 1000 in those age 75 and older. Older adults age 65 or over have foot problems almost three times more often than young adults ages 18 to 44.[5]

NAIL AND SKIN DISORDERS

Nail pathology is one of the most common of all foot conditions, affecting more than 11 million annually.

Onychomycosis

Fungal infection of the toenails is undoubtedly the most prevalent of nail and skin disorders, often involving all 10 toenails in extreme cases. Although painless and fairly benign, onychomycosis *(tinea unguium)* causes concern and frustration because it responds poorly to most treatments.[3,6] The mycotic nail is easily recognized by its typical yellowish white, opaque appearance on a thickened nail plate. On close inspection the accumulation of subungual debris is evident and often appears as a "double" nail. Most often the infection begins at the distal aspect of the nail plate and gradually spreads proximally to involve the nail matrix, nail bed, and entire nail plate. Frequently the patient had an injury in the remote past, with subungual hematoma, loss of the nail, and regrowth of the dystrophic nail. Chronic plantar and interdigital dermatophytosis is usually associated with the nail involvement. The most common infecting organisms are *Trichophyton rubrum* and *T. mentagrophytes,* although *Candida albicans* can often be cultured from moist subungual debris. Differential diagnoses include psoriatic nails, lichen planus, and posttraumatic nail dystrophy. Diagnosis can be confirmed by gathering nail and debris scrapings for dermatophyte culture or potassium hydroxide (KOH) examination. Placing the scrapings in a drop of KOH on a glass slide should reveal the fungal hyphae coursing through the epidermal cells.

Definitive treatment for onychomycosis has traditionally been disappointing, and therefore palliation with periodic debridement has most often been the treatment of choice. Only early in the course of fungal infection under the nail is topical antifungal treatment effective. Miconazole, clotrimazole, ketoconazole, and terbinafine creams may be beneficial when applied twice daily to a debrided nail for months until improvement is noted. Trials of oral ketoconazole or griseofulvin have had limited success. Liver toxicity, gastrointestinal disturbances, and blood dyscrasias frequently accompany prolonged use, with recurrence following discontinuance of the medicine. Two newer oral antifungal agents have an improved safety profile and more clinical efficacy (90%) for this recalcitrant problem. Itraconazole, a broad-spectrum agent active against dermatophytes, saprophytes, and *Candida,* is effectively administered with a pulsed dosing schedule of 200 mg twice daily for 7 days in each of 3 consecutive months. Plasma clearance occurs in 7 to 10 days, providing a depot effect in the skin and nails for 6 to 10 months. Although liver toxicity and other adverse events are rare, metabolism through the cytochrome P-450 enzyme pathway precludes use of itraconazole in patients taking cisapride, terfenadine, astemizole, and lovastatin. Terbinafine, an allylamine, is effective only against the dermatophytes and is administered for 90 days in single daily doses of 250 mg. Taste disturbances and agranulocytosis are reported, but liver toxicity is not a significant complication of terbinafine treatment.

Permanent surgical removal of the nail with matrixectomy remains the only certain method of eradicating the mycotic nail with severe dystrophy of the nail plate. This is not usually performed, however, unless the nail becomes symptomatic. Although untested by formal clinical trials, simple temporary removal of the nail (avulsion) followed by topical antifungal treatment generally is not clinically effective. Once the nail is completely infected into the matrix, total permanent removal (matrixectomy) will prevent reinfection.

Onychocryptosis

The most symptomatic of nail dystrophies, onychocryptosis *(ingrown toenail)* ranges from a simple pinching of a distal skin fold to a severely infected paronychia with granuloma formation. This painful malady is frequently self-inflicted through "bathroom surgery" on nail borders. Self-treatment of this disorder often exacerbates a relatively benign condition. Cryptotic nail borders may therefore be idiopathic, iatrogenic, or secondary to injured matrix tissue, hypertrophic nail folds, or a subungual exostosis. Tight shoes and injudicious nail care often lead to an inflamed nail fold from an offending nail border or spicule. Patients in the habit of digging out the corners of a painful nail often leave a deep portion of the nail intact, which acts as a lancet and grows forward into the distal nail groove. A paronychia then develops from the break in the skin, followed by a granuloma ("proud flesh") from the chronic irritation and inflammation (Fig. 130-1). Extremely incurvated or "tented" nails may be caused by the constant deforming pressure from a subungual exostosis on the dorsum of the distal phalanx, and exostosis must be treated as well as the nail disorder.

The primary goal of treatment for any ingrown toenail is to remove the offending nail border from the inflamed skin fold (ungualabia). Antibiotic administration and soaks may reduce inflammation and infection when present but usually are not sufficient to resolve the problem. The severity of the condition usually dictates the appropriate treatment. A simple

Table 130-3. Number of People per 1000 Who Reported Having Specific Foot Problems in the Past 12 Months, by Age, 1990

	Age (years)							
Problem	**Under 5**	**5-17**	**18-24**	**25-44**	**45-64**	**65-69**	**70-74**	**75 and older**
Toenail problems	5	20	39	44	59	78	94	123
Foot infections	5	44	45	52	52	55	46	41
Corns and calluses	*	5	23	48	72	90	105	125
Foot injuries	3	22	36	28	21	17	14	10
Flatfeet	7	14	20	20	23	25	24	23
Bunions	*	2	8	14	29	44	47	66
Arthritis of toes	*	1	3	7	30	47	68	68
Toe and joint deformities	2	3	4	6	16	24	39	41
All foot problems combined	26	100	148	179	229	281	316	336

From Greenberg L, Davis H: Foot problems in the US: the 1990 National Health Interview Survey, *J Am Podiatr Med Assoc* 83:475, 1993.
*Statistically unreliable; fewer than 10 observations in the sample.

nail debridement of the nail's distal corner usually is enough to eradicate a minor paronychia. Occasionally, packing the nail groove with cotton after trimming the nail back is helpful. In more advanced cases, especially those with granuloma formation, avulsion of the nail or nail border under local anesthesia is required to allow resolution of the process before regrowth of the nail. With chronic recurrent onychocryptosis, permanent removal of the entire nail or just the offending nail borders should be performed by a matrixectomy procedure, including phenol or sodium hydroxide chemical cauterization, surgical techniques (e.g., Zadik, Winograd, Frost), or carbon dioxide (CO_2) laser vaporization.[8]

Partial and Total Nail Avulsion. For immediate relief and drainage of any paronychia of one or both borders, a partial nail avulsion is sufficient. When the entire nail, both borders, or a deformed nail is involved, a total nail avulsion can temporarily remove the entire nail plate to allow resolution of the drainage. This is also an optimal procedure for traumatically loosened toenails or subungual hematomas that fail to respond to simple drainage procedures and soaks.[8] After performing a digital block with local anesthesia (see later section), the nail folds should be freed from the nail border(s) and proximal eponychium with a Freer elevator or spatula-like instrument. Starting centrally and distally, the nail is carefully separated from the bed, working side to side and back to the matrix area under the proximal eponychium. Once the nail is adequately loosened, a straight hemostat is used to grasp the entire plate back to its origin. A rolling motion from side to side releases any remaining lateral attachments while the toe is held firmly with the other hand (Fig. 130-2). Finally, the nail is rolled from proximal to distal to remove the nail plate from its attachment to the matrix under the eponychium. If only a partial avulsion of a border is required, the nail should be split with an English anvil or other appropriate straight-edge nail splitter approximately ¼ inch from the inflamed nail fold. Only this portion of nail needs to be freed and removed, using the same basic technique while leaving the remainder of the nail intact. An appropriate antiseptic (e.g., povidone-iodine, bacitracin) is then applied, followed by a dry, sterile dressing. Bathing is allowed within 24 hours, and the dressing is then changed twice daily until the wound heals. Usually these procedures allow a rapid, uneventful recovery, with complete healing within 1 week.

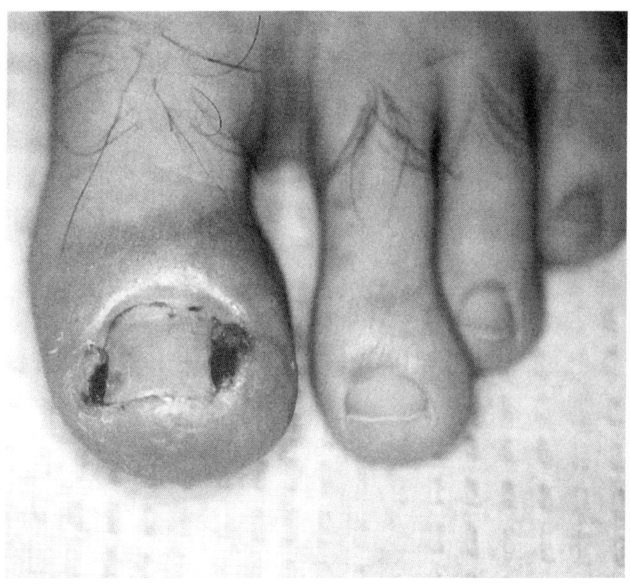

Fig. 130-1. Paronychia with granuloma formation.

COMMON SKIN DISORDERS

Tinea Pedis

Tinea pedis is a very common foot problem not specific to any particular age group, race, gender, or disease status.[3,6] Often the patient with chronic dermatophytosis also has chronic onychomycosis, which may be the source of the chronic fungal infection. *T. mentagrophytes*, *T. rubrum*, and *Epidermophyton floccosum* are the most frequent pathogens, with *C. albicans* occasionally present on fungal culture. The patient presents with an erythematous pruritic desquamating rash, usually extending up the medial and lateral borders of the foot (moccasin distribution) and frequently with maceration and peeling between the toes, which may cause secondary bacterial infection. Diagnosis is confirmed by KOH examination or culture of skin scrapings from active peripheral vesicular lesions. Dermatophytosis must be differentiated from other skin dermatoses, such as contact dermatitis, atopic dermatitis, dyshidrotic eczema, lichen planus, and psoriasis. Interdigital lesions also may be caused by simple maceration, white psoriasis, verrucae, or erythrasma *(Corynebacterium minutissimum)*.

Treatment consists of drying the moist lesions and eradicating the dermatophyte infection by applying topical antifungal agents. Systemic therapy with itraconazole or terbinafine is rarely necessary. Effective topical medications include tolnaftate, miconazole, clotrimazole, econazole, ciclopirox, and ketoconazole, and terbinafine applied twice daily. For severely inflamed cases, a combination therapy of clotrimazole with betamethasone is available. Since "athlete's foot" is produced by a warm, moist environment, proper foot hygiene is important. The feet should be bathed daily, dried between the toes, and powder applied routinely or after antifungal application. Antifungal powders or sprays are helpful as prophylactic agents but are not sufficient to treat active cases. When hyperhidrosis is a coexisting and

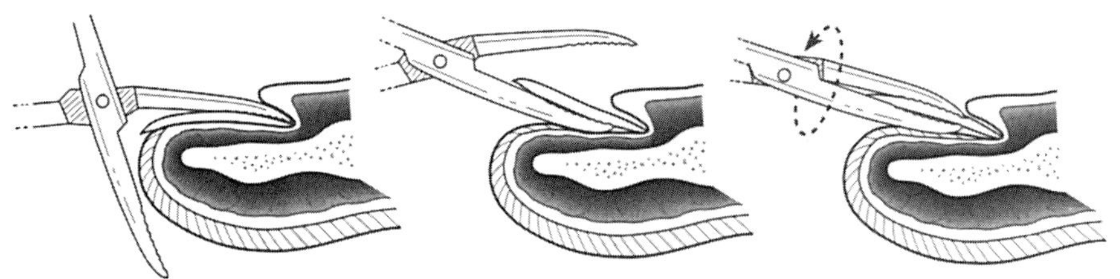

Fig. 130-2. Total nail avulsion technique. (From McGlamry ED, editor: *Comprehensive textbook of foot surgery*, Baltimore, 1987, Williams & Wilkins.)

contributing problem, absorbent socks should be worn and changed at least twice daily. Sneakers and other synthetic or rubber-soled shoes are also contributory; their use must be limited, especially during warmer months of the year.

Hyperkeratotic Lesions

Hyperkeratotic lesions (corns or calluses) are extremely common foot disorders because of their chronicity as well as frequency.[5,6] Corns and calluses are pressure-induced lesions and indicate areas of high or repetitive pressure. Dorsal, medial, and lateral lesions are almost exclusively the result of shoe pressure. Contracted hammer toes abutting against the top of the shoe are typically the etiology of very painful digital corns *(clavi)*. Plantar keratoses can be focal or diffuse callosities, usually termed *intractable plantar keratoses* (IPKs), and are extremely distressing for the patient who must walk on them. As always, pressure is the etiology. A plantar-flexed or long metatarsal is the most frequent underlying structural deformity giving rise to the hyperkeratosis.[1] When palpated, the underlying bone is immediately evident, as is pain from the chronic inflammation. On debridement, no skin lines are visible coursing through the center or core of the lesion; this often represents a plugged sweat duct lesion, referred to as a *porokeratosis*. The opaque core may be the "corn" so often mentioned by patients but is not always present in digital clavi, which are routinely called by the same name. Diffuse plantar calluses *(tylomata)* are usually biomechanical and, although possibly large, are typically not as painful as IPKs because of their more superficial nature and lack of a discrete central site of pressure, even though an IPK may be found in the center of a diffuse tyloma. Discolored lesions signify capillary hemorrhage with fluid collection under the keratosis and are usually more symptomatic or acute than normal-appearing callosities.

Simple debridement of a hyperkeratotic lesion provides immediate relief in most patients but cannot be expected to eradicate the problem, which involves correcting the underlying source (e.g., bony prominence, structural deformity, tight shoe, biomechanical imbalance). In patients unwilling or unable to undergo corrective surgery, conservative measures (e.g., shoes, orthotic therapy) combined with regular palliative care can achieve pain-free ambulation. Sneakers and cushioned walking shoes with generous toe room are advised for daily use in most patients. When necessary, cushioned insoles and prefabricated or custom-made orthoses are beneficial in relieving pressure on the sole. Although generally not successful in eradicating IPKs, such devices can provide comfort and extended periods between necessary debridements. If conservative measures fail, elective reconstructive surgery should be considered on the underlying structural deformity in the appropriate patient,[1,8] usually performed on an outpatient basis under local anesthesia (see later discussion).

Verrucae

Verruca plantaris is a common skin lesion, especially in children and adolescents, who are not particularly prone to callus development. This lesion is different from other hyperkeratotic disorders because of its viral etiology, human papillomavirus (HPV). A verruca can be distinguished from a callus by its typical pinpoint bleeding on debridement and well-defined borders. The patient may relate a history of a minor puncture wound at the site that allowed entrance of the virus. These lesions enlarge over time and frequently develop small satellites near the primary wart. HPV is ubiquitous and causes skin lesions ranging from genital warts to planar warts on the dorsum of the hand. On the foot, HPV causes several warts with distinct morphologies, probably due to different strains of the virus. The simple plantar verruca is the most common. This singular verruca can also occur on the dorsum of the foot, on the toes, adjacent to or under the toenails, or in the interdigital areas. A difficult type to manage involves multiple, small, disseminated warts across the entire sole of the foot. The most challenging verruca is the *mosaic* plantar verruca. This lesion with a mosaic pattern can consist of literally hundreds of confluent individual verrucae. Such lesions, usually evolving from longstanding or ineffectively treated single warts, can grow to several centimeters in diameter (Fig. 130-3).

Treatments for verrucae are numerous because no therapy is superior to the others or is successful on all patients for all warts.[3,6] Large clinical trials have not been performed contrasting the multiple therapies currently in use. Salicylic acids (40% or 60%) are the mainstay of treatment and are applied either once or twice a day in a paste form or as a plaster on an adhesive-backed dressing. Combinations of lactic and salicylic acids are also available over the counter in a liquid or gel form and are similarly applied by the patient each day. Such acid treatments can be effective but might require many months to show improvement. Other topical therapies include acetic acids, cantharidin, injection of sclerosing agents, formalin, and retinoic acid preparations. Care must be taken with aggressive blistering agents because of violent skin reactions and attendant pain. Dermatologists often use cryotherapy with liquid nitrogen or liquid CO_2, especially for singular lesions. Usually applied without local anesthesia, cryotherapy is uncomfortable and produces a painful blister. Repeated applications are frequently required,

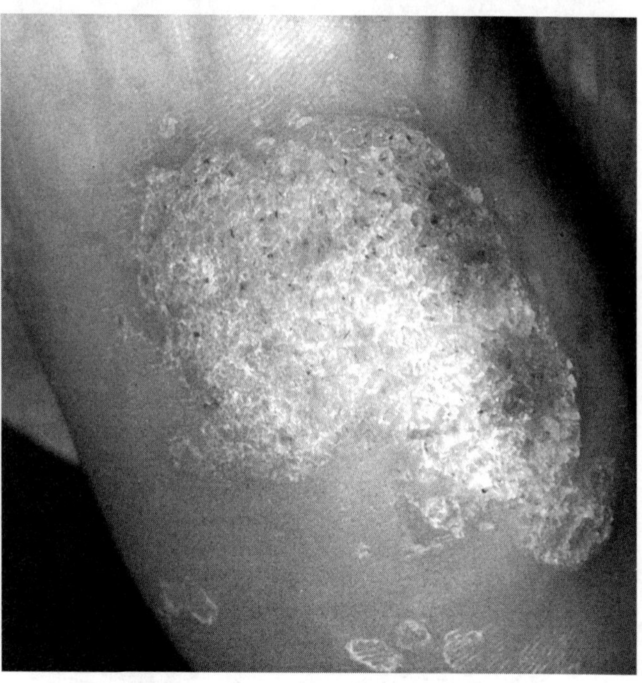

Fig. 130-3. Large mosaic verruca of the heel.

as with most modalities. Surgical treatments include electrocautery, blunt dissection, curettage, excision, and CO_2 laser vaporization. Although perhaps most effective on smaller, untreated verrucae, such methods are most frequently used on lesions recalcitrant to other, more conservative therapies. I prefer laser vaporization of recurrent or large mosaic verrucae, but success rates only approach 80% for multiple recurrent lesions. Frequently this treatment must be repeated to eradicate recurrent lesions.

These common lesions are difficult to eradicate permanently, and success can take months to years to achieve. Persistence and patience are mandatory in their management. Early recurrence or recalcitrance to therapy typically occurs, so long-term follow-up is required to assess adequacy of treatment. Recurrent lesions should be treated early to prevent regrowth. Combinations of therapies or successive changes in therapy should also be considered for unresponsive lesions.[3]

MUSCULOSKELETAL DISORDERS

Musculoskeletal problems within the foot and ankle are diagnostically challenging. Structural deformities are usually self-evident either clinically or radiographically, but soft tissue, joint, and functional abnormalities are difficult to specify and manage. Fortunately, specific diagnoses of related disorders (e.g., tendinitis, bursitis, capsulitis) are not as important as general management, since treatment regimens for the related disorders are the same. When the etiology of a problem is overuse, regardless of the specific source of pain, rest and immobilization are generally effective. Diagnostic acumen is still essential in distinguishing among infectious, metabolic, and traumatic etiologies, however, since the management of each is different (Fig. 130-4).

Forefoot: Digital and Metatarsal Disorders

Digital disorders become symptomatic primarily because of shoe pressure abutting on dorsal surfaces or squeezing the toes together. The digital deformity causing most distress is the *hammer toe,* which can affect children and adults alike. Although this term is generally used to denote any toe with a dorsal contracture, hammer toe is distinct from claw toe and mallet toe. A hammer toe has a dorsal (extensor) contraction at the metatarsophalangeal (MTP) joint and a flexion contracture at the proximal interphalangeal (PIP) joint (Fig. 130-5, *A*). The contractures can result from dynamic imbalances of tendinous structures around the joints secondary to hypermobility or neuropathy, as well as from traumatic or arthritic processes. A *claw toe,* in addition to the MTP and PIP contractures, also has a flexion contracture at the distal interphalangeal (DIP) joint (Fig. 130-5, *B*). A *mallet toe* is characterized by a single flexion contracture at the DIP joint, with weight on the tip of the toe (Fig. 130-5, *C*). In all these conditions, abnormal pressures are applied on dorsal digital surfaces from shoes and on distal toe surfaces directly. Since these sites are not protected by a fat pad, painful digital keratoses often develop. Contracted toes also can lie under or over adjacent digits, causing painful interdigital corns. Since these deformities progressively worsen over time, patients need to consider corrective surgery when conservative measures fail to provide long-term relief. A simple arthroplasty with resection of the proximal phalangeal head can permanently correct these conditions, generally with a rapid recovery.[8]

Hallux Valgus and Bunions. Metatarsal problems are often categorized into first metatarsal and lesser metatarsal disorders because of the separate axes of motion and distinguishing pathologic entities. First ray deformities comprise the most significant metatarsal complaints, with bunion deformities affecting an estimated 3.8 million people annually. *Hallux valgus,* as bunions are more properly called, refers not only to the medial prominence of the first metatarsal head, but also to the lateral drifting (abduction) and valgus rotation of the great toe.[2] The etiology of this condition, besides its strong familial predisposition, is a hypermobility of the first metatarsal, which allows it to drift progressively and medially. Hypermobility routinely accompanies a pronated foot (flatfoot) but is not specific to it. Concurrent with the adduction of the metatarsal is a lateral contracture of the hallux caused by a compensatory bowstringing effect of the long and short flexor (with sesamoids) and extensor tendons inserting into the great toe. In severe cases the great toe crowds the second toe, eventually causing a hammer toe of this digit. Progressive deformity results in not only a large bunion and abducted hallux, but a second toe that overlaps it as well (Fig. 130-6).

Although hallux valgus can be the sequela of rheumatoid, psoriatic, or gouty arthritis, degenerative joint disease eventually develops as the joint slowly becomes subluxed. Bunions are not characteristic of only an elderly population. Juvenile and adolescent hallux valgus may occur and, when left unattended, may progress to the severe deformities seen so often in geriatric patients. Bunions are not always painful, and thus patients and physicians tend to ignore them as long as a shoe can fit over them. They insidiously worsen, however, and both patient and physician should consider correcting the deformity before severe degeneration of the joint.

Conservative treatment has not been found effective in arresting the progression of hallux valgus, although orthotic therapy has been advocated. Footwear should have adequate width and depth to prevent compression of the widened forefoot. When the deformity becomes symptomatic or progresses beyond a mild stage, reconstructive surgery is indicated. Many procedures have been described for this deformity, ranging from simple excision of the medial eminence to fusion or prosthetic implantation of the first MTP joint.[2,8] The specific procedure performed should not be a matter of routine but based on the degree of deformity, presence of arthritis, age, and activity level of the patient. The goals of surgery are relief of pain and restoration of normal alignment of the first metatarsal and great toe. Rarely is a simple bunionectomy (e.g., Silver, McBride) advisable, since it does not correct the adduction of the first metatarsal. When bunionectomy is combined with a resection of the proximal phalangeal base (Keller arthroplasty), however, an excellent correction can be obtained in geriatric patients. Furthermore, most bunionectomies are easily performed under local anesthesia without the need for casts, crutches, or inpatient hospital stays.[2] With much of the morbidity previously associated with these procedures obviated by current techniques, physicians should be less reluctant to advise reconstruction of moderate or severe deformities.

Hallux Rigidus. Sometimes referred to as hallux limitus, hallux rigidus is a similar yet distinct condition of the first MTP joint. It implies a rigid great toe at the MTP joint,

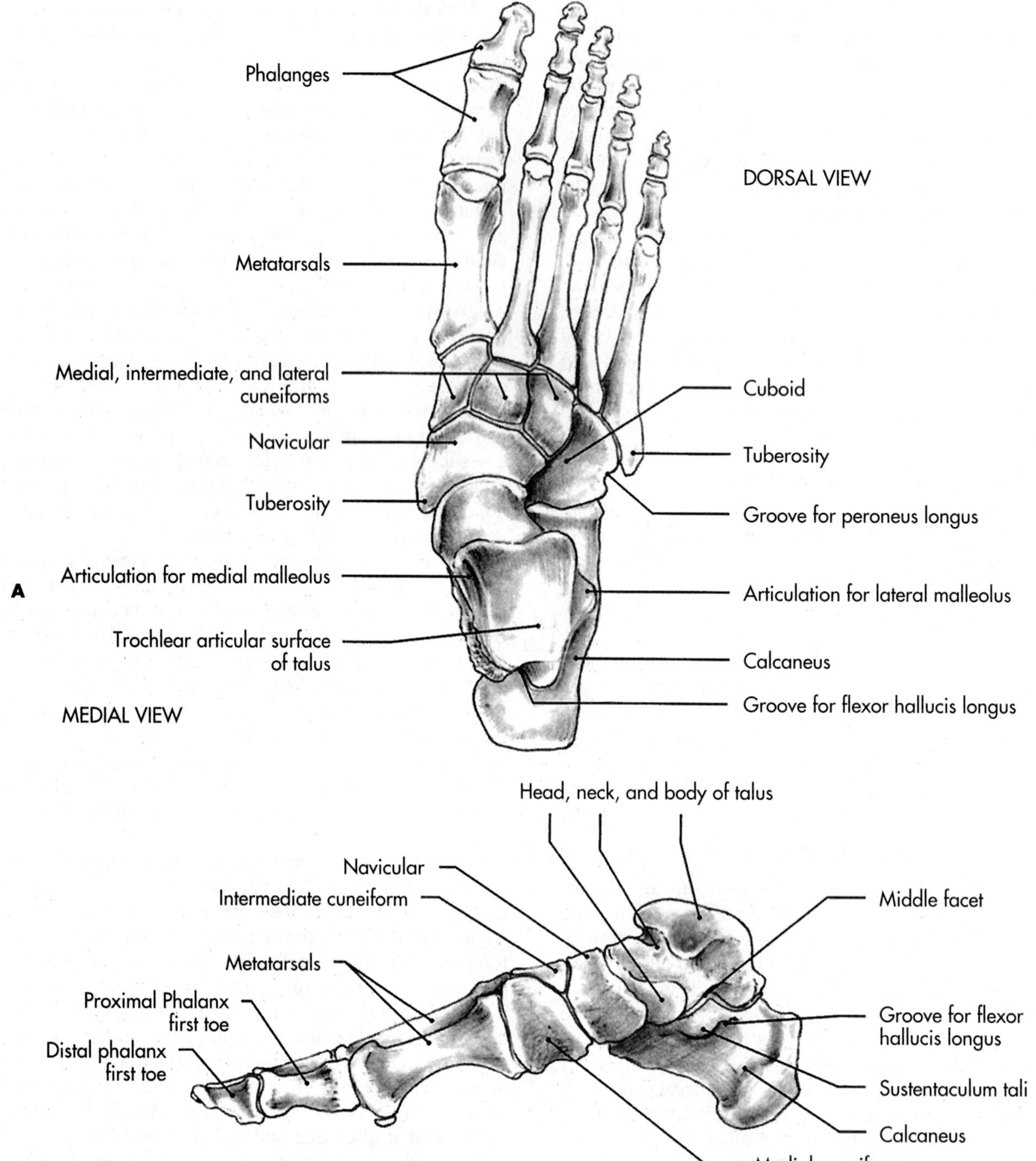

Fig. 130-4. Anatomy of the foot. **A,** Osseous structure. (From Reckling FW, Reckling JB, Mohn MP: *Orthopaedic anatomy and surgical approaches,* St Louis, 1990, Mosby.) *Continued*

whereas *hallux limitus* indicates only a limitation of motion at this joint.[6] The bunion in these patients lies dorsal to the metatarsal head and represents dorsal osteophytic proliferation secondary to abnormal function and degenerative changes within the first MTP joint (Fig. 130-7). A prior history of injury to the great toe is a common inciting event. This disorder is frequently painful, especially on range of motion, and can significantly restrict normal activity. It also can progress from a mild limitation of dorsiflexion to a severe degeneration of the joint with attendant loss of motion. Conservative care in early stages consists of wearing nonconstricting, rigid-soled footwear with low heels and a trial of orthoses. As the condition progresses, surgery is frequently required to provide relief.[6,8] Relatively mild arthrosis of the joint can be treated with cheilectomy, a debridement of the joint osteophytes. When an elevated first metatarsal is a principal component of the hallux limitus, cheilectomy is often combined with a plantar flexion osteotomy to increase the range of dorsiflexion. If severe arthritic changes are present, Keller bunionectomy, total

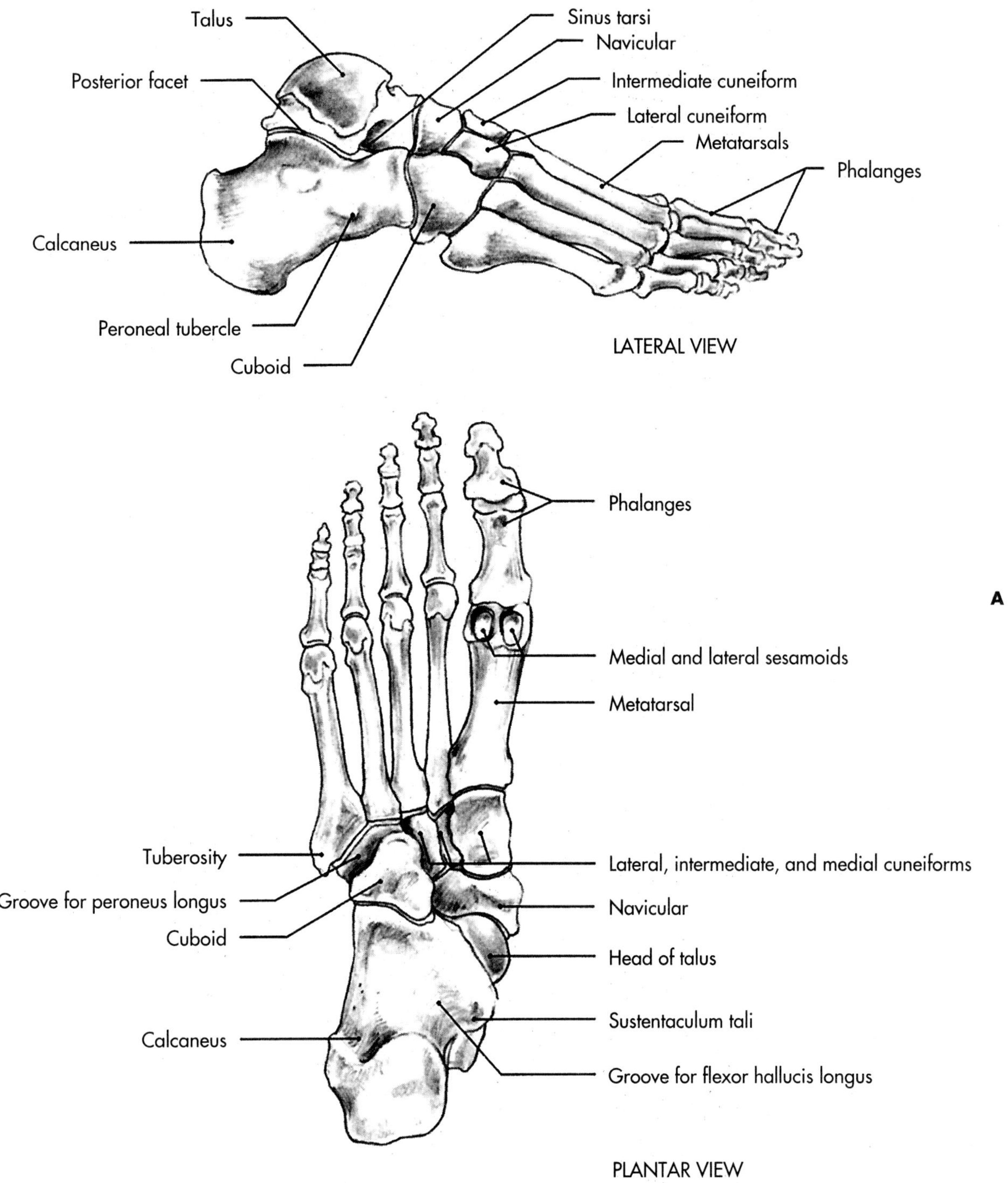

Fig. 130-4, cont'd. Anatomy of the foot. **A,** Osseous structure.

Continued

prosthetic implantation, or arthrodesis procedures should be considered.[8]

Sesamoiditis. Sesamoiditis of either the tibial or the fibular sesamoid or of both can be a very painful malady with an insidious onset and a chronic course if not diagnosed and treated early. The periosteal inflammation is usually the result of minor repetitive trauma, such as aerobic exercises or extended walking in thin-soled dress shoes or high heels. The inflammation may also involve the long flexor tendon, when the pain also extends along the central plantar aspect of the great toe. When acute trauma has occurred, sesamoid fracture or stress fracture must be ruled out. The diagnosis of sesamoiditis is made by eliciting maximal tenderness to direct palpation of the sesamoid in question. The patient usually has no swelling, erythema, or ecchymosis. Radiographs are negative, but bone scans may show signs of hyperemia and therefore may be falsely read as positive for fracture.

Treatment is based on protecting the injured part to avoid exacerbation of the inflammation. Since each step is essentially further trauma to the sesamoids, weight bearing must be limited or modified. Although crutches are rarely

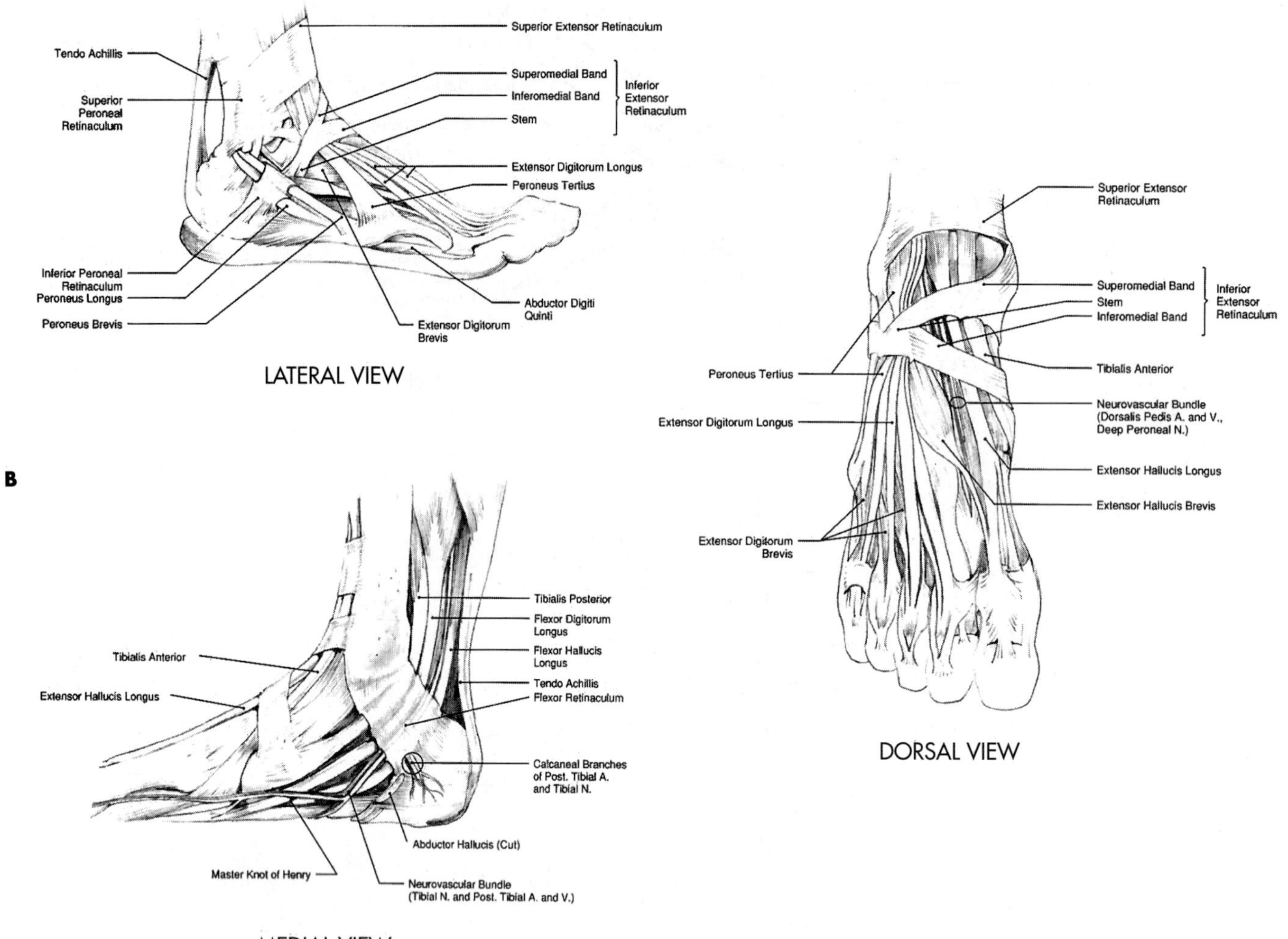

Fig. 130-4, cont'd. Anatomy of the foot. **B,** Musculotendinous anatomy. *Post.,* Posterior; *N.,* nerve; *A.,* artery; *V.,* vein. (From Reckling FW, Reckling JB, Mohn MP: *Orthopaedic anatomy and surgical approaches,* St Louis, 1990, Mosby.)

necessary, accommodative padding with rest strapping (taping) of the foot frequently provides relief. Nonsteroidal antiinflammatory drugs (NSAIDs) should be prescribed to help resolve the inflammation. The patient should wear shoes with cushioned soles and low heels and avoid activities that aggravate the condition. Frequently, soft orthoses are fabricated that can off-load the sesamoid area during gait. These should be worn on a long-term basis to prevent recurrence once the sesamoiditis has resolved. Unresolved sesamoiditis may require sesamoid excision in selected patients.

Metatarsalgia. Metatarsalgia is a nonspecific term that refers to pain in the ball of the foot around the lesser metatarsal heads.[1] This problem can be caused by bone, joint, musculotendinous, neurologic, vascular, or dermatologic pathology. The examination must therefore focus on specific sites, signs, symptoms, and history to differentiate possible causes of discomfort in the lesser metatarsal region.

Morton's Neuroma. Morton's neuroma is a classic cause of metatarsalgia that is usually centered in the third intermetatarsal and web space, between the third and fourth toes.[1] It is actually a benign enlargement of the third common digital branch of the medial plantar nerve as it passes plantar to the deep intermetatarsal ligament and between the metatarsal heads. Compression within this compartment during walking in tight shoes is considered the etiology of this painful neuralgia. Women are affected much more often than men, but no specific age ranges are predisposed in the adult population. Symptoms include burning, tingling, sharp, or shooting pains into the third or fourth toe, especially when wearing shoes or on direct compression of the interspace. Removing the shoe and rubbing the foot provide temporary relief. Symptoms are progressive, increasing in intensity and frequency over months to years. Diagnosis involves excluding osseous or other pathology in the region, as confirmed by negative radiographic findings. Magnetic resonance imaging (MRI), ultrasound, or electrophysiologic examination is usually not necessary in establishing the diagnosis.

Initial treatment of Morton's neuroma consists of a change to comfortable footwear and occasionally orthoses. Local corticosteroid injections and a course of NSAID therapy may provide additional relief in acute cases, but these measures are usually only temporizing. In time, most patients require excision of the neuroma when symptoms become too severe to enable normal daily activities. Surgery usually provides immediate relief, with a fairly benign postoperative recovery.

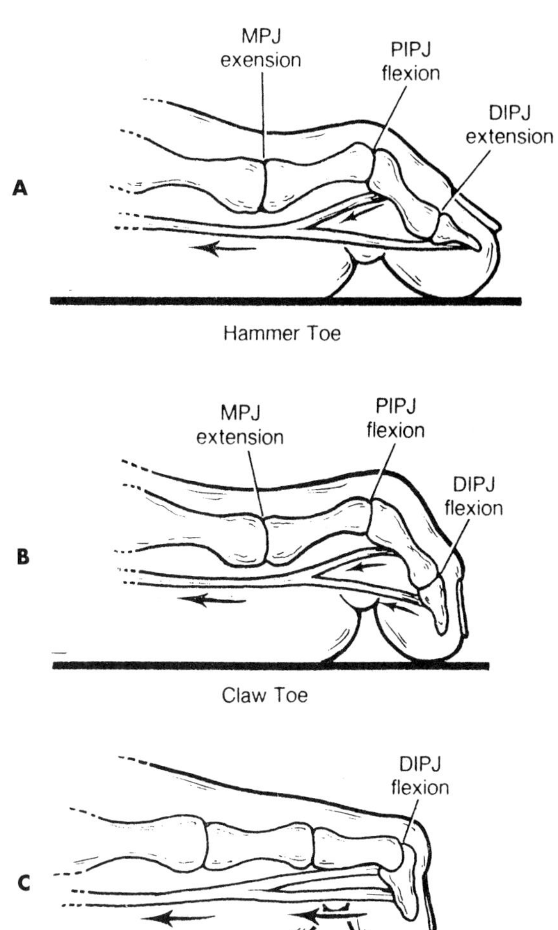

Fig. 130-5. Digital deformities. **A,** Hammer toe deformity, with extension contracture of metatarsophalangeal joint *(MPJ)* and flexion contracture of proximal interphalangeal joint *(PIPJ).* **B,** Claw toe, with additional flexion contraction of distal interphalangeal joint *(DIPJ).* **C,** Mallet toe, with single flexion contraction at distal interphalangeal joint. (From McGlamry ED, editor: *Comprehensive textbook of foot surgery,* Baltimore, 1987, Williams & Wilkins.)

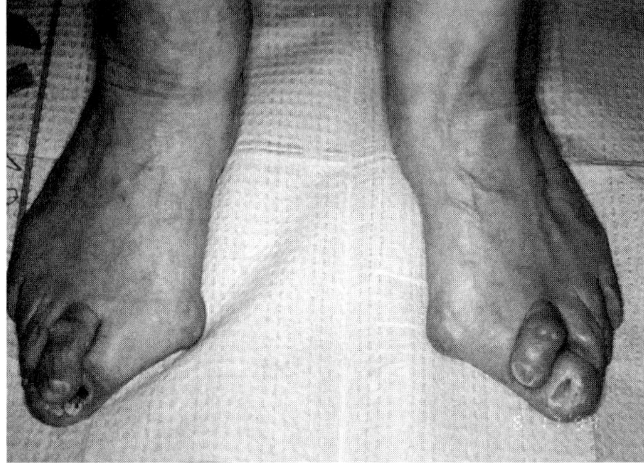

Fig. 130-6. Severe hallux valgus deformity, with overlapping second hammer toe on both feet, resulting from neglect.

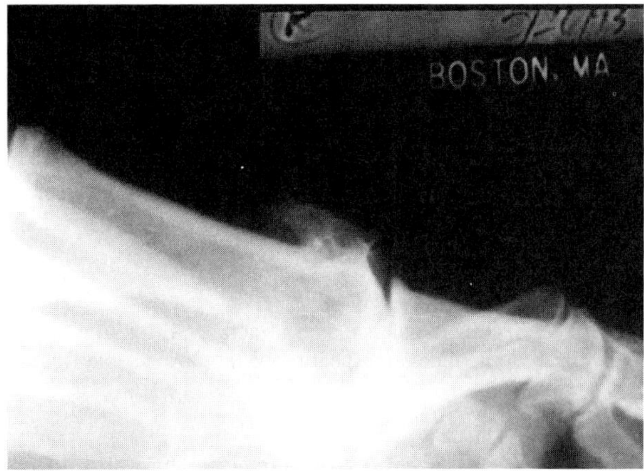

Fig. 130-7. Hallux rigidus, with dorsal osteophyte and degenerative changes of first metatarsophalangeal joint.

Plantar Keratoses and Lesser Metatarsalgia. Underlying IPKs, the physician can usually palpate the plantar surface of a prominent metatarsal head. Because of plantar displacement, excessive length (or shortened adjacent metatarsal), abnormal plantar prominence, or altered biomechanics, the metatarsal head bears more weight than adjacent bones during stance and gait. This creates excessive plantar pressure, and the IPK develops. These lesions are intractable unless the underlying bony deformity is addressed. Painful lesser metatarsal problems can be found even in the absence of a keratosis but are usually more acute in nature.[1] As with sesamoiditis, repetitive moderate stress can result in a capsulitis, tendinitis, or osteitis on the plantar surface of the metatarsal head. On occasion, stress fracture or aseptic necrosis of a lesser metatarsal (Freiberg's infraction) needs to be considered and the diagnoses differentiated through appropriate radiographic techniques.

When aberrant functioning of the metatarsal is the cause of this type of metatarsalgia, treatment should begin with custom orthoses to redistribute the weight-bearing forces properly under the foot.[3] This therapy is recommended in concert with footwear modification for almost any metatarsal problem. External bars and similar shoe alterations are employed less often than orthoses because patients generally resist such corrections. In recalcitrant cases, however, a metatarsal osteotomy can often be performed to realign or reconstruct the offending metatarsal such that all the metatarsals lie on the same transverse plane. Care must be taken, however, to prevent excessive shortening or dorsal displacement of the metatarsal head, since such errors can lead to transfer lesions on adjacent metatarsals. Although a variety of techniques are currently practiced, osteotomies are usually performed on the metatarsal neck through a dorsal approach to facilitate postoperative ambulation in a surgical shoe.[1,8]

Stress Fractures. Stress fractures of the lesser metatarsals are fairly common, especially in younger persons engaging in new activities such as running or aerobics. Older patients are equally subject to these types of fatigue fractures from common activities such as missed steps or long walks in uncushioned dress footwear. The patient presents with a mild

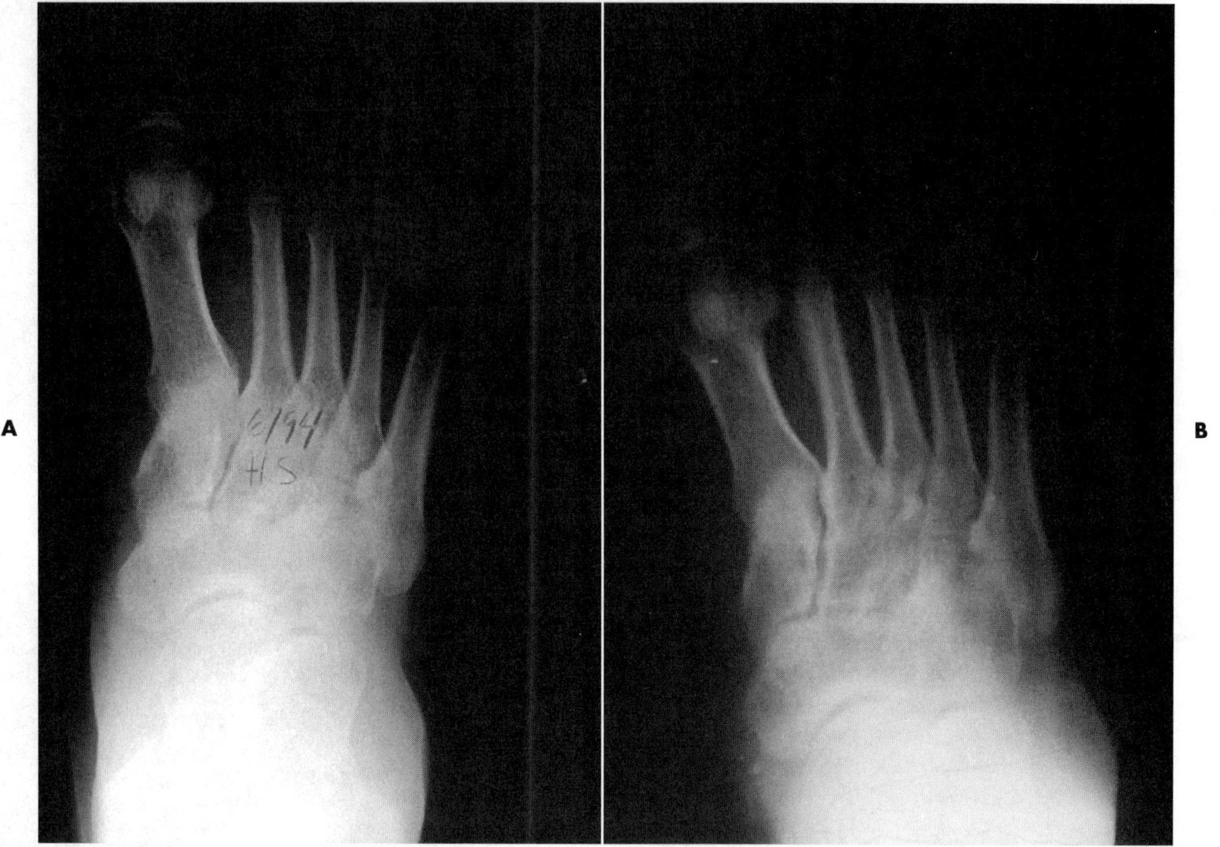

Fig. 130-8. Second metatarsal stress fracture. **A,** Initial radiograph does not show evidence of fracture. **B,** At 4 weeks' follow-up, radiograph reveals bone callus, indicating healing of the now-visible fracture.

to moderate swelling of the forefoot, perhaps with some erythema but minimal ecchymosis. Usually the pain is localized to one or two metatarsal shafts dorsally. Typically, early radiographs are negative because the bone has no complete fracture. Bone scans are positive, however, making this the diagnostic modality of choice when early stress fracture is suspected. Plain films become positive approximately 2 weeks after the injury, with evidence of periosteal proliferation at the site of maximal tenderness (Fig. 130-8). The physician can palpate a painful bony prominence, usually on the dorsum of the affected metatarsal. In some cases the relatively minor stress fracture can propagate to a complete transverse fracture of the metatarsal, especially when treatment is delayed or inadequate. In suspected cases, therefore, treatment should begin with a discontinuance of recreational activities or extended periods of walking. A standard postoperative shoe should be prescribed for exclusive use until symptoms have resolved. Usually, an Unna boot, rest strapping, or an elastic bandage is applied to provide further support and reduce swelling. Ice, rest, and elevation are warranted as well. Crutches are usually not required, and the patient can return to work if walking can be limited. Stress fractures respond quickly to these measures, with symptoms resolving within a few weeks. Strenuous activities are generally avoided for 4 to 6 weeks and then only after proper conditioning and footwear have been prescribed.

Bunionette. Bunionette, or *tailor's bunion,* is a lateral prominence or enlargement of the fifth metatarsal head not restricted to any gender or age group. The pathology includes enlargement of the metatarsal head, lateral bowing of the fifth metatarsal, or both.[6,8] Painful bunionettes can also arise from chronic shoe irritation over a normal fifth metatarsal head, causing only a soft tissue inflammation (adventitious bursitis). Similarly, a painful keratosis can develop over the lateral side of the fifth metatarsal head, indicating the role of footwear in the symptomatology of this disorder. Treatment therefore must initially be directed at providing relief from lateral shoe pressure, and when acutely inflamed, corticosteroid or NSAID therapy may be of benefit. Orthotic therapy is generally not successful. For patients with significant deformity or who are unresponsive to conservative measures, a partial metatarsal head resection or adductory fifth metatarsal osteotomy will correct the structural deformity (Fig. 130-9).

Midfoot Disorders

Disorders of the midfoot do not present as frequently as those of the forefoot but still cause considerable discomfort and contribute to deformities of the forefoot. In most patients, midfoot structural disorders are related to problems of the rearfoot or leg and represent biomechanical disturbances that can significantly affect normal gait and propulsion.

Flatfoot. Also called *pes planovalgus* or *pes planus,* flatfoot is the most significant of all midfoot disorders, affecting more than 4 million people at a rate of 18 per 1000 in the 1990 NHIS. Although this chronic structural deformity

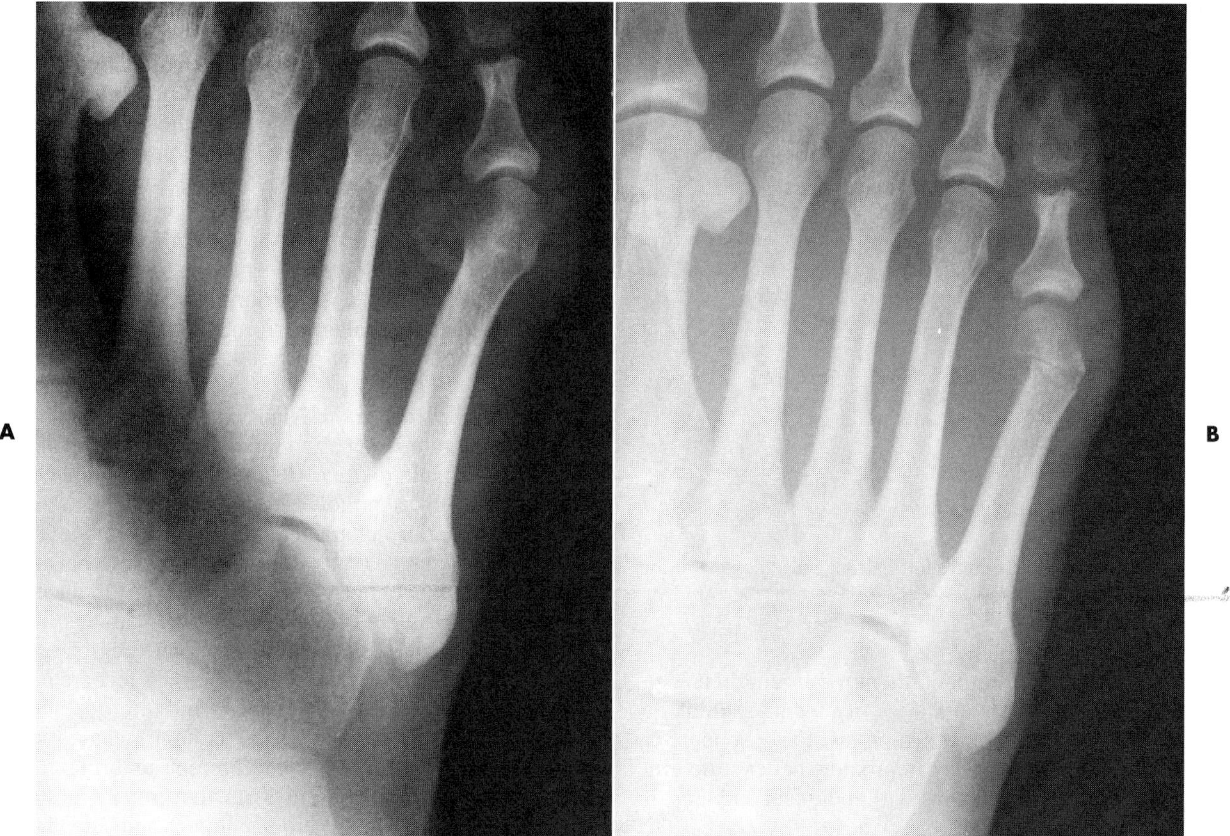

Fig. 130-9. Tailor's bunion. **A,** Preoperative view demonstrating fifth metatarsal head prominence and lateral bowing of metatarsal. **B,** Postoperative view after performing metatarsal head osteotomy.

infrequently originates in the midfoot in the absence of trauma, flatfoot usually results from more proximal disturbances of function. For example, a tight Achilles tendon (gastrocnemius equinus) restricts ankle joint dorsiflexion, and excessive pronation (including dorsiflexion) of the subtalar joint compensates for this during gait. The pronated subtalar joint allows an unlocking of the midtarsal joint (talonavicular and calcaneocuboid joints), which also results in excessive pronation.[6] This general instability is translated into a *hypermobility,* which refers to the foot's excessive motion when it should be a stable, propulsive organ. The hypermobility contributes to weakness of the foot, fatigue, hallux valgus with hammer toe formation, and inefficient forward propulsion in gait. Besides symptoms within the foot, excessive pronation frequently contributes to anterior shin splints or tendinitis, chondromalacia patellae, and chronic low back pain. These problems are particularly relevant in athletes or people in exercise programs because the forces sustained by the weakened feet are exaggerated. Overuse injuries of the lower extremities are therefore more prevalent and more difficult to resolve in patients with flatfeet.

A flatfoot is not a simple deformity and can have multiple etiologies and specific sites of involvement.[6] It can be congenital or acquired, rigid or flexible, and primary or secondary. Pes planovalgus may result from a neuromuscular disease, stroke, trauma, arthritis, primary structural deformity, or a peroneal spasm secondary to a fractured tarsal coalition. Peripheral neuropathies and other acquired or congenital disorders resulting in weakness, contracture, or paralysis of leg musculature and affecting the normal mechanics of the foot can produce a flatfoot deformity. Generally, spasticity of the gastrocnemius-soleus complex results in flatfoot, whereas flaccidity results in a high-arched foot. Weakness of the posterior tibial muscle also leads to flatfoot, whereas spasticity of the long flexors leads to a high arch. Neuromuscular disorders must be evaluated to determine muscle groups affected and the qualitative impact on foot mechanics. Congenital flatfoot results from developmental aberrations such as clubfoot (talipes equinovalgus), congenital convex pes valgus, talipes calcaneovalgus, forefoot varus, torsional disturbances of the lower extremities, or ligamentous laxity. These deformities must be properly evaluated for rigidity or flexibility, since nonreducible rigid deformities portend a poor prognosis and require surgical intervention. Minor structural or functional deviations from the norm, such as forefoot varus, accessory navicular with altered insertion of the posterior tibial tendon, flexible calcaneovalgus, or tightened heel cords, are generally considered nonpathologic or idiopathic causes of flexible pes planovalgus. Acquired flatfoot is usually the result of neurologic disorder or trauma to the foot or leg. The most common cause of acquired adult flatfoot is a rupture of the posterior tibial tendon, frequently seen in elderly rheumatic patients. This is marked by a unilateral deformity in a patient with a prior history of injury or prodromal symptoms of chronic posterior tibial tendinitis (Fig. 130-10).

Once potential pathologic causes of flatfoot have been addressed, treatment of symptomatic hypermobile pes planus

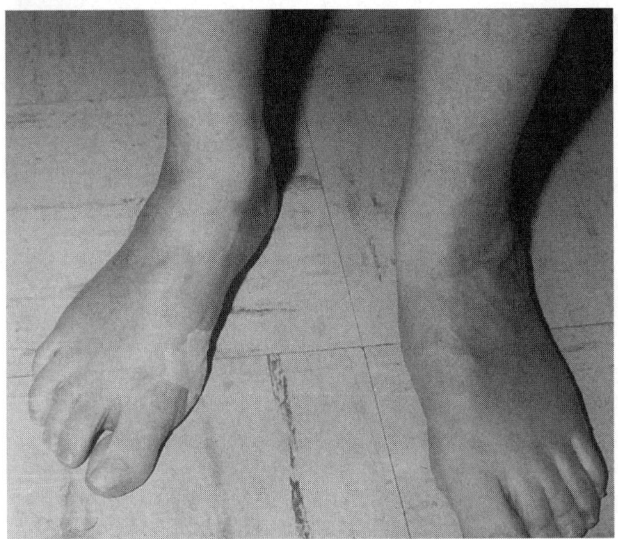

Fig. 130-10. Unilateral acquired adult flatfoot caused by posterior tibial tendon rupture of left foot.

should always begin with orthotic therapy.[6] In children with nonpathologic deformities, orthotic treatment should be initiated by age 5, even without symptoms. Early support of the flat foot in the growing child can promote better structural development and fewer symptoms within the feet and legs. It cannot be presumed, however, that orthoses will *correct* the structural deformity in either the child or the adult patient. The purpose of the orthosis is generally to relieve symptoms by providing structural support under the weakened foot, by limiting the amount of abnormal pronation, and by allowing more efficient locomotion.

Foot orthoses include prefabricated "customizable" devices and others custom made by laboratories or health-care professionals. Since treatment for pes planus is aimed at functional improvement of the pronated foot, custom-fabricated *functional* orthoses should be used. Custom orthoses are usually categorized as flexible, semirigid, or rigid designs depending on the materials used in fabrication. The specific type used depends on the patient's age, weight, and activity level as well as the deformity's severity and symptoms. Flexible orthoses, often fabricated from softer materials (e.g., Plastazote, microcellular rubbers) can provide gentle support as well as cushioning. They are useful in sports medicine and for geriatric or diabetic patients. Semirigid orthoses are traditionally fabricated from leather composites, although newer synthetic materials are less bulky and more durable. A compromise between flexible and rigid designs, semirigid devices provide good support with a degree of flexibility. Many sport orthoses fabricated in commercial laboratories fall in this category. Rigid orthoses are the gold standard of orthotic devices and provide the greatest control over foot function and abnormal pronation (or supination). Although previously made from stainless steel, rigid orthoses are currently fabricated from very durable materials such as polypropylenes and thermoplastics. Often guaranteed against fatigue and breakage, these low-profile "high-tech" devices can be computer manufactured from digital scanning of plaster cast impressions of the feet. Advances in fabrication technology have also resulted in thinner, easier-to-fit designs that are extremely comfortable and more exacting in their correction of abnormal function.

Since orthoses can control function and ameliorate symptoms in flatfeet, only the most severe of deformities usually require reconstruction. These more pathologic entities include congenital vertical talus, tarsal coalitions, and neurologic or traumatic conditions. Excessive ankle equinus secondary to triceps surae contractures often requires Achilles tendon lengthening in concert with any localized foot procedure.[8] The Kidner procedure removes the accessory navicular and tightens the pull of the posterior tibial tendon. Variations of this procedure are also performed in cases of partial or complete rupture of the posterior tibial tendon.[10]

High-arched Foot. Also known as *pes cavus,* a high-arched foot is not as common as flatfoot (pes planus) but is more difficult to treat. Classically seen with neurologic disorders such as polio or peroneal muscular atrophy, pes cavus is generally characterized by a lack of flexibility, an anterior equinus (plantar flexion) of the forefoot, and claw toes.[6] Although underlying neurologic disturbances should always be considered in evaluating such patients, idiopathic or nonpathologic pes cavus of a moderate degree is the most frequent presentation (Fig. 130-11). Cavus feet are marked by excessive supination of the rearfoot and forefoot whereby the plantar-flexed first ray (medial column) causes abnormal inversion (supination) of the forefoot to bring the lateral column (fourth and fifth rays) to the ground in stance and gait. Because of the forefoot equinus and attendant exaggeration of metatarsal declination, the toes are usually clawed due to a loss of the normal stabilizing mechanism of the intrinsic muscles around the MTP and interphalangeal joints. Hyperactivity of the peroneus longus, posterior tibial, and long flexors or weakness of the triceps surae, peroneus brevis, anterior crural, and intrinsic foot muscles can all contribute to high-arched foot in varying degrees. Multiple imbalances between agonist and antagonist muscle groups often coexist, especially in patients with documented neuromuscular diseases. Therefore detailed neuromuscular, biomechanical, and gait evaluations are required to assess both the etiology and the specific pathomechanical attributes.

In the absence of trauma or recent neurologic disease, most patients adapt well to their longstanding cavus foot deformities, except for repeated ankle sprains ("weak ankles"), persistent plantar calluses, or painful dorsal digital corns. Periodic debridement and cushioned insoles in shoes with adequate depth for the toes are usually adequate initial measures for relief of hyperkeratotic lesions. Patients with complaints of lateral or postural instability or painful metatarsalgia, however, are best treated with custom functional orthoses to limit supinatory motion during gait. In severe cases unresponsive to these measures, surgery can be performed to realign the forefoot, stabilize lateral ankles, or correct digital deformities.[6]

Rearfoot Disorders

Heel Spur and Plantar Fasciitis. Heel spur syndrome and its soft tissue analog, plantar fasciitis, are the most common disorders of the hindfoot. The painful heel can be attributed to rheumatic diseases such as rheumatoid arthritis, gout, Reiter's disease, ankylosing spondylitis, or other seronegative spondyloarthropathies (see Chapter 137).[3,6]

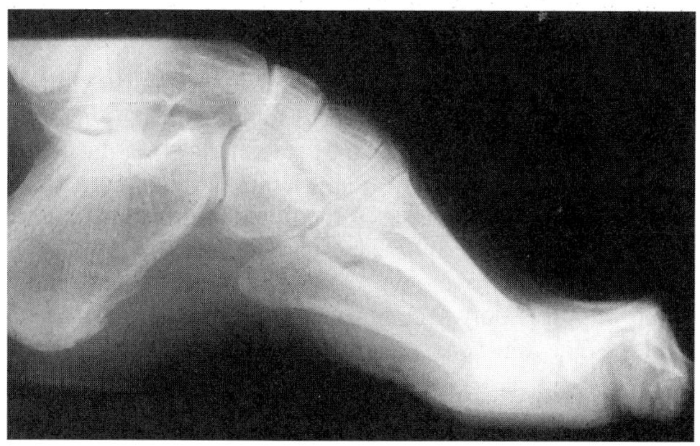

Fig. 130-11. Radiograph of pes cavus deformity with anterior metatarsal equinus and claw toes.

These arthritic entities are distinguished more by erosive changes to the heel than by spur formation. Heel spurs and plantar fasciitis, however, are generally considered to be pathomechanical. With each step the plantar fascia is drawn taut as it resists collapse of the arch, a function analogous to a windlass mechanism. Concurrently, there is a rather constant traction on the periosteal insertion point on the calcaneus. Over time or with overuse, this constant traction results in a spur formation at the anteroinferior aspect of the calcaneus. This enthesopathy is an insidious process in many cases, since patients often have rather large, asymptomatic calcaneal spurs as incidental findings on radiographs. Conversely, patients with acutely painful heels in the absence of trauma can have negative radiographs. These patients would then be considered to have a heel "bursitis" or localized plantar fasciitis at the insertion of the aponeurosis. Typical plantar fasciitis, as seen in overuse injuries to athletes, usually extends more distal along the medial band of the fascia. Excessive pronation is the underlying etiology of heel spur syndrome, except when a cavus foot type is subjected to repetitive heel trauma. Radiographs confirm a spur or rule out other causes of heel pain when plantar fasciitis is suspected. Differential diagnoses in patients with heel pain include stress fracture or bone contusion, subtalar joint pathology, tumor, rheumatic disease, nerve entrapment, plantar fascial tear, Achilles tendinitis, calcaneal apophysitis, or Sever's disease (calcaneal avascular necrosis).

Treatment for heel spur syndrome, including patients with plantar fasciitis only, initially requires attenuation of activities, NSAIDs, and rest strapping of the foot to limit pronation. Heel cups or prefabricated orthoses can be useful, as can simple heel cushions or cutouts. Night splints may provide symptomatic relief by maintaining a stretch on the fascia and preventing nocturnal contracture. Corticosteroid injection is reserved for recalcitrant cases and is usually limited to three injections from a medial approach. Athletic or cushioned walking shoes with slight heel elevation are also beneficial. When improvement is noted, a soft orthosis is usually fabricated to provide support and cushioning for the heel. This should be used on a long-term basis to improve foot function and prevent relapse. Once comfortable, patients can gradually discontinue NSAID therapy while continuing with orthotic therapy. Physical therapy modalities such as ultrasound are prescribed when these prior measures fail to provide relief. Below-knee casting or immobilization in ambulatory cast braces with or without crutches must also be considered in severe cases. Inferior calcaneal heel pain usually resolves in about 6 months. Patients who do not improve for 12 months or longer despite exhaustive efforts may consider heel spur surgery or plantar fasciotomy. Medial calcaneal nerve entrapment should also be evaluated at this stage and released as necessary. Since the great majority of patients eventually recover with conservative therapy alone, surgery should not be the initial treatment.

Posterior Tibial Tendinitis. Posterior tibial tendinitis is a very painful condition of the rearfoot often mimicking a medial ankle sprain or sometimes medial arch pain. It most frequently affects people beyond middle age who are moderately active and may have a history of other rheumatic complaints. It is also a common overuse injury in younger individuals or in people with significant degrees of foot pronation. Since the posterior tibial muscle is the major antagonist to the peroneus brevis tendon, it is the major supinator of the foot and primarily functions to resist pronation of the subtalar and midtarsal joints during gait.[6] The pronated foot alters normal anatomic relationships and vectors of force, resulting in inefficiency of the posterior tibial muscle. This insufficiency causes overuse compensation, and the muscle functions beyond its usual phasic activity, leading to both fatigue and chronic tendinitis. Chronic posterior tibial tendinitis can then lead to partial tearing, internal degeneration, or complete rupture, which is a classic cause of adult acquired flatfoot deformity. Symptoms include pain and mild swelling just below the medial malleolus as the tendon courses below this structure to insert on the navicular and plantar midfoot. Pain is exacerbated by active inversion and plantar flexion of the foot, especially when standing on the ball of the foot and toes. In cases of complete rupture the pain is usually gone, but in addition to the unilateral flatfoot, toe stance demonstrates a lack of heel and arch inversion. During stance the forefoot is greatly abducted, and when viewed from behind, the "too many toes" sign is evident. The pain from the chronic tendinitis is usually related to activity but is persistent from day to day, progressive, and almost disabling in its most severe forms.

Treatment of posterior tibial tendinitis is based on preventing pronation of the foot, resting, and reducing inflammation of the tendon and tendon sheath. Although rest strapping and resistive ankle taping are often effective, cast or cast bracing with or without crutches may be necessary to provide relief. A prolonged course of NSAID therapy is also necessary, frequently in conjunction with physical therapy. Corticosteroid injections are usually not recommended because of the risk of subsequent tendon atrophy and rupture. Custom orthotic therapy is always required to support the foot and reduce tension on the posterior tibial tendon. Rigid orthoses are preferable, but semiflexible or flexible orthoses should be fabricated as an alternative in patients who are unable to tolerate rigid support. Debridement of the degenerated tendon or repair and augmentation of the ruptured posterior tibial tendon should be reserved for patients who complain of chronic severe pain or instability.[10] Surgery in elderly patients requires prolonged immobilization without weight bearing, making such procedures inadvisable except in the most severe circumstances.

Ankle Disorders

Sprains. Ankle sprains are the most common ankle problem presented to primary care physicians. Lateral ankle sprains of the lateral collateral ligaments are the usual presentation of such disorders, since medial sprains of the deltoid ligament are frequently accompanied by lateral ankle fractures.[10] Three separate collateral ligaments of the anterolateral talocrural joint are subject to tear or partial tear on inversion injury (Fig. 130-12). The most anterior and most frequently torn of the three is the anterior talofibular ligament (ATFL). This intracapsular, fan-shaped ligament extends from the anteroinferior end of the fibular malleolus and inserts into the lateral surface of the body of the talus. Primarily resisting ankle inversion during plantar flexion, the ATFL is usually the first to be ruptured during inversion injuries because the ankle is least stable when plantar flexed. The extracapsular, cordlike calcaneofibular ligament (CFL) courses from the inferior tip of the fibula to the lateral surface of the calcaneus under the peroneal tendon sheath. The CFL primarily resists inversion during ankle dorsiflexion and usually ruptures only second to the ATFL in severe inversion injuries. The intracapsular posterior talofibular ligament

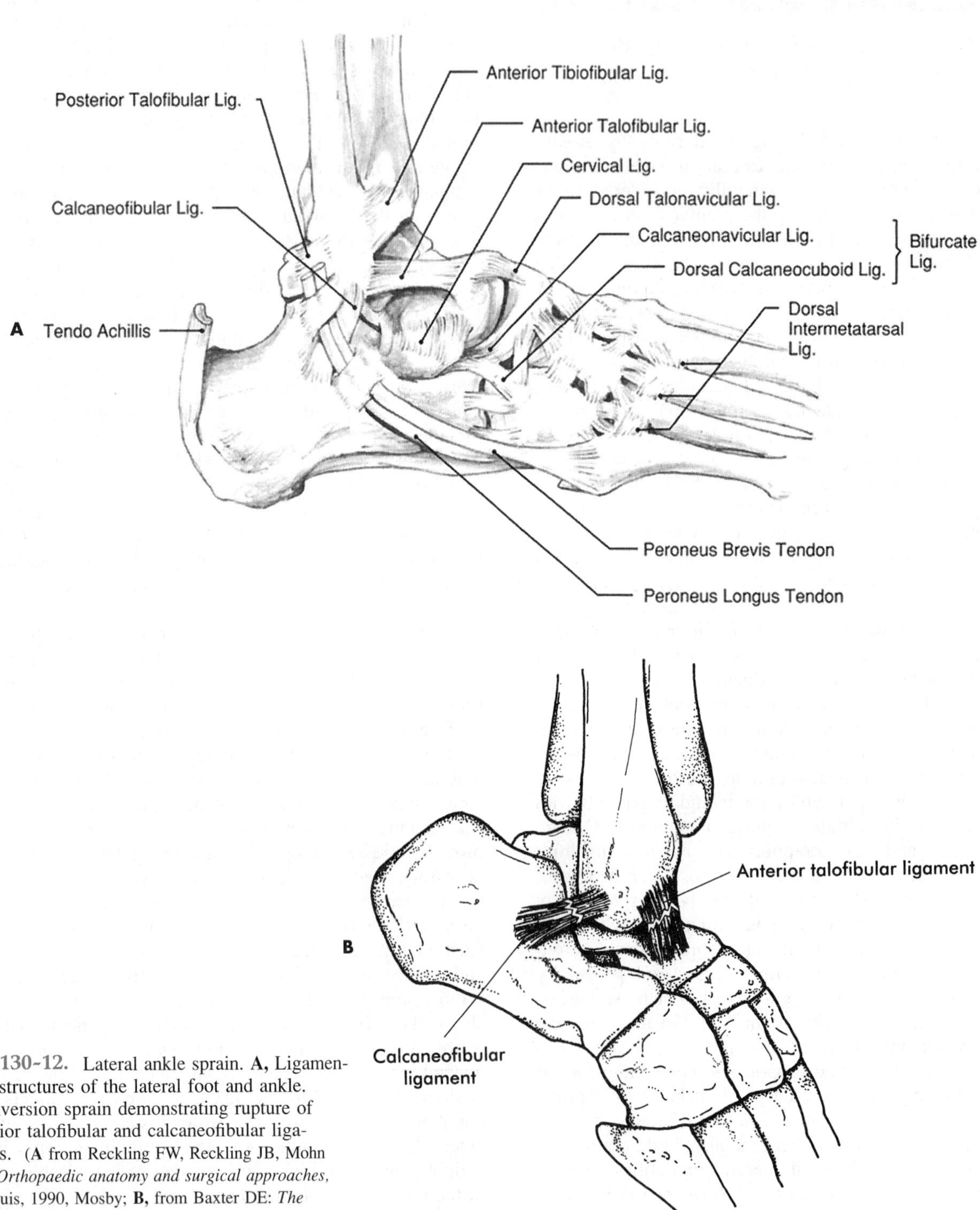

Fig. 130-12. Lateral ankle sprain. **A,** Ligamentous structures of the lateral foot and ankle. **B,** Inversion sprain demonstrating rupture of anterior talofibular and calcaneofibular ligaments. (**A** from Reckling FW, Reckling JB, Mohn MP: *Orthopaedic anatomy and surgical approaches,* St Louis, 1990, Mosby; **B,** from Baxter DE: *The foot and ankle in sport,* St Louis, 1995, Mosby.)

(PTFL), the strongest of the three, runs posteriorly from the fibular malleolus to the posterior lateral surface of the talus. The PTFL is infrequently ruptured except in cases of severe trauma with associated osseous injury to the ankle. Diagnosis of a lateral ankle sprain should be obvious by the history and signs of acute edema, ecchymosis, and pain at the anterolateral aspect of the ankle. Radiographs are taken to rule out associated lateral ankle or talar fracture. The examiner must also palpate the base of the fifth metatarsal in such injuries, since ankle sprains can often be accompanied by fracture of the styloid process or proximal fifth metatarsal shaft (Jones fracture). When present, such fractures require prolonged cast immobilization or open reduction with internal fixation.

For isolated ligamentous sprains, ice, rest, elevation, and some form of immobilization are required. Crutches should be used in acute cases when symptoms and examination warrant no weight bearing. Immobilization can be a simple elastic bandage or rest strapping in minor sprains or below-knee casting, ambulatory cast bracing, or ankle stirrup braces for more severe injuries (Fig. 130-13). For chronic ankle instability resulting from repeated sprains, an ankle stirrup or taping is recommended when patients engage in athletic activities. Severe instability, especially in competitive athletes, can be corrected with a variety of lateral ankle stabilization procedures.[8,10] Such operations attempt to restore ligamentous integrity with direct repair or by augmentation with tendon transfer. In patients with chronic ankle pain and a history of previous sprain in the absence of severe instability, the physician must consider a talar dome osteochondral lesion (osteochondritis dissecans), which can usually be detected only by computed tomography (CT) scan or MRI and which rarely heals without intervention. Arthroscopic procedures can remove or repair these osteochondral fragments and are an alternative to open ankle arthrotomy procedures.

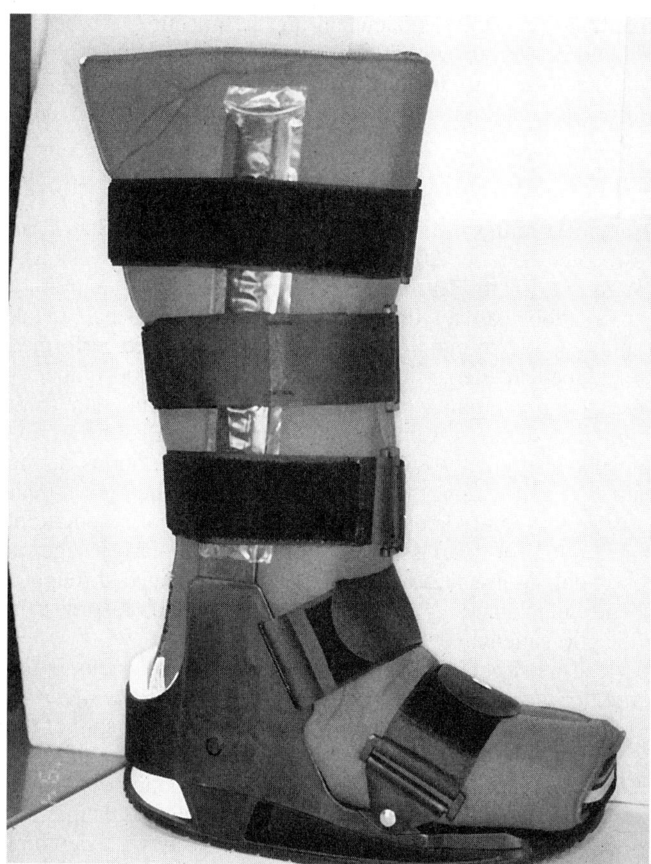

Fig. 130-13. Prefabricated removable cast brace for severe sprains or postsurgical immobilization.

LOCAL ANESTHESIA

The primary care physician may frequently need to treat an acute paronychia or toenail injury, remove a foreign body, or fulgurate a plantar verruca. Local anesthetic injection techniques augment the physician's ability to handle such foot maladies and provide comfort to patients. The injection technique used in the foot depends on the condition and its location. Techniques include local infiltration, digital block, specific nerve block, or regional anesthesia (ankle block). The basic premise is that the afferent sensory nerves must be blocked *proximal* to the site of the lesion being treated. For example, when treating a paronychia, it is *always* advisable to perform a digital block at the base of the toe and *never* to inject at the distal pulp of the toe or adjacent to the nail border. Distal toe injections are simply too painful because of the tautness of the subcutaneous tissues. Conversely, when removing a simple plantar wart, it is often easier to infiltrate under and around the lesion than to perform a nerve block. With the patient's comfort always in mind, the excision of multiple plantar lesions is best approached with a posterior tibial nerve block at the medial ankle rather than repeated injections on the sole of the foot.

Lidocaine (0.5% or 1%) is the most frequently used of the local agents because of its rapid onset. Bupivacaine (0.5%) is usually mixed with the lidocaine to provide lasting anesthesia for 8 to 12 hours. Epinephrine in combination with the anesthetic agent provides not only increased duration of activity through a delay of absorption but also vasoconstriction and intraoperative hemostasis. The use of epinephrine in digits is still controversial, although many digital blocks have employed this agent without adverse sequelae. Discretion and proper patient selection are required, however, when using epinephrine in any foot procedure.

Digital blocks are simple to perform and can be used in any patient who requires anesthesia of any part of a toe. Most digital operations should be done under local anesthesia unless a specific indication requires general or spinal anesthesia. Usually, all four digital nerves must be infiltrated to produce an adequate block of the entire toe. Either a ring block technique (Fig. 130-14) or an inverted-V block (Fig. 130-15) can be employed using a 25-gauge 1½-inch needle on a 3-ml syringe. A total of 3 ml for the great toe and 2 ml for the lesser toes is usually sufficient to provide complete digital anesthesia after about 5 minutes. When the metatarsal head or MTP joint must be anesthetized, a more proximal V block around the metatarsal neck should be used. Bunionectomy procedures usually require a digital block in combination with a circumferential segmental block of the first metatarsal proximal to the metatarsal neck.

Ankle blocks are extremely useful in providing anesthesia to the entire foot when multiple sites must be approached. The primary care physician rarely needs to perform this technique, but a general knowledge of the anatomic location and distributions of the nerves crossing the ankle is beneficial

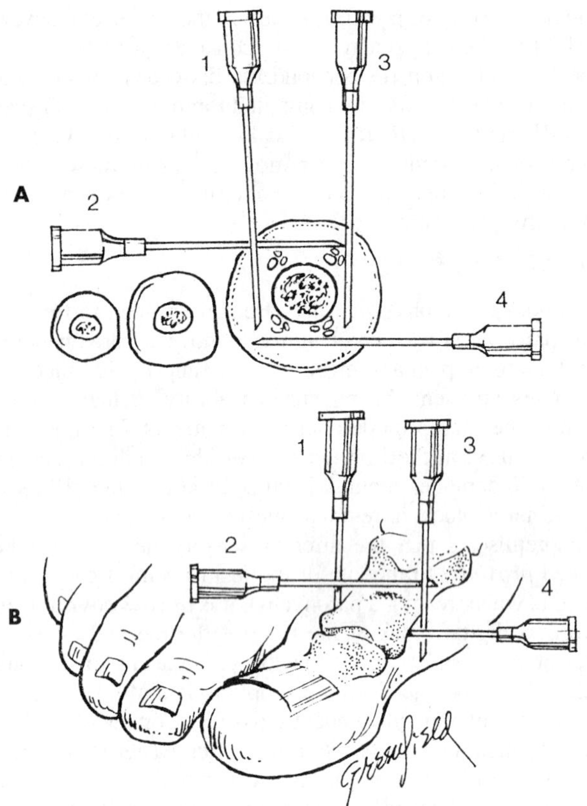

Fig. 130-14. Ring block injection technique for the great toe. **A,** Cross-sectional view. **B,** Dorsal view. (From Frykberg RG: Podiatric problems in diabetes. In Kozak GP et al, editors: *Management of diabetic foot problems,* ed 2, Philadelphia, 1995, Saunders.)

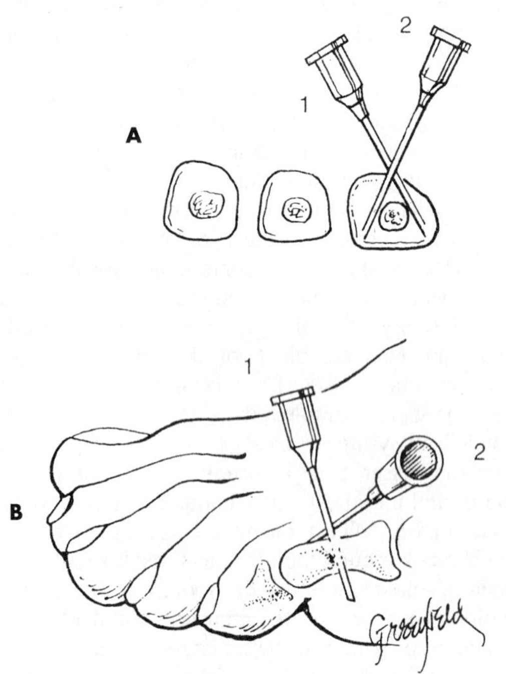

Fig. 130-15. Inverted-V block injection technique for lesser toes. **A,** Cross-sectional view. **B,** Dorsal view. (From Frykberg RG: Podiatric problems in diabetes. In Kozak GP et al, editors: *Management of diabetic foot problems,* ed 2, Philadelphia, 1995, Saunders.)

when an isolated nerve block is required. The two deep nerves that cross the ankle, the deep peroneal (anterior tibial) and the posterior tibial, run adjacent to the dorsalis pedis and posterior tibial arteries, respectively. The other four nerves are all superficial and, from lateral to anterior to medial, are the sural, intermediate dorsal cutaneous, medial dorsal cutaneous, and saphenous nerves. The sural nerve lies just behind and inferior to the lateral malleolus and innervates the lateral border of the foot and fifth metatarsal. The two branches of the superficial peroneal nerve can often be seen or palpated directly under the skin on the ankle's anterior surface; they provide sensation to the dorsum of the foot and toes. The saphenous nerve lies anterior to the medial malleolus and runs with the greater saphenous vein, providing sensation to the medial border of the foot. These four superficial nerves are easily blocked with simple subcutaneous infiltration around the nerves. The deep peroneal nerve is blocked by palpating the dorsalis pedis artery and injecting around it deep to the fascia, taking care to aspirate before injection. The large posterior tibial nerve lies deep to the flexor retinaculum and runs adjacent to the posterior tibial artery and veins. The three branches—medial calcaneal, medial plantar, and lateral plantar nerves—supply the medial and plantar heel, medial plantar sole and toes, and lateral plantar sole and toes, respectively. Anesthesia of these sites is best obtained concurrently with a block of the posterior tibial nerve behind, deep to, and just above the tip of the medial malleolus. Once again, the artery should be palpated and the needle inserted so that infiltration will occur around the vessel and nerve without penetrating either structure. Aspiration should always be performed to prevent intraarterial injection. If significant pain and paresthesias occur during the injection, the needle should be slightly withdrawn to avoid injection directly into the nerve. Approximately 6 to 10 ml is required for this difficult injection, delivered with a 25-gauge needle on a 10-ml syringe.

THE DIABETIC FOOT

Of the 16 million diabetic patients in the United States, an estimated 15% to 20% will develop serious foot lesions.[4] With a 15- to 40-fold greater risk of lower extremity amputation than for those without diabetes, one half of all nontraumatic amputations in the United States are performed on diabetic patients.[7] In 1994 more than 67,000 diabetes-related amputations were performed, not including data from military, Veterans Administration, or Indian Health Service hospitals. Typically, 80% to 85% of these amputations can be attributed to a nonhealing foot ulceration. Since the 5-year survival rate only approaches 50% after a major amputation, prevention or aggressive treatment at an early stage is essential. Many feet and limbs can be salvaged through a better understanding of the peculiarities of such disorders in diabetic patients.

The most characteristic of all diabetic foot lesions is the *plantar ulceration,* often termed a *mal perforans ulcer* or *trophic ulcer.* The underlying pathophysiology is a sum of the systemic alterations occurring in diabetes with manifestations in the lower extremities.[4,9] Most diabetic foot ulcers can broadly be categorized into neuropathic, ischemic, or neuroischemic etiologies. Further grading scales use depth of penetration, presence of infection, or degree of tissue loss, but no consensus exists on a universal classification system. The most widely used grading system is the Wagner scale, consisting of grades 0 to 5, each representing progressively deeper or more extensive loss of tissue.[4] As might be expected, higher grades portend a worse prognosis and necessitate more aggressive surgical interventions or amputations.

A triad of intrinsic systemic disorders frequently cited as contributing to diabetic foot disease includes peripheral neuropathy, peripheral vascular disease, and impaired resistance to infection. This "triopathy" does not necessarily need to coexist in order to complete a causal chain to ulceration. Some form of trauma, when applied to the high-risk diabetic foot, can result in ulceration even in the presence of a single risk factor when such injuries are neglected or undetected. Evidence indicates that neuropathy, minor precipitating trauma, and structural foot deformity (e.g., hammer toes, Charcot's foot) are the three most common causes implicated in diabetic foot ulceration. Usually, however, interactions occur among multiple contributory factors in the etiology of diabetic foot ulceration[9] (Fig. 130-16).

Peripheral neuropathy is an extremely common complication of diabetes mellitus, affecting about 50% of patients with longstanding disease.[7] Approximately 70% of diabetic foot ulcerations can be attributed primarily to this underlying permissive factor. Neuropathy can be further categorized into motor, sensory, or autonomic components, with combinations present in many patients. Motor neuropathy results in muscle weakness, atrophy, dysfunction, and gait disturbance. Clinical manifestations include footdrop from anterior crural muscle atrophy or characteristic hammer toes from intrinsic muscle atrophy *(intrinsic minus foot)*. Sensory neuropathy presents in the classic "glove and stocking" distribution, symmetrically affecting the toes first and gradually moving proximally. Losses in deep tendon reflexes, proprioception, vibratory, pain, and light touch sensation are the most common findings, collectively called "negative" symptoms. Conversely, painful neuropathy is a distressing manifestation of peripheral neuropathy consisting primarily of "positive" symptoms, such as burning, gnawing, or lancinating pains that worsen at night. The *painful-painless leg* is a descriptive term used to identify patients with positive symptoms of painful neuropathy in concert with negative symptoms characteristic of the insensate foot and limb. *Autonomic neuropathy* has gained attention in recent years as an early manifestation of neuropathy and a significant factor in foot ulceration.[4,7,9] Autonomic dysfunction of thermoregulatory mechanisms in the foot results in decreased vascular tone and increased skin blood flow. Arteriovenous shunting is widespread and diverts blood flow from the nutrient capillary beds. There is also a concomitant impairment of normal hyperemic responses to injury, putatively related to insufficient endothelial cell production of nitric oxide. Sudomotor dysfunction, manifested by anhidrosis, produces dry skin that is extremely susceptible to cracking and fissuring. These are common precursors to ulceration and infection in the diabetic population.

Peripheral vascular disease, long thought to be the primary etiology of diabetic foot ulcerations, plays a dominant role in only a third of such lesions and often coexists with neuropathy. Large-vessel atherosclerotic lesions affecting the tibioperoneal trunk of the lower leg are the hallmark of diabetic macrovascular disease, although occlusions of the aortic bifurcation, iliac, and femoral systems are also common.[7] In the typical scenario, therefore, a diabetic patient can present with a gangrenous foot in the presence of a palpable popliteal artery. A relative absence of atherosclerotic disease in the foot makes distal vascular reconstruction to the dorsalis pedis or posterior tibial arteries the limb-salvaging procedures of choice in most patients. *Diabetic microangiopathy* refers to disease of the capillaries, the hallmark being a thickening of the capillary basement membrane and a resulting impairment of leukocyte diapedesis and nutrient exchange. There is *no* intravascular occlusion of these vessels, a longstanding misconception that gave rise to the term "small-vessel disease," which should be abandoned.

Susceptibility to infection and an impairment in the ability to fight established infections have long been recognized as significant factors in the etiology of diabetic foot infections, ulceration, and gangrene.[9] Although infection is infrequently a direct cause of ulceration, ulcers can be infected and often place the limb at risk of amputation. The diabetic patients' "immunopathy" is caused by a deficiency in the phagocytic activity of leukocytes, impaired intracellular bacterial killing, and a defect in normal chemotactic mechanisms. Even common pathogens can result in overwhelming infections, especially in the presence of neuropathy and ischemia. Usually "benign" bacteria such as *Staphylococcus epidermidis* or enterococci assume extremely pathogenic roles in the diabetic milieu. Anaerobic infections with *Bacteroides* species are characteristic of diabetic foot infections, although they rarely cause infection as isolated organisms. Polymicrobial infection is the rule in most severe diabetic foot infections, with gram-positive cocci, gram-negative rods, and anaerobes being cultured simultaneously from deep specimens. Empiric antibiotic therapy for limb-threatening infections should always attempt to cover a broad spectrum of organisms until final specification and sensitivities are received. Osteomyelitis is an ever-present complication of such infections and must be suspected in deeply probing, longstanding, or recalcitrant ulcerations. Although ulcerations will not completely heal when underlying bone or joint infection exists, local bone debridement and culture-specific antibiotic therapy, with vascular reconstruction as necessary, are successful in eradicating such infections and preserving limb integrity.

Trauma is usually the precipitating event in the development of diabetic foot infections or ulcerations.[4,7,9] Although such trauma can be acute (sharp, mechanical, thermal, chemical), most foot lesions in the diabetic patient are caused by the minor repetitive trauma of walking and moderate pressures, the high pressures of a tight shoe, or any degree of abnormal pressure against a structural deformity. Altered biomechanics, including increased plantar pressures, bony abnormalities (e.g., hammer toes, bunions), and limited joint mobility have been associated with an increased risk of ulceration and amputation in the diabetic population.[7] Thus, the etiology of any lesion must be investigated with the assumption that some trauma has a role in its development. In the absence of acute trauma, dorsal, medial, and lateral lesions are usually caused by tight shoes, whereas plantar lesions are the result of repetitive moderate stress or neglected preexisting hyperkeratoses. Burns are common precursors to ulceration, especially in the insensate foot, and most often result from hot foot soaks or walking barefooted on hot sand or pavement. Acute trauma in the presence of neuropathy and abundant vascular supply can also lead

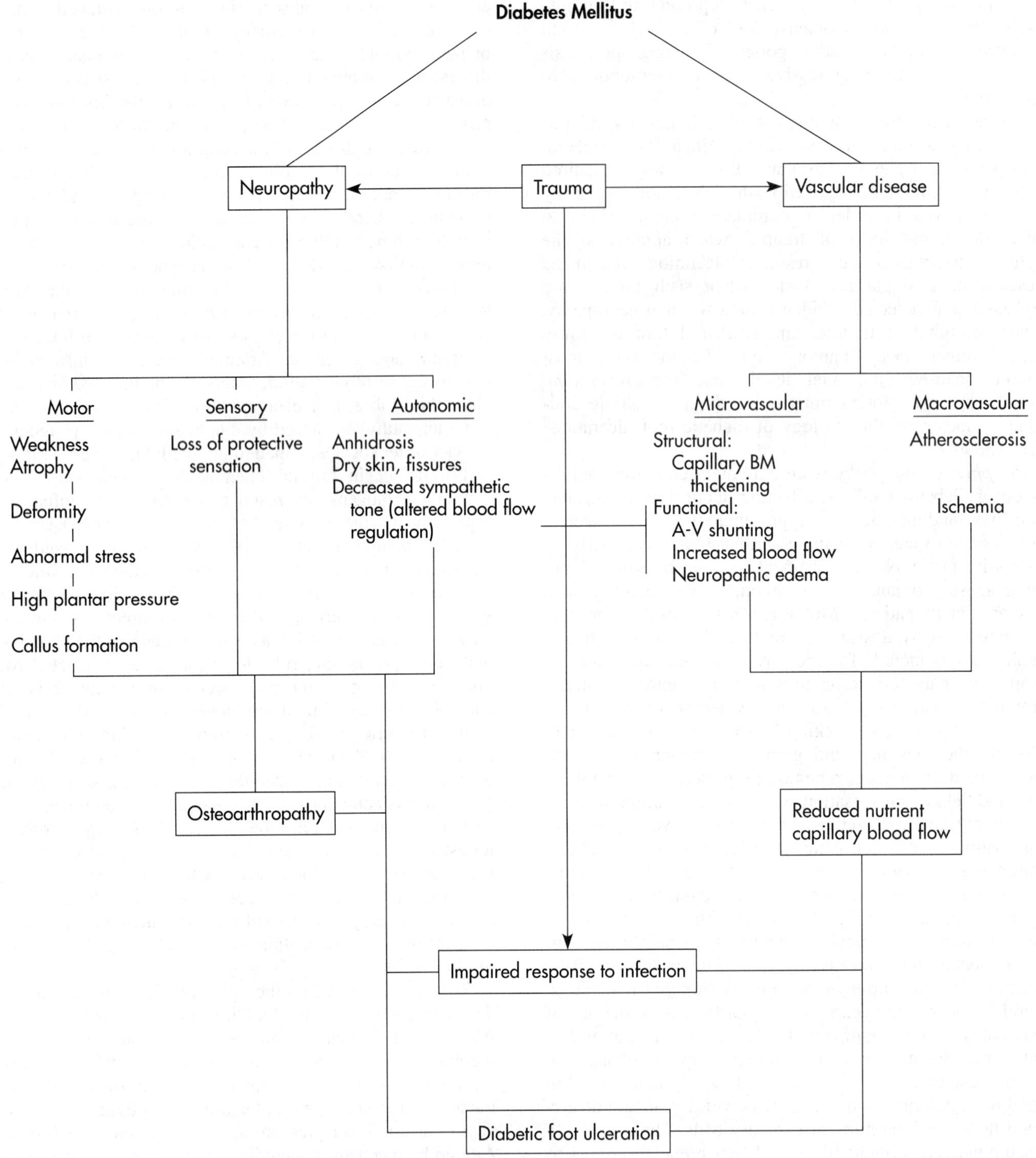

Fig. 130-16. Interactions among major contributory factors in etiology of diabetic foot ulceration. *BM,* Basement membrane, *A-V,* arteriovenous. (Modified from Boulton AJM: The diabetic foot, *Med Clin North Am* 72:1513, 1988.)

to the onset of another characteristic diabetic foot disorder, Charcot's foot or osteoarthropathy. The ensuing foot deformity creates abnormally high pressures during walking and frequently leads to chronic plantar ulceration (Fig. 130-17).

Treatment

Treatment of foot ulcerations must focus on the contributory factors and must be appropriately assessed at the onset. Acute infections are treated by culture-directed antibiotic therapy. Ischemic lesions must be recognized by their atrophic appearance and lack of pedal pulsations and referred for vascular consultation. Such lesions infrequently heal without restoration of pulsatile blood flow. Above all, non–weight bearing or attenuation of weight bearing is essential for the resolution of any ulceration.[4] The neuropathic individual, for example, will continue to walk on the ulcerated foot because of absent pain sensation or denial of the ulceration. Since

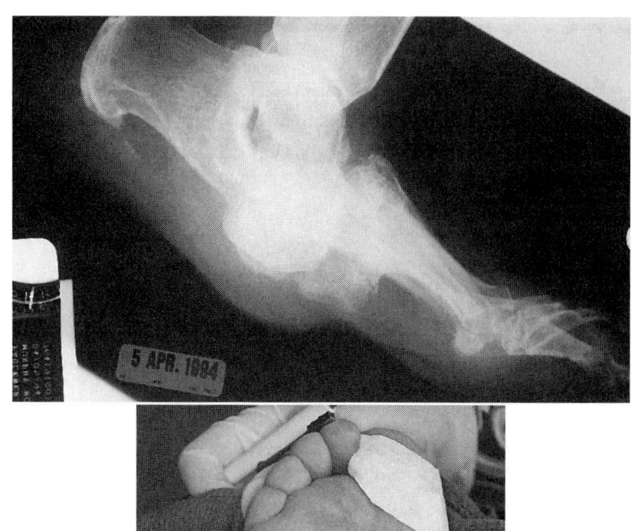

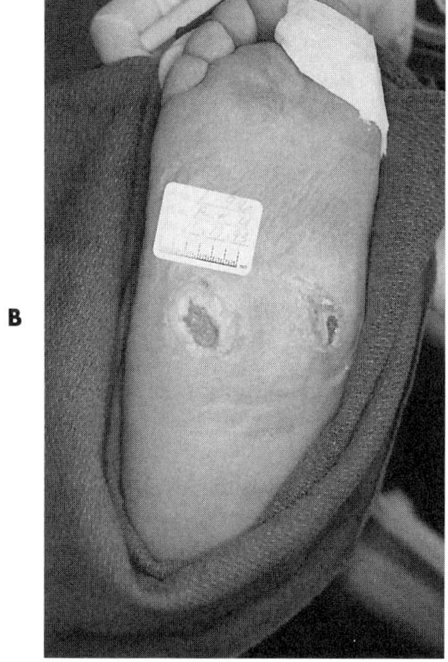

Fig. 130-17. Charcot's foot deformity. **A,** Lateral radiograph demonstrating severe midfoot osteoarthropathy with collapse of cuboid and medial cuneiform. **B,** Same foot, with plantar ulceration underlying abnormal prominences of midfoot.

walking (trauma) is a usual causative factor in ulceration, healing will not commence until walking has ceased. Although total non–weight bearing is the ideal situation, pressure-attenuating methods include foam pressure-dispersion dressings, healing sandals, surgical shoes, total contact casting, and removable cast braces. Local wound care consists of daily or twice-daily dressing changes with a topical agent of choice (e.g., quarter-strength povidone-iodine solution, saline, silver sulfadiazine cream). Topically applied growth factors (e.g., becaplermin gel, Regranex) facilitate healing of uncomplicated foot ulcerations compared with saline alone. Clinical trials are also being conducted to assess the efficacy of tissue-engineered dermal replacements. Even when proven beneficial, however, any topical agent, graft, or dressing cannot supplant the need for pressure reduction, treatment of infection, and abundant blood flow.[4]

Recurrent ulcers usually indicate a persistent bony structural deformity, shoe problem, or biomechanical foot disorder that needs attention to allow final resolution of the problem. Recalcitrant ulcers may indicate this same problem but also may suggest inadequate treatment, noncompliance, or an unrecognized infection and osteomyelitis. Overall treatment of foot ulcers therefore requires immediate attention not only to infection, circulation, and pressure reduction, but to long-term prevention as well. Prevention encompasses proper foot care, patient education, periodic examination, appropriate footwear, and prophylactic foot surgery as necessary to correct structural deformities.[4] Multiple studies from the United States and abroad indicate that more than a 50% reduction in ulcer recidivism and subsequent amputation can be realized through appropriate education, regular podiatric care, and appropriate footwear. Education can consist of simple talks or handouts regarding potential diabetic foot problems and how to recognize and avoid them. Provider education is also necessary to ensure that appropriate screening and examination techniques are reinforced as highly effective measures to detect early lesions or patients at risk of ulceration. Regular podiatric care involves bimonthly visits for examination and routine care of toenails and calluses. While serving as forums for constant patient education, such visits also provide a mechanism for early detection of potential problems and appropriate intervention. Therapeutic footwear ranges from simple molded insoles in athletic shoes to extra-depth shoes to custom-molded shoes, depending on the severity of foot lesions and the magnitude of foot deformity. When shoe therapy alone is not effective, corrective surgery is recommended in the appropriate patient and may be the best chance for permanent resolution of a recurrent problem.

As with most complex medical disorders, management of the diabetic foot should ideally be accomplished through a multidisciplinary approach.[4] The primary care physician or the podiatrist who regularly attends the patient should serve as the gatekeeper and overseer of the patient's foot health. When problems arise, an organized plan should commence for referral to the appropriate service or consultant. The emphasis is on early aggressive care and concomitant limb preservation. With such an organized approach to the high-risk foot in diabetes mellitus, the worldwide goal of a 50% reduction in lower extremity amputation can be met or exceeded within the next decade.

REFERENCES

1. American College of Foot and Ankle Surgeons: *Central metatarsalgia,* Preferred practice guidelines, Chicago, 1998, The College.
2. American College of Foot and Ankle Surgeons: *Hallux valgus in the healthy adult,* Preferred practice guidelines, Chicago, 1998, The College.
3. Birrer RB, DellaCorte MP, Grisafi PJ, editors: *Common foot problems in primary care,* Philadelphia, 1992, Hanley & Belfus.
4. Frykberg RG: Diabetic foot ulcers: current concepts, *J Foot Ankle Surg* 37:440, 1998.
5. Greenberg L, Davis H: Foot problems in the US: the 1990 National Health Interview Survey, *J Am Podiatr Med Assoc* 83:475, 1993.
6. Levy LA, Hetherington VJ, editors: *Principles and practice of podiatric medicine,* New York, 1990, Churchill Livingstone.
7. Mayfield JA, Reiber GE, Sanders LJ, et al: Preventive foot care in people with diabetes, *Diabetes Care* 21:2161, 1998.
8. McGlamry ED, editor: *Comprehensive textbook of foot surgery,* ed 2, Baltimore, 1993, Williams & Wilkins.
9. Murray H, Boulton AJM: The pathophysiology of diabetic foot ulceration, *Clin Podiatr Med Surg* 12:1, 1995.
10. Scurran BL, editor: *Foot and ankle trauma,* ed 2, New York, 1995, Churchill Livingstone.

CHAPTER 131

Idiopathic Inflammatory Myopathies

Steven R. Ytterberg

Idiopathic inflammatory myopathies (IMs) are acquired inflammatory disorders of skeletal muscle of unknown etiology. They are characterized clinically by muscle weakness that is classically symmetric, involving proximal muscles of the limbs, but may include neck and pharyngeal muscles. The chief conditions in this group are polymyositis (PM) and, when accompanied by cutaneous manifestations, dermatomyositis (DM). Several clinically defined subgroups of PM and DM have been described (Box 131-1). DM or PM may be associated with another connective tissue disease or malignancy. Inclusion body myositis (IBM) is a distinctive member of the IM group, with more frequent distal weakness and unique inclusions seen on muscle biopsy.[1] Several other less often diagnosed disorders have features of inflammatory myositis (Box 131-2).[9] Although the IMs have many similarities, they can be distinguished on clinical and histologic grounds. In addition to these IMs, a number of infectious agents and toxins can cause inflammatory myositis (see Differential Diagnosis).

Box 131-1. Classification of Polymyositis (PM) and Dermatomyositis (DM)

Idiopathic PM
Idiopathic DM
Juvenile DM or PM
DM or PM with malignancy
PM or DM with another connective tissue disease

Box 131-2. Less Common Forms of Inflammatory Myositis

Inclusion body myositis
Eosinophilic myositis
Localized nodular myositis
Proliferative myositis
Infectious myositis

EPIDEMIOLOGY

The IMs are rare disorders, with a combined annual incidence of approximately 5 to 10 per million.[3] In adult patients with IM, isolated PM and DM are each found in approximately one third of patients. PM or DM is associated with connective tissue disease in about 20% of patients and with malignancy in approximately 15%. IBM has been reported in up to 25% of adult patients with inflammatory myositis, although this estimate may be high in coming from a referral center. PM and DM have a female/male ratio of approximately 2:1. There is a greater female predominance among younger patients and among those patients who have another connective tissue disease, whereas the gender ratio is equal in patients with associated malignancy. In contrast, IBM occurs most often in middle-aged to older men. PM and DM have two peaks of incidence: during childhood and during the fifth to sixth decades. Patients with IM associated with malignancy have a mean age over 60. PM and DM are three to four times more common in blacks than whites. Seasonal variation in the onset of PM and DM has been reported, suggesting a role for environmental agents in the etiology.

The relationship between IMs and malignancy is controversial. Early observations suggested an increased frequency of malignancy in patients with PM and DM. A review of several large clinical series found malignancy in 20% of adult patients with DM, 13% with PM, and 15% overall.[5] Several case-controlled and population-based studies support the association of DM and PM with malignancy, demonstrating that patients with DM are at greater risk than those with PM. Data suggest that the relationship between IMs and malignancy is indirect, not causal. Of patients with IMs associated with malignancy, some develop malignancy first and others myositis first; no particular type of malignancy has been associated with IMs. Malignancy is more frequent in patients diagnosed with myositis after age 45. Malignancy has been reported in only a small number of patients with IBM, but experience with this condition is less extensive than with PM and DM.

PATHOPHYSIOLOGY

The etiology of the IMs is unknown. Microorganisms have long been considered as potential etiologic agents, including *Toxoplasma gondii* and several different groups of viruses, but direct evidence implicating microorganisms has been difficult to obtain. Group B coxsackieviruses and encephalomyocarditis virus, members of the Picornaviridae family, can cause inflammatory myositis in mice with similarities to human PM. Various viruses have been isolated in select patients with PM and DM, and elevated titers of antibodies to group B coxsackieviruses have been found in some children with recent onset DM. Coxsackievirus ribonucleic acid (RNA) may persist in some patients with PM and DM. No studies have shown a clear relationship of infection with IM in large groups of patients. The characteristic muscle fiber inclusions in patients with IBM resemble viral inclusions, but no virus has been linked clearly with IBM. PM and DM may be associated with retroviral infection, including human immunodeficiency virus (HIV) and human T-cell lymphotropic virus type I (HTLV-I). These viruses do not invade muscle directly.

Each of the disorders classified as IMs is characterized by clinical weakness and histologic muscle inflammation, but they have different pathophysiologic mechanisms.[3,8] Cell-mediated immunologic mechanisms are involved in the pathogenesis of PM and IBM. T cells, especially CD8 cytotoxic T cells, predominate in inflammatory infiltrates, typically in the endomysium, in PM and IBM. Activated CD8 T cells can be found invading viable muscle fibers. Humoral

Table 131-1. Autoantibodies in Patients With Idiopathic Inflammatory Myopathies (IMs)

Antibody	Approximate frequency in IMs (%)	Clinical associations
Antibodies found in other connective tissue diseases		
Antinuclear (ANA)	50-90	SLE, MCTD, scleroderma
Anti-Sm	4	SLE
Anti-nRNP	10-15	SLE MCTD
Anti-Ro (SS-A)	7-12	SLE, Sjögren's syndrome
Anti-La (SS-B)	2-10	SLE, Sjögren's syndrome
Anti-Scl-70	8	Scleroderma
Myositis-specific antibodies		
Antisynthetase antibodies	25	
Anti-Jo-1 (histidyl t-RNA)	20	Adult PM; interstitial lung disease, arthritis
Anti-PL-7 (threonyl t-RNA)	2	Interstitial lung disease
Anti-PL-12 (alanyl t-RNA)	1	Interstitial lung disease
Anti-EJ (glycyl t-RNA)	2	Interstitial lung disease
Anti-OJ (isoleucyl t-RNA)	1	Interstitial lung disease
Antisignal recognition particle (SRP)	<5	Severe PM
Anti-Mi-2	10-20	Adult DM
Anti-PM-Scl	8	PM-scleroderma overlap
Anti-Ku	<1	PM-scleroderma overlap

SLE, Systemic lupus erythematosus; *MCTD*, mixed connective tissue disease; *PM*, polymyositis; *DM*, dermatomyositis.

immune mechanisms play a greater role in DM. More CD4 T cells and a higher proportion of B cells are found, with a perivascular and perifascicular distribution. Mononuclear cells do not invade muscle fibers directly in DM, as they do in PM and IBM. In juvenile DM, vascular damage is apparent. Endothelial cell hyperplasia and vascular infarction are present, with atrophy of muscle fibers at the periphery of the fascicles (perifascicular atrophy). Immunoglobulin and the membrane attack complex of complement are found in areas of muscle necrosis, underscoring the role of humoral mechanisms in disease pathogenesis.

A variety of autoantibodies can be found in patients with IMs (Table 131-1).[4,7,10] They are infrequently found in patients with IBM. Several myositis-specific autoantibodies have been identified in patients with IMs. Most of these antibodies are directed against cytoplasmic ribonucleoproteins involved in protein synthesis. The antigens for one group of these myositis-specific antibodies are the aminoacyl tRNA synthetases, enzymes that charge the appropriate amino acid onto its corresponding tRNA. It is unclear if myositis-specific antibodies inhibit cellular function in vivo; they may be markers, rather than causes, of disease.

Muscle inflammation results in weakness and muscle tenderness. Muscle fibers demonstrate necrosis, degeneration, regeneration, and phagocytosis. The cause of weakness appears to be multifactorial. In addition to loss of muscle fibers and muscle bulk, functional abnormalities of muscle may be involved. Fibrosis and muscle atrophy may be present in later stages, also contributing to muscle weakness. Genetic factors play a role in disease, presumably through control of immunologic responsiveness.[4,7] Approximately half of white patients with PM and DM have the HLA-DR3 phenotype, usually linked with HLA-B8. In African-American patients with PM and DM, HLA-DR3 is only slightly increased, but linkage with B8 is increased over the frequency in control populations. These markers are most common in patients with anti-Jo-1 antibodies, regardless of race. In patients with IBM, HLA-DR1 is increased threefold compared with control populations. Familial cases of IBM have been described.

PATIENT EVALUATION

History

Muscle weakness is the most frequent presenting complaint in patients with IMs. Weakness is usually insidious in onset and slowly progressive, although its onset may be more abrupt, with rapid progression. Acute onset is often associated with more severe disease. Weakness is characteristically symmetric and unrelated to exercise, affecting the legs before the arms. In PM and DM, proximal limb weakness is typical; distal weakness suggests IBM. Neck, pharyngeal, and respiratory muscles may be involved. It is helpful to identify specific activities affected by weakness, such as rising from a low chair or toilet seat, getting out of a car, climbing stairs, or combing hair. Involvement of pharyngeal or esophageal muscle may result in dysphonia, dysphagia, or aspiration. Muscle tenderness and aching occur in about 50% of patients. Muscle atrophy may occur with later disease.

When a patient complains of weakness, it is important to differentiate true loss of muscle strength from fatigue or pain. Fatigue may be present in the IMs, but it is a nonspecific complaint and is seen in a variety of inflammatory diseases, as well as some noninflammatory disorders that may be confused with IMs, such as polymyalgia rheumatica and fibromyalgia. Limitation of activity by pain from articular or periarticular sources in patients with arthritis may be identified as weakness by some patients. A thorough history and muscle strength testing with elicitation of maximal effort can eliminate these possibilities and identify muscle as the source of weakness.

Box 131-3. Manual Muscle Strength Testing

0: No contraction
1: Flicker of muscle contraction but no joint movement
2: Joint movement with gravity eliminated
3: Joint movement against gravity only
4: Joint movement against gravity and resistance
5: Normal power

Skin rash may be the presenting complaint of patients with DM. Arthralgia and Raynaud's phenomenon are present in approximately 25% of patients. Systemic features can include fatigue, morning stiffness, and weight loss. In patients who have myositis associated with another connective tissue disease, features of the associated condition may be apparent. The most common associated connective tissue or autoimmune disorder is systemic lupus erythematosus (SLE); others include Hashimoto's thyroiditis, scleroderma, Sjögren's syndrome, rheumatoid arthritis, insulin-dependent diabetes mellitus, and Graves' disease. Thus arthritis, sclerodactyly, or cutaneous symptoms of SLE may be present. Occasionally, cardiac or pulmonary symptoms lead the patient to seek attention. Pulmonary involvement may lead to diminished chest wall motion or interstitial fibrosis, resulting in complaints of dyspnea or cough. Cardiac involvement may produce conduction disturbances or myocarditis with symptoms from dysrhythmia, congestive heart failure, or ischemia. Symptoms of associated malignancy may be found in some patients.

Physical Examination

Examination should exclude other causes of muscle weakness, especially neuropathic causes; identify systemic features of myositis; recognize an associated connective disease; and detect an associated malignancy. A thorough general physical examination is required, with special attention given to the neurologic examination. Muscle strength is important in a suspected IM patient. Although strength can be measured using a dynamometer, manual muscle strength testing is usually employed (Box 131-3). Manual testing has crude sensitivity but can monitor response to therapy.

Dermatomyositis is present when cutaneous manifestations accompany inflammatory myositis. A variety of skin lesions may be found in patients with DM. Two characteristic lesions are the heliotrope rash and Gottron's papules. A *heliotrope rash* is a faint, lilac-colored eruption on the upper eyelids. *Gottron's papules* are raised, red or violaceous, sometimes scaly lesions overlying the metacarpophalangeal and proximal interphalangeal joints, sparing the phalanges (Fig. 131-1). Gottron's papules may be found over the elbows or knees as well. Other nonspecific lesions, including an erythematous macular rash on the face, neck, upper chest, or shawl distribution, might be present. Vasculitic lesions may be seen at the base of the nails. Some patients have "machinist's hands." Subcutaneous calcification may be found, most often in childhood DM.

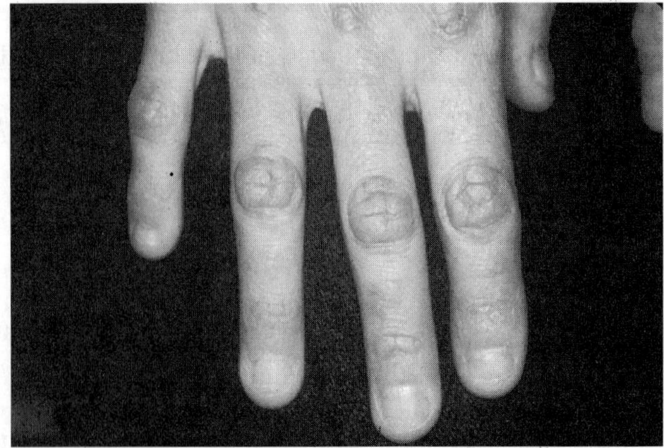

Fig. 131-1. Dermatomyositis (Gottron's papules), with erythematous papules over joints and periungual telangiectasias.

LABORATORY STUDIES AND DIAGNOSTIC PROCEDURES

Serum creatine kinase (CK) and other muscle-associated enzymes are typically elevated in patients with IMs and can be useful as indicators of response to therapy. CK levels may be modestly or markedly elevated in PM and DM; in IBM they are typically only mildly elevated. Elevation of the MB isoenzyme of CK may occur in patients with IM in the absence of myocardial involvement. A variety of pathologic and nonpathologic conditions can elevate serum CK values. Men have higher values than women, reflecting increased muscle mass. CK levels in blacks are higher than those in whites; healthy African-American subjects frequently have values that are above normal, as defined by most laboratories.[10] Elevated serum CK values can follow muscle trauma, jogging, or use of certain medications. In some patients with IMs, the CK level may be normal, whereas levels of other muscle-associated enzymes, including aldolase, lactate dehydrogenase (LDH), alanine transaminase (ALT), or aspartate transaminase (AST), are elevated.[2] Myoglobin and creatine levels may be elevated; myoglobinuria occurs in rare patients. To evaluate patients who have muscle weakness, tests for electrolytes, renal function, thyroid function, calcium, magnesium, and phosphorus are needed to exclude other causes of weakness; these tests are usually normal in patients with IM.

Autoantibodies are found in most patients with PM and DM (see Table 131-1).[4,7] Some are unique to patients with myositis, but many are seen in other connective tissue disorders as well. Serologic testing for autoantibodies can help categorize patients into subgroups and diagnose a specific connective tissue disorder.[4] Positive antinuclear antibodies (ANAs) are found in 50% to 90% of patients with IMs. The other non-muscle-specific antibodies may be seen in patients with myositis alone but occur most often in patients who have an overlap syndrome of another connective tissue disorder. Myositis-specific antibodies are found in approximately 50% of patients with PM or DM and occur infrequently in patients with IBM. The most common myositis-specific antibodies are the antisynthetase antibodies, most often anti-Jo-1 (antihistidyl tRNA synthetase). Anti-Jo-1 antibodies are found in approximately 10% of adult patients with DM and 30% to 40% with PM; they are rare in childhood disease. Anti-Jo-1 antibodies are highly specific for IMs and have a strong association with interstitial lung disease. Patients with any of the antisynthetases have a higher incidence of interstitial lung involvement and arthritis. Patients with antibodies to signal recognition particle (SRP) have the worst prognosis, often with acute onset, severe disease, and myocardial involvement.[4] To evaluate a patient with suspected IM, the primary care physician generally finds ANA, anti-Jo-1 antibody, and anti-Sci-70 antibody determinations most helpful.

Electromyography (EMG) helps differentiate myopathic from neuropathic causes of weakness and active from inactive myositis.[2,9] The myopathic pattern seen in patients with IMs is not diagnostic and is seen in other forms of active myopathy. Findings include irritability and increased insertional and spontaneous activity manifested by fibrillations, complex repetitive discharges, and positive sharp waves. With voluntary muscle activity, short-duration, low-amplitude polyphasic motor unit action potentials are observed. Patients with IBM may show neuropathic EMG changes as well. Normal EMGs are obtained in approximately 5% of patients with active IM.

Muscle biopsy is critical to establish the diagnoses of PM, DM, and IBM and to exclude other neuromuscular disorders.[3,7] Biopsy can be performed by needle technique, although many pathologists prefer open biopsies. Normal biopsies are found in approximately 7% of patients. Despite a possible false-negative result, biopsy is important before initiating therapy with significant potential for morbidity. The muscle for biopsy should be carefully selected, neither the most nor the least affected muscle. A muscle studied previously by EMG should not be biopsied because the needle may have caused pathologic changes. Magnetic resonance imaging (MRI) can help identify inflamed muscles for biopsy and can be useful in following disease progress.[8]

The key findings on muscle biopsy in patients with IMs are prominent inflammatory cells and muscle fiber changes, including degeneration, variation in cross-sectional diameter, necrosis, regeneration, and phagocytosis.[2] Biopsies are usually diffusely abnormal, but approximately 25% show only focal changes. Capillary damage and increased amounts of connective tissue and fat may be noted. In DM, inflammation tends to be perivascular and around muscle fascicles, with fiber atrophy in perifascicular areas. Perifascicular atrophy is not a characteristic finding in PM or IBM. In PM the inflammation is primarily endomysial, within muscle fascicles. Necrotic fibers are not grouped as in DM and may not be near areas of inflammation. The characteristic histologic finding in IBM is nuclear and cytoplasmic inclusions, with rimmed vacuoles.[1] These inclusions show masses of filamentous material on electron microscopy. Although inflammatory cells on biopsy are characteristic of IMs, their presence alone does not make the diagnosis. Muscle inflammation can be seen in other necrotizing conditions, including Duchenne's dystrophy and myasthenia gravis.

Other workup should be directed by specific complaints or physical findings. A chest radiograph is helpful in identifying interstitial fibrosis or associated pulmonary malignancy. If interstitial fibrosis is present, the lung diffusion capacity is often diminished. Because of the cost and potential hazards of performing tests and procedures to identify an occult malignancy, an exhaustive search for malignancy in all patients with a new diagnosis of IM is unreasonable.[1] A patient should undergo a thorough history and physical examination, chemistry panel, blood count, stool guaiac examination, and chest radiograph. Appropriate cancer screening for colon, cervical, breast, and prostate cancers is appropriate if not done recently.

Course and Prognosis

Survival rates for patients with PM and DM are approximately 80% 5 years after diagnosis and 73% after 8 years. Several clinical features correlate with poor prognosis: older age at diagnosis; cardiac involvement, dysphagia, or malignancy; long delay between symptom onset and initiation of therapy; and poor initial response to corticosteroids. Patients with antibodies to SRP or to any of the aminoacyl-tRNA synthetases have more severe disease than those without these antibodies.[4] Of patients with PM or DM, approximately half have complete or near-complete recovery. In contrast, patients with IBM often do not respond to therapy and usually follow a gradually deteriorating course.

Differential Diagnosis

The diagnosis of PM, DM, or IBM is based on muscle inflammation in a patient with muscle weakness, but the physician must consider other diseases that can cause weakness and inflammatory myositis (Fig. 131-2). Criteria for diagnosing PM and DM are widely used; preliminary criteria for diagnosing IBM are also available (Boxes 131-4 and 131-5). These criteria were established to facilitate classification of patients for study purposes rather than to be specific diagnostic criteria for individuals, but they can be useful when considering the diagnosis of IM in an individual. Before these criteria are used, other causes of weakness must be excluded. Muscle weakness can result from different disease processes (Box 131-6).[9,10] Many can be excluded by the history and physical examination, but laboratory and biopsy data may be required.

Neurologic disorders are primary differential diagnoses of patients with weakness. The presence of other neurologic abnormalities on examination strongly suggests a neuropathic rather than a myopathic etiology. IBM may have neuropathic features, however, including diminished deep tendon reflexes. Asymmetric or early distal muscle involvement or muscle hypertrophy may be clues to a diagnosis other than IM. The presence of facial or ocular complaints and unique EMG findings help identify myasthenia gravis or Eaton-Lambert syndrome. A familial history of weakness and younger age at onset may suggest a muscular dystrophy, which may increase the serum CK (e.g., Duchenne's).

Electrolyte abnormalities and metabolic disorders must be excluded. Elevation or lowering of serum sodium, potassium, or calcium levels, as well as hypophosphatemia and hypomagnesemia, should be sought. Hypothyroidism can cause weakness and marked CK elevations. Hyperthyroidism, hyperparathyroidism, Cushing's disease, and Addison's disease are other easily excluded endocrine causes of muscle weakness.

Some drugs can cause weakness, with or without CK elevation. The list of implicated agents is long, but several merit specific mention. Ethanol is probably the most common drug that produces myopathy; it can cause acute muscle swelling and pain after binge drinking or chronic progressive proximal myopathy with long-term alcohol use. Corti-

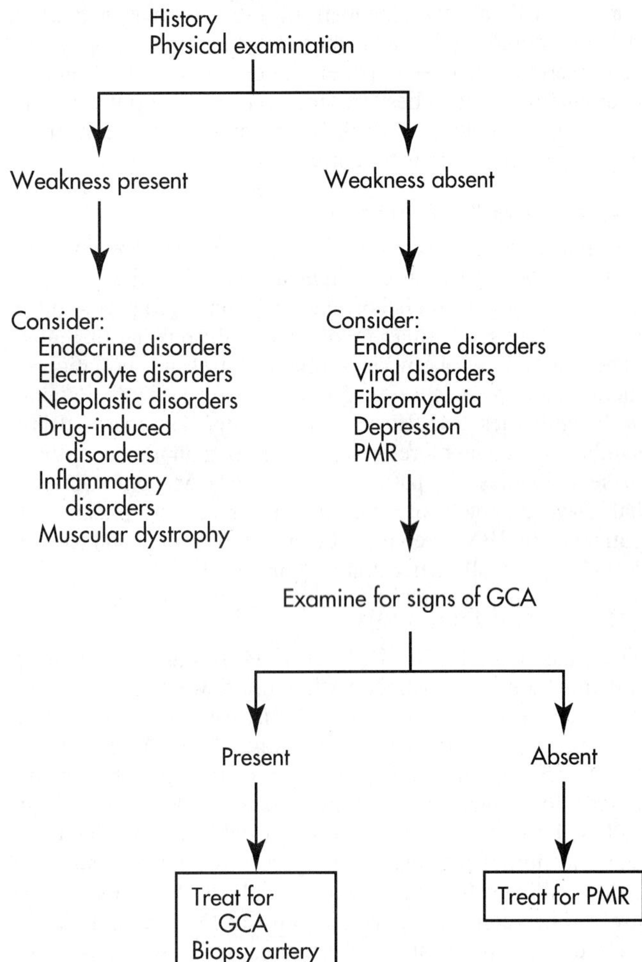

Fig. 131-2. Treatment of patient with diffuse muscle pain and stiffness. *PMR,* Polymyalgia rheumatica; *GCA,* giant cell arteritis. (From Maricic MJ: Diffuse muscle pain and stiffness: polymyalgia rheumatica and giant cell arteritis. In Greene HL, Johnson WP, Maricic MJ, editors: *Decision making in medicine,* ed 2, St Louis, 1998, Mosby, p 445.)

Box 131-4. Criteria for Diagnosis of PM and DM

1. Symmetric proximal muscle weakness
2. Elevated serum skeletal muscle enzyme levels
3. Myopathic changes on electromyography
4. Muscle biopsy showing inflammatory myositis
5. Skin rash typical of DM

Polymyositis

Definite: all of criteria 1-4
Probable: any three of criteria 1-4
Possible: any two of criteria 1-4

Dermatomyositis

Definite: criterion 5 plus three other criteria
Probable: criterion 5 plus two other criteria
Possible: criterion 5 plus one other criterion

Box 131-5. Criteria for Diagnosis of Inclusion Body Myositis (IBM)

I. Clinical Criteria

A. Proximal muscle weakness
B. Distal muscle weakness
C. Electromyographic evidence of generalized myopathy
D. Elevation of muscle enzyme levels
E. Failure of muscle weakness to improve with high-dose corticosteroids

II. Pathologic Criteria

A. Electron microscopy of muscle showing inclusions containing microtubular filaments
B. Light microscopy
  1. Intranuclear/intracytoplasmic inclusions
  2. Lined vacuoles

Classification of IBM

Definite: Clinical criterion IA plus one other clinical criterion and pathologic criterion IIA
Probable: Clinical criterion IA plus three other clinical criteria and pathologic criteria IIB1 and IIB2
Possible: Any three clinical criteria plus pathologic criteria IIB1 and IIB2

costeroids can cause proximal muscle weakness, which can be confusing in patients with IM treated with steroids, but CK levels are typically normal. Clofibrate, colchicine, D-penicillamine, chloroquine, hydroxychloroquine, ε-aminocaproic acid, and vincristine can cause weakness with CK elevation. Zidovudine (AZT) has been associated with myalgia and muscle weakness, which may produce diagnostic difficulty because HIV infection itself has been associated with PM. In primary care patients, among the most common medications to cause myopathy are the lipid-lowering HMG-coenzyme reductase inhibitors such as lovastatin, especially when combined with gemfibrozil, clofibrate, niacin, erythromycin, or cyclosporine. Cocaine may cause an elevated CK and even rhabdomyolysis.

Chronic myositis can result from parasitic infections, including toxoplasmosis, trichinosis, and schistosomiasis, and with certain viral infections, most notably coxsackieviruses and influenza virus. HIV and HTLV-I infections have been associated with PM, but these agents do not infect muscle directly. Bacterial infection of muscle usually causes acute symptoms that are usually not confused with IMs.

Metabolic myopathies can cause muscle weakness and may be confused with the IMs. Several glycogen storage diseases, including McArdle's disease (myophosphorylase deficiency), can cause elevation of the CK and muscle weakness. Symptoms exacerbated by exercise, muscle cramps, or myoglobinuria may suggest these diagnoses. Disorders of fat metabolism (e.g., carnitine deficiency, carnitine palmitoyltransferase deficiency) and purine metabolism (e.g., myoadenylate deaminase deficiency) can present with proximal weakness and CK elevation as well. Ischemic forearm muscle exercise testing can help identify some of these patients. In normal subjects, venous lactate and ammonia levels rise after

Box 131-6. Differential Diagnosis of Idiopathic Inflammatory Myopathies (IMs)

Collagen Vascular Disease
Fibromyalgia
Polyarteritis nodosa
Polymyalgia rheumatica
Rheumatoid arthritis
Scleroderma
Systemic lupus erythematosus
Temporal arteritis

Neurologic
Denervation
  Amyotrophic lateral sclerosis
Neuromuscular junction disorders
  Myasthenia gravis
  Eaton-Lambert syndrome
Muscular dystrophies
  Duchenne's
  Limb girdle
  Other
Neuropathies
  Guillain-Barré syndrome
  Diabetes mellitus
  Porphyria

Metabolic/Nutritional
Uremia
Hepatic failure
Malabsorption
Hypercalcemia or hypocalcemia
Hypernatremia or hyponatremia
Hyperkalemia or hypokalemia
Hypophosphatemia
Periodic paralysis
Vitamin E deficiency
Vitamin D deficiency

Endocrine
Hyperthyroidism or hypothyroidism
Hyperparathyroidism or hypoparathyroidism
Cushing's disease
Addison's disease
Hyperaldosteronism

Carcinomatous
Neuropathy
Neuromyopathy
Myositis
Microembolization

Drug Induced
Cimetidine
Clofibrate
Colchicine
Corticosteroids
ϵ-Aminocaproic acid
Emetine
Ethanol
Hydroxychloroquine
Ipecac
Lovastatin
Penicillamine
Vincristine
Zidovudine (AZT)

Infectious
Viral
  Influenza
  Epstein-Barr virus
  Coxsackieviruses A and B
  Human immunodeficiency virus
  Adenovirus
  Echovirus
  Rubella
Parasitic
  Toxoplasmosis
  Trichinosis
  Schistosomiasis
  Toxocariasis
  Cysticercosis
Bacterial
  Staphylococcal
  Streptococcal
  Clostridial
Rickettsial

Storage Diseases
Glycogen storage diseases
Lipid
  Carnitine deficiency
  Carnitine palmitoyltransferase deficiency
Purine
  Myoadenylate deaminase deficiency

Modified from Wortmann RL: Idiopathic inflammatory myopathies. In Bennett JC, Plum F, editors: *Cecil textbook of medicine*, ed 20, Philadelphia, 1996, Saunders.

ischemic exercise. In patients with glycogen storage disorders, ammonia, but not lactate, rises after such exercise, whereas in myoadenylate deaminase deficiency, lactate levels but not ammonia levels rise. Histochemical studies of muscle biopsy specimens are key to making the diagnosis of a storage disease.

Myositis and muscle weakness may occur with connective tissue disorders that include rheumatoid arthritis, SLE, and scleroderma. Among the more common disorders considered in the differential diagnosis of the IMs are polymyalgia rheumatica and fibromyalgia. Key features in the workup can eliminate these disorders (Table 131-2). Most notable is the presence of pain with normal muscle strength in the latter two conditions. The patient must be urged to maximal effort during the examination to demonstrate normal strength.

Table 131-2. Findings in Idiopathic Inflammatory Myopathies (IMs) and Differential Diagnoses

Finding	Disorder				
	PM	**DM**	**IBM**	**PMR**	**Fibromyalgia**
Weakness	Proximal > distal	Proximal > distal	Proximal and/or distal	No	No
Pain	No	No	No	Yes	Yes
EMG findings	Myopathic	Myopathic	Myopathic or neuropathic	Normal	Normal
Muscle enzymes	Elevated, up to 50×	Elevated, up to 50×	Elevated, up to 10× or normal	Normal	Normal
Muscle biopsy	Characteristic*	Characteristic*	Characteristic*	Normal or type II fiber atrophy	Normal
Skin rash	No	Yes	No	No	No

PM, Polymyositis; *DM*, dermatomyositis; *IBM*, inclusion body myositis; *PMR*, polymyalgia rheumatica; *EMG*, electromyographic.
*Characteristic features may be seen in these biopsies (see text).

MANAGEMENT

Given the complexity of the differential diagnosis in patients suspected of having an IM, the need to assess the overlap with other connective tissue diseases, and the potential for complications of therapy, confirmation of diagnosis and management plans should be made in consultation with a rheumatologist. Corticosteroids are the mainstay of treatment, although their use has not been tested in controlled studies.[2,3,6,7] Treatment should be started at approximately 1 to 2 mg/kg/day, given in two to three divided doses. Patients with a more acute onset and more severe disease should be treated at the more aggressive end of this range. Clinical and laboratory parameters should be monitored to assess the response to therapy. Muscle enzymes may respond before improvement in muscle strength, but evaluation of functional improvement is most important. Patience is required; unlike many other inflammatory autoimmune disorders, the IMs often respond slowly. In patients who respond to steroids, strength usually improves in 1 to 2 months but may require 3 months. As the patient responds, the dosing frequency must be consolidated, ultimately to a single daily dose. High-dose steroids should be continued for 4 to 6 weeks after strength has improved, before tapering is slowly begun. The lowest possible dosage that controls the disease should be used. Attaining a stable condition on the minimal dosage often requires 1 to 2 years. Alternate-day steroids may be effective but should be reserved for patients with mild disease.

Some patients respond initially but then have a decrease in strength while tapering steroid dosage. Coincident elevation of CK values suggests exacerbation of myositis, but if the serum CK remains normal, steroid myopathy should be considered. The EMG in steroid myopathy may show a myopathic pattern, but the fibrillations seen in IMs are not present. Muscle biopsy can help in showing type II fiber atrophy without inflammation in the patient with steroid myopathy, but this is not absolute, given the focal nature of inflammation that may occur in IMs. At times the steroid dosage may need to be raised or lowered, awaiting signs of improvement or worsening. Since high dosages are usually given over long periods, measures to prevent potential complications of corticosteroid therapy should be instituted. Prophylaxis of steroid-induced osteoporosis with calcium (1 to 2 gm/day) and vitamin D should be undertaken. In postmenopausal women, hormone replacement therapy should be considered. Bone mineral density screening can help guide measures directed at preventing or treating osteoporosis.

For patients who do not respond to corticosteroids, accuracy of the diagnosis should be questioned, with consideration of IBM or an associated malignancy, because both typically respond less well to treatment. Immunosuppressive agents may be required for patients who do not respond to steroids, who flare while the dose is being lowered, or who develop intolerable side effects from steroids. Some authors advocate early use of immunosuppressives in an attempt to minimize the potential side effects of corticosteroids. The most frequently used immunosuppressive agents are azathioprine and methotrexate; 6-mercaptopurine, cyclophosphamide, chlorambucil, and cyclosporin A are also reported to be effective.[3,6,7] Methotrexate can be administered intravenously, intramuscularly, or orally; the oral route is preferred to avoid elevation of CK values from the injections. A potential problem of methotrexate therapy is interstitial pulmonary fibrosis, which is also a potential extramuscular site of pathology in IMs.

For patients unresponsive to standard immunosuppressants, other immunosuppressive modalities have been attempted. Intravenous immunoglobulin (IVIg) appears to be the most promising, with biochemical and clinical response shown in patients with severe disease. Combinations of immunosuppressives may be needed in some patients. Patients with IBM are considered to be unresponsive to therapy with steroids, although some may respond with improvement or at least stabilization of strength and function. Thus an attempt to treat patients with IBM is warranted. For patients with IM associated with malignancy, the first step is to deal with the malignancy. If the malignancy responds to treatment, the IM may as well, but this is highly variable.

Physical therapy and other modalities are important adjuncts to the therapy of patients with IMs. During periods of active muscle inflammation, patients should be kept on bed rest. An exercise program should include daily stretching done passively or with therapist assistance to maintain range of motion and prevent contractures. With response to medical therapy, active exercise should be encouraged, avoiding overwork that can damage muscle. Adaptive aids can improve function. A raised toilet seat and grip bars can be helpful. Inspiratory muscle training can help patients with respiratory muscle weakness.

REFERENCES

1. Askanas V, Engel WK: Sporadic inclusion-body myositis and hereditary inclusion-body myopathies: current concepts of diagnosis and pathogenesis, *Curr Opin Rheumatol* 10:530, 1998.
2. Bohan A, Peter JB, Bowman RL, Pearson CM: A computer-assisted analysis of 153 patients with polymyositis and dermatomyositis, *Medicine* 56:255, 1977.
3. Dalakas MC: Polymyositis, dermatomyositis, and inclusion-body myositis, *N Engl J Med* 325:1487, 1991.
4. Love LA, Leff RL, Fraser DD, et al: A new approach to the classification of idiopathic inflammatory myopathy: myositis-specific autoantibodies define useful homogenous patient groups, *Medicine* 70:360, 1991.
5. Masi AT, Hochberg MC: Temporal association of polymyositis-dermatomyositis with malignancy: methodologic and clinical considerations, *Mt Sinai J Med* 55:471, 1988.
6. Oddis CV: Therapy of inflammatory myopathy, *Rheum Dis Clin North Am* 20:899, 1994.
7. Plotz PH, Rider LG, Targoff IN, et al: Myositis: immunologic contributions to understanding cause, pathogenesis, and therapy, NIH conference, *Ann Intern Med* 122:715, 1995.
8. Reimers CD, Finkenstaedt M: Muscle imaging in inflammatory myopathies, *Curr Opin Rheumatol* 9:475, 1997.
9. Strongwater SL: Overview and clinical manifestations of inflammatory myositis: polymyositis and dermatomyositis, *Mt Sinai J Med* 55:435, 1988.
10. Wortmann RL: Idiopathic inflammatory myopathies. In Bennett JC, Plum F, editors: *Cecil textbook of medicine,* ed 20, Philadelphia, 1996, Saunders.

CHAPTER 132

Osteoarthritis

Eric W. Jacobson

Osteoarthritis (OA, also known as osteoarthrosis or degenerative joint disease) is the most common rheumatic disease, affecting more than 50 million people in the United States. The cost to society for treatment and lost earnings is staggering. Recent advances in the understanding of the pathophysiology of OA have altered the conception of this disease. Once viewed as a slowly advancing disease with limited possibilities for medical intervention, OA is now seen as a disease that can be modified in regard to immediate treatment and long-term outcome.[7]

EPIDEMIOLOGY

Osteoarthritis is a prevalent disease of cartilage that increases steadily with age. Up to 85% of the general population has radiographic evidence of OA by age 65.[4] OA is equally distributed among men and women when all age groups are considered. In people over age 55, however, women are more often affected and tend to have more severe disease because of body habitus or genetic predisposition. Prevalence patterns of OA may be subtly different among races, but this may relate more to differences in occupations and lifestyles than directly to race.[10] Genetic predisposition involves mainly OA of the distal interphalangeal (DIP) joints of the hands, which seems to follow an autosomal dominant pattern of inheritance with variable expression. Expression is gender linked and dominant in women.

Box 132-1. Factors in Etiology of Osteoarthritis

- Age
- Genetic predisposition (distal interphalangeal joints)
- Trauma, repetitive stress
- Occupation
- Obesity
- Altered joint anatomy, joint instability
- Changes in cartilage biochemistry
- Secondary inflammation

ETIOLOGY

The etiology of OA is multifactorial (Box 132-1). Although a strong association exists between OA and aging, OA is not a natural consequence of aging. Biochemical changes in the matrix molecules of cartilage occur with age but are different from the biochemical changes that occur in osteoarthritic cartilage.[11] Aging cartilage, however, may be more prone to OA if other etiologic factors (e.g., genetic predisposition) are present.

Joints that have sustained serious trauma (e.g., fractures, ligamentous injuries) are prone to OA in later years. Joints exposed to repetitive trauma also are associated with OA, often related to occupation. Ballet dancers have an increased incidence of OA in the ankles and feet because of repetitive trauma across these joints; American football players are prone to knee OA. An exception is long-distance runners, in whom studies have failed to show an increased incidence of OA in lower extremity joints despite repetitive stress.[9] Self-selected body habitus in runners at baseline may be associated with protection against development of OA.

Obesity is also associated with OA, although studies show conflicting results. A statistically significant increase of knee OA was shown in obese women but not in obese men.[5]

Any alteration of normal joint anatomy or of joint stability is associated with an increased risk of OA in that joint, as in congenital abnormalities (e.g., congenital hip dislocation) and acquired abnormalities (e.g., chronic dislocation resulting from trauma). Altered joint anatomy leads to a change in the distribution of force across that joint. In a normal joint, force is distributed uniformly across the cartilaginous surface. If the anatomy is altered, forces across the joint may localize to one area of cartilage, leading to focal damage. This initiates the osteoarthritic process. Therefore any process leading to joint destruction predisposes to secondary OA. This includes inflammatory arthropathies (e.g., rheumatoid arthritis [RA], gout, pseudogout), metabolic conditions affecting joints (hemochromatosis, ochronosis), bleeding diatheses (e.g., hemophilia) in which recurrent hemarthrosis occurs, avascular necrosis with subsequent alteration of normal bony contour, and neurologic disorders associated with altered sensation of proprioception around a joint. Alterations in the molecular composition of cartilage and secondary inflammatory processes are also important in the development of OA.

PATHOPHYSIOLOGY

Normal articular cartilage is composed of interstitial fluid, cellular elements, and matrix molecules (Box 132-2).

Box 132-2. Composition of Cartilage

Interstitial fluid
Cellular elements
- Stationary (chondrocytes)
- Circulatory (mononuclear cells)

Proteins
- Type II collagen
- Elastin
- Fibronectin

Complex polysaccharides: proteoglycans (glycosaminoglycans plus hyaluronic acid backbone)

Approximately 70% of cartilage is water; this percentage increases with advancing stages of OA. Cellular elements may be stationary (e.g., chondrocytes) or circulatory (e.g., lymphocytes, other mononuclear cells). The chondrocyte synthesizes matrix molecules, thus possessing reparative capabilities. The major matrix molecules consist of proteins (collagen, mainly type II; elastin; fibronectin) and complex polysaccharides (proteoglycans). The proteoglycan molecule is made up of a hyaluronic acid backbone with glycosaminoglycan derivatives attached at about 90-degree angles. This composition gives cartilage strength and elasticity. Its function is to absorb impact loading across the joint and to allow smooth gliding of juxtaposed articular surfaces.

The pathogenesis of OA involves a dual process of catabolism and repair. Remodeling is ongoing in normal cartilage; matrix molecules are regularly degraded by autolytic enzymes and then replaced through production by chondrocytes. In OA this process is altered and causes an overall loss of matrix molecules despite attempts at repair. The newly synthesized matrix molecules are considered mechanically inferior to the original molecules and therefore may be more prone to injury and further damage. The process may be initiated by local trauma that leads to chondrocyte injury. Chondrocytes release proteolytic enzymes (e.g., neutral proteases, acid cathepsins, collagenase, metalloproteases), which degrade matrix molecules, including the proteoglycan aggregate, producing smaller, nonaggregating molecules. This leads to thinner, mechanically inferior cartilage. The rate of release of these enzymes and the subsequent rate of matrix molecule destruction are significantly more rapid in osteoarthritic cartilage than in normal cartilage.[1] Loss of tensile strength for load support leads to transmission of greater force to chondrocytes and subchondral bone. Chondrocytes sustain greater injury, leading to further release of degrading enzymes. Subchondral bone sustains microfractures, causing stiffening and loss of compressibility. Some of the breakdown products from cartilage and proteoglycans may stimulate a secondary inflammatory response involving polymorphonuclear leukocytes, synovial cells, and macrophages. The whole process is perpetuated in a continuous destructive cycle (Fig. 132-1).

PATIENT EVALUATION

History

Osteoarthritis is the prototype of a noninflammatory arthritis. From the history the physician should begin to differentiate OA from inflammatory arthropathies (e.g., RA). OA typically begins in the later decades of life and has a slow, insidious onset that is gradually progressive over many years. The joint distribution is distinctive, mainly involving the weight-bearing joints, the spine, and the hands. Unless the patient has a history of trauma or other predisposing factors, OA typically spares the wrists, elbows, and shoulders. Involvement of any of these joints without a history of trauma should suggest other causes of the arthritis.

The patient describes classic mechanical joint pain. The pain is typically aching in quality and is brought on by use of the joint. Early in the disease the pain is relieved by rest. In advanced disease, pain occurs at rest and with exertion. This is in contrast to inflammatory arthritis, in which pain frequently improves with activity. In classic OA, patients complain of pain, but there is no obvious swelling, redness, or warmth. With time the patient may describe progressive bony enlargement of joints and restricted joint motion. The patient describes short-term stiffness after inactivity and less than 30 minutes of stiffness in the morning. This is in contrast to the inflammatory arthritides, in which morning stiffness can be very prolonged and may correlate with disease activity. Patients may also describe a creaking or cracking of joints with motion that may worsen with progressive loss of cartilage (Box 132-3).

OA may involve the cervical and the lumbosacral spine, unlike RA, which typically involves the cervical spine but spares the lumbosacral spine. Nerve root compression may occur with spinal involvement. The patient may then complain of radiating pain down an extremity, associated with paresthesias and focal weakness. These symptoms should present in a dermatomal distribution. Osteoarthritic involvement of the lumbar spine can also lead to spinal stenosis. The classic history of spinal stenosis is leg claudication. Pain occurs with ambulation, persists with stopping and standing, but is relieved with sitting or bending forward. Vascular claudication, on the other hand, is relieved with stopping and standing still.

Inflammatory or erosive OA involves the hands, affecting proximal interphalangeal (PIP) and DIP joints, and is associated with swelling, redness, and warmth. True erosions occur, leading to joint destruction and occasionally bony ankylosis. This arthropathy may be confused with psoriatic arthritis, another erosive arthropathy often affecting DIP joints.

Physical Examination

Examination of a patient with OA requires consideration of the typical joint distribution (Box 132-4). OA tends to involve the weight-bearing joints, the spine, and the hands. Hips and knees are often affected, usually somewhat symmetrically. In the hands the classic joint involvement includes the first carpometacarpal (CMC) joint at the base of the thumb, the PIP joints, and the DIP joints. This is in contrast to RA, which involves the metacarpophalangeal joints and PIP joints but spares the DIP joints. OA also involves the first metatarsophalangeal (MTP) joints of the feet.

Joint examination in OA depends on the area being examined. In general, there is pain with motion and sometimes with palpation, limited range of motion of the joint (related to loss of articular cartilage), and bony enlargement of the joint (related to the proliferative spurs). The capsule may appear thickened. Typical OA shows no signs of active inflammation (warmth, erythema, true

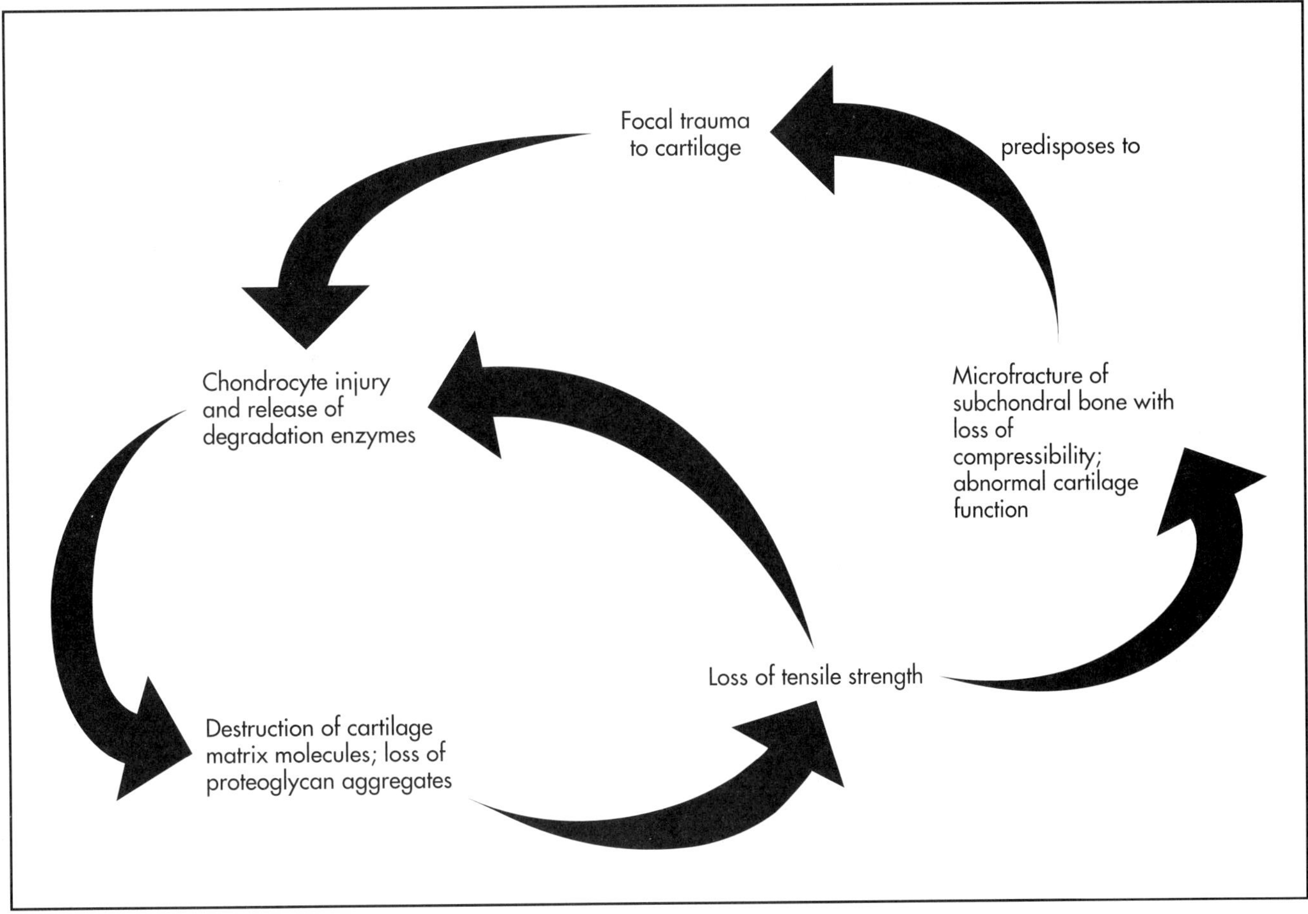

Fig. 132-1. Pathogenesis of osteoarthritis.

Box 132-3. Classic Features of Osteoarthritis

Aging population
Insidious onset over many years
Mechanical pain that worsens with activity
Bony enlargement, but *no* true swelling, warmth, or erythema
Progressive loss of joint range of motion
Short-term morning stiffness (less than 30 minutes)

Box 132-4. Joint Distribution in Osteoarthritis

- Weight-bearing joints
  - Hips
  - Knees
- Spine
  - Cervical spine
  - Lumbosacral spine
- Hands
  - Carpometacarpal joints
  - Proximal interphalangeal joints (Bouchard's nodes)
  - Distal interphalangeal joints (Heberden's nodes)
- Feet: first metatarsophalangeal joints

effusions). Lack of these signs helps distinguish OA from the inflammatory arthritides. Examination of the spine may reveal loss of range of motion, depending on the stage of the disease. When spinal involvement is present, a thorough neurologic examination of the extremities should be performed to screen for nerve root impingement syndromes. Hip examination reveals loss of range of motion and pain. Knee examination shows loss of motion and frequently crepitus (a feeling of crunching when the joint is moved). Effusions are generally absent. Bony enlargement of PIP and DIP joints leads to a knobby appearance. These changes are referred to as Bouchard's nodes in the PIP joints and Heberden's nodes in the DIP joints. CMC involvement is associated with a squaring at the base of the thumb, usually accompanied by marked pain with squeezing. MTP involvement is often associated with bunion formation.

As OA progresses, loss of articular cartilage becomes more prominent, and normal anatomy is altered. This changes the distribution of force across the joint, sometimes leading to strain across tendons, bursae, and other periarticular structures. The physician must therefore check for the presence of soft tissue rheumatism in areas in proximity to osteoarthritic joints. Trochanteric bursitis of the hip and anserine bursitis of the knee are common causes of pain, in addition to the pain caused by the OA (see Chapters 128 and 129).

LABORATORY STUDIES AND DIAGNOSTIC PROCEDURES

Laboratory studies in OA are generally unrevealing. Tests checking for systemic inflammation (e.g., erythrocyte sedimentation rate, C-reactive protein), blood counts, and general chemistries are normal. Ordering rheumatology profiles is not indicated when the history and physical examination are consistent with OA. Routine x-ray films confirm the presence of OA and are helpful in establishing extent of disease (Fig. 132-2). Radiographic findings include joint space narrowing, subchondral bony sclerosis, subchondral cysts, and osteophytes (proliferative spurs) (Box 132-5; see Chapter 123). Erosions are not seen in general OA but may be seen in the inflammatory form. Computed tomography (CT) or magnetic resonance imaging (MRI) scans of the spine may be indicated if the patient has signs or symptoms suggesting a nerve impingement syndrome. These studies rule out neuroforaminal encroachment or disk herniation leading to nerve impingement. CT and MRI also are used to assess for associated spinal stenosis.

Box 132-5. Radiographic Changes in Osteoarthritis

Joint space narrowing
Subchondral bony sclerosis
Subchondral cysts
Osteophytes (proliferative spurs)

MANAGEMENT

As with any arthritis, treatment should begin with education so the patient understands the diagnosis, prognosis, and treatment options (Box 132-6). In OA it is important to preserve joint cartilage and thus range of motion. The patient is taught joint protection and avoids activities that lead to repetitive trauma to the joint; jogging, for example, results in repetitive stress across the knee joints and may predispose cartilage to more rapid deterioration. Similarly, weight loss is an appropriate goal for patients with OA involving lower extremities and the lumbar spine.

Box 132-6. Treatments for Osteoarthritis

- Patient education
- Periodic rest
- Joint protection
- Weight loss
- Physical therapy (e.g., TENS)
- Occupational therapy (e.g., assistive devices)
- Medications
  - Analgesics
  - Nonsteroidal antiinflammatory drugs (NSAIDs)
  - Cyclooxygenase II inhibitors
  - Topical capsaicin
  - Hyaluronic acid (viscosupplementation)
  - Intraarticular corticosteroid injections
- Surgery
  - Osteotomy
  - Joint debridement
  - Arthrodesis (fusion)
  - Arthroplasty (replacement)

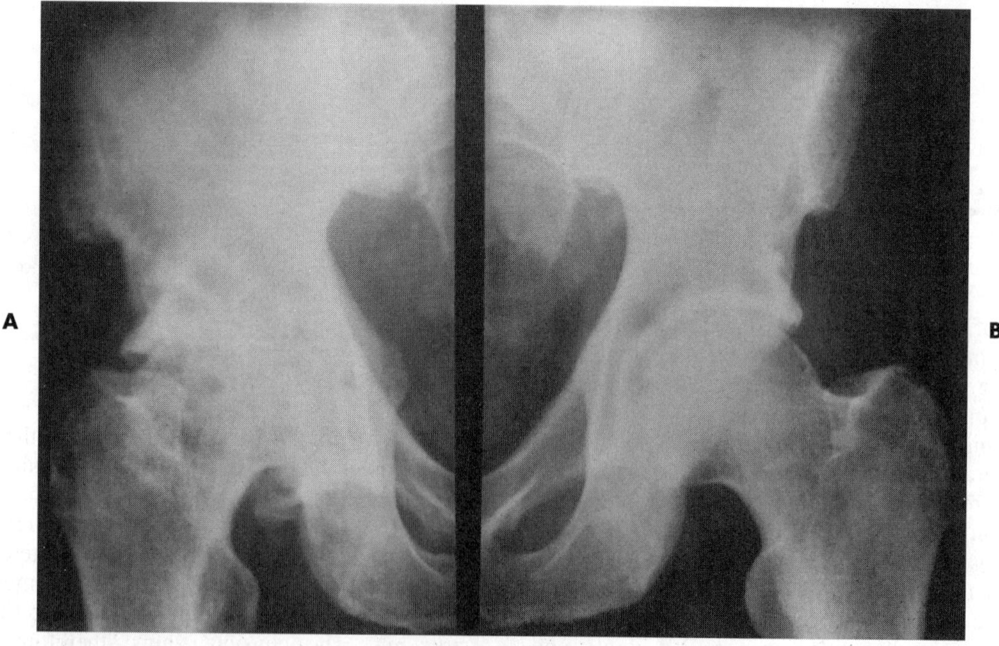

Fig. 132-2. Severe osteoarthritis of hip (**A**) compared with normal hip (**B**). (Courtesy American Rheumatism Association.)

Physical therapy and occupational therapy are useful modalities for patients with OA. Basic physical therapy should include education regarding range of motion exercises, which may preserve joint mobility. Physical therapists teach patients appropriate strengthening exercises to preserve the strength of muscle groups surrounding involved joints. This helps maintain stability of the joints, reduce pain, and prevent injury. Heat, ultrasound, and massage techniques may also reduce pain. For chronic pain unresponsive to other measures, a transcutaneous electric nerve stimulation (TENS) trial may be appropriate; the patient can wear the unit throughout the day. The TENS unit can be adjusted to maximize electric output when pain increases. This is helpful for some patients with chronic low back, hip, and knee pain related to OA. An occupational therapy evaluation is useful in assessing the patient's functional limitations. Occupational therapists provide assistive devices that allow patients to perform home or work tasks that would otherwise be difficult or impossible. Patients are also taught the principles of joint protection and energy conservation.

The main medications used for the treatment of OA are analgesics and NSAIDs; both reduce pain. NSAIDs have the added advantage of reducing any secondary inflammation. Both types of medications are comparable for short-term pain control in symptomatic OA of the knee.[2] Further studies are required to assess benefit risk of these medications for OA in general. In early disease, analgesics may be tried on an as-needed basis. As the disease progresses, regular use of analgesics or NSAIDs may be required to control symptoms. Patients taking NSAIDs chronically must be monitored closely for toxicity, especially gastrointestinal (GI) complications (e.g., gastritis, peptic ulcer disease) and renal insufficiency.

The mechanism of action of NSAIDs is to inhibit prostaglandin production by blocking a specific enzyme, cyclooxygenase. Prostaglandins are mediators of pain and inflammation but also play important roles in GI mucosal protection, maintenance of renal blood flow, and platelet aggregation. Blocking prostaglandin production is antiinflammatory, but patients are at risk for serious side effects, including GI complications. Cyclooxygenase I (COX-I) is found in all tissues and mediates the GI, renal, and platelet functions of prostaglandins. Cyclooxygenase II (COX-II) is induced mainly in areas of inflammation.[8] Thus selectively blocking COX-II over COX-I should diminish inflammation without altering the protective benefits of prostaglandins in the GI tract and other tissues. Two selective COX-II inhibitors, celecoxib (Celebrex) and rofecoxib (Vioxx), have antiinflammatory benefits similar to other NSAIDs and a better GI toxicity profile.[12]

Topical capsaicin also may be useful in the treatment of OA.[6] Capsaicin can deplete and prevent reaccumulation of substance P at the sensory nerve terminals, thus reducing pain. It is usually applied four times per day. Local burning may occur initially, but this side effect generally ceases with continued use.

Use of hyaluronic acid (viscosupplementation) for OA is a relatively new treatment option. Both hyaluronin (Hyalgan) and hylan G-F 20 (Synvisc) have been approved for treatment of knee OA.[3] Hyaluronic acid, a major component of synovial fluid, lubricates and protects the joint. In OA the amount of hyaluronic acid is reduced. Injecting hyaluronic acid–like substances into joints should restore the protective and lubricating properties. Patients receive either a five-dose (hyaluronin) or three-dose (hylan G-F 20) weekly series of injections into their affected knee. Studies comparing these compounds to placebo, intraarticular steroids, and NSAIDs have shown variable results, with improvement in pain and functional ability but uncertain long-term benefit. Benefit may be most pronounced in patients with milder disease. Currently, many rheumatologists consider viscosupplementation only for patients who have failed other treatment options.

Patients can now buy cartilage components such as glucosamine sulfate and chondroitin sulfate over the counter. These components are taken orally in various dosage regimens. Their long-term benefit is unclear, and large-scale studies are needed.

Judicial use of intraarticular corticosteroid injections can provide temporary relief of pain in some patients with OA. A long-acting corticosteroid preparation (triamcinolone hexacetonide or methylprednisolone acetate) mixed with a local anesthetic (1% lidocaine) is generally used. Patients are instructed to rest the joint for 2 to 3 days after an injection. Complications include infection (less than 0.001%), bleeding, skin atrophy, and postinjection flare. Frequent injections with corticosteroids may accelerate cartilage deterioration. For this reason the same joint should not be injected more frequently than every 3 months. If a joint is injected at this rate for more than 1 year, alternate treatment options should be explored.

The final treatment option for OA is surgery. Surgical procedures may include osteotomy, joint debridement, arthrodesis (fusion), and arthroplasty (replacement). Joint replacement should be considered for patients who have significant disability related to the OA and for whom medical treatment options have failed.

REFERENCES

1. Bland JH, Cooper SM: Osteoarthritis: a review of the cell biology involved and evidence for reversibility: management rationally related to known genesis and pathophysiology, *Semin Arthritis Rheum* 14:106, 1984.
2. Bradley JD et al: Comparison of an antiinflammatory dose of ibuprofen, an analgesic dose of ibuprofen, and acetaminophen in the treatment of patients with osteoarthritis of the knee, *N Engl J Med* 325:87, 1991.
3. Cohen MD: Hyaluronic acid treatment (viscosupplementation) for OA of the knee, *Bull Rheum Dis* 47:4, 1998.
4. Kellgren JH: Osteoarthritis in patients and populations, *Br Med J* 2:1, 1961.
5. Leach RE, Baumgard S, Broom J: Obesity: its relationship to osteoarthritis of the knee, *Clin Orthop* 93:271, 1973.
6. McCarthy GM, McCarty DJ: Effect of topical capsaicin in the therapy of painful osteoarthritis of the hands, *J Rheumatol* 19:604, 1992.
7. Moskowitz RW et al: *Osteoarthritis: diagnosis and management,* Philadelphia, 1984, Saunders.
8. Needleman P, Isakson PC: The discovery and function of COX-2, *J Rheumatol* 24(suppl 49):6, 1997.
9. Puranen J et al: Running and primary osteoarthritis of the hip, *Br Med J* 2:424, 1975.
10. Roberts J, Burch TA: *Prevalence of osteoarthritis in adults by age, sex, race and geographic area, United States—1960-1962,* US Public Health Service Pub No 1000, series 11, no 15, Washington, DC, 1966, US Government Printing Office.
11. Ryu J, Treadwell BV, Mankin HJ: Biochemical and metabolic abnormalities in normal and osteoarthritic human articular cartilage, *Arthritis Rheum* 27:613, 1984.
12. Simon LS et al: Preliminary study of the safety and efficacy of SC-58635, a novel cyclooxygenase 2 inhibitor, *Arthritis Rheum* 41:1591, 1998.

CHAPTER 133

Rheumatoid Arthritis

Tammi L. Shlotzhauer
James L. McGuire*

Rheumatoid arthritis (RA) is a chronic inflammatory arthritis characterized by symmetric, erosive synovitis. The etiology of RA is unknown, with several factors under consideration. Genetic influences are suspected because human leukocyte antigens HLA-DR4 and HLA-DR1 have been associated with RA. Many theories suggest an infectious agent acting as an environmental trigger without persisting in the host. These arthritogenic agents may induce autoimmunity in the genetically susceptible individual. The initiation and perpetuation of chronic inflammation may be influenced by other factors, including cytokine activity and hormonal influences.

Once considered as a benign disorder, RA is now known to cause significant morbidity and decreased life expectancy. Prompt aggressive treatment is warranted in patients with RA, particularly those with poor prognostic factors.[8] RA affects about 1% to 2% of the adult U.S. population, an estimated 3 to 5 million Americans. Women are three times as likely as men to develop RA. The peak onset is ages 30 to 50, with all races affected.[5]

*Deceased.

PATHOPHYSIOLOGY

Previously the pathophysiology within the joint in patients with RA was broadly divided into inflammatory and proliferative phases. It was assumed that the inflammation occurred first, usually in response to a series of external agents (infectious, hormonal, environmental) in the susceptible individual. The inflammatory response became chronic and supported the development of the proliferative phase in the synovium, which resulted in the invasive pannus. A variety of cells, especially lymphocytes (both B and T cells), macrophages, and fibroblasts, could be identified in the established lesion. However, this pathophysiologic separation is oversimplified. Both the inflammatory and the proliferative components represent a continuum of interrelated events driven by cellular interaction and disequilibrium between proinflammatory and antiinflammatory cytokines. Tumor necrosis factor and interleukin-1 are proinflammatory cytokines believed to be most responsible for rheumatoid injury. The pathophysiologic processes involved in RA have been correlated with clinical manifestations. The five phases incorporate the dominant pathophysiologic events that can be observed during the first few years of established disease (Table 133-1).[4] These events can be targeted therapeutically.

Table 133-1. Stages of Rheumatoid Arthritis

Pathogenesis	Symptoms	Physical signs	Radiographic changes
Stage 1			
Antigen presentation to T cells	Probably none	—	—
Stage 2			
T-cell proliferation B-cell proliferation Angiogenesis in synovium	Malaise Mild joint stiffness	Possible swelling of small joints of hands or wrists	None
Stage 3			
PMN leukocyte accumulation in synovial fluid Synovial cell proliferation without polarization	Joint pain and swelling Morning stiffness Malaise and weakness	Warm, swollen joints Synovial fluid in excess Soft tissue proliferation within joints Pain and limitation of motion	Soft tissue swelling
Stage 4			
Polarization of synovitis into a centripetally invasive pannus Activation of chondrocytes	Same	Same, but more pronounced swelling	MRI revealing proliferative pannus Periarticular osteopenia indicated by radiographs
Stage 5			
Erosion of subchondral bone Invasion of cartilage by pannus Chondrocyte proliferation Stretched ligaments around joints	Same, plus loss of function and early deformity (e.g., ulnar deviation at MCP joints)	Same, plus instability of joints, flexion contractures, and decreased range of motion Extraarticular complications	Early erosions and joint space narrowing

From Harris ED Jr: Mechanisms of disease: rheumatoid arthritis—pathophysiology and implications for therapy, *N Engl J Med* 322:1277, 1990.
PMN, Polymorphonuclear neutrophil; *MRI,* magnetic resonance imaging; *MCP,* metacarpophalangeal.

PATIENT EVALUATION

History

RA is a heterogenous disorder that varies in presentation and clinical course. The onset of RA may be gradual or sudden, involving one or many joints. Most often the onset is insidious, presenting as slowly progressive pain and stiffness in the joints over weeks to months. Small joints of the hands and feet are usually involved at the onset. Swelling may not be apparent initially despite significant arthralgias. The pain tends to increase slowly, and swelling eventually becomes manifest. This may take months or rarely years. In most patients, RA involves several joints symmetrically, although monoarticular or asymmetric arthritis may be the first sign.

In the geriatric population, significant morning stiffness with nonspecific muscle aching, particularly in the shoulders and hips, is a common form of onset, often mimicking polymyalgia rheumatica. It may take weeks to months before joint swelling occurs. In addition to joint and muscular complaints, fatigue is the most prominent presenting feature of RA, often more debilitating than the arthritis itself. Fortunately, the acute and intense onset of arthritis presenting with systemic features (e.g., severe fatigue, low-grade fever, anorexia, weight loss) is rare. RA that presents in this manner must be differentiated from sepsis, paraneoplastic syndromes, and hypersensitivity reactions. Although impressive in its intensity, this presentation is not predictive of a poor prognosis.

The natural history of RA is also varied and may even change over time in the same person. The presentation often helps predict the subsequent course. RA can take one of four general courses: spontaneous remission, palindromic or remitting, remitting-progressive, or progressive (Table 133-2). RA can go into a spontaneous remission over weeks to months in 10% to 20% of patients. A majority of these patients experience a recurrence of RA. Thus permanent remission without treatment is unlikely. Recurrent flare-ups of arthritis with return to normal health between attacks are the hallmark of the remitting or palindromic course. These attacks are usually treated with nonsteroidal antiinflammatory drugs (NSAIDs). Disease-modifying antirheumatic drugs (DMARDs) may not be required if signs of joint damage are absent and the patient returns to normal joint function between flare-ups. If attacks are frequent, protracted, or debilitating, DMARDs should be considered to prevent recurrences. In the remitting-progressive course, complete return to a normal state between attacks does not occur. Ongoing destructive changes result from persistent active synovitis. DMARD therapy should be strongly considered for these patients. The most common course of RA is characterized by an ongoing synovitis with progressive pain, swelling, and joint damage. The progression of synovitis is generally insidious but may result in a rapid decline of function. Early DMARD therapy is recommended in an attempt to halt the progression of arthritis in these patients.

Table 133-2. Clinical Course of Rheumatoid Arthritis (RA)

Clinical course	Comment
Spontaneous remission	Unusual without DMARD exposure
Palindromic or remitting	Classic RA developing in 50% of patients
Remitting-progressive	No return to normal baseline
Progressive	Disability proportional to duration

DMARD, Disease-modifying antirheumatic drug.

The literature of the past decade has emphasized that patients with chronic RA experience progressive disability and premature mortality. This is in contrast with previous clinical impressions that RA had a relatively benign course. Recent studies suggest that patients who develop more severe disease develop erosive lesions within the first 2 years of diagnosis. Efforts to identify and treat this subset of patients are ongoing. Prognosis is being evaluated from the per spective of genetics, earlier onset of disease, educational level, and articular cartilage damage evidenced on magnetic resonance imaging (MRI). These factors are being integrated with traditional predictors of disease severity, including positive rheumatoid factor (RF), elevated erythrocyte sedimentation rate (ESR), subcutaneous nodules, insidious onset of joint disease, and erosion of bone on plain radiographs.

Physical Examination

The examination usually reveals some synovitis. Early in the disease course, however, the classic symmetric arthritis involving the hands, wrists, knees, and feet, which is typical of well-established disease, may not be present. The examination may reveal a single swollen joint or an asymmetric pattern of oligoarthritis. Observable changes include warmth, soft tissue swelling, effusion, tenderness, and diminished range of motion in involved joints. Potentially involved joints include the neck, shoulders, elbows, wrists, metacarpophalangeal (MCP) joints, proximal interphalangeal (PIP) joints, hips, knees, ankles, metatarsophalangeal (MTP) joints, and tarsal joints. Less frequently involved joints include the sternoclavicular, acromioclavicular, temporomandibular, and cricoarytenoid joints.

Changes specific to the shoulder include rotator cuff injury with superior migration of the humeral head. Loss of full extension is an early change noted in the elbow. Early hand and wrist changes include diffuse puffiness of the digits, with MCP and PIP soft tissue swelling (Fig. 133-1). Ulnar deviation at the MCP joint is a result of connective tissue injury and mechanical factors. The swan-neck deformity is frequently observed with flexion of the distal interphalangeal (DIP) and MCP joints and hyperextension of the PIP joints. Extensor hood damage can result in fixed flexion of the PIP joint and hyperextension of the DIP joint, resulting in boutonniére deformity. Evidence of tenosynovitis may also be present, particularly in the wrists and dorsum of the hands. Patients with marked proliferative tenosynovitis may experience tendon rupture. Lower extremity signs include knee synovitis with effusion, quadriceps atrophy, and popliteal cysts. Patients often have ankle and foot deformities. Valgus of the ankle, pes planus, and forefoot varus deformity frequently exist simultaneously. MTP joints are often involved with downward subluxation of the metatarsal heads, cock-up deformities, hammer toes, and hallux valgus.

DIAGNOSIS

In 1987 the American Rheumatism Association revised criteria for the classification of RA. To make a diagnosis of

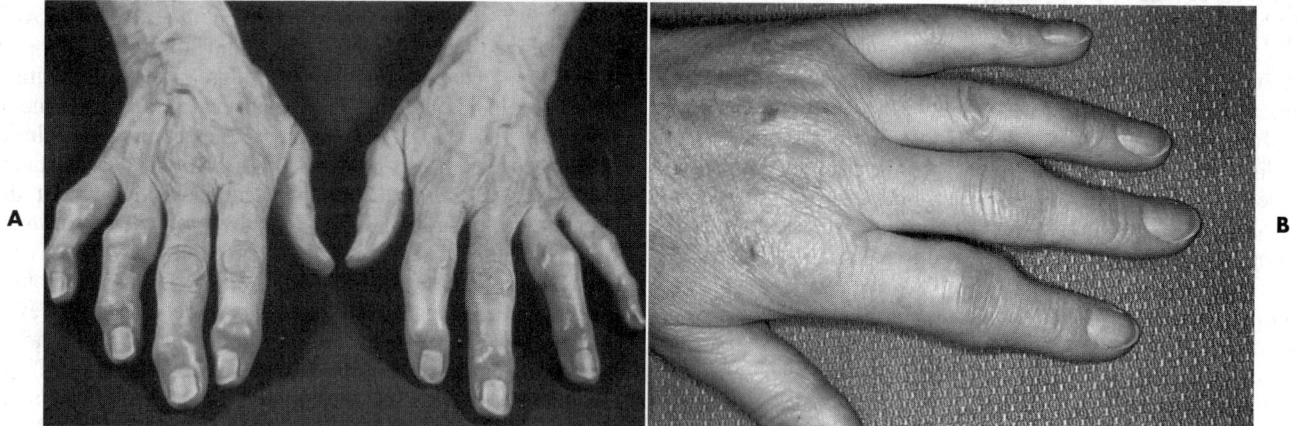

Fig. 133-1. **A,** Bony proximal interphalangeal (PIP) hypertrophy of osteoarthritis. **B,** Synovial PIP hypertrophy of rheumatoid arthritis. (Courtesy American Rheumatism Association.)

Box 133-1. Criteria for Classification of Rheumatoid Arthritis (RA)*

1. Morning stiffness lasting at least 1 hour before maximal improvement.
2. At least three joint areas simultaneously with swelling observed by physician. The 14 possible areas are right and left PIP, MCP, wrist, elbow, knee, ankle, and MTP joints.
3. Swelling in a wrist, MCP, or PIP joint.
4. Symmetric involvement of the same joint areas (as defined in 2); bilateral involvement of the PIPs, MCPs, or MTPs is acceptable without absolute symmetry.
5. Subcutaneous nodules observed by physician.
6. Demonstration of positive rheumatoid factor.
7. Radiographic changes typical of RA, including erosions of unequivocal periarticular bony decalcification, present at least 6 weeks.

Modified from Arnett FC et al: The American Rheumatism Association 1987 revised criteria for the classification of rheumatoid arthritis, *Arthritis Rheum* 31:315, 1988.
PIP, Proximal interphalangeal; *MCP,* metacarpophalangeal;
MTP, metatarsophalangeal.
*Diagnosis of RA requires 4 of 7 criteria.

RA, criteria 1 through 4 must have been present for at least 6 weeks, and four or more criteria must be met (Box 133-1).[2]

Diagnostic Procedures

Early in the course of RA, clinical history and examination may be more definitive than laboratory analysis. Nonspecific inflammatory indices are often present, such as elevations of ESR, C-reactive protein, and γ-globulins, as well as the presence of normocytic anemia, leukocytosis, and thrombocytosis. RF, frequently absent in the first year of symptoms, eventually converts to a positive status in approximately 80% of patients. Antinuclear antibody (ANA) is frequently present in RA.

Synovial fluid analysis is helpful in the diagnosis of RA and other forms of inflammatory arthritis. Synovial cell counts typically range from 2000 to 50,000/mm^3 in affected joints, with a predominance of polymorphonuclear neutrophil leukocytes (PMNs). Early in the course of RA, counts may be lower with a relative monocytosis. Synovial fluid glucose levels are usually equal to but can be lower than serum glucose levels in chronic, severely inflamed joints. Synovial fluid from these joints or from those of monoarticular presentation should also be examined with Gram's stain and culture for bacterial infection. Synovial glucose is routinely extremely low in infected joints.

Synovial tissue biopsy may be useful when the diagnosis of RA is elusive. This is particularly important in chronic monoarticular arthritis of unclear etiology. Tissue is best obtained arthroscopically but can also be obtained blindly using needle biopsy.

Differential Diagnosis

It is often difficult on initial presentation to differentiate RA from other forms of inflammatory arthritis. Frequently, laboratory analysis is not revealing, and historic clues are particularly important. Four determinants are consistently used in the differential diagnosis of arthritis: gender, age at presentation, pattern of joint involvement, and clinical course. For example, classic RA occurs in women during their fourth decade and is a symmetric, progressive arthritis.

The presence of low back and sacroiliac discomfort should suggest the HLA-B27–associated diseases, or seronegative spondyloarthropathies (see Chapter 137). Ankylosing spondylitis in women often is not accompanied by the marked back stiffness and discomfort observed in men. With Reiter's syndrome the physician should seek evidence of insertional tendinitis, fasciitis, "sausage" digits, conjunctivitis, genital lesions, or urethral symptoms. Reactive polyarthritis can also be associated with psoriasis, inflammatory bowel disease, Whipple's disease, and Behçet's disease.

The common crystal arthropathies are frequently confused with RA. Chronic gout may mimic RA, with symmetric polyarthritis, tophaceous nodules, and recurrent attacks. Calcium pyrophosphate dihydrate deposition disease or pseudogout may be difficult to differentiate from RA because both conditions can involve similar joints and develop subacutely. Radiographic evidence of chondrocalcinosis is helpful. Arthrocentesis and examination of synovial fluid for crystals usually confirm definitive diagnosis of gout and pseudogout.

Other forms of diffuse connective tissue disease, including systemic lupus erythematosus (SLE), vasculitis, scleroderma, polymyositis, and mixed connective tissue disease, may resemble RA on initial presentation. Primary Sjögren's syndrome is frequently confused with RA clinically and serologically. Significant eye and mouth dryness and the presence of ANA, including SSA and SSB (found in Sjögren's), help determine the correct diagnosis.

In the systemically ill patient with inflammatory arthritis, the physician should also consider the possibilities of bacterial endocarditis, septic arthritis, Lyme disease, and malignancy if historic or physical clues are present. Other, less acute systemic conditions that can present as polyarthritis include thyroid disease, sarcoidosis, amyloidosis, and paraproteinemias.

Three additional entities are occasionally confused with RA because of patients' similarities in age, gender, morning stiffness, and periodic joint attacks. *Fibromyalgia* is a clinical syndrome of multiple aches and pains, prominent morning stiffness, and nonrestorative sleep that occurs predominantly in middle-aged women. Synovitis is not present, but classic muscle tender points are associated with normal blood counts, ESR, and blood chemistries. Prominent myalgias and morning stiffness are also characteristic of *polymyalgia rheumatica,* but this presents almost exclusively after age 55. Synovitis can be present in some patients. The ESR is generally significantly elevated, and response to corticosteroids is almost immediate. *Palindromic rheumatism* may be a presentation of RA but can exist as an independent clinical entity. Observation over time, often years, may be necessary to make this differential diagnosis.

MANAGEMENT

Nonpharmacologic Therapy

Rehabilitation Issues: Joint Protection. When joints are inflamed, cartilage is prone to injury and irreversible damage. During this vulnerable period, it is critical that principles of joint protection are understood and practiced. MCP and wrist joints are particularly prone to deformity. Special attention to protecting these joints during daily activities is indicated. An occupational therapist can teach methods of joint protection, giving specific examples on the use of these guidelines as they relate to each joint (Box 133-2).[9]

Splinting plays an important role in joint protection. Splints can be designed to reduce inflammation through immobilization, to protect a vulnerable joint, or to improve function of a damaged joint. Splints should be worn only if they diminish pain and inflammation or improve function. No reliable evidence has documented that splints prevent deformity, but this is a common belief. Inappropriate or prolonged use of splints may cause increased stiffness, decreased strength, and decreased motion. An occupational therapist with expertise in hand therapy can be particularly helpful in devising appropriate upper extremity splints.

Assistive equipment can facilitate joint protection. Examples of equipment available for upper extremity problems include built-up handles, faucet levers, key adapters, buttonhooks, elastic shoelaces, use of Velcro in place of buttons and laces, door-opening levers, and extended handles on utensils. Useful assistive equipment for lower extremity problems includes elevated seats with armrests, raised toilet seats, shower benches, long-handled reachers, tub grab bars, and walking aids.

Box 133-2. Joint Protection Guidelines[9]

Respect pain.
Balance rest with activity to conserve energy.
Maintain muscle strength and tone to increase support to joints.
Avoid prolonged activities that cannot be interrupted.
Avoid positions that promote deformity.
Use the largest joints and the strongest muscles available to complete a task.
Avoid remaining in one position or using muscles in one stationary position for long periods.
Use assistive equipment as needed.

Proper footwear is crucial to protect the feet and ankles. RA may cause significant foot deformities and dysfunction. Swelling and secondary ligamentous laxity may result in a broad forefoot with toe deformities. A poorly fit shoe can create foot discomfort and further deformity. With mild arthritis in the feet a good supportive walking shoe or an athletic shoe usually suffices. When choosing shoes, the following features should be considered: light weight, deep enough to clear the top of toes (deeper if an insert is needed), wide enough not to pinch the toes together, 1 inch or less heel, good shock absorption, support along the inside of the shoe with an adequate arch, durable, stiff back for support, and breathable and supple uppers. If foot deformities are present, an insert or orthosis may be required. Orthotic supports are designed to relieve pressure caused by deformities or to correct foot deformity. If deformity is severe, orthopedic shoes or custom-made shoes can be fabricated from a cast of the feet.

Concepts of energy conservation should accompany principles of joint protection. Activities that cause fatigue in the patient without having an aerobic or strengthening benefit should be eliminated if possible. Discussions on the value of rest during the day are important. An occupational or physical therapist can help to teach methods of task minimization. The Arthritis Foundation has pamphlets available that review energy conservation and joint protection.

Exercise. Appropriate exercise with adequate rest is a mainstay of the treatment of RA. Exercise recommendations have changed significantly over the past 30 years. For many years, patients were treated with prolonged bed rest to reduce active arthritis. Since inflammation improves with immobilization, the practice had some merit. It has become evident, however, that the negative effects of muscle atrophy, osteoporosis, and generalized deconditioning outweigh the benefits. Range of motion (ROM), specific strengthening, and low-impact aerobic fitness exercises can be prescribed with positive effects. Appropriate exercise can improve stamina, decrease fatigue, reduce time lost from work, and enhance the level of function. Appropriate exercise can also increase joint stability, help prevent joint deformities, decrease pain, improve function, promote self-esteem, improve sleep, and lessen muscle tension and anxiety. Compliance with exercise can be increased and joint damage avoided if guidelines are followed (Box 133-3).[9]

Box 133-3. Exercise Guidelines for Patients With Rheumatoid Arthritis (RA)[9]

Review exercises in detail with a physician or a therapist who is familiar with RA, particularly if the arthritis is severe.
Perform exercise as part of a daily routine.
Perform a brief series of range of motion exercises in the morning, after immobility, and before fitness exercises.
Exercise when the energy level is at its peak.
Balance exercise with adequate rest and sleep.
Always follow principles of joint protection.
Use tactics that make exercise most comfortable:
- Wear loose clothing.
- Consider showering before exercise to decrease pain and stiffness and to increase flexibility.
- Take medications in advance, timed to be effective during exercise.

Take deep, regular breaths during exercise.
Keep movements smooth and flowing. Avoid jerking or bouncing motions.
Apply ice packs to warm joints for 20 minutes after each exercise session to limit inflammation.
Never perform a painful exercise.
Never exercise to the point of extreme muscle fatigue or weakness.
If joints hurt for more than 2 hours after exercising or if joints hurt or swell the next day, realize that the exercise program is too rigorous.
For patients with joint replacements, always review exercises with the orthopedic surgeon before proceeding.
Be adaptable to changes in condition and modify accordingly.
Keep a log of completed exercises.

The recommended amount and type of exercise depend on the degree of inflammation and the pattern of joint involvement. Gentle ROM exercises are prescribed for patients with very active inflammation. Moving affected joints through approximately five repetitions of ROM helps to maintain motion. Joints should not be stretched to the point of increased pain. Muscle setting can be performed if it does not cause significant discomfort. Muscles surrounding affected joints can be contracted, with tension maintained for 6 seconds each day to prevent muscle weakening. Moderately inflamed or subacute joints should also be taken through ROM exercise. Isometric strengthening exercise with contraction against a fixed resistance can be added. Elastic bands or other forms of fixed resistance can be used. Approximately 75% of maximum strength for 6 seconds should be used with less force when pain occurs. Slow addition of endurance exercises may be appropriate at this stage. Adding a swimming program is often recommended because the buoyancy of water tends to relieve mechanical stress on joints.

In cases of controlled synovitis, exercise recommendations vary depending on the amount of damage in the joints. General guidelines include continuing ROM exercises daily with a maximum of 10 repetitions. Isometric strengthening exercises may be performed as they would with moderately inflamed joints. Once maximum ROM and strength are achieved, more time can be devoted to aerobic exercise. Endurance exercises are most important at this stage as a means of regaining aerobic conditioning that is lost when the disease is more active. Although swimming is still the best form of exercise, other forms of low-impact aerobics (e.g., walking, bicycling, simulated ski machines, low-impact dancing) may be considered if lower extremity joints are not severely involved. Thirty minutes of aerobic exercise three times weekly increases fitness.

Nutrition. In determining whether a relationship exists between nutrition and RA, data suggest that fewer than 5% of patients with predominantly seronegative RA have a food allergy. Improvement in arthritis through elimination diets supports these data. Specific foods to avoid in various reports include milk products, lactose-containing foods, corn, cereals, shrimp, and nitrates.

The foremost nutritional question is whether diet modification can alter the abnormal immune response in RA. Studies of hypocaloric diets show improvement in symptoms of RA. This improvement is usually temporary and is poorly understood. Diets low in saturated fats and high in omega-3 fatty acids have also been shown to have some therapeutic benefit. Supplemental fish oils containing omega-3 fatty acids have been shown to have modest antiinflammatory activity in RA.

A well-balanced diet, with total caloric intake calculated to maintain lean body weight, and limited stress on weight-bearing joints are recommended. Adequate protein is advised to prevent muscle atrophy. Calcium and vitamin D supplementation, particularly for patients taking corticosteroids, should be considered in view of the increased risk of osteoporosis in patients with RA. Estrogens for postmenopausal women should also be considered. Sodium restriction may be necessary to limit fluid retention and secondary hypertension in patients who take NSAIDs or corticosteroids.

Pharmacologic Therapy

Traditionally, medical treatment for RA was outlined according to a pyramid approach, beginning with nonpharmacologic modalities and NSAIDs at the base. In the distant past, frank destructive changes on radiographs were mandated before physicians moved up the therapeutic pyramid to DMARDs. Usually, 2 to 3 years elapsed before DMARDs were even considered. It is now appreciated that cartilage erosions and resultant irreversible damage can occur within 2 years of the diagnosis of RA. Since progressive disability and premature mortality occur with RA, DMARDs are used earlier in the clinical course. Moreover, combinations of DMARDs have been advocated for progressive disease. Current rheumatology practice supports prompt, aggressive intervention with DMARDs in an effort to halt early, irreversible damage. Usually a single DMARD is initiated within weeks of a clear diagnosis of RA. If ineffective, serial DMARDs are attempted until control is achieved. Others propose that low doses of multiple DMARDs be initiated simultaneously; drug synergy may provide rapid improvement with less dose-related toxicity. After control is achieved, therapy is slowly withdrawn, and the patient is maintained on the least toxic DMARD that subdues the inflammatory process.

For the primary care physician, this information could translate into the following therapeutic plan. After 1 to 3 months of arthritis treatment with an NSAID alone, a low-toxicity DMARD such as hydroxychloroquine should be considered if the patient remains symptomatic. If, after an additional 3 to 6 months of an NSAID/hydroxychloroquine combination, evidence of significant synovitis persists, an additional DMARD should be considered. If the physician is not comfortable with the second DMARD option, a rheumatology consultation is appropriate, particularly if methotrexate, cyclosporine, leflunomide, or etanercept is considered. This aggressive approach to patients with RA may be difficult to justify because of the potential toxicity of medications and the uncertainty of the disease course. RF and subcutaneous nodules suggest aggressive disease but are often not present in early disease. HLA-DR4 has been reported to correlate with disease severity, but testing is not readily available and has not yet been incorporated into DMARD treatment decisions. Until trial genetic tests are proven to predict severity and become readily available, treatment decisions must rely on physical and radiographic evidence of progressive synovitis and on the presence of acute-phase reactants in early disease, when RF is often negative. In a managed care system the primary care physician is likely to make the diagnosis of RA and to initiate the first NSAID and DMARD based on the clinical features. This is complicated by similarities in the presentations of several different rheumatic disorders. Consultation with a rheumatologist may be helpful for cases that present diagnostic difficulty.

Agents used for treating RA are divided into four major groups: NSAIDs, DMARDs, corticosteroids, and biologic response modifiers.

Nonsteroidal Antiinflammatory Drugs.

NSAIDs are used as the first-line therapy to decrease pain and inflammation promptly. Because of significant interpatient variability in efficacy, multiple agents may need to be prescribed before the most effective NSAID is discovered for an individual. NSAID efficacy generally requires 1 to 3 weeks to assess. With few exceptions, NSAIDs work by inhibiting the production of inflammatory prostaglandins. Despite their efficacy in reducing the symptoms of arthritis, these drugs probably do not change the natural history of RA. It is important to prescribe antiinflammatory dosages of the NSAID and not analgesic dosages, which are generally lower.

Toxicity of aspirin and NSAIDs is well described (Box 133-4). The major toxicity is to the gastrointestinal (GI) tract, with potential gastritis, erosive change, and gastric ulceration. Risk factors for toxicity in RA include advanced age, concomitant corticosteroid use, tobacco, alcohol, and a history of ulcers. Patients with prominent risk factors should be strongly considered for prophylactic treatment with the synthetic prostaglandin misoprostol (Cytotec) or use of the newest class of NSAIDs, the cyclooxygenase II (COX-II) inhibitors. By blocking COX-II significantly more than COX-I, their use is expected to be associated with less GI toxicity. Celecoxib (Celebrex) and rofecoxib (Vioxx) have recently been approved, and others are expected to be available soon.

Disease-modifying Antirheumatic Drugs.

DMARDs are aimed at altering the course of rheumatoid synovitis, thus preventing joint damage.[3] These agents often need to be administered for several weeks to months before positive results can be seen. It is postulated that DMARDs are effective in modulating the immune process of RA.

The choice of initial second-line agent depends on the physician's judgment and preference as well as the severity of disease. Patients with severe, aggressive disease should be treated with methotrexate, leflunamide, or less often, injectable gold salts by a physician familiar with these medications. Patients with lesser symptoms may be treated with hydroxychloroquine, auranofin, or sulfasalazine, often by the primary care physician. When the initial DMARD does not result in the expected efficacy, a second agent may be added or may replace the first.[7] More than one DMARD may be initiated from the onset of second-line therapy, with eventual step-down to a simplified regimen once control is achieved. Three other DMARDs—penicillamine, azathioprine, and cyclophosphamide—have efficacy for RA but should be prescribed only by physicians familiar with their toxicities.

Injectable Gold Salts. Gold sodium thiomalate (GSTM) and gold sodium thioglucose (GSTG) are the two forms of injectable gold used in the United States. GSTM is a water-based solution and has limited availability; GSTG has a sesame oil vehicle and has become the preferred agent (Box 133-5). Gold was first introduced as a treatment for infections, particularly for tuberculosis, in the early 1900s. Although hailed as the DMARD of choice for several years, the efficacy of gold therapy has been questioned. Despite this controversy, many rheumatologists still believe that intramuscular (IM) gold has a role in the treatment of RA, although its use has largely been replaced by methotrexate.

Initially, IM gold is given in the form of weekly injections. Two test doses are administered; the first is a 10-mg injection, and the second weekly dose is 25 mg. Thereafter the prescribed dosage is 50 mg per week. After improvement is noted or a cumulative dose of 1000 mg is attained, the interval between injections is increased to 2 weeks. If improvement continues, the interval can be further lengthened, generally to a maximum of 1 month. IM gold therapy frequently requires 6 weeks to 6 months before maximum effectiveness is evident.

Gold therapy is often associated with toxicity, resulting in discontinuation of treatment in approximately 30% of

Box 133-4. NSAID Characteristics

Time to effectiveness: variable, generally at least 2 weeks

Toxicity

Greater than 5%: ototoxicity, rash, gastric erosions or ulcerations, platelet effect

Less than 5%: hypersensitivity, hepatic insufficiency, renal pathology, small bowel ulcerations, central nervous system effects, stomatitis, drug fever, pancreatitis, hemolytic anemia, thrombocytopenia, neutropenia, pulmonary infiltrates

Safety monitoring

Initial: CBC, Cr, U/A, and AST for baseline and frequently if abnormal

Stable: CBC, Cr, U/A, and AST every 12 months

CBC, Complete blood count; *Cr,* creatine; *U/A,* urinalysis; *AST,* asparate transaminase.

Box 133-5. Injectable Gold Characteristics

Gold sodium thiomalate (Myochrysine)
Gold sodium thioglucose (Solganal)
Generic available: no
Time to effectiveness: 6 weeks to 6 months
Administration: First week test dose, 10 mg; second week test dose, 25 mg; follow with weekly 50-mg injections to total of 1000 mg; then alternate weekly dosage for 3 months; then every third week for 3 months; then monthly
Toxicity
Greater than 5%: rash, stomatitis, nitritoid reaction*
Less than 5%: alopecia, thrombocytopenia, granulocytopenia, aplastic anemia, eosinophilia, proteinuria, pulmonary infiltrates, neuropathy, hepatic insufficiency, hematuria, enterocolitis
Safety monitoring
Initial: CBC, differential, platelet count, and U/A preinjection for the first 20 weeks
Stable: CBC differential, platelet count, and U/A before every other injection

*Nitritoid reaction may occur with gold sodium thiomalate (see text).

patients. Rash and stomatitis are reported most often. With renal toxicity, the most common problem is proteinuria. In less than 1% of patients treated with parenteral gold, serious renal insufficiency occurs. The major toxicity is nephrotic syndrome. Hematuria may also occur. The vast majority of kidney problems are reversible. Fortunately, gold-induced hematologic problems are rare. In 1% to 3% of patients, leukopenia or thrombocytopenia may develop. If no other obvious cause is found, gold therapy should be discontinued. Eosinophilia is common in RA, but a marked increase in the eosinophil count may indicate impending toxicity, and gold should be withheld until the eosinophilia resolves. In less than 0.5% of patients, aplastic anemia may result; the mortality is in excess of 50%. The most effective therapy for aplastic anemia appears to be antithymocyte globulin. Nitritoid reaction may occur with GSTM, the water-based gold preparation that is rapidly absorbed. This reaction occurs immediately or within 20 minutes after an injection. Flushing, fainting, dizziness, and sweating usually characterize it. Because of this toxicity, the oil-based GSTG is used more often.

In view of potential renal and hematologic toxicities, weekly preinjection complete blood counts (CBCs) and urinalyses (U/As) are suggested for the first 20 weeks. Since toxicity is less likely after the first 6 months, laboratory tests may be obtained before every injection or every other injection.

Oral Gold. The introduction of auranofin (Ridaura) in the 1980s allowed physicians to prescribe an oral form of gold. Many rheumatologists believe that auranofin is not as effective as injectable gold, but the compound can be effective if used for very early disease. A trial of 6 months may be required before a determination is made that auranofin is definitely not efficacious in a given patient. The recommended dosage is 3 mg twice a day. If no improvement is noted in 6 months, a trial of 3 mg three times per day may be considered. Recommended laboratory monitoring for toxicities requires CBC with manual differential and U/A every 4 to 12 weeks. Unlike injectable gold, auranofin has a low incidence of serious toxicities. The most prominent side effects are abdominal cramps, diarrhea, nausea, and changes in appetite. Most of these problems can be treated by starting with 3 mg a day administered with meals and by prescribing a high-fiber, bulk-inducing agent. Rash and stomatitis are uncommon; renal and hematologic toxicities are rare.

Antimalarial Drugs. The medicinal qualities of quinine have been recognized for more than a century. Antimalarial agents include hydroxychloroquine, chloroquine, and quinacrine. Quinacrine was introduced in the 1950s as the first antimalarial used to treat RA. Chloroquine and hydroxychloroquine are used today in the treatment of RA. Hydroxychloroquine has become the antimalarial agent of choice because of its lower toxicity profile (Box 133-6). Hydroxychloroquine is contraindicated in patients allergic to the medication or to quinine. Hydroxychloroquine is given in initial dosages of 400 mg/day (200 mg orally twice a day). If an excellent response occurs, the dosage can be decreased to 200 mg/day. A trial for a minimum of 6 to 10 weeks is required to determine efficacy.

Hydroxychloroquine is probably the safest DMARD. Patients should have a baseline ophthalmologic examination before starting therapy. Only an estimated 5% of patients discontinue hydroxychloroquine because of side effects. GI effects are reported most frequently. Thrombocytopenia and other forms of bone marrow suppression are rare. The principal concern regarding antimalarial drugs is the risk of retinopathy with long-term use. The risk of retinopathy for patients taking the standard dose of 400 mg/day of hydroxychloroquine is very low. If ophthalmologic evaluation is performed routinely every 3 to 6 months as recommended and hydroxychloroquine discontinued at the earliest sign of retinal change, the risks for permanent eye damage are negligible. When loss of vision is the first sign of damage, continued loss can progress despite drug withdrawal, emphasizing the importance of routine examination. Chloroquine has a higher risk of retinopathy than hydroxychloroquine. When hydroxychloroquine is initiated, blurring of vision may occur; this is transient and caused by smooth muscle relaxation rather than retinal pathology. Corneal deposits may also occur but do not present a risk to vision.

Penicillamine. Penicillamine is an oral preparation with a delayed onset of action and side effect profile similar to gold. Penicillamine therapy has numerous potential side effects that limit its use to uniquely refractory cases (Box 133-7). Toxicity is frequently related to dosage and generally appears in the first year of treatment. Serious side effects are similar to those of injectable gold. The chief concern is the development of hematologic toxicity. Thrombocytopenia occurs most frequently, affecting approximately 4% of patients, and leukopenia occurs in approximately 2% of patients. These side effects are largely reversible but can be life threatening in rare situations. Renal toxicity, especially nephritis with proteinuria, may occur but usually can be halted if detected early. Nephrotic syndrome is more common than with injectable gold. If significant proteinuria (greater than 1 gm) is documented by 24-hour urine evaluation, penicillamine therapy should be discontinued. The rare development of other autoimmune conditions, such as myasthenia

Box 133-6. Hydroxychloroquine (Plaquenil) Characteristics

Generic available: no
Dosage: 200 mg orally twice daily
Time to effectiveness: 6-10 weeks
Toxicity
Greater than 5%: gastrointestinal discomfort, rash, headache, irritability, skin hyperpigmentation, corneal deposits
Less than 5%: tinnitus, retinopathy, neuromyopathy, leukopenia, cardiomyopathy, alopecia, hemolytic anemia with glucose-6-dehydrogenase deficiency
Safety monitoring
Initial: baseline eye examination by ophthalmologist before start of therapy
Stable: eye examination every 3-6 months

Box 133-7. Penicillamine (Cuprimine, Depen) Characteristics

Generic available: no
Cuprimine: capsule 125 mg, 250 mg
Depen: scored tablet, 250 mg
Administration and dosage: initial dose, 125-250 mg; incremental dose increase, 125-250 mg; intervals 3 months between dose increase; maximum dose: 750 mg daily in most patients
Time to effectiveness: 2-9 months
Toxicity
Greater than 5%: hypogeusia, rash, nausea, anorexia, stomatitis, proteinuria
Less than 5%: thrombocytopenia, leukopenia, autoimmune diseases, gynecomastia, aplastic anemia, liver test abnormalities, pulmonary toxicity, immune complex glomerulonephritis
Safety monitoring
Initial: CBC with differential, platelet count, and U/A every 2 weeks until dosage stable
Stable: CBC with differential, platelet count, and U/A every 1-3 months; CPK as needed

CPK, Creatine phosphokinase.

gravis, pemphigus, Goodpasture's syndrome, and SLE, may also result from penicillamine therapy.

Penicillamine therapy is initiated with 125 to 250 mg/day taken on an empty stomach. Incremental increases of 125 to 250 mg (depending on tolerance) are made every 3 months until the desired beneficial response or a daily maximum of 750 mg is reached. Higher doses occasionally are used but generally are discouraged. CBC and U/A should be monitored every 2 weeks until dosage stable, then every 1 to 3 months.

Sulfasalazine. Sulfasalazine was originally developed in the 1930s specifically for the treatment of RA (Box 133-8). Since the 1980s, sulfasalazine use has had a resurgence because several studies demonstrated its effectiveness.

Box 133-8. Sulfasalazine (Azulfidine) Characteristics

Generic available: yes
Tablets: 500 mg
Enteric-coated tablets: 500 mg
Liquid form: available
Dosage: two or three tablets twice daily
Time to effectiveness: 2-6 months
Toxicity
Greater than 5%: gastrointestinal, rash, headache, macrocytosis
Less than 5%: leukopenia, thrombocytopenia, megaloblastic anemia, hepatic insufficiency, reduced sperm count, pulmonary toxicity, other hypersensitivities (e.g., arthralgia, angioedema, eosinophilia), hemolytic anemia with glucose-6-phosphate dehydrogenase (G6PD) deficiency
Safety monitoring
Initial: CBC and platelet count every 2-4 weeks for first 3 months; in patients at risk, G6PD
Stable: CBC and platelet count every 3 months

Sulfasalazine is usually given as 2 gm/day divided into two to four equal doses. If no benefit is noted in 3 to 6 months, the dosage can be increased to 3 gm/day for an additional 2 to 3 months. Efficacy is generally apparent after 2 to 6 months of therapy. Baseline testing should include CBC, aspartate transaminase (AST), alanine transaminase (ALT), and in patients at risk, glucose-6-phosphate dehydrogenase (G6PD). Monitoring for toxicity includes requesting CBC with differential every 2 to 4 weeks for the first 3 months, then CBC (with or without liver function tests) every 12 weeks.

Sulfasalazine is contraindicated in patients who are allergic to sulfa compounds or salicylates. The most frequently observed side effect of sulfasalazine is GI intolerance, which is reduced with the use of enteric-coated tablets taken with meals. Starting therapy at a low dose with gradual increases also improves tolerance. Rash also occurs. Serious toxicity is rare and generally occurs early in treatment. Severe hypersensitivity reactions include pneumonitis and hepatitis, and cytopenias include thrombocytopenia and leukopenia. Spermatogenesis may be affected, causing reversible sterility. Most side effects are reversed uneventfully with discontinuation of the medication.

Methotrexate. Methotrexate was introduced in the 1940s as a form of chemotherapy and later became popular in the treatment of psoriasis and psoriatic arthritis. Since the early 1980s, use of methotrexate for treatment of RA has increased dramatically (Box 133-9). This increased popularity is explained by the increased efficacy and relatively rapid onset of action of methotrexate compared with previously available DMARDs. Clinical improvement may be observed as early as 2 to 3 weeks, with 8 to 12 weeks of therapy required for full evaluation of efficacy. Administration of methotrexate is convenient; it allows a weekly dosage regimen. Routine laboratory monitoring is needed less frequently than that required for gold and penicillamine.

The dosage of methotrexate is 5 to 15 mg/week, with an average weekly dosage of 7.5 mg (three 2.5-mg tablets). Folic acid is often prescribed in a dosage of 1 mg/day to decrease

Box 133-9. Methotrexate (Rheumatrex) Characteristics

Generic: yes, but not recommended
Tablets: 2.5 mg
Injectable
Usual dosage: two to five tablets 1 day per week or one intramuscular injection per week
Time to effectiveness: 6-12 weeks
Toxicity
Greater than 5%: gastrointestinal intolerance, stomatitis, headache, liver function test abnormalities, hematologic effects
Less than 5%: rash, alopecia, hepatitis, cirrhosis, pneumonitis, nodulosis, gastrointestinal ulceration, atypical infection
Safety monitoring
Initial: CBC, platelet count, AST, alkaline phosphatase, creatinine, albumin; hepatitis B and C serology in high-risk patients; chest radiograph within past year
Stable: CBC, platelet count, AST, albumin, and creatinine every 4-8 weeks

Box 133-10. Cyclosporine (Neoral) Characteristics

Generic available: no
Neoral: soft gelatin capsule 25, 100 mg; oral solution, 100 mg/ml
Dosage: initially 2.5 mg/kg/day in two divided doses; 0.5 to 0.75 mg/kg/day titrated at 8 and 12 weeks; maximum, 4.0 mg/kg/day
Time to effectiveness: 4-8 weeks; discontinue if no benefit by 16 weeks
Toxicity
Greater than 5%: creatinine elevations, hypertension, headache, abdominal pain, diarrhea, dyspepsia, nausea, vomiting, edema, leg cramps, upper respiratory infections, hypertrichosis, rash, dizziness, paresthesia, tremor, pain, stomatitis
Less than 5%: fever, fatigue, bronchitis, pneumonia, purpura, cough, alopecia, depression, chest pain, hypomagnesemia, urinary tract infection, gum hyperplasia
Safety Monitoring
Initial: two baseline blood pressure levels and two serum creatinine levels, therapy not initiated if either is elevated; blood pressure and creatinine every 2 weeks for the first 3 months; if hypertensive or if creatinine 30% or more above baseline, cyclosporine reduced by 25%-50%
Stable: repeated measurement of BUN, serum bilirubin, liver enzymes; periodic measurement of serum lipids, magnesium, potassium, uric acid, and cyclosporine blood levels; monthly CBC and liver tests with methotrexate

BUN, Blood urea nitrogen.

potential toxicity. Safety monitoring requires baseline CBC, platelet count, renal function tests, liver function tests (LFTs), and chest x-ray studies. In high-risk patients, hepatitis B and C studies should also be evaluated. A CBC should be performed again within the first 1 to 2 weeks of therapy and monthly initially. When stable, CBC, platelet count, AST, albumin, and creatinine should be monitored every 4 to 8 weeks. Methotrexate is excreted by the kidney and should not be used in the setting of renal function impairment.

As with other immunosuppressants, methotrexate has potential side effects. Those most often reported relate to GI intolerance. Nausea, vomiting, and diarrhea can usually be minimized by dividing the weekly dosage throughout the day of administration, taking the medication with food, adjusting the dosage, or using antiemetics. IM methotrexate is better tolerated. The most frequent serious side effect is hepatotoxicity. Inflammation and fibrosis of the liver can occur with long-term use. Changes in LFTs do not always correlate with liver damage. Cirrhosis of the liver is rare but has been described, particularly in patients with psoriasis. Fibrosis and cirrhosis appear to be much less common in RA patients who take methotrexate. The risk of liver toxicity can be greatly reduced by eliminating alcohol and staying as close to lean body weight as possible. Routine surveillance liver biopsies are not recommended. Biopsy may be indicated if liver function abnormalities persist during treatment. Risk of cytopenia also exists. At the dosages used for RA, cytopenia is unusual and almost always reversible with discontinuation of methotrexate. Rare atypical infections include *Pneumocystis carinii* pneumonia caused by immunosuppressive effects. Methotrexate also may rarely cause pneumonitis, most often in smokers, with cough, shortness of breath, and interstitial infiltrates on chest films. Pneumonitis is generally reversible but can be life threatening, requiring treatment with corticosteroids.

Cyclosporine. Cyclosporine (cyclosporin A, Neoral) is indicated for the treatment of severe, active RA in patients who do not respond to methotrexate (Box 133-10). Only physicians experienced in management of systemic immunosuppressive therapy for RA should prescribe this agent. Cyclosporin A is most often prescribed in combination therapy with methotrexate but is also used as monotherapy. Patients with severe RA and only partial responses to methotrexate show improvement with a combination of methotrexate and cyclosporine. In controlled studies, side effects were not substantially increased compared with methotrexate alone.[10] Long-term evaluation of this combination is needed to assess toxicity in clinical practice.

Initial therapy with cyclosporine is 2.5 mg/kg/day taken in two divided doses. The dose is then titrated by 0.5- to 0.75-mg/kg increments every 4 to 8 weeks as indicated. The maintenance dose should be the lowest effective dose and should not exceed 4.0 mg/kg. If adverse effects occur, the dose should be reduced by 25% to 50%. Cyclosporin A should be discontinued if no benefit is seen at 16 weeks or if dose reduction does not eliminate side effects. The principal adverse reactions associated with cyclosporine in RA are renal dysfunction, hypertension, headache, GI disturbances, and hirsutism/hypertrichosis.

Azathioprine. Azathioprine (Imuran) was the first immunosuppressant approved by the U.S. Food and Drug Administration (FDA) for use in RA (Box 133-11). Although effective, toxicity issues may be prohibitive for most primary care physicians. Many rheumatologists reserve this therapy for patients who have failed treatment with other DMARDs, although azathioprine is used in many combination therapies.

Azathioprine requires 6 weeks to 6 months of use to

Box 133-11. Azathioprine (Imuran) Characteristics

Generic: no
Dosage: 50-150 mg daily (can be divided)
Toxicity
Greater than 5%: nausea, myelosuppression (thrombocytopenia, granulocytopenia, lymphopenia), macrocytosis
Less than 5%: rash, stomatitis, alopecia, atypical infections, hepatotoxicity, pancreatitis
Safety monitoring
Initial: CBC and platelet every 1-2 weeks with changes in dosage
Stable: CBC and platelet every 1-3 months

become effective. An initial dosage of 1 mg/kg/day or 100 mg for the first 3 months is generally prescribed. The dosage can be increased every 3 months in increments of 25 mg, to a maximum of 150 mg, when lower dosages prove ineffective. Baseline CBC, platelet count, creatinine, and AST should be performed. Safety screening consists of monitoring CBCs every 1 to 2 weeks with changes in dosage, then every 1 to 3 months. LFTs should be performed sporadically if indicated.

The toxicity of azathioprine largely depends on the dosage. Of most concern is the development of cytopenias, often leukopenia. As with other immunosuppressants, azathioprine frequently results in macrocytosis without anemia. Marked hepatotoxicity is rare, but low-grade liver function abnormalities are more common. Azathioprine therapy increases the risk for atypical infections, which may develop without leukopenia. Less common hematologic complications include thrombocytopenia and anemia. These complications are largely reversible. Life-threatening complications are rare when vigilant monitoring is performed. The potential increased risk of subsequent malignancy, particularly lymphoma, with prolonged use has received much attention. Recent long-term studies of RA patients taking azathioprine are reassuring. Any additional risk of cancer in patients receiving azathioprine compared with others with RA appears to be small. Well-controlled studies are lacking, however, and patients should be informed of the potential risk when considering this therapy.

Cyclophosphamide. Cyclophosphamide (Cytoxan) is the most potent and toxic immunosuppressive drug used to treat RA (Box 133-12). Although its effectiveness as a DMARD is undisputed, its potential toxicity prohibits its use in the vast majority of RA patients. Its use is limited to severe complications of RA, such as vasculitis and other severe organ involvement. Cyclophosphamide therapy should be monitored by a rheumatologist because of the seriousness of the rheumatoid and medication complications. Cytopenias appear to be related to the dosage. Risk of an atypical infection also is increased. Interstitial cystitis may occur, and adequate hydration and morning therapy are crucial to reduce cystitis. Pulmonary toxicity has been observed. Cyclophosphamide therapy is associated with an increased risk of bladder cancer and hematologic malignancy. Since cyclophosphamide is given almost exclusively for severe, unremitting RA or for life-threatening complications, this increased risk is usually justified.

Box 133-12. Cyclophosphamide (Cytoxan) Characteristics

Toxicity
Greater than 5%: gastrointestinal intolerance, stomatitis, hemorrhagic cystitis, alopecia, myelosuppression (thrombocytopenia, granulocytopenia, lymphopenia)
Less than 5%*: atypical infection, hepatotoxicity, infertility, bladder cancer, lymphoproliferative malignancy
Safety monitoring
Initial: baseline CBC, platelet count, U/A, creatinine, and AST or ALT; CBC, platelet count, and U/A every 1-2 weeks with changes in dosage
Stable: CBC, platelet count, and U/A every 4-12 weeks; urine cytology and U/A 6-12 months after cessation

*Percentage may be higher with high dosage or prolonged use.

Box 133-13. Leflunomide (Arava) Characteristics

Generic available: no
Arava: tablet; 100, 20, 10 mg
Dosage: initially 100 mg for 3 days, then 20 mg daily (can be decreased to 10 mg if poorly tolerated)
Time to effectiveness: 4-10 weeks
Toxicity
Greater than 5%: abdominal pain, hypertension, diarrhea, nausea, dyspepsia, headache, bronchitis, respiratory infection, alopecia, pruritus, rash, dry skin, dizziness
Less than 5%: anorexia, gastroenteritis, mouth ulcer, vomiting, pneumonia
Safety monitoring
Initial: monthly ALT
Stable: intermittent ALT based on individual patient

ALT, Alanine transaminase.

Leflunomide. Introduced in late 1998, leflunomide (Arava) is the newest of the DMARDs (Box 133-13). It represents a new generation of low-molecular-weight immunoregulatory agents. Leflunomide appears to have an efficacy profile similar to other DMARDs, comparing favorably with sulfasalazine and methotrexate. The onset of action may be as early as 4 weeks. Leflunomide is administered orally, with an initial loading dose of 100 mg for 3 days, usually followed by 20 mg daily as a single dose. A 10-mg tablet is available for decreased dosage. As with methotrexate, concomitant administration of folic acid (1 mg/day) is recommended to decrease GI effects. Potential toxicity includes GI symptoms, rash, reversible alopecia, weight loss, and moderate LFT elevations. Leflunomide should not be used in women or men attempting pregnancy because of maternal and male-mediated fetal toxicity. Male or female patients who wish to initiate a pregnancy should discontinue leflunomide and undergo a drug elimination procedure with cholestyramine, 8 gm three times daily for 11 days. Plasma levels less than 0.02 mg/L are verified by two separate tests at least 14 days apart. Without the elimination procedure, it may take up to 2 years to lower plasma levels adequately. Definitive guidelines for laboratory monitoring have not been confirmed. At a minimum, ALT determinations are performed.

Corticosteroids. Corticosteroids have been used for patients with RA since the 1940s (Box 133-14). Corticosteroids have prominent antiinflammatory properties that result in dramatic improvement of symptomatic arthritis and systemic complaints. The ability to modify the rheumatoid disease course with low-dose corticosteroids continues to be debated. Low-dose corticosteroids, given in a single morning dose, are popular among many rheumatologists as a form of bridge therapy after NSAIDs have been prescribed and before DMARDs become effective. During this period, corticosteroids are used to relieve symptoms while awaiting therapeutic efficacy of DMARD therapy. Corticosteroids should not be used as the sole therapy for RA in most circumstances because of their long-term toxicity. Dosage escalation for the antiinflammatory effects and a shift of dosing to the evening increases the risks of hypercortisolism. Every effort should be made to restrict the dosage to no more than 5 mg of prednisone taken in the morning.

Corticosteroid intraarticular injections are an important adjunct to therapy in RA, particularly in a persistently inflamed joint. "Depo" preparations such as methylprednisolone acetate and triamcinolone hexacetonide may give up to 1 month of relief as sole therapy. Benefits may persist much longer when the steroid injection is combined with systemic therapy. Care must first be taken to rule out a joint infection by aspiration and fluid analysis before injection. The primary care physician can often easily inject large joints (e.g., knees). Systemic absorption occurs and can temporarily suppress the hypothalamic-pituitary-adrenal axis. This may be clinically relevant in patients who have received multiple recent injections and are undergoing joint replacement or other surgery. Preoperative and postoperative corticosteroid stress dosage requires consultation with the surgeon or anesthesiologist.

Box 133-14. Corticosteroid Characteristics

Toxicity: increased appetite, osteoporosis, cataracts, impaired wound healing, diabetes, hypertension, edema, weight gain, increased risk of infection, cushingoid features, acne, easy bruising, suppression of hypothalamic-pituitary-adrenal axis, myopathy, increased intraocular pressure, subcapsular cataracts, avascular necrosis

Safety monitoring

Initial: U/A, blood glucose

Stable: U/A, blood glucose (at least yearly, but more frequently if symptoms warrant)

Biologic Response Modifiers. The role of cellular interaction and cytokine disequilibrium in rheumatoid synovitis and resultant cartilage damage is becoming more clearly defined. This opens the door for targeted biologic response modifiers (BRMs). Broadly, BRMs fall into four categories: monoclonal antibodies, soluble receptors, receptor antagonists, and antiinflammatory cytokines. Multiple trials are currently under way studying these biologic targeted treatments.

Etanercept (Enbrel). Tumor necrosis factor (TNF) has been found to be a major regulator of inflammation in the rheumatoid joint. TNF communicates its proinflammatory effects by binding to specific cell receptors on white blood cells and synovial cells. Soluble TNF receptor levels are elevated in the serum of patients with RA but not in adequate amounts to inhibit the proinflammatory effects of TNF. Etanercept (Enbrel) is a dimeric soluble form of the TNF receptor that can bind two TNF molecules, rendering them biologically inactive thus also modulating the biologic responses that are induced or regulated by TNF (Box 133-15).

Box 133-15. Etanercept (Enbrel) Characteristics

Generic available: no

Enbrel: sterile powder vial, 25 mg, requiring reconstitution to injectable solution; requires refrigeration

Dosage: manufacturer's guidelines for reconstitution; 25 mg given twice weekly as subcutaneous injection

Time to effectiveness: 2-12 weeks

Toxicity

Greater than 5%: injection site reactions, upper respiratory infections, autoantibodies

Less than 5%: dyspepsia, sinusitis, rash, pharyngitis, headache

Safety monitoring: no written guidelines; observation and early treatment for bacterial infections

In randomized, double-blind trials, this has translated into significant reductions in disease activity in patients with RA, even in those who had failed previous DMARD therapy.[6] Clinical responses can occur within 1 to 2 weeks after initiating therapy, significantly faster than most DMARDs. After discontinuation of etanercept, symptoms generally returned within a month.

Etanercept is self-administered by subcutaneous injection twice weekly and requires reconstitution by the patient. Patients may self-inject only after proper training and demonstration of appropriate injection technique. Because of the extraordinary cost of this agent, managed care guidelines will likely be forthcoming. The most frequently reported adverse effect is injection site reactions. Long-term studies are required to determine if there is significantly increased immunogenicity, chronic infections, or malignancy. Close observation for evidence of bacterial infection is suggested because treatment may increase mortality in patients with sepsis.

Surgery

RA can result in persistent inflammation and joint deformity, despite timely medical therapy. Surgical techniques provide several alternatives to ensure that patients with RA continue to maintain function. Surgical options are considered to control severe pain resulting from inflammation or damaged joints, to repair ruptured ligaments or tendons, to remove inflamed synovial tissue that has not responded adequately to medical therapy and is threatening joint damage or tendon rupture, and to retain or restore function in an affected joint.

Synovectomy facilitates the removal of proliferating pannus in an effort to preserve cartilage and surrounding soft tissue structures. Synovectomy should not be viewed as a corrective procedure, since complete resection of all synovial tissue is rarely possible and synovial tissue can grow back. Synovectomy can be performed using arthroscopy or an open procedure. Recovery from arthroscopic synovectomy is generally quite rapid. Although more invasive, open surgical synovectomy has the advantage of improved access, facilitating a more thorough removal of the inflamed synovial tissue.

RA may result in damage to and occasionally rupture of surrounding tendons and ligaments. Rupture of finger extensors secondary to dorsal tenosynovitis occurs most often. If rupture occurs, reconstruction is possible with tendon transfer. *Arthrodesis* (joint fusion) is performed only on painful and unstable joints, most often the wrists, feet, ankles, and thumbs. Although effective in decreasing pain and improving stability, fusion permanently sacrifices motion. For this reason, it is rarely performed on the shoulder or hip. With longstanding RA, atlantoaxial subluxation and other cervical instability can occur because of ligament and bone loss caused by synovitis. In severe cases with neurologic deficits, fusion may be required to increase stability. *Osteotomy* can be performed to improve joint alignment and to compensate for deformity. This procedure is rarely done now because of improved joint replacement procedures.

New techniques for joint replacement have dramatically improved the outlook for even the most severely disabled patients. Traditionally, total joint replacement was performed only in older, inactive individuals who had less chance of outliving the replacement. Current trends reveal an increased use of artificial joints in younger, more active patients. Total joint replacement is frequently performed in the knees, hips, and shoulders with excellent results. Replacements for the elbows, wrists, and ankles are available but have more variable outcomes. Newer designs will likely provide better and more consistent results.

Before surgery, several precautions must be considered. Ruling out cervical subluxation is imperative if tracheal intubation is anticipated. NSAIDs should be discontinued for at least 1 week in most patients; aspirin should be discontinued 2 weeks before surgery. Stress doses should be considered for patients taking corticosteroids or those who recently had multiple intraarticular injections. Whether to stop methotrexate is controversial, but some evidence indicates a lower postoperative infection rate if methotrexate is stopped for the surgery and held for several weeks after the procedure.

SPECIAL ISSUES

Complications

Musculoskeletal complications of RA can include significant cervical spine involvement with atlantoaxial subluxation or impaction and subaxial impaction. Cervical spine involvement should be considered in all rheumatoid patients with painless sensory loss, paresthesias, severe neck or shoulder girdle pain, or weakness in the upper extremities, particularly if deficits increase with neck motion (see Chapter 124). More serious symptoms of myelopathy, such as loss of sphincter control, dysphagia, vertigo, or syncopal episodes, require immediate intervention. MRI is the radiographic technique of choice to assess for cervical cord compression. Evaluation for cervical spine stability with plain radiographs of the lateral neck in flexion and extension is recommended for any patient with advanced RA who is being considered for general anesthesia with intubation and concomitant hyperextension of the neck. The sudden onset or progression of hoarseness should prompt laryngoscopic evaluation for cricoarytenoid joint involvement. Inspiratory stridor should be considered a medical emergency.

Extraarticular complications of RA may vary in severity. Rheumatoid nodules, generally found on extensor surfaces, are noted in up to one third of patients with RA. Nodules rarely cause more than cosmetic problems but can be painful if traumatized. Other systemic features include sicca syndrome secondary to inflammatory changes in lacrimal and salivary glands and in other exocrine glands. Diffuse lymphadenopathy may also be a feature of RA. Lymph node biopsy should be considered if malignancy is a concern.

Hematologic abnormalities include anemia of chronic disease, eosinophilia, and thrombocytosis. Felty's syndrome, a triad of seropositive RA, significant hypersplenism, and granulocytopenia, occurs infrequently. Such patients may be susceptible to infection. If infections are recurrent, corticosteroid, DMARD, or immunosuppressive therapy may be required after the existing infection is eradicated. Splenectomy has been performed on many patients without clear evidence of benefit. Drugs used to treat RA may also cause hematologic abnormalities, including anemia from GI bleeding and bone marrow suppression.

Systemic vasculitis can occur in patients with severe, deforming RA and high RF titers. Vascular damage can range from small vessel involvement, causing palpable purpura, to a necrotizing, medium-sized arteritis. Periungual nail infarcts are common and require no specific treatment. In contrast, systemic vasculitis, with signs of mononeuritis multiplex, visceral vasculitis, cutaneous ulceration, digital infarction, or other organ involvement, requires prompt aggressive treatment.

Peripheral nerve pathology can occur in addition to the structural cervical neurologic complications previously described. Compressive neuropathies, particularly carpal tunnel syndrome, are common. Peripheral nerve damage can also result from angiopathic, amyloid, and monoclonal antibody–induced inflammatory polyneuropathy.

Pulmonary involvement includes pleural diseases, interstitial fibrosis, nodules, pneumonitis, vasculitis, and airways disease. Pleural involvement is frequent but generally asymptomatic. Large pleural effusions may cause shortness of breath. In rare instances a progressive form of pulmonary fibrosis occurs. Finding large numbers of PMNs in bronchoalveolar lavage can support the diagnosis.

Symptomatic cardiac complications are rare. Pericarditis is frequently described but rarely results in cardiac tamponade. Less frequent cardiac involvement includes myocarditis, endocardial changes, arteritis, and conduction defects.

Ocular manifestations range from those that are relatively innocuous to those resulting in blindness. Severity often parallels activity, intensity, and chronicity of RA. Most common is keratoconjunctivitis sicca. Less common and more severe complications include keratitis, episcleritis, scleritis, uveitis, and retinopathy. Visual changes or eye pain should be promptly evaluated by an ophthalmologist who is familiar with RA.

Psychosocial and Family Issues

RA can have an impact on all aspects of daily living, including interpersonal relationships, family dynamics, and sexuality. The perceived loss of independence and control can create fear, anger, and loss of self-esteem. The physician should not overlook this aspect of the patient's care. Since depression directly affects outcome negatively, helping the patient cope with these issues is beneficial. Sexual issues should be addressed with frankness and sensitivity, since patients are often reluctant to share problems in this area. The Arthritis Foundation provides pamphlets concerning sexual issues, coping strategies, and other practical matters. Other resources include counselors with expertise in chronic disease, self-help groups, social workers, vocational counselors, and nurse educators. Many communities have support groups for RA patients.

Pregnancy and Childbirth

Since RA predominantly affects women of childbearing age, counseling of this group is extremely important. Fortunately, pregnancy has an ameliorating effect on rheumatoid synovitis in 75% of women with RA. Most remissions occur during the first trimester but can occur at any point. Medications can usually be discontinued without adverse sequelae. Methotrexate, with its known teratogenic effects, should be discontinued long before pregnancy is attempted. As discussed, leflunomide requires an elimination procedure. Antimalarials are generally stopped 6 to 12 months before conception because of potential neurotoxicity to the fetus. Postpartum exacerbations often occur, however, most often within the first 6 months. This often presents the most significant problem, considering the physical challenges of caring for an infant. If possible, this issue should be addressed with the prospective mother and her partner before pregnancy. Prolonged breast-feeding is not always possible because antiarthritic medication, most of which is secreted in breast milk, is frequently required in the postpartum period. However, RA activity is not associated with obstetric complications or adverse fetal health.

Disability Issues

RA can interfere with the ability to work. Stiffness, pain, decreased mobility, and particularly fatigue may present serious obstacles during an 8-hour workday. Practical advice regarding open communication with employers, increased flexibility of job hours, work-site modifications, energy conservation, and possible job-sharing programs can be a valuable resource to patients trying to remain at work. Continued employment should be encouraged for financial and health insurance benefits, as well as for self-esteem.

In certain situations, continued employment may prove impossible, especially physically demanding jobs that require repetitive motion of inflamed joints. Alternative employment, a change of job description, or an application for disability benefits should be considered. This decision is highly individualized and must consider the patient's age, work experience, educational resources, financial responsibilities, and severity of arthritis. Disability benefits vary greatly in eligibility and policy definition of disability. Many private companies offer short- or long-term disability insurance as part of their benefits packages. Some states provide short-term disability benefits. Patients may be eligible for federal Social Security benefits. This program is not designed to cover short-term or partial disability and is based on the present and projected inability to perform any form of work.

FUTURE DIRECTIONS

Current treatment of RA is multidisciplinary and is likely to remain that way. With managed care constraints, primary care physicians will be involved in initial diagnostic and therapeutic decisions, including the timing of DMARDs. It is hoped that genetic markers will predict severity of arthritis and help direct aggressiveness of therapy. The first of many BRMs has been released. Several cells and cytokines have been targeted for modification. As more of the critical cellular and cytokine interrelationships involved in the pathogenesis of RA are known, newer biologic agents will be tested. Expense will be a consideration for the use of these parenteral agents for chronic disease. The future therapy of RA will likely emphasize the timing of DMARDs already in widespread clinical practice, as well as BRMs in patients with aggressive disease. The primary care physician will become familiar with DMARDs, particularly methotrexate. The total cost of medications will be scrutinized in the managed care environment and will include the cost of monitoring for adverse effects.

REFERENCES

1. American College of Rheumatology Ad Hoc Committee on Clinical Guidelines: Guidelines for monitoring drug therapy in rheumatoid arthritis, *Arthritis Rheum* 39:723, 1996.
2. Arnett FC et al: The American Rheumatism Association 1987 revised criteria for the classification of rheumatoid arthritis, *Arthritis Rheum* 31:315, 1988.
3. Fries JF, Williams CA, Morfield D, et al: Reduction in long-term disability in patients with rheumatoid arthritis by disease-modifying antirheumatic drug–based treatment strategies, *Arthritis Rheum* 39:616, 1996.
4. Harris ED Jr: Mechanisms of disease: rheumatoid arthritis—pathophysiology and implications for therapy, *N Engl J Med* 322:1277, 1990.
5. Kwoh CK: Epidemiology of rheumatic diseases: rheumatoid arthritis, *Curr Opin Rheumatol* 4:140, 1991.
6. Moreland LW, Baumgartner SW, Schiff MH, et al: Treatment of rheumatoid arthritis with a recombinant human tumor necrosis factor receptor (p75)-FC fusion protein, *N Engl J Med* 337:141, 1997.
7. Mottonen T, Paimela L, Ahonen J, et al: Outcome in patients with early rheumatoid arthritis treated according to the "Sawtooth" strategy, *Arthritis Rheum* 39:996, 1996.
8. Pincus T, Callahan LF: Taking mortality in rheumatoid arthritis seriously—predictive markers, socioeconomic status and comorbidity, *J Rheumatol* 13:841, 1986.
9. Shlotzhauer TL, McGuire JL: *Living with rheumatoid arthritis*, Baltimore, 1993, Johns Hopkins University Press.
10. Tugwell P, Pincus T, Yocum D, et al: Combination therapy with cyclosporin and methotrexate in severe rheumatoid arthritis, *N Engl J Med* 333:137, 1995.

CHAPTER 134

Periarticular Rheumatic Disorders

Nancy Y. N. Liu
Juan J. Canoso

Periarticular rheumatic disorder, also referred to as *soft tissue rheumatism,* includes a wide range of musculoskeletal conditions often encountered by the primary care physician. In contrast to diseases that primarily affect the joint, these syndromes involve the periarticular region, which includes the tendons, bursae, fascia, nerves, and muscle (Fig. 134-1). Because of the proximity of these structures to the joint, patients often complain of "arthritis." Similarly, physicians unfamiliar with these conditions may diagnose articular rather than periarticular disease. This confusion may result in delayed or inappropriate therapy. Accurate diagnosis of periarticular rheumatic conditions requires knowledge about the various disorders, a thorough patient history to distinguish between these conditions, and musculoskeletal examination. Once a diagnosis is made, the physician can provide appropriate therapy and advice. Most of these conditions are localized to one region of the body, although some, particularly fibromyalgia, are diffuse (see Chapter 142). In addition, systemic diseases, such as rheumatoid arthritis (RA) or the spondyloarthropathies, may have associated periarticular involvement (see Chapters 133 and 137).

DEFINITIONS

Bursitis

Two forms of bursae exist in the body: the superficial bursae and the deep bursae. Superficial bursae (e.g., olecranon, prepatellar) enhance the gliding of skin over bone and are not filled with fluid unless trauma, infection, or an acute crystal event occurs. Superficial bursae do not communicate with the joint. In contrast, deep bursae (e.g., subacromial, iliopsoas, gastrocnemius-semimembranosus) often develop communication with joints as they age from constant friction and facilitate the gliding of one tendon over another tendon or bone. Pathologically, both bursae are composed of synovial lining cells and thus can become involved in systemic inflammatory disease.

Tendinitis

Tendons transmit the tension generated by muscle to move bone. The highly organized type I collagen in tendons provides tremendous tensile strength and elasticity. A sheath that is histologically identical to synovium lines some tendons. Tendinitis occurs with repetitive use, resulting in microscopic fraying of the collagen, fibrosis, and eventual limitation of tendon motion. Tendinitis may also develop secondary to systemic inflammatory disease (e.g., RA, spondyloarthropathies). Tendinopathy is associated with fluoroquinolone drugs in an estimated 15 to 20 per 100,000 patients.[9]

Enthesopathy

Enthesis is defined as the point of attachment of tendon, fascia, or ligament to bone (see Fig. 134-1). Typical areas include the Achilles tendon attachment to the calcaneus, the plantar fascia to the calcaneus, and the common origin of the

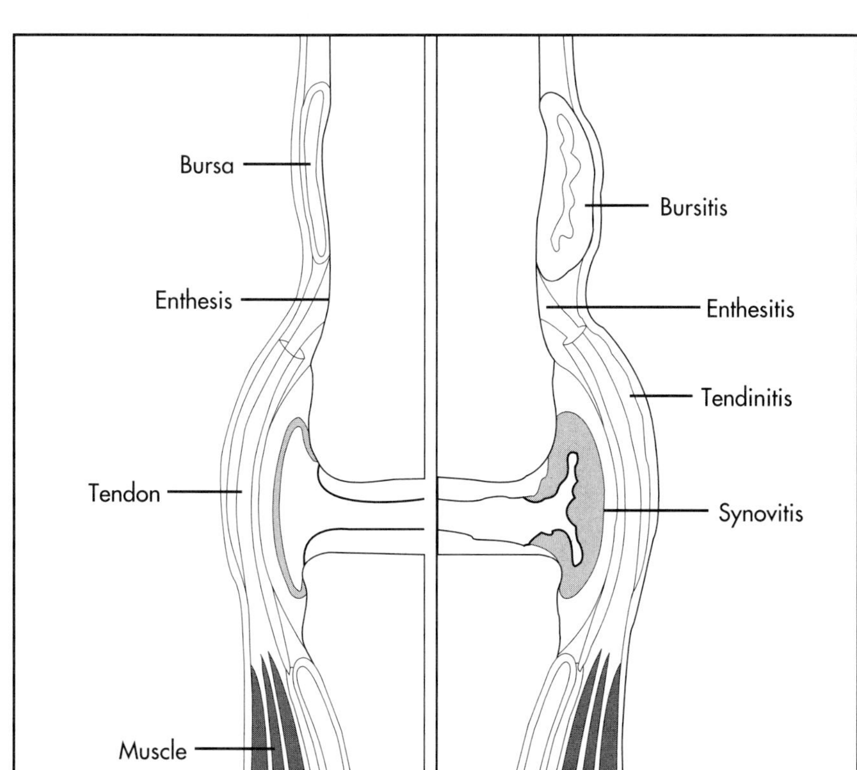

Fig. 134-1. Common structures around the joint include muscle, tendon, enthesis, and bursa.

wrist extensor muscles to the lateral epicondyle. These areas are susceptible to spur formation, calcification from hydroxyapatite deposition, and inflammatory changes from the spondyloarthropathies. Clinical findings include swelling or pain at or underneath the tendinous insertion.

Myofascial Pain

Regional myofascial syndromes are caused by localized areas of pain within muscle that often develop from overt or minor injury. Patients typically describe the pain as a vague, diffuse pain with burning. Clinically, a firm, discrete nodule or taut band, also known as a *trigger point,* can be palpated within the muscle. There is no visible swelling unless muscle spasm is present. When the trigger point is pressed, the pain radiates to a distant point in an atypical dermatomal distribution. A *twitch response* (a sudden contraction of the muscle area that has been palpated) may be pathognomonic for a trigger point. Trigger points and their zones of pain referral throughout the body most often involve the cervical, shoulder, and lower back regions[7] (Fig. 134-2). The description of myofascial pain has been mostly anecdotal. Clinical attempts to separate regional myofascial pain from fibromyalgia based on physical findings of trigger points and tender points, respectively, have not shown definitive results, although many still believe the two entities are distinct.

Nerve Entrapment

Nerve entrapment and peripheral neuropathy are discussed in Chapter 167.

REGIONAL PROCESSES

Cervical Area

Neck pain has many different etiologies, ranging from osteoarthritis to neoplastic disease (see Chapter 124). Neck pain and stiffness constitute a common complaint even in young adults. By age 45, more than 50% of the working population complains of neck stiffness and pain. History and physical examination are most helpful in differentiating the various diagnostic possibilities from myofascial neck pain.

Typically, myofascial neck pain starts after trauma, often delayed by days to weeks after the event. The patient may report no specific injury. The pain is localized to the posterior neck region and is sometimes associated with muscle contraction headaches. Patients may describe the pain beginning after prolonged sitting or sleeping. Activity may improve the pain. No neurologic symptoms are present.

Physical examination reveals well-preserved passive range of motion in the neck, although patients may be unable to move the neck actively. Palpation of the posterior cervical region reveals trigger points within the trapezius and extensor neck muscles. The ligamentum nuchae may also be very tender (see Fig. 134-2). If multiple trigger points exist, the referred area of pain can be extensive, although the neurologic examination is completely normal.

Laboratory tests may exclude other diseases but are not specific for myofascial neck pain. Radiographs may be normal or may reveal varying degrees of osteoarthritis. These latter findings, however, may not be responsible for the cervical pain. Further diagnostic tests, such as electromyography (EMG), nerve conduction studies (NCS), computed tomography (CT) scan of the neck, and magnetic resonance imaging (MRI), are not necessary at the initial stages unless the history or examination suggests other diagnoses.

The differential diagnosis of neck pain is broad and can be divided into inflammatory and noninflammatory processes (Box 134-1). Systemic inflammatory diseases include RA, spondyloarthropathies, and systemic juvenile RA. Osteoar-

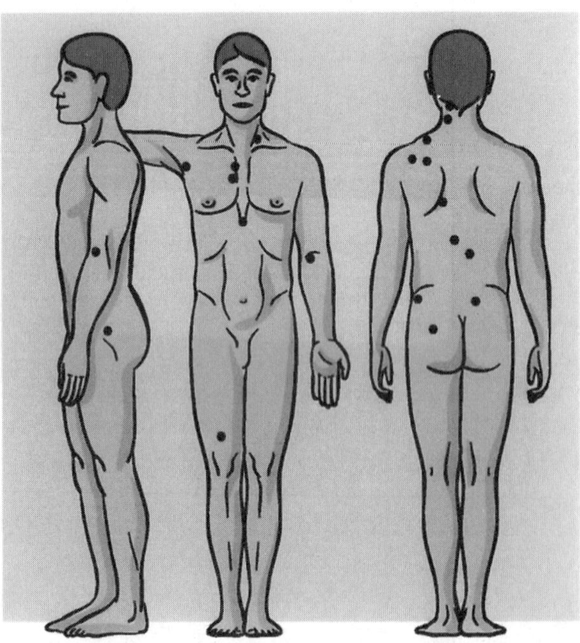

Fig. 134-2. Common myofascial trigger points.

Box 134-1. Differential Diagnosis of Cervical Neck Pain

Inflammatory Diseases

Rheumatoid arthritis (RA)
Spondyloarthropathies
Juvenile RA

Noninflammatory Disease

Cervical osteoarthritis
Diskogenic neck pain
Diffuse idiopathic skeletal hyperostosis
Fibromyalgia or myofascial pain

Infectious Causes

Meningitis
Osteomyelitis
Infectious diskitis

Neoplasms

Primary
Metastatic

Referred Pain

Temporomandibular joint pain
Cardiac pain
Diaphragmatic irritation
Gastrointestinal sources (gastric ulcer, gallbladder, pancreas)

thritis, degenerative disk disease, diffuse idiopathic skeletal hyperostosis (DISH), and fibromyalgia are common noninflammatory diseases of the cervical region. Meningitis, osteomyelitis, and infectious diskitis are infectious etiologies. Neoplastic diseases include metastatic lesions, multiple myeloma, and primary spinal cord tumors. In addition, disorders of the temporomandibular joint, heart, and gastrointestinal (GI) tract may cause pain that is referred to the cervical area.

Treatment of myofascial neck pain is similar to that outlined at the end of this chapter. In cervical neck pain, proper working and sleeping positions are crucial to rehabilitation. Appropriate height of desks, computers, and workstations should be established. At night, patients should sleep in a neutral position (lying on back with legs raised) with only a flat or cervical pillow. Appropriate exercises to stretch and strengthen the neck muscles are helpful.

Shoulder Area

Shoulder pain may arise from pathology within the true glenohumeral joint, the periarticular structures, or the distant structures that refer pain to the shoulder region. Glenohumeral processes are discussed in Chapter 125; only adhesive capsulitis is discussed here. The periarticular structures surrounding the shoulder include the rotator cuff complex, subacromial/subdeltoid bursa, and long head of the biceps. Patients can misinterpret myofascial pain as shoulder pain.

The onset, quality, location, duration, and frequency of pain are important. In addition, factors that exacerbate or improve the pain may help in the diagnosis. Acute pain after trauma suggests a tear in the rotator cuff, joint capsule, or intraarticular structures; gradual pain is less specific. Burning or radicular pain may indicate neuropathy or reflex sympathetic dystrophy. Pain localized to the anterior aspect of the shoulder is common in bicipital tendinitis, whereas rotator cuff tendinitis is more subacromial in location. Glenohumeral processes typically have constant pain referred to the lateral aspect of the upper arm; however, constant pain that is not associated with shoulder movement is an ominous symptom for malignancy or referred pain. Systemic features of fever, chills, and weight loss, visible or progressive swelling in the shoulder area, and pain aggravated by deep inspiration may indicate nonmusculoskeletal etiologies of pain. Axillary pain is usually not from a shoulder source.

Examination of the shoulder includes inspection for asymmetry between the shoulders and palpation of various anatomic regions, including the common myofascial regions of the rhomboid, trapezius, serratus, and rotator cuff muscles. Joints participating in shoulder movement include the sternoclavicular, acromioclavicular, and glenohumeral joints. Scapulothoracic motion also contributes to shoulder movement. Passive range of motion (ROM) in abduction and internal and external rotation delineates the integrity of the glenohumeral joint. In contrast, active ROM provides information not only about the joint, but also about the function of the tendons and muscles surrounding the shoulder. Thus in acute rotator cuff tendinitis, passive ROM of the shoulder is normal (if the patient can relax and avoid guarding), whereas active ROM, particularly against resistance, is limited or painful. In adhesive capsulitis, however, both passive and active ROM are limited.

A general examination also provides clues, particularly if the shoulder examination is normal. Evidence for other joint involvement may suggest an inflammatory arthropathy. Neurologic deficits point to neuropathic processes. Pain referred to the shoulder may originate in the neck, lungs, heart, or abdomen.

Rotator Cuff Disorders.

The rotator cuff complex includes the supraspinatus, infraspinatus, and teres minor muscles, which attach to the greater tuberosity of the humerus, and the subscapularis, which attaches to the lesser tuberosity (Fig. 134-3). The rotator cuff is the internal and external rotator of the shoulder and also depresses the humeral head during abduction. Most common shoulder problems are caused by rotator cuff pathology, categorized as impingement syndrome, acute tendinitis, and rotator cuff tears.

Impingement Syndrome. Impingement syndrome refers to compression of the rotator cuff (particularly supraspinatus and infraspinatus) and the long head of the biceps against the acromion, coracoacromial ligament, and sometimes the acromioclavicular joint. Impingement syndrome is divided into three different stages.[4] Stage I usually occurs in patients 15 to 25 years old who perform repetitive overhead activities. Edema and hemorrhage are present in the rotator cuff. Stage II occurs in active individuals between ages 25 and 50 and is typically associated with pathologic changes of fibrosis. Stage III occurs in older individuals when the cuff progressively degenerates or tears, and secondary bony changes develop in the acromion and humerus.

The patient typically complains of pain that is often worse at night and is exacerbated by overhead activity. Pain may be localized to the area of the subacromial region or may diffusely radiate down toward the deltoid region. The pain can be intermittent or constant. In young patients, complete tear, usually resulting from trauma, is acutely painful, whereas in older patients the condition may be less symptomatic.

Examination reveals normal passive ROM of the glenohumeral joint, but active ROM may be limited by pain. Patients often use scapulothoracic movement to help in shoulder abduction. The arc of motion is a useful test (Fig. 134-4). As the patient abducts, beginning at 45 degrees, the greater tuberosity impinges the supraspinatus tendon against the acromion or coracoacromial ligament. Once the arc is beyond 120 degrees, the greater tuberosity clears the acromion, and the impingement (or pain) ceases.[1] In a rotator cuff tear, active abduction, internal rotation, and external rotation against resistance may be weak. The drop sign is positive if the patient's arm suddenly drops or gives way at 90 degrees when the arm is brought down from overhead (180 degrees) along the side.

Radiographs in early impingement are usually normal, whereas advanced stages may reveal sclerosis and cystic changes of the distal acromion or greater tuberosity. If the rotator cuff is torn, the space between the acromion and humeral head (normally measuring greater than 5 mm) is lost, and proximal migration of the humerus occurs. Scalloping or erosions of the acromion are also present. MRI may be the most sensitive test to identify a tear, whether partial or complete.

Treatment of impingement syndrome depends on the stage. In early disease, conservative therapy with antiinflammatory medications, rest, and physical therapy to strengthen the rotator cuff muscles is usually adequate. In stages I and II,

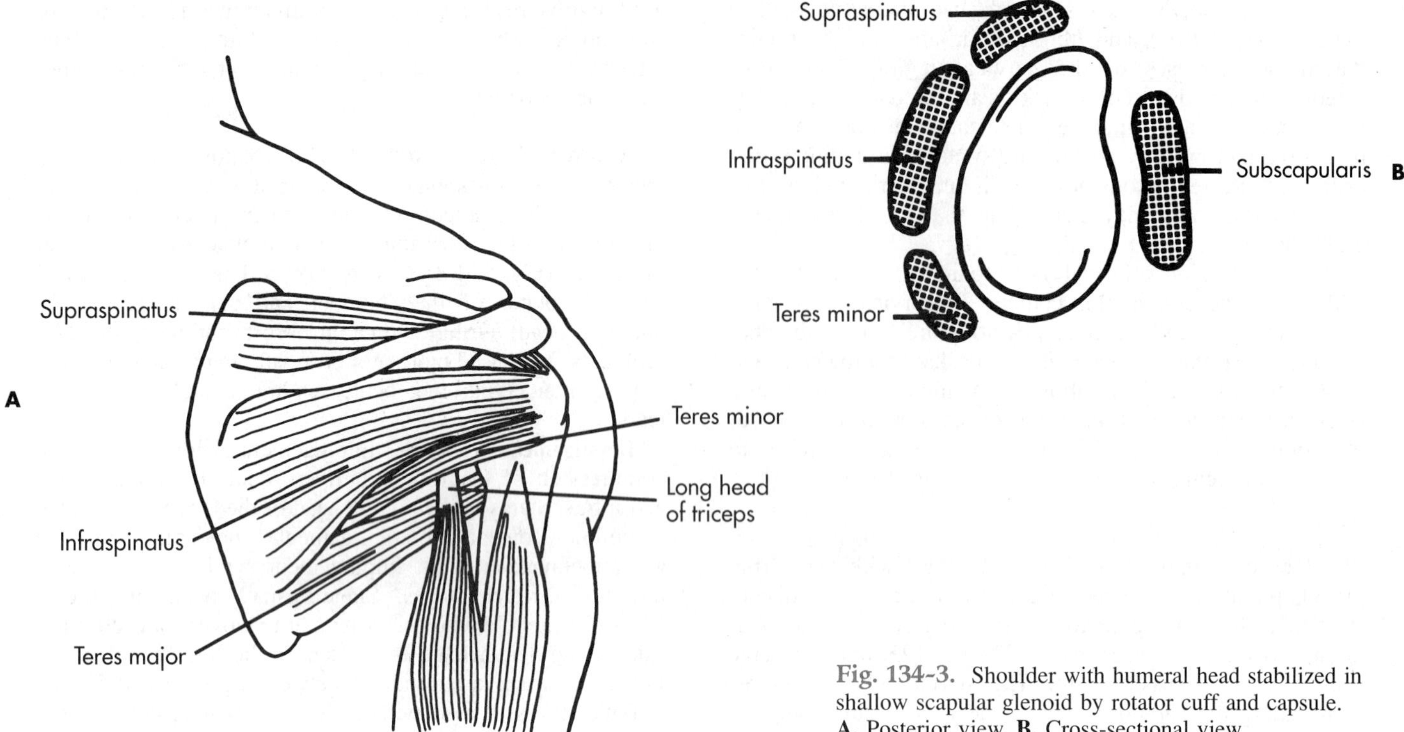

Fig. 134-3. Shoulder with humeral head stabilized in shallow scapular glenoid by rotator cuff and capsule. **A,** Posterior view. **B,** Cross-sectional view.

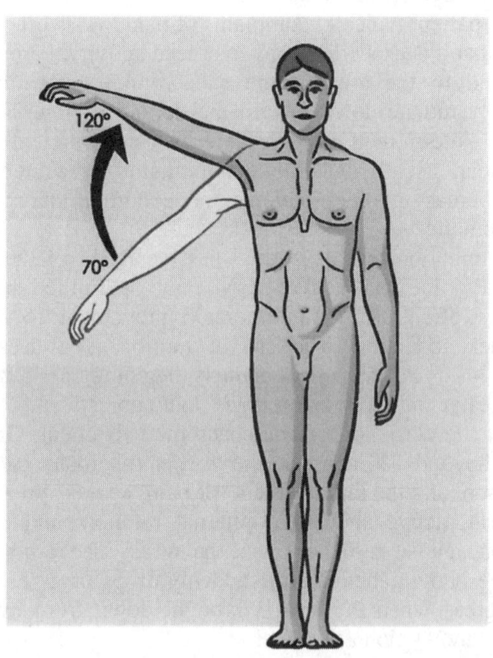

Fig. 134-4. Arc of motion test for impingement. As patient abducts, beginning at 70 degrees, greater tuberosity impinges supraspinatus tendon against acromion or coracoacromial ligament. Once arc is beyond 120 degrees, greater tuberosity clears acromion and impingement (or pain) ceases.

corticosteroid injections into the subacromial space may also be effective. Job and recreational modifications are necessary to prevent further injury. Patients unresponsive to conservative therapy that has included two or three corticosteroid injections or patients with functional impairment should be referred to an orthopedic surgeon for consultation. Arthroscopic decompression includes division of the coracoacromial ligament and acromioplasty; the latter is most successful in patients with an intact rotator cuff. The results of open and arthroscopic decompression are similar.

Acute Tendinitis. Although supraspinatus and bicipital tendinitis typically result from impingement, they may occasionally occur as separate entities. Supraspinatus tendinitis is more common. This tendon helps abduct the shoulder and maintain the strength of the arm when carrying a heavy load with the shoulder abducted; thus it is susceptible to overuse and eventual degeneration. The biceps muscle functions as a flexor of the elbow, supinator of the forearm, and forward elevator of the upper arm. Again, tendinitis occurs as a result of overuse or repetitive motion.

In supraspinatus tendinitis, pain usually localizes in the region just above the scapular spine and lateral to the acromion, near the greater tuberosity of the humerus. Active abduction against resistance elicits severe pain, but passive motion is entirely normal. In bicipital tendinitis, pain is located anteriorly in the area of the biceps tendon, and discrete swelling is sometimes palpable in the tendon area. Supination of the hand against resistance (Yergason maneuver) is painful at the shoulder. Active and passive ROM of the shoulder are normal.

Acute calcific tendinitis occurs secondary to calcium hydroxyapatite deposition in a tendon that has developed degeneration from overuse or impingement. It can involve any tendinous location, but the supraspinatus and bicipital tendons are common areas. Symptoms are usually acute, mimicking gout or pseudogout, and may resolve spontaneously over several days. Calcium deposits within the supraspinatus tendon may eventually rupture into the subacromial bursa, and secondary bursitis develops. Radiographs may reveal amorphous or well-delineated calcific deposits within the subacromial bursa, supraspinatus, or bicipital tendons. Treatment includes nonsteroidal antiinflammatory drugs (NSAIDs), local corticosteroid injection, or intramuscular adrenocorticotropic hormone (ACTH, 40 to 60 IU). Colchicine, 0.6 mg twice a day, may prevent recurrent postinjection flares. Multiple needlings, which manually disrupt the calcific deposits, and corticosteroid infiltration may help resolve resistant cases. If symptoms recur, surgical intervention may be necessary (see Chapter 125).

Bursitis. The terms "subacromial" and "subdeltoid" bursitis have often been misused to describe pain in these regions. Acute bursitis is most likely caused by impingement syndrome or calcific tendinitis. Clinical symptoms, physical findings, and treatment are identical to those previously outlined.

Rotator Cuff or Biceps Tendon Tears. See Chapters 125 and 143.

Myofascial Shoulder Pain. Myofascial pain around the shoulder region is often the result of overuse or poor positioning during work or play. The most common regions include the trapezius, the supraspinatus and infraspinatus, and the muscles along the medial border of the scapula (levator scapulae, serratus anterior, rhomboid) (see Fig. 134-2). Pain may be diffuse and may include sites distant from the myofascial trigger point. On examination a taut band may be palpable in various regions. Treatment is primarily exercises that use these muscles. NSAIDs are given in a short course. Myofascial trigger point injections may be necessary.

Adhesive Capsulitis. Adhesive capsulitis (frozen shoulder) is a slow, insidious loss of shoulder motion accompanied by varying intensities of pain. The condition is usually self-limited and resolves within 1 to 3 years unless there is an underlying disease. Often a patient is left with a 20% to 25% reduction in normal motion. Adhesive capsulitis typically develops following shoulder immobility after acute calcific tendinitis of the shoulder, acute stroke, or myocardial infarction. It is also associated with diabetes, hypothyroidism and hyperthyroidism, tuberculosis, apical lung tumors, and local primary neoplasms (Box 134-2). Women and middle-aged patients (40 to 60 years old) are at a slightly greater risk for developing adhesive capsulitis. Its pathology reveals capsular fibrosis and contracture, but it is not clear whether this is a result of inflammation or joint immobility.

Patients complain of slow, gradual onset of shoulder pain that can be severe, even at night. The pain is generalized and referred to the superolateral aspect of the shoulder and upper arm. Examination reveals no swelling at the glenohumeral joint. Passive and active ROM are greatly limited in all movements.

Diagnosis of adhesive capsulitis is based on the physical findings of limited shoulder motion. The physician should investigate associated diseases such as diabetes and thyroid disease. Laboratory studies and plain radiographs are not helpful except to exclude secondary etiologies. Shoulder arthrography can confirm the reduction of the joint cavity but is not necessary, since the diagnosis is established clinically. Routine arthroscopy is not indicated unless other processes (e.g., intraarticular pathology) are suspected or patients fail to improve from conservative therapy.

Numerous treatments for adhesive capsulitis have been described, but most studies are uncontrolled. Prevention is most important. ROM shoulder exercises are recommended for any painful shoulder. The Codman (pendulum) exercise is performed with the patient flexed forward at the waist with most of the body weight supported by the opposite arm on a table or chair back (Fig. 134-5). The affected arm is dangled perpendicular to the ground. The patient then circles the arm clockwise for a set repetition and then counterclockwise. The circles should become bigger, and the patient can progress to holding weights with the affected arm while doing the pendulum exercises. NSAIDs have inconsistent effects on the pain. Intraarticular steroids or oral prednisone (20 mg daily, tapered by 2.5 mg per week until finished) appears to be effective in controlling the nocturnal pain in early disease. To regain motion, however, an intensive physical therapy program should be initiated by a physical therapist, followed by a home program. Patients must be informed that improvement is slow; symptoms may persist for 1 to 2 years.

Some patients have intractable pain unresponsive to conservative therapy, whereas others have severe shoulder limitation, impairing activities of daily living. Further

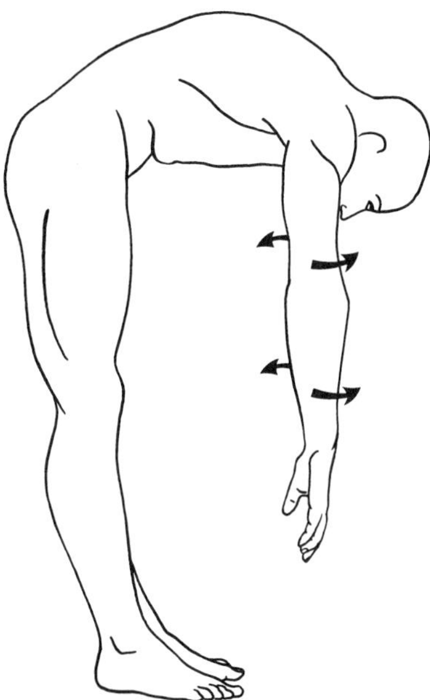

Fig. 134-5. Codman (pendulum) range of motion exercise for the shoulder.

Box 134-2. Conditions Associated With Adhesive Capsulitis

- Diabetes
- Hypothyroidism/hyperthyroidism
- Adrenal insufficiency
- Pulmonary tuberculosis
- Apical lung tumors
- Hemiparesis
- Complication after brachial cardiac catheterization
- Myocardial infarction
- Primary local tumors in humerus or chest wall

evaluation with MRI scanning may be indicated to exclude intraarticular pathology. Distention arthrography with lidocaine and saline or manipulation under general anesthesia is often performed, but the true efficacy of these interventions has not been proved in well-designed trials. Arthroscopic examination with distention and debridement of capsular adhesions appears comparable to manipulation but offers the advantage of diagnosing and repairing unsuspected rotator cuff tears.

Reflex Sympathetic Dystrophy. Reflex sympathetic dystrophy (RSD) (shoulder-hand syndrome) may present initially as shoulder pain or adhesive capsulitis. Risk factors are similar to those of adhesive capsulitis and range from traumatic soft tissue or bony injury to effects of myocardial or cerebrovascular injury. The etiology is unclear, but a disturbance of sympathetic outflow is assumed through the symptoms, physical findings, and response to treatment. RSD may also occur in the lower extremity.

In the earliest stage, patients complain of burning pain, swelling, temperature changes, and excessive perspiration in the extremity. About 3 to 6 months after the initial stage, the soft tissue swelling progresses to skin induration and muscle atrophy. Contractures of the digits, tight shiny skin, and limitation of motion characterize the late stage. Pain may extend proximally from the hand.

Radiographs in early to middle phases may be normal or may reveal patchy osteopenia, whereas late-stage findings show marked osteopenia. Triple-phase technetium bone scan classically demonstrates increased blood flow and pooling, as well as increased uptake in the periarticular structures of the affected extremity. Diagnostically, the improvement of pain and dysesthesia after regional sympathetic block is also characteristic.

The differential diagnosis of RSD includes cervical radiculopathy, carpal tunnel syndrome, the onset of systemic sclerosis, and RA. Treatment in the early phases includes high-dose systemic glucocorticoids (1 mg/kg/day) for 2 weeks. If the patient does not respond, the steroids are rapidly tapered; if improvement occurs, the steroids are tapered gradually over 4 to 6 weeks. Alternative treatments include interruption of sympathetic tone through regional ganglion block, sympathectomy, and medications. Rigorous physical therapy should follow all interventions to preserve motion. In later stages, physical therapy alone is indicated to help regain function and motion. Full recovery is limited if symptoms have been present for more than 6 months.

Differential Diagnosis. The differential diagnosis of shoulder pain is broad and can be separated into four categories (Box 134-3). Intraarticular processes include internal derangement, synovitis, osteoarthritis, infection, osteonecrosis, adhesive capsulitis, and tumor. Periarticular processes primarily involve rotator cuff pathology, bicipital tendinitis, acromioclavicular arthritis, and localized or generalized myofascial disorders. Referred pain to the shoulder often is associated with cervical radiculopathy, Pancoast's tumor, subdiaphragmatic processes, gallbladder disease, and myocardial infarction. Other considerations include RSD, brachial neuritis, suprascapular nerve entrapment, and thoracic outlet syndrome. A differential diagnosis can also be generated by the location of shoulder pain (Box 134-4).

Box 134-3. Differential Diagnosis of Shoulder Pain

Intraarticular Processes

Synovitis secondary to rheumatoid arthritis or spondyloarthropathies
Infection
Adhesive capsulitis
Osteoarthritis
Internal derangement (labral tears)
Avascular necrosis
Benign or malignant tumors (bone or synovial)

Periarticular Processes

Impingement syndrome: rotator cuff or bicipital
Calcific tendinitis
Tears of rotator cuff or biceps tendons
Myofascial pain
Acromioclavicular arthritis

Referred Pain

Sternoclavicular joint processes
Cervical radiculopathy
Pancoast's tumor
Subdiaphragmatic processes (abscess or gallbladder disease)
Myocardial infarction
Mediastinal tumors (pain localized to axilla)

Others

Reflex sympathetic dystrophy
Brachial neuritis
Thoracic outlet syndrome
Suprascapular nerve entrapment

Modified from Thornhill TS. In Kelley WN et al, editors: *Textbook of* rheumatology, ed 5, Philadelphia, 1993, Saunders.

Elbow

True articular causes of elbow pain are extremely rare except for inflammatory processes of the elbow joint. Common soft tissue syndromes include olecranon bursitis, lateral and medial epicondylitis, and nerve entrapment syndromes. Pain often localizes over a particular region. Passive and active ROM of the elbow spans 0 degrees (full extension) to 135 degrees (full flexion). With joint inflammation the patient holds the elbow in semiflexion to accommodate inflammatory fluid or cellular infiltrate. Active and passive flexion and extension are limited. With periarticular disease, however, passive ROM is usually normal.

Olecranon Bursitis. Systemic diseases such as gout, RA, and less often, pseudogout, oxalosis, and basic calcium phosphate deposition may all involve the olecranon bursa. Traumatic or infectious bursitis, however, is more common in primary care practice. Since the olecranon is a superficial bursa, it is susceptible to repetitive trauma and bacterial infection from direct skin penetration. Patients may not remember a particular event that precipitated the swelling but may have a longstanding habit of bearing pressure on the elbows. In acute crystal or infectious bursitis, pain tends to be

Box 134-4. Differential Diagnosis of Shoulder Pain by Location

Top of Shoulder (C4)
Cervical source
Acromioclavicular
Sternoclavicular
Diaphragmatic

Superolateral (C5)
Rotator cuff tendinitis
Impingement
Adhesive capsulitis
Glenohumeral arthritis

Anterior
Bicipital tendinitis and rupture
Glenoid labral tear
Adhesive capsulitis
Glenohumeral arthritis
Osteonecrosis

Axillary
Neoplasm (Pancoast's, mediastinal)
Herpes zoster

severe, and systemic symptoms (e.g., fever, sweats, chills) may be present.

An important physical finding is swelling in a discrete sac at the tip of the olecranon. The region may be warm, erythematous, and painful to palpation. Soft tissue edema distal to the elbow may be present. Occasionally, if septic bursitis is advanced, the olecranon bursa ruptures, resulting in diffuse cellulitis of the elbow and forearm. Pain may be present (sometimes severe) in flexion, but full passive extension of the elbow is possible without pain, suggesting that true elbow joint involvement is unlikely. Rheumatoid nodules or tophaceous deposits may be palpable in the olecranon bursa.

Aspiration and analysis of the olecranon bursa fluid for total and differential white blood count, crystal search, Gram's stain, and culture are important in making the diagnosis. Unlike articular infections, the septic bursal fluid may have deceptively few leukocytes (less than 10,000/mm^3). Infection cannot be excluded until culture results are final. Radiographs typically reveal only soft tissue swelling.

The differential diagnosis for swelling in the olecranon region includes traumatic, septic, gouty, and rheumatoid bursitis. In addition, superficial bursitis sometimes occurs in systemic sclerosis, systemic lupus erythematosus (SLE), and hypertrophic pulmonary osteoarthropathy.

Therapy for traumatic bursitis includes protecting the olecranon region from further trauma by consciously avoiding pressure to the elbow. Corticosteroid injection into the bursa has been successful, but skin atrophy and secondary infections may occur. Surgical resection is rarely necessary. About 80% of all septic bursitis cases are caused by *Staphylococcus aureus,* followed by *Streptococcus* organisms in 14%.[2] Rarely, gram-negative infection occurs, most often in debilitated or older patients. An oral antibiotic effective against *Staphylococcus* and *Streptococcus* organisms is the initial therapy for septic olecranon bursitis. When final cultures return, the antibiotic can be tailored. Along with antibiotic therapy, serial needle aspiration of the olecranon bursa fluid is necessary daily until culture results are negative. Antibiotics can be discontinued 5 days after the negative culture. If cultures reveal persistence of the organism despite antibiotic therapy and aspiration, surgical resection of the bursa is necessary. More aggressive initial therapy with intravenous antibiotics may be indicated for patients who are febrile, immunocompromised, or chronically debilitated.

Lateral and Medial Epicondylitis. Lateral epicondylitis *(tennis elbow)* results from trauma to the insertion of the common extensor tendon onto the lateral epicondyle. The extensor carpi radialis brevis is most often involved, at its insertion on the lateral epicondyle. Patients typically describe an aching pain in the lateral aspect of the elbow that is aggravated by grasping or turning the wrist. Pain may be present at rest. Onset ranges from acute to subacute or chronic. Despite its name, tennis elbow develops with any occupation or activity that stresses the wrist extensors.

Medial epicondylitis is the counterpart to lateral epicondylitis but results from overuse of the flexor tendons of the wrist. The point of tenderness is located over the medial epicondyle. Although termed *golfer's elbow,* this condition may occur with other sports and occupational activities.

Physical examination reveals focal tenderness in the lateral or medial epicondyle region. In addition, extension of the finger or wrist against resistance produces pain in the lateral epicondyle region, whereas flexion of the wrist against resistance produces pain in the medial epicondyle region.

Bilateral lateral epicondylitis is rare. When present, the physician should consider fibromyalgia. Entrapment neuropathies, particularly the deep branch of the radial nerve, may be confused with lateral epicondylitis, whereas compressive neuropathy of the ulnar nerve may be mistaken for medial epicondylitis. In addition, cervical radiculopathy and carpal tunnel syndrome sometimes manifest as elbow pain. Entrapment neuropathy of the deep branch of the radial nerve should be suspected in chronic refractory tennis elbow. The tenderness is anterior, on the radius, approximately 2 cm distal to the elbow crease.

Treatment of lateral and medial epicondylitis begins with avoiding the aggravating condition and modifying it to prevent recurrent injury. This may require the assistance of a professional in sports medicine or an occupational therapist. Relative rest for 3 to 4 weeks, the use of a forearm compression band, and NSAIDs are initial measures. Gentle exercises to stretch the extensor or flexor muscles should progress to strengthening exercises. The success rate of these combined conservative modalities is nearly 75%. Local corticosteroid infiltration around the lateral and medial epicondyle has been a traditional alternative when conservative therapy fails. Although corticosteroid injection is more effective than lidocaine alone for acute pain management, the outcome at 6 months is the same. Thus conservative therapy is recommended for 6 months. If pain persists after that period, surgical consultation is recommended.

Wrist and Hand

The wrist and hand are prone to traumatic injuries as well as to systemic inflammatory disease. Periarticular processes of the wrist include tenosynovitis, median and ulnar nerve entrapment, and ganglions. In the hand, tenosynovitis and Dupuytren's contracture are common periarticular conditions.

Wrist flexion normally spans 80 degrees of flexion and extension, 40 degrees of ulnar deviation, and 20 degrees of radial deviation. Palpation of the ulnar styloid and radiocarpal joints provides clues for synovitis. Muscle atrophy on examination of the hand may suggest neuropathy. Skin changes (e.g., tightening, rashes) and nail changes are helpful in diagnosing systemic inflammatory diseases. ROM of the fingers can be grossly assessed by the patient's ability to make a complete fist. If the patient cannot, the examination must focus on passive and active ROM of the fingers to distinguish an articular process from a tendinous one. If the examiner can passively move the metacarpophalangeal (MCP), proximal interphalangeal (PIP), and distal interphalangeal (DIP) joints into full flexion, the pathology resides in the tendon mechanism. If passive motion of the joint is limited, however, articular pathology is present.

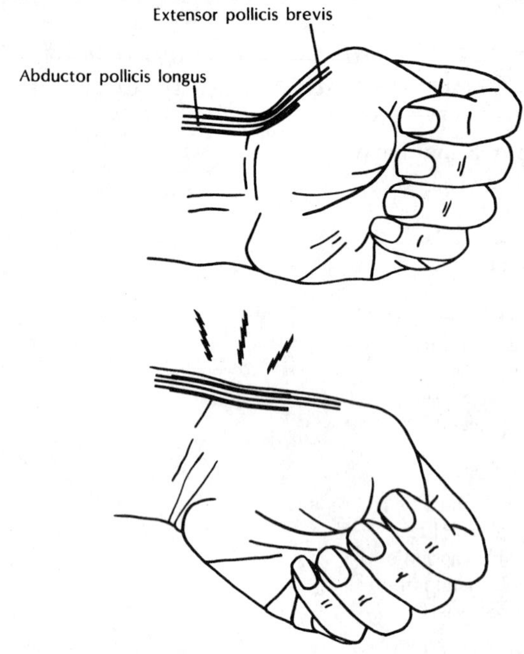

Fig. 134-6. Finkelstein's test is positive in de Quervain's stenosing synovitis. Ulnar flexion of wrist produces pain over dorsal compartment containing extensor pollicis brevis and abductor pollicis longus tendons.

Tenosynovitis. Although tenosynovitis is more common in the inflammatory arthritides (e.g., RA, psoriatic arthritis), stenosing tenosynovitis of the thumb and fingers results more often from overuse or repetitive motion.

De Quervain's Tenosynovitis. Stenosing tenosynovitis of the abductor pollicis longus and extensor pollicis brevis tendons is also known as de Quervain's tenosynovitis. It is secondary to the thickening of the fibrous sheath over the radial styloid, which impinges on the two tendons. Patients have pain over the radial aspect of the wrist, which is often exacerbated by thumb or wrist motion. Physical findings may include focal soft tissue swelling over the radial styloid region, pain on palpation of the region, or severe pain when the wrist is deviated toward the ulna while the thumb is folded within the fingers (Finkelstein's test) (Fig. 134-6). Differential diagnosis of pain in this region includes carpometacarpal disease from osteoarthritis, tendinitis of the extensors of the wrist, or tendinitis associated with systemic disease such as spondyloarthropathies or disseminated gonococcemia. Treatment includes NSAIDs, immobilization with a long thumb spica or opponens splint fashioned by an occupational therapist, and local corticosteroid injection into the tendon sheath. Activities that require repetitive motion of the thumb or wrist should be modified.

Stenosing Tenosynovitis. Stenosing tenosynovitis of the finger, also known as *trigger finger,* develops secondary to excessive forces at the fibrous rings that affix the flexor tendon in place. As a result of these forces, fibrocartilaginous metaplasia develops and obstructs the normal gliding motion of the flexor tendon. Repetitive motion of the fingers and frequent clutching of the hand are associated with this entity. Patients classically complain of the inability to open a finger from flexion in the morning without active assistance from the other hand. Other patients describe a snapping of the finger from flexion to extension. Examination reveals swelling or nodularity, often tender to palpation, along the tendon sheath in the palmar surface of the hand. If the patient actively flexes and extends the finger, crepitation is palpable through the course of the tendon within the palm. Differential diagnosis includes suppurative tenosynovitis (an acute syndrome with redness and pronounced tenderness), mycobacterial infections, systemic inflammatory diseases, Dupuytren's contracture, and sarcoidosis. If multiple fingers are involved, diabetes mellitus, amyloidosis, and ochronosis should be excluded. Local corticosteroid injection of the tendon sheath is extremely effective.[3] Modification of job or recreational activities is necessary. Referral to a hand surgeon is recommended if symptoms recur.

Median and Ulnar Nerve Entrapment. Entrapment of the median and ulnar nerves at the wrist results in carpal tunnel syndromes (see Chapter 167).

Dupuytren's Contracture. A progressive fibrotic condition involving the palmar fascia, Dupuytren's contracture leads to fixed flexion deformities at the MCP joint. This entity is painless and does not cause significant disability until the fingers develop contractures that limit function. Pathologically, fibroblasts proliferate in the palmar fascia without an inflammatory component. The flexor tendons, however, are not involved. Taut bands of fibrosis form, typically involving the fourth, fifth, and occasionally the third fingers, but rarely the thumb or index finger. Similar findings may occur in the plantar region. Men are affected more often than women. Previous reports associating Dupuytren's contracture with diabetes mellitus and alcoholism have not been consistently documented. Treatment consists of passive extension of the finger in early stages. Surgical intervention at later stages may be necessary, but recurrence is common.

Ganglions. Ganglions are cystic outpouchings of the joint capsule or tendon sheath. They often occur asymptomatically on the dorsum of the wrist and resolve or recur spontaneously. The ganglion is filled with a gelatinous fluid and transilluminates, differentiating it from solid tumors. Lipoma, neuroma, synovial cyst of RA, calcific deposits, giant cell tumor, and sarcoma may have a similar appearance. Management includes observation only, aspiration and injection with corticosteroids, or surgical removal.

Anterior Chest Wall Pain

Costochondritis, or pain in the anterior chest wall along the costosternal junction, may mimic acute cardiac or pleuritic pain. Patients describe intermittent pain that lasts for several days, radiates to the chest wall, and is exacerbated by deep breath. The costosternal junctions are often tender to palpation at one or more locations and even along the intercostal muscles. If bilateral tenderness in the costochondral regions is elicited, spondyloarthropathies and fibromyalgia should be considered in the differential diagnosis. Referred pain from cardiac, pulmonary, esophageal, and vascular sources also must be excluded.

Tietze's syndrome is a possible diagnosis if swelling is associated with pain in the costochondral regions. The etiology of Tietze's syndrome is unknown, but pathology reveals proliferation of cartilage and increased vascularity in the costochondral region. This syndrome may be acute or chronic. Differential diagnosis includes spondyloarthropathy, infection, and tumor of the bone.

Treatment of both costochondritis and Tietze's syndrome includes eliminating the factors that may aggravate the pain, administering NSAIDs, instituting physical therapy with ultrasound, or administering local corticosteroid injections. Skin atrophy in the anterior chest wall region can occur secondary to local steroid injections. This complication may be particularly undesirable for some patients.

Low Back and Pelvis

Low back pain is one of the most common complaints in a primary care practice (see Chapter 127). Although the pain is usually self-limited, loss of productivity in the working population exacts an enormous financial cost to society. Soft tissue etiologies of low back pain include myofascial pain, bursitis, and localized muscle syndromes.

Myofascial Low Back Pain. Myofascial low back pain can develop without associated conditions or can be secondary to mechanical back disease, nerve entrapment, and inflammatory diseases of the back. Patients complain of a dull, aching pain that is not well localized. Muscle spasm may be associated with the pain, and nondermatomal radicular symptoms may be present. Activity, prolonged sitting, and cool temperatures exacerbate the pain. More ominous symptoms that require further evaluation include fever, chills, weight loss, pain unrelated to position, urinary or fecal incontinence, and neurologic deficits.

Inspection of the lower back while the patient is standing may reveal asymmetry that suggests scoliosis or leg length discrepancy. Percussion of the vertebral bodies and palpation of the paravertebral musculature can localize the region of pain. Lower back ROM includes flexion, extension, lateral bending, and lateral rotation. Numerous myofascial trigger points may be palpable in the lower back (see Fig. 134-2).[7] When these points are pressed, the pain is reproduced and may radiate to distant regions.

The diagnosis of myofascial low back pain is based on the exclusion of other etiologies. The major categories include mechanical back pain secondary to degenerative disease, nerve entrapment syndromes, infection, inflammatory back disease, referred pain from abdominal or retroperitoneal sources, neoplasms, and psychogenic causes.

Treatment of myofascial low back pain includes recognition of aggravating factors at home, at work, or in recreational activities. Proper sitting, standing, and sleeping positions should be encouraged. Exercises to strengthen the abdominal musculature and back extensors, improvement of posture, and back protection are the foundation of lifelong back care.[5] Referral to a formal back school or physical therapy program is recommended if patients have chronic pain. NSAIDs may be helpful to patients with myofascial pain secondary to degenerative diseases. Muscle relaxants such as cyclobenzaprine (10 to 20 mg at night and 5 to 10 mg in the morning) are helpful if muscle spasms are present. Alternatively, low-dose tricyclic antidepressants (e.g., amitriptyline) may help patients with chronic back pain. Myofascial trigger point injections with a long-acting anesthetic followed by muscle stretching provide relief of pain. Some believe this can provide lasting benefit without the need for chronic reinjections.[5] Other modalities, including therapeutic massage and transcutaneous electric nerve stimulation (TENS), have variable results.

Piriformis Syndrome. The piriformis muscle is an external rotator of the hip that occupies the area of the greater sciatic notch. Spasms of this muscle produce symptoms of buttock pain that are aggravated by sitting and improved with standing. Symptoms may mimic sciatica, but the neurologic examination is normal. Pain can be elicited in the sciatic notch and the lateral rectal wall. External rotation of the hip against resistance may produce pain. Treatment with local corticosteroid injections can provide relief.

Ischial Bursitis. Tenderness at the ischial tuberosity results in difficulty sitting or lying down. Inflammation of the ischial bursa is assumed rather than proved. *Tailor's bottom* and *weaver's bottom* are common terms describing this condition. Although there is some association with prolonged sitting on hard surfaces, the exact etiology is unclear. Local fat atrophy is a common finding. Patients can localize the pain over the ischial prominence, which is exquisitely tender to palpation. Suppurative ischial bursitis may occur in paraplegic patients. Ischial tenderness has been associated with the spondyloarthropathies from enthesitis and can be mistaken for low back strain or even herniated nucleus pulposus. Treatment includes using foam cushions with holes cut for the two ischial tuberosities. Local corticosteroid injections should be avoided; they may result in further fat atrophy and pain.

Osteitis Pubis. Inflammation of the symphysis pubis has multiple etiologies. Septic seeding of the symphysis occurs most often after genitourinary surgery or herniorrhaphy. Spondyloarthropathies, particularly in women, and calcium pyrophosphate dihydrate (CPPD) disease may also affect this region. Trauma from sports, stress fractures, or specific injury to the gracilis or adductor longus muscles may clinically resemble osteitis pubis. Patients complain of pain in the lower anterior pelvis that may radiate into the medial thighs. Walking may be painful, and palpation over the symphysis pubis produces exquisite pain. Initial radiographs may be normal, but with advanced stages, erosions, widening of the joint space, and sclerosis are present. In CPPD disease, linear calcification in the symphysis is present. Treatment includes the use of NSAIDs during evaluation for other underlying diseases. The pain may resolve spontaneously. If infection is suspected, percutaneous aspiration must be performed. Local corticosteroid injection may be beneficial. Surgical intervention is reserved for intractable cases.

Hips

Periarticular structures and referred pain cause hip pain more often than true articular processes. In the latter, pathology in the joint results in pain localized to the groin or referred anatomically to the knee. Patients often use "hip pain" to refer to any area in the lower back, buttock, and lateral hip regions.

Inspection of the hips during weight bearing detects scoliosis or leg length discrepancy. The gait should be observed. An antalgic gait is characterized by the patient leaning over the painful hip during weight bearing to avoid contraction of the hip abductors. Alternatively, the pelvis may drop down on the opposite side when bearing weight on the affected hip (Trendelenburg's gait).

Measurement of leg lengths is performed in the supine position from the anterior superior iliac crest to the medial malleolus. Up to 1 cm of difference in length between the legs is considered normal. Passive ROM of the hip includes flexion (120 to 135 degrees), extension (20 degrees), internal rotation (35 to 45 degrees), and external rotation (45 degrees). The hips can also abduct to 60 to 70 degrees and adduct to 25 to 30 degrees. Patrick's (fabere) test involves placing the foot ipsilateral to the hip being examined onto the knee of the other leg; then the thigh is further abducted toward the table. If pain exists, intrinsic hip disease or sacroiliac disease is present. The Thomas test can detect hip contractures. With the patient supine, both hips are flexed initially, then the hip of concern is extended toward the table; the other hip remains flexed to fix the pelvis and flatten the lumbar lordosis. Limitation of full extension indicates a hip contracture on that side. Examination of the periarticular structures is detailed later.

Trochanteric Bursitis. The trochanteric bursa is located between the tendon of the gluteus maximus muscle and the posterior aspect of the greater trochanter. Bursitis classically develops from overuse or stress of the hip abductors due to hip disease, degenerative disease of the lumbar spine, leg length discrepancy, and other lower extremity conditions. The trochanteric region is a common tender point for fibromyalgia. Thus any patient with bilateral trochanteric bursitis should be examined for other tender points associated with fibromyalgia (see Chapter 142).

Patients typically complain of localized lateral hip discomfort exacerbated by rising from a chair or car seat and walking and difficulty sleeping on the affected side. Sometimes the pain is diffuse, involving the lateral hip and thigh, buttock, and even the groin or knee. Localized point tenderness on or posterior to the greater trochanter is the classic finding. Occasionally the fascia lata is also tender. Active hip abduction against resistance and passive external rotation of the hip produce pain. Passive internal rotation is normal.

Differential diagnosis of lateral hip pain includes referred pain from the spine, particularly the upper lumbar region (L2 to L4), secondary to spinal stenosis, disk herniation, and facet syndromes. Entrapment of the cutaneous branches of the iliohypogastric or subcostal nerve can produce burning pain in the lateral hip. Occult stress fractures of the femoral neck in older patients may present as lateral hip pain. Fascia lata fasciitis may mimic trochanteric bursitis, but the pain usually extends below the trochanteric region along the tensor fascia lata.

Treatment of trochanteric bursitis includes moist heat and correction of associated pathology, such as leg length discrepancy or gait abnormalities. Physical therapy referral for ultrasound may be beneficial. Local corticosteroid injection mixed with lidocaine (Xylocaine) is most effective. Patients requiring frequent injections (more than three) warrant reevaluation and surgical consultation if no underlying cause is identified.

Iliopsoas Bursitis. The iliopsoas bursa is a deep bursa located between the iliopsoas and the hip joint capsule. This bursa is in direct communication with the hip joint in approximately 15% of patients. It is not a common site for inflammation unless underlying hip pathology exists. Patients typically complain of groin or anterior hip pain. Examination may reveal a palpable mass in the middle third of the inguinal ligament. Extension of the hip produces pain. Occasionally a patient may have a pelvic mass, venous compression, secondary varices, or compression neuropathy of the femoral nerve resulting from the mass effect of the expanding bursa.[8]

Differential diagnosis of inguinal pain with or without a mass includes intrinsic hip pathology, iliopsoas tendinitis, psoas abscess, hernias, adenopathy, femoral artery aneurysm, and tumor. Treatment is directed at the underlying hip pathology when inflammation is present. Local corticosteroid injections are effective but may require radiologic guidance. Surgical resection is sometimes necessary.

Meralgia Paresthetica. See Chapter 167.

Knee

Periarticular structures of the knee contribute substantially to knee complaints in the primary care setting. Intraarticular knee pathology can be divided into inflammatory processes, degenerative processes, and internal derangement. Chapter 143 discusses sports injuries that typically produce internal derangement; Chapters 132 and 133 cover osteoarthritis and RA. The periarticular structures of the knee include the prepatellar and infrapatellar bursae, the anserine bursa, the gastrocnemius and semimembranosus bursae (which may become a popliteal cyst), and the iliotibial band.

Examination of the knee begins with the patient standing while the physician looks for evidence of genu recurvatum (hyperextension of knee, suggestive of hyperlaxity), valgus or varus deformities, posterior or anterior knee swelling, and patellar malalignment. The knee joint is palpated medial and lateral to the patella for evidence of synovitis, anterior for prepatellar bursitis, and posterior for popliteal cysts. ROM includes flexion to 140 degrees and extension to 0 degrees. Instability of the knee can be detected by several maneuvers (see Chapter 129).

Pain in the knee may be diffuse or localized. Referred pain from the hip typically is perceived medially. The differential diagnosis of knee pain can be classified according to location (Box 134-5).

Box 134-5. Differential Diagnosis of Knee Pain Based on Location

Diffuse

Articular

Anterior

Prepatellar bursitis
Patellar tendon enthesopathy
Chondromalacia patellae
Patellofemoral osteoarthritis
Cruciate ligament injury
Medial plica syndrome

Medial

Anserine bursitis
Spontaneous osteonecrosis
Osteoarthritis
Medial meniscal tear
Medial collateral ligament bursitis
Referred pain from hip and L3
Fibromyalgia

Lateral

Iliotibial band syndrome
Meniscal cyst
Lateral meniscal tear
Collateral ligament
Peroneal tenosynovitis

Posterior

Popliteal cyst (Baker's cyst)
Tendinitis
Aneurysms, ganglions, sarcoma

Prepatellar Bursitis. The prepatellar is a superficial bursa that is easily infected from direct penetration of skin surface bacteria. It can be chronically thickened by constant trauma from occupations that require kneeling. Although gout or RA may occur in this bursa, inflammation in this region is usually infectious. Patients complain of sudden onset of redness, warmth, and swelling, accompanied by variable symptoms of fever or chills. Examination reveals erythema and swelling over the patella with surrounding soft tissue edema. Palpation of the knee joint reveals no synovitis or fluid. Passive extension of the knee is painless and full, which is in marked contrast to a septic knee joint. End flexion may produce discomfort resulting from tautness of the skin over the prepatellar bursa.

Diagnosis is based on bursal fluid aspiration, and analysis is similar to that for septic olecranon bursitis. Occasionally the prepatellar bursa ruptures before the patient visits the office. Aspiration of the cellulitic region near the prepatellar bursa is still indicated, since even a drop of fluid may provide the microbiologic diagnosis.

Septic prepatellar bursa is treated similar to olecranon bursitis and requires serial drainage and antibiotic therapy against *S. aureus* and *Streptococcus* until fluid cultures become sterile. The prepatellar area is more difficult to treat, however, and initial therapy with intravenous antibiotics, whether inpatient or outpatient, is more prudent. If patients do not improve within several days (less swelling and erythema, sterile cultures), intravenous antibiotics may be necessary. In addition, the knee must be immobilized to prevent constant irritation of the bursa, but the patient should be instructed on isometric exercises to maintain quadriceps muscle tone. Early orthopedic consultation is advised so that debridement or more extensive drainage can proceed if medical therapy fails. Pigtail catheter drainage of the bursa, inserted under ultrasound or CT guidance, is an effective alternative approach to surgery. Protection of the knee with pads and avoidance of kneeling should treat chronic prepatellar bursitis that is noninfectious. Most cases require surgical excision.

Infrapatellar Bursitis. The infrapatellar bursa is located between the patellar tendon and the tibia. It is often associated with the spondyloarthropathies but can also be septic or associated with gout. Diagnosis and management are similar to those for prepatellar bursitis.

Anserine Bursitis. The pes anserine bursa is located in the medial aspect of the knee, approximately 5 cm below the medial joint line and under the tendons of the sartorius, gracilis, and semitendinosus muscles as they attach to the tibia medially. Irritation of this region is often secondary to overexertion from running, valgus knee deformities, osteoarthritis, and fibromyalgia. Patients complain of medial knee pain with weight bearing and at night if the knees touch each other. Examination reveals exquisite tenderness over the anserine region. Obese patients may have overlying fat that is also painful. The knee joint is normal unless osteoarthritis is present. Differential diagnosis includes the various causes of medial knee pain (see Box 133-5). Treatment includes NSAIDs or local corticosteroid injections with an anesthetic.

Baker's Cyst (Popliteal Cyst). Baker's cysts occur with any intrinsic pathology of the knee, including mechanical derangement, osteoarthritis, and all inflammatory arthritides, such as RA. Fluid from the knee enters the connecting gastrocnemius-semimembranous bursa but is unable to return easily to the joint space, thus mimicking a one-way valve mechanism. Patients complain of fullness or swelling in the posterior aspect of the knee with pain in the calf. The pain is aggravated by walking and relieved by rest. If the cyst has ruptured or blocks venous or lymphatic drainage through mass effect, peripheral edema of the lower extremity may be mistaken for deep venous thrombosis.

Swelling may be evident on inspection of the popliteal fossa. The Foucher sign (hardening of the mass in extension and softening of the mass in semiflexion of the knee) separates Baker's cyst from popliteal aneurysm or tumor, in which consistency is unchanged. Edema of the lower extremity with calf tenderness and a positive Homans' sign may be present if the cyst has leaked or ruptured (pseudothrombophlebitis). Other findings associated with a Baker's cyst may include secondary varices, ischemia, compressive neuropathies, and posterior compartment syndrome.

The differential diagnosis of a mass in the popliteal fossa includes popliteal artery aneurysm or cystic degeneration of the vessel wall, ganglion, lipoma, and sarcoma. Diagnosis is based on the physical examination. Ultrasonography visualizes the cyst, even if rupture has occurred, since residual fluid usually remains in the cyst.

A Baker's cyst is treated based on the underlying knee condition. Intraarticular steroids are effective if fluid is present in the knee and septic arthritis is excluded. Bed rest, heat, and elevation of the leg are necessary if the cyst has ruptured. True thrombophlebitis can develop from prolonged compression, preventing venous return, and patients then need anticoagulation.

Iliotibial Band Syndrome. The iliotibial band is the extension of the fascia lata as it attaches to Gerdy's tubercle, located on the lateral aspect of the tibia. Runners often develop pain over the lateral aspect of the knee. Pain is caused by tightness of this band as it rubs against the lateral femoral condyle during knee flexion and extension. Pain is reproduced over the lateral femoral condyle. Treatment includes NSAIDs, ice, and ultrasound, as well as exercises to stretch the hip abductors and fascia lata and correction of any mechanical factors.

Ankle and Foot

Foot and ankle problems are common in the ambulatory population. The principal motions of the ankle and foot complex include dorsiflexion, plantar flexion, inversion, and eversion. The small bones of the foot also accommodate various terrains. The true ankle joint functions in dorsiflexion (10 degrees) and plantar flexion (30 degrees). The subtalar joint allows for inversion (30 degrees) and eversion (10 degrees). The metatarsophalangeal (MTP) joints provide the greatest motion in the foot, since their major role is in the push-off action. Thus dorsiflexion of the MTP joint is at least 70 degrees. In addition, the Achilles, posterior tibialis, and peroneal tendons function to plantar flex, invert, and evert, respectively, the ankle and foot.

Examination of the ankle and foot begins with inspection of the area anteriorly and posteriorly while the patient is standing. The loss of the medial longitudinal arch is a common problem for valgus deformities. If swelling or pain is present, isolation of specific joints of the ankle is important. In true ankle arthritis, the dorsum of the ankle along the joint line is diffusely swollen. In contrast, asymmetric swelling over the medial or lateral malleolus suggests tenosynovitis of the posterior tibialis or peroneal tendon, respectively. Limitation of passive motion suggests true joint involvement. Active motion, particularly against resistance, tests the function of the tendons. The insertion of the Achilles tendon and plantar fascia should be palpated. Vascular and neurologic status completes the examination.

Achilles Tendinitis. The Achilles tendon is susceptible to acute injury, rupture, calcification, and inflammation associated with the spondyloarthropathies and RA. In addition, Achilles tendon inflammation and rupture have occurred with fluoroquinolone treatment.[9] Common symptoms are pain localized to the posterior aspect of the heel and pain exacerbated by dorsiflexion of the ankle. Acute injury usually occurs in running sports, and tendon rupture is possible. When rupture occurs, the patient describes a snapping sensation followed by the inability to stand on the toes. Acute swelling and erythema may be present in calcific tendinitis. In systemic inflammatory processes the tendon may be diffusely tender and swollen, and the retrocalcaneal bursa may also be involved. Treatment consists of rest, NSAIDs, heel inserts, and an ankle splint used at night in neutral position to prevent tendon contractures. In acute ruptures, immobilization and surgical intervention are necessary. Corticosteroid injections into the Achilles tendon are not recommended because this predisposes the patient to subsequent tendon rupture.

Posterior Tibialis Tendinitis. The posterior tibialis tendon inverts the foot and maintains the medial longitudinal arch. RA and the spondyloarthropathies often involve this tendon. Younger patients often injure the tendon while participating in high-stress activities, such as running and dancing. Older patients may note progressively flat arches and pain in the medial ankle secondary to gradual attrition of the tendon from microtrauma or degeneration. In patients with RA or other processes, acute rupture may suddenly result in a flat arch. Diagnosis is based on swelling and pain near the medial malleolus or pain and weakness with active inversion of the foot against resistance. In later stages after tendon rupture, flattening of the longitudinal arch on weight bearing is associated with hindfoot valgus deformity (Fig. 134-7).[6] MRI scans delineate the various stages of tendon degeneration. Treatment for initial stages includes rest, NSAIDs, and medial heel lift. If these approaches are ineffective, casting for a short time or local corticosteroid injection into the tendon sheath is necessary. Persistent inflammation, pain, and swelling may require surgical intervention.

Peroneal Tendinitis. The peroneal tendon everts the ankle and is susceptible to inflammatory conditions as well as mechanical injury. Examination reveals localized swelling and pain just posterior to the lateral malleolus. Active eversion against resistance is weak or painful. Therapy is similar to that for posterior tibialis tendinitis.

Retrocalcaneal Bursitis. The retrocalcaneal bursa is located posterior to the calcaneus and anterior to the Achilles tendon at its insertion site onto the calcaneus. This bursa is usually associated with systemic inflammatory diseases such as the spondyloarthropathies, RA, and gout. Pain arises in the heel at the Achilles tendon's insertion. Focal swelling may be visible in this area. Therapy is similar to that for Achilles tendinitis. Intrabursal injection or surgery may be required if symptoms persist.

Plantar Fasciitis. Inflammation of or strain on the plantar fascia is a common cause of foot pain. The plantar fascia is a thick, bandlike structure that attaches at the calcaneus and to each toe. Causes of plantar fasciitis include pes planus, prolonged standing, obesity, aerobic exercises that require jumping or bearing weight on the toes, fluoride or retinoid therapy, and the spondyloarthropathies. Patients complain of pain localized to the plantar surface of the foot that is exacerbated by pushing off with the toes. Examination with the dorsiflexed foot reveals tenderness along the plantar fascia or at the insertion of the fascia into the calcaneus. Heel spurs may be palpable or evident on radiographs. If fasciitis is associated with systemic inflammatory disease, plain films may demonstrate periostitis at the calcaneal insertion or even erosions. If clinically suspected, stress fractures of the metatarsals can be evaluated with serial radiographs or bone scan and Morton's neuroma by clinical examination. Treatment includes correction of underlying processes and

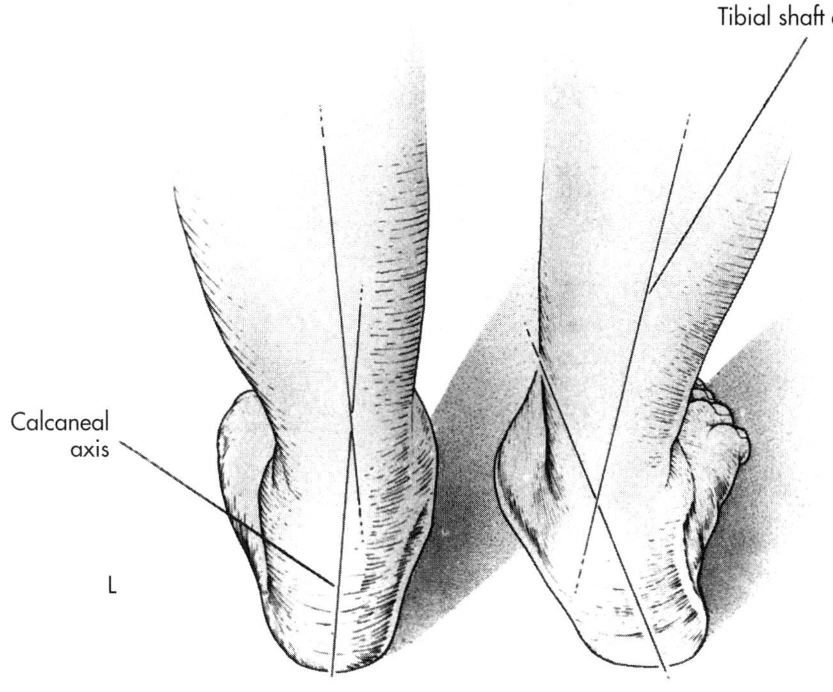

Fig. 134-7. Posterior view of normal foot *(left)* and hindfoot valgus *(right)*. Right foot also has forefoot abduction, with "too many toes" seen lateral to ankle. (From Supple KM et al: *Semin Arthritis Rheum* 22:107, 1992.)

the use of a plastic heel cup that maintains the soft tissue of the heel pad under the weight-bearing portion of the heel. Longitudinal arch support may also help. Local corticosteroid injection of the plantar fascia is also effective but must be cautiously given to avoid extensive fat pad atrophy at the heel.

Nerve Entrapment or Compression. Prominent nerve conditions include tarsal tunnel syndrome (see Chapter 167) and Morton's neuroma (see Chapter 130).

PRINCIPLES OF TREATMENT

Rehabilitation

Although treatment of the periarticular rheumatic disorders seems diverse, certain principles are applicable to tendinitis, bursitis, and myofascial pain. Overuse and injury predominate in the etiology of these processes. Thus a major focus of treatment is identifying the cause of overuse or injury and adjusting work or recreation to prevent further injury.

An occupational therapy consultation is often extremely helpful and cost-effective. An occupational therapist assesses a patient's needs and then establishes a program that maximizes joint protection, prevents disability, and optimizes joint function. Industrial rehabilitation may be required if a patient has significant limitations at work. Work hardening programs have been established to help employees with various regional soft tissue problems to return to work.

Physical therapy includes modalities that initially control pain, followed by passive and active exercises to stretch or move a joint or periarticular structure. The final step is muscle strengthening around the region to prevent reinjury or further damage.

Heat and cold are common modalities to treat various soft tissue pains. Heat from moist heating packs and ultrasound may provide relief, although usually short-lived. Since ROM improves after heat application, use of heat may be a useful adjunct and may allow patients to exercise. Cold, usually reserved for acute injuries, reduces swelling.

TENS has been used for chronic pain of the back, neck, and other regions. The mechanism of action is postulated to be interference of pain impulses to the brain by its own impulses (gate control theory of pain). The cost of a TENS unit may not be reimbursed by third-party insurance.

Exercises, both passive and active, are important to maintain ROM, strength, and function. In passive exercises the therapist or machine moves the muscle while the patient makes no muscle contraction. Active motion requires the patient to contract the muscle in an isometric (no joint motion) or isotonic (joint motion against resistance) manner. The optimal program for each patient's soft tissue problem is best gauged by a physical therapist. If the primary care physician wants to prescribe or supervise an exercise program, however, extensive exercises are available for each regional problem.[5]

Splints or orthotic devices immobilize an affected area to reduce pain, hold a particular region in an optimal position for function, or redistribute stress from a painful region to surrounding structures. Examples of these functions include a neutral wrist splint for carpal tunnel syndrome, a hindfoot orthosis to reduce valgus deformities secondary to posterior tibialis tendon dysfunction, or a forearm band for lateral epicondylitis. Properly fitting shoes are crucial in many of the periarticular disorders, and consultation with an orthopedic surgeon or podiatrist may be necessary.

Medications

Nonsteroidal Antiinflammatory Drugs. The use of NSAIDs in rheumatic diseases is discussed in Chapters 132, 133, and 137. For the periarticular entities, NSAIDs provide analgesic and antiinflammatory effects. Numerous NSAIDs are available and differ in metabolism, dosing, and toxicity profile (see Table 137-2). A particular NSAID should be prescribed for at least 10 to 14 days before the medication is discontinued for lack of efficacy. Common toxicities include GI intolerance, gastritis, and superficial ulceration. Other toxicities include renal insufficiency, elevated liver enzyme levels, hyperkalemia, headaches, mood changes, and other central nervous system alterations. NSAIDs are not as effective for myofascial pain as for inflammatory musculoskeletal disorders.

Tricyclic Antidepressants. Tricyclics are important in the treatment of chronic neck or low back pain. Possible mechanisms of action include their effect on brain neuropeptides, the direct role on stage IV sleep, endogenous opioids, and reduction of brainstem-mediated muscle spasm. In addition, these medications are helpful if there is component of depression.

Parenteral Corticosteroids. Parenteral corticosteroids may be useful in the early stages of RSD or adhesive capsulitis. ACTH can be an alternative to NSAIDs in acute calcific tendinitis. The protocol is similar to the treatment of acute gouty arthritis. Patients receive 40 to 60 IU of ACTH intramuscularly; this is repeated up to 3 days if necessary.

Corticosteroid Injections. Corticosteroid injections are a major form of treatment for the various soft tissue disorders (see Chapter 123). The primary care physician should be able to inject into common areas that include the subacromial, trochanteric, and anserine regions, along with the true knee joint. Utmost care is needed when injecting the tendon sheaths, carpal and tarsal tunnels, plantar fascia, and retrocalcaneal bursa. Injection of these regions should be referred to a rheumatologist or orthopedist if the primary care physician is not experienced. The true glenohumeral or hip joint is difficult to enter, and a specialist, or a radiologist under fluoroscopic guidance, should perform these injections.

After an injection, the area is rested or splinted for 48 to 72 hours. Patients should be informed about possible postinjection flare and its treatment with ice and analgesics. If a tendon sheath is injected, strenuous activity of that tendon should be avoided for up to 2 weeks.

Injection of trigger points in myofascial pain is based on the theory of mechanical disruption of the trigger point by saline or an anesthetic, followed by passive muscle stretch. Some studies have reported a longer duration of improvement if corticosteroids are combined with the local anesthetic. Most studies have been uncontrolled; thus corticosteroids are not recommended for injection of trigger points.

Referral

Subspecialty referrals are indicated only if patients do not respond to initial management that includes avoidance of aggravating factors, pain control, and further strengthening exercises.

REFERENCES

1. Canoso JJ: *Rheumatology in primary care,* Philadelphia, 1997, Saunders.
2. Ho G, Mikolich DJ: Bacterial infections of the superficial subcutaneous bursae, *Clin Rheum Dis* 12:437, 1986.
3. Murphy D, Failla JM, Koniuch MP: Steroid versus placebo injection for trigger finger, *J Hand Surg* 20A:628, 1995.
4. Neer CS: Impingement lesions, *Clin Orthop* 173:70, 1983.
5. Schoen RP, Moskowitz RW, Goldberg VM: *Soft tissue rheumatic pain,* ed 3, Baltimore, 1996, Williams & Wilkins.
6. Supple KM, Hanft JR, Murphy BJ, Janecki CJ: Posterior tibial tendon dysfunction, *Semin Arthritis Rheum* 22:106, 1992.
7. Travell J, Rinzler SH: The myofascial genesis of pain, *Postgrad Med* 11:425, 1952.
8. Underwood PL, McLeod RA, Ginsburg WW: The varied manifestations of iliopsoas bursitis, *J Rheumatol* 15:1683, 1988.
9. Zabraniecki L, Negrier I: Fluoroquinolone-induced tendinopathy: report of 6 cases, *J Rheumatol* 23:516, 1996.

CHAPTER 135

Systemic Lupus Erythematosus

Leslie E. Kahl

Systemic lupus erythematosus (SLE) is a chronic systemic inflammatory disorder of unknown etiology. With an unpredictable clinical course and manifestations ranging from troublesome rashes and alopecia to life-threatening cerebritis and nephritis, lupus is among the most challenging disorders to treat. The physician must not only treat acute flares of disease to minimize end-organ damage, but also distinguish manifestations of lupus from those related to adverse drug effects.

The hallmark laboratory feature of idiopathic lupus is the presence of autoantibodies, which may be nonspecific (antinuclear and anti-DNA antibodies) or tissue specific (antiplatelet and antierythrocyte antibodies). Immunoglobulin and complement deposits have been identified in involved tissues, including the skin, kidney, and brain, and are thought to be pathogenic. For this reason, many investigators consider lupus the prototypic autoimmune disease.

EPIDEMIOLOGY

Idiopathic SLE occurs predominantly in women of childbearing age. The frequency of lupus in the American population is approximately 0.1%, with higher rates seen in urban areas and among African-Americans and Asians. The ratio of women to men with lupus is approximately 11 : 1 during the childbearing years, but only about 3 : 1 in children and older adults. This gender discrepancy is thought to result from hormonal effects, as evidenced by the relative rarity of the disease before menarche and after menopause, the apparent association of disease flares with pregnancy and oral contraceptive use, and the presence of altered estrogen kinetics among women with SLE.

Etiology

SLE is a heterogenous disorder with a complex etiology rather than a single cause. Current theory suggests that in the genetically predisposed host, some stimulus (or stimuli) triggers aberrant function of T and B cells and, ultimately, increased immunoglobulin and autoantibody production. Genes encoding several different proteins, including the major histocompatibility complex (MHC), complement proteins and receptors, immunoglobulin receptors, and cytokines, are associated with an increased risk of lupus in certain ethnic groups and populations. The specific type of antibodies produced may also be influenced by these genes. The stimulus that triggers SLE probably differs from patient to patient. The potential role of sex hormones, either endogenous or exogenous, is outlined above. Environmental triggers such as ultraviolet radiation, infection, certain drugs, chemicals, and foods may play a role. Some patients associate physical or emotional stress with disease onset or with flares of established disease.

SLE is characterized by a variety of autoantibodies. Although many of the protein antigens against which these antibodies are directed play a critical role in cellular functions, little evidence indicates that the autoantibodies impede these functions. Complexes of antibodies and their antigens (immune complexes), however, may have a pathogenic role in SLE. These complexes are normally cleared from the circulation by the complement system. In lupus, however, they may be found deposited along with complement at sites of tissue injury, contributing to the inflammatory response. Complement components are consumed during immune complex clearance and tissue deposition, producing a characteristic fall in serum complement levels during disease flares.

Although the pathogenesis of most of the clinical manifestations of lupus is inflammatory, some patients also develop manifestations attributable to hypercoagulability. Vascular occlusions in both the arterial and the venous systems have been associated with antiphospholipid antibodies. Whether these antibodies are pathogenic or simply laboratory markers for this complication is unclear.

PATIENT EVALUATION

Both the presentation and the clinical course of SLE are highly variable. The initial symptoms may be nonspecific and resolve spontaneously, leading to a considerable delay in diagnosis. In many patients, only the gradual unfolding of a pattern of disease over several months leads to the correct diagnosis. In others, however, the disease is fulminant and easily recognizable at the onset.

Lupus is generally characterized by periods of remission interspersed with acute or chronic relapses. In a given patient, disease flares may involve the same organ systems each time, producing a characteristic and predictable pattern of disease. This is useful when trying to distinguish symptoms of active SLE from other conditions, such as acute infection or adverse drug reactions. However, many patients do not have such a reproducible profile of their disease flare and present a continuing diagnostic challenge.

The majority of SLE patients have fairly mild disease characterized by constitutional symptoms, arthralgias or arthritis, and rash. These individuals often lead a relatively normal life and have a normal or near-normal life span. Patients with more aggressive disease, however, may suffer considerable morbidity. The 10-year survival rate for SLE is 75% to 90%. Deaths early in the course of disease usually result from active SLE or acute infection, whereas those occurring later most often result from cardiovascular disease.

History

The clinical presentations of lupus are remarkably diverse. The American College of Rheumatology publishes classification criteria for SLE as a guideline for researchers (Table 135-1). Physicians typically use these criteria to assign the diagnosis of SLE. The criteria were specifically selected for their ability to distinguish patients with lupus from those with other connective tissue diseases and do not include many common but nonspecific features of lupus, such as arthralgias and alopecia.

Table 135-1. Revised Criteria for Classification of Systemic Lupus Erythematosus (SLE)

Criterion	Definition
Malar rash	Fixed erythema, flat or raised, over malar eminences, sparing nasolabial folds
Discoid rash	Erythematous raised patches with adherent keratotic scaling and follicular plugging
Photosensitivity	Skin rash from unusual reaction to sunlight
Oral ulcers	Oral or nasal ulcers, usually painless
Arthritis	Nonerosive arthritis of two or more peripheral joints, with swelling, tenderness, or effusion
Serositis	Pleuritis (pleuritic pain or rub, pleural effusion) *or* pericarditis (pericardial rub, typical electrocardiogram, pericardial effusion)
Renal disorder	Persistent proteinuria (>500 mg/day or >3+) *or* cellular casts
Neurologic disorder	Seizure *or* psychosis without other explanation (drug or metabolic derangement)
Hematologic disorder	Hemolytic anemia *or* leukopenia (<4000/mm^3 on two or more occasions) *or* thrombocytopenia (<100,000/mm^3 on two or more occasions)
Immunologic disorder	Positive LE cell preparation *or* anti-DNA *or* anti-Sm *or* false-positive syphilis serology
Antinuclear antibody (ANA)	Positive ANA in the absence of drugs known to cause drug-induced lupus

Modified from Tah EM, Cohen AS, Fries JF, et al: The 1982 revised criteria for the classification of systemic lupus erythematosus, *Arthritis Rheum* 25:1271, 1982.

Although nonspecific constitutional symptoms (e.g., fatigue, fever, weight loss) provide few clues to the diagnosis of SLE, they may dominate the clinical picture. The fatigue that occurs in SLE can be particularly overwhelming; patients may barely be able to get up, eat, or dress themselves. Fatigue is the chief complaint of many lupus patients whose disease is otherwise in remission.

Musculoskeletal symptoms, including myalgias, arthralgias, and frank arthritis, occur at some point in nearly all SLE patients. The arthritis is inflammatory, with prominent morning stiffness, although the symptoms are frequently out of proportion to the findings on physical examination. Joint involvement is usually symmetric and may include the small joints of the hands and feet, wrists, elbows, knees, and ankles. The patient may describe swelling of the joints that waxes and wanes over a few hours, a feature rarely found in other forms of arthritis.

Mucocutaneous features of SLE are nearly as common as those involving the joints. The characteristic butterfly rash on the cheeks and nose is present at some point in up to 50% of patients. Approximately one third note photosensitivity, with exacerbation of the rash after sun exposure. Patients may also give a history of nonscarring alopecia or unusual breakage of hair, particularly along the hairline. This history must be interpreted with caution in women using harsh coloring or curling treatments on their hair or having a tightly-braided hairstyle. Although oral or nasal ulcers occur in up to 40% of patients, they are frequently asymptomatic. Raynaud's phenomenon is present in approximately 30% of patients but also occurs in other connective tissue diseases, including scleroderma and polymyositis. Patients usually describe aching and white or bluish discoloration of the digits on exposure to cold and may also note erythema during rewarming.

Pleurisy or pericarditis (serositis) occurs in about half of SLE patients. Although occasionally manifesting only as an asymptomatic pleural effusion or globular cardiac contour on chest radiographs, serositis generally produces a characteristic sharp or stabbing pain on one or both sides of the chest. Pain referred to the left shoulder or relieved by leaning forward is more suggestive of pericarditis, whereas exacerbation of the chest pain on deep inspiration is more common with pleurisy. Pulmonary parenchymal involvement is much rarer than pleurisy in SLE. Patients with pneumonitis usually develop dyspnea suddenly and are acutely ill. They may also give a history of hemoptysis. Cough with sputum production is not typical of lung disease in lupus and should suggest a superimposed infection.

Central nervous system (CNS) manifestations of SLE may be either functional or organic.[1] The most common symptoms include mild depression, subtle cognitive deficits, and headaches. The patient may have simple tension-type headaches or classic migraines. Some patients present with short-lived focal neurologic deficits called "migraine equivalents" after structural abnormalities have been ruled out. Migraine headaches appear to be more common among patients experiencing Raynaud's phenomenon. Serious neurologic problems occur less frequently in lupus and include major affective disorders, seizures, and stroke. Patients with antiphospholipid antibodies are at particular risk for stroke.

Some of the most serious complications of lupus may be silent or present with nonspecific symptoms. Nephritis, which occurs in up to 40% of patients, may be manifest as fatigue, peripheral edema, or weight gain. Hypertension associated with nephritis is also frequently silent. Patients with hemolytic anemia may have fatigue or develop jaundice or dark urine. Thrombocytopenia is usually asymptomatic but may produce petechiae, bruising, or more serious bleeding complications.

Physical Examination

The classic physical finding in SLE is the malar or butterfly rash (Fig. 135-1). Along with the cheeks, the forehead, chin, and bridge of the nose may also be involved, but the nasolabial folds are generally spared. Involved skin is erythematous and may be slightly indurated. A maculopapular eruption with fine scaling may also be present. Unlike the classic butterfly rash that resolves without sequelae, *discoid lupus erythematosus* (DLE) involves deeper layers of the dermis and produces residual scarring. Discoid lesions are most common on the face, scalp, and ears but can also occur on the palms and soles (Figs. 135-2 and 135-3). Acute discoid lesions are annular, erythematous, indurated plaques that may

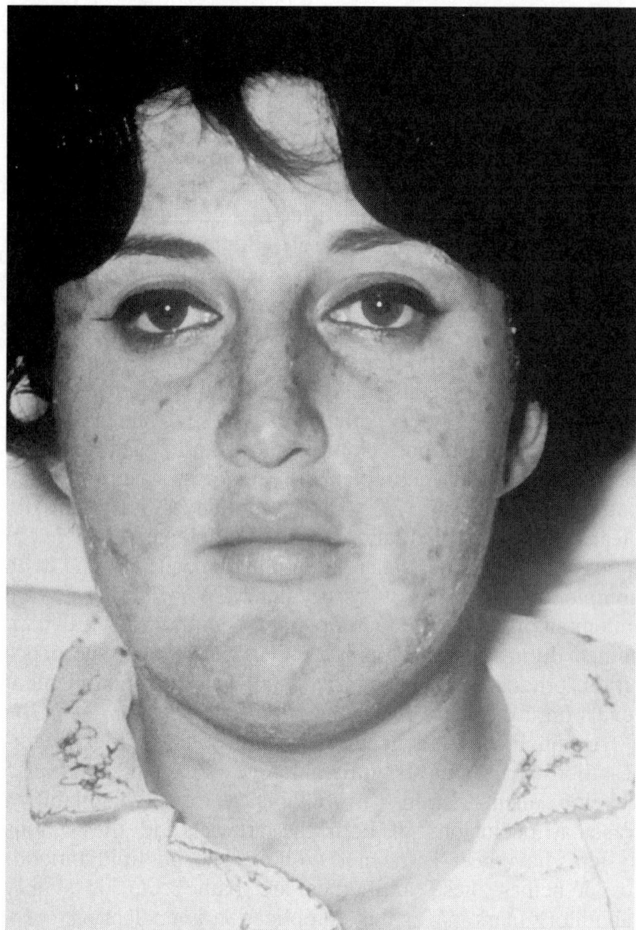

Fig. 135-1. Characteristic erythematous facial rash in systemic lupus erythematosus (SLE) may involve the forehead and chin along with the cheeks. Nasolabial fold is usually spared. (From American College of Rheumatology: *Clinical slide collection on the rheumatic diseases,* Atlanta, 1991, The College.)

be covered by an adherent scale with follicular plugging. Chronic lesions generally show central atrophy and depigmentation, with an erythematous or hyperpigmented circular border. Discoid lesions occurring in the scalp may produce well-defined areas of scarring alopecia. In contrast, the nonscarring alopecia that occurs in the absence of discoid lesions is diffuse and may be associated with breakage of hairs at the hairline or fine lanugo-like hair growth. Patients with antibodies to the Ro or SS-A antigen may have annular or psoriasiform (nonscarring) rashes, termed *subacute cutaneous lupus erythematosus* (SCLE) (Fig. 135-4). Some patients, particularly those with antiphospholipid antibodies, have livedo reticularis, a violaceous netlike pattern of vessels in the skin of the extremities.

The musculoskeletal examination may be normal in lupus, even when the patient relates a history of joint pain suggesting inflammation. Joint swelling, tenderness, and erythema may be present, but synovial effusions are usually not large. Chronic arthritis may produce deformities, particularly in the hands. Ulnar deviation of the metacarpophalangeal (MCP) joints and flexion or swan-neck deformities of the fingers are most common. In contrast to the joint abnormalities seen in rheumatoid arthritis, however, those in SLE are usually reducible, and bony erosions rarely occur.

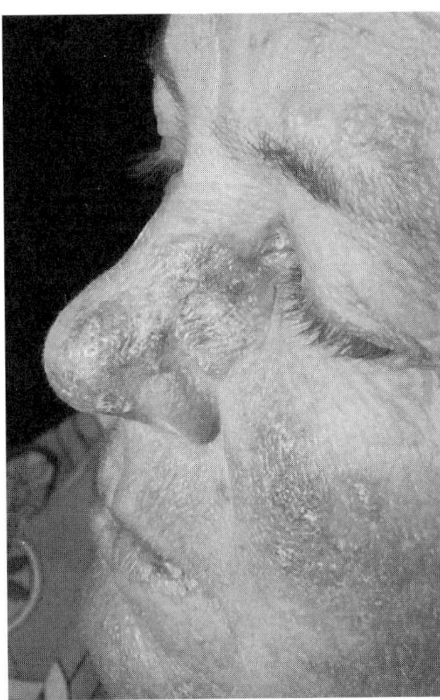

Fig. 135-2. Photodistribution of erythematous plaques in discoid lupus erythematosus (DLE). (Courtesy Frank W. Crowe, MD.)

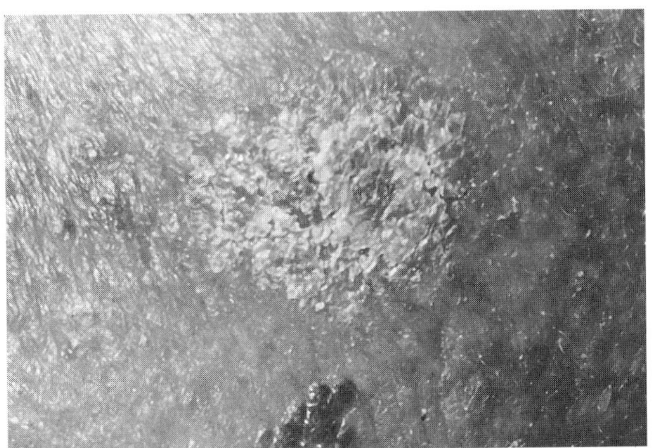

Fig. 135-3. Erythema and adherent scale in DLE.

Patients with serositis may have no abnormal physical findings; a friction rub is sometimes heard. Atelectasis may occur, producing localized findings of consolidation at the lung bases. Dullness at the lung bases may be detected if pleural effusions are large. Pericardial effusions are rarely of hemodynamic significance, and signs of congestive heart failure are not generally seen.

The neurologic examination is normal in most patients with lupus, despite the high frequency of neuropsychiatric symptoms. However, the disease may affect virtually any portion of the CNS or peripheral nervous system.[10] Stroke occurs in up to 15% of patients, producing focal deficits in the distribution of any of the cerebral vessels. Similarly, transverse myelitis may occur at any level of the spinal cord, although it is much less common than stroke. Patients with a history of headaches generally have a normal neurologic examination, but papilledema may occasionally be seen with pseudotumor cerebri. Neuropathy occurs in up to 15% of patients. Cranial nerve involvement is usually in the optic or trigeminal distribution. Peripheral nerve involvement may present as either a distal sensory neuropathy or a mononeuritis multiplex. Patients with a history of seizures generally have normal examinations between seizure events. Patients with mood disturbances may have findings consistent with an affective disorder, usually anxiety or depression. Formal testing may be necessary to detect more subtle cognitive defects.

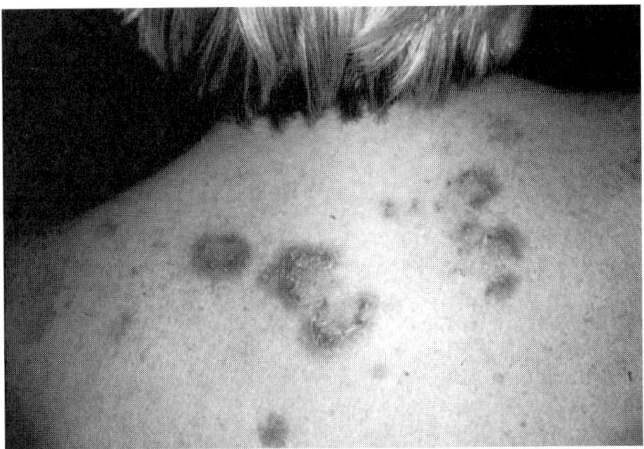

Fig. 135-4. Arcuate configuration of raised erythema and scaling in subacute cutaneous lupus erythematosus.

In addition to these findings, which would most likely be detected by using a symptom-based approach to the patient, several potential asymptomatic abnormalities should also be sought. Adenopathy occurs in up to 25% of patients, usually in the setting of active disease elsewhere, and may suggest that the other symptoms are a manifestation of lupus rather than some unrelated problem. Hypertension may be the first indication of occult renal disease. The blood pressure must be measured each visit. The prognosis of nephritis is worse for patients with persistent hypertension, who should be treated aggressively. Similarly, patients should be checked regularly for peripheral edema, which may be the presenting sign of proteinuria.

LABORATORY STUDIES AND DIAGNOSTIC PROCEDURES

The laboratory is useful in confirming a diagnosis of SLE when the clinical picture is suggestive. The classic serologic finding for SLE is the antinuclear antibody (ANA). Since ANA is present in virtually all lupus patients, it serves as a reasonable screening test for the disease. A negative ANA test makes SLE extremely unlikely. ANA is not specific for lupus, however, and is also seen in patients with rheumatoid arthritis (RA), other connective tissue diseases, and inflammatory conditions (e.g., interstitial lung disease, chronic active hepatitis), as well as in healthy elderly individuals.

A positive ANA should be interpreted on the basis of the clinical setting and the titer. Titers of less than 1:160 are more likely to be false-positive results or manifestations of nonspecific immune reactivity than are higher titers.[8] In contrast, ANA titers of 1:1280 or greater usually indicate a connective tissue disease, although not always SLE. The screening ANA detects antibody to a variety of antigenic

Table 135-2. Frequency of Autoantibodies in Connective Diseases*

Antibody	SLE	Drug-induced lupus	Rheumatoid arthritis	Sjögren's syndrome	MCTD	Diffuse scleroderma	Limited scleroderma	Polymyositis/ dermatomyositis
ds-DNA	**60**	R	R	R	R	R	R	R
Histone	70	**95**	30	20	R	R	R	R
Sm	**30**	R	R	R	R	R	R	R
RNP	40	R	R	R	**95**	15	10	15
Scl-70	R	R	R	R	R	**35**	10	R
Centromere	R	R	R	R	R	R	**70**	R
Jo-1	R	R	R	R	R	R	R	**25**
SSA/Ro, SSB/La	30	R	20	**70**	R	R	R	R

SLE, Systemic lupus erythematosus; *MCTD,* mixed connective tissue disease.
*Data are expressed as percentages.
Frequencies of antibodies with high diagnostic utility are shown in **bold** type. *R* indicates that the antibody occurs rarely.

substrates, which in turn may indicate the exact type of connective tissue disease. Thus, a positive screening ANA in a reasonable titer should be followed by more specific testing, including assays for Sm, ribonucleoprotein (RNP), SS-A/Ro, and SS-B/La. Patients with SLE frequently demonstrate different autoantibodies in their sera, whereas a single autoantibody is usually seen in other connective tissue diseases (Table 135-2).

Additional laboratory studies may be useful in diagnosing SLE (Table 135-3). The presence of antibody to double-stranded (native) deoxyribonucleic acid (DNA) is pathognomonic for lupus and in some patients may also be a marker of active disease, particularly nephritis.[3] Anti-Sm is also virtually specific for SLE. Reduced serum complement levels may be seen in any disorder mediated by immune complexes but are highly suggestive of SLE when found in the presence of a positive ANA. A positive direct Coombs' test is found in up to 60% of SLE patients, but clinically evident hemolytic anemia is usually absent. Although the normochromic normocytic anemia typically seen in lupus is a nonspecific manifestation of chronic diseases, the lymphopenia is usually mediated by antilymphocyte antibodies and serves as another indicator of the diffuse immunologic hyperreactivity that characterizes SLE. Similarly, thrombocytopenia in this setting is immune mediated. The greater the number of antibodies present, the more likely the patient has SLE.

Table 135-3. Laboratory Findings Useful in Diagnosing SLE

Finding	Cumulative frequency (%)
Antinuclear antibody (ANA)	99
Anti-DNA antibody	40-60
Anti-Sm antibody	15-30
Low C3 or C4 complement proteins	50-70
Direct Coombs' test	40-60
Lymphopenia, leukopenia	60-80
Thrombocytopenia	20-40
Antiphospholipid antibodies	20-40
Proteinuria	30-50
Cellular casts in urine	20-30

Antiphospholipid antibodies, which may be associated with thrombosis, can be detected by three tests. The classic false-positive syphilis serology has long been recognized as a marker for SLE. The lupus anticoagulant test, in which a prolonged partial thromboplastin time (PTT) is not corrected by the addition of normal plasma, also reflects antiphospholipid antibody activity. The anticardiolipin antibody test is the third assay. Antiphospholipid antibodies may be accompanied by venous or arterial thrombosis, presenting with phlebitis, stroke, or miscarriage; the risk is highest with the lupus anticoagulant[9] (Box 135-1). Antiphospholipid antibodies are not specific for SLE and are also seen in the primary antiphospholipid syndrome, with similar vascular events. A few patients with this syndrome have low titers of ANA and thrombocytopenia and may be misdiagnosed with SLE.

A urinalysis and determination of the serum creatinine level should be performed on all new patients suspected of having SLE to screen for occult renal disease. A renal biopsy may be indicated by a rising serum creatinine, new-onset proteinuria of more than 500 mg/dl, or urinary sediment containing cellular casts or red blood cells. In these patients, new-onset hypertension, reduced serum complement levels, or a positive anti-DNA antibody test should strongly increase the clinical suspicion for nephritis and lead to consultation with a nephrologist or rheumatologist. Percutaneous renal biopsy may reveal a variety of histologic patterns that cannot be accurately predicted by routine laboratory studies. The renal biopsy also provides information on the chronicity and activity of renal disease, which may have both prognostic and therapeutic implications.

DIFFERENTIAL DIAGNOSIS

The clinical manifestations of SLE are so diverse that lupus has been dubbed one of the "great imposters." When the initial presentation includes the malar rash and any of the more serious organ system manifestations, serologic testing is performed, and the diagnosis is relatively straightforward. More often, however, the patient may complain of nonspecific symptoms such as low-grade fever, fatigue, or arthralgias, and the clinical suspicion for lupus is not as high. SLE should

Box 135-1. Antiphospholipid Antibodies and Clinical Associations

Assay

False-positive syphilis serology
Lupus anticoagulant
Anticardiolipin antibody

Clinical Manifestations

Arterial or venous thrombosis (e.g., thrombophlebitis, stroke)
Miscarriage
Livedo reticularis
Thrombocytopenia

Associated Diseases

SLE
Drug-induced lupus
Primary antiphospholipid syndrome

always be in the differential diagnosis of a multisystem disease presenting in a young woman, particularly a young Black woman, and also with apparent infection in a young woman who has negative cultures and no response to antibiotics.

A lupus diagnosis is most likely to be missed when the disease presents in a single organ system. Pleurisy or pericarditis is usually attributed to a viral infection unless the ANA test is performed. The pleural fluid in SLE is typically an exudate with lymphocytic predominance in the cell count, which may be helpful in the differential diagnosis. Isolated thrombocytopenia or hemolytic anemia is generally considered idiopathic unless an ANA test is done. CNS involvement is particularly challenging to diagnose, since it often occurs without other signs or symptoms of SLE. In this setting, seizure or stroke may be regarded as idiopathic, and optic neuritis or transverse myelitis may be attributed to multiple sclerosis. Isolated synovitis may be misdiagnosed as RA. The articular findings in the two disorders have a similar character and distribution, and up to 30% of patients with RA may have positive ANA tests. Patients with these clinical scenarios may remain undiagnosed until, with time, the multisystemic nature of the disease is revealed.

Although the most common diagnostic error involving SLE is overlooking it as a clinical possibility, cutaneous lesions are probably overdiagnosed as lupus. The erythematous rash of acne rosacea may assume a malar distribution but can be differentiated from SLE by the presence of pustules. Seborrheic dermatitis also typically occurs in a malar distribution but, unlike SLE, involves the nasolabial folds. Superficial fungal infections may resemble cutaneous lupus but give positive results on examination of skin scrapings with potassium hydroxide. Photoallergic contact dermatitis and polymorphous light eruption may be difficult to distinguish from lupus clinically, but they have distinctive histopathologic pictures. Similarly, the rash of dermatomyositis may closely resemble lupus; in dermatomyositis, however, the color of the rash is more purple than red, and its scaling lesions (Gottron's papules) occur over the knuckles, whereas those of lupus occur on the dorsum of the hand between the joints. Features of other lupuslike rashes can be differentiated from SLE (Table 135-4).

Lupus must also be differentiated from other systemic inflammatory disorders, such as necrotizing vasculitis. Although cutaneous vasculitis may be a manifestation of SLE, widespread vascular involvement is unusual. Serologic studies are generally negative in vasculitis. The arthralgias or arthritis, fever, malaise, and cutaneous lesions of bacterial endocarditis may also be confused with SLE. Again, serologic studies, along with blood culture results, should clarify the diagnosis. Among the connective tissue diseases, lupus shares cutaneous features with dermatomyositis, synovitis with RA, serositis with RA and Sjögren's syndrome, and Raynaud's phenomenon with all of these disorders. In general, the clinical picture and active serologic profile of lupus are sufficient to distinguish it from these disorders. Occasionally a patient has features characteristic of several of these diseases but diagnostic of none. Antibodies to RNP are generally present, and this constellation of findings is termed *mixed connective tissue disease* (MCTD) or *overlap syndrome.*

After making the lupus diagnosis, the physician often must decide whether a new symptom represents SLE, an adverse drug effect, or an unrelated problem. For example, a patient with longstanding lupus who develops fever and pleuritic chest pain may have lupus-related serositis but may also have pneumonia or a pulmonary embolus. Signs or symptoms of active SLE in other organs may help clarify the diagnosis, along with judicious use of laboratory studies and radiographs. Similarly, a rise in the serum creatinine or new-onset hypertension is probably related to the development of nephritis, but nephrotoxicity from nonsteroidal antiinflammatory drugs (NSAIDs) must also be considered. Fatigue may be caused by SLE but also by superimposed fibromyalgia, depression, hypothyroidism, or obstructive sleep apnea from steroid-induced weight gain.

In a patient with suspected SLE the distinction must also be made between spontaneous and drug-induced lupus. Medications implicated in drug-induced lupus do not cause exacerbations of spontaneous lupus (Box 135-2). Patients with drug-induced lupus are older, are more likely to be men, and usually present with fever, malaise, serositis, and arthralgias or arthritis. Weight loss may be a prominent feature, raising the diagnostic suspicion for malignancy. More serious organ system involvement (e.g., cerebritis, nephritis, thrombocytopenia, hemolytic anemia) is rare. Serologic abnormalities are usually limited to a positive ANA test in a homogenous pattern and an elevated erythrocyte sedimentation rate (ESR); hypocomplementemia and the plethora of autoantibodies typically seen in spontaneous SLE are absent. When the offending medication is discontinued, the signs and symptoms of lupus generally resolve over several weeks, although the ANA may persist much longer. Patients who develop a positive ANA test during treatment with a lupus-inducing drug but who remain asymptomatic may continue taking the medication.

MANAGEMENT

Because SLE is not well understood by the public, treatment must begin with education. Common misconceptions about lupus are that it is always fatal, may be either contagious or strongly familial, and is a form of acquired immunodeficiency syndrome (AIDS). Reassuring lupus patients and their families about these issues may relieve many unspoken anxieties. SLE patients often look well despite overwhelming

Table 135-4. Differential Diagnosis of SLE

Disease	Cutaneous	Extracutaneous	Laboratory
SLE	Widespread, photosensitive	Multisystem renal, CNS, arthritis, serositis	ANA, 99% Anti-DNA 40%-60% Low C3 50%-70%
SCLE	Widespread, photosensitive	Less systemic involvement than SLE	ANA 60% Anti-DNA 30% Anti-SSA/Ro 30%
DLE	Localized or widespread, photosensitive	None	ANA 5%
Drug-induced lupus	Widespread	Can be multisystem	ANA 100% Anti-histone 80%-100%
Dermatomyositis	Can be widespread, photosensitive	Multisystem	ANA 50%-70% Elevated muscle enzymes (CK, aldolase, AST) Muscle biopsy

SCLE, Subacute cutaneous lupus erythematosus; *DLE*, discoid lupus erythematosus; *CNS*, central nervous system; *ANA*, antinuclear antibody; *CK*, creatine kinase; *AST*, aspartate transaminase.

Box 135-2. Agents Implicated in Drug-induced Lupus

Definite
Hydralazine
Procainamide
Isoniazid
Methyldopa
Chlorpromazine

Possible

Anticonvulsants
Diphenylhydantoin
Mephenytoin
Ethosuximide
Trimethadone

β-Blockers
Practolol
Acebutolol
Atenolol
Metoprolol

Miscellaneous
Penicillamine
Captopril
Quinidine
Sulfonamide
Tartrazine
Lithium carbonate
Propylthiouracil

fatigue and arthralgias. Frequently, this disparity leads to a lack of understanding and unrealistic expectations of family, friends, and co-workers, who also may need education. Both the Arthritis Foundation and the Lupus Foundation of America are excellent sources for educational materials regarding SLE. Many local chapters also sponsor patient support groups, allowing patients and their families to share their fears, frustrations, and successful strategies.

Nonpharmacologic Treatment

Although medications are frequently indicated in the management of lupus, several nonpharmacologic approaches also have merit. Many patients associate flares of their disease with periods of excessive fatigue. Rest is important in the daily management of SLE. Patients must learn to prioritize their daily schedules, plan ahead, and pace themselves. Because the disease tends to vary from day to day, many patients save up their chores or activities until they feel well, overdo it on that day, and are exhausted for the next several days. Other patients observe that emotional rather than physical stress is a disease precipitant, and counseling for stress management may be particularly useful.

Environmental manipulations may also help some lupus patients. The 30% to 40% of patients who are photosensitive can avoid the sun by staying indoors during midday or by wearing long sleeves and a hat. Topical sunscreens that include coverage against UVA also provide considerable protection. Patients with Raynaud's phenomenon need to avoid the cold. Most patients do not realize, however, that they must keep the whole body warm, not just the digits. Wearing a warm hat and using potholders for cold items and insulated holders for cold drinks can be helpful. They must also refrain from smoking.

Pharmacologic Treatment

No single medication is appropriate for all SLE patients (Table 135-5). Rather, the disease is managed by a problem-oriented approach. NSAIDs are the medications most widely prescribed, although the efficacy and toxicity of a particular drug in an individual patient are unpredictable. NSAIDs should generally be prescribed at the upper end of the recommended dose range. If one preparation does not provide relief after a 2- to 3-week trial, another may be prescribed. Lupus patients are subject to all the toxicities of the NSAIDs seen in other patients but to others as well. Because of subclinical or undiagnosed nephritis, SLE patients are at increased risk for NSAID-induced nephrotoxicity. This usually presents with a rise in serum creatinine, and may be accompanied by hyperkalemia and hypertension. These abnormalities are reversible once the drug is stopped but occur with sufficient frequency to merit monitoring of the serum creatinine in any patient after an NSAID is begun. Lupus patients are also probably at increased risk of mild hepatitis from NSAIDs, particularly salicylates, and serum transaminases should be monitored along with the creatinine. Aseptic meningitis, a rare complication of NSAID use, appears to be much more common in SLE and may also be caused by use of sulfa-containing antibiotics in these patients. No data are yet available on either the efficacy or the toxicity of selective cyclooxygenase II (COX-II) inhibitors in SLE but should be similar to those in RA.

Table 135-5. Drug Treatment for SLE

Drug	Indication	Adverse effects
NSAIDs	Arthritis, serositis	Gastritis, ulceration, renal toxicity
Hydroxychloroquine	Photosensitivity, rash, alopecia, oral ulcers, arthritis	Gastrointestinal intolerance, retinal toxicity
Cortocosteroids	Nephritis, cerebritis, thrombocytopenia, hemolysis, severe dermatitis	Hypertension, glucose intolerance, weight gain, osteoporosis, infection, accelerated atherosclerosis, avascular necrosis
Cyclophosphamide, azathioprine	Nephritis, vasculitis, steroid-resistant severe disease	Bone marrow suppression, infection, malignancy, infertility
Heparin, warfarin	Thrombosis (usually with antiphospholipid antibodies)	Hemorrhage

The antimalarial drug hydroxychloroquine is useful in the management of photosensitivity, rash, articular symptoms, alopecia, and oral ulcers in lupus.[6] Some patients also experience less fatigue. The usual starting dose is 400 mg daily. Clinical response may not occur for 3 months. Once symptoms are under control, the drug may be continued at a lower dose. The most common toxicity, gastrointestinal intolerance, may be ameliorated if the drug is taken before bedtime. The most serious toxicity, retinal damage, occurs in less than 1% of patients. Patients should be monitored every 6 months by an ophthalmologist. Retinal changes are generally not reversible but usually do not progress once the drug is discontinued.

Topical corticosteroids are the mainstay of treatment for cutaneous lupus. Mild to potent topical steroids may be used depending on the severity and thickness of the lesions and their location. Intralesional injections of betamethasone (6 mg/ml) or triamcinolone (5 mg/ml) may be required in well-established lesions of DLE. Antimalarial drugs are the second line of treatment of cutaneous lupus, unless lesions are widespread or occur in concert with other disease manifestations.

Systemic corticosteroids should be reserved for the more serious manifestations of lupus; however, they are also effective for milder symptoms if other therapies fail or have unacceptable toxicities. Fig. 135-5 provides a general guideline to the appropriate dose of prednisone according to disease manifestation. The lowest dose that provides control of the problem at hand should be used. Once the problem comes under control, the dose of prednisone should be gradually tapered and, if possible, discontinued. A schedule that reduces the dose by 25% every 3 to 4 weeks is generally appropriate. If the disease flares during this process, the next higher dose that controlled symptoms should be resumed and a taper reattempted once the disease has stabilized. The addition of an NSAID, hydroxychloroquine, topical steroids, or methotrexate may have steroid-sparing effects in certain patients.[11] Some manifestations of lupus, including thrombosis, end-stage or pure membranous nephritis, and occasionally thrombocytopenia or hemolytic anemia, do not respond to steroid therapy.

Rarely, when the illness is particularly fulminant or life threatening, high-dose "pulse" intravenous (IV) steroid therapy is used. This approach has met with some success in nephritis, cerebritis, pneumonitis, vasculitis, and thrombocytopenia. Methylprednisolone is generally given in a single IV dose of 500 to 1000 mg daily for 3 to 6 days, followed by 60 mg of oral prednisone daily. Patients requiring this aggressive approach should be managed with the consultation of an appropriate specialist.

Although corticosteroids may be lifesaving treatment in SLE, their use, particularly at high doses, is fraught with complications. Hypertension, weight gain, glucose intolerance, and acne are among the most common adverse effects. Osteoporosis is a major problem, especially during prolonged use. Many lupus patients also avoid the sun, and some experience premature menopause resulting from cytotoxic use, placing them at particular risk for osteoporosis. Calcium supplementation of 1500 mg daily should be prescribed when steroids are begun, along with 800 IU of vitamin D.[5]

Lupus patients are at particular risk of three potentially serious adverse effects of steroid use. *Infections* of all types occur more frequently in patients taking prednisone, particularly at higher doses. Infection is a primary or contributing factor in 30% to 50% of all deaths in SLE patients. Bacterial infections are most common, but fungal and opportunistic infections also occur and must be sought aggressively. The second unusual toxicity of steroid use in SLE is *atherosclerosis*. Both coronary artery and peripheral vascular diseases occur more often in SLE, even in young female patients, and appear to be related to long-term steroid use. Patients at highest risk are males and those with hypertension, renal disease, diabetes, hyperlipidemia, and the lupus anticoagulant. These risk factors should be vigorously addressed. *Ischemic necrosis of bone,* also referred to as *avascular necrosis* or *aseptic necrosis,* is the third type of steroid toxicity that is a particular problem in SLE. The femoral head is most often involved, although many patients have multiple sites, including the humeral heads, femoral condyles, and tali. The pain of avascular necrosis, unlike that of lupus-related synovitis, is exacerbated by use and relieved by rest. Joint stiffness is minimal.

Cytotoxic drugs are generally reserved for serious or potentially life-threatening manifestations of disease. They should be prescribed in consultation with an appropriate specialist experienced in their use. Cyclophosphamide is probably more effective than azathioprine for SLE but is also more toxic. Monthly boluses of IV cyclophosphamide are used primarily for diffuse proliferative glomerulonephritis. The initial dosage of 500 to 750 mg/m^2 is adjusted to achieve a nadir white blood cell count of 3500 to 4500, 10 to 14 days after infusion. Mesna is used with each infusion to minimize bladder irritation. Although IV therapy is associated with less bladder toxicity and a lower risk of malignancy than daily oral therapy, the risk of serious infection is similar.

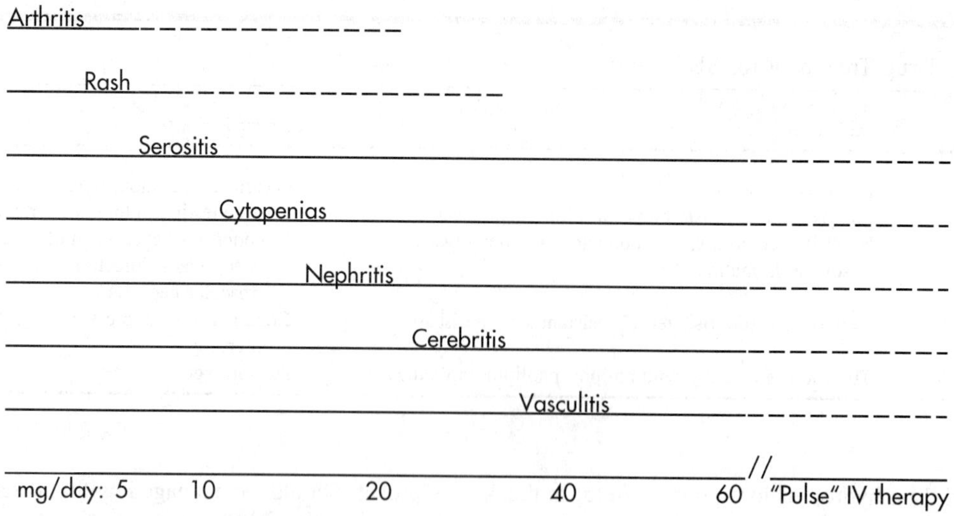

Arthritis

Rash

Serositis

Cytopenias

Nephritis

Cerebritis

Vasculitis

mg/day: 5 10 20 40 60 // "Pulse" IV therapy

Fig. 135-5. Problem-oriented guide to corticosteroid dosage: suggested minimum prednisone doses *(solid lines)* with ranges *(broken lines)*. Arthritis, rash, and serositis can often be managed without steroids.

Cyclophosphamide or azathioprine can be used in a daily oral dose of 1 to 3 mg/kg when the clinical situation is serious enough to warrant the toxicity. Patients must be monitored for marrow suppression and are at risk of infection, malignancy, infertility, and menopause.

Anticoagulants are used in the subset of patients whose disease manifestations can be attributed to thrombosis. These patients usually have one or more forms of antiphospholipid antibody. Initial therapy of the thrombosis is with IV heparin, followed by oral warfarin with a target international normalized ratio (INR) of at least 2.5. Patients with antiphospholipid antibodies who have had clear-cut thrombotic episodes are at increased risk of recurrent thrombosis. Lifelong anticoagulation must be considered, particularly if the initial event was a stroke or large-vessel occlusion. Management in this setting is the same whether the patient has SLE or the primary antiphospholipid syndrome.

Monitoring

Several laboratory tests useful in making the diagnosis of lupus are also helpful in monitoring patients with established disease. Some patients have their own distinctive pattern of laboratory abnormalities that track with clinical disease activity. For example, levels of anti-DNA antibodies may rise with flares of disease and return to negative when disease is under control. ANA titers, in contrast, are rarely useful in monitoring disease activity and should not be followed serially. Some patients reproducibly demonstrate a fall in serum complement levels or a rise in ESR or quantitative immunoglobulin levels just before a disease flare. These markers should be surveyed when the lupus is quiescent to establish each patient's normal baseline profile. When a disease flare is suspected, studies may be repeated and compared with original values. As long as the lupus is inactive, it is unnecessary to repeat these measurements. Urinalysis, serum creatinine, and complete blood count should be performed at least twice yearly, however, even if the lupus appears to be in remission, to screen for occult disease.

Reproductive Issues

One of the most problematic management areas in lupus involves issues of reproduction. Patients with active SLE should avoid becoming pregnant because of definite risks to both the mother and the fetus. Use of estrogen-containing oral contraceptive preparations may induce a disease flare. Patients taking them without difficulty are generally permitted to continue, but most rheumatologists are reluctant to allow their lupus patients to begin oral contraceptives. Barrier methods of contraception, including the diaphragm and condom with contraceptive spermicide, or progesterone-based implantable devices may be preferable. If pregnancy occurs when the disease is under control, controversy surrounds the risk of lupus flare.[4] Hypertension, proteinuria, or thrombocytopenia developing in a pregnant woman with lupus may be difficult to distinguish from preeclampsia. Serial monitoring of renal function and serum complement levels may be useful in tracking the course of the lupus. Lupus patients should be observed through their pregnancy in consultation with a high-risk obstetrician or perinatologist.

The fetus is also subject to potential dangers related to the mother's SLE. Mothers with antiphospholipid antibodies have an increased frequency of second-trimester miscarriage and stillbirth; early miscarriages may also be increased. Some women have multiple recurrent miscarriages and are unable to carry a pregnancy to term. Heparin treatment, with or without concomitant aspirin therapy, may reduce pregnancy loss in these patients but should be undertaken only with the guidance of an experienced perinatologist.

The other major risk to the fetus is neonatal lupus. This occurs in some fetuses whose mothers have anti-SSA/Ro, an immunoglobulin G that crosses the placenta to the fetus. Congenital heart block may develop, becoming evident between weeks 20 and 22 of the pregnancy. Structural cardiac defects may also occur and carry a poorer prognosis. Infants of mothers with lupus may also experience a temporary neonatal lupus syndrome, manifesting as a positive ANA test and photosensitive dermatitis. The rash and serologic abnormalities gradually disappear over the first few months of life as the infant metabolizes the maternal immunoglobulins.

Consultation and Referral

The physician caring for a patient with suspected SLE may need to consult various specialists, both to confirm the diagnosis and to assist in treatment decisions. In a patient with probable lupus and a rash, a dermatologist may be able to provide clinical or histologic confirmation of the diagnosis. For patients with more generalized problems or with a confusing serologic picture, a rheumatologist may be more appropriate. Consultation should also be sought when serious or potentially life-threatening complications develop (e.g., cerebritis, nephritis, thrombocytopenia, hemolysis). Any patient being considered for high-dose steroid therapy or cytotoxic use should also be referred for subspecialty input into management.

REFERENCES

1. Boumpas DT, Austin HA III, Fessler BJ, et al: Systemic lupus erythematosus: emerging concepts. Part 1. Renal, neuropsychiatric, cardiovascular, pulmonary and hematologic disease, *Ann Intern Med* 122:940, 1995.
2. Callen J: Management of skin disease in lupus, *Bull Rheum Dis* 46:4, 1997.
3. Hahn BH: Antibodies to DNA, *N Engl J Med* 338:1359, 1998.
4. Khamashta MA, Ruiz-Irastorza G, Hughes GRV: SLE flares during pregnancy, *Rheum Dis Clin North Am* 23:15, 1997.
5. Lukert BP, Raisz LG: ACR task force on osteoporosis guidelines, *Arthritis Rheum* 39:1801, 1996.
6. Rhynes R: Antimalarial drugs in the treatment of rheumatic diseases, *Br J Rheumatol* 36:795, 1997.
7. Tan EM, Cohen AS, Fries JF, et al: The 1982 revised criteria for the classification of systemic lupus erythematosus, *Arthritis Rheum* 25:1271, 1982.
8. Tan EM, Feltkamp TE, Smolen JS, et al: Range of antinuclear antibodies in "healthy" individuals, *Arthritis Rheum* 40:1601, 1997.
9. Wahl DG, Guillemin F, de Maistre E, et al: Risk for venous thrombosis related to antiphospholipid antibodies in systemic lupus erythematosus: a meta-analysis, *Lupus* 6:467, 1997.
10. West SG, Emlen W, Wener MH, et al: Neuropsychiatric lupus erythematosus: a 10-year prospective study on the value of diagnostic tests, *Am J Med* 99:153, 1995.
11. Wilson K, Abeles M: A 2-year, open-ended trial of methotrexate in systemic lupus erythematosus, *J Rheumatol* 21:1674, 1994.

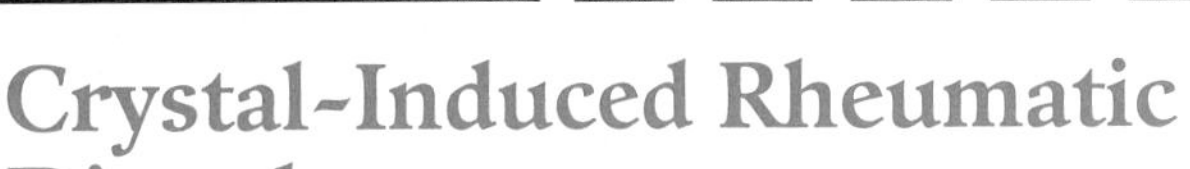

Crystal-Induced Rheumatic Disorders

David F. Giansiracusa
Leslie R. Harrold

GOUT

Gout is caused by elevated serum levels of monosodium urate, which result in deposition of urate crystals in joints and soft tissues and excessive urinary excretion of uric acid. Clinical manifestations of gout include (1) recurrent attacks of acute arthritis; (2) chronic, deforming, erosive arthritis related to deposition of large deposits of monosodium urate (tophi) in and around joints; (3) deposition of monosodium urate crystals in the kidneys, causing urate nephropathy; (4) uric acid kidney stones; and (5) uric acid crystallization in renal tubules, or acute hyperuricemic (uric acid) nephropathy.[6]

Epidemiology and Etiology

Hyperuricemia is a requisite for the development of gout. Statistically, hyperuricemia can be defined as a serum urate level greater than 2 standard deviations (SD) above the mean. Since gout represents a group of diseases that result from excessive amounts of monosodium urate, however, hyperuricemia is better defined in physicochemical terms as the level above which urate concentration exceeds the saturation point. Since the solubility of urate in plasma at 37° C is approximately 7 mg/dl, which by most chemical and automatic analyzer techniques corresponds to a serum urate level of approximately 7.5 to 8 mg/dl, hyperuricemia can be defined as a serum urate level that exceeds this concentration. Hyperuricemia may result from overproduction of urate and diminished urinary excretion of uric acid. The term *primary gout* refers to the clinical disease that results from hyperuricemia caused by a genetically determined metabolic error of excessive de novo biosynthesis and impaired excretion of uric acid.

The overproduction of uric acid is determined when a patient follows a purine-restricted diet for 5 days and excretes more than 600 mg of uric acid in 24 hours. This group of patients constitutes less than 15% of individuals with gout. In a few patients who produce too much uric acid, a primary enzymatic abnormality such as hypoxanthine guanine phosphoribosyltransferase (HGPRTase) deficiency or increased phosphoribosylpyrophosphate (PRPP) synthetase activity is responsible for excessive biosynthesis of uric acid. In approximately 75% to 90% of individuals with primary gout, hyperuricemia is the result of diminished renal clearance of uric acid. These individuals require serum urate levels 2 to 3 mg/dl higher than normal to achieve comparable uric acid excretion rates.

Secondary gout results from an acquired disease state or a drug that causes an overproduction or impaired excretion of uric acid. Secondary causes of hyperuricemia include myeloproliferative and lymphoproliferative diseases, multiple myeloma, hemolytic anemia, polycythemia vera, and psoriasis. Acquired renal disease, acidosis, and drugs are the most common causes of secondary hyperuricemia resulting from diminished renal excretion of uric acid.[10] Implicated drugs include low-dose salicylates, nicotinic acid, ethambutol, cyclosporine, and any diuretic that causes volume contraction, especially thiazides, which also compete with urate for secretion by the renal tubule.

Lead-induced renal tubular injury also impairs uric acid excretion. Alcohol consumption elevates serum urate levels because of the generation of organic acids, which compete with tubular secretion of uric acid and enhance uric acid production secondary to accelerated conversion of adenosine triphosphate to adenosine monophosphate, which is metabolized in uric acid.

Pathophysiology

Urate crystals are typically present in the synovial fluid of patients with acute gouty arthritis. Laboratory studies of crystal growth indicate that the saturation concentration varies with temperature; at temperatures below 37° C, as in the extremity joints, the saturation point for uric acid is significantly less than 7 mg/dl. This biochemical phenomenon correlates well with the clinical observations that gouty arthritis characteristically affects the joints of the feet, ankles, knees, hands, and elbows and that tophi deposit in cool sites, such as the cartilaginous helix of the external ear, the olecranon bursae, and the peripheral joints.

Acute gouty arthritis occurs when monosodium urate crystals appear in the synovial fluid as a result of shedding from articular cartilage or synovium or precipitation of new crystals. Mechanical stresses, such as twisting an ankle or stubbing the great toe, may dislodge urate crystals. Crystal shedding may also result from rapid changes in urate concentration, as in the institution of uric acid-lowering therapy (e.g., allopurinol, uricosuric agents) or the ingestion of alcohol or salicylates.[6] Once in the joint fluid, a series of processes occurs, including coating of the crystals with immunoglobulins. Polymorphonuclear neutrophil leukocytes (PMNs) ingest the crystals, releasing lysosomal enzymes and other inflammatory mediators, including toxic superoxide radicals, prostaglandins, leukotrienes, kinins, and components of the complement pathways, causing inflammation and, with repeated attacks, joint damage.

Patient Evaluation

After prolonged asymptomatic hyperuricemia, often 20 to 30 years, approximately 5% to 10% of individuals develop acute gouty arthritis, characterized by the abrupt onset of exquisite pain, tenderness, swelling, and erythema that most often affects a single joint. Approximately 50% of individuals experience their first attack in the metatarsophalangeal (MTP) joint of the great toe. Other peripheral joints, including the joints of the midfoot, ankles, knees, fingers, wrists, and elbows, may be involved in a monoarticular presentation.[6] Approximately 10% to 15% of patients present initially with polyarticular gout.[9] Gouty arthritis most frequently affects men in the fourth through sixth decades of life and, less often, postmenopausal women. Attacks often occur at night and may be associated with inflammation of the surrounding tendons, bursae, and skin, raising the differential diagnosis of joint infection and cellulitis. Even if untreated the acute attack is self-limited, generally lasting 3 to 7 days, after which the patient is completely asymptomatic. The attacks may become more frequent and more prolonged, and the individual may eventually develop chronic, persistent gout, with increasing accumulation of urate deposits, clinically evident as palpable tophi on examination, or erosions and soft tissue swelling on radiographs.

Laboratory Studies and Diagnostic Procedures

Characteristic bone radiographic features of chronic tophaceous gout include cortical indentations or erosions with sharply defined sclerotic margins resulting from tophi in adjacent soft tissues, cortical erosions with an overhanging or hooklike margin as a result of tophaceous deposits in the periosteum or cortical bones, and round or oval cysts generally with sclerotic margins in medullary bone close to joints. Relative preservation of joint space, absence of profound periarticular demineralization, and eccentric location of soft tissue swelling help differentiate tophaceous gouty arthritis from rheumatoid arthritis.

A definitive diagnosis of gouty arthritis is established by the demonstration of needle-shaped monosodium urate crystals within synovial fluid PMNs aspirated from clinically affected joints[6,9] (Fig. 136-1). Because of birefringent characteristics, urate crystals (and in pseudogout, calcium pyrophosphate crystals) are more readily visualized by polarizing microscopy than by plain light microscopy. The monosodium urate crystal appears as a bright, needle-shaped

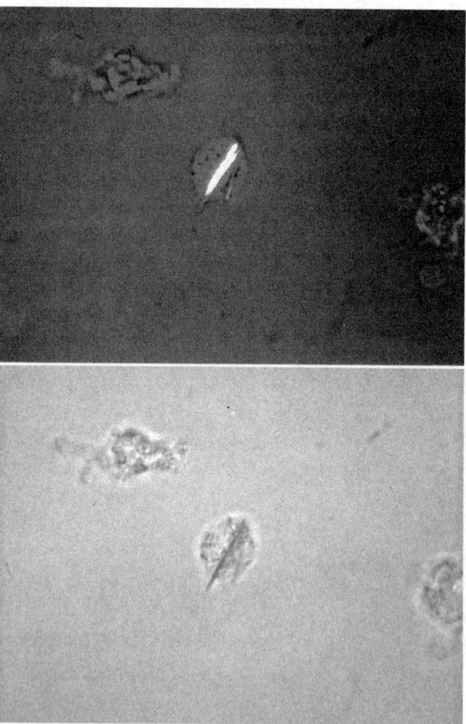

Fig. 136-1. Monosodium urate crystals phagocytosed by polymorphonuclear leukocyte in synovial fluid. *Top,* Compensated polarized light clearly demonstrates two longer crystals and one shorter one. *Bottom,* Same field under ordinary light. Comparison of two views demonstrates superiority of compensated polarized light over ordinary light microscopy when evaluating joint fluid for crystals. (From American College of Rheumatology: *Clinical slide collection on the rheumatic diseases,* 1991, The College.)

object on a dark background. With a red compensator, the negatively birefringent urate crystals are yellow when they lie parallel to the axis of the light coming through the microscope, whereas the positively birefringent, rhomboid, or square calcium pyrophosphate crystals are blue when parallel to the microscope's plane of light. The more acute the attack of gout, the more likely monosodium urate crystals are visualized within synovial PMNs.

The differential diagnosis of gout is that of an acute monoarticular or oligoarticular (four or fewer joints) arthritis (Box 136-1).

Renal Complications

Excesses of serum urate and urinary uric acid may affect the kidneys and cause a variety of medical problems, including urate nephropathy, acute hyperuricemic (uric acid) nephropathy, and uric acid urolithiasis.

Urate nephropathy manifests in the development of proteinuria, loss of maximal tubular concentrating ability, hypertension, and azotemia related to the deposition of monosodium urate crystals within the medullary and pyramidal interstitium of the kidney as a result of longstanding hyperuricemia. This condition rarely occurs in the absence of gouty arthritis and generally correlates with the severity of the joint disease. Urate nephropathy is diagnosed clinically. Pathologically the condition is characterized by urate crystal deposition in the medullary interstitium and pyramids with surrounding giant cell reaction. In most gouty patients, hypertension, heart disease, peripheral atherosclerosis, aging, diabetes mellitus, nonsteroidal antiinflammatory drug (NSAID) use, analgesic abuse, lead exposure, other intrinsic renal disease (e.g., glomerulonephritis, pyelonephritis, interstitial nephritis), and urinary obstruction are generally more important contributors to renal function impairment than urate nephropathy.

Acute hyperuricemic nephropathy (acute uric acid nephropathy) is characterized by oliguria and renal failure related to the precipitation of massive amounts of uric acid within renal tubules and collecting ducts, causing tubular obstruction. This condition most often develops during cytotoxic therapy for myeloproliferative disorders as a result of massive cell death and an increased release of uric acid. Therapy to prevent uric acid nephropathy includes vigorous hydration and the use of the xanthine oxidase inhibitor, allopurinol, generally 600 mg/day begun 2 to 3 days before the institution of cytotoxic radiation or chemotherapy.

Approximately 10% to 25% of individuals with gouty arthritis develop *urolithiasis,* usually with stones composed of a mixture of uric acid and calcium oxalate. The incidence of nephrolithiasis increases with the degree of hyperuricemia but more closely correlates with the amount of uric acid excreted in the urine (i.e., the degree of uric aciduria). Approximately 50% of individuals who excrete more than 1100 mg of uric acid in 24 hours develop stones. Other factors that predispose to uric acid urolithiasis include high urine concentration, low pH, and urinary solubility.[8] Therapeutic measures to prevent uric acid calculi include adequate hydration, alkalinization to maintain a urine pH more than 6, moderation of dietary intake of alcohol and protein, prompt treatment of any urinary tract infection, and reduction of uric acid production with allopurinol and thus reduction in the amount of uric acid excreted.

Treatment

Hyperuricemia. Asymptomatic hyperuricemia is an elevated serum urate level without gouty arthritis, tophi, urate nephropathy, or uric acid renal calculi (Box 136-2). Treatment with pharmacologic agents is rarely indicated. Arguments against treating asymptomatic hyperuricemia include the following: (1) although up to 5% of the U.S. population may have hyperuricemia, most (80% to 90%) never develop recognizable consequences; (2) gouty arthritis is a treatable condition; (3) urate nephropathy and tophaceous gout rarely develop in the absence of a history of acute gouty arthritis; (4) renal function is not adversely affected by hyperuricemia, and its normalization has little effect on renal function; and (5) treatment with an agent that lowers uric acid requires lifelong therapy, which is expensive and may be associated with potentially serious side effects. The risk of uric acid stone formation is more closely related to uric acid

Box 136-1. Differential Diagnosis of Acute Monoarticular and Oligoarticular Arthritides

- Septic arthritis
- Crystalline-induced arthritis
  - Gout
  - Pseudogout (calcium pyrophosphate arthropathy)
  - Hydroxyapatite and other basic calcium/phosphate crystals
  - Calcium oxalate
- Traumatic joint injury
- Hemarthrosis
- Monoarticular or oligoarticular flare of inflammatory polyarticular rheumatic disease
  - Rheumatoid arthritis
  - Psoriatic arthritis
  - Reiter's syndrome
  - Systemic lupus erythematosus

Box 136-2. Evaluation of Patient with Asymptomatic Hyperuricemia

- Obesity
- Alcohol consumption
- Use of salicylate, thiazide, or other diuretics
- Use of nicotinic acid, ethambutol, and cyclosporine
- Volume depletion
- Renal disease
- High cell turnover state (e.g., leukemia, hemolytic anemia, severe psoriasis)
- Evidence of hypertension or cardiovascular disease
- History of renal stones
- Previous acute attacks of arthritis
- Presence of tophi
- Family history of gouty arthritis, renal stones, and renal disease

excretion rates than to the degree of serum urate elevation. Detailed studies on cardiovascular disease indicate that hyperuricemia does not appear to be an independent risk factor for coronary artery disease (CAD) but rather is associated with other risk factors, such as obesity, hypertension, and hyperlipidemia. Conversely, no evidence supports the contention that lowering serum urate to normal levels independently reduces the risk of CAD.

Appropriate management of asymptomatic hyperuricemia consists of weight reduction for the obese patient; moderate consumption of alcohol, protein, and foods high in purine content; cessation of smoking; and treatment of hypertension and hypercholesterolemia. A diet low in purine content allows patients to reduce their serum urate levels by 1 mg/dl and the 24-hour urinary uric acid excretion by 200 to 400 mg/day. Foods rich in purines include all meats, including organ meats, seafood, meat extracts, and gravies; yeast and yeast extracts; beer and other alcoholic drinks; and beans, peas, lentils, oatmeal, spinach, asparagus, cauliflower, and mushrooms.[1] Diuretics and other drugs that contribute to hyperuricemia should be avoided if possible. Any primary condition that contributes to hyperuricemia (e.g., renal disease, high cell turnover) should be treated.

Gouty Arthritis. The goals of the treatment of gouty arthritis are termination of the acute attack, prevention of recurrent attacks, and prevention or resorption of tophi in joints and soft tissues. Pharmacologic agents used to treat gouty arthritis can be divided into antiinflammatory drugs, drugs used for prophylaxis against episodes of acute gouty arthritis, and drugs to lower urate (and uric acid) levels (Table 136-1). The earlier an acute attack of gouty arthritis is treated, the more rapidly the inflamed joints respond. Medications used to treat acute gouty arthritis include oral or intravenous

Table 136-1. Medications Used to Treat Acute Gouty Arthritis

Indication/drug	Dose	Comments
Treat acute gout (decrease inflammation and pain)		
Colchicine	0.6 mg PO qh (8-10 tablets in 24 hr) or 2 mg IV then 1 mg IV at 6-hr intervals (maximum of 4 mg in 24-48 hr)	Best if initiated within several hours of attack. Use with caution in persons with liver or renal disease or receiving concomitant therapy with cytochrome P-450 enzyme inhibitors.
Nonsteroidal antiinflammatory drugs (NSAIDs)	High dose first 2-3 days, then taper	Do not use in patients receiving anticoagulation. Use with caution in patients with peptic ulcer disease, congestive heart failure, hypertension, or renal/liver disease.
Corticosteroids	30-40 mg of prednisone, then taper by 5 mg/day 40-80 units ACTH qd up to 3 days	Can be given PO, IV, SC, or intraarticularly once septic joint ruled out. Use with caution in diabetic patients and those with concurrent infections.
Prevent acute attacks		
Colchicine	0.6 mg qd or bid	Chronic maintenance therapy for prophylaxis (cautions as above).
NSAIDs	High dose to prn dosing	Take with meals for prophylaxis (cautions as above).
Lower serum urate concentrations		
Indications include repeated attacks, tophaceous deposits, evidence of renal damage, recurrent urolithiasis, urinary uric acid excretion >1000 mg/day, and prevention of hyperuricemia in patients with malignancies.		
Allopurinol	100 mg to dosage necessary to suppress serum urate <6-7 mg/dl	Begin only after resolution of acute attack. Concurrent administration of NSAIDs or maintenance colchicine to prevent acute attack. Use with caution in patients with renal disease and those taking 6-mercaptopurine, azathioprine, or warfarin.
Probenecid	250-500 mg to 1.5 gm bid	For hyperuricemic patients who excrete less than 700 mg of uric acid per day and have normal renal function (GFR >60 ml/min). Good urine volumes required to minimize risk of urolithiasis.
Sulfinpyrazone	100-400 mg bid	As for probenecid.

PO, Orally; *qh*, every hour; *IV*, intravenously; *SC*, subcutaneously; *ACTH*, adrenocorticotropic hormone; *qd*, every day; *bid*, twice daily; *prn*, as necessary; *GFR*, glomerular filtration rate.

(IV) colchicine, NSAIDs, and systemic or intraarticular corticosteroids.

NSAIDs are generally given in high dosages for the first 2 to 3 days ("pulse" therapy) and then tapered to a lower dosage (e.g., indomethacin, 50 mg three to four times a day for 1 to 2 days with meals, followed by a taper to 25 mg three to four times a day with meals for 5 to 7 days). Other NSAIDs, including tolmetin, naproxen, ibuprofen, piroxicam, sulindac, ketoprofen, fenoprofen, and meclofenamate, may also be effective. Because of the potential adverse effects of phenylbutazone and the availability of other NSAIDs, primary care physicians should not treat patients with phenylbutazone. Intramuscular ketorolac (Toradol) has also been demonstrated to be effective. All NSAIDs may cause gastrointestinal (GI) and central nervous system (CNS) side effects as well as GI bleeding, inhibition of platelet function, fluid retention, aggravation of congestive heart failure (CHF), hypertension, and renal function impairment.

If the treatment of acute gouty arthritis is begun within several hours of the onset of the attack, oral colchicine may be effective (0.6 mg every hour for a maximum of 8 to 10 tablets or until GI side effects develop, followed by a maintenance therapy of 0.6 mg twice daily). The efficacy of oral colchicine is greatly reduced the longer that treatment is delayed after onset of the arthritis; therefore oral colchicine is not the ideal drug for the treatment of acute attacks. IV colchicine is useful for the patient who cannot take oral medications or who has a diarrheal illness (e.g., viral gastroenteritis, inflammatory bowel disease, drug-induced or dietary-induced diarrhea). IV colchicine may also be useful in the patient who should avoid NSAIDs because of other medical problems (e.g., peptic ulcer disease, anticoagulation, CHF). A total of 2 mg may be infused initially, followed by an infusion of 1.0 mg at 6-hour intervals, for a total dose of IV colchicine not to exceed 4 mg in 24 to 48 hours.[1] No more colchicine should be administered for at least 7 days. Colchicine is extremely irritating to soft tissues and may cause tissue necrosis and cutaneous slough if extravasation occurs. Colchicine should be diluted in 20 ml of normal saline and infused over 10 to 20 minutes. Although IV colchicine usually does not cause the GI side effects associated with oral administration, it may result in myelosuppression. Excessive dosing of IV colchicine may also cause disseminated intravascular coagulation, shock, renal shutdown, hepatocellular necrosis, and CNS dysfunction. Colchicine excretion is reduced in patients with chronic liver disease and impaired renal function, including older individuals who appear to have normal serum creatinine levels. Myopathy and neuropathy are associated with long-term colchicine therapy in patients with renal insufficiency; therefore colchicine either should not be used or should be used carefully (including a reduction in the dosage) in patients with significant liver or renal disease. Colchicine should not be used in patients with combined renal and liver dysfunction, biliary obstruction, or severe renal disease (creatinine clearance less than 10 ml/min).

Corticosteroids may be required in patients with particularly severe or prolonged attacks or in patients who have contraindications to treatment with other agents. After joint sepsis has been excluded, corticosteroids may be administered directly into the inflamed joint or given systematically, such as 30 to 40 mg of prednisone or its equivalent on day 1, tapered over 6 to 10 days, or 40 to 80 units of adrenocorticotropic hormone (ACTH) intramuscularly or by slow IV infusion, repeated every 24 hours for 1 to 3 days as needed.[7]

After an acute attack of gout has subsided, chronic maintenance therapy with colchicine (0.6 mg twice daily in patients with normal renal and hepatic function) or NSAIDs with meals may act as a prophylaxis against subsequent gouty attacks (see Table 136-1).

The issue of chronic uric acid–lowering therapy after one attack of gouty arthritis remains controversial. Indications for this therapy are (1) repeated attacks of disabling gouty arthritis, (2) tophaceous deposits on physical examination or radiographic studies, (3) clinical or radiographic signs of chronic gouty joint disease, (4) evidence of renal damage (glomerular filtration rate [GFR] less than 60 ml/min), (5) recurrent urolithiasis caused by pure uric acid stones or mixed stones in the setting of hyperuricosuria, (6) gross overproduction of uric acid (urinary uric acid excretion greater than 1000 mg/day), and (7) prevention of hyperuricemia and uricosuria in patients with lymphoproliferative and myeloproliferative disease before cytotoxic therapy. Allopurinol should be used for indications 4 through 7 and for indications 1 through 3 if urinary uric acid excretion on a low-purine diet exceeds 600 mg in 24 hours. Allopurinol should be instituted only after the resolution of an acute attack of gout and with the concurrent administration of NSAIDs or maintenance colchicine (0.6 mg once to twice daily) to prevent an attack of acute gout. Colchicine or NSAIDs should be continued for approximately 6 months after allopurinol has resolved all palpable tophi or, for the patient without tophi, for about 6 months after serum urate levels are suppressed below 6 mg/dl.[1] Allopurinol is generally initiated at 100 mg/day and increased every 2 to 4 weeks by 100 mg to the dosage necessary to suppress the serum urate level below 6 to 7 mg/dl. The dosage of allopurinol must be kept low in the patient with renal failure, with as little as 100 mg every other day or every third day. Since allopurinol reduces the metabolism of warfarin, 6-mercaptopurine, and azathioprine, the dosage of these medications must be appropriately reduced. With azathioprine the dosage is generally reduced to approximately 25% of the usual dosage when given in the setting of allopurinol therapy. Potential toxicities of allopurinol include nausea, diarrhea, drug fever, leukopenia, hepatotoxicity, interstitial nephritis, vasculitis, and a rash that may evolve into toxic epidermal necrolysis. Serious side effects most often occur when allopurinol is prescribed to patients with renal insufficiency, particularly with concomitant thiazide therapy.

Uricosuric agents may be prescribed in hyperuricemic patients with gout who excrete less than 700 mg of uric acid per day. Patients must have normal renal function for the agents to be effective (GFR should be greater than 60 ml/min) and should maintain good urine volumes to minimize the risk of urolithiasis. The uricosuric agents used most often are probenecid (250 to 500 mg twice a day, increased to 1.5 gm twice a day as needed) and sulfinpyrazone (100 mg twice a day, increased to 400 mg). Similar to allopurinol therapy, prophylaxis against acute gouty arthritis should be administered when a uricosuric agent is prescribed, and the prophylactic medication should be continued for at least 6 months after the serum urate level is controlled below 6 mg/dl or for 6 months after resolution of all clinically apparent tophi. Side effects of probenecid include headache, nausea, anorexia, skin rash, and rarely, nephrotic syndrome, hepatic necrosis, and aplastic anemia. Sulfinpyrazone may cause bone marrow suppression.

If a patient experiences an attack of gouty arthritis while taking allopurinol or a uricosuric agent, the dosage of the agent needed to lower the uric acid level should not be changed until after resolution of the attack.

CALCIUM PYROPHOSPHATE DEPOSITION DISEASE

Calcium pyrophosphate dihydrate (CPPD) crystal deposition disease, also referred to as *pyrophosphate arthropathy,* is a calcium crystal–induced form of joint disease that is characterized by diverse clinical manifestations associated with the deposition of CPPD crystals in and around joints.[3] The crystals most often deposit in fibrocartilage (e.g., menisci of knee, intervertebral disks, symphysis pubis) and in hyaline articular cartilage (knees, wrists, other joints). These deposits may also occur in tendons, ligaments, synovial membranes, and joint capsules.[5] The deposition of CPPD increases with aging and in osteoarthritic joints.[3] Thus pyrophosphate arthropathy is fairly common in older individuals, particularly in the acute form, called *pseudogout.* Asymptomatic articular cartilage calcifications may occur in as many as 15% of individuals 65 to 75 years of age and more than 40% of those 85 years of age and older.

Patient Evaluation

CPPD is best known for causing acute arthritis (pseudogout) because of its similarities to acute gouty arthritis. Pseudogout most often affects the knees of older women, in contrast to gout, which usually affects the joint at the base of the great toe (first MTP joint) and the joints of the instep and ankle in middle-aged men. Pseudogout may also involve the wrists and, less frequently, metacarpophalangeal (MCP) joints, ankles, shoulders, and elbows.[6]

In addition to the acute arthritis or pseudogout presentation, deposition of CPPD crystals may cause a more subacute, polyarticular presentation similar to rheumatoid arthritis (pseudorheumatoid form), a pseudoosteoarthritis form, and a destructive form, as seen with severe neuropathies (pseudoneuropathic form). CPPD crystals may be detected radiographically in an asymptomatic individual as articular chondrocalcinosis.

The most common association with CPPD deposition is aging. Other conditions are associated with CPPD deposition in articular and periarticular structures, including disorders related to elevated calcium levels (e.g., hyperparathyroidism) and metabolic disorders characterized by diminished activity of pyrophosphatases (e.g., familial hypophosphatasia and hypomagnesemia). In addition, familial hypocalciuric hypercalcemia, hemochromatosis, hypothyroidism, and Bartter's syndrome are associated with CPPD disease. Osteoarthritic degeneration of cartilage also facilitates CPPD deposition.[5]

Diagnosis

Although the diagnosis of pseudogout is suggested by an acute arthritis with radiographic evidence of articular chondrocalcinosis, definitive diagnosis requires joint aspiration with synovial fluid examination and visualization by compensated polarized microscopy of the rhomboid or square, positively birefringent CPPD crystals within synovial fluid leukocytes[6] (Fig. 136-2). Joint fluid aspirated from

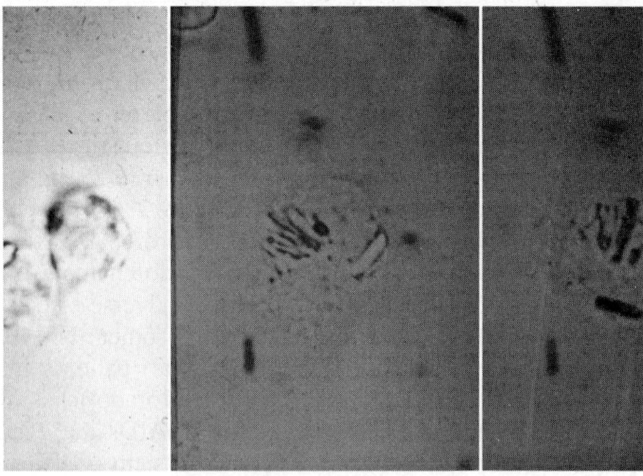

Fig. 136-2. Calcium pyrophosphate crystals phagocytosed by polymorphonuclear leukocytes in synovial fluid, demonstrating rectangular or rhomboid shapes. (From American College of Rheumatology: *Clinical slide collection on the rheumatic diseases,* 1991, The College.)

inflamed joints should also be examined for urate crystals and cultured for infectious agents (see Chapter 123).

Treatment

A fundamental component of the management of acute CPPD crystal–induced arthritis (pseudogout) is joint aspiration and synovial fluid examination to identify the crystal and exclude joint sepsis. Management of pseudogout and other forms of CPPD arthropathy includes the evaluation and treatment of underlying medical disorders and the administration of antiinflammatory medications. NSAIDs, oral and IV colchicine, and intraarticular and systemic steroids, including ACTH, may be used.[3] Screening laboratory studies may include those for calcium, phosphorus, albumin, magnesium, thyroid function, alkaline phosphatase, iron and total iron-binding capacity, and ferritin levels. The most cost-effective approach to the metabolic evaluation is to examine for hyperparathyroidism and hemochromatosis, since CPPD arthropathy may be the first clinically apparent manifestation of these conditions. Other associated metabolic diseases generally manifest with other signs and symptoms, such as liver disease in the case of Wilson's disease.

Chronic forms of pyrophosphate arthropathy are generally treated similarly to osteoarthritis, with NSAIDs, nonnarcotic analgesics, joint splinting as appropriate, and range of motion (ROM) and strengthening exercises. Joint lavage and arthroscopic irrigation may occasionally be beneficial. In severe, destructive cases of CPPD arthropathy, particularly those involving the hips and knees, joint replacement for alleviation of pain and deformity may be necessary.

CALCIUM PHOSPHATE–ASSOCIATED ARTHROPATHY

Hydroxyapatite and other calcium phosphate–containing crystals deposit in and around joints, causing acute and chronic arthropathy and periarticular inflammation.[3,5]

Periarthritis

The most familiar clinical form of hydroxyapatite-induced disease is supraspinatus tendinitis with or without calcific subacromial bursitis, presenting as shoulder pain aggravated by abduction and the radiographic evidence of amorphous calcium deposits in the region of the greater tuberosity of the humerus. The deposition of hydroxyapatite in periarticular structures (tendons, bursae, and joint capsules) may cause acute calcific periarthritis at multiple sites. The most frequently affected areas are the subacromial and trochanteric bursae, the supraspinatus tendon, the Achilles tendon, tendons of the wrists, capsules of the knees, and MCP joints. The clinical features of periarticular hydroxyapatite disease are variable, ranging from no symptoms to severe pain, tenderness, localized edema, and restricted motion. On plain radiographs, hydroxyapatite appears as amorphous, soft tissue, calcium-dense deposits or clumps, often in the anatomic sites of bursae, tendon sheaths, or joint capsules. The absence of trabeculae and the presence of the amorphous, homogenously dense deposits help to distinguish these hydroxyapatite deposits radiographically from avulsion fractures. Conditions that may predispose to calcific periarthritis include repetitive motion, diabetes mellitus, hyperthyroidism, and chronic renal failure, particularly in the setting of chronic hemodialysis.

Treatment of calcific periarthritis may include analgesics, NSAIDs, IV colchicine, aspiration and local injection of a depot steroid preparation (after excluding an infectious process), ACTH, and physical measures, including the application of heat, cold, diathermy, and ultrasound. During the initial acute stage, joint rest with splinting may help. Gentle ROM exercises should progress to a full, active ROM program to prevent the development of joint contractures and adhesive capsulitis. In recurrent and refractory cases, surgical removal of the calcium deposits may be necessary.[4]

Hydroxyapatite Crystal–Induced Arthritis

The presence of hydroxyapatite crystals may cause acute flares of osteoarthritis in joints (e.g., knees, fingers) and contribute to erosive osteoarthritis.[2] Hydroxyapatite crystals also cause a destructive arthritis, which was initially described in the shoulders, called *Milwaukee shoulder syndrome*. This form of hydroxyapatite arthropathy usually occurs in older women and results in destruction of the rotator cuff and degenerative arthritis of the glenohumeral joint. The synovial fluid is characterized by a paucity of white cells but high concentrations of prostaglandins and destructive enzymes in the setting of hydroxyapatite crystals. Since hydroxyapatite crystals are not birefringent, they cannot be detected easily by polarized microscopic examination but can be screened using calcium phosphate stains (alizarin red or von Kossa) or examining synovial fluid with x-ray diffraction and electron microscopy. The destructive process initially described as Milwaukee syndrome may also involve other joints, such as the knees and hips. Treatment of hydroxyapatite crystal–induced arthritis consists primarily of controlling inflammation with NSAIDs and colchicine and administering analgesics. Intraarticular "depo" corticosteroid preparations may provide transient benefit (see Chapter 167).

OTHER INTRAARTICULAR CRYSTALS

In addition to monosodium urate, CPPD, and hydroxyapatite crystals, cholesterol and calcium oxalate crystals and iatrogenically injected steroid crystals may play a role in rheumatic diseases. Patients with renal failure, particularly those on hemodialysis, may develop acute arthritis or periarthritis from calcium oxalate crystals. These crystals may appear on radiographs as amorphous calcifications similar to those of hydroxyapatite. The calcium oxalate crystals may be visualized under polarized light microscopy as positively birefringent crystals, thereby creating confusion with CPPD.

Injection of the intraarticular "depo" corticosteroid preparation may also result in an inflammatory arthritis termed *postinjection flare*. This occurs in approximately 5% of the patients who receive such injections and generally begins within 3 to 6 hours after the injection, lasting up to 3 days. Aspiration of synovial fluid from these patients may reveal positively or negatively birefringent crystals, thus causing confusion with CPPD or monosodium urate crystals, respectively.

In some cases the identification of crystals in synovial fluid is simply the result of synovial fluid having been placed in tubes containing calcium oxalate or lithium heparin as the anticoagulant. Since these materials are birefringent crystals, their presence may be incorrectly interpreted as diagnostic of a crystal-induced process that is the cause of joint inflammation.

Cholesterol crystals have a platelike appearance with a notch in one corner and tend to be seen in fluid aspirated from chronic joint and bursal effusions, most often in patients with longstanding rheumatoid arthritis.

REFERENCES

1. Emmerson BT: The management of gout, *N Engl J Med* 334:445, 1996.
2. Gerster JC: Intraarticular apatite crystal deposition as a predictor of erosive osteoarthritis of the fingers, *J Rheumatol* 21:2164, 1994.
3. Rosenthal AK: Calcium crystal-associated arthritides, *Curr Opin Rheumatol* 10:273, 1998.
4. Rosenthal AK, Ryan LM: Treatment of refractory crystal-associated arthritis, *Rheum Dis Clin North Am* 21:151, 1995.
5. Rull M: Calcium crystal–associated diseases and miscellaneous crystals, *Curr Opin Rheumatol* 9:274, 1997.
6. Schumacher HR Jr: Crystal-induced arthritis: an overview, *Am J Med* 100(suppl 2A):46S, 1996.
7. Siegel LB, Alloway JA, Nashel DJ: Comparison of adrenocorticotropic hormone and triamcinolone acetonide in the treatment of acute gouty arthritis, *J Rheumatol* 21:1325, 1994.
8. Simkin PA: Gout and hyperuricemia, *Curr Opin Rheumatol* 9:268, 1997.
9. Weinberger A: Gout, uric acid metabolism, and crystal-induced inflammation, *Curr Opin Rheumatol* 7:359, 1995.
10. Wise CM, Agudelo CA: Gouty arthritis and uric acid metabolism, *Curr Opin Rheumatol* 8:248, 1996.

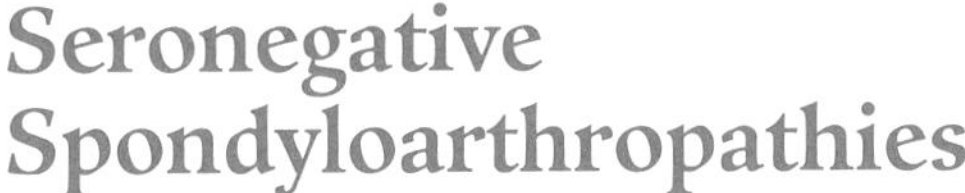

Seronegative Spondyloarthropathies

Nancy Y. N. Liu
Bruce R. Weinstein

The term *seronegative spondyloarthropathies* refers to a group of rheumatic diseases that share a number of clinical, radiologic, and pathogenetic features. These disorders are characterized by (1) inflammatory arthritis with a predilection for involvement of the axial skeleton and sacroiliac (SI) joints; (2) enthesopathy, defined as inflammation at sites of insertion of tendon, ligament, or fascia to bone; (3) asymmetric, peripheral oligoarthritis; (4) extraarticular features, most notably ophthalmologic, mucocutaneous, and urogenital involvement; (5) familial predisposition; (6) strong association with the class I HLA-B27 antigen; and (7) absence of rheumatoid factor. This group of disorders includes ankylosing spondylitis, reactive arthritis, Reiter's syndrome, psoriatic arthritis, arthropathy of inflammatory bowel disease (IBD), juvenile-onset ankylosing spondylitis, undifferentiated spondyloarthropathies, and uveitis associated with the HLA-B27 haplotype.

PATHOGENESIS

The pathogenesis of the seronegative spondyloarthropathies is unclear. The prevalence of HLA-B27 in the Caucasian population is 8%, but almost 90% of white patients with ankylosing spondylitis, Reiter's syndrome, reactive arthritis, or juvenile ankylosing spondylitis are HLA-B27 positive. The significance of this association, however, remains to be elucidated. Researchers have developed several hypotheses based on the HLA-B27 association and other clinical observations.[8] The first hypothesis is that molecular mimicry between HLA-B27 antigen and bacterial peptides results in cross-reactivity with self-peptides. In the second hypothesis, HLA-B27 binds arthritogenic bacterial peptides and elicits a cytotoxic T-cell response; subsequently the cytotoxic T cell cross-reacts with structurally similar self-peptides in articular tissue, which are also presented by HLA-B27. The third and most likely theory is that the presence of B27 molecules lacking β_2-microglobulin results in binding of B27 to exogenous bacterial peptides, which are presented to T cells. Researchers reported the spontaneous development of colitis, arthritis, psoriasiform skin lesions, and genitourinary inflammation in B27 transgenic rats. Other groups developed transgenic mice lacking β_2-microglobulin that experienced skin and joint changes in the presence of bacterial infections. Both these experiments support the direct role of HLA-B27 in the manifestation of disease.

The onset of arthritis after a urogenital or enteric infection by particular organisms (*Chlamydia, Salmonella, Shigella, Yersinia,* and *Campylobacter*) suggests that bacterial agents can initiate arthritis in a genetically susceptible host. Viable organisms are difficult to culture from joint fluid or synovium. With more sensitive polymerase chain reaction (PCR) techniques, however, bacterial ribonucleic acid (RNA) has been detected in the synovial white blood cells or tissue. Therefore the persistence of infection may induce specific synovial immune responses, particularly a cell-mediated one.

The close association of the gastrointestinal (GI) tract with the spondyloarthropathies has been supported by the presence of asymptomatic, microscopic intestinal inflammation in patients with ankylosing spondylitis, reactive arthritis, and undifferentiated spondyloarthropathies. Ileocolonoscopies and random biopsies performed on patients with these diseases revealed that 65% had subclinical IBD. Researchers therefore postulate that chronic inflammation in the intestinal tract may increase mucosal permeability and facilitate entrance of exogenous antigens into the circulation. Subsequently, these antigens initiate joint inflammation through various immune mechanisms.

It is likely that genetics (particularly HLA-B27), bacterial infections, and increased intestinal mucosa permeability make variable contributions to the pathogenesis of the spondyloarthropathies. Other possible pathogenetic mechanisms are mentioned in the following sections on specific disorders.

ANKYLOSING SPONDYLITIS

Epidemiology

Ankylosing spondylitis (AS) is often considered the prototype of the seronegative spondyloarthropathies. Although often unrecognized, AS has an overall prevalence of approximately 0.2%.[7] AS usually begins in adolescence or young adulthood, with a threefold greater incidence in men than women. Men often experience more severe axial manifestations. AS is a race-related disease, affecting whites and some Native Americans more frequently than African-Americans. Approximately 90% of patients with AS have the HLA-B27 antigen, although only 2% of B27-positive individuals have clinically detectable disease. Familial aggregation is quite pronounced. About 10% to 20% of B27-positive first-degree relatives of B27-positive patients with AS have or will develop AS.

Pathophysiology

AS is characterized by symmetric sacroiliitis and a progressive inflammatory arthritis of the axial skeleton and is often accompanied by enthesitis or inflammation at ligamentous insertions into bone. In 90% of patients the spine tends to be involved in an ascending manner, from the lumbar to the cervical region. Inflammation is followed by the formation of granulation tissue, calcification, and eventual ossification around the intervertebral disk margins, the apophyseal joint capsule insertion on bone, and the ligamentous insertions on the spine (e.g., flaval, interspinal, and supraspinal ligaments; costovertebral joints), referred to as enthesopathy.

Patient Evaluation

History. The earliest complaint in patients with AS corresponds to SI and lower axial skeleton pathology and consists of chronic, insidious low back pain and stiffness. The pain is dull and often localized in the gluteal or lower lumbar region and proximal posterior thigh. Other patients may have difficulty localizing the back pain. Morning back stiffness for more than 60 minutes is an important feature. In contrast to low back syndromes from mechanical causes, this stiffness tends to be exacerbated by inactivity and immobility and improved with exercise (see Chapter 127). Discomfort and stiffness may interrupt sleep, and the patient must arise to stretch and walk.

Nonaxial symptoms may provide the first clue to diagnosis. A young man with synovitis in a large lower extremity joint, tenosynovitis, or enthesopathy of the Achilles or supraspinatus tendon unrelated to mechanical causes should prompt the physician to consider AS in the differential diagnosis. The temporomandibular or sternoclavicular joints are less often involved. The patient may describe a pleuritic chest pain, which represents the enthesopathy at the costosternal and costovertebral joints.

Acute anterior uveitis, the most frequent and important extraarticular manifestation, is present in 25% of AS patients and is more common in patients who are HLA-B27 positive. Conversely, 50% of patients with uveitis are HLA-B27 positive; of these, one half or more have AS or reactive arthritis.[5] The onset is usually acute, starting with mild prodrome of eye discomfort or headache, followed by severe eye pain, redness, photophobia, blurry vision, and increased lacrimation. The episodes are usually unilateral, lasting several weeks to several months. Recurrences can occur in either eye.

Cardiac, pulmonary, renal, and neurologic involvement is less common in AS. Aortic regurgitation and conduction abnormalities, such as complete heart block, occur in less than 5% of patients. Restrictive lung disease, documented on pulmonary function tests, is secondary to ossification of rib and sternal articulations but is rarely clinically significant. Upper lobe pulmonary fibrosis, interstitial lung disease, and cavitation occur in less than 1% of patients. Chest radiographs are insensitive to early interstitial disease, and high-resolution computed tomography (HRCT) may be needed to evaluate AS patients with symptoms of dyspnea. Cauda equina syndrome, atlantoaxial subluxation, spinal stenosis, and spinal fractures affect less than 5% of all AS patients.

Although usually not prominent, constitutional symptoms may develop, consisting of fatigue, weight loss, and low-grade fever. A family history of spondyloarthropathy or HLA-B27 positivity should be sought.

Physical Examination. Physical findings reflect the predilection of this disease for the axial skeleton, including the SI joints, large peripheral joints, and the entheses. The apophyseal joints, which have the principal role in spinal flexion, are involved early in AS. The Shober test can detect limitation in flexion of the lumbar spine (Fig. 137-1). Lateral flexion, extension, and rotation of the back are also diminished; these measurements are part of the initial evaluation and subsequent follow-up. Limitation of neck movement tends to occur later in AS. Chest expansion, normally greater than 5 cm from full inspiration to end expiration, is often diminished. Inflammation of the SI joints can be assessed in several ways (Fig. 137-2). Palpation of inflamed entheses over the spinous processes, ischial tuberosities, greater trochanters, iliac crest, costovertebral and costochondral junctions, Achilles tendons, and plantar fascia may elicit pain. Since the hips or shoulders are involved in one third of patients, range of motion (ROM) measurements of these joints should be part of the physical examination.

Symptoms of uveitis are usually more helpful than the physical examination in differentiating uveitis from conjunctivitis. A slit-lamp examination is required to make the definitive diagnosis. The other extraarticular manifestations are relatively uncommon and are usually seen after AS is well established. The history and physical examination need to be directed toward these potential complications during routine follow-up. The most catastrophic but fortunately rare complication of AS involves neurologic sequelae. Minor trauma can fracture the cervical spine; the cervical region is the most vulnerable. Spinal cord compression and cauda equina syndrome may start with urinary and fecal incontinence. Similar to rheumatoid arthritis, general anesthesia can

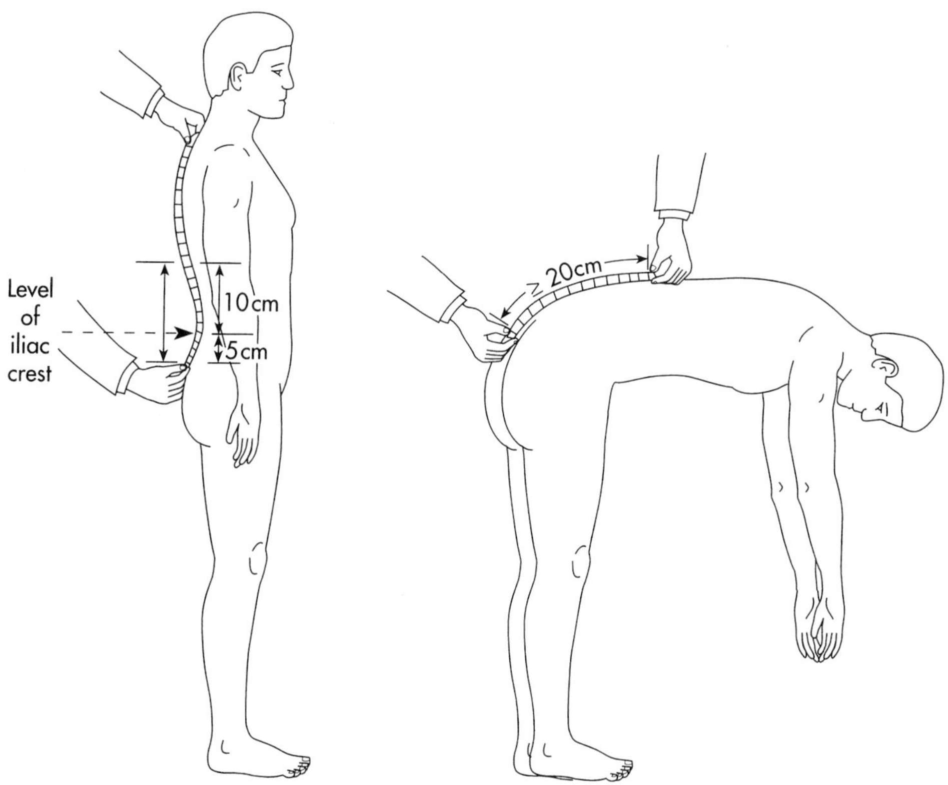

Fig. 137-1. Shober test measures forward flexion of lumbar spine and degree of separation of spinous processes. Midpoint between posterior iliac crests is marked, and measurement is made 10 cm above and 5 cm below this mark with patient in upright position. Marks are then made at upper and lower portions. In normal individuals performing forward flexion, this 15-cm distance should lengthen by at least 5 cm. In patients with ankylosing spondylitis, distraction of this distance is often reduced. (From Wise CM: In Turner RA, Wise CM, editors: *Textbook of rheumatology,* New York, 1986, Elsevier.)

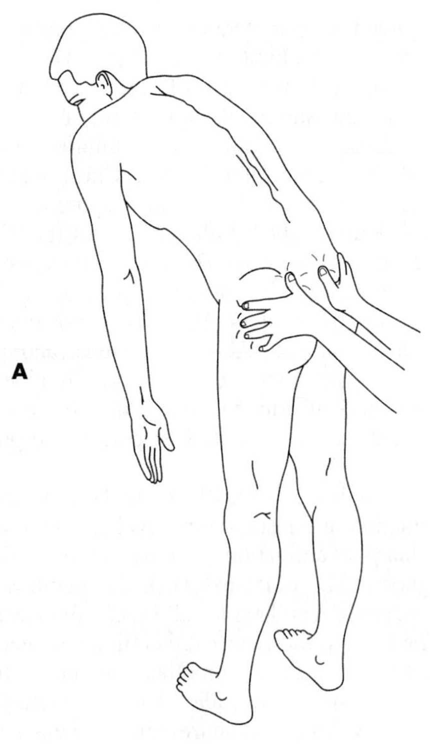
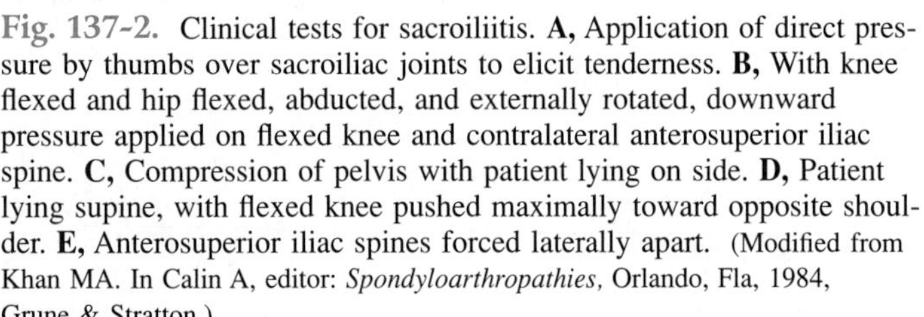
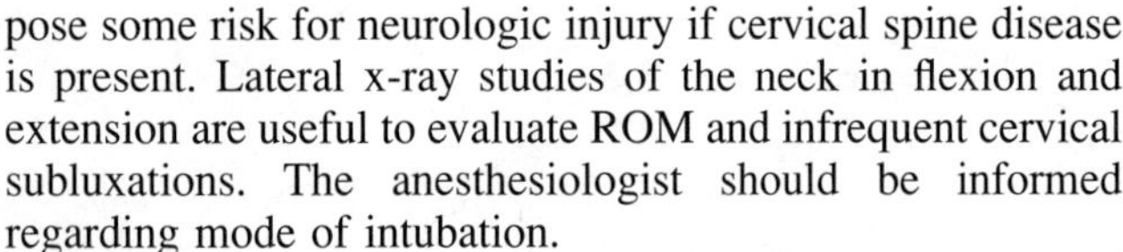
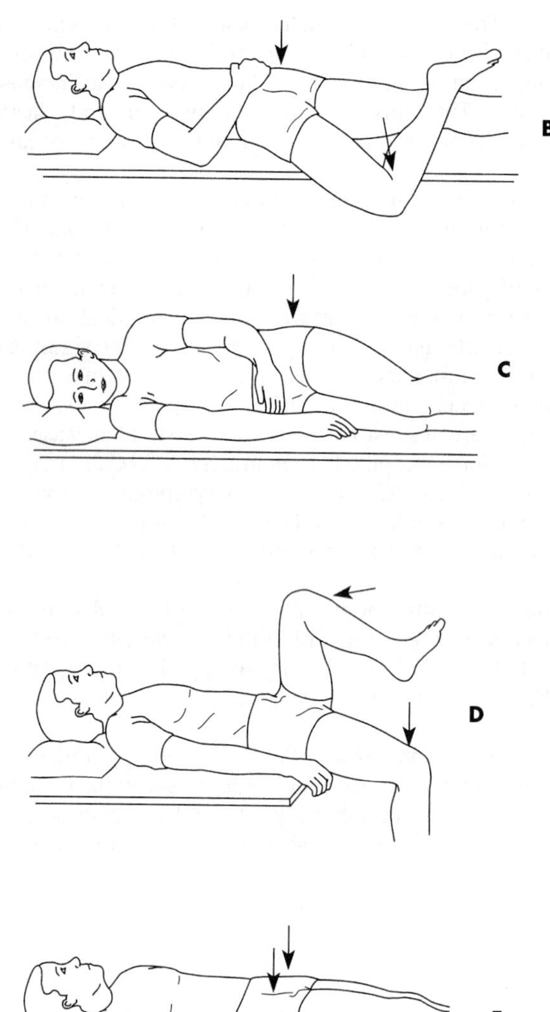
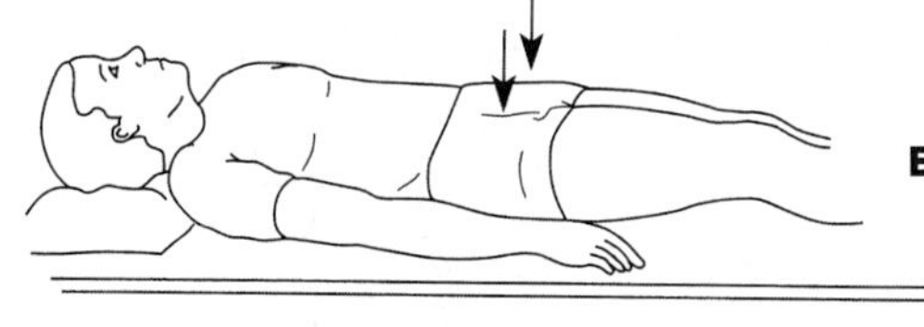

Fig. 137-2. Clinical tests for sacroiliitis. **A,** Application of direct pressure by thumbs over sacroiliac joints to elicit tenderness. **B,** With knee flexed and hip flexed, abducted, and externally rotated, downward pressure applied on flexed knee and contralateral anterosuperior iliac spine. **C,** Compression of pelvis with patient lying on side. **D,** Patient lying supine, with flexed knee pushed maximally toward opposite shoulder. **E,** Anterosuperior iliac spines forced laterally apart. (Modified from Khan MA. In Calin A, editor: *Spondyloarthropathies,* Orlando, Fla, 1984, Grune & Stratton.)

pose some risk for neurologic injury if cervical spine disease is present. Lateral x-ray studies of the neck in flexion and extension are useful to evaluate ROM and infrequent cervical subluxations. The anesthesiologist should be informed regarding mode of intubation.

Laboratory and Radiologic Studies

No laboratory tests are diagnostic. Nonspecific evidence of systemic inflammatory disease frequently includes an elevated erythrocyte sedimentation rate (ESR) and a normochromic normocytic anemia. HLA-B27 testing is most useful as a diagnostic adjunct or when a patient presents with uveitis but is generally not indicated as a screening or routine diagnostic test because of this antigen's prevalence in the general population as well as the prevalence of AS.

Routine anteroposterior (AP) x-ray study of the pelvis often demonstrates symmetric sacroiliitis (Fig. 137-3). In early disease, radiologic abnormalities may be unilateral, subtle, or inapparent. SI joint views can better demonstrate these findings in mild cases. Computed tomography (CT) and magnetic resonance imaging (MRI) scans have the greater sensitivities. Both plain SI joint views and CT scans are associated with greater radiation exposure to the gonads than are routine pelvic x-ray studies. X-ray studies of the spine and inflamed entheses can reveal bony erosions, osteitis, ossification, or syndesmophytes (Fig. 137-4). Bony ankylosis is a characteristic but late finding. Osteoporosis of the spine, kyphosis, and symmetric joint space narrowing of the hips and shoulders may be present.

Clinical Course

Expression of AS is highly variable. The course tends to progress slowly, punctuated with acute flares. Severe, unrelenting AS resulting in complete ankylosis of the spine and hips is uncommon. Life expectancy is not reduced. Most patients maintain good functional capacity and continue to work.[11] Frequently the first 10 years of AS can serve as a rough barometer of disease severity over a patient's lifetime. If the hips and other peripheral joints are not involved within the first decade of disease, they are unlikely to become affected later.

REITER'S SYNDROME AND REACTIVE ARTHRITIS

Reiter's syndrome is probably the most common cause of asymmetric inflammatory arthritis of the lower extremities in young men. The term *Reiter's syndrome* is gradually being supplanted by *reactive arthritis* (ReA). This latter term

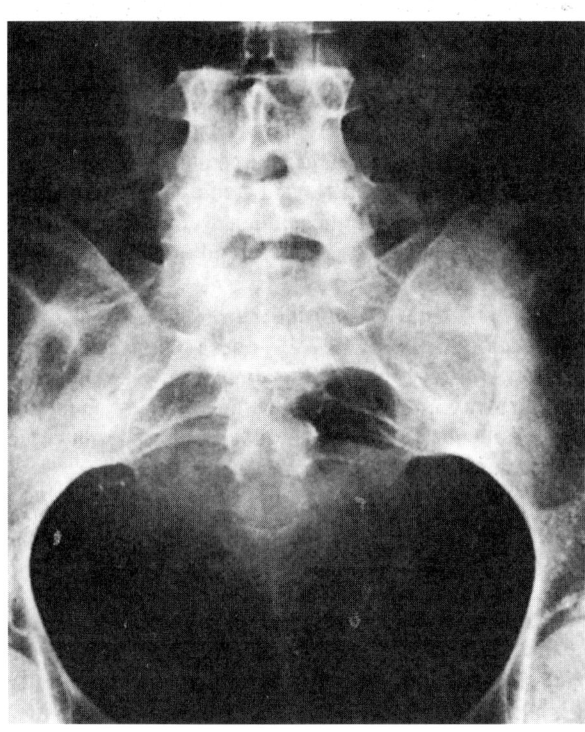

Fig. 137-3. Ankylosing spondylitis. Total ankylosis of right sacroiliac joint and moderate change in left joint. Juxtaarticular sclerosis, joint space narrowing, and irregularity, with partial fusion. (From Stein JH: *Internal medicine,* ed 4, St Louis, 1994, Mosby.)

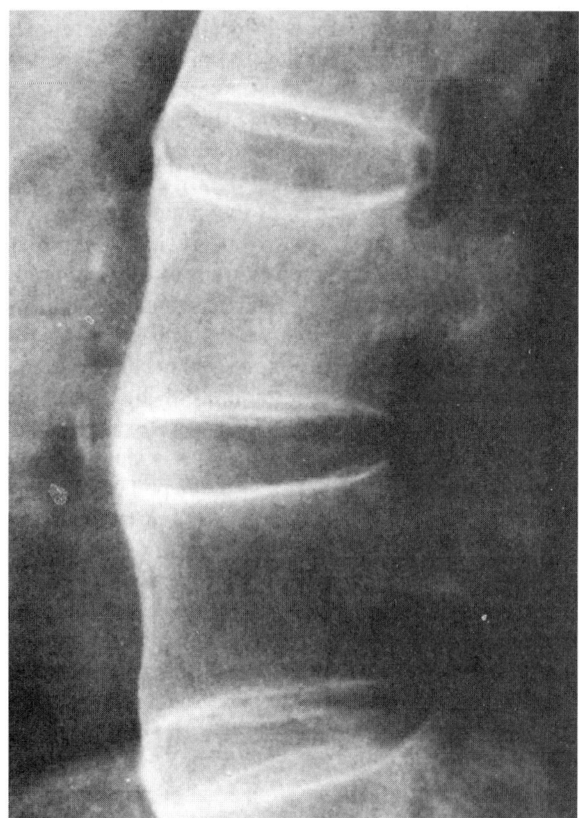

Fig. 137-4. Ankylosing spondylitis; same patient as in Fig. 137-3. Ossification in anterior fibers of anulus fibrosus between lumbar vertebrae. (From Stein JH: *Internal medicine,* ed 4, St Louis, 1994, Mosby.)

encompasses a broader group of patients, in whom inflammatory arthritis develops after an infection, usually in the genitourinary (GU) or GI tract; reactive arthritides are also distinguished on the basis of antecedent infection sites by referring to them as postvenereal (GU) and postenteric (GI). The term *B27-associated ReA* is used to emphasize the heterogeneity of these diseases and to differentiate them from other postinfectious diseases, such as rheumatic fever.[7] Reiter's syndrome is still used to describe postvenereal ReA.

Epidemiology

Approximately 1% of patients develop ReA after nongonococcal urethritis associated with *Chlamydia trachomatis.* Similarly, 2% to 3% of patients develop ReA after an enteric infection with one of the *Salmonella* species, *Shigella flexneri, Campylobacter jejuni,* or *Yersinia.*[6] *Yersinia*-associated ReA is reported more often in other countries and is rare in the United States. Approximately 60% to 80% of patients who develop ReA have HLA-B27 antigen, and conversely, approximately 20% of B27-positive individuals will develop ReA after exposure to the organisms listed. The postenteric form displays equal gender distribution, whereas the postvenereal type has a male predominance.

Patient Evaluation

ReA is a multisystem disorder and often unrecognized. The classic Reiter's syndrome triad of arthritis, urethritis, and conjunctivitis is frequently not present or is not identified. Arthritis typically develops 1 to 3 weeks after the GU or GI infection. Urethritis symptoms may be quite subtle and in women are often absent. Constitutional symptoms of fever and weight loss may be present, particularly during the acute phase, but are usually mild.

The hallmark of ReA is the development of a sterile synovitis and enthesitis similar to that seen in AS. Although ReA favors the joints of the lower extremities, especially the knees, ankles, and feet, the upper extremities may also be affected. Early in the illness, the patient complains of joint stiffness, myalgias, and low back pain. Initial physical findings may be scant. The combination of tenosynovitis, periostitis, and arthritis affecting the fingers or toes may give rise to a characteristic diffuse swelling known as *sausage digits* (Fig. 137-5). Sacroiliitis and axial involvement occur less often in ReA than in AS. Sacroiliitis is frequently unilateral and often is not identified by conventional radiology early in the illness. True spinal ankylosis occurs much less frequently than in AS. A B27-positive individual is more likely to develop inflammatory back symptoms. Urethritis, the primary feature of postvenereal ReA, can be a secondary feature in the postenteric form. Dysuria, urinary frequency, urethral erythema, and prostatitis are common in males, whereas urethritis and cervicitis are often undetected in females.

Approximately 20% of patients with the postvenereal form of ReA develop the classic skin lesion, *keratoderma blennorrhagicum* (Fig. 137-6). It is strikingly similar to

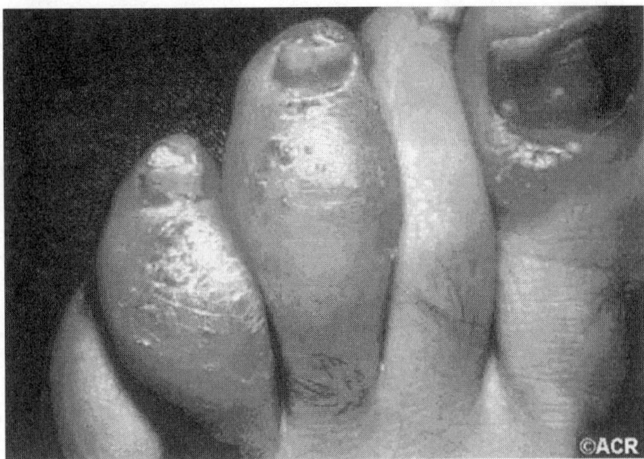

Fig. 137-5. Sausage toes, or dactylitis, in patient with psoriasis. Sausage swelling is combination of tenosynovitis, periostitis, and arthritis. It can also occur in patients with reactive arthritis. (From American College of Rheumatology: *Clinical slide collection on the rheumatic diseases*, Atlanta, 1998, The College.)

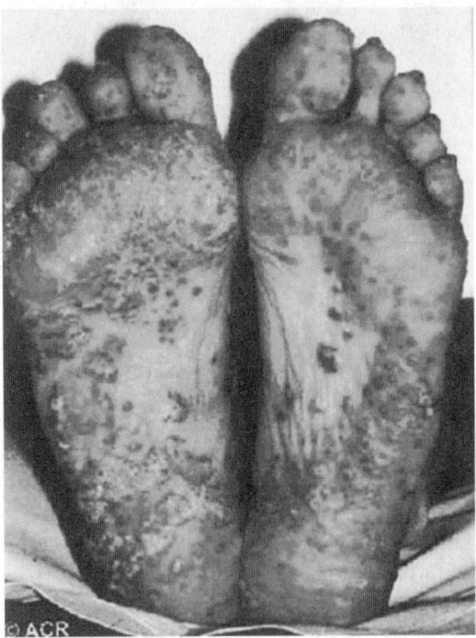

Fig. 137-6. Feet of patient with Reiter's syndrome. Vesicles on erythematous base have become sterile pustules. Development of keratotic scales (keratoderma blennorrhagicum) is most evident on right sole. (From American College of Rheumatology: *Clinical slide collection on the rheumatic diseases*, Atlanta, 1998, The College.)

pustular psoriasis and typically affects the soles of the feet but can also involve the genitalia, scalp, and trunk. Nails may show onycholysis and thickening. *Circinate balanitis* produces small, usually painless superficial erosions on the glans penis (Fig. 137-7). The oral mucosa is also frequently affected by painless, superficial ulcerations. Conjunctivitis, which can be mild and asymptomatic, occurs often, whereas acute anterior uveitis, another ocular manifestation, is strongly associated with B27-positive patients. Cardiac, pulmonary, renal, and neurologic complications may occur in similar pattern and frequency as in AS.

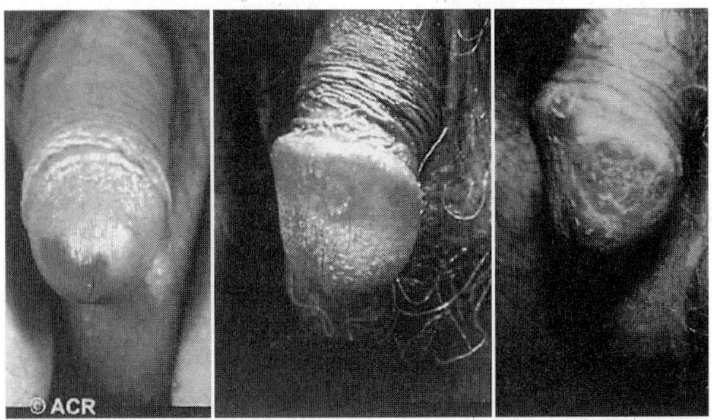

Fig. 137-7. Circinate balanitis in Reiter's syndrome. Lesion is painless, regardless of stage. *Left,* Earliest lesion is erythematous and moist. Other lesions may be pustular or vesicular initially, then progress to discrete circumscribed lesions. *Right,* Late changes are dry, scaly, and hyperkeratotic. (From American College of Rheumatology: *Clinical slide collection on the rheumatic diseases*, Atlanta, 1998, The College.)

Laboratory and Radiologic Studies

No definitive tests can establish a diagnosis of ReA. Since aggressive treatment with antibiotics may improve the natural history of postchlamydial ReA, *Chlamydia* organisms should be identified and treated accordingly.[10] It is still not clear whether aggressive treatment of the responsible bowel pathogens has the same beneficial effect on the natural history of the postenteric form.

The synovial fluid from an inflamed joint is usually inflammatory but is otherwise nondiagnostic. Analysis of the fluid is important to exclude infection and crystal disease. The ESR is often elevated. Leukocytosis and normochromic normocytic anemia may occur. HLA-B27 determination may help diagnostically in difficult cases, particularly in the evaluation of an uncharacterized chronic monoarticular or pauciarticular arthritis without other distinguishing features. This antigen can also provide prognostic information about the development of uveitis and axial disease.

The enthesopathic features of ReA may cause periostitis, erosions, and reactive new bone formation. Periosteal spurs occur most frequently in the feet and heels. Axial disease, including sacroiliitis, may be seen, although it is often not radiographically evident early in the disease.

Clinical Course

ReA is marked by bouts of exacerbation and remission. Typically, the first episode subsides in 3 to 6 months. Skin manifestations may persist longer. Severity varies considerably. The postvenereal form has a greater propensity for chronic arthritis, enthesitis, uveitis, and other extraarticular manifestations than the postenteric form. This difference may be related to degrees of arthritogenicity of the various organisms, the difficulty in completely eradicating *Chlamydia* organisms from the GU tract, or recurrent antigen exposure. A significant minority of patients develop persistent joint symptoms and chronic axial involvement similar to AS.

Human Immunodeficiency Virus

Human immunodeficiency virus (HIV) infection has been associated with a broad spectrum of cutaneous and musculoskeletal disorders, including arthritis and enthesopathies (see Chapter 32). The significance of these rheumatic associations, however, is still controversial. ReA, the first rheumatic disease associated with HIV infection, can develop before, simultaneously with, or after signs of immunodeficiency. ReA associated with HIV disease is often more severe, with pronounced constitutional symptoms and aggressive arthritis and enthesitis.[2] Involvement of the foot and ankle is common and often debilitating, altering the gait, interfering with ambulation, and leading to the "AIDS foot." Enthesopathy also affects the upper extremities. Hip and axial skeleton involvement is uncommon. Severe muscle atrophy may be prominent. Standard therapy with nonsteroidal antiinflammatory drugs (NSAIDs) is often inadequate.

The importance of HIV's association with ReA is twofold. First, the physician must consider early HIV infection in a patient presenting with Reiter's syndrome, psoriatic arthritis, or other unexplained monoarticular or pauciarticular arthritis. Second, HIV infection should be excluded before administering immunosuppressive therapy for refractory disease. Because of the severity of clinical manifestations and difficult treatment issues, a rheumatologist, a dermatologist, and infectious disease experts may be consulted to help coordinate management.

PSORIATIC ARTHRITIS

Psoriasis affects 1% to 2% of the North American white population but is less prevalent in the African-American and Native American populations. Since psoriasis is a common disease, inflammatory or noninflammatory arthritis may coexist in psoriatic patients and may not be directly related to psoriasis. Thus the true incidence of psoriatic arthritis (PsA) in patients with psoriasis is unknown, and estimates have ranged widely, from 6% to 42%. In addition, a small percentage of patients (approximately 15%) develop arthritis that may precede the onset of skin disease. PsA affects an estimated 5% to 8% of patients with psoriasis. Men and women are equally affected, but in the subsets of PsA, male predominance occurs in the spondylitic form, whereas female predominance occurs in the rheumatoid form. Onset occurs usually in the second or third decade of life but can be as late as the sixth decade. In the subset of psoriatic patients who develop spondylitis or sacroiliitis, HLA-B27 is present in 50%. The etiology of psoriasis and PsA is unknown. The causes are likely multifactorial and include genetic predisposition, with humoral and cellular abnormalities. Trauma and other environmental factors may exacerbate joint disease with the development of acroosteolysis. Infections, whether related to streptococci in the skin or to HIV, may also have some role in the pathogenesis of PsA.

Patient Evaluation

Skin disease precedes the onset of articular manifestation in 75% of patients with PsA. Concomitant presentation of skin and joint disease occurs in 10% to 15%. The remaining patients develop skin disease after the onset of inflammatory arthritis.

Five major forms of PsA have been described (Box 137-1). The most common form is an *asymmetric, oligoarticular* (i.e., fewer than five joints) *arthritis,* which affects 60% to 70% of PsA patients. Large and small joints may be affected. Dactylitis, or sausage digits, is another common feature (see Fig. 137-5). Although the majority of patients are initially categorized into this group, many progress to develop asymmetric polyarthritis.

Box 137-1. Patterns of Psoriatic Arthritis

Asymmetric, oligoarticular arthritis (60% to 70%)
Symmetric polyarticular arthritis (15% to 25%)
Isolated distal interphalangeal joint disease (5%)
Arthritis mutilans (5%)
Isolated sacroiliitis and spondylitis (5%)

Symmetric polyarthritis, clinically indistinguishable from rheumatoid arthritis (RA), is the second most common form, affecting 15% to 25% of PsA patients. Patients are rheumatoid factor (RF) negative and have no rheumatoid nodules. Distal interphalangeal (DIP) joint involvement, not typically described in RA, occurs in this form of PsA. In addition, radiographic evidence of proximal interphalangeal (PIP) or DIP joint ankylosis helps to differentiate the two diseases.

Isolated DIP joint involvement occurs in only 5% of PsA patients. This form of arthritis is associated with nail bed changes, including multiple nail pits and onycholysis (Fig. 137-8).

Arthritis mutilans, a progressively destructive form of arthritis, also occurs in 5% of patients. Starting as DIP joint disease, the arthritis progresses with osteolysis of the phalanges, resulting in telescoping of digits or pencil-in-cup deformities on radiographs. Many of these patients also have sacroiliitis and severe skin involvement.

Isolated spondylitis/sacroiliitis also affects only about 5% of PsA patients. Inflammatory back symptoms are present. Psoriatic spondylitis may be difficult to distinguish from AS except for the presence of psoriasis. Sacroiliitis is more often radiographically asymmetric than AS. In addition, the syndesmophytes are usually nonmarginal and asymmetric, in contrast to the marginal, symmetric pattern of AS.

As with all classification schemes, some patients may not be categorized easily into one of the five subsets. Others may evolve from one pattern to another or may overlap between subsets. Often, axial involvement is silent. About 20% to 40% of PA patients have sacroiliitis on plain radiographs, but almost two thirds of these patients are asymptomatic. Enthesitis also occurs in PsA, contributing to the sausage deformities, plantar fasciitis, heel spurs, and syndesmophyte formation in the axial spine.

Skin involvement is the predominant extraarticular feature of PsA. Since most patients have skin diseases that antedate or parallel the onset of their arthritis, the diagnosis is not difficult. Patients who present with only asymmetric arthritis, tenosynovitis, or inflammatory back pain, however, require a careful search for occult skin lesions, with examination of the scalp, umbilicus, intergluteal fold, groin, external acoustic

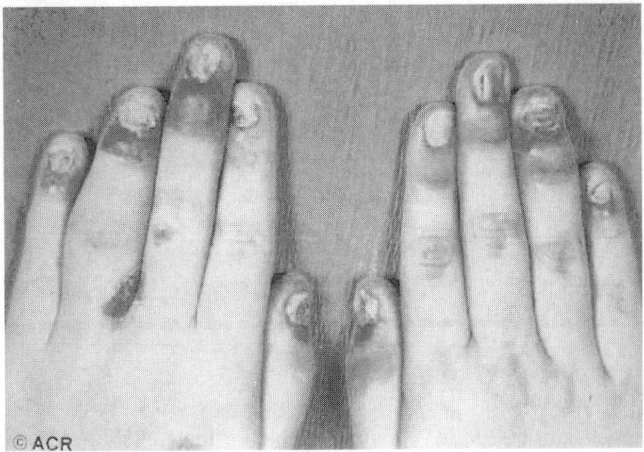

Fig. 137-8. Psoriatic arthritis with nail, skin, and joint involvement. Distal interphalangeal joint involvement in both hands is characterized by swelling and erythema. Prominent soft tissue swelling or dactylitic changes are seen at fourth proximal interphalangeal joint. Nail changes include fragmentation and lifting of nail away from the base caused by hyperkeratosis. (From American College of Rheumatology: *Clinical slide collection on the rheumatic diseases*, Atlanta, 1998, The College.)

meatus, and perineum. Extensive nail pitting (greater than 20 pits per nail) and subungual hyperkeratosis are present in 80% of PsA patients; similar nail changes are found in only 20% to 30% of patients with isolated skin disease.

Aortic insufficiency and apical pulmonary fibrosis are rare complications and are associated only with patients who have spondylitis. Inflammatory eye disease occurs in approximately 30% but usually consists of conjunctivitis rather than nongranulomatous uveitis.

Laboratory and Radiologic Studies

No specific laboratory studies can confirm the diagnosis of PsA. Nonspecific indicators of inflammation are present. RF or positive antinuclear antibodies (ANAs) are present in a small percentage of patients, but these findings are likely to reflect the baseline positive rate in the general population.

Radiographic features help distinguish PsA from some of the other inflammatory arthritides (Box 137-2). In the peripheral joints the asymmetric pattern of joint involvement, along with DIP disease, are important clues. Periarticular osteopenia, a classic finding in RA, is absent in PsA despite erosive changes. Tuft resorption, bony ankylosis, and periostitis are other common features of PsA that are uncommon in RA. Axial involvement in PsA is similar to that of ReA and can usually be distinguished from AS (Table 137-1). Asymmetric, nonmarginal syndesmophytes in the thoracolumbar region, paravertebral ossification, vertebral fusion, and disk space calcification are features of psoriatic spondylitis.

Clinical Course

Initially described as being relatively benign, PsA may be as severe and deforming as RA. Development of deformities may depend on severity of initial presentation. Poor prognostic indicators include multiple joint effusions (greater than five) at presentation, high level of medication use, low ESR, and presence of particular HLA antigens.

Box 137-2. Radiographic Findings Common to Psoriatic Arthritis and Reactive Arthritis

Erosions without periarticular osteopenia
Distal phalangeal tuft resorption
Soft tissue swelling
Pencil-in-cup deformities
Periostitis

Table 137-1. Radiographic Features of the Spondyloarthropathies

Feature	AS/IBD	ReA/PsA
Sacroiliitis	Bilateral	Unilateral
Syndesmophytes	Marginal	Nonmarginal
	Symmetric	Asymmetric
	Continuous	Skip levels
Vertebral bodies	Squaring	Less squaring
Apophyseal fusion	Common	Less common

ARTHROPATHY OF INFLAMMATORY BOWEL DISEASE

The first associations between bowel disease and arthritis were described in the early 1900s. Despite these descriptions, however, the distinct entity of inflammatory arthritis occurring in patients with IBD was not accepted in the medical community until after 1960. Currently, musculoskeletal involvement is the most common extraarticular manifestation of IBD.

The etiology of IBD arthropathy is unknown (see Chapter 108). No HLA-B27 association has been established in patients with peripheral arthritis or asymptomatic sacroiliitis. In contrast, 50% to 75% of IBD patients with symptomatic spondylitis are HLA-B27 positive. Given these genetic and clinical differences, researchers believe that a different pathogenesis may exist for each group. Since HLA-B27 is associated with spondylitis patients, the pathogenesis in this group may be similar to theories for idiopathic AS. In the peripheral arthritis subset, since clinical disease parallels bowel disease, mechanisms directly related to gut inflammation might be more applicable.

Patient Evaluation

Peripheral Arthritis. The incidence of peripheral arthropathy in IBD patients is 15% to 20%, with a more frequent occurrence in Crohn's disease (20%) than in ulcerative colitis (12%) patients. In addition, peripheral arthritis is more frequently associated with colonic than with ileal involvement in Crohn's disease. Peripheral joint involvement classically begins with or after the onset of bowel disease.[12] Subsequent flares also parallel disease activity in the bowel. Males and females are equally affected.

Joint involvement is typically asymmetric, oligoarticular, often migratory, and lasts for weeks to months but rarely becomes chronic. The most common joint affected is the knee, followed by the ankle, elbow, and wrist. Smaller joint involvement occurs less often. Enthesopathy, such as tendinitis and plantar fasciitis, may develop. Other extraarticular features of IBD, including the skin, mucous membranes, and eyes, often are concurrently active. Erosive deformities rarely develop (less than 10%) but seem to involve large joints, particularly hips and shoulders. In the few cases of erosive arthropathy, granulomatous synovitis may be responsible.

Axial Arthropathy. Two subsets of IBD-associated axial arthropathy exist: (1) asymptomatic sacroiliitis noted on plain radiographs and (2) symptomatic axial disease clinically indistinguishable from idiopathic AS. The incidence of asymptomatic sacroiliitis may be as high as 29%, but frank AS occurs in only 2% to 8% of IBD patients. In contrast to peripheral arthropathy, axial skeletal disease does not correlate with IBD activity. Spondylitis often precedes the development of active bowel disease by many years, thus making the diagnosis difficult. Unfortunately, even when IBD is under control or in remission, axial disease may persist or progress. Men are affected more often than women, but not to the degree in idiopathic AS. Classically, the symptoms of inflammatory back pain develop insidiously. Peripheral arthritis may coexist with axial disease and extraarticular features.

Laboratory and Radiologic Studies

Laboratory tests are nonspecific. RF is usually negative, and ESR and other indicators of inflammation are elevated. Chronic anemia may exist. Synovial fluid is inflammatory, with white blood cell counts varying from 5000 to 50,000/mm^3.

Radiographs of peripheral joints usually reveal only soft tissue swelling without erosive changes. The axial findings may include shoulder and hip joint space narrowing, vertebral body squaring, symmetric sacroiliitis, osteitis pubis, marginal syndesmophytes, and progressive bony bridging cephalad, beginning in the lumbar region. All these features are indistinguishable from idiopathic AS (see Figs. 137-3 and 137-4 and Table 137-1).

UNDIFFERENTIATED SPONDYLOARTHROPATHY

The current categories of spondyloarthropathies are often inadequate to encompass a spectrum of patients who may have oligoarthritis, enthesopathy, dactylitis, or inflammatory back symptoms without antecedent infection, GI symptoms, or dermatologic abnormalities. Thus the term *undifferentiated spondyloarthropathies* encompasses those patients with one or more of the features of spondyloarthropathy but who do not fulfill the criteria for established disease categories. The European Spondyloarthropathy Study Group developed criteria to broaden the definition of spondyloarthropathy (Box 137-3). Long-term follow-up of these patients reveals that 50% develop a defined spondyloarthropathy, 40% obtain remission, and only 10% continue with recurrent oligoarticular arthritis.

Box 137-3. Criteria for Spondyloarthropathy

Inflammatory spinal pain *or* synovitis (asymmetric or predominantly in lower limb) *and* one or more of the following:
- Positive family history for ankylosing spondylitis
- Psoriasis
- Inflammatory bowel disease
- Urethritis, cervicitis, or acute diarrhea within 1 month before arthritis
- Alternating buttock pain
- Enthesopathy (inflammation at ligamentous attachment to bone)
- Sacroiliitis

From Dougados M, van der Linden S, Nakache J: European Spondyloarthropathy Study Group (ESSG): Preliminary criteria for the classification of spondyloarthropathy, *Arthritis Rheum* 34:1218, 1991.)

DIFFERENTIAL DIAGNOSIS

When a patient presents with classic inflammatory back symptoms and extraarticular features, the primary care physician can easily establish the diagnosis. If the disease presents insidiously and the various symptoms and signs span many years, however, the diagnosis is less obvious and may elude the physician. The differential diagnosis of spondyloarthropathies can be separated into three categories: back pain, peripheral arthritis, and peripheral arthritis with back pain (Box 137-4). Low back pain is extremely common and has a broad differential (see earlier and Chapter 127). Osteoarthritis, infection (particularly in injection drug users), hyperparathyroidism, paraplegia and quadriplegia, and osteitis condensans ilii (primarily in multiparous women) can affect SI joints. These can usually be distinguished clinically and radiologically. Diffuse idiopathic skeletal hyperostosis (DISH) may be initially confused with AS, but DISH is a condition of older individuals, and both disorders have characteristic radiographic features.

Peripheral arthritis may be the initial or only manifestation of a spondyloarthropathy. The arthritis is classically monoarticular or oligoarticular but is sometimes polyarticular. Early RA, acute crystal disease (e.g., gout, pseudogout), acute or chronic infections (e.g., Lyme disease arthritis), osteoarthritis, sarcoidosis, and synovial neoplasm are within the differential diagnosis. Synovial fluid analysis includes crystal studies and cultures. Serologies may be helpful in the evaluation. Occasionally, synovial biopsy is necessary to exclude atypical infectious arthritis.

Disseminated gonorrheal infection (DGI) can closely resemble ReA in its articular and nonarticular features. The epidemiology of the two diseases is similar, occurring in the sexually active population. The rash of DGI is usually vesiculopustular, however, and can be easily distinguished from keratoderma blennorrhagicum. Appropriate sites (blood, joint, skin, vagina, urethra, throat, rectum) should be cultured if DGI is suspected. The diseases also may coexist in the same patient.

The symmetric pattern of PsA may be confused with RA, but PsA lacks RF, rheumatoid nodules, and swan-neck or boutonnière deformities. The involvement of DIP joints, absence of periarticular osteopenia, presence of bony ankylosis, periostitis, acroosteolysis, and bony resorption are typical for PsA or ReA but are unusual for RA. Osteoarthritis of the DIP or PIP joints, especially erosive osteoarthritis, may

Box 137-4. Differential Diagnosis for Spondyloarthropathies

Axial Arthritis

- Diskogenic back pain
- Osteoarthritis
  - Facet disease
  - Diffuse idiopathic hypertrophic osteoarthropathy
  - Osteoarthritis of sacroiliac joints
- Osteitis condensans ilii
- Infection (sacroiliitis)
  - Tuberculosis, brucellosis*
  - Bacteremia from injection drug abuse
- Others
  - Whipple's disease*
  - Behçet's syndrome*
  - Relapsing polychondritis
  - Secondary hyperparathyroidism

Peripheral Arthritis

- Other inflammatory arthritides
  - Rheumatoid arthritis
  - Crystals
- Infections
  - *Borrelia burgdorferi* (Lyme disease)
  - Gonococcal
  - Poststreptococcal, acute rheumatic fever*
  - Human immunodeficiency virus
  - Chronic fungal or tuberculous
- Noninflammatory arthritides
  - Osteoarthritis, particularly inflammatory osteoarthritis
  - Mechanical derangement
- Synovial neoplasia
  - Pigmented villonodular synovitis*
  - Osteogenic sarcoma*
  - Synovial osteochondromatosis*
- Sarcoidosis

Axial and Peripheral Arthritis

- Osteoarthritis
- Rheumatoid arthritis
- Whipple's disease*
- Behçet's syndrome*
- Relapsing polychondritis*
- Familial Mediterranean fever*

*Rare occurrences.

be confused with PsA or ReA. Bouchard's nodes (osteoarthritic involvement of PIP joints) and carpometacarpal joint disease are more consistent with osteoarthritis. Radiographically, osteophyte formation or the central erosions of erosive osteoarthritis help distinguish osteoarthritis from PsA and ReA.

The physician may not initially suspect enthesitis when a patient complains of pain or swelling in a tendon or ligamentous area. Tender areas are common in fibromyalgia. Mechanical overuse or calcific tendinitis resembles enthesopathy, particularly in the shoulder, Achilles tendon, and plantar fascia. Drugs such as retinoids or fluorides may produce plantar fasciitis or ossification, respectively. Achilles tendinitis has been associated with fluoroquinolone therapy. Recurrent or persistent tenosynovitis with inflammatory features or in atypical locations (e.g., toes, fingers, heels) should alert the physician to include spondyloarthropathies in the differential diagnosis.

Osteoarthritis and RA are common diagnoses for low back pain and peripheral joint disease. More unusual diseases that can involve both areas include Whipple's disease, Behçet's syndrome, relapsing polychondritis, and familial Mediterranean fever. Acquired immunodeficiency syndrome (AIDS) must be considered in the differential diagnosis of patients with ReA or PsA who also have risk factors for HIV infection. Fulminant psoriasis with or without arthritis and ReA has been reported as an initial presentation of HIV infections.

Finally, given the similarities among the spondyloarthropathies, each disease must be included in the differential diagnosis of the other. The separation of Reiter's syndrome (ReA) from PsA can be extremely difficult because the skin lesions and pattern of joint involvement are clinically indistinguishable. However, oral lesions, circinate balanitis, and urethritis are not features of PsA. Reports of an evolution of one spondyloarthropathy into another with time (e.g., the patient with urethritis and arthritis who later develops the skin disease of psoriasis) make the distinction between diseases less clear.

TREATMENT

Treatment for spondyloarthropathies begins with educating patients, since many of these diseases are chronic, often affecting young people during their most active and productive years. Although the pathogenesis of the disease is unknown, patients' understanding of the disease course, the potential factors that may aggravate and improve their arthritis, and the prevention measures are of utmost importance. National associations, patient newsletters, and support groups can provide educational, social, and emotional support. The Spondylitis Association of America provides mutual support, promotes research and education, and publishes useful quarterly newsletters.

Control of the associated medical conditions may have a direct benefit for the various spondyloarthropathies. Since the peripheral arthritis of IBD parallels the activity of bowel disease, treatment of the underlying bowel disease with corticosteroids, sulfasalazine, and other medications is the primary therapy. If a total colectomy is necessary for ulcerative colitis, the peripheral arthritis completely disappears. Joint disease may not resolve after total colectomy in Crohn's disease, however, perhaps because of residual or occult disease in the small intestine. Since the axial arthropathy does not correlate with bowel disease activity, management is very similar to that of idiopathic AS (see following section). Some studies on psoriasis suggest a correlation between improvement of joint disease when the skin disease is aggressively treated.

Appropriate antibiotic therapy should be instituted for patients with acute chlamydial urethritis, but antibiotics do not prevent the development of ReA. Enteric infections usually have cleared when arthritis occurs. Patients with ReA caused by *Chlamydia* may benefit from long-term therapy (3 months) with lymecycline, an antibiotic similar to tetracycline or doxycycline. It is not clear, however, if this beneficial effect results from lymecycline's antibacterial actions or another mechanism.

Nonsteroidal Antiinflammatory Drugs

NSAIDs are the mainstay of pharmacologic intervention in the spondyloarthropathies. More than 20 NSAIDs are available and differ in their half-life, routes of excretion, and interaction with other drugs (Table 137-2). The mechanism of action for all NSAIDs is based on the inhibition of both prostaglandin synthesis and neutrophil function.

Various factors influence the choice of an NSAID in a particular patient (Box 137-5). NSAIDs are contraindicated for patients with active peptic ulcer disease or chronic anticoagulation (nonacetylated salicylates can be used in some patients, if needed, and possibly the new COX-II inhibitor). Concurrent medical problems, such as history of peptic ulcer disease, congestive heart failure, renal insufficiency, hepatic insufficiency, or bleeding diathesis, make NSAIDs relatively contraindicated. The need for the NSAID must be weighed against the patient's other medical problems. Some NSAIDs interact with sulfonylureas, antihypertensives, and anticoagulants. Asthmatic patients or patients with a known allergy to aspirin can develop allergic reactions to NSAIDs. Patients' lifestyles and drug costs are other major factors to consider. Specific cyclooxygenase II (COX-II) inhibitors, which do not interfere with the constitutive effects of cyclooxygenase I on the GI mucosa, are now available (see Chapters 102 and 132). Although rheumatologists traditionally prefer indomethacin to aspirin for ReA, many other NSAIDs are equally effective. High dosages are typically necessary to control the inflammatory process (e.g., indomethacin, 150 to 200 mg/day; naproxen, 1500 mg/day).

Treatment with one NSAID should continue for at least 2 to 4 weeks before the drug is discontinued for a lack of efficacy. When one NSAID fails, another should be chosen from a different chemical class. Frequently, several different NSAIDs are prescribed before the most effective one is established for an individual. Patients should be informed of this rationale, since they often perceive this method as haphazard.

NSAIDs' toxicities are secondary to their antiprostaglandin effects; GI intolerance is the most common. *NSAID gastropathy,* a term that includes superficial gastric erosions, diffuse gastritis, and frank ulcer craters, has great morbidity. Approximately 2% to 5% of patients taking NSAIDs for more than a year may develop ulcers, bleeding, or perforation. Advanced age, additional medical problems, and a history of peptic ulcer disease are risk factors for NSAID gastropathy. Misoprostol, a prostaglandin E_1, was developed to prevent it. Proton pump inhibitors appear to be equally effective in prevention of gastric ulcers and better than misoprostol for duodenal ulcers. Thus guidelines for prevention include use of either drug in high-risk patients.[9] NSAID-induced small bowel and colon injury has also been reported. Renal toxicities include renal insufficiency from decreased renal blood flow, interstitial nephritis, and hyperkalemia. Reversible impairment of platelet aggregation may result in prolonged bleeding. Central nervous system toxicities include headaches, dizziness, mental status changes, and depression. Aseptic meningitis has been reported with ibuprofen, sulindac, naproxen, and tolmetin. Cutaneous reactions are varied. Certain NSAIDs have been reported to exacerbate psoriasis, particularly ibuprofen, indomethacin, and meclofenamate.

Box 137-5. Factors in Choice of NSAID

Age
Preexisting medical conditions
Active or history of peptic ulcer disease
Renal or hepatic insufficiency
Congestive heart failure
Asthma
Bleeding diathesis or chronic anticoagulation
Concurrent medications
Ease of drug dosing
Cost (limits of managed care formulary)

Corticosteroids

Intraarticular corticosteroids may be judiciously used in the peripheral joints of patients with spondyloarthropathies. Occasionally, injection of the plantar fascia, tendon sheath, or deep bursa is helpful if rest, NSAIDs, and orthoses have been ineffective. Systemic steroids have been used for short-term control of severe AS; however, this therapy is not recommended for routine treatment.

Second-line Agents

When NSAIDs and physical measures are ineffective in controlling symptoms or if progressive erosive disease develops in the peripheral joints, a rheumatologic referral to assist with decisions for second-line agents and monitoring for potential toxicities should be considered. Unfortunately, effective therapy to prevent ankylosis in the axial arthropathy has not been established.

Sulfasalazine, a drug initially developed for RA and subsequently used for IBD, has been studied for treatment of patients with AS, ReA, and undifferentiated spondyloarthropathies.[3] Results reveal some benefit for spondylitic symptoms in the short term, but whether the drug modifies the long-term outcome of AS is unknown. Sulfasalazine appears to be more effective for peripheral arthritis of AS or for ReA.[1] Its mechanism of actions may include reduction of intestinal mucosal inflammation and permeability or direct reduction of mediators of inflammation. Sulfasalazine has also been used in psoriasis and PsA with success. Doses range from 2 to 3 gm daily. Enteric-coated tablets given with food may reduce GI intolerance (see Chapter 133).

Methotrexate, a folate antagonist, has been used effectively for PsA since the 1960s. Initially, dermatologists used methotrexate for skin diseases, but beneficial effects on joints were coincidentally noted. Methotrexate is administered orally, subcutaneously, or intramuscularly on a weekly basis, beginning with 7.5 to 15 mg per week and titrated up to 20 to 30 mg based on response. Methotrexate has also been used for intractable Reiter's syndrome. Before instituting methotrexate, HIV infection must be excluded. Onset of AIDS has occurred in patients after methotrexate was started for severe psoriasis or ReA. Trimethoprim is contraindicated for patients who take methotrexate because of its additive antifolate effects (see Chapter 133).

Parenteral gold is also effective in the treatment of PsA. Although most studies have not been prospectively

Table 137-2. Nonsteroidal Antiinflammatory Drugs (NSAIDs) Used to Treat Seronegative Spondyloarthropathies

Drug	Metabolism/excretion	Half-life (hours)	Total daily dosage (mg)	Dosing frequency	Adverse effects: GI*	Adverse effects: Central nervous system	Adverse effects: Others
Propionic acid							
Fenoprofen	Liver	2-3	1200-3200	3-4	++		Interstitial nephritis; Papillary necrosis
Flurbiprofen	Liver, kidney	6	200-300	2-3			
Ibuprofen	Liver, kidney (1%-14%)	2	1600-3200	3-4	++	Confusion; Aseptic meningitis	Drug-induced lupus
Ketoprofen	Liver	2-4	150-300	3-4	++		
Naproxen	Kidney	13	500-1000	2-3	++	Confusion	
Oxaprozin	Liver	21	600-1800	1-2	++		
Ketorolac†	Kidney	4-9	120 (IM)	4-6	++	Sedation, headaches, somnolence (IM and PO)	
			40-60 (PO)	4-6	++		
Indoleacetic acid							
Indomethacin	Liver	2	75-200	3-4	+++	Headaches; Confusion	Thrombocytopenia
Sulindac	Enterohepatic circulation	8	300-400	2	+++	Aseptic meningitis	
Tolmetin	Liver	1-2	600-1600	3-4	++	Aseptic meningitis	
Etodolac	Kidney, bile	6-8	400-600	2	++		
Phenylacetic acid							
Diclofenac	Bile 35%, kidney 65%	2	150-200	2-4			
Enolic acid							
Piroxicam	Liver	30-86	10-20	1	+++		
Mefenamic acid							
Meclofenamate	Liver	2-3	300-400	3-4			Diarrhea; Coombs-positive hemolytic anemia
Salicylates							
Aspirin	Liver	4-15	1000-6000	2-4	+++		Tinnitus, hepatitis, thrombocytopenia
Choline magnesium trisalicylate	Liver	4-15	1500-4000	2-4	+		
Salicylsalicylate	Liver	4-15	1500-5000	2-4	+		
Diflunisal	Liver	7-15	500-1500	2	+++		
COX-II inhibitors							
Celecoxib	Liver	11	200-400	2	+		
Rofecoxib	Liver	17	12.5-25	1	+		
Other							
Nabumetone	Liver	21	1000-2000	1	++		

Modified from Liu NY, Giansiracusa DF, Strongwater SL: Collagen vascular disease in the intensive care unit. In Rippe JM et al, editors: *Intensive care medicine,* Boston, 1995, Little, Brown.

*Gastrointestinal: + mild; ++, moderate; +++, severe and may require discontinuation of drug.

[illegible] It has all the potential gastrointestinal, renal, and hematologic toxicities as other NSAIDs. *IM,* Intramuscular; *PO,* oral.

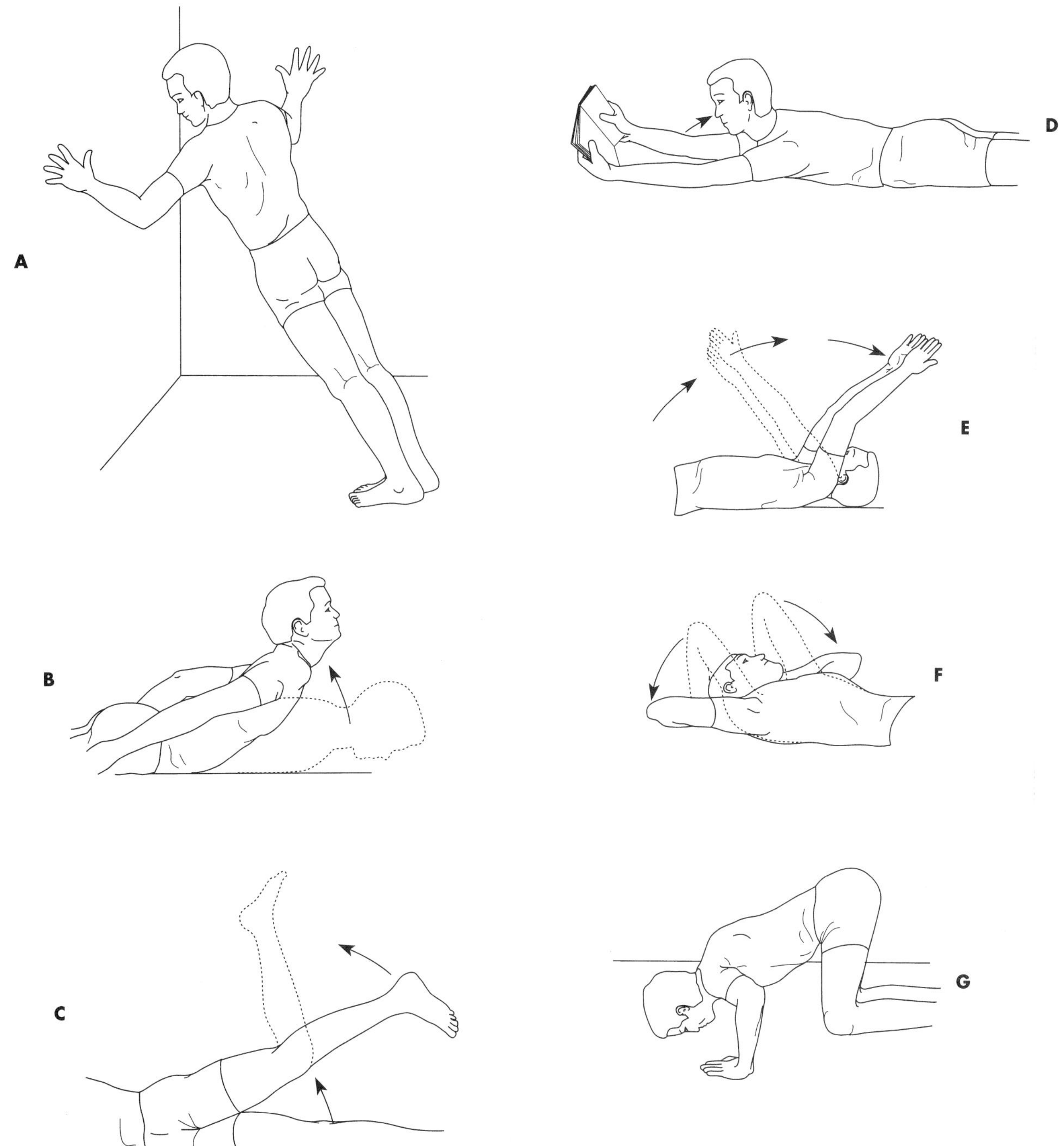

Fig. 137-9. Regular exercises for patients with ankylosing spondylitis and other spondyloarthropathies with axial involvement. Most of these exercises do not require further explanation, except "corner push-up" **(A).** Patient stands 2 feet or more from corner, places both hands on wall, and then gently leans forward toward corner, keeping heels on ground. Patient inhales (expands chest) and attempts to straighten spine when leaning toward corner, then exhales when returning to starting position. (Modified from Khan MA. In Calin A, editor: *Spondyloarthropathies,* Orlando, Fla, 1984, Grune & Stratton.)

Continued

controlled, 60% to 75% of the patients improved on parenteral gold therapy. When compared with a rheumatoid population, drug intolerance was less in PsA. Patients with peripheral arthritis responded best. Gold had no effect on the spondylitic patients. It also had no beneficial effects on the skin, although gold did not exacerbate underlying skin disease.

Hydroxychloroquine, a drug often used to treat RA and systemic lupus erythematosus (SLE), has been prescribed for PsA and Reiter's syndrome. Exacerbation of psoriasis has been reported anecdotally with hydroxychloroquine use. In recent studies, skin reaction has not been a significant problem, but any antimalarial agent should be used cautiously in psoriatic patients (see Chapters 85 and 133).

Retinoid (vitamin A) derivatives, particularly etretinate, have been studied extensively for the treatment of psoriasis; smaller studies have demonstrated etretinate's effectiveness in treating PsA. Low-dose cyclosporine can successfully and

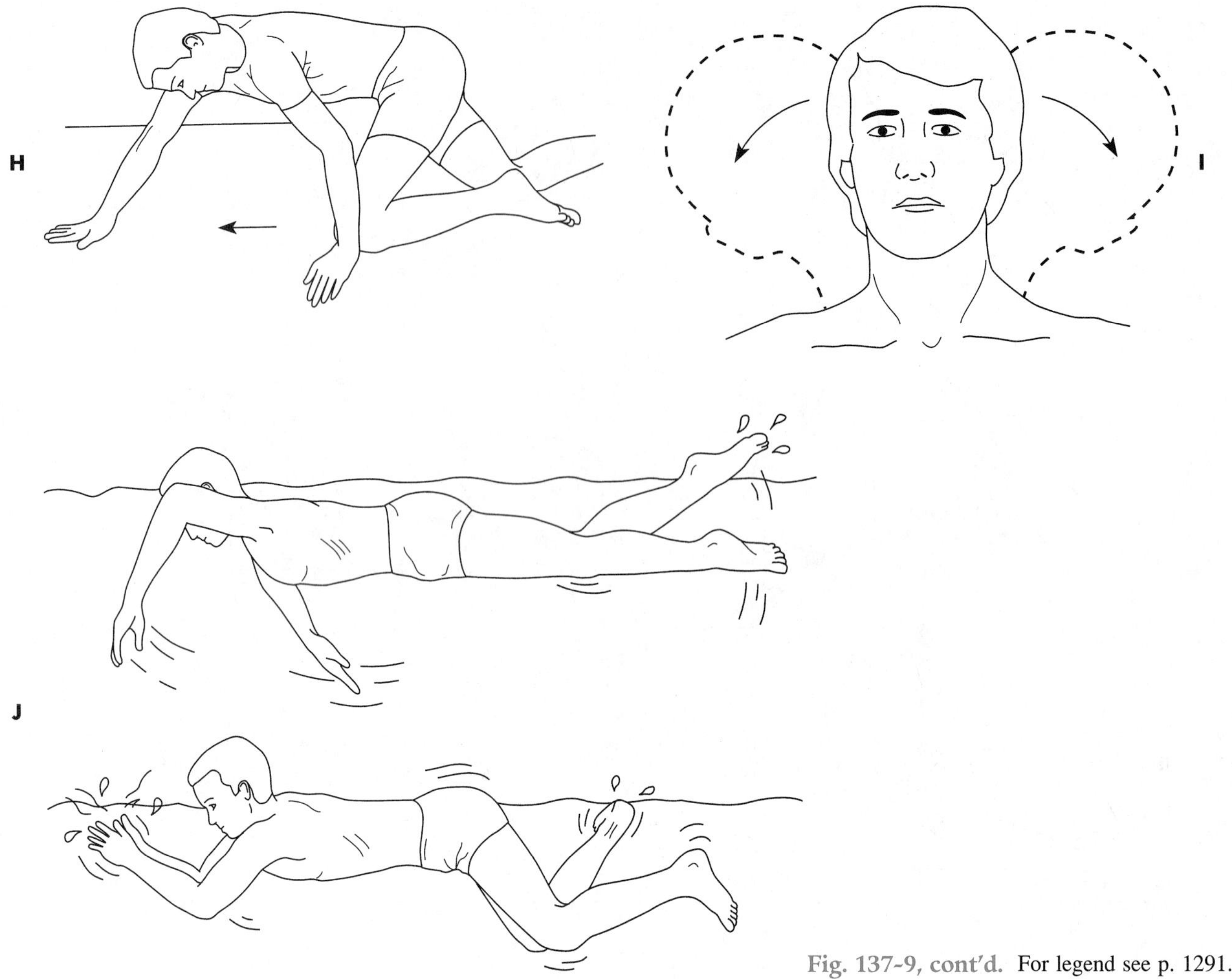

Fig. 137-9, cont'd. For legend see p. 1291.

safely treat psoriatic arthritis unresponsive to other drugs. Etretinate and cyclosporine are additional therapies to consider when methotrexate is ineffective.

Rehabilitative Management

Exercise to maintain muscle tone and function is important for patients with inflammatory arthritis. A programmed routine set by a physical therapist should be the initial step. Often, because of lower extremity disease, even low-impact weight-bearing exercises are not possible. Performing exercises in a heated pool or walking in a pool may be ideal alternatives. Judicious use of splints during acute inflammatory periods may preserve function and alignment of involved joints. Referral to an occupational therapist for splints and assessment of activities of daily living are important for patients with upper extremity involvement.

Patients with ReA or PsA often have foot and ankle involvement. Dactylitis and other small-toe joint involvement result in foot deformities that cannot be accommodated by regular shoes. Prescription shoes with extra depth or a toe box can help. Soft shoe inserts with metatarsal bars redistribute weight away from the metatarsophalangeal joints. Plantar fasciitis may also respond to soft inserts or to local corticosteroid injections. Heel cups provide extra cushioning for symptomatic heel spurs. If multiple midfoot or hindfoot joints are involved, limited periods of casting (less than 7 days) for immobilization can be ordered. Since these patients tend to ankylose joints rapidly, however, prolonged immobilization without diligent ROM exercises is not advisable. Management of Achilles tendinitis is difficult. NSAIDs are the mainstay, with cautious corticosteroid injections. Ice and immobilization may also help.

Axial involvement in any of the spondyloarthropathies should begin with referral to a physical therapist to maintain functional capacity. However, daily back and chest expansion exercises must become ingrained in patients' routines (Fig. 137-9). To minimize spinal flexion deformities, patients should sleep on a firm mattress and thin pillows. Patients should also be instructed to lie for at least 30 minutes each day or night in a prone position (belly down). In addition, protection from injury should be emphasized, since spinal fractures with minimal trauma occur in the osteoporotic spondylitic spine. Thus patients need to avoid prolonged periods of non–weight bearing, maintain adequate dietary intake of calcium and vitamin D, and refrain from sports that can result in spinal injury.

Surgery

Orthopedic intervention may be necessary for patients who have persistent peripheral arthritis despite the various interventions described. Arthroscopic or surgical synovectomy is an option in persistent synovitis of the knee. Total

Box 137-6. Managed Care Guide: Pointers on Management of Seronegative Spondyloarthropathies

1. Consultation with a rheumatologist for complex or suspicious cases, and for the consideration of second-line agents for treatment and consultation of other specialists
2. Patient education, physical and occupational therapy may significantly improve and preserve function
3. Ophthalmologic evaluation for the development of acute anterior uveitis.

joint replacement for severe hip or knee arthritis can be successful, although heterotopic bone formation may influence surgical outcome. Psoriatic patients with aggressive, small-joint arthritis should be referred to hand surgeons early for possible procedures to prevent the mutilans state. Surgical fusion of the wrist may reduce pain and preserve limited function. Persistent tendinitis of the fingers or synovitis at the wrist despite medical therapy may require synovectomy. In AS, cervical fractures at C6-7 and other levels may require stabilization. Rarely, severe flexion deformities of the spine can be corrected by osteotomies, but the procedure carries great risk.

Consultation and Referral

The seronegative spondyloarthropathies are multisystem disorders. The need for consultation depends on such factors as questions about the diagnosis, severity of the clinical manifestations, response to treatment, particular organ system involvement, and physician's familiarity and proficiency in treating these disorders (Box 137-6). Rheumatology consultation remains the cornerstone referral and should usually be sought if the diagnosis is established or suspected. The primary care physician, however, may provide most of the day-to-day management, as well as the long-term follow-up. If the disease is refractory to standard treatment with physical therapy and NSAIDs, or if second-line agents are being considered, a rheumatologist's input becomes even more important.

Patient education, exercise, and physical therapy are mainstays of therapy. A physical therapy consultation is highly recommended when the diagnosis is made. Most programs can be performed at home. A single consultation may be all that is needed.

Acute anterior uveitis, if unrecognized and untreated, can lead to severe ocular sequelae, including blindness. Urgent referral to an ophthalmologist should be made if patients have symptoms. The primary care physician must educate patients about uveitis symptoms so that medical attention is sought promptly.

Consultations with an orthopedist, podiatrist, dermatologist, cardiologist, or pulmonologist may be necessary, depending on each patient's disease manifestations.

REFERENCES

1. Clegg DO, Reda DJ, Weissman MH, et al: Comparison of sulfasalazine and placebo in the treatment of ankylosing spondylitis: a Department of Veterans Affairs cooperative study, *Arthritis Rheum* 39:2004, 1996.
2. Cuellar ML: HIV infections: associated inflammatory musculoskeletal disorders, *Rheum Dis Clin North Am* 24:403, 1998.
3. Dougados M, van der Linden S, Leirisalo-Repo M: Sulfasalazine in the treatment of spondyloarthropathy: a randomized, multicenter, double-blind, placebo-controlled study, *Arthritis Rheum* 38:618, 1995.
4. Dougados M, van der Linden S, Nakache J: European Spondyloarthropathy Study Group (ESSG): Preliminary criteria for the classification of spondyloarthropathy, *Arthritis Rheum* 34:1218, 1991.
5. Feltkamp TE, Ringrose JH: Acute anterior uveitis and spondyloarthropathy, *Curr Opin Rheum* 10:314, 1998.
6. Keat A: Reiter's syndrome and reactive arthritis in perspective, *N Engl J Med* 309:1606, 1983.
7. Khan MA, van der Linden SM: Ankylosing spondylitis and other spondyloarthropathies, *Rheum Dis Clin North Am* 16:551, 1990.
8. Khare SD, Luthra HS, David CS: HLA-B27 and the other predisposing factors in spondyloarthropathies, *Curr Opin Rheum* 10:282, 1998.
9. Lanze FL: A guideline for the treatment and prevention of NSAID-induced ulcers, *Am J Gastroenterol* 93:2037, 1998.
10. Leirisalo-Repo M: Prognosis, course of disease, and treatment of the spondyloarthropathies, *Rheum Dis Clin North Am* 24:737, 1998.
11. Ward MM: Quality of life in patients with ankylosing spondylitis, *Rheum Dis Clin North Am* 24:815, 1998.
12. Weiner SR, Clarke J, Taggart NA, Utsinger PD: Rheumatic manifestations of inflammatory bowel disease, *Semin Arthritis Rheum* 20:353, 1991.

CHAPTER 138

Vasculitis

Leslie R. Harrold
David F. Giansiracusa

The vasculitides are a group of disorders in which inflammation and necrosis of blood vessel walls result in organ system abnormalities caused by thrombosis and hemorrhage. Since vasculitis can involve any vessel in the body, it can result in a wide variety of signs, symptoms, and laboratory abnormalities. The pattern of organ involvement is one of the criteria that help differentiate between vasculitic syndromes. The current classification scheme is based on the clinical presentation, size of involved vessels, histopathology, and associated conditions. If an underlying disease is the cause of the vasculitis, such as systemic lupus erythematosus (SLE) or rheumatoid arthritis (RA), the blood vessel disorder is a secondary vasculitis. Otherwise, the vasculitis is primary (Table 138-1).

EPIDEMIOLOGY

Data on the epidemiology of vasculitic syndromes in the general population are limited. Most information is based on referral center cases, since the syndromes are sufficiently infrequent that population-based data are lacking. The incidence rates of temporal arteritis in persons over 50 years of age include 23.3 per 100,000 biopsy-proven cases in Denmark, 17.0 per 100,000 in Olmsted County, Minnesota, and 1.6 per 100,000 in Tennessee. For Takayasu's arteritis, a rare condition more often described in Asia, the estimated annual incidence in Olmsted County is 2.6 per 1 million. The annual incidence rate for polyarteritis nodosa (PAN) ranges from 4.6 per 1 million in England to 9.9 in Olmsted County,

Table 138-1. Classification of Primary Vasculitides by Vessel Size and Histopathology

Vasculitic syndrome	Pathology	Vessel size	Vessels involved
Takayasu's arteritis	Granulomatous angiitis	Large	Aorta and major branches
Temporal (giant cell) arteritis	Granulomatous angiitis	Large	Aorta and major branches, large and medium-sized arteries (predilection for extracranial branches of carotid artery)
Polyarteritis nodosa	Necrotizing vasculitis	Medium	Large, medium, and small arteries
Churg-Strauss syndrome	Granulomatous angiitis	Medium	Large, medium, and small arteries
Wegener's granulomatosis	Granulomatous angiitis	Medium	Medium and small arteries, venules, and arterioles
Microscopic polyangiitis	Necrotizing vasculitis	Medium	Medium and small arteries, venules, and arterioles
Kawasaki disease (syndrome)	Necrotizing vasculitis	Medium	Medium and small arteries, venules, and arterioles
Hypersensitivity vasculitis	Leukocytoclastic vasculitis	Small	Small vessels (capillaries, venules, arterioles)
Henoch-Schönlein purpura	Leukocytoclastic vasculitis	Small	Small vessels (capillaries, venules, arterioles)

to 77 in a hepatitis B virus (HBV) hyperendemic population. The average age of patients with PAN is 40 to 60, and there is a strong association with HBV. The annual incidence of Wegener's granulomatosis in Rochester, Minnesota, is an estimated 0.4 cases per 100,000. The incidence rate for Kawasaki syndrome varies according to race. In the United States, children 8 years old or younger have an annual incidence of 19.54 per 100,000 for Asians, 1.03 per 100,000 for blacks, and 0.45 per 100,000 for whites. Henoch-Schönlein purpura, more common in the pediatric populations, has an estimated incidence rate of 13.5 per 100,000 in the pediatric population in Belfast annually.[5] Although no population-based epidemiologic data exist on hypersensitivity vasculitic syndromes, including drug-related cutaneous vasculitis, these syndromes are likely the most common of all the vasculitides.[2]

PATHOPHYSIOLOGY

No single pathophysiologic mechanism can explain all the disease manifestations of vasculitis. Several possible mechanisms have been delineated based on animal models and more recent understanding of immunologic phenomena. In a previously immunized animal an antigenic challenge will result in vasculitis caused by an immune complex–mediated process. Also, expression of adhesion molecules may account for the different pattern of organ involvement in vasculitis. The role of antibodies other than those present in immune complexes remains unclear. Two autoantibodies, antineutrophil cytoplasmic antibody (ANCA) and antiendothelial cell antibody (AECA), have been detected in association with some forms of vasculitis. Whether they are directly involved in the pathogenesis of vasculitis is not known at this time. Cytokines and growth factors secreted by activated inflammatory cells are responsible for the clinical symptoms, such as fever, malaise, and weight loss. They also have vasoactive, prothrombotic, and fibrogenic functions responsible for the clinical findings of thrombosis, vasospasm, intimal hyperplasia, and fibrosis.[6]

PATIENT EVALUATION

History

Vasculitis should be suspected in any patient who presents with an unexplained systemic illness or has symptoms of organ-specific ischemia. Patients typically have a history of fever, fatigue, weight loss, myalgias, and arthralgias. Organ-specific symptoms depend on the size and location of the vessel involved in the vasculitic process. The involvement of large arteries may cause symptoms of headache, tongue or jaw claudication, and arm or leg claudication. When vasculitis affects medium and small arteries, hypertension, neurologic deficits suggestive of mononeuritis multiplex, abdominal pain, and hemoptysis are common manifestations. Vasculitides affecting arterioles and venules result in palpable purpura, maculopapular rash, livedo reticularis, abdominal pain, and bloody diarrhea. The one exception to the systemic vasculitides is primary angiitis of the central nervous system (CNS), which affects only blood vessels in the CNS. This entity usually presents with symptoms of severe headaches, progressive dementia, and symptoms of multifocal neurologic deficits (Table 138-2).

Physical Examination

A comprehensive examination should be performed on all patients suspected of having a vasculitis. General appearance and vital signs, including temperature, are important; hypertension may suggest vascular involvement of the kidneys. Cutaneous examination may reveal livedo reticularis, a maculopapular rash, and palpable purpura. Palpation of the sinuses is performed to assess for sinus pressure. The ophthalmologic examination should include inspection of the sclera, conjunctiva, and the fundi to assess retinal vessels. All eye structures may be involved in vasculitis, particularly temporal (giant cell) arteritis and Behçet's syndrome. Inspection of the oral mucosa may reveal ulcerations, also a sign of Behçet's disease. A detailed examination for lymphadenopathy may aid in discriminating a primary vasculitis from other diseases associated with vasculitis, such as lymphoma. Auscultation of the lungs and heart may reveal clinical abnormalities because both structures may be affected by vasculitis, as well as by conditions that mimic vasculitis, such as bacterial endocarditis and atrial myxoma, both of which may present with fever, a heart murmur, and embolic phenomena. Abdominal examination focuses on palpation for masses and hepatosplenomegaly and testing for occult blood in the stool to assess for diseases that mimic vasculitis and to examine for vasculitis of the intestines. Inspection of the genitalia may reveal ulcerations, which may be present in Behçet's syndrome, or testicular involvement, which may occur in PAN.

Specific attention should be given to the skin, joint,

Table 138-2. Summary of Vasculitic Syndromes

Vasculitic syndrome	Age range (years)	History	Physical examination	Evaluation	Treatment
Takayasu's arteritis	15-25	Females and Asians at much higher risk; arm or leg claudication	Decreased pulses, subclavian/aortic bruits	Arteriogram, vascular ultrasound, computed tomography, magnetic resonance imaging	Corticosteroids
Temporal (giant cell) arteritis	60-75	Headache, tongue or jaw claudication, scalp tenderness, hip or shoulder girdle stiffness	Tenderness, decreased temporal artery pulse	Erythrocyte sedimentation rate, temporal artery biopsy	Corticosteroids
Polyarteritis nodosa	40-60	Muscle and joint pain, abdominal pain	Hypertension, livedo reticularis, mononeuritis multiplex	Biopsy of involved tissue, mesenteric angiography, fecal occult blood	Corticosteroids, cyclophosphamide
Churg-Strauss syndrome	40-60	History of asthma or allergy, shortness of breath, abdominal pain	Pulmonary infiltrates, neuropathies, petechiae, purpura, ulcerations	Eosinophilia on differential, biopsy of involved tissue	Corticosteroids
Wegener's granulomatosis	30-50	Arthralgias, myalgias, sinusitis, bloody nasal discharge, shortness of breath	Pain over sinus areas, nasal or oral ulcers, chest pain, proptosis, cranial nerve deficits	Sinus x-rays, chest x-ray, ANCA, biopsy of affected tissue, fecal occult blood, urinalysis	Corticosteroids, cyclophosphamide
Microscopic polyangiitis	40-60	Myalgias, abdominal pain or bleeding, hemoptysis, dyspnea	Mononeuritis multiplex, rales, purpura, synovitis	ANCA, biopsy of affected tissue, fecal occult blood	Corticosteroids, cyclophosphamide
Kawasaki disease (syndrome)	1-5	Fever, skin rash	Conjunctivitis, cervical lymphadenopathy, polymorphous exanthem	Tests to rule out other diseases	Gamma globulin, aspirin
Hypersensitivity vasculitis	30-50	Exposure history (usually medication), infection	Palpable purpura	Tests to rule out other diseases	Avoidance of inciting agent
Henoch-Schönlein purpura	5-20	Preceding URI, abdominal pain, bloody diarrhea	Palpable purpura	Fecal occult blood, urinalysis	Supportive; if severe, glucocorticoids

ANCA, Antineutrophil cytoplasmic antibody; *URI*, upper respiratory infection.

vascular, and neurologic systems. A complete joint examination infrequently demonstrates frank synovitis. If polyarthritis is present, the differential is expanded to include systemic connective tissue diseases associated with vasculitis (e.g., SLE, RA). A general vascular examination is important to evaluate for atherosclerotic peripheral vascular disease, which may present as a systemic vasculitis in the setting of atheroembolization. Decreased or absent pulses may be present in Takayasu's arteritis and temporal arteritis. Full neurologic examination, including assessment of sensation, muscle strength, and cranial nerve function, is vital because mononeuritis multiplex, cranial neuropathies, and peripheral polyneuropathies are common manifestations of vasculitides and may suggest the size of the vessel involved. For example, medium-sized vasculitis tends to cause mononeuritis multiplex, whereas small-vessel involvement may cause peripheral polyneuropathies. Primary angiitis of the CNS can alter cognitive ability and cause focal deficits; mental status testing should be performed in these patients[3] (see Table 138-2).

LABORATORY STUDIES AND DIAGNOSTIC PROCEDURES

Patients with a suspected vasculitic syndrome should have routine laboratory studies, including a complete blood count, creatinine, and urinalysis. Findings such as leukocytosis, anemia of chronic disease, and thrombocytosis may be nonspecific markers of inflammation. Proteinuria, hematuria, and red cell casts suggest involvement of the kidneys. A chest radiograph may reveal pulmonary findings such as infiltrates, which may be asymptomatic. Complement levels may be suppressed by immune complex–mediated complement activation during the active phase of vasculitis. The ANCA test can also aid in making a diagnosis; 90% of patients with Wegener's granulomatosis have a positive cytoplasmic ANCA (c-ANCA), and 60% to 75% of patients with microscopic polyangiitis have a positive peripheral ANCA (p-ANCA). Positive c-ANCA is caused by antibodies to proteinase 3, a serine protease in azurophilic granules of neutrophils. Positive p-ANCA is caused by antibodies to elastase, myeloperoxidase, and other enzymes in the primary granules of neutrophils. If nerve involvement is suspected, an electromyogram (EMG) and nerve conduction studies may demonstrate mononeuritis multiplex, peripheral polyneuropathy, or myopathic process. Biopsy of affected tissues (or arteriography if biopsy is not feasible) may be necessary to confirm the diagnosis of vasculitis. Multiple arterial aneurysms on arteriography suggest a vasculitic process but are not pathognomonic. All patients should have age-specific and gender-specific cancer screening because malignancy may result in a secondary vasculitis (see Table 138-2).

DIFFERENTIAL DIAGNOSIS

It is important to differentiate between diseases that may mimic vasculitis and a true vasculitis (Box 138-1). A thorough history and physical examination help to identify the appropriate laboratory and radiographic procedures that should be pursued. Attempting to biopsy involved tissues, if feasible, should be strongly considered. In temporal arteritis, 50% of affected persons will have negative biopsies because the inflammation may not be widespread. When biopsies are negative or unattainable, treatment decisions are made based on the clinical presentation. Any atypical features need to be thoroughly investigated.

Box 138-1. Diseases that Mimic Vasculitis

Embolic Disease

Infectious or marantic endocarditis
Cardiac mural thrombus
Atrial myxoma
Cholesterol embolization syndrome

Noninflammatory Vessel Wall Disruption

Atherosclerosis
Arterial fibromuscular dysplasia
Drug effects (vasoconstrictors, anticoagulants)
Radiation
Genetic disease (neurofibromatosis, Ehler-Danlos syndrome)
Amyloidosis
Intravascular malignant lymphoma

Diffuse Coagulation

Disseminated intravascular coagulation
Thrombotic thrombocytopenic purpura
Hemolytic uremic syndrome
Protein C and S deficiencies, factor V/Leiden mutation
Antiphospholipid syndrome

Once the diagnosis of vasculitis is made, the physician must determine whether it is a primary vasculitis or secondary to an underlying condition. Systemic rheumatic conditions (e.g., RA, SLE, Sjögren's syndrome) may have vasculitis involving either medium or small vessels as one of the manifestations of the underlying condition.[1] Infection with HBV or hepatitis C has been associated with PAN and with cryoglobulinemia, which is a leukocytoclastic vasculitis similar to Henoch-Schönlein purpura. Leukocytoclastic vasculitis may also occur with inflammatory bowel disease, primary biliary cirrhosis, multiple myeloma, Waldenström's macroglobulinemia, lymphoma, leukemia, and carcinomas.

MANAGEMENT

The therapy of vasculitis depends on the size of the vessels involved and the specific clinical presentation. Treatment of patients with Takayasu's arteritis or temporal arteritis begins with prednisone, initiated at 1 mg/kg/day, about 60 mg in the typical patient. In approximately 40% of patients with Takayasu's arteritis, cytotoxic agents are necessary because of failure to respond to glucocorticoids or relapse on tapering glucocorticoids. Methotrexate and cyclophosphamide are most often used in these patients. The vast majority of patients with temporal arteritis respond to treatment with glucocorticoid therapy alone. One month after clinical parameters have returned to normal, tapering of the dose may begin. Most patients need to be treated with prednisone for 1 to 2 years.

Patients with PAN, Wegener's granulomatosis, and microscopic angiitis are initially treated with prednisone (1 mg/kg/day) and cyclophosphamide. Traditionally, cyclophosphamide is given orally (2 mg/kg/day) for 1 to 2 years after the patient is in remission. Intravenous "pulse" cyclophosphamide therapy is an option for patients at risk for side effects of the oral therapy. Churg-Strauss syndrome has been

Box 138-2. Exposures Associated With Hypersensitivity Vasculitis

Drugs

Anticonvulsants: phenobarbital and phenytoin
Antibiotics: penicillins and sulfonamides
Antiarrhythmics: quinidine and procainamide
Nonsteroidal antiinflammatory drugs
Allopurinol
Vaccines
Others (diuretics)

Infections

Acute bacterial infections
- Group A streptococci
- *Neisseria*

Chronic bacterial infections
- Subacute bacterial endocarditis
- Chronic sinusitis

Mycobacterial infections
- Tuberculosis
- Leprosy

Viral infections
- Hepatitis B and C
- Cytomegalovirus (CMV)

Fungal infections

thought to be more glucocorticoid responsive than PAN or microscopic polyangiitis. If patients with Churg-Strauss vasculitis fail treatment with glucocorticoids or relapse with tapering, however, the addition of a cytotoxic agent may be necessary. Such treatment is the same as the regimen for PAN. Azathioprine and methotrexate are alternative cytotoxic agents if patients are unable to tolerate cyclophosphamide, but are less effective.

Kawasaki disease (syndrome) is treated with aspirin and high-dose intravenous gamma globulin given over 4 or 5 days or as a one-time dose. Patients with hypersensitivity vasculitis or Henoch-Schönlein purpura usually require only symptomatic and supportive care.[4] If organ- or life-threatening visceral disease is present, however, aggressive immunosuppressive therapy is initiated.

PROGNOSIS

The prognosis of a patient with vasculitis depends on the specific type and course of the vasculitic syndrome. Approximately half of patients with temporal arteritis experience resolution within 6 to 12 months. The remainder may require 3 or 4 years of treatment. The disease course of Takayasu's arteritis is poorly understood in the United States given the rarity of the condition. Many patients have a prolonged course, however, with significant morbidity and mortality from stenosis of the vessels involved. PAN, Wegener's granulomatosis, Churg-Strauss syndrome, and microscopic polyangiitis carry a poor prognosis. Although many patients may improve with treatment and achieve a state of remission, recurrence and therapy-related morbidity often occur. In contrast, Kawasaki disease has a good prognosis, with only a 1% to 2% acute mortality rate. The overall prognosis of hypersensitivity vasculitis and Henoch-Schönlein purpura is excellent because both processes tend to be self-limited, especially in hypersensitivity vasculitis when the underlying cause, such as infection or drug use, is treated or removed (Box 138-2).

REFERENCES

1. Bacon PA, Carruthers DM: Vasculitis associated with connective tissue disorders, *Rheum Dis Clin North Am* 21:1077, 1995.
2. Calabrese LH, Duna GF: Drug-induced vasculitis, *Curr Opin Rheumatol* 8:34, 1996.
3. Calabrese LH, Duna GF, Lie JT: Vasculitis in the central nervous system, *Arthritis Rheum* 40:1189, 1997.
4. Jennette JC, Falk RJ: Small-vessel vasculitis, *N Engl J Med* 337:1512, 1997.
5. Michet CJ: Epidemiology of vasculitis, *Rheum Dis Clin North Am* 16:261, 1990.
6. Nowack R, Flores-Suarez LF, van der Woude FJ: New developments in the pathogenesis of systemic vasculitis, *Curr Opin Rheumatol* 10:3, 1998.

CHAPTER 139

Systemic Sclerosis

Virginia D. Steen
James C. Shaw

Systemic sclerosis (SSc) is a chronic, multisystem disorder of connective tissue characterized by degenerative and inflammatory changes that subsequently lead to intense fibrosis. The skin, blood vessels, synovium, skeletal muscle, and certain internal organs are affected, including the gastrointestinal (GI) tract, lungs, heart, and kidneys.

EPIDEMIOLOGY

SSc has a worldwide distribution. Approximately 20 new cases of SSc per million population occur annually, with an estimated 100,000 to 300,000 patients in the United States. Women are affected three to four times more often than men. The onset of disease usually occurs between ages 30 and 50, but younger and older adults can be affected. Childhood SSc is rare, although localized forms of scleroderma (linear, morphea) are more common in children. Familial cases have rarely been reported, and no strong genetic relationships have been found; however, other connective tissue diseases may be seen among first-degree relatives of patients with SSc.

The American College of Rheumatology's criteria for the classification of SSc require skin thickening proximal to the metacarpophalangeal joints or two of the following: sclerodactyly, digital pitting scars, or interstitial pulmonary fibrosis. These criteria have no relationship to the major clinical subsets of SSc, limited cutaneous and diffuse cutaneous scleroderma. These two major subsets have important differences in their disease onset and overall course (Box 139-1). The classic form of *diffuse scleroderma* has a rapid onset of symptoms, including Raynaud's phenomenon, polyarthritis, carpal tunnel syndrome, swollen hands and legs, and fatigue. Skin thickening progresses up the patient's arms and over the trunk, resulting in contractures and disability.

Box 139-1. Characteristics of Limited and Diffuse Cutaneous Scleroderma

Limited

Long history of Raynaud's phenomenon
Minimal constitutional symptoms except fatigue
Puffy fingers
Skin thickening restricted to distal extremities
CREST syndrome, with extensive calcinosis and telangiectasia
Isolated (vascular) pulmonary hypertension
Anticentromere antibody

Diffuse

Recent onset of Raynaud's phenomenon (but may be delayed)
Acute onset, with fatigue, weight loss, polyarthralgias, and feeling ill
Puffy fingers, hands, and lower legs
Carpal tunnel syndrome
Tendon friction rubs
Progressive skin thickening up arms and legs to trunk
Renal crisis
Antitopoisomerase and anti-RNA polymerase III antibodies

Visceral involvement, including GI tract, lung, heart, and kidney, is common, particularly in the first 4 years of disease.

Limited scleroderma, or the CREST syndrome, is at the other end of the spectrum (Fig. 139-1). These patients have a much less progressive disease and usually have Raynaud's phenomenon for a prolonged period before developing other symptoms. Puffy fingers, heartburn, and telangiectasias are clues to the diagnosis. Severe intestinal hypomotility, resulting in malabsorption and pseudoobstruction, and pulmonary hypertension are the most serious complications of limited scleroderma. Severe digital ischemia and calcinosis can cause disability. Anticentromere antibody is found in most patients.

The natural history of SSc varies considerably between the different subsets (Fig. 139-2). Even within the major subsets, survival varies significantly, depending on the extent of internal organ involvement. The 10-year cumulative survival rate from onset of symptoms is 83% for limited scleroderma and 65% for patients with diffuse scleroderma.

PATHOPHYSIOLOGY

The pathophysiology of SSc is not completely understood, but vascular and immunologic factors interact with connective tissue, causing an excessive amount of collagen production by fibroblasts (Fig. 139-3). Small arterioles show subintimal hyperplasia and hyalinization. In patients with early diffuse disease, focal collections of T-cell lymphocytes can be identified in the deep dermis. Activated T cells produce cytokines, particularly interleukin-2 (IL-2) and transforming growth factor beta (TGF-β), which stimulate fibroblast proliferation and collagen production. Endothelial cell damage may result in increased permeability and the release and activation of cell growth factors. Platelet activation, platelet-derived growth factor (PDGF), and mast cells also have major effects of stimulating the fibroblast.

The humoral immune system with B-cell activation is involved in SSc, although its relationship to endothelial cells and increased collagen production remains obscure. Several autoantibodies are specific to scleroderma and associated with unique subsets of clinical and genetic features. Because of the many toxin-induced scleroderma-like illnesses, a toxin or environmental factor could be responsible for triggering scleroderma, although none has yet been identified.

PATIENT EVALUATION

The first symptoms of scleroderma are usually Raynaud's phenomenon, puffy fingers, and polyarthritis involving the small joints of the hands. Thereafter the course and multisystem features are extremely variable. The physician must review the history and findings for each organ system to determine the expected course and best management of each patient's disease (Fig. 139-4).

Physical Examination

Raynaud's Phenomenon. Cold exposure and emotional stress may induce vasospasm, causing characteristic episodes of bilateral blanching or cyanosis of the digits (see Chapter 70). Infarction of tissue at the fingertips may lead to painful ulcerations or frank gangrene. In limited cutaneous disease, Raynaud's phenomenon usually antedates other evidence of SSc by years or even decades. In contrast, Raynaud's phenomenon is initially present in only 75% of patients with diffuse scleroderma. The finding of dilated nail fold capillaries with capillary "dropout" is typical for scleroderma and is a helpful differential finding in patients with primary Raynaud's phenomenon (Fig. 139-5).

Skin. In diffuse scleroderma an early manifestation is often bilateral symmetric swelling of the hands and legs (Fig. 139-6). Patients frequently are evaluated for cardiac, endocrine, or kidney diseases because of striking peripheral edema. After a few weeks to several months, edema is replaced by induration, resulting in thick, hard skin. An inability to elicit a wrinkle when pinching the skin is a reliable method for determining skin thickening, which spreads rapidly from the fingers, up the arms, and onto the trunk, particularly the anterior chest and abdomen. After several years the progression of skin thickening stabilizes, and spontaneous skin softening occurs to some degree in most patients. In contrast, limited scleroderma patients tend to have puffiness primarily in the fingers, and skin thickening is limited to the distal extremities and face, rarely changing throughout the illness.

After many years, numerous small macular punctate telangiectasias appear on the fingers, face, lips, and tongue (see Fig. 139-1, *D*). They occur most frequently in patients with limited scleroderma but also in those with late-stage diffuse scleroderma and disease for 5 to 10 years. Subcutaneous calcinosis is a late complication that occurs more often in limited than diffuse scleroderma (see Fig. 139-1, *B*). Sites of minor trauma are often affected, such as the fingers, forearms, elbows, and knees.

Joints and Tendons. Polyarthralgias affect both small and large joints and are especially frequent early in diffuse scleroderma. Joint pain, swollen fingers, and polyarthritis often lead to the premature diagnosis of rheumatoid arthritis. In diffuse scleroderma, rapid development of hand swelling

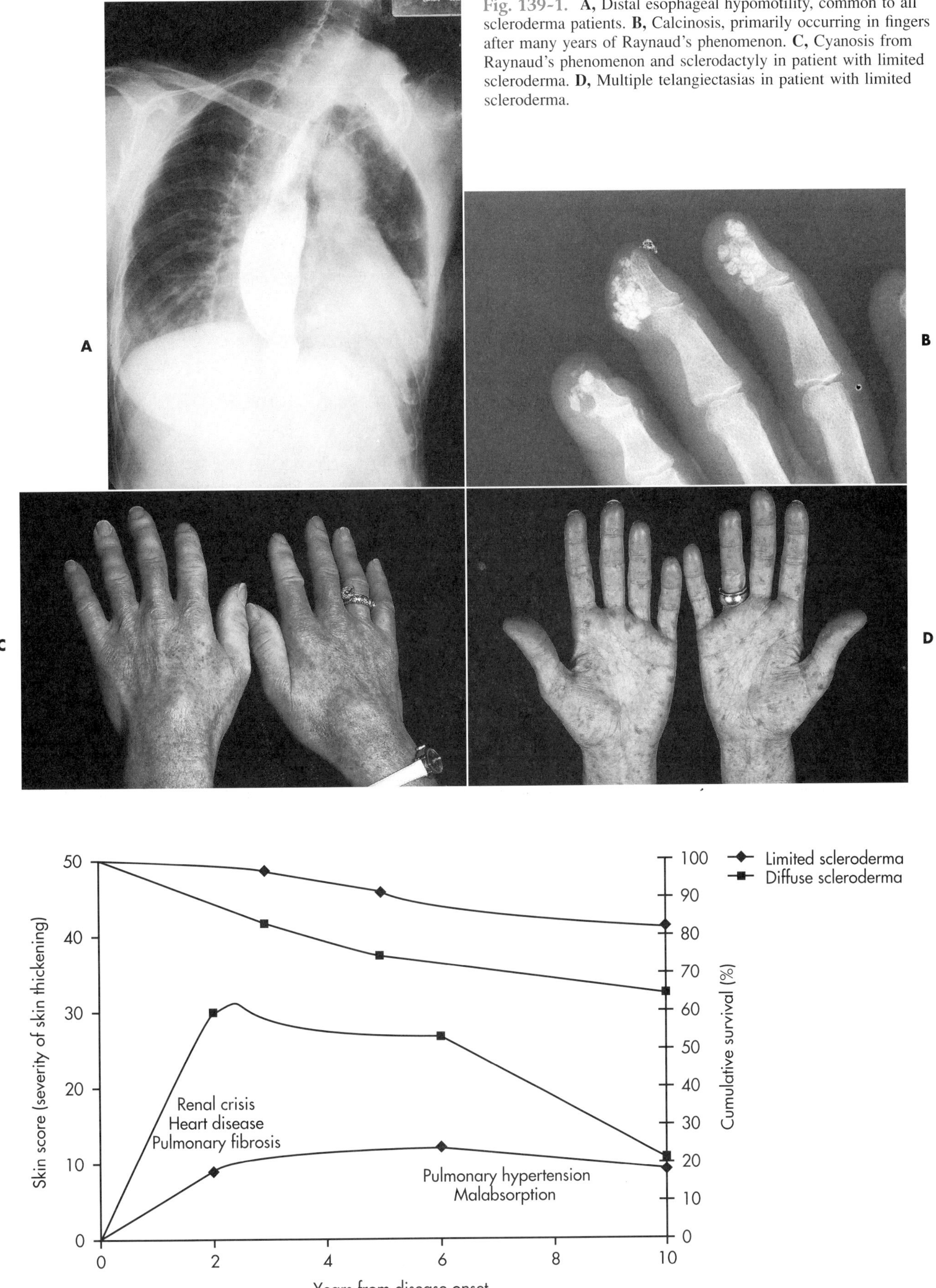

Fig. 139-1. **A,** Distal esophageal hypomotility, common to all scleroderma patients. **B,** Calcinosis, primarily occurring in fingers after many years of Raynaud's phenomenon. **C,** Cyanosis from Raynaud's phenomenon and sclerodactyly in patient with limited scleroderma. **D,** Multiple telangiectasias in patient with limited scleroderma.

Fig. 139-2. *Top,* Cumulative survival from onset of symptoms in patients with limited and diffuse scleroderma with less than 2 years of symptoms. Five-year survival is 90% for limited scleroderma and 75% for diffuse scleroderma, (p <0.001). *Bottom,* Development of cutaneous skin thickening (skin score) and other organ involvement over time in patients with limited and diffuse scleroderma.

Initial Event
Vascular
Immunologic
Connective Tissue
B-cell activation
Anticentromere
Antitopoisomerase
Mast cells
Environmental?
Toxin?
Genetic?
Autoimmunity?
Monocyte
T-cell activation
Fibroblasts
Permeability
Cytokines
Endothelial cell
TGF-β
IL-2
Increased collagen
Cytotoxic factor
Platelet activation
PDGF

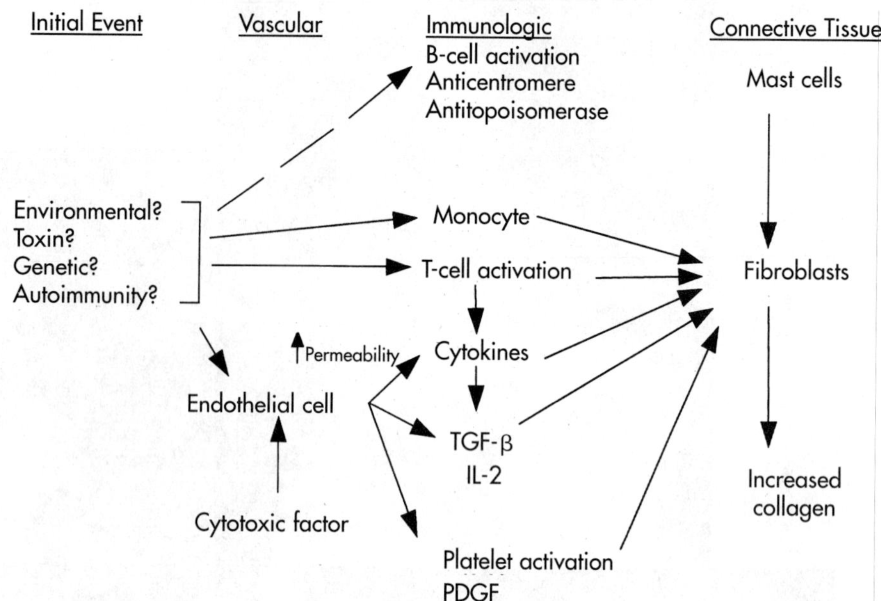

Fig. 139-3. Vascular and immunologic factors that result in increased collagen in the pathogenesis of systemic sclerosis (see text for abbreviations).

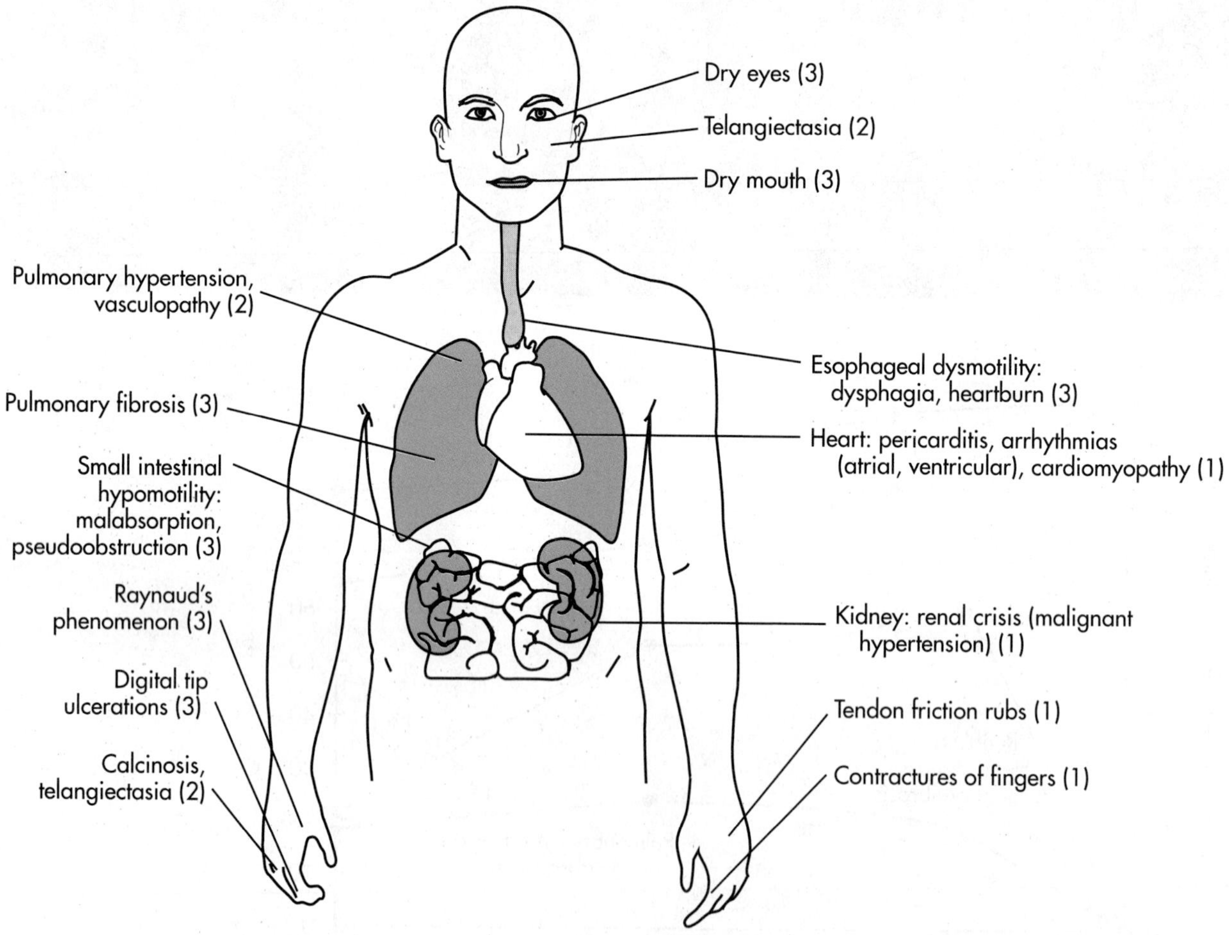

Dry eyes (3)
Telangiectasia (2)
Dry mouth (3)
Pulmonary hypertension, vasculopathy (2)
Esophageal dysmotility: dysphagia, heartburn (3)
Pulmonary fibrosis (3)
Heart: pericarditis, arrhythmias (atrial, ventricular), cardiomyopathy (1)
Small intestinal hypomotility: malabsorption, pseudoobstruction (3)
Raynaud's phenomenon (3)
Kidney: renal crisis (malignant hypertension) (1)
Digital tip ulcerations (3)
Tendon friction rubs (1)
Calcinosis, telangiectasia (2)
Contractures of fingers (1)

Fig. 139-4. Clinical manifestations of systemic sclerosis (SSc). *1,* Predominantly in diffuse scleroderma; *2,* predominantly in limited scleroderma; *3,* frequently seen in both subsets of scleroderma.

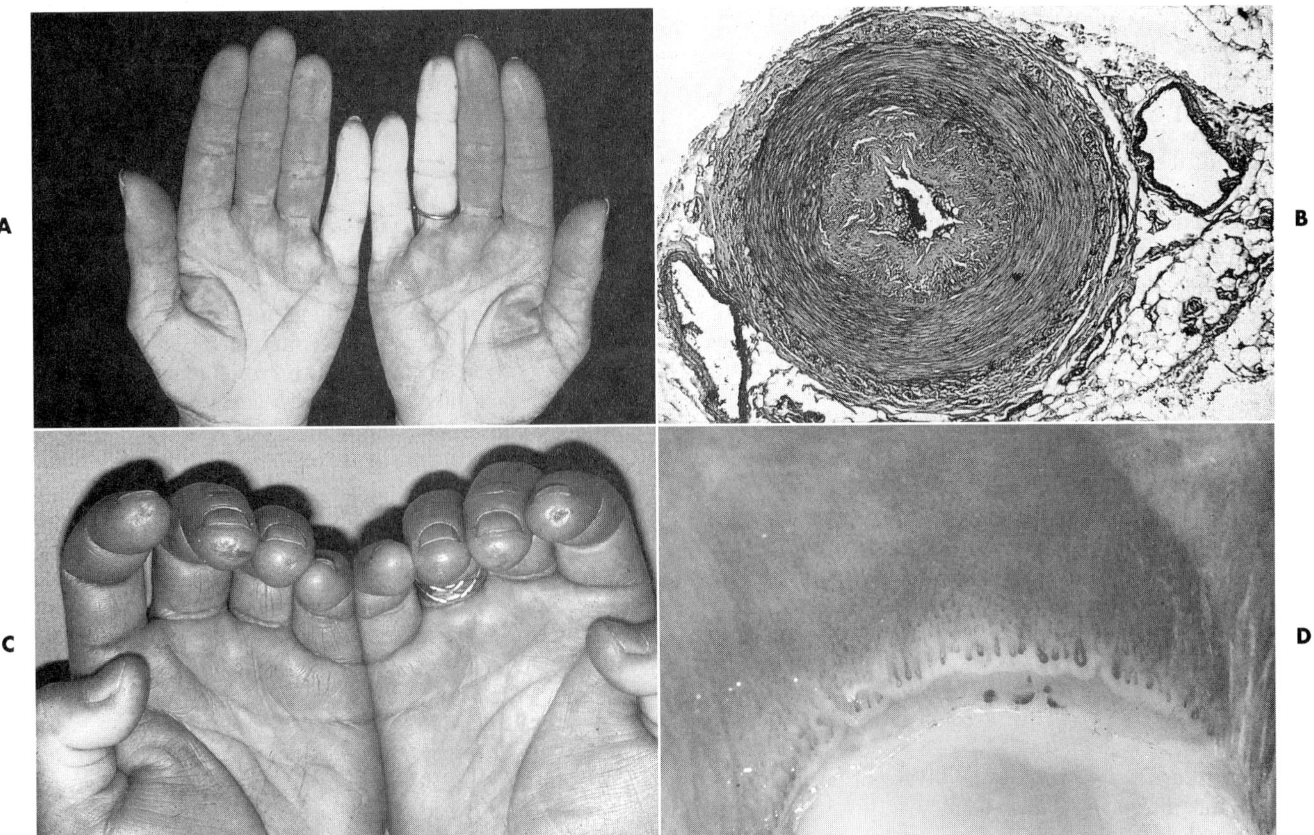

Fig. 139-5. **A,** Pallor from vasoconstriction in Raynaud's phenomenon. **B,** Digital artery from patient with scleroderma and severe digital ischemia. (Magnification ×21.) **C,** Digital pitting scars on fingertips of patient with scleroderma, one of minor criteria for scleroderma. **D,** Abnormal nail fold capillaries in patient with scleroderma. (Magnification ×4.) Note loss of capillaries and dilation of capillary loops.

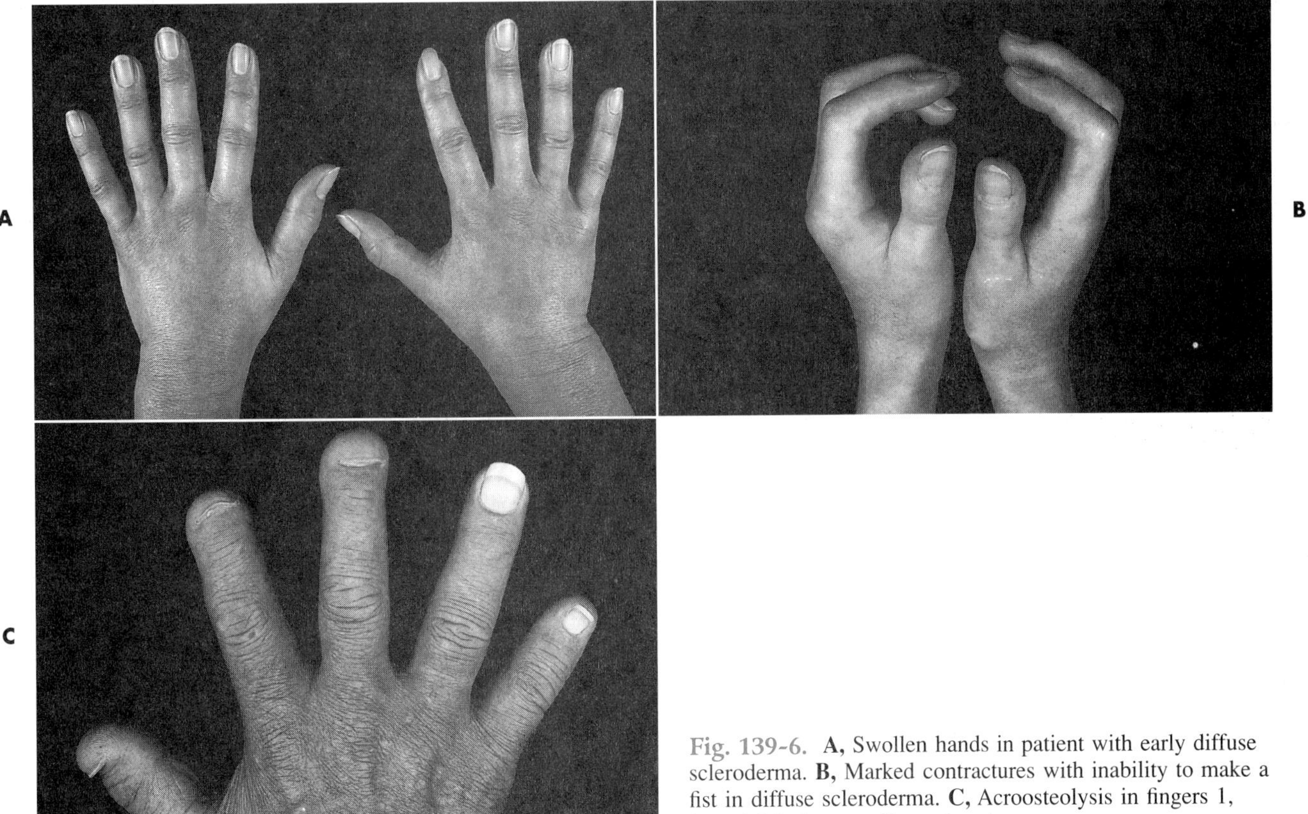

Fig. 139-6. **A,** Swollen hands in patient with early diffuse scleroderma. **B,** Marked contractures with inability to make a fist in diffuse scleroderma. **C,** Acroosteolysis in fingers 1, 2, and 3 in longstanding scleroderma.

and skin tightening often leads to severe flexion contractures, with clawlike hands and serious disability. Limited scleroderma patients have only mild, if any, contractures because the disease process is slower. Acroosteolysis, thought to be caused by hypovascularity, causes painless bone resorption, primarily of the distal phalanges (see Fig. 139-6, *C*).

Carpal tunnel syndrome is common early in diffuse scleroderma and often is the symptom that brings the patient to a physician. Coarse, leathery tendon friction rubs palpated during motion of the extensor and flexor tendons of the fingers, distal forearms, knees, and ankles are found almost exclusively in patients with diffuse cutaneous disease. Their presence can foreshadow the development of diffuse cutaneous scleroderma.

Skeletal Muscle. Patients typically have fatigue and weakness, but two specific types of myopathies exist. The most frequent is a bland, nonprogressive process characterized by mild proximal weakness, minimal elevation of serum creatine kinase (CK), and a noninflammatory fibrotic replacement of myofibrils on muscle biopsy. A second type is indistinguishable from polymyositis. These patients have impressive weakness, greatly increased CK, and classic inflammatory changes on electromyography (EMG) and muscle biopsy.

Gastrointestinal Tract. GI involvement occurs in most patients and differs little between the diffuse and limited subgroups. Distal esophageal motor dysfunction leads to distal dysphagia, and the lower esophageal sphincter musculature does not close adequately, resulting in severe reflux of gastric contents and esophagitis. This may be complicated by ulcerations, candidal infection, and stricture. Symptomatic gastric emptying malfunction and duodenal hypomotility are much less common but contribute to postprandial abdominal pain and bloating.

Loss of smooth muscle function and hypomotility of the jejunum and ileum can result in bacterial overgrowth, which interferes with normal fat absorption. Malabsorption from bacterial overgrowth is associated with persistent diarrhea, marked weight loss, and intermittent episodes of abdominal distention and vomiting. These problems and pseudoobstruction may be life threatening.

Lungs. Clinical evidence of pleural involvement, including pleurisy, pleural effusion, and pleural friction rub, is uncommon. Clinical or radiographic evidence of pulmonary interstitial fibrosis develops in most SSc patients. Common abnormalities on pulmonary function tests (PFTs) include a decline in forced vital capacity (restrictive lung disease) and a reduced diffusing capacity for carbon monoxide (DLco). Inflammatory alveolitis early in the disease results in pulmonary fibrosis, with respiratory symptoms occurring later. Progression is variable, however, and most patients have mild to moderate, nonprogressive restrictive lung dysfunction on PFTs. Serial PFTs, bronchoalveolar lavage, and high-resolution computed tomography (HRCT) scans can help to determine if alveolitis and progressive fibrosis are present early in the course.

In addition to a restrictive pattern on PFTs, patients may demonstrate an isolated decrease in the DLco, with the forced vital capacity remaining normal or near normal. Unless the DLco is less than 50%, this is not serious; however, patients with a very low DLco are at high risk of developing isolated pulmonary arterial hypertension, which develops in about 10% of patients with limited scleroderma. Histologically, the small pulmonary arteries show intense subintimal hyperplasia without inflammation. The prognosis is grave, with the mean survival only 2 years.

Heart. Clinical evidence of myocardial involvement is uncommon (less than 15%) and occurs more often in patients with diffuse scleroderma. In contrast, cardiac tests (e.g., electrocardiogram, echocardiogram, Holter monitor, nuclear studies) show evidence of asymptomatic abnormalities in a high proportion of patients. The symptomatic manifestations of myocardial disease include congestive heart failure and a variety of atrial and ventricular dysrhythmias. The mortality rate is high. Patchy replacement of the myocardium and conduction system by fibrous tissue is the rule in such cases. Interestingly, the vascular changes that occur in most other organs are not found in similar-sized blood vessels in the heart. Acute pericarditis or pericardial tamponade is more unusual than the common echocardiographic and pathologic evidence of asymptomatic pericardial involvement with effusion.

Kidneys. Renal involvement is manifested by scleroderma renal crisis, a potentially fatal event. It affects approximately 20% of individuals with diffuse disease and typically occurs early (less than 4 years after disease onset) in the setting of rapidly progressive skin thickening. This complication was once the major cause of death in patients with diffuse cutaneous involvement. In contrast, renal crisis is rare in patients with limited cutaneous involvement.

Renal crisis may present without warning. The patient develops malignant arterial hypertension with hyperreninemia and oliguric acute renal failure. It often follows a course of high-dose steroids. The urinalysis shows hematuria and proteinuria, and the serum CK rises daily. Even with aggressive treatment, these patients may develop rapidly progressive renal failure. Occasionally, the blood pressure remains normal; in these patients, microangiopathic hemolytic anemia with thrombocytopenia is prominent. This type of hemolysis also occurs with malignant hypertension and is an intravascular rather than an immune-mediated problem. The primary targets in renal crisis are interlobular and arcuate arteries and arterioles. Severe mucoid subintimal hyperplasia is evident histologically, and blood vessel walls may undergo fibrinoid necrosis. An inflammatory component and immune complex deposition are lacking.

Other Organs. Sjögren's syndrome is seen in 20% of SSc patients but symptoms of Sjögren's syndrome, including dry eyes and dry mouth, may also be caused by glandular fibrosis. Both lymphocytic inflammation (Hashimoto's thyroiditis) and fibrous replacement of the thyroid have been observed and are often associated with clinical evidence of hypothyroidism. Biliary cirrhosis is found in a few women with limited scleroderma, but hepatic involvement is otherwise rare. Trigeminal sensory neuropathy has been described.

LABORATORY STUDIES

The routine laboratory tests from a typical SSc patient are generally unremarkable. Anemia and the erythrocyte sedi-

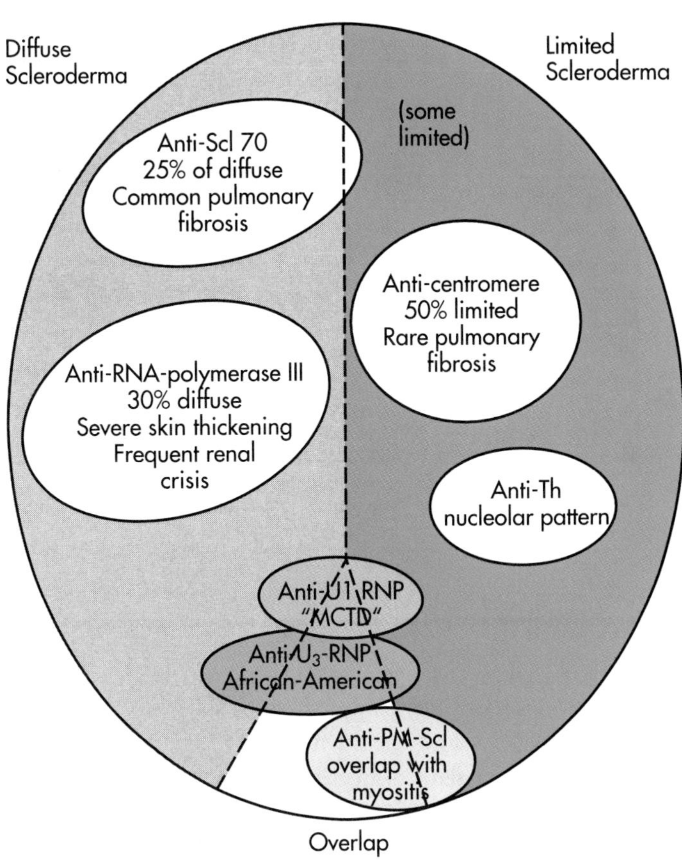

Fig. 139-7. Autoantibody subsets in scleroderma.

mentation rate (ESR) are variable. Nearly all patients with SSc have serum antinuclear antibodies (ANAs), which are highly specific for SSc and associated with distinct clinical subsets of patients (Fig. 139-7). Anticentromere antibody (centromeric staining on routine immunofluorescence) is highly specific for limited cutaneous scleroderma, and these patients rarely have pulmonary fibrosis. Antitopoisomerase I (or Scl-70) tends to identify individuals with diffuse cutaneous disease with more frequent pulmonary fibrosis and peripheral vascular difficulties. Anti-U1 ribonucleoprotein (RNP; high-titer, speckled ANA pattern) is associated with the classic mixed connective tissue disease. Also, several scleroderma-specific antibodies are not yet commercially available. Anti-RNA polymerase III identifies a large group of patients with diffuse disease who have severe skin thickening, and 25% progress to renal crisis.[1] This will be an important prognostic test when it becomes available. Several other, less common but unique nucleolar antibodies also exist. One identifies a small subset of patients with limited scleroderma (anti-Th), another is present in more than half of the black patients with scleroderma (anti-U3 RNP), and a third (anti-PM Scl) is seen in a few patients with polymyositis-scleroderma overlap syndrome.

DIFFERENTIAL DIAGNOSIS

The diagnosis of SSc is usually not difficult because of the characteristic cutaneous findings in scleroderma, except the early diffuse form. At that point, diagnosis is more difficult because of confusion with other forms of arthritis and other endocrine, cardiac, or renal diseases that result in similar types of edema. Many scleroderma-like diseases, although infrequent, can mimic scleroderma; localized forms of scleroderma, including morphea and eosinophilic fasciitis, are the most common (Box 139-2). The absence of Raynaud's phenomenon and atypical distribution of skin thickening are helpful clues. The chemically induced scleroderma-like illnesses include toxic oil syndrome and tryptophan-induced eosinophilic myalgia syndrome.

Localized Scleroderma

Localized scleroderma involves skin and subcutaneous tissue only. Three forms are recognized: morphea, generalized morphea, and linear scleroderma (Box 139-3). Lichen sclerosus is a related condition. The true incidence and mechanism of disease of localized scleroderma are unknown. It affects women three times as frequently as men, and the linear form tends to affect children and adolescents. The distribution in localized scleroderma suggests predisposed clones of fibroblasts present since birth that express their abnormal phenotype later in life. In early cases, patients may report areas of edema and pain with or without erythema. Low-grade arthralgia may also be present. Usually, however, the skin lesions are noticed because of appearance, and symptoms are absent.

In morphea, one or more patches of indurated skin have an erythematous or violaceous hue, especially at the borders. Lesions are asymmetric and favor the trunk. The epidermis is frequently atrophic, ivory white in color, with fine wrinkling (Fig. 139-8). The distinction between morphea and generalized morphea is based on the amount and depth of involvement. Generalized morphea involves the subcutaneous fat, fascia, and occasionally muscle. In linear scleroderma an indurated, depressed band is present, usually on an extremity. Hyperpigmentation is common. Subcutaneous fat

Box 139-2. Pseudoscleroderma Illnesses

Primary Cutaneous Diseases

Scleredema (see Box 139-4)
Porphyria cutanea tarda
Scleromyxedema
Lichen sclerosus

Systemic Diseases

Amyloidosis
Juvenile-onset diabetes mellitus
Acromegaly
Carcinoid syndrome
Phenylketonuria
Werner's syndrome
Graft-vs.-host disease

Chemically Induced Disorders

Polyvinyl chloride
Bleomycin (Raynaud's phenomenon, pulmonary fibrosis)
Contaminated L-tryptophan (eosinophilic myalgia syndrome)
Rapeseed oil (toxic oil syndrome)

Box 139-3. Localized Forms of Scleroderma

Morphea: cutaneous scleroderma without visceral involvement, usually localized to patches, similar to systemic sclerosis
Subcutaneous morphea: deeper, more generalized cutaneous changes similar to fasciitis
Linear scleroderma: childhood localized scleroderma that runs along extremities and occasionally on one half of face (en coup de sabre)
Eosinophilic fasciitis (see Box 139-4)

involvement may result in depressed, atrophic areas, and flexion contractures result when the process involves the skin over joints.

The ANA is positive in up to 50% of patients with localized scleroderma but is not a good predictor of disease activity. Eosinophilia and an elevated ESR may also be seen. Biopsy of involved skin shows features similar to those of SSc.

In extensive cases, differentiating between localized and systemic scleroderma is important because of differences in prognosis. Physical findings and laboratory testing usually allow a correct diagnosis. Several diseases may demonstrate sclerodermoid skin changes and need to be considered (Box 139-4).

Localized scleroderma is a self-limited disease of several years' duration. Permanent defects occur when the disease involves joints and produces contractures and when hemiatrophy of the face results from subcutaneous involvement. Physical therapy can help prevent contractures. Reconstructive dermatologic surgery, including autologous fat injections, may help correct atrophic defects of the face. Small trials with topical calcipotriene and UVA-1 have shown clinical and histologic improvement of sclerotic skin.

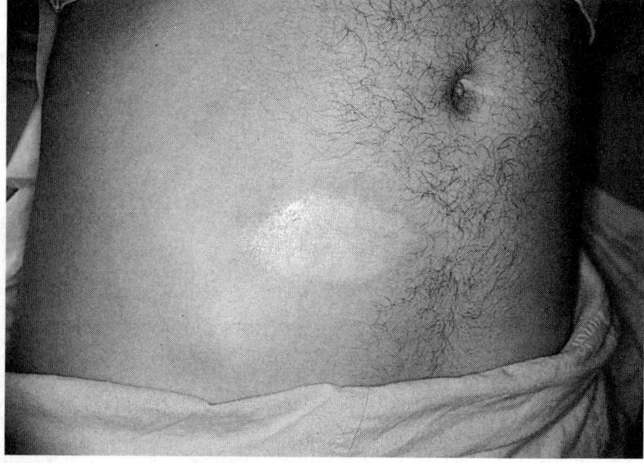

Fig. 139-8. Morphea. Note ivory color and surrounding subtle erythema.

Box 139-4. Differential Diagnosis of Scleroderma

Undifferentiated Connective Tissue Disease (UCTD)

Also called mixed connective tissue disease (MCTD)
Features of scleroderma, polymyositis, and systemic lupus erythematosus
Antibodies to ribonucleoprotein
Responds to corticosteroids
Prognosis better than systemic sclerosis

Eosinophilic Fasciitis

Resembles scleroderma, but without Raynaud's phenomenon
Affects skin and fascia of extremities, usually spares hands
Follows physical exertion in 50% of cases
Skin and fascia of extremities involved
Rarely has systemic features
Responds to corticosteroids

Chronic Graft-vs.-host Disease

History of bone marrow transplant

Scleredema

Induration and edema of skin on upper back and neck
Follows upper respiratory infection
Idiopathic form seen in diabetic patients

Porphyria Cutanea Tarda (PCT)

Sclerodermoid changes rarely
May improve with PCT treatment

Lichen Sclerosus

Lichen sclerosus (LS) is a chronic skin disease of unknown etiology, usually affecting the vulva. Women are thought to be affected more than men, although one study of 76 patients with LS showed no gender difference. A subset of patients with LS comprises prepubertal girls with involvement of the vulva and perineum. Most often, LS develops in postmenopausal women and in men between ages 40 and 60.[4]

Pruritus and a burning sensation are the most common symptoms associated with LS, especially with genital involvement. Plaques and patches of slightly sclerotic (indurated) skin, with atrophy and wrinkling of the epidermis, are typical (Fig. 139-9). The atrophic patches can become bullous and hemorrhagic or can erode repeatedly and heal with scarring.

The differential diagnosis includes localized scleroderma (morphea), atrophic lichen planus, and cutaneous diskoid lupus erythematosus. Skin biopsy for routine staining usually shows characteristic sclerosis in the upper dermis.

A potent (class I) topical corticosteroid is the treatment of choice. Topical testosterone has been shown to be less effective than clobetasol. The goal of treatment is palliation because LS tends to be chronic. Most prepubertal girls improve spontaneously at menarche. Squamous cell carcinoma can develop within the lesions in up to 10% of older patients with LS. Periodic examination and biopsy of suspicious areas are indicated.

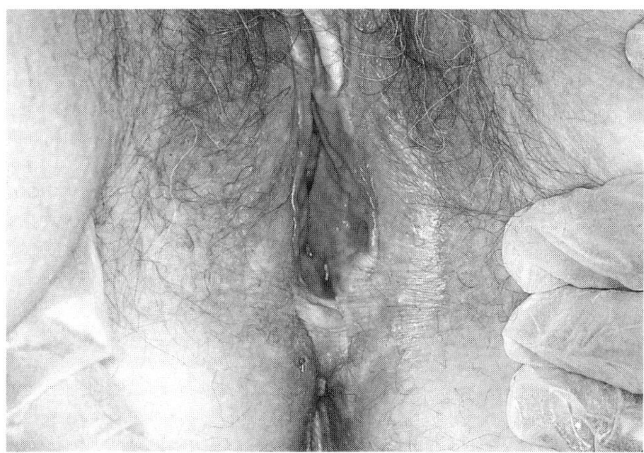

Fig. 139-9. Lichen sclerosus. Note white patches on labia minora and perineum.

TREATMENT

Treatment of SSc continues to be a major challenge. The wide spectrum of manifestations, severity, and disease courses means great interpatient variability. The relative rarity of SSc makes performing double-blind, controlled trials difficult. In addition, spontaneous improvement may occur, rendering interpretation of therapeutic results impossible without untreated comparison groups.

Disease-modifying Agents

Many drugs are being studied for SSc treatment because no single agent has been convincingly effective. Vascular abnormalities, immune mechanisms, and collagen production are possible areas for therapeutic intervention; thus far, no effective agent has been found (Fig. 139-10). The immunomodulating agent D-penicillamine interferes with cross-linking of collagen and is the most widely used drug in the treatment of scleroderma. Patients show significant improvement in skin thickening after 2 years of therapy and improved 5-year survival compared with similar untreated patients.[2] However, penicillamine, methotrexate, and photopheresis have not demonstrated consistent effectiveness. Relaxin, a biorecombinant version of the hormone, is in phase III trials, with earlier studies showing promising effects on skin thickening.

Management of Affected Organ Systems

Although no cure or remittive drug for SSc exists, patients can be treated in many ways to manage and improve different aspects of their disease. Abstinence from smoking, avoidance of cold temperatures, and common-sense measures are usually effective against Raynaud's phenomenon. More severe episodes accompanied by fingertip ulcers require calcium channel blockers, especially nifedipine and amilodopine, that relax vascular smooth muscle. Local management of fingertip ulcers includes soaking, antibiotic ointment, and oral antistaphylococcal antibiotics, as indicated. For deeper infections, surgical debridement of devitalized tissue and intravenous antibiotics may be necessary.

Nonsteroidal antiinflammatory drugs (NSAIDs) are used for joint and tendon sheath involvement. In addition to medication, early aggressive physical and occupational therapy that emphasizes stretching is important to prevent or minimize contractures. Carpal tunnel symptoms, which often occur before the diagnosis of scleroderma, can be successfully treated with resting wrist splints and local steroid injections without requiring surgery. Inflammatory myositis is treated with corticosteroids and sometimes requires the addition of immunosuppressive drugs, but the bland, fibrotic myopathy is best managed with strengthening exercises alone.

Esophageal dysmotility most often causes heartburn and lower dysphagia. The new proton pump inhibitors can completely eliminate heartburn and reflux symptoms. Prokinetic drugs are used to stimulate esophageal muscle contraction but have limited effectiveness. Primary small bowel involvement and bacterial overgrowth result in abdominal distention (or bloating), diarrhea, weight loss, and malabsorption. Broad-spectrum antibiotics (e.g., ampicillin, metronidazole, ciprofloxacin) may have a dramatic effect on these symptoms. Prokinetic agents also may be useful. Poor nutrition may require hyperalimentation. The first approach to patients with pseudoobstruction should be conservative (nonsurgical decompression) with nasogastric suction, bowel rest, and observation.

Pulmonary interstitial disease has become a major therapeutic problem in SSc. Fortunately, most patients have mild, nonprogressive involvement that does not require treatment. Attempts to reverse advanced, fixed fibrosis have been unsuccessful. In contrast, treatment of inflammatory alveolitis identified by bronchoalveolar lavage may prevent further fibrosis. When used at the appropriate time, cyclophosphamide may halt the progression of lung disease. The only option for patients with advanced end-stage pulmonary interstitial fibrosis is a lung transplant.

Isolated pulmonary arterial hypertension without significant interstitial fibrosis has the worst prognosis of all scleroderma visceral problems. Until recently, no therapy has altered the progression of this complication; it is uniformly fatal within 5 years. Continuous intravenous infusion of prostacyclins offers some hope for improving the high pulmonary artery pressures. Single-lung transplant can reverse this deadly process.

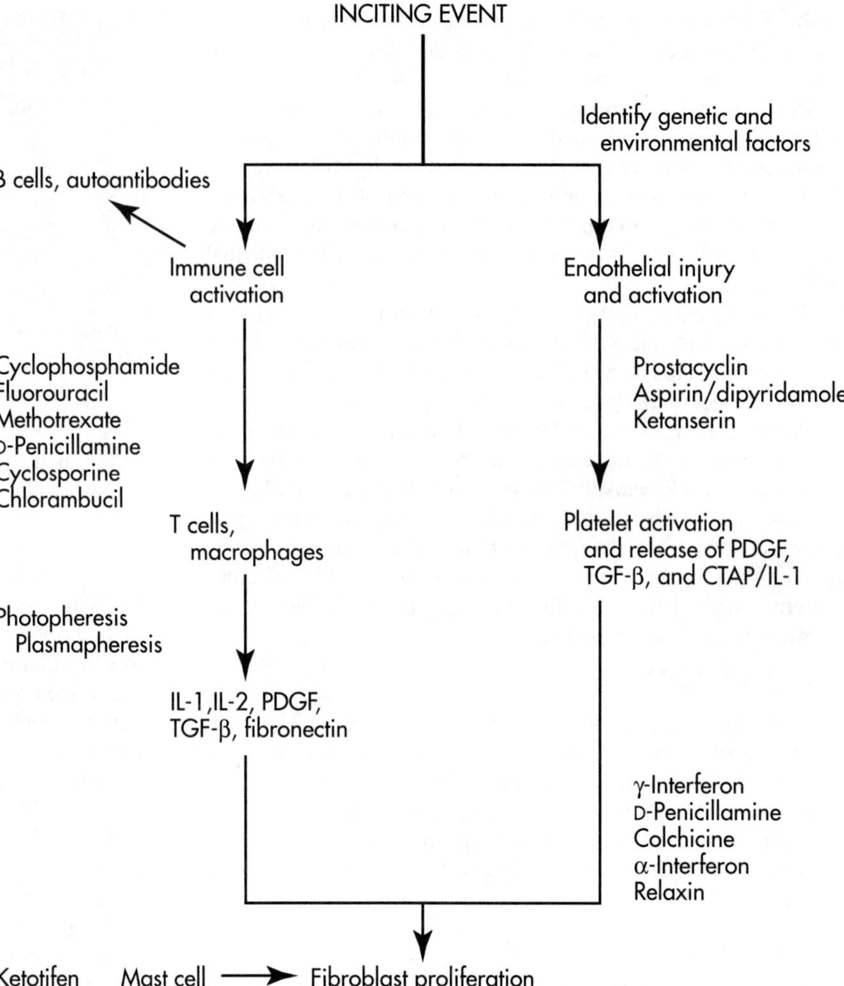

Fig. 139-10. Possible pathogenesis of systemic sclerosis (SSc) and location of possible sites where drugs might be useful for therapeutic intervention. *IL,* Interleukin; *PDGF,* platelet-derived growth factor; *TGF*-β, transforming growth factor beta; *CTAP,* connective tissue activating peptide.

Pericarditis, congestive heart failure, and serious dysrhythmias are potential complications of SSc. All are treated as they would be independent of scleroderma. Mild to moderate pericardial effusions and other asymptomatic cardiac abnormalities usually do not progress and require no treatment.

Renal crisis is treated with angiotensin-converting enzyme (ACE) inhibitors, which have dramatically improved the outcome.[3] Patients now have an 80% 1-year and 60% 5-year survival. The key to successful treatment is early detection and normalization of the blood pressure. In some cases, renal failure ensues despite early and vigorous intervention. Fortunately, however, more than 50% of those patients progressing to dialysis who remain on ACE inhibitor therapy have enough improvement in renal function to discontinue dialysis 6 to 18 months later.

Although an effective cure for scleroderma has not been determined, important advances in the management of visceral involvement have led to improved survival.

REFERENCES

1. Okano Y, Steen VD, Medsger TA Jr: Novel human serum autoantibodies reactive with RNA polymerase III: a major autoantigen in systemic sclerosis with diffuse cutaneous involvement, *Ann Intern Med* 119:1005, 1993.
2. Steen VD, Medsger TA Jr, Rodnan GP: D-penicillamine therapy in progressive systemic sclerosis (scleroderma), *Ann Intern Med* 97:652, 1982.
3. Steen VD et al: Outcome of renal crisis in systemic sclerosis: relation to availability converting enzyme (ACE) inhibitors, *Ann Intern Med* 113:352, 1990.
4. Wakelin SH, Marren P: Lichen sclerosus in women, *Clin Dermatol* 15:155, 1997.

ADDITIONAL READINGS

Follansbee WP: The cardiovascular manifestations of systemic sclerosis (scleroderma), *Curr Probl Cardiol* 11:245, 1986.

LeRoy EC: A brief overview of the pathogenesis of scleroderma (systemic sclerosis), *Ann Rheum Dis* 51:286, 1992.

LeRoy EC et al: Scleroderma (systemic sclerosis): classification, subsets and pathogenesis, *J Rheumatol* 15:202, 1988.

Masi AT et al: Preliminary criteria for the classification of systemic sclerosis (scleroderma), *Arthritis Rheum* 23:581, 1980.

Silver R et al: Cyclophosphamide and low dose prednisone therapy in systemic sclerosis (scleroderma) patients with interstitial lung disease, *J Rheumatol* 20:838, 1993.

Steen VD: Epidemiology of rheumatic disease: systemic sclerosis, *Rheum Dis Clin North Am* 16:641, 1990.

CHAPTER 140

Sjögren's Syndrome

Ann L. Parke

Sjögren's syndrome (SS) was originally defined as the presence of xerostomia (dry mouth) and xerophthalmia (dry eyes), specifically keratoconjunctivitis sicca. Dry eyes and mouth have many causes, however, which has led to confusion in defining SS (Box 140-1). A precise method of defining SS is to limit the diagnosis of SS to patients who have a specific pathologic disease process, that is, an autoimmune exocrinopathy demonstrated by the infiltration of T helper cells into exocrine glands. This chapter refers to this pathologic disease process as *Sjögren's disease* (SD). SD may be found in patients who have a well-defined rheumatologic disease, such as rheumatoid arthritis (RA) or systemic lupus erythematosus (SLE) (*secondary* SS/SD), or in patients who do not have an additional rheumatologic disease (*primary* SS/SD).

The difficulties that arose from the original definition of SS led to the development of several sets of criteria, including the European classification.[9] All these sets of criteria have limitations because they are based on subjective sicca complaints and objective investigations designed to evaluate glandular function. The criteria that require pathologic changes to demonstrate an autoimmune exocrinopathy (i.e., a positive lip biopsy) are very specific but are not sensitive, and up to 30% of lip biopsies may be falsely negative.

Box 140-1. Causes of Xerostomia and Xerophthalmia

Xerostomia

- Medications
  - Tricyclic antidepressants: amitriptyline (Elavil), doxepin (Sinequan)
  - Antihistamines: diphenhydramine (Benadryl), chlorpheniramine (Chlor-Trimeton), promethazine (Phenergan), and many cold and decongestant preparations
  - Anticholinergic agents: antiemetics such as scopolamine, antispasmodic agents such as oxybutynin chloride (Ditropan)
- Dehydration
  - Debility
  - Fever
- Polyuria
  - Alcohol intake
  - Arrhythmia
  - Diabetes
- Previous head and neck irradiation
- Systemic diseases
  - Sjögren's syndrome
  - Sarcoidosis
  - Amyloidosis
  - Human immunodeficiency virus (HIV) infection
  - Graft-vs.-host disease

Xerophthalmia

- See medications and systemic diseases listed above
- Abnormalities of eyelid function
  - Neuromuscular disorders
  - Aging
  - Thyrotoxicosis
- Abnormalities of tear production
  - Hypovitaminosis A
  - Stevens-Johnson syndrome
  - Familial diseases affecting sebaceous secretions
- Abnormalities of corneal surfaces: scarring from past injuries and herpes simplex infection

EPIDEMIOLOGY

The lack of a precise definition makes it difficult to assess the prevalence of true SS/SD. Previous estimates are based on the assumption that at least 50% of patients with RA have SS/SD and that 50% of patients with SS/SD have primary disease vs. secondary; this has led to the conclusion that SS/SD is the most common connective tissue disease, affecting more than 4 million Americans. Other reports suggest a prevalence of 1:250 individuals in the United States, whereas sicca complaints were found in up to 3% of Quebec's population. True SS/SD is more common in women than men (9:1) and is most common in postmenopausal women, for unknown reasons. Patients with earlier onset of disease and those who produce antibodies to extractable nuclear antigen Ro may develop a more aggressive systemic disease.[1] In a long-term outcome study of SS patients, malignancy was the major cause of death (56%).[6]

PATHOPHYSIOLOGY

Genetic Factors

Although the etiology of SS/SD is unknown, evidence now demonstrates the abnormal expression of autoantigen, activation of infiltrating lymphocytes, and local synthesis of autoantibodies at the primary site of pathology (i.e., the exocrine glands). These findings indicate a local immune response. HLA antigens play a vital role in individualizing the immune response because they present antigen to T cells. The presence of specific HLAs dictates the host's ability to respond to specific environmental triggers. SS/SD has been reported to be associated with DR2, DR3, and DR5 antigens. Also, production of antibodies to the Ro and La nuclear antigens is associated with DR3 and DR2. DR3 is in linkage disequilibrium with DQ2, and DR2 with DQ1. Subsequent studies have demonstrated that SS patients who are heterozygous for both DQ1 and DQ2 alleles are more likely to produce these autoantibodies.

Environmental Factors

Viruses have been implicated in the pathogenesis of various autoimmune diseases,[8] but the evidence for this association remains inconclusive. Renewed interest in this area followed the autoimmune complaints associated with human immunodeficiency virus (HIV) infection. Some HIV patients develop a diffuse infiltrative lymphocytic syndrome (DILS) and may complain of xerostomia and xerophthalmia. Biopsies of the salivary glands of these patients demonstrate lymphocytic infiltrates, but these are predominantly T suppressor cells, not the T helper cells found in SD patients.

Some retroviruses are trophic for the ductal epithelium of

salivary and lacrimal glands, and human T-cell lymphotrophic virus (HTLV-1) may be involved in the pathogenesis of SS. Epstein-Barr virus (EBV), a deoxyribonucleic acid (DNA) virus that belongs to the herpesvirus family, is secreted in saliva and is known to be associated with the development of nasopharyngeal carcinoma. EBV infects B cells and promotes B-cell proliferation and may be associated with SS. SS/SD may also be associated with hepatitis C virus (HCV) infection. HCV is secreted in saliva, and some patients with HCV infection develop sicca complaints. Rheumatic and autoimmune manifestations of chronic HCV are numerous, and chronic infection is much more prevalent than previously thought. Patients with chronic HCV liver disease may develop a sialoadenitis, with focal lymphocytic infiltrates found in salivary gland biopsy. This suggests that HCV is one of the few infections capable of producing a false-positive lip biopsy or that HCV may be directly involved in the pathogenesis of autoimmune sialoadenitis. Approximately 4% of SS/SD patients have persistent HCV ribonucleic acid (RNA) detected by polymerase chain reaction (PCR), and up to 47% of primary SS patients with cryoglobulins have antibodies to HCV.[5]

Glandular Factors

Histopathologic changes found in the salivary glands of SD patients include a benign lymphoepithelial lesion (BLEL) and focal lymphocytic sialoadenitis. BLELs are found in approximately 40% of major salivary glands from patients with SS, in whom the salivary epithelium is replaced and infiltrated with lymphocytes. Epimyoepithelial islands, remnants of ductal epithelium, are found, which help to distinguish BLEL from overt lymphoma. A pathologic feature found in the minor salivary glands of these patients is a focal lymphocytic infiltrate that consists primarily of T helper cells (Fig. 140-1). This pathology, however, is not specific for SD. Other disease entities (e.g., sarcoidosis, chronic HCV infection, graft-vs.-host disease) and HIV-positive patients with DILS may show similar pathologic changes.

Xerophthalmia and xerostomia may be consequences of senescence. Studies suggest that glandular fibrosis and atrophy are features of aging. Fatty change with some nonspecific inflammatory cell infiltrates may occur in normal salivary glands. Some believe that glandular atrophy and fibrosis are postinflammatory changes that may occur in SS/SD.

Immune Abnormalities

Autoantibody Production. Most often in SS/SD, organ-nonspecific antibodies are produced, including antinuclear antibodies (ANAs) and rheumatoid factor (RF). Many nuclear antigens exist, and therefore a variety of autoantibodies can give positive ANA tests. The ANA pattern can vary and depends somewhat on the antigenic specificity of the antibody. SS/SD patients most frequently produce a speckled ANA pattern, with the major antibody reactivity directed toward the extractable nuclear antigens Ro and La (SSA and SSB). Depending on the assay's sensitivity, approximately 60% to 90% of primary SS/SD patients have the antibody to

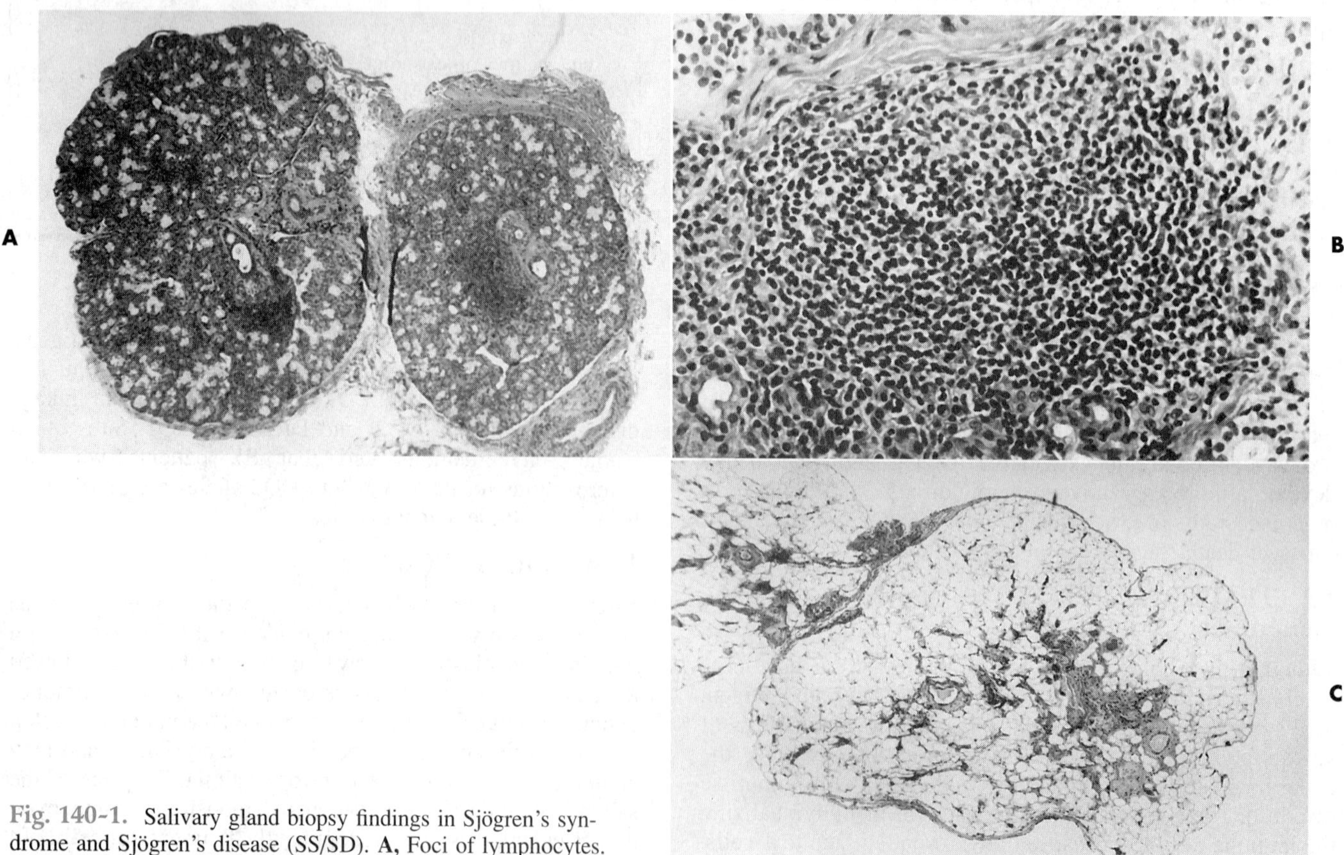

Fig. 140-1. Salivary gland biopsy findings in Sjögren's syndrome and Sjögren's disease (SS/SD). **A,** Foci of lymphocytes. (Magnification ×40.) **B,** Lymphocytic focus. (×250.) **C,** Loss of glandular tissue and atrophy with no lymphocytic foci. (×40.)

Ro, but this is not specific for SS/SD; patients with SLE (30%) and subacute cutaneous SLE (60%) also produce this antibody. Sjögren's patients and SLE patients may produce antibodies to different fractions of Ro antigen. Antibodies to the 52-kilo dalton (kD) band alone occur more often in SS patients, whereas antibodies to the 60-kD band alone occur more often in SLE patients. Ro antibodies may be associated with the more severe extraglandular complaints of SD (e.g., vasculitis). Antibodies to La rarely occur alone and are typically associated with antibodies to Ro. The finding of La antibodies in saliva suggests local glandular production of antibody that is antigen driven.

The transplacental passage of the maternal antibody to Ro and La is thought to be involved in the pathogenesis of the neonatal lupus syndrome (NLS). The clinical features of NLS are a transient photosensitive rash and a primary congenital complete heart block (CCHB). Some of these Ro-positive mothers are clinically normal during their abnormal pregnancy, but on long-term follow-up, some of these asymptomatic mothers eventually fulfill criteria for a connective tissue disease, usually SS/SD.[2]

RF is an autoantibody that is much less specific for SS/SD. Immunoglobulin A (IgA) RF may occur more often in both the blood and saliva of patients with SS/SD than in those with other autoimmune diseases. Mixed cryoglobulinemia may also be found in patients with SS/SD and is more often found in those who produce autoantibodies, especially Ro antibodies. Cryoglobulinemia may be associated with the development of vasculitis (as can any disease resulting in the production of autoantibodies). In Sjögren's patients the deposition of immune complexes with the activation of complement has been incriminated in the pathogenesis of leukocytoclastic vasculitis (perivascular infiltrate of polymorphonuclear leukocytes). In another type of vasculitis the predominant infiltrate is mononuclear, and the pathogenesis is unknown.

Hypergammaglobulinemia. Polyclonal hypergammaglobulinemia is another marker of B-cell hyperactivity. In some patients, B-cell reactivity becomes oligoclonal or even monoclonal, with the production of monoclonal spikes on immune electrophoresis and monoclonal light chains in both urine and serum. This may remain a benign gammopathy or may be associated with a B-cell malignancy.

B-Cell Malignancy. Patients with SS/SD are at an increased risk for developing non-Hodgkin's B-cell lymphoma.[11] It is estimated that fewer than 10% of Sjögren's patients develop overt malignancy. The majority of these lesions are low-grade lymphomas, and some have been noted to regress spontaneously. B-cell hyperactivity may progress from benign reactivity through a phase called *pseudolymphoma* before becoming overtly malignant. This pseudolymphomatous change must be managed aggressively if progression to true malignant change is to be averted. Some suggest that decreased titers of autoantibodies may indicate progression toward malignancy, but other studies have failed to confirm this finding.

T-cell Abnormalities. The cellular infiltrate contributing to the autoimmune exocrinopathy is predominantly an infiltration of T helper cells. This glandular lymphocytic infiltrate is secondary to some primary initiating event, but the nature of this primary event remains obscure.

PATIENT EVALUATION

History

Sjögren's syndrome is a systemic disease that requires a full patient history. Xerostomia and xerophthalmia are often late manifestations of SS/SD, and other features may precede the sicca complaints.[4] Fatigue is often a dominant symptom and is underestimated. To uncover an underlying connective tissue disease, the physician must ask questions about photosensitivity, alopecia, mucosal ulceration, Raynaud's phenomenon, and any family history. A full obstetric history is also important because an abnormal pregnancy may be an early sign of connective tissue disease.[2]

Physical Examination

Oral Component. Because the clinical manifestations of SS/SD are so diverse, a comprehensive examination must be performed for both glandular and extraglandular disease (Table 140-1). To assess for oral dryness, the tongue is examined for redness, dryness, and loss of papillae (Fig. 140-2). Sublingual pooling and overall moistness of the oral cavity should be evaluated (Fig. 140-3). Saliva production can be assessed using the Saxon test, which requires chewing on a gauze swab for 2 minutes. The difference in weight of the swab before and after chewing is a measure of the saliva produced in those 2 minutes (normally, more than 2.75 gm).

Table 140-1. Clinical Manifestations of Glandular and Extraglandular Disease Associated With Sjögren's Syndrome

Disease/site	Clinical manifestations
Glandular disease	
Salivary	Yeast infections, xerostomia, dental caries
Lacrimal	Keratoconjunctivitis sicca
Bronchopulmonary tree	Recurrent cough and infections, lymphocytic interstitial pneumonitis
Skin	Dry skin, photosensitivity, rashes
Gastrointesinal tract	Atrophic gastritis, celiac disease
Pancreas	Pancreatitis, pancreatic insufficiency, diabetes
Thyroid	Autoimmune thyroiditis
Genitourinary tract	Renal tubular acidosis, nephrolithiasis, interstitial cystitis, vaginal dryness, yeast infections, dyspareunia
Hepatobiliary tract	Chronic active hepatitis, primary biliary cirrhosis
Extraglandular disease	
Systemic inflammation	Fatigue
Arthritis, myositis	Joint swelling, muscle weakness
Vasospasm	Raynaud's phenomenon
Systemic vasculitis	Ischemia, infarction, end-organ insufficiency
Neurologic disease	Peripheral neuropathies
Abnormal pregnancy	Neonatal lupus syndrome
Cytopenia	Anemia, infection
Malignancy	B-cell lymphomas, lymphadenopathy, hepatosplenomegaly, carcinomas

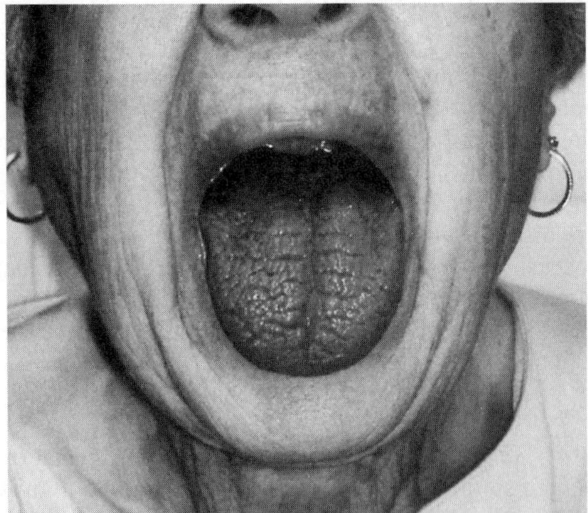

Fig. 140-2. "Crocodile tongue" in SS patient.

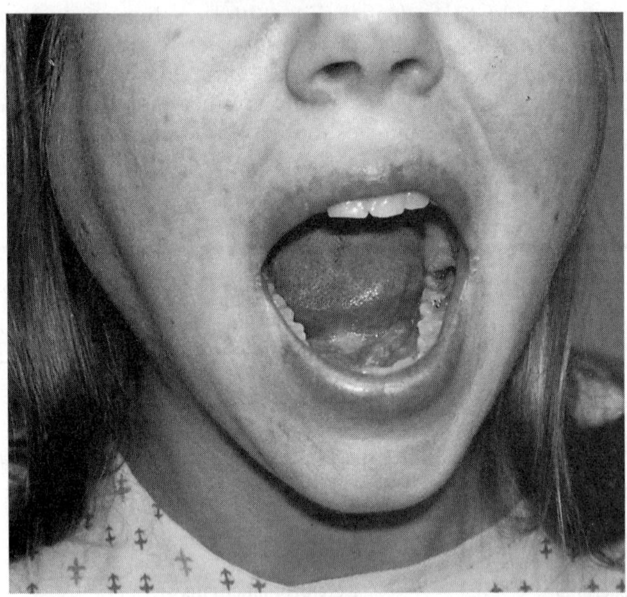

Fig. 140-3. Poor sublingual pooling and parotid swelling.

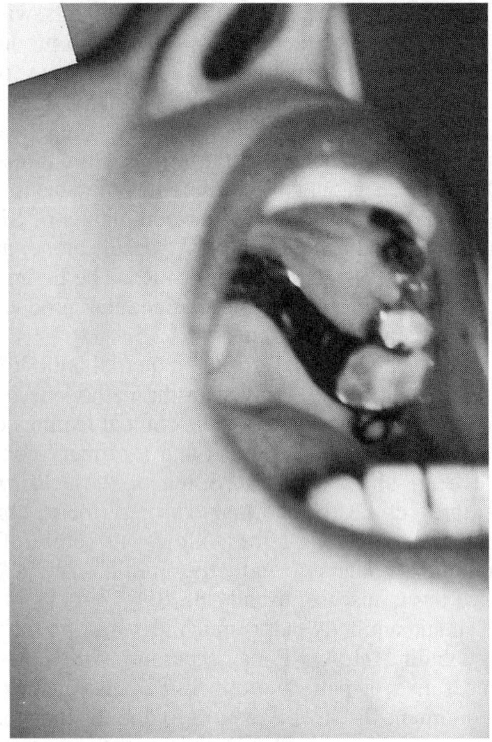

Fig. 140-4. Dental decay. (Courtesy Jason Tanzer, DMD, University of Connecticut School of Dental Medicine.)

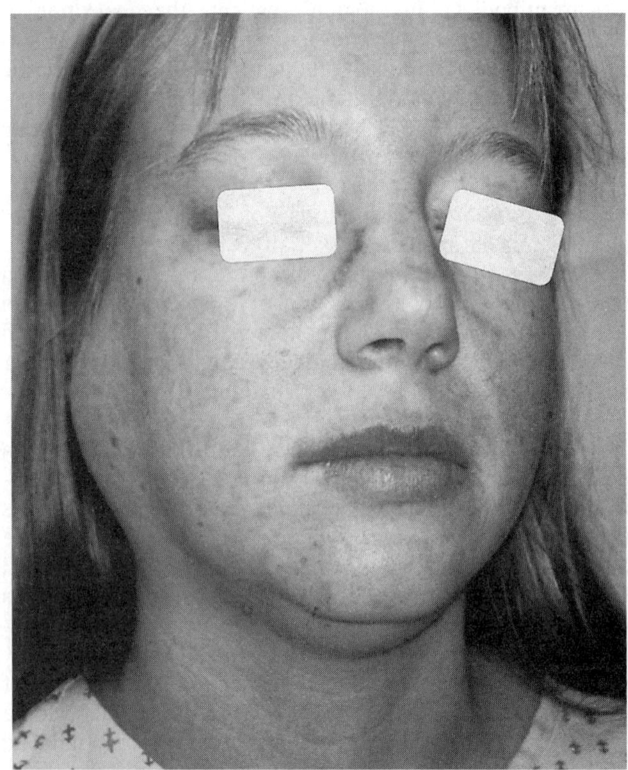

Fig. 140-5. Swollen parotids in SS patient.

Patients with dry mouths are at risk for the development of dental caries (Fig. 140-4) and oral candidiasis. These patients frequently do not show the usual white plaques typically associated with oral candidiasis. It is therefore very important to culture for *Candida* even if an oral inspection is not typical for this problem. Gingivitis, extensive dental caries, an abnormal pattern of dental caries, and burning-mouth syndrome are all complications of the dry mouth. Swollen parotids ("chipmunk facies") and swollen submandibular glands occur in some patients (Fig. 140-5). Persistent unilateral swelling is serious, and the patient should be evaluated for lymphoma (Fig. 140-6). Acute, painful swelling is a sign of infection, and milking the affected gland may produce a thick, opaque discharge into the mouth, in contrast to the usual colorless glandular secretion.

Ocular Component. Evaluating the ocular component of SS/SD can be done in the clinic with Schirmer's test. This involves placing filter papers inside the lower lid at the junction of the nasal and middle thirds of the lid for 5 minutes and measuring the length of the filter paper that is made wet by tears (normally, greater than 5 mm of wetting per 5 minutes). All other testing should be done by an ophthalmologist and includes the rose bengal test to assess conjunctival pathology (any residual staining is abnormal), examination of

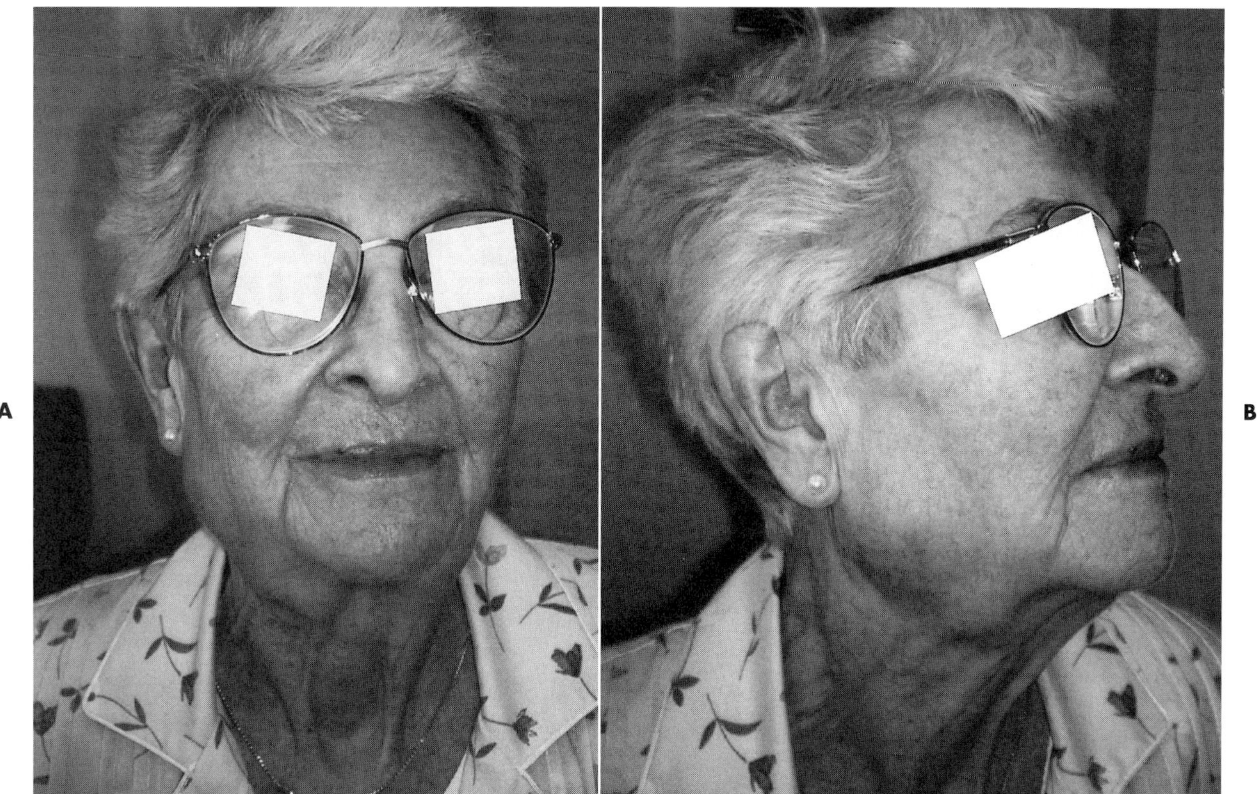

Fig. 140-6. **A,** Unilateral swelling caused by lymphoma in SS patient. **B,** Lymphoma.

the tear film and height, examination for cells and cellular debris as well as mucus and mucous debris, fluorescein staining, and a tear breakup time to assess corneal pathology. Some patients react adversely to the preservative used in rose bengal stain, so preservative-free strips should be used. A potential substitute for rose bengal is lisamine green, which does not cause pain when corneal ulcers are present. Other tests, including tear osmolality and tear lactoferrin levels, are available only in specialized centers.

Other Clinical Features. SS/SD is a multiorgan disease, and other glandular manifestations include pancreatic, hepatic, thyroid, and renal disease. More than 70% of patients with primary biliary cirrhosis and 40% with chronic active hepatitis complain of dry eyes or dry mouth. The liver is an exocrine gland, and some suggest that all these features can be explained as consequences of damage to the ductal epithelium. The relationship of SD to these autoimmune hepatic diseases, which have a fairly specific autoantibody production, is unclear, but chronic HCV infection may be one cause. Hepatitis C may also be associated with cryoglobulinemia and vasculitis (Fig. 140-7). Vasculitis occurs in SS/SD patients who do not have HCV, however, and more frequently in patients who are Ro antibody positive. Renal involvement also occurs more often in Ro antibody–positive patients. Up to 30% of SS/SD patients may develop renal tubular acidosis, most frequently type I.

LABORATORY STUDIES AND DIAGNOSTIC PROCEDURES

Laboratory tests include blood work every 6 months (Table 140-2) and a chest radiograph annually. Tests are done primarily to screen for occult lymphoma, with a full examination for lymphadenopathy and hepatosplenomegaly.

Patients complaining of xerostomia should have a lip biopsy, which can be done in an outpatient setting using local anesthesia with epinephrine to minimize blood loss. Patients who take nonsteroidal antiinflammatory drugs (NSAIDs) are usually not troubled by excessive bleeding, but patients who take anticoagulants may have additional blood loss and require suturing. Routinely, however, the mouth heals well, and the wound does not require sutures. All patients requiring antibiotic prophylaxis to prevent bacterial endocarditis must receive antibiotics when having a minor salivary gland biopsy. The biopsy involves the removal of 5 to 10 small salivary glands from inside the lower lip. A focal score greater than 1 (more than 50 cells/4 mm^2) is considered a positive biopsy, suggesting an autoimmune exocrinopathy.

Scintigraphy is used to evaluate glandular function and inflammation. Glandular uptake is evaluated by scanning the patient for 20 to 25 minutes after technetium injection. The patient is then given a lemon stimulus to promote glandular emptying and is scanned for an additional 20 to 25 minutes to measure uptake and glandular secretion. Gallium scanning is useful for assessing glandular inflammation (Fig. 140-8). The "panda sign" may also be found in patients with sarcoidosis, which can cause false-positive biopsies when evaluating patients for SS/SD. Some centers prefer to use sialography, claiming that scintigraphy with either gallium or technetium is too insensitive; however, the long-term effects of instilling contrast into chronically inflamed tissues are a concern.

DIFFERENTIAL DIAGNOSIS

The differential diagnosis of xerostomia and xerophthalmia includes many diseases (see Box 140-1). In patients with extraglandular disease and other features of an autoimmune

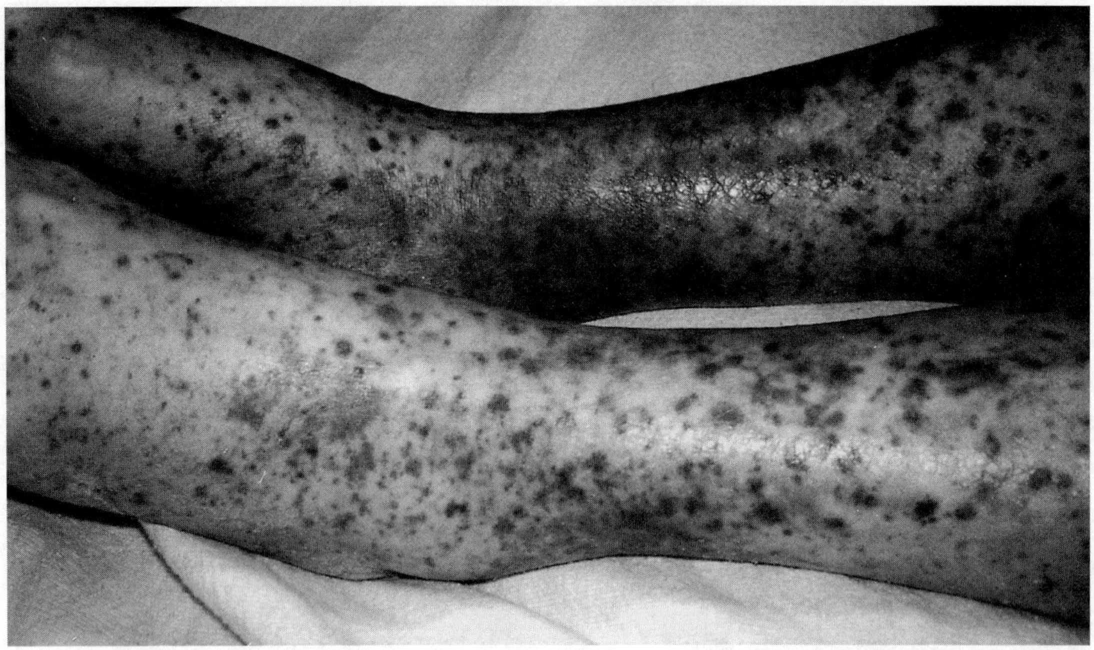

Fig. 140-7. Vasculitis in SS patient.

Table 140-2. Laboratory Evaluation for Sjögren's Syndrome

Systemic	Complete blood count, platelets, erythrocyte sedimentation rate complement levels, cryoglobulins, hepatitis C screening, HIV screening
Glandular	Amylase, lipase, aspartate and alanine transaminase, blood sugar, electrolytes, urinalysis, thyroid profile, chest radiograph
Autoantibodies	ANA (antinuclear antibody), rheumatoid factor, ENA (antibodies to Ro, La, Sm, RNP), anti-ds-DNA
	Mitochondrial, smooth muscle, and thyroglobulin antibodies; immunoglobulin levels; immunoglobulin electrophoresis

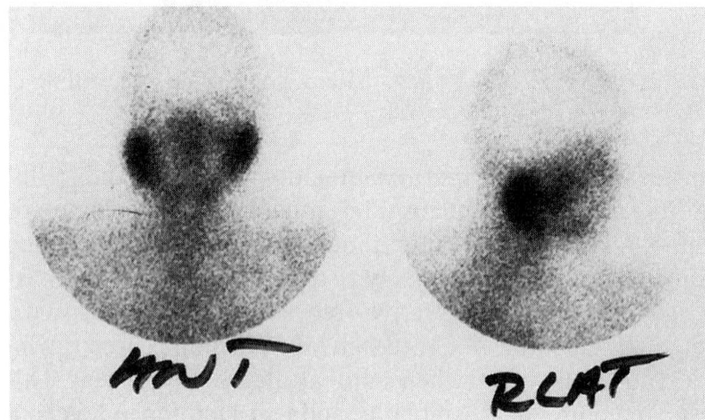

Fig. 140-8. "Panda sign" in SD patient demonstrated by uptake of gallium-67 citrate in parotid and submandibular glands. In this particular patient, uptake by lacrimal glands is not marked.

disease, it is sometimes difficult to differentiate between primary and secondary SS/SD, especially patients with SLE. The diagnosis of SLE requires the presence of 4 of 11 revised criteria, although some patients may have SLE even though they do not meet criteria at a particular time.

Sicca complaints are the end stage of SS/SD. These patients probably have had their autoimmune exocrinopathy for many years before they developed symptoms of dryness. Patients therefore may not complain of dryness but may present with other symptoms (see Table 140-1).

Diseases that can give a false-positive lip biopsy include sarcoidosis and DILS. HIV-positive patients are more likely to be young males than elderly, postmenopausal women. Patients with DILS frequently have massive glandular swelling with numerous extraglandular manifestations. The autoantibody production in classic SD occurs infrequently in these patients. HLA associations also are different, with DR5 and DR6 occurring in black DILS patients and DR6 in white patients. The usual pathology of sarcoidosis is noncaseating granulomas. Sarcoid patients may also produce RFs and have elevated immunoglobulin levels (IgG). Chest radiographs are usually abnormal in these patients, however, revealing either bilateral hilar adenopathy or diffuse parenchymal disease. Gallium scanning is positive in approximately 65% to 70% of sarcoid patients, with a positive panda sign detected as the gallium is taken up by the parotid, lacrimal, and submandibular glands.

MANAGEMENT

Although considered to be a rare disease, SS/SD is quite common. An estimated 4 million or more Americans have SS/SD, and it can take up to 10 years for patients to be diagnosed appropriately even when the sicca complaints are obvious.[4] Education of primary care physicians, nurse practitioners, and dentists is therefore a vital component in the management of this disease. Education is also probably the most important component of patient management. Patients must understand that their complaints are real and the result of a systemic inflammatory disease. Treatment is available, but not a cure.

Long-term studies of SS/SD patients suggest that up to 25% of patients will develop new clinical features, especially those with Ro antibodies.[3] Malignancy is the most common cause of death,[7] and the risk for developing a B-cell lymphoma is increased in SS/SD patients. The constant fatigue and difficulty in eating and talking are severely debilitating for SS/SD patients. This sicca complex can lead to major psychosocial and family problems. These patients should have access to support groups through the Arthritis Foundation, the Sjögren's Syndrome Foundation, or the National Sjögren's Syndrome Association (Box 140-2).

Box 140-2. Resources for Patients with Sjögren's Syndrome

Arthritis Foundation
PO Box 19000
Atlanta, GA 30326
800-283-7800

National Sjögren's Syndrome Association
PO Box 22066
Beachwood, OH 44122
216-292-3866
800-395-6772
FAX: 216-292-4955

Sjögren's Syndrome Foundation
366 North Broadway
Suite PH-W2
Jericho, NY 11753
516-933-6365 or 1-800-475-6473
FAX: 516-767-7156

Pharmacologic Treatment

The pharmacologic approach to managing SS/SD patients can be divided into two groups: agents promoting secretion (sialogogues and mucolytic agents) and antiinflammatory agents. Agents that promote the production of natural secretions have been reported to be useful.[10] Recently approved for SD/SS patients, oral pilocarpine is a positive step in management. Side effects from pilocarpine include sweating, abdominal cramping, diarrhea, bradycardia, hypotension, and bronchospasm. Pilocarpine is generally well tolerated, however, but must not be given to asthmatic patients. Sweating can be minimized if pilocarpine is taken after eating.

Mucolytic agents, such as bromhexine and acetylcysteine, have been reported to be useful, but some controlled studies have not found a benefit. Many patients report relief with bromhexine, and even though this agent is not available in the United States, some patients go to extreme lengths to obtain it.

Hydroxychloroquine (Plaquenil) is an effective agent for treating arthritis and skin disease in patients with RA and SLE. This is an extremely useful drug for patients with SS/SD, although this has not been confirmed by all studies. Some patients report that hydroxychloroquine not only improves their arthralgias and arthritis, but also reduces their overwhelming fatigue.

Corticosteroids and immunosuppressive agents should be reserved for patients with severe extraglandular disease when vasculitis and end-organ failure are potential problems. Such patients may need high-dose corticosteroids and additional immunosuppression. Methotrexate is not a well-recognized agent for managing SS/SD; however, some patients with SS/SD secondary to RA also experience an improvement in their sicca complaints as well as in their underlying arthritis when treated with methotrexate. The use of azathioprine (Imuran) should be discouraged, since these patients are already at risk for developing lymphoma. Cyclophosphamide should be used only as intermittent boluses because of the bladder toxicity (hemorrhagic cystitis and malignancy) that has been reported with daily oral therapy. Cyclosporine eye drops should soon be available.

Nonpharmacologic Treatment

Other approaches currently being developed include the use of polyunsaturated fatty acids, such as linoleic acid (the major constituent of oil of evening primrose). Ingesting these fatty acids results in the synthesis of fewer inflammatory prostanoids, and studies have demonstrated that these agents may be useful in the management of RA. Similar studies are currently being carried out in Sjögren's patients.

Complications

Glandular failure has numerous consequences. Pulmonary infections, sinusitis, glandular infections (particularly of the parotids), and eyelid infections occur frequently and require prompt treatment. Oral candidiasis results in a sore, painful mouth that further hinders eating. The usual oral preparations for treating candidiasis frequently contain sugar; therefore clotrimazole (Mycelex) troches should be prescribed for patients who are not edentulous. Patients should be treated for at least 1 month and should eat live-culture yogurt daily. Studies have demonstrated that yogurt containing lactobacilli can prevent recurrent vaginal candidiasis, which may also help to prevent yeast colonizing the mouth and esophagus.

Artificial tears and artificial saliva are important local treatments for SS to reduce the symptoms of dryness. Artificial eye drops appear to be more effective than artificial saliva. Various preparations are available, and some patients are sensitive to the preservatives used to make artificial tears. Patients frequently need to experiment to find the product best suited for them. Eye drops produced without preservatives are more expensive.

Other measures to protect the dry eye include the use of moisture chamber glasses, with a protective screen extending down the arms of the glasses. This minimizes the effects of wind and automobile heating and cooling systems blowing onto the dry eye surface. Patients who have continuing sicca problems with the cornea and who are at risk for ulceration may benefit from the use of soft contact lenses. Such patients should consider punctal occlusion in an attempt to preserve more of a tear film on the eye surface. Stents can be inserted as a temporary measure to determine if there is a benefit to the patient before surgical ablation of the punctum is performed.

Saliva substitutes do not last long enough and thus are less effective at maintaining moisture in the mouth than artificial tears are for maintaining moisture in the eyes. Patients frequently carry water bottles, and some find that mixing water and glycerin (1 L of water to 20 ml of glycerin), with lemon to taste, and using a spray bottle to apply the solution is better than simply sipping water. Constant chewing or sucking helps to stimulate salivary secretion, but a major problem is rampant dental caries if sugarless products are not used. Fluoride-containing gel used twice a day is essential.

Skin dryness may respond to moisturizers, whereas vaginal dryness may be improved with KY jelly or Replens.

Follow-up and Consultation

Patients with SS/SD must have regular follow-up with an ophthalmologist who specializes in the dry eye, a dentist who has expertise in dry mouth, and either a rheumatologist or an internist. Preventing the major medical problems associated with SS/SD is an essential aspect of care. Other exocrine glandular involvement must be identified because some patients require pancreatic supplementation and others become thyrotoxic or diabetic. Autoimmune thyroid disease may precede the sicca complaints, and therefore the physician must consider this diagnosis in all patients with any exocrine or endocrine glandular disease, chronic fatigue, or fibromyalgia syndromes.

Patients with extraglandular diseases pose additional problems. These patients generally have more severe disease and require aggressive therapy with corticosteroids or immunosuppressive agents. The development of major organ damage and associated vasculitis are of particular concern and require consultation with a rheumatologist.

The increasing awareness of SS/SD will confirm that it is a very common debilitating disease. Treatment is available, and with appropriate referrals to dentists, ophthalmologists, and rheumatologists, this disease and its complications are manageable.

REFERENCES

1. Alexander EL et al: Sjögren's syndrome: association of anti-Ro-SS-A antibodies with vasculitis, hematologic abnormalities, and serologic hyperactivity, *Ann Intern Med* 98:155, 1983.
2. Buyon JP: Autoantibodies reactive with Ro (SSA) and La (SSB) and pregnancy, *J Rheumatol* 24(suppl 50):12, 1997.
3. Kruize AA, Hene RJ, Van Der Heide A, et al: Long-term follow-up of patients with Sjögren's syndrome, *Arthritis Rheum* 39:297, 1996.
4. Manthorpe R, Asmussen K, Oxholm P: Primary Sjögren's syndrome: diagnostic criteria, clinical features and disease activity, *J Rheumatol* 24(suppl 50):8, 1997.
5. Ramos-Casals M, Cervera R, Yague J, et al: Cryoglobulinemia in primary Sjögren's syndrome: prevalence and clinical characteristics in a series of 115 patients, *Semin Arthritis Rheum* 28:200, 1998.
6. Sugai S, Cui G, Ogawa Y, et al: Analysis of the cause of death of 23 patients with Sjögren's syndrome, *Ryumachi* 36:770, 1997.
7. Sugai S, Cui G, Ogawa Y, et al: Long-term follow-up study and cause of death in patients with Sjögren's syndrome, *J Rheumatol* 24(suppl 50):39, 1997.
8. Venables PJW, Rigby SP: Viruses in the etiopathogenesis of Sjögren's syndrome, *J Rheumatol* 24(suppl 50):3, 1997.
9. Vitali C, Bombardieri S, Moutsopoulos HM, et al: Preliminary criteria for the classification of Sjögren's syndrome: results of prospective concerted action supported by the European community, *Arthritis Rheum* 36:340, 1993.
10. Vivino MD et al: Pilocarpine tablets for the treatment of dry mouth and dry eye symptoms in patients with Sjögren's syndrome, *Arch Intern Med* 159:174, 1999.
11. Zufferey P, Meyer OC, Grossin M, et al: Primary Sjögren's syndrome (SS) and malignant lymphoma: a retrospective cohort study of SS patients, *Scand J Rheumatol* 24:342, 1995.

CHAPTER 141

Infectious Agents

Bernard Zimmermann, III
Edward V. Lally
Nancy Y.N. Liu

Musculoskeletal infections constitute an important group of illnesses for which patients often seek primary care. Acute inflammation of a joint, bursa, or tendon must be identified as either infectious or noninfectious to institute proper treatment. The most common bacterial infections that affect the musculoskeletal system include septic arthritis, septic bursitis, and osteomyelitis. In addition, viral arthritis, HIV-associated musculoskeletal syndromes, and Lyme disease are associated disorders.

SEPTIC ARTHRITIS

Epidemiology and Etiology

Acute bacterial septic arthritis is an urgent medical emergency because of the potential for joint destruction and mortality if the diagnosis and treatment are delayed or overlooked. The most common presentation of septic arthritis is an acutely painful and swollen joint in the patient with preexisting arthritis. Septic arthritis is usually caused by the hematogenous spread of bacteria to a joint previously damaged by arthritis or injury. Host factors that increase the risk of septic arthritis include older age, chronic illnesses with immunodeficiency, and preexisting arthritis. A large prospective study showed that age over 80 years, diabetes mellitus, rheumatoid arthritis (RA), prosthetic joint surgery, and skin infections were important independent risk factors predisposing to the development of septic arthritis in patients with arthritis.[8] Skin flora are the most common sources of infection, but upper respiratory, gastrointestinal, and genitourinary portals of entry are also found. Rarely, septic arthritis may follow a penetrating injury or may be related to contiguous osteomyelitis, especially in children. The knee is the joint most often affected by septic arthritis, followed by, in decreasing order of frequency, the shoulder, hip, elbow, wrist, ankle, and small joints of the hands and feet. Infections of deep joints (e.g., sacroiliac) are uncommon, and the correct diagnosis often depends on the results of appropriate imaging studies.[21]

From 75% to 80% of cases of nongonococcal bacterial septic arthritis in adults are caused by gram-positive bacteria, usually *Staphylococcus* or *Streptococcus,* and 15% to 20% of these infections are caused by gram-negative organisms (Table 141-1). The incidence of gram-negative septic arthritis, particularly *Escherichia coli,* has risen in the past 25 years. These infections occur notably in elderly debilitated patients, injection drug users, and young children.[1] Septic arthritis caused by *Haemophilus influenzae* may be decreasing with the advent of vaccination of children for this organism.[14] Anaerobic joint infections, although still rare, have also increased in frequency and are most often found in association with postoperative wound infections, especially after total joint replacement.[6] A variety of unusual organisms, including fungi and mycobacteria, have been reported to

Table 141-1. Microbiology of Bacterial Septic Arthritis Related to Age of Patient*

Organism	Children (6 mo-5 yr)	Young adult	Adult	Elderly
Staphylococcus aureus	10-20	15-20	60-70	45-65
Streptococcus	5-10	1-5	15-20	10-15
Gram negative	1-5	Rare	10-15	15-35
Haemophilus influenzae	30-50	1-5	1-5	Rare
Neisseria gonorrhoeae	1-5	60-80	1-5	Rare

*Percentages compiled from several studies.

cause septic arthritis. These usually present as chronic insidious monoarticular inflammation.

Patient Evaluation

The patient usually complains of several days of progressive pain and swelling in one or more joints. Fever, sweats, or shaking chills may indicate systemic infection, and cough or dysuria may suggest an extraarticular source of bacteremia. Acute migratory polyarthritis with tenosynovitis in a young, sexually active adult suggests septic arthritis from disseminated gonococcal infection.

Physical examination may yield findings of a source of infection, such as pneumonia, otitis, pharyngitis, or cutaneous abscess. A synovial effusion is invariably present but may be difficult to discern in the obese patient. There is swelling, erythema, warmth, and limited range of motion of the affected joint. A complete musculoskeletal examination should be performed to investigate the possibility of polyarticular septic arthritis, which may be found in 20% of patients.

Laboratory Studies and Differential Diagnosis

The definitive diagnosis of septic arthritis depends on the analysis of synovial fluid obtained by arthrocentesis (Box 141-1). Septic synovial fluid appears cloudy or purulent. Gram's stain demonstrates bacteria in 50% to 75% of cases of nongonococcal bacterial septic arthritis and should be used to guide the initial choice of antibiotic therapy. Synovial fluid white blood cell (WBC) counts greater than 50,000 cells/mm^3 with more than 80% polymorphonuclear neutrophil leukocytes (PMNs) signify a high probability of infection, although gout and acute flares of RA may produce this degree of inflammation. Bacterial septic arthritis may occasionally present with a synovial fluid WBC count less than 50,000 cells/mm^3, particularly in gonococcal septic arthritis. Radiographs of the affected joints should be obtained to assess underlying arthritis, investigate for contiguous osteomyelitis, and establish a baseline for future comparison. Blood cultures are also necessary to determine the presence of bacteremia. Extraarticular sources of infection should be pursued with appropriate diagnostic studies.

The differential diagnosis includes crystalline arthritis, acute viral arthritis, and nonseptic inflammatory arthritis. The patient with preexisting RA or another chronic inflammatory arthritis presents a particular diagnostic challenge, since septic arthritis may initially be mistaken for a flare of the underlying disease. A history of pain and swelling in one joint out of proportion to the others or the presence of fever or systemic signs should suggest joint infection. The presence of monosodium urate or calcium pyrophosphate crystals on polarized microscopy establishes the diagnosis of acute crystalline arthritis in the appropriate clinical setting but does not rule out coexistent bacterial arthritis.

Box 141-1. Laboratory Studies for Septic Arthritis

Synovial Fluid

Gram's stain: positive in 50% to 75% of patients (less in gonococcal arthritis)

Culture: essential for diagnosis and treatment (may be negative in patients taking antibiotics)

White blood cell count: >50,000 is indicative of infection (lower in gonococcal arthritis)

White blood cell differential: >95% polymorphonuclear leukocytes is indicative of infection

Crystal analysis: presence of crystals does not exclude infection

Blood

White blood cell count: elevated in most patients

Blood cultures: positive in 50% of patients

Radiology

Radiograph of affected joint: preexisting arthritis, possible osteomyelitis

Gonococcal Arthritis

Disseminated gonococcal infection may present with manifestations of acute septic arthritis. The *dermatitis-arthritis syndrome* is usually seen in sexually active adults, often in females within 1 week of menstruation or in the postpartum period. Many skin and joint manifestations of the syndrome are mediated by circulating immune complexes rather than direct microbial infection.[13] The emergence of penicillin-resistant strains of gonococci requires third-generation cephalosporins in geographic areas where resistance is common (see Chapter 27). Two thirds of patients have tenosynovitis that affects the tendon sheaths of the wrists, fingers, ankles, and toes. Approximately 50% of patients have frank arthritis that is usually monoarticular but may progress to migratory or additive polyarthritis. Skin involvement occurs in as many as two thirds of patients with disseminated gonococcal infection. Cutaneous papules or pustules with an erythematous base are usually noted on the extremities and may have a necrotic center. The diagnosis must often be made on clinical grounds, since the synovial fluid WBC counts are lower than with nongonococcal bacterial infections (30,000 to 60,000 cells/mm^3), Gram's stain is often nondiagnostic, and even careful cultures plated on chocolate agar are positive in only 25% of cases. To increase the yield of positive cultures, urethral, cervical, blood, and, when appropriate, pharyngeal and rectal cultures should be performed if disseminated gonococcal infection is suspected. Studies with polymerase chain reaction (PCR) analysis have demonstrated bacterial deoxyribonucleic acid (DNA) in synovial fluid, which may be diagnostically useful.[9]

Management

The treatment of nongonococcal bacterial septic arthritis requires hospitalization for intravenous (IV) antibiotic therapy and joint drainage. Table 141-2 presents recommendations for the initial choice of antibiotics for adults based on the Gram's stain and clinical setting. Results of culture and sensitivity analysis determine the final antibiotic selection (Table 141-3). To remove inflammatory cells producing proteolytic enzymes, the joint must be thoroughly drained to minimize permanent joint damage. There are no prospective studies of the optimum method of drainage of the infected joint.[7] In many cases, such as uncomplicated knee infections, satisfactory drainage may be achieved by daily needle

Table 141-2. Antibiotic Therapy of Presumed Bacterial Arthritis in Adults (Pathogen Unknown)

Gram's stain	Presumed organism(s)	Antibiotic(s)
Positive		
Gram-positive cocci	*Staphylococcus aureus*	Oxacillin, nafcillin or cefazolin (vancomycin if MRSA suspected)
Gram-positive cocci (prosthetic joint)	*Staphylococcus epidermidis, S. aureus*	Vancomycin
Gram-negative cocci	*Neisseria gonorrhoeae*	Ceftriaxone or cefotaxime
Gram-negative bacilli	*Escherichia coli, Serratia marcescens,* other Enterobacteriaceae	Third-generation cephalosporin, imipenem, aztreonam, or ciprofloxacin* (with bacteremia or severe infection add an aminoglycoside)
Gram-negative bacilli (thin)	*Pseudomonas aeruginosa*	Ceftazidime, piperacillin, imipenem, or aztreonam, plus tobramycin or ciprofloxacin
Negative		
Noncompromised host	*S. aureus,* Enterobacteriaceae†	Nafcillin plus gentamicin *or* third-generation cephalosporin (ceftriaxone or cefotaxime) plus vancomycin if MRSA suspected
Compromised host	*S. aureus,* Enterobacteriaceae, *P. aeruginosa*†	Nafcillin (or vancomycin if MRSA suspected) plus tobramycin or ceftazidime, cefepime, piperacillin, or aztreonam plus tobramycin and vancomycin

Modified from Upchurch KS, Giansiracusa DF. In Rippe JM et al, editors: *Intensive care medicine,* ed 4, Boston, 1999, Lippencott-Raven.
*Ciprofloxacin is available for parenteral use (400 mg IV q12h).
†Treatment for both gram-positive and gram-negative pathogens must be continued until cultures return.

Table 141-3. Antibiotic Therapy of Acute Bacterial Arthritis in Adults (Known Pathogen)

Organism	Antibiotic choice	Alternatives
Staphylococcus aureus	Nafcillin 9-12 gm/day (q4h), or oxacillin 9-12 gm/day (q4h)	Cefazolin 4.5-6 gm/day (q8h), or vancomycin 2 gm/day (q12h)
S. aureus, methicillin resistant	Vancomycin 2 gm/day (q12h)	Daltopristine/quinupristin 7.5 mg/kg (q12h) or linezolid 600 mg (q12)
β-Hemolytic streptococci, Streptococcus pneumoniae	Penicillin G 12-18 million U/day (q4h)	Cefazolin or vancomycin or clindamycin 1.8 gm/day (q8h)
Neisseria gonorrhoeae	Ceftriaxone 1-2 gm/day (q24h) or cefotaxime 3-6 gm/day (q8h)	Spectinomycin 4 gm/day (q12h) *or* penicillin G if sensitive
Pseudomonas aeruginosa	Piperacillin 16 gm/day (q4h), plus tobramycin 5.1-7 mg/kg/day (q24h)	Ceftazidime 6 gm/day (q8h), or imipenem-cilastin 2-3 gm/day (q8h), aztreonam 6 gm/day (q8h), or ciprofloxacin* plus gentamicin or amikacin
Enterobacteriaceae	Third-generation cephalosporin plus gentamicin 5.1 mg/kg/day (q8h or q24h)	Aztreonam 3-6 gm/day (q8h), plus an aminoglycoside or ciprofloxacin*

Modified from Upchurch KS, Giansiracusa DF. In Rippe JM et al, editors: *Intensive care medicine,* ed 4, Boston, 1999, Lippencott-Raven.
q, Every; *h,* hours.
*Ciprofloxacin is available for parenteral use (400 mg IV q12h).

arthrocentesis. The hip is usually treated with arthrotomy because daily needle aspiration is difficult. When arthrocentesis does not achieve a good clinical response, as indicated by a rising WBC count and persistent culture positivity despite several days of antibiotic treatment, more invasive methods of drainage (e.g., arthroscopy, open arthrotomy) should be employed.

When the inflammation subsides, physical therapy with passive mobilization followed by active strengthening of periarticular structures helps to prevent joint contracture. Parenteral antibiotic therapy should continue for at least 3 to 4 weeks to ensure complete eradication of bacteria and prevent recurrence. Home IV therapy may be an effective alternative to prolonged hospitalization, particularly in the patient with infection in a non-weight-bearing joint who has responded to antibiotics and drainage.

Prognosis

The outcome of treatment for septic arthritis depends on many variables, including duration of the infection, virulence of the organism, and age and comorbidities of the patient. Virtually all patients with gonococcal arthritis recover completely, and 70% to 85% with group A streptococcal infections have a good outcome. However, up to 50% of patients who have septic arthritis from *Staphylococcus aureus* or gram-negative infections have residual joint damage. Patients with RA who develop polyarticular infection have less than a 50% chance of survival.

SEPTIC BURSITIS

Septic bursitis is a common soft tissue infection seen in outpatients. Features of the history and examination readily distinguish septic bursitis from other causes of periarticular inflammation, such as septic arthritis, traumatic bursitis, and tendinitis. The diagnosis is confirmed by bursal fluid analysis and culture. Treatment with oral antibiotics and appropriate drainage usually results in a good functional outcome.

Pathophysiology

The pathophysiology of septic bursitis differs from septic arthritis in that bacterial seeding is almost always through the transcutaneous route and is rarely associated with bacteremia. The subcutaneous olecranon and prepatellar bursae, located in the superficial tissue overlying the olecranon process and the patella, respectively, are the most frequently infected bursae. Local trauma may lead to superficial lacerations and abrasions, resulting in local cellulitis and bursal infection (Box 141-2). Infections of deep bursae (e.g., subacromial, iliopectineal) have been reported but are usually found with infection of the contiguous joint.

The vast majority (80% to 100%) of cases of septic bursitis are caused by gram-positive organisms, most often *S. aureus*. Streptococcal organisms, especially β-hemolytic streptococcus, account for 5% to 30% of infections. Case reports have described a variety of gram-negative, anaerobic, and fungal infections, but these are rare.[20]

Patient Evaluation

The presenting symptoms of septic bursitis are usually gradually progressive pain, warmth, and swelling around the elbow or knee. A history of acute or chronic antecedent trauma is often present. Fever, chills, or systemic symptoms should suggest a more serious infection. The physical examination often reveals discrete tenderness and swelling of the bursal sac, but extensive erythema and cellulitis may obscure the source of the infection. The absence of joint involvement can be inferred if there is a full passive range of joint motion. Articular fluid, if present, should be investigated for septic arthritis, but arthrocentesis may demonstrate a sterile sympathetic effusion.

Laboratory Studies and Differential Diagnosis

Needle aspiration of the inflamed bursal fluid provides both diagnostic information and relief of symptoms. The technique employs a large-bore (18- or 20-gauge) needle inserted into the bursal sac parallel to the long axis of the extremity with the joint extended. The insertion point should be away from the apex of the bursa in an area of more normal skin, if possible, to avoid poor wound healing and a chronic draining sinus tract (Fig. 141-1). Aspirated fluid should be sent for a WBC count with differential, Gram's stain, and crystal analysis. Superficial septic bursitis is often less inflammatory than septic arthritis. The bursal fluid WBC count is less than 20,000 cells/mm^3 in 50% of patients, but the range may be as high as 100,000 cells/mm^3. Gram's stain reveals organisms in approximately 75% of patients, which serves to direct initial antibiotic treatment while culture results are pending. As in the diagnosis of the inflamed joint, the presence of intrabursal crystals does not rule out a coexistent infection.

Box 141-2. Activities Associated With Septic Bursitis

Prepatellar Bursitis
- Carpet laying
- Plumbing
- Wrestling
- Crawling

Olecranon Bursitis
- Hemodialysis (dialysis elbows)

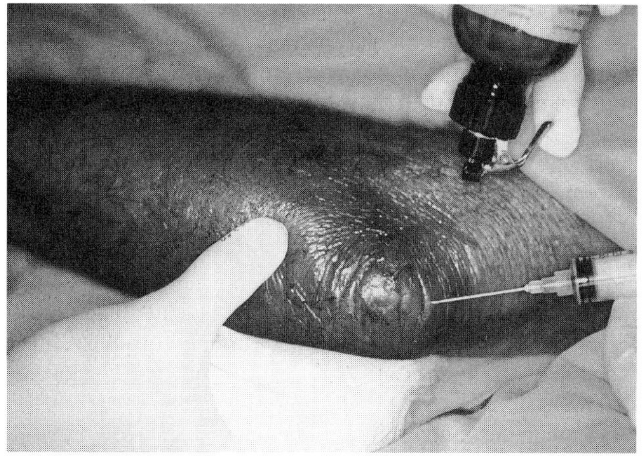

Fig. 141-1. Technique for aspirating olecranon bursa.

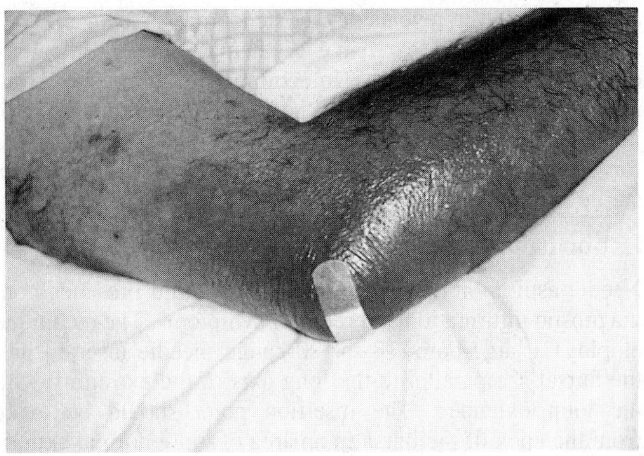

Fig. 141-2. Septic olecranon bursitis with extensive surrounding cellulitis.

Management

Treatment of septic bursitis includes appropriate antibiotic therapy, bursal drainage, and local care. An oral penicillinase-resistant antibiotic (e.g., dicloxacillin) or first-generation cephalosporin (e.g., cephalexin, 500 mg every 6 hours, or clindamycin, 300 mg every 6 hours) treats the most common pathogens and penetrates well into the inflamed bursa. A 2-week course of antibiotics is usually sufficient, but patients with extensive cellulitis require prolonged therapy. Daily needle aspiration should be performed until the fluid is sterile and no longer reaccumulating. Patients who require hospitalization for IV antibiotic therapy include those with extensive cellulitis (Fig. 141-2), a debilitated or immunocompromised state, or evidence of systemic infection. Some authors recommend inpatient therapy for all cases of septic prepatellar bursitis because of the difficulty of eradicating organisms in the thick skin overlying the knee.[15] In patients with recurrent or resistant infection, surgical consultation is advised to obtain open drainage and to consider bursectomy for definitive therapy.

The outcome of therapy for septic bursitis is generally favorable. Some patients have recurrent infections, however, especially if the behavior leading to the local trauma in the predisposed area is not modified.

OSTEOMYELITIS

The clinical spectrum of osteomyelitis varies considerably depending on age of the patient, duration of infection, anatomic location of bone involvement, host factors, rapidity of diagnosis, and adequacy of initial treatment. The ability to diagnose and adequately treat bone infections is a difficult exercise at best, but a clearer understanding of this disease has emerged in recent years.

Pathophysiology

Osteomyelitis is generally divided into adult and pediatric categories and is considered in acute, subacute, and chronic forms (Table 141-4). Furthermore, vertebral osteomyelitis is a distinctly different entity from infections of the nonaxial skeleton.

In neonates and children, hematogenous osteomyelitis most often results from a bacteremia or septicemia. In adults, hematogenous osteomyelitis is much less common and occurs most often in the vertebrae, particularly in the lumbar region. An apparent focus of infection at another site or a history of injection drug use is usually present. In the adult the arterial blood supply to the vertebrae ends at the vertebral end plate, and thus vertebral osteomyelitis is confined to the vertebral body and involves the disk only secondarily. Adult osteomyelitis most often develops secondary to trauma, contiguous infection, or surgical instrumentation. Bacteria are directly seeded into the bone at the level of the periosteum or medullary canal and produce an acute inflammatory reaction that often becomes subacute or chronic.

Table 141-4. Osteomyelitis in Adult and Pediatric Age Groups

Parameter	Pediatric	Adult
Transmission	Hematogenous	Traumatic, contiguous focus
Site	Growth plate—long bones	Diaphysis, vertebrae
Microbiology	*Staphylococcus aureus* β-Hemolytic streptococci	*S. aureus* *Staphyloccus epidermidis* Gram-negative rods Mixed (contiguous) Fungi (IV drugs)
Risk factors	Indwelling catheters Remote infection Bacteremia	Penetrating trauma Soft tissue infection Diabetes mellitus Peripheral vascular disease Injection drug abuse Immunosuppression Sickle cell disease

The microbiology of osteomyelitis varies with the mode of transmission. Aerobic bacteria or fungi are most often associated with hematogenous osteomyelitis. A single pathogen is usually responsible in both pediatric and adult patients. *S. aureus* is the most common organism in all age groups. In adult hematogenous osteomyelitis, aerobic gram-negative rods and fungal species are frequently causative, particularly in elderly patients with an extraosseous focus of infection and in injection drug users.

In contrast to the single pathogens responsible for hematogenous osteomyelitis, patients with trauma-related osteomyelitis or contiguous infection are typically infected with mixed microbial species, although *S. aureus* and *S. epidermidis* are often seen. Aerobic gram-negative bacilli and anaerobic organisms are frequently isolated from these mixed microbial infections. Unique pathogens are found under certain clinical circumstances. *Pseudomonas* species are often found in drug addicts. Osteomyelitis in patients with SC (sickle cell–hemoglobin C disease) and SS (sickle cell anemia) hemoglobinopathies is often caused by *Salmonella.* In immunocompromised patients, fungal species may be the causal agents, particularly *Candida.*

Patient Evaluation

The symptoms of osteomyelitis may reflect an acute localized infection of abrupt onset or a smoldering infectious process that is poorly localized and is associated with a paucity of systemic symptoms. Osteomyelitis is categorized as acute, subacute, or chronic based on duration of relevant symptoms. Overall, acute osteomyelitis is the most common form of the disease. The presentation is that of an acute febrile illness of a few days' duration. Localized pain in the axial or appendicular skeleton, accompanied by symptoms of acute infection, is the most common history obtained in adult osteomyelitis. Subacute or chronic osteomyelitis is usually a result of traumatic inoculation or transmission from a contiguous focus of infection. Pain is usually of longer duration, is less well localized, and frequently is not associated with systemic signs of infection.

The physical examination of acute osteomyelitis reveals signs of infection, including fever and warmth, erythema, swelling, and tenderness over the affected site. The clinical picture may be confused with cellulitis, but the localized nature of bony tenderness should suggest underlying osteomyelitis. With vertebral involvement the spine is often rigid, with localized tenderness of involved vertebrae. Signs are frequently lacking in subacute or chronic osteomyelitis. Tenderness in the axial or appendicular skeleton is often poorly localized. In cases associated with trauma or contiguous soft tissue infection, signs of osteomyelitis may be obscured by overlying inflammation. Patients with osteomyelitis contiguous with a joint may show evidence of acute septic arthritis. Careful neurologic examination should be performed, since patients with sensory peripheral neuropathies may have impaired pain perception.

Laboratory and Radiologic Studies

The ability to diagnose osteomyelitis depends on the host's ability to mount an appropriate localizing response to the osseous infection, as well as the physician's index of suspicion. An accurate diagnosis requires the documentation of a microbial species from a culture of blood or infected bone. In acute, untreated hematogenous osteomyelitis, blood cultures are positive in approximately 50% of cases, but the offending organism can be cultured from involved tissue in a much higher percentage. In chronic osteomyelitis it is usually necessary to obtain bone tissue for culture, since blood cultures are usually negative.

Radiographic abnormalities may support a diagnosis of osteomyelitis but are usually not conclusive. Plain radiographs in acute osteomyelitis usually demonstrate no bony pathology. Subacute osteomyelitis may require 2 to 3 weeks for x-ray changes to appear. These include periosteal elevation, cortical erosions, or large lytic areas.

Radionuclide imaging has been advocated as an adjunctive method to assist in the diagnosis.[16] Technetium 99m, gallium Ga 67 citrate, or indium In 111 chloride scans may become positive within 48 to 72 hours of infection, but false-positive and false-negative results are common. It is particularly difficult to interpret such scans in the presence of overlying soft tissue infection or adjacent inflammatory arthritis. The In 111–labeled leukocyte scan has significant discriminatory capacity for osteomyelitis, particularly in diabetic patients and those with overlying soft tissue infection.[12] Computed tomography (CT) and magnetic resonance imaging (MRI) are often useful to define areas of osteomyelitis more accurately.

The standard method of diagnosing osteomyelitis demands a positive culture result from a tissue specimen involved with infection; arriving at a diagnosis using any other method is presumptive. Practically, it is often difficult to make a culture-proven diagnosis, and management strategies are developed based on a high diagnostic probability for osteomyelitis. Culture of a single pathogen from blood or an overlying soft tissue infection combined with high-probability radionuclide or plain x-ray imaging studies may warrant presumptive antibiotic therapy. Less specific therapy results when diagnostic data are inconclusive. Whenever possible, a surgical or radiographically directed needle biopsy specimen of involved bone should be obtained for culture and sensitivity before initiating antibiotic therapy.

Management

Optimal treatment for osteomyelitis results from the early detection of bone infection and the isolation of a specific pathogen with known antibiotic sensitivities. In early acute osteomyelitis, IV antibiotics can be administered for a few days, then switching to oral antibiotics for up to 6 weeks. As initial therapy, antibiotics directed at *S. aureus* and β-hemolytic streptococci should be administered pending the results of culture sensitivities. Oxacillin (100 to 200 mg/kg/day), nafcillin, or benzylpenicillin (1 to 4 million U/day) are reasonable choices. Penicillin-allergic patients should receive a third- or fourth-generation cephalosporin. If the diagnosis of acute osteomyelitis is delayed for up to 2 weeks after symptoms are noted, or if the patient has chronic osteomyelitis, drainage of pus and debridement of infected bone are essential adjuncts to antibiotic therapy. Treatment of overlying soft tissue infection or removal of prosthetic devices is also necessary in most cases to eradicate infection.

Chronic osteomyelitis requires antibiotic therapy directed at identified organisms with appropriate sensitivities. In blood culture–positive adult osteomyelitis, IV antibiotics should be administered for at least 2 weeks and usually for 4 to 6 weeks. In osteomyelitis secondary to contiguous infection, broad-spectrum antibiotics that target gram-positive cocci, aerobic gram-negative organisms, and anaerobic or fungal species as appropriate should be administered.

Chronic osteomyelitis is now treated with oral antibiotics after an initial phase of parenteral medication. This approach is advocated largely because of the availability of newer antibiotics, especially the fluoroquinolones (e.g., ciprofloxacin, ofloxacin), which achieve excellent bone penetration and inhibit most strains of bacteria that cause osteomyelitis. Many patients with osteomyelitis may be treated entirely with prolonged oral courses of such agents.[5] Exceptions include patients with diabetes mellitus and severe peripheral vascular disease. Such oral therapy depends on the ability to isolate the microbial pathogen (with appropriate antibiotic sensitivities) and to achieve a complete surgical debridement or excision of necrotic tissue. Most patients with chronic osteomyelitis, however, probably should be treated with IV antibiotics for at least 2 weeks before considering oral antibiotics. For patients with unknown or uncertain bacteriology, a full course of broad-spectrum IV antibiotics is still recommended.

VIRAL ARTHRITIS

Pathophysiology

Acute viremia is often associated with severe myalgias and arthralgias, regardless of the causative viral species. Much less often, frank arthritis or tenosynovitis is associated with an acute viral infection. Acute viral arthritis may be caused by direct viral replication in the joint or synovial tissue or, more frequently, by promoting an immune complex formation that initiates an inflammatory cascade within the joint. The vast majority of acute articular syndromes (arthralgias and arthritis) are of short duration and do not lead to chronic arthritis or joint damage. However, certain viruses (e.g., human parvovirus B19) often produce polyarthritis that is subacute or chronic. A variety of viruses have been implicated in causing viral arthritis (Box 141-3).

Patient Evaluation

Patients who develop viral arthritis initially have features of a typical viral syndrome: fever, headache, malaise, myalgias, arthralgias, nausea, pharyngitis, or coryza. Such viral symptoms may occur sporadically or in association with a defined outbreak. Historically, generalized arthralgias are associated with viremia from diverse viral species. Joint swelling, severe stiffness, and redness should suggest frank arthritis. In many viral syndromes, polyarthralgias may be the only prodromal symptom. In viruses associated with characteristic rashes, articular symptoms frequently appear at or near the time of the viral exanthem. Concomitant findings associated with arthralgias include rash, oral ulcers, swollen glands, and cough.

Physical examination of patients with viral arthritis frequently reveals signs of an acute viral infection, including rash, pharyngitis, lymphadenopathy, hepatosplenomegaly, and oral ulcers. Viral arthritis may be monoarticular or oligoarticular, but it is most often symmetric and polyarticular. Most viruses lead to an arthropathy that involves large and small joints, which develops in an additive or migratory fashion. With all the viruses, involvement of the small finger joints and knees is most common. Joints in the wrists, ankles, feet, elbows, and shoulders are also frequently involved. Some viruses (e.g., hepatitis B, rubella) may involve the tendon sheath and produce tenosynovitis with swelling, erythema, and tenderness across the joint (typically the wrist or ankle), corresponding to the distribution of extensor tendons.

Specific Musculoskeletal Viruses

The three viruses that most often cause frank arthritis are human parvovirus B19, hepatitis B virus, and rubella virus.

Box 141-3. Arthritogenic Viruses

Human parvovirus B19
Hepatitis B
Rubella (natural and vaccine)
Mumps
Coxsackievirus
Echovirus
Smallpox
Vaccinia
Adenovirus
Varicella-zoster
Herpes simplex
Cytomegalovirus
Epstein-Barr
Hepatitis A
Retroviruses (e.g., HTLV-1)
Alphavirus

Human parvovirus B19, a DNA virus, is the causal agent of erythema infectiosum (fifth disease of childhood). Parvovirus is a ubiquitous virus, with 30% to 40% of adults having serologic evidence of prior exposure. In children, parvovirus infection is characterized by an evanescent rash (often a slapped-face appearance) with low-grade fever and occasional mild arthralgias (Fig. 141-3). In adults the rash is not a prominent feature of the illness. Arthralgias occur in up to 77% of patients.[11] Joints most often affected include the small finger joints, wrists, and knees, although the ankles, feet, and elbows may also be affected. The arthritis may resemble acute RA, although rheumatoid factor is usually not detected. Unlike most other forms of viral arthritis, parvovirus-associated arthritis may persist for months or even years. No evidence of chronic erosive arthritis or permanent joint damage has been documented. Parvovirus arthritis is usually documented by the identification of immunoglobulin M (IgM) anti-B19 antibodies for up to several weeks after the initial exposure.

Hepatitis B virus (HBV) is a well-known cause of articular syndromes, particularly during the prodromal phase of the illness. The incubation period for HBV is 40 to 180 days. Several features of the illness are mediated by hepatitis B surface antigen (HBsAg) and the humoral response to this agent. Prodromal symptoms include fever, headaches, malaise, anorexia, nausea, vomiting, and abdominal pain. These symptoms precede the icteric phase by 2 to 14 days. Articular symptoms are a common feature of the clinical prodrome, occurring in 10% to 25% of cases. Immune complexes with HBsAg and HBV antibody are thought to mediate this process. Arthralgia or arthritis usually precedes clinical jaundice by days to weeks and resolves before the icteric phase of HBV infection. Joint symptoms are often associated with urticarial, petechial, or maculopapular skin rashes, usually on the lower extremities. Tenosynovitis of the wrist or ankle may be noted on physical examination. Articular involvement is usually symmetric and additive and involves the large and small joints. Arthritis usually resolves completely by the onset of jaundice but persists in 5% of patients with HBV infection.

Rubella virus infection produces a characteristic maculopapular eruption and lymphadenopathy. Children have no typical prodrome. In adults, however, sore throat, headache, fever, swollen glands, and myalgias may precede the rash by

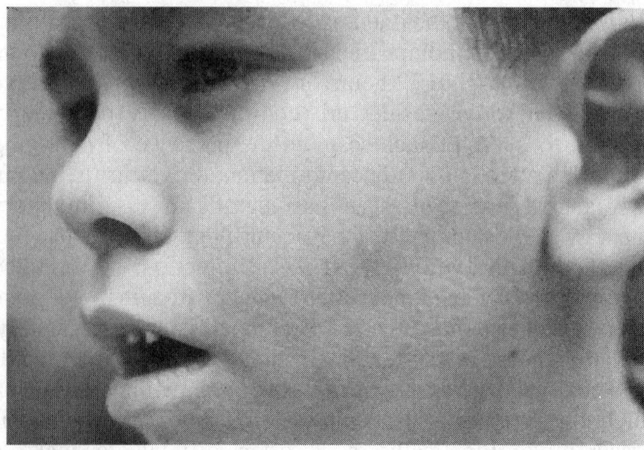

Fig. 141-3. Slapped-cheeks appearance of fifth disease.

1 to 5 days. Adult patients with rubella infection who develop joint symptoms tend to be women between ages 20 and 40. About 30% of women and 6% of men with rubella infection manifest joint symptoms. Articular symptoms may develop before or after the appearance of the rash. Polyarthralgias develop most often, but frank arthritis may occur. The joint involvement is usually bilaterally symmetric, with small and large joints affected in an additive or migratory fashion. Arthritis and arthralgias usually evolve over 7 to 10 days and most often are short-lived with complete resolution. A similar articular syndrome has been associated with rubella vaccine virus, and again, women are predominantly affected. Severe arthralgias with stiffness, particularly of the hands and knees, usually develop approximately 2 weeks after the vaccination. Unlike the articular symptoms associated with natural rubella infection, those seen with the vaccine virus may recur, but permanent joint damage does not develop.

Diagnosis

The diagnosis of viral arthritis is usually presumptive. Confirmatory tests include the demonstration of acute and convalescent viral antibody titers of the IgM and IgG classes. Accurate identification of the offending virus is usually not necessary, since the course of the joint disease is usually self-limited, and specific antiviral treatment is not indicated. Synovial fluid from joints involved with viral arthritis usually has a mild leukocytosis, although synovial fluid WBCs have a wide range, typically with a mononuclear cell predominance.

Management

The treatment of viral arthritis includes standard supportive treatment for the acute viral syndrome. Inflamed joints and tendons should be splinted in the acute setting. If arthritis persists after the resolution of the viral infection, a short course of nonsteroidal antiinflammatory drugs (NSAIDs) is indicated. More intense treatment with second-line antirheumatic drugs is rarely necessary.

Prognosis

The prognosis of viral arthritis is usually excellent. In genetically predisposed individuals a viral infection may trigger an immune response that leads to chronic arthritis. The details of such a mechanism have not been elucidated. In such patients, treatment is directed at the suppression of chronic joint inflammation.

HIV-ASSOCIATED MUSCULOSKELETAL SYNDROMES

Since 1987 a variety of rheumatic syndromes has been reported in association with human immunodeficiency virus (HIV) infection (Table 141-5). It is still not established that HIV is directly responsible for the association of these syndromes or even that HIV has a statistically significant association with these conditions (see Chapter 32).

Epidemiology and Pathogenesis

The incidence and prevalence of musculoskeletal syndromes in the HIV-infected population are unknown. Studies attempting to establish these figures suffer from ascertainment bias. Estimates vary depending on the gender, ethnicity, and risk profile of the population studied as well as the clinical stage of the HIV infection. The most common rheumatic manifestations of HIV infection probably are polyarthralgias and bone pain, which occur in up to one third of patients. Frank arthritis is noted during the infection in approximately 5% to 10% of patients. True Reiter's syndrome or psoriatic arthritis probably occurs in fewer than 5%. Sporadic cases of septic arthritis, osteomyelitis, vasculitis, Sjögren's-like syndrome, and inflammatory myopathy have been described, but incidence figures are indeterminate.[4]

Several possible mechanisms may explain the relationship between HIV infection and rheumatic disease. During a phase of viremia, HIV could produce polyarthralgias and bone pain as do other viral infections. HIV may produce a direct viral synovitis, which would explain arthritis syndrome associated with acquired immunodeficiency syndrome (AIDS). HIV has been isolated from synovial fluid, but this does not confirm an etiologic role in arthritis. Immune complexes can be found in HIV-infected individuals, but whether or not these mediate arthritis (as with HBV) is unknown. HIV infection may lead to an enhanced role for CD8 cytotoxic T cells, which have a potential pathogenetic role in the seronegative spondyloarthropathies[3] (see Chapter 137).

Patient Evaluation

When obtaining a history from an individual with known or suspected HIV infection and musculoskeletal symptoms, the physician must consider the spectrum of multisystemic rheumatic disease. In addition to symptoms of joint pain and swelling, patients with HIV should be questioned about low back and heel pain, rashes, genital ulcers, ocular inflammation, dry eyes, dry mouth, and muscle weakness.

Physical examination should include inspection for signs of ocular inflammation, lymphadenopathy, oral ulcers, skin rashes, mucocutaneous and genital ulcers, and nail changes. In addition to signs of arthritis, patients with seronegative spondyloarthropathies may have dactylitis (swelling and tenderness along an entire digit, or sausage digits). Evidence of inflammation at the entheses (points of ligamentous attachment to bones) may be particularly apparent in the heels, plantar surface of the foot, and pelvic brim. Signs of sacroiliac inflammation should also be sought on physical examination.

Diagnosis

The diagnosis of rheumatic syndromes in AIDS patients requires documentation of HIV infection. Most rheumatic syndromes are diagnosed on the basis of clinical findings. Analysis of synovial fluid obtained from involved joints demonstrates a mild to moderate inflammatory reaction with a monocytic predominance. Rheumatoid factor and antinuclear antibodies (ANAs) are typically not found in these patients and do not help to establish a specific diagnosis.

Management

The treatment of the rheumatic manifestations of AIDS requires treatment of the underlying infections. Some of the rheumatic syndromes (arthralgias, AIDS-associated arthritis) may be transient and require only analgesic medications. Syndromes associated with frank arthritis (Reiter's syndrome, psoriatic arthritis, AIDS-associated arthritis) usually require NSAIDs. Physical therapy measures may also be helpful. When these modalities are ineffective, sulfasalazine may be used for chronic arthritis. Caution should be exercised in the use of methotrexate or other immunosuppressive agents for Reiter's syndrome or psoriatic arthritis associated with AIDS,

Table 141-5. Rheumatic Syndromes Associated With Human Immunodeficiency Virus (HIV) Infection

Syndrome	Incidence	Patterns of involvement	Severity	Associated features
Arthralgias	33%	Intermittent; occurs at any stage; usually resolves in weeks to months	May be severe	Bone pain
Reiter's syndrome (RS)	1%-10%; unknown if HIV predisposes patient for RS	Usually develops around transformation to symptomatic AIDS; prominent peripheral arthritis, usually asymmetric, oligoarticular; predilection for lower extremity joint and entheses	Peripheral oligoarthritis and cutaneous manifestations often more severe than RS not associated with HIV	Severe axial involvement (sacroiliitis, spondylitis), conjunctivitis, and uveitis uncommon; hyperkeratotic skin lesions, particularly keratoderma blennorrhagicum, similar to pustular psoriasis
Psoriatic arthritis	Less common than RS	More often polyarticular than is RS; involvement of distal interphalangeal (DIP) joints		Pitting of nails, particularly adjacent to affected DIP joints: severe psoriasis
HIV-associated arthritis	Unknown	Oligoarthritis involving knees and ankles; short-lived, 1-6 weeks	Severe, incapacitating symptoms; often more severe than objective findings	Synovial fluid and synovial histology mildly inflammatory
Septic arthritis/ osteomyelitis	Not as common as might be expected	Includes opportunistic organisms		
Sicca complex	Unknown	Dry eyes and mouth at any stage of HIV infection; with parotid gland enlargement and lymphocyte infiltration of salivary glands, similar to Sjögren's syndrome; referred to as diffuse infiltrative lymphocytosis syndrome (DILS)		Many genetic, pathologic, and serologic differences between DILS and primary Sjögren's syndrome (see Chapter 140)
Polymyositis	Unknown	Myopathy at any time during HIV infection; indistinguishable from idiopathic polymyositis		Must be distinguished from the myopathy associated with zidovudine
Vasculitis	Unknown	Inflammatory vascular disease similar to polyarteritis (necrotizing, medium-sized arteritis), leukocytoclastic vasculitis, and granulomatous vasculitis		

since this form of treatment may convert AIDS-related complex or mild AIDS to a fulminant syndrome, including malignant transformation. Septic arthritis and osteomyelitis are treated as in non-AIDS patients.

Prognosis

The prognosis of AIDS-related rheumatic syndrome is directly related to the underlying disease. Reiter's syndrome may lead to chronic arthritis with deformity and disability. Cases with long-term data are insufficient to evaluate the natural history of these conditions.

LYME DISEASE

Lyme disease is a multisystem spirochetal infection secondary to *Borrelia burgdorferi*. The organism is transmitted to humans from infected deer and white-footed mice by the tick vector *Ixodes scapularis* in the northeast and north-central United States or *Ixodes pacificus* in the Pacific Northwest. These are the most endemic areas, although nearly every state has reported cases of Lyme disease.

Pathophysiology and Patient Evaluation

The clinical manifestations of Lyme disease have been divided into three stages: early localized, early disseminated, and late or persistent infection[18] (Box 141-4). Initial infection usually occurs in the late spring or early summer, when the nymphal tick is 1 to 2 mm in size. Thus the tick or tick bite may not be detected until the symptoms of early localized infection occur, usually within 3 to 32 days. Fever, malaise, myalgias, arthralgias, headache, and localized lymphadenopathy may mimic viral infections. *Erythema migrans* (EM), the classic skin lesion that develops at the site of a tick bite, occurs in 60% to 80% of patients.[10] Characteristically it is an erythematous macule or papule with expanding borders, reaching a mean size of 15 cm and often accompanied by central clearing (Fig. 141-4). The lesion resolves spontaneously without antibiotic therapy.

The early disseminated stage, representing the hematogenous spread of the spirochete, develops days to weeks after infection. Secondary skin lesions may develop and are typically smaller than the initial EM lesion. Neurologic manifestations are common (15% to 20%) and include aseptic meningitis, encephalitis, Bell's palsy (often bilateral), and radiculoneuritis that can be sensory, motor, or mixed. Cardiac involvement occurs in 4% to 8% and manifests as fluctuating degrees of atrioventricular (AV) block or myopericarditis. Migratory arthralgias in large and small joints may accompany these symptoms.

Late or persistent infection may present months to years after the initial infection. The spirochete appears to persist in the central nervous system, joints, and rarely the skin, heart, and eyes. Neurologic disease includes chronic sensorimotor polyradiculopathy, subacute encephalopathy, and rarely a meningoencephalomyelitis. The encephalopathy is characterized by cognitive abnormalities, headache, and fatigue. Cerebrospinal fluid (CSF) analysis may reveal mild pleocytosis, elevated protein, and intrathecal production of antibodies to *B. burgdorferi*.

Box 141-4. Clinical Stages of Lyme Disease*

Early Localized Infection (Stage 1)

Skin: erythema migrans (EM)
Systemic: fever, malaise, lymphadenopathy (localized)

Early Disseminated Infection (Stage 2)

Skin: secondary EM lesions
Musculoskeletal: migratory arthritis or periarthritis
Neurologic: meningitis, facial palsy or other cranial neuritis, radiculoneuritis
Cardiac: atrioventricular block, myopericarditis
Systemic: severe malaise, fatigue
Others (rare): hepatitis, myositis, inflammatory eye diseases

Late or Persistent Infection (Stage 3)

Skin: acrodermatitis chronica atrophicans (rare in United States)
Musculoskeletal: oligoarticular arthritis, intermittent or chronic
Neurologic: polyradiculoneuropathy, subacute encephalopathy, meningoencephalomyelitis
Others: keratitis, dilated cardiomyopathy

Modified from Steere AC: Lyme disease, *N Engl J Med* 321:586, 1989.
*Some patients may be totally asymptomatic after infection or may present at stage 2 or even stage 3 without other manifestations of earlier stages.

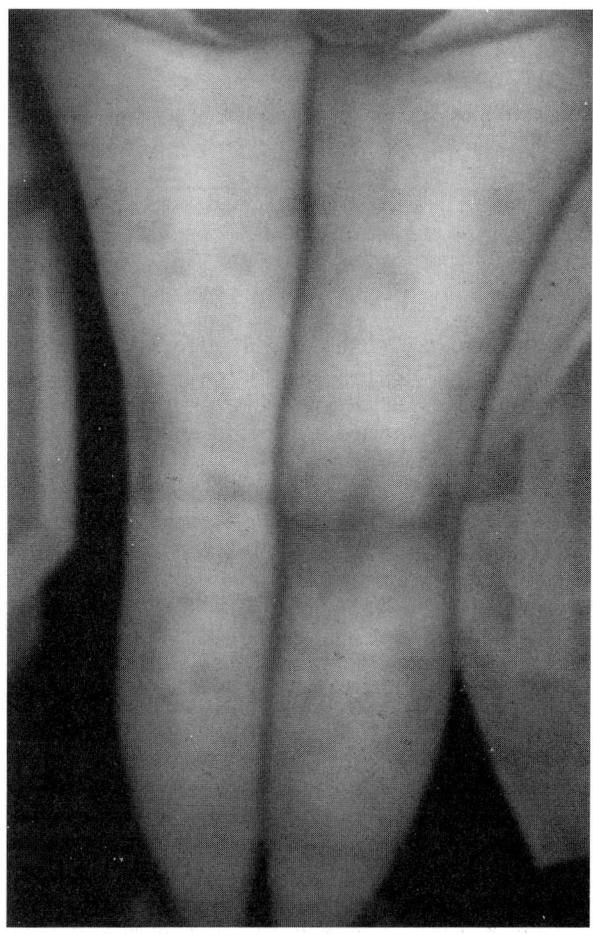

Fig. 141-4. Primary erythema migrans (EM) lesion of Lyme disease behind the knee, with multiple secondary lesions. (Courtesy Howard Keller, MD, Infectious Disease Division, Massachusetts General Hospital.)

Table 141-6. Recommendations for Treatment of Lyme Disease

Stage/pregnancy	Drug dose	Duration
1. Localized infection	Doxycycline, 100 mg PO bid *or* Amoxicillin, 500 mg PO tid *or* Cefuroxime, 500 mg PO bid	10-28 days depending on clinical response
2. Early disseminated Isolated facial palsy (without other neurologic symptoms) First-degree atrioventricular (AV) block (PR interval <0.3 sec)	Oral regimen as above may be adequate	21-28 days depending on clinical response
Meningitis, encephalitis, radiculoneuritis, other cranial neuritis High-degree AV block	Ceftriaxone, 2 gm IV daily *or* Penicillin G, 20 million U IV daily in divided doses	14-28 days
3. Late (persistent) infection Arthritis (intermittent or chronic)	Amoxicillin, 500 mg PO qid, and probenecid, 500 mg PO qid *or* Doxycycline, 100 mg PO bid Ceftriaxone, 2 gm IV daily *or* Penicillin G, 20 million U IV daily in divided doses	Oral regimen for 28 days IV therapy for 14 days
Late neurologic symptoms	Ceftriaxone, 2 gm IV daily *or* Penicillin G, 20 million U IV daily in divided doses	28 days
Pregnancy		
Tick bite or early disease	Amoxicillin, 500 mg PO tid *or* Erythromycin, 250 mg-500 mg PO tid-qid (may be less effective than amoxicillin)	21 days
Disseminated early or late	Ceftriaxone, 2 gm IV daily *or* Penicillin G, 20 million U IV daily in divided doses	14 days

Modified from Steere AC: Lyme disease, *N Engl J Med* 321:586, 1989.
bid, Twice daily; *tid,* three times daily; *qid,* four times daily; *PO,* orally; *IV,* intravenously.
*May be less effective than other oral regimens.

Joint disease occurs in 62% of untreated patients and manifests as inflammatory monoarticular or oligoarticular arthritis of the knees, ankles, and elbows. The small joints and bursae are rarely affected. Temporomandibular joint, hip, shoulder, back, and neck pain are common. Initially the pattern of joint inflammation is intermittent, lasting days to several weeks. Chronic arthritis, defined as persistent inflammation for 1 year or more, develops in 10% of untreated patients. Joint effusions may be massive; synovial fluid WBCs range from 10,000 to 20,000/mm^3 with predominantly PMNs. Cultures are usually negative.

Laboratory Studies and Diagnostic Procedures

Cultures of punch biopsies taken from the edges of EM lesions yield *B. burgdorferi* in 60% to 80% of cases, but cultures of blood, synovial fluid, and CSF are rarely successful. The diagnosis of Lyme disease is based on the clinical manifestations and serologic studies that detect antibodies to *B. burgdorferi.* The IgM response occurs 2 to 4 weeks after infection, whereas IgG is rarely detected before 4 to 8 weeks. The enzyme-linked immunosorbent assay (ELISA) is used most often; however, its sensitivity and specificity vary widely due to the lack of standardization among commercial laboratories, as well as the patient population tested. False-negative results occur because serum was obtained too early in the disease course or the patient had prior antibiotic therapy, which can abort the immune response. False-positive results may be seen in healthy individuals, autoimmune diseases, and other spirochetal and viral infections. Immunoblotting (Western blot) is useful in borderline cases or to distinguish true from false-positive results. PCR and T-cell proliferative assays are reported to be highly specific but have low sensitivity and remain primarily research techniques.

The American College of Physicians has published guidelines for laboratory evaluation in the diagnosis of Lyme disease.[19] Recommendations are based on the probability that an individual patient has Lyme disease. If probability is low, and especially if the patient has nonspecific symptoms of myalgias, arthralgias, or fatigue, then no testing should be done. When a rash typical of EM is present *and* a history of tick bite (high probability), empiric therapy is recommended without need for antibody testing. All other patients with objective clinical signs should be evaluated by two-step testing with ELISA or immunofluorescence assay followed by Western blot if results are indeterminate.

Other tests that may support the diagnosis of Lyme disease include synovial fluid analysis, lumbar puncture with CSF analysis and antibody studies, and electromyography and nerve conduction tests. MRI may show nonspecific abnormalities in 25% of patients. Neuropsychiatric testing is useful to differentiate subtle encephalopathy from depression.

Management

Antibiotics are the major treatment for Lyme disease (Table 141-6). Currently, prophylactic therapy for tick bites is not indicated unless the patient is pregnant. Oral antibiotic therapy is adequate for early disease and arthritis. Doxycycline is contraindicated in children and in pregnant or lactating women. Parenteral antibiotics are recommended for meningitis, carditis, arthritis unresponsive to oral antibiotics, and other neurologic manifestations. Patients with early neurologic symptoms improve quickly, whereas late neurologic symptoms improve slowly over months.[2]

In addition to antibiotics, management of high-degree AV block may require a temporary pacemaker. Joint aspiration and corticosteroid injections for chronic arthritis are effective but should be performed only after antibiotic therapy. Surgical synovectomy is often successful in chronic arthritis.

A minority of patients may not respond to antibiotic therapy. Patients with treated Lyme disease may have persistent fatigue or fibromyalgia symptoms that remain unresponsive to repeated courses of antibiotics. In patients with fatigue, headaches, or cognitive deficits, other useful modalities include tricyclic antidepressants, antiinflammatory medications, cognitive retraining, and behavioral modifications.

Prevention

Vaccines made of recombinant *B. burgdorferi* outer surface lipoprotein A (OspA) are now available. Effective immunity against symptomatic infections is provided after a series of three doses. The first two are given 1 month apart in the months just before nymphs are active, followed by the third dose 1 year later. Whether the third dose can be given a month after the second dose and be effective remains to be demonstrated. Side effects are minor and include local injection site irritation and influenza-like illness in a small percentage of patients. The duration of immunity and indications for vaccination have yet to be defined.

Prevention of Lyme disease should be stressed to patients traveling to endemic areas. Since most experts believe that the spirochete is not transmitted until 36 to 48 hours after tick attachment, a daily body check for ticks is crucial. If a tick is found, gentle pulling with tweezers in a steady fashion is best. In addition, wearing long sleeves, tucking pants into socks, and using insect repellent containing diethyltoluamide (deet) are effective measures against tick attachment.

REFERENCES

1. Cooper C, Cawley MID: Bacterial arthritis in the elderly, *Gerontology* 32:222, 1986.
2. Coyle PK: Neurologic complications of Lyme disease, *Rheum Dis Clin North Am* 19:993, 1993.
3. Cuellar ML: HIV infection–associated inflammatory musculoskeletal disorders, *Rheum Dis Clin North Am* 24:403, 1998.
4. Espinoza LR, Aguilar JL, Berman A, et al: Rheumatic manifestations associated with human immunodeficiency virus infection, *Arthritis Rheum* 32:1615, 1989.
5. Gentry LO: Oral antimicrobial therapy for osteomyelitis, *Ann Intern Med* 114:980, 1991.
6. Goldenberg DL: Septic arthritis, *Lancet* 351:197, 1998.
7. Ho G Jr: How best to drain an infected joint: will we ever know for certain? *J Rheumatol* 20:2001, 1993.
8. Kaandorp CJE, vanSchaardenburg D, Krijen P, et al: Risk factors for septic arthritis in patients with joint disease: a prospective study, *Arthritis Rheum* 38:1819, 1995.
9. Liebling MR, Arkfeld DG, Michelini GA, et al: Identification of *Neisseria gonorrhoeae* in synovial fluid using the polymerase chain reaction, *Arthritis Rheum* 37:702, 1994.
10. Malane MS: Diagnosis of Lyme disease based on dermatologic manifestations, *Ann Intern Med* 114:490, 1991.
11. Naides SJ: Rheumatic manifestations of parvovirus B19 infection, *Rheum Dis Clin North Am* 24:375, 1998.
12. Newman LG: Unsuspected osteomyelitis in diabetic foot ulcers: diagnosis and monitoring by leukocyte scanning with indium In 111 oxyquinoline, *JAMA* 266:1246, 1991.
13. O'Brien JP, Goldenberg DL, Rice PA: Disseminated gonococcal infection: a prospective analysis of 49 patients and a review of pathophysiology and immune mechanisms, *Medicine* 62:395, 1983.
14. Peltola H, Kallio MJT, Unkila-Kallio L: Reduced incidence of septic arthritis in children by *Haemophilus influenza* type-6 vaccination, *J Bone Joint Surg* 80B:471, 1998.
15. Raddatz DA, Hoffman GS, Franck WA: Septic bursitis: presentation, treatment and prognosis, *J Rheumatol* 14:1160, 1987.
16. Schauwecker DS: The scintigraphic diagnosis of osteomyelitis, *Am J Roentgenol* 158:159, 1992.
17. Soderquist B, Hedstrom SA: Predisposing factors, bacteriology and antibiotic therapy in 35 cases of septic bursitis, *Scand J Infect Dis* 18:305, 1986.
18. Steere AC: Lyme disease, *N Engl J Med* 321:586, 1989.
19. Tugwell P, Dennis DT, Weinstein A, et al: Guidelines for laboratory evaluation in the diagnosis of Lyme disease, *Ann Intern Med* 127:1106, 1997.
20. Zimmermann B III, Mikolich DJ, Ho G Jr: Septic bursitis, *Semin Arthritis Rheum* 24:391, 1995.
21. Zimmerman B III, Mikolich DJ, Lally EV: Septic sacroiliitis, *Semin Arthritis Rheum* 26:592, 1996.

CHAPTER 142

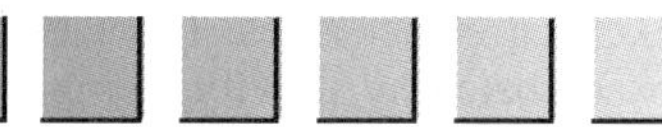

Chronic Fatigue Syndrome and Fibromyalgia

Nelson M. Gantz

Fatigue remains a common complaint, reported by 20% to 25% of patients in general medical clinics (see Chapter 21). Despite its high frequency, a standardized blood test or instrument to measure fatigue does not exist. Fatigue is the hallmark of the chronic fatigue syndrome (CFS); fatigue must be new, persistent, or relapsing and associated with a 50% reduction in a patient's premorbid activity for at least 6 months.[8] Patients are usually initially seen by their primary care physician and often are referred for diagnosis and management to a neurologist, psychiatrist, or infectious disease specialist. In the mid-1980s, reports erroneously linked CFS to Epstein-Barr virus (EBV), and CFS continues to be controversial.

Fibromyalgia is a similar disorder of widespread musculoskeletal pain and fatigue with other symptoms, such as poor sleep. CFS and fibromyalgia are overlapping disorders; about 75% of patients with CFS also meet the criteria for fibromyalgia, and vice versa.[7] The onset of CFS is often acute after an infectious illness, typically viral, whereas the onset is often gradual with fibromyalgia.

EPIDEMIOLOGY

Despite the high frequency of fatigue in the general population, CFS, as defined by the Centers for Disease Control and Prevention (CDC), may be uncommon. In a study from Australia the prevalence of CFS was 37.1 per 100,000 population, a rate similar to that for multiple sclerosis. A survey in five U.S. cities estimated the prevalence of CFS at seven per 100,000, whereas in the state of Washington the prevalence ranged from 75 to 267 cases per 100,000.[3] There is a female predominance, most patients are between ages 20 and 50 years, and all socioeconomic groups are affected. In a study of musculoskeletal pain the prevalence of fibromyalgia was 2%, affecting women seven times more often than men.[12] The disorder increases in frequency between ages 18 and 70, with a 23% prevalence in the seventh decade.

PATHOPHYSIOLOGY

The cause of CFS and fibromyalgia is unknown.[9] Patients with fibromyalgia report either a gradual onset of their disorder or an "event," such as a flulike illness or physical trauma. Patients with CFS often recall the onset after an acute viral illness. Although infectious, immunologic, neuroendocrine, metabolic, and psychiatric abnormalities have been identified in some patients with these disorders, disagreement exists as to their relevance. Some of these laboratory abnormalities may be related to chronic illness in general.

PATIENT EVALUATION

The cardinal symptom of CFS is fatigue, and the physician must carefully clarify the patient's sense of fatigue. The fatigue of CFS refers to a state of profound mental and physical exhaustion that cannot be explained by ongoing exertion or activities. The fatigue also is disproportionately exacerbated by activity and is not ameliorated by rest. If the patient is actually describing sleepiness or early-morning awakening as the main problem, attention should be directed toward the possibility of a sleep disorder, such as sleep apnea or narcolepsy.

Other characteristic symptoms of CFS include self-perceived impairments of short-term memory and concentration, sleep problems, myalgia and arthralgia, headache, dizziness, allergic symptoms, and depression. A mental status examination for abnormalities in orientation, memory, thinking, speech, mood, affect, and behavior should be routinely performed on all patients with unexplained fatigue. Attention should focus on symptoms of depression, anxiety, and self-destructive thoughts and signs such as psychomotor impairment. Evidence of an underlying or contributing psychiatric or neurologic disorder requires further evaluation.

In 1990 the American College of Rheumatology outlined guidelines for diagnosing fibromyalgia by requiring that widespread pain be present for 3 months or more.[13] *Widespread pain* refers to pain in an axial distribution involving both sides of the body and above and below the waist. In addition, to fulfill the diagnostic criteria, pain must be present in 11 or more of 18 specified tender points on digital palpation (Fig. 142-1). Other symptoms and signs include sleep problems, fatigue, stiffness, and cold intolerance. In clinical practice the diagnosis of fibromyalgia can be made when fewer than 11 tender points are present.[1]

No pathognomonic physical findings have been reported in patients with CFS. Tender points may be present in patients with fibromyalgia.

DIAGNOSIS

The CDC case definition is currently the most accepted basis for diagnosing CFS, although two similar definitions have been proposed.[4] A patient must have unexplained persistent fatigue for 6 months that is new and not caused by exertion,

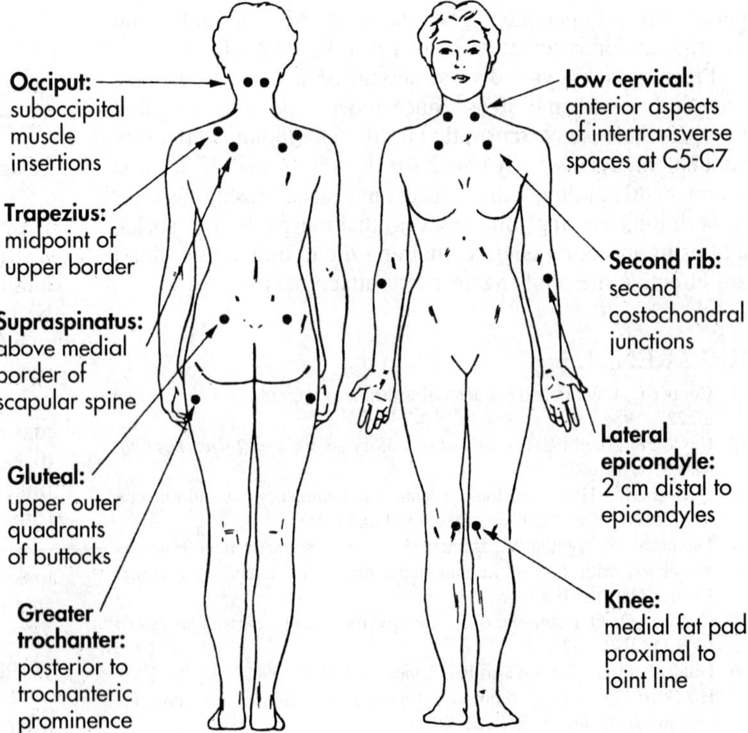

Fig. 142-1. Location of specific tender points in fibromyalgia. (From Fibromyalgia syndrome. In *Primer on rheumatic diseases*, Atlanta, 1993, Arthritis Foundation.)

Box 142-1. CDC Case Definition of Chronic Fatigue Syndrome (CFS)*

1. Clinically evaluated, unexplained, persistent, or relapsing fatigue for at least 6 months that:
   - Is of new or definite onset,
   - Is not the result of ongoing exertion,
   - Is not substantially alleviated by rest, and
   - Results in substantial reduction in previous levels of activities.
2. Four or more of the following concurrent symptoms on a persistent or recurrent basis during 6 or more consecutive months of illness, none of which may predate the fatigue:
   - Self-reported impairment in short-term memory or concentration that is severe enough to cause substantial reduction in previous levels of occupational, educational, social, or personal activities
   - Sore throat
   - Tender cervical or axillary lymph nodes
   - Muscle pain
   - Multijoint pain without joint swelling or redness
   - Headaches of a new type, pattern, or severity
   - Unrefreshing sleep
   - Postexertional malaise lasting more than 24 hours

*Both 1 and 2 are required conditions for a diagnosis of CFS.

is not relieved by rest, and results in a substantial reduction in previous levels of activity. In addition to the severe unexplained fatigue, four or more of the symptoms listed in Box 142-1 should be present concurrently for at least 6 months. This revised definition deleted the physical signs and required fewer symptoms to be present to fulfill the diagnosis. The goal was an attempt to decrease the number of patients with a somatization disorder. Patients with severe fatigue for 6 months but fewer than four other symptoms are classified as having *idiopathic chronic fatigue*. Patients with prior psychoses or behavioral disorders, such as psychotic depression, bipolar disorder, schizophrenia, or substance abuse, should be excluded, as well as patients with any prior chronic mental illness (Box 142-2).

The diagnosis of CFS is difficult and remains one of exclusion. No laboratory test can confirm the diagnosis; routine laboratory tests are normal, and the erythrocyte sedimentation rate is not elevated (Box 142-3). An evaluation to exclude other disorders should be based on the patient's history and epidemiologic exposures. Lyme disease or human immunodeficiency virus (HIV) serology is indicated only with the appropriate epidemiologic history. Similarly, antinuclear antibody or rheumatoid factor testing should be ordered only if the patient has joint complaints. Selected immunologic tests may be abnormal in patients with CFS but are indicated only for research purposes. Although symptoms of the so-called yeast connection or *Candida* hypersensitivity syndrome overlap those of CFS, no evidence indicates that the "yeast syndrome" exists, and testing for *Candida* antibodies is not indicated. Cortisol excretion is decreased in CFS patients compared with controls. This may result from a deficiency of corticotropin-releasing hormone (CRH) or another stimulus of the pituitary-adrenal axis. In contrast to

Box 142-2. Disorders that Exclude the Diagnosis of Chronic Fatigue Syndrome

- Any untreated active medical disorder that can cause chronic fatigue (e.g., untreated hypothyroidism, hepatitis C)
- Major depression
- Bipolar disease
- Schizophrenia
- Anorexia nervosa
- Bulimia
- Substance abuse
- Obesity body mass index of 45 or greater
- Any unexplained physical examination finding or laboratory abnormality that suggests another cause for the fatigue

Box 142-3. Screening Laboratory Tests for Suspected CFS/Fibromyalgia*

- Complete blood count with white blood cell differential
- Serum chemistry tests for alanine transaminase, total protein, albumin, globulin, alkaline phosphatase, calcium phosphorus, glucose, blood urea nitrogen, electrolytes, and creatinine
- Thyroid-stimulating hormone level
- Urinalysis

*Other tests based on history (e.g., epidemiologic exposures) and physical examination.

patients with CFS, cortisol secretion may be increased in patients with primary depression. Although CFS is similar to depression, these two disorders have different hormonal abnormalities. CFS has been associated with neurally mediated hypotension. In an uncontrolled trial, 30% to 89% of patients with CFS had abnormal tilt table test and responded to salt loading, fludrocortisone, β-adrenergic blockers, and disopyramide. Magnetic resonance imaging (MRI) brain scans may show multiple foci of high signal intensity in the white matter in patients with CFS compared with controls. The meaning of these findings is unknown, and an MRI brain scan is not useful as a diagnostic test. Patients complain of multiple cognitive defects, but various neuropsychologic tests have not been of value in documenting these abnormalities. Although fatigue is a hallmark of CFS, no myopathy has been identified. Similarly, patients often complain of weakness but on testing demonstrate normal muscle strength.

Widespread pain and multiple tender points are characteristic of fibromyalgia, but again, no diagnostic laboratory test exists. Patients with fibromyalgia sleep poorly, and sleep abnormalities have been identified on electroencephalograms; however, these findings are not specific for fibromyalgia. Neuroendocrine abnormalities, such as reduced excretion of urinary free cortisol and decreased levels of insulin growth

Box 142-4. Selected Differential Diagnosis of Chronic Fatigue

Habit Patterns
Caffeine habituation
Alcoholism
Other substance abuse

Psychosocial
Depression
Anxiety
Stress reaction

Pregnancy

Autoimmune Disorders
Systemic lupus erythematosus
Multiple sclerosis
Thyroiditis
Rheumatoid arthritis
Myasthenia gravis

Sleep Disorders
Sleep apnea
Narcolepsy

Infectious Diseases
Mononucleosis
 Cytomegalovirus
 Epstein-Barr virus
Human immunodeficiency virus
Chronic hepatitis B or C
Lyme disease
Fungal disease
Chronic parasitic infection
Tuberculosis
Subacute bacterial endocarditis
Occult abscess

Endocrine Disorders
Hyperparathyroidism
Hypothyroidism
Hyperthyroidism
Adrenal insufficiency
Cushing's syndrome
Hypopituitarism
Diabetes mellitus

Occult Malignancy

Hematologic Problems
Anemia
Myeloproliferative syndromes

Hepatic Disease
Alcoholic hepatitis or cirrhosis

Cardiovascular Disease
Low-output states
Silent myocardial infarction

Metabolic Disorders
Hyponatremia
Hypokalemia
Hypercalcemia

Renal Disease
Chronic renal failure

Respiratory Disorders
Chronic obstructive pulmonary disease

Miscellaneous
Medications
Sarcoidosis
Wegener's granulomatosis
Inflammatory bowel disease

Modified from Komaroff AL: Chronic fatigue. In Branch WJ Jr: *Office practice and medicine*, ed 3, Philadelphia, 1994, WB Saunders.

factor, have been reported in some patients with fibromyalgia,[1] but their role is unknown. Patients with CFS and fibromyalgia have psychologic distress, manifested by depression, anxiety, and panic attacks. These psychiatric problems probably are secondary to fibromyalgia and CFS rather than the primary problem. Most believe these disorders are not solely psychiatric diagnoses.

Differential Diagnosis

Many disorders cause chronic fatigue and should be excluded by a careful history, physical examination, and targeted laboratory testing based on epidemiologic exposures (Box 142-4).

MANAGEMENT

CFS and fibromyalgia are chronic illnesses in which the course waxes and wanes. The objectives of therapy are to educate the patient, provide symptomatic relief, and preserve or improve functional ability. Patient support groups can play an important role. Treatment can be divided into nonpharmacologic approaches (e.g., physical therapy, exercise, counseling, cognitive behavior therapy [CBT]) and pharmacologic therapy (Box 142-5).

CFS patients often avoid activity out of fear of exacerbating their symptoms. Complete bed rest should be avoided because of the problems associated with physical deconditioning. A common-sense balance between moderate levels of exercise and rest is essential, and physical activity should be gradually increased as tolerated. CBT attempts to alter attitudes, perceptions, and beliefs that can contribute to maladaptive behavior. In controlled trials using CBT and a graded exercise program, patients with CFS and fibromyalgia significantly improved compared with the placebo group.[10] Pharmacologic therapies treat symptoms such as depression, anxiety, sleep problems, allergies, and muscle and joint pains.[5,6] Antiviral drugs (e.g., acyclovir, corticosteroids,

Box 142-5. Steps in Management of CFS and Fibromyalgia

1. Establish the diagnosis and regularly reevaluate.
2. Provide emotional support and refer patient to support groups.
3. Provide nonpharmacologic therapy.
   a. Graded exercise program to prevent further disability
   b. Cognitive behavior therapy
   c. Physical therapy
   d. Counseling
4. Administer pharmacologic treatment.
   a. Treat symptoms (e.g., depression, sleep problems, muscle and joint pains) with appropriate medications.
   b. Avoid untested remedies.
5. Provide regular follow-up.

immunoglobulins) have no role. Some patients have hypotension on tilt table testing and may benefit from salt loading, fludrocortisone, or β-adrenergic blockers.[2]

Since no specific therapy exists for CFS and fibromyalgia, emotional support is critical. Patients should be followed to continue to exclude other medical problems. In more than half of patients, symptoms persist for years.[11]

REFERENCES

1. Bennett RM: The fibromyalgia syndrome. In Kelly WN, Ruddy S, Harris ED, Sledge CB, editors: *Textbook of rheumatology,* ed 5, Philadelphia, 1997, Saunders.
2. Bou-Holaigah I, Rowe PC, Kan J, et al: Relationship between neurally mediated hypotension and the chronic fatigue syndrome, *JAMA* 274:961, 1995.
3. Buchwald D, Umali P, Umali J, et al: Chronic fatigue and the chronic fatigue syndrome: prevalence in a Pacific Northwest health care system, *Ann Intern Med* 123:81, 1995.
4. Fikuda K, Straus SE, Hickie I, et al: The chronic fatigue syndrome: a comprehensive approach to its definition and study, *Ann Intern Med* 121:953, 1994.
5. Fukuda K, Gantz NM: Management strategies for chronic fatigue syndrome, *Federal Practitioner* 12:12, 1995.
6. Goldenberg D, Mayskiy M, Mossey C, et al: A randomized, double-blind crossover trial of fluoxetine and amitriptyline in the treatment of fibromyalgia, *Arthritis Rheum* 39:1852, 1996.
7. Goldenberg DL, Simma RW, Geiger A, et al: High frequency of fibromyalgia in patients with chronic fatigue seen in a primary care practice, *Arthritis Rheum* 33:381, 1990.
8. Holmes GP, Kaplan JE, Gantz NM, et al: Chronic fatigue syndrome: a working case definition, *Ann Intern Med* 108:387, 1988.
9. McKenzie R, Straus SE: Chronic fatigue syndrome, *Adv Intern Med* 40:119, 1995.
10. Scharpe M: Cognitive behavior therapy for chronic fatigue syndrome: efficacy and implications, *Am J Med* 105:104S, 1998.
11. Vercoulen JHMM, Swanink CMA, Fennis JFM, et al: Prognosis in chronic fatigue syndrome: a prospective study on the natural course, *J Neurol Neurosurg Psychiatry* 60:489, 1996.
12. Wolfe F, Ross K, Anderson J, et al: The prevalence and characteristics of fibromyalgia in the general population, *Arthritis Rheum* 38:19, 1995.
13. Wolfe F, Smythe HA, Yunus MB, et al: The American College of Rheumatology 1990 criteria for the classification of fibromyalgia: report of the Multicenter Criteria Committee, *Arthritis Rheum* 33:160, 1990.

CHAPTER 143

Sports Medicine

Lisa Rowland Callahan
Michael F. Dillingham
Alex C. Lau
James L. McGuire*

An increasing awareness of the health benefits of fitness and of sports competition has also increased the demand for state-of-the-art sports medicine. An injured athlete desires a timely return to normal function. The primary care physician can provide not only treatment and rehabilitation, but also fitness evaluation, exercise programs, and injury prevention counseling. The office physician needs to evaluate and initially treat injuries, understand the sequelae of chronic injuries, and delineate the risks of overtraining. The physician should combine the best of current aggressive and conservative approaches to treatment of the athlete, with appropriate timing of subspecialty referral.

Physicians should be prepared to guide patients in three areas. First, a regular exercise program should be encouraged for its physiologic and psychologic benefits, such as better work performance and decreased stress levels. Second, nutritional advice is important, especially for weight maintenance or reduction through exercise. This is particularly true for young women who have not yet attained maximal bone mass. Third, cardiac and arthritic risk monitoring is also an important element of total care.

GUIDELINES FOR FITNESS TRAINING

Exercise

As with a medication, exercise should be prescribed properly to attain maximum benefit. During the history and physical examination the physician should consider the patient's current level of fitness, history of medical illnesses, medications, family history, and past injuries. Laboratory testing may be necessary, including lipid screening for cholesterol levels and electrocardiogram (ECG). Formal exercise testing is generally recommended for those with known or suspected cardiovascular or pulmonary disease and should at least be considered in any sedentary patient over age 35 before initiating an exercise program. On completion of the appropriate tests, exercise recommendations consider frequency, intensity, and duration of exercise; type of activity; and need for resistance training to achieve minimum fitness levels (Box 143-1).

Each exercise session should consist of three phases: warm-up, aerobic activity, and a cool-down period. The warm-up and cool-down may simply be the same aerobic activity performed with less intensity. The warm-up usually includes stretching and activation of the aerobic mechanism, and the cool-down attempts to minimize both postexercise myalgia and the risk of cardiac events.

The goals and methods for attaining fitness in children differ significantly from those for adults. Children have a

*Deceased.

Box 143-1. Guidelines for Exercise Prescription

Frequency: 3-5 days/week
Intensity: 60%-90% of HRmax or 50%-80% of $\dot{V}O_2$ max
Duration: 20-60 minutes
Mode: any continuous aerobic activity using large muscle groups (e.g., running, cycling, swimming)
Resistance training: one set, 8 to 12 repetitions of 8 to 10 exercises (minimum recommendation)

HRmax, Maximum heart rate. This may be estimated by the formula 220 − Age = HRmax. Variation ± 10% is common.
$\dot{V}O_2$ max, Maximum oxygen uptake.

relatively inefficient metabolism, less anaerobic capacity, and less heat tolerance. They are generally motivated by having fun rather than by increasing fitness. These factors should guide the physician's recommendations for achieving fitness in children. The type of exercise recommended should be determined by the child's interests and strengths. It is clear that the more active the child, the better the gain in bone density as young adulthood is reached. Weight training in children is controversial. Children probably can achieve increases in strength through resistance training. Much work still needs to be done for clear guidelines. Adolescents may generally use the same fitness training guidelines as adults. If an adolescent's goal is to achieve excellence in a particular sport, exercise prescription should focus particularly on developing skills relative to the chosen sport (e.g., drills to develop hand-eye coordination) in addition to achieving aerobic fitness and muscular strength and endurance. This idea of sport-specific conditioning is also applicable to adults.

The opportunity to prescribe appropriate exercise for the school-age athlete may come as a preparticipation physical examination. Growing numbers of children participate in organized athletics; physicians are often asked to screen these students for conditions that might limit participation or predispose to injury. This type of examination should consist of a directed history as well as medical and orthopedic evaluations.

Nutrition and Fluid Intake

Good nutrition is essential for good health as well as for athletic success. Since athletes frequently do not practice proper eating habits, the physician should review and explain sound nutrition principles. Generally, a healthy diet should consist of 60% to 70% carbohydrate, 20% to 30% fat, and approximately 10% to 15% protein. Some athletes are too restrictive with their diets, consuming minimal amounts of fats and calories. Athletes should be screened carefully for possible eating disorders, counseled in proper nutrition, and if necessary, referred for appropriate psychologic care. In contrast, young athletes, especially those engaged in vigorous activity, require high-caloric intakes to build and maintain appropriate muscle mass. For example, high-school football players training twice daily have caloric needs of 5000 to 6000 kcal per day.

Adequate fluid intake is an essential and frequently neglected aspect of sports nutrition. Exercise greatly increases heat production. The body's thermoregulatory system dissipates this excess heat primarily by evaporation of sweat. If the fluids and electrolytes lost through sweat are not replaced, the athlete will become dehydrated. This can lead to both cardiovascular and thermoregulatory compromise, which directly affects the athlete's health and performance. To prevent this, athletes should constantly drink fluids before, during, and after competition. Adequate intake can be estimated by having the athlete monitor weight and urine color. A pound of weight lost is equivalent to 2 cups of sweat and should be replaced accordingly. If the urine volume is low and the color becomes dark yellow, dehydration probably exists, and increased fluid intake either by mouth or intravenously is immediately warranted.

Questions concerning fluid replacement with water vs. sports drink often arise. In general, water is sufficient for the recreational athlete and exercise sessions lasting 90 minutes or less. For longer exercise sessions and endurance events, a sports drink or diluted fruit juice is recommended, since it provides both glucose (carbohydrate source) and electrolytes. Cold concentrations of 2% to 6% carbohydrate are absorbed most quickly. The physician should encourage the athlete not to rely on thirst as an indicator of fluid loss because enough body water lost can adversely affect performance before the athlete becomes thirsty.

Androgenic Steroids and Other Ergogenic Aids

Maximal athletic performance depends on a complex combination of physical and psychologic factors. Competitors have tried a variety of methods to enhance performance, including psychologic techniques, vitamins, food supplements, androgens, and illicit drugs. Currently, athletes are experimenting with anabolic steroids. Because these substances are banned by all official sporting organizations, the true prevalence of their use is difficult to quantify. Despite highly publicized suspensions and loss of Olympic medals, the use of anabolic steroids in certain sports continues to increase. Also, androgen use has extended beyond the well-publicized professional and world-class amateur athlete to the high-school and community health clubs. Physicians need to be aware of the extensive risks of androgen use so that they can convey these risks, especially because athletes believe that androgens provide a competitive advantage in some sports.

Although anabolic steroids improve muscle strength through increased lean muscle mass and exercise tolerance, many hormone-related side effects result from their use. Anabolic steroids, related to the naturally produced testosterone, are available in both injectable and oral forms. Androgenic effects in males include testicular atrophy, abnormal sperm counts, cystic acne, gynecomastia, decreased sex drive, liver adenomas, and aggressive behavior. In females, masculine secondary sexual characteristics develop and are thought to be largely irreversible. These include growth of facial hair, deepening of the voice, male pattern baldness, and enlargement of the clitoris. In prepubertal athletes, anabolic steroids may cause premature epiphyseal closure, leading to growth arrest. Chronic androgen use typically results in lower high-density lipoprotein (HDL) cholesterol levels, whereas exercise usually increases this beneficial cholesterol. These serious side effects, as well as psychologic and cardiac risks, underline the danger of steroid use in athletes.

The terms *steroids, androgens,* and anabolic steroids are used interchangeably by athletes, coaches, and some sports physicians, whereas for primary care physicians, the word *steroids* usually refers to glucocorticoids.

Creatine has become a popular supplementation used by athletes to enhance their strength and aerobic exercise capacity. The oral supplement increases total muscle creatine. Short-term supplementation appears to increase body mass, although this may be caused by a concomitant increase in water. Combined with exercise, creatine may enhance muscular and work performance. Initial reports with short-term use have not shown any major health risks, but with long-term use the risks are unknown. Creatine can be purchased over the counter and is currently legal for use by athletes.

Other substances used by athletes to enhance performance include human growth hormone (HGH) and erythropoietin (EPO), two naturally occurring hormones. Some users of HGH report an increase in muscular size and strength, but others do not. Endurance athletes use EPO to increase hemoglobin concentration and thus the amount of oxygen delivered to working muscles. As the concentration of red blood cells rises (enhanced also by dehydration), so does the risk of clot formation and stroke. Death after "blood doping," as use of EPO is also known, has been reported. Androgens can be readily detected in urine, but illicit HGH and EPO injections may be difficult to detect in serum.

Specificity of Training

Proper conditioning demands specificity in training. The exercise done for the sporting contest should mimic the event itself in aspects of required endurance, motion, velocity, movement, and load. Weight training and other types of resistance training encourage development of metabolic systems that are specific to the overload and muscle size. Specificity of motion encourages neural coordination among muscle groups and within the muscles. Untrained persons cannot fully activate muscles, particularly their high-threshold muscle motor units. Specificity of training allows complete and coordinated activation of muscle with a specific task in mind. Given two muscles of equal size, the better coordinated muscle will be stronger. Thus muscular strength gains in any particular activity are achieved not only through hypertrophy of muscle, but also through better coordination of muscle activity.

Overtraining

Overtraining is a syndrome that affects athletes of all ages and abilities, resulting when an athlete's training program exceeds the body's ability to recover. Muscle growth occurs primarily as a response to muscle breakdown during bouts of exercise. Adequate rest and recovery are necessary, or muscular gains are not made. Exercise programs that emphasize endurance with high-frequency, low-resistance activity can be done every other day. Programs that focus on strength and building of muscle mass with low-repetition, high-load resistance training are generally done only every fourth day. This is true even for highly conditioned Olympic athletes. Overtraining, both in weight training and aerobic conditioning, is a common error made primarily by recreational athletes.

Overtraining manifests both psychologically and physiologically. Probably the most universal complaint is fatigue, which athletes often refer to as "staleness" or "burnout." Apathy, sleep disturbances, loss of appetite, irritability, heavy legs, sore muscles, and decreased ability to concentrate are other common complaints. Physiologic changes include increased heart rate and blood pressure. The physician should distinguish this syndrome from other causes of medical conditions that accompany fatigue, such as depression, anemia, asthma, mononucleosis, or other viral illnesses. A complete history and physical examination should be performed. Screening complete blood counts and serum chemistries should be obtained. The physician should evaluate the training regimen and consult with the coach or athletic trainer if necessary. Rest is the best treatment for overtraining. Continued activity will prevent desired gains and may even cause more harm.

ATHLETIC INJURIES

Head Injuries

Most athletic injuries involve the musculoskeletal system. However, contact sports and many so-called noncontact sports (e.g., basketball, baseball, soccer) may cause head and thoracoabdominal injuries. The physician should examine the severely injured athlete for airway and hemodynamic stability and perform any necessary stabilization and resuscitation. With a head injury, associated neck injury must always be considered, especially with a concussion.

Although different methods exist for assessing and grading concussions, the most important indicator of severity is the athlete's level of consciousness. When a head injury has occurred, five historic points are pivotal to the evaluation: (1) loss of consciousness, (2) retrograde amnesia, (3) persistent headache, (4) nausea, and (5) blurring of vision. In general the athlete can return to competition if loss of consciousness lasted less than several minutes and the athlete can remember all events or plays before the injury. A headache after the head injury should not persist. The physical examination, especially the neuromuscular evaluation, should be normal. The athlete must be asymptomatic before returning to the game. If any of these symptoms is unresolved, magnetic resonance imaging (MRI) or computed tomography (CT) may be indicated. Postconcussion headaches, especially when exercising, may occur for several weeks after the injury. During an athletic contest the primary care physician may allow the patient to reenter the game if there is no retrograde amnesia and no headache with a normal neurologic examination. When any clinical doubt remains, the physician should not allow the athlete to resume play after a concussion (Fig. 143-1).

Musculoskeletal Injuries

Evaluation of musculoskeletal injuries should include examination of bone and joint stability, deformity, and function. The most accurate examination is obtained if conducted as soon as possible after the injury. With time, muscle spasm, joint effusion, and discomfort increase, making ligamentous laxity more difficult to evaluate and dislocations more difficult to reduce. Therefore a primary care physician on the sidelines with knowledge of sports medicine can facilitate the athlete's return to play by providing an expedient and accurate assessment.

Ligamentous injury is usually called a *sprain.* Sprains are generally classified as mild, moderate, or severe, depending on the degree of disruption of the ligament's fibers: the

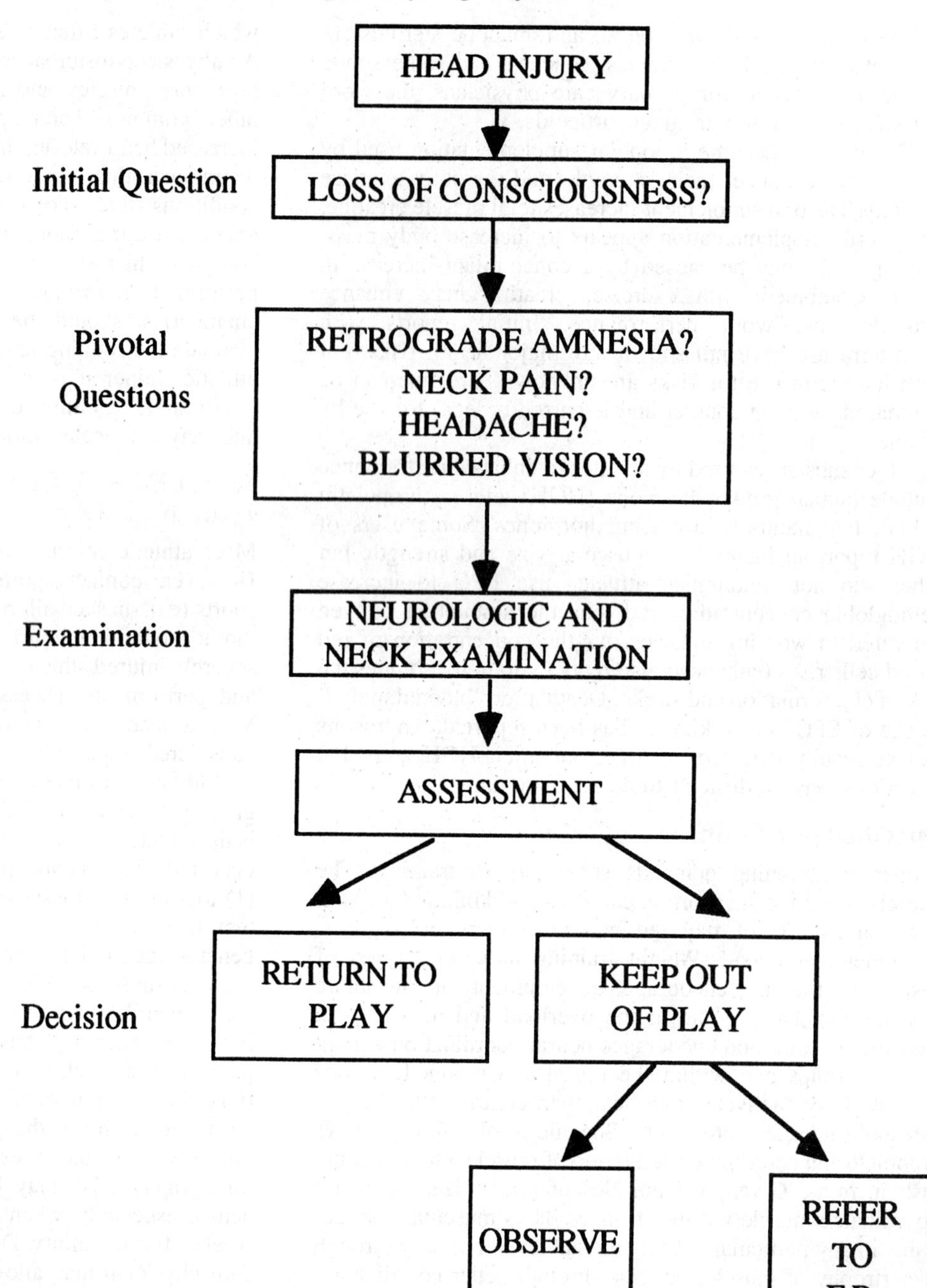

Fig. 143-1. Assessment of head injury without neck complaints.

greater the disruption, the more severe and potentially unstable the injury. A simple grading system from I to III is used to signify the degree of instability (Fig. 143-2). An injury to a musculotendinous unit is termed a *strain.* Strains are generally classified as acute or chronic, again with a grading system from I to III to describe the severity of the injury (Table 143-1).

Athletic injuries may be acute (traumatic, e.g., anterior cruciate ligament tear in a football player), chronic, or related to overuse (e.g., stress fracture in a runner). A careful history delineates the type of injury. Medical illnesses, such as rheumatologic disease, may masquerade as an athletic injury. At the first manifestation of an acute or subacute rheumatic disease, patients often attribute their joint symptoms to a recent injury. At times there may be a cause-and-effect relationship. For example, the first manifestation of rheumatoid arthritis may follow a knee or ankle injury. Premature osteoarthritis is a well-established sequela of internal derangement of the knee. Other patients attribute the early phases of a pseudogout or gout attack to a strained knee or ankle, respectively. An adolescent may attribute a swollen knee to an athletic injury. A radiograph may demonstrate a more severe bony abnormality, such as infection or tumor. Thus the physician must consider all medical possibilities when diagnosing an athletic injury (Table 143-2).

Before examining the athlete with an acute musculoskeletal injury, the examiner asks about the mechanism of injury and if a pop or snap was heard or felt, if pain or swelling was

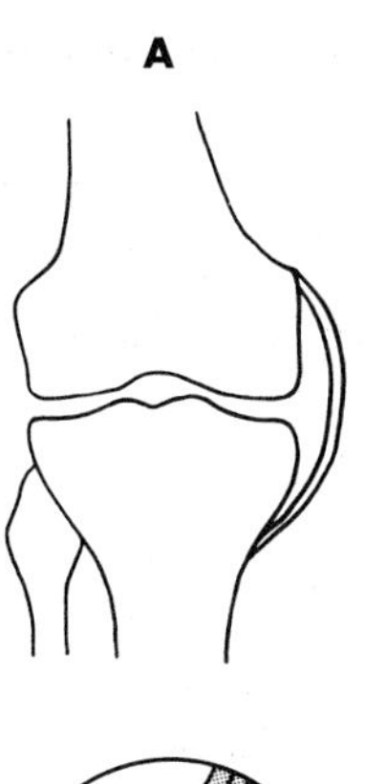

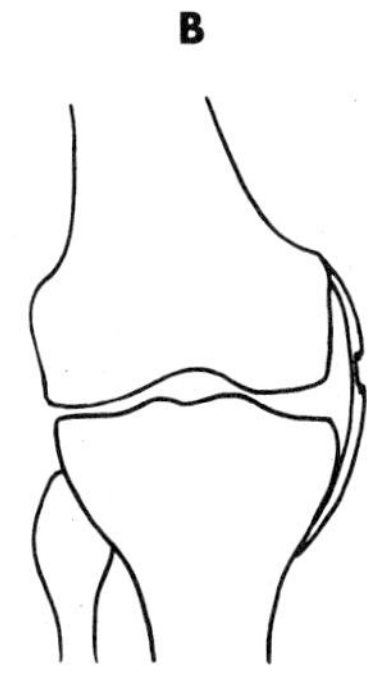

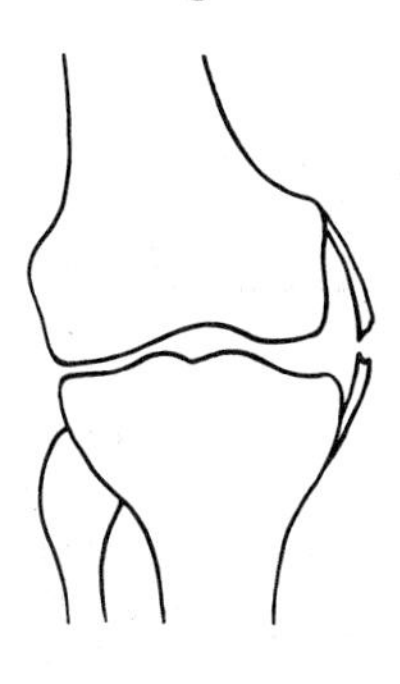

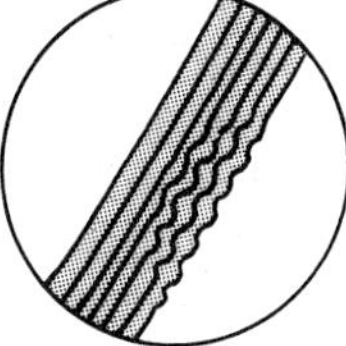

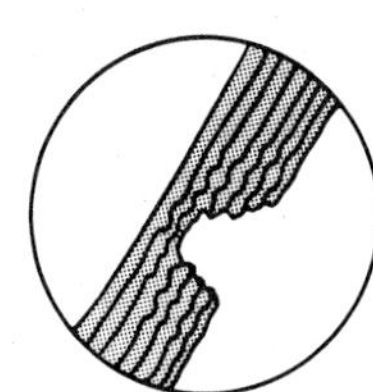

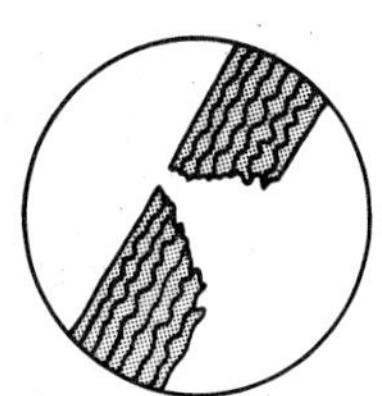

Fig. 143-2. Ligamentous sprains vary in severity. **A,** First degree. **B,** Second degree. **C,** Third-degree sprain, which indicates complete rupture.

Table 143-1. Classification of Musculoskeletal Injury

Grade	Classification	Description	Treatment
Sprains (injury to ligament)			
I	Mild	Minimal disruption of fibers, minimal or no instability	Symptomatic
II	Moderate	Mild to moderate instability	Symptomatic; consider protection with brace
III	Severe	Complete disruption of fibers, gross instability	Symptomatic; consider surgery
Strains (injury to musculotendinous unit)			
I	Mild	No gross disruption of fibers	Symptomatic
II	Moderate	Partial disruption of fibers	Symptomatic; consider protection with brace/splint or surgery for tendon tear
III	Severe	Complete disruption of fibers	Symptomatic; consider surgery for tendon tear

immediate or delayed, if the athlete was able to continue activity, and if the patient has a history of injury. Ability to bear weight on an an injured leg and injury to the dominant arm are other considerations.

Radiographs can be useful when evaluating musculoskeletal injury. At least two views, anteroposterior (AP) and lateral, should always be obtained, since injuries are not always apparent on a single view. In some cases comparison views of the contralateral extremity are helpful, especially for children who may have injured their epiphyses and for subtle dislocations of carpal bones. Additional radiographs of a specific area sometimes require special views for the sports medicine specialist at referral (Box 143-2). Other radiographic techniques, including MRI, CT, and bone scan, are helpful in certain settings.

Overuse Injuries

Overuse syndromes result from repetitive microtrauma to bones, ligaments, and musculotendinous units. Intrinsic factors include structural (e.g., leg length discrepancy) or biomechanical (e.g., poor flexibility, muscular weakness, especially eccentric weakness) abnormalities. Extrinsic factors relate to equipment (e.g., worn-out running shoes) and training errors (e.g., increasing mileage too rapidly). Training schedules and techniques often provide the reason for injury. Specifically, the type, intensity, and duration of training workouts should be evaluated for the common "too much too soon" phenomenon, especially in unconditioned high-school and college athletes and recreational runners. Consideration of these factors usually reveals the etiology of the overuse injury. The physician can then treat the injury and counsel the athlete to prevent recurrence.

Bone constantly remodels and repairs itself, but if the degree of repetitive microtrauma exceeds this capability, an overuse injury occurs as a stress fracture. Stress fractures occur most often in the weight-bearing bones of the lower extremity (e.g., tibia, metatarsals) but have also been seen in the upper extremity of the throwing athlete. The athlete presents with pain in the area of the fracture and often gives a history compatible with overuse. The physician should ask specifically about training errors, such as changes in the length, intensity, or duration of exercise. The patient may have swelling and point tenderness in the area of the fracture. Radiographs may be negative initially, but the fracture may

Table 143-2. Common Athletic Injuries

Region and injury	Sport	History/symptoms	Physical examination	Initial tests/treatment
Shoulder				
Acromioclavicular separation	Cycling, falls	Acute injury; pain and possible deformity over top of shoulder at acromioclavicular joint	Localized tenderness, possible deformity, distal clavicle displacement	X-ray; grade II: symptomatic treatment; grade III or greater: orthopedic consult
Rotator cuff tear	Contact sports	Fall on outstretched arm or acute overload of cuff; pain over lateral shoulder, occasional difficulty in abducting arm	Pain and/or weakness on external rotation and/or abduction	X-ray to rule out fracture, MRI; if complete tear, surgical repair required
Instability, anterior or posterior/ subluxation	Overhead and throwing sports, serving and swimming	Pain with overhead maneuver, possible "dead arm" when throwing, occasional sense of instability	Possibly consistent with cuff irritation or weakness; positive apprehension sign, either anterior or posterior; findings of joint laxity	Orthopedic consult to determine further treatment, including rehabilitation and surgery
Biceps tendinitis	Contact and overhead sports, weightlifting	Posttraumatic or chronic; pain with lifting or working in forward flexion	Pain with resisted forward flexion and with palpation of tendon	Diagnostic block; rest, injection, rehabilitation; rarely requires surgery
Elbow				
Epicondylitis (medial or lateral)	Throwing and racquet sports, golf	Pain with use of the forearm, wrist, or hand	Tenderness to palpation and with resistance of involved musculotendinous unit	Rest, rehabilitation, NSAIDs, possible injection
Medial ligament sprain	Throwing and racquet sports, javelin	Pain during play	Tenderness over the ligament and with valgus stress; possible clinical instability	Stress x-rays, MRI; grade I and II: rehabilitation and rest; grade III (complete or near complete tear): orthopedic consult and surgery
Navicular fracture	Contact sports	Fall on outstretched hand	Tenderness in anatomic snuffbox	X-ray; consider immobilization; if fracture present, orthopedic referral; if no fracture, but symptoms present, orthopedic referral
Lumbar spine				
Spondylolysis	Gymnastics, football (linemen), weight training, dancing, figure skating	Low back pain and stiffness; occasional buttock, leg, or thigh pain; occasionally associated with radiculopathy	Tenderness to palpation, occasional muscle spasm; pain with rotation and extension, increased lordosis	X-ray; if results equivocal, bone scan/MRI; if positive, orthopedic consult
Diskogenic pain (annular tear, disk protrusion)	Any sport	Any of the following: low back pain, buttock pain, thigh/leg pain, possible radicular pattern	Midline tenderness to palpation; possible increased pain with forward flexion; possible positive straight leg raising	X-rays, rest, ice, NSAIDs; if symptoms severe or persistent, orthopedic or physiatry referral

MRI, Magnetic resonance imaging; *NSAIDs*, nonsteroidal antiinflammatory drugs.

be apparent on repeat radiographs in 2 weeks, when healing has begun. Although not usually part of the initial evaluation, a bone scan and special MRI (STIR sequences) may be positive before the radiograph. Treatment of the uncomplicated stress fracture consists of rest for a few weeks and therapy with nonsteroidal antiinflammatory drugs (NSAIDs) and ice. Athletes frequently have difficulty complying with rest; noncompliance may delay their return to the sport. As healing occurs, substituting another activity may help increase rest compliance (e.g., swimming instead of running

Table 143-2. Common Athletic Injuries—cont'd

Region and injury	Sport	History/symptoms	Physical examination	Initial tests/treatment
Knee				
Injury to ligament				
Anterior cruciate ligament	All sports involving change of direction, jumping, or contact	Sense of "giving way," often with associated pop, subsequent swelling and pain	Effusion, positive Lachman's test; positive anterior drawer test; frequent joint line pain	Non–weight bearing and immobilization briefly for symptoms, possible MRI/ arthroscopy
Posterior cruciate ligament	All sports involving change of direction, jumping, or contact	Generally a fall onto proximal tibia, acute or subacute onset, posterior (popliteal space) knee pain	Positive posterior drawer test (may evolve over hours or days); possible effusion, possible popliteal area pain	Initial treatment is symptomatic; orthopedic consult, generally nonsurgical
Medial and lateral collateral ligaments	All sports involving change of direction, jumping, or contact	Occasional sense of tearing with acute tibial displacement and subsequent pain	Local tenderness, instability on stress testing, frequent hamstring guarding	Immobilization/crutches for comfort, possible MRI; grade I: symptomatic treatment; grade II or III: orthopedic consult
Injury to cartilage				
Meniscal tear (medial or lateral)	All sports	Usually joint line pain, occasionally clicking, popping, or locking	Joint line pain, possible effusion, possible positive McMurray's test	MRI, symptomatic treatment and possible orthopedic consult for arthroscopy
Leg				
Shin splints	Running, jumping, diving	Pain with activity	Localized tenderness if bone stress reaction or periostitis; possible muscle tenderness if compartment syndrome	X-ray; if necessary, bone scan or MRI; rest, ice, orthoses; if persistent, orthopedic referral
Foot/ankle				
Achilles tendinitis	Running, jumping, dancing, and diving	Pain with activity, subacute onset	Tenderness and possible swelling and edema over involved segment of tendon	If symptoms persist, MRI (to rule out tear); rest, rehabilitation, occasional immobilization, occasional surgery
Plantar fasciitis	Running, jumping, dancing	Usually insidious onset, occasionally acute, atraumatic onset, pain at proximal arch	Tenderness along plantar fascial insertion on calcaneus; occasionally, tight Achilles tendon/ hindfoot	Taping, orthoses, stretching, antiinflammatory modalities and NSAIDs; rarely surgery
Ankle sprain (medial-syndesmodic)	Any sport involving running or jumping	Ankle inverted, everted, and forcibly plantar flexed or dorsiflexed	Swelling and pain to palpation over involved ligaments	X-ray to rule out fracture, ice, crutches, compression, possible acute immobilization; if severe, orthopedic consult

for an athlete with a metatarsal stress fracture). After resolution of the stress fracture, a careful program is started to prevent overtraining and repetition of the injury.

Young athletes may develop the overuse syndrome known as *traction apophysitis,* which results from repeated stress at the insertion of a tendon into a growth plate center. It is most often seen at the insertion of the patellar tendon on the tibial tubercle, a condition known as *Osgood-Schlatter disease.* The young athlete presents with pain and swelling over the tubercle, which is usually enlarged and tender. Apophysitis frequently appears during rapid growth in association with tight hamstrings and quadriceps muscles. As in stress fractures, treatment is rest and NSAIDs. Prevention involves screening the athlete for contributing factors, such as tight muscles, and instruction in a stretching program, especially for the warm-up session.

Repetitive trauma at the site of tendon attachment to bone causes a common overuse syndrome of *tendinitis.* This probably results from the relatively poor blood supply of the tendon combined with tension overload. The patellar tendon, wrist flexors and extensors, and rotator cuff tendons are often affected. Ligaments may be the tissue affected by overuse, such as in breaststroker's knee, an overuse strain of the medial collateral ligament. Similarly, pitchers, golfers, and

Box 143-2. Radiographic Views for Athletic Injuries

Acromioclavicular joint
- Axillary
- Oblique
- Flexion

Shoulder/elbow
- Oblique
- Flexion

Wrist/hand
- Oblique
- Navicular view

Cervical spine
- Oblique views
- Odontoid views for C1-2

Lumbar spine
- Lumbosacral spot
- Bilateral obliques

Hip: none

Knee
- Tunnel
- Oblique
- Merchant or sunrise (patella)

Ankle
- Bilateral stress views
- Mortise

Foot
- Standing comparison AP
- Oblique views

Box 143-3. Overuse Syndromes and Associated Sports

Stress fracture or epiphyseal slip of proximal humerus: throwing sports, particularly in children and adolescents
Rotator cuff tendinitis: throwing and lifting sports
Lateral epicondylitis (tennis elbow): tennis, golf, throwing sports
Medial epicondylitis: tennis, golf, throwing sports
Strained medial collateral ligament (elbow): throwing sports
Little Leaguer's elbow: baseball
Radiocapitellar degenerative change: throwing sports, particularly in children and adolescents
Spondylolysis/spondylolisthesis: gymnastics, football
Trochanteric bursitis: running, weightlifting
Stress fracture (femoral neck): running and jumping sports
Distal iliotibial band tendinitis: running sports, cycling, hiking, climbing
Patellar tendinitis (jumper's knee): running and jumping sports, diving
Breaststroker's knee: swimming
Tibial stress fracture: running and jumping sports, diving
Tibial tubercle apophysitis (Osgood-Schlatter disease): running and jumping sports
Achilles tendinitis: running and jumping sports
Plantar fasciitis: running sports
Calcaneal apophysitis (Sever's disease): running sports

javelin throwers experience overuse strains on the medial aspect of their elbow. A complete history should uncover contributing factors. Treatment is similar to that for other types of overuse syndromes, with a similar emphasis on prevention. Overuse injuries can occur in all sports (Box 143-3).

Running Injuries

Most injuries in runners are overuse rather than acute and can be attributed to training errors. Generally, injuries are seen in those who run more than 30 miles per week or increase their mileage by more than 10% per week. The type and grade of the running surface as well as fatigue and lack of strength may contribute to injuries. Other predisposing factors include muscle tightness and accelerated training schedules.

Tendinitis of the quadriceps, patellar, or Achilles tendon is a common running injury. With a strain of the hamstring muscle group, the runner complains of localized pain, which usually increases during the run. Pain is reproduced with palpation or contraction of the involved musculotendinous unit. Posterior leg or thigh pain may be radicular. Treatment is symptomatic, emphasizing rest. The patient should understand that acute tendinitis and strains respond most favorably to rest. If allowed to become chronic, these injuries often take months to resolve.

If the runner has anterior or medial knee pain, the physician should evaluate for patellofemoral syndrome with medial facet arthritis and a synovial plica (medial shelf). A *plica* is a remnant of an embryologic wall that divides the knee into compartments and remains present in an estimated 15% to 20% of adults. It may become symptomatic with repetitive flexion and extension of the knee, such as in running. Often bilateral, a plica is frequently the source of pain in runner's knee and growing pains. It causes medial parapatellar pain, often on palpation. In a minority of cases it is palpable in flexion and extension of the knee. Symptomatic treatment of a plica is often unsuccessful; therefore arthroscopic release may be needed.

Lateral patellofemoral pain results from joint overload and is a common cause of bilateral knee pain, especially in females. Risk factors include a relatively greater angle from hip to knee, called the *Q angle* (Fig. 143-3). The Q angle increases the lateral forces on the patella, which then moves out of the normal femoral groove. The undersurface compresses against the femoral condyles in a reduced area, increasing stress. Biomechanical factors, including pes planus (flatfoot) and genu valgum (knock-knee), also contribute to the development of patellofemoral pain syndrome by increased lateralization. In a young athlete this may be caused by inflexibility. Physical findings are variable; the athlete may be apprehensive when gentle pressure is applied during lateral parapatellar palpation. Once the diagnosis is suspected and underlying causes identified, treatment generally involves NSAIDs and quadriceps stretching and strengthening. The rehabilitation program should stress eccentric strengthening and closed chain exercises. Specific knee braces and orthotic devices may also be helpful. Occasionally an arthroscopic lateral release or other procedure may be indicated.

The differential diagnosis of a runner with lateral knee pain includes *iliotibial band syndrome*. Common in cyclists and runners, this syndrome is an inflammatory condition caused by chronic friction of the iliotibial band with the bony prominence of the lateral femoral condyle. Runners with varus deformities (bowlegs) or those who run on sloped surfaces are likely to complain of lateral knee pain in association with a popping sensation. Again, treatment is symptomatic and emphasizes stretching, strengthening, and adequate warm-up exercises.

The runner complaining of foot pain should be evaluated for *plantar fasciitis*, an inflammation and strain at the origin of the plantar fascia on the calcaneus. Patients describe pain

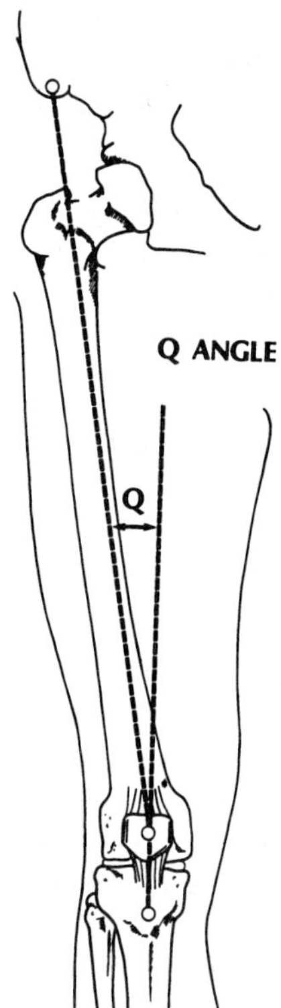

Fig. 143-3. Q angle.

on the bottom of the heel, especially on first awakening in the morning, which is relieved with activity. Frequently associated with tight heel cords of the foot and hyperpronation, plantar fasciitis can usually be controlled by heel cord stretching and orthoses. Recalcitrant cases may require injection or, rarely, surgical release.

Anterior lower leg pain is common in runners and is frequently diagnosed as shin splints. *Shin splints* refer to one of three syndromes: chronic compartment syndrome, chronic periostitis, or tibial stress fracture. Pain is generally at the medial distal tibia. Bone scan or MRI can differentiate between stress fracture and periostitis. Factors that predispose runners to shin splints include training errors, anatomic variations, and poor running techniques or equipment. Patients develop localized tenderness, which increases during running and subsides after activity. Treatment consists of rest, ice, stretching, careful warm-up, NSAIDs, and correction of predisposing factors (e.g., devices). Shin splints must be differentiated from stress fractures of the anterior tibia.

In addition to tibial stress fractures, other stress fractures are particularly common in runners. These overuse injuries are suggested when the runner complains of a persistent, dull pain while weight bearing. Although the metatarsals and tibia are probably the most common sites, the fibula, femoral neck, and pelvic bones may also sustain stress fracture. Any acute fracture should be evaluated to ensure the limb's neurovascular integrity, then splinted and the patient immediately transported to the hospital for further evaluation. Any open fracture is a surgical emergency.

Shoulder Injuries

Injuries to the shoulder are common in sports. Examination should include evaluation of the bony structures, musculotendinous units, and neurovascular system for deformity, limitation of function, and instability. Referred pain should be considered when movement of the affected joint does not change the symptom or does not elicit pain (e.g., amateur hockey player in a collision who complains of severe left shoulder pain with full range of motion). Causes of referred pain syndrome range from cervical disk herniation to a ruptured spleen with diaphragmatic irritation.

A sprain of the acromioclavicular (AC) joint is common in contact sports such as football and it often results from direct trauma to the shoulder, forcibly separating the acromion from the clavicle. The athlete usually complains of well-localized pain over the AC joint and has difficulty with cross-body adduction or abduction of the shoulder. In general, grade I (nondisplaced) and grade II (minimally displaced) reveal little or no deformity and are managed easily with NSAIDs and a sling for comfort. Athletes may return to play when their shoulder is asymptomatic, usually in 2 to 4 weeks. Grades III through VI should be placed in a sling initially, then referred to an orthopedist for further evaluation.

A fracture of the clavicle results from a direct blow to the bone and is suspected when the patient complains of pain directly over the clavicle. Radiographs confirm the diagnosis. This fracture can usually be managed with a figure-8 bandage or sling and pain medication. As with any fracture, follow-up should involve an orthopedist. Depending on the amount of displacement, most clavicular fractures heal in 6 to 8 weeks, when the athlete may return to play.

Impingement is an overuse condition often seen with overhead sports or with instability. It often results in rotator cuff tendinitis, with bursitis and compression of the cuff against the bony acromion causing pain. Depending on symptoms, impingement can be managed with NSAIDs, injections, physical therapy, and in refractory cases, surgery. Rotator cuff injuries may result from direct trauma or overuse, as seen with overhead sports. Patients complain of anterior or lateral shoulder pain and weakness. Rotator cuff tendinitis is initially managed with physical therapy and NSAIDs, but this injury is best managed by an orthopedist, potentially with surgical intervention.

Dislocation of the glenohumeral joint is also common, most often anterior dislocation resulting from an external rotation force on the abducted shoulder. The athlete complains of severe pain, limited motion of the shoulder, and a "squared off" deformity of the shoulder with anterior dislocations. The axillary nerve, which innervates the deltoid, should be evaluated before attempting reduction. The shoulder should be reduced as soon as possible, with before and after radiographs to assess for concomitant fracture. All shoulder dislocations should be managed initially with a sling and swathe for 2 to 3 weeks, then with exercises to strengthen the rotator cuff musculature. Athletes are allowed to return to play once therapy has restored their full motion and strength. Depending on the sport, specific equipment may aid in protection from the vulnerable abduction/external rotation force, which could cause a recurrent injury. The rate of redislocation is much higher in the younger athlete, who should be referred to the orthopedist for possible surgical stabilization.

Elbow, Wrist, and Hand Injuries

Most of the injuries to the elbow are from overuse, whereas wrist and hand injuries result from trauma. Fracture of the scaphoid of the wrist is often seen after a fall on the outstretched hand and should be suspected in a patient with tenderness in the anatomic snuffbox of the radial wrist, along with a distal radius fracture. The patient may have no other physical findings, and radiographs may initially be negative. With suspected injury, the wrist should be splinted and the patient referred to an orthopedist. Scaphoid wrist fractures often take up to 3 months to heal.

Gamekeeper's or *skier's thumb* is an acute sprain or tear of the ulnar collateral ligament (UCL) of the thumb (see Chapter 126). The skier or other athlete falls and forces the thumb into abduction. The metacarpophalangeal joint may appear swollen, with tenderness over the UCL. If radiographs reveal no fracture, the examiner may assess stability by stressing the UCL and evaluating for laxity. Partial or complete tears should be referred to a hand specialist. For those with persistent wrist pain, a hand surgeon should evaluate for ligamentous injury.

Knee Injuries

The knee may be the most frequently injured joint confronting the primary care physician. Accurate diagnosis and treatment depend on working knowledge of the basic anatomy, function, and topography of the knee. As with the shoulder, the knee should be evaluated for deformity, loss or limitation of function, stability, and localization of tenderness. Assessment should also be made for effusion, although aspiration is rarely performed in the acute knee injury (see Chapter 129).

The anterior cruciate ligament (ACL) is often injured by a valgus stress with external rotation or by hyperextension and internal rotation. Most athletes are injured while pivoting about their knee and often hear an audible "pop" and feel immediate pain. The knee usually swells soon after the injury, and the patient cannot bear weight on the affected leg. It is advantageous to examine the patient before the swelling. Lachman's test is the most sensitive examination, and a pivot shift is confirmatory. These tests may be difficult to perform in the patient with a swollen knee and in pain. The patient must be as comfortable as possible while the injury is examined; a pillow under the knee encourages muscle relaxation. Radiographs should be performed to rule out fractures. If an ACL injury is suspected, ice, immobilization, crutches if needed, compression, and referral to an orthopedist are recommended. If a ligament reconstruction is performed, either bone and patellar tendon autografts or patellar and Achilles tendon allografts may be used. A few centers use hamstring tendons. Many athletes return to play 6 months after reconstruction.

An injury to the meniscus may accompany an ACL tear or may occur as an isolated injury. Meniscal tear frequently results from a twisting injury. Patients complain of swelling, pain, catching, locking, and sometimes "giving way." Physical examination reveals joint line tenderness. Radiographs generally are not helpful. Arthroscopic surgery and possible repair are indicated for symptomatic athletes. Only certain meniscal tears are reparable, and partial menisectomies are performed to reduce the risk of osteoarthritis. Athletes can usually return to play in a few weeks.

Injuries to the medial (MCL) and lateral (LCL) collateral ligaments are also seen. The MCL is injured by a lateral (valgus) force to the knee, especially in sports such as football and soccer. The athlete complains of pain and swelling medially, and the ligament is tender to palpation at the site of injury. In comparison to the unaffected contralateral knee, application of a valgus stress to the knee in 30 degrees of flexion confirms laxity, along with tenderness over the MCL's origin and insertion. Radiographs may demonstrate an associated avulsion fracture if the sprain represents a complete tear. If the tear is grade I or II, protected immobilization in a brace, ice, and NSAIDs are indicated. Crutches may be used as needed. Severe tears require evaluation of other intraarticular pathology and may dictate whether surgery is required. Isolated LCL injuries are uncommon and usually associated with other ligamentous pathology. Virtually all clinically significant knee ligament injuries require physical therapy. Small tears can be protected using braces, with return to play in a few weeks. More severe tears may require 6 to 8 weeks to heal.

Foot and Ankle Injuries

One of the most common athletic injuries is the ankle sprain, and several other injuries may mimic this condition (see Chapter 130). A true sprain is a stretching or tearing of the ligaments. The most common type of ankle sprain is an *inversion sprain,* where the plantar surface of the foot rolls in, resulting in damage to the lateral ligaments, especially the anterior talofibular. This occurs frequently in running and jumping sports, such as basketball, where one player might jump for a rebound and land unevenly on another player's foot. The athlete complains of pain over the lateral ankle, and swelling usually develops quickly in the area anterior to the lateral malleolus. If there is prominent swelling or difficulty with weight bearing, radiographs should be obtained to evaluate for a fracture. On examination the most important finding is point tenderness over the injured ligament. Tests for stability, including the anterior drawer and talar tilt maneuvers, can be gently performed to aid in the diagnosis. Initial treatment should consist of elevation, ice, and compression. If the sprain is determined to be mild, this treatment, followed by appropriate rehabilitation, should be sufficient. More severe sprains, especially if unstable, require referral. Braces are available for use while a sprain is acute and also during rehabilitation. Any type of immobilization should effectively brace the injury while accommodating the patient's lifestyle. Three phases characterize subsequent rehabilitation to return to sport: immobilization and rest to control swelling and pain, training to increase strength and range of motion, and finally the athlete's return to the desired activity.

Less often, sprains to the deltoid ligament (medial) and tibiofibular ligaments (syndesmosis) occur. A deltoid injury usually is caused by an eversion injury, as opposed to the more common inversion injury. Depending on the sprain's severity, these injuries are treated similarly, with short-term immobilization and physical therapy. Syndesmosis injuries occur while the foot is planted and an external rotatory force is applied around the ankle. These patients have a positive squeeze test, which involves gently squeezing the tibia and fibula together. Tenderness is assessed over the proximal fibular area. The syndesmosis tear may have traveled proximally and caused a proximal fibular fracture. Full-length tibiofibular and ankle radiographs may reveal severe ligament or syndesmosis sprain, and orthopedic referral is warranted.

Similar to the ankle sprain affect an Achilles tendon injury may occur in a basketball or tennis player who forcefully pushes off the foot. Frequently the athlete hears a pop. Pain may be variable; the patient may infrequently continue walking but cannot stand on the toes with a complete tear. Thompson's test confirms the diagnosis. The athlete either sits with the leg dangling or lies prone while the examiner gently grasps and squeezes the calf muscle. If the tendon is intact, the foot passively plantar flexes; lack of passive flexion indicates Achilles tendon rupture. Immobilization with referral for further treatment is recommended.

Also mimicking an ankle sprain, subluxation of the peroneal tendon, which runs posteriorly to the lateral malleolus, occurs when the foot is fixed and the leg is forcibly rotated, as in cross-country skiing. The peroneal tendon tears free of its anchoring retinaculum and subluxates over the malleolus. If the examiner holds the foot in neutral position and asks the athlete to resist eversion, the peroneal tendon may subluxate, causing pain along its course. If the diagnosis is made promptly, before further damage occurs, several weeks of casting may be sufficient. If the diagnosis is delayed or the disorder recurs, surgery may be required.

The acute onset of pain in the middle to lower calf can represent a tear of the musculotendinous junction of the gastrocnemius, not of the Achilles tendon. The onset of sharp pain behind the knee may indicate rupture of the plantaris tendon. MRI can assist in the diagnosis. Both injuries are treated symptomatically.

In general, acute athletic injuries of the foot are much less common than overuse injuries. An exception is hyperextension injury of the metatarsophalangeal joint of the great toe, known as *turf toe* and often seen in football players playing on artificial turf. The athlete complains of pain; tenderness and swelling of the joint confirm the diagnosis. Radiographs are usually normal. Treatment is symptomatic with NSAIDs and rest; shoe inserts are useful in recurrent or severe cases. The midfoot sprain is often a partial subluxation of the tarsometatarsal joints requiring referral to a specialist for possible cast immobilization or surgery. Comparison between standing AP radiographs and MRI may be helpful.

Spinal Injuries

Athletic injuries of the spine fall into two major groups: the neck and lower back. Neck, or cervical spine, injuries are potentially the most serious and life-threatening athletic injuries. The most severe injuries occur with the neck in flexion, as in the now-banned tackling technique known as "spearing." This can lead to quadriplegia and death. Any question of a possible severe neck injury should be treated as a medical emergency, even if this involves suspension of the athletic event until the neck can be protected and the patient safely transported (see Chapter 124).

An injury to the cervical spine can result in transient neurapraxia, most often seen in football. The athlete may complain of altered sensation and motor function in the upper extremity, although the lower extremity may also be involved. Radiographs are often negative but are required to rule out a fracture. The paresthesias resolve spontaneously, usually within minutes. Referral to a neurologist or an orthopedist is warranted.

The *burner* or *stinger syndrome,* often seen in contact sports, is a stretching injury of the brachial plexus or a compression of nerve roots at the foramen. The athlete has burning pain radiating into the shoulder, upper arm, and hand and associated with muscle weakness (e.g., deltoid, biceps). Symptoms generally resolve spontaneously over minutes or hours. The athlete should not return to play until normal strength and sensation have returned.

Myofascial sprains occur but are overdiagnosed. Many neck and trapezial pain syndromes are facet or neurogenic, with associated disk or root pathology. Frequently the mechanism of such injuries is hyperextension in contact athletes, who are treated symptomatically, usually with NSAIDs, rest, and physical therapy. Occasionally, electromyography (EMG) and MRI are useful in refractory cases.

The lumbar spine is frequently a site of pain and injury for both athletes and nonathletes. Participants in virtually every sport, including gymnastics, football, weightlifting, wrestling, and figure skating, are at risk for low back injury. Lumbar injury is frequently diagnosed as muscle strain; although muscle strain does occur, it is important to look for other common causes of pain. Disk herniation or annular tears have been reported in athletes of all ages and are frequently associated with radiculopathy. The patient may have pain on flexion or with midline palpation of the spine at the involved level. Patients with *spondylolysis,* a stress fracture of the pars interarticularis, may also present with low back pain. This is most common in teenage athletes involved in gymnastics, football, or weightlifting. The onset of pain is associated with a specific activity and is often nonradicular. Physical findings may include pain on spinal extension, while standing on the single leg on the side of the defect (positive one-legged hyperextension test), on rotation, and during palpation over the irritated area. Radiographs confirm a defect of the pars interarticularis in spondylolysis seen on oblique view (fracture of the neck of the "Scotty dog"). Rest is the treatment of choice; immobilization is occasionally required. If the defect has progressed to become a spondylolisthesis, consultation with a spine specialist is advised (see Chapter 127).

Hip and Thigh Injuries

Acute injuries to the hip and thigh are most often contusions or muscle strains. For example, a groin pull usually involves the adductors of the thigh, and a common contusion is the *hip pointer,* resulting from a direct blow to the ilium with pain and swelling. Examination may be difficult due to painful range of motion. The affected area is extremely tender. Treatment entails immediate application of pressure, then ice and rest. *Osteitis pubis* involves a combination of groin or abductor rectus strain, pubic ramus stress, and pubic symphysis osteolysis. Treatment consists of rest, NSAIDs, and orthopedic referral. Fractures of the pelvis and femur are rare in athletes (see Chapter 128).

REHABILITATION

Once an injury has occurred and the initial treatment plan has been instituted, the physician should plan for rehabilitation. If the injury results in time lost from activity, rehabilitation must be considered. The primary goal is to return the athlete to activity as soon and as safely as possible. In the initial 24 to 48 hours after injury, acute treatment is performed according to the mnemonic PRICE. *P*rotection from further injury is accomplished by keeping the athlete from playing and using a splint for immobilization. *R*est prevents further injury and allows healing to begin. *I*ce decreases swelling, pain, and muscle spasm and should be applied for 10 to 30 minutes, with an equal period without ice. *C*ompression limits swelling and may provide some support to the injured tissue. *E*levation helps to decrease swelling.

Rehabilitation should be sport and athlete specific, that is, individually designed for each athlete depending on the sport. When an athlete is injured, it is not a "knee injury" or "shoulder injury," but rather an athlete with a specific knee injury or shoulder injury. Therefore general conditioning is important as well as local rehabilitation of the injured limb. Flexibility, strength, proprioception, and endurance must be addressed. Modalities include ice and heat, ultrasound, electric stimulation, and iontophoresis. An athlete's return to play depends on progress during rehabilitation and should be delayed until the athlete is symptom free and has regained confidence in the injured limb.

SPECIAL NEEDS

Female Athletes

Women are participating in athletics in increasing numbers. Considerable differences in the male and female anatomy and physiology affect exercise. Females have less dense bone, less muscle mass, a lower center of gravity, shorter limbs, and a gynecoid pelvis. These and other factors affect body mechanics and influence the ability to perform exercise. The female pelvis, because of its relative width, results in different running biomechanics than in males and has been associated with knee injury and overuse syndromes. Female bone is possibly at greater risk for stress fracture because it is less dense than male bone.

Back disorders such as spondylolysis and spondylolisthesis, as well as pubic ramus and femoral neck stress fractures, may be more prevalent in female athletes. ACL injuries occur four times more often in women than men, possibly because of intercondylar notch anatomy as well as muscle strength and training. Patellofemoral problems are common in the female athlete.

Nutritional considerations also differ for women. Because of menstruation, women have a greater need for iron than men. Competitive female athletes often restrict calories, leading in extreme cases to such complications as the *female athlete triad,* characterized by disordered eating, amenorrhea, and osteoporosis. Inadequate caloric intake reduces peripheral fat, which can result in decreased conversion of androgens to estrogen. This hypoestrogenic state contributes to amenorrhea and is associated with osteoporosis. Inadequate calcium intake exacerbates the effects of this syndrome.

The primary care physician should also be aware of the prevalence and appropriate treatment of eating disorders in athletes. Although most common in females, an estimated 5% of those with eating disorders are male. Between ages 10 and 20, young women must maintain sufficient caloric intake to ensure adequate bone density. Surveys indicate that about one third of female athletes have disordered eating and obsessions about food. An uninformed coach, especially in sports such as gymnastics, figure skating, and diving, which are scored in part on appearance, may contribute to the dietary problem and increase the athlete's risk of further psychologic and physiologic damage.

For the pregnant woman, exercise is generally regarded as safe, although controversy surrounds the degree of recommended endurance and intensity. Certain anatomic and physiologic changes may affect the pregnant athlete's ability to perform exercise, and therefore the physician should individualize the exercise prescription and consult the obstetrician as appropriate. In general, exercise should be carefully monitored for exacerbation of back pain, which is common in pregnant women.

Young Athletes

Children and adolescents have rapidly changing anatomic and physiologic characteristics that affect their ability to participate in various sports. The young athlete's skeletal immaturity predisposes to injuries not encountered in the older athlete. The epiphyseal plate, the cartilaginous growth center, is the weakest portion of growing bone and is often injured. Such injuries can affect growth and thus require careful evaluation. Physical examination should always include palpation of the epiphysis. Epiphyseal injuries are generally described by the Salter-Harris classification system. Depending on the type of and extent of epiphyseal injury, therapy ranges from closed reduction with excellent prognosis to open reduction and potential growth impairment.

In response to injury or trauma, young children and adults generally sustain ligament injuries, whereas adolescent patients usually have fractures. These injuries reflect the maturity of the musculoskeletal system and the relative strength of the ligament or epiphysis, not the patient's chronologic age (Box 143-4). As in the adult athlete population, tennis elbow, AC separations, and ACL tears are seen in athletic children. Certain fractures, however, such as those of the distal radius and clavicle, are seen more often in children. Developmental abnormalities, including patellofemoral dysplasia, Osgood-Schlatter disease, spondylolysis, and shoulder instability, can result in injuries or symptoms during participation in sports. Injury may precipitate these conditions, but there appears to be some predisposition based on preexisting abnormalities of growth and connective tissue, such as joint laxity in shoulders and patellar dislocations.

Older Athletes

The athlete over age 65 has the same injury profile as younger athletes, except in three areas. First, active weight-bearing exercise such as jogging is associated with better bone density in the general skeleton. This in turn offers some

Box 143-4. Pediatric Orthopedic Injuries Requiring Referral

- Ankle sprains and fractures
- Osgood-Schlatter disease (tibial tubercle)
- Shoulder instability (more likely in teenagers)
- Elbow tendinitis and osteochondritis (Little Leaguer's elbow)
- Clavicular fractures (typical playground injury)
- Acromioclavicular joint separation
- Anterior cruciate ligament tears
- Distal radius fractures
- Patellofemoral and plica syndromes (anterior knee pain syndromes)
- Spondylolysis

protection against compression fractures of the vertebral spine and hip, especially compared with the risks of fracture in a sedentary age-matched group. However, fractures of the wrist and sprained ankles are more common in the geriatric running population because of falls. To avoid falls, patients should run on level surfaces, such as tracks, rather than on the side of the road.

Second, a warm-up period is mandatory for the older population to minimize tendon injuries. The combination of degenerative processes may predispose to higher rates of musculotendinous injuries than in younger athletes, particularly with sports involving sudden acceleration and deceleration (e.g., as tennis). The same degenerative predisposition probably accounts for some back injuries in golf. A complete warm-up is essential to facilitate injury prevention.

Third, exercise can aggravate existing osteoarthritis of the knee, hip, and lower spine in older patients. However, exercise-induced weight control and increased muscle strength usually offset this, ultimately protecting the joints. As discussed earlier, the cardiovascular system needs to be carefully evaluated before beginning any incremental exercise regimen.

Sports-specific Injuries

Primary care physicians may treat patients participating in a variety of sports (Table 143-3). The incidence of previous neck injuries in wrestlers, gymnasts, and football players is especially important. This information is most relevant during a preparticipation examination, when athletes can be screened for these injuries. Continued participation in sport might expose them to further neck injury.

MEDICAL CONSIDERATIONS

The primary care physician is in the position to integrate the athlete's care. Athletes are susceptible to the same illnesses as the general population but may require special treatment considerations. Communicability of an infectious disease, control of asthma and diabetes, and risks imposed by certain conditions (e.g., dysrhythmia) may have special implications for an athlete's health and subsequent return to safe participation.

Infectious Disease

A common infectious disease is acute febrile illness, such as an upper respiratory tract infection. Although treatment of an athlete's acute infection does not differ, the physician must address ability to practice and return to play. It is generally advisable to avoid strenuous activity while acutely ill, febrile, and experiencing myalgias, although the athlete does not need to be symptom free before returning to play. Adequate fluid intake is especially important for an athlete recovering from illness. The athlete with infectious mononucleosis should not resume contact sports until the spleen has returned to normal size. Resolution of splenomegaly can be confirmed with palpation.

In wrestlers, transmission of herpes simplex virus type I (HSV-I), known as herpes gladiatorum, occurs primarily through skin-to-skin contact. Coaches and parents should be advised to exclude any wrestlers with active skin lesions from competition or practice. Similarly, skin lesions of impetigo caused by streptococci should also preclude athletic participation.

The physician who treats athletes may be questioned about communicability of certain diseases, such as the human immunodeficiency virus (HIV). Patients must understand that the risk of contracting HIV through intact skin by infected blood or saliva is extremely low. Moreover, in the asymptomatic HIV-positive patient, no evidence indicates that exercise activates HIV into clinical acquired immunodeficiency syndrome (AIDS). The physician should stress safe sexual techniques through condom use in all sexually active patients. All health personnel, including trainers, should use universal precautions (e.g., gloves) when treating injured athletes, despite the extremely low risk of contracting HIV through intact skin. Regulatory agencies, including the National Collegiate Athletic Association (NCAA), are recommending the immediate changing of blood-stained uniforms in basketball. These highly publicized communica-

Table 143-3. Approximate Frequency Distribution of Musculoskeletal Injuries in High-school Sports

Sport	Wrist/hand	Shoulder	Elbow	Lumbar spine	Knee	Foot/ankle	Neck
Football/rugby	+++	+++	+	+++	+++	+++	+++
Baseball/softball	++	+++	+	+	+	++	+
Soccer/field sports	+	+	+		+++	+++	
Volleyball	+	+++		+	+	++	+
Basketball	+	+		+	++	+++	+
Swimming		+++		+	+		+
Gymnastics	+++	++	+	+++	+++	++	+++
Tennis/racquet sports	+	++	+++		++	+	++
Weight training	+	+++	+	++	++		+
Running				+	++	+++	
Wrestling	+	++		+	++		+++
Skiing/snowboarding	++	+			+++	+	
Ice hockey	+	+	+	++	+++	+	+
Cycling	+	++		++	++		+

+, Mild concern; ++, moderate concern; +++, high concern.

tions in the media urge physicians to transmit realistic information and precautionary guidelines to their patients.

Diabetes

Studies of diabetic athletes have shown the positive effects of fitness on diabetes. Training seems to improve glucose tolerance, aid in weight control, and decrease insulin requirements. Monitoring of glucose levels in insulin-dependent patients is crucial, since insulin requirements vary with exercise. The insulin-dependent athlete must be aware of hypoglycemia and have glucose readily available. Although exercise is generally beneficial, the poorly controlled diabetic patient may become more hyperglycemic and ketotic with activity. Therefore diabetes should be fairly well controlled with diet and insulin before initiating an exercise program. Rarely in the type II diabetic patient (adult onset) taking oral hypoglycemic agents, blood sugar will decrease during sustained exercise over hours, such as golf. Such patients should carry a glucose source when playing.

Asthma

Asthma is common among athletes, especially exercise-induced asthma (EIA). EIA does not interfere with ability to perform if precautions are followed. Patients with EIA develop cough, dyspnea, or wheezing after several minutes of moderately intense exercise. Symptoms are worse in cold, dry air but improve with warm, humid air. Swimming may therefore be more appropriate for a patient with EIA than running. In cold-weather sports such as downhill and cross-country skiing, cold-induced bronchospasm may occur, but its relationship to EIA is controversial.

Prophylaxis includes a warm-up period before vigorous exercise as well as medications. The two most important agents are the β-agonists and cromolyn, which should be administered 10 to 15 minutes before exertion. The physician must be careful to comply with prescribing and disclosure guidelines of the applicable athletic organization. The list of medicines that are allowed by the NCAA and the U.S. Olympic Committee (USOC) includes NSAIDs, antihistamines, antibiotics, insulin, topical steroids, and antiulcer medicines.

Cardiovascular Conditions

Interest in cardiac disease and the athlete has largely resulted from sudden deaths among high-profile athletes. *Sudden death* is defined as death that is unexpected, nontraumatic, and instantaneous. Over age 30 the most common etiology is coronary artery disease. Before age 30 the most common etiology is a congenital condition, such as abnormal coronary arteries, valve disease, or hypertrophic cardiomyopathy. Hypertrophic cardiomyopathy is suggested by a midsystolic crescendo-decrescendo murmur, heard best at the left sternal border and without an accompanying ejection sound, that increases in duration and intensity with tests that reduce ventricular filling (e.g., standing Valsalva's maneuver). The physician must also consider *Marfan syndrome,* which is associated with thoracic aortic aneurysm and dissection. Family history or typical physical features, including long limbs and fingers, may suggest the diagnosis. Although these entities are relatively uncommon, they are emphasized because of their potential for fatal outcomes. More common cardiac problems, such as mitral valve prolapse, can be associated with exercise-induced dysrhythmias. A history of troublesome palpitations, syncope, or presyncope should suggest a preexcitation syndrome, requiring a formal cardiac evaluation. The most important clues to a cardiac abnormality include history of syncope, chest pain, and family history of sudden death.

The condition known as *athletic heart syndrome* is a constellation of physiologic adaptations of the heart to exercise. It improves cardiac function and is a benign condition characterized by bradycardia, an irregular pulse, and a flow murmur. This asymptomatic syndrome is not associated with syncope or other ominous findings and does not place the athlete at risk for cardiac events.

Referral

Provision of high-quality care to address athetic injuries depends on timely and appropriate specialty referral. Individualized testing and exercises are important (Box 143-5). The trend toward a more complete approach to care of the injured athlete is an opportunity for primary care physicians to help patients make healthy lifestyle choices.

Box 143-5. Exercises and Tests Associated with Sports Medicine and Athletic Injuries

Closed chain exercises: exercises done with the limb in contact with a surface; examples include leg presses and push-ups. This type of strengthening requires contraction of all muscles in the limb in a coordinated manner (co-contraction).

Concentric strengthening: musculotendinous unit shortens during contraction; examples are biceps curls and leg extensions (quadriceps).

Eccentric strengthening: musculotendinous unit lengthens during contraction; examples are squats (quadriceps) and elbow extensions (biceps).

Lachman's test: to determine competence of the anterior cruciate ligament; performed with the patient supine and the knee in 15 degrees of flexion. Examiner stands on side of the affected extremity; thigh is held immobile in one hand while the opposite hand grasps the proximal tibia and attempts to move it anteriorly, avoiding rotation. Examiner looks and feels for anterior tibial translation compared with the opposite, normal knee. Quality of end point should also be evaluated; it should be firm, not soft or mushy.

McMurray's test: to determine meniscal injury. Positive test produces increased joint line pain with forced flexion and rotation of the knee; there may be an audible or palpable click or pop along the joint line in conjunction with the motion. Its presence is not necessary to diagnose meniscal derangement. Joint line pain to palpation is a more sensitive means of diagnosing meniscal injury.

Pivot shift test: to assess integrity of the anterior cruciate ligament. Beginning with the knee fully extended and the foot internally rotated, examiner applies a valgus stress while progressively flexing the knee, watching and feeling for translation of the tibia on the femur, which is the type of luxation that occurs when a knee gives way in an episode of anterior cruciate incompetence or anterior cruciate tearing.

ACKNOWLEDGMENTS

The authors would like to thank Kathryn M. Peuvrelle, Gerald P. Keane, MD, and George Thabit III, MD, of Sports, Orthopedic and Rehabilitation in Menlo Park, California, for their contributions to this chapter.

ADDITIONAL READINGS

American College of Sports Medicine: Position stand on the recommended quantity and quality of exercise for developing and maintaining cardiorespiratory and muscular fitness in healthy adults, *Med Sci Sports Exerc* 22:265, 1990.

American College of Sports Medicine: Position stand on the use of anabolic-androgenic steroids in sports, *Med Sci Sports Exerc* 19:534, 1987.

Belongia EA et al: An outbreak of herpes gladiatorum at a high school wrestling camp, *N Engl J Med* 325:906, 1991.

Clark N: How to approach eating disorders among athletes, *Top Clin Nutr* 5:41, 1990.

Fuentes RJ, Rosenberg JM, Davis A: *Allen and Hanbury's Athletic drug reference '94,* Durham, NC, 1994, Glaxo.

Grana WA, Kalenak A, editors: *Clinical sports medicine,* Philadelphia, 1991, Saunders.

Greenspan A: *Orthopedic radiology: a practical approach,* ed 2, New York, 1992, Raven.

Hoppenfeld S: *Physical examination of the spine and extremities,* East Norwalk, Conn, 1976, Appleton-Century-Crofts.

Johnston CC Jr et al: Calcium supplementation and increases in bone mineral density in children, *N Engl J Med* 327:82, 1992.

Lane NE et al: The risk of osteoarthritis with running and aging: a 5-year longitudinal study, *J Rheumatol* 20:461, 1993.

Lane NE et al: Running, osteoarthritis and bone density: initial 2-year longitudinal study, *Am J Med* 88:452, 1990.

Strauss RH, editor: *Sports medicine,* ed 2, Philadelphia, 1991, Saunders.

Swander H, editor: *Preparticipation physical evaluation,* 1992.

Teitz CC et al: The female athlete: evaluation and treatment of sports-related problems, *J Am Acad Orthop Surg* 5:87, 1997.

Thabit G III, Micheli L: Orthopedic disorders of the extremities. In Burg FD, Ingelfinger JR, Wald ER, editors: *Current pediatric therapy,* Philadelphia, 1993, Saunders.

Williams MH, Branch JD: Creatine supplementation and exercise performance: an update, *J Am Coll Nutr* 17:216, 1998.

X NEPHROLOGY

Generalist's Guide to Diagnostic Tests

James A. Delmez
David W. Windus

GLOMERULAR FILTRATION RATE

Although the kidney regulates a complex array of physiologic functions, the general health of the kidney is currently assessed with estimates of glomerular filtration and the urinalysis. Loss of glomerular filtration roughly correlates with histologic changes resulting from a variety of kidney diseases. Plasma creatinine concentration and creatinine clearance are clinically useful means of estimating the true glomerular filtration rate (GFR). Optimal use of these clinical tools requires knowledge of factors affecting metabolism and the renal excretion of creatinine. Additional structural and functional information about the kidney can be obtained with imaging tests and the kidney biopsy.

Concepts

The concept of plasma clearance by the kidneys, developed in the 1920s, refers to the volume of plasma freed of a substance by renal activity per unit time (usually 1 minute). Depending on the substance studied, the renal clearance may be achieved by glomerular filtration, net tubular secretion, or a combination of the two. For clinical purposes, the focus of interest is the volume of plasma cleared per minute of a substance solely by the process of glomerular filtration. If a substance is freely filtered by glomeruli and not subsequently altered by tubular reabsorption or tubular secretion, its plasma clearance represents the GFR. Accurate measurement of GFR is probably the most critical index of renal function. Unfortunately, it is also one of the most difficult.

Measurements

A number of substances fulfill the criteria as accurate markers of GFR. These include inulin, ^{125}I-iothalamate, and ^{99m}Tc-diethylenetriamine penta-acetic acid (DTPA). The disadvantages of these are that they must be administered exogenously as an intravenous bolus, usually followed by a constant infusion to maintain steady-state plasma levels. During the infusion, four urine collections are obtained over 30-minute intervals to calculate the GFR. These are costly and labor-intensive tests whose use is usually restricted to research protocols at major medical centers.

Estimations

The endogenous substance used most commonly in the clinical assessment of GFR is creatinine. Creatinine is a waste product derived from the spontaneous degradation of creatine and creatine phosphate. The production and renal excretion of creatinine are constant and proportional to muscle mass. Accordingly, muscular athletes and men produce more creatinine than women, children, and elderly people. Wide-spread acute necrosis of skeletal muscle from any cause will also increase the production rate of creatinine.

Creatinine is freely filtered by the glomerulus but also enters the urine through secretion by the proximal tubule. The component resulting from this secretion causes the GFR to be overestimated. In patients with a normal GFR, the overestimation is only 5% to 10%. As renal function deteriorates, the contribution of creatinine secretion to creatinine clearance assumes a major role. In some subjects with renal insufficiency, the creatinine clearance may exceed the GFR by 70%. Unfortunately, the magnitude of the tubular secretion of creatinine varies from patient to patient and even within a given patient at different times. Another potential problem in assessing creatinine clearances is the use of drugs that interfere with its tubular secretion. Cimetidine and trimethoprim commonly increase serum creatinine levels and decrease creatinine clearance without affecting the GFR.

Despite its limitations, the creatinine clearance is the simplest and standard method for the evaluation of renal function. Nonetheless, it is critical that the urine sample be

Box 144-1. Formulas for Calculating Creatinine Clearance

$$\text{Creatinine clearance} = \frac{\text{Urine creatinine level (mg/dl)} \times \text{Urine volume flow rate (ml/min)}}{\text{Serum creatinine level (mg/dl)}}$$

$$\text{Creatinine clearance for a 24-hour collection period} = \frac{\text{Urine creatinine (mg/dl)} \times \text{Urine volume (ml)}}{\text{Serum creatinine (mg/dl)} \times 1440 \text{ min}}$$

collected in a complete and precisely timed fashion. The patient should be instructed to void on awakening and discard the urine sample. All subsequent urine should be collected in the next 24 hours. The collection ends when the bladder is emptied at exactly 24 hours, and the final urine specimen is included in the collection. The normal daily creatinine excretion is 18 to 21 mg/kg for men and 15 to 18 mg/kg for women. Values below these may represent an inadequate urine collection, except in individuals with either decreased muscle mass or advanced renal insufficiency. The urine container should be refrigerated during this period to avoid overgrowth of bacteria, which may promote the conversion of creatinine to creatine and therefore spuriously lower the creatinine clearance. The patient's serum may be analyzed for the concentration of creatinine at either the start or the end of urine collection. The formula for creatinine clearance is shown in Box 144-1. The results should be expressed per 1.73 m^2 (body surface area). The normal ranges depend on the chemical assay used for creatinine. In general, they are:

Women	75 to 115 ml/min/1.73 m^2
Men	85 to 125 ml/min/1.73 m^2

Measurement of the serum creatinine level is probably the first and easiest test in estimating renal function. The wide range of normal values (usually 0.6 to 1.4 mg/dl) reflects differences in muscle mass from subject to subject. The "rule of thumb" is that for every doubling of serum creatinine values, the GFR decreases by 50%. Thus a healthy but frail subject may have a baseline serum creatinine level of 0.6 mg/dl. If half the renal function is then lost, the corresponding serum creatinine concentration would be only 1.2 mg/dl, still within the normal range (Fig. 144-1, *solid line*). In this example, a further rise to 2.4 mg/dl would represent loss of 75% of renal function. In contrast, the dashed line shows this relationship in a subject with a baseline serum creatinine level of 1.0 mg/dl. Loss of half the renal function results in a serum creatinine value of 2.0 mg/dl, which is outside the normal range. Because of enhanced tubular secretion of creatinine and increased extrarenal metabolism of creatinine with renal failure, the rule of thumb may greatly underestimate the decline in GFR. If there is any question of a possible impairment of renal function despite a normal serum creatinine level, a creatinine clearance should be done. Although creatinine levels are not as affected by protein intake as urea values, a meal with meat (containing creatinine) increases serum creatinine levels by as much as 0.4 mg/dl for up to 10 to 12 hours. To avoid misinterpretation of changes in serum creatinine levels, the clinician should measure values after an overnight fast. Another potential source of error in interpreting creatinine values is the presence of substances in the serum that falsely elevate the values. These include acetoacetate (ketoacidosis)

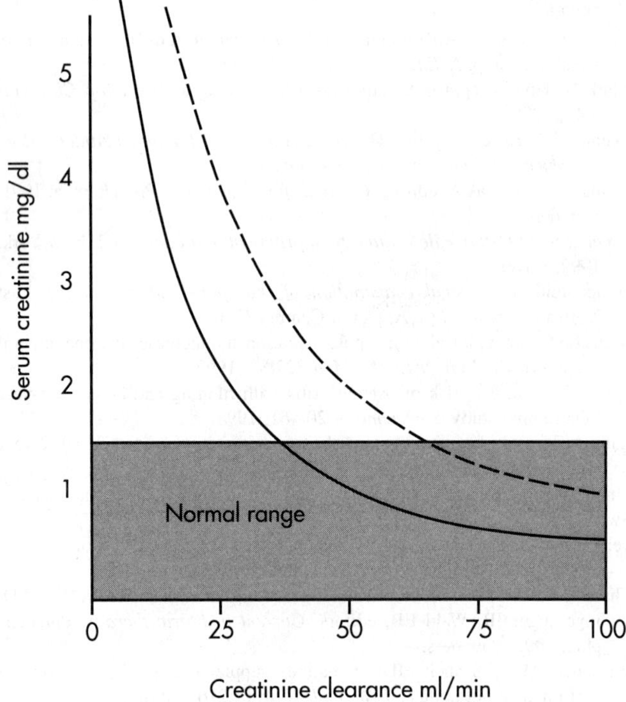

Fig. 144-1. Relationship between serum creatine level and creatine clearance in two patients with different baseline values for serum creatine.

and some cephalosporins (e.g., cephalothin, cefazolin, cefoxitin, cefamandole).

Approximately 1 ml/min of GFR is lost per year after the age of 30. Yet the serum creatinine value does not increase with age. This is due to the decreased muscle mass accompanying aging. Thus perceived minor abnormalities in the serum creatinine level in the elderly may represent severe impairment of renal function.

Various nomograms that attempt to estimate creatinine clearance from serum levels of creatinine have been published. The most accepted formulas are those of Cockcroft and Gault, which incorporate the variables of age, gender, and weight (Box 144-2).

In the equations in Box 144-2, age is in years, weight is in kilograms, and creatinine levels are in milligrams per deciliter. There are a number of limitations to these equations. They overestimate creatinine clearance if the subject is obese or edematous. Also, the patient must have relatively stable renal function. Thus these formulas should not be used for a patient experiencing acute renal failure.

The measurement of serum urea as an index of renal function has largely been supplanted by the measurement of

Box 144-2. Formula for Estimating Creatinine Clearance

Men

Creatinine clearance = (140 = age) × Weight/(Creatinine × 72)

Women

Creatinine clearance = (140 = age) × Weight/(Creatinine × 85)

creatinine because urea levels are more affected by the intake of protein in the diet. In addition, urea levels may rise with gastrointestinal bleeding, accelerated protein catabolism, and glucocorticoid therapy. Nonetheless, many nephrologists feel that urea levels correlate better than creatinine with uremic symptoms, so they monitor both values.

The clinician should know the GFR in patients with severe renal failure. This allows for the orderly planning of transplantation or dialysis. As previously discussed, creatinine clearance may cause the GFR to be greatly overestimated in this situation. The average of simultaneous creatinine and urea clearances provides a more accurate estimate of renal function when the GFR is less than 30 ml/min. Both substances are freely filtered. Creatinine, however, is secreted, whereas urea is reabsorbed by the tubules. These two events tend to offset each other, and the average is fairly accurate.

Occasionally, it is important to determine whether the function of one kidney is significantly different from the function of the other. This issue is usually raised when the consequences of a surgical nephrectomy are being weighed. A renal scan is the test of choice, but there is no agreement concerning the best radiopharmaceutical agent. ^{99m}Tc-DTPA, ^{99m}Tc-glucoheptonate (GHA), and ^{99m}Tc-dimercaptosuccinic acid (DMSA) are widely used. The general procedure is to inject the agent by vein and compare the radioactivity of the two kidneys within the first 3 minutes of the scan.

MEASUREMENTS OF URINE PROTEINS

Plasma proteins are prevented from entering the urine because of the permselectivity and negative charge of the glomerulus. In addition, much of the protein traversing the glomerulus into the urine space is reabsorbed by the renal tubules. Thus the kidneys normally excrete less than 150 mg/day of protein. Approximately 60% is derived from plasma, with the remainder produced by the kidneys and lower urinary tract. The measurement of urine proteins is often helpful in determining the presence, severity, and prognosis of renal diseases. In addition, a decline in proteinuria may indicate a response to therapy.

The urine dipstick is the simplest and most common way to measure urine proteins. It is fairly sensitive to the presence of negatively charged proteins such as albumin. However, it is insensitive to positively charged proteins such as some immunoglobulin light chains. The lower limit of detection by the standard dipstick is 10 to 20 mg/dl. Assuming a 24-hour urine output of 2 L/day, the dipsticks may not detect proteinuria of up to 200 to 400 mg/day. The dipstick should always be positive for protein in the case of nephrotic-range proteinuria (>3.5 g/day) and no paraproteinuria. Because the dipstick measures only the concentration of proteins in the urine, it is not a useful quantitative test of proteinuria.

The gold standard for quantifying proteinuria is the measurement of a 24-hour urine collection performed in the same manner as a creatinine clearance. The interpretation of proteinuria should always be in the context of renal function. As renal function deteriorates, there is decreased delivery of protein available for filtration, and proteinuria often declines with moderate to severe renal failure. A very low serum albumin level may also cause a decline in proteinuria by similar mechanisms.

An alternative to collecting a 24-hour urine for protein determination is a spot urine test measuring the protein/creatinine ratio. In the presence of stable renal function a protein/creatinine ratio of more than 3.5 (mg/mg) indicates nephrotic-range proteinuria, whereas a ratio of less than 0.2 is within normal limits. The best correlation is found when samples are collected after the first morning void and at bedtime. The estimation of proteinuria by this method should be reserved for those in whom a 24-hour urine sample is not possible or when multiple tests of proteinuria are obtained to monitor treatment.

Nephrotic-range Proteinuria

Nephrotic-range proteinuria is defined as a urine protein excretion of more than 3.5 g/day. When it is present, there is usually a defect in the permselectivity and/or negative charge of the glomeruli (see Chapter 148 for further discussion). Most of the protein in nephrotic-range proteinuria is albumin. Determining the individual types of urine protein in adults with this condition is of little value in the absence of multiple myeloma.

Non–Nephrotic Range Proteinuria

Non–nephrotic range proteinuria is defined as a urine protein excretion between 150 mg and 3.5 g/day. Proteinuria within this range renders little information about the etiology of the defect. However, urine protein excretion of less than 2 g/day suggests a tubulointerstitial disease characteristically seen in cystic diseases of the kidney, interstitial nephritis (including pyelonephritis), hypertensive nephrosclerosis, and toxic nephropathies.

Microalbuminuria

Microalbuminuria is defined as an elevated rate of urinary albumin excretion, with a daily total protein excretion rate of less than 150 mg. A timed specimen or a 24-hour urine collection is used to assess albumin excretion rates. The upper limit of albumin excretion usually ranges between 15 and 30 µg/min depending on the laboratory. A dipstick test is also available for testing for microalbuminuria; it can detect concentrations as low as 2 mg/dl. These tests are used primarily to determine which patients with diabetes are at risk of developing overt diabetic nephropathy (see Chapter 96).

Paraproteinuria

The normal excretion of immunoglobulin light chains is 1 to 7 mg/day. An increased amount of light chains in the urine is always due to overproduction and warrants a search for a lymphoproliferative disorder. Immunofixation electrophore-

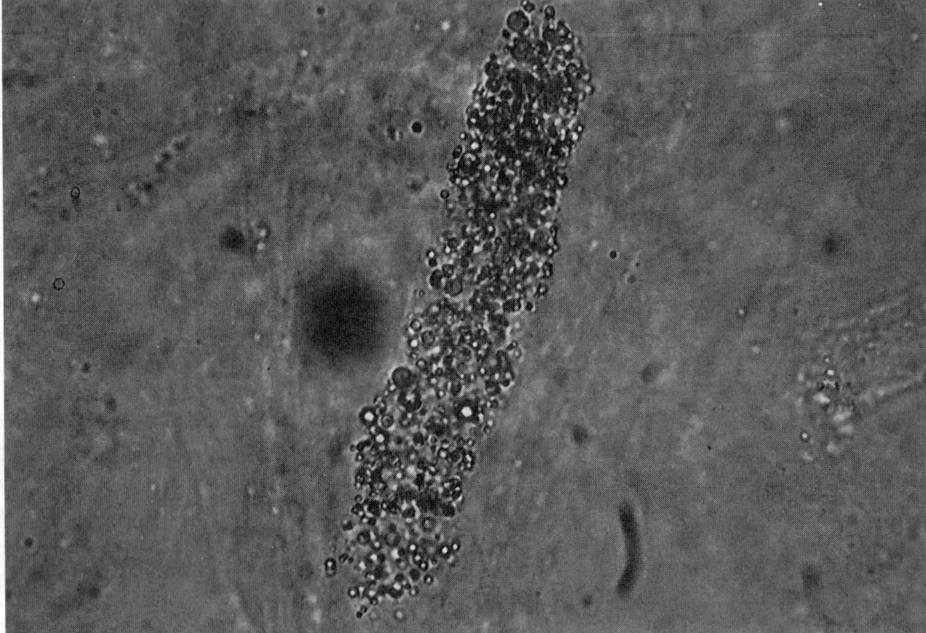

Fig. 144-2. Hyaline cast with fatty inclusions. This microscopic finding suggests the presence of the nephrotic syndrome. (×400.) (From Piccoli G, Varese D, Rotunno M: *Atlas of urinary sediments: Diagnosis and clinical correlations in nephrology,* New York, 1984, Raven.)

sis is the most sensitive test for detecting and classifying urinary paraproteins.

URINALYSIS

A careful examination of the urine often provides useful information about diseases of the urinary tract as well as metabolic or systemic diseases not directly related to the kidney. Like all laboratory procedures, the tests should be carefully performed in a standardized fashion. For chemical (dipstick) and microscopic examination, *a clean-catch, midstream urine collection* is optimal. Urine is a hazardous material and should be handled while wearing gloves. The urine should be visually assessed for color and clarity. The "unspun" urine should then be subjected to a dipstick analysis performed according to the manufacturer's specifications. A sample of the urine (10 to 15 ml) should then be centrifuged in a capped urine tube for 5 minutes at 450 g. The supernatant is poured out and the bottom pellet resuspended by gentle suction pipetting. Cellular elements begin to break down within 2 hours at room temperature. Microscopic examination using a high-power lens should therefore be done promptly. It is important to identify the type and number of cells and casts per high-power field (HPF, ×400) as well as the presence of microorganisms and crystals. Cells may originate from any tissue in the urinary system. Casts are formed only in the renal tubules because of the gelation of Tamm-Horsfall glycoprotein and are most easily seen at the edge of the coverslip. The type of cast refers to the material (cells, fat, filtered proteins) trapped within the cast at the time of formation. The presence of casts of any type strongly suggests significant renal disease. For example, if fatty inclusions are found within a hyaline cast (Fig. 144-2), it is likely that the patient has nephrotic syndrome. Epithelial cell casts (Fig. 144-3) comprise desquamated renal tubular cells embedded in a protein matrix; their presence suggests an active renal process such as glomerulonephritis or interstitial nephritis. Cellular casts may degenerate into granular casts (Fig. 144-4) wherein the outlines of the cells are lost. Brown, muddy granular casts (Fig. 144-5) suggest the presence of acute tubular necrosis.

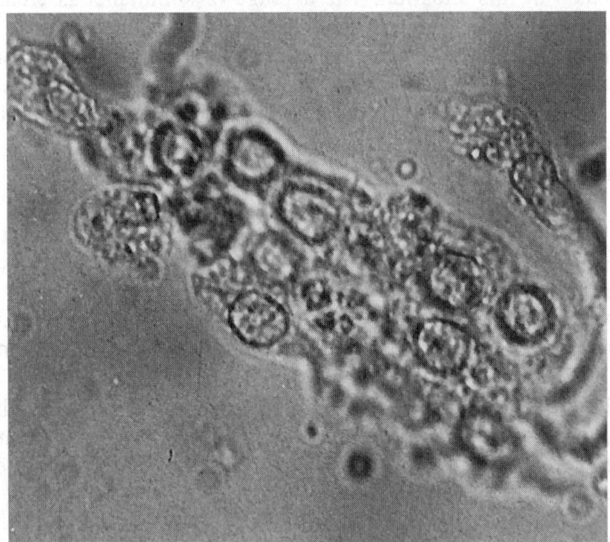

Fig. 144-3. Epithelial cell cast. (×400.) (From Piccoli G, Varese D, Rotunno M: *Atlas of urinary sediments: Diagnosis and clinical correlations in nephrology,* New York, 1984, Raven.)

Hematuria

Gross hematuria is the most frequent cause of an alteration in the color of urine. The color may range from pink to black. The lower the pH and the longer the hemoglobin is in contact with the urine, the darker the color. Hemoglobinuria and myoglobinuria also may cause red-tinged urine. The presence of hemoglobin turns the urine dipstick blue or green in two different patterns. Speckled activity indicates intact erythrocytes whereas a uniform pattern signifies free hemoglobin. Free hemoglobin in the urine is usually the result of the lysis of erythrocytes in the urine as a result of a high pH or a low

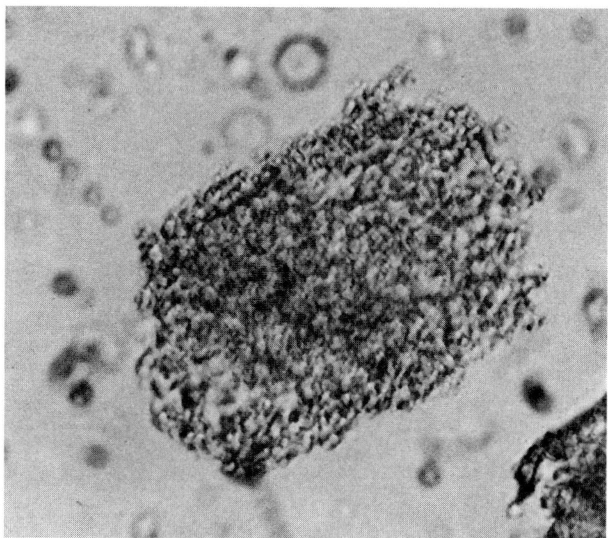

Fig. 144-4. Granular cast. (×400.) (From Piccoli G, Varese D, Rotunno M: *Atlas of urinary sediments: Diagnosis and clinical correlations in nephrology,* New York, 1984, Raven.)

specific gravity. The dipstick also detects urine myoglobin. The normal spun urine contains less than one erythrocyte per HPF. The presence of more than three per HPF suggests bleeding anywhere along the urinary tract. It has been suggested that erythrocytes of glomerular origin have a more distorted (dysmorphic) appearance than those arising elsewhere, but this is controversial. The finding of an erythrocyte cast (Fig. 144-6), however, almost always suggests that the hematuria is due to glomerulonephritis or vasculitis (see Chapter 148). The urine is often contaminated with blood during menses, so urinalysis should preferably be postponed to avoid menstrual blood.

Pyuria and Bacteriuria

The dipstick measures the esterase enzyme of neutrophils and correlates well with the number of these cells in the urine. The presence of cephalexin or cephalothin or high concentrations of oxalic acid may decrease the test result. The most common contamination is vaginal discharge. Overall, however, false-positive and false-negative results are quite low. A positive nitrite test by dipstick indicates the presence of bacteria that reduce urinary nitrate to nitrite. Most Enterobacteriaceae (90%) convert nitrate to nitrite, but some bacteria (e.g., enterococci) cannot. In addition, because it takes up to 4 hours for the conversion to nitrate in the bladder, a sample from the first voiding of the morning is preferable. Thus a positive nitrite test by dipstick, especially when accompanied by pyuria, is very suggestive of a urinary tract infection. A negative test, however, does not rule out the diagnosis.

The normal number of leukocytes is probably less than one per HPF. When present in greater numbers, there is probably inflammation somewhere in the urinary system. If leukocytes are found in casts (Fig. 144-7), the inflammation is in the renal parenchyma. Leukocyte casts can be differentiated from epithelial cell casts by the lobulation of the nuclei. Most leukocytes in the urine are neutrophils; however, in certain conditions, such as allergic interstitial nephritis, pyelonephritis, vasculitis, and atheroemboli to the kidneys, the cells may be eosinophils. A Hansel's or Wright's stain (see Chapter 148) of the sediment should be performed if pyuria is present and one of these diagnoses is being considered. Bacteria are often seen with unstained urine specimens in the presence of infection. In women, the presence of squamous epithelial cells, which are large, are flat, and have a small central nucleus (Fig. 144-8), suggests vaginal contamination. Transitional epithelial cells (Fig. 144-9) lining the bladder and ureter are smaller, with a relatively larger nucleus. These may be normally present or may represent some form of irritation of the urinary tract.

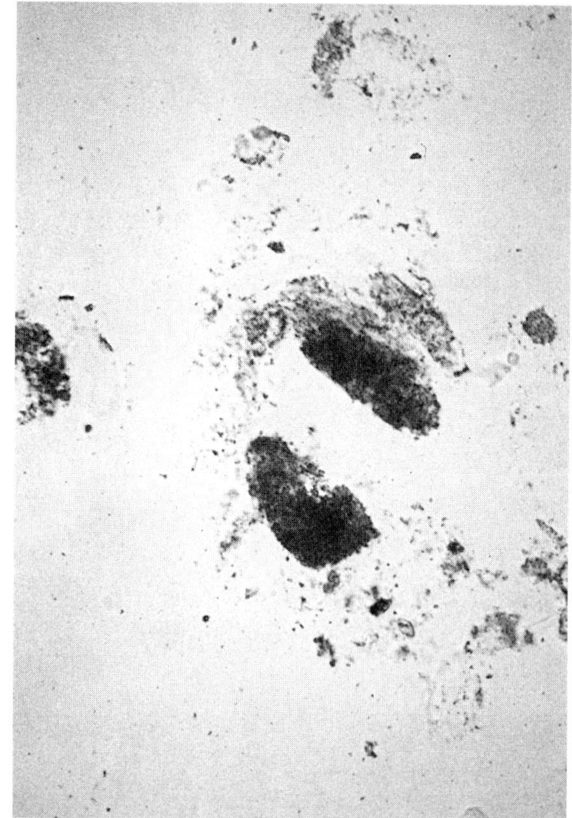

Fig. 144-5. Brown, muddy granular cast (×160.) (Courtesy Steve Miller, MD.)

Glycosuria

Glucose does not usually appear in the urine until the serum glucose levels exceed 180 to 200 mg/dl. Thus diabetes is by far the most common cause of glycosuria. In pregnancy, however, glycosuria with normal glucose levels is common. In addition, disorders that disrupt the proximal tubules' reabsorption of glucose may lead to glycosuria. These include lead poisoning, myeloma, galactosemia, and cystinosis. Finally, glycosuria may occur as part of a more generalized disorder of tubular transport. With Fanconi's syndrome, there is also impaired reabsorption of sodium, amino acids, bicarbonate, phosphate, and water. The assay for glucose varies according to the manufacturer, but most can detect a urine glucose concentration of 100 mg/dl.

Crystalluria

A wide variety of crystals may be seen in the urine. However, only the crystals of cystine (Fig. 144-10), leucine, tyrosine,

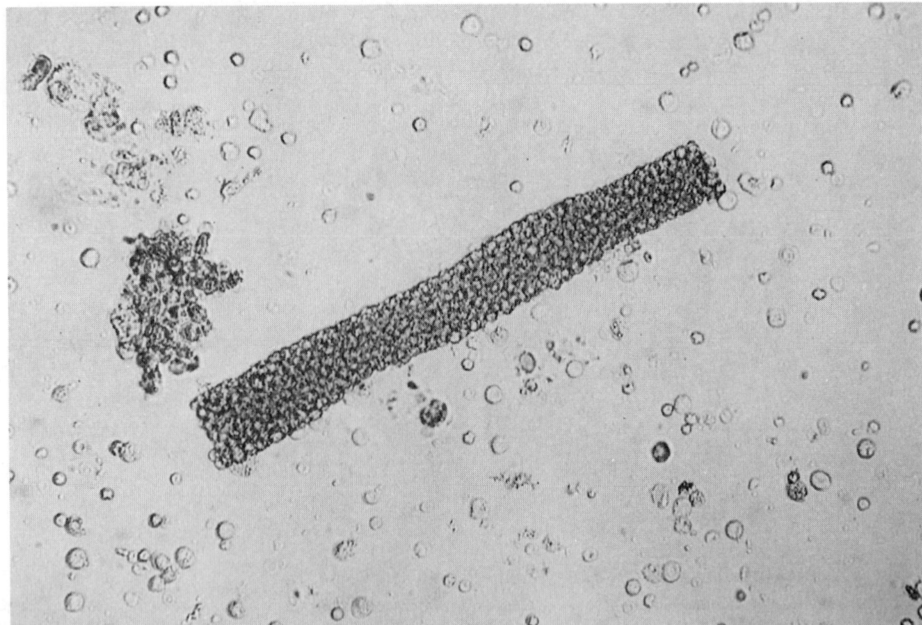

Fig. 144-6. Red cast, which strongly suggests a glomerulonephritis or vasculitis. (×160.) (From Piccoli G, Varese D, Rotunno M: *Atlas of urinary sediments: Diagnosis and clinical correlations in nephrology,* New York, 1984, Raven.)

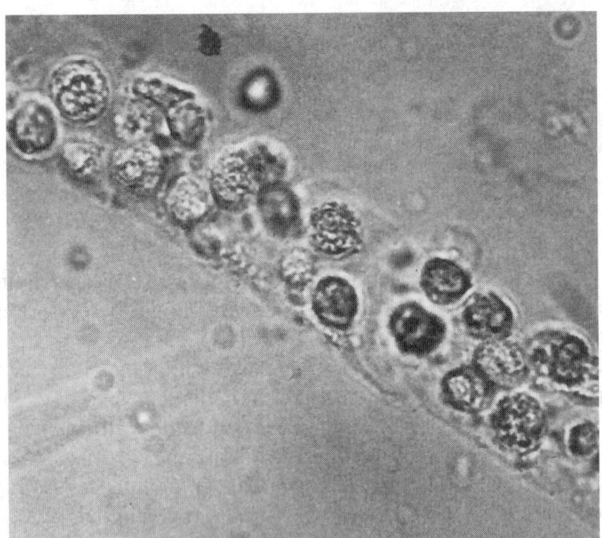

Fig. 144-7. Granulocyte cast, which indicates inflammation within the renal parenchyma (×400.) (From Piccoli G, Varese D, Rotunno M: *Atlas of urinary sediments: Diagnosis and clinical correlations in nephrology,* New York, 1984, Raven.)

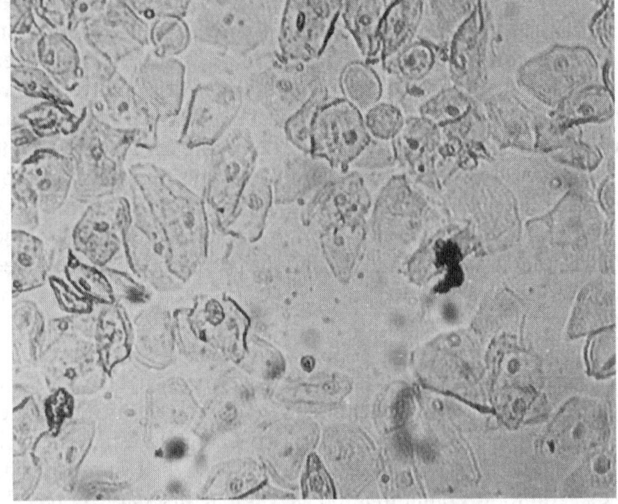

Fig. 144-8. Vaginal squamous cells, which indicate that the urine sample was not collected properly and the diagnosis of urinary tract infection cannot be made with certainty. (×100.) (From Piccoli G, Varese D, Rotunno M: *Atlas of urinary sediments: Diagnosis and clinical correlations in nephrology,* New York, 1984, Raven.)

and cholesterol have pathologic significance. In patients whose kidneys form stones repeatedly, urinary crystals may assist in predicting the type of stone being produced (see Chapter 147). This is particularly true with ammoniomagnesium phosphate crystals (coffin-lid shaped), whose presence suggests struvite stones made by urease-producing bacteria such as *Proteus* (Fig. 144-11).

Measurement of Urine Acidity

The dipstick measures the urine pH, usually within the range of 5 to 8.5. A urine pH greater than 6.5 indicates bicarbonaturia or ammonium production resulting from urease-producing organisms. A urine pH less than 5.5 indicates an absence of bicarbonate in the urine. At times, urine pH determination assists in the evaluation of acid-base disorders (see Chapter 145) and renal stone diseases (see Chapter 147).

Urinary Concentrating Ability

The volume and concentration of the urine reflect the renal adaptation for maintaining normal water and solute balance. A urine specific gravity of 1.010 corresponds to an osmolality of about 285 mOsm/L (i.e., the same osmolality as that normally measured in plasma). For this reason, urine with an osmolality of around 1.010 is referred to as *isosthenuric*. Adults with a normal diet generally have a urine specific

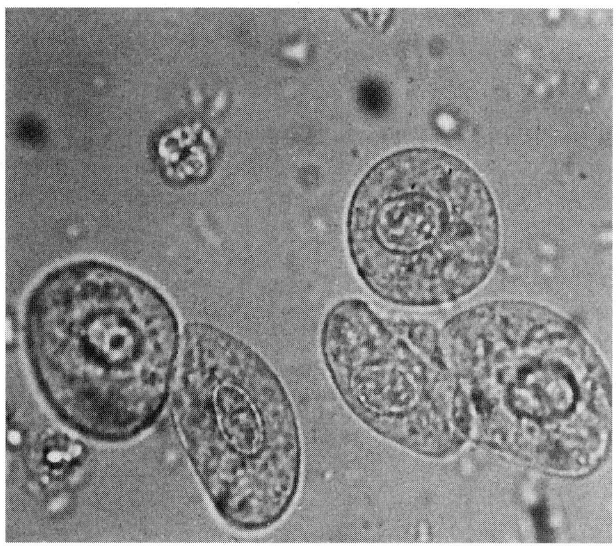

Fig. 144-9. Transitional epithelial cells. (×400.) (From Piccoli G, Varese D, Rotunno M: *Atlas of urinary sediments: Diagnosis and clinical correlations in nephrology,* New York, 1984, Raven.)

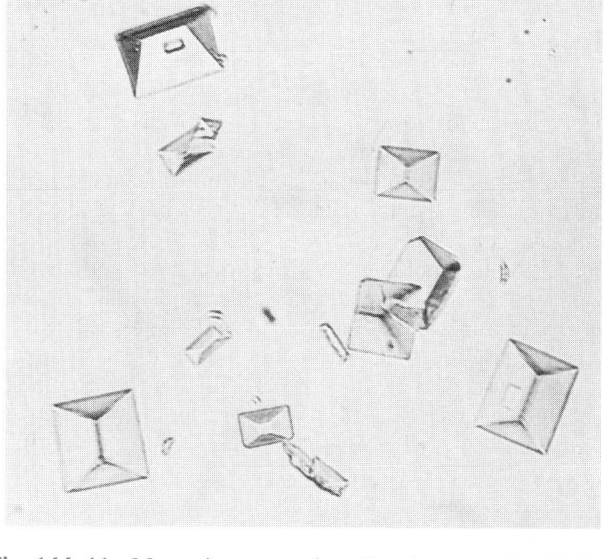

Fig. 144-11. Magnesium ammonium phosphate crystals with their typical "coffin-lid" appearance. (×400.) (From Piccoli G, Varese D, Rotunno M: *Atlas of urinary sediments: Diagnosis and clinical correlations in nephrology,* New York, 1984, Raven.)

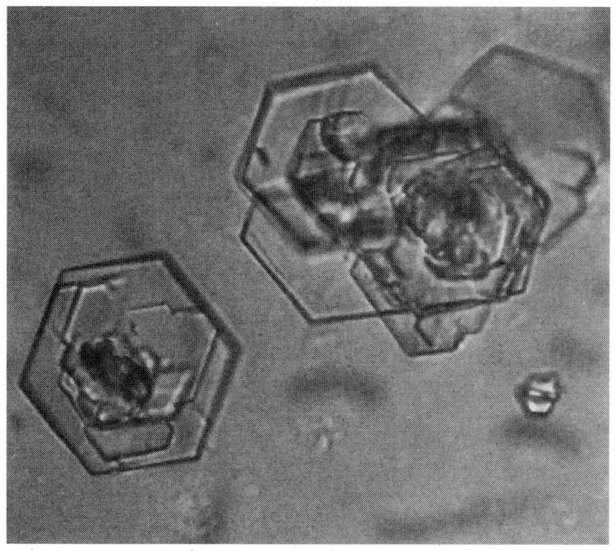

Fig. 144-10. Hexagonal cystine crystals, which indicate cystinuria. (×400.) (From Piccoli G, Varese D, Rotunno M: *Atlas of urinary sediments: Diagnosis and clinical correlations in nephrology,* New York, 1984, Raven.)

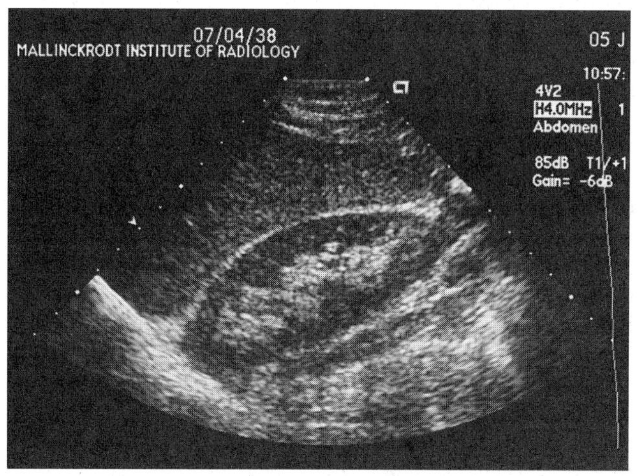

Fig. 144-12. Ultrasound of a normal kidney.

gravity of 1.016 to 1.022. The urine specific gravity after a 12-hour overnight fast should be 1.022. If the diagnosis of central or nephrogenic diabetes insipidus is being considered, more sophisticated tests of urine and plasma osmolality may be necessary (see Chapter 99).

IMAGING STUDIES

Renal Ultrasonography with Doppler Echography

In some institutions, ultrasound (US) has supplanted an intravenous pyelogram (IVP) as the most common imaging test for evaluating urologic structures. The advantages of US over IVP are that it requires no intravenous injection of contrast and does not expose the patient to radiation. The size of the kidneys is easily determined by US. The normal length varies according to body size and age, with the right kidney ranging between 8 and 14 cm and the left between 7.5 and 12.5 cm. A US image of a normal kidney is shown in Fig. 144-12. Large kidneys are associated with poorly controlled diabetes, acromegaly, acute glomerulonephritis, and infiltrative processes such as amyloidosis, leukemia, and lymphoma. The presence of small kidneys suggests that there has been irreversible renal damage, and further evaluation may not be warranted. Increased echogenicity of the renal cortex relative to that of the liver is an abnormal but nonspecific finding. Doppler flow studies can often detect patency and the direction of flow of the main renal arteries and veins. Doppler studies may also be useful in the evaluation of renal artery stenosis.

Unlike some other imaging tests (i.e., IVP), US relies exclusively on structural changes such as dilated calyces (Fig. 144-13) to detect obstructive uropathy. Hydronephrosis is diagnosed with a sensitivity rate of 98% to 100% and a specificity rate of 90% to 93%. Causes for false-positive and false-negative results are listed in Box 144-3.

Renal US is also the first-line test in evaluating inherited and acquired cysts of the kidneys. With established autosomal dominant polycystic kidney disease, the renal size is large because of the multiple cysts destroying the normal renal parenchyma. The early diagnosis of autosomal dominant polycystic kidney disease may be missed before the age of 30 years because the cysts may be too small to detect. Benign cortical cysts (Fig. 144-14) are the most commonly encountered renal masses. Cysts must meet four criteria to be considered benign (Box 144-4). If these criteria are fulfilled, the accuracy of diagnosis of a benign cyst is greater than 95%, and no further workup is warranted. Cysts that do not meet the criteria have a 37% chance of being a neoplasm and must be further evaluated, often by computed tomography (CT). Suggested criteria for the CT diagnosis of a simple cyst include a homogeneous attenuation value of mean water density, no enhancement with intravenous contrast, no measurable thickness of the cyst wall, and smooth interface with renal parenchyma. The probability of a correct diagnosis with CT is quite high. Therefore, if these criteria are not met, many centers do no further testing (i.e., percutaneous cyst puncture and angiogram) but proceed with a surgical exploration. Structures that are poorly evaluated by US include solid renal masses and nondilated ureters.

Intravenous Pyelography

An IVP may be helpful in evaluating the location of the obstruction in a patient passing a renal stone. For routine imaging of a renal stone, a plain film of the abdomen is often satisfactory, since 85% of stones are radiopaque. It is controversial whether US or IVP should be chosen for the initial renal imaging evaluation of persistent, isolated hematuria.

An IVP requires the administration of intravenous contrast. This may lead to idiosyncratic reactions ranging from mild urticaria (up to 10%) to severe anaphylaxis (1:3000 to 1:4500). Up to 10% of patients also report nausea and a transient sensation of warmth. Acute renal failure may result from contrast with preexisting impaired renal function, with volume depletion, or after multiple contrast studies. The nonionic contrast agents may decrease the incidence of adverse events.

Computed Tomography and Magnetic Resonance Imaging

If a solid renal mass has been suggested by prior US or IVP, a CT scan should be considered. US detects only 26% of CT-proven solid lesions smaller than 1 cm in diameter. Some 85% of lesions 3 cm or larger are detected. The overall accuracy of CT is 95% to 99% for solid renal masses. This is higher than that of magnetic resonance imaging (MRI). However, with the addition of Gd-DTPA for contrast-enhanced MRI, the accuracy is similar to that of CT. MRI is of little value in evaluating renal stones.

Renal Scans

Renal scans may be of some value in evaluating renovascular disease, in determining whether mild obstruction is physiologically significant (see Chapter 147), or in assessing the leakage of urine from the urinary system. They, however, provide little structural information about the kidneys that cannot be obtained by US. They also provide little valuable information about renal function except when there are marked differences between the two kidneys.

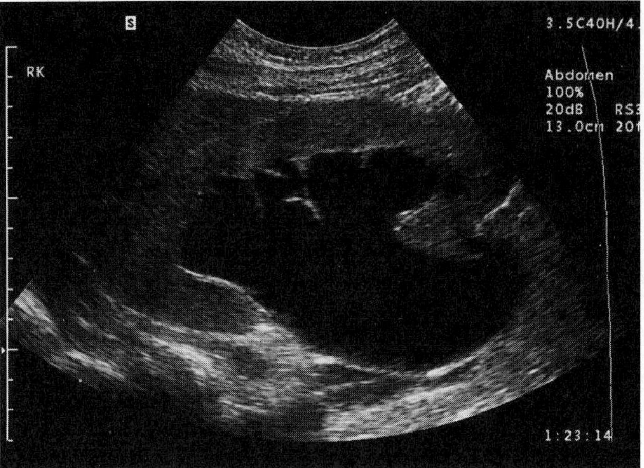

Fig. 144-13. An ultrasound of an obstructed kidney with dilated calyces.

Box 144-3. Ultrasound and Obstruction of the Urinary Tract: Causes of False-Positive and False-Negative Tests

False Positive

1. Cystic diseases of the kidneys
2. Full bladder
3. States of increased urine output
4. Extrarenal pelvis
5. Vesicoureteral reflux
6. Renal sinus lipomatosis
7. Papillary necrosis

False Negative

1. Acute obstruction without dilatation
2. Hypovolemia
3. Staghorn calculi
4. Renal cysts and obstruction, interpreted only as renal cysts
5. Intermittent obstruction

RENAL BIOPSY

Percutaneous renal biopsies are routinely performed on patients with renal diseases. Biopsies have greatly increased knowledge of the classification, prognosis, epidemiology, and treatment of a variety of renal disorders. An experienced nephrologist or radiologist should perform the renal biopsy. The usual procedure is to have the patient lie prone and to localize the lower pole of either kidney with the assistance of US. After the establishment of a sterile field and the administration of local anesthesia, several cores of renal cortex may be obtained via a variety of biopsy needles. The

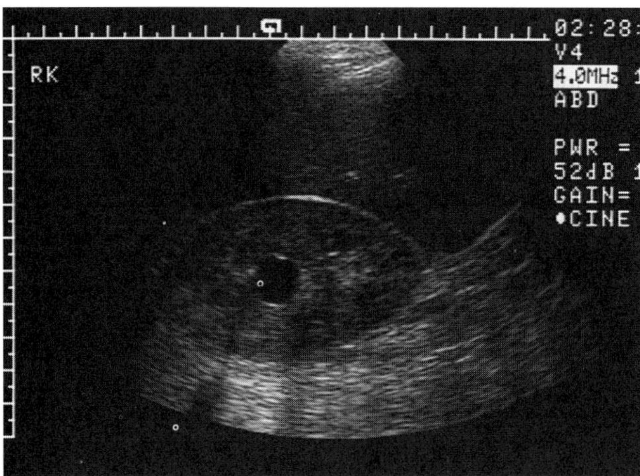

Fig. 144-14. An ultrasound of a kidney with simple cysts.

Box 144-4. Ultrasound Criteria for the Classification of Benign Renal Cysts

1. Lack of internal echoes
2. Round or oval shape
3. Clearly demarcated far wall
4. Acoustic enhancement of tissue next to far wall

Box 144-5. Information Gained from Renal Imaging Studies and Biopsies

Ultrasound/Doppler Flow Studies

1. Size
2. Structural changes
   a. Stones
   b. Obstruction
   c. Masses
   d. Cysts
3. Thrombosis of main renal artery or vein

Intravenous Pyelography

1. Size and structure
2. Site of obstruction

Computed Tomography and Magnetic Resonance Imaging

1. Evaluation of suspicious renal masses noted on previous ultrasound or intravenous pyelogram

Renal Scan

1. Renovascular disease
2. Leakage of urine (renal trauma)
3. Differential renal function

Renal Biopsy

1. Diagnosis of primary glomerular disease
   a. Severity
   b. Degree of irreversibility
2. Diagnosis of systemic disease
3. Evaluation of unexplained decline in renal function

specimens are then analyzed by light, immunofluorescence, and electron microscopy.

The decision to proceed with a renal biopsy is made after considering the impact of the results on further management of the patient balanced against the risks. Common indications are the nephrotic syndrome and unexplained renal failure (see Chapter 148). The renal biopsy provides information concerning the type of primary glomerular disease, as well as its severity and degree of irreversible scarring. In addition, a renal biopsy sometimes aids in the diagnosis or management of a systemic disease such as amyloidosis, systemic lupus erythematosus, or vasculitis. The information gained from renal imaging studies and biopsies is summarized in Box 144-5.

The main risk of a renal biopsy is hemorrhage. Although almost 90% of patients have evidence of perirenal hemorrhage as shown on CT, less than 5% require a transfusion. Severe renal hemorrhage is usually successfully treated by selective embolization of the involved vessels. Less than 1% of patients require an emergency nephrectomy. Some patients complain of pain at the site of the biopsy, but this usually resolves within 1 week. Gross hematuria may be observed in about 5% of patients, but this too usually resolves without specific treatment. An open (surgical) renal biopsy is considerably more invasive than a closed (percutaneous) renal biopsy. It should never be considered when a percutaneous biopsy is possible.

The major contraindication to renal biopsy is a coagulopathy. The criteria for exclusion vary but generally involve patients with a platelet count below 100,000 cells/mm^3, an elevated prothrombin time or partial thromboplastin time, and a history of ingesting aspirin within the previous week. Relative contraindications include a solitary kidney, an active urinary tract infection, uncontrolled hypertension, and an uncooperative patient.

ADDITIONAL READINGS

Ginsberg JM, Change BS, Matarese RA, et al: Use of single voided urine samples to estimate quantitative proteinuria, *N Engl J Med* 309:1543-1546, 1983.

Hilbrands LB, Artz MA, Wetzels JFM, et al: Cimetidine improves the reliability of creatinine as a marker of glomerular filtration, *Kidney Int* 40:1171-1176, 1991.

King AJ, Levey AS: Dietary protein and renal function, *J Am Soc Nephrol* 3:1723-1737, 1993.

Kohler H, Wandel E, Brunck B: Acanthocyturia: a characteristic marker for glomerular bleeding, *Kidney Int* 40:115-120, 1991.

Levey AS: Measurement of renal function in chronic renal disease, *Kidney Int* 38:167-184, 1990.

MacKenzie W, Drew HH, LaFrance ND: Creatinine measurements often yield false estimates of progression in chronic renal failure, *Kidney Int* 34:412-418, 1988.

Nolan CR III, Anger MS, Keheller SP: Eosinophiluria: a new method of detection and definition of the clinical spectrum, *N Engl J Med* 315:1516-1519, 1986.

O'Reilly PH, George NJR, Weiss RM, editors: *Diagnostic techniques in urology,* Philadelphia, 1990, WB Saunders.

Piccoli G, Varese D, Rotunno M: *Atlas of urinary sediments: diagnosis and clinical correlations in nephrology,* New York, 1984, Raven.
Roubenoff R, Drew H, Moyer M, et al: Oral cimetidine improves the accuracy and precision of creatinine clearance in lupus nephritis, *Ann Intern Med* 113:501-506, 1990.
Shemesh O, Golbetz H, Kriss JP, et al: Limitations of creatinine as a filtration marker in glomerulopathic patients, *Kidney Int* 28:830-838, 1985.

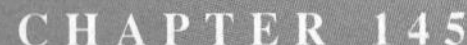
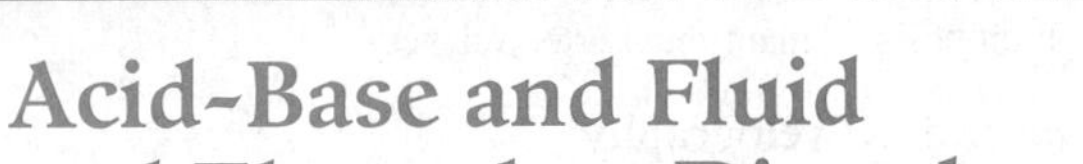

CHAPTER 145

Acid-Base and Fluid and Electrolyte Disorders

Saulo Klahr

ACID-BASE DISORDERS

Acid-Base Balance in Health

The pH of blood is kept within a narrow range of 7.37 to 7.42. The range of plasma pH compatible with life is approximately 6.8 to 7.8. The pH of body fluids in humans is maintained despite the large production of acid from two major sources: (1) volatile carbonic acid (H_2CO_3), derived from carbon dioxide (CO_2), the end product of oxidative metabolism; and (2) a variety of nonvolatile acids produced from dietary substances, mainly protein. The pH of plasma is the ratio of bicarbonate (HCO_3^-) to carbonic acid (dissolved CO_2), as formulated in the Henderson-Hasselbach equation:

$$pH = pK + \log \frac{HCO_3^-}{H_2CO_3 \ or \ \alpha \cdot Pco_2}$$

where α, the solubility constant for CO_2, has a value of 0.03 at 37°C (98.6°F). In a normal individual, this expression has the following numeric values:

$$7.4 = 6.1 + \log \frac{26 \text{ mmol/L}}{1.3 \text{ mmol/L}}$$

The denominator of the equation, the plasma carbon dioxide tension (Pco_2), is maintained within narrow limits by the excretion of CO_2 by the lungs. Although pH changes are minimized through changes in extracellular fluid (ECF) Pco_2, the integrity of plasma pH depends on the availability of HCO_3^- in the ECF. The kidneys participate in stabilizing the concentration of HCO_3^- in plasma (the numerator of the Henderson-Hasselbalch equation). A normal individual ingesting 1 to 2 gm of protein per kilogram of body weight generates daily about 60 mmol of nonvolatile acid. The same amount of HCO_3^- is consumed in the ECF to buffer this surplus acid. The restoration of serum HCO_3^- consumed in buffering either metabolically produced or exogenous acid loads occurs both by virtually complete reabsorption of filtered HCO_3^- (reclamation) and by the regeneration of HCO_3^- formed in conjunction with the excretion of titratable acid and ammonium (de novo synthesis of HCO_3^-). Both the reabsorption and the regeneration of HCO_3^- result from the secretion of hydrogen ions (H^+) into the nephron's tubular lumen. A rise in ECF HCO_3^- levels is corrected by the renal excretion of a larger-than-normal fraction of the filtered HCO_3^-.

Laboratory Considerations

Evaluation of a patient's acid-base status requires the measurement of two of the three values (pH, Pco_2, HCO_3^-) in the Henderson-Hasselbalch equation.[9] The third value can be calculated or read directly from a nomogram (Fig. 145-1). The initial test for evaluating a patient's acid-base status should be the measurement of the total CO_2 content of plasma or serum. This value reflects the total number of moles of CO_2 liberated from both HCO_3^- and H_2CO_3. Because of the relatively small amounts of H_2CO_3 (1.3 mmol at a Pco_2 of approximately 40 mm Hg), the value for the CO_2 content approximates the HCO_3^- concentration of plasma. Normal values for CO_2 content are 26 to 28 mmol/L and can be measured in venous blood. Because the H_2CO_3/HCO_3^- pair is the ECF's principal buffer system, measurement of the two components provides a meaningful and convenient expression of the organism's acid-base status. Two types of pathophysiologic events alter the pH: metabolic and respiratory. Metabolic acid-base disturbances result from processes that alter fluid pH primarily by changing the concentration of plasma HCO_3^- (numerator of the Henderson-Hasselbach equation). Respiratory acid-base disorders result from primary changes in the respiratory component (denominator of the equation), which is measured as Pco_2. A series of overlapping defense mechanisms maintain the pH of the ECF within narrow limits. These mechanisms consist of at least three well-defined systems:

1. Extracellular and intracellular buffers provide an almost instantaneous, first line of defense against changes in pH.
2. Respiratory compensation of fairly rapid onset constitutes a secondary defense in metabolic disorders.
3. The kidneys not only maintain plasma HCO_3^- constant under normal circumstances but also modify HCO_3^- excretion in respiratory acid-base disorders. The renal compensatory mechanism is slower to respond (several hours).

Metabolic Acidosis

Clinical Features and Systemic Effects. The clinical manifestations of metabolic acidosis in part may reflect the primary disorder responsible for the acidosis. The manifestations directly attributable to severe metabolic acidosis include depressed left ventricular function and decreased peripheral vascular resistance.[9] This may lead to hypotension, pulmonary edema, arrhythmias (particularly ventricular fibrillation), and tissue hypoxia. The depth and rate of respirations increase; Kussmaul's respiration is especially prominent when plasma HCO_3^- levels are below 15 mEq/L. Central nervous system manifestations include changes in mentation, confusion, and sometimes convulsions. Prolonged chronic metabolic acidosis may cause osteopenia and osteoporosis as a result of the buffering of H^+ by calcium carbonate ($CaCO_3$) in bone. This may contribute to bone disease, particularly in patients with chronic renal failure or renal tubular acidosis.

Laboratory Findings. Metabolic acidosis occurs when the addition of H^+ to the extracellular space exceeds its rate

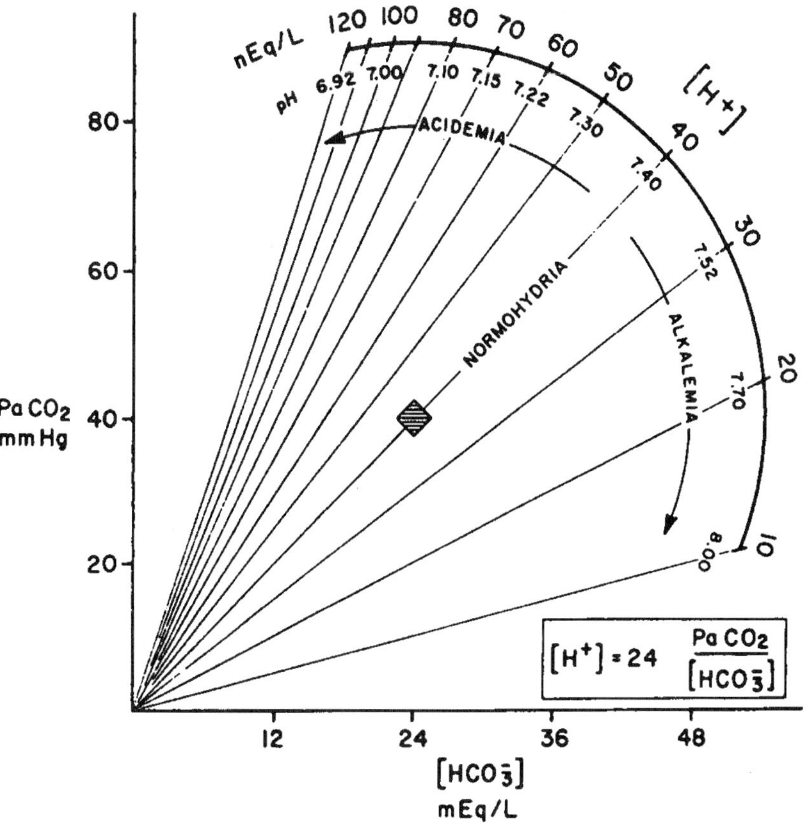

Fig. 145-1. Acid-base nomogram.

of excretion, or when base is lost from the body in excess of its rate of replenishment. The hallmark of metabolic acidosis is a high H^+ concentration (low pH and low HCO_3^- in plasma). Metabolic acidosis may also be suspected when a wide plasma anion gap (>15 mEq/L) exists, even in the absence of a pH or HCO_3^- change. The anion gap is calculated by subtracting the sum of chloride (Cl^-) plus HCO_3^- concentrations from the sodium (Na^+) concentration in plasma or serum:

$$\text{Anion gap} = Na^+ - (Cl^- + HCO_3^-)$$

Normally a difference of 8 to 12 mEq/L exists, made up predominantly by plasma proteins, phosphate, and sulfate.

Causes. Metabolic acidosis caused by a gain of H^+ is usually manifested by an increased anion gap (Table 145-1). Quantitatively the increased anion gap in plasma equals the decrease in plasma HCO_3^- concentration. Metabolic acidosis resulting from loss of HCO_3^- is characterized by a normal anion gap. In metabolic acidosis, the expected adjustment is a lowering of plasma P_{CO_2} levels to minimize the decrease in pH. This is accomplished by an increase in the depth and rate of respiration. Quantitatively, the decrease in P_{CO_2} from 40 mm Hg should equal the decrease in plasma HCO_3^- from 26 mmol/L. Compensation at the level of the kidneys involves the excretion of increased amounts of ammonium to increase the de novo synthesis of HCO_3^-. Normally the kidneys excrete 40 mmol of ammonium daily. During severe metabolic acidosis, ammonium excretion can reach 200 mmol daily.

Metabolic Acidosis Associated With Normal Anion Gap

Renal Loss of Bicarbonate

Use of carbonic anhydrase inhibitors. Carbonic anhydrase inhibitors increase HCO_3^- excretion in the urine by inhibiting the enzyme responsible for the hydration of CO_2. This process is key in the secretion of H^+ and consequently in HCO_3^- reabsorption from the renal tubule. Such an inhibitor is acetazolamide (Diamox), a diuretic used to decrease intraocular pressure in patients with glaucoma.

Renal tubular acidosis. Renal tubular acidosis (RTA) is a metabolic hyperchloremic acidosis that occurs in patients with a nonazotemic renal acidification defect. RTA is characterized by decreased H^+ excretion in the urine. The two major types of RTA are proximal and distal.[9]

Distal RTA. Distal, or classic, RTA is characterized by a defect of the distal nephron to excrete H^+. The normal kidney can lower the urine pH to 4.7, a urine/plasma concentration ratio for H^+ of approximately 800 : 1. In contrast, in patients with distal RTA, the urine pH cannot fall below 6 regardless of the severity of the systemic acidosis. A urine pH of 6 limits the amount of H^+ excreted as ammonium or titratable acid (H^+ bound mainly to phosphate). The inability to excrete H^+ at a rate comparable to the rate of formation and consequently the failure to regenerate the HCO_3^- consumed daily in the buffering process causes metabolic acidosis. Distal RTA is characterized by increased urine excretion of cations (sodium, potassium, calcium) and anions (sulfate, phosphate). This results in depletion of these cations with reduction of the ECF volume, hypokalemia, and rickets or osteomalacia. The increased calcium and phosphate excreted into the alkaline

Table 145-1. Causes of Metabolic Acidosis

Cause	Clinical comments
Normal anion gap	
Renal loss of bicarbonate	
Carbonic anhydrase inhibitors	Use of acetazolamide in patients with glaucoma
Renal tubular acidosis, proximal or distal	
Gastrointestinal loss of bicarbonate	
Diarrhea or loss of other gastrointestinal fluids with high bicarbonate content through fistulas or surgical drainage	
Ileal loop conduit	
Administration or ingestion of hydrochloric acid, ammonium chloride, or arginine hydrochloride	
Increased anion gap	
Uncontrolled diabetes mellitus (ketoacidosis)	Hyperglycemia usually present
Lactic acidosis	In hypoxic patients or those with decreased hepatic blood flow
Administration, ingestion, or intoxication	
Ethyl alcohol, with "starvation" and production of ketoacids	
Salicylate	Initial event a respiratory alkalosis
Methyl alcohol	Increase in plasma osmolality (osmolal gap)
Paraldehyde	
Ethylene glycol	Central nervous system disturbances, acute renal failure
Renal failure (acute and chronic)	Elevated serum creatinine and blood urea nitrogen levels

Modified from Klahr SK, Hamm L. In Klahr S, editor: *Renal and electrolyte disorders,* ed 2, Norwalk, Conn, 1984, Appleton-Century-Crofts.

urine often cause renal stones or nephrocalcinosis. Distal RTA is seen in (1) a sporadic congenital primary form; (2) certain hypergammaglobulinemic states; (3) nephrocalcinosis, which may result from various genetic and metabolic disorders; (4) distal tubule nephrotoxicity caused by drugs such as amphotericin B, excessive vitamin D, and toluene; (5) medullary sponge kidney; and (6) interstitial renal disease (e.g., pyelonephritis, collagen disorders). Distal RTA may also develop after renal transplantation.

Proximal RTA. Proximal RTA is characterized by a large excretion of HCO_3^- in the urine. Alkaline urine is excreted, and hyperchloremic metabolic acidosis develops. Proximal RTA may be suspected by the presence of concomitant defects in proximal reabsorption, such as aminoaciduria, glycosuria, and phosphaturia. The hallmark of proximal RTA is normal acidification of the urine in the presence of normal renal function when plasma HCO_3^- concentrations are low; excretion of an alkaline urine as plasma HCO_3^- is raised by the administration of exogenous $NaHCO_3^-$.

Gastrointestinal Loss of Bicarbonate. HCO_3^- loss through the gastrointestinal tract may lead to normal-anion-gap metabolic acidosis. *Diarrhea* may result in loss of fluid containing HCO_3^- in excess (30 to 50 mmol/L) of the concentrations present in plasma. Large amounts of potassium may also be lost, and metabolic acidosis with hypokalemia may occur. Secretions from *fistulas, the small bowel, the pancreas,* or the *biliary tract* may be rich in HCO_3^-. Losses of such fluids to the exterior may cause hyperchloremic acidosis. Patients with total cystectomies require the construction of artificial bladders in the form of an ileal loop conduit. Although hyperchloremic acidosis is uncommon in patients with ileal bladders, it may occur when the ileal segment is extremely long, when an antiperistaltic loop has been constructed, or when the stoma of the ileal loop is obstructed. Prolonged exposure of the urine to the ileal mucosa results in the exchange of chloride for HCO_3^-, leading to loss of HCO_3^- from body fluids.

Other causes of normal-anion-gap metabolic acidosis include expansion of the extracellular space with solutions not containing HCO_3^- (dilutional acidosis) and the administration of hydrochloric acid, ammonium chloride, arginine, or lysine hydrochloride. Sometimes during hyperalimentation, amino acid infusions containing inorganic cations in excess of organic anions may cause a metabolic acidosis with hyperchloremia.[9]

Metabolic Acidosis Associated With Increased Anion Gap. An excess of acid is characterized by an increase in the anion gap. The acids that accumulate under these conditions are (1) keto acids, in insulin-deficiency diabetes; (2) lactic acid, in conditions characterized by tissue hypoxia; (3) acetylsalicylic acid (aspirin); and (4) toxic acids or substances that can be metabolized to them. Example of such substances are methanol, which leads to the formation of formic acid; ethylene glycol, which results in the formation of glyoxylic acid; paraldehyde, which is converted to acetic acid; and toluene, which is converted to hippuric acid. Patients with renal failure have increased-anion-gap metabolic acidosis (mainly caused by phosphate and sulfate), not because acid production is increased but because the kidney fails to regenerate enough HCO_3^-.

When an increased anion gap occurs in metabolic acidosis, the diagnosis of ketoacidosis can be made if there are hyperglycemia, large concentrations of serum ketones, and a wide anion gap. Patients who fulfill these criteria usually have ECF volume contraction, hyperventilation, and the smell of acetone on their breath. The treatment includes insulin to decrease the production of H^+ and sodium chloride to restore ECF volume.

Lactic acid, the end product of glycolysis, may accumulate in several conditions in which hypoxia is present (e.g., circulatory insufficiency, hypotension). Lactic acidosis can also occur during extreme exercise or the administration of phenformin or other uncouplers of oxidative phosphorylation. Loss of liver tissue may increase lactic acid levels as a result of decreased conversion of this acid to glucose. This also occurs when gluconeogenesis is impaired because of drugs or inborn errors of metabolism.

Finding an increased osmolar gap in the plasma of patients with metabolic acidosis should raise the suspicion of ethanol, methanol, isopropyl alcohol, or ethylene glycol intoxication. The osmolar gap is the difference between the measured serum osmolality and the calculated osmolality, as follows:

$$\text{Calculated osmolality} = 1.87\,([Na] + [K]) + BUN/2.8 + glucose/18$$

Treatment. The ideal treatment of metabolic acidosis corrects or ameliorates the cause. Only when acidosis accounts for severe physiologic disturbances is treatment of the acidosis itself required. Historically, the therapy has involved the administration of sodium bicarbonate ($NaHCO_3$). At present, such treatment is somewhat controversial, although the judicious use of $NaHCO_3$ has been advocated. It is appropriate to administer HCO_3^- if the blood pH is less than 7.1.

Chronic metabolic acidosis, which is caused by RTA or chronic renal failure, requires treatment in children to allow normal growth and in adults to ameliorate or prevent gastrointestinal or neurologic symptoms of acidosis and bone disease. $NaHCO_3$ can be given to maintain plasma HCO_3^- levels at about 20 mmol/L. Sodium overload should be avoided. In chronic metabolic acidosis, $NaHCO_3$ may be given orally as tolerated. The 1-gm tablets contain 12 mmol of $NaHCO_3$.

Metabolic Alkalosis

The hallmark of metabolic alkalosis is an elevated blood pH resulting from an increase in the concentration of plasma HCO_3^-. The increased plasma HCO_3^- concentration may result from (1) the net loss of H^+ from the extracellular space or (2) the net addition of HCO_3^- or its precursors to the extracellular space or loss of ECF-containing chloride in a concentration greater than HCO_3^-. Therefore metabolic alkalosis results from abnormal loss of acid, excessive retention of base, or both. Normally, uncomplicated metabolic alkalosis is short-lived because the kidneys promptly excrete the excess HCO_3^-. In established metabolic alkalosis, two mechanisms should be considered: the events responsible for the development of metabolic alkalosis (i.e., the *generation* of such an acid-base disorder) and the factors that allow this disorder to persist (i.e., the *maintenance* of metabolic alkalosis). The maintenance of metabolic alkalosis relates to an inability of the kidney to excrete HCO_3^-. The factors that promote the renal tubular reabsorption of HCO_3^- include contraction of the ECF volume, chloride deficit, decreased levels of plasma and intracellular potassium, and increased mineralocorticoid levels in plasma.[9]

Clinical Features and Systemic Effects. Metabolic alkalosis should be suspected in patients with a history of vomiting, surgery and gastric drainage, diuretic therapy, muscle cramps, and weakness and hypertension (primary hyperaldosteronism). Physical examination may reveal neuromuscular irritability such as tetany or hyperactive reflexes. These signs are more prominent if hypocalcemia is present, since the ionized calcium concentration decreases further as the pH rises.

Laboratory Findings. Blood pH and plasma HCO_3^- levels are increased, and arterial PCO_2 rises as a compensatory mechanism.[9] The PCO_2 values, however, seldom exceed 50 mm Hg because the hypoventilation required to elevate the PCO_2 further would also reduce arterial PO_2. The increased PCO_2 and reduced PO_2 in arterial blood stimulate the respiratory center, thereby tending to restore ventilation and blood gas levels toward normal. Occasionally, patients with metabolic alkalosis have marked hypercapnia (CO_2 retention) that cannot be ascribed to accompanying pulmonary disease or neuromuscular weaknesses. The elevated PCO_2, sometimes in excess of 75 mm Hg, may be caused by alveolar hypoventilation from depression of the respiratory center.

Patients with metabolic alkalosis have an elevated total CO_2 content, hypochloremia, and almost invariably, hypokalemia. Renal loss of potassium is the predominant cause of the last factor. Volume depletion may increase blood urea nitrogen (BUN) and creatinine concentrations in metabolic alkalosis. The hematocrit may be increased as a result of hemoconcentration. The anion gap may increase by as much as 5 to 6 mmol/L, partly because of higher concentrations of lactic acid and undefined anions.

The concentration of chloride in the urine is a useful test in the differential diagnosis of metabolic alkalosis. It may help distinguish metabolic alkalosis with volume expansion, which is mainly related to pathologic conditions of the adrenal gland, from metabolic alkalosis with volume depletion, which is mainly related to loss of fluid caused by vomiting or the use of diuretics. A urine chloride concentration below 10 mmol/L suggests avid reabsorption of NaCl by the renal tubule. A urine chloride concentration greater than 20 mmol/L in a patient with metabolic alkalosis indicates that neither ECF volume depletion nor chloride availability is a critical factor in perpetuating the metabolic alkalosis and points to excess mineralocorticoid activity as the cause of the disorder. In the analysis of chloride concentrations in patients who received diuretics 24 to 48 hours before a "spot" urinalysis, the validity of the previous assumptions is questionable.

Causes. Box 145-1 presents the causes of metabolic alkalosis. Clinically, it is helpful to divide metabolic alkalosis into two categories: (1) with ECF volume contraction and (2) with ECF volume expansion, which is usually caused by excessive mineralocorticoid secretion. The latter form is often accompanied by hypertension. This hypertension may be accompanied by high plasma levels of renin and aldosterone, low renin and high aldosterone levels, or even low renin and low aldosterone levels. (In this case, other mineralocorticoids play a primary role in the expansion of the ECF and the increased excretion of potassium and hydrogen in the urine.) Patients with ECF volume contraction, except possibly for those with Bartter's syndrome, have low chloride

Box 145-1. Causes of Metabolic Alkalosis

ECF Volume Contraction (Urinary Cl^- <10 mmol/L)

Gastrointestinal loss of H^+: vomiting, gastric drainage, villous adenoma of the colon, diarrhea with high chloride content
Renal loss of H^+: diuretic therapy—current or remote; other—Bartter's syndrome

ECF Volume Expansion with Mineralocorticoid Excess (Urinary Cl^- >20 mmol/L)

Primary or secondary aldosteronism, Cushing's syndrome, licorice abuse, Liddle's syndrome

Excessive HCO_3^- Loads (Particularly with Advanced Renal Insufficiency)

Excessive intake of HCO_3^- or alkalinizing salts
Conversion of accumulated or administered organic acids (lactate, acetate) to HCO_3^-
Glucose-induced alkalosis during fasting
Posthypercapnic state

Modified from Klahr SK, Hamm L. In Klahr S, editor: *Renal and electrolyte disorders*, ed 2, Norwalk, CT, 1984, Appleton-Century-Crofts.

concentrations in the urine. Excessive HCO_3^- loads may cause metabolic alkalosis, but this occurs mainly in the setting of advanced renal insufficiency.

Several questions must be asked when evaluating a patient with metabolic alkalosis: Is the ECF volume contracted? Why is the ECF volume contracted? If ECF volume contraction exists, is the renal response appropriate? If ECF volume is normal or expanded, what should be done?

Treatment. The underlying disease process causing the metabolic alkalosis should be treated. Treatment should also be directed at increasing renal HCO_3^- excretion. Restoration of ECF volume in the form of NaCl plus potassium will increase the excretion of HCO_3^- and retain NaCl and potassium in most varieties of metabolic alkalosis. Treatment of the excess mineralocorticoid varieties of metabolic alkalosis requires the removal or ablation of secretory tumors or the blockade of the renal tubular effects of the mineralocorticoids with spironolactone. Patients with severe potassium depletion and NaCl-resistant alkalosis may require large amounts of KCl before NaCl can be effective in correcting the alkalosis.

Respiratory Acidosis

Respiratory acidosis is characterized by an increase in P_{CO_2} and a decrease in blood pH. It represents an imbalance between CO_2 production and CO_2 excretion by the lungs.[5] The rise in P_{CO_2} increases the concentration of H_2CO_3 in body fluids. Since CO_2 production from metabolism (13,000 to 15,000 mmol/day) tends to be constant, the increase in P_{CO_2} is usually due to decreased excretion of CO_2 via the lung. The first line of defense in respiratory acidosis is a chemical reaction in which the increased H_2CO_2 resulting from increased P_{CO_2} is buffered mainly by intracellular proteins and phosphate to mitigate a marked fall in pH. The second line of defense relates to increased H^+ excretion by the kidney and thus increased production of HCO_3^-. In the initial phases of respiratory acidosis, the increased P_{CO_2} stimulates the generation and secretion of H^+. Increased excretion of titratable acid and particularly ammonium results in de novo generation of HCO_3^-.

Clinical Features and Systemic Effects. Respiratory acidosis can be acute or chronic. In acute respiratory acidosis, there is a marked and sudden decrease in the excretion of CO_2. The acute onset of hypercapnia (increased P_{CO_2}) is usually accompanied by hypoxemia. The patient may have signs or symptoms of acute respiratory distress with marked restlessness, tachypnea, and dyspnea. As the process progresses, further manifestations include fatigue, weakness, confusion, hyperactivity and even manic periods, and headache. Coma occurs at levels of P_{CO_2} from 70 to 100 mm Hg, depending on arterial pH and on the rapidity of elevation of P_{CO_2}. Physical signs include tremor, asterixis (similar to hepatic encephalopathy), weakness, incoordination, occasional cranial nerve signs, abnormal pyramidal tract signs, papilledema, and retinal hemorrhages.

Patients with chronic respiratory acidosis have few, if any, signs or symptoms related directly to hypercapnia. The signs and symptoms of chronic pulmonary disease with or without cor pulmonale usually predominate.[5]

Laboratory Findings. There is a marked increase in P_{CO_2} and sometimes a moderately elevated plasma HCO_3^-. In acute respiratory acidosis, plasma HCO_3^- concentrations rarely exceed 30 mmol/L. However, in chronic compensated respiratory acidosis, levels of HCO_3^- may be as high as 40 mmol/L. In both chronic and acute varieties, the P_{O_2} is generally decreased. The total plasma CO_2 content is increased, usually with normal concentrations of sodium and potassium. Urine pH is usually acidic. In chronic respiratory acidosis, the plasma chloride value is greatly decreased.

Causes. Box 145-2 summarizes the causes of respiratory acidosis. The differential diagnosis of acute vs. chronic respiratory acidosis relies on both the clinical and the laboratory criteria previously discussed.

Treatment. The main goal in the treatment of acute respiratory acidosis is to restore effective ventilation. If a delay prevents achieving this goal, oxygen should be given at once. Modest amounts of $NaHCO_3$ may be given intravenously to mitigate severe acidosis (blood pH <7.2).

Chronic respiratory acidosis can be treated effectively only by restoring or improving the lung's ability to excrete CO_2. This may be impossible because of irreversible lung changes. However, airway drainage (e.g., clearing secretions), relief of bronchospasm, and treatment of pulmonary infections and congestive heart failure may result in significant improvement.

Respiratory Alkalosis

Increased alveolar ventilation augments CO_2 excretion, resulting in decreases in P_{CO_2}, HCO_3^- concentration, and H^+ concentration (reflected as a rise in blood pH). Since the production of CO_2 from metabolism is usually constant, a negative CO_2 balance can be achieved only through increased

Box 145-2. Causes of Respiratory Acidosis

Acute Respiratory Acidosis

Airway obstruction
- Aspiration (vomiting, food), foreign body
- Severe bronchospasm, laryngeal edema

Suppression of respiratory center: hypnotics, sedatives, other drugs

Hypoventilation from muscular or neuromuscular disorders: myasthenia gravis, brainstem or high cord injury, Guillain-Barré syndrome, botulism, hypokalemia

Disease of lung or thoracic wall
- Flail chest, pneumothorax, pneumonia, smoke inhalation
- Severe cardiogenic pulmonary edema, massive pulmonary embolization

Chronic Respiratory Acidosis

Lung disease: chronic obstructive lung disease and chronic bronchitis, end-stage interstitial lung disease

Neuromuscular abnormalities: poliomyelitis, diaphragmatic paralysis, myasthenia gravis

Chronic suppression of respiratory center
- Chronic use of narcotics
- Obesity with decrease in alveolar ventilation (pickwickian syndrome)
- Primary or idiopathic alveolar hypoventilation

Modified from Klahr SK, Hamm L. In Klahr S, editor: *Renal and electrolyte disorders*, ed 2, Norwalk, CT, 1984, Appleton-Century-Crofts.

alveolar ventilation. Hyperventilation may be caused by (1) increased neurochemical stimulation of the respiratory center and (2) iatrogenically assisted or controlled mechanical ventilation. Maintaining blood pH within normal limits as arterial P_{CO_2} and thus H_2CO_3 decrease requires that plasma HCO_3^- decrease. The release of H^+ from body buffers reduces plasma HCO_3^- levels. Changes in cellular metabolism also increase the production of lactic acid and probably other organic acids. In general, plasma HCO_3^- levels decrease about 2.5 mmol/L for each decrement of 10 mm Hg in arterial P_{CO_2} below normal. In respiratory alkalosis, HCO_3^- values may occasionally decrease to as low as 15 mmol/L or arterial P_{CO_2} to as low as 15 mm Hg, but metabolic acidosis should always be suspected when the plasma HCO_3^- value is less than 18 mmol/L. The other line of defense in respiratory alkalosis is a diminished rate of H^+ secretion into the tubular fluid, leading to a HCO_3^- diuresis that tends to restore pH toward normal. Ammonium excretion decreases, resulting in decreased de novo synthesis of HCO_3^-. This renal adaptation to respiratory alkalosis occurs rapidly and is usually complete within 24 hours.[5]

Clinical Features and Systemic Effects. Respiratory alkalosis may cause neuromuscular irritability. Vasoconstriction of the cerebral circulation occurs, with reduced blood flow to the brain. Blood pressure and pulmonary vascular resistance are decreased, and pulmonary flow and cardiac output are increased. Patients may complain of paresthesias in the perioral region and extremities, muscle cramps, and tinnitus. In some patients, tetany and seizures occur, and an increase in deep tendon reflexes is present. Marked alkalosis may result in cardiac arrhythmias.[5]

Laboratory Findings. There is a decrease in the P_{CO_2} of body fluids. Thus the arterial pH is elevated, and the plasma HCO_3^- value decreases as a compensatory mechanism. The serum electrolyte levels remain within normal limits unless another disorder is present. The electrocardiogram (ECG) may show flattening or inversion of ST segments or T waves. The impaired release of oxygen from hemoglobin, caused by the shift in the oxyhemoglobin dissociation curve, may account for the ECG abnormalities in hypocapnia. A rise in blood concentrations of lactic acid and pyruvic acids in response to the reduction in P_{CO_2} has been frequently observed. The clinician should consider the development of an HCO_3^- deficit in the presence of a simultaneous rise in the concentrations of lactic and pyruvic acids in patients with respiratory alkalosis, since this HCO_3^- deficit may be confused with the findings seen in metabolic acidosis with an increased anion gap.

Causes. Box 145-3 lists the causes of respiratory alkalosis. It is important to note that the acid-base disorder produced by pulmonary disease depends on the severity of that disease.

Treatment. Effective therapy corrects or ameliorates the basic disorder responsible for the hyperventilation. The correction of hypoxemia is critical. If the respiratory alkalosis is related to mechanical ventilation, decreasing the minute ventilation or increasing the dead space may be effective. If this cannot be done without compromising oxygenation, the use of an inhaled mixture containing 3% CO_2 may be helpful.

Mixed Acid-Base Disorders

The entities described—metabolic acidosis or alkalosis and respiratory acidosis or alkalosis—represent simple acid-base disturbances. They denote the presence of one primary process and its appropriate physiologic response. A *mixed acid-base disturbance* refers to the coexistence of two or more primary processes.[4] Since these processes may have either additive or nullifying effects on plasma pH, mixed acid-base disturbances may produce dramatically extreme deviations of H^+ concentration or disarmingly minor or undetectable deviations.

The coexistence of two or more simple acid-base disturbances is quite common in hospitalized patients.[1,4] A mixed acid-base disturbance is frequently suspected from a careful analysis of the acid-base values. When the magnitude of the secondary change in P_{CO_2} or HCO_3^- concentrations (in metabolic and respiratory disorders, respectively) is inappropriate with respect to the magnitude of the initiating process, the presence of a mixed disturbance should be considered (Table 145-2). Even when a seemingly appropriate relationship exists between an initiating disturbance and an anticipated secondary response, such a relationship may merely be the consequence of a dual or even a triple acid-base abnormality. To avoid this diagnostic pitfall, the clinician should seek clues to the presence of complicating acid-base disturbances from a close examination of other laboratory data and particularly from the patient's history.[1,4]

Chronic respiratory acidosis may coexist with metabolic alkalosis, particularly in patients with pulmonary insufficiency and cor pulmonale treated with diuretics and a low-salt diet. This disturbance can also emerge when longstanding hypercapnia is partially corrected by mechanical ventilation or another means.[1,4]

A combination of chronic and acute respiratory acidosis may be seen in patients with moderately severe CO_2 retention caused by chronic obstructive lung disease who also experience a sudden worsening of pulmonary function from the use of sedatives capable of depressing the respiratory center, correction of their hypoxia by oxygen therapy, or concomitant acute pulmonary infections.

Metabolic acidosis plus acute respiratory acidosis is common in patients with acute cardiopulmonary arrest and results from lactic acidosis (triggered by poor tissue perfusion) and CO_2 retention. A similar presentation may be seen in patients with severe, acute pulmonary edema. Extreme decreases in plasma pH may be seen under these conditions.

Box 145-3. Causes of Respiratory Alkalosis

Central Nervous System

Voluntary hyperventilation, anxiety-hyperventilation syndrome
Cerebrovascular accident, infection, trauma, tumor

Hypoxia

High altitude, hypotension
Inequality of ventilation/perfusion ratio

Drugs or Hormones

Salicylates, nicotine, xanthines
Pressor hormones
Progesterone

Pulmonary Diseases

Interstitial fibrosis, pneumonia, pulmonary edema, pulmonary embolism

Miscellaneous

Anemia
Pregnancy
Hepatic failure
Gram-negative septicemia
Exposure to heat
Mechanical overventilation

Modified from Valtin H, Gennari EJ. In *Acid-base disorders: basic concepts and clinical management,* Boston, 1987, Little, Brown.

FLUID AND ELECTROLYTE DISORDERS

Disorders of Potassium: Homeostasis

Potassium is a cation located predominantly in the intracellular space. Total body potassium values approximate 3600 mmol, with the extracellular space containing only 65 to 70 mmol. Approximately 100 mmol of potassium is ingested daily in the average American diet. Under normal circumstances, 90% of this amount is excreted in the urine (80 to 90 mmol daily) and 10% in the stools (8 to 15 mmol daily). Because potassium is located primarily in the intracellular space (98%), it is difficult to accurately monitor changes in body stores of this cation. The distribution of potassium between the intracellular and extracellular fluids affects the potassium concentration in the plasma. Potassium homeostasis is regulated mainly by the kidney. Potassium excretion by the kidney is influenced by acid-base status, anion excretion, urine flow rate, potassium intake, and levels of mineralocorticoids.[8]

Hypokalemia

Hypokalemia is usually defined as a plasma potassium concentration below 3.5 mEq/L. Hypokalemia may be relative or absolute.[8] Acid-base changes may shift potassium into cells, causing relative hypokalemia (lower plasma concentration) when in fact total body potassium concentrations may be normal. Absolute hypokalemia is a decrease of both intracellular and extracellular potassium concentrations. For a decline of 1 mmol/L in plasma potassium levels, the total potassium deficit may be 100 to 400 mmol.

Clinical Features and Systemic Effects. The organs usually affected by hypokalemia include skeletal muscle, heart, kidneys, and gastrointestinal tract. Clinical manifestations of mild hypokalemia may be subtle. A high degree of suspicion (history of vomiting, use of diuretics or laxatives, diarrhea) helps identify patients at risk. Most patients with plasma potassium levels below 2.5 mmol/L complain of moderate muscle weakness. When the potassium concentration falls below 1.5 mmol/L, areflexic paralysis may occur, and respiratory depression may be a threat to survival. Potassium also affects cardiac function. Acute potassium losses may cause hyperpolarization, since intracellular potassium levels may remain normal as extracellular potassium levels fall. This situation may cause premature ventricular

Table 145-2. Usual Magnitude of Compensatory Mechanism in Acid-Base Disorders

Disorder	Compensatory mechanism
Metabolic acidosis	Pco_2 should decrease by 1.0-1.5 mm Hg for every 1 mEq/L fall in HCO_3^-.
Metabolic alkalosis	Pco_2 should increase by 0.5-1.0 mm Hg for every 1 mEq/L rise in HCO_3^-.
Acute respiratory acidosis	HCO_3^- concentration increases but seldom above 30 mEq/L.
Chronic respiratory acidosis	HCO_3^- concentration should increase by 4 mEq/L for every 10 mm Hg rise in Pco_2.
Respiratory alkalosis	HCO_3^- concentration should decrease by 2.5 mEq/L for every 10 mm Hg fall in Pco_2; HCO_3^- seldom falls below 16-18 mEq/L.

From Klahr S, Hamm L. In Klahr S, editor: *Renal and electrolyte disorders,* ed 2, Norwalk, Conn, 1984, Appleton-Century-Crofts.

contractions, frequent ectopic tachycardias, and widening of the QRS complex. With small changes in the intracellular potassium concentration, which is related to myocardial contractility, cardiac output begins to fall. Significant changes in the ECG, including early depression of the ST segment with a decreased amplitude of the T wave, may be present. U waves, as well as first-degree atrioventricular block, may also be present. As intracellular potassium values decrease further, contractility progressively declines, leading to marked ventricular irregularity and profound heart failure. Potassium depletion also decreases gastric and small intestinal motility and may cause paralytic ileus. Severe prolonged potassium depletion causes histologic changes in the kidney and an inability to concentrate the urine, resulting in polyuria, polydipsia, and nocturia.

Causes. Box 145-4 lists the causes of hypokalemia. In hypokalemic patients, it is important to assess blood pressure and the ECF volume status. Also, when hypokalemia is severe (plasma potassium level below 3 mmol/L), the clinician should consider causes other than, or in addition to, diuretic therapy. The determination of potassium excretion in the urine is important. Usually, individuals with hypokalemia caused by losses of potassium via the gastrointestinal tract have a urine potassium concentration less than 15 mmol/day. Magnesium depletion also may cause hypokalemia. Fig. 145-2 outlines the evaluation of hypokalemia.

Treatment. In most patients, correction of the potassium deficit is advised. Since potassium is located mainly intracellularly, it is difficult to judge the total deficit of potassium. The rapidity of potassium replacement depends on the chronicity of the disorder, the presence of other fluid and electrolyte abnormalities, and the presence and severity of end-organ sequelae of the hypokalemia. Specific salt use to replace a potassium deficit is important. With alkalosis, potassium must be replaced as potassium chloride. When hypokalemia is associated with metabolic acidosis, as in RTA or diabetic ketoacidosis, potassium replacement by potassium bicarbonate ($KHCO_3$) or a $KHCO_3$ equivalent (potassium citrate or gluconate) can be effective. When derangements of hypokalemia are not life threatening, oral replacement of potassium is usually indicated. When intravenous potassium replacement is required, a rate of 10 mmol/hr without monitoring is safe. However, doses of 40 mmol/hr or higher should be given only with close ECG monitoring. Hypokalemia related to diuretic use, when diuretic therapy is necessary, may require the administration of potassium-sparing drugs such as triamterene or amiloride. These are usually more effective in correcting hypokalemia than potassium supplementation alone and also prevent concurrent magnesium loss by diuretics.

Hyperkalemia

Hyperkalemia is defined as a plasma potassium level higher than 5 mmol/L. It is a relatively uncommon clinical entity but has potentially lethal consequences.[2,6] Hyperkalemia can be classified as relative or absolute. Relative hyperkalemia occurs with shifts of intracellular potassium to the extracellular fluid space without an increase in total body potassium values. Absolute hyperkalemia is present when both intracellular and extracellular potassium concentrations are increased.

Box 145-4. Causes of Hypokalemia

Gastrointestinal Causes

Decreased potassium intake: starvation, anorexia nervosa
Loss of hydrochloric acid: vomiting from pyloric stenosis or gastroenteritis, gastric aspiration without adequate replacement
Defective potassium absorption
- Fistulas: biliary, pancreatic, gastrocolic
- Zollinger-Ellison syndrome, malabsorption
- Postgastrectomy dumping syndrome
- Inflammatory bowel disease: regional enteritis, ulcerative colitis

Increased intestinal secretion of potassium: diarrhea (usually infectious), villous adenomas
Iatrogenic lesions: laxative use, repeated enemas, use of exchange resins

Renal Causes

Diuretic therapy: loop diuretics, thiazides, carbonic anhydrase inhibitors
Antibiotic therapy: carbenicillin, gentamicin, amphotericin B
Renal tubular or parenchymal diseases: renal tubular acidosis; proximal and distal types; Fanconi's syndrome; chronic pyelonephritis

Renal Causes

Magnesium depletion
Adrenal steroids
Primary hyperaldosteronism (aldosteronism): adrenal adenomas, adrenal hyperplasia, 17-α-hydroxylase or 11-β-hydroxylase deficiencies, dexamethasone or glucocorticosteroid-suppressible hyperaldosteronism
Secondary hyperaldosteronism: associated with decreased "effective plasma volume" cirrhosis, congestive heart failure, or hypoalbuminemia; Bartter's syndrome; associated with malignant hypertension
Cushing's syndrome: excessive adrenocorticotropic hormone (ACTH) production from anterior pituitary gland, exogenous ACTH production (malignancy), exogenous cortisol production (malignancy)
Adrenal steroid therapy
Licorice ingestion

Miscellaneous Causes Related to Intracellular Shifts of Potassium

Systemic alkalosis, either respiratory or metabolic
Infusion of large amounts of glucose or insulin therapy
Familial hypokalemic paralysis
Ingestion of barium salts
Vitamin B_{12} therapy in patients with pernicious anemia

Modified from Harter H. In Klahr S, editor: *Renal and electrolyte disorders*, ed 2, Norwalk, CT, 1984, Appleton-Century-Crofts.

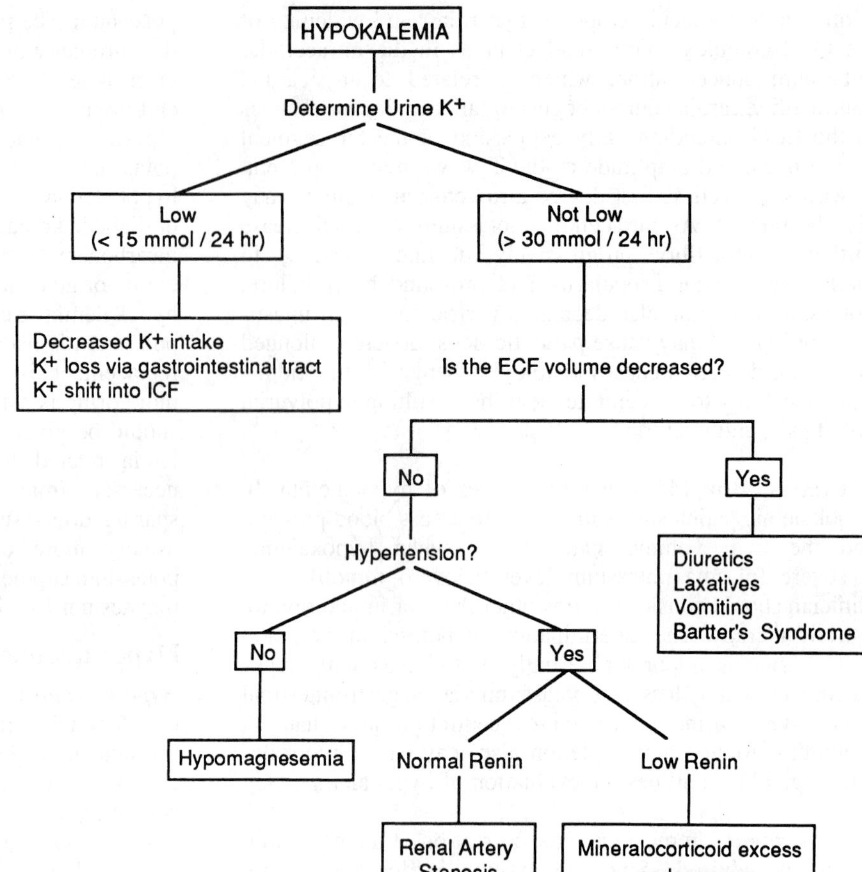

Fig. 145-2. Evaluation of hypokalemia.

Clinical Manifestations and Systemic Effects. Patients with hyperkalemia develop cardiovascular and neuromuscular abnormalities. Cardiac contractility is not affected by hyperkalemia, but significant arrhythmias may occur because of changes in conduction. ECG changes usually occur when plasma potassium levels exceed 7 mmol/L. With modest increases in plasma potassium, tall, peaked T waves are seen with a normal QT interval, and decreased amplitude of the P waves occurs with a prolonged PR interval. As hyperkalemia progresses, atrial asystole is seen, with widening of the QRS complex leading to a sine wave. Finally, plasma potassium concentrations higher than 10 mmol/L lead to ventricular standstill. The effects of hyperkalemia on cardiac function can occur with smaller increases in plasma potassium values when hyponatremia, hypocalcemia, or acidosis is present. Changes in muscle strength or nerve conduction velocity also occur, particularly when potassium levels exceed 8 mmol/L. Muscular weakness develops, usually beginning in the lower extremities and ascending to the upper extremities. Respiratory depression may occur.

Causes. Box 145-5 lists the most common causes of hyperkalemia. Acute and chronic renal failure account for most cases. Since the kidney is the major organ responsible for potassium excretion, a marked loss of renal function may cause hyperkalemia if dietary intake of potassium is not curtailed.[2,6] Increased catabolism also plays a role in the development of hyperkalemia in patients with acute renal failure. Hyperkalemia is usually not seen in patients with chronic renal failure unless excessive potassium is administered. Hyperkalemia may occur as a result of translocation of potassium from the intracellular to the extracellular space. This may be caused by acidosis, severe tissue catabolism, muscle breakdown (rhabdomyolysis), and familial hyperkalemic periodic paralysis. Since aldosterone is a major regulatory hormone of potassium homeostasis, its absence may lead to hyperkalemia. Although isolated aldosterone deficiency is exceedingly rare, primary adrenal insufficiency (Addison's disease) may be associated with severe depression of plasma aldosterone levels.

Addison's disease resulting from hypopituitarism is not associated with hyperkalemia, since aldosterone secretion rates remain normal. Addison's disease resulting from pathologic conditions of the adrenal gland may lead to hyperkalemia. In addition, patients with this condition may have hyperpigmentation, decreased appetite, hypoglycemia, and hypotension (see Chapter 98). Hyponatremia and renal sodium wasting may also be observed. In hyporeninemic hypoaldosteronism, hyperkalemia may occur because of deficient aldosterone secretion and decreased secretion of potassium in the distal tubule. Approximately 50% of patients with hyporeninemic hypoaldosteronism have associated diabetes. About 50% of these patients achieve lower potassium levels with improved diabetic control. Spironolactones, aldosterone antagonists, or potassium-sparing diuretics may also cause hyperkalemia.

Box 145-5. Causes of Hyperkalemia

Acute or Severe Chronic Renal Failure

Continued potassium intake, acidosis, increased catabolism, administration of potassium-containing solutions, gastrointestinal bleeding, hemolysis, volume depletion

Translocation of Potassium from Intracellular to Extracellular Fluid Space

Acidosis, severe catabolism, rhabdomyolysis, familial hyperkalemic periodic paralysis, depolarizing muscle paralysis (succinylcholine therapy)

Mineralocorticoid Deficiency States

Addison's disease, hyporeninemic hypoaldosteronism

Aldosterone Antagonists or Potassium-sparing Diuretics

Spironolactone, triamterene

Other Medications

Nonsteroidal antiinflammatory drugs (NSAIDs), β-blockers, angiotensin-converting enzyme (ACE) inhibitors, trimethoprim

Miscellaneous

"Pseudohyperkalemia" of myeloproliferative disorders (hyperkalemia associated with thrombocytosis or granulocytosis), hemolysis at blood sampling, intravenous potassium

Modified from Harter H. In Klahr S, editor: *Renal and electrolyte disorders*, ed 2, Norwalk, Conn, 1984, Appleton-Century-Crofts.

Treatment. The treatment of hyperkalemia differs based on the level of plasma potassium, the chronicity of the hyperkalemic state, and clinical manifestations. In acute hyperkalemia, if the potassium concentration is less than 6.5 mmol/L and there are no ECG changes, potassium intake should be decreased and drugs that compromise potassium excretion discontinued. With greater levels of potassium or pertinent ECG changes, other measures are necessary. Calcium administration may reverse several effects of hyperkalemia. The effects of calcium therapy are seen within minutes, but they are short-lived, about half an hour. The redistribution of potassium from the extracellular to the intracellular space is also an effective treatment for hyperkalemia. This can be accomplished by the administration of $NaHCO_3$, one or two ampules (44 to 88 mmol) given intravenously, or by the infusion of glucose and insulin. A solution of 500 ml of 10% glucose with 10 units of regular insulin is an adequate dose for the latter treatment. The effects of glucose and insulin therapy are seen within 30 minutes and last for several hours. A β-agonist such as albuterol used as a nebulizer at doses of 10 to 20 mg lowers the serum potassium concentration by approximately 0.6 mmol/L. The effect of albuterol occurs within 30 minutes and persists for at least 2 hours. Restoration of extracellular volume may correct hyperkalemia. Potassium can be removed from the body using exchange resins such as sodium polystyrene sulfonate (Kayexalate), which can be administered orally or rectally. Hemodialysis or peritoneal dialysis can also be used to remove potassium. The effect of dialysis on plasma potassium is seen within hours, and its duration depends on the rate of the endogenous release of potassium.

Hyponatremia

Hyponatremia is defined as a serum sodium concentration below 135 mmol/L. It does not necessarily indicate a decrease in total body sodium levels.[10] Since the concentration of sodium depends on the relative amounts of sodium and water in the ECF, a low serum sodium concentration indicates only that there is relatively more water than sodium in this space. This may occur when ECF sodium content is decreased, such as with diarrhea, in which losses of both sodium and water occur but the sodium losses are greater than those of water. When the ECF sodium content is normal (e.g., with excess administration of water) or when the ECF sodium content is increased (e.g., with edema), increases in both sodium and water content occur. Fig. 145-3 summarizes an approach to the patient with hyponatremia.

Hyponatremia may occur in the setting of an expanded, normal, or contracted ECF volume.[10] Excess water in the ECF may result from excessive intake or reduced excretion of water. Increased ingestion of water may occur as a result of compulsive polydipsia, acute psychosis, excessive parenteral administration of fluids, use of tap water enemas, or postoperative irrigation of the prostatic bed with hyponatremic solutions. Reduced excretion of water may result from intrinsic renal disease or extrinsic factors that modify the kidneys' ability to excrete water, such as the syndrome of inappropriate antidiuretic hormone (SIADH) (see Chapter 99), congestive heart failure, and cirrhosis. The first step in the evaluation of hyponatremia is to rule out hyperglycemia, hyperproteinemia, and hyperlipidemia as potential reasons for the pseudohyponatremia. With true hyponatremia, the osmolality of plasma is low. If sodium loss is the cause of the hyponatremia, urine sodium and chloride concentrations are less than 20 mmol/L. If the major reason for the hyponatremia is water excess, the excretion of a volume of 1 L hourly of dilute urine, 50 to 75 mOsm/kg water, is to be expected.

Clinical Manifestations and Systemic Effects. Patients with hyponatremia rarely have symptoms unless the plasma sodium level is below 125 mmol/L and unless hyponatremia has developed rapidly. The typical symptoms relate to osmotic swelling of brain cells and vary from mild lethargy to convulsions and coma. There may also be gastrointestinal symptoms such as anorexia and nausea.

Treatment. Treatment depends on whether the condition is acute or chronic. In acute hyponatremia, neurologic symptoms are more often seen in young female patients in the postoperative state, in elderly people receiving thiazide diuretics, and in patients with psychogenic polydipsia. These patients should be treated promptly to prevent cerebral edema and seizures. Rapid correction through the intravenous administration of sodium, 1.5 to 2.0 mM/L/hr in this setting, may be associated with a lower mortality rate than slower correction (0.6 mM/L/hour). However, central pontine myelinolysis may occur with too-rapid correction of marked hyponatremia.[7] The correction can be accomplished with hypertonic saline, preferably given with furosemide to prevent sodium overload and to enhance water excretion. Symptomatic chronic hyponatremia is best

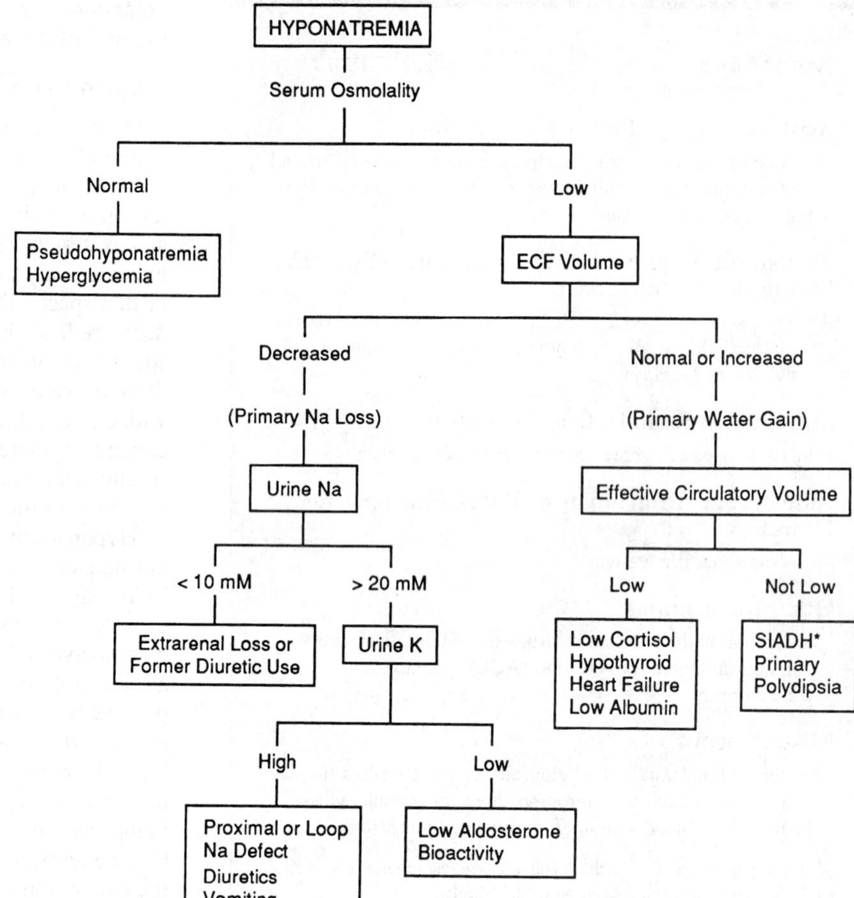

Fig. 145-3. Evaluation of hyponatremia. *SIADH*, Syndrome of inappropriate antidiuretic hormone (ADH) release.

managed conservatively with water restriction even when the serum sodium concentration is very low. Prolonged water restriction may be difficult to enforce, and therefore agents that antagonize the renal action of ADH have been used. Demeclocycline is safer and more effective than lithium in the treatment of SIADH.

Hypernatremia

Hypernatremia is marked by plasma sodium concentrations in excess of 145 mmol/L. Disturbances of either sodium or water metabolism cause hypernatremia.[3] This usually results from sodium gain or water loss. Physiologically, hypernatremia results in a decrease in cell volume. Hypernatremia is not a specific clinical entity. The clinician should look for the underlying cause of the increase in serum sodium concentration. Most often, hypernatremia is caused by water loss from renal or extrarenal sources. Daily obligatory fluid loss is related to evaporative losses through the lungs and skin plus the amount of water necessary to excrete the solutes in the urine. These obligatory fluid losses amount to about 1300 ml/day, or approximately 10% of the ECF volume. Obligatory sodium losses are much smaller. Daily losses of sodium in sweat and feces normally are less than 20 mmol. Urine sodium concentration can be reduced to below 5 mmol daily so that sodium loss can be reduced if necessary to an amount equal to less than 1% of the sodium pool in the ECF. If the daily losses of sodium and water are not replaced, the negative water balance exceeds that for sodium, and the sodium concentration in the extracellular space increases progressively. If the patient has fever or is in a high environmental temperature, the situation is aggravated because all these conditions increase evaporative water losses more than sodium loss. Water is not replaced in patients with nausea, vomiting, or dysphagia, who experience thirst consequent to the hypernatremia and are unable to increase their fluid intake appropriately. Comatose patients or those with cerebrovascular accidents (strokes) may not be aware of thirst or may not be able to communicate their needs. They depend on others for adequate fluid intake. Infants are particularly susceptible to hypernatremia. Their surface area per unit of body mass is much greater than that of the adult, so their evaporative water losses are greater. In addition, infants' ability to concentrate their urine is incompletely developed, increasing obligatory water losses.

When the major problem is loss of water in excess of sodium loss, volume contraction usually occurs, and laboratory studies show evidence of hemoconcentration with increasing hematocrit and serum protein concentrations. BUN and serum creatinine concentrations may be elevated. Unless the patient has coexistent renal disease, the urine output is low, less than 500 ml/day, and the urine is hyperosmolar, in excess of 1000 mOsm/kg water, with a very low urine sodium concentration. Failure to find a very low urine volume and a maximally concentrated urine suggests a renal problem.

The major renal causes of hypernatremia are diabetes insipidus (see Chapter 99) and an osmotic diuresis. These two disorders can be distinguished by measuring urine osmolality.

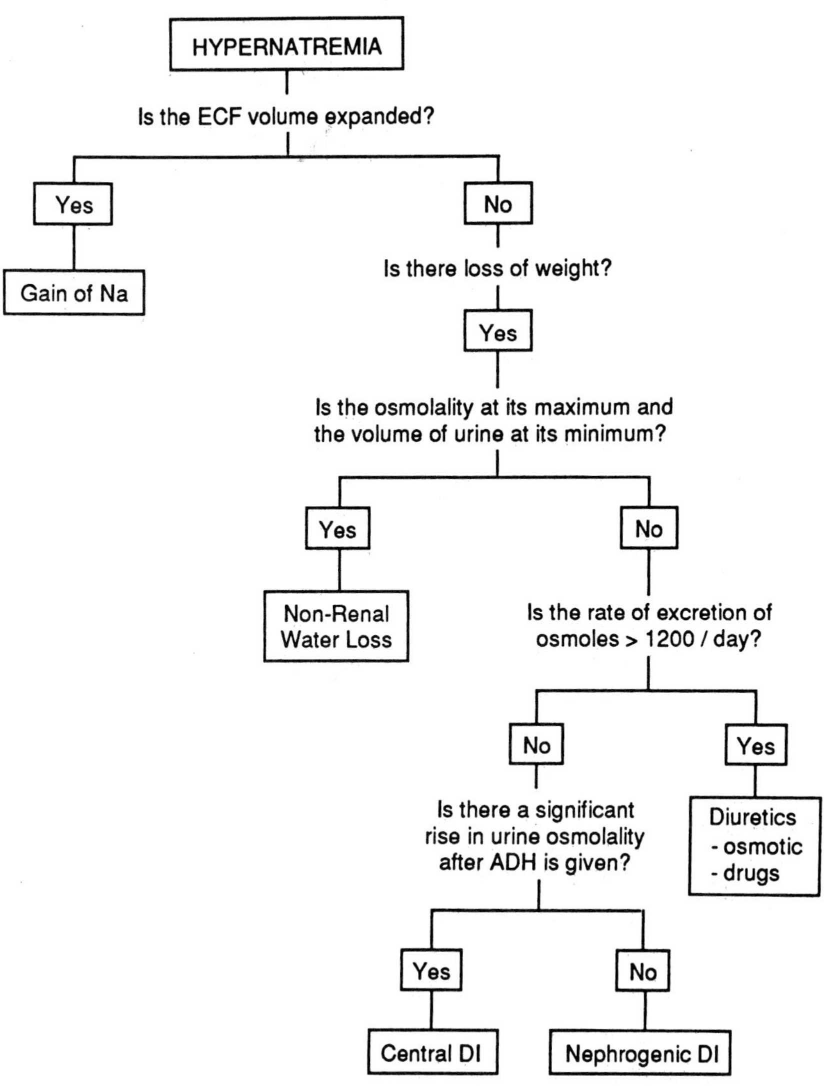

Fig. 145-4. Evaluation of hypernatremia.

When thirst is absent in patients with hypernatremia, a central nervous system lesion should be considered. Hypernatremia caused by sodium excess is rare. Usually, it is characterized by ECF volume expansion, thirst, and the excretion of small volumes of very concentrated urine. If the hypernatremia results from water loss of extrarenal origin and the patient does not have access to water, he or she will be thirsty and excrete a minimal volume of maximally concentrated urine. If the cause of the hypernatremia is loss of water via the kidney, the urine will not be concentrated and the urine volume will not be decreased. In this setting, two major diseases may be present: diabetes insipidus (central or nephrogenic) or diuretic-induced water loss (usually osmotic diuresis from glucose or urea). Fig. 145-4 summarizes an approach to the patient with hypernatremia.

Clinical Manifestations and Systemic Effects. As with hyponatremia, the principal clinical manifestations relate to osmotic effects on the brain. In hypernatremia, there is dehydration of brain cells, which leads to symptoms ranging from confusion to convulsions and coma. The intensity of the symptoms correlates with both the severity and the rapidity of development of the hypernatremia.

Treatment. The primary goal is the restoration of serum tonicity. The following principles are helpful. If the patient is hypervolemic and hypernatremic, excess sodium should be removed, which can be achieved by the intravenous administration of diuretics along with 5% dextrose. If renal function is impaired, dialysis may be needed. If the patient has a low total body sodium concentration, isotonic NaCl should be given until systemic hemodynamics are stabilized. Hypernatremia is then treated with half-normal saline or 5% dextrose. The patient who is hypernatremic but euvolemic and therefore has sustained water losses almost exclusively requires replacement of water with a 5% dextrose infusion.

REFERENCES

1. Abelon B: *Understanding acid base,* Baltimore, 1998, Williams & Wilkins.
2. Allon M: Hyperkalemia in end-stage renal disease: mechanisms and management, *J Am Soc Nephrol* 6:1134, 1995.
3. Feig PU: Hypernatremia and hypertonic syndromes, *Med Clin North Am* 65:271, 1981.
4. Ham L: Mixed acid-base disorder. In Kokko JP, Tannen RL, editors: *Fluids and electrolytes,* ed 3, Philadelphia, 1996, WB Saunders, pp 343–357.

5. Molony DA, Schiess MC, Dosekun AK: Respiratory acid base disorders. In Kokko JP, Tannen RL, editors: *Fluids and electrolytes,* ed 3, Philadelphia, 1996, WB Saunders, pp 267–342.
6. Peterson LN, Levi M: Disorders of potassium metabolism. In Schrier RW, editor: *Renal and electrolyte disorders,* ed 5, 1997, Lippincott-Raven, pp 192–240.
7. Sterns RH, Cappuccio JD, Silver SM, et al: Neurologic sequelae after treatment of severe hyponatremia: a multicenter perspective, *J Am Soc Nephrol* 4:1522, 1994.
8. Sterns RH, Spital A: Disorders of internal potassium balance, *Semin Nephrol* 7:206, 1987.
9. Toto RD, Alpern RJ, Metabolic acid-base disorders. In Kokko JP, Tannen RL, editors: *Fluids and electrolytes,* ed 3, Philadelphia, 1996, WB Saunders, pp 201–266.
10. Verbalis JG: Hyponatremia epidemiology, pathophysiology and therapy, *Curr Opin Nephrol Hypertens* 2:636, 1993.

CHAPTER 146

Urinary Tract Infections

Bahar Bastani

Urinary tract infection (UTI) is the most common bacterial infection affecting humans. Up to one third of all female patients experience at least one episode of UTI in their lives. UTIs occur in all ages, neonatal to geriatric; they have a particular impact on female patients, male patients at the two extremes of life (infancy and after 50 years of age), and anyone with functional or structural abnormalities of the urinary tract. The infection may be limited to one part of or extend throughout the urinary tract and may involve the perinephric tissues. Although the bacteriology and pathogenesis of UTI may be the same, the clinical features, the risk of acute or chronic complications, and the treatment vary depending on where the infection is and whether functional or structural abnormalities are present.

EPIDEMIOLOGY AND ETIOLOGY

Definitions and Terminologies

Despite the pitfalls and difficulties in determining bacteriologic localization, the UTIs have conventionally been classified into those involving the upper vs. the lower urinary tract. Each category is further divided into uncomplicated vs. complicated UTI, depending on the absence or presence of host conditions known to promote infection, account for persistence of infection, or promote recurrence of infection. Although the majority of the uncomplicated UTIs occur in young women and are community acquired, complicated UTIs occur in patients with anatomic or urologic abnormalities or with recent urinary catheterization or instrumentation, involve both sexes, and are often hospital acquired. The complicated UTIs are associated with a higher incidence of antimicrobial resistance, a poorer response to therapy, and a higher risk of renal damage, urosepsis, and abscess formation.[10,11,13]

The lower UTIs include cystitis, prostatitis, and urethritis (Box 146-1). Atrophic vaginitis; sexually transmitted diseases caused by *Chlamydia trachomatis, Neisseria gonorrhoeae,* or herpes simplex; and vaginal infections caused by *Candida albicans* or *Trichomonas* species can also present with dysuria and urinary frequency but are not considered UTIs (see Chapters 29 and 46).

Box 146-1. Classification of Urinary Tract Infections (UTIs)

Lower UTI: cystitis, urethritis, prostatitis
Upper UTI: acute or chronic pyelonephritis, renal or perirenal abscess
Uncomplicated lower or upper UTI
Complicated lower or upper UTI (risk of renal damage, urosepsis, abscess formation): presence of functional or anatomic abnormalities, obstruction, calculi/catheter/stent, pregnancy, hospitalization, immunosuppression, diabetes mellitus, sickle cell disease, analgesic/NSAID abuse
Acute urethral syndrome: dysuria/frequency with less than 10^5 colonies/ml of urine
Asymptomatic bacteriuria: asymptomatic with more than 10^5 colonies of the same bacteria per milliliter of clean-catch mid-stream urine

NSAID, Nonsteroidal antiinflammatory drug.

The upper UTIs, which are much less common, include acute or chronic pyelonephritis and renal or perirenal abscess. Acute pyelonephritis is a clinical diagnosis based on the presence of fever, flank tenderness, and bacteriuria. However, the diagnosis of chronic pyelonephritis is based on radiologic demonstration of calyceal clubbing and deformity associated with renal scarring, typically a sequela of bacterial infection superimposed on an anatomic abnormality of the urinary tract (e.g., obstruction, more often vesicoureteral reflux).

The term *acute urethral syndrome* (also called the *dysuria-pyuria syndrome*) describes women with signs and symptoms suggestive of lower UTI but less than 10^5 colonies/ml of urine. Between 30% and 50% of all patients with dysuria have this condition. *Asymptomatic bacteriuria* refers to the presence of more than 10^5 colonies of the same bacterial species per milliliter of urine in two consecutive midstream urine cultures and in the absence of any signs or symptoms of UTI.

Incidence and Prevalence

Except during the newborn period, when the incidence of UTI in both symptomatic and asymptomatic infants is much greater in boys than in girls, in all other age groups, UTIs occur much more frequently in female patients. The incidence of UTI, which only occasionally occurs in prepubertal girls, greatly increases in late adolescence and during the third and fourth decades of life. Approximately one third of women 20 to 40 years of age develop signs and symptoms suggestive of UTI. During the reproductive years, women are 20 to 50 times more likely to acquire UTI than men. It is more common in sexually active women, and its incidence increases with age. The difference in the incidence of UTI between men and women diminishes in later life. In the older age group, hospitalization for other illnesses is frequently associated with urinary catheterization and the acquisition of nosocomial UTI. Hospitalization and catheterization increase the risk of infection in both sexes.

Uropathogenic Bacteria

Most UTIs are caused by bacteria that originate from flora in the lower gut.[10,11,13] *Escherichia coli,* normally present in large quantities in the feces, accounts for 80% to 90% of uncomplicated community-based UTIs. The same strain of *E. coli* recovered from infected urine is usually also recovered from the patient's periurethra, vagina, and rectum. However, not all *E. coli* strains are uropathogenic, and a relatively small number of strains that possess certain virulence factors cause most UTIs.

Other enteric gram-negative bacteria (such as *Klebsiella pneumoniae, Enterobacter aerogenes,* and *Proteus* species) and gram-positive bacteria (such as *Enterococcus faecalis* and *Staphylococcus saprophyticus*) are also common uropathogens. However, anaerobic bacteria, which are present in much greater abundance in the gut flora, only rarely produce UTI.

Although the urethra, periurethra, introitus, and vagina do not normally contain significant quantities of the uropathogenic bacteria, in women with recurrent UTI, a heavy colonization with the uropathogenic bacteria precedes or is associated with the episodes of UTI. Table 146-1 shows the frequency of different uropathogenic bacteria in uncomplicated community-acquired and complicated hospital-associated UTIs.

S. saprophyticus is the second most common pathogen isolated from young women. It accounts for 10% to 15% of uncomplicated lower UTIs, especially during summer and autumn. The bacterial counts with this organism are often less than 10^5 colonies/ml of urine. Its pathogenic role at this low titer has been supported by the finding of 10^2 to 10^4 colonies/ml in bladder urine obtained via suprapubic aspiration in symptomatic young women.

Among gram-negative microorganisms, *Proteus mirabilis* is particularly important because it produces the enzyme urease, which splits urea into carbon dioxide and ammonia. This process results in alkalinization of urine and leads to the formation of struvite stones that entrap the bacteria, protecting them from antimicrobial agents (see Chapter 147). The continued growth of bacteria leads to further urinary alkalinization and the precipitation of struvite crystals, resulting in the formation of massive staghorn stones.

Since the contamination of urine samples by bacteria normally present in the anterior urethra or periurethra occurs often, especially in women, a bacterial count of greater than 10^5 colonies/ml from a clean-catch midstream urine has been traditionally used to distinguish genuine bladder bacteriuria from contamination. In men, since contamination of carefully collected urine is less common, a count greater than 10^4 colonies/ml of urine with the same organism has been considered adequate for diagnosing bladder bacteriuria. However, prospective studies of women with recurrent UTI have shown that bacterial counts of less than 10^5 colonies/ml may be responsible for symptoms on some occasions. Moreover, some recent studies have demonstrated that in about one third of women with acute lower UTI caused by *E. coli, S. saprophyticus,* and *Proteus* species, there are of 10^2 to 10^4 colonies/ml in midstream urine. Similarly, acute pyelonephritis has been reported in association with low bacterial counts in voided urine. Thus many cases of the acute urethral syndrome are in fact bacterial UTIs with low colony counts, and they respond to the usual antibiotics.

Genuine mixed infections with a significant number of different microorganisms occur infrequently except in catheterized patients and those with ileal conduit, stones, neurogenic bladder, or vesicocolonic fistula. The presence of mixed infection is best confirmed by culture of urine samples obtained via sterile catheterization or suprapubic aspiration.

Table 146-1. Prevalence of Microorganisms in Uncomplicated Outpatient vs. Complicated Hospital-associated UTIs

Microorganism	Uncomplicated (%)	Complicated (%)
Escherichia coli	80.0	32.0
Klebsiella species	2.0-5.0	7.5
Enterobacter species	2.0	4.5
Proteus species	2.0	7.5
Pseudomonas aeruginosa	0	12.5
Citrobacter species	0	1.5
Serratia species	0	1.0
Enterococci	1.0	15.0
Staphylococcus epidermidis	0	3.5
Staphylococcus saprophyticus	10.0-15.0	0
Staphylococcus aureus	0	1.5
Group B streptococci	0	1.0
Bacteroides and other anaerobes	0	Very rare
Candida species	0	5.0

Host Susceptibility and Bacterial Virulence Factors

Several systemic and local factors increase host susceptibility for developing UTI.[10,11,13] Malnutrition, diabetes mellitus, an altered immune system, local receptor characteristics of uroepithelial cells, the presence of foreign bodies (stone, stent, catheter), urine stasis (obstruction or neuromuscular dysfunction such as neurogenic bladder), and congenital or acquired abnormalities (ureterovesical reflux, bladder diverticula) all predispose patients to develop UTI. Other risk factors include lack of circumcision in infants and young sexually active men, insertive anal intercourse, and the use of diaphragm and spermicides by sexually active women.

Bacterial virulence factors are bacterial characteristics that facilitate infection of the urinary tract. These include bacterial adherence, capsular K antigens, endotoxins, resistance to serum bactericidal effects, hemolysin production and iron-binding proteins, and finally the ability to produce urease enzyme.

Bacterial selective adherence to genitourinary mucosal surfaces can influence the degree of colonization by rendering the organisms resistant to being washed out by the urinary flow. The presence of adhesins on the bacterial fimbriae (pili), which recognize their specific receptors in some humans' uroepithelial cells, plays the most important role in bacterial adherence and colonization leading to infection.

E. coli elaborates a capsular antigen also called *K antigen.* Certain K antigens, when expressed in high quantities, can determine the degree of virulence of the strain (i.e. whether the organisms can produce pyelonephritis or only cystitis).

The toxic properties of gram-negative bacteria relate to the endotoxins present in the bacterial wall called *lipopolysaccharide-containing lipid A*. Lipid A is immunogenic and induces antibodies that cross-react among different gram-negative bacteria and thus decrease the frequency of shock and death in patients with gram-negative sepsis.

Many strains of gram-negative bacteria are killed in the presence of fresh human serum via a process that involves the activation of complement pathways. *E. coli* strains isolated from patients with acute pyelonephritis or acute cystitis have been found to be significantly more serum resistant than strains normally found in the feces.

Since bacteria require iron, their ability to release hemolysin, resulting in hemolysis of the host erythrocytes and release of hemoglobin, and their iron-binding protein content are the other two important virulence factors.

Normal Defense Mechanisms of the Urinary Tract

A variety of specific and nonspecific mechanisms protect the urinary tract against microbial invasion. One of the nonspecific resistant mechanisms is the lactobacilli of the normal vaginal and introital flora, which interfere with the adhesion and thus colonization with the uropathogenic *E. coli*. Another mechanism is a hydrophilic glycocalyx protein on the surface of the bladder epithelium, rendering it resistant to bacterial adherence. Moreover, Tamm-Horsfall glycoprotein in the urine binds to *E. coli* receptors and facilitates the removal of *E. coli* in the urine. Finally, the normal slow shedding of bladder epithelial cells is greatly increased during episodes of UTI, resulting in removal of a greater number of organisms from the urinary tract.

The specific immune responses in the urinary tract consist of urinary secretory immunoglobulin A (IgA), half of which originates in the urethra, providing a barrier to the ascent of bacteria, and IgG excretion, which is increased during acute pyelonephritis.

PATHOPHYSIOLOGY

Routes of Infection

Bacteria generally do not enter the urinary system by filtration. The three well-recognized routes of infection are (1) ascending infection, as with fecal microorganisms colonizing the periurethral area and subsequently entering the bladder via the urethra; (2) hematogenous spread, as in staphylococcal bacteremia and bacterial seeding of the renal cortex, resulting in abscess formation; and (3) direct extension, as with enterovesical fistula.[10,11,13]

Ascending transurethral infection is the most common route. The short female urethra offers little obstacle to the passage of uropathogenic bacteria, which have colonized the periurethral area, to the bladder. Sexual intercourse forces bacteria into the bladder, accounting for the increased incidence of UTIs in sexually active women. In male patients, the length of the urethra, the distance between the external urethral orifice and the perianal area, and the presence of antibacterial factors in prostatic secretions are all responsible for the reduced risk of infection. The presence of a foreskin, fecal incontinence, and poor toilet habits promote colonization by the fecal bacteria and contribute to the higher prevalence of infection seen in uncircumcised infants and young, sexually active men as well as elderly men with poor anal sphincter control. Catheterization or other instrumentation in either sex increases the risk of UTI, which has been reported to occur with a frequency of 1% after an acute bladder catheterization. In patients with indwelling bladder catheters and an open drainage system, infection invariably occurs within a few days.

Hematogeneous spread of bacteria, fungi, and mycobacteria from a distant focus of infection may invade the kidneys, bladder, or prostate. Renal cortical and perirenal abscesses caused by staphylococci or group A streptococci are frequently the result of bacteremia with a primary focus of infection in another organ.

Direct extension of bacteria from the gut into the bladder may occur via a colovesical fistula secondary to diverticulitis or colon cancer or via an enterovesical fistula, as in Crohn's disease. These infections are usually recurrent, polymicrobial (high titers of several different species of enteric bacteria present), and accompanied by pneumaturia (air in the urine) or fecaluria (fecal material in the urine).

HISTORY AND PHYSICAL FINDINGS

Symptoms and Signs of Lower vs. Upper UTI[10,11,13]

Acute bacterial cystitis produces inflammation of the bladder and urethra. The typical symptoms of uncomplicated lower UTI include dysuria, frequency, urgency, nocturia, voiding of small urine volumes, incontinence, and suprapubic or pelvic pain. Hematuria may occur and is usually at the termination of voiding; however, women may have total gross hematuria and may even pass clots. Patients may also complain of a foul-smelling or cloudy urine. Fever and flank tenderness occur infrequently in these patients.

With acute pyelonephritis, patients are generally sicker with flank or low back pain, chills, fever, sweats, nausea, vomiting, headache, and malaise. Patients often have symptoms of cystitis. Gross or microscopic hematuria is present in 10% to 15% of patients. Acute pyelonephritis may cause either a mild or a very severe illness that may include gram-negative septicemia, papillary necrosis, oliguric or anuric acute renal failure, and intrarenal or perirenal abscess formation. In 20% of these patients, bacteremia can be documented.

With complicated UTI, such as in hospitalized patients or those with indwelling catheters, the clinical manifestations can range from asymptomatic bacteriuria to a severe gram-negative sepsis with shock. Most of the catheter-associated UTIs are asymptomatic. Similarly, a high percentage of elderly patients who are institutionalized or community based without an indwelling bladder catheter may have asymptomatic bacteriuria. Complicated UTI can also present with signs and symptoms of acute cystitis or acute pyelonephritis. The hallmark of complicated UTI is the broader spectrum of microorganisms involved, which are generally more virulent and antibiotic resistant, have a lower clinical response rate to antimicrobial therapy, and tend to recur. It should be emphasized that in hospitalized patients who suddenly develop signs and symptoms of septic shock, urosepsis should be considered, even in the absence of urinary symptoms, particularly after a recent instrumentation or catheterization. Patients with complicated UTI are particularly prone to develop urosepsis, papillary necrosis, and renal or perirenal abscess.

Although clinicians usually use patients' signs and symptoms to differentiate upper from lower UTI, diagnosing the site of infection based on clinical signs can be quite inaccurate. Approximately one half of women with asymptomatic bacteriuria may have infection originating in the upper tract. Also, as many as one third of women with characteristic symptoms of uncomplicated acute cystitis may have subclinical infection of the upper urinary tract. Moreover, flank pain and tenderness with fever may be present in up to one third of patients documented to have lower UTI.

In some patients with recurrent infection, particularly the elderly, symptoms may be much less obvious, and the patient may only notice a slight change in frequency or "smelly urine" or may develop urinary incontinence or some vague abdominal pain.

Both acute and chronic bacterial prostatitis are associated with UTI. The diagnosis is often made on the basis of symptoms of dysuria; frequency; perineal, groin, or low back pain; and difficulty in urination and the finding of an enlarged, tender prostate gland. Relapsing UTI in men is highly suggestive of chronic bacterial prostatitis.

Physical Examination

With acute cystitis, about 10% of patients may have suprapubic tenderness, but there is generally no flank tenderness.

With acute pyelonephritis, the patient's temperature may rise to 104° F (40° C), the abdomen may be distended with hypotonic bowel sounds, and there is severe tenderness in the lumbar region. In bacteremic patients, signs of septic shock may be evident.

Except for women with clear-cut signs and symptoms of upper or lower UTI associated with significant pyuria and bacteriuria and a prompt response to the appropriate antimicrobial treatment, all other women need a careful pelvic examination to rule out other conditions presenting with acute dysuria and frequency or as acute pyelonephritis (see Differential Diagnosis).

In men with UTI symptoms, physical examination should include inspection and palpation of the genitals (including retraction of the foreskin in an uncircumcised man) for evidence of urethral discharge, meatal erythema, inflammation of the glans penis, penile lesions, enlarged or tender epididymis or testicle, and inguinal lymphadenopathy. A rectal examination with palpation of the prostate gland should be a standard part of the physical examination in all men with UTI symptoms. Evidence for prostate infection has been found in one half of men with relapsing UTI. In patients with acute bacterial prostatitis, the prostate gland is swollen, warm, and tender, whereas in those with chronic bacterial prostatitis, the gland is usually but not always tender and may feel slightly irregular. Massage of the prostate gland in patients with acute bacterial prostatitis may result in bacteremia and should be avoided.

Natural Course

In most women, acute cystitis is an isolated event that may never or rarely be repeated. The onset of sexual activity or change in sexual partner may coincide with the attack. In a small number of women, UTI may be recurrent, and the episodes may chronologically coincide with coitus. In many women, symptoms may disappear spontaneously as a result of high fluid intake. The response to antimicrobial agents is usually prompt. Acute symptoms disappear within 2 to 3 days. If untreated, in some patients, especially pregnant women or patients with obstruction, the infection may extend to the upper tract. Although lower UTI does not predispose the patient to kidney damage, the quality of life of the affected women can be seriously impaired.

With upper UTI, the presence or absence of complicating factors is critical in defining the natural course and renal sequelae. Uncomplicated upper UTI generally leaves no residual damage and can easily be treated with antimicrobial agents. Although severe renal infection can result in cortical scars, its long-term functional significance is not clear. The presence of complicating factors such as obstruction, particularly with diabetes, sickle cell disease or trait, or abuse of analgesics or nonsteroidal antiinflammatory drugs, can result in severe bacterial nephritis, papillary necrosis, life-threatening septicemia, and renal or perirenal abscess.

LABORATORY STUDIES AND DIAGNOSTIC PROCEDURES

A number of biochemical screening tests have been developed to detect significant bacteriuria. The most frequently used, the Griess test, depends on the bacterial reduction of nitrate normally present in the urine into nitrites, the latter being detected by a chemical reaction. Preferably, first-morning urine specimens should be used. This test is reasonably accurate in identifying Enterobacteriaceae but does not detect gram-positive organisms and *Pseudomonas* species. False-negative results may be caused by lack of dietary nitrate, low urine pH, ascorbic acid, or urobilinogen or may occur during diuresis, since bacteria require some time to reduce nitrate into nitrites in the bladder urine. False-positive results usually result from contamination of urine with the vaginal flora. This test and the leukocyte esterase test (detects pyuria), combined on a single inexpensive dipstick test, have greatly increased the usefulness of this approach. Bacterial counts higher than 10^5 Enterobacteriaceae/ml of urine with concomitant pyuria can be detected by this method. Overall, the combined test has a sensitivity and specificity of approximately 85% and 75%, respectively.[13]

Microscopic examination of centrifuged urine can detect the presence of significant pyuria (greater than four white blood cells per high-power field), hematuria (greater than four red blood cells per high-power field), or both. This provides further support for the diagnosis of UTI. Although the presence of pyuria does not differentiate upper from lower UTIs, leukocyte casts strongly support the diagnosis of pyelonephritis. Documentation of pyuria is especially valuable in supporting the diagnosis of UTI in symptomatic patients who have low bacterial counts (10^2 to 10^4 colonies/ml of urine). Vaginitis may result in significant pyuria because of the contamination of vaginal secretions with the voided urine and should be ruled out in abacteriuric symptomatic patients who demonstrate pyuria.

Pyuria alone is not specific for bacterial infection. It can occur with nephrolithiasis, allergic interstitial nephritis, papillary necrosis, and renal tuberculosis. The persistence of pyuria after a UTI or genital infection has been eradicated requires further investigation. The presence of a significant number of squamous epithelial cells in the urine of women highly suggests that the white blood cells may be of vaginal origin. Although pyuria is present in all patients with UTI, microscopic hematuria is present in only one half of them. Pyuria in the absence of bacteriuria (sterile pyuria) should raise the possibility of renal tuberculosis or allergic interstitial nephritis. The demonstration of significant eosinophiluria would support the latter diagnosis.

Urine culture remains the "gold standard" in documenting significant bacteriuria and the presence of UTI, as well as identifying the pathogenic microorganism. To reduce the chance of contamination, clean-catch midstream urine samples should be used for culture purposes. Casual collection of urine samples often leads to heavy contamination, which makes the interpretation of microbiologic findings very difficult, if not impossible. In a few, often obese, women it may be almost impossible to obtain uncontaminated urine samples. To minimize the chance of contamination in males, the urine sample should be collected after retraction of the foreskin. To obtain a clean-catch midstream urine, the female patient with a full bladder should stand legs apart over the toilet, separate the labia with the left hand, and clean the vulva front to back with a sterile swab. The patient should then void downward into the toilet until half through without interrupting the stream, catch urine in a sterile cup, and complete voiding. In symptomatic patients with low bacterial counts in midstream urine samples, the first-morning urine sample after awakening may increase the yield, since overnight stasis of urine in the bladder allows bacteria to proliferate and be present in higher concentrations. The presence of more than one bacterium per high-power field on a Gram-stained film of uncentrifuged urine correlates with greater than 10^5 bacterial colonies/ml in 90% of patients. Approximately 50% of patients with dysuria have fewer than 10^5 bacterial colonies/ml, and in 30% the urine is sterile, leading to the diagnosis of acute urethral syndrome.[5]

Suprapubic aspiration and bladder catheterization should be used only in patients in whom it is impossible to obtain uncontaminated urine samples or in symptomatic patients with low (10^2 to 10^4 colonies/ml) bacterial counts. For suprapubic aspiration of urine, the bladder should be full and percussible. This can be facilitated by the oral administration of 300 ml of fluids and 20 mg of furosemide given 1 hour before the procedure. In very obese patients, localization of the bladder by ultrasound (US) may help. With the patient in the supine position and after appropriate sterilization of the area, at the midline 1 inch above the symphysis pubis, the skin is penetrated with a 21-gauge, 4-inch-long needle.[13]

Catheterization of the bladder should be avoided if possible, since it can introduce bacteria into the bladder, resulting in false-positive cultures as well as a 1% chance of developing a UTI.

Radiologic imaging techniques have undergone major technologic improvement in the last decade, especially in regards to the study of the genitourinary tract. Whereas the intravenous pyelogram (IVP) was formerly the gold standard, computed tomography (CT) and US are now the preferred modalities for assessing genitourinary infections. US is sensitive in detecting obstruction, perinephric and intrarenal abscesses, tumors, and cysts. Patients with pyelonephritis should have CT with contrast or US to assess the presence of foci of pyelonephritis in the renal cortex or cortical or perinephric abscesses. Although US is extremely sensitive, it is operator dependent. Thus CT with contrast may be the preferred modality in centers that do not have special competence in US. Immediately after a CT scan with contrast, it is possible to obtain the equivalent of an IVP by taking a kidney, ureter, and bladder (KUB) film in the prone position and observing the anatomic structures of the collecting system and ureters as the contrast is cleared into the bladder.[13]

IVP is essential for visualizing the ureters, the details of calyceal anatomic structures, and the presence of stricture, calyceal dilatation, stones, or obstruction. Demonstration of calyceal details is required for an accurate diagnosis of reflux nephropathy as well as papillary necrosis. Pyelonephritis complicated by intrarenal or perinephric abscess formation is best studied by US, followed by US-guided aspiration and drainage. Coupled with appropriate antibiotic therapy, this is often a lifesaving procedure for many patients.

An US is generally indicated in patients who are hospitalized because of severe bacteremic pyelonephritis, especially if they have a slow response to intravenous antibiotic therapy. In this setting, it is imperative to rule out obstruction. In patients with septic shock caused by presumed urosepsis, an US should be performed on an emergency basis because these patients often do not respond to therapy unless obstruction, if it is the underlying pathologic problem, is relieved by a drainage procedure. In centers that do not have special competence in US, a CT with contrast may be the preferred imaging study, which similarly allows CT-guided abscess drainage. IVP is rarely indicated during an acute episode of pyelonephritis because of the poor quality of the results. Patients with clinical pyelonephritis not requiring hospitalization should have an US examination or IVP. (The IVP should be deferred at least 4 weeks to optimize its quality.) The costs of these studies are shown in Table 146-2.

Most men with bacterial UTI have some anatomic abnormality in the urinary tract. Obstruction at the prostate level may be caused by benign hypertrophy, prostate cancer, cysts or stones in the ejaculatory ducts or vas deferens, or other prostatic problems (see Chapter 152). Transrectal US is the procedure of choice for imaging these pathologic conditions in the prostate and abnormalities in the bladder. New US technology permits a quantitative assessment of prostatic enlargement, detailed imaging of anatomic abnormalities, and the option to perform biopsy at the same time. An IVP may demonstrate prostatic enlargement and postvoiding residuals. It is also useful in diagnosing abnormalities in the bladder.

In women, it is generally accepted that the first episode of UTI does not require any urologic evaluation. However, the management of recurrent infection remains controversial. Multiple studies indicate a lack of cost-effectiveness of urologic studies in the evaluation of women, even those with recurrent UTIs. Therefore the routine anatomic evaluation of women with recurrent UTI cannot be strongly recommended.

Table 146-2. Comparison of the Cost of Radiologic Investigations in a University Hospital*

Test	Cost ($)
Intravenous pyelogram (IVP)	88
Ultrasound (US)	166
Computed tomography (CT) scan (with and without contrast)	382

*Medicare allowable charges.

However, the patient's response to antimicrobial therapy may be used as a guide. Patients with relapsing infection who are cured by a 6-week course of an antibiotic and patients with recurrent reinfection who are successfully managed with a low-dose prophylactic regimen do not require anatomic evaluation. In contrast, those who fail to respond to these regimens require radiologic imaging, typically an US. Another indication for radiologic imaging is persistence of pyuria and flank pain. IVP should not be carried out during pregnancy because of the risk of irradiation to the fetus or within 6 weeks after delivery because of the pregnancy-related changes of the urinary excretory system.

When gross hematuria occurs, there is a significant risk of genitourinary cancer. US is particularly sensitive for identifying small renal cell carcinomas, especially when performed with Doppler flow analysis, which may identify tumor vascularity in the lesion.

In children with the first or second episode of UTI, particularly in those younger than 5 years of age, IVP or US as well as a voiding cystourethrogram (VCUG) should be obtained to detect obstruction or other abnormalities such as posterior urethral valve, renal scarring, or vesicoureteral reflux.[9]

Cystoscopy is only rarely indicated. It should be reserved for the workup of older patients with gross hematuria in whom bladder cancer may be suspected. Cystoscopy may also be used in patients with recurrent or persistent unexplained urinary frequency and dysuria who have no bacteriuria on repeated testing.

DIFFERENTIAL DIAGNOSIS

Although several techniques such as ureteral catheterization, bladder washout, serum antibody response, and the antibody-coated bacteria test have been used to differentiate upper vs. lower UTI, lack of sensitivity of most of these procedures and the associated morbidity and cost have precluded their routine use in clinical practice. As mentioned earlier, the clinical signs and symptoms are not accurate for distinguishing between the two entities. Thus it is generally accepted that distinction between upper and lower UTI is better assessed by the response to treatment. Since uncomplicated UTIs do not produce kidney damage, emphasis has recently swayed from localization studies toward distinguishing between complicated and uncomplicated infections.[10,11,13]

Between 10% and 30% of women with sexually transmitted diseases or other forms of vaginitis have frequency and dysuria. Therefore acute bacterial cystitis should be differentiated from vulvovaginitis caused by yeast, *Trichomonas* species, or bacterial infections, as well as sexually transmitted infections that involve the urethra and the cervix, such as those caused by *C. trachomatis, N. gonorrhoeae,* and herpes simplex virus.[13]

In patients with vulvovaginitis, the discomfort on urination is generally felt externally (external dysuria) when urine flows over the inflamed labia. These patients may also complain of soreness of the vulva, malodorous vaginal discharge, pruritus, and dyspareunia. In these patients, pyuria and hematuria are very rare, and the urine culture typically reveals less than 10^2 colonies/ml.

Urethritis caused by sexually transmitted pathogens usually causes milder symptoms with a more gradual onset of dysuria without other urinary symptoms. These patients may also complain of vaginal discharge or bleeding (from concomitant cervicitis) or lower abdominal pain. They usually have pyuria but only rarely hematuria, and their urine culture shows less than 10^2 colonies/ml. The presence of gross hematuria suggests bacterial cystitis.

In postmenopausal women, atrophic changes in the mucosa of the vulvovagina and urethra caused by hormone deficiency may result in persistent or recurrent frequency and dysuria. These patients generally respond to hormone-replacement creams. Renal and other genitourinary neoplasms must also be seriously considered in differential diagnosis of the older individual who has symptoms of a UTI and hematuria for the first time.

In young, sexually active men, the uropathogenic strains of *E. coli* can result in an acute uncomplicated cystitis. However, some patients may develop urethral discharge and urethral leukocytosis, which mimic *N. gonorrhoeae* urethritis and *C. trachomatis* infections.

Acute pyelonephritis in a young female patient should be differentiated from other intraabdominal conditions such as pelvic inflammatory disease, appendicitis, atopic pregnancy, and ruptured ovarian cyst.

MANAGEMENT

The treatment of UTI depends on what the patient's symptoms are, whether the infection is located in the upper or lower urinary tract as judged by clinical signs and symptoms, and whether it is an isolated episode or a recurrent problem.[2-4,6,7,10-13]

A young woman with the first episode of an acute uncomplicated cystitis does not require urinalysis or urine culture and may be treated with a short course of antibiotics on an empiric basis. No follow-up visit or culture after therapy is recommended unless symptoms persist or recur. In recent years, there has been considerable interest in the use of single-dose therapy on the basis of convenience, cost, compliance, and reduction in side effects. Trimethoprim-sulfamethoxazole (TMP-SMZ) (320/1600 mg, two double-strength tablets), amoxicillin (3 gm), cephaloridine (2 gm), gentamicin (5 mg/kg), and doxycycline (300 mg) have all been used as a single-dose regimen. In general, cure rates of 85% to 90% or even higher have been reported. Among these agents, TMP-SMZ is the preferred drug. With single-dose therapy, urinary symptoms may persist for 1 to 2 days, and a higher incidence of early recurrent infection occurs compared with a short-course treatment using the same antibiotics.

A more common practice is a short-course (3 to 5 days) treatment with either trimethoprim (100 to 200 mg every 12 hours), TMP-SMZ (one double-strength tablet, 160/800 mg every 12 hours), nitrofurantoin (100 mg every 8 or 6 hours), amoxicillin (250 mg every 8 hours), ciprofloxacin (250 to 500 mg every 12 hours), or norfloxacin (400 mg every 12 hours) (Table 146-3). Among these regimens, TMP-SMZ is considered the drug of choice because it effectively reduces the fecal, vaginal, and periurethral colonization. There has been an increasing trend in using less ampicillin, amoxicillin, and first-generation cephalosporins because there is frequent in vitro resistance and because these medications are not being very effective in the elimination of vaginal and periurethral colonization. Nitrofurantoin should not be used in patients with renal impairment because effective urinary concentrations may not be achieved and because there is an increased risk of peripheral neuropathy in these patients. Symptomatic improvement is usually obtained within 1 to 2

Table 146-3. Cost Comparison of 3- or 10-Day Treatment Course for Uncomplicated Cystitis

Antibiotic	Regimen	3 day ($)*	10 day ($)*
Trimethoprim	100-200 mg q12h	1.20-2.00	4.00-6.40
Trimethoprim-sulfamethoxazole	160 mg/800 mg q12h	2.22	7.40
Nitrofurantoin	100 mg q8h/q6h	10.23/13.64	34.10/45.46
Amoxicillin	250 mg q8h	2.25	7.50
Ciprofloxacin	250-500 mg q12h	21.30-25.00	71.00-83.10
Norfloxacin	400 mg q12h	23.00	76.00

*Average wholesale price per *Red Book,* Montvale, NJ, 1993, Medical Economics Data Production.

days of therapy. The recurrence of symptoms after short-course therapy indicates the need for a urine culture and retreatment of the patient for a longer period (10 to 14 days), with the choice of antibiotic based on the urine culture results. Empiric treatment with TMP-SMZ may be instituted until the culture result is available.

Pregnant women with acute uncomplicated cystitis may be treated for 7 to 10 days with oral amoxicillin (250 mg every 8 hours), ampicillin (250 mg every 6 hours), macrocrystalline nitrofurantoin (100 mg every 6 hours), or an oral cephalosporin.

Young, healthy men with acute cystitis and no discernible complicating factor can be treated with a 7- to 10-day regimen of TMP-SMZ (one double-strength tablet, 160/800 mg every 12 hours), trimethoprim (100 to 200 mg every 12 hours), or a fluoroquinolone (norfloxacin [400 mg every 12 hours] or ciprofloxacin [250 to 500 mg every 12 hours]). A pretreatment urine culture is recommended in these patients. A urologic evaluation is usually unrewarding in those who respond to treatment.

About 20% of young women with an initial episode of acute cystitis develop recurrent infections. In patients with recurrent lower UTI, it is critical to distinguish between relapse and reinfection.

RECURRENT URINARY TRACT INFECTIONS

Relapses with the same microorganism highly suggest that the source of bacteriuria is the upper tract and are usually associated with renal stones, scars, or polycystic kidneys. A relapse would be suggested if the same microorganism is recultured and has the same antibiotic sensitivities. In men, a high chance exists that a concomitant chronic bacterial prostatitis may be responsible for these relapses. When relapse occurs despite a 2-week course of appropriate antimicrobial therapy, the treatment should be extended to 4 to 6 weeks with the hope of eradicating the microorganisms from the kidney while determining potential complicating factors such as stones, papillary necrosis, and partial obstruction with an IVP or US.

Reinfection causes more than 90% of recurrent lower UTIs in women. When one or two episodes occur per year, each acute attack should be treated with either a single dose or a short course of antibiotic therapy, as with a single infection. However, if attacks of infection are more frequent, the patient may be treated with short-course antibiotic therapy followed by a long-term (12-month), low-dose, prophylactic antibacterial regimen.

Table 146-4. Cost Comparison of 12 Months of Low-dose Prophylactic Antibiotic Regimen

Antibiotic	Regimen (bedtime)	Cost ($)*
Trimethoprim	100 mg	70
Trimethoprim-sulfamethoxazole	40-80 mg/200-400 mg	57-115
Nitrofurantoin	50-100 mg	244-415
Norfloxacin	200 mg	695
Cephalexin	250 mg	208

*Average wholesale price per *Red Book,* Montvale, NJ, 2000, Medical Economics Data Production.

The antibiotics frequently used for low-dose prophylaxis are trimethoprim (100 mg), TMP-SMZ (half to one single-strength tablet, 40 to 80 mg/200 to 400 mg), nitrofurantoin (50 to 100 mg), norfloxacin (200 mg), and cephalexin (250 mg) taken at bedtime (Table 146-4). Trimethoprim with or without sulfamethoxazole has been a preferred regimen because it reduces the development of periurethral colonization. Side effects and the emergence of resistant strains are unusual. Patients with recurrence of infection after sexual intercourse should be encouraged to void and to use a single prophylactic dose of an antibiotic (TMP-SMZ, 80/400 mg; cephalexin, 250 mg; or nitrofurantoin, 50 to 100 mg) after each sexual intercourse. They should also be informed that the use of a diaphragm and spermicides may predispose them to recurrent UTI and that other forms of birth control are available. In general, all the patients with recurrent UTI should also be encouraged to maintain a high fluid intake and to void completely at 2- to 3-hour intervals during the day.

Postmenopausal women may develop recurrent lower UTIs (reinfections), which may result from residual urine after voiding (often associated with bladder or uterine prolapse) or from lack of estrogen, which causes changes in the vaginal flora (loss of lactobacilli and increased colonization by *E. coli*). Prophylactic antibiotic treatment, topical estradiol cream, or hormone-replacement therapy is beneficial in these patients.

ACUTE URETHRAL SYNDROME

Patients with the acute urethral syndrome may have fewer than 10^5 colonies/ml on routine bacterial cultures. They may have positive isolates when viral, gonococcal, chlamydial, or other special cultures are obtained. Vaginitis and sexually transmitted diseases, including trichomoniasis, must be considered.

No obvious cause is found for the acute urethral syndrome in 10% to 30% of women with dysuria. Suggestions for management include the following: (1) wearing of cotton underwear to decrease moisture in the perineal area; (2) sitz baths followed by careful drying of the perineum; (3) weight loss and exercise; (4) urinary tract analgesia with phenazopyridine (Pyridium), 200 mg tid for 2 to 3 days (advise patient that the urine will have an orange color); and (5) referral to a urologist if symptoms persist.

ASYMPTOMATIC BACTERIURIA

Patients with asymptomatic bacteriuria with or without an indwelling catheter do not require antimicrobial treatment.[1,4,7] The indication for treatment in these patients is the development of clinical symptoms and signs of UTI, the presence of leukopenia, renal transplantation, urea-splitting bacteria (particularly *Proteus mirabilis,* which can cause infection stones), the presence of some degree of upper urinary tract obstruction, pregnancy, or conditions predisposing to papillary necrosis (e.g., diabetes mellitus, sickle cell disease or trait, abuse of analgesic or nonsteroidal antiinflammatory drugs). As many as 40% of elderly men and women, especially those in nursing homes, have asymptomatic bacteriuria. However, since it only rarely leads to symptomatic infection, including pyelonephritis or sepsis, routine screening and antibiotic treatment are not advocated. Asymptomatic bacteriuria in pregnant women is an exception and should always be treated. There is an approximately 30% risk of developing acute pyelonephritis in the second or third trimester, with attendant complications for both mother and fetus (prematurity and low birth weight). Moreover, asymptomatic bacteriuria by itself has been suggested to increase the incidence of premature labor. All pregnant women should be screened for bacteriuria in the first trimester, and if it is present, they should be treated with a short course (3 to 5 days) of amoxicillin (250 mg every 8 hours), ampicillin (250 mg every 6 hours), macrocrystalline nitrofurantoin (100 mg every 6 hours), or an oral cephalosporin. After successful treatment, monthly urine cultures should be performed to detect recurrent bacteriuria. Pregnant women with recurrent asymptomatic bacteriuria can be managed safely with low-dose nitrofurantoin prophylaxis.

ACUTE PYELONEPHRITIS

Acute uncomplicated pyelonephritis can generally be treated on an outpatient basis if the patient does not have nausea or vomiting, is not severely volume depleted, has no evidence of septicemia, and is not a risk for medication nonadherence.[3,4,8,12] All other patients with acute uncomplicated upper UTI, including pregnant women, should be hospitalized for an initial 2 to 3 days of parenteral therapy. A urine culture should be obtained in all patients with suspected pyelonephritis. In 20% of patients, the culture shows less than 10^5 colonies/ml of urine. A blood culture should be obtained in patients who are hospitalized. A positive blood culture is obtained in 15% to 20% of these patients. For outpatient management, a 2-week course of TMP-SMZ (160/800 mg every 12 hours), trimethoprim (200 mg every 12 hours), amoxicillin (500 mg every 8 hours), norfloxacin (400 mg every 12 hours), or ciprofloxacin (500 mg every 12 hours) is recommended. For inpatients, empiric parenteral therapy with TMP-SMZ (160/800 mg every 12 hours), ciprofloxacin (200 to 400 mg every 12 hours), gentamicin (1 mg/kg every 8 hours) with or without ampicillin (1 gm every 6 hours), or a third-generation cephalosporin (e.g., intravenous [IV] or intramuscular [IM] ceftriaxone, 1 to 2 gm daily) should be initiated until the patient becomes afebrile and there is evidence of clinical improvement, usually within 48 to 72 hours. Subsequently, the patient may be switched to oral therapy based on the sensitivity of the microorganism. Patients with uncomplicated upper UTI with or without documented bacteremia are best treated with a 2-week course of antibiotics, and in those who show evidence of relapse, a longer course (6 weeks) should be adopted. If fever and flank pain persist after 72 hours of therapy, blood and urine cultures should be repeated and US or CT of the kidneys obtained to rule out obstruction, urologic abnormalities, and renal or perirenal abscesses. A follow-up urine culture 2 weeks after the completion of antibiotic therapy is indicated. In patients with UTI complicated by stones, renal scars, diabetes, or papillary necrosis, a 6-week course of antibiotic treatment is usually necessary. However, these patients may initially be treated for only 2 weeks, and only those who show evidence of relapse may be retreated for an extended 6-week course.

All pregnant women with acute pyelonephritis should be hospitalized and initially treated with parenteral antibiotics. The choice of antibiotic may be ceftriaxone (1 to 2 gm IV or IM daily), gentamicin (1 mg/kg every 8 hours) with or without ampicillin (1 gm every 6 hours), aztreonam (1 gm every 8 to 12 hours), or TMP-SMZ (160/800 mg every 12 hours), until fever resolves. The patient should subsequently be treated with oral amoxicillin (500 mg every 8 hours), TMP-SMZ (160/800 mg every 12 hours), or a cephalosporin for 14 days. The antimicrobial therapy should be specifically targeted to the infecting microorganism as soon as the results of urine culture and antimicrobial sensitivity tests become available. Fluoroquinolones should not be used in pregnancy. TMP-SMZ is not approved for use in pregnancy, especially in the third trimester, because sulfonamides reduce the binding of bilirubin to albumin and may cause neonatal hyperbilirubinemia, but it is widely used. Gentamicin should be used with caution because of its possible toxicity to eighth-nerve development in the fetus.

In patients with symptomatic complicated upper UTI, the relatively broad array of bacterial species responsible for the infection and the severity of the patient's illness should be considered while choosing the appropriate empiric antimicrobial agents. For septicemia in hospitalized patients, IV broad-spectrum antibiotics covering *Pseudomonas* organisms and enterococci should be initially instituted. Ampicillin (1 gm every 6 hours) and gentamicin (1 mg/kg every 8 hours), a third-generation cephalosporin with anti-*Pseudomonas* activity (e.g., ceftriaxone [1 to 2 gm IV or IM daily]), aztreonam (1 gm every 8 to 12 hours), ticarcillin-clavulanate (3.2 gm every 8 hours), ciprofloxacin (400 mg every 12 hours), and imipenem-cilastatin (250 to 500 mg every 6 to 8 hours) are reasonable initial choices. After the cause of infection has been identified, antimicrobial therapy should be specifically targeted to the infecting agent. In patients who are less ill, outpatient oral therapy with ciprofloxacin or norfloxacin is appropriate. If the infecting pathogen is known

Table 146-5. Recommended Empiric Therapy for Bacterial Urinary Tract Infections (UTIs)*

Condition	Circumstances	Empiric treatment†	Duration
Acute uncomplicated cystitis	Young woman, first episode	TMP-SMZ preferred over amoxicillin, cephaloridine, doxycycline	Single dose
		TMP ± SMZ, amoxicillin, nitrofurantoin, ciprofloxacin, norfloxacin	3-5 days
	Diabetes mellitus, symptoms >7 days, age >65 yr, diaphragm	TMP ± SMZ, amoxicillin, nitrofurantoin, ciprofloxacin, norfloxacin	7-10 days
	Pregnancy	Amoxicillin/ampicillin, nitrofurantoin, oral cephalosporin	7-10 days
	Young healthy man	TMP ± SMZ, ciprofloxacin, norfloxacin	7-10 days
Recurrent cystitis	Relapses	Based on sensitivity results; rule out renal stone/scar/cyst or chronic bacterial prostatitis	14 days; if relapse, 4-6 wk
	Reinfection:		
	≤2 episodes/yr	Treat each episode as first episode in young woman	Single dose or 3-5 days
	≥3 episodes/yr	TMP ± SMZ, amoxicillin, nitrofurantoin, ciprofloxacin, or norfloxacin, followed by low-dose antibiotic prophylaxis	3-5 days, then 1 yr of prophylaxis
	Temporally related to coitus	TMP ± SMZ, nitrofurantoin, cephalexin; voiding after intercourse	Postcoital prophylaxis
	Postmenopause	Topical estradiol cream ± low-dose antibiotic prophylaxis	
Asymptomatic bacteriuria	With/without catheter	No treatment unless symptomatic, neutropenic, renal transplant, urea-splitting bacteria, obstruction, diabetes mellitus, sickle cell disease/trait, NSAID/analgesic abuse	10-14 days
	Pregnancy	Amoxicillin/ampicillin, nitrofurantoin, oral cephalosporin	3-5 days
Acute uncomplicated pyelonephritis	Very sick or septic	Parenteral: TMP-SMZ, ciprofloxacin, ceftriaxone, or gentamicin ± ampicillin until afebrile, then oral regimen	14 days; if relapse, 6 wk
	Not very sick	Oral: TMP ± SMZ, amoxicillin, ciprofloxacin, norfloxacin	14 days; if relapse, 6 wk
	Pregnancy	Parenteral: ceftriaxone, gentamicin ± ampicillin, aztreonam, or TMP-SMZ until afebrile, then oral regimen	14 days
Symptomatic complicated upper UTI	Very sick or septic	Parenteral: gentamicin + ampicillin, ceftriaxone, aztreonam, imipenem-cilastatin, ciprofloxacin, ticarcillin-clavulanate	2-3 wk; if relapse, 6 wk
	Not very sick	Oral: ciprofloxacin, norfloxacin, or TMP-SMZ (if sensitive)	2-3 wk; if relapse, 6 wk

TMP, Trimethoprim; *SMZ*, sulfamethoxazole; *NSAID*, nonsteroidal antiinflammatory drug.
*Therapy should be targeted to infecting organism as soon as it is identified.
†For more details on antibiotics and their doses, see text.

to be susceptible, TMP-SMZ is a reasonable and less costly choice.

The duration of initial therapy for complicated upper UTI is 2 to 3 weeks depending on the clinical circumstances. A follow-up urine culture should be obtained 1 to 2 weeks after the completion of therapy. With symptomatic relapse of the infection, a longer course (6 weeks) of appropriate antimicrobial therapy should be instituted. It should be emphasized that (1) complicated UTIs tend to recur unless the underlying anatomic or functional defect is corrected, (2) infections with *Pseudomonas* species and enterococci are more prone to recur, and (3) chronic or recurrent complicated upper UTIs result in renal damage with loss of renal function. Bacteriuria and UTI tend to recur in patients with chronic indwelling bladder catheters despite treatment of individual infections. The use of aseptic techniques, a closed catheter system, and continuous "downhill" drainage can reduce the incidence of catheter-associated UTI. Antimicrobial prophylaxis has no value for chronically catheterized patients. It has been suggested that intermittent catheterization results in lower rates of bacteriuria than a long-term indwelling catheter. Oral nitrofurantoin or TMP-SMZ prophylaxis may reduce the incidence of bacteriuria in patients undergoing intermittent catheterization but not in those with a long-term indwelling catheter. Table 146-5 summarizes empiric therapy of different UTI syndromes.

REFERENCES

1. Boscia JA, Abrutyn E, Kaye D: Asymptomatic bacteriuria in elderly persons: treat or do not treat? *Ann Intern Med* 106:764, 1987.
2. Carlson KJ, Mulley AJ: Management of acute dysuria: a decision-analysis model of alternative strategies, *Ann Intern Med* 102:244, 1985.
3. Johnson JR, Stamm WE: Urinary tract infections in women: diagnosis and treatment, *Ann Intern Med* 111:906, 1989.
4. Kim ED, Schaeffer AJ: Antimicrobial therapy for urinary tract infections, *Semin Nephrol* 14:551, 1994.
5. Komaroff AL: Urinalysis and urine culture in women with dysuria, *Ann Intern Med* 104:212, 1986
6. Lipsky BA: Urinary tract infection in men: epidemiology, pathophysiology, diagnosis and treatment, *Ann Intern Med* 110:138, 1989.
7. Nicolle LE: Urinary tract infection in the elderly, *J Antimicrob Chemother* 33(suppl):99, 1994.
8. Roberts JA: Pyelonephritis, cortical abscess and perinephric abscess, *Urol Clin North Am* 13:637, 1986.
9. Ross JH: The evaluation and management of vesicoureteral reflux, *Semin Nephrol* 14:523, 1994.
10. Rubin RH, Cotran RS, Tolkoff-Rubin NE: Urinary tract infection, pyelonephritis, and reflux nephropathy. In Brenner BM, Rector FC, editors: *The kidney,* ed 5, Philadelphia, 1996, WB Saunders.
11. Schaeffer AJ et al: Urinary tract infection. In Jacobson HR, Striker GE, Klahr S, editors: *The principles and practice of nephrology,* ed 2, St Louis, 1995, Mosby.
12. Stamm WE, Hooton TM: Management of urinary tract infection in adults, *N Engl J Med* 329:1328, 1993.
13. Sussman M, Cattell WR, Jones KV: Urinary tract infection. In Cameron S et al, editors: *Oxford textbook of clinical nephrology,* ed 2, New York, 1998, Oxford University Press.

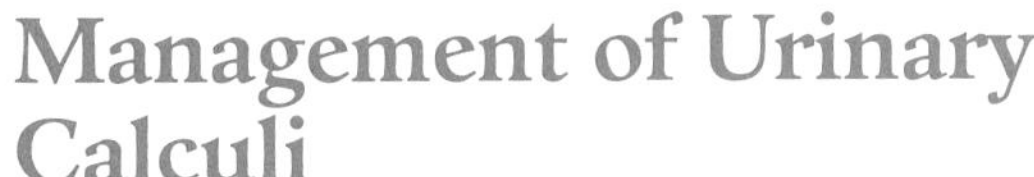

Management of Urinary Calculi

Fernando Coste Delvecchio
Glenn M. Preminger

EPIDEMIOLOGY

Nephrolithiasis is a relatively common disorder affecting 1% to 5% of the population in industrialized countries; it has a reported annual incidence rate as high as 1% in middle-aged Caucasian men. The most common type of renal calculus seen in industrialized countries contains primarily calcium oxalate occurring alone or in combination with hydroxyapatite. The frequency of stone composition is depicted in Table 147-1.

In several unselected population surveys, the life-time risk for stone formation in Caucasian men approaches 20%, whereas for Caucasian women, it is approximately 5% to 10%. In addition, the recurrence rate of nephrolithiasis has been reported to be as high as 50% within 5 years from the first stone occurrence. Overall, stone disease in African-American men is one-third to one-fourth less common than in Caucasian men. However, African-Americans demonstrate a higher prevalence of stones associated with infection by urea-splitting organisms.

Table 147-1. Kidney Stone Composition

Crystal composition	Percentage
Calcium oxalate	60
Calcium phosphate	20
Uric acid	10
Cystine	3
Struvite	7

Recent expansion in knowledge regarding the pathophysiologic mechanisms of calculus formation, paralleled by technologic advances, has allowed the identification of the physiologic or environmental causes of renal calculi in more than 97% of patients. Various diagnostic categories and their relative frequency are shown in Table 147-2. Low urinary volume is by far the most common combined abnormality and the single most important factor to be corrected to avoid recurrences of stones.[5]

PATHOPHYSIOLOGY OF CALCIUM NEPHROLITHIASIS

Hypercalciuria

Hypercalciuria encountered in nephrolithiasis is heterogeneous in origin and comprises several entities. This condition is defined as the excretion of urinary calcium exceeding 200 mg in a 24-hour collection (or a calcium excess of 4 mg/kg/24 hours). Box 147-1 summarizes the causes of secondary hypercalciuria and Table 147-3 the hypercalciuric states.

Absorptive Hypercalciuria. The basic abnormality in absorptive hypercalciuria (AH) is the intestinal hyperabsorption of calcium,[4] the exact cause of which is unknown. The resulting increase in the circulating concentration of calcium enhances the renal filtered load and suppresses parathyroid function. Hypercalciuria results from the combination of increased filtered load and reduced renal tubular reabsorption of calcium caused by parathyroid suppression. The excessive renal loss of calcium compensates for high calcium absorption from the intestinal tract and helps maintain serum calcium levels in the normal range. AH type I (AH-I) is a severe form, and the type II presentation (AH-II) is a mild to moderate form. Whereas urinary calcium levels are increased on both high- and restricted-calcium intakes in AH-I, hypercalciuria is present only during a high calcium intake in type II. (That is, in AH-II, a low-calcium diet corrects the hypercalciuria.)

Renal Hypercalciuria. The primary abnormality in renal hypercalciuria is believed to be an impairment in the renal tubular reabsorption of calcium.[4] The resulting reduction in the serum calcium concentration stimulates parathyroid function. There may be excessive mobilization of

Table 147-2. Classification of Nephrolithiases

	Sole Occurrence (%)	Combined Occurrence (%)
Absorptive hypercalciuria	20	40
Type I		
Type II		
Renal hypercalciuria	5	8
Primary hyperparathyroidism	3	8
Unclassified hypercalciuria	15	25
Hyperuricosuric calcium nephrolithiasis	10	40
Hyperoxaluric calcium nephrolithiasis	2	15
Enteric hyperoxaluria		
Primary hyperoxaluria		
Dietary hyperoxaluria		
Hypocitraturic calcium nephrolithiasis	10	50
Distal renal tubular acidosis		
Chronic diarrheal syndrome		
Thiazide-induced		
Idiopathic		
Hypomagnesiuric calcium nephrolithiasis	5	10
Gouty diathesis	15	30
Cystinuria	<1	
Infection stones	1	5
Low urine volume	10	50
No disturbance and miscellaneous	<3	
	100	

calcium from bone and enhanced intestinal absorption of calcium because of parathyroid hormone (PTH) excess and the ensuing stimulation of the renal synthesis of 1,25-hydroxyvitamin D, or 1,25-$(OH)_2D$. These effects increase the circulating concentration and renal filtered load of calcium, often causing significant hypercalciuria. Unlike primary hyperparathyroidism, the serum calcium concentration in renal hypercalciuria is normal, and the state of hyperparathyroidism is secondary.

Resorptive Hypercalciuria. Resorptive hypercalciuria is characterized by primary hyperparathyroidism. The initial event is excessive resorption of bone resulting from the hypersecretion of PTH. The intestinal absorption of calcium is frequently increased because of PTH-dependent stimulation of the renal synthesis of 1,25-$(OH)_2D$. These effects increase the circulating concentration and renal filtered load of calcium, often causing significant hypercalciuria. Abnormally high levels of PTH enhance renal reabsorption of calcium and phosphate excretion. Fasting urinary calcium levels are elevated in spite of the enhanced calcium reabsorption because of the large increase in the filtered calcium load.

Box 147-1. Causes of Secondary Hypercalciuria

With Hypercalcemia

Primary hyperparathyroidism
Sarcoidosis*
Granulomatous diseases
Lymphoma
Multiple myeloma
Paget's disease of bone*
Metastatic bone disease
Prolonged immobilization

Endocrine Disorders

Hyperthyroidism
Cushing's syndrome

Medications

Furosemide
Acetazolamide
Excessive calcium ingestion
Vitamin D intoxication
Milk-alkali syndrome

Renal Tubular Acidosis

Medullary Sponge Kidney

*May be associated with normocalcemia.

Pathogenesis of Other Causes of Calcium Stones

Hyperuricosuria. Hyperuricosuria may be the only recognizable physiologic abnormality, occurring in about 10% of patients with calcium nephrolithiasis (hyperuricosuric calcium oxalate nephrolithiasis). Box 147-2 lists the possible etiologies of this condition.

It is believed that monosodium urate or uric acid is formed in the supersaturated environment of hyperuricosuric subjects. Monosodium urate or uric acid (colloidal or crystalline) may then initiate calcium oxalate stone formation by the direct induction of heterogeneous nucleation of calcium oxalate or by the adsorption of certain macromolecular inhibitors.

Gouty Diathesis. The term *gouty diathesis* describes the formation of renal stones composed of uric acid or calcium oxalate in patients with primary gout, either manifesting fully with gouty arthritis and hyperuricemia or appearing in a latent form. The invariant feature of this condition is the passage of unusually acidic urine (pH below 5.5) in which uric acid is sparingly soluble in the absence of intestinal alkali loss or

Table 147-3. Summary of Hypercalciuric States

	Serum calcium level	Parathyroid function	Fasting urinary calcium level	Intestinal calcium absorption
Absorptive	Normal	Normal or decreased	Normal	Increased (primary)
Renal	Normal	Increased (secondary)	Increased	Increased (secondary)
Resorptive	Increased	Increased (primary)	Increased	Increased (secondary)

Box 147-2. Clinical Conditions Associated With Hyperuricosuria

Gout
Increased purine intake, excess dietary purine
Increased turnover of nucleic acids
- Hematologic malignancies: leukemia, lymphoma, myeloma
- Hemolytic anemias
- Polycythemia
- Psoriasis

Increased uric acid synthesis, alcohol consumption
Inborn errors of metabolism
Uricosuric agents

dietary acid load. Stone analysis discloses uric acid alone or in combination with calcium oxalate or calcium phosphate. In some patients the signs and symptoms of gouty diathesis, except for the lack of uric acid on stone analysis, may appear. The stones may be made up of only calcium oxalate or calcium phosphate. No specific cause has been detected for the unusually low urinary pH. The formation of uric acid stones is caused by undue acidity of urine, and that of calcium stones is caused by urate-induced crystallization of calcium salts.

Hyperoxaluria. Hyperoxaluria is usually due to the intestinal hyperabsorption of oxalate. The major cause of increased intestinal absorption of oxalate (and subsequent hyperoxaluria) is ileal disease (enteric hyperoxaluria). This disturbance may be encountered in patients with inflammatory bowel disease, gastric or small bowel resection, or jejunoileal bypass.[2]

Two factors probably act in concert to cause intestinal hyperabsorption of oxalate. Intestinal transport of oxalate may increase because of the action of bile salts and fatty acids on the permeability of intestinal mucosa to oxalate. The intestinal fat malabsorption characteristics of ileal disease may exaggerate calcium-soap formation, limit the amount of "free" calcium to complex oxalate, and thereby raise the amount of oxalate available for absorption. Stone formation in enteric hyperoxaluria is due to hyperoxaluria as well as other factors. Urinary output may be low as a result of fluid losses from the intestinal tract. The urinary citrate level is usually reduced due to hypokalemia and metabolic acidosis. Low urinary magnesium concentrations may result from impaired intestinal magnesium absorption. Other causes of hyperoxaluria include substrate excess (increased vitamin C ingestion), low calcium intake, and rarely, enzymatic disturbances in oxalate biosynthesis (primary hyperoxaluria).

Hyperoxaluria is defined by urinary oxalate excretion in excess of 45 mg/day. With levels higher than 80 mg/day, primary or enteric hyperoxaluria is probably present. A mild to moderate elevation (45 to 80 mg/day) may result from dietary noncompliance regarding oxalate-rich foods.

Hypocitraturia. Among the factors that affect the renal handling of citrate, acid-base status probably plays the most important role. Acidosis reduces urinary citrate levels both by enhancing renal tubular reabsorption and by reducing the synthesis of citrate. This mechanism accounts for the occurrence of hypocitraturia in distal renal tubular acidosis, enteric hyperoxaluria, hypokalemia (from intracellular acidosis), strenuous physical exercise (from lactic acidosis), high-animal-protein diet (from elevated acid-ash content), and sodium excess (from bicarbonaturia). Hypocitraturia occurs with other causes of calcium nephrolithiasis (50%) and may exist as a solitary abnormality (10%).

Citrate lowers the urinary saturation of calcium salts by forming soluble complexes with calcium. Moreover, citrate directly inhibits the crystallization of calcium salts. Thus in the setting of low urinary citrate levels, the urinary environment is more supersaturated with respect to calcium salts; nucleation, growth, and aggregation are promoted.

PATHOPHYSIOLOGY OF NONCALCAREOUS STONES

Uric Acid Stones

Critical determinants for pure uric acid lithiasis are a urinary pH less than the dissociation constant for uric acid (5.5), hyperuricosuria, or both. In addition to gouty diathesis, uric acid stones may develop during secondary causes of purine overproduction, such as myeloproliferative states, glycogen storage disease, and malignancy (see Box 147-2). Chronic diarrheal syndromes (e.g., ulcerative colitis, regional enteritis) or jejunoileal bypass surgery may cause uric acid lithiasis by inducing net alkali deficit and lowering urine volume (thereby reducing urinary pH and augmenting urinary concentration of uric acid, respectively).

Cystine Stones. Cystinuria is an inborn error of metabolism characterized by a disturbance in renal and intestinal handling of dicarboxylic acids, including cystine. Stone formation, occurring in a minority of patients, is the result of the excessive renal excretion of cystine and its low solubility in urine. Cystine solubility is pH dependent, with the lowest solubility at the low range of urinary pH, gradual in increase solubility with a rise in pH to 7.5, and rapid increase in solubility above a pH of 7.5. The main determinant of cystine crystallization is urinary supersaturation. Once the urinary saturation of cystine exceeds 250 mg/L, cystine will precipitate out of solution. If the cystine concentration can be maintained under 200 mg/L, cystine stones should not occur. Moreover, recent studies have demonstrated that 18% to 44% of patients with cystinuria have associated metabolic defects (e.g., hyperuricosuria, hypocitraturia), which may complicate their cystine stone disease.

Infection (Struvite) Stones. Infection of the urinary tract with urea-splitting organisms may be associated with renal stones composed of struvite (magnesium-ammonium phosphate) or calcium carbonate apatite. The critical determinant is the formation of ammonia in urine resulting from the enzymatic degradation of urea by bacterial urease. The ammonia undergoes hydrolysis to form ammonium and hydroxyl ions. The resulting alkalinity of the urine augments dissociation of phosphate to form triphosphate ions, which reduce the solubility of struvite. Thus the urinary environment becomes supersaturated with struvite. Certain bacterial species, most commonly *Proteus, Klebsiella, Pseudomonas,* and *Staphylococcus,* produce urease. However, *E. coli* does not. Struvite stones are most common in patients with chronic infections and in those with anatomic or functional abnormalities of the urinary tract that favor the stasis of urine, such as urinary diversions, neurogenic bladder, strictures, and diverticuli.

PATIENT EVALUATION

History and Physical Evaluation

A thorough past medical history may provide clues to the etiology of stone disease. A history of skeletal fracture and peptic ulcer disease suggests primary hyperparathyroidism. Intestinal disease such as chronic diarrheal states, ileal disease, or intestinal resection may predispose the patient to enteric hyperoxaluria or hypocitraturia, resulting in calcium oxalate stones. Patients with gout may form uric acid stones or calcium oxalate stones. A history of recurrent urinary tract infections may suggest infection nephrolithiasis. A physical examination should be performed but is rarely helpful unless the etiology of the stone disease has extrarenal manifestations (such as band keratopathy in hypercalcemia and tophi or gout in hyperuricemia).

A family history of stones is obtained to ascertain etiologies that express a familial tendency (e.g., AH, cystinuria, renal tubular acidosis, primary hyperoxaluria). Medical regimens that have been attempted in the past for stone disease should be discussed in detail. The failure of certain therapeutic modalities may indicate that the etiology is different than that initially suspected and that a more specific approach to treatment is needed.

A careful history of dietary habits, fluid ingestion, and over-the-counter and prescription drug use is obtained. Foods high in calcium, oxalate, and purines can aggravate existing stone disease, as can inadequate fluid ingestion. Implicated medications include vitamins A and D, calcium supplements, and antacids (hypercalciuria), acetazolamide (hypercalciuria, hypocitraturia, and pH increase), vitamin C (hyperoxaluria), furosemide (hypercalciuria), triamterene and indinavir (triamterene and indinavir stones), and hyperuricosuric drugs.

Radiologic Evaluation

A thorough radiologic evaluation is one of the most important aspects of the overall investigation of urinary stone disease. These studies are necessary for determining stone burden and location, urinary tract anatomy, and renal function. Information about these three factors must be obtained before an appropriate treatment can be selected.

Kidney, Ureter, and Bladder X-Ray Studies. Over 90% of stones within the urinary tract are radiopaque. Calcium phosphate and calcium oxalate are the most radiodense stones. A plain film of the abdomen (kidney, ureter, and bladder [KUB]) should be the initial image obtained in all patients with nephrolithiasis. A KUB study should be performed before any subsequent films that use contrast media, since contrast may obscure the presence of even large calculi.

Abdominal films are obtained to document the number, size, and location of all stones within the urinary tract. The radiopacity of any existing stones may suggest the type of stones present. The plain abdominal film is also useful in identifying nephrocalcinosis (suggestive of renal tubular acidosis, sarcoidosis, hyperparathyroidism, or primary hyperoxaluria).

It is important not to overlook stones that may be obscured when they overlie bony structures such as the sacrum or transverse processes of the lumbar vertebrae. These stones can be more easily identified using oblique or anteroposterior views. In addition, nephrotomograms can also be used to assist in the identification of small, less radiopaque calculi within the kidneys.

Intravenous Pyelogram. The intravenous pyelogram (IVP) is instrumental in defining the relationship of the calculus to the pyelocaliceal system and ureter. The exact location of stones, the presence or absence of obstruction, hydronephrosis, caliectasis, and renal and ureteral anomalies are all important pieces of information that must be gleaned from the IVP. In addition, the IVP can approximate the function of an affected or "normal" contralateral kidney as suggested by the promptness of contrast excretion, thickness of renal parenchyma, and amount of pyelocaliectasis. (For more precise information on renal function, a differential renal scan should be performed.) In patients with an apparent obstructing ureteral calculus, it is imperative that delayed films be obtained as long as necessary to specifically identify the location of small obstructing calculi. Finally, an IVP may confirm the presence of radiolucent stones and also identify anatomic abnormalities that may be responsible for stone formation, such as a ureteropelvic junction obstruction or calyceal diverticulum.

Renal Ultrasound. Ultrasonography (US) can be used as a screening tool for hydronephrosis or stones within the collecting system. Additional information provided by sonographic examination of the kidneys is the amount of parenchyma present in an obstructed kidney and identification of radiolucent calculi. The classic "sonographic shadow" clearly identifies stones that may not be visualized on radiographic examinations. However, the middle and distal ureter are not satisfactorily seen on US because of the presence of bowel gas anteriorly and bony pelvis posteriorly.

US may be helpful in the acute setting to rule out other causes of abdominal pain and during follow-up of patients with recurrent nephrolithiasis to avoid excessive x-ray exposure.

Computed Tomography. Computed tomography (CT) is particularly useful in helping identify the etiology of radiolucent filling defects within the renal pelvis or ureter. In addition, anatomic abnormalities, obstruction, and other conditions that mimic ureteral colic can be easily identified.

Nonenhanced spiral CT is currently being used as the preferred diagnostic tool in the assessment of patients with acute flank pain.[8] This technique is more sensitive than simple radiography and US. All stones, independent of their composition, are visualized by this fast and cost-effective method. Moreover, other manifestations of obstructive stones, such as periureteric and perinephric stranding and periureteric edema and hydronephrosis, are easily visualized. Finally, a spiral CT scan can identify other causes of acute flank or abdominal discomfort, such as appendicitis and diverticulitis.

Radionuclide Evaluation. Renal radionuclide studies provide rapid and safe information about total and differential renal function. These tests are specifically advantageous because the radionuclide evaluation is not invasive, requires no bowel preparation or specific preoperative preparation, subjects the patient to only minimal radiation exposure, and is apparently free of allergic complications.

METABOLIC EVALUATION

The decision to investigate thoroughly a first-time stone former should ideally be shared by the physician and the patient. One approach is to gauge the extent of evaluation according to the estimation of the potential or the risk for new stone formation (Fig. 147-1). Patients at high risk might be middle-aged, Caucasian men with a familial history of stones or those with intestinal disease (chronic diarrheal states), pathologic skeletal fractures, osteoporosis, urinary tract infection, or gout. In these patients, an extensive evaluation is recommended. Any patients with stones composed of cystine, uric acid, or struvite should undergo a complete metabolic workup. Because stone disease is uncommon in African-Americans, a search for underlying derangements in these individuals is recommended.

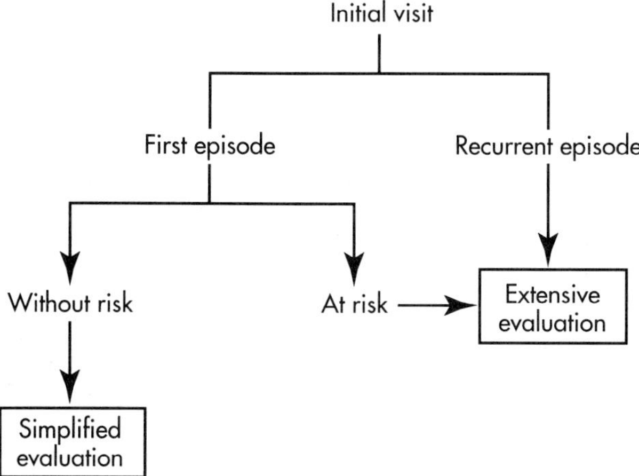

Fig. 147-1. Schema for diagnostic evaluation.

Abbreviated Protocol for Low-Risk Single-Stone Formers

In single-stone formers without risk, the following abbreviated protocol may be applied. A multichannel blood screen can be helpful in identifying certain systemic problems, including primary hyperparathyroidism (high serum calcium and low serum phosphorus levels), renal phosphate leak (hypophosphatemia), uric acid lithiasis (hyperuricemia), and distal renal tubular acidosis (abnormalities in the serum electrolytes [e.g., low serum bicarbonate and potassium levels]).

Voided urinary specimens should be obtained for comprehensive urinalysis and culture. The urinalysis should include pH determination (by electrode), since a pH of greater than 7.5 is compatible with possible infection lithiasis, whereas a pH of less than 5.5 may suggest uric acid lithiasis. The urine sediment is also examined for crystalluria, since particular crystal types may give a clue as to the composition of stones. Urine cultures positive for urea-splitting organisms such as *Proteus, Pseudomonas,* and *Klebsiella* are suggestive of infection lithiasis. In addition, urine should be examined for the presence of cystine using a qualitative examination (nitroprusside test). Abdominal x-ray films should be obtained to search for residual stones within the urinary tract.

Finally, all available stones should be analyzed to determine their crystalline composition. The presence of uric acid and cystine crystals suggests the presence of gouty diathesis and cystinuria, respectively. The finding of carbonate apatite or magnesium ammonium phosphate suggests infection lithiasis. A predominance of hydroxyapatite suggests the presence of distal renal tubular acidosis or primary hyperparathyroidism. A finding of stones composed purely or predominantly of calcium oxalate is less useful diagnostically because such stones may occur in several entities, including AH, renal hypercalciuria, hyperuricosuric calcium nephrolithiasis, enteric hyperoxaluria, hypocitraturic calcium nephrolithiasis, and low urine volume.

Extensive Diagnostic Evaluation

A metabolic evaluation directed at the identification of underlying physiologic derangements should be performed in patients with recurrent nephrolithiasis as well as in stone formers at increased risk for further stone formation or with evidence of multisystem involvement.

Before and during the evaluation, the patient is instructed to discontinue any medication that is known to interfere with the metabolism of calcium, uric acid, or oxalate. Three 24-hour urine samples are collected. Two are obtained with the patient on a random diet, which is reflective of usual dietary intake. The third 24-hour sample is collected after a week of a diet restricted in calcium (less than 400 mg/day), sodium (less than 100 mEq/day), and oxalate (less than 50 mg/day). This dietary restriction is imposed to standardize the diagnostic tests, to better assess the etiology of hypercalciuria, and to prepare for the "fast and calcium load" test, which is performed on the second visit. Blood samples are obtained on both visits (Table 147-4).

The fasting urinary calcium level is expressed in milligrams per deciliter of glomerular filtrate, since it is

Table 147-4. Outline of Extensive Ambulatory Protocol

	Blood					Urine						
	Complete blood count	SMA	PTH	Calcium	Uric acid	Calcium creatinine	Oxalate sodium	pH	Total volume	Uric acid	Citrate	Qualitative cystine
Visit 1*	X	X		X	X	X	X	X	X	X	X	X
Visit 2†		X	X	X	X	X	X	X	X	X	X	
Fast				X		X			X			
Load				X		X			X			

SMA, Multi-channel blood screen (electrolytes, calcium, phosphorus, uric acid); *PTH,* parathyroid hormone.
*History and physical examination, diet history, radiologic evaluation, two 24-hour urine tests on a random diet are performed and dietary instruction for a restricted diet is given.
†The 24-hour urine tests after restricted diet (400 mg of calcium and 100 mEq of sodium a day), or the fast-and-load-test, is performed.

reflective of renal function. To obtain this unit of measurement, the urinary calcium level (in milligram per milligram of creatinine) is multiplied by the serum creatinine level (in milligram per deciliter). The normal fasting urinary calcium level is less than 0.11 mg per deciliter of glomerular filtrate. A calcium load of 1 gm is then administered orally. The post-load urinary calcium level is best expressed in milligrams per milligram of creatinine because it is a function of a fixed oral calcium load. The normal value for this measurement is less than 0.2 mg of calcium per milligram of creatinine.

MANAGEMENT

Acute Stone Episode

Classic symptoms associated with an acutely obstructing urinary stone include colicky flank pain with radiation to the groin, ipsilateral testicle, or labia, and hematuria (gross or microscopic). Stones in the distal ureter may also present with frequency, urgency, and dysuria. Nausea and vomiting are common. If the obstruction is infected, high-grade fevers or even sepsis may ensue.

If a patient demonstrates these classic findings and has a previous history of recurrent radiopaque nephrolithiasis, a KUB study is warranted to address the size and location of the stone to decide the best course of treatment. Stones no more than 4 mm in size (largest diameter) have a rate of spontaneous passage greater than 90% with conservative measures alone; however, stones larger than or equal to 6 mm pass alone only 10% of the time.[3]

In patients who lack the classic findings, who are experiencing their first stone episode, or who are known to form radiolucent stones, either a nonenhanced spiral CT or an IVP should be performed. US may be used to assess hydronephrosis and intrarenal calculi but is not very accurate for the diagnosis of ureteral stones.

If the patient is clinically stable and there is no evidence of systemic infection, complete obstruction leading to renal deterioration, or obstruction of a solitary kidney, then conservative management may be offered with pain medication alone (usually nonsteroidal antiinflammatory drugs and narcotic analgesics). However, in the presence of such impending problems, urinary drainage should be performed on an emergency basis, either as ureteral stent placement or percutaneous nephrostomy. In the case of infection, antibiotics should be started promptly. The size of the stone on imaging studies determines the need for intervention. If there is no evidence of movement or passage of a ureteral stone that has been treated conservatively after 3 to 4 weeks or if pain is intractable, surgical intervention is warranted.

PREVENTION OF STONE RECURRENCES

Medical Management of Nephrolithiasis

Conservative Medical Treatment. Certain conservative recommendations are made for all patients regardless of the underlying etiology of the stone disease. These measures include increased fluids to maintain a urine output above 2000 ml/day. In addition, all patients should be placed on a diet limited in oxalate and sodium, which should help decrease the urinary excretion of oxalate and calcium. In patients with suspected AH without evidence of bone loss, a dietary limitation of dairy products may also be enforced. A restriction of animal proteins in patients with "purine gluttony" and hyperuricosuria should be encouraged.

After 3 to 4 months on conservative management, patients should be reevaluated. If the metabolic or environmental abnormalities have been corrected by the conservative dietary and fluid manipulations alone, conservative therapy should be continued and the patient followed every 6 months with 24-hour urine testing. Follow-up is essential not only for monitoring the efficiency of treatment but also for encouraging patient compliance. If, however, a metabolic or environmental defect persists while the patient is on conservative therapy, more selective medical therapy may be instituted.

Selective Medical Treatment

Sodium Cellulose Phosphate. Currently, no treatment program is capable of correcting the basic abnormality of AH-1. When sodium cellulose phosphate (SCP) is given orally, this nonabsorbable ion-exchange resin binds calcium and inhibits calcium absorption. However, this inhibition is caused by limiting the amount of intraluminal calcium available for absorption, not by correcting the basic disturbance in calcium transport.

The aforementioned mode of action accounts for the three potential complications of SCP therapy. First, this medication may cause a negative calcium balance and parathyroid stimulation when used in patients with normal intestinal calcium absorption or with renal or resorptive hypercalciuria. Second, the treatment may cause magnesium depletion by binding magnesium. Third, SCP may produce secondary hyperoxaluria by binding divalent cations in the intestinal tract, reducing divalent cation-oxalate complexation, and making more oxalate available for absorption. These complications may be overcome by using the drug only in documented cases of AH-I, providing oral magnesium supplementation (given independent from SCP), and imposing a moderate dietary restriction of oxalate.

When these precautions are followed, SCP, 10 to 15 gm/day (given with meals), reduces urinary calcium levels and the saturation of calcium salts (calcium phosphate as well as calcium oxalate), maintains stable bone density, and is clinically effective.

Thiazide. Thiazide is ideally indicated for the treatment of renal hypercalciuria. This diuretic corrects the renal leak of calcium by augmenting calcium reabsorption in the distal tubule and by causing extracellular volume depletion and stimulating proximal tubule reabsorption of calcium. The ensuing correction of secondary hyperparathyroidism restores normal serum 1,25-$(OH)_2D$ levels and intestinal calcium absorption. Thiazide provides a sustained correction of hypercalciuria commensurate with a restoration of normal serum 1,25-$(OH)_2D$ levels and intestinal calcium absorption for up to 10 years of therapy. Physiochemically, the urinary environment becomes less saturated with respect to calcium oxalate and brushite during thiazide treatment, largely because of the reduced calcium excretion. Moreover, urinary inhibitor activity, as reflected in the limit of metastability, is increased by an unknown mechanism. These effects are shared by hydrochlorothiazide, 50 mg twice a day; chlorthalidone, 50 mg/day; or trichlormethiazide, 4 mg/day. Potassium supplementation (approximately 40 mEq/day) is required to prevent hypokalemia and attendant hypocitraturia with all of these agents. Potassium citrate is effective in averting hypokalemia and in increasing urinary citrate when administered to patients with calcium nephrolithiasis who are taking thiazide. Concurrent use of triamterene, a potassium-sparing agent, should be undertaken with caution because of recent reports of triamterene stone formation. Thiazide is contraindicated in primary hyperparathyroidism because of a potential aggravation of hypercalcemia.

Thiazide is not considered a selective therapy for absorptive hypercalciuria, since it does not decrease intestinal calcium absorption in this condition. However, it has been used widely to treat absorptive hypercalciuria because of its hypocalciuric action and the high cost and inconvenience of alternative therapy (SCP).

Current studies indicate that thiazide may have a limited long-term effectiveness in AH-I.[6] Despite an initial reduction in the urinary calcium excretion rate, the intestinal calcium absorption rate remains persistently elevated. These studies suggest that the retained calcium level may be accreted in bone at least during the first few years of therapy. Bone density may increase during thiazide treatment in absorptive hypercalciuria. With continued treatment, however, the rise in bone density stabilizes, and the hypocalciuric effect of thiazide becomes attenuated. The results suggest that thiazide treatment has caused a low turnover state of bone that interferes with continued calcium accretion in the skeleton. The "rejected" calcium would then be excreted in urine. In contrast, bone density is not significantly altered in renal hypercalciuria in which thiazide causes a decline in intestinal calcium absorption commensurate with a reduction in urinary calcium.

Guidelines for the use of sodium cellulose phosphate or thiazide in absorptive hypercalciuria type I. Neither SCP nor thiazide corrects the basic, underlying physiologic defect in AH. SCP might be used in patients with severe AH-I (urinary calcium level greater than 350 mg/day) or in those resistant to or intolerant of thiazide therapy. In patients with AH-I who may be at risk for bone disease (growing children, postmenopausal women) or who already have bone loss, thiazide may be the first choice. When thiazide loses its hypocalciuric action (after long-term treatment), SCP may be temporarily substituted for approximately 6 months; thiazide treatment may then be resumed.

Allopurinol. Allopurinol is the drug of choice in patients with hyperuricosuria (with or without hyperuricemia) because of its ability to reduce uric acid synthesis and lower urinary uric acid levels by inhibiting the enzyme xanthine oxidase. Allopurinol is preferred in patients with marked hyperuricosuria (higher than 1,000 mg/day), especially if hyperuricemia coexists. The usual dose is 300 mg/day, but it should be lowered in patients with renal insufficiency.

Potassium Citrate. Potassium citrate is used as a treatment for primary hypocitraturia and hypocitraturia secondary to metabolic acidosis (i.e., renal tubular acidosis, chronic diarrheal states) and as an alkali in patients with uric acid and cystine stones. It is also used in the prevention of potassium depletion and hypocitraturia induced by thiazides.

The use of potassium citrate in hypercalciuric and hyperuricosuric calcium nephrolithiasis is warranted, since citrate has an inhibitory activity with respect to calcium oxalate (and calcium phosphate) crystallization, aggregation, and agglomeration.

The administration of potassium citrate (30 to 60 mEq/day in divided doses) to patients with hypercalciuric calcium oxalate nephrolithiasis may reduce the urinary saturation of calcium oxalate (by complexing calcium) and inhibit the urate-induced crystallization of calcium oxalate. Potassium citrate may be particularly useful in patients with mild to moderate hyperuricosuria (less than 800 mg/day) and uric acid lithiasis in whom hypocitraturia is also present. It is the drug of choice in the management of patients with gouty diathesis, in whom the major goal of management is to increase the urinary pH above pH 5.5, preferably to approximately 6.5. Potassium citrate is capable of maintaining urinary pH at approximately 6.5 at a dose of 30 to 60 mEq/day in two divided doses. Attempts at alkalinizing the urine to a pH of greater than 7.0 should be avoided. At a higher pH, there is a possibility of precipitating calcium phosphate (hydroxyapatite) and therefore increasing the risk of calcium stone formation.

Calcium. The oral administration of large amounts of calcium (0.25 to 1.0 gm four times a day) or magnesium has been recommended for the control of enteric hyperoxaluria. Although urinary oxalate levels may decrease (probably from binding of oxalate by divalent cations), the concurrent rise in urinary calcium levels may obviate the beneficial effect of this therapy, at least in some patients.

Calcium citrate may theoretically have a role in the management of enteric hyperoxaluria. This treatment may lower urinary oxalate concentrations by binding oxalate in the intestinal tract. Calcium citrate may also raise the urinary citrate values and pH by providing an alkali load. Finally, calcium citrate may correct the malabsorption of calcium and adverse effects on the skeleton by providing efficiently absorbed calcium. If hypercalciuria develops during calcium citrate treatment, thiazide (e.g., trichloromethiazide 2 to 4 mg/day) may be added.

α-Mercaptopropionylglycine. The object of treatment for cystinuria is to reduce the urinary concentration of cystine to below its solubility limit (200 to 250 mg/L). The initial treatment program includes a high fluid intake and oral administration of soluble alkali (potassium citrate) at a dose sufficient to maintain the urinary pH at 6.5 to 7.0. When this conservative program is ineffective, D-penicillamine or α-mercaptopropionylglycine (1000 to 2000 mg/day in divided doses) has been used. This treatment increases cystine solubility in urine via the formation of a more soluble mixed-disulfide. Penicillamine has been associated with frequent side effects, including nephrotic syndrome, dermatitis, and pancytopenia. This profile appears to be less marked with α-mercaptopropionylglycine.

Captopril. Recent studies have suggested that captopril may work in the same way as penicillamine and α-mercaptopropionylglycine, forming a captopril-cysteine disulfide that is 200 times more soluble in urine than cystine. However, further investigations are needed to confirm the long-term effectiveness of captopril for the management of cystinuria.

Acetohydroxamic acid. The gold standard for the treatment of infection stones is complete surgical removal and treatment of infection with adequate antibiotics. When the former therapies are contraindicated or unsuccessful, acetohydroxamic acid (AHA) may be used. AHA, a urease inhibitor, reduces the urinary saturation of struvite and retards stone formation. When given at a dose of 250 mg three times a day, AHA may prevent the recurrence of new stones and inhibit the growth of stones in patients with chronic urea-splitting infections. In addition, in a limited number of patients, AHA has caused the dissolution of existing struvite calculi. However, some patients on chronic AHA therapy have experienced minor side effects, and a few developed deep venous thrombosis. Additional long-term studies must be done to determine the benefit risk ratio of AHA.

SURGERY

Surgical Management

Indications for the surgical management of urinary stones include symptomatic calculi, obstruction, staghorn calculi (even if asymptomatic), and stones in high-risk patients who must not experience an episode of kidney colic (i.e., airplane pilots) or infection (patients who have undergone transplants and patients receiving prostheses). Surgical therapy for urinary tract calculi has changed significantly over the previous 10 years. The advent of shock wave lithotripsy (SWL) and advances in fiberoptics with the subsequent development of flexible instruments as well as small-caliber rigid endoscopes have allowed minimally invasive treatment of urinary calculi and the development of the subspecialty of endourology ("the closed, controlled manipulation of the entire urinary tract"). Determination of the composition, location, and burden of the stone, and renal function and anatomic structures are all important factors in planning the appropriate approach for stone removal.

Selecting the Adequate Treatment Strategy

Shock Wave Lithotripsy. Currently, most symptomatic renal and proximal ureteric stones are treated by SWL. This procedure uses high-energy shock waves that are transmitted through water and are directly focused onto renal and ureteral stones with the aid of fluoroscopy or US. The change in tissue density between the soft renal tissue and the hard stone causes a release of energy at the stone surface, with subsequent stone fragmentation. Multiple shock waves applied to the stone ideally pulverize the stone into small pieces (between 2 and 3 mm), which can then be passed down the ureter and out of the body with the urine.

To diminish the incidence of postprocedural residual fragments and of procedures aimed at treating complications caused by retained fragments, SWL should be reserved for stones that are highly likely to be broken into small, easy-to-pass fragments. Several authors have already proved the long-term negative impact on stone recurrence of untreated residual fragments after surgery.[7]

Therefore SWL should not be considered in cases in which the stone is associated with an obstruction (i.e., primary or secondary ureteropelvic junction obstruction, ureteral stricture, the presence of a distally impacted second stone). Other relative contraindications to SWL treatment are severe hydronephrosis, impaired renal function, and stones within calyceal diverticulum or hydrocalyxes, since stone fragments may not pass in these clinical settings, even when adequately fragmented. SWL should not be considered for stones larger than 1 cm when renal anomalies are present (e.g., pelvic kidney, horseshoe kidney, malrotated kidneys) or in transplanted kidneys.

SWL therapy provides poor results with stones composed of calcium oxalate monohydrate or cystine, since their hard composition may preclude adequate fragmentation. Using other treatment modalities (i.e., percutaneous stone removal, ureteroscopy) may salvage inadequate fragmentation after a technically sound SWL.

Similarly, SWL management of lower-pole kidney stones may not be successful because of inadequate drainage of stone fragments within a gravity-dependent calyx. Other contraindications to SWL are uncontrolled hypertension and bleeding diathesis, since SWL in this setting may cause bleeding around the kidney.

In properly selected patients, SWL should be the procedure of first choice for low-volume stone disease of the upper urinary tract because of its reduced patient morbidity, noninvasiveness, and cost-efficiency.

Percutaneous Nephrostolithotomy. The technique of percutaneous nephrostolithotomy (PNL) relies on access to the intrarenal collecting system through a percutaneous nephrostomy tract (Fig. 147-2). A fiberoptic telescope is passed directly into the renal collecting system, where stones are visualized, fragmented, and extracted. For stones located in calyces that cannot be reached using rigid fiberoptic telescopes, a flexible fiberoptic endoscope and instruments can be used.

PNL is ideally suited for all patients who have renal stones and who are not candidates for SWL. PNL is currently indicated for the treatment of hard calculi, stones larger than 2 cm, stones within the lower-pole calyx or within a calyceal diverticulum, and staghorn calculi; it is also used as a salvage procedure after failed SWL.

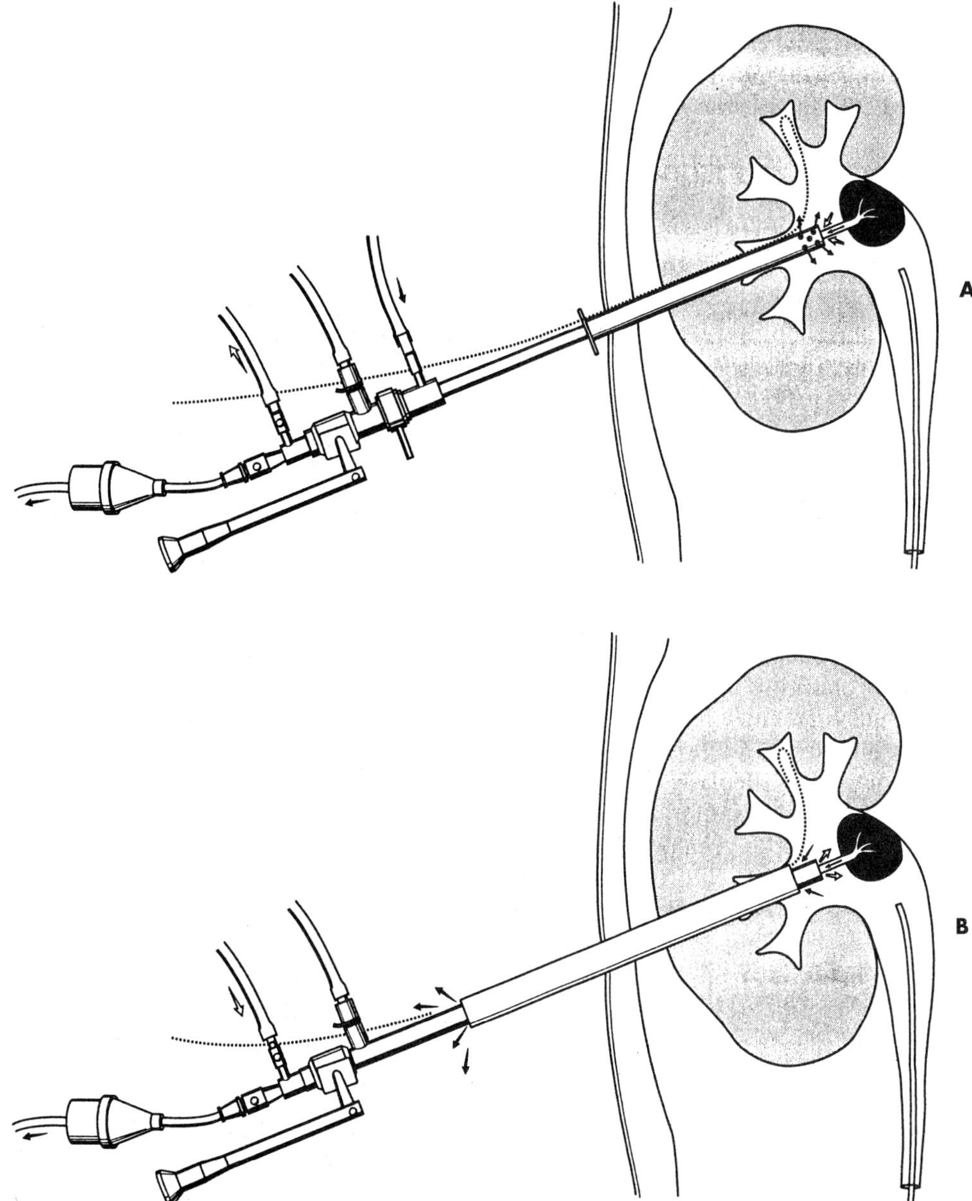

Fig. 147-2. Percutaneous ultrasonic stone disintegration. **A,** Nephroscopic sheath with a closed, continuous-flow irrigation system: using the working channel as an outflow port *(open arrows)* keeps the fragments around the tips of the sonotrode, even if it is clogged. **B,** Open system with a nephrostomy sheath; debris is flushed out continuously alongside the nephroscope. (From Krane R, Siroky M, Fitzpatrick J, editors: *Clinical urology,* Philadelphia, 1994, JB Lippincott.)

Ureterorenoscopy. Another endourologic method for the management of ureteral and renal calculi uses rigid or flexible ureteroscopes. These instruments can be advanced under direct vision or fluoroscopic guidance directly to the level of the stone, which may be fragmented or extracted intact. Various modalities of intracorporeal stone fragmentation, such as electrohydraulic lithotripsy, pneumatic lithotripsy, and laser lithotripsy, may be used to break up stones too large for intact extraction.

Although ureteroscopy requires specific expertise and specialized equipment, its major advantage is decreased morbidity and trauma for the patient undergoing stone removal. Most ureteroscopies are performed as out-patient procedures, with the patient returning to work within 1 to 2 days.

Ureteroscopy is a versatile technique that can be used to treat stones throughout the urinary tract. As with all calculi, the location and size of stones are the most important factors in planning the approach for ureteral stone removal (Fig. 147-3). Upper ureteral calculi can be approached by direct SWL, antegrade percutaneous stone extraction, or ureteroscopy. However, the success rate of SWL treatment for ureteral stones has not been as good as with stones located within the renal pelvis. Current experience reveals that lower ureteral calculi may be best approached with a ureteroscopic technique.

Open Surgery. For only a very small number of patients (less than 1%) with extremely large or complex calculi, an open surgical procedure, most commonly an anatrophic nephrolithotomy, can be used for stone removal.

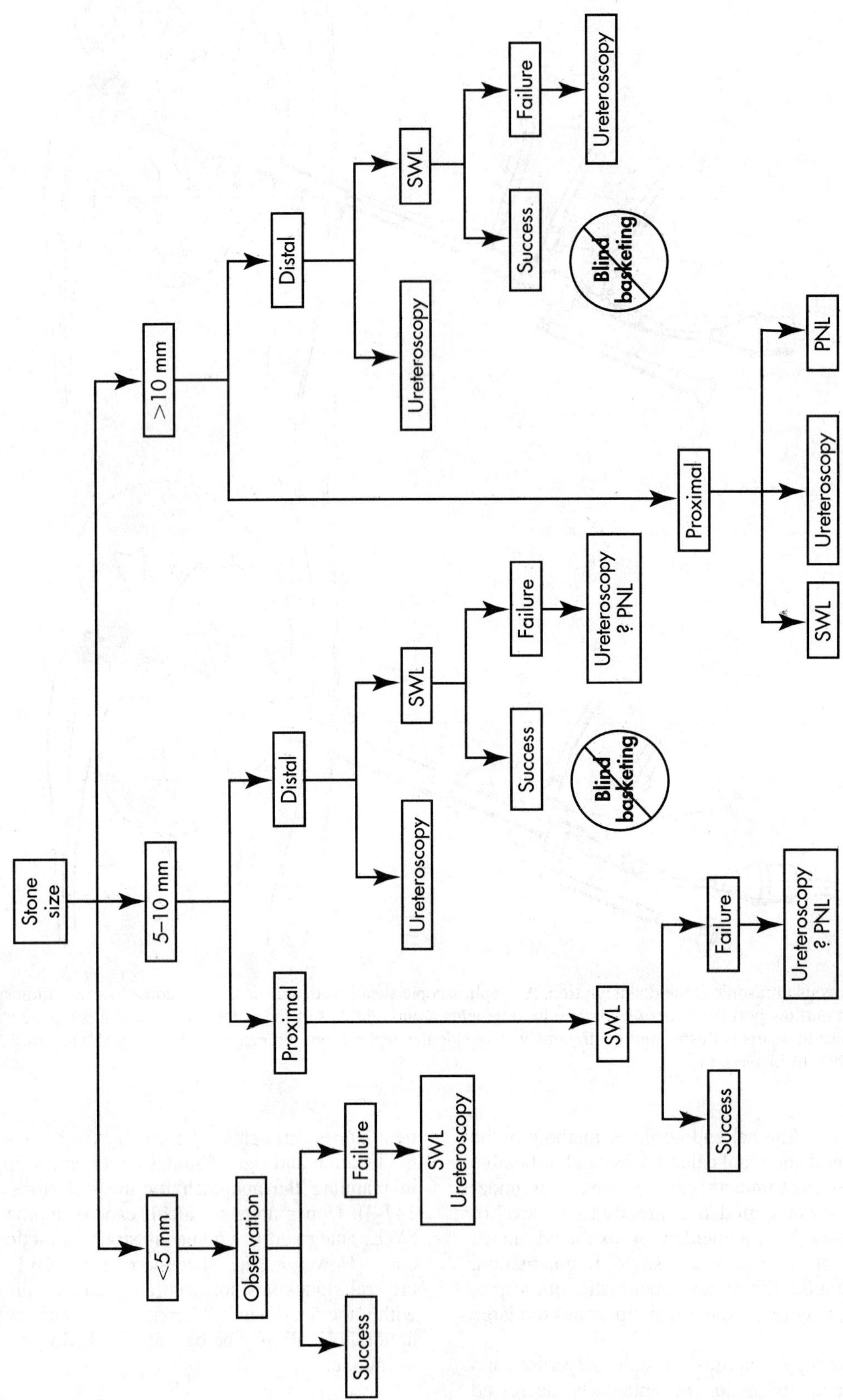

Fig. 147-3. Management of ureteral calculi. *SWL*, Shock wave lithotripsy; *PNL*, percutaneous nephrostolithotomy.

REFERENCES

1. Chow GK, Streem SB: Medical treatment of cystinuria: results of contemporary clinical practice, *J Urol* 156:1576, 1996.
2. Clayman RV, Buchwald H, Varco RL, et al: Urolithiasis in patients with a jejunoileal bypass, *Surg Gynecol Obstet* 147:225, 1978.
3. Morse RM, Resnick MI: Ureteral calculi: natural history and treatment in an era of advanced technology, *J Urol* 145:263, 1991.
4. Pak CY: Physiological basis for absorptive and renal hypercalciurias, *Am J Physiol* 237:F415, 1979.
5. Pak CY, Sakhaee K, Crowther C, et al: Evidence justifying a high fluid intake in treatment of nephrolithiasis, *Ann Intern Med* 93:36, 1980.
6. Preminger GM, Pak CY: Eventual attenuation of hypocalciuric response to hydrochlorothiazide in absorptive hypercalciuria, *J Urol* 137:1104, 1987.
7. Streem SB, Yost A, Mascha E: Clinical implications of clinically insignificant stone fragments after extracorporeal shock wave lithotripsy, *J Urol* 155:1186, 1996.
8. Vieweg J, Teh C, Freed K, et al: Unenhanced helical computerized tomography for the evaluation of patients with acute flank pain, *J Urol* 160:679, 1998.

CHAPTER 148

Glomerular and Tubulointerstitial Disease

Paul G. Schmitz

ETIOLOGIC CLASSIFICATION

Glomerular and tubulointerstitial diseases are the most common causes of chronic renal insufficiency. A precise understanding of the relationship between clinical features and histopathologic features is necessary to classify glomerular and tubulointerstitial renal disease correctly.

Glomerular Disease

The clinical hallmark of glomerular disease is proteinuria, hematuria, or both conditions. Proteinuria in the nephrotic range or the presence of red blood cell (RBC) casts in the urine sediment is virtually pathognomonic for glomerular disease. More important, most glomerular diseases can be conveniently classified into those with a "nephrotic" urine sediment vs. those with a "nephritic" urine sediment (Figs. 148-1 and 148-2). Thus examination of the urine is a crucial initial step in the clinical evaluation of glomerular disease. Glomerular disease can be further classified into primary

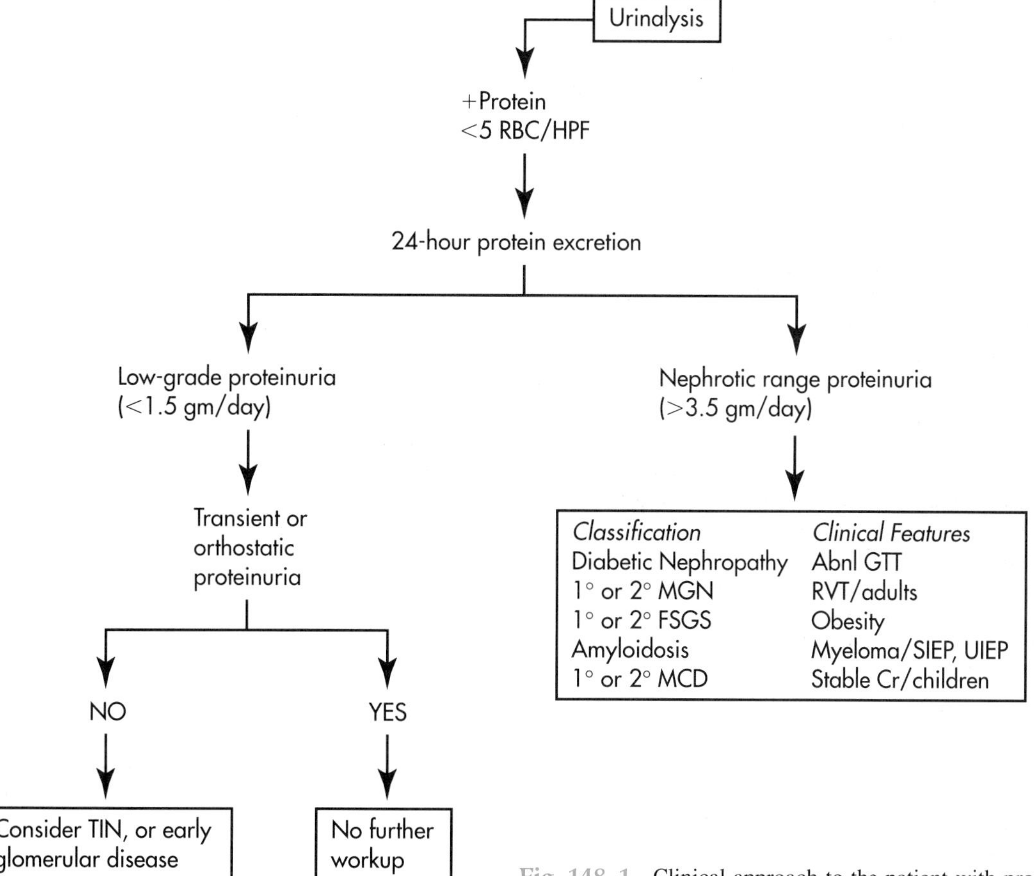

Fig. 148-1. Clinical approach to the patient with proteinuria.

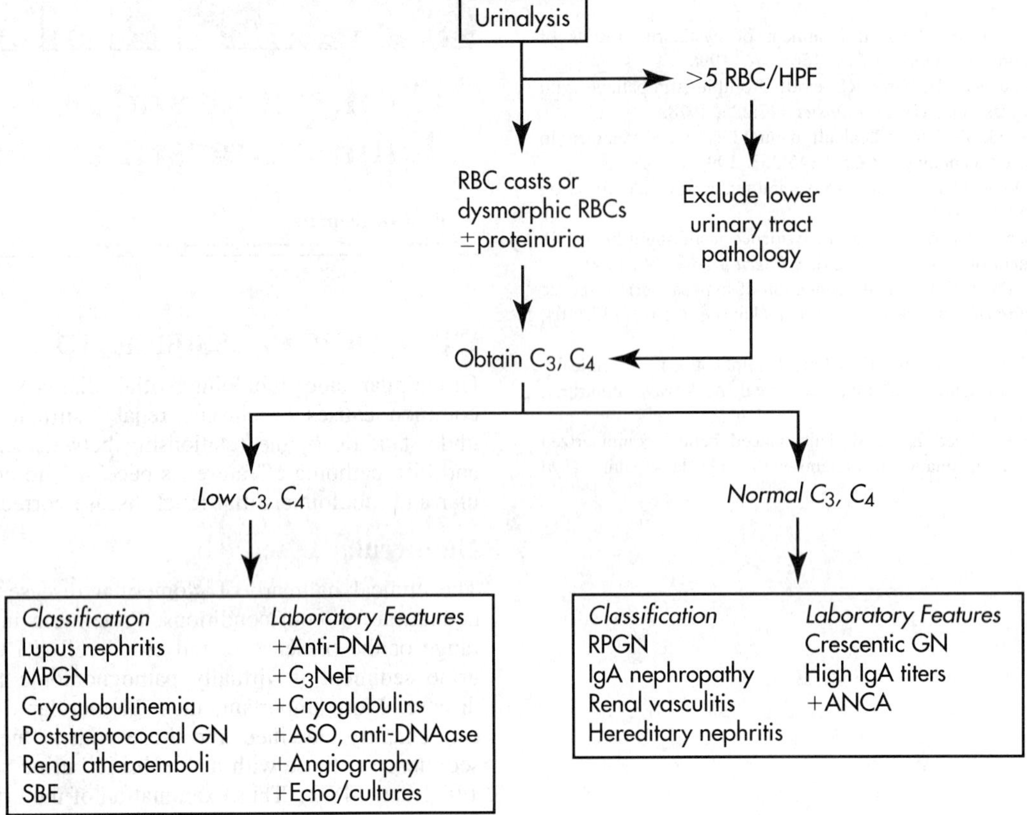

Fig. 148-2. Clinical approach to the patient with hematuria.

(idiopathic) and secondary (e.g., systemic lupus erythematosus [SLE], amyloidosis) causes. Since the clinical presentation may not accurately predict the underlying histologic features, a renal biopsy is often indicated in the evaluation of suspected glomerular involvement.

Tubulointerstitial Disease

Although scarring of the tubules and interstitium often occurs with glomerular disease, primary tubulointerstitial injury can occur as the principal manifestation of a variety of toxic, metabolic, and genetic diseases (Fig. 148-3). Acute tubular necrosis secondary to ischemic or toxic injury is the most common cause of hospital-acquired acute renal insufficiency. Other common causes include drug-induced interstitial nephritis, cystic kidney disease, infectious pyelonephritis, and urinary tract obstruction. In contrast to glomerular involvement, tubulointerstitial disease is characterized by mild proteinuria (usually less than 1 gm/24 hr) and impaired distal or proximal tubular function (renal tubular acidosis, glucosuria, aminoaciduria, defective urinary concentration). Although acute tubulointerstitial injury is often characterized by an active urine sediment (white blood cells [WBCs], WBC casts, and RBCs), a "bland" urinalysis is the rule in chronic tubulointerstitial disease.

PATHOPHYSIOLOGY

Normal Anatomy and Function

The glomerulus is a specialized vascular structure that functions as the basic filtering unit of the kidney (Fig. 148-4). Glomerular cells are composed of endothelial cells, visceral epithelial cells (podocytes), mesangial cells, and resident macrophages. These cells have different functions, including regulation of renal blood flow and intraglomerular pressure, synthesis and degradation of extracellular matrix, modulation of glomerular permeability for various macromolecules, and phagocytosis. An important function of the normal glomerulus is to restrict passage of certain plasma constituents while allowing filtration of endogenous waste products. The glomerular filtration barrier is composed of three layers: an inner fenestrated endothelium, a middle basement membrane, and an outer visceral epithelial cell. These elements form a physical barrier limiting the passage of molecules with molecular weights exceeding 50,000 daltons. Moreover, the visceral epithelial cell and basal lamina contain negatively charged sialoglycoproteins, which impede the filtration of negatively charged substances (e.g., albumin).

The renal interstitium is composed of interstitial cells embedded within the extracellular matrix. Interstitial cells provide physical support for the renal tubules embedded within the interstitium. Moreover, peritubular interstitial fibroblasts are believed to secrete endogenously produced erythropoietin. Toxins (lead), drugs (antibiotics), and genetic diseases (polycystic kidney disease [PKD]) may produce interstitial injury and progressive loss of renal function.

Pathogenesis of Glomerular and Tubulointerstitial Injury

A variety of factors have been implicated in the initiation and progression of glomerular and tubulointerstitial disease.[2] Glomerular injury is frequently associated with the deposition of immunoglobulins within the glomerulus. Antibody deposition presumably leads to the recruitment of inflamma-

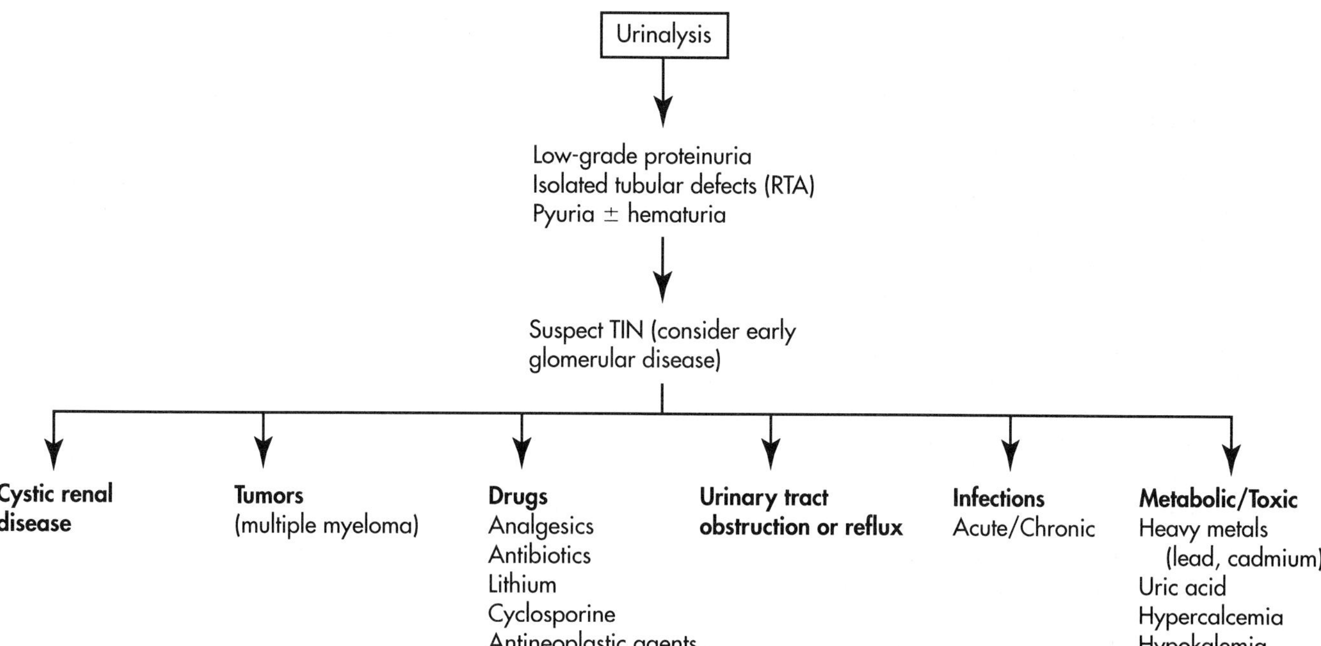

Fig. 148-3. Clinical approach to the patient with suspected tubulointerstitial disease.

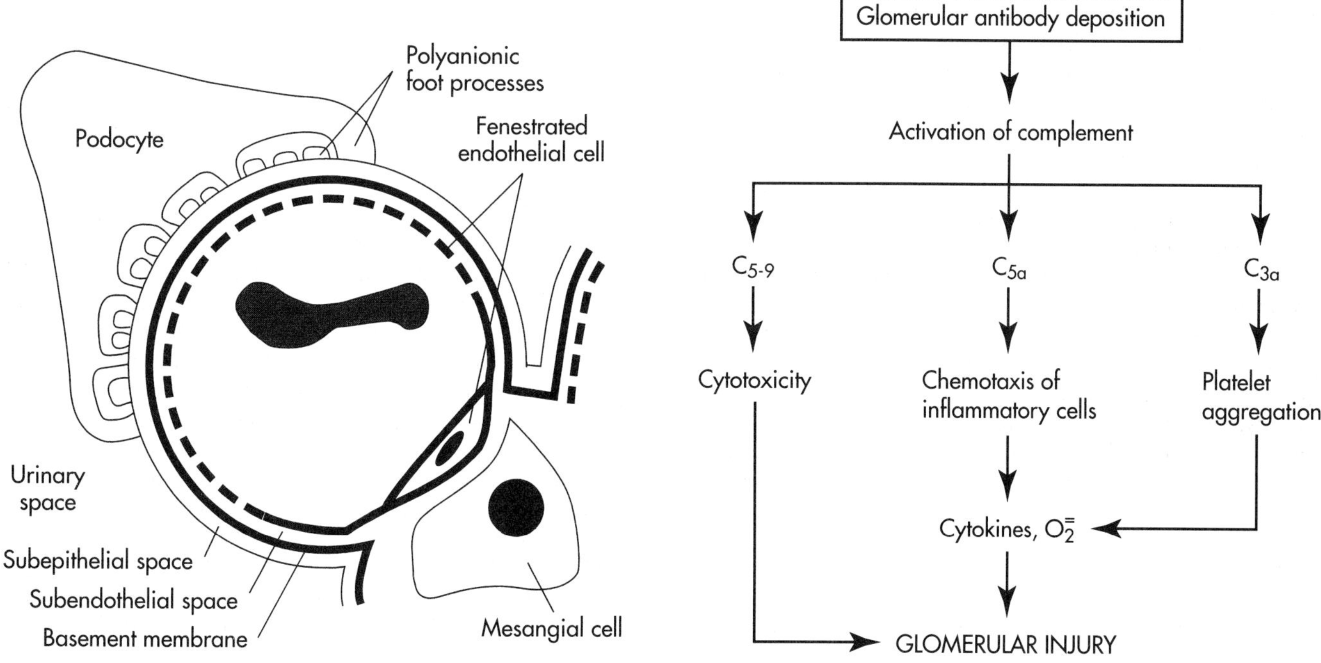

Fig. 148-4. Normal glomerular anatomy.

Fig. 148-5. Pathogenesis of immune-mediated renal injury.

tory cells and the release of serum complement components and other mediators of cell injury (interleukins, chemokines, reactive oxygen metabolites) (Fig. 148-5). The direct activation of the T-lymphocytes may also contribute to glomerular injury. Two mechanisms may give rise to antibody deposition within the glomerulus: (1) circulating antibody bound to a fixed glomerular antigen and (2) passive glomerular entrapment of circulating immune complexes. Analogous mechanisms of renal injury have been proposed in tubulointerstitial diseases.

A variety of nonimmune mechanisms may also contribute to the initiation and progression of chronic renal insufficiency. The significance of nonimmune-mediated renal injury is underscored by the absence of immune deposits in common renal disorders such as diabetic nephropathy and hypertensive nephrosclerosis. Animal models of experimental renal disease have demonstrated that a significant reduction in nephron mass leads to adaptive changes in the remaining (remnant) nephrons that may potentiate the progression of renal disease. For example, the removal of five sixths of the renal mass in a rat results in glomerular capillary hypertension and progressive renal injury. Several studies have demonstrated that a dietary reduction in protein as well as converting-enzyme inhibition (e.g., captopril) attenuate the glomerular hemodynamic and ultrastructural changes occurring in remnant nephrons.[7,9] Although hemodynamic mechanisms of renal injury have received considerable attention, a variety of other factors have also been postulated to be important in the progression of renal injury (Fig. 148-6). These include (1) proteinuria, (2) abnormalities in circulating lipids and hormones, (3) enhanced renal synthesis of eicosanoids, (4) mesangial cell proliferation, (5) enhanced extracellular matrix deposition, and (6) secretion of growth factors and other cytokines (transforming growth factor-β). Treatment strategies aimed at correcting these factors may provide a novel approach to treating medical renal disease.

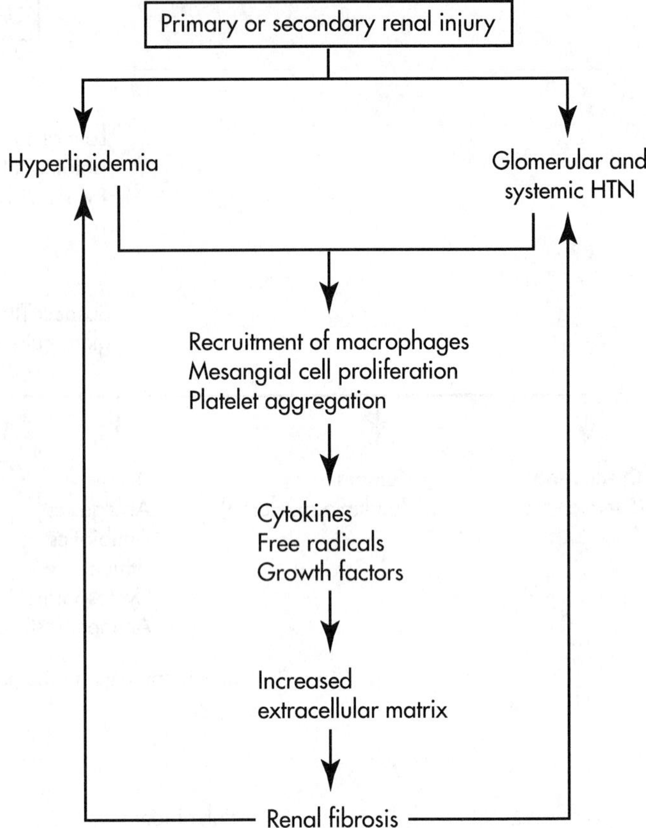

Fig. 148-6. Pathogenesis of nonimmune-mediated renal injury.

Pathophysiology of the Nephrotic Syndrome

The nephrotic syndrome is a urine protein excretion rate exceeding 3.5 gm/24 hr coupled with hypoalbuminemia, edema, and hyperlipidemia[11] (Fig. 148-7). The mechanisms underlying the nephrotic syndrome remain poorly understood; however, an abnormality of glomerular permeability is the hallmark of this syndrome. Altered glomerular permeability may be secondary to injured epithelial cells and loss of anionic sialoglycoproteins (minimal change disease [MCD]) and/or physical disruption of the glomerular filtration barrier (necrotizing glomerulonephritis). The magnitude of proteinuria is influenced by changes in the glomerular filtration rate (GFR), plasma albumin concentration, and dietary intake of protein.

Renal sodium and water retention leading to edema formation invariably occurs in patients with the nephrotic syndrome. The mechanism of enhanced tubular sodium and water reabsorption has been attributed to a reduced effective circulating volume caused by vascular redistribution of fluid. However, recent evidence suggests that plasma volume is not contracted in the nephrotic syndrome. Furthermore, the gradient of plasma to interstitial oncotic pressure is unchanged. Other studies suggest that disturbances in intrarenal physical factors, atrial natriuretic peptides, or sympathetic nervous system activity may account for the changes in tubular sodium and water reabsorption in the nephrotic syndrome.

Since the hepatic synthesis of albumin can normally increase several-fold (exceeding 30 gm/day), the mechanism of hypoalbuminemia in the setting of nephrotic-range proteinuria continues to generate much debate. Possible factors contributing to hypoalbuminemia include (1) enhanced degradation of albumin by the kidney, (2) impaired hepatic synthesis of albumin, and (3) extrarenal changes in albumin catabolism. Hyperlipidemia also accompanies urinary loss of protein and is thought to be secondary to the increased hepatic synthesis of very-low-density lipoproteins. An increase in low-density lipoproteins is also common in patients with the nephrotic syndrome and is probably the result of the catabolism of very-low-density lipoproteins. The increased incidence of cardiovascular disease noted in patients with the nephrotic syndrome is believed to be induced by changes in serum lipid levels. Indeed, the results of preliminary studies indicate that patients with unresponsive nephrotic syndrome benefit from the treatment of hyperlipidemia.

There is an increased incidence of arterial and venous thrombosis in the nephrotic syndrome. Urinary loss of endogenous anticoagulants, particularly antithrombin III, protein C, and protein S, may account for the hypercoagulable state. Indeed, plasma levels of these substances are often decreased in patients with the nephrotic syndrome. Whether systemic anticoagulation should be initiated prophylactically in all patients with severe proteinuria remains controversial.

Finally, there is an increased incidence of infection in the nephrotic syndrome. The mechanism responsible for this phenomenon is believed to be secondary to loss of immunoglobulins in the urine. Serum immunoglobulin G (IgG) levels that remain persistently below 600 mg/dl portend a high risk of infection, which may be amenable to treatment with intravenous (IV) IgG (10 to 15 gm per month).

HISTORY AND PHYSICAL EXAMINATION

A careful history can provide important clues for ascertaining the etiology of glomerular or tubulointerstitial disease. For example, childhood nephrotic syndrome is most likely secondary to MCD, whereas adult nephrotic syndrome is often a consequence of idiopathic membranous glomerulonephritis (MGN). IV drug abuse has been described in association with focal glomerulosclerosis and the nephrotic syndrome. Eliciting information about the duration of the illness is helpful in establishing the chronicity of the process. The presence of comorbid conditions such as diabetes, cancer, SLE, or viral hepatitis may also provide an important clue to the underlying renal histology. For example, MGN has been described in various malignant disorders, particularly

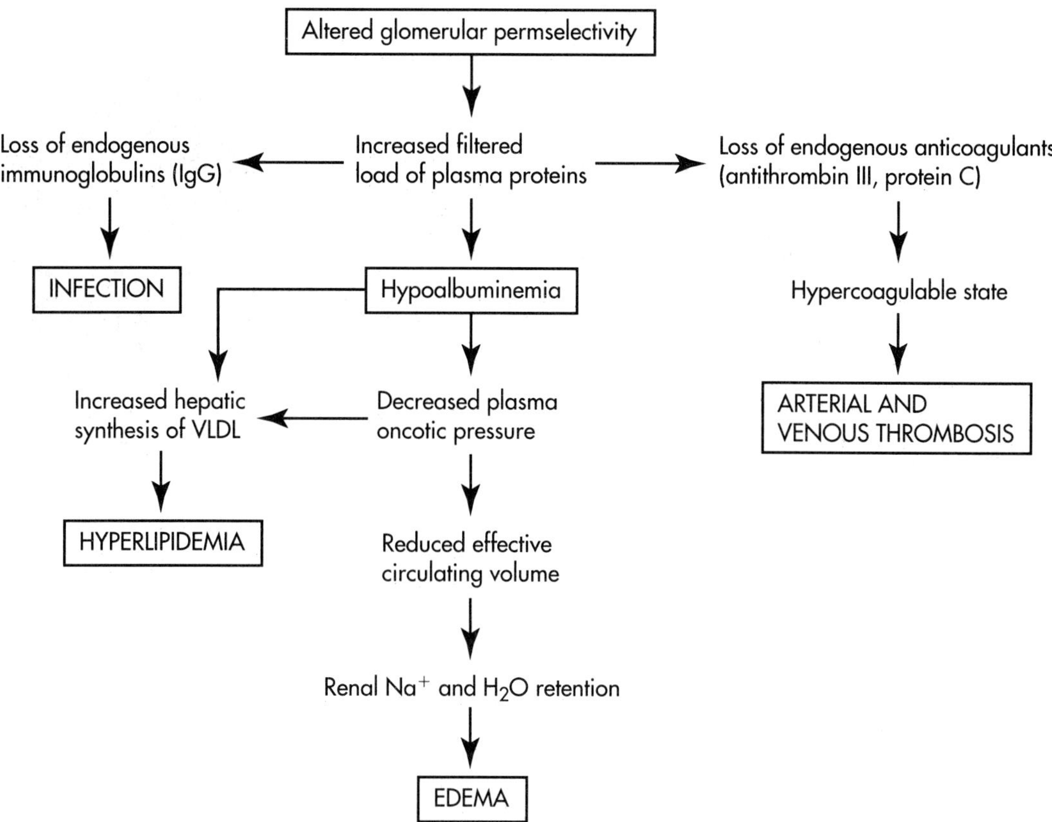

Fig. 148-7. Pathophysiology of the nephrotic syndrome.

solid tumors of the gastrointestinal tract. Finally, obtaining a detailed family history is an essential step in the evaluation of hereditary nephritis or PKD.

The physical examination may also provide important information in the evaluation of the patient with renal disease. Hypertension, edema, and generalized fatigue are nonspecific findings observed in a variety of renal diseases. All patients should be carefully examined for the presence of skin rashes, arthritic changes, lymphadenopathy, and peripheral neuropathy. The presence of a malar rash in a patient with renal insufficiency, proteinuria, and hematuria strongly suggests renal involvement secondary to SLE. In contrast, peripheral neuropathy in an elderly patient with proteinuria and an elevated serum globulin level should prompt an investigation for systemic amyloidosis. The presence of livedo reticularis in a patient recently undergoing cardiac catheterization should raise the possibility of cholesterol embolization. Abdominal pain and a purpuric rash in an adolescent with renal failure would strongly support the diagnosis of Henoch-Schönlein purpura. In addition, palpation of the abdomen may reveal the presence of irregular or enlarged kidneys consistent with PKD or renal cell carcinoma.

LABORATORY STUDIES AND DIAGNOSTIC PROCEDURES

Patients with clinically significant renal disease most often have an abnormal urinalysis (hematuria, proteinuria, casts), a decline in GFR, or both problems. Therefore examination of a freshly voided urine specimen and determination of the serum creatinine level provide the basis for the initial evaluation of renal disease. Isolated or transient abnormalities in the urinalysis must be distinguished from abnormalities secondary to glomerular or tubulointerstitial disease.[12] Moreover, false-positive elevations in the serum creatinine level must be differentiated from a true reduction in GFR.

Examination of Urine

Transient proteinuria may occur in up to 10% of otherwise healthy individuals. The magnitude of proteinuria is typically mild but can rarely be severe (more than 3 gm/24 hours). Transient proteinuria is particularly common in patients with congestive heart failure, infection, and other stress-related illnesses. The mechanism responsible for transient proteinuria in these settings is poorly understood but may involve changes in the circulating levels of stress hormones (angiotensin II, epinephrine). These hormones alter glomerular permeability for protein and modulate intrarenal blood flow and glomerular pressure. More important, transient episodes of proteinuria are not associated with the presence of significant glomerular diseases and thus are considered benign.

Postural, or orthostatic, proteinuria is noted only during upright posture and not during recumbency. The magnitude of proteinuria is generally mild (less than 1 gm/day) but can rarely exceed 3 gm/day. It is more common in adolescents and is rare in patients over 30 years of age. The diagnosis rests on establishing the relationship of posture to the presence of protein in the urine. However, postural changes in urine protein excretion can sometimes occur in serious renal diseases. Therefore benign orthostatic proteinuria should be diagnosed only when the recumbent protein excretion rate is less than 50 mg/day.

In contrast to proteinuria, hematuria can arise anywhere within the urinary tract. The most common cause of hematuria in an adult is urinary tract disease (e.g., prostatitis, renal calculi, cystitis). In the absence of RBC casts or a rising creatinine level, a thorough urologic evaluation (IV pyelography, renal ultrasonography, and cystoscopy) should be performed. RBC morphology has been used to distinguish renal parenchymal from lower urinary tract causes of hematuria. Typically, extrarenal hematuria is characterized by uniform RBC morphology, whereas glomerular hematuria is usually accompanied by dysmorphic RBCs as a result of their passage through the renal tubule and the hypertonic medullary interstitium.

Measurement of Glomerular Filtration Rate

The hallmark of significant renal disease is a reduction in GFR. At steady state the serum creatinine measurement inversely correlates with GFR. Thus a doubling of the serum creatinine value indicates a 50% reduction in the GFR. The clearance of endogenous creatinine is the most widely used method of determining GFR. (See Chapter 144 for a detailed discussion on GFR.)

Serologic Studies

Determination of serum complement components (C_3, C_4, CH_{50}) constitutes an important step in the evaluation of patients with suspected glomerular disease (see Fig. 148-2). Other serologic markers useful in the evaluation of glomerular disease include serum cryoglobulin levels (essential mixed cryoglobulinemia), hepatitis B and C serologic tests (MGN and membranoproliferative glomerulonephritis [MPGN]), human immunodeficiency virus (HIV) testing (focal glomerulosclerosis), serum and urine immunoelectrophoresis (myeloma, amyloidosis), and quantitative determination of antinuclear antibodies (lupus nephritis).

In addition the presence of circulating antibodies to specific cytoplasmic antigens (antineutrophil cytoplasmic antibodies [ANCAs]) has been described in association with renal vasculitis.[10] These antibodies possess several different antigenic specificities, although two major classes are routinely reported using indirect immunofluorescence staining. Antibodies with a cytoplasmic pattern of staining (C-ANCA) are directed toward proteinase-3 and are commonly found in granulomatous vasculitis (Wegener's granulomatosis). In contrast, antibodies with specificity to myeloperoxidase demonstrate a perinuclear staining pattern (P-ANCA). P-ANCAs are often noted in patients with systemic vasculitis (microscopic polyangiitis) (Fig. 148-8). These antibodies have also been described in several nonrenal diseases such as inflammatory bowel disease and therefore cannot be considered absolutely specific for renal disease. Antiglomerular basement membrane antibodies (anti-GBMAb) are found in Goodpasture's syndrome and are sometimes noted in association with circulating ANCAs, implying a nonspecific disturbance in immune regulation.

Radiologic Studies

Ultrasonic determination of kidney size can be useful in the evaluation of unexplained renal insufficiency. Kidneys measuring less than 10 cm in length are highly suggestive of a chronic process and would tend to mitigate against further evaluation. An asymmetric kidney size suggests the possibility of renal vascular disease. Abnormal renal scintigraphy is seen in virtually all patients with significant glomerular or tubulointerstitial disease and thus adds little in establishing the correct diagnosis. Magnetic resonance imaging (MRI) may be used to evaluate the renal artery and veins (e.g., renal vein thrombosis). The use of computed tomography (CT) is particularly beneficial in the evaluation of suspected analgesic nephropathy, showing microcalcifications at or near the papillary tip.

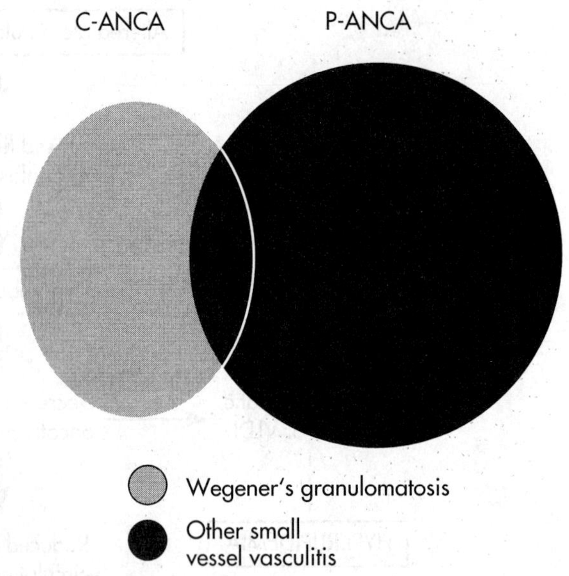

Fig. 148-8. Incidence of C-ANCA and P-ANCA in the two principal types of renal vasculitis.

Renal Biopsy

The renal biopsy remains the "gold standard" for establishing the diagnosis of glomerular and tubulointerstitial renal disease. Often the clinical description and laboratory features of renal disease may be insufficient to arrive at a definitive diagnosis. In these circumstances, a renal biopsy is necessary for delineating the underlying disease.

DIFFERENTIAL DIAGNOSIS

Glomerular Disease Associated With a Nephrotic Pattern

Classifying glomerular disease according to the urinary findings (nephrotic vs. nephritic) is a useful strategy for formulating a differential diagnosis (see Figs. 148-1 and 148-2). Five clinical entities account for most cases of the nephrotic syndrome in an adult: (1) diabetic nephropathy, (2) MGN, (3) focal segmental glomerulosclerosis (FSGS), (4) amyloidosis, and (5) MCD.

Diabetic Nephropathy. Diabetic nephropathy accounts for the majority (up to 40%) of patients receiving dialysis for end-stage renal disease (ESRD). The incidence of diabetic renal disease is greater in Mexican-Americans and African-Americans and in some Native American populations in North America. Microalbuminuria (30 to 300 mg/day of albumin in the urine) is the hallmark of incipient diabetic renal disease and is predictive of progression to ESRD (Fig. 148-9).[1] "Hyperfiltration" (GFR >140 ml/min) is frequently observed in insulin-dependent diabetes mellitus

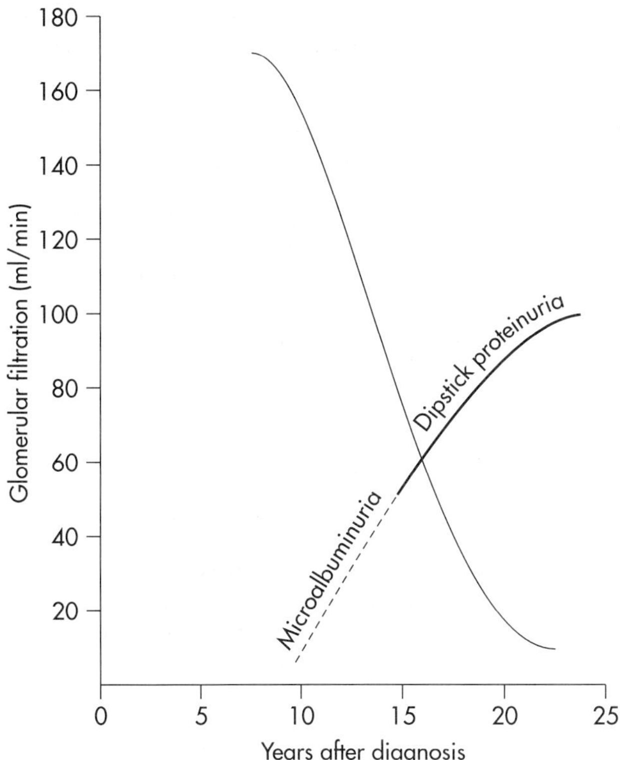

Fig. 148-9. Clinical course of diabetic nephropathy. Note that microalbuminuria precedes overt proteinuria by 5 to 10 years. Once proteinuria is diagnosed based on dipstick testing, renal function slowly declines over 10 to 15 years.

(IDDM) in the early stages of the disease; however, microalbuminuria develops in less than 40% of these patients. The identification of specific risk factors for the development of microalbuminuria in patients with IDDM has remained uncertain; however, poor glycemic control, abnormal intrarenal hemodynamics, and hyperlipidemia have been implicated in the progression of latent hyperfiltration to overt proteinuria. With the onset of microalbuminuria, renal function slowly deteriorates over 15 to 20 years, ultimately progressing to ESRD. Uncontrolled hypertension and poor glycemic control accelerate the progression to ESRD. Recent evidence suggests that patients with non-IDDM evolve through similar stages of hyperfiltration and microalbuminuria, although the incidence of nephropathy in non-IDDM is less well established. Indeed, the incidence of nephropathy may be similar to that of IDDM, although many patients die because of other clinical disorders with advancing age. Nephropathy is strongly associated with other complications of diabetes (retinopathy, neuropathy). Indeed, in the absence of retinopathy, the clinician should question the diagnosis of diabetic nephropathy.

Systemic hypertension plays an important role in the progression of diabetic nephropathy, since antihypertensive therapy can significantly attenuate the progression of renal disease. Angiotensin-converting enzyme inhibitors ameliorate renal injury and proteinuria in humans independent of alterations in systemic blood pressure. In patients intolerant of converting-enzyme inhibitors, the use of nondihydropyridine calcium channel antagonists and possibly angiotensin receptor antagonists may provide reasonable alternatives based on several preliminary reports. A protein-restricted diet (0.6 gm/kg/day) also slows the rate of progressive renal disease in diabetic nephropathy. However, many patients find these diets unpalatable, and frequent assessment of nutritional status is necessary.

Membranous Glomerulonephritis. As many as 40% of adults with the idiopathic nephrotic syndrome are found to have MGN. The pathologic hallmark of MGN is the presence of glomerular subepithelial immune deposits on electron microscopic examination. A variety of underlying conditions have also been described in association with this clinicopathologic syndrome. These include chronic hepatitis B and C, SLE (lupus nephritis type V), malignancies, and some drugs (gold, penicillamine). For unknown reasons, the incidence of thrombotic events is more common in MGN than in other causes of the nephrotic syndrome. The natural history of MGN varies depending on the underlying cause, but in idiopathic MGN, up to 50% of patients remain in partial or complete remission 10 to 15 years after the original diagnosis. Less than 25% of cases progress to ESRD. Because of the variable clinical course, controversy exists regarding the optimal treatment for these patients. Some series report striking benefits with a combination of chlorambucil and prednisone, whereas other investigators have been unable to confirm these findings.

Focal Segmental Glomerulosclerosis. FSGS accounts for up to 10% to 15% of cases of adult nephrotic syndrome. Unfortunately, many cases progress to ESRD within 5 years of the diagnosis. Although most appear to be idiopathic, many cases have been reported in patients after IV drug abuse (heroin) and with HIV infection. HIV nephropathy differs from idiopathic FSGS in that it typically follows a more virulent course, frequently progressing to ESRD in a matter of months. Although some investigators recommend a course of steroid administration in patients with idiopathic FSGS, definitive studies regarding the optimal treatment for these patients do not exist.

Amyloidosis. Renal amyloidosis accounts for a small percentage of cases of adult nephrotic syndrome. Massive proteinuria (>10 gm/day), severe edema, and hypoalbuminemia are frequently noted on clinical presentation. In some patients, multiorgan involvement, as well as hepatosplenomegaly, congestive heart failure, peripheral neuropathy, macroglossia, and carpal tunnel syndrome, is present. The overall prognosis is poor, and often the mean survival time is less than 1 year, with most patients dying from renal failure or infection. Light-chain deposition disease (LCDD) involves a similar pathogenesis; however, the fibrils detected on electron microscopy are distinct from those of amyloid. More than 80% of patients with renal amyloidosis or LCDD demonstrate a circulating or urinary monoclonal protein. Thus serum and urine immunoelectrophoresis is invaluable in establishing the proper diagnosis. The diagnosis can be made with a rectal biopsy (60%) or a transcutaneous fat aspiration (90%). Up to 25% of patients with renal amyloidosis or LCDD demonstrate the presence of a malignant plasma cell clone (e.g., myeloma). Melphalan and prednisone appear to offer promise in the management of these patients, even in the absence of a plasma cell malignancy.[8]

Chronic inflammatory disorders such as rheumatoid arthritis may occasionally be complicated by renal deposition of amyloid. The amyloidogenic protein in these disorders is distinct from light chains and appears to be derived from a circulating protein synthesized in the liver. Treatment for these conditions is directed at the underlying disease process.

Minimal Change Disease. The most common histology detected in the childhood nephrotic syndrome is MCD, also known as *lipoid nephrosis* or *nil disease*. Up to 20% of adults with the nephrotic syndrome may also have MCD. Generally, only "fusion" of the glomerular epithelial cell foot processes is observed with electron microscopy. The results of light microscopy and immunofluorescent studies are unremarkable. The pathogenesis appears to be secondary to diffuse injury of the epithelial cell and loss of polyanionic sialoglycoproteins. Patients with this syndrome typically have edema, hypoalbuminemia, hyperlipidemia, and a normal GFR. Rarely, patients may develop acute renal failure, presumably secondary to profound volume depletion. Although most cases are idiopathic, MCD has occasionally been noted in association with hematologic malignancies (Hodgkin's disease) or drug administration (nonsteroidal antiinflammatory drugs, gold, lithium). Most patients with idiopathic MCD respond to corticosteroid therapy, although remissions are less frequent in adults. Although an excellent response is usually detected within 2 weeks of initiating therapy, some individuals may require up to 12 weeks to respond. Frequent relapses and resistance may occur in some individuals, and long-term administration of low-dose steroids (up to 1 year) may be required to induce a permanent remission. Occasionally, a patient with refractory disease may respond to immunotherapy with either cytotoxic agents (cyclophosphamide and chlorambucil) or cyclosporine.

Glomerular Disease Associated With a Nephritic Urinary Sediment (see Fig. 148-2)

Hereditary Nephritis. Hereditary nephritis, or Alport's syndrome, is characterized by lenticular opacities, renal insufficiency, and sensorineural hearing loss. Three modes of inheritance have been described: X-linked dominant, autosomal dominant, and rarely, autosomal recessive. The differing modes of inheritance are associated with the expression of different phenotypes. For example, X-linked dominant families have renal insufficiency and deafness, which is usually less severe in female patients (Lyon hypothesis). In contrast, autosomal dominant or recessive inheritance results in renal insufficiency but usually no auditory or eye involvement. The pathologic hallmark in the kidney consists of thinning and splitting (lamination) of the GBM. Urinary findings frequently include hematuria and proteinuria; the latter can be severe. Most male patients with this disorder progress to ESRD by age 40; female patients typically follow a less virulent course, although some may progress to ESRD by age 30. The pathogenesis of this disorder is poorly understood, although considerable evidence suggests that patients have a mutated GBM antigen. Unfortunately, no specific therapy exists for hereditary nephritis.

Postinfectious Glomerulonephritis. Poststreptococcal glomerulonephritis (PSGN) is the most common form of postinfectious glomerular injury. Certain strains of "nephritogenic" streptococci (type 12 and type 49 β-hemolytic streptococci) are associated with glomerular inflammation. Electron microscopy reveals granular deposits ("humps") of immune complexes (IgG and complement) in the subepithelial space. Affected glomeruli usually show diffuse proliferation of inflammatory cells and in some cases, crescent formation. Epidemiologic studies suggest that glomerulonephritis may occur in up to 25% of patients infected with nephritogenic strains of β-hemolytic streptococci. Serum complement components, particularly C_3, are low, and circulating antibodies to antistreptolysin O and DNAase B are usually elevated. The clinical manifestations of PSGN range from florid nephrotic syndrome to asymptomatic hematuria and proteinuria. Although most patients spontaneously recover, some may exhibit mild urinary abnormalities for several years. Sporadic reports of patients with chronic renal insufficiency and severe intrarenal scarring occurring 30 to 40 years after an acute episode have been described. The mechanism of progression to ESRD is uncertain in these patients. Other infectious causes of diffuse proliferative glomerulonephritis and immune complex deposition include infected ventriculoatrial shunts and subacute bacterial endocarditis. These disorders typically resolve after appropriate antimicrobial therapy, removal of the infected shunt, or both treatments.

Membranoproliferative Glomerulonephritis. MPGN is often associated with a combination of nephrotic-range proteinuria and hematuria. The clinical course of renal disease ranges from a fulminant, rapidly progressive glomerulonephritis to a slowly progressive course dominated by the symptoms and signs of the nephrotic syndrome. Two histologic subtypes have been characterized: type 1 is associated with mesangial hypercellularity and interposition, resulting in the characteristic "tram track" appearance on light microscopy, whereas type 2 (dense deposit disease) is characterized by heavy deposits of immune complexes along the entire length of the GBM. Both types are associated with hypocomplementemia, although type 1 is characterized by activation of the classic pathway (low C_3 and C_4 values), whereas type 2 is characterized by activation of the alternative pathway (low C_3 values). The latter is thought to occur as a consequence of the persistent activation of C_3 via an antibody (C_3 nephritic factor, C_3NeF), which stabilizes and prolongs the half-life of C_3 convertase. Although most cases of MPGN are idiopathic, an association with SLE, chronic hepatitis B and C, chronic lymphocytic leukemia, cryoglobulinemia, IV drug abuse, and transplant rejection has also been reported.

The treatment of idiopathic MPGN is controversial. An investigation of childhood MPGN demonstrated a beneficial effect of long-term administration of low-dose corticosteroids. However, there is no evidence in adults that steroid use is beneficial. A controlled trial of aspirin and dipyridamole for 1 year in adult MPGN appeared to slow the progression of renal injury when compared with placebo. However, other studies have not confirmed the benefits of antiplatelet drugs.

Systemic Lupus Erythematosus. Renal disease in the setting of SLE is extremely common. Approximately 90% of patients have abnormalities on a renal biopsy. In many instances, pathologic abnormalities are present in the absence of clinical or urinary findings. Five histologic subtypes of renal disease have been described in patients with SLE

Table 148-1. Classification, Prognosis, and Therapy for Lupus Nephritis

Histology	Prognosis*	Therapy
Type I (normal)	++++	NA
Type II (mesangioproliferative GN)	+++	N
Type III (focal proliferative GN)	++	Y/N
Type IV (diffuse proliferative GN)	+	Y
Type V (membranous GN)	+++	Y/N

NA, Not applicable; *GN*, glomerulonephritis; *N*, marginal or no evidence to support therapy; *Y/N*, some evidence to support therapy; *Y*, strong evidence to support therapy.
*Prognosis (untreated): +, worst; ++++, best.

(Table 148-1). Hypocomplementemia frequently accompanies active lupus nephritis. Serum complement levels may be used to follow disease progression and response to treatment. Rarely, lupus nephritis may present without systemic involvement. The natural history of lupus nephritis is poorly understood. Spontaneous conversion from one histologic subtype to another is the rule rather than the exception. The uncertain natural history has complicated treatment strategies and the interpretation of interventional studies. Treatment has been best defined for the diffuse proliferative class of lupus nephritis, in which the response to combined prednisone and cyclophosphamide is clearly superior to that to placebo or steroids alone.[5] However, it is uncertain whether treatment for other histologic subtypes of lupus nephritis offers similar benefits.

Rapidly Progressive Glomerulonephritis. The pathologic hallmark of rapidly progressive glomerulonephritis (RPGN) is the presence of cellular crescents in more than 60% of the glomeruli examined in a renal biopsy specimen. Three major subtypes of RPGN have been described based on the pathologic distribution of immune deposits.

Type 1 RPGN has linear deposits of IgG along the glomerular capillary basement membrane. Anti-GBM Ab are also detected in serum. Pulmonary hemorrhage may also occur (classic Goodpasture's syndrome), or the immune deposits may be limited to the kidneys.

Type 2 RPGN is characterized by immune complex deposition along the glomerular capillary basement membrane. In most cases the inciting antigen is unknown; however, some individuals may have an underlying immune complex disorder (e.g., SLE, PSGN).

Type 3 RPGN (pauci-immune) is characterized by the absence of immune deposits within the kidney. Many patients have an underlying vasculitis. Interestingly, type 3 RPGN is frequently associated with the presence of circulating ANCAs. Serologic evaluation in patients with RPGN can provide an important clue to the pathogenesis of the underlying disease process.

The prognosis and treatment for all three subtypes of RPGN are similar. Early initiation of cytotoxic therapy (2 to 4 mg/kg/day of oral cyclophosphamide) and prednisone (1000 mg methylprednisolone IV each day for 3 days, followed by 1 mg/kg oral prednisone daily) leads to dramatic improvement in renal function and overall mortality rates. However, response rates are substantially less when treatment is delayed (creatinine level >5.0 mg/dl). Plasma exchange therapy may be beneficial in patients with high titers of circulating anti-GBM Ab.

IgA Nephropathy. IgA nephropathy is the most common cause of glomerulonephritis worldwide. Its pathogenesis remains poorly understood, but the presence of increased circulating levels of IgA suggests increased synthesis or decreased degradation of IgA. Although elevations in circulating levels of IgA are found in as many as 50% of affected patients, the nonspecific nature of this finding precludes its usefulness as a diagnostic test. The presence of mesangial deposits of IgA is pathognomonic. Gross or microscopic hematuria is the most common presenting feature and is often preceded by a viral syndrome. Most patients have normal renal function, and their disease follows a benign course. However, progression to ESRD with nephrotic-range proteinuria may occur in up to 20% of affected individuals. Treatment remains controversial, although some studies suggest that sustained use of angiotensin-converting enzyme inhibitors may be helpful. A large multicenter trial assessing the efficacy of fish oils (ω-3 fatty acids) in IgA nephropathy suggests that these agents ameliorate the progression of renal disease.[3]

Systemic Vasculitis. The classification of vasculitis is frequently perplexing, largely because of the varying causes of this syndrome and a lack of understanding of the underlying pathophysiologic mechanisms. A reasonable classification system is based on the size of the artery involved (Fig. 148-10). Although systemic vasculitis can present with multiorgan involvement, renal-limited forms have been recognized. The vasculitides can be conveniently classified into three major categories: (1) large vessel, (2) medium vessel, and (3) small vessel. Renal involvement is more common when small or medium-sized vessels are involved. The most common disorders associated with renal injury are Wegener's granulomatosis and microscopic polyangiitis.

Wegener's granulomatosis affects the small and medium-sized arteries and is associated with granuloma formation in the respiratory tract. A sinus biopsy in a patient with sinusitis and renal disease can often yield a diagnosis. Renal biopsy specimens are characterized by segmental necrotizing glomerulonephritis with or without crescent formation. Immune deposits are conspicuously absent. Affected patients may have either renal-limited disease or pulmonary hemorrhage and/or sinusitis. Response rates as high as 90% are obtained with a combination of cyclophosphamide and prednisone. Microscopic polyangiitis is a systemic vasculitis that typically involves the small arterioles and capillaries. The clinical presentation is similar to that of Wegener's granulomatosis without granuloma formation and sinus involvement.

Other causes of small-vessel vasculitis include Henoch-Schönlein purpura, essential mixed cryoglobulinemia, and serum sickness. Henon-Schönlein purpura is characterized by purpuric lesions of the upper and lower extremities, arthralgias, abdominal pain, and renal failure. Classically, this syndrome is seen in children and resolves spontaneously with supportive care. Adults appear to have less favorable outcomes. Deposits of IgA in the mesangium and mesangial cell proliferation are the hallmarks of this disorder.

Essential mixed cryoglobulinemia is characterized by the presence of circulating cryoglobulins. These complexes

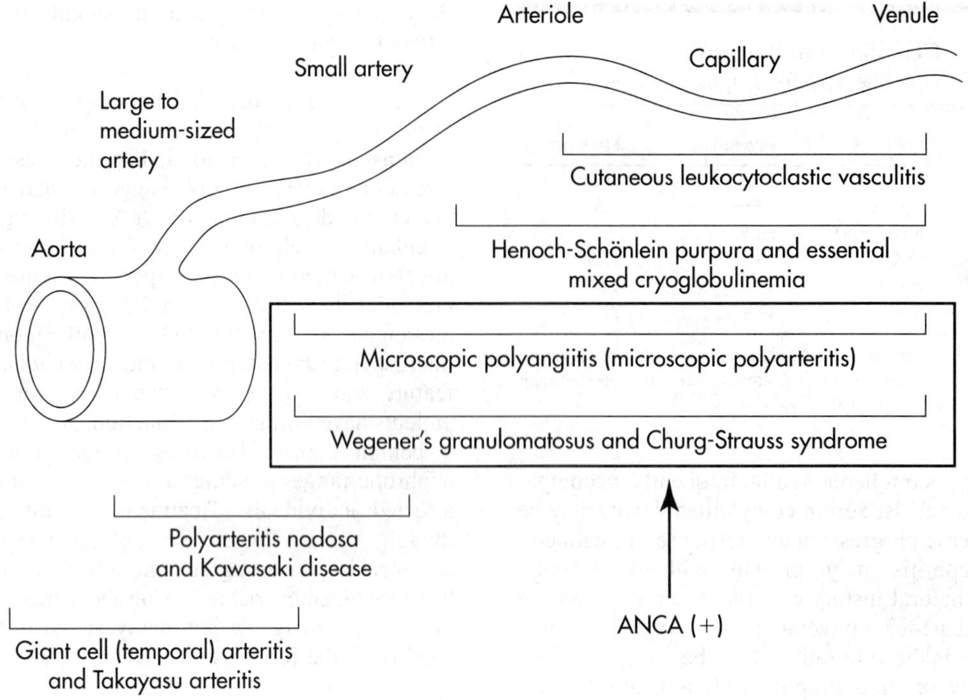

Fig. 148-10. Classification of renal vasculitides based on the size of the vessel involved. (From Jennette JC, Falk RJ: *N Engl J Med* 337:1512-1523, 1997.)

consist of an antigen, an antibody of the IgG type to the antigen, and a rheumatoid factor IgM antibody to the IgG. The inciting event that stimulates the synthesis of these antibodies is uncertain. In many cases, there is an underlying hepatitis B or C infection. A recent report also implicated HIV. Up to 60% of patients with circulating cryoglobulins have renal involvement. Characteristic findings include arthralgias, fatigue, purpuric rash, lymphadenopathy, Raynaud's phenomenon, and hepatosplenomegaly. Hypocomplementemia frequently accompanies disease activity. Pathologically, essential mixed cryoglobulinemia is characterized by the presence of intraluminal thrombi of precipitated cryoglobulins in the kidney. Treatment is similar to that for other vasculitis syndromes (cytotoxic agents and corticosteroids) but may also include plasmapheresis to remove circulating cryoglobulins. The administration of interferon-α to treat hepatitis B or C may result in a renal remission.

Serum sickness is rarely observed in clinical practice. Classically reported after the administration of heterologous antisera, most cases occur after the administration of an antibiotic (commonly a penicillin) or an acute viral syndrome. For example, acute viral hepatitis has been associated with a serum sickness–like syndrome. Circulating antibody-antigen complexes are the hallmark of these disorders. Clinical manifestations include fever, urticaria, rash, and lymphadenopathy. When the kidneys are involved, the urinalysis is dominated by red blood cells and cellular casts. Infrequently a rapidly progressive glomerulonephritis may ensue. Virtually all patients respond to removal or treatment of the inciting event (e.g., discontinuance of drugs, resolution of viremia, effective treatment of viral hepatitis).

Renal Atheroemboli. Renal atheroembolic disease may occur in association with invasive angiographic procedures. Virtually all patients with atheroemboli also have an ulcerated atherosclerotic aorta. Clinical findings that distinguish renal atheroemboli from contrast nephropathy include embolic findings in the lower extremities, livedo reticularis, hypocomplementemia, and peripheral eosinophilia. Many individuals also experience labile hypertension. The mechanism of hypertension appears to be renin mediated, perhaps because of the occlusion of small renal vessels. A biopsy of the affected tissue may disclose the presence of a microthrombus, with needle-shaped crystals representing dissolved cholesterol. Occasionally, examination of the retina reveals refractile bodies consistent with cholesterol embolization. Systemic anticoagulation may exacerbate atheroemboli and thus should be avoided.

Thrombotic Microangiopathies. The thrombotic microangiopathies are characterized by thrombocytopenia, microangiopathic hemolytic anemia, and renal insufficiency. In adults, neurologic complications secondary to thrombotic occlusion of the cerebral vessels may also occur (thrombotic thrombocytopenic purpura). In contrast, renal insufficiency is typically severe in the childhood form of the disease (hemolytic uremic syndrome). Indices of disseminated intravascular coagulation (thrombin time, fibrin split products, fibrin monomers, prothrombin time, partial thromboplastin time) are not increased in these syndromes.

Thrombotic microangiopathy may occur spontaneously or in association with cyclosporine administration, combination chemotherapy (especially mitomycin C), malignant hypertension, vasculitis, postpartum acute renal failure, and HIV infection. Recent outbreaks of hemolytic uremic syndrome have been associated with verotoxin-producing *Escherichia coli* (serotype 0157:H7). The pathologic hallmark of these syndromes includes endothelial cell injury and swelling (endotheliosis) with platelet and fibrin thrombi of the microvasculature. The pathogenesis remains poorly understood, but recent studies suggest that endothelial injury results in abnormalities in circulating von Willebrand's factor that predispose to platelet aggregation. Children with the disorder frequently recover spontaneously with supportive care alone. In adults or children who do not recover within 1 to 2 weeks, treatment should be initiated without delay because the mortality rate can exceed 90%. Infusions of fresh-frozen plasma alone can induce a remission in up to 50% of patients. If no response is noted within 24 hours, plasma exchange therapy should be instituted. Occasionally, patients with refractory disease respond to IV infusions of IgG; the administration of aspirin, dipyridamole, or corticosteroids; and rarely, splenectomy.

Tubulointerstitial Disease

Tubulointerstitial disease represents a broad group of renal diseases that predominantly affect the tubules and interstitium (see Fig. 148-3). In contrast to glomerular disease, heavy proteinuria (more than 2 gm/day), RBC casts, lipiduria, and oval fat bodies are usually not found. More often, either the urine sediment is normal or it demonstrates pyuria with or without WBC casts (allergic or infectious interstitial nephritis). In some instances, discrete tubular defects such as renal tubular acidosis may be the presenting feature (e.g., multiple myeloma).

Allergic Interstitial Nephritis. The most common cause of tubulointerstitial disease is drug-induced allergic interstitial nephritis (AIN). A variety of drugs have been implicated in the pathogenesis of AIN, although the exact mechanism responsible for renal injury is uncertain (Box 148-1). An immune basis for injury seems likely because antibody deposition, complement activation, and infiltration of inflammatory cells (especially eosinophils) are frequently noted in the renal interstitium. The clinical features of AIN include peripheral eosinophilia, rash, fever, renal insufficiency, and pyuria. The urine sediment may also demonstrate WBC casts and hematuria. The presence of eosinophils in the urine can be helpful in establishing the correct diagnosis. In this regard, Hansel's stain of the urine sediment appears to offer greater sensitivity for detecting the presence of eosinophils (about 90%) compared with the traditional Wright's stain (about 25%). Although a renal biopsy may be required for a definite diagnosis, in many patients with AIN the classic symptoms of a rash, fever, eosinophilia, and renal insufficiency after exposure to a known offending agent are sufficiently diagnostic to obviate the need for a renal biopsy. Unfortunately, the classic clinical syndrome is noted in fewer than 60% of patients with AIN. Gallium scintigraphy has been used to noninvasively determine the presence of interstitial inflammation. However, radiologic evaluation of AIN with gallium is highly subjective, and considerable overlap exists among various renal diseases. Nonetheless, it is imperative to establish the proper diagnosis of AIN, since the clinical and laboratory findings are largely reversible on removal of the offending agent. Several uncontrolled trials suggest more rapid resolution of symptoms and improved recovery of renal function with corticosteroid therapy. However, randomized controlled clinical trials have yet to establish the role of corticosteroids in the treatment of AIN.

Box 148-1. Drugs Associated With Acute Interstitial Nephritis

β-Lactam Antibiotics
Methicillin*
Penicillin G
Ampicillin
Flucloxacillin
Oxacillin
Nafcillin
Carbenicillin
Amoxicillin
Mezlocillin
Piperacillin
Cephalothin
Cephalexin
Cephradine
Cefotaxime
Cefoxitin
Cefaclor
Cefazolin
Cefotetan

Other Antibiotics
Sulfonamides*
Trimethoprim-sulfamethoxazole*
Rifampin*
Polymyxin B sulfate
Ethambutol
Vancomycin
Chloramphenicol
Gentamicin?
Isoniazid?
Minocycline
Aminosalicylic acid
Ciprofloxacin
Nitrofurantoin
Norfloxacin
Erythromycin
Spiramycin
Acyclovir
Foscarnet

Diuretics
Thiazides*
Furosemide
Chlorthalidone
Triamterene
Indapamide

Nonsteroidal Antiinflammatory Drugs
Fenoprofen*
Indomethacin
Naproxen
Ibuprofen
Mefenamic acid
Tolmetin
Diflunisal
Piroxicam
Diclofenac
Ketoprofen
Suprofen
Sulindac

Other Drugs
Phenytoin*
Cimetidine*
Omeprazole
Sulfinpyrazone*
Allopurinol*
Aspirin
Carbamazepine
Clofibrate
Azathioprine
Phenylpropanolamine
Methyldopa
Phenobarbital
Interferon-α
Floctafenine
Haloperidol
Warfarin
Diazepam
Valproate
Chlorprothixene
Captopril
Propranolol
Amphetamines
Doxepin
Quinine
Ranitidine
Interleukin-2
Propylthiouracil

Modified from Appel GB: Subsection VIII: Tubulointerstitial diseases, Section 10: Nephrology. In Dale D, Federman D, eds: *Scientific American Medicine,* New York, 1999, Scientific American.
*Most common causative agents of AIN. ?May cause AIN.

Analgesic Nephropathy. Analgesic-induced chronic renal insufficiency probably accounts for less than 1% of all cases of ESRD. There are geographic variations in the incidence of this disorder. In some European countries, such as West Germany, the incidence may be as high as 18%. In the southeastern regions of the United States, it may be as high as 10%. The specific analgesic or combination of analgesics necessary to initiate this process remains controversial. Epidemiologic data suggest that a combination of phenacetin with a nonsteroidal antiinflammatory drug such as ibuprofen or aspirin may be the most nephrotoxic combination. Most patients have ingested at least 1 gm of analgesic per day for several years before renal disease becomes apparent. Renal biopsy reveals severe interstitial fibrosis associated with mild infiltration of inflammatory cells. Papillary necrosis is the hallmark of analgesic nephropathy. Its pathogenesis is uncertain, but the inhibition of vasodilator prostaglandins may lead to ischemia of the interstitial cells and surrounding tubules. CT is useful in establishing the diagnosis, since most patients have microcalcifications in the inner medulla near the papillary tip.[4]

Reflux Nephropathy and Chronic Pyelonephritis. Reflux nephropathy results from the abnormal backflow of urine from the urinary bladder to the renal parenchyma. It is unclear whether the mechanism of tubulointerstitial scarring is a direct consequence of high-pressure reflux or is secondary to chronic, repeated urinary tract infections (UTIs). Children with chronic reflux usually have symptoms and signs of UTI, such as dysuria, pyuria, flank pain, and fever. In later stages, glomerular involvement may occur, manifested by focal scarring and heavy proteinuria (more than 3.5 gm/day). The diagnosis of urinary tract reflux can be established with a voiding cystourethrogram. The management of reflux nephropathy depends on the severity of the reflux. Mild abnormalities generally respond to conservative measures such as the long-term administration of low-dose antimicrobial agents. Many patients have spontaneous remission with time. More severe grades of reflux may require surgical intervention. The hallmarks of advanced reflux nephropathy are interstitial scarring, tubular atrophy, and mild inflammatory cell infiltration (e.g., chronic pyelonephritis). Although chronic pyelonephritis is most frequently described in association with chronic UTI with or without reflux, it has also been reported with chronic lithium exposure, cisplatin administration, cyclosporin use, hyperoxaluria, cadmium exposure, hypercalcemia and hypercalciuria, chronic hypokalemia, and hyperuricemia.

Polycystic Kidney Disease. PKD is a clinical disorder with two distinct inheritance patterns. The infantile variety is transmitted via an autosomal recessive gene, whereas adult PKD is transmitted in an autosomal dominant fashion. Infantile PKD usually follows a fulminant course, resulting in ESRD early in childhood. More than 90% of patients with adult PKD have an abnormal gene on the short arm of chromosome 16 (PKD1). Most of these patients have a family history of PKD. Other forms of adult PKD (non-PKD1) also may occur. The abnormal gene in some of these variants has been localized using linkage analysis. In general, patients with non-PKD1 appear to have a more favorable prognosis than those with the PKD1 locus. The abnormal gene in PKD1 encodes for a large protein referred to as *polycystin;* its function, however, remains a mystery.

The mechanism of cyst formation in this disorder remains poorly understood. Cyst enlargement results in the compression of adjacent normal tissue, causing scarring and progressive renal insufficiency. The demonstration of multiple renal cysts using ultrasonography confirms the diagnosis. Most of these patients develop ESRD by age 55 to 60. Cysts may also occur in the liver, pancreas, and spleen.

Significant cystic involvement of the kidney may not be apparent until early adulthood. Thus screening high-risk patients with ultrasonography may reveal nothing early in the course of PKD. However, by age 30 virtually all patients have multiple cysts on ultrasonography. However, the natural history of this disease is quite variable and seems to depend on a combination of genetic and environmental factors. Approximately 35% of patients have hematuria.

Complications of PKD include infection and bleeding into cysts, usually accompanied by severe pain. Infections can be treated symptomatically with antimicrobial therapy, but cyst drainage may be necessary for the resolution of symptoms. The most ominous complication is a ruptured intracerebral berry aneurysm. This complication has been reported in up to 4% of affected patients. Guidelines for screening patients for intracranial aneurysms have not been clearly established, although patients with a family history of intracranial aneurysm should undergo routine testing with MR angiography. Patients at high risk for developing a ruptured aneurysm (previous rupture, large aneurysms, bleeding diathesis) should be considered for invasive repair. Other complications include renal calculi (20%), colonic diverticuli (70%), cardiac valvular abnormalities (25%), and hepatic cysts (75%). No specific therapy exists for this disorder.

MANAGEMENT

In addition to the immunosuppressive regimens outlined for specific renal syndromes, several nonspecific measures are useful in the management of patients with progressive renal injury. These include dietary protein restriction,[7] treatment of hypertension, and management of associated metabolic disorders (hyperphosphatemia, hypocalcemia, metabolic acidosis, hyperlipidemia). Abundant evidence indicates that angiotensin-converting enzyme inhibition lessens proteinuria and retards progression of diabetic[9] and nondiabetic renal disease. In addition, the role of hypertension in accelerating the progression of renal disease is well established. Other metabolic complications contributing to renal injury include hyperlipidemia, hyperphosphatemia, and secondary hyperparathyroidism. The treatment of these complications may attenuate progressive renal scarring in addition to reducing the risk of various comorbid events such as atherosclerotic vascular disease and renal osteodystrophy. Since the cardiovascular risk of hyperlipidemia is well established, it seems prudent to initiate antihyperlipidemic therapy in patients with renal disease who are at high risk for cardiovascular events.

REFERENCES

1. Bennett PH, Haffner W, Kasiske BL, et al: Screening and management of microalbuminuria in patients with diabetes mellitus: recommendations to the Scientific Advisory Board of the National Kidney Foundation from an ad hoc committee of the Council on Diabetes Mellitus of the National Kidney Foundation, *Am J Kidney Dis* 25:107-112, 1995.
2. Couser WB: Pathogenesis of glomerular damage in glomerulonephritis, *Nephrol Dial Transplant* 13(suppl 1):10-15, 1998.
3. Donadio JV Jr, Bergstralh EJ, Offord KP, et al: A controlled trial of fish oil in IgA nephropathy: Mayo Nephrology Collaborative Group, *N Engl J Med* 331:1194-1199, 1994.
4. Elseviers MM, De Schepper A, Corthouts R, et al: High diagnostic performance of CT scan for analgesic nephropathy in patients with incipient to severe renal failure, *Kidney Int* 48:1316-1323, 1995.

5. Gourley MF, Austin HA III, Scott D, et al: Methylprednisolone and cyclophosphamide, alone or in combination in patients with lupus nephritis: a randomized, controlled trial, *Ann Intern Med* 125:549-557, 1996.
6. Jennette JC, Falk RJ: Small-vessel vasculitis, *N Engl J Med* 337:1512-1523, 1997.
7. Klahr S, et al: The effects of dietary protein restriction and blood-pressure control on the progression of chronic renal disease, *N Engl J Med* 330:877, 1994.
8. Kyle RA, Gertz MA, Greipp PR, et al: A trial of three regimens for primary amyloidosis colchicine alone, melphalan and prednisone, and melphalan, prednisone, and colchicine, *N Engl J Med* 336:1202-1207, 1997.
9. Lewis EJ, et al: The effect of angiotensin-converting enzyme inhibition on diabetic nephropathy, *N Engl J Med* 329:1456, 1993.
10. Merkel PA, Polisson RP, Chang Y, et al: Prevalence of antineutrophil cytoplasmic antibodies in a large inception cohort of patients with connective tissue disease, *Ann Intern Med* 126:866-873, 1997.
11. Orth SR, Ritz E: The nephrotic syndrome, *N Engl J Med* 338:1202-1211, 1998.
12. Yamagata K, Yamagata Y, Kobayashi M, et al: A long-term follow-up study of asymptomatic hematuria and/or proteinuria in adults, *Clin Nephrol* 45:281-288, 1996.

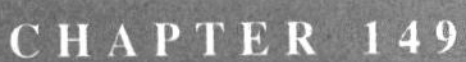

CHAPTER 149

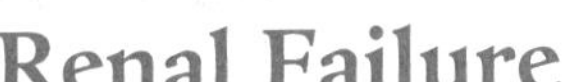

Renal Failure

Sanford T. Reikes
Kevin J. Martin

EPIDEMIOLOGY AND ETIOLOGY

Acute renal failure is a commonly encountered problem characterized by a sudden reduction in function that limits the kidney's ability to maintain homeostasis and eliminate nitrogenous waste. Traditionally, causes of acute renal failure have been categorized into those resulting from impaired perfusion of the kidney, those resulting from injury to the nephron itself, and those resulting from the obstruction of urine flow. These broad categories have been termed *prerenal, intrinsic,* and *postrenal acute renal failure,* respectively. Clinical setting influences the frequency and etiology of acute renal failure, which complicates 2% to 5% of hospitalizations[3,12] and is most often due to intrinsic factors, primarily acute tubular necrosis. In contrast, acute renal failure was found in 1% of patients at admission to the hospital, and these cases were most often of a prerenal etiology.[5]

Chronic renal failure is a syndrome characterized by a slow, progressive decline in glomerular filtration rate (GFR) and other kidney functions. Various adaptations of the diseased kidney limit the clinical manifestations until the loss of kidney function is severe. In practice, it is convenient to divide chronic renal failure into stages such as mild, representing GFRs between 70 ml/min and the normal 120 ml/min; moderate renal insufficiency, representing GFRs from 30 to 70 ml/min; severe renal failure, with GFRs less than 30 ml/min; and end-stage renal disease (ESRD), representing GFRs less than 10 ml/min.

Uremia is the clinical syndrome associated with the retention of the end products of nitrogen metabolism that occurs with severe reductions in renal function. In uremia, the presence of symptoms is unusual before the blood urea nitrogen (BUN) level reaches 60 mg/dl or when the serum creatinine level is 8 mg/dl.

Uremic symptoms are more frequently associated with a BUN level higher than 100 mg/dl and a serum creatinine level higher than 12 mg/dl; the BUN value typically correlates most strongly with uremic symptoms. The metabolic derangements encountered in acute or chronic renal failure result in the dysfunction of several organ systems highlighting the kidney's central role in maintaining the internal environment of the body as a whole.

The overall incidence of new cases of ESRD in the United States is approximately 280 patients per million population annually and has been steadily increasing over the past decade. Approximately 304,000 Americans were receiving chronic dialysis treatment and almost 19,500 renal transplants were performed in 1997. Fig. 149-1 depicts the causes of ESRD in the United States, with diabetes mellitus being the most common.[13]

PATHOPHYSIOLOGY

Acute Renal Failure

Classically in acute renal failure, the GFR is reduced to 1 to 5 ml/min and is associated with a marked fall in urine output to less than 500 ml in 24 hours. The terms *oliguria* and *anuria* refer to urine output of less than 500 and 100 ml/day, respectively. Many patients, however, do not have such severe reductions in GFR, and severe acute renal failure may occur without significant reductions in urine output, giving rise to the term *nonoliguric acute renal failure.*

Renal function is assessed through measurement of the GFR. The normal GFR is 90 to 120 ml/min/1.73 m^2 of body surface area. Although the measurement of insulin clearance is the "gold standard" for measuring GFR, it is usually more convenient to measure serum creatinine levels and creatinine clearance. An elevated serum creatinine value is frequently the first indication of renal failure, often preceding any overt symptoms. However, serum creatinine measurements must be interpreted with caution, since the proportion of creatinine secreted into the tubule increases as the GFR decreases,

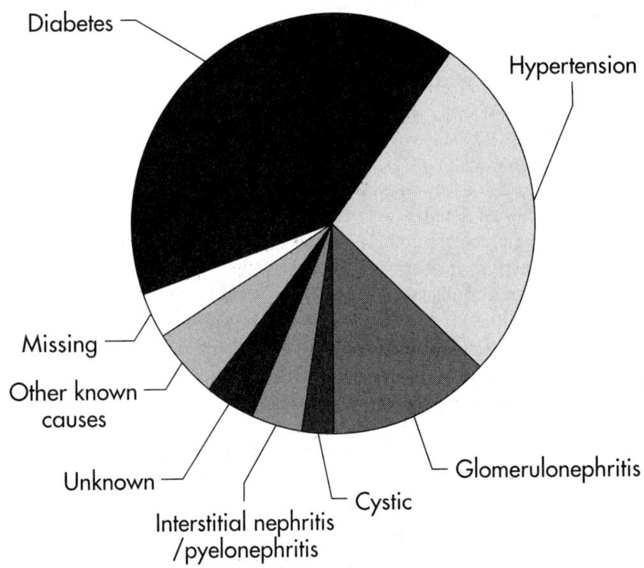

Fig. 149-1. Causes of end-stage renal disease.

resulting in a nonlinear relationship between serum creatinine and GFR and in the overestimation of GFR by the creatinine clearance in the setting of renal impairment. Furthermore, the normal levels of serum creatinine depend on age, sex, and muscle mass, and thus a given level of serum creatinine may reflect a normal GFR in one patient but significant renal failure in another. (See Chapter 144 for further discussion of assessment of renal function.)

Differentiation of the principal causes of acute renal failure (Box 149-1)—prerenal, intrinsic renal, and postrenal—is of extreme importance, since the prognosis and treatment are radically different for each of the three causes. Thus severe acute renal failure from obstruction of the urinary tract requires relief of the obstruction. Acute renal failure caused by a marked reduction in intravascular volume requires treatment with replenishment of the extracellular fluid volume. Analysis of the specific intrinsic renal causes of acute renal failure is also important, since various conditions may be associated with this type of renal failure and require specific evaluation and treatment.

Most cases of acute renal failure occur in the hospital and are related to losses of extracellular fluid volume, the use of nephrotoxic drugs, sepsis or radiographic contrast diagnostic agents, or the effects of surgery or anesthesia. Cases of acute renal failure that occur outside the hospital often produce a great diagnostic challenge; these cases are often serious, and if a definite cause is not readily identifiable (see following discussion) or if the clinical course cannot be easily monitored, prompt referral to a nephrologist for detailed evaluation is required.

The laboratory assessment of acute renal failure is important for distinguishing between prerenal and intrinsic renal causes. In the presence of oliguria, the measurement of the concentrations of sodium and creatinine in serum and urine can provide valuable information regarding the cause of the renal insufficiency. In prerenal acute renal failure, the kidney's normal response is to conserve sodium and water. The conservation of sodium is manifested by a low concentration of sodium in the urine. Water conservation is manifested by an elevated concentration of the nonreabsorbable solute creatinine in the urine compared with the concentration of this solute in plasma; that is, the ratio of urine creatinine to plasma creatinine (U/P creatinine) is high. In the presence of intrinsic renal disease, these adaptations may not occur. Thus the finding of a relatively high urine sodium concentration and a low U/P creatinine ratio usually indicates intrinsic renal disease but is not invariable. These two parameters can be combined to yield the fractional sodium excretion (FE_{Na}), which has improved diagnostic value and is extremely useful in supporting the diagnosis of prerenal azotemia. The FE_{Na} is calculated from measurements of serum and urine concentrations of sodium and creatinine as follows:

$$FE_{Na} = \frac{\text{Urine sodium} \times \text{Serum creatinine} \times 100}{\text{Serum sodium} \times \text{Urine creatinine}}$$

As illustrated in Table 149-1, an FE_{Na} less than 1 suggests prerenal conditions, whereas an FE_{Na} greater than 1 in the presence of oliguria indicates intrinsic renal insufficiency. Certain clinical situations may result in misleading FE_{Na} values. For example, in urinary tract obstruction a wide range of urine sodium concentrations may be found, so obstruction must be excluded directly. In acute glomerular disease, the urinary excretion of sodium may be low, reflecting the marked decrease in GFR with preservation of tubular reabsorption of sodium. Prior administration of diuretics increases the urine sodium levels and renders the value of such determinations useless. If there is preexisting renal disease, the diseased kidney may not be able to reduce the urine sodium concentration maximally in conditions of

Box 149-1. Causes of Acute Renal Failure

Prerenal Causes of Acute Renal Failure

1. Decreased intravascular volume
   Hemorrhage, vomiting, diarrhea, burns
2. Increased intravascular capacity
   Sepsis, vasodilators, anaphylaxis
3. Myocardial failure
   Myocardial infarction, pulmonary embolism, congestive heart failure
4. Hepatorenal syndrome

Intrinsic Renal Causes of Acute Renal Failure

1. Ischemic
   Same conditions as in prerenal causes, postoperative shock
2. Nephrotoxic
   Aminoglycosides, contrast agents, heavy metals
3. Pigment release
   Rhabdomyolysis, hemolysis
4. Inflammatory
   Interstitial nephritis, acute glomerulonephritis, vasculitis
5. Pregnancy related
   Septic abortion, abruptio placentae, eclampsia, postpartum hemorrhage
6. Renovascular disease
   Renal artery thrombosis and embolism, dissecting aneurysm
7. Miscellaneous
   Uric acid nephropathy, hypercalcemia

Postrenal Causes of Acute Renal Failure

1. Obstruction to ureters
   Stones, papillary necrosis, tumors, lymph nodes, fibrosis
2. Obstruction to bladder outlet
   Prostatic hypertrophy, carcinoma

Table 149-1. Urinary Chemistries in Acute Renal Failure*

	Prerenal	Renal
Urinary sodium (U_{Na}) level	<20	>20
Urine to plasma creatinine ratio	>20	<20
Fractional sodium excretion (FE_{Na})	<1	>1

*Although these laboratory tests are extremely useful, urine is not diagnostic in the following conditions: urinary tract obstruction, acute glomerulonephritis, prior administration of diuretics, preexisting chronic renal disease, and metabolic alkalosis.

decreased perfusion, resulting in an elevated FE_{Na} despite prerenal pathophysiologic conditions. Finally, in metabolic alkalosis with alkaline urine, sodium bicarbonate excretion may raise urine sodium levels, so measurement of urine chloride may yield more useful physiologic information in this circumstance. Some cases of acute renal failure caused by allergic interstitial nephritis or secondary to radiographic contrast or cyclosporine toxicity may have low values for FE_{Na}.

Chronic Renal Failure

Although chronic renal failure may occur as a result of many disorders, the same signs and symptoms occur irrespective of the primary cause of nephron loss, and many of the pathophysiologic adaptations are similar. As the nephrons become damaged, the remaining nephrons undergo compensatory hypertrophy. Thus each tubule undergoes several adaptations in an effort to maintain the composition of the extracellular fluid. Although these adaptations maintain the constancy of the internal environment, the capacity of the residual nephrons to cope with the extremes of salt, water, or potassium excess or deficiency is limited. Thus, until renal insufficiency is severe, adaptations of tubular function can allow the excretion of relatively normal amounts of salt and water.

Serum potassium can be maintained within the normal range until renal insufficiency is severe (GFR <10 ml/min), and phosphorus excretion can be maintained by increasing the levels of parathyroid hormone. Although the increases in parathyroid hormone maintain the levels of phosphorus within the normal range, there are additional consequences of the high levels of this hormone on the skeleton, such as the development of hyperparathyroid bone disease (renal osteodystrophy).

As renal function decreases, the kidney's endocrine functions also become limited. Erythropoietin, which is essential for normal red blood cell (RBC) production, is produced in the kidney. The development of anemia is associated with progressive renal disease as erythropoietin production diminishes. Anemia may occur with reductions of renal function of 30% to 50% of normal values and tends to be progressive unless treated with recombinant erythropoietin.

An additional major endocrine function of the kidney is the production of calcitriol, the active form of vitamin D. As calcitriol levels decrease during progressive renal insufficiency, further stress is placed on efforts to maintain calcium and phosphorus homeostasis, which exaggerates the development of secondary hyperparathyroidism.

Impaired acid excretion by the kidney results in the demineralization of bone tissue directly and through the stimulation of osteoclasts and the inhibition of osteoblasts.[1] Since alkali is then released from the skeleton, serum pH and bicarbonate concentrations may change little despite the significant dissolution of bone tissue. Since chronic metabolic acidosis and secondary hyperparathyroidism have a synergistic effect resulting in skeletal damage, patients with chronic renal failure are at particular risk for fractures, bone pain, and disfigurement.

HISTORY

Evaluation of the patient should include a comprehensive clinical history of not only the present complaint but also a previous history of systemic diseases, including those of childhood; a history or family history of hypertension or diabetes; and a careful history of drug ingestion, including over-the-counter medications such as analgesics, nonsteroidal antiinflammatory drugs, herbal or other naturopathic remedies, and other potential nephrotoxins. In women a full gynecologic and obstetric history is also required, including hypertension, proteinuria, or preeclampsia during pregnancy. The occupational history for exposure to potential nephrotoxins may be relevant in certain instances (see Chapter 11). Hospitalized patients should be evaluated for recent hypotensive episodes, sepsis, exposure to radiocontrast media or nephrotoxic drugs, and procedures that subject the patient to atheroemboli such as arteriography or surgery of the aorta.

Both acute and chronic renal insufficiency may present in a variety of ways, and the initial manifestations are often mistaken for primary problems in the affected organ system (Box 149-2). Thus patients may have nausea and vomiting

Box 149-2. Symptoms of Renal Insufficiency

Symptoms Referable to the Urinary Tract

Nocturia
Polyuria
Hematuria
Anuria

Routine Urinalysis

Proteinuria
Hematuria

Routine Physical Examination

Symptoms
- Nausea
- Dyspepsia
- Malaise
- Lassitude
- Weakness
- Pruritus
- Bruising
- Halitosis

Signs
- Hypertension
- Edema
- Congestive heart failure
- Skin abnormalities
- Corneal calcifications

Routine Laboratory Testing

Increased blood urea nitrogen level
Increased creatinine level
Acidosis
Hyperphosphatemia

Presence or History of Systemic Disease Associated with Renal Insufficiency

Hypertension
Diabetes
Connective tissue disorders
Multiple myeloma
Hereditary renal diseases

that may be evaluated as peptic ulcer disease but might represent manifestations of uremia. Presentations with vague symptoms such as weakness and tiredness can easily be attributed to anemia, the basis of which could be renal insufficiency. Difficulties with salt and water homeostasis, such as edema or dyspnea on exertion, may be mistaken for a primary cardiac problem. At the other end of the spectrum, significant renal disease may be present without significant clinical manifestations and may be detected only by routine urinalysis, which may reveal the presence of hematuria or proteinuria and should prompt further evaluation. Moderate to severe renal insufficiency may occur in the absence of symptoms. The patient should be asked questions to determine the etiology of acute renal failure (see Box 149-1) as well as its systemic effects.

PHYSICAL EXAMINATION

A complete physical examination should be performed to evaluate the patient with regard to the etiology of the renal disease and the assessment of complications (Box 149-3). Clues to the etiology of renal disease may be elicited by searching for manifestations of systemic problems such as hypertension, dehydration, diabetes, vasculitis, or leukemia and lymphoma. Hearing impairment may be associated with the hereditary Alport's syndrome. Large bilateral abdominal masses may indicate polycystic kidney disease. Peripheral vascular disease or the presence of abdominal bruits may raise the possibility of atheroembolic renal disease or renal artery stenosis. An enlarged bladder or abnormal prostate or pelvic examination may suggest obstructive uropathy. A rash may point to acute interstitial nephritis, and livedo reticularis is commonly seen in atheroembolic acute renal failure.

The physical examination should strive to assess complications of the chronic renal disease. Assessment of the extracellular fluid volume is important; the patient should be examined for elevation of neck veins, the presence or absence of edema, and ascites. Determination of blood pressure should be performed with the patient lying and standing, and cardiac and lung examinations should be performed. The optic fundi should be examined for evidence of hypertension or diabetes, the skin for bruising or signs of vasculitis, and the bones for tenderness or fracture. Gynecomastia may be seen in men with chronic renal failure, but the incidence of this complication appears to have decreased in recent years. Pericarditis, asterixis, Kussmaul's respirations, ecchymoses, uremic fetor (malodorous breath), and encephalopathy are manifestations of severe uremia.

Some of the presentations of renal disease are serious and require emergency management. Examples of such emergencies would include malignant hypertension; marked decreases in urine output; severe abnormalities in serum chemistries, including hyperkalemia, hypocalcemia, and acidosis; the presence of systemic vasculitis; acute pericarditis; pulmonary edema; encephalopathy; or the development of fever in the presence of urinary tract obstruction.

Box 149-3. Clinical Consequences of Advanced Renal Failure

Cardiovascular
1. Expansion of extracellular fluid
2. Pulmonary edema
3. Hypertension
4. Cardiac arrhythmias
5. Peripheral edema

Metabolic
1. Hyponatremia
2. Hypocalcemia
3. Hyperphosphatemia
4. Hyperuricemia
5. Hyperkalemia
6. Azotemia
7. Acidosis

Neurologic
1. Somnolence
2. Asterixis
3. Seizures
4. Coma
5. Confusion

Hematologic
1. Anemia
2. Platelet dysfunction

Gastrointestinal
1. Nausea
2. Vomiting
3. Gastrointestinal bleeding

Infectious
1. Pneumonia
2. Urinary tract infection
3. Septicemia

LABORATORY STUDIES AND DIAGNOSTIC PROCEDURES

If renal insufficiency is suspected, laboratory evaluation is indicated to assess the degree of the insufficiency and to monitor complications. Microscopic examination of the urine may reveal the presence of moderate numbers of hyaline and fine granular casts in prerenal azotemia. The presence of RBC casts indicates glomerular diseases such as glomerulonephritis or vasculitis. The presence of large amounts of cellular debris or brown muddy, coarsely granular casts is suggestive of ischemic or nephrotoxic acute renal failure.

As previously noted, the GFR may be estimated by measuring the creatinine clearance. Further laboratory evaluation should include a chemistry profile to evaluate serum electrolyte, calcium, phosphorus, uric acid, serum protein, cholesterol, and creatine kinase levels. Anemia and thrombocytopenia should be assessed with a complete blood count and evaluated further as appropriate. Serologic evaluation is useful when vasculitis is a consideration, whereas serum and urine protein electropheresis can detect multiple myeloma. As previously noted, the measurement of FE_{Na} can aid in the diagnosis of acute renal failure.

Imaging of the kidneys and urinary tract, initially by ultrasound, is often helpful for evaluating the size of the kidneys and for excluding the possibility of urinary tract obstruction, which can be reversed with appropriate intervention. Small kidneys indicate chronic renal insufficiency with little possibility of reversal of renal dysfunction, whereas normal-sized kidneys in the presence of severe renal insufficiency should prompt urgent further evaluation for the possibility of reversal of renal dysfunction. Specific diagnoses such as polycystic kidney disease may be revealed by these techniques. In certain patients, renal biopsy is indicated for the specific diagnosis, particularly if a specific treatment might improve or stabilize renal function.

DIFFERENTIAL DIAGNOSIS AND DIAGNOSTIC EVALUATION

When a patient has renal insufficiency, the initial consideration should be to distinguish whether he or she has acute or chronic renal failure. This may be difficult in certain patients, and previous history and laboratory determinations may be useful. Factors that suggest chronicity include long duration of symptoms, severe anemia, bone disease (renal osteodystrophy), sexual dysfunction, skin pigmentation or calcification, neurologic complications, and small kidneys on imaging. Alternatively, patients with chronic renal failure may have few symptoms despite a very high BUN or serum creatinine level as a result of the gradual onset and worsening of renal failure.

In any patient with acute or chronic renal failure, factors must be sought that may exacerbate the degree of renal insufficiency, especially those that may be reversible (Box 149-4). Such reversible factors may represent the activity of the primary renal disease, which may require specific treatment. One common problem is contraction of the extracellular fluid volume because of overdiuresis or fluid loss from vomiting or diarrhea. The development of congestive heart failure as a result of primary cardiac disease or as a manifestation of an expanded extracellular fluid volume may result in decreases in cardiac output, leading to decreases in renal perfusion and worsening of renal insufficiency. Patients with underlying renal disease are predisposed to iatrogenic acute exacerbations of renal failure from angiotensin- converting enzyme (ACE) inhibitors, angiotensin receptor blockers (ARBs), aminoglycosides, and radiocontrast media. Box 149-5 lists other risk factors for contrast-induced renal failure.

Urinary tract infections may lead to pyelonephritis and decreased renal function. Obstruction to the urinary tract may result from stones or sloughed renal papillae, in addition to prostatic disease. Allergic interstitial nephritis as a result of drug therapy may also cause decrements in renal function in the presence of preexisting renal disease (see Chapter 148). The development of metabolic derangements, such as hyperuricemia or hypercalcemia, may also result in a worsening of renal function. Vascular complications, such as the persistence of atheroembolic disease or cholesterol emboli to the kidneys, are often associated with generalized vascular disease and also the possible development of renal vein thrombosis in patients with heavy proteinuria. Acute renal failure in the setting of thrombocytopenia and hemolytic anemia suggest renal involvement in either hemolytic uremic syndrome or thrombotic thrombocytopenia purpura, known collectively as *thrombotic microangiopathy.* Finally, urinary tract obstruction by tumor, fibrosis, prostatic hypertrophy, or infection can result in acute or chronic renal failure. The underlying cause must be carefully sought in any patient with a sudden or unexpected decrement in renal function, since prompt correction of the abnormality may be successful in returning renal function to baseline.

Box 149-4. Factors that May Aggravate Renal Insufficiency

1. Active primary disease
2. Extracellular fluid volume contraction
3. Congestive heart failure and volume overload
4. Drugs
5. Radiographic contrast agents
6. Infections
7. Obstruction
8. Acute interstitial nephritis
9. Hyperuricemia
10. Hypercalcemia
11. Renal vein thrombosis
12. Atheroembolic disease and cholesterol embolism

Box 149-5. Risk Factors for Contrast Nephrotoxicity

1. Underlying renal insufficiency (serum creatinine level >2 mg/dl)
2. Diabetes mellitus, especially with renal insufficiency
3. Congestive heart failure
4. Volume contraction
5. High doses of contrast
6. Multiple myeloma
7. Advanced age

MANAGEMENT

Acute Renal Failure

Acute renal failure is a serious condition has a considerable mortality rate ranging from 30% to 50%. If acute renal failure is suspected, prompt referrals should be made to specialized centers for specific diagnosis and management if resolution does not occur promptly or if the etiology is in doubt. Since the course of acute renal failure ranges from 7 to 21 days, dialysis may be required until renal recovery can occur. Absolute indications for prompt referral include volume overload with congestive heart failure, hyperkalemia, severe acidosis, bleeding, and uremic symptoms. If hyperkalemia is present with the electrocardiographic changes of peaked T waves, flattened P waves, prolongation of the PR interval, or widening of the QRS complex, urgent treatment is required. Immediate therapy should include the administration of calcium gluconate intravenously, followed by the correction of acidosis with the administration of intravenous bicarbonate. Additional therapy should include 50 ml of 50% dextrose with 10 units of regular insulin to shift extracellular potassium into the cells. Potassium removal from the body can be accomplished by the use of sodium polystyrene sulfonate (Kayexalate) given orally or as a retention enema. If renal failure is severe, arrangements should be made for the prompt institution of dialysis.

In patients with oliguric renal failure, a trial of diuretics may be undertaken to attempt to convert this situation to nonoliguric failure through the use of loop diuretics. In this way, fluid balance can be improved, and there may be some therapeutic benefit by increasing tubular urine flow.

Chronic Renal Failure

Box 149-6 lists the general principles of the management of chronic renal failure. In addition to monitoring the progression of renal failure and evaluating the response to specific therapies, complications of renal failure must be successfully anticipated and promptly treated. Chronic renal failure subsequent to systemic illness mandates attention to the underlying illness as well. Furthermore, routine medical

Box 149-6. Chronic Renal Insufficiency: Principles of Management

Prevention of or Delay in Progression to End-Stage Renal Disease

1. Blood pressure control
2. Glycemic control
3. Drug therapy
4. Protein restriction

Nutrition

1. Prevention of malnutrition
2. Prevention of electrolyte imbalance
3. Prevention of uremic symptoms

Psychosocial

1. Adjustment to chronic illness
2. Employment and disability issues
3. Family support

Anemia

1. Erythropoietin
2. Iron supplementation

Bone and Mineral Metabolism

1. Dietary phosphate restriction
2. Phosphate binding therapy
3. Calcium supplementation
4. Bicarbonate supplementation
5. Vitamin D therapy

Preparation for Renal Replacement Therapy

1. Education
2. Selection of renal replacement modality
   - Dialysis
     - Peritoneal dialysis vs. hemodialysis
     - Home hemodialysis vs. in-center hemodialysis
   - Transplantation
     - Living donor vs. cadaveric donor
     - Living related donor vs. living unrelated donor
3. Dialysis access placement
4. Psychosocial preparation
5. Pretransplant testing

issues such as appropriate drug dosing and infection management must be approached within the context of the deranged physiology of renal failure. Finally, preparation for dialysis or transplantation involves attention to the special medical, social, emotional, and psychologic needs of the patient and the family. To accomplish these goals, a consensus conference of the National Institutes of Health[11] has recommended referral to a nephrologist as soon as the creatinine level reaches 1.5 mg/dl in women and 2.0 mg/dl in men; the nephrologist can facilitate the management of the case with the primary care physician.

As already discussed, the mainstay of monitoring for the progression of renal failure is the measurement of serum creatinine levels supplemented with occasional determination of creatinine clearance. Some have advocated the use of plots of the reciprocal of the serum creatinine over time to monitor progression of renal failure, since a linear relationship often is found, making it possible to predict the time at which dialysis might be required and to evaluate deviations from the predicted course.

Serial serum chemistry determinations are important in the assessment of complications so that compliance with the diet can be evaluated and levels of potassium, bicarbonate, serum albumin, cholesterol, and uric acid and parameters of renal function can be monitored. This is also important in evaluating the efficacy of efforts to control serum phosphorus values and to maintain the levels of serum calcium. In diabetic patients, serial assessment of glycosylated hemoglobin determinations is useful for obtaining an index of the efficacy of blood sugar control between office visits. It is important to realize that renal insulin clearance decreases with increasing renal insufficiency. Therefore diabetic patients typically have decreasing insulin requirements as renal disease progresses.

As renal failure progresses, modest restriction of protein intake to 0.8 gm/kg/day can ameliorate symptoms of uremia and in some but not all studies has been shown to slow the progression of renal failure. It may become necessary to restrict phosphorus to 700 to 800 mg/day and potassium to 60 mmol/day based on frequent surveillance of the serum chemistry values. Sodium retention with signs of volume overload and sodium depletion with signs of dehydration and volume contraction are common in patients with chronic renal failure; therefore attention to salt and water intake is extremely important in their management. In general, only moderate salt restriction should be prescribed except with clear evidence of volume overload. Patients with chronic renal failure are usually able to maintain normal serum potassium levels until the GFR falls below 10 ml/min.

The incidence of hypertension increases with the increasing degree of renal failure, reaching 95% in patients with a GFR of 10 ml/min or less.[9] Control of blood pressure in patients with renal disease prevents not only further deterioration in renal function but also the development of vascular complications of hypertension. The National High Blood Pressure Education Program Working Group[10] recommends treating hypertension to a goal of 130/85 mm in patients with chronic renal failure. A target pressure of 125/75 Hg should be used for patients with urinary protein levels higher than 1 gm/day. Measurements of blood pressure with the patient both lying and standing are useful in diabetic patients, who may have autonomic dysfunction, and in patients receiving drug therapy for the evaluation of potential postural hypotension. This may also be valuable in patients with suspected extracellular volume contraction.

Although lowering the systemic blood pressure is beneficial, the choice of antihypertensive drugs may have an impact on the progression of renal disease. Data from numerous studies have demonstrated that ACE inhibitors slow the progression of renal failure independent of their effects on reducing blood pressure in several types of renal disease, with the most pronounced effects in patients with diabetes types I and II with urinary protein levels higher than 1 gm/day.[4,7,8] Blood pressure measurements should be followed closely after the institution of antihypertensive therapy so that excessive reductions in renal blood flow do not further compromise renal function, especially in the presence of renal vascular disease. This may be seen with any agent that effectively lowers the blood pressure, but the use of ACE inhibitors has been particularly implicated in such effects. Serum potassium levels should be checked several days after the start of therapy with ACE inhibitors to exclude hyperkalemia. This is particularly important in diabetic patients and those using β-blockers and nonsteroidal antiinflammatory drugs, who may be particularly susceptible to the development of hyperkalemia. Although few studies have been undertaken, data suggest that calcium channel blockers, particularly verapamil and diltiazem, may attenuate the progression of diabetic nephropathy.[2] These agents may be used as second-line antihypertensives for patients unable to tolerate ACE inhibitors. In animal models of renal failure, like ACE inhibitors, angiotensin II receptor antagonists such as losartan delay the progression of renal failure, but it must be stressed that long-term human trials have yet to be performed. As with ACE inhibitors, hyperkalemia may complicate therapy with angiotensin receptor blockers in patients with renal insufficiency.

Diuretics are often necessary in combination with other antihypertensives to control blood pressure in patients with renal insufficiency. Loop diuretics are used most commonly because thiazides tend to be ineffective at a GFR less than 25 ml/min and the use of potassium-sparing diuretics is frequently contraindicated as a result of predisposition for hyperkalemia in patients with chronic renal failure.

Hyperlipidemia is often associated with chronic renal failure and is often more severe in patients who have nephrotic syndrome or diabetes. Since cardiovascular complications are common in chronic renal disease and since experimental evidence shows that hyperlipidemia may have a deleterious effect on the progression of renal disease,[6] the clinician should attempt to treat hypercholesterolemia. This can be done by attention to the diet, but many patients require drug intervention.

Histologic changes of hyperparathyroidism occur relatively early in the course of chronic renal failure. Early surveillance of intact parathyroid hormone levels and a low-phosphorus diet are the initial steps. Most patients eventually require therapy with phosphate binders such as calcium carbonate, calcium acetate, or cross-linked polyallylamine hydrochloride, also called Sevelamer or RenaGel, taken with meals, as well as calcium salts taken on an empty stomach to increase serum calcium levels in the setting of hypocalcemia. The use of aluminum-containing antacids as phosphorus binders is no longer recommended. The use of calcitriol, the physiologically active form of vitamin D, is also useful in treating mild to moderate hyperparathyroidism but often causes hypercalcemia, so such therapy should be undertaken with caution. Newly developed vitamin D analogs have the potential to reduce PTH levels without causing hypercalcemia.

Acidosis should be treated, if possible, with the awareness that bicarbonate supplementation may also lead to excessive sodium intake. Citrate-containing alkali salts should be avoided in advanced renal failure because of the possibility of enhancing the absorption of aluminum from the intestine.

The anemia of chronic renal failure is due primarily to low erythropoietin levels. When measured, erythropoietin levels are typically within the "normal" range of 15 to 30 mU/mL, reflecting an inappropriately low response to anemia. Intervention includes the institution of therapy with recombinant human erythropoietin (rHuEPO) with a target hematocrit of 33% to 36%.[13] Supplementation of iron is frequently necessary in patients taking rHuEPO. Such therapy requires careful supervision because aggravation of hypertension and development of polycythemia may occur.

Since many drugs required for general medical management are handled by the kidneys for excretion, it is imperative that the dosing of any prescribed drug be verified for the degree of renal insufficiency.

End-stage Renal Disease. It is usual to initiate dialysis when the creatinine clearance is less than 10 to 12 ml/min, which would usually correlate with a serum creatinine concentration of 8 to 12 mg/dl. Often, however, the initiation of dialysis depends on the development of symptoms of uremia. Excessive delay in starting dialysis can result in malnutrition and may delay ultimate recovery and rehabilitation. Most facilities provide hemodialysis and peritoneal dialysis and either perform transplantation or can refer to a transplantation center. The involvement of the nephrologist is important in the choice of dialysis modality and in the consideration for renal transplantation. Thus the patient may become both educated about the various forms of therapy and acquainted with the personnel involved in the management of the ESRD program.

Hemodialysis requires safe and reliable vascular access. The preferred access is through a primary arteriovenous fistula, which can usually be created under local anesthesia. The fistula requires 2 to 6 months of maturation before use. If the patient's vessels are inadequate, synthetic grafts can be inserted in the arm. These grafts can generally be used within 4 weeks of placement. The major complications of such vascular-access procedures are clotting and infection. It is usual to perform hemodialysis three times a week, with each session lasting approximately 4 hours. The annual mortality rate for hemodialysis patients is approximately 20% to 25%. This estimate varies according to comorbid conditions (e.g., diabetes, cardiovascular disease).[4]

Continuous ambulatory peritoneal dialysis is an alternative treatment in which dialysis fluid is inserted through a catheter into the abdominal cavity, where exchange of solute occurs between blood and fluid. After a period of time, the fluid containing waste products and extra water is then removed through the catheter and discarded. A modified form of such therapy is the use of an automated cycling machine during the night. This continuous cycling peritoneal dialysis can be helpful to patients with limited mobility. Continued ambulatory peritoneal dialysis requires a minimum of four dialysis exchanges per day. The advantages of this form of dialysis is that it provides greater flexibility to patients, enabling them to work or travel and set their own schedules. Peritonitis is a potential complication of peritoneal dialysis, so strict attention to sterile technique is necessary. Since repeated connections of tubing are required, it is desirable that the patient's vision and fine-motor coordination be satisfactory; however, some devices can facilitate these connections. Although comparative survival statistics between hemodialysis and peritoneal dialysis are somewhat difficult to interpret in view of the unmatched patients, it would appear that under most conditions, survival rates are comparable.

Of the therapies for ESRD, a successful renal transplant provides the most complete correction of the uremic syndrome. Kidney transplantation from living related donors now has 1-year success rates above 90%, and that of transplantation with cadaveric kidneys now routinely exceeds 80%. Long-term success rates are somewhat lower, and some kidneys fail because of chronic rejection, but median graft survival in living donor transplants is 15 to 16 years and 9 to 10 years in cadaveric donor transplants.[14]

REFERENCES

1. Alpern RJ, Khashayar S: The clinical spectrum of chronic metabolic acidosis: homeostatic mechanisms produce significant morbidity, *Am J Kidney Dis* 29:291-302, 1997.
2. Amann K, et al: Effect of ACE inhibitors, calcium channel blockers and their combination on renal and extrarenal structures in renal failure, *Nephrol Dial Transplant* 10(suppl):9:33, 1995.
3. Hou SH, et al: Hospital-acquired renal insufficiency: a prospective study, *Am J Med* 74:243, 1983.
4. Kasiske BL, et al: Effect of antihypertensive therapy on the kidney in patients with diabetes: a meta-regression analysis, *Ann Intern Med* 118:129, 1993.
5. Kaufman J, et al: Community-acquired acute renal failure, *Am J Kidney Dis* 17:191, 1991.
6. Keane WF: Lipids and the kidney, *Kidney Int* 46:910, 1994.
7. Lewis EJ, et al: The effect of angiotensin-converting-enzyme inhibition on diabetic nephropathy, *N Engl J Med* 329:1456, 1993.
8. Maschio G, et al: Effect of the angiotensin-converting-enzyme inhibitor benazepril on the progression of chronic renal insufficiency, *N Engl J Med* 334:939, 1996.
9. Modification of Diet in Renal Disease Study Group (prepared by Buckalew VM, et al): Prevalence of hypertension in 1,795 subjects with chronic renal disease: the Modification of Diet in Renal Disease Study baseline cohort, *Am J Kidney Dis* 28:811, 1996.
10. National High Blood Pressure Education Program Working Group: 1995 update of the working group reports on chronic renal failure and renovascular hypertension, *Arch Intern Med* 156:1938, 1996.
11. National Institutes of Health Consensus Developmental Conference on Morbidity and Mortality of Dialysis: Morbidity and mortality of renal dialysis: an NIH consensus conference statement, *Ann Intern Med* 121:62, 1994.
12. Shusterman N, et al: Risk factors and outcome of hospital-acquired acute renal failure: clinical epidemiologic study, *Am J Med* 83:65, 1987.
13. US Renal Data System: Incidence and Prevalence of ESRD. In *USRDS 1999 annual data report,* Bethesda, Md, 1999, The National Institutes of Health, National Institute of Diabetes and Digestive and Kidney Diseases.
14. US Renal Data System: Renal transplantation: access and outcomes. In *USRDS 1999 annual data report,* Bethesda, Md, 1999, The National Institutes of Health, National Institute of Diabetes and Digestive and Kidney Diseases.

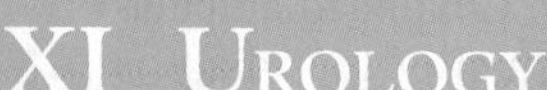

XI UROLOGY

CHAPTER 150

Male Infertility

Robert D. Oates

Infertility affects approximately 15% of couples trying to conceive. This may be higher or lower depending on the age of the female partner because her fertility potential declines after the age of 35. Male factors contribute to at least 50% of cases of infertility. The traditional definition of *infertility* is the inability to conceive after 1 year of unprotected intercourse, but this time frame has been substantially shortened over the last several years as couples seek evaluation and treatment sooner and sooner. The fertility evaluation should begin as soon as the couple comes to medical attention. Couples may first seek help from their primary care physician when they become concerned about their inability to conceive. A basic history and physical examination may reveal an obvious cause for either partner, but a referral to a gynecologist or urologist is most appropriate, even at this point. However, the primary care physician may play a critical role in predicting a possible problem with fertility or in preventing future difficulties.

This chapter reviews the most common etiologies of male infertility and provides a list of physical examination findings that may be detected by the primary care physician. Infertility is a "couple" issue, and both partners should be evaluated, even if a dramatic finding (anovulation, azoospermia) is discovered early.

EPIDEMIOLOGY OF MALE REPRODUCTIVE DYSFUNCTION

Primary infertility is the inability to conceive for the first time within 12 months. However, many couples become concerned after just a few months and initiate conversations with the primary care physician or gynecologist. For many, there are no real limitations to achieving pregnancy. For others, a prior history (e.g., chemotherapy), a present problem (e.g., anovulation), or a female age issue (age >38 years) may be of concern. These types of issues justify an early evaluation because patients are often on target and their chances of natural conception are indeed low. Today, many couples are delaying childbearing, and a woman's fertility potential begins to decline after age 35, with a more precipitous slope after age 38 to 39.

BASIC ANATOMY AND PHYSIOLOGY OF THE MALE REPRODUCTIVE SYSTEM

The finely tuned interplay of the spermatogenic axis and the androgenic axis is crucial to maximal sperm production. Spermatogenesis occurs in the millions of seminiferous tubules that make up the bulk of the testicular parenchyma. As mature sperm are released into the tubule lumen, they travel to the intratesticular rete testis, a series of widened tubules in the mediastinum of the testis. The rete testis gives rise to six to eight efferent ductules that exit the testis to form the head (caput) of the epididymis. Here the efferent ducts merge to form one continuous epididymal tubule, which is highly coiled and serpentine as it makes up the body (corpus) and the tail (cauda) of the epididymis. The epididymis is not a storage organ for sperm, since the spermatozoa generally make the complete journey in just a few days.[5] The epididymal tubule thickens and develops more of a muscularis as it becomes the convoluted portion of the vas deferens. The vas straightens out in the scrotal portion as it enters the external ring and emerges through the internal ring and then takes a course down, posterior to the base of the bladder. There, it becomes even wider and corkscrew in shape at the ampullary region. The seminal vesicle joins the vas on its lateral aspect to create the ejaculatory duct just outside the capsule of the prostate. The ejaculatory duct pierces the substance of the prostate, traversing the parenchyma obliquely to open into the urethra at the verumontanum.

The process of ejaculation is a complex neurologic event

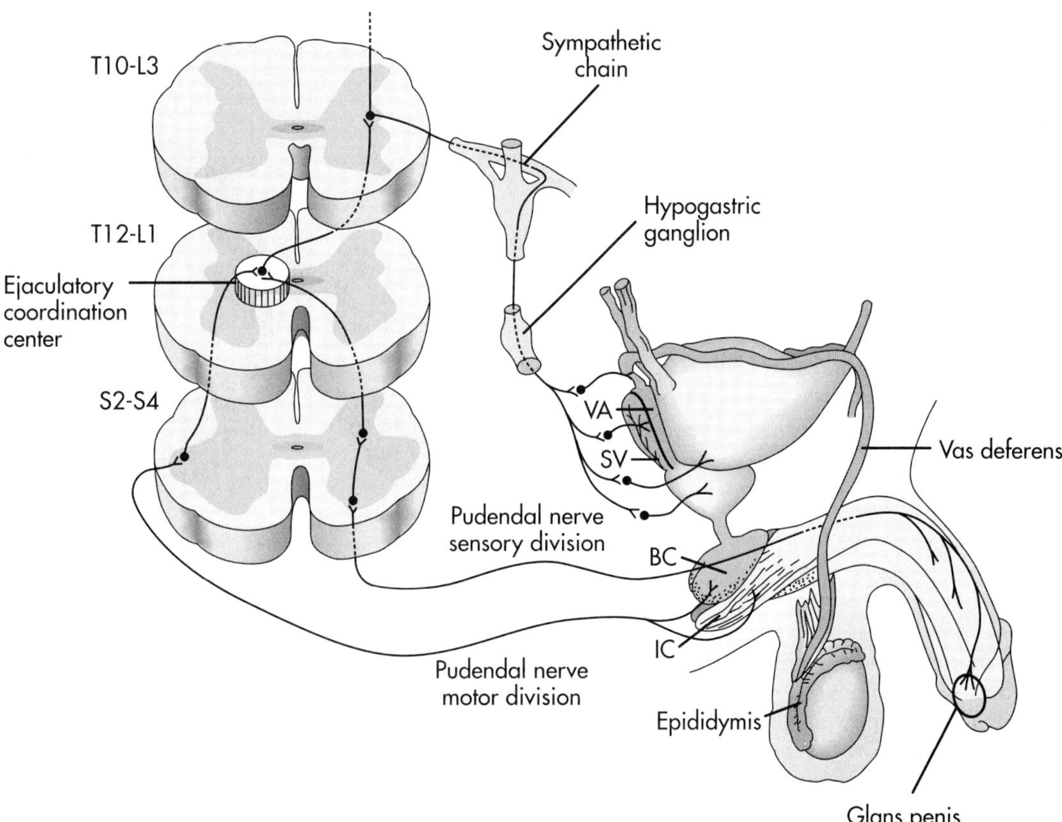

Fig. 150-1. Neuroanatomy of the ejaculatory reflex. Sympathetic fibers originate from the thoracolumbar cord to innervate the vas deferens, seminal vesicle *(SV)*, prostate, and bladder neck. Somatic fibers control contraction of the periurethral musculature and arise from the sacral cord. The ejaculatory reflex center integrates the phases of emission and antegrade ejaculation and is located at T12-L1. Sensory fibers travel from the penis to the sacral cord at S2-S4. *BC*, Bulbocavernosus muscle; *IC*, ischiocavernosus muscle; *VA*, vasal ampulla.

consisting of two distinct but integrated phases (Fig. 150-1). Emission is a sympathetically mediated contraction of the seminal vesicles, vasal ampullae, and prostate that delivers the various seminal fluid components into the prostatic urethra. Simultaneously, the bladder neck closes, a process controlled by these same sympathetic fibers. This prevents the ejaculate bolus from flowing backward into the bladder. Periurethral musculature contraction is the next phase of the ejaculatory event and propels the fluid contained within the prostatic urethra in an antegrade direction. The rhythmic contraction of this musculature is controlled through somatic efferents emanating from S2-S4 and traveling with the pudendal nerve. The sympathetic outflow originates from spinal segments T10-T12. Within the cord (T12-L1) exists an ejaculation reflex center that coordinates and temporally integrates the ejaculatory event. Any interruption of the sympathetic fibers, as may occur during pelvic surgery, an anterior approach to thoracolumbar disk disease, or a retroperitoneal lymph node dissection, may impair emission, bladder neck closure, or both processes. This may result in complete failure of emission (a dry ejaculate) or retrograde seminal fluid flow. The sensation of orgasm is intact, but no ejaculate is visible to the patient. Spinal cord injury above the sympathetic outflow and reflex center disrupts any augmentation that may arise in the cerebral cortex from visual, auditory, or conceptual stimuli.

The hypothalamus releases gonadotropin-releasing hormone (GnRH), which stimulates the secretion of luteinizing hormone (LH) and follicle-stimulating hormone (FSH) from the anterior pituitary (Fig. 150-2). LH stimulates intratesticular Leydig cells to produce testosterone that feeds back negatively on the hypothalamus and pituitary to regulate the secretion of LH. Exogenous androgenic compounds (e.g., anabolic steroids) suppress LH secretion and consequently shut down intratesticular testosterone production, which is necessary for spermatogenesis to occur. This is why most men taking illegal anabolic steroids are azoospermic. FSH acts directly on Sertoli cells to stimulate spermatogenesis. Inhibin is released from Sertoli cells to negatively regulate FSH secretion. As spermatogenic ability declines, inhibin levels drop, and FSH output increases. There is no defined cut-off for FSH values below which spermatogenesis is normal and above which it is abnormal. It is a gradual rise, correlated with spermatogenic capability. The "normal" range of FSH, as documented by the manufacturer of the assay machine being used, is really not relevant in clinical practice because the FSH concentration rises steadily as spermatogenesis declines. However, there is no strict correlation. In an azoospermic patient with primary spermatogenic failure, the FSH value is higher than that seen in men with completely adequate sperm production but does not need to be two to three times the upper limit of the assay range. Measurement of FSH, LH, and testosterone levels needs to be performed only in the azoospermic or severely oligospermic patient and has no influence on the diagnostic impressions or therapeutic decisions in a patient with a

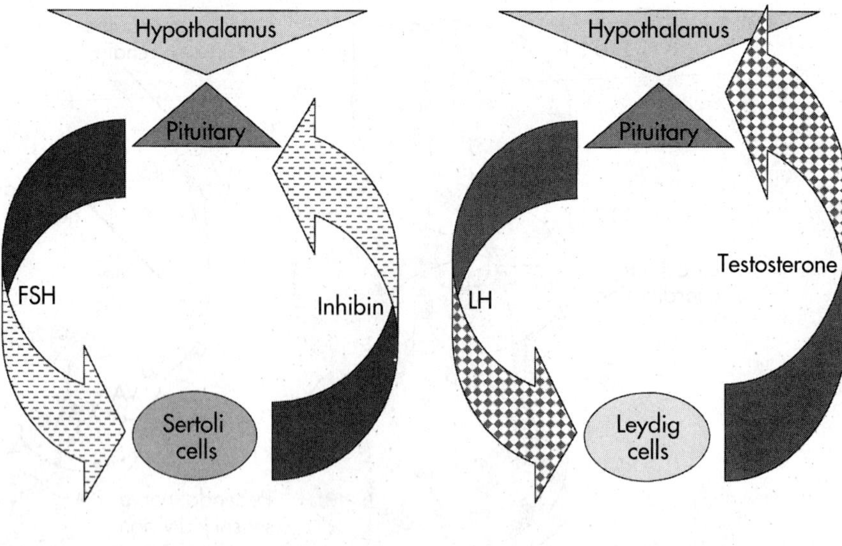

Fig. 150-2. The hypothalamic-pituitary-gonadal axis. Gonadotropin-releasing hormone is secreted by the hypothalamus to induce the formation and secretion of follicle-stimulating hormone *(FSH)* and luteinizing hormone *(LH)*. FSH stimulates spermatogenesis via its action on Sertoli cells and is negatively regulated by inhibin, a product of Sertoli cells (the spermatogenic axis). LH activates interstitial Leydig cells to produce and elaborate testosterone, which negatively controls LH release via feedback on both the pituitary and hypothalamus (the androgenic axis).

slightly low count or somewhat impaired motility (mild to moderate oligoasthenospermia).

Spermatogenesis is a complex, highly ordered process with three goals (Fig. 150-3). The first is the reduction in the number of chromosomes from a diploid (2n) complement to a haploid (1n) state. When fertilization occurs, the haploid sperm pronucleus joins with the female pronucleus, recreating a diploid chromosomal constitution. The second purpose of spermatogenesis is to allow recombination events to occur between homologous chromosomes, which leads to diversification of the genome, an evolutionary advantage. These first two processes are inherent features of the meiotic process that drives the alteration of spermatogonia to spermatids. The final goal of the spermatogenic cell cycle is accomplished in spermiogenesis, in which profound morphologic changes create a functional spermatozoan, the vehicle that delivers the genetic material to and breaks through the barriers of the waiting oocyte.

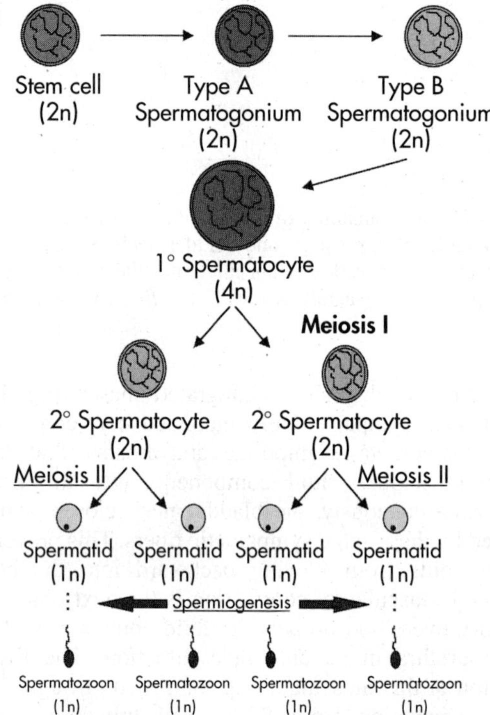

Fig. 150-3. Spermatogenic cell cycle. Spermatogonia divide mitotically to either renew themselves or begin down a course of sperm development. Type B spermatogonia, primary spermatocytes, secondary spermatocytes, and spermatids are successive stages in the meiotic process resulting in a haploid cell. Spermiogenesis is the morphologic transformation of the spermatid to the spermatozoan.

MALE REPRODUCTIVE HISTORY

It is important to review with the couple the elements of the menstrual cycle, proper coital timing, and the necessity of a concomitant female evaluation. Many men and women have poor knowledge of reproductive anatomy and physiology. Education may be all that is required to help them achieve pregnancy. There is no optimal frequency of intercourse; it may occur every day or every other day. Ideally, sperm should be in the female reproductive tract at the time of ovulation because the oocyte is viable for only a short time. Couples who wait until they believe ovulation has occurred may be missing their "window" of opportunity. Ovulation-predictor kits may be used to more precisely pinpoint when ovulation will occur.

Pediatric Issues (Box 150-1)

Cryptorchidism may be found in up to 9% of men seeking care for infertility. A history of bilateral cryptorchidism puts men at significant risk of severe oligospermia or azoospermia. Most men with unilateral cryptorchidism have sperm in the ejaculate, but their natural fertility rate may be reduced compared to those without such a history.

Hernias and hydroceles in infancy may be associated with testicular maldescent. Therefore hernia and hydrocele repairs, along with orchidopexy, may have been performed, even though the patient is not aware of it. Vasal injury at the level of the internal ring may be a consequence of infant hernia repair and may be the cause of unilateral or bilateral vasal occlusion.

Box 150-1. Etiology of Male Reproductive Dysfunction: Pediatric

Cryptorchidism
Hernia repair
Hypospadias
Bladder exstrophy
Cystic fibrosis
Malignancies
  Genitourinary
  Lymphoreticular
Testis torsion
Hydrocele repair
Posterior urethral valves
  Myelomeningocele
  Prune-belly syndrome
  Chemotherapy
  Radiotherapy

Male patients with cystic fibrosis (CF) are born without vasa deferentia and are azoospermic. Congenital bilateral absence of the vas deferens (CBAVD) is a milder phenotype of CF.

Hypospadias of significant degree may impair the delivery of semen. After the repair of hypospadias, male patients may have strictured areas that impede the force of seminal fluid release, again potentially inhibiting seminal fluid and thus sperm contact with the cervical mucus. Testicular torsion that is not surgically corrected in time leads to loss of that testis and functional compromise of the remaining testis as a result of unexplained immunologic effects. Other rare conditions of development can interrupt the ejaculatory process or cause spermatogenic compromise (e.g., bladder exstrophy, prune-belly syndrome). Any malignancy that is treated with chemotherapy may lead to permanent spermatogenic damage.

Adult Issues

Any neurologic disturbance may impair ejaculatory function (Box 150-2). This may be at the level of the spinal cord (traumatic injury, transverse myelitis, myelodysplasia) or the peripheral neuroanatomy (retroperitoneal surgery disrupting the afferent sympathetic fibers or the autonomic dystrophy consequent to diabetes mellitus). With a malignancy that involves the testis (germ cell tumor) or the prostate or bladder, posttreatment functional and anatomic problems can interfere with ejaculation or sperm production. Chemotherapy acutely suppresses spermatogenesis and may also have significant long-term effects, even to the point of producing permanent azoospermia. The final outcome depends not only on the inherent spermatogenic ability of the individual but also on the exact chemotherapeutic regimen used. Radiotherapy to the pelvic area also has an immediate effect, although long-term consequences are typically not as severe.

Toxin exposure may lead to the suppression of spermatogenesis (Box 150-3). Cigarette smoking should be discontinued to reduce any possible detrimental effects on the sperm count, motility, and fertilizing ability. Excessive alcohol should be avoided. Marijuana use may lead to alterations in the hormonal axis as well as impaired fertilization. The possible consequences on human spermatogenesis of most medications have not been well explored or investigated. Drugs such as azulfidine and colchicine are known spermatotoxins, and with other pharmaceuticals, there may be ill effects that have not yet been fully realized. If a patient can safely be taken off a medication, then it makes sense to

Box 150-2. Etiology of Male Reproductive Dysfunction: Ejaculatory Disrupters

Spinal cord injury
Transverse myelitis
Retroperitoneal surgery
Multiple sclerosis
Diabetes
Prostate or bladder surgery

Box 150-3. Etiology of Male Reproductive Dysfunction: Adult Toxin Exposure

Cigarette smoking
Illicit drugs
Medications
  Azulfidine
  Colchicine
  Calcium channel blockers
Alcohol abuse
Marijuana use
Occupational toxins
  Organic solvents
  Heavy metals
  Pesticides and herbicides

discontinue that medication in case it is having a subtle effect on sperm production or function.

Anabolic steroid use is becoming an epidemic among high school and college athletes. Any exogenous testosterone or derivative feeds back on the hypothalamus and pituitary and suppresses the secretion of LH and FSH, thereby inhibiting the intratesticular testosterone production required for spermatogenesis. These men are severely oligospermic or azoospermic. An occupational history may elicit exposure to chemicals that can impair sperm production. The patient should be counseled to take all precautions recommended by the Occupational Safety and Health Administration (OSHA). Other problems such as epididymitis (possible epididymal tubule occlusion) or prostatitis (possible ejaculatory duct cyst) may be revealed in the genitourinary history. All of the information must be integrated with the semen analysis, physical examination, and simultaneous female evaluation.

Genetic syndromes can have male factor infertility as a part of their phenotypic spectrum (Box 150-4). For example, males with myotonic dystrophy often have reduced spermatogenesis for an unknown reason. Males with CF have bilateral vasal agenesis. Men with Klinefelter's syndrome typically possess markedly impaired spermatogenesis and a compromised androgenic axis. The immotile cilia syndrome may be first recognized because of the respiratory illness often associated with this diagnosis; as the ciliated cells of the lower and upper airway system are paralyzed, so are the spermatozoa, and infertility is the rule. These and other genetic disorders are discussed in later sections.

MALE REPRODUCTIVE PHYSICAL EXAMINATION

As in all disease processes, the physical examination may reveal the reason for infertility or may predict male reproductive dysfunction (Box 150-5). The general appearance of

Box 150-4. Etiology of Male Reproductive Dysfunction: Genetic Disorders

Cystic fibrosis
Klinefelter's syndrome
Immotile cilia syndrome
Androgen receptor deficiency
Y chromosomal microdeletions
Congenital absence of the vas deferens
Kallmann's syndrome
Myotonic dystrophy
Prune-belly syndrome
Translocations

Box 150-5. Physical Examination Findings that May Predict Infertility

Decreased testis size
Firm epididymides
Varicocele
Inguinal incisions
Penile deformity
Extreme obesity
Decreased testis consistency
Absent vasa deferentia
Hypospadias
Scrotal incisions
Poor virilization
Anorexia

the individual is important, since profound obesity may affect spermatogenesis. The patient may be undervirilized with poor beard growth and minimal muscular development, potentially indicating conditions such as Kallmann's or Klinefelter's syndrome. Gynecomastia may be seen when the testosterone/estradiol ratio deviates from the norm. The penis should be examined carefully for hypospadias or phimosis. The testes should be oblong and measure approximately 3.5 by 2.5 cm. Their consistency should be slightly firm. Decreased testis size and consistency are signs of depressed spermatogenic ability because most of the bulk of the testis consists of the spermatogenic epithelium within the seminiferous tubules. The vasa deferentia are easily palpable in most men. Their presence must be documented, especially in the azoospermic man in whom congenital vasal aplasia is a distinct possibility. Only the caput and cauda epididymis are typically palpable, since the corpus is generally flat in the unobstructed system. When the entire epididymis can be appreciated and it is firm, distal obstruction may be present, as occurs in the patient who has had a vasectomy. A distended pampiniform plexus is easily felt, usually in the left hemiscrotum, and defines a varicocele. Approximately 15% of men have a clinically palpable left varicocele, and it is one of the most frequent causes of male infertility. Another finding to note is the presence of any inguinal or scrotal incisions, which may implicate infant genitourinary surgery of which the patient was unaware.

BASIC PARAMETERS OF THE SEMEN ANALYSIS (Table 150-1)

The sperm count is the most important sperm parameter but is not very predictive of pregnancy achievement. Even though the lower limit of normal is considered to be 20×10^6 sperm/ml, this does not mean that patients are necessarily sterile with counts below this level or fertile with counts above it.[9] The "normal" limit is just a number that allows classification of patients in terms of sperm count. The lower the count, the less likely pregnancy will occur, but the couple's entire situation must be taken into account. The same holds true for motility (the percentage of sperm that are moving), forward progression (how well the motile sperm are moving), and morphology (the percentage of "normally" shaped sperm as defined by a number of criteria).[7] The semen volume is especially relevant when creating a differential diagnosis for the azoospermic patient. In patients with a volume greater than 2 ml and a pH higher than 7.0, seminal vesicle fluid is present in the ejaculate, since it makes up 70% of the total ejaculate volume and is alkaline. This overwhelms the small amount of acidic contribution from the prostate (20% of the total) and creates an alkaline milieu for the spermatozoa. If there is less than 1.5 ml of fluid and it is acidic (pH, 6.5), then seminal vesicle fluid will not be in that ejaculate. (See the later section for a discussion of the differential diagnosis of azoospermia.) *Oligospermia* is defined as a count below 20×10^6 sperm/ml. Asthenospermia occurs when the motility is below the limits of normal and teratospermia when the morphology is so categorized. Therefore a sample with a low count, motility, and morphology is considered to be oligoasthenoteratospermic and have the so-called OAT syndrome.

Table 150-1. Semen Analysis: Normal Ranges

Parameter	Value
Ejaculate volume	1.5-5.0 ml
Sperm density	>20 million/ml
Sperm motility	>60%
Forward progression	>2 (scale of 1-4)
Morphology	>30% (WHO criteria) >14% (Strict criteria)

Data from *WHO laboratory manual for the examination of human semen and sperm—cervical mucus interaction,* ed 4, Cambridge, UK, 1997, Cambridge University Press.

DIFFERENTIAL DIAGNOSIS OF OLIGOASTHENOTERATOSPERMIA

No one specific etiology gives rise to the OAT syndrome or to a lowering of only the sperm count, motility, or morphology. All of the factors listed in the sections on history and physical examination need to be considered. That is, a varicocele might be present, drug use might be harming sperm production, or cryptorchidism might be in the history and indicate less of a potential for normal spermatogenic capability.

DIFFERENTIAL DIAGNOSIS OF AZOOSPERMIA

In the case of azoospermia, the differential diagnosis is greatly dependent on the semen volume and pH as well as on the findings of the physical examination. If the volume and pH are low, indicating the absence of seminal vesicle fluid, then either the patient has complete ejaculatory duct obstruction bilaterally or he has CBAVD. In ejaculatory duct obstruction, the seminal vesicles and vasal ampullae are

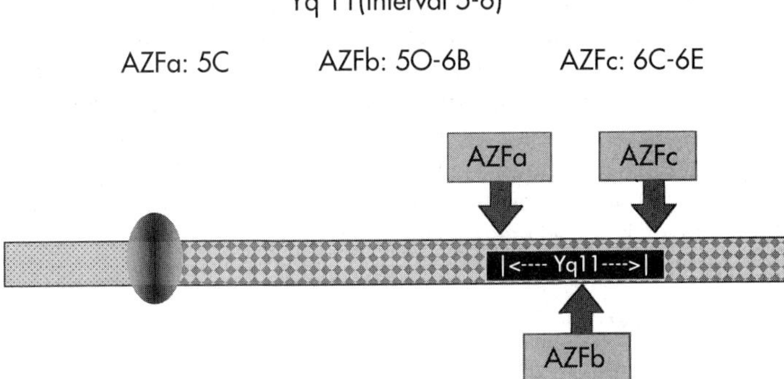

Fig. 150-4. Y chromosomal azoospermia factor (AZF) region, which is located on the long arm of the Y chromosome (Yq11) and has been divided into three subregions: AZFa, AZFb, and AZFc. AZFc is the best characterized and contains a cluster of genes involved in sperm production. AZFc is deleted in approximately 13% of men with nonobstructive azoospermia.

unable to empty their contents into the posterior urethra during emission because the ejaculatory ducts are occluded. However, the prostate is able to contribute to the ejaculate, so the antegrade fluid is acidic and of low volume, generally 0.5 ml. Obviously, the patient has the sense of orgasm. In CBAVD, the seminal vesicles are most often aplastic or completely dysfunctional. If the vasa are not palpable in the scrotum, the diagnosis is secure.

If the semen volume is normal and the pH is alkaline, the diagnosis cannot be bilateral complete ejaculatory duct obstruction. If these semen parameters exist coupled with palpation of the vasa, CBAVD cannot be the diagnosis. In the azoospermic patient with a normal semen volume, the differential diagnosis then focuses away from the distal ductal system and turns to the scrotum. Most commonly, the spermatogenic ability of the testes is severely compromised (nonobstructive azoospermia [NOA]), or vasal or epididymal occlusion prevents sperm flow. In the case of NOA, the testes may be small and soft and the FSH elevated. In the situation of epididymal occlusion, the testes are normal in size and consistency, the FSH value is adequate, and the epididymides may feel full and firm. In general, a testis biopsy is not required to distinguish between NOA and obstructive azoospermia.

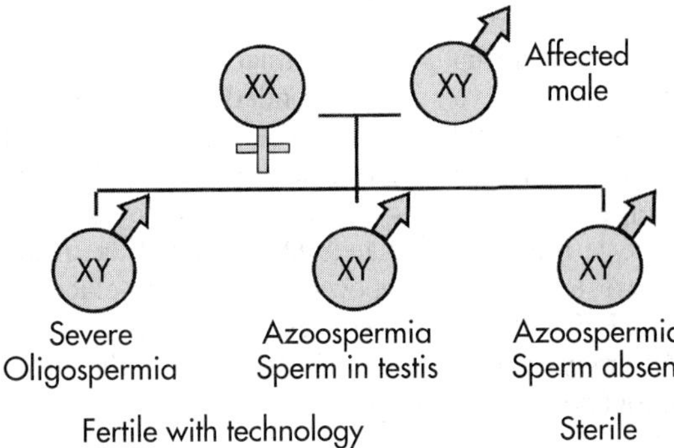

Fig. 150-5. Transmission possibilities of an AZF region microdeletion. If a male has a microdeletion in the AZF region, such as AZFc, he will pass along this microdeleted Y chromosome to all male offspring. These sons would display the known phenotypic spectrum of AZF region deletions with significantly reduced, if not absent, spermatogenesis when they reach reproductive age.

Genetic Basis of Azoospermia

CBAVD is a mild phenotypic form of CF.[2] Patients need to be screened for mutations in the CF gene. Most have at least one recognized mutation, but many demonstrate a second known mutation or a polymorphism on the opposite allele that has an impact on the quantity or the quality of the CF gene protein product known as *CFTR*. Once the patient's CF gene status is known, his immediate family also needs genetic counseling. It is mandatory that the patient's wife be screened also to help define and determine their risk, as a couple, of having an offspring with CF or CBAVD. If the spouse is a carrier of a CF gene mutation, the couple is clearly at risk of generating children that may be affected by CF or CBAVD.

NOA may be caused by a karyotypic anomaly such as 47,XXY Klinefelter's syndrome; 46,XX male syndrome; a translocation; or an anomaly of the Y chromosome. In all patients with NOA, a karyotypic analysis should be performed and the couple should be counseled before therapy is instituted because translocations, depending on their exact nature, may confer a risk of poor reproductive outcome if sperm can be found in the testis tissue (see later section). In certain situations, couples may choose not to pursue therapy based on this information. NOA is most often due to microdeletions of the Y chromosome in areas where important genes regulate sperm production. So far, three such regions have been defined, AZFa, AZFb, and AZFc (Fig. 150-4). AZFc contains the *DAZ* gene cluster and is found to be deleted in 13% of patients with NOA. Any sperm that are found and that bear the Y chromosome will also be missing this critical region. Any male child conceived by the couple will later in life have either severe oligospermia or azoospermia and may be sterile (Fig. 150-5). This is a heavy burden for the couple to consider and may lead to a decision not to undertake therapy but to use donor sperm instead.

TREATMENT OF OLIGOASTHENOSPERMIA

The removal of all spermatotoxins is mandatory in the treatment of any patient with any deficiency in the semen. Surgical correction of varicoceles is certainly indicated because improvement in the semen analysis parameters can be seen in approximately 70% of patients after surgery. As long as the patient is living a healthy lifestyle and all potential suppressive factors have been altered, removed, or corrected, he will be able to realize his full spermatogenic potential. If at that time the couple is still not pregnant or if no change is anticipated or has been seen in sperm quality or function, additional procedures may be instituted. These include intrauterine insemination (sperm are placed into the uterine cavity timed with ovulation), in vitro fertilization (IVF) (sperm are placed next to each oocyte in a Petri dish after multiple oocytes are harvested following ovulation-induction therapy), and intracytoplasmic sperm injection (ICSI) (a single sperm is placed into a single oocyte after harvesting as in IVF).[1,3] The number of sperm required for ICSI is extremely low. ICSI is also a tremendous treatment advance for a man with spermatozoa that do not fertilize well, since the fertilization process is almost completely bypassed.

Although empiric medical therapy is generally unsuccessful, specific medical treatment may be beneficial. This may include replacement of FSH and LH for men with hypothalamic or pituitary hypogonadism. α-Agonist, sympathomimetic medications can be used to augment emission, which is often helpful for patients with such failure secondary to diabetes mellitus or retroperitoneal lymph node dissection. Penile vibratory stimulation can be used to help approximately 60% of men with spinal cord injuries to reflexively ejaculate. The semen specimen can be used for home insemination or intrauterine insemination. For those anejaculate men who have not responded to penile vibratory stimulation or in whom this type of stimulation is not successful, rectal probe electroejaculation will allow recovery of a semen specimen for use with whatever adjunctive technique is most appropriate.[8] Discontinuation of anabolic steroid use leads to the renewal of pituitary elaboration of FSH and LH, with consequent resumption of spermatogenesis. This may take several months because the process of spermatogenesis is a long one.

TREATMENT OF AZOOSPERMIA

If obstruction exists, reconstructive surgery is carried out to restore sperm to the ejaculate, thereby giving the couple an opportunity to achieve conception naturally. For the patient who has had a vasectomy, sperm return to the ejaculate occurs in approximately 90% after reconstruction. The most important determinant is the time that has elapsed since the vasectomy (Fig. 150-6). If reconstruction is not possible, as in CBAVD, microsurgical epididymal sperm aspiration may be used to provide sperm (either fresh or cryopreserved) to be used in conjunction with ICSI. For men with NOA, approximately 50% have a tiny amount of spermatogenesis, and individual spermatozoa can be found in pieces of the testis tissue. Even azoospermic men with Klinefelter's syndrome may have sperm in the testis tissue.[6] Surgery is similar to a testis biopsy but may involve extraction of many pieces. The tissue can be frozen and the sperm used at a later date. For men with a midline cystic structure or dilation of the ejaculatory ducts as imaged by transrectal ultrasonography, transurethral resection is carried out to allow the free flow of seminal fluid into the posterior urethra. As previously discussed, testing is carried out before any therapy for patients in whom a genetic basis may exist. Couples may choose not to proceed with the use of the male partner's sperm if there may be major genetic consequences in their children.[4]

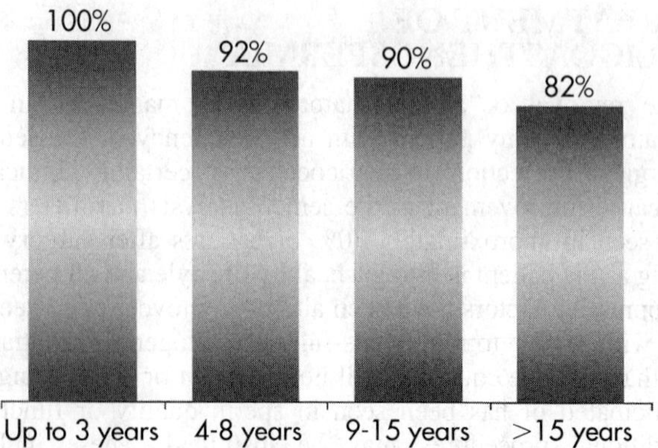

Fig. 150-6. Patency of vasectomy reversal according to the time from vasectomy (years). In general, the success rate declines steadily with no precipitous drop-off. (Unpublished data of RD Oates.)

SUMMARY

The primary care physician is often the first person that a male partner in an infertile marriage asks for assistance. An immediate referral to a urologist is most appropriate in these circumstances, but at least some of the information obtained from the history and physical examination can direct these initial conversations. Most important, the primary care physician is in a position to prevent or predict reproductive dysfunction. Large varicoceles, anabolic steroid use, small and soft testes, and a history of childhood chemotherapy should lead to a discussion of either the possible or definite effects of these conditions on fertility potential. The primary care physician can help identify factors that can be altered or corrected and can help preserve or improve a couple's ability to conceive and become parents.

REFERENCES

1. Dickey RP, Pyrzak R, Lu PY, et al: Comparison of the sperm quality necessary for successful intrauterine insemination with World Health Organization threshold values for normal sperm, *Fertil Steril* 71(4):684, 1999.
2. Dohle GR, Veeze HJ, Overbeek SE, et al: The complex relationships between cystic fibrosis and congenital bilateral absence of the vas deferens: clinical, electrophysiological and genetic data, *Hum Reprod* 14(2):371, 1999.
3. Edwards RG: Widening perspectives of intracytoplasmic sperm injection, *Nat Med* 5(4):377, 1999.
4. Giltay JC, Kastrop PM, Tuerlings JH, et al: Subfertile men with constitutive chromosome abnormalities do not necessarily refrain from intracytoplasmic sperm injection treatment: a follow-up study on 75 Dutch patients, *Hum Reprod* 14(2):318, 1999.
5. Jones RC: To store or mature spermatozoa? The primary role of the epididymis, *Int J Androl* 22(2):57, 1999.
6. Ron-el R, Friedler S, Strassburger D, et al: Birth of a healthy neonate following the intracytoplasmic injection of testicular spermatozoa from a patient with Klinefelter's syndrome, *Hum Reprod* 14(2):368, 1999.
7. Szczygiel M, Kurpisz M: Teratozoospermia and its effect on male fertility potential, *Andrologia* 31(2):63, 1999.
8. Taylor Z, Molloy D, Hill V, et al: Contribution of the assisted reproductive technologies to fertility in males suffering spinal cord injury, *Aust N Z J Obstet Gynaecol* 39(1):84, 1999.
9. Ulstein M, Irgens A, Irgens LM: Secular trends in sperm variables for groups of men in fertile and infertile couples, *Acta Obstet Gynecol Scand* 78(4):332, 1999.

CHAPTER 151

Bladder Dysfunction and Urinary Incontinence

Kathleen C. Kobashi
Gary E. Leach

Urinary incontinence affects an estimated 13 million adults in the United States. The prevalence varies with the profile of the group considered. Some 10% to 20% of women aged 15 to 64 years and 40% of women over 60 years of age have urinary incontinence. Some 56% of institutionalized patients of both sexes, or 1.06 million individuals, are incontinent of urine. In 1995, the cost of treatment of urinary incontinence in patients over 65 years of age was approximately $26 billion, amounting to $3565 per individual. Incontinence is a prevalent and costly problem that affects not only patients' physical health (infection and physical debility) but also their psychologic and social status. Incontinence can clearly have a devastating impact on quality of life.

The treatment modalities used for urinary incontinence can, in themselves, cause complications. Chronic indwelling catheters place a patient at risk for infection, stones, tumors, and urethral and meatal damage. Condom catheters and diapers lead to chronic infections, skin breakdown, and decubiti.

Since many patients find it humiliating and difficult to express the inconveniences associated with urinary incontinence, appropriate diagnosis and treatment are often not administered as readily as they should be. Patient, family, and caretaker education is one of the most important issues to be addressed when instituting proper treatment for urinary incontinence. Throughout this chapter *incontinence* refers to *urinary* incontinence.

NORMAL PHYSIOLOGY

An intricate control system regulates bladder function. Normal bladder physiology involves both a storage phase and an evacuation phase, which must be coordinated. Both these phases depend on interaction between the bladder and the sphincteric mechanism, which allows for low-pressure storage and the maintenance of continence. Subsequent voiding is accomplished by detrusor muscle contraction accompanied by essentially simultaneous relaxation of the sphincteric mechanism.

The detrusor is composed of smooth muscle. The sphincteric mechanism has two well-defined components in the male patient. The bladder neck and proximal prostatic urethra form the internal sphincteric mechanism, which is a smooth muscular structure. The external sphincter is formed by skeletal muscle contributions from the pelvic floor and a second component arising from the urethral wall. A third component of the distal mechanism is an intrinsic urethral, smooth muscular component.

In female patients the continence mechanism is formed predominantly by the bladder neck and proximal urethra. This mechanism is further augmented by the urethral submucosal tissues, which create a "seal" effect in the urethra, thus potentiating continence. Estrogens enhance this seal by mechanisms that may involve the maintenance and proliferation of the urethral submucosal vascular plexus and by promotion of the function of the adrenergic receptor population that exists in this area and is crucial to urethral mucosal closure. Failure of this seal results in intrinsic sphincteric deficiency or type III urinary incontinence.

The motor nucleus controlling detrusor function is located in the sacral spinal cord between the S2 and S4 cord levels (spinal column levels T11 to L1) (Fig. 151-1). Parasympathetic afferents from this motor nucleus course in the hypogastric nerve to synapse with ganglia located within the detrusor wall. Postganglionic afferents carry impulses that cause detrusor excitation and bladder contraction. Receptors in the detrusor muscle are predominantly parasympathetic in mediation, with primarily muscarinic and to a lesser extent cholinergic receptors being identified. These receptors mediate detrusor contraction. Also present within the detrusor muscle are adrenergic receptors that are responsible for muscular relaxation. Efferent fibers transmit impulses from the bladder back to the detrusor nucleus. These impulses convey information, including degree of bladder distention. In the bladder base and proximal urethra, the predominant type of neuroreceptor is α-adrenergic. These receptors mediate contraction and are intimately involved in the continence mechanism.

The nucleus controlling external sphincteric function is also located in the sacral cord. Extensive neural interconnections between these two cell groupings provide continual interplay between these entities and allow coordination between them.

The sacral cord is tonically inhibited by descending impulses carried by the spinal cord that arise in the pontine mesencephalic reticular formation located in the midbrain. A specialized neural grouping that governs voiding is located in this area of the pons. This micturition center in turn receives descending input from the cerebral cortex, cerebellum, and limbic system.

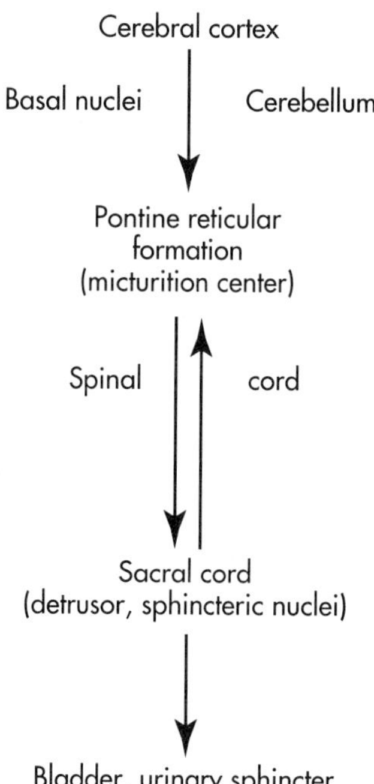

Fig. 151-1. The bladder and urinary sphincter are controlled by an intricate neurologic system.

When the detrusor reaches capacity, the higher centers cease to inhibit the sacral cord. Through descending paths, the pons potentiates the initiation of voiding and the coordination of detrusor contraction and sphincteric relaxation. Voiding is completed by a detrusor contraction, which is facilitated until emptying is complete.

PATHOPHYSIOLOGY

Dysfunction of any element of this mechanism produces some loss of regulation of voiding and may result in urinary incontinence or retention. Interruption by pathology above the midbrain center results in loss of inhibitory influences on the midbrain. This may be reflected in the appearance of uninhibited bladder contractile activity, causing urgency symptomatology and urgency incontinence. Two notable exceptions to this statement should be considered. Cerebrovascular accidents (CVAs) may rarely result in retention but only in the acute phase. Parkinson's disease often results in uninhibited and poorly sustained detrusor contractile activity. However, this activity is usually accompanied by sphincteric dysfunction, which results in poor coordination between detrusor and sphincter (sphincter bradykinesia).

Injury or disease of the midbrain or descending spinal pathways results in loss of coordination between the bladder and the urinary sphincter, as well as loss of descending inhibitory input on the detrusor nucleus. The resulting clinical picture is that of uninhibited detrusor contractile activity associated with a nonrelaxing urinary sphincter. The result of this process is a high-pressure, poorly emptying bladder that is prone to decompensation. This high pressure is subsequently transmitted to the kidneys, resulting in hydronephrosis and eventual azotemia. The most common setting for this scenario is a spinal cord injury (trauma or infection), tumor, or vascular event.

Injury or disease of the sacral cord, or peripheral neural projections from this level, results in ablation of detrusor and sphincteric nuclei function. Initially, this is manifested by an areflexic (noncontractile) detrusor. Low-pressure, large-volume urinary retention results. With chronicity, however, the characteristics of the bladder wall that produce a low-pressure, high-capacity reservoir (compliance) are altered. This alteration results in part from the loss of innervation and also from changes in the composition (increasing fibrosis) of the bladder wall. Higher pressures ensue, which may be deleterious to renal function and may also produce spontaneous urine loss.

In the discussion of any pathologic process involving the nervous system, it is important to note that the resultant clinical picture infrequently reflects a "complete" lesion. More often, an incomplete neural lesion results. Frequently, some function is preserved in the absence of other functions, which cannot be predicted by the level or degree of injury. Another aspect of importance that further obfuscates the clinical presentation is that neural lesions also may be present at multiple levels.

EVALUATION

Data regarding an individual's bladder dysfunction should be gathered in an orderly manner so as to delineate all appropriate historic and physical examination elements crucial to establishing a diagnosis and treatment plan. These elements are supplemented by urinary evaluation and further urologic tests as indicated.

History

The patient history should include a notation of the duration of symptoms. Whether the patient has experienced symptoms since childhood or only relatively recently yields information regarding the potential for congenital disorders. Symptoms noted only recently may indicate a potentially reversible cause of bladder dysfunction or incontinence. The presence of irritative symptoms, including nocturia and frequency, is recorded. Dysuria or pain with bladder filling may indicate infectious or inflammatory conditions. Obstructive symptoms include hesitancy, straining to void, intermittency of stream, and incomplete emptying. These symptoms may further complicate overflow incontinence. The presence of intercurrent urinary tract infection or gross hematuria is established. Diurnal and nocturnal frequency should be recorded. The volume of fluid ingested also should be evaluated. If necessary, patient home logs of intake and output should be kept to evaluate the appropriateness of fluid ingestion.

Incontinence should be classified to better define possible etiologies. The failure to store urine or the failure to empty provides an easily reproducible method by which to categorize bladder function. This system conceptualizes lower urinary tract function as depending on the interaction of the bladder and bladder outlet (sphincter) for normal urine storage and expulsion. A defect in either bladder or sphincteric function can result in either failure to store or failure to empty. Mixed bladder and sphincteric dysfunction may also be responsible for the clinical scenario (Box 151-1).

Incontinence may be considered as fixed or transient. Transient incontinence usually has a definable, sudden onset and often has a discrete cause. A simple mnemonic summarizes the differential diagnosis of transient incontinence (Box 151-2).

Fixed or established causes of incontinence may be subdivided into several broad headings with differential considerations on the basis of patient sex. These etiologic possibilities may affect storage, emptying, or both functions of the lower urinary tract (Box 151-3).

Urge incontinence is characterized by the patient experiencing a strong desire to void and doing so precipitously without the ability to suppress the urinary loss. This type of incontinence results from overactivity of the detrusor, resulting in uncontrollable bladder contractions. The patient may experience this loss related to a particular activity or exposure or may note no inciting etiology. This is the most common type of incontinence noted in elderly populations. Urge incontinence frequently complicates central disorders such as Parkinson's disease, Alzheimer's disease, CVA, and brain tumor. Urge incontinence is also noted with local bladder disorders such as outlet obstruction, carcinoma in situ, and infection.

Reflex incontinence is another category of incontinence related to urge incontinence. This type of incontinence is manifested by the precipitous loss of urine with no sense of urgency. This category is most often noted in patients with suprasacral spinal cord lesions, in whom midbrain inhibitory influences are ablated. Failure of the storage component of bladder function ensues.

Overflow incontinence is caused by the chronic retention of urine, with small volumes being frequently voided. Overflow incontinence may result from detrusor hypocontractility, as seen in tabes dorsalis, diabetes mellitus, or vitamin B_{12} deficiency. Overflow incontinence may also

Box 151-1. Etiologic Classification of Incontinence

Failure to store
- Bladder dysfunction
- Outlet dysfunction

Failure to empty
- Bladder dysfunction
- Outlet dysfunction

Combination of failure to empty and failure to store

Box 151-2. Etiologies for Transient Urinary Incontinence: "Diapers" Mnemonic

Drugs: hypnotics, sedatives, anticholinergic agents, diuretics, adrenergic agents
Delirium: or altered mental status
Infection
Atrophy: of vagina or urethra
Psychologic disorder: functional depression
Endocrine: hyperglycemia or hypercalcemia
Restricted mobility
Stool impaction

From Resnick NM, Yalla SV: Management of urinary incontinence in the elderly, *N Engl J Med* 313(13):800, 1985.

result from bladder outlet obstruction, which is caused by prostatic or urethral pathology, with subsequent bladder decompensation.

Continuous incontinence implies total and unabated leakage of urine, unrelated to activity. This situation is identified when a fistula of the urinary tract is present. The most common etiology for urinary tract fistula in a woman is prior hysterectomy.

Stress incontinence is manifested by urinary loss with physical activity or sudden increases in abdominal pressure, as encountered with coughing or lifting. This type of incontinence arises from a deficiency of the bladder outlet resulting either from hypermobility of the urethra and bladder neck in women or from intrinsic damage in either sex.

A mixed category of incontinence also should be considered because in many cases, especially those noted in elderly persons, more than one type of incontinence is present (see Box 151-3). An example of this situation arises in women with stress urinary incontinence. In this group, a significant incidence of coexistent urge incontinence is identified, which may confuse the presenting symptomatic complaints. The need for and use of protective garments should be established.

Symptomatic history, although important in establishing the magnitude and extent of the condition, is often inaccurate in predicting the ultimate bladder or sphincter dysfunction defined by more involved testing. However, in institutionalized elderly patients, simple algorithms based on patient symptoms and bedside assessment have been reported to have a diagnostic accuracy of greater than 80% when verified by urodynamic testing.

Significant neurologic symptoms are also important in the evaluation of urinary tract dysfunction. Prior cranial or spinal surgical procedures should be ascertained. Symptoms of lower extremity motor or sensory deficit are significant. Diplopia, vertigo, and gait disturbance indicate central neurologic pathology, including multiple sclerosis and neoplasm. Voiding dysfunction associated with neurologic abnormalities noted on a screening examination may be the

Box 151-3. Types of Incontinence

Female

Failure to store

Bladder dysfunction
- Detrusor instability or detrusor hyperreflexia
- Decreased bladder compliance
- Fistula
- Urgency-related bladder decompensation

Outlet dysfunction
- "Typical" stress incontinence (anatomic urethral hypermobility)
- Intrinsic sphincteric deficiency

Failure to empty

Bladder dysfunction
- Detrusor decompensation
- Bladder denervation resulting in absent or poorly sustained contraction

Outlet dysfunction
- Neurogenic sphincter dysfunction
- Iatrogenic urethral obstruction

Combined

Detrusor instability with poorly sustained contraction

Male

Failure to store

Bladder dysfunction
- Detrusor instability or detrusor hyperreflexia alone
- Detrusor instability secondary to outlet obstruction
- Decreased bladder compliance
- Bladder decompensation with overflow incontinence

Outlet dysfunction
- Stress urinary incontinence
  - Iatrogenic (after prostatectomy)
  - Neurogenic denervation

Failure to empty

Bladder dysfunction
- Bladder decompensation
- Bladder denervation

Outlet dysfunction
- Benign prostatic hyperplasia with obstruction
- Neurogenic sphincter dysfunction

Combined

Detrusor hyperreflexia with poorly sustained contraction
- Detrusor hyperreflexia with impaired contractility
- Parkinson's disease
- Cerebrovascular accident

first indication of multiple sclerosis. Perineal or genital anesthesia associated with impotence indicates involvement of the cauda equina and interruption of the sacral nerves (S2 to S4) or their roots. Fecal incontinence or chronic constipation further indicates neural pathology, related either to specific nervous system lesions or to more global systemic processes such as diabetes mellitus. Any recent or chronic change in mentation or sensorium could indicate dementia, CVA, or other demyelinating disease. All have an impact on bladder dysfunction.

Other components of the medical history are also essential. The presence of systemic diseases such as diabetes mellitus or autonomic neuropathy should be noted. A history of cancer and therapies rendered for malignancy, including radiotherapy and chemotherapy, can give important diagnostic clues regarding metastases or injury resulting from therapy. Renal disorders may lead to neuropathy or bladder dysfunction related to increased urine production resulting from concentration defects. In women, a prior gynecologic and obstetric history is crucial. Hysterectomy can cause detrusor denervation when performed for uterine or cervical carcinoma. Prior therapy for endometriosis indicates the potential for recurrent disease and associated symptoms. If the patient is perimenopausal or postmenopausal, relative lack of estrogenic supplementation can lead to vaginal atrophy and susceptibility to urinary tract infection and incontinence.

Previous surgical history is extremely important. As noted, prior neurosurgical procedures involving the back or cranium can directly contribute to bladder dysfunction. Any prior urologic or gynecologic procedure may also contribute to current symptoms.

Elucidation of the patient's current drug regimen is extremely important. Medications in many categories affect the bladder and voiding function. Antihypertensive agents, including sympatholytics, ganglionic blocking agents, and calcium channel blockers, affect bladder physiology. α-Adrenergic antagonists may worsen preexisting stress urinary incontinence in women. Tranquilizing agents and psychotropic drugs can result in retention because of decreased appreciation of bladder filling or parasympatholytic effects. Similarly, many medications used in the therapy of Parkinson's disease can worsen bladder function as a result of anticholinergic side effects. Decongestants, as a result of sympathomimetic side effects, can exacerbate borderline voiding in men with bladder outlet obstruction caused by benign prostatic hyperplasia. The recent addition or change of diuretic medication can result in substantial urinary volume increases and decompensation of a borderline obstructive situation. Opiates, including antidiarrheal agents, may inhibit detrusor contraction. Antiarrhythmic agents, such as disopyramide, may also have a negative impact on detrusor contraction. The physician should note not only the drug and dose but also any possible relationship to the onset of the current symptoms.

Physical Examination

Physical examination includes a general examination with special attention to the genitourinary system. Blood pressure evaluation should be included.

Inspection of the back should be performed to identify an overt spinal deformity such as scoliosis. Attention to the base of the spine should exclude the identification of sacral skin discoloration or tufts of hair as well as an overt skin deformity such as a pit. These stigmata indicate the presence of spinal dysraphism and the possibility of a coexistent neurogenic bladder. The sacrum should be palpated to ensure bony integrity.

Abdominal examination should include palpation of the flanks for a mass or tenderness. The suprapubic area is evaluated for pain, and an attempt to palpate and percuss the bladder is made to identify distention.

Examination of the genitalia often indicates the presence of longstanding incontinence, with skin irritation and fungal infestation easily identifiable. Rectal examination reveals not only mucosal evaluation but also the presence and degree of resting and augmented sphincter tone. The size and consistency of the prostate gland are evaluated at this time. The covert presence of prostatic carcinoma can be manifested by symptomatic voiding dysfunction.

Pelvic examination must be performed to evaluate the adnexal structures for mass or tenderness. Speculum examination of the vaginal vault may reveal vulvar or cervical malignancy. Atrophy of the epithelial lining of the vagina is often present in postmenopausal women. Also, the presence of significant pelvic prolapse (cystocele, rectocele, uterine prolapse, vault descent) should be identified. Pelvic examination should be performed with the patient in both the supine and the standing positions to better elucidate the degree of uterine prolapse. This prolapse may be significantly underestimated if the examination is performed only while the female patient is supine. Significant bladder prolapse may result in hydronephrosis because of traction on the bladder base. Speculum examination of the vagina documents other forms of vaginal prolapse. A cystocele can be identified as a protrusion of the anterior vaginal wall that is accentuated when the patient strains. The coexistence of urinary loss associated with Valsalva's maneuvers or coughing should also be identified. A cystocele represents prolapse of the bladder base and proximal urethra and is frequently seen as a component of the hypermobility associated with uncomplicated stress urinary incontinence (Fig. 151-2). This defect arises from weakness of the supporting (pubocervical) fascia of the bladder base.

A rectocele can be identified as a posterior vaginal wall protrusion composed of the rectum, which can also be accentuated by Valsalva's maneuver (Fig. 151-3). This form of prolapse arises from a defect in the pelvic floor (pubococcygeus muscles) allowing anterior "herniation" of the rectum.

An enterocele represents a defect at the vaginal apex usually seen after hysterectomy (Fig. 151-4). This entity contains peritoneal contents. If a woman has previously undergone hysterectomy, the entire vaginal vault may prolapse to or through the introitus as a result of surgical damage to the supporting structures of the upper vagina (uterosacral ligaments).

Evaluation of the sacral cord can be enhanced further by eliciting the bulbocavernosus reflex, which reflects the integrity of the S2 to S4 levels of the cord. Compression of the glans penis (male) or mons pubis clitoris (female) produces anal sphincter contraction if the sacral cord is intact. Approximately thirty percent of neurologically normal women and five percent of normal men do not exhibit this reflex.[1] The sacral dermatomes in the perianal area (S2, S3) should be tested for anesthesia or diminished sensation.

Neurologic examination is crucial to the initial patient

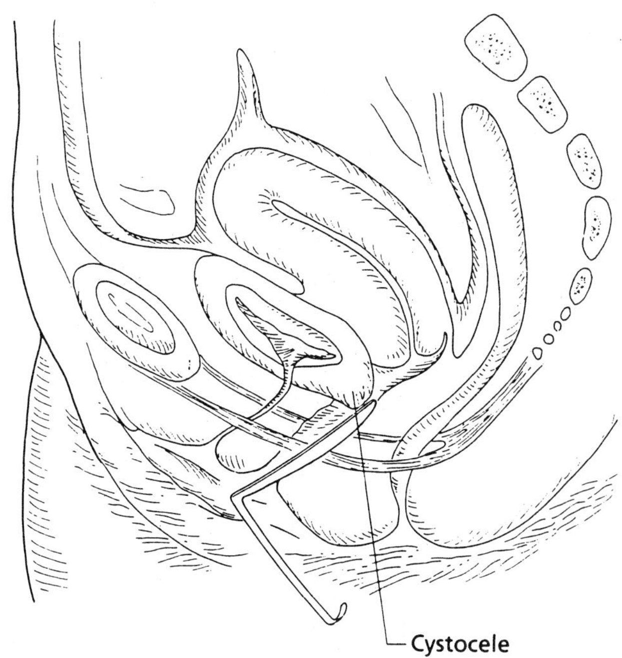

Fig. 151-2. A cystocele appears as a large bulge in the anterior vaginal wall that may be exacerbated when the patient strains. (From Webster GD, et al, editors: *Reconstructive urology,* Cambridge, Mass, 1993, Blackwell.)

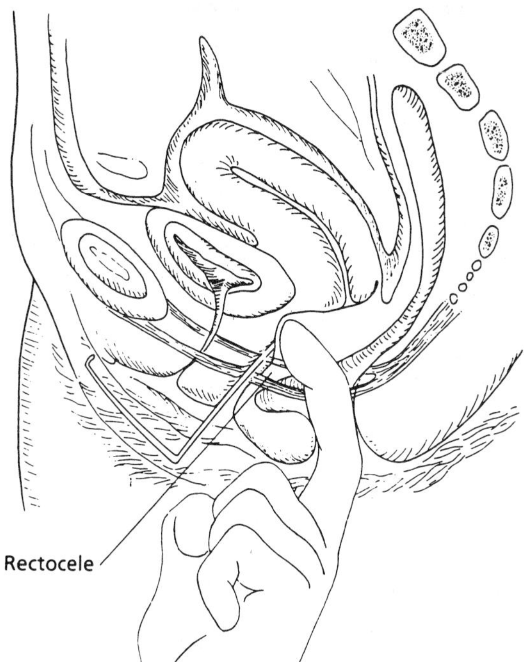

Fig. 151-3. Rectoceles are confirmed by placing a finger in the rectum and applying anterior pressure. Any weakness of the posterior vaginal wall is demonstrated. (From Foote JE, Zimmerman PE, Leach GE: Vaginal reconstruction for pelvic floor laxity. In Webster GD, et al, editors: *Reconstructive urology,* Cambridge, Mass, 1993, Blackwell.)

evaluation. Mental status should be documented. Gait and balance are observed. Gross abnormalities of the cranial nerves and upper extremity function can yield information regarding systemic neurologic disease. Reflex testing of the knee (L2, L3) and ankle (L5, S1) is performed. The presence of Babinski's reflexes and clonus indicating upper motor neuron disease is also identified. Sensory evaluation of the lower extremities for fine touch, pinprick, vibratory, and positional sensation is performed. Gross motor weakness of the lower extremities is documented.

The initial examination includes an assessment of postvoiding residual urine volume. Difficulty in passing a small urethral catheter for this purpose may indicate the presence of urethral stricture, prostatic enlargement, or another abnormality. The presence of overflow incontinence or large volumes of retained urine can be a significant and often overlooked etiology to the presenting symptom complex, especially in the patient with urge incontinence.

Laboratory Evaluation

Urinary examination includes urinalysis, culture, and voided cytology. Microscopic inspection of the urine reveals hematuria, pyuria, or bacteriuria, which may coexist with pathology of the urinary system. Urinary tract infection may present with urgency or urge incontinence as the primary symptom. A voided urine cytology identifies malignant cells reflective of transitional carcinoma, which symptomatically can cause urgency and frequency.

Hematologic evaluation includes a serum creatinine analysis to estimate renal function. Evaluation of serum glucose and calcium may be indicated in patients with large urine volumes. Other testing is determined on the basis of any specific disease entity that is identified.

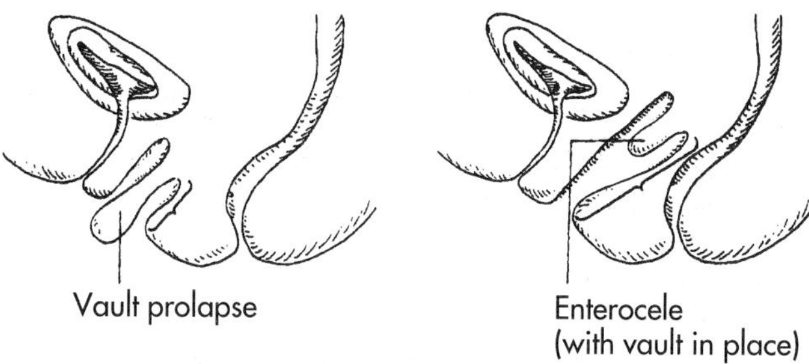

Fig. 151-4. An enterocele can be differentiated from vaginal vault prolapse by assessing the length of the posterior vaginal wall. The posterior wall is shortened in vault prolapse but retains its length with an enterocele. (From Webster GD, et al, editors: *Reconstructive urology,* Cambridge, Mass, 1993, Blackwell.)

Radiographic Evaluation

Radiographic evaluation should be tailored according to symptomatology. Plain films of the abdomen (kidneys, ureters, and bladder) give information regarding soft tissues and any radiopaque urinary tract calculous disease. These radiographs are useful if the patient has a history of prior stones and or symptoms suggestive of this diagnosis. Ultrasound of the kidneys and abdomen is particularly useful in identifying hydronephrosis, calculous disease, and soft tissue pathology of the kidneys (tumor, abscess, medical renal disease). Renal ultrasound is indicated in the presence of azotemia to rule out any obstructive component. It is also indicated in the evaluation of neurogenic dysfunction of the bladder as a baseline study for longitudinal follow-up of ongoing therapy.

Box 151-4. Referral Criteria for Urologic Evaluation

History
- History of pelvic or lower urinary tract surgery within 6 months
- Rapid recurrence of urinary tract infection after appropriate therapy

Physical examination
- Significant pelvic prolapse
- Suspicion of prostatic carcinoma or significant enlargement of the prostate

Diagnostic tests
- Postvoiding residual urine volume greater than 100 ml
- Marked urinary hesitancy or intermittency of urine stream
- Symptomatic stress urinary incontinence in a woman who is a candidate for surgery when treatment attempts have failed
- Symptomatic stress incontinence in a man
- Obstruction to the passage of a 14 Fr urinary catheter

Urinalysis
- Microhematuria without bacteriuria or pyuria

Lack of diagnostic certainty after initial evaluation

Failure of a therapeutic trial for urge or stress incontinence to have a response

From Ouslander J, et al: Prospective evaluation of an assessment strategy for geriatric urinary incontinence, *J Am Geriatr Soc* 37:715, 1989.

Further testing is predicated on diagnostic suspicions and often occurs after urologic referral. Criteria for referral have been established. This simplified system uses six categories to delineate factors that may indicate the presence of complicated urologic disease. These criteria arise from data easily obtainable from the history, physical examination, and simple diagnostic tests (Box 151-4).

Further radiographic imaging of the urinary tract may include an intravenous urogram to define urinary tract anatomy or to evaluate hematuria. Voiding cystourethrography (VCUG) is selectively performed to identify vesicoureteral reflux, the presence and degree of cystocele in the standing position, postvoiding residual, and any urethral abnormality.

Urodynamic Evaluation

Bladder storage function is evaluated by cystometrogram. Cystometry may be modified in several ways. The bedside cystometrogram is the most basic form of cystometry. This involves the insertion of a 12 or 14 Fr urinary catheter into the bladder. A 50-ml syringe, without the piston, is then attached to the end of the catheter. Sterile water is poured into the syringe in 50-ml aliquots while the syringe is held 15 cm above the symphysis pubis. Filling is continued until the column of water in the syringe rises, indicating a bladder contraction. The study is also terminated in the presence of patient discomfort or an infused volume greater than 500 ml.

More formal cystometry involves multichannel recording of bladder and rectal pressures. This study identifies the compliance (volume-related pressure changes) of the bladder. Fluid is instilled through a urethral catheter at a constant rate with continuous pressure monitoring. During recording, the patient's first urgency to urinate is identified, as is the sensation of bladder fullness. Failure to store urine appropriately is identified during this stage of the study. The presence of detrusor contractions that occur involuntarily during filling is noted. If this type of activity is noted, the contractions are referred to as *detrusor instability* (in the absence of overt neurogenic disease) or *detrusor hyperreflexia* (in the presence of nervous system pathology). Carbon dioxide has also been used as the infusant for cystometry. However, gas cystometry is difficult to interpret and prone to artifact. Findings are also not as reproducible as with water cystometry.

Failure to store urine on the basis of outlet dysfunction is also evaluated. During this phase of the study, the patient is asked to perform Valsalva's and stress maneuvers, which may identify stress incontinence. Failure to store urine as a result of combined defects in bladder storage and outlet resistance is elucidated by this simultaneous monitoring of bladder and bladder outlet events.

When the characteristics of the individual's voiding are to be determined, the patient is asked to void, and pressure and flow monitoring is continued. This simultaneous evaluation gives additive information to that obtained by uroflowmetry, which is usually performed at the same session. Failure to empty because of poor bladder contraction is identified during this segment of the evaluation. High-pressure, low-flow voiding identifies outlet obstruction as the cause of failure to empty resulting from outlet obstruction.

Infusion with radiographic contrast allows the study to be monitored fluoroscopically, and real-time evaluation of bladder events may be made. Videourodynamics represents the most complex form of urodynamic evaluation. This type of evaluation is used to document the presence of bladder outlet dysfunction. It also identifies continuous loss of urine across the sphincteric mechanism in the absence of bladder contraction, which is seen in intrinsic sphincteric deficiency.

Cystourethroscopy

Outpatient urologic evaluation also includes cystoscopy. This reveals any overt pathology of the urethra or bladder, such as tumor, stone, stricture, or foreign body.

THERAPEUTIC INTERVENTIONS

Therapeutic options for voiding dysfunction include medical, surgical, and biofeedback and behavioral therapy. The primary goals of the treatment of bladder dysfunction are preservation of renal function, alleviation of urinary tract infection, and improved quality of life.

Failure to Store

Failure of the bladder to store urine at low pressures is treated according to whether the cause is secondary to a problem with the bladder, a problem with the bladder outlet, or a combination thereof. Incontinence may be caused by transient or chronic factors, and it is important to determine all potential etiologies to provide proper management. Remediable etiologies for incontinence include urinary tract infection, drug interactions, bladder tumors or stones, and problems related to changes in mental status. If the incontinence persists once these issues have been addressed, therapy for more chronic etiologies can be administered as indicated.

Secondary to Problems With the Bladder. The true incidence of bladder overactivity in the general population has been estimated to be approximately 8%.[4] In the geriatric patient population, failure to store urine is due to detrusor overactivity in more than 70% of patients. Treatment is optimally nonsurgical, with surgical therapy used only as a last resort. Therapeutic options include various medications, behavioral therapy, biofeedback, neuromodulation, and acupuncture, the last of which is not routinely used in the United States.

Detrusor instability or hyperreflexia may coexist with impaired contractility (DHIC) in up to 33% of cases.[7] Despite overactivity of the bladder, the patient is unable to sustain a contraction sufficient for complete bladder emptying. DHIC may be suspected when instability is identified in the presence of significant postvoiding residual urine volumes. Anticholinergic medications to control the symptoms of urgency and clean intermittent catheterization to ensure complete bladder emptying are indicated in the treatment of DHIC. Regular catheterization not only helps avoid the complication of urinary tract infection that may be seen as a result of poor emptying but also contributes to alleviation of the symptoms of urgency associated with higher vesical volumes.

Medications. Agents that inhibit bladder contractility can thereby increase bladder capacity and may also decrease intravesical pressures. Sustained elevation of intravesical pressures above 40 cm H_2O, seen especially in patients with myelodysplasia, puts the patient at risk for upper tract damage. Renal ultrasound should be performed to rule out the presence of hydronephrosis in these patients.

Anticholinergic medications competitively inhibit acetylcholine at the postganglionic autonomic (muscarinic) receptors. *Musculotropics* act directly on smooth muscle contractility by a papaverine-like action and also have varying anesthetic properties. Medications and their respective dosages are listed in Table 151-1.

The adverse effects of these medications vary with the systemic absorption and tend to be the most pronounced with oxybutynin (Ditropan). Effects include dry mouth, constipation, blurred vision, tachycardia, drowsiness, precipitation of urinary retention, and confusion. Narrow-angle glaucoma is an absolute contraindication to the use of this group of medications. The adverse effects often result in poor compliance by patients. The hepatic metabolites of oxybutynin are responsible for the severity of its side effects. Once-a-day slow-release oxybutynin (Ditropan XL) recently became available. Although the efficacy of immediate-release oxybutynin appears to be equivalent to that of Ditropan XL, the incidence of dry mouth is significantly lower for the latter. The incidence of other anticholinergic adverse effects was similar in both groups. Patients who are unable to tolerate the adverse effects of oral oxybutynin, patients in whom other oral therapies have failed, and patients who are willing to undergo catheterization are all candidates for intravesical oxybutynin. Intravesical instillation of oxybutynin bypasses the liver, and therefore the tolerance of this route of administration is better.[2] Tolterodine (Detrol) is a competitive muscarinic antagonist that was released for use in the United States in mid-1998; it is administered at 2 mg twice a day. Because of its higher specificity for bladder muscarinic receptors (as compared to the salivary gland muscarinic receptors), its systemic and central side effects are significantly decreased and it is far better tolerated than oxybutynin.[6]

Table 151-1. Anticholinergics and Musculotropics

Medication	Dosage
Anticholinergics	
Probantheline bromide (Probanthine)	15-30 mg QID
Hyoscyamine sulfate (Levsin, Levsinex)	#1 BID (available in capsule, slow-release, elixir)
Musculotropics	
Oxybutynin	2.5-5.0 mg QD to TID, may try intravesical instillation
(Ditropan)	
(Ditropan XL)	5-10 QD
Dicyclomine hydrochloride (Bentyl)	20-30 mg TID
Flavoxate hydrochloride (Urispas)	100-300 mg TID
Belladonna/opium (B & O Suppository)	⅓-1 per rectum TID
Tolterodene (Detrol)	2 mg BID

QID, Four times a day; *BID*, twice a day; *QD*, every day; *TID*, three times a day.

Tricyclic antidepressants (TCAs) have both anticholinergic and local anesthetic effects, which make them a good choice for the treatment of detrusor instability. In addition, the increase in norepinephrine increases α-stimulation at the bladder neck to increase bladder outlet resistance. The primary agent in this category is imipramine (Tofranil), which is administered at 10 to 25 mg two or three times a day and may be increased up to 150 mg/day. Higher doses are used for the treatment of depression.

The adverse effects of TCAs can be divided into α-adrenergic and anticholinergic effects. The medication is generally well tolerated but is contraindicated in patients with cardiac arrhythmias or heart block. α-Adrenergic side effects include tachycardia, restlessness, blood pressure elevation, and exacerbation of heart block. Anticholinergic effects include orthostatic hypotension, dry mouth, ataxia, tachycardia, restlessness, hallucinations, and mental status changes. The latter effects are typically only seen at the higher doses used for antidepressive therapy.

The administration of an agent such as 1-desaminocystine-8-D-arginine vasopressin (DDAVP), a synthetic analog of the antidiuretic hormone, vasopressin, decreases urine production. In this manner, the problem of bladder instability may be eluded altogether, although it is not treated. This drug is used primarily in patients with nocturnal enuresis and diabetes insipidus and is not routinely administered in the therapy of detrusor instability. Adverse effects are rare and usually occur within the first few weeks of therapy.[9] The main risk includes water intoxication and hyponatremia, and therefore the drug must be used with caution in the elderly, particularly in patients with a history of congestive heart failure.

Behavioral Modification, Bladder Training, and Biofeedback. All patients deemed to be mentally and physically fit for active participation are candidates for behavioral modification. Patients must also be dedicated to compliance to the program to benefit maximally from it. Instructional teaching materials to assist patient education, such as those from *H*elp for *I*ncontinent *P*eople, or HIP, are available. Fluid restriction to 30 to 40 oz/day with avoidance of caffeine and alcohol is imperative. Fluid restriction is particularly important in patients who experience urgency and urge incontinence only at higher bladder volumes. Often, patients increase fluid intake in response to the dry mouth they experience when on anticholinergic medications and must be counseled strongly to avoid drinking more fluid. Candy, gum, artificial saliva, or small sips of fluid can be used to overcome the dry mouth. In addition, the constipation experienced by many patients can be treated with polycarbophil (Mitrolan), a wafer laxative that does not require the intake of the large amounts of fluid required by some fiber supplements.

Biofeedback is a method that uses monitoring equipment to facilitate the development of conscious control of various body functions of which the patient is unaware. It allows patients to take an active role in the management of their own health care. In combination with behavioral modification, biofeedback is used to train patients to postpone urination and void according to the clock rather than according to the urge to void. Using biofeedback, they are taught to inhibit or resist the sensation of urgency. Initially, the goal is set for urination every 1 to 2 hours; then it is gradually increased to 3 to 4 hours. For patients with instability only at high volumes, timed voiding every 2 to 3 hours may be helpful in avoiding the uninhibited contractions that result in the symptoms of urgency.

Electrical Stimulation. Sacral nerve stimulation is currently increasing in use in the United States.[8] The postulated mechanism of action is via activation of spinal or β-adrenergic nerves. A success rate of 60% to 70% is being reported in the initial studies.

Augmentation Cystoplasty and Urinary Diversion. Surgery is the last resort for the treatment of urge incontinence. It may be offered to patients who have poor results with medications or are unable to continue medications because of the adverse effects. A patch of ileum or colon may be used to augment the bladder to decrease intravesical pressure and instability and increase bladder capacity. The authors counsel their patients that lifelong intermittent catheterization may be expected in 100% of patients after surgery. Urinary diversion or augmentation cystoplasty with creation of an abdominal stoma is a logical consideration for patients who may have difficulty accessing the urethra for catheterization.

Secondary to Problems With the Bladder Outlet. When counseling patients about treatment alternatives for stress urinary incontinence, all options must be considered. Most patients wish to try noninvasive therapy before surgery. The goal, regardless of treatment choice, is to improve the patient's quality of life. Standard nonsurgical treatments include medications, biofeedback and behavioral therapy, and periurethral collagen injection.

Continuous incontinence or leakage of urine from the vagina may result from urinary-vaginal fistula. Fistulas tend to occur in patients who have had recent pelvic surgery or have a history of pelvic radiation. If a fistula is suspected, referral to a urologist should be obtained.

Medications. α-Agonists stimulate the α-receptors at the bladder neck and proximal urethra, resulting in smooth muscle stimulation and increased bladder neck and proximal urethral resistance. α-Stimulators are useful in the treatment of mild to moderate stress incontinence but are usually not sufficient for treating this condition when it is severe. For maximal results, α-agonists should be used in conjunction with pelvic floor exercises and estrogens (see later paragraphs).

α-Stimulants should be used with caution in the elderly population, especially in patients with cardiac disease, hypertension, or hyperthyroidism. α-Agonists can cause drowsiness, anxiety, weakness, insomnia, headache, tremor, palpitations, cardiac arrhythmias, respiratory difficulty, and blood pressure elevation. Tachyphylaxis may be seen. Ephedrine and pseudoephedrine stimulate both α- and β-receptors and induce the release of norepinephrine. Phenylpropanolamine is a pure α-agonist with less central stimulation than ephedrine and pseudoephedrine; therefore the adverse effects of anxiety, insomnia, and headache tend to be minimized.

Because *TCAs* increase bladder outlet resistance and have anticholinergic and musculotropic effects and a strong direct inhibitory effect on the detrusor, they are ideal for treatment of mild stress incontinence, urge incontinence, and mixed stress and urge incontinence (see TCA discussion in previous section).

Estrogen supplementation plays an important role in the therapy of incontinence in women by enhancing the mucosal seal effect in the urethra. Intravaginal administration of ⅓ applicator three times a week amplifies the local effect of the estrogen over the effect of oral estrogen on the urethral and vaginal epithelium.[3] Estrogen is usually used with other medications, pelvic floor exercises, and behavioral modification to get maximal benefit.

Behavioral Therapy and Biofeedback. Patients who appear to benefit the most from behavioral therapy alone are those who suffer from only mild stress urinary incontinence. Concomitant use of biofeedback is an excellent treatment option for patients who would benefit from nonsurgical therapy based on either individual preference or clinical situation. A vaginal probe measures the activity of the levator ani musculature, and surface electrodes detect contractions of the abdominal or gluteal muscles, which might otherwise be mistaken by the patient as contraction of the pelvic floor musculature. Patients are taught to tighten the sphincter muscle without increasing abdominal pressure, and the biofeedback equipment relays auditory or visual feedback to patients regarding the physiologic activity.

Injection Therapy. Various materials have been used in periurethral injection therapy for the treatment of ISD. Only collagen and fat are approved for use in the United States. The theory behind injection therapy is to bulk up the urethra to create a degree of outlet obstruction to facilitate continence.

Surgical Options. Innumerable surgical techniques have been described for the treatment of stress urinary incontinence in the female patient, including pubovaginal slings, retropubic suspensions (e.g., Marshall-Marchetti-Krantz, Burch), needle suspensions (e.g., Raz, Stamey, Pereyra), anterior colporrhaphy, and variations thereof. For male patients, surgical treatment involves the placement of an artificial urinary sphincter.

The authors prefer to use pubovaginal slings for all female patients with stress urinary incontinence who opt for surgical therapy. Slings are placed beneath the proximal urethra and bladder to provide a "hammock" for support and direct urethral compression. The sling serves as a "backstop" to prevent urethral descensus and opening when increased intraabdominal pressure occurs. Slings and retropubic suspensions maintain an 83%-84% success rate beyond 48 months as compared to that for the needle suspensions, which decreases to 67% at that point. Overall, slings appear to be the most efficacious treatment over time.

Pubovaginal slings have been created from a variety of materials, including synthetic, autologous, allogenic, and xenogenic tissues. The authors use cadaveric fascia lata, placed via a transvaginal approach (*C*adaveric *T*ransvaginal *S*ling, or *CaTS*), which achieves better cosmesis and affords a significantly shorter operative time, hospital stay, and recovery period than the combined transvaginal/transabdominal approach or when harvesting of fascia is necessary. CaTS also results in less postoperative pain, typically requiring only acetaminophen for adequate analgesia in the experience of the authors.

In male patients, the artificial urinary sphincter is a successful therapeutic option. The device involves a fluid-filled cuff placed around the bulbous urethra to provide occlusion. When the patient wishes to void, a pump located in the dependent portion of the scrotum is pumped to move the fluid from the cuff to a pressurized suprapubic reservoir. Deflation of the cuff temporarily relieves the obstruction of the urethra, allowing the urine to pass. The cuff automatically refills in 3 to 5 minutes.

Failure to Empty

Failure to empty the bladder is also treated according to whether the pathology is due to the bladder, the outlet, or a combination. First, the patient's medication profile is reviewed for the possibility of urinary retention secondary to the anticholinergic or α-adrenergic side effects of medications. When possible, any medications that could be contributing to the problem is discontinued.

When there is persistent retention or when discontinuation of contributing medications is not feasible, the patient should be placed on intermittent catheterization.

Secondary to Problems With the Bladder. In theory, medications that increase detrusor contractility, such as bethanechol (Urecholine), should promote bladder emptying if there is no concomitant outlet obstruction. However, there is no evidence to support that any medication this satisfactorily accomplishes this action.[5]

Clean intermittent catheterization is the treatment of choice for incomplete bladder emptying with or without overflow incontinence. However, this option requires compliant patients (or caretakers) with the mental capacity and manual dexterity to perform catheterization. Indwelling catheters are a last resort because of the risks of complications from long-term catheterization. Complications include urethral damage, infections, stones, and tumor. If a long-term indwelling catheter is necessary despite these risks, a suprapubic cystostomy is preferred to avoid urethral damage. Catheters should be changed monthly.

Surgical therapy for the treatment of the acontractile bladder, including continent urinary diversion or the creation of a conduit with an external drainage device, is infrequently performed. Indications include patients who are unable to perform catheterization because of problems with manual dexterity or difficulty accessing the urethra.

Secondary to Problems With the Outlet. Bladder outlet obstruction secondary to prostatism is commonly encountered in male patients. First-line therapy is α-blockers such as terazosin (Hytrin), doxazosin (Cardura), prazosin (Minipress), and tamsulosin (Flomax). Tamsulosin is more specific for the α_{1a}-receptors found in the prostate and therefore theoretically causes fewer side effects, such as dizziness and headache, than the other nonspecific α_1-antagonists. Anticholinergic medications may be added to control the urgency at the discretion of the clinician. Obviously, in patients with outlet obstruction, the addition of medications to relax the bladder may exacerbate urinary retention. In patients in whom medical therapy fails and who demonstrate a low flow rate despite adequate bladder function, prostate surgery is an option. Transurethral incision of the prostate is highly successful in small glands with minimal risk of incontinence, erectile dysfunction, or retrograde ejaculation. Larger glands may require resection (transurethral resection of the prostate) or open simple prostatectomy. Other therapies, such as microwave treatment or laser ablation of the prostate, are also widely used.

Bladder outlet obstruction is rarely seen in female patients and is most commonly due to periurethral scarring or suture "kinking" the urethra after antiincontinence surgery. Other causes include pelvic prolapse and very rarely, urethral malignancy. Release of the sutures and the scar tissue around the urethra or prolapse repair may be performed as indicated to relieve the obstruction.

SUMMARY

Bladder dysfunction and urinary incontinence are common and affect patients of all ages. Only about 2% of patients with incontinence actually receive treatment; therefore physicians should educate patients and other practitioners about the successful treatment options that are available. Incontinence is a problem with which no individual should live. A systematic approach to evaluation can lead to successful treatment and significant improvement in a patient's continence and quality of life.

REFERENCES

1. Blaivas JG, Zayed AA, Labib KB: The bulbocavernosus reflex in urology: a prospective study of 299 patients, *J Urol* 126(2):197, 1981.
2. Buyse G, Waldeck K, Verpoorten C, et al: Intravesical oxybutynin for neurogenic bladder dysfunction: less systemic side effects due to reduces first pass metabolism, *J Urol* 160:892, 1998.
3. Cervigni M: Hormonal influences in the lower urinary tract. In Raz S, editor: *Female urology*, Philadelphia, 1996, WB Saunders.
4. Diokno AC, Brown MB, Brock BM: Clinical and cystometric characteristics of continent and incontinent non-institutionalized elderly, *J Urol* 145:567, 1988.
5. Finkbeiner AE: Is bethanecol chloride clinically effective in promoting bladder emptying? A literature review, *J Urol* 134(3):443, 1985.
6. Gillberg PG, Sundquist S: Tolterodine, *Eur J Pharm* 349(2-3):285, 1998.
7. Resnick NM, Yalla SV: Detrusor hyperactivity with impaired contractile function: an unrecognized but common cause of incontinence in elderly patients, *JAMA* 257(22):3076, 1987.
8. Shaker HS, Hassouna M: Sacral nerve root neuromodulation: an effective treatment for refractory urge incontinence, *J Urol* 159(5):1516, 1998.
9. Vandersteen DR, Husmann DA: Treatment of primary nocturnal enuresis persisting into adulthood, *J Urol* 161:90, 1998.

CHAPTER 152

Prostate Disorders: Benign and Malignant

Ronald A. Morton
Herbert Lepor

BENIGN PROSTATIC HYPERPLASIA

Benign prostatic hyperplasia (BPH) is a benign proliferative process of the stromal and epithelial elements of the prostate. Macroscopic enlargement of the prostate often results from the proliferative process. The macroscopic prostatic enlargement may be associated with bothersome urinary symptoms, bladder outlet obstruction, or both problems. Until recently, the treatment options for BPH were limited to watchful waiting or prostatectomy. Now, however, medical and minimally invasive surgical strategies are presently available. Four drugs have FDA approval for the treatment of BPH. Three are α-blocking agents (terazosin [Hytrin], doxazosin [Cardura], and tamsulosin [Flomax]), and one is a blocker of 5α-reductase (finasteride [Proscar]). In addition, a number of minimally invasive strategies have been designed to heat the prostate. These include transurethral microwave therapy (TUMT) and transurethral needle ablation (TUNA). The diagnosis and treatment of BPH are complex and cannot be reduced to a simple flow chart. This chapter provides the primary care physician with a practical overview of the management of this condition.

Epidemiology and Natural History

The prevalence of microscopic BPH has been determined from reported autopsy data. One study reported that microscopic BPH was rarely identified in male patients younger than 40 years of age. The prevalence of microscopic BPH was observed to be age dependent: 50% and 90% of men developed histologic BPH by age 60 and 80 years, respectively. The prevalence of macroscopic BPH has been determined from the database of the Baltimore Longitudinal Study of Aging (BLSA). Approximately 50% of men were observed to have prostatic enlargement by age 70 based on a digital rectal examination (DRE). The BLSA also revealed that the prevalence of clinical BPH is age dependent. Approximately 70% of men also developed symptoms of prostatism by age 70 years. Although microscopic, macroscopic, and clinical BPH are age-dependent events, no compelling evidence indicates that these phenomena are causally related.

The natural history of BPH is poorly understood. Several cohort studies have followed groups of patients with clinical BPH retrospectively and prospectively. The available natural history data strongly indicate that clinical BPH is not always a progressive process; in fact, in some series only 30% to 40% of cases progressed symptomatically over a 5-year period. Based on the natural history data, patients should not be encouraged to pursue intervention solely to prevent the ravages of untreated BPH. It is difficult to determine from the existing literature whether race is a determinant for the development of BPH, since a universally accepted definition of *clinical BPH* does not exist. Although sporadic case-controlled studies have implicated dietary factors, smoking, body habitus, sexual history, and socioeconomic status in the pathogenesis of BPH, these associations are tenuous.

Pathogenesis

The development of BPH depends on aging and the presence of testes. The testes represent the primary source of circulating androgens. The embryologic development of the prostate and the development of BPH depend on dihydrotestosterone (DHT). The enzyme catalyzing the conversion of testosterone to DHT is 5α-reductase. Male individuals affected with a genetic deficiency of the enzyme 5α-reductase have a rudimentary prostate. BPH also rarely develops in male patients castrated before puberty. It is generally believed that androgens play a permissive role in the pathogenesis of BPH. The specific biochemical events initiating the hyperplastic process, however, remain unknown. Although many growth factors have been identified in the prostate, their precise role in the pathogenesis of BPH is unknown.

Pathophysiology

The clinical manifestations associated with BPH include obstructive and irritative urinary symptoms, incomplete bladder emptying, detrusor instability, urinary tract infection (UTI), bladder calculi, urinary retention, renal insufficiency, and hematuria (Box 152-1). The most prevalent clinical manifestation of BPH is urinary symptoms. The obstructive urinary symptoms are hesitancy and straining to initiate urination, diminished caliber of and interrupted urinary stream, and postmicturition dribbling. The irritative symptoms are diuria, nocturia, urinary urgency, incontinence, and dysuria. These symptoms collectively are referred to as *prostatism*. Several symptom indices have been developed to quantify the severity of prostatism. The International Prostate Symptom Score (I-PSS) has been validated and has gained the greatest level of clinical application. The I-PSS is self-administered and provides an excellent instrument for assessing baseline severity, response to therapy, and disease progression (Fig. 152-1). The numeric score of symptoms provides an objective assessment of the degree of prostatism.

The pathophysiology of urinary symptoms is unclear. Because prostatic enlargement and urinary symptoms are age-dependent events, it has been assumed that these phenomena are causally related. The presumed mechanism for the development of symptoms was the bladder outlet

Box 152-1. Clinical Manifestations of Benign Prostatic Hyperplasia

Urinary symptoms
Incomplete bladder emptying
Detrusor instability
Urinary tract infection
Urinary retention
Bladder calculi
Hematuria

International Prostate Symptom Score (I-PSS)

Patient name:	Not at all	Less than 1 time in 5	Less than half the time	About half the time	More than half the time	Almost always	Your score
1. Incomplete emptying Over the past month, how often have you had a sensation of not emptying your bladder completely after you finished urinating?	0	1	2	3	4	5	
2. Frequency Over the past month, how often have you had to urinate again less than two hours after you finished urinating?	0	1	2	3	4	5	
3. Intermittency Over the past month, how often have you found you stopped and started again several times when you urinated?	0	1	2	3	4	5	
4. Urgency Over the past month, how often have you found it difficult to postpone urination?	0	1	2	3	4	5	
5. Weak stream Over the past month, how often have you had a weak urinary stream?	0	1	2	3	4	5	
6. Straining Over the past month, how often have you had to push or strain to begin urination?	0	1	2	3	4	5	

	None	1 time	2 times	3 times	4 times	5 or more times	
7. Nocturia Over the past month, how many times did you most typically get up to urinate from the time you went to bed at night until the time you got up in the morning?	0	1	2	3	4	5	
Total I-PSS Score =							

Quality of Life due to Urinary Symptoms

	Delighted	Pleased	Mostly satisfied	Mixed-about equally satisfied and dissatisfied	Mostly dissatisfied	Unhappy	Terrible
If you were to spend the rest of your life with your urinary condition just the way it is now, how would you feel about that?	0	1	2	3	4	5	6

The International Prostate Symptom Score (I-PSS) is based on the answers to seven questions concerning urinary symptoms. Each question allows the patient to choose one out of five answers indicating increasing severity of the particular symptom. The answers are assigned points from 0 to 5. The total score can therefore range from 0 to 35 (asymptomatic to very symptomatic).

Furthermore, the International Consensus Committee (ICC) recommends the use of only a single question to assess the quality of life. The answers to this question range from "delighted" to "terrible" or 0 to 6. Although this single question may or may not capture the global impact of BPH symptoms or quality of life, it may serve as a valuable starting point for a doctor-patient conversation.

The ICC strongly recommends that all physicians who counsel patients suffering from symptoms of prostatism utilize these measures not only during the initial interview but also during and after treatment in order to monitor treatment response.

Fig. 152-1. International Prostate Symptom Score (I-PSS).

obstruction resulting from the enlarged prostate. Recent studies have challenged these assumptions. The examination of several large BPH clinical databases has demonstrated unequivocally that no direct relationship exists between prostate size and symptom severity or prostate size and degree of bladder outlet obstruction.

Incomplete bladder emptying is often attributed to bladder outlet obstruction secondary to BPH. The presumed consequences of incomplete bladder emptying include bladder calculi and UTI. Although the postvoid residual (PVR) can be measured precisely by catheterization or ultrasonography, the residual volume in a single patient is highly variable. Another limitation of PVR is that no consensus exists regarding the amount that represents a clinically or pathologically significant level. For example, no data suggest that the threshold PVR is associated with the development of irreversible bladder damage, urosepsis, or urinary retention.

Although no direct relationship exists between prostate size and bladder outlet obstruction, BPH has been implicated as a cause of obstruction. Several mechanisms unrelated to prostate size may cause obstruction. A prominent median lobe, a noncompliant prostatic capsule, and predominantly stromal hyperplasia have been implicated as prostate-dependent factors causing bladder outlet obstruction. Bladder outlet obstruction can be measured noninvasively by uroflowmetry or invasively by multichannel urodynamics. Uroflowmetry simply measures the maximum urinary flow rate. A reduced rate indicates bladder outlet obstruction. The primary limitation of uroflowmetry is that an acontractile bladder may also result in a decreased urine flow rate. Multichannel urodynamics allows for the simultaneous determination of both the bladder pressure at the time of voiding and the urine flow rate. A decreased urine flow rate at elevated detrusor pressures is pathognomonic for outlet obstruction. Although multichannel urodynamics quantifies bladder outlet obstruction, the precise clinical and pathologic significance of these measurements is equivocal. For example, it is unknown what level of obstruction is associated with the development of irreversible bladder dysfunction or the predisposition to develop life-threatening complications of BPH. Furthermore the irritative voiding symptoms associated with prostatism may also be unrelated to the degree of obstruction.

Evaluation of the Patient with BPH

History. A detailed urologic history and focused general medical history are essential in the evaluation of male patients with BPH (Box 152-2). The severity of symptoms should be quantified using a validated instrument such as the I-PSS. Validated questionnaires such as this offer a means of quantifying symptoms, following up on therapy, and determining when therapy is indicated. The history should also determine the level of "bother" and the impact of the urinary symptoms on quality of life. It is not unusual for patients with identical symptom scores to have very different perceptions of the degree of bother resulting from the symptoms.

Other urologic and nonurologic conditions may masquerade as prostatism. Adult-onset diabetes mellitus (AODM) may result in diuria and nocturia because of the obligatory loss of urine associated with glucosuria. AODM may also cause neuropathic bladder dysfunction. Primary neurologic disorders such as Parkinson's disease and secondary neurologic conditions such as cerebrovascular accidents (CVAs) often cause detrusor instability, resulting in urinary frequency, urgency, and urge incontinence. Prostate cancer and transitional cell carcinoma of the bladder may also cause irritative urinary symptoms. Older women suffer irritative voiding symptoms similar to those of older men, in whom these symptoms are ascribed to prostatism. More recent data appear to imply that aging and ischemia of the detrusor muscle may be responsible for some of these voiding problems.

Box 152-2. Pertinent History in the Evaluation of Benign Prostatic Hyperplasia

Urologic History

International Prostate Symptom Score (I-PSS)
Family history of prostate cancer
History of hematuria or urinary tract infection
Prior urologic instrumentation

Nonurologic History

Adult-onset diabetes mellitus
Neurologic conditions
- Primary: Parkinson's disease
- Secondary: cerebrovascular accident

Medications

Anticholinergics
α-Adrenergic agonists

The role of the bladder is to store urine under low pressure and empty urine in socially acceptable circumstances. Medications may affect bladder emptying and storage and therefore may interfere with bladder function and cause symptoms of prostatism. Bladder contraction is a parasympathetic event mediated by muscarinic cholinergic receptors, whereas bladder outlet resistance is a sympathetic function mediated predominantly by the α_1-adrenoceptor. Therefore muscarinic cholinergic antagonists such as propantheline (Probanthine) or α-adrenergic agonists such as phenylephrine may impede bladder emptying and exacerbate or independently cause BPH-like symptoms.

Physical Examination. The physical examination should include careful palpation of the prostate (Box 152-3). The DRE should focus on identifying stony hard nodules, induration, tenderness, or asymmetric enlargement. Although the size is often estimated, this observation has limited clinical significance. The rectal tone should be assessed to identify an underlying neurologic condition. The suprapubic region may be percussed for a large PVR.

Laboratory Assessment. A urinalysis is a simple and often informative screening test for genitourinary diseases (Box 152-4). It is recommended that all men with BPH undergo this simple test. The presence of glucosuria may be the initial presentation for AODM. The presence of microscopic hematuria requires additional imaging and

Box 152-3. Physical Examination for Benign Prostatic Hyperplasia

Digital rectal examination
- Nodules, induration, tenderness
- Rectal tone

Percussible and palpable bladder

Box 152-4. Laboratory Assessment for Benign Prostatic Hyperplasia

Urinalysis
- Glucosuria
- Hematuria, pyuria, bacteriuria

Serum creatinine level
- Serum level of prostate-specific antigen

diagnostic studies to exclude genitourinary malignancies or benign conditions such as nephrolithiasis. The presence of pyuria or bacteriuria indicates the need for a urine culture. Additional testing is required to determine the etiology of the UTI. A serum creatinine test is often recommended to identify significant renal disease resulting from bladder outlet obstruction. This recommendation is not based on data defining the specificity and sensitivity of a serum creatinine test to identify BPH-dependent renal dysfunction. If the serum creatinine level is elevated, the PVR should be determined.

The role of serum prostate-specific antigen (PSA) determination for screening prostate cancer has become less controversial. The controversy involves not whether screening increases detection but whether increased detection achieves increased survival. Although the data to resolve this controversy are not available, individuals with BPH should routinely undergo a baseline PSA determination. Where appropriate, men with elevated PSA levels should be evaluated for prostate cancer.

Uroflowmetry, multichannel urodynamics, and PVR have already been discussed. Although these studies may provide valuable information related to the level of obstruction or the indications for intervention, the data derived from these studies are often too nonspecific to establish definitive treatment recommendations (Box 152-5). Therefore these studies may be considered options. Uroflowmetry offers a simple noninvasive baseline that can easily be followed to determine the results of therapy. Cystoscopy and imaging of the upper urinary tract by intravenous pyelography (IVP), ultrasound, and computed tomography (CT) scans should not be routinely obtained as part of the evaluation of BPH. If the history, physical examination, or laboratory studies suggest specific abnormalities, these tests may be indicated.

Box 152-5. Optional Diagnostic Studies for Benign Prostatic Hyperplasia

Uroflowmetry
Postvoid residual determination
Multichannel urodynamics
Cystoscopy
Imaging of upper urinary tracts

Box 152-6. Indications for Intervention in Benign Prostatic Hyperplasia

Absolute

Urinary retention
Recurrent urinary tract infection
Refractory gross hematuria
Bladder calculi
Renal insufficiency secondary to benign prostatic hyperplasia

Relative

Urinary symptoms
Incomplete emptying
Urodynamic obstruction

Indications for Intervention

The indications for therapeutic intervention in BPH may be stratified as absolute vs. relative (Box 152-6). Absolute indications imply that the patient's overall well-being is compromised if treatment is not rendered. Urinary retention, refractory hematuria, and UTIs secondary to BPH are widely accepted absolute indications for intervention. Only a small subset of patients with BPH have these absolute indications for intervention.

The relative indications for intervention include bothersome urinary symptoms, incomplete bladder emptying, and bladder outlet obstruction. Severe symptoms in the absence of absolute indications for intervention do not jeopardize the patient's health status. It is imperative to determine both the level of bother and the risk that the patient is willing to assume to alleviate the urinary symptoms. Physicians cannot impart their own perception of risk/benefit for patients. Although incomplete bladder emptying and urodynamic evidence of bladder outlet obstruction may exacerbate urinary symptoms and lead to UTI and irreversible bladder dysfunction, no data precisely define the clinical, physiologic, and pathologic implications of these findings. Therefore the treatment recommendations by different physicians vary and reflect individual bias.

Treatment

Prostatectomy. There are several surgical and minimally invasive approaches for the treatment of BPH (Box 152-7). The prostatic tissue may be removed by open enucleation or by transurethral resection of the prostate (TURP). The surgical approach is based on the size of the prostate and the surgeon's preference. Approximately 90% of prostatectomies are performed via the transurethral route. Open prostatectomy requires a lower abdominal incision and hospitalization ranging from 5 to 7 days. TURP requires no surgical incision, and the hospital stay is approximately 2 to 3 days. Table 152-1 presents the risks associated with TURP. Although the complications after prostatectomy are rarely life-threatening, the inherent risks may discourage patients with relative indications from pursuing surgical intervention. Approximately 80% to 90% of patients achieve marked to moderate symptom improvement after TURP and are very satisfied with the treatment outcome. The mean improvement in the urine flow rate is approximately 100%.

Laser energy has recently been advocated as another method for removing the obstructing prostatic tissue. The primary advantage of laser ablation over prostatectomy is that irrigation fluid is not resorbed and therefore the risks of hyponatremia and fluid overload are alleviated. Bleeding is negligible, and transfusions are rarely, if ever, required.

Retrograde ejaculation is also a rare outcome. The patients are often discharged on the day of surgery. The preliminary data suggest that the prostatic defect after laser ablation is far less than that achieved with TURP and that many patients experience irritative symptoms for several months. The improvements in symptom score, bladder emptying, and urine flow rate approximate, but are not equivalent to, those with TURP. The reduced cost from shorter hospitalization is balanced by the cost of the laser fiber and the new technology. The long-term effectiveness of laser ablation has yet to be defined. It is likely that patients will choose a less invasive and safer procedure such as laser ablation even if the level of improvement is slightly less than with TURP.

Transurethral incision of the prostate (TUIP) is an alternative surgical procedure that is less invasive than TURP. The bladder neck and prostatic adenoma are deeply incised without resecting prostatic tissue. Randomized studies have demonstrated that the effectiveness of TURP and TUIP are comparable. The intraoperative time, blood loss, and complications are less with TUIP. TUIP is not recommended if the prostate is larger than 30 gm. Approximately half the patients undergoing TURP are candidates for TUIP.

Box 152-7. Surgical and Minimally Invasive Interventions for Benign Prostatic Hyperplasia

Prostatectomy
- Open enucleation
- Transurethral resection of the prostate (TURP)

Laser ablation
Transurethral incision of the prostate (TUIP)
Balloon dilation
Prostatic stents
Microwave thermotherapy

Table 152-1. Morbidity Associated With Transurethral Prostatectomy (TURP)

Complication	Incidence (%)
Epididymitis	4.8
Urinary tract infection	8.4
Impotence	10.2
Incontinence	3.3
Transfusion	10.5
Transurethral resection syndrome	—
Death	—

Minimally Invasive Intervention. Balloon dilation of the prostate (BDP) has been advocated for the treatment of BPH. Although the initial uncontrolled reports were encouraging, a randomized, double-blind study reported that BDP and cystoscopy achieve equivalent therapeutic benefit. This study suggested that the observed effectiveness of BDP is likely a placebo response.

Permanent indwelling prostatic stents are endoscopically positioned in the prostatic urethra and eventually become covered by transitional epithelium. Occasional stone formation on the uncovered stent and severe irritative voiding symptoms are the primary limitations of the procedure.

Heating the prostate with microwave energy (transurethral microwave therapy [TUMT]) is another method used to destroy prostatic tissue. The microwave energy is delivered to the prostate by a transurethral catheter. The urethra is cooled to improve patient tolerance. Longitudinal studies have shown excellent symptomatic relief with modest change in the peak urinary flow rate. Sham controlled studies have shown statistically significant differences between TUMT and sham groups in terms of both urinary flow rates and symptom scores on questionnaires. The cost of the microwave energy machine is presently about $120,000. Prostatic heating strategies are usually used after oral medical therapy has failed.

Medical Therapy

α-Blockade. The rationale for α-blockers in BPH is based on several morphologic, physiologic, and pharmacologic observations. Double immunoenzymatic staining and color-assisted image analysis have revealed that smooth muscle accounts for 40% of the tissue volume of the prostate. In vitro isometric tension studies have demonstrated that the contractile properties of prostate smooth muscle are mediated primarily by α_1-adrenoceptors. Radioligand receptor binding studies have shown that the human prostate contains a relative abundance of α-adrenoceptors. Based on the physiologic and pharmacologic observations just mentioned, α_1-adrenergic blockers should decrease the resistance along the prostatic urethra by relaxing the smooth muscle component of the prostate.

Several different α-blockers have been investigated for the treatment of BPH. These α-blockers can be subgrouped according to the α-adrenoceptor subtype selectivity and the duration of serum elimination half-lives (Box 152-8). Phenoxybenzamine antagonizes α_1- and α_2-adrenoceptors, whereas prazosin, alfuzosin, indoramin, terazosin, doxazosin, and tamsulosin are selective α_1-antagonists. The advantage of the selective α_1-antagonists is that the incidence and severity of adverse events are far less than with the nonselective α-blockers. Terazosin (Hytrin), doxazosin (Cardura), and tamsulosin (Flomax) are FDA approved for the treatment of BPH in the United States. The advantages of the long-acting, once-a-day α-blockers are improved compliance and tolerance. The most common adverse events associated with selective α_1-blockers include dizziness, lightheadedness, and asthenia. The administration of a once-a-day formulation at bedtime appears to reduce the incidence and severity of these adverse events.

Lepor et al reported the results of a phase III multicenter, double-blind, parallel-group, randomized, placebo-controlled study of once-a-day administration of terazosin to patients with symptomatic BPH. A total of 285 patients received either placebo or 2, 5, or 10 mg of terazosin once daily. The level of improvements in the symptom scores were dose dependent (Table 152-2). The percentages of patients exhibiting a greater than 30% improvement in the total symptom scores for the placebo and 2-, 5-, and 10-mg treatment groups were 40%, 51%, 57%, and 60%, respectively. The changes in peak urine flow rate were also dose dependent. The percentages of patients experiencing a greater than 30% increase in the peak flow rate in the placebo and 2-, 5-, and 10-mg treatment groups were 26%, 40%, 35%, and 52%, respectively. A significantly greater proportion of patients in the 10-mg treatment group exhibited a more than 30% improvement in symptom scores compared with the placebo group. An interim analysis of an open-label study evaluating the long-term safety and effectiveness of terazosin for BPH indicates that improvements in symptom scores and urine flow rates are maintained throughout a 2-year follow-up.

Box 152-8. α-Blockers Investigated for Therapy of Benign Prostatic Hyperplasia

Nonselective α-blockers
Phenoxybenzamine

Selective α-blockers
Prazosin
Alfuzosin
Indoramin

Selective long-acting α_1-blockers
Terazosin
Doxazosin
Tamsulosin

Overall, the adverse events in the four treatment groups were minor and reversible. Although a higher incidence of asthenia, influenza syndrome, and dizziness were observed in the terazosin treatment groups, the differences from placebo were not statistically significant. Only one patient in the 10-mg treatment group developed syncope at the 5-mg dose.

One of the presumed limitations of α-blockers for the treatment of BPH was the consequences of lowering blood pressure in relatively elderly normotensive patients. The observed effect of terazosin on baseline systolic blood pressure in normotensive and hypertensive patients was 3 mm Hg and 14 mm Hg, respectively. These data demonstrate that terazosin lowers blood pressure in patients with BPH when it is a desired physiologic outcome.

Three multicenter, randomized placebo-controlled studies have evaluated the safety and effectiveness of doxazosin for the treatment of BPH. A long-term open-label doxazosin study demonstrated that the level of its effectiveness is similar to that of terazosin.

Tamsulosin, an α_1-blocker, has the benefit of no need for dose escalation and an improved safety profile in that it causes much less orthostatic hypotension. It does, however, cause more retrograde ejaculation. Men treated with tamsulosin appear to have the same results in terms of symptom score and peak flow rate changes as those treated with the other α-blocking agents.

There is a definite physiologic and pharmacologic rationale for a blockade in BPH. Multicenter, randomized placebo-controlled studies have consistently and unequivocally demonstrated the ability of α-blockers to relieve symptoms of BPH and increase urine flow rates. The clinical response is rapid and durable. The presumed advantages of the long-acting selective α_1-blockers include better compliance and tolerance. Selective α_1-blockers lower blood

Table 152-2. Effectiveness of Terazosin (TRZ) for Benign Prostatic Hyperplasia

Outcome measures	Baseline	12 weeks	% Δ*	*p* value†
Symptom score‡				
Placebo	9.7	7.4	−23.5	<0.001
TRZ (10 mg)	10.1	5.5	−45.1	
Peak flow rate (ml/sec)				
Placebo	10.1	10.2	+10.4	
TRZ (10 mg)	8.8	12.2	+34.0	0.009

*Values correspond to the means of the changes from baseline in each man and therefore cannot be derived from the baseline and 12-week results.
†Comparison between mean %Δ placebo vs. TRZ.
‡Boyarsky symptom score.

pressure in these patients when it is a desired clinical outcome. Since approximately 50% of men with BPH are also hypertensive, the ability to treat BPH and hypertension simultaneously and effectively with a single drug is a distinct advantage of selective α_1-blockers.

Androgen Suppression. The reduction of prostate volume after castration in male patients with BPH was observed 100 years ago. Castration never gained widespread acceptance for the treatment of BPH because of the psychologic impact of removal of the testes and the subsequent development of impotence, loss of libido, and hot flashes resulting from the imbalance of androgens and estrogens. Medical castration can be achieved by drugs that block the action or synthesis of either testosterone or DHT. The morbidity associated with the drugs lowering serum testosterone levels often counterbalances the therapeutic benefit, especially in BPH therapy. Since the maintenance of prostate volume depends on tissue levels of DHT, a drug that selectively blocks the production or action of DHT would achieve involution of the prostate without the problematic adverse events associated with castrate levels of serum testosterone. Finasteride, a 5α-reductase inhibitor, lowers serum and prostatic levels of DHT without lowering serum testosterone levels. Finasteride is the only hormonal therapy that is FDA approved for BPH.

A multicenter, randomized, placebo-controlled, double-blind study recently evaluated the safety and effectiveness of finasteride in men with BPH. A total of 895 patients were randomized to receive daily placebo or 1 or 5 mg of finasteride for 12 months. Table 152-3 summarizes the improvements in symptom scores, flow rate, and prostate volume. The effect of finasteride on these outcome measures was statistically significant.

Adverse events were rare in the placebo and treatment groups. The differences between decreased libido (4.7% vs. 1.3%) and ejaculatory dysfunction (4.4% vs. 1.7%) in the 5-mg and placebo groups were statistically significant. The percentages of patients who developed an adverse event resulting in premature withdrawal in the placebo and 5-mg treatment groups were only 6% and 5%, respectively. The short-term safety profile of finasteride is exceedingly favorable. The durability of the therapeutic response is maintained at 36 months in a subset of patients.

A definite rationale exists for androgen suppression in the treatment of BPH. Finasteride represents the only drug that has been studied in a multicenter trial with sufficient numbers of patients and adequate follow-up. Androgen suppression causes prostate involution primarily by affecting prostatic epithelium. It is not surprising that only a relatively modest reduction in prostate volume occurs, since only 10% of the prostate volume is accounted for by the epithelium. Although the differences between placebo and 5 mg of finasteride are modest, the differences are statistically significant. The adverse events associated with finasteride are minimal and reversible. Finasteride is likely to benefit a relatively small subset of patients with clinical BPH. More recent studies have shown that finasteride works best in patients with larger prostates. It probably should not be used in patients with small prostates (PSA values < 3). Longitudinal studies have shown that men with larger prostates who are treated with finasteride have a statistically lower potential to develop urinary retention.

Summary

Enlargement of the prostate secondary to BPH is essentially an inescapable phenomenon for the aging male population. The pathophysiology of clinical BPH is poorly understood. Evaluation of men with clinical BPH is targeted to identify other conditions that may masquerade as BPH. Prostatectomy, thermotherapy, and medical therapy represent the treatment strategies presently accepted for the treatment of clinical BPH.

Individuals with absolute indications should be offered prostatectomy, although recent data demonstrate a reasonable success rate in treating patients in urinary retention with thermotherapy. Most patients who do not have life-threatening consequences of BPH and who are bothered by their symptoms should be offered medical therapy. When medical therapy fails or is not well tolerated, the patient usually goes on to receive more invasive therapy. The treatment decision should be based on the patient's perception of bother from the symptoms and the risks the patient is willing to incur to achieve the desired therapeutic response.

PROSTATE CANCER

Prostate cancer is now the most frequently diagnosed cancer in American men, accounting for 32% of all diagnosed male

Table 152-3. Effectiveness of Finasteride for Benign Prostatic Hyperplasia

Outcome measures	Baseline	52 weeks	% Δ*	*p* value†
Symptom score‡				
Placebo	9.8	8.8	−2	<0.05
Finasteride (5 mg)	10.2	7.5	−21	
Peak flow rate (ml/sec)				
Placebo	9.6	9.8	+8	<0.001
Finasteride (5 mg)	9.6	11.2	+22	
Prostate volume				
Placebo	61.0	59.8	−3	<0.001
Finasteride (5 mg)	58.6	47.5	−19	

*Values correspond to the means of the changes from baseline in each man and therefore cannot be derived from the baseline and 52-week results.
†Comparison between mean %Δ placebo vs. finasteride.
‡Modified Boyarsky score.

cancers. Prostate cancer is second only to lung cancer as a cause of male cancer deaths. In 1997, there were approximately 180,000 new cases of prostate cancer diagnosed and 36,000 deaths from prostate cancer. In addition to this critical number of clinically manifested prostate cancers, autopsy studies forecast that 11 million men in the United States over age 45 harbor histologic (clinically silent) prostate cancer. African-American men represent a particularly high-risk group. The incidence of prostate cancer in African-American men is 50% higher than in Caucasian Americans. Moreover, the 5-year survival rate from 1983 to 1989 for Caucasian Americans was 79%, whereas for African-Americans it was 64%. Patients with hereditary prostate cancer characterized by early age at onset and autosomal dominant inheritance represent a second high-risk group.

The etiology of this exceedingly common cancer is unknown. Unlike other solid tumors such as colon and breast cancer, no candidate genes or genetic loci have been identified to explain the hereditary form of the disease.

Clinical Presentation

The presentation of prostate cancer depends on the stage at the time of diagnosis. In its early stages, prostate cancer is asymptomatic. Early cases are often diagnosed by DRE during routine physical examination or during examination for another illness (Box 152-9). PSA has had a profound impact on the clinical presentation of prostate cancer. In 1988, PSA became widely available as a serum marker for prostate cancer. It is a serine protease produced only by prostatic epithelium. Although produced by both normal and malignant cells, the contribution to serum levels differs greatly for these two cell populations. The contribution to serum PSA by BPH tissue is 0.3 ng/ml/cm^3 of tissue. Elevations in PSA levels correlate with increasing clinical stage and pathologic grade and stage of prostate cancer. However, a wide variation in prostatic epithelial/stromal ratios among patients limits the predictive value of a single PSA measurement in a given individual. The normal reference range for serum PSA is also age dependent. Nevertheless, PSA can assist in differentiating between benign and malignant conditions of the prostate.

The normal reference range for PSA is up to 4 ng/ml. Values between 4 and 10 ng/ml fall into the indeterminate range. Values greater than 10 ng/ml are highly suggestive but not diagnostic for prostate cancer. Three observations have provided guidelines for interpreting PSA data in the ambiguous middle range. Ultrasound has been used to measure prostate volume and then calculate the amount of PSA per unit volume of tissue. This value has been termed *PSA density (PSAD)*. A PSAD value of 0.15 or greater in association with a PSA value between 4 and 10 suggests that a needle biopsy of the prostate is indicated regardless of DRE findings. Such biopsies should be performed with transrectal ultrasound guidance (TRUS). Researchers with the BLSA measured the change in serial PSA levels on historic samples from men with known outcomes. This has been termed *PSA velocity (PSAV)* or *rate of PSA change*. The researchers were able to establish that a PSAV of 0.75 ng/ml/yr correlated with the development and diagnosis of clinically significant prostate cancers. This value has been confirmed by two larger studies. Consequently, men with a PSA level of 4 to 10 ng/ml and serial PSA measurements demonstrating a PSAV of 0.75 ng/ml/yr should undergo a full evaluation for prostate cancer. Age-associated reference ranges for PSA also have been described. The following normal values have been recommended for PSA: up to 2.5 ng/ml for men age 40 to 49, up to 3.5 ng/ml for men age 50 to 59, up to 4.5 ng/ml for men age 60 to 69, and up to 6.5 ng/ml for men age 70 and older. More recently, it has been shown that measurement of the unbound or free PSA (PSA II) may be helpful in interpreting PSA levels of 4 to 10 ng/ml. If the free PSA is greater than 25%, the condition is usually benign disease. Conversely, when the free PSA is less than 10% the patient usually has an underlying malignancy. Unfortunately, most patients do not have a free PSA in either extreme, thereby making the test not helpful in many patients. It does become one of the variables along with PSAD, age-related PSA, and PSAV that is used to determine the need for repeated biopsies. More recently a study looking at the use of the bound PSA has been published that shows only a modest increase in sensitivity.

Each of these PSA derivatives has certain disadvantages. PSAD is hampered by the inability of current radiologic techniques to measure prostate volume precisely and by the wide variance in prostatic epithelial/stromal ratios. The age-specific reference ranges were determined in a single community consisting only of Caucasians. Attempts to generalize these data to other populations have yielded inconsistent results. The optimal interval between PSA measurements necessary to calculate PSAV has yet to be determined. In general, most urologists perform TRUS-guided prostate biopsies (usually 6 to 12 biopsies are taken from prescribed areas of the prostate) in patients with abnormal rectal examination or PSA values higher than 4 ng/ml (in the 50- to 75-year-old age group). The PSA derivatives already described can be used to obviate a prostate biopsy but are usually used to determine the need for subsequent biopsies when follow-up PSA determinations are obtained. For example, a patient may have a PSA value of 5 ng/ml and undergo a negative biopsy. He may return 1 year later with a PSA determination of 5.6 ng/ml. Should he have another biopsy? Should he be worried? Here one can take into account his prostate volume, PSAV, and even his free PSA to answer these questions.

There have been recent technologic improvements in radiologic techniques for imaging prostate cancer. These include TRUS, pelvic magnetic resonance imaging (MRI), and improved radionuclide bone scan. Despite these advances before routine PSA screening, only approximately 40% of men thought to have clinically localized prostate cancer did not have organ-confined disease at the time of radical prostatectomy. This number has improved in more recent studies. In fact the majority of radical prostatectomies are

Box 152-9. Clinical Presentation of Prostate Cancer

- Abnormality found with screening digital rectal examination or serum prostate-specific antigen determination
- Urinary symptoms (prostatism)
- Hematuria
- Bony metastasis

now performed on men with stage T1c disease (normal rectal examination and elevated PSA level). The realization that PSA can help detect prostate cancer at an earlier stage than was previously thought possible has led to the use of PSA as a screening test for prostate cancer. In five large studies of screening PSA, the sensitivity ranged from 46% to 89.5% and the specificity from 59% to 91.2%. These studies encompass both office- and community-based populations. Because of the low sensitivity of PSA in these studies, the value of PSA screening has come into question. It has also been the impetus for the development of the PSA variants. PSA screening will not be universally accepted until the death rate from this disease decreases. Because of the slow progression of prostate cancer, this is not likely to occur until 2004 or 2005.

Despite growing efforts to identify men with early stage prostate cancer, patients continue to come to medical attention with advanced-stage disease (although the authors have seen a stage migration in that a lower percentage of patients come to medical attention with advanced disease). At presentation, these men may have hematuria, lower urinary tract obstruction, or pain from bone metastasis. The axial skeleton, particularly the pelvis and lumbar spine, is most susceptible to metastatic spread of prostate cancer. Other sites of metastasis include the seminal vesicles by local extension and lymphatic spread to the obturator and external iliac nodes.

Diagnosing and Staging

Patients identified at risk for having prostate cancer by DRE, PSA, or TRUS should undergo transrectal biopsy of the prostate. This can be performed as an outpatient procedure, with oral antibiotic prophylaxis initiated the night before the procedure (fluoroquinolone). Biopsies in the setting of an elevated PSA level without obvious findings on DRE should be performed with TRUS guidance. Prostate cancer sometimes appears as a hypoechoic lesion on ultrasound. The presence of a hypoechoic lesion on ultrasound is not pathognomonic for prostate cancer, and its absence does not rule out the disease. Biopsies should therefore be taken from each sextant of the prostate to ensure maximal diagnostic accuracy. Once the presence of prostate cancer is confirmed with a biopsy specimen, the tumor is assigned a grade. The most common grading system in use today is the Gleason grading system. This system is based on the glandular architecture of the two most frequently seen patterns in the tumor. Each pattern is given a Gleason grade from 1 to 5, with a grade of 1 being the most differentiated. The sum of the two grades is the Gleason score. Therefore the Gleason score can range from 2 to 10.

Clinical staging is used to determine the initial mode of therapy. Radiologic modalities (e.g., pelvic CT scan) for evaluating pelvic lymph nodes are of little benefit in the staging of prostate cancer unless the pelvic lymph nodes are enlarged, which usually will not occur until the PSA level is 20 ng/ml or higher. Enlarged nodes on CT scan may be biopsied by skinny needle to aid in clinical staging. The clinical staging of prostate cancer can be accomplished with DRE, radionuclide bone scan, PSA analysis, and findings on transurethral prostatectomy when appropriate. As with pelvic CT scan, the bone scan is usually not "positive" until the PSA value is significantly elevated. At present the TNM staging of prostate cancer has been adopted worldwide (Table 152-4). Organ-confined tumors are designated either T1 or T2; the ability to palpate the tumor on DRE is the feature that separates these groups. T1 tumors are nonpalpable tumors diagnosed via TURP (T1a, T1b) or biopsy performed for an elevated PSA level only (T1c). T1 tumors detected during TURP are subdivided into two groups based on the percentage of resected tissue that is cancerous: T1a is 5% or less, and T1b is greater than 5%. This distinction has prognostic significance: 16% of men with untreated T1a disease develop metastatic disease at 10 years, whereas 35% of men with T1b disease have metastatic disease at 5 years and 20% die of prostate cancer in 5 to 10 years. Palpable T2 tumors are further stratified with respect to the size of the nodule. T2a disease is tumor involving half a lobe or less, T2b

Table 152-4. Staging of Prostate Cancer: TNM Classification

Primary tumor stage	Clinical findings	Corresponding Whitmore classification
T0	No evidence of tumor	
T1	Nonpalpable disease	
T1a	Tumor found at TURP ≤5% of resected tissue	A1
T1b	Tumor found at TURP >5% of resected tissue	A2
T1c	Tumor on needle biopsy for elevated PSA level only	
T2	Palpable tumor confined to the prostate	
T2a	Tumor involves half a lobe or less	B1
T2b	Tumor involves more than half a lobe, not both lobes	B2
T2c	Tumor involves both lobes	
T3	Tumor extends through prostatic capsule	C
T3a	Unilateral extracapsular extension	
T3b	Bilateral extracapsular extension	
T3c	Tumor invades seminal vesicle(s)	
T4	Tumor is fixed or invades other adjacent structures	
T4a	Tumor invading bladder neck or rectum	
T4b	Tumor fixed to pelvic side wall	

disease is tumor in more than half a lobe but not both lobes, and T2c disease is tumor involving both lobes. T3 disease encompasses local spread outside the prostate. T3a are tumors with unilateral extracapsular extension, and T3b tumors have bilateral extracapsular extension. T3c represents seminal vesicle involvement. T4 stage tumors have greater degrees of local extension with involvement of contiguous organs (see Table 152-4).

Treatment

The treatment of prostate cancer is dictated by the clinical stage at presentation, the patient's age, and the patient's general health. The optimal treatment is highly controversial (Box 152-10). Treatment options include watchful waiting, hormonal therapy, radical prostatectomy, radiation therapy, TURP, and chemotherapy. The objectives of treatment depend on the stage and realistic expectations. The goals of therapy include cure, increased survival, relief of urinary retention and bothersome urinary symptoms, and palliation of systemic metastasis (Box 152-11).

Radical prostatectomy and radiation therapy are offered with the intent to cure T1 and T2 disease. The limitations of treatment result in part from the limitations of clinical staging, since approximately half of the patients with clinically localized disease do not have pathologically organ-confined disease. The morbidity of treatment also is a factor. Moreover, 60% to 75% of patients treated with radiation therapy have positive results from prostate needle biopsies 18 months after treatment. A more recent addition to external beam radiation therapy has been brachytherapy using radioactive seeds. A recent study reported that 79% of men who had PSA levels less than 10 ng/ml and a Gleason grade 6 or less enjoyed a 79% biochemically disease-free survival (no rise in PSA) 8 years after radioactive seed implantation. These numbers are similar to those for radical prostatectomy outcomes; however, they essentially come from one center and represent a relatively short follow-up period, especially with respect to the existing radical prostatectomy data. The major morbidities related to the surgical treatment of localized prostate cancer are erectile dysfunction and urinary incontinence. Postoperative erectile dysfunction occurs in essentially 100% of patients undergoing a standard radical prostatectomy, in which both cavernosal nerves are cut. After a nerve-sparing radical prostatectomy, the rate is 10% to 60%. It should be mentioned that for Viagra to successfully work for postoperative erectile dysfunction, at least one cavernosal nerve must be spared. The incontinence rate for radiation therapy is approximately 2%, whereas for radical prostatectomy, it ranges from 2% to 10%. The incontinence rate after radical prostatectomy is likely to be reduced in academic centers where greater numbers of prostatectomies are performed. After brachytherapy, the rate of erectile dysfunction is 25%, and the incontinence rate is less than 2%.

Box 152-10. Treatment Options for Prostate Cancer

Watchful waiting
Radical prostatectomy
Radiation therapy
Transurethral resection of the prostate (TURP)
Hormonal therapy
Chemotherapy

Box 152-11. Objectives of Therapy for Prostate Cancer

Cure
Increased survival
Relief of bladder outlet obstruction
Relief of bothersome urinary symptoms
Palliation of systemic metastasis

With the widespread availability of PSA testing, prostate cancer is now diagnosed earlier and with greater frequency. Autopsy studies consistently show that 15% to 30% of men over age 50 harbor histologically identifiable prostate cancer cells. This percentage increases to 50% to 60% of men older than 90 years of age. These types of studies document the presence of a large population of asymptomatic men with prostate cancer who never have any adverse effects from the disease. These data had prompted some to advocate that cancers diagnosed via PSA level alone (T1c) may be clinically insignificant and not require treatment; however, a recent study reviewed the pathologic findings of 157 consecutive patients with clinical stage T1c disease and found that 84% of tumors were significant and that definitive treatment was justified in most patients. At present, studies imply that watchful waiting is adequate for men with stage T2 cancers or less. Although of interest, these studies have been imperfect in that some men received hormonal therapy; the mean age of patients in these studies was generally 70 or older (patients who would not be treated aggressively under standard guidelines); and the studies were biased toward patients with low-grade disease. Watchful waiting is used in older patients (usually older than 70 years) with Gleason 6 or less tumors. Watchful waiting does not mean "benign neglect." It implies that periodic PSA determinations are obtained, and if the PSA is rising, appropriate therapy is started. At present, the biologic potential of a given tumor cannot be reliably predicted. Furthermore, no consistent data have been presented suggesting that young healthy patients do not benefit from aggressive treatment of prostate cancer. In general, patients younger than 70 years of age are preferentially offered surgery, whereas those over 70 years are offered radiation therapy. Obviously, many other issues such as other health problems and patient preference must be taken into consideration before determining a treatment for clinically localized prostate cancer.

Stage T3 tumors extend through the prostatic capsule, and 50% to 80% of these patients have lymph node metastases. Because there is no proven adjuvant therapy for prostate cancer, these patients do not benefit from radical prostatectomy. To achieve local control of their disease, external beam radiation therapy may be offered.

At this time, patients with known distant metastases cannot be cured, and treatment efforts for this group are largely palliative. Hormonal therapy aimed at decreasing serum testosterone levels via castration or luteinizing hormone–releasing hormone (LHRH) agonist therapy should be begun with the development of symptoms of metastatic disease. An antiandrogen must be given for approximately 3 to 4 weeks in conjunction with LHRH agonist therapy to avoid the testosterone flare response. The benefit of long-term combination therapy (LHRH agonist and antiandrogen) remains moot. In patients with asymptomatic metastatic prostate cancer, it is not known whether there is a survival benefit from early vs. delayed hormonal manipulation.

To date, efforts to develop chemotherapeutic regimens for prostate cancer have been disappointing. Since all tumors may eventually acquire a hormonally insensitive phenotype, hormonal therapy inevitably fails. Many single agents, combinations of chemotherapy agents, and various vaccines are being tested in clinical trials for relapsing or hormonally refractory disease.

ADDITIONAL READINGS

Barry MJ: Epidemiology and natural history of benign prostatic hyperplasia, *Urol Clin North Am* 17:495, 1990.

Barry MJ, et al: The Measurement Committee of the American Urological Association: The American Urological Association symptom index for benign prostatic hyperplasia, *J Urol* 148:1549, 1992.

Benson MC, et al: The use of prostate specific antigen density to enhance the predictive value of intermediate levels of serum prostate specific antigen, *J Urol* 147:817, 1992.

Berry SJ, et al: The development of human benign prostatic hyperplasia with age, *J Urol* 132:474, 1984.

Boring CC, et al: Cancer statistics, *CA Cancer J Clin* 44:7, 1994.

Carter HB, Pearson JD: PSA velocity for the diagnosis of early prostate cancer, *Urol Clin North Am* 20:665, 1993.

Catalona W, et al: Evaluation of percentage of free prostate specific antigen to improve specificity of cancer screening, *JAMA* 274:1214, 1995.

Critz F, et al: Prostate specific antigen nadir achieved by men apparently cured of prostate cancer by radiotherapy, *J Urol* 161:1199, 1999.

De la Rosette JJMC, et al: Transurethral microwave thermotherapy (TUMT) in benign prostatic hyperplasia: placebo versus TUMT, *Urology* 44:58, 1994.

Djavan B, Roehrborn K, et al: Prospective randomized comparison of high energy transurethral microwave thermotherapy vs. α-blocker treatment of patients with benign prostatic hyperplasia, *J Urol* 161:139, 1999.

Epstein JI, et al: Pathologic and clinical findings to predict tumor extent of nonpalpable (stage T1C) prostate cancer, *JAMA* 271:368, 1994.

Fowler FJ, Barry MJ, et al: Effects of radical prostatectomy for prostate cancer on patient quality of life: results of a Medicare survey, *Urology* 45:1007, 1995.

Gormley GJ, et al: The effect of finasteride in men with benign prostatic hyperplasia, *N Engl J Med* 327:1185, 1992.

Guess HA, et al: Cumulative prevalence of prostatism matches the autopsy prevalence of benign prostatic hyperplasia, *Prostate* 17:241, 1990.

Holtgrewe HL, et al: Transurethral prostatectomy: practice aspects of the dominant operation in American urology, *J Urol* 141:248, 1989.

Lepor H: Medical therapy for BPH, *Urology* 42:483, 1993.

Lepor H, et al: The efficacy of terazocin, finasteride, or both in benign prostatic hyperplasia, *N Engl J Med* 335:533, 1996.

Lepor H, et al: A randomized multicenter placebo controlled study of the efficacy and safety of terazosin in the treatment of benign prostatic hyperplasia, *J Urol* 148:1467, 1992.

Oesterling JE, et al: Influence of patient age on the serum PSA concentration: an important clinical observation, *Urol Clin North Am* 20:671, 1993.

Ragde H, et al: Interstitial iodine[125] radiation without adjuvant therapy in the treatment of clinically localized prostate cancer, *Cancer* 80:442, 1997.

Ramos C, et al: Retrospective comparison of radical retropubic prostatectomy and iodine[125] brachytherapy for localized prostate cancer, *J Urol* 161:1212, 1999.

Schulman C, Zlotta AR: Transurethral needle ablation of the prostate for treatment of benign prostatic hyperplasia: early clinical experience, *Urology* 45:28, 1995.

Walsh P, et al: Cancer control and quality of life following anatomical radical retropubic prostatectomy: results at 10 years, *J Urol* 152:1831, 1994.

CHAPTER 153

Bladder and Kidney Cancer

Michael J. Droller

BLADDER CANCER

Bladder cancer generally refers to malignancy of the transitional cell epithelium, which comprises more than 90% of all forms of urothelial cancer. Squamous cell cancer is seen in approximately 5% of cases, whereas adenocarcinoma is diagnosed in 2% to 3%. Approximately 54,000 new cases of bladder cancer are diagnosed annually. Men are affected three to four times as often as women. At least 75% of new cases are categorized as superficial (see Tumor Staging) and are usually amenable to conservative treatment. Whereas 75% of these may recur, only 10% to 15% may become progressive or life-threatening. In contrast, 25% of bladder cancers when initially diagnosed are deeply invasive of the bladder wall. These are potentially life-threatening and require prompt aggressive surgical treatment for there to be any chance of success.

Epidemiology

In 1895, Rehn suggested an association between urothelial cancer and exposure to aniline dye, based on his observations that several factory workers had developed bladder cancer. Subsequent studies correlated exposure to aromatic amines and to related substances in other industries (e.g., rubber manufacturing, hairdressing) with an increased risk for urothelial cancer. This led to the institution of various guidelines and regulations designed to minimize these risks.

Probably the greatest and most clearly characterized associative risk for urothelial cancer and carcinogen exposure has been that observed with cigarette smoking. Cigarette smoking produces a threefold to fourfold increase in the risk for developing bladder cancer. Correlations have been made between the intensity of exposure (number of cigarettes smoked, degree of inhalation) and the increased risk of developing bladder cancer. Unfortunately, these have not received widespread publicity, and public awareness of this needs to be increased.

Correlations between the use of artificial sweeteners, coffee intake, and tryptophan (as a health food additive) and the risk for development of bladder cancer have also been suggested. However, these associations have been called into question and remain unproven. Urinary infections with certain organisms capable of converting urinary metabolites to carcinogens have also been proposed as risk factors.

Genetic risk factors for urothelial cancer have not yet been clearly identified. Although recent studies have associated several specific genetic changes with the development of particular types of bladder cancer, they have not clarified any genetic predisposition to the development of urothelial cancer. On the other hand, a growing body of evidence suggests the existence of populations with distinct urothelial enzymatic profiles that may be associated with an increased or decreased likelihood of cancer development, depending on whether carcinogens are activated or detoxified by the urothelium. Whether this may be associated further with specific types of cancer development is unknown.

Presenting Signs and Symptoms

The most common presenting symptom in patients with bladder cancer is gross painless hematuria. Such hematuria is characteristically observed throughout the urinary stream. If hematuria in men occurs only at the beginning or end of urination, it is more likely associated with a prostatic problem. However, urothelial cancer still needs to be excluded. Often, hematuria may not be visualized grossly but may be seen only on urinalysis. Here too, the possible presence of urothelial cancer must be evaluated, since the amount of hematuria is not an indication of whether a transitional cell cancer may be present.

Occasionally, patients complain of an increasing sense of urgency or discomfort while urinating. Although these symptoms are often indistinguishable from those associated with acute bacterial cystitis, their persistence in the absence of a positive culture should prompt an evaluation for bladder cancer.

The most common presenting sign of bladder cancer is microscopic hematuria. In many instances, the patient may not have seen blood in the urine. However, there is no association between the amount of blood and the likelihood that a bladder cancer is present. Therefore the occurrence of blood in the urine, at least the first time, should always prompt an evaluation to diagnose or exclude bladder cancer. At the same time, microscopic hematuria is common in the general population in the absence of any diagnosable abnormality. There is no consensus regarding the frequency with which such hematuria should be evaluated. However, it does not seem unreasonable to consider a screening evaluation with urinary cytology and kidney and bladder ultrasound (see Diagnostic Evaluation) every 2 to 3 years for such individuals above the age of 50 years and perhaps more frequently for those with risk factors (cigarette smoking, other environmental exposures).

Diagnostic Evaluation

Standard examinations to evaluate gross or microscopic hematuria when urothelial cancer is suspected include intravenous pyelography, cystoscopy, and urinary cytology. Upper tract imaging is necessary both to exclude the possibility of upper tract disease (renal cell carcinoma, urothelial cancer, kidney stones) and to determine whether upper tract obstruction by a bladder tumor is present. Sonography may be used instead of pyelography as an initial screening tool but does not permit as full a visualization of the entire collecting system. Retrograde pyelography may be performed if a patient is allergic to intravenous contrast. This permits both direct visualization of the bladder by cystoscopy and imaging of the entire upper tract.

Cystoscopy is used to examine the urothelium that lines both the urethra and the bladder. Abnormal areas can be characterized, and the type of tumor that may be present can be defined. Although the cystogram phase of the intravenous pyelogram can be occasionally used to visualize a bladder tumor, it is generally of insufficient sensitivity to definitively exclude the presence of either a small or a flattened bladder cancer (i.e., carcinoma in situ).

A voided urine sample should be sent for cytologic assessment. Catheterized specimens should be avoided at first, since instrumentation may produce false-positive readings. On the other hand, barbotage (bladder wash) specimens can be obtained to provide a more cellular sample that can facilitate analysis using cytologic testing or flow cytometry. More recently, urine nuclear matrix protein-22 (NMP-22) (see Superficial Disease) has been used at initial diagnosis and in follow-up for patients with bladder cancer.

The sine qua non of bladder cancer diagnosis is histologic examination of tissue removed by transurethral biopsy of the bladder epithelium and resection of the bladder tumor. Biopsies should be obtained of any areas in the bladder that appear abnormal to assess the urothelium for the presence of epithelial dysplasia or carcinoma in situ (see Tumor Staging). Bladder tumors should be fully resected so that the tumor configuration can be characterized, the grade of cells that make up the tumor can be determined, and the depth of tumor penetration into the bladder wall can be measured.

Tumor Staging

A staging system has evolved based on correlations between the depth to which a particular bladder cancer has penetrated the bladder wall and its potential behavior. Bladder cancers have traditionally been classified as either "superficial" or "deeply invasive." Superficial tumors are either confined to the mucosal layer or have penetrated through the epithelial basement membrane into the underlying connective tissue (lamina propria). Deeply invasive tumors have extended into the superficial or deep muscle layer or extended even more deeply into the perivesical fat. An increased depth of penetration has been correlated with a greater likelihood of metastatic disease.

The most common form of bladder cancer is a papillary, mucosally confined tumor that generally appears as a solitary lesion resembling a clustering of raspberry-shaped fronds on a fibrovascular stalk. Even when multiple tumors are seen, they tend to be of low or moderate grade. These tumors may recur in 75% of instances after the initial lesion has been resected. However, less than 3% of such tumor diatheses are associated with the later development of progressive disease. Though occasionally multiple, these lesions are rarely associated with either atypia or frank carcinoma in situ either at their margin or at other sites in the bladder. Such tumors rarely present a life-threatening risk.

In contrast, superficial tumors that have infiltrated the epithelial basement membrane and underlying lamina propria have been associated with subsequent progression in as many as 30% of instances. These tumors are often of a higher grade than their mucosally confined counterparts and are often seen in association with atypia or flat carcinoma in situ at their margin or at other sites in the bladder. Although they may appear endoscopically to have a papillary configuration (as do the mucosally confined lesions), they may also have a more solid or nodular appearance, especially when part of a more diffuse malignant diathesis.

There are two types of muscle-infiltrative bladder cancers: those that are invasive of only the superficial muscle and those that penetrate more deeply either into the deep muscle or perivesical fat. The former have been characterized as invading in a broad front and involve the bladder wall vasculature and lymphatics in approximately one third of instances. They may have a less progressive course than their more deeply infiltrative counterparts, which present with a more nodular configuration, appear to penetrate the bladder wall in a more tentacular pattern, and may involve the bladder wall vasculature and lymphatics in two thirds of cases.

The more superficial muscle-infiltrative cancers have been associated with a 40% to 65% 5-year survival rate, and a variety of bladder-conserving approaches have been applied with some success in treating these types of tumors (see Treatment). The more deeply muscle-infiltrative cancers have generally been associated with a 10% to 15% 5-year survival rate despite aggressive surgical therapies; 50% of these patients have metastatic disease within 2 years of diagnosis despite their having undergone prompt cystectomy. These forms of disease may therefore already be systemic at the time of the initial clinical diagnosis. Although deeply invasive tumors have undoubtedly proceeded through progressive phases of infiltration into the bladder wall, only 10% to 15% clinically arise from earlier superficial cancers. The majority have already reached an advanced stage at their earliest clinical presentation.

Carcinoma in situ is an entity that consists of neoplastic cells that are confined to and may undermine the urothelial layer, are high grade, and generally do not produce papillary lesions. In as many as 30% of instances, cancer cells in these lesions infiltrate microscopically into the lamina propria. These cancer diatheses may ultimately demonstrate aggressive infiltration of the bladder wall at varying intervals after initial diagnosis, especially when carcinoma in situ is found in the context of papillary tumors that have penetrated the lamina propria. Nodular or solid tumors may arise directly in areas of carcinoma in situ and infiltrate the bladder wall before any evidence of cancer is clinically evident. Whether aggressive treatments need to be applied in all of these situations or whether some of the tumors can be controlled with conservative measures requires further study.

Endoscopically, areas of carcinoma in situ may appear reddened, velvety, and "inflamed," and therefore this condition is sometimes misdiagnosed as cystitis. While carcinoma in situ is often accompanied by irritative symptoms, superficial or deeply infiltrative cancers are generally asymptomatic. The presence of carcinoma in situ generally indicates a more diffuse tumor diathesis with an often more aggressive potential behavior. Urinary cytologic testing may be particularly useful in suggesting its existence.

In addition to stage, the grade of a bladder cancer is also useful in determining the prognosis of a particular tumor diathesis. Grade is determined by the degree of differentiation of cells that make up the tumor. Cells in well-differentiated (grade 1) tumors maintain a normal appearance with regularly shaped nuclei and a normal nuclear/cytoplasmic ratio. Although the number of cell layers in such tumors is often greater than in the normal epithelium, the normal polarity of these cell layers is generally maintained. Cells in higher-grade tumors (grades 2 and 3) have a more irregular nuclear shape, clumped chromatin, prominent nuclei, and a very high nuclear/cytoplasmic ratio. Cell polarity is generally lost. The higher the grade, the more deeply invasive a particular bladder cancer is likely to be. The exception is carcinoma in situ, which is generally composed of high-grade cells that have remained confined to the epithelium without grossly penetrating the bladder wall. Nonetheless their biologic potential for aggressive behavior is high, and the cells in carcinoma in situ may progress to deep muscle invasion over variable intervals.

Treatment

Superficial Disease. Transurethral resection, which is used to obtain tissue for pathologic diagnosis, is generally successful in fully excising a tumor when it is the type that is mucosally confined and low grade. Although recurrence is frequently seen (50% to 75% of instances), repeat transurethral resection will again restore a normal epithelium. Transurethral resection has little morbidity, and in this setting, there is minimal risk for progressive disease to occur. When rapid recurrence is seen or a multiplicity of tumors does not permit effective resection, instillation of chemotherapeutic agents may facilitate elimination of disease.

Transurethral resection is also an effective treatment for the superficial papillary tumors that may have infiltrated the lamina propria. However, if extensive infiltration has occurred, transurethral resection may not remove all of the cancer. It is therefore common to instill adjunctive intravesical agents to eradicate any tumor cells remaining after resection. This may be especially appropriate in situations when lamina propria–infiltrative tumors are high grade and are associated with carcinoma in situ elsewhere in the urothelium.

The most common intravesical agents used as adjuncts to transurethral resection for the treatment of superficial disease are thiotepa, mitomycin-C, and doxorubicin, all chemotherapeutic agents, and bacillus Calmette-Guérin, an immunotherapeutic agent. The former have been most effective in preventing the recurrence of mucosally confined papillary transitional cell tumors. The latter has been most effective in preventing the recurrence of carcinoma in situ and in the adjunctive treatment of high-grade lamina propria–invasive tumors. Morbidities associated with these treatments have generally been rare. Continued surveillance with cystoscopy and urinary cytologic testing is necessary for detecting treatment failure early so that intervention can be more aggressive.

The greatest risk associated with high-grade lamina propria–infiltrative cancers, especially when accompanied by carcinoma in situ, is the possibility of rapid progression. Radical cystectomy may be important to consider in these instances, since many of these cancers, once they have progressed to the bladder wall musculature, are found to be metastatic and beyond the realm of regional cure.

Interest has grown in the identification of substances that might serve as markers to detect tumor recurrence or indicate the possibility of tumor progression. Despite the promise of initial reports on a variety of substances for which the urine has been assayed (bladder tumor antigen [BTA] [BTA Stat or BTA Trak test]; NMP-22; telomerase; fibrin degradation products [Acudiff]; ImmunoCyt; hyaluronidase) validation of their clinical usefulness and reliability remains to be determined.

Muscle-infiltrative Cancer. The current standard of treatment for muscle-infiltrative bladder cancer is radical cystectomy. The 5-year survival rates, or "cures," have been reported to be as high as 70% to 80% when the muscle-infiltrative cancers are more superficial. The 5-year survival rates for deeply infiltrative cancers have been only 10% to 15%. Although occasional long-term survival rates have been described in patients with cancers that have involved one or two pelvic lymph nodes microscopically, gross involvement of the pelvic lymph nodes or extension of disease beyond the pelvic lymphatics have in most instances not been associated with cure by radical surgery.

Occasionally, bladder cancers that have invaded only the superficial musculature have been amenable to treatment by transurethral resection or by partial cystectomy. Such patients, however, need to be selected carefully, and these approaches are generally reserved for patients who are not candidates for cystectomy and who may require palliation rather than cure. Those with deep muscle invasion who are not candidates for cystectomy may undergo deep transurethral resection and adjunctive radiation therapy and chemotherapy. Although 5-year estimated survival rates with these approaches have been suggested to approximate those seen with cystectomy and control of regional disease has been satisfactory, such patients seem best served by cystectomy for long-term disease-free survival.

Additional treatments have been applied to enhance response rates. These have included preoperative radiation therapy, preoperative chemotherapy, and adjunctive chemotherapy. Although occasional long-term responders have been seen, these have largely comprised anecdotal events, and predictably effective regimens remain to be defined. In essence, deeply infiltrative bladder cancer in most instances is likely to represent a systemic disease. No predictably effective systemic chemotherapeutic regimen has yet been discovered.

Recent studies have suggested that certain molecular markers (p53, Rb) may be associated in muscle-invasive tumors (and some lamina propria–invasive tumors) with the likelihood of progression. Further studies are needed to validate these relationships before they can be applied routinely in clinical management.

Because removal of the bladder remains the standard therapy for deeply infiltrative bladder cancer, urinary diversion is an important component of treatment of patients with this condition. Major advances have been made in using segments of bowel to create continent reservoirs and even to attach these reservoirs to the urethra. Generally, the ileum, or segments of colon, has been used in creating these reservoirs. Although no reservoir is perfect in replacing the normally functioning bladder, this imaginative use has led to dramatic improvement in the quality of life in both men and women undergoing cystectomy.

Summary

Much remains to be learned about the biology and natural history of bladder cancer. Increased use of molecular analysis is providing information about the different pathways of bladder cancer development and may ultimately offer the opportunity to apply distinct treatments for specific types of bladder cancer based on molecular profile. In the future it may be possible to reverse the carcinogenic progress by applying knowledge of the molecular events that underlie the development of various types of bladder tumor to change their course through the restoration of the normal genetic complement. In addition, more effective systemic therapies may be identified that will not only treat regional bladder cancer but also deal effectively with sites of metastasis.

KIDNEY CANCER

Kidney cancer, or renal cell carcinoma, is a malignancy thought to arise from the proximal tubule cells of the kidney. It is most commonly seen in men and women between 40 and 60 years of age, affecting men more commonly than women (1.5:2). It is estimated that 28,500 new cases of renal cell cancer will be diagnosed in the United States in 2000 (17,000 males; 10,500 females), and that 11,000 will die of their disease (6500 males; 4500 females).

Little is known about the carcinogenic process or epidemiologic factors that account for the development of renal cell carcinoma. Associations have been suggested between exposures to heavy metals such as mercury and cadmium and the development of kidney malignancies. Similar associations between cigarette smoking or environmental pollutants and renal cancer have not been described. Patients on chronic dialysis who develop multicystic disease are at risk for the development of renal cell cancers. The mechanism underlying this phenomenon is not understood. Some forms of renal cancer have a genetic basis. A hereditary basis in the predisposition to develop renal cell cancer in the majority of cases, however, remains to be determined.

Presenting Signs and Symptoms

The triad of hematuria, flank pain, and palpable abdominal mass that has traditionally been associated with the presence of renal cell cancer is now rarely seen. A patient may have only gross or microscopic hematuria without other symptoms. Patients with sudden-onset gross hematuria should always be evaluated for renal cell cancer.

Renal colic may occur if a blood clot obstructs the ureter. Rarely is an abdominal mass palpated unless the cancer has grown very large. Renal cell cancer is most often diagnosed when imaging studies are performed in the evaluation of asymptomatic microscopic hematuria. In addition, it is becoming more common for a renal mass to be diagnosed coincidentally when imaging studies are performed for unrelated symptoms (see Diagnostic Studies).

Physical examination rarely elicits any abnormality associated with renal cell cancer. The ability to palpate a renal mass is limited by both the size of the mass and the location of each kidney under the rib cage. Flank tenderness is rarely demonstrated. Occasionally, the development or enlargement of a scrotal varicocele is observed. However, this may be seen only if the cancer has involved the renal vein on the left or has extended into the vena cava on the right.

Paraneoplastic syndromes occasionally accompany the development of renal cell cancer. Fevers of unknown origin, anemia, and polycythemia have been reported in approximately 1% to 3% of renal cell cancers.

Diagnostic Studies

Imaging studies are critical in documenting the presence of a renal mass. Previously, the most commonly used diagnostic imaging study was intravenous pyelography. This has now been largely replaced by sonography. Sonography avoids the use of intravenous contrast materials to which patients may be allergic and permits distinctions to be made between masses that are solid and those that are cystic. In general, renal cell cancers are solid masses. It is rare to see a renal cell cancer involving a simple renal cyst. This may not be the case, however, if a cyst is multiseptated, is thick-walled and irregular, or contains irregular calcifications in its wall.

The presence of a solid mass or complex cyst on ultrasound generally indicates the need for a computed tomography (CT) scan. This should be performed both with and without intravenous contrast to determine both the character of the lesion and the presence of enhancement with contrast. Enhancement generally indicates a malignancy, and this appearance on CT scan is virtually pathognomonic of a renal cell cancer. Some mass lesions such as oncocytoma may be indistinguishable radiographically from a renal cell cancer. Others such as angiomyolipoma can be distinguished easily because of the characteristic low density of fat.

CT and ultrasound studies are also useful in determining whether the renal vein and vena cava have tumor thrombi. Lymph nodes at the renal hilum and around the great vessels may also be assessed for increased size and the possible presence of metastatic disease. Magnetic resonance imaging (MRI), nuclear scanning, and arteriography rarely aid in the evaluation of renal cell cancer, although the latter may occasionally be useful in planning the surgical approach when a partial nephrectomy is being considered.

It has become more common to diagnose kidney cancer as an incidental finding on sonograms or CT scans that have been performed for symptoms (back or abdominal pain) that are entirely unrelated to the presence of the cancer. Tumors that are diagnosed under these circumstances are often far smaller than those that have been seen previously when imaging studies were performed for signs or symptoms associated directly with these mass lesions.

Once a diagnosis of renal cell cancer has been made, a nuclear bone scan and a pulmonary CT scan are generally performed to exclude metastases to these sites.

Staging of Kidney Cancer

A staging system for kidney cancer has evolved on the basis of correlations that have been observed between extent of the malignancy, likelihood of metastatic disease, and amenability to cure by surgical excision. Smaller lesions (those smaller than 3 cm in diameter) have generally been called *adenomas* to distinguish them from renal cell cancers on the assumption that the likelihood of these lesions metastasizing is small. Recent studies have disputed the validity of these suggestions.

Given the increased frequency with which small solid masses are now diagnosed, such observations must be considered in the management of these cancers. Smaller cancers are more likely to be confined within the renal capsule and appear to have the best prognosis. Once a cancer has extended beyond the renal capsule, survival for 5 years is far less likely. Kidneys that have extended beyond Gerota's fascia have an even poorer likelihood of cure. Such tumors often involve adjacent structures or have metastasized to adjacent lymph nodes and distant sites. Renal cell cancers occasionally extend tumor thrombi into the renal vein and vena cava. The prognosis for these patients is generally far better than it is for those who have involvement of the regional lymph nodes.

Treatment

Surgical excision is the only treatment that is predictably effective for kidney cancers. "Radical" nephrectomy involves removal of the kidney and the surrounding fat contained within Gerota's fascia. The adrenal gland, often contained in its own compartment within Gerota's fascia, may be removed with the kidney. Hilar lymph nodes are often also removed, but this serves largely a diagnostic purpose rather than one that enhances therapy. Many urologists now favor leaving the ipsilateral adrenal gland if CT scan or MRI demonstrates it to be normal.

Some have suggested that simple enucleation or segmental nephrectomy may be the appropriate approach for smaller renal masses. Earlier studies in which such procedures were performed in the setting of a solitary kidney, bilaterally poorly functioning kidneys, or multiple cancers in both kidneys (such that preservation of renal tissue was an important objective in managing the patient) documented that renal-sparing approaches were as successful in achieving equivalent 5-year survival rates for low-stage, low-grade disease as was radical nephrectomy.

The likelihood that microscopic disease is present at multiple sites in the affected kidney is only 10% to 15%. The risk for developing recurrent tumor in the original cancer bed may be only as great as 10%, depending on the size and conformation of the original cancer. Although each of these considerations has prompted the conclusion that radical nephrectomy should remain the standard approach in most patients with renal cell cancer (especially since the likelihood of cancer development in the contralateral kidney is small), the smaller size at which kidney cancers are diagnosed, in association with the increasing rate of their coincidental discovery, has prompted the suggestion that partial nephrectomy should be considered more often, especially when clinical conditions justify attempts to preserve normal renal tissues, even in the setting of bilaterally normal functioning kidneys. Because there may be increased risks associated with partial nephrectomy and because most patients experience little consequence from removal of the entire kidney, radical nephrectomy remains the standard approach to treatment. However, the use of partial nephrectomy as more acceptable standard therapy is growing, especially when the tumor is smaller than 4 cm in diameter.

Surgery is not an effective therapeutic modality in the setting of metastatic disease. Although nephrectomy has been associated anecdotally with the resolution of metastatic lesions in 1% to 2% of cases, documentation has for the most part been inadequate, and the outcome has been poor. Angioinfarction before surgery, presumably to stimulate an immune response that might lead to resolution of metastatic deposits, has also not been found to be an effective approach.

In the setting of a concurrent solitary metastasis, removal of both the primary kidney cancer and the metastatic lesion has generally been followed by the appearance of multiple additional metastases within a year of surgery. On the other hand, when a solitary metastasis has appeared after nephrectomy has been performed, its removal has occasionally been associated with long-term survival. This may reflect the occasionally unpredictable biology of the primary disease rather than an expression of surgical efficacy.

Radical nephrectomy in the setting of metastatic disease has largely been reserved for palliation. Flank pain seen in association with a large renal mass, uncontrollable hemorrhage (despite attempts at angioinfarction), and unremitting fever or hypercalcemia have been used as indications for radical nephrectomy even though metastatic disease may be present. Such patients ultimately die from their disease, often with limited survival times.

Radiation therapy has not been effective in the treatment of renal cell cancer. Currently, no single chemotherapeutic agent or combination of agents has been found to be effective in producing durable responses in renal cell cancer. The use of progestational agents (e.g., Megase) has produced only anecdotal responses.

Isolated reports of "spontaneous" remissions of metastatic lesions have led to suggestions that the immune response may play a role in the control of renal cell cancer. A variety of attempts have therefore been made to recruit immune response mechanisms in the design of novel approaches in the treatment of this problem.

Vaccines, cytokines, lymphokines, and immune effector cells have been used to treat patients with metastatic renal cell cancer. These approaches have at best produced mixed results with response rates ranging between 15% and 20%. These results have generally been of very limited durability.

Most recently, the efficacy of interferons, interleukin-2 (IL-2), lymphokine-activated killer (LAK) cells, tumor-infiltrating lymphocytes (TIL cells), and various combinations of these, either alone or together with cytotoxic chemotherapeutic agents, has been investigated. Although some have been reported to produce variable remissions of metastatic diseases at several sites, these responses have generally not been durable, and survival rates have remained largely unimproved. High-dose IL-2 remains the only FDA-approved treatment for metastatic renal cancer. It has a 5% complete response rate.

The unpredictable natural history of renal cell cancer, even when metastatic, has made interpretation of these results difficult and controversial. Because of this and because of the morbidity associated with many of these treatments, these approaches cannot be depended on to predictably palliate the disease or prolong survival rates in patients with metastatic renal cell cancer, and therefore they remain in the realm of investigation.

ADDITIONAL READINGS

Bubowski RM: Natural history and therapy of metastatic renal cell carcinoma: the role of interleukin-2, *Cancer* 80:1198, 1997.

Ghoneim MA, et al: Radical cystectomy for carcinoma of the bladder: critical evaluation of the results in 1,026 cases, *J Urol* 158:393, 1997.

Krishnamurthi V, Novick AC, et al: Nephron sparing surgery in patients with metastatic renal cell carcinoma, *J Urol* 156:36, 1996.

Lundholm C, et al: A randomized prospective study comparing long-term intravesical instillations of mitomycin C and BCG in patients with superficial bladder carcinoma, *J Urol* 156:372, 1996.

Novick AC, et al: Conservative surgery for renal cell carcinoma: a single center experience with 100 patients, *J Urol* 141:835, 1989.

Rosenberg SA, et al: Experience with the use of high dose interleukin-2 in the treatment of 652 cancer patients, *Ann Surg* 210:474, 1989.

Shipley WU, Zietman AL, et al: Invasive bladder cancer: treatment strategies using transurethral surgery, chemotherapy and radiation therapy with selection for bladder conservation, *J Radiat Oncol Biol Phys* 39:937, 1997.

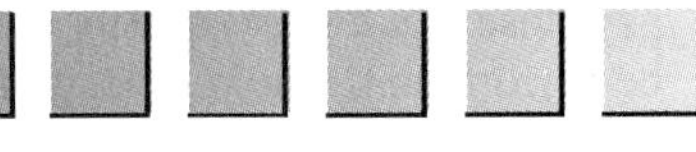

Male Sexual Dysfunction

Michael D. LaSalle
Irwin Goldstein
Robert J. Krane

MALE DYSFUNCTION

Erectile dysfunction is the consistent inability to obtain or maintain a penile erection of sufficient rigidity for satisfactory sexual performance.[6] Erectile dysfunction is a significant health problem for many reasons. According to the Massachusetts Male Aging Study, a community-based survey of men aged 40 to 70 years, the prevalence of erectile dysfunction is 52%.[2] Extrapolating this data to the general population, it has estimated that more than 20 million American men suffer from some form of this disorder. Erectile dysfunction also appears to be an age-related phenomenon. At 40 years of age, approximately 40% of men have some degree of dysfunction, whereas at 70 years, the prevalence approaches 70%. With the increasing aging population demographics, the numbers of men complaining of erectile dysfunction and seeking treatment will continue to grow.

Psychologic problems such as depression and poor self-esteem were once believed to be primary causes of most cases of erectile dysfunction. However, erectile dysfunction is now viewed as a very common and reversible health-related problem, often with an organic etiology. Medical risk factors associated with erectile dysfunction include hypertension, hypercholesterolemia, diabetes, cigarette smoking, alcoholism, atherosclerosis, neurologic disorders, and peripheral vascular disease.

Historically, the urologist was the sole physician diagnosing and treating erectile dysfunction. Now, the primary care physician is the first to diagnose and treat such disorders. This shift is a direct result of many factors. First, the managed care environment exposes large numbers of patients to the primary care physician for treatment, thereby diminishing referrals to specialists. Second, an expanding aging population presents more patients to their primary care physicians for other health-related problems. Finally, erectile dysfunction issues are no longer viewed as "taboo" by the public, allowing patients to willingly and openly discuss them with their doctors. Given these reasons, primary care physicians must now be more comfortable with (1) discussing sexuality issues with their patients, (2) identifying when a problem exists, and (3) offering appropriate therapy when indicated. More important, the physician must understand that the presenting complaint of erectile dysfunction may signal an underlying and potentially threatening concurrent illness.

This section emphasizes the basic elements for understanding normal penile anatomy and erectile physiology as well as the pathophysiology associated with erectile dysfunction. Coordinated functioning of these anatomic and physiologic systems is needed for the initiation and maintenance of an erection. A detailed medical history, psychosexual history, and focused physical examination must be performed by the physician. In addition, diagnostic testing can be used to establish an etiology, and then appropriate therapeutic options can be offered to the patient for successful treatment.

Penile Anatomy

Anatomically, the penis contains three chambers. These chambers include two paired dorsal erectile bodies (i.e., corpora cavernosa) and a ventrally located spongy tissue cylinder (i.e., corpus spongiosum). Each chamber has an arterial blood supply, a venous drainage system, and neural innervation that contribute to normal physiologic function.

Corpora Cavernosa. Each corpus cavernosum is surrounded by a thick fascial investment called the *tunica albuginea*. The tunica albuginea has two concentric layers (an inner circular and an outer longitudinal layer) that, along with its elastic fibers, allows it to stretch when filled with arterial blood. Each cylinder contains venous sinusoids that trap blood when filled. These venous sinusoids are surrounded by trabeculae consisting of connective tissue and smooth muscle. After blood enters the penis, each cylinder increases in volume. When each cylinder has reached maximal volume, pressure rises, and the penis gains rigidity. Penile rigidity (both axial and radial components) is what ultimately facilitates vaginal penetration.

Corpus Spongiosum. The corpus spongiosum is the chamber located ventrally within the penis and contains the urethra. This chamber mushrooms out distally on the penis, forming the glans. Although the corpus spongiosum lacks a tunica albuginea covering, its tissues still become engorged with blood during sexual arousal. Venous communications often exist between the corpus spongiosum and the corpora cavernosal bodies.

Penile Arterial Blood Supply. Branches of the iliohypogastric-pudendal arterial system supply blood to the sexual organs. The internal pudendal artery is the main blood supply to each cavernosal body of the penis. One branch, the common penile artery, further bifurcates into the dorsal penile artery and the cavernosal artery (Fig. 154A-1). Each cavernosal artery enters the corpus cavernosum at the penile hilum. Helicine arteries branch along its course and provide the blood supply to the sinusoidal tissue. The cavernosal artery and the deep dorsal penile artery often communicate. This is important for understanding penile revascularization surgery because a new blood supply is brought into the cavernosal bodies via the deep dorsal artery. Blood flow can travel either retrograde into the corpora cavernosa from the cavernosal artery or antegrade via branches off the dorsal penile artery that penetrate directly through the tunica albuginea to supply the cavernosal bodies.

Penile Venous Blood Supply. The cavernosal bodies contain numerous venous sinusoids that coalesce and drain into one another. Blood progressively moves outward toward the most peripheral sinusoids. Small venules drain these sinusoids and then travel below the tunica albuginea, forming the subtunical venular plexus. These subtunical venules drain into the emissary veins, which pierce through the tunica albuginea. During an erection, the tunica albuginea stretches,

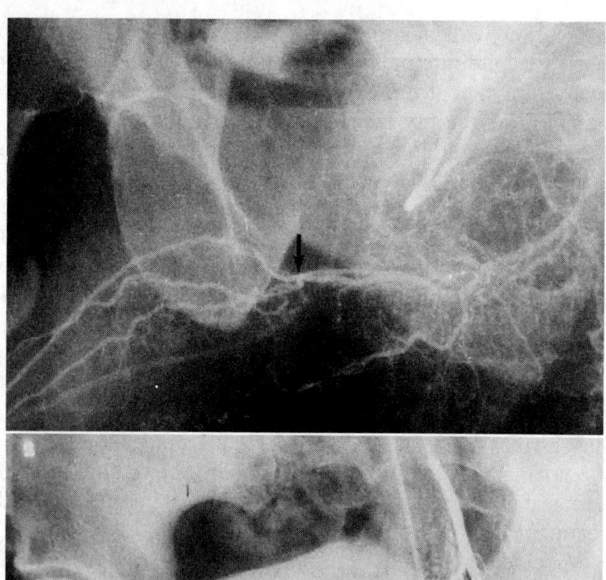

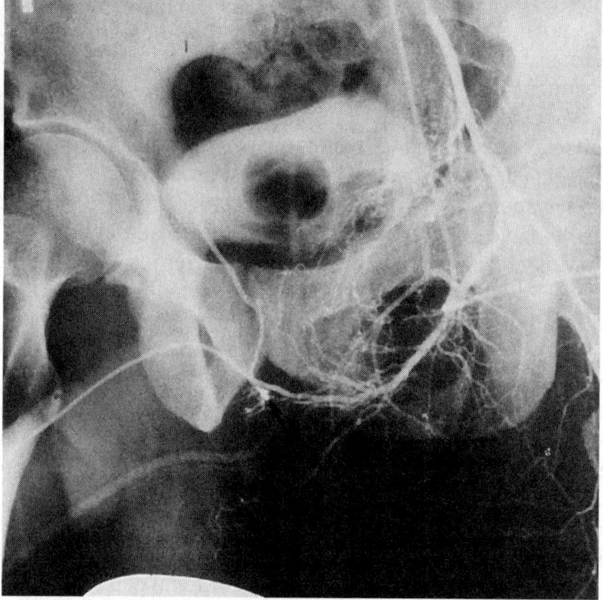

Fig. 154A-1. **A,** Normal pudendal arteriogram showing a patent pudendal-penile artery bifurcating *(arrow)* into normal dorsal and corporal arteries. **B,** Arteriogram showing a diseased pudendal artery and obstruction at the takeoff of the corporal artery *(arrow)*. In this case the dorsal artery is well visualized.

and the subtunical and emissary veins become elongated, causing a functional closure of their lumina. This venoocclusive mechanism acts like a valve during an erection, preventing the release of blood from the penis back into the general circulation. This mechanism is very important in establishing and maintaining penile rigidity.

Penile Neuroanatomy. The penis is innervated by both the autonomic and somatic nervous systems. The erectile autonomic nerve fibers are known as the *cavernous nerves*. The parasympathetic nerve components originate in the second, third, and fourth sacral vertebrae (S2, S3, and S4 [the spinal erection center]). The preganglionic parasympathetic fibers enter the pelvic plexus and are subsequently joined by sympathetic nerves to form the cavernous nerves. The cavernosal nerves enter the penile hilum anterior to the bulbous urethra. Stimulation of the cavernous nerves induces an erection.

The parasympathetic nerves are responsible for initiating tumescence. The most potent neurotransmitter for the erectile process is nitric oxide. Postganglionic nerves secrete nitric oxide (NO), which subsequently causes cavernosal smooth muscle relaxation. Smooth muscle relaxation allows for increased blood flow into the penis. In contrast, stimulation of the sympathetic plexus causes an increase in vascular smooth muscle tone that results in a decrease in arterial blood flow into the penis. Detumescence occurs primarily through the action of the neurotransmitter norepinephrine.

Somatic sensory innervation of the penile shaft and glans is derived from the dorsal penile nerve. These afferent nerves coalesce into the internal pudendal nerve (S2 to S4), which travels along the ischiopubic ramus of the pelvis through Alcock's canal. Crushing of this nerve can cause penile and glandular numbness. Such injuries can result from blunt pelvic trauma or chronic compression to the perineum (i.e., a motor vehicle accident with fracture of the ischiopubic ramus or perineal compression from a bicycle seat).

Afferent stimulation of the penis causes erection via spinal pathways. The pudendal nerve is responsible for initiating most erections, but psychologically and centrally mediated erections do occur. Psychogenic erections are caused by signals from the brain that are transmitted to the spinal erection center. The pudendal nerve also carries the somatic motor innervation to the bulbocavernosus and ischiocavernosus muscles. Contraction of these muscles occurs during sexual excitation and compresses the corpora cavernosal muscles further, increasing overall intracavernosal pressure. The somatic component of the pudendal nerve also is important in the ejaculatory process, causing the bulbocavernosus muscles to contract rhythmically, resulting in propulsion of semen through the urethra.

Erectile Physiology and Pathophysiology

An erection is primarily a hemodynamic phenomenon. Two processes must be intact and functionally coordinated for a successful erection to occur. First, blood flow must increase to the corpora cavernosa via the internal pudendal artery. When blood volume increases, tissues expand, and intracavernosal pressure rises. Second, venous outflow resistance must increase as a direct result of the trapping of blood via an intact venoocclusive mechanism. Further increases in blood inflow without venous outflow allow higher intracavernosal volume and pressure, increased penile length, and ultimately, penile rigidity.

Anatomically, smooth muscle cells line both the cavernosal sinuses and the afferent arterioles. When the smooth muscle relaxes, the lumina increase in size, and blood flow increases. When the smooth muscle lining the cavernosal sinuses relaxes, the sinuses can accommodate more blood. Thus they increase in size with subsequent compression of the subtunical venules, causing venous trapping. If inadequate blood flow reaches the penis, inadequate rigidity is achieved. If inadequate venous trapping occurs, even with good inflow, the penis does not become rigid. Therefore smooth muscle relaxation and a normal venoocclusive mechanism are the key factors in achieving an erection. Often, explaining this concept to a patient can be difficult. A simple analogy of attempting to fill a tire connected to an air hose helps the physician describe this process more easily to patients. If the tire does not become full after inflating, there can either be a kink in the air hose (i.e., an arterial problem) or a leak in the tire (i.e., a venous trapping problem).

In addition to having a functional hemodynamic system, the patient must also be neurologically intact to receive afferent stimuli and transmit autonomic signals for initiation of an erection. Neurologic disorders resulting in decreased cavernosal nerve function diminish the patient's spontaneous erections even though the hemodynamic vascular system is intact. The psychologic and hormonal milieus are also significant factors affecting erection. Disorders such as depression, anger, and hypogonadism can disrupt erectile function. Patients may not be satisfied with the quality of their erectile potency either in terms of performance or in comparison with previous performance. Therefore in addition to all other factors that affect potency, the quality of the erection must be evaluated in terms of rigidity or sustaining ability.

Rigidity is highly dependent on penile geometry (its dimensions), its biomechanical properties, and intracavernosal pressure for proper function. The achievement of intracavernosal pressure depends on hemodynamic factors and proper smooth muscle relaxation. Rigidity has two major components: radial and axial. Axial rigidity (i.e., the columnar component) is needed for vaginal penetration.

Erectile Dysfunction Evaluation

The primary purposes for erectile dysfunction evaluation are to determine an etiology and to direct a method of therapy. Although some patients may require a comprehensive evaluation, other patients may need only basic screening before treatment. For example, an explanation of etiology may be unnecessary for older patients with known risk factors for erectile dysfunction, since they may simply want to regain potency without specifically identifying an etiology. For many other patients, the evaluation may simply provide a better means of understanding why they developed erectile dysfunction. Many patients and their partners are relieved to know that the problem is not necessarily psychologic.

The physician must realize that at least a minimal evaluation is needed before treatment. Erectile dysfunction may be the presenting complaint of a previously undiagnosed illness (e.g., hypertension, hypercholesterolemia, diabetes mellitus, vascular disease). The patient's medical and psychosexual history and physical examination provide the basis for diagnosis and management; they may also result in the identification of other conditions.

Patient History. As in many medical disciplines, the diagnosis of erectile dysfunction is frequently apparent from the patient history. The first goal of the history is to determine exactly what type of problem exists. The physician must distinguish among problems with libido, ejaculation, orgasm, and erection. These other disorders should be treated independently of erectile dysfunction issues.

One simple way to assess whether a patient has erectile dysfunction is the administration of a validated erectile dysfunction questionnaire such as the International Index of Erectile Function (IIEF).[7] This questionnaire not only acts as a screening device but can also be used for a baseline index comparison of function before treatment starts. Such questionnaires may identify patients who cannot specifically identify which aspects of erection are problematic. Next, the effects of the erectile dysfunction on the patient and his partner must be assessed. Such issues may have a significant impact on the form of treatment recommended. Finally, the physician must understand the patient's goals for receiving treatment.

The medical history can often direct the physician to the etiology of erectile dysfunction. The onset of the problem may help differentiate between psychologic and organic etiologies. If the erectile problems are of acute onset after some traumatic event and occur during sexual encounters but not during sleeping or masturbation, a psychologic etiology may be suspected (but is not necessarily ensured). Psychosexual assessment is important in determining what psychologic factors could be affecting the patient's erections and what psychologic effects the patient's erections have had on him. A psychologic cause can be associated with an organic etiology in up to 90% of cases.

When the onset of erectile dysfunction is slow and is not associated with a specific event or life situation, an organic etiology is more likely. The medical history often plays a more crucial role in the evaluation of such cases of organic erectile dysfunction. Medical disorders such as diabetes, atherosclerosis, neurologic disease, hypercholesterolemia, hypertension, and sickle cell disease are frequently associated with erectile dysfunction. Many medications have adverse effects on erections. Antihypertensive medications often cause erectile dysfunction not directly at the penile level, but by lowering systemic blood pressure and thus decreasing intracavernosal pressure. Surgical history can also indicate a potential iatrogenic etiology. Previous pelvic surgery or abdominal surgery may have injured the neurologic innervation of the penis or its vascular supply. Arterial or venoocclusive dysfunction may be associated with a prior history of penile or perineal trauma.

Physical Examination. A comprehensive physical examination should be completed on each patient with erectile dysfunction. This examination should not differ significantly from a routine physical performed by a primary care physician. However, it should emphasize evaluation of the genitourinary, vascular, and neurologic systems. Vital signs, including blood pressure and peripheral pulse measurements, may reveal problems with hypertension, heart disease, or peripheral vascular disease. Aneurysmal disease can be detected by listening and palpating for abdominal bruits. Secondary sexual characteristics such as sparse hair growth and gynecomastia may indicate an endocrinologic disorder. The genitalia should be assessed for testicular size, penile length, penile geometry, curvature, or other penile deformities such as Peyronie's plaques. Sensory neurologic assessment can be easily performed by evaluating sensory changes in the genitalia. The digital rectal examination not only screens for prostate cancer but also detects the integrity of the neurologic innervation of the external anal sphincter (S2 to S4). Although the physical examination provides a source of valuable information for the physician, it also provides a great opportunity for patient education and reassurance.

Laboratory Tests. Screening for systemic medical disorders, endocrine disease, and vascular risk factors is appropriate in the workup for erectile dysfunction. Complete blood counts, standard serum chemistry analysis (including a fasting glucose test), and a cardiac profile (fasting cholesterol, low-density lipoprotein, high-density lipoprotein, and triglyceride tests) should be obtained. If libido is diminished, serum testosterone and prolactin levels should be measured. This assessment determines the integrity of the pituitary-gonadal axis. Serum determinations for prostate-specific antigen (PSA) should be performed after the screening tests done according to the American Urological Association or AFP guidelines. Tests for thyroid disease, such as thyroid-stimulating hormone levels, should be used in highly selected cases.

Diagnostic Testing

Nocturnal Penile Tumescence. Nocturnal penile tumescence testing uses a strain gauge placed around the penile shaft. It measures changes in penile circumference and erectile activity during a night of sleep. Normally, a male subject will have three to five physiologic erections lasting approximately 25 to 35 minutes every night. Men with psychogenic erectile dysfunction usually have normal sleeping erections. On the other hand, men with an organic etiology to their erectile dysfunction usually have abnormal nocturnal erections. The most notable exception to this is patients who have neurologic impotence that affects their afferent sensory nerves. Thus this test is a useful screening tool for aiding in the differentiation between psychogenic and organic erectile dysfunction. It is a simple test that may be performed at home or in a sleep laboratory. A portable machine measuring both circumferential penile size changes and rigidity (Rigiscan) is available for home use. One major limitation to this test is that it only measures radial rigidity and not axial rigidity.

Neurologic Testing. Neurologic disorders producing erectile dysfunction may be present in either the peripheral or central conduction pathways. Ultimately, some interference within the motor efferent autonomic nerves to the penis must allow smooth muscle relaxation to occur. Many devices for neurologic assessment are available for the evaluation of the patient with neurogenic erectile dysfunction. Biothesiometry is a simple screening tool that assesses the ability to sense vibration and peripheral afferent nerve transmission. A vibratory device is placed on the penis and on the extremities to detect whether sensory deficits exist between the different areas tested. Dorsal nerve conduction velocity testing or bulbocavernosus reflex latency testing can be used to detect sacral or peripheral nerve pathology. Other tests using needle electrodes (intracavernosal electromyography) or patch electrodes on the penile shaft can determine the electrical activity of the cavernosal nerve as transmitted to corporal smooth muscle. For evaluation of the central nervous system, a genitocerebral evoked potential study can determine conduction times after electrically stimulating the penis and recording the sensory input to the cerebral cortex.

Psychologic Testing. Psychologic aspects in the diagnosis of erectile dysfunction are often difficult to identify, since multifactorial etiologies are often present. Each patient evaluated for erectile dysfunction should have a psychosexual evaluation. This evaluation not only helps differentiate between psychogenic and organic causes of erectile dysfunction but also helps determine the effects of the problem on the patient and his partner as well as their goals in seeking treatment.

Erections can be initiated with or without direct penile stimulation. Therefore positive psychologic stimuli can create or enhance an erection, and negative psychologic stimuli can inhibit them. Negative psychologic input can inhibit the sacral cord–mediated reflexogenic erections. In addition, excessive adrenergic states associated with disorders such as anxiety can increase penile smooth muscle tone. Such psychologic disturbances can oppose the normal smooth muscle relaxation needed for an erection.

Hormonal Testing. The role of testosterone in the evaluation of erectile dysfunction remains unclear. Patients with decreased libido or poor virilization often undergo serum testosterone screening. Since serum testosterone levels vary throughout the day, early morning specimens are optimally measured. If morning testosterone levels are consistently low, luteinizing hormone and prolactin levels are then obtained. Low serum testosterone levels have been associated with disorders such as hyperprolactinemia. However, if serum prolactin levels remain elevated, potency is restored in only half the patients whose testosterone concentrations are normalized by exogenous replacement. When hyperprolactinemia is identified on screening, it requires its own investigation. Pituitary adenomas can be manifested first by symptoms such as erectile dysfunction. Often magnetic resonance imaging of the pituitary is required.

Hyperthyroidism can also be associated with diminished libido and occasionally with erectile dysfunction. Hypothyroidism may cause erectile dysfunction secondary to associated low testosterone and elevated prolactin levels.

Vascular Testing. As stated previously, an erection is a complex hemodynamic event requiring both adequate arterial inflow and venous trapping. Vascular testing allows the physician to identify which system is functionally disrupted. It is important to distinguish between these two components for two reasons: first, quantifying which component is faulty helps direct appropriate therapy, and second, identification of the indicated therapy improves clinical outcomes. For instance, isolated blockages in the penile arterial tree (as opposed to diffuse disease) are often surgically corrected by microvascular arterial bypass procedures. On the other hand, disorders such as diffuse arterial disease and venous leakage are not amenable to corrective therapy. Therapy under these circumstances may attempt to override (penile injection therapy) or completely circumvent (prosthesis or vacuum erection devices) the problem.

Arterial testing. Penile arterial testing can be performed in either the erect or flaccid state. As in any hemodynamic system, more accurate information is obtained in the active state. However, the flaccid state may give some clues as to the etiology of the problem. Intracavernosal injection of vasoactive agents such as papaverine, phentolamine, prostaglandins, and combinations thereof have been used for vascular testing during the erect state.

Penile brachial index. The systolic pressure of all arteries should be theoretically the same. Thus if there is no arterial blockage, the systolic pressure in the arm (brachial pressure) should be similar to the systolic pressure in the penis. The penile pressure may be measured by placing a small cuff around the base of the penis and inflating it until the arterial pulse, as determined by Doppler ultrasound, disappears. The penile brachial index (PBI) is the ratio of penile systolic pressure to brachial systolic pressure. Normal PBI values should be greater than 0.85.

Duplex ultrasonography. Duplex ultrasonography is a noninvasive method for evaluating the arterial system's ability to deliver blood to the erectile chambers during an erection. Medications injected intracavernosally during arterial testing can cause smooth muscle relaxation with subsequent increases in arterial blood flow. Ultrasound can detect changes in both the cavernosal arterial diameter and blood velocity. When these findings are normal, arterial insufficiency can be ruled out to the level of the vessels tested. One limitation to vascular testing is the adrenergic inhibition of smooth muscle relaxation, which can override intracavernosal vasoactive medications. Excessive adrenergic tone can be induced by the anxiety of an office visit, a needle injected into the penis, or embarrassment over speaking about issues associated with erectile dysfunction. If the patient can achieve an erection that closely approximates his best erections at home, however, he can be presumed to have achieved complete smooth muscle relaxation. Many times, excessive adrenergic tone can be reversed with re-dosing of intracavernosal medications. Most investigators believe that cavernosal arterial velocities greater than 30 cm/sec are within the normal range.

Corporal venoocclusive function testing. The ultimate test for evaluating erectile hemodynamics is the dynamic infusion cavernosometry and cavernosography test (DICC).[4] Both cavernosal arterial insufficiency (CAI) and venoocclusive dysfunction (CVOD) are tested by this procedure using the intracavernosal injection of smooth muscle relaxants. DICC consists of two needles being placed into the cavernosal bodies of the penis. One needle is attached to a pressure transducer, which measures intracavernosal pressure, and the second is attached to an infusion pump for heparinized saline infusion.

During this procedure, it is possible to test the integrity of the cavernosal arteries by determining a PBI. Discrepancies in the PBI with a normal trapping mechanism suggest sluggish blood flow to the penis, which may be secondary to a blockage in the cavernosal/common penile arterial bed. In younger individuals with erectile dysfunction, the DICC procedure is needed as a screening device before evaluating an anatomic blockage by an arteriogram.

In addition, the DICC evaluates the venoocclusive function by determining the amount of flow required to maintain a given intracavernosal pressure. Normally in this study, only 2 to 3 ml/min of flow is required to maintain a rigid erection at 120 to 150 mm Hg. Leakage can be visualized by injecting contrast via one of the needles during this active test. In a normal penis with normal trapping, minimal to no contrast should be seen escaping from the corpora. In CVOD, there often can be an adequate arterial blood flow into the penis, but the trapping mechanism does not allow the blood to remain in the erectile cylinders long enough to maintain an erection.

Selective pudendal arteriogram. In younger patients who demonstrate focal proximal arterial obstruction but no evidence of venous leak, penile revascularization may be considered. The patient's arterial system must be evaluated before a penile revascularization procedure can be performed. Since this is an invasive and expensive test, it is almost exclusively used for patients considering microsurgical penile revascularization procedures.

Classification of Erectile Dysfunction

Failure to Initiate. Decreased libido may result from endocrine or psychologic disorders. Hypogonadism with low testosterone levels may cause a decrease in libido. However, men with low to normal testosterone levels are not generally treated with testosterone replacement. Patients may have a psychologic loss of libido, which is a response to their erectile problems; that is, they would be interested in increasing their sexual activity if their erections were not unreliable. Some psychologic element with or without an organic etiology can play a role in erectile dysfunction in up to 90% of cases. Orgasmic and ejaculatory disorders also can have a psychologic etiology, but any neurologic process that interferes with the somatic or sympathetic neural innervation to the pelvic structures can also contribute to these problems.

Failure to Fill. The integrity of both the arterial and the venoocclusive systems must be intact for successful potency. Most often, arteriogenic insufficiency can be a direct result of a traumatic event or atherosclerotic disease. A proper history may provide a clue for diagnosing a failure to fill. A young man who achieves an erection, but very slowly, and who has a history of trauma would most typically have an arterial blockage causing arterial insufficiency. On the other hand, an older patient with several risk factors for vascular disease who indicates a prolonged time to obtain an erection may have diffuse arterial blockage associated with diffuse atherosclerotic disease. Some patients may have an element of both arteriogenic and venoocclusive dysfunction, which cannot be determined by history alone. Often, diagnostic testing can help differentiate etiologies.

Failure to Store. Venous leakage can result from many etiologies (i.e., trauma, diabetes, Peyronie's disease, corporeal fibrosis, penile ischemia). The patient history may also provide a clue about the diagnosis of failure to store (venoocclusive dysfunction). For example, a man who achieves a rigid erection rapidly but loses it quickly would most typically have a venoocclusive problem. Again, diagnostic testing helps differentiate etiologies.

Failure to Achieve Rigidity or Penetration. Failure to achieve rigidity or penetration is commonly associated with disorders affecting penile geometry and the ability to attain rigidity. Congenital penile curvature and Peyronie's disease are two such disorders. These disorders can be identified by asking the patient if there is pain with erection, penile curvature, penile lumps or plaques, or a history of penile trauma. Peyronie's disease is thought to be secondary to penile trauma (either chronic or acute) with resultant scarring of the tunica albuginea. This condition causes not only penile curvature but also in many cases an inability to achieve complete venoocclusion. In these cases, loss of rigidity and sustaining capability are noted. Documentation by a photograph of the penis in the erectile state is often clinical proof of the extent to which a deformity can be associated with erectile dysfunction.

Treatment

Many forms of treatment now exist for the patient with erectile dysfunction (Box 154A-1). Some treatments are directed solely at the underlying etiology of erectile dysfunction, whereas others are more directly focused on the patient's goals.[5]

Psychologic Therapy. Traditionally, most cases of erectile dysfunction were considered to be caused primarily by psychologic causes. Previously the main form of therapy, psychotherapy is now focused on correcting the immediate causes of the problem: (1) decreasing performance anxiety, (2) providing alternative methods of giving pleasure, and (3) dealing with the secondary problems that the erectile dysfunction has created. Although the etiology is psychologic in origin for some patients, oral erectogenic agents or penile injections can be used as an adjunct to help them overcome otherwise untreatable performance anxiety.

Box 154A-1. Treatment for Erectile Dysfunction

- Psychosexual therapy
- Hormonal therapy
  - Testosterone replacement
- Nonhormonal medical therapies
  - Oral therapies
    - Yohimbine
    - Apomorphine
    - Phentolamine
    - Sildenafil citrate
  - Intraurethral suppository
    - Prostaglandin E_1
  - Intracavernosal injection agents
    - Papaverine
    - Phentolamine
    - Prostaglandin E_1
- Vacuum constriction devices
- Penile prosthesis
  - Malleable
  - Inflatable
- Vascular surgery
  - Penile revascularization
  - Venous ligation surgery

Hormonal Therapy

Testosterone. Serum testosterone levels usually decrease as a man ages. Only men with hypogonadal disorders are candidates for testosterone replacement. A hypogonadal disorder is either hypogonadotropic hypogonadism (pituitary or hypothalamic in origin) or hypergonadotropic hypogonadism (testicular failure). Testosterone replacement can restore libido and improve potency. Treatment should be given only to patients with multiple low serum levels of testosterone levels in the morning. Unfortunately, oral testosterone replacement has side effects of hepatotoxicity. The recommended therapy is via an intramuscular injection of 200 to 300 mg of testosterone enanthate every 2 to 3 weeks. One serious problem with testosterone replacement is its potential to induce growth of a prostate carcinoma. Given the increasing incidence of prostate cancer, all men should be screened with a rectal examination and PSA testing before beginning treatment. If either value is abnormal, a transrectal ultrasound-guided biopsy should be performed.

Prolactin. Hyperprolactinemia is usually treated by the administration of bromocriptine or by surgical ablation of a pituitary prolactin-secreting tumor. Medications causing hyperprolactinemia, including estrogens and methyldopa, should be stopped. High levels of prolactin seem to inhibit erections, since simply replacing testosterone in patients with continued hyperprolactinemia does not always restore potency.

Nonhormonal Medical Therapies. Nonhormonal medical therapies are now the most frequently used form of first-line therapy for patients suffering from erectile dysfunction. In the past, oral agents such as yohimbine hydrochloride were prescribed with limited efficacy. Yohimbine, a centrally acting α_2-adrenergic blocking agent, showed improvement over placebo in controlled studies with patients with psychogenic erectile dysfunction. For the majority of patients, however, it did not represent an effective solution to the problem.

Newer forms of nonhormonal medical therapy with different methods of delivery and pharmacologic action have been approved by the FDA. An intraurethral suppository of alprostadil (Medicated Urethral System for Erection [MUSE]) and direct intracavernosal injection agents (prostaglandin E_1 [PGE_1] [Caverject, Edex]) have clinical efficacy of between 70% and 90%. Penile pain associated with the use of a needle for injection and exposure to prostaglandins are among some of the side effects experienced with these medications (see Intracavernosal Injection).

Recently, clinical trials with multiple oral agents with specific action on erectile activity (i.e., phentolamine, apomorphine, and phosphodiesterase type 5 inhibitors) have shown promise. Phentolamine, a competitive α-adrenergic antagonist, causes smooth muscle relaxation and increases arterial blood flow into the penis. Apomorphine, a central dopamine receptor agonist, has also shown improvement in erectile function in patients. Both agents are undergoing clinical trials but have not been approved for clinical application by the FDA in the United States.

To date, the only U.S. FDA-approved oral medication for the treatment of erectile dysfunction is sildenafil citrate, a selective phosphodiesterase type 5 inhibitor. Sildenafil citrate (Viagra), has been extensively studied in clinical trials with overall clinical efficacy in the range of 60% to 80%.[3] Sildenafil's mechanism of action is by blocking the breakdown of cyclic guanosine triphosphate to guanosine monophosphate, thereby allowing calcium to be removed from the smooth muscle cells, resulting in smooth muscle relaxation. As previously discussed, smooth muscle relaxation is very important for increasing blood flow into the penis.

Sildenafil comes in blue tablets: 25, 50, and 100 mg. Usually, 50 mg is first prescribed, and if the results are not positive, 100 mg will be tried. The drug is taken 30 to 60 minutes before expected coitus. One must be sexually stimulated for the drug to work. Patients with significant renal or hepatic disease should begin with 25 mg. Some side effects are headaches, nausea, altered vision, and nasal congestion. Oral sildenafil is contraindicated with use of nitrates because of profound lowering of blood pressure when the two drugs are combined.

The side effects just mentioned increase with increasing dosages. In the studies performed for Food and Drug Administration (FDA) approval, only 2% to 3% of patients stopped taking sildenafil because of side effects. In addition, dosages over 100 mg do not improve erectile responses.

There were 130 sudden deaths in Viagra users by November 1998. A small percentage were in patients taking nitrates. At the moment, there is no known direct effect on the heart by Viagra that can explain the rest of the sudden deaths reported. It is recommended that an exercise tolerance test be performed in patients with heart disease or on multidrug antihypertensive therapy.

Vacuum Constriction Devices. For many years, a variety of external penile appliances have been used for the management of erectile dysfunction. Although many different devices are now manufactured, the majority have three components, including a vacuum chamber, a vacuum pump that creates negative pressure within the chamber, and a constriction ring or tension band that is applied to the base of the penis after erection is achieved. The constriction ring provides an artificial means of venous outflow obstruction.

A vacuum-induced erection is significantly different than a physiologically induced erection. A physiologically induced erection causes rigidity along the entire length of the corpora, in contradistinction to a vacuum-induced erection, which only causes rigidity distal to the constricting band, allowing for the penis to pivot at its base. Because the constriction ring limits arterial inflow as well as venous outflow, the erect state is also an ischemic one. In most cases, manufacturers recommend that the vacuum-induced erection be maintained for less than 30 minutes.

Vacuum constriction devices (VCDs) can be considered for any patient with erectile dysfunction except those whose penis has significant intracorporal scarring and thus cannot fill with blood to achieve rigidity. VCDs are specifically used in patients with severe venous leak who are unresponsive or poorly responsive to intracavernosal injections and do not wish to consider penile prosthesis surgery. The advantages of the VCDs include a relatively low cost, noninvasiveness, and few long-term complications. Patients may experience the inability to achieve adequate rigidity, difficulty with ejaculation (secondary to the constricting ring around the urethra), or penile pain, petechiae, and ecchymoses. To date, these complications have been minor and self-limited. Patients taking aspirin or warfarin (Coumadin) are more likely to develop vascular complications. Many of the devices manufactured have a valve that limits the vacuum pressure (<250 mm Hg), which might aid in decreasing the complication rate.

Patient acceptance and satisfaction with VCDs have been reported to range from 68% to 83%, but this form of treatment has lost considerable favor in the past several years secondary to other available forms of therapy. Other reasons for discontinuing VCD use have included premature loss of penile tumescence and rigidity, penile pain, pain during ejaculation, and inconvenience.

Intracavernosal Injection of Vasoactive Agents and Penile-erection Program. Intracavernosal injection of vasoactive agents causing pharmacologic erections has been one of the largest advances in the field of the diagnosis and treatment of erectile dysfunction. By causing localized smooth muscle relaxation, blood flow increases into the penis. Approximately 80% of patients respond to intracavernosal pharmacotherapy. Patients responding are usually those with an arteriogenic, psychologic, endocrinologic, or neurologic etiology, but not those with a pathologic condition causing a venous leak. Although patients with venous leakage may be able to overcome their leakage with increased arterial blood flow, the majority of patients with significant leakage will not respond to such therapy.

Medications. Numerous medications have been tried as intracavernosal injection agents for the treatment of erectile dysfunction.[1] The main medications used for intracavernosal injection include papaverine, phentolamine, and prostaglandin E_1 (PGE_1), and phentolamine. Each of these agents can be used individually or in combination.

Papaverine acts by relaxing the smooth muscle cells of the lacunar trabeculae and the penile arteries (primarily the helicine arteries). Thus more blood is brought into the penis via the arteries. As long as the venoocclusive mechanism is intact, an increase in blood flow will potentiate an erection. Although rare, side effects include hypotension, nausea, vomiting, flushing, dizziness, weakness, and sinus tachycardia. Rare elevations in liver transaminase levels have also been reported.

PGE_1 is an endogenously produced eicosanoid. It also causes smooth muscle relaxation. Side effects are all local (probably because the drug is metabolized in the penis) and include penile discomfort and pain, redness, and a burning sensation of the penile skin.

Phentolamine is an α-adrenergic antagonist and blocks sympathetic vasoconstrictive activity by blocking both α_1- and α_2-adrenergic receptors. Because it does not directly create smooth muscle relaxation, phentolamine does not work by itself to produce an erection. Rather, it is used as an adjunct to papaverine and PGE_1. Phentolamine's side effects include hypotension, tachycardia, cardiac arrhythmias, weakness, dizziness, nasal stuffiness, nausea, and vomiting.

Penile-erection Program. Before being enrolled in a penile erection (injection) program, all patients must sign an informed consent. An explanation of the procedure, including all potential side effects, should be thoroughly understood by the patient. Although many of the medications are approved by the U.S. FDA for other medical uses, patients must understand that most medications have not been approved by the FDA for penile injection therapy. The only FDA-approved intracavernosal injection agents include Caverject and Edex (both PGE_1 medications). These medications should usually be offered as first-line intracavernosal injection agents.

The program consists of two phases. The titration phase includes injections given in the office. This phase determines how much medication the patient needs and teaches him to perform the injection. The home-trial phase includes prefilled syringes given to the patient for injections administered to himself in the privacy of his home. Once a proper dosage has been achieved, the patient is given a supply of the medication for each time he desires an erection.

Side effects of intracavernosal injections include hematomas, penile pain with injection, infection, penile fibrosis, and penile curvature. One major side effect is the potential to develop priapism. Priapism is a prolonged erection lasting longer than 4 hours. If not treated promptly, priapism may lead to severe scarring of the corpora cavernosa. This scarring is a direct result of penile ischemia and may result in a worsened erectile dysfunction that is unresponsive to future intracavernosal injections. The development of priapism almost always occurs during the dosage-determination phase, and patients should be instructed to call their physician if an erection after injection lasts for more than 4 hours. Patients with priapism are usually treated with an intracavernosal injection of an α-agonist to produce detumescence. Phenylephrine or ephedrine is the agent of choice for reversing the process. One side effect, painless fibrotic nodules within the corpora cavernosa, can develop secondary to the trauma of injection or inadequate manual compression of the injection site. Nodules usually develop after prolonged use and rarely require cessation of therapy. On rare occasions, these nodules may lead to penile curvature (Peyronie's disease).

Patient satisfaction rates with injection therapy are relatively high, and side effects are relatively few. For these reasons, intracavernosal injection of vasoactive drugs is one of the most frequently used and successful modalities available for the treatment of erectile dysfunction.

Penile Prosthesis. The penile prosthesis is an artificial device that is implanted within the corpora cavernosa and that can provide sufficient rigidity for penetration during intercourse. Ideally, a prosthesis should mimic a normal penis, being erect only when desired; be comfortable; be infection and pain free; and have no mechanical failures.

The original prostheses were semirigid. This meant that although the length of the penis was always the same, the angle of penile protrusion could be altered by bending it. Subsequently, many variations in design have been developed, with current models being of the inflatable type (Fig. 154A-2). The inflatable penile prosthesis consists of two cylinders that are placed in the patient's corpora cavernosa. Each cylinder is connected to a pump, which is placed in the scrotum. The pump is connected to a reservoir, usually placed in the prevesical space. When the pump is compressed, it takes the fluid from the reservoir and pushes it into the cylinders. The cylinders fill and become rigid, making the penis around it larger and rigid. When the erection is no longer desired, the pump can be deactivated and cylinders deflated. For patients with severe erectile tissue leakage, this option may be the only viable one.

Certain disadvantages of the prosthesis insertion are clear. Insertion requires a surgical procedure. A definite mechanical failure rate exists depending on the device implanted, which over time probably approaches 30%. With the invention and introduction of devices with less compliant materials and fewer connections, this rate has fallen. Prosthesis infection rates range from 1% to 8%. In these patients the prosthesis is almost always removed. The infection usually causes severe corporitis, leading to fibrotic changes in the corpora and making subsequent prosthesis placement, although definitely possible, more difficult. Once a prosthesis is placed, the patient's corporal tissue is no longer intact, and thus the patient may not reverse the procedure and subsequently obtain normal erections. For patients with no other viable options, the prosthesis remains an excellent way to regain potency. Given all the newer treatment alternatives available, the percentage of patients requesting penile prosthesis insertion is diminishing.

Vascular Surgery. Vascular surgery may be divided into arterial and venous techniques. Unfortunately, venous surgery does not appear to be effective in stopping venous leakage in most patients. The leak is usually secondary to a diffuse process with multiple collaterals, and simply ligating the leak does not usually correct the problem.

Arterial Surgery. Candidates for penile revascularization include those with localized blockages in the pudendal-penile arterial tree. The ideal candidate is a younger man with a history of pelvic or perineal trauma and isolated lesions of the pudendal artery, the common penile artery, or both arteries. These patients have the greatest chance of success after reestablishing blood flow by revascularization. Erectile

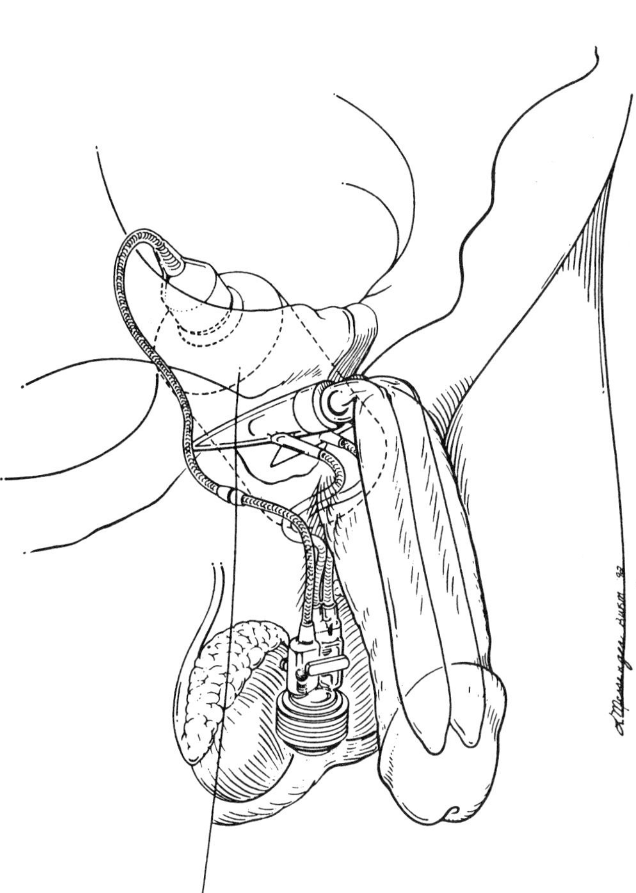

Fig. 154A-2. After placement of an inflatable penile prosthesis, the two cylinders are within the corpora, the pump is in the scrotum, and the reservoir is in Retzius space just posterior to the pubic bone. This can all be accomplished through a scrotal incision. (From Krane RJ, Siroky MB, Fitzpatrick JM, editors: *Clinical urology,* Philadelphia, 1994, JB Lippincott.)

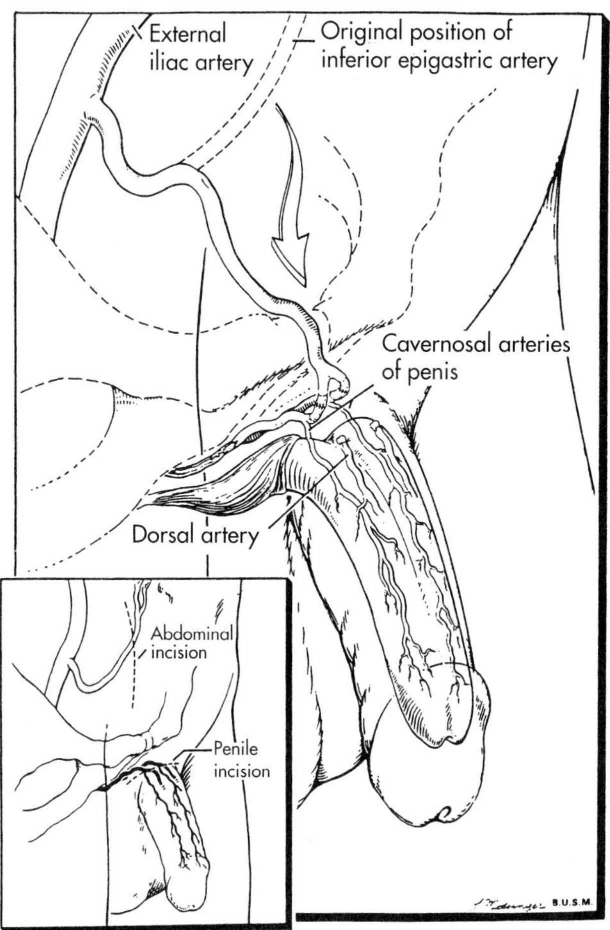

Fig. 154A-3. Schematic representation of a penile revascularization procedure. In the inset, note that two incisions are required. Initially, the inferior epigastric artery is harvested through a vertical abdominal incision. This neoarterial source is then brought through an incision at the base of the penis. The inferior epigastric artery can then be anastomosed in a retrograde end-to-end fashion to the dorsal arteries of the penis. (From Krane RJ, Siroky MB, Fitzpatrick JM, editors: *Clinical urology,* Philadelphia, 1994, JB Lippincott.)

dysfunction may occur immediately after trauma, or it may be delayed. Complaints that are delayed are most likely secondary to damage to the vascular endothelium and subsequent atherosclerotic changes over time in the regions of injury. The inferior epigastric artery is the usual neoarterial source for penile revascularization procedures (Figs. 154A-3 and 154A-4). The arterial blockage is bypassed by anastomosing this artery to the dorsal artery of the penis. Patient selection and significant surgical experience are prerequisites for performing this technique.

The preoperative patient evaluation is complex and includes DICC to ensure that venous leakage is not a component and to confirm that a gradient does exist between the brachial systolic pressure and the cavernosal artery pressure. Patients also must have a selective internal pudendal arteriogram to outline their arterial anatomy. The recipient dorsal penile artery must demonstrate evidence of branching collaterals to the cavernosal tissue on preoperative arteriogram to maximize postoperative outcomes. Appropriately selected patients have a 50% to 70% success rate with these techniques and thus may have their potency fully restored.

Venous Surgery. Venous surgery involves the surgical removal or ligation of the veins leaving the corpora cavernosa. This is usually accomplished by removing the deep dorsal vein and ligating the cavernosal veins with or without plication of the penile crura. Intuitively, venous leak should be correctable. Although in vogue for a long time, venous leak surgery has had a poor success rate, and the authors no longer routinely perform this procedure.

Summary

Over the past few decades, the knowledge and understanding of the anatomy and physiology of the penis, as well as the pathophysiology of erectile dysfunction, have evolved. Technologic advances in the areas of biochemical research have led medical personnel into a new era in the development of less invasive and more efficacious treatment modalities. Many diagnostic tests have been developed to identify the etiology of erectile dysfunction and thus target appropriate

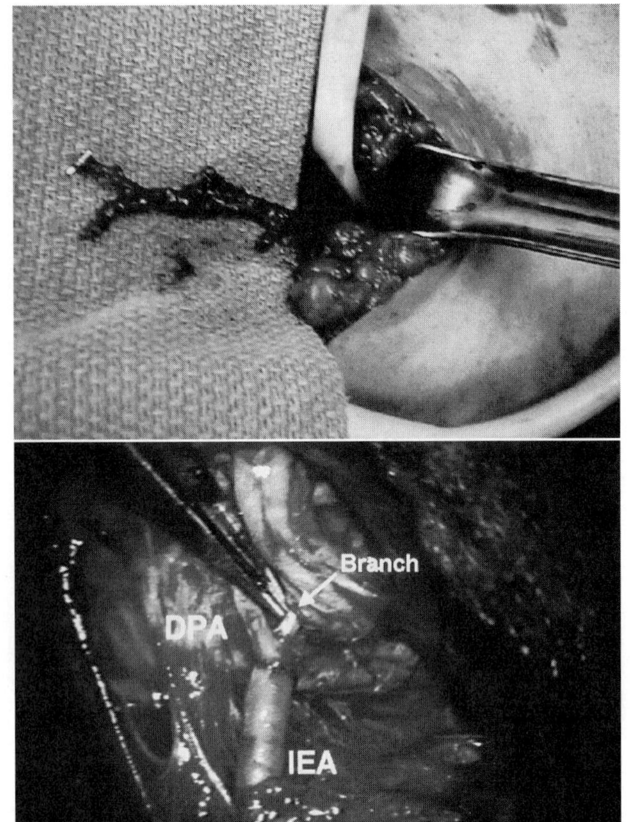

Fig. 154A-4. **A,** The harvested donor vessel, the inferior epigastric artery, is used for a neoarterial blood supply for penile revascularization procedures. **B,** Penile revascularization procedure using the inferior epigastric artery *(IEA)* supplying blood to the dorsal penile artery *(DPA)*. Note the branch off the dorsal penile artery, which travels through the tunica albuginea, supplying new blood to erectile bodies.

treatment. These advances, as well as the heightened awareness of erectile dysfunction issues by both physicians and patients, help prevent the adverse social and behavioral changes afflicting men and their partners.

REFERENCES

1. Fallon B: Intracavernous injection therapy for male erectile dysfunction, *Urol Clin North Am* 22:833, 1995.
2. Feldman HA, Goldstein I, Hatzichristou DG, et al: Impotence and its medical and psychosocial correlates: results of the Massachusetts Male Aging Study, *J Urol* 151:54, 1994.
3. Goldstein I, Lue TF, Padma-Nathan H, et al: Oral Sildenafil in the treatment of erectile dysfunction, *N Engl J Med* 338:1397, 1998.
4. Goldstein I, Padma-Nathan H: Venous evaluation of impotence. In Rajfer J, editor: *Infertility and impotence,* Chicago, 1990, VBMP, pp 269-275.
5. Lue TF: Impotence: a patient's goal directed approach to treatment, *World J Urol* 67-74, 1990.
6. NIH Consensus Panel on Impotence: Impotence, *JAMA* 270:83, 1993.
7. Rosen RC, Riley A, Wagner G, et al: The International Index of Erectile Function (IIEF): a multidimensional scale for assessment of erectile dysfunction, *Urology* 49(6):822, 1997.

CHAPTER 154B

Female Sexual Dysfunction

Jennifer R. Berman
Sapana P. Adhikari
Irwin Goldstein

FEMALE SEXUAL FUNCTION AND DYSFUNCTION

Epidemiology

Sexuality plays an important role in every individual's life. Female sexuality, in particular, encompasses a variety of disciplines involving various anatomic, physiologic, psychologic, social, and emotional factors. Until recently, little research or attention has focused on female sexual function. As a result, the knowledge and understanding of the anatomy and physiology of the female sexual response and the pathophysiology of female sexual dysfunction are limited. Based on understanding of the physiology of the male erectile response, recent advances in modern technology, and recent interest in women's health issues, the study of female sexual dysfunction is evolving at a rapid pace.

Female sexual dysfunction is an age-related, progressive, and highly prevalent problem affecting 30% to 50% of women.[23] Based on the National Health and Social Life Survey, 43% of 1749 women experienced sexual dysfunction.[9] U.S. population census data reveal that 9.7 million American women aged 50 to 74 self-report complaints of diminished vaginal lubrication, pain and discomfort with intercourse, decreased arousal, and difficulty achieving orgasm. Female sexual dysfunction is clearly an important health issue that affects the quality of life of many women.

Female Sexual Response Cycle

Masters and Johnson first characterized the female sexual response in 1996 as consisting of four successive phases: excitement, plateau, orgasmic, and resolution phases.[10] In 1979, Kaplan proposed the aspect of "desire" and the three-phase model consisting of desire, arousal, and orgasm.[7a] This three-phase model is the basis for the *Diagnostic and Statistical Manual of Mental Disorders,* 4th edition, or *DSM-IV,* classifications of female sexual dysfunction, as well as the recent reclassification system made by the American Foundation of Urologic Disease (AFUD) Consensus Panel in October 1998.[1a]

1998 AFUD Consensus Panel Classifications and Definitions of Female Sexual Dysfunction

Hypoactive Sexual Desire Disorder. Hypoactive sexual desire disorder is the persistent or recurring deficiency (or absence) of sexual fantasies and thoughts about and/or receptivity to sexual activity, which causes personal distress.

Sexual aversion disorder. Sexual aversion disorder is the persistent or recurring phobic aversion to, and avoidance of, sexual contact with a sexual partner, which causes personal distress. This disorder may result from psychologic or emotional factors or may be secondary to physiologic problems such as hormone deficiencies and medical or surgical interventions. Any disruption of the female hormonal milieu caused by natural menopause, surgically or medically induced menopause, or endocrine disorders can result in inhibited sexual desire. Sexual aversion disorder is generally a psychologically or emotionally based problem that can result from a variety of causes such as physical or sexual abuse or childhood trauma.

Sexual Arousal Disorder. Sexual arousal disorder is the persistent or recurring inability to attain or maintain sufficient sexual excitement, causing personal distress. It may be experienced as a lack of subjective excitement or lack of genital lubrication or swelling or other somatic responses.

Disorders of arousal include, but are not limited to, lack of or diminished vaginal lubrication, decreased clitoral and labial sensation, decreased clitoral and labial engorgement, and lack of vaginal smooth muscle relaxation. These conditions can occur secondary to psychologic factors; however, often there is a medical or physiologic basis such as diminished vaginal or clitoral blood flow, prior pelvic trauma, pelvic surgery, or medications (i.e., selective serotonin reuptake inhibitors [SSRIs]).

Orgasmic Disorder. Orgasmic disorder is the persistent or recurrent difficulty in, delay in, or absence of attaining orgasm after sufficient sexual stimulation and arousal, which causes personal distress.

This may be a primary (never-achieved orgasm) or secondary condition resulting from surgery, trauma, or hormone deficiencies. Primary anorgasmia can be secondary to emotional trauma or sexual abuse; however, medical and physical factors can certainly contribute to the problem.

Sexual Pain Disorders

The classifications of sexual pain disorders are subtyped as lifelong vs. acquired, generalized vs. situational, and organic vs. psychogenic or mixed. The etiology of any of these disorders may be multifactorial, occurring alone or in combination. At present, sexual arousal disorder is the focus of clinical and basic science research, as well as treatment interventions.

Dyspareunia. Dyspareunia is recurrent or persistent genital pain associated with sexual intercourse. Dyspareunia can develop secondary to medical problems such as vestibulitis, vaginal atrophy, or vaginal infection. It can be either physiologically or psychologically based or a combination of the two.

Vaginismus. Vaginismus is recurrent or persistent involuntary spasms of the musculature of the outer third of the vagina that interferes with vaginal penetration and that causes personal distress. Vaginismus usually develops as a conditioned response to painful penetration or develops secondary to psychologic or emotional factors.

Other sexual pain disorders. Other sexual pain disorders cause recurrent or persistent genital pain induced by noncoital sexual stimulation.

Female Sexual Anatomy

A formal understanding of female pelvic anatomy is necessary to adequately evaluate and treat female sexual dysfunction. Although female pelvic anatomy is composed of a continuum of organs and structures interrelated in both structure and function, it is helpful to group them into two categories: external genitalia and internal genitalia.

External Genitalia.

The organs of the external genitalia are collectively known as the *vulva*. The vulva is bound anteriorly by the bony symphysis pubis, posteriorly by the anal sphincter, and laterally by the ischial tuberosities. The vulva consists of three general structures: the labial formation, the interlabial space, and the erectile tissues.

Labial Formation. The labial formation is located posterior to the mons pubis and anterior to the anal sphincter. The mons pubis is the rounded eminence located anterior to the pubic symphysis and lower abdominal wall. It is made up of a pad of fatty connective tissue that changes in size and texture throughout life. During puberty, the mons pubis increases in size and becomes covered with coarse pubic hair; after menopause, it decreases both in size and in amount of hair.

The labial formation consists of two pairs of symmetrical skinfolds designed to protect the urethral and vaginal orifices that both open into the vestibule of the vagina. The outer fold, the labia majora, is composed of subcutaneous fat that is covered by hair-bearing skinfolds that fuse with each other anteriorly at the anterior labial commissure and posteriorly connect to a bridge of skin called the *posterior labial commissure*. The thin inner fold, the labia minora, consists of a fat-free spongy tissue punctuated by sebaceous and sweat glands along with many blood vessels. It is covered by a hairless skin. The pinkish medial side of the labia minora is continuous with the vaginal mucosa and contains many sensory nerve endings. The labia minora fuse with each other anteriorly, forming the prepuce of the clitoris, and fuse with each other posteriorly as the frenulum. In young women, this area is easily torn during childbirth or during an episiotomy.

Innervation. The innervation of the labial formation consists of the perineal branch and posterior labial branches of the pudendal nerve (Fig. 154B-1).

Blood Supply. The rich arterial supply arises from the inferior perineal and posterior labial branches of the internal pudendal artery. Superficial branches of the femoral artery also supply the labial formation (Fig. 154B-2).

Interlabial Space. The interlabial space is the area medial to the labia minora. It is bound anteriorly by the clitoris and posteriorly by the frenulum. The greater vestibular glands, the urethral orifice, and the vaginal orifice all open into this space.

The greater vestibular glands are oval and lie under the bulbs of the vestibule. During sexual arousal, these glands secrete a small amount of lubricating mucus into the vestibule of the vagina (Fig. 154B-3).

Female Erectile Organs. The female erectile organs include the clitoris and the vestibular bulbs. The clitoris is an erectile organ located posterior to the anterior labial commissure and is usually hidden by the labial formations when nonengorged. The part of the labia minora that passes anterior to the clitoris forms the prepuce of the clitoris, and the part that passes posterior to the clitoris forms the frenulum of the clitoris. Cylindric in shape, the clitoris is made up of three parts: the outermost glans, the midline corpus or body, and the innermost crura. The glans clitoris can be visualized as it emerges from the labia minora. The body of the clitoris extends under the skin and gives rise to bilateral crura, which sit posterior and lateral to the body. These paired crura, called *corpora cavernosa*, are composed of erectile tissue and are separated by a septum of connective tissue. The distal

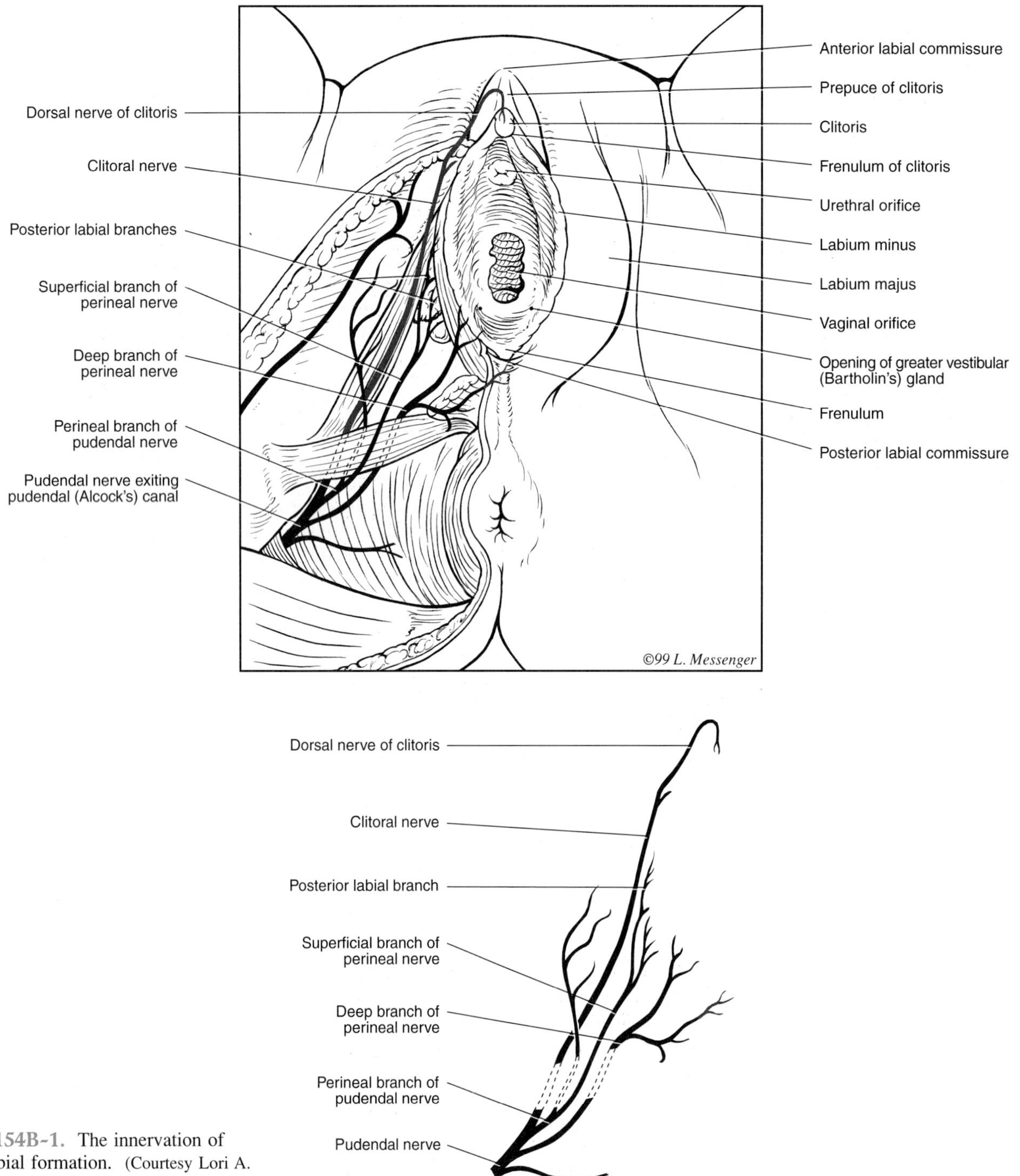

Fig. 154B-1. The innervation of the labial formation. (Courtesy Lori A. Messenger, CMI.)

segments of the two separate crura attach bilaterally to the undersurface of the pubis along the ischiopubic rami (see Fig. 154B-3).

Like the penis, the clitoris is suspended to the anterior abdominal wall by a suspensory ligament, and its corpora cavernosa has similar tissue organization. The paired crura are homologous to the male corpora and composed of a trabecula of vascular smooth muscle, a complex area of lacunar sinusoids, and a collagen connective tissue surrounded by a thick fibrous sheath of tunica albuginea.

Innervation. The clitoris has many nerve endings and is highly sensitive to touch, pressure, and temperature. The autonomic innervation of the clitoris arises from the pelvic and hypogastric plexuses. These plexuses carry sympathetic (T1-L3) and parasympathetic (S2-S4) fibers and join together to form the uterovaginal plexus, which lies in the base of the broad ligament on each side of the supravaginal part of the cervix. This plexus sends direct fibers to both the vagina and the clitoris (Fig. 154B-4). The clitoris exhibits a dense collection of pacinian corpuscles innervated by rapidly adapting myelinated afferents as well as Meissner's corpuscles, Merkel's tactile disks, and free nerve endings. Somatic sensory innervation to the clitoris arises in the skin, travels via the dorsal nerve of the clitoris, and

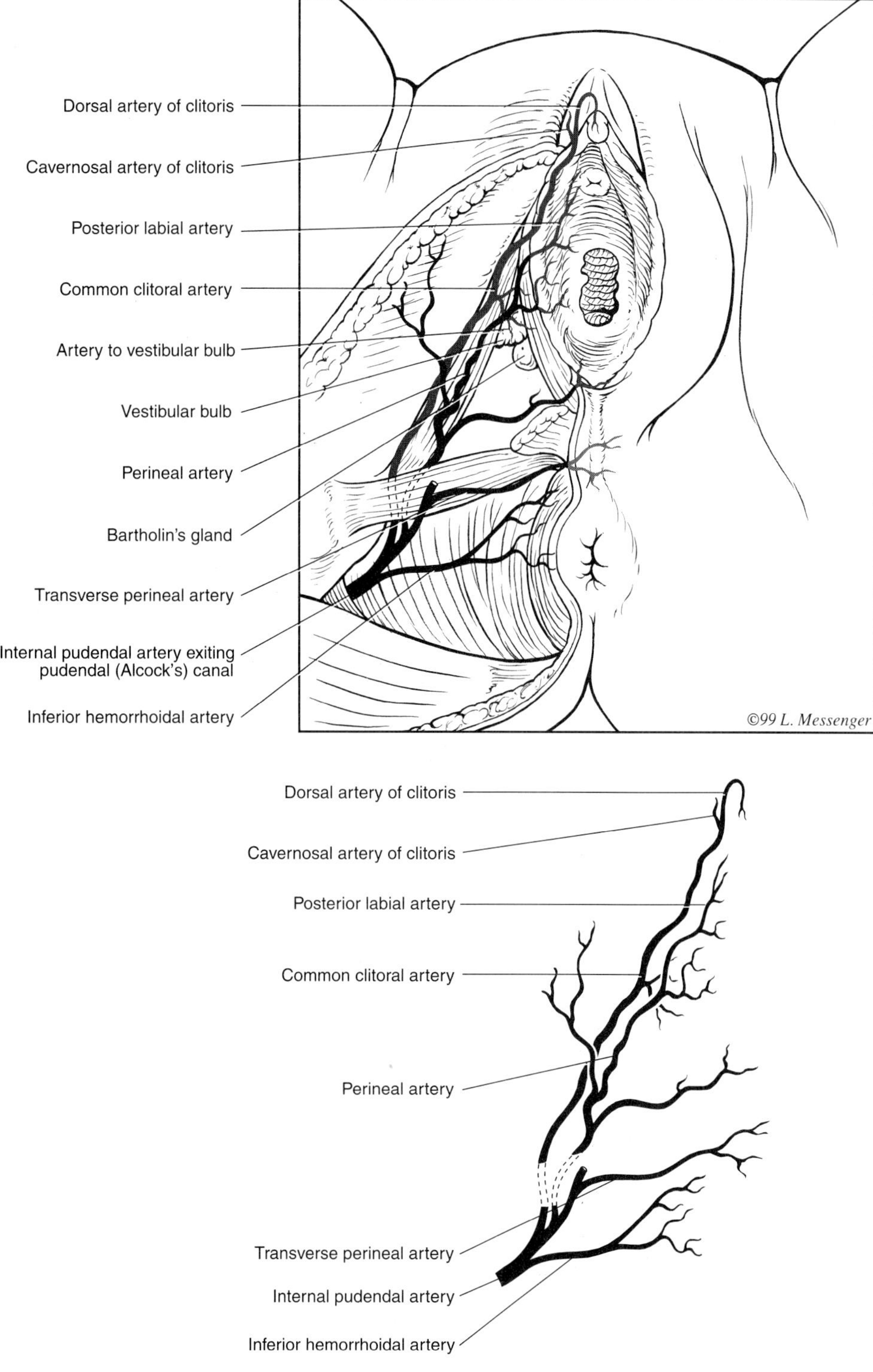

Fig. 154B-2. Superficial branches of the femoral artery. (Courtesy Lori A. Messenger, CMI.)

continues within the pudendal nerve to reach the sacral spinal cord.[20]

Blood supply. The main arterial supply to the clitoris is via the iliohypogastric pudendal arterial bed. After the internal iliac artery gives off its last anterior branch, the internal pudendal artery, it traverses Alcock's (pudendal) canal and terminates as the common clitoral artery, which then gives off the dorsal clitoral artery and clitoral cavernosal arteries. On sexual stimulation and arousal, the corporal bodies become engorged with blood (see Fig. 154B-2).

The other erectile tissues of the female are the vestibular bulbs. These 3-cm-long paired structures lie along the sides of the vaginal orifice, directly beneath the skin of the labia. Although they are homologous to the corpus spongiosum of the penis, they are distinct in that they are separated from the clitoris, urethra, and vestibule of the vagina. The main arterial supply to the vestibular bulbs is via bulbar and posterior labial branches of the internal pudendal artery. Recent cadaver dissections reveal that in young, premenopausal women, the bulbs lie on the superficial aspect of the vaginal

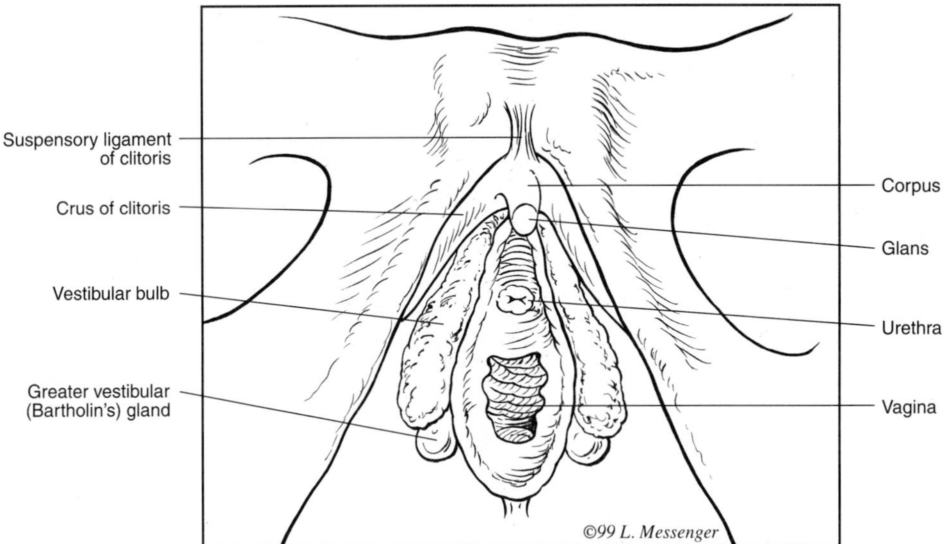

Fig. 154B-3. The interlabial space. (Courtesy Lori A. Messenger, CMI.)

wall and do not form the core of the labia minora.[13] Furthermore, there are considerable age-related variations in the dimensions of the erectile tissue between young, premenopausal specimens and older, postmenopausal specimens.[13]

Internal Genitalia. The organs of the internal genitalia of the female consist of the vagina, uterus, uterine tubes, and ovaries.

Vagina. This midline cylindric organ about 7 to 9 cm in length extends from the vestibule of the vagina to the cervix of the uterus. The vaginal wall consists of three layers: an inner glandular layer, a lamina propia, and a muscularis. The inner layer consists of a mucous membrane type of stratified squamous cell epithelium that undergoes hormone-related cyclical changes. During the menstrual cycle, a slight keratinization of the superficial cells takes place. Beneath the thick middle lamina propia layer lies the muscularis. This layer is composed of outer longitudinal and inner circular smooth muscle fibers. The surrounding fibrous layer, rich in collagen and elastin, provides structural support to the vagina, and allows for expansion of the vagina during intercourse and childbirth.

Innervation. The autonomic innervation of the vagina originates from two separate plexuses, the hypogastric plexus and the sacral plexus, which gives rise to the uterovaginal nerves that contain both parasympathethic and sympathethic fibers. These fibers travel within the uterosacral and cardinal ligaments to supply the proximal two thirds of the vagina and the corporal bodies of the clitoris. Somatic sensory innervation is provided by the pudendal nerve, which reaches the perineum through Alock's canal. Studies show that there is an abundance of nerve fibers in the distal, as compared to more proximal, parts of the vagina.[22b] It is important to recognize this uterovaginal plexus, which plays a major role in sexual function, as a potential site of injury when performing female pelvic surgeries such as hysterectomy. Neurovascular injury to this area may cause sexual dysfunction. Currently, nerve-sparing pelvic procedures similar to those now routinely performed in men are being developed for women.

Blood Supply. The arterial supply to the superior aspect of the vagina arises from the vaginal branches of the uterine artery and the hypogastric artery, which supplies the middle aspect of the vagina. Branches of the middle hemorrhoidal and clitoral arteries supply the distal aspect of the vagina (Fig. 154B-5).

Uterus. This midline, very mobile organ is located between the rectum and urinary bladder. It is suspended posteriorly by the uterosacral ligaments and suspended laterally by the cardinal ligaments. The round ligaments, which prevent the uterus from retroversion, also provide lateral support. The uterine wall consists of three distinct layers: the endometrium, the myometrium, and the perimetrium layers. The myometrium is by far the largest component; three layers of smooth muscle fibers form it.

Innervation. The autonomic innervation comes from the ovarian and hypogastric plexuses. These plexuses carry sympathetic (T12-L1) fibers and parasympathetic fibers (S2-4).

Blood supply. The main arterial supply comes from three major arteries: the uterine artery, a branch of the hypogastric artery; the ovarian artery, which give rise to uterine branches that anastomose with the uterine artery; and the round ligament artery, a branch of the epigastric artery (see Fig. 154B-5).

Female Sexual Response: Physiology of Sexual Arousal

The female sexual response cycle, associated with neurotransmitter-mediated vascular and nonvascular smooth muscle relaxation, results in increased vaginal lubrication, vaginal wall engorgement, and luminal diameter as well as increased clitoral length and diameter.[7] These mechanisms are mediated by a combination of vasocongestive and neuromuscular events. Engorgement results secondary to increased pelvic blood flow to the iliohypogastric pudendal arterial bed and concomitant relaxation of the vaginal wall and clitoral cavernosal smooth muscle.

In the labia minora, blood flow increases, particularly to the vestibular bulbs that directly underlie the skin of the labia.

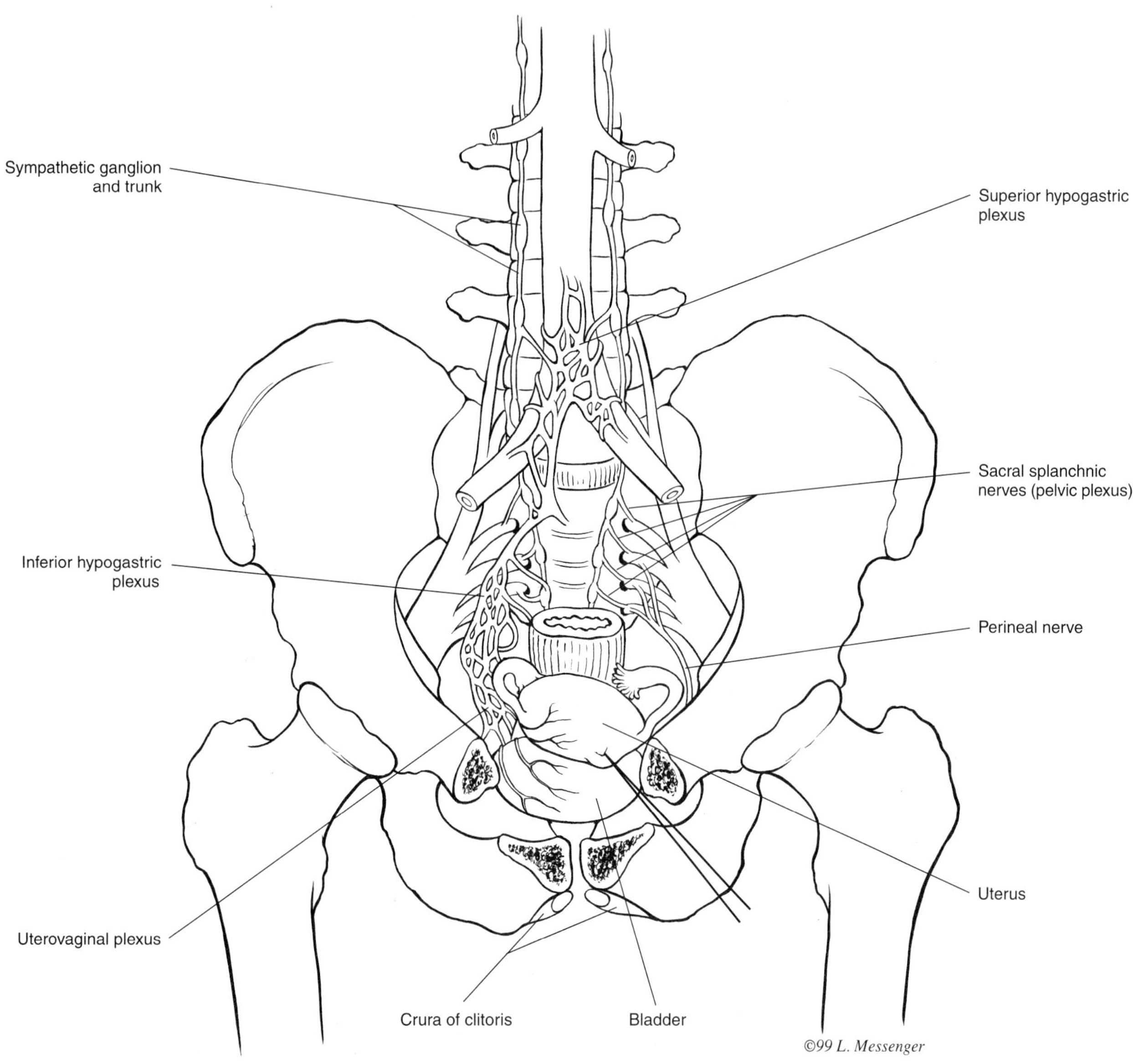

Fig. 154B-4. The uterovaginal plexus. (Courtesy Lori A. Messenger, CMI.)

This causes a twofold to threefold increase in the diameter and eversion of the labia with exposure of its inner surface. Vaginal blood flow also increases during sexual excitement. The extensive tree of blood vessels of the middle muscularis layer of the vagina becomes highly infiltrated with blood. As this happens, the outer supportive fibrous mesh composed of elastin and collagen fibers provides structural support. In the clitoris, increased blood flow to the clitoral cavernosal arteries results in an increased clitoral intracavernous pressure, leading to tumescence and extrusion of the glans. Studies show that, unlike the penis, the clitoris lacks a subalbugineal layer between the erectile tissue and the tunica albugineal layer.[13] In the man, this layer possesses a rich venous plexus that, during sexual excitement, expands against the tunica albuginea, reducing venous outflow and making the penis rigid. The absence of this venous plexus in the clitoris suggests that this organ achieves tumescence but not rigidity during sexual arousal.

Increased lubrication during sexual arousal is a direct result of increased blood flow. The vaginal canal is lubricated principally via two mechanisms: secretions from the uterine glands and transudate originating from the subepithelial vascular bed that is passively transported through intraepithelial spaces or intercellular channels. Vaginal engorgement enables a process of plasma transudation to occur, allowing a flow through the epithelium and onto the vaginal surface. Vascular engorgement within the vaginal wall increases pressure within the blood vessel, helping transudate to form. This vaginal lubricative plasma flows through the epithelium onto the surface of the vagina, initially forming sweatlike droplets that coalesce to form a lubricative film covering the vaginal wall. Additional moistening during intercourse comes from secretions of the paired greater vestibular or Bartholin's glands, although some believe that these glands have a more primal function of emitting an odoriferous fluid to attract the male.

Enhanced sensation during sexual activity results from an activation of the somatic sensory nerve endings; these

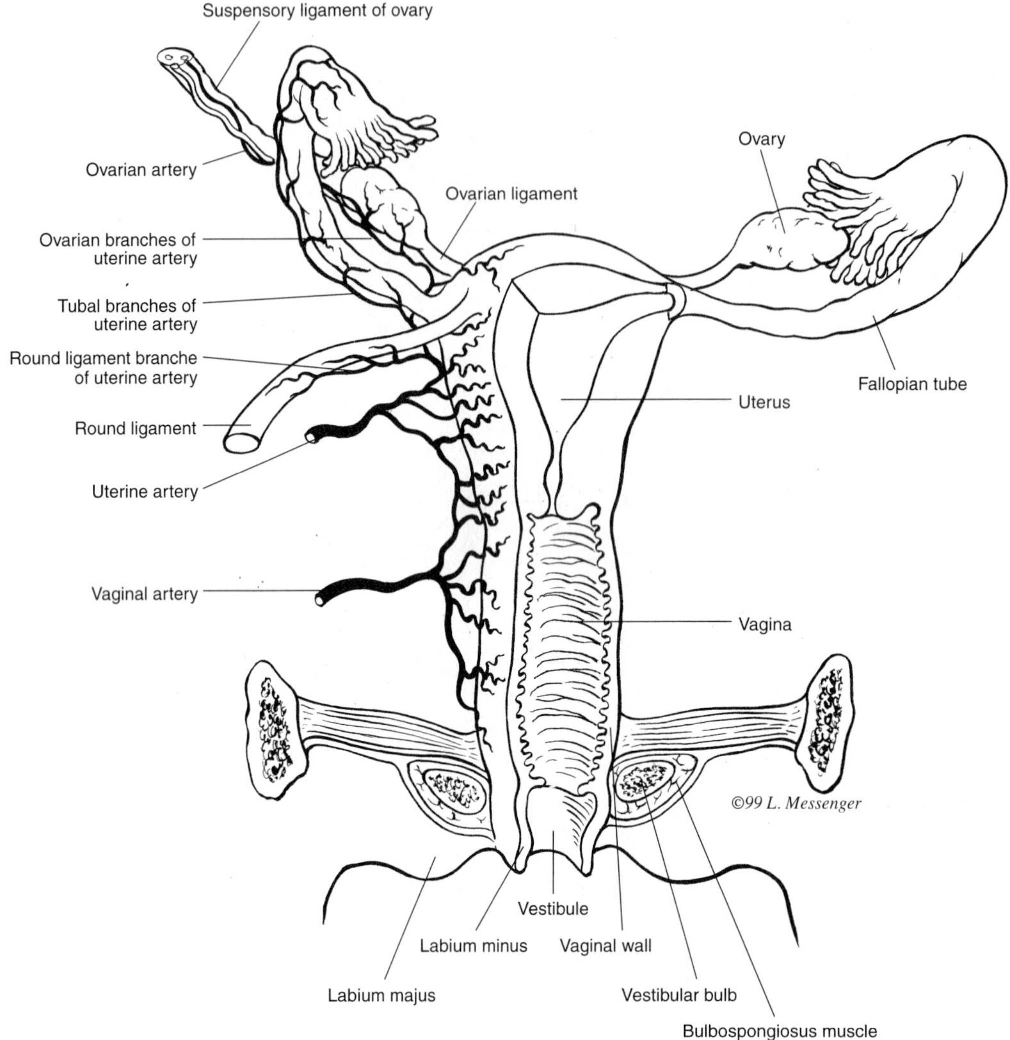

Fig. 154B-5. Branches of the middle hemorrhoidal and clitoral arteries. (Courtesy Lori A. Messenger, CMI.)

endings are abundant in the clitoris and labia minora and elsewhere within the female sexual anatomy.

Neurogenic Mediators of the Female Sexual Response. Within the central nervous system, the medial preoptic, anterior hypothalamic region and related limbic-hippocampal structures are responsible for sexual arousal. On activation, these centers transmit electrical signals through the parasympathethic and sympathetic nervous system.

The neurotransmitters that modulate vaginal and clitoral smooth muscle tone are currently under investigation. Recently, NO and phosphodiesterase type V, the enzyme responsible for both the degradation of cyclic guanosine monophosphate and NO production, have been identified in clitoral and cavernosal smooth muscle.[4,15]

Other studies suggest that vasoactive intestinal polypeptide in combination with NO is involved in modulating vaginal relaxation and secretory processes.[14] This polypeptide is a nonadrenergic, noncholinergic neurotransmitter that enhances vaginal blood flow, lubrication, and secretions.[14] Although the exact identity of the relaxatory nonadrenergic, noncholinergic neurotransmitters remains unclear, from these initial observations, NO does seem to have a potential role as mediator of the female sexual response.

Hormonal Regulators of Female Sexual Response. Hormone levels in the body affect female sexual function.

Estrogen. Levels of estradiol influence both central and peripheral nerve transmissions. In animal models, the administration of estradiol results in expanded touch receptor zones along the distribution of the pudendal nerve, suggesting that estrogen affects sensory thresholds.[19] Aside from the neurologic effects, estrogens also have vasoprotective and vasodilatory effects that increase vaginal, clitoral, and urethral arterial flow.[19] This results in the maintenance of the female sexual response by preventing atherosclerotic compromise to the iliohypogastric arterial bed.

Estrogen also regulates the expression of nitric oxide synthase (NOS), the enzyme responsible for the production of nitric oxide. A decline in circulating estrogen levels resulting from aging or surgical castration results in decreased vaginal NO levels and increased vaginal wall fibrosis.[2] Estrogen replacement therapy restores vaginal mucosa, increases vaginal NO levels, and decreases vaginal mucosal cell death.

This suggests a positive correlation among the expression of vaginal NOS, cyclic guanosine monophosphate, and estrogen levels. Animal studies also show that aging and surgical castration result in decreased vaginal NOS levels, vaginal fibrosis, and increased apoptosis, or death of vaginal mucosal and smooth muscle cells. Estrogen replacement restores vaginal mucosa, increases vaginal NOS expression, and decreases vaginal apoptosis.[2]

Estrogen is important in the maintenance and function of the vaginal epithelium, stromal cells, and smooth muscles of the muscularis as well as the thickness of the vaginal rugae and vaginal lubrication. A decline in the level of estrogen results in thinner vaginal walls that are more easily damaged and a drier, less acidic environment in the vaginal canal. This ultimately results in complaints of female sexual dysfunction such as vaginal dryness and dyspareunia.[5]

A majority of women experience some degree of change in sexual function with the decline in circulating estrogen levels observed during aging and menopause. Common sexual complaints include loss of desire, painful intercourse, decreased frequency of sexual activity, difficulty achieving orgasm, diminished sexual responsiveness, and decreased genital sensation. In 1966, Masters and Johnson first published their findings of the physiologic changes related to sexual function occurring in menopausal women.[10] Currently, studies show that symptoms related to alterations in genital sensation and blood flow are, in part, secondary to declining estrogen levels. There is a direct correlation between the presence of sexual complaints and levels of estradiol below 50 pg/ml.[2] Symptoms markedly decrease with estrogen replacement therapy; therapy is designed not only to restore hormonal levels but also to restore genital vibration and pressure sensation to premenopausal levels.[1,6,17]

Testosterone. Decreased sexual arousal, libido, sexual responsiveness, genital sensation, and orgasm can also be associated with low levels of testosterone. Studies show that menopausal women respond better to parenteral estrogen-androgen combinations than estrogen alone with regard to enhanced sexual desire, libido, energy, sexual motivation, and overall sense of well being.[21] Women on this therapy noted significant improvement in sexual desire, sexual arousal, number of sexual fantasies, enjoyment of sex, and number of orgasms.[21] Testosterone treatment with estrogen is also successfully used to treat dyspareunia or lack of vaginal lubrication in menopausal women. However, there are conflicting reports regarding the benefit of methyltestosterone for the treatment of inhibited desire or vaginismus in premenopausal women.[17] Topical testosterone cream is currently used in treating vaginal lichen planus. Potential benefits of this therapy include increased clitoral sensitivity, increased vaginal lubrication, increased libido, and heightened arousal. All androgens carry the risk of inducing virilization in women. Early reversible manifestations include acne, hirsutism, and menstrual irregularities. Long-term side effects such as male-pattern baldness, worsening of the hirsutism, voice changes, and hypertrophy of the clitoris are largely irreversible. However clinical studies are under way assessing the potential benefits of testosterone for the treatment of female sexual dysfunction.

Pathophysiology of Female Sexual Dysfunction

The female sexual response is a complex, integrating process that involves several factors. Disruptions of one or any combination of these factors may cause female sexual dysfunction. These factors are vasogenic, neurogenic, hormonal, and psychogenic.

Vasculogenic Factors. Male impotence and more recently female sexual arousal have been associated with medical conditions, including high blood pressure, high cholesterol levels, smoking, and heart disease. The recently named clitoral and vaginal vascular insufficiency syndromes are, in fact, directly related to diminished genital blood flow secondary to atherosclerosis of the iliohypogastric/pudendal arterial bed.[11] Aortoiliac or atherosclerotic disease causes a diminished pelvic blood flow resulting in vaginal wall and clitoral smooth muscle fibrosis. This can ultimately result in symptoms of vaginal dryness and dyspareunia.[16] It is possible that conditions other than those of a vasculogenic origin may manifest in decreased vaginal and clitoral engorgement. These may include conditions that have a psychologic or physiologic/organic basis. However, arterial insufficiency is one etiology that should be considered. In addition, traumatic injuries to the iliohypogastric/pudendal arterial bed can also result in symptomatic diminished vaginal and clitoral blood flow and complaints of sexual dysfunction. Such injuries can result from pelvic fractures, blunt trauma, surgical disruption, or chronic perineal pressure from bicycle riding.

Neurogenic Factors. The same neurogenic etiologies that cause erectile dysfunction in men may also cause sexual dysfunction in women. Female sexual dysfunction can result from spinal cord injuries or disease of the central or peripheral nervous system such as diabetes. Women with complete upper motor neuron injuries affecting sacral spinal segments are unable to achieve psychogenic lubrication and have significantly more difficulty achieving orgasm.[22] Women with incomplete injuries retain that capacity for psychogenic lubrication.[24] A recent study demonstrated that sildenafil partially reverses the sexual dysfunction commonly associated with spinal cord injury in women.[22a]

Hormonal-endocrine Factors. Hypothalamic-pituitary axis dysfunction, surgical or medical castration, menopause, premature ovarian failure, and chronic birth control pill intake are the most common causes of hormonal- and endocrine-related female sexual dysfunction. The symptoms include, but are not limited to, decreased desire and libido, vaginal dryness, and lack of sexual arousal.

Psychogenic Factors. Emotional, self-esteem, body image, and relational issues, in the presence or absence of organic disease, can significantly affect sexual arousal. In addition, psychologic disorders such as depression and anxiety disorders are associated with female sexual dysfunction. Patients are often treated for these disorders by taking psychotropic drugs such as SSRIs. SSRIs have been associated with decreased desire, decreased arousal, decreased genital sensation, and difficulty achieving orgasm. However, several recent studies document improvement in SSRI-induced sexual dysfunction in women treated with sildenafil.[12,18]

Evaluation

In the clinical setting, female sexual responses have been difficult to quantify objectively because the changes that occur are difficult to measure and are not readily visible or recognized by the patient. In the past, psychotherapists and physiologists have evaluated women with sexual dysfunction primarily by estimating vaginal engorgement with photoplethysmography.[8] Although validated, this method is subject to movement artifact, making it unsuitable for recording during stimulation or orgasm. In addition, it is adequate only during low to moderate levels of arousal and provides arbitrary rather than absolute units of measurement. It provides no anatomic information.

Currently, a collaborative approach is suggested for evaluating female sexual dysfunction, taking both physiologic and psychologic aspects into consideration. For every patient, a full history and physical examination, including a pelvic examination and hormonal profile (follicle-stimulating hormone, luteinizing hormone, testosterone, and estradiol levels), is crucial. Any deviation may clue the investigator in to possible medical etiologies for the patient's complaint. In addition, it is important to assess physiologic changes that occur during the sexual response. Measurements of vaginal pH, vaginal wall compliance, genital vibratory perception thresholds, and genital hemodynamics can be recorded before and after sexual stimulation in the clinical setting.[3] Blood flow assessment, especially in the clitoral, labial, urethral, vaginal, and uterine arteries, is recorded, and a comparison between blood velocity and venous pooling, both before and after stimulation, should be made. In many patients, observations show that despite complaints of sexual dysfunction, sexual stimulation does in fact result in significant increases in genital blood flow.[3a] Currently, normative data are being gathered to determine normal physiologic responses. Evaluating the female sexual response in the clinical setting both validates the patient's problems and potentially diagnoses organic disease such as vascular insufficiency, hormonal abnormalities, and neurologic disorders.

In addition to the medical and physiologic evaluation, it is important to assess psychologic factors that may be contributing to the dysfunction. Possible factors include emotional or relational issues, the context in which the patient experiences her sexuality, the patient's self-esteem and body image, and the patient's ability to communicate her sexual needs to her partner. In addition, medications that adversely affect libido or sexual function are noted. For example, β-adrenergic blockers, central nervous system depressants, and anticholinergics negatively affect female sexual function. Antidepressant medications, especially SSRIs, as previously noted, are associated with female sexual dysfunction.

Treatment

The treatment of female sexual dysfunction is gradually evolving as more clinical and basic science studies are dedicated to evaluating the problem. Aside from hormone replacement therapy, the medical management of female sexual dysfunction remains in the early experimental phases. Nonetheless, medical and health care professionals should realize that not all female sexual complaints are psychologically based. Studies are currently assessing the effects of vasoactive substances on the female sexual response.[22a] Aside from hormone replacement therapy, all medications listed subsequently, although useful in the treatment of male erectile dysfunction, are still in experimental phases for use in women.

Estrogen Replacement Therapy. Estrogen replacement therapy is indicated in menopausal women (either spontaneous or surgical). Aside from relieving hot flashes, preventing osteoporosis, and lowering the risk of heart disease, estrogen replacement results in improved clitoral sensitivity, increased libido, and decreased pain during intercourse. Local or topical estrogen application relieves symptoms of vaginal dryness, burning, and urinary frequency and urgency. In menopausal or oophorectomized women, complaints of vaginal irritation, pain, or dryness secondary to vaginal atrophy can be relieved with topical estrogen cream. A vaginal estradiol ring (Estring) is now available that delivers low-dose estrogen locally, which may benefit patients with breast cancer and other women unable to take oral or transdermal estrogen.[1]

Methyltestosterone. Methyltestosterone is often used in combination with estrogen for inhibited desire, dyspareunia, or lack of vaginal lubrication in menopausal women. There are conflicting reports regarding the benefit of methyltestosterone for the treatment of inhibited desire) or vaginismus in premenopausal women.[17a] Topical testosterone cream is an approved treatment of vaginal lichen planus. Potential benefits of this therapy include increased clitoral sensitivity, increased vaginal lubrication, increased libido and heightened arousal. Potential side effects of testosterone administration, either topical or oral, include weight gain, clitoral enlargement, increased facial hair, and hypercholesterolemia.

Sildenafil. Functioning as a selective type 5 phosphodiesterase inhibitor, sildenafil (Viagra) decreases the catabolism of cyclic guanosine monophosphate, the second messenger in the NO-mediated relaxation of clitoral and vaginal smooth muscle.[1] Sildenafil may prove useful alone or possibly in combination with other vasoactive substances for the treatment of female sexual arousal disorder. Clinical studies evaluating the safety and efficacy of this medication in women with sexual arousal disorder are currently in progress. Several published studies demonstrate the efficacy of sildenafil for treating female sexual dysfunction secondary to SSRI use.[1,12] Another recent study describes the subjective effects of sildenafil in a population of postmenopausal women.[1,7b]

L-Arginine. The amino acid, L-arginine, functions as a precursor to the formation of NO, which mediates the relaxation of vascular and nonvascular smooth muscle. L-Arginine has not been used in clinical trials in women; however, preliminary studies in men appear promising.

Prostaglandin E_1. An intraurethral application absorbed via mucosa (MUSE), PGE_1 is now available for male patients. A similar application of PGE_1 delivered intravaginally is currently under investigation for use in women. Clinical studies are necessary to determine the efficacy of this medication in the treatment of female sexual dysfunction.

Phentolamine (Vasomax). Currently available in an oral preparation, phentolamine functions as a nonspecific α-adrenergic blocker and causes vascular smooth muscle relaxation. This drug has been studied in male patients for the treatment of erectile dysfunction. A pilot study in menopausal women with sexual dysfunction demonstrated enhanced vaginal blood flow and improved subjective arousal with the medication.[18a]

Apomorphine. Initially designed as an antiparkinsonian agent, apomorphine, a short-acting dopamine agonist, facilitates erectile responses in normal men, men with psychogenic erectile dysfunction, and men with organic impotence. Data from pilot studies in men suggest that dopamine may be involved in the mediation of sexual desire as well as arousal. The physiologic effects of this drug have not been tested in women with sexual dysfunction, but it may prove useful either alone or in combination with vasoactive medications.

Summary

The physiologic mechanism underlying the female sexual response cycle is beginning to be better understood because of the recent expanses in clinical research, the increased interest in female sexual function, and the advent of modern technology. In particular, advances in the technology used to assess sexual function have resulted in a growing body of evidence indicating that women with sexual dysfunction commonly have physiologic abnormalities such as decreased pelvic blood flow.

Although there are significant anatomic and embryologic parallels between men and women, the multifaced nature of female sexual dysfunction is clearly distinct from that of the male. Thus physicians must approach female patients and their sexual function problems like they do male patients and their sexual function problems—in a systematic and scientific manner. The ideal approach to treating patients with female sexual dysfunction is a comprehensive effort between therapists and physicians. The patient's emotional needs and feeling of her own sexuality should be evaluated and treated. Psychosocial issues need to be determined before beginning medical therapies or attempting to determine treatment efficacies. Whether current therapy such as vasoactive agents or treatments currently being used in men are found to be predictably effective in women remains to be seen. At the very least, discussions about female sexual function and dysfunction are leading to heightened interest and awareness as well as more clinical and basic science research in this area.

REFERENCES

1. Ayton RA, Darling GM, Murkies AL, et al: A comparative study of safety and efficacy of continuous low dose estradiol released from a vaginal ring compared with conjugated equine estrogen vaginal cream in the treatment of postmenopausal vaginal atrophy, *Br J Obstet Gynaecol* 103:351, 1996.

1a. Basson R, Berman JR, Burnett A, et al: Report on the International Consensus Development Conference of Female Sexual Dysfunction: definitions and classifications, *J Urol* 163:888-893, 2000.

2. Berman J, McCarthy M, Kyprianou N: Effect of estrogen withdrawal on nitric oxide synthase expression and apoptosis in the rat vagina, *Urology* 44:650, 1998.

3. Berman JR: Female sexual dysfunction: incidence, pathophysiology, evaluation and treatment options, *Urology* 9:385, 1999.

3a. Berman JR, Berman LA, Werbin T, et al: Clinical evaluation of female sexual function: effects of age and estrogen status on subjective and physiologic responses, *Int J Impot* Res 11:31-38, 1999.

4. Burnett AL, Calvin DC, Silver RI, et al: Immunohistochemical description of nitric oxide synthase isoforms in human clitoris, *J Urol* 158:75, 1997.

5. Carson C, ed: *Textbook of erectile dysfunction,* Oxford, England, 1999, ISIS Medical Media, pp 627-638.

6. Collins A, Landgren BM: Reproductive health, use of estrogen and experience of symptoms in perimenopausal women: a population based study, *Maturitas* 20(2):101, 1994.

7. Goldstein I, Berman JR: Vasculogenic female sexual dysfunction: vaginal engorgement and clitoral erectile insufficiency syndromes, *Int J Impot Res* 10:S84, 1998.

7a. Kaplan HS: *The new sex therapy*, London, 1974, Bailliere Trindall.

7b. Kaplan S: *J Urol,* 1998.

8. Laan E, Everaerd W: Physiological measure of vaginal vasocongestion, *Int J Impot Res* 10:S107, 1998.

9. Laumann E, Paik A, Rosen R: Sexual dysfunction in the United States: prevalence and predictors, *JAMA* 281:537, 1999.

10. Masters EH, Johnson VE: *Human sexual response,* Boston, 1966, Little, Brown.

11. Myers LS, Morokof PJ: Physiological and subjective sexual arousal in pre- and post-menopausal women taking replacement therapy, *Psychophysiology* 23:283, 1986.

12. Nurnberg HG, Lodillo J, Hensley P, et al: Sildenafil for iatrogenic seratonergic antidepressant medication-induced sexual dysfunction in 4 patients, *J Clin Psych* 60(1):33, 1999.

13. O'Connell HE, Hutson FM, Anderson CR, Plenter R: Anatomic relationship between the urethra and clitoris, *J Urol* 159:189-192, 1998.

14. Ottesen B, Pedersen B, Nielesen J, et al: Vasoactive intestinal polypeptide provokes vaginal lubrication in normal women, *Peptides* 8:797, 1987.

15. Park K, Moreland RB, Goldstein I, et al: Characterization of phosphodiesterase activity in human clitoral corpus cavernosum smooth muscle cells in culture, *Biochem Biophys Res Com* 249:612, 1998.

16. Park K, Goldstein I, Andry C, et al: Vasculogenic female sexual dysfunction: the hemodynamic basis for vaginal engorgement insufficiency and clitoral erectile insufficiency, *Int J Impot Res* 9:27, 1988.

17. Pearce MJ, Hawton K: Psychological and sexual aspects of menopause and HRT, *Baillieres Clin Obstet Gynecol* 10(3):385, 1996.

17a. Rako S. Testosterone deficiency and supplementation for women: matters of sexual health, *Psychiatric Ann* 29(1):23-26, 1999.

18. Rosen RC, Lane R, Menza M: Effects of SSRI on sexual dysfunction: a critical review, *J Clin Psychopharmacol* 19(1):67, 1999.

18a. Rosen RC, Phillips NA, Gendrana N: Oral phentolamine and female sexual arousal disorder: a pilot study, *J Sex Marital Ther* 25:137-144, 1999.

19. Sarrel PM: Ovarian hormones and vaginal blood flow using laser Doppler velocimetry to measure effects in a clinical trial of post-menopausal women, *Int J Impot Res* 10:S91, 1998.

20. Schiavi RC, Segraves RT: The biology of sexual function, *Psychiatr Clin North Am* 18:7, 1995.

21. Sherwin BB, Gelfand MM: The role of androgen in the maintenance of sexual functioning in oophorectomized women, *Psychosom Med* 49:397, 1987.

22. Sipski ML, Alexander CJ, Rosen RC: Sexual response in women with spinal cord injuries: implications for our understanding of the able-bodied, *J Sex Marital Therap* 25:11, 1999.

22a. Sipski ML, Rosen RC, Alexander CJ, et al: Sildenafil effects on sexual and cardiovascular responses in women with spinal cord injury, *Urology* 55(6):812-815, 2000.

22b. Sjoberg I: Morphological, functional and etiological aspects, *Acta Obstet Gynecol Scand* 71-84, 1992.

23. Spector I, Carey M: Incidence and prevalence of the sexual dysfunction: a critical review of the empirical literature, *Arch Sex Behav* 19:389, 1990.

24. Tarcan T, Park K, Goldstein I, et al: Histomorphometric analysis of age-related structural changes in human clitoral cavernosal tissue, *J Urol* 161(3):940, 1999.

CHAPTER 155

Testicular Disorders and Disorders of the Scrotal Contents

Grannum R. Sant
Kenneth A. Kingsly

Diseases of the scrotum and its contents usually lead affected individuals to seek medical attention. Most scrotal conditions are benign and self-limiting, although malignant testicular tumors can be life-threatening. The clinician evaluating scrotal lesions should differentiate benign from malignant diseases, pursue an efficient cost-effective diagnostic evaluation, and initiate prompt and appropriate urologic referral.

Pain and swelling are the cardinal symptoms of scrotal disease: congenital or acquired, benign or malignant. Accurate diagnosis requires a careful history and a structured physical examination, including urinalysis. Radiologic studies such as scrotal ultrasonography, radionuclide studies, and Doppler blood flow studies are performed in selected patients with uncertain diagnosis.

ANATOMY AND PHYSICAL EXAMINATION

The scrotum is partitioned into two sacs, each containing a testis, epididymis, and the lower portion of the spermatic cord. The scrotal wall consists of skin, dartos muscle, and several fascial layers.[7]

Examination of the scrotum is best performed with the patient standing. A warm room and warm examining hands are encouraged because cold temperatures cause contraction of the dartos and cremaster muscles and elevation of the testis toward the external inguinal ring. The left testis usually lies lower than the right, and the scrotal sac is hypoplastic when its gonad is absent. Palpation is carried out by systemically examining the testis, epididymis, and cord for size, consistency, and other factors (Fig. 155-1). The epididymis is adherent to the posterolateral aspect of the testis, and the spermatic cord is palpable in the upper portion of the scrotum. Fig. 155-2 illustrates common epididymal abnormalities.

Scrotal masses should be evaluated by careful palpation (Box 155-1 and Fig. 155-3). The exact nature and location of the mass should be noted. Is it hard and firm or cystic and fluid filled? Does it arise from the testis or the other intrascrotal structures? Does it change with straining or Valsalva's maneuver? When transilluminated, fluid-filled structures (e.g., hydroceles) radiate a reddish glow. Tables 155-1 and 155-2 outline the physical signs and symptoms of mass lesions of the scrotum and the common causes of scrotal swelling.

INFLAMMATORY DISEASES

Fungal skin diseases are treated with topical or systemic fungicides and furuncles. Minor lacerations of the scrotum are treated as they would be elsewhere in the body.

Purulent fistulous drainage in the scrotum requires prompt management. Causes include urethral stricture with formation of urethrocutaneous fistulas, tuberculosis, or syphilis of the testis or epididymitis with abscess formation and fistulization. Pus should be examined and cultured for acid-fast bacilli and spirochetes. Scrotal fistulas require surgical drainage. Fistulas from inflammatory bowel diseases (e.g., Crohn's disease) may occur in the perineoscrotal area.

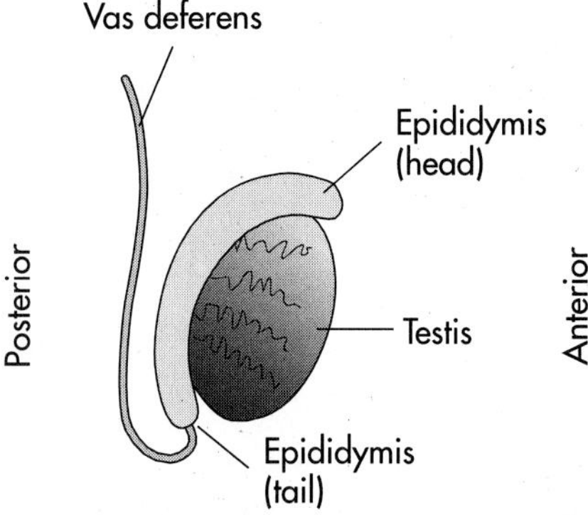

Fig. 155-1. Lateral view of the right testis, epididymis, and vas deferens. (From Krane RJ, Siroky MB, Fitzpatrick JM, editors: *Clinical urology,* Philadelphia, 1994, JB Lippincott.)

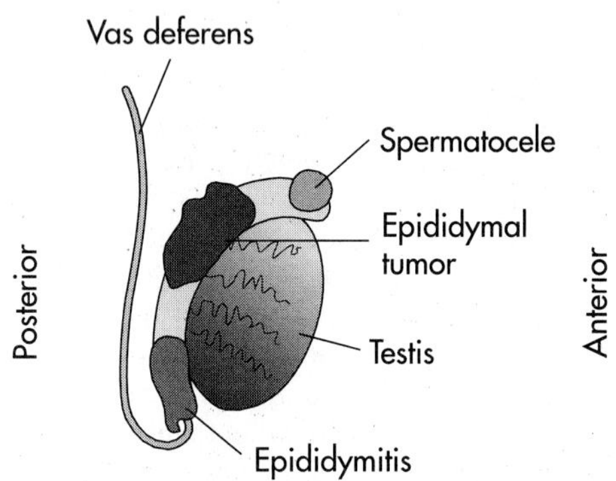

Fig. 155-2. Various abnormalities of the epididymis, including spermatocele, epididymal tumor, and epididymitis. (From Krane RJ, Siroky MB, Fitzpatrick JM, editors: *Clinical urology,* Philadelphia, 1994, JB Lippincott.)

Fournier's Gangrene

Fournier's gangrene, an uncommon but potentially life-threatening infection of the scrotal, perineal, and inguinal areas, can be a urologic emergency. It causes tissue and fascial necrosis (necrotizing fasciitis) and is usually secondary to perirectal, ischiorectal, or periurethral infection. Initially, erythema and edema of the scrotum and a small patch of dry gangrene develop. Gangrene may then extend rapidly along fascial planes into the lower abdominal wall, especially in diabetic and immunocompromised patients. A complete blood count, platelet count, and Gram's stain with cultures (aerobic and anaerobic) of the gangrenous area are performed.

Prompt treatment of suspected Fournier's gangrene is mandatory because patients require hospitalization, intravenous (IV) antibiotic therapy, close monitoring and observation, and early, aggressive, urgent surgical debridement. Combination antibiotic therapy (high-dose penicillin, gentamicin, and clindamycin) is indicated until the causative

Box 155-1. "Structured" Physical Examination of the Scrotum

Cystic or solid
Tender or nontender
Confined to scrotum or extending into inguinal region
Anatomic position
- Testis, spermatic cord
- Epididymis
- Surrounding testis (hydrocele)
- Inguinoscrotal (hernias, hydroceles)

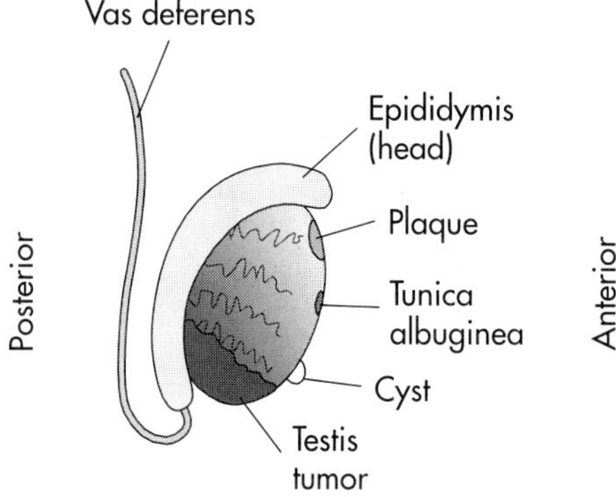

Fig. 155-3. Intratesticular abnormalities, including testis tumor, fibrous plaque, and cyst of the tunica albuginea. (From Krane RJ, Siroky MB, Fitzpatrick JM, editors: *Clinical urology*, Philadelphia, 1994, JB Lippincott.)

Table 155-1. Common Intrascrotal Conditions

	Testicular torsion	Epididymitis	Testis tumor	Appendiceal torsion
Age	Neonate to early 20s	Childhood to old age	15 to 35 years	Prepubertal
Onset	Acute	Insidious	Gradual	Subacute
Degree of pain	Severe	Variable	Absent or mild	Variable
Urinalysis	Negative	Pyuria, bacteruria	Normal	Negative
Cremasteric reflex	Negative	Positive	Positive	Positive
Treatment	Surgical exploration	Antibiotics	Orchiectomy	Bed rest/surgery

organism or organisms are identified. Fournier's gangrene is associated with significant mortality in elderly, diabetic, or immunocompromised patients.

Epididymitis

Epididymitis, a common condition in younger men, is usually unilateral and is associated with "scrotal heaviness." Some men have urethral discharge or symptoms of urinary tract infection, and others develop pyrexia, chills, and malaise. A severely inflamed and indurated epididymis may be indistinguishable from the testis, and this can lead to difficulty in differentiating epididymitis from testicular torsion and testicular tumor.

Epididymitis is caused by infection from bladder urine, prostate infection, or an ascending urethral infection that spreads via the ejaculatory duct into the epididymis. In men under 35 years of age, epididymitis is usually chlamydial in origin and is associated with symptoms of urethritis (e.g., urethral discharge). In men over 35 years of age, infection is usually due to coliform organisms.[6] Signs and symptoms of cystitis, prostatitis, or prostatism are common. "Sterile" epididymitis associated with vigorous physical activity can be caused by vasal reflux of sterile urine and chemical inflammation of the epididymis. In boys, epididymitis may be the presenting feature of congenital urologic abnormalities (e.g., ectopic ureter, posterior urethral valves). Evaluation with IV urography, cystourethroscopy, and voiding cystourethrography is indicated in boys with epididymitis. Careful clinical and radiologic evaluation may be needed to distinguish epididymitis from testicular torsion.

Table 155-2. Causes of Scrotal Swelling

Structure	Pathology
Scrotal wall	Urinary extravasation
	Trauma
	Edema from cardiac, hepatic, or renal failure
	Fungal infection
Testis	Carcinoma
	Torsion of testis or appendix testis
	Infection
Epididymis	Infection
	Tumors (usually benign)
	Torsion of appendix epididymis
Spermatic cord	Hydrocele
	Hematocele
	Hernia
	Varicocele
	Lipoma of cord
	Spermatocele

The epididymis lies posterior to the testis, and this demarcation is preserved in all but the most severe cases of epididymitis. A "reactive" hydrocele may make palpation of the intrascrotal structures difficult. Transillumination usually confirms the presence of hydroceles, although ultrasonography is more accurate and may be needed for confirmation. When in doubt, surgical exploration is required to exclude torsion and should be done within 4 to 6 hours to preserve testicular viability.

Epididymitis from syphilis, gonorrhea, or tuberculosis is uncommon (Box 155-2). "Chronic" epididymitis may follow acute epididymitis. However, this diagnosis most frequently represents mild, chronic, nonspecific (i.e., noninfectious) epididymitis associated with dull scrotal ache and mild induration of the epididymis. Tuberculosis epididymitis has reemerged as a health care problem in the increasing number of immunosuppressed men with acquired immunodeficiency syndrome.

Epididymitis is usually treated on an outpatient basis with scrotal elevation, bed rest, and appropriate antibiotics. Patients with leukocytosis and high fevers may require hospitalization for parenteral antibiotics and vigorous supportive treatment. Nonsteroidal antiinflammatory drugs (e.g., ibuprofen) and antipyretics (e.g., acetaminophen, aspirin) are usually prescribed. Severe pain may necessitate spermatic cord anesthetic block.

In younger men, epididymitis is usually caused by *Neisseria gonorrhoeae* or *Chlamydia trachomatis*. A Gram's stain of the urethral discharge may reveal the characteristic gram-negative intracellular diplococci of gonococcal urethritis. Gonococcal epididymitis is much less common, however, than chlamydial epididymitis. Nongonococcal urethritis is usually treated with doxycycline (Vibramycin), 100 mg orally twice a day, or minocycline (Minocin), 100 mg twice a day for 10 to 14 days. In older men with pyuria and bacteriuria, third-generation quinolones such as ciprofloxacin (Cipro), 500 mg twice a day, or trimethoprim-sulfamethoxazole (Septra, Bactrim), one double-strength tablet twice a day for 10 days, are recommended. The newer fluoroquinolones (e.g., ofloxacin, levofloxacin) also merit consideration. Antimicrobial therapy should be continued for 4 weeks if bacterial prostatitis is suspected. Hospitalized patients require parenteral antibiotic therapy (e.g., an aminoglycoside or a cephalosporin) before they are switched to oral antibiotics. The fluoroquinolones can obviate the need for parenteral antibiotics because of their broad-spectrum activity and the high tissue levels achieved after oral administration (see Box 155-2).

Most patients feel better within 48 hours, but swelling and discomfort may persist for weeks or months. Persistent fever despite suitable antimicrobial therapy suggests abscess formation and is an indication for ultrasound evaluation. Surgical drainage, epididymal orchiectomy, or both, treatments are required for abscesses. Epididymitis can be complicated by testicular necrosis, testicular atrophy, or infertility. Chronic inflammation and fibrosis can block the ductal cord structures and impair sperm production, especially in severe bilateral epididymitis. Swelling and edema may compromise blood flow and cause testicular atrophy. A urologist should be consulted when there is concern regarding the diagnosis of testicular torsion vs. epididymitis or testicular cancer (Box 155-3).

Box 155-2. Epididymitis

Types

"Sterile" (noninfectious)
Infectious (chlamydia, coliform bacteria)
- Acute
- Chronic (tuberculosis, syphilis)

Physical Examination

Tender enlarged epididymis posterior to testis
Associated orchitis (minority)

Clinical Groups

Age <35 years
- Chlamydial etiology
- Signs and symptoms of urethritis
- Pyuria
- Treatment with doxycycline/minocycline/fluoroquinolones

Age >35 years
- Enterobacteriaceae
- Signs and symptoms of cystitis/prostatitis
- Pyuria, bacteriuria
- Positive urine culture
- Treatment with trimethoprim-sulfamethoxazole (TMP-SMX), fluoroquinolones

Box 155-3. Managed Care Guide: Epididymitis

Presentation

Common

Scrotal pain
Swelling (usually unilateral)

Uncommon

Urethral discharge
Fever, chills

Baseline Information Required (History, Screens, etc.)

Duration symptoms
History trauma
Medical conditions—diabetes, immunosuppression
History instrumentation—Foley catheter, cystoscopy

Recommended Laboratory Tests/Diagnostic Procedures

Urinalysis, urine culture
Digital rectal examination
Urethral swab for Gram's stain
Scrotal ultrasound
Intravenous pyelography, voiding cystourethrography in selected cases (boys, elderly men)

Approximate Duration of Care

10-14 days

Frequency of Follow-Up

1 month

Indications for Consultation/Referral

Abscess formation
Lack of response to therapy
Doubtful diagnosis

Comments

Testicular tumor must not be misdiagnosed as epididymitis.

BENIGN SCROTAL MASSES

Most scrotal masses are benign and due to inflammation, trauma, and congenital defects. Testicular tumors, however, must be included in the differential diagnosis of all scrotal masses.[4]

Hydrocele and Spermatocele

Hydroceles and spermatoceles are common paratesticular lesions caused by fluid accumulation. A *hydrocele* is an abnormal collection of fluid between the tunical layers and is congenital or acquired. Congenital or pediatric hydroceles are found in approximately 10% of boys and result from nonclosure of the processus vaginalis during embryologic testicular descent. Congenital hydroceles vary in size during the day, becoming larger with fluid accumulation, and most resolve by 1 year of age. Surgical treatment is indicated for persistent hydroceles beyond this age. Acquired "reactive" hydroceles are secondary to intrascrotal infection, regional or systemic disease, inguinal or scrotal surgery, trauma, or neoplasm.

Adult hydroceles are usually asymptomatic and enlarge slowly or remain unchanged. Occasionally, a pulling or dragging sensation is associated with large hydroceles. The hydrocele is a nontender, cystic, transilluminating mass that lies anterior to the testis. If the underlying testis cannot be palpated because of the size of the fluid-filled mass, a scrotal ultrasound should be performed to exclude a testicular tumor.

A *spermatocele* is a cystic dilation of the epididymis that frequently involves the upper pole or epididymal head. It is usually small and painless and may follow an episode of epididymitis. Physical examination reveals a transilluminating cystic mass located above and separate from the testis. The cyst fluid contains dead spermatozoa in retention cysts. Ultrasonography easily differentiates spermatoceles from hydroceles and other testicular lesions.

Surgical treatment of hydroceles and spermatoceles is reserved for men with pain and discomfort or lesions that are cosmetically embarrassing. Aspiration and sclerotherapy are useful nonsurgical treatment modalities in small to moderate-sized lesions. Sclerotherapy is successful in 80% to 90% of patients, but multiple treatments may be necessary. Surgery is indicated for large hydroceles and spermatoceles, and a variety of techniques (e.g., excision, exertion) are available.

Varicocele

A varicocele can be easily recognized by the presence of spermatic cord or scrotal enlargement caused by dilation of the pampiniform venous plexus. The exact etiology of varicoceles is unknown, although valvular incompetence is common. Clinically obvious varicoceles present as a "bag of worms" in the spermatic cord and are more prominent when the patient stands. The incidence of varicoceles in healthy males is approximately 20%, and the left side is involved in more than 80% (Box 155-4).

Varicoceles occasionally cause scrotal pain and heaviness, especially if large. Varicoceles are the most common surgically correctable cause of male infertility, occurring in 30% of infertile men. Infertile men with varicoceles are oligospermic (have low sperm counts) with "a stress pattern" of reduced sperm motility and abnormal morphology.

Ipsilateral testicular atrophy may occur with varicoceles. Size is best assessed by ultrasound or calibrated orchidometers. The exact role of the varicocele in male subfertility has not been clearly ascertained, although an elevated scrotal temperature and reflux of adrenal metabolites (e.g., steroids) may contribute to the pathogenesis.

Asymptomatic men without a history of infertility should be observed. For patients with concomitant testicular atrophy (especially young boys), infertility, or both conditions, various treatment modalities are available.[3] Several techniques, including retroperitoneal, inguinal, laparoscopic, or scrotal, may be used for surgical ligation of the spermatic vein. Nonsurgical treatment can be achieved by percutaneous spermatic vein embolization. However, a skilled interventional radiologist is needed, and a small radiation risk exists. Improvement in semen parameters (improved motility and number of sperm) occurs in 50% to 60% of patients, with successful pregnancy in 30% to 40% of patients' significant others.

BENIGN TUMORS OF THE TESTIS AND EPIDIDYMIS

Benign tumors of the testis are rare (Box 155-5) and can be diagnosed by ultrasound evaluation. Scrotal exploration, when indicated, ascertains the diagnosis. Paratesticular masses account for 7% of all intrascrotal tumors, with 60% to 70% originating in the spermatic cord and the remainder in

Box 155-4. Varicoceles

Features

Present in 15% of healthy, fertile men
Associated with:
- Infertility (80%)
- Pain (20%)

Most common treatable cause of male infertility
Dilated pampiniform venous plexus in spermatic cord

Diagnosis

Palpation (standing position, Valsalva's maneuver)
Ultrasound (>3-mm vein diameter)
Semen analysis ("stress" pattern: low count, low motility)

Treatment

Radiologic embolization
Surgical division of spermatic vein
Transperitoneal laparoscopic ligation

Results

Semen improvement in 60%-70%
Pregnancy in 30%-40%

Box 155-5. Benign Solid Intrascrotal Tumors

Cord lipoma
Adenomatoid tumor (spermatic cord)
Cystadenoma of epididymis
Fibrous pseudotumors
Testicular cysts

the epididymis. The most common paratesticular mass is a benign cord lipoma, which accounts for approximately 25% of all cord tumors. Cord lipomas arise from preperitoneal fat remnants in the spermatic cord.

Intratesticular epidermoid cysts can be confused with malignant testicular lesions on physical examination. These rare lesions can be confidently diagnosed by scrotal ultrasound. A common finding on physical examination or testicular self-examination (TSE) is tunical cysts or calcifications on the surface of the tunica albuginea of the testis. These lesions are nonmalignant, and their etiology is uncertain. Ultrasound is diagnostic, and surgical exploration can usually be avoided.

MALIGNANT TUMORS OF THE TESTIS

Testicular cancer is the most frequent cancer in young men (15 to 35 years of age) and is rare in African-Americans. Cryptorchidism is a well-known risk factor even after orchiopexy. Testicular tumors usually present as painless lumps, but some men (20% to 25%) develop scrotal pain as a result of bleeding caused by rapid tumor growth and necrosis. Most tumors are discovered as hard testicular lumps during TSE. Gynecomastia is an unusual manifestation associated with chorionic gonadotropin or estrogen production. Occasionally, patients may present with metastatic disease (e.g., retroperitoneal, mediastinal, and supraclavicular lymphadenectomy or pulmonary metastases). Unfortunately, a painful testicular tumor can be misdiagnosed as epididymitis, leading to delayed diagnosis with the risk of advanced disease and a poor prognosis.

Diagnosis and Staging

Physical examination usually reveals a hard testicular lump. "Reactive" hydrocele may make palpation of the lesion difficult. The testicular tumor may be small (e.g., a choriocarcinoma) and not easily palpable through the thick, overlying tunica albuginea. Scrotal ultrasound is an excellent imaging modality for the assessment of testicular masses. Testicular microcalcifications are associated with a high propensity for developing seminomas, and patients should be screened by ultrasound every 6 months. Testicular cancers are typically nonhomogenous with hypoechoic areas on ultrasound (Fig. 155-4).

Lymphatic spread of testicular tumors is predictable. The "first-echelon" nodes are the paraaortic and paracaval nodes at the level of the renal vessels. The primary drainage area of right-sided tumors is the interaortocaval nodes, and left-sided cancers spread initially to the left paraaortic nodal area. This is explained by the embryologic descent of the testis and vascular and lymphatic vessels from the abdomen into the scrotum. Avoidance of scrotal skin violation is mandatory when treating testicular tumors. The scrotal skin lymphatics drain into the inguinal nodes, and violation leads to nonretroperitoneal lymphatic tumor dissemination. Transscrotal needle biopsy or orchiectomy is therefore contraindicated. Suspected testicular tumors should be explored via an inguinal incision with early control of the spermatic cord to prevent vascular or lymphatic dissemination of tumor cells.

Tumor markers are helpful in the diagnosis, staging, and management of malignant testicular tumors. α-Fetoprotein (α-FP) and the β-subunit of human chorionic gonadotropin (β-hCG) are the clinically useful markers. α-FP is often associated with embryonal carcinoma, whereas β-hCG ele-

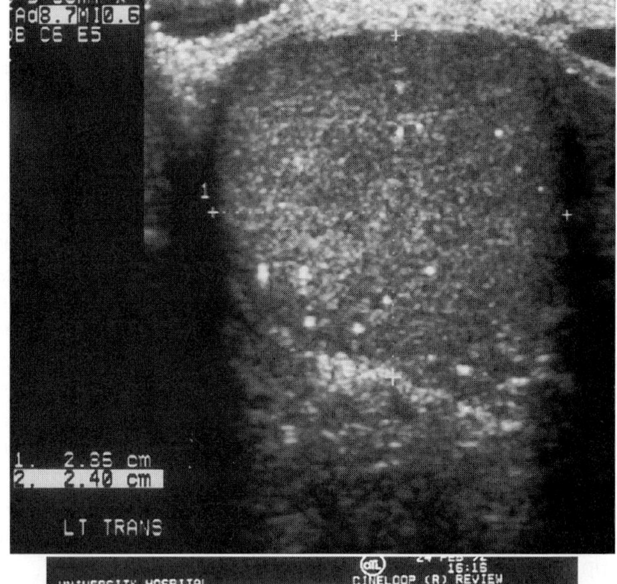

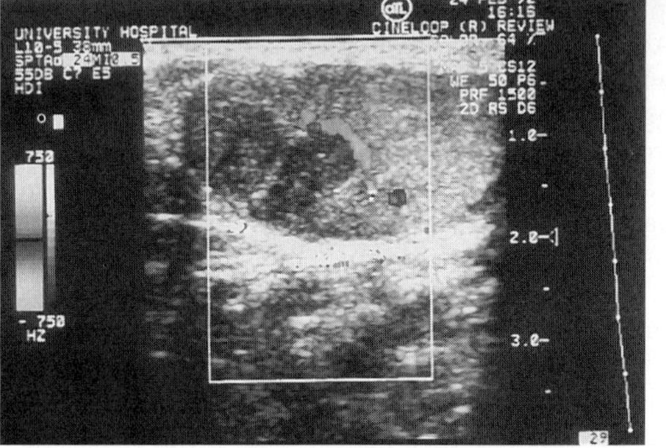

Fig. 155-4. **A,** Microcalcifications visualized on an ultrasound of the testis. This condition is often a premalignant sign of seminoma and requires ultrasound screening at 6-month to 1-year intervals. **B,** Seminoma of testis noted on ultrasound and by color Doppler.

vations occur with choriocarcinoma. However, many testicular cancers are of mixed germ cell origin (e.g., seminoma, embryonal cell carcinoma, choriocarcinoma, teratoma), and tumor marker elevation is variable. Persistent tumor marker elevation after "radical" inguinal orchiectomy suggests the presence of metastatic disease. However, there is a 25% false-negative marker elevation rate. Thus serum tumor markers are not completely reliable for staging, especially when their levels are normal.

Computed tomography (CT) scanning and chest x-ray studies are used for staging (Box 155-6). A false-negative rate of 20% to 25% occurs in the presence of nonenlarged (smaller than 1.5 cm) but microscopically involved retroperitoneal nodes. Stage A disease is confined to the testis, whereas stage B disease is associated with retroperitoneal lymphatic metastases below the diaphragm but an absence of visceral metastases. Stage B is subdivided into B1, B2, and B3 stages according to tumor extent (B1 smaller than 5 cm, B2 larger than 5 cm, B3 smaller than 10 cm). Stage C disease indicates metastases (usually visceral) beyond the retroperitoneum.

Histology

Most testicular tumors are of germ cell origin—seminoma, embryonal cell carcinoma, teratoma, and choriocarcinoma—

Box 155-6. Initial Approach to Testicular Cancer

Step 1

Suspicion on physical examination
Confirmation by scrotal ultrasound (optional)
Serum tumor markers (α-FP, β-hCG)
Chest x-ray study

Step 2

Inguinal exploration
"Radical" inguinal orchiectomy
Histologic examination
- Pure, "mixed" tumor
- Vascular space invasion (lymphatic)
- Extension into epididymis, cord

Step 3

Staging
- Abdominal computed tomography scan
- α-FP and β-hCG levels

Treatment selection
- Seminoma vs. nonseminoma
- Surgery vs. chemotherapy vs. radiation
- Surveillance protocol (selected patients)

but 40% are "mixed," containing more than one cell type. Choriocarcinoma is the most aggressive testicular cancer, with a propensity for rapid growth and early hematogenous spread.

Non–germ cell testicular tumors are rare and usually benign. Interstitial cell (Leydig's cell) tumors in prepubertal male patients may secrete androgens and estrogens and cause gynecomastia. Sertoli's cell tumors are extremely rare. The testis can be the site of metastatic spread from other primary tumors (e.g., lymphoma, leukemia, and lung, prostate, and gastrointestinal cancers).

Treatment

Whenever a testicular tumor is suspected on physical examination, the next step is confirmation of the diagnosis by orchiectomy. Inguinal exploration with ligation of the spermatic cord at the level of the internal inguinal ring is recommended. Serum tumor markers (α-FP, β-hCG) and a chest x-ray study are obtained before surgical exploration.

Further treatment is based on histologic assessment of the tumor and staging (Box 155-7). Microscopic examination identifies tumor type (pure or mixed), tumor extent (involvement of epididymis or spermatic cord), and vascular space (lymphatic and venous) tumor invasion (Box 155-8).

Nonseminomatous Germ Cell Tumors

Stage A nonseminomatous germ cell tumors are treated by modified, unilateral lymphadenectomy, which spares the sympathetic chain and preserves ejaculation (see Box 155-7). If the nodes are negative, further therapy is unnecessary, and cure rates approach 95%. Recent improvements in chemotherapy for metastatic disease have led to the emergence of surveillance protocols for selected patients with stage A disease (i.e., those with negative tumor markers, normal abdominal CT scans, and lack of vascular space invasion). However, strict selection and meticulous clinical and radiologic follow-up are needed. The overall tumor relapse rate with surveillance protocols is 20% to 30%.

Box 155-7. Treatment of Testicular Cancer: Stage and Cell Type

Clinical Stage A

Seminoma
- External beam radiation to the retroperitoneum

Nonseminomas
- Retroperitoneal lymphadenectomy
  - Chemotherapy if nodes or markers are positive (20%)
- Surveillance protocols
  - Meticulous follow-up (markers, CT, chest x-ray studies)
  - Chemotherapy for relapses (20%)

Clinical Stages B and C

Seminoma, nonseminoma
Combination-drug chemotherapy
- Salvage lymphadenectomy for nonseminomas

Box 155-8. Managed Care Guide: Testicular Cancer

Presentation

Common

Scrotal mass or lump

Uncommon

Scrotal pain
Pulmonary/retroperitoneal metastases

Baseline Information Required (History, Screens, etc.)

History of trauma

Recommended Laboratory Tests/Diagnostic Procedures

Chest x-ray study
Tumor markers (α-FP, β-hCG)
Scrotal ultrasound
Radical inguinal orchiectomy

Approximate Duration of Care

Variable

Frequency of Follow-up

Every 1-3 months

Indications for Consultation/Referral

All testicular masses

Comments

Early diagnosis is the key to successful treatment.
Testicular cancer should not be confused with epididymitis or testis torsion.

Microscopic lymph node involvement or tumor marker elevation after lymphadenectomy are indications for multidrug combination chemotherapy with vinblastine, bleomycin, and cisplatin. Cure rates for stage B and C testicular tumors exceed those for any other human solid-organ neoplasm. Five-year survival rates in excess of 90% are now achievable. The keys to the optimistic outlook in nonseminomatous testis cancer are early diagnosis, prompt inguinal orchiectomy, modified retroperitoneal lymphadenectomy, and combination chemotherapy.

Seminomas

The usual treatment for testicular seminoma is "radical" inguinal orchiectomy and external beam radiation to the retroperitoneum (see Box 155-6). Pure seminomas are exquisitely radiosensitive. Patients with stage A seminoma undergo postorchiectomy radiation to the paraaortic and ipsilateral iliac nodes. Patients with stage B disease receive additional "boosts" to involved areas and prophylactic radiation to the mediastinal and supraclavicular nodes. Radiation therapy is less effective in "bulky" stage B or C

Box 155-9. Differential Diagnosis of Scrotal Pain

- Torsion
  - Appendages
  - Spermatic cord
- Infection
  - Orchitis (mumps)
  - Abscess
  - Epididymitis
- Neoplasia
  - Benign
  - Malignant
- Incarcerated hernia
- Trauma
- Hydrocele
- Spermatocele
- Varicocele

Box 155-10. Testicular Torsion

Surgical emergency
Common in pubertal boys and adolescents
Ischemia >6 hours irreversible
When in doubt, exploration indicated
Doppler/radionuclide studies in selected cases
Early manual detorsion
Exploration with orchiopexy/orchiectomy

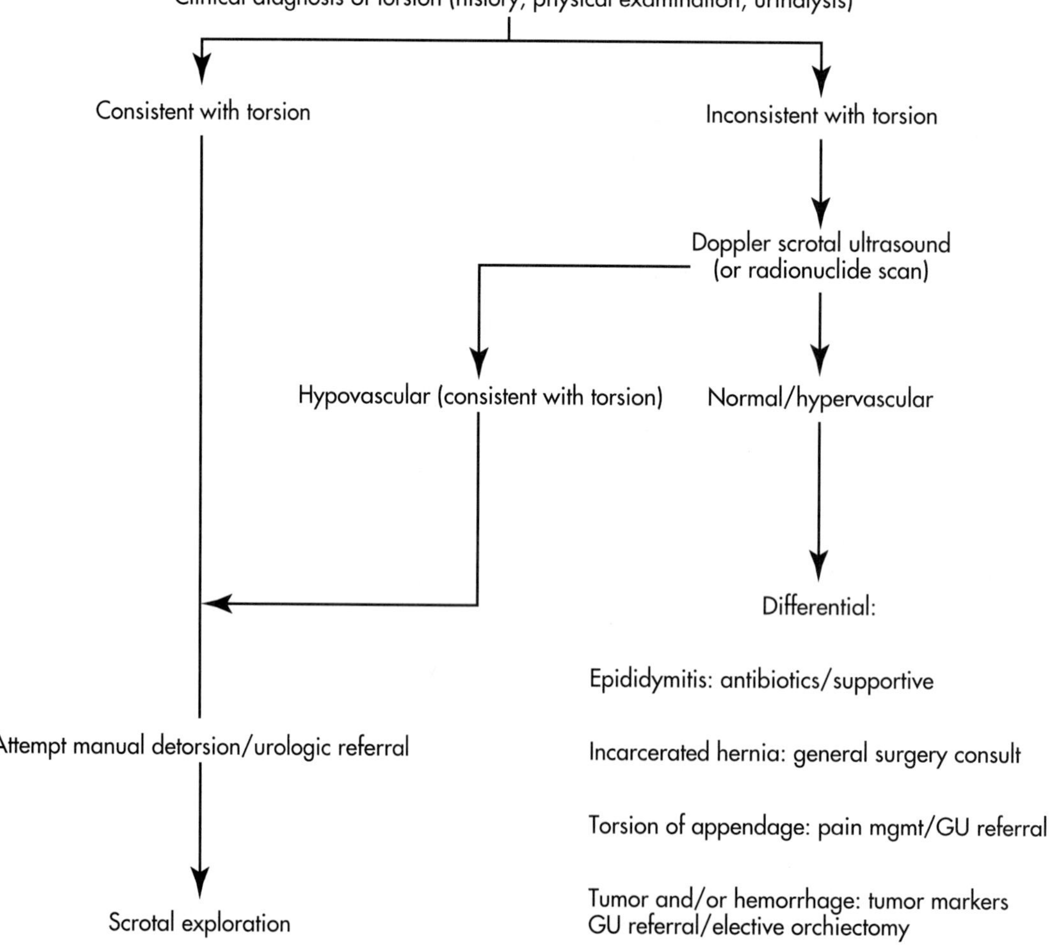

Fig. 155-5. Acute scrotum: management algorithm.

disease. The success of combination chemotherapy for nonseminomatous germ cell tumors has led to its use for the treatment of "bulky" seminomas (i.e., stages B and C).

ACUTE SCROTUM

Testicular pain should always be considered an emergency.[2] Evaluation should not be delayed if testicular damage from torsion of the spermatic cord and subsequent ischemia are to be avoided.[5] Box 155-9 outlines the differential diagnosis of scrotal pain. Differentiation between testicular torsion and epididymitis is usually possible on the basis of the presentation and physical findings (see Box 155-1).

Testicular torsion is a surgical emergency (Box 155-10). Testicular loss can be avoided only by prompt diagnosis and early treatment (either manual or surgical detorsion). Torsion, a disease mainly of adolescents and young adults, can be confused with epididymitis, especially in postpubertal boys. A teenager with a sudden onset of scrotal pain and a normal urinalysis most likely has testicular torsion. Unrelieved torsion (longer than 6 hours) leads to testicular ischemia and atrophy, and early treatment is therefore imperative.[1] Some 90% of testicular torsions occur in patients younger than 30 years of age.

A delay in the diagnosis of testicular torsion beyond 12 hours causes progressive testicular ischemia and irreversible damage. A technique for early manual detorsion of the spermatic cord is available. Under IV sedation, detorsion can be performed in the emergency department by rotating the testis toward the respective thigh for approximately 1½ turns. Relief of pain can be dramatic, and return of testicular blood flow can be documented by color Doppler ultrasound.

Testicular torsion can be confirmed by Doppler ultrasound (greater than 90% sensitive, 70% specific) and nuclear scanning (greater than 90% sensitive, 80% specific). However, if any doubt exists, scrotal exploration and detorsion should be performed. A management algorithm for the acute scrotum is outlined in Fig. 155-5. The common anatomic defect in testes that undergo torsion is high "investment" (or attachment) of the tunica vaginalis—the so-called bell-clapper deformity (Fig. 155-6). This inherited defect is usually bilateral, and detorsion should always be followed by testicular fixation (orchiopexy) of the affected gonad as well as its contralateral mate.

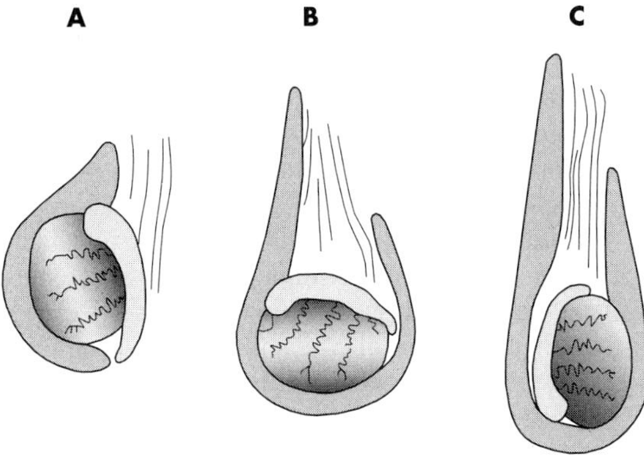

Fig. 155-6. Attachment of the testicular mesentery to the testis. **A,** Normal peritoneal disposition around the testis. **B,** Capacious tunica vaginalis surrounding the cord; the testis lies horizontally. **C,** Inverted testis, which most easily twists because of its narrow attachment, the bell-clapper deformity. (From Krane RJ, Siroky MB, Fitzpatrick JM, editors: *Clinical urology,* Philadelphia, 1994, JB Lippincott.)

If, after intraoperative detorsion, the testis remains dusky and cyanotic, irreversible ischemia is probable, and an orchiectomy is indicated. Torsion of an appendix testis or an acutely incarcerated scrotal hernia may mimic the symptoms of testicular torsion. Torsion of the appendix testis can be diagnosed by the presence of localized pain in the upper pole of the testis and the presence of a "blue dot" on transillumination; this blue dot is caused by the ischemic appendage seen through the skin. An incarcerated hernia causes thickening of the spermatic cord and is associated with peritoneal signs of intestinal obstruction (Box 155-11).

SCROTAL TRAUMA

Penetrating gunshot or knife wounds can involve the scrotum. Emergency surgical debridement and exploration are required for hemostasis and testicular repair, if indicated. Severe blunt injuries of the scrotum may cause testicular dislocation or rupture. Palpation and examination of the scrotum are extremely painful, and ultrasound imaging can be misleading. Surgical exploration with repair or orchiectomy is indicated.

Minor trauma can cause scrotal pain or hematoma formation. Testicular tumors are more likely to bleed after minor trauma compared with normal testes. Occasionally, a

Box 155-11. Managed Care Guide: Testicular Torsion

Presentation

Common

Scrotal pain (usually acute)
Swelling

Uncommon

Nausea
Vomiting
Fever

Baseline Information Required (History, Screens, etc.)

History of trauma
Prior history of scrotal pain

Recommended Laboratory Tests/Diagnostic Procedures

Urine culture
Attempt early manual detorsion
Scrotal ultrasound
Doppler imaging } in selected patients
Radionuclide studies }

Approximate Duration of Care

Detorsion within 6 hours

Frequency of Follow-up

Variable

Indications for Consultation/Referral

Refer on initial suspicion

Comments

Early diagnosis is the key to testicular and fertility preservation.

testicular tumor may present in this manner, with the degree of trauma not being commensurate with the degree of pain or hematoma formation.

CRYPTORCHIDISM

The absence of the testis in the scrotum warrants a careful search for the missing gonad by palpation of the upper scrotum and groin. Testicular maldescent or cryptorchidism is common, affecting 0.8% of all males. Surgical repositioning of a cryptorchid testis is recommended in the pediatric age group. However, patients who have not undergone such a procedure and still have a malpositioned testis should undergo removal of that gonad because of the high incidence of testicular tumors (usually seminomas) in cryptorchid testes (8% to 10%). If no testis is found on physical examination, surgical exploration is indicated. Transabdominal laparoscopic evaluation of patients with nonpalpable testes is now the recommended modality for localization of cryptorchid testis. Testicular absence can be confirmed and first-stage orchidopexy performed if intraabdominal testes are discovered.

Atrophy of the testis may result from neonatal torsion or prior injury. Surgical removal of the testis is not mandatory. However, associated masses or abnormalities should be excluded by scrotal ultrasound. A number of patients have compensatory, contralateral testicular hypertrophy.

REFERENCES

1. Bartsch G, Mikuz G, et al: Testicular torsion. In Resnick MI, Kursh ED, editors: *Current therapy in genitourinary surgery,* Philadelphia, 1992, BC Decker, pp 436-440.
2. Galejs LE, Kass EJ: Diagosis and treatment of the acute scrotum, *Am Fam Physician* 59(4):817, 1999.
3. Kass EJ: Pediatric varicocele. In O'Donnell B, Koff SA, editors: *Pediatric urology,* ed 3, Oxford, England, 1997, Butterworth-Heinemann, pp 608-615.
4. Kogan SA: Acute and chronic scrotal swellings. In Gillenwater JY, et al, editors: *Adult and pediatric urology,* ed 2, St Louis, 1999, Mosby, pp 2189-2215.
5. Lewis AG, Bukowski TP, Jarvis PD, et al: Evaluation of acute scrotum in the emergency department, *J Pediatr Surg* 30:277, 1995.
6. Meares EM: Nonspecific infections of the genitourinary tract. In Tanagho EA, McAninch JW, editors: *Smith's general urology,* ed 14, Norwalk, Conn, 1995, Appleton & Lange, pp 237-238.
7. Rowland RG, Donohue JP: Scrotum and testis. In Gillenwater JY et al, editors: *Adult and pediatric urology,* ed 2, St Louis, 1991, Mosby.

XII NEUROLOGY

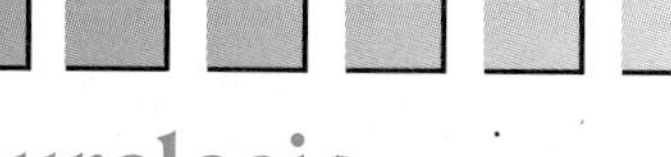

CHAPTER 156

Relevant Neurologic Problems in Primary Care

T. Jock Murray

Neurologic problems are frequent in daily primary care practice. About 10% of patients consulting a primary care physician have a neurologic symptom and 1% to 2% of such complaints result in a definite neurologic diagnosis. Most patients can be effectively managed by the general physician; others can be managed with a single neurologic consultation for advice on diagnosis or management, and only a few require ongoing management by a neurologic consultant. This presupposes that the general physician has knowledge of some basic concepts about the nervous system, has an effective and efficient neurologic examination that is used routinely, and has an understanding of the common, emergent, and treatable neurologic conditions. The following chapters focus on these conditions.

Most primary care physicians manage neurologic patients well, but studies have shown that they may lack confidence in the neurologic examination, the interpretation of the results of the examination, or determinations of which investigations are necessary.[1,2] In these studies, when the physician was not confident of the assessment, the outcome was not usually referral to a neurologist but a tendency to dismiss the patient as quickly as possible. The physicians in such instances indicated they did not like diagnosing and treating neurologic conditions. Developing competence in the assessment and management of common and treatable neurologic conditions leads to a positive attitude about a very interesting and rewarding aspect of primary care medicine.[3,4]

The primary care physician should have competence in the following four areas:

1. Background concepts and knowledge of the nervous system that allow understanding and localization of neurologic disorders
2. Appropriate attitudes toward people with neurologic diseases
3. A neurologic examination that is brief and efficient
4. Conditions that are common, that require emergency management, and that are treatable[5]

The important conditions in which the primary care physician should have confidence and ability to assess and manage, even if the management is to recognize when referral is required, are listed in Box 156-1.

The array of neurologic problems seen in the primary care physician's office can be tabulated according to an emphasis score, with varying emphasis scored on the basis of frequency of the problem, potential seriousness, and the effect of intervention on the outcome (Table 156-1).

Box 156-1. Important Neurologic Problems in Primary Care

Problems that Require Emergency Management

Coma
Meningitis
Seizures
Stroke
Status epilepticus
Increased intracranial pressure
Acute visual failure
Any rapidly progressing neurologic deficit

Neurologic Conditions that Are Common

Headaches
Seizures
Strokes
Vertigo and dizziness
Sleep disorders
Multiple sclerosis
Neuropathies
Altered consciousness
Parkinson's disease
Dementia
Mental retardation
Pain syndromes

Problems that Are Treatable

Seizures
Meningitis
Migraine
Transient ischemic attacks
Parkinson's disease
Pernicious anemia
Temporal arteritis
Polymyositis
Subdural hematoma
Myasthenia gravis
Tourette's syndrome
Wilson's disease

Problems that Illustrate New Developments in the Neurosciences

Creutzfeldt-Jakob disease
Prion diseases

Table 156-1. Emphasis Score for Neurological Conditions in Primary Care Practice

Neurologic condition	Score*
Headache	4 × 3 × 4 = 48
Stroke	2 × 4 × 5 = 40
Transient ischemic attacks	2 × 5 × 4 = 40
Sleep disorders	4 × 3 × 3 = 36
Epilepsy	3 × 5 × 2 = 30
Dementia	3 × 5 × 2 = 30
Vertigo and dizziness	3 × 3 × 3 = 27
Meningitis	1 × 5 × 5 = 25
Subdural hematoma	1 × 5 × 5 = 25
Temporal arteritis	1 × 5 × 5 = 25
Meningitis	1 × 5 × 5 = 25
Delerium tremens	1 × 5 × 5 = 25
Pernicious anemia	1 × 5 × 5 = 25
Multiple sclerosis	2 × 4 × 3 = 24
Memory problems	3 × 4 × 2 = 24
Head injury	2 × 4 × 3 = 24
Low back pain	4 × 3 × 2 = 24
Weakness	2 × 4 × 3 = 24
Acute pain	4 × 2 × 3 = 24
Parkinson's disease	1 × 5 × 4 = 20
Trigeminal neuralgia	1 × 4 × 5 = 20
Cervical spondylosis	3 × 2 × 3 = 18
Syncope, blackouts	2 × 3 × 3 = 18
Conversion reaction	2 × 3 × 3 = 18
Chronic pain	2 × 4 × 2 = 16
Sensory symptoms	4 × 2 × 2 = 16
Coma	1 × 5 × 3 = 15
Organic psychosis	1 × 5 × 3 = 15
Peripheral neuropathy	2 × 3 × 2 = 12
Brain tumor	1 × 5 × 2 = 10
Bell's palsy	1 × 2 × 4 = 8
Herpes zoster	2 × 2 × 2 = 8
Muscle cramps	2 × 1 × 3 = 6
Cerebral palsy	1 × 4 × 1 = 4
Mental retardation	1 × 4 × 1 = 4

*A score of 1 to 5 is given for each factor. The emphasis score is determined by multiplying the three factors: *frequency* × *seriousness* × *effect of intervention*.

REFERENCES

1. Murray TJ: Concepts in undergraduate neurological teaching, *Clin Neurol Surg* 79:273, 1976.
2. Murray TJ: Relevance in undergraduate neurological teaching, *Can J Neurol Sci* 4:131, 1977.
3. Murray TJ: The neurologist as educator, *Can J Neurol Sci* 10:230, 1983.
4. Murray TJ: What should a family physician know about neurology? *Can Fam Physician* 36:297, 1990.
5. Pryse-Phillips W, Murray TJ: *Essential neurology,* ed 4, New York, 1992, Medical Examination Publishers.

CHAPTER 157

Alterations in Mental State: Coma and Acute Confusional States

Harold B. Schiff
Thomas D. Sabin

COMA

Coma is a disturbance of consciousness in which the patient cannot be aroused by any stimulus, no matter how vigorous. With the return of any form of responsiveness, coma ends. The recovering patient then progresses through various levels of disordered consciousness until finally attaining a clear sensorium. An understanding of the pathogenesis is essential to the clinical management of the comatose patient.

Pathogenesis

The ascending reticular activating system (RAS) is a highly complex polysynaptic region in the core of the upper pons and midbrain. These isodendritic fibers extend from the midbrain into the thalamic regions bilaterally and ultimately become widespread within the hemispheres. Specific afferent systems contribute some portion of their neuronal activity to the RAS as they pass through these brainstem structures. Specific neurotransmitter function in the RAS is not fully understood.[4] GABAergic fibers and cholinergic systems play a role in controlling consciousness (GABA, γ-aminobutyric acid).[13] A pathologic decrease in consciousness results from either a local anatomic or a general biochemical disturbance of the RAS.

If the brainstem is sectioned below the level of the upper pons, a disturbance in alertness does not occur. Once the ascending RAS has reached the level of the thalamus and becomes bilaterally distributed, a unilateral destructive lesion does not cause obtundation. Although extramedullary distortion of the ascending RAS in the midbrain is the major anatomic basis for disordered arousal, critically located small focal lesions from the upper pons to the mesencephalic-diencephalic junction may also produce this clinical picture. Thus small infarcts that destroy the reticular core of the brainstem may cause states of prolonged coma. In unilateral supratentorial space-occupying lesions, the medial or uncal portion of the temporal lobe is forced through the tentorial notch beside the midbrain. This distorts the reticular-activating substance in the core of the midbrain and thereby causes decreased alertness. The herniated uncus also causes compression of the oculomotor nerve. Parasympathetic pupillomotor fibers are superficially placed, and the compression may result in an ipsilateral dilated pupil that is unresponsive to light.

When the herniated uncus forces the midbrain against the rigid, contralateral tentorial margin, motor fibers within the midbrain may be affected, and signs of upper motor neuron deficits appear on the same side as the supratentorial mass lesion. Pupillary dilation, however, is a more accurate predictor of the side of supratentorial mass lesion than the side of the hemiparesis. When there is bilateral herniation of supratentorial structures, the midbrain is forced caudally and elongated in the anteroposterior direction.

The pharmacologic and biochemical vulnerability of the RAS is also well recognized. This vulnerability is reflected in the appearance of obtundation in almost every variety of severe metabolic disturbance. The most common causes of obtundation are endogenous or exogenous toxins. The numerous synapses in the ascending RAS may be the basis for the striking vulnerability of the RAS to so many classes of drugs and toxins.

Making the distinction between an intracranial structural lesion and an extracranial toxic-metabolic encephalopathy is the primary diagnostic step in evaluating the comatose patient.

Early Management of the Comatose Patient

If patients with transient loss of consciousness are excluded and coma persists for 6 hours or more, the chance of either a sedative/toxic or a hypoxic/ischemic etiology is 40%; of a cerebrovascular etiology (stroke, hemorrhage, or subarachnoid bleed), 35%; and of a metabolic etiology (e.g., diabetes, infection, renal/hepatic), 25%. The overriding concern in the early management of the comatose patient is the immediate treatment of any remedial cause of brain damage. Several steps should be taken even before a full diagnostic assessment is made.

The patient must be guaranteed an adequate airway, respiratory exchange, circulation, and metabolic substrate, glucose, and thiamine (which acts as a cofactor in the metabolism of glucose).[11] After blood is obtained for various diagnostic studies (including glucose levels), the patient should be given 100 mg of thiamine intravenously followed by a 50-ml 50% glucose solution. Thiamine must be administered before the glucose, since a glucose load in a thiamine-deficient patient may precipitate acute Wernicke's encephalopathy and may cause sudden death from circulatory collapse. If narcotic ingestion is suspected, naloxone (Narcan) should be administered.

If ingestion of benzodiazepines is suspected, flumazenil can be used and is often effective. In cases in which the ingested substance is unknown, flumazenil can be used empirically. If there is a positive response, albeit short-lived, repeat injections can be used. The safe use of flumazenil is, however, an important factor to consider in each clinical situation.[14]

The patient should be positioned to prevent aspiration but nevertheless should be handled as if a cervical spinal fracture is present until more is known about the patient's history and more diagnostic studies can be performed. As soon as these initial urgent needs are satisfied, a rapid general medical and neurologic examination should be performed.

Evaluation of the Comatose Patient

The neurologic examination of the comatose patient is quite different from the routine neurologic evaluation.[10] In most common conditions associated with coma, a rostral-caudal deterioration in nervous system function tends to occur as the process worsens. This is generally the case for both structural intracranial processes and toxic metabolic encephalopathies. *Rostral-caudal deterioration* refers to the sequential loss of certain functions, beginning with the cerebral cortex and followed by the diencephalon, midbrain, pons, and finally the medulla. A rapid assessment of the anatomic level of a given patient can be made by examining the state of consciousness, pupils, eye movements, respirations, and remaining motor functions (Table 157-1). Before this evaluation, the physician should make a quick assessment for evidence of head trauma. An ecchymosis that surrounds the eye ("raccoon sign"), a hemotympanum, and "bogginess" with or without ecchymosis on the mastoid process just behind the ear (Battle's sign) are evidence of a basal skull fracture. The importance of looking for subtle signs of head injury must be emphasized. Slight bogginess with an area of petechiae on the scalp, which can only be identified if the patient's hair and scalp are carefully searched, may be the sole evidence for head trauma. Certain injuries, such as a blow to the head from a stocking filled with sand, can create devastating brain lesions with minimal external signs.

The level of consciousness is evaluated by repeated efforts to wake the patient and gain his or her attention. Terms such as *light coma, semicoma,* and *stupor* as defined in the literature are of little value in clinical practice and are best avoided. A clear description of the patient's behavior and clinical status is preferred.[2]

Examination of the pupils should include size, symmetry, and response to light. In the diencephalic stage of the rostral-caudal deterioration, both pupils tend to be small. This may be noted in an expanding supratentorial mass or with widespread edema that causes midline herniation. A magnifying glass may be necessary to see if the pupillary response to light has been preserved. A unilateral supratentorial mass that causes the uncus to herniate through the tentorial notch is signaled by compression of the parasympathetic motor fibers surrounding the third cranial nerve, producing loss of constriction and thus progressive pupillary dilation and finally a widely dilated, unreactive pupil. The pupillary signs of third nerve dysfunction appear before the paralysis of extraocular muscles. The diencephalic stage is thus characterized by either unilateral pupillary dilation (with unilateral herniation syndromes) or symmetric, small pupils that respond to light (in midline herniation or most toxic metabolic encephalopathies).

Once the deterioration involves the midbrain, the pupils are no longer reactive to light; they tend to be in the midposition and may not change with progression of the syndrome to the pontine and medullary phases of deterioration. The agonal dilation of unresponsive pupils has been attributed to a widespread release of norepinephrine throughout anoxic body tissues.

Examination of the extraocular movements is another important means of assessing the anatomic level of brainstem involvement. Before the specific findings at each anatomic level and its significance in assessing coma are discussed, some of the normal physiology is reviewed. Conjugate gaze is important in the initial assessment, even before extraocular movements are assessed. In drowsiness, mild squints, which are not seen in the awake patient, may become obvious; that is, phorias become manifest tropias. Divergent squints are most common and are exaggerated with upward deviation of the eyes. These signs reflect a decreased level of consciousness, but do not have specific anatomic localization value.

With coma and depending on the level, these oculocephalic reflexes may become overly facile or disappear completely despite maximal stimulation (Fig. 157-1). When a normal conscious individual has the head passively turned to the right, the eyes move to the right. In an obtunded individual, they move to the left. This release of vestibular reflexes is believed to be the basis for the doll's head maneuver. With further involvement of the diencephalon a stronger stimulus may be necessary. Conjugate deviation of the eyes to the stimulated side can be induced by instilling cold water to the external ear canal. The maximal stimulus consists of 40 ml of ice water instilled over 30 seconds. No perforation of the drum or other process in the external ear that might be adversely affected by this irrigation should be present. In the diencephalic stage of coma, the so-called doll's head eye maneuvers become overly facile, and with rotation of the head the reflex is brisk. In the mesencephalic stage of dysfunction, the eyes can still be conjugately drawn to the side of the stimulation, although if third nerve connections are sufficiently damaged, there may be a deficit in adduction. In the mesencephalic stage, cold-calorics are almost invariably required. Once the pons and medulla have been destroyed, the lateral eye movements do not respond to the doll's head maneuver or ice water–caloric stimulation. When the patient's head is at 35 degrees to the horizontal and both ears are simultaneously stimulated with warm water at 44° C

Table 157-1. Major Neurologic Signs Reflecting Anatomic Levels of Rostral-Caudal Progression in Coma

	Motor response to deep pain stimuli	Pupils	Extraocular movement	Respirations
Diencephalic	Spontaneous movements: limbs/face/eye to loud hand clap Limb withdrawal to deep pain Decorticate posturing	Small/reactive Unilateral dilation in uncal herniation	Overly facile (brisk) Doll's eye reflexes May need cold-calories to elicit doll's eye reflex	Normal or Cheyne-Stokes
Mesencephalic	Decerebrate posturing, or fragments of it, to deep pain	Unresponsive	Need cold-calories to elicit Doll's eye reflexes	Central neurogenic Hyperventilation
Pontine	Flaccid tone/lack of motor response to deep pain	Unresponsive	No response to oculocephalic stimulation	Return of "normal" apneustic respiratory rhythm
Medullary	Flaccid tone/lack of motor response to deep pain	Unresponsive	No response to oculocephalic stimulation	Ataxic/irregular respiration Respiratory arrest

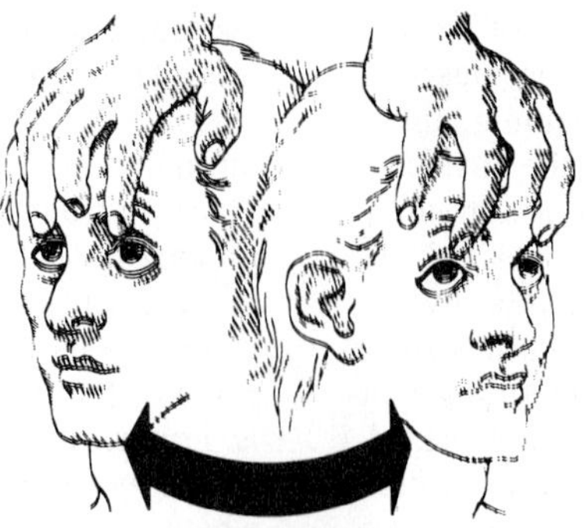

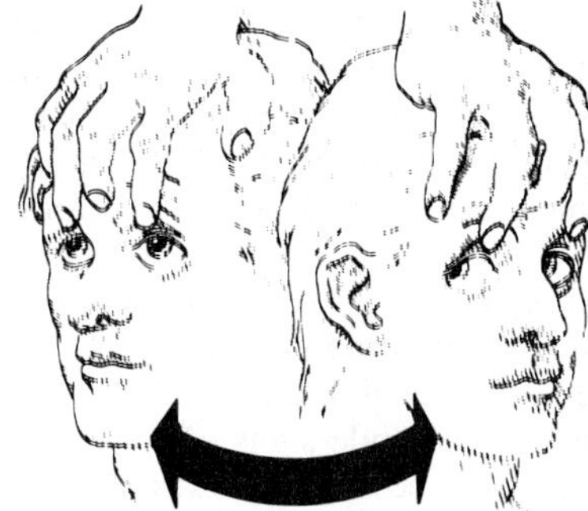

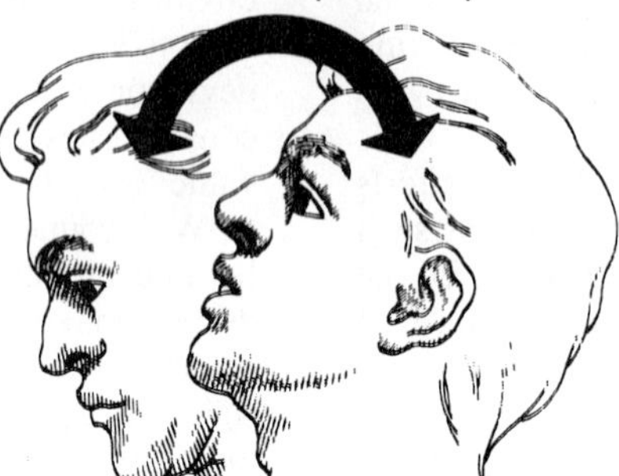

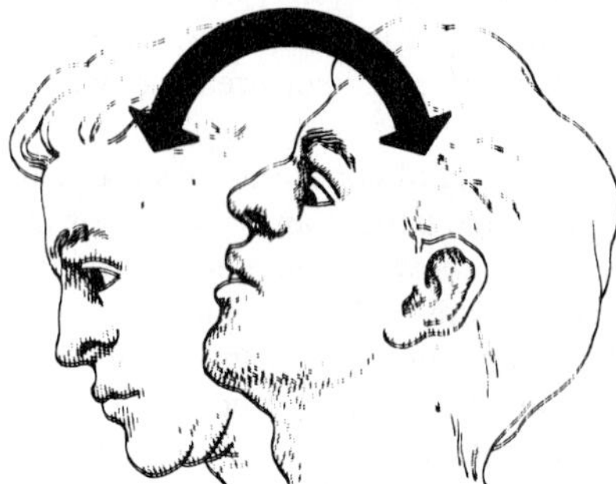

Fig. 157-1. Doll's head maneuver. This maneuver consists of rapidly turning the head from side to side (*top*) or flexing and extending the neck (*bottom*). Conjugate movement of the eyes to the side opposite the direction of the head movement demonstrates that brainstem centers for eye movement are intact. In the bottom drawing, as in the top drawing, the eyelids are held open because the patient is comatose. (From Geller AE, Sabin TD: *Med Times* 106:47, 1978.)

(111° F), conjugate upward deviation of the eyes occurs if the midbrain centers for vertical gaze are intact.

The comatose patient may have tonic conjugate deviation of the eyes. In an acute hemispheric lesion, destruction of the fibers from the frontal gaze center for contralateral conjugate gaze occurs. This results in a relative overactivity of the contralateral intact center, causing deviation of the eyes toward the injured hemisphere. If an associated hemiplegia exists, the eyes deviate away from the side of the hemiplegia and toward the side of the lesion (Fig. 157-2). With lesions in the brainstem, these fibers have already crossed in the midbrain, and the eyes may conjugately deviate away from the side of the lesion and toward the hemiplegia.

The respiratory pattern is another useful marker for determining the level of remaining nervous system function. Respirations at the diencephalic stage of rostral-caudal deterioration may be normal or show periodic respiration, including Cheyne-Stokes respirations. Central neurogenic hyperventilation with continued respiratory rates of about 40 breaths/min (with appropriate changes in blood gas values) may occur with midbrain dysfunction. When pontine damage is superimposed on the midbrain syndrome, central neurogenic hyperventilation disappears and may be replaced by breathing that is apparently more normal. A pause at inspiration (apneustic breathing) is characteristic of pontine-level lesions. As the pons is destroyed, breathing becomes ataxic, irregular, and unpredictable. At this point, respiratory arrest is imminent.

Testing of motor system function in obtunded patients is different from the usual neurologic examination. Simple observation of spontaneous movements or the movements in relation to painful stimuli is done. In the diencephalic stage an associated hemiplegia is easily recognized, and bilateral decorticate posture may rarely be seen. Decorticate posturing consists of adduction at the shoulder and flexion at the elbows, wrists, and fingers, with extensor posturing of the lower extremities. A stage occurs before decorticate posturing in which fairly facile movement is away from painful stimuli, but the range of passive movement in these limbs is often limited by counterholding (gegenhalten or paratonia).

In the midbrain state of deterioration, decerebrate postures appear. Decerebration rarely appears in a florid, full-blown form but is seen more often as only fragments of the posture in response to noxious stimulation. The examiner should place the semiflexed upper extremities across the patient's abdomen and then provide a painful stimulus to the sternum. If the patient consistently reacts to the painful stimulus with only one limb, the opposite side is hemiplegic. If the patient's forearms extend away from the painful stimulus or pronate even slightly, decerebration and thus dysfunction at the mesencephalic level should be suspected. When the patient moves the limb toward the painful stimulus at the sternum, a second stimulus at the iliac crest confirms that the patient is not simply demonstrating decorticate posturing but is actually reaching for the noxious stimuli.

As the midbrain is destroyed and pontine dysfunction appears, decerebration disappears, and the limbs become flaccid. No movement appears with noxious stimulation. Disappearance of decerebration is often mistaken for improvement. The limbs remain flaccid in the medullary phase of deterioration.

With these parameters of examination in mind, the physician can quickly localize the level of nervous system dysfunction and begin consideration of the major diagnostic categories.

Differential Diagnosis

The initial diagnostic consideration is to determine whether the alteration in consciousness is caused by a primarily intracranial structural lesion or a systemic toxic or metabolic disorder.

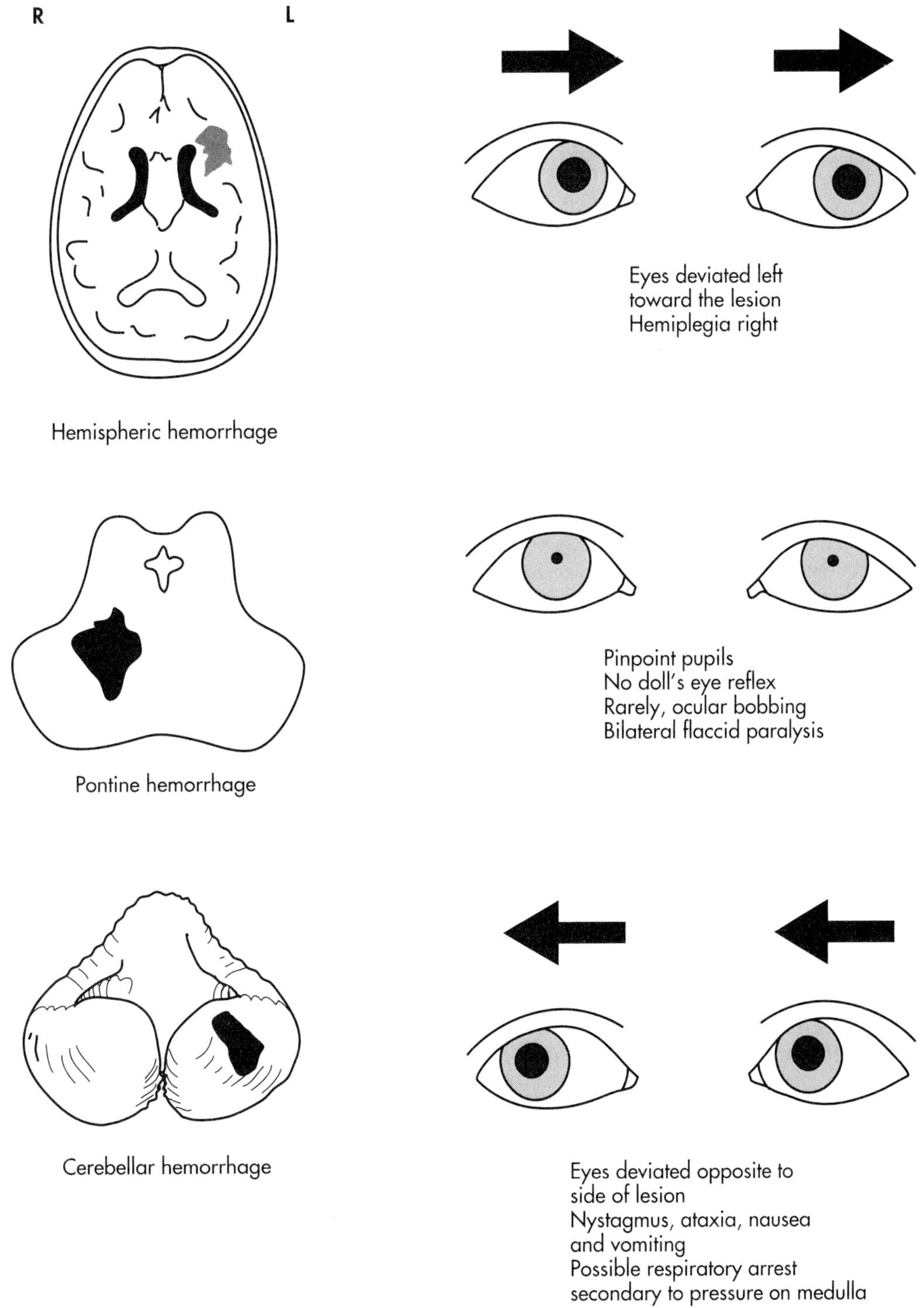

Fig. 157-2. Hemispheric, pontine, and cerebellar hemorrhage demonstrating the accompanying eye movement and pupillary responses.

Structural Central Nervous System Lesions. The intracranial processes are subdivided into those in which focal signs are likely vs. those in which no focal signs may be anticipated. The major categories of intracranial processes with focal brain dysfunction include trauma, intraparenchymal hemorrhages, tumors, certain forms of infection, and brain infarction.

With Focal Signs

Trauma. *Concussion* refers to a transient loss of consciousness. If there is associated brain contusion, unconsciousness may be more lasting. Focal signs such as hemiplegia, aphasia, or other signs of cortical injury are usually obvious. In addition, blood may be found in cerebrospinal fluid (CSF).

Frequent consequences of closed-head trauma are hematomas in the subdural or epidural space or in the brain parenchyma. Neuroimaging has greatly simplified the diagnosis of this problem. However, an apparently negative computed tomography (CT) scan in an appropriate clinical setting should not dissuade the physician from diagnosing subdural hematoma, since this lesion may be isodense with brain tissue but is seen on the more sensitive magnetic resonance imaging (MRI). Since the mass lesion produces a widely dispersed force over the convexity of one side of the brain, there are often no focal cortical signs. However, the distortion of the ascending RAS, secondary to the mass effect, causes abnormal drowsiness, which may be the only feature present.

Hemorrhage. Spontaneous hemorrhages into brain parenchyma are occurring less frequently as the assiduous treatment of hypertension becomes more widely practiced. Brain hemorrhages may occur in a variety of disorders, such as anticoagulation, end-stage leukemias, hepatic disease, amyloid angiopathy, and intracranial aneurysms; however, the major association is still with hypertension. Symptoms and signs usually appear suddenly, but occasionally the onset of these hemorrhagic syndromes may progress in severity, taking several days to develop. Hypertensive hemorrhages tend to occur in five sites (see Fig. 157-2). The lateral ganglionic or putaminal areas of the hemisphere are most often affected. Hemorrhage at these sites results in severe headache, hemiplegia, conjugate deviation of the eyes away from the hemiplegia, and signs of progressive uncal herniation with rostral-caudal deterioration.

The thalamus is a second common site of hypertensive hemorrhage and also produces headache and hemiplegia. The hemorrhage frequently dissects into upper midbrain structures, which may explain why the eyes are often conjugately deviated toward the hemiplegia. A rarer but highly characteristic tonic downward convergence of the eye has also been reported with thalamic hemorrhage (see Fig. 157-2).

Pontine hemorrhage is usually fatal within 48 hours. Since the initial lesion is in the pons, the clinical picture is different from that seen with rostral-caudal deterioration. There is bilateral flaccid paralysis of the limbs, and the doll's head maneuver or the ice water–caloric test fails to cause lateral conjugate eye deviation, although some vertical gaze may remain because of intact midbrain centers. Peculiar vertical conjugate eye movements known as *ocular bobbing* may be witnessed. The eyes drift downward and then more rapidly elevate upward, slightly above the resting level, before descending once again to the resting level. The movements often occur in brief bursts. Pontine hemorrhage is usually also associated with pinpoint pupils, resulting from destruction of the descending sympathetic fibers at a time when midbrain parasympathetic fibers are still functioning. The pinpoint pupils respond to light but so minimally that a magnifying glass may be necessary to see the constriction (see Fig. 157-2).

The prompt diagnosis of hypertensive cerebellar hemorrhage is most important because of the urgency of surgical intervention as a lifesaving procedure. Cerebellar hemorrhage presents with acute ataxia, nausea, vomiting, and severe headache. On examination, both truncal ataxia and hemiataxia may be present. Nystagmus usually occurs, and there may be forced deviation of gaze opposite the side of the hematoma (see Fig. 157-2). An acute cerebellar mass can compress medullary respiratory centers and cause sudden death. Surgical evacuation of cerebellar hemorrhages can be lifesaving.

Tumors. Most intracranial tumors are now diagnosed early enough that patients do not come to medical attention in a coma. However, one should keep certain situations in mind.

Tumors in the midline of the neuraxis either within or outside the ventricular system may cause minimal neurologic symptoms or signs until CSF flow is obstructed, and then obtundation occurs with acute hydrocephalus and a rapid deterioration in clinical status. Patients with posterior cranial fossa lesions may have respiratory arrest as the first manifestation of foramen magnum herniation. The evaluation of patients suspected of having posterior fossa mass lesions should reflect this possibility. Papilledema is usually present in these patients. Since papilledema takes about 24 hours to develop fully, it is not seen in massive acute hemorrhages, but if the patient has a slowly growing tumor, he or she is more apt to have papilledema when seen with an acute deterioration in level of consciousness. Midline, posterior fossa or intraventricular tumor–associated hydrocephalus should be treated with emergency ventricular drainage or ventriculostomy.

Patients with pituitary adenomas can lapse into acute coma when spontaneous hemorrhagic necrosis of the tumor occurs. Patients with pituitary apoplexy have headaches, visual loss, stiff neck, obtundation, extraocular palsies, and acute hypotension. The recognition and treatment of the acute hypoadrenal state caused by the failure of adrenocorticotrophic hormone (ACTH) production are essential lifesaving maneuvers. An enlarged sella seen on plain skull films is an important clue to the diagnosis of pituitary apoplexy. MRI or CT scans have proved to be extremely useful in diagnosing most intracranial tumors.

Cerebellar abscess usually presents as a mass lesion. The appearance is often characteristic on MRI or CT scan. A small bubble of air in the low-density center of a lesion with a ringlike enhancement is diagnostic of abscess. Brain abscesses alone do not necessarily result in fever, and the CSF may be normal.

Infarction. Hemispheric infarcts may produce lethargy or confusion acutely, but unilateral lesions seldom cause complete coma. An exception occurs when a massive, acute hemispheric infarction results in severe brain edema; herniation and fatal rostral-caudal deterioration of brain function can occur in 1 to 2 hours. Small infarcts of the brainstem can interrupt the RAS and produce lasting coma. In the "locked-in" syndrome, extensive paralysis occurs because of bilateral destruction of the motor pathways in the basis pontis. The patient is conscious, but the medical staff may not realize it. These patients are able to develop a code, using eye blinks to communicate.

Without Focal Signs. In certain other intracranial processes that cause coma, such as meningitis, encephalitis, and subarachnoid hemorrhage, no focal signs may be present. The physician depends greatly on careful examination of the spinal fluid for the correct diagnosis. Focal signs may be present but are a bonus for the diagnostician. Aneurysms of the posterior communicating artery often cause an acute third nerve palsy. Bacterial meningitis may cause cerebral thrombophlebitis with hemiplegias and focal seizures. Similarly, the predilection of the herpes simplex virus for the temporal lobe often assists in the diagnosis of that variety of viral encephalitis.

This category of intracranial processes without obvious focal signs should serve as a forceful reminder that every comatose patient must have a CSF examination performed unless lumbar puncture is contraindicated. If the patient is deemed too ill for a lumbar puncture, some other diagnostic procedure must be substituted on an emergency basis. An MRI or CT scan before lumbar puncture is advisable in many circumstances. Standard CSF studies may be complemented by brain creatine kinase and neuron-specific enolase tests, which may be useful in prognostication.

Toxic-Metabolic Causes. The differential diagnosis of endogenous metabolic derangement is extensive and includes disturbances in all organ systems. Box 157-1 presents a logical schema for the approach to the differential diagnosis of endogenous metabolic encephalopathies.

The toxic encephalopathies are most often caused by drug overdose, and some patients, especially elderly ones, may be unusually sensitive to the side effects of many drugs, even at standard dosages.

Some sedative drugs have special effects on the eyes that may help with the diagnosis. Glutethimide (Doriden) may cause large pupils that are unresponsive to light. Morphine produces pupilloconstriction. Atropine-like effects cause dilated, fixed pupils. Severely obtunded patients with drug overdose may be capable of brushing away painful stimuli and even muttering a few sounds but may have no eye movements even with ice water–caloric stimulation. This disparity of rostral-caudal localization is highly suggestive of sedative drug overdose. A toxic screen and an electroencephalogram (EEG) that shows characteristic effects of sedative medication are useful in confirming the diagnosis.

Patients with endogenous metabolic encephalopathies usually have no focal signs, but exceptions occur when clinically inapparent, earlier neurologic lesions once again become manifest as metabolic derangement occurs. Hemiplegia may reappear when a patient who has had a previous cerebral infarct with complete recovery begins to develop, for example, carbon dioxide narcosis of chronic pulmonary disease. Focal seizures apparently arising from the supplementary motor area, with fencing postures and groping movements of the extended arm, have proved to be highly suggestive of nonketotic hyperglycemic coma.

One of the most important practical distinctions between the toxic-metabolic encephalopathies and the structural intracranial processes relates to the pupillary light response. In all the toxic-metabolic encephalopathies except anoxic encephalopathy and those caused by drugs that have specific effects on the pupil, pupillary response to light is spared regardless of the rostral-caudal involvement. The clinical differentiation of structural from metabolic causes of coma pivots around a clearly progressive anatomic localization of the rostral-caudal syndrome. Intracranial mass lesions usually follow this syndrome exactly, whereas the signs of the toxic-metabolic encephalopathy may be much more patchy, such as pontine involvement without prior mesencephalic involvement and no clear-cut rostral-caudal progression.

Decerebration does occur in the toxic-metabolic encephalopathies and should not be considered diagnostic of structural brain disease. Metabolic encephalopathy is often accompanied by widespread, involuntary, small-amplitude myoclonic jerks. The patient should be examined with an oblique light for several minutes, since the muscle twitches are often not otherwise apparent.

Clearly, a full discussion of all the causes of coma is beyond the scope of this chapter, which serves only as a model for an approach to the comatose patient.

Box 157-1. Toxic-Metabolic Causes of Coma

Exogenous Intoxications

Alcohol, barbiturates
Tranquilizers
Belladonna derivatives
Psychomimetics
Others: ergot, salicylates, caffeine, heavy metals
Withdrawal syndromes

General Medical Diseases

Disturbances of hydration, electrolytes, osmolarity
Cardiovascular disturbances (hypotension, congestive heart failure, hypertensive encephalopathy)
Pulmonary failure (carbon dioxide narcosis, anoxia)
Hepatic encephalopathy
Uremia and the postdialysis syndrome
Endocrine disorders: hypoglycemia; thyroid, adrenal, and pituitary syndromes
Porphyria
Vasculitides
Acute infections outside the central nervous system
Toxemia of pregnancy

Outcome and Prognostication

A body of literature exists on the outcome of coma, but the most reliable data stem from studies of posttraumatic coma.[12] The Glasgow Coma Scale and the Glasgow Outcome Scales are most helpful in the monitoring and prognostication of traumatic coma but are less reliable in other forms of coma. Only 10% of patients with nontraumatic coma, who do not demonstrate spontaneous eye movements at 6 hours, will make a moderate to good recovery.[7] Eye opening to painful stimuli at 6 hours raises the chances of moderate to good recovery. Some 85% die, remain in a vegetative state, or recover to a state of significant dependency.[3]

BRAIN DEATH

Guidelines for the determination of brain death recommended by the President's Commission in 1981 are now used widely; however, state and local laws or practices may modify their applications (Box 157-2).

Patients are not brain dead if they have reactive pupils, corneal or gag reflexes, or decerebrate or decorticate posturing (Box 157-3). The pupils are generally midposition and dilated in brain death. Small pupils are uncommon and should be checked for reactivity because of possible drug overdose. Spinal reflexes (deep tendon and Babinski's) may persist in the presence of brain death. And, in the 15- to 30-minute interval after ventilatory assistance is withdrawn, unusual movements of the extremities may occur, most likely resulting from terminal ischemia of the spinal cord.

Hypothermia, drug intoxication, and viral encephalitis may all produce an isoelectric EEG. Thus the presence of an

Box 157-2. Managed Care Guide: Brain Death in Adults*

I. Cessation of all function of the entire brain
   A. Unresponsive coma
   B. Absent brainstem reflexes
      1. Pupillary light reflex
      2. Corneal reflex
      3. Cephalic (caloric) reflexes
      4. Oropharyngeal (gag) reflex
      5. Respiration (apnea testing)
II. Irreversibility
   A. Coma of known cause without potential for
   B. reversibility
   C. Exclusion of contributory, reversible condition
      1. Drug intoxication
      2. Neuromuscular blockade
      3. Hypothermia (<32.2° C, 90° F)
      4. Shock
      5. Major metabolic disturbance
   D. Persistence for an appropriate period (6-24 hours, depending on cause of coma and local practice)
III. Confirmatory investigations (may be optional or required)
   A. Electrocerebral silence (isoelectric EEG)
   B. Absence of circulation to the brain

Adapted from *JAMA* 246:2184, 1981.
*Local and institutional rules are superseding.

Box 157-3. Clinical Features of Brain Death

Hemisphere death
- Deep coma
- Absence of purposeful movement, well-defined posturing, or convulsions
- Corroboration by EEG, brain scan, or angiography*

Brainstem death
- Unreactive midposition or enlarged pupils
- Absent eye movements with oculocephalic ("doll's eyes" and oculovestibular (caloric) stimulation)
- Absent corneal responses
- Absence of spontaneous breathing with apnea testing

Exclusions
- Sedative drugs
- Severe hypothermia
- Time immediately preceding circulatory arrest

*Brain death is a clinical diagnosis: laboratory confirmation may be used in special circumstances.

isoelectric EEG alone is not sufficient to serve as a criterion for brain death.

ACUTE CONFUSIONAL STATES

Acute confusion, also known as *acute encephalopathy, acute toxic psychosis,* or *delirium,* can be thought of as an acquired incapacity to think with customary speed and clarity. The major feature of this syndrome is the failure to maintain

Box 157-4. Diagnostic Criteria for Acute Confusional Syndrome

1. Clouding of consciousness, that is, a reduced capacity to shift, focus, and sustain attention to environmental stimuli
2. At least two of the following: (a) perceptual disturbances (i.e., misinterpretations, illusions, hallucinations), (b) incoherent speech, (c) disturbances of the sleep-wake cycle, or (d) increased or decreased psychomotor activity
3. Disorientation and memory disturbance
4. Clinical features that develop over a short period and tend to fluctuate over the course of the day
5. Elements from the history and physical examination and laboratory tests that suggest a specific organic factor, judged to be etiologically related to the disturbance

Data from the Diagnostic and statistical manual of mental disorders (DSM-IV), ed 4.

normal, sequential thought, reflecting an inability to rank the priority of stimuli. Patients thus are unable to maintain a coherent stream of thought. The consequent failure in the designation of behavioral priorities causes an immediate and drastic disintegration of the adaptational interaction with the environment. Patients' general behavior and speech reflect an inappropriate sequencing of ideas, and patients exhibit a wide range of abnormal behaviors, including assaultiveness, motor hyperactivity, hallucinations, somnolence, and extreme states of panic or fear.[8]

The diagnosis of an acute confusional syndrome is often not entirely objective, and most physicians rely to some degree on intuition. A clear definition has not been established, but the fourth edition of the *Diagnostic and Statistical Manual of Mental Disorders (DSM-IV)* provides specific diagnostic criteria that may serve as a point of departure in defining the clinical features of this syndrome (Box 157-4).

Clinical Features

The diagnosis of confusion depends on the recognition of specific disturbances in the processes of attention, thought, and perception.

Attentional Deficits. Disordered attention is a major feature of confusion.[1] Disturbances include difficulties in attaining and maintaining attention. This disturbance is apparent in the evaluation of patients with confusion; it is often very difficult to attract the attention of these individuals, who may appear relatively unresponsive to external stimuli. Furthermore, maintaining their attention may also prove difficult. Patients respond equally to all auditory, visual, and kinesthetic stimuli and are unable to filter out irrelevant stimuli. They may be extremely distractible and thus unable to sustain any goal-directed behavior.

Thought Disorder. Disordered thought is most frequently recognized as an incoherent stream of thought. The patient may be aware of this and complain of being "confused," "unable to think straight," or "unable to get it together." Some patients, however, may be unaware of their deficit.

The term *thought disorder* is used here to encompass the various cognitive deficits that result in an incoherent stream of thought. Although memory disturbance and disorientation are invariably present, the patient may respond appropriately on formal memory and orientation testing. The patient does have significant difficulty in organizing recent and remote memories into an orderly sequence. Thus features of spatial disorientation may be expressed as symptoms of reduplicative paramnesia. This usually involves the reduplication of place; for example, the patient insists that the hospital room is duplicated and shifted in place so that "a branch of the main hospital is in my home." Temporal disorientation is obvious when events from the past are directly related to the present. This association of unrelated events may lead to a diagnosis of confabulation. Indeed, the patient may exhibit frank confabulation; this may be concrete and obviously related to surrounding visual and auditory cues; alternatively, it may be quite bizarre, apparently generated from inner thought processes.

Thought content may have a dreamlike quality. The patient may find it difficult to separate fact from fantasy or dreams from reality. Delusions may occur, are usually fleeting, and may be modified by environmental stimuli. Vague feelings of apprehension are often crystallized into persecutory delusional beliefs. Delusions are often concrete; the classic schneiderian delusions of thought insertion, withdrawal, control, and broadcasting are only rarely seen.

Perceptual Disturbances. Perceptual disturbances are perhaps the most dramatic manifestations of acute confusion. Illusions range from simple to more complex misinterpretations of environmental stimuli. For example, markings on the wall are interpreted as crawling insects, folds in the bedclothes as snakes or wild animals, and sounds as fire alarms or gunshots. In more complex illusions the hospital room might be mistaken for a prison or the door for a window. The patient may act on these misinterpretations, resulting in inadvertent accident or death.

Hallucinations may occur in all sensory modalities. Visual and auditory hallucinations are more frequent than tactile, kinesthetic, olfactory, and gustatory hallucinations. However, no characteristic type of hallucination exemplifies the acute confusional state. The content of these hallucinations varies greatly and is usually interpreted by the patient as real.

Language Disturbances. Language is often vague, circumlocutory, and perseverative. Word-finding difficulty may take the form of approximations. A pitcher may be called a *glass* or a bedrail a *gate*. Reading is often preserved, whereas writing is very abnormal. The patient demonstrates poor penmanship, starting off well but ending with micrographia. The patient characteristically shows no regard for paper space or lines and neglects to dot the *i*s and cross the *t*s (Fig. 157-3). Misspellings and perseverations or overdrawings on letters and words are common.

Disturbance in the Sleep-Wake Cycle. Disturbance in the sleep-walk cycle is an invariable feature of confusional states. Some patients are hypersomnolent, whereas others remain awake for days at a time. The patient may not offer this information, but it is the most common complaint of family or friends.

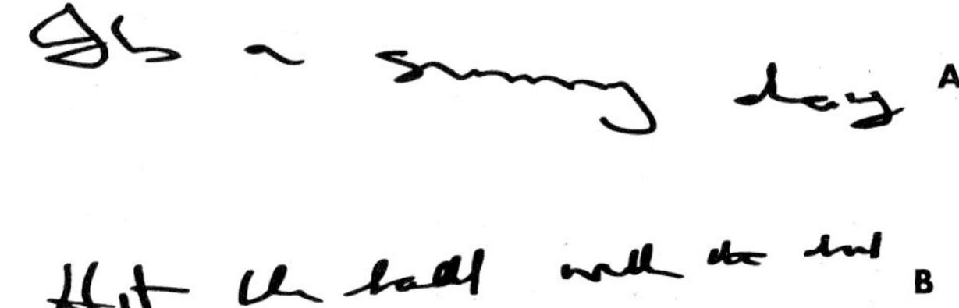

Fig. 157-3. **A,** "It's a sunny day." The down-slant of the sentence, the uncrossed *t,* and the perseveration of the *n* of *sunny* illustrate the dysgraphic features of the confusional state. **B,** "Hit the ball with the bat." The up-slant of the sentence, the uncrossed *t,* and the generally sloppy orthography further illustrate the dysgraphic features of the confusional state.

Fluctuations in Symptomatology. The patient shows fluctuations in cognitive function over a 24-hour cycle and also from day to day. The patient usually functions worse in the early morning, after a nap, or at sundown. However, the patient has periods of surprising lucidity. Such fluctuation is rarely seen in any other disorder of the mental status.

Arousal: Psychomotor and Autonomic Activity. The degree of psychomotor activity in acute confusion varies. Two distinct syndromes have been described. In the hypoactive syndrome, patients have diminished psychomotor activity and are generally quiet and withdrawn. Verbal output is restricted, varying from complete mutism to empty, vague speech. In the hyperactive syndrome, on the other hand, patients appear to be hyperaroused, and there is psychomotor and autonomic overactivity. These patients tend to require minimal sleep and constantly thrash about in bed or pace the halls. Speech output is increased and emotional tone heightened. Most often, however, the physician encounters a clinical syndrome that contains elements of both the hyperactive and the hypoactive variants, with unpredictable changes over the course of the day. No evidence indicates that the hypoactive syndrome is a milder form of, and will progress to, the hyperactive variant, and no obvious relationship exists between the specific cause of acute confusion and a particular variant of this syndrome.

Pathophysiology

The pathophysiologic mechanisms underlying the confusional states remain to be established. Some researchers have suggested that acute confusional states may result from decreased cerebral metabolism. However, in studies of patients with delirium tremens and delirium associated with hyperthermia, the cerebral metabolic rate is normal. Likewise, regional cerebral blood flow studies have thus far been inconclusive.[1]

Studies of endocrine function and delirium tremens have shown abnormalities of thyroxine (T_4), ACTH, and growth hormone; however, these disturbances are not considered to be of clinical significance.[1] Similarly, EEG and polygraphic sleep studies have not been helpful in understanding the pathophysiology of acute confusional states. The most common EEG abnormality is general slowing with activity in the theta and delta ranges. Bifrontal delta activity and triphasic waves have also occasionally been noted. However, the EEG is not invariably abnormal in confusion and is not directly correlated to mental status or behavior abnormalities.

In studies of the CSF metabolites of confused patients, abnormalities of 5-hydroxyindoleacetic acid, homovanillic acid, serotonin, and dopamine breakdown products have been documented.[6]

An acute confusional state associated with infarction in the area of the right middle cerebral artery involving the parietal and frontal lobes has been reported. Similarly, other case reports have demonstrated lesions associated with confusion in the right fusiform and calcarine regions, the fusiform and lingual gyri, and the hippocampal formation.[5]

No unified hypothesis for the pathophysiology of confusional states has yet emerged from these diverse observations. However, a discussion on consciousness and selective attention postulated a central nervous system (CNS) network, involving a disturbance in the integration of stimuli at one or more of several specific sites, the RAS, the limbic system, and the polymodal association areas of the cortex.[9] Such an elaborate network might be vulnerable to the wide range of etiologic agents reported to result in acute confusional states. The biochemical disturbances that are by far the most common causes of confusional states would probably act at the RAS level. This hypothesis would also encompass the less common focal cortical lesions associated with this disorder. This theory could explain various issues concerning the etiology, clinical signs, treatment, and outcome of confusional states.

Etiology

Acute confusional states can be divided into those of CNS origin and those caused by toxic-metabolic disorders. The common CNS disorders are trauma, seizures, infections, dementing diseases, nutritional problems, and mass lesions.

In head trauma a period of loss of consciousness may be followed by an agitated confusional state, even in the absence of obvious focal deficit.

A variable period of confusion may follow a seizure. In most instances, however, the duration of this confusional state is short. Occasionally, continuous psychomotor seizures manifest as an acute behavioral syndrome with profound confusion. Close observation of the patient may reveal clonic twitches, mouthing, or lip-smacking movements; an EEG may be needed to elucidate the diagnosis.

Encephalitis, especially when caused by herpes simplex and purulent meningitis, is an important infectious cause of the acute confusional syndrome and is one reason for performing a lumbar puncture in all patients with acute confusion in whom no clear contraindication exists.

Elderly patients or patients with dementia seem particularly prone to episodes of acute confusion. Acute confusion occurs in elderly patients most often when they develop congestive heart failure, a slight electrolyte imbalance, mild carbon dioxide retention, or constipation with fecal impaction. A relatively asymptomatic pyelonephritis or pneumonia may also manifest with acute confusion as the presenting problem.

Nutritional disorders such as Wernicke-Korsakoff syndrome (encephalopathy) are not rare. Patients with this syndrome have acute confusion, ataxia, bilateral sixth nerve palsies, and nystagmus. The disorder is most common in alcoholics, but food faddists and recluses may also develop thiamine deficiency. The policy of discharging increasing numbers of patients from state mental institutions has resulted in an increased incidence of Wernicke-Korsakoff encephalopathy in nonalcoholic patients. Some of these patients become recluses and severely neglect their nutrition. Pellagra caused by niacin deficiency is much rarer in Western society; confusion, irritability, insomnia, and photosensitive rash with diarrhea suggest this diagnosis.

Intracranial space-occupying lesions may cause confusional states as a nonfocal manifestation of distortion of the intracranial contents. The mass may be a neoplasm, hematoma, cyst, or granuloma. In all these instances, gadolinium-enhanced MRI or contrast CT is the major diagnostic test for sorting out these possibilities.

As previously discussed, occasionally, a patient with an acute, agitated confusional state may have only a small area of infarction, presumably in one of the multimodal cortical areas.

Drug intoxication is the most common cause of the acute confusional state in older adolescents and young adults. Amphetamines, lysergic acid, cocaine, and phencyclidine (angel dust) often produce an excited, hyperalert confusion with hallucinations (see Chapter 52). The belladonna alkaloids can cause a dramatic acute confusion in the elderly patient being treated for Parkinson's disease. Many prescription drugs in common use can cause acute confusional states, and this should be a prime consideration in any individual recently beginning medical treatment. Cimetidine has been found to be a fairly common cause of confusion in recent years, but many other frequently used drugs also seem capable of producing acute confusion.

The paradigm of the hyperalert, acute confusional state is that associated with alcohol withdrawal. In this condition, confusion, tremulousness, illusions, and hallucinations with restlessness appear within 10 to 72 hours after the cessation of drinking (see Chapter 51). Withdrawal seizures consistently occur before the onset of mental symptoms.

The range of alcohol-withdrawal syndromes is wide. The most severe form is delirium tremens, in which simultaneous mental, motor, and autonomic abnormalities occur. It is a life-threatening disorder with a significant mortality rate. Major withdrawal syndromes and seizures with confusion may also develop 2 to 8 days after withdrawal from chronic use of many sedatives and tranquilizers, including the barbiturates, glutethimide, and paraldehyde.

The metabolic encephalopathies are partially listed (Box 157-5). The clinical appearances of the mental syndrome in almost all disorders may be indistinguishable from one another. The distinction must be based on a careful, general medical evaluation and appropriate laboratory investigations for these disorders. The encephalopathy caused by endogenous derangements in metabolism usually causes a hypoalert or sleepy confusion with progression to coma. Some interesting exceptions to this rule include the hyperalert, agitated mental syndromes that may be seen in acute porphyria and hyperthyroidism. The finding of asterixis (metabolic flaps) or widespread, small-amplitude myoclonic jerks is characteristic of metabolic encephalopathies.

A full discussion of the psychiatric disorders that may be associated with acute confusional states is beyond the scope of this chapter. Acute schizophrenia and manic-depressive illness in the manic phase are the two most common problems. Physicians should be very wary of making the diagnosis of a psychiatric disorder in a somnolent or obtunded, confused patient.

The cause of confusional states appears to be nonspecific.

Box 157-5. Etiologic Agents in Acute Confusional States

A. Injury by physical agents
   1. Head trauma
   2. Heatstroke
   3. Radiation
   4. Electrocution
B. Infections
   1. Systemic pneumonia, typhoid, typhus, acute rheumatic fever, malaria, influenza, diphtheria, brucellosis, infectious mononucleosis, infectious hepatitis, subacute bacterial endocarditis, bacteremia, septicemia, Rocky Mountain spotted fever legionnaires' disease.
   2. Intracranial: acute, subacute, and chronic
      a. Viral encephalitis, aseptic meningitis, rabies
      b. Bacterial meningitis: meningococcal, pneumococcal, *Haemophilus influenzae,* etc.
      c. Postinfectious and postvaccinial encephalomyelitis
      d. Tuberculous meningitis
      e. Neurosyphilis
      f. Fungal infections: cryptococcosis, coccidioidomycosis, histoplasmosis, candidiasis (moniliasis), mucormycosis
      g. Protazoal infections: *Toxoplasma* encephalitis, cerebral malaria
      h. Trichinosis
C. Intoxication by drugs and poisons and withdrawal syndrome
   1. Drugs: anticholinergics, sedative-hypnotics, digitalis derivatives, opiates, corticosteroids, salicylates, antibiotics, anticonvulsants, antiarrhythmics and antihypertensives, antineoplastic agents, cimetidine, lithium, antiparkinsonian agents, disulfiram, indomethacin, bismuth salts, phencyclidine
   2. Alcohol: ethyl and methyl
   3. Addictive inhalants: gasoline, glue, ether, nitrous oxide, nitrates
   4. Industrial poisons: carbon disulfide, organic solvents, methyl chloride and bromide, heavy metals, organophosphorus insecticides, carbon monoxide
   5. Snakebite
   6. Poisonous plants and mushrooms
D. Metabolic disorders: nutritional and hormonal
   1. Hypoxia
   2. Hypoglycemia
   3. Hepatic, renal, pancreatic, and pulmonary insufficiency (encephalopathy)
   4. Avitaminosis: nicotinic acid, thiamine, cyanocobalamin (vitamin B_2), folate, pyridoxine
   5. Hypervitaminosis: intoxication by vitamins A and D
   6. Hormonal disorders: hyperinsulinism, hyperthyroidism, hypothyroidism, hypopituitarism, hyperparathyroidism
   7. Disorders of fluid and electrolyte metabolism
      a. Dehydration, water intoxication
      b. Alkalosis, acidosis
      c. Hypernatremia, hyponatremia, hyperkalemia, hypercalcemia, hypocalcemia, hypermagnesemia, hypomagnesemia
   8. Errors of metabolism
      a. Porphyria
      b. Carcinoid syndrome
      c. Hepatolenticular degeneration (Wilson's disease)
E. Vascular disorders
   1. Migraine
   2. Cerebrovascular disorders
      a. Transient ischemic attacks
      b. Hypertensive encephalopathy
      c. Thrombosis, embolism
      d. Subarachnoid hemorrhage
   3. Cardiovascular disorders
      a. Myocardial infarction
      b. Congestive heart failure
      c. Cardiac arrhythmias
   4. Vasculitis
      a. Polyarteritis nodosa
      b. Systemic lupus erythematosus
      c. Rheumatoid vasculitis
      d. Temporal arteritis
   5. Hematologic disorders
      a. Pernicious anemia
      b. Erythema
      c. Thrombotic thrombocytopenic pupura
F. Cerebral degenerative disorders: multiple sclerosis
G. Extracranial neoplasms and intracranial space-occupying lesions
H. Hypersensitivity and autoimmune disorders
   1. Serum sickness
   2. Food allergy

Modified from Lipowski ZJ: *Delirium,* Springfield, Ill, 1980, Charles C Thomas.

Almost any disturbance of body function may result in this syndrome. Box 157-5 presents an etiologic classification as an example of the long list of agents associated with confusional states.

Differential Diagnosis

The differential diagnosis of acute confusional states includes both "organic" and "functional" disorders. Although acute confusion is a distinctive syndrome, the varied symptomatology may cause difficulty in differentiating acute confusion from closely related disturbances.

Dementia. Dementia is an important consideration in the differential diagnosis of confusional states (see Chapter 158). The two conditions are similar in that they both involve a diffuse impairment of intellectual functioning. The confused patient, however, has what appears to be a specific disturbance of consciousness, whereas dementia occurs in the context of a "clear sensorium." The nature of onset and course of the illness are most valuable in separating these two conditions. Dementia is usually insidious in onset with a progressive deterioration, whereas confusion usually begins abruptly and shows little progression. Confusional states are relatively short-lived. If treated appropriately, and in some patients even if left untreated appropriately, spontaneous clearing may occur. Most cases of dementia, on the other hand, do not improve unless a specific treatable cause exists. Other features that help differentiate the two conditions are (1) fluctuation in symptoms, (2) disruption of the sleep-wake cycle, and (3) autonomic overactivity. These features, if present, usually favor a diagnosis of acute confusion. Periods of acute confusion, however, may be noted in the course of dementia. Dementia sometimes becomes much worse, and a stable dementia may exhibit a sudden deterioration. Frequently, this deterioration in the mental status is the result of a superimposed confusional state for which a reversible cause may be identified and corrected.

Korsakoff's Psychosis. Korsakoff's psychosis is an amnesic syndrome associated with features of disorientation and confabulation and dominated by memory disturbance. Confusional states should be easily differentiated, since Korsakoff's psychosis occurs in the setting of a clear sensorium.

Psychiatric Disorders. If the criteria in the *DSM-IV* are followed, the physician should have no difficulty in differentiating delirium from illnesses such as schizophrenia, mania, and depression.

Laboratory Investigations

The workup of the acutely confused patient is similar to that of the patient in coma: routine chest x-ray study; complete blood count; sedimentation rate, along with determination of serum glucose, electrolyte, calcium, and blood urea nitrogen levels and a toxic screen. Arterial blood gas values, serum ammonia tests, liver function studies, serum cortisol and T_4 levels, antinuclear antibodies, serum protein electrophoresis, and a urine test for porphyrins and heavy metals may be required in certain patients. An EEG may offer important evidence of a continuous complex partial seizure disorder or demonstrate the widespread symmetric slowing with triphasic activity that characterizes metabolic encephalopathies (e.g., hepatic encephalopathies). Rapid, frontally distributed EEG activity may signify the presence of sedative drugs.

A lumbar puncture should be performed on every patient who is acutely confused unless a distinct contraindication exists. Contraindications consist of two possibilities: (1) the patient may be seen in a phase marked by extremely rapid, ongoing improvement, as in the treatment of a bout of hypoglycemia, or (2) a lumbar puncture may be deferred, a circumstance that arises in a patient with signs of increased intracranial pressure from a mass lesion. In this second situation, it is not satisfactory simply to defer a lumbar puncture; urgent alternative diagnostic measures, usually neuroimaging, should be performed.

Neurologic and neurosurgical consultation should be obtained for advice and guidance regarding the selection of procedures or further diagnostic tests. The role of other noninvasive examinations, such as isotope brain scanning, flow scans, and the EEG, remains a matter of judgment that must take into account both the rate of progression of the patient's clinical status and the likelihood of diagnostic yield. Both EEG and neuroimaging may be difficult if the patient is restless or combative.

Management

Treatment largely depends on correcting the specific underlying abnormality. Since medication is frequently a cause of confusional states, the most effective approach is to discontinue the medication whenever possible while correcting any underlying metabolic disturbance. In most instances the etiology is clear, but in the more difficult cases a full workup is essential because attempts at simply controlling the behavior may result, for example, in not recognizing a case of fatal meningitis.

The management of the behavior disturbance could be accomplished by pharmacotherapy; however, most confused patients benefit more from specialized nursing care. For the more belligerent patients, it is often necessary to use geriatric chairs or padded bedrails or to glove and partially restrain the patient limbs. Generally, however, patients do best unrestrained but contained in an environment where strict limits are set. Large calendars, constant reassurance, and positive reinforcement from the staff are invaluable orienting stimuli and often improve behavior. The bedside lamp and radio are helpful aids when the patient awakens at night. Only when these measures have failed should pharmacotherapy be used.

Antipsychotics are the most popular drugs in the treatment of confusional states. No evidence has shown that one is superior to any other. Haloperidol is frequently used. Loxapine is more sedating and in some patients might be preferable. Most of the sedative-hypnotic agents, such as barbiturates, chloral hydrate, and flurazepam, are less helpful and may even exacerbate the confusional state. The anxiolytics are sometimes effective. Chlorazepam and oxazepam have relatively short half-lives with little buildup of active metabolites. β-Adrenergic blockers such as propranolol have been reported to be effective in agitated and belligerent patients and may be particularly effective in elderly patients. Antihistamines are sedating and sometimes useful. Initial dosages of all drugs should be low and should increase only in gradual increments, since all these medications may precipitate a paradoxical reaction with greatly increased behavioral disturbances. Disturbances in the sleep-wake cycle are often difficult to correct. Prevention of "catnaps" during the day may help promote a full night of sleep. Sedation, however, is rarely effective; the sleep-wake cycle usually normalizes only as the confusional state clears.

REFERENCES

1. Adams RD, Victor M: Delirium and other acute confusional states. In Adams RD, Victor M, editors: *Principles of neurology,* New York, 1981, McGraw-Hill.
2. Adams RD, Victor M: *Principles of neurology,* ed 4, New York, 1989, McGraw-Hill.
3. ANA Committee on Ethical Affairs: Persistent vegetative state: report of the American Neurological Committee on Ethical Affairs, *Ann Neurol* 33:386, 1993.
4. Defeudis FV: Cholinergic roles in consciousness. In Defeudis FV, editor: *Central cholinergic systems and behavior,* London, 1974, Academic.
5. Horenstein S, Chamberlain W, Conomy J: Infarction of the fusiform and calcarine regions: agitated delirium and hemianopia, *Trans Am Neurol Assoc* 92:85, 1967.
6. Jouvet M: The role of monoamines and acetyl choline containing neurons in the regulation of the sleep/wake cycle, *Rev Physiol* 64:166, 1972.
7. Levy DE, et al: Prognosis in non-traumatic coma, *Ann Intern Med* 94:293, 1981.
8. Lloyd GG: Acute behavior disturbances, *J Neurol Neurosurg Psychiatry* 56:1149, 1993.
9. Mesulam M: A cortical network for directed attention and unilateral neglect, *Ann Neurol* 10:309, 1981.
10. Plum F, Posner JB: *The diagnosis of stupor and coma,* ed 3, Philadelphia, 1980, FA Davis.
11. Sabin TD: Coma and the confusional state in the emergency room, *Med Clin North Am* 65:15, 1981.
12. Teasdale G: Prognosis of coma after head injury. In Turnbridge WMG, editor: *Advanced medicine,* London, 1981, Pittman Medical.

13. Tinuper P: Idiopathic recurring stupor: a case with possible involvement of the gamma aminobutyric acid (GABA)ergic system, *Ann Neurol* 31:503, 1992.
14. Weinbroum A, Rudick V, Sorkine P, et al: Use of flumazenil in the treatment of drug overdose: a double blind and open study in 110 patients, *Crit Care Med* 24:199, 1996.

CHAPTER 158

Cognitive Change and Dementia

Claire A. Levesque

Dementing illnesses occur often, particularly in elderly persons, and are major causes of devastating losses of function, leading to institutionalization. Dementia, a syndrome resulting from many etiologies, is a slow loss of previously acquired intellectual or behavioral function without alteration in level of awareness. At least two areas of cognitive function, such as memory, language, personality, visuospatial abilities, or judgment, are impaired in dementia, and the disabilities affect independent daily living.[22]

Dementia differs from delirium. Delirium, or an acute confusional state, is an acute or subacute onset of disorientation with alterations in levels of awareness, including hyperalert and drowsy states. It often disrupts day/night cycles and can be accompanied by delusions (see Chapter 157). Delirium may coexist with dementia. Dementia also differs from normal aging. In elderly persons, short-term memory may be impaired in tasks requiring the manipulation of material such as digit spans backward or in memory tasks requiring divided attention. Response time can increase, and memory for proper names may be affected. This "benign senescent forgetfulness" is a gradual process that does not impair daily living or disrupt social skills.

Dementia is a common disorder in elderly persons, occurring in all ethnic groups. There may be some variabilities in etiologies based on ethnic background and other precipitant factors. People in all ethnic groups show an increasing prevalence of dementia with increasing age. Alzheimer's disease (AD) is the most common cause of dementia, and the estimated prevalence of probable AD in those over 84 years old in one study was 47.2%.[9] These statistics are sobering in the context of a predicted population of 4.6 million over age 85 in the United States in the year 2000.

Dementia is truly a devastating disease that robs patients of their personalities and their ability to interact. It is also the fourth or fifth most common cause of death, although it rarely appears on death certificates. The economic impact of this problem is staggering. The annual cost of the formal and informal care for one patient with AD is estimated at $47,000 in 1990 dollars, with the annual cost for all forms of dementia at $58 billion.[19] The cost of a full diagnostic evaluation (usually less than $2000) is clearly cost-effective even if a treatable form of dementia is found only occasionally. Also, the difference in the quality of life is vast. Unfortunately, many patients have progressive irreversible forms of dementia. Families often keep their loved ones in the home in the face of staggering caregiver burden. Behaviors most likely to lead to institutionalization include wandering, aggressive outbursts, sleep disturbances, and incontinence. Home care can be practical and cost-effective in the early stages of dementia, but levels of service vary depending on the latest insurance regulations, and the burden on family is immense. In later stages, nursing home care provides relief to the overburdened caregiver and can also be less costly than formal and informal home care costs.

Multiple studies have been done on the risk factors for the development of dementia. Many have focused on AD, the most common progressive neurodegenerative cause. Some studies have implicated factors such as history of head trauma or lower educational level, but no definitive risk factors have been identified. Hypertension and diabetes are major risk factors for vascular forms of dementia, such as multiinfarct dementia and Binswanger's disease. Since the differential diagnosis of dementia is so broad, other risk factors can be found specific to particular etiologies, such as alcohol abuse and subdural hematomas or exposure to the transmissible agents and the development of Creutzfeldt-Jakob disease. Genetic factors also play a role in some dementing illnesses, such as Huntington's disease, the familial form of AD, and perhaps even in "sporadic" cases of AD.

Most causes of dementia lead to the death or metabolic dysfunction of neurons, producing losses in cognitive function. The location of the cell loss is a critical factor. In AD the cell loss is most prominent in the cortex, hippocampus, and amygdala, disrupting connections critical for memory and other cognitive function. In multiinfarct dementia, small strokes placed in strategic locations can lead to the loss of memory, visuospatial abilities, language, and personality. Dementia can also occur because of a change in the overall chemical milieu of the brain; common examples include endocrine disturbances such as hypothyroidism and toxic encephalopathies resulting from medications. These and other "reversible" dementias are less common but are critically important to diagnose. Patients with a definitive neurodegenerative cause of dementia often have a coexisting treatable factor at initial presentation or later in the course of the disease. For instance, a patient with AD may have a rapid functional deterioration caused by problems such as depression or endocrine disturbances.

HISTORY

In a dementing illness, it is critically important to obtain history from the caregiver as well as the patient. In addition to questions about the changes in the patient's behavior, specific questions should be asked about difficulties with activities of daily living such as eating, dressing, and toileting. Some standardized questions have been developed to assist in this history taking, such as the Blessed dementia scale (Box 158-1). All medications, including over-the-counter (OTC) medications, folk remedies, alcohol, and street drugs, should be carefully reviewed. A change in drinking pattern may go unnoticed by family members, especially if the patient lives alone, and may represent self-treatment of depression. Currently, a history of street drug use occurs infrequently in elderly persons but may be expected to increase in prevalence in the ensuing years and is a risk factor for dementia related to acquired immunodeficiency syndrome

Box 158-1. Blessed Dementia Scale

Name ____________________
Total incompetence = 1
Variable incapacity = ½

Changes in Performance of Everyday Activities

1. Inability to perform household tasks, handle money	1	½	0
2. Inability to cope with small sums of money	1	½	0
3. Inability to remember short list of items, (e.g., in shopping)	1	½	0
4. Inability to find way about indoors	1	½	0
5. Inability to find way about familiar street	1	½	0
6. Inability to interpret surroundings (e.g., to recognize whether in hospital or at home, to discriminate among patients, physicians, nurses, relatives, hospital staff)	1	½	0
7. Inability to recall recent events (e.g., recent outings, visits of relatives or friends to hospital)	1	½	0
8. Tendency to dwell in the past	1	½	0

Changes in Habits

9. Eating	
a. Cleanly with proper utensils	0
b. Messily with spoon only	1
c. Simple solids, (e.g., biscuits)	2
d. Has to be fed	3
10. Dressing	
a. Unaided	0
b. Occasionally misplaced buttons, etc.	1
c. Wrong sequence, often forgetting items	2
d. Unable to dress	3
11. Complete sphincter control	0
a. Occasional wet beds	1
b. Frequent wet beds	2
c. Doubly incontinent	3

Changes in Personality, Interests, Drive

No change	0
12. Increased rigidity	1
13. Increased egocentricity	1
14. Impairment of regard for feelings of others	1
15. Coarsening of affect	1
16. Impairment of emotional control (e.g., increased petulance and irritability)	1
17. Hilarity in inappropriate situations	1
18. Diminished emotional responsiveness	1
19. Sexual misdemeanor (appearing de novo in old age)	1
20. Hobbies relinquished	1
21. Diminished initiative or growing apathy	1
22. Purposeless hyperactivity	1

Subtotal ____________

Information-Memory-Concentration Test

Positive score for each correct item; 37 points maximum (intact)

Name ____________	1
Age ____________	1
Time (hour) ____________	1
Time of day ____________	1
Day of week ____________	1
Date ____________	1
Month ____________	1
Season ____________	1
Year ____________	1
Place: Name ____________	1
Street ____________	1
Town ____________	1
Type of place (home, hospital, etc.) ____________	1
Recognition of persons (cleaner, physician, nurse, patient, relative; any two available) ____________	1

Memory

1. Personal	
a. Date of birth	1
b. Place of birth	1
c. School attended	1
d. Occupation	1
e. Name of siblings/spouse	1
f. Name of any town where patient had worked	1
g. Name of employer	1
2. Nonpersonal	
a. Date of WWI	1
b. Date of WWII	1
c. President	1
d. Vice-President	1
3. Name and address (5-minute recall) Mr. John Brown 42 West Street Cambridge, MA	5

Concentration

Months of year backward	2	1	0
Counting 1 to 20	2	1	0
Counting 20 to 1	2	1	0

Subtotal ____________

Total dementia score ____________

Modified from Blessed G et al: *Br J Psychiatry* 114:797, 1968.

(AIDS). A medical review of systems should focus on a history of hypertension, diabetes, thyroid disease, vitamin B_{12} deficiency (including history of gastric surgery), and syphilis and on an evaluation of the risk factors for disease related to the human immunodeficiency virus (HIV). The family history of dementia is vital for certain diagnoses such as Huntington's disease and familial AD. Prior psychiatric illnesses in the patient or other family members should be recorded. The patient's educational and occupational history allows an estimation of premorbid cognitive functioning.

PHYSICAL AND NEUROLOGIC EXAMINATION

In addition to a general medical examination, including cardiac and thyroid examinations plus evaluation for carotid bruits, orthostatic blood pressures are determined for any patient with vascular risk factors. Because of incorrect answers, "covering" of memory lapses, and overreliance on empty social comments, open-ended discussion with the patient often suggests a diagnosis of dementia. The mental status examination should include a range of questions to assess multiple cognitive spheres. The Folstein minimental status examination (see Chapter 8) and the Blessed dementia scale (see Box 158-1) include scales of information, memory, concentration, language, and visuospatial abilities. Testing for apraxia can include imitation of gestures and demonstrations of complex movements, such as saluting or brushing hair. Vision can be tested with a hand-held card with patients wearing eyeglasses, if applicable. Hearing can be tested by whispering numbers in each ear. The remainder of the neurologic examination should focus on finding focal abnormalities. Hemiparesis, reflex asymmetries, and sensory changes may be signs of previous strokes or mass lesions. Patterns of sensory loss may represent peripheral neuropathy suggestive of vitamin B_{12} deficiency, alcohol-related causes of dementia, neurosyphilis, and multiple other reversible causes. These focal signs suggest the need for further neurologic consultation.

DIFFERENTIAL DIAGNOSIS

Evaluation of the patient with dementing illness, particularly in the mild to moderate stages, must emphasize a search for potentially reversible causes. Patients may also have multiple causes for dementia, and even when the clinical impression strongly suggests a neurodegenerative process, coexisting reversible causes should be investigated. The primary care physician should consider neurologic consultation when the dementing process is accompanied by elementary neurologic findings, when atypical features emerge, or when therapeutic questions arise. The differential diagnoses listed here emphasize the most common and the most treatable causes.[5,16]

Alzheimer's Disease and Familial Alzheimer's Disease

AD is the most common cause of devastating progressive dementia.[9,32] The characteristic neuropathologic change consists of senile plaques (Fig. 158-1), neurofibrillary tangles (Fig. 158-2), and atrophy. Although some of these changes can be seen with normal aging, both the distribution and the extent of the senile plaques and tangles are different.[14]

Many neurotransmitters are decreased in brains of AD patients. The cholinergic system shows consistent involvement and has been a target of various therapeutic approaches, including tacrine and donepezil. Multiple lines of research implicate β-amyloid or its processing as a key event in causation. The β-amyloid protein is a major constituent of the plaque seen in brains of AD patients (see Fig. 158-1), and mutations have been found in some pedigrees of familial AD on chromosome 21 near the gene encoding amyloid precursor protein. However, other pedigrees have mutations in other loci on chromosomes 14 and 19. These genetic data, plus the variability in age at presentation and extrapyramidal features, point to heterogeneity even in familial cases.[4] A potential

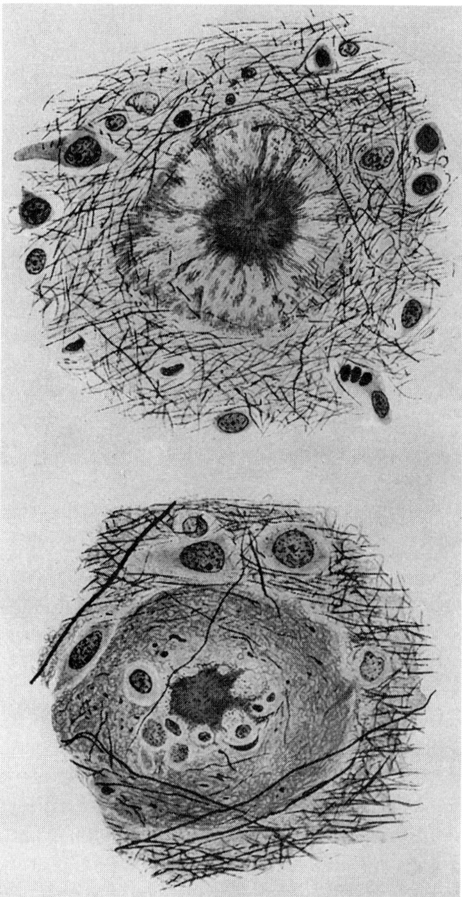

Fig. 158-1. Senile plaque appears to be made up of degenerating neural processes with a central accumulation of amyloid. (From Spielmeyer W: *Histopathologie des Nervensystems*, Berlin, 1922, Springer.)

genetic link for sporadic cases has been identified with an association with the E4 allele for apolipoprotein E (the basis for APOE testing), which is involved in lipoprotein metabolism and binds to the β-amyloid protein.[4,7,29] Environmental toxins have also been considered in AD, and studies have demonstrated aluminum in the neurofibrillary tangles.

In patients with both sporadic and familial AD, mental changes are gradual and progressive. Sometimes, the changes are first noted by family members or health care providers after a major event in the patient's life, such as the death of a family member, surgery, or another medical illness. The mental change usually begins with impaired recall of recent events, word-finding difficulty, and inability to perceive spatial relationships. A series of words may be correctly done with immediate repetition if the patient is attentive, but the patient is unable to perform accurately if an interval of 3 to 4 minutes is interposed. Complaints by family members that the patient is "living in the past" reflect the relative preservation of remote memory. The attentive examiner often is able to detect difficulty in word finding as the patient makes word substitutions and circumlocutions. Asking the patient to name a series of common objects and their parts confirms this finding. Difficulty in drawing a simple map of a familiar intersection, an outline map of the United States, or a geometric shape reveals the associated difficulty with spatial

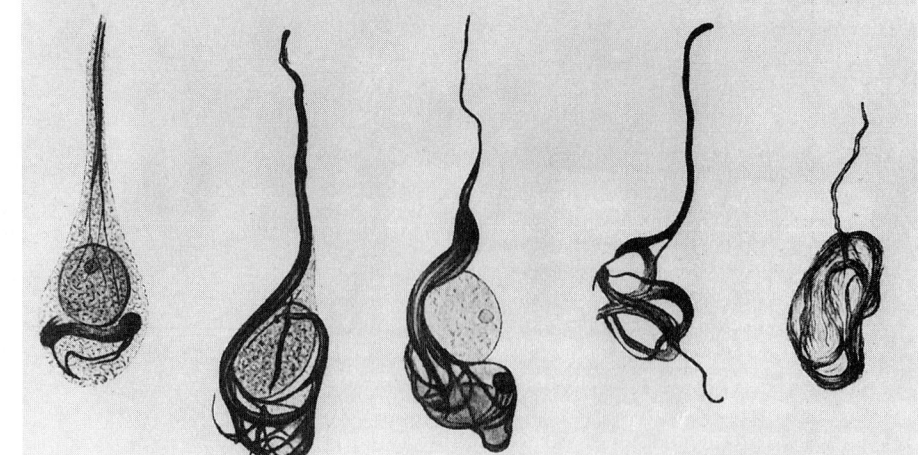

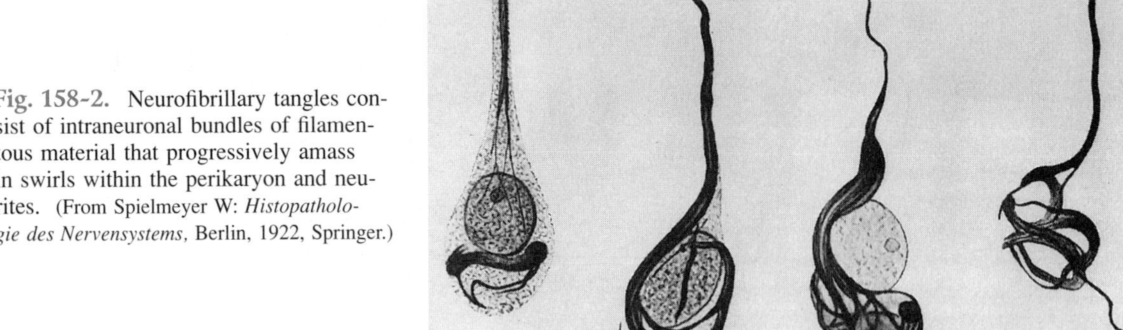

Fig. 158-2. Neurofibrillary tangles consist of intraneuronal bundles of filamentous material that progressively amass in swirls within the perikaryon and neurites. (From Spielmeyer W: *Histopathologie des Nervensystems,* Berlin, 1922, Springer.)

relationships. A patient with this problem often becomes lost when driving alone or walking even in a familiar area.

These three features—retentive memory, spatial difficulties, and word-finding problems—are usually well established before frontal lobe dysfunction occurs. With progression, inappropriate behavior with neglected personal hygiene develops. The episodic outburst, sometimes called a *catastrophic reaction,* can involve aggressive behavior toward family members. These outbursts by a patient with dementia are very frightening to caregivers and consist of an outpouring of negative emotions unresponsive to reassurance or redirection. Wandering is another behavior that is very difficult for family members. Patients may leave the home inappropriately attired and lose their way. Wandering patients with dementia unfortunately may be found dead because of exposure to the environment or traumatic injury. Sleep disturbances also occur, and patients wake in the middle of the night and wander in the home. This can be particularly dangerous, since the patient can drop burning cigarettes, turn on the gas stove, or engage in other potentially dangerous activities while the caregiver sleeps. Disrobing and inappropriate sexual advances occur in some individuals as the disinhibition progresses. These behaviors are poorly tolerated in both the family home and nursing home and do respond to a combination of behavioral techniques and medications.

Even the most severe abnormalities in these higher functions are not ordinarily accompanied by elementary neurologic findings. The motor abnormalities occur only in advanced cases and include hyperreflexia, spasticity, or upgoing toes. Most patients have paratonic rigidity with a tendency toward flexed immobility in the upper and lower extremities. Frontal release signs, such as grasp, suck, and snout reflexes, develop in later stages. This state is preceded by a deterioration in gait, which has been attributed to grasp reflexes in the feet. Initiating gait becomes difficult, and the patient takes many small steps before moving forward. Seizures may occur very late in the course of AD. A patient with focal neurologic signs or early onset of seizures should be evaluated by a neurologist because other causes of dementia may be present.

Patients with AD usually die 2 to 10 years after diagnosis, although some live longer. Pneumonia is a common cause of death. There is no "gold standard" test for AD. The only definitive test is neuropathologic evaluation of the brain at biopsy or at postmortem examination. Since no curative treatment currently exists for AD, brain biopsy is not recommended. Computed tomography (CT) scans or magnetic resonance imaging (MRI) of the head shows widespread atrophy with a predilection for the temporal lobes and helps exclude other causes. Biparietal hypoperfusion is seen on single-positron emission computed tomography (SPECT) scanning, although this finding is not specific and has not been well documented pathologically. Genotypes for the E4 allele of apolipoprotein E (APOE) are commercially available and may be used as supportive data if the clinical syndrome is present. APOE testing is not indicated in presymptomatic individuals at this time. Other peripheral markers in blood, skin, and cerebrospinal fluid (CSF) have been investigated, but none is definitive currently. The use of potential diagnostic tests for AD, especially those felt to predict future risk, is fraught with potential problems, particularly in the absence of preventive or curative treatments. Test results may have a negative impact on employment and insurance status and cause emotional trauma.[7,29]

Although no gold standard test exists for AD, clinicopathologic correlations have shown that experienced clinicians correctly diagnose AD in most cases. This accuracy is improved by an initial evaluation by a clinician specializing in dementia and a clinical reevaluation about 6 to 12 months after the diagnostic evaluation. Although previously underdiagnosed, AD may now be overdiagnosed, and reversible causes may be missed. In addition, AD sometimes does not occur in isolation. Overlap of AD and vascular dementia is relatively common, and treatable causes such as depression, drug effects, vitamin B_{12} deficiency, and coexisting chronic infections can occur. AD is slowly progressive, and rapid deteriorations in function or additional focal neurologic signs should always prompt evaluation for other causes, such as intercurrent pneumonia, urinary tract infection, or chronic subdural hematoma.

Alzheimer's Disease and Down Syndrome

The pathologic changes seen in AD have been found in the brains of adults with Down syndrome.[36] However, many of these individuals do not develop the clinical syndrome. In some, no cognitive deterioration is apparent. In others the presentation is atypical. Diagnosis is also hindered by the lack of an appropriate neuropsychologic instrument to delineate cognitive deficits across the intelligence quotient (IQ) spectrum found in Down syndrome.[2] APOE testing is unlikely to be helpful, since the distribution of alleles in a population with Down syndrome appears to be similar to that in the general population. However, the presence of the E4 allele may correlate with earlier onset of the disease.[26] Other potentially treatable causes of dementia, particularly hypothyroidism and depression, are also common and must always be considered.

Other Neurodegenerative Diseases

Frontal lobe dementias are syndromes characterized by frontal atrophy with prominent behavioral features. The most common is Pick's disease, a neurodegenerative disorder that is sometimes difficult to differentiate from AD. The temporal and frontal lobes are selectively involved in this disease. Features that support a diagnosis of Pick's disease include early onset of personality change, disinhibition, increased oral behaviors (e.g., eating, smoking, drinking), and onset before age 65. A very severe and unusual form of aphasia may be an early manifestation and is often combined with behavioral disturbances. This disorder may occur more often than previously thought. The course of Pick's disease appears to be more rapid than that of AD. Imaging studies may show preferential enlargement of the temporal horns with focal frontal and temporal atrophy. SPECT scanning also shows a preferential hypoperfusion of the frontal lobes with relative sparing of parietal lobes. Definite diagnosis requires examination of the brain, which reveals "knife-edge" atrophy of the superior temporal gyrus, absence of the characteristic plaques and tangles of AD, and the presence of Pick's cells and Pick's bodies. No known treatment exists for Pick's disease, and patients with this condition often require earlier nursing home placement because of the behavioral disturbances.[23]

Dementia with Lewy bodies is now felt to be more common than previously thought.[21] Although a positive diagnosis is possible only by biopsy or at autopsy, certain clinical features support the diagnosis. The presence of visual hallucinations and Parkinson's disease must prompt consideration of this form of dementia. The course is progressive, although cognitive performance can vary. This disorder is also marked by an acute sensitivity to neuroleptic agents, and these medications must be used with great caution and careful monitoring, if at all.[21]

Other primary neurologic causes of dementia have associated elementary neurologic findings accompanying the changes in mental status. Huntington's disease is an autosomal dominant disorder with dementia, chorea, and psychiatric changes. The average age of onset is the fourth decade, although dementia may appear more than a year before any movement disorder is present. During this time, diagnosis may be difficult if a positive family history has not been determined. CT or MRI shows marked atrophy of the caudate nucleus. Wilson's disease is an autosomal recessive disorder of copper metabolism characterized by behavioral disturbances, tremors, other abnormal movements, Kayser-Fleischer rings, and liver disease. The onset is usually in adolescence or young adulthood but may be as late as the fifth decade of life.

Multiple sclerosis may present as a dementing disease because of the development of bilateral periventricular demyelination. In such a case the evaluation should include a detailed search of the medical history for evidence of a previous demyelinating episode in an atypical cause of dementia, especially with early, severe frontal lobe features. Examination of the spinal fluid for oligoclonal banding and for immunoelectrophoresis and MRI of the brain showing the characteristic white-matter changes are diagnostic in the appropriate clinical setting.

The tremor, rigidity, and bradykinesias present in Parkinson's disease eliminate diagnostic difficulties in this cause of dementia. The treatment of Parkinson's disease and any associated depression often temporarily improves these patients' cognitive function. Olivopontocerebellar degeneration is a progressive disorder and is often associated with very slow, progressive dementia. Characteristic shrinkage of the pons and cerebellum can be best seen on MRI and is always present at the time mental changes supervene. No effective treatment is available for this disorder. A mild dementia, compounded by extreme slowness in expression, language, and movement, accompanies progressive supranuclear palsy. Loss of vertical eye movements and development of truncal rigidity are characteristic features of this rare disease. These patients do not respond to dopaminergic drugs.

Cerebrovascular Disease

In the past, dementia was commonly thought to result from "hardening of the arteries." This misconception resulted in the widespread use of cerebrovasodilators for dementia, a treatment of dubious value. Cerebrovascular disease, however, does produce dementia if lesions are strategically placed. One series demonstrated a 38.7% prevalence of vascular dementia in a white Northern European cohort of 85-year-old people,[32] which is even higher than previously reported. Also, vascular causes of dementia can also coexist with AD. A patient who has several strokes in areas important for cognitive function (e.g., deep temporal lobe, frontal lobes) can be easy to diagnose. However, in other patients, multiple small lacunar infarcts can occur, often in "silent" areas of the brain. Hypertension or diabetes significantly increases the risk for lacunar infarctions. A careful history may elicit several episodes of clear-cut deterioration in function. Since multiinfarct dementia can be difficult to distinguish from AD, a scoring system called the *Hachinski ischemic score* (Table 158-1) can be a useful reminder of features that suggest vascular disease.[12] MRI can also be helpful in this diagnosis because very small infarctions can be seen using this modality. This diagnosis is important to make, since careful control of hypertension while maintaining adequate perfusion and avoiding episodic hypotension may be the key to preventing further deterioration. Another dementing cerebrovascular disorder is Binswanger's encephalopathy. The dementia in this case is accompanied by bilateral pyramidal signs (weakness, increased reflexes) and intense frontal lobe signs. The patient may appear abulic and have diffusely increased muscle tone. Prominent palmar and plantar grasp reflexes are often present, and urinary incontinence and a slow, unsteady gait are common. MRI shows multiple white-matter infarcts in a periventricular distribution becoming confluent. Unfortunately, MRI also shows this pattern in patients who do not exhibit a clinical syndrome. The diagnosis of Binswanger's disease and other forms of dementia are in evolution, and several criteria have recently been proposed.[8,15,28]

Table 158-1. Hachinski Ischemic Score to Distinguish Cerebrovascular Dementia from Alzheimer's Disease

Feature	Score*
Abrupt onset	2
Stepwise deterioration	1
Fluctuating course	2
Nocturnal confusion	1
Relative preservation of personality	1
Depression	1
Somatic complaints	1
Emotional incontinence	1
History of hypertension	1
History of cerebrovascular accidents (strokes)	2
Evidence of associated atherosclerosis	1
Focal neurologic symptoms	2
Focal neurologic signs	2

Modified from Hachinski VC, et al: Cerebral blood flow in dementia, *Arch Neurol* 32:632, 1975.
*A total score less than 4 means that vascular dementia is unlikely, whereas scores greater than 7 indicate that vascular dementia is probable.

Vasculitis

Systemic vasculitides, such as systemic lupus erythematosus, can involve the brain and cause a confusional state. These patients can be diagnosed by the systemic signs and symptoms. Vasculitis involving the brain occurs infrequently in other systemic illnesses, such as sarcoidosis and AIDS. Less often, isolated central nervous system (CNS) vasculitis occurs without involvement of other organs and without increases in sedimentation rate or antibody titers. Cerebral angiography may show beading of blood vessels and other changes in vessel caliber, but often the results are normal. Biopsy of meningeal vessels can show vasculitic changes in some cases. Although CNS vasculitis is a challenging diagnosis, patients do respond, at least transiently, to immunosuppressive agents.

Depression and Psychiatric Disorders

Depression can cause a syndrome termed *pseudodementia,* which can be difficult to distinguish from other causes of dementia.[35] Depression can also coexist in AD, usually in the early stages in patients with enough retained insight. A depressed affect may be present in some of these patients but is not universal. As with other forms of depression in elderly patients, agitation or psychotic features can occur. During cognitive testing, these patients frequently answer, "I don't know," and often give up easily. The examination reveals inconsistencies in performance. The failures tend to occur in all areas of testing, unlike the more selective deficits seen in other dementias. A previous history of depression in the patient or a positive family history can be helpful. Patients with mild or moderate dementia can still answer questions about their mood, and statements can be corroborated by caregivers. Formal testing by a qualified neuropsychologist may be helpful, but even then, the patient's condition may be indistinguishable from that of true dementia. Extensive and repeated interdisciplinary assessments may be necessary.

If depression is a serious consideration, a trial of antidepressant treatment should be given. However, this treatment should have clear end points with reevaluations because long-term use of antidepressants, particularly those with anticholinergic side effects, can cause confusion. The pharmacologic options for the treatment of depression include the serotonin reuptake inhibitors and tricyclic antidepressants and related compounds. The medication chosen should have the least potential for serious side effect and the most potential for improvement. Close follow-up is essential. Methylphenidate, a stimulant drug, may be helpful in depressed elderly patients with psychomotor retardation but should be started at low doses, gradually increased, and continued only if improvement is noted. Electroconvulsive therapy is sometimes beneficial and safe even in the fragile elderly patient, especially when medication side effects prohibit drug use (see Chapter 48). Referral to a psychiatrist or behavioral neurologist should be considered to confirm the diagnosis in atypical cases if symptoms persist after first line treatment or if side effects limit therapy.

Patients with chronic schizophrenia can also appear cognitively slowed in their older years. It is important to remember the potential effects of long-term use of neuroleptic agents on motor function and response time. Episodic periods of institutionalization can also produce limits on knowledge of current and historical information, making some memory testing more complicated. Patients with schizophrenia are also naturally at risk for all causes of dementia, and a careful diagnostic evaluation is warranted if a cognitive deterioration is suspected. Reduction of medication doses and changes to the newer atypical antipsychotic medications should also be considered.

Normal-Pressure Hydrocephalus

In normal-pressure hydrocephalus (NPH), the clinical triad of dementia, incontinence, and gait disorder is associated with enlarged cerebral ventricles out of proportion to any atrophy present. This is a disorder of CSF circulation or absorption, with normal or high-normal opening pressure on lumbar puncture. The syndrome may develop after inflammatory states within the subarachnoid space, such as meningitis, encephalitis, or subarachnoid bleeding, but most are idiopathic. The dementia associated with NPH does not appear to have any characteristic features. CT or MRI of the head shows enlargement of ventricles out of proportion to the amount of atrophy, transependymal fluid, and rounding of the ventricular horns. On MRI, a signal void caused by moving CSF has been described in the third ventricle. Radioisotope cisternography demonstrates the absence of isotope flow in the subarachnoid space over the hemispheric convexities. Another test that may be helpful is removing a large amount (20 to 30 ml) of CSF, followed by a careful observation for transient improvements in cognitive status and gait. Cognitive and timed-gait testing is then repeated after the lumbar puncture at intervals over several days. An improvement in clinical status after a high-volume lumbar puncture has been felt to be predictive of a positive response to lumboperitoneal shunting, although this has been challenged.[18] Unfortunately, none of the diagnostic tests has been effective in demonstrating a high probability of favorable response to shunting. Therefore the risk-benefit ratio of shunting must be carefully considered in consultation with the patient, the family, and the neurosurgeon.[3,34]

Nonconvulsive Status

Most seizures are dramatic events with sudden alteration in consciousness, stereotyped behaviors, and jerking movements. However, in some instances, subclinical seizures can occur and may be almost continuous, resulting in a state called *nonconvulsive status* or *complex partial status*. This state of continuous nonclinical seizures can continue for prolonged periods. It is readily diagnosed by electroencephalography (EEG), with a characteristic ictal pattern. This syndrome occurs infrequently but is treatable with anticonvulsants. It may occur with metabolic or toxic disruptions or with no apparent precipitant. A prior seizure history is not necessary.

Infections

At the turn of the twentieth century, neurosyphilis would have been one of the most common reasons for chronic progressive dementia. Although the widespread use of penicillin has made CNS syphilis a rare disorder, it has been more prevalent since the onset of AIDS. The CSF in active cases always contains increased numbers of white blood cells and produces positive results from the Venereal Disease Research Laboratories (VDRL) test. Patients tend to have a progressive frontal-type dementia associated with bilateral pyramidal signs and distal and perioral tremors, along with delusions of grandeur and Argyll Robertson pupils. Treatment with intravenous (IV) penicillin is indicated.[30,31]

Several diseases traditionally classified as degenerative are now known to be caused by prions; the prime example is Creutzfeldt-Jakob disease. This disorder affects middle-aged individuals, who develop severe dementia, widespread myoclonic jerking, and rigidity, with a fatal outcome usually in weeks to months. Some patients have survived for several years and have had a more chronic course. This disease has been transmitted to nonhuman primates, and human-to-human transmission has been documented via corneal transplants, injection with growth hormone extracted from human pituitary glands, human cadaveric dura mater implants, and indwelling brain electrodes. Usual methods of sterilization are not adequate to destroy the agents responsible for this disease; common household bleach is most effective. Tissue may remain infectious for years, and the transmissible agent appears to be a prion. Brain biopsy is required to prove the diagnosis. The clinical syndrome and an EEG showing characteristic periodic complexes support the diagnosis of Creutzfeldt-Jakob disease. Rare familial forms of prion diseases (e.g., Gerstmann-Sträussler disease) appear to represent a situation in which the genome can manufacture an infectious polypeptide. The recent outbreak of "mad cow disease" in the United Kingdom has raised concerns of possible transmission to humans by the ingestion of affected meat products. There have been a limited number of atypical cases of Creutzfeldt-Jakob disease with prominent psychiatric and sensory symptoms in younger individuals in the United Kingdom, but to date none has been conclusively linked to the ingestion of meat products.[13]

Other infectious causes of dementia include frontal or temporal lobe brain abscesses and chronic meningitides, such as cryptococcal meningitis, which is spread by ubiquitous spores. Although most common in immunosuppressed patients, cryptococcal meningitis is one of the only fungal meningitides that occurs in an otherwise healthy adult.

HIV encephalopathy must also be considered in the initial evaluation of dementia. Inquiries about risk factors for HIV disease are often neglected in elderly persons. Consent for HIV testing can be difficult to obtain in patients with dementia. Low T-cell counts are surrogate markers of HIV disease but can raise ethical questions if performed without consent. Neuroimaging such as MRI or CT with contrast delineates many of the mass lesions associated with deterioration in cognitive function in this population or the atrophy and white-matter changes seen in HIV encephalopathy. Fortunately the advent of new medications has decreased the prevalence of HIV encephalopathy. However, some patients, particularly the elderly, are not diagnosed in early asymptomatic stages or are not taking antiretroviral treatment and present with dementia (see Chapter 32).

Metabolic Disorders

Metabolic disorders may cause gradual changes in mental status, and the aged brain is extremely vulnerable to a host of changes in the metabolic state. Mild degrees of pulmonary, renal, hepatic, or cardiac failure that would not cause mental changes in younger individuals seem capable of causing mental disease in older persons. Small imbalances in endocrine function, particularly hypothyroidism and the apathetic form of hyperthyroidism, are frequently associated with change in mental status as the dominant clinical feature. Disturbances in electrolyte or acid-base balance and mild anemia or anoxia may also present with mental changes. Laboratory examinations are available to confirm or deny clinical suspicion of most of these metabolic, endocrine, or deficiency states. Even chronic constipation causes decreased mental acuity and confusion in elderly persons. Hepatic encephalopathy, common in alcoholic patients but found in patients with other forms of liver disease or with various medications such as valproic acid, produces a drowsy confusional state that sometimes may be misinterpreted as dementia.

Nutritional deficiencies are a prominent problem in elderly persons, who may lead isolated lives on inadequate incomes. This, combined with depression, may result in severe neglect of dietary intake of vitamins. The most common vitamin disorder that can produce dementia is vitamin B_{12} deficiency. Most traditional American diets are rich in vitamin B_{12}, but occasionally, strict vegetarians can become deficient. Gastric surgery or pernicious anemia may be the cause. Signs of a peripheral neuropathy and myelopathy are often present. Neuropsychiatric manifestations of B_{12} deficiency can occur in the absence of anemia or macrocytosis. A vitamin B_{12} level should be performed routinely in evaluation of dementia. In patients with other signs of B_{12} deficiency, it is important to remember that tissue stores can be depleted before the serum level falls. If B_{12} deficiency is strongly suspected, a normal B_{12} level should prompt a request for methylmalonic acid assay, a metabolite of vitamin B_{12} that is increased in B_{12} deficiency.

Thiamine deficiency can produce an acute Wernicke's encephalopathy, sometimes followed by Korsakoff's psychosis, also known as alcoholic amnestic syndrome (see Chapter 51). Although most often seen in alcoholic patients, patients with thiamine malabsorption caused by surgery (e.g., gastric plication) or severe malnutrition have occasionally been reported to develop thiamine deficiency with neurologic effects. The classic patient is apathetic and has marked impairment of immediate and short-term memory and relative preservation of more distant memory. These patients repeat a list of three objects and then cannot recall them after a 10-second distraction. Confabulation may occur but is not necessary for the diagnosis, and it can be induced in some patients who want to please the examiner. Recovery of memory function is variable and slow. Peripheral neuropathy, cerebellar degeneration, and other signs of neurologic damage from alcoholism are often present.

Tumors

Dementia can be a presenting feature of certain tumors that develop in the frontal or temporal lobes, especially when they are situated medially and impinge on the limbic system without causing elementary neurologic signs. Some are benign and easily resected, even in elderly people. A subfrontal meningioma that distorts and compresses the frontal lobes in the olfactory tracts causes loss of sense of smell and lends itself to surgical treatment. Certain tumors in the midline fail to cause lateralizing signs but often result in deterioration of behavior, which may be caused by direct effects on the limbic, hypothalamic, or endocrine system or by hydrocephalus. The mental status of patients with hydrocephalus improves dramatically with CSF shunting, even if the tumor cannot be removed. Neoplasms can also cause dementia through more distant effects. Meningeal carcinomatosis with spread of neoplastic cells to CSF can present as dementia. Neoplasms also produce multiple metabolic disturbances that can affect mental status. Limbic encephalitis can occur as a result of antibody to neuronal cells produced as part of a paraneoplastic syndrome. In tumors involving the brain, imaging studies may provide a diagnosis. In some cases, stereotactic biopsy of the mass may be necessary for a definitive answer. Indirect effects of tumors can be more challenging. CSF studies with cytology, serum samples for neuronal antibodies, and metabolic studies should be considered in the evaluation and may need to be repeated to establish a diagnosis.

Trauma

Trauma to the nervous system occurs frequently, particularly in patients with a history of alcohol or drug abuse. Traumatic injuries to the brain are easy to diagnose near the time of the event if the patient remembers it. However, minor head injuries can produce chronic subdural hematomas, particularly in elderly and alcoholic patients. The normal loss of brain volume in aging causes a slight stretching of the veins that bridge the subdural space, allowing relatively trivial trauma to tear a vein with accumulation of blood in the subdural space. When the accumulation is unilateral, early herniation may cause somnolence, sometimes without other focal neurologic deficits. Bilateral subdural hematomas (about 20% of cases) may not present with focal signs, and mental changes often occur without drowsiness. These patients may show an extreme degree of apathy and immobility, which is sometimes mistaken for advanced depression. These chronic subdural hematomas can be missed because they are isodense with brain tissue on a CT scan of the head. This is a particular problem when the hematomas are bilateral and do not produce a shift of the brain. MRI of the head can be extremely helpful in these cases (Fig. 158-3).

In addition to subdural hematomas, repetitive traumatic head injury can cause widespread damage and present like dementia. Imaging studies may show traces of the past trauma, but the deficits can be expected to remain stable or perhaps to improve with rehabilitation. The elderly brain is more sensitive, and responses are often less robust.

Alcohol-Related Dementia

In addition to Wernicke-Korsakoff syndrome, which is specific to thiamine deficiency, another less clearly delineated

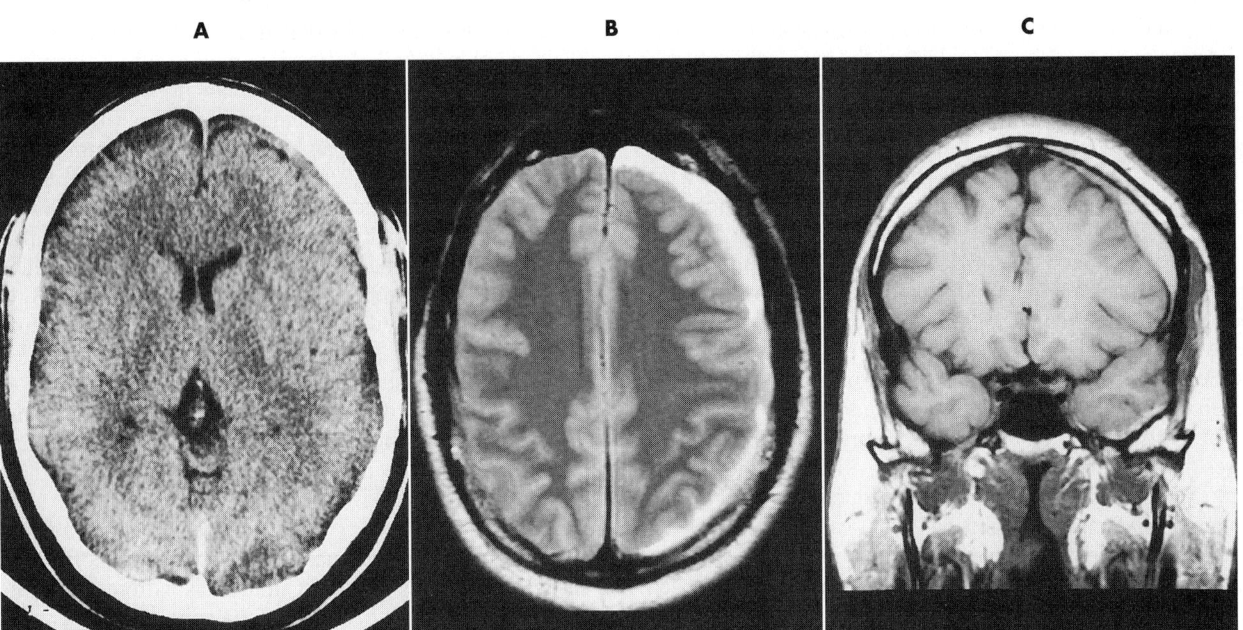

Fig. 158-3. Subacute subdural hematoma. **A,** Head computed tomography scan shows a nearly isodense subdural hematoma. **B** and **C,** With magnetic resonance imaging the hematoma is much more apparent. **C,** Sagittal image demonstrates the mass effect of the lesion.

disorder is called alcohol-related dementia. This disorder is likely a result of the combined effect of alcohol on the brain, poor nutrition, and multiple traumatic insults. The cognitive disabilities are more varied than in Wernicke-Korsakoff syndrome and include loss of memory function, visuospatial abilities, and naming. Precise clinical criteria are lacking.[25] Head CT or MRI shows diffuse cerebral atrophy. Abstinence from alcohol and good nutrition may result in essentially complete recovery of cognitive function in some of these patients. The cognitive losses in the active alcoholic patient can pose considerable challenges for the clinician. The patient may be essentially incompetent while drinking and highly functional when abstinent. Alcohol rehabilitation services are critical to the treatment of these patients. In the acute phases, the retention of material related to alcohol avoidance is minimal because of cognitive impairment, and patient education sessions need to be repeated later.

Toxic Causes

The most important toxic cause of dementia is prescription or OTC medications. A good dementia workup must include complete cataloging of the patient's medications and careful consideration of their possible adverse effects on the brain. Any drug used to treat behavioral or psychiatric disorders, such as benzodiazepines, antipsychotic medications, and antidepressants, can depress cognitive abilities. When possible a trial off of these medications is warranted in the evaluation of cognitive decline, using slow tapers in those that can cause withdrawal symptoms.

Various drugs often used for general medical illnesses are capable of causing mental changes. Some examples are antihypertensives, analgesics, and H_2 blockers. In addition, drugs that may be well tolerated as monotherapy have prolonged half-lives, and their side effects are potentiated when used in combination with other medications. The average elderly patient takes multiple medications and has a higher likelihood of experiencing significant side effects. After careful review of medications, all potentially unnecessary drugs should be discontinued. In the medications deemed necessary, the lowest possible dose should be given. It is important to remember that low doses in elderly patients may produce the intended result and dramatically reduce side effects.

OTC medicines, home remedies, and folk remedies must also be considered during the evaluation of patients. Patients and their families often neglect to mention the use of OTC antihistamines, sleeping preparations, and analgesics that may alter sensorium. A home visit by health care providers can be helpful if the patient allows a review of the medicine cabinet. This may also reveal a stash of expired medications that the patient may use intermittently. Patients with dementia may also use overdoses or underdoses of their medications. Calendar-type drug boxes may be helpful, but often the caretaker must dispense medications.

Sensory Deprivation

Losses in hearing ability and visual acuity are common in elderly persons and when undetected or minimized by the patient can present as confusion. With treatment, improvements are noted, even in those with neurodegenerative disease.

LABORATORY INVESTIGATIONS

The evaluation of any patient with dementia should be tailored to the patient's clinical history, risk factors, and examination. The evaluation must stress the search for the most probable disorder but must also contain an evaluation for less common but highly treatable etiologies.[5] It is also important to remember that dementia can be multifactorial.

Laboratory Studies

In mild to moderate dementia, all patients should have a complete blood count with differential, thyroid-stimulating hormone level, vitamin B_{12} level, syphilis testing (VDRL), liver function tests, and urinalysis. These laboratory tests should be supplemented by the analysis of other endocrine functions, if necessary, or arterial blood gas concentrations, ceruloplasmin levels, erythrocyte sedimentation rate, or antinuclear antibody testing. The physician should consider HIV testing, remembering that this disease occurs in elderly as well as young persons. Testing for the apoprotein E E4 allele in a patient with clinical features suggesting AD can be considered.[4,7,29] If familial AD is considered, the physician can look for the common mutations found in this disorder, but it may be best to refer the patient to a consultant with expertise in the genetics of neurologic disorders.[7]

Lumbar Puncture

A lumbar puncture is an appropriate examination for patients with early or moderate dementia. Although positive studies occur infrequently, they often reveal the presence of a treatable etiology. The spinal tap should be deferred until imaging is performed to avoid possible brain herniation and to guide any special CSF studies. CSF should be collected with careful note of the opening pressure and the fluid's appearance. Cell count, protein, and glucose levels, a VDRL test, cryptococcal antigen, and cultures should be performed. If multiple sclerosis is suspected, oligoclonal bands should also be sent. High-volume lumbar puncture is indicated in NPH. If AIDS is possible, testing for viral load and other atypical infections is warranted.

Imaging Studies

All patients should have an imaging study at the time of the initial diagnosis of dementia. A repeat of the imaging study should be considered in patients with acute deterioration in function, particularly with development of new focal neurologic signs or any history of head trauma. A CT scan of the head or an MRI should be performed. The determination of the most appropriate test depends on the likely diagnosis, the level of patient cooperation, and any contraindications. CT scan of the head, particularly with contrast, demonstrates most mass lesions, cerebrovascular accidents, subdural hematomas, and atrophy. However, isodense subdural hematomas may be missed or underestimated (see Fig. 158-3), and small lesions of all types may also be inapparent. Temporal lobe lesions and atrophy may be difficult to diagnose with CT. Head CT with contrast carries the risk associated with the contrast agent and cannot be performed in patients who have renal insufficiency.

For the evaluation of dementia, MRI can usually be performed without contrast. However, the MRI procedure is very difficult for claustrophobic patients and requires a higher level of cooperation than CT scanning. MRI cannot be performed in patients who have any metal in their body, including many surgical clips and metal fragments from occupational injuries (e.g., welding-related eye injuries). Pacemakers are also an absolute contraindication for MRI. The anxiety associated with MRI can be ameliorated by reassurance by the technologists, but this may sometimes need to be supplemented by a low dose of a sedating agent (e.g., a benzodiazepine) with a short half-life.

SPECT scanning may also have a role in the evaluation of patients with dementia. Characteristic patterns have been described in AD and Pick's disease but have not been fully substantiated with clinicopathologic correlations. The test involves the infusion of a radionucleotide followed by a relatively brief period of imaging. It again requires some patient cooperation, but most patients can tolerate the procedure. At this stage, results should be considered supportive but not diagnostic. SPECT scans are not part of a routine evaluation at this stage.

Electroencephalography

An EEG should be considered in some patients with dementia. This test is diagnostic in nonconvulsive status, showing a pattern of continuous ictal discharges. Also, a characteristic pattern is usually present in Creutzfeldt-Jakob disease. In other cases the EEG may suggest a mass lesion by showing high-voltage slow-wave activity in the area involved. However, imaging studies make this indication rarely useful. The low-voltage fast activity present with the use of sedatives may indicate a toxic encephalopathy. The EEG in certain metabolic derangements shows slowing and highly suggestive triphasic waves. However, in both these instances, other hints from the history or laboratory studies are more definitive in making the diagnosis.

Neuropsychologic Testing

Formal neuropsychologic testing consists of a battery of standardized tests of cognitive functions such as memory, visuospatial abilities, and language function. IQ testing is a well-known example. Neuropsychologists can be particularly helpful in establishing a diagnosis of dementia in early cases and in patients with high premorbid IQs. They can sometimes be helpful in supporting a diagnosis of depression by demonstrating variability in performance and patterns of losses inconsistent with a neurodegenerative process. Neuropsychologic evaluations are sometimes also performed before and after a course of treatment to help determine response or before and after high-volume lumbar puncture to diagnose NPH and potential response to shunting.

Summary

Dementia is the result of many common and uncommon disorders. The clinician's skills and judgment are important in delineating the most likely cause and in evaluating for all potentially present, treatable causes.

MANAGEMENT

A full account of treatments for disorders that may cause dementia would be inappropriate. These treatments may range from penicillin for neurosyphilis to shunting for NPH to discontinuation of medications. Some of these therapies are described in the section on differential diagnosis. This section presents common treatable features and an approach to the neurodegenerative disorders.

Therapy for all treatable causes must be maximized. However, treatable causes rarely reverse totally, but they can be arrested. In all patients, medications known to cause confusion should be discontinued if possible. The essential medications should be used in the lowest possible dosage. Alcohol use should be discouraged in patients who have a long history of frequent alcohol use; even small amounts may require detoxification. Hearing and vision correction should be prescribed when necessary, even for patients with neurodegenerative causes such as AD, which may be worsened by visual or auditory misperceptions.

Multiple nonpharmacologic interventions are helpful for patients and their caregivers. One of the first measures is to ensure safety at home by making sure outside doors cannot be opened by the patient and stoves can be disconnected intermittently when necessary. Home visits by clinicians who have trained as dementia specialists can provide valuable assistance to the family by providing safety hints and activity suggestions. Patients with wandering habits should be enrolled in the National Alzheimer Wanderers Alert Registry sponsored by the Alzheimer's Association, which enters patients into a national database, provides labels for them and their clothing, and ensures access to recent, high-quality photographs of patients. Driving by the patient can be a concern. Families may hide the keys or disable vehicles if the patient has moderate dementia. In early dementia the patient and caregiver can avoid adversarial roles by finding an objective third party to arbitrate. Some state motor vehicle departments or rehabilitation hospitals retest patients at the request of a physician or family member. In other cases the patient can be referred to a driving school for a safety evaluation.

Some general measures are also helpful in improving the level of functioning of patients with dementia. Patients do better if their environment and daily routines are stable. In nursing homes, color coding of the room, stripes leading along the hallway to various shared areas, and large-print calendars with a single day on each page are all simple measures that help the patient retain orientation. *Sundowning* is a term often used to describe the agitated, confused state that may be brought on in demented patients when the level of light is reduced in the evening. This problem is sometimes resolved by leaving the light on. Even during the day, many patients do better if present in a room where some activities are occurring. Frequent recreational activities keep the patient occupied, decrease the number of catastrophic reactions, and increase the number of positive interactions between the patient and caregiver. Activities may include reminiscence sessions, singing of old favorites, art activities, and continued involvement in household duties. It is important to tailor the task to the level of the patient's cognitive abilities. When frustration occurs over inability to perform the task, a simpler activity should be substituted.

The ability to perform activities of daily living eventually deteriorates, and the patient gradually requires more and more assistance. The ability to eat with silverware deteriorates, and substituting finger foods is helpful. Bath time may be stressful, with the patient becoming fearful of the running water. Preparing the bath in advance may help, and sponge baths can be substituted. Dressing can be facilitated by providing each item in a stepwise fashion and eliminating choices. Incontinence is a significant stress for caregivers and often prompts nursing home referrals. Frequent trips to the bathroom can minimize accidents in early stages, and adult diapers can be used later in the course. A workup for urinary tract infections, benign prostatic hypertrophy, and prostate cancer is indicated for new-onset incontinence.

Support groups are important for the patient in the early stages and for the caregiver throughout the disease and are available through local chapters of the Alzheimer's Association. If the family understands the symptoms to be expected, the patient can often be maintained in the home setting for much longer. This is particularly true when an interdisciplinary approach is available, including access to nurses, social workers, and physicians. Literature available from the Alzheimer's Association and books written specifically for families of patients (e.g., *The 36-Hour Day* by Mace and Rabins[17]) can be of enormous value. A book called *Living in the Labyrinth,*[10] written by a person with dementia, also provides insight. Adult day-care programs can allow family members to continue working or provide them with free time for other errands and respite. Overnight respite programs are unfortunately rare, and the financial burden for these usually falls on the family. As the disease progresses, the focus becomes the caregiver, who needs additional assistance with care and emotional support, especially when the often heart-rending decision about nursing home placement approaches.

Health care proxy forms and durable power of attorney decisions should preferably be made in the early stages of the disease when the patient can participate. Decisions regarding resuscitation attempts and other aggressive measures can be difficult for family but are best discussed before a crisis. In late stages, decisions about nutritional support are emotionally difficult for family members.

PHARMACOLOGIC INTERVENTIONS

In treatable causes of dementia, treatment for the target disease is naturally the first approach. However, it is important to remember that cognitive abilities may not return to baseline and there may be permanent deficits. It is particularly important to advise patients and family that recovery of function may not be complete.

Only two medications (tacrine and donepezil) have been approved by the Food and Drug Administration for use in AD, and both are cholinesterase inhibitors developed to increase the availability of acetylcholine. Both drugs slow progression of cognitive deficits, but their effects are modest. Positive effects on behavior are also reported but have been more difficult to prove objectively.[27,33] Both agents require a gradual titration of dose, and neither has immediate effects. Side effects include nausea, vomiting, and diarrhea, which are usually self-limited. Tacrine was the first drug released, and widespread use has been hindered by the need for dosing four times a day and the possibility of hepatotoxicity, necessitating close monitoring of liver function. Although elevations of alanine aminotransferase occur in about 25% of patients, they seem to be reversible if the administration of tacrine is stopped.[11] The starting dose of tacrine is 10 mg four times a day; it is increased in 6 weeks to 20 mg, then 30 mg 6 weeks later, and finally 40 mg, four times a day. Donepezil is given once a day with a starting dose of 5 mg at bedtime, increasing to 10 mg. Liver function tests do not seem to be affected, and no monitoring of blood work is needed. Therefore it is currently the preferred agent. It is reasonable to consider a trial of donepezil in all patients in the early or moderate stages of AD, since it can delay the later stages and the need for nursing home placement. Both tacrine and donepezil have been tried in other progressive dementias, but the published literature is currently too limited to develop guidelines for other uses.

Multiple other medications are being promoted to either slow or prevent the development of AD. It is important for the physician to note that the data on most of these treatments are limited, the studies are often flawed, and the improvements are often small. Vitamin E is frequently recommended, but a review of the literature indicates small studies and no available meta-analysis. The major complication appears to be rare instances of bleeding complications. Since so many patients now take vitamin E without a physician's recommendation, it may be difficult to perform the necessary studies to gauge its effect. A meta-analysis of studies of *Gingko biloba* revealed a modest improvement at doses of 120 to 240 mg, but most of the reviewed studies were excluded because of flaws in design or incomplete information.[24] Nonsteroidal antiinflammatory drugs appear to have a protective effect for AD.[1,20] Estrogen therapy in women may also have a protective effect, but there are conflicting results and flawed studies.[37] Since estrogen therapy can have considerable risk, it is prudent to wait for more convincing data before recommending estrogen for the treatment or prevention of dementia.

Treatment also focuses on the behavioral symptoms of dementia. In all patients a trial of an antidepressant should be considered in the early stages. It is important to remember that the presentation of depression can be atypical in this population. Sleep disruptions are common and can sometimes be treated with attention to sleep routines. Short-acting benzodiazepines and trazodone can also be used. Agitation is a major problem, and the initial assessment must first exclude medical causes, particularly pain and infection. Next, it is important to look at the patterns of agitation, and the other signs and symptoms to guide medication use. Agitation can come from many causes, including depression, mania, and psychosis. Treatment targeted to the most likely etiology used in the lowest effective dose has the highest chance for success.[6]

The treatment of a patient with dementia can be disheartening to a physician. However, the support of a knowledgeable and caring physician can make tremendous improvements in quality of life for both the patient and the caregiver.

EBM EVIDENCE-BASED MEDICINE

Primary sources for this chapter were found using MEDLINE with searches dating back to 1966. Review articles, meta-analyses, and consensus statements were stressed, and the last search was done in January 1999.

SUPPORT GROUPS

Alzheimer's Association National Office
919 North Michigan Avenue, Suite 1000
Chicago, IL 60611-1676
(800) 272-3900
www.alz.org

REFERENCES

1. Beard CM, et al: Nonsteroidal anti-inflammatory drug use and Alzheimer's disease: a case-control study in Rochester, Minnesota, 1980-1984, *Mayo Clin Proc* 73:951, 1998.
2. Burt DB, et al: Dementia in adults with Down syndrome: diagnostic challenges, *Am J Ment Retard* 103:130, 1998.
3. Caruso R, et al: Idiopathic normal-pressure hydrocephalus in adults: result of shunting correlated with clinical findings in 18 patients and review of the literature, *Neurosurg Rev* 20:104, 1997.
4. Clark RF, Goate AM: Molecular genetics of Alzheimer's disease, *Arch Neurol* 50:1164, 1993.
5. Consensus Conference: Differential diagnosis of dementing diseases, *JAMA* 258:3411, 1987.
6. Consensus Report: Treatment of agitation in older persons with dementia, *Postgrad Med* Spec No 1, April 1998. Available on the internet at www.psychguides.com.
7. Consensus report of the Working Group on Molecular and Biochemical Markers of Alzheimer's Disease, The Ronald and Nancy Reagan Research Institute of the Alzheimer's Association and the National Institute on Aging Work Group, *Neurobiol Aging* 19:109, 1998.
8. Erkinjuntti T: Clinical criteria for vascular dementia: the NINDS-AIREN criteria, *Dementia* 5:189, 1994.
9. Evans DA, et al: Prevalence of Alzheimer's disease in a community population higher than previously reported, *JAMA* 262:2251, 1989.
10. Friel McGowin D: *Living in the labyrinth,* San Francisco, 1993, Elder Books.
11. Gracon SI, et al: Safety of tacrine: clinical trials, treatment IND, and postmarketing experience, *Alzheimer Dis Assoc Disord* 12:93, 1998.
12. Hachinski VC, et al: Cerebral blood flow in dementia, *Arch Neurol* 32:632, 1975.
13. Johnson RT, Gibbs CJ: Creutzfeldt-Jakob disease and related transmissible spongiform encephalopathies, *N Engl J Med* 339:1994, 1998.
14. Kemper TL: Neuroanatomical and neuropathological changes in normal aging and dementia. In Albert M, editor: *Clinical neurology of aging,* Oxford, England, 1984, Oxford University Press.
15. Konno S, et al: Classification, diagnosis and treatment of vascular dementia, *Drugs Aging* 11:361, 1997.
16. Larson EB, et al: Diagnostic evaluation of 200 elderly outpatients with suspected dementia, *J Gerontol* 40:536, 1985.
17. Mace NL, Rabins PV: *The 36-hour day,* 2nd rev ed., New York, 1992, Warner Books.
18. Malm J, et al: The predictive value of cerebrospinal fluid dynamic tests in patients with idiopathic adult hydrocephalus syndrome, *Arch Neurol* 52:783, 1995.
19. Max W: The economic impact of Alzheimer's disease, *Neurology* 43(suppl 4):S6, 1993.
20. McGeer PL, Schulzer M, McGeer EG: Arthritis and anti-inflammatory agents as possible protective factors for Alzheimer's disease: a review of 17 epidemiologic studies, *Neurology* 47:425, 1996.
21. McKeith IG, et al: Consensus guidelines for the clinical and pathologic diagnosis of dementia with Lewy bodies (DLB): report of the consortium on DLB international workshop, *Neurology* 47:1113, 1996.
22. McKhann G, et al: Clinical diagnosis of Alzheimer's disease: report of the NINCDS-ADRDA Work Groups under the auspices of Department of Health and Human Services Task Force on Alzheimer's Disease, *Neurology* 34:939, 1984.
23. Neary D, Snowden J: Fronto-temporal dementia: nosology, neuropsychology, and neuropathology, *Brain Cogn* 31:176, 1996.
24. Oken BS, et al: The efficacy of *Gingko biloba* on cognitive function in Alzheimer disease, *Arch Neurol* 55:1409, 1998.
25. Oslin D, et al: Alcohol related dementia: proposed clinical criteria, *Int J Geriatr Psychiatry* 13:203, 1998.
26. Prasher VP, et al: ApoE genotype and Alzheimer's disease in adults with Down syndrome: meta-analysis, *Am J Ment Retard* 102:103, 1997.
27. Qizilbash N, et al: Cholinesterase inhibition for Alzheimer's disease: a meta-analysis of the tacrine trials: Dementia Trialists' Collaboration, *JAMA* 280:1777, 1998.
28. Rockwood K, et al: Diagnosis of vascular dementia: Consortium of Canadian Centres for Clinical Cognitive Research consensus statement, *Can J Neurol Sci* 21:358, 1994.
29. Roses AD: Genetic testing for Alzheimer disease: Practical and ethical issues, *Arch Neurol* 54:1226, 1997.
30. Scheck DN, Hook EW III: Neurosyphilis, *Infect Dis Clin North Am* 8:769, 1994.
31. Simon RP: Neurosyphilis, *Arch Neurol* 42:606, 1985.
32. Skoog I, et al: Population based study of dementia in 85-year-olds, *N Engl J Med* 328:153, 1993.
33. Stewart A, et al: Pharmacotherapy for people with Alzheimer's disease: a Markov-cycle evaluation of five years' therapy using donepezil, *Int J Geriatr Psychiatry* 13:445, 1998.
34. Vanneste J, et al: Shunting normal pressure hydrocephalus: do the benefits outweigh the risks? A multicenter study and literature review, *Neurology* 42:54, 1992.
35. Wells CE: Pseudodementia, *Am J Psychiat* 136:895, 1979.
36. Wisniewski KE, et al: Occurrence of neuropathological changes and dementia of Alzheimer's disease in Down's syndrome, *Ann Neurol* 7:278, 1985.
37. Yaffe K, et al: Estrogen therapy in postmenopausal women: effects on cognitive function and dementia, *JAMA* 279:688, 1998.

CHAPTER 159

Epilepsy and Seizures

R. Mark Sadler

Seizures are a very common manifestation of cerebral cortical dysfunction. Seizures occur when there is an abnormal, excessive, and synchronous electrical discharge of cortical neurons. An important concept to remember is that the central nervous system (CNS) is inherently susceptible to seizures. The fundamental neural circuitry and neurochemistry of the brain are such that there exists a "built in" tendency for seizures to occur that is normally suppressed by a balance of excitatory and inhibitory influences. The basic mechanisms of seizures are incompletely understood and are different for different seizure types and varieties of epilepsy. Simplistically, seizures can be viewed as occurring in circumstances of excessive excitation and/or impaired inhibition.

Epilepsy, as distinct from a *seizure,* is usually defined as a chronic condition characterized by the occurrence of recurrent, apparently unprovoked seizures. Thus the patient who experiences a generalized tonic-clonic seizure as the result of hypoglycemia is not considered to have epilepsy.

EPIDEMIOLOGY AND ETIOLOGY OF EPILEPSY

Population-based studies report the prevalence of epilepsy (number of active cases per unit population) at approximately 1%. The incidence (number of new cases per year in a given population) is approximately 40 to 70/100,000. Age-specific incidence rates show the highest figures in the first decade, a decline to a steady level in the 20- to 60-year age range, and a sharp rise again in the last decades of life.[7] These incidence figures reflect the various etiologies of epilepsy at different ages.

The *cumulative incidence* of acquiring epilepsy is 2% to 4%. The cumulative incidence of having at least one seizure during one's lifetime is estimated at 8% to 10%.

Virtually any pathologic process that can affect the cerebral cortex may give rise to a seizure or epilepsy. Large population-based studies, however, continue to demonstrate that of patients with epilepsy, up to 60% are of unknown etiology. Genetic varieties of epilepsies are included in the "unknown" group because the precise genetic basis for inherited epileptic disorders is still unknown. Commonly recognized causes of epilepsy include developmental disorders, cerebrovascular disease, trauma, the sequelae of intracranial infection, tumor, and degenerative disorders. The relative proportion of these causes will depend on the age group under study. Thus cerebrovascular disease, degenerative disorders, and tumors are more common in the older population and developmental disorders represent a higher proportion in the pediatric population. The causes of epilepsy are also related to geographic areas. For example, cerebral cysticercosis is an extremely prevalent cause of epilepsy in Africa, South America, Central America, and India.

CLASSIFICATION

There have been many proposed classification systems of seizures and types of epilepsy. Some systems have used terminology that emphasizes an anatomic basis (e.g., temporal lobe seizures), behavioral aspects (e.g., psychomotor seizures), or etiology (e.g., posttraumatic epilepsy). The most widely used systems in current use are those developed by the International League Against Epilepsy (ILAE). The ILAE has developed a classification of *seizures* and a separate classification of *epilepsies and epileptic syndromes.*

ILAE CLASSIFICATION OF EPILEPTIC SEIZURES

The components of the ILAE seizure classification are listed in Box 159-1.[4] This system was developed by reviewing the clinical and electroencephalographic (interictal and ictal) features of epileptic seizures demonstrated by simultaneous videotape and electroencephalogram monitoring.

The ILAE system is clinically weighted, and the first important consideration is the distinction of seizures that have the initial clinical and EEG features indicating activation of a restricted portion of one cerebral hemisphere (partial seizures) from those seizures that initially display bilateral cerebral involvement (generalized seizures).

The term *partial* is used synonymously with *focal* and does not imply an incomplete variety of seizure.

Within the general category of partial seizures a distinction is made between simple and complex seizures. The term *simple* indicates that the patient has no impairment of consciousness, whereas *complex* means that during the seizure consciousness is impaired.

Simple partial seizures have a variety of clinical features that depend on what part of the cortex is involved during the seizure. When *motor* phenomena occur, clonic movements (jerks) may involve a restricted body part (e.g., the hand or face) and may spread to adjacent body parts (a Jacksonian march). *Tonic features* refer to relatively pure stiffening (without clonic movements) or sustained postures, such as head and/or eye deviation (version). There may be transient weakness of the body part involved during the seizure after a motor seizure (Todd's paresis). *Sensory* seizures cause hallucinations or illusions. Somatosensory seizures typically cause numbness or tingling in a body part. Illusions or hallucinations of any of the senses can occur when specialized sensory cortex is involved: olfactory or taste (typically from seizures of mesial temporal lobe structures), visual (occipital cortex), hearing or vestibular (superior temporal gyrus). *Autonomic* seizures can cause symptoms of sweating, piloerection, palpitations, and, very commonly, an unpleasant, rising epigastic sensation. These autonomic features are usually seen in association with temporal lobe–originating seizures. *Psychic* phenomena refer to a panoply of sensations, including changes in emotions (fear, depression), déjà vu, depersonalization, memory flashbacks, and a "dreamy" state. These difficult-to-describe experiences most often evolve to partial complex seizures (see below) and probably infer seizure involvement of limbic structures in the temporal lobe.

Partial complex seizures are, by definition, associated with an impairment of consciousness. These seizures start in a restricted part of the brain and spread to other neuroanatomic structures involved with attention and consciousness. Typically the patient will have an arrest of behavior, a blank or "wide-eyed" stare followed by automatisms (e.g., lip smacking or chewing movements), or may continue a complex motor task (such as riding a bicycle). The patient is relatively unresponsive to the environment during a partial complex seizure. The patient will appear "out of touch" for a period of time (usually 30 to 90 seconds). Frequently there is postictal confusion and sleepiness. The postictal confusion can be brief and the patient may be unaware that he or she experienced any type of altered behavior. The patient will be

Box 159-1. ILAE Classification of Epileptic Seizures

I. Partial (focal, local) seizures
   A. Simple partial seizures
      1. With motor signs (focal motor without march, focal motor with march, versive, postural, phonatory (vocalization or arrest of speech)
      2. With somatosensory or special sensory symptoms (including visual, auditory, olfactory, gustatory, and vertiginous)
      3. With autonomic symptoms or signs
      4. With psychic symptoms (including dysphasic, dysmnesic, cognitive, affective, illusions, and structured hallucinations)
   B. Complex partial seizures
      1. Simple partial onset followed by impairment of consciousness
      2. With impairment of consciousness at onset
   C. Partial seizures evolving to secondarily generalized seizures
      1. Simple partial evolving to generalized seizures
      2. Complex partial evolving to generalized seizures
      3. Simple partial evolving to complex partial to generalized seizures
II. Generalized seizures
   A. Absence
      1. Absence (typical)
      2. Atypical
   B. Myoclonic
   C. Clonic
   D. Tonic
   E. Tonic-clonic
   F. Atonic
III. Unclassified epileptic seizures

amnestic for the event but may be able to describe some features that occurred at the beginning of the seizure (i.e., the simple partial component before spread of the seizure to contralateral cortical structures). Partial complex seizures often begin in the temporal lobe but may be initiated from any lobe, propagate to temporal lobe structures, and give rise to clinical features indistinguishable from temporal lobe–originating attacks. Therefore a careful inquiry of the initial features of the seizure may give clues to the true origin. An important concept to appreciate is that although a partial complex seizure starts in one area, the seizure may spread very quickly, resulting in impaired consciousness from the outset. Therefore the patient will not be able to give any history of a warning for the attack. Partial complex seizures must be distinguished from absence seizures (see below), with which they are often confused. Partial complex seizures are a focally originating seizure disorder (absence attacks are generalized), they usually last longer than absence seizures, and they commonly have postictal confusion that is lacking with absence attacks. Partial complex seizures are secondary to a variety of focal cortical structural pathologies and have different drugs of choice as initial treatment.

As indicated in Box 159-1, partial seizures may evolve to secondarily generalized seizures. An important concept is that the form of a secondarily generalized seizure is usually a tonic-clonic seizure (convulsion) and not one of the other varieties of generalized seizures (e.g., absence, atonic, or myoclonic). Propagation (spread) of the seizure can occur with such rapidity that there may be no indication of the partial (focal) onset. Seizures that arise focally and spread very rapidly may not be clinically distinguishable from primary generalized tonic-clonic seizures, and an accurate diagnosis will depend on laboratory investigations, including EEG and neuroimaging studies.

Generalized seizures have in common the property of bihemispheric onset from the beginning of the attack. Therefore none of the primary generalized seizures will have a warning.

Absence seizures (formerly called *petit mal*) are brief (5 to 15 seconds) episodes of impaired awareness that usually consist of an arrest of behavior and a blank stare. There is no postictal confusion. In the untreated patient, these seizures commonly occur multiple times per day and almost always begin in childhood (although they may persist to adulthood). During the seizure a diagnostic, generalized spike-and-wave pattern is seen on the EEG. Approximately 50% of patients will have, or will eventually develop, other primary generalized seizure types, including tonic-clonic (grand mal) seizures and myoclonus. *Atypical absence* seizures are characterized by a less precise onset and offset, they last longer than typical absence seizures, they may be associated with motor features such as a loss of body tone, and they usually occur in patients with intellectual handicaps and other seizure types.

Myoclonic seizures consist of brief shocklike jerks that in the primary generalized epilepsies consist of bilateral movements of the head, neck, and often the proximal arms and legs. This seizure type can occur alone but more commonly is associated with other primary seizure types and can occur in many different epilepsy syndromes of diverse etiology.

A pure *clonic* seizure resembles a sequence of myoclonic jerks. *Tonic* seizures are characterized by brief episodes (usually less than 20 seconds) of bilateral stiffening of the body and extremities. These seizures are characteristic of Lennox-Gastaut syndrome (see Box 159-2), in which tonic seizures occur predominantly during sleep.

Atonic seizures consist of an abrupt, brief (seconds) loss of body tone. Typically the head will droop or the patient will fall to the ground; if consciousness is lost it is very brief. Patients with this seizure type often sustain multiple injuries from their falls. Almost invariably, patients with this seizure type develop their epilepsy in childhood and are cognitively impaired; thus atonic seizures are not usually within the differential diagnosis of drop attacks of a previously neurologically intact adult.

Generalized tonic-clonic seizures (formerly called *grand mal*) begin with a loss of consciousness and a tonic phase consisting of a generalized stiffening of the body and extremities. A vocal "cry" or "scream" sometimes occurs as the result of air being expelled through the contracted vocal cords. The tonic phase gradually merges with the clonic phase by an evolution from a low-amplitude, high-frequency vibration to bilaterally symmetric clonic jerks of higher amplitude that gradually slow in frequency. The motor component of the seizure typically ends with one to two violent, generalized jerks. The tonic-clonic phase is accompanied by cyanosis and prominent salivation. Tongue biting (on the lateral aspect) and urinary incontinence are common. Musculoskeletal injury (including spinal compression fractures and dislocation of the shoulders) from the force of muscular contraction may occur. Most convulsions last 1 to 2 minutes. The postictal state is characterized by transient stupor, sleepiness, confusion, headache, and muscular soreness later that day or the next. Some patients complain of a postictal memory disturbance lasting hours or, occasionally, a day or two.

The unclassified category of seizures is reserved for any seizure type that does not correspond to one of the other categories and/or whose nature is unclear (e.g., some neonatal seizures).

THE INTERNATIONAL CLASSIFICATION OF THE EPILEPSIES AND EPILEPTIC SYNDROMES

The ILAE has created a classification of the epilepsies and epileptic syndromes that must be distinguished from the classification of epileptic seizures described earlier. The list of disorders in Box 159-2[5] is extensive and contains a number of relatively unusual disorders, but it is included because primary care physicians will receive correspondence from consultants using the terminology in this box.

An epileptic syndrome is a disorder characterized by a cluster of signs and symptoms that include factors such as the seizure type, etiology, anatomic onset, precipitating factors, age of onset, severity, chronicity, diurnal cycling, and prognosis.

The major divisions of this classification are those epilepsies with generalized seizures and those characterized by partial (focally originating) seizures. Each of these groups is further subdivided into *idiopathic* (in which a genetic component is usually assumed) and *symptomatic* types. *Symptomatic* refers to the epilepsies and epileptic syndromes that are the result of a known or suspected disorder of the CNS. In Box 159-2 the term *cryptogenic* is also employed and indicates an epileptic disorder that is symptomatic but the etiology is unknown. It should be appreciated that not all patients are easily classified within this system.

Box 159-2. Classification of the Epilepsies and Epileptic Syndromes

1. Localization-related (focal, local, partial) epilepsies and syndromes
1.1 Idiopathic (with age related onset)
- Benign childhood epilepsy with centrotemporal spikes
- Childhood epilepsy with occipital paroxysms

1.2 Symptomatic
- Chronic progressive epilepsia partialis continua of childhood
- Syndromes characterized by seizures with specific modes of precipitation
- Temporal lobe epilepsies
- Frontal lobe epilepsies
- Parietal lobe epilepsies
- Occipital lobe epilepsies

1.3 Cryptogenic
2. Generalized epilepsies and syndromes
2.1 Idiopathic (with age related onset)
- Benign neonatal familial convulsions
- Benign neonatal convulsions
- Benign myoclonic epilepsy in infancy
- Childhood absence epilepsy
- Juvenile absence epilepsy
- Juvenile myoclonic epilepsy
- Epilepsy with grand mal seizures on awakening
- Other generalized idiopathic epilepsies not defined above
- Epilepsies with seizures precipitated by specific modes of activation

2.2 Cryptogenic or symptomatic
- West syndrome (infantile spasms)
- Lennox-Gastaut syndrome
- Epilepsy with myoclonic-astatic seizures
- Epilepsy with myoclonic absences

2.3 Symptomatic
2.3.1 Nonspecific etiology
  - Early myoclonic encephalopathy
  - Early infantile epileptic encephalopathy with burst suppression
  - Other symptomatic generalized epilepsies not defined above

2.3.2 Specific syndromes
3. Epilepsies and syndromes undetermined, whether focal or generalized
3.1 With both generalized and focal features
- Neonatal seizures
- Severe myoclonic epilepsy in infancy
- Epilepsy with continuous spike waves during slow wave sleep
- Acquired epileptic aphasia (Landau-Kleffner syndrome)
- Other undetermined epilepsies not defined above

3.2 Without unequivocal generalized or focal features
4. Special situations
4.1
- Febrile convulsions
- Isolated seizures or isolated status epilepticus
- Seizures occurring only when there is an acute toxic or metabolic event

One of the common syndromes is described here to convey the concept of an epilepsy syndrome.

Juvenile myoclonic epilepsy (JME) is one of the common generalized epilepsy disorders. Patients with JME are usually intellectually and neurologically intact. The seizure disorder begins in the preadolescent or adolescent years and is characterized by myoclonic jerks (usually of the head and upper extremities) that typically occur upon awakening. The majority of patients have tonic-clonic seizures that may follow a burst of the myoclonic jerks. Approximately one third of patients have a history of absence attacks during childhood. Myoclonic jerks and generalized tonic-clonic seizures often are precipitated by sleep deprivation. The interictal EEG demonstrates bursts of generalized polyspike and wave discharges at 4 to 6 cycles per second. Many patients also demonstrate photic sensitivity to intermittent strobe light stimulation. The drug of choice for treatment is valproic acid. The majority of patients find their seizures are well controlled with medical therapy. There is a high relapse rate if medication is discontinued, even if the patient has been seizure free for many years.

DIFFERENTIAL DIAGNOSIS

The diagnosis of a seizure remains a clinically based decision. The most common event that is misconstrued as a generalized seizure is a syncopal attack. Neurocardiogenic (vasovagal) syncope is the most commonly encountered variety among the many causes of syncope.[9] The distinction of a seizure from syncope can be troublesome if the syncopal attack progresses to a brief tonic phase or includes myoclonic jerks. Clinical features to be sought in the history include a prodrome of nausea, hunger, "feeling hot," yawning, an erect position (or sudden standing after prolonged recumbency), and a brief loss of consciousness (usually 30 seconds or less). An extremely important component to obtain from a witness is whether the patient was pale (which will not occur in a convulsion). The diagnosis of syncope is secured if the patient returns to consciousness, attempts to stand, but promptly loses consciousness a second time. Patients with neurocardiogenic syncope often give a history of presyncope or complete syncope in association with emotional factors (such as the sight of blood or syringes) or with acute pain. A family history of similar phenomena is frequently obtained.

Disorders with an associated impairment of consciousness that less commonly are confused with seizures include posterior circulation transient ischemic attacks, unwitnessed trauma with retrograde amnesia, episodic metabolic disturbances (such as hypoglycemia), sleep disorders (e.g., narcolepsy), and abrupt elevations of intracranial pressure caused by obstruction of cerebrospinal fluid (CSF) flow.

Psychogenic pseudoseizures commonly have a superficial resemblance to a generalized tonic-clonic seizure but typically lack the relatively stereotypic phases of an epileptic convulsion as described above. A prior psychiatric history is often present and a history of sexual and other physical abuse is typical. Panic attacks with prominent hyperventilation may lead to a transient loss of consciousness. Occasionally, partial complex seizures with bizarre automatisms may be misdiagnosed as a psychiatric disorder and expert assessment will be required. Clues that the spells are epileptic in nature will be the repetitive, stereotypic nature of the attacks and their occasional progression to unequivocal secondarily generalized tonic-clonic seizures. The clinician should also be aware of the possibility of the coexistence of epilepsy and psychogenic pseudoseizures.

A variety of disorders presenting with paroxysmal motor or sensory phenomena may simulate partial motor or partial sensory seizures, respectively. Migraine attacks with prominent visual features may resemble occipital lobe–originating seizures, but generally the visual phenomena last much longer in migraine than those associated with occipital seizures. Similarly, the sensory "numbness and tingling" attacks encountered with migraine tend to be much longer in duration than sensory seizures of parietal lobe origin. Movement disorders (including tics, tremor, and intermittent dystonic posturing) may resemble partial motor seizures, but careful attention to the actual details of the motor phenomena will usually distinguish these events from seizures.

HISTORY TAKING AND PHYSICAL EXAMINATION

The most common cause of misdiagnosis of a seizure is a failure to obtain an accurate and complete history. It is essential to obtain a history from two sources: the patient and a witness. For patients with "repeated spells" it is most useful to obtain a detailed description of a recent typical event that the patient and a witness can describe in detail.

Frequently the partial (focal) nature of the seizure is overlooked in patients who have rapid secondary generalization to a tonic-clonic seizure. It is important to ask the patient "what happened just before you lost consciousness?" "Do you ever have a warning or a feeling that you are going to have a seizure?" "Do you ever think you are going to have a seizure and it doesn't occur?" An affirmative answer to these questions will often divulge the focal nature of the seizure, with the "aura" representing the simple partial component of the seizure.

The patient's state after the ictus is important. For example, the patient with absence attacks will instantaneously return to awareness, in contrast to most patients with partial complex seizures who gradually awaken. Postictal limb paralysis (Todd's paresis) or dysphasia favors a focal onset.

The neurologic functional inquiry should emphasize potential causes, including a history of head injury and an estimate of its severity, previous intracranial sepsis (meningitis or encephalitis), birth and developmental milestones, and a family history of seizures or other neurologic disorders. A history of febrile convulsions in early childhood should be distinguished from the patient's habitual seizure disorder.

The general medical functional inquiry should be directed toward a search for clues of systemic illnesses that secondarily involve the CNS. Examples of the latter include malignancies with a high predisposition for CNS invasion, such as lung and breast cancers and melanoma.

The purpose of the neurologic examination is to look for clues to etiology and site of seizure onset. A careful assessment of visual fields (as an indicator of occipital lobe pathology) is mandatory if the seizure begins with visual phenomena. Patients with temporal lobe–originating seizures should be examined for a contralateral superior quadrant visual field defect (because the visual pathway subserving this visual field traverses part of the temporal lobe).

INVESTIGATION

A careful history and physical examination will dictate the appropriate choice of serum tests. Certainly a variety of metabolic and systemic disorders may present with seizures, but extensive tests of blood counts, electrolytes, serum calcium, and hepatic and renal function are not indicated in the otherwise uncomplicated patient.

Most patients with a suspected seizure disorder will have an EEG as part of their investigation. Unfortunately, many physicians expect the EEG to answer the question as to whether the patient has epilepsy or not. Epilepsy is a clinical diagnosis, and the EEG cannot produce a diagnosis with certainty unless the patient has a seizure during the recording. This occurrence is relatively unusual except for patients with very frequent seizures, such as absence attacks. The predominant role of the outpatient EEG is to provide laboratory support for a clinical impression. The interictal (between seizure) EEG abnormality of generalized spike waves or focal spikes may provide clues to the mechanism of the seizures (generalized or partial, respectively).

The frequency of interictal spikes is highly variable and therefore a single normal EEG does not rule out the possibility of a seizure disorder. Some patients require multiple recordings (including recording during sleep) before definitive interictal spikes are noted. At least 80% of patients with undoubted epilepsy will eventually demonstrate EEG interictal spikes. The specificity of definite interictal spikes is relatively high because less than 2% of the population will have spikes without an accompanying seizure disorder. However, it must be emphasized that accurate identification of EEG abnormalities is very dependent on the experience and skills of the electroencephalographer. There is no indication for repeated EEGs after a diagnosis of epilepsy is established (e.g., on a yearly basis as a checkup or follow-up).

The EEG is useful for guiding further studies. For example, an adolescent or young adult who presents with generalized tonic-clonic seizures, lacks risk factors for focally originating seizures, has a normal physical examination, and whose EEG demonstrates generalized spike wave discharges has a diagnosis of one of the primary generalized epilepsy syndromes (Fig. 159-1). No neuroimaging tests are required. Conversely, the presence of focal EEG spikes (Fig. 159-2) suggests the presence of focal pathology (note the exception of the childhood benign localization-related syndromes listed in Box 159-2) and neuroimaging studies are indicated. A computed tomography (CT) scan is a minimal neuroimaging study for focally originating seizure disorders. A CT scan may be the only imaging study required for patients who have a history of a brain insult that could explain the etiology of the seizure disorder (e.g., ischemic cerebral infarction, trauma). However, a magnetic resonance imaging (MRI) scan is the neuroimaging study of choice for focally originating seizures, particularly for those patients with seizures of unknown etiology and whose CT scans are normal. Examples of epileptogenic lesions well seen with MRI that are poorly imaged during a CT scan include mesial temporal sclerosis (the most common neuropathology of patients with temporal lobe epilepsy), low-grade primary brain tumors, vascular lesions (such as cavernous angiomas), and neuronal migration disorders (Figs. 159-3 and 159-4).

Continuous video–EEG telemetry has become increasingly available in specialized centers. This technique involves the acquisition of EEG signals that are synchronized with simultaneous videotaping of the patient's behavior. Patients are typically recorded for long periods (days) in an attempt to capture their paroxysmal events. This technique may be very useful in clarifying the diagnosis in patients with frequent spells of an unknown nature (e.g., distinguishing epileptic seizures from psychiatrically based pseudoseizures). Video–EEG telemetry is an obligatory part of the investigation of patients with medically resistant epilepsy who may be candidates for epilepsy surgery.

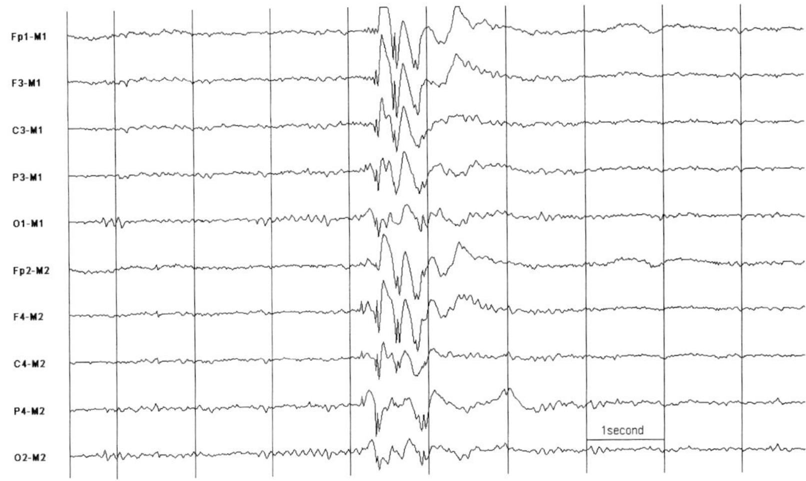

Fig. 159-1. Ten channels from a 32-channel EEG recording are shown. The top five channels are from scalp electrodes over the left hemisphere; the bottom five channels are from the homologous electrode positions overlying the right hemisphere. The recording is from a 20-year-old female with a history of two generalized tonic-clonic seizures. The demonstrated interictal abnormality is a generalized spike-and-wave discharge; note the bilaterally synchronous nature of the EEG abnormality. This finding would support a clinical impression that the patient has one of the primary generalized epilepsies.

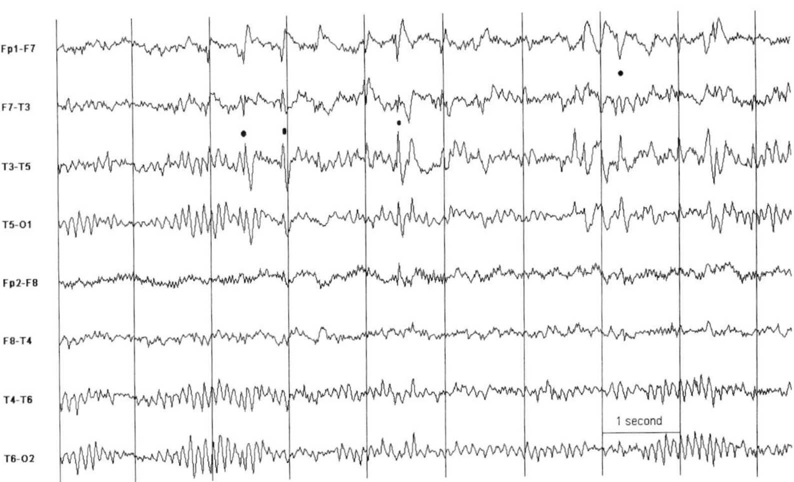

Fig. 159-2. Eight channels from a 32-channel EEG are shown. The top four channels are derived from scalp electrodes overlying the left temporal lobe; the bottom four channels are from the homologous electrodes overlying the right temporal lobe. Several left temporal interictal spikes are shown *(black circles)*. This recording is from an 18-year-old male who came to medical attention after a convulsion in sleep. Further history revealed a several-month history of partial complex seizures. Further neuroimaging studies with particular attention to the left temporal lobe are indicated.

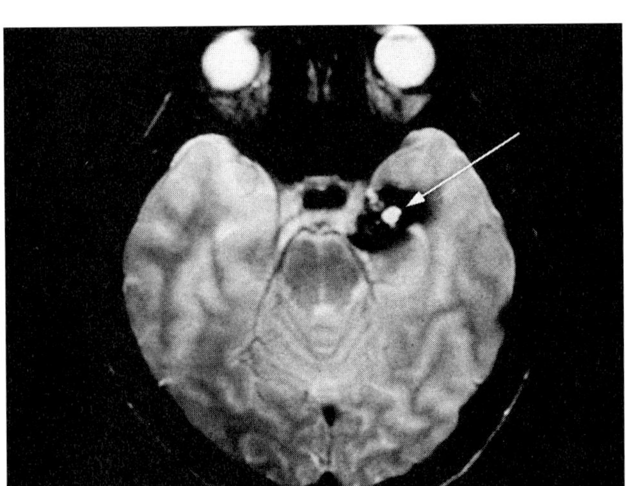

Fig. 159-3. Axial MRI scan showing a collection of abnormal blood vessels (cavernous angioma) in the temporal lobe *(arrow)*. This scan is from a 25-year-old male with longstanding partial complex seizures; the CT scan was normal. Neurosurgical excision of this lesion rendered the patient seizure free.

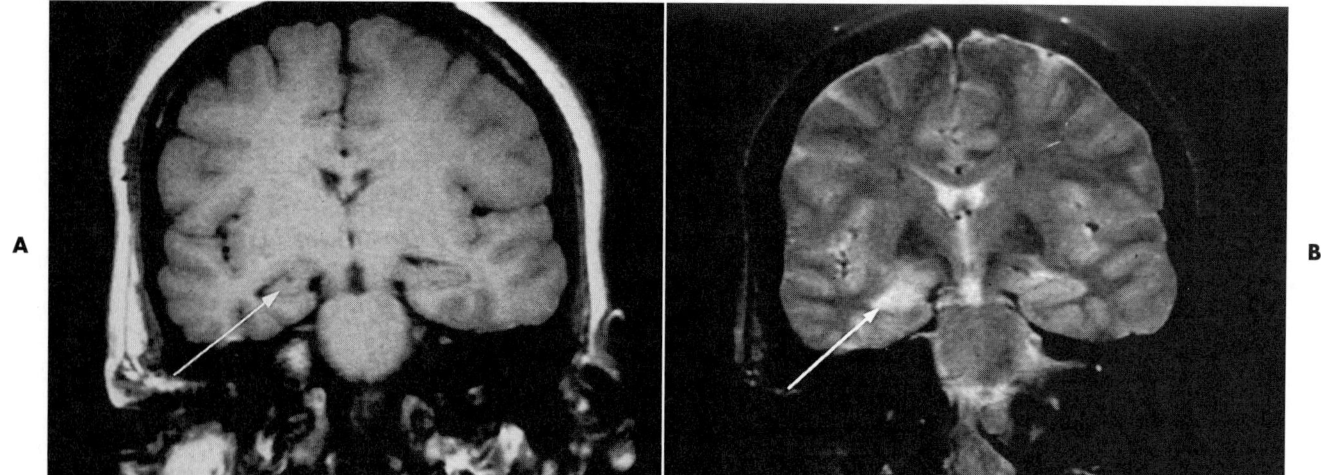

Fig. 159-4. Coronal MRI scans from a 24-year-old female with medically resistant partial complex seizures that began 6 years after an episode of febrile status epilepticus in early childhood. The T1 weighted image (**A**) shows atrophy of the right medial temporal structures *(arrow)*. The T2 weighted image (**B**) shows increased signal (as indicated by the brighter white area, *arrow*) in the right medial temporal area. These MRI scan abnormalities are characteristic of the pathology known as *mesial temporal sclerosis*. This is the most common pathologic finding in patients undergoing epilepsy surgery for refractory temporal lobe epilepsy. The precise mechanism of temporal lobe damage in these patients is debated but may be related to neuronally mediated cell death during status epilepticus.

GENERAL MEASURES IN THE MANAGEMENT OF EPILEPSY

Patients with a diagnosis of epilepsy face a number of burdens that are relatively unique in medicine. Patients continue to encounter remarkable prejudices from society because of a number of misperceptions and preconceived notions about the nature of epilepsy. When initially informed of the diagnosis, many patients need to be reassured that they do not have a mental illness and that a progressive decline in cognitive function is not the typical course for the vast majority of patients with seizure disorders.

Friends and relatives of the patient should be instructed in the first aid management of generalized tonic-clonic seizures, including admonitions to avoid placing objects in the mouth of the patient to prevent them from swallowing their tongue.

The physician should be aware of local regulations governing the operation of motor vehicles by persons who experience seizures. There are considerable worldwide differences in the obligations of the physician (mandatory vs. nonmandatory reporting) and the length of time required for a patient to be seizure free before operating a motor vehicle. Additional attention should be given to local regulations concerning professional drivers.

Patients may find that certain employment situations are unsuitable or may be prohibited, though not necessarily with validity. Career counseling, particularly for adolescents, may be required. For example, an individual considering a career in the military is well advised to determine if he or she may be disqualified because of a history of seizures. A common-sense approach should be used pertaining to recreational activities. Most sports are acceptable, but activities in which an abrupt loss of consciousness could lead to major physical injury (such as hang gliding or scuba diving) and those sports carrying a substantial risk of head injury (such as boxing) should be discouraged.

Patients should be encouraged to take showers, as opposed to tub baths. An unattended seizure in a bathtub can lead to a catastrophe.

Excessive alcohol intake should be discouraged, but small amounts of alcohol usually can be consumed without adverse effects. Recreational drug use of substances with potent proconvulsant properties (notably cocaine) must be forbidden.

Sleep deprivation is a potent activating effect for some seizures and therefore adequate sleep should be encouraged.

Patients should be made aware of the potential for drug interactions of their antiepileptic medications with other prescription medications. Antiepileptic medication compliance must be emphasized. Strategies include the simplest possible dosing schedules, linking the taking of medication to other regular daily activities (e.g., tooth brushing), and pill reminder containers.

Caregivers with active epilepsy who supervise very young children should be instructed to change and feed babies on the floor and never to bathe a baby alone.

MEDICAL MANAGEMENT

Antiepileptic drug (AED) treatment should be considered after a confident diagnosis of epilepsy (recurrent, unprovoked seizures) is made. In general, treatment should not be initiated until a diagnosis is reasonably established. A therapeutic trial should not be undertaken with an AED to prove if a patient does or does not have epilepsy.

The goals of therapy should be made clear to the patient and may include complete control of seizures with minimal adverse effects from the AEDs. It is important to recognize that some seizure types and epilepsy syndromes are notoriously difficult to bring under complete control. It may be preferable to accept, for example, occasional simple partial seizures rather than complete seizure control at the expense of medication toxicity. Conversely, simple partial seizures that occur exclusively in sleep may not require any AED treatment at all. In general, patients with normal cognition and without neurologic deficits require complete seizure control and no or few adverse effects from AEDs to obtain optimal quality of life and psychosocial development.

The patient should understand that AEDs treat symptoms and do not remove the underlying cause of epilepsy. Similarly, there is no compelling evidence that any of the currently available AEDs prevent the development of epilepsy in patients who are destined to do so (i.e., prophylactic AED treatment is not indicated after head injury in an attempt to prevent the development of epilepsy).

Prospective randomized trials have failed to demonstrate major differences in AED efficacy for most seizure types. Differences in successful treatment of epilepsy have been accounted for predominantly by differences in toxicity among AEDs.

Additional considerations in the initial selection of an AED include the presence of other medical conditions that could interfere with the metabolism of AEDs (e.g., hepatic and renal disease) and the presence of concomitant medication (of which there are multiple potential interactions with AEDs). Cost of medication is a consideration in AED selection because there are marked differences in price among the AEDs, particularly when comparing the traditional AEDs (phenobarbital, phenytoin, carbamazepine, valproic acid) to the new AEDs (gabapentin, lamotrigine, vigabatrin, and topiramate).

Suggestions for initial AED selection for specific seizure types are listed in Table 159-1. A detailed discussion of doses, adverse effects, and drug interactions is beyond the scope of this chapter, but selected aspects are listed in Table 159-2. The product monograph for each medication should be carefully consulted before initiating treatment. The recent published reviews of AEDs cited at the end of this chapter are highly recommended.[1,6]

Virtually all modern AED treatment is initiated as monotherapy (single drug). With the exceptions of phenytoin and phenobarbital, which may be started at their maintenance dose, AEDs are started at a fraction of the ultimate maintenance dose and slowly titrated upward. The patient should be assessed after achieving the initial desired maintenance dose to monitor efficacy and toxicity. If seizures continue but the drug has been well tolerated, the dose should be slowly increased to the maximally tolerated amount before abandoning treatment with that drug. One of the alternate monotherapy choices should be introduced if seizure control cannot be achieved with the maximally tolerated dose of the first-choice medication. The first drug should be slowly withdrawn if seizure control is achieved with the second drug. Although commonly practiced, there are very few clinical data to support polytherapy for most patients with epilepsy. Polytherapy combinations are probably best used after consultation with a physician experienced in epilepsy management.

Table 159-1. Suggested Choices for AEDs*

Seizure type	First choice monotherapy	Alternate monotherapy or add-on drug
Generalized tonic-clonic	Carbamazepine Phenytoin Valproic acid	Clobazam† Lamotrigine Topiramate
Absence	Ethosuximide Valproic acid	Clobazam† Lamotrigine Topiramate
Myoclonic and atonic	Valproic acid	Clobazam† Lamotrigine Topiramate
Partial (simple or complex) with or without secondary generalization	Carbamazepine Phenytoin	Clobazam† Felbamate† Gabapentin Lamotrigine Phenobarbital Primidone Topiramate Valproic acid Vigabatrin

Modified from Guberman A, Bruni J: *Essentials of clinical epilepsy,* Boston, 1999, Butterworth/Heinemann.

*AEDs are listed alphabetically; the order in the list does not imply a rank order.

†Clobazam is not available in the United States; felbamate is not available in Canada.

DRUG LEVELS: HEMATOLOGY AND LIVER FUNCTION MONITORING

Most laboratories can monitor the serum levels of the traditional AEDs. The ability to measure AED levels has demonstrated that there are substantial differences in dose and the resultant serum level from patient to patient. These variations can be attributed to individual differences in absorption, metabolism, and excretion. Serum AED levels may also be altered considerably by the presence of some other AEDs and other concomitant medications.

Serum AED levels are reported by most laboratories in the context of a therapeutic range. This range implies that there is a minimal drug concentration required for the antiepileptic effect and an upper limit that indicates the presence of dose-related (serum level) toxicity. However, in reality, there are relatively few studies that have substantiated the therapeutic ranges for any of the AEDs. There are considerable difficulties in conducting clinical trials that would establish minimal drug concentrations for seizure control because of the considerable spectrum of epilepsy severity. Consequently, patients with relatively mild epilepsy may have seizure control with drug concentrations below the usually quoted therapeutic range. Some patients with moderate to severe epilepsy may require AED serum levels above the usually quoted therapeutic range (provided there is no clinical toxicity) to obtain satisfactory seizure control.

The clinical data describing the relationship of drug level to toxicity are somewhat better than those supporting the antiepileptic effect, but they are still imperfect. The upper end of the therapeutic range is a statistical measure indicating that at this upper limit most patients will have some manifestations of toxicity. However, because this is only a statistical probability, there will be patients who display unequivocal toxicity at relatively low serum levels and patients who can tolerate higher levels without difficulties. Dose-related toxicity can take many forms, and not all toxic manifestations occur at the same serum level. When using AEDs it is prudent to adhere to the adage that "there are no toxic drug levels, only toxic patients."

Measurement of serum AED levels may be useful in certain circumstances. Some experts will check the AED level after sufficient time has elapsed for the drug to achieve steady-state pharmacokinetics to determine if a "reasonable" serum level has been achieved. AED levels can be used as a measure of patient compliance, although an open

Table 159-2. Some Characteristics of Antiepileptic Drugs*

Drug (mg/day)	Selected adverse effects†	Advantages	Disadvantages	Comments	Cost (approximate per month)
Carbamazepine (800-1200)	Rash 5%-10%, rarely can be very serious Liver enzyme elevation Blood dyscrasia common; transient neutropenia; extremely rare aplastic anemia Low serum sodium	BID dose for controlled release preparations Linear pharmacokinetics	Liver enzyme inducer Drug interactions Only oral form available May worsen absence seizures; may produce or exacerbate myoclonus	Start at 100 mg BID and increase by 200 mg/day q 3-4 days Use "CR" (controlled-release preparation)	$$
Clobazam (20-40)	Irritability Depression	Very safe OD or BID dosing Broad spectrum Rapid onset Few interactions	Tolerance (initial good response followed by loss of seizure control)	Can be very useful as "add-on" for patients "nearly" seizure free	$$
Ethosuximide 750-1000	GI upset	Few drug interactions	For absence seizures only	Confers no protection for generalized tonic-clonic seizures	$-$$
Gabapentin (1200-3600)		No drug interactions Well tolerated Very safe	Narrow spectrum of efficacy Predominantly for partial and secondarily generalized seizures TID dosing	Very expensive at high doses Best used as "add on" drug	$$$$
Lamotrigine (300-400)	Rash 5%-10%, rarely can be very serious Insomnia	BID dosing Broad spectrum No enzyme induction (few interactions) Some patients more "alert"	Very slow dose titration (see product monograph) Metabolism markedly inhibited by valproic acid Only oral form	Very expensive at high doses (when used with enzyme enhancing AEDs) Increasing use as monotherapy Increasing use for primary generalized seizures	$$$$
Phenobarbital (90-120) Primidone (500-1000)	Sedative properties prominent Skin rash 5% Some patients intolerant of low-dose primidone Depression Diminished libido	Long half life OD dosing for phenobarbital Extremely inexpensive (phenobarbital) Parenteral form of phenobarbital easy to use (emergencies)	Potent liver enzyme inducers Metabolism inhibited by valproic acid QID dosing for primidone (to maintain high primidone/phenobarbital ratio) Slow dose titration (primidone)	Declining use because of adverse effect profile Primidone metabolized to phenobarbital, but parent compound has significant antiseizure properties	$

Phenytoin (300-400)	Skin rash 5%-10%, rarely very serious Liver enzyme elevation Blood dyscrasias Gingival hyperplasia Dose-related encephalopathy	OD or BID dosing Parenteral form Inexpensive Easy-to-give loading dose, but follow manufacturer's instructions carefully	Saturation kinetics Enzyme inducer Drug interactions Long-term cosmetic effects	Saturation kinetics can create dosing problems for some physicians	$
Topiramate (200-400)	Relatively common cognitive problems Kidney stones Weight loss Headache Fingers/toes paresthesia	BID dosing Broad spectrum Very safe Few drug interactions	Slow titration Decreased effectiveness of oral contraceptive efficacy Expensive	Potent AED with broad spectrum of activity, but cognitive effects commonly limit use Very expensive at high doses	$$$$
Valproic acid (750-1500)	Nausea Weight gain Tremor Hair loss Blood dyscrasias Rare hepatotoxicity Rare edema Menstrual irregularities Spina bifida teratogenic effect (1%-2%)	Often may use BID dosing Broad spectrum No enzyme induction Very low incidence of rash Cognitive effects generally less than other older AEDs	Drug interactions (but does not reduce oral contraceptive efficacy)	Drug of first choice for patients with mixed primary generalized seizures (generalized tonic-clonic, myoclonus, absence)	$$$
Vigabatrin (2000-4000)	Low incidence of psychosis; depression Low incidence of irreversible visual field problems	BID dosing Generally well tolerated Few drug interactions Easy to use; linear pharmacokinetics Safe from skin, blood, liver adverse effects	May worsen absence seizures; myoclonus Can be expensive at high doses	Recent concern of visual field effects has limited use of this drug by some physicians	$$$$

$, <$25; *$$*, 25-50; *$$$*, 50-100; *$$$$*, 100-200.

*Consult product monograph for details of dosing, preparations, titration schedules, drug interactions, and a complete list of adverse effects; felbamate is not listed because it is not available in Canada and the lack of experience with this drug by the author.

†Virtually all AEDs can produce sedation, fatigue, cognitive impairment, dizziness, and ataxia in a dose-dependent fashion.

patient-physician relationship and direct questioning of the patient will probably be as effective. AED levels may be useful in guiding therapy when a patient continues to have a substantial number of seizures despite relatively high serum levels. In this situation, change to a different medication should be considered because it is unlikely that a marginal increase in serum levels will abruptly transform the patient to a seizure-free state. AED levels can be used as a guide to which medication is likely to be responsible for toxic symptoms when the patient is taking multiple AEDs. Drug levels may be helpful in guiding initial dose requirements and subsequent dose adjustments in complex metabolic situations (e.g., hepatic or renal failure and pregnancy).

An area of controversy is the required frequency of checking hematologic and hepatic function studies in patients taking AEDs. Among the traditional AEDs, this issue relates to treatment with carbamazepine, valproic acid, and to some extent, phenytoin. Virtually all of the older AEDs have been associated with idiosyncratic hematologic toxicity (e.g., aplastic anemia, thrombocytopenia, neutropenia) and hepatic dysfunction (hypersensitivity reactions and possibly direct toxic effects by an AED or its metabolites). Some manufacturers have recommended that complete blood counts (CBCs) and hepatic function studies be performed on a regular basis throughout the period of treatment with the drug. This position has been challenged on the basis that testing of asymptomatic patients will create unnecessary medical costs, some patients may be withdrawn from effective therapy on the basis of trivial laboratory abnormalities, and there may not be a presymptomatic phase before the adverse effect can be detected by laboratory tests.[2] One suggested approach is to provide informed consent of the major adverse effects, baseline CBC and liver function studies, a follow-up of these investigations in 4 to 12 weeks (since most of the major idiosyncratic effects develop in the first several weeks of therapy), and only investigate patients further if they are symptomatic. Minor elevations of hepatic transaminase levels (e.g., less than twice the baseline level) and modest reductions of blood counts are common with AED treatment, but they do not predict impending catastrophe and are not indications to stop otherwise successful therapy.

With the notable exception of felbamate, the most recently marketed AEDs appear to be relatively safe with respect to hepatic and hematologic difficulties.

TREATMENT OF MEDICALLY RESISTANT EPILEPSY

Approximately 30% of all patients with epilepsy will be resistant to treatment with a single drug. Polytherapy (the addition of one or more AEDs) may improve seizure control in approximately 10% of these patients.

Surgery for epilepsy has become increasingly available at specialized centers. Prerequisites for epilepsy surgery generally include an unequivocal failure of reasonable AED therapy, demonstration of a surgically accessible focus that can be removed without substantial risk, and a motivated patient.

Patients considered for epilepsy surgery will be admitted to a specialized monitoring unit for video–EEG telemetry monitoring. The epileptogenic zone is delineated by assessment of the interictal and ictal EEG abnormalities and recording the patient's behavior during seizures. Detailed neuropsychology testing is performed to identify language areas and to assess cognitive functions. High-quality MRI scans are used to search for structural lesions. Optimum surgical results are obtained when there is congruence of information from the various investigations (i.e., structural and functional studies demonstrate abnormalities in the same brain region and this region can be resected without creating a major neurologic deficit).

The most common type of epilepsy surgery performed is a temporal lobe resection. A resection may result in a seizure-free or markedly improved outcome in at least 60% to 80% of patients with disease confined to one temporal lobe. The results for epilepsy surgery outside the temporal lobe are not as impressive but are still worthy of consideration in individual circumstances.

Epilepsy surgery need not be deferred until all possible AEDs and AED combination therapies have been explored. Optimal psychosocial outcome, employability, and contribution to society are more likely to be achieved with early eradication of the seizures.

Patients with multifocal epilepsy, and particularly those with akinetic (drop) attacks, may receive palliative benefits from other surgical procedures, including a corpus callosum section.

Other nonsurgical and nonpharmacologic therapies have attracted recent attention. A unique ketogenic diet may be successful for severe forms of epilepsy that are resistant to conventional AEDs. This therapy has been most widely used in children; it is a very difficult diet to initiate and maintain in adults. Vagal nerve stimulation (with a device similar to a cardiac pacemaker implanted in the chest wall) delivers intermittent electrical stimulation to the vagus nerve. This therapy may be considered for those patients with medically resistant epilepsy who are not candidates for other forms of surgical therapy.

SPECIAL SITUATIONS

The First Seizure

An area of some controversy is the management of the patient who presents with the first seizure.[3] This situation will usually arise in the setting of a convulsion (either primary generalized or secondarily generalized). An important factor to ascertain is whether the presentation is truly the first seizure. A careful inquiry for features of prior unrecognized nocturnal seizures (e.g., awakening in the morning with a chewed tongue, unexplained episodes of incontinence, musculoskeletal injury) or partial complex seizures and simple partial seizures is mandatory. Similarly, in the child and adolescent, a careful line of inquiry should be conducted to determine if there have been absence attacks or myoclonic jerks. Patients rarely come to medical attention after their first partial complex seizure and virtually never with the first absence seizure.

Most epilepsy experts do not recommend treatment after a single convulsion, particularly if the patient has an otherwise unremarkable history, normal neurologic examination, and negative investigations. The risks of treatment must be weighed against the likelihood of seizure recurrence. It has been estimated that a patient with an idiopathic seizure and normal EEG has a recurrence risk of 24% by 2 years. A significantly increased risk of seizure recurrence has been noted in patients who have a clear, remote, known cause for a seizure. Some studies have suggested an increased risk of recurrence if one or more of the following features are present: (1) a focally originating seizure, (2) presence of an abnormal neurologic examination, and (3) an abnormal EEG, particularly if the EEG demonstrates epileptiform discharges.

It should be noted that most studies that have evaluated recurrence rates after a first seizure do not include patients with "active" intracranial disease such as acute stroke and brain tumor. Therefore, the decision to treat patients with AEDs after a single seizure must be individualized.

Epilepsy and Women[10]

It has long been recognized that some women have an exacerbation of seizures in relationship to their menstrual cycles. Close scrutiny of seizure calendars with recording of menstrual cycles does not always corroborate the impression of a tight linkage of these phenomena. However, there is a relatively small subset of women who have an increased tendency for seizures in the days immediately preceding and after the onset of menstrual flow. The precise mechanisms of this so-called *catamenial epilepsy* have not been determined but likely relate to the ratio of the proepileptic effects of estrogen and the antiepileptic effects of progesterone. Specific treatment with hormonal manipulation (such as exogenous progesterone) has been suggested for catamenial epilepsy but does not appear to be widely used.

There are no contraindications to women with epilepsy receiving estrogen in the form of oral contraceptives or as postmenopausal therapy from the perspective of these hormones exacerbating epilepsy. It is important to appreciate that the hepatic enzyme–enhancing AEDs (phenobarbital, primidone, carbamazepine, phenytoin, and topiramate) confer an increased risk of "pill failure" in women taking oral contraceptives. The failure rate has been estimated to increase from 0.7 per 100 women years to 3.1 when enzyme-enhancing AEDs are used. Experts have recommended that women taking enzyme-enhancing AEDs should use an oral contraceptive containing a minimum of 50 μg of estrogen. Women concurrently taking oral contraceptives and enzyme-enhancing AEDs and who experience midcycle breakthrough bleeding may be at risk of ovulation and require an increase in their estrogen dose.

Epilepsy in pregnancy is a complex topic, and the ideal time to discuss the various issues surrounding epilepsy and pregnancy is before conception occurs. In women whose epilepsy has been well controlled for several years it may be advisable to discontinue AED therapy before embarking on a planned pregnancy. The rationale of this approach relates to the potential teratogenic effect of AEDs on the developing fetus (see below).

Some authorities recommend continuous folic acid supplementation (a minimum dose of 0.4 mg daily) for all women taking AEDs who are of childbearing potential.[10] Folate may reduce the incidence of major malformation in the offspring in this population.

Recent studies suggest that a relatively minor increase in seizure frequency may occur during pregnancy. Most authors have attributed the seizure exacerbations to changes in the pharmacokinetics of the AEDs (including increased metabolism and volume of distribution) but contributions from the sex hormones, other metabolic changes in pregnancy, sleep deprivation, and psychologic stress have all been implicated. Several authors recommend following AED serum levels throughout the pregnancy, with dose adjustment accordingly.

Studies of the outcome of pregnancy in women with epilepsy who are taking antiepileptic drugs have demonstrated a number of adverse outcomes. There is a twofold to fourfold increase in complications, including preeclampsia, placenta previa, and abruptio placentae. Some studies have demonstrated a twofold to fourfold increase in prematurity and low birth weight.

A major concern of prospective parents is the potential for teratogenic effects of the AEDs. In general, the overall risk of malformations in the offspring of women with epilepsy taking AEDs is 4% to 6%. Some studies have found an increased risk of malformations in women with untreated epilepsy. This finding, if confirmed, would suggest that genetic factors also play a role in teratogenesis. There are probably few specific malformations that are directly related to an individual AED. Examples of minor malformations associated with AED use include digital nail hypoplasia, hypertelorism, and abnormally shaped ears. The most common "major" malformations associated with AED use include congenital heart disease (including cardiac septal defects) and a variety of clefting disorders of the face and palate. Valproic acid appears to confer a 1% to 2% risk of producing spina bifida. Carbamazepine may also be associated with a small risk of a similar malformation. The major malformations take place very early in embryogenesis (even before the woman may know she is pregnant), thus the recommendation for folic acid supplementation to all women of childbearing potential. The majority of spinal closure defects and many cardiac abnormalities can be very reliably detected early in pregnancy with modern ultrasound techniques. The diagnostic algorithm for detecting these defects may vary from center to center; expert consultation is recommended for appropriate timing and type of ultrasound.

Among the commonly used AEDs, there is no overwhelming evidence that any particular AED is safer in pregnancy than another. Most authorities do not recommend changing one AED to another in women whose seizures are well controlled and are planning a pregnancy. However, some physicians discontinue valproic acid if there is a positive family history of spinal closure defects. In general, it is best to use the AED that is most suitable for the patient's seizure disorder. Monotherapy should be achieved before conception if at all possible.

The experience with the new generation of AEDs is insufficient to make any recommendations pertaining to their safety in pregnancy. Most of the traditional AEDs have the potential to reduce vitamin K levels, and it is recommended that oral vitamin K supplementation (20 mg/day) be given during the 4 weeks before the expected delivery date.

There is no strict contraindication to breastfeeding, although babies born to mothers taking barbiturates may be somewhat sedated.

Women whose AED dose has been increased during the pregnancy are at risk of rather precipitously developing AED dose-related toxicity in the first 2 to 4 weeks postdelivery as enzymatic deinduction occurs. The dose of the AED should be reduced to the prepregnancy level soon after delivery.

It should be emphasized to prospective mothers that over 90% of pregnancies in women with epilepsy who are taking AEDs have a satisfactory outcome and that a number of steps can be taken to maximize the probability of a healthy baby and mother.

Status Epilepticus

Status epilepticus (SE) is a state of continuous or rapidly repeating seizures. Recent publications have suggested a working definition of SE as a state of continuous seizures lasting at least 20 minutes; a more conservative definition has been proposed suggesting that SE consists of more than two seizures between which there is an incomplete return to consciousness. Most review papers discuss predominantly the management of "convulsive" SE, although it should be appreciated that all of the seizure types listed in Box 159-1 may manifest as a form of a status.

Myoclonic SE is a relatively unusual form of primary generalized seizure disorder. A number of rare neurologic degenerative disorders and some toxic-metabolic disorders may produce myoclonic SE. Notable among the latter is myoclonic SE occurring in association with anoxic-ischemic encephalopathy (particularly after cardiac arrest). This form of SE is extremely difficult to treat, is often associated with a very poor prognosis for neurologic recovery, and is viewed by some authorities as an agonal brain event.

The two major forms of nonconvulsive SE are *partial complex SE* and *absence SE*. Patients with these disorders present with an alteration of consciousness that ranges from subtle confusion to an unresponsive state. Absence SE may last for hours or occasionally days to weeks; the diagnosis is confirmed by an EEG that discloses abundant or continuous runs of generalized spike and wave discharges. Absence SE should be in the differential diagnosis of any patient who presents with an acute onset confusional state, particularly when he or she has a history of one of the primary generalized epilepsy syndromes. The SE may be spectacularly terminated with intravenous benzodiazepines that are best administered during simultaneous EEG recording. In its classic form, partial complex SE consists of a continuous twilight state alternating with episodes of more typical partial complex seizures. The distinction of absence SE from partial complex SE usually will require an EEG.

Emotionally based pseudoseizures may occur as "status" with recurrent attacks that superficially resemble generalized tonic-clonic seizures that are unresponsive to the usual initial treatments. Conversely, patients with absence SE and partial complex SE are easily misdiagnosed as having "hysteria" or a "conversion disorder."

The remainder of this section on SE will concentrate on convulsive SE. At least 80% of cases of convulsive SE are of the secondarily generalized variety; close clinical observation at the onset of the attack may disclose the focal onset (e.g., head and eye deviation to one side, clonic jerks beginning in one limb). In other patients, particularly those with a frontal lobe focus, the propagation may be of such rapidity that an EEG is required to recognize the focal onset.

Virtually any process that affects the CNS can lead to SE. In the pediatric age group the most common causes are secondary to congenital structural lesions, infections (including febrile SE), trauma, and consequences of anoxia. In adults the most common causes are cerebrovascular disease, anoxic injury, trauma, decrease in AEDs, and ethanol and other recreational drug use. Additional causes of SE common to both adults and children include toxic-metabolic disturbances (e.g., disorders of fluid and electrolytes, glucose, and calcium) and neoplasm.

The overall mortality rate of convulsive SE is approximately 20%. The major determinants of mortality relate to the etiology and duration of SE. Animal models of SE and some data from human studies suggest that brain damage occurs with SE lasting more than 30 to 45 minutes. Some studies suggest that the longer status is allowed to continue, the more difficult it is to terminate. The injury to brain (especially the hippocampus) is separate from the underlying process that initiated the SE and appears to be mediated by excitotoxic neurotransmitters. Therefore prompt termination of the seizures and correction of the underlying cause offer the best hope to diminish mortality and morbidity.

The initial care of patients with convulsive SE consists of attention to the airway (patients require an oral airway and often intubation and ventilation), administration of oxygen, electrocardiographic monitoring, and blood work as noted in Table 159-3. All patients should receive 50 ml of 50% dextrose and 50 to 100 mg of thiamine. A large-bore intravenous catheter should be inserted in each arm (one for the administration of a rapidly acting benzodiazepine, the other to begin an infusion of phenytoin or phenobarbital). A benzodiazepine alone may be sufficient if the underlying cause of the status is quickly correctable.[8,11] Most published protocols for treating SE recommend using diazepam or lorazepam as initial therapy. These benzodiazepines are potent and have a rapid onset of action. Lorazepam has become increasingly popular and a recent prospective randomized trial attests to its efficacy.[11]

Simultaneous to the administration of a benzodiazepine, either phenytoin or phenobarbital is started in the second intravenous line. An adequate loading dose of either of these

Table 159-3. Initial Management of Convulsive Status Epilepticus

Time (minutes)	Management
0-5	History, physical examination Oral airway, oxygen Consider intubation Venous blood (glucose, blood counts, electrolytes, calcium, renal function, liver function, antiepileptic blood levels, consider drug screen) Arterial blood gases Monitor ECG, pulse oximetry, blood pressure
5-10	Start two large-bore intravenous saline infusions Use 50 ml of 50% dextrose Inject 50-100 mg thiamine intramuscularly Start intravenous lorazepam, 0.1 mg/kg at 2 mg/min (usual dose = 4 to 8 mg) or Intravenous diazepam 5 mg/min (usual dose = 10 to 20 mg)
10-30	Intravenous phenytoin 17-18 mg/kg (50 mg/min) or Intravenous phenobarbital 20 mg/kg (50-75 mg/min)
30-60	If seizures persist after initial phenytoin, start phenobarbital If seizures persist after initial phenobarbital, use phenytoin Admit patient to critical care unit, arrange for EEG Obtain expert consultation

AEDs must be given. Phenytoin cannot be given in glucose-containing solutions; it should be given at a dose of 17 to 18 mg/kg at a rate not exceeding 50 mg/minute. The infusion rate should be slowed if hypertension or cardiac arrhythmias develop. A water-soluble prodrug of phenytoin (fosphenytoin) and a parenteral preparation of valproic acid have recently been released for use; the precise roles for these agents are yet to be determined. If phenytoin fails, phenobarbital (20 mg/kg at 50 to 75 mg/minute) should be infused while careful monitoring of respiratory function and blood pressure is maintained. Most episodes of convulsive SE can be terminated with adequate doses of benzodiazepines, phenytoin, and/or phenobarbital (see summary in Table 159-3). Expert consultation should be sought urgently if these therapies are unsuccessful, with consideration of treatment with propofol, midazolam, pentobarbital, or thiopental. Further details of the management of therapy-resistant SE can be obtained in the literature cited at the end of this chapter.

REFERENCES

1. Brodie MJ, Dichter MA: Antiepileptic drugs, *N Engl J Med* 334:168-175, 1996.
2. Camfield P, Camfield C, Dooley J, et al: Routine screening of blood and urine for severe reactions to anticonvulsant drugs in asymptomatic patients is of doubtful value, *Can Med Assoc J* 140:1303-1305, 1989.
3. Chadwick D: Epilepsy after first seizure: risks and implications, *J Neurol Neurosurg Psychiatr* 54:385-387, 1991.
4. Commission on Classification and Terminology of the International League Against Epilepsy: Proposal for revised clinical and electroencephalographic classification of epileptic seizures, *Epilepsia* 22:489-501, 1981.
5. Commission on Classification and Terminology of the International League Against Epilepsy: Proposal for revised classification of epilepsies and epileptic syndromes, *Epilepsia* 30:389-399, 1989.
6. Dichter MA, Brodie MJ: New antiepileptic drugs, *N Engl J Med* 334:1583-1590, 1996.
7. Hauser WA, Annegers JF, Rocca WA: Descriptive epidemiology of epilepsy: contributions of population-based studies from Rochester, Minnesota, *Mayo Clin Proc* 71:576-586, 1996.
8. Lowenstein DH, Allredge BK: Status epilepticus, *N Engl J Med* 338:970-976, 1998.
9. Pedley TA: Differential diagnosis of episodic symptoms, *Epilepsia* 24 (Suppl 1):S31-S34, 1983.
10. Report of the Quality Standards Committee of the American Academy of Neurology: Practice parameter: management issues for women with epilepsy (summary statement), *Neurology* 51:944-948, 1998.
11. Treiman DM, Meyers PD, Walton NY, et al: A comparison of four treatments for generalized convulsive status epilepticus, *N Engl J Med* 339:792-798, 1998.

Headache

William Pryse-Phillips
T. Jock Murray

Nothing in clinical neurology exceeds the demands on the clinician more than diagnosing and managing the patient with headache, a process that demands a combination of clinical skill and good interpersonal relationships. The physician dealing with the patient who presents with headache will by the history determine the likely diagnosis; by the brief, structured examination receive some reassurance that there is no lurking lesion causing the problem; and by his or her ability to see past the patient's naive words of complaint, recognize a pattern of symptomatology, allowing a confident diagnosis that will allow equally confident management. As always, the physician must determine during the interview what the patient wants—is it pain relief, reassurance that no serious disease underlies the symptoms experienced, or simply an explanation?

The classifications of headaches that will be discussed in this chapter and other types of headaches are listed in Box 160-1.

MECHANISMS OF CRANIAL PAIN

The extracranial and intracranial pain-sensitive structures all project pain sensation to the cranial surface, usually fairly near to the source of pain. Because many such sources register their pain in the same general area, a pain in any location may represent disordered function in any of several structures, intracranial or extracranial. Some common sites at which cranial pain is felt and the anatomic structures that may be the source of referral to these areas are shown in Fig. 160-1. The sensory pathways responsible for pain from various areas of the cranium are shown in Fig. 160-2.

Common mechanisms of cranial pain are illustrated in Fig. 160-3 and include the following:

- Nerve irritation, as with the neuralgias
- Pressure or traction on pain-sensitive structures (Fig. 160-3, *B*)
- Vasodilation of pain-sensitive vessels (anoxia, hypercapnea, fever, histamine injection, nitroglycerin ingestion, and sudden rise in blood pressure)
- Prolonged contraction of cranial muscles
- Inflammation of pain-sensitive structures
- Nonorganic pain (a diagnosis of last resort)

Common causes of acute severe headaches are listed in Box 160-2.

Danger Signals

The following features of a headache should raise concern about a potentially sinister underlying cause for the headache and suggest the need for further investigation:

- The first or worst headache of the patient's life, particularly if of rapid onset (subarachnoid hemorrhage?)
- A change in frequency, severity, or features of the headache attack from that commonly experienced in the past (any new pathology?)
- The new onset of headache in middle age or later, or a significant change in any long-standing headache pattern (new pathology?)
- The appearance of a progressive or new daily, persistent headache (medication-induced headache?)
- The precipitation of head pain with coughing, sneezing, or bending down (mass lesion, Chiari malformation?)
- The presence of systemic symptoms such as myalgias, fever, malaise, weight loss, scalp tenderness, or jaw claudication (cranial arteritis?)
- The presence of focal neurologic symptoms or any abnormalities on neurologic examination, or of confusion, seizures, or any impairment in the level of consciousness (mass lesion?)

Box 160-1. Classification of Headaches

1. Migraine
    - Without aura
    - With aura
        - Typical
        - Prolonged
        - Familial hemiplegic migraine
        - Basilar migraine
        - Aura without headache
    - Ophthalmoplegic
    - Retinal
    - Precursors
        - Benign paroxysmal vertigo of childhood
        - Alternating hemiplegia of childhood
    - With intracranial disorder
    - Complications
        - Status migrainous
        - Migrainous infarction
    - Unclassifiable
2. Tension-type
    - Episodic tension with and without pericranial muscle disorder
    - Chronic tension with and without pericranial muscle disorder
3. Cluster headache
    - Cluster headache
        - Episodic, chronic
    - Chronic paroxysmal hemicrania
    - Unclassifiable
4. Posttraumatic
5. Vascular
    - Ischemic vascular disease
    - Hemorrhagic vascular disease
    - Unruptured arteriovenous malformation
    - Arteritis
    - Hypertension
    - Other: Carotidynia, postendarterectomy
6. Associated with nonvascular intracranial disease
    - Raised intracranial pressure
    - Cerebrospinal fluid leakage
    - Intracranial infection
    - Intracranial tumor
7. Substance withdrawal
    - Monosodium glutamate, alcohol, nitrites, carbon monoxide
    - Ergot, analgesics, chronic toxic exposure
    - Alcohol/ergot withdrawal
8. Systemic/focal infection
9. Metabolic abnormality
    - Hypoxia, dialysis
10. Referred
    - From cranial bones, neck, eyes, teeth, jaws, nose and sinuses, ears, temporomandibular joints
11. Cranial neuralgias
    - Persistent
        - Cranial nerve distortion, demyelination, infarction, or inflammation (herpes zoster, post-herpes zoster)
        - Tolosa-Hunt syndrome
    - Trigeminal neuralgia (idiopathic, symptomatic)
    - Glossopharyngeal neuralgia
    - Central causes
        - Anesthesia dolorosa
        - Thalamic pain
12. Other
    - Ice-pick pains
    - Cold stimulus headache
    - Benign cough
    - Benign exertional
    - Coital cephalalgia
    - Atypical facial pain
13. Psychogenic headache
14. Not classifiable

Physical Examination

The physical examination performed at the first consultation for a headache problem should at least evaluate blood pressure, heart rate, cardiac status, sinuses, scalp arteries, cervical paraspinal muscles, the temporomandibular (TMJ) joints, and the range of motion of and presence of pain in the cervical spine. A screening neurologic examination capable of detecting most of the abnormal signs likely to occur in patients with headaches caused by intracranial or systemic disease should include evaluation of the following:

- Neck flexion (for evidence of meningeal irritation)
- The presence of bruits over the cranium, orbits, or neck
- The optic fundi, visual fields, pupillary reactions, fifth cranial nerve sensory function, and corneal reflexes
- Motor power in the face and limbs, muscle stretch reflexes, plantar responses, and gait

The presence of any such abnormalities is unusual in uncomplicated migraine and suggests the need for further investigation.

Investigations

The history is the most important step in the management of a headache patient. Profiles both of an individual attack and of the behavior of this form of headache over years should be drawn, and if the patient has more than one type of headache, separate profiles for each must be formulated. Pointers to serious organic causes are indicated above.

The electroencephalogram (EEG) is not useful in the routine evaluation of patients with headache unless the patient has associated symptoms suggesting a seizure disorder, such as atypical migrainous aura or episodic loss of consciousness. An EEG is inadequate to exclude a structural cause for headache. Many patients with migraines have dysrhythmic EEGs, and when this is reported the physician may become unnecessarily concerned and initiate further tests and consultation.

Lumbar puncture (LP) may have value if the headache is the first or worst in the patient's life; in the presence of severe, rapid onset, recurrent headache, or progressive headache without signs of raised intracranial pressure; with atypical, chronic, and intractable headache; or when headache is associated with fever. We suggest that LP should be performed only if meningitis, encephalitis, subarachnoid hemorrhage, or high-pressure or low-pressure headache syndromes are considered possible. If subarachnoid hemorrhage is the concern, a CT scan will rule out or confirm the diagnosis.

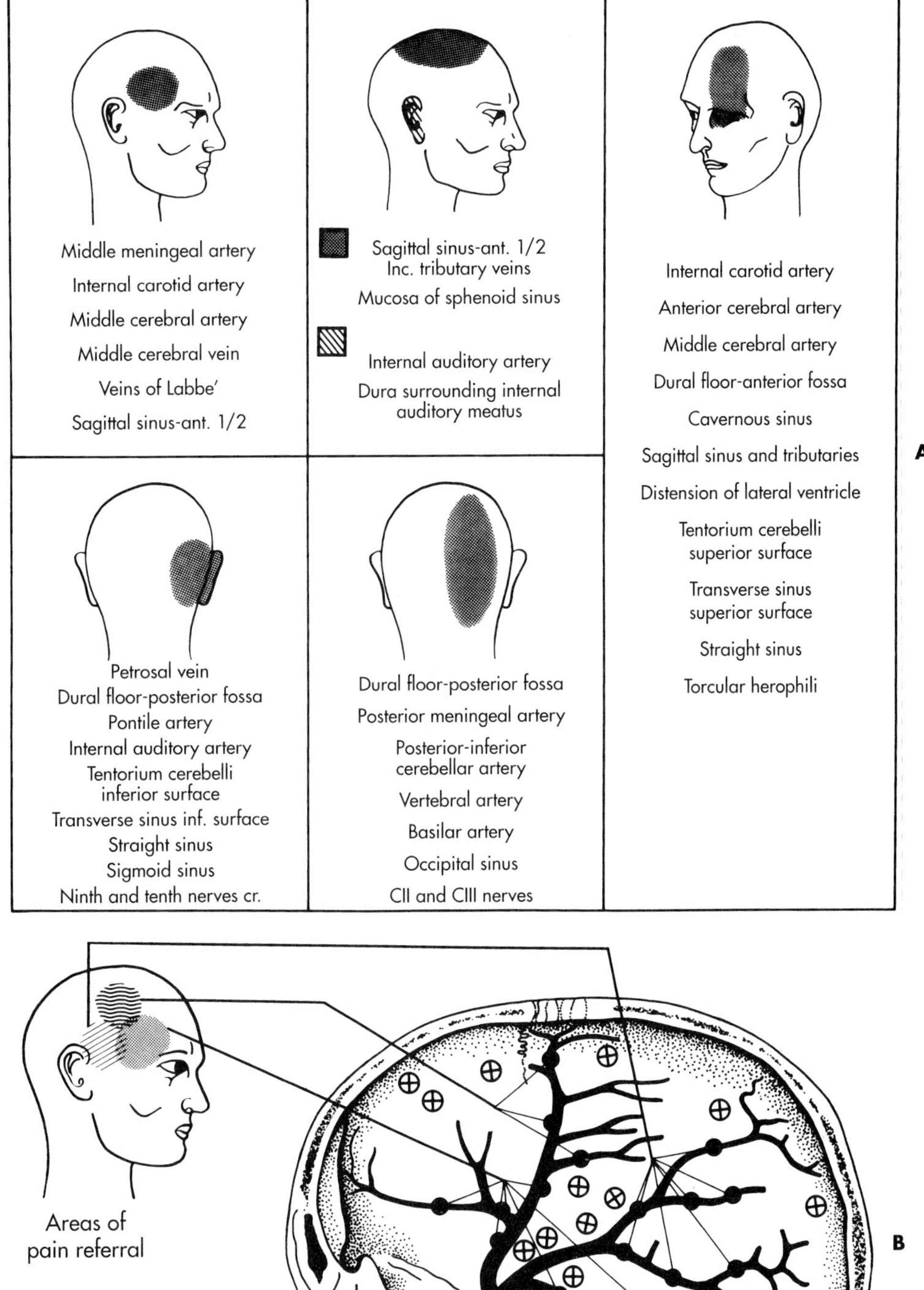

Fig. 160-1. Some areas of the head to which pain is referred (**A**) by stimulation of certain cranial structures (**B**). (From Wolff HG: In Dalessio DJ, Silbers SD, editors: *Headche and other head pain,* ed 6, New York, 1993, Oxford University Press.)

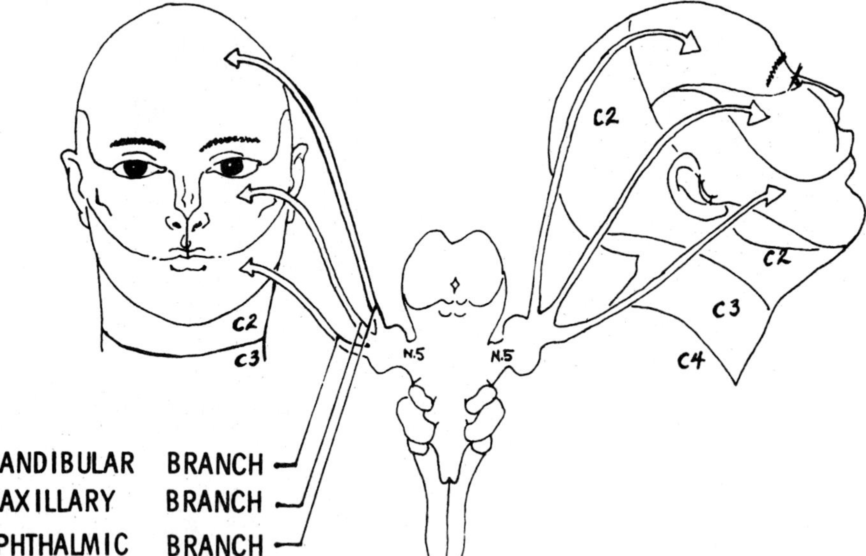

Fig. 160-2. Sensory pathways for cranial pain. (From Pryse-Phillips W, Murray TJ: Essential neurology: a concise textbook, ed 4, New York, 1992, Medical Examination Publishing.)

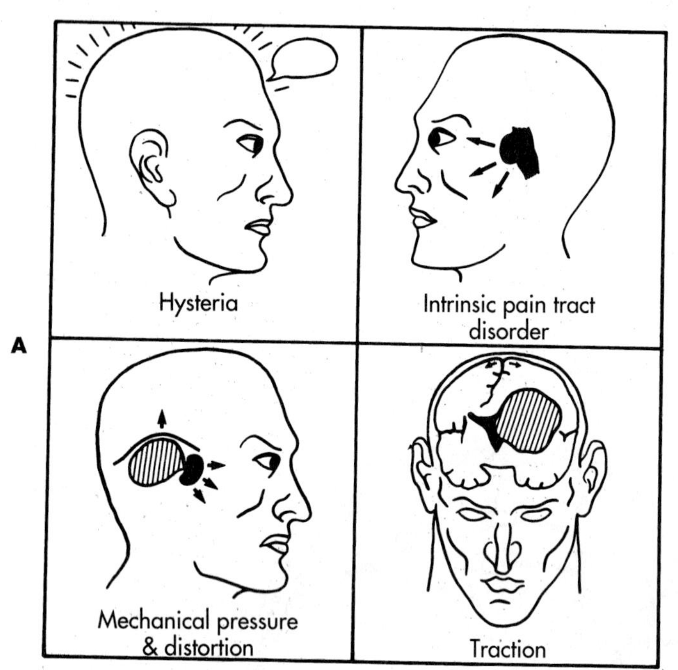

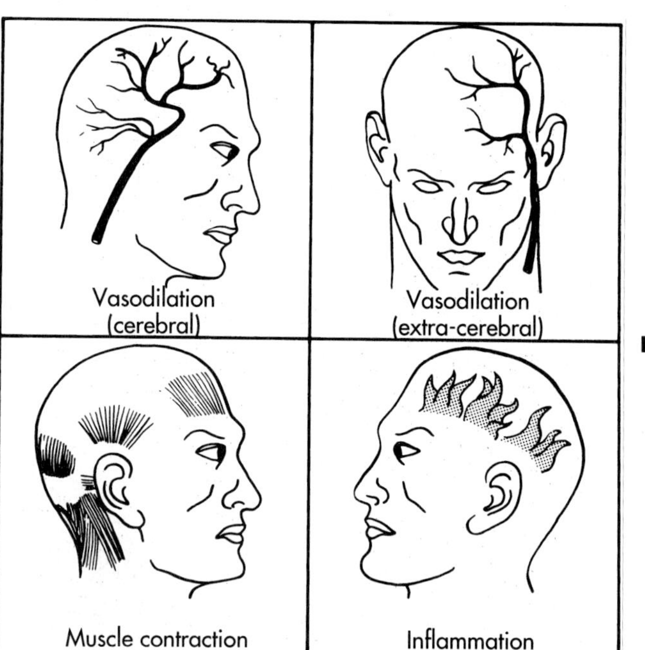

Fig. 160-3. **A** and **B,** Mechanisms of cranial pain.

Computed tomography (CT) or magnetic resonance imaging (MRI) scans are only warranted in adult patients whose headaches fit a broad definition of recurrent migraine if there is also any recent substantial change in headache pattern, a history of seizures, or the presence of focal neurologic symptoms or signs.

MIGRAINE

Migraine is a common clinical disorder that is underdiagnosed and inadequately managed. It affects about 1 in 20 men and 1 in 5 women, most of whom suffer some headache-related disability.

Migraine Without Aura

The International Headache Society (IHS) criteria of 1988 provide a reliable diagnostic tool for migraines without an aura (Box 160-3), but they do not mention therapy, unlike the Canadian Headache Society guidelines, which do.

No one should expect that a single patient will have a "full-house" of the symptoms listed in Box 160-3, but the more there are, the more likely is the diagnosis of migraine to be correct. The following features also suggest migraine:

- The headaches occur more or less regularly in perimenstrual or periovulatory periods

Box 160-2. Causes of Acute Severe Headaches

Meningitis, encephalitis
Cerebral abscess
Intracerebral bleed/subarachnoid hemorrhage/acute subdural hematoma
Acutely raised intracranial pressure from other causes (e.g., ball-valve III ventricle cyst)
Migraine, cluster headache
Triggering agents with MAOIs (cheese, monosodium glutamate, alcohol, chocolate, red wine)
Nitrites
Hypertensive encephalopathy
Pheochromocytoma
Postseizure headache

- Food, odors, change in the weather, stress, or let-down after stress consistently precipitate headaches
- Headaches are relieved by sleep
- Irritability or other mood variations, hyperactivity, inability to concentrate, food cravings, or hyperosmia precede the headaches

The painful headache phase during attacks of migraine lasts for 2 to 6 hours and is typically accompanied by phonophotophobia, hyperacusis, hyperosmia, nausea, and vomiting. The pain is usually steady, with an added throbbing character, and it is worse on bending over or walking about. Attacks may recur consistently on one side of the head but often swap sides in different attacks. Persistence on one side may raise the suspicion of organic causes and should stimulate investigation to rule out vascular malformation or other structural disease.

Migraine With Aura

The diagnostic criteria for migraine with aura are the same as those listed above but include symptoms of neurologic dysfunction (including visual disturbance) occurring before or during the headache. If such symptoms persist after the pain has gone, referral for a neurologic consultation is wise. This form of migraine (Fig. 160-4, *A*) was described in the writings attributed to Galen and Hippocrates. Its hallmark is the neurologic prodrome to the headache phase (though sometimes this occurs alone). The aura usually has a sharp beginning and ending, lasts for 10 to 60 minutes (most often about 20 minutes), and is followed by the beginning of the headache. A visual aura in the form of a scintillating scotoma (Fig. 160-4, *B*) is the most common type. It starts as a small, twinkling, corrugated circle of tiny white, golden, or colored lights that form a pattern similar to medieval fortifications (Fig. 160-4, *C*). The lights appear in one homonymous field, spread peripherally, and are followed by visual loss in the area where the scintillating lights had been (Fig. 160-4, *D*). Gradually the apparition disappears, vision returns, and the headache begins. Patients are irritable during the prodromes, but during the headache phase they withdraw to some degree, seeking a place free of light, noise, problems, and children.

The next most common and equally characteristic prodrome is the development of prickling in the fingers of one hand that creeps or "marches" up the arm to the face, especially around the mouth, followed by hypoesthesia and/or complete anesthesia of the same area that has been "prickled," until the whole process clears and the headache begins. Fig. 160-5 shows spreading cerebral hypoperfusion correlated with the evolution of a scintillating scotoma and migraine headache demonstrated during a cerebral blood flow study. Less frequent are spots of flashing lights, "seeing through heat waves" (Fig. 160-6), aphasia, confusion, fuguelike states, distortion of the size of objects seen (micropsia), and even sensations of another person being present at one side or the other of the patient.

Prodromes are usually homonymous and seldom bilateral. The headache that follows them can be on either side. Rarely, they recur during the headache or continue after the headache has ceased. In such cases, thorough neurologic investigation should be performed to rule out organic disease.

Many patients have migraines both with and without aura. Attacks without aura are probably about 20 times more

Box 160-3. Suggested Diagnostic Criteria for Migraine Without Aura

A. At least five attacks fulfilling criteria B-D below shall have occurred. (One should recall in this context that migraine seldom occurs more frequently than 4 times per month.)
B. Headache attacks lasting 2 to 72 hours (untreated or unsuccessfully treated).
C. The headache has at least two of the following characteristics:
   1. Unilateral location: 30% to 40% of migraines cause bilateral pain. Ask if the patient feels pain on one or both sides. If one-sided, is it always on the same side or maximal on one side?
   2. Pulsating quality: Over half of all patients with migraines report nonthrobbing pain during some attacks, and a third of patients with tension-type headache report pulsating pain. Ask about the character of the pain—tightening, pressing, throbbing, pounding, pulsating, burning, etc.
   3. Moderate or severe intensity (i.e., the severity of the headache inhibits or prohibits daily activity).
   4. Aggravation by walking stairs or similar routine physical activity. Ask if the patient tries to avoid even slight movements (walking, head movement, or bending down) during a headache.
D. During a headache, at least one of the following should be present:
   1. Nausea and/or vomiting.
   2. Photophobia and phonophobia. The presence of osmophobia (aversion to odors) is also a highly sensitive and specific feature of migraine.
E. There is no evidence, on history or examination, of any other disease that might cause headaches.

Modified from the Headache Classification Committee of the International Headache Society: Classification and diagnostic criteria for headache disorders, cranial neuralgias, and facial pain, *Cephalagia* 8(suppl 7):9-97, 1988.

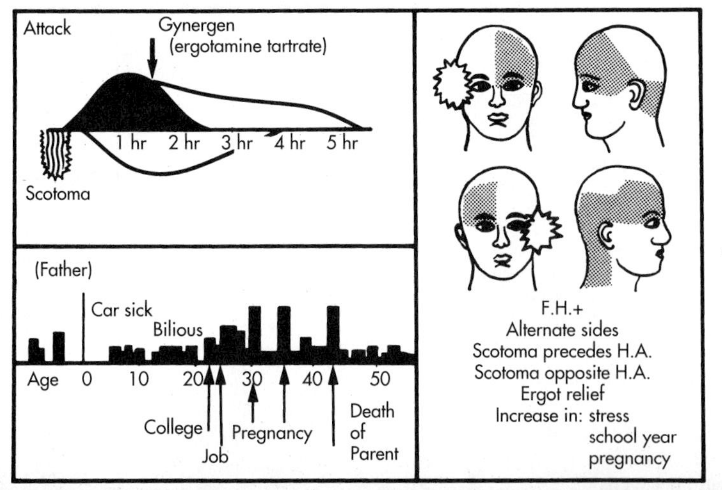

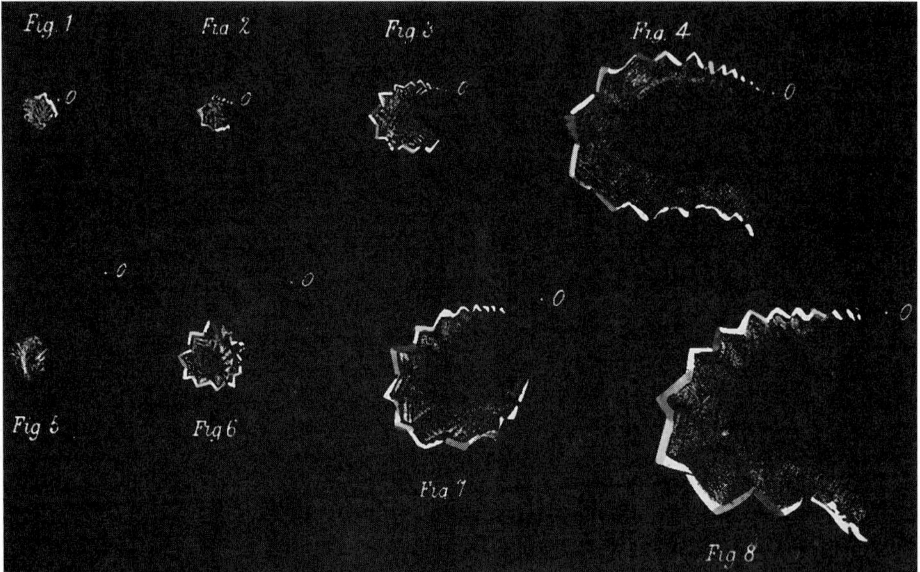

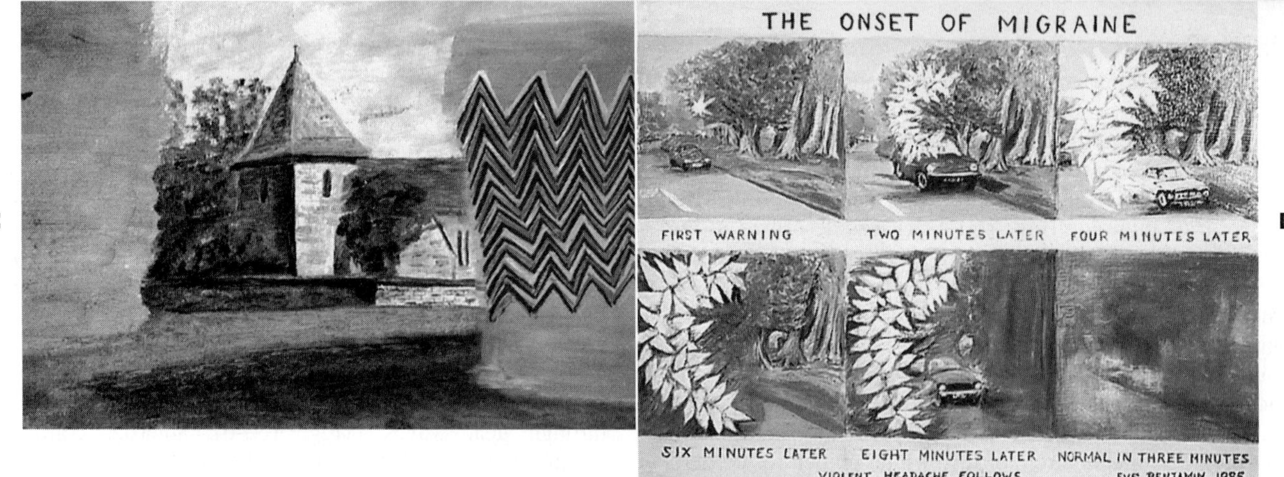

Fig. 160-4. **A,** Classic migraine. Profile of attack, profile of life history of headache, and "portrait." On this and similar diagrams the physician may register (above the line) the attack profile—duration, speed of onset and offset, severity, effect of therapy on the attack—and (below the line) the accompaniments of the attack—prodromes, nausea and vomiting, polyuria, etc. In the life profile the frequency and severity of attacks are recorded in relation to milestones in the patient's life (including family history). The portrait shows the location of the symptoms on a diagram of the patient's head and *(bottom right)* a list of key points in diagnosis. It is suggested that each physician create a similar diagram for patients. **B,** Scintillating scotomas tend to enlarge and occupy a central portion of the field of vision. This progression was drawn by P.W. Latham for his description of the "Nervous or Sick Headache" in 1873. **C,** Scintillating scotomas form a pattern like medieval fortifications. See CD-rom for color reproduction. **D,** Patient artistically depicts visual distortions and scintillating scotoma during aura of migraine headache that may relate temporally with spreading cerebral hypoperfusion. See CD-rom for color reproduction. (**C** courtesy the Migraine Action Association and Boehringer Ingelheim.)

frequent than migraine with aura and are more disabling. Migraine attacks commonly diminish in frequency and severity after about age 40 in both males and females, but as patients enter the 60s and 70s, the syndrome may reappear in the form of prodromes without subsequent headache (late-life migraine) and resemble transient ischemic attacks (TIAs). Recurrence of similar phenomena, the march, and occurrence of scintillating scotomas usually serve to identify it as a migrainous "equivalent" rather than as an ischemic process. Occasionally, however, migrainous scotomas in older patients cause a permanent deficit.

A variant characterized by unilateral, constant, steady, or throbbing pain in the lower half of the face, the carotid sheath, and suboccipital areas was once known as *lower-half*

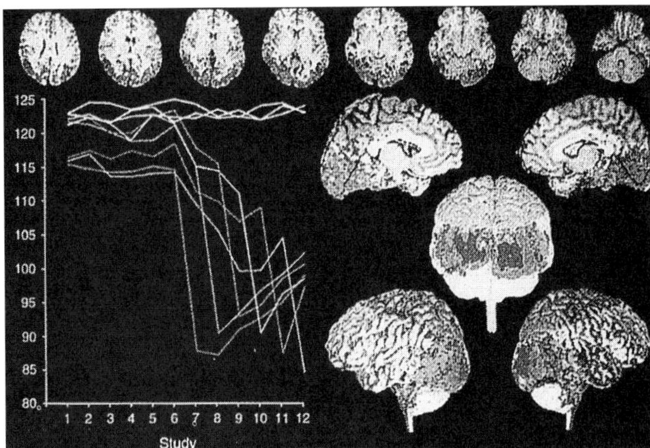

Fig. 160-5. Spreading cerebral hypoperfusion demonstrated by cerebral blood-flow measurement using intracarotid Xenon-133 technique. Patient spontaneously developed migraine during procedure. See CD-rom for color reproduction. (From Woods RP, et al: *N Engl J Med* 331(25):1689, 1992.)

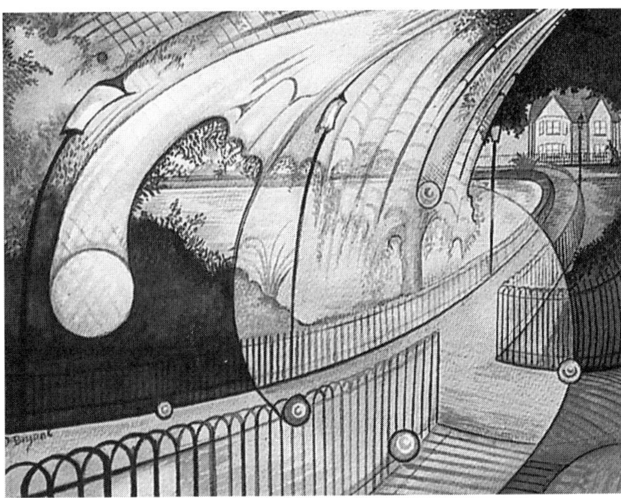

Fig. 160-6. Visual distortion of light and objects experienced by some patients with the aura of migraine. See CD-rom for color reproduction. (Courtesy the Migraine Action Association and Boehringer Ingelheim.)

headache. Its first appearance may be in the form of intermittent attacks resembling migraine, but attacks increase in frequency and duration until they become continuous with dull or moderate pain, by which time anxiety, depression, and dependence on analgesics are common. This type is unusually difficult to relieve with current medications.

Familial Hemiplegic Migraine

Familial hemiplegic migraine is a severe, if uncommon, form of migraine characterized by the appearance of motor paralysis of central origin during headache attacks accompanied by striking sensory, mood, orientation, and speech phenomena. It is commonly inherited as a dominant characteristic.

The attacks usually begin with the headache, which is followed by dramatic neurologic symptoms, an order of events that is the reverse of the usual in attacks of migraine with aura. Sensory phenomena, motor paralysis, dysarthria, aphasias, ataxia, tinnitus, vertigo, transient global amnesia, confusion, and fever may occur and usually outlast the headache, sometimes for days or even weeks; focal EEG abnormalities may persist even longer. Many patients who have marked sensory disturbances during classic migraine report that they are "paralyzed" during the attacks, but careful questioning shows that actual paralysis is not present. In hemiplegic migraine, however, it is.

Basilar Migraine

In basilar migraine there are symptoms of occipital lobe, cerebellar, and brainstem dysfunction, these areas being supplied by the basilar artery and its branches. Features include vertigo, ataxia, total blindness, total sensory or motor paralysis ("locked-in syndrome"), and unconsciousness. The disorder is more common in young women in whom attacks occur several weeks or months apart. Menstruation, tense life situations, prolonged mental strain, and use of oral contraceptives seem to bear some relation to the frequency and severity of the attacks, which usually decrease over the years, but in a few patients they reappear in middle or old age, and severe episodes occasionally leave a permanent deficit caused by cerebral infarction.

Treatment of basilar migraine attacks is difficult. Use of triptans is ineffective and also contraindicated. Breathing 90% O_2 with 10% CO_2 for 5- to 10-minute intervals is an old remedy but is not easily accessed. Oral prednisone, 50 mg, repeated twice at 4-hour intervals (or given parenterally), and the use of a calcium channel blocker are of unproven benefit. Prophylaxis of attacks is the same as for other forms of migraine.

Ophthalmoplegic Migraine

In ophthalmoplegic migraines, headache attacks are associated with a third nerve palsy that outlasts the headache and may become permanent. Some form of arterial imaging angiography is necessary to exclude an aneurysm on the circle of Willis or of the posterior communicating artery. Whether the pain is caused by arterial pressure on the third nerve or a lesion at the level of the III nerve nucleus is unknown. CT scans rarely demonstrate local bleeding or a vascular anomaly and may miss a small aneurysm that may be detected only by contrast or magnetic resonance angiography (MRA). Once organic causes have been ruled out, attacks may be treated symptomatically and prophylactically, similar to migraine without aura. Steroids have been recommended for paralysis outlasting the headache (prednisone tapered from 40 mg daily over several days).

Retinal migraine is characterized by the occurrence of any pattern of visual loss in one eye, with all the usual features of auras and followed by the headache.

Symptomatic Treatment

Symptomatic treatment is appropriate when the headaches are more than a mild pain and disrupt the patient's ability to function normally. Attacks of differing severity require different levels of therapy.

Acute Therapy

Mild Attacks. The buffered or soluble forms of acetylsalicylic acid (ASA) and ibuprofen or naproxen are effective in mild attacks but may cause gastrointestinal side effects. Acetaminophen is widely used, but often in subanalgesic doses (i.e., less than 1 gm for an adult). Neither dimenhydrinate nor domperidone has been shown to confer advantage as an adjunctive medication, but metoclopramide alone may relieve both the headache and the nausea and will enhance the effect of any analgesic by improving its absorption.

Moderate Attacks. Nonsteroidal antiinflammatory drugs may relieve some moderate attacks, but the specific drugs are much better. Sumatriptan, a selective 5HT1 agonist, relieves up to 70% of migraine headaches within an hour. If the 50-mg oral dose is ineffective, a 100-mg dose should be used subsequently. Subcutaneous injection (6 mg) gives relief rates of up to 77% at 1 hour, and an intranasal preparation is also available. The drug is effective when taken at any time during the attack, but in the case of migraine with aura, it should not be taken during the aura phase. The same dosage may be repeated once subcutaneously or twice orally within 24 hours if the headache was relieved initially but recurred. Sumatriptan should not be taken within 24 hours of dihydroergotamine (DHE) or ergotamine.

Zolmitriptan, 5 mg; rizatriptan, 2.5 mg; and eletriptan, 80 mg, are other powerful agents for the relief of pain and other symptoms of the acute migraine attack. Their speeds of onset, relief rates, success in maintaining the patient's headache-free status over 24 hours, and side-effect profiles are more similar than different, and the preparation eventually favored by any one patient is likely to be a personal decision based on his or her sampling of the different drugs available. Naratriptan, 2.5 mg, is somewhat different, having a slower time to maximum effect but a substantially longer period of action and an unusually favorable side-effect profile. Though potentially successful for some patients with severe headaches, our experience is that naratriptan is of particular value for those patients with mild-to-moderate migraines who are happy to trade early for consistent and prolonged relief.

The unwanted effects of all the triptans include chest heaviness, tightness, or pain; pain in the throat; tingling in the head or limbs; and nausea, all of which are usually self-limiting. Patients with cardiac disease or uncontrolled hypertension must not take triptans, and those with hepatic problems should limit the dose. Sumatriptan acts faster and causes less nausea than DHE, but headaches recur more often within 24 hours.

DHE is a nonselective 5HT1 agonist that is effective in providing headache relief with subcutaneous, intramuscular, intravenous, or intranasal use. Its side effects are similar to those of sumatriptan, except that it causes more nausea but is less likely to induce chest and throat discomfort. The duration of action of DHE is longer than that of sumatriptan, so recurrence rates are lower.

Ergotamine has been used for many years in various forms. Its unwanted effects are similar to those of DHE, but nausea is usually more severe. Ergotamine may produce more side effects than benefit, but some patients consider it to be useful, particularly if taken with an antiemetic. Because of slow gastric absorption during migraine, the suppository form of ergotamine is more effective and rapid acting when a headache begins.

Combination medications such as acetaminophen with codeine, ASA with codeine and caffeine, or ASA with butalbital and caffeine (with or without codeine) can be used in patients with mild or moderate migraines who do not respond to the initial choices, or when vasoconstrictors are contraindicated. However, frequent use of such combinations is a prominent cause of medication-induced (rebound) headache, and they should be taken only intermittently and for short periods.

Severe Attacks. For severe attacks, the choice of medications is DHE or a triptan, although a weaker alternative is the use of metoclopramide, 10 mg intravenously. If this is ineffective within 20 minutes, it may be followed with DHE, 0.5 to 1.0 mg intravenously, repeated to a maximum of 2 mg over 3 hours, or by sumatriptan, rizatriptan, eletriptan, or zolmitriptan. Another option is chlorpromazine (0.1 mg/kg intravenously over 20 minutes and repeated after 15 minutes to a maximum dose of 37.5 mg). The patient must be pretreated with normal saline, 5 ml/kg body weight, to prevent hypotension. Prochlorperazine (25 mg rectally, or 5 to 10 mg intravenously or intramuscularly) is another option. If no relief is obtained with the above treatments, ketorolac, 30 to 60 mg intramuscularly, or dexamethasone, 12 to 20 mg intravenously, may be effective. The place of butorphanol, a mixed opioid agonist-antagonist, in acute migraine management is still to be determined. We regard butorphanol, meperidine, and all narcotics as treatments of last resort.

Ultrasevere Attacks (Status Migrainosus). Prolonged severe headaches should be treated on an in-patient basis so the diagnosis can be confirmed, investigations performed as required, and therapies administered according to the patient's response. Patients vomiting repeatedly during severe migraine attacks need rehydration with normal saline, to which 1 gm magnesium sulfate may be added once daily, because there is evidence of its positive effect in treatment of acute headache, especially for menstrual migraine attacks.

DHE in a 0.5- to 1.0-mg subcutaneous injection (each dose preceded by metoclopramide, 10 mg, to prevent nausea) is the medication of choice, but it may have to be repeated intravenously every 8 hours for 24 hours or more. Zolmitriptan, 5 mg orally, and sumatriptan, 100 mg orally or 6 mg subcutaneously, are often effective (if available in the hospital setting). One repeat dose after 4 hours is allowed, but the agents should not be mixed. In cases still resistant, potentially useful medications, given alone or in combination, include the following:

- Promethazine, 50 mg, and chlorpromazine, 50 mg, intramuscularly, or prochlorperazine, 5 mg intramuscularly
- Prochlorperazine, 10 mg, and diphenhydramine, 10 mg, intravenously every 4 to 6 hours as needed until relief is obtained
- Chlorpromazine, 10.0 to 12.5 mg (0.1 mg/kg), intravenously after an intravenous bolus of 500 ml normal saline
- Dexamethasone, 8 to 20 mg intramuscularly or intravenously, or methylprednisolone, 100 to 250 mg intravenously
- Dexamethasone, 8 mg; meperidine, 75 to 100 mg; and promethazine, 50 mg given intramuscularly

Management of Menstrual Migraine

Menstrual migraine headaches are associated with reduction in sex hormone levels. In pregnancy, migraines tend to increase in the first trimester and to decrease thereafter. In true menstrual migraine, the headaches occur exclusively just before or during the menses as a result of estrogen withdrawal, mediated in part by prostaglandins (PG). Treatment options include the following:

- NSAIDs (inhibit prostaglandin synthesis or block PG receptors)
- Subcutaneous DHE
- Increase usual prescription premenstrually
- Magnesium pyrrolidine carboxylic acid, 360 mg/day on days 15 to 30 of the menstrual cycle
- Pyridoxine orally
- For extremely severe headaches, oral steroids, DHE, or chlorpromazine may be required. Some hormonal therapies have been used in prophylaxis, including danazol, tamoxifen, estrogen, parlodel (in the luteal phase), the combination of estradiol and an androgen, and, as a last resort, artificial menopause.

Prophylactic Treatment

The diagnosis of migraine should be clearly and confidently given after the appropriate history-taking, clinical examination, and (when necessary) investigations have been completed. The patient should be reassured that he or she does not have a serious underlying cause for the headaches, such as a brain tumor. Patients should be provided with a basic interpretation of migraine as a physiologic disorder—a genetically based, neurochemical instability of the nervous system triggered by various intrinsic and/or extrinsic factors. A brief description of what is known of the central and peripheral vascular and humoral mechanisms may aid motivation and an understanding of the treatment plan. Wherever possible, printed materials should be used to reinforce the practitioner's orally presented educational advice. Ideally, patients will be interviewed on at least a second occasion so that their learning can be reviewed. Practitioners should establish realistic goals and expectations of treatment, explaining the possible treatment options available (including their benefits and limitations) and describing the concept of control as opposed to cure. The patient should be encouraged to be an active partner in the treatment plan and share a responsibility for managing the disorder with the physician. Patients may be referred to the local Migraine Association in their country for information, and support and possible referral to local self-help groups.

Before drug prophylaxis is considered, all patients should have been instructed to keep a diary noting potential precipitants of their migraines. They should also follow the monoamine oxidase inhibitor (MAOI) diet, with the added proscription of foods containing aspartame, monosodium glutamate (MSG), or nitrites. Medications known to induce headache should be discontinued. Ideally, the patient should keep a calendar to record headache characteristics, treatment, and response to therapy and should be educated about the general nature of migraine, the action of the medications prescribed, and their interactions, side effects, and contraindications. Any medication prescribed should be continued for an adequate period, usually several months, and withdrawn slowly to prevent exacerbations of headache. If patients do not respond to the initial treatment, or treatment eventually fails, different medications may be tried in sequence, starting with a low dose and building to a maximally effective tolerable dose. Dosages may need adjustment over time. Prophylactic medications are often ineffective while patients are concurrently ingesting analgesics but may work well when the analgesics are withdrawn. The cost of the medications should be considered in the choice of prophylactic agents. Patients must be educated about the diagnosis and nature of migraine, the existence of helpful nonpharmacologic therapies (such as the avoidance of triggers), and the nature of the medications prescribed, as well as their potential side effects, interactions with other medications, and any circumstances that make the ingestion of the drug inadvisable (e.g., pregnancy). The patient should be encouraged to keep a diary of the doses and response to all medications used, and their side effects, and should inform the physician if she becomes pregnant or is contemplating pregnancy.

Trigger Factors. The stimuli that trigger migraine attacks may be external, physiologic, or psychologic (Box 160-4). It is essential for the physician to recognize these stimuli and to teach the patient to do so as well. The same triggers have been recorded as relevant in patients with tension-type headaches. The role of dietary factors is uncertain in the absence of published randomized controlled trials, but clinical experience indicates that ingestion of foods containing nitrites, aspartame, or MSG, and the cumulative effects of eating foods with a high content of neurotransmitter precursors such as tyramine, tyrosine, or phenylalanine are associated with the precipitation of migraine headaches and that their avoidance leads to a reduction in headache frequency or severity, although this observation has not been subjected to randomized clinical trial. The vulnerability of the patient to these stimuli varies from time to time in relation to the cyclic behavior of migraine itself and the life-stress situation of the patient. Thus at one time a single stimulus from any one of the three major areas mentioned may set off the explosion of an attack, whereas at other times several stimuli from more than one category may need to appear together to precipitate an attack.

Drug Prophylaxis. Drug prophylaxis is indicated when the headaches are severe enough to impair the patient's

Box 160-4. Potential Triggers of Migraine Attacks

Emotional stress
Changes in behavior
Missing a meal, hypoglycemia, sleeping more or less than usual
Environmental factors
Bright or flickering light, loud noise, weather changes, odors, allergens
Foods and beverages
Chocolate, cheese, cured meats (hot dogs, bacon), caffeine-containing beverages, alcoholic beverages (especially red wine), and other individually recognized dietary factors
Chemicals
Aspartame, MSG, benzene, insecticides, nitrites
Drugs
Caffeine (and caffeine withdrawal), nitroglycerin, reserpine, hydralazine, nonsteroidal antiinflammatory drugs, oral contraceptives, H_2 blockers, nifedipine

quality of life, or if the patient has three or more severe migraine attacks per month that fail to adequately respond to symptomatic treatment.

β-Blockers. Propranolol, nadolol, metoprolol, and atenolol have each been proven efficacious, but β-blockers are contraindicated in patients with asthma, chronic obstructive pulmonary disease, insulin-dependent diabetes, heart block or failure, or peripheral vascular disease, and are relatively contraindicated in pregnancy. Nadolol and atenolol, excreted by the kidneys, may have fewer CNS side effects than propranolol. One β-blocker may not work whereas another does, so trials of different agents in this class are appropriate. Medication should be tapered because sudden withdrawal may cause rebound headaches and adrenergic side effects. In prescribing these medications, the physician should always begin therapy with a low dose and titrate upward as required.

Calcium Channel Blockers. Calcium channel blockers may have a long latency-to-action period (up to several months) and produce many side effects. Flunarizine and verapamil are most commonly used but are contraindicated in patients with hypotension, congestive heart failure, arrhythmias, depression, and pregnancy and must be used cautiously in those with Parkinson's disease and in patients receiving βblockers. Flunarizine is not recommended for patients with depressive illness or extrapyramidal symptoms.

5-HT2 (Serotonin) Blockers. Pizotyline, a serotonin receptor antagonist with mild antihistaminic and anticholinergic properties, is somewhat effective in the treatment of migraine but its side effects include weight gain and sedation. Methysergide (an ergot derivative) may be used for the prophylaxis of severe, recurrent migraine unresponsive to other medications. Contraindications include hypertension; cardiac, lung, liver, kidney, and collagen diseases; thrombophlebitis; peptic ulcers; and pregnancy. Side effects are numerous and include nausea, muscle cramps and aching, claudication, weight gain, and hallucinations. Methysergide should not be used for more than 6 months without a 1- to 2-month drug holiday to reduce the risk of retroperitoneal fibrosis. The dosage should be decreased gradually before discontinuation.

Tricyclic Analgesics. Tricyclic analgesics are the so-called *antidepressants*. Amitriptyline is a useful prophylactic in the treatment of migraine, quite independent of its antidepressant activity and especially in patients who also have tension-type headaches. Oral doses of 10 mg each night should be used initially, with the dose being increased by 10 mg every week up to a maximum of 50 mg, although higher doses are sometimes required. Nortriptyline and desipramine (in similar dosages) produce less sedation and anticholinergic effects. Contraindications to all of these agents include significant cardiac, kidney, liver, prostate, or thyroid disease; glaucoma; hypotension; seizure disorders; and MAOI usage. The use of tricyclics in elderly patients is difficult because of anticholinergic side effects.

Selective Serotonin Reuptake Inhibitors. The selective serotonin reuptake inhibitors (SSRIs) have no demonstrably useful role in migraine prophylaxis.

Sodium Valproate/Valproic Acid/Divalproex Sodium. Valproic acid and its congeners have been found to be effective for migraine prophylaxis but should be used cautiously in patients taking ASA or warfarin because they affect hemostasis. ASA may displace valproic acid from its protein-binding sites and may lead to valproate toxicity. Side effects include nausea, alopecia, tremor, and weight gain, and their use has been associated with hepatotoxicity, particularly in children. It may also cause neural tube defects and should not be given to women who are pregnant or considering pregnancy. Women with a potential for reproduction should have this risk minimized by the use of appropriate contraception.

Nonsteroidal Antiinflammatory Drugs. Both naproxen and naproxen sodium are useful in the prevention of perimenstrual attacks, but it is recommended that nonsteroidal antiinflammatory drugs (NSAIDs) be used only for intermittent prophylaxis because of their gastrointestinal side effects.

Prophylactic medications that are ineffective while patients are concurrently ingesting analgesics regularly can become effective when the analgesics are withdrawn. Some prophylactic medications (especially the calcium channel blockers) may take 1 to 2 months to work. Except in the most resistant cases, only one preventive agent should be used at a time. In the case of lack of response to a combination of prophylactic agents from different groups (such as propranolol plus amitriptyline), neurologic consultation should be obtained. Headache medications other than those prescribed, including medication obtained without prescription, should not be used because the excessive use of other medications may reduce the effectiveness of prophylactic therapy. The cost of medications should be considered in the choice of all therapies.

Biobehavioral Prophylaxis

Biofeedback. Biofeedback refers to the use of monitoring instruments to detect, amplify, and display internal physiologic processes online so the patient may learn to accomplish the alteration of these processes at will. The preferred technique is thermal control, in which the patient learns to elevate finger temperature during therapy sessions using a digital temperature reading device. A meta-analysis of 25 controlled studies of biofeedback indicated that its efficacy is comparable to that of prophylactic medications, and sustained improvement has been demonstrated. Although relaxation therapy and biofeedback probably confer equal therapeutic benefit, there appears to be no advantage to combining them. If biofeedback is locally available, it may be considered as an alternative or adjunct to pharmacologic therapy for patients intolerant of medications.

Relaxation Therapy. A biobehavioral approach to migraine using relaxation techniques (including progressive muscular relaxation, breathing exercises, or directed imagery) may reduce attack frequency. Meta-analytic reviews have suggested that relaxation is as effective as biofeedback. Where a treatment effect has been reported, it may be enhanced by the addition of prophylactic agents such as β-blocking drugs. The usual goal of relaxation therapy is the development of long-term prophylaxis rather than the reduction of the pain during an acute event. Relaxation may be taught one-on-one or in a group setting by an appropriately trained physician, psychologist, or other therapist. As with biofeedback, patient acceptance, availability, and the time commitment involved may limit its use. Self-instruction, using audiotapes, may be used. The physician should determine if relaxation therapy is available locally and should select only motivated patients for such training, instructing them that relaxation therapy is intended to provide long-term prevention of headaches rather than short-term pain relief, although other measures may be combined.

Cognitive-Behavioral Therapy. Cognitive-behavioral therapy (CBT) is designed to help patients identify and modify those maladaptive responses that may trigger or aggravate a migraine event. The role of emotional reactivity as a trigger for migraine is considered to be pertinent in many patients. CBT is based on the principle that anxiety and distress are aggravators of an evolving migraine; it attempts to introduce a more adaptive approach and to help develop a specific action plan. Stress-management training is often part of this approach. As with other behavioral therapies, factors such as availability, cost, patient acceptance, and the time commitment required may restrict their use. These techniques are usually combined with biofeedback, although uncontrolled studies have shown their efficacy in reducing intensity, duration, and frequency of headaches when used alone.

Other Approaches. Psychiatric referral of patients with migraine is indicated solely for the presence of a comorbid psychiatric disorder, although referral to a psychologist to improve stress management may be appropriate in selected cases. Hypnosis may reduce distressing sensory input and may have a placebo effect, as it does in other pain disorders. It was more effective than prochlorperazine in one randomized controlled trial, and a meta-analysis of largely uncontrolled studies also suggested benefit when combined with CBT. Physical measures such as physiotherapy, chiropractic, or other manipulations have rarely been subjected to trial, and evidence for the superiority of any one form of cervical manipulation is lacking. In two randomized studies, one with follow-up, chiropractic manipulations reduced migraine frequency and severity. Aerobic training may reduce the number but not the severity of migraines. Transcutaneous electrical nerve stimulation (TENS) and acupuncture have also been shown to provide some relief. Oral magnesium has been shown to be an effective prophylactic in a single trial. In an open pilot study followed by a small, randomized placebo-controlled trial, riboflavin (400 mg daily) was found to be effective for migraine prophylaxis and could be a promising option. Two small randomized controlled trials have demonstrated the efficacy of the herb *feverfew* in migraine prophylaxis. Because feverfew appears to have a relatively benign side-effects profile (occasional mouth ulceration, contact dermatitis) it may be considered as an option for migraine prophylaxis, although there are no studies documenting its long-term safety or efficacy. Other treatments, including herbal therapy, naturopathy, and homeopathy, have not been subjected to sufficient critical study to allow appropriate evaluation.

TENSION-TYPE HEADACHE

Tension-type headache is the most common headache type of all in western populations. The diagnostic criteria are shown in Box 160-5. Muscle contraction is not always the basis of this headache. Pressure on sensory nerves, interference with blood supply of muscles and other tissues, and alterations in the threshold to pain from changes in the central nociceptive system may also be relevant. The headache is described as a tight band around the head, a pressure or fullness, a feeling that the head is in a vise, or a feeling that the head will explode. The whole head and often the neck and upper shoulders are typically involved, as may be the temples, the face, and the region of the upper trapezius (Fig. 160-7).

Box 160-5. Diagnostic Criteria for Tension-Type Headache

A. Average headache frequency greater than 15 days/month (180 days/year) for greater than 6 months. Headaches fulfilling criteria B-D
B. Duration 2 to 168 hours
C. At least two of the following pain characteristics:
   - Pressing/tightening quality
   - Mild or moderate severity
   - Bilateral location
   - No aggravation by walking stairs or similar routine physical activity
D. No vomiting and not more than one of the following: nausea, photophobia, or phonophobia

Tension-type headaches are benign and hard to treat. The physician should look for evidence of neck injuries and of TMJ dysfunction (especially if the pain is unilateral) and search for clues in the history as to why a person may show the effects of physical, psychologic, or social stress in this way. There are no physical signs other than tenderness in the craniocervical muscles.

Physical and emotional pressures, including states of depression or anxiety, are often considered responsible for tension-type headaches, but if the headache is unilateral, TMJ dysfunction should be considered. Therapy (if no local cause is discovered) might include amitriptyline or nortriptyline, muscle relaxants, psychotherapy (seldom), or other approaches as described under treatments for migraine and in Box 160-6. Such headaches are sometimes treated successfully by physical measures, such as local heat and massage, ultrasonic stimulation, or acupuncture. Relaxation techniques provided by courses of instruction and aided by tapes and biofeedback are often useful.

Combined Headache

Combined or mixed headache is thought to be related to both vascular and muscle contraction mechanisms. It presents as a constant tightness and pressure, with an added pulsatile component, and at times with nausea and vomiting. The treatment is the same as for migraines. It is common for someone who has had migraine headaches for many years to evolve to a headache that has features of both tension and migraine.

CLUSTER HEADACHE

The pain associated with cluster headache is said to be the worst known to mankind and it requires prompt diagnosis and management. Diagnostic criteria are shown in Box 160-7. The pain uniquely makes the patient move about in his or her distress. The basic mechanism of cluster headache is unknown.

Each episode of pain is manifest by sudden, very severe pain with a relatively short duration of an hour or two, one or more times per day or night, but usually with the first REM sleep period (Fig. 160-8). Marked autonomic features (ipsilateral sweating, flushing, tearing, enophthalmos, miosis, nasal blocking, and rhinorrhea) accompany the pain. Attacks

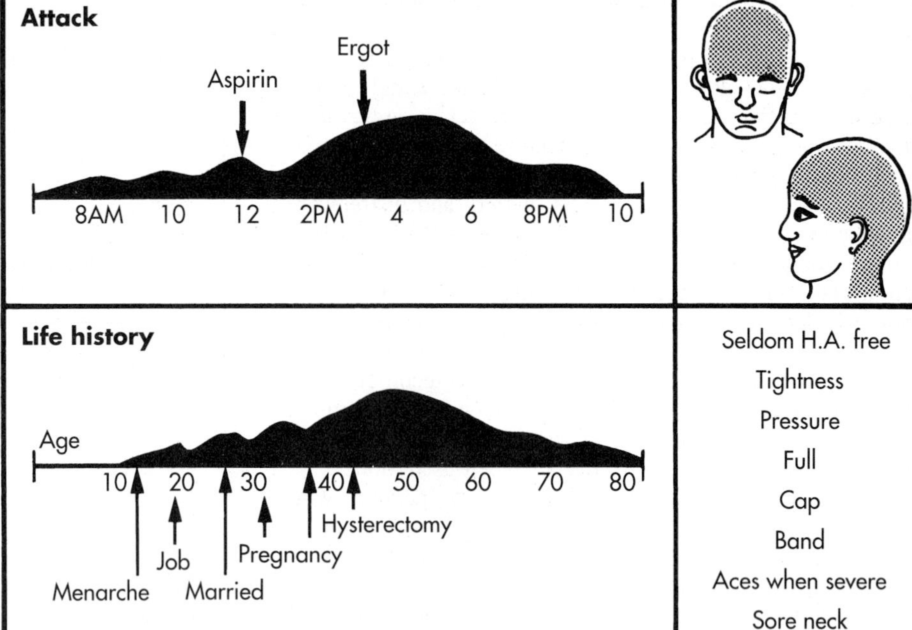

Fig. 160-7. Profile of muscle contraction headache.

frequently occur with clocklike regularity during or immediately after REM sleep. During the attacks the patients are up and about, pacing, stamping, locking themselves into rooms, violently resisting help, at times screaming, begging for relief, occasionally going into a trancelike state for short periods. Sometimes patients threaten suicide during an attack, but they rarely if ever perform it. Many patients explain that the pain is worse than that experienced with a fracture, surgery, or childbirth, or that associated with passing a kidney stone. Although the attacks of pain usually remain limited to a given side of the head and face during a given cluster, in some patients the attacks may switch to the other side before the cluster is over and, in a few rare instances, may involve both sides at once during one or several individual attacks.

During the clusters, which may last weeks or months, the patient is extremely vulnerable to vasodilating stimuli (e.g., alcohol, nitrites, histamine) and great changes in pace (e.g., weather, time, and activity), such as occur during naps or REM sleep, travel, seasonal changes, and work. Once the cluster has passed, these stimuli are no longer active until the next cluster supervenes.

Cluster headache patients, mostly men, are said to have an athletic build, including increased height, a leonine facies characterized by thick "orange peel" skin; deep furrows in forehead, cheeks, and chin, and telangiectasia, especially on the cheeks and bridge of the nose (Fig. 160-9 and Box 160-8). Clusters may begin during childhood or more often in young adulthood, or they may not occur until middle and late middle age. They may persist over a lifetime into the 70s and 80s, but more often they tend to decrease during the 60s. Intervals between clusters may range from a few weeks to a few months or a few years. The headaches recur occasionally after 10, 15, or even 35 years of freedom.

Chronic Cluster Headache

A few unfortunate individuals may remain in a constant or chronic cluster state almost daily for more than a year or even for several years. Usually, chronic clusters result from the gradual compression of periodic clusters closer together until a continuous or chronic state results. Rarely, clusters are chronic or classified as primary chronic cluster from the beginning.

Differential Diagnosis

Cluster headache is most often confused with tic douloureux or trigeminal neuralgia. However, unless secondary to multiple sclerosis or tumor, tic first appears in patients over 60 years of age, whereas cluster headache begins even during childhood and most frequently during the second, third, and fourth decades of life. Tic pain is described in Chapter 162. Rarely, cluster pain is accompanied by short shocks or jolts of pain similar to that of tic superimposed on the constant steady pain, creating the so-called *cluster-tic syndrome*.

Keratitis, corneal abrasions, and glaucoma cause pain and redness of the eye, but the eye examination should confirm the diagnosis. Raeder and Tolosa-Hunt syndromes sometimes present with recurring steady pain in the eye and face lasting days, weeks, or occasionally months (see Chapter 165). Malignant growths of the nose and throat may also mimic the pain of cluster headache, even presenting at first with intermittent bouts of pain associated with Horner's syndrome, pain in the cheek and eye, and nasal blockage. Radiographs and CT scans of the nasofacial bones and sinuses may reveal organic lesions in the nasopharynx and sinus areas, with destructive lesions in the hard palate and floor of the skull (Fig. 160-10).

Treatment

Treatment for the pain of the individual acute attack of cluster headache must be immediately available and quick in its action. Patients should always have their treatment with them or within easy reach because the pain develops rapidly. Although it does not last long, the pain is devastating, giving rise to the term *suicide headaches*. Strenuous exercise for 5 to

Box 160-6. Managed Care Guide: Stepwise Treatment of Tension Headaches*

I. Over-the-counter antiinflammatory medications
  A. Ibuprofen (Advil and others), 400-800 mg initially up to 2400 mg daily
  B. Aspirin, 650 mg every 4 hours as needed
  C. Acetaminophen (Tylenol and others), 650-1000 mg every 4 hours as needed
II. Prescription nonsteroidal antiinflammatory medications
  A. Naproxen sodium (Anaprox), 550 mg bid
  B. Ketorolac tromethamine (Toradol), 10 mg qid as needed
  C. Diflunisal (Dolobid), 1000 mg initially followed by 500 mg bid as needed
  D. Mefenamic acid (Ponstel), 500 mg initially followed by 250 mg every 6 hours as needed
III. Combination analgesic-sedative medications (1 or 2 tablets or capsules every 4 hours as needed up to 8 daily)
  A. Acetaminophen, caffeine, and butalbital (Esgic, Fioricet, Medigesic)
  B. Aspirin, caffeine, and butalbital (Fiorinal)
  C. Aspirin and butalbital (Axotal)
  D. Acetaminophen and butalbital (Bancap, Phrenilin)
  E. Isometheptene mucate, dichloralphenazone, and acetaminophen (Midchlor, Midrin)
IV. Prophylactic medications
  A. Tricyclic antidepressants†
    1. Amitriptyline HCl (Elavil, Endep), 10-50 mg tid
    2. Nortriptyline HCl (Aventyl, Pamelor), 25 mg tid
    3. Desipramine HCl (Norpramin, Pertofrane), 25 mg tid
    4. Doxepin HCl (Adapin, Sinequan), 10-50 mg tid (often, daily dose given at bedtime to avoid sedation)
    5. Imipramine HCl (Janimine, Tofranil), 10-50 mg tid
  B. β-Adrenergic blockers
    1. Propranolol HCl (Inderal), 160-240 mg daily in divided doses or single time-released dose
    2. Nadolol (Corgard), 20-240 mg daily

Modified from Trachtenbarg DE: *Headache: home study self assessment,* No. 138. Kansas City, Mo, 1990, American Academy of Family Physicians.
*Agents listed in order of the author's preference.
†Daily dose may also be given once at bedtime.

Box 160-7. Diagnostic Criteria for Cluster Headache

A. At least five attacks fulfilling B-D below
B. Severe unilateral orbital, supraorbital, and/or temporal pain lasting 15 minutes to 3 hours untreated
C. Headache is associated with at least one of the following signs, present on the painful side:
  - Conjunctival injection
  - Lacrimation
  - Nasal congestion, rhinorrhea
  - Forehead and facial sweating
  - Miosis
  - Ptosis
  - Eyelid edema
D. Frequency of attacks from 1 every other day to 8 per day

10 minutes at onset and ice-cold or very hot applications to the affected area are of questionable value. Acute abortive therapy today comprises breathing 100% oxygen by nasal mask at 7 to 10 L/minute for 10 to 15 minutes at onset of attacks; the intranasal instillation of 4% lidocaine into the nostril on the affected side, with the head dependent; or subcutaneous sumatriptan, 6 mg, or DHE, 1 mg.

The best prophylactic agent is prednisone (or equivalents), 40 to 60 mg/day, reduced by 5 mg/day every 2 or 3 days. The total period of therapy should be no longer than 6 to 8 weeks—preferably 4 weeks—because of possible chronic steroid side effects. Lithium and verapamil are appropriate long-term therapies. One of these drugs should be started at the same time as the steroids are given. The usual dose is 900 mg of lithium carbonate/day in three doses, to achieve a blood lithium level of 0.5 to 1.0 mEq/L. Thyroid function, blood counts, and renal function are monitored as they are in other patients taking lithium. As the patient improves, the dose may be gradually reduced. In chronic cluster headache, it may be wise to continue one dose of lithium per day for many months or even permanently. When headache cycles break through, the dosage may be raised appropriately. Ergot or steroids may be added to the lithium regimen if recurrence takes place.

The calcium channel blocker verapamil (240 mg/day) must be taken for at least a month to obtain full effect. Other drugs that can be used include cyproheptadine (Periactin), 4 mg orally one to four times daily; tricyclics such as amitriptyline (Elavil) and doxepin (Sinequan); and methysergide, 2-mg tablets one to four times daily. This last drug is an effective preventative agent but its side-effect profile includes potentially lethal complications (it must be stopped at 3-month intervals for at least 2 weeks), which lead us to consider it a drug of last resort.

Finally, surgery may be necessary if cluster headache has failed to respond to medical treatment and is seriously affecting the patient's life. Sphenopalatine ganglion block or excision, greater superficial petrosal neurectomy, and nervus intermedius neurectomy by radiofrequency, surgical transection, and/or glycerol injection are other techniques to be considered.

Chronic Paroxysmal Hemicrania

Chronic paroxysmal hemicrania is a rare variant of cluster headache characterized by its occurrence most often in women (in 90% of cases), the short duration of the attacks (minutes), and their frequent occurrence (perhaps 15 attacks or more per day). The pain resembles that of cluster headache in its unilaterality; its involvement of the eye, cheek, and temples; and the associated autonomic dysfunction. A remarkable feature of this condition is its specific rapid response to indomethacin, 150 to 200 mg daily. Within a few hours of the first dose, attacks usually cease completely. Some patients with this syndrome have multiple daily attacks for several years without relief from any of the ordinary cluster headache remedies.

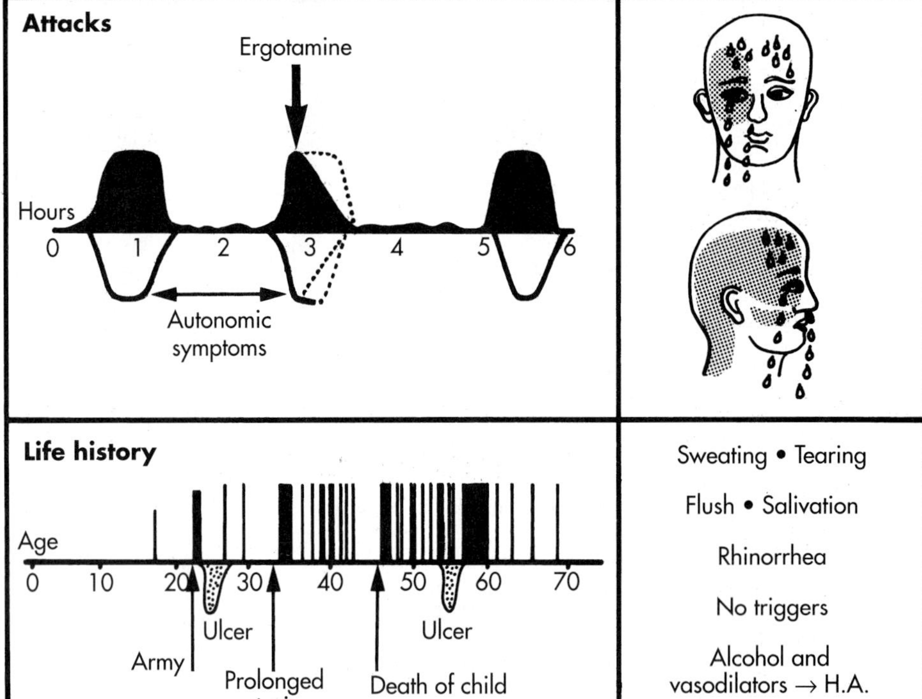

Fig. 160-8. Profile of a cluster headache.

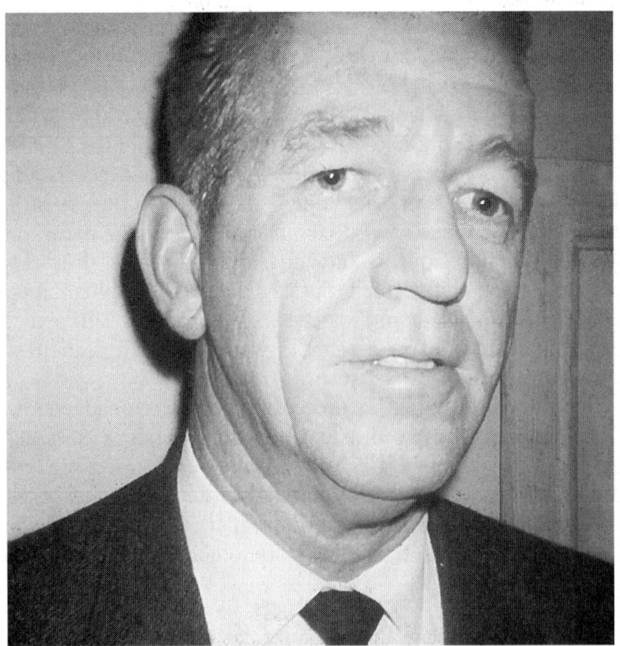

Fig. 160-9. Leonine facies of a cluster headache patient. Note the thick vertical and horizontal furrows, extra crease in the cheek, thick "orange peel" skin, and telangiectasis on the nostril.

Box 160-8. Physical Characteristics Often Observed Among Cluster Males

Facial

Ruddy complexion
Deep furrows
Orange peel skin
Telangiectasia
Narrowed palpebral fissures
Asymmetric creases
Broad chin, skull
Leonine appearance

General

Rugged appearance
Tall, trim
Obesity rare
Hazel eye color (one third of patients)

POSTTRAUMATIC HEADACHE

The simplest form of posttraumatic headache results from injury to a specific cervical or cranial nerve, leading to causalgic pain. The territory of the pain is denoted by marked skin tenderness on gentle pinching. Such pains may be briefly relieved by local anesthetic infiltration; more permanent relief is obtained from drugs such as dilantin, carbamazepine, or neurontin, or by surgical neurectomy.

Other posttraumatic symptoms are more complicated; a blow to the head involves also a blow to the person and to the state of his or her life, with psychologic consequences. The characteristics of posttraumatic headache are too varied to make their description here of any value, except insofar as the pain is usually felt in the approximate area of the trauma and is almost completely unresponsive to any drug therapies presently available. Other forms of therapy, often psychologic or at least nonpharmacologic, should be considered. The

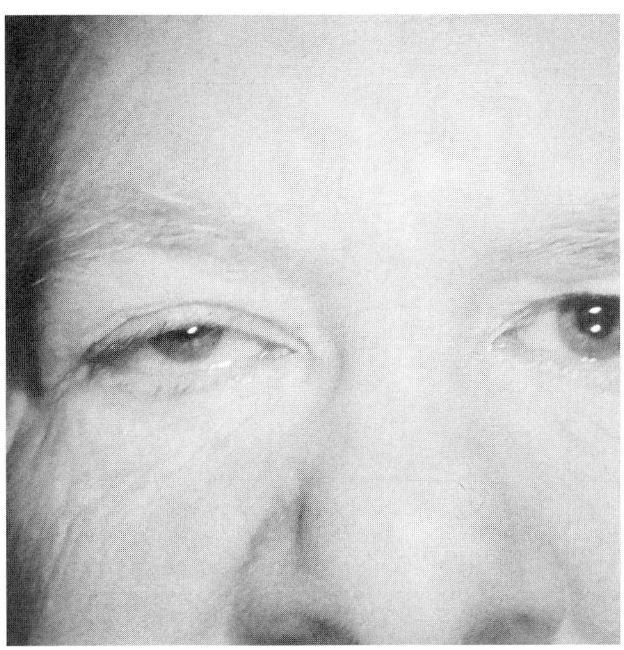

Fig. 160-10. Horner's syndrome, causing drooping eyelid and small pupil in the right eye of a 60-year-old woman with a history of cluster headaches increasing in intensity over 3 months. Sinus radiographs revealed destruction of the floor of the maxillary sinus by a nasopharyngeal carcinoma.

following words of the late Dr. J.R. Graham, the author of this chapter in its first two editions, address these headaches in more detail:

> Accidents that happen at home or because of one's own carelessness or foolishness are much less likely to produce significant prolonged headache syndromes than those related to circumstances in which someone else is at fault or in some way responsible. The time required for recovery and return to work is much shorter with home accidents than with industrial or motor vehicle accidents. This shorter interval results from not only litigious aspects of the incident, but also from what has been called the "antitherapy factors" that surround industrial accidents and those caused by someone else's neglect. When an industrial accident was caused by work in certain circumstances or with certain machinery, the patient should return to the same situation or should have a lead-in time and perhaps experience in another department or situation to allow regaining of confidence. Settlement of the "case," although highly desired, may not end the problem because much has happened to this injured individual. The person has been knocked off his or her perch in life, not just "hit on the head." Such factors are difficult for some physicians, juries, and judges to understand, partly because some individuals with personal gain as an objective take advantage of these situations and provide fuel that leads to distrust of others who have really had a major blow to themselves as well as their head.

VASCULAR HEADACHES

Cranial Arteritis

Cranial arteritis, a form of giant cell arteritis, involves the branches of arteries arising from the thoracic aorta, such as the temporal and ophthalmic arteries, and the ophthalmic and intracranial vessels. The condition only affects people over the age of 60 years. If untreated, it leads to blindness in half of the cases. The leading symptom—a mild to moderate, constant, unilateral temporal pain—moves between head regions and is associated with local tenderness and redness over the scalp. The temporal arteries are typically tender, cordlike, and often pulseless. Accompanying the headache may be painful "angina" of the jaw muscles or tongue when chewing or swallowing or dental pain that may lead to misguided extractions. Confusion, impaired concentration, aphasia, and other focal signs reflect intracranial artery involvement. Repeated episodes of blurry or blotted-out areas of vision may precede complete loss of vision in one or both eyes. The patient often feels unwell, with low-grade fever, anorexia, malaise, and symptoms such as morning muscle stiffness and weight loss. An elevated erythrocyte sedimentation rate (ESR) and positive antinuclear antibody (ANA) titers are almost always present. The differential diagnosis includes depression, hypertension, cervical degenerative joint disease, and recurrent migraine.

Temporal artery biopsy is not essential but can be obtained from the most tender and inflamed area of an artery to confirm the diagnosis, even after treatment has been started. Delay in therapy may allow serious vascular events (e.g., retinal artery occlusion) to occur. The value of having a biopsy may be appreciated after several months, when the potential complications of steroid therapy threaten and questions arise as to the veracity of the diagnosis. Doppler flow studies may also help identify areas in the superficial cranial circulation where occlusion is taking place and the process is active.

Immediate treatment with steroids is essential; prednisolone (100 mg/day initially, reduced gradually to a maintenance dose of 5 mg/day) with medication to prevent gastric ulceration (such as ranitidine, 150 mg bid) is appropriate. Gradual tapering of this dose is indicated over weeks and months (and occasionally years) in relation to symptoms and the decreasing ESR. If steroid therapy is contraindicated (active infection, active gastrointestinal ulceration or perforation, serious CNS reaction to steroids), other NSAIDs may be tolerated and prove useful. In some patients the arteritis may continue to be active over 3 to 4 years, with symptoms recurring whenever the steroid dose falls below a certain level. In patients with long-term arteritis, alternate-day steroid therapy to reduce side effects may be practical.

Hypertension

In hypertensive encephalopathy and crises related to pheochromocytoma and preeclampsia, a sudden rise in blood pressure leads to headache. Hypertension associated with Cushing's syndrome or with aldosterone-producing tumors may also cause headache of a vascular type resembling migraine in a few patients.

Dialysis Headache

Almost all patients on dialysis experience headache if the dialysate contains too little sodium. Dialysis headache is related to reduction in osmolality caused by large sodium decreases and worsens as blood pressure drops (Fig. 160-11). Headache also is one of the first symptoms of transplant rejection.

Headache from Dissection of the Carotid Artery

Acute carotid dissection may cause sudden, severe, unilateral neck pain and headache radiating to the ear, temple, and eye.

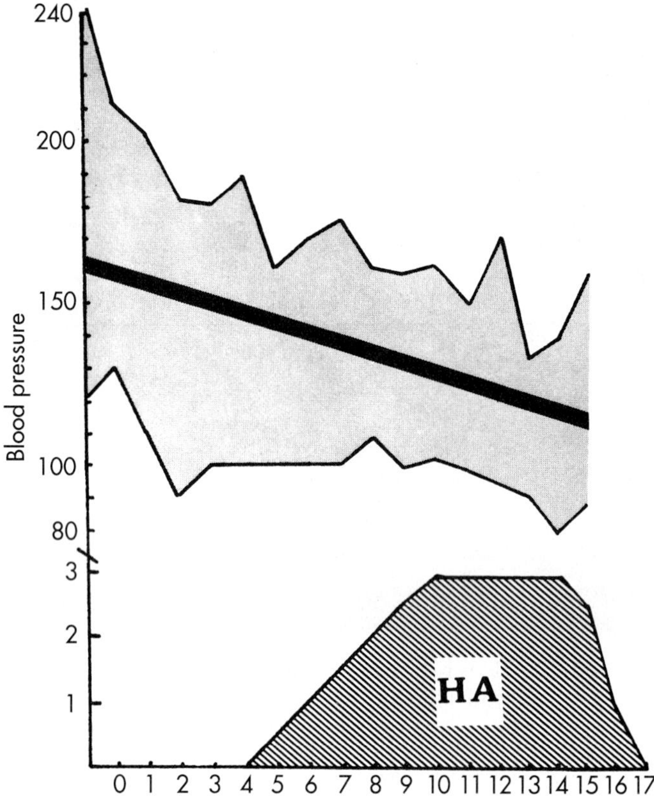

Fig. 160-11. Dialysis headache. Headache *(HA)* appears as blood pressure falls during renal hemodialysis. (From Graham JR, Bara DS, Yap AU: *Res Clin Stud Headache* 6:147, 1978.)

An ipsilateral Horner's syndrome is the only physical sign unless there is evidence of a TIA or stroke from embolism. During the acute phase the carotid sheath is tender, the pulse is poorly felt, and a carotid bruit may be heard. The patient should be referred for MRA or angiography. There is no evidence to support the use of anticoagulants, but they are commonly prescribed.

Migraine and Mitral Valve Prolapse (Barlow's Syndrome)

Patients with migraine have an increased incidence of mitral valve prolapse (MVP), which may be responsible for the increased frequency of paroxysmal cardiac arrhythmias reported in patients with migraines. Small cerebral emboli in patients with MVP may simulate classic migraine attacks. Some patients have positive anticardiolipin antibody tests and need specialized assessment. Propranolol is used to treat MVP and so may serve a double purpose. Antiplatelet agents are also used in prophylaxis.

Headache after Ischemic Cerebral Infarction

After a stroke, many patients complain of a headache that has a vague resemblance to migraine without aura, as first described by Thomas Willis in the seventeenth century. A possible reason is the increase in blood flow in the scalp vessels when a major artery such as a carotid has been occluded. Analgesics are appropriate as therapy in the short term. In many cases the headache fades spontaneously over months. Use of vasoconstrictors is obviously inappropriate.

Headache Caused by Intracranial Bleeding

The profile of an attack of headache resulting from intracranial hemorrhage from aneurysms or arteriovenous malformations (AVM) is shown in Fig. 160-12. Such lesions rarely cause headache except when they bleed, although in exceptional cases headache may result from pressure of an aneurysm on pain-sensitive structures. The usual presentation is acute: the patient experiences sudden posterior head pain that feels like a hammer blow without apparent cause, although it may occasionally be related to physical stress such as sexual intercourse or weight lifting. In other cases the headache is only minor and may recur repeatedly before a major, perhaps fatal event. If the bleeding is into the subarachnoid space, stiff neck, fever, backache, and severe, sudden headache result. If it extends intracerebrally, local neurologic deficits result. In severe cases, such as subarachnoid hemorrhage caused by rupture of an aneurysm, spread of blood into the ventricles is often fatal. Smaller leaks from an AVM tend to recur and are far less dangerous. Differentiation of either of these from benign exertional headaches is clinically impossible and, at least on the first occurrence, full investigation is essential.

Any acute, severe headache, even without stiff neck or other physical signs, should be regarded as evidence of subarachnoid hemorrhage until proved otherwise by CT scan and perhaps LP. Immediate consultation with a neurologist or neurosurgeon is indicated in all such cases. A small subarachnoid leak (producing a "sentinel headache") will lead to such a severe headache without physical signs.

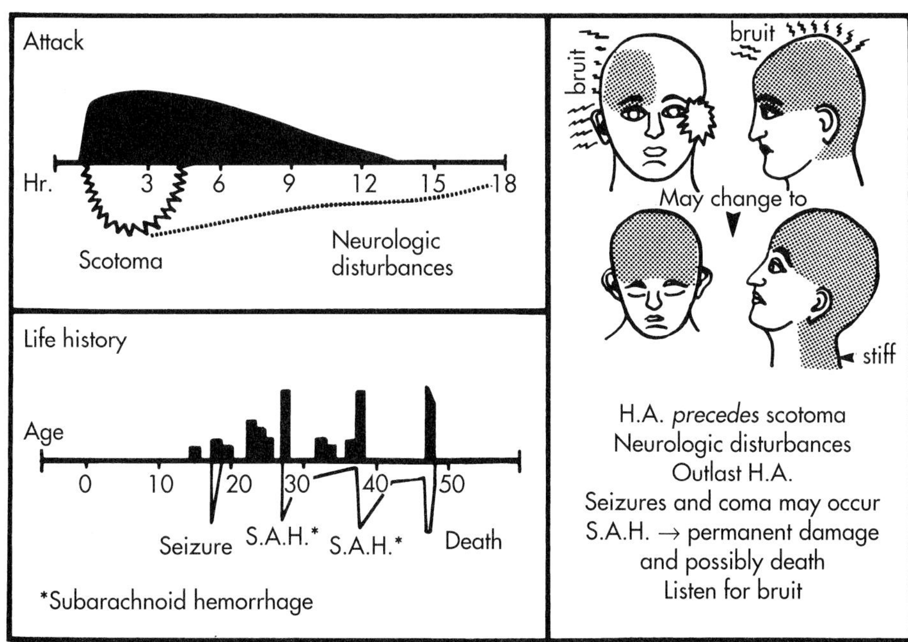

Fig. 160-12. Profile of subarachnoid hemorrhage from a vascular anomaly.

Initially, this should be managed exactly as would a full-blown subarachnoid hemorrhage.

A condition similar to headache caused by intracranial bleeding is *exertional headache* (including "coital cephalgia" and "weight-lifters headache"), which is manifest by the occurrence of a severe, acute, usually posterior head pain at times of maximal muscular activity—as suggested by the alternate names for the condition. The first time this happens should be the occasion for full investigation (CT scan of the head, and perhaps LP) to exclude a small subarachnoid bleed. If these rule out subarachnoid hemorrhage, and the activity is to be repeated, indomethacin, 25 mg tid, is an effective prophylactic.

The nature of *cough headache* is unexplained. Its characteristics are those of exertional headache and it occurs at times of violent coughing or during the performance of Valsalva's maneuver. In such cases, the presence of an intracranial mass lesion is possible and must be excluded by appropriate examination and scanning. The Chiari malformation is another, more benign cause.

TRACTION HEADACHE

Traction headache is a relatively uncommon type of headache that results from traction on the pain-sensitive structures inside the head—the V, VII, IX, and X cranial nerves; the basal meninges; the intracranial venous sinuses; and the intracranial arteries up to their second branch off the circle of Willis. Inflammatory and mass lesions are the most common causes (Fig. 160-13). The pain arising from distortion of intracranial pain-sensitive structures is not as characteristic as one would like and is often described just as a steady, dull, bursting or pressure sensation felt deep within the head that is not as severe as migraine. Unfortunately, patients with other headaches use the same words occasionally, so this description is not diagnostic. The pain has no rhythm to it, but tends to be continuous and is seldom throbbing. It is often relieved by aspirin or cold packs applied to the skull, giving a false sense of security. It is poorly localized and may be referred to the eyes or neck. Special times of occurrence include the early morning, with some relief being obtained from the upright posture as the day goes on. Any further increase in intracranial pressure, as with stooping, coughing, or bending, makes the headache worse. A history of head and/or neck injury during recent months, especially in elderly patients, should raise suspicion of subdural hemorrhage.

The site of the headache may have some diagnostic value because most subjects with brain tumors complain of pain over or near to the region of the underlying mass. Those with posterior fossa lesions often have occipital headaches; unfortunately, associated neck muscle tension and neck stiffness or tenderness may suggest muscle contraction headache unless the other characteristics are noted. Another danger is that this headache is often not very bad in the early stages, and the patient's description may not be precise, leading to a false sense of security. Some growing tumors merely accentuate the patient's "usual" headache (e.g., of muscle contraction or migraine). Thus the diagnosis is indeed difficult and this situation points up the need for a careful neurologic examination in all patients with head pain.

The symptoms associated with traction headache depend on the rate of expansion of the mass and its site more than its actual size. Vertigo, nausea, vomiting, drowsiness, pain on ocular movement, and irritability are commonly found in association. If high pressure causes herniation of intracranial contents, then hypertension, drowsiness, bradycardia, and such localizing signs as VI or III nerve palsies may appear, as may any other focal disturbances of brain function. The causes are those of increased intracranial pressure. Idiopathic intracranial hypertension (see below), obstructive hydrocephalus, intracranial infections, cerebral edema, tumor, and hemorrhage are examples. Treatment is determined by the cause, or by temporary reduction of increased pressure using mannitol or steroids.

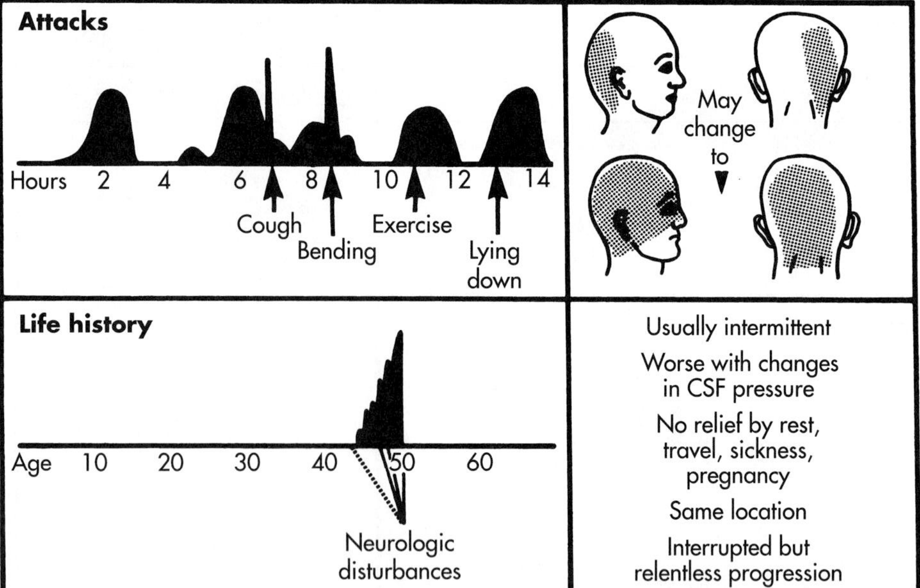

Fig. 160-13. Profile of a brain tumor.

Idiopathic Intracranial Hypertension

When a patient (most often a young woman who is obese) presents with complaints of the onset of a new headache and has papilledema without other physical signs, the diagnosis is straightforward. Without such evidence of increased pressure, however, these patients may be labeled as suffering from a functional headache. The headache features are not specific and may resemble those of migraine, traction headache, or both. They are usually worse in the mornings and with any activity that raises intracranial pressure. Patients taking large amounts of vitamin A or hormonal therapy are also at risk. Neurologic referral is suggested in all such cases.

Low Pressure Headache

Low cerebrospinal fluid (CSF) pressure also may cause headache, especially when the patient sits or stands up. This is usually caused by a leak of CSF after LP. In the presence of a CSF leak, headache manifests when the patient stands up and goes away when he or she lies flat. A repeat study shows that the CSF pressure is very low, perhaps unmeasurable. Eventually the hole in the dural sac will heal and CSF will no longer leak. This type of headache may be avoided by using a small needle for LP with the bevel horizontal (thus splitting rather than cutting the longitudinal fibers of the dura mater) and by requiring the patient to lie flat for 2 hours after the procedure. Occasionally, true "drainage" headaches persist over days, in which case treatment requires the injection of a few milliliters of the patient's own blood into the lumbar spinal canal, "patching" the leaky dural hole. Fluid ingestion and tight abdominal binders are quite useless.

CSF leaks resulting in chronic postural headache occur also as a result of congenital defects, neoplastic invasion of the meninges, or vigorous athletic activity. In these conditions a dural tear opening a passage between the cranial and nasal cavities may have occurred. Constant dripping of clear fluid from the nose is a useful symptom; some of the fluid must be collected for evaluation of glucose content. If glucose is present, the fluid is probably CSF. When such a leak is strongly suspected, a radioimmunosorbent assay (RISA) scan is performed, with pledgets placed in the nose and sinus areas to detect radioactivity from the leaked CSF.

Patients with congenital defects in the cribriform plate and other areas of the skull where CSF can escape into the nasopharynx may have repeated bouts of meningitis. These episodes are often mild but are potentially dangerous.

HEADACHE ASSOCIATED WITH SUBSTANCE USE OR WITHDRAWAL

Medication-induced Headache ("Transformed Migraine")

A medication-induced headache occurs in people whose chronic tension-type headaches or migraines have worsened, in response to which they have ingested increasing amounts of medication (more than three times/week) for 3 months or more. All patients with chronic headaches are prone to this form of chemical dependency, one of the commonest headache types seen in referral practice. The drugs prescribed (or bought over the counter) for management of such headaches and able to induce this syndrome include muscle relaxants, benzodiazepines, ergot preparations, simple analgesics (often with codeine), NSAIDs, and caffeine. The intermittent use of these agents is appropriate but their frequent use leads to down-regulation of nociceptor pathways in the brain, creating the vicious cycle of medication-induced headache. Narcotics should not be prescribed again for these patients.

Typically the headaches are present daily or nearly every day, are present on waking, and are *reduced* but not *removed* by ingestion of the usual medication taken. Nausea, malaise, anergia, depression, and sleep disturbances are almost invariable accompaniments, with the production of a syndrome of daily or near-daily "rebound" headaches that are worse on waking in the morning, briefly reduced by the next dose of the usual medication(s), and inhibiting the useful effects of oral prophylactic agents. Many patients utilize several sources of supply for their medications.

The best treatment strategy is to discontinue all of the analgesics the patient has taken, supplying instead DHE, 0.5

to 1.0 mg every 8 hours whether the subject has a headache or not, for three days (nine doses), with metoclopramide, 10 mg, preceding each dose if required to control nausea. This treatment may require hospitalization, but in some cases the use of DHE nasal spray (Migranal) every 8 hours for three days is sufficient.

The second stage of the treatment plan is just as important. After the subject is off the daily analgesics, it is likely that prophylactic medications will be effective again and they should be restarted, even if they had failed before in competition with the analgesics. Behavioral modification with biofeedback, hypnosis, counseling, and, occasionally, formal psychologic or psychiatric therapy may be needed to help remodel lifestyles that are detrimental. When true migraine attacks do occur in the future, specific therapies (the triptans) or DHE should be prescribed rather than the analgesics that got the patient into trouble in the first place.

Headache Associated With Medication Ingestion

Drugs that may cause headaches when ingested are listed in Box 160-4. Nitrites can precipitate headaches that are often migrainelike in nature. Substitution of β-blockers or calcium channel blockers may eliminate the problem, though calcium channel blockers can also cause headaches if they are also vasodilators. Rebound headache may also follow prolonged use of caffeine, ergotamine, the triptans, and methysergide.

Withdrawal from Steroids

Withdrawal from prolonged steroid therapy may be accompanied by the first appearance of headaches, probably caused by idiopathic intracranial hypertension. Reinstatement of the previous dose, with subsequent slower reduction of the dose, is the best solution.

HEADACHE FROM METABOLIC DISORDERS

Medical conditions causing headaches include systemic infections, usually with fever; hypoxia; carbon monoxide poisoning; postconvulsive states; foreign protein reactions; hypoglycemia; hypercapnia; acute pressor reactions; and renal failure. In most of these instances, the headache is a temporary and easily diagnosed problem, but a few conditions warrant comment.

Headache from Overt Cranial Inflammation

Inflammation caused by infectious agents (bacterial, viral, parasitic) or chemical or autoimmune processes and involving pain-sensitive cranial structures may produce headache. The headache is likely to be a secondary symptom, and diagnosis should be achieved on the basis of the major manifestations of the condition.

Headache Caused by Chemical Inflammation of the Meninges

Spinal anesthetics, contrast media, antineoplastic drugs, and antibiotics can cause allergic or chemical inflammation in the CNS, with headache, stiff neck, low-grade fever, and sterile pleocytosis in the CSF. The headache is present in all positions, unlike the headache after LP. Analgesics and antihistamines or corticosteroids are helpful, as long as it is ensured that no bacterial infection is present.

Headache With Systemic Symptoms

Pulsatile headaches and flushing occur rarely in mastocytosis, carcinoid syndrome, and gastrointestinal conditions in which vasoactive peptides are involved. Mastocytosis looks at first like common freckles, but biopsy of new freckles may confirm the diagnosis. Carcinoid tumor may cause flushing, wheezing, diarrhea, and headache. Alcohol, epinephrine, and histamine may induce headaches in both carcinoid tumor and mastocytosis. Bronchogenic carcinoid tumor causes headache before metastasizing to the liver, but liver metastases usually are necessary for gastrointestinal carcinoid tumors to produce these symptoms.

Headaches associated with flushing or pallor, sweating, and acute hypertension require exclusion of pheochromocytoma by blood and urinary catechol tests and appropriate CT or MRI scanning. It is important to examine the patient during such episodes so that blood pressure measurements may be recorded and the physician can make sure that the urine in the patient's bladder at the time of the hypertensive episode is included in the collection to be tested for vanillylmandelic acid (VMA), catechols, and metanephrine.

Endocrine Conditions

Hypothyroidism, Cushing's syndrome, Addison's disease, and pituitary tumors (especially prolactinomas) may induce headaches of any type until the primary underlying condition is diagnosed and treated.

REFERRED HEAD PAINS

Refractive Errors

When headache is caused directly by refractive errors, it usually occurs while the patient is engaged in using the eyes for reading or other fine work, not hours later. Strain from prolonged use of the eyes if refraction or accommodation is imperfect may lead to tension-type headaches. However, this is very generally known, and few patients present for diagnosis of their headaches without having had their eyes tested already. However, any of these patients may later develop migraines.

Glaucoma

Mild glaucoma can be a cause of recurring pains in one or both eyes and forehead and will be missed unless ocular tensions are measured.

Temporomandibular Joint Pain

Headache resulting from disorders of the TMJ requires evaluation by very conservative oral surgeons and dentists. Abnormalities of the bite and of the joint and its meniscus can be a source of local pain around the TMJ in the cheek, mouth, ear, and temple, especially if patients also have bruxism. The pain may be felt in the face and may be misidentified as trigeminal neuralgia. Local TMJ tenderness, asymmetric opening and closing of the mouth, the presence of notable overbite, and the patient's response to the relatively cheap bite plates fitted by a dental surgeon all suggest the diagnosis. The presence of any other source of pain, such as TMJ dysfunction, is also a stimulus to an increased number of attacks of migraine in those who suffer from that condition.

Nasopharyngeal Tumors

Tumors of the nasopharynx that involve the eustachian tube or the hard palate may cause prolonged facial or ear pain or pain resembling chronic cluster headache. Impaired hearing, Horner's syndrome, and altered facial sensation and power are other features. Diagnosis is best made by CT or MRI scans.

Cervicogenic Headache

The upper three cervical nerves carry pain sensation from the posterior half of the head and neck. These areas must be evaluated when considering any head-pain problems. Disturbances in one neck area may often also cause spasm and physical alterations of positioning of other neck areas, sending afferent pain impulses to the descending tract of the fifth nerve. Attention may be especially called to the neck when downward pressure on the head precipitates head pain and upward traction brings relief, when head pain extends into the neck and down the arm, or when it is associated with ipsilateral Horner's syndrome.

Cervical traction may relieve symptoms in some cases but just as often seems to aggravate them. Skilled cervical manipulation may help, as may injection of the zygapophyseal facet joints. NSAIDS are usually helpful in reducing the discomfort. Cervical collars are sometimes useful for treatment of cervical degenerative disease that is painful, but they work better if used intermittently. Theoretically, continual use of collars can weaken cervical muscles, which may aggravate the problems.

Whiplash Injuries

Whiplash injuries resulting in sprain and injury to multiple tissues in the neck (regardless of radiographic findings that may show no significant abnormalities) sometimes precipitate bouts of headache or accentuate previous migraine-type headaches. Recommended treatment includes short-term use of physical therapy, a soft collar, night-time tricyclic use to assist with muscle relaxation, analgesia, and explanation of the injury in terms of muscle strain and stretching of ligaments rather than rupture of joints or bones with the potential for spinal cord damage. Strong encouragement should be given to the subject to continue graded increases in activity and early return to work. The longer a person is disabled, the greater the likely legal settlement in cases involving litigation. Most people, however, do not malinger. If an opinion is given that restoration of near-normal motility will eventually be possible and that there is no evidence of damage to the spinal cord, litigation may be concluded relatively early and one more source of stress removed from the patient.

Greater Occipital Neuralgia

Greater occipital neuralgia is a condition of presumed stretch injury to one or both of the greater occipital nerves, sometimes caused by trauma but usually without known cause. A constant dull or boring pain is felt at the back of the head. It may radiate as far forward as the forehead (Kerr's sign). Examination reveals tenderness of the nerve (felt midway between the mastoid process and the cervical spinous processes) and possibly subjective alteration in light touch or pin sensation over the back of the head as far forward as the vertex. As in the case of other sources of cranial pain, preexisting migraine or tension-type headaches may be exacerbated by this lesion.

Local injection of the nerve with Marcaine or another local anesthetic is both a diagnostic test and good therapy; if successful, repeated injections with or without methylprednisolone may be given. For long-term relief, surgical avulsion of the nerve is sometimes advocated.

ACKNOWLEDGMENTS

A group of acknowledged experts on headache prepared a state-of-the-art summary of headache for the continuing education program of the American Academy of Neurology, which was consulted in preparation of this chapter: Silberstein SD, et al: *Headache and facial pain, part A and B*, Volume 1, Number 5, Cleveland, Ohio, 1995, Continuum, American Academy of Neurology, Advanstar Communications.

ADDITIONAL READINGS

Classification Committee IHS: Classification of headache disorders, cranial neuralgias and facial pain, and diagnostic criteria for primary headache disorders: *Cephalalgia* 8(suppl):1-96, 1988.

Pryse-Phillips WEM, Dodick DW, Edmeads JG, et al: Guidelines for the diagnosis and management of migraine in clinical practice, *Can Med Assoc J* 156:1273-1287, 1997.

Silberstein SD, et al: Headache and facial pain, Part A and B, Continuum, American Academy of Neurology, Advanstar Communications, Cleveland, Ohio, Volume 1, Number 5, 1995.

CHAPTER 161

Sleep Disorders

William Pryse-Phillips
T. Jock Murray

Sleep is a normal, complex, cyclical physiologic state in which consciousness and activity are altered. It is composed of non-rapid eye movement (NREM) sleep (divided into stages 1, 2, 3, and 4, according to its depth) and rapid eye movement (REM) sleep, characterized by profound muscular relaxation and by alterations of blood pressure, pulse rate, respiration, and electroencephalographic activity when compared with wakefulness. Despite the muscle inactivity, there are repetitive darting eye movements. If awakened in this stage, the subject will recall a vivid dream.*

When falling asleep, a person without a sleep disorder passes from a state of alertness to drowsiness and then into stage 1 NREM sleep, characterized by muscle relaxation and the appearance on the electroencephalogram (EEG) of low-amplitude, fast-frequency waves. During this stage the patient often denies having been asleep if asked. As the patient falls deeper asleep, he or she enters stage 2 sleep, with spindles of 12 to 16 Hz waves on the EEG, and then in turn stages 3 and 4, which are characterized by higher amplitude slow waves, profound muscle relaxation, and difficulty in

*Despite tremendous advances in understanding the physiology of sleep, our interpretation of the meaning of dreams has not advanced since Joseph, son of Jacob, counseled the Pharaoh (Genesis, 41:25).

rousing the subject. A healthy young adult going to bed at night rapidly passes through drowsiness with mental fantasies into stages 1 and 2 and then into longer periods of stages 3 and 4 sleep. After about 90 minutes of NREM sleep, the first REM sleep episode occurs. This is usually associated with a dream lasting 5 to 10 minutes, but during the night four to five further REM periods occur, each becoming progressively longer as the night continues. After the first REM period the subject again drops down through the NREM sleep stages and oscillates about every 90 minutes between one type of sleep and the other. Infants spend much of their time in stages 3 or 4 sleep but half of their sleep is of REM type. By the age of 5, REM sleep takes up about one fourth of sleep time, which is comparable to a young adult pattern. Approximately 5% to 10% of sleep is in stage 1, 50% in stage 2, and 20% in stages 3 and 4. REM sleep decreases somewhat after age 50, as does the time spent in the deeper stages of NREM (slow wave) sleep.

The major disorders of sleep are classified as dyssomnias, parasomnias, and sleep disorders associated with medical psychiatric disorders.

DYSSOMNIAS

Dyssomnias are disorders associated with difficulty in initiating or maintaining sleep, or with excessive sleep.

Intrinsic sleep disorders are sleep disorders that either originate or develop within the body or arise from causes within the body, such as psychophysiologic and idiopathic insomnia, narcolepsy, recurrent idiopathic and posttraumatic hypersomnia, sleep apnea, central alveolar hypoventilation syndrome, periodic limb movement disorder, and restless legs syndrome.

Extrinsic sleep disorders are those caused by some other stimulus arising from outside the body. The more common are altitude insomnia, insufficient sleep syndrome, and various sleep disorders resulting from exposure to hypnotics, stimulants, alcohol, or toxins.

Circadian rhythm sleep disorders include those problems related to changes in sleep schedules (e.g., time-zone change, shift work), and will not be discussed here.

Insomnia

Insomnia is the classic disorder of initiating and maintaining sleep and is the most common sleep complaint. It is also one of the most common complaints patients bring to a primary care physician. Insomnia is the inability to get to sleep or stay asleep for the time expected by the individual and is only an abnormality when the patient complains about it, because a person who sleeps for only 3 hours a night may accept this as his or her normal pattern. Insomnia is only a symptom; during the interview the physician must search for the underlying cause. Because many physicians lack understanding of sleep physiology and of the drugs that affect sleep, insomnia is also commonly mismanaged.

In most cases of insomnia there is an underlying psychologic disturbance. Over 85% of insomniacs have one or more major pathologic scores on the Minnesota Multiphasic Personality Test (MMPI), particularly on the scales for depression, sociopathy, obsessive-compulsive features, and schizophrenia. It is common for patients to concentrate on their sleep disturbance and ignore or deny the underlying emotional problem. Poor sleepers have been found to spend less time in REM and more time in NREM sleep stages 1 and 2. They also have an increased heart rate, peripheral vasoconstriction, and a higher body temperature during sleep, suggesting a higher level of physiologic arousal, which demonstrates that their sleep is different not only in quantity but also in quality from that of persons without sleep disorders.

The management of insomnia consists of improving sleep hygiene and often the use of drugs for a limited period. Alcohol, nicotine, and caffeine should be eliminated, emotional or medical problems (especially those causing dyspnea or pain or affecting bladder or bowel function) treated, and the bedroom made conducive to sleeping by reducing noise and light. The patient should use the bedroom for sleep only; if not asleep after 15 minutes, he or she should get up and go to another room and read until tired. Watching television is not recommended because the light and content are arousing. The patient should rise at the same time each morning regardless of how little sleep there was the previous night. Sleep restriction therapy requires that subjects stay in bed only for as long as they usually sleep, although the time is increased by 15 minutes per week as sleep time increases.

When medications are needed, the lowest effective dose should be employed, and dosing should be intermittent—perhaps 3 to 4 nights per week. Discontinuation should be gradual. Geriatric patients need only about half the dose normally used for younger adults. The use of barbiturates is obsolete because in the long term they disturb sleep even further, cause excessive daytime sleepiness, and may lead to rebound effects on discontinuation. Tryptophan is a natural, if weak, sleep promoter; a hot malted drink is the best thing to take as a late-evening beverage. Melatonin has anecdotal evidence for use as a sleeping aid but few controlled clinical trial results support its use. Tricyclic drugs, such as amitriptyline, frequently work well in cheerful insomniacs, but may lead to atropinic effects and daytime sleepiness.

Flurazepam induces normal patterns of sleep but its long half-life (5 days) may lead to excessive daytime sleepiness. Other benzodiazepines, such as triazolam (Halcion), temazepam (Restoril), lorazepam (Ativan), and diazepam (Valium), are acceptable medications for insomnia, but all are best used intermittently because with many, active metabolites accumulate, a constant blood level is attained, and cognitive impairment, sleepiness by day, incoordination, and sometimes depression may result.

Triazolam (Halcion) has a short action and limited "hangover" effect, but its short half-life may lead to the patient waking during the night, and its rapid action causes some to have impaired memory for the period while they remain awake after taking it.

Idiopathic Hypersomnia

Idiopathic hypersomnia is an uncommon condition characterized by a periodic or chronic tendency to sleep deeply for prolonged periods and to take frequent naps. Unlike narcolepsy, the tendency to sleep in hypersomnia is not irresistible and the onset of sleep is slower.

Characteristically, these patients feel confused on awakening and have difficulty becoming completely alert ("sleep drunkenness"). Like the patients who describe themselves as poor sleepers, hypersomniacs show a sleep pattern suggesting a more aroused or lighter type of sleep. Fatigue, lethargy, and poor motor and intellectual performance by day result. In the chronic hypersomniac, attention must be paid to the psychologic mechanisms underlying the symptoms, particularly depression. Stimulant drugs such as methylphenidate may be effective, but tricyclic drugs are usually better. Amphetamines should be avoided.

Kleine-Levin Syndrome

Kleine-Levin syndrome is characterized by bulimia (a tendency to eat excessively), hypersexuality, and prolonged sleeping. The patients are usually young men who sleep excessively for a number of weeks, awakening only to eat voraciously any food put in front of them. They also have a tendency to act out sexually during this state. The disorder usually clears spontaneously after a few years.

Central Alveolar Hypoventilation Syndrome

Central alveolar hypoventilation syndrome (Pickwickian syndrome*), a disorder of periodic ventilatory insufficiency caused by gross obesity, is characterized by chronic sleepiness and a tendency to fall asleep easily when at rest.

Sleep Apnea

Sleep apnea is a condition in which repetitive nocturnal apneic spells result in recurrent hypoxemia and sleep disruption. When 15 or more apneic episodes occur per hour of sleep, symptoms appear, including complaints of restless nocturnal sleep with attacks of choking and repeated awakenings, excessive daytime sleepiness, morning headaches, nocturia, and irritability. Clinically, the condition presents most often with snoring, abnormal sleep behavior, excessive daytime sleepiness, intellectual deterioration, personality change, morning headache, and sleep disturbances. It occurs in association with a wide range of primary neurologic diseases, most of which affect the brainstem or the brain in a diffuse manner. There are two major types of sleep apnea; in each, the clinical diagnosis is confirmed by polysomnographic monitoring.

In *central sleep apnea syndrome* all ventilatory movements cease during sleep because of prolonged pauses in the central brainstem motor output to the ventilatory muscles. There are frequent episodes of shallow or absent breathing during sleep, associated usually with gasps, grunts, or choking during sleep; frequent body movements; and cyanosis. The result of this reduced ventilatory effort is oxygen desaturation. Patients commonly complain of excessive sleepiness and associated headache, but are sometimes unaware of the underlying problem. Avoidance of sedative drugs, alcohol, steroids, and diuretics is helpful prophylaxis. Medroxyprogesterone acetate and aminophylline or caffeine may stimulate the respiratory centers, reducing the number of spells. If these treatments are ineffective, mechanical ventilatory assistance may be required during sleep; this may require phrenic nerve stimulation or positive pressure ventilation through a tracheostomy. Cervical cordotomy, Chiari malformation, kyphoscoliosis, bulbar polio, and brainstem infarct or tumor are other causes of central sleep-related apnea, which may be accompanied by disturbed sleep with abnormal movements, hypnagogic hallucinations, enuresis, and somnambulism.

In *obstructive sleep apnea syndrome* there are repetitive episodes of upper airway obstruction during sleep, usually with a reduction in blood oxygen saturation. In this form, the diaphragm and chest wall move with variations in intrathoracic pressure, but there is no air flow at the nose or mouth. The problem is usually due to collapse of the muscular wall of the pharynx and less commonly to facial/palatal malformations or upper airway disease. Patients are commonly unaware of the apneic spells and of the "snorting and/or snoring" that signals the beginning of the respiratory phase, so a history from the bed partner is needed to confirm suspicions.

Many patients with sleep apnea are obese males who smoke and drink alcohol excessively. Their usual complaints are of excessive daytime sleepiness; morning headaches and a dry mouth on awakening; personality change, especially irritability; and some cognitive alteration. Milder cases of the condition may respond to losing weight, stopping smoking and drinking, and to the drug protriptyline. In more severe cases, because of the respiratory obstruction during sleep, surgical reconstruction of the pharynx (uvulopalatopharyngoplasty) may be needed. A permanent tracheostomy was once used in some cases, but nasal continuous positive airway pressure (CPAP) using a mask or nasal prongs (which act as a pneumatic splint providing the pressure to keep the nasopharyngeal air passages open) is now advised instead. Some therapy should be encouraged, because sleep apnea carries an increased risk of systemic and pulmonary hypertension, stroke, right heart failure, and polycythemia.

Excessive Daytime Sleepiness

Excessive daytime sleepiness is usually a symptom of chronic sleep loss, sleep apnea syndrome, narcolepsy, or such psychologic disorders as depression.

Narcolepsy

The full narcolepsy syndrome consists of a tetrad of symptoms: sleep attacks, cataplexy, sleep paralysis, and hypnagogic hallucinations (waking dreams). The sleep attacks are characterized by irresistible, brief (5 to 10 minute) sleep episodes that occur at times of decreased sensory stimulation. The patients may fall asleep at their desks, at the table, at the movies, in front of television, or in front of their house guests. They awake feeling quite refreshed. Some patients feel perpetually drowsy and have superimposed sudden sleep attacks of either REM or NREM type. Although sleep attacks may occur many times a day, there is usually a refractory period of a number of hours after each one.

Cataplexy is a sudden relaxation of muscle tone, usually precipitated by emotion, which causes the patient to slump, often falling on the floor but remaining conscious during this brief episode. Narcoleptics often learn to steel themselves against extremes of emotion (particularly laughing) to avoid these episodes. Some patients get only a partial weakness, exhibited by the sudden sagging of the jaw, face, and head, or their arms may drop to their sides. Rarely, a patient will experience slowing of speech or of all movements for a brief period.

Sleep paralysis usually occurs in the interval between sleep and wakening, often on awakening in the morning or after a sleep attack, when the patient finds that he or she is completely unable to move. Even though it may have occurred many times before, it is frightening, but seldom lasts

*Named after the Fat Boy in Dickens' *The Pickwick Papers*, who was usually asleep.

longer than 60 seconds. Even a gentle touch terminates an attack.*

Hypnagogic hallucinations are vivid auditory or visual hallucinations or illusions that occur, like sleep paralysis, when the patient is in the state between wakefulness and sleep, or when coming out of a sleep attack. The patient is aware of what is going on around him or her but also experiences a vivid hallucination (e.g., the sight, sound, or voice of a long-dead parent) at the same time.

Although narcolepsy is classically a tetrad of symptoms, some patients also manifest symptoms of sleep drunkenness and disturbed nocturnal sleep. Narcoleptic symptoms appear to be normal components of REM sleep that occur at abnormal times. The sleep attacks are episodes of REM sleep in people who have the other components of the tetrad; but patients who have only sleep attacks may experience NREM sleep during the episodes. Both cataplexy and sleep paralysis appear to represent the motor inhibition that characterizes REM sleep. Hypnagogic hallucinations are vivid dreams as the person falls asleep. Unlike the memory of a dream, the dream is on while the person is awake and aware of his or her surroundings. These hallucinations are also different from the sleep fantasies that normally occur as a person falls asleep. Hypnopompic hallucinations† represent a vivid dream such as would be normal during REM sleep but not when occurring in the drowsy stage as they do in this case. The night sleep of a narcoleptic patient is not normal but is disrupted, with frequent wakenings. In most cases, the first period of REM sleep has an unusually short latency (minutes rather than an hour or two).

Narcolepsy has to be differentiated from other causes of excessive sleepiness, such as idiopathic hypersomnia, hypothyroidism, depression, vertebrobasilar ischemia, and medication ingestions. The best diagnostic method is a careful history, but searching for the human leukocyte antigen (HLA) may be helpful because the prevalence of HLA-DR2, DQw1 in patient with narcolepsy is nearly 100%; thus if the patient lacks HLA-DR2, the diagnosis of narcolepsy may well be wrong. Pupillography is a research tool that may be used as an objective test for narcolepsy and is based on the facts that the pupil is large when the patient is alert, small when asleep, and intermediate when drowsy. It is an accurate way to evaluate a patient's ability to stay awake and has been used in evaluating sleepy drivers. Narcoleptic patients are a great risk on the highway because 77% report being drowsy when driving, 40% have fallen asleep at the wheel, and 16% have actually had accidents because of the narcolepsy.

After a definite diagnosis of narcolepsy has been made, the situation should be explained fully to the patient, to his or her family, and often to the patient's employer. The patient should not drive until therapy has been successful. Therapy may begin with methylphenidate, 10 mg tid, increased as required. The average patient takes 30 to 60 mg per day to control sleep attacks. Modafinil 200 to 400 mg/day, selegiline (up to 40 mg/day), and pemoline (37.5 mg po od) are alternatives. Amphetamines, once the mainstay of therapy, are rarely used now because of the problems of addiction, tolerance, and medicolegal complexities associated with their long-term use. Cataplexy, sleep paralysis, and hypnagogic hallucinations may not be helped by methylphenidate but may respond to imipramine or clomipramine (25 mg daily, increasing to 25 mg tid, if required). The selective serotonin reuptake inhibitor (SSRI) fluoxetine, 20 mg/day, is also effective against cataplexy.

PARASOMNIAS

Sleeptalking

Sleeptalking is the utterance of speech or sounds during sleep without subjective detailed awareness of the event. Such talking during REM sleep may represent the vocal expression of dream experiences, but it also occurs during transient arousals from non-REM sleep. In some cases, anxiety disorders or febrile illness are associated, and sleepwalking, obstructive sleep apnea syndrome, or REM sleep behavior disorder may also occur.

Sleepwalking

Sleepwalking is a sequence of complex behaviors during clouded consciousness that are seen mainly in prepubertal children and that tend to disappear spontaneously as they get older. It occurs during the first nocturnal periods of NREM sleep stages 3 or 4, with subsequent amnesia. It is hard to arouse the child during an episode, which may end with confused awakening or with a return to normal sleep. The person is able to perceive the world around to some extent because he walks around people and furniture. Sitting up in bed, perseverated simple movements, and complex automatic activities such as walking, going down stairs, and opening doors may occur. Attempts to restrain the subject usually lead to avoidance behavior.

Sleepwalking is seen less in adults than in children, among whom it may be associated with enuresis and sleep terrors. Although there is little evidence of psychologic disturbance in children who sleepwalk, there is some evidence that adults with this problem do have some underlying psychopathology.

Management of sleepwalking includes protection of the sleepwalker from injury, because he or she may wander into areas of danger or fall down stairs. A nightly dose of amitriptyline, clonazepam, or flurazepam may help sleepwalkers, although patients sometimes return to their sleepwalking patterns after 3 to 6 months despite the medication.

Sleep Terrors

A sleep terror is characterized by sudden awakening from sleep with intense anxiety, autonomic overstimulation, movement, and crying out. Despite the appearance of terror, the child has no memory for the event later, except for the feeling that something strange has just happened. The child with night terrors may also have enuresis or sleepwalking. Night terrors arise during stage 4 NREM sleep, often within the first hour. The child shows an impaired arousal response but a waking alpha EEG pattern, extreme motility, sleepwalking, and vocalization in the form of terrified screams or moaning. Pulse and respiratory rates increase but the episode is over within a minute or two. The child then has a feeling of intense fear and anxiety, respiratory restriction (hence the medieval image of a devil—an "incubus"—on the chest), and an overwhelming sensation of doom. Sleep

*The fable of Sleeping Beauty may have been based on this syndrome, with the touch of the prince's kiss unlocking her immobility. Mundane stimuli, however, are equally effective.

†Hypnopompic hallucinations are the same thing as hypnagogic, except that they occur on waking up.

terrors, like sleepwalking and other disorders of sleep, may be primarily disorders of arousal. Children with sleep terrors seldom require psychotherapy or medication.

Sleep-Wake Transition Disorders

Sleep starts may lead patients to complain either of difficulty falling asleep or of an intense body movement at sleep onset. These sudden, brief jerks at sleep onset, mainly affecting the legs or arms, are often associated with a subjective feeling of falling, a sensory flash, or a hypnagogic dream. They last less than a quarter of a second, mainly affect the legs, resemble the startle reaction of wakefulness, and occur in many people, usually during sleep onset. A positive family history is frequently found. Sleep starts represent a partial arousal response, are not associated with clinical or EEG abnormalities, and are of no pathologic significance.

Physiologic hypnic myoclonus is the condition of small, irregular twitches that occur normally in sleep and are of no significance. Virtually everyone has experienced these occasionally when just falling asleep. Brief attacks of dystonic, dyskinetic posturing during the night, lasting up to 2 minutes, have also been described and they respond well to carbamazepine.

Parasomnias Usually Associated With Rapid Eye Movement Sleep

Sleep paralysis is a dissociated REM sleep inhibitory process characterized by periods of flaccid paralysis of all but the respiratory and extraocular muscles with areflexia. Sleep paralysis occurs for minutes during the waking stage immediately preceding or succeeding sleep and is terminated by sleep or by sensory stimulation. The experience is frequently frightening, and some episodes are associated with hypnagogic hallucinations or dreamlike mentation. It may represent the tonelessness of normal REM sleep occurring in the conscious state. Cataplexy is the equivalent in the waking state. The syndrome may occur in isolation or as a component of the narcolepsy syndrome.

Dreams occur in both light NREM and REM sleep. A *nightmare* (or dream anxiety attack) is a normal but frightening dream, and the subject often has good recall of the episode initially if aroused from REM sleep. Nightmares are most common in childhood but may be induced in adults by the REM rebound that occurs after stopping a course of drugs such as benzodiazepines. The first step in management consists of determining the characteristics of the sleep disturbance. In adult cases, nightmares require only explanation and reassurance, but it is important to recognize that many medications used at bedtime may actually increase nightmares, L-dopa and propranolol for example. If treatment is required (when these drugs must be continued), then benzodiazepines in small doses may be helpful.

REM sleep behavior disorder is a striking behavior pattern related to REM sleep in which the patients (who are often older men) manifest vigorous and sometimes aggressive and dangerous activity associated with excessive limb or body jerking and dreams. They may jump from bed, damage furnishings, and injure (even murder) their bed partner or hurt themselves in the midst of an attack. It is important to remove objects and alter the room to minimize the danger of injury. Clonazepam, 0.5 mg at bedtime, usually suppresses the activity, but higher doses may be required.

Sleep-related painful erections are prolonged, painful erections that subside over minutes and often recur during the same night, usually during REM sleep periods. There are no associated deficits in sexual functioning, and erections during wakefulness are painless.

Other Parasomnias

Restless legs syndrome (RLS) is a common condition that particularly affects middle-aged people. In this disorder, the subject complains of a strong desire—almost a compulsion—to move the legs, often accompanied by paresthesias and dysesthesias in the legs; motor restlessness, worsening at rest and with temporary relief from activity; and worsening in the evening or at night. The clinical examination is usually normal, although the syndrome may also complicate pregnancy, peripheral sensory neuropathies from any cause, and iron-deficiency anemia. In most of the idiopathic cases there is a positive family history suggesting dominant inheritance. In addition to the conscious urge to move the legs, periodic limb movements are commonly associated during the lighter stages of NREM sleep. These are stereotyped patterns of flexion movements, always including dorsiflexion of the hallux, that occur repetitively once or twice per minute. The movements resemble akathisia, but their timing allows the differential. Vespers curse (lumbosacral and leg pain with leg cramps and fasciculations waking the patient from sleep) resembles RLS but occurs in patients with lumbar spinal stenosis and cardiac failure.

Therapy for RLS rests on the three pillars of benzodiazepines, opioids, and dopaminergic drugs. Levodopa-carbidopa (100 to 200 mg of levodopa) is the treatment of choice and is valuable for many patients. The controlled-release preparation reduces the tendency for a rebound increase in movements in the latter part of the night. Bromocriptine, 2.5 to 5 mg at bedtime, is almost as effective. Clonazepam, 0.5 mg at bedtime, is a reasonable initial therapy, and the dose can be increased to 2 mg if necessary. Clonidine, baclofen, carbamazepine, and pramipexole (0.125 mg at night, increasing slowly to 1 mg at bedtime if necessary) have also been used with some success. Methadone, 10 mg, codeine, 30 mg, or propoxyphene, 65 mg, may be effective but are preferably used only when other treatments have failed.

Nocturnal leg cramps are a common problem in the elderly, to whom they are a source of great misery. The calf pain is relieved only by standing up out of bed, but may still persist for some minutes. Prevention is easily accomplished, using small doses of quinine, 200 mg daily, dilantin, 200 mg at bedtime, and sometimes calcium lactate, 200 to 400 mg daily.

Primary enuresis refers to enuresis that continues after infancy, without any prolonged dry periods occurring. About one out of every six children are bedwetters at age 5, but up to 3% of healthy young adults still wet the bed occasionally. Primary enuresis is usually idiopathic, or may have a genetic basis in some cases, but sometimes results from organic diseases such as urethral obstruction, ectopic ureter, diverticulum of the anterior urethra, epispadias, or chronic urinary tract infection. *Secondary enuresis* is the recurrence of enuresis after a prolonged period of dryness and may be due to psychologic disturbance or to organic disease such as infection or diabetes.

Enuresis occurs in any stage of NREM sleep, most often in the first third of the night. The episode often begins in stage 4 sleep and is associated with a burst of rhythmic delta waves on the EEG, after which the sleep pattern switches to stage 2 or 1 and micturition occurs.

It is important to determine whether enuresis is primary or secondary. If primary, then reassurance and explanation are helpful, particularly because many other family members may have had and outgrown the same problem. One must look for organic problems in both primary and secondary cases. Careful attention must also be paid to psychologic factors. An understanding and empathetic approach must be taken with the children or they may see the encounter as a form of punishment. It is important to recognize not only psychologic cases of enuresis but the psychologic trauma and lowered self-image that can result. Parents often take a punitive attitude toward the child. Not only is this ineffective but it may augment the psychologic factors that worsen secondary enuresis. Therapy of primary enuresis begins with a reassuring explanation to the parents and the child based on an interview and examination. The child is advised to restrict fluids after supper, and on weekends and after school try to see how long he or she can hold urine in his or her full bladder. A parent should awaken the child late at night, usually when the parents are retiring, to have the child void again.

Imipramine, a tricyclic, is a moderately effective treatment for enuresis, but children are often made irritable by this drug. Its effect could be through decreasing stage 4 sleep or there may be a more direct effect on bladder innervation. An alternative method of therapy is the conditioning approach, using a mild electric shock pad that awakens the child at the first drop of urine. The Mozes detector has shown excellent results in clearing enuresis in 80% of children within 3 months. One has to be aware of the psychologic effect of this type of machine, and it has to be explained to the child with understanding and encouragement. Intranasal vasopressin (DDAVP) is a highly effective symptomatic remedy. Its remarkable ability to control enuresis suggests that the problem may sometimes be related to some failure of nocturnal secretion of this hormone by the posterior pituitary.

Sleep drunkenness is a parasomnia of adult life characterized by clouding of the sensorium with confusion and inappropriate impulsive behavior that occurs during an abnormally prolonged period of transition between the states of being asleep (commonly in a deep NREM sleep stage) and of being awake. Tiredness, impaired concentration, ataxia, headache, and drowsiness are also described.

Sleep bruxism is nocturnal grinding of the teeth, usually in the lighter stages of NREM sleep. It often runs in families and has no psychologic basis. Although dental malocclusion is thought to be associated, orthodontic treatment is expensive and generally useless as a remedy. A rubber mouthguard may be helpful.

Headbanging consists of rhythmic, rocking movements of the head and trunk that occur before or in the early stages of NREM sleep, usually in children.

Cluster headache (see Chapter 160) characteristically awakens the patient from sleep in the earliest hours of the morning during the first REM sleep period.

Infantile sleep apnea is the occurrence in infants of central or obstructive apneas during sleep. The clinical presentation includes noisy breathing during sleep, an episode of cessation of breathing during sleep characterized by pallor or cyanosis, and limpness, but rarely stiffness.

Nocturnal paroxysmal dystonia, sudden unexplained nocturnal death syndrome, sudden infant death syndrome, and primary snoring are other parasomnias described.

SLEEP DISORDERS ASSOCIATED WITH MEDICAL/PSYCHIATRIC DISORDERS

Sleep disturbances may also be associated with medical diseases such as sleeping sickness, chronic obstructive pulmonary disease, sleep-related gastroesophageal reflux, peptic ulcer disease, and fibrositis syndrome.

Medical Conditions Associated With Sleep

The list of medical conditions associated with sleep disturbance is very long, and only a few will be discussed here.

Myocardial infarction and episodes of angina commonly occur at night. There may be some relationship to the physiologic changes of REM sleep, but this has not been a consistent finding in all studies. It is now recognized, however, that sleep is not a quiet state of suspended animation, but a period with variable and often increased electrophysiologic, biochemical, physiologic, and psychologic activity—almost an "autonomic storm." Such stresses may also induce cerebrovascular accidents.

Patients with duodenal ulcers secrete more gastric acid at night than normal subjects, primarily during REM sleep. This probably explains the common nocturnal pain and discomfort in such patients. *Asthmatic attacks* commonly occur at night, particularly in the early morning during stage 2 but rarely in stage 4.

Hypothyroid patients complain of excessive drowsiness, and sleep laboratory studies show that they mainly experience only the lighter stages of sleep. With replacement therapy, these patients regain a more normal sleep pattern. *Pregnant women* spend less time in the deeper stages of sleep. There may be increased sleeping and drowsiness during the first trimester of pregnancy, but increased wakening occurs as pregnancy continues. In *encephalitis* and *dementing illnesses,* reversal of the normal sleep pattern may occur, with sleeping during the day and alertness during the night.

Sleep disturbance in mental illness is well known. Depressed patients may oversleep, have difficulty getting to sleep because of superimposed anxiety, and experience early morning awakening. They take longer to get to sleep and spend twice as much time in light stages, often claiming they are not asleep at all. A disturbance in sleep patterns may predict deterioration in some mental illnesses; thus in schizophrenia acute episodes are often preceded by increasing insomnia, restlessness, and excessive rapid eye movements during REM sleep, suggesting overstimulation of the arousal system. In chronic organic brain syndromes, some patients have excessive REM sleep and others experience little.

Nocturnal seizures are common, especially in the epilepsies with focal origin. They usually occur in stage 2 NREM or in REM sleep periods. Both random and regular discharges may be recorded because of a decrease of inhibition, which leads to the jerking, twitching, or myoclonic movements that may be seen at the onset of sleep (very often in normal subjects as well) and may also initiate focal or generalized seizure activity. Vascular headaches commonly begin between 5 and 8 AM. In fibrositis (fibromyalgia) syndrome, the muscle pains and headache are associated with disturbed sleep, and it has been suggested that the sleep disorder is primary.

ADDITIONAL READINGS

ASDA Diagnostic Classification Steering Committee: *The international classification of sleep disorders diagnostic and coding manual,* Rochester, Minn, 1990, American Sleep Disorders Association.

Guilleminault C, editor: *Sleep and its disorders in children,* New York, 1987, Raven Press.

Kupfer DJ, Reynolds CF: Management of insomnia, *N Engl J Med* 336:341-346, 1997.

Mahowald MW, Chokroverty S, Kader G, Schenck CH, editors: *Sleep disorders: Continuum: Lifelong learning in neurology,* Part A, Vol 3, 1997.

Schapiro C, editor: *ABC of sleep disorders,* London, 1994, British Medical Association.

CHAPTER 162

Facial Palsy, Pain, and Numbness

T. Jock Murray
William Pryse-Phillips

Of the many ills that may affect us, disorders involving the face are of particular importance. One can sometimes be dispassionate about pain, numbness, or weakness of a limb—a seemingly distant portion of our bodies—but the face has strong significance in our concept of "self." It is a mirror to the world and a sounding board for ourselves. Disorders in the face have much greater personal significance than disorders occurring elsewhere.

FACIAL PALSY

The muscles of the upper part of the face obtain innervation from the motor cortex on each side. Thus the right frontalis and orbicularis oculi in the upper quadrant of the face are supplied by motor fibers running in the right VII nerve, whose nuclear cell bodies receive corticopontine fibers from *both* the left and the right cortical motor areas. The nerve supply to the muscles of the *lower* face on the right, however, comes from other cells in the VII nerve nucleus that *only* receive impulses from the opposite (left) cerebral cortex.

With a unilateral left cortical lesion, therefore, the frontalis and orbicularis oculi on the right will still function but the orbicularis oris and platysma will not. A unilateral upper motor neuron lesion produces only a lower quadrant facial weakness. If the nerve is damaged at the nucleus, in the cerebellopontine angle, within the facial canal, or immediately after leaving the canal, *all* of the muscles on that side of the face will be paralyzed. Therefore one can decide whether the cause of weakness is an upper or lower motor neuron lesion by seeing whether the frontalis and orbicularis oculi muscles are involved (lower motor neuron lesion) or not (upper motor neuron lesion). In the latter case, weakness of the hand and arm on the same side are also likely to be found.

Localization of Lesions

Supranuclear

Cortical Lesions. Paresis of the lower half of the face can result from a contralateral cortical lesion in the motor area controlling facial movement. Usually, such a lesion will give rise to typical upper motor neuron weakness in the arm as well.

Corticospinal Tract Lesions. Corticospinal tract lesions may occur anywhere between the cortex and the facial nuclei and although cerebral infarction is the most common cause, this type of paresis can result from a tumor or other compressive lesions, from multiple sclerosis, or from motor neuron disease.

Nuclear. If the lesion involves the facial nucleus in the pons, other signs may be found, indicating involvement of nearby brainstem structures, including the medial lemniscus and the nuclei and fibers of the V, VI, or VIII (vestibular) nerves. Possible lesions within the pons include a tumor, multiple sclerosis, and infarction. Congenital absence of the facial nuclei or nerves is also possible (Mobius syndrome) and is characterized by bilateral facial paralysis from birth, palsy of the VI nerves, and sometimes deafness.

Infranuclear

In the Subarachnoid Space. When the VII nerve leaves the brainstem it crosses the subarachnoid space at the cerebellopontine angle and enters the internal auditory meatus in close company with the VIII nerve and the nervus intermedius and lies adjacent to the middle cerebellar peduncle. Lesions here may affect all or any of these structures. Complaints of vertigo, tinnitus, or deafness, reduction in facial sensation, loss or diminution of the corneal reflex, VI nerve palsy, facial weakness, and/or cerebellar signs on the same side may be found.

In the Meatus. A lesion of the nerve in the internal auditory meatus and its continuation, the facial canal, may be determined by the presence of associated damage to the following (Fig. 162-1):

1. Greater superficial petrosal nerve (loss of tear formation in that eye)
2. VIII nerve (tinnitus, deafness, vertigo)
3. Nerve to the stapedius (hyperacusis in that ear)
4. Chorda tympani (diminution of taste in the anterior two thirds of the tongue)

The most common lesion here is a tumor, infection, or fracture of the petrous temporal bone after trauma.

At the Genu. With the lesion at the genu, there will be associated damage to the VIII nerve fibers and also to the nerves to the stapedius and chorda tympani. Signs will be as suggested above for lesions in the meatus. The most common causes here are trauma, mastoiditis, the presence of a neoplasm (usually benign), and herpes zoster. Facial pain is common with this latter disorder *(Ramsay Hunt syndrome),* and a herpetic vesicular eruption on the fauces or in the external auditory meatus will be visible. Patients sometimes complain of deafness or vertigo related to involvement of the VIII nerve as well.

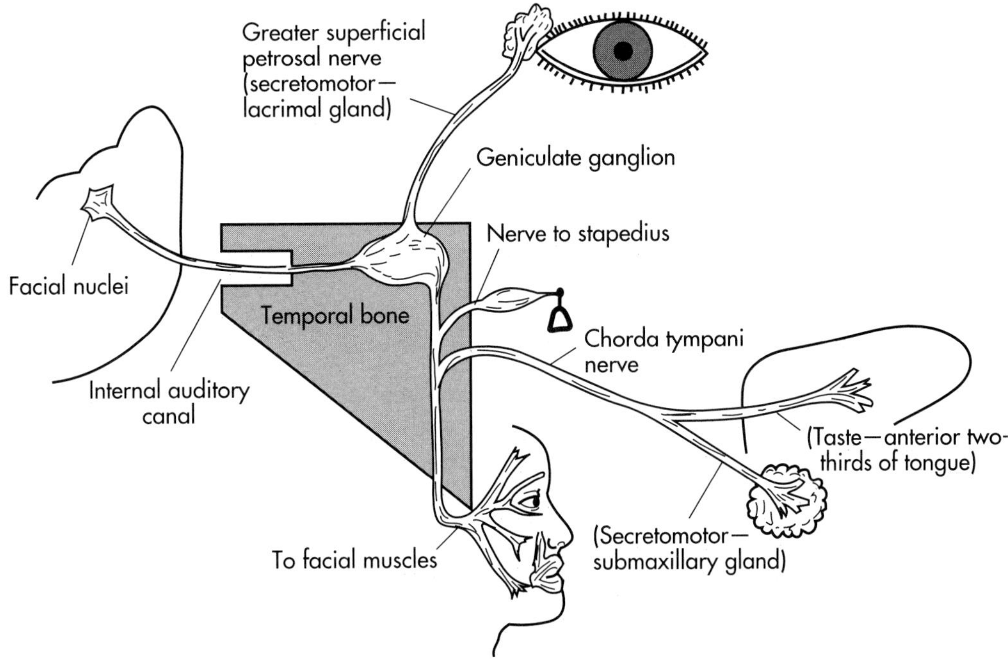

Fig. 162-1. Schematic representation of the facial nerve and its branches.

In the Facial Canal. At the facial canal, only the chorda tympani will be involved with the facial nerve because everything else has branched off at a higher level. If the lesion is very low down in the canal, even the chorda tympani will be spared. The most common causes here include infections of the middle ear and mastoid area that involve the nerve because of local extension of the inflammation. Facial paralysis is probably often caused by herpesvirus infections and sometimes occurs in diphtheria, mumps, measles, chickenpox, Epstein-Barr virus infection, and tetanus. Sarcoidosis causes facial paralysis, often bilaterally, because of involvement of the nerve in the canal and not in the parotid gland (although this may also be affected). Guillain-Barré syndrome may produce bilateral facial weakness, and in these cases the lesion probably affects all or any part of the nerve.

Trauma (e.g., skull fracture) may damage the nerve either as it runs in the petrous bone or facial canal, or after the nerve has left the stylomastoid foramen. Direct stab, surgical, or gunshot wounds to the face, ear, or parotid gland may produce facial paralysis. Less common causes of facial paralysis include lead poisoning, thiamine deficiency, and polyarteritis nodosa, but the most common cause of all (3 in 4) is Bell's palsy.

During assessment of the patient with apparent facial palsy, the first question to ask is whether both the upper and the lower face are involved. If they are, then the cause is a lower motor neuron lesion. If the pathology involves the VII nerve nucleus, full examination will almost always show other signs of a brainstem lesion, but usually the site of damage is distal. Assessment of tear formation, hearing, and taste, as well as general neurologic examination and blood pressure recording, should allow accurate localization.

BELL'S PALSY

Bell's palsy is a common peripheral facial paralysis of unknown cause that affects perhaps 20 out of 100,000 persons per year. The onset is always sudden, never progressive, and the paralysis is almost always unilateral. Although most causes will recover spontaneously, the severity of the cosmetic effects, the complications during the course of the illness, and the dangers of incomplete recovery warrant some form of therapy. Many patients relate the onset to exposure to cold temperatures or wind. It has been suggested that it is more common in taxi drivers, and during World War II it was seen in Army personnel driving trucks with the windows open. Hereditary factors may play a role because one third of the patients have a positive family history of Bell's palsy. Because the disease sometimes occurs in epidemics, a viral etiology has been suggested; the herpes group of viruses has been implicated in some cases (herpes simplex, Epstein-Barr), suggesting that Bell's palsy is only part of a generalized viral inflammatory disease. Whatever the initiating cause, the nerve becomes further damaged by edema and ischemia because it is entrapped within the bony facial canal at a site usually below the geniculate ganglion.

Clinical Features. At the onset, the acute, unilateral, lower motor neuron flaccid paralysis of the face is accompanied, or preceded in half of the cases, by pain behind the ear that reaches a peak within 2 or 3 hours. There may be associated fever, dizziness, tinnitus, decreased hearing, or a mildly stiff neck. All of the functions of the facial nerve will probably be affected, producing motor weakness of all facial muscles on that side and frequently loss of taste on the anterior two thirds of the tongue. There will be inability to wrinkle the forehead and close the eye related to weakness of the frontalis and orbicularis oculi. Eversion of the lower eyelid, loss of the nasolabial fold, and dropping of the corner of the mouth, with drooling of saliva, are common effects. In some cases, there is only partial palsy, which may make the diagnosis more difficult. Hyperacusis caused by paralysis of the stapedius muscle and reduced lacrimation and salivation indicate a lesion proximal to the end of the canal, sometimes even proximal to the geniculate ganglion, but these are less common in Bell's palsy.

Bell's palsy usually involves the VII nerve only; evidence of other neurologic deficits suggests some other disorder such as a stroke, tumor, infection, or multiple sclerosis. Occasionally the V and other cranial nerves are involved too, usually subclinically, and the disorder can be a manifestation of a more generalized but mild peripheral neuropathy. It is a good rule, however, to suspect a more sinister central nervous system (CNS) disorder if more than the VII lesion is evident.

Treatment

General supportive measures, such as mild analgesics and warm coverings for the face and ear, can be started immediately. The eyelid should be taped shut if blinking is not possible; artificial tears may be instilled twice daily to prevent drying of the conjunctiva. Medical therapy for Bell's palsy has in the past included a variety of treatments, from reassurance to vasodilators. Most are useless; only steroids started early reduce the chance of some residual paralysis. A suggested course of therapy for an adult consists of 60 mg of prednisone per day for 5 days, tapering to zero over a further 6 days. The patient should be evaluated weekly for the first 2 weeks and then again in 4 weeks.

If the symptoms worsen when the steroids are reduced, or if the postauricular pain returns, then the treatment course may be repeated once. Surgical decompression of the nerve is not indicated; the only surgical procedure that may be of benefit in these patients is late surgical autografting of the hypoglossal to the VII nerve if spontaneous recovery has not taken place.

Complications and Prognosis

Although at least 85% of patients with Bell's palsy will recover spontaneously in 2 months, the physical and social disability of those who do not warrants the use of immediate prednisone therapy in all cases seen before the third day. Patients more likely to be left with some paresis are those with complete paralysis of the nerve initially, those with pain other than that in the ear, those with diabetes or hypertension, and those over 60 years of age. In most cases, however, recovery starts within 2 weeks of onset, with the upper facial muscles recovering first. Complete restoration of function may not be achieved over a year. If there is no improvement by the eighteenth day, some permanent disfigurement may be expected.

The occurrence of crocodile tears (shedding of tears when salivating) from a month or so after the initial palsy is caused by aberrant regeneration of some fibers that grow out to the lacrimal gland instead of the salivary gland. If other regenerating fibers reach the wrong muscles, then abnormal movements may be seen, such as winking when the jaw is opened. If recovery is slow, contractures of the facial muscles can occur, and incomplete recovery may lead to the condition of clonic hemifacial spasm.

HEMIFACIAL SPASM

Hemifacial spasm is an abnormal movement disorder characterized by repetitive jerky contractions of the face on one side so that the eye closes and the mouth is drawn up toward the ear. The most common cause is the presence of a long loop of the anterior inferior cerebellar artery that impinges on the VII nerve in the posterior fossa, producing electrical "chatter." This results in the involuntary contraction of the muscles of one side of the face, which is both uncomfortable and socially embarrassing. The condition may be treated by injection of botulinum toxin into the motor end points of the affected facial muscles, or more radically (but permanently) by exposure of the VIII nerve roots in the posterior fossa and dissection of the nerve from the impinging artery, very much in the same way as the V nerve is decompressed in some patients with trigeminal neuralgia.

FACIAL MYOKYMIA

Discontinuous but repetitive involuntary twitching or writhing of the periorbital muscles is common in everyone when tired or otherwise stressed, and it presumably occurs as a result of excessive activity in some generator within the brainstem. The movements are small, usually unilateral, and brief, with each set of contractions lasting only a few seconds. Rarely, brainstem lesions as seen in multiple sclerosis or tumors cause the same thing.

FACIAL PAIN

The pain-sensitive structures in the face and the anterior part of the head are mostly innervated by the V or IX cranial nerves, although referred pain from other areas may also be felt in the lower part of the face. The major causes of facial pain may be conveniently subdivided under four headings:

1. Local structural changes in craniofacial tissues
2. Irritation of nerves (the neuralgias)
3. Referred pain
4. Atypical facial pain

Clinical Approach

Quality of the Pain. The pains in facial neuralgias are brief, knifelike, or lancinating in character, whereas the postherpetic neuralgias are classically described as burning. Pain described with an exuberance of phraseology, marked anguish, and great intensity may be associated with depression ("atypical facial pain"). Severe boring pain felt unilaterally behind the eye and radiating into the face occurs in cluster headache. Toothache, ocular disease, and sinusitis produce crescendos of pain or continuous aching, frequently with a throbbing component. Constant pains may also be felt in association with an infiltrating carcinoma at the base of the skull, usually arising in the nasopharynx, and also with brainstem vascular disease. Central irritation of the V nerve fibers by demyelination, for example, produces a pain indistinguishable from that of trigeminal neuralgia, but other neurologic signs should be present.

Site. Trigeminal neuralgia is felt in the V nerve territory, usually in the second or third divisions and very seldom in the first. Glossopharyngeal neuralgia is felt in the back of the throat, lower jaw, gums, and neck on the involved side. Postherpetic neuralgia is usually in the first division of the nerve, whereas cluster headache is felt largely in or just posterior to the eye. The pain may also extend up into the frontotemporal area and occasionally more diffusely below the eye. Referred pain is usually felt in the lower part of the face, often bilaterally, and the same is true of atypical facial pain. Trigger zones on the cheek or in the mouth are characteristic of the classic neuralgias.

Timing. The classic neuralgias are brief, repeated, knifelike stabs of pain described as "lancinating" and each lasting seconds, with no pain between the jabs; pain of much longer duration, perhaps even continuous, occurs in all of the other types of facial pain. With cluster headache, 40 to 60 minutes of acute pain often occurs at night, waking the patient from sleep, unlike the classic neuralgias, which hardly ever do so. Constant or long-lasting pains occur with infiltration or irritation of the V nerve by, for example, nasopharyngeal tumors, aneurysm of the posterior communicating artery, or chronic basal meningitis. Atypical facial pain tends to be constant.

Cluster headache occurs in bouts lasting a few weeks (hence the name) with months of freedom in between. There is also a periodicity with the classic neuralgias: repeated paroxysms of pain over the space of 1 or 2 weeks, often followed by a remission lasting up to months. Postherpetic pain usually goes away within 2 years but is almost constant while it is present and is accompanied by excessive pain reaction with simple touch. Spontaneous complete remission seldom occurs with the classic neuralgias.

Chewing and recent dental work may produce pain from the temporomandibular joint (TMJ) that is usually associated with over-closure of the bite, which is susceptible to orthodontic treatment. Chewing and the presence of hot or cold fluids in the mouth may produce glossopharyngeal neuralgia and accentuate the pain of toothache. Touching the skin may intensify the continuous background pain of postherpetic neuralgia and may trigger neuralgia.

Associated Symptoms. Associated symptoms of facial pain are of great importance. Mucosal and periosteal lesions producing primary facial pain may be associated with symptoms of sinusitis (nasal discharge, sometimes bloody; postnasal discharge; a history of recent upper respiratory infection). Cluster headaches are often associated with a small pupil, conjunctival engorgement, and severe lacrimation and nasal congestion, with an outpouring of sweat on the same side of the face and of clear fluid from the nostril. The whole episode looks rather like an intense, localized parasympathetic discharge.

Central (brainstem) lesions producing "symptomatic trigeminal neuralgia" include vascular disease, neoplasm, syringobulbia, and multiple sclerosis. Other clinical signs of these conditions will probably be found and almost always will be associated with a loss of the corneal reflex and perhaps subjective or objective alteration in sensation in the territory of the affected nerve. Peripheral infiltrating or compressive lesions of the nerve are also associated with sensory change, which rules out the diagnosis of trigeminal neuralgia. Posterior communicating artery aneurysm, nasopharyngeal carcinoma, cerebellopontine angle tumor, and chronic basal meningitis may all be expected to produce at least some signs in other cranial nerve territories. Evidence of depressive illness should be sought in patients with atypical facial pain.

In the classic neuralgias (trigeminal and glossopharyngeal), in cluster headache, and in atypical facial pain there are no physical signs on examination of the cranial nerves (although unilateral ptosis and miosis are seen in some cases of cluster headache). With dental, sinus, or jaw lesions, at least local signs will be detected, whereas with irritation of the V or IX nerves, postherpetic neuralgia, and brainstem disease, neurologic signs are likely.

In the absence of physical signs, referred pain from the heart, jaw, or other structures; atypical or depressive pain; and classic neuralgias will be most likely. In the presence of any physical signs, however, full investigation is required, perhaps including radiographic studies of the nasopharynx and of the skull, including the internal auditory meatus; lumbar puncture; and in many cases, contrast radiography and computed tomography (CT) or magnetic resonance imaging (MRI).

Clinical Presentations

Local Facial Pain Syndromes

Facial Pain Caused by Local Pathology. Any infection or tumor in the facial region or in the nose, pharynx, or ear may cause pain in the face. Common causes are toothache, nasopharyngeal tumors, trauma to the face, and vascular lesions, probably the most important of which is cranial arteritis, the inflammation of the scalp vessels being felt as a pain over the temporal region and posterior facial area, especially with chewing (so-called *jaw claudication*). The arteries are typically reddened, pulseless, and tender. These patients may go blind if the diagnosis is not made and the condition is not immediately treated with steroids.

Vascular Causes of Facial Pain. Cluster headache is a very severe eye and head pain that originates in the ocular, frontal, or frontotemporal regions and often spreads over the side of the head and face. The pain is associated with watering of the eye and nasal discharge on the same side, conjunctival suffusion, and sometimes ptosis and miosis (Horner's syndrome), which often remains after the acute pain has gone. The condition is most commonly seen in males and its timing is peculiar, frequently waking the patient from sleep in the early hours of the morning. The pain recurs daily over the course of a few weeks before disappearing, only to return weeks or months later in another bout (or "cluster"). Whether this is a neuralgia or a form of migraine is not clear.

Migraine headaches are usually experienced in the side of the head but sometimes patients feel pain in the face as well. The differential diagnosis should not be difficult because migraines usually have a throbbing, aching quality, as opposed to the sharp, lancinating, or burning sensation characteristic of most types of neuralgia.

The Neuralgias

Major Neuralgias

Trigeminal neuralgia. Trigeminal neuralgia is characterized by recurrent paroxysms of sharp, stabbing pain in one or more branches of the nerve on one side of the face, occurring in persons over age 50 who show no physical signs of V nerve dysfunction. The cause is uncertain; the disorder has often been referred to as "idiopathic trigeminal neuralgia" or "tic dauloureux," but examination of the trigeminal nerve has disclosed microneuromas and vascular compression in some cases. Other V nerve lesions that may result in pain include compression by an aneurysm or tumor, trauma, and multiple sclerosis, but these are often accompanied by physical signs and are regarded as symptomatic rather than idiopathic trigeminal neuralgia. Because the latter occurs only in the older age group (patients are almost always over the age of 50), one should suspect multiple sclerosis if it develops in a younger person. There is a reported association between trigeminal neuralgia and diabetes.

Trigeminal neuralgia is the commonest of the classic neuralgias. It is more common in women and, for some reason, on the right side of the face. The pain comes on in paroxysms; individual jabs of pain last only seconds, but a paroxysm may last for up to 15 or 20 minutes. These attacks of "lightning" pain may recur daily or several times a month. Patients are pain-free between the paroxysms. Over half of the cases will have remissions of 6 months or longer during the course of the disorder.

The term *tic doloureux* refers to the grimace that is often made with each jab of pain. Patients usually recognize trigger points, stimulation of which will precipitate the pain. These are commonly over the malar area, at the base of the nose, or along the gums. Because of aggravation of the pain with eating or chewing, many patients fast when a bout develops. The facial pain rarely occurs on both sides and never affects both sides at the same time, a useful point in differentiating it from other types of pain that may spread to the other side of the face; any pain that crosses the midline warrants a different diagnosis.

The differential diagnosis includes a number of disorders that cause sudden jabbing pain in the side of the face, but these can usually be eliminated by a careful history and examination. There may be confusion over pain from dental problems or from those arising from the nasal sinuses. Costen's syndrome, caused by a disorder of the TMJ, can cause jabbing pain that radiates into the face; however, this can be differentiated by tenderness in the TMJ and by the dull aching pain remaining in the background when the jabs have gone. In trigeminal neuralgia there is no pain at all between the paroxysms. Another confusing disorder is *cluster headache,* not because it is very similar but because this very severe, localized eye and head pain is often unrecognized, whereas everybody knows about trigeminal neuralgia and physicians tend to make the more familiar diagnosis. Herpes zoster will eventually show the typical skin vesicles, and one can establish the diagnosis of glossopharyngeal neuralgia by spraying the tonsillar region with local anesthetic, which should abolish the pain for a period. If one does find neurologic signs, such as loss of sensation over the face or weakness of the masseter or temporalis muscles, one must consider a compressive lesion of the trigeminal nerve. The muscle contraction headaches that refer from the occipital region are often felt as a pressing ache behind the eyes, which draws attention away from the cervical muscles where the problem originates. The distribution of atypical facial pain is often over the central part of the face, quite unlike that seen with trigeminal neuralgia.

Treatment of all of the classic neuralgias is started with oral carbamazepine, a drug that gives excellent results in most patients in a dosage slowly increasing from 100 mg twice a day to a maximum of 1 gm daily.[1] In most patients the result is so dramatic within hours that it almost serves as a diagnostic test. However, about 20% of the elderly have side effects such as ataxia, drowsiness, and confusion and cannot tolerate the drug. Marrow depression has also been recorded, although rarely. Before carbamazepine was available, about half of the patients responded to oral diphenylhydantoin. If the patient does not respond to these agents, then baclofen or clonazepam are often helpful in controlling the pain. Recent publications have suggested some newer agents may also be beneficial, including misoprostol, gabapentin, and lamotrigine.

The pain may also be relieved by radiofrequency heating, glycerol injection, or ultrasonic lesions of the trigeminal rootlets in the posterior fossa. These techniques are about 90% effective, although they may have to be repeated. A few patients still complain of pain in a totally anesthetic area even after nerve block or surgical section (anesthesia dolorosa). Trigeminal root section was once performed, but now more selective lesions can be placed and such an approach can be considered only in patients who do not respond to drugs.

Based on the observation that many patients have V nerve irritation from the pulsation of an artery abutting the nerve, a very successful surgical treatment has been to separate the two using a small sponge during open operation. The drawback is that this involves a major operation. Although it provides excellent relief with less sensory loss than the radiofrequency or injection techniques, most patients prefer to try the latter first.

Glossopharyngeal neuralgia. Glossopharyngeal neuralgia is characterized by paroxysmal bursts of sharp, stabbing pain localized to the region of the ear, throat, tongue, and jaw. It is much less common than trigeminal neuralgia and may be bilateral. The trigger zones are usually in the tonsillar area, tongue, or external auditory meatus so the patient may precipitate the pain by swallowing, talking, yawning, or placing a finger in his ear. There is no neurologic deficit on examination.

This is the only neuralgia that is a significant hazard to the life of the patient. Because the glossopharyngeal nerve innervates the carotid sinus, syncope, convulsions, or even cardiac arrest can occur as a result of the paroxysmal discharge. Atropine prevents bradycardia and hypotension but does not affect the pain. Dehydration and wasting are also significant problems in the patient who is unwilling to swallow because he or she knows that it may lead to agony.

Spraying local anesthetic onto the tonsillar region and the posterior pharynx is a useful way of differentiating this disorder from trigeminal neuralgia. Glossopharyngeal neuralgia occasionally results from tumors, aneurysms, or systemic inflammatory disease affecting the nerve. The drug treatment is the same as that for trigeminal neuralgia; if it fails, intracranial section of the nerve proximal to the ganglion is required.

Minor Neuralgias

Occipital neuralgia. There is some confusion between occipital neuralgia and muscle contraction headache caused by tension or cervical spondylosis as both can produce long-lasting pain over the back of the neck and occiput with radiation bifrontally. In the more usual presentations of occipital neuralgia, however, sharp lancinating pains occur in the occipital region only, and tapping over the nerve (exactly half way between the mastoid process and the cervical spinous processes) causes a paroxysm of pain. Relief can be obtained by injecting the nerve with procaine and hydrocortisone; if this is only effective for a short time, than an alcohol block can be done, or the nerve can be sectioned.

Geniculate neuralgia. Geniculate neuralgia, a neuralgia of the sensory portion of the VII nerve, results in lancinating pain around the ear, sometimes radiating to the external ear, the mastoid region, the soft palate, or the neck. The explanation for these areas of radiation is probably based on central connections between the V, VI, and IX nerves in the spinal nucleus and tract. The cause is seldom determined; the pain usually responds to carbamazepine.

Vagal neuralgia. Vagal neuralgia may occur in the territory of the superior laryngeal nerve, causing unilateral neck pain aggravated by movements of the neck and by swallowing or speaking. The paroxysmal pain radiates from the side of the larynx up behind the ear to the gums, or even down over the shoulder and breast. Most patients are female and middle-aged or older. Many have a trigger point near the pyriform fossa. Massage of the neck may relieve the neuralgia temporarily, but carbamazepine is of more lasting value.

Postherpetic neuralgia. Herpes zoster may cause two painful facial syndromes. The first is the Ramsay Hunt syndrome, characterized by pain in or behind the ear associated with herpetic vesicles in the external auditory meatus or throat. There may be weakness or paralysis of the masseter or facial muscles and decreased salivation on that side. Sometimes vesicles can also be seen over the eardrum, tongue, uvula, or external ear, or in the auditory canal.

The second syndrome is herpes zoster ophthalmicus with supraorbital neuralgia. This results in a severe, burning, aching, or stabbing pain around and above the eye; often it becomes a long-lasting pain syndrome. One often sees cutaneous scarring, redness, or edema around the eye and there is often hyperesthesia in that area. Corneal ulceration with infection can result in blindness.

Only 2% of patients with ophthalmic herpes get this type of neuralgia, but the incidence increases with age. Treatment is unsatisfactory, but the pain spontaneously improves after 2 years. Acyclovir has been found effective for treatment of the acute-stage pain; it hastens healing but has no effect on the incidence of postherpetic neuralgia. Famciclovir may also be beneficial. Some patients respond to massage of the area, to the use of a vibrator, or to spraying ethyl chloride locally, particularly if done frequently to start with and then daily, protecting the eye while spraying. Tricyclic drugs such as amitriptyline are the most helpful agents of all. Nortriptyline has the same analgesic action as amitriptyline but with less sedative effect. Avulsion of the supraorbital nerve or undercutting of the skin of the area may give relief if all else fails.

Referred Facial Pain. Pain felt in the face may originate from the eye, ear, nose, throat, teeth, sinuses, TMJs, heart, or muscles of the head and neck. Patients often feel that any pain in the face originates in their teeth or sinuses. If it is around their eyes, they will initially have their eyes tested, and it is all too common for patients presenting with specific facial pain syndromes to have bought an expensive pair of glasses, had their sinuses drained and a few teeth removed, and invested in a new set of dentures. The cosmetic results are excellent but the analgesic results poor.

One common form of referred facial pain is that resulting from TMJ disorders. Pain from the joint caused by excessive biting, malocclusion, or arthritis is referred to the frontal and parietal areas of the skull or to the face. The patient may relate the pain to the ear and often experiences sharp pains radiating toward the jaw and tongue. The mechanism in most cases is that of chronic jaw clenching caused by tension and anxiety, and often a self-perpetuating spasm of the muscles of mastication occurs. Many of these patients have bruxism (nocturnal tooth-grinding), suggesting an underlying chronic tension state.

On examination, there is tenderness anterior to the ear over the TMJ, and one may feel crepitus on mouth opening. Jaw opening is often limited and closure is asymmetric. The discomfort can be relieved by putting a tongue depressor between the back teeth and asking the patient to bite gently on it, which removes pressure from the joint. The existence of this syndrome has been questioned; it has been suggested that it represents a watered-down version of atypical facial pain (see below), and it often responds to tricyclic drugs.

The eyes are not a common source of pain in the face despite common opinion. An exception is probably glaucoma, which can cause severe pain around the eye. Sinusitis as a cause of facial pain is attested to by television commercials, but it is rare. Otitis is another cause, particularly in the young. Angina pectoris is an unusual cause of facial pain. Cardiac pain is usually referred from the chest to the jaw region but we have seen some patients with angina complaining of pain in the anterior face or posteriorly as far as the ear.

Atypical Facial Pain. Atypical facial pain syndrome is characterized by a constant aching, throbbing, or burning in the facial region. It may be mild or severe and is often experienced bilaterally. The pain may spread over the scalp, neck, and even to the shoulder or arm. It is often worse at night. There are usually no trigger zones, and examination shows no sensory loss nor any other neurologic abnormalities.

The syndrome is usually seen in middle-aged women and is aggravated or precipitated by illness, surgical procedures, social problems, or depression of mood. By the time such patients reach the neurologist, they are usually truly depressed and it is important to recognize this emotional component of the disease. Psychiatric evaluation and social assessment are both important.

Treatment consists of tricyclic drugs and supportive psychotherapy. Carbamazepine is not of value, and surgery is unhelpful.

FACIAL NUMBNESS

Any complaint of continuous numbness of the face should raise concern. Although patients who are depressed may have this symptom and it may occur in migraine, most cases of persisting facial numbness are due to an underlying structural disease process, usually situated in the brainstem or in the V nerve itself and seldom cortical. The major differentiation between brainstem and V nerve lesions is difficult, but if all three modalities (pain, temperature, and touch) are involved, this suggests a nerve lesion, whereas if there is dissociation of sensation a brainstem lesion may be suspected. If all three divisions of the nerve are involved, again the lesion is likely to be either in the cranial cavity as the nerve leaves the brainstem and runs toward the gasserian ganglion or in the ganglion itself. A lesion that is more distal will affect only one of its three divisions. Such a lesion is usually at the cerebellopontine angle but may be a primary or secondary tumor at the base of the skull or, rarely, a pontine glioma. In the case of basal skull tumors, the mandibular division may also be involved, causing weakness of the masseter, temporalis, and pterygoids on that side. Complaints of numbness of the chin mandate a search for malignancy.

Cerebellopontine angle tumors usually cause complaints of sensorineural hearing loss and tinnitus. Headache, vertigo, balance and gait disturbance, facial numbness, pain, and weakness are less common symptoms. Examination reveals involvement of the auditory or cochlear branches of the VIII nerve and a decreased corneal reflex. Other evidence of V or VII damage occurs in about half of the cases seen, and cerebellar signs occur in over half. Evidence of raised intracranial pressure, corticospinal tract involvement, and VI cranial nerve involvement is less commonly found. It is interesting that facial pain is an unusual finding with compression of the V nerve by a tumor or aneurysm.

In perhaps a fifth of the patients no cause is ever found. Such patients are described as having trigeminal sensory neuropathy of benign type because it may clear spontaneously. Pain is sometimes felt by these patients but it is seldom, if ever, an initial symptom. The corneal reflex is frequently retained and there is no motor weakness.

About 10% of patients with facial numbness have multiple sclerosis, diagnosed on the basis of the later appearance of signs of involvement of other areas of the nervous system. Other conditions, accounting for some 20% of cases, include viral encephalitis of the brainstem, presenting as an acute illness with involvement of the V and often also of the VI and VII nerves and signs of meningeal irritation; dental and facial trauma; chronic pansinusitis; and, rarely, such conditions as basal meningitis, syringobulbia, peripheral neuropathy, collagen-vascular disease, and the rare neuroma of the gasserian ganglion.

Therefore a patient who is seen with clinical evidence of V nerve sensory involvement must be examined carefully to see whether he or she has dissociated sensory loss, and whether one, two, or three divisions of the nerve are involved (with or without additional motor involvement). The corneal reflex must be tested with great care.

Investigation should include radiographs of the skull base, nasopharynx, and internal auditory meatus, and CT or MRI scans of the posterior fossa. Serologic tests for syphilis and lumbar puncture may be necessary because demonstration of a raised level of protein, IgG, or cells in the cerebrospinal fluid will assist diagnosis. An electromyographic (EMG) study of brainstem reflexes may confirm involvement of the ophthalmic division of the V nerve and may also indicate damage to the VII nerve. Brainstem evoked potentials will be of value in cerebellopontine angle tumors, and if there is any doubt about the diagnosis an ear, nose, and throat specialist should be asked to examine the posterior nasal space. Only if all of these investigations are negative can an exclusion diagnosis of benign trigeminal neuropathy be made and the patient observed for recovery over the course of the ensuing months or years.

REFERENCES

1. Tenser RB: Trigeminal neuralgia: mechanisms of treatment, *Neurology* 51:17-19, 1998.

ADDITIONAL READINGS

Fromm GH, Sessle BJ: *Trigeminal neuralgia*, London, 1990, Butterworth-Heinemann. 1990.

Mamdani FS: Pharmacologic management of herpes zoster and postherpetic neuralgia, *Can Fam Phys* 40:321-332, 1994.

Spruance SL: Bell's palsy and herpes simplex virus, *Ann Int Med* 120:1045-1046, 1994.

Taha JM, Tew JM: Treatment of trigeminal neuralgia by percutaneous radiofrequency rhizotomy, *Neurosurg Clin North Am* 8:31-39, 1997.

Watson CPN: Nortriptyline versus amitriptyline in postherpetic neuralgia: a randomized trial, *Neurology* 51:1166-1171, 1998.

CHAPTER 163

Movement Disorders

Nagagopal Venna

This chapter is devoted to disorders characterized by excessive abnormal involuntary movements (Box 163-1). Parkinson's disease and related conditions are discussed elsewhere. Recent advances in molecular genetics, neuropharmacology, and stereotactic neurosurgery have invigorated this long-neglected area of neurology, as evidenced by the emergence of movement disorder clinics worldwide. The biologic substrate of the various hyperkinetic movement disorders is not well understood. Current evidence suggests that perturbations in the complex neural networks of the basal ganglia, subthalamic nuclei, inferior olivary nuclei of the medulla, and dentate nuclei of the cerebellum, driven by neurochemical imbalances, underlie these disorders, which are illustrated in video demonstration on the CD-rom published with this edition.

TREMORS

Tremors are rhythmic, involuntary oscillations of body parts caused by abnormal synchronous or alternating contractions of antagonistic muscles. They are common manifestations of many neurologic and systemic diseases (Box 163-2).[6] Tremors can be focal or multifocal and usually affect the hands, head, lips, jaw, and tongue but only infrequently involve the legs and trunk. They may occur at rest or only on maintaining certain postures or with certain voluntary movements and cease during sleep. Tremors are sources of social embarrassment and occasionally are incapacitating. Their clinical characteristics and other abnormalities accompanying them, such as rigidity or ataxia, help determine the nature and etiology of the tremor.

Box 163-1. A Clinical Classification of Hyperkinetic Disorders

- Tremors
  - Enhanced physiologic tremors
  - Essential tremor
  - Tremors caused by focal or multifocal brain disorders (multiple sclerosis, stroke)
- Dyskinesia
  - Chorea, choreoathetosis
  - Hemiballismus
  - Tardive dyskinesias
- Dystonia
  - Focal
  - Segmental
  - Hemidystonia
  - Generalized dystonia
- Mixed movement disorders
  - Wilson's disease

Enhanced Physiologic Tremor

The normal oscillations of voluntarily moving body parts cause a fine 8 to 12 Hz tremor, becoming clinically noticeable when exaggerated by toxic and metabolic causes and drug and alcohol withdrawal states (Box 163-3). The tremor is brought on by holding the arms outstretched with fingers extended and stops when limbs are at rest. The tremor has small amplitude and is most prominent in the fingers. A history of drug and alcohol use, a review of current medications, and, in the appropriate clinical context, laboratory tests for hyperthyroidism, hypoglycemia, and pheochromocytoma help in determining the etiology. Drug and alcohol withdrawal tremors are transient. Toxic tremors usually resolve after decreasing or stopping the drug, although they may be persistent in the case of lithium and amiodarone. Anxiety-related tremors in musicians and other performers may be suppressed by propranolol, 20 to 40 mg taken 1½ hours before a performance. Similarly, tremor of thyrotoxicosis is lessened by propranolol as antithyroid drugs take hold.

Box 163-2. Clinical Classification of Tremors

- Enhanced physiologic tremors
  - Metabolic causes
  - Toxic causes
  - Drug and alcohol withdrawal states
- Essential tremor
- Tremors as part of specific neurologic diseases
  - Parkinson's disease
  - Cerebellar disease (multiple sclerosis)
  - Wilson's disease
  - Rare cases of peripheral neuropathy

Box 163-3. Causes of Enhanced Physiologic Tremor

- Anxiety, fear, stage or performance fright
- Fatigue from exercise
- Hypoglycemia
- Hyperthyroidism
- Pheochromocytoma
- Related to drugs and alcohol
  - Alcohol withdrawal
  - Beta adrenergic drugs (Terbutaline)
  - Valproate
  - Lithium
  - Methylxanthines (caffeine theophylline)
  - Tricyclic antidepressants
  - Hormonal drugs (thyroid supplements and adrenocorticosteroids)
  - Metrizamide used as contrast agent
  - Amiodarone
  - Cyclosporine

Essential Tremor

A community-based study from Canada showed prevalence of 14% for essential tremor (ET) in persons over the age of 65 years compared with a rate of 3% for Parkinson's disease. Onset peaks in the second and fifth decades, and in about 30% of patients it is inherited as an autosomal dominant trait. The etiology of ET is unknown. Brain imaging and pathologic studies are normal, but positron emission tomography (PET) studies reveal hypermetabolism in the cerebellum, red nuclei, and thalamic and inferior olivary nuclei. These studies, and tremor suppression by thalamic stimulation, suggest a putative deep-brain pacemaker for the generation of the tremor. Tremor appears in the fingers and hands while holding a posture or with other voluntary movements. Using utensils or drinking from a cup brings on the tremor, and writing becomes distorted. Tremor may spread to the head as a side-to-side nod and to the jaw, tongue, and voice, but lower limbs are rarely affected. When arms are held outstretched, adduction and abduction, flexion and extension of fingers, and less often, pronation and supination of forearm emerge. A writing sample and copy of a spiral are an easy way of monitoring the tremor. In contrast to Parkinson's disease, there is no rigidity, bradykinesia, or postural instability. In some, the tremor is markedly decreased by even small amounts of alcohol. The diagnosis of ET is clinical, and neuroimaging is not indicated. ET as a risk factor for Parkinson's disease remains unproven although they often coexist.

Reassurance that the tremor is not caused by Parkinson's disease often suffices for patients with mild tremor. When it interferes with social, occupational, recreational, or day-to-day activities, moderately effective treatment is available (Box 163-4).[1] Over 25 randomized, placebo-controlled studies have established propranolol as the most effective treatment to decrease the amplitude of the tremor of the hands and tongue in about 50% to 60% of the patients. From 20 to 40 mg of propranolol 1½ hours before a social gathering, professional meeting, or public performance may be adequate in some cases. For continuous suppression, propranolol, titrated from 60 mg up to 320 mg/day, either in single dose of the long-acting preparation or in three divided doses, is recommended. Tolerance does not develop in long-term use. Metoprolol and nadolol have been shown to be effective in one controlled study each. They are indicated when propranolol is effective but not tolerated because of adverse side effects or asthma. Metoprolol, 100 to 200 mg/day in

Box 163-4. Treatments for Essential Tremor

- Beta-adrenergic blocking drugs
  - Propranolol
  - Metoprolol
  - Nadolol
  - Primidone
  - Clonazepam
- Botulinum toxin injection
- Stereotactic thalamic stimulation

divided doses, is relatively safe despite bronchospasm. Nadolol has the advantage of once-a-day dosing at 120 to 240 mg. Incidentally, atenolol is ineffective and pindolol may worsen ET. After a serendipitous observation in a patient with epilepsy and ET, long-term efficacy of primidone, a barbiturate antiseizure drug, has been confirmed in several controlled trials and is similar in magnitude to propranolol. It is started at a dosage of 25 mg at bedtime and increased gradually up to 250 to 750 mg/day in three doses to minimize early drowsiness and ataxia. Severe ET may need combinations of primidone and propranolol. An uncontrolled study demonstrated marked benefit from clonazepam in a subset of ET predominantly seen with goal-directed movement (kinetic tremor). In one placebo-controlled study, alprazolam improved ET in 24 patients at doses of 0.75 mg to 2.75 mg/day. One well-designed study showed no benefit from gabapentin. A good short-term study showed that theophylline was as effective as propranolol. A recent double-blind study confirmed modest reduction of ET of the hand with minor finger weakness after forearm intramuscular injection of botulinum toxin. The benefit lasted up to 12 weeks after each injection. Another study of botulinum injections in 43 patients showed benefit in head tremor, a component of ET less responsive to propranolol. Several small series have demonstrated significant amelioration of contralateral hand tremor and improvement in disability with a recently FDA-approved treatment by stereotactically implanted electrical stimulator in the thalamus, comparable to the benefit in Parkinson's disease tremor, in selected incapacitating cases.

CHOREA AND CHOREOATHETOSIS

Chorea and choreoathetosis are involuntary movements caused by dysfunction of the networks of the caudate nuclei and putamen, resulting in excessive dopaminergic and decreased inhibitory γ-aminobutyric acid (GABA) neurotransmitter function. Many brain diseases, as well as systemic and toxic factors, can induce choreoathetosis (Box 163-5).[5] In chorea, movements are quick, brief, nonrhythmic, and usually affect the proximal parts of the limbs, although the head, neck, and trunk may also be involved. Movements are often incorporated into voluntary activity to mask them, as in brushing the hair when the arm jerks. Axial chorea causes lurching gait. Limbs may be hypotonic, with pendular tendon reflexes best seen at the knees. Voluntary movements, although strong, may be unsustained. When a patient grips the examiner's fingers, intermittent give in the grip feels like milking movements ("milk maid grip"). Athetosis causes slow, writhing, twisting movements, most evident in hands and feet, although the trunk can be affected. Frequently there is a mixture of chorea and athetosis (choreoathetosis). Like most hyperkinetic movements, these are increased by anxiety, fatigue, and stress, decreased by relaxation, and cease in sleep.

Drug-induced Choreoathetosis

Many drugs induce reversible choreoathetosis (Box 163-6).[3] A few drugs cause chorea regularly, whereas with most it is a rare side affect. Levodopa is a common cause of choreoathetosis when used to treat advanced Parkinson's disease, and cocaine is an under-recognized cause of chorea ("crack dance"). With some drugs there is an underlying individual susceptibility for chorea. Oral contraceptive drugs cause chorea, particularly in women with a history of rheumatic fever, chorea gravidarum, systemic lupus erythematosus (SLE), and the antiphospholipid antibody syndrome. Phenytoin brings out choreoathetosis in persons with cerebral palsy.

Chorea Caused by Systemic Disease

Choreoathetosis is the most frequent movement disorder in systemic diseases (Box 163-7).[5] About 4% of patients with SLE develop chorea in the course of known disease or as a presenting symptom. The abnormal movements may last a few days to as long as 3 years and may remit and relapse, with relapses usually coinciding with systemic flare-up of SLE.

Box 163-5. Causes of Choreoathetosis

- Drugs and toxins
- Systemic diseases
  - Systemic lupus erythematosus
  - Polycythemia
  - Thyrotoxicosis
  - Rheumatic fever
  - Cirrhosis of the liver (acquired hepatocerebral degeneration)
  - Diabetes mellitus
  - Wilson's disease
- Primary degenerative brain diseases
  - Huntington's chorea
  - Olivopontocerebellar atrophies
  - Neuroacanthocytosis
- Focal brain diseases
  - Hemichorea
  - Stroke
  - Tumor
  - Arteriovenous malformation

Box 163-6. Drug-induced Choreoathetosis

- Parkinson's disease drugs
  - Levodopa
- Epilepsy drugs
  - Phenytoin
  - Carbamazepine
  - Phenobarbital
  - Gabapentin
  - Valproate
- Psychostimulant drugs
  - Cocaine
  - Amphetamine
  - Methamphetamine
  - Dextroamphetamine
  - Methylphenidate
  - Pemoline
- Psychotropic drugs
  - Lithium
  - Tricyclic antidepressant drugs
- Oral contraceptive drugs
- Cimetidine

Magnetic resonance imaging (MRI) scans of the brain may be normal or show nonspecific change. Some patients with SLE and chorea have antiphospholipid antibodies and are at risk for arterial and venous thrombosis, including cerebral infarction. Microvasculopathy or antineuronal cytotoxic autoantibodies are proposed pathogenic mechanisms. Treatment is with prednisone for lupus activity and haloperidol for chorea. Chorea is a feature of the recently recognized primary antiphospholipid antibody syndrome, especially with use of oral contraceptives or pregnancy. Thyrotoxicosis presenting with chorea in young women has long been recognized and may remit and relapse with the hyperthyroidism and responds to dopamine-blocking haloperidol. Excess exogenous thyroxine can provoke chorea. Paroxysmal unilateral or generalized choreoathetosis has been reported with idiopathic hypoparathyroidism and is reversed by correcting the hypocalcemia. Polycythemia vera is a well-documented cause of buccolingual and limb choreoathetosis, principally in women over the age of 50 years. The chorea may last weeks to years and fluctuate, with no clear relations to hematocrit level, although treatment of the polycythemia does ameliorate the chorea. Chorea caused by rheumatic fever (Sydenham's chorea) is still prevalent outside the United States and Western Europe. Generalized chorea develops in about 20% of children with rheumatic fever, often as a presenting symptom and mostly in girls. Encephalopathy with emotional lability is a common accompaniment. In 75% of the patients the movements remit spontaneously in about 6 months, but about 20% have recurrences. Oral contraceptives and pregnancy may induce relapse even several years after the rheumatic fever. MRI scans may show reversible abnormalities in the caudate, putamen, and globus pallidus. The chorea is probably caused by autoantibodies provoked by the streptococcal infection cross reacting with caudate neurons. Haloperidol and valproic acid help control the chorea as natural remission occurs over several months. Diabetic nonketotic hyperglycemia is recently recognized as a cause of acute hemibody chorea, sometimes with hemiballismus, in women over the age of 50. MRI scans show abnormalities in the contralateral striatum consistent with petechial hemorrhages or demyelination. The chorea stops in a few days to a month with correction of metabolic derangement and a short course of haloperidol or diazepam.

Paroxysmal Choreoathetosis

Paroxysmal choreoathetosis is a rare episodic disorder that has been better delineated in recent years. In this disorder, bursts of generalized chorea/dystonia lasting minutes, hours, or a few days occur spontaneously or are triggered by sudden or sustained voluntary movements. Most cases are idiopathic or familial but it can be caused by multiple sclerosis, stroke, brain trauma, or encephalitis. Affected persons are often misdiagnosed as psychogenic. Carbamazepine, phenytoin, clonazepam, and acetazolamide reduce the paroxysms in some cases.

Box 163-7. Choreoathetosis in Systemic Diseases

Systemic lupus erythematosus
Primary antiphospholipid antibody syndrome
Hashimoto's thyroiditis–related encephalopathy
Thyrotoxicosis
Hypoparathyroid hypocalcemia
Polycythemia
Rheumatic fever (Sydenham's chorea)

Hemiballismus

Hemiballismus is a dramatic syndrome that usually appears in elderly patients with hypertension and diabetes mellitus as a result of small infarctions or hemorrhages in or around the subthalamic nucleus. Metastases and toxoplasmosis in AIDS are occasional causes. Violent flinging of the limbs on one side, accompanied by continuous hemibody choreoathetosis, appears abruptly. Injuries may occur as the limbs strike surroundings or because of falls. The MRI may show the lesions in the contralateral basal ganglia or subthalamic nucleus. Frail elderly patients become exhausted by the incessant hyperactivity, which abates only in sleep. Stroke-related hemiballismus gradually subsides within a few weeks to a few months. Dopamine-blocking haloperidol and GABA-ergic clonazepam ameliorate the movements in most cases and can be synergistic. Valproic acid and progabide, both GABA-ergic drugs, may also be helpful. The rare refractory hemiballismus cases may benefit from stereotactic pallidotomy.

Huntington's Chorea

Huntington's chorea is an autosomal dominant neurologic disease caused by mutation of a gene on chromosome 4 with expansion to above 40 CAG triplets coding for glutamine. By unknown mechanisms, this causes a progressive loss of GABA-ergic and substance P interneurons of the striatum. A combination of involuntary movements and neuropsychiatric changes appears insidiously and worsens steadily. Onset is in the fourth and fifth decades, with an incidence of 2 to 7/100,000. Chorea of the face, tongue, head and neck, trunk, and limbs is the dominant symptom, accompanied by lurching gait and early impairment of voluntary eye saccades. Irritability, paranoia, and antisocial behavior are common and occur early, followed by cognitive deterioration. Depression and suicide are prevalent. Rigidity and bradykinesia eventually supervene. Diagnosis is based on the clinical picture and family history and is supported on MRI scans by selective atrophy of the heads of caudate nuclei and confirmed by DNA testing. Unfortunately there is no specific treatment. Chorea, when functionally disabling, can be improved by dopamine blockers such as haloperidol, low-dose dopamine agonist bromocriptine, or benzodiazepines such as clonazepam. Depression and the commonly observed obsessive-compulsive behaviors may respond to serotoninergic drugs such as fluoxetine.

TARDIVE DYSKINESIA

Tardive dyskinesia (TD) has emerged as a common hyperkinetic syndrome with the widespread use of antipsychotic dopamine-blocking drugs (Box 163-8).[8] Most patients with TD have schizophrenia but it can develop in patients with depression or anxiety. Approximately 20% of patients on chronic treatment with antipsychotic drugs develop TD, but prevalence is as high as 36% in institutionalized patients. Risk factors for TD are age over 40 years, high dose, early

Box 163-8. Drugs Associated With Tardive Dyskinesia

Neuroleptic drugs (conventional)
- Haloperidol
- Chlorpromazine
- Thioridazine
- Fluphenazine
- Perphenazine
- Trifluoperazine
- Thiothixene

Nonneuroleptic drugs causing tardive dyskinesia

Anti-emetics
- Metoclopramide
- Prochlorperazine
- Promethazine

Calcium channel blockers
- Flunarizine
- Cinnarizine

Cardiac antiarrhythmic drugs
- Flecainide

Sympathomimetic drugs
- Clenbuterol

occurrence of drug-induced Parkinson's disease, and female gender. Routine chronic use of anticholinergic drugs to offset drug-induced parkinsonism and diabetes mellitus are other predisposing factors.

Clinical experience shows that TD is rare with the new atypical antipsychotic drugs such as clozapine, although long-term observation is needed to confirm this. TD is increasingly reported with chronic use of drugs to treat nausea, gastroesophageal reflux, and gastroparesis of diabetes. Certain calcium channel blockers with dopamine agonist properties are also implicated. Drugs with high incidence of TD block the D2 receptors almost exclusively, whereas the new atypical antipsychotics cause more equal D2 and D1 receptor blockade, suggesting the possible pathogenesis.

Restless protrusions and twisting movements of the tongue, smacking and puckering of lips, and chewing movements appear insidiously and progress to increased blinking and blepharospasm. Movements become continuous and stereotyped. Hyperkinesia spreads to limbs, causing abrupt jerky movements, piano-playing hand movements, and foot tapping. Pelvic thrusts and grinding movements may appear. Some patients develop breathing dyskinesias that cause grunting, sighing, irregular noisy breaths, shortness of breath, and even respiratory alkalosis. Persistent TD can cause abrasions of the lips and tongue; truncal dyskinesia can cause sacral ulcers and exhaustion. Diagnosis is clinical in the context of chronic antipsychotic drug treatment. In persons not currently on these drugs, careful inquiry into recent or remote exposure should be made. In patients without psychiatric history, exposure to drugs such as metoclopramide should be sought. In the absence of such drug exposure, other causes of choreoathetosis, such as Huntington's disease, need to be considered. If the neuroleptics are continued, TD is likely to persist indefinitely, or worsen, but may rarely improve (17%). When the drug is stopped, however, most patients get better in the long term, despite a temporary

Box 163-9. Treatment of Tardive Dyskinesia

Switching drug to clozapine

Dopamine-depleting drugs
- Reserpine (1 to 8 mg/day)
- Tetrabenzine (25 to 150 mg/day)

GABA-enhancing drugs
- Clonazepam (1 to 4 mg/day)
- Valproate
- Vigabatrin
- Baclofen

Antioxidants
- Vitamin E 800 IU/bid

Presynaptic DA autoreceptor stimulators
- Low-dose bromocriptine

increase in the dyskinesia. Remission of TD may occur in 30% to 60% of patients by 5 years, but in some TD has been permanent. The smallest effective dosage for the shortest possible time and periodic reevaluation of the need to continue the drugs are prudent. If TD does emerge, decreasing the dose or discontinuation of drug should be considered whenever feasible. For patients with moderate to severe disability, switching to clozapine—the atypical antipsychotic—has been effective both for the psychosis and for TD, based on several large series and several case reports, in doses of 200 mg/day to 900 mg/day (Box 163-9).

DYSTONIA

Dystonia is the least common but the most disabling of the hyperkinetic movement disorders. It is defined by twisting involuntary movements and abnormal postures. The biologic substrate of most forms of dystonia is poorly understood, but hypofunction of the medial globus pallidus and thalamus appears to be a common theme. Major advances in molecular genetics and neurochemistry, highlighted by the recent discovery of L-dopa–responsive dystonia, new therapies with botulinum toxin, and deep brain stimulation are driving the resurgence of interest in these disorders.

Acute Dystonic Reaction

Acute dystonic reaction is an alarming syndrome that is commonly seen in psychiatric practice and affects 2% to 12% of patients taking neuroleptics. Less well recognized is its occurrence with drugs used to treat nausea and migraine (Box 163-10). Acute blockade of dopamine receptors (D2 type) and relative hyperactivity in the cholinergic environment of the basal ganglia appear to mediate the abnormal movements. The greatest risk of this reaction is with high doses of high-potency neuroleptics. Young age, male gender, previous reactions, cocaine addiction, and dementia related to acquired immunodeficiency syndrome (AIDS) are other risk factors. In over 90% of cases dystonia occurs within 5 days. With sumatriptan, used for migraine, it may appear within 3 to 6 hours.

The movements are acute, dramatic, and often bizarre and are likely to be mistaken for hysterical behavior. Blepharospasm, forced eye deviation (oculogyric crisis), torticollis or

Box 163-10. Drugs Causing Acute Dystonia

Psychotropic drugs
Dopamine receptor-blocking antipsychotics
- Phenothiazines
- Haloperidol

Serotonin agonist anxiolytic
- Buspirone

Dopamine receptor-blocking drugs used to treat nausea/migraine
- Metoclopramide
- Prochlorperazine
- Domperidone
- Sulpiride

Serotonin agonists in migraine
- Sumatriptan

retrocollis, trismus, slurred speech, and even opisthotonus may occur. Rarely, laryngeal and pharyngeal spasms may cause difficulty with breathing. Anxiety is a common accompaniment. Even though the dystonia is self limited, it can recur for several days after withdrawal of the causative drug. Treatment with anticholinergic medications such as benztropine or diphenhydramine or with a benzodiazepine such as lorazepam quickly arrests the dystonia (Box 163-11). The treatment should be continued orally for several days to prevent recurrences. Exceptionally, laryngeal/pharyngeal dystonia requires repeated intravenous medications, close monitoring of breathing, and, rarely, tracheal intubation. Subsequently, decrease of the dose of the drug or replacement with a lower-potency neuroleptic is needed.

Generalized Chronic Dystonia

The striking clinical syndromes of generalized chronic dystonia (Box 163-12) present with contortions of the limbs, head, neck, and trunk and disintegration of voluntary movements by the dystonia. Many begin in the limbs and eventually become generalized. Despite grossly normal strength and sensation the patients often eventually become chair or bedbound, with difficulty in speech and swallowing. In Rochester, Minnesota, the incidence is estimated to be 2 per million per year.

Drug-induced Chronic Tardive Dystonia

Chronic treatment with commonly used dopamine receptor-blocking neuroleptic drugs can result in a generalized dystonia with opisthotonus, retrocollis, and oromandibular dystonia. Despite discontinuation of the drugs, movements persist for a long time. This disorder is about one tenth as common as TD and tends to affect young adults in particular. The clinical picture may be readily mistaken for primary generalized dystonias. Treatment consists of decreasing the dose or discontinuing the neuroleptic drug whenever feasible and treating the residual dystonia symptomatically (Box 163-13). Clozapine, the new antipsychotic drug, may also alleviate TD.

Generalized dystonia is common in congenital encephalopathy caused by perinatal trauma, or cerebral palsy. Dystonia appears in early childhood and may worsen over the years. History of difficult birth, floppy baby syndrome, or delayed developmental milestones indicates the diagnosis. The treatment is symptomatic. Primary generalized dystonias, whether sporadic or inherited, have a similar clinical picture. The vast majority of these belong to Oppenheim type DYT-1, an autosomal dominantly inherited dystonia (dystonia musculorum deformans) prevalent in Ashkenazi Jews. Recent

Box 163-11. Treatment of Acute Dystonic Reaction

Anticholinergics
- Benztropine 2 mg intramuscularly (IM) or intravenously (IV)
- Diphenhydramine 50 mg IM or IV
- Benzodiazepines
- Lorazepam 1 mg IM or IV
- Diazepam 5 to 10 mg IM or IV

Oral therapy continued for a few days to prevent recurrences

Box 163-12. Etiology of Chronic Generalized Dystonia

Symptomatic dystonia
- Drug induced: Neuroleptics (conventional)

Congenital static encephalopathies (cerebral palsy)
- Kernicterus
- Perinatal brain injury

Dystonia as part of multisystem neurologic syndrome
- Wilson's disease
- Neuroacanthocytosis
- Olivopontocerebellar atrophy
- Hallerverden-Spatz disease
- Non-Wilsonian hepatocerebral degeneration

Primary dystonia
- Sporadic (idiopathic torsion dystonia)

Inherited dystonia
- Oppenheim's (classic, DYT-1) L-dopa–responsive dystonia (DYT-5)

Box 163-13. Symptomatic Treatment for Generalized Dystonia

Withdrawal of neuroleptic drugs
Trial of L-dopa/decarboxylase inhibitor
Anticholinergic drugs (trihexyphenidyl)
Benzodiazepines
Baclofen: oral or intrathecal infusion pump
Botulinum injection
Pallidotomy (globus pallidus)
Deep brain electrical stimulation
Supportive/physical therapy

studies have identified the abnormal gene on chromosome 9 and the gene product as torsin-A, similar to heat shock proteins and proteases. The mechanism by which the gene lesion causes dystonia is not known. Dystonia frequently begins in the legs and becomes generalized over a few years. Intelligence is unaffected. The disease can be identified by family history and confirmed by DNA testing. No specific treatment is available but significant advances have occurred in the symptomatic treatment (Box 163-13).

L-Dopa Responsive Dystonia (Segawa Disease, DYT-5)

The identification of a generalized dystonia relieved by L-dopa has been the most dramatic recent discovery in the field of dystonia. Symptoms appear in childhood with toe walking, foot and leg dystonia, and disturbed gait, and slowly spread to the upper limbs and trunk. Bradykinesia and rigidity are often superimposed. The lower limb dystonia may be nearly absent in the morning but be severe in the evening and with exercise. Many are misdiagnosed as having static cerebral palsy. The condition is inherited as an autosomal dominant trait caused by a mutant gene on chromosome 14 encoding an enzyme needed for the synthesis of biopterin, a cofactor for tyrosine hydroxylase required for dopamine synthesis. The result is severe deficiency of dopamine in the striatum. Striking reversal of the dystonia by L-dopa is a defining feature.[7] Because of atypical presentations, a therapeutic trial of L-dopa is worthwhile in any dystonia of uncertain etiology.

Chronic Focal Dystonia

Torticollis (Cervical Dystonia). Torticollis is the most common focal dystonia of adults, with an incidence of about 24/1 million/year as estimated in Rochester, Minnesota. Most cases are idiopathic and monosymptomatic, with a presumed neurophysiologic perturbation in the basal ganglia and upper brainstem. It typically begins as intermittent torticollis between 30 and 50 years of age and slowly becomes continuous. Only about 10% of patients have remissions, but relapse is the rule. Forceful rotation of the neck to one side is the chief symptom. Characteristically, this is temporarily relieved by sensory tricks such as supporting the back of the head on a wall, touching the chin, or lying down. Dystonia ceases in sleep and worsens with stress. After years of dystonia, cervical spondylosis and radiculopathy may develop, with neck and arm pain. Rarely, hypertrophy of the trapezius can cause thoracic outlet neurovascular compression. Lateral bending and retrocollis are less common. Diagnosis is clinical, and brain imaging is normal. Initially, drug-induced and other symptomatic dystonias should be considered. Rarely, pseudotorticollis occurs because of structural disorders of the neck (Box 163-14).

Before botulinum toxin treatment, high doses of anticholinergic drugs were the mainstay of treatment for torticollis and were unsatisfactory. The symptomatic treatment of torticollis has been dramatically improved with the use of botulinum toxin injections into the dystonic muscles and is now the treatment of choice except in the mildest cases.[4] The toxin acts on the intramuscular nerve ending, causing presynaptic blockade of acetylcholine release (chemical denervation). Numerous open-label and double-blind controlled trials have established the efficacy and safety of botulinum toxin for cervical dystonia. About 80% of patients experience major relief lasting about 3 months, but repeated injections over many years continue to provide benefit. In the few patients not responding to botulinum, selective peripheral surgical denervation can be helpful by sectioning the spinal accessory nerve branch to the sternomastoid muscle. Support through dystonia organizations is also very helpful in coping with such a chronic and disfiguring condition (website *www.wemove.org*).

Box 163-14. Causes of Pseudotorticollis

- Peritonsillar abscess
- Trochlear nerve palsy
- Acute labyrinthitis
- Atlantoaxial subluxation
- Cervical syringomyelia
- Klippel-Feil syndrome
- Dystonic seizures with head turning

COMPLEX HYPERKINETIC MOVEMENT DISORDERS

Wilson's Disease

Many varieties of abnormal movements occur in Wilson's disease, singly in the beginning and in complex combinations later. It should be considered in the diagnosis of any movement disorder of uncertain cause (Box 163-15). This rare but global autosomal recessive genetic disease is caused by heterogeneous mutations of a gene on chromosome 13. Copper deposition is most dense in the putamen, but many other basal ganglia and the cerebellum are affected by copper-induced neuronal destruction years after copper overload of the liver.

Neurologic symptoms begin in childhood to about age 50, with or without overt liver disease. Combinations of chorea, dyskinesia, dystonia, and tremor occur, along with bradykinesia and rigidity. Dystonia of face and bulbar muscles is early, with distortion of facial expression, dysarthria, and drooling. A proximal, postural tremor of the arms ("wing-beating" tremor) is characteristic. Neuropsychiatric symptoms range from subtle alteration, with irritability and impaired social judgment, to aggressive behavior and cognitive decline. Syndromes resembling manic-depression and schizophrenia may be seen. Over 90% of cases of Wilson's disease with neurologic abnormalities have diagnostically critical Kayser-Fleischer rings. In about 40% of cases they are grossly visible as golden brown rings around the corneal limbus, but slit-lamp examination is the most sensitive method of detection. MRI scans show nonspecific abnormal signals in the putamen, caudate, and white matter. Diagnosis is confirmed by a battery of tests of copper metabolism, with a serum ceruloplasmin level of less than 20 mg/dl, free serum copper of more than 8 μmol/L, and liver copper of over 250 μg/g of dry weight.

Treatment early in the course of neurologic symptoms can reverse brain dysfunction in 20% of cases and produce marked improvements in about 60% (Box 163-16).[2] Early diagnosis is critical to preserve and restore brain function.

Box 163-15. Complex Hyperkinetic Movement Disorders

Wilson's disease
Olivopontocerebellar atrophy
Neuroacanthocytosis
Ataxia/telangiectasia

Box 163-16. Treatment of Wilson's Disease

Copper chelation
- D-Penicillamine
- Trientine

Reduction of intestinal absorption of copper
- Zinc

Orthotopic liver transplantation
Symptomatic treatment
- L-dopa, dopamine agonists
- Amantadine

Treatment is best done by specialists in this disease because of its rarity and complexity. In several cases of advanced disease, liver transplantation produced sustained dramatic improvement of cerebral function.

REFERENCES

1. Bain PG: The effectiveness of treatments for essential tremor, *The Neurologist* 3:305-321, 1997.
2. Brewer GJ: Practical recommendations and new therapies for Wilson's disease, *Drugs* 50:240-269, 1995.
3. Diedrich NJ, Goetz CG: Drug-induced movement disorders, *Neurol Clin* 16:125-139, 1998.
4. Jankovic J, Brin MF: Therapeutic uses of botulinum toxin, *N Engl J Med* 324:1186-1194, 1991.
5. Jonvas JL, Aminoff MJ: Dystonia and chorea in acquired systemic disorders, *J Neurol Neurosurg Psychiatry* 65:436-445, 1998.
6. Koller WC: Diagnosis and treatment of tremor, *Neurol Clin* 2:499-514, 1992.
7. Nygaarad TG, Marsden CD, Fahn S: L-Dopa responsive dystonia: long term treatment, response and prognosis, *Neurology* 41:174-181, 1991.
8. Trugman JM: Tardive dyskinesia: diagnosis, pathogenesis and treatment, *The Neurologist* 4:180-187, 1998.

RESOURCES

Patient support group website: *www.wemove.org*

Tremors

The International Tremor Foundation
833 West Washington Blvd.
Chicago, IL 06607
312-733-1893

Tardive Dyskinesia

Tardive Dyskinesia/Tardive Dystonia National Association
PO Box 45732
Seattle, WA 45732
206-522-3166
e-mail: Skaertd/tdna@aolnet.com

Huntington's Disease

Huntington Disease Society of America
158 W. 29th Street
7th Floor
New York, NY 10001
800-345-4372
Website: *http://hdsa.mgh.harvard.edu*

Dystonia

Dystonia Medical Research Foundation
1 E. Wacher Drive
Suite 2430
Chicago, IL 60601-1905
800-377-3978
Website: *http://www.dystoniafoundation.org*

Torticollis

National Spasmodic Torticollis Association
PO Box 5849
Orange, CA 92863-5849
800-487-8385
Website: *http://www.blueheronweb.com.nsta/NSTA/htm*

Wilson's Disease

Wilson's Disease Association
4 Navaho Drive
Brookfield, CT 0680
800-399-0266
e-mail: Stork#2@aol.com

Physician Website

www.movementdisorders.org

CHAPTER 164

Stroke

William Pryse-Phillips
T. Jock Murray

A stroke is a focal neurologic disorder that develops acutely because of a pathologic process affecting the blood vessels that results in ischemic damage to cells. Strokes are the third most common cause of death in our population (10.6% of deaths), with an annual incidence of about 200 cases per 100,000 population. Death caused by stroke is only one aspect of the problem, however, as a disturbing number of stroke patients survive but are severely disabled. These are people who were frequently quite well until the moment they were stricken. About 20% of them have their first stroke between the ages of 45 and 65 years.

CEREBROVASCULAR FLOW DYNAMICS

There are a few basic concepts important in understanding the dynamics of cerebrovascular disease. We stress the term

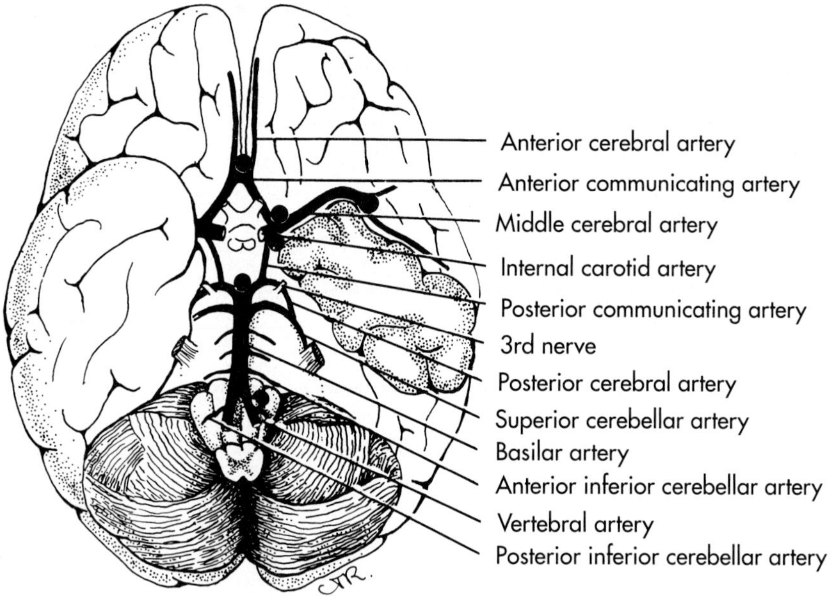

Fig. 164-1. Location of major arteries as seen from the base of the brain. The illustration also demonstrates the most common location of congenital aneurysms.

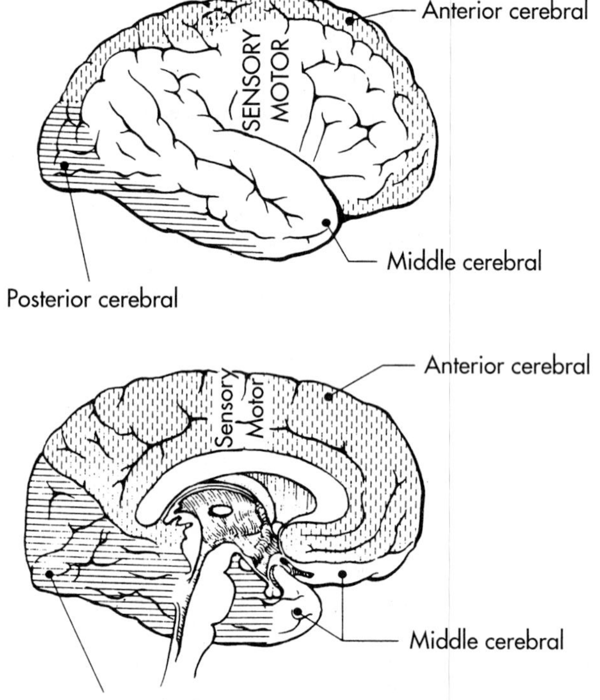

Fig. 164-2. Major vascular supply to brain. (From Barsan WG, Kothari R: Stroke. In Rosen P, et al: *Emergency medicine: concepts and clinical practice,* ed 4, St. Louis, 1998, Mosby.)

dynamics because the older idea that the brain is supplied by a number of end-arteries is incorrect. Three factors that must be considered in understanding cerebral blood supply are the anatomy of the cerebral circulation, cerebral blood flow, and collateral blood supply.

Anatomy of the Cerebral Circulation

Two systems supply the brain—the carotid and the vertebrobasilar—connected by the circle of Willis. The textbook picture of this anastomotic circle is unusual because congenital variations are seen in perhaps 85% of people. The circle may not be complete, or some of its major vessels may be absent or extremely small. The normal anatomy will not be considered here, but the major arteries are shown in Fig. 164-1.

Collateral Supply

Many collateral vessels connect the major arteries (anterior, middle, and posterior cerebral and vertebrobasilar system) supplying the cerebrum and brainstem (Fig. 164-2). The circle of Willis acts as a collateral connection between the carotid and vertebrobasilar systems and the other collaterals connect the extracranial with the intracranial vessels.

The branches of the major intracerebral vessels form an extensive collateral bed. Thus despite occlusion of a middle cerebral (MCA) and the posterior cerebral (PCA) arteries, blood supply to much of their territories may yet be maintained through their collateral connections. As a result, most infarctions do not exactly demarcate the anatomic distribution of a vessel involved. Occasionally this anastomotic area between two cerebral arteries (the "watershed") is the site of infarction when both vessels are partially occluded and this border zone becomes ischemic.

An occlusion of a major intracerebral artery may be compensated for by redirection of the blood flow within the circle of Willis. For example, one anterior cerebral artery can be supplied from the other side through the anterior communicating artery.

Extracranial anastomoses can also supply intracranial structures. Carotid occlusion seldom causes blindness on that side because of the collateral connections between the external carotid and the ophthalmic arteries. The meningeal, occipital, thyrocervical, costocervical, and caroticotympanic arteries can reverse their flow and dilate, thus supplying the brain if an appropriate vessel obstruction has occurred.

This potentially extensive collateral system can come into play almost immediately, which explains many peculiarities about strokes, such as why they do *not* occur in some situations. The efficiency of the collaterals depends on the following:

- *Their anatomy.* Some congenital anomalies remove potential collateral patterns. Thus agenesis of the posterior communicating artery will make infarction of the occipital lobe on that side more likely if there is an occlusion of the vertebrobasilar system. If the posterior communicating artery is not functioning, the carotid system cannot deliver blood back to that side.
- *The cross-sectional area of the lumina of the collateral supply.* If the total area is equal to that of the occluded vessel, then the anastomoses will probably be adequate.
- *The location of the collateral vessels.* If the site of anastomosis is nearer to the heart and proximal to the occlusion, it tends to be more efficient. This of course depends on the number of anastomotic channels.
- *The general state of the vascular system.* Atherosclerotic lesions, for example, will impair the potential for the opening of collaterals.
- *Timing.* A sudden occlusion will allow little time for the collateral circulation to adapt to the altered flow patterns, whereas gradual occlusions can be compensated for by an efficient collateral circulation, with perhaps little or no neurologic deficit developing.

Cerebral Blood Flow

The cerebral vessels differ from those in the periphery. The sympathetic fibers anatomically present appear to have little functional significance except perhaps to regulate blood pressure effects in the larger vessels around the circle of Willis. The control of cerebral blood flow depends mainly on autoregulation, an intrinsic mechanism regulating vessel diameter, to keep cerebral blood flow constant in spite of a variety of anatomic and metabolic variations. Thus if blood pressure is reduced, dilation of the cerebral vessels occurs to maintain blood flow at a constant rate. Conversely, as in hypertension, cerebrovascular constriction keeps flow constant. Only in extreme situations do the vessels fail to compensate, allowing cerebral blood flow to fall.

Cerebral blood flow is, however, dramatically changed by altering the arterial CO_2 content, CO_2 being the most powerful cerebral vasodilator known. An increase in arterial oxygen tension causes vasoconstriction, as does alkalosis, but these factors and blood pressure are both weak in comparison to the effect of carbon dioxide. Drugs have little effect on cerebral blood flow. Intracranial pressure, sleep, the pH level of cerebrospinal fluid (CSF), and body temperature also have little effect in comparison.

Ischemia inhibits the process of *cerebral autoregulation,* and the presence of collaterals cannot compensate. Autoregulation may also be lost if there is a fall in diastolic blood pressure below 50 mm Hg or a rise above 150 mm Hg in the area of a cerebral infarction, or when there is severe vascular disease, such as widespread atherosclerosis or intracranial arteritis. When autoregulation fails, the cerebral blood flow has a linear relationship to the blood pressure. Elderly patients tend to lose some of this autoregulatory compensation and so are abnormally prone to the effects of hypotension and hypertension.

CLASSIFICATION OF STROKE

When considering the pathologic basis for strokes, the first essential differentiation to be made is between ischemic infarction and hemorrhage. (Sometimes, however, these occur together, as when spasm of cerebral vessels occurs distal to the site of a ruptured aneurysm that has produced hemorrhage; the spasm itself may produce ischemia and perhaps infarction.) The following four classes of ischemic stroke are defined according to their time-line and severity:

- *Transient ischemic attack (TIA).* Brief ischemia, most often caused by an embolus, producing focal symptoms and signs lasting (quite arbitrarily) less than 24 hours (and usually less than 6 minutes)
- *Reversible ischemic neurologic deficit (RIND).* The same as TIA, except that the signs persist for longer than 24 hours but less than 7 days before full clinical recovery occurs
- *Evolving stroke.* The term used for ischemic or hemorrhagic stroke that worsens under clinical scrutiny, usually in a step-wise fashion
- *Completed stroke.* An ischemic or a hemorrhagic stroke that has caused a maximal deficit and that may now start to show improvement

The lesion causing *cerebral ischemia* may be within the vessel (embolus), in the wall (e.g., spasm, arteritis, or atherosclerosis), or entirely extracranial (hypoxemia or reduced cardiac output). Anoxia may produce relatively minor, transient symptoms and signs, or it may lead to infarction, an irreversible state of ischemic damage from which the brain cells cannot completely recover.

Intracranial hemorrhage may occur because of rupture of either of the smallest vessels deep in the substance of the brain or of an aneurysm, which is usually situated at the base of the brain and close to the circle of Willis. Less common causes of hemorrhage are bleeding from an arteriovenous malformation (AVM) or hemorrhagic infarction resulting from an embolus. These are intracerebral, but extracerebral bleeding can also occur (e.g., subdural or extradural hemorrhages).

The relative frequency of *ischemic strokes* (thrombotic or embolic) and of the various types of cerebral hemorrhage is in some dispute. For many years, thrombosis was considered to be by far the most common cause; for instance, the middle cerebral artery syndrome was thought to be due to occlusion of the MCA, until it was shown that almost half of these patients had a significant thrombotic lesion in a large vessel in the neck, usually in the internal carotid artery. We now recognize that emboli from these sites rather than decreased blood flow because of arterial narrowing or occlusion are the commonest cause of TIAs and strokes. The heart is also important in the pathogenesis of stroke, either because an arrhythmia reduces flow or as a result of cardiac emboli, as has been made plain by long-term cardiac monitoring and telemetry. In many cases of cerebral infarction in which no significant arterial disease is found at autopsy, there is evidence of a cardiac origin of an embolism unsuspected in life; this probably accounts for the strokes that previously had been ascribed to arterial spasm or hypotension. It seems that "atherosclerotic occlusive thrombosis," a time-honored diagnosis in clinical neurology, might actually be quite unusual.

Although the syndrome of MCA infarction is the most common clinical stroke pattern, only 4% of cases can be shown at autopsy to have an actual occlusion of that vessel, embolism from the internal carotid artery or from cardiac lesions being much more common. Interest in the pathogenesis of stroke has therefore shifted outside of the head to the large vessels in the neck and to the cardiovascular system.

PATHOGENESIS OF STROKES
Thrombosis and Embolism

Atheromatous occlusion of the great vessels in the neck is more common at sites of bifurcation or change in course of the vessels (Fig. 164-3). Thus the origins of the innominate, carotid, subclavian, and vertebral arteries; the bifurcations of the carotid arteries; and the more tortuous portions of the cerebral and carotid arteries are the major sites of atherosclerotic plaques, ulcers, and stenosis. Exposed collagen at these sites causes platelets to adhere to the wall because of a difference in electrical charge. These platelets release ADP, which results in their aggregation and the formation of a friable platelet thrombus that may either increase in size, ultimately occluding the vessel, or may break up to form emboli.

Cerebral emboli are usually composed of platelets, fibrin, cholesterol, and atheromatous material from ulcerated plaques if they arise from extracranial vessels. Emboli arising from the other sites listed in Box 164-1 are rare, in comparison. Except for infective emboli, which may produce a mycotic aneurysm, the clinical features of all emboli are more or less similar. These will be discussed in the next section.

Emboli may cause either transient ischemia in an area of brain, or infarction. If the blood supply is reinstituted by the opening of collateral vessels, or if the emboli break up, allowing blood to flow again, then the ischemia is transient and function is restored; in many instances emboli are completely asymptomatic.

Atherosclerosis is primarily a disorder of larger arteries. It is unusual to find typical changes of the condition more distal than the major branches of the arteries arising from the circle of Willis. This is in contrast with the vascular changes typical of hypertension, which are primarily found in arterioles.

Risk Factors. The risk factors that predispose to the development of atherosclerosis in the cerebrovascular system are essentially the same as those for coronary and peripheral vascular disease (see Boxes 164-2 and 164-3). Virtually all can be treated. The most important include hypertension (both systolic and diastolic), hyperlipidemia, and diabetes. Obesity, ischemic heart disease, peripheral vascular disease, and (in younger people) oral contraceptives, migraine, cardiac lesions, and aneurysms are also important. Smoking and hyperlipidemia seem to pre dispose to ischemic heart disease. In the case of cerebral emboli, atrial fibrillation (from any cause), cardiomyopathy, valve prostheses, recent myocardial infarcts, and prolapsed mitral valve are the major risk factors.

TIAs are usually embolic, but other mechanisms can also produce brief ischemia. These include vascular spasm in migraine and severe hypertension and severe generalized reduction in cerebral blood flow caused by cardiac arrhythmias or hypotension. Ischemia is particularly likely to occur if there is any preexisting obstruction in the cerebral vessels. Ischemia may also occur when an obstruction causes blood flow to be "stolen" from another area. A classic example of this is the *subclavian steal syndrome.* To compensate for stenosis or occlusion of the first part of a subclavian artery, blood is diverted from one vertebral artery down the other one so it supplies the occluded subclavian at a point distal to the obstruction and prevents the normal flow of blood from the healthy vertebral artery into the basilar artery. Ischemia can also result from polycythemia because of slowed circulation or occlusion caused by the sludging effect of high-viscosity blood, or from marked anemia or vasculitis.

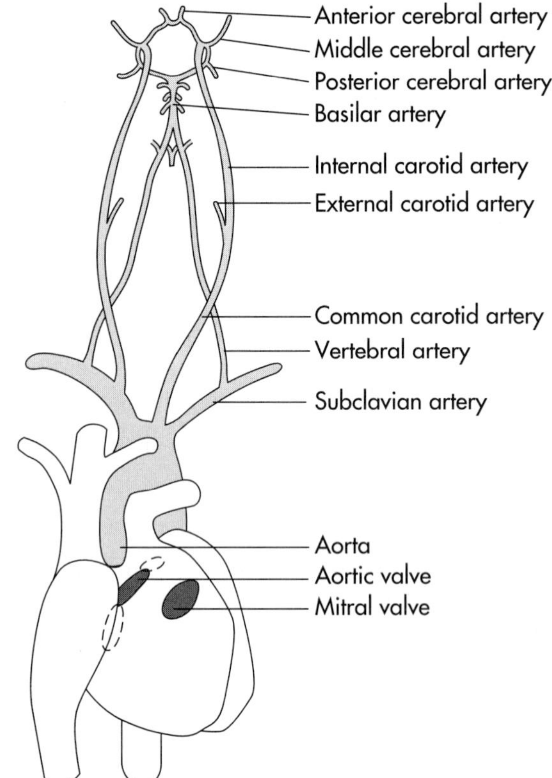

Fig. 164-3. Common sites of atheromatous stenosis or ulceration in the neck vessels. (From Pryse-Phillips W, Murray TJ: *Essential neurology: a concise textbook,* ed 4, New York, 1992, Medical Examination Publishing.)

Box 164-1. Origins of Cerebral Emboli

Cardiac
- Atrial fibrillation
- Mural thrombi after myocardial infarction
- Acute and subacute bacterial endocarditis
- Aortic and mitral valve disease; prolapsing mitral valve
- Nonbacterial thrombotic endocarditis
- Paradoxical embolism
- Complications of cardiac surgery and prosthetic valves
- Atrial myxoma

Noncardiac
- Atheroma of aorta, carotids, and vertebrals
- Atheroma of largest intracranial vessels
- Pulmonary vein thrombi
- Fat emboli
- Tumor emboli
- Air emboli
- Complications of pulmonary and neck surgery

Uncertain

From Pryse-Phillips W, Murray TJ: *Essential neurology: a concise textbook,* ed 4, New York, 1992, Medical Examination Publishing.

Box 164-2. Risk Factors for Stroke

Advanced age
Cardiac disease
Hypertension (diastolic and systolic)
Hyperlipidemia
Diabetes mellitus
Family history of vascular disease
Smoking
Physical inactivity
Oral contraceptive pills
Abnormal electrocardiogram (ECG)
Polycythemia
Severe anemia

From Pryse-Phillips W, Murray TJ: *Essential neurology: a concise textbook*, ed 4, New York, 1992, Medical Examination Publishing.

Box 164-3. Causes of Hemorrhagic Strokes

Intracerebral hemorrhage
- Hypertensive intracerebral hemorrhage
- Trauma
- Hematologic disorders
- Anticoagulant therapy
- Hemorrhage into tumors
- Septic embolism or mycotic aneurysms
- Amyloid angiopathy
- Vasculitis
- Vasopressor drugs
- Encephalitis and postinfectious encephalopathy

Subarachnoid hemorrhage
- Ruptured saccular aneurysm
- Ruptured angioma
- Trauma
- Anticoagulant therapy

From Pryse-Phillips W, Murray TJ: *Essential neurology: a concise textbook*, ed 4, New York, 1992, Medical Examination Publishing.

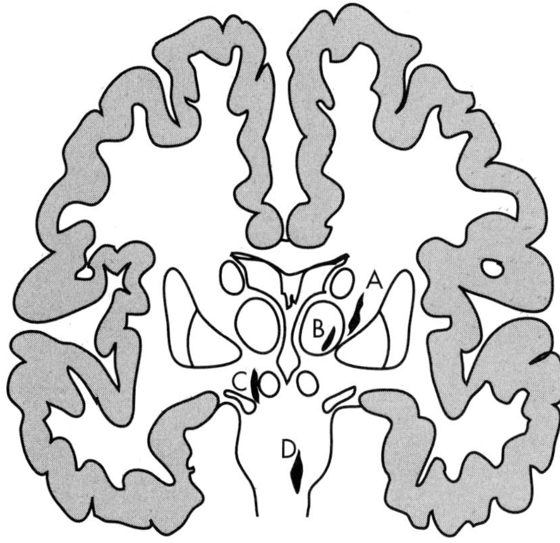

Fig. 164-4. Usual sites of lacunar infarcts in the deep white matter. **A,** Internal capsule/putamen; **B,** Thalamus, **C,** Mesencephalon; **D,** Pons. (From Pryse-Phillips W, Murray TJ: *Essential neurology: a concise textbook*, ed 4, New York, 1992, Medical Examination Publishing.)

Intracranial Hemorrhage

Hypertension has been mentioned as a risk factor in the development of atherosclerosis and of thrombotic or embolic cerebrovascular disease, but it also predisposes to the development of intracranial hemorrhage. In a large majority of cases, one of two pathologic lesions is present. In the first, fibrinoid necrosis of arterioles deep in the white matter causes weakening of the arteriolar wall, with the production of tiny aneurysms bound by glial tissue (Charcot-Bouchard aneurysms). With continuing arteriolar damage and disruption of its muscular coat, further weakening of the wall may lead to hemorrhage that cannot be prevented by arteriolar constriction. The severity of a hemorrhage is widely variable. On the one hand, there may be no more than a few milliliters of blood released, splitting local white-matter fibers and producing a smaller area of local damage. Later, a small cavity may result called a *lacune*. If the hemorrhage is more severe it will act as a quickly expanding mass lesion, producing compressive brain destruction (Fig. 164-4). The blood will track further afield and often enters the CSF or the ventricles. The sudden hemorrhagic mass lesion produces widespread pressure increase that may compress the brainstem structures, causing hemorrhages in the pons (Duret hemorrhages). Most intracranial hemorrhages occur in the deep white matter of the brain, both they and the small lacunae being found in the putamen, the internal capsule, the corona radiata, and in the pons and deep white matter of the cerebellum.

The second major disorder causing intracerebral hemorrhage is a *ruptured aneurysm*. An aneurysm is a dilation of an artery, varying from a few millimeters to 2 or 3 cm in diameter. They occur at the bifurcation of a vessel where the media is weakest. In the presence of hypertension, raised pressure produces dilation at these sites, and in time ruptures the aneurysm, with bleeding into the subarachnoid space and often into the brain itself. Local vascular spasm caused both by vessel rupture and the presence of blood in the subarachnoid space results in further widespread vasospasm, increasing the risk of brain damage from ischemia. Thus, although the bleeding may remain within the subarachnoid space, a pale infarct in the distribution of the vessel intracerebrally may also be caused (Fig. 164-5).

The other causes of intracranial hemorrhage listed in Box 164-3 are comparatively rare. About 90% of subarachnoid hemorrhages are due to ruptured berry aneurysms. For more complete lists of causes see Boxes 164-1, 164-2, and 164-4. Only the more common among these pathologies will be described here.

CLINICAL ISCHEMIC STROKE SYNDROMES

Transient Ischemic Attacks

TIAs are brief, transient, focal disturbances of neurologic function that clear without significant residual deficit within 24 hours. We have not been as strict in this definition as some authors (who regard any mild residual deficit after 24 hours as representing a cerebral infarction rather than a TIA), because

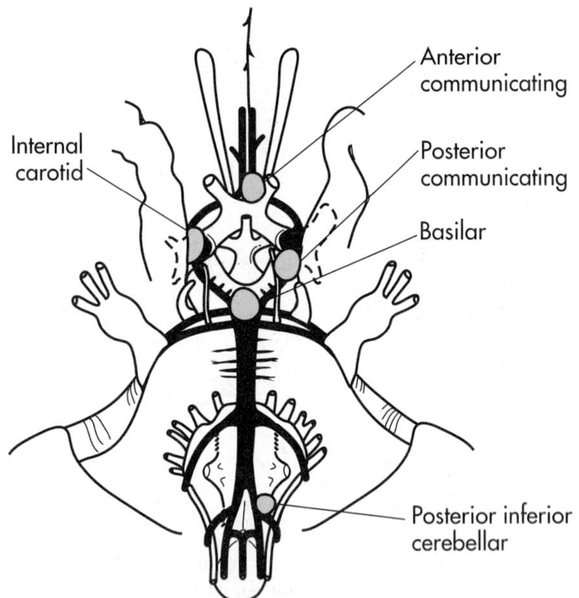

Fig. 164-5. Common sites of aneurysm formation at base of the brain. All but mycotic aneurysms tend to occur on the vessels of the circle of Willis or before the second branch of the vessels arising from it. (From Pryse-Phillips W, Murray TJ: *Essential neurology: a concise textbook,* ed 4, New York, 1992, Medical Examination Publishing.)

Box 164-4. Causes of Transient Cerebral Ischemia

Emboli (see Box 164-1)
- Cardiac origin
- Noncardiac origin
- Uncertain origin

Carotid artery stenosis or occlusion
Subclavian steal syndrome
Polycythemia, anemia
Carotid sinus sensitivity
Hypertensive crises
Other causes of syncope
Migraine
Cerebral hypoperfusion (cardiac failure, acute hypovolemia, abnormal blood viscosity, or coagulability)

From Pryse-Phillips W, Murray TJ: *Essential neurology: a concise textbook,* ed 4, New York, 1992, Medical Examination Publishing.

our management of the patients with minimal deficit is the same as that for those with TIAs.

TIAs used to be referred to as *"little strokes,"* but they are harbingers of more serious ones. A careful history in stroke patients will elicit evidence of previous transient disturbances of function in about half of the cases. If a group of patients who have had TIAs is followed long term, 5% to 10% each year will have a major infarction or die; the greatest risk is in the 3 months after the first TIA. Overall, a patient has about a 40% chance of a major cerebral infarction within 5 years.*

Clinical Features. Symptoms associated with TIA may involve either the carotid or the vertebrobasilar system. Typical symptoms in the carotid territory include *amaurosis fugax,* a monocular visual disturbance consisting of abrupt, painless loss of function, "like a curtain being drawn" over part of the visual field, reaching maximum deficit within minutes or less, and clearing progressively over minutes or hours. During this period a pale embolus may be visible in a retinal arteriole.

Other classic symptoms of TIA include the following:
- Monoparesis, hemiparesis, or clumsiness of one limb
- Numbness, loss of sensation, or paresthesias involving one or both limbs on one side
- Dysphasia
- Homonymous hemianopia
- Ipsilateral blurring of vision

Vertebrobasilar TIAs usually present with multiple symptoms; it is unwise to diagnose vertebrobasilar disease when only one is present. Vertebrobasilar symptoms include the following:
- Numbness, loss of sensation, or weakness involving one or both sides of the face, arm, or leg
- Complete or partial loss of vision in both eyes, often with vertigo or dizziness
- Homonymous hemianopia
- Diplopia
- Ataxia, imbalance, or staggering
- Drop attacks (sudden collapse with loss of muscle tone but without prolonged loss of consciousness, though brief unconsciousness can occur)
- Transient amnesic attacks
- Alternating hemiplegia (involvement of the face on one side and the arm and leg on the other)

Although in perhaps 40% of cases the attacks stop spontaneously, the chances of stroke are still high and an aggressive attitude toward therapy is warranted. The various causes of TIAs are shown in Box 164-4. All of the pathologies that may lead to TIAs should be considered, as should the conditions that may masquerade as them, before a diagnosis of TIA caused by platelet embolism is made (Box 164-5).

An atherosclerotic basis is suspected if there is evidence of vascular disease elsewhere, such as intermittent claudication, angina, or a history of myocardial infarction. The physician should also look for atherosclerotic changes in the fundi, an absence of peripheral pulses, and hypertension. The presence of a number of the risk factors mentioned earlier should also point in this direction. A bruit may be heard, localized to the carotid bifurcation in the neck, but this is an overrated sign of carotid vascular disease; many patients with carotid stenosis do not have a bruit, because occluded carotid vessels are silent, and because people can have bruits of no significance.

Embolic and Thrombotic Infarction

Embolic and thrombotic infarctions are together known as *atherothrombotic brain infarcts* and are classed together here, first because a clinical differentiation is often impossible, second because both are often operational in a patient, and

*Actually, the major cause of death is not a stroke but a myocardial infarction (MI), which affects 20% of patients with TIA within 5 years. In fact, a TIA is a better predictor of MI than is angina.

Box 164-5. Leading Causes of Transient Neurologic Dysfunction

Migraine
Transient ischemic attacks (see Box 164-4)
Seizures
Acute hyperventilation syndromes
Cerebral tumor or subdural hematoma
Multiple sclerosis
Hypoglycemia
Labyrinthine vertigo including Ménière's syndrome
Cataplexy
Leaking intracranial aneurysm or arteriovenous malformation
Ingested drugs or toxic agents

From Pryse-Phillips W, Murray TJ: *Essential neurology: a concise textbook,* ed 4, New York, 1992, Medical Examination Publishing.

Box 164-6. Causes of Cerebral Infarction

Atherosclerosis
Arteritis
- Infections (syphilis, meningitis)
- Collagen-vascular diseases (cranial arteritis, lupus)

Hematologic disorders
- Polycythemia
- Sickle-cell disease
- Thrombotic thrombocytopenia
- Macroglobulinemias

Trauma to the carotid artery
Complications of angiography
Dissecting aortic aneurysm
Hypotension
Migraine (vasoconstrictive phase)
Hypoxia
Radiation
Closed head injury

From Pryse-Phillips W, Murray TJ: *Essential neurology: a concise textbook,* ed 4, New York, 1992, Medical Examination Publishing.

last because thrombotic strokes are uncommon compared with embolic strokes (Box 164-6).

Clinical Features. In acute infarction the onset may be sudden, progressive over a short period of hours, or step-wise over a day or more. A history of TIAs can be elicited in half of the cases.

Most patients are over 55 years old, but strokes can occur at any age. There is frequently evidence of atherosclerotic disease in the peripheral or cardiac vessels by history or examination, and risk factors may be expected.

Many of these patients do not lose consciousness unless the brainstem reticular activating system is involved, but drowsiness, confusion, or stupor is common if strokes involve large areas or cause a rise in intracranial pressure. Typically the patient suffers the event during the night and awakes with the deficit, whereas intracerebral hemorrhages tend to occur during the day.

The focal abnormalities that result from a stroke depend entirely on which area of the brain has suffered ischemic damage. Some common syndromes are described here but there are many variations on these patterns, and partial syndromes are very common. Remember that an infarction in the distribution of a vessel does not necessarily mean that there is any pathologic process in that vessel itself. The problem is often in the neck vessels or heart, or the ischemia may be due to hemodynamic change from hypotension, cardiac arrhythmia, anemia, or polycythemia.

Carotid Syndromes

Middle Cerebral Territory Infarction. The most common pattern of stroke is a middle cerebral territory infarction. Signs include homonymous hemianopia indicating involvement of the optic radiation. Typically the eyes are deviated *toward* the infarcted hemisphere* and there is lower quadrant facial weakness and a spastic hemiparesis on the opposite side, the arm being involved more than the leg. Tone in the affected limbs may initially be decreased, but spasticity develops over days or weeks. Sometimes the leg has neither significant sensory nor motor involvement and the face and arm are involved in isolation. Hemisensory loss in the face and arm is common on the side opposite the infarction, but the trunk and leg tend to be much less involved. If the dominant hemisphere is involved, an expressive and/or receptive dysphasia may occur, whereas nondominant hemisphere lesions cause a parietal lobe syndrome that includes complex sensory find ings and sensory perceptual difficulties. Right hemisphere lesions often induce a confusional state, and those on the left cause a depressive syndrome in the later stages.

Brain swelling may cause coning and occlusion of one or both PCAs, producing hemianopia or cortical blindness. MCA infarct is illustrated in Fig. 164-6.

With occlusion of the internal carotid artery (ICA) in the neck, the anterior cerebral artery usually gets enough blood from the opposite side through the anterior communicating artery, which prevents infarction in the frontal and medial portions of the hemisphere; the PCA should get an adequate supply from the vertebrobasilar system. Thus carotid occlusion often manifests as an infarction in the territory of the MCA but not in the entire carotid distribution.

Although the presence of a localized bruit over the bifurcation of the carotid may indicate a stenotic lesion, palpation of the vessel is of dubious value because the presence of the external carotid artery (ECA) may allow one to feel a normal pulse in that area. If there is a marked difference in the carotid pulses on the two sides, however, this may indicate common carotid artery occlusion on the side of the reduced pulse. Occlusion of the ICA may be suggested by relatively increased pulses in the facial or superficial temporal vessels on that side because these are branches of the ECA, which is now receiving all the carotid blood supply. This is a difficult judgment to make, however. Orbital bruits may suggest ICA stenosis.

*The pattern is the other way around with brainstem strokes, in which the eyes are deviated away from the side of the infarct (when it is unilateral).

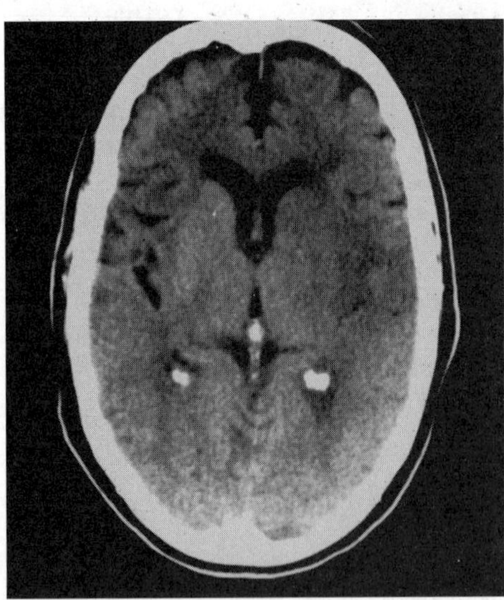

Fig. 164-6. MCA territory infarction. Scan taken shortly after the onset of patient's symptoms demonstrates the following structures are hypodense because of infarction: basal ganglia, insula (loss of insular stripe), and temporal lobe. (From Cwinn AA, Grahovac SZ: *Emergency CT scans of the head: a practical atlas,* St. Louis, 1998, Mosby.)

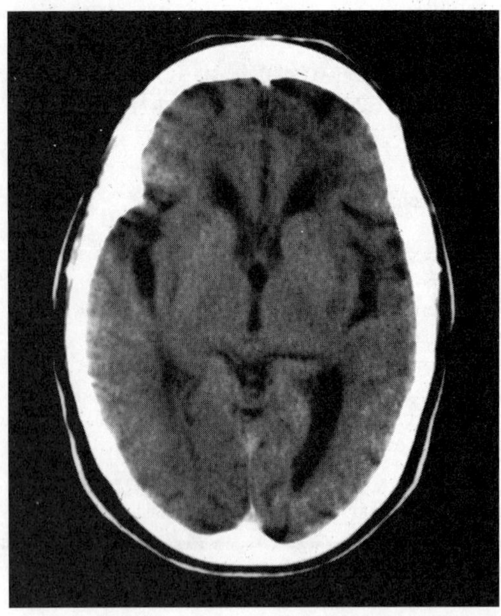

Fig. 164-7. Occipital lobe infarct (posterior cerebral artery territory). Note the large right occipital hypodensity with mass effect caused by infarction. (From Cwinn AA, Grahovac SZ: *Emergency CT scans of the head: a practical atlas,* St. Louis, 1998, Mosby.)

Anterior Cerebral Territory Infarction. Infarction in the anterior cerebral territory is a much less common type of stroke and is characterized by more marked weakness of the leg than of the arm. The face is usually spared, but the patient's head and eyes are deviated toward the infarcted hemisphere. Sensory changes in the leg are minimal or absent. Urinary incontinence and personality changes may develop. If the dominant hemisphere is involved, an expressive dysphasia is common, whereas with the nondominant hemisphere apraxia of the opposite limbs or of all limbs may be found. Occasionally a syndrome suggesting cerebellar disease results from disruption of fibers connecting the frontal lobes to the cerebellum. Incoordination and ataxia on the side opposite the infarction are the chief signs; nystagmus and speech abnormalities are less common than with true cerebellar lesions. Another clue to the frontal localization is the finding of unilateral cerebellar signs on the same side as pyramidal changes.

Cerebral Hypoperfusion. Generalized cerebral hypoperfusion syndromes occur in patients with severe extracranial arterial disease affecting more than one vessel, especially when there is an abrupt reduction in cardiac output and thus of cerebral perfusion pressure. Patients most often complain of light-headedness, imbalance, and weakness of the limbs, and examination reveals such nonspecific findings as poverty of speech, mild dementia, and impaired memory. There is no orthostatic hypotension, but the symptoms improve with recumbency and naturally with restoration of cardiac output. In more severe cases, *watershed infarcts* occur. These comprise 10% of all infarcts and usually are due to an abrupt and severe fall in cerebral perfusion pressure or to ICA occlusion; they lead to ischemia of those parts of the brain situated between the territories of supply of the middle and anterior or middle and posterior cerebral arteries and the subcortical white matter. The most characteristic syndromes include transcortical dysphasia, hemianopia, and sensory or motor deficits.

Vertebrobasilar Syndromes

Posterior Cerebral Territory Infarction. The clinical picture of posterior cerebral territory infarction is variable, depending on whether the infarction occurs in the distal or more proximal distribution of the artery (Fig. 164-7). With a *distal infarct,* a homonymous hemianopia results. If the artery is occluded *proximally* near its origin, then branches to the thalamus and brainstem may be involved, producing a mild hemiparesis and a thalamic syndrome of contralateral sensory loss and pain. In other cases, cerebellar ataxia, receptive dysphasia (if the infarction is on the dominant side), and transient confusion and memory loss are the main features. If ischemia occurs in the territory of *both* posterior cerebral arteries, as from hypotension or basilar artery occlusion, the patients often develop cortical blindness, sometimes with denial (Anton's syndrome) and agitated delirium. Variable visual field defects can be documented as the patient progressively improves.

Brainstem Infarction. The vertebral arteries give rise to the posterior inferior cerebellar arteries, which supply the lateral medulla and inferior cerebellum. Occlusion or ischemia in this area will give rise to a classic *lateral medullary syndrome*. In this syndrome, damage to the inferior cerebellar peduncle produces a homolateral cerebellar ataxia; damage to the nucleus ambiguus causes dysarthria and dysphonia, and involvement of the descending sympathetic fibers causes Horner's syndrome on the same side. The descending nucleus and tract of the V nerve will be involved, producing loss of pinprick and temperature sensation on the same side of the face, whereas involvement of the adjacent ascending lateral spinothalamic tract produces similar findings in the arm, trunk, and leg on the opposite side of the body. Vertigo, caused by ischemia of the vestibular nuclei, and hiccup are also frequent symptoms. Because the pyramidal tracts and the medial lemniscus are centrally placed and are supplied by paramedian branches of the vertebral and basilar arteries, they are not affected in this condition.

Other brainstem ischemic syndromes probably will cause alternating hemiplegia and signs indicating damage to, for example, the reticular activating system (RAS), cerebellum, and sensory tracts, with marked changes in blood pressure, pulse and respiratory rates, and possibly homonymous hemianopia due to PCA occlusion.

Occlusion of the basilar artery is often fatal. Because so many ascending and descending tracts and cranial nerve nuclei are closely applied in a small volume of the brainstem, symptoms and signs will be severe, extensive, and bilateral (although not necessarily symmetric). Involvement of any of the cranial nerves from III to XI, of the cerebellum, of corticospinal and corticobulbar tracts, and of the reticular system is the result. These patients are usually admitted to the hospital in coma and seldom survive.

Vertebrobasilar Insufficiency. The term *vertebrobasilar insufficiency* (VBI) is used for the syndrome of brainstem ischemia caused by generalized decreased perfusion, hypertension or hypotension, atherosclerosis, or steal syndromes. (Cardiac emboli usually land in the carotid territory.) Cervical spondylosis predisposes to VBI by compressing the vertebral arteries as they run through the bony canals of the cervical vertebrae. Symptoms sometimes can be produced by extending or rotating the head and neck to one side or the other; turning the head occludes one vertebral artery even in normal people.

Clinical features. Symptoms of VBI resemble those of TIAs in that territory (see p. 1539). They include nausea and vomiting, vertigo, transient paresthesias in the face or limbs, tinnitus, diplopia, blurring of vision, hemianopia or even total blindness, ataxia, limb weakness, and occipital headache. Transient reduction in consciousness, deafness, and unilateral or bilateral limb weakness are other possible complaints. Typical signs include nystagmus and various other signs of cranial nerve involvement, patchy pyramidal tract signs, and cerebellar incoordination. There may be a subclavian bruit or differences between the systolic blood pressures in the arms of 20 mm Hg or more. In the event of cerebellar infarction, the same symptoms are accompanied by signs of a mass lesion compressing the brainstem and raising intracranial pressure.

The prognosis with small infarctions in the vertebrobasilar territory is better than with those in the carotid territory, and recovery from a mild vertebrobasilar infarction is usually excellent. Angiography is seldom warranted in patients with VBI because surgery in this area is less well developed than in the carotid system and a specific lesion is less often found in this territory; therefore management is seldom altered by the angiographic findings. However, brainstem and cerebellar infarcts are well shown by computed tomography (CT) scans, and surgery may be lifesaving if a swollen, infarcted cerebellum is causing compression of the brainstem.

Spinal Cord Infarction. Thrombosis of the anterior spinal artery is rare and is usually secondary to trauma or cervical spondylosis. Infarctions of the spinal cord are usually caused by global decrease in perfusion pressure, and they usually occur in thoracic regions. Occlusion of a radicular artery by an atherosclerotic plaque, a ruptured intervertebral disk, direct trauma, or (more commonly) by atheroma or aortic aneurysm blocking the supplying arteries as they leave the aorta can cause infarcts at other sites, and infarction can also occur during aortic surgery.

Clinical features. The clinical features of spinal cord infarction indicate involvement of the anterior two thirds of the spinal cord in the distribution of the anterior spinal artery, because the posterior third of the cord is supplied by the two posterior spinal arteries, which have more extensive anastomoses. Damage to the corticospinal tracts produces paraplegia and a spastic bladder. Spinothalamic involvement gives rise to loss of pain and temperature sensation up to the level of the infarction, and damage to the anterior horn cells produces a lower motor neuron lesion with fasciculations at the level of the lesion. Pain is usually not a feature because the posterior sensory roots are supplied by the posterior spinal arteries.

Venous infarcts of the cord occur in patients already predisposed to venous embolism (e.g., in cases involving pregnancy, thrombophlebitis, or polycythemia); spinal pain with sensory and motor long tract signs are characteristic features.

Cerebral Venous Infarction. The major cerebral venous sinuses and veins can become thrombosed, usually due to infection; hemorrhage and edema result from the obstruction to venous outflow from the brain. Cavernous sinus obstruction may cause a distinctive syndrome of chemosis, proptosis, and painful ophthalmoplegia, which can be unilateral or bilateral. With obstruction to other venous sinuses the features may be less specific and the patient may show focal deficits, headache, decreasing consciousness, seizures, and papilledema, and may progress to death. The headache of cerebral venous thrombosis (CVT) is a common feature but varies from a moderate pressure sensation to a severe pain and is usually sensitive to aggravation by coughing or bending. The onset can be sudden or slow over weeks. Suspicion should be raised when the headache is constant and increasing, the patient's condition is worsening, and focal neurologic signs appear. CVT can also present initially with an encephalopathic picture, especially in children and in the elderly and cachectic.

On CT images, the changes may be minimal or nonspecific, but if contrast is used 20% will have features that suggest the diagnosis, such as the "empty delta sign" in the posterior sagittal sinus caused by contrast in the collateral veins in the sinus wall but lack of contrast in the sinus because of clotting. Magnetic resonance imaging (MRI) is more helpful because it will show the thrombus in the sinus and can be used to follow the progress of the condition.

A search for the underlying cause should be made as soon as the diagnosis is made, looking for local infection, trauma, general infection, dehydration, malignancy, and hematologic disorders such as polycythemia, sickle cell disease, and coagulation disorders. The disorder is frequently associated with pregnancy or the use of oral contraceptives. In about 20% of cases no cause will be found.

DIFFERENTIAL DIAGNOSIS OF STROKES

In assessing any acute cerebral catastrophe we must consider the differential diagnosis of ischemic and hemorrhagic strokes from other common nonvascular pathologies that may also cause the sudden appearance of neurologic signs. *Epileptic seizures with Todd's paralysis* are sometimes indistinguishable from strokes when first seen, particularly because emboli and hemorrhages may sometimes present with seizures. *Tumors, cerebral abscesses,* and *extradural* or *subdural hematomas* can all mimic stroke, and one should never assume without question that an elderly patient with the sudden onset of a grave neurologic disorder is necessarily suffering from a stroke. In younger patients, diseases of the arterial wall that are not atherosclerotic (but caused by, for example, *infection, diabetes, dissection of the arterial wall* or *collagen-vascular disease*) also have to be considered.

CLINICAL FEATURES OF HEMORRHAGIC STROKE SYNDROMES

Intracerebral hemorrhages may be small (producing a small lacune) or large (producing a sudden increase in intracranial pressure caused by the enlarging clot, as well as signs of focal brain destruction). Both of these types of hemorrhage are associated with hypertension, which can produce strokes in a number of ways. In malignant hypertension, intracranial arteriospasm and cerebral edema sometimes produce reversible focal and general ischemic damage characterized by decreasing consciousness, seizures, fundal hemorrhages, and papilledema *(hypertensive encephalopathy).* Congenital berry aneurysms bleed when the blood pressure is elevated. Hypertension also accelerates the development of atherosclerosis.

Lacunar Strokes

Lacunar strokes may be the most common vascular lesions occurring in the brain. These small, cystic spaces resulting from healed ischemic infarcts can be found in many routine autopsies, particularly in patients who have had hypertension. They are most commonly located in the thalamus, striatum, internal capsule, and pons and occasionally in the cerebellum and corona radiata. A large majority are asymptomatic, but in about 20% of cases a stroke syndrome occurs. Representative syndromes (from about 20 defined) include the following:

- A *pure motor hemiplegia.* Here the lesion is in the internal capsule or in the base of the pons.
- A *pure hemisensory syndrome.* The lesion is in the ventrolateral nucleus of the thalamus.
- Cerebellar and pyramidal signs occurring together in the same leg (and less obviously in the arm). The lesion involves the superior cerebellar peduncle fibers after they have crossed and the corticospinal fibers at the level of the midbrain.
- A syndrome of slurred speech, facial weakness, and clumsy hand *(dysarthria-clumsy hand syndrome)* caused by a lacune in the base of the pons. Involvement of the face and tongue accounts for the dysarthria, while the clumsy hand is a manifestation of a pyramidal lesion or of a mild cerebellar syndrome.
- Unilateral third nerve palsy with contralateral hemiplegia *(Weber syndrome).*
- Cerebellar ataxia and crossed third nerve palsy *(Claude syndrome).*
- *Hemiballismus* from a lesion in the subthalamic nucleus.
- A *"locked in syndrome"* caused by bilateral lesions of the ventral pons.
- A *"top of the basilar syndrome"* with unilateral or bilateral third nerve palsies, paralysis of downward gaze, and drowsiness caused by infarction in the territory of a penetrating arteriole arising from the distal part of the artery.

These syndromes are relatively mild and often transient; they have a good prognosis, particularly if the patient's blood pressure is controlled in the future. If they are recognized, these syndromes usually do not require extensive investigation because the angiogram is usually normal. CT scans show a small area of infarction in 25% of cases and evidence of bleeding in a few.

Parenchymal Hemorrhage

In contrast to the relatively benign lacunar syndromes, primary hypertensive intracerebral hemorrhage is frequently fatal. In this situation a Charcot-Bouchard aneurysm or a small artery ruptures, causing a fiber-splitting hemorrhage that can be small but is more usually moderate or massive. The intracerebral bleeding stops only when the blood pressure falls, pressure within the clot rises, or vasospasm in the artery prevents further bleeding.

Parenchymal hemorrhage occurs in hypertensive patients in the same sites that lacunar strokes develop (putamen 55%, thalamus 25%, cerebellum 10%, subcortical 10%, pons 7%). The most common area is that supplied by the deep penetrating vessels branching from the MCA around the internal capsule.

Clinical Features. Symptoms of parenchymal hemorrhage are usually severe, with a sudden onset, most often during the day. The deficit is maximal within minutes of the onset of hemorrhage, and the patient often loses consciousness after complaining of a severe headache with nausea and vomiting. This is one of the most common causes of sudden death.

A grand mal seizure may occur, with or without a focal onset. Such a combination of headache and vomiting strongly suggests an intracerebral or a subarachnoid hemorrhage. In those patients who do not immediately lose consciousness, confusion, headache, oculomotor pareses, and hemiparesis are common, as are signs of raised intracranial pressure eventually.

The focal signs that might allow one to localize the lesion are at times clouded by the presence of coma, meningism, or raised intracranial pressure. With hemorrhage into the *putamen,* both eyes deviate conjugately to the side of the cerebral lesion and away from the hemiparesis, whereas with *thalamic* hemorrhage, the eyes are deviated downward, the pupils are small and sluggish to reaction, and there may be aphasia and sensorimotor deficit. If the patient is conscious, unilateral sensory loss is likely to be detected.

With *pontine* hemorrhage the patient is usually comatose, with Cheyne-Stokes or neurogenic hyperventilation, pinpoint pupils, hyperpyrexia, facial weakness, and flaccid quadriplegia. Decerebrate rigidity is typical. With *cerebellar* hemorrhage there may be conjugate deviation of the eyes (toward the other side) or a VI nerve palsy without pupillary signs; often there is no hemiparesis either. These patients may have only a transient period of unconsciousness, after which they awaken with vomiting and severe occipital headache. When they can cooperate, facial weakness, cerebellar signs, and meningism will usually be present.

There is a particular danger of tonsillar herniation caused by raised intracranial pressure; however, if the syndrome is recognized, immediate neurosurgical intervention may allow excellent recovery. Although angiography can demonstrate the mass effect of a hemorrhage in the cerebellum, it is best shown by a CT scan that is angled to see the cerebellum and brainstem.

The differentiation of bleeding at other sites is probably less important, but the recognition and removal of any large intracerebral clot can result in excellent improvement if there is no evidence of brainstem compression.

Hemorrhages sometimes occur from AVMs, in bleeding diatheses, after trauma, or because of disease of the vessel wall such as cerebral amyloid angiopathy. In many of these conditions, the CT scan shows that the bleed is in or just beneath the cortex—a very atypical site for primary intracerebral hemorrhage.

Subarachnoid Hemorrhage

Most patients with subarachnoid hemorrhage (SAH) bleed from a ruptured berry aneurysm. Such intracranial aneurysms are usually found on the vessels around the circle of Willis or on the arteries directly leading from it (Fig. 164-8) at sites of bifurcation, where the muscular medial coat is deficient and the elastica and intima may be damaged by hypertension.*

Under these circumstances the intima is unable to withstand the increased intraluminal pressure and bulges out. Because the intracranial vessels are not covered by adventitia, the aneurysm expands, and those over 10 mm in diameter often rupture. Before doing so, they may compress local structures, such as the III nerves. The risk of SAH is also much increased in smokers and in women taking oral contraceptives.

Clinical Features. When an aneurysm ruptures into the subarachnoid space it produces sudden, severe, explosive headache, with transient or prolonged loss of consciousness in about half of the patients (Fig. 164-9). Occasionally a grand mal seizure occurs. If the patient is awake, severe headache and meningism are the major complaints. Examination shows meningism, confusion, preretinal (subhyaloid) hemorrhages on funduscopy, Babinski's signs, and other focal neurologic deficits.

Monocular blindness and a severe confusional state may attend the rupture of an aneurysm on the anterior communicating artery, whereas a III nerve palsy is commonly found with an aneurysm on the posterior communicating artery. Apart from these, few signs exist to help one locate the site of the aneurysm clinically, although motor asymmetries may assist in lateralization. Minor bleeding may have occurred in the past, producing only a "sentinel headache," nuchal rigidity, or evidence of transient mild central nervous system (CNS) dysfunction, symptoms that were ignored.

*The sites of bleeding aneurysms are quite easy to remember; about one third occur on the MCA, one fourth on the anterior cerebral artery/anterior communicating artery, one fifth on the internal carotid artery/posterior communicating artery, and one sixth on the basilar artery or its branches. One in five patients will have multiple aneurysms.

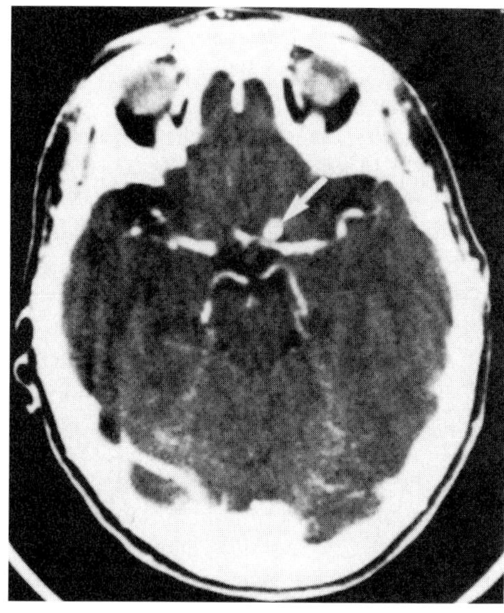

Fig. 164-8. Enhanced CT scan of a berry aneurysm demonstrates an 8-mm left ophthalmic artery aneurysm *(arrow)*. (From Little N, Eelkema EA: Headache. In Rosen P, et al: *Diagnostic radiology in emergency medicine*, St. Louis, 1992, Mosby.)

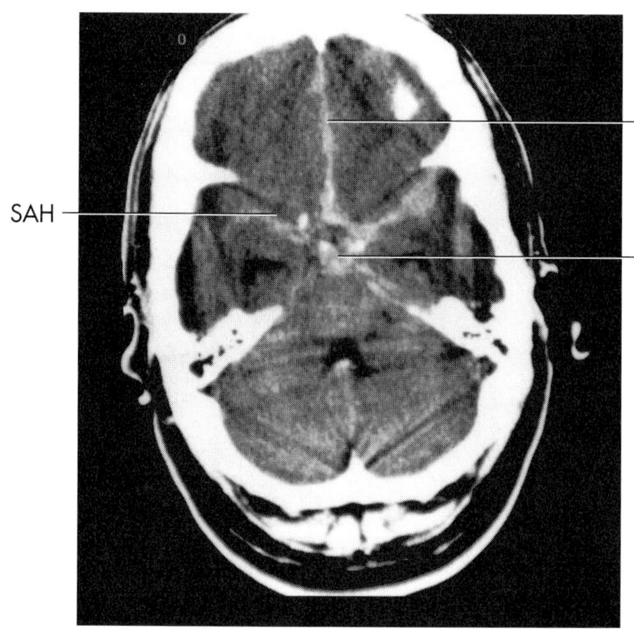

Fig. 164-9. Subarachnoid hemorrhage. Note blood in the basal cistern and interhemispheric fissure. (From Cwinn AA, Grahovac SZ: *Emergency CT scans of the head: a practical atlas*, St. Louis, 1998, Mosby.)

Metabolic changes associated with SAH frequently include diencephalic stimulation with alteration of sympathetic function. Both blood sugar levels and blood pressure tend to be elevated, and ECG abnormalities are common. The latter may be due to alteration in sympathetic tone and include bradycardia with a prolonged QT interval and large upright or deeply inverted T waves. The ECG changes often suggest a myocardial infarction, and appropriate treatment may therefore be withheld if it is not recognized that such changes are extremely common in SAH.

In patients who have had an acute onset with coma, the diagnosis from primary intracerebral hemorrhage can be difficult. In any case in which intracerebral bleeding is likely, CSF examination is potentially dangerous, but it is particularly so in the patient with an intracerebral clot. If the diagnosis of SAH can be made clinically, there is no point in performing a lumbar puncture, especially because the CT scan can determine the presence of blood in the brain, subarachnoid space, and basal cisterns. The absence of blood in the cisterns on the CT scan is a good prognostic sign. In patients with an acute severe headache that could have been caused by a small bleed—a warning leak—the CT may be negative and lumbar puncture will be required, but it may take at least 4 hours after the bleed for red cells in the CSF to reach the lumbar region.

Differential Diagnosis. Other conditions may be confused with SAH or sentinel headache. Meningitis or encephalitis of sudden onset may mimic it, and if there is any doubt about the diagnosis and the question of meningitis has been raised, lumbar puncture is justifiable. Some red cells may be found in the CSF in cases of herpes simplex encephalitis and also with embolic infarction, because of migration of red cells from the damaged brain into the subarachnoid space. These conditions do not give rise to frank blood in the CSF, however. Patients taking monoamine oxidase inhibitors (MAOIs) and who eat foods containing tyramine may have symptoms and signs similar to SAH, with increased blood pressure and severe headache without any actual bleeding, although SAH has also complicated this situation. Severe migraine headaches (particularly in patients who have not had migraine before), coital cephalgia, and severe cluster headache may resemble SAH, but these patients will have clear CSF. Acute neck strain, pituitary infarction, hypertensive encephalopathy, and severe systemic infections may also cause difficulty in diagnosis.

About 1 in 10 cases of SAH are due to bleeding from an AVM (Fig. 164-10). Such patients may have a history of previous subarachnoid bleeding, and there is a history of recurrent seizures in 30%, recurrent vascular headaches in 10%, and focal neurologic findings in 50%. These patients are usually in a much younger age group than those with SAH caused by a ruptured aneurysm. Any premonitory features preceding the typical signs of a subarachnoid hemorrhage in a young person should make the physician consider the diagnosis of AVM. Patients with bleeding disorders and those on anticoagulants may rarely bleed into the CSF, but in these cases bleeding is seldom severe and the correct diagnosis is often suggested by the history, physical examination, and initial laboratory values.

Spinal subarachnoid hemorrhage is distinctly uncommon. The clinical features include sudden severe root pain with incapacitating backache and meningism. This triad is virtually diagnostic and early transfer to a neurosurgical unit is mandatory.

Prognosis. The prognosis for patients with SAH is not good. About half of the patients who have a bleed die within the first month; by the end of the first year well over half have died. The greatest mortality is within the first 10 days, but there is a further chance of rebleeding when the clot around the ruptured aneurysm lyses at the end of the second week. If the patient survives the first 3 months, the mortality rate for the next 5 years is only about 10%. Death in the

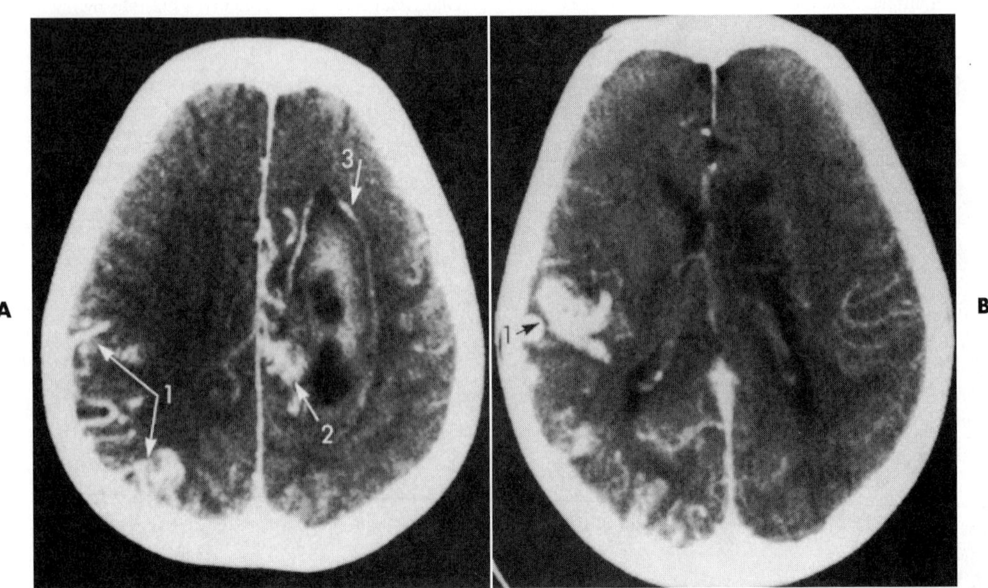

Fig. 164-10. **A** and **B,** Enhanced CT scans of bilateral arteriovenous malformations. With intravenous enhancement, the right *(arrow 1)* and left *(arrow 2)* arteriovenous malformations undergo dense enhancement. There is rim enhancement of the hematoma *(arrow 3)*. (From Little N, Eelkema EA: Headache. In Rosen P, et al: *Diagnostic radiology in emergency medicine,* St. Louis, 1992, Mosby.)

first month is usually due to brain destruction or distortion, rebleeding, raised intracranial pressure, or brainstem compression.

Vasospasm is one cause of secondary deterioration of consciousness with increasing physical signs. It is usually treated with blood volume repletion and calcium channel blockers. Hyponatremia, hydrocephalus, infarcts, cardiac dysrhythmias, seizures, and rebleeding are the other leading causes of deterioration. Epsilon aminocaproic acid reduces rebleeding but may increase the risk of ischemic complications. The prognosis for patients with AVMs is much better, although they tend to bleed again.

Prognosis and Complications. The management of SAH is considered below. Given successful surgical intervention after a SAH and good control of blood pressure in the future, an additional SAH is not likely. However, the patient always has a slightly increased risk, particularly if there is another aneurysm present, which is why asymptomatic aneurysms are attacked surgically if possible. The long-term complications of blood in the CSF include both acute and normal pressure hydrocephalus, and the patient may be left with some deficit after the initial episode. However, these complications are not common. In about 25% of cases, no cause for the bleeding is ever diagnosed; these patients may have an even better prognosis than those who undergo surgery. It is possible that in many of these cases, the aneurysm was destroyed by the bleed, or arteriospasm prevented further loss of blood, and spontaneous healing occurred. Sometimes, a repeat angiogram after 2 weeks will show an aneurysm that was not seen during the first study, probably because of vasospasm.

MANAGEMENT OF STROKES

Some details of management have already been given but the following material provides a general outline for the acute, postacute, and long-term or chronic stages.

Acute Management

The initial history and findings are particularly important in determining those specific measures that must be taken for each individual patient. An assessment of the patient's general status (including pulse rate, blood pressure, respiratory rate and pattern, and hydration) and of neurologic signs (level of consciousness, speech, pupils and other brainstem reflexes, and limb movements) is essential. Observation for changing signs is far more useful than any single evaluation, however precise.

In all patients who are comatose, supportive measures must be provided, including the establishment of an airway and, if necessary, assisted ventilation. An intravenous (IV) line should be put in to maintain fluid and electrolyte balance, and all patients need intermittent catheterization.

Investigations in the acute stage need be but few. The purpose is to prove the diagnosis of stroke rather than, for example, tumor; to assess its extent; and to note any complications at this stage. ECG, radiographs of the chest, and routine hematologic and biochemical tests will be required, and an early CT scan will be of value, particularly in cases of diagnostic doubt, to rule out hemorrhage, to show cerebellar infarction or bleeding, or in cases of unexplained deterioration. Angiography may be useful in certain circumstances but this decision will be made by a neurologist. Cardiac monitoring may be indicated when there is clinical evidence of a dysrhythmia.

The use of anticoagulants is discussed later. Steroids are prescribed more to assuage the anxiety of the physician than to provide effective reduction in intracranial pressure, because in cases of cytotoxic cerebral edema (the type that occurs in stroke) they are ineffective.

In the acute stage the awake patient may be supported by reassurance and explanation of the nature of his disease; the patient's family should be told of the diagnostic possibilities and the likely prognosis, although prognoses given at an early stage are often embarrassingly wrong. The uncertainty of the situation, however, should be recognized by the family.

If the patient is seen within 3 hours after the stroke begins, therapy with tissue plasminogen activator (t-PA) may be considered. The patient must be assessed, a CT scan performed, and the therapy administered within 3 hours. Rapid management and decision making are mandatory for successful thrombolytic therapy. Patients cannot be considered if the onset is uncertain, such as when the patient awakens with a stroke. If there is a hemorrhage on the CT scan, t-PA is contraindicated. Patients are not considered for t-PA if they have minor symptoms or are clearly recovering, or if they have a history of recent trauma, neurosurgery, clotting disorder, seizure, hyperglycemia, or hypertension. There is a risk of cerebral hemorrhage from the therapy, but despite that, the treated patients have better outcomes in terms of mortality and major deficit, indicating that selected patients can have brain tissue preserved by the t-PA.

Postacute Stage

Transient Ischemic Attacks. Because the symptoms and signs are transient, the patient experiencing a TIA requires explanation and reassurance about the nature of the problem to be convinced of the need for further investigations. These investigations are indeed necessary, both to assess the various risk factors and to determine the nature of the TIA that has occurred. We use as routine tests a complete blood count, including platelet estimation and ESR; BUN; syphilitic serology; uric acid; AC and 2-hour PC sugar; serum lipid profile and electrophoresis; chest radiograph and ECG; and we order a glucose tolerance test in some cases. The CT scan is negative in TIAs but positive within a day of a completed stroke. Doppler studies are used to determine whether carotid obstruction means surgery. One must also look for evidence of the conditions listed in Boxes 164-4 and 164-5.

The treatment of TIAs is evolving as studies more clearly define who will benefit from the therapeutic options. If severe (over 75%) localized atherosclerotic stenosis of a carotid (or subclavian) artery can be identified, surgical endarterectomy is appropriate treatment. However, the value of this procedure over "medical" forms of therapy in preventing a future stroke when the stenosis is less than 75% is less convincing. Operable lesions are more common in patients with prior TIAs, hypertension, claudication, and a carotid bruit. However, only half of the patients with TIAs actually have any demonstrable ipsilateral lesion at all.

Anticoagulant therapy diminishes or completely stops TIAs in 80% of cases but as yet there is no good evidence that anticoagulants significantly reduce the ultimate mortality rate, although they may prevent strokes in the most dangerous period, namely the 3 months after the first TIA. In assessing surgery and use of anticoagulants, we must recall that many patients with TIAs are not candidates for either option because other serious medical disease is present.

Because most TIAs appear to be due to platelet emboli, therapy with platelet-inhibiting agents such as clopidogrel or aspirin is used. Both have been shown to reduce strokes and deaths. Aspirin cannot be tolerated by about one third of patients because of gastric upset or ulceration. Although these side effects are less often a problem with clopidogrel, that drug is more expensive and thrombocytopenia has been described as a rare complication. Results with an aspirin and dipyridamole combination (Aggvenox) are the best to date. Therefore patients who present with transient episodes of neurologic dysfunction of sudden onset and brief duration should be referred for further investigation. If a localized area of arterial disease can be demonstrated on arteriography, then either surgical therapy or antiplatelet drugs should be considered.

Infarction. Most patients with strokes should be admitted to the hospital. Many will have an altered state of consciousness, and continued attention to the airway, ventilatory function, blood pressure, skin, bladder and bowel care, fluid and electrolyte balance, and calorie and vitamin intake will all be necessary. Patients do better in specialized stroke units. Investigations of value are the same as for TIAs but in all cases a CT scan is indicated, if only to determine the extent of the infarct and to rule out intracranial bleeding.

When the type and site of the lesion have been diagnosed and as soon as the patient is stable, conscious, and rational, he or she should be allowed initially to sit up in bed and later in a chair, and physiotherapy begun. Active physiotherapy should replace passive therapy as early as possible, and ambulation should be encouraged, with emphasis on gait training and use of the limbs. Hemiparesis also causes some diminution in ventilation, so chest physiotherapy may be required. As soon as it is practical, urinary catheterization should be stopped if it has been necessary at all. Antiepileptic drugs are not routinely given because seizures follow strokes in only about 10% of cases, usually as a late complication.

An isotope scan during the first 3 or 4 days after the stroke should be negative, but it becomes positive at about 6 days. If it is positive on the first day, the physician should suspect a cerebral tumor or AVM. If the diagnosis is in doubt, an angiogram may be performed, but it is otherwise not indicated in a completed infarct. A lumbar puncture is only indicated if meningeal infection is suspected. The required history, examination, and investigation for risk factors are the same as those performed for patients with TIAs.

The place of anticoagulants in therapy remains ill-defined. If the stroke is due to an embolism from a cardiac lesion, and if the infarct is not large and the blood pressure not grossly raised, then heparin may be given after 24 hours. We also give anticoagulants to patients whose stroke deficit is evolving under observation and whose CT scan shows no hemorrhage. In all other cases we advise against anticoagulant use in the acute or postacute stages, but may use them (with little experimental support) for a flurry of TIAs not prevented by antiplatelet agents. After a completed stroke, clopidogrel or aspirin and dipyridamole will likely reduce the likelihood of further infarcts, and one of these agents appears to be indicated in all such cases.

Bad prognostic factors are increased age, reduced conscious level, and severe hemiplegia, hemianopia, or higher cerebral dysfunction. Female patients and those with hypertension or past myocardial infarcts also do less well.

Parenchymal Hemorrhage. The management of patients with parenchymal hemorrhage is almost exactly the same as those with infarct. Greater attention must be paid, however, to reduction of blood pressure to normal levels, always attempting to keep the diastolic pressure below 100 mm Hg, and preferably lower than 90 mm Hg. A CT scan will be positive immediately. If there is any suggestion of cerebellar hemorrhage, lumbar puncture must be avoided and a neurosurgeon should be called immediately. Patients with lacunar strokes diagnosed by CT scan can be managed in the same way as those with TIAs, except that angiography is usually negative.

Subarachnoid Hemorrhage. When patients with suspected SAH arrive in the emergency room, the physician should order urinalysis, ECG, routine hematology, biochemistry, and a coagulation profile, and arrange for an urgent CT scan. Patients who are awake and in pain should be sedated with phenothiazines or demerol. Hypertension above 100 mm Hg diastolic should be treated. Fluids should be restricted and the patient catheterized. The earlier an angiogram can be done and the aneurysm surgically attacked, the better.

The patient should be transferred to a neurosurgical unit when his or her condition is stable (signs are static or improving and the blood pressure is normal). In a neurosurgical unit, CT scanning and four-vessel angiography should be performed. In 20% of cases the patient has multiple aneurysms and it is important to note those angiographic changes indicating which aneurysm has bled. Aneurysms in most sites are susceptible to either direct or indirect surgical treatment, with the approaches varying from tying the carotid artery in the neck to a direct attack, clipping the aneurysm itself, wrapping it with muscle or plastic resins, or thrombosing it with foreign material. The chance of rebleeding may be lessened by a number of regimens, including the use of epsilon aminocaproic acid; therapy for arteriospasm (calcium channel blockers) and for raised intracranial pressure will also be required in a number of patients.

Long-term Management

There are three important aspects of late management that are often overlooked. The first is the availability of many rehabilitation services. Speech therapists may assist the patient's recovery to some degree of useful language communication and may also provide a great psychologic boost to the patient who is continually frustrated by difficulties in communicating. Physiotherapists may aid in gait and arm retraining, and occupational therapists develop competency in the activities of daily living. Social services can greatly help the patient to realize those benefits to which he is entitled by his sickness, and they may arrange suitable placement. Home care and social and nursing services may also be called in to assist the patient in returning home, and they may provide follow-up assessments of his or her ability to function in the home and reliability in taking prescribed medication.

A second factor is the importance of continuing therapy for the prevention of further strokes. The use of antiaggregants, proper treatment for hyperlipidemia, weight reduction, diets, and specific treatment for hypertension,

Box 164-7. Quality of Life at the End of Life

I. Importance of quality of life at the end of life
  A. Patient's perception of the illness and how it affects daily living
  B. Reflects individual's dimensions of life affected by the disease or treatments
  C. Influences treatment decisions
  D. Influences patient status
II. Physical well-being (symptoms)[2]
  A. Multiple symptoms due to disease progression, debility, organic and metabolic changes
  B. Ability of self-care
  C. Pain
  D. Nausea, vomiting
  E. Lack of appetite
  F. Dyspnea
  G. Delirium, restlessness, agitation
  H. Fatigue, weakness, immobility, sleep changes
  I. GI disturbances (constipation/diarrhea)
  J. Urinary incontinence
III. Psychologic well-being (mood states)[2]
  A. Anxiety, fear
  B. Depression
  C. Loneliness
  D. Suffering
  E. Dependency, lack of independence
  F. Decreased self-esteem, self-respect
  G. Guilt, anger
  H. Adjustment to the disease, prognosis
  I. Satisfaction with care
  J. Despair
  K. Acceptance of loss
  L. Denial/acceptance
IV. Social well-being (roles)[2]
  A. Sense of burden on family
  B. Loss of control over life
  C. Relationships with others
  D. Changing family roles, status, family structure
  E. Family interactions
  F. Fear of abandonment or isolation
  G. Financial concerns
  H. Declined leisure activities
  I. Employment status, workplace relations
  J. Sexuality
V. Spiritual well-being (own sense of self)[1,2]
  A. Religion (rituals, practices, prayers, meditation)
  B. Relatedness to God (Superior Being)
  C. Meaning of life/existential
    1. Reason for events
    2. Purpose of life
    3. Belief in a primary force in life
  D. Hope (realistic-based)
  E. Forgiveness/acceptance
  F. Transcendence
    1. Redefines views of life
    2. Redefines relationships
  G. Spiritual needs vary and fluctuate with changes in physical symptoms
  H. Feelings of uselessness
VI. Ways to help enhance quality of life at the end of life
  A. Effective communication/listening
  B. Stress management, effective coping mechanisms
  C. Available resources, support available
  D. Support in decision making
  E. Resolve conflicts
  F. Complete unfinished business
  G. Maintain "non-illness–related aspects of life"
  H. Changing perception of space, span, or focus of time (take one day at a time)
  I. Coping with anticipatory grief
  J. Define attainable goals
  K. Engage in spiritual practices
  L. Conserve energy with demands (use resources)
  M. Help the individual explore losses and their meanings

diabetes, and other risk factors have a large part to play in the prophylaxis of further attacks. In cases where there may be familial risk factors such as hyperlipidemia, hypertension, or diabetes, other family members should be assessed to prevent vascular disease occurring in them as well. It has been well shown that the prognosis in patients after a stroke can be dramatically improved if all risk factors are continually monitored. In one study the 5-year mortality rate in those who were followed carefully by managing all risk factors was about 15%, compared with 65% in the patients who were not so treated.

The third factor that always warrants careful attention is the presence of depression. A stroke is well named, for it often strikes down men and women in their years of greatest achievement and happiness, devastating their ambitions and chilling them with the fear of impending renewed disaster. Depression is not just a neurotic tilt at the windmill of an unkind world, nor is it purely an expression of chemical dysfunction in the limbic system. It is, in part, both of these; in addition, depression is a near-universal response of the mind to damage of its own substrate, the brain. When the stroke patient seems to perform well on formal examination but does not go to work, can climb the stairs to his bedroom but will not visit across the road, and writes his will but will not read a book, then the physician must search for other somatic and mental symptoms of depressive illness. When they are found, these symptoms should not be regarded as the inevitable and immutable consequences of brain damage, but rather a further challenge to the diagnostic and therapeutic skills that every physician can, and must, meet.

END OF LIFE CARE

The challenge to achieve the best quality of life for patients with advanced or major illnesses requires attention not only to the treatment of the disease and related symptoms, but also to factors that influence the quality of a person's life. A good place to start is to help patients retain their identity by reinforcing those aspects of their lives that have defined who they are and to not reinforce the relative anonymity often conveyed by seriously debilitating illness. Secondly, meaningful stimulation should be provided to help them keep going and to eliminate the boredom of empty hours dragging by. Finally it is important to remove causes of stress and to provide support that conveys caring and security.

Goal	*Antithesis*
Identity	Anonymity
Stimulation	Boredom
Security	Stress

Goals for a plan of management may be based on these factors and the many aspects of daily life outlined in Box 164-7. Guidelines for critical areas of end of life care were published by the project entitled *Strengthening Nursing Education to Improve End of Life Care.* Extensive website resources that address end of life care are listed below.

REFERENCES

1. Kemp C: *Terminal illness: a guide to nursing care,* Philadelphia, 1995, Lippincott.
2. Pickett M, Yancey D: Symptoms of the dying. In McCorkle R, Grant M, Frank-Stromborg M, et al, editors: *Cancer nursing: a comprehensive textbook,* ed 2, Philadelphia, 1996, WB Saunders, pp 1157-1182.

ADDITIONAL READINGS

Adams HP Jr: Treating ischemic stroke as an emergency, *Arch Neuro* 55:457-461, 1998.

Clark WM, Albers GW: The ATLANTIS rt-PA (Alteplase) acute stroke trial: final results, *Stroke* 30:234, 1999.

Ferrell BR, Virani R, Grant N: Analysis of end of life content in nursing textbooks, *Oncol Nurs Forum* 26:869-876, 1999.

Wolf PA: Prevention of stroke, *Lancet* 352(suppl III):15-18, 1998.

End of Life Care

Carroll-Johnson RM, Gorman LM, Bush NJ, editors: *Psychosocial nursing care,* Pittsburgh, 1998, Oncology Nursing Press.

Cella DF: Measuring quality of life in palliative care, *Semin Oncol* 22:73-81, 1995.

Cella D: Quality of Life: the concept, *J Palliat Care,* 8(3):8-13, 1992.

Clinch JJ, Dudgeon D, Schipper H: Quality of life assessment in palliative care. In Doyle D, Hanks GWC, McDonald N, editors: *Oxford textbook of palliative medicine,* ed 2, Oxford, UK, 1998, Oxford Medical Publication, pp 83-94.

Cohen SR, Mount BM: Quality of life in terminal illness: defining and measuring subjective well-being in the dying, *J Palliat Care* 8(3):40-45, 1992.

Cohen SR, Mount BM, Strobel MG, et al: The McGill quality of life questionnaire: a measure of quality of life appropriate for people with advanced disease. A preliminary study of validity and acceptability, *Palliat Med* 9:207-219, 1995.

Donnely S, Walsh D: Quality of life assessment in advanced cancer, *Palliat Med* 10:275-283, 1996.

Ferrans CE: Development of a quality of life index for patients with cancer, *Oncol Nurs Forum* 17:15-21, 1990.

Ferrans CE, Powers MJ: Development of a quality of life index: development and psychometric properties, *Adv Nurs Sci* 8(1):15-24, 1985.

Field MJ, Cassel CK, editors: *Approaching death: improving care at the end of life,* Washington, DC, 1997, National Academy Press.

Lynn J: An 88-year-old woman facing the end of life, *J Am Med Assoc* 277(20):1633-1640, 1997.

McMillan SC, Mahon M: Measuring quality of life in hospice patients using a newly developed hospice quality of life index, *Qual Life Res* 3:437-447, 1994.

Skeel RT: Measurement of outcomes in supportive oncology: quality of life. In Berger AM, Portenoy RK, Weissman DE, editors: *Principles and practice of supportive oncology,* Philadelphia, 1998, Lippincott-Raven, pp 875-888.

Smeenk FW, de Witte LP, van Haastregt JC, et al: Transmural care of terminal cancer patients: effects on the quality of life of direct caregivers, *Nurs Res* 47(3):129-136, 1998.

WEBSITES

Agency for Health Care Policy and Research *www.achpr.gov*
American Academy of Hospice and Palliative Medicine *www.aahpm.org*
American Association for Therapeutic Humor *www.aath.org*
American Board of Internal Medicine—Care for the Dying, Physician Narratives *www.abim.org/pubs/narr001.html*
The American Geriatrics Society *www.americangeriatrics.org*
American Massage Therapy Association *www.amtamassage.org*
American Medical Association *www.ama-assn.org:80/about.htm*
American Music Therapy Association *www.namt.com*
American Pain Society *www.ampainsoc.org*
American Society for the Advancement of Palliative Care *www.asap-care.com*
American Society for Bioethics and Humanities *www.asbh.org*
American Society of Law, Medicine, and Ethics *www.aslme.org*
ABCD Americans for Better Care of the Dying *www.abcd-caring.com*
Approaching Death: Improving Care at the End of Life *www2.nas.edu/hcs/21da.html*
Association of Cancer Online Resources *www.acor.org; www.medinfo.org*
Association of Death Education and Counseling *www.adec.org*
Before I Die: Medical Care and Personal Choices *www.wnet.org/archive/bid*
Bereavement and Hospice Support Netline *www.ubalt.edu/www/bereavement*
Better Health *www.BetterHealth.com*
Breast Cancer Information Clearinghouse *www.nysernet.org/bcic*
Cancer Net *Cancernet.nci.nih.gov/*
Caregiver Network *www.caregiver.on.ca/index.html*
Caregiver Survival Resources *www.caregiver911.com/*
Catholic Health Association of the United States *www.chausa.org*
Center to Improve Care of the Dying *www.gwu.edu/~cicd*
Center for Medical Ethics and Mediation *www.wh.com/cmem*
Choice in Dying *www.echonyc.com/~choice/*
The Compassionate Friends *www.jjt.com*
Death, Dying and Grief Resources *www.katsden.com/webster/index.html*
Death Net *www.rights.org/deathnet/*
Department of Health and Human Services, Healthfinder *www.healthfinder.gov*
Dying Well *www.dyingwell.com/*
Elizabeth Kubler Ross, M.D., "On Death and Dying" *www.doubleclickd.com/kubler.html*
Growth House *www.growthhouse.org*
History of Body Donation *www.com.uci.edu/~anatomy/willed_body/wbpol.htm*
Hospice Foundation of America *www.hospicefoundation.org*
Hospice Hands *hospice-cares.com*
International Association for the Study of Pain *www.halcyon.com/iasp*
The International Work Group on Death, Dying and Bereavement *www.wwdc.com/death/iwg/iwg.html*
Last Acts *www.lastacts.org*
Lindesmith *www.lindesmith.org/about_tlc/pain.html*
Medical College of Wisconsin Bioethics *www.mcw.edu/bioethics/*
Medical College of Wisconsin Palliative Care Programs *www.mcw.edu/pallmed/*
Memorial Sloan Kettering Cancer Center *www.mskcc.org*
The Nathan Cummings Foundation *www.ncf.org/ncf/aboutncf/about.html*
National Association for Home Care *www.nahc.org/*
National Center for Health Statistics *www.cdc.gov/nchswww/about/about.htm*
National Conference of State Legislatures *www.ncsl.org/programs/pubs/endoflife.htm*
National Family Caregivers Association *www.nfcacares.org*
National Hospice Organization *www.nho.org*
National Institute of Aging *www.nih.gov/nia/*

CHAPTER 165

Infectious Diseases of the Nervous System

T. Jock Murray
William Pryse-Phillips

The central nervous system (CNS) has no lymphatic system as such, and although usually well protected from direct infection, its resistance to any infection that does occur is low. The patterns of infective illness are relatively few, but the organisms that can produce disease are many. In this chapter we will outline the features of those kinds of infection more commonly seen (Box 165-1).

MENINGITIS

Although the word *meningitis* suggests an inflammation of the meninges only, there is always some involvement of the most superficial parts of the brain that are contiguous to the meninges. Often there are also alterations in the flow of cerebrospinal fluid (CSF). An occlusive arteritis is common in the subpial cortex, so meningitis is properly considered as a meningoencephalitis in all cases. Causative organisms include bacteria, spirochetes, viruses, fungi, and protozoa; sometimes carcinomatous invasion of the meninges produces meningeal inflammation that is hard to clinically differentiate from infective meningitis.

The most common organisms responsible for bacterial meningitis in people over the age of 2 months are *Neisseria meningitidis, Streptococcus pneumoniae, Haemophilus influenzae,* and *Listeria monocytogenes,* but other organisms such as *Escherichia coli* and group B streptococci must be considered in neonates. Any of the above organisms and also staphylococci, anaerobes, and mixed infections can be identified in patients with CNS defects or local infections and in those taking immunosuppressants. Most cases of meningitis are associated with infection in the upper respiratory tract, but one should always consider whether the patient may have a lowered resistance to infections or an abnormal portal of entry for organisms to reach the nervous system.

When managing a patient with possible meningeal inflammation, the first step is to confirm the diagnosis and the second is to start appropriate therapy (even before the results of the Gram's stain are available) selected on the basis of an educated guess as to the most likely organism. One has also to consider why this patient developed this infection at this time.

Meningitis may present as an acute, subacute, chronic, or recurrent inflammation of the meninges. It is classed as bacterial (or septic or purulent) when organisms are isolated by routine culture methods. With bacterial infection, polymorphonuclear leukocytes predominate in the CSF. Viruses usually cause an aseptic meningitis in which mononuclear cells predominate and routine cultures do not grow the organism.

Certain pathologic conditions consistently predispose to CNS infections (meningitis, abscess, and encephalopathy) and they must be considered in all patients, if not in the acute stage at least immediately after it. Thus immunosuppressed patients (those with leukemia, lymphoma, or acquired immunodeficiency syndrome [AIDS]; those receiving immunosuppressive drugs including steroids; or after splenectomy) are at risk of infection by measles, herpes zoster, cytomegaloviruses (CMVs), fungi, streptococci, Listeria, or gram-negative bacilli. Skull defects and cranial trauma, including brain surgery, make pneumococcus, staphylococcus, and gram-negative infections more likely. Progressive multifocal leukoencephalopathy is always associated with impaired immune responsiveness, and toxoplasmosis is a common infecting agent in patients with AIDS.

In children, prematurity, perinatal complications, and neural tube defects are predisposing factors for meningitis, which in such cases is usually due to gram-negative organisms.

Box 165-1. Overview of CNS Infections

- Meningitis*
  - Acute
  - Subacute
  - Chronic
  - Recurrent
- Encephalitis
  - Viral (e.g., herpes simplex, rabies, polio, arbor)
  - Fungal
  - Parasitic
- Acquired immunodeficiency syndrome
- Abscess
  - Epidural (intracranial, spinal)
  - Subdural
  - Intracerebral
- Other
  - Herpes zoster
  - Cytomegalovirus
  - Poliomyelitis
  - Coxsackievirus
  - Infectious mononucleosis
  - Influenza
  - Tick paralysis
  - Tetanus
  - Botulism
  - Toxoplasmosis
  - Syphilis
  - Lyme disease
  - Rabies
  - Behçet's syndrome
- Slow virus infections
  - Creutzfeldt-Jakob disease
  - Subacute sclerosing panencephalitis
  - Progressive multifocal leukoencephalopathy
- Neurologic complications of other infections
  - Acute toxic encephalopathy
  - Acute postinfectious encephalomyelitis
  - Epidemic myalgic encephalomyelitis
  - Bacterial endocarditis
  - Cerebral thrombophlebitis

From Mandell GL, Bennett JE, Dolin R, editors: *Principles and practice of infectious diseases,* ed 4, New York, Churchill Livingstone, 1995.
*These may be bacterial, viral, fungal, or parasitic.

Acute Meningitis

Acute meningitis is a neurologic emergency. It is most common in the earliest years of life, particularly in premature infants, of whom up to half may die as a result. The peak incidence is in the first 2 years and about three fourths of all cases occur before the age of 10. The death rate in older patients has decreased to about 20%, but continuous developments in therapy do not seem to have lowered it further. *H. influenzae* vaccine has almost eliminated this agent as a cause of childhood meningitis.

Acute Bacterial Meningitis

Clinical Features. Acute meningitis evolves over hours or, at most, days. Patients who have been quite healthy or have only had an upper respiratory infection now begin to complain of the symptoms of meningeal irritation and of raised intracranial pressure (ICP). Malaise; fever; headaches of traction type; nausea; vomiting; anorexia; stiff, painful neck; and photophobia are the usual initial symptoms. Depression in the level of consciousness, delirium, seizures, and various focal neurologic signs may follow. The association of fever and any form of mental deterioration must make one consider meningoencephalitis as a possible diagnosis. Inflammatory cells in the CSF and accompanying cerebral edema may cause a rapid rise in ICP and produce false localizing signs.

Examination usually shows meningism, with stiff neck and resistance to flexion of the spine or to straight leg raising. Such signs may be absent in overwhelmingly ill adults and in neonates, who may just show the features listed in Box 165-2, such as a bulging fontanelle, neck stiffness, and drowsiness. Children may also show head retraction, which can be so marked as to warrant the term *opisthotonos*.

General examination may show a rash (particularly if the meningococcus is involved or echovirus or coxsackievirus is involved); signs of infection in the ears, joints, bones, chest, or heart; and sometimes purpura and hypotension. Shock is common if a gram-negative organism is the cause of septicemia with secondary meningitis and in meningococcal septicemia causing adrenal infarction (Waterhouse-Friderichsen syndrome). The combination of fever and purpura in this context can occur with *N. meningitidis*, echovirus, *E. coli, Pseudomonas, Proteus, L. monocytogenes*, streptococcus, gonococcus, or *Staphylococcus aureus* infections.

Evaluating the Cerebrospinal Fluid. Whenever there is evidence of meningeal inflammation, a lumbar puncture (LP) must be done eventually, even though some patients with meningitis show early papilledema. Intracerebral abscess or expanding mass lesions, particularly in the posterior fossa, must be ruled out by physical examination, although in the presence of any focal signs an emergency computed tomography (CT) scan is necessary. In this situation an expert opinion should be requested if available. LP should be performed when any such masses are excluded because identification of the organism and determination of its sensitivities are essential; however, if a bacterial process is suspected, antibiotics should be started as soon as blood cultures are drawn and before an LP is done. A patient may be transferred to specialist care from remote areas, with the CSF sample kept warm beside him or her and after the first dose of antibiotic. In infants, LP is indicated in the investigation of pyrexia of unknown origin and may be indicated in any ill child with fever or septicemia, with or without neurologic signs and in the investigation of failure to thrive or seizures.

If the result of the first LP is not conclusive (i.e., no organisms are seen and the cells present are not polymorphonuclear neutrophil leukocytes [PMNs]) the patient can be carefully observed for a period without antibiotics and the test repeated in 12 to 18 hours with a greater chance of finding organisms or diagnostic cell patterns.

The CSF pressure need not be taken if the initial fluid is cloudy or bloodstained because knowledge of the pressure does not contribute to diagnosis in these circumstances. The fluid may be turbid or clear; microscopy may show any number of mononuclear or polymorphonuclear cells. PMNs almost always predominate in acute bacterial meningitis. Mononuclear cells usually predominate in the other forms of meningitis (due to *Mycobacterium tuberculosis*, viruses, or fungi).

CSF protein levels are raised in all forms of meningitis, particularly those of longer duration or with very high cell counts. Apart from Gram's and Ziehl-Neelsen stains, auramine stains for *M. tuberculosis*, India ink preparations for fungi, special stains for other organisms, and specific antigen or antibody studies may be needed. The sample should be examined immediately. Many of the above tests are being replaced by DNA amplification techniques. Current polymerase chain reaction (PCR) technology (using the LightCycler) can identify the causative organism within 30 minutes. In many instances a physician will have to rely on the conventional Gram's stain, and occasionally may have to do this personally (Boxes 165-2 and 165-3).

A simultaneous estimation of the CSF blood sugar is mandatory when the LP is done. With most viral meningitides and parameningeal foci of infection, CSF sugar values are often normal. Values will be low (i.e., less than 50% of the blood level) in bacterial meningitis. High PMN counts are to

Box 165-2. Signs of Meningitis in Infants and Children

Neonates	Older Infants	Over Age 2
Fever	Fever	Fever
Lethargy	Vomiting	Drowsiness
Anorexia	Irritability	Headache
Vomiting	Drowsiness	Stiff neck
Respiratory distress	Convulsions	Vomiting
Convulsions	Bulging fontanelle	Convulsions
Irritability		
Jaundice		
Bulging fontanelle		

From Mandell GL, Bennett JE, Dolin R, editors: *Principles and practice of infectious diseases*, ed 4, New York, Churchill Livingstone, 1995.

Box 165-3. How to Do a Rapid Gram's Stain

A rapid Gram's stain can be performed by drying and fixing the centrifuged deposit of CSF and staining it with fresh gentian violet for 2 seconds and Gram's iodine for 2 seconds. The sample is then rinsed in water. 95% ethyl alcohol is dripped onto the slides until the gentian violet is completely eluted (up to 3 seconds), and the slide is then rinsed in water, counterstained with 2% safranin O or carbol, fuchsin for 3 seconds, and then again rinsed in water. (Use fresh reagents with little or no precipitated granules of gentian violet.)

be expected in all cases—over 50,000/mm^3 if the meningitis is due to rupture of an abscess.

If there is clinical uncertainty as to whether the patient has bacterial or aseptic meningitis and the patient is not seriously ill, the physician may properly maintain careful observation, withhold antibiotics, and repeat the LP in 12 to 18 hours. With aseptic meningitis, the second CSF sample will almost always show a shift toward mononuclear cell predominance, whereas later examinations will show the eventual disappearance of all PMNs. In bacterial meningitis, PMNs increase quickly, CSF sugar falls, and the protein level rises (Box 165-4).

Organisms. Specific organisms that cause meningitis may be suspected from certain clinical features. Thus (apart from the clinical features of meningitis in general) meningococcal meningitis has a peak appearance between the ages of 2 and 25, tends to occur in epidemics (Table 165-1), and may lead to disseminated intravascular coagulation, a purpuric skin rash, and shock from adrenal hemorrhage. Pneumococcal meningitis is mainly a disease of adult life, with a peak incidence in old age. It is particularly common in subjects with an obvious focus of infection elsewhere (e.g., ears, chest, recent skull fracture with CSF leak, or ear, nose, and throat [ENT] operation), in patients with immunologic deficiency, and in alcoholics. *H. influenzae* infection is common in children up to the age of 2 years in countries in which the vaccine is not used, but it is far less common after the age of 6 years. Patients have often had recent otitis or upper respiratory infection. Adults infected with *H. influenzae* are likely to have otitis or another parameningeal infection, a CSF leak, or immunologic deficiency.

Staphylococcal and gram-negative meningitis are usually complications of endocarditis or prior head trauma. In such cases the CSF may not show many leukocytes and may be sterile; **a blood culture is mandatory in all cases of meningitis,** however, so the correct diagnosis should not be missed. *L. monocytogenes* infections occur in neonates, the elderly, and patients with compromised host defenses. The abrupt onset of signs suggesting meningitis, encephalitis, or abscess in such patients should make one consider this organism. In the first 3 months of life, other commonly responsible organisms include streptococcus (group B), *S. aureus, E. coli,* and other Enterobacteriaceae.

Management. Urgent management of bacterial meningitis is vital because severe cortical damage or death can result from delay. Blood cultures should be obtained and any skin lesions swabbed before the antibiotic is started. Having obtained the CSF, the physician should hold it up to the light to see if it is cloudy (over 500 cells/ml) or clear, and then take it to the laboratory, where a Gram's stain, culture, cell count, and differential should be performed and the protein and sugar levels estimated. Virus cultures and cytology might be indicated if septic meningitis is excluded by these tests.

Antibiotics should be started at once if the CSF is cloudy and bacterial infection is suspected. In many instances the physician won't know the exact organism until the cultures return, but treatment cannot be delayed that long. Unless clinical clues suggest one particular organism, the patient should begin an empirical regimen likely to be effective against the most common organisms (Table 165-2). The smear will indicate the type of organism responsible and thus the correct therapy. If meningococcal meningitis is suspected, intravenous benzylpenicillin should be given even before the patient is transferred to the hospital; the organism may still be grown from the CSF, and this is no time for diagnostic niceties.

For the choice and doses of antibiotics commonly used to treat meningitis see Table 165-3. Seventy-five percent of adult cases of meningitis will be due to meningococcus or pneumococcus organisms. Penicillin-resistant D. pneumonia is now common in many countries, including the United States and Canada. This has changed our approach to the

Box 165-4. When to Suspect Meningitis

Immediate referral to a specialist is necessary in the following circumstances:

- When a patient has both fever and meningism
- Ill patients with a petechial rash or impaired consciousness
- Adults with the combination of fever and seizures
- Babies with fever and a bulging fontanelle, especially if they have been vomiting; dehydration would normally lead to depression of the fontanelle, and bulging now indicates intracranial pathology
- Patients with fever who have been in contact with persons with meningococcal infection

Table 165-1. Occurrence of Organisms in Bacterial Meningitis in Adults*

Organisms	%
N. meningitidis	30-40
H. influenzae	5
S. pneumoniae	40-50
Other organisms	10

From Mandell GL, Bennett JE, Dolin R, editors: *Principles and practice of infectious diseases,* ed 4, New York, 1995, Churchill Livingstone.

*In about 10% of cases, usually caused by prior antibiotic treatment, no organism can be cultured.

Table 165-2. Treatment of Meningitis of Uncertain Etiology in Adults*

Antibiotic	Dosage
Ampicillin	1 gm intravenously every 3 hours
Ampicillin and chloramphenicol†	1 gm intravenously every 6 hours
Penicillin	1-2 megaunits intravenously q2h
Penicillin and sulfadiazine	2-4 gm intravenously stat and every 6 hours
Penicillin and chloramphenicol	1 gm intramuscularly or intravenously every 6 hours

From Mandell GL, Bennett JE, Dolin R, editors: *Principles and practice of infectious diseases,* ed 4, New York, Churchill Livingstone, 1995.

*What to give until the cultures come back.

†The authors' preference.

Table 165-3. Doses of Antibiotics Commonly Used to Treat Meningitis

Drug	Child*	Adult
Aqueous penicillin G†	50,000-75,000 units/kg every 4 hours	3-4 megaunits intravenously every 4 hours
Ampicillin†	200-300 mg/kg/day in 4-6 doses intravenously	2 gm intravenously every 4 hours
Cloxacillin‡	40 mg/kg intravenously every 4 hours	2 gm intravenously every 4 hours
Cefotaxime	50 mg/kg intravenously every 8 hours	2 gm intravenously every 6 hours
Ceftriaxone	75 mg/kg loading dose; then 50 mg/kg every 12 hours	2 gm every 12 hours
Ceftazidime	50 mg/kg every 8 hours	2 gm every 12 hours
Chloramphenicol	25 mg/kg every 6 hours (not in neonates)	1-2 gm intravenously every 6 hours to a maximum of 6 gm/day
Gentamicin	1.5 mg/kg intravenously every 8 hours	

From Mandell GL, Bennett JE, Dolin R, editors: *Principles and practice of infectious diseases,* ed 4, New York, Churchill Livingstone, 1995.
*Different doses will be needed in neonates.
†If the patient is allergic to penicillin, use chloramphenicol.
‡Vancomycin should be used in patients allergic to penicillin.

Table 165-4. Initial Antibiotic Therapy for Suppurative Meningitis of Unknown Cause

Patient group	Suspected pathogen	Preferred therapy	Alternative therapy
Neonate (1 month or younger)	Group B streptococci, *E. coli, Listeria*	Ampicillin plus cefotaxime	Ampicillin and gentamicin
Child	*S. pneumoniae, H. influenzae*	Ampicillin plus cefotaxime or ceftriaxone plus dexamethasone	Chloramphenicol plus gentamicin plus dexamethasone
Adult	*N. meningitidis, S. pneumoniae, H. influenzae, Listeria*	(Ampicillin or penicillin G) plus ceftriaxone	Chloramphenicol or cefotaxime
Adult or child resident in a community with >2% high level (≥2 μg/ml) penicillin resistant *S. pneumoniae*	Penicillin resistant *S. pneumoniae, N. meningitidis*	Vancomycin plus cefotaxime or ceftriaxone	Possible meropenem
Immunocompromised adult (e.g., older than 60, with cirrhosis or neoplastic disease)	*Listeria, Pseudomonas, S. pneumoniae, N. meningitidis*	Cefotaxime plus ampicillin	Trimethoprim-sulfamethoxazole (TMP-SMX) plus chloramphenicol
Postcraniotomy patient	*Staphylococcus aureus, Staphylococcus epidermidis, Pseudomonas,* Enterobacteriaceae	Nafcillin plus cefotaxime plus gentamicin	Vancomycin and cefotaxime and gentamicin
	H. influenzae	Cefotaxime or chloramphenicol	Ampicillin only if isolate is susceptible
	N. meningitidis	Aqueous penicillin G or cefotaxime	Chloramphenicol
	E. coli, Klebsiella, Proteus, and similar organisms	Gentamicin plus cefotaxime	Chloramphenicol
	Pseudomonas	Ceftazidime plus gentamicin	—

empiric treatment of meningitis. In children, when Haemophilus infection is at all likely, the treatment plan must take into account the occurrence of ampicillin-resistant strains. The antibiotics usually used against each organism are listed in Tables 165-4 and 165-5.

Chloramphenicol and the sulfonamides always cross the blood-brain barrier, whereas penicillin and cephalosporins cross well only when there is inflammation of the meninges. Even with inflammation, however, penetration into the CSF is poor with tetracyclines, streptomycin, kanamycin, gentamicin, polymyxin, and colistin. Thus the choice of agents is crucial. The dose should be arrived at by consideration of the severity of the infection and the age of the patient.

Gram-negative meningitis in adults usually complicates trauma, surgery, spinal anesthesia, or chronic debilitating diseases, but is uncommon. Pseudomonas is the organism most often cultured. Ciprofloxacin, 400 mg every 6 hours intravenously, is probably the best agent, but all such cases should be referred to a specialist in infectious diseases.

The duration of antibiotic therapy varies with the organism, the age of the patient, and the clinical course but is usually at least 10 days (2 weeks with pneumococcal

Table 165-5. Adjunctive Therapy for Bacterial Meningitis

Therapy	Comments
Dexamethasone 0.15 mg/kg every 6 hours for 4 days	Best studied in children with meningitis. Resulted in decreased incidence of sensorineural hearing loss and other neurologic sequelae
Control of increased intracranial pressure (ICP)	Patients with signs of increased ICP may benefit from insertion of an ICP measuring device and treatment of the ICP
Plasmapheresis	Has proven useful in fulminant meningococcemia
Supportive care	Meticulous attention to fluid and electrolyte balance, high index of suspicion for complications such as subdural empyema
Eradication of nasopharyngeal carriage of *N. meningitidis* and *H. influenzae*	Mucosal colonization may persist despite successful treatment of the meningitis; rifampin should be given to eradicate this colonization

infections). Isolation of patients with undiagnosed or meningococcal disease is wise for the first 24 hours after treatment is started.

Steroids are recommended as adjunctive therapy in patients with meningitis who are in a coma or who have markedly raised ICP, and in children with *H. influenzae* meningitis, in whom there is evidence that deafness can be prevented.

Prophylaxis should be used for all household contacts and others closely associated with patients suffering from meningococcal disease (e.g., children in the same nursery school). Rifampin, 600 mg bid for 2 days, is a recommended treatment for adult contacts, whereas in children the dose is 10 mg/kg bid, and in infants 3 months to 1 year of age, 5 mg/kg bid. Prophylaxis is also recommended in contacts of cases of *H. influenzae* meningitis; rifampin is recommended at a dosage of 20 mg/kg/day (not to exceed 600 mg/day) for adults and children in households or day care centers containing children 4 years of age and younger. The index case should also receive rifampin at the end of the definitive course of treatment. Vaccination against meningococcal disease is also available and is an important public health measure. At diagnosis, the public health service should be informed of all cases of meningitis.

Acute Aseptic Meningitis

Clinical Features. Acute aseptic meningitis is characterized by fever, headache, and meningeal signs. Change in consciousness and localizing neurologic signs are rare. Patients with this disease look and feel wretched but are not severely ill. CSF examination will usually show an increase in mononuclear cells to fewer than 500/mm^3 (although PMNs may be increased in the early stages); the protein is normal or only slightly elevated, and the CSF sugar is usually normal, except with mumps infection.

As can be seen from Box 165-5, 70% of the known causes of aseptic meningitis are common viral infections (coxsackievirus, echovirus, Epstein-Barr virus, mumps, and lymphocytic choriomeningitis [LCM]). In about 25% of the cases the virus is not defined. The remaining long list of viruses identified includes measles, chickenpox, and influenza. Rarely, the clinical picture of aseptic meningitis may be seen in the preicteric stage of infectious hepatitis or in uremia and in patients with inadequately treated bacterial meningitis.

Management. Management of acute septic meningitis requires only analgesics and reduction in fever; the prognosis here is much better than in bacterial meningitis—the patient is seldom as ill and usually recovers readily. One may attempt to identify the virus by culture of the CSF or by PCR. A chest radiograph, tuberculosis skin test, syphilis serology, blood cultures, and a collagen-vascular screen are commonly ordered. A CT scan may be required to rule out a parameningeal focus. Acute and convalescent antibody titers may implicate enteroviruses or other viruses, but usually no agent is incriminated.

Subacute Meningitis

Inadequately treated bacterial meningitis, fungal infections, and tuberculous meningitis (TBM) are the more common causes of subacute meningitis; viral causes are much less common. TBM is the prototype and will be discussed at greatest length.

Tuberculous Meningitis. Tuberculosis is most likely to occur in North America among the native and immigrant populations, among alcoholics, and in those patients with immunologic deficiency or generalized illness. A third of the cases occur before the age of 10. About half of the patients will be known cases of tuberculosis. The illness usually occurs in the active stage of primary infection but may present years later. Tuberculin skin tests are positive in 85% of cases. The organism may be recovered in the sputum as well as from CSF.

Clinical Features. Moderate but increasing signs of meningeal inflammation develop over days or weeks. Children present with lethargy, failure to thrive, anorexia, irritability, nausea, and vomiting. In adults, similar symptoms lead to a mild and gradual reduction in consciousness, with confusion and headaches, occasionally seizures, but only moderate evidence of meningeal irritation. Symptoms may have been precipitated by an initial flulike illness or measles.

If untreated, there occurs the slow but relentless progression of extraocular palsies, deafness, cerebellar signs, convulsions, optic atrophy, pupillary abnormalities, delirium, and possibly dementia. In the latest stages decerebrate rigidity occurs. The CSF contains mononuclear cells mainly, up to 500/mm^3; the protein is high and the sugar is low.

Unusual presentations include a single seizure in infants and children, isolated focal neurologic signs, the picture of acute meningitis, transverse myelopathy, or a preponderance of psychiatric symptoms in adults. Complications include blindness, deafness, hydrocephalus, spinal block, hypotha-

Box 165-5. Causes of Aseptic Meningitis*

Common Viral Causes[†]	Less Common Viral Causes	Nonviral Causes	Noninfectious Causes
Mumps	Measles	Tuberculosis	Chemical meningitis
Coxsackievirus	Rubella	Brucellosis	Collagen-vascular disease
Lymphocytic choriomeningitis	Chickenpox	Syphilis	Malignancy
Echovirus Epstein-Barr	Herpes simplex	Lyme disease	
	Influenza	Leptospirosis	
	Inectious mononucleosis	Fungi	
	Arbovirus	Parameningeal infections (e.g., intracerebral, epidural abscess)	
	Encephalomyocarditis	Mycoplasma	
	Behçet's disease	Infectious hepatitis	
	Polio	Bacterial endocarditis	
		Bacterial meningitis, inadequately treated	

From Mandell GL, Bennett JE, Dolin R, editors: *Principles and practice of infectious diseases,* ed 4, New York, Churchill Livingstone, 1995.
*Routine cultures negative.
†70% of cases.

lamic abnormalities, focal signs from persistent arachnoiditis, and cortical damage caused by subpial vasculitis and predisposing to seizures.

The lesion is essentially a basal meningitis with secondary vasculitis. An accumulation of purulent cellular infiltrate over the inferior surface of the brain and brainstem, blocking CSF flow through the fourth ventricle roof foramina, is responsible for the nerve palsies and raised ICP. In meningococcal and pneumococcal meningitis the purulent material is seen over all of the brain surface.

Cerebrospinal Fluid Studies. In subacute meningitis, laboratory studies of CSF find large numbers of lymphocytes and elevated protein levels. In TBM, PMNs may predominate in the early stages, and the glucose level is almost always depressed, even to zero. The chance of finding the organism varies with the time taken looking for it on the Ziehl-Neelsen smears. PCR has revolutionized the diagnosis of TBM. Other causes of lymphocytic meningitis are listed in Box 165-5.

Treatment. TBM can be treated successfully in almost all cases if therapy is started before the patient becomes unconscious. The generally accepted antibacterial regimen consists of quadruple therapy, with isoniazid, rifampin, pyrazinamide, and ethambutol (Table 165-6).

There is disagreement about the use of intrathecal therapy, particularly with antibacterial agents, but it is a good general rule not to inject anything into the intrathecal space if possible. Perhaps the use of steroids intrathecally in TBM is an exception, because this tends to reduce the fibrotic reaction that may block CSF pathways as healing takes place. However, as better antituberculous agents are developed, the need for intrathecal steroids is decreasing.

Cryptococcal Meningitis. Cryptococcal meningitis also has an insidious onset, with evidence of a confusional state, focal signs, and raised ICP. Although a smoldering meningitis is the usual presentation, abscesses may form. This condition also occurs in those with immunologic deficiencies, AIDS, diabetes, or chronic alcoholism.

A clinical point of interest in cryptococcal meningitis is

Table 165-6. Treatment of Tuberculous Meningitis in the Adult

Drug	Dosage
Isoniazid*	10-20 mg/kg/day orally up to 300 mg/day
Rifampin	10 mg/kg/day orally (usual dose 600 mg/day)
Ethamutol	25 mg/kg/day orally for 2 months; then 15 mg/kg/day orally
Pyrazinamide	25 mg/kg/day up to 2.5 gm/day maximum

From Mandell GL, Bennett JE, Dolin R, editors: *Principles and practice of infectious diseases,* ed 4, New York, Churchill Livingstone, 1995.
*The usual regimen comprises isoniazid and two of the three other drugs listed. Pyridoxine, 40 mg daily, should be added to prevent neuropathy caused by isoniazid.

the prolonged and severe nature of the headache that precedes cranial nerve palsies, meningism, or increased ICP. The sequential loss of cranial nerve function may be both dramatic and devastating. Diagnosis may be made with India ink–stained CSF preparations, but cryptococcal antigen should be detected in the blood and CSF.

Treatment is with amphotericin B, 0.6 mg/kg/day intravenously to a total dose of 2.5 gm with oral 5-fluorocytosine, continued for 6 weeks. Patients with AIDS need long-term suppressive treatment with fluconazole.

Other Causes. Secondary syphilis, brucellosis, sarcoidosis, and infiltration of the meninges by carcinoma, lymphoma, larval cysts, or fungi are uncommon causes of a similar subacute syndrome.

The term *meningismus* refers to the condition of meningism without any actual infection of the meninges. Tonsillitis, cervical adenitis, pyelonephritis, and lobar pneumonia are common causes. Other sources of meningeal irritation include blood in the CSF from any cause: otitis, sinusitis, spinal osteomyelitis, and epidural abscess (all parameningeal foci).

Chronic Meningitis

Chronic meningitis is uncommon, although it is produced by the same organisms that cause subacute meningitis. The characteristic symptoms include mild fever, headache, depression, lethargy and malaise, and subtle personality change progressing to confusion. Signs include meningism and, frequently, cranial nerve palsies and evidence of raised ICP.

The CSF may show a persistent lymphocytosis with high protein and low glucose levels. In such cases viruses, fungi, bacteria (including leptospira, treponema, and acid-fast bacilli), or malignant cells have variously been found. In sarcoidosis, a chronic basal meningitis may cause focal neurologic signs and, rarely, hydrocephalus, cranial nerve palsies, paraplegia, optic atrophy, or seizures. Meningeal carcinomatosis and leukemias cause headaches and cranial nerve palsies, but seldom long tract signs.

The appropriate treatment of chronic meningitis depends, naturally enough, on its cause and will not be detailed here.

Chronic Spinal Arachnoiditis. Chronic spinal arachnoiditis is a variant of chronic meningitis. It usually follows intrathecal injection of contrast media, steroids, anesthetics, or antibiotics, but spinal injury or surgery, prolapsed intervertebral disks, and numerous infections (e.g., tuberculosis, syphilis, or viral) have also been held responsible. The thickened meninges, usually in the lumbar region, entrap the nerve roots, causing bilateral burning leg pain at many root levels and local backache. Signs of multiple root lesions are usually detectable, and there may be loss of bladder function. If symptoms begin acutely after spinal surgery, fever may also occur.

Myelography (even though suspected to be a cause) and magnetic resonance imaging (MRI) scanning will confirm the diagnosis. Treatment is surgical, but it is not very effective and the condition tends to recur.

Recurrent Meningitis

Recurrent acute or subacute meningitis should lead one to search for the reason why repeated infections have involved the CNS. Although spontaneous repeated infection by different organisms is possible, some defect opening up a pathway allowing organisms to penetrate the nervous system is far more likely. In such cases a midline sinus running to the meninges from the upper respiratory tract or from the skin of the head, neck, or spine should be carefully sought, possibly using a magnifying glass. Chronic mastoiditis, sinusitis, agammaglobulinemia, and immunodeficiency syndromes are other possibilities. The condition may occur after splenectomy, in infancy, and also in association with skull fractures, particularly if there has been CSF leakage. Pneumococcus is the most common organism cultured.

Differential Diagnosis of Meningitis

Acute meningitis may be mimicked by subarachnoid hemorrhage, encephalopathy of bacterial endocarditis, malignant hypertension, lead poisoning, porphyria, migraine, or viral encephalitis. It may also be hard to differentiate bacterial meningitis from autoallergic acute postinfectious (disseminated) encephalomyelitis (described below). Cerebral abscesses usually have a less acute onset, but thrombophlebitis in association with chronic mastoid or sinus infection and the toxic encephalopathy associated with bacterial endocarditis may present similarly, except that focal signs and evidence of increased ICP are usual in all of these latter conditions.

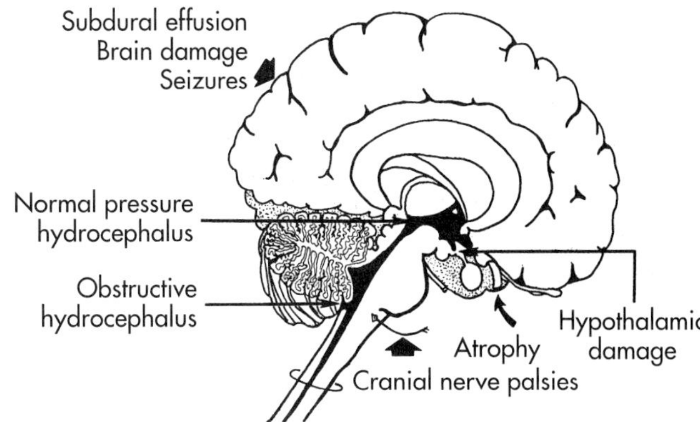

Fig. 165-1. Diagram of complications of meningitis. (From Mandell GL, Bennett JE, Dolin R, editors: *Principles and practice of infectious diseases*, ed 4, New York, Churchill Livingstone, 1995.)

Certain causes of endarteritis, such as collagen-vascular disease, may also present a similar but milder picture, as may slow virus infections, neoplasms seeding throughout the CSF, and local infections such as spinal osteitis or cranial osteomyelitis (parameningeal foci).

Subacute or chronic meningitis can be confused with cerebral tumor, subdural hematoma, a rapidly progressive dementing illness such as Creutzfeldt-Jakob disease (CJD), or the paraneoplastic encephalopathy of carcinoma.

Complications of Meningitis

In patients who recover from meningitis there may be evidence of significant focal residua caused by bacterial vasculitis, cortical infarction, or hydrocephalus. Seizures occur in 10% of those recovering. In infants, subdural effusions and deafness may be associated with *H. influenzae* and pneumococcal infections, whereas acute or chronic obstructive or normal pressure hydrocephalus may follow meningitis from any cause. Obstructive hydrocephalus is particularly common with TBM, as are deafness or other lower cranial nerve palsies, which occur in 15% of patients with meningitis. Hypothalamic damage and optic atrophy are much less common, except in chronic basal meningitis (Fig. 165-1).

Small infants and children who recover from meningitis may show signs of cerebral palsy, and such upper motor neuron signs may occur temporarily in adults recovering from severe meningitis. Because of the dangers of serious neurologic impairment, early diagnosis and appropriate specific therapy are essential to prevent such tragedies.

ENCEPHALITIS

Infection of the brain parenchyma is most commonly viral. When the infection is bacterial, the condition is known as *cerebritis*, which may progress to abscess formation. Viral encephalitis may be widespread or focal. Both DNA and RNA viruses may be responsible, certain viruses in each group having a particular affinity for the nervous system. These neurotropic viruses include polio, rabies, herpes zoster, and arboviruses. Viruses that are usually nonneurotropic but that sometimes still involve the nervous system include herpes simplex, mumps, measles, coxsackievirus, echovirus,

Box 165-6. Causes of Encephalitis

Viruses
- Sporadic
  - Herpes simplex*
  - Herpes zoster
  - Monkey B
  - Cytomegalovirus
  - Epstein-Barr (mononucleosis)*
  - Mumps*
  - Lymphocytic choriomeningitis*
  - Rabies
  - Human immunodeficiency virus
- Epidemic
  - Arboviruses (California, E* and W equine, St. Louis)
  - Enteroviruses (polio, coxsackievirus, and echovirus)
  - Measles*
- Slow viruses

Bacteria, rickettsiae, and spirochetes
- Bacterial endocarditis
- Cerebritis (early cerebral abscess)
- Syphilis
- *Coxiella burnetii*

Fungi
- Cryptococcus neoformans
- Histoplasmosis
- Aspergillosis

Protozoa and Metazoa
- Malaria
- Toxoplasmosis
- Amoebas (Naegleria, Acanthamoeba)
- Echinococcus, cysticercosis, and trichinosis
- Schistosomiasis, trypanosomiasis

Possible viral
- Encephalitis lethargica
- Behçet's syndrome
- Encephalomyocarditis

From Mandell GL, Bennett JE, Dolin R, editors: *Principles and practice of infectious diseases,* ed 4, New York, Churchill Livingstone, 1995.
*The more common conditions in North America.

CMVs, and Epstein-Barr virus. Finally, measles, the papovaviruses, and perhaps others may give rise to slow virus infections. Other organisms causing encephalitis are listed in Box 165-6.

In the following discussion, the classical picture of encephalitis in general and that caused by herpes simplex in particular will be discussed. Other viral infective syndromes will be mentioned in brief. Most of the viruses causing encephalitis cannot be clinically differentiated, however, and specific identification techniques are needed to determine which virus is involved.

Typical Encephalitis

Causative Organisms. Arboviruses are found in ticks and mosquitos. They include Eastern and Western equine, Venezuelan, St. Louis, Japanese B, Powassan, California, La Crosse, Jamestown Canyon, Snowshoe hare, Rift Valley, and Orbivirus 1 agent of Colorado tick fever. Enteroviruses such as polio, coxsackievirus, and echovirus, and the viruses responsible for rubella, measles, chickenpox, mononucleosis, mumps, viral hepatitis, and influenza can all produce a more or less similar clinical picture because of direct parenchymal invasion of the nervous system and the subsequent antibody reaction.

In North America, herpes simplex, enteroviruses (polio, echovirus, and coxsackievirus), and arboviruses are the most common causative agents, with LCM and mumps the next most frequently identified causes. The prognosis in mumps and LCM is excellent, but arbovirus and herpes simplex infections are sometimes lethal or result in severe sequelae. Epstein-Barr virus is another cause of encephalitis, especially in younger subjects.

Enteroviral infection is most common in the summer months; the arbovirus infections spread by ticks occur mainly in the spring and those by mosquitos in the late summer. Mumps is the most common cause of encephalitis in the earlier part of the year, whereas LCM is more common in the fall and winter. During the great influenza pandemic of 1917, many patients developed the syndrome of von Economo encephalitis characterized by marked drowsiness (sleeping sickness), which often developed years later into a form of Parkinson's disease with oculogyric crises. It is not certain whether such an illness still exists sporadically because the virus was never isolated.

In North America, arboviruses other than St. Louis and Eastern and Western equine (see Box 165-3) are rare indeed, as are protozoal and metazoal infections. Bacteria, meningovascular syphilis, and fungi cause encephalitis usually only in association with frank meningitic signs. Although herpes and other arbovirus infections are often exceedingly severe, most other viruses produce a milder illness. Tertiary neurosyphilis smolders to produce the features of general paresis or tabes or meningovascular syphilis. Obviously many of the causative agents listed are unlikely causes of encephalitis in, for example, Eastern Canada, but one always must ask about visits a patient may have made to another country in these days of frequent air travel.

Clinical Features. Typical features of encephalitis include fever, meningism, and signs of raised ICP. Reduction in consciousness level from drowsiness to coma, seizures that are often focal, and various other focal signs also occur, depending on which areas of brain are affected by the inflammatory process. As with cerebral abscesses, the combination of fever and meningism with evidence of cerebral dysfunction, either generalized (delirium, seizures, coma) or focal (hallucinations, hemiparesis, and so forth) must make one consider encephalitis.

Major pathologic features include edema and petechiae within the brain, with mononuclear perivascular cuffing and neuronal degeneration, mainly in the grey matter, cortex, and deep nuclei of the brainstem.

Differential Diagnosis. The list of differential diagnoses is rather long. Any form of meningitis may be accompanied by evidence of cortical inflammation. Abscesses, septic emboli, cortical septic thrombophlebitis, and postinfectious and toxic encephalopathies may be hard to distinguish from encephalitis; all are described here. Subdural and subarachnoid hemorrhage, bleeding into a tumor, porphyria, poisoning, and even multiple sclerosis can produce encephalopathy with meningism and sometimes fever.

Encephalopathy without actual invasion of the brain substance occurs with bacterial endocarditis, pertussis, and typhoid. These cannot be differentiated by their neurologic signs from viral encephalitis, but other clinical findings may allow diagnosis.

Laboratory Findings. CSF taken during the acute stage of encephalitis shows a moderate rise in protein and contains lymphocytes up to about 250/mm^3. The sugar level is usually normal, except in mumps (and occasionally in herpes simplex virus [HSV] and LCM) encephalitis, when it is low, as it is in bacterial, fungal, and carcinomatous meningitis.

Specific laboratory diagnosis requires a fourfold increase in the level of viral antibody titers between acute and convalescent sera or virus isolation from the CSF or brain. Specimens must be frozen immediately after collection and shipped on dry ice to a laboratory for direct virus isolation, whereas acute and convalescent paired serum specimen can be sent unfrozen. If enterovirus infection is suspected, feces, CSF, or throat washings may be used for virus isolation. Throat washings and CSF are used for mumps identification, blood and CSF are used to detect LCM, and CSF or occasionally brain biopsy material is used to check for herpes simplex. Other viruses may be isolated from blood or CSF, and CMV can be found in the urine, saliva, or liver biopsy specimens. Cryptococcal or other fungal antigens may need to be sought as well. The heterophile test and tests for IgM antibody to viral capsid antigen should be positive in cases of Epstein-Barr virus encephalitis.

PCR is so sensitive for the diagnosis of herpes simplex virus encephalitis that brain biopsy is now rarely, if ever, necessary to diagnose this serious infection.

Treatment. The treatment of encephalitis is improving. General measures include maintaining the patient's hydration and metabolic status, reducing fever, and preventing seizures. Antiviral agents are now available for treatment of herpes simplex (see below) and varicella-zoster forms of encephalitis.

Herpes Simplex Encephalitis

In North America, herpes simplex is the most common single cause of acute, sporadic, severe encephalitis. Both human and monkey types of herpesvirus occur, and both can cause severe neurologic infection, although the latter is usually seen only in laboratory workers or monkey handlers. Infections occur at any age, but particularly in the first three decades. Of the two serologic types of human herpesvirus, type I causes sporadic encephalitis and oral ulcers, whereas type II produces aseptic meningitis and genital ulceration. In adults, nearly all cases of herpes simplex virus encephalitis (HSVE) are caused by type I virus.

Clinical Features. Herpes simplex encephalitis may have an acute or subacute onset. Typically, a few days of malaise, fever, headache, anorexia, nausea, and other nonspecific symptoms progress to a subtle change of personality, with evolving depression, paranoia, or abnormal behavior and confusion. Photophobia, signs of raised ICP, meningeal irritation, and focal signs appear next; the latter include hemiparesis, facial weakness, dysphasia, dysarthria, decerebrate rigidity, ocular palsies or nystagmus, seizures, and in the late stages stupor or coma. Although the whole brain is involved, the temporal lobes are particularly affected.

Laboratory Findings. With herpes simplex encephalitis, the CSF shows an increase in pressure and protein levels; lymphocytes and red cells are often present. A characteristic electroencephalogram (EEG) pattern (diffuse, mainly temporal-region slow activity with periodic discharges) is described but is not specific. The CT scan may demonstrate swelling and enlargement of the temporal lobes (usually asymmetrically), although MRI scans show this even better. The specific methods of diagnosis are PCR of the CSF, fluorescent antibody staining, or culture of a brain biopsy specimen. Because of the mass effect of the lesion, LP may be dangerous and CT or MRI should be done first to rule out the presence of a pressure cone.

Treatment. Acyclovir reduces mortality and morbidity if it is given early, and the low toxicity of this drug has led to its use empirically in most cases of acute, sporadic encephalitis. Acyclovir, 10 mg/kg given intravenously every 8 hours for 10 days, reduces mortality to about 20%; half of the patients completely recover.

Herpes simplex virus can also cause aseptic meningitis or a sacral plexopathy, with perineal numbness, impotence, and retention of urine and feces.

RABIES

The virus of rabies is introduced into the body through the bite of an infected dog, fox, vole, bat, or other wild animal (see Chapter 101). It travels centrally along peripheral nerves, producing a focal encephalitis that mainly involves the cervical cord, the brainstem, and the temporal lobes. The latent period between the bite and the clinical features of the disease may be as long as a year.

Clinically, early irritability and agitated delirium progress to muscle hypertonia, especially affecting the pharyngeal muscles, which go into spasm—hence the term *hydrophobia*. Convulsions and death usually occur within 10 days of the onset.

Human diploid rabies virus vaccine has been found to be strongly immunogenic, and its introduction is an important breakthrough in the prevention of rabies. Rabies immune globulin should be given as soon as possible after a bite. Usually, 50% of the dose is infiltrated at the bite site and the remainder is given intramuscularly.

ACQUIRED IMMUNODEFICIENCY SYNDROME

Infection with the human immunodeficiency virus (HIV) ultimately results in profound deficits in function of the immune system, predisposing the infected individual to severe opportunistic infections and to certain malignancies. In addition to the neurologic involvement caused by HIV itself, these patients are also susceptible to a variety of CNS infections. Ten percent of patients with AIDS present with neurologic problems, but these ultimately occur in at least 75% of cases.

Syndromes of encephalopathy, aseptic meningitis with cranial neuropathy, myelopathy, or multiple mononeuropathy may occur at the time of initial infection with the virus; recovery occurs within a week or so in most cases.

Toxoplasma encephalitis is the most common cause of mass lesions in the brains of patients with AIDS. Headache, confusion, lethargy, focal deficits, seizures, fever, and coma result; chorea, dystonias, myoclonus, and tremor are less common. Mass lesions in patients with AIDS are due either to such opportunistic infections or to tumors. A CT scan typically shows ring-enhancing lesions when toxoplasma, tubercular, candida, or CMV infection is present and with primary CNS lymphoma.

AIDS dementia is a manifestation of the subacute encephalitis that occurs in one third of HIV-infected patients, and it is accompanied by a host of neurologic signs. Apart from the major cognitive symptoms, such as forgetfulness, impaired concentration, confusion, and slowing of thought processes, signs such as apathy, organic psychoses, headache, depression, seizures, myoclonus, cerebellar and pyramidal deficits, neuropathy, and retinopathy are common.

Vacuolar myelopathy leads to paraparesis with spastic weakness, ataxia, and paresthesias in the legs. It is considered to represent the effect of direct HIV infection of the spinal cord.

Cryptococcal and tuberculous meningitis, CMV retinitis, toxoplasma chorioretinitis, herpes simplex myelitis, and spirochetal or viral encephalomyelitis are other frequent complications, as are progressive multifocal leukoencephalopathy, CNS lymphomas, and a painful symmetrical sensorimotor peripheral neuropathy. Again these entities are probably related to direct infection with the HIV virus.

AIDS remains a fatal disease, but prompt diagnosis and treatment of the opportunistic infections have prolonged survival. Toxoplasmosis is treated with pyrimethamine, 200 mg as a loading dose, then 50 to 75 mg daily, with sulfadiazine, 4 gm/day, or clindamycin. All patients who are treated with pyrimethamine or sulfadiazine should also receive folinic acid, 10 mg orally each day.

ABSCESS

Abscesses may occur in the epidural or subdural spaces or within the substance of the brain, in which case they are examples of suppurative bacterial encephalitis.

Epidural Abscess

Intracranial Epidural Abscess. Intracranial epidural abscess is usually associated with a local skull fracture, osteomyelitis, or inflammation of the transverse or sagittal sinuses. The abscess is frequently situated over the convexity of the brain, and the clinical features are those of a generalized infection, of a local destructive lesion compressing the brain, and of raised ICP.

Spinal Epidural Abscess. The usual organism found in spinal epidural abscesses is *Staphylococcus aureus* in the lumbar region or tuberculosis at thoracic levels. In tuberculosis, granulation tissue, pus, and the products of vertebral body and disk collapse to cause cord compression and local pain. Acute angulation *(angular kyphosis)* may result from the local infection and should be treated first by the usual antituberculous agents to render the contents of the abscess sterile; it can then be surgically drained, with later stabilization of the spine. Should the abscess cause neurologic signs, emergency surgical intervention will be required.

Differential Diagnosis. Problems may arise in the differential diagnosis of acute lumbar spinal epidural abscess and acute transverse myelopathy that is usually of viral origin (and eight times as common). Both cause root pain in girdle distribution, stiff neck, marked muscle spasms, and local tenderness of the spine, with the usual neurologic deficit of paraparesis with a sensory level, fever, and increased cells and protein in the CSF. However, the erythrocyte sedimentation rate (ESR) is always high in epidural abscesses, but not necessarily with transverse myelitis. Evidence of block of CSF passage, radiographic findings of osteomyelitis of the appropriate vertebrae, recent bacterial infection elsewhere, and perhaps slower clinical development (so that the maximal deficit is not reached until the third or fourth day) are all factors in favor of epidural abscess. Transverse myelitis is also more common at thoracic levels and less so at lumbar levels. In children, transverse myelitis sometimes presents without any pain in the back.

Subdural Abscess (Empyema)

Causes. The underlying cause in at least 80% of cases of subdural abscess is disease of the nasal sinuses or of the middle ear, whether by direct extension or as a result of thrombophlebitis leading to focal intracranial infection. Paranasal infection commonly results in frontal abscesses, and otitis causes posterior cerebral and cerebellar abscesses. Subdural abscesses also occur when a subdural hematoma or effusion (particularly if secondary to meningitis in infants) becomes infected, when a cerebral abscess ruptures into the subdural space, or after a penetrating wound.

Organisms. The bacteria responsible for subdural abscesses are usually mixed aerobic and anaerobic streptococci, less commonly staphylococci, gram-negative cocci, or Clostridia. The disease occurs particularly between the ages of 10 and 20 years with paranasal infection and after the age of 40 with an otitic origin.

Clinical Features. The usual features of subdural abscess include evidence of skull osteomyelitis (local tenderness, swelling, and cellulitis), systemic signs of infection, altered consciousness, headache, fever, meningism, and focal signs appropriate to the area of cerebral involvement. These patients are severely ill, and seizures of any type are common. The diagnosis is suggested by the findings of nasal sinus or middle ear infection in the presence of the above signs.

Laboratory Findings. An EEG will show local slow wave activity, and plain skull radiographs may show sinus opacity or osteomyelitis (and sometimes a shift of the pineal gland). An enhanced CT scan localizes the abscess precisely.

Treatment. The abscess should be surgically drained. Cloxacillin and metronidazole are recommended in the same regimen as for intracerebral abscess (see below), and the treatment should be continued for 1 month. The mortality rate in subdural abscess is about 10%; residual seizures and focal neurologic deficits are common, so anticonvulsants are routinely prescribed. Consultation and referral are mandatory to ensure timely and optimal treatment for all intracranial abscesses.

Intracerebral Abscess

Causes. Over half of all cases of intracerebral abscess complicate an ear or paranasal sinus infection. Skull fractures, facial or dental infections, and congenital heart disease also predispose, and hematogenous spread of infection from chronic lung disease (bronchiectasis, lung abscess) is responsible for another 20%. The intracerebral abscess is truly a local purulent encephalitis and although it is usually single and well-localized to frontal or temporal regions when the infection extends from an adjacent source, multiple abscesses can occur with hematogenous spread (Fig. 165-2). This usually occurs in elderly patients, particularly those with diabetes, among whom multiple staphylococcal microabscesses are becoming more common.

Neonates, diabetics, immunocompromised patients, heroin and alcohol addicts, patients with prosthetic or congenitally damaged heart valves, and those with lymphomas are especially at risk. Immunocompromised patients may develop candidal abscesses with intracerebral vasculitis; they present with fever but few focal signs. In many patients the infection can be traced to endocarditis or other septic foci.

An abscess may spread directly or as a result of septic thrombophlebitis, in which the infected clot may extend backwards along a large vein to infect other areas of the brain. The organisms most frequently cultured include streptococci, staphylococci, klebsiella, proteus, bacteroides, pneumococcus, and anaerobic organisms.

Clinical Features. The symptoms of intracerebral abscess may for a time be vague and nonspecific; they include fever, mild drowsiness, and headache, followed by evidence of focal brain destruction, meningism, and raised ICP.

A

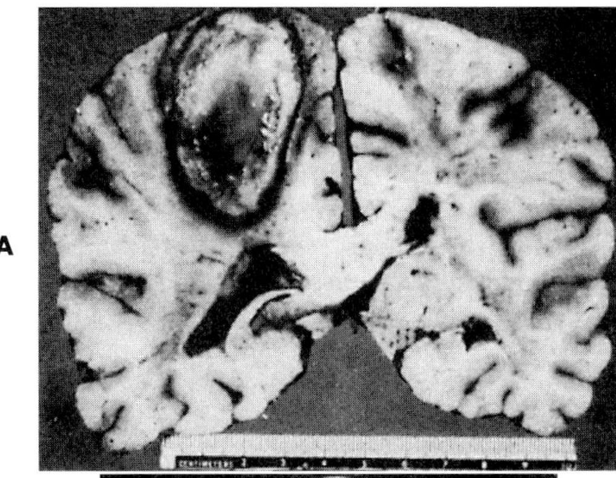

B

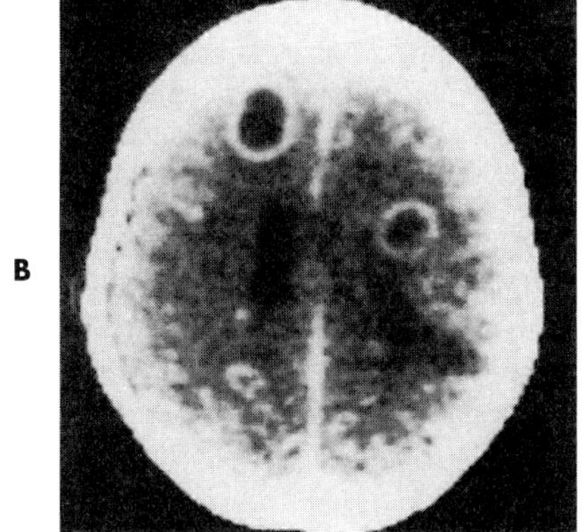

Fig. 165-2. **A,** Coronal section of brain showing a chronic right frontal lobe abscess. **B,** Enhanced CT scan; multiple abscesses with ring enhancement. (From Mandell GL, Bennett JE, Dolin R, editors: *Principles and practice of infectious diseases,* ed 4, New York, Churchill Livingstone, 1995.)

Seizures are particularly common with cerebral abscesses in the frontal, temporal, and parietal regions. Often there is little systemic evidence of sepsis, and the patient presents in lethargic delirium. However, cerebellar abscesses produce rapidly rising ICP and brainstem signs.

Diagnosis. Diagnosis of an intracerebral abscess should be suggested by the clinical pictures of lung, ear, or sinus disease with signs of intracranial infection and seizures; meningitis with a focal deficit; stroke with fever; or raised ICP with no obvious cause. The EEG is invariably abnormal, with prominent focal slow waves. A CT or MRI scan will localize the abscess and will determine the degree of capsule formation. LP is potentially lethal.

Treatment. Initial treatment consists of surgical aspiration of pus from the abscess cavity; this will allow identification of the organisms and use of appropriate intravenous antibiotics in high doses.

If the origin of the abscess is sinusitis, anaerobic streptococci will grow in culture and penicillin and chloramphenicol or metronidazole should be given to the patient. Otitic abscesses imply mixed organisms and will respond to gentamicin, as well as the above drugs. Traumatic abscesses usually yield staphylococci, for which cloxacillin is recommended. Multiple broad-spectrum antibiotic therapy is required for abscesses of metastatic origin; cloxacillin 12 g/day, with metronidazole, 500 mg every 8 hours, and a third-generation cephalosporin might be employed.

ICP is likely to be raised as a result of vasogenic edema around the abscess; steroids may be expected to help relieve it, but antibiotic treatment should be started before steroids are given. Patients who have recovered from an acute cerebral abscess frequently go on to have seizures. If it is likely that the abscess developed by hematogenous spread, congenital heart disease with a right-to-left shunt, pulmonary disease such as bronchiectasis, and sepsis elsewhere in the body must be excluded. The physician should look for needle marks and other signs of intravenous drug use; many younger patients use dirty syringes to mainline drugs.

Cerebral abscesses are serious emergencies and require rapid diagnosis so that antibiotic therapy can begin and surgical intervention is expedited. Even in these days of new antibiotics, steroids, and CT scanning, these abscesses still carry a 10% mortality rate.

OTHER NEUROLOGIC INFECTIONS

Herpes Zoster

The varicella-zoster virus is neurotropic. After many years of latency, it may be reactivated (by unknown mechanisms) and primarily affects the dorsal root ganglion cells of spinal nerves and the sensory ganglia of cranial nerves, certainly the gasserian (V) ganglion and perhaps the geniculate (VII). At the spinal level, the involvement is usually unilateral, and 75% of cases occur in the abdominal or upper thoracic regions. The virus occasionally attacks anterior horn cells of the spinal cord. Edema, monocytic infiltration, and perivascular cuffing with neuronal degeneration are seen histologically, with later fibrosis and secondary degeneration of the distal part of the nerve fiber.

Among elderly patients, recurrent herpes should put one on guard for the presence of an underlying malignancy, lymphoma, or immune deficiency syndrome. Chickenpox itself may be complicated by acute allergic encephalomyelitis (see below), polyradiculitis, and cerebellar ataxia.

Clinical Features. With herpes zoster viruses, burning or shooting pain with local hyperalgesia within the affected dermatomes is followed in 3 or 4 days by a typical vesicular eruption that fades over the next few days, with scarring and depigmentation of the skin. Within the affected area the skin may be anesthetic but at the same time painful or itchy. Motor involvement may affect the face, eye, diaphragm, or limb musculature. Postherpetic neuralgia is exceedingly painful. During the acute phase, valacyclovir and famciclovir both reduce the rate of postherpetic neuralgia.

Herpes Zoster Ophthalmicus

Herpes zoster ophthalmicus may produce the feared complications of corneal damage and secondary infection. The eye should be treated immediately with topical idoxuridine. The region of the forehead and eye may be exceedingly painful at the time of diagnosis, and postherpetic neuralgia may follow. When herpes zoster attacks the VII nerve, the V nerve is often involved as well, which explains why there are vesicles in the auricle and inside the mouth. Intracranial CNS involvement is uncommon, but arteritis causing stroke, and meningoencephalitis do occasionally occur.

Cytomegalovirus

CMVs are members of the herpesvirus family. They may cause eye and brain damage in utero, and adults (especially if immunocompromised) may develop meningoencephalitis, retinitis, or polyneuropathy. Ganciclovir has been used to treat serious CMV infections.

Poliomyelitis

Poliomyelitis is still prevalent throughout much of the world, and children who have not been immunized in the most advanced nations are susceptible to infection. Thus primary care physicians must remain informed about its clinical presentation and acute management. The neurotropic poliovirus has three serotypes, of which type 1 is the most common. Spread from person to person is by fecal contamination. After entering the gastrointestinal (GI) tract, the virus passes into the blood stream to invade the nervous system. The incubation period is 7 to 14 days, and in nonimmunized populations the disease may be either epidemic or sporadic. Subclinical infection frequently occurs and produces immunity; this is also the basis of live virus immunization.

If the poliovirus invades the nervous system, a minor illness occurs, with headache, drowsiness, fever, and mild GI symptoms. The illness may stop at that stage, or after 1 or 2 days of apparent remission severe muscle pains, meningism, and delirium progress within 24 hours to sudden asymmetric or generalized paralysis (the paralytic form of the major illness). The muscles are tender, and fasciculations may be seen (and felt) in the earliest stages. After a week, some degree of improvement usually begins. Truncal and bulbar involvement may give rise to severe respiratory and bulbar paralysis that requires artificial ventilation and skilled nursing attention in an intensive care unit. The lower motor neuron lesions produced may eventually progress to contractures, trophic changes, failure of limb growth, and eventual joint disorganization.

A nonparalytic form of the major illness also occurs, with signs of meningoencephalitis (as in the paralytic form) but without anterior horn cell involvement.

Diagnosis. In the earliest stages, the disease can only be easily diagnosed during an epidemic because the mild symptoms resemble many other nonspecific viral illnesses. A paretic illness can also be caused by other enteroviruses, in which case the prognosis is much better. Weakness may also occur in association with other inflammatory bone or joint diseases.

Other fast-advancing peripheral motor neuropathies include those caused by porphyria, Guillain-Barré syndrome, and polyarteritis nodosa. Lower motor neuron lesions seldom complicate other CNS infections, although mumps may rarely produce encephalomyelitis. Even in these days, however, the presence of an acute infective illness associated with signs of anterior horn cell involvement must always make one suspect poliomyelitis.

The development of new weakness, muscle atrophy, fatigue, and pain decades after acute poliomyelitis, accompanied by a mixed picture of active and chronic denervation on an electromyogram (EMG), suggests the diagnosis of postpolio syndrome. This condition appears to be due to the late death of neurones that regrew or sprouted after the initial illness, but the reason why they die at this late stage remains unknown.

Coxsackievirus

Although coxsackievirus infection may cause aseptic meningitis, epidemic myalgia (Bornholm disease) is a more common manifestation. In this condition, the sudden onset of acute chest pain, with severe tenderness of the intercostal muscles in one or more spaces and great difficulty in breathing because of pleuritic pain, frequently raises suspicion of pulmonary embolism, pneumonia, or even myocardial infarction. The pain may occur so acutely that patients sometimes fear that they may have had a heart attack. Very few systemic signs are associated, and after a few days of useless symptomatic treatment, complete recovery occurs.

Infectious Mononucleosis

About 5% of patients with infectious mononucleosis develop neurologic complications as a result of inflammatory infiltrates and neuronal degeneration in the nervous system. The most common of these complications is aseptic meningitis, a benign and relatively transient disorder. Encephalitis and encephalomyelitis present with seizures, reduction in level of consciousness, raised ICP, focal neurologic signs, and meningism. A generalized peripheral neuropathy indistinguishable from Guillain-Barré syndrome is well recognized, but patients may also have mononeuropathies, and virtually every cranial nerve has been reported as affected. Less commonly, illnesses resembling Reye's syndrome, dysautonomia, brachial neuropathy, movement disorders, or a syndrome such as multiple sclerosis have been described.

Influenza

The neurologic complications of influenza are usually indirect, taking the form of an acute postinfectious encephalomyelitis. Depression frequently occurs after influenza, and some patients with multiple sclerosis may have a relapse after even a mild attack. Neuralgic amyotrophy is another occasional complication (see Chapter 167).

Tick Paralysis

Particularly in western North America, wood ticks may attach themselves to persons exploring the undergrowth, especially children. The tick can be found attached to the head or to any other hairy body parts. Its toxin may block neuromuscular transmission, causing a rapidly progressive, symmetric, flaccid paralysis, with signs resembling a severe myasthenic crisis.

The weakness may be so severe that respiratory and bulbar paralysis occur and the patient may die of respiratory insufficiency. The sudden onset of such profound weakness over the course of a day or less should make one think of tick paralysis. Treatment consists of removal of the tick, but it may be difficult to find and may require shaving the child or searching through the hair with a fine comb. With supportive measures, recovery should occur within a few days.

Tetanus

Although *Clostridium tetani* is not as widespread now as it was in the days of horse-drawn transport, tetanus still constitutes an important disease despite a fairly high level of immunization in Western communities. The organism enters a wound (which may be very small) or follows surgical procedures, otitis media, or puerperal or umbilical sepsis. Its toxin then ascends the peripheral motor nerves to block inhibitory postsynaptic potentials affecting the anterior horn cells.

After an incubation period of up to 3 weeks, patients develop pain and stiffness of the muscles (especially in the neck, back, and abdominal wall). Trismus, dysphagia, and reflex spasms are common, often beginning in the back, neck, and jaw muscles and lasting up to 30 seconds. The strong muscular contractions may induce hyperpyrexia, and respiratory arrest may occur. Laryngospasm, chest infections, and cardiac arrest are occasional lethal complications. Diagnosis is only achieved early if a high index of suspicion is maintained.

Treatment. Treatment for tetanus is along several lines.

1. Human antitetanus immunoglobulin has replaced horse serum antitoxin, and 2000 to 4000 units are given intramuscularly, after which a course of intramuscular penicillin is necessary.
2. Tetanus toxoid is required to achieve active immunization.
3. The wound must be excised and cleaned, with all dead tissue removed.
4. Symptomatic treatment depends on the severity of the case. Mild cases will need only diazepam and sedatives. Respiratory difficulty requires tracheostomy and possibly curarization, as well as the above measures. The most severe cases must be anesthetized and paralyzed, so all patients must be transferred urgently to an intensive care unit. Many metabolic and urinary problems complicate the acute illness, and close nursing attention is essential.

Even in the best facilities, about 10% of patients with tetanus die, mainly because of complications. The most seriously affected patients are those with cephalic tetanus infection from invasion in the head and neck area, and those in whom symptoms begin within a few days of wounding.

Botulism

The toxin of *Clostridium botulinum* impairs acetylcholine release at motor nerve endings. The source of this toxin is often improperly canned foods, although wounds are sometimes the portal of entry. In infants, progressive weakness, hypotonia, poor gag and suck reflexes, and constipation are the main signs. In adults, extraocular muscle, respiratory, facial, and bulbar palsies occur; the limbs are flaccid and paretic, and reflexes are lost. The pupils usually dilate and are poorly responsive. Treatment consists of urgent ventilatory support with neutralization of toxin using the specific trivalent (ABE) antiserum, penicillin, and cathartics.

Toxoplasmosis

Toxoplasmosis may occur as a congenital infection or may be acquired later in life, usually in immunosuppressed patients. This protozoan organism commonly affects the nervous system and produces an inflammatory reaction with formation of miliary granulomas. These may later calcify or undergo necrosis, resulting in hydrocephalus, or they may be completely asymptomatic.

Congenital toxoplasmosis may be evident shortly after birth. Failure to thrive, convulsions, spasticity, opisthotonos, and eye defects such as chorioretinitis or microphthalmos are possible presentations. Optic atrophy is a common later development, as is hydrocephalus. Some children do not develop symptoms until the age of 4 or 5, when hepatomegaly and splenomegaly are found. Radiographs of the skull often show scattered calcifications.

Acquired toxoplasmosis is often traceable to infected animals. Clinical features include skin lesions, pulmonary and lymphatic involvement, acute meningitis, encephalitis, myositis, and chronic granulomatous meningitis.

Laboratory findings will depend on the type and extent of involvement. The CSF may be under increased pressure, and the protein will usually be increased with a slight or moderate increase in mononuclear cells. Skull radiographs and funduscopy are often extremely helpful in making a diagnosis, but more definitive support comes from complement-fixation and fluorescent antibody tests.

Children with symptomatic congenital toxoplasmosis often have significant mental and neurologic defects, if they survive. In the adult form (which is much less common), the prognosis depends on the severity of the infection; patients with overt encephalitis do poorly. Treatment is with sulfonamides combined with pyrimethamine.

Syphilis

Although a request for specific serology is (or should be) routine on all patients admitted to neurologic wards, the overall return on these tests is relatively small. The request is still important because the prevalence of syphilis is probably increasing (in part associated with the spread of AIDS) but the number of patients who are coming for treatment is not, suggesting that we are going to be faced with an increasing number of cases of late and congenital syphilis in the future (see Chapter 29).

Serodiagnostic tests for syphilis may be classified as *reagin tests* and *specific antitreponemal antibody tests.* In the former group, the one most commonly used in North America is the rapid plasma reagin (RPR), a slide test that detects the presence of cardiolipin antigens. This is positive in between 75% and 95% of patients with primary, secondary, late, or latent syphilis. Unfortunately, false positive tests are common with reagin tests, being seen in conditions accompanied by abnormal globulins or excessive normal globulins. These include almost all of the collagen-vascular diseases, pregnancy, vaccination for smallpox, Hansen's disease (leprosy), infectious mononucleosis, measles, and atypical pneumonia. Narcotic addicts and patients with chronic rubella, viral hepatitis, viral pneumonia, hemolytic anemia, and the tropical diseases yaws and pinta may show such biologic false-positive reactions (Box 165-7).

The specific antitreponemal antibody test in common use is the microtreponema pallidum hemagglutination test (MTPHA). It is the first to react in syphilis and is positive in about 95% of cases of primary, secondary, late, and latent syphilis. It can be performed on the CSF and the blood and is seldom positive in the conditions causing false-positive RPR reactions (except for yaws and pinta, when it may give a weak positive reaction).

One single positive serologic test for syphilis does not make the diagnosis, however, and clinical evidence or repeat testing by different methods is always necessary. In the following discussion, the classical patterns of syphilis are described (Box 165-8), but today the intercurrent use of penicillin has changed the clinical picture of syphilis, and seizures, strokes, confusional states, depression, and visual field alterations may be the sole presenting signs.

Box 165-7. Causes of Biologic False-positive Serologic Test Results for Syphilis

Transient (negative after 3 months)
- Recent vaccination, typhoid inoculation
- Infective hepatitis
- Infectious mononucleosis, measles, varicella-zoster
- Viral encephalitis
- Pregnancy
- Undetermined (30%)

Persistent (positive after 3 months)
- Collagen-vascular diseases
- Hashimoto thyroiditis
- Rheumatic heart disease
- Hepatic cirrhosis
- Hemolytic anemia
- Chronic nephritis
- Peripheral vascular disease
- Undetermined (50%)

From Mandell GL, Bennett JE, Dolin R, editors: *Principles and practice of infectious diseases*, ed 4, New York, Churchill Livingstone, 1995.

Box 165-8. Forms of Syphilis

Latent

Primary
- CSF lymphocytosis

Secondary
- Acute syphilitic meningitis

Tertiary
- *Meningovascular:* cerebral or spinal endarteritis, cerebral or spinal leptomeningitis, meningomyelitis
- *Parenchymatous:* tabes dorsalis, general paresis, isolated optic atrophy, gummas

Congenital

From Mandell GL, Bennett JE, Dolin R, editors: *Principles and practice of infectious diseases*, ed 4, New York, Churchill Livingstone, 1995.

Primary Syphilis. The chancre is the only lesion that occurs in primary syphilis. This lesion, classically on the pudenda, appears after an incubation period of 3 weeks to 3 months. There may be some increase in CSF lymphocytes at this time, but no clinical signs appear.

Secondary Syphilis. The secondary syphilis stage follows immediately after the primary stage, 2 or 3 months after the appearance of the chancre. Constitutional symptoms are those of fever in association with a symmetric, nonitchy skin rash over all of the body, but particularly on the palms and soles. Snail-track ulcers (mucous patches on the mucosa of the mouth and genitalia), generalized lymphadenopathy, loss of hair, and iritis may occur. A meningoencephalitis presenting the usual features of fever, meningeal irritation, raised ICP, and occasionally with focal signs including seizures, is the main neurologic problem. The CSF shows a small increase in protein but a marked increase in lymphocytes, reduced glucose levels, and positive serologic reactions.

Tertiary (Late) Syphilis. After the lesions of secondary syphilis clear, a latent stage occurs, even in untreated cases in which there are no signs of the underlying infection. Tertiary syphilis may appear years later and involves the skin, mouth, eyes, bones, joints, gut, or genitourinary system. Cardiovascular problems related to tertiary syphilis include aortitis, granulomas of the myocardium or arterial walls (gummas), or a generalized vasculitis; the nervous system may also show a variety of abnormalities. The three most common syndromes are described below. The diversity of involvement led to the old adage that syphilis is the great mimicker of virtually every known medical disease; lupus erythematosus and AIDS now have the same distinction.

Meningovascular Syphilis. In the meningovascular form of tertiary syphilis, a chronic basal meningitis results in increased ICP, cranial nerve lesions, or cerebral infarction. The CSF will show positive serology, increased protein and lymphocytes, and occasionally decreased sugar levels.

Tabes Dorsalis. Tabes dorsalis is characterized by degenerative changes in the posterior roots and root entry zone of the spinal cord (Fig. 165-3). This results in numerous sensory signs. Because of the atrophy of the large sensory fibers in the posterior roots and dorsal columns, the patients show poor proprioception, loss of deep pain, absent reflexes, hypotonia, a "stamping" gait, and a positive Romberg's test. Lancinating lightning pains may be felt in girdle distribution or in the smooth muscles of the bowel, bladder, or larynx. They are much diminished by carbamazepine. The loss of "thick fiber" or "dorsal column" sensation may result in ulcers of the feet and painless destruction of joints *(Charcot's joints)*. Impotence and bladder dilation caused by deafferentation are also common; optic atrophy, ptosis, and Argyll Robertson pupils complete the clinical picture.

General Paresis. General paresis is a subacute meningoencephalitis and is characterized by progressive dementia with major frontal lobe signs and evidence of involvement of the

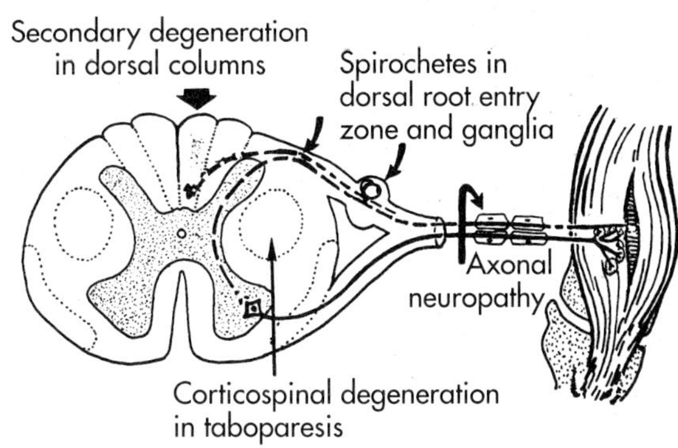

Fig. 165-3. Sites of primary pathology in tabes dorsalis. (From Mandell GL, Bennett JE, Dolin R, editors: *Principles and practice of infectious diseases,* ed 4, New York, Churchill Livingstone, 1995.)

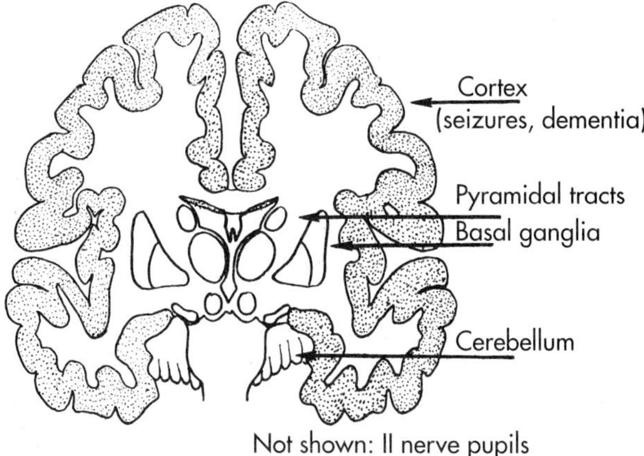

Fig. 165-4. Sites of primary pathology in general paresis. (From Mandell GL, Bennett JE, Dolin R, editors: *Principles and practice of infectious diseases,* ed 4, New York, Churchill Livingstone, 1995.)

motor cortex and the parietal and temporal lobes (Fig. 165-4). Tremors and a parkinsonian picture may also result from basal ganglion involvement.

Optic atrophy and Argyll Robertson pupils are usually found. Seizures are frequent and may be the presenting problem. The basal ganglion and corticospinal lesions combine to produce severe dysarthria, with tremors of the tongue and lips and variable motor disturbances in the arms and legs (Fig. 165-5). These patients often show marked emotional changes and mental deterioration and typically have delusions of grandeur. It is the patient with general paresis who has been typified as the "insane" patient who believes that he is God, Napoleon, or Batman.

Gummas. Syphilitic gummas may be single or multiple. If they occur intracerebrally, they may mimic a brain tumor. If they are multiple and involve the meninges, the patient may present with dementia and focal neurologic signs.

Congenital Syphilis. In about 10% of cases, the children of mothers who have seropositive syphilis have nervous system involvement. Either meningovascular or parenchymatous (general paresis, tabes, optic atrophy) syndromes may occur. Seizures, mental retardation, gummas of the musculoskeletal system, bilateral painful joint effusions, osteochondritis, skin lesions, and abnormalities of the teeth are characteristic signs.

Management of Syphilis. Given a positive RPR test on a patient, a further history and examination are required, with the specific aim of finding evidence of any disease that may cause a biological false-positive reaction. One should also seek historical evidence of a previous syphilitic infection. The RPR should be repeated and the MTPHA performed to have two separate positive serologic tests at different times. The CSF should be examined for cells, serology, sugar, and protein. Any abnormality of the CSF should suggest the possibility of neurosyphilis.

If the CSF serology is positive, CSF must be rechecked every 6 months after treatment for 2 years to ascertain that the infection has cleared, the best indicators of which are the levels of cells and protein in the CSF.

For early syphilis (primary, secondary, or latent for less

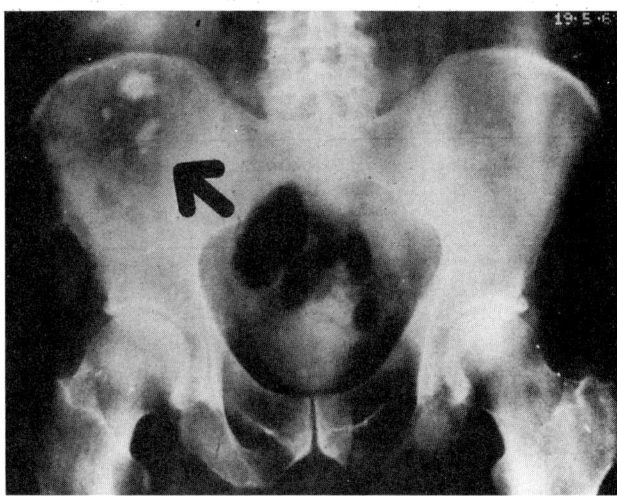

Fig. 165-5. Radiograph of pelvis of patient with general paresis, formerly treated with injection of bismuth. (From Mandell GL, Bennett JE, Dolin R, editors: *Principles and practice of infectious diseases,* ed 4, New York, Churchill Livingstone, 1995.)

than 1 year), a single injection of benzathine penicillin, 2.4 megaU intramuscularly or procaine penicillin, 600,000 units intramuscularly daily for 8 days is adequate treatment.

In late latent stages, however, benzathine penicillin, 2.4 megaU intramuscularly weekly for 3 weeks is required. CNS syphilis requires intravenous benzylpenicillin therapy for at least 10 days. In patients allergic to penicillin, tetracycline or erythromycin, 500 mg qid for 30 days, may be used. The latter is the drug of choice in women who are pregnant and in young children.

Lyme Disease

Lyme disease is caused by the spirochete *Borrelia burgdorferi* and is transmitted by a tick endemic in North America and Europe. Most cases occur in summer; the first manifestations are in the skin: a red macule or papule extending outward from the site of the tick bite, with central clearing (erythema chronicum migrans). Fatigue, malaise, and a mild meningoencephalitis may occur in this stage, but the CSF is normal. Within the next 1 to 6 months, 1 in 10 patients develop recurrent or chronic lymphocytic meningitis with cranial and/or peripheral neuropathies or painful radiculopathies. The CSF then contains lymphocytes and plasma cells and the protein level will be high. IgG and oligoclonal bands may be detected. Half of these patients also have mild encephalopathy, but severe focal signs are uncommon.

Chronic arthropathy is the usual feature of the late stages of the disease, but chronic progressive meningoencephalitis with multifocal signs also occurs at a late stage. A raised ESR, increased serum IgM, and the presence of serum cryoglobulins suggest the diagnosis, which may be confirmed by finding high Borrelial antibody levels in the serum or CSF. Early diagnosis is important because treatment with oral antibiotics may be effective then. When neurologic features are present, high-dose penicillin or ceftriaxone is the treatment of choice.

Slow Virus Infections of the Nervous System

In 1957 an unusual disease (kuru) was described in the Fore tribe of New Guinea. Its cause was traced to cannibalism and to the ceremonial rubbing of the blood and brains of the deceased over the bodies of those taking part in the ritual. Brain material from those who had died of kuru was injected into chimpanzees; some 19 months later they developed evidence of the disease.

Using a concept developed by Siggurdson, a Scandinavian veterinarian, the researchers postulated a slow virus infection—one caused by a transmissible agent presumed to be a virus particle, with a very long incubation period and slow course to death. Other conditions in this category have now been recognized.

In retrospect, it need not surprise us that an infection may produce disease months or years later. It has long been known that warts are caused by a virus with a similarly prolonged latent phase, rabies is recognized as having a prolonged incubation period, and herpes zoster remains in dorsal root ganglia, often causing no clinical disease for many years. Other viruses capable of behaving thus include CMV, HIV, rubella, and infectious hepatitis.

Creutzfeldt-Jakob Disease

Creutzfeldt-Jakob disease (CJD) is an unusual condition, clinically and pathologically almost identical with kuru; it is characterized by a spongiform degeneration of the cerebellar cortex, some subcortical structures, and the cerebellum in older adults.

Clinical features include the subacute onset in later middle age of malaise, headache, weight loss, ataxia, twitching, behavioral disturbances, and personality change progressing to obvious dementia. Slowly progressive spasticity, dysphasia, cerebellar and extrapyramidal signs, fasciculations, and myoclonus, with marked "startle" effect, appear later. Ninety percent of patients die akinetic, cortically blind, mute, and eventually decorticate within a year. In this condition, the EEG is of diagnostic value because periodic abnormal discharges appear eventually in 75% of cases.

Gajdusek and others have been successful in transmitting the disease to chimpanzees through five consecutive passages, but the agent that is transmitted has not been isolated, although it is presumed to be a virus particle. There is no effective treatment.

New Variant of Creutzfeldt-Jakob Disease

There are three epidemiologic types of CJD known. Sporadic CJD, described in this chapter, accounts for 90% of the cases and may result from the spontaneous somatic mutation of a prion protein gene within the host. Familial CJD results from the inheritance of a defective form of the prion protein gene and accounts for 5% to 10% of cases. An unusual form, the infective form of CJD, accounts for less than 1% of cases. It can result from the transmission of infective material from a CJD case to another person via transplantation, cadaveric human growth hormone and gonadotrophin, and through contaminated neurosurgical instruments.

In the late 1980s and through the 1990s cases of a variant form of CJD disease have been reported from the United Kingdom. Epidemiologic evidence suggests that these cases are linked to bovine spongiform encephalopathy (BSE), perhaps as a result of consumption or other exposure to BSE-infected tissues. Patients with new variant CJD (nv-CJD) are younger than those with classic CJD (age range for nv-CJD is 19 to 41 years). This disease is progressive, leading to death in 7 to 23 months. Early and prominent behavioral changes dominate the clinical picture. Myoclonus and progressive dementia occur late. The typical EEG pattern of classic CJD is not seen in nv-CJD. Spongiform changes and prion protein plaques are distributed extensively throughout the cerebrum and cerebellum.

In the United Kingdom there was about one case per million population per year of nv-CJD. It has been theorized that nv-CJD might be the result of ingesting material from cows suffering from BSE, but this has not been proven. Although it is speculation, the theory closed down the British beef industry, which is now struggling to return, and has affected the blood donation system. Canada, again based on theory, now refuses to accept blood donations from those who have visited the United Kingdom in the last 16 years.

Subacute Sclerosing Panencephalitis

Subacute sclerosing panencephalitis (SSPE) is a delayed measles encephalitis associated with a defective immune response in the host. It is becoming less common, perhaps because of widespread measles immunization. Typically, children or young adults show mental and behavioral changes that lead to progressive dementia, myoclonic jerking, seizures, and increasing motor disability. The patients deteriorate and die in 1 to 3 years.

The EEG characteristically shows periodic slow wave and sharp wave discharges (Fig. 165-6), and the CSF contains excessive IgG; positive oligoclonal banding and a high titer of antimeasles antibody are also found. The paramyxovirus has been isolated from the brains of many such patients.

In most cases, the measles infection probably occurred up to 10 years before the onset of SSPE, so this condition is a convincing argument for the existence of persistent virus-induced autoimmune diseases of the nervous system. Children born with the congenital rubella syndrome may develop a similar disease, as do immunosuppressed patients (e.g., those with lymphomas).

Progressive Multifocal Leukoencephalopathy

Progressive multifocal leukoencephalopathy (PML) is a fatal brain disease seen only in immunosuppressed patients, in whom progressive demyelination occurs in the white matter of the cerebellar hemispheres and sometimes that of the brainstem, cerebellum, and spinal cord. The patchy areas of

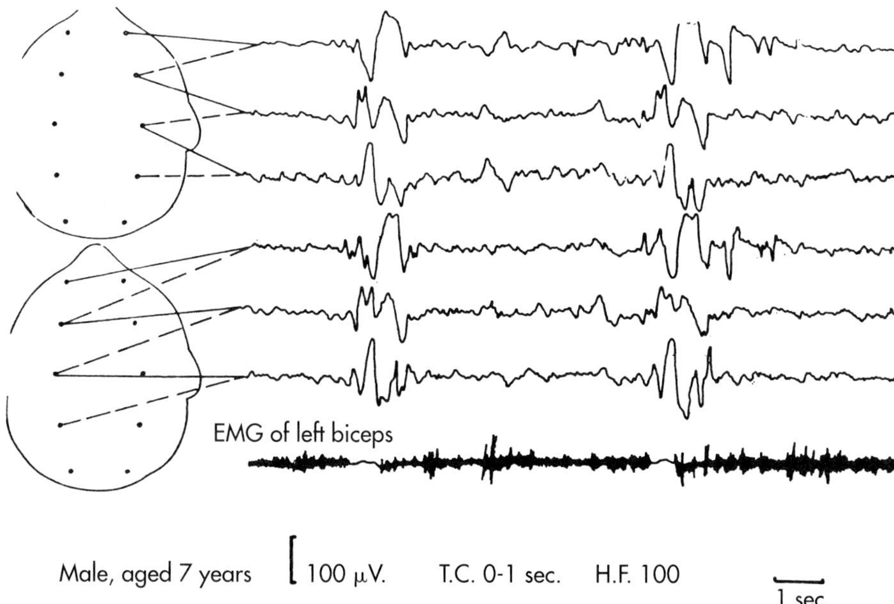

Fig. 165-6. EEG of a patient with subacute sclerosing panencephalitis, showing typical periodic complexes. (From Mandell GL, Bennett JE, Dolin R, editors: *Principles and practice of infectious diseases,* ed 4, New York, Churchill Livingstone, 1995.)

demyelination show preservation of axis cylinders, and the astrocytes are large with abnormal nuclei and many mitoses. The supportive oligodendrocytes are reduced in number and contain inclusion bodies. Crystalline arrays of Papova virions are seen at the periphery of the lesions.

This disorder is often a terminal event in patients with Hodgkin's disease or lymphoma, and occasionally in sarcoidosis, tuberculosis, and other conditions marked by immunologic incompetence. It is due to a polyoma viral infection acting as a slow virus. Patients die within 3 years after a progressive downhill course characterized by behavioral change and developing ataxia, aphasia, blindness, paralysis, and ultimately coma.

These are just a few examples of disease that had been considered to be degenerative in nature but are now known to be due to viruses acting in an unusual way. It appears that the virus can stay in the nervous system for prolonged periods before causing a progressive disease. It is also of interest that the brain lesions often look more degenerative than inflammatory or infective under the microscope, and one naturally begins to wonder about other "degenerative" processes, such as Alzheimer's disease, motor neuron disease, Parkinson's disease, and multiple sclerosis.

NEUROLOGIC COMPLICATIONS OF OTHER INFECTIONS

The classification of the parainfectious encephalopathies has been clarified by Ropper, who suggests four categories of disorder:

1. Encephalitis caused by direct viral invasion of the brain
2. Acute toxic encephalopathy, with brain swelling rather than inflammation
3. Postinfectious or postvaccinal encephalopathy (also called *acute disseminated* or *acute allergic* encephalomyelitis) is a multifocal demyelinating disease with an immunologic basis
4. An inflammatory encephalitis occurs with Epstein-Barr virus, influenza, and mycoplasma infections that cannot be clinically distinguished from ordinary viral encephalitis, but the agent is not recoverable from the brain

The findings in encephalitis have already been discussed; we will describe the encephalopathies named above under the older, popular headings.

Acute Toxic Encephalopathy

Fever and acute neurologic signs may suddenly appear during or within 2 weeks of acute specific (e.g., measles) or nonspecific infections in children, during the acute illness in bacterial endocarditis in adults, or after vaccination in anyone. Typical signs include meningism, acute obtundation and delirium, seizures, myoclonus, cerebellar signs, chorea, and evidence of raised ICP. The CSF is usually normal. A few patients recover completely but most are left with significant residual neurologic deficits or epilepsy. No infective agent has ever been isolated from the brain in these cases, and the etiology is presumed to be an allergic vasculitis.

Reye's syndrome is a form of acute toxic encephalopathy that occurs in children and young adults, possibly as a complication of a preceding influenza or varicella infection, or use of acetylsalicylic acid (ASA) in children. Encephalopathy (delirium, seizures, coma, and inconstant focal signs) follows a period of malaise and fever with persistent vomiting. Fatty degeneration of the liver and cerebral edema with a marked rise in ICP are the pathologic basis of these signs. Because intensive metabolic therapy may be lifesaving, immediate referral is essential whenever even drowsiness follows prolonged vomiting in young people.

Acute Postinfectious Encephalomyelitis

Alternative names for acute postinfectious encephalomyelitis are *allergic* or *postvaccinal encephalomyelitis.* These are a group of similar disorders characterized by a monophasic course after a febrile illness or vaccination. Multiple perivenular foci of demyelination and lymphocytic infiltration appear in the nervous system with secondary damage to axons. Thus, unlike the acute encephalitides, the white rather than the grey matter is primarily affected.

Characteristically, this disorder occurs 1 to 2 weeks after an acute infection or an immunologic challenge. The presumed pathogenesis is an autoimmune reaction to brain myelin, after either vaccination (e.g., against rabies or smallpox) or infection with measles, rubella, chickenpox, smallpox, mumps, leptospirosis, etc. Injections of antitetanus serum may result in the same clinical picture. About one third of the cases diagnosed as encephalitis may in fact be of this type.

Clinical Features. The incubation period is 8 to 15 days, after which there is an abrupt onset of headache, with signs of raised ICP and drowsiness that may progress to coma. Before coma develops, the patient may have nausea, vomiting, high fever, meningism, myoclonus or seizures, flaccid paralysis, and variable sensory loss. Cerebellar ataxia is sometimes the main feature. The brunt of the disease may be borne by the brain, the spinal cord, or occasionally by the spinal nerve roots (producing a radiculopathy). The CSF is under increased pressure and contains excess protein and sometimes increased mononuclear cells, but no virus is isolated.

Treatment. Steroids in high dosage in the early stages of this disease are probably effective in reducing the immunologic reaction, and concern about spreading a viral infection is probably unjustified. At the other end of the scale, the clinical picture may be identical with that of epidemic myalgic encephalomyelitis, and illnesses of any intermediate stage of severity are also possible. Despite therapy, a majority of the patients will either die or be left with serious neurologic deficits. Others recover, often with some neurologic sequelae.

Differential Diagnosis. The distinction from multiple sclerosis is made by the presence of fever, the monophasic character of the illness without any past history of neurologic symptoms, a painful radiculopathy in many cases, and the flaccid paresis. The EEG shows bilateral delta activity in a high proportion of patients but is not diagnostic, although such recordings are not commonly seen in multiple sclerosis.

Bacterial Endocarditis

Over one third of the patients with bacterial endocarditis present with neurologic signs. Half of these appear to have cerebrovascular disease (usually an infarct, but occasionally a hemorrhage). In the later stages, mycotic aneurysms may rupture and cause a subarachnoid hemorrhage. Acute toxic encephalopathy with delirium can occur, and some patients have a clinical presentation indistinguishable from acute meningitis or cerebral abscess. In these cases the CSF usually contains mononuclear cells but no organisms, although *S. aureus* is the most common infecting agent. Other complications of bacterial endocarditis include retinal hemorrhages, seizures, and recurring headaches (Table 165-7).

Children with bacterial endocarditis often show a rash in association with fever and delirium, and this picture must be differentiated from that caused by the acute specific fevers such as scarlet fever, measles, enterovirus and adenovirus infections, and rubella and by allergic and drug reactions. Purpura with fever may occur in mononucleosis, rickettsial disease, Henoch-Schönlein purpura, and in other types of allergic vasculitis.

Table 165-7. Neurologic Complications of Bacterial Endocarditis

Complications	%
Cerebrovascular disease	
Infarct	40
Hemorrhage	10
Acute toxic encephalopathy	20
Acute meningitis	5
Headache, seizures, coma, retinal changes, etc.	25

From Mandell GL, Bennett JE, Dolin R, editors: *Principles and practice of infectious diseases,* ed 4, New York, Churchill Livingstone, 1995.

Box 165-9. Causes of Intracranial Venous Thrombosis

Cachexia
Dehydration
Mastoiditis, sinusitis
Trauma
Polycythemia, sickle cell anemia
Superior vena caval obstruction
Cardiac failure
Pregnancy, postpartum
Oral contraceptive use

From Mandell GL, Bennett JE, Dolin R, editors: *Principles and practice of infectious diseases,* ed 4, New York, Churchill Livingstone, 1995.

Cerebral Thrombophlebitis

Causes. Cerebral abscesses in association with sinus infection or otitis usually occur as a result of direct extension of the infection within or alongside the dural sinuses and the other large intracranial veins. Sometimes the brain is not directly involved itself, but the infection in the walls of the veins causes venous thrombosis with venous infarction of the portions of the brain drained by the occluded vessels. In children, sinus thrombosis can occur without local infection at all, as in marked dehydration or high fevers. Sinus thrombosis may also complicate sickle cell anemia and severe cachexia, in which case the superior sagittal sinus is usually involved. It may also occur in women in the postpartum period or those who are taking oral contraceptives. An association with polycythemia and with lymphomas has also been recognized.

Clinical Features. Clinical features include those of local ear or sinus infection complicated by seizures, raised ICP caused by failure of venous drainage, meningism, and sometimes focal neurologic findings as a result of venous infarction. Otitis usually produces thrombophlebitis in the transverse sinuses, and there may be little in the way of focal signs. General examination may show evidence of systemic disorders such as those listed in Box 165-9.

Sinus thrombosis complicating mastoiditis may also present subacutely with raised ICP without meningism, a condition described as *otitic hydrocephalus.* Cavernous sinus thrombosis (Fig. 165-7) may complicate infections of the face or nasal sinuses; signs include raised ICP, exophthalmos with marked edema of the conjunctiva, chemosis, and often ophthalmoplegia and bilateral optic nerve damage. There may

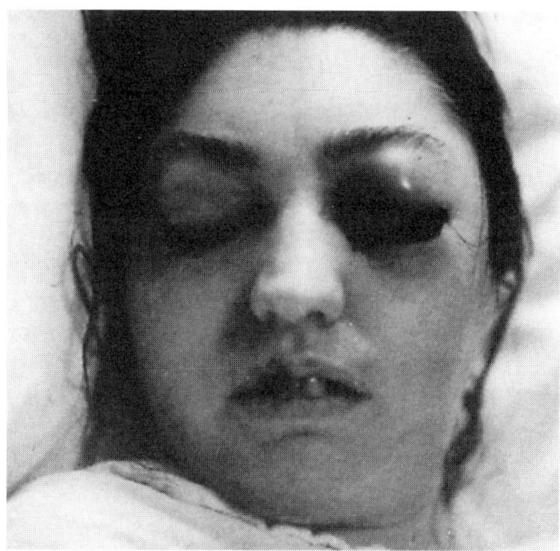

Fig. 165-7. Cavernous sinus thrombosis; bacterial panophthalmitis was followed by septic thrombophlebitis. (From Mandell GL, Bennett JE, Dolin R, editors: *Principles and practice of infectious diseases,* ed 4, New York, Churchill Livingstone, 1995.)

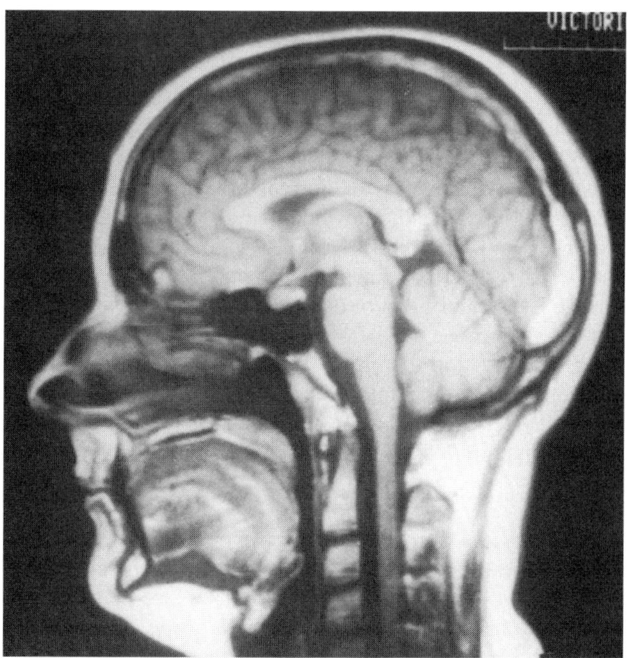

Fig. 165-8. MRI scan showing superior sagittal sinus thrombosis. The increased signal from the superior sagittal and straight sinuses is due to the presence of methemoglobin in the clot. (From Mandell GL, Bennett JE, Dolin R, editors: *Principles and practice of infectious diseases,* ed 4, New York, Churchill Livingstone, 1995.)

also be evidence of meningitis. This condition has a grave prognosis. With superior sagittal sinus occlusion, seizures and unilateral or bilateral corticospinal signs in the legs are to be expected because the territory infarcted is the motor strip region representing the lower limbs (Fig. 165-8).

Differential Diagnosis. Distinction between sinus thrombophlebitis and cerebral abscess or meningitis may be difficult, although brain scanning and EEG will probably not show the clear-cut localizing features to be expected with cerebral abscesses. The diagnosis is probably best made by MRI and carotid arteriography. The CSF pressure, lymphocyte count, and protein level are high. Red cells may be present with thrombophlebitis, but organisms are not detected and are only cultured from the blood.

If cerebral abscess seems clinically likely, however, LP is best deferred until the patient is in a neurologic center, because it is dangerous and often is unnecessary when a CT scanner is available.

Treatment. Treatment consists of attempts to lower the ICP with steroids or dehydrating solutions and the use of high doses of broad-spectrum antibiotics. Ligation of the infected veins is of questionable value. Where specific underlying medical disease is found, this may be treatable. Anticoagulants are of doubtful value in sinus thrombosis.

ADDITIONAL READINGS

King AA, Turner GS: Rabies: a review, *J Comp Pathol* 108(1):1, 1993.

Mandell GL, Bennett JE, Dolin R, editors: *Principles and practice of infectious diseases,* ed 4, New York, Churchill Livingstone, 1995.

Ropper AH: Case records of the Massachusetts General Hospital, *N Engl J Med* 305:507-514, 1981.

CHAPTER 166

Toxic Damage to the Nervous System

William Pryse-Phillips
T. Jock Murray
James Boyd

Many chemicals, drugs, and other agents may cause permanent or reversible damage to the central nervous system (CNS). When it is recalled that over 10% of inpatients at any one time have primary symptoms related to toxicity from treatment agents (as opposed to intrinsic disease), it will be understood that a knowledge of intoxications is of great importance. Sometimes the CNS symptom results from the normal pharmacologic actions of a drug (e.g., coma with sedative overdose). Sometimes it will be due to direct damage to neurons (e.g., lead or carbon monoxide poisoning). Competition for enzymes in the nervous system or in the liver may also produce symptoms; thus phenothiazines may produce dyskinesias, phenytoin induces rickets, and isoniazid induces neuropathy through pyridoxine deficiency. Other methods include alterations in the secretion or drainage of cerebrospinal fluid (CSF), producing intracranial hypertension, and in the membrane potential on the neurons, with resultant epilepsy. Other toxic effects still cannot be explained, such as the production of glare photophobia related to tridione use.

Box 166-1. Drugs and Toxins That Can Cause Encephalopathy

Alcohols
  Ethyl, methyl, propyl, ethylene glycol
Analgesics, narcotics
  All
Anticonvulsants
  Diphenylhydantoin, bromides, all barbiturates, primidone, all benzodiazepines, sodium valproate
Antidepressants
  Tricyclic drugs, lithium
Antineoplastic drugs
  L-Asparaginase, methotrexate, mitotane, nitrogen mustards, procarbazine, vidarabine, vinca alkaloids, interferon alpha-*n1*, recombinant IL-2 (aldesleukin)
Diuretics
  All
Sedatives and Hypnotics

Miscellaneous

Acetaminophen	Carbon disulfide	Gold	Prajamalium
Amantadine	Carbon monoxide	Heroin	Propranolol
Aminophylline	Chloroquine	Isoniazid	Rifampin
Amphetamines	Chymopapain	Insulin	Steroids
Arsenic	Cimetidine	Interferon	Streptomycin
Aspirin	Cycloserine	Lead	Strychnine
Atropine/belladonna alkaloids	Cyproheptadine	Methyl bromide	Sulfonamides
Baclofen	Disulfiram	Methyl mercury	Sulfonylureas
Bismuth	L-Dopa	Metrizamide	Thallium
Bromocriptine	Digitalis	Organophosphorus	Toluene
Calcium salts	Gasoline	Penicillin	

DRUGS DIRECTLY AFFECTING CENTRAL NERVOUS SYSTEM FUNCTION

Encephalopathy

Many drugs and toxins can result in alteration in consciousness, personality change, delirium, seizures, lethargy, raised intracranial pressure (ICP), or coma with or without focal signs of neurologic dysfunction and with evidence of intact brainstem function (Box 166-1).

Seizures

Epileptic seizures may occur in patients taking a variety of drugs, sometimes in normal dosage; but in other situations, seizures only occur in the presence of toxic levels of a given drug or if the patient has a preexisting low threshold for seizures (Box 166-2). Usually, the manifestation is of generalized epilepsy, but if there is any preexisting brain disease that had not formerly produced seizures, the reduction of threshold caused by the toxic agent may produce a focal seizure.

Dementia

Dementing syndromes are usually regarded as being irreversible, but in the case of drug-induced dementia this is incorrect. Focal neurologic signs referable to the frontal lobe, the cerebellum, or the basal ganglia may also be present along with the altered mental state. It is even more common for patients with organic brain syndromes to have their conditions worsened by drugs, particularly sedatives, hypnotics, and tranquilizers; dialysis is another cause. In recent years progressive dementia caused by solvent sniffing (e.g., glue, gasoline) has become an increasing problem (Box 166-3).

Insomnia

Insomnia is obviously to be expected with stimulants such as methylphenidate and caffeine, but other agents are also able to produce insomnia (Box 166-4).

Reduction in Levels of Consciousness

Patients who are comatose as a result of drugs and toxins ingested show evidence of normal brainstem function with retained doll's head movements and ice-water caloric responses and with normal pupillary reactions. This is not true with drugs that have an anticholinergic effect (Box 166-5). Respiratory and/or cardiovascular depression may be marked and cause further brain damage from hypoxia. In severe intoxication the electroencephalogram (EEG) may be isoelectric; this is not a sign of brain death in this circumstance. Almost any drug in sufficient quantity can cause coma.

Stroke

Indirect causes of stroke are legion, operating as risk factors through the mechanism of accelerated atherosclerosis or induction of hypertension. Direct causes are few; cocaine (especially in the form of "crack") is a prime example. Oral contraceptives may increase the risk of stroke, especially in women with migraine headaches.

Extrapyramidal Syndromes

Chorea. Some patients who have had Sydenham's chorea in childhood, usually women, may again develop abnormal jerking movements if they are given L-dopa or phenytoin. Choreic movements in patients with Parkinson's disease treated with L-dopa are a common toxic manifestation. Agents that may cause chorea are listed in Box 166-6.

Parkinsonism. The four classic features of parkinsonism (tremor, rigidity, akinesia, and postural changes) are produced by a number of agents. Tremor, however, is less prominent in drug-induced parkinsonism. Drugs may also induce oculogyric crises, which are otherwise only seen in the postencephalitic form of parkinsonism. The effects are reversible when the drug is withdrawn. Responsible agents are listed in Box 166-6.

Box 166-2. Drugs That Can Cause Seizures

Alcohol (and withdrawal from alcohol)
Aminophylline
Amiodarone
Amphetamines
Analeptic agents
Anticholinesterase agents (organophosphates, physostigmine)
Antihistamines
Antipsychotics
Aqueous iodinated contrast agents
Baclofen
Beta-blockers (propranolol, oxprenolol)
Camphor
Carbon monoxide
Chlorambucil
Cisplatin
Cocaine
Corticosteroids
Cycloserine
Cyclosporine
Deanol
Ergotamine
Ergonovine
Folic acid
Furosemide
General anesthetics (ketamine, halothane, althesin, enflurane, propanidid)
Heroin
Hyperbaric oxygen
Hypoglycemic agents
Hyposmolar parenteral solutions
Imipenem
Insulin
Intravenous iron
Ioniazid
Iron (intramuscular injection)
Lidocaine
Lithium
Local anesthetics (bupivacaine, lidocaine, procaine, etidocaine)
MAO inhibitors
Marijuana
Mefenamic acid
Methyl bromide
Methylxanthines
Metrizamide
Metronidazole
Misonidazole
Nalidixic acid
Narcotic analgesics (fentanyl, meperidine, pentazocine, propoxyphene)
Oral contraceptives
Oxytocin (water intoxication)
Pemoline
Penicillin
Phencyclidine
Phenobarbital
Phenothiazines
Phenylpropanolamine
Phenytoin
Physostigmine
Prednisone (intravenous, with hypocalcemia)
Reserpine
Strychnine
Sympathomimetics (amphetamines, ephedrine)
Terbutaline
Theophylline
Tolbutamide
Tricyclic drugs
Vincristine (perhaps because of excess antidiuretic [ADH] secretion)
Vitamin K

Box 166-3. Drugs and Toxins That Can Cause Dementia

Alcohol
Barbiturates
Benzodiazepines
Bromides
Carbon monoxide
Gasoline
Lead
Manganese
Mercury
Organic substances (e.g., CCl_4, CS2, TOCP)
Phenytoin
Toluene

Following MPTP, cyanide, CS2, or CO poisoning, and with most other causes of severe hypoxia, a parkinsonian syndrome may occur, but without oculogyric crises and due to permanent neuronal damage in the basal ganglia. It should be noted that although tricyclic drugs may produce a parkinsonian syndrome rarely, they are also of value in treatment of depression in Parkinson's disease.

Acute Extrapyramidal Symptoms. The severe disorders of movement included under this heading include dystonias, facial tics and spasms, and akathisia. The symptoms usually occur in young males given bromocriptine, butyrophenones, phenothiazines (with a piperazine ring), phenytoin, or metoclopramide and also in people stung by insects. In older patients, methyldopa, tricyclics, and levodopa produce severe extrapyramidal symptoms of this type. Cyanide is an unusual cause of dystonia.

Akathisia and other dyskinesias may also occur with benztropine, which is otherwise a reasonable choice among synthetic anticholinergic agents used to treat parkinsonism and which can be given intramuscularly in doses of 1 to 2 mg for acute extrapyramidal symptoms. Intramuscular diphenydramine or intravenous diazepam, 10 to 20 mg given slowly,

Box 166-4. Agents That Can Cause Insomnia

Antihypertensives (clonidine, alpha methyldopa, reserpine)
Beta-blockers (propranolol, timolol, atenolol)
Bronchodilators (terbutaline, albuterol, salmeterol, metaproterenol, theophylline and other methylxanthines)
Decongestants (phenylpropanolamine, pseudoephedrine)
Hormones (oral contraceptives, cortisone, progesterone, thyroid hormone)
Sympathomimetics (amphetamines, epinephrine, ephedrine, pseudoephedrine)
Antineoplastics (alpha interferon, goserelin acetate, leuprolide acetate, medroxyprogesterone, pentostatin, daunorubicin)

Others:
Levodopa
MAO inhibitors
Manzidol (imidazo-isoinodole)
Methylphenidate
Nicotine
Phenytoin
Quinidine
Selective serotonin reuptake inhibitors (SSRIs)
Tacrolimus

Box 166-5. Drugs and Toxins That Can Cause Coma

Alcohol (ethyl and methyl)
Analgesics
Anticholinergic agents
Anticonvulsants
Antihistamines
Baclofen
Bromides
Calcium salts
Digoxin
Methyl bromide
Organophosphates
Orphenadrine
Phenylbutazone
Psychoactive drugs
Sedatives

Box 166-6. Drugs and Agents That May Cause Extrapyramidal Syndromes

Chorea

- Amphetamines
- Anticholinergics
- Calcium salts
- Carbamazepine
- CO_2 narcosis
- Dopamine agonists
- Methylphenidate
- Opiates
- Oral contraceptives
- Pemoline
- Phenytoin
- Primidone

Parkinsonism

- Alpha methyldopa
- Butyrophenones
- Carbon tetrachloride
- Cinnarizine
- Cyanide
- Diazoxide
- Diltiazem
- Disulfiram
- Flunarizine
- Lithium
- Manganese
- Mercury
- Methanol
- Metoclopramide
- Paroxetine
- Phenothiazines
- Reserpine
- Tetrabenazine
- Tricyclic drugs

Acute Extrapyramidal Symptoms

- Benztropine
- Bromocriptine
- Butyrophenones
- Levodopa
- Methyldopa
- Metoclopramide
- Phenothiazines
- Phenytoin
- Tricyclics

Tremor

- Amiodarone
- Beta-agonists, oral
- Cyclosporine
- Ephedrine
- Epinephrine
- Lithium
- Metoclopramide
- Sodium valproate
- Sympathomimetics
- Tacrolimus
- Theophylline and other methylxanthines
- Thyroxine
- Tricyclics
- Vidarabine

Cerebellar Ataxia

- Amiodarone
- Benzodiazepines
- BCNU
- Carbamazepine
- Clioquinol
- Ethyl alcohol gasoline
- 5-Fluorouracil
- Lamotrigine
- Lithium
- Mercury
- Methsuximide
- Nabilone (antiemetic, synthetic cannabinoid)
- Phenobarbitone
- Phenytoin
- Perhexiline maleate
- Polymyxin B
- Procarbazine
- Toluene
- Topiramate
- Zopiclone

Nystagmus

- Amiodarone
- Barbiturates
- Carbamazepine
- 5-Fluorouracil
- Glucose (in vitamin B_1-deficient subjects)
- Phenytoin
- Primidone

Myelopathy

- Clioquinol
- Deep x-ray therapy
- Electric shock
- Halogenated organophosphateseroin
- Hydroxyquinolines
- Mercury
- Methylene blue (intrathecal)
- Intrathecal methotrexate
- Metrizamide
- Phenytoin
- Tricyclic drugs
- Vaccination

usually stops the acute symptoms in these cases, but it must be coupled with withdrawal or reduction in the dose of the drug. Intravenous diazepam is most safely given when respiratory support is available, should it be required.

Tremor. Regular and repetitive tremor, usually fast and of small amplitude (thus not very much like that of Parkinson's disease), can be produced by amiodarone, oral beta-agonists, cyclosporine, ephedrine, epinephrine and all sympathomimetics, lithium, metoclopramide, sodium valproate, tacrolimus (an immunosuppressant), theophylline and other methylxanthines, thyroxine, tricyclics, and vidarabine.

Cerebellar Ataxia. The usual cerebellar syndrome with horizontal jerk nystagmus, limb or truncal ataxia, and failure of motor control may be due to such agents as seen in Box 166-6.

Nystagmus. Toxicity may cause both horizontal and vertical jerk nystagmus to occur without other evidence of a cerebellar syndrome. Cerebellar connections are probably involved, but there may also be damage to the medial longitudinal fasciculus. Substances incriminated include amiodarone, barbiturates, phenytoin, carbamazepine, primidone, glucose (in vitamin B_1-deficient subjects), and 5-fluorouracil.

Myelopathy. Spinal diseases are discussed in Chapter 127. Upper motor neuron and long tract signs, usually without a discrete cord level and with or without evidence of anterior horn cell or dorsal root ganglion cell involvement, can occur with the agents listed in Box 166-6. Tetracycline and colchicine may induce vitamin B_{12} deficiency with resulting myelopathy.

DRUGS AFFECTING OTHER INTRACRANIAL COMPONENTS

Meningism

Stiff neck with positive Kernig's and Brudzinski's signs, fever, and photophobia may occur as a drug reaction. The CSF usually contains either no cells or only a few mononuclear cells, but the pressure may be slightly raised. The CSF should be sterile on culture. Agents responsible for causing meningism are listed in Box 166-7.

Chemical Meningitis. Meningism may occur after intrathecal injection of a number of agents, in which case the CSF contains many mononuclear cells, increased protein, and

Box 166-7. Drugs and Agents Affecting Other Intracranial Components

Meningism

MAO inhibitors (and tyramine)
Heroin
Ibuprofen
Sulfonamides
Tridione

Chemical Meningitis

Amphotericin
Contrast media
Local anesthetics
Penicillin
Polymyxin B (intrathecally)
Radioiodinated serum albumin
Steroids
Streptomycin

Idiopathic Intracranial Hypertension

Carbon dioxide
Nalidixic acid
Oral contraceptives
Organic insecticides
Perhexiline maleate
Steroid withdrawal in children
Steroids
Tetracyclines
Vitamin A

Migrainous and Other Vascular Headaches

Baclofen
Chloroquine
Ergot derivatives
Estrogen-androgen therapy (testosterone and estrogen)
Ethosuximide
Indomethacin
Isosorbide dinitrate/-5-mononitrate
Nitroglycerin
Oral contraceptives
Organophosphates
Perhexilene maleate
Verapamil

sometimes reduced sugar levels. Agents responsible for causing chemical meningitis are listed in Box 166-7.

Fungal Meningitis. The picture of acute or chronic meningitis with markedly raised protein, low sugar, mainly mononuclear cells, and the presence of fungi (usually *Candida albicans*) may complicate treatment with immunosuppressive agents and steroids. Fungal meningitis may also be seen in patients with diabetes or with alcoholism.

Idiopathic Intracranial Hypertension

Idiopathic intracranial hypertension is characterized by papilledema unaccompanied by focal neurologic signs and investigations are negative. A computed tomography (CT) scan shows the ventricles to be normal or small in size. The patient's usual complaint is headache, sometimes with visual obscurations. Substances that can produce this syndrome are listed in Box 166-7.

Migrainous and Other Vascular Headaches

Typical vascular headaches may occur de novo, or preexisting migraine may be made more severe or more frequent if the patient takes substances listed in Box 166-7. Headaches caused by a sudden marked rise in systolic blood pressure may occur in patients who eat foods high in tyramine while they are taking MAO inhibitors. Other causes of vascular headache include ingestion of alcohol by patients who are taking disulfiram. Withdrawal from caffeine is a common but poorly recognized cause of headaches.

DRUGS AFFECTING NERVES

Cranial Nerves

Parosmia is a common result of the chronic use of nasal decongestant sprays and drops, which causes severe damage to the unmyelinated fibers of the first nerve. In time, loss of olfactory acuity supervenes. Toluene also causes hyposmia.

Optic Atrophy. Pallor of the optic discs may be caused by the agents in Box 166-8, from which it will be seen that many are either derivatives of the original sulfonamide drugs or are agents used in the treatment of rheumatoid arthritis. Visual acuity may not be greatly affected despite marked primary optic atrophy.

Subacute Myeloopticoneuropathy. A virtual epidemic of a disease marked by optic neuropathy, encephalopathy, and transverse myelopathy has occurred in Japan and in the Western world in the last 10 years. The distinction from multiple sclerosis is hard to make, but the CSF is normal. Toxicity from halogenated hydroxyquinolines (Entero-Vioform) and/or a herpes-related virus are incriminated.

Miosis. Small pupils that do not appear to react but are not usually associated with any subjective complaint may occur with the use of opiates, pilocarpine, organophosphates, sedatives, and physostigmine.

Mydriasis. Dilation of the pupils bilaterally, with subjective difficulty in accommodation and focusing and sometimes with photophobia, may occur as a drug effect. In such cases, pupillary constriction to light may be reduced. Drugs responsible include: amphetamines, antihistamines, cocaine, disopyramide, glutethimide, haloperidol, L-dopa, muscarinic blockers (e.g., atropine), phenothiazines, phenytoin, and tricyclics.

Ophthalmoplegia. Carbamazepine and tricyclic drugs have been incriminated as causes of ophthalmoplegia in cases of overdose. Beta-blocking drugs may cause diplopia. Chymopapain has been the cause of a third nerve palsy.

Trigeminal Sensory Loss. Trigeminal sensory loss is usually unilateral but can extend to both sides of the face in any of the three divisions of the nerve. Apart from the patient's subjective complaint of numbness, which is objectively verifiable, no motor signs and no other sensory changes are usually detected. The agents that are responsible include stilbamidine, trilene (a solvent), and streptomycin.

Box 166-8. Agents That Can Cause Optic Atrophy

Alcohol (methyl and ethyl)	INAH
Arsenic	Phenylbutazone
BCNU	Quinine
Chloramphenicol	Quinidine
Chloroquine	Salicylates
Chlorpropamide	Streptomycin
Disulfiram	PAS
Digitalis	Penicillamine
Ethambutol	Sulfonamides
Heavy metals (Au, Hg)	Tobacco
Methyl bromide	Toluene

VII Nerve Palsy. Unilateral facial palsy is more common in women taking oral contraceptives. Angiotensin-converting enzyme (ACE) inhibitors, clarithromycin, cisplatin, penicillamine, synthetic thyrotropin-releasing hormone (TRH), and zopiclone may alter taste sensation.

VIII Nerve Involvement. Different agents affect the cochlear and vestibular components of the VIII nerve to a different extent. The typical picture is of vestibular impairment with streptomycin, compared with the primarily cochlear damage caused by dihydrostreptomycin, neomycin, cisplatin/carboplatin, kanamycin, and valproic acid. However, both divisions are involved to some extent with most of the drugs listed in Box 166-9.

Impairment of Taste Sensation. Agents that can impair taste sensation include ACE inhibitors, cisplatin, clarithromycin, penicillamine, synthetic TRH, and zopiclone.

Recurrent Laryngeal Palsy. Recurrent laryngeal palsy is an uncommon complication of the vinca alkaloids.

Peripheral Nerves

Most of the agents listed in Box 166-10 have been shown to produce neuropathy. In some, the association is less certain. In almost all cases, the pathology is primary axonal degeneration with secondary demyelination, but primary Schwann-cell damage is a possible cause. The clinical picture produced is of distal symmetric polyneuropathy. In patients with diabetes or rheumatoid arthritis and associated neuropathy, steroids seem to worsen the condition, perhaps by damaging the small vasa nervorum. Steroid withdrawal may be involved in the severe neuropathy that occurs in some patients with rheumatoid arthritis. Sensory functions are almost invariably affected first, and motor involvement is seen less severely and at a later stage.

Autonomic Nerves

Impotence. Most drugs that cause impotence are either ganglion blockers or specific parasympatholytics, but most antihypertensives, including thiazide diuretics, are causal. Other responsible agents include anticholinergic drugs, barbiturates, ganglion blockers, guanethidine, haloperidol, phenothiazines, primidone, thioridazine, tricyclic drugs, and vasodilators.

Box 166-9. Agents That Can Affect VIII Nerve

Carbamazepine	Lithium	Quinine
Ethacrynic acid	Mercury	Salicylates
Furosemide	Mitotane	Streptomycin (and all aminoglycosides)
Heroin	Nabilone	Toluene
Lead	Quinidine	

DRUGS AFFECTING MUSCLE

Myopathy

The usual features of primary proximal muscle disease with atrophy and weakness and usually without pain can occur in patients who have taken drugs listed in Box 166-11.

Hypokalemia secondary to the administration of diuretics, liquorice, or amphotericin B may also be associated with severe proximal weakness, pain, and wasting. Intramuscular paraldehyde, phenytoin, and lidocaine cause local pain, muscle fibrosis, and atrophy. Clofibrate and the other drugs above may cause elevation of serum creatine kinase (CK) levels. Phenytoin may cause metabolic bone disease associated with proximal myopathy. L-Tryptophan can cause the newly diagnosed eosinophilia-myalgia syndrome.

Neuromuscular Blockade

The cardinal symptom of myasthenia is fatigability, particularly seen in the ocular bulbar and proximal limb muscles. Patients with myasthenia may have an exacerbation of their symptoms, or a myasthenia-like syndrome may occur in patients without previous evidence of that condition in the presence of hypokalemia from any cause, such as steroids, muscle relaxants, or ether, or after enemas or wasp stings. Botulinum toxin is designed to induce this symptom, but may diffuse away from the region injected to produce systemic fatigability. The drugs listed in Box 166-12 tend to increase neuromuscular block and should not be given to patients with myasthenia gravis. In the event of myasthenic symptoms being produced or exacerbated when these agents are administered, intravenous calcium may reverse the immediate severe weakness and fatigability.

Acute Muscle Necrosis

Acute muscle necrosis, an uncommon complication of a number of drugs, produces a rise in serum CK levels and myoglobinuria with pain and proximal weakness. It is more likely to happen in patients who are dehydrated. Agents incriminated include alcohol, amphetamines, amphotericin, barbiturates, carbenoxolone, diazepam, epsilon amino caproic acid (EACA), heroin, INH, methadone, and phencyclidine.

Muscle Cramps

Drugs that can cause muscle cramps are listed in Box 166-13.

Malignant Hyperpyrexia

Malignant hyperpyrexia is a genetically determined syndrome that may be precipitated by a number of drugs in susceptible patients who have subclinical myopathy but often

Box 166-10. Agents That May Cause Neuropathy

2-4, D
Acrylamide
Alcohol
Amiodarone
Aniline
Anticoagulants
Antimalarials
Antimony
Antineoplastic agents
Antitetanus serum
Arsenic
Barbiturates
Bismuth
Bush tea
Butazolidine
Carbamazepine
Carbon disulfide
Carbon tetrachloride
Carbon monoxide
Cc14
Chloral hydrate
Chloramphenicol
Chloroquine
Chlorpropamide
Cisplatin
Clioquinol
Clofibrate
Colchicine
Copper
CS2
Cyclosporine
Dapsone
DDT
Didanosine (antiretroviral)
Dinitrobenzol
Dinitrophenol
Diphenylhydantoin
Disopyramide
Disulfiram
Electric shock
Emetine
Ergotamine
Ethionamide
Ethyl alcohol
Ethylene oxide
Gasoline
Glue
Glutethimide
Gold
Hexachlorophene
Hydralazine
Imipramine
Indomethacin
Industrial solvents
Ipecacuana
Isoniazid
Lacquer thinners
Lead
Lindane
Lithium
Mercury
Methaqualone
Methylbutylketone
Metronidazole
Misonidazole
n-Hexane
Nitrofurantoin
Nitrogen mustard
Nitrous oxide
Organophosphates (TOCP)
Pentachlorophenol
Perhexiline
Phenylbutazone
Phenytoin
Podophyllin
Polychlorinated biphenyls (PCBs)
Polymyxin B
Procainamide
Procarbazine
Prolonged cold
Propylthiouracil
Pyridoxine (high dose)
Sodium cyanate
Stilbamidine
Streptomycin
Sulfonamides
Suramin
Tacrolimus
Taxol
Tetrachloroethane
Thalidomide
Thallium
Tolbutamide
Toluene
Topiramate
Trichloroethylene
Tricyclic drugs
Triorthocresyl phosphate
Vermouth
Vinca alkaloids
Zalcitabine (antiretroviral)

Box 166-11. Agents That May Cause Myopathy

Amphetamines
Bretylium
Chloroquine
Cimetidine
Clofibrate
Colchicine
EACA
Emetine
Guanethidine
Heroin
Hydralazine
Ipecac
Imidazole
Immunosuppressants
Lithium
Penicillamine
Pentazocine
Phencyclidine
Phenytoin
Procainamide
Propranolol
Quinidine
Rifampin
Spironolactone
Steroids (fluorinated)
Succinylcholine
Triamterene
Vincristine

raised serum CK levels. These drugs include anesthetics (inhalational and local), tricyclic drugs, MAO inhibitors, and succinylcholine.

Fasciculations

Brief rippling, irregular contractions of motor units occur in patients poisoned with organophosphorus compounds and patients undergoing anesthesia who are given succinylcholine as a muscle relaxant. Neuromyotonia may be caused by penicillamine.

Box 166-12. Drugs That Can Increase Neuromuscular Blockade

Aminoglycoside antibiotics
Chloroquine
Clindamycin
Colistin
Erythromycin
Lidocaine
Lincomycin
Lithium
Penicillamine
Phenytoin
Polymyxin B
Propranolol
Quinine
Quinidine
Tetanus antitoxin
Tetracyclines
Thyroxine
Trimethaphan

Box 166-13. Drugs That May Cause Muscle Cramps

Adrenergic agonists
Amphotericin B
Anticholinesterases
Bumetanide
Carbenoxalone
Cimetidine
Clofibrate
Cytotoxics
Danazol
Diuretics
Labetalol
Liquorice
Lithium
Metolazone
Neostigmine
Nifedipine
Purgatives
Pyridostigmine
Salbutamol

DRUGS WITH AN INDIRECT EFFECT ON THE CENTRAL NERVOUS SYSTEM

Inappropriate ADH Syndrome

Inappropriate ADH syndrome may be induced by carbamazepine, carbenoxolone, chlorpropamide, cyclophosphamide, fluphenazine, oxytocin, thiothixene, thioridazine, theophylline (and other methylxanthines), and vincristine.

Hypoglycemia

Propranolol may mask the signs and symptoms of hypoglycemia and must be carefully used in diabetics. The usual symptoms and signs of hypoglycemia may be induced by alcohol, insulin, and sulfonylureas (especially if used with phenylbutazone or salicylates).

Alterations in Blood Pressure

The clinical manifestations of hypotension and hypertension will not be described here, nor shall we attempt to list any of the huge range of drugs that affects blood pressure. Any patient with abnormal blood pressure readings, or even symptoms of postural hypotension, should be questioned carefully about all drugs taken because these drugs are often at least partly responsible for the abnormality. The dangers of taking sympathomimetic drugs (including cold remedies), meperidine, phenothiazines, methyldopa, and numerous foods at the same time as MAO inhibitors may be mentioned again in this context because headaches, subarachnoid or intracerebral hemorrhage, delirium, or severe hypertension may result. Carbamazepine may cause Stokes-Adams attacks with loss of consciousness.

Hypercoagulability

The increased susceptibility to venous (and possibly to arterial) thrombotic occlusions in women taking oral contraceptives has been noted.

Vasculitis

Vasculitis may complicate ingestion of organic arsenicals, iodides, DDT, mercurial diuretics, gold, phenothiazines, hydantoins, and sulfonamides and their derivatives. These same agents, along with those that follow, have been incriminated in the production of the syndrome of onset of systemic lupus erythematosus (SLE): carbamazepine, griseofulvin, hydralazine, isoniazid, methyldopa, PAS, phenylbutazone, phenytoin, procainamide, streptomycin, and tetracycline.

MISCELLANEOUS ASSOCIATIONS

Neoplasia

Lymphoma has been described in patients who have been given immunosuppressive agents after renal transplantation and in patients taking phenytoin. Although lymphoma is an uncommon neurologic malignancy, lymphomas may present with features of chronic basal meningitis, scattered demyelination, and, rarely, intracranial mass lesions.

Photophobia

Complaints of pain in the eyes and excessive glare may be heard in any patient with dilated pupils caused by the use of mydriatics, and in patients taking lithium. Glare photophobia is commonly associated with the use of trimethadione, an antiepileptic drug of slight value in true petit mal epilepsy.

INTERACTIONS INVOLVING DRUGS USED IN NEUROLOGY

Enzyme Induction

Through enzyme induction, warfarin and phenytoin may be mutually antagonistic and less clinically effective. Phenytoin, phenobarbitone, and valproic acid induce hepatic microsomal enzymes. Although a reduction in the availability of each drug would be expected, serum levels nevertheless usually change but little. Drugs that inhibit oral anticoagulants include barbiturates, tranquilizers, meprobamate, and tricyclics.

Interactions between anticonvulsants are many and involve increased or decreased metabolism, substrate competition, and reduced absorption. In addition, serum phenytoin levels may be markedly increased or decreased by other drugs, and phenytoin, phenobarbital, or carbamazepine may reduce other drug levels.

The Serotonin Syndrome

The serotonin syndrome is a constellation of symptoms that occur after the use of serotonomimetic agents, alone or in combination with MAOIs, that are typically seen soon after initiation, dose increase, or addition of another agent. It was originally detected in animals given L-tryptophan and MAOIs or other 5HT precursors, producing a hypermetabolic state with fever, myoclonus, involuntary movements, and autonomic overactivity. Hyperstimulation of 5HT 1a receptors in the brainstem and spinal cord can lead to the following clinical features:

- Change in mental status (confusion, disorientation, impaired judgment and planning, agitation)
- Headache, coma
- Myoclonus, rigidity, multifocal myoclonus, incoordination, hyperreflexia
- Dysautonomia (dilated pupils, sweating, low-grade fever, nausea, diarrhea, tachycardia, tachypnea, increased blood pressure, flushing, shivering)
- Rarely, high fever, nystagmus, oculogyric crises, dysarthria, pyramidal syndrome, myoglobinuria, renal failure, disseminated intravascular coagulation (DIC), cardiac arrhythmia, death

Mild and partial manifestations of the syndrome (e.g., slight confusion, occasional myoclonus, headache, restlessness, impaired concentration) are probably rather common and underdiagnosed (Box 166-14).

Often no treatment is needed because symptoms usually remit after withdrawal of the selective serotonin reuptake

Box 166-14. Drug Combinations Reported to Cause Serotonin Syndrome

L-Tryptophan and SSRIs or MAOIs
SSRIs and carbamazepine, pentazocine, or MAOIs (or alone)
Clomipramine and MAOIs (or alone)
Bromocriptine and L-dopa
Demerol and MAOIs or iproniazid
Dextromethorphan and MAOIs

inhibitor (SSRI) or the other drug. In general, one should observe electrolytes and vital signs and treat deviations from normal levels (e.g., cooling if required using aspirin and intravenous fluids). Serotonin antagonists such as cyproheptadine, 4 mg orally tid, or methysergide and propranolol may be useful but their value is unproven. For muscle rigidity and myoclonus, clonazepam, lorazepam, benztropine, diphenhydramine, or chlorpromazine should be of benefit.

Many of the drugs listed in Box 166-14 enhance serotonin activity by blocking its reuptake and increasing presynaptic release. Bromocriptine is a 5HT agonist. L-Dopa myoclonus likely is due to serotonomimetic activity. Lithium is able to enhance all aspects of the syndrome, but it has not so far been reported with 5HT1b/d agonists such as the triptans, although the package insert lists many of its components as potential side effects. One should not prescribe SSRIs and MAOIs within 2 months of each other.

An imbalance of 5HT and dopamine may cause a relatively hypodopaminergic state capable of inducing neuroleptic malignant syndrome, which is characterized by changes in mental state; muscle rigidity; severe hyperthermia; autonomic nervous system dysfunction; hypertension or hypotension; fever; cardiac arrhythmias; and a huge rise in CK levels. Treatment is with dantrolene and muscle paralysis. The overlap of the two conditions is notable.

THE NEUROLOGIC COMPLICATIONS OF ALCOHOL

The complications of alcohol abuse include those related to acute intoxication, withdrawal, and nutritional disease in chronic alcoholism, but there is also a group of CNS disorders that occurs in alcoholics that is due to unknown causes. A chronic alcoholic is a person whose dependence on alcohol interferes with his health, interpersonal relationships, social adjustments, job, or economic efficiency. About 5% of the adult population are so classifiable, constituting one of the major health problems in North America.

Intoxication

Acute Drunkenness. The symptoms of acute alcoholic intoxication are well known. Initial exhilaration, relaxation, and excitement are followed by signs of decreased inhibition, slurred speech, ataxia, irritability, combativeness, and drowsiness. After very heavy drinking, the person may pass into a state of stupor and possibly even into coma. Because 90% of the ingested alcohol is oxidized by the liver at a fairly constant rate, the time taken to recover from the bout is variable. However, the next morning the ghost of the evening past may return in the form of a vascular headache with its accompanying irritability, nausea, hyperacusis, photophobia, and anorexia. Although eating increases the metabolism and slows absorption of alcohol somewhat, most methods of treating a hangover are probably ineffective.

Pathologic Intoxication. Occasionally a person develops a marked excitatory response to even a small amount of alcohol. Symptoms of this acute psychosis include excessive excitement, combativeness, destructive behavior, and motor restlessness. The patient should be sedated and protected until the episode has passed, usually in a few hours.

Alcoholic Coma. Because alcohol depresses both subcortical (brainstem) and cortical structures in the same way as do anesthetics, a patient who ingests a large amount may pass through a state of stupor to actual coma. With high blood levels of ethanol (300 mg/dl), reduction in consciousness is usual, but this may also occur at lower levels. A comatose patient with alcohol on his breath may have any number of different problems, and the coma may have nothing to do with drinking. He or she could be comatose from alcohol, but also from a seizure, a head injury, a subdural hematoma, hypoglycemia, or a cerebral infarction. He or she may have ingested other drugs with the alcohol in a suicide attempt. Occasionally a well-meaning bystander tries to revive an unconscious person with brandy or whiskey, so the patient arrives in the emergency room with the smell of alcohol on his breath. Meningitis, pneumonia, liver failure, or gastrointestinal hemorrhage may be present in an alcoholic who has a decreased level of consciousness. The patient will require intravenous glucose and saline. Thiamine should be added to glucose because Wernicke-Korsakoff syndrome can be precipitated by glucose infusion in someone who is thiamine deficient. Gastric lavage is not helpful because alcohol is absorbed too rapidly from the gastrointestinal tract. The patient should be placed in a semiprone position to avoid aspiration: failing that, intubation may be needed.

Alcohol Withdrawal Symptoms

Alcoholic Tremulousness. In a chronic alcoholic, even one night without alcohol may produce the early symptoms of withdrawal, including tremulousness, irritability, headache, anorexia, sweating, depression, and anxiety. An alcoholic quickly learns that another drink in the morning will relieve "the shakes." If he or she cannot get any alcohol, the tremulousness increases to a peak at 24 hours and is associated with general irritability, nausea, and vomiting. The face is flushed and the conjunctivae are injected. He or she appears generally weakened, with a rapid pulse and an irregular gross tremor that involves the hands and forearms, though it can be generalized and so marked that the patient has difficulty walking, speaking, or eating. Alcoholics are extremely susceptible to startle and tend to remain preoccupied with their own misery and relatively inattentive to those around them. They should be encouraged to eat and drink fluids and should be given moderate doses of chlordiazepoxide, lorazepam, or chlorpromazine. A multivitamin preparation should be given, particularly to provide vitamin B_1.

If hospitalized for a few days an alcoholic patient will get over the most uncomfortable period of withdrawal and may be able to accept long-term help, but to discharge an alcoholic from the emergency room will almost certainly send him or her back to alcohol as a form of relief.

Alcoholic Hallucinosis. The tremulous patient in withdrawal may develop fearful visual or auditory hallucinations similar to bad dreams that result from rebound after the deprivation of rapid eye movement (REM) sleep that occurs while drinking. This state is treated like acute tremulousness. An unusual variant of this is the more persistent *auditory hallucinosis*. In this form, the hallucinations are of voices that are often reproachful, critical, or threatening. The episode usually lasts about a week but occasionally much longer. Although initially the alcoholic lacks insight, he or she begins to question the voices' reality as the episode ends and thereafter can discuss the contents of these abnormal experiences.

Alcohol Withdrawal Seizures. The withdrawal seizures of alcoholism are of generalized type. Ninety percent of them occur within 48 hours of the last drink. Usually there is only one seizure. Tremulousness and hallucinosis also occur and may be followed by delirium tremens (the "DTs"), but seizures do not follow the appearance of delirium. Seizures caused by the withdrawal of alcohol have been termed "rum fits," but it is important to remember that people with a low convulsive threshold for other reasons may have seizures provoked by alcohol or its withdrawal. Thus some epileptic persons may have seizures whether they drink a little alcohol or a lot. If the seizure is focal ("partial") in type, then a focal lesion is present and the patient does not have rum fits. Respiratory alkalosis and a low serum magnesium level may be factors in the advent of withdrawal seizures. Alcohol can also induce hypoglycemia in 6 to 12 hours, possibly caused by a reduction in the amount of glycogen stored in the liver through a reduction in the capacity for hepatic gluconeogenesis; this may be another cause of seizures.

Anticonvulsants are not usually required after a single withdrawal seizure, and long-term anticonvulsants are neither logical nor practical because both cause and prevention lie in the alcoholism. However, prophylactic carbamazepine may prevent seizure occurrence and decrease withdrawal symptoms. In rare instances status epilepticus develops.

Delirium Tremens

Clinical Features. After 12 to 24 hours without alcohol, the chronic alcoholic may become irritable, nauseated, sweaty, restless, sleepless, and tremulous, with the dramatic appearance of delusions, confusion, irritability, vivid hallucinations, and marked agitation. Other evidence of increased autonomic activity includes fever, dilated pupils, hypertension, and tachycardia. In this state it is hard to keep the patient calm because his or her agitation reflects confusion, fear of delusions, and hallucinations. An irregular tremor involves the hands, face, and tongue and is increased with activity. A tendency to tug at clothing and bedclothes is also characteristic. Speech becomes more difficult to understand, and screaming, whimpering, and mumbling of garbled sentences may follow.

The DTs may clear after a week, almost as quickly as they developed, leaving the patient with little memory of the delirious period. Patients may die during the acute stage because of hyperthermia, hypokalemia, and peripheral circulatory collapse, but the cause of death cannot always be determined.

Management of these cases includes a search for other underlying problems, including infection, subdural hematoma, and meningitis. Correction of fluid and electrolyte imbalance and the addition of thiamine are vital steps. Shock should be treated immediately with fluids and vasopressor drugs, and if hyperthermia develops, ice packs, fans, and a cooling mattress should be used. The patient's room should be well-lighted because he or she will be fearful of every shadow. Sound should be kept to a minimum, and the patient requires continuous reassurance. Family members are sometimes helpful in keeping the patient calm. High doses of chlordiazepoxide (25 to 50 mg every 6 hours), lorazepam, or chlorpromazine help to reduce agitation and consequent exhaustion. Steroids should not be used except in the event of shock, but propranolol may be useful for the agitated, tremulous patient with autonomic overactivity. Small doses of alcohol have been used as a temporary measure.

Nutritional Disorders

Wernicke-Korsakoff Syndrome. In 1881 Karl Wernicke described three patients with similar symptoms. Two were alcoholic and one was a young woman with chronic vomiting after a suicide attempt in which she had ingested sulfuric acid. Symptoms included in the Wernicke syndrome are ophthalmoplegia, ataxia, and mental disturbance resulting from edema, petechiae, and demyelination in the walls of the third and fourth ventricles and aqueduct and in the medial dorsal nucleus of the thalamus and mammillary bodies. It can occur with any chronic cause of thiamine deficiency but is more common in alcoholism. *Korsakoff psychosis* refers to the loss of ability to record new data, sometimes seen in (mainly male) chronic alcoholics. Korsakoff also described a peripheral neuropathy accompanying this memory loss. *Korsakoff syndrome* is a residuum from an episode of Wernicke encephalopathy, which may not have been evident clinically in its acute stages, and one designates the term *Wernicke-Korsakoff syndrome* to encompass both the acute syndrome and its residua. The odd distribution of the demyelination and petechiae is probably because the oligodendroglia in these areas contain thiamine-dependent transketolase enzymes.

The clinical features of Wernicke-Korsakoff syndrome are first of headache, nausea, vomiting, and depression, and are followed by delirium. This may be a typical agitated and excited DT or a quiet confusional state that occurs with a decreasing level of consciousness, sometimes amounting to coma. The brainstem involvement accounts for both ocular muscle and gaze palsies, but the pupils are normal. Nystagmus and poor caloric responses probably result from lesions around the vestibular nuclei, and truncal ataxia results from involvement of the cerebellum or vestibular nuclei. Most of these patients have a peripheral neuropathy caused by thiamine deficiency, but cardiac involvement is unusual. Complications in the acute stage include hyperthermia, seizures, and a syndrome of inappropriate ADH secretion.

The picture of Korsakoff psychosis becomes apparent as the patient recovers. The ataxia and eye signs improve relatively quickly in the first few days or weeks after treatment but the memory abnormality becomes more evident and may never be entirely clear. It may be so bad that the patient remembers nothing that happened more than 45 seconds ago, although he or she retains previously learned skills. Confabulation is usual; that is, the patient tends to answer with incorrect statements any question that the examiner puts forth. The patient is not lying in order to cover up poor memory, but rather his or her answers are disjointed memories from the past that are out of temporal sequence. Confabulation is not always present in Korsakoff syndrome and it clears fairly rapidly, so one should not depend on it to make the diagnosis. The lesion responsible is probably in the medial dorsal nucleus of the thalamus, rather than the mammillary bodies.

Wernicke-Korsakoff syndrome is an emergency because the patient can die if untreated, or he or she may be left at least with serious memory loss. Initial treatment should be 50 mg of thiamine intravenously and another 50 mg intramuscularly; larger doses are unnecessary. Sedation with phenothiazines or diazepam may be necessary during the early stages. Oral thiamine must be continued. Treated as above, the eye signs begin to improve within 12 hours. Rehabilitation starts thereafter.

Alcoholic Peripheral Neuropathy. The neuropathy of chronic alcoholism is due to chronic deficiency of thiamine. There is a degeneration of both sensory and motor peripheral nerves distally with destruction of both the myelin sheath and axon (see Chapter 167). Although sensory symptoms are common, the chronic alcoholic usually does not complain unless motor changes are marked or a burning feet syndrome develops. Examination shows a distal loss of all modalities of sensation, with mild motor weakness or atrophy in most cases. Reflexes are absent distally. Treatment (alcohol withdrawal, vitamins) leads to a very slow improvement; residual sensory and sometimes motor losses are common.

Alcoholic Amblyopia. Some alcoholics develop blurring of vision with decreased acuity caused by central scotomas. Examination shows mild hyperemia of the disc or, later, optic atrophy. There may be a relationship with tobacco amblyopia in these patients, but alcoholic amblyopia is due to nutritional deficiency and is not a toxic effect of alcohol or tobacco. Treatment is by a balanced diet and B vitamins.

Pellagra. Nicotinamide deficiency results in mental changes, insomnia, irritability, and depression. Advanced cases have dementia, dermatitis, and diarrhea. Neurologic signs include posterior and lateral column involvement and peripheral neuropathy.

Alcoholic Cerebellar Degeneration. Some chronic alcoholics develop bilateral cerebellar incoordination and instability in the legs. There is little abnormality in the arms, and evidence of nystagmus or cerebellar speech difficulty is unusual. This involvement is due to selective atrophy of the anterior lobe or vermis of the cerebellum, best shown by magnetic resonance imaging (MRI) scans. Occasionally the syndrome can be reversed by stopping the intake of alcohol, but in the chronic form this is not so, although at least it should not get worse. This chronic cerebellar degeneration may represent a residuum from a previous Wernicke-Korsakoff syndrome, suggesting it is due to a nutritional deficiency.

Complications of Alcoholism of Uncertain Origin

Marchiafava-Bignami Disease. Marchiafava-Bignami disease is a rare complication of alcoholism that is characterized by degeneration of the corpus callosum, leading to a progressive decrease in mental function, convulsions, tremor, rigidity, paralysis, akinetic mutism, and coma. Some contaminant in the alcohol or a nutritional deficiency may be the cause.

Central Pontine Myelinolysis. Central pontine myelinolysis is characterized by rapidly progressing demyelination in the central pons, which results in pseudobulbar palsy and spastic quadriplegia with a decreasing level of consciousness leading to coma and often death. Although usually seen in alcoholics, it also occurs with underlying malignancy, chronic renal disease, and other debilitating disorders. This syndrome is usually caused by the inappropriately fast restoration of a low serum sodium level after a prolonged period during which the serum level had been low (below 120 mmol/L). The syndrome of inappropriate ADH secretion and any condition producing severe hyponatremia are other causes.

Cerebral Cortical Atrophy. Many chronic alcoholics show evidence of diffuse cortical atrophy, especially of the frontal lobes, with enlargement of the ventricles. This is evidenced by an organic mental deficit, even long after they have stopped drinking. CT scans suggest, however, that some reexpansion can occur.

Alcoholic Myopathy. Three myopathies are associated with alcoholism. The acute syndrome is characterized by painful, swollen, and tender muscles, occasionally with myoglobinuria and renal damage. Another type shows subacute girdle weakness and atrophy with aching pains; a third resembles McArdle disease, with muscle cramps and a flat lactic acid curve after ischemic exercise. Alcoholic cardiomyopathy, sometimes associated with hyperkinetic heart failure, is probably part of a deficiency syndrome, but one outbreak was traced to the use of cobalt as a preservative in beer.

Other Complications of Chronic Alcoholism

Chronic alcoholics who develop hepatic insufficiency may show evidence of encephalopathy or coma.

Pressure palsies are common in alcoholics. One common variation affects the radial nerve when the drunk person falls asleep with his or her arm hanging over the back of a chair (Saturday night palsy). Half of the patients in any large series of subdural hemorrhages will be alcoholics. The hematomas may be bilateral. Occasionally, chronic alcoholics may show an enlarged sella turcica on skull radiographs. Nobody knows why. They also have an increased incidence of carcinoma of the stomach, and some show evidence of B_{12} deficiency caused by chronic gastritis, gastrectomy for ulcers, or poor dietary intake. Dupuytren's contractures in the hands, chronic infections, venereal disease, and tuberculosis are all much more common in alcoholics than in the general population.

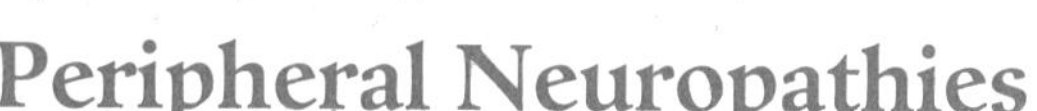

Peripheral Neuropathies

William Pryse-Phillips
T. Jock Murray

The site of primary damage to peripheral nerves may be any of their four components: the cell body and its axon (neuronal or axonal neuropathy), the Schwann cell sheath (demyelinating neuropathy), the supporting tissue (infiltrative neuropathy), or the vascular supply (ischemic neuropathy). To classify neuropathies as primarily caused by damage to one of these four components is of diagnostic value, but because the differences are not always easy to clinically determine, nerve conduction studies and nerve biopsies are necessary in most cases.

NEURONAL (AXONAL) NEUROPATHIES

In neuronal neuropathies the damage is to the cell body or to the axon itself. On the motor side, damage to the anterior horn cell clinically manifests as weakness, wasting, and perhaps fasciculations. If the process is severe or long-standing, diminution or loss of muscle stretch reflexes occurs; but this is seen at an early stage if the reflex arc is interrupted on the sensory side. Anterior horn cell damage means that the pathology is actually operating in the spinal cord, but the condition is still referred to as a neuropathy because the clinical effects are almost entirely related to peripheral nerve dysfunction. Sensory axonal neuropathies tend to affect the various modes of sensation more or less equally.

Both Wallerian degeneration and "dying-back" neuropathies lead to secondary redundancy of Schwann cells, which may disappear or become markedly reduced in numbers. This *secondary demyelination* must, however, be distinguished from *primary demyelination* in which the major damage is caused to the Schwann cells in the first place. The Schwann cells perform the same function vis-a-vis the axon as the oligodendroglia perform in the CNS; that is, they have nutritive and insulating functions. In the case of the peripheral axon, the presence of Schwann cells with interspersed nodes of Ranvier allows saltatory conduction to occur, and their absence causes a marked reduction in the speed of the passage of the nerve impulses.

DEMYELINATING NEUROPATHIES

If there is significant Schwann cell damage, the first axons to have their function impaired will be those that rely most on the insulating action of these Schwann cells, namely those with the thickest layer of myelin, the fastest conducting fibers. Clinically, the first and most severe modalities of sensation lost will be vibration, joint position sense, and tactile discrimination, although there will usually also be some diminution in thin-fiber function, too. In the case of axonal sensory neuropathies, the different sensory modes tend to be affected to a similar extent.

Demyelinating neuropathies lead to early loss of muscle stretch reflexes. Both motor and sensory nerves are commonly involved, although in most cases the sensory effects overshadow the motor findings. Spontaneous pain is not uncommon but it is not a strong diagnostic indicator of any particular type of neuropathy (nor indeed of neuropathy itself, as spontaneous pain and tenderness in muscles may occur with both neuropathy and primary muscle disease).

INFILTRATIVE NEUROPATHY

In infiltrative neuropathy, the appearances are hardly distinguishable from demyelinating types. Accumulation of extraneous material within the nerves enlarges them, causing secondary Schwann cell damage. Examples include sarcoidosis, myelomatosis, amyloidosis, and the leukodystrophies.

ISCHEMIC NEUROPATHY

Schwann cells tolerate ischemia badly because they have a high metabolic rate and are dependent on the small vasa nervorum for their blood supply. If this supply fails, the insulating capacity of the Schwann cell is damaged as it becomes metabolically embarrassed, leading to conduction block. Such failure of blood supply may occur because of occlusion of the vasa nervorum from compression, or in diabetes, collagen-vascular diseases, atheroma, or paraneoplastic vasculitis. The result is an ischemic mononeuropathy, which may affect multiple nerves. The diabetic forms are typical of them all.

APPROACH TO THE PATIENT WITH NEUROPATHY

The clinical features of greatest relevance in the diagnosis of neuropathies are included in Box 167-1.

The clinical history should focus on the speed of onset or development of symptoms, family history, occupation and exposure to toxins/drugs, preexisting systemic illness, and trauma.

Sensory symptoms consist of paresthesias and numbness, beginning in the feet and spreading to the legs and hands. There may be dysesthetic sensations in the same distribution in the form of burning, prickling, coldness, and heaviness. Limb pain is poorly localized, often lancinating, and especially severe at night. At times, however, severe sensory loss may develop silently.

Sensory loss develops according to axonal length, so the sensory impairment is chiefly distal in the extremities in a symmetric stocking-and-glove distribution. The likely reason for this is that based on the effect of the inciting agent, the metabolism of the cell body is impaired so that it cannot easily pump axoplasm to the most distant parts of its axon. The process of "dying back" then occurs, and it is the "Outposts of the Empire" rather than the regions close to the nerve cell body that are first affected, at least as clinically seen. Afferent fibers in the legs can be over 3 feet long,

Box 167-1. Clinical Features of Neuropathy

Distribution of weakness and modes of sensory loss
Distribution of atrophy and sensory change
Symptoms of numbness, bandlike tightness, burning, paresthesias, pain, dysesthesia, unsteadiness, and stumbling
Physical signs
- Weakness
- Atrophy
- Deformity
- Clumsiness
- Cramps
- Fasciculations
- Hyporeflexia or areflexia
- Trophic changes
- Impotence
- Postural hypotension
- Sphincter disturbance
- Constipation/diarrhea
- Sweating/dryness
- Raynaud's phenomenon
- Other evidence of autonomic involvement

whereas in the arms the distance is a good deal less; thus the first symptoms usually appear in the lower limbs. By the same token, the face is seldom affected, although stilbamidine and trichloroethylene do impair V nerve sensory function selectively. Cutaneous sensory loss extends to about the knee before it appears in the fingers. In more advanced stages it extends to the trunk so that there is hypoesthesia to pinprick on either side of the midline of the abdominal wall and lower part of the anterior chest in the shape of a teardrop.

Motor abnormalities generally follow the same distribution, with weakness or clumsiness appearing in the feet and extending to the legs and hands and, in the most severe cases, involving the proximal muscles; however, as a rule, muscles innervated by cranial nerves are spared. Eventually the wasting and weakness of affected muscles may lead to disabling bilateral footdrop and wristdrop.

In long-standing cases of polyneuropathy with sensory loss (e.g., in hereditary sensory or diabetic polyneuropathy), trophic changes appear in the feet and less often in the hands. The best known are Charcot's joints or neuroarthropathy, in which the joints undergo insidious, painless disorganization, leading to swelling and gross deformity. The foot and ankle joints are most frequently affected, but neuroarthropathy can also occur in the knee, wrist, elbow, and shoulder. Even more common are the consequences of recurrent injury to insensitive parts of the body; corns and calluses break down to punched-out chronic ulcers over the feet that may penetrate down to the bone, setting the stage for serious infection of foot spaces and gangrene. Cigarette burns are a telltale sign in the hands. Muscle stretch reflexes are typically lost early and symmetrically. In some demyelinating and infiltrative neuropathies there is visible or palpable enlargement of the greater auricular nerve on the lateral side of the neck, the superficial cutaneous branch of the radial nerve at the wrist, and the ulnar and peroneal nerves.

Autonomic disturbances coexist with many chronic polyneuropathies, such as chronic diabetic and hereditary neuropathies and primary amyloidosis. The dysautonomia is often asymptomatic, but postural hypotension, urinary retention or incontinence, impotence, generalized or regional anhidrosis, cardiac irregularities, gastroparesis, diarrhea, and impaired pupillary motility are notable manifestations. A battery of tests can be performed at the bedside to document autonomic impairment.

The diagnosis of chronic polyneuropathy is readily made on clinical grounds, although it is clear that in many patients it is subclinical. The preservation of ankle reflexes in what appears otherwise to be symmetric polyneuropathy should arouse suspicion that one is dealing with a myelopathy. Exceptionally, ankle reflexes are preserved in some familial polyneuropathies and others that preferentially affect the thin fibers subserving pain and temperature, as in amyloidosis, porphyria, and rare cases of diabetes.

The etiologic diagnosis of chronic symmetric polyneuropathy may be obvious on clinical examination and a limited routine biochemical screening. About 40% of polyneuropathies will be due to some chronic systemic medical disorder (e.g., diabetes, malignancy, collagen-vascular disease, organ failure, B_{12} deficiency, alcoholism or other toxic exposure, acquired immunodeficiency syndrome [AIDS], occult malignancy, or plasma cell dyscrasia), in 30% a hereditary cause will be found, and inflammatory disease will account for another 20%. AIDS is now an important cause of mononeuropathies as well.

A significant number of patients with polyneuropathy lack a specific diagnosis even after extensive investigation. Many will eventually be found to have inherited neuropathies, so examination of family members for skeletal deformities (e.g., kyphoscoliosis, pes cavus and hammer toes, and enlarged nerve trunks) and nerve conduction studies provide important clues. Nerve biopsy is a useful way of determining the etiology of some polyneuropathies, such as amyloidosis, leprosy, sarcoidosis, certain toxic neuropathies that cause giant swellings of axons, and vasculitic neuropathies.

Although classification of neuropathies by clinical presentation alone is fallacious because the same pathologic process may create different manifestations, methodical clinical evaluation can point one toward a pathologic diagnosis.

When the question of neuropathy is raised, the physician should decide first whether this is a *mononeuropathy,* in which the symptoms are confined to the distribution of a single nerve; *a multiple mononeuropathy,* in which discrete nerves are involved at various sites; or a *polyneuropathy,* a symmetric (usually distal) pattern of involvement. The first two groups usually are due to nerve compression or inflammation.

The clinical approach to diagnosis in the case of a patient with polyneuropathy continues with the second differentiating question: *is the neuropathy motor, sensory, or mixed?* After this has been decided, the fields of possible etiologies are smaller but still quite long, so further branches of the tree must be explored.

The physician should next determine whether the *progression of symptoms has been acute* (over hours to days), *subacute* (over days to weeks), *or chronic* (over months). Acute neuropathies, developing in less than a week, are almost all motor; porphyria, poliomyelitis, and poisoning are the most common causes. Uncommon acute sensory neuropathies are usually caused by toxic agents but sometimes occur in association with underlying malignancy. Chronic neuropathies make up the majority of cases (Boxes 167-2 to 167-4). When there is more motor than sensory involvement, the physician should think first of motor neurone disease (e.g., amyotrophic lateral sclerosis [ALS]), poliomyelitis, hereditary motor and sensory neuropathies, chronic infectious polyneuropathy, and toxic causes. With more sensory than motor involvement, axonal neuropathies such as those caused by toxicity, vitamin B_{12} deficiency, hereditary sensory neuropathy, or other systemic disease, and demyelinating neuropathies related to diabetes, uremia, myelomatosis, and dysproteinemia should be considered first.

The fourth question to consider is *whether the polyneuropathy is of axonal or of demyelinating/infiltrating type.* This can usually be answered using nerve conduction studies, although the findings of marked thick-fiber function loss (e.g., vibration and joint position sense) and of enlarged nerves would strongly suggest that the pathology is demyelinating or infiltrative. Boxes 167-2 to 167-4 list the more likely causes of polyneuropathies with these pathologies and whether they are motor, sensory, or mixed; acute/subacute or chronic; and axonal or demyelinating. At this point in the investigation, the list of likely causes should have been narrowed to a reasonable length, allowing efficient planning of further investigations.

Box 167-2. Causes of Sensory Neuropathies by Clinical Type

Acute/Subacute

Axonal
- Herpes zoster
- Lymphoma
- Acute sensory neuropathy
- Cisplatin
- Carcinoma
- Polycythemia

Demyelinating
- Diabetes

Chronic

Axonal
- Hereditary sensory neuropathies, types 1-4
- Spinocerebellar degenerations
- Tabes dorsalis
- Acromegaly
- Malabsorption syndromes
- Primary biliary cirrhosis
- Carcinoma, lymphoma, myeloma
- Arsenic, hydralazine, N_2O, metronidazole, cisplatin, pyridoxine
- B_{12} deficiency
- Hypothyroidism
- Polycythemia

Demyelinating
- Diabetes
- Leprosy
- Hypothyroidism
- Polyclonal gammopathy
- Rheumatoid

From Pryse-Phillips W, Murray TJ: *Essential neurology*, ed 4, 1996, Appleton-Lange.

Finally, more precision may be obtained by considering if the condition is painful and whether there is evidence of autonomic involvement or thickening of the peripheral nerves.

MONONEUROPATHIES

Asymmetric Proximal Neuropathies

Distinctive clinical syndromes of rapidly evolving painful weakness in the arm and shoulder or thigh and hip frequently occur because of involvement of the brachial or lumbosacral plexus. The pathology and pathogenesis, however, are ill-understood.

Neuralgic Amyotrophy (Idiopathic Brachial Plexus Neuropathy, Parsonage-Turner Syndrome). Neuralgic amyotrophy is well characterized clinically, although the cause and pathogenesis are not known. It may follow immunizations and rarely is familial. The process seems to cause an acute dysfunction of multiple nerves of the brachial plexus or more distal nerve branches, usually unilaterally but occasionally bilaterally. Otherwise healthy patients between 20 and 40 years of age are usually affected. The onset is abrupt, with intense pain over the shoulder and upper arm that persists for days or a few weeks. As pain abates, weakness and atrophy appear rapidly, most often affecting the serratus anterior, deltoid, supraspinati and infraspinati, rhomboids, sternomastoids, biceps, triceps, brachioradialis, and extensors of the wrist in various combinations. Sometimes only one or two of these muscles are affected. If any sensory impairment occurs, it is confined to an area over the deltoid in the distribution of the axillary nerve.

Box 167-3. Causes of Sensorimotor Neuropathies by Clinical Type

Acute/Subacute

Axonal
- Nutritional/alcohol
- Carcinoma
- 2,4-D, gold, As, thallium, disulfiram
- Porphyria
- Leukemia
- Trauma

Demyelinating
- Diphtheria
- Polyarteritis
- Diabetes
- Buckthorn berry
- Acquired amyloid
- Fabry's disease
- Carcinoma

Chronic

Axonal
- Hereditary motor and sensory neuropathies, type 2
- Sarcoid
- Malabsorption syndromes
- Diabetes
- Carcinoma
- Amyloid (primary systemic)
- Cryoglobulinemias and macroglobulinemias (IgA, IgM)
- Acrylamide, As, amiodarone, CS_2, dilantin, disulfiram, hexacarbons, isoniazid, nitrofurantoin, organophosphates, perhexilene, thalidomide, thallium, vinca alkaloids
- Uremia
- Nutritional
- Myeloma
- Leukemia

Demyelinating
- Hereditary motor and sensory neuropathies, types 1, 3, 4
- Chronic (relapsing) inflammatory polyneuropathy
- Leukodystrophies
- Diabetes
- Genetic amyloid
- Carcinoma
- Macroglobulinemia
- Monoclonal and polyclonal gammopathies
- Amiodarone
- Myelomatosis
- Leprosy
- Hepatic disease
- Fabry disease

From Pryse-Phillips W, Murray TJ: *Essential neurology*, ed 4, 1996, Appleton-Lange.

The diagnosis is clinical. Cerebrospinal fluid (CSF) studies are unwarranted. In the acute phase of pain the diagnosis is

Box 167-4. Causes of Motor Neuropathies by Clinical Type

Acute/Subacute

Axonal
- Poliomyelitis
- Porphyria
- Dapsone, *n*-hexane, organophosphates, lead, thallium
- Lymphoma
- Hypoglycemia

Demyelinating
- Acute inflammatory polyneuropathy
- Polyarteritis nodosa
- Mercury, *n*-hexane
- Rheumatoid arthritis
- Diphtheria

Chronic

Axonal
- Hereditary motor neuropathies
- Motor neuron disease
- Multiple system atrophy

Demyelinating
- Chronic (relapsing) inflammatory polyneuropathy
- Myelomatosis
- Metachromatic leukodystrophy
- Dapsone, hydralazine, mercury
- Globoid cell leukodystrophy

From Pryse-Phillips W, Murray TJ: *Essential neurology*, ed 4, 1996, Appleton-Lange.

difficult, with referred pain from gallbladder disease, local disease such as bursitis of the shoulder, or cervical disk prolapse entering into the differential diagnosis. Unlike acute disk protrusions, there is no neck spasm or limitation of neck movement. No specific treatment is available. It is a clinical impression that a short course of steroids decreases the duration of pain but does not seem to alter the course of the disease otherwise. Recovery occurs in most instances but may take up to 2 or 3 years.

Idiopathic Lumbosacral Plexopathy. Idiopathic lumbosacral plexopathy is most often caused by diabetes, but retroperitoneal tumors, aneurysm, abscess, or vasculitis in elderly patients can produce the same picture. Patients with vasculitis will complain of severe root pain and focal deficits in the distribution of the femoral, obturator, and/or sciatic nerves. The diagnosis is seldom possible without the aid of electromyography and computed tomography (CT) scanning, but a clue may be obtained from the high erythrocyte sedimentation rate (ESR) that is generally found.

Lumbosacral Polyradiculopathy (Cauda Equina Syndrome) in Acquired Immunodeficiency Syndrome. A rapidly evolving cauda equina syndrome may occur in patients with AIDS as a result of necrotizing vasculitis of the lumbar and sacral nerve roots of the cauda equina from cytomegalovirus (CMV) infection. Clinically, patients are in the later stages of human immunodeficiency virus-1 (HIV-1) infection and complain of numbness in the feet or sacral areas, beginning asymmetrically and progressing rapidly to areflexic, hypotonic paraparesis and urinary retention. The CSF shows a predominantly granulocytic pleocytosis of up to 1000 cells/cm with raised protein and decreased glucose. CMV can usually be cultured from the CSF. The clinical picture is supported by evidence of other foci of CMV infection, such as retinitis, pneumonitis, or encephalitis. Prompt therapy with ganciclovir based on the clinical and CSF picture while awaiting confirmation by CSF culture is essential to prevent worsening to paraplegia. A similar syndrome may evolve in a slower, subacute fashion in patients with AIDS and can be caused by leptomeningitis localized to the cauda equina from cryptococcosis, syphilis, and tuberculosis. A rare cause of a similar syndrome in which CSF abnormalities are found has been recognized in otherwise normal persons resulting from industrial exposure to dimethyl-aminoproprionitrite (DMAPN), a catalyzer in the manufacturing of polyurethane foam.

Diabetic Amyotrophy. In diabetes, the VI, III, and IV cranial nerves and the femoral and obturator nerves are those most often affected by neuropathy. The diabetic femoral neuropathy (diabetic amyotrophy) is really a lumbosacral plexopathy. This is a syndrome caused by microinfarcts of the lumbrosacral plexus. It is seen in middle aged or elderly patients with undiagnosed or mild diabetes and a history of recent marked weight loss. The patients present with severe, persistent, deep pain in the thigh accompanied by marked weakness and wasting of the hip and thigh muscles. It is usually unilateral; when bilateral, it is asymmetric. There is severe weakness of the iliopsoas and quadriceps femoris and often there is some weakness in other muscles innervated by the femoral, gluteal, and obturator nerves. The knee jerk reflex is lost, but sensation is normal. There is often considerable weight loss, which raises the suspicion of malignancy.

The condition is easily misdiagnosed as an L4 root lesion. However, that would not produce weakness of the iliopsoas and quadriceps muscles, and sensory impairment over the inner aspect of the leg would be notable, whereas in diabetic amyotrophy, weakness spills over to muscles supplied by the obturator and sciatic nerves, outside the territory of the L4 root. The condition must be distinguished from acute femoral neuropathy caused by retroperitoneal hematoma in patients with bleeding disorders.

Treatment is symptomatic, but symptoms may last from 3 to 18 months. Initially the main problem is to provide pain relief. Diphenylhydantoin and carbamazepine are helpful for some patients, whereas others respond to amitriptyline; in intractable cases amitriptyline is combined with fluphenazine. These agents are given along with nonnarcotic analgesics such as aspirin or ibuprofen. Aspirin is preferable, when tolerated, because it has the advantage of inhibiting platelet aggregation, which might be involved in the pathogenesis. When paralysis is severe, the patient may benefit from bracing the knee.

More Distal Mononeuropathies

Diabetic Ischemic Neuropathies

Diabetic III Nerve Palsies. Diabetic III nerve palsies frequently spare the pupil,* perhaps because the parasympathetic fibers are situated around the outside of the nerve,

*But so do aneurysms sometimes. The Golden Rule is that there are no Golden Rules.

where they can receive some blood supply from the local pia-arachnoid vessels. The initial complaints are of eye pain, headache, and diplopia that have sudden onset but usually clear after weeks or months. In diabetes, such ischemic neuropathies are often superimposed on a preexisting metabolic polyneuropathy. In forms with any of these etiologies, single or multiple nerves show acute loss of motor and sensory function, often with pain, and recovery occurs slowly as long as the original disease is successfully treated.

Diabetic Truncal Radiculopathy. In diabetic truncal radiculopathy the thoracic nerve roots are asymmetrically affected, causing a deep burning pain felt over the upper abdomen or side of the chest for some weeks. It is often associated with anorexia and weight loss so most patients are investigated for occult malignancy without result. Diagnosis is made primarily by an awareness that this syndrome occurs in diabetic patients. Electromyography of thoracic and lumbar paraspinal muscles shows extensive signs of denervation, usually bilaterally. A myelogram may occasionally be required to rule out compressive or inflammatory lesions of the roots. This neuropathy differs from the painless form of truncal neuropathy, which is bilateral, symmetric, and causes sensory impairment over the anterior abdominal wall. In these patients there is also severe sensory loss in the limbs and often evidence of visceral autonomic neuropathy. These cases represent a very advanced stage of the common diabetic distal symmetric polyneuropathy. The pain resolves spontaneously over months, but may be alleviated as outlined under the treatment of diabetic amyotrophy.

Compression and Traction Neuropathies

Although nerve compression produces dysfunction partly through the mechanism of ischemia, compression neuropathies will be described separately because they are so common and distinctive. Any superficial nerve in the body may be stretched or compressed; even comparatively minor pressure will prompt long-lasting symptoms if the nerves have been damaged already and are thus "at risk." This may occur in the presence of any subclinical neuropathy and also when another lesion is situated proximally (such as cervical spondylosis), where it is already decreasing axoplasmic flow from a higher level. Superficial nerves are especially liable to injury by external pressure where they overlie bone. The radial nerve in the spiral groove of the humerus, the ulnar nerve in the cubital tunnel, and the common peroneal nerve at the neck of the fibula are especially vulnerable to compression, occupationally or resulting from deep sleep or coma. Patients with generalized wasting diseases and loss of fat will have less of a subcutaneous buffer between nerves and external objects. Because patients may be lying in bed for long periods, compression neuropathies are common in such cases. Rarely, the condition is inherited.

The mechanism is one of chronic pressure on a segment of the nerve that lies in a fibroosseous tunnel close to the joint where it is vulnerable to recurrent microtrauma. The compressed segment of the nerve shows areas of demyelination chiefly affecting the thickly myelinated fibers. In most patients, the axons are preserved and remyelination eventually occurs.

The anatomic diagnosis is made by clinical examination. Measurement of nerve conduction velocities, however, is a sensitive and easy laboratory test that shows slowing across the entrapped nerve segment. In general, sensory conduction is impaired earlier than motor conduction, although the latter is more easily tested. Electromyographic examination of the muscles supplied by the affected nerve may add more data because evidence of muscle denervation indicates a substantial degree of compression.

The etiologic diagnosis is usually evident from the history of occupational, habitual, or hobby-related trauma, but diabetes, hypothyroidism, and generalized (sometimes subclinical) polyneuropathy should be excluded, which may require laboratory tests.

Awareness of the possibility of nerve injury and careful technique should obviate nerve compression resulting from the application of a tourniquet or plaster cast to limbs. Every effort should be made to prevent or minimize prolonged local pressure in patients undergoing general anesthesia and in comatose patients (Fig. 167-1). The regions of the limbs in which nerves are vulnerable to pressure must be protected. If the arm is to be immobilized on a board for intravenous (IV) infusion, it should be placed in a supine position. If it is not immobilized, it should be kept half-flexed at the elbow and across the chest so that elbows are clear of the bed. If the arm is to be kept by the side, soft pads under the arm and forearm will protect the nerve from pressure. The unconscious patient should be turned frequently so that the weight of the body does not press on the limbs for any length of time. The elbow should be prevented from pressing against the metal edge of the bed or operating table and should not be allowed to hang over the edge of the bed to avoid pressure over the radial

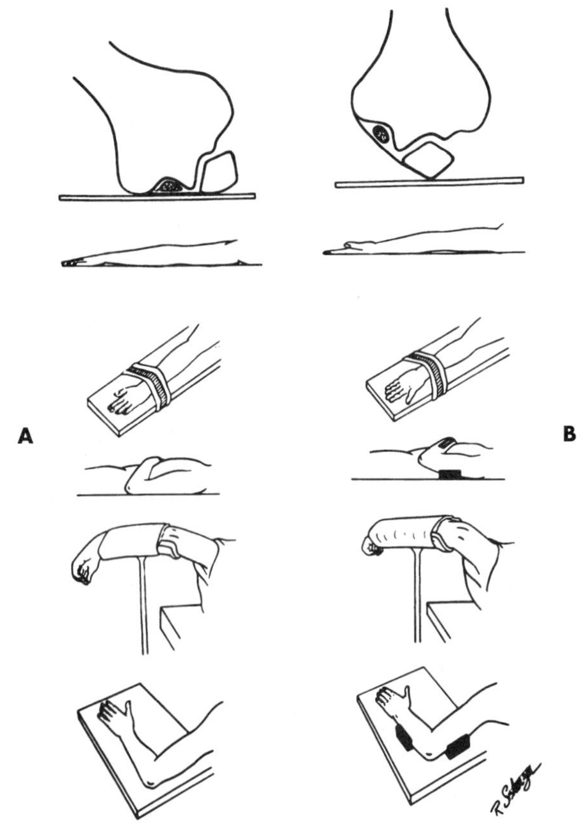

Fig. 167-1. Ulnar nerve compression. **A** illustrates positions that put the ulnar nerve behind the elbow at risk for external compression. **B** illustrates positioning of the upper extremity that minimizes this risk. (From Wadsworth TG: *Anesth Analg* 53:303, 1974.)

nerve. In the legs, the peroneal nerves can be protected by soft cushions, avoiding crossing of the legs, and by care in using stirrups for the lithotomy position.

Treatment. Treatment of hypothyroidism, acromegaly, or gout often relieves an associated carpal tunnel syndrome, but decompression is effective in a majority of cases of compressive neuropathy. Conservative therapy is attempted in most instances and is the rule in self-limited neuropathies such as the carpal tunnel syndrome of pregnancy. Occupational and habitual modification is important. Rest from heavy work with hands and wrists in a patient with carpal tunnel syndrome is helpful, but this may call for a change of jobs. The avoidance of habitual trauma is essential. For instance, the patient with ulnar entrapment must not lean on the elbows nor sleep with them flexed. Physical medicine has a useful role. A 20-degree wrist cock-up splint may abolish the nocturnal pain in carpal tunnel syndrome. A soft pad behind the elbow may ease the pain and paresthesia of mild ulnar neuropathy. Local injection of steroids (usually methylprednisolone) may decrease the interstitial edema of the nerve and of the synovial membranes surrounding it when injected in the vicinity of the entrapped nerve segment, not into the nerve itself. The techniques of injecting the carpal tunnel, for which it is most frequently used, can be learned quickly and performed in the clinic. When successful, the injection can be repeated, but if it is required more than every 2 or 3 months, surgery should be considered.

Surgery is indicated for failure of conservative measures and the presence of enduring sensory loss or weakness. The procedures are simple and direct and in principle involve decompressing the affected nerve segment by sectioning the flexor retinaculum for the carpal and tarsal tunnel syndromes. Surgery for ulnar nerve entrapment should be decompression rather than transposition, which further damages its blood supply. Surgery effectively relieves pain and paresthesia and in most cases leads to gradual recovery of sensation. Muscle weakness, if already established before surgery, is the last to recover. Disability resulting from some palsies can be minimized before natural recovery occurs. The use of appropriate splints for wrist drop and a brace for foot drop is helpful for patient comfort and for prevention of contractures. If a minor causalgic syndrome develops, the burning pain and trophic changes can last for months and can be quite distressing. The symptoms are treated with nonnarcotic analgesics, transcutaneous electrical nerve stimulation (TENS), carbamazepine or tricyclic drugs, and, in recalcitrant cases, with sympathetic blockade. There is seldom any indication for surgery in the acute phase because the palsies usually recover spontaneously. An occasional patient with postoperative ulnar neuropathy may continue to have severe weakness for 1 to 2 years, and surgical decompression of the nerve is then advisable.

Cranial Nerves. Because all the cranial nerves leave the skull through foramina, they are also liable to compression (e.g., the VII as in Bell's palsy, the VIII in a cerebellopontine angle tumor or Paget's disease, and the III with a temporal lobe expanding lesion producing uncal herniation syndrome). Pressure on the lower cranial nerves from inflammatory, neoplastic, or vascular lesions may occur as well. Pressure on spinal nerve roots by tumors, disks, or osteophytes and so on could also be regarded as compression neuropathies.

Facial Palsy. Facial palsy is the most common cranial mononeuropathy seen in general practice and is discussed in Chapter 162.

Brachial Plexus. The usual cause of Erb's palsy is a stretching injury to the C5 and C6 roots. Weakness and wasting of the deltoid, spinati, biceps, and periscapular muscles are found (Erb's palsy); lymphedema is common, but pain is unusual. Weakness of shoulder abduction and external rotation, elbow flexion and supination, and wrist and finger dorsiflexion lead to the classical Porter's tip appearance. For some reason, myokymia in the proximal muscles is also common in this condition. The upper fibers of the brachial plexus may also be compressed by fibrous tissue after radiation therapy.

The lower fibers of the brachial plexus may be infiltrated by malignant tissue, producing Horner's syndrome, pain, and mainly distal signs, such as wasting and weakness of the thenar and hypothenar muscles and reduced sensation in the distal upper limb. Damage to these fibers also occurs with acute abduction injuries of the shoulder (Klumpke's palsy), which stretch the C8 and T1 roots.

Thoracic Outlet Syndrome. Thoracic outlet syndrome is a much disputed condition that is more a vascular than neurologic entity; although the diagnosis is often made, objective neurologic or electrical signs are rare. Symptoms ascribed to the disorder include pain in the arm, especially with heavy lifting or carrying; coldness, color change, and pain in the hands; and weakness of the forearm and hand. Symptoms may be produced or exacerbated by downward traction on the arm and sometimes by hyperabduction at the shoulder, when a diminution of the radial pulse may be found (which may be the key to the whole matter if the problem is venous or arterial compression rather than stretching of the lower fibers of the brachial plexus). Objective physical signs, such as C8-T1 sensory loss or small hand muscle wasting, are rare but many of these patients have long necks and droopy shoulders, suggesting that the symptoms stem from a disorder of posture—the *droopy shoulder syndrome*.

When physical signs are actually found, even if radiographs do not show cervical ribs, a fibrous band may be present between the (often large) C7 transverse process and the first rib. The scalenus anticus muscle is inserted into the first rib, just anterior to the subclavian artery and the lower trunk of the brachial plexus, and it has been suggested that hypertrophy or abnormal contraction of this muscle can be a cause of compression. In the presence of even minor vascular changes, the potential damage to the subclavian artery (dilation or thrombosis) makes surgical exploration advisable. Resection of the scalenus anticus or of the first rib, a cervical rib, or a band between them is now seldom done and it is best to advise all patients to practice shoulder-girdle strengthening exercises and to avoid surgery.

Axillary (Circumflex) Nerve. The axillary (circumflex) nerve may be damaged when the head of the humerus is dislocated posteriorly and is less often by direct trauma. The same nerve is severely involved in the condition of neuralgic amyotrophy. Weakness and wasting of the deltoid and a small patch of sensory loss over the outer part of the shoulder are the only signs resulting from selective axillary nerve damage. This condition must be differentiated from a C5 root lesion, which will also show signs of a lower motor neuron lesion affecting the rhomboids and the supraspinati and infraspinati, as well as other muscles supplied in part by C5.

Other Brachial Plexus Branches. Other brachial plexus branch nerves may be damaged in isolation. The long thoracic nerve to the serratus anterior fixes the scapula to the chest wall when forward pressure is exerted on the upper limb. It also brings the scapula forward when the arm is thrust forward, as in a fencer's lunge, causing injury in healthy young people who have been exercising heavily. Injury may produce pain in the shoulder that is referred to the scapular and periscapular muscles. Causes include shoulder trauma, carrying heavy weights, and neuritis after a viral respiratory illness such as coxsackievirus infections. The patient may complain of winging of the scapula when asked to push the arm forward against resistance and of pain when rotating or extending the neck, and will be unable to raise the arm over the head in the forward position. Conservative treatment with rest leads to a resolution of symptoms in most cases. Restorative surgery is possible in patients with persisting deficits. The suprascapular nerve is sometimes compressed or locally traumatized, which results in weakness of shoulder abduction and external rotation.

Ulnar Nerve. The ulnar nerve is vulnerable in its subcutaneous position in the ulnar groove behind the elbow, behind the medial epicondyle where it is liable to compression, as well as being involved in lesions affecting the lower trunk. The most frequent site of damage is where the nerve passes under the common origin of the flexor muscles at the elbow. Everyone has experienced the disagreeable pain and electric shock sensation of banging the "funny bone" and of paresthesia in the hands when leaning on the elbows. When the elbow is flexed, the nerve is partially stretched and rises superficially, where it may well be damaged when the elbow rests on a hard surface. Weakness of the ulnar half of the flexor digitorum profundus, all of the interossei, the hypothenar muscles, and the adductor pollicis and sensory symptoms (diminution of common sensation in the little finger and the ulnar half of the ring finger) may be expected, and the Tinel's sign will be positive at the elbow. Striking wasting of the dorsal and palmar interossei may be seen.

Patients may present with tingling and numbness on the inner aspect of the palm and on the little and ring fingers, or with the gradual onset of wasting of the muscles of the hand, with clawlike deformity of the fingers but with little pain or paresthesia. Wasting and weakness of dorsal and palmar interossei and hypothenar muscles and decreased sensation over the little finger and ulnar half of the ring finger are found. The nerve may be tender at the elbow and may be enlarged above the ulnar groove.

Tardy ulnar palsy appears years after an injury to the elbow, such as supracondylar fracture of the humerus. The elbow is deformed and its movements restricted. Idiopathic ulnar palsy is the most common variety and occurs with a normal elbow. Recurrent trauma to the nerve during elbow flexion (as with frequent vigorous "arm curls" with weights for fitness training) may cause the neuropathy. Recurrent subluxation of the ulnar nerve, in which the nerve snaps out of the ulnar groove frequently with elbow flexion, is usually asymptomatic, but may cause pain and paresthesia.

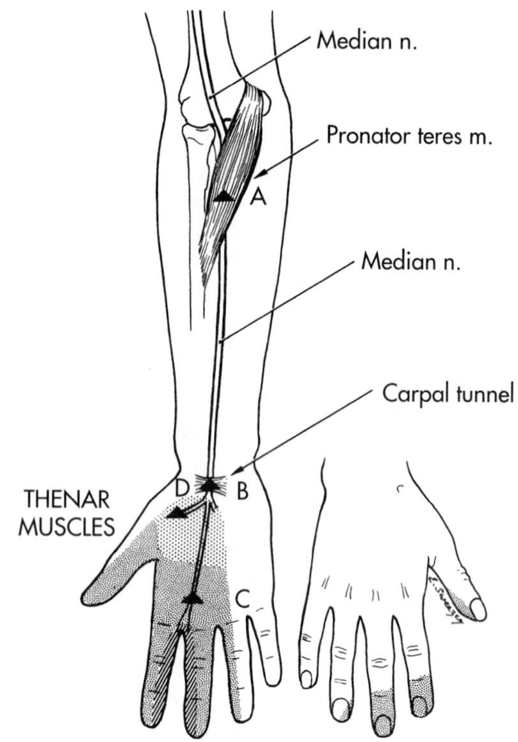

Fig. 167-2. Carpal tunnel syndrome. *B* points to the level where the median nerve is compressed in the carpal tunnel. The pronator teres muscle *(A)* and the transverse intermetacarpal ligaments *(C)* are less common sites of median nerve compression. The motor branch innervates the thenar muscle *(D)*. The lightly stippled area shows the sensory supply of the palmar cutaneous branch, which arises proximal to the carpal tunnel and thus is spared in the carpal tunnel syndrome. The densely stippled zone represents the cutaneous sensory area of the median nerve distal to the carpal tunnel. The hatched area shows the sensory supply of the interdigital branch of the nerve. (From Dyck PJ, Thomas PK, Lambert EH: *Peripheral neuropathy,* Philadelphia, 1975, WB Saunders.)

In carpenters and shoemakers who use palm pressure on awls and screwdrivers, or in heavy equipment operators and truck drivers who push gears with the palm of the hand, the deep palmar branch of the nerve may be compressed medial to the pisiform bone at the wrist. This is below the origin of the superficial sensory branch to the fingers and that of the motor branch to the hypothenar eminence, so interosseous wasting and weakness of the adductor pollicis are the only signs.

Median Nerve. Carpal tunnel syndrome, the most common compression neuropathy, is due to entrapment of the nerve in the carpal tunnel under the flexor retinaculum, where it is surrounded by the tendons and synovial sheaths of the long flexors of the fingers (Fig. 167-2).

The syndrome is particularly common in people with tenosynovitis of the flexor tendons, which lie with the nerve under the flexor retinaculum of the wrist. Synovial herniation or a simple ganglion or a lipoma may be present. Those with any abnormal degree of fluid retention (e.g., related to hypothyroidism, pregnancy, or chronic renal disease) are also susceptible, and the syndrome may also complicate Paget's disease, myelomatosis, acromegaly, and obesity. The problem is frequently bilateral, in which case it is worse in the dominant hand. The leading symptom is recurrent, painful numbness, usually worst at night. It often affects all fingers rather than being restricted to the thumb, index, and middle fingers. Pain is less evident but when it occurs it may spread up the arm, even to the shoulder. Patients may also complain of dropping objects from the hand. In the early stages, examination may be normal despite prominent symptoms.

Patients are more frequently women than men. They complain of pain in the hand that rises up the arm as far as the shoulder and characteristically awakens them at night. The syndrome also is associated with paresthesia of at least 3½ fingers (although patients sometimes may complain of tingling throughout the whole hand). When the patient wakes up early in the morning, he or she tends to rub or flick the hand to try and restore feeling. Any heavy exertion during the day, such as housework, knitting, or gripping a steering wheel, or repetitive use of the wrist at work tends to worsen the symptoms. Weakness of the thumb is manifested as clumsiness and difficulty with some fine movements. Examination reveals weakness of the thenar muscles, especially of the opponens (but not the adductor) and possibly of the two radial lumbricals so that extension at the interphalangeal joints of the second and third fingers is impaired; sometimes there is hypoesthesia of the radial side of the palm and of the palmar aspects of the first 3½ digits, a positive Tinel's sign at the wrist, and worsening of symptoms with passive compression of the volar aspect of the wrist (Phalen's sign).

Precise electrophysiologic criteria for the diagnosis of carpal tunnel syndrome have been defined, and most surgeons prefer to operate after the diagnosis has been confirmed by nerve conduction studies. The best long-term results are achieved by incision of the flexor retinaculum under regional anesthesia to relieve the pressure on the nerve. Alternatively, splints worn at night that hold the wrist in 20 degrees of extension, or an injection of 20 mg of prednisone under the flexor retinaculum may produce temporary relief. Conservative measures such as these are correctly used in pregnant women because the condition often clears after delivery.

Radial Nerve Palsy. In radial nerve palsy the radial nerve is compressed as it lies in the spiral groove (Fig. 167-3). With damage at that site, the branches to the triceps are spared so the patient can still extend the elbow, but there is wrist drop and failure of finger extension. A small patch of sensory loss can sometimes be detected between the thumb and first finger on the dorsum of the hand. The condition is common among alcoholics, in whom there is often the added factor of preexisting alcoholic neuropathy, and in the male partner of a courting couple, as well as from improper positioning under anesthesia, wherein the arm is allowed to hang over the edge of the operating table. Rarely, it appears after heavy exertion in a very muscular individual. The patient complains of weakness of the hand, without pain, that is noted on awakening and often misconstrued as a stroke. The chief abnormality is weakness of dorsiflexion of the wrist and fingers, but sensation and the triceps reflex are usually intact.

A common pitfall is the apparent weakness of the muscles of the hand that are innervated by the ulnar and median nerves in addition to those supplied by the radial nerve, so that the entire hand appears weak. This pseudoparesis is

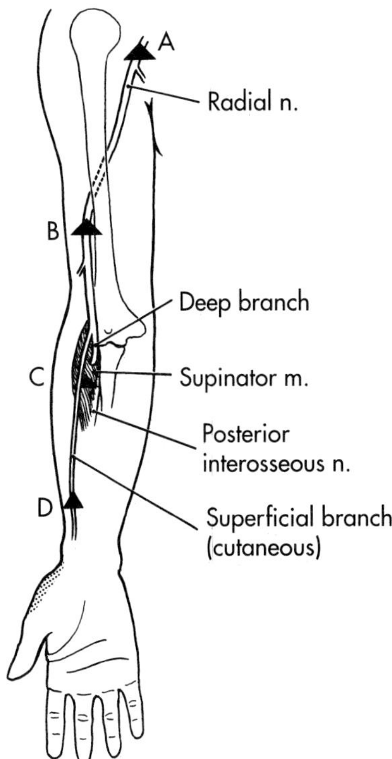

Fig. 167-3. Radial nerve compression. The radial nerve can be compressed in the axilla *(A)* or, more often, as it winds around the humerus *(B)* in the spiral groove. Its deep motor branch may become entrapped at the supinator muscle *(C)*, whereas the superficial cutaneous branch *(D)* may be injured along the forearm or wrist, causing sensory symptoms over the dorsum of the hand *(stippled area)*. (From Dyck PJ, Thomas PK, Lambert EH: *Peripheral neuropathy*, Philadelphia, 1975, WB Saunders.)

caused by the lack of normal fixation of the wrist and fingers by the extensor muscles necessary for the optimal use of other hand muscles. The confusion can be resolved by demonstrating that these movements are in fact normal when the wrist and fingers are supported by laying them on a firm, flat surface.

When radial nerve palsy is bilateral or appears subacutely, the possibility of lead poisoning should be considered. In patients with rheumatoid arthritis, symptoms should be differentiated from those of rupture of the extensor tendons.

The posterior interosseous nerve is a major terminal branch of the radial nerve. It may be compressed by a fibrous band or by a posterior dislocation of the radial head, where it passes underneath the origin of the extensor carpi radialis longus and supinator, or it may be damaged more distally after forearm fractures. Patients complain of pain in the forearm and of tenderness just below the lateral epicondyle, as with lateral epicondylitis. Examination shows weakness of extension of the thumb and index finger, but there is no change in sensation. After electrodiagnostic confirmation of the diagnosis, surgical decompression should relieve the symptoms.

Femoral Neuropathy. One cause of femoral neuropathy is compression of the nerve by a hematoma in the iliopsoas muscle (Fig. 167-4), although the bleeding rarely occurs directly into the nerve. Most often it affects patients receiving

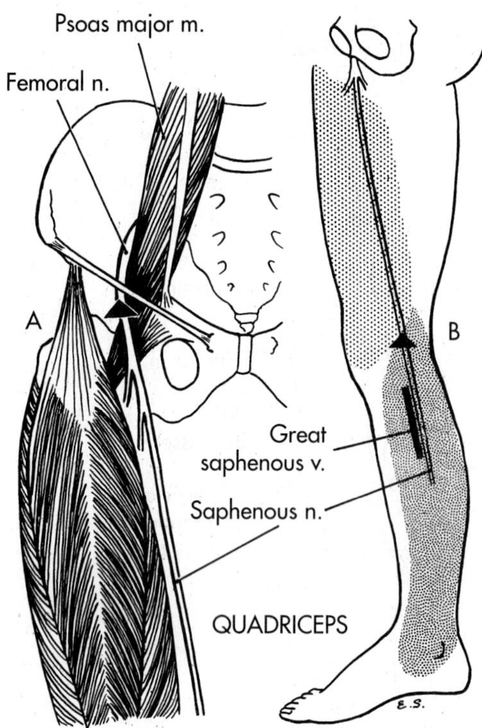

Fig. 167-4. Femoral nerve compression. This nerve has a close anatomic relation with the psoas muscle and inguinal ligament *(A)*. Compression at the groin may cause quadriceps weakness and sensory impairment in the nerve's distribution at the thigh *(lightly stippled area)* and in the saphenous branch *(heavily stippled area)*. Pressure at the knee *(B)* or surgery to the saphenous veins may affect the saphenous nerve. (From Dyck PJ, Thomas PK, Lambert EH: *Peripheral neuropathy,* Philadelphia, 1975, WB Saunders.)

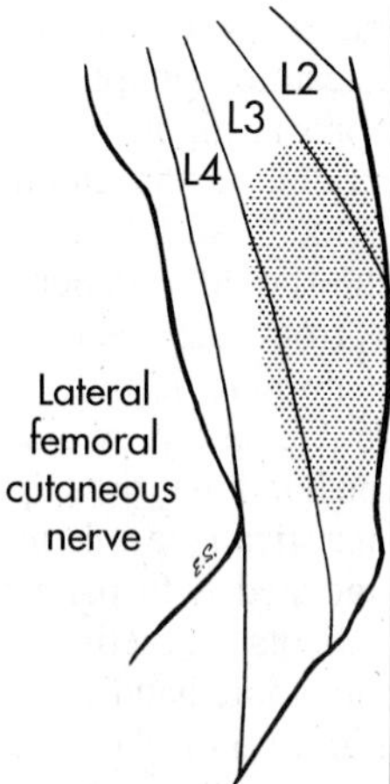

Fig. 167-5. Meralgia paresthetica. The sensory supply of the lateral cutaneous nerve of the thigh is shown. Note how this area overlaps with the distribution of upper lumbar innervations. (From Dyck PJ, Thomas PK, Lambert EH: *Peripheral neuropathy,* Philadelphia, 1975, WB Saunders.)

anticoagulant treatment or those with hemophilia. Typically, pain in the thigh and weakness of flexion of the hip and extension of the knee rapidly evolve over hours or days. The knee jerk reflex is diminished or lost. Sensation is diminished over the anterior aspect of the thigh, and bluish discoloration may be seen in the inguinal region. In patients with coagulation disorders, there should be a high degree of suspicion for this complication; CT scan of the retroperitoneal region readily visualizes an iliopsoas hematoma.

With conservative therapy of rest, discontinuation of anticoagulation, or correction of bleeding disorder in hemophiliac patients, the neuropathy should improve, recovering fully in a few weeks, although mild residual disability may remain in some patients. The role of early surgical evacuation of hematoma is unproven.

Lateral Femoral Cutaneous Nerve. The lateral femoral cutaneous nerve (Fig. 167-5) is sometimes compressed as it passes underneath the outer edge of the inguinal ligament. Such an occurrence is common in pregnancy and in obese people, in whom the nerve is compressed by a pad of fat. Pain, burning paresthesia in the anterolateral thigh, and a small area of local sensory loss characterize this condition, known as *meralgia paresthetica*. Treatment includes explanation and reassurance as to the benign nature of the otherwise baffling symptoms, weight loss if appropriate, local injection of the nerve with hydrocortisone and local anesthetic, or surgical decompression if such measures fail.

Obturator Nerve. Occasionally damage to the obturator nerve occurs in the obturator canal, usually caused by the pressure of the fetal head during parturition, or after the imprecise application of forceps. The main features are pain in the inner side of the thigh, with some sensory loss in that area, and weakness of the hip adductors.

Sciatic Nerve. Damage to the sciatic nerve may follow a posterior dislocation of the hip or a misplaced intramuscular injection. The initial result will be paralysis of all muscles in the leg except for those innervated by the obturator and femoral nerves. Sensory loss will be complete below the knee.

Common Peroneal Nerve. Compression of the common peroneal nerve as it winds around the neck of the fibula is a common problem. Perhaps because of the anatomic arrangement of its fibers, those that pass in the deep peroneal branch to form the anterior tibial nerve (which innervates the space between the hallux and the second toes) are sometimes spared. Those carrying sensation from the outer edge of the calf and the dorsum of the foot in the superficial peroneal nerve are usually involved, with diminution or loss of sensation in that area. The motor fibers running to the peronei and the anterior tibial muscles are also affected, producing a foot drop and failure of eversion of the foot. If foot drop is pronounced, there may be apparent weakness of inversion and plantar flexion of the foot caused by lack of fixation of the ankle, a situation analogous to that in severe radial palsy. Tinel's sign will be positive, initially at the neck of the fibula when regeneration begins. Patients placed in stirrups in the Trendelenburg's position, those who have ill-fitting plaster casts or braces applied, those who are wasted and who lie long in bed, and especially those who sit with their legs crossed for a long time are likely to develop peroneal nerve palsy.

An acute fifth lumbar (L5) root lesion causes back pain, and straight leg raising is painfully restricted. When an L5 root lesion is suspected, evidence of denervation is sought in muscles supplied by L5 but not by the peroneal nerve, such as the posterior tibial, hamstring, and gluteus medius muscles.

Posterior Tibial Nerve. The posterior tibial nerve may be compressed when it runs behind the medial malleolus under the flexor retinaculum to supply the small foot muscles (as the medial and lateral plantar nerves) and the skin of the sole of the foot on the medial side. Some cases occur idiopathically but in most it complicates a previous fracture with deformity of the ankle. A ganglion or neurofibroma is an occasional cause. Pain, tingling, and numbness in the sole of the foot are the main manifestations, often with nocturnal exacerbations. The nerve is usually tender behind the medial malleolus, and the Tinel's sign may be elicited on tapping it. In established cases there is wasting of the abductor hallucis, causing a hollowing out of the normal bulge on the medial margin of the foot. Apart from these motor and sensory changes, pain may also be a dominant feature. Surgical decompression is usually effective.

Rather more distally, a lateral plantar nerve may be compressed by a neuroma between the heads of the third and fourth metatarsals, producing very little in the way of clinically definable sensory loss or motor weakness but causing a lot of pain. The patient has a characteristic pattern of pain in the foot while walking, often stopping to take off the shoe and rub the foot. This condition, known as *Morton's metatarsalgia,* is also helped by surgery.

MULTIPLE NEUROPATHIES

Multiple Mononeuropathies

In multiple mononeuropathy syndrome, palsies of individual peripheral nerves appear acutely or subacutely and are scattered over the body in an irregular pattern (e.g., a wrist drop may appear caused by radial nerve palsy, followed in a few days by a foot drop from peroneal nerve injury and later by an ulnar neuropathy or cranial nerve palsy such as facial paralysis). Rarely, multiple mononeuropathy evolves gradually over months or years. In the Western world, the syndrome is most often caused by diabetes mellitus, vasculitis, or sarcoidosis; worldwide, however, leprosy is the most common cause. The vasculitides responsible include polyarteritis nodosa, Wegener's granulomatosis, rheumatoid arthritis, and systemic lupus erythematosus (SLE). The syndrome also occurs in Waldenström's macroglobulinemia and cryoglobulinemia, but the nerve ischemia in these disorders is due to hyperviscosity of the blood. Finally, multiple mononeuropathies may be manifestations of HIV-1 infection and of Lyme disease.

Pain is a noticeable feature in many cases. Sensory perineuritis is an uncommon variant, but it is of interest because it causes recurrent, migrating, painful numbness in different parts of the body, yields no abnormal investigative results, and eventually disappears.

The diagnosis in most cases is aided substantially by the relatively limited number of causes. Nerve biopsy may show vasculitis of the vasa nervorum, granulomas of sarcoidosis, or the bacilli of leprosy. In the appropriate clinical and epidemiologic circumstances, serologic tests for HIV-1 infection and Lyme disease should be obtained. A mononuclear CSF lymphocytosis is common to both disorders.

The treatment and prognosis are of the underlying diseases. In the acute vasculitides of polyarteritis nodosa and in Wegener's granulomatosis, the neuropathy may respond to steroids and immunosuppression, but the overall prognosis is poor. In macroglobulinemia and cryoglobulinemia, the mononeuropathies may recover fully. Antibiotic therapy is essential in Lyme disease; plasmapheresis and intravenous immunoglobulin may alleviate HIV-related neuropathies.

Polyneuropathies

When a patient has symptoms of weakness, numbness, tingling, and/or pain, and shows evidence of wasting, objective loss of power, fasciculations, and sensory loss in distal centripetal distribution, the diagnosis of neuropathy is relatively easy. The next stage is to determine the etiology, and the many potential causes make this a harder task.

The approach suggested at the start of this chapter has the merit of reducing the etiologic possibilities and thus makes investigation more efficient. Differentiation between acute and chronic is the first step, and the physician should always remember that some of these disorders evolve over days, which disallows an easy determination. Clinical evidence will give a fast answer to the question of whether the neuropathy is of motor, sensory, or mixed origin.

The third step (axonal or demyelinating?) is aided by the following: enlarged nerves, little wasting, hyporeflexia or areflexia, and major deficits in thick-fiber functions (vibration, joint position sense, tactile discrimination) point toward a demyelinating cause. Marked wasting, fasciculations, lancinating pains, no loss of reflexes, and major deficits in thin-fiber function (pinprick pain, crude light touch, scratch, temperature) indicate axonal loss. However, combinations are frequently seen, and the speed of nerve conduction may be the simplest and fastest way of making the determination.

Mainly Motor Neuropathies

Acute Motor Axonal Neuropathies. Acute acquired neuronal motor neuropathies include poliomyelitis (see Chapter 165), porphyria, the severe neuronal variant of acute inflammatory polyneuropathy (see below), and less commonly lymphoma and recurrent hypoglycemia. Poisoning with dapsone, n-hexane, organophosphates, lead, and thallium are other causes.

Porphyric Neuropathy. Recurrent bouts of acute polyneuropathy are a major and serious feature of the recessively inherited hepatic porphyrias—the acute, intermittent, variegate coproporphyric types. The principal pathologic abnormality is axonal degeneration affecting the nerve roots and proximal parts of nerves, including the autonomic fibers. The pathogenesis of nerve injury is not known, although it has been suggested that the large amounts of delta-amino levulinic acid (ALA) and porphobilinogen (PBG) produced in the acute attack may be neurotoxic.

Attacks are heralded by prominent and persistent abdominal and limb pain and constipation followed by symmetric, mainly proximal limb weakness. In severe cases, bulbar and respiratory paralysis occurs. General areflexia is present, although curiously, ankle reflexes may remain intact. A distinctive feature is sensory impairment, which often takes the form of broad bands around the thighs or arms or the shape of an old-fashioned bathing suit affecting the trunk. Autonomic disturbance is a constant feature, manifested by persistent tachycardia, ileus, hypertension, postural hypotension, and cardiac arrhythmias. The neuropathy is often accompanied or preceded by neuropsychiatric disturbances in the form of emotional lability, intense anxiety, depression, or frank psychosis with seizures.

Of great importance is the precipitation of acute attacks of porphyria by drugs, especially barbiturates. Other precipitants include starvation, acute infection, and possibly menstruation. Diagnosis is established by examining urine for PBG and ALA, both of which are present in great abundance in the acute phase. The urine typically turns port-wine color on standing in light. Relatives must be screened also.

Because of the cognitive and emotional features of acute attacks, patients in the early phases of neuropathy with bilateral limb pain are often misdiagnosed as hysterical. Another common and potentially tragic situation is that of a patient with acute abdominal pain in whom an exploratory laparotomy is performed under anesthesia using barbiturates; as the patient recovers from the anesthesia, a catastrophic barbiturate-induced neuropathy develops.

Symptomatic therapy is needed for maintenance of respiratory autonomic and metabolic functions. Propranolol is well tolerated, is an effective therapy for tachycardia and hypertension, and may also suppress the overproduction of porphyrins. Specific measures include avoidance of drugs that are known to exacerbate porphyria (Box 167-5) and the provision of an adequate amount of carbohydrates that seem to suppress porphyria precursor production and have a protective effect on neuropathy. Dextrose or levulose is given via nasogastric tube or intravenously. Hematin given early in the course of the acute attack consistently suppresses the overproduction of ALA by feedback inhibition of ALA synthetase and is of major benefit in minimizing neurologic damage.

Recovery from severe attacks of porphyric neuropathy is slow and often leaves substantial chronic neurologic disability. Thus prevention and early treatment assume great importance. This is especially true because the patient with porphyria is at continual risk of attacks of neuropathy throughout life. It is vital to identify relatives who may be affected and caution them against factors that could induce attacks of porphyria, especially anesthesia and drugs.

Biologic Toxins: Shellfish and Ciguatera Fish. The ingestion of certain shellfish and ciguatera fish in endemic coastal areas can cause severe acute peripheral neuropathy. The fish accumulate potent, flagellate-elaborated neurotoxins but are themselves unaffected by them. The usual offenders among ciguatera are barracuda and red snapper along the reefs off Florida, Hawaii, and the West Indies. Among the shellfish, oysters, mussels, clams, and scallops along the coasts of New England, Alaska, and the West Coast have been implicated. The toxins directly affect the axonal nerve membrane.

Ingestion is followed by nausea and vomiting and within a few hours by an explosively evolving neuropathy. Paresthesia occurs around the face and spreads to the limbs and is accompanied in severe cases by quadriparesis with bulbar and respiratory weakness. Bizarre sensations, such as the "feeling that teeth are coming loose" or "the body is floating away" have been noted.

The diagnosis is based on clinical evidence of rapid evolution of a neuropathy shortly after ingestion of marine food in endemic areas. One should be aware that respiratory paralysis can swiftly occur. No specific treatment exists, but supportive therapy is lifesaving and neuropathy recovers over many months.

Box 167-5. Drugs and Porphyria

Drugs to Be Avoided	Drugs That Are Safe
Analgesics	**Analgesics**
Pentazocine	Codeine
Sedatives	Meperidine
Barbiturates	Methadone
Chlordiazepoxide	Morphine
Glutethimide	Propoxyphene
Meprobamate	**Sedatives**
Psychotropics	Chloral hydrate
Imipramine	Diazepam
Amphetamines	Diphenhydramine
Anticonvulsants	**Psychotropics**
Barbiturates,	Chlorpromazine
including primidone	Meclizine
Phenytoin	Promazine
Mephenytoin	Promethazine
Methsuximide	Trifluoperazine
Antibiotics	Prochlorperazine
Sulfonamides	Valproic acid
Griseofulvin	**Antibiotics**
Cardiovascular	Ampicillin
Ergot	Cloxacillin
Methyldopa	Nitrofurantoin
Endocrine	Penicillin
Estrogen	Tetracycline
Progesterone	Streptomycin
Tolbutamide	**Cardiovascular**
Chlorpropamide	Digoxin
	Propranolol
	Reserpine
	Warfarin sodium (Coumadin)

Triorthocresyl Phosphate Poisoning. Triorthocresyl phosphate (TOCP) is a synthetic organophosphate compound used in the manufacture of hydraulic fluids, lubricants, and plastics. It is a potent neurotoxin, and thousands of cases of neuropathy have occurred from its consumption. Most outbreaks have resulted from contamination or adulteration of foods, cooking oils, or alcohol with TOCP. One of the best-known examples is the Jamaica ginger paralysis, which affected thousands in the United States during Prohibition years, when TOCP was found in illicit liquor.

Similar neuropathies occur with exposure to organophosphates used as pesticides in agriculture, such as chlorophos and mipafox (see Chapter 11). In these cases, a predominantly motor neuropathy evolves in a few days, leading in severe cases to flaccid quadriplegia. A distinctive feature is the latency of 1 to 2 weeks from the time of ingestion of the organophosphate to the onset of neuropathy. In the case of pesticide ingestion, cholinergic crisis precedes the neuropathy, with diarrhea, sweating, fasciculations, and convulsions. Although the acute neurologic picture is one of severe generalized polyneuropathy, as patients recover, signs of upper motor neuron dysfunction emerge. No specific therapy is available. Patients with mild or moderately severe disease make a gradual and often incomplete recovery. Severely involved patients are left with spastic weakness.

Thallium Poisoning. Poisoning with thallium, a heavy metal, is distinctly unusual today. The most common sources are thallium-containing rodenticides such as Gizmo mouse killer, Zelio paste, or Senco corn mix, ingested accidentally by children or for suicidal purposes. The neuropathy that evolves closely resembles acute inflammatory polyneuropathy with autonomic disturbances. Nausea and vomiting may precede the neuropathy. Some patients are encephalopathic, with clouded consciousness and seizures. Alopecia, the telltale sign of thallium intoxication, appears 2 to 4 weeks after ingestion. The diagnosis is established by detecting thallium in a 24-hour collection of urine, and it can also be found in the blood and saliva.

Vigorous supportive therapy is the mainstay of treatment, as outlined in the section on acute inflammatory polyneuropathy. The chelating agents helpful in treating poisoning by other heavy metals are not effective for thallium. However, Prussian blue (potassium ferric ferrocyanote II), an ion exchange resin, is said to help prevent or minimize evolution of the neuropathy, although it is not useful once the neuropathy is established. Prussian blue forms a complex with thallium in exchange for potassium, and the complex is excreted in the gut, thus decreasing the absorption of thallium. This treatment should be combined with a laxative. Early treatment with Prussian blue has decreased severe residual neurologic disability. Alopecia recovers fully and spontaneously.

Polyneuropathy of Critical Illness. An acute, severe, generalized axonal polyneuropathy may occur in patients critically ill with prolonged sepsis, multiple organ failure, and hypoalbuminemia. Failure to wean the patient off the ventilator often brings the weakness to attention. Examination reveals generalized areflexic quadriparesis with muscle atrophy; nerve conduction studies show an axonal neuropathy, and CSF remains normal. With supportive therapy, surprisingly good recovery of the neuropathy is the rule, although improvement may take several months. The pathogenesis is uncertain but appears to be related to complex toxic-metabolic systemic derangements.

Acute Motor Demyelinating Neuropathies

Acute Inflammatory Polyneuropathy (Guillain-Barré Syndrome). The other important demyelinating peripheral neuropathy, and the most common form of acute polyneuropathy encountered, is that described by Landry and later by Guillain, Barré, and Strohl, and which is known as *Guillain-Barré syndrome, postinfectious polyneuropathy,* or *acute inflammatory polyneuropathy (AIP).*

Etiology. This condition commonly follows a viral or mycoplasmal illness affecting the upper respiratory or alimentary tracts, vaccination, or surgery, or it may complicate an underlying malignancy such as Hodgkin's disease. Because infections seem to have occurred in the preceding 2 weeks in about half of the cases seen, the term *postinfectious polyneuropathy* is preferred by some. Increased titers of IgM antibodies to Epstein-Barr virus, CMVs, and other viruses have been reported and, rarely, connective tissue diseases such as SLE and polyarteritis nodosa and malignancies such as Hodgkin's disease trigger the autoimmune process. The syndrome has also heralded HIV-1 seroconversion. The enteric infection *Campylobacter jejuni* is the cause of an identical but usually very severe syndrome, with neuronal degeneration rather than demyelination as the basis. Both genders are equally involved. AIP occurs at any age but most commonly in adults over age 40. It is a polyradiculopathy, which means that the brunt of the acute allergic response is seen in the spinal (or cranial) nerve roots. Here, intense round cell infiltration is seen, extending distally in the nerves with accompanying demyelination caused by Schwann cell damage.

Clinical features. The onset is acute or progressive over a week or two. Complaints of paresthesia, numbness, muscle tenderness, and weakness appear in that order, initially in the legs. There is no fever. Weakness is usually but not always symmetric and may progress to any degree of severity, from minimal weakness in the legs to profound quadriparesis with respiratory and bulbar failure, which occurs in about 10% of cases. The distal muscles are usually involved first and the disease normally spreads centrally, although rarely the reverse is the case. The bladder is never much affected, and although facial involvement is common, the eyes are seldom involved.

Examination shows mainly motor findings consisting of flaccid weakness peripherally with areflexia. The face is especially affected, with at least weakness of eye closure. Power also may be lessened or lost proximally in the girdle muscles, trunk, and bulbar muscles, or these areas may escape entirely. Wasting occurs early in the affected limbs. Sensory findings are minimal, but pain may be severe.

Autonomic features represent a dangerous complication. Tachycardia, postural hypotension, pupillary disturbances, hyperhidrosis, and lack of variation in the inter-beat interval (measured by the R-R interval on an electrocardiogram [ECG] with deep breathing) signifying the need for ECG and blood pressure monitoring are the most common, but paroxysmal atrial or ventricular tachycardia and various bradyrhythmias and wide swings of blood pressure have been documented. Sphincter control and mental clarity are usually retained.

In a malignant form of AIP, there is early involvement of the cranial nerves and trunk with bulbar palsies and respiratory failure. In all, up to 20% of patients develop some degree of ventilatory inadequacy caused by involvement of the diaphragm and intercostal muscles. Because it cannot be predicted who will develop this severe form of the disease and who will not, all patients with AIP must be admitted to the hospital until at least the first signs of recovery appear.

Uncommon variants of AIP produce ophthalmoplegia, ptosis, facial weakness, limb ataxia, and areflexia with little systemic weakness (Miller Fisher syndrome); an acute sensory neuropathy; acute dysautonomia; or acute ataxia of gait and limbs without weakness or sensory loss, presumably from denervation of muscle spindles.

Investigations. The CSF protein level is initially normal but rises as the disease progresses. Protein values are often above 2 g/L eventually, but the cell count is normal, a fact serenaded by the euphonious French term *dissociation cyto-albuminologique*. In cases associated with HIV-1 seroconversion, moderate lymphocytosis may be found. Occasionally, the protein level exceeds 10 g/L, producing a *Froin's syndrome* of xanthochromic, acellular CSF that clots spontaneously. Electrodiagnostic studies show slowing or loss of late responses; later in the illness there is marked slowing of motor nerve conduction velocities.

Course. The recovery period is prolonged; over half of the patients are completely better by 6 months and three fourths within 1 year. But continuous weakness, malaise, and easy fatigability trouble the remainder, and in a few patients recurrent attacks occur. Those patients who begin to recover in the first 2 weeks after onset usually do so completely.

Fatalities occur in 5% of cases because of ventilatory failure, pneumonia, cardiac arrhythmias, or autonomic failure. These deaths should be preventable with intensive nursing and medical care; one must be vigilant for any hint of respiratory involvement during the early stages. In any patient diagnosed as having AIP, the vital capacity should be repeatedly measured.

Differential diagnosis. The syndrome of AIP is the most important cause of acute severe progressive motor peripheral neuropathy. Other causes include acute porphyria, diphtheria, tick paralysis, hypokalemia and hyperkalemia, and organophosphate and lithium toxicity. Note also that myasthenia gravis may present in a similar way.

Management. In the acute stages, attention to the airway, prevention of respiratory infections, and watchfulness for autonomic disturbances (such as acute hypertension) are the most important measures. Frequent passive limb movement to prevent contractures, subcutaneous heparin injections to prevent deep vein thrombosis, and oral quinine (300 mg daily for pain) are useful. Steroids are of no benefit (they may be harmful), but both intravenous immunogammaglobulins (IVIg; 0.4 mg/kg/day, repeated over 5 days) and plasma exchange are valuable therapies. All patients with significant weakness should be considered for IVIg therapy, and if there is still progression of weakness after the treatment, plasma exchange should be considered.

Monitoring of vital functions is essential at all times in the evolution of the disease, and patients should be cared for at least within easy distance of an intensive care unit because ventilatory support is essential for the severely affected patient. A fall in vital capacity to 25% of the predicted value, or below 1000 ml, is an indication for intubation. One must also pay attention to fluid and electrolyte status and monitor for such complications as cardiac arrhythmias, inappropriate ADH secretion, and hypertension or hypotension. The latter should *never* should be treated with sympathomimetics because of the denervation hypersensitivity present. Endotracheal intubation should be performed promptly when pulmonary function shows deterioration or bulbar paralysis occurs. Even with modern endotracheal tubes, tracheostomy may be necessary if the ventilatory weakness persists beyond 10 days.

Nutrition is best provided through a nasogastric tube if there is any bulbar weakness. For all patients, psychologic support is essential. Some patients are unable to move at all and need tremendous attention, support, and repeated assurance that they will indeed regain muscle power. Successful management of such a case is a triumph of medical and nursing care.

In all cases, positioning of the weakened patient is important to protect against pressure palsies of the ulnar, peroneal, and sciatic nerves; otherwise the patient recovers from AIP only to be left with a drop foot or hand weakness from secondary compression. Similar care must be taken to maintain the feet in dorsiflexion to prevent contractures.

Other Acute Motor Neuropathies. In diphtheria, lead poisoning, and porphyria the signs are almost entirely motor and often proximal.

Chronic Motor Axonal Neuropathies

Hereditary Neuropathy. *Hereditary motor neuropathy* (HMN) is the term now used for what used to be called the *spinal muscular atrophies,* also known by the terms *Werdnig-Hoffmann disease* and *Wohlfart-Kugelberg-Welander syndrome*.

HMNs are common, have varied modes of inheritance, and share degeneration of the lower motor neuron as their primary pathology. Severity of the disorder varies with the age of onset. Infantile onset presages rapid progression and early death; the later the onset, the more benign the course.

Evidence of the condition may appear before birth. Mothers of affected infants often comment on reduced fetal movements in the last trimester of the pregnancy. The infant will show proximal or distal symmetric weakness and wasting with hypotonia and anergy, respiratory and feeding problems being marked. Fasciculations are seen in only half of the babies because the fat layer obscures them. Reflexes are depressed. Muscle contractures and aspiration pneumonitis are common complications. When the onset is in childhood, pelvic girdle weakness causes a waddling gait and problems in climbing stairs; arm weakness is due to involvement of the shoulder girdle muscles, and scoliosis is related to trunk weakness. In adults, girdle weakness and wasting with fasciculations and hyporeflexia produce similar features but progress slowly.

Diagnostic confirmation depends on muscle biopsy; an electromyogram (EMG) is of confirmatory value, but serum creatine kinase (CK) levels are only slightly elevated. Only supportive treatment is available. Without muscle biopsy, HMN is easily misdiagnosed as limb girdle dystrophy. Uncommonly, other patterns of weakness and wasting in HMN mimic fascioscapulohumeral or distal myopathies. In all adult cases, differentiation from motor neuron disease such as amyotrophic lateral sclerosis (ALS), syringomyelia, and other conditions that affect the cord, such as trauma, myelitis, and tumor (these latter damaging the anterior horn cells in the cord), is necessary. Most of these conditions are considered elsewhere in this book. The history or accompanying evidence of central nervous system (CNS) dysfunction allows a reasonable chance of making the correct diagnosis clinically, but in other cases, diagnosis is only possible with time and with the detection of corticospinal tract signs.

Acquired Neuropathy. Acquired chronic axonal motor neuropathies are few; multiple system atrophy (see Chapter 169) and motor neuron disease (see Chapter 170) are discussed elsewhere.

Subacute Motor Neuropathy. Subacute motor neuropathy is a rare disorder that is a mirror image of paraneoplastic sensory neuropathy. It is associated with lymphoma, rather than lung cancer, and with Waldenström's macroglobulinemia. A subacute weakness affects distal and proximal muscles of limbs and sometimes of the neck with areflexia but without sensory impairment. In contrast to the bleak prognosis of the sensory form, this neuropathy often spontaneously recovers over 1 to 3 years, independent of the activity of the underlying neoplasm.

Chronic Demyelinating Motor Neuropathies. Motor polyneuropathies may occur in rheumatoid arthritis and polyarteritis nodosa, but multiple mononeuropathy is a more common presentation. Chronic inflammatory demyelinating neuropathy is a variant of the acute form, in which there is either recurrence after successful initial treatment or impaired response to that therapy. Multifocal motor neuropathy with conduction block presents in a manner very similar to ALS, from which it is differentiated by nerve conduction studies that show scattered slowing of motor nerve conduction velocities. The syndrome has been defined in young adults and is associated with high serum levels of antibodies against GM1 ganglioside (anti-GM1 antibodies). There are no upper motor neuron or bulbar signs, and the course is indolent. Intravenous cyclophosphamide therapy has produced significant improvement.

Mainly Sensory Neuropathies

Acute Axonal Sensory Neuropathies. The prototype of acute axonal sensory neuropathy is the acute inflammation of dorsal root ganglion cells that occurs with herpes zoster, but this form usually affects the V nerve or a few dermatomes at most and so is really a radiculopathy or mononeuropathy. Systemic causes include polycythemia, lymphoma, carcinoma, and acute sensory neuropathy, a form of acute inflammatory polyneuropathy with mainly sensory rather than motor changes. Poisoning with cisplatin and inflammation of the dorsal root ganglion cells as a toxic effect of penicillin, Adriamycin, or mercury are other causes.

Chronic Axonal Sensory Neuropathies

Hereditary. In most hereditary forms of chronic axonal sensory neuropathies mild but progressing centripetal sensory loss that affects thin-fiber and thick-fiber functions brings the patient to the doctor. Complaints of girdle pains, atrophic changes in the feet, and imbalance are also common. In the uncommon hereditary sensory and autonomic neuropathies (HSAN) either all forms of sensation are absent from birth (recessive variety, type 2) or pain and temperature loss develop insidiously in the second decade (dominant form, type 1). Numerous other variants with added neurologic problems are described. Lancinating pains are common in the early stages but respond to dilantin, carbamazepine, or a tricyclic. The loss of pain and position sense can lead to terrible mutilation. Motor weakness and wasting may accompany the sensory loss in the dominant form. Obsessive care of the feet and hands is the only prophylactic measure available.

Friedreich's ataxia and the other spinocerebellar degenerations involve the dorsal root ganglia also, and the degeneration of the peripheral axons could be regarded as a neuropathy.

Acquired. When the dorsal root ganglion cells are primarily involved, one must consider tabes dorsalis, vitamin B_{12} deficiency (subacute combined degeneration of the cord), and a paraneoplastic syndrome (usually from an oat-cell carcinoma of the bronchus, carcinoma of the breast, or lymphoma). Acromegaly, hypothyroidism, malabsorption syndromes, polycythemia, primary biliary cirrhosis, uremia, Lyme disease and poisoning with arsenic, hydralazine, N_2O, metronidazole, misonidazole, cisplatin, and pyridoxine are other causes.

Polyneuropathy of Vitamin B_{12} Deficiency. Peripheral neuropathy is one neurologic syndrome resulting from vitamin B_{12} deficiency. The initial symptoms are sensations of pins and needles and numbness in the feet and later (seldom initially) in the hands. The initial impression is of a peripheral neuropathy, because of the depressed or absent ankle reflexes and a stocking-distribution impairment of touch and pinprick. However, there are also signs of myelopathy with loss of proprioception and pyramidal signs in the legs. Romberg's sign is positive.

The diagnosis is established if the plasma B_{12} levels are low and if there is a macrocytic megaloblastic anemia, although there may be no anemia at all and the syndrome can exist with normal blood and bone marrow examination.

The response to injections of vitamin B_{12} is dramatic, except in long-established cases. Paresthesia may improve within days of injection, and the neuropathy recovers completely if therapy is started within a few weeks of onset of symptoms. Treatment must be lifelong.

Paraneoplastic Polyneuropathy. Asymmetric polyneuropathies are common in patients with malignancy as a side effect of chemotherapy (vincristine, procarbazine, cisplatin, misonidazole) because of neoplastic infiltration of multiple spinal and cranial nerve roots; meningeal carcinomatosis or lymphomatosis (which typically produces an asymmetric, patchy, multiple monoradiculopathy); or as a true paraneoplastic polyneuropathy.

The most distinctive of these syndromes is subacute sensory neuropathy, in which the dorsal root ganglia are symmetrically affected. The condition is most often associated with bronchogenic carcinoma, which may be occult and not evident for a year or more. Patients present with the subacute onset of pain, paresthesia, and dysesthesia in the limbs and face, and show ataxia of gait and limbs. There is a striking loss of all modalities of sensation over the limbs, sometimes extending to the face and buccal mucosa. A sensory ataxic gait is present, with a prominent Romberg's sign. Weakness is minimal, but areflexia is universal. A similar syndrome can occur in Sjögren's syndrome. The prognosis is poor, although in the rare case associated with lymphoma, treatment of the lymphoma produces a remission.

Polyneuropathy of Endocrine Disease: Hypothyroidism. The most common neuropathy in hypothyroidism is bilateral carpal tunnel syndrome, but a demyelinating, mainly sensory neuropathy with paresthesia and cramps in the feet and legs is described, sometimes accompanied by mild myelopathy. An excellent response to thyroid replacement can be expected.

Vitamin E Deficiency Neuropathy. A chronic myeloneuropathic syndrome similar to that caused by vitamin B_{12} deficiency may develop insidiously in patients with longstanding fat malabsorption and resultant low levels of vitamin E. Supplementation with large doses of vitamin E may produce some improvement in neurologic function.

Acute Demyelinating Sensory Neuropathies. The only types of acute demyelinating sensory neuropathies described are the rare variant of AIP in which there is pure sensory involvement and the rapid development of sensory loss in patients with diabetes, usually in association with recent rapid weight loss. Thick-fiber function (joint position, vibration, and discriminatory light touch) are the modalities especially affected.

Chronic Sensory Demyelinating Neuropathies. Chronic sensory demyelinating neuropathies are common in those diabetic patients in whom motor signs are minimal in the early stage of the development of their sensorimotor disease. Other causes include rheumatoid arthritis (particularly if treated with steroids), gammopathy, leprosy, and hypothyroidism.

Sensorimotor Neuropathies

Acute Axonal Sensorimotor Neuropathies. Damage to the axon can follow trauma to the nerve. With mild compression or stretching, function may be only temporarily interrupted. In the stage called *neurapraxia* there is no damage to the anatomic integrity of the nerve. With pressure having produced only local ischemia and edema, recovery occurs over minutes, days, or a few weeks, depending on the severity of the pressure. With more severe but briefly applied trauma, such as a severe stretch or a heavy blow to the nerve, the axons may be interrupted (axonotmesis) but the Schwann cell sheaths remain in continuity. Wallerian degeneration will occur distally and for one or two segments proximally, after which axonal sprouting occurs. Sprouts will grow down the still-present Schwann cell tubes to reach their end-plates or sensory receptors at the rate of about 1 mm daily. With yet more severe trauma (neurotmesis), the whole anatomic nerve is lacerated and divided, again producing distal Wallerian degeneration. This leads to inefficient axonal sprouting because some motor nerve fibers may grow down tubes leading to the wrong muscle, or into tubes formerly occupied by sensory nerves, for example.

Chronic Axonal Sensorimotor Neuropathies. Many metabolic and toxic neuropathies (particularly those caused by exogenous chemicals or drugs) produce major damage both to the axons and to the cell body. Examples include deficiency of vitamins B (beriberi, pellagra), B_{12}, and E; sprue; alcoholism; uremia; and many toxins. Neuropathy from glue sniffing is progressive, primarily affects motor functions, and is caused by the organic solvents n-hexane and toluene in the glue. However, most other toxic agents affect sensory function more than motor, and the clinical presentation is more frequently a subacute or chronic, symmetric, distal sensorimotor neuropathy. Dysglobulinemias are also associated with an axonal sensorimotor neuropathy. Estimation of immunoglobulins is an important test in the investigations of unexplained neuropathies of this type. This syndrome can also occur as a paraneoplastic syndrome. A neuronal form of HMSN (Charcot-Marie-Tooth disease) is described; clinically it differs little from the more common demyelinating form. Alcoholic polyneuropathy is the prototype of this class.

Alcoholic Polyneuropathy. Deficiencies of multiple B complex vitamins, especially vitamin B_1, seem to be critical for the alcoholic polyneuropathy form of axonal degeneration, although other deficiencies and the direct effects of alcohol may contribute. Other toxic neuropathies to which the alcoholic patient might be exposed include lead, triorthocresyl phosphate from drinking illicit liquor, and disulfiram.

The neuropathy is symmetric, distal, and predominantly sensory. Painful hypersensitivity of the feet to contact is common. In severe cases there is weakness of the distal parts of the limbs. Pressure palsies are sometimes superimposed, causing foot drop or wrist drop. Abstinence from alcohol, supplementation with B complex vitamins, and a well-balanced diet lead to gradual improvement of the neuropathy.

Drug-induced Neuropathies. Many drugs cause subacute or chronic axonal polyneuropathy (Box 167-6), although procainamide and perhexiline maleate are exceptions because they cause demyelination. The mechanisms of damage are usually obscure, but isoniazid-related neuropathy results from the pyridoxine deficiency that it induces, especially in slow acetylators, and vinca alkaloids interfere with nerve cell body metabolism. These two agents produce neuropathy in a dose-related manner, whereas with others the neuropathy is unpredictable.

The clinical picture is typically one of a chronic symmetric sensorimotor polyneuropathy that can be of any degree of severity. Autonomic neuropathy is an added feature with some drugs such as vincristine, which can also cause facial or laryngeal nerve palsies and ophthalmoplegia. Cisplatin can cause sensorineural hearing loss. Physicians should be alert to this complication in relation to all drugs, especially those that are newly introduced. Improvement of neuropathy with discontinuation of the suspect drug and relapse when the drug is reintroduced provide the only confirmation under these circumstances. The crucial step in treatment is recognition and withdrawal of the culprit drug. In most cases, the neuropathy will slowly recover. When the neurotoxicity is dose related (e.g., vincristine), the drug may be continued or resumed at a lower dose. Certain drug-induced polyneuropathies are preventable. For instance, supplementation of isoniazid with daily pyridoxine obviates the danger of neuropathy, whereas nitrofurantoin should be avoided in patients with renal failure. Boxes 167-6 and 167-7 list drugs used to treat neuropathic pain and drugs that cause neuropathy.

Polyneuropathy Caused by Industrial Chemical Exposure. Severe peripheral neuropathies can result from exposure to industrial and household chemicals. The industrial solvent n-hexane is abused by teenagers in glue sniffing, which can cause severe neuropathy, as can the grouting agent acrylamide. In neuropathy caused by n-hexane, methylbutylketone, acrylamide, and solvent mixtures, the nerves show characteristic giant swellings of the axons (Table 167-1).

The typical presentation is of a subacute, symmetric, distal sensorimotor polyneuropathy; however, there are some

Box 167-6. Pharmacotherapy of Neuropathic Pain

- Antidepressant drugs
  - Amitriptyline
  - Desipramine
  - Trazodone
  - Fluoxetine
- Anticonvulsant drugs
  - Carbamazepine
  - Phenytoin
  - Clonazepam
- Antiarrhythmic drugs
  - Tocainide
  - Mexiletine
  - Nifedipine
  - Baclofen (trigeminal neuralgia)
- Antiserotonin agent
  - Cyproheptadine
- Anti–substance P agent
  - Topical capsaicin (Zostrix, Axsain)
- Opioids
  - Morphine, codeine, and analogs
  - Transdermal opioids

characteristic variations, such as the cauda equina syndrome seen with dimethylaminoproprionitrile poisoning, which causes urinary retention, impotence, and paresthesia in the limbs that progresses to paraparesis. A severe sensory neuropathy associated with blisters on the hands suggests acrylamide poisoning. The diagnosis rests on a high degree of suspicion and a careful history (e.g., seeking exposure occupationally or in the pursuit of a hobby). Although these chemicals can seldom be measured in the body as proof of exposure, with volatile hydrocarbons and acrylamide poisoning, nerve biopsy may provide supportive evidence for the diagnosis.

Treatment is by removal from further exposure. The neuropathy may continue to worsen for a few months but usually improves slowly in the end.

Polyneuropathy Caused by Heavy Metal Intoxication. Intoxication with heavy metals occupationally or by accident has become less common in western countries because of public health measures but is still seen (Table 167-2). Lead, arsenic, and thallium each cause a multisystem illness by interfering with cellular enzymes; axonal degeneration is the principal pathologic change, with clinical evidence of florid neuropathy. The metals cannot be rapidly excreted and thus they accumulate in the peripheral and central nervous systems, skin, hair, nails, and other organs. Intermittent exposure to toxins may lead to the puzzling picture of a neuropathy that remits and relapses.

Typically, a sensorimotor polyneuropathy appears subacutely or chronically, but arsenic and thallium can also induce an acute neuropathy that resembles AIP. Characteristic patterns of neuropathy include that of lead poisoning in adults, which is predominantly motor and often asymmetric, frequently presenting with bilateral radial or peroneal palsies. Arsenical neuropathy tends to be predominantly sensory and painful. Thallium neuropathy is associated with autonomic disturbances and with generalized and striking alopecia. Diagnostic clues are also provided by changes in skin, hair, and nails. Transverse white lines (Mees' lines) occur in both arsenic and thallium poisoning. Hyperkeratosis of the palms and soles and hyperpigmentation of the skin suggest arsenic intoxication.

Another characteristic feature of heavy metal poisoning is the occurrence of encephalopathy and multiple system dysfunction simulating other endogenous diseases. Fortunately, the intoxications can be reliably and readily diagnosed

Box 167-7. Drugs That Cause Polyneuropathy

- Drugs used in oncology
  - Vincristine
  - Procarbazine
  - Cisplatin
  - Mesonidazole
  - Metronidazole
  - Taxol
- Drugs used to treat infectious diseases
  - Isoniazid
  - Nitrofurantoin
  - Dapsone
  - ddC (Dideoxycytidine)
  - ddI (Dideoxyinosine)
- Drugs used in cardiology
  - Amiodarone
  - Hydralazine
  - Perhexiline maleate
  - Procainamide
  - Disopyramide
- Drugs used in rheumatology
  - Gold salts
  - Chloroquine
- Drugs used in neurology and psychiatry
  - Diphenylhydantoin
  - Glutethimide
  - Methaqualone
- Miscellaneous
  - Disulfiram
  - Vitamin B_6: pyridoxine (megadoses)

Table 167-1. Sources and Modes of Exposure to Industrial Chemicals

Chemical	Occupational	Abuse/accidental
n-Hexane	Hexacarbon solvent widely used in adhesives, glues, laminated products, shoes, cabinet finishing	Glues containing n-hexane inhaled in enormous quantities, principally by teenagers
Methylbutylketone (MBK)	Hexacarbon used as an industrial solvent in color printing, furniture finishing, plastic-coated fabrics	Cleaning and washing with lacquer thinner containing MBK
Solvent mixtures	Lacquer thinners containing several solvents such as acetone, methylisobutylketone, methylethylketone	Abused for euphoriant effect ("huffer neuropathy")
Nitrous oxide	Used in dental offices as anesthetic; food propellant	Abused by dentists and related health workers for euphoriant effects and as an unconventional remedy for hangover
Acrylamide	Widely used chemical grouting agent for waterproofing in tunnels, water conduits, sewers	Outbreaks possible from contamination of water supplied from sewers recently grouted with acrylamide
Dimethylaminoproprionitrile (DMAPN)	Catalyzer in polyurethane foam manufacture	

Table 167-2. Sources and Modes of Exposure to Heavy Metals

Metal	Occupational	Abuse/accidental
Lead	Use of lead-based paint in automobile industry; manufacture of storage batteries and printing	Drinking of bootleg whiskey distilled in lead-containing pipes; burning of batteries as cheap fuel; hand mixing of lead-based paints by artists
Arsenic	Exposure in farming to arsenic-containing sprays, pesticides, weed killers	Accidental ingestion of arsenic-containing rodenticides such as Antrol, Paris Green, Rat-Doom; rare source is old medicinal solutions such as Fowler's; still occasionally abused for suicidal and homicidal purposes
Thallium	Manufacture of optic glass, prisms, industrial diamonds, fuel additive in internal combustion engines	Accidental ingestion still occurs from thallium-containing rodenticides such as Gizmo mouse killer, Zelio paste, etc.

by estimation of the metal levels from hair, urine, and blood. Identification and removal from exposure usually allow slow recovery. The accumulated metal can be eliminated faster by chelators such as Ca-EDTA, dimercaprol, or penicillamine, and in the case of thallium by Prussian blue, an ion exchanger that complexes with thallium, preventing its absorption from the gut.

Polyneuropathy of Acquired Immunodeficiency Syndrome. Acquired immunodeficiency syndrome is now a leading cause of chronic polyneuropathy in young adults. Its pathogenesis is not established but it appears to be parainfectious rather than directly related to HIV-1 infection. It appears in the advanced phase of immunodeficiency with prominent pain and intolerable dysesthetic sensations aggravated by standing, walking, and pressure. The course is indolently progressive but may stabilize after months. Treatment remains symptomatic, and many patients require long-term narcotic analgesics to alleviate the neuropathic pain. Various other neuropathic syndromes have been described in association with HIV-1 infection (Box 167-8).

Box 167-8. Peripheral Neuropathies Caused by HIV-1 Infection

- Mononeuropathies
  - Bell's palsy
  - Peroneal nerve palsy
- Lumbosacral radiculopathy: cauda equina syndrome
  - Cytomegalovirus radiculitis
  - Cryptococcosis, tuberculosis, syphilis
- Mononeuritis multiplex
- Generalized symmetric polyneuropathies
  - Acute Guillain-Barré syndrome
  - Chronic inflammatory demyelinating polyneuropathy (CIDP)
  - Chronic polyneuropathies
    - AIDS-related painful neuropathies
    - Drug-induced neuropathy (e.g., ddI, ddC, vincristine)
- Autonomic neuropathy

Acute Demyelinating Sensorimotor Neuropathies. A variety of peripheral nerve abnormalities occur often in the course of Lyme disease, typically following the phase of erythema marginatum and polyarthropathy but sometimes without such antecedents (see Chapter 166). In a subgroup of patients, facial palsy appears and may become bilateral and spread to involve the sixth, fifth, and eighth cranial nerves (cranial polyneuritis). Widespread peripheral neuropathy often appears about 6 weeks after a tick bite or erythema marginatum with prominent pain, paresthesia, and dysesthesia in the limbs and trunk, followed in days to weeks by asymmetric, spreading, multifocal, areflexic paralysis in the limbs that follows the pattern of multiple mononeuropathy. Sometimes the picture evolves into an acute inflammatory polyneuropathy syndrome, but with prominent mononuclear pleocytosis in the CSF. Electrodiagnostic tests show a combination of axonal and demyelinating multifocal neuropathy. The diagnosis is confirmed by antibodies to *Borrelia burgdorferi* in the serum and CSF in the course of disease or a fourfold increase in the acute and convalescent titers in the appropriate clinical context.

Chronic Demyelinating Sensorimotor Neuropathies

Hereditary Motor and Sensory Neuropathies (HMSNs). Most of the HMSNs (e.g., Charcot-Marie-Tooth disease, peroneal muscular atrophy) are of the demyelinating type, but a neuronal form is described. They may be inherited in any manner (autosomal dominant or recessive or sex-linked recessive) and also occur sporadically. In youth, patients complain of foot deformity (high arches), difficulty in getting shoes to fit, hammer toes, drop foot, and the insidious progression of wasting and weakness of the distal musculature of the leg and much later of the arms. Atrophy of the lower one third of the thigh and calf is said to give the leg an "inverted champagne bottle" appearance. The muscle stretch reflexes are usually lost in the legs but are present in the arms until a late stage. Minor sensory symptoms and signs (diminution of vibration, light touch, and joint position sensations) are also later findings.

Other associated problems may include optic atrophy, retinal changes, cerebellar signs, upper motor neuron or extrapyramidal signs, scoliosis, spinal dysraphism, or autonomic features. Circulatory insufficiency is common, and thickened nerves may be visible or palpable. Pes cavus is caused by this condition in about one third of cases but occurs alone just as frequently.

The family pedigree frequently contains evidence of similar neuropathies and of spinocerebellar degenerations of one kind or another often referred to as "arthritis." The disease is slowly progressive but there is extreme variability and although some patients die with cardiac conduction defects in the fourth and fifth decades, others are still working at the ordinary age of retirement.

Motor nerve conduction velocities are markedly slowed, and sensory nerve action potentials are diminished or absent. In most cases, nerve biopsy shows a hypertrophic neuropathy with "onion bulb" laminations of Schwann cells caused by episodes of demyelination and remyelination.

No specific treatment is possible, but physiotherapy may delay contractures and assist the patient to use his remaining motor skills in the most efficient way. Bracing, special shoes, and orthopedic procedures to improve mobility or stability of the ankle may be helpful.

Other Hereditary Motor and Sensory Neuropathy Variants. One HMSN variant is a neuronal form (HMSN II). In HMSN III, the neuropathy is accompanied by pyramidal and cerebellar signs, choreiform movements, nystagmus, miosis, raised CSF protein levels, kyphoscoliosis, and marked enlargement of the peripheral nerves. A fourth variant (HMSN IV) is Refsum's disease. In this condition, a high level of circulating phytanic acid is found, which can be reduced (and to some extent symptoms are reduced) by restricting the amount of animal fats and foods containing chlorophyll that the patient eats. Some of the leukodystrophies of childhood manifest optic atrophy, seizures, amentia or dementia, and various motor signs, as well as a chronic hypertrophic demyelinating neuropathy.

There are also some inherited multisystem disorders associated with specific biochemical lesions in which neuropathy is part of the syndrome. Most are recessively inherited, but Fabry disease and adrenomyeloneuropathy have sex-linked recessive inheritance. This group of diseases, although rare, is significant because biochemical manipulations may be potentially therapeutic.

Refsum's Disease (HMSN Type IV). A nonspecific sensorimotor polyneuropathy, Refsum's disease appears in the second to fourth decades, is sometimes associated with enlarged nerves, and follows a chronic or relapsing course over years. Bilateral nerve deafness, retinitis pigmentosa, ichthyosis, corneal and lens opacities, cardiomyopathy, and epiphyseal dysplasia complete the picture, although only retinitis pigmentosa invariably occurs. Diagnosis is established by the finding of elevated levels of serum phytanic acid. Lowering of the phytanic acid content of blood and tissues following a long-term low-phytanic-acid diet, perhaps combined with plasmapheresis, is of major benefit for all effects of the disease, including neuropathy.

Bassen-Kornzweig Syndrome. Bassen-Kornzweig syndrome is a chronic sensorimotor polyneuropathy that begins in childhood or adolescence, is associated with ataxia, and is preceded by steatorrhea in infancy. Retinitis pigmentosa is universal. Plasma lipoprotein analysis shows the diagnostic abnormality of very low cholesterol and low triglycerides; betalipoprotein is absent. Another characteristic abnormality is the presence of spiculated red blood cells in peripheral blood (acanthocytosis). Treatment with large doses of vitamins A and E may improve the neuropathy.

Tangier Disease. The neuropathy of the rare Tangier disease is clinically distinctive and resembles syringomyelia, with dissociated sensory loss for pain and temperature and segmental atrophy and areflexia that affect the face, upper extremities, and/or lower limbs. Eventually the whole body may be anesthetic. The telltale sign of this disease is the presence of orange discoloration and enlargement of the tonsils. Plasma lipoprotein analysis shows very low cholesterol levels with normal or high triglycerides and absence of alphalipoproteins.

Fabry's Disease. Neuropathy associated with Fabry's disease—an extraordinary syndrome affecting only boys—is evident by curious and disabling episodes of pain in the extremities and abdomen with few signs on examination. The paroxysms of excruciating burning or lightninglike pains are precipitated or aggravated by fever or hot weather. Progressive anhidrosis may occur. Clusters of dark-red, punctate telangiectases around the umbilicus, buttocks, groin, knees, and elbows are diagnostic. Decreased activity of α-galactosidase in serum or leukocytes or skin fibroblasts establishes the diagnosis. The enzyme deficiency leads to tissue accumulation of the lipid ceramide. No specific treatment is yet available, but the disabling pain can be relieved or suppressed by diphenylhydantoin.

Adrenomyeloneuropathy. The spectrum of sex-linked recessive adrenoleukodystrophy has been expanded to include patients with a chronic neuromyelopathic syndrome but without cerebral manifestations. The neuropathy is chronic, symmetric, sensorimotor, and associated with spastic paraparesis. Primary hypoadrenalism may be subclinical, and hypogonadism often accompanies this syndrome. The diagnosis is usually established by the finding of a marked increase in serum long-chain fatty acids. Testicular or adrenal biopsy, and less consistently sural nerve or conjunctival biopsy, shows specific cytoplasmic inclusions on electron microscopy. The role of bone marrow transplantation and efforts to decrease blood levels of long-chain fatty acids are still under investigation.

Metachromatic Leukodystrophy. The polyneuropathy that is invariable in metachromatic leukodystrophy is overshadowed by cerebral dysfunction in the infantile and juvenile forms. The demonstration of metachromatic material in nerve biopsies and of deficiency of arylsulfatase A in serum, white cells, and skin fibroblasts establishes the diagnosis. No effective treatment is available.

A sensorimotor neuropathy occurs sometimes in association with carcinoma, usually of the bronchus or ovary, and in secondary amyloidosis. But far more common are two other conditions that deserve discussion in some detail.

Diabetes. Various types of neuropathy are found in both type I and type II diabetes mellitus. The most common is a subacute or chronic distal, symmetric, sensorimotor demyelinating neuropathy that is probably related to the duration (but not to the degree of control) of the diabetes. The peripheral nerves show a combination of nonspecific segmental demyelination, axonal degeneration, and sometimes a vasa nervorum plugged with platelets. Rarely, evidence of the neuropathy precedes clinical or significant biochemical evidence of diabetes. The neuropathy is predominantly sensory and varies in severity from asymptomatic loss of ankle reflexes to severe sensory loss and weakness of all limbs. Other patients may have proprioception impairment that is so severe that combined with diminished pupillary light reflexes, it has been called *diabetic pseudotabes*. Persistent pain in the limbs, with nocturnal exacerbation, is a problem in a few patients. Signs include a diminution of vibration, deep pain and joint position sensations, and of touch, with reduction of distal reflexes and some distal wasting at a later stage. In most cases the neuropathy is a minor problem; but when it is severe an autonomic component may result in poor healing, and the lack of deep pain sensation and unawareness of trivial trauma may in time produce skin ulcers and disorganization of joints—the *Charcot joints* also described in patients with syringomyelia, HSANs, and tabes dorsalis. A rare variant is the painful "small-fiber neuropathy" in which there is dissociated loss of pain and temperature sensation with relative preservation of touch and proprioception and intact tendon reflexes.

Diabetes may also cause a pure sensory neuropathy that leads to mutilating acropathy, with damage to the distal parts of the body caused by cumulative trauma and lack of care of the relatively painless denervated areas. Unfortunately, control of diabetes is poorly related to the severity of the neuropathy and no effective treatment is known.

Ischemic diabetic neuropathies are multiple mononeuropathies. The cranial nerves and thoracic roots are most commonly affected, but signs tend to remit slowly when the diabetes is well controlled. Diabetics with nerves "at risk" because of metabolic factors are unusually susceptible to pressure palsies.

A syndrome of proximal, asymmetric pelvic girdle wasting and weakness may occur in diabetes because of lumbosacral plexopathy (diabetic amyotrophy). This usually happens only when diabetes control has been poor. In such cases, thigh pain is often severe, and quadriceps and adductor wasting is marked, with loss of the knee jerk reflex. Recovery occurs slowly with improved control, which almost always means insulin. The pain is best treated with a combination of amitriptyline (up to 75 mg at night) and fluphenazine 1 to 2 mg tid. A painful thoracic radiculopathy may also be a manifestation of diabetes.

The autonomic nervous system is often involved with diabetes-related neuropathy. Postural hypotension, nocturnal diarrhea, acute gastric dilation, impotence, bladder atony, lack of sweating (anhidrosis), and a loss of vasomotor and axon reflexes in the skin and trophic changes in the extremities are typical features. Argyll Robertson pupils may occur in diabetes because of involvement of the parasympathetic fibers to the eye. This neuropathy may prevent the patient from being aware of the symptoms of hypoglycemia. Sudden cardiorespiratory arrest has been reported in those with autonomic neuropathy in association with pulmonary infections, respiratory depressant drugs, and anesthesia. Autonomic neuropathy can abolish the awareness of hypoglycemia by blunting the anxiety, tremor, sweating, and hunger mediated by the autonomic system.

The CSF may show a moderate elevation of protein to about 100 to 200 mg/dl but is otherwise normal. Treatment is symptomatic for pain, insensitivity, and autonomic dysfunction, as outlined in the section on chronic symmetric polyneuropathies.

Uremic Polyneuropathy. With improved methods of dialysis better removing bloodborne toxins, serious symmetric, distal sensorimotor axonal neuropathies are now less common in patients with chronic renal failure. Mild autonomic dysfunction is manifest by postural hypotension. Some patients have troublesome limb pains or restless legs syndrome, which compels them to move the legs or walk about because of a peculiar distress in the legs.

Severe established neuropathy responds only to renal transplantation, but then often remarkably well. Curiously, the neuropathy may also be improved by bilateral nephrectomy performed to control malignant hypertension of renal failure. Nitrofurantoin can cause severe neuropathy, especially in the presence of renal failure, and should be avoided.

Chronic Relapsing Dysimmune Polyneuropathy. Chronic relapsing dysimmune polyneuropathy (CRDP) is very similar to the acute form of the disease, from which it can only be differentiated in retrospect by its slower onset and steady or remittent course over months. It is a sensorimotor polyneuropathy with both proximal and distal involvement in which the CSF protein level is markedly raised and the motor nerve conduction velocities are equally reduced. Unlike AIP, CRDP responds well to immunosuppression with azathioprine or steroids; some patients have shown a good response to plasma exchange.

Polyneuropathy With Peripheral Nerve Antibodies. A chronic demyelinating sensorimotor polyneuropathy may affect middle-aged men who have high serum titers of antibodies against peripheral nerve myelin-associated glycoprotein (anti-MAG). Improvement occurs with combinations of plasmapheresis, intravenous immunoglobulin, and immunosuppressants.

Nerve Infiltration. Infiltration of nerves with myeloma, amyloid, sarcoid, xanthoma, or carcinoma may cause Schwann cell dysfunction and visible enlargement of the nerves. In leprosy, excessive collagen produces ischemia and Schwann cell damage in both the lepromatous and tuberculoid forms. In the former, a distal, symmetric, sensory neuropathy or a multiple mononeuropathy is seen, and many acid-fast bacilli will be detected in the hypertrophic skin lesions. The anesthetic areas are typically in the colder, distal parts of the body such as the digits, nose, and chin. In the tuberculoid form, the skin atrophies, loses pigment, and becomes anesthetic. The nerves are nodular and thickened. This form usually presents as a slowly progressive multiple mononeuropathy. Leprosy is the most common cause of neuropathy worldwide.

Polyneuropathy With Plasma Cell Dyscrasias. A chronic, unremitting, severe sensorimotor polyneuropathy occurs with little systemic impairment as a complication of a solitary plasmacytoma in a vertebral body, the pelvis, or a clavicle. The CSF protein is often strikingly elevated to 1 to 2 g/ml; there is sometimes papilledema, but otherwise the general examination is normal. Regression of the neuropathy may follow surgical or radiation therapy.

In the rare syndrome of *P*olyneuropathy, *O*rganomegaly, *E*ndocrinopathy, *M*onoclonal gammopathy, and *S*kin changes (POEMS syndrome), severe subacute or chronic polyneuropathy is associated with pigmentation of skin, hypertrichosis, hypogonadism, hypothyroidism, and hepatosplenomegaly. Immunoelectrophoresis shows monoclonal gammopathy, and a skeletal survey reveals solitary or multiple areas of myeloma. Radiotherapy of the tumors improves both the neuropathy and the systemic features.

Atypical myeloma is much more common than either of these two conditions and may also be associated with a severe polyneuropathy, high CSF protein levels, and a monoclonal gamma globulin spike in the serum. Compared with classic multiple myeloma the condition is less aggressive, patients are not systemically ill, and the degree of plasmacytosis in bone marrow is mild. The neuropathy does not respond to therapy. A chronic sensorimotor polyneuropathy is a significant clinical problem in Waldenström's macroglobulinemia. Chemotherapy with chlorambucil may improve it.

Primary systemic (nonhereditary) amyloidosis, a plasma cell dyscrasia, is a progressive multisystem disease in which infiltration of the peripheral nerves with amyloid is common, producing a relatively selective loss of thinly myelinated fibers (small-fiber neuropathy). Carpal tunnel syndrome is a common presentation, but often a disabling chronic polyneuropathy occurs with pain and paresthesia in the legs and dissociated loss of sensation in a stocking-and-glove distribution (more loss of pinprick and temperature than of touch and proprioception initially). Neuropathic ulcers and Charcot's joints may result. As the disease progresses, severe motor impairment and a prominent autonomic neuropathy appear, the latter causing impotence, bowel and bladder incontinence, severe postural hypotension, and cardiac denervation. Most patients have a monoclonal gammopathy or immunoelectrophoresis of serum and/or urine. No specific treatment exists and death results usually from renal failure.

Autonomic Neuropathy. In elderly patients, mild autonomic nervous system (ANS) degeneration is common, but in diabetes, tabes dorsalis, multiple sclerosis, myelopathies, AIP, Wernicke's encephalopathy, amyloidosis, and rare degenerative diseases such as multiple system atrophy the ANS is markedly involved. Drugs that cause autonomic neuropathy are considered in Chapter 166.

Patients with ANS degeneration may complain of postural hypotension; diarrhea, especially nocturnally; impotence; and the consequences of incomplete bladder emptying. Demonstration on the ECG of a lack of "overshoot" tachycardia on standing up, of variations in pulse rate with Valsalva's maneuver or in the cold pressor test, and of blood pressure to increase more than 10 mm systolic with sustained hand grip all suggest autonomic involvement.

Treatment of postural hypotension and the other features of autonomic failure is difficult. One may try getting the patient to eat more salt than usual and, if necessary, may prescribe fludrocortisone, but this is seldom very effective. Elastic stockings are often prescribed, again seldom with great help to the patient. An anti-G suit may be useful, but if the postural blood pressure fall is extreme, even this will be inadequate. Cholinergic drugs may reinforce bladder contraction. In Shy-Drager syndrome (idiopathic hypotension complicated by basal ganglion and cerebral degeneration), fludrocortisone, indomethacin, and occasionally propranolol may be helpful, but the course is relentlessly progressive.

INVESTIGATIONS IN PATIENTS WITH NEUROPATHY

For the patients in whom no causative pathology can be found and in those in whom more than one cause may be operating, investigations are best carried out by a neurologist with access to EMG because electrodiagnostic studies are an extension of the clinical examination. A full family history must be obtained because it may indicate at the outset whether this is a hereditary or an acquired disease. In the case of hereditary neuropathies, examination of serum proteins and lipoproteins and an estimation of such substances as phytanic acid and porphyrins may be indicated.

Depending on the clinical findings already discussed, the usual battery of screening tests in hematology and biochemistry in addition to a glucose tolerance test, urine microscopy, renal and liver function tests, serum folic acid and B_{12} estimations, and serum protein electrophoresis might be of value in acquired neuropathies. If there is any suggestion of previous infection, viral studies and examination of CSF for protein and cells will also be required, whereas with diphtheria bacteriologic proof must be obtained. A suspicion of such general medical conditions as carcinoma, myeloma, reticulosis, amyloidosis, collagen-vascular disease, and ingestion of toxic chemicals and drugs will direct other appropriate investigations.

Electrodiagnostic studies are very helpful and are called for in the case of any peripheral neuropathy in which the diagnosis is not absolutely clear. In primary axonal disorders, one can obtain an indication of severity (e.g., partial vs. complete axonal interruption) by conduction studies, which are also of great value in localizing the precise site of nerve compression in the entrapment neuropathies and in giving an early indication of reinnervation of denervated muscles. In selected cases, nerve biopsy will give direct information about the pathologic process involved. In the case of infiltrations, such tests may be diagnostic.

In acute neuropathies, serum lead and porphyrins and urinary delta ALA levels should be requested if the neuropathy is mainly proximal and motor. It will have been seen already, however, that a good start in the differentiation of neuropathies can be made if the pathologic basis can be determined (Box 167-9).

TREATMENT

Since specific treatment cannot be given to nerves (except when they are compressed) but only to the causes leading to their dysfunction, therapy is really dependent on the diagnosis and treatment of the causative disease. Patients with AIP, however, must be observed intensely in case they should pass into a stage of respiratory inadequacy, as described earlier. Management in or close to an intensive care unit is also essential in patients with diphtheria or botulism, in

Box 167-9. Potential Investigations in the Diagnosis of Polyneuropathy

Examine the family; interrogate about alcohol consumption and diet
Investigate hobby and work exposures
Electrodiagnosis (nerve conduction studies, EMG)
CBC, ESR, serum protein electrophoresis
IgA, IgG, IgM levels
Liver and thyroid function tests, BUN and creatinine levels
Vitamin B_{12} and folate levels, AC and 2 hr PC sugars
Chest radiographs
Autonomic testing, sural nerve biopsy
CSF analysis
Collagen-vascular screen (SS, SS-A, SS-B)
Heavy metal screen
Antiganglioside GM1 antibodies
Vitamin E and cholesterol levels; heavy metals, porphyrins, delta ALA levels
Malignancy search
HIV, Lyme disease serology
Genetic studies

whom bulbar paralysis may be life threatening so that ventilatory support is essential.

The management of the patient with hereditary neuropathies was discussed earlier. Patients with symptomatic compressive neuropathies need decompression if the site of the lesion can be determined accurately by clinical and electrodiagnostic methods. A search for other causes of subclinical neuropathy should be instituted in patients without an obvious cause for the compression.

In all remaining types of neuropathy, treatment is determined by the cause. Thus replacement of vitamin deficiencies, removal of toxic agents, and treatment of such medical conditions as diabetes and other endocrine disorders, collagen-vascular disease, and cancer will often lead to improvement in the neuropathic symptoms. Chelating agents can accelerate the elimination of lead, arsenic, and mercury. Polyneuropathy associated with plasma cell dyscrasia is rare, but it is important to consider because the syndrome of severe neuropathy in association with solitary plasmacytoma usually regresses with excision or radiation therapy to the plasmacytoma. Immunosuppressive drugs improve the rare neuropathy associated with benign monoclonal gammopathy. In metabolic polyneuropathies, early use of hemodialysis has made severe uremic neuropathy a rarity. Unfortunately, the neuropathies associated with diabetes mellitus are resistant to current modalities of treatment, and one can only suggest rigorous control of hyperglycemia. Some inherited polyneuropathies can be substantially alleviated by specific therapy. Thus in Refsum's disease, long-term dietary reduction of phytols and intermittent plasmapheresis to remove phytanic acid is of real benefit. The neuropathy and myelopathy of the Bassen-Kornzweig syndrome (abetalipoproteinemia) respond to large doses of vitamin E. Last, the substantial group of chronic inflammatory demyelinating polyneuropathies with recurrent and relapsing course over many years often responds to treatment with corticosteroids or azathioprine combined with intermittent plasmapheresis and intravenous immunoglobulin therapy (Table 167-3).

Symptomatic Therapy

Symptomatic therapy is the mainstay of the long-term management of many chronic polyneuropathies for which no specific therapy exists; it helps the patient cope with the disorder, adds comfort, and most importantly, serves to prevent certain serious complications of the neuropathy.

In the case of sensory neuropathies, prevention is the key to the management of trophic changes and their complications. Patients should be reminded that their hands and feet are vulnerable to mechanical and thermal injury that is likely to go unrecognized because of lack of pain sensitivity. The need for long-term deliberate steps to avoid this problem should be emphasized so that these steps become routine. The feet should be kept clean and inspected daily for abrasions and other injuries. When feet are dry because of loss of sweating, they should be soaked for 15 minutes in tepid water daily, lightly dabbed, and petroleum jelly applied so that moisture is kept in and cracking of skin is prevented. The use of properly fitting shoes with reinforced toecaps is essential because poorly fitting shoes are the most common cause of ischemic ulcers of the feet. Corns and calluses should not be pared by the patient, keratolytic agents should be avoided, and the patient should see a podiatrist regularly. Precautions are necessary to avoid thermal injury by, for instance, wearing gloves in the kitchen, using pots with long wooden handles, and avoiding cigarette smoking.

Once a foot ulcer develops, it should be vigorously treated from the outset. If there is evidence of acute ulceration or infection, bed rest with elevation of the foot and appropriate antibiotics are necessary. Once the acute phase subsides, walking can be allowed, but it is crucial to avoid weight bearing on the foot. Although this is a self-evident principle and patients with normal sensation will not bear weight on an ulcerated foot, much exhortation is needed for the patient with anesthetic limbs to follow this direction. A total-contact cast to the foot and leg is the best method, but in conscientious patients who decline the cast, crutches may be used. It is remarkable that with such care even patients with severe, inherited sensory neuropathies can protect their limbs for years.

Management of Motor Disabilities

Physical medicine and rehabilitation departments can help the patient make the best use of remaining strength. Braces for dropped feet, special shoes, and attachments to utensils, tools, and cutlery can aid disabled patients in activities of daily living.

Management of Chronic Neuropathic Pain

Persistent pain is a relatively uncommon problem, but it is difficult to treat and requires special strategies. Chronic pain may be a distressing feature of some cases of diabetic, alcoholic, or uremic polyneuropathy. It is a common manifestation of amyloid neuropathy and an outstanding aspect of Fabry's disease.

The first step is to make sure that the pain is indeed neuropathic and not ischemic. Musculoskeletal and joint pain secondary to weakness and uneven distribution of body weight should be excluded. Depression may frequently masquerade as chronic pain.

Narcotic analgesics should be avoided because of the danger of addiction in these chronic situations. Treatment should be initiated with simple analgesics such as aspirin or with nonsteroidal antiinflammatory drugs (NSAIDs) such as ibuprofen. The next choice is a trial of diphenylhydantoin or carbamazepine. In resistant cases, amitriptyline or other tricyclic drugs may be effective, occasionally combined with a neuroleptic drug such as fluphenazine (Prolixin). The use of neuroleptics, however, should be a last resort because of the risk of tardive dyskinesia. Occasional reports indicate success with such drugs as propranolol, cyproheptadine, small doses of levodopa (L-dopa), and clonazepam-mexiletine. Topical application of 10% Xylocaine ointment or capsaicin ointment (Axsain, Zostrix) may bring modest relief in some cases (see Box 167-6). TENS is sometimes helpful. No single drug is consistently effective in every patient, and one must work to find a suitable agent for a given patient. The painful states usually remit, although it takes several months.

Management of Chronic Autonomic Neuropathy

Chronic autonomic neuropathy is a challenging therapeutic problem typically encountered in diabetic and amyloid polyneuropathy. Many patients may be disabled by orthostatic symptoms. Elastic thigh-length stockings and elevation of the head end of the bed while the patient is recumbent may suffice for mild postural hypotension but in more severe cases

Table 167-3. Treatments for Neuropathies

Treatments	Neuropathies
Immunotherapies	
Plasmapheresis	Guillain-Barré syndrome CIDP
Intravenous immunoglobulin	Guillain-Barré syndrome Demyelinating neuropathies associated with HIV-1 infection
Cytotoxic immunosuppressive drugs	
Prednisone	Bell's palsy CIDP Vasculitic neuropathies
Cyclophosphamide (often in combination with prednisone)	Vasculitic neuropathy of polyarteritis nodosa Wegener's granulomatosis Motor neuropathy associated wtih multifocal conduction block and anti-GM1 ganglioside antibodies
Antiinfectious agents	
Penicillin, ceftriaxone, doxycycline	Lyme disease–associated neuropathies
Ganciclovir	Cytomegalovirus lumbosacral radiculitis in AIDS
Dapsone, rifampin, clofazimine	Leprosy
Replacement therapies	
Thyroxine	Hypothyroid carpal tunnel syndrome Hypothyroid meralgia paresthetica
Vitamin B_1	Nutritional neuropathies
Vitamin B_6	Nutritional neuropathies Isoniazid-induced neuropathy (preventive)
Vitamin B_{12}	Pernicious anemia myeloneuropathy
Vitamin E	Malabsorption syndrome with myeloneuropathy
Toxic-metabolic modulations	
Identification, chelation, and prevention of reexposure	Alcohol Heavy metal neuropathies of arsenic, mercury, and lead Drug-induced neuropathies
Hematin	Neuropathy of acute intermittent porphyria
Low phytanic acid diet and plasmapheresis	Refsum's disease
Hemodialysis/renal transplantation	Uremic polyneuropathy
Local corticosteroid injection	Carpal tunnel syndrome
Surgical treatment	Entrapment neuropathies: carpal tunnel syndrome, cubital tunnel (ulnar nerve) syndrome, tarsal tunnel syndrome
Radiation therapy	Polyneuropathy associated with plasmacytoma

CIDP, Chronic inflammatory demyelinating polyneuropathy.

the most consistently effective treatment is fludrocortisone, although it is far from ideal. A variety of pharmacologic agents have been tried singly or in combination and include indomethacin, ephedrine, propranolol, monoamine oxidase (MAO) inhibitors, and even drugs that affect atrial tachypacing. Holter monitoring may identify intermittent heart block that requires a pacemaker. The gastroparesis of diabetes may be eased by metoclopramide. Small-bowel dysautonomia may cause intermittent diarrhea that responds to antidiarrheals or tetracyclines.

The neurogenic bladder predisposes to bladder and upper urinary tract distention, infection, and eventual renal impairment. Pharmacotherapy should be directed by the physiologic abnormalities found on cystometrography. The detrusor stimulant bethanechol (urecholine) is the mainstay of treatment. In selected cases, resection of the bladder neck is effective.

The vexing problem of impotence can now be proved to be neuropathic and not primarily psychogenic, ischemic, or endocrinologic by flow studies and measures of nocturnal penile tumescence. Neuropathic impotence is permanent, and the recently introduced agent Viagra is a significant advance in selected patients.

NEUROPATHIC PAIN SYNDROMES

Neuropathic pain syndromes are a group of syndromes in which chronic intense pain is the outstanding manifestation. The pain arises from injury to one or more nerves, such as the trigeminal, glossopharyngeal, intercostal, or any limb nerve. Sometimes the cause of the nerve injury is clear, such as acute infection by herpes zoster and herpetic neuralgia, or a partial injury to a major nerve trunk in causalgia. In others, the etiology is obscure. Diagnosis rests chiefly on the characteristic features of the pain itself, and therefore these conditions are often misdiagnosed. The treatment of these disorders is challenging and difficult.

Causalgia

Causalgia occurs most often from partial injury to major nerve trunks, especially of the sciatic and median nerves and the medial cord of the brachial plexus. Most cases are the result of knife or gunshot wounds, or high-velocity missile injuries. The pathogenesis is ill-understood, but regional sympathetic neural dysfunction plays a major role.

The clinical picture is dominated by burning pain felt diffusely in the limb with the injured nerve. This pain is spontaneous, continuous, excruciating, and characteristically intensified by emotional upset, light touch, exposure to cold, manipulation of the limb, or even by noise. Patients often go to extraordinary lengths to protect the limb and resent physical examination. The deterioration of behavior secondary to chronic intense pain often leads to a psychiatric diagnosis. The skin of the affected part is shiny, moist, either warm or cool, and often edematous. Enforced immobility often leads to contracture. Light touch and pinprick may induce excruciating diffuse pain, and neurologic examination other than the observation of trophic change, weakness, and atrophy may be impossible.

The syndrome usually resolves spontaneously in less than 12 months but may persist for years. Treatment is very difficult. Simple analgesics are ineffective and although narcotics may relieve the pain temporarily, they should not be used for more than a few weeks. Various other measures are available to be tried in order. The principal aim is to suppress the pain and begin exercising the limb so that no permanent changes occur from disuse. TENS of the nerve trunk proximal to the injury is simple, safe, and sometimes adequate. Sympathectomy is the most consistently effective measure and should be done as early as possible to avoid the sequelae of causalgia. A stellate ganglion block is first performed for arm causalgia, with block of the lumbar ganglia used for causalgia of the leg. Repeated injections may be needed, but if each is temporarily effective, surgical sympathectomy may be offered. A vigorous program of massage, range of movement, and active exercise should be instituted from the earliest stage and pursued with perseverance. Squeezing a ball of putty is a helpful way of encouraging active exercises for the hand.

Minor Causalgia and Reflex Sympathetic Dystrophy

Minor causalgia and reflex sympathetic dystrophy (RSD) are much more common in civilian practice than is full-blown causalgia. Minor causalgia refers specifically to the painful syndrome associated with a nerve injury, whereas RSD is similar but results from soft tissue injury to the limb, such as a sprain, or a fracture, without actual nerve damage.

The predominant symptom of minor causalgia is burning pain in the distribution of the nerve. The nerve injury itself is often trivial (e.g., mild ulnar compression caused by improper positioning of the arm under anesthesia) and the pain is less profound and less affected by emotional, tactile, or temperature stimuli than in causalgia. The affected limb shows signs of partial nerve injury and sympathetic dysfunction, seen as reddened, smooth, shiny skin with excessive sweating and marked increase of pain with limb manipulation. RSD shows similar features but without neurologic deficit.

The pain of RSD is distressing, lasts weeks to months, and impedes rehabilitation of the limb. Treatment with narcotic drugs should be avoided. TENS may be sufficient, but often carbamazepine is needed to reduce the pain. If conservative measures fail, sympathectomy is consistently effective. Regional postganglionic sympathetic blockade using intravenous guanethidine or reserpine may be effective, and some patients have responded to oral propranolol. Vigorous physical therapy is important.

Trigeminal Neuralgia

Trigeminal neuralgia is described in Chapter 162.

Glossopharyngeal Neuralgia

Glossopharyngeal neuralgia is described in Chapter 162.

Postherpetic Neuralgia

The pain of acute herpes zoster usually subsides in a few weeks but in about half of the patients over age 60, persistent pain felt in the dermatomal distribution of the affected nerve root follows resolution of the acute symptoms, especially at trigeminal and the upper thoracic root levels. The pain is spontaneous, continuous, and burning, with superimposed paroxysms of stabbing pain. The affected skin may be hyperesthetic to touch or the friction of clothes. Many patients become insomniac and depressed and may contemplate suicide.

Because elderly people so often develop this distressing complication, a 3-week course of oral steroid therapy may be prescribed to decrease the risk. This is indicated in patients without malignancies, immune deficiency, severe diabetes, or active peptic ulcer disease. There is some evidence that treating acute herpes zoster with the antiviral drugs acyclovir or famciclovir decreases the incidence of postherpetic neuralgia.

There is no single consistently effective therapy for established postherpetic neuralgia. Use of different methods and combinations tailored to individual patient requirements, with realistic expectation of alleviation but not abolition of pain, is necessary. TENS is simple and may be effective in some patients. Local subcutaneous injection of corticosteroids in the area of zoster is also helpful. When local measures fail, the most consistently useful medical therapy is the use of tricyclic drugs such as amitriptyline, beginning with 10 mg at bedtime. If this is not sufficient alone, fluphenazine, carbamazepine, phenytoin, baclofen, or clonazepam may be added. However, although these agents are useful in the treatment of trigeminal neuropathy they are of less benefit in postherpetic neuralgia by themselves and may be more useful in combination with tricyclic drugs.

Throughout the illness, one should provide psychologic support, be aware of suicidal potential, and reassure the patient that eventually the pain will resolve.

ADDITIONAL READINGS

Brown MJ, Asbury AK: Diabetic neuropathy, *Ann Neurol* 15:2-12, 1984.

McLeod JG: Investigation of peripheral neuropathy, *J Neurol Neurosurg Psychiatry* 58:274-283, 1995.

Medical Research Council: *Aids to the diagnosis of peripheral nerve injuries*, London, 1987, Bailliere Tindall.

Stewart JD: Focal peripheral neuropathies, New York, 1987, Elsevier.

Subramony SH: Neuralgic amyotrophy, *Muscle Nerve* 11:39-44, 1988.

CHAPTER 168

Muscle Diseases

Timothy J. Benstead

PRESENTING SYMPTOMS OF MYOPATHY

Primary muscle diseases, or myopathies, include a broad range of disorders with many etiologies but with common presentation patterns. Most myopathic disorders affect only muscle fibers, producing symptoms and signs confined to the muscle. A few myopathies are accompanied by pathology of other tissues resulting in non-muscle manifestations. A good example of a myopathy with many non-muscle manifestations is myotonic dystrophy, which will be discussed later in this chapter.

The most frequently encountered manifestation of myopathy is weakness (Box 168-1). Weakness can occur because of failure of diseased muscle fibers to contract effectively, or in more severe processes the loss of muscle fibers. Some myopathies produce very little weakness and the manifestations may be restricted to other indicators of muscle fiber disease, such as myalgia, muscle cramps, and fatigue. Most myopathies produce symmetric symptoms and signs, unlike some nerve or motor neuron diseases, which can be highly asymmetric. There are a few exceptions to this rule, such as inclusion body myositis, but in general myopathies are highly symmetric. Myopathies also usually present with proximal muscle weakness and may remain confined to proximal muscles throughout the course of the illness. Again, not all myopathies follow this rule, but the majority do, and a disorder with distinctly proximal muscle weakness should always raise the concern for a myopathy.

The facial, palatal, cervical, and respiratory muscles are all quite proximal, and these muscle groups are often targets of muscle disease. Myasthenia gravis is not considered a primary muscle disease, although its pathologic process occurs at the acetylcholine receptor on the muscle fiber. Myasthenia gravis also usually affects proximal muscle most severely and will often be included in the differential diagnosis of a patient presenting with myopathic symptoms. Muscle fibers are the most distal aspect of the motor unit, which originates at the motor neuron and includes the nerve axon and neuromuscular junction. The muscle therefore is a component of the lower motor neuron complex. A lower motor neuron pattern of muscle weakness should be expected in muscle disease. In many ways this is true. Babinski's signs are absent in muscle diseases, and the muscle tone is often reduced. However, muscle stretch reflexes are usually not reduced as much as in peripheral nerve disease for the degree of weakness present. Also, muscle wasting is usually a later feature of myopathy than neuropathy. When sensory loss accompanies weakness this usually excludes myopathy as a possible etiology. These clinical features can be helpful in differentiating clinically between muscle and nerve disease, although a definite differentiation is not always clinically possible and laboratory evaluation is very important for establishing whether myopathy is the cause of a patient's weakness as well as determining the type of muscle disease.

Box 168-1. Clinical Indicators of Myopathy

- Weakness, myalgia, fatigue, and/or muscle cramps
- Proximal upper and lower extremity distribution of weakness
- Symmetric weakness
- Weakness of cranial nerve innervated muscles
- Absent sensory disturbance
- Absent upper motor neuron signs

LABORATORY INVESTIGATIONS FOR MYOPATHY

There are many investigations that may be helpful in accurately diagnosing a muscle disease, but the core investigations helpful for establishing whether a myopathy is present include measurement of serum muscle enzyme levels, electromyography, and muscle biopsy (Box 168-2). Many additional tests may be helpful in clarifying a more precise diagnosis, such as genetic analysis and evaluation of other organ systems, but the triad of investigations noted above remains the cornerstone of myopathy investigation.

The serum creatine kinase (CK) measurement is the most useful enzyme analysis in the diagnosis of muscle disease. Other serum enzymes that can be derived from skeletal muscle, such as lactate dehydrogenase (LD), aspartate aminotransferase (AST), and alanine aminotransferase (ALT), may also be elevated in myopathy, but they do not increase as readily or dramatically as does CK in response to muscle pathology. It should be remembered that these serum enzymes can arise from other organs, and clinical acumen needs to be exercised to avoid attributing CK elevation to cardiac disease or LD, AST, and ALT elevation to liver disease when they may all be rising from skeletal muscle. Serum CK analysis is critical because isoenzyme analysis of CK can determine the source of the enzyme elevation and CK will not rise in response to liver disease.

In myopathy the CK elevation can range from mild to very severe. The degree of elevation tends to reflect the degree of muscle fiber necrosis that is occurring and the tempo of the disease. Disorders with widespread necrosis of muscle fibers, such as Duchenne's muscular dystrophy, have high CK

Box 168-2. Core Myopathy Investigations

- Serum CK: May require isoenzyme analysis to confirm skeletal muscle source. Elevation usually associated with disorders producing muscle fiber necrosis.
- EMG: Look for small, polyphasic motor unit potentials. Fibrillations suggest muscle fiber necrosis.
- Muscle biopsy: It is important to perform special histochemical stains and electron microscopy as well as routine hematoxylin and eosin staining.

levels. Disorders producing myoglobinuria, which have a very rapid onset of necrosis, will have the highest CK levels, often increasing to the many thousands. More slowly progressive disorders, such as some toxic myopathies, may have a CK elevation level in the hundreds. Many static muscle diseases, such as congenital myopathies, may have normal CK levels. If the disease process does not produce muscle fiber necrosis or some instability of muscle membrane, then CK levels do not usually increase. Elevated CK levels will sometimes occur in disorders affecting nerves. Usually this is in rapidly progressive disorders, such as amyotrophic lateral sclerosis (ALS) in which rapid denervation of many muscle fibers leads to enough muscle membrane leakage of CK to elevate the serum level. Usually this is a relatively minor CK elevation, unlike the much higher elevation that would be expected in a primary muscle disease of equivalent severity.

Electromyography will aid investigation of myopathy in two ways. Electromyograms (EMGs) are very helpful in confirming the presence of disease of the motor unit. The technique will usually differentiate between disorders of nerve, muscle, and the neuromuscular junction. Once features of myopathy are detected on an EMG, the results will sometimes point to specific subtypes of myopathy. However, it should be remembered that the EMG changes of many myopathies overlap and are nonspecific. Other assessments will usually be required to firmly establish a diagnosis. The motor unit forms the core structure that is being assessed with EMG techniques. During EMG a recording needle electrode is inserted into a muscle and the electrical activity generated by muscle fibers adjacent to the needle is recorded. Because many myopathies affect muscles in variable degrees, needle EMGs entail a survey of several muscles. Through this approach, insight is obtained into the distribution of changes, enhancing the ability to diagnose neurologic disease through pattern recognition. With the EMG electrode in place in a muscle, motor unit potentials can be recorded by asking the patient to voluntarily contract the muscle. Muscle fibers within a motor unit are always activated as a group. Thus the electrode will record potentials that are the summated electrical discharges of several muscle fibers within a motor unit firing simultaneously. Many motor units will recruit with strong muscle contractions, but by asking for a graded muscle contraction the electromyographer is usually able to distinguish the features of individual motor unit potentials and compare them to expected normals. Myopathies affect muscle fibers in many motor units with indiscriminate selection of which motor units are affected. In this way, the number of effectively working muscle fibers within a motor unit will be reduced, leading to fewer summated responses in the motor unit potential. The recorded motor unit potentials in myopathy are usually smaller than normal, and this is the electromyographic hallmark of muscle disease. Similar changes do not occur in neuropathy or motor neuron disease. During the course of the disease there may be partial repair of muscle fibers within a motor unit, but the normal architecture of the motor unit is often not recovered and this can lead to other motor unit potential changes, such as an increased complexity or polyphasia. When muscle disease leads to muscle fiber necrosis, spontaneous discharges in the absence of voluntary contraction of the muscle called *fibrillations* can occur. Fibrillations are also seen in nerve and motor neuron disease, but in the presence of small motor unit potentials they imply a myopathy with active muscle fiber necrosis—a finding that has major implications for diagnosis. Diseases in which muscle fiber necrosis is a characteristic feature, such as polymyositis and muscular dystrophy, will almost always have fibrillations seen during an EMG. Alternatively, myopathies that usually do not produce muscle fiber necrosis, such as steroid myopathy, will usually be free of fibrillations.

The muscle biopsy is a critical aspect of precise diagnosis in myopathy. Because many myopathies have overlapping clinical and EMG findings, the biopsy is often the crucial diagnostic test. Choosing the appropriate muscle to biopsy is always important in improving diagnostic yield of this procedure. The clinical and EMG examinations can usually guide the choice of muscle. It is important to choose at least a moderately affected muscle and one easily accessible to the surgeon. A muscle with severe weakness and atrophy may yield only fatty replacement tissue on biopsy and therefore it is usually better to choose a lesser-affected muscle when end-stage disease is present in some muscles. A muscle that has recently been examined with a needle during EMG should be avoided because the needle track can produce microscopic changes in the muscle. The laboratory reviewing the biopsy should be experienced in the special preparation and evaluation techniques of muscle biopsy, including histochemical stains for fiber typing, mitochondria, glycogen, lipid and selected enzymes, and electron microscopic evaluation of muscle. Except for inflammatory muscle diseases and a few other selected myopathies, routine hematoxylin and eosin (H and E) staining alone will not be adequate to be certain of the pathologic diagnosis of the myopathy.

DIAGNOSING A MYOPATHY

The approach to myopathy diagnosis can be conducted systematically and will lead to an accurate diagnosis in most cases. The diagnostician must be aware of the many symptoms that can result from muscle disease and the broad range of disorders that produce myopathy. Myoglobinuria always indicates a pathologic muscle process. Weakness, myalgia, fatigue, and muscle cramps should trigger a suspicion of myopathy. These symptoms can occur in nonmyopathic neurologic disorders or as a general reaction to medical or psychiatric illness. Deciding which patients require a more thorough evaluation of possible myopathy can be difficult. In many patients, co-morbid conditions or indications of a psychologic disorder will eliminate the need for further muscle investigation. If the pattern of muscle weakness is proximal, then myopathy is more likely, although myasthenia gravis should be considered because it can produce a similar pattern of weakness. Evidence of sensory disturbance or upper motor neuron signs on neurologic examination will usually eliminate myopathy as a cause of weakness. Though some myopathies will not elevate the serum CK, it is increased in the majority, and this simple investigation should be performed as soon as myopathy is suspected. When muscle fatigue and myalgia are prominent symptoms, a serum lactate in the rested patient may be informative. If the examination and blood tests are suggestive of myopathy, then an EMG will be helpful in confirming the presence of myopathy and may provide information regarding the type of muscle disease.

Box 168-3. Initial Steps for Investigating Myopathy

- Review all drugs and toxic exposure for potential muscle toxicity
- Take a detailed family history for muscle disease
- Search for non-muscle stigmata of muscle diseases (e.g., cardiac disease, rash, endocrine dysfunction, rheumatologic manifestations)
- Do blood screening for thyroid disease and collagen-vascular diseases
- Use clinical clues to guide other blood testing
- Perform genetic tests when a specific inherited myopathy is suspected
- Perform muscle biopsy when less invasive investigations are uninformative

Patients with confirmed myopathy should have several screening procedures (Box 168-3). A careful review of medications and toxic exposures should be performed. The patient's family history should be carefully reviewed for similar problems. The general medical history and examination should search for nonskeletal muscle stigmata of myopathies, such as cardiac disease, collagen-vascular disease manifestations, rashes, and evidence of an endocrinologic disorder. Patients should have blood screening for thyroid disease and collagen-vascular diseases. Additional blood screening can be directed toward evaluation of other clues apparent in the history and examination. If a specific inherited myopathy is apparent, then genetic testing may be possible. When a diagnosis cannot be made through less invasive means, a muscle biopsy should be strongly considered. Many myopathic disorders cannot be diagnosed properly without the aid of muscle biopsy. If a muscle biopsy is performed, then the laboratory analyzing the tissue should be experienced in performance and interpretation of the many special histochemical stains and electron microscopy necessary for a complete assessment of muscle tissue.

Referral to a Specialist

The primary care physician can perform much of the initial screening for myopathy. As noted earlier, the proper management of myopathy may only require the removal of a toxic substance or the treatment of an underlying medical disorder. The patient should be referred to a physician with specialized training in myopathy when initial evaluation fails to yield a specific diagnosis, or if the diagnosing physician is not experienced with the diagnosis and management of specific muscle disorders.

DIFFERENTIAL DIAGNOSIS OF MYOPATHY

Myopathy can be divided into several large categories of muscle disease, based on etiologic factors and clinical presentation. A complete discussion of myopathy is well beyond the scope of this chapter, but is presented elsewhere.[2] Box 168-4 lists the major categories of muscle disease.

Box 168-4. Classification of Primary Muscle Diseases

Inherited myopathies
- Congenital myopathies
- Muscular dystrophies
- Inherited channelopathies
- Periodic paralysis
- Inherited metabolic myopathies
  - Disorders of glycolysis
  - Disorders of oxidative metabolism
    - Lipid myopathies
    - Mitochondrial myopathies

Acquired myopathies
- Inflammatory myopathies
- Acquired metabolic myopathies
- Toxic myopathies

INHERITED MYOPATHIES

Congenital Myopathies

Several usually nonprogressive presumed inherited disorders of muscle exist, most of which are distinguishable primarily by the appearances of the muscle biopsy. As a group these myopathies are called the *congenital myopathies,* and they should be distinguished from the more clearly progressive muscular dystrophies. Children with congenital myopathy may present as floppy infants with mild feeding difficulty, but serious weakness and feeding or breathing problems would be uncharacteristic of most congenital myopathies. Some of the congenital myopathies may have marked variability of clinical expression and more severe infantile forms. Usually this would not be suspected until the specific muscle biopsy abnormalities were detected. Many patients with congenital myopathy present as thinly muscled, mildly weak children, with the problem often becoming apparent when walking begins or as the child begins to attempt more physically demanding tasks, such as climbing. It may be difficult sometimes to distinguish when this truly represents a pathologic process. Functional testing of muscles can be helpful in determining when the muscle is more likely to be abnormal. Difficulty in rising from the floor, climbing up on a chair, or a history of inability to perform common childhood physical activities should be clues that muscle disease is present. The weakness will be lifelong in congenital myopathy, but marked progression of weakness over time with loss of motor milestones should lead to consideration of a more progressive disorder.

On biopsy it may be possible to distinguish the subtypes of congenital myopathy, including central core disease, nemaline myopathy, centronuclear myopathy, multicore disease, and congenital fiber type disproportion. In some disorders dysmorphic physical features may be present, including elongated facies, kyphoscoliosis, congenital hip dislocation, and foot deformities. Central core disease was the first described congenital myopathy and in many ways is typical of the group. Small muscles and mild to moderate proximal muscle weakness are apparent usually in early childhood. The CK level is usually normal, or at most only mildly elevated, attesting to the relatively nonprogressive nature of the disorder. The family history may be positive for a similar disorder. On muscle biopsy the predominant feature is circular cores that are apparent running through the center of the long muscle fibers. The cores are densely packed myofilaments. Other features of muscle fiber necrosis are usually absent. The other congenital myopathies all have distinctive pathologic features, generally denoted by the myopathy name, but many have overlapping clinical features. An important distinguishing feature of central core disease is that this congenital myopathy also results in susceptibility to malignant hyperthermia. This susceptibility can be life threatening during anesthesia and is very important to identify for the patient.

Muscular Dystrophies

Duchenne's Muscular Dystrophy. Many myopathies fall within the diverse category of muscular dystrophy. The clinical features, inheritance patterns, and prognosis vary widely within this group, but all have some common features. The dystrophies are all inherited primary muscle diseases that are progressive and have pathologic features of muscle fiber degeneration and attempted regeneration. The most dramatic condition within this group is Duchenne's muscular dystrophy (DMD), the most prominent of the muscle diseases with an inherited defect of dystrophin. Dystrophin is a muscle membrane protein essential for membrane integrity. With complete dystrophin deficiency, the full expression of DMD occurs. Inherited partial dystrophin deficiencies can produce a variety of more benign presentations, of which Becker's muscular dystrophy (BMD) is the most frequently encountered.

DMD is an X-linked recessive disorder. Male children with the abnormal gene express the disorder. Females who are carriers do not manifest DMD, although female carriers can sometimes demonstrate mild abnormalities such as an elevated CK level or minimal weakness. Most boys with DMD are first noted to be weak before the age of 3. Increased frequency of falling, difficulty climbing, or regression of motor milestones may indicate the first change. These children develop difficulty in rising from the ground early and adopt the Gowers' maneuver to accommodate (Fig. 168-1). With the Gowers' maneuver the child uses his hands to "climb" up the legs, allowing him to get his trunk into the upright position. Once upright, the child may need to swing the legs out at the hip to walk as opposed to a more normal stride. This gait has the appearance of waddling and is called a *Trendelenburg gait.* Most children with DMD have pseudohypertrophy of the calves. The calves appear disproportionately large compared to proximal leg muscles and have a rubbery, firm consistency. During the later half of the first decade of life, patients with DMD become progressively weaker, and most have lost the ability to ambulate by age 12. Joint contractures and scoliosis develop during this period and worsen as mobility declines. DMD frequently involves cardiac muscle and produces electrocardiographic and echocardiographic abnormalities early and may lead to heart failure late in the patient's disease. Some patients with DMD will have abnormalities of the brain, which will present as a static cognitive delay. The ultimate prognosis of DMD relates to the unrelenting skeletal muscle weakening, with eventual involvement of respiratory function or cardiac disease. Respiratory or cardiac failure are the most

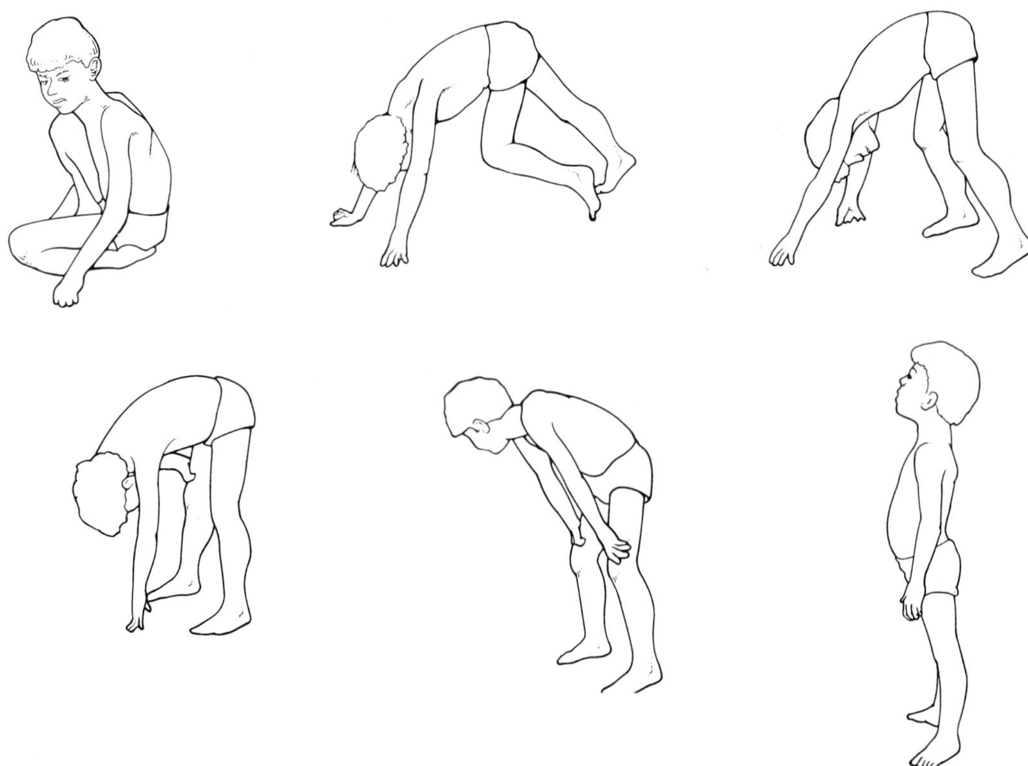

Fig. 168-1. Gowers' sign. Child must use his hands to rise from sitting position. (Redrawn from Siegel IM: Clinical management of muscle disease. In Canale: Campbell's Operative Orthopedics, ed 5, London, 1977, William Heinemann.)

common causes of death in DMD. The mean age of survival is approximately 20 years.

DMD can be inherited from a female carrier or as a new mutation. Approximately one third of boys with the disease appear to have a new mutation. The diagnosis can be confirmed through DNA analysis in about 70% of carriers or affected patients. If DNA analysis is positive, prenatal diagnosis and counseling will be possible for future pregnancies or relatives at risk for carrying the abnormal gene. Even without positive DNA analysis, dystrophin staining of muscle will be absent. This is a highly reliable test to confirm diagnosis, but it is impractical for many aspects of potential carrier screening or prenatal diagnosis. Another useful tool to screen potential carriers is measurement of CK levels because elevations will be present in about 50%.

The management of DMD depends heavily on the utilization of physical therapies, bracing, and surgery. As the disease progresses the physical devices used to maintain ambulation progress from splints through walking aids. Passive stretching will slow contracture development. Surgery can help prevent contracture formation, but it may also be needed to relieve discomfort from progressive scoliosis. Alternate-day steroids have been shown to slow progression for at least a few years and are now a well-accepted management tool for this group.[5] A number of experimental therapies have been evaluated, but none have significantly affected the prognosis of this severe myopathy.

Becker's Muscular Dystrophy. Inherited disorders of dystrophin can present with conditions less severe than DMD. The most frequently encountered is BMD. In DMD dystrophin is completely absent from immunohistochemical staining of muscle tissue. Dystrophin staining is partially lost in BMD, and this partial disorder of dystrophin produces a clinical phenotype that has many similarities to DMD but presents at a later age and is less severe. Patients with BMD typically develop symptoms later than those with DMD. The mean age of first symptom is 12, but the range is marked and some patients will first note problems in later adult life. The inheritance is X-linked similar to DMD, and some of the clinical clues to the diagnosis are similar, such as calf hypertrophy. Although BMD is a less severe muscular dystrophy than DMD, it is still a disabling condition, with gradual progression and a high risk of loss of ambulatory ability. The diagnosis can be confirmed through appropriate histochemical staining of muscle tissue. Genetic counseling issues are important both for parents of patients with BMD and for the patients themselves because most will survive to reproductive age.

Myotonic Dystrophy. For physicians with numerous subspecialty interests, knowledge of myotonic dystrophy is important. In addition to the muscle manifestations of myotonic dystrophy, a number of other body systems can be affected in this condition. Myotonic dystrophy is inherited as an autosommal dominant disorder with highly variable expression of the disease phenotype. The molecular abnormality is an expansion of a CTG nucleic acid triplet repeat sequence on the nineteenth chromosome.[1] Similar to a number of other triplet repeat disorders, the longer the expansion of the repeating triplet sequence, the more profound the phenotypic expression of the disorder. Over generations there tends to be a progressive increase in the length of the expansion sequence, which accounts for the phenomenon of "anticipation" that results in the children of carriers expressing the disease more severely.

The muscle weakness of myotonic dystrophy can be quite mild in some patients, but it often produces marked facial weakness, ptosis, and greater distal extremity weakness than is often seen in other myopathies. The myotonic manifestations of the disorder are noted by the patient as a stiffness of muscles or a difficulty in releasing his or her hand grip. At the bedside, myotonia is best demonstrated either by watching the release of a firm hand grip or by percussion of the thenar eminence with a reflex hammer. Myotonia will appear as a slow release of the grip or a sustained contraction of the muscle after percussion.

The systemic manifestations of myotonic dystrophy can be key to the initial consideration of the diagnosis. Frontal balding is a frequent manifestation. It is usually more prominent in men but is also seen in women. A patient complaining of weakness and who has marked thinness of facial and neck muscles, ptosis, and balding has a high likelihood of having myotonic dystrophy. Some of the systemic manifestations have important health implications and are important to monitor. Premature cataracts will often occur, even in patients without very many muscle manifestations. Cardiac arrhythmias, diabetes, and testicular atrophy will also occur in this disorder. Follow-up of patients with myotonic dystrophy should include periodic electrocardiograms (ECGs), fasting glucose measurements, and ophthalmologic assessment.

Myotonia can be a disturbing symptom in some patients, but often it does not affect function. If the patient has disabling myotonia, quinine and phenytoin can be helpful. Mexiletine is more effective but should not be used if cardiac manifestations are present.

Limb-Girdle Muscular Dystrophy. The molecular basis of many of the adult-onset muscular dystrophies has now been described. Limb-girdle muscular dystrophy (LGMD) often presents in adult life with slowly progressive weakness and wasting of proximal muscles of the legs and arms. The disorder can be autosomal dominant or recessive. Patients with LGMD can be severely disabled, but the prognosis is generally better than DMD. Molecular abnormalities have been described of the sarcoglycan complex, which is an important muscle membrane protein complex that interacts with dystrophin. Histochemical staining of the muscle biopsy will often lead to a specific diagnosis of the subtype of LGMD.

Inherited Channelopathies

Myotonia Congenita. Muscle diseases that result from inherited dysfunction of muscle membrane ion channels produce two main varieties of muscle symptom: myotonia and periodic paralysis. The two symptoms are sometimes found in the same patient. Myotonic dystrophy differs from other myotonic disorders by the presence of weakness and the manifestations outside of the skeletal muscle. Myotonia congenita (Thomsen's disease) is inherited as an autosomal dominant condition. A recessive form (Becker myotonia) is usually more severe. Dominantly inherited myotonia congenita may lead to muscle hypertrophy caused by the frequent, excessive contraction of the muscle, producing a heavily muscled appearance although the patient is not usually excessively strong. Unlike myotonia in myotonic dystrophy, the symptom is often very bothersome to the patient, who may require pharmacologic management. Treatment is similar to the management of myotonia for myotonic dystrophy, although mexiletine is less likely to cause cardiac side effects. Myotonia congenita occurs because of an inherited defect of calcium channel function on the muscle membrane.

Paramyotonia Congenita. Paramyotonia congenita can lead to both myotonic symptoms and periodic paralysis. The myotonia is different in paramyotonia congenita in that it worsens the more a muscle is used, which is the opposite of other myotonic disorders. Patients with paramyotonia congenita also have cold-sensitive symptoms (e.g., in the cold they experience paralysis of muscles). The genetic defect is on the same chromosome as hyperkalemic periodic paralysis and affects the function of K^+ ion channels in muscle membrane.

Periodic Paralysis

Periodic paralysis episodically results in severe weakness of extremity and trunk muscle, but it usually spares respiratory and bulbar muscles. The subtypes of periodic paralysis include hypokalemic, hyperkalemic, and normokalemic periodic paralysis. These patients do not have sensory manifestations and are often mistaken for patients with conversion reaction. Large meals or exercise in patients with the hypokalemic form can trigger the episodes of weakness. A positive family history is extremely helpful for suspecting the diagnosis. The serum K^+ levels should be measured during attacks to facilitate diagnosis. The hypokalemic form can be diagnosed through provocative tests using glucose loading with or without additional insulin to promote hypokalemia. This test needs to be performed under carefully controlled circumstances to recognize hypoglycemia and treat it promptly if it occurs. The EMG in hyperkalemic periodic paralysis will often demonstrate myotonia, which will be a clue to the diagnosis. Acetazolamide is useful as a prophylactic agent for hypokalemic and hyperkalemic periodic paralysis, although dietary manipulation can also help avoid attacks. Potassium supplementation with a low-carbohydrate diet may prevent attacks in hypokalemic periodic paralysis. Eating a carbohydrate-rich substance may abort milder hyperkalemic periodic paralysis attacks. If periodic paralysis first occurs in adult life, then a secondary form should be considered, such as thyrotoxic periodic paralysis or periodic paralysis caused by loss of K^+ from the kidneys or gastrointestinal tract from medication or disease.

Inherited Metabolic Myopathies

The inherited metabolic myopathies are a large and diverse group of disorders, each of which is due to an abnormality of muscle energy metabolism. The two primary sources of energy in muscle are sugars and fats. Thus the two major categories of inherited metabolic myopathy are disorders of glycolysis and lipid metabolism. Lipid metabolism leads to oxidative phosphorylation to produce ATP for high-energy utilizing tissues such as muscle. Oxidative phosphorylation occurs within mitochondria; therefore mitochondrial disorders are a subtype of lipid metabolism disorders that lead to muscle manifestations.

Myoglobinuria. The most dramatic presentation of an inherited metabolic myopathy is with myoglobinuria, which develops when massive muscle fiber necrosis, or rhabdomyolysis, occurs very quickly and muscle fiber contents are spilled into the blood stream in large amounts. The serum CK level is always markedly elevated in patients with myoglobinuria. Myoglobin is filtered through the kidney and appears as a tea-colored discoloration of the urine. The large protein load on the kidneys induced by myoglobinuria can lead to acute renal failure and needs to be promptly managed.

Disorders of glycolytic and lipid metabolism can lead to myoglobinuria. McArdle's disease is caused by a deficiency of myophosphorylase and is a good example of a disease of glycolysis. Myophosphorylase deficiency impairs the ability of the muscle to metabolize glycogen as an energy source. This is particularly important during anaerobic muscle activity, when oxidative phosphorylation cannot be depended on because of reduced oxygen delivery to the muscle tissue. Exercise-induced myalgia is the most frequent symptom of patients with McArdle's disease. The exercise intolerance is most noticeable during the beginning stages of muscle activity or when isometric exercise is performed. In both situations glycolytic pathways are more important as an energy source for the muscle. Most patients with McArdle's disease describe a "second wind" phenomenon. If symptoms develop after a brief exercise and patients stop exercising briefly, when they restart the exercise they usually perform better. During exercise the muscle normally switches from being glycolytic pathway dependent to oxidative phosphorylation dependent for its energy source. "Second wind" represents that transition (i.e., the patient with McArdle's disease functions much better when oxidative phosphorylation is the predominant source of muscle energy). If McArdle's disease is suspected, the ischemic forearm test will provide strong evidence of the disorder. With a blood pressure cuff on the upper arm inflated above systolic blood pressure, the patient exercises forearm muscles by repeatedly squeezing the hand. Blood is drawn to evaluate the serum lactate level before the exercise and several times after its completion. Normally, at least a threefold increase in serum lactate levels is detected immediately after the exercise and lasts for several minutes. In McArdle's disease, the lactate fails to rise because of the inability of muscle to utilize glycolytic pathways even under ischemic conditions. Myophosphorylase staining of the muscle biopsy will confirm the diagnosis. Currently, no effective treatment is available for McArdle's disease, but accurate diagnosis is important to appropriately counsel patients regarding the need for prompt treatment of episodes of myoglobinuria.

Myoglobinuria will also occur with carnitine palmityl transferase (CPT) deficiency, which is an enzyme deficiency impairing transport of free fatty acids across the membrane of the muscle mitochondria. Because oxidative phosphorylation is the metabolic pathway altered in CPT deficiency, the exercise intolerance tends to occur after a longer duration of aerobic exercise than was encountered in McArdle's disease. The manifestations of myoglobinuria and the importance of prompt treatment are the same regardless of the underlying diagnosis.

Acid maltase deficiency is also a disorder of glycolysis and can present in childhood or adult life. The key clinical clue is the early and severe involvement of respiratory muscles in this disorder, often leading to the need for assisted ventilation. Management may be aided by biphasic positive airway pressure (BIPAP) or continuous positive airway pressure (CPAP) at night, but these patients often need to consider the possibility of long-term home ventilation.

Mitochondrial Myopathy. Muscle is dependent on mitochondria to produce adenosine triphosphate (ATP) through oxidative phosphorylation. Many defects of mitochondrial function have been detected and most are associated with muscle disease, although other body tissues may also be affected. Several muscle syndromes are associated with mitochondrial dysfunction. The mitochondrial syndromes can include progressive external ophthalmoplegia, progressive extremity weakness often associated with exercise-induced myalgia, or a combination of myopathy and neuropathy. Other neurologic manifestations can occur in mitochondrial disorders, such as stroke at a young age, myoclonic seizures, migraine, sensorineural hearing loss, ataxia, and dementia.[3] Nonneurologic manifestations of mitochondrial disorders can include lactic acidosis, diabetes mellitus, pigmentary retinopathy, cardiac conduction disorders, short stature, and Fanconi's syndrome. Several syndromes have been described that combine groups of manifestations of mitochondrial disease. The MELAS syndrome consists of *m*itochondrial myopathy, *e*ncephalopathy, *l*actic *a*cidosis, and *s*troke-like episodes. *MERRF* refers to *m*yoclonic *e*pilepsy with *r*agged *r*ed *f*ibers. The muscle biopsy of mitochondrial myopathy often demonstrates an excessive accumulation of mitochondria, forming clumps adjacent to the muscle membrane. The mitochondria likely proliferate in an attempt to compensate for abnormal function. Using a Gomori's trichrome stain, these mitochondria appear as red granular deposits leading to the ragged red muscle fiber description. Ragged red fibers are a pathologic feature common to many of the mitochondrial myopathies. The genetic defects of some mitochondrial syndromes have been described, facilitating diagnosis in some patients. Muscle can also be evaluated for the components of oxidative phosphorylation, allowing detection of the specific defect of energy metabolism in some patients. No effective treatment is yet available for mitochondrial diseases, although some manifestations may be effectively managed, such as diabetes, cardiac conduction defects, migraine, and others.

ACQUIRED MYOPATHIES

Inflammatory Myopathies

The inflammatory myopathies are an important treatable group of muscle diseases. There are several inflammatory myopathy syndromes with different treatment options for each. This subject is discussed in detail in Chapter 131. It is always important to consider the diagnosis of an inflammatory myopathy in a newly acquired myopathy, but it is equally important to recognize the differential diagnosis as outlined in this chapter to ensure the management plan for the patient with myopathy is correct.

Acquired Metabolic Myopathies

Endocrine Myopathies. Myopathy is common in many endocrine disorders, although the severity and clinical significance of the myopathy will vary according to the endocrine disorder. Box 168-5 lists endocrine causes of myopathy.

Box 168-5. Endocrine Causes of Muscle Disease

- Thyroid disease
  - Hypothyroid myopathy
  - Hyperthyroid myopathy
  - Thyroid ophthalmopathy
  - Thyrotoxic periodic paralysis
- Pituitary and adrenal disease
  - Cushing's syndrome
  - Steroid myopathy
  - Adrenal insufficiency
  - Primary hyperaldosteronism
  - Acromegaly
- Parathyroid diseases
  - Hyperparathyroidism
  - Hypoparathyroidism

Thyroid Myopathy. Evidence of myopathy is commonly found with hyperthyroidism and hypothyroidism, although the muscle disease is often subclinical or only mildly symptomatic. Patients with hypothyroidism commonly have a striking elevation of serum CK levels, with only mild weakness or fatigue and myalgia. The delayed tendon reflexes found in hypothyroidism reflect a slowness of muscle relaxation. Weakness is typically proximal and slowly improves with thyroid hormone replacement.

Although the serum CK levels in hyperthyroid myopathy are often only mildly increased or normal, weakness is frequently much greater than encountered in the hypothyroid state. In thyrotoxicosis, weakness can develop abruptly and can be severe, but the usual course is a gradual worsening of weakness over several months. Thyrotoxicosis is also a secondary cause of periodic paralysis and is described later. Hyperthyroid myopathy produces proximal weakness, and fatigue can be a prominent symptom. The differential diagnosis of myopathy in the presence of thyroid disease includes myasthenia gravis, which has a strong association with autoimmune thyroid diseases. Myasthenia produces fatigable muscle weakness, and bulbar muscles are more commonly affected in myasthenia gravis. The distinction between hyperthyroid myopathy and myasthenia gravis associated with hyperthyroidism can be difficult on clinical grounds alone and investigations such as EMG, measurement of serum CK levels and acetylcholine receptor antibodies. The Tensilon test is often required to clarify the diagnosis. Serum CK levels will be elevated in most myopathies, and acetylcholine receptor antibodies will be present in most patients with myasthenia gravis. Repetitive nerve stimulation during EMG will demonstrate decrement of the motor response in many myasthenia patients. Intravenous injection of 10 mg of Tensilon will temporarily correct the weakness in myasthenia gravis. The Tensilon test should be performed cautiously because of the potential for bradycardia and syncope. In addition, the subjective nature of the test can result in false interpretation. Dependence on the more objective investigations is recommended.

Thyroid Ophthalmopathy. Thyroid eye disease is most commonly associated with hyperthyroidism but will occur in hypothyroid or, occasionally, in euthyroid patients (see Chapter 97). The most frequent manifestation is lid lag as the patient looks down and eyelid retraction, giving the impression of protuberant eyes. This is almost always associated with thyrotoxicosis. In a small number of patients with thyroid disease the extraocular muscles and soft tissues of the orbit gradually swell, producing proptosis, diplopia, and abnormalities of extraocular movement on examination. The swelling can increase intraorbital pressure, which has the potential to damage vision. Because the eye disease is likely related to the autoimmune process associated with thyroid disease, inducing a euthyroid state will not always correct the eye problem. Treating the underlying thyroid disease may help the eye disease, but some patients will require surgical decompression of the eye and steroid treatment.

Pituitary and Adrenal Disease

Steroid Myopathy. *Cushing's syndrome* refers to a variety of conditions in which excessive corticosteroid activity produces clinical manifestations. The syndrome can occur because of Cushing's disease (see Chapter 98). The myopathies caused by the various forms of Cushing's syndrome are similar. Steroid myopathy is the most important toxic myopathy and the most common cause of myopathy. Steroid myopathy usually occurs in the presence of long-term, high-dose steroid treatment, but it can also develop with lower doses during long-term treatment or as a complication of very-high-dose acute treatment in critically ill patients. Most steroid myopathies produce proximal muscle weakness and should always be considered in patients on steroids who complain of new weakness. Unlike many other myopathies, steroid myopathy is usually not accompanied by an elevated serum CK level and the EMG usually has relatively little change. In particular, there is usually an absence of fibrillations on EMG. The muscle pathology in steroid myopathy is a type 2 muscle fiber atrophy without evidence of muscle fiber necrosis or loss of muscle membrane integrity, which explains the lack of CK elevation and fibrillation on EMG. The diagnosis can be particularly difficult in patients being treated with steroids for polymyositis or dermatomyositis and who appear to have a late deterioration in their condition. A normal serum CK level and absence of evidence of active muscle fiber necrosis on EMG will point to steroid myopathy as a complication of management and will be helpful in guiding therapeutic decisions. Steroid myopathy improves readily with withdrawal of the steroid treatment. Because muscle fiber necrosis has usually not occurred, the recovery is generally complete and reasonably prompt. In patients who cannot have steroids withdrawn, myopathy can be minimized by using the smallest possible dose of steroid, treating with alternate-day steroids, avoiding protein deprivation in the diet, and increasing physical activity. Myopathy related to Cushing's syndrome other than that due to steroid treatment should be suspected if the myopathy is accompanied by a cushingoid facial appearance, truncal weight distribution, or other physical features of corticosteroid excess.

Intensive Care Unit–Associated Myopathy. Critically ill patients are at risk for developing a variety of neuromuscular problems. The polyneuropathy of critical illness is associated with multiorgan failure. The mechanism of intensive care unit (ICU)–associated myopathy is still incompletely understood, although high-dose steroid treatment—often in the presence of paralyzing agents—is usually associated with the disorder.[6] Patients with ICU-associated myopathy develop a fulminant paralyzing illness, usually equally affecting distal and proximal muscles. These patients cannot be weaned from the ventilator because of the muscle weakness. Pathology studies have improved our understanding of the pathogenesis of ICU-associated myopathy. Some patients will have inflammatory changes, but the usual pathologic abnormality is an absence of myosin (or thick filaments) in the muscle fiber. Myosin is part of the structure that contracts to shorten muscle; thus without myosin the muscle fiber will fail to work even in the absence of fiber necrosis. Electromyography is an essential component of investigation of ICU patients with apparent neuromuscular weakness because polyneuropathy, myopathy, and other causes of weakness can usually be distinguished by an EMG. If the EMG suggests myopathy, muscle biopsy will confirm the disorder. Myosin filament loss is reversible. Patients with ICU-associated myopathy should be appropriately supported while the disorder corrects itself.

Other Pituitary and Adrenal Disorders. Adrenal insufficiency, acromegaly, and primary aldosteronism can all cause weakness in the pattern of a myopathy. The serum CK level in these disorders is usually normal or only minimally increased and each disorder usually corrects with the appropriate endocrine treatment.

Parathyroid Diseases. The most frequently encountered myopathy related to parathyroid dysfunction occurs in patients with chronic renal failure who develop secondary hyperparathyroidism. The myopathy in this disorder is similar to primary hyperparathyroidism caused by parathyroid adenoma. Patients complain of muscle weakness and stiffness, which is more marked in the lower extremities. Serum CK levels are usually normal, but the EMG will demonstrate myopathic motor unit potential changes. Primary hyperparathyroidism myopathy will correct with parathyroidectomy, but in patients with secondary hyperparathyroidism myopathy does not respond well to intervention other than renal transplantation.

Myopathic weakness is only rarely associated with hypoparathyroidism, but hypocalcemia associated with hypoparathyroidism will lead to muscle tetany. Myopathy can also occur in other parathyroid-related conditions, such as osteomalacia.

Toxic Myopathies

As pharmacologic management of disease advances, the list of agents capable of producing muscle disease is constantly growing. Some agents have a greater impact on modern medical management because of the frequency the agent is used. For example, although steroid myopathy only occurs in a small percentage of patients taking steroids, the broad list of indications for oral steroid treatment leads to the disorder being encountered by physicians with many different interests. Box 168-6 lists several agents that can provoke myopathy. Some of these are used in the treatment of diseases and some result from poisoning or ingestion of recreational agents toxic to muscle.

Box 168-6. Toxic Substances Capable of Causing Muscle Disease

Abused substances
- Alcohol
- Cocaine
- Heroin
- Aromatic hydrocarbons and ketones (used recreationally)

Therapeutic agents
- Corticosteroids
- Vecuronium
- Zidovudine (AZT)
- HMG-CoA reductase inhibitors
- Anesthetic agents (cause malignant hyperthermia)
- Neuroleptics (cause neuroleptic malignant syndrome)
- Chloroquine
- Colchicine
- D-Penicillamine
- Interleukin-2
- Cyclosporine
- Retinoids
- Taxol
- Amiodarone
- Lithium

Other exposures
- L-Tryptophan (causes eosinophilic myalgia syndrome)
- Organophosphates
- Snake venoms

Box 168-6 is only a partial list of agents capable of producing a toxic reaction in muscle. The agents listed are examples of muscle syndromes associated with toxic agents and are those that may be more frequently encountered or appear to have a particularly potent reaction on muscle. Many other drugs and toxins have been associated with muscle disease, and if a patient develops evidence of muscle disease the adverse reaction profile of agents taken by the patient should be carefully reviewed. Details of some toxic myopathies are outlined below.

Alcoholic Myopathy. Alcohol can affect muscle in many ways. Chronic alcoholism with associated protein-calorie malnutrition can produce muscle wasting and weakness, which is often attributed to neuropathy, but muscle biopsy also demonstrates primary muscle degeneration. Alcohol is likely toxic to muscle through many mechanisms, including the production of toxic metabolites such as acetaldehyde and impairment of muscle metabolism. Acute severe alcohol intoxication can produce widespread necrosis of muscle associated with myoglobinuria and the associated complications of myoglobinuria. Dehydration and compression injury to muscle in obtunded patients will contribute to rhabdomyolysis secondary to alcohol intoxication. Abstention from alcohol and proper nutrition will reverse the muscle damage in this disorder.

Antiretroviral Agent–Associated Myopathy. Myopathy is a less commonly occurring complication of antiretroviral therapy than neuropathy and is most often detected in patients taking zidovudine (AZT). Myopathy related to AZT therapy of the human immunodeficiency virus (HIV) can be difficult to differentiate from the wasting and weakness associated with acquired immunodeficiency syndrome (AIDS) but it should be considered when myopathic symptoms are prominent. Patients with AZT-related myopathy develop a steadily progressive, painful muscle weakness. The muscle biopsy demonstrates mitochondrial abnormalities, suggesting a toxic disruption of oxidative metabolism in the muscle. AZT-related myopathy may improve after withdrawal of the drug, but if the myopathy worsens, the muscle disease may be more likely related to the HIV infection.

HMG-CoA Reductase Inhibitors (Statin-Type Lipid-Lowering Agents). HMG-CoA reductase inhibitors used in the treatment of hyperlipidemia increase serum CK levels in approximately 0.5% to 1.0% of patients on long-term therapy. Most of these patients will not have significant clinical symptoms of myopathy. However, if the chronic CK elevation has not been documented, confusion can arise if the patient is assessed for chest pain with enzyme testing. The CK elevation caused by statin drugs is skeletal muscle in origin. Isoenzyme testing should clarify the origin of the muscle enzyme elevation.

Much less commonly statin drugs will produce myalgias and weakness. Occasionally, rhabdomyolysis will develop. Concurrent use of some medications, including cyclosporine and gemfibrozil, increases the incidence of severe myopathy associated with statin drugs. Patients presenting with muscle pain or weakness should be evaluated promptly for evidence of myopathy because withdrawal of the medication will be necessary if there is evidence of muscle fiber necrosis.

Malignant Hyperthermia. Malignant hyperthermia is a potentially fatal reaction to anesthetic agents. Succinylcholine, halothane, and other agents used during general anesthesia can induce the disorder. The condition begins shortly after induction of anesthesia, with severe contraction of jaw and extremity muscles. The heat production from massive muscle fiber activity elevates the body temperature. Acidosis, hypertension, and cardiac arrhythmias will develop quickly. Untreated, the mortality rate is about 70%. Intravenous dantrolene started early in the development of malignant hyperthermia will relax muscles adequately in most patients to reverse the process. Malignant hyperthermia is an inherited disorder with autosommal dominant inheritance. The gene locus responsible for malignant hyperthermia in some families is on chromosome 19. Determining susceptibility can be difficult. Patients at risk because of family history should be counseled regarding the potential for this life-threatening disorder, and treating physicians need to be aware of the risk because some anesthetic agents will be safer to use in susceptible patients. CK testing can help determine risk. A patient with elevated CK levels who is genetically at risk for the disorder should follow all of the precautions for patients with known susceptibility to the disorder. If the CK level is normal, a special evaluation of the muscle biopsy by performing the contracture test will assess risk. This test is only available in selected muscle biopsy centers.

Neuroleptic Malignant Syndrome. Several features of neuroleptic malignant syndrome are similar to malignant hyperthermia. This disorder occurs sporadically in patients treated with neuroleptic agents, such as haloperidol and chlorpromazine. Patients develop muscle rigidity, elevated body temperature, tachycardia, and elevated CK levels. The disorder begins gradually over a few weeks and is not inherited. As the disorder progresses, the patient may develop dehydration related to reduced intake and greater loss of fluids from the hyperthermia. Withdrawal of the neuroleptic, general medical support, bromocriptine, and dantrolene will improve the condition, but it may take several weeks to completely reverse.

Cocaine and Other Abused Drugs. Cocaine and less frequently heroin and amphetamines have been associated with episodes of rhabdomyolysis, sometimes producing myoglobinuria. With all of these agents, coma and prolonged pressure from lying on muscle can lead to muscle fiber necrosis. Cocaine also may damage muscle through vascular injury. A chronic myopathy may occur because of repeated injury from chronic use of cocaine.

Eosinophilic Myalgia Syndrome (L-Tryptophan). L-Tryptophan has been used as a dietary supplement and is sold without prescription. L-Tryptophan–induced eosinophilic myalgia syndrome is an example of the effects of widespread contamination of a dietary product.[4] The condition was first detected in the early 1980s but increased dramatically in incidence in 1989. A similar event occurred in 1981 when thousands of people in Spain developed an eosinophilic myalgia syndrome related to the ingestion of contaminated rapeseed oil. The L-tryptophan contamination resulted in a gradual onset of fatigue, muscle pain, fever, and skin rash. Skin and muscle biopsies demonstrated inflammatory infiltrates. Some patients died from the illness, and the offending product has now been withdrawn.

REFERENCES

1. Brook JD, McCurrach ME, Harley HG, et al: Molecular basis of myotonic dystrophy: expansion of a trinucleotide (CTG) repeat at the 3' end of a transcript encoding a protein kinase family member, *Cell* 68:799-808, 1992.
2. Engel AG, Franzini-Armstrong C, editors: *Myology,* ed 2, New York, 1994, McGraw-Hill.
3. Johns DR: Mitochondrial DNA and disease, *N Engl J Med* 333:638-644, 1995.
4. Kamb ML, Murphy JJ, Jones JL, et al: Eosinophilia-myalgia syndrome in L-tryptophan–exposed patients, *JAMA* 267:77-82, 1992.
5. Mendell JR, Moxley RT, Griggs RC, et al: Randomized, double-blind six-month trial of prednisone in Duchenne's muscular dystrophy, *N Engl J Med* 320:1592-1597, 1989.
6. Showalter CJ, Engel AG: Acute quadriplegic myopathy: analysis of myosin isoforms and evidence for calpain-mediated proteolysis, *Muscle Nerve* 20:316-322, 1997.

CHAPTER 169

Parkinson's Disease

William Pryse-Phillips
T. Jock Murray

Parkinson's disease is a disorder of the basal ganglia and its connections of unknown etiology, characterized by tremor at rest, rigidity, akinesia or bradykinesia (slowness and poverty of movement), postural disorders, and autonomic abnormalities. Parkinson's disease is the most prevalent movement disorder after essential tremor. Its incidence is distributed unevenly throughout the world, being more common in highly industrialized countries than in agricultural societies and more frequent in Europe and North America than in the Far East. The prevalence in North America is 100 cases per 100,000 population, therefore about 500,000 people are affected in the United States, although over the age of 65 the prevalence may be as high as 1%. There is a slight (1.5:1) male predominance, and Caucasian people may be affected more than blacks. The role of hereditary factors in the idiopathic variety is uncertain, although there is a small subset of hereditary Parkinson's disease.

Parkinsonism is a pathophysiologic state caused by degeneration or dysfunction of the dopaminergic nigrostriatal system. This system includes the substantia nigra, caudate nucleus, putamen, and globus pallidus. The cell bodies are in the substantia nigra, and their axons run to the upper basal ganglion structures where dopamine normally acts as an inhibitory neurotransmitter, balancing an excitatory cholinergic system. Neuronal loss in this system leads to the depigmentation of the substantia nigra that is typical in Parkinson's disease. The disorder may be more complex than this, as other biochemical changes are also apparent and neuronal degeneration occurs not only in the substantia nigra but also more widely within the basal ganglia and sometimes diffusely in the cerebral cortex.

Features of Parkinson's disease occur in four major groups of disorders: idiopathic Parkinson's disease, secondary Parkinson's disease, Parkinson's plus syndromes, and degenerative drain disorders. The idiopathic form (once known as *paralysis agitans*) may be due to a viral infection, as suggested by the presence of inclusion bodies in the degenerating neurons of the substantia nigra (Lewy bodies). However, the exact replication of the pathology and clinical features in subjects poisoned with industrial chemicals, manganese, pesticides, herbicides, or MPTP (a narcotic derivative) has led to the hypothesis of a toxic cause.

CLINICAL FEATURES

The clinical features of Parkinson's disease vary with the cause (Box 169-1) but essentially the major signs occur without other clinical evidence of damage to other major structures within the central nervous system (CNS). The onset is usually after the age of 50. Early signs that help to distinguish Parkinson's disease from other parkinsonian disorders are asymmetry of signs, marked rest tremor, a clinically significant response to levodopa, and the relative absence of balance problems in the first years of the disease.

Box 169-1. Features of Parkinson's Disease

Major Features

1. Rest tremor (slow) and action tremor (fast)
2. Rigidity
3. Bradykinesia
4. Poor postural reflexes

Other Features

Decreased blinking
Blepharospasm
Impaired convergence
Dysphonia, dysarthria, dysprosody, palilalia
Drooling
Stooped simian posture
Trunk tilt, akathisia, gait disorder (retropulsion and propulsion)
Ulnar deviation of the fingers
Micrographia
Foot inversion
Distal dystonic movements (inversion of the foot, extended hallux)
Oily skin
Depression
Organic mental changes

The leading symptoms as the disease progresses are rigidity, tremor, bradykinesia, and difficulty with balance and in walking, and these are the most disabling. Other symptoms include depression, sleep disturbances, dementia, blepharospasm, hypophonia, dysphagia and drooling, constipation, difficulty voiding, dizziness, stooped posture, ankle swelling, and impotence.

The development of symptoms in the idiopathic variety is often slow, and their insidious onset may puzzle both patients and physicians, particularly if the tremor is not yet present and the patient's description of the symptoms is unclear. It is common for patients to use words such as "tiredness" for the slowing, and "pain" and "arthritis" for the difficulty with their legs.

Early nonspecific symptoms include weakness, tiredness, and fatigue; complaints of slowness of movements, impaired fine motor control, a posture characterized by flexion, and vague heaviness and stiffness or aching in the limbs, all likely related to a subclinical increase in muscle rigidity. Other early symptoms include difficulty in starting to walk or in getting into and out of a chair or car, difficulty turning over in bed, reduction in the size of the patient's handwriting (micrographia), depression, and drooling, especially at night.

Patients with moderate disease experience increased difficulty with balance and walking. Some of these complaints suggest arthritis, depression, or normal aging as the reason until rest tremor appears. As time goes by, more obvious postural disturbances appear, such as generalized flexion, a loss of associated movements (e.g., arm swing while walking), and difficulties in maintaining balance.

In the developed case, examination of the cranial nerves shows a mask-like facies with a blank stare and infrequent blinking. Voluntary and emotional facial movements are both limited and slow. If the glabella is tapped repeatedly, blinking continues, whereas normally, adaptation to the tapping will stop the blinking after three or four taps (glabellar tap sign). However, this abnormal response also occurs with other causes of diffuse cerebral dysfunction and is not specific. Speech is low, monotonous, and as the disease progresses, hard or impossible to understand. The problem is compounded by drooling of saliva.

Bradykinesia is one of the most disabling symptoms. It is characterized by a delay in starting all movements, by slowness and poverty of movements, and by the arrest of ongoing movements. It may contribute to imbalance, gait disturbance, and falls. The gait problems include difficulties in starting to walk; a decrease in the natural arm swing; short, shuffling steps; difficulty in turning; and freezing spells.

Motor examination in patients with developed disease shows that strength is normal but voluntary and spontaneous tasks are made difficult by the rigidity and slowness in initiation of movements. The patient may sit motionless, even if in an uncomfortable position, and not make those minor postural adjustments that normal people do automatically. When he or she does move, each action is performed in a series of separate steps rather than in a smooth continuum. Handwriting changes are often useful diagnostic early signs because the writing is shaky and small, tending to get even smaller as the sentence continues. Micrographia is later seen in which the writing may not be read without a magnifying glass in some instances (Fig. 169-1). Rigidity is found in most muscles, although initially it may be confined to one limb. At first, only a slight, consistent increase in tone may be felt within the muscles on movement, but eventually one can detect a ratchet-like jerking (*cogwheel rigidity*) that is accentuated by having the opposite arm perform rapid alternating movements, or clenching the opposite fist while tone is tested in the first limb. In the trunk, the increase in tone can be felt over the paraspinal muscles if the patient flexes and extends his or her back.

Parkinsonian tremor is characteristic when present, but it may be absent in up to 25% of patients. At first confined to one hand, it spreads eventually to all limbs. It is commonly a 4 to 6 per second alternating flexion-extension or rotatory movement, most noticeable in the thumb and index finger. This last characteristic led to the old term *pill-rolling tremor*, ascribed to the motion in the days when pharmacists rolled pills by hand. It rarely occurs in the head (visible head shaking usually indicates essential tremor rather than parkinsonism), but it may be seen in the closed eyelids, the tongue, or the chin. It is characteristically best seen when the limb is maintaining a posture, and it is absent when the limb is at complete rest, as during sleep. At a later stage there is sometimes an added action component, so the tremor occurs during the whole range of a voluntary movement, and the leverage effect from extending the arm may make it appear that the tremor is actually worse during movement. Any form of emotional stimulation increases tremors of all types. Tremors usually decrease when the hands are stretched out in front of the patient or when the hands are moving. In some patients, however, the tremor may increase when the hands are in this position (postural tremor).

Apart from the stooped, flexed, and shuffling gait disturbance, *propulsion* and *retropulsion* may be found. When these are present, patients who managed to start walking forward or backward find themselves unable to stop

CLINICAL TESTS IN MONITORING PATIENTS WITH PARKINSON'S DISEASE

Writing sample ________________________________

Draw a spiral

right hand examiner left hand

A Timed motor performances

turn over in bed
sit up in bed
get up out of chair
drink from a cup with both hands
take off and put on a shoe
walk the length of the room

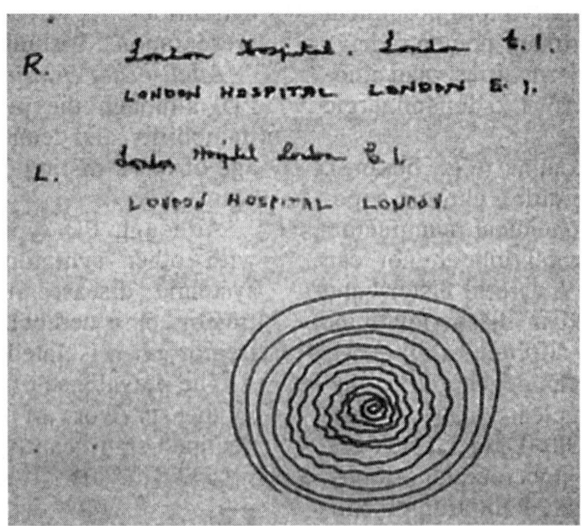

B

Fig. 169-1. **A,** Clinical tests in monitoring Parkinson's disease. **B,** The handwriting of a patient with Parkinson's disease shows micrographia and the tremulous spiral. (From Trend P,et al: *Neurology: colour guide,* Edinburgh, 1992, Churchill-Livingstone.)

so that it is as if they were chasing their own centers of gravity (festinating gait). This inability to halt may be extremely dangerous. Patients may begin to lean backwards when standing for awhile and begin to take rapid steps backwards. Because the normal reactions to stop the movements are not taken, the patients fall and often sustain a head injury. This loss of normal postural responses, corrective actions usually made automatically, causes these patients to fall easily, often toppling like a tin soldier, when they start to go off balance. This is common when turning or when they are on an uneven terrain. To test the postural reflexes, the examiner stands behind the patient and pulls back on his or her shoulders, putting the patient off balance slightly. Normally one would put a foot back and correct the imbalance. Patients with Parkinson's disease may begin to take the small, rapid, festinating backward steps and keep going until they fall into the arms of the examiner. Loss of postural reflexes is one of the most serious symptoms of Parkinson's disease because of the danger of injuries such as subdural hematomas and fractured hips. In fact, one of the paradoxical complications of levodopa therapy when it was first introduced was an increase in the number of fractured hips as the patients suddenly became more mobile but still had poor postural reflexes and thus had an increase in falls.

In Parkinson's disease, all motor actions are performed slowly and with effort, so to get ready in the morning, patients may need an hour or two for toilet purposes, shaving, and dressing. There are no sensory changes but patients often complain of stiffness and *aching in the muscles.* Reflexes, including the plantar responses, are normal unless there is evidence of other generalized brain disease.

Abnormalities of the *autonomic nervous system* result in excessive sweating, oily skin, abnormal gastric motility, and slight bladder disturbances in some cases. Impotence is probably caused by the motor disabilities as much as by autonomic changes. Initial insomnia and frequent night-time awakenings that leave the patient exhausted in the morning are common problems. Vivid dreaming and myoclonus may be due to levodopa therapy, in which case eliminating the evening dose may suffice. However, in some patients withdrawal of levodopa makes them so rigid that they cannot turn over in bed.

In the earlier stages of the disease, intellectual abilities are unaffected despite the patient's appearance, but some degree of *dementia* (manifest as difficulty with memory, recognition, abstraction, and calculation) occurs eventually in at least one third of the patients. Levodopa, anticholinergics, and dopamine agonists also may cause delusions, confusion, paranoia, or hallucinations, which disappear within a few days when the drugs are stopped or the dose reduced.

Many patients are depressed, perhaps in part as a result of their encasement within a body with high inertia, but undoubtedly also because of biochemical disturbances. In about one fourth of the patients, frank hallucinatory and psychotic features occur.

Sialorrhea with drooling results from the mild to moderate dysphagia that is common in the later stages of the disease. This is especially a problem at night when the patient is recumbent and gravity is no longer available to assist swallowing. Anticholinergics decrease saliva production and may be helpful if taken in the evening.

Speech impairments consist of monotony, with the usual expressiveness of speech being impaired; impaired articulation; decreased volume, so that the patient speaks more softly and the volume fades through the utterance of sentences; and slowing of speech. Initially, these problems are most obvious on the telephone. Speech therapy and amplification devices may be helpful here.

Dysphagia is a late symptom and affects both solids and liquids. The difficulty arises either from an inability to force the food down the throat or rigidity of the voluntary muscles of the throat and leads to complaints of food getting stuck in the throat. Ingestion of only small portions of food and careful chewing, one morsel being swallowed before the next is taken, may help. The problem is important because of the risk of aspiration.

Weight loss may be related to dysphagia, depression, or the energy used up by the involuntary movements, or it may be a central, hypothalamic effect.

Constipation is a common problem, often as a result of decreased intestinal peristalsis induced by anticholinergics. Increased fluid intake, use of bulk formers such as bran or methylcellulose, glycerine suppositories, small doses of senna laxatives, or Fleet enemas may be tried. Urinary hesitancy is a common side effect of anticholinergics, but when it occurs in men, prostate gland disease should be excluded first.

Orthostatic hypotension is both a feature of the disease and a side effect of levodopa, dopamine agonists, hypotensives, and antidepressants. It is also a symptom of multiple system atrophy (see below).

Edema of the feet usually occurs at the end of the day (but disappears overnight) as a result of the inability of the rigid leg muscles to maintain venous circulation in patients with decreased mobility. Cardiac failure must be excluded. Amantadine and dopamine agonists also can cause ankle edema. If the edema is severe, elevation of the feet for 1 hour twice a day and elastic support stockings or diuretics may be tried.

A decrease in the desire for sexual activity may result from the nonspecific effects of a chronic illness, from fear of being unable to perform satisfactorily, as a symptom of depression, or because of medications. Parkinson's disease itself is not a cause of impotence. Levodopa only increases sexual function activity in relation to the patient's general improvement.

Current treatments have also led to the awareness of certain features of the disease that may have always been present but were not recognized or occur as a result of the drugs used. These include the following motor fluctuations.

Most commonly, a decline in motor performance occurs near the end of the effective period of each dose of medication. Patients change gradually from showing a good response to the medication (the "on" period) into an "off" period that occurs approximately 1 hour before the next dose is due. Involuntary dyskinetic movements (dyskinesias) may occur either when the drug levels peak after each dose is taken or when the levels are falling off.

A sudden *freezing* of movements is another late-stage complication in treated patients, who may be unable to walk through a doorway without a brief involuntary stop, or on sitting down may stay suspended just above the seat for a few seconds before plopping down into the chair. At its worst, freezing halts the patient while standing or walking, with the likely consequence of a fall.

SECONDARY PARKINSON'S DISEASE

The many secondary causes of parkinsonism all affect the neurons involved in basal ganglion function. The classic secondary cause was the worldwide pandemic of influenza beginning in 1917 that often resulted in *von Economo's encephalitis.* Many of these patients developed parkinsonism even years later, with typical degenerative changes in the basal ganglia and substantia nigra.

Parkinsonian features may be seen in acquired immunodeficiency syndrome (AIDS) and general paralysis of the insane (GPI), but they are hardly ever found in association with multiple sclerosis or cerebral tumor. Cerebral anoxia from any cause, including "successful" resuscitation after cardiac arrest, repeated hypoglycemic attacks, and repeated head injuries (as in boxers) also produce parkinsonian signs. Rigidity and akinesia, but not true Parkinson's disease, may follow multiple cerebral infarcts and have been seen in patients with normal pressure hydrocephalus and Wilson's disease.

Parkinsonism may be induced or unmasked by numerous drugs and other chemicals (see Chapter 166). Neuroleptic drugs are dopamine antagonists and frequently induce parkinsonism, especially the piperazines such as haloperidol and fluphenazine. Metoclopramide, the antidepressant amoxapine, some calcium channel blockers (e.g., flunarizine and cinnarizine), and amiodarone can all cause tremor or other parkinsonian features. A number of toxins can induce parkinsonism, including the illicit narcotic designer drug known as MPTP, manganese, and petroleum wastes.

In postencephalitic and phenothiazine-induced forms of secondary Parkinson's disease, severe autonomic disturbances and oculogyric crises are seen, but the latter do not occur in other types. Rigidity is severe in postencephalitic patients but is not marked in idiopathic Parkinson's disease until a late stage. Tremor is prominent in idiopathic and postanoxic forms, but may not be at all marked in postencephalitic parkinsonism nor in that caused by phenothiazine drugs, in which *bradykinesia* is the most striking of the four major features. Postural disturbances occur in all forms.

DIFFERENTIAL DIAGNOSIS

Diagnosis is not always easy and can require perception and acumen in the early case when signs are minimal and symptoms vague. Early signs of value include infrequent blinking, the lack of arm swinging, and cogwheel or plastic rigidity accentuated when the opposite side is stressed. The history must concentrate on those possible causes of secondary parkinsonism mentioned above, in particular recent anoxia or drug ingestion, and a family history is sometimes of value (although more commonly so in cases of essential tremor, the condition with which, in the early stages at least, it is most likely to be confused). In this disorder, however, the tremor is present with maintenance of a posture and with voluntary activities but hardly ever at rest. It is reduced by alcohol ingestion and disappears at rest. Moreover, the head and voice are often involved, and the family history suggests an autosomal dominant inheritance in half of the cases.

Juvenile Parkinson's disease is a rare familial variety of the disease.

Parkinsonism-plus is a term that includes conditions in which there are other signs of CNS dysfunction in addition to those of parkinsonism. These include hypotension, autonomic insufficiency, ocular palsies, dementia, cerebellar signs, and lower motor neuron lesions. One cluster of these conditions is *multiple system atrophy.* Subtypes of this condition are *progressive supranuclear palsy,* in which there are impairment of vertical gaze and unusual extensor rigidity of the neck; *olivopontocerebellar atrophy,* characterized by limb and gait ataxia and rigidity, dyssynergia, and kinetic tremor; and *striatonigral degeneration,* which should be suspected when features of parkinsonism such as rigidity, slowness, speech hesitancy, pyramidal signs, slow chewing and swallowing, hypomimia, slow flexed gait, and occasionally a resting tremor are accompanied by memory loss, hallucinations, insomnia, and eventually delirium. Finally *idiopathic autonomic failure* (Shy-Drager syndrome) produces dysautonomia that leads to crippling orthostatic hypoten sion, dryness of the skin, impotence, and sphincter disturbances.

Early dementia with hallucinations is a feature of *diffuse cortical Lewy body disease.* In *hemiatrophy-hemiparkinsonism* the parkinsonian features occur in young adults who show a degree of hemibody atrophy on the involved side and in whom contralateral brain hemiatrophy is seen on computed tomography (CT) scans. A positive family history of dystonia may indicate that the parkinsonian patient actually has the condition of *dopa-responsive dystonia.* All but the last of these parkinsonism-plus syndromes are poorly responsive to levodopa.

Parkinson's disease also has to be differentiated from severe, retarded depression and from certain rare neurodegenerative disorders. The rigid forms of *Huntington's disease* and *Wilson's disease* (see below) usually present in children and young adults in whom the family history or serum copper and ceruloplasmin levels should indicate the diagnosis. *Creutzfeldt-Jakob disease* is characterized by parkinsonian and pyramidal signs, myoclonus, dementia, and distal muscle atrophy. *Lytico-Bodig* is a disorder peculiar to Guam that is characterized by signs of parkinsonism, dementia, and amyotrophic lateral sclerosis (ALS).

PROGNOSIS

Before the advent of levodopa, the mortality rate for Parkinson's disease was substantially increased, but this has been reduced, although not normalized, by this drug. The development of dementia or the appearance of any of those physical signs indicating that the condition is actually one of the Parkinson's-plus syndromes indicates a worse prognosis for both the quality and the duration of life.

TREATMENT

General Measures

As with all conditions, the patient and his or her family should be made aware of the nature of the disorder and the possible courses it may take. The best source of printed materials is the National Parkinson Disease Association (1-800-362-3479) or other national organizations.

Physiotherapy is of value to maintain mobility and optimal activity. Massage, exercises, and posture and gait training have been found to be helpful, the latter particularly if propulsion or retropulsion is present. Falls are a particular problem in patients with parkinsonism, and physical and occupational therapy assessment is valuable and can provide gait training and appropriate ambulation aids to prevent these complications.

Many patients with Parkinson's disease benefit from deferring protein intake until the evening meal. This phenomenon is due to the fact that certain amino acids, the components of proteins, compete with levodopa for metabolism in the brain. Therefore all medications for parkinson's disease lose some effectiveness if taken with protein. Patients with fluctuations in their response to antiparkinsonian medications often benefit from a low-protein diet. Ordinarily the total protein content of breakfast and lunch is restricted to under 5 gm, and the remaining daily protein requirement (usually 50 to 100 gm) is eaten after 6 PM. There is little clinical evidence that any vitamin supplements help patients with Parkinson's disease.

Simple things, such as eating more fruits and vegetables, are best. Bran cereals are good unless the subject is taking levodopa, although patients should be careful about adding milk to their cereal because of the protein content. Commercial psyllium or methylcellulose compounds can also be helpful, but some of these compounds contain a lot of sugar. Docusate compounds are marketed as stool softeners and can be added to the above therapies. It is best to avoid laxatives such as cascara or senna because their effectiveness tends to wane with continued use and side effects can be severe.

Drug Therapy

Drug therapy is based on the observation that dopamine is depleted in the nigrostriatal tracts and the excitatory cholinergic effects are relatively increased.

Anticholinergic drugs such as trihexyphenidyl at 2 to 6 mg/day, benztropine at 0.5 to 4 mg/day, procyclidine at 2.5 to 5 mg tid, and orphenadrine at 100 to 300 mg/day are recommended. Antihistamine drugs such as diphenhydramine are used with variable results; they have more effect on the tremor than on rigidity or akinesia. If these drugs are used for any time they must not be stopped abruptly or a rebound effect with increased symptoms may occur.

Selegiline, a monoamine oxidase inhibitor (MAOI), reduces the metabolism of levodopa, the uptake of dopamine at synapses, and the production of free radicals. As an adjunctive therapy, it reduces motor fluctuations and may delay the onset of disability, but it requires a reduction in the dose of levodopa to prevent dyskinesias or hallucinations. The dose is fixed at 5 mg in the morning and again at midday. At present, this drug's place in the management of the disease is still undetermined.

Amantadine hydrochloride is less effective than levodopa in improving symptoms but is relatively free of serious side effects. It may be used alone or in conjunction with levodopa. It was originally developed and prescribed as an antiviral agent and its method of action in Parkinson's disease is unclear. Amantadine is given in oral doses of 100 mg one to two times daily. Its action on bradykinesia, rigidity, and gait disturbance is rapid but decreases over a few months. Significant side effects are not common, but depression, confusion, hypotension, and cardiac failure can occur. If patients stay on amantadine for a long time they will usually develop mottling of the skin of their lower legs (livedo reticularis) with some ankle swelling.

Propranolol (best given as the long-acting preparation at 60 to 240 mg/day) reduces the tremor and some of the psychologic effects of anxiety but is contraindicated in patients with concomitant cardiac failure or bronchospasm.

Tricyclic drugs such as amitriptyline may increase activity and lighten the frequently added depression; nocturnal antihistamines (e.g., diphenhydramine) are sedative, dry up secretions, and reduce tremor slightly.

All of the above agents can be considered before levodopa is given and may be given concurrently.

The subcutaneous injection of apomorphine (a dopamine receptor agonist) reduces parkinsonian signs, fluctuations in response, and the unpleasant features of the "off" periods. A self-injection regimen, in which the invariable nausea caused by this agent is controlled by domperidone, is occasionally used.

There are three classes of drugs more or less specific for the treatment of Parkinson's disease.

Levodopa. A combination drug such as Sinemet, levodopa plus carbidopa, which inhibits dopa-decarboxylase and diminishes the extracerebral breakdown of levodopa, is a most effective agent. It should be started at a small dose (one 100/10 mg tablet bid) and slowly increased to a qid or 4-hourly dose when the patient starts to respond. The average dose is one 250/25 tablet tid. If the effect is variable during the day, with swings in response and a tendency for the effects of the drug to wear off before the time for the next dose, the controlled-release preparation should be used; the dosage increased; the frequency of doses increased (e.g., to every 3 or even 2 hours); or an agonist added. The long-acting preparations are often preferable to the standard formulation.

Long-term results over the years have not been encouraging because the symptoms progress despite continued therapy. It has been suggested that the prescription of levodopa should be delayed and not given on diagnosis because it appears to lose its effect after a few years. It has also been observed that many patients on long-term levodopa develop significant mental changes, although this may be due either to the therapy or to the natural history of the disease. Thus the question of when to start treatment with levodopa is vexing. In favor of early treatment is the likelihood that the patient would maintain a better quality of life, for example being able to continue to work during the latter part of his or her career, or to carry out more leisure activities and hobbies. In addition, mortality may be less in patients treated early with levodopa. On the other hand, the spectre of chronic levodopa neurotoxicity has been raised to account for that loss of efficacy and increase in side effects (especially dyskinesias) commonly seen as the disease progresses.

It has been estimated that the drug loses a third of its effect in two thirds of patients within 3 years. Because dyskinesias are most likely to develop in young-onset Parkinson's disease patients, levodopa is generally not prescribed for those age 40 years or less.

The main early complications of levodopa are nausea caused by stimulation of the vomiting center in the brain and possible direct gastric irritation; postural hypotension; anorexia; depression and confusion; abnormal movements such as retrocollis, dystonic postures, and akathisia; and cardiac arrhythmias. After long-term therapy with levodopa, an "on-off" effect, with variability in the signs and symptoms throughout the day, may be seen in which an abrupt increase of symptoms such as freezing or rigidity occurs as the serum levels of levodopa decline. In many patients dyskinesias also occur at the time when the highest drug levels are attained, usually 2 to 3 hours after ingestion. Reduction of the dose or addition of an agonist or an anticholinergic may reduce these involuntary movements. End-of-dose deterioration (wearing off), fatigue, and loss of efficacy of the drug are other problems, usually appearing after 3 to 5 years of use. The former may be helped by changing to the controlled-release preparation, by the addition of a COMT inhibitor or dopamine agonist, or by reducing the spacing between doses of levodopa. All such problems support the view that levodopa should not be used until it is really needed.

A less common complication is hip fracture caused by over-enthusiastic resumption of physical activity as the benefits of levodopa therapy appear. The formerly publicized aphrodisiac effect of the drug is probably due mainly to an increase in physical freedom rather than to stimulation of sexual appetites. In all patients given levodopa in any form, protein intake should be concentrated in the evenings because of the reduction in available dopamine when given with protein, and foods high in pyridoxine (an antagonist to levodopa) should be restricted.

Dopa-Receptor Agonists. Direct dopamine D2 receptor agonists stimulate striatal receptors without affecting dopamine metabolism. In early or mild Parkinson's disease, these agents have been used as monotherapy, and in more advanced disease they enhance the effects of levodopa. As well as improving the overall effect of the levadopa, they can also reduce motor fluctuations. Four agents are currently available—bromocriptine, pergolide, pramipexole, and ropinirole—each with a unique profile in terms of its effects on D1, noradrenergic, and serotonergic receptor activity. One common practice is to start patients with low-dose levodopa (up to about 600 mg/day) and to add an agonist when control of symptoms is lost. Another is to start with the agonist, adding levodopa when its effect is inadequate.

Bromocriptine may reduce some of the long-term complications of levodopa, but when it is used the dosage of levodopa will need to be reduced by 10% to 50% over many weeks, or toxicity may be expected. Initial dosages should be low (2.5 mg once a day), slowly increasing by 2.5 mg weekly to a maintenance dosage of 5 mg three times a day, although side effects such as hypotension, dyskinesia, and hallucinations are to be expected in most cases at the highest dose.

Ropinirole should be given at 0.25 mg tid and increased by 0.25 mg/day each week to a maximum of 24 mg/day in divided doses. This agent is not related to ergot, so it has a good side-effect profile.

Pergolide is a longer-acting drug; it is begun at 0.05 mg per day and increased weekly to a maximum of 9 mg/day.

Pramipexole can be prescribed as monotherapy or as adjunctive treatment to carbidopa/levodopa for all stages of Parkinson's disease and may be helpful for levodopa-induced motor fluctuations. The initial dose should be 0.125 mg tid and increased weekly by 0.125 mg/day to a maximal dosage of about 4.5 mg/day. This dopamine agonist binds only to the dopamine receptors and stimulates the D2 subfamily of receptors. Again, it is not related to ergot, so it has a good side-effect profile; the occurrence of somnolence, nausea, and hallucinations is not significantly different from that resulting from placebo use.

Cabergoline is a new dopamine agonist that has a longer duration of action than the currently available drugs in this class. Cabergoline is currently used to treat certain endocrine disorders and is not yet approved for Parkinson's disease.

Drugs Delaying Levodopa Metabolism. Two catecholamine-O-methyl transferase inhibitor agents increase the bioavailability of levodopa. Entacapone acts primarily extracerebrally and will soon be available. The dose is one 200 mg tablet with each levodopa dose. Tolcapone (100 to 200 mg tid) acts both extracerebrally and intracerebrally and inhibits the metabolism of dopamine within the brain, but it has been withdrawn from the market because of the occurrence of hepatic necrosis as a rare side effect and is now available only after administrative supplication. Both agents reduce motor fluctuations and daily levodopa requirements.

Other Agents

Some patients with Parkinson's disease who cannot tolerate levodopa because of intolerable psychiatric side effects, such as hallucinations, paranoia, or confusion, may benefit from neuroleptic medications such as clozapine or olanzapine, both of which have a slight beneficial effect on parkinsonian symptoms as well as an antipsychotic effect. Traditional neuroleptic medications are usually avoided in patients with Parkinson's disease because of their induction of unwanted motor effects.

Patients with hallucinations or psychotic features may respond well to risperidone at 0.5 to 4 mg/day or to clozapine, an antipsychotic that has significant depressant effects on the bone marrow that necessitate frequent hematologic monitoring.

Surgery

Surgical interventions in advanced Parkinson's disease include destruction or high-frequency stimulation of the thalamic nuclei, the globus pallidus, the subthalamic nucleus, or the ventrointermediate thalamic nucleus. The latter procedures require electrode implantation into the brain and are used for patients with an inadequate response to traditional antiparkinsonian therapy and in those with severe symptoms before the age of 40.

Thalamotomy is primarily beneficial for uncontrolled tremor but does not affect the bradykinesia, which is the single most disabling symptom of all. Although safe and effective in an experienced neurosurgeon's hand, ventrolateral thalamotomy is accompanied by significant morbidity, especially when done bilaterally, and it has been performed much less frequently since the advent of levodopa.

Unilateral pallidotomy can improve the duration of "off" periods, tremor, dyskinesias, and the daily levodopa requirement. Major morbidity and mortality are less than 1%, but side effects include visual field deficits, intracerebral hemorrhage, and behavioral changes.

We regard the experimental grafting of autologous adrenal tissue, fetal extracts, and other tissues into the basal ganglia as effective stimuli for further research into other methods of therapy.

WILSON'S DISEASE (HEPATOLENTICULAR DEGENERATION)

Early in this century a "pseudosclerosis" was described with changes in the lenticular (putaminal and pallidal) nuclei of the basal ganglia. In 1902 Kayser described the characteristic golden brown corneal ring, and the next year Fleischer noted the association with pseudosclerosis. In 1912 Kinnear Wilson noted the association with cirrhosis of the liver. Eventually it became clear that this disorder was due to accumulation of copper in the affected areas due to a genetic deficiency of ceruloplasmin, the enzyme that binds copper.

Wilson's disease is an autosomal recessive genetic disease with a prevalence of one in 35,000 in the population. One in a hundred people carry the abnormal gene, which has been assigned by linkage analysis to the esterase D locus on chromosome 13.

The disease usually begins in the teen years, and rarely after age 30. Tremor and slowness of movement (bradykinesia) in the tongue, lips, and larynx are early symptoms, causing dysarthria and dysphagia, and there may be a wing-beating tremor, chorea, or dystonia of the limbs. Some patients look Parkinsonian, but the involvement follows a different spread, moving from the bulbar muscles and later to the limbs, and in a very young person. As the disease progresses they become slower, rigid, and with a fixed facies, drooling, and mental deterioration. A Kayser-Fleischer ring can be seen in each cornea, best seen with a slit lamp.

Laboratory investigation shows a low serum ceruloplasmin level (below 20 mg/dl), low serum copper, increased copper excretion, high copper in the liver biopsy, and abnormal liver function tests. The CT and MRI will show widened brain sulci, slightly enlarged ventricles, and hypodensity in the posterior lenticular nuclei, with changes in the subcortical white matter, midbrain, pons, and cerebellum.

Treatment must be started early to avoid permanent damage, which is preventable. Copper intake is restricted to less than 1 mg/day by avoidance of copper-rich foods (liver, cocoa, chocolate, mushrooms, nuts, shellfish) and giving an agent to deplete copper, such as D-penicillamine (with supplementary pryidoxine to avoid anemia), zinc acetate, or triethylene tetramine (trientene). If instituted early, all changes can reverse. Some patients may show initial worsening when the drugs are instituted, perhaps because of release of a lot of copper into the system. Treatment is lifelong.

ADDITIONAL READINGS

Adams RD, Victor M: *Principles of neurology,* ed 5, New York, 1993, McGraw-Hill.

Lang AE, Lozano AM: Parkinson's disease, *N Engl J Med* 339:1044-1053, 1130-1143, 1998.

Olanow CW, Koller WC: An algorithm (decision tree) for the management of parkinson's disease: treatment guidelines, *Neurology* 50(3)Suppl 3;S1-S57, 1998.

Stern MB: Parkinson's disease, *Neurology* 49(Suppl 1) S2-S9, 1997.

Waters CH: *The diagnosis and management of parkinson's disease,* Los Angeles, 1998, Professional Communications, Inc.

Wilson SAK: Progressive lenticular degeneration: a familial nervous system disease associated with cirrhosis of the liver, *Brain* 34:1295, 1912.

CHAPTER 170

Amyotrophic Lateral Sclerosis

T. Jock Murray

William Pryse-Phillips

Amyotrophic lateral sclerosis (ALS) is also called the motor neuron disease, or Lou Gehrig's disease after the baseball player who died of the disease in 1941 (Box 170-1). In ALS, the anterior horn cells and corticospinal tracts are usually affected at many levels, although a few patients have clinical manifestations of involvement at only one level.

According to the pattern of involvement, different names have been employed, e.g., *progressive muscular atrophy* (anterior horn cell degeneration only); *primary lateral sclerosis* (pyramidal tract degeneration only); *progressive bulbar palsy* (brainstem motor nuclear degeneration); and

Box 170-1. Who Was Lou Gehrig?

ALS has become known to the public as Lou Gehrig's disease. Lou Gehrig was one of the greatest baseball players of all time, a New York Yankee from 1923 to 1939, until his career was stopped by a progressive neurologic disease. Nicknamed "the Iron Man," the "Iron Horse," and "the Pride of the Yankees," he was on his way to surpassing Babe Ruth for many records when his game seemed to go into a slump, starting in 1938 and noticed by all in 1939. In an emotional tribute to his impressive career and his stature as a respected sportsman, he told a packed Yankee Stadium that he felt he was the luckiest man alive. Although the illness took his life in June 1941 at the age of 38, he has become the symbol not only for ALS but also for hope and strength by those who suffer with the disease.

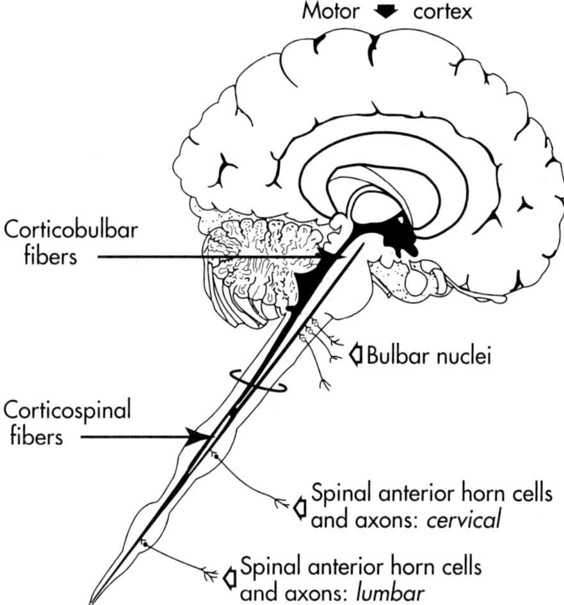

Fig. 170-1. Sites of the lesions in ALS. (From Pryse-Phillips WM, Murray TJ: *Essential neurology: a concise textbook,* New York, 1992, Medical Examination Publishing, p 660.)

pseudobulbar palsy. The most common picture, however, is a mixture of these features: the patient has both upper and lower motor neuron signs and symptoms often with bulbar involvement as well. Because the disease eventually generalizes to involve both upper and lower motor neurons at both cranial and spinal levels, many authors use the term *ALS* for all forms. At death, some patients who have had clinical evidence of degeneration at only one level may show pathologic changes at other levels not evident clinically.

PATHOLOGY

The pathologic features are primarily degeneration of motor cells in the spinal cord, brainstem, and to a lesser extent the cerebral cortex, with secondary degeneration of pyramidal tracts. The anterior horn cells and pyramidal tracts are more or less severely affected; the cellular destruction is greatest in the cervical and lumbar regions of the cord (Fig. 170-1). There is some diffuse loss of myelin in all areas of the spinal cord except the posterior columns, but the loss in the pyramidal tracts is striking, giving the cord a characteristic picture on myelin staining.

In the brainstem, degeneration occurs in the motor nuclei of the cranial nerves but the three oculomotor nuclei are spared; this feature is worthy of careful investigation, as we might learn more about this enigmatic disease from the few nuclei that are never involved than the many that usually are. Degeneration is found in the pyramidal tracts and sometimes in other fiber tracts in the brainstem. Pyramidal degeneration can be traced into the internal capsule in about one-half of cases, and in one-third the number of Betz cells in the motor cortex is decreased and there is a variable loss of medium-sized motor cortical cells.

CLINICAL FEATURES

The overall incidence of ALS is 2 per 100,000 population. The onset is usually between the ages of 50 and 70 years, and twice as many men develop the disease as women. The disease appears as a dominant character in some families. It accounts for 1 in 1000 deaths.

Although ALS is a disease of the motor neurons and the findings are entirely motor, secondary degeneration in nerves and muscles may give rise to vague pains and paresthesias in a quarter of the patients, particularly at the onset of the disease, but the clinical findings will be entirely motor. Most patients first notice weakness in their legs or arms, sometimes mentioning atrophy as well but seldom commenting on fasciculations (Box 170-2).

In *progressive muscular atrophy* the clinical features are those of degeneration of the anterior horn cells of the spinal cord. The patient notes weakness in the hands and legs, and on examination is found to have atrophy of the small muscles of the hands and of the more distal muscles of the arms and legs. Fasciculations can be seen in these areas and often over the shoulder girdle, trunk, tongue, and face as well. Although about 20% of patients show this picture at the onset, in only 8% does it remain as a "pure form" throughout the course of the disease. Other causes that must be ruled out include hexosaminidase A deficiency, multifocal motor neuropathy, and inherited adult-onset spinal muscular atrophies (Box 170-3).

In *primary lateral sclerosis* the manifestations are of pyramidal tract degeneration, with weakness and spasticity of the legs and later of the arms. Hyperactive muscle stretch reflexes including the jaw jerk, palmomental and pouting reflexes, and Hoffmann's and Babinski's signs are commonly found. This is a difficult diagnosis, however, as many more common causes of paraplegia must first be excluded. Although the existence of this rare form has been disputed, cases have been confirmed by autopsy.

In *progressive bulbar palsy* the degeneration is primarily of the motor nuclei of the brainstem. The patient complains of slurred speech and later has difficulty in swallowing and coughing, so aspiration is a constant danger. There are atrophy and fasciculations of the tongue, poor palatal movement, and sometimes fasciculations and weakness of the facial muscles. Although less than 10% of cases have pure progressive bulbar palsy, most ALS patients show some bulbar involvement eventually. Pseudobulbar palsy can also

Box 170-2. Signs and Symptoms of ALS

Lower Motor Signs

Muscle weakness
Fasciculations
Dyspnea
Atrophy
Slurred speech
Muscle cramps
Fatigue
Swallowing difficulty

Upper Motor Signs

Weakness
Babinski's sign
Pseudobulbar palsy
Spasticity
Dysarthria
Swallowing difficulty
Hyperactive reflexes
Pathologic laughing and crying
Fatigue

Absent Features

Sensory signs
Bowel and bladder symptoms
Dementia
Pain

Box 170-3. Conditions That May Mimic ALS

Myasthenia gravis
Cervical myelopathy
Multifocal motor neuropathy
Hexosaminidase A deficiency
Hypoparathyroidism
Inclusion body myositis
Bulbospinal neuronopathy (Kennedy's syndrome)
Lymphoma
Postradiation syndrome

occur with signs of spastic weakness of the bulbar muscles, but no evidence of an upper motor neuron lesion elsewhere.

Amyotrophic lateral sclerosis (ALS) is the term applied to the most common form, in which there is evidence of both anterior horn cell and pyramidal degeneration, usually at both bulbar and spinal levels. On examination these patients have atrophy, weakness, and fasciculations in their limbs, indicating a lower motor neuron lesion, combined with hyperactive reflexes and Babinski's signs. It is this combination of upper and lower motor neuron signs in all limbs that is the hallmark of ALS.

FAMILIAL ALS

In a small number of cases (5% to 10%) there is a positive family history of ALS. One in five of those have a defective superoxide dismutase 1 (SOD1) gene. The pattern of inheritance is autosomal dominant with penetrance of up to 90% by age 70. The clinical picture is similar to sporadic ALS except that the male to female ratio is 1:1, whereas there are more males in the sporadic form, and this form occurs 10 years earlier on average. A rare juvenile-onset familial form has also been described in African families.

DIAGNOSTIC CRITERIA

The El Escorial ALS Diagnostic Criteria (1994) tried to refine the diagnosis. The system recognizes that the problem involves the peripheral and central nervous system (CNS) in four regions: bulbar, cervical, thoracic, and lumbosacral. To make the diagnosis of ALS the following should be present:

1. Progression of disease (confirmed by examinations 6 months apart).
2. Clinical and/or electrical evidence of involvement of two regions (probable ALS) or three or four regions (definite ALS).
3. No other disease that could mimic the presentation (see Box 170-3).

ASSOCIATED DISEASES

ALS has been associated with recurrent hypoglycemia, hyperthyroidism, poliomyelitis, and carcinoma, and it has also been reported in pregnancy and after gastrectomy. ALS has also been associated with acromegaly, electric shock injury, and heavy metal poisoning. With most of these conditions, the association is rare and probably coincidental. However, malignant tumors, particularly carcinoma of the lung, have been noted in about 10% of the patients. An ALS-like syndrome (postpolio syndrome) sometimes occurs many years after an episode of poliomyelitis, but this syndrome is unrelated and is much more benign. An ALS syndrome with associated parkinsonism and dementia occurs on the island of Guam.

COURSE AND PROGNOSIS

The course of the disease is variable, but the average life expectancy is 3.5 years from onset; only 20% survive over 5 years. We have seen patients who died in as short a time as 9 months, and others who had a slow course over 15 to 20 years and more, with long periods without change. To some extent, survival depends on the type of ALS but there is great variation even within the same type.

Although bulbar palsy is regarded as an ominous form of the disease, some patients survive for up to 15 years, while in contrast, other patients with this form of the disorder may die within months of developing brainstem symptoms. In general, those with bulbar palsy have a more rapid course than those with primary lateral sclerosis, in whom the prognosis is markedly better.

DIFFERENTIAL DIAGNOSIS

ALS must be differentiated from other conditions that produce a combination of upper and lower motor neuron lesions. The most obvious of these are disorders of the cervical cord, such as skull base deformities, syringomyelia, cord tumors, and cervical spondylosis. In such cases, however, there should not be any evidence of anterior horn cell involvement in the legs or trunk, but only in the upper limbs. Any signs of disease due to a lesion above the foramen magnum (such as bulbar signs or V or VII nerve involvement) would rule out a cervical cause.

Lower motor neuron lesions may be predominant with spinal arachnoiditis (usually syphilitic) and radiculitis, cervical ribs, and peripheral nerve lesions, including the postpolio syndrome previously mentioned. Weakness and wasting are typical of all forms of hereditary motor neuropathy, some of which occur first in adult life, and in hereditary motor and sensory neuropathy. The same findings, although without fasciculations, are also seen in primary muscle disease, rheumatoid arthritis, and myotonic dystrophy. If there is doubt about evidence of anterior horn cell disease in the trunk or legs, electromyography (EMG) should be able to demonstrate that which cannot be seen clinically.

LABORATORY STUDIES

Although the diagnosis is usually evident clinically, there are a few investigations that can be used to confirm the diagnosis or to rule out other diseases or associated disease. Nerve conduction studies yield results that are normal or only slightly slowed, making demyelinating neuropathies unlikely. EMG shows evidence of denervation and reduced numbers of motor unit potentials among which are giant units and polyphasic potentials, as well as fasciculations. The cerebrospinal fluid (CSF) protein is elevated, in the range of 45 to 95 mmol/L in one-third of cases. Decreased urinary creatinine and increased urinary creatine levels are found but are not useful diagnostic tests. Muscle biopsy demonstrates the characteristic features of a neurogenic muscular atrophy but is seldom needed, unless a condition such as inclusion body myositis is suspected.

Investigations should be undertaken to rule out underlying malignancy if there is any atypical feature on examination or investigation, such as marked slowing of motor nerve conduction velocities. Cervical myelopathy can look like ALS if cord compression is combined with root involvement. The lower motor neuron findings are only in the arms, an important diagnostic feature, and this situation can be confirmed by imaging of the cervical cord and using EMG to show fasciculations in the legs. Most other mimics can be excluded by history (hereditary neuropathy; prior gastrectomy, polio, or electrical injury); by examination (hyperthyroidism, acromegaly); or by laboratory tests (lead or other metal poisoning, recurrent hypoglycemia, hexosaminidase deficiency, and anti-GM_1 ganglioside antibody if multifocal neuropathy is suspected).

MANAGEMENT

Treatment of this disease is disappointing, despite some new agents that may make a slight difference in the course of the progression. Riluzole (Rilutek), a glutamate-blocking agent, has shown a statistical improvement in the rate of progression, but this is of minor clinical significance since the difference translates to a prolongation of death by 3 months or so. Despite its minor effect, the release of this drug, the first to make any difference in the disease, has had a much greater effect on the sense of hope for these patients, who have had little before. A number of other agents are under study, but none as yet has shown much promise. With such first steps, however, there is always the hope of the next steps.

Other studies have suggested some effect from brain-derived neurotrophic factor (BDNF), insulin-like growth factor (IGF-1), and gabapentin, but further trial and experience are required to assess whether they have any place in the treatment of this disease.

Despite limited therapy for the underlying disease, help with the major symptoms of ALS can be offered in the following, which outlines some of the approaches to symptomatic therapy:

Slurring, Choking, and Drooling. Anticholinergics can dry secretions, and paradoxically, neostigmine may be helpful to increase muscle power temporarily. The patient should decide how liquid his food should be, and how large the mouthfuls. Cricopharyngeal myotomy can be performed to aid swallowing.

Involuntary Limb Jerks. Phenytoin, carbamazepine, baclofen, and clonazepam may be helpful.

Cramps and Aching Limb Pains. Quinine, phenytoin, or carbamazepine may be helpful, but major pain is usually not a problem.

Insomnia and Problems Turning in Bed. Special beds can be leased or borrowed. Family and friends may organize a roster of people to sleep over, sparing the spouse from waking every 3 hours to turn the patient.

Frustration and Boredom. Family and volunteers can be mobilized from neighborhood groups, such as church or social groups, to visit to talk, listen, play cards, turn pages or read, or just to be there for a while. Occupational therapists can advise on a number of communications aids.

Motility and Posture. Occupational therapy assessment can be arranged for the home environment, providing rails, hoists, or supports; eliminating stairs where possible; and advising on helpful devices for feeding, shaving, dressing, recreation, and ambulation. Posture may be improved with a collar, a brace, or spring-loaded splints.

Leg Swelling. The legs should be elevated, and elastic stockings used if leg swelling is a problem. Avoid using diuretics for leg swelling.

Cachexia. As mentioned, swallowing can be improved, but a nasogastric tube may become necessary when weakness and atrophy advance. Gastrotomy can be used but often just adds misery to the last days of the patient.

Constipation. Constipation is due to weak abdominal muscles and reduced activity. Bulk purgatives, laxatives, and enemas are helpful. Avoid manual evacuations if possible.

Sexual Frustration. Sexual frustration is common and is not often discussed. The clinician should do so freely and without embarrassment with both the patient and spouse; the problems are mainly matters of method. The partner may need counseling to understand that he or she needs to take the active role and to learn effective techniques that overcome weakness and muscle spasms.

Pneumonia. Respiratory infections become a risk as chest movement is restricted and the patient is bedridden.

Treatment is as for any patient, but there comes a time when this may fail because of the respiratory failure.

Respiratory Failure. When there are early signs of respiratory failure the patient may be made more comfortable, especially at night, by noninvasive positive pressure ventilation (NIPPV) methods such as bi-level positive air pressure (BiPAP). Tracheotomy and machine ventilation may become necessary. The clinician should not embark on measures that only prolong distress, unless the patient clearly wishes to prolong the course of the disease. With a tracheostomy and ventilator the patient may have a year of passive, uncommunicating existence, and that may be important to him or her, but many do not wish this. It is crucial to determine if the patient is willing to accept this state well before it occurs, by means of early discussions and by having a living will. The patient should appoint a trusted person to act with power of attorney on his or her behalf.

Management of problems such as these demands a team approach, but the team has to be led by someone who can identify the needs, prescribe for them, and coordinate their delivery. Ideally, that person should be a physician but a rehabilitation specialist is not always available. The patient's primary care physician is perhaps best of all for he or she is available, knows the family, and can properly take the responsibility for relieving the symptoms and suffering during the course of the disease. The primary care physician can comfort the patient to the end.

The Multidisciplinary Approach

The management of an ALS patient through the course of the disease requires many professionals with diverse backgrounds and skills, each bringing important components to the overall care (Table 170-1).

At the outset the primary care physician should recognize that the patient has a progressing neurologic disease and refer the patient to a neurologist for confirmation of the diagnosis. The neurologist is responsible for the neurologic assessment and the EMG tests that confirm the diagnosis. The neurologist is often the best person to explain the diagnosis, the nature of the disease and its meaning to the life of the patient, and expectations for the future. The neurologist will usually administer the initial treatments, explain research on therapies, and explain the availability of any clinical trials. There may be a multidisciplinary ALS clinic in the area to begin to coordinate the care.

The nurse coordinator in the ALS clinic is usually responsible for coordinating care and involvement of other health professionals, but in other settings where such a clinic is not available the primary care physician usually is responsible for this role. Other professionals who are needed as the disease progresses are a physical therapist, an occupational therapist, a dietitian, a speech pathologist, and a social worker. Since the weakness affects pulmonary function, a pulmonologist becomes very important. A counselor and spiritual advisor may be needed, if wished by the patient and family, and early involvement is recommended in most instances.

Table 170-1. Multidisciplinary Approach to ALS Care

Problem	Approach
Weakness	Physical therapy Exercise program
Ambulation	Braces and walking aids Battery-operated scooter or wheelchair
Depression	Physician counseling Antidepressants Psychiatrist or psychologist Family counseling
Activities of daily living	Occupational therapist Adaptive devices
Home assistance	Home health aids Health service agencies
Swallowing difficulty	Swallowing evaluation Speech pathologist or physical therapist Surgical gastrostomy
Pulmonary failure	Periodic forced vital capacity measurement Positive pressure ventilation Tracheostomy and ventilator
Advanced directives	Durable power of attorney for health care Living will
Pain	Analgesics and physical therapy Antispasticity agents

End-of-Life Care

Every patient with ALS and their families have to come to grips with the many end-of-life decisions that confront them. These include the need to get the many events in life in order, come to terms with relationships, and decide how forthcoming disabilities will be handled. Should a ventilator be used if it just prolongs the inevitable? If it is used, will there be other decisions about how and who would discontinue the ventilator at the end? When nursing care increases, will care be at home or in a nursing facility? Should there be an advance directive? A living will? Power of attorney? Patients may raise the question of suicide or assisted suicide, and the physician should be comfortable not only talking about these issues but also calling on others who may have more expertise and experience in discussing these issues. It makes things more difficult for the patient and family if the physician avoids these sensitive areas and talks only about the disease and medical management.

Further information can be found at The ALS Association, 21021 Ventura Blvd, Suite 321, Woodlawn Hills, California 91364-2206, USA.

In addition, information on ALS resources can be found in the *Cleveland Clinic ALS Care Manual,* 1996; write to the ALS Coordinator, CCF—Department of Neurology, 9500 Euclid Avenue, Cleveland, Ohio 44195, USA.

A group of acknowledged experts on ALS (Mitsumoto et al) prepared a state-of-the-art summary of ALS for the continuing education program of the American Academy of Neurology, which was extensively used in the preparation of this chapter. See Additional Readings for details.

ADDITIONAL READINGS

Brooks BR: El Escorial World Federation of Neurology criteria for the diagnosis of amyotrophic lateral sclerosis, *J Neurol Sci* 124(suppl):96-107, 1994.

Mitsumoto H, Norris FH, editors: Amyotrophic lateral sclerosis: a comprehensive guide to management, New York, 1994, Demos Publications.

Mitsumoto H, Cwik VA, Neville H, et al: *Motor neuron diseases:* CONTINUUM, *Am Acad Neurol* 3:48-77, 1997.
Mitsumoto H, Chad DA, Pioro EP: *Amyotrophic lateral sclerosis* Philadelphia, 1996, F.A. Davis Co.
Rowland LP, editor: *Amyotrophic lateral sclerosis and other motor neuron diseases,* New York, 1991, Raven Press.
Williams DB, Windebank AJ: Motor neuron disease (amyotrophic lateral sclerosis), *Mayo Clin Proc* 66:54-82, 1991.
Yuen EC, Mobley WC: Therapeutic potential of neurotrophic factors for neurological disorders, *Ann Neurol* 40:346-354, 1996.

CHAPTER 171

Multiple Sclerosis

T. Jock Murray
William Pryse-Phillips

Multiple sclerosis (MS) is a recurrent and progressive neurologic disorder characterized by signs and symptoms due to plaques of demyelination in the white matter of the brain, brainstem, and spinal cord of the central nervous system (CNS). Magnetic resonance imaging (MRI) scans demonstrated that there is continuing activity even though the patient is unaware of new symptoms. Although MS is defined as a demyelinating disease, it is the changes in the blood-brain barrier that initiate new lesions, and axonal damage is likely responsible for progression.

PATHOLOGY

The plaques of demyelination within the CNS are characterized by breakdown of myelin, perivascular edema and inflammation, and later gliosis (scarring). The axons are preserved initially but may be damaged eventually. Although the multifocal involvement suggests a random process, lesions tend to occur in the brainstem and periventricular regions and within the thickly myelinated areas of the brainstem (e.g., medial longitudinal fasciculi). Such lesions may occur suddenly and then apparently heal, perhaps because of remyelination (thin layers of new myelin being formed by oligodendrocytes) and compensation. The remyelinated nerves conduct more slowly, as shown in evoked-potential studies, and are likely to show conduction block with heat. Thus symptoms that have disappeared can reappear with a hot bath or exercise or on a hot, humid day.

EPIDEMIOLOGY

One case of MS per 500 population probably occurs in temperate climates, where the disease has an incidence rate of about 5 per 100,000, but due to its chronicity, prevalence is high, about 200 per 100,000. MS occurs rarely in children or the elderly; most patients develop their first symptoms between ages 20 and 40, with 30 the average age of onset. The disease is two to three times more common in women.

Latitudes

The most intriguing finding in the epidemiology of MS is the increasing prevalence at latitudes farthest from the equator, both north and south. Thus it is a rare disease in tropical countries but is a common serious neurologic disorder in the northern United States, Canada, Great Britain, and central Europe. Isolated areas of increased prevalence have been found in New England, the Orkney Islands, Washington State, Nova Scotia, and Alaska.

Migration Studies

Migration studies have demonstrated that the risk factor in MS is carried along if a person moves from an area of high incidence to one of low incidence. Conversely, if one moves from an area of low incidence to an area of high incidence, one takes on the greater risk of the new country, but this is age related; a critical age of 15 years has been calculated, suggesting that some environmental risk factor for developing MS may be acquired at about the time of puberty. Studies of migration to Israel suggested that the disease has an incubation period of 3 to 23 years.

Many factors have been considered to explain the world distribution of MS, including temperature, solar radiation, local infections, diet, and other environmental factors, but none is convincing. Under consideration is the role of genetic factors, because the concordance rate in identical twins is about 40% but is about 5% for fraternal twins and nontwin siblings. Some suggest that the disease originated in central Europe and that the world distribution corresponds to the areas to which these peoples migrated. Degenerative, vascular, biochemical, infectious, and allergic theories explain MS. Although a viral infection might explain the disease trigger and continuation in a susceptible person, no virus has been isolated consistently, and only weak evidence suggests Epstein-Barr virus (EBV), canine distemper viruses, measles, and herpesvirus type 6. A slow virus with a long incubation period, causing progressive neurologic deficits many years later, would be a plausible explanation, but all transmission experiments have been negative. Different viruses may initiate demyelination in predisposed patients, because it was noted that MS populations have slightly elevated levels of antibody to various viruses compared with control groups. However, this may merely reflect abnormalities in the immune system.

An immunologic reaction in the CNS mediates the neurologic events, as shown by assessment of the cerebrospinal fluid (CSF) and by examination of the plaques. In the CSF the gamma globulin fraction is increased; this appears to be active antibody produced within the CNS, appearing as oligoclonal IgG bands on CSF immunoelectrophoresis.

Genetics

About 20% of patients with MS have a family history of this disorder, which is strong evidence for genetic influences in MS. A first-degree relative of an MS patient has about a 2% risk of also developing the disease, about 10 times the risk in the normal population. In identical twins the risk is one in three, but still not 100%, so some environmental factor must also be involved. HLA typing in MS patients has shown an overrepresentation of the A3, B7, Dw2, and DR2 haplotypes. A person seems genetically predisposed to the disease; then another factor determines whether they develop the clinical picture of MS.

Clinical Course

The following categories are usually defined in the course of MS.

Relapsing-remitting MS. Patients with relapsing-remitting MS have discrete motor, sensory, cerebellar, or visual attacks that come on over 1 to 2 weeks, resolving in 4 to 8 weeks.

Relapsing-progressive MS. Patients with relapsing-progressive MS have attacks but eventually have progression of disability, with or without continuing attacks.

Progressive-relapsing MS. Patients with progressive-relapsing MS begin with a slowly progressive course, then have attacks occasionally during their course. Ninety percent of patients with these latter two forms eventually go on to primary progressive MS.

Primary Progressive MS. Primary progressive MS is characterized by progressive worsening without periods of stability. The primary form has no initial relapsing-remitting course, as does the secondary form. The primary form has less female preponderance, affects mainly middle-aged males, and involves especially the cervical or thoracic cord. Visual and sensory symptoms are less common. MRI studies show less "activity" and "disease burden," and more axonal loss. The prognosis is worse. The disorder may differ fundamentally from the usual forms of MS.

Stable MS. In stable MS there is no clinical disease activity nor worsening of state in the previous 12 months. When this is obtained for over 10 to 15 years, the term *benign MS* is sometimes used, even though these patients usually show some progression late in the course of the disease.

Attacks and Remissions. By the end of the first 5 years it is usually clear which pattern the patient's disease is following, although it may take much longer to know whether the course will continue to be benign. About 80% of patients begin as relapsing-remitting, but by 5 years, half have become relapsing-progressive. Most frequently an attack occurs without any obvious precipitant, but two factors have been shown to be related to attacks: acute infections and the 6-month postpartum period. Patients often relate an exacerbation of the disease to physical or emotional stress, but little evidence indicates that these are related; this may reflect only the attempt of patients to find some reason for an attack. Although there is a 70% increase in attacks in the 6-months postpartum over a 9-month period without pregnancy, a similar 70% decrease in attacks occurs during the pregnancy itself. Again, most attacks occur without any evident cause, and the mechanism is undoubtedly internal.

The course varies in individual patients. An occasional patient has an acute onset with a rapidly progressive course to disability within a few months (Marburg disease) or years. Most patients have a much more benign course, however, and may remain functioning normally 30 years later. The most common pattern, particularly among those with onset in early adulthood, is acute attacks and remissions that slowly change to a more progressive course. When the onset is in the 40s and 50s or later, a gradual onset with a slow but relentless course, particularly of progressive paraplegia, is characteristic.

It is common for the first attack to be followed by complete remission. As attacks recur, however, more and more deficit is left. Despite this, about 10% of the patients with MS have a benign course. The prognosis is much better than previously thought, and most patients have a normal life span, although usually with disability. About 32% are functioning well at work 10 years after the onset of the disease. At 25 years, 75% of patients were alive in one study, and two thirds of the original group were still able to walk.

Clinical Features

MS is a condition with a multiplicity of lesions and a variable course, but it is progressive over the long term. A *monosymptomatic* onset occurs in about 40% of cases, although other sites are affected within the nervous system as time progresses. Initial events that cause difficulty in diagnosis when they occur alone include the appearance of eye pain and visual impairment due to retrobulbar neuritis, vertigo, facial myokymia, facial numbness, extraocular palsy, or facial weakness, resembling Bell's palsy. Internuclear ophthalmoplegia, long tract motor or sensory signs, and Lhermitte's sign are other presentations that may occur entirely alone and recover spontaneously. Later, they are replaced by combinations of symptoms that suggest the diagnosis of MS (Box 171-1).

The scattered plaques of demyelination may affect most nerve fiber pathways in the spinal cord, brainstem, or hemispheres, but the common patterns of deficit result from lesions in the motor and sensory systems, the brainstem nuclei, and the optic nerves. Involvement of the pyramidal tract anywhere along its course results in spasticity with the characteristic findings of hyperreflexia, clonus, loss of abdominal reflexes, and Babinski's signs, eventually developing into progressive limb weakness. Cerebellar involvement typically produces nystagmus, incoordination, dysarthria, and ataxia. Numbness, tight feeling in the limbs, paresthesias, and impaired sensation are common symptoms and at the onset of MS often have a distribution similar to that of peripheral neuropathy, but the reflexes are usually increased. Involvement of the posterior columns is often associated with a Lhermitte's sign, as well as the usual diminution in vibration and joint position sense.

Any of the brainstem nuclei may be involved by the plaques of MS. Thus ocular muscle weakness is common, causing diplopia and mild facial numbness; weakness or fine rippling of the facial muscles (myokymia) may occur. Involvement of the vestibular system results in vertigo, nausea, and unsteadiness. Nystagmus is common, but an ataxic nystagmus is particularly important, greater in the

Box 171-1. Prevalence of MS Symptoms

Fatigue	88%
Walking problems	87%
Bowel/bladder problems	65%
Pain and other sensations	60%
Visual disturbances	58%
Cognitive problems	44%
Tremors	41%

Data from Aronson BGW: Interferon beta in the treatment of multiple sclerosis. In Abramsky O, Ovadia H: Proteins in multiple sclerosis: clinical research and therapy, London, UK, 1997, Martin Dunitz, pp 223-228. et al, 1996.

abducting eye and associated with poor adduction of the other eye. This *internuclear ophthalmoplegia* results from a lesion in the medial longitudinal fasciculus, which coordinates movements of all the oculomotor muscles. This common finding in MS is almost diagnostic in young people, particularly when bilateral. In patients less than 50 years old who complain of pain in the face resembling that of trigeminal neuralgia, MS should always be suspected.

The optic nerves are often involved, resulting in blurring, dimming or loss of vision, and alteration of visual fields. A common problem is acute optic neuritis (retrobulbar neuritis), presenting with pain on eye movement, blurring or loss of vision, altered visual fields, or scotomas. About 4% of patients with MS develop optic neuritis at some time, and 75% of those presenting with optic neuritis develop signs of MS. After one attack of optic neuritis, the patient is examined for evidence of any other neurologic signs and kept under watchful review.

Mental changes may occur but usually only late in the disease. Patients may note subtle problems in learning new information, identifying this as a memory problem, although memory may be normal on testing. Euphoria was once said to be the most common emotional abnormality, but depression is more common. The development of marked emotional changes in a patient with MS should always suggest demyelination involving the periventricular areas and the frontal lobes. After years, neuropsychologic testing may show intellectual changes, but these may be missed on standard tests and only recognized by tests specially designed for MS.

The quality of patients' coping skills and their attitude are very important in determining how well they manage their MS. In all patients, personal characteristics, experiences, and personality strongly affect their response. Not surprisingly, anxiety and depression may occur in these patients. Even numbness of a hand has ominous meaning for the patient. Conversion symptoms may occur and may be difficult to differentiate from another attack of demyelination. A mistaken diagnosis of "hysteria" is often made in these patients because the fleeting signs of MS are not recognized.

Grand mal seizures occur in about 6% of MS patients during the course of the disease. They respond well to the usual anticonvulsants. Patients with bilateral corticospinal lesions may have a spastic bladder, with complaints of urgency, frequency, and incontinence. Such symptoms may be caused by detrusor muscle or sphincter spasticity, dyssynergia of these, or some other change; a full urologic assessment is required to choose appropriate therapy. Impotence occurs in about half the men with MS, usually in association with progressing spasticity. When this first occurs, a strong psychogenic reaction is common.

LABORATORY TESTS AND DIAGNOSTIC PROCEDURES

MS is a diagnosis made clinically or by autopsy, but some tests support the presence of plaques of demyelination throughout the CNS with accompanying immunologic changes. MRI scans may show scattered lesions in the white matter as a result of inflammation with swelling and subsequent demyelination. The CSF may contain increased gamma globulins, often in an oligoclonal band pattern, indicating immunologic activity. Evoked-potential tests may show slowing of conduction in the optic nerves, the auditory system, or the posterior columns, but these are all nonspecific in that such impaired conduction may also be caused by other conditions. The most definitive diagnostic method is still the clinical assessment, and tests merely support or confirm the diagnosis.

Cerebrospinal Fluid Findings

Until MRI provided better and noninvasive test results in confirming MS, tests of CSF were sometimes helpful. Cell counts are usually in the normal range, although up to 30% of samples may contain increased lymphocytes. About half the patients show slight elevation of total CSF protein, usually 0.45 to 0.70 gm/L, and again about half have an increase in the CSF IgG; a greater than 13% increase in total CSF protein supports a diagnosis of MS. The test's accuracy is compromised by the need to concentrate the CSF. An improvement in gamma globulin assessment is the technique of oligoclonal banding of the CSF protein, which may be positive in up to 90% of "definite" cases in a laboratory with experience. Unfortunately the "possible MS" cases most require an accurate test, and patients with "possible MS" often have a negative test. The level of myelin basic protein may measure the degree of demyelination activity, but this test is nonspecific and not routinely done.

Scanning Techniques

MRI is a powerful noninvasive tool assisting in the diagnosis of MS, showing scattered white matter lesions in about 90% of cases of confirmed MS. Few of these lesions are visible even on an enhanced computed tomography (CT) scan. MRI is the best test to confirm a clinical suspicion and is now done routinely (Box 171-2). If the patient is known to have MS, however, MRI is of little value because treatment approaches should not be altered based on whether the scan shows few or many lesions. In clinical trials of the interferons and glatiramer (Copaxone) the MRI has shown that the number of new lesions can be dramatically reduced, but these findings do not correlate well with the patient's clinical condition. Care must be taken in the interpretation of lesions seen in the white matter, since they are not pathognomonic of MS and can be seen in ischemia and other conditions (Box 171-3).

Evoked-potential Tests

When demyelination lesions remyelinate, with variable gliosis, the new myelin is thinner and conducts impulses more slowly than normal. This slowing can be detected by measuring the time for a stimulus (to the eye, ear, or peripheral nerve) to reach the cerebral cortex. Visual, auditory or brainstem, and somatosensory evoked potentials can indicate the presence of lesions scattered within the CNS in the absence of symptoms, helping clinical diagnosis.

Box 171-2. MRI Criteria for MS

Four lesions, or three lesions, one of which is periventricular: sensitivity 94%, specificity 57%

Two of the following: lumpy ventricular surface, one lesion >6 mm, and at least one infratentorial lesion: sensitivity 88%, specificity 90%

Box 171-3. Diseases With MRI Appearances Resembling MS

Angiitis	Lacunes
Trauma	HIV infection
Amyotrophic lateral sclerosis	Deep x-ray therapy
Hydrocephalus	Whipple's disease
Ischemia	Sarcoid
Acute disseminated encephalomyelitis	Sjögren's syndrome
	Fat embolism
Lyme disease	Cerebral autosomal dominant arteriopathy with sub-cortical infarcts and leukoencephalopathy
Progressive multifocal leukoencephalopathy	
Behçet's syndrome	
HTLV-1 infection	Migraine
Adrenoleukodystrophy	Lymphoma
Phenylketonuria	Systemic lupus erythematosus

MANAGEMENT

At present, no specific cure exists for MS. Therapy is directed at the acute attacks, at the underlying disease mechanisms, and at the symptoms of the disease and its complications.

Acute Attacks

Steroids marginally improve the symptoms and signs of acute attack, as long as the disease is active. No evidence indicates that increased benefits result from continuous therapy, and patients usually develop complications from the steroids if they are used long term, but the steroid-induced sensation of well-being may convince them they are benefiting from the therapy. Such treatment is difficult to stop in these patients, since they feel worse from withdrawal and are then convinced the drug helps. Intrathecal steroids were used in the past, but the effects were transient, and the complication of arachnoiditis led to abandonment of this therapy.

High-dose intravenous methylprednisolone is often used to treat acute attacks of MS. Doses of 500 to 1000 mg intravenously are well tolerated when given over an hour each day for 3 to 5 days (pulsed therapy). Such treatment can be given in an outpatient setting. Cimetidine or ranitidine is also prescribed for a total of 10 days.

Underlying Disease

Various immunosuppressants have been tried in MS but none has proved to produce appreciable benefit to the patient, and the potential side effects and complications of these drugs are a concern.

Azathioprine suppresses cell-mediated hypersensitivity reactions. A meta-analysis of 22 trials concluded that although it was effective in reducing disease progression, the effect was not statistically significant, although its ability to reduce the relapse rate was significant. The drug has the convenience of easy oral use. Long-term trials have shown no substantial risk of malignancy; this is the concern preventing its wide use in North America, although it is a common drug in Europe. Azathioprine may be used in relapsing-remitting MS if the interferons or Copaxone cannot be given.

Cyclophosphamide is an alkylating agent with cytotoxic and immunosuppressant functions. Its short-term effect is marginal, its side effects are potentially life-threatening, and it may be indicated only in patients with rapidly progressive MS.

Cyclosporine inhibits helper T cells. In one trial there was a statistically significant reduction in disease progression, but the clinical effects were slight. Methotrexate inhibits cell-mediated and humoral immunity. A dose of 7.5 mg weekly by mouth significantly slowed disease progression over 2 years in a small trial of subjects with secondary progressive MS, with minimal adverse effects; another study found it to be ineffective. When effective, cyclosporine helps mainly arm function. Mitoxantrone and cladribine reduce the MRI "lesion burden" but have not been shown to affect disability.

A trial producing almost total immunosuppression with antilymphocytic serum, cyclophosphamide, steroids, and thoracic duct drainage showed that acute attacks may be reduced. The frequency of relapse was reduced in the short term, but efficacy was minimal and side effects serious, so the regimen is not used. Total lymphoid irradiation produces some immediate benefit in rapidly progressing patients, but further studies need to be evaluated before this approach can be recommended. Studies on bone marrow replacement are in progress. Hyperbaric oxygen treatment (widely promoted but very expensive) and plasmapheresis are not helpful.

Interferons have been shown to be beneficial in MS and were the first agents shown to alter the course of the disease. *Interferon beta-1a* (Avonex, Rebif) reduces the number and severity of attacks and also may modestly alter the progression of the disease. Avonex is given by weekly intramuscular injection and Rebif by subcutaneous injection three times a week. *Interferon beta-1b* (Betaseron) reduces the number and severity of attacks by 30% and may reduce progression; it is administered by a subcutaneous injection every second day. The reduction of attacks is only by about one third; their severity is reduced by about half, but attacks still occur in many patients. Betaseron should not be expected to improve current problems or stop the disease. Patients should be aware of the reasonable expectations for the treatment, or they will discontinue therapy.

The most troublesome side effects from the interferons are a flu-like reaction soon after the injection and local injection site reactions. The flu-like symptoms can be managed by ibuprofen or acetaminophen, and in most they decrease and disappear within 2 months. Glatiramer (Copaxone) is a designer drug, synthesized to mimic myelin basic protein, which also reduces the number and severity of acute attacks, as well as the progression to some extent. It is injected subcutaneously daily. Glatiramer has fewer side effects than the interferons, although rashes, allergic reactions, and injection site reactions occur. An acute sensation of chest tightness can occur, although this is infrequent, benign, and may not recur if the drug is continued.

Numerous other agents are currently under study, and the future of therapy is promising but a slow process.

Treatment of Symptoms

Spasticity. Spasticity is overall the most disabling problem in MS and is particularly difficult to manage. Many simple muscle relaxants have been used with poor results. Diazepam can reduce spasticity, but the doses required for good effect are so high that drowsiness is a major problem, which makes it impractical. Baclofen is the most effective drug, but it is more useful for treating spasms and pain than for the underlying disability and the functional change induced by spasticity. Thus patients may have relief from spasms, but they do not walk any better. It is best to start with a low dose of baclofen, 5 to 10 mg per day, increasing to a maintenance of 10 mg four times a day. Patients should be warned that they may experience weakness and a "washed-out" feeling at higher doses; they can skip one day and go back to the previous dose if this occurs. Baclofen pumps inserted under the skin allow higher doses to be given directly into the intrathecal space. This is helpful in severe spasticity when the patient is having difficulty staying mobile, but the procedure is complicated and expensive and takes a dedicated staff to monitor the patient, refill the pump, and manage the complications.

Tizanidine (Zanaflex) is a new antispasticity agent that can be used alone (4 mg one to four times daily) or with baclofen. Dantrolene (25 mg daily, slowly increasing to 100 mg four times daily) is sometimes used but has limited utility. The use of cannabis for the treatment of spasticity is controversial; studies have shown that the patients felt better but all measures of their performance, such as balance, mobility, alertness, and concentration, were worse.

Ataxia. Another disabling feature of some MS cases is cerebellar ataxia. Ataxia is probably the most disabling feature of MS, since training and effort do not improve the incoordination, imbalance, and gait disturbance. Weighting of the wrists with 250- to 350-mg increases inertia and reduces tremor slightly. A number of agents have been tried, including high doses of INH, β-blockers, glutethimide, neurontin, and primidone, but the results are disappointing and the side effects disturbing.

Temperature Sensitivity. Many patients notice that a warm room, a muggy day, sitting in front of a hot fire, or taking a hot bath causes an increase in symptoms. Conversely, treatment with ice packs or submerging in a cool swimming pool sometimes improves symptoms and allows the patient 2 or 3 hours of painless increased mobility and strength, far outlasting the cooling effect of the ice or cold water. The cooling suits available give some relief for the 60% to 80% of MS patients who find this a troublesome symptom. The use of 4-aminopyridine and 3,4-aminopyridine in heat-sensitive patients is growing, although their place in therapy is uncertain; side effects include dizziness and seizures.

Contractures. Surgical procedures are done for contractures, spasticity, and deformities. The major thrust has been in reducing spasticity and muscle spasms by various destructive procedures on nerves, roots, and spinal cord or by phenol or alcohol injections into the intrathecal space.

Incontinence. Urologic assessment is needed to clarify what type of bladder dysfunction is present when the MS patient begins to complain of frequency, urgency, or incontinence. Mild degrees of upper motor neuron bladder dysfunction may respond to anticholinergic drugs such as oxybutynin (Ditropan) or propantheline (Pro-Banthine). Patients should schedule their fluid intake and activities in relation to bladder function. If necessary with a more significantly spastic bladder with incontinence, a condom drainage system can be used. A catheter should be avoided if possible because of the great dangers of infection, but if a catheter must be used, intermittent catheterization should be tried. The patient should have a high intake of fluid, urine cultures must be performed regularly, and appropriate antibiotics must be used if significant infection develops. In a few cases an indwelling catheter is needed. In the male the penis should be taped to the abdominal wall to avoid a penile-scrotal junction fistula.

Constipation. Inactivity predisposes to constipation, and MS patients should be on a high-fiber diet, with regular bran and adequate fluids. When constipation is a problem, other agents may be needed, such as psyllium hydrophilic colloid (Metamucil).

Sexual Dysfunction. Impotence is common in males after years with pyramidal involvement from MS. Understanding and support are important. Sensation changes may also alter sexual responses and prevent orgasms in women. Oral sildenafil (Viagra) is likely to become the treatment of choice for impotence. Formerly, injection of papaverine into the penis with a fine needle was useful to produce satisfactory erections and was reasonably well tolerated. Penile implants may produce satisfactory results but are less often needed with the advent of Viagra.

Pain. Pain is much more common in MS than thought; symptomatic trigeminal neuralgia, muscle spasms, and dermal hyperesthesias or dysesthesias are examples. Carbamazepine (Tegretol) is effective for trigeminal neuralgia and other lancinating pains in MS, whereas spasms in the back and limbs are often relieved by local cooling, massage, hydrotherapy, and exercise. Limb spasms, trigeminal neuralgia, and other pains also respond to baclofen (Lioresal), clonazepam (Klonopin), and gabapentin (Neurontin), which are useful in patients who cannot tolerate carbamazepine. Tricyclic drugs are also useful in chronic diffuse pain, but transcutaneous electrical stimulation (TENS) was found to be helpful only in those with muscular pains.

Fatigue. Fatigue is the most common complaint of MS patients, occurring in 80%, and is their major complaint in 40% of cases. It is an unusual fatigue, consisting of a feeling of inertia as if the subject's mainspring had broken rather than increasing weakness with persisting muscular activity; it can be very severe and disabling. Rest periods and naps may help, but the fatigue often continues despite adequate rest and good sleep. Amantadine (Symmetrel), 100 mg twice a day, helps about half of the patients, dramatically in some. In the long term, many patients develop livedo reticularis, although this is not a serious side effect and clears when the drug is stopped. Pemoline (Cylert), methylphenidate (Ritalin), and fluoxetine (Prozac) have less effect but may be useful.

Psychologic Problems. MS patients must be educated about their disease to gain any confidence about their future. Most have many conflicts and problems related to their families, income, and future, many of which can be resolved by a caring physician. Tranquilizers and antidepressants are effective when used in appropriate situations, but they should not be used to replace the personal impact of the physician. Patients often relate acute exacerbations to periods of physical or emotional strain. They cannot avoid all these situations but should recognize the importance of avoiding such stresses when possible; the family should understand this as well. The physician should not overemphasize the need to reduce stress, since the relationship between stress and exacerbation is not that clear. When an attack occurs, it tends to evoke guilt in the patient and family. MS societies are active in North America and in Europe. Community chapters are able to provide information, expertise, companionship, reassurance, social benefits, and health care aids (Box 171-4).

Diet. Many diets have been used in MS with various rationales, but none has yet proved to benefit patients permanently. The diet undergoing most careful evaluation at present is low in cholesterol and supplemented by linoleic acid (sunflower seed, evening primrose oil, or corn oil). Linoleate may be an immunosuppressant or may be necessary to maintain the integrity of myelin against immunologic challenge.

Aids to Improve Function. The many aids to assist the MS patient overcome problems include prisms for double vision; adapted cutlery; canes and walkers for gait difficulty; braces for foot drops; wheelchairs and electric scooters for mobility in the community; lifts and special beds for bedridden patients; and house, kitchen, and bath adaptions. Occupational therapists are important advisors on how to adapt the environment to cope with handicaps.

Primary Care Needs

With a chronic illness, the patient, family, and physician tend to focus on the problems of MS as the patient's only health needs. This leads to neglect of the health and wellness needs. Although MS is usually diagnosed and managed by neurologists, the general needs of an MS patient are best managed by a primary care physician. MS patients do not experience more diseases but do experience the same diseases as other people. Patients with chronic disease may receive inadequate management of other conditions. Symptoms possibly caused by other disorders may be dismissed as diverse manifestations of MS.

Self-assessment of health status is encouraged. Women should examine their breasts monthly; if hand dexterity or sensation is a problem, a partner assists. Men also need to perform self-examination of the testicles for any changes or lumps. General health care should include regular general checkups by the physician. Assessment of symptoms and problems, blood pressure assessment, Pap smears, prostate examination, and tests and examinations appropriate for age are indicated. Vision should be checked regularly, and visual effects that can be corrected with lenses should be managed normally. MS visual problems are not corrected by lenses, but the incidence of glaucoma, uveitis, cataract, and other disorders is the same as for other people.

Although most women with MS do not notice a change in their symptoms with their periods, some may notice increased fatigue or numbness or other symptoms just before menses, improving as the period begins. If this is a significant problem, oral contraceptives may alleviate these symptoms. Pregnancy does not aggravate MS. Slight amelioration of symptoms may even occur but the number of attacks increases 6 to 9 months postpartum. An attack is managed as is any attack. Even if no additional problems occur during pregnancy or postpartum, the MS patient experiences all the symptoms of pregnancy with the additional stress of increased fatigue and other MS symptoms. Prenatal and postnatal counseling and support are important to guarantee adequate rest, avoidance of infection, and management of stress. First-time parents need education and advice, and the experienced mother needs additional support. Since MS patients are prone to osteoporosis because of inactivity, hormone replacement therapy (HRT) may be important to reduce symptoms and possible fractures in addition to menopausal symptoms.

MS symptoms can be aggravated by heat in about 80% of patients; this can mistakenly be identified as an attack, even though the symptoms may disappear as soon as the person moves to a cool place. Patients may become so weak after a hot bath that they must lie down to rest; they may even have difficulty climbing from the bath. On a hot, muggy day, MS patients may feel dizzy, weak, and ill. These are not attacks, and patients must be advised about avoiding heat, drinking cold liquids, taking cool showers, and using air conditioning.

Exercise is important for MS patients, but some note increasing symptoms and weakness when their body heat increases. An unusual symptom is increased blurring of vision during exercise, with improvement as the person cools off (Uhthoff's sign). MS patients do well with exercises in a swimming pool because water cools the body during exercise, increasing their exercise tolerance. Patients should learn to cope with the heat problem and exercise as much as possible, with a reasonable balance between the benefits of exercise and the resulting fatigue.

Infections can increase symptoms by increasing body temperature. Patients must be assessed carefully to see if this is a transient episode related to the temperature and symptoms of the infection or a longer-lasting attack that needs treatment with steroids. MS patients are not more prone to infection, except when they develop bladder involvement or when inactivity or being bedridden makes them less resistant to respiratory infections. Viral infections not only make the patient weaker but also may precipitate an attack of MS. Because viral infections do not respond to antibiotics, prevention is the best plan. Vaccinations to prevent influenza are helpful for MS patients and do not pose a significant risk for acute attacks from the injection. Amantadine, an antiviral agent that can prevent influenza, also can help treat the fatigue so common in MS patients. General management of infections includes fluids, acetaminophen, nonsteroidal anti-inflammatory drugs (NSAID), and rest until the infection has passed.

Pseudorelapses may occur when the MS patient first begins interferon therapy, when the side effects and

Box 171-4. Internet Links

www.nmss.org
www.infosci.org/MS-UK-MSSoc
www.infosci.org/IFMSS/ifmsswel.html
www.mssoc.ca

aggravation of spasticity may resemble an acute attack. A reduction in dosage, with a gradual increase as the patient adjusts to the drug, usually manages this situation. Some patients may switch to glatiramer if the side effects continue to be intolerable.

Other Diseases

Other illnesses in MS patients can be divided into three categories: (1) unrelated to MS, (2) complications of MS, and (3) complications of MS treatments. Illnesses can be difficult to identify, especially if the symptoms are similar to MS. Hypothyroidism can cause slowing down, fatigue, weight gain, slowing of thinking, and even neurologic symptoms. Hypertension must be assessed in MS patients as in any patient and treated if blood pressure remains high. The aches and pains of arthritis and fibromyalgia are often attributed only to MS; nonspecific pain occurs in about half of MS patients and requires careful assessment to determine the best treatment. Insomnia is another common problem that can make dealing with other symptoms of MS difficult, especially fatigue.

Bladder infection is a common complication of the neurologic involvement of the bladder. Adequate fluids, cranberry juice, and local hygiene are important in preventing infections, and prophylactic antibiotics may be necessary. Decubiti (pressure sores) can be prevented by good skin care and turning of the patient, with attention to the mattresses, pillows, and chair seats. Pressure palsies develop with pressure on a peripheral nerve, and the sensory loss or weakness can be mistakenly attributed to the MS. Trigeminal neuralgia occurs in a few patients with MS and responds to carbamazepine, baclofen, or local neurosurgical procedures on cranial nerve V. Epilepsy occurs in 5% of MS patients and responds to the usual treatments for seizures.

Many of the treatments for MS also cause drug side effects and complications. Physicians should outline common side effects and complications for patients. Interferons can aggravate symptoms when initiated and can cause allergic responses, as can glatiramer. Steroids can cause cushingoid features if used for weeks or more, which is not recommended. Repeated steroid administration may result in aseptic necrosis of the hip.

Few diseases are associated with MS. Although MS has an immunologic aspect, little evidence indicates an association with other immunologic diseases. With 50,000 MS patients in the United States, many diseases occur due to the natural incidence of these conditions.

Principles of and resources for end of life care are described and extensively referenced in Chapter 164.

ADDITIONAL READINGS

Compston A, et al: *McAlpine's multiple sclerosis,* ed 3, Edinburgh, 1998, Churchill Livingstone.

Cook SD, editor: *Handbook of multiple sclerosis,* New York, 1991, Marcel Dekker.

Halper J, Murray TJ: Primary care needs of multiple sclerosis patients. In van den Noort S, Holland N, editors: *Multiple sclerosis in clinical practice,* New York, 1999, Demos.

Paty DW, Ebers GC: *Multiple sclerosis: contemporary neurology series,* volume 50, Philadelphia, 1998, F. A. Davis Co.

Redelmeier DA, Tan SH, Booth GL: The treatment of unrelated disorders in patients with chronic medical disease, *N Engl J Med* 338:1516-1520, 1998.

Sibley WA: *Therapeutic claims in multiple sclerosis,* ed 3, New York, 1995, Demos.

Siva A, Kesselring J, Thompson AJ: *Frontiers in multiple sclerosis,* London, 1998, Martin Dunitz.

OPHTHALMOLOGY XIII

CHAPTER 172

Primary Care of the Eye

Keith Doram
Yehia Mishriki

The eye is the most accessible and informative bi-directional "window" known to man. From the inside looking out, most of our daily wakeful activities significantly rely on visual input. From the outside looking in, the physical examination of the eye yields more useful information per unit area (or per unit weight) than any other organ in the body (Fig. 172-1). For example, direct inspection of the retina can often detect evidence for systemic disease—in some cases even before there are other obvious signs, symptoms, or laboratory abnormalities. Since the eye and the visual system are the most complex and developed sensory mechanisms of the body, primary care clinicians must be competent in the evaluation and management of the eye and eye-related disorders.

The Association of University Professors of Ophthalmology (AUPO) issued a policy statement regarding the areas of ophthalmology in which all physicians should be competent. These areas include visual acuity, red eye, traumatized eye, strabismus and abnormal eye movements, abnormal pupillary response, optic nerve and fundi abnormalities, initial management, and referral guidelines. Adequate competency

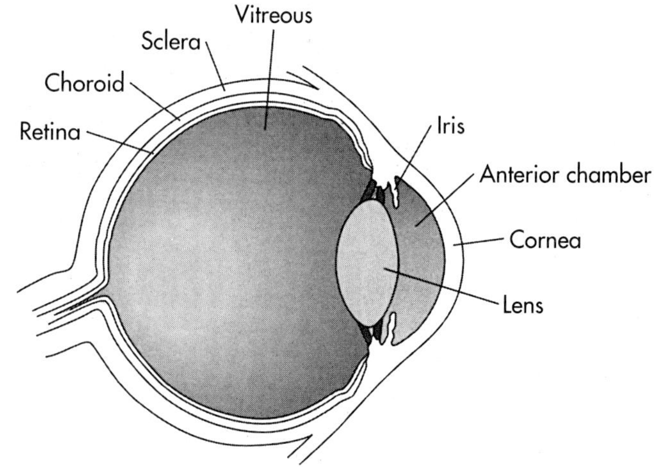

Fig. 172-1. Sagittal section showing the major structures of the eye.

Box 172-1. Common Mistakes Made During the Eye Examination

- Failure to look in both eyes
- Failure to examine the cornea and lens
- Failure to do adequate visual acuity testing and note acute visual acuity changes
- Failure to dilate the pupils or inappropriate dilation of the pupils
- Failure to note the presence of spontaneous retinal venous pulsations
- Failure to diagnose a penetrated or ruptured globe and placing too much pressure on a ruptured globe
- Failure to recognize multiple floaters or new flashes as emergencies representing possible retinal detachment
- Failure to adequately document the eye findings
- Failure to recognize an infectious cause of "red eye" and inappropriately prescribing topical corticosteroid eye drops
- Failure to give oral analgesics rather than prescribing topical anesthetic agents
- Failure to differentiate preseptal cellulitis from orbital cellulitis—the latter can lead to death
- Failure to order a head CT scan with direct coronal views instead of an MRI in a patient with proptosis

Box 172-2. The Four Cardinal Eye Complaints

- Change in vision
- Change in appearance
- Pain or discomfort
- Trauma

helps ensure that many of the common mistakes made during the eye examination do not occur (Box 172-1).

This chapter presents practical information that will better enable the primary care clinician to gain and maintain an acceptable level of competency in the evaluation and management of the eye and eye-related disorders. The main outline of information includes how to obtain an adequate directed ophthalmologic history and physical, as well as the recognition and implications of the four cardinal complaints related to the eye: change in vision, change in appearance, pain, and trauma (Box 172-2). The AUPO's core competencies, effective prevention measures, and treatment/referral guidelines are be incorporated. Additional information on the ocular manifestations of systemic disease, ophthalmologic procedures, and other special topics of interest to primary care clinicians are presented.

OPHTHALMOLOGY ABBREVIATIONS

Often the primary care clinician can be confused by the cryptic abbreviations used in ophthalmology consultations. Box 172-3 includes some of the more commonly used abbreviations; these abbreviations are used throughout this chapter.

HISTORY

It is important to first determine the primary (cardinal) eye problem (see Box 172-2). The next step is to assess the eye complaints by time course, precipitating factor(s), palliative or exacerbating variables, and course history.

Adequate characterization of any discomfort is important. For example, is there any pain, a sensation of "something in the eye," itching, excessive tearing, or burning? Often a person can accurately localize the foreign body and help direct the focus of the ophthalmoscopic examination. Itching and excessive tearing can suggest an allergic cause.

If there were any changes in vision, it should be noted whether there was painless or painful loss of vision. It is also important to determine the extent of the visual change and whether it involves one or both eyes. Bilateral visual loss usually implies a primary neurologic etiology and not a primary ophthalmologic problem. The presence of multiple new flashes or floaters could represent a retinal tear or vitreous hemorrhage, whereas a single floater is probably a benign condition. The rate of onset of visual impairment may give a clue as to the etiology. In general, rapid deterioration of vision points to a vascular cause, whereas more gradual loss of vision suggests causes such as cataracts.

The tetanus immunization status is important in patients with a history of eye trauma. Also knowing the acidity or alkalinity of any fluid/chemical eye exposure is essential.

A detailed ocular history should also include information on any type of corrective lenses (i.e., glasses, contact lenses); any acute or chronic eye problems (e.g., glaucoma); any eye medications (e.g., antiglaucoma medications, topical antibiotics); any eye surgery history (e.g., cataract removal, refractive surgery); any associated systemic symptoms like headaches, nausea, or vomiting; and finally any relevant systemic diseases (e.g., diabetes, hypertension, and HIV disease).

PHYSICAL EXAMINATION

The eye examination should ideally proceed in a sequential fashion. The suggested order of the examination is shown in Box 172-4.

Vision Testing

Assessing VA should be the first step in essentially all ophthalmologic examinations. The severity of any eye disorder is greatly determined by its effect on VA. VA testing is the most fundamental component of evaluating a patient's visual function. In essence, VA testing is the "vital sign" of the eye. The examiner should measure vision using a standardized Snellen distance VA chart (Fig. 172-2 *A*) or a near acuity card (Fig. 172-2, *B*). If these tools are unavailable, newsprint, the patient's chart, or other legibly printed materials can be used. In all physical eye examination procedures, each eye must be evaluated individually. This is especially important in cases of trauma, where the treating clinician often fails to recognize injury in the "uninjured" eye.

VA testing should always be done with the patient wearing his or her corrective lenses when possible. Patients may have preexisting myopia (nearsightedness), hyperopia (farsightedness), or astigmatism (unequal corneal or lenticular curvatures). The examiner should note whether corrective lenses were used during the visual testing, and each eye's VA should be documented separately. Patients over 40 years of age may require bifocals or reading glasses to compensate for the

Box 172-3. Common Ophthalmologic Abbreviations

A-1: Atropine 1%
*AC: Anterior chamber
ACIOL: Anterior chamber intraocular lens
AION: Anterior ischemic optic neuropathy
ALT: Argon laser trabeculoplasty
ARMD: Age-related macular degeneration
BDR: Background diabetic retinopathy
BRAO: Branch retinal artery occlusion
BRVO: Branch retinal vein occlusion
C-1: Cyclopentolate 1%
CA: Corneal abrasion
CAI: Carbonic anhydrase inhibitor
cat: Cataract
*CC: With correction
C/D: Cup-to-disc ratio
CF: Counts fingers vision
CL: Contact lens
CME: Cystoid macular edema
CNVM: Choroidal neovascular membrane
*Conf: Confrontational visual field
CRAA: Central retinal artery occlusion
CSM: Central steady and maintained fixation
D: Diopter
*D + C: Deep and clear
DCR: Dacryocystorhinostomy
dil: Dilate
D + N: Distance and near
DVD: Dissociated vertical deviation
E: Esophoria
ECCE: Extracapsular cataract extraction
EOM: Extraocular muscle
*EOMI: EOM intact
EUA: Examination under anesthesia
FA: Fluorescein angiogram or angiography
FB: Foreign body
FBS: Foreign body sensation
F + F: Fix and follow vision
FTFC: Finger-to-finger counting
GPC: Giant papillary conjunctivitis
gtts: Drops
HM: Hand motion
HT: Hypertropia
ICCE: Intracapsular cataract extraction
IOL: Intraocular lens
ION: Ischemic optic neuropathy
*IOP: Intraocular pressure
IVFA: Intravenous fluorescein angiography
J: Jaeger (card for near vision)
K: Keratometry
LET: Left esotropia
LL: Lower lid
LP: Light perception
LUL: Left upper eyelid
LXT: Left exotropia
M1: Tropicamide 1% (Mydriacyl)
MG: Marcus Gunn pupil
MR: Manifest refraction
N: Near vision
NFL: Nerve fiber layer
NLD: Nasolacrimal duct
NLP: No light perception; total blindness
NPA: Near point of accommodation
NS: Nuclear sclerosis
NVD: Neovascularization of the disc
NVG: Neovascular glaucoma
*OD: Right eye *(oculus dexter)*
ON: Optic nerve
OR: Over-refraction
*OS: Left eye *(oculus sinister)*
*OU: Both eyes *(oculi uerque)*
PBK: Pseudophakic bullous keratopathy
PC: Posterior capsule (or posterior chamber)
PCAG: Primary closed-angle glaucoma
PDR: Proliferative diabetic retinopathy
*PERRLA: Pupils equal, round, and reactive to light and accommodation
*PH: Pinhole
PI: Peripheral iridectomy
PK: Penetrating keratoplasty
POAG: Primary open-angle glaucoma
PPDR: Preproliferative diabetic retinopathy
PRP: Panretinal photocoagulation
PSC: Posterior subcapsular cataract
PVD: Posterior vitreous detachment
*RAPD: Relative afferent pupillary defect
RD: Retinal detachment
RET: Right esotropia
RGP: Rigid gas-permeable contact lens
RHT: Right hypertropia
RLL: Right lower eyelid
RXT: Right exotropia
sc: Without correction
SCH: Subconjunctival hemorrhage
SCL: Soft contact lens
SI: Sector iridectomy
SLE: Slit-lamp examination
Sph: Sphere
SPK: Superficial punctate keratitis
SRNVM: Subretinal neovascular membrane
T: Tension
*T: Tonometry
Trab: Trabeculectomy
*TT: Tactile tension
*VA: Visual acuity
*VF: Visual field
Vit: Vitreous
XT: Exotropia at distance
W: Glasses worn by patient (wear)
*5 → 2: Pupil constricts from 5 mm to 2 mm in response to light

*Abbreviations used to document eye examination findings.

Box 172-4. Suggested Order of the Physical Examination

1. VA/vision testing (the "vital sign" of the eye)
2. Pupillary reactions (check before dilating the pupils)
3. External examination
4. Ocular motility
5. VF testing
6. SLE (usually done per ophthalmologist)
7. OP measurement (if able to perform accurately and safely)
8. Direct ophthalmoscopy

age-related stiffening of the crystalline lens (presbyopia) and the accompanying loss of focusing ability. If a patient's glasses or contact lenses are not available, pinhole testing of the visual acuity can correct any refractive error. (An 18-g needle or a sharp pencil can be used to punch holes in a 3 × 5-inch note card if a premade pinhole device is not available.) Pinhole testing generally corrects any uncorrected refractive errors. If correction is not seen, the examiner should look for other pathologic causes such as cataracts, optic nerve disease, or retinal diseases.

The use of a Snellen chart at 20 feet is a time-honored method for determining VA. The patient stands 20 feet from the chart and covers one eye. (Or when using the pocket-sized near chart, it is held 14 inches from the patient's face.) The patient begins reading from the top line down. The examiner notes the acuity by the line where most (more than half) of the characters are read correctly. The first eye is then covered (with an eye cover or the palm) and the opposite eye is tested in the same manner. VA is reported as two numbers separated by a slash, followed by a minus sign and the number of characters missed on that line. The first number, usually "20," is the standard distance from the chart to the individual being tested. The second number is the distance, in feet, at which the letter subtends 5 minutes of an arc on the retina. For example, if a patient has 20/40 vision, he or she can see

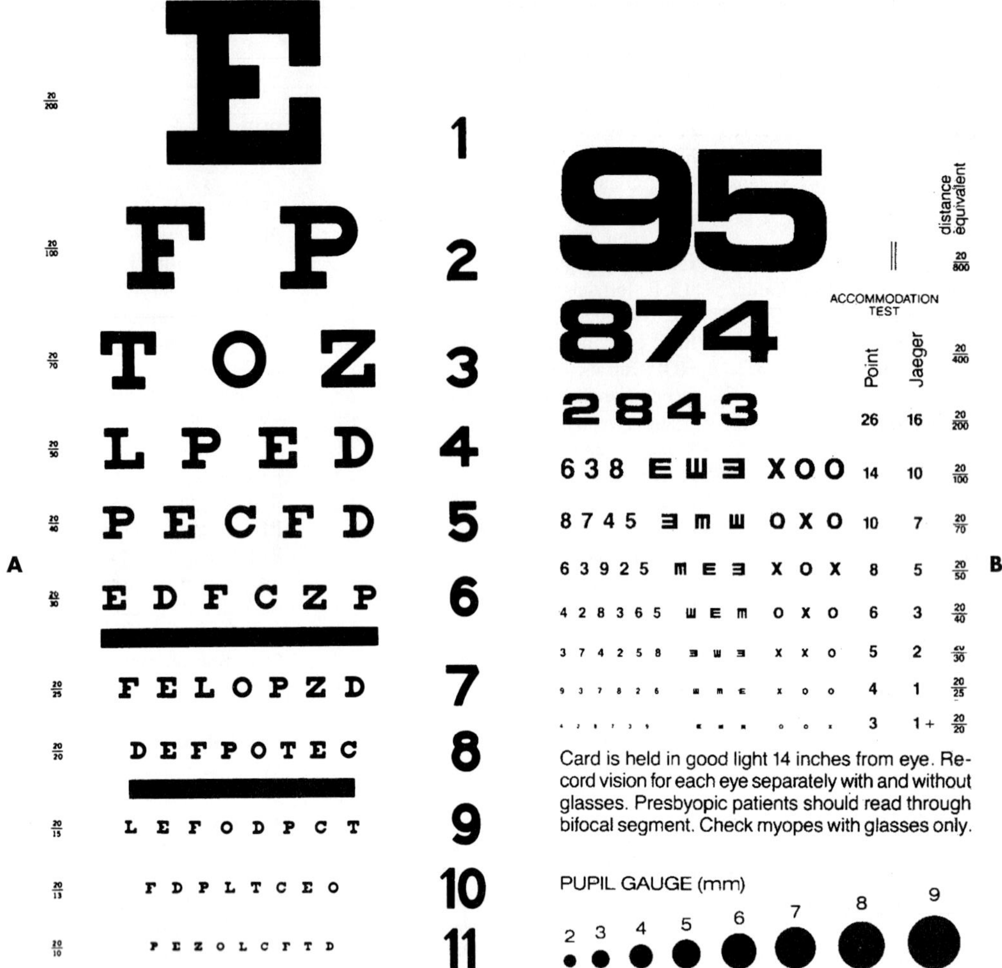

Fig. 172-2. **A,** Snellen distance acuity chart. **B,** Snellen near acuity card. (From Soley WA, Broocker G: General eye exam. In Palay DA, Krachmer JH: *Ophthalmology for the primary care physician,* St. Louis, 1997, Mosby.)

at 20 feet what a "normal" person can see at 40 feet. If the patient can read some but not all of the letters on a line, VA is recorded as the acuity for that line "minus" the number of letters missed (e.g., 20/40 – 2). For patients with less than 20/400 vision, the examiner can use the notations "CF," "hand motions," "LP," and "NLP" vision. Illiterate patients and small children can use other charts with "E" shapes or pictures (e.g., Allen chart).

Pupil Examination

Assessing the shape, size, and reactivity of the pupils is essential in determining the integrity of the anterior visual pathway. Pupillary dilation agents, of course, should not be used before pupil testing. Pupillary function testing is critical to evaluation of both the neurologic and the ophthalmologic status of the patient. Mistakenly, PERRLA is noted and substituted for an accurate assessment of pupil function. Both pupils should be round on examination. Irregularly shaped pupils are probably a result of prior ocular surgery, although it could be due to ocular rupture, laceration, or scarring from a previous inflammatory process of the iris or ciliary body. The pupils should be tested individually and in a dim light with the patient fixating on a distant object. Discrepancy in pupillary size is called *anisocoria.* A difference in pupillary size of ½ to 1 mm is common, and in the absence of any symptoms or other signs, does not necessarily indicate any pathology. The examiner directs a penlight at each pupil and notes the rapidity and amount of pupil constriction in each eye. As a general rule, a difference in pupil size greater than 1 mm or in the pupil that reacts poorly to direct light is abnormal. When confronted with a dilated pupil, the examiner must search for other signs of a third nerve palsy such as ptosis, diplopia, or ocular motor paresis. Even when these conditions are not present, a significantly dilated pupil is considered a medical emergency, particularly when accompanied by headache or other neurologic signs. The "swinging light" test helps determine if there is integrity of the visual pathways. A bright light is moved back and forth from one eye to the other eye quickly enough not to allow the pupil to dilate. If a pupil does dilate when the light is shined on it, a defect along that visual pathway is present. A RAPD or MG pupil is due to a defect anywhere in the visual pathway from the lens to and including the optic nerve. The pupil constricts consensually (due to the crossing neural fibers in the midbrain) when light is shined in the opposite eye but paradoxically dilates when the light is brought back and shined on the affected eye. This reaction must not be mistaken for a rhythmic wavering pupil (hippus), which is a normal finding. Also, if there is severe bilateral disease, both eyes may react equally. Therefore no RAPD exists. Cataracts and macular degeneration do not normally cause RAPD unless they are very advanced. In *Horner's syndrome,* sympathetic innervation of the pupil and levator palpebrae superioris muscle is interrupted. There is ptosis, miosis of the affected eye, and anhydrosis of the ipsilateral half of the face. The pupil is small but reacts to light. (Anhydrosis may be difficult to detect and is more easily assessed by looking for small droplets of sweat at the vermilion border of the upper lip using the ophthalmoscope set at +40 diopters.) A pupil that constricts very slowly and incompletely, or not at all, to direct light but is otherwise normal is called an *Adie's tonic pupil.* It may also constrict better to near light than to direct light. This is due to degeneration of the ciliary ganglia and the postganglionic parasympathetic fibers that constrict the pupil and effect accommodation. Adie's pupil is supersensitive to dilute solutions of pilocarpine and can be positively identified if 0.1% pilocarpine constricts the pupil. Patients with Adie's pupil may complain of difficulty reading because of accommodative paresis, but usually the dilated pupil is an incidental finding. Similar Adie's pupil findings can often be a manifestation of a mild dysautonomia and can also be associated with Shy-Drager syndrome, diabetes mellitus, and amyloidosis.

The much-taught Argyll Robertson pupil is uncommon. It was classically described in patients with tertiary syphilis, but today is more likely to be seen in diabetics. It has also been described in the meningoradiculitis of Lyme disease. The pupils are usually small, unequal, and irregular. They do not react to light but constrict on accommodation. Mydriatics cause an incomplete dilation.

External Examination

Examination of the eyelids, lid margins, periorbital position, and globe position is the next step in a comprehensive examination. In cases of trauma it is critical not to palpate the globe. Observe for proptosis or exophthalmos (protruding eye), which may indicate orbital disease (e.g., retrobulbar hemorrhage, orbital cellulitis, orbital tumor, Graves' disease). A sunken eye (enopththalmos) is often seen in fractures of the orbital floor (especially if associated with ecchymosis, point tenderness, and a palpable step-off around the orbital rim). These conditions can best be identified by observing the patient above the head and looking downward toward the eyes.

Examine the eyelids for any crusting, irregularity, lash loss, or lesions. A hordeolum (stye) is a painful localized infection of the lash follicle. A chalazion is a more chronic inflammatory painful lesion of the meibomian gland. The hordeolum is at the lid's edge, while the chalazion is not. Note any ectropion (out-turned lower lid margins)—commonly seen in elderly patients, entropion (in-turned lower lid margins), and trichiasis (posteriorly misdirected eye lashes).

The inferior aspects of the conjunctiva can be examined by pulling down the lower eyelid from the inferior orbital rim and have the patient look up. To see the inner aspect of the upper eyelid and the superior conjunctiva and cul-de-sac, a lid eversion procedure should be performed. The examiner should grasp the upper eyelash, pull the upper lid away from the globe, and use a small, slender object (e.g., applicator stick) to press the region of the superior tarsal plate inferiorly (Fig. 172-3). Never invert the lid if rupture of the globe is suspected. Look carefully in these areas for any suspected retained foreign body. Next examine the bulbar conjunctiva. Look for subconjunctival hemorrhage (spontaneous or due to trauma)—this is usually a harmless condition. However, globe rupture is more likely in cases of trauma and when the subconjunctival hemorrhage encircles the entire cornea. Conjunctival injection due to conjunctivitis is a common cause of "red eye." If the injection is just around the cornea, the inflammation could be the result of keratitis (corneal infection), iritis, or acute glaucoma. Ocular pain relieved by topical anesthetic is due to conjunctival or corneal disruption. Pain unrelieved by topical anesthetic is due to deeper eye structures.

Ocular Motility

Six eye muscles move the eyes in conjugate fashion (see Chapter 177). The six extraocular muscles are intact (EOMI) if they properly perform the cardinal movements as shown in Fig 172-4. Cranial nerve III innervates the medial rectus (adducts the eye), inferior rectus (depresses the eye), superior rectus (elevates the eye), and inferior oblique (abducts, elevates, and outwardly rotates the eye) muscles. Cranial nerve IV innervates the superior oblique (abducts, depresses, and inwardly rotates the eye) muscles. Cranial nerve VI innervates the lateral rectus (abducts the eye).

The extraocular movements involve complex coordination via neuropathways located in the frontomesencephalic and cerebellomesencephalic areas—the visual, vestibular, and ocular motor centers. Eye movements are responsible for capturing and locking onto a visual object of interest and for maintaining fixation on that object even during head and body movements. Any disturbance in intracranial processing, midbrain or cranial nerve function, or intraorbital muscle abnormalities may result in an ocular position imbalance. The examiner must carefully note the position of the eyes and their excursions relative to each other in patients with complaints of diplopia (double-vision), strabismus (misalignment), blurred vision, jumpy vision, those with more general complaints of unsteadiness, dizziness, or vertigo, and those with suspected neurologic or orbital disease. Abnormalities may be seen in the primary gaze (straight ahead) or congruity of gaze in the six cardinal positions (left, right, up and right, up and left, down and right, down and left).

A large degree of misalignment of the eyes is easily determined by inspection. In patients with subtle degrees of strabismus, the position of the corneal light reflexes can help determine if there is any squint or not, since these reflexes are normally located in identical positions on each eye (Hirchberg test). Fixation maintenance and smooth pursuit mechanisms are tested by asking the patient to fixate on a target, while slowly moving the target to extreme positions of gaze. During this process, it is important to observe the steadiness of eye position and fixation. The patient should be asked to look in each cardinal position and asked if diplopia develops and if so, in which direction of gaze. Inability to abduct the eye suggests a sixth cranial nerve (abducen's) palsy. This can be seen in patients with diabetes and is due to infarction of the nerve. It is also seen in patients with increased intracranial pressure, and in such a case, it is accompanied by papilledema. An abducen's palsy can also be seen with tumors, meningitis, or compression by an aneurysm. In a patient with a complete lateral gaze palsy, one

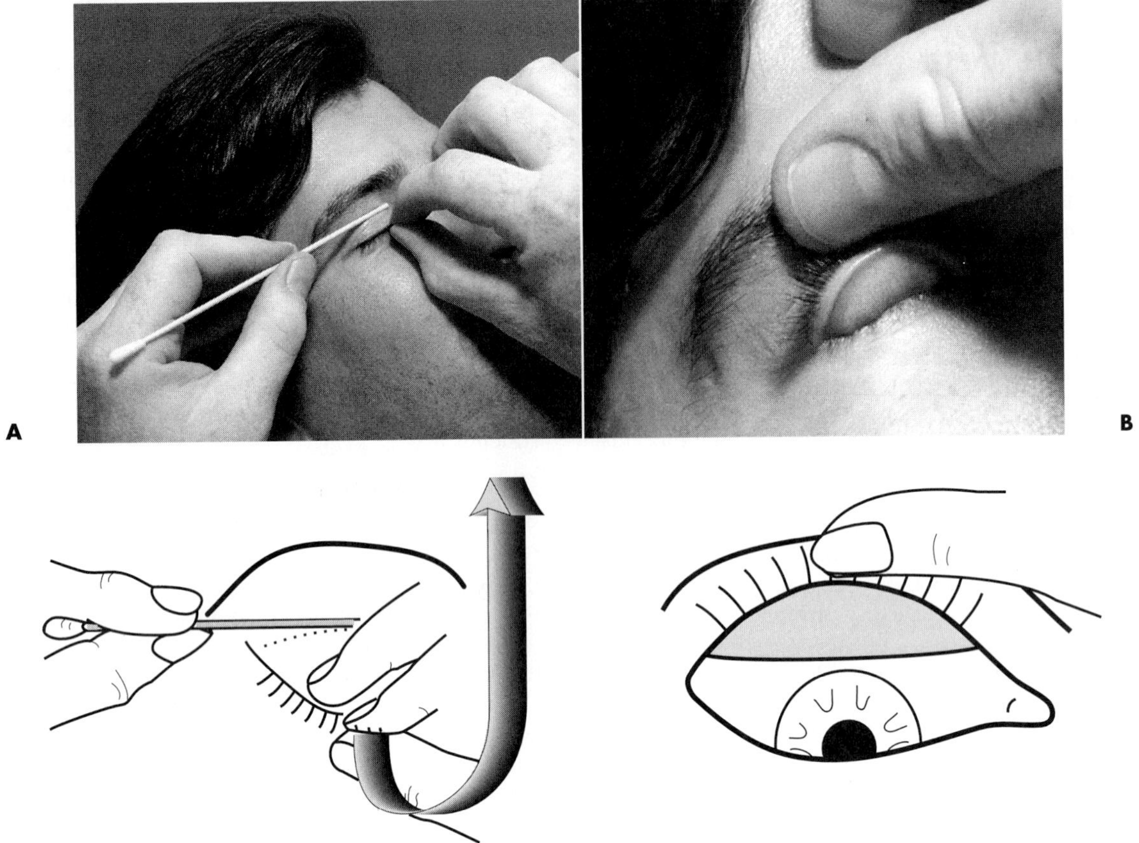

Fig. 172-3. **A,** For eversion, the examiner places a wooden applicator stick at the superior edge of the superior tarsal plate, firmly grasps the lashes of the upper eyelid, and gently moves the applicator stick inferiorly while pulling up on the lashes slightly. **B,** The examiner removes the stick while holding the eyelid in place (often with the cotton-tipped end). Administration of a topical anesthesia (proparacaine) may make this a slightly more comfortable procedure but is not essential. (From Soley WA, Broocker G: General eye exam. In Palay DA, Krachmer JH: *Ophthalmology for the primary care physician,* St. Louis, 1997, Mosby.)

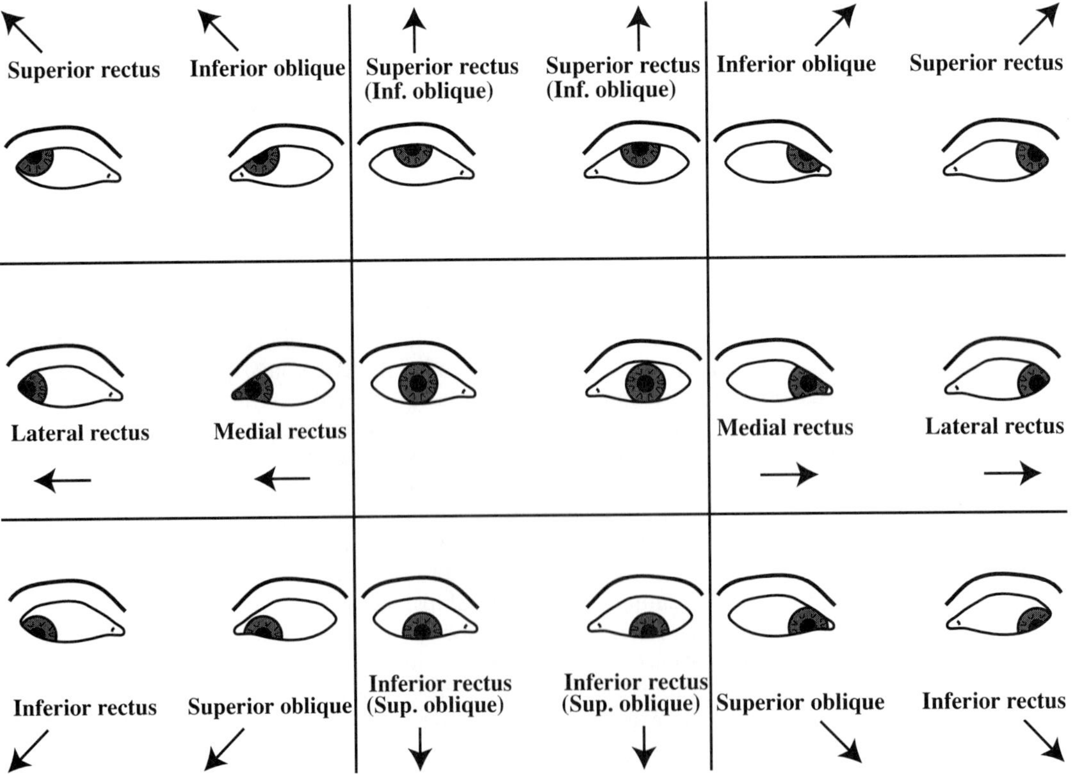

Fig. 172-4. The principal actions of the extraocular muscles. (From Soley WA, Broocker G: General eye exam. In Palay DA, Krachmer JH: *Ophthalmology for the primary care physician,* St. Louis, 1997, Mosby.)

should suspect a lesion of the abducen's nucleus since the nucleus contains interneruons that project via the medial longitudinal fasiculus (MLF) to the contralateral medial rectus. An eye that is "down and out" and is associated with ptosis is seen in patients with third cranial nerve (oculomotor) palsy. If the pupil is also dilated, one should suspect an aneurysm of the circle of Willis, especially if accompanied by pain. Sparing of the pupil suggests an infarction of the nerve. This is primarily seen in patients with diabetes. Patients with fourth cranial nerve (trochlear) palsy complain of vertical or oblique double vision, which worsens as they look downward. They may assume a characteristic head posture in which their head is turned and titled away from the affected side. Because of its close anatomic relationship to the tentorium, the fourth nerve is subject to physical injury during head trauma. For this reason, fourth nerve palsies are most frequently associated with trauma. However, microinfarctions along the nerve are also common. Complex eye movement deficits suggest myasthenia gravis or thyroid eye disease.

Nystagmus, which are involuntary rhythmic oscillations of the eyes, can be seen in a variety of disorders. Jerk nystagmus is characterized by a slow drift away from the visual target followed by a rapid correction. It can be downbeat, horizontal, or torsional. Acquired nystagmus is usually of the jerk form and can be divided into two major subcategories: nystagmus due to disorders of the peripheral vestibular apparatus and nystagmus due to disorders of the central nervous system (CNS). Peripheral nystagmus develops with vestibular dysfunction. It is usually purely horizontal, or horizontal and rotatory. It is often associated with severe vertigo. Symptoms can be recurrent, transient, and last days to weeks; but they usually resolve with time. Associated postural effects and hearing deficits are often noted. The common causes are infectious disease of the labyrinth (labyrinthitis) or the vestibular nerve (neuronitis), Ménière's disease, or trauma. Central nystagmus is much more variable and is not usually associated with severe vertigo. Symptoms may be transient or permanent. Central nystagmus often is a result of a brainstem or cerebellar lesion caused by demyelinating disease, vascular infarction, or tumor. Subtle nystagmus can sometimes be detected during funduscopic examination at which time one observes nystagmoid movements of the optic disc. End-gaze nystagmus is common even in patients without ocular or neurologic pathology and usually occurs for only a few beats. Exaggerated-gaze nystagmus can be caused by drugs (anticonvulsants, sedatives, alcohol), myasthenia gravis, demyelinating disease, and cerebellopontine angle, brainstem, and cerebellar lesions. Spontaneous nystagmus suggests labyrinthine vestibular disease or cerebellar disease. A torsional component is usually seen with labyrinthine disease. Vertical nystagmus implicates the pontomedullary or pontomesencephalic areas as the source. Vertical nystagmus of the upbeat type is seen in patients with demyelinating disease, brainstem vascular disease, tumors, or Wernicke's disease. Downbeat nystagmus may be seen in Wernicke's disease but is characteristic of syringobulbia. In pendular nystagmus, the to-and-fro oscillations are of nearly equal rate. It is usually observed in individuals in whom central vision has been compromised early in life (i.e., albinism, congenital diseases of the retina). This type of nystagmus is always bilateral and in one plane. Head oscillation may accompany the nystagmus and is felt to be compensatory.

Visual Field Testing

The usual techniques used in VF testing by confrontation are crude, and if there is any suspicion that the patient may have a VF defect, formal testing should be sought. The usual technique is as follows:

- Sit 2 feet from the patient.
- Ask the patient to cover one eye and fixate on your eye that is directly in front of him or her (i.e., if the patient were to fixate with his or her right eye, he or she would look at your left eye, and vice versa).
- Begin by first checking to see if there is a central field defect. Ask the patient if he or she sees your entire face with his or her uncovered eye. If the patient can only see your hair and chin but not your eye or nose, he or she has a central defect.
- Stretch your arms out in a plane that is equidistant from the patient and at the outermost periphery of your vision.
- Wiggle the index and middle fingers on one hand and ask the patient if he or she sees movement, and if so, on which side.
- Move your hands to different positions, checking the patient's superior, inferior, nasal, and temporal fields. Randomly change fingers that are wiggled.

Some ophthalmologists recommend that patients identify the number of fingers being held outstretched rather than whether or not the examiner's finger is being wiggled. Since red vision is affected earliest, using a red object to test VFs increases the sensitivity of the test. A lesion affecting the visual pathway anterior to the optic chiasm will produce a monocular VF defect. A central scotoma (blind spot) usually represents optic nerve or macular pathology. The visual system and VF defects resulting from lesions at various points in the visual pathway are shown in Fig. 172-5.

Slit-Lamp Examination

An ophthalmologist (or optometrist) usually is the examiner who has the slit lamp along with the necessary expertise and training to use it. The SLE is essential in any condition requiring an accurate and highly magnified view of the anterior and posterior segments of the eye.

Intraocular Pressure

The IOP of the eye is analogous to the systemic blood pressure of the cardiovascular system in that both pressures should be periodically assessed and maintained in the optimal range (see Chapter 173). As in systemic hypertension, the risk for IOP elevation increases with age—especially 35 years and older. Normal IOP is 8 to 21 mm Hg, but in pathologic states can range from 0 (in cases of ruptured globe, after glaucoma surgery, and severe intraocular inflammation) to 70 or 80 (in cases of angle-closure glaucoma). However, most primary care examiners do not have the necessary equipment to safely and accurately directly measure the IOP. The primary care examiner must rely on the recommended glaucoma screening guidelines, crude manual techniques, and other observational methods (e.g., optic nerve cupping, unexplained blurred monocular vision) to determine if more formal testing for IOP should be performed.

The IOP can be measured in a variety of ways. The applanation tonometer (found on most slit lamps, although there is a Perkins handheld version) and the pneumotonometer are not available for most primary care examiner usage. The Schiøtz tonometer (see Fig. 173-3), although easily available, is not the preferred method because of its

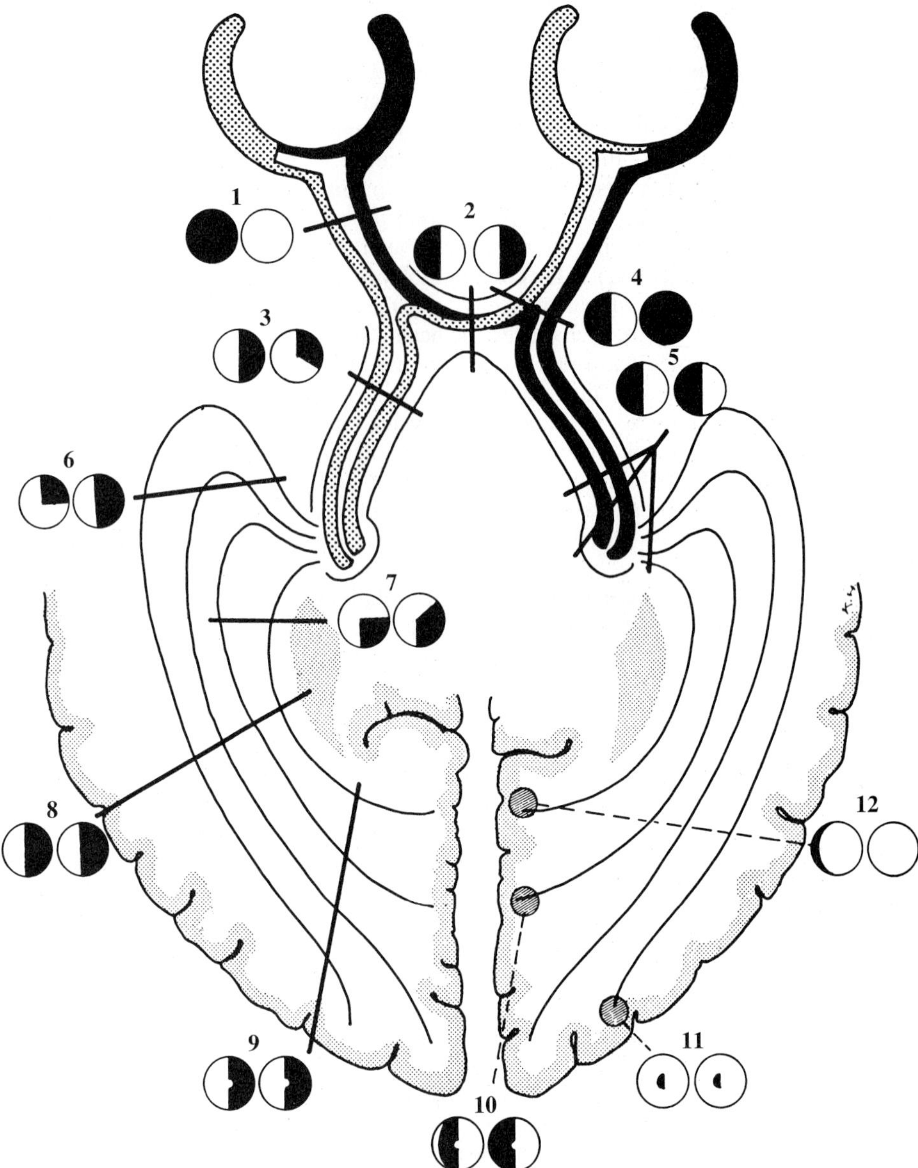

Fig. 172-5. The visual system and VF defects resulting from lesions at various points in the visual pathway. An optic nerve lesion only affects the visual field of one eye *(1)*. However, bilateral optic nerve lesions are not uncommon. Lesions of the body of the chiasm tend to produce bilateral temporal VF defects *(2)*. Optic tract lesions (and all lesions posterior) produce defects that are homonymous on the same side in both eyes *(3)*. Lesions at the junction of the optic nerve and chiasm severely affect vision in the ipsilateral eye but produce an often asymptomatic temporal peripheral VF defect in the contralateral eye *(4)*. Complete homonymous hemianopic VF defects are nonlocalizing; that is, they can occur anywhere from the optic tract to the occipital lobe (*5* and *8*). A unilateral homonymous hemianopia does not decrease VA. Lesions in the temporal lobe produce superior homonymous defects *(6)*. Parietal lesions cause inferior homonymous defects (7). Occipital lobe lesions are highly congruous (*9* to *11*). Bilateral occipital infarctions can profoundly affect VA and VF bilaterally, with normal-appearing fundi and normal pupillary responses. (From Martin TJ: Neuro-ophthalmology. In Palay DA, Krachmer JH: *Ophthalmology for the primary care physician*, St. Louis, 1997, Mosby.)

disadvantages (increased risk in spreading infection, cumbersome, can cause injury). The tonometer pen (see Fig. 173-4) is the preferred device for the primary care examiner. It is easy to use and is fairly accurate. Table 172-1 compares the advantages and disadvantages of each IOP testing modality.

FUNDUSCOPIC EVALUATION

The final part of the comprehensive eye examination is direct ophthalmoscopy—it is invaluable diagnostic tool for the primary care clinician. Ideally, after vision and pupillary testing, dilation of the pupils should be done, especially if an abnormality in the posterior eye is suspected. Funduscopic evaluation is best accomplished after the pupils are dilated with a weak mydriatic agent such as tropicamide 0.5% to 1% or phenylephrine 2.5% (both reverse effects in 4 to 6 hours). Always document the time of dilation and the agents used for dilation. Atropine drops should not be used because they produce dilation for up to 1 to 2 weeks. The pupils should not be dilated if serial neurologic examinations are required, in elderly patients who have had cataract surgery (can cause artificial lens displacement), or if acute angle-closure glaucoma is suspected. One can do a simple screen for angle-closure glaucoma by shining a handlight obliquely across the anterior chamber. If a shadow on the iris is noted on the opposite side of the illuminator, there may be narrowing of the anterior chamber and the presence of angle-closure glaucoma (see Fig. 173-6). Although trying to view the fundi without pupillary dilation has been likened to trying to view the contents of a room while looking through a keyhole, for practical and logistic reasons primary care clinicians do not dilate the pupils in the vast majority of their patients. Therefore it is important to refer all patients to an ophthalmologist if a more sensitive and complete funduscopic evaluation is deemed necessary.

However, even in undilated eyes, examination with the direct ophthalmoscope can give useful information on both the anterior and posterior aspects of the eye. The examination should be done in dim light. The examiner's right eye should be used to examine the patient's right eye, and visa versa. Begin at a distance of 1 to 2 feet from the patient's eye,

Table 172-1. Intraocular Pressure Testing Modalities

Modality	Advantages	Disadvantages
Applanation tonometer	Very accurate, easy to use	Expensive, requires direct contact to cornea and globe, ineffective on abnormal corneal surfaces and irregular tear films
Tonometer pen (Tono-pen)	Relatively accurate, easy to use, has disposable covers to prevent infection	Accuracy diminishes outside the normal IOP range; pens are fragile and expensive
Pneumotonometer (Air-puff tonometer)	Accurate, easy to use, effective on abnormal corneal surfaces and irregular tear films	Expensive to maintain, not portable, must be calibrated often
Schiøtz (indentation) tonometer	Inexpensive, accurate to ±3 mm Hg	Cumbersome, can spread infection, prone to false-positive elevations of IOP, more likely to cause corneal injury
Manual assessment	Does not require instrumentation	Extremely inaccurate if performed by persons who are not ophthamologists, only rough approximations can be made

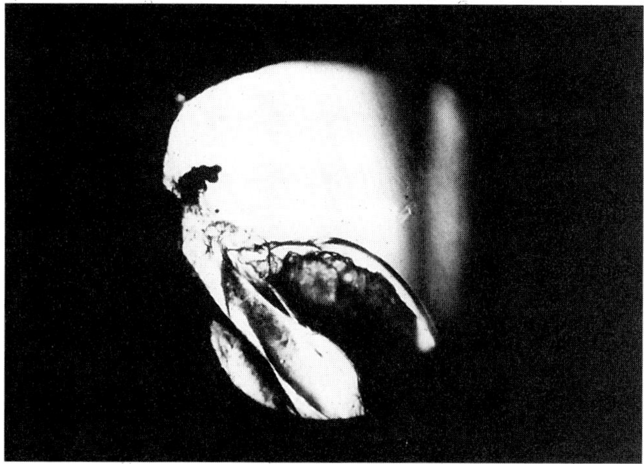

Fig. 172-6. Abnormal red reflex. (See CD-rom for color reproduction of all figures depicting retinal conditions.)

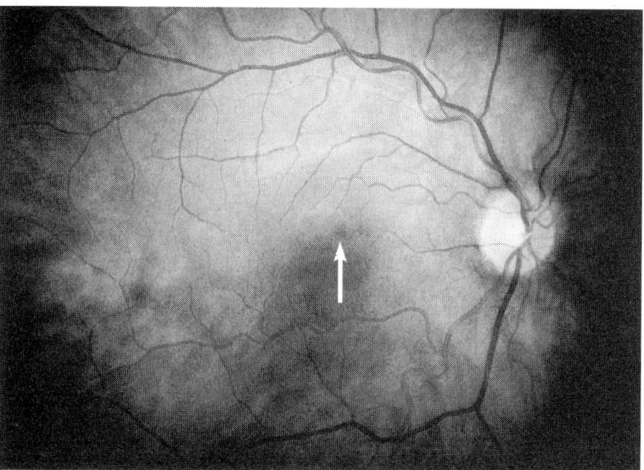

Fig. 172-7. Macular region of retina. The arrow identifies the area of the fovea and the foveola.

standing slightly to the side of the patient. The patient should be asked to focus on a distant object. Usually setting the ophthalmoscope diopter lens to −2 to −3 (the red 2 or 3) will generate a comfortable view of the fundus. Black numbers focus anteriorly and red numbers focus posteriorly (toward the reddish retina). Focus anteriorly on the lids, cornea, conjunctiva, and iris. A diminished red reflex or irregularities in the red reflex may result from cloudy media (e.g., corneal or lens opacities, vitreous blood) and unusual refractive errors (Fig. 172-6). Next focus posteriorly toward the vitreous humor. With the red reflex in view, aim the ophthalmoscope toward the opposite mastoid process and then move as close to the eye as possible to bring the optic disc into view. (The small aperture setting allows for an easier fundus view through an undilated pupil.) If you do not visualize the disc, just follow the vessels in the right direction until you see the disc. The green (or red-free) light aids in viewing vessels and hemorrhages, which appear almost black (the veins appear bluer). Follow the outlines of the vessels in each quadrant.

The optic disc should have sharp margins and the vessels should appear crisp as they cross the edge of the disc. If the margins are indistinct or seem elevated above the rest of the fundus, the patient may have papilledema. The examiner notes any hemorrhages or infarctions of the nerve fiber layer (cotton-wool spots) near the nerve head. Pale optic discs may indicate atrophy and should be evaluated by an ophthalmologist. Marked or asymmetric cupping of the nerve is a possible sign of glaucoma.

The macula is very sensitive to light, so it should be examined last. The best view of the macula occurs when the patient looks directly at the examining light (Fig. 172-7). The presence of the foveal light reflex is one indicator of normal foveal anatomy. Systemic diseases, such as diabetes mellitus and hypertension, can often result in funduscopic microvascular abnormalities (e.g., exudates, arteriovenous nicking, hemorrhage, microaneurysms, and edema). In significant carotid atherosclerosis, cholesterol emboli (Hollenhorst plaques) may lodge in the retinal arterioles at their bifurcations. If a patient has experienced a significant change in vision, the examiner should look specifically for a central retinal artery occlusion (pale fundus with cherry-red spot at macula), a retinal vein occlusion (diffuse venous dilation and retinal hemorrhages), or a retinal detachment (a "billowing sail" retinal appearance) or tear (Fig. 172-8).

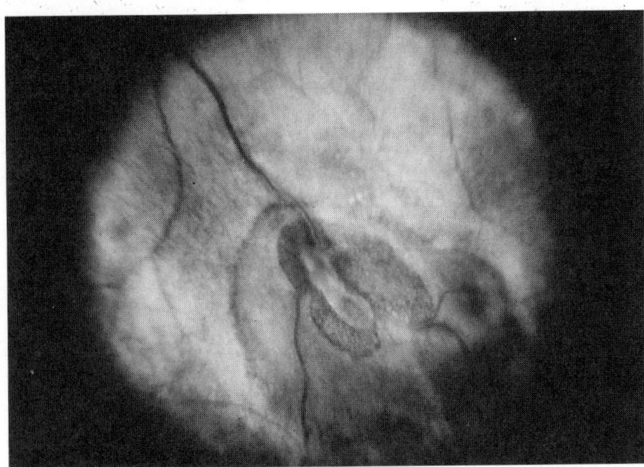

Fig. 172-8. Retinal tear.

Box 172-5. Categories of Eye Complaint Severity

Emergent	Requires immediate ophthalmologist consultation (sudden vision loss, retinal artery occlusion, chemical burns perforation, rupture, acute angle-closure glaucoma, vitreous hemorrhage).
Urgent	Needs ophthalmologist follow-up in 1 day or less (acute glaucoma, orbital cellulitis, hyphema, corneal ulcer or abrasion, retinal detachment, sudden congestive proptosis, macular edema or hemorrhage, ischemic optic neuropathy).
Nonurgent	Follow-up with ophthalmologist within 2 days or as needed.

Documentation of the Eye Examination

The many abbreviations that are used in ophthalmology have been considered by many primary care physicians to be rather cryptic. However, there are many aspects to the eye examination, and abbreviations are necessary to aid in succinct documentation. Some of the more common abbreviations used in documenting the eye examination findings are included in Box 172-3.

Assessment and Management Stratification

Since it is often the primary care physician who initially evaluates patients with any of the four cardinal eye complaints, it is very important that the examiner knows what is *emergent* (requiring immediate ophthalmologic consultation); *urgent* (needing ophthalmologic follow-up in 1 day or less; and *nonurgent* (follow-up with ophthalmology within 2 days or as needed) (Box 172-5).

CHANGE IN VISION

There is often a discrepancy between the patient's perceived degree of visual loss and the examiner's objective determination of vision, thus formal testing of visual acuity is essential. In addition, because a field defect may be perceived as visual loss, testing of VFs by confrontation is imperative. Finally, testing of color vision is also indicated as impairment of color discrimination suggests disease of the optic nerve or central retina. The rapidity with which the patient has had impairment of vision determines the urgency of the need for evaluation. Impairment of vision in one eye implicates the eye itself or disease of the optic nerve anterior to the optic chiasm. Bilateral, symmetric visual field defects suggest a central etiology.

Visual loss can be separated into categories based on anatomic location. Refractory problems can usually be corrected with a pinhole device to 20/25 or 20/30. Opacities in the media (cornea, aqueous humor, lens, vitreous humor) can result in an abnormal red reflex that does not correct with a pinhole device. Examples include cataracts, corneal ulceration, and vitreous hemorrhage. Retinal diseases, such as central retinal artery occlusion, retinal detachment, macular degeneration or hemorrhage, diabetic retinopathy, cytomegalovirus (CMV), central retinal vein occlusion, and "ocular migraine," can be seen on ophthalmoscopic examination. Optic nerve diseases can result in anterior ischemic optic neuropathy (e.g., temporal arteritis, glaucoma, papilledema, neuroretinitis, optic neuritis). Chiasmal diseases can be inferred from abnormal findings during the pupil, optic disc, and VF tests. Advanced disease is associated with bilateral enlarged, sluggish pupils and pale optic discs. VF deficits ultimately define the chiasmal disease. Pituitary adenomas can result in bitemporal field defects. Cortical blindness is the result of bilateral lesions in the occipital cortex that produce bilateral homonymous hemianopia. A unilateral cortical lesion produces a VF loss on one side only and the visual acuity is not affected. Functional visual loss is a diagnosis of exclusion after comprehensive ocular and neurologic examinations are found to be normal. Various techniques are used that can help determine if a patient is feigning blindness. For example, it is possible to bring one's outstretched hands together or legibly and neatly sign one's name—even if totally blind. Patients with functional total or near-total blindness often show an inability to do these tasks. Fig. 172-9 depicts serious causes of acute vision loss that every primary care physician should be able to recognize.

Acute, Painless Loss of Vision

The inner, posterior, nonconjunctival aspects of the eye are usually involved in acute, painless loss of vision. The following information gives key history and physical examination characteristics of each entity.

Vitreous Hemorrhage

History. There is often a sensation of seeing through a "spider web" or of having had floaters. Associated diseases include diabetes mellitus, retinal tears and detachments, sickle cell anemia, and blood dyscrasias.

Examination. The red reflex may be decreased or nonhomogeneous, and there may be difficulty focusing on the retina. Smaller, vitreous hemorrhages may not be visible with direct ophthalmoscopy.

Treatment. The head must be elevated, as well as immediate referral to an ophthalmologist. Delayed vitrectomy may be required for blood that does not clear with time.

Retinal Detachment

History. The patient may experience flashes and floaters before the detachment. There may be a sense of loss of part of the VF or of looking through a sheer curtain. Trauma,

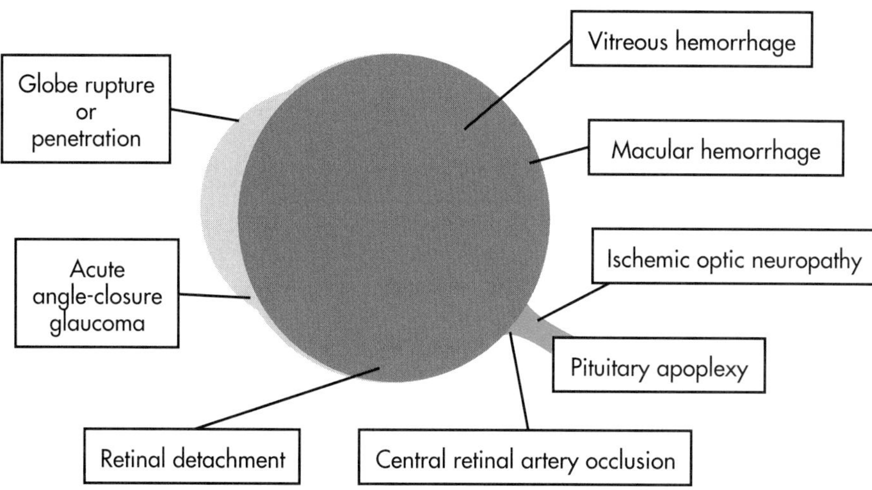

Fig. 172-9. A "Don't Miss" emergent/urgent list of causes of acute vision loss.

severe myopia, and eye surgery are all predisposing conditions. Elderly males are predisposed to retinal detachment.

Examination. Visual field testing discloses a unilateral defect that may be sectoral, quadrantal, hemifield, or total. On funduscopic examination, one may see retinal hydration lines, or rugae, which have the appearance of a "ripple on a pond" or a "billowing sail." A relative afferent pupillary defect may be present. Unfortunately, visualization of a peripheral detachment may not be possible with direct ophthalmoscopy (Fig. 172-10).

Treatment. Immediate referral to an ophthalmologist is a priority. Treatment includes various surgical options including photocoagulation, cryotherapy, diathermy, scleral buckling, or air/silicon oil injections.

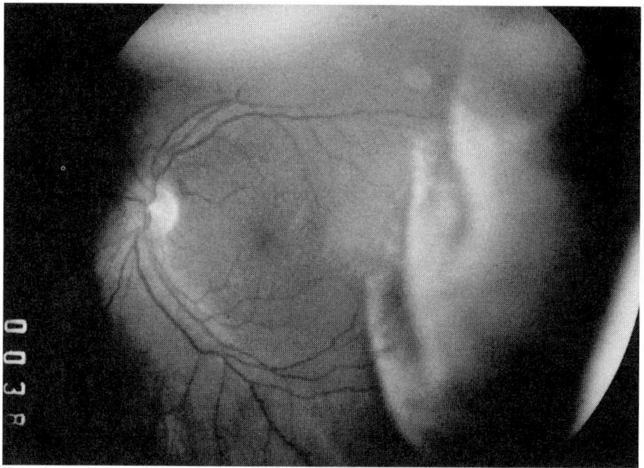

Fig. 172-10. Retinal detachment.

Retinal Artery Occlusion

History. Loss of vision is quite abrupt and nearly complete if the central retinal artery is involved. There may be an antecedent history of transient loss of vision sometimes described as a curtain coming down over the VF, which resolves completely within a short time (amaurosis fugax). Giant cell arteritis should be considered in an elderly patient, especially if they have had headaches, jaw or lingual claudication, or proximal musculoskeletal pain. In addition, patients with migraine headaches, particularly if they have had focal neurologic signs or symptoms associated with their headaches, are at risk for retinal artery occlusion. Young women taking oral contraceptives, elderly males, and patients with cardiac valve abnormalities (i.e., emboli prone) also have an increased risk.

Examination. There is severe impairment of visual acuity often limited to hand motion or light perception. Visual field may be restricted to a small island in the temporal field. On ophthalmoscopy, a refractile object within one of the arterioles may be visualized (Hollenhorst plaque). With central retinal artery occlusion, the retina is diffusely pale and attenuated. A "cherry-red spot" may be seen in the fovea (an area of thin retina overlying the "reddish" choroidal layer) (Fig. 172-11).

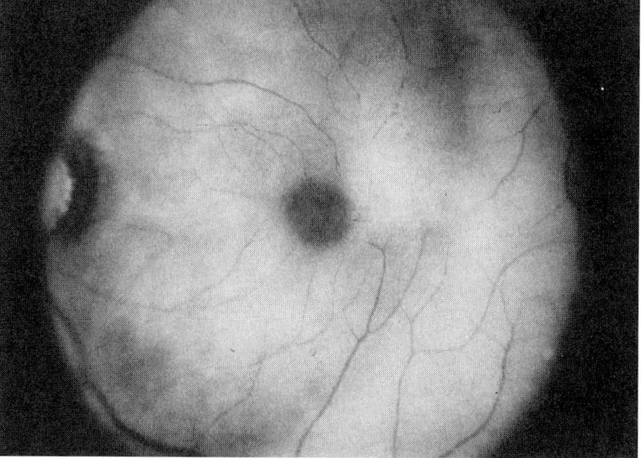

Fig. 172-11. Central retinal artery occlusion.

Treatment. Patients should be immediately referred to an ophthalmologist. In the interim, the patient should be made to lie down and the globe should be gently massaged intermittently (few seconds on and off) in an attempt to dislodge the embolus. Permanent damage can often ensue if the visual loss persists for 2 or more hours. Other interim measures include having the patient breathe into a paper bag every 10 to 15 minutes per hour (increases P_{CO_2} and artery dilation) or alternatively, inhalation of 95% oxygen and 5%

CO_2 (also increases vasodilation). If available, a 250-mg dose of acetazolamide (Diamox) should be given intravenously.

Retinal Vein Occlusion

History. The patient complains of prolonged visual obscurations. Although most often idiopathic, hypertension, diabetes, hyperviscosity syndromes, and glaucoma are risk factors.

Examination. The retinal veins are distended and appear "phlebitic." Multiple retinal hemorrhages are often present and one may see cotton-wool spots. If the thrombosis does not resolve spontaneously, extensive retinal bleeding may occur ("blood and thunder" appearance). Despite the striking retinal picture, the visual loss is often slight and limited to a mild decrease in central visual acuity due to macular hemorrhage and edema (Figs. 172-12 and 172-13).

Treatment. There is no proven effective therapy. Naturally, any underlying hypercoaguable/hyperviscous state should be corrected (e.g., polycythemia, thrombocytosis).

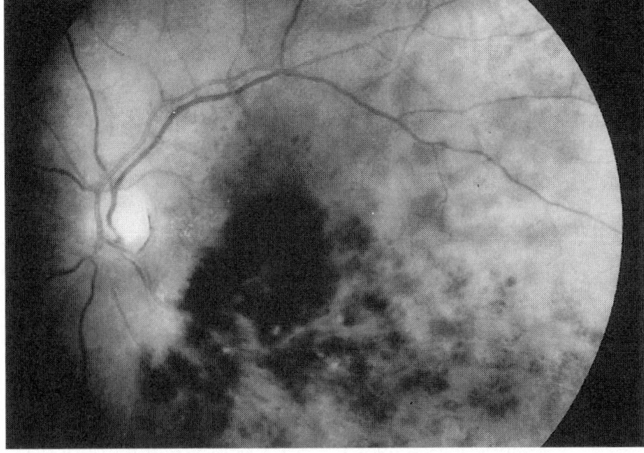

Fig. 172-12. Branch retinal vein occlusion.

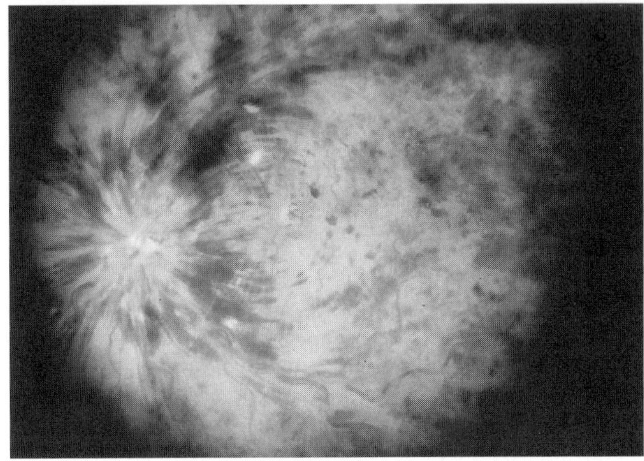

Fig. 172-13. Central retinal vein occlusion.

Anterior Ischemic Optic Neuropathy

History. Anterior ischemic optic neuropathy (AION) is caused by decreased blood flow through the posterior ciliary arteries that supply the optic disc. Two forms are (1) arteritic—most commonly due to giant cell (temporal) arteritis and (2) nonarteritic (the more common form)—the specific cause is unknown but hypertension and diabetes are risk factors. The vision loss is sudden, although patients may on occasion describe premonitory obscurations. If associated with giant cell arteritis, patients may have myalgias, headaches, low grade fever, jaw claudication, weight loss, and anemia.

Examination. An afferent pupil defect (MG pupil) is present. The optic disc is swollen and surrounded by nerve fiber layer splinter hemorrhages.

Treatment. No treatment is available. However, if giant cell arteritis is suspected, glucocorticoid therapy should be started pending determination of a sedimentation rate and temporal artery biopsy to prevent loss of vision in the contralateral eye.

Optic Neuritis

History. Optic neuritis most often occurs in young women and in patients with multiple sclerosis. Vision loss is gradual, occurring over several days. There may be ocular pain, especially with eye movement.

Examination. An afferent pupillary defect is present. Since the demyelinating process is retrobulbar most of the time, the optic disc appears normal at presentation. One third of patients have optic disc pallor and edema at presentation. Many but not all patients, later develop multiple sclerosis.

Treatment. Nearly all patients gradually or spontaneously recover most of their vision after a single episode of optic neuritis. If not, the initial diagnosis should be reconsidered. Administration of glucocorticoids in patients with monocular optic neuritis is controversial, and consultation with a neurologist or neuroophthalmologist is strongly recommended. In patients with bilateral disease, the case for systemic glucocorticoids is much stronger.

Exudative, Age-related Macular Degeneration

History. Exudative, age-related macular degeneration occurs in elderly patients greater than 60 years. Visual blurring is gradual but may suddenly worsen over several days. Patients have diminished central vision, as well as distortion of images (metamorphopsia). Often both eyes are affected, although one eye may be more severely affected than the other.

Examination. Testing with an Amsler grid detects the distortion of images in the central VF. Retinal hemorrhage can sometimes be seen in the macula, although the neovascular membrane (associated with "wet" macular degeneration) may be difficult to see because of its subretinal location. Fluorescein angiography is often needed for its detection (Figs. 172-14 and 172-15).

Treatment. Supplementation with various vitamins and minerals has not been shown to be beneficial. Laser ablation of the choroidal neovascular membrane can arrest the exudative process.

"Ocular Migraine"

History. The patient may or may not have a headache. However, he or she often has a personal or family history of migraine. The loss of vision is fairly rapid but is not sudden.

Examination. On occasion, the retinal arterioles may be attenuated. In some patients, disc edema and peripapillary hemorrhages may be seen. Vision may only partially recover over the course of several months.

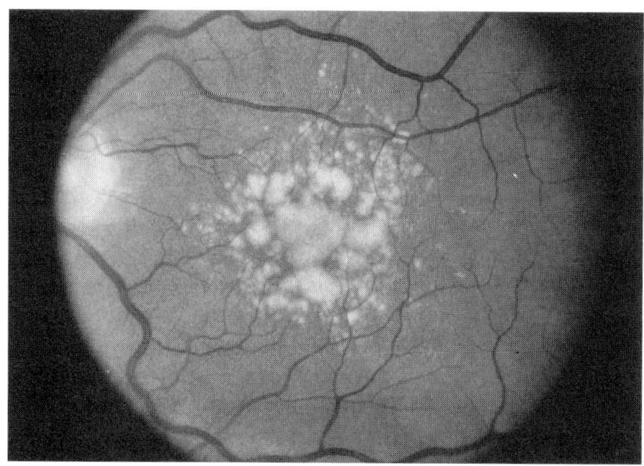

Fig. 172-14. Dry macular degeneration.

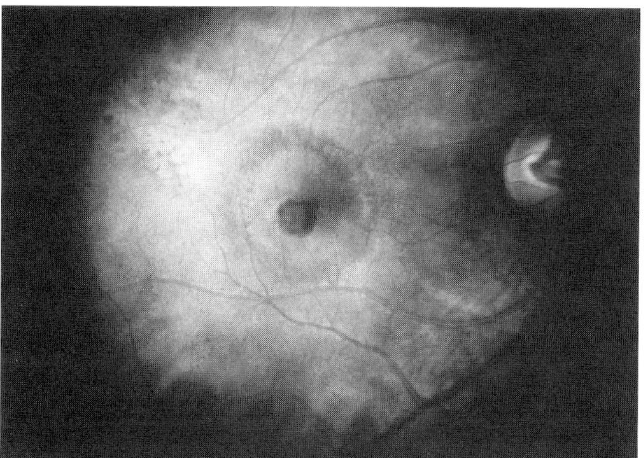

Fig. 172-15. Wet macular degeneration.

Treatment. Vasoconstrictive medications should be avoided. There is anecdotal support for use of rapid-acting calcium channel blockers (e.g., sublingual nifedipine).

Cerebral Infarction

History. Vision loss is sudden and usually bilateral. The nature of the VF deficit depends on the location of the infarction as it relates to the optic radiations. Patients often have a history of or risk factors for arteriosclerotic disease.

Examination

- Homonymous hemianopia: Interruption of the optic radiations after the chiasm.
- Superior quadrantanopia: Involvement of Myerson's loop as the postchiasmal fibers dip into the temporal lobe.
- Inferior quadrantanopia: Involvement of the more cephalad fibers of the postchiasmal within the parietal lobe.
- Homonymous hemianopia with macular sparing: Infarction within one of the visual cortices.

Treatment. Aside from rehabilitation, there is no treatment for the completed stroke. Rapid response to acute stroke syndromes and controlling the risk factors for stroke are important prevention strategies.

Functional Visual Loss

History. The history may be atypical and there is inconsistency of responses on repeated questioning. Secondary gain may be appreciable.

Examination. Pupillary reflexes and funduscopic findings are normal. Optokinetic nystagmus is also present. Normal visual-evoked responses confirm the intactness of the retinooccipital pathways. The patients may not perform doable tasks that even totally blind patients should be able to perform (e.g., writing their name legibly).

Treatment. Psychiatric consultation is indicated.

Acute Painful Loss of Vision

In contradistinction to conditions causing painless loss of vision, patients with pain accompanying their vision loss often have conjunctival injection due to ocular inflammation.

Corneal Ulcer

History. There is often a history of eye trauma or of wearing contact lenses. Patients unable to completely close one or both eyes are also at risk (i.e., severe nerve VII palsy, proptosis, severe ectropion). A painful, vesicular rash in the distribution of the first division of the fifth cranial nerve may be present. In addition, strangely, herpes simplex corneal ulcers are not very painful.

Examination. Observing the cornea with the ophthalmoscope set at +40 diopters (in effect fixing a 10× magnifying lens) may reveal the corneal ulcer. However, staining the cornea with fluorescein is more sensitive in identifying early ulcers. With more advanced infections, a layering of white cells in the anterior chamber (hypopyon) may be seen. This is best appreciated by SLE. With herpes zoster, involvement of the cornea (herpes zoster ophthalmicus) is more likely if the rash involves the tip of the nose (Hutchinson's) as both areas are supplied by the nasociliary branch of the first division of the trigeminal nerve.

Treatment. If the corneal ulcer is small and due to trauma, antibiotic drops and patching the eye for a few days may be all that is needed. In patients with corneal ulcers due to impaired closure of the eye, patching and frequent application of a lubricating ointment allows the ulcer to heal and prevent recurrence. The patient should then be referred to an ophthalmologist for possible definitive treatment of the predisposing condition. If the corneal ulcer is due to herpes zoster, the patient should be prescribed any of the available oral herpes zoster antivirals, have his or her eye patched, and be referred immediately to an ophthalmologist.

Uveitis. In general, inflammation of the iris or ciliary body is termed *anterior uveitis,* whereas involvement of the vitreous, retina, or choroid is termed *posterior uveitis.* Iritis describes involvement of the iris only and iridiocyclitis describes involvement of the iris-ciliary complex. Endophthalmitis describes inflammation predominantly of the vitreous body. Although inflammation of the unveal tract (iris, ciliary body, and choroid) is often idiopathic, it may be associated with many systemic disorders including sarcoidosis, tuberculosis, syphilis, Lyme disease, Behçet's disease, and various seronegative spondyloarthropathies—the HLA-B27–associated disorders (e.g., Reiter's syndrome, ankylosing spondylitis, inflammatory bowel disease, psoriasis).

Distinguishing which segment of the uveal tract is involved is often beyond the skill of most primary care physicians, but is important as it determines the differential diagnosis, work-up, and treatment.

Anterior Uveitis (Iritis)

History. The onset is usually subacute or insidious. Pain as well as photophobia, is present. Vision may be normal or blurred. Extraocular symptoms are present, if the uveitis is part of a systemic disorder.

Examination. One or both eyes may be involved. The conjunctiva is injected, especially at the limbus (ciliary flush). The pupil may be constricted and, if adhesions (synechiae) have developed between the iris and the lens, the pupil may be irregular. On funduscopic examination, deposits may be seen on the posterior surface of the cornea (keratic precipitates). Floating inflammatory cells and protein are not usually seen with the direct ophthalmoscope but if the inflammation is severe enough, these cells may layer out in the lower portion of the anterior chamber (hypopyon).

Treatment. No work-up is necessary for the patient with a first attack of unilateral, nongranulomatous anterior uveitis and an unremarkable comprehensive history and physical, but the patient should be referred to an ophthalmologist within 24 hours. A topical cycloplegic agent (homatropine hydrobromide 5%, atropine sulfate 1%) should be administered 2 to 3 times a day. If the patient has bilateral disease, recurrent disease, or granulomatous inflammation, a search for a systemic disorder is warranted.

Posterior Uveitis

History. Either one or both eyes can be involved. Vision is decreased or blurred. Floaters are common. Onset may be acute or insidious. Again, if the eye is involved as part of a systemic disease, other symptoms referable to that disease may be present. As toxoplasmosis is the most common cause, a history of cat exposure or of AIDS (a significant risk factor) may be elicited.

Examination. The conjunctivae and sclerae are clear. On ophthalmoscopy, the fundus may appear hazy due to inflammation of the vitreous. The optic disc appears swollen and indistinct. There may be retinal and choroidal hemorrhages, exudates, and vascular "sheathing," although these may be difficult to see with direct ophthalmoscopy.

Treatment. A complete history and physical are mandatory with attention being paid to identify any of the disorders associated with posterior uveitis. If there is associated anterior segment inflammation, topical cycloplegic/mydriatic agents (e.g., 1% cyclopentolate, 2% homatropine) should be prescribed. The patient should be referred to an ophthalmologist within 24 hours. If a systemic disorder is present, work-up and treatment of that disease should occur concurrently.

Acute Angle-closure Glaucoma. The ciliary body (located at the inner base of the iris next to the lens—the PC) produces the clear liquid aqueous humor that fills the AC and PC of the eye. The aqueous humor flows from the PC (just behind the iris and in front of the lens) through the pupil into the AC and into the trabecular meshwork. The meshwork functions as a one-way valve and filter. The ciliary muscle inserts on this meshwork and helps pump the aqueous humor through and increase the rate of drainage. The aqueous humor primarily drains into Schlemm's canal (located at the AC angle) and drains into episcleral veins. Any process that significantly disrupts this flow/drainage process may result in a significant increase in IOP. Predisposing risk factors for angle-closure glaucoma (see Chapter 173) usually involve any condition that reduces (narrows) the flow/drainage channels, e.g., hypermetropia (because of corneal shape), aging (lens thicken and push iris forward), or pupillary dilation (increases contact of the iris and the lens).

History. Acute angle-closure glaucoma occurs most often in older individuals, particularly those who have hyperopia. Women are affected 3 to 4 times more often than men. Patients usually present with sudden onset of blurred vision and eye pain. There may be antecedent blurring of vision, halos about lights, and eye pain brought on by being in the dark or in dimmed ambient lighting. During an attack, the patient will have a headache and be nauseated and diaphoretic due to increased IOP. These symptoms may predominate and focus attention away from the eyes as their cause.

Examination. The patient is obviously in pain and is photophobic. During an acute attack, only one eye is affected. Vision is decreased. There may be edema of the eyelids and the conjunctiva is injected. The pupil is midpoint and not reactive to light. There is corneal edema, which blurs the red reflex, and the IOP is elevated, often to a shallow AC.

Treatment. Immediate referral to an ophthalmologist is indicated. The initial IOP-lowering therapies include decreasing aqueous humor production (using topical β-adrenergic antagonists and acetazolamide), reducing vitreous humor volume (using systemic hyperosmotic agents like intravenous mannitol), and facilitating aqueous humor outflow (using miotic agents like pilocarpine that pull the iris from the iridocorneal angle). In most cases, laser iridectomy (creating an alternative pathway for the egress of aqueous humor) reopens a portion of the angle with marked lowering of the IOP.

Endophthalmitis

History. Endophthalmitis is most often related to recent eye surgery and can occur as a complication of a full-thickness wound to the globe. Infrequently, this condition is due to metastatic infection from a distant source (i.e., endogenous endophthalmitis). Pain is not always present. Vision is diminished, and the patient experiences floaters. Intravenous drug users, immunocompromised individuals, and patients with chronic indwelling intravenous lines are a risk for endogenous endophthalmitis. These patients are often very ill and septic.

Examination. Conjunctival injection is present. The red reflex may be diminished and there may be a hypopyon. The vitreous may be hazy or the posterior pole of the fundus may be obscured due to inflammation of the vitreous. Patients with candidal endophthalmitis may have small focal areas of localized retinitis that enlarge into large vitreous opacities.

Treatment. Immediate consultation with an ophthalmologist is indicated. In patients with endogenous endophthalmitis, treatment of the primary source of infection is necessary.

CHANGE IN APPEARANCE

The Red Eye

Aside from VA problems (i.e., myopia and hyperopia), the red eye is the most common presenting ophthalmologic problem encountered by primary care physicians (see Chapters 173 and 175). The history should focus on vision, degree of discomfort, and the presence or absence of discharge. The presence of significant pain suggests possible serious pathology such as acute glaucoma, iritis, scleritis, or a foreign body or corneal ulcer. The causes range from a benign nonurgent form of conjunctivitis to an emergent acute closed-angle glaucoma. This section describes the various causes, manifestations, and treatments of the red and inflamed eye.

Acute Closed-angle Glaucoma. Patients usually present with sudden onset of blurred vision and eye pain. See previous section on acute closed-angle glaucoma for the clinical presentation and treatment guidelines.

Corneal Abnormalities. Corneal problems cause immediate discomfort because of the rich sensory innervation of the corneal epithelium. Corneal abrasions due to small ocular foreign bodies or inadvertent direct trauma from fingernails or makeup brushes are a common occurrence. Tearing and conjunctival injection are apparent. The VA may be impaired if the abrasion is near the central axis.

A short-acting topical anesthetic (e.g., 0.5% tetracaine) is used to facilitate the examination. Corneal fluorescein staining (visualized using a Wood's lamp or a cobalt-blue slit lamp) can be used if the defect or foreign body is not readily apparent. If a foreign body is located, careful sterile saline irrigation (or water in a prehospital setting) directed from the sclera over the cornea is the safest method. Eversion of the lids and copious irrigation of both superior and inferior fornices is important. (See section on removal of foreign body.) Topical antibiotics should be used, and oral (not topical) analgesics may be useful. Close follow-up is necessary, usually within 1 to 3 days. Although soft pressure patches are often used they are usually not necessary. Additionally, patients who wear contact lens should not receive eye patches at all because this can promote corneal/conjunctival infection (e.g., *Pseudomonas*).

Conjunctivitis. Conjunctivitis (an inflammation of the conjunctiva) is usually readily apparent on history and physical examination. The inflammation involves the anterior ocular sclera, the bulbar conjunctiva, the inner surfaces of the eye and lids, and the palpebral conjunctiva. Conjunctivitis, as opposed to scleritis and episcleritis, usually involves the entire conjunctiva, is usually associated with a discharge, and is usually not associated with pain.

Conjunctivitis is usually classified as noninfectious or infectious. Noninfectious causes are mostly allergic (with intense "itchy eyes") and include allergic rhinoconjunctivitis (associated with sneezing, and other hay fever symptoms), vernal (a hypersensitivity reaction characterized by giant cobblestone papillae of the upper palpebral conjunctiva), atopic (associated with eczematous skin lesions), giant papillary (associated with contact lens wearers and inner lid 1- to 2-mm diameter papillae), and contact allergy (secondary to chemical agents). Infectious causes are bacterial (mucopurulent, purulent—acute and chronic), viral (adenovirus, acute hemorrhagic, herpes simplex/zoster, molluscum contagiosum), fungal (candidal), and chlamydial.

Conjunctivitis in children is approximately 50% bacterial and 50% adenoviral (the so-called pink eye). A bacterial cause should be suspected if there is more mucopurulent discharge, less adenopathy, and no other viral symptoms. The three most common organisms are *Staphylococcus aureus, Streptococcus pneumoniae,* and *Haemophilus influenzae* (especially in young children). Because adenoviral conjunctivitis is self-limiting, and topical antibiotics are safe, most cases of pediatric conjunctivitis are treated as bacterial (using 10% sulfacetamide four times a day for 7 to 10 days). The authors do not recommend the use of Polymyxin B because of the significant risk of adverse allergic eye reaction. Patients should be advised they may get worse for 1 to 2 days before they get better. Adenoviral infections are very contagious; infected children should not attend school, and adults who deal with the public should not attend work. Family members should use separate washcloths to avoid transmission, and frequent handwashing is advised. Hot or cool compresses may provide symptomatic relief.

Conjunctivitis in adults is approximately 85% adenoviral and 15% bacterial, so routine antibiotic treatment is not indicated. Topical antibiotics should only be considered in patients presenting with more purulent discharge, no nodes, and no conjunctival follicles (small white bumps on conjunctiva that represent lymphocytic displacement of adjacent blood vessels).

Table 172-2 depicts common ophthalmic disorders that manifest primarily as a conjunctivitis.

Anterior Uveitis (Iritis). See section on uveitis.

Episcleritis/Scleritis. The episclera and sclera form a protective coat of connective tissue for the eye. The episclera overlies the primarily avascular sclera and supplies nutrition to the sclera. Inflammation of the episclera and sclera is not common in clinical practice. Misdiagnosis and delay in proper treatment commonly occur because it is confused with the more common causes of red eye. Episcleritis is characterized by the acute onset of redness and dull, aching eye pain. The VA, pupil, and cornea are usually normal. No discharge is present. Nonurgent referral to an ophthalmologist is recommended for confirmation. Most cases are self-limited and resolve without treatment. Scleritis has an insidious onset but has severe pain that may radiate to the temple or jaw. Photophobia is present and tearing occurs. Vision is usually normal but may be mildly decreased. The globe may be tender to palpation. Most of the patients have an associated systemic disease (e.g., systemic lupus erythematosus, rheumatoid arthritis, gout). Nonurgent referral to an ophthalmologist is required. The initial treatment consists of nonsteroidal antiinflammatory drugs or systemic corticosteroids. A drop of phenylephrine 2.5% in the eye causes the episcleral vessels (as opposed to the deeper scleral vessels) to blanch. This test is useful in determine whether it is episcleritis or scleritis. Also, if a patient's eye is viewed in normal lighting, an eye with scleritis may have a bluish hue when seen in daylight (signifying a thinning of the sclera).

Subconjunctival Hemorrhage. Subconjunctival hemorrhage (SCH) is caused by the rupture of small subconjunctival vessels that stain the bulbar conjunctiva. Commonly, minor trauma or violent Valsalva maneuvers (coughing, vomiting, or straining) can cause SCH. Less commonly, poorly controlled hypertension and coagulopathies can be associated with SCH, especially if recurrent and bilateral. Once hyphemas (blood in the anterior chamber) and foreign bodies are excluded, the treatment is with cool compresses. The conjunctiva usually clears in 2 to 3 weeks.

Table 172-2. Ophthalmic Disorders Associated With Conjunctivitis

Acute or chronic	Unilateral or bilateral	Key symptoms	Degree of injection	Discharge type	Other features
Viral conjunctivitis					
Acute	Bilateral, possibly asymmetric	Itching, burning, soreness	4+	Watery	Preauricular lymphadenopathy
Bacterial conjunctivitis					
Acute	Unilateral or bilateral	Burning, general irritation	3+	Heavy, mucopurulent	Lids possibly adherent
Herpes simplex conjunctivitis					
Acute	Unilateral	Photophobia, mild irritation	1-2+	None	Dendrite on the cornea or vesicles on the lid possible
Adult chlamydial conjunctivitis					
Subacute/chronic	Usually unilateral	Burning, general irritation	2+	Scant, mucopurulent	Usual occurrence in young, sexually active adults
Allergic conjunctivitis					
Chronic	Bilateral	Itching	2+	Stringy, mucoid	Usual occurrence in atopic individuals, possible seasonal symptoms
Blepharitis					
Chronic	Bilateral	Itching, burning, foreign body sensation	1-2+	Usually none	Inflammation and crusting of lid margins
Dry eye					
Chronic	Bilateral	Foreign body sensation	1+	Mucoid in severe cases	Punctate fluorescein staining of the cornea
Cavernous sinus AV fistula					
Chronic	Unilateral	Double vision, audible bruits	1-4+	None	Elevated IOP, proptosis, possible vision loss

From Palay DA: Ophthalmic differential diagnosis. In Palay DA, Krachmer JH: *Ophthalmology for the primary care physician,* St. Louis, 1997, Mosby.
AV, Arteriovenous.

The White Eye

Pinguecula are elevated, fleshy conjunctival masses located in the interpalpebral region, most commonly on the nasal side. They are yellow or light brown. The patients are asymptomatic and no treatment is usually necessary. Pterygium is also fibrovascular tissue that begins on the epibulbar conjunctiva; but in contradistinction to pinguecula, it grows slowly onto the cornea and can eventually affect the vision. Its unsightly appearance and propensity to become inflamed on occasion often brings it to a physician's attention. Both conditions appear to be related to ultraviolet (UV) exposure, repeated trauma, and dry and windy conditions. Clear indications for excision are a lesion that encroaches on the visual axis, one that induces significant irregular astigmatism causing loss of acuity, and a lesion that affects eye movement enough to cause double vision.

Keratoconjunctivitis sicca (dry eye) is often seen with connective tissue disease (e.g., associated with xerostomia is classified as Sjögren's syndrome). Several drugs, including antihistamines, nasal decongestants, analgesics, sedatives, and tricyclic antidepressants, decrease lacrimation.

Corneal dystrophies are inherited abnormalities of the cornea unassociated with systemic disease or prior inflammation. Penlight examination may reveal (at most) a value loss of corneal luster or clarity. SLE is necessary to make the diagnosis. Several corneal degenerations lead to corneal thinning (e.g., keratoconus, keratoglobus). The resulting ectasia causes an irregular astigmatism. Referral to an ophthalmologist for slit-lamp examination is necessary.

The Pigmented Eye

Pigmented lesions of the conjunctiva or sclera may be either melanocytic or nonmelanocytic. Nonmelanocytic pigmentation may be due to thinning of the sclera, allowing visualization of the underlying pigmented choroid (scleromalacia), metabolic disorders, or deposition of pigment (Box 172-6). Melanocytic lesions, on the other hand, arise from melanocytes, which produce the pigment melanin. "Physiologic" causes of increased melanocytes include ethnicity (African-Americans naturally have melanosomes that are larger in size and number) and long-term exposure to sunlight, which increases the number of melanocytes both in the skin and in the eye. Pigmented lesions of melanocytic origin can be classified into four groups—congenital melanosis, nevi, acquired epithelial melanosis, and conjunctival melanoma (Box 172-7).

Box 172-6. Nonmelanocytic Ocular Pigmentation

Scleral Disorders

Blue sclera (osteogenesis imperfecta, iron deficiency anemia)
Staphyloma
Scleromalacia
Senile hyaline plaque

Metabolic Disorders

Ochronosis
Gaucher's disease
Jaundice

Pigment Deposits

Epinephrine
Argyria
Mascara
Quinoline
Iron
Hemosiderin

Box 172-7. Melanocytic Conjunctival Lesions

Congenital Melanosis

Benign epithelial melanosis of conjunctiva
Subepithelial lesions
- Melanosis oculi
- Oculodermal melanosis (nevus of Ota)
- Pigmented episceral spot

Nevi

Intraepithelial (junctional)
Subepithelial
Compound
Spindle epithelioid (juvenile melanoma)
Blue nevus
Cellular blue nevus

Acquired Epithelial Melanosis

Primary acquired melanosis
Secondary acquired melanosis (bilateral)

Melanoma of Conjunctiva

From nevi, acquired melanosis, or de novo
From metastatic or intraocular extension

Congenital Melanosis. *Benign epithelial melanosis* is associated with skin pigmentation (complexion-associated conjunctival pigmentation) and, therefore, seen most commonly in African-Americans or darkly pigmented Latino individuals. This pigmentation is usually bilateral but may be asymmetric and most often located in the limbal area. There is no associated inflammation. It is probably due to UV light exposure or as a response to conjunctival inflammation.

Melanosis oculi is associated with diffuse or localized, irregular pigmentation of the episclera. This is usually unilateral and may be associated with increased pigmentation of the iris and choroid. It is seen more commonly in African-American and Asian individuals. Depending on the location of the melanocytes, the episclera may be blue, gray, or brown. Since the pigmentation is in the episclera not the conjunctiva, it does not move with movement of the conjunctiva. There is a small risk in whites of developing a choroidal melanoma.

Oculodermal melanosis (nevus of Ota) has eye findings similar to those of melanosis oculi except that there is associated hyperpigmentation of the periocular skin, including the eyelid. Once again, the pigmentation does not move with the conjunctiva and the condition is usually unilateral.

A small risk exists for developing a uveal melanoma or an ocular melanoma. There is no risk of developing a conjunctival melanoma but an increased risk for developing in whites only a choroidal melanoma.

Pigmented episcleral spot (Axenfeld's nerve loop) is a slightly raised, hyperpigmented spot 3 to 4 mm from the limbus. Occasionally, more than one spot may be seen. The lesion may be tender and is much more common in African-American individuals. It represents an intrascleral nerve loop that penetrates the sclera, carrying with it a branch of the anterior ciliary artery or nerve or both. Choroidal pigment migrates along the nerve and deposits in the episcleral space. There is no increased risk of degeneration into a melanoma.

Conjunctival Nevi. Conjunctival nevi originate from melanocytes and represent hamartomas of the conjunctiva. They are classified as congenital or acquired and tend to occur at the limbus, eyelid margin, caruncle, or plica semilunaris. Although most are flat and circumscribed, there can be thickening of the conjunctiva. Since they originate from the conjunctiva they are freely movable, except near the limbus where the conjunctiva is fixed. Attachment to the sclera or episclera should raise suspicion of a melanoma. Conjunctival nevi are lightly colored before puberty but tend to get darker with puberty, pregnancy, use of hormones, UV light exposure. As many as 30% of conjunctival nevi never acquire pigmentation. Occasionally, they can develop clear cystic spaces. Although conjunctival nevi progress through certain levels of maturation, they uncommonly lead to melanoma. The accurate diagnosis of these lesions is beyond the skill of most generalists. It is prudent to refer any patient with a pigmented conjunctival lesion that has changed in size or color or has developed associated inflammation. In addition, any pigmented conjunctival lesion adherent to the underlying episclera or sclera should also be referred.

Acquired Melanosis. *Primary acquired melanosis* is a diffuse, poorly circumscribed lesion with variegation of pigmentation affecting the conjunctiva near the limbus. The pigment may extend beyond the eye to involve the skin of the eyelids. The condition is unilateral but the lesions can be multifocal, and hence the examiner must visualize the entire conjunctiva, both bulbar and tarsal. In contradistinction to most other disorders of pigmentation of the external eye, these lesions are more common in white individuals. There can also be mild pigmentation of the corneal epithelium.

These lesions can wax and wane or even disappear completely. Lesions with greater proliferation of cells and cellular atypia can progress to malignant melanoma. Since this requires a conjunctival biopsy, all such lesions should be referred to an ophthalmologist, preferably one with experience in dealing with pigmented eye lesions.

Secondary acquired melanosis is considered a physiologic or irritant-induced increase in pigmentation of the conjunctiva. This occurs in response to hormonal changes (i.e., Addison's disease, pregnancy), chemical effects (i.e., arsenic, chlorpromazine), chronic inflammatory conjunctival disorders (i.e., vernal keratoconjunctivitis, trachoma), or radiation. The lesions are often bilateral, discrete, and restricted to the conjunctival epithelium. They are nonproliferative and thus do not have the potential of malignant transformation.

Malignant Melanoma. *Primary conjunctival melanomas* are rare tumors that may arise de novo from a conjunctival nevus or from primary acquired melanosis. The clinical features are not distinctive enough to allow early diagnosis. Palpebral, forniceal, and caruncle-based melanoma tend to have a worse prognosis than melanomas of the limbus. In fact, any pigmented lesion arising in the palpebral or forniceal areas should be considered potentially malignant, since benign pigmented lesions rarely involve these areas. Deep pigmentation of the eyelid margins also worsens the prognosis of conjunctival melanomas. Conversely, conjunctival melanomas are very rare in African-Americans. Naturally, individuals with multiple nodules have a greater chance of developing metastases and have a worse prognosis.

Secondary conjunctival melanomas are lesions that usually originate in the intraocular uveal tract or ciliary body and extend through the emissary channels of the sclera or migrate along Axenfeld's nerve loop. Rarely, conjunctival melanomas may be metastatic deposits from a primary skin melanoma.

Eyelid, Lash, and Lacrimal Abnormalities

The surrounding maintenance structures that protect and support the globe are shown in Figure 172-16. These structures help protect the eye from foreign bodies, infections, injuries, and maintain a moist corneal surface. Note the innervations of the orbicularis muscle (VII nerve)—responsible for closing the eye—and the levator muscle (III nerve)—responsible for opening the eye.

Eyelid Infections and Inflammation. An external *hordeolum* (stye) is a furuncle at the lid margin involving a lash follicle and gland of Zies or Moll. It presents with painful lid swelling that becomes localized, often pointing through the skin at the lash line. Treat with warm compresses and topical antibiotic drops (e.g., fluoroquinolones) 3 to 4 times a day. Incision and drainage is performed if the more conservative measures are ineffective. Follow-up is important to ensure that preseptal cellulitis does not occur.

An internal hordeolum (chalazion) involves a meibomian gland. It presents with minimal discomfort and firm inflammatory nodule located away from the lid margin. Early treatment consists of 5 days of warm compresses to open the inflamed gland. The ophthalmologist may need to do steroid injections or marsupialization of the encysted meibomian gland using a conjunctival approach.

Blepharitis is an inflammation of the lid margins with an associated thickening and possible scaling, crusting, and ulceration. The three distinct types are seborrhea (associated with dandruff of the brows and scalp), staphylococcal infection (often associated with styes), and meibomian gland dysfunction (often associated with chalazia). It presents with irritation, burning, excessive tearing (epiphora), photophobia, and intermittent blurred vision. Treatment includes scrubbing the lid margins with a cotton-tipped application dipped in dilute baby shampoo and massage of the lid margins to help express the abnormal meibomian secretions. Topical antibiotics (e.g., erythromycin) are applied to the lid margins at night if lid scrubs are ineffective. A 6-week course of doxycycline (50 to 200 mg/day) is added to improve meibomian gland function. Blepharitis is often recurrent and refractory to treatment.

Orbital cellulitis can cause eyelid swelling and can lead to blindness, cranial nerve palsies, brain abscesses, and life-threatening infection. Preseptal cellulits/periorbital cellulitis and other infections located around the globe (e.g., ethmoid sinusitis, styes), eyelid injury, or intraorbital surgery can be predisposing conditions leading to orbital cellulitis. Preseptal cellulitis and orbital cellulitis present with similar symptoms (e.g., warm, red, and swollen eyelids that may extend over the nasal bridge to the opposite side). However, vision, pupillary reflexes, and extraocular movements are normal in preseptal cellulitis as opposed to orbital cellulitis (Figs. 172-17 and 172-18).

Eyelid dermatitis (acute, chronic, or contact) is very common and is associated with itching and swelling. Rubbing and exposure to irritants, such as cosmetics, aerosol hair sprays, and deodorant soaps, can be causative agents. For treatment, patients should stop any exposure to eyelid irritants and use cool compresses four times daily. Once improvement begins, a weak topical steroid like hydrocortisone 0.5% can be massaged into the skin three to four times daily until resolution.

Common viral infections include the pox viruses (molluscum contagiosum), wart viruses (verruca vulgaris, plana, digitata, and filiformis), and the herpes viruses (herpes simplex, varicella-zoster). The herpes viruses manifest as crops of vesicles that may attack the lid margins and conjunctiva. In varicella-zoster virus infections the pain is often severe and may develop into a postherpetic neuralgia. Treatment of herpes virus infections includes using oral acyclovir.

Fungal infections of the eyelid are rare but can be caused by blastomycosis, coccidioidomycosis (known as valley fever or San Joaquin fever in the southwestern United States), cryptococcosis, and sporotrichosis. Blastomycosis often affects the eyelid, producing gradually enlarging, hyperkeratotic, verrucous plaques that may become confluent, ulcerate, and crusted. Coccidioidomycosis, cryptococcosis, and sporotrichosis may produce chronic lid margin and periocular ulceration. Oral itraconazole or intravenous amphotericin are used in treatment.

Parasitic infections involving the eyelid include phthiriasis palpebrarum (crab lice), demodicosis (*Demodex* species—the hair follicle and sebaceous gland mite), myiasis (spread by fly larvae especially in Central and South America), *Dirofilaria tenuis* (a raccoon parasite spread by mosquito bites that produce a solitary nodule), leishmaniasis, and cysticercosis. The itchy crab lice blepharitis may reveal few or multiple nits

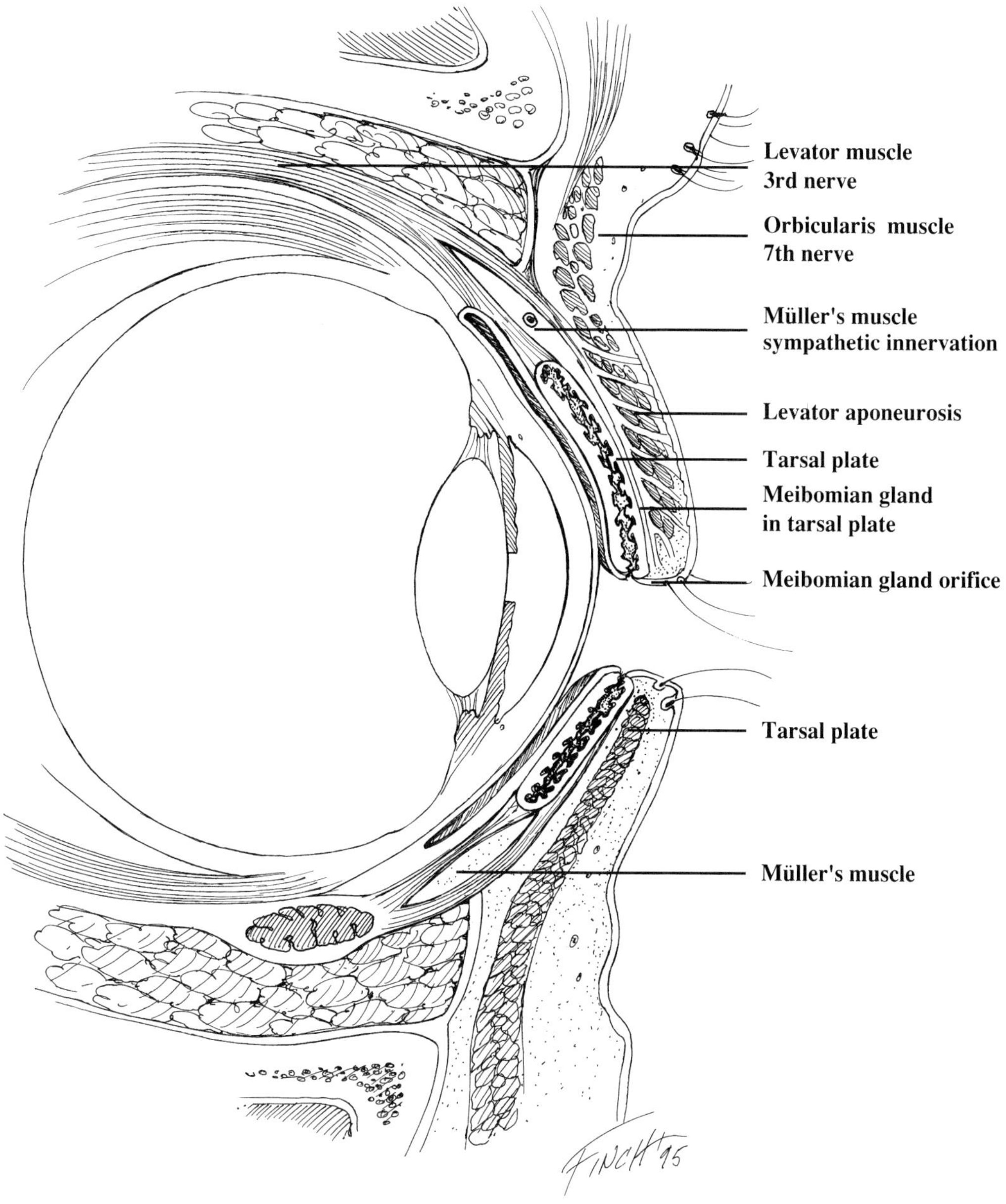

Levator muscle
3rd nerve
Orbicularis muscle
7th nerve
Müller's muscle
sympathetic innervation
Levator aponeurosis
Tarsal plate
Meibomian gland
in tarsal plate
Meibomian gland orifice
Tarsal plate
Müller's muscle

Fig. 172-16. Side view of eyelid anatomy. (From Wojno TH: Eyelid abnormalities. In Palay DA, Krachmer JH: *Ophthalmology for the primary care physician,* St. Louis, 1997, Mosby.)

(eggs) glued to the lash bases and several lice crawling about the shafts. Treatment of the lice includes washing all clothes and bed linen in hot, soapy water, using antilice shampoo, and picking off the nits and lice.

Other Eyelid Lesions. Xanthelasma is the most common cutaneous xanthoma. It occurs in middle-aged and elderly persons, one third of whom are hyperlipidemic. These slightly raised, yellowish tan, soft plaques are usually bilateral and located at the inner canthi. Other lesions include foreign body granulomas, hidrocystomas (retention cysts of the apocrine or eccrine sweat glands), pilosebaceous cysts (milia and sebaceous cysts), epidermal inclusion cysts, seborrheic keratosis, actinic keratosis, and other tumors (basal cell carcinoma, squamous cell carcinoma, sebaceous gland adenoma).

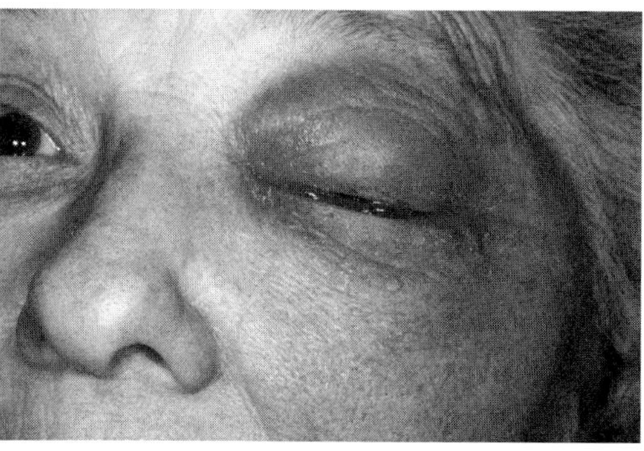

Fig. 172-17. Orbital cellulitis resulting from ethmoid sinusitis. (From Wojno TH: Orbital disease. In Palay DA, Krachmer JH: *Ophthalmology for the primary care physician,* St. Louis, 1997, Mosby.)

Eyelid (and Eyelash) Malpositions and Injuries. The diagnosis and management of eyelid malpositions and the treatment of eyelid lacerations are shown in Box 172-8 and Table 172-3.

Lacrimal Abnormalities. Tears aid in the supply of essential nutrients, antibacterial substances and the flushing of microorganisms, oxygen, and lubrication of the eyes. Tear film is composed of three layers. The outer lipid layer is produced form the meibomian sebaceous glands. The middle layer is the most plentiful and is produced by the lacrimal gland. The innermost layer of tear film is produced by the conjunctival globlet cells and allows the tear film to spread evenly over the cornea. Vitamin A deficiency can decrease mucin production and induce severe dryness and corneal scarring. Tearing is stimulated by the first division of the trigeminal nerve and from sympathetic and parasympathetic innervation.

Alacrima (dry eye syndrome/keratoconjunctivitis sicca) is often caused by systemic diseases and systemic medication. Basic palliative measures include avoiding low humidity,

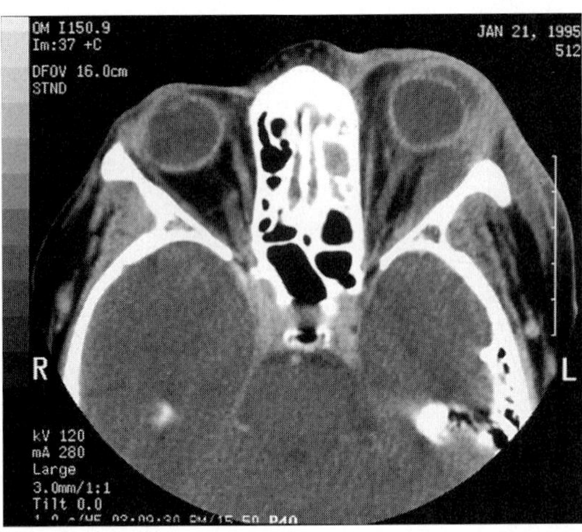

Fig. 172-18. An axial CT scan of the patient in Fig. 172-17 shows diffuse infiltration of the left orbital structures. (From Wojno TH: Orbital disease. In Palay DA, Krachmer JH: *Ophthalmology for the primary care physician,* St. Louis, 1997, Mosby.)

Box 172-8. Eyelid Lacerations

Repair

Nonmarginal lacerations that do not involve:
- Canthal tendons
- Levator
- Lacrimal drainage system
- Extensive tissue loss

Close
- Clean carefully
- Debride conservatively
- Repair meticulously
- 6-0 or 7-0 nonabsorbable sutures
- Do not fix the lid to the orbital rim by including orbital septum in the repair

Refer to an Ophthalmologist*

Nonmarginal eyelid lacerations involving canthal tendons
Nonmarginal eyelid lacerations involving levator or aponeurosis
Eyelid lacerations involving eyelid margin
Lacerations with significant tissue loss
Canalicular lacerations
Any eyelid laceration about which there is any doubt

*Cover with a high, moist dressing and refer.

Table 172-3. Eyelid Malpositions

Malposition	Symptoms	Signs	Management
Trichiasis: normal lid position, but lashes directed posteriorly	Irritation, tearing red eye	Eyelid: no entropion, scarring, inflammation Eyelash: against the eye Eye: red, corneal ulcer	Lid scrubs, hot compresses, antibiotics For lash: temporary epilation, permanent epilation Electroepilation: excision of root(s), cryodestruction
Entropion: can be congenital, acquired, cicatricial, mechanical, senile	Intermittent (?), irritation, tearing, red eye	Eyelid: lid flipped in lashes and skin against the eye Eye: red, corneal ulcer	For lid: temporary or permanent tape, restore anatomy For eye: lubricate
Ectropion: can be congenital, acquired, cicatricial, paralytic, senile	Irritation, tearing, red eye, red lid	Eyelid: eyelid flipped out, irritated, exposed conjunctiva Eye: dry, irritated	For lid: surgically restore anatomy
Blepharoptosis Neurogenic Neuromuscular junction: myogenic, aponeurotic, mechanical	Upper lid droop	Frontalis contraction, brow elevation, excess skin, high lid crease, droopy lid	Surgically restore, suspend lid
Retraction: Graves' disease?	Stare, eye too big, irritation, tearing	Lid: upper > up, lower > down Eye: red, exposed	Surgically lower upper and/or raise lower
Blepharospasm	Eyes close involuntarily	Lid spasms, facial twitches	Botulinum toxin, surgery

smoking, wind fans, and all air pollution. Artificial tears during the day and lubricant ointment at night can also be helpful.

Excessive tearing is often due to conjunctival, corneal, or eyelid margin irritation from a foreign body or inflammation. Epiphora is present if overflow of tears onto the cheek occurs. Excessive tearing, popularly known as "crocodile tears," is due to the rare abnormal linkage of the salivary and lacrimal glands so that stimuli that produce salivation also produce lacrimation. Bell's palsy and facial trauma with aberrant regeneration of the facial nerve can be predisposing risk factors.

Dacryoadenitis (infection of the lacrimal system) may be acute (viral or bacterial) or chronic (bacterial). Acute viral dacryoadenitis produces a fullness or pain in the upper outer orbit with an inflammatory, abscesslike, firm, tender, and lateral lid swelling, an S-shaped upper lid margin, a mechanical ptosis, sometimes inferonasal proptosis, and preauricular lymphadenopathy. Resolution takes 1 to 2 weeks. Viral causes include mumps, infectious mononucleosis, herpes zoster, measles, influenza, and dengue fever. Acute bacterial dacryoadenitis, although rare, is more severe and may suppurate, draining through the conjunctiva or skin. Causative organisms include *Staphylococcus, Streptococcus, Pneumococcus,* and *Gonococcus.* Systemic antibiotics are indicated.

Chronic bacterial dacryoadenitis produces a superotemporal orbital mass with diplopia on looking toward it, inferonasal proptosis, and often dry eye. Causes include trachoma, tuberculosis, leprosy, lymphoma, leukemia, syphilis, and actinomycosis. Daily ophthalmologic follow-up is required. Canaliculitis presents with chronic unilateral tearing and irritation and redness and swelling of the area over the canaliculus. *Actinomyces, Candida,* and *Aspergillus* are causative agents. Dacryocystitis, a common condition due to nasolacrimal duct obstruction, presents in middle-aged adults (females more than males) with acute or chronic lacrimal sac swelling (below the medial canthal tendon), irritation, and tearing. Common bacterial organisms are similar to those associated with acute bacterial dacryoadenitis. Titrate the treatment to the clinical picture, with appropriate systemic antibiotics (oral or intravenous), hot compresses, abscess drainage, and dacryocystorhinostomy.

EYE PAIN OR DISCOMFORT

Pain or discomfort in the eye or periorbital region may be difficult to localize or interpret. Generally, the outer eye and supporting structures are more pain sensitive (e.g., cornea, sclera, etc.) than the inner eye (e.g., retina). The primary structures of the eye and periorbital region that have significant sensory innervations (conveying pain/discomfort sensations) include the sclera, the cornea, the eyelids (from the ophthalmic and maxillary divisions of the trigeminal nerve), and conjunctiva. Refer to the other sections that discuss clinical syndromes that are associated with eye pain or discomfort (e.g., acute closed-angle glaucoma).

TRAUMA

Evaluating the Traumatized Eye

The primary care physician is frequently asked to evaluate patients with severe ocular trauma but may often be confronted with the patient with mild or moderate trauma. Assessing the severity of the trauma and referring those patients with sight-threatening injuries is the first priority. In addition, identifying and addressing concurrent nonocular injuries is of paramount importance. Careful and detailed documentation of the history, the physical findings, and any procedures or interventions is especially important in case of legal action either against the physician or other parties.

The mechanism of injury is important to elucidate. High velocity injuries, as when using a hammer and chisel, may lead to penetration of the globe by a foreign object. Blunt trauma of moderate-to-severe intensity can cause a "blow-out" fracture. The *size* of the object causing the trauma is also important—larger objects transfer most of their energy to the orbital rim, whereas smaller objects may directly strike the globe itself. In evaluating the patient with ocular trauma, one follows the same pattern in the examination as when performing a routine eye examination—vision testing, VF assessment, extraocular muscles, eyelids, conjunctivae and sclerae, cornea, AC, lens, optic nerve and, finally, retina. In addition, attention is paid to periocular structures, such as the orbital bones (including the zygoma) and the maxillary, frontal and ethmoid sinuses. It may be necessary to use a local anesthetic to facilitate the examination, and fluorescein must be used to not to miss a corneal abrasion or laceration.

Fractures and Soft Tissue Injuries

Zygomatic Fracture. The zygoma bone is composed of two portions—the zygomatic arch and the body. The arch forms the lateral and inferior portions of the orbit, whereas the body gives rise to the malar eminence.

History. The patient has experienced blunt trauma of moderate force. There may be pain on opening the mouth since the temporalis muscle inserts into the arch.

Examination. There may be flattening of the malar eminence; this is best seen by standing behind a seated patient and looking down his or her face. Palpation of the zygoma may reveal a "step-off" deformity. There is edema and often an ecchymosis of the soft tissues of the temple or infraorbital area. Hypesthesia of the infraorbital area suggests damage to the infraorbital nerve. Impairment in gaze suggests entrapment of one of the extraocular muscles in an orbital "blow-out fracture."

Diagnostic Studies. A Waters' view and a "jug-handle" view (a submental to vertex view of the zygomatic arches) reveal most zygomatic fractures. If there is suspicion of damage beyond a simple zygomatic fracture, a CT scan should be obtained immediately.

Treatment. The patient should be given an immediate referral to an ophthalmologist or plastic surgeon.

Periorbital or Ocular Contusion

History. The patient has experienced a blunt trauma and has mild-to-moderate pain. Vision may be slightly blurred or decreased. *Diplopia* and sometimes an ipsilateral nose bleed suggest a blow-out fracture of the orbit. As mentioned, the size of the striking object determines the likelihood of injury to the periocular soft tissues vs. the globe itself.

Examination. Slight diminution of vision can result from traumatic iritis or a corneal abrasion. More marked disturbance of vision suggests a hyphema (i.e., blood in the AC), vitreous hemorrhage, traumatic optic neuropathy, or a lens subluxation. Periorbital edema and ecchymosis may be present. SCH may be present. Diminished sensation in the infraorbital area suggests a blow-out fracture of the floor of the orbit (which is thin and poorly supported) with damage or swelling of the infraorbital nerve. The physician should look for a laceration of the margin of a lid. Ocular motility is normal unless there has been a blow-out fracture. In such a case, there may be restriction of ocular movement due to entrapment of the rectus muscles, usually the inferior rectus. The pupillary sphincter may be damaged and the pupil may therefore react poorly to light. Pharmacologic dilation of the pupil is mandatory. The red reflex may be diminished or inhomogeneous if there has been bleeding into the vitreous or if the lens has been dislocated. There may be a hyphema or the iris may have been torn, giving a crescent-like defect at its periphery.

Treatment. If the injury is mild or moderate and is limited to the periocular tissue, application of cool compresses and moderate strength analgesics is all that is immediately necessary. The patient should be nonemergently referred to an ophthalmologist for a careful funduscopic examination. Moderate-to-severe diminution of vision, eyelid laceration, hyphema, or restriction of ocular range of motion should be immediately referred to an ophthalmologist.

If the patient returns with pain, severe photophobia, excessive tearing and blurred vision 2 or 3 days after blunt trauma to the eye, traumatic iritis should be suspected. This is a result of intraocular inflammation induced by the trauma. The patient should be referred to an ophthalmologist for SLE and dilated fundus examination.

Corneal Abrasion

History. The patient with corneal abrasion usually has a history of blunt trauma. There is significant eye pain and photophobia. Involuntary lid closure may occur due to *blepharospasm.* There may be a foreign body sensation. Vision may be decreased or blurred. (See also Chapter 175.)

Examination. The patient is obviously uncomfortable, tearing excessively and keeping his or her eye closed. If the abrasion is central, then there may be significant diminution in vision (i.e., 20/80 to 20/200). If the patient has a foreign body sensation, the upper and lower tarsal conjunctivae should be inspected carefully; the upper lid should be inspected by eversion. A foreign body imbedded in the upper tarsal conjunctiva can repeatedly scratch the cornea as the eye is opened and closed. These corneal abrasions are linear and are named "ice skate tracks." The eyelids may be edematous, and the conjunctiva is significantly injected. If the cornea is hazy, bacterial superinfection should be suspected. Fluorescein dye will be taken up by the areas of the cornea devoid of epithelium. A topical anesthetic brings immediate relief, although this should be used for diagnosis and not as a treatment modality.

Treatment. Patients with *contact lens–associated corneal abrasions* should be referred immediately to an ophthalmologist since a significant risk of gram-negative bacterial infection exists, particularly with *Pseudomonas*. An eye patch should not be used because it can accelerate the damage caused by a gram-negative infection. Corneal abrasion that is not associated with contact lens use should be treated with the following:

- A cycloplegic (i.e., homatropine 5%) is instilled three times a day. This relieves ciliary spasm and eases the pain.
- Antibiotic ointment twice daily and at bedtime. For abrasions caused by vegetable matter or tree branches, an antibiotic with extended gram-negative coverage is necessary (i.e., tobramycin).
- An eye patch is applied for larger (i.e., 5-10 mm) abrasions, or if the patient is in severe pain. It should not be worn for more than 48 hours and the eye should be uncovered several times in the interim as bacteria otherwise thrive in the warm, moist environment created by a patch.
- Oral analgesics are often necessary due to the severity of the pain. A short course of a moderately potent narcotic analgesic is not unreasonable.

The patient should be seen daily until the abrasion has healed. Patients with large abrasions or those with central abrasions should be referred to an ophthalmologist.

Foreign Bodies. It is vital to remove corneal or conjunctival foreign bodies as soon as possible since they may become more imbedded and may cause ongoing local damage. A metal foreign body can leave a permanent "rust stain" in the cornea if not removed quickly. (See also Chapter 175.)

History. The patient may or may not recall having had a foreign body enter the eye. A foreign body sensation, excessive tearing, and pain may be present. These symptoms tend to be worse if the foreign body is imbedded in the cornea rather than in the conjunctiva. A blurring of vision that is not improved with blinking to clear excessive tears suggests that the cornea is affected.

Examination. There is conjunctival injection and tearing. Instillation of a topical anesthetic may facilitate vision testing and the patient's cooperation with the examination. Using the ophthalmoscope set at +40 D and held close to the eye may disclose a foreign body imbedded in the conjunctiva or cornea. A small conjunctival laceration can be present, as can a subconjunctival hemorrhage, in the case of a conjunctival foreign body. Linear, vertical abrasions (ice skate tracks), can be seen if the foreign body is in the superior tarsal conjunctiva. As mentioned, eversion of the superior eyelid is mandatory when evaluating a patient with an ocular foreign body. A dilated fundus examination is also indicated.

Diagnostic Testing. Diagnostic testing usually is not necessary with the exception of high speed missile or "metal on metal" injuries. In such circumstances, a CT scan of the orbits with 2-mm axonal/coronal cuts should be obtained in search of an intraorbital or intraocular foreign body.

Treatment. Removal of the foreign body is indicated if it is not deeply imbedded and if it is seen in full (i.e., no portion of it penetrates the sclera into the intraocular space). If the foreign body is very superficial, irrigation of the eye with normal saline may dislodge the object. If it is adherent, a sterile, saline-soaked cotton-tipped swab can be used to remove it. The remaining epithelial defect is then treated as an ocular abrasion with a topical antibiotic ointment and artificial tears, if needed.

Patients with globe penetrating or deeply imbedded foreign bodies, conjunctival lacerations, or numerous foreign bodies should have a light patch placed and referred immediately to an ophthalmologist.

Acute Ultraviolet Radiation Injury

History. Acute UV radiation injuries occur typically after welding without the use of protective eyewear. It can also occur after exposure to large amounts of reflected sunlight while sunbathing or skiing (i.e., "snowblindness") or exposure to an indoor sunlamp. Patients are in moderate-to-severe pain, have photophobia, excessive tearing, blurred vision, and may have blepharospasm. Symptoms occur 6 to 12 hours after the exposure.

Examination. There is mild conjunctival injection and edema. Fluorescein staining shows dense punctate staining of the cornea with greater involvement of the central cornea. Both eyes should be examined, and the superior lids should be everted and scrutinized.

Treatment. Treatment is the same as that for corneal abrasions:

- A cycloplegic (i.e., homatropine 5%) is instilled 3 times a day.
- Antibiotic ointment is applied 2 to 3 times per day.
- For severe damage, both eyes may need to be patched.
- Oral analgesics of moderate strength are necessary.

After 24 hours, the patches are removed and if the condition has improved, the antibiotic ointment is continued for another 3 days. If there is no improvement after 1 to 2 days, the patient should be referred to an ophthalmologist.

Subconjunctival Hemorrhage

History. SCH is often associated with blunt trauma to the eye or can occur spontaneously. SCH can be associated with a primary bleeding diathesis or with the use of oral anticoagulants, accelerated hypertension, or with large and sudden rises in venous pressure as with Valsalva maneuver, coughing, sneezing, weight lifting, and so on. Infrequently, SCH may complicate an infectious conjunctivitis, especially due to adenovirus or pneumococcus.

Examination. Typically, a bright red collection of blood is seen underneath the conjunctiva that does not extend beyond the limbus and does not appreciably raise the conjunctiva. In very severe cases, there may be hemorrhagic suffusion of the conjunctiva that may also be edematous.

Diagnostic Tests. Most often, no diagnostic tests are needed. Blood pressure should be checked in all patients. If there is a history of recurrent, unprovoked SCH, a bleeding diathesis should be considered and coagulation studies should be obtained. If the trauma has been moderate to severe and the hemorrhage is temporally located, a fracture of the zygomatic arch should be considered and appropriate x-rays or CT scan should be obtained.

Treatment. In the uncomplicated hemorrhage that is not associated with any significant trauma or bleeding diathesis, no intervention is necessary, and reassurance is all that is needed. If the hemorrhage is significant and has been associated with trauma to the eye, the physician should consider the possibility of an underlying globe rupture and should immediately refer the patient to an ophthalmologist. Obviously, if a predisposing disorder is discovered, it should be handled in whatever manner is appropriate.

Chemical Injury

History. A chemical injury is usually caused by inadvertent or intentional splashing of the eye with an acid, alkali, or other chemically active substance such as mace and tear gas. The patient experiences severe pain, blurring of vision, and blepharospasm.

Examination. Physical findings may vary depending on the severity of the injury.

Mild-to-moderate injuries:

First-degree burn of the periorbital skin.

Injection and edema of the conjunctiva (chemosis), occasionally with SCH.

Episcleral and conjunctival vessels are visible and intact.

Cornea is hazy.

Severe injuries:

Periocular skin involvement may be significant (i.e., second- or third-degree burn).

Loss of episcleral and conjunctival vessels; the sclera appears white.

Significant conjunctival edema.

Cornea is edematous and opacified.

Treatment. In the case of severe chemical injuries, the following treatment takes precedence over evaluation:

- Anesthetic drops are instilled initially and every 10 to 15 minutes thereafter to facilitate eye lavage. The possibility of a ruptured globe must be kept in mind and ruled out if a consideration.
- Eye is lavaged with 2 L of normal saline over the course of 1 hour. Lid retractors may be necessary if there is significant blepharospasm.
- Fornices of the eye should also be swept with a moistened, cotton-tipped applicator to remove any particulate material. In the meantime, arrangements are made for an urgent ophthalmologic referral.

In the case of less severe exposure, the following is done:

- Fornices are also swept with a cotton-tipped applicator, and the eyelids are everted and inspected for any retained chemical material.
- The pH of the conjunctiva is assessed using litmus paper or urine dipsticks. The eye is lavaged with normal saline until the pH normalizes to 7.3 to 7.6 on 2 or 3 consecutive measurements each 15 minutes apart.
- A cycloplegic (i.e., homatropine 5%) is instilled 3 times a day.
- Antibiotic drops are instilled and the eye is patched.
- The patient is then emergently referred to an ophthalmologist.

Thermal Injury

History. There is exposure to an intense heat source (e.g., curling iron, tobacco ash, electric arc). The patient experiences pain, a foreign body sensation, excessive tearing, and decreased vision.

Examination. There is diminished VA. Burns of the eyelids, eyelashes, and periorbital tissues are usually present. The conjunctiva is injected and edematous. The cornea may be whitened, indicating an epithelial or stromal burn.

Treatment. Antibiotic eyedrops should be instilled and the eye patched. The patient is emergently referred to an ophthalmologist.

Glue Injury

History. Accidental application of cyanoacrylate (Super Glue) to the eye or eyelashes has occurred. The patient has a foreign body sensation and excessive tearing.

Examination. The eyelids are usually held fixed in a partially closed position with dried glue seen at their margins.

The conjunctiva is injected, and fluorescein staining, if possible, shows a diffuse uptake of the dye (i.e., toxic epitheliopathy).

Treatment. The eyelids should not be pried apart since this is painful and further injures the eyelid margins. Solvents are not to be applied to the eyes in an attempt to dissolve the glue.

- Warm compresses are applied to the closed eye and the eyelids are gently massaged.
- Warmed topical antibiotic ointments are applied on the eye and gently rubbed onto the lid margins three times daily.
- Artificial tears are instilled as often as necessary for comfort.
- If, after 3 to 4 days, the lids have not separated, the patient is referred to an ophthalmologist for possible surgical separation. *Note:* The glue usually adheres only to the corneal epithelium and therefore does not cause severe scarring.

THE EYES AND SYSTEMIC DISEASE

Anatomic Correlations in the Eye

Table 172-4 provides specific systemic diseases and clinical findings by anatomic correlations of the eye. Box 172-9 includes ocular manifestations found in various systemic diseases (Figs. 172-19 and 172-20). See specific chapters for the clinical description of the diseases.

EYE DISORDERS IN HYPERTENSION, DIABETES, AND ACQUIRED IMMUNODEFICIENCY SYNDROME

Hypertension

Hypertension is very prevalent in the U.S. population, affecting over 60 million individuals. Unfortunately, many of these individuals are either not diagnosed or do not have their blood pressure adequately controlled. Many who are hypertensive have no symptoms and therefore do not come to medical attention until a complication becomes clinically evident. The Joint National Committee on Detection, Evaluation, and Treatment of High Blood Pressure has recently issued its sixth report, which should be carefully read by all clinicians who care for patients with hypertension.

This section summarizes ocular findings in hypertension. The fundus is the only anatomic structure in which blood vessels can be seen directly. Changes in these vessels reflect the effects of a chronically elevated blood pressure, not only in the eye but possibly in the heart and other vascular beds, such as in the kidney and the central nervous system.

A detailed funduscopic examination, preferably through a dilated pupil, is mandatory in every patient with hypertension. The Keith-Wagener-Barker classification of retinal arteriolar and background changes in chronic hypertension is a useful guide for describing the changes that occur in hypertension (Table 172-5). A modification of Schleie's classification has also been described but is not as well known as the Keith-Wagener-Barker classification. Hayreh and colleagues suggested that hypertensive fundal changes be categorized as vascular or nonvascular, while Tso and co-workers divide hypertensive retinopathy into vasoconstrictive, exudative, scleroritic, and complications of sclerotic categories. Sapira is careful to distinguish arteriolar sclerosis, the change seen in fundal vessels of hypertensive patients, which is due to chronic wear and tear on arterioles, from atherosclerosis, which is a process associated with lipid deposition in intimal and smooth muscle cells of blood vessel walls. Five major categories of findings in retinal arteriolar sclerosis are described.

Arteriovenous Crossing Changes. For AV changes (i.e., AV nicking) to be significant, they must be seen at least two disc diameters away from the optic disc and there must be "complete nicking," meaning that a clear space must be seen on either side of the arteriole. This gives the illusion that the vein has been compressed with resulting obstruction of venous blood flow, but contrary to common belief, these changes are not due to compression of the vein by the arteriole but by sclerosis of the wall of the arteriole. As the arteriolar wall thickness increases, more light is reflected from the walls obscuring the more posterior vein.

Changes in the Arteriolar Light Reflex. With sclerotic changes in the arterioles there is a greater reflection of light from the arteriole, while the column of blood is less well seen. At some point, the reflected light is golden red in color and the arteriole appears as a "copper wire." With increasing arteriolar wall thickness and opaqueness, the reflected light appears silver in color (i.e., "silver wiring").

Tortuosity of the Arterioles. With sustained, moderately severe elevations of blood pressure, the arterioles become more tortuous. If the tortuosity is extreme, the arterioles cross the veins at 90 degrees. According to Sapira, this change is not dependent on arteriolosclerois and thus can help distinguish hypertensive retinal changes from those in older but normotensive individuals.

Focal Arteriolar Narrowing. The etiology of focal arteriolar narrowing is controversial, but it is the one finding that may arise from atherosclerosis of arterioles in addition to chronic hypertensive changes.

Diffuse Arteriolar Narrowing. A wide variety of ratios of the diameter of the arteriole to the diameter of the vein (i.e., AV ratio) have been suggested as normal, but these ratios are arbitrary. In assessing the AV ratio, one cannot know for certain that it is the arteriole that is narrowed and not the vein that is engorged. Nevertheless, the AV ratio is entrenched in the literature and is part of the Keith-Wagener-Barker classification.

In addition to the arteriolar changes in hypertension, background changes also occur. Flame-shaped hemorrhages are not specific for hypertension and can be seen in other retinal vascular diseases such as retinal vein thrombosis. The "flame" shape of the hemorrhage is due to the fact that when blood extravasates from the retinal blood vessels it does so into the retinal nerve fiber layer. The retinal nerve fibers that emanate from the optic disc and course outward in a radial fashion trap the extravasated blood between them and give the hemorrhage its distinctive shape.

Cotton-wool "exudates" are another feature of hypertensive retinopathy that is not specific for hypertension. They can be seen in systemic lupus erythematosus, proliferative diabetic retinopathy, and other retinal diseases. In fact, these exudates are not true exudates but represent clusters of ganglion cell axons in the nerve fiber layer that have undergone bulbous dilation at the site of retinal ischemia or infarction. On histopathologic examination, the area affected

Table 172-4. The Eyes in Systemic Disease: Anatomic Correlations

Disease	Clinical findings
Eyelids	
Amyloidosis	Periorbital ecchymosis, classically after being placed head down during rigid sigmoidoscopy. Waxy, flat papules about the eyelids.
Basal cell nevus syndrome	Multiple basal cell carcinomas.
Cowden's syndrome	Multiple trichilemommas.
Diabetes mellitus	Xanthelasma. May be found in the presence of hyperlipidemia, usually of the medial upper and lower eyelids.
Dermatomyositis	Periorbital edema. Heliotrope discoloration of the upper eyelid.
HIV/AIDS	Molluscum contagiosum. Kaposi's sarcoma. Lice infestation of the eyelashes in patients with poor hygiene.
Hyperlipidemia	Xanthelasma. Note that most patients with xanthelasma do not have hyperlipidemia. The association of xanthelasma and hyperlipidemia is stronger for patients under the age of 50.
Lymphoma	Enlargement of the lacrimal glands, which may be seen as a swelling in the lateral aspects of the upper eyelids.
Myasthenia gravis	Unilateral ptosis, although it can on occasion be bilateral.
Myotonic dystrophy	Bilateral ptosis.
Muir-Torre syndrome	Multiple keratoacanthomas or sebaceous adenomas.
Nephrosis	Edema of the eyelids.
Neurofibromatosis	Neuroma, often plexiform, of the eyelid.
Sarcoidosis	Enlargement of the lacrimal glands, which may be seen as a swelling in the lateral aspects of the upper eyelids. Granulomatous nodules may be found on the eyelids.
Thyroid ophthalmopathy	Upper eyelid retraction (Dalrymple's sign) and lid lag on downward gaze (von Graefe's sign).
Trichinosis	Edema of the eyelids and periorbital tissues.
Conjunctiva	
Ataxia telangiectasias	Telangiectasias and petechial hemorrhages.
Bacterial endocarditis	Petechial hemorrhages.
Hereditary hemorrhagic telangiectasia	Telangiectasias and petechial hemorrhages.
Reiter's syndrome	Nonspecific conjunctivitis, usually without a significant follicular or papillary response.
Sarcoidosis	Granulomatous nodules may involve the conjunctiva.
Thyroid disease	Edema of the conjuctiva (chemosis). Deep injection, especially of the temporal conjunctival vessels (Goldzieher's sign).
Uncontrolled hypertension, bleeding diathesis, or scurvy	Recurrent SCHs.
Vitamin A deficiency	Drying of the conjunctiva (xerosis). Small gray plaques with foamy surface (Bitot's spot).
Sclera	
Inflammatory bowel	Scleritis or episcleritis.
Osteogenesis imperfecta	Blue sclera (the color varies from slate to dark blue).
Reiter's syndrome	Scleritis and/or episcleritis (diffuse or sectoral injection may be seen).
Rheumatoid arthritis	Necrotizing scleritis. Scleromalacia perforans.
Syphilis	Scleritis or episcleritis.
Systemic lupus erythematosus	Scleritis or episcleritis.
Wegener's granulomatosis	Scleritis.
Cornea	
Ehlers-Danlos syndrome	Keratoglobus, also known as keratoconus (thinning and protrusion of the cornea) may be seen in type VI.
Fabry's disease	Light colored, whorl-shaped corneal opacities.
Hyperlipidemia	Arcus juvenilis, usually seen in patients younger than 50 years of age.
Hypercalcemia, chronic, of any cause	Band keratopathy, a degenerative process that develops in a band-shaped distribution across the middle of the cornea.
Mucopolysaccharidosis (MPS)	Clouding of the cornea due to diffuse, fine punctate stromal opacities that are homogeneous and bilateral. Seen in types IH (Hurler's syndrome), IS (Scheie's syndrome), IV (Morquio's syndrome), VI (Maroteaux-Lamy syndrome), and VII (Sly's syndrome).
Osteogenesis imperfecta	Keratoglobus (keratoconus) due to thinning of the cornea.
Rheumatoid arthritis	Dry eye with fine, punctate fluorescein staining of the corneal epithelium.
Sarcoidosis	Dry eye with fine, punctate fluorescein staining of the corneal epithelium. "Mutton-fat" keratic precipitates may be seen on the corneal endothelium as a result of a granulomatous uveitis.

Continued

Table 172-4. The Eyes in Systemic Disease: Anatomic Correlations—cont'd

Disease	Clinical findings
Sjögren's syndrome	Dry eye with fine, punctate fluorescein staining of the corneal epithelium.
Syphilis, congenital	Interstitial keratitis.
Systemic lupus erythematosus	Fine, punctate fluorescein staining of the corneal epithelium.
Wegener's granulomatosis	Peripheral sclerokeratitis (intense inflammation of the peripheral cornea and perilimbal sclera), which may lead to ulceration.
Wilson's disease	Kayser-Fleischer ring at the periphery of the cornea, representing deposition of copper in Descemet's membrane (while this may sometimes be seen with the naked eye or the ophthalmoscope, it often requires SLE for visualization).
Lens	
Ehlers-Danlos syndrome	Lens dislocation.
Homocysteinuria	Lens dislocation.
Hypoparathyroidism	Cataracts.
Marfan's syndrome	Lens dislocation.
Iris and uveal tract	
Ankylosing spondylitis	Anterior uveitis.
Behçet's disease	Anterior uveitis.
Juvenile rheumatoid arthritis	Anterior uveitis.
Lyme disease	Anterior uveitis.
Neurofibromatosis (von Recklinghausen's disease)	Increased number of nevi of the iris. Lisch nodules—smooth, round, and translucent hamartomas.
Psoriatic arthritis	Anterior uveitis.
Reiter's syndrome	Anterior uveitis.
Sarcoidosis	Anterior uveitis. Posterior synechiae (attachment of the posterior iris to the lens as a result of chronic inflammation).
Syphilis, secondary or tertiary	Anterior uveitis, especially granulomatous iritis. Posterior synechiae.
Syphilis, tertiary	Argyll Robertson pupil.
Tuberculosis	Anterior uveitis.
Vitreous, retina, or choroid	
Bacterial endocarditis	White-centered retinal hemorrhages (Roth spots).
Behçet's syndrome	Posterior uveitis. Retinal vasculitis.
Dermatomyositis	Retinal cotton wool spots.
Ehlers-Danlos syndrome	Angioid streaks (breaks in Bruch's membrane).
GM_2 gangliosidoses (e.g., Tay-Sachs disease and Sandhoff's disease)	Cherry red spot.
Hemoglobin C disease	Retinal neovascularization at the periphery.
Histiocytic lymphoma	Posterior uveitis.
Leukemia	White-centered retinal hemorrhages (Roth spots).
MPS IIIA (Sanfilippo A syndrome)	Pigmentary retinopathy manifests as a "salt and pepper" appearance of the retina, no associated clouding of the cornea.
Niemann-Pick disease	Macular degeneration. Cherry red spot in type A.
Paget's disease	Angioid streaks (breaks in Bruch's membrane).
Polyarteritis nodosa	Posterior uveitis.
Pseudoxanthoma elasticum	Angioid streaks (breaks in Bruch's membrane).
Sarcoidosis	Posterior uveitis. Retinal vasculitis with secondary neovascularization. "Candle wax-type" drippings may be seen on the retinal in a linear pattern along the retinal vessels.
Sickle cell hemoglobin	Angioid streaks (breaks in Bruch's membrane). Retinal neovascularization at the periphery.
Syphilis	Posterior uveitis. Retinal vasculitis. Retinal edema adjacent to the disc, which may extend to the macula.
Systemic lupus erythematosus	Cotton wool spots. Blotchy retinal hemorrhages of the posterior pole. White-centered retinal hemorrhages (Roth spots).
Tuberculosis	Posterior uveitis.
Vogt-Koyanagi-Harada syndrome	Posterior uveitis.
Optic nerve	
Multiple sclerosis	Optic neuritis.
Syphilis	Optic atrophy.
Temporal arteritis	Optic atrophy accompanied by swelling of the disc.

Box 172-9. Ocular Manifestations in Various Diseases

Ankylosing Spondylitis (see Chapter 137)
Ocular manifestations

1. Anterior uveitis in 25% to 30% of cases.

Behçet's Syndrome (see Chapter 138)
Ocular manifestations

1. Anterior uveitis.
2. Retinal vasculitis may occur.
3. Optic atrophy.

Diabetes Mellitus
See next section on eye disorders in diabetes.

Hypertension
See next section on eye disorders in hypertension.

Hyperthyroidism (see Chapter 97)
Ocular manifestations

Can be divided into spastic and mechanical. Often, the infiltrative disease manifests shortly after treatment for the hyperthyroidism has been instituted. Patients should be referred to an ophthalmologist for any mechanical involvement of the eyes.

Spastic:

1. Lid lag and lid retraction (due to the hyperadrenergic state).

Mechanical:

1. Periorbital edema.
2. Conjunctiva injection.
3. Congestive oculopathy with chemosis.
4. Proptosis with or without ophthalmoplegia (Figs. 172-19 and 172-20).
5. Optic neuritis and optic atrophy.

Inflammatory Bowel Disease (see Chapter 108)
Ocular manifestations

1. Episcleritis and scleritis.
2. Anterior uveitis.
3. Recurrent iritis.
4. Cataracts as a complication of long term systemic corticosteroid use.
5. Xerophthalmia and night blindness may occur due to longstanding malabsorption of vitamin.

Marfan's Syndrome
Ocular manifestations

1. Myopia.
2. Ectopia lentis.
3. Increased risk of glaucoma.

Myotonic Dystrophy (see Chapter 168)
Ocular manifestations

1. Bilateral ptosis and weakness of the orbicularis oculi muscles.
2. Sluggish reaction of pupils.
3. Fine punctate corneal staining on fluorescein staining.
4. Cataracts
5. Pigmentary granules may be seen in the macula and at the periphery of the retina.

Neurofibromatosis (von Recklinghausen's Disease)
Ocular manifestations

1. Neuromas (especially plexiform) of the lid.
2. Buphthalmous (enlargement of the globe) may occur.
3. Juvenile posterior subcapsular lenticular opacities, a form of cataracts, may be seen in NF2.
4. Glaucoma.
5. Nevi (Lisch nodules) of the iris; smooth, round, and somewhat translucent.
6. Optic gliomas.
7. Optic atrophy due to optic glioma or glaucoma.

Reactive Arthritis (Reiter's Syndrome) (see Chapter 123)
Ocular manifestations

1. Conjunctivitis.
2. Episcleritis or scleritis (extremely rare).
3. Anterior uveitis.

Rheumatoid Arthritis (see Chapter 133)
Ocular manifestations

1. Dry eyes (due to Sjögren's syndrome)—one may see punctate staining of the cornea.
2. Episcleritis/scleritis—in its most severe manifestation, may lead to scleromalacia perforans.

Sarcoidosis (see Chapter 78)
Ocular manifestations

1. Lacrimal gland enlargement and tenderness. May be accompanied by keratoconjunctivitis sicca.
2. Conjunctival injection and/or yellowish nodules.
3. Band keratopathy due to chronic hypercalcemia.
4. Corneal drying and fine punctate staining on fluorescein staining.
5. Nodular lesions of the iris.
6. Granulomatous uveitis. One sees "mutton-fat" large keratic precipitates on the corneal epithelium.
7. Cataracts.
8. Retinal vasculitis which may be complicated by retinal neovascularization.

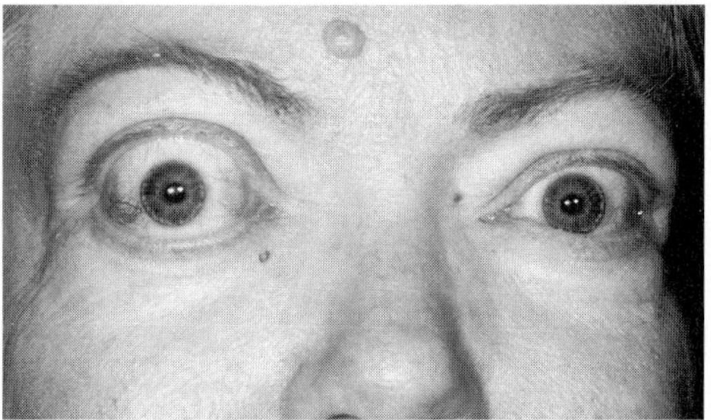

Fig. 172-19. A patient with thyroid eye disease showing both exophthalmos and lid retraction. Note the dilated conjunctival blood vessels over the medial and lateral rectus muscles. (From Wojno TH: Orbital disease. In Palay DA, Krachmer JH: *Ophthalmology for the primary care physician,* St. Louis, 1997, Mosby.)

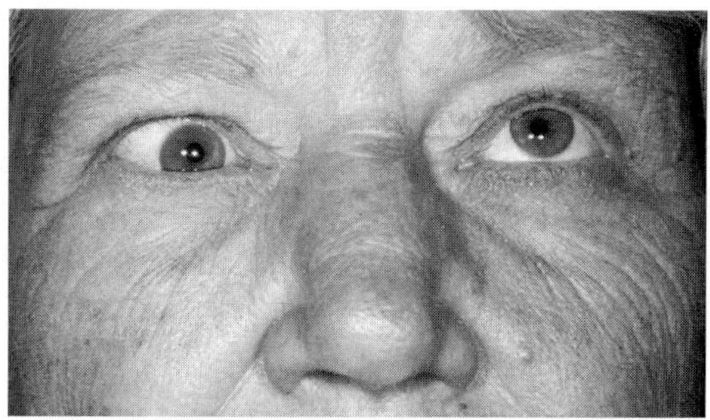

Fig. 172-20. A patient with severe ocular motility disturbance resulting from thyroid eye disease. The patient is attempting to look up. (From Wojno TH: Orbital disease. In Palay DA, Krachmer JH: *Ophthalmology for the primary care physician,* St. Louis, 1997, Mosby.)

Table 172-5. Keith-Wagener-Barker Hypertensive Retinopathy Classification

Degree	General narrowing AV ratio	Focal narrowing	Hemorrhage	Exudate	Papilledema	Light reflex	AV crossing changes
Normal	3:4	1:1	None	None	No	Fine, yellow Full blood column	None
Grade I	1:2	1:1	None	None	No	Broad, yellow Thin blood column	Mild depression of the vein
Grade II	1:3	2:3	None	None	No	"Copper wire," blood column not visible	Depression or humping of the vein
Grade III	1:4	1:3	Present	Present	No	"Silver wire," blood column not visible	"Complete" AV nicking
Grade IV	Fine, fibrous cords	Obliteration of distal flow	Present	Present	Present	Fibrous cords, blood column not visible	"Complete" AV nicking

by a cotton-wool change resembles a cell and has been termed a *cytoid (cell-like) body.*

Diabetes Mellitus

Diabetic retinopathy is one of three microvascular complications of diabetes mellitus (the other two being nephropathy and neuropathy). It can be insidious and asymptomatic until significant damage has occurred. In the United States, diabetes is responsible for almost 14% of all new cases of blindness each year and is the leading cause of adult blindness. Vision-affecting retinopathy does not occur in type 1 diabetes for the first 3 to 5 years after diagnosis, whereas as many as 20% of patients with type 2 diabetes may be found to have retinopathy at the time of diagnosis. Early detection is important, since strong evidence exists that surgical intervention (i.e., laser photocoagulation) can decrease the risk of vision loss in patients with high risk eye disease. The progression of retinopathy is typical, advancing from mild nonproliferative changes to moderate or severe nonproliferative retinopathy to proliferative retinopathy. Puberty, pregnancy, and cataract surgery can accelerate the changes of diabetic retinopathy.

Diabetes may affect the eyes through (1) cataracts, (2) nonproliferative retinopathy, (3) proliferative retinopathy, (4) macular edema, (5) macular ischemia, (6) cranial nerve palsy due to infarction of one of the cranial nerves subserving the extraocular muscles (i.e., cranial nerve III, IV, VI) (Fig. 172-21), and (7) glaucoma. Loss of sight usually results from proliferative retinopathy, macular edema, or macular ischemia. Vision loss may occur from one or more processes—macular edema due to retinal ischemia, retinal detachment due to contraction of fibrous tissue associated with neovasculature, or vitreous hemorrhaging.

Retinal disease is a consequence of disease of the microvasculature that leads to impaired perfusion and oxygenation of the retinal tissues. Initially, one sees thickening of the basement membrane of the retinal vascular endothelium with hyalinization and gradual occlusion of the precapillary arterioles. This is followed by loss of pericytes and weakening of the arteriolar wall, which leads to microaneurysm formation. Rupture of the microaneurysms gives rise to "dot and blot" and "flame" hemorrhages. In addition, infarction of the nerve layer of the retina produces cotton wool spots (soft exudates). Intraretinal microvascular abnormalities (IRMA) are areas of dilation of capillaries in regions of ischemia and do not represent new vessel formation. These vascular lesions remain within the retina, do not have significant leakage, and do not cross over major existing retinal vessels. With continued ischemia, the blood-retinal barrier is lost, and proteins and lipids leak onto the retina, giving rise to hard exudates. All of these changes are characteristic of nonproliferative retinopathy (also known

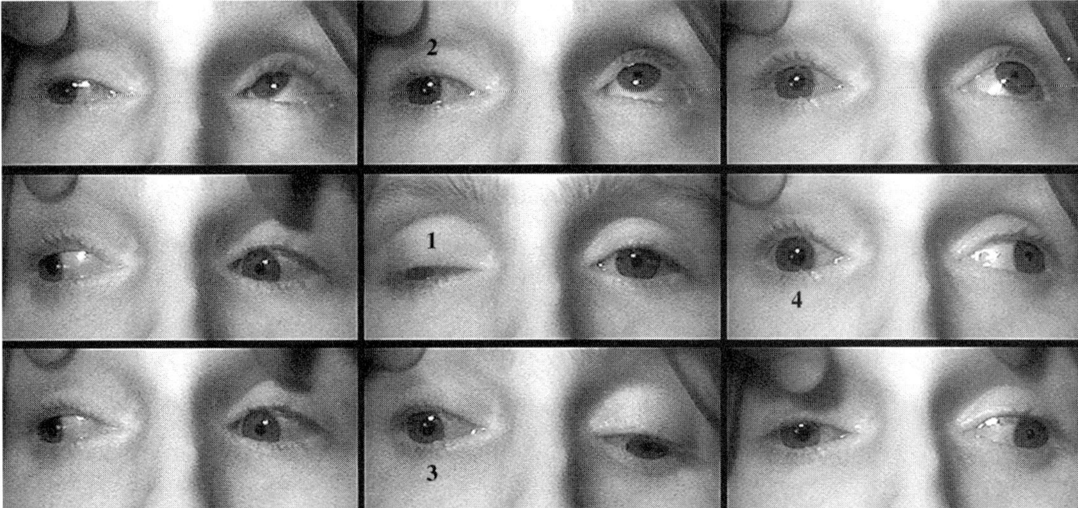

Fig. 172-21. Third cranial nerve paresis with pupil involvement. Note the profound right ptosis (lid droop) and the down-and-out position of the right eye *(1)*. Gaze positions demonstrate poor elevation *(2)*, depression *(3)*, and inability to turn the eye inward (adduction) *(4)*. Note the dilated pupil in the affected right eye. (From Martin TJ: Neuroophthalmology. In Palay DA, Krachmer JH: *Ophthalmology for the primary care physician*, St. Louis, 1997, Mosby.)

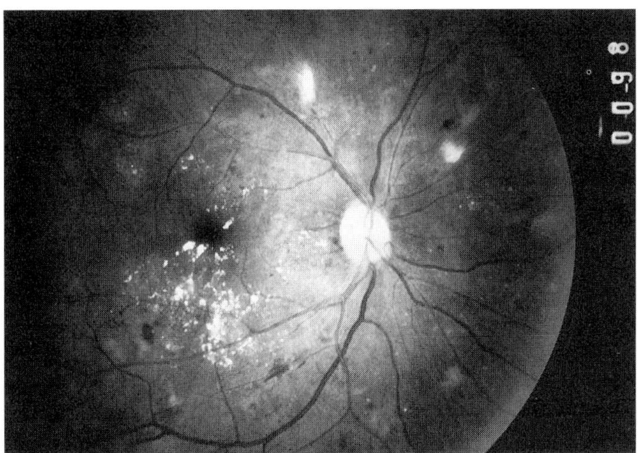

Fig. 172-22. Background diabetic retinopathy.

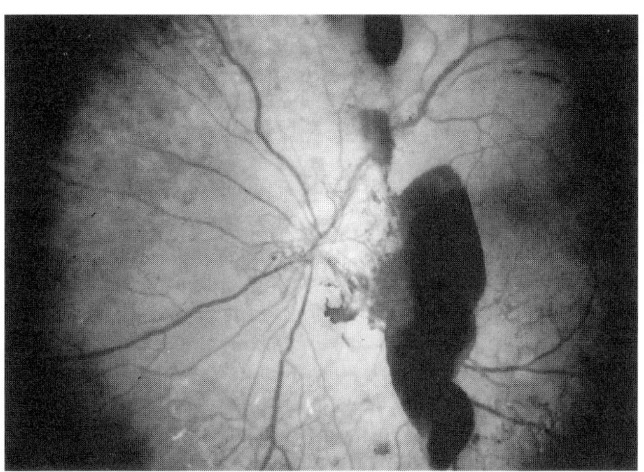

Fig. 172-23. Proliferative diabetic retinopathy.

as background diabetic retinopathy). As the ischemia and acidosis worsen and become chronic, new blood vessels arise from the retina and optic disc (neovascularization). This is the hallmark of proliferative retinopathy. These tufts of vessels have a propensity to bleed spontaneously, giving rise to preretinal or vitreol hemorrhages that can lead to fibrosis as they are resorbed. These new vessels may also involute and give rise to fibrosis between the vitreous and the retina, which in turn can lead to vitreol or retinal detachment (Figs. 172-22 and 172-23).

Diabetic macular edema occurs as a result of leakage of intravascular fluid into the macula. It may occur in patients with nonproliferative, as well as proliferative, retinopathy and is the leading cause of visual impairment in diabetics. Patients may experience unilateral or bilateral decrease in VA or may be asymptomatic, highlighting the importance of regular screening. On examination, the usual nonproliferative changes as described are seen, as well as graying or slight opacification of the retina as a result of edema. There may be cystoid changes of the fovea.

In addition to the microvascular complications, diabetics may develop two different types of cataracts. The more common is the usual "senile" cataract, which occurs earlier and progresses faster in patients with diabetes than in others. The second type is less common and is a "true" diabetic cataract. It develops as a consequence of osmotic imbalances, can mature in a few days or weeks, and has occurred as early as 1 year of age. Patients with diabetes are also at increased risk of developing primary open-angle glaucoma. They may also develop neovascular vessels in the anterior chamber that can acutely block egress of the aqueous humor from the AC. This leads to neovascular glaucoma (NVG), a particularly rapid and destructive form of glaucoma that can be resistant to treatment.

Up until recently, it was believed but not proved that tight control of blood glucose reduced the risk of diabetic eye disease. Recently a landmark study, the Diabetes Control and Complications Trial (DCCT), showed a 34% to 76% reduction in significant diabetic retinopathy in patients with type 1 diabetes placed on intensive therapy as opposed to those randomized to standard diabetic care. There was also a significant reduction in diabetic nephropathy, manifested as microalbuminuria, and peripheral neuropathy. This was, however, at a cost of a three-fold increase in the incidence of severe hypoglycemia. More recently, the United Kingdom Prospective Diabetes Study (UKPDS) showed a similar relationship between glycemic control and diabetic retinopathy (as well as nephropathy and possibly neuropathy) in patients with type 2 diabetes. In this study, there was a continuous relationship between microvascular complications and glycosylated hemoglobin so that a 1% percent decrease in HbA_{1C} led to a 35% reduction in microvascular complications. It is important to note that while tight control of blood glucose lessens the risk of diabetic retinopathy, it does not eliminate it. Hypertension and hyperlipidemia have also been shown to be associated with an increased risk of diabetic retinopathy as have smoking and renal failure. Therefore, control of all of these factors is required to reduce the risk of developing diabetic retinopathy.

In addition to the efficacy of primary prevention of diabetic retinopathy, two large trials have shown the benefit of detecting established diabetic retinopathy before loss of vision. The Diabetic Retinopathy Study (DRS) evaluated the efficacy and benefit of scatter (panretinal) laser photocoagulation in patients with proliferative diabetic retinopathy. At the end of 2 years, severe vision loss (i.e., best acuity 5/200) was seen in 15.9% of untreated patients vs. 6.4% of treated patients. The benefit was greatest in patients with the most severe retinopathy. The Early Treatment DRS evaluated the benefit of argon laser photocoagulation and aspirin in patients with early proliferative diabetic retinopathy, moderate-to-severe nonproliferative diabetic retinopathy, and diabetic macular edema. This study established the benefit of focal laser photocoagulation in patients with macular edema. Aspirin was of no benefit in retarding the progression of diabetic retinopathy. It did not, however, lead to an increase in the incidence of vitreous of preretinal hemorrhage.

Based on these data, the American Diabetes Association issued the following position statement regarding ophthalmologic screening (Table 172-6) of patients with diabetes:

1. Patients greater than or equal to 10 years of age with diabetes should have an initial dilated and comprehensive examination by an ophthalmologist or optometrist within 3 to 5 years after the onset of diabetes. In general, screening for diabetic eye disease is not necessary before 10 years of age. Patients with type 2 diabetes should have an initial dilated and comprehensive eye examination by an ophthalmologist or optometrist shortly after the diagnosis of diabetes is made.
2. Subsequent examinations for patients with both type 1 and type 2 diabetes should be repeated annually by an ophthalmologist or optometrist who is knowledgeable and experienced in diagnosing the presence of diabetic retinopathy and is aware of its management. Examinations will be required more frequently if retinopathy is progressing.
3. When planning pregnancy, women with preexisting diabetes should have a comprehensive eye examination and should be counseled on the risk of development or progression of diabetic retinopathy. Women with diabetes who become pregnant should have a comprehensive eye examination in the first trimester and close follow-up throughout pregnancy.

Table 172-6. Ophthalmologic Screening in Patients With Diabetes

Patient group*	Recommended first examination	Minimum routine follow-up†
29 years or younger	Within 3-5 years after diagnosis of diabetes once patient is 10 years or older	Yearly
30 years or older	At times of diagnosis of diabetes	Yearly
Pregnancy in preexisting diabetes	Before conception and during the first trimester examination	Physician discretion pending results of the first examination

From American Diabetes Association: Position Statement, *Diabetes Care,* Vol. 22, Supplement 1, 1990.

*These are operational definitions of type 1 and type 2 diabetes based on age (age <30 years at diagnosis: type 1; age >30 years at diagnosis: type 2) and not a pathogenetic classification.

†Abnormal findings may necessitate more frequent follow-up.

Acquired Immunodeficiency Syndrome and Human Immunodeficiency Virus Disease

As many as 40% to 75% of patients with acquired immunodeficiency syndrome (AIDS) experience an ophthalmic complication sometime during their infection. Although not well appreciated by generalists, eye involvement in AIDS affects the external eye, as well as the posterior segments (i.e., retina and choroid). Approximately 10% of the serious complications of AIDS first present in the eye. Therefore, a careful eye examination at each visit is necessary in all patients with AIDS who are immunocompromised.

Eyelids. In addition to the usual eyelid disorders that can affect the general population, individuals who are positive for human immunodeficiency virus (HIV) are also predisposed to other afflictions of the eyelids. In addition, common disorders in HIV-positive patients often progress more quickly and are more difficult to treat than in patients who are not immunocompromised.

Molluscum contagiosum is a primary skin infection caused by the molluscum contagiosum virus, a member of the poxvirus group. It presents with multiple, small, round, and waxy white papules 2 to 4 mm in diameter, often with a central umbilication. The umbilication may be filled with a white "cheesy" material. Lesions close to the globe can release toxic byproducts onto the eye and cause a follicular conjunctivitis with a fine punctate, epithelial keratitis. If chronic, this can lead to corneal scarring or pannus formation. In patients with AIDS, these lesions can be larger and more numerous than in immune-competent individuals. They also tend to resist treatment by the usual modalities and may require hyperfocal cryotherapy for control.

Verrucae are warts caused by the human papilloma virus. They can affect the skin surrounding the eye and cause a subacute catarrhal conjunctivitis if near the eyelid margins.

Kaposi's sarcoma is the most common neoplasm affecting the eye in patients with AIDS. Eyelid lesions may be nodular or plaquelike. In general, these lesions tend to be more of a nuisance than to cause significant symptoms or debility.

Herpes zoster may on occasion involve the skin of the forehead and upper eyelid without any involvement of the eye itself. Patients present with pain, fever, and headache. On examination, vesicles, erythema, and edema of the surrounding skin are seen. There may be regional adenopathy. The vesicles become pustules, crust over, and eventually resolve, at times with scarring of the affected skin.

Conjunctiva. *Bacterial and viral conjunctivitis* do not occur more frequently in patients with AIDS but tend to be more severe and difficult to control. The microbiology is for the most part the same as that for immune-competent individuals.

Bacterial Conjunctivitis. Bacterial conjunctivitis can be caused by *S. aureus, S. epidermidis,* and *Streptococcus pneumoniae.* Occasionally, coliform bacteria, *Neisseria gonorrhoeae,* and *Haemophilus* are indicated. Gonococcal conjunctivitis is a medical emergency since the bacteria can invade the cornea and lead to a severe keratitis with ulceration and vision loss within a short time.

Viral Conjunctivitis. Viral conjunctivitis can be caused by adenovirus and enteroviruses. Herpes simplex virus is a rare cause.

Kaposi's sarcoma has conjunctival lesions that are violaceus to red in color and can be confused with a SCH. In herpes zoster, in addition to involvement of the skin surrounding the eye, the reactivated varicella zoster virus can at times also cause a conjunctivitis.

Keratoconjunctivitis Sicca. As many as 25% of patients with HIV/AIDS suffer from symptoms of dry eyes (e.g., burning, stinging, and blurred vision), which might predispose them to conjunctivitis, keratitis, or trophic ulceration.

Cornea

Keratitis. *Herpes simplex keratitis* is the most common infectious cause of blindness in the United States and the second most common cause of unilateral visual loss due to corneal disease. There may or may not be any skin involvement. Patients present with blurred vision, injection, burning, and tearing. A distinctive characteristic on examination is of branching epithelial dentrites with terminal bulbs that stain with fluorescein or Rose-Bengal.

Recurrent ocular herpes simplex can also occur and may be infectious or immune. In the infectious type, there is epithelial viral, dentritic, or geographic ulceration. In the immuneform, nonviral, trophic (i.e., postinfectious) ulceration is seen.

Microbial keratitis does not occur more frequently in patients with AIDS but as mentioned for other conditions tends to be more severe in these patients. In addition, *Candida albicans* may be the cause in as many as 35% of patients. The infections may also be polymicrobial or bilateral. Apical or central ulcers are sight threatening and can progress very rapidly. Organisms include *S. aureus, S. pneumoniae, Pseudomonas* sp, and *Moraxella.* Coliform bacteria, such as *Proteus, Escherichia, Serratia,* and *Klebsiella,* can also affect the eye. These organisms require antecedent damage to the corneal epithelium. In contradistinction, *Neisseria, Haemophilus aegyptius,* and *Diphtheria* sp can invade the cornea through an intact epithelial layer. Capnocytophaga, a part of the mouth flora, has been described as causing an ulcerative keratitis in AIDS patients with poor oral hygiene.

Microsporidial keratitis is an opportunistic organism that can invade both the corneal and conjunctival epithelia. Patients present with photophobia, blurred vision, dry eyes, and a foreign body sensation. On examination, diffuse, punctate epithelial corneal deposits with mild conjunctival injection are seen. The infection tends to run a chronic course. Diagnosis requires Giemsa or Gram's stain of conjunctival scrapings.

Herpes Zoster Ophthalmicus. Herpes zoster ophthalmicus is due to reactivation of a latent varicella zoster virus infection. The virus travels along the path of a nerve to cause a skin eruption in that nerve's dermatome. The supraorbital branch of the first (ophthalmic) division of the trigeminal nerve is most commonly affected. If the rash involves the tip of the nose (Hutchinson's sign), this implies involvement of the nasociliary branch of the first division of the trigeminal nerve and increases the patient's risk for infection of the deeper structures of the eye (i.e., cornea, iris, ciliary body, choroid). Patients also experience a low grade fever, malaise, headache, and local adenopathy. In patients with AIDS, the virus often affects the cornea (keratitis) or the uveal tract (anterior uveitis). The infection is usually severe and prolonged and the virus may remain in the cornea for weeks to months.

Uveal Tract. Anterior uveitis may be in response to an ongoing keratitis or may be secondary to a posterior infection (i.e., posterior uveitis, retinitis). The causes of keratitis have been outlined previously. Isolated anterior uveitis may be due to herpes simplex, herpes zoster, tuberculosis, or syphilis. Diagnosis is made based on the clinical history and findings on funduscopic examination, indirect ophthalmoscopy, and SLE and supported by appropriate laboratory testing (e.g., chest x-ray, PPD).

Posterior Segments. Vitritis or retinitis may be caused by toxoplasmosis, CMV, herpes zoster (acute retinal necrosis), syphilis, tuberculosis, histoplasmosis, candida, or rarely cryptococcus. The disease may be unilateral or bilateral and often requires indirect ophthalmoscopy after pupillary dilation.

CMV retinitis affects 30% to 40% of patients with AIDS whose CD4 cell count has fallen below 50/mm.^{3} Retinal detachment occurs in 25% to 40% of these patients.

History. Patients may be asymptomatic or may experience floaters. Vision may be blurred or acuity may be decreased. Scotomas may occur.

Examination. Stellate-shaped keratic precipitates may be seen on the cornea. The vitreous is hazy and contains inflammatory cells. One may see patchy areas of retinal whitening with surrounding areas of hemorrhage (Fig. 172-24).

Treatment. Immediate referral to an ophthalmologist is crucial. After the diagnosis is definitively made, the patient is begun on appropriate anti-CMV therapy. This may include one of the following options:

1. *Ganciclovir* is an analogue of acyclovir and is administered for a 14- to 21-day induction period at a dose of 5 mg/kg intravenously twice a day followed by an indefinite maintenance phase at a dose of 5 mg/kg

intravenously once daily or 6 mg/kg a day for 5 days a week. Bone marrow suppression is the main side effect of ganciclovir and requires that blood counts be obtained on a regular basis. If the patient has responded well to ganciclovir but has developed neutropenia or severe anemia, G-CSF (neupogen) or erythropoietin (epogen) may need to be administered to continue it.

2. *Foscarnet* (sodium phosphonoformate) drug inhibits viral DNA but does not require phosphorylation to become active as does ganciclovir. Thus it is effective against ganciclovir-resistant CMV. It is administered for an induction period of 2 weeks in a dose of 60 mg/kg every 8 hours followed by a maintenance phase at a dose of 90 to 120 mg/kg once daily. Foscarnet's main toxicity is renal since it can cause renal dysfunction, hypokalemia, hypocalcemia, and hypomagnesemia. These side effects can be prevented or reduced by vigorously hydrating the patient before the foscarnet infusion. Foscarnet can also cause genital ulcers, dysuria, nausea, and paresthesias.
3. *Cidofovir* is a third-line drug since there is a significant incidence of renal insufficiency (53%). To limit toxicity, vigorous hydration and concomitant administration of probenecid are necessary.
4. In patients with very mild CMV retinitis the intraocular implantation of a ganciclovir-impregnated pellet that slowly discharges its contents, along with the administration of oral ganciclovir has been used with some success. The oral ganciclovir is given to reduce the risk of infection of the unaffected eye.

Recent studies have suggested that maintenance infusions of anti-CMV medications may be discontinued in patients who have had a sustained rise in CD4 cell count >100/mm^3 and whose HIV viral loads are undetectable.

Some experts recommend that patients with CD4 cell counts of <100/mm^3 undergo regular dilated funduscopic examinations and possibly fundus photography. The lower the CD4 cell count, the more frequent the examinations. In our institution, we recommend ophthalmic evaluation every 6 months for patients with CD4 cell counts ≤50/mm^3 and yearly examinations for patients with CD4 cell counts between 50 and 100 cells/mm^3. It has also been recommended that patients with low CD4 cell counts regularly use the Amsler grid to detect early changes in central vision. More recently, entoptic perimetry testing was found to be an effective and inexpensive alternative to fundus photography in detecting early CMV retinitis in patients with AIDS.

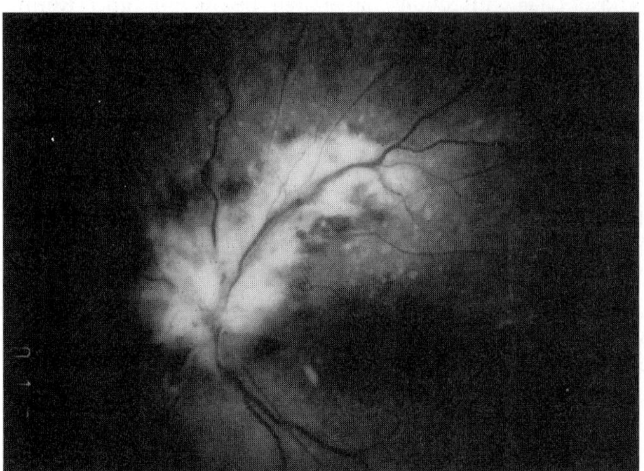

Fig. 172-24. CMV retinitis.

PREVENTION AND EARLY DIAGNOSIS OF EYE DISORDERS

Visual impairment is common, affecting nine million Americans. The incidence rises with increasing age. Although vision testing and screening for eye diseases is a standard of care in children, guidelines in adults are usually empiric and without substantial scientific basis and they tend to vary widely depending on the issuing organization. Nevertheless, it is felt that early detection of visual impairment in adults may improve functional status and prevent injuries from falls, automobile crashes, and other unintentional trauma. One study attributed as many as 18% of hip fractures to impaired vision.

Visual Acuity Testing Guidelines

Periodic screening for impaired VA is appropriate in older adults, but there is no scientific evidence regarding the optimal interval. School-age children should receive periodic VA testing. Asymptomatic adolescents and young adults do not require routine VA screening. In addition, a one time testing of VA at the first office visit for an adult who has not had vision testing in the previous 2 years or who wears corrective lenses is reasonable. Patients who wear corrective lenses should be asked to bring them to their first office visit.

Screening Tool. A 25-question Visual Function Questionnaire (VFQ 25) has been developed by the National Eye Institute. This questionnaire is intended to screen older individuals for possible eye disease. Specifically, it asks questions related to overall vision, near vision, distance vision, peripheral and color vision, ocular pain, social functioning as it relates to vision, psychologic effects of visual impairment, role limitations, degree of dependence on others, and driving difficulties. The questionnaire takes 4 to 5 minutes to complete either by the patient alone or with the help of an interviewer. The examiner should measure vision using a standardized Snellen distant VA chart or a near acuity card. (For more information, write to the National Eye Education Program, Box 20/20, Bethesda, MD 20892 or call 301-496-5248.)

Age-related Macular Degeneration. Individuals with a family history of age-related macular degeneration (ARMD) or early pigmentary changes in the macular area can be given an Amsler grid to help detect early disease of the macula. The Amsler grid is a graph paperlike pattern composed of 5 mm squares with a dot in the center. The patient is asked to hold the grid at reading distance and to stare at the dot. The patient is then asked to cover one eye and to continue looking at the dot. Do the squares around the dot become distorted (i.e. wavy, blurred, or discontinuous) or disappear? If so, this may be a sign of macular disease. Naturally, the process is repeated with the opposite eye.

Counseling

- Older adults should be counseled that while a decrement in VA is common with increasing age, it is not necessarily normal. They should report any such decreases in VA to their primary care physician.
- Patients at risk for retinal detachment (e.g., those with severe myopia) should be instructed on the symptoms that can accompany retinal detachment and told to immediately report any such symptoms.

- Patients who participate in certain sports in which eye injuries are more likely (e.g., racquetball) should be encouraged to wear protective eyewear when competing. Similarly, individuals who engage in activities in which high velocity projectiles are produced (e.g., hammering metal, using electric saws, using motorized weed wackers) should be counseled to wear protective eyewear.
- Individuals who spend significant time outdoors and are exposed to direct or reflected sunlight should wear sunglasses designed to block UV light as such exposure has been linked to the development of cataracts. In addition, patients who have undergone cataract extraction with IOL implantation should also wear sunglasses that block UV light as the IOL lets in a greater amount of UV light than does the natural lens. Exposure to light and windblown debris may also lead to pingueculae or pterygiae.

Patient Education. Free patient education publications are available to health care professionals from the National Eye Institute as part of its National Eye Health Education Program (NEHEP). These include the "Don't Lose Sight Of" series for individuals at risk for cataracts, glaucoma, diabetic eye disease, or age-related macular degeneration, as well as information for patients diagnosed with these diagnoses. To order these materials, call NEHEP at 1-800-869-2020 or visit the NEHEP website at www.nei.nih.gov.

Phacomatoses (Table 172-7)

Angiomatosis Retinae (von Hippel-Lindau Disease). A rare syndrome with no sexual or racial predilection, angiomatosis retinae usually presents sporadically, with no familial grouping. Presenting symptoms usually relate to the eyes or CNS. A cerebellar hemangioblastoma, the classic CNS lesion, can present with the usual signs of increased intracranial pressure. Spinal cord tumors also occur. Cysts and tumors of the kidney, epididymis, and other viscera are often seen. The ocular manifestations include retinal angiomas, which are often multiple and are bilateral in over 50% of cases. On ophthalmoscopic examination a smooth, dome-shaped tumor with an engorged vascular supply is seen. An exudative retinal detachment can develop around these lesions, which may become total and, if untreated, lead to absolute glaucoma and a blind, painful eye.

Ataxia-telangiectasia (Louis-Bar Syndrome). An autosomal recessive disorder, Louis-Bar syndrome can involve the skin and CNS, and ocular, hematologic, and lymphatic systems. Neurologic dysfunction includes a progressive and ultimately severe cerebellar ataxia with mental retardation. The immune system of these patients is incompetent, and thus they are subject to an increased rate of infections, lymphomas, and leukemias. The classic ocular finding is marked telangiectasia of the conjunctiva. Various oculomotor abnormalities also are seen.

Encephalotrigeminal Angiomatosis (Sturge-Weber Syndrome). The hallmarks of the Sturge-Weber syndrome are a facial port-wine stain (nevus flammeus) and leptomeningeal angiomas. The syndrome also includes characteristic intracerebral calcifications, seizures, mental retardation, and ocular dysfunction. The three major eye findings are glaucoma ipsilateral to the port-wine stain, choroidal hemangiomas, and an ipsilateral darker iris (heterochromia).

Glaucoma is seen in 30% of patients and is often thought to be secondary to increased episcleral venous pressure due to the vascular malformations. The choroidal hemangiomas, seen in about 40% of patients, can be confused with metastatic lesions. Secondary retinal detachments with severe ocular complications can develop.

Neurofibromatosis (von Recklinghausen's Disease). Probably the most common of the phacomatoses, neurofibromatosis occurs in about 1 in 3,000 births. It is autosomal dominant, with a highly variable penetrance. The skin, CNS, and eye are the primary sites of abnormality. The presence of more than five cutaneous café au lait spots is pathognomonic; the neurologic hallmark of the disorder is the neurofibroma, which can occur anywhere in the peripheral or central nervous system.

Numerous possible ocular and orbital findings are possible. A marked distortion of the upper lid can occur if a neurofibroma develops inside it. This distortion in turn produces ptosis and a typical S-shaped contour to the upper lid. Proptosis and pulsatile exophthalmos can occur secondary to congenital bony malformations of the skull, particularly the absence of the orbital roof or the greater wing of the sphenoid bone. The herniation of brain tissue into the orbit causes proptosis, which can also occur secondary to neurofibromas or meningiomas arising from any of the orbital nerves, optic nerve, or meninges. Therefore any child presenting with proptosis should be evaluated for neurofibromatosis.

Up to 50% of patients with lid and facial involvement in neurofibromatosis develop glaucoma on the ipsilateral side due to various mechanisms. Also characteristic are thickened corneal nerves and neurofibromas on the surface of the iris.

Table 172-7. Phacomatoses

Disease entity	Lids and adnexa	Conj. & sclera	Cornea	Cataract	Glaucoma	Retina & opt. nerve	Extra-oc muscles	Orbit	Uveitis	Visual CNS
Angiomatosis retinae						XX				XX
Ataxia-telangiectasia		XX					XX			
Encephalotrigeminal angiomatosis	XX				XX	XX				
Neurofibromatosis	XX		XX		XX			XX		
Tuberous sclerosis	XX					XX				XX
Wyburn-Mason syndrome						XX		XX		XX

Tuberous Sclerosis (Bourneville's Syndrome). Both autosomal dominant and sporadic forms of tuberous sclerosis exist. About 60% of patients are mentally retarded. Epilepsy and skin lesions are also key findings. Fifty percent of patients have intracranial astrocytic hamartomas containing calcium. Hamartomas in the kidneys, heart, lungs, and liver have been reported. The classic cutaneous finding is the adenoma sebaceum, which are angiofibromas that appear as small nodules on the sides of the nose and across the face.

About 50% of patients have ocular findings, the most common being a large astrocytic hamartoma of the optic disc, with a multinodular appearance resembling fish eggs, tapioca, or mulberries. Bilateral in about 15% of cases, visual field defects can be seen.

Wyburn-Mason Syndrome. A syndrome of unknown etiology, Wyburn-Mason can present with either ocular or neurologic symptoms. The major pathology is arteriovenous malformations (AVM) in the retina and the brain. AVMs can occur in the orbit, leading to pulsatile exophthalmos. The retinal AVMs can vary from small vessels in a localized area to extensive, racemose lesions covering the retina and creating a "bag of worms" fundus appearance. Cranial nerve palsies also have been reported.

OPHTHALMIC PROCEDURES

"Pinhole" Correction of Refractive Errors

Emmetropia is the refractive state of the eye in which light rays are focused exactly onto the retina. Myopia (nearsightedness) occurs when the image comes to focus in front of the retina. Most commonly this is due to an elongated globe. A "minus" lens (concave) placed in front of the pupil helps focus the light rays directly onto the retina. Hyperopia (farsightedness) is the condition in which the image comes into focus posterior to the retina. This may be due to an abnormally short globe, a flat retina, or a lens that is too weak to bring the image in focus at the right distance. A "plus" lens (convex) corrects this defect. In the patient with poor VA, retest VA with the patient looking through "pinholes" in a specialized instrument or small holes punched in an index card with a sharp pencil. Significant improvement of VA with pinhole testing implies an uncorrected refractive error. Minimal or no correction of VA should prompt a search for another cause of the diminished vision.

Measuring Proptosis (Exophthalmos)

Proptosis is measured with the Luedde exophthalmometer, which is a clear, short, plastic rod with gradations on opposing sides. The proximal part of the exophthalmometer is nestled into the lateral orbital notch (the posterior-most part of the lateral orbit) and the anterior-most edge of the cornea is sighted through it from a lateral vantage point. The 99th percentile for white men is 21 mm; for white women is 19 mm; for black men is 24 mm and for black women is 23 mm. Unilateral exophthalmos is defined by a difference between the two eyes of 2 mm in white individuals and 3 mm in black individuals.

Assessing the Depth of the Anterior Chamber

Before dilating the eye for the first time, it may be prudent to assess the depth of the AC. A patient with a shallow AC may develop an attack of acute narrow-angle glaucoma after dilation as this further narrows the angle and impairs egress of aqueous humor.

- The patient sits and stares straight ahead.
- A bright light is shined tangentially across the AC from the temporal side toward the nose. The iris should be completely but barely illuminated.
- If a shadow is cast on the medial portion of the iris, this implies that the iris is displaced forward and that the AC is shallow. Dilation of the iris in a patient with a positive test is relatively contraindicated.

Note that a positive test does not make a diagnosis of narrow angle glaucoma but merely indicates that the anterior chamber is shallow.

Eversion of the Upper Eyelid

Careful inspection of the tarsal conjunctivae is essential in a patient complaining of a foreign body sensation or who has vertical corneal abrasion (see Fig. 172-3). The lower tarsal conjunctiva is easily visualized by downwardly displacing the lower lid with one's examining finger. The upper tarsal conjunctiva is not as easily visualized. To do so:

- Carefully wash hands.
- Ask patient to close his eyes and relax.
- Place untipped end of a cotton applicator across the upper eyelid crease.
- Grasps the eyelashes of the upper eyelid and while exerting a slight inward and downward pressure with the cotton applicator, pull up on the eyelashes to evert the upper eyelid.

Schirmer Test

Schirmer test is used to check the adequacy of tearing. A strip of special filter paper is bent at one end and the bent portion is placed between the lower palpebral and scleral conjunctivae. After 5 minutes the distance that tears have migrated is measured. In patients under 40 years of age, a normal distance is at least 15 mm. Migration for fewer than 10 mm is suspicious for inadequate tear formation. Migration for fewer than 5 mm is abnormal.

Primary Dye Test

Primary dye test evaluates tear drainage function including patency of the nasolacrimal puncta, canaliculi, lacrimal sac, and nasolacrimal duct. A drop of fluorescein dye is placed in each lower cul-de-sac, and a cotton-tipped applicator is placed 3.5 to 4 cm posterocephalad into each nasal passageway. The cotton-tipped applicators are then examined 2 minutes later. Staining of the cotton tip implies a patent system. Absence of staining is either due to blockage of the system somewhere along its course or improper positioning of the cotton-tipped applicator. Absence of staining, however, does not pinpoint the exact level of obstruction, and the patient should be referred to an ophthalmologist for further testing.

Eye Patching

Patching of the eye is usually recommended for individuals with large corneal abrasions or in patients who have significant photophobia from a corneal abrasion. The patch must be snug to prevent the eye from opening beneath the patch.

- The patient reclines at 30 to 45 degrees.
- Antibiotic ointment is placed in the lower conjunctival sac and the patient is asked to blink several times to spread the material.
- The patient firmly closes both eyes.
- An eye patch is applied against the affected eye either lengthwise or folded in two.

- A second patch is placed lengthwise over the first patch.
- Paper tape is applied diagonally across the patch from the mid-forehead toward the ipsilateral angle of the jaw.

ADDITIONAL READINGS

Brody JM: AIDS and the external eye, *AIDS Reader* May/June 1996, pp 94-107.

Diabetic Retinopathy Research Group: Indications for photocoagulation treatment of diabetic retinopathy: DRS report 14, *Int Ophthalmol Clin* 27(4):239, 1987.

Dunn JP, Holland GN: Human immunodeficiency virus and opportunistic ocular infections, *Infect Dis Clin North Am* 6(4):909-923, 1992.

Early treatment Diabetic Retinopathy Research Group: Early photocoagulation for diabetic retinopathy: ETDRS report 9: *Ophthalmology* 98(5 suppl):766, 1998.

Fauci AS, Braunwald E, Isselbacher KJ, et al, editors: Harrison's principles of internal medicine, ed 14, New York, 1998, McGraw-Hill.

Folber R, Jakobiec FA, Bernardino VB, et al: Benign conjunctival melanocytic lesions: clinicopathologic features, *Ophthalmology* 96:436-461, 1989.

Frank KJ, Dieckert JP: Diabetic eye disease: a primary care perspective, *South Med J* 89(5):463-70, 1996.

Grossniklaus HE, Green WR, Luckenbach M, et al: Conjunctival lesions in adults: a clinical and histopathologic review, *Cornea* 6:78-116, 1987.

Hemady RL: Microbial keratitis in patients with the human immunodeficiency virus, *Ophthalmology* 102:1026-1030, 1995.

Jabs D, Green W, Fox R, et al: Ocular manifestations of acquired immune deficiency syndrome, *Ophthalmology* 96:1092-1099, 1989.

Katzman M, Carey JT, Elmets CA, et al: Molluscum contagiosum and the acquired immunodeficiency syndrome: clinical and immunological details of two cases, *Brit J Dermatol* 116:131-138, 1987.

Khaw PT, Elkington AR: *ABC of eyes,* ed 2, London, 1994, BMJ Publishing Group.

Kirkendall WM, Armstrong ML: Vascular changes in the eye of the treated and untreated patient with hypertension, *Am J Cardiol* 9:663, 1962.

Liesegang TJ: Pigmented conjunctival and scleral lesions, *Mayo Clin Proc* 69:151-161, 1994.

Morris WR: The eyes give the clue. Ocular manifestations of systemic disease, *PGM* 91(1):195-199, 202, 1992.

Munter DW, McGuirk TD: Head and facial trauma. In Knoop KJ, Stack LB, Storrow AB, editors: *Atlas of emergency medicine,* New York, 1997, McGraw-Hill.

Olk RJ, Akduman L: What you need to know about diabetic retinopathy, *Intern Med* 19(6):18-26, 1998.

Olsen TW: Retina. In Palay DA, Krachmer JH (eds): *Ophthalmology for the primary care physician* St. Louis, 1997, Mosby.

Palay DA, Krachmer JH, editors: *Ophthalmology for the primary care physician,* St. Louis, 1997, Mosby.

Palestine A, Rodrigues M, Macher A, et al: Ophthalmic involvement in acquired immunodeficiency syndrome, 91:1092-1099, 1985.

Pavan-Langston D: Diagnosis and therapy of common eye infections: bacterial, viral, fungal, Compr Ther 9:33-42, 1983.

Pavan-Langston D, Foulks G: Cornea and external disease. In Pavan-Langston D, editor: *Manual of ocular diagnosis and therapy,* ed 3, Boston, 1991, Little, Brown.

Plummer DJ, Banker A, Taskintuna I, Azen SP, et al: The utility of entoptic perimetry as a screening test for cytomegalovirus retinitis, *Arch Ophthalmol* 117(2):202-207, 1999.

Polis MA, Masur H: Promising new treatments for cytomegalovirus retinitis, *JAMA* 273:1457-1459, 1995.

Position statement: American Diabetes Association, *Diabetes Care* 22(1): 1999.

Progression of retinopathy with intensive versus conventional treatment in the Diabetes Control and Complications Trial. Diabetes Control and Complications Trial Research Group, *Ophthalmology* 15(8):647, 1995.

Report of the US Preventive Services Task Force: *Guide to clinical preventive services,* ed 2, Philadelphia, 1996, Williams & Wilkins.

Sapira JD: *The art and science of bedside diagnosis,* Baltimore, 1990, Urban & Schwarzenberg.

Woolf SH, Lawrence RS: The physical examination: where to look for preclinical disease. In Woolf SH, Lawrence RS, editors: *Health promotion and disease prevention in clinical practice,* Baltimore, 1996, Williams & Wilkins.

CHAPTER 173

Glaucoma

G. Robert Lesser
Deborah A. Darnley-Fisch
Talya H. Kupin
Rhett M. Schiffman

Glaucoma is a term used for a group of diseases characterized by damage to the optic nerve and visual field loss, usually associated with an elevated intraocular pressure (IOP). The optic nerve becomes pale and cupped, and other abnormalities may be noted as well (Fig. 173-1). Once the optic nerve has been damaged, the visual loss is irreversible. For this reason early detection and prompt treatment are essential.

EPIDEMIOLOGY

Glaucoma is one of the leading causes of blindness in the United States, affecting at least 2 million people, and is the leading cause of blindness among African-Americans. The Baltimore Eye Survey revealed that more than half of these individuals are unaware that they have the disease.[4] Another 5 million to 10 million are at risk of developing the disease over their lifetime. The medical and financial implications of the disease and its treatment are staggering, and delayed diagnosis is a major component of glaucoma-induced blindness.

PATHOPHYSIOLOGY

Damage to the axons of the retinal ganglion cells as they course through the optic nerve results in cell death and characteristic optic atrophy. The pattern of the atrophy is determined by the anatomy of the optic nerve, but it is not clear whether the damage is due to mechanical compression of the axons from elevated IOP or due to indirect damage from vascular compromise. Most intervention has been directed toward lowering IOP, as well as modifying blood flow to the optic nerve. An exciting new development is the use of neuroprotective agents to protect the retinal ganglion cell axons from damage.

KEY RISK FACTOR: INTRAOCULAR PRESSURE ELEVATION

The key risk factor for losing vision is elevated IOP. The normal range of IOP is 11 to 21 mm Hg, with a mean of 15.5 mm Hg. The normal pressure curve in the general population is not a normal gaussian distribution, but is skewed toward the higher pressures (Fig. 173-2).

Almost 80% of patients with glaucoma eventually have a documented elevation of IOP. Although a direct prospective study of treated vs. untreated glaucoma patients has not been formally conducted, there appears to be a direct correlation between the magnitude and duration of IOP elevation and subsequent visual loss.

Up to 20% of patients with typical optic nerve and field changes have IOP measurements completely in the normal range. In these patients other unknown factors such as vasospasm, hemodynamic perturbations, or structural abnormalities appear to contribute to the optic nerve damage.

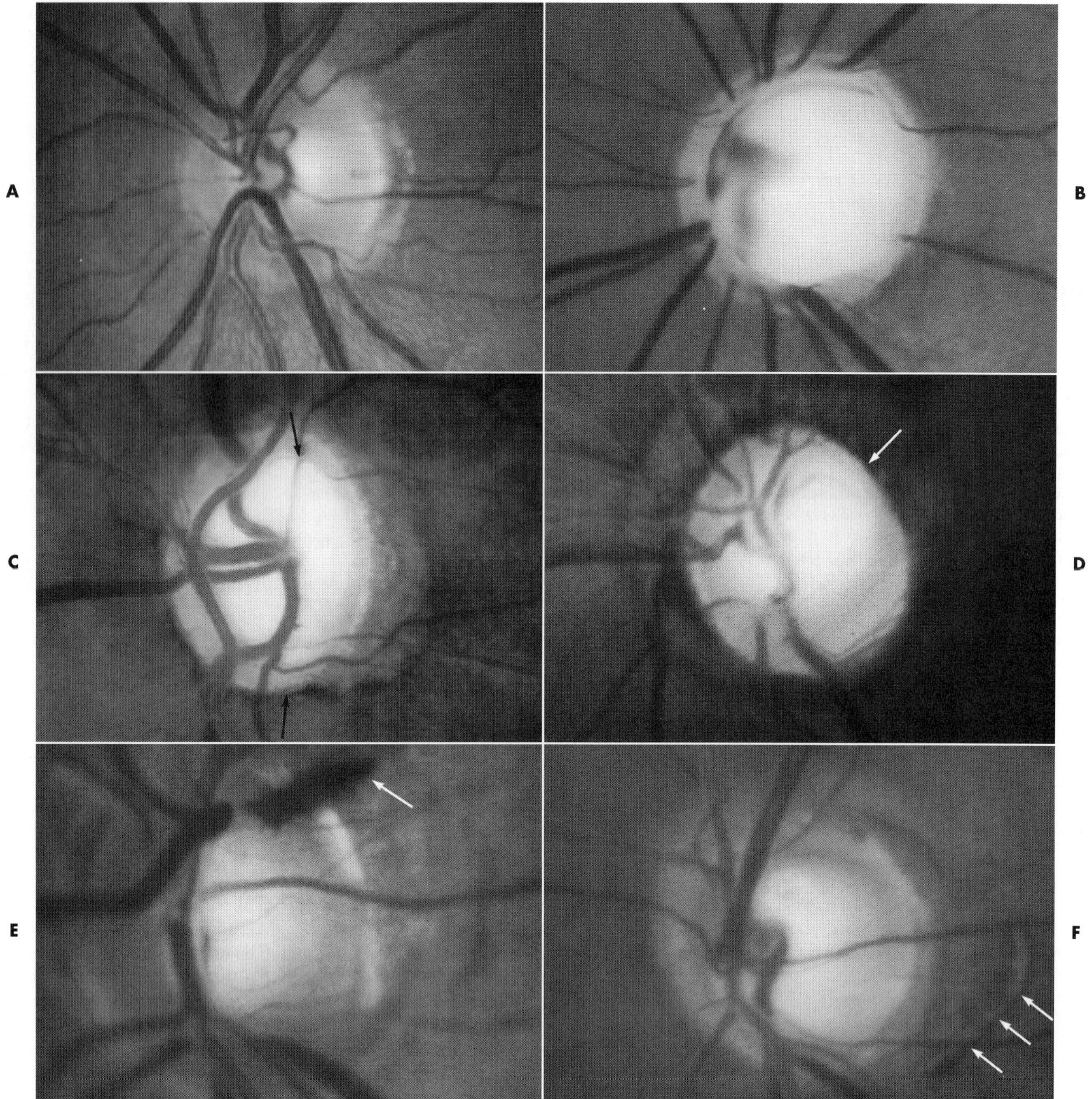

Fig. 173-1. Optic nerve damage from glaucoma. **A,** Normal optic nerve. **B,** Enlarged cup, undermining of the rim. **C,** Verticalization of the cup. **D,** Focal notching of the rim. **E,** Superficial nerve fiber hemorrhage. **F,** Peripapillary atrophy.

Approximately 5 million to 10 million Americans have elevated IOP without optic nerve or visual field damage, a condition called *ocular hypertension*. It is not known how many of these people with ocular hypertension progress to actual glaucoma, but current estimates are approximately 1% per year. The rate of conversion of ocular hypertension to glaucoma, as well as the benefit of prophylactic treatment to lower IOP, is being studied in a 10-year prospective trial by the National Institutes of Health (NIH).

Many factors influence the IOP. It varies throughout the day and is often higher early in the morning. This pressure fluctuation is subject to the individual's diurnal rhythm and may vary greatly between patients. The IOP increases slightly when the patient is supine but may be lowered during sleep. Mean IOP increases with age and is higher in African-Americans.

Although IOP rises only slightly with increased systemic hypertension, it may be lowered by medications administered systemically to lower blood pressure, such as β-blockers and calcium channel blockers. There are conflicting reports with respect to the effect of caffeine, smoking, and exercise on IOP. There is also a small group of people who are steroid

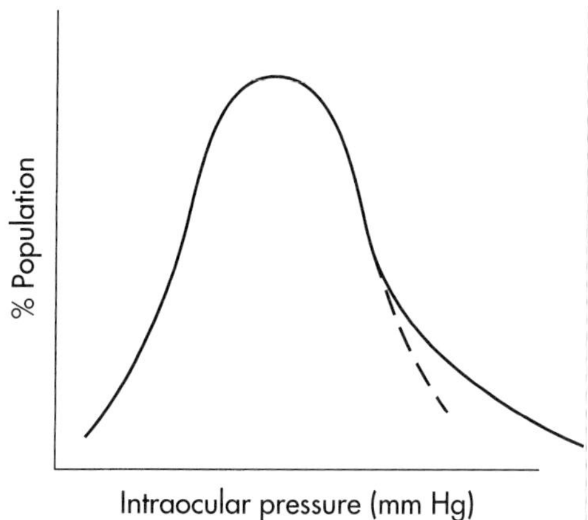

Fig. 173-2. Normal intraocular pressure.

responders. In these individuals there can be a large elevation of IOP in response to systemic steroids, topical ocular steroids, and in rare instances the use of topical dermatologic steroid preparations close to the eyes.

This marked variability makes an isolated measurement of IOP a poor indicator for predicting the risk of glaucoma, and seriously limits any diagnosis that relies on IOP alone. When 10,444 individuals in East Baltimore were examined, 194 cases of open-angle glaucoma were found, but 59% of those individuals eventually diagnosed with the disease actually had normal pressures during screening.[4]

OTHER RISK FACTORS

There is now evidence of a genetic component to many of the glaucomas, and glaucoma should be suspected in all patients with a positive family history, especially after age 40. The disease is also more common in patients with diabetes, high myopia, systemic hypertension, cardiovascular disease, and possibly vasospasm (Box 173-1). The risk of optic nerve damage increases with age. African-Americans are at particularly high risk because they tend to develop visual loss at an earlier age (in their thirties), and their disease can be very aggressive. It has been estimated that one in 10 elderly African-Americans has glaucoma, a rate five times higher than elderly white patients.

PATIENT EVALUATION

General

Patients with early and moderate primary open-angle glaucoma are asymptomatic. Only when there is advanced optic nerve damage may they notice dimmed or blurred vision. Rarely can they detect peripheral vision loss, and usually monocular patching is necessary for patients to be aware of their visual defect. Conjunctival injection, ocular pain, or halo vision may be noted by patients with intermittent angle-closure glaucoma. In addition to these symptoms, nausea and vomiting can be dramatic during acute angle-closure attacks.

Because symptoms may be lacking, subtle, or generalized, it is important to obtain a careful ocular and general medical history. Ocular history may reveal recent or remote ocular trauma or intraocular surgery. Previous ocular inflammatory diseases such as herpes zoster ophthalmicus or uveitis also indicate patients at higher risk for glaucoma. The general medical history may reveal associated systemic diseases such as diabetes, hypertension, herpes zoster, sarcoidosis, and ankylosing spondylitis.

A review of patient medications is vital, since steroids may cause a marked elevation of IOP in susceptible individuals. Anticholinergics, such as atropine, tropicamide, and scopolamine, may precipitate acute angle-closure glaucoma. Other relatively common medications have some anticholinergic effects as well, including antihistamines, antipsychotics, and antiparkinsonian medications (Box 173-2).

Finally, a family history of glaucoma should be sought from every patient in whom the disease is suspected. The risk for glaucoma is at least 10 times higher in individuals with a first-degree relative with the disease.

IOP Determination

IOP is measured by determining the force needed to indent the eye. The most common device available to the general practitioner for measurement of IOP has been the Schiøtz tonometer (Fig. 173-3). With the patient in the supine position, a metal footplate plunger is gently placed on the anesthetized cornea and the IOP is determined by the displacement of a weighted plunger that protrudes through the footplate. The advantage of this technique is the durability and portability of the device. It is, however, sometimes difficult to apply and may be uncomfortable for the patient. Moreover, it underestimates IOP in highly myopic patients due to decreased scleral rigidity.

Optometrists may use a noncontact air puff tonometer in which the eye is indented with a rapid impulse of air. This technique has the advantage of not requiring topical

Box 173-1. Risk Factors for Glaucoma

Family history
African-American
Increasing age
Diabetes
Myopia
Vascular disease
Elevated IOP

Box 173-2. Drugs That May Precipitate Angle-closure Glaucoma

Phenothiazines
Antihistamines—H_1 antagonists
Stimulants
- Amphetamines
- Caffeine
- Methylphenidate

Vasodilators
Sympathomimetic agents
- Epinephrine
- Ephedrine
- Norepinephrine
- Dopamine
- Naphrazoline

Tetrahydrozoline
Methoxamine
Hydroxyamphetamine
Parasympathomimetic agents
Parasympatholytic agents
- Cyclopentolate
- Tropicamide
- Atropine
- Homatropine
- Scopolamine

Cocaine
Clonidine
Antiparkinsonian agents

Modified from Mandelkorn RM, Zimmerman TJ. In Ritch R, Shields MB, editors: *The secondary glaucomas,* St Louis, 1982, Mosby.

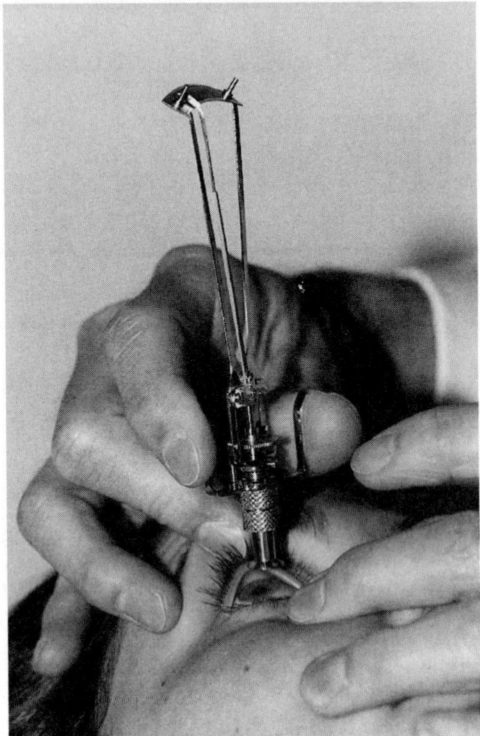

Fig. 173-3. Use of Schiøtz tonometer.

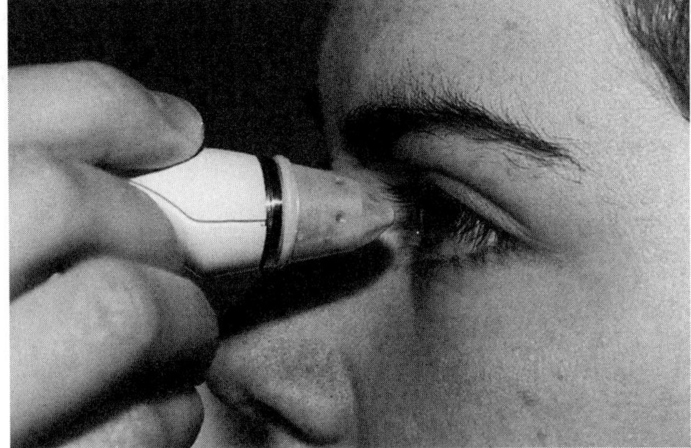

Fig. 173-4. Use of Tonopen device.

anesthetic drops and minimizes the chance of cross-contamination between patients, since only the stream of air actually touches the cornea. It is somewhat uncomfortable for patients, requires moderately expensive equipment, and tends to give measurements higher than actual. Many public health screenings are conducted with this device, and the results should not be used to establish a diagnosis or follow a patient.

Ophthalmologists usually use Goldmann's applanation tonometry, in which a small plastic device mounted on a slit lamp indents the cornea, and the pressure is determined by displacement of the tear film. This requires a topical anesthetic and is very accurate and reproducible. The technique requires special equipment and training.

A newer device for measuring IOP is the Tonopen (Fig. 173-4), a handheld device in which a 1.02-mm central plunger is connected to a microprocessor that measures the applied force. This device and its successors offer the general practitioner a convenient way of screening for elevated IOP. The device is portable and battery operated, and pressures may be taken with the patient in any position. After instillation of a topical anesthetic, proparacaine HCl (Alcaine), the tip of the Tonopen is gently applied to the central cornea until an audible tone is heard, and the pressure measurement is immediately available on a small display within the handle. A disposable sterile cap is used on the tip of the Tonopen. Although significantly more expensive than a Schiøtz tonometer, the Tonopen is easy to use with limited training and much more comfortable for both the patient and physician. The Tonopen tends to overread pressures below 5 mm Hg and underread pressures over 30 mm Hg, but for screening purposes these limitations are not significant.

Visual Fields

Measurement of peripheral vision loss requires specialized equipment. Ophthalmologists often use automated perimeters

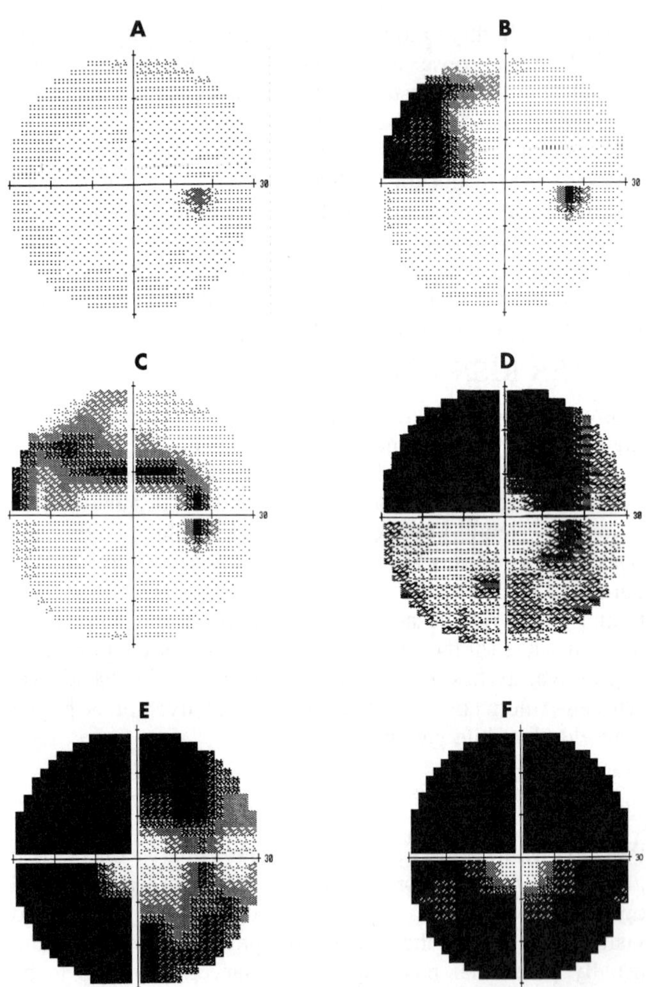

Fig. 173-5. Common pattern of progressive glaucomatous visual field loss. **A,** Normal visual field. **B,** Early nasal step. **C,** Superior scotoma. **D,** Complete loss of superior field. **E,** Additional inferior field loss. **F,** Small remaining central island of vision with decline in central acuity.

with standardized parameters. Examples of common patterns of visual field loss with glaucoma are shown in Fig. 173-5.

Optic Disc Abnormalities

The optic nerve can usually be visualized with a direct ophthalmoscope, even through an undilated pupil, and is thus accessible to the general practitioner. Findings suggestive of glaucoma include a large cup/disc (c/d) ratio (only 6% of the normal population has a c/d ratio greater than 0.50), narrowed optic disc neural rim, asymmetric cupping between the two eyes, vertical elongation of the cup, focal notching, disc pallor, and superficial disc hemorrhages (see Fig. 173-1).

GLAUCOMA SCREENING

The general practitioner needs to screen for glaucoma during routine physical examinations if risk factors are present (see Box 173-1). If the IOP is elevated or the optic nerve appears abnormal (see Fig. 173-1), a patient should be referred for formal ophthalmologic testing. If either factor cannot be assessed adequately or if the patient has additional risk factors, the patient should also be referred. A recently developed device called a frequency doubled perimeter (FDP) has been shown in several studies to allow for rapid (2 to 3 minutes) assessment of moderate to severe visual field loss and may prove useful as a screening device in a primary care setting.

DIFFERENTIAL DIAGNOSIS

The general practitioner may encounter patients with glaucoma in two clinical settings. The first is a patient with a white, quiet eye, in whom the disease is suspected because of risk factors, elevated IOP found during screening examination, optic disc cupping and pallor found during routine funduscopic examination, or painless visual loss. Commonly encountered glaucomas in this setting are shown in Box 173-3. In the second setting the patient presents with an inflamed red eye, and an elevated IOP is found during the evaluation (Box 173-4). The treatment varies according to which setting is encountered.

Primary Open-angle Glaucoma

Primary (chronic) open-angle glaucoma is the most common form of glaucoma. Patients initially have no symptoms until the disease is far advanced, at which time they have sustained significant field loss close to fixation. There is blockage of aqueous outflow in the trabecular meshwork. The pressure is usually elevated above 21 mm Hg and is often over 30 mm Hg. There is considerable variation in the amount of damage to the optic nerve for a given pressure. This is also true for normal tension glaucoma, in which the IOP is consistently in the normal range but the patients sustain optic nerve and visual field change identical to that seen with primary open-angle glaucoma.

Treatment consists of a stepwise progression of drops, pills, laser surgery, and filtration surgery, modified to take into account the overall health of an individual and side effects from the medications (Box 173-5).

Acute Angle-closure Glaucoma

Angle-closure glaucoma usually occurs in hyperopic individuals, those with thick convex glasses that magnify images. Acute angle-closure glaucoma occurs when the pupillary margin of the iris is pushed against the surface of the lens, a configuration called pupillary block. Aqueous fluid can no longer flow forward through the pupil, resulting in an increase in the pressure behind the iris. The iris is then pushed forward, blocking the trabecular meshwork. This results in a raised IOP. As the IOP increases, the lens is then pushed further forward, increasing the pupillary block, resulting in an upward spiral of increasing IOP over several hours.

Box 173-3. Elevated IOP and the White Eye

Chronic open-angle glaucoma
Steroid-induced glaucoma
Chronic angle-closure glaucoma
Old trauma or previous inflammation

Box 173-4. Elevated IOP and the Red Eye

Angle-closure glaucoma
Neovascular glaucoma
Herpes zoster and other uveitic glaucomas
Acute ocular or orbital trauma

Box 173-5. Therapy for Primary Open-angle Glaucoma

Topical β-blockers (e.g., timolol maleate)
Topical prostaglandin analog (e.g., Xalatan)
Topical α-agonist (e.g., Alphagan)
Topical carbonic anhydrase inhibitor (e.g., Trusopt)
Argon laser trabeculoplasty
Systemic carbonic anhydrase inhibitors
Glaucoma surgery

Pupillary block is often precipitated in predisposed individuals by pupillary dilation. This can occur several hours after patients have been pharmacologically dilated for examination, when pupils dilate in the dark, or as a result of dilation from medications with anticholinergic effects such as antihistamines and some cold remedies (see Box 173-2). This sudden rise in IOP often results in severe ocular pain and can be accompanied by referred gastrointestinal pain with nausea and vomiting. The vision is often very blurred, and patients may complain of halos around lights.

When examined with a handlight, the cornea appears cloudy or steamy from corneal edema and the anterior chamber is often very shallow. The pupil is commonly mid-dilated, fixed, and can be slightly eccentric. The sclera is injected and there can be profuse reflex tearing. The eye may feel firm to touch, and the IOP is very elevated; pressures of greater than 50 mm Hg are often seen. The fundus is difficult to see through the cloudy cornea. Examination of the opposite eye should demonstrate shallowing of the anterior chamber as well (Fig. 173-6).

If left untreated, acute angle-closure glaucoma can lead to permanent blindness. The optic nerve may be severely damaged and a secondary retinal vascular occlusion can occur. Damage to the corneal endothelium may result in

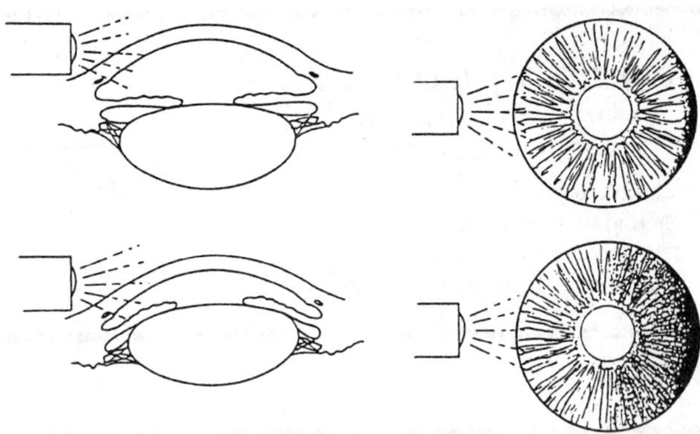

Fig. 173-6. Angle-closure glaucoma. Anterior chamber depth can be estimated using oblique illumination with a handlight.

thickening and clouding of the cornea (bullous keratopathy), and cataract formation is accelerated.

When the patient is first seen, the immediate goal is to reduce the IOP. Corneal indentation with an anesthetic (proparacaine)-soaked cotton applicator may help break the pupillary block. Medications to acutely lower IOP are shown in Box 173-6. Definitive treatment for angle-closure glaucoma is an iridectomy to bypass the mechanical blockage of the iris. This usually can be achieved with a YAG or argon laser, although occasionally a surgical iridectomy is necessary. Following an acute attack a patient may have persistently elevated pressures despite adequate iridectomies as a result of damage to the trabecular meshwork and may require chronic medication or surgery.

Box 173-6. Medical Therapy for Angle-closure Glaucoma

Miotics (pilocarpine 2%)
β-Adrenergic blockers (timolol maleate 0.5%)
α-Adrenergic agonists (apraclonidine [Iopidine, Alphagan])
Carbonic anhydrase inhibitor (acetazolamide [Diamox] 500 mg PO or IV)
Hyperosmotic agents (Osmoglyn, mannitol)

Box 173-7. Treatment for Neovascular Glaucoma*

Panretinal photocoagulation ASAP
β-Adrenergic blockers (timolol maleate 0.5%)
α-Adrenergics (Iopidine, Alphagan)
Carbonic anhydrase inhibitors (acetazolamide)
Topical atropine 1%
Topical prednisolone acetate 1%
Glaucoma surgery
- Glaucoma drainage device
- Filtration surgery with antimetabolites

*Do not use miotics.

Neovascular Glaucoma

Patients with extensive ischemia to the retina from diabetic retinopathy or following a central retinal vein occlusion are at risk for developing neovascular glaucoma, a particularly devastating disease that often results in blindness and is difficult to treat. The ischemic retina releases an unidentified angiogenic factor(s), which causes proliferation of new vessels in the retina and on the surface of the iris (rubeosis iridis). These vessels eventually grow across the trabecular meshwork, resulting in mechanical closure of the angle and elevation of the IOP.

The eye may initially be white and quiet, but eventually it becomes inflamed with bulbar injection, corneal edema, and elevated IOP. Fine vessels are invariably present on the surface of the iris but may be difficult to see with a handlight. Occasionally the fibrovascular membrane on the surface of the iris contracts, pulling the darker posterior layer of the iris through the pupil, which is easily visible as ectropion uveae.

Treatment is directed toward reducing IOP and inflammation and removing the underlying stimulus to neovascularization with retinal laser photocoagulation (Box 173-7). In addition to the poor visual prognosis, patients with this diagnosis have a higher incidence of death than age-matched controls, often from cerebral vascular and cardiac causes within 6 to 12 months from the time of diagnosis.

Herpes Zoster Ophthalmicus

Herpes zoster affecting the first division of the trigeminal nerve has a high incidence of ocular involvement and is frequently found when there are lesions on the tip of the nose (Hutchinson's sign). Secondary glaucoma often occurs with ocular involvement. The pressure elevation may be asymptomatic. Therefore IOP should be checked in every patient during the acute phase of the disease and probably rechecked 1 to 2 weeks later. The mechanism of the glaucoma is probably direct inflammation of the trabecular meshwork, and the treatment includes systemic acyclovir or Famvir, topical steroids, and antiglaucomatous medications (Box 173-8).

Acute Trauma

Blunt and penetrating trauma to the eye may cause elevated IOP and glaucoma acutely by several different mechanisms. Bleeding directly into the orbit can cause acute proptosis and a very high IOP. The fundus should be visualized immediately to rule out spontaneous arterial pulsations (best seen on the optic nerve), which indicates impending vascular occlusion from the high IOP. The orbit needs to be decompressed immediately, usually with a lateral canthotomy or a controlled fracture of the orbital floor into the maxillary sinus.

Intraocular bleeding may also cause an acute elevation of IOP. Blood and inflammatory debris can plug the trabecular meshwork, and a large clot in the anterior chamber (hyphema) can result in pupillary block glaucoma. The pressure is usually controlled with aqueous suppression (β-blockers and/or carbonic anhydrase inhibitors) and if necessary osmotic agents (Osmoglyn, mannitol). If the pressure is persistently elevated, the anterior chamber can be washed out in the operating room. Patients with sickle cell

Box 173-8. Treatment for Glaucoma in Association With Herpes Zoster

β-Adrenergic blockers (timolol maleate 0.5%)
α-Adrenergics (Iopidine, Alphagan)
Carbonic anhydrase inhibitors (acetazolamide)
Topical atropine 1%
Topical prednisolone acetate 1%
Systemic antivirals (acyclovir [Zovirax, Famvir])

trait or disease are at increased risk from these anterior segment bleeds, and early surgical intervention is often recommended.

After the acute episode, patients with ocular trauma are at long-term risk for secondary glaucoma. The trabecular meshwork may be permanently damaged, and a laceration into the ciliary body (angle recession) is associated with an elevated IOP. These patients are often completely asymptomatic with white, quiet eyes, and as in chronic open-angle glaucoma, may not be aware of their visual loss until it is far advanced.

MANAGEMENT OF ELEVATED IOP

Although there are many different types of glaucoma, there are only a limited number of modalities currently available to lower IOP. They are used in a stepwise progression, analogous to the treatment of systemic hypertension.

Pharmacologic Agents

In the United States, the initial treatment for glaucoma is usually the use of drops to lower the IOP. These drops work by decreasing aqueous production and/or increasing aqueous outflow, and they may be used in combination. When these drops are applied to the eye, a significant portion flow through the nasolacrimal duct, where they are absorbed through the mucous membranes into the systemic circulation. The clinician therefore needs to be aware of the potential side effects of these medications (Table 173-1). The most commonly prescribed antiglaucomatous medications used are β-blockers, which may have adverse cardiovascular and bronchopulmonary effects, such as worsening chronic obstructive pulmonary disease (COPD) and congestive heart failure, precipitation of asthmatic attacks, and increasing sinus bradycardia or heart block. These medications may also raise serum triglycerides and lower high-density lipoprotein (HDL) cholesterol, which may have serious cardiovascular implications, since these medications could be taken for decades. Less obvious effects include impotence in men and confusion in elderly patients.

Newer topical medications include a prostaglandin analog, two different α-agonists that are clonidine derivatives, and two topical carbonic anhydrase inhibitors. Fatigue, local allergy, and dry mouth are their most common side effects.

When drops fail to adequately lower IOP, carbonic anhydrase inhibitors may be added, such as acetazolamide (Diamox) and methazolamide (Neptazane). They decrease aqueous production in the ciliary body and commonly cause side effects such as generalized fatigue, loss of appetite, and paresthesias in the hands and feet. They may also be associated with renal stones and aplastic anemia and should not be used for patients with a sensitivity or allergy to sulfonamides. Of particular interest to the general practitioner is a transient hypokalemia, which can be severe and may require adjustment of a concurrent diuretic or other antihypertensive medications, as well as potassium replacement.

Lasers

When the IOP is not controlled with medications, argon laser trabeculoplasty may be used to lower pressure. The procedure is done in an outpatient setting and consists of using a mirrored contact lens to place 80 to 100 small burns on the trabecular meshwork. The exact mechanism by which argon laser trabeculoplasty works is not known, but the procedure is initially effective in almost 80% of patients. Unfortunately, at 5 years almost 50% of patients who initially responded to the laser are no longer controlled. A prospective study of 203 patients demonstrated that argon laser trabeculoplasty as the initial treatment was equally efficacious as medical therapy[2] and does diminish the systemic risks by reducing the medications needed.

Surgery

The IOP can be effectively controlled with glaucoma filtration surgery, in which a fistula is created between the anterior chamber and the subconjunctival space. The procedure is 85% to 90% effective but does carry significant potential complications, including cataract formation. When successful, the procedure may reduce or eliminate the need for glaucoma medications and does not depend on the compliance of patients with their medications. In the United States surgery is done when medications and lasers are not effective. The Scottish Glaucoma Trial and the Moorfields Primary Treatment Trial showed lower pressures and better visual fields when surgery was used as the initial intervention.[3] An NIH trial is currently underway to study this question as well.

Much of the success of modern glaucoma surgery can be attributed to the use of the antimetabolites 5-fluorouracil and mitomycin, which in prospective clinical trials showed substantial improvement in surgical success in high-risk cases.[1] They prevent scarring of the fistula. However, the poorly healed fistula may serve as an entry portal for bacteria, and as many as 8% to 10% of these patients may be at serious risk for developing an intraocular infection (endophthalmitis) over their lifetime. Therefore even a simple conjunctivitis should be treated as a significant medical emergency for a patient who has had glaucoma surgery.

SPECIAL ISSUES

Preoperative and Postoperative Surgical Management

The glaucoma patient may be sent to a general practitioner before glaucoma filtering surgery for medical evaluation. Unlike cataract surgery, these procedures are often not elective, and prolonged delays may be vision threatening.

The surgery may be done under local anesthesia, particularly in elderly patients with significant cardiovascular and/or pulmonary disease. Lidocaine (Xylocaine) and bupivacaine (Marcaine) are often used for regional blocks, and epinephrine may be added for hemostasis and prolonga-

Table 173-1. Medication Actions and Side Effects

Medication	Strength	Frequency	Action	Side effects
β-Blockers			Reduces aqueous secretion	Local allergy and irritation, bradycardia, heart block, bronchospasm, decreased libido, depression
Timolol (Timoptic)	0.25%-0.5%	qd-bid		
Levobunolol (Betagan)	0.25%-0.5%			
Carteolol (Ocupress)	1%			
Metipranolol (Optipranolol)	0.3%			
Betaxolol (Betoptic)	0.25%-0.5%			
Sympathomimetics			Improves aqueous outflow	Ocular irritation and allergy, adrenochrome deposits, rebound hyperemia, mydriasis, cystoid macular edema in aphakia, hypertension, extrasystoles, headache
Epinephrine (Glaucon)	1%-2%	bid		
Dipivefrin (Propine)	0.1%	bid		
α-Adrenergic agonist			Reduces aqueous secretion	Ocular irritation and allergy, upper lid elevation, mydriasis, bradycardia, dry mouth
Apraclonidine (Iopidine)	0.5%	tid		
Direct- and indirect-acting parasympathomimetics				
Pilocarpine (Isopto Carpine)	0.5%-6%	qid	Improves aqueous outflow	Miosis, decreased night vision, variable induced myopia, brow ache, exacerbation of cataract, induced-angle closure, retinal tear or detachment
Carbachol (Isoptocarbachol)	0.75%-3%	tid	Improves aqueous outflow	Intense miosis, iris pigment epithelial cysts, induced myopia, cataract, retinal detachment, paradoxic angle closure, punctal stenosis, intense bleeding and inflammation with ocular surgery, abdominal cramps, diarrhea, enuresis, prolonged recovery from succinylcholine
Echothiophate iodide (Phospholine Iodide)	0.03%-0.25%	bid		
Carbonic anhydrase inhibitors			Reduces aqueous secretion	Paresthesias, malaise, lethargy, abdominal cramps, diarrhea, nausea, renal stones, loss of libido, anorexia, depression, hypokalemia, acidosis, aplastic anemia, thrombocytopenia
Acetazolamide (Diamox)	125-250 mg	qid		
Acetazolamide (Diamox Sequels)	500 mg	bid		
Methazolamide (Neptazane)	25-50 mg	bid-tid		
Hyperosmotic agents			Reduces vitreous volume	Congestive heart failure, headache, subdural and subarachnoid hemorrhages, diabetic ketoacidosis (glycerol)
Mannitol	1-2 gm/kg	IV or PO q8-12h		
Isosorbide (Ismotic)	1.5 gm/kg			
Glycerin (Omoglyn)	2-3 ml/kg			
Prostaglandin agonist				
Latanoprost (Xalatan)	0.003%	QHS	Increased uveoscleral outflow	Conjunctival hyperemia, increased iris and eyelid skin pigmentation, hypertrichosis, ocular irritation and allergy
α-Adrenergic agonist				
Brimonidine tartate (Alphagan)	0.2%	bid-tid	Reduces aqueous secretion; increased uveoscleral outflow	Conjunctival hyperemia, increased iris and eyelid skin pigmentation, hypertrichosis, ocular irritation and allergy, drowsiness, fatigue
Topical carbonic anhydrase inhibitor				
Dorzolamide hydrochloride (Trusopt) (Azopt) Dorzolamide hydrochloride and timolol in combination (Cosopt)	2.0%	bid-tid	Reduces aqueous secretion	Ocular irritation and allergy, superficial punctate keratitis, blurred vision and photophobia, same systemic reactions as oral CAI's possible but much less frequent

tion of the block. Allergies to these medications need to be noted, and contraindications to epinephrine use need to be explicitly conveyed to the operating surgeon.

Occasionally, general anesthetics are used. A particular problem arises if the patient has been using long-acting parasympathomimetics such as echothiophate iodide (Phospholine Iodide) to control glaucoma. If succinylcholine is used as a paralyzing agent during intubation, there may be prolonged apnea because of the pseudocholinesterase inhibition by the echothiophate. In addition, succinylcholine may also cause a transient rise in IOP due to sustained extraocular muscle contraction.

Since vascular disease is one of the risk factors in glaucoma, it is not surprising that some of these patients may be taking anticoagulation medication. Anticoagulation can create several problems during glaucoma surgery, including a retrobulbar hemorrhage during the local block and an increased risk of an intraoperative sudden massive hemorrhage from a suprachoroidal blood vessel, which usually results in blindness. Therefore, if possible, anticoagulation medications such as aspirin and Coumadin should be discontinued, if medically safe, before surgery. The IOP may be very low for several days following the surgery, and the anticoagulation medications can be safely restarted once the IOP returns to the normal range.

Close attention needs to be taken to control systemic hypertension and to suppress severe coughing during the procedure. Identifiable sources of infection such as an active upper respiratory tract infection need to be cleared if possible before surgery.

Postoperatively, patients often have very blurred vision until the IOP stabilizes. The eye is often patched or covered with a protective metal shield, and care needs to be taken to avoid falls. Strenuous activity such as heavy lifting should be avoided. Other activities such as a physical rehabilitation program might need to be modified for a limited time, and employed individuals may request temporary disability because of their blurred vision and the limitation of activity that is required during their convalescence.

REFERENCES

1. The Fluorouracil Filtering Surgery Study Group: Five-year follow up of the fluorouracil Filtering Surgery Study, *Am J Ophthalmol* 121:349-366, 1996.
2. Glaucoma Laser Trial Research Group: The Glaucoma Laser Trial (GLT) and Glaucoma Laser Trial Follow-up Study: 7, Results, *Am J Ophthalmol* 120:718-773, 1995.
3. Migdal C, Gregory W, Hitchings R: Long-term functional outcome after early surgery compared with laser and medicine in open-angle glaucoma, *Ophthalmology* 101:1651-1657, 1994.
4. Sommer A, Tielsch J, Katz J, et al: Racial differences in the cause-specific prevalence of blindness in East Baltimore, *N Engl J Med* 325:1412-1417, 1991.

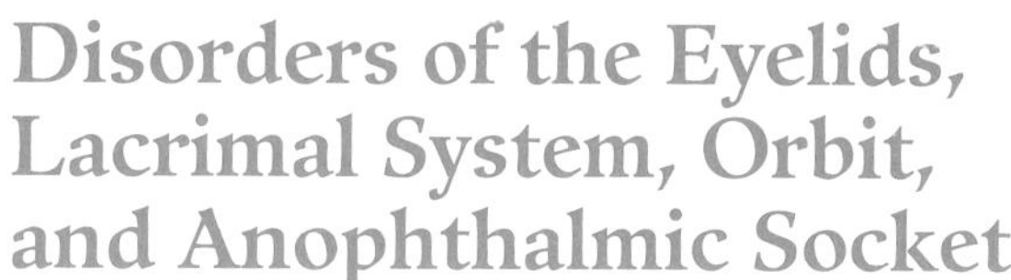

Disorders of the Eyelids, Lacrimal System, Orbit, and Anophthalmic Socket

Murray D. Christianson

DISORDERS OF THE EYELIDS

Anatomy and Physiology

The eyelids protect the eyes and, with each blink, smooth an optically important film of tears over the cornea.

Eyelid skin is the thinnest in the body. The subcutaneous tissue is thin and areolar, swelling easily with injury or infection. The orbicularis oculi muscle is sphincterlike, closing the lid aperture when it contracts. With a facial palsy, the lids do not protect the cornea.

Near the lid margins, just posterior to the muscle, are the tarsi, tough fibrous tissue plates that extend horizontally from the lacrimal puncta to the lateral canthal angle. They are attached to bone by the medial and lateral canthal tendons, continuations of the pretarsal and preseptal orbicularis. Full-thickness lid tears are usually through the medial canthal tendons that are weakened by the lacrimal canaliculi passing through them.

Each tarsus has about 25 large, vertical meibomian glands that secrete sebum onto the lid margin just anterior to the posterior lid margin. Modified sebaceous glands (of Zeis) and modified sweat glands (of Moll) empty into or beside the eyelash follicles.

The eyelashes (cilia), 100 to 150 in the upper lid and half that number in the lower, form two or three rows at the anterior lid margins. They curve anteriorly away from the cornea. Each has an average life span of about 5 months; its replacement is fully grown in 10 weeks.

The conjunctiva has three parts: bulbar, covering the globe; tarsal, lining the eyelids; and forniceal, in the cul-de-sacs inferiorly and superiorly. The bulbar portion is exposed to sunlight and may develop degenerative and neoplastic conditions. When the tarsal conjunctiva scars and shrinks, it rotates the margin of the eyelid posteriorly causing cicatricial entropion. The forniceal conjunctiva may prolapse between the eyelids with orbital swelling.

The eyelids are richly vascularized. Lymphatic drainage is to the preauricular and submandibular nodes.

Mueller's muscle and the levator muscle lift the upper lid. Blepharoptosis occurs when Mueller's muscle is denervated, or when the levator muscle is denervated, diseased, damaged by age or injury, or congenitally fibrotic.

The capsulopalpebral fascia connects the inferior rectus muscle capsule to the inferior border of the tarsal plate. In Graves' disease, pull on the capsulopalpebral fascia by the diseased inferior rectus muscle often causes lower eyelid retraction. The orbital septum extends from the periosteum at the orbital rim into the upper and lower eyelids, separating the "eyelid" from the orbit, holding back orbital fat and acting as a barrier to infection.

Table 174-1. Eyelid Malpositions

Malposition	Symptoms	Signs	Treatment
Trichiasis (normal lid position, but lashes directed posteriorly)	Irritation; tearing; red eye	Eyelid: no entropion; scarring; inflammation Eyelash: against the eye Eye: red; corneal ulcer	For inflammation: lid scrubs; hot compresses; antibiotic drops For lashes: epilation (temporary); electroepilation (permanent); excision of root(s); cryodestruction
Entropion Congenital; acquired (cicatricial, mechanical, senile)	Off and on? Irritation; tearing; red eye	Eyelid: lid flipped in, lashes and skin against the eye Eye: red; corneal ulcer	For lid: tape (temporary); surgical repair (permanent)
Ectropion Congenital; acquired (cicatricial, paralytic, senile)	Irritation; tearing; red eye; red lid	Eyelid: eyelid flipped out; irritated, exposed conjunctiva Eye: dry, irritated	For eye: lubricate For lid: surgical repair
Blepharoptosis (neurogenic neuromuscular junction; myogenic; aponeurotic; mechanical)	Upper lid droop	Frontalis contraction; brow elevation; excess skin; high lid crease; droopy lid	For underlying disease For lid (surgically): restore anatomy; suspend lid
Lid retraction (Graves' disease?)	Stare; eye bigger; irritation; tearing	Lid: upper pulled up; lower pulled down Eye: red, exposed	For underlying disease For lid: surgically lower upper lid and/or raise lower lid
Blepharospasm	Eyes close; can't see	Lid spasms; facial twitches	Botulinum toxin Surgery

Orbital fat is packed around the globe, extraocular muscles, nerves, and blood vessels, cushioning and supporting them. The eyebrows normally sit at or above the bony superior orbital rim.

Clinical Evaluation of Eyelid Disease

Clinical evaluation of eyelid disease should begin with a personal, occupational, and social profile; past medical history; list of medications and allergies; and family history. Obtain a careful chronologic history of the disorder, inquiring about inciting factors, associated symptoms and signs, and response to treatments. Examine the face from the top down, noting: frontalis use in attempting to raise the lids; position and asymmetry of the brows; upper lid skin irritation, redundancy, or tumors; position of the upper lid skin crease; lash orientation; upper lid level and contour; lid excursion measurements from full down-gaze to full up-gaze (normally about 15 millimeters); vertical palpebral aperture measurements; lower lid position and contour; herniated orbital fat pockets in both upper and lower lids; lacrimal punctal position; lower lid skin laxity, inflammation, or tumor; and cheek abnormalities. Sketch the pathology. Examine, with magnification if available, the lid margin, and palpebral and bulbar conjunctiva. When indicated, palpate the preauricular and submandibular lymph nodes.

Eyelid Malpositions

See Table 174-1.

Eyelid Defects and Reconstruction

Cosmetic Eyelid Surgery. With age, forehead and eyelid skin and subcutaneous supporting structures sag. The brows may fall below the superior orbital rims, and the upper lid skin may hang down, obstructing vision, or push the lashes into the cornea. The upper lid crease may collapse, and orbital fat may herniate through orbital septal defects, giving lid bags. Lower lids may sag. Dramatic improvement in function and appearance may result from lifting the brows, removal of excess eyelid skin and prolapsing fat, re-creation of the upper lid crease, and eyelid tightening.

Lower and Upper Eyelid Defects. Skin defects may be repaired with flaps or free, full-thickness skin grafts from the upper eyelid or behind the ear. Full-thickness lid repairs replace skin, tarsus, and conjunctiva with local flaps, and free grafts of skin, tarsus, cartilage, and mucous membrane are options.

Canthal Tendons: Medial and Lateral. After tumor resection, the canthal tendons must be reanchored to bone.

Eyelid Injuries

After injury, assess and treat more pressing systemic problems, then protect the eye and vision. Marked eyelid swelling and bruising are the rule. They usually resolve over 1 to 2 weeks. Unless exposure threatens the cornea, eyelid repair can usually wait 24 to 36 hours (Box 174-1). The necessary expertise, instruments, lighting, magnification, and anesthetic must be available.

Gently clean thermal eyelid burns and apply light, moist dressings. Aggressively, immediately, and copiously irrigate chemical burns and refer as emergencies.

Infections, Infestations, and Inflammations

Eyelid lumps can be infectious, inflammatory, cystic, xanthomatous, or neoplastic. *Lid infections* can be viral, bacterial, or fungal; *lid infestations* can be from lice or mites (Table 174-2). *Lid inflammations* include marginal blepharitis and associated disorders, dermatitis, and foreign body granulomas (Table 174-3).

Box 174-1. Eyelid Lacerations

May Repair Without Referral

Nonmarginal lacerations that do not involve:
- Canthal tendons
- Levator
- Lacrimal drainage system
- Extensive tissue loss

Laceration repair:
- Clean carefully
- Debride conservatively
- Repair meticulously
- 6-0 or 7-0 nonabsorbable sutures
- Do not fix the lid to the orbital rim by including orbital septum in the repair

Refer to an Ophthalmologist

Cover with a light, moist dressing and refer:
- Nonmarginal eyelid lacerations involving canthal tendons
- Nonmarginal eyelid lacerations involving levator aponeurosis
- Eyelid lacerations involving eyelid margin
- Lacerations with significant tissue loss
- Canalicular lacerations
- Any eyelid laceration about which there is any doubt

Table 174-2. Eyelid Infections and Infestations

Lid infection	Symptoms	Signs	Treatment
Viral			
Molluscum contagiosum	Mildly contagious; bumps on lids; more bumps coming; itchy eyes	One or many dome-shaped, skin-colored, umbilicated nodules, 1-3 mm diam; cheesy, sebum-like material expressed; may give follicular conjunctivitis	Incise Excise Curet Swab with alcohol
Verruca	Warty lid bumps; often from inoculation from warts on hands	Verruca vulgaris: round, warty Verruca plana: flat Verruca digitata: fingerlike, horny, capped filaments, grouped on narrow base Verruca filiformis: threadlike, normal skin covering	Excise
Herpex simplex	Spread by kissing, two infection peaks—6 mo-4 yr, 16-25 yr; blisters on lids; "cold sore" on lid	Primary: subclinical or unilateral crop of pinhead-sized vesicles on swollen, slightly red base, usually lower lid; may have fever; resolve in 7 days, leave no scars; may give keratitis or conjunctivitis; in atopic patients, may give severe systemic infection, Kaposi's varicelliform eruption Recurrent herpes (cold sore) may affect the eyelids; benign unless eye infected	Refer Acyclovir 300 mg po five times daily Vidarabine 3% ointment five times daily
Herpes zoster	Headache, sudden fever, malaise; in 3-4 days swelling and blistering on lid and forehead; usually adults and aged, sometimes the young; at increased risk are immuno-suppressed patients; post-herpetic neuralgia may be helped with antidepressants	Vesicles in V1 or V2 distribution, respect midline, one third involve lids and eye; vesicles filled with clear, then turbid fluid, quickly burst, giving eschar in nerve distribution, inviting secondary infection, healing in a week or two; may be marked eye inflammation; pain often severe, may persist for years (*postherpetic*) in elderly; skin often left mildly numb, yet giving pain on the slightest provocation (anesthesia dolorosa)	Refer If early diagnosis: oral antiviral for 7 days (acyclovir, famciclovir, valacyclovir)

Continued

Table 174-2. Eyelid Infections and Infestations—cont'd

Lid infection	Symptoms	Signs	Treatment
Bacterial			
Hordeolum (much less common than chalazia)	Stye: pain and lid margin swelling and redness	Rapidly forms abscess, may point and drain, often secondary to staphylococcal blepharitis External hordeolum, furuncle of lash follicles and adjacent glands Internal hordeola involve meibomian glands	Refer Hot compresses Oral penicillinase-resistant antibiotics Surgical drainage if necessary
Fungal			
Tinea corporis	Often spreads from face; red spot	Red spot with centrifugal extension and central healing; ring shape	Topical antifungal twice daily, continue for 10 days after lesions disappear
Infestation			
Crab lice (*Phthirus pubis*)	Often in children; chronic, itchy blepharitis	Blepharitis Dramatic: multiple nits (eggs) glued to lash bases, several lice gripping lash bases or crawling about the shafts Subtle; only one or two nits	Refer Wash all clothes and bed linen in hot, soapy water Use an anti-lice shampoo on all affected individuals Pick off the nits and lice at the slit lamp
Demodex mites	Red, itchy lids; infest the lid margin pilosebaceous units	Chronic blepharitis and meibomianitis	Lid scrubs Antibiotic ointment

Marginal blepharitis is a common chronic condition associated with staphylococcal infection, seborrhea, acne rosacea, and dry eyes. It eventually gives secondary lid margin scarring, with misdirection of lashes causing corneal damage. Patients complain of chronic burning, itching, and redness of their lids, which are often worse in the morning. Symptoms are often out of proportion to signs. Although often a mixed staphylococcal/seborrheic condition, each type has its hallmarks.

Eyelid Neoplasms

Epithelial Neoplasms. See Table 174-4.

Melanocytic Neoplasms. Nevi (moles) vary in size and pigmentation, and can be flat, elevated, papillomatous, dome-shaped, and pedunculated. Appearing and growing rapidly in childhood, they grow more slowly during adolescence, and become stable in adulthood. They should be excised if troublesome.

Freckles (ephelides) are little, circumscribed, brown spots, seen usually in adolescents following sun exposure. They may be transient or permanent and need no treatment.

Lentigo senilis occurs in 90% of elderly Caucasians and resembles seborrheic keratosis, giving multiple, dark-brown macules with irregular outlines. It should be observed.

Malignant melanoma of the eyelid skin is rare.

Sebaceous Neoplasms. Sebaceous carcinoma arising from the meibomian glands or the glands of Zeis or the caruncle is the third most common eyelid malignancy, occurring usually in the elderly or in younger patients with irradiated lids. Presentation varies, with the sebaceous carcinoma appearing as: a small, firm nodule like a chalazion; an atypical or recurrent chalazion; a diffuse, plaquelike tarsal thickening; a fungating or papillomatous growth; or a persistent unilateral conjunctivitis, blepharitis, or meibomitis (masquerade syndrome). Spread is local, lymphatic, and hematogenous. Prognosis is good unless diagnosis is late. The physician should biopsy and excise widely.

Vascular Eyelid Lesions

See Table 175-5.

Neurogenic Neoplasms

Neurogenic neoplasms occur with neurofibromatosis, type 1. Plexiform neurofibromas are unencapsulated, diffuse, intertwining bundles of Schwann cells, axons, and endoneural fibroblasts in a perineural sheath that usually grow along sensory nerves. The most common and complex orbital peripheral nerve tumors, they give elephantiasis neuromatosa, with hypertrophic skin, lid, and face; proptosis and disfigurement; and on palpation, a "bag of worms." The patient should be referred to an ophthalmologist.

Molluscum fibrosum usually occur in great numbers over the body and involve the lids, they occasionally become pedunculated and hang down over the cheek. They should be excised if indicated.

Miscellaneous Eyelid Lesions

Xanthomatous Lesions. Xanthelasma is the most common cutaneous xanthoma, and the only common lid xanthoma. It occurs in the middle-aged and elderly patients, two thirds of whom are *normolipemic*. Usually bilateral and at the inner canthi, they are flat or slightly raised, yellowish-tan, soft plaques. The patient should be referred to an ophthalmologist or the xanthelasma should be excised with care.

Table 174-3. Eyelid Inflammations

Inflammation	History	Signs	Treatment
Staphylococcal marginal blepharitis	Often begins in childhood; may last a lifetime; women > men; irritated, red, crusting eyelids; recurrent styes, often associated with seborrhea and acne rosacea	Dilated skin vessels; brittle, yellow crusts at lash roots leaving a bleeding ulcer when removed; recurrent hordeolum If chronic may give entropion or ectropion, lid thickening or notching; lash loss, misdirection or whitening; papillary conjunctivitis, keratitis	Dandruff shampoo if seborrheic Wash with warm, soapy water twice a day "Eyelid scrubs" with face cloth or cotton-tipped applicator twice a day; remove all crusts Flare-ups or resistant cases: scrubs, then massage antibiotic ointment into lid margin If severe: antibiotic/corticosteroid ointment; oral tetracycline
Seborrheic marginal blepharitis	Associated seborrheic dermatitis of the scalp, nasolabial folds, brow, retroauricular area, and presternum	Reddened lid margins, soft, greasy scales, not clustered at the lash roots, and not giving bleeding microulcers when removed, foamy tear meniscus, meibomian orifices swollen or plugged by oil globules, chalazia, secondary chronic papillary conjunctivitis, interpalpebral corneal epithelial punctate erosions	As above
Chalazion	Stye; one or many; variable growth rate; variable pain, less than hordeolum; sebaceous gland inflammation from duct obstruction, spontaneous or secondary lid margin disease; associated with seborrheic dermatitis or acne rosacea	Usually painless, rounded, slowly enlarging, subcutaneous lid mass that may wax and wane in size; may rupture posteriorly, giving a polypoid, conjunctival mass of granulation tissue on the conjunctiva, or anteriorly, giving a subcutaneous mass	For acne rosacea or seborrheic dermatitis For lids: hot, moist compresses for 15 min, four times a day For resistant or chronic chalazia: incision and curettage, with subconjunctival triamcinolone injection Marginal chalazia resist conservative treatment
Dermatitis	Common Acute: red, itches, burns, swollen, flakes; blisters if severe Chronic: itchy, thick, scaling skin	Red, irritated, thickened, scaling lid skin	Remove irritant Cool compresses Hydrocortisone 0.5% in Aquaphor four times a day Dermatologic referral if widespread
Atopic dermatitis	Personal or family history of asthma, hay fever, atopic dermatitis	As above	As above
Contact dermatitis	Cosmetics, aerosols, nail polish, soap, eye drops—especially neomycin	As above	As above
Foreign body granuloma	Lid lump, grows slowly; old injury	Quiet lid lump	Excise

Cystic Lesions of the Eyelids. See Table 174-6.

Involvement of the Eyelids in Systemic Diseases

Eyelid lesions occur in primary systemic amyloidosis, sarcoidosis, leprosy, and mycosis fungoides.

DISORDERS OF THE LACRIMAL SYSTEM

Anatomy and Physiology

The lacrimal glands, both primary (orbital and palpebral lobes in the superotemporal orbit) and secondary (Krause's and Wolfring's), secrete tears except during sleep. These enter the conjunctival sac superotemporally through the lacrimal ductules. The eyelids close from medial to lateral and milk the tears toward the medial canthus. The lacrimal puncta are normally turned posteriorly into the lacrimal lakes. Capillary attraction draws tears from the lid margin menisci into the puncta, and blinking pumps them the 10 millimeters through the canaliculi to the lacrimal sac. The lacrimal sac empties under the inferior turbinate into the nose through the nasolacrimal duct. The duct's inferior end is often not yet open at birth, giving tearing and chronic purulence that usually clears when the duct opens during the first few months of life.

Clinical Evaluation of Lacrimal Diseases

Begin with a careful chronologic history of the complaint, usually moistness, or tears running down the cheek (true epiphora).

If there is no true epiphora, suspect dry eyes, with secondary irritation and reflex tearing. Ask about variations in

Table 174-4. Primary Epithelial Neoplasms of the Eyelids

Neoplasm	History	Signs	Treatment
Benign			
Squamous cell papilloma (most common benign eyelid lesion)	Chronic lid bump	Sessile or pedunculated, skin colored, often multiple, often involve lid margin	Observe or excise
Seborrheic keratosis (dermatosis papulosa nigra, in Blacks)	Common eyelid and facial skin lesions in the middle-aged or older	Caucasians: tan to light brown, sharply circumscribed, wartlike, soft, friable, "stuck on" the skin Blacks: darkly pigmented lesions	Curettage Cryotherapy Excise if pedunculated
Keratocanthoma	Uncommon; in aged; grows rapidly	Begins as a reddish papule, grows rapidly over weeks or a few months into a firm nodule with a keratin-filled crater	Excisional biopsy
Precancerous			
Actinic keratosis (solar, senile keratosis; untreated, about 12% develop squamous cell carcinoma)	Most common precancerous skin lesion; older Caucasians; sun-exposed skin	Scaly, keratotic, flat or warty, brownish, circumscribed Cutaneous horns (also from squamous papillomata, seborrheic keratosis, inverted follicular keratosis, and verruca vulgaris)	Consider biopsy Exfoliative agents Curettage Excision
Cancers			
Basal cell carcinoma (Jacob's ulcer; most common eyelid malignancy)	Fair-skinned; commonly lower lids and medical canthi; often other facial lesions; almost never metastasizes; slowly grows, invading and destroying ("rodent ulcer")	Varies, often misleading Common types: 1. Noduloulcerative: raised, firm, pearly nodule with telangiectatic vessels, central ulcer, and bleeding with minor trauma 2. Pigmented: noduloulcerative with pigment 3. Sclerosing or morpheaform: pale, firm plaque with ill-defined borders 4. Superficial: erythematous scaling patches with a fine pearly border	Look for second lesions Biopsy Excise with frozen section control Mohs' Radiation
Squamous cell carcinoma (second most common lid malignancy; in the upper eyelid and lateral canthal areas, more common than basal cell; arises de novo or from actinic keratosis)	Elderly, fair-skinned; lower eyelid margin	Elevated, firm plaque or nodule, often ulcerates, irregular borders; grows faster than basal cell, invades and destroys locally, may metastasize to regional lymph nodes	Biopsy and wide excision Radiotherapy

the symptoms from day to day with aggravation by winds, cigarette smoke, automobile defrost fans, and low relative humidity from central heating. Obtain a complete medication history looking for drying medications. Inquire about systemic diseases associated with dry eyes (rheumatoid arthritis, Sjögren's syndrome, sarcoidosis). Ask about dry mouth and dry skin. If there is true epiphora, suspect nasolacrimal duct obstruction, which is more common in women. Ask about previous facial injuries, sinus or nasal surgery, or previous bouts of dacryocystitis.

Examine the eyes looking for an irritant causing hypersecretion, debris in the tear film, normal lid tautness, punctal position, and patency. Press on the lacrimal sac and look for reflux from the puncta.

Diagnosis and Treatment

Dry Eyes. The diagnosis should be explained to the patient in some detail. Treat any treatable systemic diseases. Change any contributing systemic medication. Recommend avoiding winds, fans, low humidity, smoking, and all air pollutants. Suggest artificial tears during the day and lubricant ointment at night. Consider temporary lacrimal punctal occlusion with punctal plugs, or permanent occlusion with cautery.

Epiphora or Tearing. Identify and treat the cause by surgically correcting lid laxity, punctal atresia, punctal ectropion, canalicular disease or obstruction, lacrimal sac, and nasolacrimal duct disease. A dacryocystorhinostomy

Table 174-5. Vascular Lesions of the Eyelids

Lesion	History	Signs	Treatment
Capillary hemangioma	Develops just after birth, grows rapidly for about 1 year, then stabilizes, then involutes until about age 5 years	Raised, dimpled, intensely red "strawberry mark"; bulges with Valsalva's maneuver; blanches with pressure	Observe and await involution if possible Treat if amblyopia threatens Local injections of steroid Excision
Nevus Flammeus or port-wine stain (may be part of Sturge-Weber syndrome)	Always present at birth; does not enlarge; often becomes darker with time	Flat, port-wine colored mark of varying size; no bulging with Valsalva's maneuver; no blanching	Cosmetics Photoablation Check for ocular and intracranial involvement if Sturge-Weber syndrome
Cavernous hemangioma	Usually develops in the second to fourth decade; grows slowly; does not involute	Raised, red or purplish lesion	Excise
Pyogenic granuloma (most common acquired eyelid lesion)	Follows minor trauma or surgery; grows rapidly; bleeds easily	Scarlet, brown, or blue-black nodule; friable surface	Excise
Varices	Grow slowly; often with other facial venous anomalies	Dark blue, deeper, soft lesions	Debulk as necessary Often recur
Lymphangiomas	Grow slowly; no spontaneous regression; intralesional bleeding may cause enlargement	Yellowish-tan or reddish swelling; deep component	Observe Excise Often recur
Kaposi's sarcoma	In patients with AIDS	Reddish vascular nodule of conjunctiva or lid	Treat AIDS Biopsy and excise as necessary

Table 174-6. Cystic Lesions of the Eyelids*

Lesion	History	Signs	Treatment
Hidrocystomas (retention cysts either of the apocrine [Moll's gland] or eccrine sweat glands)	Common; chronic, painless lid margin cyst	Occasionally multiple, but usually solitary; lid margin translucent, cystic nodule; often bluish, transilluminates	Excise
Pilosebaceous cysts, milia	Asymptomatic, multiple white lid bumps	Rounded, white; sharply circumscribed, pinhead-sized, pearly nodules	Excision, diathermy, or electrolysis
Pilosebaceous cysts, sebaceous or pilar cysts	Subcutaneous lid bump; stable or grow slowly	Globular, subcutaneous masses, attached to skin, often of brow; plugged pore at the summit often	Excise
Epidermal inclusion cysts	After trauma or surgery; grow slowly	Firm, globular, painless, mobile, dermal or subcutaneous masses; skin intact	Excise

*Other cystic lesions include dermoid cysts, pilomatrixoma, cystic basal cell carcinoma, and dacryops (cysts from dilated ducts of accessory lacrimal glands from scarring or chronic inflammation).

(DCR) has a 97% success rate in primary cases, can be done as an outpatient case under local anesthetic, and leaves little scarring.

Infections. Dacryoadenitis may be acute (viral or bacterial) or chronic (bacterial) (Table 174-7).

Injuries. Facial lacerations may cut the canaliculi. Medial canthal tendon avulsions, medial to the punctum, may tear the canaliculus, displacing the punctum laterally. Repair should be meticulous to avoid permanent tearing. The sac and nasolacrimal duct are often disrupted in midfacial fractures and by sinus surgery. The normal anatomy should be restored.

Tumors. Lacrimal gland tumors are discussed in the orbital section below. Lacrimal sac tumors are rare.

DISORDERS OF THE ORBIT

Many orbital diseases are uncommon, and patients with them are best referred to an ophthalmologist with a special interest in these conditions.

Table 174-7. Infections of the Lacrimal System

Infection	History	Signs	Treatment
Lacrimal gland			
Acute viral dacryoadenitis (dacryoadenitis from mumps, infectious mononucleosis, herpes zoster, measles, influenza, and dengue fever)	Fullness or pain in the upper outer orbit	Abscesslike, firm, tender lateral lid swelling, S-shaped upper lid margin; mechanical ptosis; sometimes inferonasal proptosis; preauricular lymphadenopathy; lid eversion shows gland swelling with localized chemosis	Observe Resolves in 1 week
Acute bacterial dacryoadenitis (from staphylococci, streptococci, pneumococci, gonococci)	Severe pain and fullness in the upper outer orbit	Abscess in upper outer orbit; may suppurate, draining through the conjunctiva (palpebral lobe) or skin (orbital lobe)	Refer Systemic antibiotic Drainage Support
Chronic bacterial dacryoadenitis (from trachoma, tuberculosis, leprosy, syphilis, actinomycosis)	Slow-growing orbital mass, up and out	Superotemporal orbital mass; diplopia on looking toward it, inferonasal proptosis, dry eye	Refer Specific therapy
Canaliculus			
Canaliculitis (from actinomyces)	Chronic unilateral tearing and irritation, resistant to topical antibiotics	Redness and swelling over canaliculus; pouting punctum	Canaliculotomy, stone removal, painting with iodine
Lacrimal sac			
Dacryocystitis (from staphylococcus, streptococcus)	Middle-aged (females:males 3:1); acute or chronic swelling below the medial canthal tendon; irritation and tearing	From nasolacrimal duct obstruction; lacrimal sac swelling; tearing	Systemic antibiotic (oral/IV) Hot compresses Abscess drainage Dacryocystorhinostomy (DCR)

Anatomy and Pathophysiology

The orbit is the bony socket containing the globe; extraocular muscles; sensory, motor, and autonomic nerves; blood vessels; and lacrimal gland. They are all packed in orbital fat. The bony orbit is pear-shaped, with the "stem" entering the optic canal, and is wider just behind its anterior opening than at the opening itself. Its adult volume is about 30 cc, although it is much shallower in children. Space-occupying lesions may push the globe anteriorly, up or down, or nasally or temporally, or may invade orbital structures, restricting globe movement.

Epidemiology and Disease Patterns

Age Distribution. Congenital malformations are most common in the first decade; orbital neoplasia in the first, sixth, and seventh decades; and thyroid-associated ophthalmopathy (TAO) in the fourth, fifth, and sixth decades. Structural and degenerative disease prevalence gradually increases with age, whereas prevalence of inflammatory and vascular diseases remains stable.

Clinical Presentation

History. Onset may be hyperacute (trauma and hemorrhage), acute and subacute (inflammation, a few neoplasms), or chronic (most neoplastic and structural defects).

Physical Examination. Presentation can be dominated by inflammation (specific and nonspecific infection, neoplasia, structural defects, vascular disorders), mass effect (low-grade inflammations such as granulomas and sarcoid, neoplasia, structural defects, vascular conditions such as varices and arteriovenous [A-V] shunts), vascular disturbances (A-V shunt, varix, ophthalmic vein thrombosis, lymphedema), or infiltration (sclerosing inflammation, neoplasia, amyloid deposition, linear scleroderma).

Clinical Evaluation

During the clinical evaluation of orbital disease the following questions should be considered:

1. Where is the lesion?
2. What is it doing?
3. How quickly?
4. What is the pathology?
5. What should be done?

Answering these questions, in order, directs the history, examination, investigations, and analysis, giving a diagnosis and management plan.

History. A detailed, chronologic story should be obtained. When and how did the trouble start? Was progression catastrophic (hemorrhage, fulminant infection), less rapid but steady (inflammation, fulminant neoplasm), or insidious (low-grade inflammation, slowly growing benign or malignant neoplasm)? Does it vary (lid swelling from TAO)? Does it increase with Valsalva's maneuver (venous anomaly)? Does it pulsate (arteriovenous fistula, orbital wall defect)? Previous photographs, investigations, and treatments should be reviewed.

Examination. A complete general examination should be done. Findings such as goiter, hair loss, tremor,

Table 174-8. Clinical Differential Diagnosis of Orbital Diseases

Clinical signs	Differential diagnosis
Bilateral axial proptosis	TAO, acute and subacute idiopathic inflammation, craniofacial disorders, high myopia, lymphomas, leukemias, metastases, A-V shunts
Pseudoproptosis	Facial asymmetry, contralateral enophthalmos, ptosis, lid retraction, buphthalmos, high myopia
Nonaxial proptosis	Implicates the quadrant opposite the displacement
Superior	Maxillary neoplasm, lymphoma, contralateral globe ptosis, lacrimal sac tumor, lower eyelid capillary hemangioma, childhood neoplasm (rhabdomyosarcoma, Ewing's sarcoma)
Inferior	Lacrimal gland fossa tumors, sphenoid wing meningioma
Temporal	Frontoethmoidal mucocele, secondary sinus and nasopharyngeal tumors, reactive and neoplastic midline lesions, large intraconal masses, metastases, lymphomas, lacrimal sac tumors
Nasal	TAO, frontal mucocele, medial dermoid cysts, reactive and dysplastic bone lesions, neurofibromata, rhabdomyosarcoma, neuroblastoma
Enophthalmos	Bone defects: fractures, facial asymmetry, neoplastic destruction, sphenoid wing absence)
	Fat atrophy: (trauma, irradiation, lipodystrophy, recurrent variceal swelling)
	Cicatrization: trauma, inflammation, sclerosing metastatic carcinoma (breast, stomach, lung, prostate)
	Postsurgical muscle shortening, nystagmus retractorius, sympathetic paresis, linear scleroderma
Dynamic orbital diseases	Pulsate or vary with position or Valsalva's maneuver
	Movement transmitted from brain or temporalis through bony defect: sphenoid wing absence (neurofibromatosis or meningoencephalocele); destructive lesions (massive frontal mucocele, aneurysmal cyst, reparative granuloma, xanthomata, posttraumatic/surgical dehiscence, dermoid, metastatic lytic tumors, histiocytosis X)
	Globe pulsations from vessels: varies during Valsalva's maneuver; shunts (capillary hemangioma, A-V shunts, and vascular tumors [nephroblastoma, thyroid, prostate])

TAO, Thyroid-associated ophthalmopathy.

hyperreflexia, pretibial myxedema, finger clubbing, tachycardia, wide pulse pressure, breast lumps, prostatic malignancy, abdominal masses, pulmonary lesions, testicular masses, and skin lesions may be associated with orbital diseases, and may help guide management.

The face should be inspected for asymmetry, proptosis, and signs of inflammation. Measure the best visual acuity, both near and far; assess eye movements; and examine the fundi. Decide on the level of urgency and refer to an ophthalmologist.

Investigations. Thyroid function studies, computed tomography (CT), and magnetic resonance imaging (MRI) are often indicated. A biopsy may be required.

Differential Diagnosis

Limit the differential diagnosis using clinical and imaging findings (Tables 174-8 and 174-9). Orbital imaging includes ultrasound, plain films, CT, and MRI.

Management

Tailor a plan to the individual, with good communication and coordination among all involved. One physician must take charge, orchestrating care with regard to scheduling, costs, and potential dangers. Optimum care requires conscious effort in planning, communication, and coordination, and judicious, customized application of support, local treatment, medications, radiotherapy, plasmapheresis, hyperbaric oxygen, surgery, and any other treatments available.

Diagnosis and Management of Specific Diseases

Structural Defects. See Table 174-10.

Atrophies, Degenerations, and Depositions. See Table 174-11.

Circulatory Disturbances. Hemodynamics determine the pathophysiology and clinical picture of orbital vascular diseases. Flow may be lively or intermediate (A-V shunts, venous anomalies), or sluggish (cavernous hemangioma). High-flow shunts may have pulsatile bruits, visible and palpable orbital pulsations, and increased venous pressure, with dilated episcleral veins, elevated intraocular pressure (IOP), chemosis, orbital tissue swelling, and retinal engorgement. Low-flow shunts are milder, with nonpulsatile exophthalmos, no bruit, and less IOP elevation. They are prone to venous thrombosis that may help or aggravate the symptoms. Venous anomalies may distend with Valsalva's maneuver, bruise and swell episodically from spontaneous hemorrhage, and give enophthalmos when emptied.

Orbital Edema. In orbital edema tissue fluid raises the intraorbital pressure, giving proptosis and/or optic atrophy. It may be inflammatory (reactive) or noninflammatory (static, toxic, allergic, or vasomotor). Inflammatory or reactive edema from an inflamed paranasal sinus or lacrimal gland gives proptosis, lid edema, chemosis, and mild limitation of eye movements. It may be hard to differentiate from orbital cellulitis. The physician should apply hot compresses and treat the cause. Noninflammatory edema is static (venous obstruction), toxic (exogenous [renal disease], endogenous [iodine or paraphenylenediamine poisoning], acute illnesses [trichinosis, typhus, acute myelitis, malaria, and tonsillitis]), allergic, or vasomotor (urticaria, Quincke's disease, and angioedema).

Venous Congestion and Thrombosis. Venous congestion and thrombosis commonly accompany orbital inflammatory and neoplastic diseases, but rarely occur alone. Idiopathic thrombosis of the orbital veins without cavernous sinus thrombosis is rare and confusing, with dilation of the lid and conjunctival and episcleral veins, proptosis, retinal vein congestion with hemorrhages, and glaucoma. Idiopathic

Table 174-9. Imaging Differential Diagnosis of Orbital Diseases

Defect	Differential diagnosis
Isolated discrete lesions	Benign: low-grade orbital or lacrimal inflammation, cavernous or capillary hemangioma, peripheral nerve sheath tumors, fibrous histiocytoma, hemangiopericytoma Malignant: nodular lymphomas, carcinoid, rhabdomyosarcoma, occasionally metastatic tumors
Cysts	Abscesses: microbial, parasitic (echinococcosis) Degeneration in neoplasms: lymphangioma, pleomorphic adenoma, schwannoma, isolated neurofibroma, rhabdomyosarcoma, melanoma, metastasis Structural abnormalities: microphthalmos with cyst, conjunctival, sweat gland, lacrimal, dermoid
Isolated infiltrative lesions	Inflammations: nonspecific or specific Neoplastic: benign (plexiform neurofibromas, lymphangiomas, capillary hemangiomas) or malignant (metastatic, fibrous histiocytomas, some lymphomas, leukemia) Depositions: amyloid
Extraocular muscle enlargement	Inflammatory: thyroid myopathy (muscle belly enlarged, tendon spared); myositis (muscle belly and tendon swollen) Neoplastic: breast (nodular enlargement, with reticular infiltration of adjacent orbit); melanoma (uniform enlargement); lymphoma (often marked enlargement of levator, superior or medial rectus) Vascular: A-V shunts (uniform enlargement) Amyloid deposition: smooth, nodular enlargement
Bone destruction	Solid: primary (reparative granuloma, aneurysmal bone cyst, Ewing's sarcoma, Wegener's granulomatosis, osteogenic sarcoma, osteoblastoma, fibrosarcoma); secondary (sinusitis, histiocytosis X, plasmacytoma, sinus and nasopharyngeal malignancies, lytic meningiomas); metastatic (neuroblastoma, prostate) Cystic: dermoid, mucocele, reparative granuloma, xanthomatous Hyperostotic: osteomyelitis, meningioma, prostate metastases; primary bone tumors (fibrous dysplasia, osteoma, ossifying fibroma, osteosarcoma, chondrosarcoma)
Optic nerve enlargement	Inflammation gives uniform expansion Infarction gives a central, low density Neoplastic: glioma, meningioma, plexiform neurofibroma, angiomeningioma, metastasis, leukemia, meningeal spread Nonneoplastic: sheath expansion (pseudotumor cerebri, chronic papilledema, subarachnoid hemorrhage, or apical crowding of thyroid orbitopathy); nerve expansion (optic neuritis, toxoplasmosis, tuberculosis, sarcoidosis, or infarction)
Calcified lesions without bone destruction	Dystrophic calcification: chronic inflammation, cartilage within dysgenic and malformed globes, phthisis bulbi, choroidal osteoma, optic nerve drusen, hyaline plaque, phlebolith, varix, lymphangioma, old thrombosis in A-V shunt or malformation, old hemorrhage, in the trochlea Neoplasia: malignant and, occasionally, benign epithelial lacrimal gland tumors, extraosseous chondrosarcoma, meningioma, schwannomas, and occasionally lymphomas and neuroblastomas, osseous and cartilaginous soft tissue tumors Cysts: epithelial, dermoid, mucocele Displaced, fractured bone
Calcified lesions with bone destruction	Not limited by suture lines: fibro-osseous tumors, epidermoids, mucoceles Limited by suture lines: ruptured dermoids

thrombosis of the cavernous sinus may affect the healthy patient, sometimes after surgical treatment for trigeminal neuralgia and internal carotid aneurysm, but usually occurs in marasmic infants and the elderly with anemia, dehydration, low blood pressure, and increased blood coagulability. Findings depend on collateral flow. Patients may have acute, sometimes pulsatile proptosis; V1 pain; III, IV, and VI palsy; dilation of retinal veins; glaucoma; and decreased vision. Spread to the other side is common. Treatment is uncertain; prognosis is variable but usually grave.

Orbital Hemorrhages. Orbital hemorrhages result from weakened vessel walls (arteriosclerosis, scurvy, rickets), abnormal coagulability (anticoagulation, hemophilia, myelogenous leukemia), increased pressure (systemic hypertension, thoracic compression, strangulation, violent coughing, straining), or trauma (birth injury, retrobulbar injection, penetrating injury, blunt injury with or without fracture). They give sudden, painful proptosis that is axial if bleeding is into tissue, eccentric if subperiosteal; nausea and/or vomiting; mydriasis; decreased vision; retinal vascular compromise; and delayed bruising. Vision decreases transiently or permanently. Treatment is usually conservative, but orbital decompression or CT-guided aspiration or surgical drainage of a subperiosteal hematoma or blood cyst must be done if vision is threatened or resolution is delayed.

Orbital Varices. Orbital varices give transient or intermittent proptosis. Primary varices, often with other venous anomalies, present after birth or later in life. Secondary varices result from an A-V shunt. Onset is dramatic with transient proptosis, lasting from a few seconds to a few days, recurring at intervals from a few hours to a few years, and producing proptosis from a few to 30 mm. They are always unilateral and usually left-sided, and may be produced by bending the head forward, less commonly backward or from side to side, particularly to the right; pressure on the jugular veins; stooping; a tight collar; coughing; taking a deep breath; holding the breath; and Valsalva's maneuver. Findings include pain, nausea, bruit, visible pulsations, "visual black-outs," blindness, mydriasis, retinal engorgement, and phleboliths on plain films. Resection is difficult; prognosis is

Table 174-10. Orbital Structural Defects

Structural defect	Clinical presentation	Treatment
Dermoid cysts	Usually in infancy; at the orbital rim, usually superotemporally; rounded, painless, firm, nonfluctuant, immobile, 1-2 cm diameter mass	Excision using a lid crease incision if possible If not excised, may rupture, causing brisk inflammation
Dermolipoma	Present from birth or infancy; have fine hairs or subepithelial dermal structures; painless, stable, smooth, yellow, soft subconjunctival masses; usually against the globe superotemporally	Observe Excise only if irritating or a significant blemish
Herniated orbital fat	In men older than 60 years; more common in Blacks or after weight gain; painless, gradually enlarging, smooth, yellow, soft subconjunctival masses; usually against the globe superotemporally	Observe Excise only if irritating or a significant blemish
Mucocele	Age 30-80 yr, history of facial fractures, sinusitis; sinus drainage block—slowly push the eye down, laterally, and anteriorly	Remove the mucocele and obliterate the sinus or restore sinus drainage
Orbital fractures	Orbital rim with or without displacement; blow-out (of floor +/– medial wall; always suspect after orbital trauma; may have lid emphysema, restriction of vertical gaze with diplopia, enophthalmos); children may have no ocular inflammation	CT scan with axial and positioned coronal views Repair a significantly displaced rim fracture Repair within 2 weeks a blow-out fracture with persistent diplopia or enophthalmos; consider repair urgently in children
Orbital foreign bodies	Always suspect with every open orbital wound; the mechanism of injury may raise the clinical suspicion	Suspect CT scan with axial and coronal views and bone windows Remove vegetable and other reactive or potentially infective material Inert metallic fragments such as BB's are usually best left
Orbital puncture wounds	Suspect from the history of injury; sharp objects may cause orbital injuries or pass through the orbital roof with immediate hemorrhage and brain edema or delayed meningitis or brain abscess	Suspect them CT scan of orbits and brain with axial and coronal views and bone windows Most need to be removed; some inert, nonreactive materials can be left

Table 174-11. Orbital Atrophies, Degenerations, and Depositions

Condition	Classification
Pseudoproptosis (appearance of proptosis without anterior displacement)	Eyelid asymmetry: lid retraction as in TAO; blepharoptosis not from orbital causes Unilateral globe enlargement: buphthalmos (congenital glaucoma); congenital cystic eye; scleral ectasia (scleral thinning alone); staphylomata (fused scleral and uveal thinning); high myopia Orbital asymmetry: unilateral bony hypoplasia (linear scleroderma [coup de sabre]); hemifacial atrophy of Parry-Romberg; previous trauma; radiotherapy in childhood
Atrophy and enophthalmos	Microphthalmos Bone loss: tumor, trauma, surgery Fat atrophy: age, lipodystrophy, facial hemiatrophy, varices; trauma (irradiation, inflammation hemorrhage, tumor removal) Cicatrization: scirrhous breast carcinoma; trauma, inflammation, surgery
Oculomotor defects	Nystagmus retractorius, Duane's syndrome, muscle shortening after strabismus surgery; scarring from inflammation; progressive external ophthalmoplegia
Mass effect	Amyloidosis: systemic (primary—abnormal immunocytes, secondary—from inflammatory disease); localized (primary—no known local disorder, secondary—local inflammation, degeneration Orbital fat prolapse

guarded. In the Klippel-Trenaunay-Weber syndrome, orbital venous varicosities may be associated with hypertrophy of soft tissues and bone.

Orbital Aneurysms. Orbital aneurysms give pulsatile exophthalmos, as do vascular tumors, varices, A-V shunts, and bony defects (meningoceles, sphenoidal mucoceles, sphenoidal hypoplasia in neurofibromatosis). Ophthalmic artery aneurysms are fusiform or, less often, saccular. Pulsating proptosis, optic nerve dysfunction, and diplopia may occur. Angiography should be used for diagnosis; treat with ligation or excision. Lacrimal, ethmoidal, and internal maxillary artery aneurysms occur less commonly.

Arteriovenous Fistulas. A-V shunts, the most common cause of pulsating exophthalmos, are congenital, traumatic or spontaneous (caroticocavernous or dural), and usually in the cavernous sinus. Congenital shunts are rare, occurring alone or with Wyburn-Mason's and Rendu-Osler-Weber syndromes. Traumatic cases (males > females) are due to penetrating, contrecoup, or blunt injuries with basal skull fractures. Onset may be delayed or gradual but is usually sudden, with unilateral or bilateral pulsating proptosis, a swishing noise in the head, pain, and decreased vision. Spontaneous cases (females > males, 25% in pregnancy), resulting when an aneurysm bursts into the cavernous sinus, begin dramatically with vomiting, vertigo, unconsciousness, and sometimes death. Dural shunts (postmenopausal women) have a chronic, fluctuating course with exacerbations, due to thrombosis, and spontaneous resolution in 40%. In all shunts, the degree of proptosis, pulsation, lid swelling, chemosis, venous engorgement, corneal exposure, glaucoma, cranial nerve (III, IV, V-1, VI) palsy, retinal involvement, and bruit varies from slight to marked. The proptosis, bruit, and thrill are increased on stooping or exertion, and diminished with carotid compression on the affected or both sides. CT may show proptosis, extraocular muscle and superior ophthalmic vein enlargement, and a nonenhancing, superior ophthalmic vein or cavernous sinus defect, suggesting thrombosis. Arteriography, often with superselective catheterization, is essential for diagnosis. Prognosis is poor, although some resolve spontaneously. Detachable balloon-catheter occlusion and a multidisciplinary approach have improved the outlook for high-flow cases.

Orbital Inflammations, Infections, and Infestations.

In a busy orbital clinic, 57% of cases were inflammations, infections, or infestations: 47% dysthyroid, 4.7% nonspecific, 3.7% specific infective, and 1.6% other specific. Inflammations may be nonspecific or specific; infections may be viral, bacterial, or fungal; and infestations may occur with protozoa, roundworms, flatworms, or arthropods.

Nonspecific Inflammations

Acute and subacute idiopathic inflammatory syndromes (pseudotumors). These have a varying and confusing presentation, outcome, and histopathology. Onset is acute or subacute with pain, dilated vessels, and edema, with or without malaise. CT shows an irregular margin by the primary focus, swelling, and contrast enhancement. It may resolve rapidly with treatment or be chronic with progressive infiltration, destruction, and fibrosis. Histopathology shows fibroblasts, neutrophils, lymphocytes, plasma cells, and macrophages. Location may be anterior, diffuse, apical, myositic, or lacrimal (Table 174-12). Treatment for all these inflammations requires biopsy unless very difficult, intralesional steroids at biopsy, then oral prednisone 80 mg daily. Most respond rapidly. If recurrent with rapid tapering, restart prednisone and taper more slowly. If again recurrent with tapering, or unresponsive, biopsy is mandatory. If benign, consider radiation, with 1000 to 3000 centigray (cGy), or chemotherapy.

Idiopathic sclerosing inflammation. Idiopathic sclerosing inflammation entraps orbital structures in scar. Sometimes part of multifocal fibrosclerosis, usually unilateral, it gives diplopia, proptosis, progressive visual loss, lid retraction, mild inflammation, and pain. CT scan shows homogeneous, dense lesions, often contrast-enhancing, with regular margins, infiltrating orbital fat and muscles. Histopathology shows scarring with scattered inflammatory cells. Differential diagnosis includes chronic inflammations (Wegener's and other granulomatous inflammations), secondary and metastatic cancers (especially sclerosing types), and lymphomas. Initial response to steroids may be good, but later, relentless progression is the rule. Biopsy, then treat with prednisone (80 mg daily) plus radiotherapy (2500 to 3000 cGy).

Idiopathic noninfectious granulomatous inflammation. Idiopathic noninfectious granulomatous inflammation is defined by its histopathology (nonnecrotizing granuloma or lipogranuloma), affecting orbital soft tissues without specific localization or systemic associations. It presents with mild inflammation, a palpable mass, and a slow onset. Treat with excision or prednisone 80 mg daily.

Specific Inflammations. Specific inflammations include TAO, sarcoidosis, Sjögren's syndrome, vasculitides, other granulomatous and histiocytic diseases, and orbital inflammation secondary to ocular disease (Table 174-13).

Infections. Infections may be viral, bacterial, or fungal. Viral orbital infections produce acute dacryoadenitis. Bacterial and fungal orbital infections produce acute and chronic dacryoadenitis, and acute, subacute, and chronic orbital cellulitis (Table 174-14).

Infestations. Infestations include those with protozoa (amebiasis), roundworms (nemathelminthes: filariasis, dracontiasis, trichinosis), flatworms (platyhelminthes: schistosomiasis, paragonimiasis, sparganosis, echinococcosis, cysticercosis), mollusks, and arthropods (orbital ophthalmomyiasis). Knowledge of the patient's geographic location and the life cycle of the parasite aids diagnosis.

Protozoa. Amebiasis is a very rare cause of an orbital inflammatory mass.

Nemathelminthes. The roundworms *Wuchereria bancrofti* and *Dirofilaria conjunctivae* can cause chronic granulomatous orbital cysts mimicking orbital tumors. *Dracunculus medinensis* can infest the orbit. About 11 days after an individual eats infested meat, *Trichinella spiralis,* during dissemination, produces a doughy edema of the eyelids, especially the upper, occasionally with chemosis and a reddish rash. Extraocular muscle invasion is early, limiting eye movement because of pain and causing a transient, pale, lemon-jelly chemosis, usually bilateral, over the insertions of the horizontal rectus muscles. Later generalized aches and systemic symptoms supervene. Death from myocarditis, encephalitis, meningitis, bronchopneumonia, or nephritis may follow. The physician should diagnose from the clinical picture, high eosinophilia, positive serology, and biopsy.

Platyhelminthes. Flatworms *Schistosoma haematobium* and *Paragonimus westermani* may give orbital cysts. *Sparganum mansoni* may produce painful proptosis, lid edema, and

Table 174-12. Orbital Inflammatory Syndromes: Anatomic Patterns

Syndrome	Presentation	Investigations	Differential diagnosis
Anterior	Young, pain, proptosis, lid swelling, ptosis, injection, and decreased vision from uveitis, sclerotenonitis, papillitis, or exudative retinal detachment	CT: diffuse anterior orbital infiltration against the eye, scleral and choroidal thickening, globe–optic nerve junction blurring, nerve sheath extension Ultrasound: irregular, uniform anterior infiltrate, sclerotenonitis with Tenon's space accentuation, optic nerve shadow doubling (T sign)	Orbital cellulitis, a sudden event in a preexisting lesion (dermoid cyst rupture, vascular lesion hemorrhage), ocular inflammation (scleritis, uveitis), collagen vascular diseases, and, in children, rhabdomyosarcoma, neuroblastoma, and leukemia
Diffuse	More severe: ocular movement limitation, papillitis, exudative retinal detachment	CT: soft tissue infiltration from apex to globe, blurring of optic nerve and muscles	As for anterior
Apical	Pain, minimal proptosis, restricted eye movements, often decreased vision	CT: irregular apical infiltration with extension along the extraocular muscles or the optic nerve	Optic neuritis, tumors, Tolosa-Hunt syndrome
Myositic	Lid swelling, ptosis, chemosis and injection over the affected muscles, diplopia, restricted eye movement, and pain, worse when the affected muscles act Forced duction test may be positive; often unilateral; one or more rectus, usually superior or medial; may be recurrent	CT: irregular extraocular muscle swelling including the tendon (unlike Graves' disease), and localized fat infiltration	Graves' disease, Lyme disease, metastases
Lacrimal	Female > male, any age, pain, inferonasal proptosis, S-shaped upper lid, temporal lid and conjunctival fornix injection, little motility disturbance, a tender, palpable lacrimal gland, pouting of lacrimal ducts Chronic: few inflammatory signs, may be bilateral, recurrent, and associated with alopecia or colitis	CT: infiltration in the superolateral orbit Ultrasonography: mass with internal reflectivity, an echolucent area next to the sclera, anterior thickening of adjacent muscle	Viral and bacterial dacryoadenitis, dermoid cyst rupture, sarcoidosis, Sjögren's syndrome, cysts, neoplasms

Table 174-13. Specific Orbital Inflammations*

Inflammation	History	Findings	Treatment
Thyroid-associated ophthalmopathy (TAO) 1. Most common cause of both unilateral and bilateral proptosis 2. An organ-specific, autoimmune-mediated inflammation of the extraocular muscles and perhaps the periorbital connective tissue 3. Muscles swell, pushing the globe forward, tethering the levator and rectus muscles, and squeezing the optic nerve	Variable and unpredictable; 90% mild, noninfiltrative disease; 10% severe, infiltrative disease; 30% + family history; associated with diabetes mellitus and myasthenia gravis; TAO occurs within 18 mo of diagnosis of thyroid disease; bulging eyes, pressure behind eyes, irritated eyes, lid pulled up, lid swelling, tearing, double vision, decreased vision	Variable; exophthalmos; eye movement restriction; lid swelling; more pigment; lid lag, retraction with "scleral show," and stare; conjunctival injection and chemosis, especially over insertion of rectus muscles; cornea exposure; compressive optic neuropathy; lacrimal gland enlargement and prolapse, tearing; CT enlarged muscles; laboratory: T3, T4, TSH, antibodies	Chronic, depressing disease, give support Stop smoking Treat thyroid disease Lubricants Corticosteroids: buy time; avoid chronic use Surgery: fix retracted lids; strabismus correction; decompress orbit Radiation Immunosuppressive drugs

*Other granulomatous and histiocytic diseases include eosinophilic granuloma (histiocytosis X), juvenile xanthogranuloma, Erdheim-Chester disease, necrobiotic xanthogranuloma, pseudorheumatoid nodules, and fibrous histiocytoma.

Continued

Table 174-13. Specific Orbital Inflammations*—cont'd

Inflammation	History	Findings	Treatment
Sarcoidosis (multisystem, immunologic disorder, with noncaseating granulomas involving many tissues [especially hilar lymph nodes and pulmonary parenchyma] with symptoms dependent on site and degree of involvement)	Highest risk in black women age 20-40 yr in southern United States; dry eyes, swollen upper lids, lid bumps	Eyelid nodules or papules, uveitis, chorioretinitis, dry eye, lacrimal gland enlargement, conjunctival nodules, neuropathies, and, very rarely, deep orbital disease	Treat systemic disease Local corticosteroids Surgery as indicated
Sjögren's syndrome (chronic, systemic inflammatory disorder, unknown cause, with dry mouth, eyes, and other mucous membranes, associated with autoimmune diseases)	Dry irritated eyes, dry mouth, epistaxis, reduced sense of smell, hoarseness, recurrent bronchitis, and increased risk of malignant lymphoma and pseudolymphoma	Dry eyes, filamentary keratopathy, enlarged tender lacrimal and parotid glands, anti SS-A antibodies positive	Local lubricants Systemic with systemic steroids and immunosuppressives
Vasculitides: (1) periarteritis nodosa (classical polyarteritis nodosa, allergic angiitis and granulomatosis [Churg-Strauss], and systemic necrotizing vasculitis "overlap syndrome"), (2) hypersensitivity (leukocytoclastic) angiitides (orbital vasculitis, vasculitides with connective tissue disorders, Cogan's syndrome); (3) Wegener's granulomatosis; (4) other respiratory vasculitides; and (5) giant cell arteritis. Early cases mimic nonspecific inflammations. Diagnosis can be difficult and treatment specialized.			
Orbital Inflammation Secondary to Ocular Disease: These include: endophthalmitis, severe uveitis, and scleritis. The diagnosis is usually clear, but posterior scleritis can mimic other acute and subacute orbital inflammations. Suspect it in older patients, usually those with collagen-vascular diseases, presenting with orbital inflammation, severe aching pain, and typical ultrasound and CT findings.			

*Other granulomatous and histiocytic diseases include eosinophilic granuloma (histiocytosis X), juvenile xanthogranuloma, Erdheim-Chester disease, necrobiotic xanthogranuloma, pseudorheumatoid nodules, and fibrous histiocytoma.

chemosis resembling cellulitis. Treat with excision. In endemic areas suspect a hydatid cyst from *Taenia echinococcus* as a potential cause of unilateral proptosis of insidious onset in a young person. Treat with excision. *Cysticercosis cellulosae* from *T. solium* is the most common helminthic ocular infection in man. Subretinal, vitreous, and conjunctival involvement is frequent; orbital disease is rare, producing pea-sized anterior cysts. Treat with excision.

Arthropoda. Various species of the fly family Calliphoridae Arthropoda produce orbital ophthalmomyiasis. Risk factors include tropical climates, poor hygiene, poverty, debilitation, malodorous gonococcal conjunctivitis, ulcerated periorbital cancer, and the extremes of age. Tissue destruction may be extensive. Treatment is difficult.

Orbital Cysts. Except for dermoids and mucoceles, orbital cysts are rare. They include lacrimal cysts (simple palpebral and orbital lobe cysts, multiple cystic degeneration, parasitic cysts, Krause's glands' cysts) and orbital cysts (simple epithelial cysts [primary cutaneous epithelial cysts or epidermoid cysts, primary conjunctival epithelial cysts, primary respiratory epithelial cysts, implantation epithelial cysts, and sudoriferous cysts or Moll's gland cysts]; dermoid cysts; teratomas; congenital cystic eye; colobomatous cysts; meningocele; meningoencephalocele; primary optic nerve sheath cysts; mucoceles; hematoceles; hematic cysts; parasitic cysts [*W. bancrofti, T. echinococcus, T. solium,* and *Multiceps*]; and dentigerous cysts). Most of these have been discussed.

Acquired lacrimal cysts are cystic swellings of the excretory ducts. They are blue-domed; usually single, although sometimes multiple or bilateral; and visible through the conjunctiva that transilluminates. Resect carefully without damage to other ducts.

Orbital Tumors. Orbital tumors can be congenital, primary, secondary, or metastatic. Congenital tumors and malformations will not be discussed. Primary tumors can be neurogenic, mesenchymal, vascular, lacrimal, lymphoproliferative, or leukemic. Secondary tumors can spread from nasopharynx and paranasal sinuses, bones, intracranial tissues, eyelids, conjunctiva, lacrimal sac, or eye. Metastatic tumors commonly spread from the breast, lung, adrenal gland, prostate, GI tract, kidney, thyroid, skin, and bone.

Primary Orbital Tumors

Neurogenic tumors. Neurogenic tumors include those of the optic nerve, meninges, peripheral nerves, and rare neuroectodermal tumors (Table 174-15).

Primary mesenchymal tumors. Primary mesenchymal tumors include those of bone and cartilage, striated and smooth muscle, fibrous tissue, histiocytes, and fat. Most are osseous, with striated muscle and histiocytic tumors next, and fat and fibrous tumors being rare. In one series primary mesenchymal tumors made up 3% of orbital cases and 16% of orbital neoplasia.

Orbital bone tumors, all rare, include dysplasia and related fibro-osseus lesions, reactive lesions, and neoplasms. Patterns of presentation include:

1. A slowly growing, noninfiltrative tumor, seldom-eroding bone, with nonaxial proptosis and facial disfigurement (e.g., fibrous dysplasia, osteoma, chordoma, or low-grade chondrosarcoma).
2. Bleeding into a bone-eroding dysplasia giving acute proptosis (e.g., reparative granuloma, aneurysmal bone

Table 174-14. Orbital Infections*

Infection	History	Findings	Treatment
Acute orbital cellulitis (usually from sinus; *threatens vision and life;* non-sinus sources include: face, teeth, meninges, ear, conjunctiva, eye, lacrimal sac or gland, bacteremia, foreign body; may be preseptal or postseptal [orbital]; cavitate forming a subperiosteal or orbital abscess, or spread, causing cavernous sinus thrombosis, intracranial abscess or thrombophlebitis, or temporalis fossa abscess)	Younger children: viral coryza, spread from the ethmoid and maxillary sinuses (not frontal), and infection with aerobes (*H. influenzae*) Adults: sinusitis, polyps, allergy, trauma, or recent dental extraction, spread from frontoethmoidal sinuses, and multiple microbial infection, often anaerobic	Preseptal cellulitis (usually *S. aureus* or *S. pyogenes*) gives pain, lid swelling, chemosis, and systemic toxicity with fever and leukocytosis Orbital (postseptal) cellulitis adds proptosis, limited eye movement, and decreased vision Subperiosteal abscesses, usually superior or retrobulbar, are poorly defined masses showing homogeneous, heterogeneous, or ring enhancement on CT with contrast; infrequent in children, when treated, usually resolve without drainage or sequelae; more common in adults, often require sinus drainage, and have more severe sequelae Osteomyelitis may result	Adult preseptal cellulitis: hot compresses and oral dicloxacillin 500 mg qid All others: admit, IV antibiotics, infectious diseases consultation, drain abscesses as necessary
Subacute and chronic orbital infections			
Orbital tuberculosis: periostitis	>20 yr, involves the zygomatic bone	Painless, indolent, red swelling that points and drains	Biopsy Drugs Generous debridement
Orbital tuberculosis: tuberculoma	Most common in women 40-60 yr; TB elsewhere	Painless, slowly enlarging mass, often on superomedial orbital wall	Biopsy, debulk, and treat with antituberculosis drugs, expecting steady improvement
Orbital syphilis: marginal periostitis (orbital syphilis, in tertiary disease, presents as a diffuse hyperplastic periostitis involving the margin, walls, or apex)	Most commonly involves superior rim, indolent inflammatory swelling, tenderness, intractable headache, radiating neuralgia most marked at night	Bony thickening with boss formation may be marked or the gumma may break down, leaving a persistent fistula with a depressed scar leading down to softened bone; bony absorption may be marked, especially in congenital cases	Antisyphilitic antibiotics Expect rapid improvement
Orbital syphilis: periostitis of the orbital walls			Antisyphilitic antibiotics
Orbital syphilis: gummatous apical periostitis			Antisyphilitic antibiotics
Fungal infections			
Rhinoorbital mucormycosis or phycomycosis	Immunocompromised patients with diabetic ketoacidosis or AIDS, or those receiving corticosteroids systemically or as nasal sprays; sinusitis, pharyngitis, and nasal discharge; it presents with a boring orbital pain	Dramatic cellulitis, proptosis, cranial nerve pareses, visual loss, and general deterioration; thrombosing arteritis with gangrene of the nasal mucosa, turbinates, and palate, septal perforation, and intraluminal spread into the brain	Treat underlying disease, biopsy stat: ask for rapid histologic processing Start IV amphotericin B Positive biopsy, generously debride, post-operative drainage Local amphotericin B irrigation; possibly hyperbaric oxygen (controversial) Grave prognosis
Orbital aspergillosis (allergic and invasive)	Immunocompromised patients living in hot, humid climates; a slowly enlarging mass	Spreads to the orbit from a paranasal sinus or the lacrimal sac; biopsy: long septate filaments with dichotomous branches that stain with hematoxylin-eosin stain as well as Gomori methenamine silver	Excise Amphotericin B
Orbital actinomycosis	Slowly increasing proptosis and nasal obstruction	Spreads into the orbit from the mouth, nose, paranasal sinuses conjunctiva, lids, or canaliculus	Debridement and penicillin

*For acute viral dacryoadenitis and acute and chronic bacterial dacryoadenitis see Table 174-7.

Table 174-15. Primary Orbital Neurogenic Tumors

Tumor	History	Findings	Management
Optic nerve tumors*			
Juvenile optic nerve glioma; low-grade pilocytic astrocytomas	Females > males; 75% <10 yr; neurofibromatosis; decreased vision; proptosis	Chiasmal, orbitocranial, orbital, and diffuse or multifocal; grow slowly and intermittently	Excision and/or radiation is controversial
Malignant optic glioma/ glioblastoma of adulthood	Middle aged; visual loss early; rapid progression	Decreased vision, disc edema; CT shows enlargement of nerve or chiasm	Poor prognosis
Meningioma			
Intracranial meningiomas	Women/men = 3/1; at risk–neurofibromatosis; most common in fifth decade; vision loss, palsies, mass effect	Sphenoid ridge, suprasellar, olfactory groove; CT: bony hyperostosis and/or lysis; well-defined, homogeneous, soft-tissue mass with uniform post-contrast enhancement; a "tumor blush"	Excision, debulking, radiation, hormonal manipulation
Optic canal meningiomas	Women/men = 3/1; at risk–neurofibromatosis; early visual loss from optic nerve compression	CT or MRI demonstration difficult; spread over the planum sphenoidale to the opposite optic nerve	Excise before chiasm involved
Orbital optic nerve meningiomas	Women/men = 2/1; at risk–neurofibromatosis; bimodal peak second and fifth decade, second more aggressive; early transient visual obscurations in gaze extremes, but otherwise minimal visual impairment; later: mild proptosis, progressive field constriction	Increasing disc edema with gliosis and refractile bodies, optociliary shunts, and choroidal folds ; finally, vision is lost, nerve head gliosis and atrophy increase, and the refractile bodies disappear; CT: diffuse, fusiform swelling	Excise the lesion using: a lateral orbitotomy, if it clearly spares the posterior one third of the nerve, or a neurosurgical approach otherwise Consider optic canal decompression or radiotherapy when the remaining eye is involved
Peripheral nerve tumors			
Neurofibromas, isolated (generally dermal) tumors	90% do not have neurofibromatosis; often multiple; middle age	Solitary, slow-growing mass, anesthesia, paresthesia, hypesthesia	Resect, being careful not to damage a motor nerve
Neurofibromas, plexiform lesions	Neurofibromatosis: most common and complex orbital peripheral nerve tumors; elephantiasis neuromatosa	Hypertrophic skin, lid, and face, proptosis and disfigurement; palpation: "bag of worms"	Debulking difficult Recurrence common
Orbital amputation neuromas	Previous injury, neuralgic pain	May be very small; sensitive, trigger point	Pain cured by excision
Schwannomas, neurilemomas	Adults age 20-50, 18% have neurofibromatosis	Intraconal: proptosis, lid swelling, globe indentation, diplopia in extremes of gaze, and central scotomata, vision fluctuation on lateral gaze; extraconal: hypesthesia	Excise Prognosis good
Malignant peripheral nerve sheath tumors (perineural fibrosarcoma, malignant schwannoma, neurofibrosarcoma, and neurogenic sarcoma)	Adults age 20-60 yr, males > females: 50% neurofibromatosis	Painful superonasal mass growing over weeks to months, with paresthesia and tenderness	Biopsy and treat with exenteration or more radical "craniofacectomy"

*Others: medulloepitheliomas/neuroepitheliomas, secondary and metastatic tumors, primary CNS tumors, and pseudoneoplasms.

cyst, reactive xanthomatous lesions, or brown tumor of hyperparathyroidism).

3. A relentless, infiltrative neoplasm with pain, hypesthesia, muscle restriction, and optic neuropathy (e.g., osteogenic sarcoma, Ewing's sarcoma, malignant fibrous dysplasia, histiocytoma, histiocytosis X, lymphoma, or plasmacytoma).

The histopathologic diagnosis of bony tumors is difficult, requiring correlation with radiographs.

In childhood, rhabdomyosarcoma is both the most common soft tissue malignancy and the most common primary orbital malignancy (70% in first decade; most < age 7 years; male:female ratio, 5:3; 50% retrobulbar, 25% suprabulbar, 12% infrabulbar). Seldom familial, it is subacute, acute, or often fulminant, with inferolateral proptosis, no pain or decreased vision, but ptosis, lid injection, and swelling.

The histology tends to change with age: embryonal in childhood, alveolar in adolescence, and pleomorphic in adults. Embryonal and alveolar types arise in soft tissue, not extraocular muscles. Pleomorphic lesions arise from dedifferentiation of, and are associated with, adult muscles. Embryonal lesions make up two thirds of cases. Alveolar lesions, more common in the inferior orbit, have the poorest prognosis; adult pleomorphic lesions, the least common, have the best. A new classification divides them into three groups: anaplastic (ANA), monomorphous round cell (MRC), and mixed (MX), the last having the best prognosis.

Differential diagnosis includes progressive, rapidly developing tumors and inflammations, including neuroblastoma, chloroma, lymphangioma, infantile hemangioma, ruptured dermoid cysts, cellulitis, and nonspecific inflammations. Management involves biopsy, staging, limited resection, radiation (4000 to 5000 cGy), and chemotherapy, and is best done in centers with experience. Five-year survival is 65% for all rhabdomyosarcomas occurring anywhere, but 95% with lesions limited to the orbit, because of early detection and lack of lymphatic metastases. Treatment morbidity includes cataracts, keratopathy, retinopathy, ptosis, enophthalmos, lacrimal duct stenosis, facial asymmetry, bone hypoplasia, leukemia, and behavioral problems.

Smooth muscle tumors (leiomyoma and leiomyosarcoma), fibrous tissue tumors (fibroma, nodular fasciitis, fibromatoses, fibrosarcoma, congenital and infantile fibrosarcoma, myxoma), and adipose tumors (lipomas, liposarcomas) are very rare, and should be excised.

Histiocytic tumors and tumorlike lesions include fibrous histiocytoma and juvenile xanthogranuloma. Fibrous histiocytoma, the most common adult mesenchymal orbital tumor, presents in middle age as a slow-growing or aggressive mass, rarely metastasizing, that is commonly found in the upper nasal quadrant or lacrimal sac or gland. The physician should biopsy and resect. Radiotherapy is not useful. Orbital juvenile xanthogranuloma is rare.

Vascular tumors and malformations. Vascular tumors and malformations include primary vascular tumors, A-V shunts and venous anomalies, congenital vascular anomalies (phakomatoses), aneurysms, obstructions, and unclassified hemorrhages. Mass effect, vascular engorgement, orbital pulsation, and intermittent exophthalmos suggest this diagnosis.

Primary vascular tumors. Primary vascular tumors include hamartomas, choristomas, and neoplasms. Infantile hemangiomas have high flow, cavernous hemangiomas have low flow, and lymphangiomas and some solid tumors have "no" flow.

Hamartomas include infantile capillary hemangiomas and cavernous hemangiomas. Infantile capillary hemangiomas can occur in the orbit as well as in the eyelids, and can mimic other orbital tumors. They should be treated with observation unless the behavior requires exploration. Cavernous hemangioma, the most common primary orbital tumor of adults, is a benign, well-encapsulated, slow-growing, usually intraconal, and well-tolerated orbital mass. It may give proptosis, posterior pole indentation, choroidal striae, optic nerve compression, diplopia, orbital pain, or transient gaze-induced amaurosis. CT scan shows a smooth, well-defined, oval or rounded, intraconal, poorly enhanced mass. Most are lateral, may bow the lateral orbital wall, and occasionally extend extraconally. A- and B-scans are pathognomonic. These should be observed or resected. The plump, nodular, plum-colored, relatively avascular, encapsulated mass with surface vascular channels is usually easily removed in toto or pieces.

Choristomas include lymphangiomas. Most common between ages 1 and 15 years, they are worse with upper respiratory tract infections, are sometimes associated with face and neck lesions, are relatively avascular, and may present as superficial, deep, or combined. Superficial lymphangiomas give a clear, yellowish, blood-filled, or bluish lid or conjunctival cyst or cysts that can be transilluminated. They should be resected if unsightly. Deep lymphangiomas present, usually in childhood, with intralesional hemorrhage and sudden proptosis that may gradually increase, perhaps from osmosis, and may compress orbital structures (*chocolate cyst*). There is no arterial or venous connection. CT scan shows low-density, cystlike masses behind orbital septum, with a thin rim of enhancement, focal-enhancing areas outside the cysts, and orbital enlargement. Combined superficial and deep lymphangiomas present, usually in infancy, sometimes with oral or intracranial lesions; enlarge slowly over many years, sometimes becoming massive; and bleed repeatedly with recurrent subconjunctival hemorrhages, periorbital ecchymoses and swelling, and progressive optic nerve damage. Resection of deep and combined lesions when indicated may be difficult because they are poorly circumscribed in a mass of orbital scar. A CO_2 laser may help. Recurrence is common.

Vascular neoplasms include hemangiopericytoma, malignant hemangioendothelioma, Kaposi's sarcoma, angiolymphoid hyperplasia, and vascular leiomyoma (angiomyoma).

Arteriovenous shunts and venous anomalies. Arteriovenous shunts and venous anomalies are discussed in Circulatory Disturbances.

Congenital vascular anomalies (phacomatoses) *(see Chapter 172).* Congenital vascular anomalies are neurocutaneous syndromes with cutaneous or mucosal nevi, hamartomas, or neoplastic growths that usually involve the central nervous system (CNS) and the eyes. They have the following orbital manifestations: Sturge-Weber syndrome (port-wine stains, glaucoma, and buphthalmos), hereditary hemorrhagic telangiectasia (CNS vascular malformations, telangiectasia of the conjunctiva or optic nerve), Wyburn-Mason's syndrome (sudden or gradual visual loss, pulsatile proptosis from optic nerve and orbital A-V shunts, hemianopia from A-V shunts at or behind the chiasm, hemiparesis, hemiplegia, seizures, and subarachnoid hemorrhage), Klippel-Trenaunay syndrome (orbital varices, conjunctival telangiectasia, retinal varicosities, and angiomas of the conjunctiva, sclera, and choroid), are neurofibromatosis (see Disorders of the Eyelids).

Aneurysms, obstructive lesions, and unclassified spontaneous and posttraumatic orbital hemorrhages. These are discussed in Circulatory Disturbances.

Lacrimal gland tumors. The normal lacrimal gland, a minor salivary gland, is seldom palpable in Caucasians, but can often be felt in Blacks. Masses may be intrinsic or extrinsic, and each of these may be inflammatory, structural, or neoplastic. (For inflammatory and structural lesions see above.)

Intrinsic primary lacrimal gland neoplasms. Intrinsic primary lacrimal gland neoplasms include epithelial tumors and lymphomas.

About 50% of epithelial tumors are benign (mixed cell tumors or pleomorphic adenomas) and 50% are malignant. Of the carcinomas, 25% are adenoid cystic and 25% are malignant mixed cell tumors (pleomorphic adenocarcinomas), or, rarely, mucoepidermoid and squamous carcinomas. Most arise in the orbital lobe, are large when detected, but do not affect gland function.

Benign lesions give painless masses that grow for more than 1 year. They excavate, without infiltrating, bone. Malignant lesions grow more rapidly (6 to 12 months), give pain (about 40%), and on CT scan show bone infiltration, with irregular or serrated margins, and calcification (also seen with choristomas, dermoid and implantation cysts, plasmacytoma, and lymphoma).

Benign mixed tumors, which usually occur between ages 17 to 77 years (mean age 39 years) and have a male:female ratio of 2:1, are well-circumscribed, bosselated masses with a pseudocapsule invaded by fingers of tumor. A high recurrence rate, occasionally with malignant transformation, is likely with incisional biopsy, pseudocapsular rupture, or incomplete removal. If suspected, *do not biopsy,* but excise completely. From 15 to 80 years (mean age 50 years), a benign mixed cell tumor may develop areas of malignancy (male:female ratio, 2:1), usually poorly differentiated adenocarcinoma (male: female ratio, 3:1), but also adenoid cystic (female:male ratio, 2:1) or squamous carcinoma, or even sarcoma. It suddenly expands with pain and bony infiltration. Radical excision should be offered. Prognosis is poor, with a 70% recurrence rate, often delayed 10 or more years. At death 50% have intracranial extension and 30% distant metastases.

Adenoid cystic carcinoma, a subtype of adenocarcinoma, is the most common lacrimal gland epithelial malignancy. It affects males and females equal and occurs at any age, with peaks in the second and fourth decades. It gives a mass growing for <1 year, with pain (9% to 40%), ptosis, diplopia, formication, paresthesia, and bone expansion or erosion. At diagnosis it has often spread along orbital nerves and vessels into the cavernous sinus, precluding excision. It may metastasize early or late. Prognosis for cure is dismal, although some patients may coexist for years with their carcinoma.

Adenocarcinoma may arise de novo (7%) or within a benign mixed tumor. It occurs in older patients (between 40 and 60 years), but otherwise behaves as adenoid cystic carcinoma. Mucoepidermoid carcinoma, rare in the lacrimal gland, arises from ductal epithelium. Squamous carcinoma is a very rare primary lacrimal gland tumor.

Lacrimal gland lymphomas develop over several months in older patients between ages 50 and 60 years, and give smooth, painless mass, sometimes with a pink, salmon-colored subconjunctival mass. Many present as isolated orbital lesions, but go on to develop systemic disease. All require a systemic assessment. CT scan shows molding to adjacent structures without soft tissue invasion, bone excavation, or globe flattening.

Other intrinsic neoplasms of the lacrimal gland fossa include spindle cell sarcoma, cavernous hemangioma, melanomas, and peripheral nerve tumors.

Extrinsic lacrimal gland neoplasms. Extrinsic lacrimal gland neoplasms include myeloma, sclerosing Hodgkin's lymphoma, eosinophilic granuloma, and brown tumor of hyperparathyroidism.

Optimum management of lacrimal gland fossa masses demands accurate, timely diagnosis with early incisional biopsy unless a benign mixed cell tumor is suspected, or the mass is obviously a viral or bacterial infection, requiring only observation or antibiotic treatment.

Lymphoproliferative and leukemic tumors. Lymphoproliferative and leukemic tumors are immune cell disorders including lymphocytic, plasma cell; other lymphocytic and leukemic lesions; and the histiocytoses.

Lymphocytic tumors. Lymphocytic tumors include reactive lymphoid hyperplasia, atypical dysplastic lymphoid hyperplasia, and frank lymphomas. Reactive lymphoid hyperplasia or idiopathic inflammations may be acute, subacute, or chronic, with inflammatory histopathology showing polymorphic infiltrates, fibrosis, and granulomas. Atypical dysplastic lymphoid hyperplasia has a dense mildly dysplastic infiltrate, but not frank malignancy. Frank lymphomas are anaplastic. They give four clinical syndromes: (1) insidious, painless masses, (2) more fulminant (weeks to months) infiltrating masses, (3) spread from adjacent tissues, and (4) neuro-ophthalmic disease.

Insidious, painless, often anterior masses are most common, disrupting function little, and are from low-grade disorders whether benign, atypical, or malignant. More fulminant infiltrating masses, usually less well-differentiated lymphomas, acute leukemias, and histiocytoses, are prone to secondary infections. Spread of adjacent disease of bone (multiple myeloma, Burkitt's lymphoma), sinuses, or skin may give rapid onset of orbital masses with bone destruction, suggesting metastatic carcinoma or aggressive lacrimal gland malignancies. With improved survival and the limitations on chemotherapy posed by the *blood-brain barrier,* ocular and CNS invasion by end-stage lymphomas and leukemias is common. Orbital lymphocytic tumors parallel those seen in other extranodal and extramedullary sites, with a progression from benign to malignant, involving lymphoid hyperplasia, atypical lymphoid hyperplasia (dysplastic category), and frank lymphomas. Lymphoid lesions of the conjunctiva, where the fornices normally host lymphocytes, tend to be benign both histologically and clinically, 90% being localized and not associated with systemic disease. Lymphoid lesions of the orbit, where there are no lymphatics or lymph nodes, are very abnormal, 50% being associated with systemic disease.

Reactive lymphoid hyperplasia is benign, giving an indolent, painless, rubbery, nodular, usually anterior, orbital infiltration, sometimes with a fleshy subconjunctival mass. There may be associated lesions in the salivary gland, GI tract, or respiratory tract. Malignant transformation is possible. If localized, it should be treated with oral prednisone. If unresponsive, give local irradiation, 2000 cGy. If multifocal, chemotherapy should be considered.

Atypical lymphoid hyperplasia (dysplastic category) behaves like low-grade lymphomas, may be chronic, is often bilateral or disseminated, is often resistant to corticosteroids, and may undergo malignant transformation.

Frankly malignant, non-Hodgkin's lymphomas, the most common orbital lymphoproliferative disorders, are rare in children, usually presenting in the sixth or seventh decade as a unilateral (75%), smooth, nontender, anterior mass that molds to the globe, often having a salmon-pink subconjunctival mass. CT scan shows a well-defined, usually extraconal, anterior, superior, and lateral mass, often involving the lacrimal gland, and seldom showing bony involvement or globe distortion. Of the two thirds presenting as localized disease, all are monoclonal B cell lymphomas. Of these, 85% remain localized. Poorly differentiated lesions have extraorbital disease in half. All must be followed carefully for the rest of the patient's life; late development of systemic disease is always possible. Other systemic disorders are common, include chronic lymphocytic leukemia, Sjögren's syndrome, Waldenström's macroglobulinemia, collagen vascular diseases, and other neoplasms. They should be treated with biopsy, careful pathologic study, systemic oncologic review, staging, and orbital radiotherapy and/or systemic chemotherapy.

Orbital plasma cell tumors. Orbital plasma cell tumors present with: (1) most commonly, a bony tumor, either a solitary plasmacytoma or a local lesion of multiple myeloma, (2) a solitary soft tissue plasmacytoma or reactive plasmacytic granuloma, or (3) a fulminant orbital infiltration from multiple myeloma or concurrent infection. Most orbital plasma cell tumors have systemic involvement.

Solitary plasmacytomas may be polyclonal or monoclonal. The polyclonal tumors usually present subconjunctivally as indolent, well-circumscribed masses. They should be biopsied, characterized as polyclonal or monoclonal, staged, debulked, and irradiated. Solitary monoclonal plasmacytomas occur extremely rarely in the orbit, are most frequently seen in the sixth and seventh decades, and have a male:female ratio of 3:1. They should be biopsied, staged, and irradiated (4000 to 5000 cGy). Orbital involvement in multiple myeloma is rare, but when it occurs, it is often the initial finding. It gives an orbital mass, usually in a man in his seventh or eighth decade with bone pain, fatigue, recurrent infection, pathologic fractures, anemia, hyperglobulinemia, Bence Jones proteinuria, and an abnormal serum immunoelectrophoresis. Conjunctiva shows a discrete mass, diffuse thickening, or conjunctivitis. CT scan shows a mass eroding bone and expanding into the orbit. It should be treated with biopsy (note risk of renal failure from intravenous contrast and dehydration during anesthesia), staging, systemic chemotherapy, and local radiation. IgG and IgA myelomas have a better prognosis than IgD and light-chain disease.

Other lymphoproliferative and leukemic lesions. Other lymphoproliferative and leukemic lesions include Burkitt's lymphoma, granulocytic sarcoma (chloroma) and leukemia, Hodgkin's disease, and T-cell lymphomas.

Undifferentiated lymphoma, Burkitt's type, endemic in Central Africa, occurs worldwide. The Epstein-Barr virus and chronic exposure to malaria are suspected etiologic factors. The African type gives a solitary, fulminant facial mass in a boy (median age, 7 years; male:female ratio, 2:1). The non-African type more commonly presents in an older child (median age, 11 years) with an abdominal mass. They should be treated with biopsy, staging, chemotherapy, and radiotherapy. Younger children and localized disease have a better prognosis.

Granulocytic sarcoma (chloroma) is a localized, usually extramedullary, form of acute myeloblastic leukemia or of chronic granulocytic leukemia entering blast crisis, which occurs in 3% of patients with myeloid leukemia. Unlike true lymphoma, chloroma has a predilection for the orbit in children, presenting as a rapidly growing soft tissue or bony mass, usually in the non-Caucasian boy (median age 7 years; male:female ratio, 3:2). It should be treated with local irradiation and systemic chemotherapy. Prognosis is poor.

After rhabdomyosarcoma, leukemia is the most common malignancy causing unilateral proptosis in children. It is usually a late, sudden manifestation of acute, especially lymphoblastic, leukemia and is secondary to soft tissue infiltration or hematoma; it carries a grave prognosis, despite radiation and chemotherapy.

Orbital Hodgkin's disease occurs extremely rarely, usually occurring in the disease's terminal stages. It should be treated with local irradiation.

T-cell lymphomas include mycosis fungoides, Sézary syndrome, lymphoma cutis, and adult T-cell leukemia. Mycosis fungoides has three progressive stages: *erythematous,* with a superficial, eczematous, psoriasiform lesion; *plaque;* and *tumor,* with ulcerating tumors involving the eyelid, conjunctiva, and orbit. Usually secondary to spread from adjacent skin, orbital and ocular diseases include lid, conjunctival, and caruncular lesions; keratitis; uveitis, and optic nerve lesions.

Histiocytoses (Langerhans cell granulomas). Histiocytoses include histiocytosis X and malignant histiocytosis. Histiocytosis X includes Letterer-Siwe disease, a fulminant systemic disorder occurring before 3 years; Hand-Schüller-Christian disease, most commonly involving the lungs and several bones of children and rarely giving the triad of bone defects, exophthalmos, and diabetes insipidus; and eosinophilic granuloma, occurring most commonly between ages 20 and 40, usually with localized bone involvement, but occasionally with lung infiltration only. There are ophthalmologic manifestations in about 10% of cases, with a male:female ratio of 2:1. When localized it presents as an indolent, progressive bony orbital mass. Eosinophilic granuloma may affect the superolateral orbit with focal, bony lysis, and soft tissue expansion. Hand-Schüller-Christian disease with multifocal bone involvement may produce fibrosis, with sclerosis and failure of bony development, with a shallow orbit and flattened forehead. There may be a pruritic, eczematous, yellow-red infiltration of the scalp skin. Malignant histiocytosis is a fulminant neoplastic disorder affecting all age groups. It may give skin, conjunctival, and orbital soft tissue infiltrates. Stage and treat with local radiotherapy and local and systemic steroids. Prognosis in multifocal cases in young children is poor.

Secondary Orbital Tumors. Secondary orbital tumors constitute one third of orbital neoplasias and spread from nasopharynx and paranasal sinuses, skin and conjunctiva, bones, intracranial tissues, eye, and lacrimal sac (Table 174-16). Metastases commonly present with painless, axial

Table 174-16. Secondary Orbital Tumors

Tumor	Symptoms	Signs	Treatment
Nasopharyngeal and paranasal sinus tumors (70% from maxillary sinus; 60% squamous cell carcinomas; others: Schneiderian papillomas, adenoid cystic carcinomas)	40-60 yr, male : female, 2 : 1; maxillary lesions: infraorbital nerve pain or paresthesia, facial swelling, trismus, toothache, tearing; ethmoid lesions: inferolateral proptosis	Maxillary lesions: superior proptosis, lower lid fullness; CT: solid mass, with sinus epicenter, bone destruction	Radical surgery and radiotherapy Prognosis poor
Eyelid malignancies (see Disorders of the Eyelids)			
Basal cell carcinoma	If neglected, a recurrence, morpheaform or sclerosing variants, a medial canthal location where undertreatment attempts to avoid lacrimal drainage damage	Grows along medial orbital wall, into ethmoid sinus and posterior orbit, fixing the eye	Cure: extirpation Palliation: radiation or ? cisplatin
Squamous cell carcinoma	Pain, ulcerating lid, diplopia; more aggressive, spreads along nerves and tissue planes, metastasizes to preauricular and submandibular lymph nodes	Skin lesion, orbital mass	Cure: extirpation Palliation: radiation
Sebaceous adenocarcinoma (one third of epithelial lesions invading orbit)	Old age, chronic recurrent chalazion or unilateral blepharoconjunctivitis; metastases most often local and then cervical nodes; hematogenous to lung, liver, brain, skull	May mimic chalazion, conjunctivitis, basal cell carcinoma	Cure: early recognition, extirpation, and lymph node dissection Palliation: radiotherapy
Conjunctival tumors			
Squamous cell carcinoma (chronic sun exposure)	Male > female; 50-70 yr; conjunctivitis and limbal leukoplakia or gelatinous, telangiectatic epibulbar masses	Invade orbit if neglected or extensive	Conjunctival: histologically controlled cryotherapy or resection Orbital extension: exenteration Nodal metastases: with radical dissection Radiation: palliative
Malignant melanoma	Middle age, from primary acquired melanosis (50%), preexisting nevus (25%), de novo (25%)	Change in (usually) pigmented conjunctival lesion	Repeated cryotherapy, radiotherapy, or extirpation with lymph node dissection if indicated Prognosis variable
Bony tumors (see Primary Mesenchymal Tumors)			
Intracranial tumors*			
Ocular tumors			
Retinoblastoma (most common intraocular malignancy in childhood)	Child: birth to 7 years; ? family history; white "cat's eye" pupil, "crossed eyes," red eye	Leukocoria, strabismus; ocular inflammation, hyphema, glaucoma; intraocular tumor	Chemotherapy and radiation Mortality is 67% to 91% with orbital extension
Uveal melanoma	Caucasian, adult; decreased vision, sore eye	Intraocular tumor	Palliation 80% mortality with orbital extension
Ciliary body medulloepitheliomas and carcinomas	Children: mean 5 yr; poor vision, pain, white "cat's eye" pupil	Leukocoria, ciliary body mass	Poor prognosis with orbital extension
Lacrimal sac tumors (25% inflammatory; 75% neoplasms [75% malignant, usually carcinomas])	Tearing, bloody tears, pain, mass at medial canthus, dacryocystitis	Mass above the medial canthal tendon	Treatment depends on behavior and histology

*Meningiomas most common. See Table 174-15.

Box 174-2. Metastatic Orbital Tumors

In Children*

Neuroblastoma: 90% <5 yr, second most common malignant orbital tumor in early childhood; 40% bilateral proptosis; "raccoon eye" lid ecchymoses; abdominal or thoracic mass; prognosis guarded

Nephroblastoma: Wilms' tumor, most <5 yr, smooth flank or abdominal mass; prognosis guarded

Ewing's sarcoma: 10-20 yr; pain or swelling at long bone or soft tissue primary site; prognosis guarded

In Adults†‡

Breast carcinoma: most common orbital (33%) metastasis; up to 30% present with orbital disease; 40-50 yr; gives proptosis or enophthalmos; CT- > mass in muscle; poor prognosis

Lung carcinoma: men, 30-70 yr; rapidly growing orbital mass; palliate

Prostate carcinoma: men >80 yr; involves soft tissue or bone (osteosclerosis) and high serum acid phosphatase

Gastrointestinal carcinoma: male > female; peak, sixth decade; primary usually scirrhous stomach carcinoma or colonic adenocarcinoma; may give enophthalmos or hyperostosis

Renal cell carcinoma: male > female; 40-60 yr; aggressive orbital mass, often with an occult primary; may pulsate

Thyroid carcinoma: female > male; peak 50-60 yr, more common in women in the sixth decade

Skin melanoma: commonly gives orbital metastasis; CT- > smooth extraocular muscle enlargement

*Usually embryonal sarcomas.
†Usually postembryonal carcinomas.
‡Incisional or fine-needle aspiration biopsy.

proptosis, whereas secondary tumors give nonaxial proptosis; infiltration with pain, paresthesia, decreased vision, chemosis, injection, and reduced eye movements; nasal obstruction, chronic sinusitis, or epistaxis; and tearing.

Metastatic Orbital Tumors. Tumors metastatic to the orbit (1/10 eyeball metastases) are blood-borne; in children they are most often embryonal sarcomas from the adrenals, bone, brain, or kidney, whereas in adults they are postembryonal carcinomas from breast, lung, adrenal gland, prostate, GI tract, kidney, thyroid, skin, or bone. Unrestricted growth in the vascular target tissues (choroid, extraocular muscles, lacrimal gland, and bone) produces unilateral or bilateral progressive vision loss, strabismus, diplopia, ptosis, dull pain, paresthesia, proptosis, palpable masses, and sometimes enophthalmos (scirrhous breast carcinoma, lung, and GI carcinoma), periorbital hemorrhage (neuroblastoma), or pulsation (from vascular renal cell or thyroid carcinoma, or transmission of brain pulsations after orbital wall destruction). As cancer patients live longer, metastases are increasing, and are now 2% to 10% of orbital tumors. They are the presenting problem in 20% to 30% of patients with primaries elsewhere. Most from solid tumors occur in patients between 40 and 80 years. They are more common in women because of the frequency of metastatic breast carcinoma. In men, primaries are in lung, GI tract, and kidney, and in old age, prostate. Skin melanoma and breast carcinoma frequently metastasize to extraocular muscles, and prostatic carcinoma to bone. Seminoma can cause a nonmetastatic reversible proptosis. CT scan shows extraocular muscles that are knobby, focally swollen, or have excrescences; a circumscribed mass; or an infiltrating mass, often with bone destruction. The physician should diagnose (consider fine-needle aspiration) and palliate.

Specific Metastases. See Box 174-2.

Orbital Operations

At operation, the orbit may be approached from anteriorly, laterally, or superiorly, or some combination of these (Table 174-17).

DISORDERS OF THE ANOPHTHALMIC SOCKET

When an eye is absent from birth or is removed because it contains a tumor, or is blind and painful, the goal of socket rehabilitation is symmetry with the remaining eye, matching shape, color, and movement. Close cooperation between the ophthalmologist and the ocularist who crafts the artificial eye gives the best results.

In congenital anophthalmos the socket and eyelids are often small, leaving no place to fit an artificial eye. The socket can usually be expanded with progressively larger conformers until an eye can be fit. Enlarging the lids may be impossible.

A person who loses an eye requires practical advice and psychologic support. Techniques for coping with the loss of visual field and of binocular depth perception must be learned. Socket rehabilitation requires several steps.

First, the orbital volume deficit following enucleation is corrected by placement of a buried ocular implant. Once healing has occurred, a custom-molded and painted plastic prosthetic eye (artificial eye) is fashioned by an ocularist. This sits in the conjunctival sac like a large contact lens. The extraocular muscles are left after both evisceration and enucleation. The movement of these muscles must be transmitted to the intraorbital ocular implant, and then to the overlying artificial eye. The muscles are attached to the intraorbital ocular implant, either by being passed through holes in it or by being sewn to it. Achieving good movement of the ocular implant has been largely successful. However,

Table 174-17. Orbital and Socket Operations

Procedure	Indications	Technique
Anterior orbitotomy		
Transconjunctival	Optic nerve sheath fenestration; limited exposure to anterior lesions	Through the conjunctival fornices or bulbar conjunctiva
Transseptal	Lacrimal gland and anterior lesion biopsy	Through the skin, orbicularis, and orbital septum, usually in the upper lid
Extraperiosteal	More posterior dissection before exposing orbital fat that obscures the field	Through the skin down to the orbital rim, through periosteum, then posteriorly between periosteum and bone
Lateral orbitotomy		
Kronlein	More posterior tumors, benign mixed cell tumors of lacrimal gland	Through skin and muscle with removal of lateral orbital wall
Transcranial Orbitotomy	Apical tumors or those with intracranial involvement	Through frontal cranial flap, and roof of orbit
Orbital Decompression	Graves' disease with optic nerve compression or marked proptosis	Removal of the medial, lateral, and inferior orbital walls
Evisceration	Blind, painful eye; unsalvageable eye after injury	Removal of the contents of the globe, leaving the sclera attached to the muscles
Enucleation	Blind, painful eye; unsalvageable eye after injury, intralocular malignancy	Removal of the whole eye, including its coats; usually an intraorbital spherical or other shaped implant is placed
Exenteration	Malignancy spread to eye and orbital tissues	Removal of all of the orbital contents leaving only a bony socket, spectacle mounted prosthesis may be fit

transmitting that movement to the artificial eye in the conjunctival sac has been a continuing problem. Since 1941, various forms of mechanical and magnetic coupling of the implant and artificial eye have been tried, and abandoned, usually because of implant extrusion. The newest technique being evaluated involves placement of an implant made of porous hydroxyapatite (from sea coral), waiting for vascularization, then drilling a well in the implant, and inserting a plastic peg that fits into a depression on the back of the artificial eye.

The patient should know how to remove and insert his or her artificial eye, but, ordinarily, should remove it only if the socket is irritated and the prosthesis needs cleaning. The patient's physician should remove the prosthesis and examine the socket when indicated and as part of every complete examination. The prosthesis should have an annual cleaning and polishing by the ocularist. Consider a new prosthesis every 7 or 8 years. Manipulating the socket causes irritation and increased mucus discharge. The artificial eye should not be left out, especially if the socket is inflamed, because the socket can quickly contract and the prosthesis cannot be replaced. Reconstruction of a contracted socket with such techniques as oral mucous membrane or dermis-fat grafting can be difficult or impossible. With time, the weight of the artificial eye may stretch the supporting lower eyelid. The lower lid, eye, and upper lid all sag as a unit, giving blepharoptosis and a deep upper lid sulcus, with loss of symmetry. Correction requires some combination of remaking the artificial eye, tightening the lower lid, correcting the upper lid ptosis, and adding orbital volume.

After orbital exenteration, a prosthetician can fashion a remarkably lifelike, spectacle-mounted or bone-fixed replacement for the eye, lids, and brow.

ADDITIONAL READINGS

Albert DM, Jakobiec FA, editors: *Principles and practice of ophthalmology* Philadelphia, 1994, WB Saunders.

Collin JRO: *A manual of systematic eyelid surgery,* ed 2, Edinburgh, 1989, Churchill-Livingstone.

Duke-Elder S, MacFaul PA: The ocular adnexa, volume XIII. In Duke-Elder S, editor: *System of ophthalmology,* London, 1974, Kimpton.

Duke-Elder S, MacFaul PA: Injuries, volume XIV. In Duke-Elder S, editor. *System of ophthalmology,* London, 1972, Kimpton.

Hart WM, editor: *Adler's physiology of the eye,* ed 9, St Louis, 1992, Mosby.

Henderson JW: *Orbital tumors,* ed 3, New York, 1994, Raven Press.

McCord CD, Tanenbaum M, Nunery WR, editors: *Oculoplastic surgery,* ed 3, New York, 1995, Raven Press.

Miller NR, Newman NJ, editors: *Walsh and Hoyt's clinical neuro-ophthalmology,* ed 5, Baltimore, 1998, Williams and Wilkins.

Rootman J: Frequency and differential diagnosis of orbital disease. In: *Diseases of the orbit,* Philadelphia, 1988, JB Lippincott.

Whitnall SE: *Anatomy of the human orbit and accessory organs of vision,* facsimile of 1921 edition, Robert E. Krieger, New York, 1979, Huntington.

Yanoff M, Fine BS: *Ocular pathology,* ed 4, London, 1996, Mosby-Wolfe.

CHAPTER 175

Diseases of the Cornea

Thomas J. Byrd

Although only 12 mm across and less than 1 mm thick, the cornea is optically transparent and has no blood supply, but it is far more complex than a simple "watch crystal" crowning the globe.

ANATOMY

The cornea is composed of five layers: epithelium, Bowman's layer, stroma, Descemet's membrane, and endothelium. The *epithelium* is five or six cell layers thick and richly supplied with free nerve endings only, since specialized receptors would compromise corneal clarity. *Bowman's layer* is a collagenous layer 8 to 10 μg thick to which the basal epithelial cells adhere via hemidesmosomes. The *stroma* constitutes about 90% of the total corneal thickness. It consists almost entirely of an extracellular matrix of collagen (and other glycoproteins), interspersed with fibroblasts and keratocytes. The regularity and organization of the collagen fibril orientation are responsible for corneal clarity. The cornea becomes cloudy when edema or new collagen synthesis alters the spacing of these fibrils. The *endothelium* is a monolayer of hexagonal cells rich in cytoplasmic organelles, especially mitochondria. These cells actively pump fluid across an osmotic gradient from the corneal stroma to the aqueous cavity and thus are responsible primarily for maintenance of corneal clarity. These cells do not replicate and therefore steadily decrease in number with advancing age or disease.

Cellular mediators of infection must migrate in from adjacent limbal vessels unless the cornea has been vascularized by an earlier process. Corneal physiology is best summarized by the renowned corneal specialist Dr. Herbert E. Kaufman: "The cornea breathes air and eats aqueous."

DIAGNOSTIC APPROACH

As with all ocular disease, a thorough history and eye examination are the keys to accurate diagnosis of corneal disease (see Chapter 172). The physician should document the presence of protective eyewear, contact lens type and wearing schedule, photophobia, decreased vision, or type of foreign body. Unilaterality, bilaterality, and time course may be important. Lids matted shut in the morning suggests conjunctivitis. Autoimmune disease can cause lacrimal insufficiency. Severe pain on opening the eyes in the morning is diagnostic of recurrent erosion.

Visual acuity with optical correction must be measured, noting any improvement from looking through a pinhole. A pinhole compensates for uncorrected refractive errors and can limit visual degradation due to diffraction from corneal (or lens) opacities or irregularities. Improved acuity through a pinhole therefore suggests the cornea or lens as the etiology for visual disturbance. Intraocular, inflammatory, hemorrhagic, retinal, optic nerve, or cortical causes of decreased acuity are not correctable with a pinhole.

Conjunctival injection helps to define the process as either inflammatory or noninflammatory. The lids should be evaluated for signs of inflammation and the lash bases examined for dried scales, which may indicate staphylococcal infection. Fingertip pressure at the lid margin should elicit clear, oily, meibomian gland secretions, not white strands that resemble toothpaste.

Although gross corneal foreign bodies or opacities may be visible with a penlight, a slit lamp is essential for any detailed examination of the cornea. The optical cross section combined with high magnification allows comprehensive assessment of the multiple layers of the cornea. Contour irregularities, stromal thinning, and epithelial hypertrophy are readily detected. Fluorescein dye highlights areas where the epithelium is disrupted or missing. Useful information can be difficult to obtain, however, if too much dye is applied. Decreased corneal sensation can be measured using a wisp of cotton if herpes simplex virus is suspected. Corneal disorders can be categorized first based on whether they generally cause a red eye (Fig. 175-1).

THE RED EYE

Anterior Blepharitis

Bacteria (overwhelmingly *Staphylococcus*) colonize the lash bases, form a crusty scale where lash meets skin, secrete toxins into the tear film, and can cause a red eye and possible corneal infiltrates. Blepharitis is usually bilateral, with the chief complaint of itching of lid margins, which may be injected. Lash whitening (poliosis) or loss (madarosis) can occur. Foam often forms on the lid margins as the toxins saponify the tear lipids, and conjunctival injection is common. When a sebaceous gland at the base of a lash becomes acutely infected and forms a painful localized purulent abscess, it is known as a *hordeolum* or *stye*.

Initial treatment is simple hygiene twice daily. A 5-minute hot washcloth soak softens the scales. The area is then cleansed by scrubbing the lash bases with a cotton ball soaked in a 50:50 mixture of baby shampoo and water, followed by rinsing and patting dry. For initial treatment, local or systemic antibiotics usually are not warranted, although severe styes may require incision and drainage. If significant debris persists for 2 months, erythromycin ointment is applied to the lash bases at the end of treatment. This chronic problem usually requires chronic treatment.

Allergic Blepharitis

The predominant symptom of ocular allergy is itching, often accompanied by lid edema, mucoid discharge, conjunctival hyperemia, burning, lacrimation, and conjunctival edema (chemosis). Eosinophils are seen on Giemsa staining of conjunctival scrapings, except in mild cases. Brief episodes of these symptoms with nasal involvement are often seen in hay fever conjunctivitis after exposure to airborne allergens. Acute treatment consists of cool compresses, topical vasoconstrictor-antihistamine combinations, or topical nonsteroidal antiinflammatory drugs (NSAIDs). Prophylactic treatment may include topical mast-cell stabilizing agents such as cromolyn sodium or lodoxamide tromethamine. Topical steroids may be indicated in severe cases.

Vernal conjunctivitis causes severe itching, photophobia, and a heavy, ropy mucous discharge. Symptoms begin in the first two decades of life, are bilateral, and typically recur in

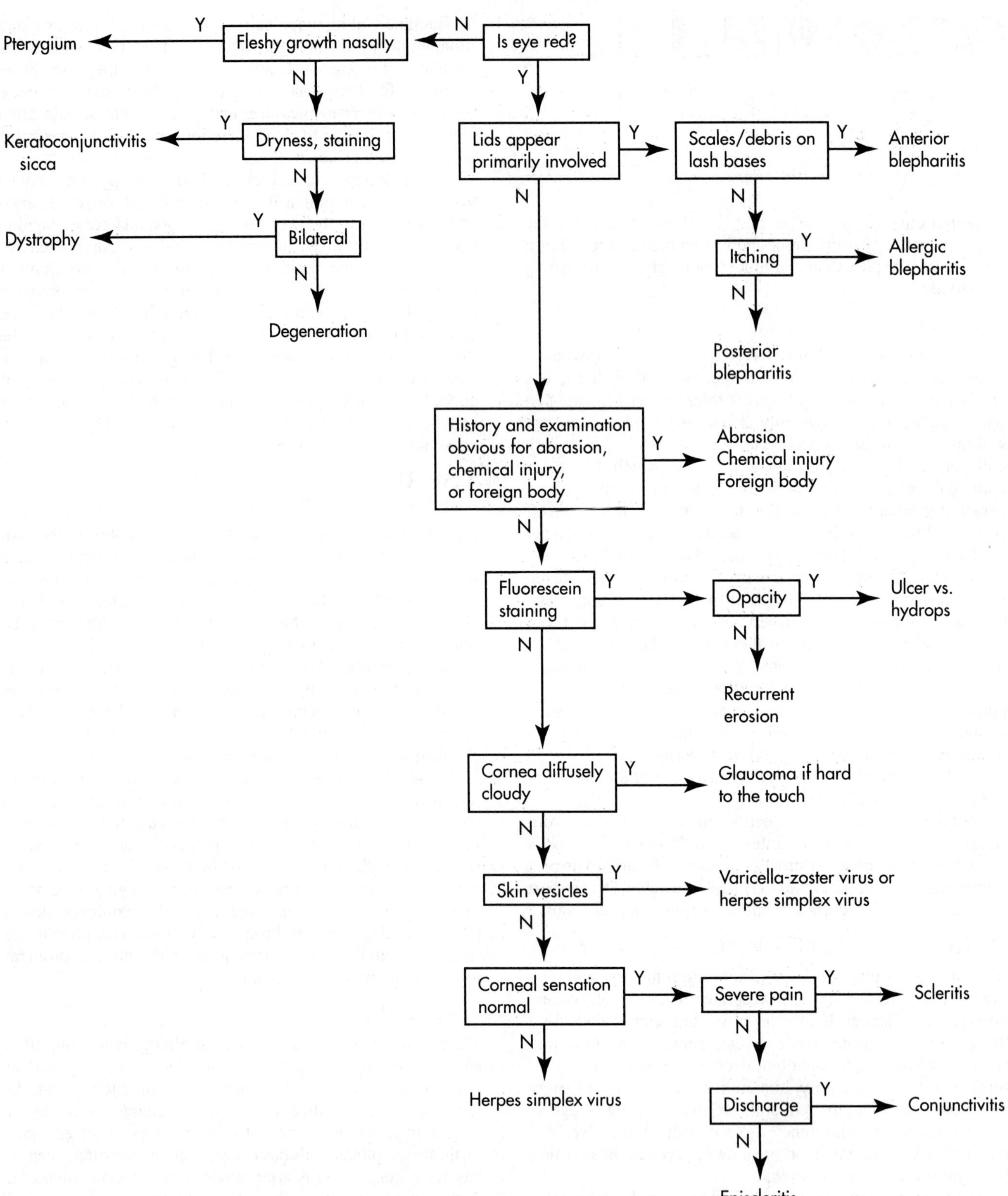

Fig. 175-1. Approach to the patient with corneal disorders. *Y*, Yes; *N*, no.

the spring months in nontropical climates. About 90% of patients have a history of atopy. Giant cobblestone papillae are characteristically found on the superior tarsal conjunctiva and cause corneal complications in severe cases. Environmental control of allergens is the best initial treatment, followed by therapy for hay fever conjunctivitis. Treatment seldom eradicates symptoms altogether, and the physician must be cautious to avoid steroid-induced ocular complications in this generally self-limited disease.

The incidence of ocular involvement in atopic dermatitis is

approximately 25%. *Atopic keratoconjunctivitis* causes a moist, erythematous skin eruption that becomes vesicular and then crusts. The lid skin ultimately becomes scaly and excessively wrinkled. Although sometimes difficult to differentiate from vernal conjunctivitis, atopic symptoms are perennial, the tarsal conjunctival papillae are smaller, and corneal involvement tends to be more severe. Treatment is similar to that of vernal conjunctivitis, with the same caution to avoid chronic steroid use.

The delicate and distensible lid tissues are particularly susceptible to irritants, including environmental allergens, cosmetics, topical medications, and some chemicals. Eczematoid inflammation of the lids is characteristic of *contact dermatitis*. Topical steroid ointment is used to treat the acute inflammation, while elimination of the offending agent is the definitive treatment.

Posterior Blepharitis

Meibomian glands are responsible for secreting the oily layer of the tear film. When they become inspissated and plugged, an acute chalazion may develop if the lipid is extruded into the surrounding tissues. In most cases the secretions are merely thick and of poor quality, causing tear film instability and ocular irritation symptoms.

Initial treatment is simple hygiene twice daily. A 10-minute hot soak is needed to heat the meibomian glands sufficiently to thin the secretions. Vigorous fingertip compression of the eyelid against the globe then forces the fluids to flow and avoid stagnation. If symptoms are not relieved after 2 months of this hygiene regimen, oral tetracycline is added for its effect on lipid metabolism, not for its antibiotic effect; 250 mg is given four times daily for a month, then once daily. The thinner secretions then cause fewer symptoms.

Conjunctivitis

Conjunctival injection is a nonspecific indicator of inflammation. Follicles are small white bumps in the conjunctiva that represent collections of lymphocytes that have displaced adjacent blood vessels. They suggest a viral or chlamydial cause of conjunctivitis. Papillae are velvety red conjunctival bumps with a central vessel that are nonspecific indicators of conjunctival inflammation. Papillary conjunctivitis is more likely bacterial in origin. Examination also should note the presence of preauricular adenopathy. Because the lower conjunctiva drains there, the presence of tender preauricular nodes suggests adenoviral conjunctivitis.

Conjunctivitis is approximately 50% bacterial and 50% adenoviral in children. The bacterial cases tend to have a more mucopurulent discharge, less adenopathy, and no other viral symptoms. The three most common agents are *Staphylococcus aureus, Streptococcus pneumoniae,* and *Haemophilus influenzae,* with the latter most often affecting young children. Because adenoviral conjunctivitis is self-limiting and topical antibiotics are safe, virtually all cases of pediatric conjunctivitis are treated as bacterial. Either sulfacetamide 10% or trimethoprim–polymyxin B (better *H. influenzae* coverage) is given four times a day for a week to 10 days. Patients may worsen for 1 or 2 days before they improve. The infection may spread to the other eye. Family members should use separate washcloths to avoid transmission, and frequent handwashing is advised. Infected children should not attend school, and adults who deal with the public should not attend work. Hot or cool compresses may provide symptomatic relief. Conjunctivitis in adults is approximately 85% adenoviral and 15% bacterial, so routine antibiotic treatment of all patients is unnecessary. Antibiotics are used for patients with a more purulent discharge, no nodes, and no follicles, since the latter two suggest a viral etiology. Any conjunctivitis that does not improve in 7 to 10 days merits ophthalmologic evaluation.

Episcleritis

Ocular redness without irritation is characteristic of episcleritis. Transient and self-limited, it affects adults and lasts approximately 1 to 3 weeks, with spontaneous resolution. Episcleritis is generally not related to systemic immunologic disease. The redness is often in the interpalpebral zone, with inflammation of the straight episcleral vessels perpendicular to the limbus. Unlike the vascular injection of scleritis, these vessels are salmon pink in sunlight, can be moved over the underlying sclera with a cotton-tipped applicator, and blanch with topical phenylephrine 10% solution.

Simple episcleritis usually requires no treatment, although the nodular form is more severe, lasts longer, and requires topical steroids. The redness of simple episcleritis may be treated with topical vasoconstrictors. When present, pain may be relieved with topical NSAIDs or mild topical steroids.

Scleritis

Scleritis is much more serious than episcleritis and is usually associated with a systemic immunologic disease (see Chapter 172). Patients complain of severe, deep pain, and the eye is often tender to palpation. Examination in sunlight reveals a blue or violet hue to the affected sclera. The vessels are not straight and radial, cannot be moved with a cotton-tipped applicator, and do not blanch with topical phenylephrine 10% solution. The patient may have significant visual morbidity.

Scleritis is divided anatomically into anterior and posterior forms. Anterior scleritis is further divided into three clinical subtypes: diffuse, nodular, and necrotizing. *Diffuse anterior scleritis* is the most benign form of the disease. The vascular injection is nonfocal without nodularity or avascularity. It is associated with connective tissue disease in approximately 30% of cases. Heavy topical steroids are often sufficient to control the inflammation. As in all scleritis, subconjunctival steroid injection is contraindicated because of the propensity for the sclera to melt at the injection site. *Nodular anterior scleritis* consists of single or multiple, deep-red or purple nodules of immobile scleral tissue with overlaying edematous episclera. Half the patients have an autoimmune disorder. *Necrotizing anterior scleritis* can result in vision and life-threatening complications. The lesion is usually inflammatory with a pale center, but scleral necrosis without inflammation (scleromalacia perforans) can also occur, usually in patients with longstanding rheumatoid arthritis. In most cases, symptoms of severe, boring pain are out of proportion to inflammatory signs. The sclera thins, and the dark underlying uveal tissue becomes visible as the disease progresses. About 60% of necrotizing scleritis patients develop bilateral disease, and approximately 30% die within 5 years of diagnosis, usually from complications of vasculitis.

Only 10% of patients with *posterior scleritis* have had an associated systemic disease. The diagnosis can be easily missed in the absence of anterior inflammation, especially if the pain is referred elsewhere in the head. Pain, proptosis, and visual loss are common complaints. Visual consequences may ensue from exudative retinal detachment and optic disc edema.

Topical steroids are seldom sufficient to control more severe scleritis. Systemic NSAIDs often can control the inflammation in diffuse or nodular scleritis. Control of the pain is a useful guide to therapy. Oral corticosteroids are used in severe or necrotizing cases, with the addition of systemic cytotoxic immunosuppressive therapy as needed (e.g., cyclophosphamide, azathioprine, methotrexate). Patients with systemic autoimmune disease often receive prednisone for its rapid effect while waiting a week or more for immunosuppressant therapy to become effective.

Chemical Injury

Chemical injury is one of only two true ophthalmic emergencies, the other being central retinal artery occlusion. Minutes or even seconds of delay in treatment can result in irreparable tissue damage and loss of vision. Chemical injury is the only condition when treatment may be initiated before assessing visual acuity.

The first priority is immediate and copious irrigation with any noncaustic liquid. Although sterile irrigating solution or saline is preferable once the patient arrives at the office, tap water is usually most practical at the time of injury. Fifteen minutes of continuous irrigation at home or a liter of fluid irrigation in a medical setting is recommended, with the emphasis on rapid dilution of the offending agent. Topical anesthetic drops and a lid speculum make irrigation more comfortable and effective. Tears should be tested with pH paper a few minutes later. If not within the 7.2 to 7.8 range, another liter of irrigation should be administered after inspection of the everted lids to detect retained particulate matter.

A good history with an exact description of the agent should be obtained after irrigation. The container that identifies the chemical is helpful. Documentation of protective eyewear is important, particularly for work-related accidents. Alkali burns are generally worse than acid, although either can be blinding. Acid is precipitated and inactivated by the tissue proteins it destroys, whereas alkali saponifies collagen and damages underlying tissue. Hydrocarbons can be quite irritating but usually cause much less tissue damage. The epithelium should be assessed with fluorescein stain, realizing that "all off" is easily confused with "all on" when no clear demarcation line is present. Prophylactic topical antibiotics are used three or four times a day, and some physicians omit a patch for the first 24 hours to permit additional clearing of any retained chemical.

Steroid-antibiotic combinations are often used to help decrease inflammation. "Clean" chemical injuries and bilateral ocular allergies are two of the very few indications for topical ocular steroid use by the nonophthalmologist. Aminoglycoside antibiotics impair epithelial healing and should be avoided. Oral analgesia and sedatives enhance patient comfort, whereas topical nonsteroidals such as ketorolac provide effective pain control in an unpatched eye when used four times a day for up to 4 days. When present, epithelial defects must be healed, and daily examinations to rule out infection and monitor progress are mandatory. Healing is slower than with a comparable abrasion for the first 1 or 2 days because the remaining epithelium has also been chemically damaged. The physician should apply ointment and patch an epithelial defect daily. Having the patient remove and reapply the patch at home is not effective, so patients should not apply topical medications when patching. Steroid-antibiotic drops to reduce inflammation are continued for approximately a week after epithelialization is complete.

Severe chemical burns, large epithelial defects, any suspicion of infection or tissue thinning, slow healing, and the development of conjunctival adhesions are indications for immediate referral to an ophthalmologist. Ultimate prognosis is related to the degree of limbal ischemia as well as symblepharon (conjunctival adhesion) formation.

Foreign Body

After a thorough history, including use of protective eyewear, visual acuity is assessed in the patient with a foreign body before other examination or placement of eyedrops. Proparacaine drops are then used to facilitate further examination. Both upper lids should always be everted to look for additional foreign bodies, and their absence should be documented to prevent patching over a retained foreign body. Multiple vertical, linear, superficial abrasions indicate a foreign body trapped under the upper lid. Eversion is simple and painless when performed properly with consideration of the tarsal plate, which makes the inferior 10 mm of the upper lid rigid and unfoldable. The patient is asked to look down, and the upper lashes are grasped with the fingers. A cotton-tipped applicator (or any small, blunt instrument) is then placed 10 to 12 mm superior to the lash margin, and the lid is everted using the applicator as a fulcrum. When the examination is completed, the lid will right itself if the patient is asked to look up and blink.

Although using a slit lamp is preferable, a hand light may be used to look for a corneal foreign body. If not readily visible, a small particle can sometimes be detected by observing its shadow cast on the iris. Vigorous irrigation or a moistened cotton-tipped applicator are the only methods that should be used to remove a superficial foreign body without the assistance of a slit lamp. Many ophthalmologists routinely dilate such patients with a mid-acting mydriatic such as homatropine 5% or scopolamine 0.25% to prevent pain from iritis. The presence of "consensual photophobia" (pain in the injured eye when a light is shone only in the opposite eye) is a good indication for dilation.

With daily follow-up and patching, healing should be steady and rapid over 1 or 2 days. No steroids are used. Inability to remove the particle, the presence of a rust ring or infiltrate, worsening vision, and failure to heal are indications for immediate ophthalmologic evaluation.

Corneal Abrasion

The examination of a corneal abrasion begins with a thorough history, including protective eyewear. Visual acuity measurement is followed by proparacaine drops to ease the examination. The lid is everted to detect a foreign body. A small quantity of fluorescein outlines the defect, and charting a diagram with a size estimate simplifies follow-up. The general principles of monitoring and facilitating epithelial healing are identical to those used for chemical injuries, with daily patching and follow-up with or without cycloplegia. Antibiotic ointment without steroid use is appropriate for these presumably contaminated wounds. The presence of an infiltrate, worsening vision, and failure to heal are indications for immediate ophthalmologic referral. Nonhealing epithelial defects are one of the most frustrating ophthalmologic maladies. Treatment options restricted to ophthalmologists and corneal subspecialists include bandage soft contact lenses, placement of collagen shields, mechanical or excimer laser debridement, anterior stromal micropuncture, tarsorrhaphy, and placement of a conjunctival flap.

Recurrent Corneal Erosion

A good history is the key to diagnosis and treatment of recurrent corneal erosions. Patients present with symptoms (and often signs) of a corneal abrasion but without acute trauma. Patients almost always report being asymptomatic when going to bed and awakening with severe pain as the eye is first opened. Symptoms subside gradually over several hours, but recur another morning several days or weeks later. The pathophysiology is based on a defect of epithelial adhesion. Patients often have a history of prior traumatic abrasion, classically a paper cut or fingernail injury. The injury causes defects in Bowman's layer. During the 6 to 8 weeks required for re-formation of hemidesmosomal complexes, the epithelium is often separated from the underlying Bowman's layer by a thin fluid layer. This separation occurs at night, when evaporative loss is diminished by closed lids. The epithelium then sticks to the inside of the upper lid and is torn off when the eyes open in the morning. Treatment therefore must focus on eliminating the fluid layer, so that hemidesmosomes may form, and preventing adhesion between the epithelium and lid.

Clinically, this corneal erosion often appears identical to a corneal abrasion on hand light examination. The edges often are more loose and ragged. Initial treatment is for an abrasion, with patching, pain control, and optional cycloplegia. Once epithelialized, hyperosmotics become the mainstay of treatment. Five percent sodium chloride ointment is used at bedtime for a full 8 weeks after the most recent erosive episode. This agent both dehydrates the subepithelial space and lubricates the epithelial surface. Simple lubricating ointment often works but is less effective because it does not have a dehydrating effect. Concomitant use of 5% NaCl drops four times a day for 2 weeks after an acute episode is also helpful. Patients must know why ointment is necessary for 8 weeks so they will not stop treatment and precipitate another erosion.

Patients with recurrent erosion but without a prior history of trauma usually have Cogan's anterior basement membrane dystrophy, an abnormality of Bowman's layer that includes reduplication of the layer and the presence of epithelial inclusion cysts. Fortunately, their initial treatment is identical to that of those with traumatic erosion because the dystrophy cannot be detected without a slit lamp.

Referral indications include recurrence during hyperosmotic treatment, as well as those for corneal abrasion. Ophthalmologic treatment options are those used for corneal abrasions.

Corneal Ulcer

Corneal ulcer is a keratitis accompanied by an overlying epithelial defect. Most are bacterial, with *Staphylococcus, Streptococcus,* and *Pseudomonas* the most common agents. This medical urgency requires ophthalmologic evaluation and initiation of treatment within hours of diagnosis to prevent permanent visual loss. Because the cornea has no blood supply and is less than 1 mm thick, certain virulent collagenolytic organisms can penetrate the full thickness and perforate in less than 24 hours. The primary care physician's role is early diagnosis, differentiation from nonurgencies, and immediate referral once the diagnosis is suspected.

A good history includes questions about trauma and contact lens wear. Patients who sleep wearing lenses have an eightfold increased risk of ulceration compared with those who do not sleep wearing lenses; the latter are at increased risk over nonlens wearers. Patients complain of pain, tearing, and photophobia similar to abrasion patients. A bacterial ulcer causes a red eye and a localized corneal opacity containing bacteria, inflammatory cells, and edema. Other, noninfectious causes of a corneal opacity in a red eye cannot be differentiated without a slit lamp, experience, and often diagnostic testing. Any such lesion is a bacterial ulcer until proved otherwise. Patients should be instructed to bring their contact lenses and the case (for culture) on referral. Antibiotic treatment should not be started without prior approval of the consultant. The antibiotics used by nonophthalmologists are seldom adequate for treatment and usually only prevent obtaining good cultures. If consultation must be delayed, treatment should consist of ciprofloxacin 0.3% every half hour around the clock until the patient can be evaluated.

Ophthalmologic treatment of corneal ulceration consists of thorough culturing directly onto culture plates, followed by frequent doses of specially formulated topical cephalosporin and aminoglycoside antibiotics. Recent reports of effective monotherapy with commercially available fluoroquinolones are the rationale for the ciprofloxacin recommendation, and many ophthalmologists still treat small ulcers with such monotherapy. Emerging concern about the effectiveness of these agents against *Streptococcus* species (common causes of ulceration) have prompted most ophthalmologists to retain the cephalosporin-aminoglycoside combination in severe cases.

Herpes Simplex Virus

The possibility of herpetic keratitis is the reason no practitioner should treat a red eye with steroids without first performing a slit-lamp examination. Such unwitting treatment can hasten the demise of an eye with an already severe and recurrent problem. The medicolegal consequences can be severe as well.

More than 95% of cases of clinical herpetic disease are recurrences that develop long after the primary infection. Although primary infection usually occurs by 5 years of age, most adults do not have a history of clinical herpetic disease. The cervical and trigeminal ganglia become host to the latent herpes simplex virus (HSV), which is reactivated intermittently and travels via the neuronal network to the end organ. Corneal nerves are thought to shed reactivated HSV into the tears, which may cause corneal disease. Herpetic blepharitis is most likely to occur with a primary infection, exhibiting classic vesicles on the eyelids and surrounding skin. Although most patients will not develop ocular disease, many ophthalmologists recommend prophylactic treatment with an ocular antiviral agent. Recurrent follicular conjunctivitis can be caused by HSV, even without corneal disease, and should be considered before initiating steroid treatment of a chronic conjunctivitis of undetermined etiology.

Herpetic epithelial and stromal keratitis (HSV keratitis) are potentially blinding disorders that require care by an ophthalmologist. Dendritic staining patterns with fluorescein or rose bengal and decreased corneal sensation are classic signs of HSV keratitis but are not always present. As with syphilis, HSV is "the great mimic" in the eye and must be included in many differential diagnoses. Epithelial, endothelial, and stromal forms of herpetic keratitis are described. Treatment with assorted combinations of topical and systemic antivirals and corticosteroids is complicated and often chronic.

Varicella-Zoster Virus

Ocular involvement during primary varicella infection occurs infrequently. Lid lesions begin as papules, become vesicular and pustular, and then crust. Conjunctivitis is the most common ocular involvement. Recurrent varicella-zoster virus (VZV) infection in the trigeminal distribution is more likely to cause corneal disease. The ophthalmic division is most often involved (herpes zoster ophthalmicus). Because the nasociliary branch of the trigeminal nerve innervates both the tip of the nose and the cornea, the presence of herpetic vesicles on the nose tip (Hutchinson's sign) often suggests corneal disease. Lid edema impairs proper closure (lagophthalmos) and leads to the most common cause of permanent ocular damage from zoster. Liberal use of lubricating ointments can prevent this complication. Epithelial dendrites are the next most common type of VZV ocular involvement. These eyes lose sensation much more often than those with HSV and frequently have chronic surface problems that are challenging to manage.

Antivirals are of little use in treating active VZV corneal infections, although oral acyclovir decreases the incidence and severity of dendritiform keratopathy, stromal keratitis, and uveitis when taken within 72 hours of onset of the skin lesions. Acyclovir therefore should be given to any patient with herpes zoster ophthalmicus as early as possible.

Acute Glaucoma

Acute glaucoma can overwhelm the endothelial ability to maintain corneal stromal deturgescence in the presence of an elevated intraocular pressure (IOP). A hot, red eye and cloudy cornea (with or without epithelial defects) may ensue. Palpation of the globe through the closed lid will reveal a unilateral increase in IOP, which establishes the underlying diagnosis of acute glaucoma. Treatment focuses on the glaucoma (see Chapter 173). The corneal problems usually resolve spontaneously, with restoration of normal IOP.

Acute Hydrops in Keratoconus

Keratoconus is a degenerative corneal ectasia characterized by noninflammatory stromal thinning that is most pronounced at the apex of the cone. Patients have progressive myopia and increasing astigmatism that becomes irregular and uncorrectable with glasses. Hard or gas-permeable contact lenses are required to correct vision adequately, and corneal transplantation is required when lenses can no longer be worn or when central scarring prevents useful vision.

Acute corneal hydrops can cause a red painful eye, with corneal clouding in a patient with keratoconus. Tears in Descemet's membrane can violate the endothelial barrier and lead to acute stromal edema (hydrops) in the region of the cone. The clinical scenario is a patient wearing contact lenses who has a unilateral red, painful, photophobic eye with decreased acuity and a corneal opacity. This presentation is similar to that of an infectious corneal ulcer. Because keratoconus patients are at increased risk of ulceration from epithelial instability at the cone apex, they presumably have an infectious ulcer and should be referred immediately to an ophthalmologist. Once ulceration has been ruled out, watchful waiting will allow the edema to resolve in about 4 months.

THE WHITE EYE

Keratitis Sicca

Keratoconjunctivitis sicca (dry eye) is seen frequently in patients with connective tissue disease. Keratoconjunctivitis sicca plus xerostomia is classified as a primary Sjögren's syndrome; the addition of a connective tissue disease is secondary Sjögren's syndrome. A wide variety of drugs (e.g., antihistamines, nasal decongestants, analgesics, sedatives, tricyclic antidepressants) decrease lacrimation. Patients complain mainly of chronic "dryness" and foreign body sensation. A dry cornea can cause blurring of vision. Many patients report increased mucus in the cul-de-sacs. Examination reveals decreased tear strips along the lower lid margins, as well as punctate staining of the ocular surface with fluorescein. Tear film deficiency can cause severe problems (e.g., ulceration, perforation) for an ocular surface designed to function as a wet system. Artificial tear substitutes (drops by day and ointments at night) are the mainstay of treatment. Referral to an ophthalmologist is indicated if symptoms persist with artificial tears used four times daily. Plugging of the lower lacrimal punctae (tear drains) with silicone plugs or hot cautery can provide dramatic relief. Heavier ointments or partial lid closure (tarsorrhaphy) can be used in severe cases.

Corneal Dystrophies

As corneal anatomy suggests, a variety of dystrophies affect the epithelium, basement membrane, Bowman's layer, stroma, Descemet's membrane, and endothelium. These inherited, bilateral abnormalities of the cornea are not associated with systemic disease or prior inflammation. Most dystrophies present in the first few decades of life and demonstrate autosomal dominant inheritance. Basement membrane and Bowman's layer dystrophies manifest through the faulty epithelial adhesion of recurrent erosion. Stromal dystrophies generally cause blurriness and glare trouble, although some anterior stromal dystrophies cause epithelial adhesion problems. Endothelial dystrophies lead to corneal decompensation through failure of the pump function. The history may reveal a family member with similar complaints. Penlight examination may reveal (at most) a vague loss of corneal luster or clarity. The diagnosis requires an experienced observer using a slit lamp, so any patient suspected of having a dystrophy should be referred for complete ophthalmologic evaluation.

Corneal Degenerations

Several corneal stromal degenerations lead to corneal thinning (e.g., keratoconus, keratoglobus, pellucid marginal degeneration). The resulting ectasia causes a visual disturbance from irregular astigmatism. Degenerations tend to have a later onset, more rapid progression, and unilateral occurrence, distinguishing them from the dystrophies. Because physical findings are unremarkable on penlight examination, all patients must be referred to an ophthalmologist for slit-lamp evaluation. In some early cases, changes are not visible on slit-lamp examination. New computerized topographic mapping systems can diagnose many more subtle disorders of corneal contour in these patients.

Pterygium

Pterygium is a triangular wedge of fibrovascular tissue that begins on the epibulbar conjunctiva and grows slowly onto the cornea. Its unsightly appearance and occasional inflammation often bring it to a physician's attention. Prevalence of pterygium is directly related to the proximity to the equator; the incidence is negligible beyond the 40th parallel. Ultraviolet exposure seems to be the primary factor; with such exposure, only surgery can arrest growth. The variety of available surgical techniques and reported recurrence rates, ranging from 3% to 40%, illustrate the propensity for pterygium to recur. Because growth often stops spontaneously and surgery may stimulate a fast-paced regrowth, excision is delayed until necessary. Clear indications for excision are lesions that encroach on the visual axis, induce significant irregular astigmatism causing loss of acuity, and restriction of eye movement enough to cause double vision. A "soft" but valid indication is cosmesis. Any lesion causing concern to the patient should be referred to an ophthalmologist for a detailed discussion of prognosis and treatment options.

ADDITIONAL READINGS

Brightbill FS: *Corneal surgery: theory, technique, and tissue,* ed 2, St Louis, 1993, Mosby.

Casey TA, Sharif KW: *A colour atlas of corneal dystrophies & degenerations,* Aylesbury, England, 1991, Wolfe.

Grayson M: *Diseases of the cornea,* St Louis, 1979, Mosby.

Kaufman HE, Barron BA, McDonald MB, Waltman SR: *The cornea,* New York, 1988, Churchill Livingstone.

Roy FH: *Ocular differential diagnosis,* ed 5, Philadelphia, 1993, Lea & Febiger.

Tasman W, Jaeger EA: *Clinical ophthalmology,* vol 4, rev ed, Philadelphia, 1993, Lippincott.

CHAPTER 176

Retinal and Choroidal Diseases

Uday R. Desai
Julian J. Nussbaum

Referrals to the ophthalmologist are often necessary because of the need for specialized examination modalities, including slit-lamp biomicroscopy, tonometry, and ophthalmoscopic examinations. In patients with vitreoretinal or choroidal disease, adequate examination requires the indirect ophthalmoscope and perhaps ophthalmic ultrasonography. Therefore suspected vitreoretinal or choroidal disease always mandates a referral to a vitreoretinal specialist. Awareness of the more common vitreoretinal abnormalities helps the primary care physician judge the urgency of different referrals. By identifying the patient's condition as vitreoretinal, the physician also may be able to refer the patient directly to the retinal specialist.

ANATOMY

The adult human eye averages 24 mm in diameter and consists of the anterior segment and posterior segment (Fig. 176-1). The posterior segment contains the retina, choroid, sclera, and vitreous body. The three layers of the posterior segment are the retina, choroid, and sclera (Fig. 176-2). The retina consists of the neurosensory retina, which is the sensory component of the ocular system, and the retinal pigment epithelium (RPE), which provides metabolic support. The retina has a vascular network that supplies the inner three fourths of the neurosensory retina. The choroid is composed of Bruch's membrane, choriocapillaris, middle and outer choroidal vascular layers, and the suprachoroidal space. Bruch's membrane is located adjacent to the RPE and is composed of basement membrane, collagen, and elastic layers. The vascular layers proceed outward from the choriocapillaris to the outer choroidal layer. This vascular network supplies the outer one fourth of the neurosensory retina and the RPE. The choroid contains connective tissue, melanocytes, and the short posterior ciliary nerves, which are responsible for pain sensation in this portion of the globe. Outside the choroid lies the sclera.

The three layers of the posterior segment surround the vitreous body, which has an average volume of 4 ml. The vitreous is a gel-like substance, the composition of which is 99% water. Other components include hyaluronic acid, which provides elasticity, and collagen, which provides strength. The vitreous is attached to the overlying retina early in life. The strongest attachments are at the vitreous base, which attaches to the peripheral retina, optic nerve, macula, and retinal vessels.

The vitreous can be visualized with slit-lamp biomicroscopy. The retina and choroid are seen with direct and indirect ophthalmoscopy (Fig. 176-3). The most prominent structure is the optic nerve, which is 1.5 mm wide and 1.75 mm high. It is seen as the yellow-red oval structure located nasal to the visual axis. From this nerve emerge the retinal arterioles and venules. Four pairs of vessels extend to each one of the

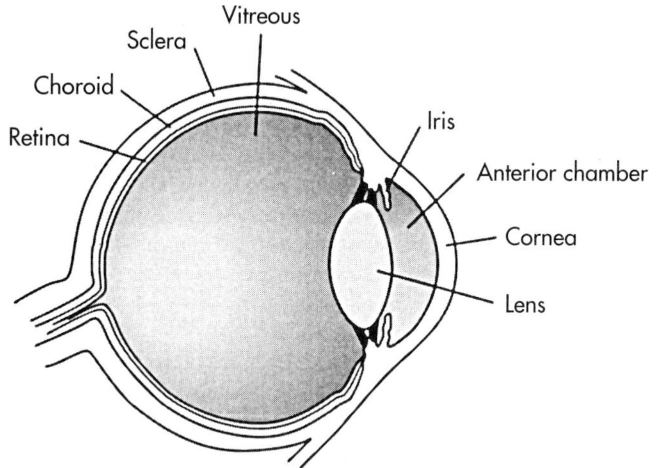

Fig. 176-1. Sagittal section showing major structures of the eye.

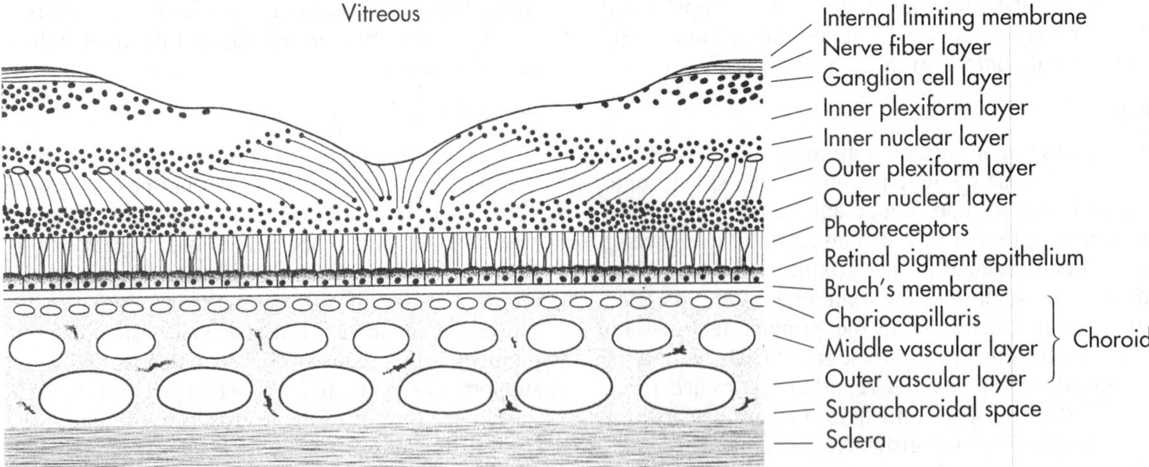

Fig. 176-2. Posterior segment layers of the eye. (From Johnson RN, et al: Fluorescein angiography: basic principles and interpretation. In Ryan SJ et al: *Retina*, ed 3, St Louis, 2001, Mosby.)

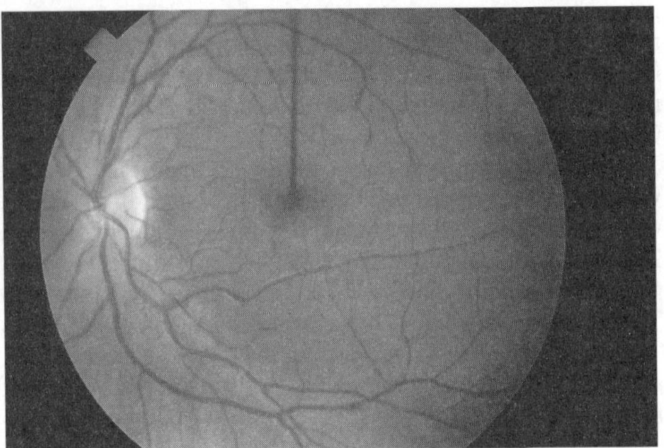

Fig. 176-3. Macular region of retina. Pointer identifies fovea.

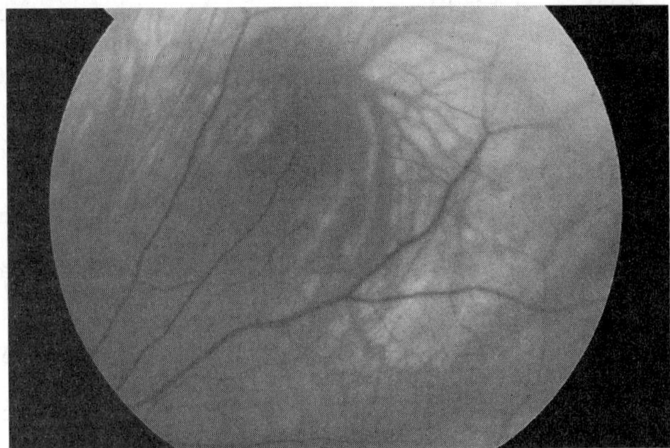

Fig. 176-4. Vortex veins.

following quadrants: superonasal, inferonasal, inferotemporal, and superotemporal. The superotemporal and inferotemporal arcades outline the retinal structure known as the *macula*. Within the macula is a 1500-μm-wide depression called the *fovea centralis*. Within the fovea is a 350-μm-wide area called the *foveola*, which contains only cone photoreceptors. Because cone photoreceptors have potential for good vision, the foveola is the only area of the retina with 20/20 visual potential.

The choroid lies deep to the retinal structures. The most visible of the choroidal structures are the four to seven vortex veins, which are the efferent arm of the choroidal circulation (Fig. 176-4). These orange vessels are located 2 to 3 disc diameters (1 DD about 1.5 mm) posterior to the equator of the eye. The other vascular structures of the choroid can be seen in lightly pigmented patients or those with RPE atrophy.

PHYSIOLOGY

The sensory function of the eye is performed by the neurosensory retina. The eye is capable of photopic and scotopic vision. *Photopic vision* is used in bright illumination and includes the recognition of colors; it is a function of the cone photoreceptors. *Scotopic vision* is used in dim illumination and does not include color recognition; it is a function of the rod photoreceptors. Cone photoreceptors are located primarily within the macula; rod photoreceptors are located in the peripheral retina. The macula therefore provides color vision as well as central visual acuity; the peripheral retina is responsible for peripheral vision and night vision.

The photoreceptors are located in the deepest portion of the retina. They contain light-sensitive pigment molecules in the 11-*cis*-retinal configuration. Once stimulated, they convert to the *trans* configuration, which initiates an electrical potential that spreads from the photoreceptor cell to the bipolar cell. The bipolar cells stimulate the ganglion cells, the axons of which form the nerve fiber layer. This nerve fiber layer exits the eye as the optic nerve. The optic nerve transmits the visual information back to the brain. The information that began at the photoreceptors ultimately ends in the visual cortex of the occipital lobe (see Fig. 176-2).

PATIENT EVALUATION

History

Specific symptoms, including painless visual disturbances, indicate retinal pathology (Table 176-1). Disorders of the peripheral retina impair peripheral vision and night vision. Disorders of the central retina affect central visual acuity and

Table 176-1. Ocular Symptoms and Associated Retinal Disorders

Symptom	Disorder
Decreased vision	Macular abnormality or obscuration
Poor color vision	Macular abnormality
Poor night vision	Peripheral retinal dysfunction
Peripheral field loss	Peripheral retinal dysfunction
Entopsias (floaters)	Vitreous opacity
Photopsias (flashes)	Traction or inflammation of retina or choroid
Metamorphopsia (micropsia, macropsia)	Macular abnormality

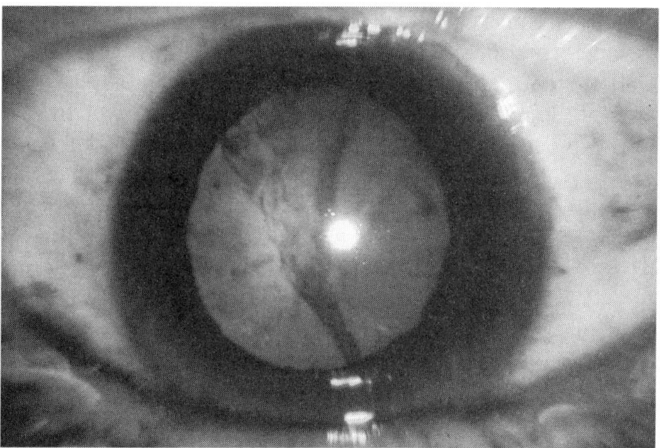

Fig. 176-5. Abnormal red reflex.

color vision. Decreased visual acuity suggests an abnormality within the macula or a media opacity (e.g., hemorrhage, inflammation) that is obscuring the macula. Abnormal color vision also may be associated with retinal disease. Congenital color defects may indicate cone photoreceptor abnormalities; acquired color defects may result from acquired macular disease. Unilateral peripheral field loss suggests peripheral retinal disease. Poor night vision may indicate rod photoreceptor dysfunction or generalized peripheral retinal disease. Entopsias (floaters) usually represent vitreous opacities. Photopsias (flashes) that are unilateral usually indicate retinal irritation. Causes of unilateral photopsia include vitreous traction, retinal detachment, and retinal or choroidal inflammation or infection. Metamorphopsia, including micropsia and macropsia, usually indicates macular dysfunction. Finally, monocular diplopia (double vision with one eye closed) also suggests macular dysfunction.

Physical Examination

Media opacities in the vitreous cavity can be visualized by the direct ophthalmoscope. Retroillumination of the fundus reveals dark opacities within the red reflex. A dull or absent red reflex may indicate a retinal detachment, vitreous opacity, or intraocular tumor (Fig. 176-5).

Abnormalities in the retina or choroid may be differentiated by the color of the lesions. Most abnormalities are red, yellow, white, gray-white, brown, or black (Box 176-1). Red lesions in the retina typically represent hemorrhage. The location of the hemorrhage, both topographically on the retina and depth within the retina, helps narrow the differential diagnosis. For example, a sector of retina with hemorrhages may contain a branch vein occlusion, whereas midperipheral and macular hemorrhages suggest a systemic vasculopathy such as hypertensive or diabetic retinopathy. In addition, the depth of the hemorrhages suggests different entities. An intraretinal hemorrhage is characteristic of diabetic retinopathy, whereas a subretinal hemorrhage is classic for a choroidal neovascular membrane. Vascular tumors (e.g., hemangiomas) and vascular abnormalities (e.g., telangiectasias) also appear red.

The most common yellow lesions are probably the deep subretinal lesions known as *drusen* ("bumps"). Seen in elderly patients, drusen are a risk factor in the development of age-related macular degeneration. Hard exudates also are a common yellow lesion seen in the retina. They have

Box 176-1. Fundus Lesions by Color With Associated Disorder

Red

Hemorrhage
Hemangioma
Telangiectasia

Yellow

Drusen
Hard exudates
Chorioretinal scars
Heredodegenerative conditions

White

Soft exudates (cotton-wool spots)
Myelinated nerve fibers
Coloboma
Fibrosis
Gliosis
Astrocytic hamartoma
Retinoblastoma
Retinitis or chorioretinitis

Gray-White

Retinal edema
- Retinal arterial occlusion
- Vascular leakage

Retinal elevation
Retinal detachment
- Tractional
- Rhegmatogenous
- Exudative

Brown and Black

Migration of pigment into retina
- Hereditary (retinitis pigmentosa)
- Retinal trauma
- Intraocular inflammation

Chorioretinal scarring
Congenital pigment epithelial hypertrophy
Choroidal nevus
Choroidal melanoma

numerous causes, but the common pathophysiology is the presence of incompetent vasculature, which allows the exudation of extracellular material into the outer plexiform layer of the retina. Because the outer plexiform layer forms a radiating pattern from the central foveola, lipid exudates may form a so-called macular star if the incompetent vessels are located close to the macula. Atrophic chorioretinal scars also may appear yellow. Finally, heredodegenerative conditions may present with retinal or subretinal yellow lesions within the macula, periphery, or both.

White lesions include soft exudates, or cotton-wool spots. These focal areas of retinal ischemia block the retrograde axoplasmic flow, resulting in accumulation of axoplasmic material. Cotton-wool spots suggest different diagnoses but are not a diagnosis. They usually occur in retinal diseases characterized by retinal ischemia. Another white lesion consists of myelinated nerve fibers, are usually adjacent to the optic nerve and with feathering borders. Although they may be confused with cotton-wool spots, these lesions are whiter and persistent rather than transitory. Colobomas, which are a congenital absence of retinal and choroidal structures, also appear as white lesions. Fibrosis, which occurs with disciform scars, causes a white-appearing retinal lesion. Gliosis also can appear white and is impossible to differentiate from fibrosis without histology. Tumors such as astrocytic hamartomas and retinoblastomas can appear white. Finally, infectious retinitis or chorioretinitis can lead to the accumulation of inflammatory cells, which can give the retina a whitish appearance.

Gray-white lesions of the retina occur with edema or elevation of the retina. These lesions are usually associated with loss of the choroidal details. A retinal arterial occlusion can cause edema of the retina with a resultant gray-white discoloration. In addition, vascular leakage (e.g., diabetic maculopathy, retinal telangiectasia) can cause edema of the retina before the development of lipid exudation. Elevation of the retina can occur with retinal detachment from a tractional, rhegmatogenous, or exudative cause. Any of these etiologies of retinal detachment can cause the retina to appear gray-white.

Brown and black lesions indicate alterations in the pigment of the retina and choroid. Normally, pigment is seen only in the RPE and the choroidal stroma. Migration of pigment into the retina can occur with hereditary conditions such as retinitis pigmentosa. Migration also can be caused by retinal trauma or intraocular inflammation. Chorioretinal scarring can result in RPE hyperplasia, which appears as irregular brown-black lesions in areas usually with adjacent atrophy. Well-demarcated areas of black pigmentation usually signify congenital RPE hypertrophy. When pigmented lesions occur within the choroid, the lesions may have a subtle greenish hue. The most common lesion is a choroidal nevus. Another serious lesion is a choroidal melanoma, which is also elevated.

The retina and choroid respond in only a few ways to different pathologic insults. These signs, however, may vary considerably in their location, duration, fluctuation, and associated history.

VITREOUS ABNORMALITIES

The vitreous body is normally attached to the retinal surface early in life. The consistency of the vitreous changes from gel-like to liquid with age (Box 176-2). As this change occurs, condensations of collagen can present to the patient as floaters. These structures may be described as hairlike or cobweb shaped. They also may appear to the patient as insectlike. Floaters, although annoying, are not a threat to vision. With increasing liquefaction, liquid vitreous may insinuate between the posterior vitreous surface and the inner retinal surface, a condition known as a *posterior vitreous detachment*. An acute presentation is associated with photopsias. As the vitreous surface separates from the retina, the stimulated retinal surface produces the sensation of flashing lights. As the separating vitreous moves anteriorly, the collagen fibers condense even further, producing a more noticeable vitreous floater. A vitreous detachment alone is not a visual risk, but because vitreous detachments can be associated with retinal tears and vitreous hemorrhage, a referral within a week is warranted.

Box 176-2. Vitreous Abnormalities

Liquefaction
Posterior detachment
Hemorrhage
Inflammation or infection (vitritis)
Asteroid hyalosis
Synchysis scintillans

Vitreous detachments can be associated with vitreous hemorrhage when the retina or superficial retinal vessel is torn. More common causes of vitreous hemorrhage include diabetic proliferative disease and sickle cell disease. The bleeding comes from active neovascular tufts on the retinal surface. The patient presents with painless loss of vision. Initially the patient sees numerous floaters and may see a "waterfall," representing a stream of blood. The blood would then clot, and the patient may see a cobweb or a dense floater if the bleeding is not excessive. With a large amount of blood the complaint may be acute loss of vision. The patient should avoid aspirin and aspirin-like medicines, remain in a strict head-up position, and sleep with the head elevated at least 45 degrees to allow the blood to settle in the inferior vitreous cavity. A retinal specialist should be consulted within 24 hours.

Floaters and loss of vision also may be associated with vitritis, an inflammation of the vitreous. The inflammation spills into the vitreous from either the retina or posterior uvea (choroid or ciliary body). Any infectious or noninfectious inflammation of the choroid or retina produces similar symptoms. Generally, this posterior inflammation does not produce pain, and the eye also does not look inflamed. The red reflex is dulled, and ophthalmoscopy reveals obscured or absent details. Vitritis associated with recent ocular surgery may indicate bacterial endophthalmitis and warrants immediate referral to an ophthalmologist (Fig. 176-6). Vitritis not associated with previous ocular surgery may be referred to the ophthalmologist within 24 hours.

Other, uncommon vitreous conditions include synchysis scintillans and asteroid hyalosis (Fig. 176-7). These two conditions are characterized by the presence of crystals within the vitreous cavity. Asteroid hyalosis is a primary condition that presents with calcium crystals in the vitreous

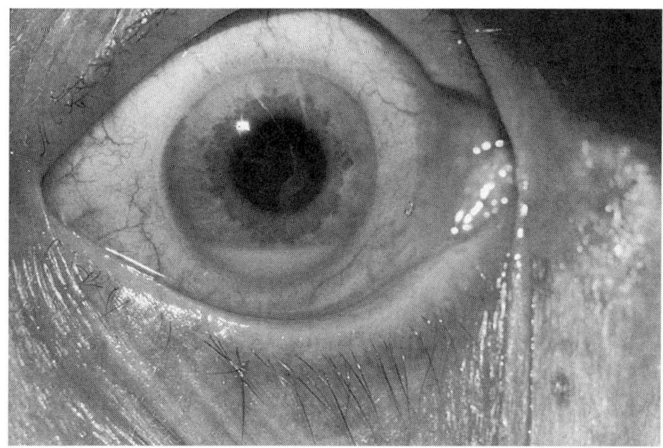

Fig. 176-6. Bacterial endophthalmitis.

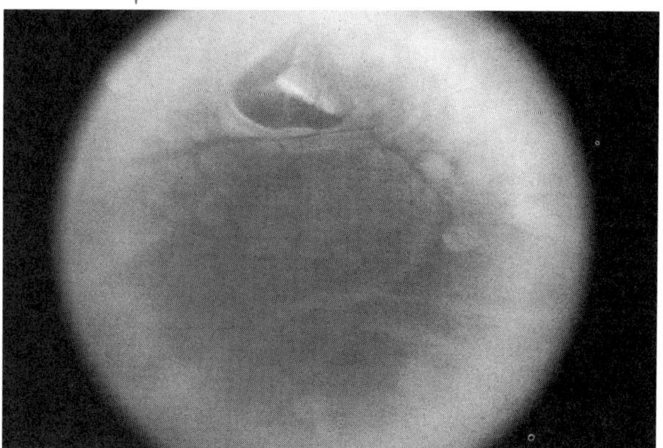

Fig. 176-8. Retinal tear.

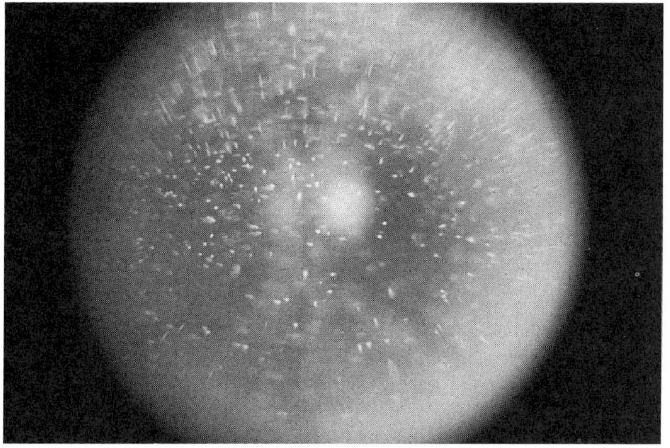

Fig. 176-7. Asteroid hyalosis.

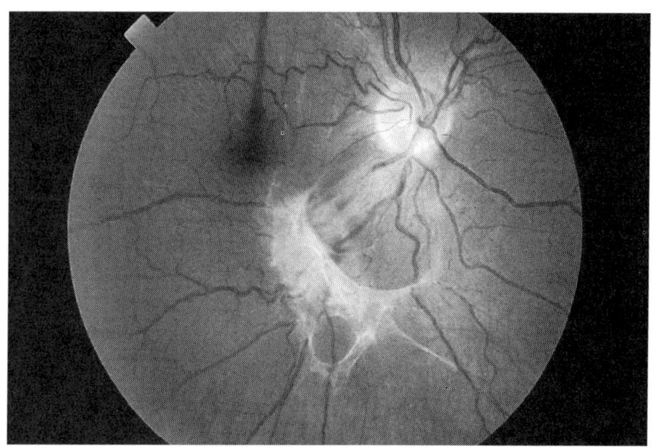

Fig. 176-9. Epiretinal membrane.

cavity. Synchysis scintillans is a secondary condition in which previous vitreous hemorrhage results in the deposition of cholesterol crystals in the vitreous cavity.

VITREORETINAL INTERFACE ABNORMALITIES

The vitreoretinal interface may be the location or the cause of ocular pathology (Box 176-3). Vitreous separation is the primary cause for these abnormalities. In the process of posterior vitreous separation, areas of tight vitreoretinal adhesion may become sites of retinal tear formation (Fig. 176-8). The symptoms of tears are not different from symptoms of posterior vitreous separation. Floaters and photopsias are often noted. Decreased vision related to vitreous hemorrhage also may be present. Since retinal tears may cause retinal detachment, patients with such symptoms should be seen within 24 hours.

Vitreous separation may also cause epiretinal membranes. The separation of the posterior hyaloid may cause microscopic dehiscence of the retinal internal limiting membrane. This dehiscense may give glial cells, metaplastic RPE cells, and fibrocytes access to the inner surface of the internal limiting membrane. The growth and ultimate contraction of this tissue result in distortion of the retinal surface (Fig. 176-9). Patients may complain of decreased vision and metamorphopsia. These complaints are chronic because the epiretinal membranes are slow growing. Visual impairment may be mild. If the visual acuity is better than 20/60 Snellen visual acuity, intervention is not warranted. For vision worse then 20/60, pars plana vitrectomy with removal of the epiretinal membrane is recommended. Because the progression of epiretinal membranes is slow and because many patients do not have significant visual impairment, the referral is not urgent. An appointment within 3 weeks is reasonable.

When vitreous liquefaction causes retention of posterior cortical vitreous, this layer may exert horizontal traction on the retina. This horizontal or tangential traction may cause a full-thickness foveal dehiscence called a *macular hole* (Fig. 176-10). The formation of a macular hole may be associated

Box 176-3. Vitreoretinal Interface Abnormalities

Retinal tears
Epiretinal membrane
Macular hole

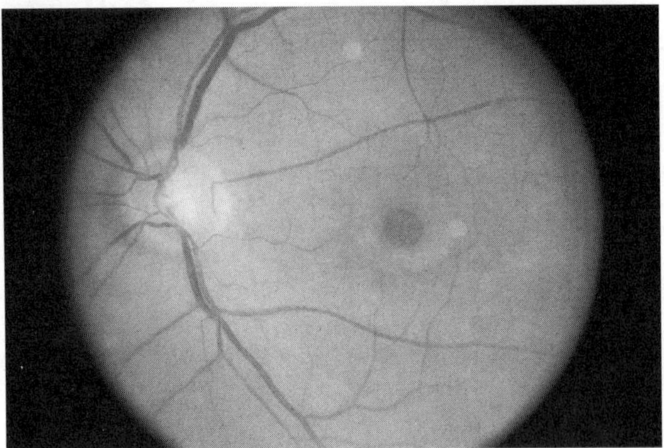

Fig. 176-10. Macular hole.

with a rapid drop in visual acuity, which may not be appreciated by the patient because vision in the other eye remains good. On discovering the affected eye, the patient will notice a central scotoma with poor acuity. Certain macular holes may be treated surgically to remove the posterior cortical vitreous. Sincc this procedure can be attempted even years after the formation of a macular hole, an ophthalmic referral is not urgent. Consultation within 3 weeks is appropriate.

RETINAL ABNORMALITIES

Vascular Disorders

Systemic hypertension can cause ocular changes that primarily affect the neurosensory retina (Box 176-4). Fundus examination may reveal focal or generalized attenuation of the retinal arterioles. Breakdown of the endothelial tight junctions may result in intraretinal hemorrhages and exudation. Hard exudates may be seen within the neurosensory retina. In severe cases these hard exudates may form a star within the macula. Focal areas of retinal ischemia may be seen as cotton-wool spots. Severe hypertension also may cause edema of the optic nerve. Recognition of hypertensive retinopathy may allow better control of hypertension and thereby lessen ocular complications (e.g., retinal vascular occlusions) and systemic complications (e.g., coronary artery disease, neurologic disease). The primary goal after diagnosis of hypertensive retinopathy is control of blood pressure. Once this is established, an ophthalmic referral may be made to rule out ocular complications.

Diabetic retinopathy has many of the retinal findings seen in hypertensive retinopathy because both cause similar breakdown in the vascular endothelial tight junctions. Intraretinal hemorrhages, hard exudates, cotton-wool spots, and microaneurysms may be seen on fundus examination. These findings indicate *background diabetic retinopathy* (BDR, Fig. 176-11). BDR is not a threat to vision except when retinal capillary ischemia or neurosensory retinal edema affects the fovea. In patients with foveal ischemia, vision is irreversibly damaged. Prevention of ischemia is the only approach. Tight control of blood glucose and blood pressure may prevent progression of ischemia. Neurosensory retinal edema, if located within 500 μ of the center of the foveal, is called *clinically significant macular edema* (CSME), and the patient is at risk for losing vision. This risk can be decreased by applying laser photocoagulation to the areas of retinal edema. Resolution of edema may take 3 to 4 months. If residual edema is present after this time, additional photocoagulation may be performed. With worsening retinal ischemia, growth of neovascular tissue can be seen on the optic nerve or elsewhere on the retina; this clinical picture is known as *proliferative diabetic retinopathy* (PDR, Fig. 176-12). Because bleeding may occur from these neovascular fronds, recognition of such vessels by the physician should be followed by prompt referral within 24 hours; otherwise, referral within 3 weeks is appropriate. Bleeding from neovascular fronds and formation of tractional bands that emanate from neovascular fronds cause decreased vision in patients with PDR. Patients with any three of the following four conditions are at high risk of losing vision and should be treated with panretinal laser photocoagulation: (1) any neovascular frond, (2) frond within 1 DD of the optic nerve, (3) large frond (large defined as ½ disc diameter if it is within 1 disc diameter of the optic nerve or greater than ½ disc diameter if elsewhere), and (4) associated vitreous or preretinal hemorrhage. If vitreous hemorrhaging does not

Box 176-4. Retinal Abnormalities

Vascular Disorders
Hypertensive retinopathy
Diabetic retinopathy
Sickle cell retinopathy
Venous occlusions
Arterial occlusions

Retinal Pigment Epithelial Disorders
Central serous retinopathy
Age-related macular degeneration

Inflammatory Conditions
Retinal pigment epitheliitis
Acute posterior multifocal placoid pigment epitheliopathy
Multiple evanescent white-dot syndrome
Acute macular neuroretinopathy
Birdshot chorioretinopathy

Infections
Toxoplasmosis
Toxocariasis
Human immunodeficiency virus (HIV)
Cytomegalovirus (CMV)

Neoplasms
Retinoblastoma
Astrocytoma
Capillary hemangioma
Cavernous hemangioma
Congenital pigment epithelial hypertrophy

Hereditary Conditions
Retinitis pigmentosa
Cone dystrophy

Detachment
Rhegmatogenous
Tractional
Exudative

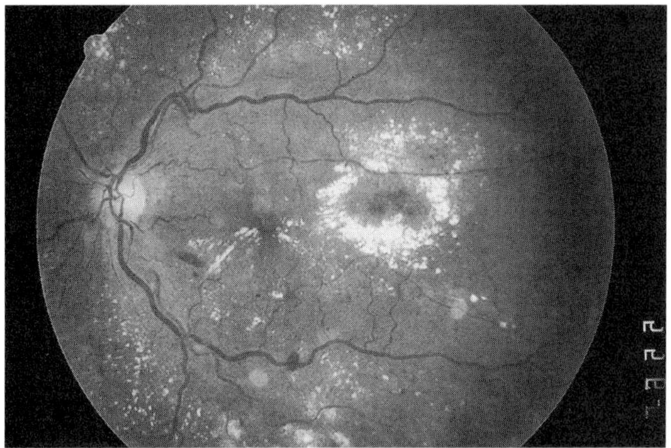

Fig. 176-11. Background diabetic retinopathy.

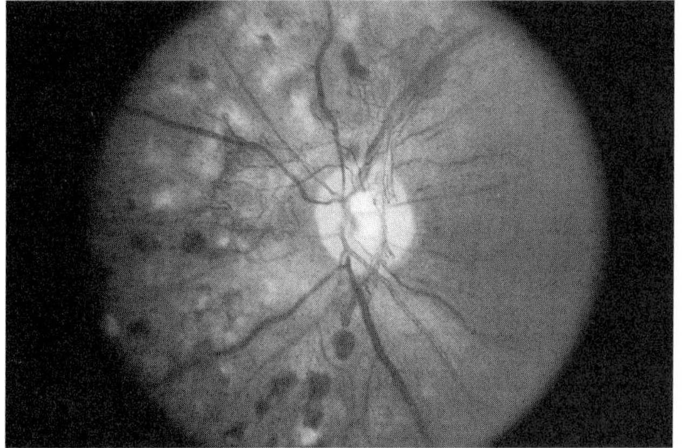

Fig. 176-12. Proliferative diabetic retinopathy. Note new vessels on optic nerve and peripheral laser scars.

clear, pars plana vitrectomy can be performed to clear the vitreous cavity. The time to wait before proceeding to vitrectomy is 2 months in type I and 4 months in type II diabetic patients. Vitrectomy can also be performed in diabetic patients who develop tractional retinal elevation that involves the fovea. Sickle cell disease can also be associated with neovascular fronds.

Retinal venous occlusion can occur in either the central retinal vein or one of its branches (Figs. 176-13 and 176-14). If the fovea is involved, the patient presents with acute visual loss. Funduscopic examination reveals venous dilation, tortuous retinal veins, intraretinal hemorrhages, hard exudates, and cotton-wool spots in the affected quadrants. If the fovea is not involved, the patient may be asymptomatic or may present with only peripheral visual field loss. This diagnosis does not require acute intervention, but referral should be made within 24 hours to confirm the diagnosis.

Retinal arterial occlusions also may occur within the central retinal artery or any of its branches. Arterial occlusion manifests as an ischemic, opaque retina in the affected quadrants, which may be associated with visible emboli within the arterial circulation and a cherry-red spot, or prominent red color in the fovea (Fig. 176-15). If the fovea is involved, vision drops acutely, creating one of the few extreme emergencies in ophthalmic practice. Once this diagnosis is suspected, the patient should be referred immediately to the ophthalmic specialist. A delay of even a few minutes may adversely affect visual outcome.

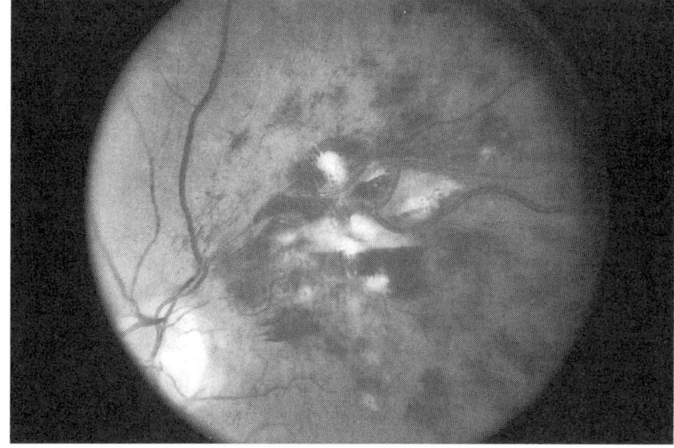

Fig. 176-13. Branch retinal vein occlusion.

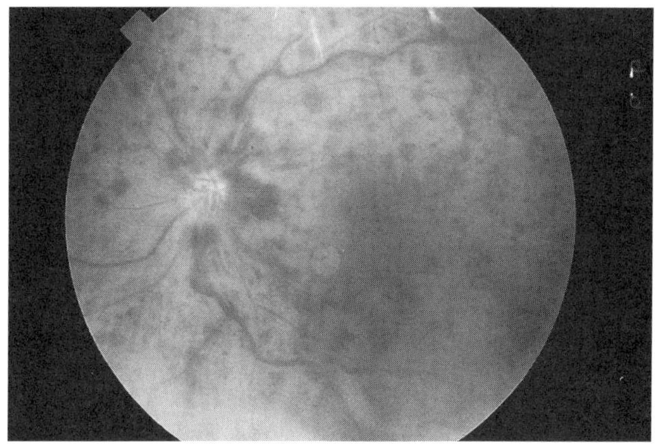

Fig. 176-14. Central retinal vein occlusion.

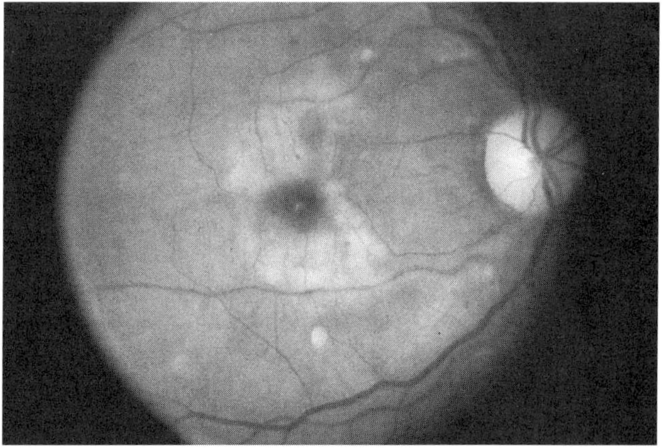

Fig. 176-15. Central retinal artery occlusion. Note macular whitening with center cherry-red spot.

Retinal Pigment Epithelial Disorders

Two conditions of the RPE are central serous retinopathy and age-related macular degeneration. Central serous retinopathy generally occurs in patients less than 50 years of age, whereas macular degeneration occurs in older patients. The pathogenesis of *central serous retinopathy* probably involves misdirected fluid transport by the RPE. The epithelium transports fluid underneath the neurosensory retina, causing a neurosensory retinal elevation. The patient complains of acute loss of vision with metamorphopsia, usually micropsia. Examination of the fundus reveals a dulled foveal reflex and neurosensory retinal elevation. This condition is generally self-limited; within 4 months the neurosensory elevation resolves. If not, laser photocoagulation may be necessary. Referral can be made within 3 weeks.

Dry macular degeneration results from loss of RPE cells, giving the macula a mottled appearance (Fig. 176-16). The RPE has atrophic as well as hypertrophic regions. Subretinal accumulations of waste products (drusen) are yellow-white and primarily occur in the macula. Dry macular degeneration causes gradual central visual loss and has no definitive treatment at this time. Some speculate that exposure to visible and ultraviolet light may lead to formation of reactive oxygen species in the outer retina or choroid. This presumably could lead to dysfunction of the photoreceptor-RPE-choriocapillaris complex and hasten macular degeneration, which has led some to advocate use of antioxidants. Results of studies are inconclusive, but wearing sunglasses is encouraged. The role of diet and nutritional supplementation in managing patients with macular degeneration is not clear. The Age-Related Eye Disease Study (AREDS) may be able to answer these questions. Until then, a well-balanced diet and daily multivitamins are recommended for patients with macular degeneration.

In 10% of patients with macular degeneration, new vessels grow underneath the retina. These abnormal extensions of choroidal vasculature are called *choroidal neovascular membranes* (CNVMs). These new vessels change the diagnosis from dry macular degeneration to *wet-macular degeneration*. The vessels have a propensity to grow close to the fovea and predispose the eye to subretinal exudation and subretinal hemorrhage (Fig. 176-17), both of which can cause rapid decrease in central visual acuity with accompanying metamorphopsia. If CNVMs are not immediately under the fovea, laser photocoagulation may allow closure of the vessels with retention of good visual acuity. Because the vessels show continued growth without treatment, urgent referral within 24 hours is mandated. CNVMs are visualized using intravenous fluorescein angiography (IVFA). This allows localization of the neovascular complex; the location in relation to the fovea is important to determine the available management options. If the CNVM is *not* under the fovea, laser photocoagulation is the best option, obliterating the CNVM with thermal energy. The effectiveness of therapy is determined by repeating IVFA 10 to 14 days after treatment. Any residual CNVM is re-treated with photocoagulation. Patients with CVNMs under the fovea are at risk for losing vision after laser photocoagulation. In select patients (smaller CNVM, worse starting vision), laser photocoagulation is still the preferred treatment modality. When the subfoveal CNVM is associated with moderately good vision, observation or photocoagulation that spares the fovea may be recommended. Other modalities being investigated for use in patients with subfoveal CNVM include photodynamic therapy using photosensitive dyes and surgical extraction of the CNVM using pars plana vitrectomy and subretinal surgery.

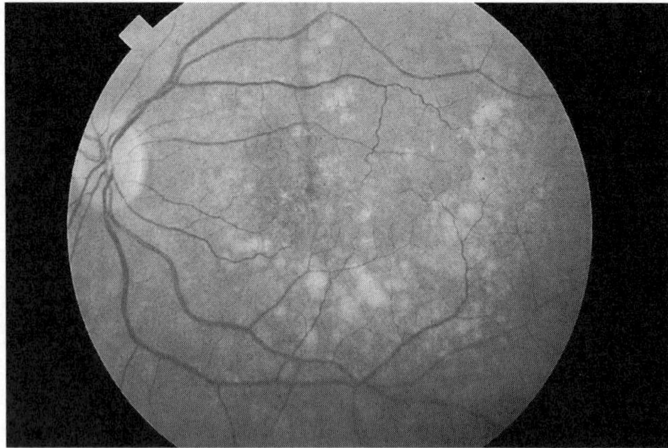

Fig. 176-16. Dry macular degeneration.

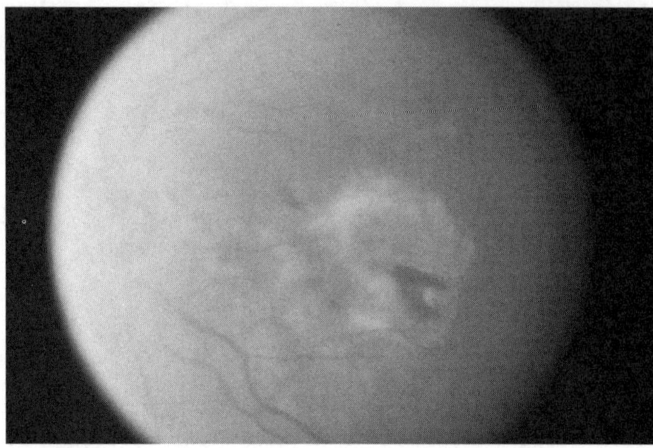

Fig. 176-17. Wet macular degeneration. Note subretinal hemorrhage and subretinal scar.

Inflammatory Conditions

Retinal inflammatory conditions affect the RPE or inner retina and include retinal pigment epitheliitis, acute posterior multifocal placoid pigment epitheliopathy (Fig. 176-18), multiple evanescent white-dot syndrome, acute macular neuroretinopathy, and birdshot chorioretinopathy. These conditions primarily are acute in onset and occur in younger patients. The etiologies are presumed to be viral. They are usually self-limiting, and treatment is not warranted. Referral is semiurgent, with no immediate therapy necessary. Patients have acute loss of vision, and the affected eyes display yellow inflammatory lesions.

Infectious Conditions

Agents that infect the retina include the parasites *Toxoplasma gondii* and *Toxocara canis* as well as human immunodeficiency virus (HIV) and cytomegalovirus (CMV). *Toxoplasmosis* is acquired congenitally and results in large, bilateral, pigmented and depigmented chorioretinal scars, which contain the dormant organism that may reactivate later in adolescence or young adulthood. Reactivation results in marked retinal and vitreous inflammation and causes floaters and decreased vision. *Toxocariasis* also occurs in younger children and results in granuloma formation, primarily

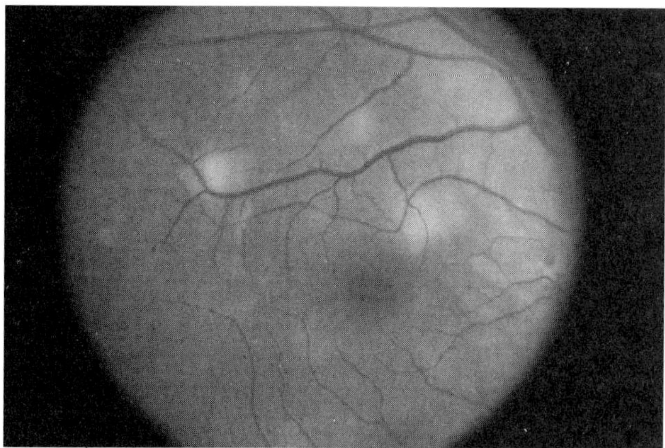

Fig. 176-18. Acute multifocal placoid pigment epitheliopathy.

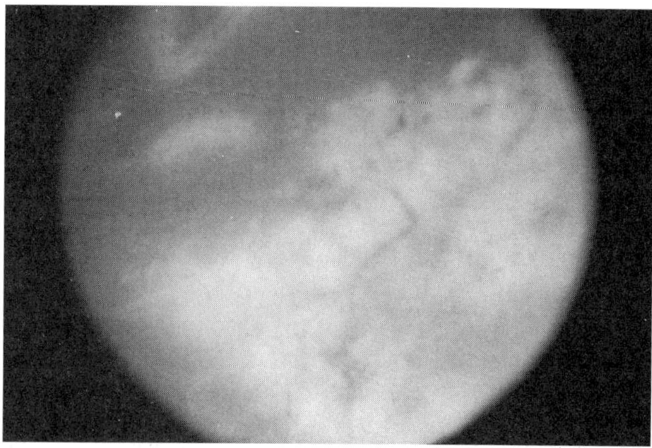

Fig. 176-19. Cytomegalovirus (CMV) retinitis.

affecting the optic nerve, macula, or peripheral retina. The granulomas that affect the optic nerve and the macula usually are associated with decreased vision and a white pupillary reflex. They may result in retinal detachment and significant vitreal inflammation.

Viruses also may result in infectious retinitis. HIV may lead to formation of cotton-wool spots in the retina, which are white with soft margins. Cotton-wool spots are transitory and are not associated with a decrease in vision. When HIV-positive patients present with a white retinal lesion, the most devastating etiology is *CMV retinitis,* which initially may be indistinguishable from a cotton-wool spot. With time, the retinitis, which begins around retinal arterioles, acquires a cheeselike consistency and becomes associated with intraretinal hemorrhages (Fig. 176-19). The retinitis spreads rapidly and, if it involves the optic nerve or macula, is associated with sudden visual loss. HIV retinopathy necessitates every 2- to 3-month examinations for the detection of CMV retinitis. Once CMV retinitis is diagnosed, the patient needs lifelong treatment with ganciclovir, foscarnet, or a combination of the two. When CMV retinitis is suspected, immediate referral for confirmation is necessary.

Neoplastic Conditions

Retinal neoplasms may be pedunculated or sessile. The shape, color, and associated findings may help differentiate them. Because of its potentially fatal outcome, retinoblastoma should be ruled out immediately. *Retinoblastomas* are pedunculated white vascular tumors that may grow into the vitreous cavity or outward toward the choroid. Retinoblastoma is the most common intraocular malignancy of childhood, diagnosed mainly between ages 12 and 18 months, when a young child presents with a white pupil (Fig. 176-20) or new onset of ocular misalignment (strabismus). Because of the risk of metastatic spread, the child should be referred immediately for the possibility of enucleation.

Retinal astrocytomas may be mistaken for retinoblastomas. *Astrocytomas* are pedunculated white lesions that extend into the vitreous cavity. They are benign growths of glial astrocytes and are primarily avascular. They have a "mulberry" shape and may be unilateral or bilateral and multifocal. Patients with tuberous sclerosis and neurofibromatosis may manifest retinal astrocytomas, but this tumor is usually not associated with systemic syndrome.

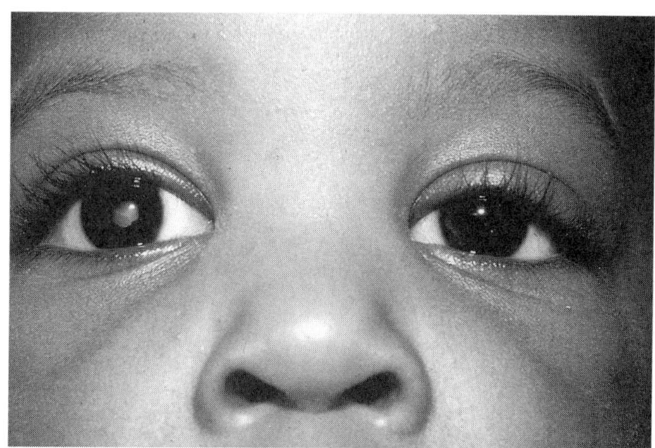

Fig. 176-20. Leukokoria (leukocoria, cat's eye reflex).

Retinal capillary hemangiomas are pedunculated vascular lesions that begin as small, red intraretinal lesions. With time they grow and can be recognized by the presence of a feeding retinal vessel. These hemangiomas may result in bleeding, exudation, and tractional retinal detachment. They may occur as a part of the autosomal dominant von Hippel–Lindau syndrome or on a nonfamilial basis. Because the larger tumors are more difficult to treat, hemangiomas should be diagnosed when they are small and can be treated with laser photocoagulation or retinocryopexy.

Retinal cavernous hemangiomas are sessile lesions that appear as a "cluster of grapes" on the retinal surface. They may be associated with similar skin and central nervous system lesions. Unlike retinal capillary hemangiomas, these lesions do not exhibit marked hemorrhage or exudation.

Congenital RPE hypertrophy is a jet-black lesion with well-defined margins (Fig. 176-21). RPE hyperplasia is an acquired condition with a mottled appearance and results from inflammation, trauma, or vitreoretinal traction. With the exception of suspected retinoblastomas, retinal tumors can be seen on a nonurgent basis.

Hereditary Conditions

Three factors should be considered when a hereditary retinal condition is part of the differential diagnosis. First, the condition tends to occur in younger patients, with most

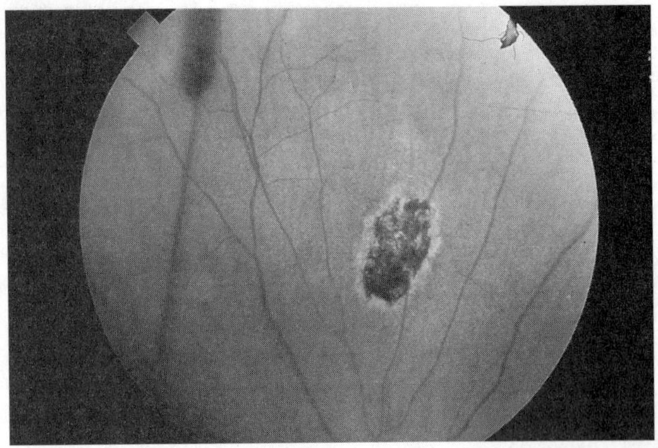

Fig. 176-21. Congenital retinal pigment epithelial hypertrophy.

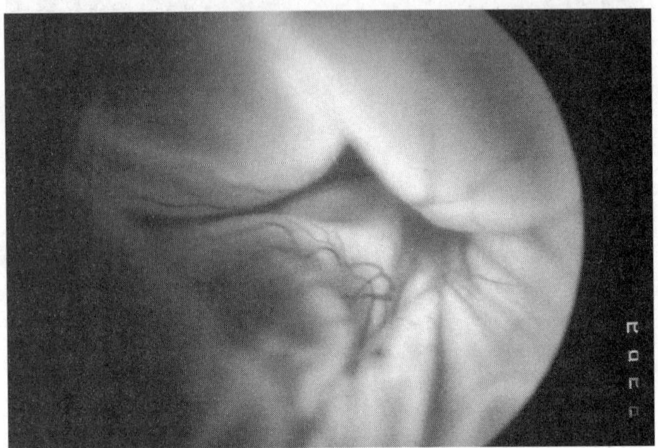

Fig. 176-22. Rhegmatogenous retinal detachment.

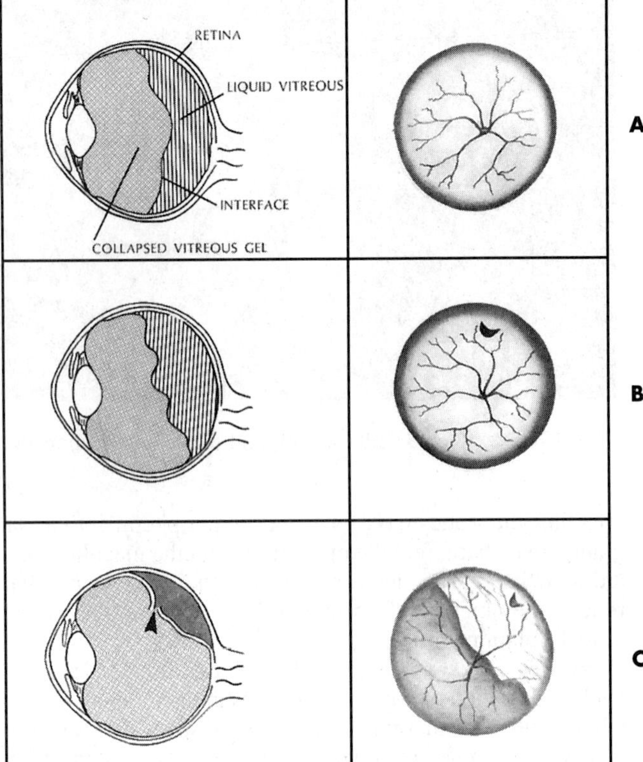

Fig. 176-23. Vitreous detachment, retinal hole, and retinal detachment. **A,** Vitreous body has collapsed and pulled away from retina in posterior half of eye. Retina remains intact. **B,** Vitreous body has detached from retina in posterior portion of eye. Superiorly, strong adhesion between vitreous and retina remains, with retinal tearing caused by vitreous detachment. Retinal tear usually has "horseshoe" appearance when viewed through ophthalmoscope. **C,** Vitreous has detached as in **A** and **B** and has caused a retinal tear as in **B.** Fluid from area of liquid vitreous posteriorly has coursed through retinal hole, and retina has detached from eye wall, with a balloon shape on ophthalmoscopy.

entities manifesting changes in adolescence or young adulthood. Second, the condition is usually bilateral, with symmetric involvement. Third, the patient may have other affected family members, and a specific genetic transmission pattern may be discovered. These entities may affect primarily the periphery and result in decreased peripheral vision and night vision or may affect the macula and result in early central visual loss. The most common peripheral entity is retinitis pigmentosa, and the most common central entity is cone dystrophy.

Retinal Detachments

Three pathogenic mechanisms can result in the retina being elevated off the RPE: rhegmatogenous detachments result from a break in the retina, tractional detachments from tractional fibrosis within the vitreous cavity, and exudative detachments from exudation of fluid under the retina. *Rhegmatogenous* retinal detachments, the most common type, result from posterior vitreous separation (Figs. 176-22 and 176-23). The subsequent retinal break allows liquid vitreous to enter the subretinal space and cause a retinal detachment. The patient generally presents with photopsias and entopsias. With detachment of the fovea, central vision greatly decreases. When the fovea is not detached, central vision can be quite good, even though peripheral vision is limited. When a patient has symptoms of a detachment and good vision, the referral should be made urgently. If vision is decreased, the patient can be seen semiurgently. The primary goal should be to prevent foveal detachment. Once the fovea detaches, surgery to reattach the retina may be performed within a week for equivalent results.

The most common cause of *tractional* retinal detachment is diabetic retinopathy. The proliferative stage results in growth of vascular and fibrous components into the vitreous cavity. The fibrous component may cause tractional forces to develop between the retina and vitreous. These forces may cause the retina to be pulled off the underlying RPE. Unlike rhegmatogenous detachments, tractional detachments do not produce acute symptoms, and the earliest detectable symptom may be visual loss once the fovea detaches. Tractional detachments are slow to form, and thus referral is semiurgent. Treatment involves vitrectomy surgery to remove the tractional components; this procedure is performed only if the fovea is detached or if foveal detachment appears imminent.

Exudative retinal detachments result from subretinal inflammatory and neoplastic conditions that cause the accumulation of fluid under the retina. The fluid has the ability to "shift" under the retina, with different portions of the retina detaching with alterations in position. Once the fluid reaches the fovea, vision decreases. These detachments tend to be inferior in primary position because of gravity. Consultation should be urgent.

CHOROIDAL ABNORMALITIES

Choroidal neovascular membranes occur when normal choroidal vasculature extends into the subretinal space through breaks in Bruch's membrane (Box 176-5). Several conditions may result in such a break. *Angioid streaks* result in Bruch's membrane cracks that radiate from the optic nerve. These orange-red streaks may occur in patients with pseudoxanthoma elasticum, sickle cell disease, and Paget's disease. *High myopia* may result in attenuations of Bruch's membrane, or lacquer cracks, which occur primarily in the macula. Trauma can result in ruptures of the choroid, including Bruch's membrane. These ruptures usually occur concentrically around the optic nerve. Presumed ocular histoplasmosis syndrome results in circular, yellow-white chorioretinal scars. These scars have breaks in the overlying Bruch's membrane. All these conditions may result in green-gray extensions of the choriocapillaris under the retina, resulting in subretinal exudation and hemorrhage. Depending on the location of CNVMs, central visual acuity may be greatly affected. If no predisposing factor is present, the CNVM is considered idiopathic. Once the diagnosis is suspected, urgent referral is made for possible laser photocoagulation to obliterate the CNVM.

Inflammatory Conditions

As with retinal inflammatory conditions, choroidal inflammatory conditions have unknown etiologies. The entities are diagnosed because of the constellation of signs that accompany each disorder. All the choroidal inflammatory disorders may present with photopsias and decreased vision that is sudden in onset. *Serpiginous choroidopathy* occurs in a peripapillary location. The choroid is actively inflamed, and the leading edge has a snakelike shape. *Multifocal choroiditis* and *punctate inner choroidopathy* both have characteristic inflammatory inner choroidal lesions. The eye usually has lesions in different stages of evolution. The acute lesions have a yellowish, thickened appearance, whereas the chronic lesions resemble typical chorioretinal scars that are circular with pigmented and depigmented components. The difference between the two conditions is that multifocal choroiditis has intravitreal inflammation, whereas punctate inner choroidopathy does not.

Neoplastic Conditions

Choroidal neoplastic conditions present as melanotic or amelanotic, unifocal or multifocal subretinal lesions. The most common entity is the choroidal nevus (Fig. 176-24). This benign accumulation of melanocytic cells presents as a flat, greenish brown lesion. This congenital lesion may become more pigmented with time, and its size varies from less than 1 mm to many millimeters. The patient has no overlying retinal involvement and is asymptomatic. These patients should be referred semiurgently. Follow-up consists of yearly observation because of the small risk of malignant transformation into a malignant melanoma.

A choroidal malignant melanoma may arise from a choroidal nevus or may arise de novo (Fig. 176-25). Although amelanotic melanomas are present, the more common presentation is a melanotic subretinal lesion. The color may range from green to brown; a jet-black lesion is rare. A melanoma is differentiated from a nevus by its height (2 to 15 mm). Melanoma may be associated with neurosensory retinal elevation, subretinal exudation, and subretinal hemorrhage.

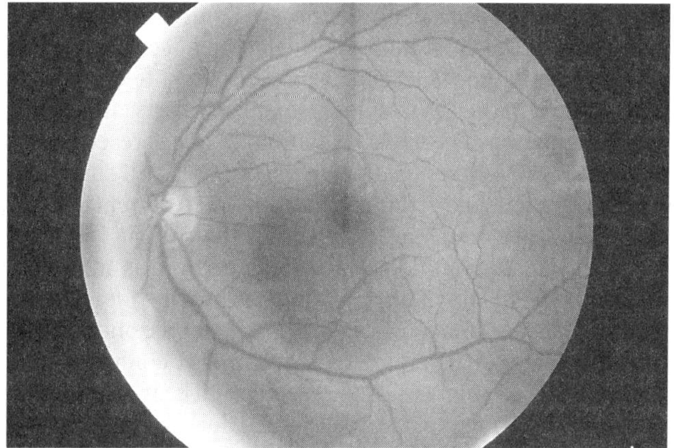

Fig. 176-24. Choroidal nevus.

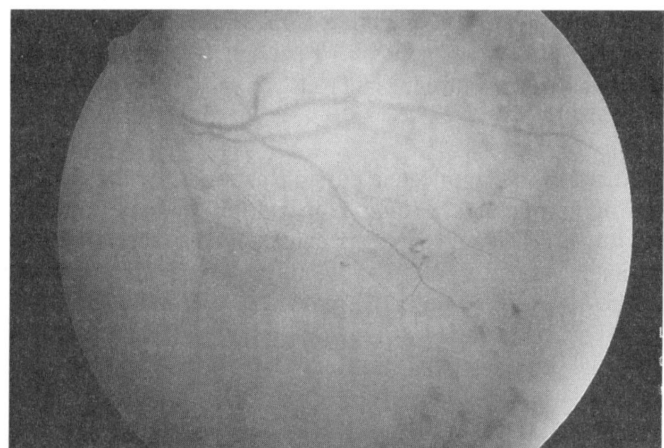

Fig. 176-25. Choroidal melanoma.

Box 176-5. Choroidal Abnormalities

Choroidal Neovascular Membranes (CNVMs)
Angioid streaks
High myopia
Choroidal rupture
Choroidal scar
Idiopathic form

Inflammatory Conditions
Serpiginous choroidopathy
Multifocal choroiditis
Punctate inner choroidopathy

Neoplasms
Nevus
Malignant melanoma
Choroidal metastasis

Large melanomas can show extension through the sclera. Metastatic spread of a choroidal melanoma occurs primarily to the liver and lungs. Once metastasis occurs, life expectancy is less than 1 year. Treatments include observation, laser photocoagulation, cryopexy, radiation, surgical resection, or enucleation. Urgent referral while the tumor is still small may afford the patient and retina specialist more treatment options, which may save some sight as well as the patient's life.

Another malignant condition of the choroid is metastatic disease. Choroidal metastases are primarily amelanotic, multifocal lesions that occur in the posterior pole and result in visual decline. Bilateral involvement is common. The condition affects men and women equally. The most common primary tumors are in the breasts and lungs; less common sites include the kidneys, testicle, prostate, and gastrointestinal tract. Ocular involvement may be the first sign of lung cancer, whereas patients with choroidal metastases from breast cancer usually have already been diagnosed. Although systemic treatment is essential in metastatic disease, ocular radiation may be beneficial in patients whose vision has decreased from choroidal metastases.

REFERRAL

Once symptoms implicate a possible abnormality in retinal or choroidal structures, examination can be directed appropriately. If a confident diagnosis can be made, referral should be made urgently or semiurgently. When the diagnosis cannot be made confidently, referral to the ophthalmologist should be made emergently, within minutes, if the symptoms are acute, or urgently, within 24 hours, if the symptoms are chronic.

ADDITIONAL READINGS

American Academy of Ophthalmology: *Basic and clinical science course,* Section 4, Retina and vitreous, San Francisco, 1987, The Academy.

Davis MD: The natural history of retinal breaks without detachment, *Trans Am Ophthalmol Soc* 71:343, 1973.

Diabetic Retinopathy Study Report Number 3: Four risk factors for severe visual loss in diabetic retinopathy, *Arch Ophthalmol* 97:658, 1979.

Early Treatment Diabetic Retinopathy Study Report Number 2: Treatment techniques and clinical guidelines for photocoagulation of diabetic macular edema, *Ophthalmology* 94:761, 1987.

Endophthalmitis Vitrectomy Study Group: Results of the Endophthalmitis Vitrectomy Study: a randomized trial of immediate vitrectomy and of intravenous antibiotics for the treatment of postoperative bacterial endophthalmitis, Arch Ophthalmol 113:1479, 1995.

Hilton GF, McLean EB, Chuang EL: *Retinal detachment,* San Francisco, 1989, American Academy of Ophthalmology.

Johnson RN, Gass JD: Idiopathic macular holes: observation, stages of formation, and implications for surgical intervention, *Ophthalmology* 95:917, 1988.

Klein R, Klein BEK, Linton KLP: Prevalence of age-related maculopathy: the Beaver Dam Eye Study, *Ophthalmology* 99:933, 1992.

Macular Photocoagulation Study Group: Argon laser photocoagulation for neovascular maculopathy: five-year results from randomized clinical trials, *Arch Ophthalmol* 109:1109, 1991.

Pilkerton AR, Gilbert WS, Perrant LE, et al: Idiopathic preretinal fibrosis: a review of 237 cases, *Ophthalmol Surg* 23:113, 1992.

Schachat AP, Cruess AF: *Ophthalmology,* Baltimore, 1984, Williams & Wilkins.

Shields JA: Counseling the patient with a posterior uveal melanoma, *Am J Ophthalmol* 106:88, 1988.

CHAPTER 177

Neuro-Ophthalmology

Barry Skarf

Vision, and thus the discipline of ophthalmology, involves more than just the eyes and their supporting structures. The eyes form extensive connections with the brain, and normal visual function depends on the development and maintenance of connections to visual, sensory, and motor centers. The field of neuro-ophthalmology deals with those disorders of neurologic function that can affect vision: diseases of the central nervous system (CNS) and of the cranial nerves as well as systemic conditions that affect the CNS. Representative conditions that affect vision through their CNS action include multiple sclerosis, cerebrovascular disease, intracranial and intraorbital tumors, and generalized systemic diseases (e.g., syphilis, sarcoidosis).

Neuro-ophthalmology is divided into two broad divisions: sensory and motor. The *sensory visual system* directly subserves sight; disorders affecting it can cause profound visual disturbances. This system is made up of the retinas, the optic nerves and chiasm, the optic tracts, both lateral geniculate nuclei of the thalamus, the optic radiations (which connect the lateral geniculate nucleus to the visual cortex), and those regions of the cerebral cortex, primarily in the occipital lobe, that subserve vision. Neuro-ophthalmology deals with diseases that affect all portions of this pathway, excluding disorders that involve only the eye and retina. The second division of neuro-ophthalmology involves the *ocular motor system* and its disorders. Essential to the normal function of vision is the ability to execute appropriate, coordinated eye movements. Disturbances of eye movements and of ocular alignment can seriously degrade vision and visual function. The ocular motor system includes the eye muscles and the nerves that control them, as well as the brainstem and cortical centers, which direct eye movements. The principal symptoms that result from ocular motor system disorders are blurring of vision, diplopia, and difficulty achieving or maintaining appropriate fixation.

The neuro-ophthalmologist is concerned with conditions causing visual disturbances for which no obvious intraocular pathology exists. This category includes a variety of transient visual disturbances, functional complaints, and factitious visual loss, as well as conditions that cause optic nerve swelling (edema) and systemic conditions that affect vision and CNS structures.

SENSORY VISUAL SYSTEM

Patient Evaluation

History. Visual loss is the principal manifestation of disease involving the sensory visual system. Patients who note an unexplained change in vision will present to their primary care physician, optometrist, or ophthalmologist. When the change in vision is sudden and dramatic or accompanied by a headache or other systemic disturbance, the physician is consulted preferentially. Usually the visual loss is spontaneous, but a history of trauma and antecedent ocular, neurologic, or systemic disease should be elicited. The visual loss may be transient or persistent and may affect one or both eyes. Loss of central vision and a decrease of peripheral vision may occur. Most important, visual loss may be acute, having occurred instantaneously or over a few days, or it may have developed much more gradually.

Patients with true sensory pathway dysfunction often complain of blurred vision, dim vision, or a decrease in the brightness of colors. Although a detailed history is essential, care must be taken in its interpretation, since patients are often unclear or even incorrect about the nature of their visual loss. For example, a patient with a right homonymous hemianopsia may describe visual loss in the right eye. In fact, the patient has lost vision in the right hemifield of *both* eyes, but this can be determined only through appropriate examinations. Also, a patient claiming acute visual loss in one eye may have been unaware of a gradual loss of vision in the eye until this loss is "discovered" when the good eye is inadvertently covered. The nature of the visual loss, whether transient or permanent, can be invaluable in making a diagnosis and determining suitable management.

Frequently, patients present with transient photopsias or complaints of seeing flashing lights or various other positive visual phenomena not associated with visual loss. These complaints must be taken seriously because they could relate to incipient retinal detachment or retinal tear, migrainous visual auras, or more serious CNS diseases (e.g., arteriovenous malformations, brain tumors).

Examination. Objective clinical findings may be difficult to obtain in neuro-ophthalmic disease. The most reliable sign of monocular visual loss caused by neuro-ophthalmic disease is the relative afferent pupillary defect (Marcus Gunn pupil), as determined by the swinging flashlight test. When this clinical sign is absent in a patient complaining of persistent uniocular visual loss, the examiner should look for an abnormality of the eye itself (e.g., refractive error, media opacity, mild retinal edema). If tests for these conditions are negative, factitious visual loss must be considered. The presence of a relative afferent pupillary defect, however, confirms the patient's visual deficit and is usually indicative of a serious problem (see Chapter 172).

Optic Nerve Disease

Funduscopic examination of the optic nerve heads is an established part of any complete medical examination, especially in patients who complain of headaches, other neurologic problems, or visual disturbances. Abnormal optic nerves can reflect a variety of local, neurologic, and systemic diseases. It is important to emphasize, however, that the optic nerve head may be *abnormal* in only one of three ways: (1) swollen (edematous); (2) pale in color, which is usually a sign of optic atrophy; and (3) morphologically or structurally abnormal or anomalous, such as optic disc cupping in glaucoma and optic disc drusen (calcific bodies embedded within the optic nerve substance). The primary care physician must determine whether the appearance of each optic nerve is normal or abnormal and categorize them appropriately. When visual loss is caused by retrobulbar optic neuropathy (neuritis), the optic nerve head may appear normal. Because optic nerve pathology can be difficult to recognize, consultation with an ophthalmologist or neuro-ophthalmologist should be obtained whenever the appearance of the optic nerve heads is suspect.

Optic Disc Swelling. Disorders associated with optic disc swelling can be divided into those without significant visual loss and those with visual loss.

No Visual Loss. Patients complaining of headache associated with transient visual disturbances may have bilateral disc swelling or edema. Bilateral disc edema usually implies *papilledema,* a term reserved exclusively for disc edema secondary to elevated intracranial pressure (ICP). Visual function is usually preserved, except for enlarged blind spots. Patients may describe shadows or photopsias in the temporal portion of the visual field. Central vision may be slightly disturbed, but patients can usually achieve normal or near-normal acuity. Although true papilledema is usually bilateral, it may be asymmetric. Papilledema should be considered a medical emergency requiring computed tomography (CT) or magnetic resonance imaging (MRI) to rule out an intracranial mass lesion. The patient's medical history must include detailed information on trauma, illness, infection, and other neurologic symptoms. Because papilledema can result from severe hypertension, blood pressure must be checked.

Another common cause of papilledema is pseudotumor cerebri, or *benign intracranial hypertension* (BIH). BIH typically affects middle-aged, overweight women who have had children. Patients with BIH often have headaches, although BIH may occur without headache and may be discovered only when a routine examination reveals papilledema. Because BIH is a diagnosis of exclusion, patients must have MRI or CT scan to rule out an intracranial mass. If a space-occupying lesion is not found, the patient should have a lumbar puncture to obtain cerebrospinal fluid (CSF) for laboratory studies as well as to determine CSF pressure.

Unfortunately, many normal optic nerves appear elevated with blurred margins, giving them a "swollen" appearance. When exaggerated, prominent disc elevation and blurred disc margins represent *pseudopapilledema,* a congenital variation that mimics true papilledema. This anomaly is often associated with intrapapillary calcium deposits known as *optic disc drusen.* The examining physician must distinguish between pseudopapilledema, a benign condition, and papilledema, as well as among other causes of disc edema.

True disc edema, including papilledema, can be recognized because the swollen edge of the optic disc obscures some of the small and medium-sized vessels that transverse the disc margin. This clinical picture can occur relatively early in the development of disc edema before elevation of the disc is obvious. If the optic discs show marked elevation with blurred margins, but all vessels traversing the disc margin (including small capillaries) are well defined and are not obscured by edema, the patient probably has pseudopapilledema. Fluorescein angiography of the fundus, which results in leakage of dye into and around the optic disc, can help distinguish true edema.

Occasionally, unilateral disc swelling, indistinguishable from papilledema, is noted; in rare cases, this can be true papilledema caused by elevated ICP. More frequently, however, it is caused by localized optic nerve disease. Unilateral causes of optic disc edema in the absence of significant visual loss include (1) *compressive optic neuropathies* (i.e., tumor compression of the optic nerve obstructing venous drainage and causing disc swelling) and (2) *papillophlebitis,* an idiopathic condition that usually causes only slight visual loss and mild to moderate disc swelling, mainly in young, otherwise healthy patients. Unilateral optic disc swelling may also result from *ocular hypotony,* which can occur after a perforating injury of the globe, including ocular surgery. This condition is seen most frequently after cataract extraction.

Visual Loss. Patients presenting with visual loss (usually in one eye) and mild to moderate swelling of the optic disc may have a number of different disorders. *Papillitis* is the most common cause of visual loss associated with disc swelling in patients younger than 40. In this form of optic neuritis the anterior portion of the optic nerve becomes inflamed and the optic nerve head is swollen. Occasionally the disc swelling may be accompanied by retinal swelling and exudates, a condition known as *neuroretinitis.* Retrobulbar optic neuritis presents acutely without any change in the appearance of the nerve head. Neuroretinitis, papillitis, and retrobulbar optic neuritis, however, are essentially the same type of inflammatory condition involving different segments of the optic nerve.

Anterior ischemic optic neuropathy (AION) is the most common cause of visual loss associated with optic disc swelling in patients older than 50. This condition represents an acute infarction of the optic nerve head. Typically, patients present with sudden, painless loss of vision in one eye, but mild orbital pain may precede or accompany the event. Both eyes are rarely involved simultaneously. Usually the visual loss is central or altitudinal, but patients may complain of seeing a shadow to one side, above, or below their fixation. The typical fundus appearance shows a swollen optic disc; a portion of the disc is hyperemic, with the remaining portion somewhat paler in appearance. Frequently, one or a few streaky nerve fiber layer hemorrhages surround the disc.

The two major pathologic types of AION are the idiopathic, nonarteritic form and the arteritic form, associated with temporal arteritis. In addition, a variety of vasculitides, coagulopathies, and systemic diseases can contribute to the development of AION (Box 177-1). Occasionally, ischemic optic neuropathy develops within a few days of cataract surgery. All patients with ischemic infarction of the optic disc should undergo the following laboratory tests: complete blood count (CBC), platelets, erythrocyte sedimentation rate (ESR), glucose, antinuclear antibody (ANA), Venereal Disease Research Laboratories (VDRL), prothrombin time (PT), partial thromboplastin time (PTT), and cardiolipin antibodies. Neuroimaging studies are not indicated.

Idiopathic AION is more common than the arteritic form and generally occurs in patients older than 45. Hypertension is an accepted risk factor, a diabetic relationship exists and persons with small, crowded optic discs seem predisposed. AION affects men more than women and results in a permanent visual deficit. Approximately one third of patients experience progressive visual loss, and another one third improve. Recovery is usually modest, although if central vision is involved, substantial improvement in visual acuity can occur.

Although no treatment for AION has proved successful, patients should take one tablet of aspirin daily. Risk factors such as hypertension should be treated appropriately. With time, optic disc swelling subsides, but the patient has residual sectoral optic atrophy. Once visual loss stabilizes, there is little chance of recurrent infarction in the same optic nerve head. Bilateral involvement occurs in approximately 25% of affected individuals, although the second eye may not succumb for months or years.

Box 177-1. Causes of Anterior Ischemic Optic Neuropathy (AION)

Giant cell arteritis
Hypertension
Diabetes mellitus
Atherosclerosis
Migraine
Systemic lupus erythematosus
Polyarteritis nodosum
Syphilis
Carotid occlusive disease
Buerger's disease
Allergic vasculitis
Postviral vasculitis
Postimmunization
Radiation necrosis
Takayasu's disease
Polycythemia vera
Sickle cell disease (trait)
Acute hypotension (shock)
Glucose-6-phosphate dehydrogenase deficiency

AION associated with temporal (giant cell) arteritis is a treatable medical emergency; without appropriate medical management, visual loss can progress rapidly in both eyes, resulting in blindness. This arteritic form of AION occurs in elderly patients, who often appear cachectic. Although known to occur in younger individuals, temporal arteritis is unusual in patients younger than 65. Visual loss in the arteritic form of AION frequently develops in stages and becomes catastrophic with severe reduction in field and acuity. The entire optic disc is swollen and pale. Untreated patients have increased risk of rapid progression with involvement of the second eye.

To identify this treatable condition and to help establish the diagnosis of AION, the primary care physician should obtain an immediate ESR on every patient over 50 who presents with sudden visual loss and a swollen optic disc. The patient should be questioned carefully about constitutional symptoms suggesting temporal arteritis (Box 177-2). Persons in their 70s or 80s are particularly vulnerable, and it is always best to obtain an ESR, even when the diagnosis of AION is uncertain. If temporal arteritis is suspected based on the ESR or clinical history, immediate therapy with oral prednisone (1 mg/kg/day) must be initiated. If the diagnosis is uncertain, it is best to begin treatment (unless steroids are contraindicated) and arrange for a temporal artery biopsy. Histopathologic examination of a segment of the superficial temporal artery usually confirms the diagnosis; in rare situations, however, a normal biopsy may be obtained in a patient with temporal arteritis. Once again, clinical judgment is crucial. The principal goal of therapy is to prevent further visual loss and to preserve vision in the second eye. Unfortunately, high-dose corticosteroids do not promote recovery once vision is lost.

Several features of retinal vein occlusion, which occurs mainly in patients over 40, resemble those seen in AION. Acute visual loss is common, although patients often

Box 177-2. Symptoms and Signs of Temporal Arteritis

- Visual loss
- Amaurosis fugax
- Diplopia
- Headache
- Scalp tenderness
- Jaw claudication
- Tongue claudication
- Difficulty talking
- Numbness, burning dysesthesias of tongue
- Intermittent arm claudication
- Myalgias
- Anorexia
- Weight loss
- Fever
- Malaise
- Vertebrobasilar insufficiency
  - Vertigo
  - Deafness
  - Tinnitus
  - Ataxia
- Dementia
- Angina pectoris
- Ischemic optic neuropathy
- Central retinal artery occlusion
- Ocular motor paresis
- Cyanosis, blanching necrosis of tongue
- Swollen, tender temporal artery
- Absent temporal artery pulse
- Decreased upper extremity blood pressure or pulse

complain of a "sputtering" of their vision before they develop a persistent visual deficit. Fundus examination reveals a swollen disc with peripapillary hemorrhages. The veins are extremely dilated, but unlike AION, the hemorrhages extend along the affected vascular tree outward toward the periphery. If the central vein is involved, multiple hemorrhages are scattered along both upper and lower arcades of the fundus. If a branch vein is occluded, hemorrhage is found only in the territory of the involved branch.

Papillophlebitis is a milder form of vein occlusion that occurs in younger individuals. It is characterized by moderate swelling of the optic discs, moderate engorgement of the veins, and a few hemorrhages. Visual deficits are usually minimal.

All patients with retinal venous occlusive disease should be examined for causes of increased serum viscosity, including dysproteinemia, polycythemia, hemoglobinopathy, diabetes, and leukemia. These patients are at risk for developing a secondary form of glaucoma and must be followed closely by an ophthalmologist.

Neoplasms can cause optic nerve swelling and loss of vision through a variety of mechanisms. Externally, they compress the optic nerve causing venous congestion, which in turn leads to disc swelling. Primary optic nerve tumors (meningiomas or gliomas) can produce the same effect (see later). Leukemia, lymphoma, and meningeal carcinomatosis may infiltrate the optic nerve causing optic disc swelling either by direct tumor extension into the optic nerve head or by producing venous congestion. Visual loss occurs rapidly with optic nerve infiltration but may be gradual and insidious when there is optic nerve compression. Optic nerve swelling and visual loss also can occur in advanced dysthyroid ophthalmopathy when greatly enlarged extraocular muscles compress the optic nerve at the apex of the orbit. Any patient with optic nerve swelling and visual loss who does not fit a typical description of optic neuritis or ischemic optic neuropathy should undergo neuroimaging studies, as should any patient with a history of slowly progressive visual loss over weeks to months.

Leber's hereditary optic neuropathy superficially resembles papillitis. It tends to occur in young healthy individuals, who present with subacute visual loss and optic nerve swelling. Several features, however, differentiate this condition from optic neuritis. Visual loss is always painless and optic nerve hyperemia is marked, with engorgement of the peripapillary capillaries and small retinal vessels. The contralateral optic nerve may appear swollen as well, even when visual function is normal. At a minimum the small vessels in the contralateral peripapillary region are prominent. Leber's neuropathy is transmitted by mitochondrial deoxyribonucleic acid (DNA) from mothers to their children (never through the paternal line). Men are twice as likely to be affected as women. Several markers on mitochondrial DNA have been linked to Leber's hereditary optic neuropathy. Patients with bilateral visual loss from optic neuropathy have tested positive for these markers, even in the absence of the characteristic fundus appearance. The second eye is almost always affected within weeks to months; however, the visual loss may be asymmetric. Patients tend to have permanent central visual loss, although some improve several years after the acute episode. Patients may have a cardiac myopathy, and an electrocardiogram (ECG) should be obtained to rule out a preexcitation syndrome. No effective treatment exists for Leber's hereditary optic neuropathy.

Optic Atrophy. *Retrobulbar optic neuritis* is one of the most common causes of subacute visual loss in young adults, especially young women ages 18 to 45, although it also occurs in older individuals. Pain and discomfort in or around the affected eye, often exacerbated by eye movements, are common symptoms. A few days after the onset of ocular discomfort, the patient generally notes progressively decreasing visual acuity. This disturbance can vary from mild blurring or dimming of vision, with colors taking on a washed-out appearance, to complete blindness. Visual field deficits and an afferent pupillary defect are present in the affected eye. In acute retrobulbar optic neuritis, examination of the fundus is completely normal, with no evidence of swelling or pallor of the optic disc. Papillitis and neuroretinitis are also forms of optic neuritis, but in adults these forms occur much less frequently than the retrobulbar form. Clinically, however, all forms of optic neuritis have similar natural histories. After a few weeks, most patients notice improving vision, followed by slow recovery for up to 1 year. Optic atrophy usually develops after a few weeks.

Retrobulbar optic neuritis is closely associated with multiple sclerosis. Frequently, questioning reveals a relationship to systemic demyelinating disease. Other patients may have no previous history, but MRI shows multiple small lesions scattered in the brain's white matter. A positive MRI may indicate the development of multiple sclerosis in otherwise idiopathic cases of optic neuritis.

Treatment of retrobulbar optic neuritis is still controversial. Results of the Optic Neuritis Treatment Trial sponsored by the National Institutes of Health (NIH) have shown that oral steroids are of no value but that intravenous (IV) methylprednisolone can promote a more rapid recovery and may delay the development of multiple sclerosis. The established dose is 250 mg of IV methylprednisolone every 6 hours for 3 days, followed by 11 days of oral prednisone (1 mg/kg/day). The prednisone is then tapered. Vision usually begins to improve within 1 month with or without treatment. Patients who do not improve within 6 weeks or who continue to worsen after the first 2 weeks should be investigated fully for other causes of optic neuropathy.

Gliomas of the visual pathway, including optic nerve and chiasm, are primarily childhood phenomena frequently associated with neurofibromatosis. Proptosis, visual loss, disc swelling, or optic atrophy may occur; however, not all optic nerve and chiasmal gliomas produce visual deficits. Some cause asymptomatic optic nerve enlargement that can remain stable for many years.

Optic nerve sheath meningiomas are the second major primary tumor of the optic nerve. They are most prevalent in young to middle-aged women but can occur in older individuals. Although they tend to occur in an older population than gliomas and usually have a distinct radiologic appearance, occasionally it may be difficult to differentiate between the two tumors. Patients with optic nerve sheath meningiomas usually present with proptosis and slowly progressive visual loss. Optic disc swelling, optic atrophy, and optociliary shunt vessels on the optic disc are common.

Treatment of primary optic nerve tumors remains controversial and depends on the extent of visual loss and location of the tumor. Management of these tumors is best referred to a neuro-ophthalmologist or neurosurgeon familiar with current treatment.

Intracranial meningiomas growing along the sphenoid ridge or plane frequently involve the chiasm and optic nerves. They may infiltrate the orbit along the optic nerve sheath and can compress optic nerve, causing swelling and visual loss similar to that seen with primary optic nerve sheath meningiomas. En plaque meningiomas are particularly common in women between 40 and 60 years of age. They may be associated with hyperostosis, which can lead to proptosis, often the presenting sign. Neuroimaging is mandatory, and the patient should be referred to a neurosurgeon once the diagnosis is made.

Optic atrophy is thought to be present from birth. Mild to moderate reduction in visual acuity and decreased color vision are common. Both eyes usually are affected symmetrically, but some variation may be present. Family members are affected in a dominantly inherited pattern. Expression of the abnormality is variable, with some patients manifesting only a mild color vision deficit and better than 20/100 vision. Those with more severe disease may develop nystagmus.

Nutritional optic neuropathy is typically associated with inadequate B-complex vitamins and folate in the diet. These nutritional factors are frequently exacerbated by excessive consumption of alcohol and use of tobacco products, producing classic tobacco-alcohol amblyopia. Most significant, however, is the nutritional inadequacy that usually accompanies a diet in which most calories are obtained from alcohol. Resultant visual loss, usually central, can be rapid or insidious.

Toxic optic neuropathy can result from exposure to a variety of drugs and toxic substances. The extensive list of causative medications and environmental substances includes many chemotherapeutic agents (e.g., vincristine, mevatricate, BCNU), ethambutol, fluoroquinolones, isoniazid, quinine, streptomycin, and sulfacetamides. Among the environmental toxins are ethylene glycol mercury and methyl alcohol. To diagnose toxic optic neuropathy, patients must be questioned carefully about their working environment, medications, and drug and alcohol use.

Toxic and nutritional optic neuropathies are typically bilateral and symmetric. If unilateral involvement occurs, another diagnosis should be suspected. In addition to central visual loss, there may be generalized constriction of the visual field. Optic atrophy can develop, color vision is lost, and visual acuity may decrease to recognition of hand movements only. In nutritional amblyopia, visual acuity can improve if proper diet is restored.

Traumatic optic neuropathies occur after closed head injuries or skull fractures. Although the ocular examination may be normal, sudden or subacute visual loss occurs. Visual loss in closed head injury is attributed to shearing forces at the optic canal or microfractures in the skull base that produce optic nerve ischemia and swelling in the canal. When visual loss is sudden, recovery is unlikely. Visual recovery is more likely with subacute visual loss, which can develop within hours to days after injury. Aggressive treatment with IV corticosteroids or surgical decompression of the optic canal may benefit patients with progressive visual loss documented over time.

Radiation optic neuropathy occurs months to years after radiotherapy treatment for primary or secondary intracranial tumors. Because visual loss is typically delayed, a relationship to radiation therapy is not always apparent. Usually the only finding is decreased vision, with a field defect and mild optic disc pallor indicating atrophy. In acute cases, disc pallor may be absent initially. Physicians should consider radiation optic neuropathy in any patients with a history of radiotherapy to the head. When the eyes have been included in the irradiated field, the diagnosis becomes easier because characteristic radiation retinopathy, with neovascularization, microaneurysms, soft exudate, and arteriolar narrowing, is associated with optic disc pallor. Usually the dose of radiation must exceed 5000 cGy. No effective treatment can reduce radiation injury to the optic nerves.

Optic Nerve Anomalies. Congenital anomalies that alter the appearance of the optic nerve head can create diagnostic confusion. Some of these anomalies are associated with reduced vision or visual field defects, complicating the diagnosis even more. The most common and important anomaly is *pseudopapilledema* (see earlier), in which the optic nerve head appears elevated and enlarged with blurred margins. Moderate blind spot enlargement and subtle field defects also may be present. Unlike papilledema, however, pseudopapilledema is not associated with elevated ICP, the retinal venules are not distended, and spontaneous venous pulsations are frequently present. In pseudopapilledema, hemorrhages around the optic nerve are very unusual. Pseudopapilledema is usually bilateral and benign, reflecting a local process at the optic nerve head and not intracranial pathology. Often, optic disc drusen are noted, and the diagnosis is straightforward; otherwise, distinguishing pseudopapilledema from papilledema can be difficult. An expert opinion should be obtained before proceeding with an extensive neuroradiologic investigation.

Other congenital anomalies that affect the shape and size of the optic disc develop when the eye and optic nerve are formed. These include tilted optic discs, optic nerve colobomas and pits, and hypoplasia (congenitally underdeveloped optic nerves). Each anomaly has a characteristic morphology and spectrum of severity. Eyes with the worst anomalies also may be associated with developmental CNS abnormalities and usually have poor vision. Mildly anomalous optic nerves are compatible with normal acuity and mild to moderate peripheral visual field defects. An optic disc anomaly should be suspected when the optic discs appear abnormal in an otherwise healthy individual with no complaints, especially when the rest of the examination is unremarkable and the condition is bilateral and fairly symmetric. Except for the unusual optic disc appearance, the fundus shows no evidence of swelling, hemorrhage, infarct, or edema.

Chiasmal Compression and Syndrome

Most lesions at the optic chiasm are compressive, producing visual loss in both eyes. The most common cause of chiasmal compression is a pituitary tumor arising from within the sella turcica and extending upward to stretch and compress the chiasm. Most pituitary tumors are adenomas. In premenopausal women they cause amenorrhea and are discovered early, usually before producing any visual loss. In contrast, nonsecreting pituitary tumors and those in men and postmenopausal women are usually not detected until they produce visual loss. Other tumors (e.g., craniopharyngiomas, meningiomas, gliomas, aneurysms) also cause a similar pattern of visual loss by compressing the chiasm. Pituitary tumors cause slowly progressive, painless, usually asymmetric visual loss and characteristic bilateral, typically bitemporal and asymmetric visual field defects that assume several forms. Occasionally, if hemorrhage or infarction occurs within a pituitary tumor, visual loss can be rapid and associated with severe headache and even loss of consciousness (pituitary apoplexy).

Patients with pituitary tumor often present with endocrinologic disturbances such as amenorrhea and galactorrhea (women) or impotence and decreased libido (men). A hormonal workup, particularly for prolactin levels, is critical in evaluating patients with suspected pituitary tumor. Patients must be asked about endocrine functions (e.g., menstrual cycles), symptoms of acromegaly, and thyroid dysfunction. When the condition has evolved slowly, the optic nerves appear atrophic, and occasionally a characteristic horizontal band of atrophy may be noted across the optic disc. Changes in the optic nerve may be subtle, even in the presence of a large visual field defect. A normal-appearing optic nerve suggests a good potential for visual recovery, often after surgical decompression in patients with a chiasmal syndrome. Occasionally, tumors of this region may extend into the patient's cavernous sinus, causing palsies of the third, fourth, and sixth cranial nerves and resulting in diplopia.

All patients suspected of having chiasmal syndrome must undergo formal perimetry. If perimetry confirms a characteristic pattern of visual field loss, usually bitemporal, with some portion of the field deficit in at least one eye respecting the vertical meridian, the next step is neuroimaging. MRI is generally more effective than CT in evaluating lesions of the chiasmal region. If a pituitary tumor is demonstrated, management depends on tumor size and whether it secretes prolactin. Prolactin-secreting adenomas can be treated with bromocriptine, which should shrink the tumor and improve symptoms. When this treatment is inappropriate or inadequate, however, a neurosurgeon should be consulted. Most pituitary tumors, even those with marked suprasellar extension, can be decompressed via a transsphenoidal approach. Depending on the degree of optic atrophy and type of tumor involved, vision often improves after treatment. Some patients, however, require lifetime hormonal replacement.

Although chiasmal compression by extrinsic tumor is the most common cause of the chiasmal syndrome, visual loss at the chiasm also may result from compression by an aneurysm, mucocele, abscess, or glioma (chiasmal or hypothalamic). Demyelinating lesions of the optic chiasm, ischemic and traumatic lesions, traction from chiasmal arachnoiditis, postradiation neuropathy, and prolapse of the chiasm into an empty sella may also be associated with visual loss.

Postchiasmatic Disease

Retrochiasmal lesions involving the optic tract, optic radiations, and cerebral cortex produce *homonymous hemianopsia.* These lesions can be caused by stroke, tumor, vascular malformations, demyelinating lesions, and abscesses. Patients who develop a partial or complete homonymous hemianopsia may be unaware of the extent of their visual loss. They may have a vague sense of visual disturbance on the affected side, which they may attribute to a problem with the ipsilateral eye. They may complain of difficulty reading or of bumping into objects on that side. Visual acuity is unaffected in unilateral hemispheric lesions. Occasionally, patients with a tumor or an arteriovenous malformation will experience visual hallucinations contralateral to the affected hemisphere. These may resemble migrainous aura but are always present on the same side. Visual field examination is mandatory in the diagnosis of retrochiasmal disease. Thus patients with normal visual acuity should be referred for visual field testing if they complain of difficulty reading or difficulty with vision to one side. A visual field obtained on confrontation often can establish the diagnosis with minimal effort.

Although a complete homonymous hemianopsia is nonlocalizing, partial hemianopsias can localize the lesion to the temporal, parietal, or occipital lobes. Visual field defects produced by occipital lesions are exquisitely congruent in both eyes. Patients with occipital lobe lesions also may demonstrate macular sparing; that is, they may have a complete hemianopsia except for a small region of the hemifield extending from central fixation into the hemianopic field. This condition occurs when an infarction of the occipital cortex spares the most posterior portion of the occipital lobe, which is quite common in strokes of this region. Macular sparing is virtually pathognomonic for an infarction of the occipital cortex. Cortical blindness can result from bilateral occipital lobe lesions. When the patient denies blindness, the condition is termed *Anton's syndrome.* Temporal lobe lesions tend to produce visual field defects that are more dense superiorly in the visual field; parietal lobe lesions tend to produce defects that are denser inferiorly. Temporal and parietal defects are less congruent than those produced by occipital lobe lesions and are usually associated with other neurologic deficits. The least congruent homonymous hemianopsias result from lesions of the optic tract, which occur infrequently.

CT scan, or preferably MRI, is required in any patient who has a complete or partial homonymous hemianopsia. These examinations usually demonstrate an infarct, tumor, or other CNS lesion. Appropriate management of these neurologic conditions can then be arranged.

Transient and Subjective Visual Disturbances

Patients frequently complain of transient, temporary, and vague visual disturbances that frighten or concern them. It is important to distinguish potentially serious disturbances from the multitude of symptoms that are usually benign. Because objective signs are rare and symptoms frequently have passed, physicians must rely on the patient's history of the event(s).

The duration of the visual disturbance is critical. Momentary spots or flashes of light indicate vitreous traction or a retinal tear but are not characteristic of pathology along the retrobulbar visual pathway. Transient visual obscurations lasting less than a minute can occur in papilledema. Transient monocular visual loss that results from vascular occlusion of the retinal or optic nerve circulation (amaurosis fugax) usually lasts several minutes but may last a half hour. The positive and negative visual disturbances that accompany migraine typically last 15 to 20 minutes. They rarely last less than 5 minutes or more than 45 minutes.

Although it is crucial to determine whether the visual loss is monocular or binocular, patients often are unable to make this determination. Patients may also attribute visual loss in one hemifield to a visual disturbance in the ipsilateral eye. For these reasons, care must be taken in interpreting patient descriptions.

The mode of onset and evolution of the visual disturbance further define the pathophysiology. Common symptoms in patients with visual disturbances include dimming or darkening of vision in all or part of the visual field, photopsias, shimmering lights, rings, and arcs of light that can obscure vision. The patient's activity at the onset, changes during the visual loss, and nature and duration of the recovery help define the visual disturbance. Also, neurologic symptoms (e.g., lightheadedness, weakness, numbness, paresthesias, dizziness, unsteadiness) can help localize the disturbance to the anterior or posterior visual pathway.

Amaurosis fugax usually is caused by carotid artery stenosis, which produces decreased vascular perfusion of the retina and optic nerve. The carotid artery also can be a source of platelet-fibrin emboli, which may obstruct the central retinal artery or any of its branches. Patients complain of "darkening" or dimming of vision. They often describe a curtain or shade that may rise or fall to obscure part or all of the vision in the affected eye. The onset is usually rapid, and the episode may last seconds or minutes. On examination, whitish Hollenhorst plaques may be seen in the retinal circulation. When amaurosis fugax is suspected, patients should report any symptoms suggestive of other transient ischemic attacks, with or without visual loss. Frequently, vascular risk factors, including stroke, are present. Transient neurologic symptoms (paresthesia, weakness) or a carotid bruit may indicate a high-grade stenosis of the carotid artery. These patients are at significant risk of stroke and permanent visual loss. Management requires a complete cardiovascular and cerebrovascular workup and possible treatment with antiplatelet agents, anticoagulants, or endarterectomy.

When similar episodes of transient monocular visual loss occur in a young person in the absence of any risk factors, they can be attributed to retinal migraine. Transient visual loss in retinal migraine is thought to be produced by vasospasm of the retinal artery and is rarely associated with risk of permanent deficit. Carotid artery dissection, which can cause similar transient visual loss, must be excluded. Patients presenting with transient photopsias describe flashing lights or spots of light in one eye that last moments but occur sporadically. They should be asked whether their symptoms are more noticeable in the dark and whether they are aggravated by head or eye movement. Movements that induce flashes suggest vitreous traction on the retina or, more seriously, retinal tear or detachment. These patients should be referred immediately for dilated ophthalmologic examination, even when they have normal vision and no other complaints.

Photopsias that last from 5 to 45 minutes more typically represent migrainous phenomena. They usually are binocular but can be monocular if caused by retinal migraine. Patients typically refer binocular photopsias occurring in one hemifield to the ipsilateral eye. A typical history for a migraine is a scintillating scotoma or fortification scotoma that expands or contracts, lasts 15 to 40 minutes, and is followed by a headache. Patients not currently experiencing headache must report any history of migrainelike headaches. In older patients, migrainelike symptoms can be caused by vertebrobasilar insufficiency, although this problem is usually associated with other neurologic symptoms (e.g., dizziness, ataxia, diplopia). If the episodes are always unilateral, an arteriovenous malformation or other intracranial pathology must be suspected, and neuroimaging studies should be ordered.

Patients who complain of blurred vision that changes from day to day may have diabetes, with a fluctuating, poorly controlled blood sugar level. Other causes of bilateral blurred vision are vasculopathies, hyperviscosity and hypercoagulation syndromes, and seizures.

Patients may report a variety of visual experiences in which they see distorted or illusory objects as well as hallucinations. Visual illusions and distortions are the altered visual perception of real objects. These phenomena can arise from optical as well as central mechanisms. *Hallucinations,* on the other hand, are visual perceptions that have no basis in reality. They are generated centrally, although they may be triggered by an external sensory stimulus. They may be related to seizure disorders, intake of a variety of medications and toxic substances, various disease processes, or altered states of consciousness.

Occasionally a patient presents with factitious visual loss, which may be psychogenic or may represent malingering. Differentiation of factitious visual loss from true deficits caused by organic disturbances can be difficult. Primarily the physician must demonstrate that the pattern of visual loss is inconsistent with normal physiologic constraints by uncovering various inconsistencies in the pattern and degree of visual dysfunction. The physician must rule out an underlying organic defect and demonstrate that visual function exceeds that claimed by the patient.

OCULAR MOTOR SYSTEM

An intact ocular motor system is essential for normal vision. Eye movements are responsible for capturing and locking onto a visual object of interest and for maintaining fixation on that object even during head and body movements. This requires an elaborate supranuclear control system involving extensive connections among the visual, vestibular, and oculomotor centers. Disturbances of this system profoundly affect vision and bring patients to their physicians with complaints of double vision, blurred vision, jumpy vision, and more general complaints of unsteadiness, dizziness, and vertigo.

Functions

The functions of the ocular motor system can be categorized into five subgroups: saccades, fixation, smooth pursuit movements, vestibuloocular mechanism, and vergence mechanism. *Saccades* are rapid eye movements that are used to refixate from one object of regard to another. They rapidly execute a foveation reflex, which captures items of interest onto the fovea. The *fixation mechanism* enables the maintenance of foveation or fixation on an object once it has been "captured." *Smooth pursuit movements* are slow movements that allow an object to be followed as it moves from place to place. The *vestibuloocular mechanism* produces reflex eye movements driven by the semicircular canals, which detect head movement. A combination of the smooth pursuit, fixation, and vestibuloocular mechanisms allows continued steady fixation of moving targets during head or whole body movement. All these mechanisms generate conjugate eye movements; that is, they move both eyes equally and symmetrically in the same direction. In contrast, the *vergence mechanism* produces disconjugate movement, principally horizontal, which adjusts the position of the two eyes with respect to each other so that fixation is maintained by both eyes on the object of interest. During normal activity, all these mechanisms operate simultaneously to produce a seamless pattern of eye movements.

Evaluation. To evaluate oculomotor function clinically, it is best to test each of these mechanisms separately. Fixation maintenance and smooth pursuit mechanisms are tested by asking the patient to fixate on a target while slowly moving the target to extreme positions of gaze. During this process it is important to observe the steadiness of eye position and fixation. If the target motion is slow and steady, any instability in eye movement is abnormal, except in the most extreme positions, where physiologic nystagmus can occur. Saccades can be tested by having patients refixate back and forth from a central to a peripheral target held successively up, down, and to each side. The vestibuloocular reflex can be tested by having the patient make rapid head movements (side to side and up and down) while fixating on a distant target. This test does not rely only on the vestibuloocular reflex because visual feedback exists; if head movements are rapid, however, the principal mechanism driving the eye movements is vestibular. Vergence mechanisms can be tested by having a patient refixate between distant and near targets. When evaluating the oculomotor system, ocular alignment must also be tested by covering first one eye and then the other while looking for movement of the uncovered eye. This test should be performed with the eyes in the primary position and to the left, right, up, and down.

Symptoms

Double vision, or *diplopia,* is one of the most frequent complaints related to the oculomotor system. Diplopia can be monocular or binocular; therefore the physician should determine whether double vision disappears when one eye is covered. If double vision persists with monocular viewing, the patient has *monocular diplopia,* which is never caused by an oculomotor disturbance. Various optical and ocular diseases can combine to cause monocular diplopia; infrequently it can result from CNS pathology. True *binocular diplopia* always disappears when either eye is covered. Occasionally, patients do not recognize diplopia and simply complain of blurred vision or of letters, print, or sentences running together.

Once it is determined that a patient has true binocular diplopia, the patient should be asked (1) whether two perceived images are displaced horizontally, vertically, or obliquely; (2) whether one image is tilted with respect to the other; (3) which direction of gaze results in the greatest separation of the images and which produces the least; and (4) whether the diplopia is worse at distance or at near. Typically, lateral rectus muscle weakness produces an *esodeviation* (inturning eye), which is worse at distance; weakness of the medial rectus muscle produces an *exodeviation* (outturning eye), which is worse at near. However, patients may be troubled more by double images close to each other than by those widely separated. Diplopia is most frequently caused by a benign process and often resolves spontaneously; however, it also can be a medical emergency. Therefore any patient who presents with acute diplopia must be evaluated immediately by a neuro-ophthalmologist or neurologist.

Nystagmus (an involuntary rhythmic oscillation of the eyes) is a cardinal sign of oculomotor dysfunction. Often, patients do not recognize that they have nystagmus, which is discovered by friends or family. These patients typically complain of blurred vision or actual jumpiness of objects, a phenomenon termed *oscillopsia.*

Oculomotor dysfunction and diplopia also may cause unsteadiness or a sense of dizziness or may be associated with true vertigo. In certain oculomotor disorders, patients may have difficulty looking to either side or up or down and difficulty looking at their feet or at a plate of food. Appropriate questioning is often necessary to reveal a history of this type of disorder. The patient may complain of difficulty reading, but when tested, visual acuity at distance and near will be perfect. Reading is adversely affected by the patient's inability to make precise movements from one word to another. This problem can occur with oculomotor disturbances that affect saccadic eye movements.

Disorders of Ocular Motility

Disturbances of eye movement can be divided topographically into two categories: infranuclear disorders and central or supranuclear disorders. Infranuclear disorders result from lesions in the cranial nerves, extraocular muscles, or the tissue supporting the eyes and their muscles. They frequently affect only one eye and generally present with diplopia. Central disorders upset the control of eye movements and create problems with conjugate gaze. That is, they affect the saccadic, pursuit, or convergence movements of both eyes and may upset the balance or alignment between them.

Infranuclear Disorders

Orbital and Systemic Diseases. Diseases that involve the orbital contents can cause disturbances in ocular motility. They can restrict the range of normal eye movements both mechanically and physiologically, producing diplopia.

Thyroid ophthalmopathy is the most common disease affecting orbital tissues and resulting in oculomotor symptoms. This condition occurs in a high percentage of patients with Graves' disease; however, approximately 10% of patients with thyroid ophthalmopathy are clinically euthyroid. Typical signs of thyroid ophthalmopathy include exophthalmos, lid retraction, lid lag, and limitation of eye movement, particularly on attempted upgaze. Patients may or may not have a previous history of thyroid disease. Thyroid ophthalmopathy may simulate other causes of ophthalmoplegia. Typically, however, the abnormal eye movement cannot be explained on the basis of a single or even multiple oculomotor nerve palsies. The diagnosis is established by endocrine investigation, by other signs of hyperthyroidism, and by restriction of eye movements and enlargement of the eye muscles on CT scan of the orbits. Thyroid ophthalmopathy can pose difficult management problems. Sensory visual function and diplopia must be monitored carefully by an ophthalmologist with experience in managing and treating this condition.

Besides thyroid disease, other causes of mechanically restricted eye movements include orbital trauma, most often an orbital floor fracture and entrapment of the inferior rectus muscle. The medial rectus muscle also can be caught in a medial wall fracture. Infiltrative diseases (inflammatory or neoplastic) can enlarge one or more orbital muscles, causing limitation of eye movement. Orbital myositis can involve one muscle or several muscles and is associated with pain and discomfort. Orbital pseudotumor is a more extensive inflammatory condition affecting the eye muscles, as well as other orbital soft tissue, causing severe pain and limitation of movement. Less frequently the muscles and soft tissues of the orbit may become infiltrated with lymphoma or an inflammatory process such as sarcoidosis, polymyositis, or Wegener's granulomatosis. Neoplasm can infiltrate the orbit by direct extension from adjacent sinuses and periorbital tissues or by metastatic spread from distant sites.

Chronic Progressive External Ophthalmoplegia (CPEO). CPEO is a group of syndromes that result in gradual loss of eye movements. Progressive bilateral ptosis is an early sign, with patients developing a generalized ophthalmoplegia over many years. Diplopia may not occur because the eyes can remain aligned in the primary position, although their movements become extremely limited. A variety of associated conditions coexist with CPEO, including heart block, pigmentary retinopathy, ataxia, myopathy, and weakness elsewhere. Patients may complain only of bilateral ptosis and may have a vague sense of difficulty looking to the side. Most forms of chronic, progressive external ophthalmoplegia are related to mitochondrial disease, and muscle biopsy reveals ragged red fibers characteristic of mitochondrial myopathy. Because a risk of heart block and sudden death exists, CPEO is potentially life threatening.

Myasthenia Gravis. A condition that can affect all skeletal muscles, myasthenia gravis is prone to affect the extraocular muscles, particularly those that elevate the eyelids. Isolated ocular myasthenia occurs in 20% of patients and can pose a diagnostic challenge to physicians. Myasthenia gravis can mimic almost any oculomotor disorder, from single-nerve palsies to complete ophthalmoplegias. Its distinguishing characteristics, however, are fatigability and variability. The ptosis that occurs in myasthenia varies with the time of the day and usually worsens toward evening. Patients often relate that their lids open normally in the mornings but become increasingly ptotic as the day progresses. Diplopia, when present, may also worsen later in the day. Fatigue is demonstrated when the examiner has the patient look steadily upward for several minutes, without blinking. The eyelids will gradually descend over the globe in affected individuals. Diplopia, when present, may also worsen later in the day.

Myasthenia gravis results from defective synaptic transmission at the motor end plates because of antibodies to the acetylcholine receptors. The diagnosis can be confirmed by (1) demonstrating an elevation of circulating acetylcholine receptor antibodies; (2) testing with Tensilon, which produces a transient improvement in lid position; or (3) having the patient rest the eyes for a half hour and noting improvement in lid position and ocular alignment. Further confirmation can be obtained by demonstrating characteristic electromyographic disturbances in skeletal or ocular muscles. Definitive diagnosis and treatment are best handled by a neurologist. Treatment is usually oral pyridostigmine (Mestinon), but in resistant cases, corticosteroids or azathioprine can be added. A CT scan of the chest determines whether the thymus gland is enlarged. If it is, surgical resection is recommended.

Oculomotor Palsies. Three paired cranial nerves are responsible for innervating the extraocular muscles and producing eye movements. A dysfunction in any of these nerves can cause diplopia in one or more positions of gaze. Of the numerous causes of such dysfunction, some affect more than one of the nerves, whereas others are specific for a particular nerve. Patients may present with single or multiple nerve palsies that affect movements in one or both eyes.

Sixth nerve palsy. The most easily recognized isolated ocular nerve palsy involves the sixth cranial nerve producing weakness in the ipsilateral lateral rectus muscle. Patients complain of horizontal double vision that worsens when they look toward the side of the affected nerve. On examination a limitation of abduction is seen when the patient looks in the direction of the weak lateral rectus muscle. Lateral rectus weakness can be caused by any of the orbital diseases already described; however, if no evidence suggests orbital involvement, a diagnosis of sixth nerve palsy can be made.

The sixth nerve passes through the cavernous sinus and can be compromised by diseases of this region. Intracavernous carotid artery aneurysm or fistula, meningioma, metastatic disease, infection, and inflammation (e.g., the Tolosa-Hunt syndrome) can cause sixth nerve dysfunction. Nasopharyngeal carcinoma and pituitary tumors also can invade the cavernous sinus from adjacent regions. Tracing the course of the sixth nerve proximally, it turns caudally to descend down the clivus toward the pons. This segment of the nerve can be compromised by tumor, head trauma, or elevated ICP. Meningeal carcinomatosis can also involve the sixth nerve in the prepontine portion of its course. Gradenigo's syndrome, which develops when an otitis media spreads to involve the sixth nerve, occurs principally in children. Finally, CNS disease (e.g., tumor, stroke, multiple sclerosis) can affect the sixth nerve fasciculus within the pons; usually other brainstem structures are involved, with coexisting oculomotor and neurologic abnormalities.

The most common etiology of an acute isolated sixth nerve palsy is idiopathic. Presumably, these cases result from small-vessel infarction along the course of the sixth nerve, most probably in its intracavernous portion. This infarction occurs more frequently in patients with vasculopathic histories, including diabetes and hypertension. Usually, idiopathic sixth nerve palsies resolve spontaneously within 2 to 3 months.

Congenital abnormalities and those acquired early in childhood can sometimes be confused with sixth nerve palsies. Patients with Möbiuss' syndrome may appear to have bilateral sixth nerve palsies, but they also have facial diplegia, clubfoot, branchial malformations, and abnormalities of pectoral muscles. Patients with Duane's syndrome have unilateral or occasionally bilateral absence of the sixth nerve, with limitation of abduction and sometimes adduction. The globe retracts on attempted adduction.

Fourth nerve palsy. The fourth nerve is the only cranial nerve to exit from the dorsal surface of the brain. It leaves the posterior midbrain, crosses to the opposite side, and travels beneath the tentorium and then through the cavernous sinus to innervate the contralateral superior oblique muscle.

Patients with fourth nerve palsy complain of vertical or oblique double vision, which becomes worse when they look downward. They may assume a characteristic head posture in which their head is turned and titled away from the affected side. Because of its relationship to the tentorium, the fourth nerve is subject to physical injury during head trauma, and palsies are often associated with trauma.

Idiopathic fourth nerve palsies, attributed to microvascular infarction along the nerve, usually resolve spontaneously with time. Tumors rarely cause fourth nerve palsy, although myasthenia and orbital disease can occasionally mimic this disorder. Patients with congenital fourth nerve palsies have a long history of abnormal head posture, which can be revealed by examining old photographs. The fourth nerve also can be compromised by the same cavernous sinus and brainstem diseases that produce sixth nerve palsies.

Third nerve palsy. The third nerve is the largest and most important cranial nerve involved with eye movements. It innervates the superior, inferior, and medial rectus muscles, as well as the inferior oblique and levator palpebrae. It also innervates the pupil and ciliary body, producing pupillary constriction and accommodation. Thus a complete third nerve palsy immobilizes most eye movements, although patients often develop a partial third nerve palsy that does not affect all its components. Patients usually complain of horizontal or oblique diplopia but may not have diplopia if the ptotic eyelid covers the eye. In partial third nerve palsies, myasthenia gravis or orbital disease must be considered, especially if the pupil is spared.

Orbital or cavernous sinus diseases can cause third nerve palsies, but typically one or more of the fourth, fifth, or sixth cranial nerves are also involved. Of greatest concern, third nerve palsies may result from compression by an aneurysm of the posterior communicating artery or from uncal herniation. Strokes, demyelinating disease, and brainstem tumors can cause lesions of the third nerve nucleus or fasciculus in the midbrain. These lesions usually produce other neurologic abnormalities. Nuclear lesions produce bilateral ptosis and weakness of the contralateral superior rectus muscle.

One of the most common causes of third nerve palsy is microvascular infarction, which typically spares the pupil; however, some patients can have partial pupillary involvement. Small-vessel infarction tends to affect the interpeduncular or intercavernous portions of the nerve and generally resolves within 2 to 3 months. It is much more common in patients with diabetes, hypertension, and other vasculopathies.

Multiple oculomotor nerve palsies. As previously stated, diseases affecting the cavernous sinus and orbital apex frequently cause multiple oculomotor nerve palsies. The optic nerve and trigeminal nerve also may be involved. These diseases may mimic myasthenia gravis and other orbital diseases that cause multiple extraocular muscle dysfunction. In the absence of clinical signs of these diseases, however, evaluation of the cranial nerves traversing the cavernous sinus and neuroimaging are mandatory when a combination of oculomotor palsies occur. If there is associated pain, inflammatory disease of the cavernous sinus (Tolosa-Hunt syndrome) should be suspected.

Another condition that may produce multiple oculomotor nerve palsies is the Fisher variant of the Guillain-Barré syndrome. Patients develop acute onset of diplopia and ptosis, often after an upper respiratory tract infection, resulting from involvement of multiple extraocular muscles bilaterally. Pupillary involvement is variable and distinguishes this condition from myasthenia gravis. Associated neurologic abnormalities include ataxia and loss of the deep tendon reflexes. The condition resolves spontaneously but may last several months.

Evaluation. Isolated fourth and sixth nerve palsies are rarely emergencies. Microvascular infarction is the most frequent cause in the absence of a history suggesting trauma. Tests include a blood glucose to rule out diabetes and an ESR to check for temporal arteritis in patients older than 50. If myasthenia gravis is considered in the differential diagnosis, a Tensilon test should be arranged and acetylcholine antibodies measured. Neuroimaging studies should be performed only in patients with other cranial nerve involvement or other neurologic abnormalities or with suspected orbital disease. Acute third nerve palsies, on the other hand, can be much more serious, particularly when they are caused by aneurysm. If the pupil is involved, neuroimaging studies and cerebral angiography should be obtained immediately in acute cases. If the pupil is spared, and particularly with a history of diabetes or hypertension, the patient may be observed and a broader differential diagnosis considered. As already indicated, multiple oculomotor nerve palsies are virtually synonymous with cavernous sinus disease. Multiplanar MRI with gadolinium can uncover cavernous sinus involvement that is otherwise difficult to demonstrate. Consideration also must be given to myasthenia gravis and thyroid disease, which mimic multiple oculomotor nerve palsies.

Central (Supranuclear) Disorders. CNS disorders (e.g., stroke, brain tumor) affect the conjugate movements of both eyes and also may disturb the balance or alignment between the eyes and the coordination of eye movements. In contrast, peripheral oculomotor nerve disorders generally affect one eye or, if they involve both eyes, tend to affect them asymmetrically. Eye movement abnormalities produced by lesions in the CNS include disorders of both horizontal and vertical conjugate gaze, skew deviations, ocular dysmetria, and many forms of nystagmus.

Disorders of Conjugate Gaze. Conjugate gaze depends on a flow of impulses from centers in the brain, including the cerebral hemispheres, midbrain, pons, and cerebellum, as well as the pathways that connect them. Thus lesions of the CNS frequently produce disorders of eye movement.

The inability to move both eyes to one side is called a *horizontal gaze palsy;* it results from a lesion in the pons that damages either the ipsilateral paramedian pontine reticular formation (PPRF) or the ipsilateral sixth nerve nucleus. Bilateral lesions in the pons can cause a complete bilateral horizontal gaze palsy while leaving vertical movements preserved. Less complete lesions in this region may result in partial horizontal gaze palsies or in gaze-evoked nystagmus, that is, nystagmus on attempted gaze with rapid beats in the direction of gaze. Usually, other neurologic deficits are present. Hemispheric disorders and those involving the upper brainstem can produce similar horizontal gaze palsies. These are typically transient, however, and usually can be overcome by reflex horizontal eye movements generated by the vestibular nuclei with head movement (doll's eye reflex) or by caloric stimulation.

Vertical gaze depends on intact centers in the midbrain. Diseases that affect the dorsal midbrain produce up-gaze paresis and may also produce light/near dissociation of the pupils and characteristic convergence-retraction nystagmus. In the young patient this condition is typically caused by a pinealoma or hydrocephalus, whereas infarction is more common in older patients. Down-gaze paresis occurs less frequently than up-gaze and results from a bilateral midbrain lesion in the region of the red nuclei. Infarction may precipitate a sudden down-gaze palsy, but difficulty with down-gaze frequently develops slowly in association with Parkinson's disease, progressive supranuclear palsy, and a variety of diffuse neurodegenerative diseases.

Midbrain lesions also can cause a vertical misalignment between the two eyes (skew deviation). *Skew deviation* is a term reserved for vertical oculomotor imbalances that result from supranuclear (i.e., central) disorders. A skew deviation may resemble a fourth nerve palsy superficially but usually does not have all the characteristics. In addition, skew deviations rarely occur in isolation and usually are accompanied by other central disorders of ocular motility and other neurologic signs.

Internuclear ophthalmoplegia (INO) is a common central disorder of ocular motility that results from a lesion of the medial longitudinal fasciculus between the pons and midbrain. It causes weakness of the medial rectus muscle on the ipsilateral side and produces a partial or complete adduction palsy accompanied by abducting nystagmus of the contralateral eye. INO can be unilateral or bilateral and may occur in relative isolation. In young adults and especially women, acute bilateral INO is highly suggestive of multiple sclerosis. Unilateral INO in elderly patients is more typical of a small lacunar infarct and is frequently associated with diabetes, vasculitides (e.g., systemic lupus erythematosus), aneurysm, and other conditions.

Central disorders can selectively disrupt rapid or slow eye movements. Disturbances of rapid refixation eye movement (saccades) produce ocular *dysmetria,* which can cause the patient to undershoot or overshoot the intended visual target. More severe disorders of saccadic movement can generate ocular *flutter* (brief bursts consisting of reversing saccades) and, in the worst cases, *opsoclonus* (back-to-back, continuous unrestrainable saccades, "saccadomania"). Saccadic dysmetria, flutter, and opsoclonus occur in cerebellar and brainstem disease. Specifically, opsoclonus can be a component of a paraneoplastic syndrome such as neuroblastoma in children or oat cell carcinoma in adults. Loss of rapid eye movements occurs in a variety of degenerative disorders, such as Wilson's disease, spinocerebellar degenerations, and progressive supranuclear palsy.

Children may manifest a congenital absence of rapid eye movements called *congenital ocular motor apraxia.* During the first 2 years of life, these children develop head thrusts that compensate for their inability to make normal refixation movements. As indicated earlier, saccadic palsies that occur with lesions in the cerebral hemispheres and brainstem, whether partial or incomplete, also may result in an inability to initiate refixation movements or in slowed or hypometric saccades.

Disorders impairing slow eye movements used in smooth pursuit result in jerky movements termed *saccadic pursuit.* This finding is not always indicative of disease but may be caused by fatigue, drugs, or lack of attention. When asymmetric, saccadic pursuit is likely caused by an organic disease of the brainstem, cerebellum, or parietooccipital junction of the cerebrum.

Vergence system dysfunction is frequently psychogenic, and it may be difficult to separate organic disease from a factitious abnormality. A paresis of convergence can occur after infarction, demyelination, or head trauma. Patients complain of diplopia at near range only and have no obvious limitation or abnormality in their eye movements, except for the inability to converge. When this symptom is of long duration and associated with longstanding reading difficulties, it may be a true convergence insufficiency, which is congenital and not caused by neurologic disease.

Patients who continue to converge, even when attempting to fixate at a distance, may have spasm of the near reflex, which includes convergence spasm, excessive accommodation, and pupillary constriction. Excessive accommodation causes these patients to complain of blurred vision. Although convergence spasm is associated with organic diseases (e.g., neurosyphilis, trauma, encephalitis), it is also related to stress and psychogenic causes.

Divergence palsy occurs rarely and results in the acute onset of esotropia and diplopia, with full preservation of eye movements. It may follow systemic illness and is usually benign and self-limited; however, it also can be caused by demyelinating disease, neurosyphilis, encephalitis, and trauma.

Evaluation. Patients with central disorders of ocular motility may present with vague symptoms that may not easily characterize their oculomotor disturbance. Diplopia may be a prominent symptom, but other patients may complain of blurred vision, difficulty looking to one side, difficulty reading, running together of words, blurred vision when looking to one side, difficulty focusing at near gaze, or jumpiness of targets (oscillopsia). Any time a patient's symptoms suggest a central disorder affecting eye movements, the physician should assess for other neurologic symptoms. A complete oculomotor examination is essential. Fixation must be observed in all positions and a cover test performed to evaluate ocular alignment. The range of eye movements in all directions, steadiness of fixation, saccadic refixations, smooth pursuit movements, and convergence should be tested. Finally, reflex eye movements should be evaluated by observing the doll's head response to head rotation and Bell's phenomenon (elevation of the globe during forced eye closure).

Nystagmus

The term *nystagmus* describes a group of involuntary ocular movements that are rhythmic and oscillatory. The two major categories of nystagmus are *jerk nystagmus,* which consists of a slow phase in one direction followed by a fast phase in the opposite direction, and *pendular nystagmus,* in which movements in both directions are equal in velocity. Ocular oscillations that are involuntary and recurrent but not rhythmic also occur; these are called *nystagmoid movements.*

Physiologic Nystagmus. Extreme gaze in any direction can result in *end-point nystagmus,* a jerk nystagmus with fast phase in the direction of gaze. *Optokinetic nystagmus* is a jerk nystagmus that develops when a subject views a repetitive visual stimulus. The slow phase of the nystagmus occurs when the subject follows the moving target; this phase is interrupted by fast phases as the eyes return to refixate on to another target entering the visual field. *Vestibular-induced nystagmus* can result from the effect of whole-body rotation or caloric stimulation on the semicircular canals.

Congenital Motor Nystagmus. Resulting from a primary oculomotor system abnormality, congenital motor nystagmus may be pendular or jerk. Typically, complex cycles of repetitive eye movements are generated. The amplitude of the nystagmus decreases with convergence. Acuity is mildly reduced, and patients do not complain of oscillopsia.

An early infantile form of nystagmus can result from sensory (visual) deprivation. This sensory form of "congenital" nystagmus usually develops between 2 and 3 months of age in a child with abnormally decreased central vision. Sensory deprivation nystagmus is typically pendular and also may decrease with convergence.

Latent Nystagmus. Demonstrated only when one eye is occluded, latent nystagmus is a jerk form that beats away from the occluded eye. It is seen frequently in children with strabismus and amblyopia and may be bilateral or unilateral.

The physiologic, congenital, and latent forms of nystagmus are benign and differ from the pathologic forms. Patients with congenital or physiologic nystagmus may be unaware of their condition and do not have symptoms of oscillopsia. They may have decreased central vision, but this is longstanding.

Acquired Nystagmus. Most forms of acquired nystagmus produce ocular oscillations that involve both eyes about equally; however, some forms of nystagmus may produce asymmetric nystagmus or exclusive involvement of only one eye. Acquired nystagmus is usually of the jerk form and can be divided into two major subcategories: nystagmus caused by disorders of the peripheral vestibular apparatus and nystagmus caused by disorders of the CNS.

Peripheral nystagmus develops after loss of vestibular function and is usually purely horizontal or horizontal and rotatory. Purely vertical or tortional nystagmus is unusual with peripheral vestibular disease. Peripheral nystagmus is frequently acute in onset and associated with severe vertigo. Symptoms can be recurrent, transient, and last days to weeks but usually resolve with time. Postural effects and hearing deficits can occur. The common causes are infectious disease involving the labyrinth (labyrinthitis) or the vestibular nerve (neuronitis), Meniere's disease, or trauma.

Central nystagmus is much more variable and usually is not associated with severe vertigo. Symptoms may be transient or permanent. The nystagmus may beat in both directions depending on eye position, and in some forms the direction may change over time. Central nystagmus often is a result of a brainstem or cerebellar lesion caused by demyelinating disease, vascular infarction, or tumor.

The pattern of nystagmus has many variations, some of which have particular pathognomonic or localizing significance. Acquired nystagmus should always be investigated by a neurologist, ophthalmologist, or otolaryngologist familiar with its variations. Many rhythmic oscillations, including vertical forms, can affect the eyes and are usually pathognomonic for lesions in specific regions of the brainstem. These special forms of nystagmus include up-beating and down-beating vertical nystagmus, ocular myoclonus, ocular bobbing, convergence-retraction nystagmus, rebound nystagmus, and periodic alternating nystagmus. Some forms of nystagmus respond to medications, but most are resistant to therapy.

The Pupil

Pupillary Response. Observation of the pupillary response is one of the most important components of the routine physical and ophthalmic examinations (see Chapter 172). Pupil size should be evaluated in both bright and dim illumination while the patient fixates on a distant object. Any difference in pupil size *(anisocoria)* should be noted, with particular attention to whether the difference increases in bright or dim light. The light response of each pupil should then be evaluated independently. Next, the pupils are examined for a relative afferent pupillary defect (Marcus Gunn pupil) by alternating a flashlight between eyes while noting pupillary responses. Both eyes must be stimulated equally and symmetrically. If the pupils are unequal initially, it may be helpful to observe the reaction of one pupil to stimulation of the ipsilateral and contralateral eyes during the swinging flashlight test. The examiner also observes pupillary reaction when the eyes converge and accommodate onto a near target. Use of eyedrops and oral medications may affect pupillary response and size.

Dilated or Nonreacting Pupil. If a patient's larger pupil does not constrict well to a light stimulus and the anisocoria increases with greater light levels, the patient has a form of pupillary sphincter palsy. Once local disease in the eye is ruled out (e.g., history of trauma, ocular inflammation), only three causes for dilated pupil remain: (1) compression or other lesion of the third cranial nerve, (2) parasympathetic denervation of the pupil due to injury or lesion in the ciliary ganglion that produces an Adie's pupil, and, (3) pharmacologic block of the pupillary sphincter. Therefore, when confronted with a dilated pupil, the physician must search for other signs of a third nerve palsy, such as ptosis, diplopia, or oculomotor paresis. Even when these conditions are not present, a dilated, sluggish, or nonreactive pupil can be a sign of third nerve compression, which can result from uncal herniation or posterior communicating artery aneurysm. Therefore, if recent in onset or acute, a dilated pupil is considered a medical emergency, particularly when accompanied by headache or other neurologic signs. If the pupil has been dilated for at least a few weeks, however, and the reaction to a near stimulus produces slow constriction, followed by an even slower redilation after the near stimulus is removed, the diagnosis is likely *Adie's pupil,* or *tonic pupil.* This benign condition is usually unilateral but may be bilateral. Adie's pupil is supersensitive to dilute solutions of pilocarpine and can be positively identified if 0.1% pilocarpine constricts the pupil. Patients with tonic pupil may complain of difficulty reading because of accommodative paresis, but usually the dilated pupil is an incidental finding. The condition is believed to result from damage to the ciliary ganglion caused by infectious (viral) or vascular disease.

Sometimes patients introduce substances into the eye that dilate the pupil pharmacologically. These pupils react poorly to both light and near stimulation and do not react to 1% pilocarpine. Thus they can be distinguished from Adie's pupil and the dilated pupil seen with lesions of the third nerve, both of which constrict with pilocarpine. A dilated pupil may also result from direct or indirect trauma. The pupillary sphincter may be damaged during surgery or by penetrating injury or blunt trauma to the globe. Trauma to the iris usually can be detected by slit-lamp examination. Depending on the extent of damage, the pupil may constrict to pilocarpine. Occasionally the pupil remains dilated as a result of previous intraocular disease (e.g., inflammation, rubeosis, trauma, surgery). Other less common causes of an unreactive pupil are congenital anomalies, central iris atrophy, and tumors involving the anterior chamber.

Constricted or Small Pupil. If the two pupils are unequal in size and the pupillary light reaction appears normal, the anisocoria is physiologic or the patient may have Horner's syndrome. Physiologic anisocoria occurs in 20% of the normal population. Also, many elderly individuals have involutional ptosis, which also may be asymmetric.

Horner's syndrome is characterized by a slight ptosis of the ipsilateral upper lid and a minor elevation of the lower lid causing narrowing of the palpebral fissure. Patients may complain that their eye appears smaller. In addition to the ptosis and miosis, patients with Horner's syndrome may have anhydrosis (decreased sweating on the ipsilateral forehead region). Horner's syndrome is suspected by observing an increase in anisocoria in dim light and a decrease in bright light. Pharmacologic testing for Horner's syndrome is performed by instilling 4%, 5%, or 10% cocaine drops in both eyes. Normal pupils dilate over 40 minutes, but in Horner's syndrome the pupil dilates much less, if at all. Thus the anisocoria increases. The response to cocaine may be minimal in both eyes of patients with dark irides. If the anisocoria does not increase with the cocaine test, the patient does not have Horner's syndrome. If the anisocoria increases after instillation of cocaine, the diagnosis of Horner's syndrome is confirmed, implying a lesion of the sympathetic pathway. Hydroxyamphetamine (1% drops) can be used on a subsequent visit to determine whether the lesion in the sympathetic pathway is preganglionic or postganglionic. Postganglionic lesions are distal to the superior cervical ganglion, whereas preganglionic lesions are more proximal or central. Hydroxyamphetamine does not dilate a miotic pupil resulting from a postganglionic lesion but does dilate the pupil if there is a preganglionic lesion.

Horner's syndrome is frequently observed in asymptomatic patients and may be longstanding. It is helpful to review old photographs of the patient to determine the duration of the ptosis and the anisocoria. Congenital Horner's syndrome can result from birth trauma, but it is also associated with a lightly pigmented iris on the affected side. In the absence of a history of birth trauma, a child with Horner's syndrome should undergo radiologic studies to exclude the presence of a tumor in the mediastinum or cervical region. In adults a postganglionic Horner's syndrome is almost always benign and is frequently associated with a history of migraine headaches. Preganglionic lesions are more ominous and are often a result of neoplasm affecting the cervical region or brainstem. Because preganglionic lesions can be a sign of internal carotid dissection, a high order of suspicion is appropriate when a patient presents with severe radiating neck pain, headache, and new-onset Horner's syndrome.

When caused by a central lesion, Horner's syndrome usually is associated with other neurologic abnormalities. Patients with preganglionic lesions therefore require a complete neurologic examination, including neck and thyroid gland. Imagining studies of the mediastinum, neck, and brain are recommended to rule out neoplasm. If carotid dissection is suspected, magnetic resonance angiography selective cerebral arteriography is required. If old photographs establish that the Horner's syndrome has been present for years, however, investigation is not indicated, even in preganglionic cases.

Other Pupillary Abnormalities. Episodic dilation of the pupil lasting minutes to hours can occur in otherwise healthy patients. It may be associated with headache, blurred vision, or photophobia. Patients are rarely seen during episodes but usually are normal when examined. The condition is considered benign, and further investigation is not indicated.

Patients with severe neurologic lesions or taking certain drugs may have small but reactive pupils. Light/near dissociation, or a good response to an accommodative target but a poor response to light stimulation, can affect any patient with severe visual impairment. With normal vision, however, dissociation occurs in patients who have midbrain lesions, a long history of diabetes, alcoholism, or late syphilis (Argyll-Robertson pupils).

ADDITIONAL READINGS

Burde RM, Savino PJ, Trobe D: *Clinical decisions in neuro-ophthalmology,* ed 2, St Louis, 1992, Mosby.

Hedges TR III: *Consultation in ophthalmology,* Philadelphia, 1987, Decker.

Heuven WAJ, van Zwaan JT: *Decision making in ophthalmology,* Philadelphia, 1992, Decker.

Newman NM: *Neuro-ophthalmology: a practical text,* New York, 1992, Appleton & Lange.

XIV OTOLARYNGOLOGY

CHAPTER 178

Common Problems of the Ear

Michael D. Seidman
George T. Simpson, II
Mumtaz J. Khan

Primary care physicians encounter many disorders that affect the ear, and thus they must understand common otologic problems and know basic anatomy and physiology of the ear (Fig. 178-1). Physicians also must be able to examine and evaluate disorders of the ear. They should know routine management for common otologic diseases and when to refer to an otolaryngologist.

FOREIGN BODIES

Foreign bodies in the external auditory canal are a common problem, particularly in children. The foreign bodies include peanuts, plastic beads, pins, paper, and pencil erasers, virtually anything that can be placed in the canal. Insects may become trapped in the canal and produce irritating symptoms. Unless the ear canal is traumatized, these foreign bodies may be asymptomatic. When retained for some time, however, infection may develop and produce edema and inflammation of the canal wall itself, as well as purulent and foul-smelling discharge. The true etiology of the problem may be obscured.

The first step in evaluation and treatment of a foreign body in the ear is a complete examination of the head and neck, including the opposite ear and the nose to rule out the presence of multiple foreign bodies. In the absence of a clear history of foreign body placement, a foreign body may not be suspected or detected on the initial examination because of severe inflammation and swelling, which can sometimes mimic that of acute or chronic mastoiditis. This situation requires otolaryngology consultation.

Removal should never be attempted by the patient or the family, because it will usually be unsuccessful and may exacerbate the problem. Removal requires complete cooperation by the patient or immobilization to prevent movement of the patient's body and head. Sometimes, particularly in young children, immobilization will require brief general anesthesia. When a live insect is trapped in the ear canal, it may be killed by filling the canal with mineral oil or alcohol.

The basic principle of removal is to apply pressure behind the object so as to pull it from the canal. Instruments such as clamps or alligator forceps should not be used routinely, since they may push the foreign body further into the canal and may traumatize both the canal and the tympanic membrane. Small soft objects that are not occluding the canal may be removed using syringe irrigation, as in removing wax. The water should be at body temperature (lukewarm) to avoid inducing pain or caloric response with vertigo and nausea. Water irrigation should not be used with hygroscopic foreign bodies such as beans or other vegetable material, since they will swell with the absorption of water and make removal more difficult.

A small instrument such as a wax or wire-loop curet or a blunt hook can be passed through the canal until it is beside the foreign body, then used to pull the object from the canal. Because removal is most easily accomplished under direct vision through a binocular operating microscope, an otolaryngologist should be consulted if difficulty is encountered. If the foreign body is near the tympanic membrane, an audiogram may be obtained first to ensure hearing is not

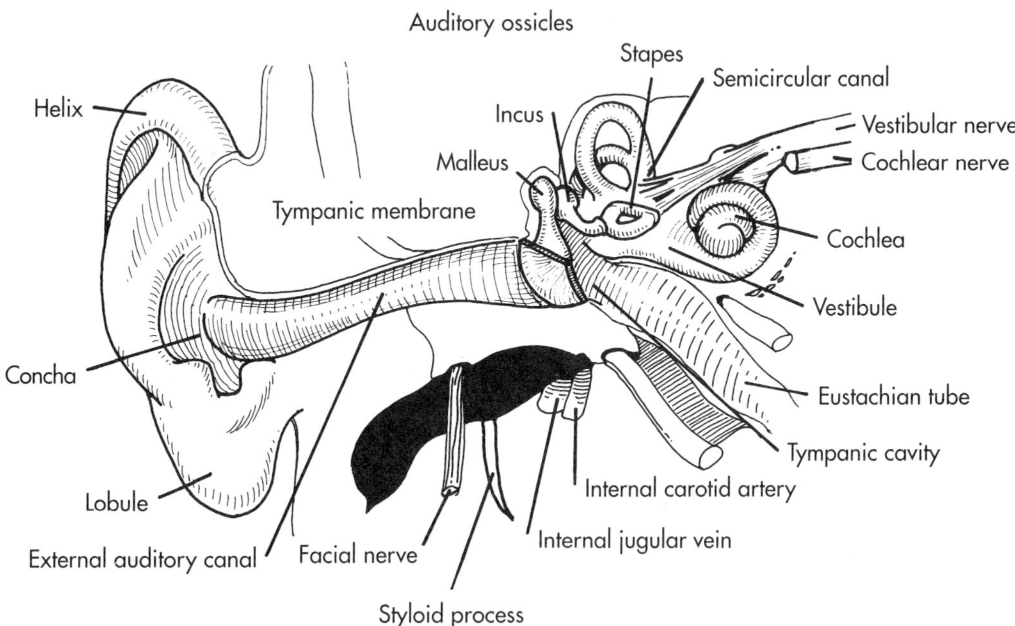

Fig. 178-1. Anatomy of the external, middle, and internal ear.

already compromised. If the foreign body has perforated the tympanic membrane, the patient should be seen by an otolaryngologist.

If no gross contamination has occurred, with no signs of inflammation or infection of the middle ear, medication is not usually necessary. An obvious infection should be treated as outlined later (see Otologic Infections). For lacerations of either the canal or the tympanic membrane, the ear canal should be kept dry to allow healing. This means preventing water from entering the ear canal while showering, bathing, and hair washing. Cotton balls coated with petroleum jelly may be placed in the external meatus to prevent the entry of water.

Any object in the ear canal that bleeds on manipulation should be suspected of being a mucosal polyp from the middle ear. These polyps occur in the presence of chronic middle ear infections. Their removal should not be attempted because they may be attached to the facial nerve or ossicles of the middle ear. An otolaryngologist must be consulted for this condition.

TRAUMA

External Ear Injuries

Trauma to the external ear may produce superficial abrasions, contusions, hematomas, lacerations, or partial or complete avulsion. Superficial abrasions are managed as elsewhere in the body. The ear must be inspected for other signs of injury.

Contusions may occur in the postauricular muscles and the muscles of mastication, such as the temporalis. Hematomas may occur when the perichondrium is torn. The accumulation of blood between the perichondrium and the cartilage will produce avascular necrosis and provide an excellent site for soft tissue infection and abscess formation. If untreated, these infections can result in a loss of portions of the cartilaginous skeleton of the ear, producing a severe cosmetic deformity: the classic "cauliflower ear" seen in wrestlers, boxers, and others with blunt ear trauma. Temporary treatment with petroleum jelly or collodion-soaked gauze may help to compress the swelling. Protective headgear is now available and should be worn to avert hematoma formation during athletic events. Large hematomas of the external ear must be treated immediately by incision and drainage, including saline irrigation to remove clots, placement of drains, compression dressings, and systemic antibiotics. An otolaryngologist should be contacted for urgent consultation and surgery if necessary.

Lacerations of the external ear may be minor and require only a few simple sutures for closure. Fine sutures produce excellent results but should be removed in several days. The earlobe may be lacerated when earrings are torn away; repair uses simple sutures with an excellent result. If not closed primarily, these lacerations require more complex plastic repair later. When small lacerations extending through skin and cartilage are closed, care is taken to avoid penetration of the cartilage by sutures passing through the skin. This complication may lead to infection of the cartilage. More extensive lacerations and avulsions require an otolaryngologist.

The external ear canal is occasionally lacerated by a fingernail, cotton-tipped swab, hairpin, or other instrument. These lacerations usually do not cause problems and do not require repair. Antibiotic drops may be indicated if a laceration involves more than half the external canal, and larger lacerations, the risk for stenosis significantly increase. Placement of an otowick and application of antibiotic drops may be necessary. Water must be kept out of the ear. The physician must determine that the tympanic membrane is intact and that hearing function is normal. Laceration of the external canal skin may be associated with a fracture of the temporal bone; if the patient has been struck on the ear, such a fracture becomes more likely.

Trauma may produce injury to the tympanic membranes, including perforations or tears. Blows to the outer ear and explosive barotrauma may produce a tear in the tympanic membrane. Foreign bodies in the external canal also can cause membrane injury. Most tympanic membrane perforations or tears heal spontaneously without intervention. Unless the tympanic membrane is grossly contaminated by dirty water, antibiotics are not usually necessary, although they may be used prophylactically. Occasionally the otolaryngologist places a small paper patch over the perforation or laceration to speed the rate of healing. The examiner must assess and document the hearing status and other functions of the middle and inner ear at the initial examination. An audiogram should be obtained. If any question remains regarding healing of the injury, an otolaryngology consult must be sought.

Middle Ear Injuries

Middle ear injuries result when physical forces are transmitted to structures within the tympanic space. Such injuries may result from loud noises, pressure injuries, and the introduction of foreign objects through the tympanic membrane. Head trauma with basilar skull fracture may include facial paralysis, fracture, and dislocation of the ossicles with discontinuity of the ossicular chain and conductive hearing loss. The stapes may be subluxated out of position in the oval window. Forces may be transmitted from the stapes through the cochlea and may rupture the round window membrane. Ossicular injury and blood in the middle ear space result in conductive hearing loss. A leak of perilymph may produce symptoms of vertigo and sensorineural hearing loss, which may result from a displaced stapes or ruptured round window membrane. Such ruptures usually close spontaneously, and they may not be diagnosed as often as they occur. If they persist, a fistula may result with gradual deterioration of hearing. Perilymph fistulas are considered an otolaryngologic emergency.

Inner Ear Injuries

Structures of the inner ear may be injured by sudden forces associated with acceleration, deceleration, or blows to the head. Hydraulic forces transmitted by the ossicles may cause ruptures between the fluid cavities within the labyrinth, disruption or tearing of labyrinthine structures, and bleeding within the labyrinth. Symptoms may vary from hearing loss to dizziness, vertigo, and disequilibrium. These symptoms may be profound, immediate, and incapacitating. They may be irreversible. Significant inner ear injuries usually involve both the vestibular and the cochlear systems and may be associated with fractures of the temporal bone in the base of the skull.

Vertigo, hearing loss, and tinnitus constitute the syndrome of the *labyrinthine concussion.* The most common symptom is positional vertigo, with a brief attack of vertigo and nystagmus caused by a change in head position. The syndrome is similar to benign paroxysmal positional vertigo. The prognosis for this type of vertigo is good, with spontaneous remission usually occurring in 6 months but occasionally not until more than 2 years after the injury.

In evaluating ear trauma, computed tomography (CT) scanning for bony detail is helpful. Ear function after trauma must be evaluated by audiologic testing. With significant likelihood of major injury or significant sequelae, consultation with an otolaryngologist is mandatory on an urgent basis.

HEARING IMPAIRMENT

Hearing is one of the primary special senses. Hearing impairment not only compromises communication but also may result in inappropriate responses to environmental dangers and induce a sense of isolation with profound emotional effects. An estimated 10% to 15% of the population has some degree of hearing impairment, which means about 30 million persons in the United States have hearing difficulty. Hearing loss is frequently overlooked as a major problem despite its common occurrence. Primary care physicians must understand hearing impairment and its socioeconomic ramifications. They have an important responsibility for identifying hearing difficulties and obtaining appropriate consultation and treatment (Fig. 178-2).

Causes of Hearing Loss

Hearing impairment implies a defect in the appropriate identification of acoustic information in the external environment. It may involve any portion of the transducer mechanism of the ear. That is, hearing impairment may result from a defect in the mechanical conduction of sound from the external environment, in sensorineural coding, in transmission of signals to the central nervous system (CNS), or from a mixture of these defects.

Conductive Hearing Loss. Conductive hearing losses are characterized by mechanical defects or a relative inefficiency in the mechanical portion of the auditory system (Fig. 178-3). Any or all anatomic portions of the external or middle ear may be involved.

External Ear. In the external ear, any problem or condition that prevents sound energy from reaching the middle ear will result in a hearing loss. The most common

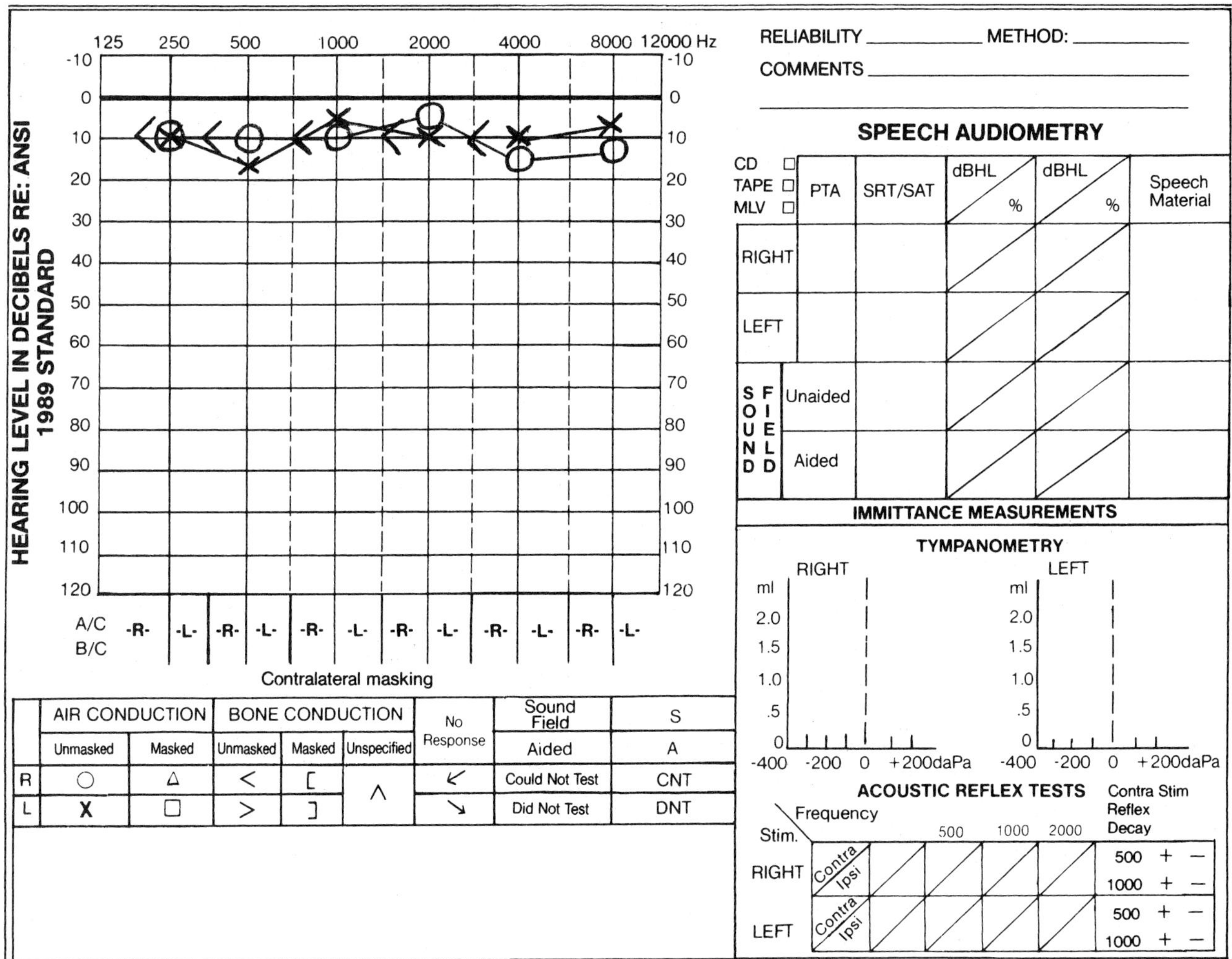

Fig. 178-2. Normal audiogram. Pure tone audiograms are graphic representations of the thresholds of perception for tones of various frequencies. Loudness of the tone is measured in decibels (dB), and frequency or pitch of the tone is measured in hertz (Hz) or cycles per second.

condition that produces a hearing loss is occlusion of the external ear canal by cerumen. A buildup of cerumen gradually occludes the canal. Most frequently, cerumen becomes impacted in the ear canal through misguided attempts to clean the ear canal using a fingertip or a cotton-tipped applicator. Rather than migrating externally, the cerumen is pushed more medially in the canal, eventually occluding it. Hearing may be restored by removing the cerumen from the canal.

Infection of the soft tissues of the external ear canal produces a conductive hearing loss by closing the canal with edema and retained secretions. Effective management requires removal of all secretions and use of medical therapy.

Overgrowth of the bony wall of the external ear canal may result from contact with cold water while swimming, as in long-distance swimmers, surfers, and scuba divers. The bony knobs may close the ear canal and contribute to retention of the cerumen, fluid, and local inflammation. Occlusion may produce a conductive hearing loss. This condition is called *external canal bony exostosis.* Exostoses do not require treatment when they are small. When they become large and symptomatic, however, they must be removed surgically by an otolaryngologist.

Rare conditions that produce a conductive hearing loss through occlusion in the external ear canal include tumors and congenital atresias of the canal. Occasionally, multiple recurrent external canal infections can produce a fibrotic or cicatricial stenosis of the canal that requires surgical treatment.

Tympanic Membrane. When movement of the tympanic membrane is impaired, a mild to moderate mechanical or conductive hearing loss results. Impaired mobility may result from middle ear infection with a buildup of fluid or effusion. A perforation after infection or trauma impairs mobility of the tympanic membrane. The membrane's mechanical efficiency may be compromised by scar tissue formation and deposition of calcium, a condition called *tympanosclerosis,* or by a healed perforation with hypermobility of the tympanic membrane at the site of healing. Eustachian tube dysfunction, barotrauma, or barotitis (middle ear inflammation associated with diving injuries or flying) results in negative middle ear pressure and impairs mobility of the tympanic membrane.

Middle Ear. Besides those involving the tympanic membrane (e.g., middle ear effusion, otitis media, barotitis, tympanosclerosis), other conditions affect structures of the middle ear and result in a conductive hearing loss. *Otosclerosis,* a bony fusion of the stapes, reduces the motion of the ossicle, resulting in hearing loss. It is inherited in an

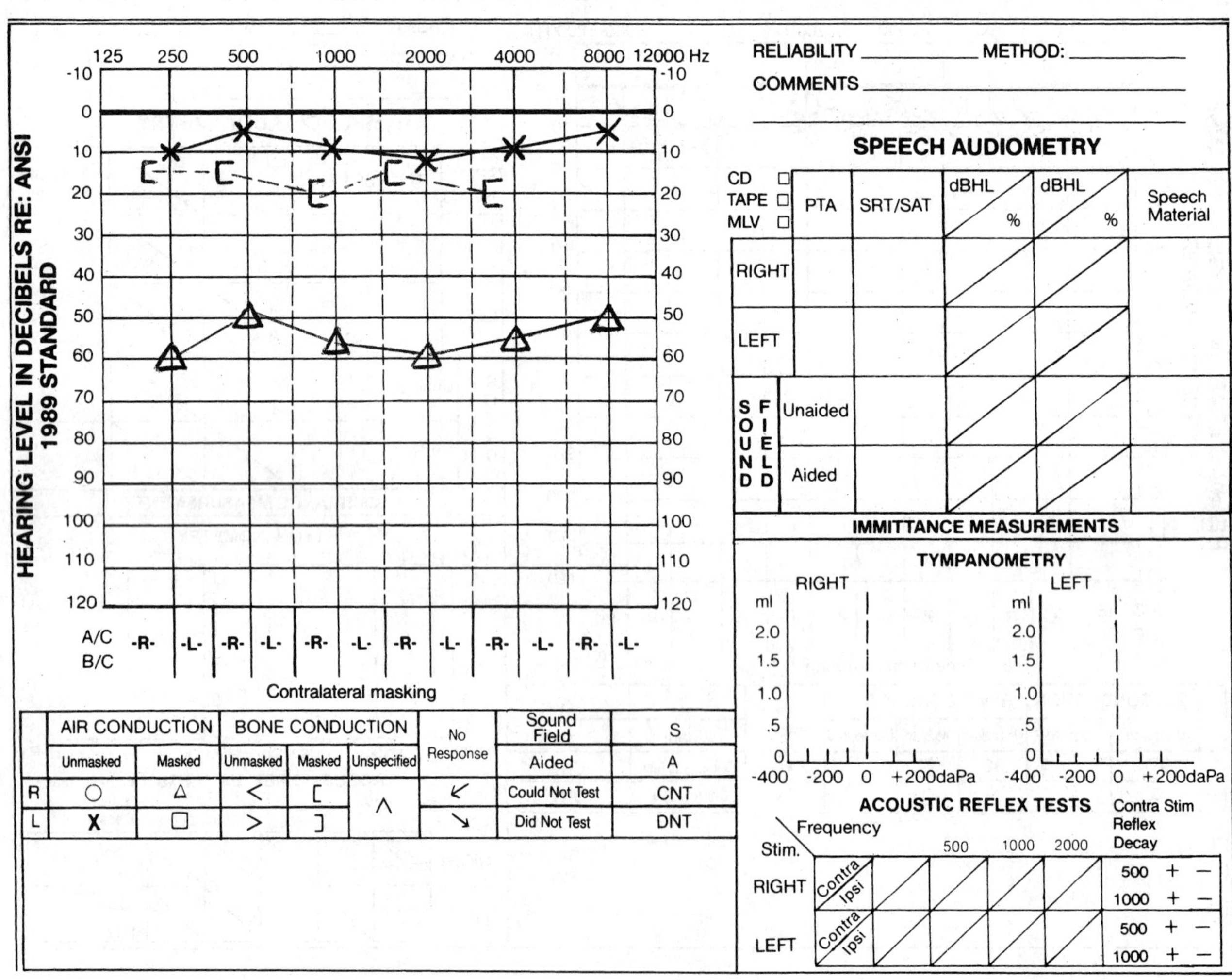

Fig. 178-3. Audiogram illustrating moderate conductive hearing loss characterized by air-bone gap in the right ear.

autosomal dominant pattern with variable penetrance. Otosclerosis occurs (but frequently is not detected) in 10% of the population and is treatable with surgery. Ossicular discontinuity, fracture, or subluxation may result from trauma and interfere with the middle ear sound conduction mechanism. Congenital malformations also may produce conductive hearing loss. *Cholesteatoma* (keratoma), a collection of normal squamous epithelium occurring within a sac or forming a ball, also affects sound conduction in the middle ear. Cholesteatomas usually follow a perforation or retraction pocket in the tympanic membrane. The ball of squamous epithelium gradually enlarges over time and, through direct pressure and enzymatic resorption, can cause the destruction of the ossicles and erosion of structures within the inner ear or cranial cavity. If communication with the outside exists, chronic infection and drainage may occur and induce otitis media or disseminated infection, with serious sequelae. The degree of destruction may not be appreciated initially, since the collection of squamous cells may become a mechanical transmission device to the inner ear, even when extensive destruction has already occurred.

Mechanical (conductive) hearing loss frequently can be improved or eliminated safely by surgery. Underlying disease must be treated. If surgery is not possible or desired, hearing aids may significantly improve hearing.

Sensorineural Hearing Loss. Disorders within the cochlea, including the auditory nerve and its connections in the brainstem, produce hearing loss that is classified as sensorineural. Sensorineural hearing losses are divided into those involving the cochlea and those involving the retrocochlear region (the eighth cranial nerve and central pathways).

Several disorders within the cochlea produce hearing loss. A common and increasingly recognized form of hearing loss is that induced by *noise trauma* (Fig. 178-4). This trauma can be explosive noise, but most often it is prolonged exposure to excessive levels of noise above 85 dB. Mechanical stress on structures of the inner ear may produce temporary injury and, if prolonged, result in permanent injury and increasing hearing loss. The most easily damaged structures are the hair cells in the organ of Corti, which is attached to the basilar membrane in the basal turn of the cochlea. Since hair cells in this region of the cochlea are involved in the perception of high-frequency sounds, the initial hearing loss is about 4000 Htz but gradually progresses to involve higher and lower

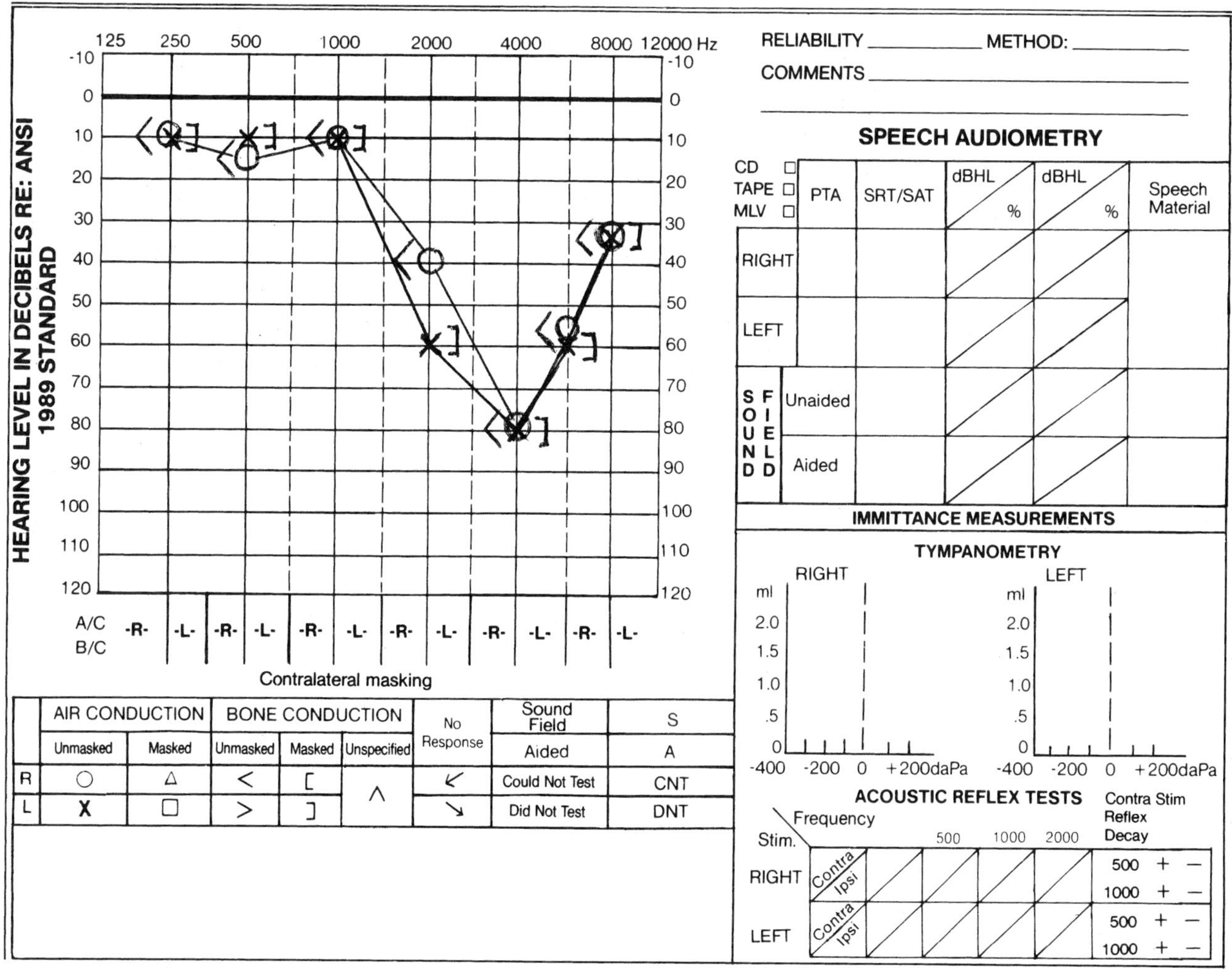

Fig. 178-4. Audiogram of bilateral noise-induced sensorineural hearing loss. Typically, it is a high-frequency hearing loss, with normal audition at lower frequencies.

frequencies. Temporary hearing loss from loud noise exposure is called a *temporary threshold shift*. Such a hearing loss typically improves over 24 to 72 hours. Repeated or persistent noise exposures produce an irreversible hearing loss.

The most common form of sensorineural hearing loss after traumatic noise exposure is *presbycusis*. This hearing loss of aging represents gradual, progressive degeneration of cochlear structures and central neural connections. Some degeneration of the mechanical portion of hearing may also occur. Typically, hearing loss is most severe in the highest frequencies and is less in lower frequencies (Fig. 178-5). Presbycusis may have a hereditary component involving sensitivity to a variety of factors that produce degeneration. The ability to attenuate presbycusis using dietary restriction and antioxidant therapy shows promise.[1,2]

Sensorineural hearing loss may result from viral or bacterial infections of cochlear structures. Such hearing loss is usually rapidly progressive and frequently total. Similar hearing loss results from labyrinthitis of any etiology but is usually associated with vestibular symptoms (vertigo and disequilibrium). Syphilitic (luetic) involvement of the labyrinth produces a fluctuating hearing loss and disequilibrium. Symptoms gradually progress, and hearing deteriorates without treatment.

Ménière's disease may be present in patients who experience fluctuating hearing loss. It comprises the syndrome of fluctuating sensorineural hearing loss, tinnitus, pressure symptoms in the ear, and vertigo. The ultimate etiology is unknown, but the pathology involves the buildup of intralabyrinthine pressure, called *endolymphatic hydrops*. The increased pressure distends structures of the labyrinth in episodes associated with a sudden onset of cochlear and vestibular symptoms. Therapies have had varying success, including salt-restricted diet and vasodilator agents, including nicotinic acid, histamine, 5% carbon dioxide inhalations, diuretic, and diazepam. The symptoms may be associated with periods of increased stress. Symptoms wax and wane and may be absent for months to years and then return. Occasionally, profound hearing loss and loss of vestibular function may result. The majority of patients benefit from diuretics and salt restriction. Approximately 15% to 20% fail medical management, and several surgical options are available (see Vertigo).

Although usually associated with conductive hearing losses, otosclerosis also may produce intralabyrinthine

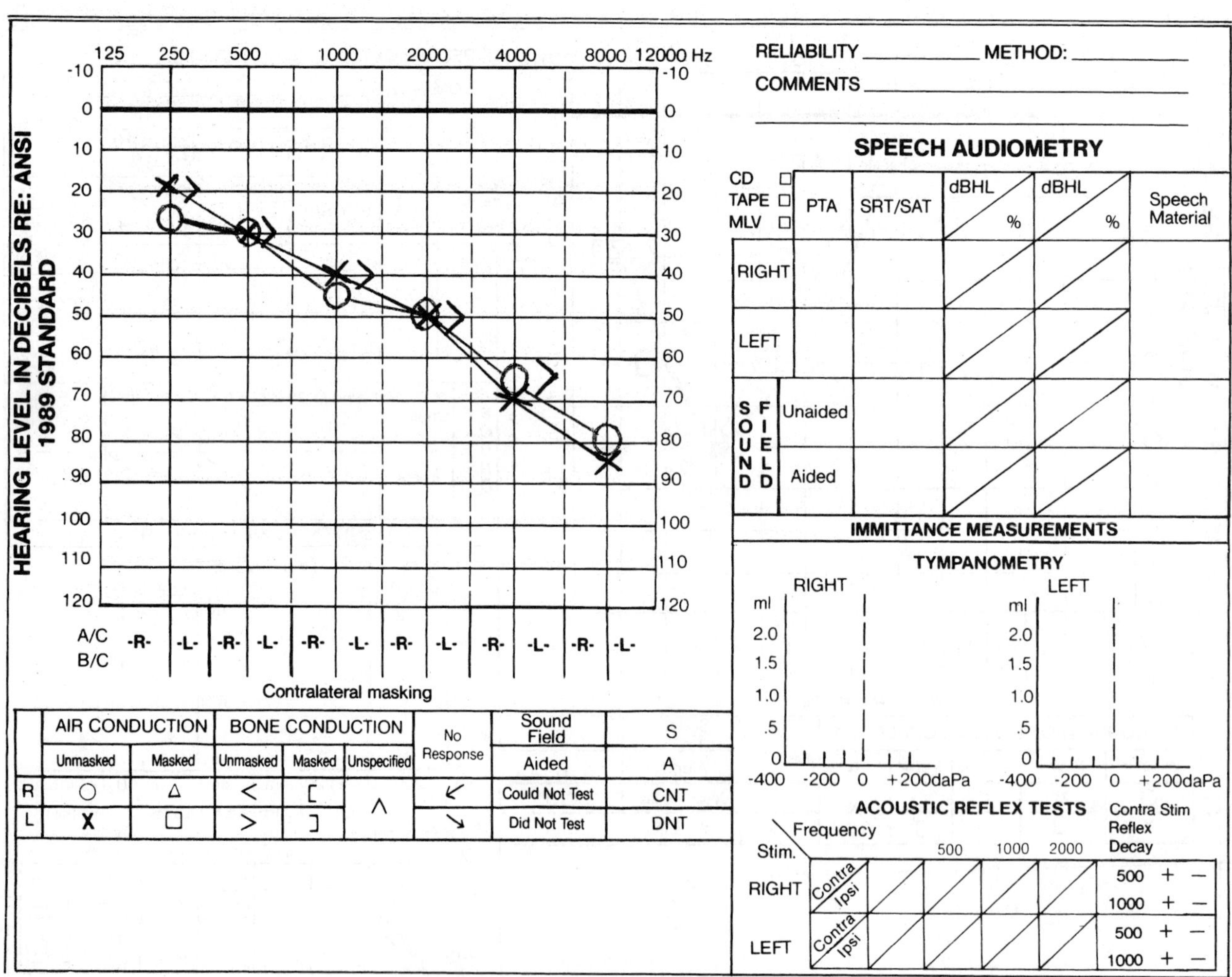

Fig. 178-5. Audiogram of mid- to high-frequency sensorineural hearing loss consistent with presbycusis. Hearing loss is most severe at the highest frequencies and is less at lower frequencies.

symptoms, particularly tinnitus and sensorineural hearing loss. Surgery in otosclerosis, while improving hearing, may not affect the other symptoms. Medical treatment with sodium fluoride occasionally leads to stabilization of hearing.

Fistulas involving leakage of perilymphatic fluid from the middle ear or mixing of perilymphatic fluid with endolymphatic fluid may be associated with sudden hearing loss. The symptoms do not usually persist but may be variably present and may occur episodically. Fistulas are usually associated with physical activity or sudden barotrauma; they may follow external trauma to the ear and head. Bed rest with the head elevated must be begun immediately, with otolaryngologic consultation. Surgical correction is occasionally required.

Ototoxic effects of medication are of increasing importance. Most often, Salicylates produce ototoxic drug effects, including tinnitus, hearing loss, dizziness, and disequilibrium. The hearing loss involves all frequencies. Symptoms rapidly disappear after cessation of medication. Other drugs producing ototoxic effects include ethacrynic acid and furosemide. Quinine-related antimalarial compounds cause a progressive irreversible hearing loss, sometimes of delayed onset. Malarial infections, however, may produce permanent sensorineural hearing loss if the labyrinth has been infected. Quinine and its analogs may cause fetal injury and congenital deafness. Nitrogen mustard and cisplatin, as used in chemotherapy, also can produce significant hearing loss.

Clinically, the most significant agents producing ototoxicity are the aminoglycosides, all of which produce varying degrees of auditory and vestibular damage. Streptomycin and gentamicin have their greatest effects on the vestibular end organ; kanamycin, tobramycin, and neomycin cause more damage to the cochlear end organ. Patients receiving aminoglycosides rarely complain of vertigo but experience unsteadiness of gait, particularly in darkness. A sensorineural hearing loss is produced, beginning in the high frequencies and progressing to a flat, moderately severe loss across all frequencies. Serial audiograms must be obtained for any patient receiving a prolonged course of these agents. Aminoglycosides produce their effects by damaging the hair cells of the inner ear. Unlike other common antibiotics, aminoglycosides are concentrated in both the perilymph and endolymph so that the hair cells are exposed to high concentrations. The ototoxicity of aminoglycosides does not correlate well with serum drug levels. If the total dose is limited to less than 2 gm, however, and the duration of therapy is less than 10 days, the incidence of ototoxicity is low. Because these drugs are eliminated almost exclusively by the kidneys, they must be used with caution in renal failure.

Several congenital disorders may produce a sensorineural hearing loss. When they are not identified at an early age, the acquisition of language skills is severely impaired. Many individuals have been misdiagnosed with mental impairment when their only problem was impaired hearing. Such events have profound and devastating lifelong consequences for education and quality of life. For this reason, hearing screening should begin at a young age, and full audiologic testing should be used when any child appears to have a significant problem in interacting appropriately with the environment.

Currently, the only effective treatment for sensorineural hearing loss is the use of amplification devices. Research studies have been designed to regenerate cochlear hair cells, and avian models have had some success. All cases of suspected hearing loss should be evaluated by an otolaryngologist.

Retrocochlear Hearing Loss. When the site of the hearing disorder involves the auditory nerve, brainstem, or CNS, it is defined as a retrocochlear hearing loss. Common causes include CNS sequelae of infection or cerebrovascular injuries such as a stroke, intracranial bleed, or concussion. Other CNS disorders include demyelinating and other degenerative diseases or neoplasms. A common site of retrocochlear pathology involves the eighth cranial nerve, either within the internal auditory canal or within the posterior fossa in the cerebellar pontine angle near the brainstem. Tumors here are rare but must not be overlooked. Within the auditory canal or near its opening, the most common neoplasm is the vestibular schwannoma, a benign tumor arising in the perineurium of the cochleovestibular nerve. Occasionally, congenital keratomas may occur in this area. Other benign tumors are meningiomas. Primary intracranial malignancies or metastases may produce similar symptoms. Vestibular schwannoma and the cerebellar pontine angle tumors have an insidious onset and thus may be encountered in a primary care practice. Early symptoms may include tinnitus, hearing loss, and disequilibrium.

Mixed Hearing Loss. A mixed hearing loss is present when a conductive hearing impairment occurs simultaneously with sensorineural hearing loss. A mixed or combined hearing loss may follow injury involving structures of the external, middle, and inner ears. Infection may produce acute and chronic changes in the structure of the ear, including acute inflammation and nerve injury, as well as tympanosclerosis. Congenital disorders may involve structures in any or all parts of the ear. A mixed hearing loss may produce variable and confusing signs on physical examination and requires more specialized testing for proper identification.

DIAGNOSIS OF HEARING LOSS

The diagnosis of hearing loss requires a suspicion of its presence, either by the patient or the examining physician. In moderate to severe hearing loss, communication clearly is impaired, and a hearing loss is likely. In mild degrees of hearing loss, however, a high index of suspicion is necessary. The patient may not be aware of the gradual onset of the loss and may use the psychologic defense of denial to avoid facing the realities of aging and altered body image. Because of the socially isolating effects of impaired communication, what may initially appear to be depression or even irrational behavior may actually be the result of hearing loss. Severe or profound hearing loss of long duration prevents proper self-assessment of accurate pronunciation and may result in slurred speech, which can be misinterpreted as resulting from other pathology (Table 178-1). Family members may become frustrated and angry with the person who has the hearing impairment if the nature of the problem is not recognized. Communication problems may be attributed to antisocial tendencies or impaired mental status. For all these reasons, awareness of possible hearing impairment and suspicion of its presence are essential.

Sudden sensorineural hearing loss is a relatively rare entity that accounts for varying degrees of hearing impairment. The etiology is elusive, but vascular, viral, or autoimmune causes may be most common. Treatment is controversial, and medications have included vasodilators, anticoagulants, steroids, and Hypaque. Treatment is much more likely to be efficacious if instituted early in the course (i.e., within 24 hours and preferably earlier).

With a thorough examination of the ear, the primary care physician usually can recognize the presence of a hearing loss even if the problem cannot be diagnosed more accurately. The physician may have the patient undergo an audiologic evaluation. In most cases of hearing loss, a consultation from an otolaryngologist is essential. During this consultation a complete audiogram may be obtained and appropriate therapy arranged. The physician must understand the process involved in audiologic testing to interpret a report directly from the audiologist or an otolaryngologic consultation.

TINNITUS

Tinnitus is noise heard by the patient in the absence of any external stimulation. Recent estimates suggest that approximately 40 million Americans are affected by tinnitus. Rarely, the sound can be heard by the examiner.

Objective Tinnitus

Objective tinnitus can be heard when the examiner places a stethoscope (with the bell removed) in the patient's external auditory canal or places the bell around the ear on the neck. A blowing sound that coincides with inspiration and expiration can result from an abnormally patent (patulous) eustachian tube. The history may indicate this type of tinnitus because of the association with respiration. Objective tinnitus most frequently follows rapid weight loss or may occur during a debilitating illness.

Sharp clicking sounds that occur in bursts and last for several seconds or minutes may be produced by tetanic contractions of the muscles of the soft palate or the tensor tympani muscle. This phenomenon is known as *palatal myoclonus*. Occasionally the palatal contractions can be observed by the examiner when the tinnitus is audible. Disturbances in the vascular blood flow produce a pulsatile sound that is synchronous with the heartbeat. Aneurysms, vascular neoplasms, and arteriovenous malformations may produce this tinnitus. A venous hum produced by turbulence within the internal jugular vein can produce a "whooshing" or continuous machinelike sound synchronized with the pulse. The examiner may eliminate the sound by occluding the distal jugular vein while avoiding obstructing arterial flow. Carotid bruits may also manifest as pulsatile tinnitus. Radiologic studies with contrast may reveal an enlarged jugular bulb or carotid vascular disease. Ligation of the internal jugular vein may be curative in some patients.

Recent studies have shown that highly sensitive recording techniques can detect the sound produced by the normal motion of cochlear hair cells. This sound represents mechanical effects produced by the stiffening of the basilar membrane within the cochlea and are called *otoacoustic emissions*. Although these sounds are found in patients with normal hearing without any symptoms, they may produce subjective tinnitus.

Subjective Tinnitus

Subjective tinnitus is a sound in the ears or head heard only by the patient. Tinnitus may be produced by lesions or conditions within the external ear canal, tympanic membrane, middle ear structures, cochlea, auditory nerve, brainstem, and cerebral cortex. Patients may describe the noise as an ill-defined buzzing, ringing, whistling, or hissing or may identify a specific noise associated with insect or motor sounds. This description can be diagnostically valuable. Ménière's syndrome produces a low-pitched, continuous tinnitus similar to an ocean roar and frequently becomes very loud immediately preceding an acute attack of vertigo. It may then disappear after the attack. In otosclerosis, tinnitus is usually low pitched and continuous but can be intermittent. Cerumen, foreign bodies, or loose hairs in the external ear canal may rub against the tympanic membrane and produce a variety of sounds. Noise or physical trauma, including acoustic trauma from an explosion, produces a high-pitched tinnitus that usually subsides after a few hours, although occasionally it can persist if permanent hearing loss has occurred. Continuous, bilateral, high-pitched tinnitus frequently accompanies hearing loss from chronic noise exposure, presbycusis, and ototoxic chemicals or drugs. A continuous, unilateral, high-pitched tinnitus may be the first symptom of a vestibular schwannoma and may precede loss of hearing or distortion of hearing by several years.

Cochlear and retrocochlear lesions producing tinnitus are usually associated with sensorineural hearing loss or distortion of sounds. The perceived pitch of the tinnitus frequently corresponds to the frequency of greatest hearing

Table 178-1. Hearing Threshold Levels and Associated Handicaps

Hearing threshold	Probable handicap*
<40 dB	Has difficulty hearing faint or distant speech; needs favorable seating, and may benefit from lip reading instruction; may also benefit from a hearing aid.
40-55 dB	Understands conversational speech at 3 to 5 feet; needs hearing aid, lip reading, favorable seating, and speech correction.
55-70 dB	Conversation must be loud to be understood, with great difficulty in group and classroom discussion; needs all the above plus language therapy and perhaps special class for those with difficulty hearing.
70-90 dB	May hear a loud voice about 1 foot from the ear; may identify environmental noises, may distinguish vowels but not consonants; child who needs special education for deaf persons with emphasis on speech, auditory training, and language may enter regular classes later.
>90 dB	May hear loud sounds; does not rely on hearing as a primary channel for communication; needs special class or school for the deaf; some of these children enter regular high schools.

*Assumes all medical or surgical treatment has been applied. If the hearing loss is detected in childhood, special education may be required.

impairment. CNS lesions producing tinnitus may not be associated with hearing loss but are almost always associated with other neurologic signs and symptoms. Although some patients with tinnitus do not have associated hearing loss, this finding may represent limitations in testing equipment that typically does not measure hearing beyond 8000 Hz. Many drugs produce tinnitus without associated hearing loss, including salicylates, indomethacin, quinidine, propranolol, levodopa, carbamazepine, aminophylline, and caffeine. The exact anatomic site where tinnitus is produced by the actions of these drugs in unknown, but the drugs probably have both peripheral and central effects.

The treatment of tinnitus may be frustrating. All efforts should be made to diagnose associated, treatable conditions. Several medications taken systemically may suppress tinnitus temporarily, but treatment requires high doses that may be near the toxic range. No drugs are available to "cure" tinnitus, but amitryptyline and alprazolam may reduce the severity of tinnitus. These medications are typically reserved for patients with severe tinnitus because they may have significant side effects. Ambient or environmental noise is most helpful in suppressing tinnitus. Wide-band, or white, noise suppresses tinnitus, not only while the noise is present but for some time after its cessation. Maintaining background noise from a radio or television set or from a device generating the sound of the ocean or falling rain may be helpful, particularly before sleep. A hearing aid may not only improve hearing but also suppress tinnitus. Tinnitus masking devices worn by the patient may be helpful. These devices are similar to hearing aids, but they produce a lower level of continuous white noise for tinnitus suppression. The patient with tinnitus is helped most by the physician's reassurance that no underlying condition exists. Proper evaluation and tests are necessary and can readily be obtained. Consultation with an otolaryngologist is often indicated.

OTOLOGIC INFECTIONS

Ear infections and their sequelae are relatively common problems in all age groups and represent one of the largest categories of illness in the pediatric population. Effective treatment depends on the specific anatomic structures involved, the agents responsible for infection, and appropriate treatment strategies. Ear infections may involve structures of the external ear, the tympanic and mastoid cavities, or even the labyrinth and temporal bone. Infectious agents may be viral, bacterial, or fungal.

External Ear Infections

External ear infections involve the skin lining, the external auditory ear canal, and the periosteum of the bone immediately beneath the skin. After cleansing the ear canal, the diagnosis is established by the presence of characteristic diffuse inflammation of the ear canal skin, with or without involvement of the tympanic membrane. Edema may occur, and frequently moist otorrhea is present. If the tympanic membrane cannot be seen or otitis media cannot be ruled out, treatment must be directed at both external and middle ear infection. Use of a systemic agent is required (see Middle Ear Infection). Absorbent wicks (otowicks) that expand in the external auditory canal are often used when the edema is severe (Table 178-2).

The infected ear must be kept dry. No swimming is allowed, and care must be taken while bathing or hair washing to keep water out of the ear. The external meatus can be temporarily occluded with a cotton ball coated with petroleum jelly. All secretions and debris must be removed at least once or twice a week until the infection resolves. Specific treatments are directed at the infecting organisms (most often *Pseudomonas aeruginosa*) and inflammatory effects. Cortisporin Otic suspension or Col-Mycin usually eradicates the infection; 3 or 4 drops in the ear four times a

Table 178-2. External Ear Infections

	Etiology	Clinical findings	Common microbiologic agents	Management
Bacterial				
Diffuse otitis externa	Swimming, trauma, metabolic disorders (diabetes)	Severe otalgia, tragal tenderness, diffuse inflammation of ear canal	*Pseudomonas, Staphylococcus aureus, Streptococcus, Escherichia coli*	Aural cleansing; topical antibiotic; Burow's solution
Localized otitis externa	Furuncles	Otalgia, otorrhea, localized tenderness, furuncle in outer third of ear canal	*Staphylococcus*	Aural cleansing; topical antibiotic; Burow's solution, oral antistaphylococcal agent
Malignant otitis externa	Diabetes, immunosuppression	Diffuse external otitis, necrotizing granulation tissue, facial nerve paralysis	*Pseudomonas*	Systemic antibiotic; necrotic tissue debridement
Viral	Unknown	Otalgia, vesicles on ear canal; facial nerve paralysis	Herpes zoster (Ramsay Hunt syndrome); varicella; measles	Analgesics
Fungal	Diabetes, tropical climate	Pruritis, minimal otalgia; black, white, or yellow spores	*Aspergillus, Candida*	Aural cleansing; Burow's solution

day for 7 to 10 days is the typical course. Other medications include Vasocidin, Cetapred, VoSol, Domeboro, Garamycin, and boric acid with alcohol.

Viral Agents. Viral infections of the external ear are rare. They include varicella, measles, and occasionally herpesvirus. Unless secondary bacterial infections develop, treatment is essentially supportive and specific only for symptoms (e.g., pain). In patients with weeping lesions or edema, astringent agents such as Burow's solution are applied liberally every 4 hours in drops or soaks. Use of steroids is controversial. Symptoms of herpes zoster oticus (Ramsay Hunt syndrome) include severe otalgia, facial paralysis or paresis, decreased lacrimation on the involved side, loss of taste on the anterior two thirds of the tongue, and vesicles on the external ear canal and posterior surface of the auricle. The likelihood of good facial function after Ramsay Hunt syndrome is 40%. Treatment with acyclovir and occasionally steroids has been advocated but is controversial. Occasionally, surgical decompression of the facial nerve is necessary to preserve nerve viability and function. Symptomatic treatment for pain and provision of artificial tears are required pending the resolution of symptoms. Any patient with facial nerve paresis or paralysis should be seen in an urgent consultation with an otolaryngologist, who will evaluate the viability of the nerve and determine whether decompression is required.

Bacterial Agents. The most common pathogen involved in an external ear infection is *P. aeruginosa.* Its frequency of involvement, however, may represent opportunistic contamination within the environment in a moist ear. Other bacterial agents include *Staphylococcus aureus* and *Streptococcus* species. Occasionally, enteric organisms may be present. External ear infections are painful; the pathognomonic sign is pain with manipulation of the auricle. Analgesia must be adequate. Codeine may be required, as appropriate for age and weight. In general, analgesic eardrops are not effective because inflamed tissue resists local anesthetic agents. All moist infected ears should be swabbed to obtain specimens for culture and sensitivity determinations. All foreign materials, debris, and secretions must be removed.

In general the most effective antibiotic agents are those applied topically, but occasionally systemic agents may be required. Some of the most effective topical antibiotic agents currently available are mixtures: neomycin and bacitracin or polymyxin with hydrocortisone. Since neomycin is ototoxic, some suggest that it should not be used with a coexistent perforation; however, most otolaryngologists have used neomycin for many years without difficulty. Steroid compounds are included in topical medications to decrease inflammation. A small percentage of patients have an idiosyncratic sensitivity to neomycin and develop erythema, swelling, and pain at the site of application. If these or other severe external ear symptoms develop or persist for more than 1 or 2 weeks after starting the medication, it should be discontinued and another medication substituted. Alternative medications for treatment of otitis externa include Vasocidin, Cetapred, Domeboro, chloramphenicol otic solution, acetic acid solutions with or without hydrocortisone, and Burow's solution. These agents have either a bacteriostatic effect or the ability to reduce the pH of the external canal, thus restoring an acid pH to the milieu of the canal skin. Some of these medications also have a mildly astringent effect that aids in drying the skin and decreasing edema. All medications are given in a dosage of 3 or 4 drops three or four times per day. Burow's solution used alone should be applied every 2 to 3 hours for the first 48 hours. Acetic acid, in the form of white vinegar, may be used alone; it is painful if it enters the middle ear. All medications are instilled into the ear canal with the ear up to allow the medication to contact all portions of the ear canal. The patient should keep the head turned to the side or lie on the side with the treated ear up for 2 to 5 minutes after instillation. Then the medication is allowed to run out by turning the head the opposite way.

External ear infections rarely may extend to involve external ear structures and surrounding tissue. Systemic antibiotics are then necessary. Unless culture and sensitivity reports suggest other treatment, penicillinase-resistant penicillin (dicloxacillin orally or oxacillin or cephalosporins parenterally) is usually best. Occasionally, hospitalization is necessary; applying continuous Burow's solution soaks to the affected area is soothing and helps reduce inflammation, swelling, and pain.

An external ear infection that may have lethal consequences is *necrotizing otitis externa* (malignant otitis externa). This soft tissue infection, which usually affects elderly, diabetic, or immunocompromised patients, is typically caused by *Pseudomonas* alone or with other organisms. It may begin with an indolent course, have minimal symptoms (e.g., otorrhea, inflammation), and appear benign. This course progresses relentlessly, if untreated, to invasion and necrosis of contiguous soft tissue structures, including the auricle, scalp, and parotid gland. Further extension occurs to structures of the middle and inner ear with eventual extension to the brain. Facial nerve paralysis may be an early sign. Diagnosis requires a high index of suspicion and the demonstration of granulation tissue. Effective treatment involves a prolonged course of systemic antibiotics and aggressive debridement of necrotic tissue and drainage to prevent further progression. Without treatment, the disease is uniformly fatal, but with aggressive treatment the majority of patients survive.

Fungal Agents. Fungal infections of the external ear frequently elicit pruritus. Black, white, or yellow spores may be seen. Contact sensitivity reactions to the fungus may be present. Pain is usually minimal. Mild fungal infections are best treated by general aural hygiene, which includes removal of all cerumen and debris. A dry ear with a normal mildly acidic pH is restored with Burow's solution, VoSol, Domeboro or boric acid, and alcohol irrigations two to four times a day. Persistent mycoses may benefit from a brief course of tincture of cresylate, 3 or 4 drops twice a day for 1 to 2 weeks; cresylate should not be used if the eardrum is perforated. Clotrimazole, 1% lotion in a similar dosage, may also be effective. If systemic mycotic allergy is present and associated with local inflammatory changes in the external ear, immunotherapy with desensitization injections can produce dramatic relief of symptoms.

Middle Ear Infections (Table 178-3)

Bullous Myringitis. Small blebs or blisters are present on the tympanic membrane in this extremely painful condition. Bullous myringitis, once thought to result from a *Mycoplasma* infection, is caused by a bacterial middle ear infection. Treatment is both supportive and antibacterial.

Table 178-3. Middle Ear Infections

	Etiology	Clinical findings	Common microbiologic agents	Management
Acute suppurative otitis media	Bacterial contamination with possible eustachian tube dysfunction	Bulging or retracted TM, air-fluid level, pulsatile discharge	*H. influenzae, S. pneumoniae, Mycoplasma,* GAS, *C. diphtheriae,* gram-negative bacilli; parainfluenza virus, RSV	Aural cleansing, oral antibiotic, analgesia
Acute and serous otitis media	Eustachian tube dysfunction, barotrauma, nasopharyngeal tumor	Thickened retracted TM, gray or amber fluid in middle ear, impaired mobility of TM, conductive hearing loss	Rare	Nasal decongestant, autoinflation exercises
Chronic suppurative otitis media	Bacterial contamination	Mucopurulent otorrhea, perforated TM, conductive hearing loss, cholesteatoma	Mixed aerobic and anaerobic flora: *S. aureus, E. coli, Pseudomonas, Bacteroides fragilis*	Aural cleansing, topical antibiotic, surgery

TM, Tympanic membrane; *GAS,* group A streptococci; *RSV,* respiratory syncytial virus.

Medications used to alleviate pain include acetaminophen (Tylenol), ibuprofen, and possibly codeine. Erythromycin, penicillin, or amoxicillin (30 to 50 mg/kg/day) is given. Resolution or rupture of the bulla should not be induced unless the pain is severe; lancing the bulla promptly alleviates the pain.

Acute Suppurative Otitis Media. Acute middle ear infections are one of the most common problems seen by the pediatrician or family physician. Infections typically develop as a result of bacterial contamination through the eustachian tube in the presence of preexisting inflammation in the middle ear. This inflammation results from eustachian tube dysfunction, and oxygen is absorbed from the air in the middle ear space. A negative partial pressure results, which induces an inflammatory response. This response in turn produces a sterile transudate within the middle ear, which may evolve into an exudative process. Concurrent or subsequent contamination of the middle ear from infective nasopharyngeal contents may occur by aspiration or insufflation during nose blowing or crying. In infancy it may be produced by the flow of milk or other liquids into the eustachian tube while the infant is lying supine with a bottle propped in the mouth to induce sleep. The major bacterial pathogens in acute suppurative otitis media include *Streptococcus pneumoniae, Moraxella catarrhalis, Haemophilus influenzae,* and group A *S. pyogenes. Staphylococcus aureus, Mycoplasma pneumoniae, Corynebacterium diphtheriae,* and gram-negative bacilli are less frequent causes. The most frequent viruses producing otitis media are the parainfluenza viruses, respiratory syncytial virus, adenoviruses, and coxsackieviruses.

Nontypable *H. influenzae* (nonencapsulated) strains constitute most middle ear isolates. These strains are not associated with invasive or disseminated infections and are responsible for a small but significant proportion of middle ear infections in older children and adults. Their frequency appears to be increasing. The drug of choice, as recommended by the American Academy of Otolaryngology, is amoxicillin. The resistance of *H. influenzae* type B to amoxicillin is increasing and averages approximately 30% in the United States. Augmentin, cefaclor, Biaxin, or Lorabid is used to treat amoxicillin-resistant *H. influenzae.*

Diagnosis. Examination and confirmation of otitis media are best accomplished using a pneumatic otoscope. When fluid is present in the middle ear space, mobility of the tympanic membrane is reduced. Additional signs include a bulging, inflamed tympanic membrane or a severely retracted tympanic membrane. Bubbles or an air-fluid level may be seen. With a perforated membrane a pulsatile discharge may be seen, usually in the anteroinferior segment of the membrane. Although otalgia is present, pain or tenderness is not present on manipulating the auricle. Pain is intensified by the insufflation of air with the pneumatic otoscope.

Tympanometry is an objective test in which the mobility of the tympanic membrane is assessed by means of a signal reflected from it while the pressure against the eardrum is continuously changed. The test can be performed by an audiologist, a technician, a nurse, or a physician with only brief training. The margin for artifact and error is less than 10%. Common tympanograms include type A (normal), type B (flat, consistent with middle ear effusion), and type C (retracted, consistent with negative middle ear pressure). Less common tympanograms include type Ad, consistent with a disarticulated ossicular chain leading to hypermobility of the tympanic membrane (Fig. 178-6). This test has a higher reliability in identifying middle ear fluid than many physicians and can be helpful in supporting a clinical diagnosis.

In most cases, tympanocentesis or myringotomy is not indicated in the diagnosis of otitis media. These procedures remove secretions from the middle ear to allow bacteriologic studies and are rarely necessary for diagnosis and treatment. Almost all cases of otitis media respond quickly to proper management and may even resolve spontaneously. Virtually all bacteria implicated in middle ear infections are sensitive to common antibiotics. For these reasons, the risk associated with myringotomy cannot be justified in the typical patient. These procedures are usually performed by an otolaryngologist using a binocular operating microscope. Tympanocentesis or myringotomy can be helpful, however, in middle ear infections in neonates, immunocompromised or immunosup-

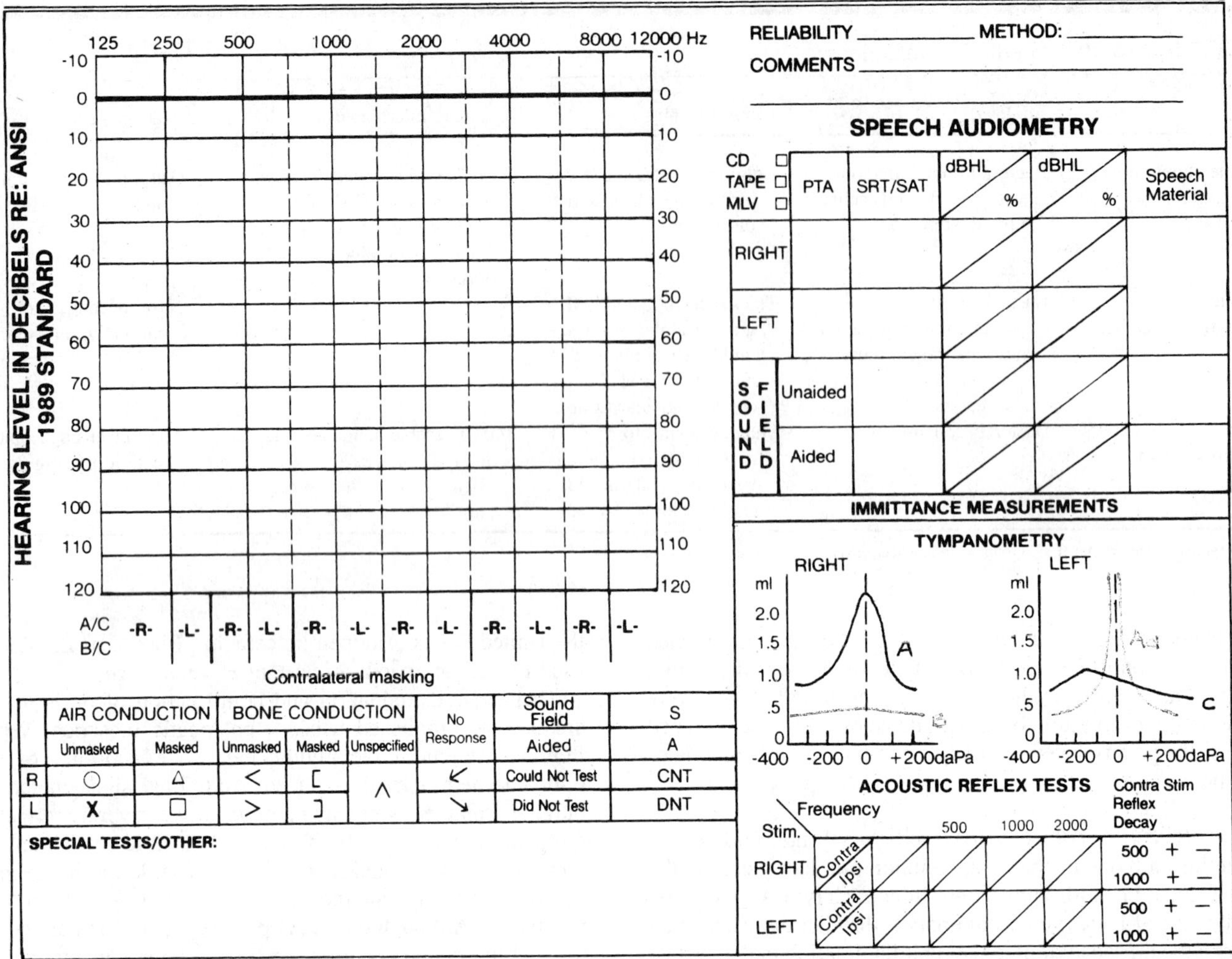

Fig. 178-6. Tympanometry. Typical tympanograms include types *A*, normal; *B*, flat, consistent with middle ear effusion; *C*, retracted, consistent with negative middle ear pressure; and *Ad*, consistent with disarticulated ossicular chain.

pressed and leukemic patients, patients who do not respond to adequate doses of antibiotics, and patients who have developed a complication such as meningitis. Tympanocentesis may offer specific identification of the etiologic organism and thereby promote an effective choice of antibiotic.

Therapy. Antibiotics are the most effective measure in all cases of acute otitis media. Depending on allergic history and the patient's age, any of several antibiotics can be used. Amoxicillin, 20 to 40 mg/kg/day in divided doses by mouth for 10 days, effectively manages most infections in all age groups. The usual dosage in older children and adults is 250 to 500 mg every 8 hours. If there is a high local prevalence of amoxicillin resistance, amoxicillin plus clavulanate (Augmentin), cefaclor, clarithromycin (Biaxin), or loracarbef (Lorabid) should be substituted. The combination of trimethoprim (8 mg/kg) and sulfamethoxazole (40 mg/kg) in two divided doses per day covers most pathogens implicated in otitis media, including *H. influenzae*. Some physicians have recommended avoidance of this medication because of the potential for aplastic anemia. All medications are given for at least 10 days. A longer course of antibiotic treatment may satisfactorily resolve otitis media and prevent chronic middle ear effusions (serous otitis media), reducing the need for myringotomy and pressure-equalizing tubes.

Satisfactory analgesia usually can be provided with acetaminophen or ibuprofen, supplemented by low doses of codeine as necessary. Codeine should be avoided in very young children, and aspirin is typically avoided because of the potential for Reye's syndrome. Antihistamines and decongestants are usually of no help in acute otitis media except for relieving associated coryza symptoms. Antihistamines may actually impair middle ear clearance by interfering with mucociliary flow through the eustachian tube, but this theory is controversial.

Each patient should be evaluated in 2 weeks. If an effusion persists beyond 4 weeks, the patient is treated for chronic serous otitis media and chronic middle ear effusion (see later). Repeated episodes of acute bacterial otitis media with clearing of middle ear effusions between each attack usually can be managed by chronic, low-dose prophylactic amoxicillin. Alternatives to antibiotic therapy exist. If acute bacterial otitis media develops in a patient receiving prophylactic therapy, a myringotomy and insertion of a ventilation tube may be indicated to restore middle ear ventilation and function.

If the tympanic membrane is perforated and drainage is present, this drainage can be cultured for guidance in treatment. Most perforations heal spontaneously. If perforation persists longer than 3 months, the patient should be referred to an otolaryngologist for consultation and treatment.

Acute Mastoiditis. Virtually all cases of bacterial otitis media have an associated medical mastoiditis, an infection of the soft tissue surrounding the air spaces in the mastoid bone. Since this air cell system is confluent with the middle ear space, medical mastoiditis is treated concurrently with therapy for otitis media. No radiographs are indicated or necessary but usually reveal clouding of the mastoid air cell system when otitis media is present.

Surgical mastoiditis is an osteitis and periostitis (occasionally associated with thrombophlebitis of the horizontal and sigmoid venous sinuses) that follows acute otitis media. Surgical mastoiditis can be diagnosed clinically by the marked swelling, pitting edema, erythema, and percussion tenderness of the skin over the mastoid bone. Occasionally, edema and displacement of the posterosuperior external canal wall may occlude the canal. The swelling produces an anterior and inferior displacement of the auricle. Facial nerve paresis or paralysis may be present and typically signifies the need for more aggressive management. A fever of 104° to 105° may have a spiking pattern. Surgical mastoiditis is a medical and surgical emergency. Intravenous cephalosporins or ampicillin, in divided doses appropriate for weight, is begun immediately. An antistaphylococcal antibiotic should be given if *S. aureus* is suspected, pending culture results. Antibiotics are continued for 21 days. An otolaryngologist should be consulted on an urgent basis because surgery is often necessary, including myringotomy, mastoidectomy, incision and drainage of any abscess, and debridement of devitalized bone. These procedures must be performed as soon as possible.

Acute and Serous Otitis Media. As discussed, middle ear effusion develops with persistent negative intratympanic pressure. This condition results from eustachian tube dysfunction, which may be associated with such conditions as upper respiratory infection, chronic rhinosinusitis of bacterial or allergic origin, dysfunction of the soft palate (from clefts or surgical defects), and masses in the nasopharynx from adenoid hypertrophy or benign or malignant tumors. When an effusion persists beyond a few days or weeks, its character changes from a serous transudate to an increasingly mucoid, protein-laden exudate with an increasingly gluelike consistency. Although their role is not clear, bacteria are present in approximately one third of persistent effusions.

The diagnosis of middle ear effusion is established on examination. The tympanic membrane is classically thickened, with a gray or amber fluid seen in the middle ear. Sometimes a fluid meniscus, air bubbles, or bluish fluid may appear behind the tympanic membrane. Mobility of the membrane is always impaired. The membrane is frequently retracted by negative pressure, and if this condition is prolonged, retraction of the pars flaccida area may lead to the formation of a cholesteatoma (keratoma). Tympanometry is helpful in supporting the clinical impression of serous otitis media, especially in young children. Hearing may be evaluated by tuning forks and audiograms.

Chronic middle ear effusions represent a special problem in young children because effusions are most common in the early years, when significant speech development occurs. Persistent effusions and mild conductive hearing losses are associated with prolonged impairment of language acquisition skills, and these deficits may last for years. The patient's speech is less well developed than in peers of a similar age. Therefore, if medical management does not resolve middle ear effusions within 3 to 4 months, surgical intervention with myringotomy and possibly tubes should be considered.

Chronic middle ear effusions in adults may be secondary to a nasopharyngeal tumor, most often a poorly differentiated squamous cell carcinoma. This diagnosis must be suspected, actively sought, and then ruled out in every adult with a chronic unilateral middle ear effusion. Although the most common causes of middle ear effusions in adults are allergies, eustachian tube dysfunction, and barotrauma, nasopharyngeal tumor must be considered.

Therapy. In general, acute effusions are self-limited, resolving in about 2 weeks. A brief course of decongestants (e.g., pseudoephedrine, three or four times a day) or topical nasal spray may be helpful. If their use is prolonged, however, topical medications may promote reactive mucosal edema and prolong eustachian tube dysfunction. Typically, we do not recommend use of over-the-counter nasal sprays for more than 2 to 4 days. Antihistamines are of no proven benefit, except in the management of coryza or allergic symptoms. If bacterial infection is suspected or cannot be ruled out, antibiotics are used as in acute bacterial otitis media.

Certain measures can sometimes prevent the more severe manifestations in patients prone to develop acute effusions during air travel or diving. Young patients should be awakened when the airplane begins descent and given a bottle or other drink or chewing gum to promote eustachian tube opening with deglutition. Older patients can be instructed in autoinflation exercises. These exercises should be mastered before the flight. The ingestion of alcohol must be avoided, since the vascular dilation in the nasopharyngeal mucosa produces some edema and impairs eustachian tube opening. Patients of any age should be awake during the descent to promote eustachian tube activity by chewing, swallowing, or practicing autoinflation exercises. Topical decongestant medications such as nose sprays work rapidly and should be applied before short flights or just before descent. They are used similarly before diving.

Reestablishing proper aeration of the middle ear is the ultimate therapeutic goal in the management of chronic effusion. Effective therapy depends on establishing, if possible, the cause of eustachian tube dysfunction. Likely causes include chronic rhinosinusitis of bacterial or allergic origin, palatal dysfunction, and hypertrophied adenoid tissue or nasopharyngeal tumors. In infants, milk or other fluids may produce local irritation and flow into the eustachian tube with bacteria.

In older children and adults, autoinflation exercises may be helpful. These exercises include blowing the nose forcefully while the mouth and nares are kept closed. A hand-held nasal balloon "toy" that children enjoy using can be quickly constructed with a soft, flexible plastic tube such as a disposable medicine dropper. The tip of the bulb is removed with scissors, and the balloon or a rubber finger cot is secured over the opposite end with rubber bands. The tube is then placed in one nostril while the other is pinched closed, and the balloon is inflated through the nose. This procedure is repeated several times on both sides. Swallowing and motion of the palate (enhanced by the patient producing a "gunk" sound) while simultaneously maintaining balloon pressure or blowing the nose may open the eustachian tube. Once the patient has mastered such exercises, they should be repeated four to ten times a day.

When autoinflation exercises are unsuccessful or cannot be performed, medical therapy may be helpful. Most cases of chronic effusion resolve spontaneously over several weeks. Although antihistamines and decongestants have been widely used, their efficacy is not supported in clinical studies. Antihistamines and decongestants, however, may be efficacious in the allergic patient. In other patients, these medications may inhibit resolution of the effusion by producing more viscid secretions. A 7- to 10-day course of tapered steroids also may greatly reduce allergic effusions.

A chronic, low-grade, "steady-state" infectious process may be involved in one third of chronic effusions, as shown by the finding of bacteria in the chronic effusion fluids and the response of effusions to antibiotic treatment. The initial therapy for chronic effusions persisting beyond 3 to 4 weeks should be the same as for acute otitis media. Effective medications include amoxicillin, Augmentin, cefaclor, trimethoprim-sulfamethoxazole, erythromycin, clarithromycin, and loracarbef over a 14- to 21-day course and then, if necessary, once nightly at bedtime for 4 to 6 weeks. The effusions frequently resolve with this treatment, which may implicate low-grade bacterial infections in chronic effusions.

If the effusion persists more than 10 to 12 weeks despite adequate medical therapy and autoinflation exercises, an otolaryngologist should be consulted. This recommendation is also true when multiple recurrent episodes of effusion are present, especially if complicated by acute otitis media. In these situations, myringotomy and insertion of ventilation tubes may be considered. This treatment is especially important whenever conductive hearing loss is present. The ventilation tube allows equalization of middle ear pressure. Conductive hearing loss secondary to the effusion and impaired tympanic membrane mobility usually is greatly improved immediately after surgery.

Chronic effusions may produce tympanic atelectasis when the membrane touches the medial wall of the middle ear space. Retraction pockets may form in the tympanic membrane, and a thick adhesive effusion with chronic inflammation and mucosal hypertrophy may impair its function. Myringotomy and ventilation tubes prevent further progression of these problems. Tubes reverse these conditions and help to prevent chronic hearing loss, cholesteatoma formation, and chronic suppurative otitis media.

In occasional patients with adenoidal hypertrophy, the adenoidal tissue may occlude the eustachian tube orifices. Chronically infected adenoid tissue also may produce local edema that interferes with tubal function and, with lymphatic drainage from the middle ear, contributes to recurrent ear infections. Adenoidectomy may be helpful in resolving the effusion and recurrent infection problem.

Chronic Suppurative Otitis Media. Chronic suppurative otitis media always involves a tympanic membrane perforation or defect with chronic purulent otorrhea and middle ear inflammation. A mild to moderate conductive hearing loss is present. In general the condition is otherwise asymptomatic unless it progresses to involvement of the inner ear and produces sensorineural hearing loss, vertigo, and disequilibrium or facial nerve palsy. Cholesteatoma (keratoma) is the presence of normal squamous epithelium within the middle ear and may occur from retraction of the pars flaccida of the tympanic membrane with chronic negative pressure, with a sac being formed and gradually enlarging to enclose the trapped dead cells of desquamated skin. Alternatively, squamous epithelial tissue may migrate through a perforation of the tympanic membrane and slowly extend to form a large mass within the middle ear. The dead desquamated skin cells form an ideal medium for bacterial growth. The enlarging keratoma or cholesteatoma causes local destruction of bone and the ossicles and may progressively erode into the cranial cavity or inner ear, producing associated symptoms of meningitis and labyrinthitis. Epidural abscesses also may occur, since the ear and paranasal sinuses are the most common sites for these abscesses.

Chronic suppurative otitis media is characterized by a more complex bacteriology than simple otitis media. Cultures frequently reveal a mixed flora of aerobic and anaerobic organisms. The aerobic pathogens usually found include *Escherichia coli, S. aureus, Proteus mirabilis, P. aeruginosa,* and diphtheroid bacilli. Common anaerobes include *Bacteroides fragilis, Bacteroides melaninogenicus,* and *Peptococcus magnus.*

The diagnosis is established by examination and requires removal of secretions, crusts, and debris from the external canal and from against the tympanic membrane. Mucopurulent otorrhea is usually seen, and secretions may have a foul odor. After cleansing, the tympanic membrane is examined as previously described. A defect usually is seen in the superior, posterior, or inferior portion of the tympanic membrane. Mucopurulent fluid may be seen draining through the defect. The middle ear mucosa is extremely inflamed.

The initial treatment for chronic suppurative otitis media is medical. Topical antibiotics as given for external ear infections are helpful. In general, follow-up is by an otolaryngologist, who also should direct therapy. Surgery may be required for closure of a tympanic membrane defect or for exploration of the ear and mastoidectomy to eradicate chronic sources of infections, such as necrotic bone and cholesteatoma. The goal is to create a safe ear. A secondary but important consideration is improvement of hearing.

Inner Ear Infections (Table 178-4)

Acute Labyrinthitis. Labyrinthitis is an inflammation of inner ear structures of the resulting from invasion of microorganisms or irritation of the inner ear by the passage of toxic products from middle ear infections.

Viral Labyrinthitis. Many viruses may produce a labyrinthitis, but the most common is the mumps virus. If labyrinthitis occurs, the infection may produce a sudden unilateral inflammation of the cochlea with severe and total sensorineural hearing loss. Vertigo is uncommon with mumps. If the hearing loss is limited to one ear, no specific measures are required. Bilateral hearing losses are unusual but, when persistent, require amplification. Although some advocate systemic corticosteroid therapy to diminish inner ear destruction from viral infection, no clear evidence supports its efficacy.

Viral labyrinthitis involves damage to both the cochlea and the vestibular system. This condition is permanent and needs

Table 178-4. Inner Ear Infections

Labyrinthitis	Etiology	Clinical findings	Common microbiologic agents	Management
Viral	Middle ear infection Meningitis	Unilateral inflammation of cochlea, sensorineural hearing loss, vertigo	Mumps	Symptomatic
Bacterial	Acute or chronic otitis media Meningitis	Severe vertigo, nausea, vomiting, hearing loss	Agents causing acute and chronic otitis media	Myringotomy, intravenous antibiotic, mastoidectomy
Vascular	Occlusion of anteroinferior cerebellar artery or labyrinthine artery	Severe vertigo, hearing loss	Vascular insult	Symptomatic, possibly antiplatelet medications

to be differentiated from the transient vertigo that occurs in vestibular neuronitis.

Bacterial Labyrinthitis. Bacterial labyrinthitis may represent a complication of acute or chronic otitis media or of meningitis. Typical symptoms include hearing loss and severe vertigo associated with nausea and emesis. Labyrinthitis complicating acute otitis media requires more aggressive therapy than oral antibiotics. An otolaryngology consultation must be obtained on an urgent basis. Treatment requires myringotomy and intravenous (IV) administration of appropriate antibiotics, as determined by culture, sensitivity, and Gram's stain studies of the middle ear exudate. These tests must be performed immediately and before the the institution of the IV medication. If chronic suppurative otitis media is associated with a sudden development of labyrinthitis, effective therapy requires surgical debridement of the diseased tissue by mastoidectomy, in addition to the appropriate use of IV antibiotics, as determined by a culture and Gram's stain.

VERTIGO

Vertigo is the cardinal symptom of a disturbance of the vestibular system. The word refers to any hallucination of movement, whether a sensation of spinning, tilting, swaying, or falling. The pathology may exist anywhere in the vestibular pathway, from the vestibular end organs to the highest cerebral representation of the vestibular system in the temporal lobe. Thus the major priority in the management of the vertiginous patient is anatomic localization. With careful history taking and methodic physical examination the physician can select the most useful tests.

Normal equilibrium requires accurate information from the vestibular system as well as sensory input from the proprioceptive, visual, and cerebellar systems. Thus, although disequilibrium is often associated with vertigo, many disorders of balance may occur in the absence of vertigo. For instance, a lesion of the dorsal columns, which relay proprioceptive sensation, may cause marked disequilibrium but will not be associated with vertigo. Vertigo is the result of a conflict between the input to the brain from the vestibular system and from other systems concerned with the maintenance of normal balance.

The vestibular system may be divided anatomically into two parts, peripheral and central. The *peripheral* system comprises the vestibular end organs (semicircular canals, utricle, saccule, endolymphatic sac) and their first-order neuronal supply (afferent fibers, Scarpa's ganglia, centrally connected fibers). The *central* system is formed by the vestibular nuclei and their central projections. The examining physician must be familiar with the important practical differences between lesions of these two divisions of the vestibular system.

History

Obtaining an accurate history from the vertiginous patient is essential. Many patients have considerable difficulty in describing their symptoms, and such descriptions are often charged with emotion. Taking a careful history is tantamount in developing a clinical plan to diagnose and treat the problem efficiently.

Otologic History. The date and circumstances of onset should always be ascertained, as well as the frequency, severity, and duration of attacks. Peripheral lesions cause the greatest systemic upset because they are often associated with pallor, sweating, nausea, and vomiting. Episodic vertigo lasting a few seconds and associated with position changes is typically associated with benign positional vertigo. Vertigo lasting 30 minutes to 12 hours typically is seen in Ménière's disease, whereas that lasting several days suggests vestibular neuronitis or labyrinthitis (Table 178-5). Vertigo of psychogenic origin may have been present for several years. Factors that precipitate or aggravate attacks should be determined, such as association with a particular position or movement. The patient should be asked what he or she does to alleviate symptoms.

Because of the close anatomic relationship between the hearing and vestibular systems, vertigo may be associated with auditory symptoms. Such symptoms often provide valuable information about the localization of a lesion within the vestibular system (Table 178-6). Even the most subtle impairment of hearing, particularly if unilateral, is important because it may be the presenting feature of vestibular schwannoma. Tinnitus may accompany vertigo and may sometimes change character before or during a vertiginous episode. Other derangements of hearing, such as *diplacusis* (hearing the same pitch differently in each ear) or *paracusis* (distortion), are useful because they tend to suggest cochlear pathology. Symptoms suggestive of suppurative ear disease (e.g., earache, discharge) should be investigated. An expanding cholesteatoma (a collection of keratinizing squamous epithelium) may erode the bony labyrinth and cause a fistula in the semicircular canal.

Table 178-5. Typical Duration of Vertigo in Common Ear Problems

Condition	Duration of vertigo
Benign positional vertigo	Few seconds
Ménière's disease	30 minutes to 12 hours
Vestibular neuronitis	2-3 days
Labyrinthitis	3-10 days
Psychogenic	Several years

Table 178-6. Usual Hearing Status in Syndromes Associated With Vertigo

Hearing loss usual	Hearing loss unusual
Ménière's disease	Vestibular neuronitis
Labyrinthitis	Multiple sclerosis
Cholesteatomatous ear disease	Vertebrobasilar ischemia
Labyrinthine membrane rupture	Benign positional vertigo
Ototoxicity	Basilar migraine
Vestibular schwannoma	

Ototoxicity as a cause of vertigo is likely to be determined only by direct questioning. The vestibulotoxic effects of some drugs may not become apparent until several weeks after administration. Labyrinthine membrane rupture (oval or round windows) is an often unrecognized cause of vertigo that is eminently treatable. It should be suspected in patients whose symptoms occur after head injury, barotrauma (flying or diving), or unusual physical exertion. Patients should be referred without delay to an otolaryngologist. Previous otologic surgical procedures (e.g., mastoidectomy, stapedectomy) may have a direct effect on a patient's symptoms.

General History. Assessment of the vertiginous patient demands evaluation of other systems integrally related with the vestibular system. Patients should be questioned about certain symptoms that may suggest disease within the CNS or cardiovascular system. For example, loss of consciousness during an episode of vertigo strongly suggests a CNS lesion. It is important, however, not to confuse double vision with the disordered visual sensations that are a feature of vertigo. Numbness or weakness in the arms or legs and difficulty with swallowing or speech suggest CNS disease. Syncopal attacks associated with vertigo may be of cardiogenic origin, and such patients need cardiologic evaluation.

Disorders of equilibrium may signal an underlying stress phenomenon, often marital or employment difficulties. The old adage that "for every mistake made by not knowing, ten are made by not looking" can be aptly applied to the examination of the vertiginous patient. Particular attention must be paid to the otologic, neurologic, and cardiovascular systems, since the underlying disorder frequently resides in one of these areas.

Otologic Examination

The primary care physician should be able to perform a basic examination of the auditory and vestibular systems. The examination is initiated by inspecting the pinna for stigmata of previous surgery (e.g., postauricular incision scars) or for ecchymosis or hematoma (Battle's sign) in injured patients. The ear canal is examined by gently retracting the pinna upward and backward and gently introducing an otoscope. Cerumen may be removed with a wax hook or by syringing gently. The irrigation device is not aimed directly at the tympanic membrane because perforation can occur. The tympanic membrane is inspected in its entirety. Signs of an effusion are sought, and the mobility of the membrane is tested with the pneumatic otoscope. The physician should scrutinize the uppermost portion of the tympanic membrane (Shrapnell's membrane, or pars flaccida) because cholesteatomas frequently develop here. A cholesteatoma may cause a fistula into the lateral semicircular canal; increasing the pressure in the external canal (e.g., by tragal pressure or with a pneumatic otoscope) may induce vertigo (a positive fistula sign). Patients with this clinical presentation require urgent referral to an otolaryngologist.

Deafness. It is mandatory to test hearing in the vertiginous patient. Each ear should be tested separately while masking the opposite ear (placing a sound into the nontest ear). The patient is asked to repeat phonetically balanced words (e.g., send, thick, daybreak). In general, the patient should not miss more than one word in ten; otherwise, referral to an otolaryngologist should be arranged.

Tuning fork tests (Weber's and Rinne) should never be omitted (Table 178-7). They are simple to perform and can help differentiate between normal hearing and conductive and sensorineural hearing loss. *Weber's test* is performed by placing a vibrating tuning fork at the center of a patient's forehead. If the patient has a unilateral conductive hearing loss, the sound localizes to that ear because the better ear is being masked, or "distracted," by the ambient noise. Alternatively, if the patient has a unilateral sensorineural hearing loss, the sound localizes to the opposite ear, which has a better cochlear reserve. A patient who senses the sound in the midline may have normal hearing or bilateral hearing loss (either conductive or sensorineural) of equal severity.

The *Rinne test* compares the patient's hearing by air and bone conduction. In normal circumstances, sounds are better perceived by air conduction. A vibrating tuning fork is placed on the patient's mastoid process; the examiner should be sure that the patient is hearing it in the test ear. Then the tuning fork is placed opposite the patient's ear canal, and the patient is asked in which position the sound was heard clearest and longest. Patients with normal hearing or with sensorineural loss hear the sound better by air conduction (positive Rinne test). In conductive hearing loss, bone conduction is heard better than air conduction (negative Rinne response).

Nystagmus. Nystagmus and ataxia are the most objective signs of vertigo. Nystagmus refers to involuntary, repetitive movements of the eye and may be spontaneous or induced. A wide variety of disordered patterns of eye movement have been described; only those forms of nystagmus often encountered in primary practice are discussed here.

Table 178-7. Types of Hearing Loss Associated With Vertigo

Site of lesion	Example	Type of deafness	Tuning fork tests
Middle ear	Cholesteatoma	Conductive	Rinne-negative Weber's to affected ear
Cochlea	Ménière's disease	Sensorineural	Rinne-positive Weber's to better cochlea
Eighth nerve	Vestibular schwannoma	Sensorineural	Rinne-positive Weber's to better cochlea

Table 178-8. General Characteristics of Peripheral and Central Nystagmus

Peripheral nystagmus	Central nystagmus
Conjugate	Dysconjugate
Unidirectional	Multidirectional
Never vertical	May be vertical
Temporary	May be permanent
Associated with vertigo	May not be vertigo
Enhanced by loss of visual fixation	Unaffected by loss of visual fixation

Peripheral Nystagmus. Disease of the labyrinth or of its central connections may cause a jerky or "sawtooth" nystagmus, in which the eyes move slowly in one direction (the vestibular component) and rapidly return to a midline position (the central component). By convention, the direction of a nystagmus is the direction of the fast component or the central component. Knowledge of the features of this type of vertigo are of the utmost importance (Table 178-8).

To assess spontaneous nystagmus, the patient should sit opposite the examiner in a well-illuminated room. Vestibular nystagmus is enhanced by loss of optic fixation and may be achieved by having the patient use a Fresnel lens. These glasses have +20 diopter lenses, which prevent the patient from focusing and have the advantage of giving the observer a clear view of ocular movements. A simple hand lens may be helpful if Fresnel lenses are not available. While holding a finger at least 18 inches from the patient, the examiner asks the patient to follow it through an arc within 30 degrees of the primary position. Only sustained nystagmus within this range should be considered pathologic. Outside the range of 30 degrees, nystagmus is a finding in normal subjects and is associated with loss of binocular vision.

Central Nystagmus. The essential features of central nystagmus should be carefully contrasted with those of peripheral nystagmus (Table 178-8). Multidirectional or vertical nystagmus is a sinister finding indicating brainstem pathology. Nystagmus only in the abducting eye when the adducting eye is weak indicates internuclear ophthalmoplegia. This finding strongly suggests multiple sclerosis. Nystagmus occurring in the absence of vertigo is most likely caused by a central lesion.

Positional Nystagmus. Spontaneous nystagmus may be induced by the Dix-Hallpike maneuver. While the subject sits on a couch or examination table, the head is rapidly lowered to below the horizontal and turned to either side. The examiner should check the mobility of the cervical spine before performing this maneuver. In labyrinthine disorders, nystagmus is induced after a latent period of a few seconds, when the affected ear is undermost, and has all the hallmarks of a peripheral nystagmus. Further, the nystagmus is fatigable, since it diminishes in severity each time the test is repeated. Positional nystagmus caused by central pathology may be vertical or multidirectional, is not fatigable, and may not be associated with vertigo.

Caloric Testing. This test is performed with the patient lying supine on an examination couch with the head raised 30 degrees (in this position, the lateral semicircular canals are in the vertical plane). Each ear is irrigated with cold and warm water. Cold water causes nystagmus to the opposite side, whereas warm water results in nystagmus to the same side as the irrigated ear (COWS: cold, opposite, warm, same). Caloric testing evaluates impaired responsiveness of a labyrinth to caloric stimuli and assessment of the involved side.

Physical Examination

Every patient with vertigo requires a full physical examination. Blood pressure should be determined in both arms and in the lying and standing positions. The neck should be auscultated carefully for bruits and for evidence of a subclavian steal syndrome. In the neurologic examination, all the cranial nerves should be tested, signs of cerebellar dysfunction sought, and the peripheral nervous system evaluated, with particular reference to the maintenance of posture and gait (Table 178-9). Complete blood count, erythrocyte sedimentation rate, glucose tolerance testing, blood urea nitrogen, and thyroid function tests are done as indicated by the primary care physician. It is important to consider neurosyphilis as a cause of vertigo; in suspected cases a fluorescent *Treponema* antibody absorption test should be obtained (VDRL misses congenital syphilis in about 50% of cases). Examination of the cerebrospinal fluid may be valuable in multiple sclerosis (elevated levels of IgG or oligoclonal bands, which are suggestive but not pathognomonic of the diagnosis).

The radiologic investigations should be appropriate to the nature of the suspected underlying pathology. When a lesion of the internal auditory canal is suspected, an auditory brainstem response is typically obtained. This test is accurate in 96% of cases and has a false-negative rate of approximately 1% to 2%. It is considered an excellent screening test to evaluate for tumors on the cochleovestibular nerve. In either case, magnetic resonance imaging (MRI) with gadolinium may reveal subtle pathology in exquisite detail and currently is the procedure of choice. In patients who

Table 178-9. Outline of Neurologic Examination

Cranial nerve	Test
I	Sense of smell
II	Fundi, visual acuity, visual fields, light reflexes
III, IV, VI	Eye movements; check for spontaneous nystagmus (may need Fresnel lenses)
V	Corneal reflexes, facial sensation
VII	Check for palsy or spasm
	Test sensation on posterior wall of ear canal
VIII	Hearing and vestibular testing
IX	Tonsilar sensation
X	Gag reflex, soft palate movements, vocal cord movements
XI	Sternomastoid and trapezius contractions
XII	Tongue movements
Test of equilibrium	Romberg's
	Gait
Cerebellar tests	Evaluate for dysmetria (past pointing), dysdiadochokinesia (inability to perform successive movements), rebound and gait (usually wide based)

cannot undergo MRI, CT with dye enhancement may be necessary.

Disorders Associated With Vertigo (Table 178-10)

Ménière's Disease. Ménière's disease consists of four main symptoms: vertigo, hearing loss, tinnitus, and fullness. Classically, all these symptoms must be present for the correct diagnosis to be made. Ménière's disease has been further subclassified into *cochlear* and *vestibular* forms to differentiate patients who have only cochlear symptoms from those with only vestibular symptoms. The symptoms are generally attributed to distention of the membranous labyrinth (endolymphatic hydrops). The vertigo may be violent and is usually associated with nausea and vomiting. It rarely lasts less than a half hour or persists for more than 12 hours. The deafness in Ménière's disease is of a fluctuating sensorineural type, most marked initially in the low tones, and is accompanied by loudness recruitment. Hearing loss may be permanent. Every patient with suspected Ménière's disease should be evaluated by an otolaryngologist early.

The treatment of Ménière's disease is controversial. In the natural history of the disease, spontaneous remission occurs in 50% to 60% of patients, making it difficult to evaluate the true efficacy of any treatment modality. After full evaluation, reassurance is sufficient for many patients. Salt-restricted diets and triamterene with hydrochlorothiazide (Dyazide) may be beneficial. The most frequently used vestibular suppressants are the antihistamines, such as meclizine (Antivert) and cyclizine (Marezine). Diazepam (Valium) is a valuable adjunct to treatment in the acute attack and in patients with anxiety. These drugs should be used only for a limited period. Surgical therapy is indicated when symptoms are disruptive to a patient's life and persist despite appropriate medical therapy. The procedure undertaken depends on the level of hearing and whether the disease is unilateral or bilateral. Some procedures decompress the labyrinth (endolymphatic sac surgery, cochleosacculotomy) and strive to preserve hearing. Total destruction of the labyrinth (labyrinthectomy) is an effective procedure in an ear with total or near-total sensorineural hearing loss. Vestibular nerve section has the advantage of treating vertigo while preserving cochlear function. Recently, there has been a renewed interest in the transtympanic use of oto/vestibulotoxic drugs such as gentamicin and less frequently streptomycin.

Vestibular Neuronitis. The cause of vestibular neuronitis is uncertain, but some evidence implicates a viral or vascular etiology. The symptoms, severe vertigo with nausea and vomiting, usually last for 2 to 3 days. An important feature is the absence of cochlear symptoms or signs. After the acute episode subsides, the patient may experience minor episodes of disequilibrium over the ensuing months to years. The condition is self-limiting, and symptomatic initial treatment with vestibular suppressants followed by vestibular rehabilitation with vestibular exercises is usually sufficient.

Multiple Sclerosis. The diagnosis of multiple sclerosis may be difficult, and suspected cases should be referred to a neurologist. A plaque of demyelination in the brainstem may cause an acute vertiginous episode. Patients typically are young, healthy adults with no previous neurologic history. The accompanying nystagmus, which may persist after the vertigo has abated, is central. The finding of nystagmus in the abducting eye, with weakness in the adducting eye (internuclear ophthalmoplegia), strongly suggests the diagnosis. Auditory brainstem response may show changes in the auditory system that are not detectable by conventional testing. MRI may demonstrate pathognomonic plaques within the brain and spinal cord.

Benign Positional Vertigo (Cupulolithiasis). Patients with cupulolithiasis complain of vertigo when they adopt particular positions (e.g., turning in bed, bending, stooping). It often occurs after head injury. Cupulolithiasis may be caused by release of otoconia (statoconia) from a disrupted utricle into the endolymph. Otoconia then become deposited on the cupula of the posterior semicircular canal, making it unduly sensitive to head movement. It is important to distinguish this condition from postural hypotension, in which there are no auditory symptoms and the vertigo lasts only a few seconds.

Positional testing is extremely useful in differentiating those cases caused by end-organ pathology (usually the posterior semicircular canal or utricle) and those due to brainstem pathology. The diagnosis of benign positional vertigo clearly depends on the correct interpretation of the observed nystagmus. Treatment formerly was avoidance of provocative positions; however, current recommendations strongly suggest vestibular habituation exercises known as Cawthorne exercises. These exercises are a program of progressive movements of the head, neck, and upper body that provoke vertigo initially but over time attenuate the symptoms in approximately 90% of patients. Another conservative possibility includes a maneuver to reposition the otoconia. Of the 10% who fail conservative management, singular neurectomy (section of the posterior ampullary nerve that innervates the posterior semicircular canal) or surgical occlusion of the posterior semicircular canal may be beneficial. Referral to an otolaryngologist is indicated if

Table 178-10. Disorders Associated With Vertigo

	Etiology and contributing factors	Clinical findings	Diagnosis	Management
Ménière's disease Cochlear Vestibular	Idiopathic; distention of membranous labyrinth (endolymphatic hydrops)	Vertigo, fluctuating sensorineural hearing loss, roaring tinnitus, fullness in ear	Clinical; audiologic and vestibular testing	Reassurance, salt-restricted diet, triamterene and diazepam, vestibular suppressants, surgical therapy
Vestibular neuronitis	Viral or vascular (?)	Severe vertigo, nausea, vomiting (absence of cochlear signs)	Clinical	Symptomatic-vestibular sedatives, vestibular exercises
Multiple sclerosis	Demyelinating plaque in brainstem	Central nystagmus, internuclear ophthalmoplegia	MRI	Symptomatic
Benign positional vertigo (cupulolithiasis)	Deposits of otoconia on cupula, after head injury, positional changes	Vertigo (no auditory symptoms)	Clinical; positional testing	Cawthorne exercise, repositioning maneuver, singular neurectomy Posterior semicircular canal occlusion
Vertebrobasilar ischemia	Episodic ischemia of brainstem due to vasospasm, hemodynamic factors, or platelet aggregation	Vertigo, tinnitus, signs of brainstem ischemia Subclavian steal syndrome		Neurologic and cardiovascular management
Vestibular schwannoma (acoustic neuroma)	Benign neoplasm	Mild vertigo, sensorineural hearing loss with poor speech discrimination, involvement of cranial nerves, increased intracranial pressure	MRI	Surgical

MRI, Magnetic resonance imaging.

patients do not improve significantly after 1 month of exercises.

Vertebrobasilar Ischemia. Vertebrobasilar ischemia due to episodic ischemia of the brainstem is caused by a circulatory disturbance in the distribution of the vertebrobasilar artery and is a form of transient ischemic attack. Such episodes may result from hemodynamic factors, vasospasm, or platelet aggregation. Vertigo and tinnitus are the outstanding symptoms but must be accompanied by symptoms or signs of brainstem ischemia, such as diplopia, homonymous hemianopia, facial dysesthesias, dysarthria, or ipsilateral ataxia. Exercising an arm may rarely induce ischemia of the vertebrobasilar system (subclavian steal syndrome). Patients with these transient ischemic attacks should be referred for neurologic and cardiovascular assessment.

Vestibular Schwannoma (Acoustic Neuroma). A benign neoplasm, vestibular schwannoma may vary from the most subtle audiovestibular disturbance to increased intracranial pressure (ICP), constituting a medical emergency. The vertigo caused by these neoplasms is usually mild or completely absent. The patient usually has unilateral sensorineural hearing loss with tone decay and poor speech discrimination. Caloric stimulation may show a canal weakness on the affected side. Involvement of the fifth cranial nerve may be inferred from an impaired corneal reflex or by a disturbance of facial sensation. Large tumors may cause a sixth nerve palsy, facial paralysis, ipsilateral cerebellar deficits, and ultimately, increased ICP and papilledema. Prognosis is directly related to tumor size, which in turn depends on early diagnosis. Thus patients with even minimal audiovestibular dysfunction, particularly unilateral, should always be referred for otolaryngologic evaluation.

FACIAL PARALYSIS

Facial paralysis is a symptom of an underlying disease. The physician must localize the site of nerve injury, assess its severity, establish its nature, and, if possible, treat the underlying causes (Box 178-1). The ability to localize the site of facial nerve injury follows directly from a knowledge of the nerve's anatomy (Fig. 178-7). Simple tests (topognostic tests) have been devised to evaluate the various branches of the facial nerve. Interpretation of results may be performed best by an otolaryngologist. These tests are not always routinely performed but may include tests to determine lacrimation (Schirmer's test), salivation (electrogustometry), and audiologic parameters (stapedial reflex testing).

The diagnosis of facial paralysis rarely presents any difficulty. Because facial paralysis has many causes, however, thorough history taking and physical examination are essential (Box 178-2). The single most important structure that may be affected by facial paralysis is the eye; without appropriate care, blindness may result. Several measures to

Box 178-1. Etiology of Facial Paralysis

Infection

Bacterial
- Otitis media
- Mastoiditis
- Chronic suppurative otitis media (especially with cholesteatoma)
- Meningitis
- "Malignant otitis media"

Viral
- Infectious mononucleosis
- Herpes zoster
- Varicella
- Rubella
- Mumps

Mycobacterial
- Tuberculous meningitis
- Leprosy

Miscellaneous
- Syphilis
- Malaria

Trauma

Temporal bone fracture
Facial lacerations
Surgical

Neoplasm

Malignant
- Squamous cell carcinoma
- Basal cell and adenocystic tumors
- Leukemia
- Parotid neoplasms
- Metastatic tumors

Benign
- Vestibular schwannoma
- Congenital cholesteatoma
- Facial nerve neuroma

Immunologic

Guillain-Barré syndrome
Reaction to tetanus antiserum
Periarteritis nodosa

Metabolic

Pregnancy
Hypothyroidism
Diabetes mellitus

protect the cornea temporarily or permanently can be performed by an otolaryngologist or ophthalmologist. Eyedrops, protective eyeglasses, and moisture chambers may be sufficient in milder cases. In some patients, the eyelids may need to be taped together, with care that the tape does not touch the cornea. Surgical procedures such as tarsorrhaphy or the implantation of a palpebral spring or gold weight are needed if paralysis is permanent or likely to be prolonged. An ophthalmologist should be consulted early in the course of a facial paralysis.

Idiopathic Facial Paralysis (Bell's Palsy) (see Chapter 162)

Although the etiology of Bell's palsy is an enigma, support favors the viral inflammatory immune concept based on serologic findings in patients with Bell's palsy and the isolation of herpes simplex type I virus from the epineurium of biopsy specimens. Immune complexes found in the chorda tympani are of viral origin. The vascular theory for Bell's palsy suggests that edema of the nerve (possibly initiated by vasospasm or viral infection) causes further ischemia of the nerve within its narrow, unyielding, bony canal.

Treatment of Bell's palsy is controversial and should consider the natural history. Spontaneous recovery of full function can be expected in 80% of patients; 10% have mild sequelae. The remainder, about 10% or less, have severe sequelae and poor return of facial function. Steroid therapy is used in Bell's palsy, although support is lacking; prednisone (1 mg/kg/day) is recommended. Surgical decompression of the nerve has limited application.

Suppurative Ear Disease

Acute Otitis Media. The widespread use of antibiotics in acute otitis media has considerably lessened the frequency of facial paralysis as a complication of otitis media. When it occurs, the nerve is usually dehiscent (incompletely covered by bone), and its sheath becomes involved in the inflammatory process. The paralysis is caused by neuropraxia. Treatment requires the judicious use of antibiotics, myringotomy, and culture of the middle ear aspirate. In acute mastoiditis a cortical mastoidectomy should be performed. Exploration of the nerve is generally not indicated.

Chronic Otitis Media. Facial paralysis complicated by chronic ear disease is most often the result of an expanding cholesteatoma, which may exert direct pressure on the nerve. It may also occur in noncholesteatomatous ear disease as a result of a low-grade osteitis involving the nerve sheath. The prognosis for return of facial nerve function depends on the degree of nerve degeneration. Timely surgical intervention may avert permanent facial paralysis, emphasizing the need for early referral to an otolaryngologist.

Temporal Bone Fracture

The most frequent temporal bone fracture (about 90% of cases) occurs in the long axis (longitudinal fractures). Fortunately, the facial nerve is involved in only about 10%. Fractures in the transverse axis of the temporal bone occur less often (about 10% of cases), but about half are complicated by facial paralysis. The time of onset of the facial paralysis is of prime importance. If the onset immediately follows the injury, severe injury to the nerve is likely to occur; if it occurs several hours or days after the injury, nerve continuity is ensured and the prognosis for spontaneous recovery is good. Basilar skull fractures usually are managed primarily by a neurosurgeon, and the decision to explore the facial nerve is made in consultation with an otolaryngologist. The decision is clearly influenced by the patient's general condition, the time of onset of the paralysis (immediate or delayed), and the presence or absence of degeneration, as evidenced by electrophysiologic testing.

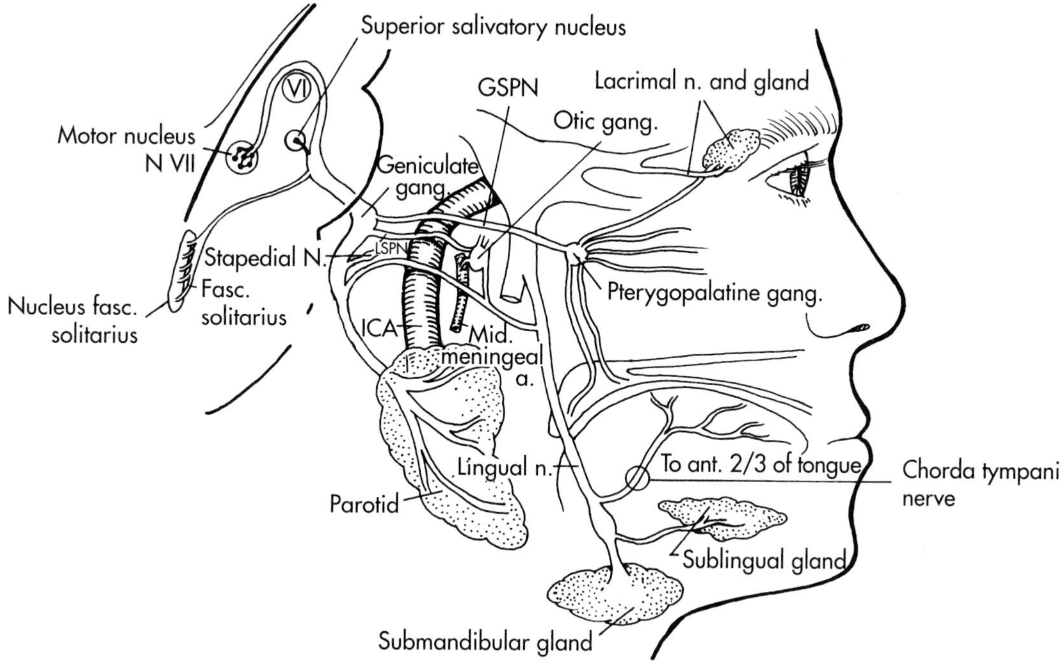

Fig. 178-7. Facial nerve anatomy. *GSPN*, Greater-nerve; *ICA*, internal carotid artery; *LSPN*, lesser-nerve; *n.*, nerve; *fasc.*, fasciculus; *a*, artery; *gang.*, ganglion; *ant.*, anterior.

Box 178-2. Diagnostic Workup in Facial Paralysis

Examination
- Otolaryngologic and neurologic evaluation
- Photographic records of facial movements
- General physical examination

Topognostic studies: Schirmer's test stapedial reflex testing taste testing

Electrophysiologic studies: nerve excitability testing, electromyography, electroneuronography

Audiology: pure tone audiometry and impedance tests, electronystagmography

Radiology: MRI and CT scanning as indicated

Hematology: complete blood count, sedimentation rate, other investigations (glucose tolerance thyroid function tests) as indicated

Herpes Zoster Oticus (Ramsay Hunt Syndrome)

The Ramsey Hunt syndrome comprises a triad of clinical findings: vesication of the auricle, facial nerve paralysis, and audiovestibular disturbances. In many cases, vesicular eruption may be seen in the areas of distribution of the cervical, trigeminal, glossopharyngeal, or vagus nerves, thus the term *cephalic herpes zoster.* Steroids have unproven value but are often used. Acyclovir also has been advocated. (For other etiologies in facial nerve paralysis, see a general otolaryngology text.)

REFERENCES

1. Seidman MD, et al: Mitochondrial DNA deletions associated with aging and presbycusis, *Arch Otolaryngol Head Neck Surg,* 123, 1997.
2. Seidman MD: The effects of dietary restrictions and antioxidants on presbycusis, *Laryngoscope* 110(5):727-738, 2000.

ADDITIONAL READINGS

Otolaryngology

Bluestone CD, Stool S, editors: *Pediatric otolaryngology,* Philadelphia, 1983, Saunders.

English GM, editor: *Otolaryngology,* Hagerstown, Md, 1976, Harper & Row.

Goodhill V, editor: *Ear diseases, deafness and dizziness,* Hagerstown, Md, 1979, Harper & Row.

Paparella MM, Shumrick DA, editors: *Otolaryngology,* ed 2, Philadelphia, 1980, Saunders.

Sade J: *Secretory otitis media and its sequelae,* New York, 1979, Churchill Livingstone.

Vertigo

Epley JM: The canalith repositioning procedure for treatment of benign positional vertigo, *Otolaryngol Head Neck Surg* 107:399, 1992.

Gibson WPR: The functional and physical examination of the vestibular system. In Ballantyne J, Groves J, editors: *Scott Brown's Diseases of the ear, nose and throat,* ed 4, vol 2, London, 1979, Butterworth.

Parnes LS, Price-Jones RG: Particle repositioning maneuver for benign paroxysmal positional vertigo, *Ann Otol Rhinol Laryngol* 102:325, 1993.

Schuknecht HF: Cupulolithiasis, *Arch Otolaryngol* 90:765, 1969.

Facial Paralysis

Esslen E: *The acute facial palsies: investigations on the localization and pathogenesis of meatolabyrinthine facial palsies,* New York, 1977, Springer-Verlag.

Fisch U, Felix H: On the pathogenesis of Bell's palsy, *Acta Otolaryngol (Stockh)* 95:532, 1983.

Graham MD, House WF, editors: *Disorders of the facial nerve,* New York, 1981, Raven.

May M: Facial nerve disorders, *Am J Otolaryngol* 4:77, 1982.

CHAPTER 179

The Nose and Paranasal Sinuses

Samuel A. Mickelson
Michael S. Benninger

The nose and paranasal sinuses provide for the diverse functions of respiration, conditioning and purifying inspired air, and olfaction. Although healthy individuals are not necessarily conscious of these functions, they may be significant sources of discomfort and lifestyle interruption when dysfunctional. In fact, nasal sinus–related disorders are the most common reason that patients now visit physicians in the United States. This chapter concerns the more common disorders affecting these sites and suggests approaches to management of patients with nasal and sinus disorders.

MEDICAL HISTORY

Symptoms and Their Significance

Many disorders affecting the nose and paranasal sinuses can be diagnosed by history and physical examination alone. Most laboratory testing is confirmatory only. It is important to obtain a thorough history and have an understanding of the various symptoms and their significance. The major symptoms related to the nose are nasal obstruction (congestion), drainage, facial pain or headache, epistaxis, and change in smell or taste.

Nasal Obstruction

Nasal obstruction (congestion or stuffy nose) can be caused by a deflected nasal septum, enlargement of turbinates, or polyps or mass lesions within the nose. Nasal obstruction is the most common symptom, since turbinate hypertrophy can result from many disorders. It is important to assess whether the nasal obstruction is unilateral, bilateral, or alternating in sides and determine if it is constant or intermittent. If unilateral, a fixed anatomic problem such as a deviated septum, polyp, or mass lesion is likely. Any intermittent or alternating obstruction must relate to variations in the turbinate size. When bilateral, the obstruction is due to a bilateral process such as polyps or allergy, or from a complex deflection of the septum.

Nasal Drainage and Postnasal Drip

Drainage from the nose is one of the most helpful symptoms in determining the nature of the disorder. It is important to determine if rhinorrhea is unilateral or bilateral, clear or discolored, and watery, mucoid, or tenacious. Unilateral drainage represents a localized process such as unilateral sinusitis or cerebrospinal fluid (CSF) leak, whereas bilateral drainage is due to a more systemic or general process. Clear drainage suggests a diagnosis of vasomotor, nonallergic, or allergic rhinitis, whereas thick and discolored (yellow, green, or brown) drainage suggests bacterial or viral infection. The sensation of postnasal drainage is influenced more by the thickness of the drainage than the quantity. Though many patients complain that swallowing large amounts of drainage causes nausea, it is unclear if they are causally related. A sense of mucus in the throat, hoarseness, and chronic throat clearing are rarely, if ever, caused by sinus drainage since the normal swallowing mechanism clears the mucus without laryngeal contact. The exceptions are during an allergic or viral episode where both nasal sinus and laryngeal inflammation occur simultaneously.

Facial Pain and Headache

Facial pain and headache are not useful symptoms in differentiating disorders because of the multiple different disorders that can cause pain. These include many of the nasal and sinus disorders, tension headache, migraine headache, myofacial pain syndrome, temporomandibular joint syndrome, tic douloureux, and dental caries. Pain overlying the sinuses is not necessarily due to pathology in the underlying sinus. When pain is related to nasal or sinus pathology, it is usually due to ostial obstruction or mucous membrane contact with referred pain to other areas of the face. Severe facial pain associated with swelling over the sinuses and purulent drainage is generally related to sinusitis. Many patients with allergic or nonallergic rhinitis complain of intermittent facial pressure or headache associated with changes in the weather, humidity, or other environmental factors. Malignant tumors are to be considered in patients with persistent unilateral facial pain without purulent rhinorrhea.

Epistaxis

Epistaxis is a nonspecific symptom that may accompany almost any pathology in the nose, nasopharynx, or paranasal sinuses. The most common cause of bleeding is breaks in the prominent capillary vessels along the anterior septum (Kiesselbach's plexus or Little's area). This occurs frequently with local trauma such as frequent nose blowing, sneezing, or digitally caused trauma. Once bleeding occurs, it may spontaneously recur if the scab becomes dislodged. Patients with a septal deviation may bleed along the deflected portion of the septum, which becomes dry and excoriated. Blood mixed with purulent drainage generally suggests acute sinusitis. Blood will exit anteriorly if the head is leaned forward and posteriorly if the head is straight or leaned backward. Tumors are rare causes of nasal bleeding.

Changes in Olfaction

Anosmia is the complete loss of olfaction, and hyposmia is a decrease in the sense of smell. Parosmia and dysosmia are conditions resulting in an altered sense of smell. Cacosmia, the sensation of unpleasant smell, can occur with acute sinusitis, when recovering from anosmia after influenza or head trauma, or with the use of tetracycline or streptomycin. Phantosmia is the hallucination of smells and can be seen in schizophrenia and temporal lobe seizures.

Anosmia or hyposmia can occur in any condition that affects nasal air flow to the region of the cribriform plate bilaterally. Therefore an alteration in smell thresholds is common in patients with nasal polyps or severe chronic sinusitis, whereas unilateral anosmia usually goes unnoticed. Anosmia without nasal obstruction is most frequently caused by viral upper respiratory tract infections or severe head trauma. Certain industrial chemicals, such as formaldehyde, can also lead to anosmia. Lead poisoning, vitamin A deficiency, tobacco use, and radiation therapy have been associated with hyposmia or anosmia. Hyposmia occurring in hypogonadal females or during pregnancy is relieved with hormonal treatments or the completion of pregnancy. Rarely, an anterior cranial fossa meningioma can cause slowly progressive anosmia. Other rare causes of anosmia include diabetes, hypothyroidism, pernicious anemia, and amphetamine toxicity.

Congenital or genetic causes of anosmia include Turner syndrome, pseudohypoparathyroidism, and congenital hypogonadotrophic eunuchoidism. A decreased sense of smell frequently occurs with increasing age (presbyosmia).

In patients with anosmia but a normal nasal examination, a thorough history and directed laboratory and radiologic tests usually determine the etiology. Treatment of the loss of olfaction should be directed at the cause. Postviral anosmia often spontaneously resolves. Use of oral zinc supplements has recently been advocated for persistent anosmia but benefit has not been proved. Patient counseling is of utmost importance with regard to use of smoke detectors in the home, avoidance of excessive perfumes or colognes, control of bodily odors, and attention to expiration dates on food products.

Allergic Symptoms

Characteristic symptoms of seasonal allergic rhinitis include sneezing, nasal or ocular pruritus, bilateral clear watery or mucoid nasal drainage, and nasal congestion. Patients also complain of pruritus of the upper palate and ears, and dry, scratchy and erythematous conjunctiva. These symptoms are associated with elevations of specific pollen counts. Springtime allergies typically relate to tree pollens, midsummer symptoms to grasses, and fall symptoms to weed pollens.

Dust and mold perennial allergies are less distinct because nasal congestion and clear drainage frequently occur without sneezing and pruritus. Patients with dust or mite allergies are more symptomatic in the morning and with exposure to upholstered furniture, mattresses, pillows, and carpeting. Mold allergies vary significantly through the year depending on the particular mold sensitivities.

Tobacco, Medications, and Chemical Exposures

Tobacco smoke is an irritant causing congestion of the turbinates, destruction of cilia, and alteration in the mucus-secreting cells of the nasal mucosa. Smokers have increased symptoms of nasal congestion and thick postnasal drainage and may be predisposed to sinusitis.

A variety of medications can also affect the nose. After just a few days of using topical phenylephrine or oxymetazoline, there is rebound swelling of the turbinates (rhinitis medicamentosa) in which the nose becomes chronically congested. Treatment is the discontinuation of the offending agents. Diuretics cause thicker and more tenacious secretions. Turbinate hypertrophy is caused by many drugs, including β-blockers, reserpine, and exogenous estrogens. Although most medication effects are temporary, long-term use of these drugs can have irreversible effects on the nose.

Many chemicals used in industry cause mucosal edema and increased mucoid secretion from the turbinates. Use of intranasal cocaine can cause large septal perforations with resultant bleeding and crusting from the edges. Wood dust and asbestos exposure can also have irritant effects on the nose with secondary congestion of the turbinates.

Systemic Disorders and Their Effects

Systemic conditions can affect the nose either directly or indirectly. Rhinitis of pregnancy due to elevated estrogen levels causes turbinate engorgement and resolves at the end of pregnancy. When severe it can be treated with an oral decongestant.

Sarcoidosis and Wegener's granulomatosis can affect the nose and are covered in more detail later.

EXAMINATION AND DIAGNOSTIC STUDIES

Physical Examination

The nasal examination is important in the diagnostic work-up of any nasal or sinus disorder because most pathologic conditions can be visualized without special studies (Fig. 179-1). Otolaryngologists typically examine the nose before and after use of a topical decongestant to allow a better view of the nasal cavity. Anterior rhinoscopy with a nasal speculum and headlight allows delineation of the septum, the inferior and middle turbinates, and portions of the nasopharynx and may allow a limited view into the middle meatus. Posterior rhinoscopy with a tongue blade, nasopharyngeal mirror, and headlight allow examination of the posterior choana, nasopharynx, eustachian tubes, and posterior edges of the septum and inferior turbinates. Although examination of the anterior nares with an otoscope is easy, the view is limited to the first 2 or 3 cm of the nose. If this technique is to be used, the nose should at least be decongested first with a topical decongestant.

Flexible and rigid nasal endoscopes have recently been reintroduced for use in the nose in the office setting. The procedure is done after application of a topical decongestant and anesthetic agent. Nasal endoscopy is a sensitive way to evaluate the nose for gross or subtle changes associated with sinusitis. The scope can frequently identify small polyps, erythema, and purulent drainage coming from sinus ostia that would not be visible by routine anterior or posterior rhinoscopy. The maxillary sinuses can also be examined with the endoscope via a sinus puncture, which can assist in the diagnosis of sinus malignancies. Due to the high cost of the instrumentation, nasal endoscopy should not be used for the routine examination of the nose.

Transillumination is a simple technique whereby a bright light (in a darkened room) is applied to the frontal or maxillary sinuses. Transillumination occurs in a sinus with normal or slightly thickened mucosa, whereas the light does not transmit in an opacified or fluid-filled sinus. Transillumination can be used instead of a radiograph before treating acute sinusitis.

Laboratory Studies

Nasal and nasopharyngeal cultures are generally not useful because pathologic bacteria (*Staphylococcus aureus, Streptococcus pneumoniae, Haemophilus influenzae,* and *Moraxella catarrhalis*) are present in both normal and sinusitis patients. Cultures from a sinus tap or from an endoscopic-guided culture through the sinus ostia are more precise.

Nasal smears are simple and inexpensive studies that can help differentiate sinusitis from allergic or nonallergic rhinitis by determining the type of white blood cells present. A predominance of eosinophils suggests allergic rhinitis, whereas predominance of leukocytes suggests an infection.

Serum immunoglobulin (Ig) levels can be helpful in the diagnosis of allergic rhinitis (elevated IgE level). Immunoglobulin G (IgG) subclass studies are performed when an immune deficiency is suspected as a cause for persistent

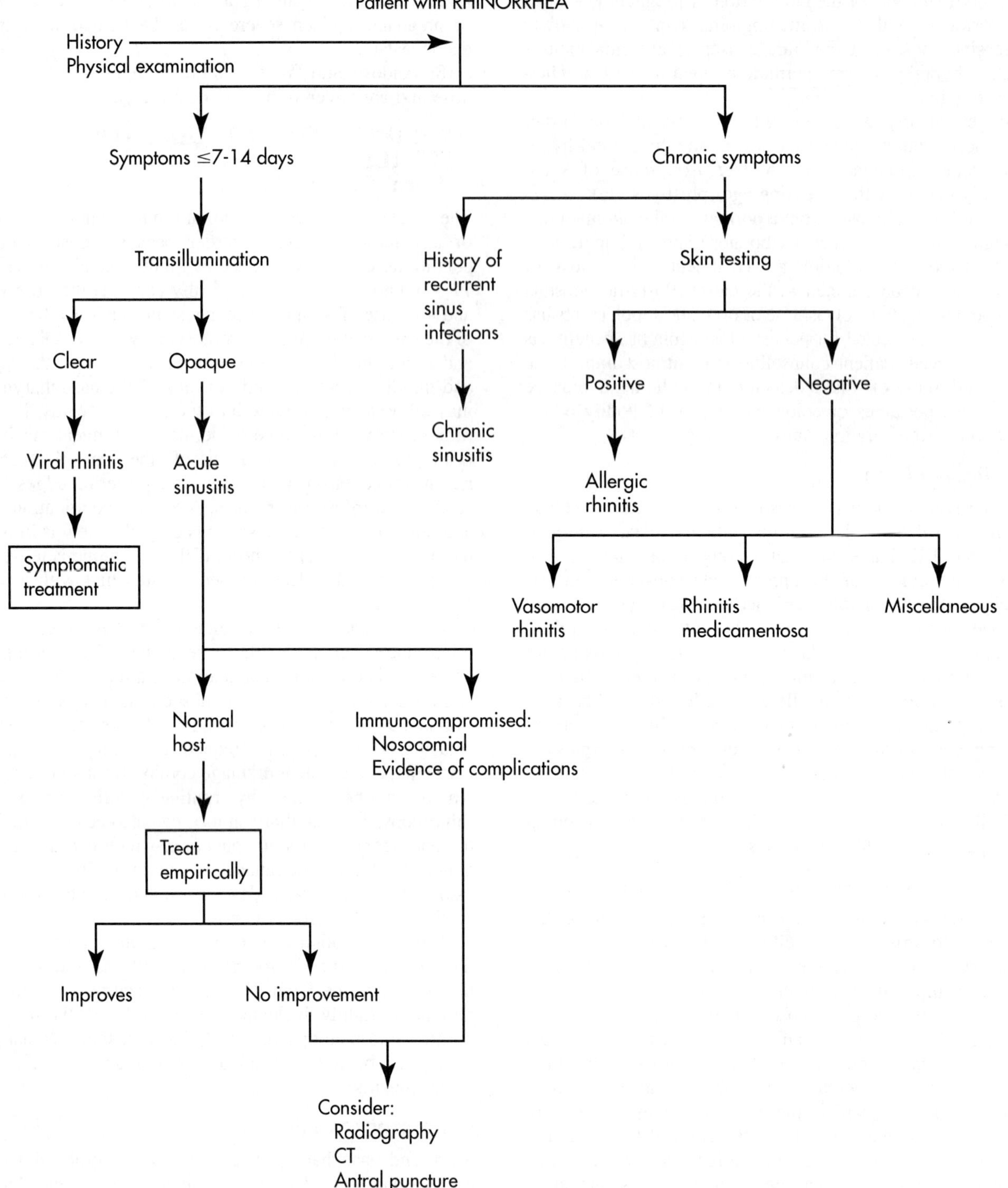

Fig. 179-1. Algorithm describing the treatment of a patient with rhinorrhea.

sinusitis. The patient's immunologic response to a pneumococcal vaccine can confirm or eliminate a functional immune deficiency. A complete blood count is useful to help differentiate bacterial sinusitis (elevated neutrophil count) from viral rhinitis (elevated lymphocyte count).

Radiographic Tests

Routine sinus films are useful to help confirm a suspicion of sinusitis and to follow disease resolution following a course of treatment. They are sensitive for air-fluid levels (Fig. 179-2) in the maxillary or frontal sinuses and for moderate to severe mucosal thickening or complete opacification in the maxillary sinuses (Fig. 179-3). However, their ability to identify mild ethmoid, sphenoid, maxillary, or frontal mucosal thickening is severely limited.

Computed tomography (CT) is the most useful of all radiographic studies for the paranasal sinuses. Axial and coronal views give detailed information about the osseous

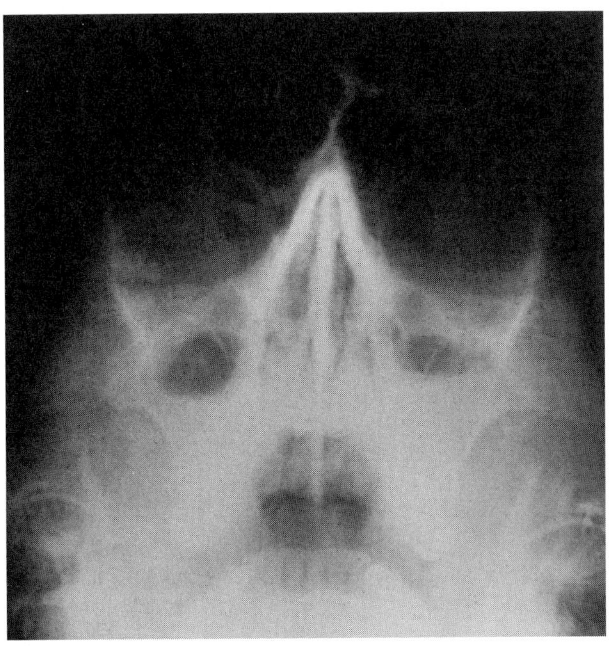

Fig. 179-2. Waters' view of maxillary sinus with air-fluid level.

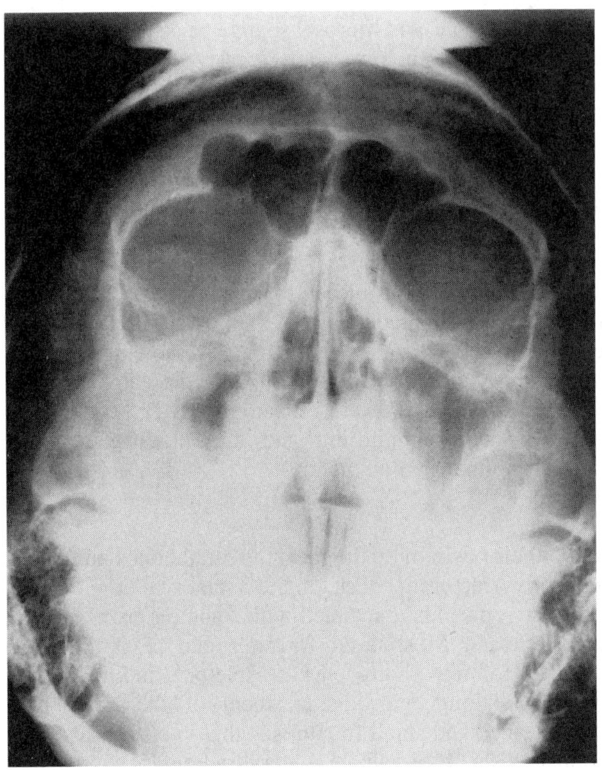

Fig. 179-3. Waters' view of maxillary sinus with mucosal thickening.

and soft tissues of the nose and paranasal sinuses, as well as the region of the osteomeatal complex. While some centers perform screening CT scans at a fee comparable to routine sinus films, they should rarely be ordered by primary care physicians, since their major roles are in assessing patients refractory to medical therapy, evaluating the extent of disease, and preoperative planning.

Magnetic resonance imaging (MRI) is very accurate in determining the extent of sinusitis and tumors. However, at this time, cost and availability preclude it from use in the routine management of sinus disease.

Allergy Testing

Allergy testing is useful in patients who have significant symptoms related to seasonal or perennial allergic rhinitis. Radioallergosorbent test (RAST) is a serum test that determines the amount of IgG-mediated immunoglobulin against a specific allergen or allergen group. Prick or scratch skin testing measures the clinical responses to inoculation with various allergens and is mediated by release of histamine and other chemicals. Intradermal testing is more sensitive than prick tests, yet poses a higher risk of anaphylaxis and is performed if prick testing is negative or not diagnostic.

EVALUATION OF COMMON DISORDERS

The Common Cold

The common cold is an acute viral rhinosinusitis with inflammation of all mucosa of the nose and paranasal sinuses. Generalized symptoms include malaise, fatigue, low-grade fever, chills, and sore throat. The nasal symptoms include nasal obstruction, anterior and posterior clear rhinorrhea, diffuse pressure over the paranasal sinuses, and occasionally plugged ears associated with eustachian tube dysfunction. On the second or third day of infection an increase of neutrophils in the nasal secretions may cause the drainage to be more discolored, but within 1 to 2 days the drainage becomes clear again. The white blood cell count may be slightly elevated, with a predominance of lymphocytes or atypical lymphocytes. Sinus radiographs are normal or show mild mucosal thickening.

Management

Management is supportive with antipyretics, analgesics, and oral decongestants; hydration and saline nasal sprays aid in mucus clearance. Although a topical decongestant is helpful for the symptoms, one needs to be cautious about the potential for rebound effects from excessive use. Symptoms usually resolve in 5 to 8 days without other treatment.

Epistaxis

The etiologies of epistaxis include both local and systemic factors. Local causes are most common in children and are usually associated with nose picking, excessive blowing, sneezing, or rubbing. Bleeding frequently occurs with the common cold, acute sinusitis, or allergic rhinitis. Recurrent bleeding may occur if a scab forms at the bleeding site and becomes dislodged. Although tumors are rare causes of epistaxis, they should be included in the differential diagnosis, especially with profuse bleeding in adolescent males (juvenile nasopharyngeal angiofibroma) or in adults without other known etiologies. In adults, bleeding tends to be more profuse and may be from the posterior nasal cavity. Systemic causes of epistaxis include acquired coagulopathies, hereditary blood dyscrasias, and the use of aspirin, coumadin, or heparin. Patients with hypertension are not more likely to have a nosebleed, although elevated blood pressure can result in more profuse bleeding and makes it more difficult to control. Antihypertensive agents should be administered to hypertensive patients with epistaxis.

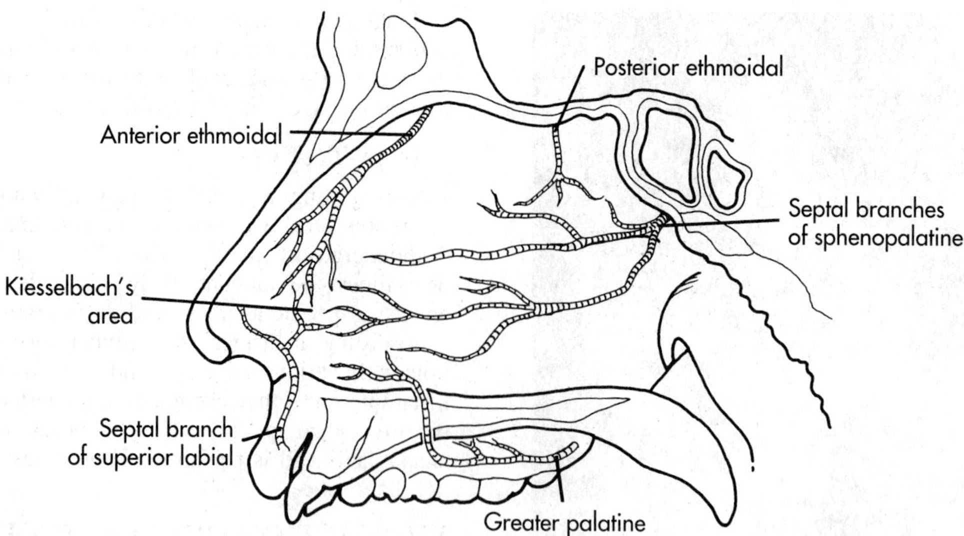

Fig. 179-4. Kiesselbach's plexus on the anterior septum derives blood supply from the superior labial, descending palatine, and sphenopalatine arteries.

The most common site of bleeding is from Kiesselbach's plexus (Fig. 179-4) on the anterior septum. Posterior epistaxis is less common but can be a serious problem in adults. A posterior bleed is defined as bleeding far enough posterior that the site of bleeding cannot be seen by anterior rhinoscopy.

Evaluation of epistaxis is primarily by physical examination. Anterior rhinoscopy with a nasal speculum and Fraser suction (to remove clots and fresh blood) are usually sufficient to identify the site of bleeding. Areas with prominent vessels or scabs should be examined with caution because manipulation may start up active bleeding. Sinus radiographs should be done only when tumors are suspected as the cause of bleeding. When a severe posterior bleed cannot be controlled by packing, carotid artery angiography may help to delineate the source of bleeding.

The management of epistaxis depends on the site of bleeding, the severity, and the etiology. Patients with coagulopathies should have the nose packed with dissolvable packing materials (Oxycel cotton or Gelfoam), since any localized trauma such as pack removal will cause bleeding from multiple sites in addition to the original site. Attempts should be made to correct the coagulopathy.

Conservative measures can be helpful in all patients. These include improving the humidity of inspired air, moisturizing the nose with saline sprays 6 to 10 times a day, and applying antibiotic ointments to reduce scabbing and speed healing of the excoriated areas. Long-term care with an unscented water-base lotion twice a day along with saline sprays usually prevents recurrences.

Recurrent bleeding along the anterior septum is best treated conservatively. When these measures fail, application of silver nitrate or electrocautery can be helpful. This should be performed after application of a topical decongestant and anesthetic agent (4% cocaine or 1% tetracaine). Silver nitrate cautery should be performed from the periphery toward the site of bleeding. When done in the opposite direction, there is a risk of precipitating active bleeding that may be difficult to control. A cotton-tip applicator helps remove excessive silver nitrate from the rest of the nose.

Active bleeding from the anterior nasal cavity is best treated with an anterior nasal pack left in place for 2 to 5 days. Vaseline gauze packing impregnated with an antibiotic ointment can be layered in the nose to apply pressure to the bleeding site. Other packing materials include commercially available balloons and Merosel sponge packs. Oral antibiotics should be given to help prevent excessive bacterial growth in the packing and subsequent bacterial sinusitis. A posterior pack is indicated for more posterior bleeding that fails to respond to anterior packing. Posterior packs may be fashioned from gauze materials, Foley catheters, or commercially available balloon packs. Patients with posterior packs are usually admitted to the hospital and given supplemental oxygen, since significant hypoxemia can occur.

Alternative methods of controlling severe posterior bleeds include arterial ligation of the internal maxillary or ethmoidal vessels and occasionally even ligation of the external carotid artery. Arteriography with embolization has also been used for posterior bleeds. Posterior bleeding may be severe enough to require ICU monitoring and multiple transfusions to maintain normal hemodynamics.

Trauma

Due to their position on the face, the nasal bones are the most frequently fractured bones of the facial skeleton. There is frequently epistaxis associated with fractures from intranasal mucosal tears. Most nasal fractures can be diagnosed by palpation of the bony nasal skeleton finding pinpoint tenderness along with displacement of the nasal bones. Nondisplaced and small fractures at the tip of the nasal bones are more difficult to palpate. Lateral radiographs can confirm a displaced fracture but should be used with caution, since normal suture lines can look like nondisplaced fractures.

Initial management is supportive with head elevation and cold compresses to diminish swelling. Epistaxis usually stops spontaneously or with a topical decongestant spray. Nondisplaced fractures require no active treatment. Nasal fractures are repaired for either functional (nasal obstruction) or cosmetic reasons. Reduction of the nasal fracture is generally done 4 to 8 days after injury. This allows the soft tissue swelling to diminish, allowing for a better reduction of the displaced nasal bones. A comparison to the preinjury state in a recent photograph helps assess the need for reduction. Although management of the fracture is not emergent, it is important to examine and palpate the nasal septum at the time of the initial evaluation to be sure there is no widening and softening that would be suggestive of a septal hematoma. Untreated septal hematomas cause disruption of the blood supply to the septum and can lead to a subsequent saddle nose deformity. When a septal hematoma is suspected, an emergency consultation with an otolaryngologist is in order. All other fractures may be assessed 3 to 4 days after injury, allowing for a better assessment of subtle deformities. Nondisplaced fractures do not require further evaluation.

Acute Sinusitis

Acute sinusitis represents an acute bacterial infection involving the mucosal surfaces of the paranasal sinuses and nasal cavity. It usually occurs after an upper respiratory tract infection. Less common causes include swimming in contaminated water, nasal foreign bodies, and spread from dental infections. Indwelling nasotracheal and nasogastric tubes also predispose to acute sinusitis. When of dental origin, the causative tooth is usually the first or second maxillary molar whose roots extend toward the floor of the maxillary sinus.

Acute sinusitis typically presents with unilateral or bilateral nasal obstruction, purulent rhinorrhea, facial pain, and pressure overlying the paranasal sinuses. There is exacerbation of pain with bending over or straining, and the maxillary teeth may be tender. In contrast to the clear secretions of viral infections, the secretions in acute sinusitis are purulent.

The diagnosis can be made by history, along with a physical examination finding tenderness over the paranasal sinuses, congestion of the turbinates, and purulent drainage in the nose, nasopharynx, or posterior oral pharynx. After decongesting with a topical agent, purulent drainage may be seen in the middle meatus and a nasal endoscope may help in identifying swelling, erythema, and purulence coming out of sinus ostia. Transillumination of the sinuses usually shows a decrease in light transmission of the involved sinus. Radiographic studies are generally needed only to support a questionable history or physical examination. Routine sinus films show mucosal thickening or an air-fluid level in the sinuses. Acute bacterial sinusitis is caused by *S. pneumoniae, H. influenzae,* and *M. catarrhalis.*

Acute sinusitis is usually treated empirically without cultures with a 10- to 14-day course of an appropriate antimicrobial agent, saline nasal sprays, oral decongestants, and analgesic agents. Topical decongestants should be used for 2 to 3 days only and then switched to oral agents to prevent potential rebound. Antihistamines should be avoided unless there is also a history of allergic rhinitis. Good first-line agents are amoxicillin, erythromycin plus a sulfonamide, and amoxicillin with clavulanate. Alternatives include cefuroxime, cefprozil, cefpodoxime, doxycycline, and trimethoprim with sulfamethoxazole. Though there is evidence of increasing β-lactamase activity in bacterial pathogens, antibiotics that cover these organisms are generally used as second-line drugs due to their increased cost and potential side effects. When acute sinusitis is from a dental source, the causative tooth should be treated with root canal or drainage of periapical abscess.

Sinus irrigation is indicated when there is severe pain and the maxillary sinus is not draining. The sinus tap obtains a culture and clears the purulent material from the sinus, giving significant symptomatic relief. Surgery is indicated when there is spread of infection to adjacent areas. External ethmoidectomy is used for ethmoiditis with periorbital abscess and frontal sinus trephination for frontal sinusitis with spread to the intracranial cavity. Endoscopic sinus surgery may benefit patients who have sinusitis that recurs more often than three times per year.

The goals of treatment are not only the resolution of symptoms but also the elimination of mucosal thickening that could narrow the ostiomeatal complex and predispose to recurrent or persistent infection. Since sinus radiographs and computed tomography are not routinely performed at the completion of treatment, it would seem prudent to treat the patient for 5 to 7 days after resolution of symptoms. The patient should be referred for otolaryngology evaluation in cases of recurrent infections greater than two to three per year, severe infection that fails to respond to antibiotics, or persistent infection despite a few courses of antibiotics.

Chronic Sinusitis

Chronic sinusitis represents a persistent low-grade infection involving the paranasal sinuses with persistent mucosal thickening. Pansinusitis or multifocal sinusitis is usually due to nasal polyposis or dysfunction of mucociliary transport (Fig. 179-5), whereas more localized infection is due to ostial obstruction. Patients present with persistent low-grade infection with intermittent acute exacerbations more typical of acute sinusitis. The chronic symptoms are persistent nasal obstruction associated with chronic nasal drainage. The drainage is usually discolored, thick, and copious in the morning, slowly clearing by afternoon. Anosmia is not uncommon, and nasal obstruction is also worse in the morning. Facial pain and sinus headaches may occur daily or only with exacerbations of acute sinusitis.

The diagnosis of chronic sinusitis is made by the classic symptoms associated with radiographic findings of mucosal thickening on routine films or sinus CT scans. Allergy testing is helpful, since perennial allergic rhinitis can mimic sinusitis symptoms. Chronic sinusitis is a polymicrobial disease with cultures usually growing multiple pathogens. The most common pathogens are *M. catarrhalis, H. influenzae, S. pneumoniae, S. aureus,* and a variety of anaerobes.

Chronic sinusitis is treated with decongestants and intranasal steroid preparations. Since the cause of infection is ostial obstruction, antibiotics alone frequently do not result in resolution. Antimicrobials of choice for empiric primary treatment include antistaphylococcal penicillin, clindamycin, cephalosporins, and doxycycline. Treatment should be for at least 3 to 4 weeks before surgery is considered. In patients with nasal polyposis, administration of oral or intramuscular steroids can also be helpful in controlling infection. Injection of the polyps with steroids must be done with caution to avoid complications of blindness. Patients with chronic sinusitis and allergic rhinitis should undergo maximal treatment for the allergies to reduce nasal inflammation. Antihistamines should be avoided unless there is an allergic diathesis to avoid thickening of the mucus blanket and slowing of mucociliary transport. Patients with chronic sinusitis should be referred for surgical intervention if symptoms persist despite 1 to 2 months of treatment with intranasal steroids, decongestants, and a trial of antibiotics. Surgery is directed at relieving the obstruction at the sinus ostia.

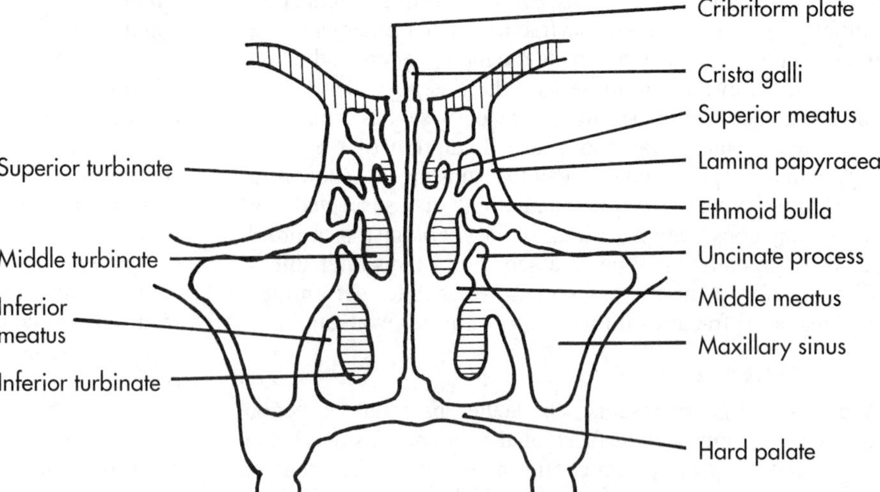

Fig. 179-5. Coronal view of nasal cavity, turbinates, and meati and their association with the paranasal sinuses.

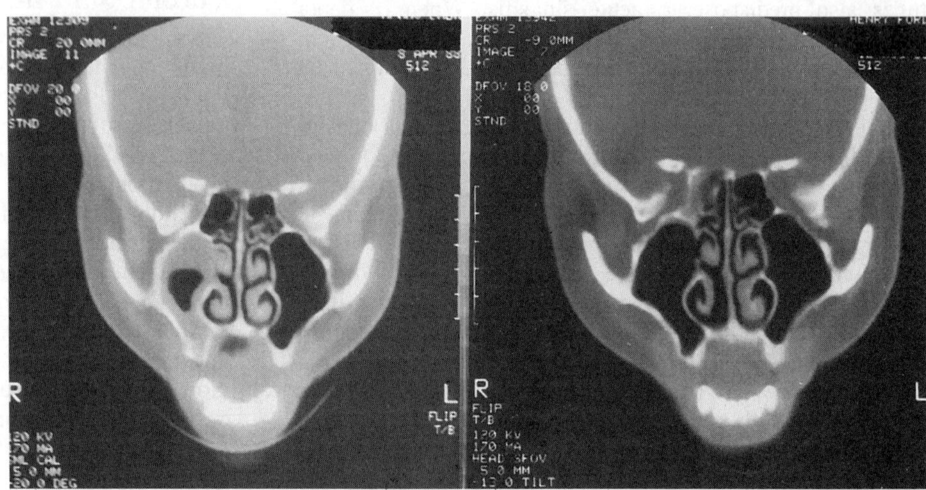

Fig. 179-6. Coronal CT of patient before *(left)* and after *(right)* endoscopic anterior ethmoidectomy and enlargement of the maxillary ostium. Maxillary mucosal thickening has resolved following surgery.

Chronic infection in the maxillary, anterior ethmoid, and frontal sinuses can be caused by ostiomeatal complex obstruction. Endoscopic sinus surgery can frequently relieve this obstruction, allowing the return of normal function of the sinuses and resolution of the chronic infection (Fig. 179-6). Older surgical options included the nasal antral window, which creates a new opening into the maxillary sinus under the inferior turbinate. This procedure improves aeration of the maxillary sinus but is limited because of a high incidence of closure over time. The Caldwell-Luc procedure involves a sublabial approach to the maxillary sinuses with removal of all mucosa. This procedure is generally reserved for patients with irreversibly damaged, nonfunctioning mucosa. Surgery on the frontal sinuses is indicated for mucoceles or chronic osteomyelitis (Pott's puffy tumor) in which the infectious process has eroded through the anterior or posterior walls of the sinus. Treatment of these patients includes systemic antibiotics plus frontal sinus obliteration with fat following debridement of infected bone and removal of all mucosa. Reconstruction of the patient's frontal nasal duct may have merit when performed with the nasal endoscope.

Deviated Septum

Deviation of the nasal septum from the midline occurs either from trauma or from disproportionate growth rates between the facial skeleton and nasal septum. Patients with a deviated septum have chronic unilateral or bilateral nasal obstruction without any other significant symptoms. Although most patients have nasal obstruction on the side of the deflection, some have a worse airway on the opposite side due to compensatory turbinate hypertrophy.

Diagnosis of a deviated septum is made by history and physical examination. Even small anterior cartilaginous deflections tend to cause worse symptoms than posterior deflections. The more common posterior septal spurs rarely cause significant nasal obstruction. Septal deflections may predispose to recurrent sinusitis due to focal ostial edema, increased turbulence of airflow, or bacterial deposition.

Correction of a septal deformity is a minor elective surgical procedure that is performed under local anesthesia with sedation in the ambulatory setting. In patients who have external nasal deformities, a rhinoplasty may be performed in conjunction with septoplasty to improve both the functional and cosmetic problems. Occasionally a functional rhinoplasty is necessary along with the septoplasty to correct a severe septal deflection.

Turbinate Hypertrophy

The nasal turbinates may enlarge for a variety of reasons, including allergic rhinitis, nonallergic rhinitis, septal deflec-

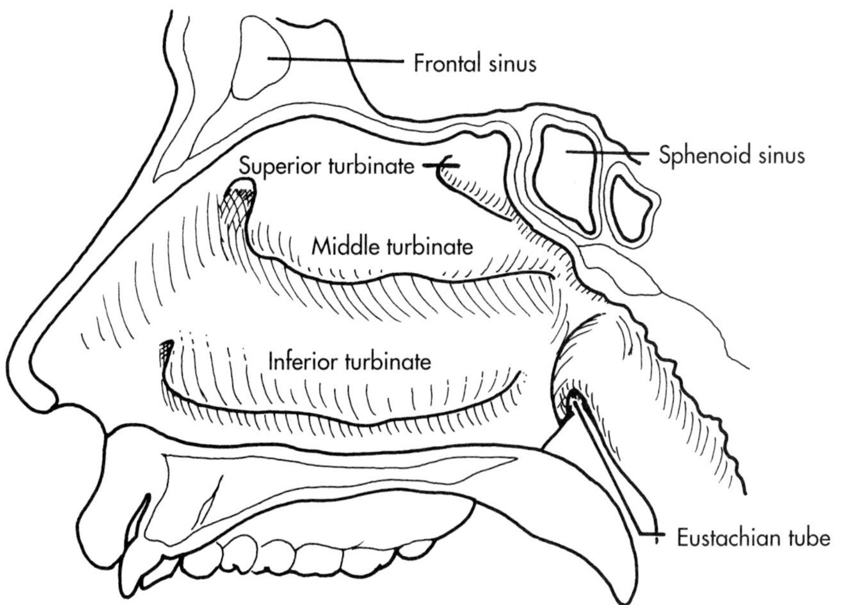

Fig. 179-7. View of the lateral nasal wall.

tion, exposure to tobacco smoke, irritants and pollutants, and use of certain drugs (Fig. 179-7). Prescription drugs that cause turbinate hypertrophy include β-blockers, reserpine, and hormones such as estrogen. Frequent cocaine use may cause turbinate congestion similar to the rebound effect associated with overuse of topical decongestants. Compensatory turbinate hypertrophy frequently occurs on the side opposite a septal deviation. Aeration of the middle turbinates (concha bullosa) occurs in 10% of adults and, when large enough, can lead to significant nasal obstruction.

The diagnosis of turbinate dysfunction is based on a history of chronic nasal obstruction associated with examination findings of turbinate hypertrophy. Reexamination after a topical decongestant can help differentiate enlargement due to osseous or soft tissue changes. Patients with turbinate hypertrophy that fails to respond to decongestants, antihistamines, or intranasal steroids may be candidates for surgical reduction. A variety of surgical techniques have been used to reduce turbinate size. Cautery of the inferior turbinates causes scarring in the submucosa and limits edema from allergic and nonallergic rhinitis. Lateral turbinate fracture is commonly performed with septoplasty to displace the turbinates away from the septum. Submucosal resection of the turbinate bone with preservation of the mucosa is useful when the bone is the primary cause of enlargement. Turbinoplasty involves removal of a portion of the turbinate bone and mucosa and leads to a greater reduction than submucous resection. Total resection of the inferior turbinates is rarely performed due to the risk of atrophic rhinitis and ozena (foul smelling mucus accumulating underneath large crusts).

Nasal Vestibulitis

Nasal vestibulitis is a common problem caused by *S. aureus* infection around a hair follicle in the nasal vestibule. The infection is associated with excessive nose blowing or picking. Management is directed at limiting digitally induced nasal trauma, application of an antistaphylococcal antibiotic ointment (mupirocin) to help prevent scabbing around hair follicles, and use of an antistaphylococcal oral antibiotic. Patients with diabetes, immune deficiency, or progressive infection despite antibiotics should be placed on intravenous antibiotics due to the potential of spread to the cavernous sinus.

Nasal Polyposis

Nasal polyps represent an inflammatory disorder of the nose and paranasal sinuses of unknown etiology. They usually originate from sinus mucosa and protrude through the ostia, appearing as gray translucent pedunculated masses above or below the middle turbinate. Although patients with allergic rhinitis have an incidence of nasal polyps similar to that of the general population, those with nasal polyps have a 30% incidence of allergy. The growth and persistence of nasal polyps may be exacerbated by inflammatory reactions and release of histamine and other mediators of inflammation. Solitary nasal polyps may be caused by acute or chronic sinusitis, and diffuse nasal polyposis may cause secondary sinusitis. Antral choanal polyps originate from the maxillary sinus and may fill the nasal cavity and nasopharynx and hang into the oral pharynx.

Symptoms of nasal polyps include nasal obstruction, hyposmia or anosmia, and symptoms associated with secondary infection. The diagnosis is made by anterior rhinoscopy or nasal endoscopy after nasal decongestion. Nasal endoscopy allows detection of smaller polyps that may not be visible without magnification. A biopsy should be taken from unilateral or solitary polyps to rule out a benign or malignant tumor. Isolated asymptomatic polyps or retention cysts occurring in the floor or roof of the maxillary sinuses do not require any treatment or evaluation. These lesions should be biopsied only if symptomatic or suspicious for malignancy.

The management of nasal polyps is directed at the control of symptoms. When secondary sinusitis occurs, broad-spectrum antibiotic therapy is beneficial. When polyps produce nasal obstruction or anosmia, topical steroid sprays may reduce the size of the polyps and improve the airway. Large obstructive polyps may require oral steroids, intramuscular steroid injections, or injection of steroid suspensions into the polyps. When medical management fails to adequately control the symptoms, surgical intervention is warranted.

Nasal polypectomy alone can improve the nasal airway but rarely relieves sinusitis or anosmia, since it fails to open the sinuses, which are the source of polyp growth. Office polypectomy is generally used for diagnosis or for limited or solitary lesions. Sinus surgery with an endoscope or an open approach is used to remove polyps along with enlargement of sinus ostia and removal of the origins of the polyps (Fig. 179-8). This can improve the efficacy of topical steroids and can be beneficial in long-term management of the disorder. Antral choanal polyps are removed by direct visualization of the maxillary sinus through an endoscope or through a Caldwell-Luc approach.

The triad of nasal polyps, asthma, and aspirin sensitivity (Sampters triad) is a particularly difficult combination to treat. Chronic sinusitis from polyp growth and ostial obstruction may cause exacerbation of the asthma. Although surgical intervention is generally not curative, it can be very beneficial for the nasal symptoms and can be helpful in controlling wheezing in selected patients in whom the sinusitis is an exacerbating factor for the asthma. Asthma has been reported to improve after sinus surgery in 40% to 98% of patients.

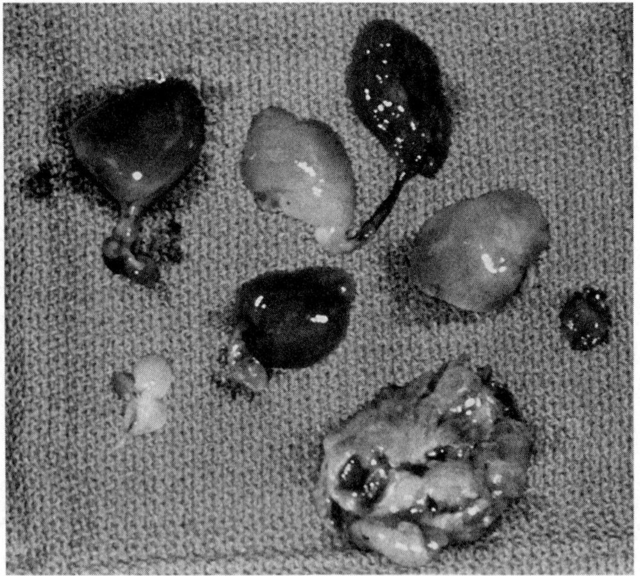

Fig. 179-8. Multiple nasal polyps removed from nose and paranasal sinuses.

Allergic, Nonallergic, and Vasomotor Rhinitis

Allergic rhinitis typically includes symptoms of intermittent nasal obstruction, clear rhinorrhea or postnasal drainage, frequent sneezing, watery eyes, and pruritus of the nose, eyes, and palate (Fig. 179-9). In North America the seasonal allergies are triggered by tree pollens in the spring, grasses in midsummer, and weeds in the fall (typically August 15 until the first frost). Allergies also occur in response to exposure to animal danders. Dust, mite, and mold allergies produce perennial symptoms, with less pruritus and sneezing than seasonal allergies. Dust or mite allergy is worse in the morning from exposure to upholstered furniture, pillows, and mattresses, which have high mite populations. The diagnosis is confirmed with serologic (RAST), epidermal (prick or scratch), or intradermal skin testing. Nasal smears frequently demonstrate an increase in eosinophils in nasal secretions, and serologic testing shows an increase in IgE levels.

Nonallergic rhinitis has symptoms similar to perennial allergic rhinitis but fails to show responses on allergy skin testing. Vasomotor rhinitis is a form of nonallergic rhinitis with exacerbation of symptoms from changes in temperature and humidity, exposure to hot or cold foods, anxiety, or the ingestion of vasoactive substances in foods or drinks. Nonallergic rhinitis with eosinophilia (NARE) is an entity of chronic rhinitis and nasal eosinophilia without evidence of atopy. Nasal polyps have been found more frequently in patients with NARE than in the general population, but symptoms may be more recalcitrant to medical therapy.

The treatment of allergic and nonallergic rhinitis is directed at the control of symptoms. Allergic rhinitis responds to combined oral decongestant and antihistamine preparations, whereas nonallergic rhinitis is better treated with a decongestant without antihistamine. For tenacious mucus, mucus thinners and expectorants such as guafenesin can be helpful. Both conditions may benefit from intranasal steroid sprays, and allergic rhinitis may also improve with topical cromolyn sodium. Cromolyn is used as a preventive agent only. Traditional antihistamines are useful in the primary treatment of allergic rhinitis. When excessive sedation occurs despite use of a reduced dose (pediatric dosage), the nonsedating antihistamine preparations should be considered.

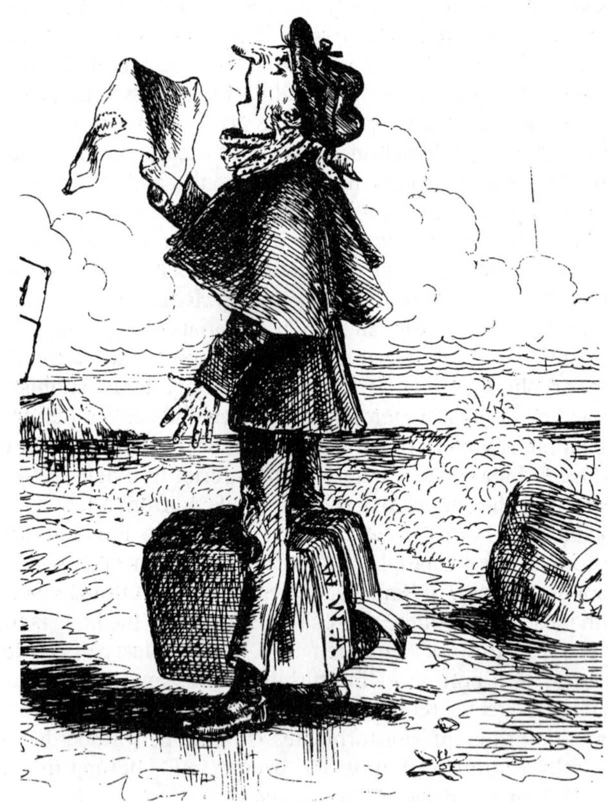

Fig. 179-9. Severe pollen allergy as depicted in 1873. (From Augustas Hoppin: *Hay fever,* plate XIII, Boston, 1873, JS Osgood.)

When medications fail to adequately control allergic rhinitis, hyposensitization can be beneficial in symptom control. While hyposensitization is most effective for seasonal allergic rhinitis, avoidance of causative allergens is

Table 179-1. Granulomatous Diseases Affecting the Nose

Disease	Symptoms	Diagnosis	Treatment
Sarcoidosis	Nasal obstruction	1-3 mm septal nodules, noncaseating granulomas on biopsy	Systemic steroids
Wegener's granulomatosis	Nasal obstruction, bloody drainage	Septal ulcers and turbinate hypertrophy vasculitis, acute and chronic inflammation on biopsy; elevated antinuclear cytoplasmic antibody and sedimentation rate	Systemic steroids, cyclophosphamide, methotrexate; oral trimethoprim and sulfamethoxazole
Syphilis	Foul smelling drainage and gummatous mass, chondritis, osteitis, saddle nose deformity	Positive FTA-ABS test and VDRL, treponeme on smear	Long course of penicillin
Tuberculosis	Beefy red mucosa with ulcerations and exudate, granulomas on septum	Positive PPD, *Myobacterium* spp. on smear, caseating granulomas on biopsy	Isoniazid, rifampin, streptomyocin, and ethambutol
Rhinoscleroma	Painless submucosal plaques causing airway obstruction	Biopsy and culture grow *Klebsiella* rhinoscleromatous	High dose ampicillin
Lethal midline granuloma	Rapidly progressive septal ulceration and perforation	Biopsy similar to lymphoepithelioma	Radiation therapy
Leprosy	Red granular ulcers, septal perforations with crusting, bleeding, and atrophic rhinitis	Biopsy and culture show *Mycobacterium leprae*	Dapsone and other sulphone antibiotics, saline and mineral oil sprays for atrophic rhinitis

FTA-ABS, Fluorescent treponemal antibody absorption; *PPD*, purified protein derivative.

important for all patients. Surgical reduction of the turbinates is used only for patients with severe symptoms despite maximal medical therapy.

MANAGEMENT OF UNCOMMON DISORDERS

Benign and Malignant Tumors

Benign and malignant tumors are discussed in Chapter 183.

Granulomatous Disorders

The granulomatous disorders represent systemic diseases with local manifestations. Referral to an otolaryngologist is indicated for nasal symptoms occurring in any patient with a known systemic granulomatous disease. The most common symptoms are persistent nasal obstruction, crusting and bleeding, and secondary sinusitis. Examination may show small nodular areas involving the nasal mucosa, diffuse thickening of the septal and turbinate mucosa, and septal ulceration, granulation tissue, or perforation. The granulomatous diseases that affect the nose, their presenting symptoms, diagnostic criteria, and treatments are listed in Table 179-1.

Mycotic Infections

Mycotic infections are rare, occurring almost exclusively in patients with diabetes or immunocompromised patients in either an invasive or superficial form. The invasive form is a rapidly progressive and destructive infection that causes necrosis of facial soft tissues and the nose. If not contained, infection spreads to the orbit and intracranial cavity, leading to rapid death. Presenting symptoms are severe facial pain, bloody discharge, fever, and facial swelling. A gray or black nonsensate avascular area of nasal mucosa or facial skin is due to fungal vascular invasion with secondary avascular necrosis. Treatment is with aggressive and repeated debridement of avascular tissue along with systemic antifungal agents. *Mucor* and *Aspergillus* are the most common fungi to cause the invasive form.

The superficial form is most likely from aspergillosis but can also be caused by histoplasmosis, blastomycosis, cryptococcosis, rhinosporidiosis, mucormycosis, and sporotrichosis. These infections are most common in hot and humid climates, presenting in an indolent manner or occurring along with chronic bacterial sinusitis due to overgrowth of fungi in retained secretions. Recommended treatment is to surgically open the sinus and remove the infected material. Systemic antifungal treatment is not necessary.

ADDITIONAL READINGS

Axelsson A, Brorson JE: The correlation between bacteriologic findings in the nose and maxillary sinus in acute maxillary sinusitis, *Laryngoscope* 83:2003, 1973.

Benninger MS: Rhinitis, sinusitis, and their relationship to allergies, *Am J Rhinol* 6(2):37, 1992.

Benninger MS, Mickelson SA, Yaremchuk K: Functional endoscopic sinus surgery: morbidity and early results, *Henry Ford Hosp Med J* 38(1):5, 1990.

English GM: Nasal polypectomy and sinus surgery in patients with asthma and aspirin idiosyncrasy, *Laryngoscope* 96:374, 1986.

Fairbanks DNF: *Pocket guide to antimicrobial therapy in otolaryngology—head and neck surgery,* ed 7, Alexandria, VA, 1993, American Academy of Otolaryngology—Head & Neck Surgery Foundation.

Leopold DA: Physiology of olfaction. In Cummings CW et al, editors: *Otolaryngology—head and neck surgery,* vol 1, ed 2, St Louis, 1993, Mosby.

Rosnagle RS, Yanagisawa E, Smith HW: Specific vessel ligation for epistaxis: survey of 60 cases, *Laryngoscope* 83:517, 1973.

Weiss NS: Relation of high blood pressure to headache, epistaxis, and selected other symptoms: the United States health examination survey of adults, *N Engl J Med* 287(13):632, 1972.

CHAPTER 180

Oral Cavity and Salivary Gland Disease

Dennis D. Diaz

The oral cavity consists of the lips, cheeks, and oral cavity proper, including the tongue and teeth. The lips and cheeks are essentially similar in structure, consisting primarily of an external layer of skin, a middle muscular layer (orbicularis oris for the lips and buccinator for the cheeks), and an internal layer of mucous membrane.

The parotid gland is the largest salivary gland opening into the oral cavity via Stensen's (parotid) duct, which penetrates the buccinator muscle. The duct opens bilaterally out the parotid papilla, which is situated at the level of the second upper molar. The submandibular gland is located in the submandibular triangle. Wharton's duct, which is the opening for this salivary gland, extends forward and empties through the floor of the mouth just lateral and on each side of the lingual frenulum at the sublingual caruncle. The sublingual gland is the smallest of the major salivary glands and lies above the mylohyoid muscle immediately below the mucosa of the floor of mouth. This gland opens via a series of small, minor ducts along the sublingual fold. Sometimes a major sublingual duct may open into Wharton's duct. Scattered throughout the oral cavity are numerous minor salivary glands. Small superficial yellow sebaceous glands are often seen close to the free borders of the lips.

The hard palate is primarily a bony plate covered with mucous membrane that separates the oral cavity from the nasal cavity. The soft palate, part of the oropharynx, is muscular tissue covered by mucous membrane. It plays an active role in swallowing and vocal resonance. The oropharynx, with the soft palate, also includes the anterior and posterior tonsillar pillars, tonsils, base of the tongue, and posterior pharyngeal walls. The tongue helps to form the floor of mouth. Muscles, nerves, and vessels enter through the base of the tongue. It is divided into anterior two thirds and posterior one third at the V-shaped sulcus terminalis. The tongue's bumpy appearance is caused by numerous lingual papillae, the largest of which are the circumvallate papillae. They are arranged in a V-shaped row just anterior to the sulcus terminalis. The fungiform papillae are irregularly scattered over the tongue.

Examination of the oral cavity and its structures is relatively easy and requires only a strong light source (a head light allows free use of both hands) and two tongue blades. Most conditions are diagnosed from history and physical examination alone. With these tongue blades, tissue can be spread and manipulated, allowing complete inspection and visualization of all areas of the oral cavity and oropharynx. Attention should be directed to the lips, buccal mucosa, teeth, gingiva, floor of mouth, tongue, hard and soft palate, and oropharynx. The base of tongue and posterior oropharynx may be seen, but this area often requires a mirror for improved visualization. Systemic examination of the oral cavity ensures that no abnormalities are overlooked. Dentures, if present, should be removed. Palpation of the oral cavity, especially if an abnormality is noted, provides important information. Palpation is extremely helpful in assessing the salivary glands because normal glands are not palpable.

Tables 180-1 to 180-5 summarize common disease processes seen in otolaryngology–head and neck surgery as they present in the oral cavity, oropharynx, and salivary glands. Box 180-1 lists diseases rarely or infrequently associated with these structures.

Box 180-1. Uncommon Processes of the Oral Cavity

Vascular
Hemangioma
Lymphangioma
Cystic hygroma

Infectious
Blastmycosis
Actinomycosis
Tuberculosis
Histoplasmosis
Cat-scratch fever
Coccidioidomycosis
Gonorrhea
Syphilis

Toxic/Trauma
Agranulocytosis
Drug related
Inhalant allergy
Food allergy
Contact allergy
Caustic injury
Thermal injury

Collagen Vascular
Wegener's granulomatosis
Scleroderma
Systemic lupus erythematosus
Dermatomyositis
Midline granuloma

Metabolic
Drug related
Myxedema
Acromegaly

Idiopathic
Pemphigus
Erythema multiforme
Angioneurotic edema
Melkersson-Rosenthal syndrome
Epidermolysis bullosa
Sarcoidosis
Hairy tongue

Neoplasms
Sarcoma
Kaposi's sarcoma
Midline granuloma

Table 180-1. Common Disease Processes Affecting the Oral Cavity

Disease	Cause	Symptoms	Patients	Appearance	Course	Treatment
Herpangina	Coxsackievirus A (fall and summer months)	Severe sore throat, odynophagia, sudden high fever, malaise	Primarily children, adolescents	Initially, numerous small vesicles with red halos; flat ulcers later	Usually less than 1 week	Self-limiting; supportive and symptomatic
Aphthous stomatitis	Herpes simplex virus	Multiple, yellowish erosions/vesicles, high fever, oral pain	Primarily infants, small children	Lesions localized to anterior oral cavity and gums	1-2 weeks	Tetracycline syrup as mouthwash
Recurrent aphthous ulcer	Unknown	No stomatitis; ulcers tender when touched; eruptions at mucosal folds	Older children, adults	Reddened, raised, millet seed to pea-sized bumps; ulcerated at center, covered by yellowish fibrinous exudate	7-10 days; history of recurrence	Supportive and symptomatic; tetracycline 250 mg mouthwash four times daily for 5-7 days
Herpes zoster	Varicella-zoster virus	Extremely painful; burning pain; may have fever, malaise	Elderly adults with impaired host defenses	Unilateral vesicles on buccal mucosa, tongue, uvula, pharynx, larynx; erosions noted when vesicles rupture	7-14 days	Antiviral drugs, otherwise symptomatic
Herpes simplex labialis	Herpes simplex virus type I	Itching, tension, or neuralgiform complaints as prodromes; painful when ulcers form	Children, adults	Recurrent, episodic eruptions of yellowish fluid–filled vesicles on upper/lower lip, nose	7-14 days; history of recurrence	Supportive and symptomatic
Cheilitis sicca	Exogenous damage by weather, drying, solar radiation	Itching, burning, or "cracked" lips	Children, adults	Dry, fissured, reddened or scaling lip mucosa		Symptomatic
Angular cheilitis	Infection, genetic, neoplasm, others	Dryness and burning sensation at corners of mouth	Children, adults	Macerated, deep fissures or cracks at corners of mouth	Resolve; exacerbation common	Empiric based on etiology
Burning tongue	Variety of local and systemic disorders	Pain, burning, itching, or stinging of mucous membrane	Adults, rare in children	Tissues usually normal	Remission rare	Supportive and symptomatic
Kaposi's sarcoma	AIDS (HIV infection)	Purplish tender or painful nodules on mucous membrane	Can occur at any age	Purplish macules; can also be raised, nodular, or ulcerated		Diagnosis established by biopsy or HIV serology
Hand-foot-and-mouth disease	Viral	Sore mouth, low-grade fever, coryza	Young children, 6 months to 5 years	Maculopapular exanthemous and vesicular lesions of skin; small, multiple, vesicular and ulcerative oral lesions	Self-limiting; usually regresses within 1-2 weeks	No specific treatment; local measures
Candidiasis	*Candida albicans* (found on 15%-20% of normal mucous membrane surfaces)	White to yellow lesions in cheek, at folds, and on tongue; seen at any age, especially in debilitated or chronically ill patients	Newborns; persons with impaired host defenses or poor oral hygiene	Soft, white to yellow, slightly elevated plaques; "milk curds;" wiping reveals erythematous mucosal surface	Can be persistent	Specific antifungal agents

AIDS, Acquired immunodeficiency syndrome; *HIV,* human immunodeficiency virus.

Table 180-2. Common Disease Processes Affecting the Oropharynx

Disease	Cause	Symptoms	Patients	Appearance	Course	Treatment
Acute tonsillitis	Group A β-hemolytic streptococci most important treatable pathogen	Sudden-onset intense throat pain, odynophagia, fever, chills, malaise; painful "glands" in neck; cough, coryza, and rhinorrhea suggestive of viral etiology	Children, adults	Sickly; pharyngeal erythema with intensely red palatine tonsils and faucial arch; yellow exudate; painful cervical adenopathy; rapid strep test or throat culture helpful	7-14 days of medical therapy; risk of serious sequelae in inadequately treated cases	Penicillin, clindamycin; alternatives: cephalexin, cefadroxil, erythromycin; local and symptomatic measures
Peritonsillar abscess	Inflammatory infiltration and abscess formation	Despite initial antibiotic therapy, worsening severe unilateral throat pain, fever, malaise, difficulty eating, drooling, fetid breath, "hot potato" voice	Any age, peak occurrence in second to fourth decades	Marked erythema and bulging of peritonsillar area; deviation of uvula to unaffected side; fluctuance of soft palate, exudate; painful cervical adenopathy; trismus	Initial sore throat, followed by symptom-free interval, then worsening	Needle aspiration, incision and drainage of abscess, tonsillectomy; appropriate antibiotic therapy
Infectious mononucleosis	Epstein-Barr virus	Severe sore throat most common symptom; odynophagia, high fever, malaise, headache	Primarily adolescents and young adults	Bilateral tender cervical adenopathy; huge tonsils; gray-white fibrinous deposit on tonsils; leukocytosis with increased monocytes	Usually runs course in 10-21 days	Monospot test; specific treatment not available; antibiotics for sore throat complicated by group A streptococci
Chronic tonsillitis	Group A β-hemolytic streptococci chronic inflammation, microabscesses	Frequent sore throats, "scratchy" throat, oral fetor, "swollen glands"	Children, adults	Redness around tonsils; fissured tonsils; yellowish concretions expressed with pressure	Waxing and waning, painful flare-ups	Antibiotics, local measures; surgery if four or more infections of tonsils per year despite medical therapy
Tonsillar hypertrophy	Excessive reactive proliferation of tonsil tissue	Mouth breathing, eating difficulties, snoring, sleep disorder, change in speech resonance	Children most often; adults	Increase in volume of palatine tonsils; cervical adenopathy; unilateral hypertrophy referred for head and neck evaluation by otolaryngologist	Progressive with worsening upper airway symptoms	Surgery if dental malocclusion, impaired orofacial growth, upper airway obstruction, severe dysphagia, sleep disorders
Acute pharyngitis	Primary viral infection followed by bacterial superinfection	Raw, dry burning throat with odynophagia; in children, associated with fever and cervical adenopathy; adults, milder course; rhinorrhea, cough	Children, adults	Dry, red, thickened pharyngeal mucosa; exudate	7-14 days	Analgesics, local measures, antibiotics for group A β-hemolytic streptococci
Chronic pharyngitis	Chronic mucosal inflammation by numerous etiologies	Habitual throat clearing, globus sensation, cough; thick colorless phlegm; no fever, no malaise	Usually adults	Varying degrees of pharyngeal irritation with mucosal thickening; thick, colorless to yellow secretions	Waxing and waning for years	Underlying cause (e.g., infection, GERD, tobacco); local measures

Table 180-3. Lesions and Morphologic Changes of the Oropharynx and Oral Cavity

	Cause	Symptoms	Appearance	Course	Treatment
Papilloma	Human papillomavirus	Nonpainful mass	Single or multiple raspberry-like masses	Predilection for mucocutaneous junctions	Excisional biopsy with histologic examination
Torus palatinus or mandibularis	Exostosis or outgrowth of bone	Usually none; incidental finding	Hard bony growth with intact mucosa unless traumatized	Incidence: Palatinus, 20%-25% Mandibularis 6%-8%	No treatment needed
Basal cell carcinoma of lips	Prolonged exposure to sunlight	Lesion ulcerates, heals over, then breaks down again; history of ultraviolet light exposure	Crusting ulcer with heaped or rolled borders; induration	Untreated lesions: enlarge, infiltrate adjacent and deeper tissues	Biopsy for diagnosis; each lesion considered separately when choosing therapy
Squamous cell carcinoma					
Oral cavity, floor of mouth, anterior tongue	Lack of specific etiology Tobacco, alcohol, poor oral hygiene, syphilis implicated	Usually painless ulcer unless nerves or periosteum involved; fetid breath	Ulcerated lesion with raided borders; bimanual palpation of mouth and tongue mandatory; deep invasion if trismus noted	Comprise about 90% of oral cancer; no barriers to extension in oral cavity; regional metastasis in neck	Biopsy for diagnosis; therapy depends on staging: surgery, radiation, photodynamic, chemotherapy, combined modalities
Oropharynx (tonsil)	Lack of specific etiology; tobacco, alcohol implicated	Usually painful ulceration; dysphagia, odynophagia, weight loss present; referred otalgia possible	Angry looking; ulcerated enlarged mass involving one or both tonsils; tongue base and palate, bimanual palpation	Early involvement of regional lymph nodes	Biopsy for diagnosis; depends on staging but usually combined therapy
Leukoplakia	Multifactorial (e.g., tobacco use, trauma, lupus, lichen planus, irritative reactions)	Painless white patch or plaque on surface of mucosa	White patch, with predilection for lips, tongue, palate, floor of mouth, and buccal mucosa	Not all are precancerous but complete evaluation for diagnosis suggested	Often incidental finding; biopsy, especially if risk factors in history (e.g., tobacco use, alcohol)

Table 180-4. Common Disease Processes Affecting the Salivary Glands*

	Cause	Symptoms	Appearance	Course	Treatment
Bacterial sialadenitis	Streptococci or staphylococci most common	Severe pain, fever, overlying skin warm; trismus; parotid most often affected	Swollen, tender, firm gland; purulent discharge from punctum of involved gland; absent or decreased salivary flow	Acute, progressive if not treated; often seen in debilitated, hospitalized patients	Local and symptomatic measures; hydration; sialogogues; antistaphylococcal penicillin; alternatives: clindamycin, cephalosporin, vancomycin
Mumps	Paramyxovirus	Mild temperature elevation, malaise; sudden onset of acute distention, pain	Painful, diffuse, doughy swelling over parotid gland; gland feels tense and tender; usually bilateral; puncta congested; expressed saliva clear	Self-limited	Local and symptomatic measures; hydration; analgesia
Sialolithiasis	Formation of calculus in excretory duct; foreign body	Sudden painful swelling of affected gland initiated by eating; usually reduces in size once meal complete; submandibular gland most common	Tender, swollen gland may be detected; bimanual palpation may detect calculus; Panorex or bite wing radiographs may identify stone in affected submandibular gland	Recurrent; if obstruction not relieved, complications include infection, fistula, abscess, strictures	Stones may pass spontaneously; if not, intraoral removal attempted if stone within 1 cm of puncta; hydration, analgesics, antibiotics; surgical treatment for chronic recurrence
Radiation sialadenitis	Injury to salivary gland parenchyma by ionizing radiation	Burning, dry mouth with decreased taste; xerostomia with atrophy of mucosa	Dry, violaceous mucosa with thick secretions	May improve after radiation therapy	Local and symptomatic; sialogogues; hydration; dietary consult recommended; oral pilocarpine (Salagen)
Sjögren's syndrome	Autoimmune; classic triad; xerostomia, keratoconjunctivitis sicca, connective tissue disorder (rheumatoid arthritis most common)	Gradual swelling and enlargement of parotid/submandibular gland; usually bilateral; increasing xerostomia; dry eye when lacrimal gland involved; arthritis; laryngitis	More common in women; dry lips or mouth; diminished salivary flow; parotid/submandibular glands enlarged bilaterally; viscous mucus when expressed from salivary ducts	Progressive; rheumatology evaluation	Local and symptomatic; humidification and hydration; biopsy for diagnosis; no medications that decrease salivary flow
Pleomorphic adenoma	Most common benign salivary gland tumor	Painless, slow-growing, salivary gland mass (parotid most common)	Firm, nontender mass without fixation to overlying skin; more common in women	Slow growing; enlarges greatly if ignored	Surgical excision with preservation of facial nerve
Warthin's tumor (adenolymphoma)	Almost exclusively in parotid gland	Painless, slow-growing, palpable mass	Soft, nontender, mobile mass; frequently bilateral	Primarily males, fifth to sixth decades	Surgical excision with preservation of facial nerve
Mucoepidermoid carcinoma	Most common malignancy of parotid gland; 3:1 female predominance	Low grade: slow-growing, painless mass; high grade: fast-growing, painful mass; facial nerve paralysis, regional spread	Low grade: circumscribed nodule with variable consistency; high grade: fixed, painful mass; facial nerve paralysis, cervical adenopathy	Usually fourth to fifth decades; most common malignant salivary gland tumor in children	Surgical excision with or without facial nerve preservation depending on degree of invasion
Adenoid cystic carcinoma	Most common malignancy of submandibular gland	Slow growth initially; pain or paresthesia later	Hard fixed mass; facial paralysis fairly common; regional and distant spread common	Spread of tumor along perineural and perivascular spaces	Surgery

*Salivary gland neoplasms are uncommon in children. For children, most common benign tumor of salivary gland is hemangioma; most common malignant tumor is mucoepidermoid carcinoma; most common benign epithelial tumor is

Table 180-5. Disorders of the Tongue

	Cause	Symptom	Appearance	Course	Treatment
Ankyloglossia	Developmental variation of lingual frenulum	Incidental finding; restriction of elevation and protrusion	Thick, fibrous lingual frenulum; usually does not affect speech; little interference with infant's feeding	If speech delay present, other cause	Frenotomy, often to relieve mother's anxiety, not child's
Fissured tongue	Differential: syphilis, tuberculosis, myxedema, acromegaly	Usually painless, except if food debris in grooves leads to irritation	Numerous small furrows of dorsal and lateral surfaces of tongue	Of no concern unless evaluation reveals other underlying disease	Hygiene; stretch/flatten fissures, clean surface with toothbrush/ gauze sponge
Geographic tongue	No specific cause; may be stress related	25% report tenderness and burning	Discrete, irregular areas of desquamation, white to yellow in color, resembling a map; "migrates"	Regression and recurrence	No specific treatment necessary
Median rhomboid glossitis	Congenital	Food and debris accumulation with inflammation, pain	Ovoid or rhomboid fissured or smooth, red mass in midline of tongue; anterior to V location	More common in men	No specific treatment; hygiene; biopsy if diagnosis uncertain or malignancy suspected
Macroglossia	Multiple etiologies	Nothing specific except for large tongue; dysphagia or feeding difficulties in newborn	Large tongue; malocclusion; scalloping of lateral tongue edge		Treat primary cause, surgical debulking
Tongue carcinoma	Associated with tobacco, alcohol use, syphilis	Initial painless mass or ulcer ultimately becomes painful; difficulty with speech, eating; referred ear pain; weight loss	Ulcer or mass with induration and raised borders; fetid breath; firm tongue; neck mass	Metastasis common	Staging biopsy for diagnosis; depending on stage, combined surgery and radiotherapy most beneficial

ADDITIONAL READINGS

DeWeese DD, Saunders WH: *Textbook of otolaryngology,* ed 6, St Louis, 1982, Mosby.

English GM, editor: *Otolaryngology,* vol 3, *Diseases of the larynx, pharynx, and upper respiratory tract,* Philadelphia, 1992, Lippincott.

Fairbanks DNF: *Pocket guide to antimicrobial therapy in otolaryngology–head and neck surgery,* Washington, DC, 1987, American Academy of Otolaryngology–Head and Neck Surgery Foundation.

Lee KJ: *Essential otolaryngology–head and neck surgery,* ed 3, New York, 1983, Medical Examination.

Naumann HH: *Differential diagnosis in otorhinolaryngology,* New York, 1993, Thieme.

Shafer WS, Hine MK, Levy BM: *Textbook of oral pathology,* ed 4, Philadelphia, 1983, Saunders.

Strome M, Kelly JH, Fried MP, editors: *Manual of otolaryngology diagnosis and therapy,* Boston, 1985, Little, Brown.

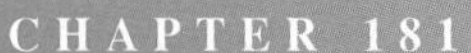

CHAPTER 181

Laryngeal and Upper Airway Disease

Andrew Shapiro
James Malone

The larynx is a complex organ designed to serve several functions, most notably as the instrument of human voice. Because of its tenuous location at the junction of the respiratory and digestive tracts, the larynx also protects the lower airway during swallowing, ensures airway patency during inspiration, and provides sufficient resistance during expiration to prevent atelectasis. These disparate functions demand complex sensory and motor capabilities and close interactions with other organ systems.

The larynx is generally divided into three regions (Fig. 181-1). The *supraglottis* comprises the epiglottis, aryepiglottic folds, arytenoids, and false vocal folds and provides a dynamic valve mechanism that occludes the lower airway during swallowing. The *glottis,* or true vocal folds, consist of an underlying muscular layer, a surface squamous epithelium, and an intervening loose connective tissue layer that allows for a flowing mucosal "wave" to maintain normal voice quality. The *subglottis* extends from the vocal cords to the upper trachea, largely corresponding to the cricoid cartilage, the only complete cartilaginous ring within the airway. Sensory and motor innervation is provided by two branches of the vagus nerve, the superior and recurrent laryngeal nerves.

PATIENT EVALUATION

The evaluation of patients with airway disorders begins with a complete history and physical examination. Although the duration, severity, and concurrent symptoms of airway disorders may vary depending on the underlying etiology, certain similarities prevail. In adults, hoarseness or a change in the quality of the voice is often the earliest symptom. Other common features include cough, hemoptysis, and pain with swallowing or speech. Dyspnea and airway obstruction are late indicators and demand immediate intervention. Essential components of the history include concurrent medical problems and therapy, occupational or recreational voice use and abuse, prior surgeries or intubations, and tobacco and alcohol use.

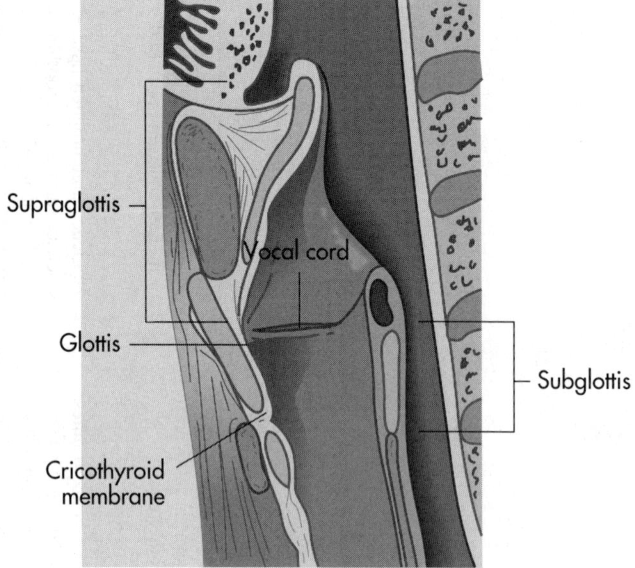

Fig. 181-1. Sagittal view of larynx.

The physical examination is comprehensive but emphasizes particular aspects of the head and neck. The oral and nasal mucosa are examined for acute or chronic inflammatory changes. Palpation of the neck may identify cervical masses, thyromegaly, deviation, or tenderness of the larynx or trachea. Direct inspection of the larynx and hypopharynx presents a challenge in a primary care setting. Specialized training and experience are required even to visualize this area, let alone identify subtle pathologic changes in an active larynx. Thus consultation with an otolaryngologist may be beneficial when patients have either severe or persistent (e.g., more than 3 weeks) symptoms.

Indirect transoral examination using a head light and mirror is a useful technique in adults and some children. An overactive gag reflex or anatomic variations may limit this method. Flexible fiberoptic nasopharyngeal laryngoscopy allows a more prolonged and comprehensive examination of laryngeal morphology and function. Patients with disorders of voice quality may benefit from a stroboscopic examination of the larynx. This technique provides detailed stop-action visualization of mucosal lesions and evaluation of the waveform morphology. Laryngeal electromyography is useful in the diagnosis of neuromuscular disorders of the larynx, such as paralysis or focal dystonia. Finally, cross-sectional imaging with computed tomography (CT) or magnetic resonance imaging (MRI) plays an important role in the management of laryngeal and extralaryngeal neoplasms.

PEDIATRIC CONSIDERATIONS

Stridor

Children are subject to numerous congenital, inflammatory, and even neoplastic diseases that may produce upper airway symptoms. The cross-sectional area of the airway lumen in children is smaller than that of the adult, and a small amount of edema produces a greater degree of airway compromise (Fig. 181-2). In contrast to adults, in whom diseases of the

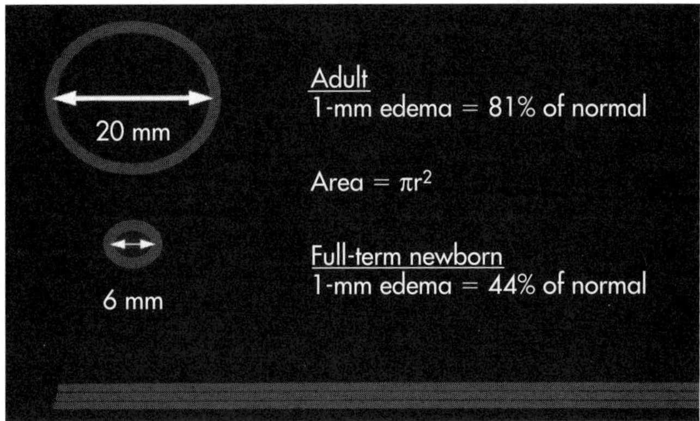

Fig. 181-2. Effect of edema on cross-sectional airway diameter.

airway usually manifest as hoarseness, infants and young children with airway disorders most often present with obstructive symptoms, in particular, stridor, a harsh sound produced by abnormal turbulence in the airway. Unlike respiratory distress, which may result from disease in a variety of systems, stridor always implies obstructive disease of the airway. Stridor is loudest over the site of obstruction. In contrast, *wheezing* is produced by the small airways and is therefore loudest over the chest. *Stertor* is a coarse inspiratory sound from a pharyngeal source (e.g., snoring). Distinguishing these characteristic sounds allows rapid localization of the site of the problem. The quality and timing of stridor can further define the site of disease within the larynx or trachea. Disorders above the larynx produce stridor on inspiration. Disorders of the subglottis result in biphasic (inspiratory and expiratory) stridor, whereas intrathoracic pathology usually produces stridor on exhalation. Any child with stridor and concurrent signs of respiratory distress (e.g., tachypnea and tachycardia, intercostal or substernal retractions, nasal flaring) should be transferred immediately to an emergency room for airway support.

Disorders in the Infant

Congenital lesions are the most common cause of infantile stridor (Box 181-1). The three most common problems are likely to be seen in a primary care setting.

Box 181-1. Causes of Stridor and Respiratory Distress in Infants and Children

Nasal/Nasopharyngeal/ Oropharyngeal
Choanal atresia
Rhinitis
Tonsil/adenoid hypertrophy
Craniofacial anomalies
Retropharyngeal abscess
Macroglossia

Laryngeal
Laryngomalacia
Vocal cord paralysis
Subglottic stenosis
Croup
Intubation injury
Reflux laryngitis
Epiglottitis
Angioedema
Foreign bodies
Papillomata

Tracheal
Tracheomalacia
Tracheal stenosis
Vascular compression
Foreign bodies
Mediastinal masses

Laryngomalacia. Laryngomalacia is the most common cause of stridor in infants. The supraglottic structures collapse into the airway lumen on inspiration, producing a coarse to musical sound. The noise begins in the first few weeks after birth and is often accentuated in the supine position. Eating, crying, and sleep increase the intensity in some infants. Gastroesophageal reflux (GER) appears to be strongly related to laryngomalacia. In most patients the disease is self-limited and should resolve by 18 months of age. Approximately 5% of patients have serious sequelae, such as failure to thrive or episodes of respiratory distress and cyanosis. Medical therapy for GER is helpful in some patients. Rarely, surgical therapy is required for symptom relief.

Subglottic Stenosis. Defined as a narrowing in the area of the cricoid cartilage, subglottic stenosis may be congenital but results more often from an intubation injury. The subglottic anatomy is unique because it represents both the narrowest segment of the neonatal airway and the only complete cartilaginous ring. Infants with subglottic stenosis manifest biphasic stridor and a characteristic barking cough. Milder cases may present as recurrent episodes of "croup." Children who experience croup before 6 months of age may also benefit from an airway evaluation. Depending on the severity of the stenosis, treatment ranges from observation to medical therapy to endoscopic or external procedures to widen the subglottis.

Vocal Cord Paralysis. Most cases of *unilateral* vocal cord paralysis result from injury to the recurrent laryngeal nerve. A weak, breathy voice and choking with feedings are the most common presenting symptoms. A difficult delivery can lead to traction on the cervical portion of the nerve, and injury is particularly common after pediatric heart surgery. *Bilateral* vocal cord paralysis presents with respiratory distress and inspiratory stridor. The voice may be surprisingly strong in these patients, which may delay recognition, with disastrous results. The most common cause of bilateral vocal cord paralysis is central nervous system (CNS) disease, especially the Arnold-Chiari malformation.

INFECTIOUS AND INFLAMMATORY DISORDERS

Laryngitis

Laryngitis refers to any inflammatory process involving the larynx and may result from infections, environmental irritants, or other inflammatory processes involving the pharynx. Laryngitis also may result from habitual factors, such as voice abuse, coughing, or throat clearing.

Acute Laryngitis. Viral laryngitis is probably the most common inflammatory disorder of the larynx. The patient usually has an associated prodrome of low-grade fever, myalgias, and upper respiratory congestion. The voice is characteristically hoarse, with breaks and reduced pitch. A number of viruses are responsible. Treatment is supportive, with an emphasis on voice rest and humidification.

Noninfectious Laryngitis. Chronic noninfectious laryngitis may result from prolonged exposure to tobacco smoke and alcohol, which are strongly associated with the development of laryngeal cancer. More recently, GER has also been noted to play a similar role in laryngeal disease.

Croup

Croup *(acute laryngotracheobronchitis)* is most common in children between 1 and 3 years of age. After a 24- to 72-hour prodrome of upper respiratory symptoms, a characteristic nonproductive seal-like cough is associated with stridor and sometimes wheezing. Illness is most common in the late fall and winter and may progress to respiratory distress. Parainfluenza virus is the most common cause. Treatment varies with severity and includes cool mist humidification, racemic epinephrine, systemic steroids, and rarely intubation.

Spasmodic Croup. A common cause of stridor in children 1 to 3 years of age, spasmodic croup has an unknown etiology, but viral infection, allergies, and GER are suspected. Typically, barking cough and stridor begin suddenly at night, with no prodromal symptoms. Humidity and cold air seem to alleviate the symptoms, but racemic epinephrine and glucocorticoids may be required to provide relief.

Epiglottitis

Acute epiglottitis is a rapidly progressing infection of the supraglottic larynx most often caused by *Haemophilus* influenza type B (HIB). This disease can be distinguished from croup by the sudden onset of stridor, dysphagia, drooling, high fever, and the absence of a cough. The voice is muffled. Patients characteristically hold the neck in extension to maintain airway patency. Although this disease most often affects children 2 to 7 years of age, adults may be affected. Emergency airway support is essential, and patients in distress should be kept comfortably in their parents' arms until the airway can be assured, forgoing examination of the throat or radiologic studies. The use of conjugated vaccine for HIB has significantly reduced the incidence of epiglottitis, but the disease may be associated with other organisms.

Diphtheria

Diphtheria is fortunately a rare disorder in the United States because of widespread immunization. Infection by *Corynebacterium diphtheriae* leads to inflammation and membrane formation in the oropharynx and larynx that can result in airway obstruction and death.

Fungal Infections

Fungal infection of the larynx typically occurs in the setting of disseminated disease and results in hoarseness and cough. Treatment with amphotericin B typically produces satisfactory results. *Histoplasmosis* is endemic to the Ohio and Mississippi River valleys, where 80% to 90% of the population is infected. Painful granulomas are noted, particularly on the anterior aspect of the larynx. *Blastomycosis* is most common in the southeastern United States. Laryngeal infection results in a granular laryngitis. Biopsy often demonstrates thickened squamous epithelium, which may be confused with squamous cell carcinoma. *Coccidioidomycosis* is endemic to the southwestern United States and may occur in any age group. Laryngeal involvement occurs less often than lung disease.

Granulomatous Diseases

Granulomatous diseases of the larynx most often occur in the setting of systemic disease. The most common cause is tuberculosis. Syphilis, sarcoidosis, Wegener's disease, leprosy, and rhinoscleroma are also associated with granuloma formation in the larynx, although definitive diagnosis may be difficult.

Angioedema

Angioedema is an acute inflammatory process affecting the soft tissue of the face, oropharynx, and larynx. It may be precipitated by insect bites and stings, irritants, and medications. Hereditary angioedema is a relatively rare disorder that may be associated with a deficiency in C1 esterase. Treatment for acute events includes racemic or subcutaneous epinephrine, antihistamines, and steroids.

Gastroesophageal Reflux Disease

Gastroesophageal reflux disease (GERD), also known as *laryngopharyngeal reflux,* is a well-known clinical entity involving reflux of gastric acid into the esophagus and upper aerodigestive tract (see Chapter 102). Upper airway manifestations of GERD are common, and up to 25% of patients with GERD may have symptoms isolated to the head and neck region. Although symptoms vary in frequency and severity, the patient typically describes a lump in the throat, "globus" sensation, throat tightness, burning or sore throat, hoarseness, and odynophagia. The patient may describe symptoms of dysphagia or food sticking in the throat. GERD should be considered in patients with postnasal drip, chronic cough, and throat clearing. Patients may awaken during the night with a coughing episode, and symptoms may be worse in the morning hours after recumbency. In addition to underlying anatomic or medical disorders, reflux of gastric contents may be exacerbated by various lifestyle behaviors. The use of caffeine, alcohol and tobacco products, meals less than 2 hours before bedtime, tight clothing, obesity, stress, and depression are just a few of the factors that promote GERD in adults. Vomiting, failure to thrive, apnea, laryngospasm, and respiratory distress are seen in infants with acid reflux, and GERD has been documented in approximately 50% of infants presenting with life-threatening events.

Physical examination of the larynx in patients with laryngopharyngeal reflux reveals mucosal erythema and edema of the posterior commissure and arytenoid processes. The vocal cords may be inflamed or edematous. In more severe cases, vocal cord ulcers or granulomas may form posteriorly on the vocal process of the arytenoid cartilages. The posterior pharyngeal wall and hypopharynx may be erythematous and have a cobblestone appearance.

The diagnosis of GERD can often be made based on history and physical examination. The gold standard in diagnostic testing is a 24-hour pH probe for continuous monitoring of esophageal pH at both the upper and the lower esophageal sphincters. This test provides useful information about the pH of the environment around the larynx and upper aerodigestive tract.

The treatment of GERD involves medical therapy with antacids, H_2 blockers, and proton pump inhibitors. In addition, patients should be counseled in necessary lifestyle changes to eliminate factors that aggravate or promote GERD. Adherence will result in elimination of symptoms and reversal of laryngeal mucosal and vocal cord changes.

MISUSE AND ABUSE OF THE VOICE

Misuse or abuse of the voice occurs in avocational and professional speakers or singers and may result in structural changes to the vocal folds. These changes produce alterations in vocal quality with loss of pitch and intensity, often leading to a monotonous, harsh, or breathy voice. Attempts to overcome poor vocal quality frequently lead to further voice misuse. A speech pathologist, speech therapy, and behavioral modifications are key in restoring normal vocal cord form and function.

Reinke's Space Edema

Structural changes on the vocal cords due to abuse or misuse of the voice begin with edema of Reinke's space. This is a potential space between the vocal cord epithelium and underlying lamina propria. Reinke's edema results in a lower fundamental voice frequency that the patient perceives as a lower vocal pitch. The edematous changes in Reinke's space are reversible if appropriate compensatory techniques are instituted to eliminate vocal misuse. Speech therapy and elimination of contributing factors (e.g., smoking, GER) are essential for successful long-term management. If Reinke's space edema persists despite these interventions, evaluation for an underlying disease process should be pursued (e.g., hypothyroidism). Progression of Reinke's edema may lead to more permanent pathologic changes of the vocal cords, including vocal cord nodules and polyps.

Vocal Cord Nodules

Chronic vocal abuse from yelling, talking, or using an unnaturally low-pitched voice can lead to hyalinization of Reinke's space and the development of vocal fold nodules. Most often seen in boys and women, these lesions are often referred to as "singer's," "preacher's," or "screamer's" nodules. The history reveals chronic hoarseness and difficulty attaining high notes with singing. A harsh or breathy vocal quality is observed depending on the nodule's size. The nodules are usually bilateral and symmetric and originate at the junction of the anterior one third and posterior two thirds of the vocal cord. In children, vocal cord nodules may spontaneously regress with puberty. In adults, the nodules are best managed conservatively by maintaining adequate hydration and controlling sources of laryngeal irritation (e.g., smoking, GER). With speech therapy, behavior modification, and a speech-language pathologist, most nodules are reversible. If conservative therapies fail, the nodules may be removed surgically, followed by voice rest and further speech therapy. Failure to correct abusive vocal behaviors will likely lead to recurrence.

Vocal Cord Polyps

The etiology of vocal cord polyps is similar to that of vocal cord nodules. Chronic allergic reactions and inhalation of irritants may serve as contributing factors. The patient typically reports persistent hoarseness and difficulty maintaining adequate vocal intensity or loudness when speaking. A breathy quality to the voice may also be noted. Polyps are the result of subepithelial edema that may be localized or extend along the entire length of the vocal fold's free edge. Unlike vocal cord nodules, polyps are frequently unilateral, although both cords may be involved depending on the underlying cause. Abrupt or forceful voice abuse may rupture capillaries or ectatic vessels on the surface of the vocal fold and lead to the formation of a hemorrhagic polyp. Surgical removal of the polyps using microlaryngoscopy under general anesthesia is necessary to restore vocal function. Speech therapy before and after surgery is essential in eliminating patterns of vocal abuse to prevent polyp recurrence. Concomitant therapy for other inciting factors, such as allergies, GER, and inhalational irritants (e.g., smoking), should be initiated.

Vocal Cord Granulomas

Vocal cord granulomas, or contact ulcers of the larynx, result from misuse and abuse of the voice or mucosal injury from endotracheal intubation. Symptoms consist of hoarseness and pain with swallowing or phonation. The lesions may be unilateral or bilateral and usually form over the vocal process of the arytenoid cartilage. GER may predispose or contribute to the development of granuloma formation. Treatment for vocal cord granulomas is dictated by the underlying etiology. Granulomas from intubation trauma are readily managed by surgical excision. In contrast, surgical removal of granulomas due to vocal abuse or misuse often results in rapid recurrence. Therefore, as directed by a speech pathologist, voice therapy and voice rest are important. Additional treatment includes GER medication and antireflux precautions, such as elevating the head of the bed on blocks, avoiding alcoholic beverages and caffeinated products, and avoiding meals at least 2 hours before bedtime.

Vocal Cord Cysts

Vocal abuse may lead to the development of vocal cord cysts. These lesions are classified as either *mucous retention cysts*, caused by an occluded mucous gland duct, or *epidermoid cysts* containing keratin. The patient has a similar history and symptoms as the patient with vocal cord nodules. Epidermoid cysts are more common and are best managed with voice therapy. Patients with mucous retention cysts may also be treated with speech therapy, but in the absence of voice abuse, surgical removal by microlaryngoscopy typically results in improvement. Occasionally the cysts rupture spontaneously. Adjunctive measures such as adequate hydration, antireflux management, and smoking cessation are helpful in obtaining resolution.

NEUROMUSCULAR LARYNGEAL DYSFUNCTION

Alterations in the form and function of the vocal cords present as changes in voice or speech patterns. These changes may be caused by abnormalities of the intrinsic or extrinsic laryngeal musculature, neurologic dysfunction, or the aging process.

Vocal Cord Paralysis

Diseases affecting the vagus nerve or its laryngeal branches result in vocal cord paralysis and impaired laryngeal sensation. Although the exact incidence of vocal cord paralysis is unknown, unilateral vocal cord paralysis accounts for approximately 75% of all cases. The left vocal cord is more frequently affected, presumably because of its longer length and more circuitous route. The etiology of vocal cord paralysis can be divided into CNS lesions and peripheral lesions involving the vagus nerve (Box 181-2). Approximately 90% of the lesions are peripheral. In adults, neoplasm is the most common cause of unilateral vocal cord paralysis, followed by postsurgical, idiopathic, medical/inflammatory, traumatic, and central lesions.

The symptoms associated with vocal cord paralysis vary depending on the nerves involved. Hoarseness is probably the most common complaint, but stridor, shortness of breath, changes in vocal quality, cough, and aspiration may also be noted. Some cases may be asymptomatic. The goal in evaluating vocal cord paralysis is to identify the underlying cause. A detailed history should include pulmonary or thyroid neoplasms, previous neck or chest surgery, endotracheal intubation, neck trauma, systemic diseases, recent viral infection, and previous hoarseness. Physical examination requires complete laryngeal examination by flexible laryngoscopy to assess vocal cord function and position and to evaluate laryngeal sensation. Cranial nerve examination may reveal other cranial neuropathies associated with the underlying etiology. Imaging begins with a chest radiograph. CT scan or MRI of the brain, neck, and chest can demonstrate the entire length of the recurrent laryngeal nerves in patients with vocal cord paralysis of unknown origin. Direct laryngoscopy and bronchoscopy are useful to assess the mobility of the cricoarytenoid joints and to evaluate for occult neoplasm. Laboratory tests (e.g., thyroid function tests, erythrocyte sedimentation rate, complete blood count) are of relatively low yield given the previous approach.

The management of vocal cord paralysis consists of surgical and nonsurgical interventions, depending on the cause and degree of laryngeal dysfunction. Every attempt is made to identify and treat the underlying etiology. Patients with minimal changes in voice and no evidence of aspiration may benefit from speech therapy alone. This provides the patient with appropriate vocal techniques to avoid the sequelae associated with vocal abuse and misuse. In patients with more severe vocal dysfunction or signs and symptoms of aspiration, surgical intervention is usually warranted.

Bilateral vocal cord paralysis is uncommon and results in inability to abduct the vocal cords. The causative factors include CNS abnormalities (e.g., Arnold-Chiari malformation, hydrocephalus, meningomyelocele) and postsurgical injury (e.g., total thyroidectomy). Symptoms include severe stridor, cyanosis, and respiratory distress, with the need to secure the airway urgently by endotracheal intubation or tracheotomy. Because both vocal cords remain adducted, patients with bilateral vocal cord paralysis may have a normal or near-normal voice.

Box 181-2. Etiology of Vocal Cord Paralysis

Neoplasm (35.8%)

Pulmonary
Laryngeal
Thyroid, parathyroid
Jugular foramen tumors
Central nervous system tumors
Carotid sheath and parapharyngeal space tumors
Mediastinal

Postsurgical (24.6%)

Thyroidectomy
Parathyroidectomy
Cervical spine surgery
Carotid endarterectomy
Neck dissection
Cervical esophageal surgery
Cardiac surgery

Idiopathic (14.3%)

Medical/Inflammatory (13.3%)

Rheumatoid arthritis
Toxic neuropathy
Viral and bacterial infection
Congestive heart failure (Ortner's syndrome)

Trauma (6.0%)

Intubation injury
Blunt or penetrating neck or chest injury
Birth trauma

Central Nervous System (6.0%)

Arnold-Chiari malformation
Hydrocephalus
Meningomyelocele
Stroke, vascular insufficiency
Multiple sclerosis
Parkinson's disease

Spasmodic Dysphonia

Spasmodic dysphonia is a focal dystonia involving the laryngeal musculature. It is similar to other focal dystonias (e.g., blepharospasm, torticollis, writer's cramp) and may coexist with them. Spasmodic dysphonia occurs in adulthood, frequently after an upper respiratory tract infection or a period of emotional stress. Spasm of the laryngeal muscular adductors or abductors produces a strained or choked voice quality with abrupt breaks in phonation and a staccato-like pattern. The voice is decreased in loudness or hypophonic, and speech intelligibility often is poor. Accurate assessment involves evaluation by a speech pathologist with videostroboscopic examination. At rest the larynx appears normal, but during phonation, spasms of the true and false vocal cords are intermittently observed. In addition to speech therapy, treatment of spasmodic dysphonia may require percutaneous injection of botulinum toxin to eliminate muscle spasm. This is performed safely in the outpatient setting every 3 to 4 months.

Paradoxic Vocal Cord Motion

Paradoxic vocal cord motion (PVCM) is characterized by adduction of the vocal folds on inspiration and abduction on expiration. It typically occurs in young women and health care workers, often with a history of psychologic disorders. Presenting symptoms include inspiratory stridor, dyspnea, weak voice, and poor cough, which may be preceded by an upper respiratory tract infection. Patients with severe stridor from unrecognized PVCM occasionally undergo endotracheal intubation and tracheotomy. PVCM is a functional dyskinesia, and symptoms resolve with sleep but promptly return when the patient awakens. Diagnosis can only be made by visualization of vocal cord motion during an attack using indirect or flexible laryngoscopy. Routine laboratory studies, including an arterial blood gases, should be obtained to eliminate underlying organic etiologies for vocal cord dysfunction. The treatment for PVCM is mainly supportive, consisting of speech therapy and psychiatric counseling.

Presbyphonia

As part of the normal aging process, structural changes occur in the vocal cords and laryngeal musculature, including calcification of the laryngeal cartilage, loss of vocal cord elasticity, and decrease in muscle bulk. Presbyphonia is characterized by a breathy, weak, tremulous voice with alterations in pitch and early fatigability. Examination of the presbyphonic larynx typically reveals a posterior glottic gap, bowing of the vocal cords, and muscle atrophy. The physician must rule out any underlying medical problems that may be contributing to voice changes. Treatment strategies include voice therapy to eliminate vocal strain and maximize the functional capacity of the larynx. In addition, surgery to augment the thyroarytenoid muscles and vocal folds may be considered.

Parkinson's Disease

Patients with Parkinson's disease may develop vocal dysfunction secondary to bradykinesia and difficulty initiating voluntary muscle activity (see Chapter 169). The parkinsonian voice is characterized as breathy, hypophonic, tremulous, and of monotonous quality. The vocal folds are adynamic and bowed. Treatment is aimed at increasing vocal intensity and reducing vocal tremor through intensive speech therapy. Systemic treatment of Parkinson's disease with dopamine replacement for limb tremor may help to reduce vocal tremor as well.

Myasthenia Gravis

A disorder involving the neuromuscular junction, myasthenia gravis is characterized by weakness and fatigue of skeletal muscle. All age groups may be affected. The disorder typically presents with ocular involvement, including diplopia and ptosis of the eyelids. The voice may be altered by fatigue and weakness of the laryngeal muscles. Patients may note difficulty speaking and vocal fatigue, particularly with prolonged voice use. Vocal quality improves after a brief rest. Dysphagia and difficulty breathing may progress and require intubation and mechanical ventilation. Diagnosis of myasthenia gravis involves an anticholinesterase test and electrodiagnostic testing.

Amyotrophic Lateral Sclerosis

Amyotrophic lateral sclerosis (ALS) is caused by progressive degeneration of anterior horn cells in the spinal cord, resulting in wasting and weakness of skeletal muscle (see Chapter 170). Laryngeal involvement produces a raspy, monotonous voice, and involvement of the tongue may cause difficulty speaking. The gag reflex is depressed, and pooling of secretions in the hypopharynx and larynx may be observed. Aspiration of oral secretions occurs as the disease progresses. ALS is ultimately fatal primarily because of respiratory insufficiency and aspiration pneumonia. In the later stages, tracheotomy may be required to assist with ventilation, protection from aspiration, and pulmonary toilet.

LARYNGEAL TRAUMA

Endotracheal intubation is associated with a spectrum of injuries, ranging from mild mucosal inflammation to complete ulceration and necrosis of the underlying cartilage. The damage begins within hours of intubation; the degree of injury depends on duration and frequency of intubation, endotracheal tube size, presence of nasogastric tubes, and overall status of the patient. The cuff causes injuries in the subglottis, whereas the tube tends to damage the posterior glottis. Granulomata and ulcerations are common, and permanent sequelae may include stenosis and impaired vocal cord movement.

Blunt trauma is usually the result of motor vehicle injuries or "clothesline" injuries in which the unprotected neck is struck focally by a horizontal object. Strangulation causes a widespread but usually less severe laryngeal injury. The evaluation and management of laryngeal trauma varies with the mechanism of injury. Patients with signs and symptoms of acute airway compromise must have airway support in the form of endotracheal intubation or tracheotomy. The larynx is then examined endoscopically, with direct repair of fractured cartilage and mucosal injuries. Patients with a stable airway and mild symptoms (e.g., hoarseness) should undergo flexible laryngoscopy to identify hematomas or mild mucosal injuries. Airway obstruction in patients with relatively mild laryngeal trauma may be delayed up to 24 hours, and careful observation is required. Patients with intermediate injuries should undergo flexible laryngoscopy and CT scan of the larynx to identify cartilaginous injuries. Treatment is based on the specific injury.

Penetrating trauma from knives and projectiles may result from "urban warfare." Exploration of the wounds and repair of the larynx and trachea are indicated.

Burns

Thermal injury to the larynx may occur even in the absence of significant pulmonary insult because of protective mechanisms resulting in glottic closure. Steam tends to deliver more thermal injury than heated air. Patients with carbonaceous sputum and erythema of the laryngeal mucosa benefit from early airway control with intubation rather than observing while edema and inflammation may progress.

Accidental or purposeful ingestion of caustic substances also results in esophageal and airway injuries. Patients with stridor after caustic ingestion should have the airway assured as quickly as possible, because the inflammatory process can progress rapidly.

RESPIRATORY FOREIGN BODIES

Aspiration of foreign bodies is a relatively common cause of respiratory symptoms in children and is associated with approximately 3000 deaths per year in the United States. Vegetable material (e.g. peanuts) and toy parts are the most common objects aspirated by children. Foreign body aspiration should be suspected in any patient who suddenly develops localized wheezing with diminished breath sounds and cough. Although a witnessed choking episode provides supporting evidence, such a history is not required.

Inspiratory and expiratory chest radiographs may demonstrate air trapping in cases of major airway obstruction. Both rigid and fiberoptic techniques are used for foreign body removal. Rigid endoscopy provides the advantage of controlled airway and ventilation. In skilled hands the risks of a missed foreign body exceed the risks of a negative endoscopic evaluation. Therefore it is reasonable to proceed to endoscopy if foreign body aspiration cannot be eliminated from the differential diagnosis of a persistently wheezing child.

LARYNGEAL NEOPLASIA

The larynx may be involved with a variety of benign and malignant neoplastic lesions (Box 181-3). Manifestations of laryngeal neoplasia may include hoarseness, dysphagia, odynophagia, and aspiration depending on the site and extent of involvement.

Recurrent Respiratory Papillomatosis

Recurrent respiratory papillomatosis (RRP) is the most common benign neoplastic process involving the larynx (Fig. 181-3). This disease is caused by infection with human papillomavirus (HPV), most often types 6 and 11. Affecting both children and adults, RRP is characterized by the recurrent growth of exophytic warty lesions. Patients usually present with hoarseness, stridor, and cough. Typically, children have a more aggressive course, with numerous recurrences. Treatment is primarily surgical, with repeated endoscopic excision and vaporization of the papillomatous growth. Medical therapy is typically reserved for severe cases; at present only interferon has been conclusively demonstrated to impact the pattern of the disease, and this effect ends with cessation of therapy. Other medical therapies have been used, and new protocols are currently under investigation. Currently, neither surgical nor medical therapies are curative.

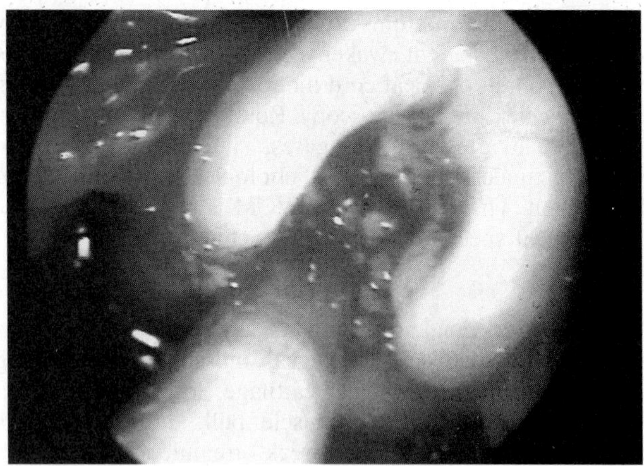

Fig. 181-3. Recurrent respiratory papillomatosis of the larynx.

Box 181-3. Laryngeal Neoplasms

Benign	Malignant
	Primary
Recurrent respiratory papillomatosis	Squamous cell carcinoma
Oncocytic tumor	Verrucous carcinoma
Granular cell tumor	Adenocarcinoma
Hemangioma	Sarcoma
Lymphangioma	
Paraganglioma	***Metastatic***
Nerve sheath tumor	Melanoma
Lipoma	Kidney
Chondroma	Prostate
Pleomorphic adenoma	Breast
Nodular fasciitis	Lung
Fibrous histiocytoma	Stomach
Fibromatosis	
Rhabdomyoma	

Leukoplakia

Leukoplakia is a clinical term denoting a white patch or plaque on the mucous membrane of the larynx or other sites of the upper aerodigestive tract. The most common inciting agent for the development of leukoplakia of the larynx is cigarette smoking. These lesions may be asymptomatic or may present with hoarseness or voice changes depending on location and extent of laryngeal involvement. Leukoplakia may be isolated to the vocal cord or may involve the larynx diffusely. Histologically, keratinization of the mucosa with or without dysplastic epithelial changes is observed. Leukoplakia is not necessarily a premalignant lesion, but carcinoma may develop in up to 3% of these lesions. Because of the risk of malignant degeneration, especially in a patient with a history of tobacco and alcohol abuse, excisional biopsy is both diagnostic and therapeutic. Close follow-up with indirect or flexible laryngoscopy is important to observe for recurrence or progression of the lesion.

Laryngeal Cancer

Recent epidemiologic data indicate that the incidence of laryngeal cancer in the United States is about 11,100 new cases per year, with 4300 deaths. The most common type is squamous cell carcinoma, which accounts for more than 90% of all head and neck cancers. Laryngeal cancer has a male/female ratio of 5:1 to 10:1 and most often affects patients in the sixth to seventh decades of life. Major risk factors are tobacco and alcohol use. Ionizing radiation, viruses (e.g., HPV), occupational exposure (e.g., nickel), and GER are also implicated as risk factors.

The signs and symptoms of laryngeal cancer include hoarseness, stridor, dysphagia, odynophagia, hemoptysis, weight loss, and referred otalgia. Cancers arising from the true vocal cords present the earliest because of hoarseness, and a patient with hoarseness longer than 2 weeks should have careful inspection of the larynx to rule out a glottic carcinoma. In contrast, patients with supraglottic cancers tend to present with advanced disease because these lesions may grow to considerable size before becoming symptomatic. In addition to a patient history, accurate diagnosis requires a thorough head and neck examination with full visualization of the larynx, hypopharynx, oropharynx, and tongue base by indirect mirror examination or flexible endoscopy. The neck should be palpated for the presence of lymphadenopathy to assess for regional metastasis. Ultimately, direct laryngoscopy, bronchoscopy, and esophagoscopy with biopsies need to be performed to obtain a histologic diagnosis, document the extent of tumor involvement, and rule out synchronous primary lesions.

Treatment modalities for laryngeal cancer consist of surgery, radiation, and chemotherapy alone or in combination. Despite recent advances, no significant change in 5-year survival has occurred over the past 20 to 30 years. In general, for less extensive tumors, radiation alone is as effective as surgery. Larger or more extensive tumors typically require surgery with or without radiation therapy. Chemotherapy as a single-modality treatment is not very effective for laryngeal cancer. Multimodality therapy using induction chemotherapy with radiation therapy is currently in clinical trials and showing promising results. Chemoradiation holds the prospect of cure rates similar to surgery while preserving laryngeal function. Ultimately, treatment plans must be individualized by taking into account tumor stage and location, underlying medical problems, and socioeconomic factors.

EMERGENCY AIRWAY MANAGEMENT

Patients with disorders of the larynx or upper airway, such as acute epiglottitis, laryngeal cancer, or head and neck trauma, may present with severe upper airway obstruction and respiratory distress. Obtaining an adequate and secure airway is of paramount importance in the treatment of these patients. When routine orotracheal or nasotracheal intubation is unsuccessful or contraindicated, a surgical airway must be established. The preferred method for an emergent surgical airway is a *cricothyroidotomy.* This may be safely and rapidly performed by creating a vertical, midline incision through the cricothyroid membrane between the thyroid and cricoid cartilages and inserting an endotracheal or tracheostomy tube. The cricothyroidotomy site may be used for approximately 3 to 5 days, after which the site should be converted to a tracheotomy to avoid the risk of subglottic injury and stenosis.

An alternative to cricothyroidotomy is emergent *tracheotomy.* This procedure involves greater risks and is technically more difficult to perform in an emergency setting. Emergent tracheotomy should be performed only by those with sufficient surgical experience and expertise.

ADDITIONAL READINGS

Bastian RW: Benign vocal cord fold mucosal disorders. In Cummings CW et al, editors: *Otolaryngology–head and neck surgery,* St Louis, 1998, Mosby.

Koufman JA: The otolaryngic manifestations of gastroesophageal refluz disease: a clinical study of 225 patients using ambulatory 24-hour pH monitoring and an experimental investigation of the role of acid and pepsin in the development of laryngeal injury, *Laryngoscope* 101(suppl 53), 1991.

Leach JL, Schaefer SD: *Diagnosis and treatment of cancer of the glottis and subglottis,* 1993, American Academy of Otolaryngology–Head and Neck Surgery.

Snow JB: Surgical therapy for vocal dysfunction, *Otolaryngol Clin North Am* 17:91, 1984.

Terris DJ, Arnstein DP, Nguyen HH: Contemporary evaluation of unilateral vocal cord paralysis, *Otolaryngol Head Neck Surg* 107:84, 1992.

CHAPTER 182

Evaluation of Neck Masses

Fred G. Fedok
Michael Burnett

The differential diagnosis for a neck mass is extensive. The primary care physician should establish an orderly, streamlined approach based on historic and anatomic considerations to diagnose and treat neck masses. The history and physical examination provide the diagnosis for most neck masses and guide an expedient workup for the remainder.

ANATOMY AND AGE

An understanding of fundamental anatomic considerations can greatly simplify the diagnosis and treatment of a neck mass. Most neck masses fit into one of the following diagnostically salient locations: (1) midline: suggests thyroglossal duct cyst, dermoid, or teratoma; (2) anterior to the sternocleidomastoid muscle: suggests branchial cleft remnant anomalies; (3) associated with thyroid gland: suggests diffuse thyroid enlargement or thyroid nodule; (4) areas of major salivary glands (preauricular region or angle of the jaw): suggests pathology of the parotid or submandibular glands, including sialoadenitis vs. salivary neoplasms; and (5) routes containing clusters of lymph nodes: suggests inflammatory or neoplastic lymphadenopathy (Fig. 182-1).

Neck masses may be divided into three broad etiologic categories: congenital, inflammatory, and neoplastic (malignant or benign). The earliest branch point used in formulating a differential diagnosis, in order of probability, may be the patient's age. Regarding neck masses, patients can be grouped by age into children ages 15 and younger, young adults ages 16 to 40, and adults over 40. Statistically, there is a dramatic rearrangement in the order of likelihood of a given diagnosis based on these groupings. In children and young adults an inflammatory condition is the most likely etiology of a neck mass, with congenital masses second and neoplastic diagnoses least likely. In adults over 40, however, a persistent neck mass should be considered a malignant neoplasm, generally metastatic, until proven otherwise (Fig. 182-2).

PATIENT EVALUATION

History

The physician approaches the history of the neck mass as any other physical complaint. The physician determines when the mass was first noticed, what brought it to the patient's attention, and if the mass is progressively increasing in size or following a crescendo/decrescendo pattern of growth. Associated pain and discharge are noted, as well as constitutional symptoms such as fevers, weight loss, and night sweats. Any patient with a neck mass should be specifically questioned about the presence or absence of hoarseness or changes in voice, odynophagia, dysphagia, otalgia, decreased hearing or aural fullness, nasal fullness or discharge, cough, and hemoptysis. The patient reports any history of cancer or lesions removed from the head or neck, as well as any recent dental work, dental complaints, or upper respiratory tract infections. Relevant exposure history

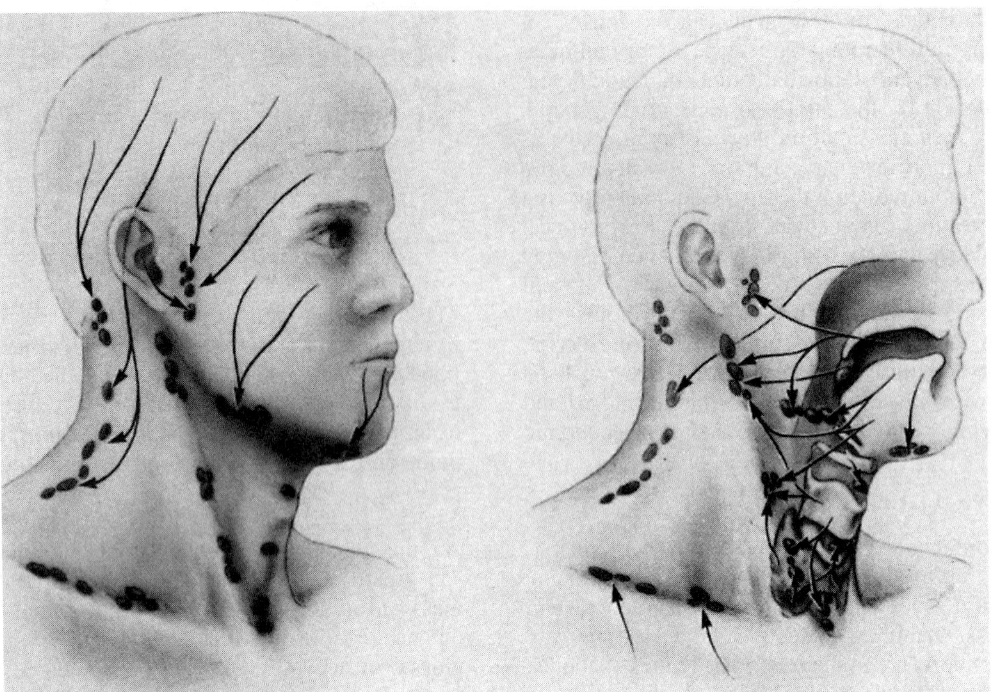

Fig. 182-1. Lymphatic drainage of external *(left)* and internal *(right)* areas of head and neck. Arrows indicate lymphatic drainage pathways. (From McGuirt FW. In Cummings CW, et al, editors: *Otolaryngology: head and neck surgery,* ed 2, St Louis, 1998, Mosby.)

includes tuberculosis exposure during travel, animal exposures (e.g., cat or dog scratches), radiation exposure, and occupational exposures to substances implicated in head and neck cancer (e.g., nickel, woodworking). A family history of head and neck cancer might suggest one of the familial syndromes of endocrine neoplasia. Social history is extremely important, including tobacco and alcohol use, which are significant risk factors for head and neck carcinoma. If the mass is in the supraclavicular region, the pulmonary, gastrointestinal, and genitourinary systems are reviewed, with a history of mammograms and their results, since the supraclavicular node often represents a metastasis from a primary neoplasm below the clavicles.

Physical Examination

Any patient with a neck mass requires a thorough physical examination. The etiology of a neck mass in the adult involves a search for a primary site of disease in the head and neck that may have lead to either inflammatory or neoplastic change in a neck lymph node. Thus the head and neck examination must be methodic, not focusing solely on the mass.

The skin of the head and neck is examined for suspicious skin lesions. The ears are examined, including pneumatic otoscopy. A unilateral middle ear effusion might be a clue to a mass obstructing the eustachian tube orifice. The nasal mucosa is examined for lesions. The oral cavity and oropharynx are best examined using a head mirror or head light, thus freeing both hands to perform the examination. The palate, tonsils, tonsillar pillars, and posterior pharyngeal wall are examined. The tongue examination includes the lateral surfaces and underneath the tongue on the floor of the mouth, which are more likely to contain mucosal malignancies than the dorsum. The tongue and floor of mouth should be palpated in search of submucosal lesions, which would otherwise be missed. Bimanual examination can often better delineate and size discrete structures, including normal anatomy (e.g., submandibular glands) and pathologic masses. The gingiva is examined throughout the lingual and buccal surfaces. A mirror examination inspects the nasopharynx above and the larynx and hypopharynx below.

The mass is palpated for texture. Rock-hard masses are more typical of carcinoma, whereas fluctuance usually denotes a fluid-filled or pus-filled entity. A mass fixed to the overlying skin or deeper tissues might indicate invasion of the surrounding tissues. A mass that moves up and down on swallowing indicates tethering to either the strap muscles or tongue base, typically seen with thyroid-associated entities (e.g., thyroid nodule, thyroglossal duct cyst). Signs of inflammation include tenderness and overlying erythema and warmth. The position within the neck may suggest the primary site of pathology.

The remainder of the neck is palpated along the major lymph drainage routes for adenopathy (see Fig. 182-1). The thyroid gland is palpated for nodules, and the trachea's position is noted with respect to the midline. The cranial nerves should be specifically challenged for deficits.

A thorough head and neck examination often identifies the primary site of pathology, thereby guiding the remainder of the workup and treatment plan.

INFLAMMATORY NECK MASSES

Lymphadenopathy

Lymphadenopathy simply implies enlarged lymph nodes, without specifically indicating pathology or disease. Palpable lymph nodes are a common and frequently normal finding in children. About 50% of children have palpable lymph nodes 1 to 1.5 cm in size and not associated with obvious infection

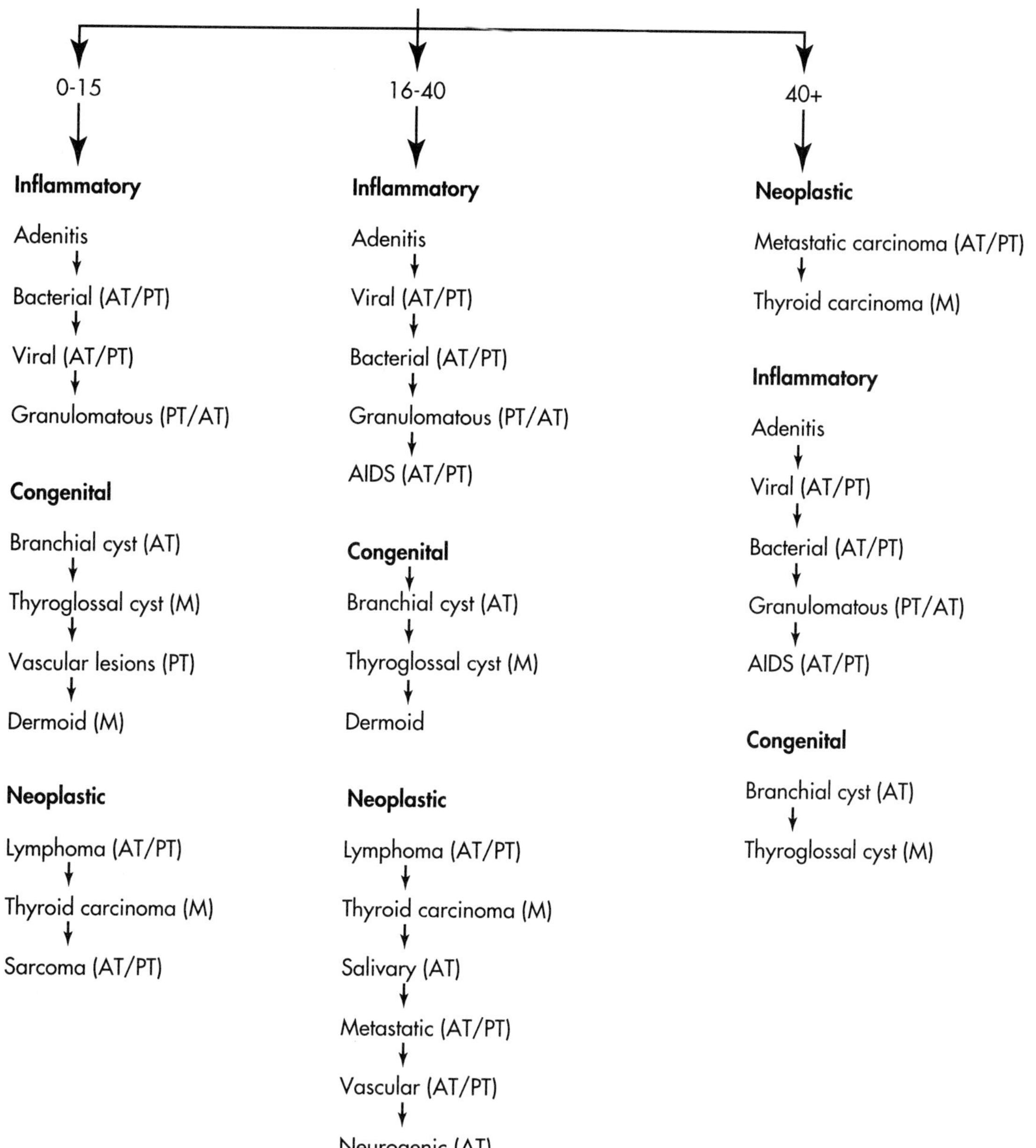

Fig. 182-2. Relative frequency of specific neck masses within causative groups by age. *AT,* Anterior; *PT,* posterior; *M,* midline; *AIDS,* acquired immunodeficiency syndrome. (From McGuirt FW. In Cummings CW, et al, editors: *Otolaryngology: head and neck surgery,* ed 3, St Louis, 1993, Mosby.)

or systemic illness. Cervical lymphadenopathy should prompt a search for a primary site of head and neck pathology that may have caused the adenopathy. Odontogenic sources and pharyngitis are common etiologies. *Lymphadenitis* implies signs of inflammation of lymph nodes, including enlarged, tender, warm, erythematous nodes. *Suppurative lymphadenitis* further denotes purulent change within the lymph nodes. The varying etiologies for lymphadenitis generally have distinct patterns. Important differentiating characteristics in diagnosing the etiology of cervical lymphadenitis include acute vs. chronic presentation, number of nodes involved (single, unilateral, bilateral, generalized), signs of inflammation, fluctuance, associated head and neck or dental disease, exposure history, and age.

Acute cervical lymphadenitis is most often caused by regional or generalized viral infections. Seasonal viral upper respiratory tract infections (e.g., rhinovirus, adenovirus, enterovirus) are common causes. Herpes simplex virus (HSV) gingivostomatitis, roseola infantum (exanthema subitum, HSV-6), Epstein-Barr virus (EBV), cytomegalovirus (CMV), and human immunodeficiency virus (HIV) are common etiologies of acute cervical lymphadenitis. With viral causes, enlarged lymph nodes are generally found bilaterally, frequently with signs of inflammation such as tenderness and overlying erythema and warmth, but without fluctuance. Often, concomitant constitutional symptoms can be elicited.

Acute suppurative lymphadenitis, in contrast, is typically a unilateral infection of bacterial origin. The involved nodes may be mildly tender and fluctuant, although otherwise not particularly inflamed. Group A β-hemolytic streptococci and *Staphylococcus aureus* are the most common organisms and may be primary infectors or may superinfect a viral lymphadenitis. As many as 25% of such infections involve anaerobes, with gram-negative organisms occasionally identified.[2] Suppuration tends to occur within 2 weeks of symptom onset. Up to 40% of patients present with antecedent upper respiratory symptoms.[7] Systemic signs and toxemia are uncommon unless there is an overlying cellulitis or clinically apparent primary focus of infection.

In *chronic cervical lymphadenitis* (longer than 3 weeks), viruses again are the most common etiologies, and patients typically present with bilaterally enlarged lymph nodes. When unilateral and fluctuant, lymphadenitis is usually of bacterial origin and should suggest bacteria found in acute suppurative lymphadenitis or in common granulomatous diseases (e.g., *Mycobacterium tuberculosis,* atypical mycobacteria, cat-scratch disease, toxoplasmosis).

Granulomatous Diseases

Mycobacteria. Mycobacteria may cause chronic granulomatous lymphadenitis, typically within the nodal network of the major salivary glands. *M. tuberculosis* lymphadenitis occurs after spread from a primary pulmonary focus. Patients may have associated constitutional symptoms of weight loss, night sweats, or fevers, although their absence is not unusual. The diagnosis is strongly suggested by a positive response to purified protein derivative (PPD) skin testing. Treatment involves a full course of antituberculous medications.

Atypical mycobacteria are common colonizers in the mouths of children. They invade locally to cause infection, manifesting as a chronic, unilateral, firm mass in the submandibular or preauricular areas, generally in children younger than 5 years old and rarely after age 12. Atypical mycobacteria lymphadenitis does not respond to systemic medications; definitive therapy involves surgical excision. Incisional biopsy should be avoided because of the potential for persistently draining infections. Diagnosis of mycobacterial infection may be made on acid-fast staining or culture of an aspirated specimen, although the yield on culture may be less than 60%.[8] Approximately 50% of patients with atypical mycobacteria infection will mount a weak response to a PPD skin test.

Cat-scratch Disease. Cat-scratch disease represents another granulomatous lymphadenitis. The putative causative organism is *Bartonella henselae.* The typical patient presents with tender lymphadenopathy in the head and neck, particularly in the regions of the parotid and submandibular glands, developing within 2 weeks after a cat scratch. The primary site of inoculation often manifests a skin lesion such as a pustule. Approximately 75% of patients are able to recall an antecedent cat scratch, with another 15% reporting exposure to a cat.[4] In a small percentage of patients canine exposure is responsible. Needle aspiration yields sterile pus. A cat-scratch disease skin test is available. The majority of cases will resolve without treatment in 2 to 3 months. Symptoms include fever and usually are mild in immunocompetent patients. Treatment is generally supportive, with antipyretics and analgesics as needed. More severe cases can be treated with erythromycin or doxycycline.

Toxoplasmosis. Toxoplasmosis is caused by the organism *Toxoplasma gondii,* usually carried by a domestic cat host. It is typically transmitted to humans through eating infected food products. Although immunocompromised patients are at risk for the more severe disseminated forms of the disease, immunocompetent patients are more likely to develop only mild symptoms, including lymphadenopathy, particularly in the head and neck. The diagnosis can be ascertained through acute and convalescent titers. Effective treatment is provided by a course of pyrimethamine and trisulfapyrimidine, which is especially important in immunocompromised hosts and pregnant women. In the otherwise healthy adult the infection is usually self-limited.

Actinomyces. Poor oral hygiene and mucosal trauma are risk factors for *Actinomyces* infections, as are diabetes and impaired immune function. Infection with these organisms typically manifests as a painless, indurated neck mass, which may mimic a neoplasm. This is not a lymphadenitis, and the infection usually does not cause lymphadenopathy. The diagnosis is made by needle aspirate to identify characteristic sulfur granules, which represent conglomerations of organisms. The infections can reach the skin surface to cause chronic, draining cutaneous fistulas. Treatment is with high-dose penicillin, since no penicillin resistance has been identified to date.

Miscellaneous Infections. Other, less common infectious causes of cervical lymphadenitis include secondary syphilis, a sexually transmitted disease caused by the spirochete *Treponema pallidum;* brucellosis, which may be acquired by drinking infected unpasteurized milk; and Lyme disease, caused by the organism *Borrelia burgdorferi,* through inoculation by a bite from the carrier tick *Ixodes dammini,* endemic to many regions in the northeastern and midwestern United States.

Salivary Gland Origin

Sialolithiasis. Sialolithiasis, or calculi within the system of salivary gland ducts, is principally a disease of the submandibular gland (90% of cases), although it can occur in the parotid or minor salivary glands.[1] The majority of submandibular sialoliths are radiopaque, whereas this applies to only a minority of parotid calculi. Stones may be revealed because of recurrent swelling and pain that may be exacerbated by superimposed infection. The diagnosis may be made by bimanual palpation, plain radiographs, sialography, or computed tomography (CT) scan. Transoral removal of an obstructing stone may be accomplished if the stone is situated near the duct orifice. Recurrent symptoms caused by salivary calculi may require surgical excision of the involved salivary gland.

Acute Suppurative Sialoadenitis. Acute suppurative infection can affect the parotid, submandibular, or sublingual salivary glands, although the most common scenario is an acute parotitis. The typical patient is an adult, over age 50, generally with one or more reasons for decreased salivary secretions and poor oral hygiene. Volume depletion from any cause, debilitation leading to decreased fluid intake, and medications with anticholinergic side effects are factors that reduce the flow of saliva through the salivary ducts, allowing for retrograde infection of the salivary gland. A common scenario is in the postoperative setting. The usual symptom complex is acute onset of pain and swelling of the affected salivary gland, often associated with fevers or other constitutional symptoms. Examination reveals a swollen, tender gland with overlying erythema. A few patients present with bilateral parotid involvement. Regional adenopathy may be noted. Suppurative parotitis rarely impairs facial nerve function, and such a finding suggests an alternative or concomitant diagnosis, including malignancy. The physician should assess for pus at the orifice of the parotid duct, found opposite the upper second molar, or at the submandibular duct orifice, found adjacent to the frenulum of the tongue. A discharge sample, if obtainable, can be sent for Gram's stain and culture. The most common offending organism is *S. aureus,* although streptococci, and occasionally gram-negative or anaerobic organisms, can be cultured.

Treatment consists of (1) empiric antibiotics to cover β-lactamase-resistant *S. aureus;* (2) measures to improve salivary flow, including sialogogues (e.g., lemon drops); (3) volume repletion; and (4) cessation of anticholinergic medications, if possible. Analgesics and warm compresses alleviate pain. If tolerated by the patient, manually "milking" the affected salivary gland may assist with drainage and resolution of the infection. If no significant improvement is noted after 2 to 3 days of therapy, a CT scan may be considered to rule out abscess, mass lesion, or impacted sialolith, all of which may require surgical intervention. Sialography is specifically contraindicated in the setting of acute infection. In the patient with recurrent acute episodes or unresolving infection, a consult with an otolaryngologist is indicated.

Acute Nonsuppurative Sialoadenitis. Acute nonsuppurative sialoadenitis (sialadenitis) is typically a viral infection, the most common cause of which is mumps, although EBV, coxsackievirus, HIV, and other viruses may also involve the salivary glands. Mumps typically presents in children, manifesting as a viral syndrome with fevers, arthralgias, malaise, and parotid swelling, which is frequently bilateral. Treatment is generally supportive, although steroids or gamma globulin may be given to patients with severe disease. Parotid swelling usually resolves within 2 weeks.

Human Immunodeficiency Virus. Patients with HIV infection may develop multiple lymphoepithelial cysts within the major salivary glands, especially the parotid gland, which may become infected. Parotid enlargement is usually diffuse and symmetric. Asymmetric rapid enlargement of a salivary gland in HIV patients suggests a need to rule out lymphoma.

Miscellaneous Masses. Noninflammatory painless swellings of the salivary glands, especially the parotid gland, can be seen with nutritional deficiencies, alcoholism, anorexia or bulimia, and endocrinopathies (e.g., diabetes). Sjögren's disease is an autoimmune disorder frequently characterized by nontender swelling of the parotid glands and less often the submandibular glands. It may be a primary disease or associated with a systemic collagen vascular disease. Diagnosis is often made with a biopsy of a minor salivary gland of the lip, revealing a lymphocytic infiltrate.

Thyroid Masses

Thyroid masses make up a large percentage of anterior neck masses (Box 182-1). The differential diagnosis includes parathyroid tumors and several congenital neck masses (see later section). Enlarged thyroid glands or palpable thyroid nodules are common findings in clinical practice; 6.4% of women and 1.5% of men in the Framingham Study had palpable thyroid nodules. An even greater percentage of patients have thyroid nodules when imaging studies are employed.

Box 182-1. Thyroid Masses

Nodular Thyroid Disease

- Solitary nodule
  - Benign cyst
  - Benign neoplasm
  - Malignant neoplasm
- Multinodular goiter
  - Toxic
  - Nontoxic

Autoimmune Disease

- Graves' disease

Inflammatory Disease

- Hashimoto's thyroiditis (chronic lymphocytic)
- Subacute lymphocytic thyroiditis (sporadic or postpartum)
- De Quervain's thyroiditis (subacute granulomatous)
- Acute suppurative thyroiditis (Reidel's)

Clues to the diagnosis that a mass either represents or is associated with the thyroid gland include identifying its paratracheal position, palpating its intimacy with identifiable thyroid tissue, appreciating a bilaterality to the mass, and observing it move vertically with swallowing. The nature of the mass can often be identified with further testing, including radiologic imaging, generally ultrasound or CT scan.

Goiter refers to an enlarged thyroid gland. Iodine deficiency is uncommon in the United States but is the most common cause of goiter worldwide, called *endemic goiter.* In the United States the most common cause of goiter is the autoimmune disorder, Hashimoto's thyroiditis. Thyroid masses must be categorized both functionally and anatomically. Functionally, thyroid masses are labeled as toxic or nontoxic, based on whether an excess of thyroid hormone is released. Anatomically, a thyroid mass is categorized as displaying diffuse, multinodular or uninodular enlargement of the gland. To narrow the differential diagnosis further, the enlarged thyroid is classified as painful or painless. Pain suggests an inflammatory thyroiditis, hemorrhage into an existing cyst or nodule, or a rapidly expanding thyroid malignancy.

Along with a history of the mass itself, its onset, rate of growth and associated local symptoms, the history should include eliciting signs and symptoms of hypofunctioning or hyperfunctioning of the gland. Cold intolerance, lethargy, constipation, a deep voice, and cool dry skin suggest hypothyroidism. In contrast, heat intolerance, irritability, diarrhea, tachycardia, diaphoresis, and weight loss suggest hyperthyroidism. Prior radiation exposure, extremes of age (children, elderly), and associated hoarseness are all associated with increased risk of a thyroid mass being malignant.

The thyroid gland is best evaluated with the examiner standing behind the patient and reaching around each side to palpate the gland, felt just adjacent to the trachea, from approximately the level of the laryngeal cartilages to just above the level of the thoracic inlet. When the patient swallows, the thyroid sweeps under the examining fingers in the vertical dimension. More prominent thyroid glands are obvious on visual inspection. The examiner should search for signs of inflammatory enlargement of the gland, such as tenderness and overlying erythema.

Before ordering further laboratory or imaging studies, the physician should know what the test will reveal and how the results will affect the treatment plan. In assessing a patient with a neck mass of thyroid origin, the physician should (1) determine any functional thyroid abnormality resulting in altered hormone levels, (2) diagnose malignancies, and (3) evaluate local compressive symptoms or cosmetic disturbances. Thyroid-stimulating hormone (TSH) is the most effective screening test for thyroid functioning, with a full set of thyroid function tests for patients with an abnormal TSH. Approximately 5% to 10% of solitary nodules or dominant nodules in a multinodular goiter are malignant.[5,9] No imaging study is sensitive or specific enough to diagnose or rule out malignancy. In contrast, fine-needle aspiration (FNA) biopsy is a safe and reliable means to assess for malignancy. In a large review of 18,000 FNA biopsies, 70% of patients were diagnosed with benign thyroid conditions, 4% with malignancy, and the remainder with indeterminate, nondiagnostic, or suspicious findings.[6] If the initial biopsy is negative, repeating the biopsy improves the diagnostic yield by 50%. The false-positive and false-negative rates are less than 5%.[6,9] The results of FNA biopsy can be used to guide a treatment plan, either observation for benign biopsies or referral and possible surgery for biopsies positive or suggestive of malignancy or for indeterminate biopsies. With simple cysts, FNA can even be therapeutic, with the nodule vanishing after aspiration.

Ultrasound or CT scan is best used to determine if the mass is truly thyroid in origin rather than distinguish a malignant vs. nonmalignant etiology. A thyroid nuclear uptake scan helps determine whether a hyperthyroid state is caused by a toxic multinodular goiter, functioning adenoma, or release of thyroid hormone from inflammation. The test may also have a role in treatment planning for the patient with a nondiagnostic FNA biopsy. If the nodule is hyperfunctioning ("hot nodule") on nuclear uptake scan, it is unlikely to be malignant, and often the patient can be safely observed. The lack of uptake of nuclear tracer ("cold nodule"), however, is not sufficiently predictive for malignancy to be useful in clinical decision making.

NEOPLASTIC NECK MASSES

Head and neck cancers make up approximately 5% of new cancers diagnosed annually in the United States.[3] In adults over age 40 a neck mass that persists for more than 4 weeks must be considered malignant until proved otherwise. The workup begins with a detailed history and physical examination; the physician should not rush to obtain excisional or incisional biopsies, since both are associated with an increased rate of local recurrence for most types of head and neck cancer. Rather, the physician searches for a potential primary site of cancer. A patient with a mass suspicious for head and neck cancer should be referred to an otolaryngologist.

If a suspected site for the primary lesion is identified, the lesion is biopsied. CT scan or magnetic resonance imaging (MRI) from skull base to thoracic inlet is obtained to explore the extent of the tumor and assess for occult metastases in the neck. A chest radiograph is an effective screen for pulmonary metastases. FNA biopsy of a neck mass can be obtained to confirm a diagnosis of malignancy. In contrast to excisional or incisional biopsies, FNA is not associated with increased rates of tumor recurrence, although FNA is much less capable of making a diagnosis of lymphoma. A suspected diagnosis of lymphoma is one of the few indications for an excisional lymph node biopsy in an adult. If a supraclavicular lymph node is involved, a mammogram for women and evaluation of the gastrointestinal and genitourinary tracts must be considered. If the primary site remains occult, the patient undergoes direct laryngoscopy, bronchoscopy, esophagoscopy, and nasopharyngoscopy, with appropriate random biopsies to find a primary site.

The treatment of head and neck cancer is site specific and depends on appropriate staging. As with other cancers, treatment modalities include surgery, with or without adjuvant radiation or chemotherapy, and primary radiation with or without chemotherapy. For children, in contrast to adults, only 10% of neck masses prove to be malignant. Thus the workup is more likely to focus initially on inflammatory and congenital etiologies of neck masses (see Chapter 183).

CONGENITAL NECK MASSES

In children and young adults, neck masses of congenital origin are second only to inflammatory neck masses in frequency of occurrence. The two most common categories of congenital neck masses are branchial cleft cysts and thyroglossal duct cysts, each of which constitutes about one third of congenital neck masses. Most congenital neck masses are recognized by the third decade of life.

Branchial Cleft Cysts

The branchial apparatus consists of five paired *arches* in the lateral wall of the embryo foregut, separated by invaginations called *clefts*. This system of arches and clefts normally gives rise to the varying components of the head and neck, and the arches and clefts themselves are obliterated in the process. Remnants of these embryologic precursors may persist, however, and result in cysts, sinuses, and fistulas. These lesions appear most often along the anterior border of the sternocleidomastoid muscle or in the periauricular region. Branchial cysts are blind pouches that may open to the skin or internally into the aerodigestive tract. In contrast, branchial fistulas extend all the way from skin to the aerodigestive tract. Branchial cleft abnormalities typically become evident in childhood or early adulthood, presenting as nontender, fluctuant masses. They may contain rests of lymphoid tissue and may become inflamed in the setting of an upper respiratory tract infection. Superinfection can occur, requiring treatment with broad-spectrum antibiotics. Definitive therapy requires complete surgical excision, ranging from minimal to extensive surgical dissection, depending on the extent of the tract involved. Diagnosis is supplemented by radiologic imaging, which may include CT scan and fistulogram.

Thyroglossal Duct Cysts

Thyroglossal duct cysts represent remnants of the thyroid's descent from the foramen cecum at the base of tongue to its final position in the neck. These embryologic remnants are cysts, not sinuses or fistulas, and do not drain to the outside spontaneously. They typically present as an asymptomatic neck mass in the midline near the hyoid bone. As with branchial cleft cysts, they can rapidly enlarge in the setting of infection. Effective surgical treatment, which minimizes chance for recurrence, requires excising the entire tract of thyroid descent, including the center portion of the hyoid bone. Before a suspected thyroglossal duct cyst is excised, the physician must ensure that the mass does not represent ectopic thyroid tissue, which is frequently the only thyroid tissue in the neck.

Vascular Anomalies

Hemangiomas and vascular malformations represent different pathologies, as determined by their cellular features and clinical behavior. Hemangiomas represent endothelial proliferation at abnormally rapid rates causing a vascular tumor. They are usually first noted in the immediate postnatal period, not at birth, with nearly all hemangiomas apparent by 6 months of age. Most undergo spontaneous regression over the first several years of life. Occasionally they require treatment with steroids, interferon-α, or surgical excision if they result in significant disability, as with aerodigestive tract compressive symptoms.

Unlike hemangiomas, vascular malformations are present at birth and typically grow at a rate commensurate with the child's overall growth. These may be capillary, venous, or lymphatic subtypes or a combination. Vascular malformations can be triggered into a rapidly accelerated growth phase by infection, trauma, or hormonal changes. When disfiguring or causing local compressive symptoms, they may require surgical excision.

Teratomas and Dermoid Cysts

Teratomas and dermoid cysts arise from rests of pluripotential cells, which persist from embryogenesis. They always occur in the midline of the neck, typically as painless masses. Dermoid cysts are attached to and move with the skin. This distinguishes them from thyroglossal duct cysts, which are also found in the midline but which move vertically underneath the skin with swallowing. In contrast to dermoid cysts, which are composed of two of the three germ layers, teratomas are composed of all three germ layers and therefore can give rise to any type of differentiated tissues, even hair or teeth.

Laryngocele

Laryngocele is an abnormal outpouching from the larynx, arising from the space between the true and false vocal cords known as the *ventricle.* This outpouching can pierce through the thyrohyoid membrane to reach the lateral neck. Activities such as glass blowing or trumpet playing, which cause prolonged increases in intralaryngeal pressure, can predispose to laryngoceles. The patient can often make the neck mass more apparent by performing maneuvers that increase laryngeal pressures. The diagnosis can be made on plain x-ray film, which shows an air-filled pouch. These lesions can be surgically excised.

REFERENCES

1. Batsakis JG: Salivary glands: physiology. In Cummings CW et al, editors: *Otolaryngology–head and neck surgery,* ed 3, St Louis, 1998, Mosby.
2. Brook I: Oropharyngeal anaerobes. In Johnson JT, Yu VL, editors: *Infectious diseases and antimicrobial therapy of the ears, nose and throat,* Philadelphia, 1997, WB Saunders.
3. Davis WE, Zitsch RP III: Statistics of head and neck cancer. In Thawley SE et al, editors: *Comprehensive management of head and neck tumors,* ed 2, Philadelphia, 1999, WB Saunders.
4. Gayner SM et al: Infections of the salivary glands. In Cummings CW et al, editors: *Otolaryngology–head and neck surgery,* ed 3, St Louis, 1998, Mosby.
5. Hermus AR, Huysmans DA: Treatment of benign nodular thyroid disease, *N Engl J Med* 338:1438, 1998.
6. Gharib H, Goellner J: Fine-needle aspiration biopsy of the thyroid: an appraisal, *Ann Intern Med* 118:282, 1993.
7. Kellner JD, Wang EL: Cervical lymphadenitis. In Johnson JT, Yu VL, editors: *Infectious diseases and antimicrobial therapy of the ears, nose and throat,* Philadelphia, 1997, WB Saunders.
8. Littlejohn MC et al: Granulomatous diseases of the head and neck. In Bailey BJ, Calhoun KH, editors: *Head and neck surgery–otolaryngology,* ed 2, Philadelphia, 1998, Lippincott-Raven.
9. Singer PA: Evaluation and management of the solitary thyroid nodule, *Otolaryngol Clin North Am* 29:577, 1996.

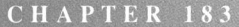

Head and Neck Oncology

Dennis H. Kraus
David G. Pfister

The head and neck contain a variety of tissues and organs. Accordingly, a broad spectrum of malignant lesions can occur in this region. Carcinomas, lymphomas, sarcomas, and melanomas arise in the head and neck; salivary gland, thyroid, ocular, and brain tumors are all technically head and neck malignancies. When nonmelanoma skin cancers are excluded, approximately 80,000 such cancers are diagnosed in the United States each year.

Most often, however, the term head and neck cancer (HNC) refers to squamous cell carcinoma (SCC) arising from the surface epithelium of the upper aerodigestive tract, including the oral cavity, pharynx, larynx, and nasal cavity/paranasal sinuses (Box 183-1). When so defined, approximately 45,000 new cases of HNC are diagnosed each year, or 4% to 5% of all newly diagnosed invasive cancers. SCC or one of its variants is the histologic type in 95% of these cases. HNC comprises a heterogenous group of neoplasms, with important site-specific differences in etiology, clinical presentation, staging, prognosis, treatment, and survival. Unless otherwise specified, HNC refers to cancers of this location and histology. Despite their heterogeneity, certain general principles of management can be identified.

EPIDEMIOLOGY AND RISK FACTORS

The incidence of HNC has shown a minimal increase over the last 30 years. Patients with HNC are predominantly male (3 : 1) and have a median age of approximately 60 years. An increasing proportion are women, reflecting increased tobacco use in this population. The oral cavity and the larynx are the two most common primary sites. Marginal improvements in survival have occurred over the last 30 years.

Box 183-1. Primary Sites of Head and Neck Cancer

Oral Cavity
Lip
Buccal mucosa
Floor of mouth
Alveolar ridge (lower, upper)
Retromolar trigone
Hard palate
Tongue

Pharynx
Oropharynx
  Base of tongue
  Tonsil
  Lateral wall
  Posterior pharyngeal wall
  Inferior surface of soft palate, uvula
Hypopharynx
  Pyriform sinus
  Posterior pharyngeal wall
  Postcricoid
Nasopharynx

Larynx
Supraglottis
  False vocal cords
  Epiglottis
  Arytenoids
Glottis: true vocal cords
Subglottis

Nose and Paranasal Sinuses
Maxillary sinus
Sphenoid sinus
Ethmoid sinus
Nasal cavity

HNC is associated with several etiologic factors, especially tobacco and alcohol use. Inhaled tobacco smoke is probably the most important. It affects most sites, although the association is strongest for laryngeal cancer. The risk increases with the number of cigarettes smoked each day. In individuals who stop smoking, it takes over a decade for their risk of HNC to approach that of a nonsmoker. Other tobacco products besides cigarettes, including cigar, pipe, and smokeless tobacco, are associated with a significant increase in HNC. The popularity of smokeless tobacco in adolescents and young adults has been associated with increases in oral cavity (especially buccal mucosa) and oropharyngeal cancers. Alcohol consumption is a major risk factor for HNC, especially of the oral cavity, oropharynx, and hypopharynx. As with tobacco, the subsequent incidence of cancer is dose related. When tobacco and alcohol are both used by a patient, the two risk factors appear to be synergistic.

Nasopharyngeal cancer is especially prevalent in the Far East, where the incidence is 20 to 25 times higher than in Western countries. The increased risk is diminished but still present in American descendants of Chinese origin. The exact roles played by genetic and environmental factors, however, remain controversial. Epstein-Barr virus (EBV) is a potential etiologic agent. Patients with nasopharyngeal carcinoma have a greater elevation in their EBV viral capsid titers compared with control patients without the disease, and the level of these titers correlates with the tumor burden present. The EBV genome can be demonstrated in nasopharyngeal cancer tissue. Human papillomavirus (HPV) is also an etiologic agent for the development of SCC throughout the upper aerodigestive tract.

PATHOPHYSIOLOGY

Certain lesions, although not invasive carcinoma, are important to recognize as precursors of SCC. Since a different histologic diagnosis can dramatically affect prognosis and treatment, direct interaction with the pathologist under these circumstances is crucial. *Leukoplakia* clinically appears as a white patch, which reflects epithelial thickening. It can be distinguished from a candidal infection in that the leukoplakia plaque cannot be removed with direct contact. Leukoplakia most often occurs on the buccal mucosa, dorsal tongue, and alveolar ridges. Most of these lesions are not associated with significant cellular atypia and spontaneously regress in about 25% of patients; longitudinal follow-up of patients with leukoplakia documents a low incidence of malignant transformation (5% to 10%). *Erythroplasia,* on the other hand, is an ominous mucosal change. Clinically, it appears as a velvety red patch, most often affecting the floor of mouth, ventral tongue, soft palate, and tonsil. This lesion is associated with a high rate of severe dysplasia or in situ/invasive carcinoma at biopsy (80% to 90%). The risk of malignant conversion over time is also significant. As such, erythroplasia always requires biopsy.

Verrucous carcinoma is a low-grade variant of SCC, most often found in the oral cavity and larynx. Clinically it resembles a wart and has an indolent growth pattern. Biopsies of the lesion reveal no invasive cancer. Verrucous carcinoma can be locally aggressive. True verrucous carcinomas rarely develop lymph node metastases.

In the nasopharynx and nasal cavity/paranasal sinuses, the frequency of SCC is slightly less than in other sites (80% to 85%). The incidence of the different types of epidermoid carcinoma of the nasopharynx shows marked geographic variation. Well-differentiated SCC, or World Health Organization (WHO) type I, which is more common in North America, occurs in older patients and is more closely linked to traditional carcinogens of the upper respiratory tract, with less association with EBV. Poorly differentiated carcinomas (WHO types II and III), including those with heavy lymphocytic infiltration (so-called lymphoepithelioma), occur in younger patients, with major endemic areas in Asia and the Mediterranean.

CLINICAL PRESENTATION AND NATURAL HISTORY

HNC is best described as a local and regional disease. In the majority of patients, symptoms and signs related to the primary tumor or its spread to regional (neck) lymph nodes are the primary manifestations of the disease. Asymptomatic cervical adenopathy may be the presenting complaint. An isolated neck mass in an adult should be considered cancer until proved otherwise. Spread of disease to regional lymphatics generally occurs in a predictable manner. For example, tumors of the oral cavity most often involve the

Table 183-1. Clinical Presentation of Head and Neck Cancer

Primary site	Clinical presentations
Oral cavity	Pain, mouth ulcers, poorly fitting dentures, premalignant lesions, change in speech, foul mouth odor, trismus
Oropharynx	Sore throat, neck mass, ear pain, dysphagia, change in speech, trismus
Hypopharynx	Sore throat, ear pain, dysphagia, odynophagia, neck mass, hoarseness, foreign body sensation
Nasopharynx	Neck mass, hearing loss, otitis media, diplopia, epistaxis, nasal stuffiness, cranial neuropathies (esp. VI)
Supraglottic larynx	Odynophagia, sore throat, ear pain, neck mass, hemoptysis, cough, hoarseness, stridor
Glottic larynx	Hoarseness, sore throat, dysphagia, dyspnea
Paranasal sinuses	Sinusitis, toothache, loose teeth, poorly fitting dentures, epistaxis, proptosis, cheek swelling, hypoesthesia, pain

submandibular and upper jugular nodes; tumors of the larynx, hypopharynx, and oropharynx involve the upper and middle jugular nodes; and nasopharynx cancer affects the retropharyngeal, jugulodigastric, and spinal accessory nodes. The frequency of lymph node metastases at presentation is related to the amount of capillary lymphatics draining the primary site. Sites with a rich supply of capillary lymphatics (e.g., nasopharynx, hypopharynx) typically present with enlarged lymph nodes, relative to sites with few lymphatic channels (e.g., glottic larynx, paranasal sinuses). The size of the lesion, its grade, and the depth of tumor invasion are also important in predicting the frequency of lymph node involvement. Large, high-grade, and deeply infiltrating tumors are more likely to have involved lymph nodes.

Tumors most often present as a mass or ulcer. Since much of the mucosal surface is not immediately accessible, symptoms are often ignored, leading to a delay in diagnosis. Symptoms that fail to respond to conservative treatment (antibiotics) in 4 weeks necessitate evaluation by a trained otolaryngologist–head and neck specialist. The symptoms and signs associated with these lesions vary with the primary site and are best understood in the context of the anatomy of the area (Table 183-1).

Distant metastases are uncommon at presentation in HNC, occurring in less than 10% of patients. Ultimately, 20% to 30% of patients manifest distant spread of the disease. Autopsy studies suggest that distant metastases are more frequent but do not manifest clinically because the local and regional aspects of the disease are more prominent. The risk of distant metastases increases with involvement of neck nodes. The most common sites of distant spread are lung, liver, bone, and skin. Hypercalcemia occurs in 3% to 5% of patients and generally reflects recurrent or advanced disease.

Given the central roles tobacco and alcohol abuse play in the development of HNC, other problems stemming from their excessive use are associated with these tumors. An estimated 50% to 60% of patients with HNC show significant signs of malnutrition. Many patients with HNC have comorbid ailments that complicate their management, including alcoholic liver disease and cirrhosis, chronic obstructive pulmonary disease, and vascular disease. Second primary cancers are increasingly appreciated in these patients, arising in other head and neck sites, lung, and esophagus. The terms *field defect, field cancerization,* and *condemned mucosa* have been used to describe this phenomenon. The estimated risk is at 3% to 5% each year, although it is much higher in patients who continue to smoke and drink. Ultimately, 10% to 40% of patients develop a second primary cancer.

All smokers and users of smokeless tobacco products should have routine screening examinations of the oral cavity (Fig. 183-1 and Box 183-2).

PATIENT EVALUATION AND STAGING

A careful history documenting symptoms, potential risk factors, and other comorbid medical problems is important. The percentage of total body weight lost in the last 6 months and the patient's performance status, as defined by a well-recognized scale, quantitate disease impact and symptom severity. Physical examination is central to patient evaluation, with a thorough inspection of the head and neck. Palpation of the parotid, submandibular, and thyroid glands is essential. Although the name of specific nodal groups can be used, a leveling system is now applied at many centers and is clinically reproducible (Fig. 183-2). *Level I* refers to lymph nodes in the submental region and submandibular triangle; *levels II, III,* and *IV* refer to the upper, middle, and lower thirds of the internal jugular chain, respectively; and *level V* refers to nodes in the spinal accessory and transverse cervical chains. Many oral cancers involve the ventral surface of the tongue, and this area is carefully assessed. At certain sites, such as the floor of the mouth and the base of the tongue, visual inspection alone either misses or underestimates the size of a lesion, and palpation or bimanual examination allows a better assessment. The nasopharynx warrants careful scrutiny. Visualization is facilitated by the use of mirrors and rigid and flexible scopes. Flexible scopes are especially useful in patients who continue to have a hyperactive gag reflex after adequate local anesthesia. Vocal cord mobility and facial nerve function are assessed.

Medical imaging with computed tomography (CT) and magnetic resonance imaging (MRI) is increasingly used in the evaluation of these patients. A barium swallow may be useful, especially in patients complaining of dysphagia. CT scan has the advantage of lower cost, faster scanning time, and decreased motion artifact. MRI scan has the advantage of better differentiation of soft tissues and may be the preferable study at certain sites (e.g., nasopharynx, base of tongue). Routinely obtaining both studies is unnecessary; they should be ordered by the otolaryngologist–head and neck surgeon only when appropriate.

Because of the low frequency of distant metastases at presentation, an extensive search for distant metastatic disease is not routinely indicated. A chest radiograph is important, as much to document a possible synchronous lung primary or chronic lung disease in this smoking population as to demonstrate metastatic disease. Liver function abnormalities usually reflect alcohol abuse or some other nonmalignant process. Formal imaging of the liver and bones is necessary only if appropriate biochemical abnormalities or symptoms are present. A complete blood count may suggest nutritional

Date_________Male___Female____
Provider #______Location/Site______

A. *Risk Factors*

1. Do you smoke cigarettes now?	no__	yes__	pks/day _____yrs __
2. Did you ever smoke cigarettes?	no__	yes__	pks/day _____yrs __
3. Do you use cigar/pipe/snuff/chewing tobacco?	no__	yes__	which? _________
4. Do you drink alcohol now?	no__	yes__	
5. If no, did you ever drink alcohol?	no__	yes__	when quit? ________

B. *Symptoms* (as answered by the patient)

			≥2 weeks' duration? no	yes	unknown
1. Do you have any soreness or pain in					
throat	no__	yes__	__	__	__
mouth	no__	yes__	__	__	__
ear	no__	yes__	__	__	__
jaw	no__	yes__	__	__	__
neck	no__	yes__	__	__	__
teeth	no__	yes__	__	__	__
on swallowing	no__	yes__	__	__	__
2. Has your voice changed?	no__	yes__	__	__	__
3. Is your voice hoarse?	no__	yes__	__	__	__
4. Have you felt any masses or lumps?	no__	yes__	__	__	__
5. Have you had trouble swallowing?	no__	yes__	__	__	__
6. Have you had trouble chewing?	no__	yes__	__	__	__
7. Have you lost >10 lb in the past 2 months?	no__	yes__	how much? ________		
8. Have you coughed up blood?	no__	yes__	when? __________		

C. *Physical Examination*

Shortness of breath	no__	yes__
Hoarseness	no__	yes__
Nose: blood in nares	no__	yes__
Oral cavity:		
caries	no__	yes__
blood in mouth	no__	yes__
edentulous	no__	yes__
white patches	no__	yes__
red patches	no__	yes__
bleeding areas	no__	yes__
tenderness	no__	yes__
mucosal lesion	no__	yes__
Neck:		
pain	no__	yes__
masses	no__	yes__
nodes	no__	yes__

Locate positive findings below:

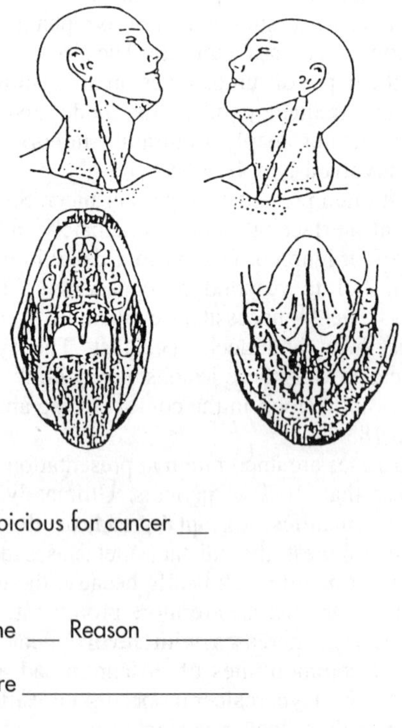

D. Were the above signs and symptoms the reason for this visit? no__ yes__

E. *Conclusion* (check one):
Normal __ Abnormal, cancer not suspected __ Abnormal, suspicious for cancer __

F. *Action* (check one):
None required__ Refer for follow-up because of: Screening exam __ Other __ Exam not done __ Reason ________

Signature _________________

Fig. 183-1. Oral cancer screening form. (From Prout MN et al: *J Cancer Educ* 7:139, 1992.)

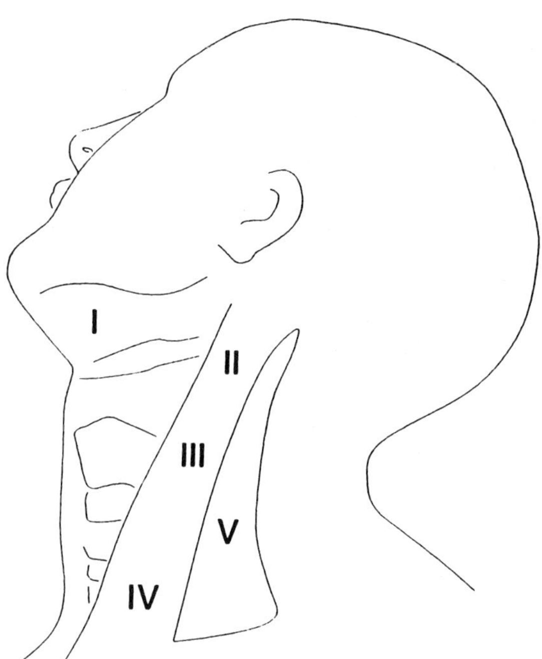

Fig. 183-2. Level *I*, lymph nodes in submental region and submandibular triangle; levels *II, III, IV*, lymph nodes in the upper, middle, and lower thirds of the internal jugular chain; level *V*, lymph nodes in the spinal accessory and transverse cervical chains.

Box 183-2. Managed Care Guide: Criteria for Positive Head and Neck Cancer Screen*

Simple leukoplakia: white patch that does not scrape off
Recommended action: oral examination, elective referral to ENT
Complex leukoplakia: mixed white and red patches
Erythroplakia: red velvety patches
Mucosal lesion with gross appearance of cancer
Hoarseness or voice change persistent throughout the day for 2 weeks
Mucosal lesion of uncertain type in high-risk anatomic area: floor of mouth, ventrolateral tongue

From Prout MN et al: *J Cancer Educ* 7:139, 1992.
*Established for "abnormal, suspicious for cancer sign and/or symptom" found at primary screening. Recommendation is immediate referral to ear-nose-throat (ENT) specialist.

deficiency or chronic blood loss. Pulmonary function tests and electrocardiogram (ECG) are incorporated into preoperative assessment and may necessitate additional management.

Endoscopy under anesthesia is especially useful in patients with tumors of the larynx and pharynx. The routine use of so-called triple endoscopy (laryngoscopy, esophagoscopy, bronchoscopy) in the evaluation of these patients is controversial. Proponents emphasize the 5% or higher incidence of synchronous primary cancers that affect prognosis and management. Triple endoscopy is appropriate in two groups: patients at high risk for multiple primaries with clinical evidence of diffuse mucosal abnormalities and patients who have cervical adenopathy without an identifiable primary site.

As with all malignancies, histologic proof is obtained from the primary site. When the primary is occult, histologic confirmation of a suspicious neck node is required. Initially, fine-needle aspiration (FNA) is preferred instead of an open biopsy. FNA is well tolerated and accurate, especially for SCC, with no significant risk of seeding the needle tract. Multiple endoscopies should be performed to exclude an occult primary arising in the nasopharynx, base of tongue, tonsil, or pyriform sinus. If the FNA biopsy is noncontributory, an excisional biopsy is indicated, with the incision part of the usual neck dissection. Preoperative counseling of the patient facilitates rapid neck dissection when malignancy is confirmed on frozen section. When followed over time, 30% of these patients have their primary tumor identified. Interestingly, the patients in whom the primary site is found generally do worse than those in whom it remains occult (30% vs. 60% long-term survival, respectively).

The goal of this evaluation is to stage the cancer appropriately, which helps define prognosis and management and facilitates uniform reporting of treatment results. The staging used for HNC is the tumor-node-metastasis (TNM) system, as determined by the American Joint Committee on Cancer and the International Union Against Cancer (Box 183-3). The T stage depends on the site, size, and extent of invasion at the primary site. Tumors of the oral cavity and oropharynx use the same criteria; other sites are different. The N stage is defined by the number, size, and location relative to the primary lesion of the regional lymph nodes. The M stage refers to the presence or absence of distant metastases. The N (except for the nasopharynx) and M formulations are the same for all primary sites. The respective T, N, and M stages are then combined to create four stages. Stage I is the best prognostic group; stage IV is the worst prognostic group. Clinical staging (excluding information obtained at surgery) is the type most often used, since clinical decisions are typically based on this information.

MANAGEMENT

Patients with HNC present a challenge on many levels. Ongoing tobacco and alcohol abuse are common, as are other medical comorbidities. The disease and its treatment can cause dysfunction and disfigurement. Optimal treatment and rehabilitation of these patients therefore requires close interdisciplinary cooperation not only among the treating surgical, radiation, and medical oncologists, but also among other health professionals, including dentists and prosthodontists, speech and swallowing therapists, audiologists, nutritionists, occupational and physical therapists, and psychiatrists. Plans for rehabilitating patients should start before treatment.

Control of disease at the primary site and in the neck is the primary goal. Historically, surgery and radiation therapy have been the principal treatment modalities. Chemotherapy's role is best established in the palliative setting but is being actively investigated in combination with surgery and radiation, with important implications for the development of function preserving therapy and the treatment of patients with unresectable disease. In general, treatment is determined by the TNM stage at presentation, although there are site-specific variations (Table 183-2). Management of the primary site and

Box 183-3. TNM System of Cancer Staging

Tumor (T): Varies With Primary Site

Oropharynx/oral cavity

T_1 Tumor ≤2 cm in greatest dimension
T_2 Tumor >2 cm but ≤4 cm in greatest dimension
T_3 Tumor >4 cm in greatest dimension
T_4 Tumor with massive invasion of adjacent structures

Supraglottic larynx

T_1 Tumor limited to one subsite of supraglottis with normal vocal cord mobility
T_2 Tumor invades more than one subsite of supraglottis or glottis, with normal vocal cord mobility
T_3 Tumor limited to larynx with vocal cord fixation and/or invades postcricoid area, medial wall of pyriform sinus, or preepiglottic tissues
T_4 Tumor invades through thyroid cartilage and/or extends to other tissues beyond the larynx

Lymph Node (N): Same for All Primary Sites*

N_0 No regional lymph node metastasis
N_1 Metastasis in a single ipsilateral lymph node, ≤3 cm in greatest dimension
N_{2a} Metastasis in a single ipsilateral lymph node, >3 cm but ≤6 cm in greatest dimension
N_{2b} Metastasis in multiple ipsilateral lymph nodes, none >6 cm in greatest dimension
N_{2c} Metastasis in bilateral or contralateral lymph nodes, none >6 cm in greatest dimension
N_3 Metastasis in a lymph node >6 cm in greatest dimension

Distant Metastasis (M): Same for All Primary Sites

M_0 No distant metastasis
M_1 Distant metastasis

TNM Stage*

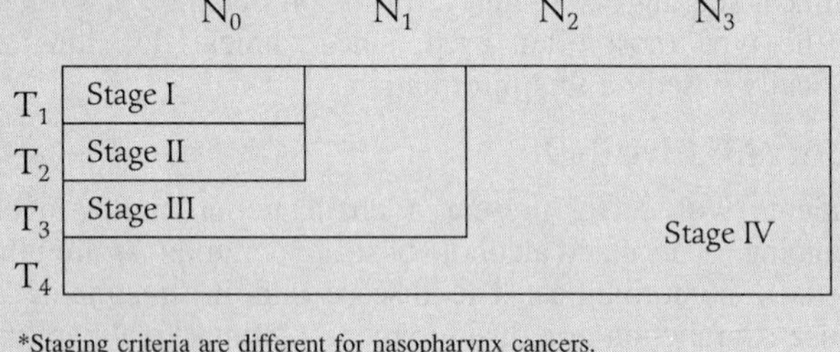

*Staging criteria are different for nasopharynx cancers.

that of the neck are related but also present separate concerns. Treatment plans should consider both survival and quality of life.

For limited disease (T_1-T_2, N_0-N_1, M_0) single-modality treatment with surgery or radiation is associated with equivalent results (60% to 90% cure rate). The choice of modality depends on a variety of factors, including primary site, patient age and general health, local expertise, functional concerns, and patient preference. Patients with an N_0 stage can have their necks treated electively depending on the risk of occult nodal disease. This estimate is based on T stage, primary site, differentiation of the tumor, evidence of vascular and lymphatic invasion, and depth of invasion of the primary tumor. If the estimated risk of neck failure is greater than 15%, elective neck staging or treatment is advisable. Obviously, the results of treatment with one modality may require the immediate addition of the other. A positive margin after resection or the finding at neck dissection of multiple positive lymph nodes or extracapsular extension necessitates postoperative radiation therapy; a persistent or growing mass after radiation therapy requires resection.

Patients with bulky, advanced resectable disease (T_3-T_4, N_2-N_3, M_0) require treatment with a combination of surgery and radiation, since this approach has improved local and regional disease control compared with unimodality therapy. The expected cure rate in this group is 10% to 60%. Chemotherapy has been studied in combination with standard local and regional treatment to improve tumor control and/or functional outcome. In patients with unresectable disease, radiation therapy alone has been the standard treatment. The integration of chemotherapy with radiation appears to improve response rates and potentially survival.

If a patient has recurrent disease after primary treatment, attempts are made to salvage the patient with surgery and radiation, depending on previous therapy. If a patient previously received definitive radiation therapy, the options of receiving further radiation are limited. Patients undergoing salvage therapy are at higher risk for disease recurrence compared with similarly staged, untreated patients. Patients with recurrent disease that is not amenable to further surgery or radiation and patients with distant metastatic disease (M_1) at presentation or recurrence are treated with palliative chemotherapy.

Five-year survival rates are generally reported for HNC. However, most relapses occur within the first 2 years after treatment. Involved regional lymph nodes reduce the

Table 183-2. Head and Neck Cancer Treatment by Category and Stage

Disease category	Stage	Standard therapy	Cure rate
Limited	I, II, III (T_1/T_2, N_0/N_1, M_0)	Surgery or RT	60%-90%
Advanced	III, IV (T_3/T_4, N_2/N_3, M_0)	Surgery and RT; RT; chemotherapy and RT*	10%-60%
Metastatic	IV (M_1)	Chemotherapy; other palliative treatment	Rare
Recurrent	Variable	Surgery and/or RT if feasible	Selected patients salvaged
		Chemotherapy; other palliative treatment	Rare

RT, Radiation therapy.
*The choice among these options will depend on many factors, including but not limited to disease extent, primary site, a patient's clinical/performance status, and the anticipated outcomes (e.g., disease control, functional, cosmetic) associated with a given approach.

anticipated cure rate within each T stage by approximately 50%. Anticipated survival rates depend on the stage and primary site. For example, hypopharyngeal primaries have a worse prognosis, stage for stage, than laryngeal primaries, even though the structures are immediately adjacent to each other.

The treatment of patients with an occult primary and metastatic SCC in a cervical node depends on the clinical presentation. Patients with an N_1 neck diagnosis can be treated with primary radiation or a neck dissection with equivalent local control. Patients with an N_2 or N_3 neck diagnosis probably require treatment with neck dissection and radiation therapy. Patients with advanced neck disease have a worse prognosis. Elective irradiation of the potential primary mucosal sites should sterilize the low-bulk disease. However, radiation to the mucosal surfaces will increase the morbidity of treatment in the form of xerostomia and potentially complicate subsequent salvage therapy.

Surgery

Certain advantages are associated with surgical treatment of HNC. The treatment time is shorter, and surgery is limited to those tissues at greatest risk of tumor invasion. The immediate and long-term sequelae of radiation are avoided. Pathologic information found at surgery is useful in predicting prognosis and in planning postoperative treatment with radiation.

An adequate surgical procedure requires margins free from tumor. In more advanced lesions this may necessitate a procedure associated with significant functional or cosmetic morbidity. In patients with laryngeal and pharyngeal tumors a total laryngectomy may be required. Tumors of the oral cavity and oropharynx may require a composite resection, with removal of part of the mandible and en bloc resection of the primary tumor and regional lymph nodes. Patients with extensive oropharyngeal tumors often require total laryngectomy, not to remove the primary tumor but to prevent the sequelae of chronic aspiration. Patients with advanced paranasal sinus tumors may require a radical maxillectomy, which occasionally includes orbital exenteration.

Function-preserving procedures adhere to sound surgical oncologic principles. Supraglottic laryngectomy and hemilaryngectomy are examples that spare laryngeal function. Successful application of these procedures requires both surgical expertise and careful patient selection. The use of a variety of skin and bone grafts can optimize the functional and cosmetic results. A prosthodontist can customize obturators and other prostheses that facilitate speech and swallowing.

Certain features of a tumor indicate that it is unresectable. The distinction between technically unresectable and unresectable for medical reasons is important. Contraindications for resection include massive skull base involvement, prevertebral fascia invasion, carotid artery encasement, and skin infiltration. CT scan and MRI can be helpful in assessing some of these issues.

The traditional radical neck dissection involves removal of the cervical lymphatic tissues, the sternocleidomastoid muscle, the internal jugular vein, and the eleventh cranial nerve. The procedure can be associated with pain, shoulder weakness, and paresthesia. Because of these potential morbidities, a variety of modified and selective procedures that preserve function have evolved. The clinical decision to use one of these modified or selective techniques requires careful patient selection.

Radiation Therapy

Compared with surgery, radiation is associated with certain advantages. In some instances (e.g., early laryngeal cancer) the functional results are better. When elective therapy to high-risk lymph nodes is indicated, this treatment can easily be incorporated into patient management. This option is especially relevant in patients who are at risk for bilateral neck node involvement. Treatment-related mortality rarely occurs.

The ability of radiation therapy to control local and regional disease as a single modality is inversely related to tumor bulk. The probability of tumor control is dose dependent. Large total doses are required to sterilize SCC. The dose and portals of treatment depend on the primary site and goals of therapy. When single-modality, definitive radiation is used, doses of 6600 to 7000 cGy are necessary. The dose is generally administered over 6 to 7 weeks, with daily fractions of 180 to 200 cGy. These are optimally delivered either by a megavoltage linear accelerator or ^{60}Co unit. The dose to the spinal cord must be monitored, since its radiation tolerance is considerably lower.

Radiation therapy can be combined with surgery using preoperative or postoperative dosing. The customary preoperative dose is 5000 cGy; the difficulty of subsequent surgery and the frequency of serious postoperative complications increase when the radiation dose exceeds this level. The postoperative dose to the primary site and neck are influenced by the findings at surgery and range from 5000 to 7000 cGy, depending on factors such as surgical margins and the presence of residual gross disease. Postoperative radiation is currently the usual approach. The local and regional control rate appears to be higher with postoperative treatment, although no survival advantage has been proved. Radiation therapy generally starts 2 to 4 weeks after resection, at which time the wounds are satisfactorily healed.

Adverse effects of radiation in the head and neck can occur both early and late. Mucositis and edema lead to dysphagia, hoarseness, and otitis media. These toxicities are generally managed with conservative measures and resolve with time. Occasionally, temporary placement of a feeding tube, tracheostomy, or myringotomy with pressure-equalizing tubes may be necessary. Fibrosis and induration of irradiated tissues develop to a variable extent. Xerostomia and loss of taste are related to salivary gland dysfunction. Long-term return of function varies, depending in part on dose and portals. The use of certain drugs may ameliorate this toxicity (e.g., amifostine, pilocarpine). Because of the reduction of saliva, dental caries and periodontal disease can be considerable. Dental evaluation before radiation therapy, with extraction of damaged teeth, optimization of oral hygiene, and fluoride treatments, is essential and can prevent long-term complications. Lhermitte's sign, which is characterized by shocklike sensations in the spine, arms, and legs with neck flexion, occurs when the spinal cord is irradiated and is self-limiting. Varying degrees of thyroid dysfunction may develop, and thyroid function tests should be closely monitored in those patients undergoing surgery and radiation to the neck, larynx, or pharynx. Two serious late complications are myelopathy due to overdosing of the cervical spinal cord and osteoradionecrosis of the mandible.

Several techniques aimed at improving the therapeutic index of radiation therapy are under active clinical evaluation and investigation. Radiation implants (brachytherapy) are placed within the tumor bed. The implant can either be permanent (e.g., ^{125}I) or temporary via afterloading catheters (e.g., ^{192}Ir). These can be used either alone or in combination with external beam treatment. Their use is associated with excellent local control in selected tumors of the oropharynx (base of tongue) and oral cavity. Hyperfractionated radiation (using more than one fraction per day) has yielded encouraging results in patients with advanced tumors. Conformal radiation more precisely delivers treatment to the tumor and facilitates dose escalation.

Chemotherapy

By itself, chemotherapy is not curative in HNC. A number of chemotherapy agents cause a major shrinkage of tumor in 20% to 40% of HNC patients. Combinations with the drug cisplatin are thought to have the highest response rates. The exact response rate depends on the tumor bulk and previous treatment. Large, previously treated tumors have the lowest response rates.

Historically the prime role of chemotherapy has been in the palliation of patients who have largely exhausted surgical and radiation treatment options or in patients with distant metastatic disease. Under these circumstances the gold standard drug is methotrexate. In general, the treatment is well tolerated, but possible toxicities include mucositis, myelosuppression, hepatotoxicity, nephrotoxicity, and fatigue. Cisplatin is considered to be as active but is associated with more toxicity and greater difficulty of administration. Toxicities include nausea and vomiting, myelosuppression, nephrotoxicity, neurotoxicity, and ototoxity. Other drugs, such as 5-fluorouracil, carboplatin, paclitaxel, and docetaxel, also have activity. Unfortunately, the median duration of response with these agents remains short and the median overall survival poor. In hopes of improving these results, a variety of combination chemotherapy regimens have been compared to treatment with a single agent. These trials have revealed no improvement in survival.

The response rates in patients with previous untreated HNC are higher than in those with recurrent or metastatic disease. Indeed, cisplatin-based combination chemotherapy yields response proportions in the 60% to 90% range, with complete responses in 20% to 60% of patients. Despite these high response rates, induction chemotherapy, adjuvant chemotherapy, or combination therapy integrated with standard surgery and radiation has not improved survival in these patients compared with results from surgery and radiation alone.

The use of chemotherapy in a treatment scheme that does not improve survival may still be useful, if the functional result is superior to that after standard surgery and radiation therapy. Since radiation is most effective when the tumor burden is small, chemotherapy may decrease the tumor bulk before definitive therapy. In one trial, patients with stage III and IV laryngeal cancer received either standard total laryngectomy with postoperative radiation or induction chemotherapy with radiation; total laryngectomy was reserved for patients who had no chemotherapy response or who relapsed. The survival in both treatment groups was equivalent, and more than 60% of surviving patients in the chemotherapy/radiation group had their larynx preserved. Similar data are available for patients with advanced hypopharynx cancer.

The use of chemotherapy concomitantly with radiation has been intensely investigated. The emphasis has been on choosing chemotherapeutic agents that have independent activity in HNC but can also serve as radiation enhancers or sensitizers. Randomized trials suggest this approach yields a higher response rate and improves local control compared with radiation alone. Local mucocutaneous toxicity is generally increased. The potential utility of concomitant chemotherapy and radiation may be a significant part of a functional preservation treatment approach and is often applied to patients with unresectable disease, including advanced nasopharynx cancers, and more recently in patients with advanced oropharynx cancer.

PREVENTION

Since tobacco and alcohol use are the primary risk factors for HNC, any prevention program must focus on the cessation or modification of these behaviors. Tobacco cessation is most successful when a counseling program is combined with the use of a tapering nicotine patch. Even in patients who stop smoking and consuming alcohol, however, the risk for second malignancy persists for years. Accumulating evidence suggest the retinoids may be important in the prevention of epithelial carcinogenesis, as evaluated in a study of 13-*cis* retinoic acid (50 to 100 mg/m^2/day orally) vs. placebo in patients who were disease free after primary treatment for HNC. No difference was seen in the number or pattern of relapses or the overall survival in the two groups of patients, but the rate of second primary tumors in the treatment group was significantly decreased. Toxicities associated with the 13-*cis* retinoic acid included skin dryness, cheilitis, hypertriglyceridemia, and conjunctivitis. Approximately 20% of patients did not complete treatment because of toxic effects. Less toxic schedules and less toxic substances (β-carotene, vitamin E) are being investigated.

SPECIFIC SITES

Salivary Glands

Cancer of the major and minor salivary glands is uncommon, accounting for about 7% of head and neck malignancies. They arise from the three paired major salivary glands (parotid, submandibular, sublingual) and the approximately 700 minor salivary glands that are distributed throughout the upper aerodigestive tract. There may be an association with previous low-dose radiation exposure, such as that used for acne or lymphoid hypertrophy. An association also may exist between salivary gland tumors and patients with a history of breast cancer, cancer of the male genital tract, HNC, and skin cancer.

A variety of benign and malignant histologic changes occur in the salivary glands. Approximately 80% of all salivary gland tumors arise in the parotid, 10% to 15% in the submandibular gland, and the remainder in the sublingual and minor salivary glands. The odds of a salivary gland neoplasm being malignant are inversely related to the size of the gland. It is estimated that 20% to 30% of parotid, 40% to 60% of submandibular, and the majority of sublingual and minor salivary gland tumors are malignant. The distinction between benign and malignant tumors can be difficult. The parotid is a potential site for regional and distant metastases, particularly for skin cancer arising on the face.

Salivary gland tumors grow by direct extension and infiltration and generally present as a painless swelling. Rapid growth and facial nerve involvement are both associated with a malignant histology and a poor prognosis. The clinical aggressiveness of the tumors varies with size, histology, and grade. The incidence of clinical and subclinical neck node metastases is lower than with HNC. Distant metastases are uncommon. The risk of distant failure is highest for adenoid cystic tumors, the lung being the most common site.

The use of FNA biopsy in the management of salivary neoplasms is controversial. The information does not change therapy in most cases but may be useful in treatment planning for certain patients (e.g., with unresectable tumors). Excisional biopsy should be discouraged, since it only complicates subsequent definitive therapy. CT scan or MRI may provide additional useful information. These modalities distinguish between intrinsic and extrinsic glandular masses, extraglandular extension, and the presence of occult metastatic cervical disease. Sialograms were used more often in the past but have been replaced by these newer technologies.

Surgery is the treatment of choice for salivary gland neoplasms. Enucleation of salivary gland tumors leads to local recurrence, even with benign tumors, and should be avoided. Excision of the superficial or deep lobe of the parotid gland with facial nerve preservation is performed depending on the tumor's location. The entire gland is removed in submandibular and sublingual tumors. Elective neck dissections are generally not performed, although sampling adjacent lymph nodes based on histology and size may have a role. Depending on the location and extent of the parotid tumors, resections may include part of the temporal bone, mandible or zygoma, and the facial nerve. Placement of an immediate nerve graft for facial nerve resection has shown success. Management of the eye, including a moisture chamber at night and the use of artificial preparations for replacement of tears, is mandatory to prevent exposure keratopathy, which can accompany facial paralysis. Postoperative radiation is generally indicated for high-grade, large, deeply invasive tumors with positive or close margins and positive nodes. Doses are similar to those used with HNC. Primary radiation is generally limited to patients with unresectable tumors; neutron beam therapy is under investigation. Chemotherapy has no standard role in the management of salivary gland tumors.

Parotid tumors are associated with better survival than lesions at other sites. Adenoid cystic cancers often have indolent growth, even when distant metastases are present. Ten-year survival statistics are a more accurate estimate of treatment results for many of these tumors because of their long natural histories.

Thyroid

Cancer of the thyroid accounts for approximately 12,000 new cases per year and 1000 deaths, with an increased incidence in females and whites. Prognosis is improved in women and in patients with disease onset at a younger age. Exposure to radiation therapy places patients at an increased risk for thyroid cancer. Approximately 10% of medullary carcinomas of the thyroid are inherited as an autosomal dominant gene. Medullary thyroid cancer is associated with the multiple endocrine neoplasia (MEN) syndromes.

Thyroid neoplasms represent an array of benign and malignant processes. The most common thyroid mass represents either multinodular goiter or benign follicular adenomas. The well-differentiated thyroid carcinomas—papillary and follicular adenocarcinomas—represent almost 90% of all thyroid malignancies. Papillary adenocarcinoma (50% to 60%) is nearly twice as common as follicular adenocarcinoma (25% to 35%). The high-grade variants include medullary (5%) and undifferentiated/anaplastic (5%) carcinomas.

Thyroid malignancies most often present as a painless thyroid mass. Cervical lymphadenopathy is consistent with lymph node metastases. Unlike HNC, cervical metastases do not adversely affect long-term survival; distant metastases, however, are associated with reduced long-term survival. Hoarseness may represent recurrent laryngeal nerve paralysis. (See Chapter 181 for diagnosis and management.)

ADDITIONAL READINGS

Deiter M et al: Modern management of cervical scrofula, *Head Neck* 11:60, 1989.

de Visscher JGAM, van der Wal KGH, de Vogel PL: The plunging ranula: pathogenesis, diagnosis, and management, *J Craniomaxillofac Surg* 17:182, 1989.

Dillon WP, Harnsberger RH: The impact of radiologic imaging on staging of cancer of the head and neck, *Semin Oncol* 18:64, 1991.

Friedman M et al: Nodal size of metastatic squamous cell carcinoma of the neck, *Laryngoscope* 103:854, 1993.

Harrison LB, Sessions RB, Hong WK, editors: *Head and neck cancer: a multidisciplinary approach,* Philadelphia, 1999, Lippincott-Raven.

Jacobs C: The internist in the management of head and neck cancer, *Ann Intern Med* 113:771, 1990.

Johns ME, Goldsmith MM: Incidence, diagnosis, and classification of salivary gland tumors, *Oncology* 3:47, 1989.

Johns ME, Goldsmith MM: Current management of salivary gland tumors, *Oncology* 3:85, 1989.

Lindberg RD: Distribution of cervical lymph node metastases from squamous cell carcinoma of the upper respiratory and digestive tracts, *Cancer* 29:1446, 1972.

Lucente FE: Impact of the acquired immunodeficiency syndrome epidemic on the practice of laryngology, *Ann Otol Rhinol Laryngol* 102(suppl 161), 1993.

McGuirt WF: Panendoscopy as a screening examination for simultaneous primary tumors in head and neck cancer: a prospective sequential study and review, *Laryngoscope* 92:569, 1982.

Mulliken JB, Glowacki J: Hemangioma and vascular malformations in infants and children: a classification based on endothelial characteristics, *Plast Reconstr Surg* 69:412, 198.

Pfister DG et al: The role of chemotherapy in the curative treatment of head and neck cancer, *Surg Oncol Clin N A* 6:749, 1997.

Rice DH, Spiro RH, editors: *Current concepts in head and neck cancer,* Atlanta, 1989, American Cancer Society.

Silverman S, editor: *Oral cancer,* Atlanta, 1990, American Cancer Society.

Witterick IJ et al: Nonpalpable occult and metastatic papillary thyroid carcinoma, *Laryngoscope* 103:149, 1993.

Work WP: Hemangiomas of the head and neck, *Ann Otol Rhinol Laryngol* 87:633, 1978.

Zangwill KM et al: Cat scratch disease in Connecticut: epidemiology, risk factors, and evaluation of a new diagnostic test, *N Engl J Med* 329:8, 1993.

Index

E

H

I

M

HEMATOLOGIC NORMAL VALUES (cont'd.)

Acid hemolysis test (Ham)	No hemolysis	
Carboxyhemoglobin		
Nonsmoker	<1%	
Smoker	2.1%-4.2%	
Cold hemolysis test (Donath-Landsteiner)	No hemolysis	
Complete blood count (see Table 3)		
Erythrocyte life span		
Normal	120 days	
^{51}Cr-labeled half-life	28 days	
Erythropoietin by radioimmunoassay	9-33 mU/dl	
Ferritin, serum		
Male	15-200 µg/L	
Female	12-150 µg/L	
Folate, RBC	120-670 ng/ml	
Fragility, osmotic		
Hemolysis begins 0.45%-0.38% NaCl		
Hemolysis completed 0.33%-0.30% NaCl		
Haptoglobin, serum	100-300 mg/dl	
Hemoglobin		
Hemoglobin A_{1c}	0%-5% of total	
Hemoglobin A_2 by column	2%-3% of total	
Hemoglobin, fetal	<1% of total	
Hemoglobin, plasma	0%-5% of total	
Hemoglobin, serum	2-3 mg/ml	
Iron, serum		
Male	75-175 µg/dl	
Female	65-165 µg/dl	
Iron-binding capacity, total serum (TIBC)	250-450 µg/dl	
Iron turnover rate (plasma)	20-42 mg/24 hr	
Leukocyte alkaline phosphatase (LAP) score	30-150	
Methemoglobin	<1.8%	
Reticulocytes (see Table 3)		
Schilling test (urinary excretion of radiolabeled vitamin B_{12} after "flushing" intramuscular injection of B_{12})	6%-30% of oral dose within 24 hr	
Sedimentation rate	*Male*	*Female*
Wintrobe	0-5 mm/hr	0-15 mm/hr
Westergren	0-15 mm/hr	0-20 mm/hr
Transferrin saturation, serum	20%-50%	
Volume	*Male*	*Female*
Blood	52-83 ml/kg	50-75 ml/kg
Plasma	25-43 ml/kg	28-45 ml/kg
Red cell	20-36 ml/kg	19-31 ml/kg

Table 3. Complete blood count

Parameter	Male	Female
Hematocrit (%)	40-52	38-48
Hemoglobin (gm/dl)	13.5-18.0	12-16
Erythrocyte count ($\times 10^{12}$ cells/L)	4.6-6.2	4.2-5.4
Reticulocyte count (%)	0.6-2.6	0.4-2.4
MCV (fL)	82-98	82-98
MCH (pg)	27-32	27-32
MCHC (gm/dl)	32-36	32-36
WBC ($\times 10^9$ cells/L)	4.5-11.0	4.5-11.0
Segmented neutrophils	1.8-7.7	1.8-7.7
Average (%)	40-60	40-60
Bands (cells)	0-0.3	0-0.3
Average (%)	0-3	0-3
Eosinophils (cells $\times 10^9$/L)	0-0.5	0-0.5
Average (%)	0-5	0-5
Basophils (cells $\times 10^9$/L)	0-0.2	0-0.2
Average (%)	0-1	0-1
Lymphocytes (cells $\times 10^9$/L)	1.0-4.8	1.0-4.8
Average (%)	20-45	20-45
Monocytes (cells $\times 10^9$/L)	0-0.8	0-0.8
Average (%)	2-6	2-6
Platelet count (cells $\times 10^9$/L)	150-350	150-350

Coagulation Normal Values

Template bleeding time	3.5-7.5 min
Clot retraction, qualitative	Apparent in 30-60 min; complete in 24 hr, usually in 6 hr
Coagulation time (Lee-White)	
Glass tubes	5-15 min
Siliconized tubes	20-60 min
Euglobulin lysis time	120-240 min
Factors II, V, VII, VIII, IX, X, XI, or XII	100% or 1.0 unit/ml
Fibrin degradation products	<10 µg/ml or titer ≤1.4
Fibrinogen	200-400 mg/ml
Partial thromboplastin time, activated	20-40 sec
Prothrombin time (PT)	11-14 sec
Thrombin time	10-15 sec
Whole blood clot lysis time	>24 hr

PULMONARY FUNCTION TESTS

Abbreviations

P_B = barometric pressure (mm Hg)
F_IO_2 = inspired oxygen fraction (0.21 = room air)
$PaCO_2$ = partial pressure of carbon dioxide in arterial blood (mm Hg)
P_ACO_2 = partial pressure of carbon droxide in alveolar gas (mm Hg)
PaO_2 = partial pressure of oxygen in arterial blood (mm Hg)
P_AO_2 = partial pressure of oxygen in alveolar gas (mm Hg)

Alveolar-arterial oxygen gradient ($F_IO_2 = 0.21$)
$P(A - a)$ in adolescents = <10 mm Hg
adults <40 years = 10 mm Hg
>40 years = 10-15 mm Hg

Alveolar oxygen partial pressure (sea level, $F_IO_2 = 0.21$)
$P_AO_2 = 150 - (1.2 \times PaCO_2)$

Blood gases ($F_IO_2 = 0.21$)

	Arterial	*Alveolar*
PO_2	80-105 mm Hg	90-115 mm Hg
PCO_2	38-44 mm Hg	38-44 mm Hg
pH	7.35-7.45	

Spirometric volumes and lung volumes are size-dependent. Typical normal values for adults are provided.

Lung volumes	*Male*	*Female*
Total lung capacity (TLC)	6-7 L	5-6 L
Functional residual capacity (FRC)	2-3 L	2-3 L
Residual values (RV)	1-2 L	1-2 L
Measures of air flow		
Forced vital capacity (FVC)	4.0 L	3.0 L
1 sec forced vital capacity (FEV_1)	>3.0 L	>2.0 L
Pulmonary resistance (RL)	<3.0 cm H_2O/sec/L	
Airway resistance (Raw)	<2.5 cm H_2O/sec/L	
Other		
Pulmonary compliance (CL)	0.2 L/cm H_2O	
Diffusing capacity (DLCO)	25 ml CO/min/mm Hg	

RENAL FUNCTION TESTS

Anion gap

$Na^+ - HCO_3^- + Cl^- = 12 \pm 2$ mEq/L

Osmolality

$$\text{Osmolality (serum)} = 2\ \text{Na (mEq/L)} + \frac{\text{BUN (mg/dl)}}{2.8} + \frac{\text{glucose (mg/dl)}}{18}$$

Bicarbonate deficit

HCO_3^- deficit = body weight (kg) × 0.4 (desired HCO_3^- – observed HCO_3^-)

Glomerular filtration rate

$$GFR = \frac{Ucr \times V}{Pcr}$$

$= 130 \pm 20$ ml/min in males

$= 120 \pm 15$ ml/min in females

$$\cong \frac{Ucr}{Pcr} \times 70$$

where

Ucr = urine creatinine (mg/dl)

Pcr = plasma creatinine (mg/dl)

V = urine volume/24 hr (ml/min)

Renal plasma flow

$$RPF = \frac{Upah \times V}{Ppah}$$

$= 700 \pm 130$ ml/min in males

$= 600 \pm 100$ ml/min in females

where

Upah = urine para-aminohippuric acid (mg/dl)

V = urine volume/24 hr (ml/min)

Ppah = plasma para-aminohippuric acid (mg/dl)

SEMEN NORMAL VALUES

Liquefaction	Complete in 15 min
Morphology	>50% normal forms
Motility	>75% motile forms
pH	7.2-8.0
Spermatocrit	10%
Spermatocyte count	>50 million/ml
Volume	2.0-6.6 ml

SERUM NORMAL VALUES

Acetoacetate	0.3-2.0 mg/dl
Acid phosphatase	0-0.8 U/ml
Acid phosphatase, prostatic	2.5-12.0 IU/L
Albumin	3.0-5.5 gm/dl
Aldolase	1-6 IU/L
Alkaline phosphatase	
15-20 years	40-200 IU/L
20-101 years	35-125 IU/L
Alpha-1 antitrypsin	200-500 mg/dl
ALT	0-40 IU/L
Ammonia	11-35 µmol/L
Amylase, serum	2-20 U/L
Anion gap	8-12 mEq/L (mmol/L)
Ascorbic acid	0.4-1.5 mg/dl
AST	5-40 IU/L
Bilirubin	
Total	0.2-1.2 mg/dl
Direct	0-0.4 mg/dl
Calcium, serum	8.7-10.6 mg/dl
Carbon dioxide, total	18-30 mEq/L (mmol/L)
Carcinoembryonic antigen, serum	<2.5 µg/L
Carotene (carotenoids)	50-300 µg/dl
C3 complement	55-120 mg/dl
C4 complement	14-51 mg/dl
Ceruloplasmin	15-60 mg/dl
Chloride, serum	95-105 mEq/L (mmol/L)
Cholesterol, total	
12-19 years	120-230 mg/dl
20-29 years	120-240 mg/dl
30-39 years	140-270 mg/dl
40-49 years	150-310 mg/dl
50-59 years	160-330 mg/dl
Copper	100-200 µg/dl
Creatine kinase, total	20-200 IU/L
Creatine kinase, isoenzymes	
MM fraction	94%-95%
MB fraction	0%-5%
BB fraction	0%-2%
Normal values in	
Heart	80% MM, 20% MB
Brain	100% BB
Skeletal, muscle	95% MM, 2% MB
Creatinine, serum	
Female adult	0.5-1.3 mg/dl
Male adult	0.7-1.5 mg/dl
Delta-aminolevulinic acid (ALA)	<200 µg/dl
α-Fetoprotein, serum	<40 µg/L
Folate, serum	1.9-14.0 ng/ml
Gamma glutamyl transpeptidase	
Male	12-38 IU/L
Female	9-31 IU/L
Gastrin	150 pg/ml
Glucose, serum (fasting)	70-115 mg/dl
Glucose-6-phosphate dehydrogenase	5-10 IU/gm Hb
G6PD screen, qualitative	Negative
Haptoglobin	100-300 mg/dl
Hemoglobin A_2	0%-4% of total Hb
Hemoglobin F	0%-2% of total Hb
Immunoglobulin, quantitation	
IgG	700-1500 mg/dl
IgA	70-400 mg/dl
IgM	
Male	30-250 mg/dl
Female	30-300 mg/dl
IgD	0-40 mg/dl
Insulin, fasting	6-20 µU/ml
Iron-binding capacity	250-400 µg/dl
Iron, total, serum	40-150 µg/dl
Lactic acid	0.6-1.8 mEq/L
LDH, serum	20-220 IU/L
LDH isoenzymes	
LDH_1	20%-34%
LDH_2	28%-41%
LDH_3	15%-25%
LDH_4	3%-12%
LDH_5	6%-15%
Leucine aminopeptidase (LAP)	30-55 IU/L
Lipase	4-24 IU/dl
Magnesium, serum	1.5-2.5 mEq/L
5′-Nucleotidase	0.3-3.2 Bodansky units
Osmolality, serum	278-305 mOsm/kg serum water
Phenylalanine	3 mg/dl
Phosphorus, inorganic, serum	2.0-4.3 mg/dl
Potassium, plasma	3.1-4.3 mEq/L
Potassium, serum	3.5-5.2 mEq/L
Protein, total, serum	
2-55 years	5.0-8.0 gm/dl
55-101 years	6.0-8.3 gm/dl
Protein electrophoresis, serum	
Albumin	3.2-5.2 gm/dl
Alpha-1	0.6-1.0 gm/dl
Alpha-2	0.6-1.0 gm/dl
Beta	0.6-1.2 gm/dl
Gamma	0.7-1.5 gm/dl
Sodium, serum	135-145 mEq/L
Sulfate	0.5-1.5 mg/dl
T_3 uptake	25%-45%
T_4	4-11 µg/dl
Triglycerides	
2-29 years	10-140 mg/dl
30-39 years	20-150 mg/dl
40-49 years	20-160 mg/dl
50-59 years	20-190 mg/dl
60-101 years	20-200 mg/dl

Labelled overleaf

CEREBROSPINAL FLUID NORMAL VALUES

Bilirubin	0
Cells	0-5/mm^3, all lymphocytes
Chloride	110-129 mEq/L
Glucose	48-86 mg/dl or ≥60% of serum glucose
pH	7.34-7.43
Pressure	7-20 cm water
Protein, lumbar	15-45 mg/dl
Albumin	58%
α_1-globulins	9%
α_2-globulins	8%
β-globulins	10%
γ-globulins	10 (5-12)%
Protein, cisternal	15-25 mg/dl
Protein, ventricular	5-15 mg/dl

ENDOCRINOLOGIC NORMAL VALUES

Hormone and Metabolite Normal Values

Adrenocorticotropin (ACTH), serum	15-100 pg/ml
Aldosterone (mean ± standard deviation)	
Serum	
210 mEq/day sodium diet	
Supine	48 ± 29 pg/ml
Upright (2 hr)	65 ± 23 pg/ml
110 mEq/day sodium diet	
Supine	107 ± 45 pg/ml
Upright (2 hr)	532 ± 228 pg/ml
Urine	5-19 μg/24 hr
alcitonin, serum	
Basal	0.15-0.35 ng/ml
Stimulated	<0.6 ng/ml
atecholamines, free urinary	<110 μg/24 hr
horionic gonadotropin, serum	
Pregnancy	
First month	10-10,000 mIU/ml
Second and third months	10,000-100,000 mIU/ml
Second trimester	10,000-30,000 mIU/ml
Third trimester	5000-15,000 mIU/ml
Nonpregnant	<3 mIU/ml
ortisol	
Serum	
8 AM	5-25 μg/dl
8 PM	<10 μg/dl
Cosyntropin stimulation (30-90 min after 0.25 mg cosyntropin intramuscularly or intravenously)	>10 μg/dl rise over baseline
Overnight suppression (8 AM serum cortisol after 1 mg dexamethasone orally at 11 PM)	≤5 μg/dl
Urine	20-70 μg/24 hr
peptide, serum	0.28-0.63 pmol/ml
-Deoxycortisol, serum	
Basal	0-1.4 μg/dl
Metyrapone stimulation (30 mg/kg orally 8 hr prior to level)	>7.5 μg/dl
nephrine, plasma	<35 pg/ml
radiol, serum	
Male	20-50 pg/ml
Female	25-200 pg/ml

	Male	*Female*
rogens, urine (increased during regnancy; decreased after nenopause)		
Total	4-25 μg/24 hr	5-100 μg/24 hr
Estriol	1-11 μg/24 hr	0-65 μg/24 hr
Estradiol	0-6 μg/24 hr	0-14 μg/24 hr
Estrone	3-8 μg/24 hr	4-31 μg/24 hr

ocholanolone, serum	<1.2 μg/dl
icle-stimulating hormone, serum	
Male	2-18 mIU/ml
emale	
Follicular phase	5-20 mIU/ml
Peak midcycle	30-50 mIU/ml
Luteal phase	5-15 mIU/ml
Postmenopausal	>50 mIU/ml
thyroxine index, serum	1-4 ng/dl
Gastrin, serum (fasting)	30-200 pg/ml
Growth hormone, serum	
Adult, fasting	<5 ng/ml
Glucose load (100 gm orally)	<5 ng/ml
Levodopa stimulation (500 mg orally in a fasting state)	>5 ng/ml rise over baseline within 2 hr
17-Hydroxycorticosteroids, urine	
Male	2-12 mg/24 hr
Female	2-8 mg/24 hr
5′-Hydroxyindoleacetic acid (5′-HIAA), urine	2-9 mg/24 hr
Insulin, plasma	
Fasting	6-20 μU/ml
Hypoglycemia (serum glucose <50 mg/dl)	<5 μU/ml
17-Ketosteroids, urine	
Under 8 years old	0-2 mg/24 hr
Adolescent	0-18 mg/24 hr
Adult	
Male	8-18 mg/24 hr
Female	5-15 mg/24 hr
Luteinizing hormone, serum	
Male adult	2-18 mIU/ml
Female adult	
Basal	5-22 mIU/ml
Ovulation	30-250 mIU/ml
Postmenopausal	>30 mIU/ml
Metanephrines, urine	<1.3 mg/24 hr
Norepinephrine	
Plasma	150-450 pg/ml
Urine	<100 μg/24 hr
Parathyroid hormone, serum	
C-terminal	150-350 pg/ml
N-terminal	230-630 pg/ml
Pregnanediol, urine	
Female	
Follicular phase	<1.5 mg/24 hr
Luteal phase	2.0-4.2 mg/24 hr
Postmenopausal	0.2-1.0 mg/24 hr
Male	<1.5 mg/24 hr
Progesterone, serum	
Female	
Follicular phase	0.02-0.9 ng/ml
Luteal phase	6-30 ng/ml
Male	<2 ng/ml
Prolactin, serum	
Nonpregnant	
Day	5-25 ng/ml
Night	20-40 ng/ml
Pregnant	150-200 ng/ml
Radioactive iodine (^{131}I) uptake (RAIU)	5%-25% at 24 hr (varies with iodine intake)
Renin activity, plasma (mean ± standard deviation)	
Normal diet	
Supine	1.1 ± 0.8 ng/ml/hr
Upright	1.9 ± 1.7 ng/ml/hr
Low-sodium diet	
Supine	2.7 ± 1.8 ng/ml/hr
Upright	6.6 ± 2.5 ng/ml/hr
Diuretics and low-sodium diet	10.0 ± 3.7 ng/ml/hr
Testosterone, total plasma	
Bound	
Adolescent male	<100 ng/dl
Adult male	300-1100 ng/dl
Female	25-90 ng/dl
Unbound	
Adult male	3-24 ng/dl
Female	0.09-1.30 ng/dl
Thyroid-stimulating hormone, serum	<10 μU/ml
Thyroxine (T_4), serum	
Total	4-11 μg/dl
Free	0.8-2.4 ng/dl
Thyroxine-binding globulin capacity, serum	15-25 μg T_4/dl
Thyroxine index, free	1-4 ng/dl
Tri-iodothyronine (T_3), serum	70-190 ng/dl
T_3 resin uptake	25%-45%
Vanillylmandelic acid (VMA), urine	1-8 mg/24 hr

Endocrine Function Tests

Adrenal gland	
Glucocorticoid suppression: overnight dexamethasone suppression test (8 AM serum cortisol after 1 mg dexamethasone orally at 11 PM)	≤5 μg/dl
Glucocorticoid stimulation: cosyntropin stimulation test (serum cortisol 30-90 min after 0.25 mg cosyntropin intramuscularly or intravenously)	>10 μg/ml more than baseline serum cortisol
Metyrapone test, single dose (8 AM serum deoxycortisol after 30 mg/kg metyrapone orally at midnight)	>7.5 μg/dl
Aldosterone suppression: sodium depletion test (urine aldosterone collected on day 3 of 200 mEq day/sodium diet)	<20 μg/24 hr
Pancreas	
Glucose tolerance test* serum glucose after 100 gm glucose orally)	
60 min after ingestion	<180 mg/dl
90 min after ingestion	<160 mg/dl
120 min after ingestion	<125 mg/dl
Pituitary gland	
Adrenocorticotropic hormone (ACTH) stimulation. See Adrenal gland, Metyrapone test	
Growth hormone stimulation: insulin tolerance test (serum growth hormone after 0.1 U/kg regular insulin intravenously after an overnight fast to induce a 50% fall in serum glucose concentration or symptomatic hypoglycemia)	>5 ng/ml rise over baseline
Levodopa test (serum growth hormone after 0.5 gm levodopa orally while fasting)	>5 ng/ml rise over baseline within 2 hr
Growth hormone suppression: glucose tolerance test (serum growth hormone after 100 gm glucose orally after 8 hr fast)	<5 ng/ml within 2 hr
Luteinizing hormone (LH) stimulation: gonadotropin-releasing hormone (GnRH) test (serum LH after 100 μg GnRH intravenously or intramuscularly)	4- to 6-fold rise over baseline
Thyroid-stimulating hormone (TSH) stimulation: thyrotropin-releasing hormone (TRH) stimulation test (serum TSH after 400 μg TRH intravenously)	>2-fold rise over baseline within 2 hr
Thyroid gland	
Radioactive iodine uptake (RAIU) suppression test (RAIU on day 7 after 25 μg tri-iodothyronine orally 4 times daily)	<10% to <50% baseline
Thyrotropin-releasing hormone (TRH) stimulation test. See Pituitary gland, Thyroid-stimulating hormone (TSH) stimulation	

*Add 10 mg/dl for each decade over 50 years of age.

HEMATOLOGIC NORMAL VALUES

Table 2. Differential cell count of bone marrow

Myeloid cells	
Neutrophilic series	
Myeloblasts	0.3%-5.0%
Promyelocytes	1%-8%
Myelocytes	5%-19%
Metamyelocytes	9%-24%
Bands	9%-15%
Segmented cells	7%-30%
Eosinophil precursors	0.5%-3.0%
Eosinophils	0.5%-4.0%
Basophilic series	0.2%-0.7%
Erythroid cells	
Pronormoblasts	1%-8%
Basophilic normoblasts	
Polychromatophilic normoblasts	7%-32%
Orthochromatic normoblasts	
Megakaryocytes	0.1%
Lymphoreticular cells	
Lymphocytes	3%-17%
Plasma cells	0%-2%
Reticulum cells	0.1%-2.0%
Monocytes	0.5%-5.0%
Myeloid/erythroid ratio	0.6-2.7